D1716715

# OPERATIVE PEDIATRIC SURGERY

# OPERATIVE PEDIATRIC SURGERY

## SECOND EDITION

**Moritz M. Ziegler, MD**
*Retired, Surgeon-in-Chief and the Ponzio Family Chair*
*Children's Hospital of Colorado*
*Professor of Surgery*
*University of Colorado School of Medicine*
*Cincinnati, Ohio*

**Richard G. Azizkhan, MD, PhD (Hon)**
*Surgeon-in-Chief*
*Lester W. Martin Chair of Pediatric Surgery*
*Professor of Surgery and Pediatrics*
*Cincinnati Children's Hospital Medical Center*
*University of Cincinnati College of Medicine*
*Cincinnati, Ohio*

**Daniel von Allmen, MD**
*Frederick C. Ryckman Chair of Pediatric Surgery*
*Professor of Surgery*
*Cincinnati Children's Hospital Medical Center*
*University of Cincinnati College of Medicine*
*Cincinnati, Ohio*

**Thomas R. Weber, MD**
*Professor, Pediatric Surgery*
*Department of General Surgery*
*Rush University Medical Center*
*Chicago, Illinois*

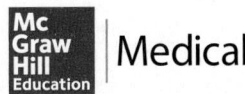

New York   Chicago   San Francisco   Athens   London   Madrid
Mexico City   Milan   New Delhi   Singapore   Sydney   Toronto

**Operative Pediatric Surgery, Second Edition**

1 2 3 4 5 6 7 8 9 0   CTP/CTP   20 19 18 17 16 15 14 13

ISBN 978-0-07-162723-8
MHID 0-07-162723-5

This book was set in Minion Pro Regular by Thomson Digital.
The editors were Brian Belval and Peter J. Boyle.
The production supervisor was Richard Ruzycka.
Project management was provided by Ritu Joon, Thomson Digital.
The interior designer was Alan Barnett.
The cover designer was Anthony Landi.
China Translation & Printing Services, Ltd. was printer and binder.

This book is printed on acid-free paper.

**Cataloging-in-publication data for this book is on file at the Library of Congress.**

McGraw-Hill Education books are available at special quantity discounts to use as premiums and sales promotions, or for use in corporate training programs. To contact a representative, please visit the Contact Us pages at www.mhprofessional.com.

The editors would like to dedicate this volume of *Operative Pediatric Surgery*, second edition, to two of the most contributing as well as recognizable pediatric surgeons in the world, the late **Charles Everett Koop, MD, DSc (1916-2013)** and the late **M. Judah Folkman, MD (1933-2008)**.

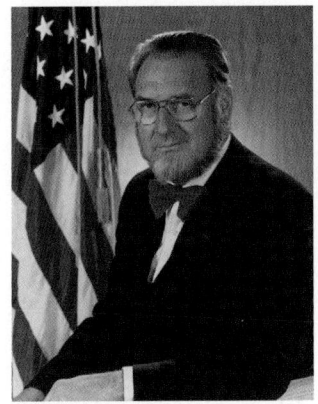

Dr. Koop received his undergraduate degree at Dartmouth, his medical degree at Cornell, and his surgical training at the Hospital of the University of Pennsylvania. At the young age of 32, Dr. Koop was appointed to the position of Surgeon-in-Chief, Children's Hospital of Philadelphia (CHOP). Koop's accomplishments were many: development of the first neonatal intensive care unit; development of a skilled multidisciplinary surgical service; development of an internationally renowned training program in pediatric surgery; development of operative approaches that emphasized speed and simplicity; and a remarkable attention to detail for procedures that ranged from the simple to the highly complex; and he was an international leader in the prolonged task of attaining recognition for the emerging field of pediatric surgery. Dr. Koop was the first editor of the *Journal of Pediatric Surgery*.

At the age of 65 in 1982, Dr. Koop was appointed by President Reagan first as Deputy Assistant Secretary of Health and subsequently as Surgeon General of the U.S. Public Health Service. The recognition and respect that his actions and uniformed dress generated for the PHS were legendary. His policy challenges included a position of anti-tobacco, promoting smoking cessation education, and the benefits of limiting the effects of second-hand smoke; the education of America about the newly recognized transmissible HIV/AIDS virus epidemic; a strong position for life preservation in the "Baby Doe" case; and an anti-obesity and prevention of traumatic injury campaigns.

Dr. Koop also was a devout Christian with a strong commitment to the sanctity of human life, a position widely respected, yet controversial. His principles were strongly reflected in his surgical service at CHOP, in his role as mentor and friend to his trainees and colleagues, and in his respect for the importance of family, spouses, and children—either those in his own life, children under his care and their families, or those in the lives of his mentees.

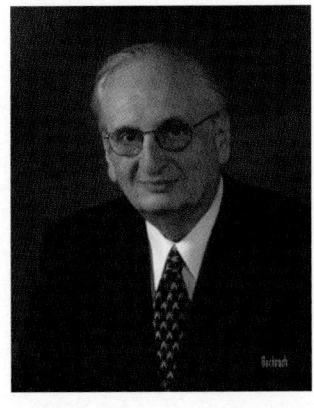

M. Judah Folkman, MD, received his undergraduate degree from Ohio State University and his medical degree from Harvard. He did his surgical residency at Massachusetts General Hospital. In 1960, Folkman was drafted into the U.S. Navy, a fate that brought him to the National Naval Medical Center, where, in association with David Long, he first reported the use of silicone rubber implantable polymers for the sustained release of drugs, a discovery that launched the field of controlled-release technology. Also, during this time, he made his first experimental observation that tumor-related or environmental factors were essential for tumor growth, the founding principle of "tumor angiogenesis."

An appointment at Boston City Hospital followed, and at age 34, he was appointed Surgeon-in-Chief, Boston Children's Hospital. He spent six months of additional pediatric surgical training under Dr. Koop in Philadelphia before returning to the position he held in Boston for 14 years. Dr. Folkman then turned his full attention to research. His laboratory proved that the inhibition of tumor-feeding blood vessels would inhibit growth of the tumor, whether benign or malignant, primary or metastatic. A class of angiogenic inhibiting agents followed that propelled the laboratory work from cancer to diabetic retinopathy, macular degeneration, inflammatory bowel disease, and vascular benign tumors. Angiogenesis inhibition therapy became a worldwide research and treatment focus.

In 1968, Folkman was appointed the Julia Dyckman Andrus Professor of Pediatric Surgery at Harvard Medical School. He was the founder and director of the Boston Children's Hospital Vascular Biology Program and the Vascular Anomalies Center.

Folkman founded an entirely new field of biology and a new approach to understanding and treating cancer and other diseases. He was a stimulator of thought, an educator whether one-on-one or in a formal lecture whose presentations were spectacular in content and clarity, an empathetic, compassionate surgeon, and a friend and colleague.

It is for these reasons that we dedicate this second edition of *Operative Pediatric Surgery* to the late Charles Everett Koop and the late M. Judah Folkman, our colleagues, mentors, and friends, whose impact on this earth extended from the life of an individual infant to the betterment of the health of an entire nation as well as the world.

# Contents

Contributors                                                    xi
Preface                                                         xxiii
Acknowledgments                                                 xxv

## PART I

### GENERAL PRINCIPLES                                          1

1   History of Pediatric Surgery                                3
    *Moritz M. Ziegler*

2   Ethical Considerations in Pediatric Surgery                 16
    *Donna A. Caniano*

3   Fetal Surgery, Diagnosis, and Intervention                  22
    *Jesse D. Vrecenak and Alan W. Flake*

4   Gastrointestinal, Pulmonary, Cardiac,
    and Neurologic Developmental Physiology
    of the Premature and Term Newborn                           42
    *Brian T. Bucher and Brad W. Warner*

5   Renal Developmental Physiology and
    Pediatric Fluid and Electrolyte Management                  54
    *Scott J. Keckler and David W. Tuggle*

6   Metabolic Response to Illness and Operation                 60
    *Tom Jaksic, Stephen B. Shew, and
    Ivan M. Gutierrez*

7   Pediatric Surgical Critical Care:
    Cardiopulmonary Monitoring,
    Advanced Hemodynamic Monitoring,
    Acute Cardiopulmonary Resuscitation,
    Pharmacology, Respiratory Failure, and ECMO                 70
    *Ronald B. Hirschl, Steven L. Moulton, Jane Mulligan,
    Victor A. Convertino, Pamela D. Reiter,
    Steven L. Moulton, Artur Chernoguz,
    and Jason S. Frischer*

8   Nutritional Supplementation
    in Pediatric Surgery                                        129
    *Walter J. Chwals*

9   Vascular Access Procedures                                  137
    *Kristen A. Zeller and John K. Petty*

10  Pediatric Anesthesia and Analgesia                          150
    *Alan Bielsky and David M. Polaner*

11  Transfusion Medicine and Coagulation
    Disorders                                                   172
    *Gregory T. Banever*

12  Wound Healing                                               180
    *Stig Sømme*

13  Surgical Infection: Classification, Diagnosis,
    Treatment, and Prevention                                   189
    *John R. Gosche and Samuel Smith*

14  Office-Based Ambulatory Surgery                             207
    *Wallace W. Neblett III and Joshua B. Glenn*

## PART II

### THE HEAD AND NECK                                           215

15  Head and Neck Lesions                                       217
    *Richard G. Azizkhan*

## PART III

### CHEST WALL AND THORACIC DISEASE                             241

16  Breast Disease                                              243
    *Leslie Ann Taylor and Richard G. Azizkhan*

17  Pectus Excavatum                                            254
    *Frazier W. Frantz, Michael J. Goretsky, and
    Robert C. Shamberger*

18  Pectus Carinatum and Other Deformities
    of the Chest Wall                                           270
    *Jennifer Bruny*

19  Ectopia Cordis and Sternal Defects                         277
    *Jonathan I. Groner*

20  Airway Endoscopy and Pathology,
    and Tracheotomy                                             292
    *Alexandros Georgolios, Charles Johnson III,
    and Charles Bagwell*

21 Posterior Laryngeal Cleft 307
*Michael J. Rutter and Richard G. Azizkhan*

22 Tracheal Stenosis and Tracheomalacia 317
*Patricio Herrera, Priscilla P. L. Chiu, and Peter C. W. Kim*

23 Gastrointestinal Endoscopy, Caustic Ingestions, and Foreign Bodies 328
*Robert A. Cina and Andre Hebra*

24 Esophageal Atresia 342
*Paolo De Coppi and Agostino Pierro*

25 Esophageal Replacement 349
*Richard G. Azizkhan*

26 Achalasia 359
*Philip K. Frykman and Richard G. Azizkhan*

27 Gastroesophageal Reflux Disease 366
*Stephen G. Jolley and J. Brent Roaten*

28 Mediastinal Cysts, Tumors, and Myasthenia Gravis 393
*Steven Teich, Jennifer H. Aldrink, and Jonathan I. Groner*

29 Congenital Lung Malformations: CPAM, Bronchopulmonary Sequestration, Congenital Lobar Emphysema, and Bronchogenic Cyst 407
*Steven Rothenberg and Timothy M. Crombleholme*

30 Lung Infections: Lung Biopsy, Lung Abscess, Bronchiectasis, and Empyema 422
*Harsh Grewal and Barry Evans*

31 Thoracoscopy for Sympathectomy and Spine Exposure 434
*Katherine P. Davenport and Timothy D. Kane*

32 Pleural Disease: Pneumothorax and Chylothorax 438
*Anthony C. Chin and Marleta Reynolds*

33 Diaphragmatic Hernias and Eventration 447
*Thomas Tracy Jr and Francois I. Luks*

## PART IV

ABDOMINAL DISEASE **469**

34 Abdominal Wall Defects: Omphalocele and Gastroschisis 471
*Saleem Islam*

35 Umbilical and Supraumbilical Disease 483
*Evan Kokoska and Thomas R. Weber*

36 Hernias of the Inguinal Region 489
*Michael W. L. Gauderer and Robert A. Cina*

37 Stomach: Obstruction, Microgastria, Foreign Body, and Peptic Ulcer 510
*Michael G. Caty and Mauricio A. Escobar Jr*

38 Gastrointestinal Tract Feeding Access 517
*Shannon Acker and David A. Partrick*

39 Bariatric Surgery in Adolescents 523
*Mark Holterman, Allen Browne, and Ai-Xuan Holterman*

40 Pyloric Stenosis 534
*Edward M. Barksdale Jr and Todd A. Ponsky*

41 Intestinal Rotation Abnormalities 540
*Emily Christison-Lagay and Jacob C. Langer*

42 Intestinal Atresia 549
*Eric D. Strauch and J. Laurence Hill*

43 Meconium Ileus 558
*Brent E. Carlyle, Drucy S. Borowitz, and Philip L. Glick*

44 Hirschsprung Disease 571
*Daniel H. Teitelbaum, Mark L. Wulkan, Keith E. Georgeson, and Jacob C. Langer*

45 Intussusception 592
*Brad A. Feltis and David J. Schmeling*

46 Necrotizing Enterocolitis 597
*Shannon L. Castle, Allison L. Speer, Tracy C. Grikscheit, and Henri Ford*

47 Intestinal Stomas 609
*Thomas R. Weber*

48 Appendicitis 613
*Rebeccah L. Brown*

49 Inflammatory Bowel Disease 632
*D. Dean Potter and Christopher R. Moir*

50 Short Bowel Syndrome 643
*Megan K. Fuller, Jeffrey J. Dehmer, and Michael A. Helmrath*

51 Gastrointestinal Duplications 651
*Mark F. Brown*

52 Cystic Abdominal Disease: Mesenteric, Omental, Solid Organ 664
*Harry Applebaum and Roman Sydorak*

53 Anorectal Malformations 669
*Marc A. Levitt and Alberto Peña*

54 Common Acquired Anorectal Problems of Childhood 694
*Robert M. Arensman and Daniel J. Stephens*

55 Gallbladder Disease 699
*David Juang and George W. Holcomb III*

56 Biliary Atresia and Choledochal Cyst 710
*Stephanie A. Jones and Frederick M. Karrer*

57 Portal Hypertension 724
*Jaimie D. Nathan, Kathleen M. Campbell, Frederick C. Ryckman, Maria H. Alonso, and Greg M. Tiao*

CONTENTS

58  Chronic Pancreatitis in the Pediatric Population  733
    *Alex Bondoc and Greg M. Tiao*

59  The Spleen  741
    *Michael J. Allshouse*

60  Conjoined Twins  752
    *John H.T. Waldhausen and Mary Hilfiker*

## PART V

UROLOGY FOR THE
PEDIATRIC SURGEON  **767**

61  The Acute Scrotum  769
    *Heidi A. Stephany and J. Patrick Murphy*

62  Cryptorchidism  775
    *Wolfgang Stehr and James M. Betts*

63  Circumcision  784
    *Marc S. Arkovitz*

64  Hypospadias  790
    *Sean Primley and Duncan Wilcox*

65  Urinary Tract Obstruction  800
    *Michael C. Carr and Howard M. Snyder III*

66  Vesicoureteral Reflux  818
    *Prem Puri and Manuela Hunziker*

67  Bladder Exstrophy  828
    *Douglas A. Canning, Lisa Parrillo,
    Kavita Gupta, and Howard M. Snyder III*

68  Cloacal Exstrophy  846
    *Charles G. Howell Jr and Jeffrey Donohoe*

69  Urinary Tract Reconstruction for
    Continence and Renal Preservation  857
    *Curtis A. Sheldon and Eugene Minevich*

70  Pediatric and Adolescent Gynecology  880
    *Lesley Breech and Akilah Weber*

71  Disorders of Sexual Differentiation  899
    *Mary E. Fallat and Jeannie Chun*

## PART VI

VASCULAR SYSTEM ANOMALIES  **927**

72  The Surgical Treatment of Patent
    Ductus Arteriosus and Aortic
    Coarctation  929
    *Andrew C. Fiore, Michael Hines,
    and D. Glenn Pennington*

73  Vascular Compression Syndromes  943
    *Peter B. Manning*

74  Abdominal Aortic Pathology  952
    *Jaimie D. Nathan*

75  Vascular Anomalies  963
    *Richard G. Azizkhan, Aliza P. Cohen,
    Roshni Dasgupta, and Denise Adams*

## PART VII

NEUROSURGERY FOR THE
PEDIATRIC SURGEON  **999**

76  Neurosurgery for the Pediatric Surgeon  1001
    *Daniel von Allmen*

## PART VIII

TRAUMA  **1027**

77  Trauma Epidemiology, Scoring and
    Triage Systems, and Injury Prevention  1029
    *Thane A. Blinman and Michael Nance*

78  Child Abuse  1042
    *Arthur Cooper, Leslie Ann Taylor,
    and David Merten*

79  Head Injury  1055
    *Charles B. Stevenson and Kerry R. Crone*

80  Thoracic Injuries  1067
    *Marianne Beaudin and
    Richard A. Falcone Jr*

81  Abdominal Trauma  1082
    *Alex Stoffan and David P. Mooney*

82  Extremity Injuries  1098
    *Roger Cornwall, James C. Gilbert,
    Peter F. Sturm, Robert S. Hatch,
    Richard M. Schwend,
    William W. Robertson Jr, and
    Douglas G. Armstrong*

83  Burn Injury  1118
    *John P. Crow*

84  Animal Assaults: Bites and Stings  1129
    *Marcene R. McVay and Charles Wagner*

## PART IX

SURGICAL ENDOCRINOLOGY  **1139**

85  Neonatal Hypoglycemia  1141
    *Daniel von Allmen*

86  Disorders of the Thyroid, Parathyroid,
    and Adrenal Glands  1147
    *Corey W. Iqbal and David C. Wahoff*

## PART X

ONCOLOGY  **1165**

87  Principles of Adjuvant Therapy
    in Pediatric Cancer  1167
    *Rebecca J. McClaine and Daniel von Allmen*

88  Nephroblastoma (Wilms Tumor)  1177
    *Andrew M. Davidoff*

**89** Neuroblastoma     1187
*Eric Long and Dai H. Chung*

**90** Teratoma     1198
*Frederick J. Rescorla*

**91** Diagnosis and Treatment
of Rhabdomyosarcoma     1211
*Felicia N. Williams and David A. Rodeberg*

**92** Nonrhabdomyosarcoma Soft
Tissue Sarcomas     1221
*Andrea Hayes-Jordan*

**93** Liver Tumors     1228
*Rebecka L. Meyers and Greg M. Tiao*

**94** Gastrointestinal Polyps/Intestinal Cancer     1249
*Artur Chernoguz and Jason S. Frischer*

**95** The Lymphomas     1260
*Peter Ehrlich*

**96** Pigmented Lesions and Melanoma     1270
*Brian S. Pan and David A. Billmire*

# PART XI

SOLID ORGAN TRANSPLANTATION     **1281**

**97** Immunology and Transplantation     1283
*Sara K. Rasmussen and Paul M. Colombani*

**98** Surgery and End-Stage Renal Disease     1293
*Khashayar Vakili and Craig W. Lillehei*

**99** Liver Transplantation     1306
*Greg M. Tiao*

**100** Intestine Transplantation     1317
*Jorge Reyes*

Index     1327

CONTENTS

x

# Contributors

**Shannon Acker, MD** [38]
Research Fellow in Pediatric Surgery
Department of Surgery
Children's Hospital of Colorado
University of Colorado School of Medicine
Aurora, Colorado

**Denise Adams, MD** [75]
Professor of Pediatrics and Surgery
Medical Director of the Hemangioma Vascular
    Malformation Center
Marjory J. Johnson Chair of Vascular Tumor Translation
    Research
Cancer Blood Disorders Institute
Cincinnati Children's Hospital Medical Center
Cincinnati, Ohio

**Jennifer H. Aldrink, MD** [28]
Assistant Professor of Clinical Surgery
Department of Pediatric Surgery
Nationwide Children's Hospital
Columbus, Ohio

**Michael J. Allshouse, DO, FACS, FAAP** [59]
Medical Director
Department of Pediatric Surgery and
    Pediatric Trauma Program
Children's Hospital Central California
Madera, California

**Maria H. Alonso, MD** [57]
Associate Professor of Surgery
Surgical Assistant Director, Liver Transplantation
Division of Pediatric General and Thoracic Surgery
Cincinnati Children's Hospital Medical Center
Cincinnati, Ohio

**Harry Applebaum, MD** [52]
Clinical Professor of Surgery
Division of Pediatric Surgery
David Geffen School of Medicine at UCLA
Los Angeles, California

**Robert M. Arensman, MD** [54]
Professor of Surgery
Department of Surgery
University of Illinois at Chicago
Chicago, Illinois

**Marc S. Arkovitz, MD** [63]
Surgeon
Department of Pediatric Surgery
Tel Hashomer Medical Center, Safra Children's Hospital
Ramat Gan, Israel

**Douglas G. Armstrong, MD** [82]
Director of Pediatric Orthopedic Surgery,
    Edwards P. Schwentker Professor
Department of Orthopaedics and Rehabilitation
Penn State Hershey Bone and Joint Institute
Hershey, Pennsylvania

**Richard G. Azizkhan, MD, PhD (Hon)** [15, 16, 21, 25, 26, 75]
Surgeon-in-Chief
Lester W. Martin Chair of Pediatric Surgery
Professor of Surgery and Pediatrics
Cincinnati Children's Hospital Medical Center
University of Cincinnati College of Medicine
Cincinnati, Ohio

**Charles Bagwell, MD, FACS, FAAP** [20]
Professor of Surgery and Pediatrics
Chairman, Division of Pediatric Surgery
Medical College of Virginia/Virginia
    Commonwealth University
Richmond, Virginia

**Gregory T. Banever, MD** [11]
Assistant Professor of Surgery
Department of Surgery
Division of Pediatric Surgery
Tufts University School of Medicine,
    Baystate Medical Center
Springfield, Massachusetts

**Edward M. Barksdale Jr, MD** [40]
Robert J. Izant Professor and Surgeon-in-Chief
Department of Surgery
Division of Pediatric Surgery
Rainbow Babies and Children's Hospital/University Hospitals
Case Western Reserve School of Medicine
Cleveland, Ohio

**Marianne Beaudin, MD** [80]
Pediatric Surgery Trauma Fellow
Department of Surgery
Division of Pediatric and Thoracic Surgery
Cincinnati Children's Hospital Medical Center
University of Cincinnati College of Medicine
Cincinnati, Ohio

**James M. Betts, MD** [62]
Surgeon-in-Chief
Clinical Professor of Pediatric Surgery and Urology
Department of Outpatient Center
Children's Hospital and Research Center Oakland
University of California San Francisco - East Bay
Children's Hospital Oakland
Oakland, California

**Alan Bielsky, MD** [10]
Assistant Professor of Anesthesiology
Department of Anesthesiology
Children's Hospital Colorado
University of Colorado School of Medicine
Aurora, Colorado

**David A. Billmire, MD, FACS, FAAP** [96]
Professor of Surgery
Division of Pediatric Plastic Surgery
Cincinnati Children's Hospital Medical Center
Cincinnati, Ohio

**Thane A. Blinman, MD** [77]
Assistant Professor of Surgery
Department of Surgery
Children's Hospital Philadelphia
Philadelphia, Pennsylvania

**Alex Bondoc, MD** [58]
Pediatric Surgery Fellow
Department of Pediatric and Thoracic Surgery
Cincinnati Children's Hospital Medical Center
University of Cincinnati
Cincinnati, Ohio

**Drucy S. Borowitz, MD** [43]
Professor of Clinical Pediatrics
Director, Cystic Fibrosis Center
Women and Children's Hospital of Buffalo
University at Buffalo
State University of New York
Buffalo, New York

**Lesley Breech, MD** [70]
Division Director
Division of Pediatric and Adolescent Gynecology
Cincinnati Children's Hospital Medical Center
Cincinnati, Ohio

**Mark F. Brown, MD** [51]
Pediatric Surgeon
Department of Surgery
Louisiana State University-Shreveport
Willis-Knighton Health System
Shreveport, Louisiana

**Rebeccah L. Brown, MD** [48]
Associate Professor of Clinical Surgery and Pediatrics
Division of Pediatric General and Thoracic Surgery
Cincinnati Children's Hospital Medical Center
Cincinnati, Ohio

**Allen Browne, MD** [39]
Clinical Professor
Department of Surgery
University of Illinois College of Medicine–Peoria
Children's Hospital of Illinois
Peoria, Illinois

**Jennifer Bruny, MD** [18]
Assistant Professor of Surgery
Department of Surgery
Colorado Children's Hospital
University of Colorado School of Medicine
Aurora, Colorado

**Brian T. Bucher, MD** [4]
Resident
Department of Surgery
Washington University School of Medicine
St. Louis, Missouri

**Kathleen M. Campbell, MD** [57]
Assistant Professor of Pediatrics
Division of Gastroenterology, Hepatology and Nutrition
Pediatric Liver Care Center
Cincinnati Children's Hospital Medical Center
Cincinnati, Ohio

**Donna A. Caniano, MD** [2]
Professor Emeritus
Surgeon-in-Chief Emeritus
Department of Surgery
The Ohio State University College of Medicine
Nationwide Children's Hospital
Columbus, Ohio

**Douglas A. Canning, MD** [67]
Chair and Professor of Urology
Division of Pediatric Urology
Children's Hospital of Philadelphia
University of Pennsylvania School of Medicine
Philadelphia, Pennsylvania

**Brent E. Carlyle, MD**  [43]
University at Buffalo
State University of New York
Buffalo, New York

**Michael C. Carr, MD, PhD**  [65]
Associate Director
Professor of Urology
Department of Pediatric Urology
Children's Hospital of Philadelphia
University of Pennsylvania
Philadelphia, Pennsylvania

**Shannon L. Castle, MD**  [46]
Research Fellow
Department of Pediatric Surgery
Children's Hospital Los Angeles
Los Angeles, California

**Michael G. Caty, MD, MMM**  [37]
Robert Pritzker Professor and Chief Program Director
Surgeon-in-Chief
Department of Pediatric Surgery
Yale-New Haven Children's Hospital
New Haven, Connecticut

**Artur Chernoguz, MD**  [7, 94]
Research Fellow
Division of Pediatric General and Thoracic Surgery
Cincinnati Children's Hospital Medical Center
Cincinnati, Ohio

**Anthony C. Chin, MD, MS**  [32]
Assistant Professor of Surgery
Department of Surgery
Northwestern University Feinberg School of Medicine
Ann and Robert H. Lurie Children's Hospital of Chicago
Chicago, Illinois

**Priscilla P. L. Chiu, MD, PhD, FRCSC, FACS, FAAP**  [22]
Paediatric Surgeon
Assistant Professor
Division of Pediatric Surgery
Department of Surgery
Hospital for Sick Children
University of Toronto
Toronto, Ontario

**Emily Christison-Lagay, MD**  [41]
Assistant Professor of Pediatric Surgery
Division of General and Thoracic Surgery
Yale-New Haven Children's Hospital,
    Yale School of Medicine
New Haven, Connecticut

**Jeannie Chun, MD**  [71]
Assistant Professor of Surgery
Department of Surgery
University of Maryland
Baltimore, Maryland

**Dai H. Chung, MD**  [89]
Professor and Chairman
Department of Pediatric General and Thoracic Surgery
Vanderbilt University Medical Center
Nashville, Tennessee

**Walter J. Chwals, MD, FACS, FCCM, FAAP**  [8]
Professor of Surgery and Pediatrics
Surgeon-in-Chief
Director of Trauma
Department of Surgery
Tufts University School of Medicine
Floating Hospital for Children
Kiwanis Pediatric Trauma Institute
Boston, Massachusetts

**Robert A. Cina, MD**  [23, 36]
Assistant Professor of Surgery and Pediatrics
Department of Surgery
Division of Pediatric Surgery
Medical University of South Carolina
Charleston, South Carolina

**Aliza P. Cohen, MA**  [75]
Medical Writer
Surgical Services
Cincinnati Children's Hospital Medical Center
Cincinnati, Ohio

**Paul M. Colombani, MD**  [97]
Robert Garrett Professor of Pediatric Surgery
Pediatric Surgeon-in-Charge
Department of Pediatric Surgery
Johns Hopkins University Hospital
Baltimore, Maryland

**Victor A. Convertino, PhD**  [7]
Senior Research Physiologist
Director of the Human Physiology Laboratory
Manager of the Tactical Combat Casualty Care Research
    Task Area
US Army Institute of Surgical Research
Fort Sam Houston, Texas

**Arthur Cooper, MD, MS**  [78]
Professor of Surgery
Director of Trauma and Pediatric Surgical Services
Department of Surgery
Columbia University College of Physicians and Surgeons
Harlem Hospital Center
New York, New York

**Roger Cornwall, MD**  [82]
Associate Professor of Orthopedic Surgery
Department of Orthopedic Surgery
Cincinnati Children's Hospital Medical Center
Cincinnati, Ohio

**Timothy M. Crombleholme, MD, FACS, FAAP** [29]
Ponzio Family Chair for the Surgeon-in-Chief
Vice Chair of Pediatric Surgical Programs
Director, Center for Children's Surgery
Professor of Surgery
Director, Colorado Institute for Maternal Fetal Health
Director, Colorado Fetal Care Center
Department of Surgery at the University of Colorado
    School of Medicine
Colorado Children's Hospital
Aurora, Colorado

**Kerry R. Crone, MD** [79]
Professor of Neurosurgery and Pediatrics
Division of Pediatric Neurosurgery
Cincinnati Children's Hospital Medical Center
Cincinnati, Ohio

**John P. Crow, MD** [83]
Chairman of Surgery
Clinical Professor of Surgery
Department of Pediatric Surgery
Northeastern Ohio Universities College of Medicine
Akron Children's Hospital
Akron, Ohio

**Roshni Dasgupta, MD, MPH** [75]
Associate Professor of Surgery
Division of Pediatric General and Thoracic Surgery
Cincinnati Children's Hospital Medical Center
Cincinnati, Ohio

**Katherine P. Davenport, MD** [31]
Joseph E. Robert Jr Research Fellow
Sheikh Zayed Institute for Pediatric Surgical Innovation
Children's National Medical Center
Washington, DC

**Andrew M. Davidoff, MD** [88]
Chairman
Department of Surgery
St. Jude Children's Research Hospital
Memphis, Tennessee

**Paolo De Coppi, MD, PhD** [24]
Head of Surgery Unit
Institute of Child Health
University College London
Great Ormond Street Hospital for Children
NHS Foundation Trust
London, United Kingdom

**Jeffrey J. Dehmer, MD** [50]
Surgical Resident
Department of Surgery
University of North Carolina at Chapel Hill
Chapel Hill, North Carolina

**Jeffrey Donohoe, MD** [68]
Chief, Pediatric Urology
Department of Surgery
Children's Hospital of Georgia
Augusta, Georgia

**Peter Ehrlich, MD, MSC** [95]
Associate Professor of Surgery
Vice Chair Surgery Hodgkin's Lymphoma Children's
    Oncology Group
Section of Pediatric Surgery
University of Michigan School of Medicine
Ann Arbor, Michigan

**Mauricio A. Escobar Jr, MD, FACS, FAAP** [37]
Pediatric Trauma Medical Director
Clinical Instructor
Department of Pediatric Surgery
MultiCare Health Systems
UW Medicine
University of Washington
Tacoma, Washington

**Barry Evans, MD, FACCP, FAAP** [30]
Associate Professor of Pediatrics
Department of Pediatrics
Temple University School of Medicine
Philadelphia, Pennsylvania

**Richard A. Falcone Jr, MD, MPH** [80]
Associate Professor
Division of Pediatric General and Thoracic Surgery
Cincinnati Children's Hospital Medical Center
University of Cincinnati College of Medicine
Cincinnati, Ohio

**Mary E. Fallat, MD** [71]
Hirikati S. Nagaraj Professor
Division Director Pediatric Surgery
Surgeon-in-Chief
Department of Surgery
University of Louisville
Kosair Children's Hospital
Louisville, Kentucky

**Brad A. Feltis, MD, PhD** [45]
Pediatric Surgical Associate
Department of Surgery
Children's Hospitals and Clinics of Minnesota
Minneapolis, Minnesota

**Andrew C. Fiore, MD** [72]
Director, Pediatric Cardiac Surgery
Professor of Surgery
Division of Cardiac Surgery
Cardinal Glennon Children's Hospital
St. Louis University
St. Louis, Missouri

**Alan W. Flake, MD**   [3]
Professor of Surgery
Director, Center for Fetal Research
Department of Pediatric, Thoracic, and Fetal Surgery
Children's Hospital of Philadelphia
Philadelphia, Pennsylvania

**Henri Ford, MD, MHA**   [46]
Professor
Department of Pediatric Surgery
Children's Hospital Los Angeles
Los Angeles, California

**Frazier W. Frantz, MD, FACS**   [17]
Associate Professor of Clinical Surgery and Pediatrics
Pediatric General and Thoracic Surgery
Children's Hospital of The King's Daughters
Norfolk, Virginia

**Jason S. Frischer, MD**   [7, 94]
Assistant Professor of Surgery and Pediatrics
Division of Pediatric General and Thoracic Surgery
University of Cincinnati College of Medicine
Cincinnati Children's Hospital Medical Center
Cincinnati, Ohio

**Philip K. Frykman, MD, PhD, MBA, FACS, FAAP**   [26]
Associate Director, Pediatric Surgery
Associate Professor of Surgery and Biomedical Sciences
Department of Surgery
Cedars-Sinai Medical Center
Los Angeles, California

**Megan K. Fuller, MD**   [50]
Surgical Resident
Department of Surgery
University of North Carolina at Chapel Hill
Chapel Hill, North Carolina

**Michael W. L. Gauderer, MD, FACS, FAAP**   [36]
Professor of Pediatric Surgery and Pediatrics
Children's Hospital, Greenville Hospital System University
   Medical Center
University of South Carolina School of Medicine
   (Greenville)
Greenville, South Carolina

**Keith E. Georgeson, MD**   [44]
Specialist in Pediatric Surgery
Department of Surgery
Providence Pediatric Surgery Center
Spokane, Washington

**Alexandros Georgolios, MD**   [20]
Resident, Otolaryngology
Department of Otolaryngology, Head and Neck Surgery
VCU Medical Center
Virginia Commonwealth University
Richmond, Virginia

**James C. Gilbert, MD**   [82]
Clinical Associate Professor of Pediatric Surgery
Department of Pediatric Surgery
Tennessee Valley Pediatric Surgery
Huntsville, Alabama

**Joshua B. Glenn, MD**   [14]
Assistant Professor Surgery
Director of Pediatric Surgery
Department of Surgery
Mercer University School of Medicine
Medical Center of Central Georgia
Macon, Georgia

**Philip L. Glick, MD, MBA**   [43]
Vice Chairman
Professor of Surgery
Department of Surgery
University at Buffalo
State University of New York
Buffalo, New York

**Michael J. Goretsky, MD, FACS**   [17]
Associate Professor of Clinical Surgery and Pediatrics
Pedaitric General and Thoracic Surgery
Children's Surgery Specialty Group
Norfolk, Virginia

**John R. Gosche, MD, PhD**   [13]
Professor of Surgery and Pediatrics
Division of Pediatric Surgery
University of South Alabama
Mobile, Alabama

**Harsh Grewal, MD, FACS, FAAP**   [30]
Professor of Surgery
Division Head, Pediatric Surgery
Division of Pediatric Surgery
Cooper Medical School and Cooper University Health Care
Camden, New Jersey

**Tracy C. Grikscheit, MD**   [46]
Assistant Professor
Department of Pediatric Surgery
Children's Hospital Los Angeles
Los Angeles, California

**Jonathan I. Groner, MD**   [19, 28]
Professor of Clinical Surgery
Department of Surgery
Ohio State University College of Medicine
   and Nationwide Children's Hospital
Columbus, Ohio

**Kavita Gupta**   [67]
Student, Division of Pediatric Urology
Children's Hospital of Philadelphia
Student, George Washington University
Washington, DC

**Ivan M. Gutierrez, MD** [6]
Research Fellow
Department of Surgery
Children's Hospital Boston
Boston, Massachusetts

**Robert S. Hatch, MD** [82]
Orthopedic Surgeon
Department of Orthopedics
Hatch Orthopedics
Ormond Beach, Florida

**Andrea Hayes-Jordan, MD** [92]
Associate Professor and Director of Pediatric Surgical
   Oncology
Department of Surgical Oncology
University of Texas MD Anderson Cancer Center
Houston, Texas

**Andre Hebra, MD** [23]
Professor of Surgery and Pediatrics
Department of Surgery
Division of Pediatric Surgery
Medical University of South Carolina
Charleston, South Carolina

**Michael A. Helmrath, MD** [50]
Professor of Surgery
Division of Pediatric General and Thoracic Surgery
Cincinnati Children's Hospital Medical Center
Cincinnati, Ohio

**Patricio Herrera, MD** [22]
Head of OR
Department of General Surgery
Hospital Dr. Exequiel González Cortés and Clínica Alemana
Santiago, Chile

**Mary Hilfiker, PhD, MD, MMM** [60]
Professor of Surgery
Department of Surgery
UCSD School of Medicine and
   Rady Children's Specialists of San Diego
San Diego, California

**J. Laurence Hill, MD** [42]
Professor Emeritus of Surgery
Department of Surgery
Division of Pediatric Surgery
University of Maryland School of Medicine
Baltimore, Maryland

**Michael Hines, MD** [72]
Director
Assistant Professor Cardiothoracic Surgery and Pediatrics
Department of General Heart Surgery
Section of Medicine
Brenner Children's Hospital
Wake Forest University
Winston-Salem, North Carolina

**Ronald B. Hirschl, MD** [7]
Professor, Department of Pediatric Surgery
C.S. Mott Children's Hospital
University of Michigan
Ann Arbor, Michigan

**George W. Holcomb III, MD, MBA** [55]
The Katharine B. Richardson Professor of Surgery
Surgeon-in-Chief
Department of Surgery
Children's Mercy Hospital
Kansas City, Missouri

**Ai-Xuan Holterman, MD** [39]
Professor
Department of Surgery
University of Illinois College of Medicine–Peoria/
   Children's Hospital of Illinois
Peoria, Illinois

**Mark Holterman, MD, PhD** [39]
Professor
Department of Surgery
University of Illinois College of Medicine–Peoria/
   Children's Hospital of Illinois
Peoria, Illinois

**Charles G. Howell Jr, MD** [68]
Surgeon-in-Chief
Professor of Surgery and Pediatrics
Chairman, Department of Surgery
Medical College of Georgia
Children's Hospital of Georgia
Augusta, Georgia

**Manuela Hunziker, MD** [66]
Senior Research Fellow
National Children's Research Centre
Our Lady's Children's Hospital
Dublin, Ireland

**Corey W. Iqbal, MD** [86]
Chief and Assistant Professor of Surgery
Section of Fetal Surgery
Children's Mercy Hospitals and Clinics
University of Missouri Kansas City
Kansas City, Missouri

**Saleem Islam, MD, MPH**  [34]
Associate Professor
Department of Surgery
University of Florida
Gainesville, Florida

**Tom Jaksic, MD, PhD**  [6]
W. Hardy Hendren Professor of Surgery
Department of Pediatric Surgery
Harvard Medical School
Boston Children's Hospital
Boston, Massachusetts

**Charles Johnson III, MD**  [20]
Professor of Surgery
Chair of the Division of Pediatric Otolaryngology
Department of Otolaryngology, Head and Neck Surgery
Medical College of Virginia/Virginia
    Commonwealth University
Richmond, Virginia

**Stephen G. Jolley, MD**  [27]
Pediatric Surgeons of Alaska
Anchorage, Alaska

**Stephanie A. Jones, DO**  [56]
Resident in Pediatric Surgery
Children's Hospital of Colorado
Department of Surgery
Children's Hospital of Central California
Madera, California

**David Juang, MD**  [55]
Assistant Professor of Surgery
Director, Surgical Critical Care
Department of Surgery
Children's Mercy Hospital
Kansas City, Missouri

**Timothy D. Kane, MD, FACS, FAAP**  [31]
Division Chief, General and Thoracic Surgery
Sheikh Zayed Institute for Pediatric Surgical Innovation
Children's National Medical Center
Washington, DC

**Frederick M. Karrer, MD**  [56]
Professor of Surgery
Chief of the Division of Pediatric Surgery
Department of Surgery
University of Colorado School of Medicine
Colorado Children's Hospital
Aurora, Colorado

**Scott J. Keckler, MD**  [5]
Resident in Pediatric Surgery
Department of Pediatric Surgery
University of Oklahoma College of Medicine
Oklahoma City, Oklahoma

**Peter C. W. Kim, MD, PhD**  [22]
Vice President
Associate Surgeon-in-Chief
Professor of Surgery, Pediatrics and Systems Integrative
    Biology
Department of Surgery
Sheikh Zayed Institute for Pediatric Surgical Innovation
Children's National Medical Center
George Washington University School of Medicine
Washington, DC

**Evan Kokoska, MD**  [35]
Clinical Associate Professor of Surgery
Division of Pediatric Surgery
Indiana University School of Medicine
Peyton Manning Children's Hospital
Indianapolis, Indiana

**Jacob C. Langer, MD**  [41, 44]
Professor of Surgery
Division of General and Thoracic Surgery
University of Toronto
Hospital for Sick Children
Toronto, Ontario

**Marc A. Levitt, MD**  [53]
Colorectal Center for Children
Professor of Surgery
Division of Pediatric General and Thoracic Surgery
Cincinnati Children's Hospital Medical Center
University of Cincinnati College of Medicine
Cincinnati, Ohio

**Craig W. Lillehei, MD**  [98]
Associate Professor of Surgery
Department of Surgery
Harvard Medical School
Boston Children's Hospital
Boston, Massachusetts

**Eric Long, MD**  [89]
Pediatric Surgical Research Fellow
Department of Pediatric General and Thoracic Surgery
Vanderbilt University Medical Center
Nashville, Tennessee

**Francois I. Luks, MD, PhD**  [33]
Professor of Surgery, Pediatrics and
    Obstetrics and Gynecology
Department of Surgery (Pediatric Surgery)
Alpert Medical School of Brown University/Hasbro
    Children's Hospital
Providence, Rhode Island

**Peter B. Manning, MD** [73]
Professor of Surgery
Division of Pediatric Cardiothoracic Surgery
Washington University in St. Louis School of Medicine
St. Louis Children's Hospital
St. Louis, Missouri

**Rebecca J. McClaine, MD** [87]
Assistant Professor of Surgery
Department of Surgery
University of Cincinnati
Cincinnati, Ohio

**Marcene R. McVay, MD** [84]
Pediatric Surgeon
Department of Pediatric Surgery
Arkansas Children's Hospital
Little Rock, Arkansas

**David Merten, MD** [78]
Emeritus Professor of Radiology and Pediatrics
University of North Carolina at Chapel Hill
Chapel Hill, North Carolina

**Rebecka L. Meyers, MD** [93]
Professor of Pediatric Surgery
Primary Children's Medical Center
University of Utah
Salt Lake City, Utah

**Eugene Minevich, MD, FAAP, FACS** [69]
Professor
Division of Pediatric Urology
Cincinnati Children's Hospital Medical Center
Cincinnati, Ohio

**Christopher R. Moir, MD** [49]
Professor of Surgery
Division of Pediatric Surgery
Mayo Clinic Rochester
Rochester, Minnesota

**David P. Mooney, MD, MPH** [81]
Director, Trauma Center
Assistant Professor of Surgery
Department of Surgery
Boston Children's Hospital and Harvard Medical School
Boston, Massachusetts

**Steven L. Moulton, MD, FACS, FAAP** [7]
Professor of Surgery
Director
Department of Trauma and Burn Services
University of Colorado, School of Medicine
Children's Hospital Colorado
Aurora, Colorado

**Jane Mulligan, PhD** [7]
Chief Scientific Officer
Flashback Technologies, Inc.
Boulder, Colorado

**J. Patrick Murphy, MD** [61]
Chief, Section of Urology
Professor of Surgery
University of Missouri Kansas City School of Medicine
Clinical Professor Surgery
University of Kansas School of Medicine
Children's Mercy Hospital
Kansas University Medical Center
Kansas City, Missouri

**Michael Nance, MD** [77]
Professor of Surgery
Department of Surgery
Children's Hospital Philadelphia
Philadelphia, Pennsylvania

**Jaimie D. Nathan, MD** [57, 74]
Assistant Professor of Surgery
Division of Pediatric General and Thoracic Surgery
Cincinnati Children's Hospital Medical Center
Cincinnati, Ohio

**Wallace W. Neblett III, MD** [14]
Professor of Surgery
Department of Pediatric Surgery
Vanderbilt University Medical Center
Monroe Carell Jr, Children's Hospital at Vanderbilt
Nashville, Tennessee

**Brian S. Pan, MD, FAAP** [96]
Assistant Professor of Surgery
Division of Pediatric Plastic Surgery
Cincinnati Children's Hospital Medical Center
Cincinnati, Ohio

**Lisa Parrillo, MD** [67]
Resident
Division of Urology, Department of Surgery
Perelman School of Medicine
University of Pennsylvania
Philadelphia, Pennsylvania

**David A. Partrick, MD** [38]
Associate Professor of Surgery
Department of Surgery
University of Colorado School of Medicine
Colorado Children's Hospital
Aurora, Colorado

**Alberto Peña, MD** [53]
Professor of Surgery
Division of Pediatric General and Thoracic Surgery
Founding Director Colorectal Center for Children
Cincinnati Children's Hospital Medical Center
University of Cincinnati College of Medicine
Cincinnati, Ohio

**D. Glenn Pennington, MD** [72]
Professor of Surgery
Department of Surgery
East Tennessee State University
Johnson City, Tennessee

**John K. Petty, MD** [9]
Director of Pediatric Trauma
Associate Professor of Surgery and Pediatrics
Department of General Surgery
Brenner Children's Hospital
Wake Forest School of Medicine
Winston-Salem, North Carolina

**Agostino Pierro, MD, FRCS (Engl), FRCS (Ed), FAAP** [24]
Robert M. Filler Professor of Surgery
Head, Division of General and Thoracic Surgery
The Hospital for Sick Children
University of Toronto
Toronto, Canada

**David M. Polaner, MD, FAAP** [10]
Professor of Anesthesiology and Pediatrics
Department of Anesthesiology
Children's Hospital Colorado
University of Colorado School of Medicine
Aurora, Colorado

**Todd A. Ponsky, MD, FACS** [40]
Associate Professor of Surgery and Pediatrics
Division of Pediatric Surgery
Northeast Ohio Medical University
Akron Children's Hospital
Akron, Ohio

**D. Dean Potter, MD** [49]
Clinical Associate Professor of Surgery
Division of Pediatric Surgery
University of Iowa Hospitals and Clinics
Iowa City, Iowa

**Sean Primley, MD** [64]
Resident
Division of Urology Academic Office One Building
Children's Hospital of Colorado
Aurora, Colorado

**Prem Puri, MS, FRCS, FRCS (ED), FACS, FAAP (Hon)** [66]
Newman Clinical Research Professor
President of National Children's Research Centre
Consultant Pediatric Surgeon
National Children's Research Centre
University College Dublin
Our Lady's Children's Hospital
Beacon Hospital Dublin
Dublin, Ireland

**Sara K. Rasmussen, MD, MSC** [97]
Assistant Professor of Surgery
Department of Surgery
Division of Pediatric Surgery
University of Virginia School of Medicine
Charlottesville, Virginia

**Pamela D. Reiter, PharmD** [7]
Clinical Associate Professor
Clinical Pharmacy Specialist in Pediatric ICU and Trauma
Department of Pharmacy
University of Colorado, School of Pharmacy
Aurora, Colorado

**Frederick J. Rescorla, MD** [90]
Surgeon-in-Chief
Department of Surgery
Division of Pediatric Surgery
Riley Hospital for Children
Indiana University School of Medicine
Indianapolis, Indiana

**Jorge Reyes, MD** [100]
Professor of Surgery and Adjunct Professor of Pathology
Chief Division of Transplant Surgery
University of Washington
Seattle Children's Hospital
Seattle, Washington

**Marleta Reynolds, MD** [32]
Head, Department of Surgery and Surgeon-in-Chief
Lydia J. Fredrickson Professor of Pediatric Surgery
Northwestern University Feinberg School of Medicine
Ann and Robert H. Lurie Children's Hospital of Chicago
Chicago, Illinois

**J. Brent Roaten, MD, PhD** [27]
Pediatric Surgeons of Alaska
Anchorage, Alaska

**William W. Robertson Jr, MD** [82]
Field Representative
Clinical Professor of Orthopaedic Surgery
Orthopaedic Surgery and Pediatrics
Accreditation Council for Graduate Medical Education
George Washington University School of Medicine
Washington, DC

**David A. Rodeberg, MD**  [91]
Professor of Surgery
Chief, Division of Pediatric Surgery
Department of Pediatric General and Thoracic Surgery
Pitt County Memorial Hospital East Carolina University
Greenville, North Carolina

**Steven Rothenberg, MD**  [29]
Chief of Pediatric Surgery
Rocky Mountain Hospital for Children
Clinical Professor of Surgery
Department of Surgery
Columbia University College of Physicians and Surgeons
Denver, Colorado

**Michael J. Rutter, FRACS**  [21]
Professor of Pediatric Otolaryngology
Department of Otolaryngology–Head and Neck Surgery
University of Cincinnati College of Medicine
Cincinnati Children's Hospital Medical Center
Cincinnati, Ohio

**Frederick C. Ryckman, MD**  [57]
Professor of Surgery
Sr. Vice President, Medical Operations
Department of Surgery
Division of Pediatric and Thoracic Surgery
University of Cincinnati
Cincinnati Children's Hospital Medical Center
Cincinnati, Ohio

**David J. Schmeling, MD**  [45]
Department of Surgery
Pediatric Surgical Associates, Ltd
Minneapolis, Minnesota

**Richard M. Schwend, MD**  [82]
Director of Orthopaedic Research
Clinical Professor of Orthopaedic Surgery
Department of Orthopaedic Surgery
Children's Mercy Hospital
Kansas City, Missouri

**Robert C. Shamberger, MD**  [17]
Robert E. Gross Professor of Surgery and Chief of Surgery
Department of Surgery
Harvard Medical School
Boston Children's Hospital
Boston, Massachusetts

**Curtis A. Sheldon, MD**  [69]
Professor of Surgery
Division of Pediatric Urology
Cincinnati Children's Hospital Medical Center
Cincinnati, Ohio

**Stephen B. Shew, MD**  [6]
Associate Professor of Surgery
Division of Pediatric Surgery
Mattel Children's Hospital
David Geffen School of Medicine at UCLA
Los Angeles, California

**Samuel Smith, MD**  [13]
Boyd Family Chair Professor of Surgery
Chief of Pediatric Surgery
Department of Surgery
University of Arkansas for Medical Sciences
Arkansas Children's Hospital
Little Rock, Arkansas

**Howard M. Snyder III, MD**  [65, 67]
Senior Surgeon
Professor of Urology
Department of Pediatric Urology
Children's Hospital of Philadelphia
University of Pennsylvania
Philadelphia, Pennsylvania

**Stig Sømme, MD**  [12]
Assistant Professor of Pediatric Surgery
Department of Surgery
University of Colorado School of Medicine
Children's Hospital Colorado
Aurora, Colorado

**Allison L. Speer, MD**  [46]
Research Fellow
Department of Pediatric Surgery
Children's Hospital Los Angeles
Los Angeles, California

**Wolfgang Stehr, MD**  [62]
Attending Surgeon
Assistant Clinical Professor
Department of Surgery
Division of Pediatric Surgery
Children's Hospital and Research Center Oakland
University of California San Francisco—East Bay
Oakland, California

**Heidi A. Stephany, MD**  [61]
Staff Surgeon
Department of Urology
University of Pittsburgh
Assistant Professor of Pediatric Urology
University of Pittsburgh School of Medicine
Pittsburgh, Pennsylvania

**Daniel J. Stephens, MD**  [54]
General Surgery Resident
Department of General Surgery
University of Minnesota
Minneapolis, Minnesota

**Charles B. Stevenson, MD** [79]
Assistant Professor of Neurosurgery and Pediatrics
Division of Pediatric Neurosurgery
Cincinnati Children's Hospital Medical Center
Cincinnati, Ohio

**Alex Stoffan, MD, MPH** [81]
Department of Surgery
Wayne State University
Detroit, Michigan

**Eric D. Strauch, MD** [42]
Assistant Professor of Surgery
Department of Surgery
Division of Pediatric Surgery
University of Maryland School of Medicine
Baltimore, Maryland

**Peter F. Sturm, MD** [82]
Professor of Pediatric Orthopedic Surgery
Alvin H. Crawford Chair of Spine Surgery
Director of Crawford Spine Center
Department of Orthopedic Surgery
Cincinnati Children's Hospital Medical Center
Cincinnati, Ohio

**Roman Sydorak, MD, MPH** [52]
Pediatric Surgeon
Department of Pediatric Surgery
Kaiser Permanente Medical Center
Los Angeles Medical Center
Los Angeles, California

**Leslie Ann Taylor, MD** [16, 78]
Professor, Chief of Pediatric Surgery
Department of Surgery
East Tennessee State University
Johnson City, Tennessee

**Steven Teich, MD** [28]
Associate Professor of Clinical Surgery
The Ohio State University College of Medicine
Department of Pediatric Surgery
Nationwide Children's Hospital
Columbus, Ohio

**Daniel H. Teitelbaum, MD** [44]
Professor of Surgery
Department of Surgery, Section of Pediatric Surgery
C.S. Mott Children's Hospital
University of Michigan Medical Center
Ann Arbor, Michigan

**Greg M. Tiao, MD** [57, 58, 93, 99]
Associate Professor of Surgery
Surgical Assistant Director, Liver Transplantation
Professor of Surgery
Division of Pediatric General and Thoracic Surgery
Cincinnati Children's Hospital Medical Center
Cincinnati, Ohio

**Thomas Tracy Jr, MD, MS, FACS, FAAP** [33]
Professor of Surgery and Pediatrics
Department of Pediatric Surgery
Hasbro Children's Hospital
Alpert Medical School of Brown University
Providence, Rhode Island

**David W. Tuggle, MD, FACS, FAAP, FCCM** [5]
Professor and Vice-Chairman
Department of Surgery
University of Oklahoma College of Medicine
Oklahoma City, Oklahoma

**Khashayar Vakili, MD** [98]
Instructor in Surgery
Department of Surgery
Harvard Medical School
Boston Children's Hospital
Boston, Massachusetts

**Daniel von Allmen, MD** [76, 85, 87]
Frederick C. Ryckman Chair of Pediatric Surgery
Professor of Surgery
Cincinnati Children's Hospital Medical Center
University of Cincinnati College of Medicine
Cincinnati, Ohio

**Jesse D. Vrecenak, MD** [3]
Research Fellow, Center for Fetal Research
Center for Fetal Diagnosis and Therapy
Children's Hospital of Philadelphia
Philadelphia, Pennsylvania

**Charles Wagner, MD** [84]
Retired Professor of Surgery and Pediatrics
Department of Surgery
University of Arkansas for Medical Sciences
Little Rock, Arkansas

**David C. Wahoff, MD, PhD** [86]
Assistant Clinical Professor of Surgery
Department of Surgery
Mayo Clinic College of Medicine
Pediatric Surgical Associates
Minneapolis, Minnesota

**John H.T. Waldhausen, MD** [60]
Professor of Surgery
Department of Surgery
Division of Pediatric General and Thoracic Surgery
University of Washington School of Medicine
Seattle Children's Hospital
Seattle, Washington

**Brad W. Warner, MD** [4]
Jessie L. Ternberg, MD, PhD, Distinguished
   Professor of Pediatric Surgery
Department of Surgery
Division of Pediatric Surgery
Washington University School of Medicine
St. Louis, Missouri

**Akilah Weber, MD** [70]
Assistant Professor
Department of Obstetrics and Gynecology
UT Southwestern
Dallas, Texas

**Thomas R. Weber, MD** [35, 47]
Professor, Pediatric Surgery
Department of General Surgery
Rush University Medical Center
Chicago, Illinois

**Duncan Wilcox, MD** [64]
Professor of Pediatric Urology
Chair, Department of Pediatric Urology
Children's Hospital of Colorado
Aurora, Colorado

**Felicia N. Williams, MD** [91]
Assistant Professor
University of Texas Medical Branch
Pitt County Memorial Hospital
East Carolina University
Houston, Texas

**Mark L. Wulkan, MD** [44]
Professor of Surgery and Chief
Division of Pediatric Surgery
Department of Surgery
Children's Healthcare of Atlanta
Emory Children's Center
Atlanta, Georgia

**Kristen A. Zeller, MD** [9]
Assistant Professor of Surgery and Pediatrics
Department of General Surgery
Brenner Children's Hospital
Wake Forest School of Medicine
Winston-Salem, North Carolina

**Moritz M. Ziegler, MD** [1]
Retired, Surgeon-in-Chief and the Ponzio Family Chair
Children's Hospital of Colorado
Professor of Surgery
University of Colorado School of Medicine
Cincinnati, Ohio

CONTRIBUTORS

# Preface

Ten years ago, the first edition of *Operative Pediatric Surgery* was published by McGraw-Hill. The "editorial purpose" of the book was to consolidate into a single volume a pediatric surgical textbook that would include a limited introduction of the topic's history and a thorough discussion of diagnostic and therapeutic principles, with the generous use of artistic illustrations, radiographs, and photographs that emphasize the authors' preferred operative techniques, all in an atlas format. Also included, where appropriate, would be diagnostic and treatment algorithms or care guidelines. In this second edition, our authors have presented a contemporary update of each topic, and where relevant we have admixed minimally invasive operative techniques with the open approach, rather than separating laparoscopy and thoracoscopy into a separate topic as in the first edition. This should bring greater clarity to the current operation(s) preferred by each author.

This textbook is divided into 11 parts that include a total of 100 chapters. The critical care chapter has been expanded to be as current as possible, including the application of new monitoring techniques. There are also new chapters on the topics of hypospadias, adolescent bariatric surgery, vesicoureteral reflux, non-rhabdomyosarcoma sarcomas, and gastrointestinal polyps and cancer. In short, this second edition of *Operative Pediatric Surgery* represents a completely new book that preserves the structural format of the first.

Pediatric surgery remains the life's calling of the four editors as well as our authors. It represents a surgical enterprise that provides operative care to our most vulnerable population, our children. It is hoped that this textbook will provide comprehensive information for trainees, practicing pediatric surgeons, and those surgeons—whether adult general surgeons or other specialty surgeons—who provide operative care for children.

# Acknowledgments

When developing one's commitment as well as expertise in a field of medicine and surgery, there are multiple levels of teaching, mentoring, and even nurturing involved that shape this personal evolution. Leading the list of influences would be the patients and their families; and to each and every one of them for whom we were privileged to know and provide care, we give our ultimate in recognition and gratitude. Our teachers and mentors were many but for each of us the following deserve thanks and special recognition: for MMZ: Clyde Barker, C. Everett Koop, Harry Bishop, Louise Schnaufer, John Templeton, and Lester Martin; for RGA: M. Judah Folkman, Bradley M. Rodgers, J. Alexander Haller, J. Laurance Hill, George F. Sheldon, and James M. Anderson; for TRW: C. Gardner Child, William J. Fry, Judson Randolph, and R. Peter Altman; and for DVA: Moritz Ziegler, Frederick Ryckman, Josef Fischer, and Anthony Meyer. We also acknowledge with extreme gratitude and respect our fellow faculty members, our nursing and administrative teams, and most importantly our trainees themselves—those future leaders, educators, researchers, and clinicians who will carry pediatric surgery forward.

However, the most important advocates for each of us have been our families, who encouraged, supported, and sacrificed the element of family time so that this project and our careers could progress—acts of sincere unselfishness. For MMZ: these family members include Barbara, my wife of 43 years who accompanied me through four career moves, and our sons Matthew Ziegler, MD, and David Ziegler, both of whom have provided us with great joy through their personal career developments. I would like to recognize my late parents, Max and Elsa Ziegler, whose sacrifices permitted me to pursue my career. For RGA: my wife, Geralyn, and my son, Aaron, who have always given me unconditional love and much joy. I am also very grateful to my loving parents Dr. R. George and Helga Azizkhan for being my most important role models in both my professional and personal life. For TRW: these critical people are my wife of 44 years, Suzanne, and my children, Amy, Jill, and Patrick. And, for DVA: my wife, Emily, and sons, Douglas and Karl. They are the foundation of my life.

We also want to acknowledge our collective thanks for the skill and dedication of medical illustrator Jan Warren, who, while working in the Cincinnati Department of Pediatric Surgery, contributed the lion's share of the drawings depicted in this book. In addition, we would like to recognize Charlotte Bath and Aliza Cohen, who worked with several of the authors to make their contributions both elegant and refined. We are indebted to several key individuals who made this book production possible: most important was Brian Belval, Senior Editor, Clinical Medicine, for McGraw-Hill, who was with this project since its inception. We are also grateful to Marsha Loeb and Jennifer Orlando of McGraw-Hill, freelance editors Sarah M. Granlund and Portia Levasseur, and, finally, Ritu Joon of Thomson Digital for bringing the project to a close.

# PART I

GENERAL PRINCIPLES

# CHAPTER 1

# History of Pediatric Surgery

*Moritz M. Ziegler*

## KEY POINTS

1. The successful development of the field of pediatric surgery has depended on the personal devotion of the founding fathers to a lifelong exclusive commitment to the surgical care of children.

2. As diagnostic and treatment approaches have been refined for childhood disease, the principles have been disseminated by publications, presentations, and communication among like-minded colleagues, and through professional organizations and journals.

3. Key to the perpetuation of the field of pediatric surgery has been the worldwide codification of content for a rational training program for future pediatric surgeons, assuring their competence and their future leadership of the field.

4. Although surgical research may still be the least well-developed aspect of this field, there have been significant contributions by pediatric surgeons in the specific treatment of congenital and acquired pediatric disease, improvements in cancer care treatment and outcomes, our understanding of fetal development and the potential for in utero treatment, and disease-specific treatment outcomes.

5. The continued success of pediatric surgery will require a commitment to clinical care excellence that assures institutional and individual surgeon competence, optimal education, research that is designed to improve child health outcomes, and a strong commitment to advocacy for children that ensures their access to optimal surgical care.

The history of pediatric surgery has developed sequentially and simultaneously along 4 complementary pathways. First, individual pioneering surgeons declared their interest by confining their practice to the surgical diseases of children. Second, the Boston school of Ladd and Gross provided the legacy and leadership by establishing principles for the surgical care of children and by training the majority of the subsequent training program leaders in pediatric surgery. The third

critically important development was the evolution of organized pediatric surgery, the initiation of the *Journal of Pediatric Surgery* as a specialty journal, and the eventual evolution of a board certification process. Finally, the fourth pathway was the evolution of the field from a collection of anecdotal clinical observations to one of scientific achievement based on sound laboratory and clinical research. This chapter sequentially reviews these 4 topics as they collectively impact on the development of both international and American pediatric surgery.

## THE PIONEERS OF PEDIATRIC SURGERY

### William E. Ladd (1880-1967)

William E. Ladd (Fig. 1-1) was born in Milton, Massachusetts, and was raised locally. At Harvard College he rowed crew. After graduation from Harvard Medical School (1906), he was a surgical intern at the Boston City Hospital. Thereafter, in addition to his general surgery and gynecologic surgery practice, he joined the staff of the Boston Children's Hospital in 1910 to do an occasional surgical procedure on a child.

On December 6, 1917, the French munitions ship *Mont Blanc* collided with the Norwegian vessel *Imo* in the narrows of Halifax harbor. The result was the most powerful man-made explosion in history to that time. The resulting destruction of life and property was massive: 2000 men, women, and children were killed, 9000 were injured, 6000 lost their homes, and 25,000 were left without adequate shelter. Multiple medical care teams poured into Halifax, and Ladd organized and led such a team from Boston. Witnessing the plight of burned and disabled children in this disaster so moved Ladd that he resolved to change the direction of his career and devote himself exclusively to the surgical care of the pediatric age group. Thereafter, Ladd fulfilled this resolve, and in 1927 he was named Surgeon-in-Chief at the Boston Children's Hospital, succeeding James S. Stone, MD. Over the next decade, Dr Ladd applied his meticulous operative skills and attention to detail, and he began to recruit individuals who would eventually lay the foundation for the Boston School of Pediatric Surgery, culminating in the recruitment of Robert Gross as resident in 1938 and fellow staff member in 1939. Ladd ascended to the first endowed chair in pediatric surgery at the

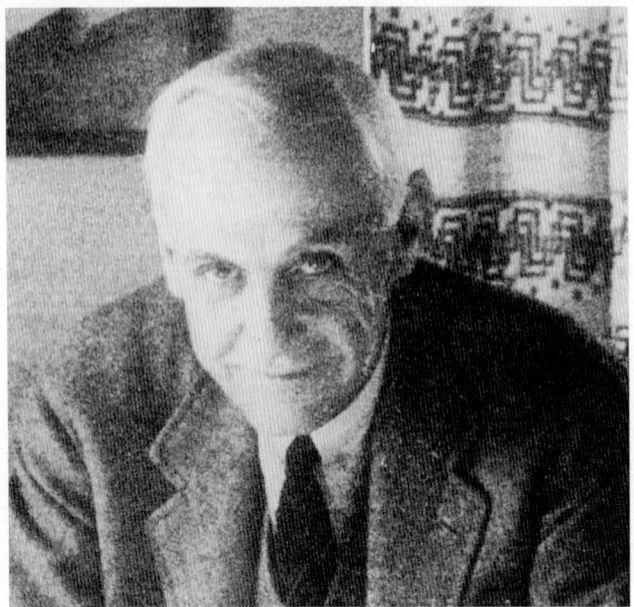

**FIGURE 1-1** William E. Ladd (1880-1967).

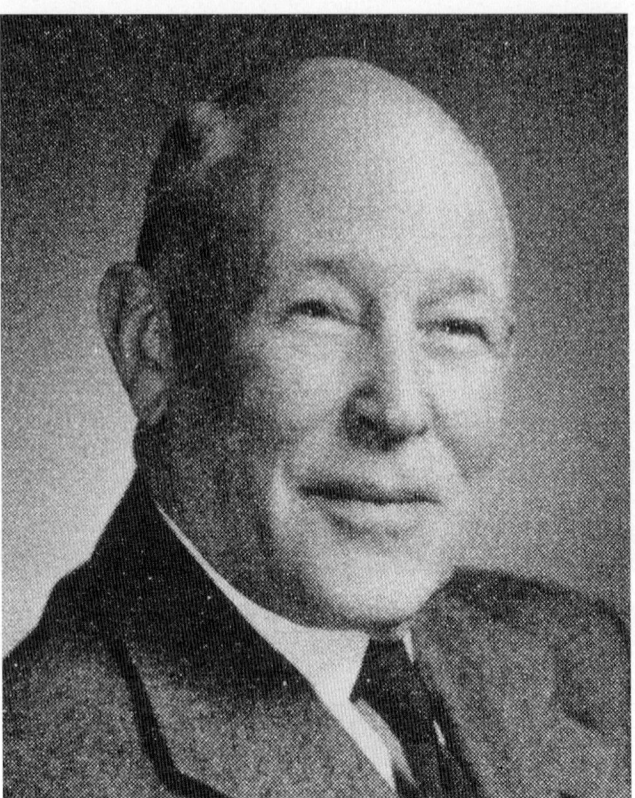

**FIGURE 1-2** Herbert E. Coe (1881-1968).

Boston Children's Hospital and the Harvard Medical School in 1941, and he retired as Surgeon-in-Chief in 1945.

Ladd's lasting contributions included his surgical leadership, his authorship with Gross of *Abdominal Surgery in Infants and Children* (1940), and his classic description of the treatment of malrotation of the colon, the "Ladd operation."

## Herbert E. Coe (1881-1968)

Herbert Coe (Fig. 1-2) was born in Michigan in 1881 to a physician father; his family moved to Seattle in 1888, where he was raised. He returned to college and medical school at the University of Michigan, earning his MD in 1906. After an internship at Allegheny, Pennsylvania, he returned to Seattle in 1908 and joined the staff of the Children's Orthopaedic Hospital.

In addition to pediatric surgery, Coe focused early on infectious diseases. In 1919, after World War I had ended, he went to Boston to spend time with Ladd, focusing on the surgical care of the pediatric age group. When Coe returned to Seattle, he restricted his work to the surgical care of children, including operations on the abdomen, chest, skeletal muscular system, and nervous system, concentrating especially on plastic and reconstructive surgery. This concentration on the pediatric age group antedates that of Ladd, such that Coe is generally acknowledged as the first exclusive surgeon of children in the United States.

Coe's most lasting contributions include the organization of the first outpatient surgery effort for children in the United States and the development of a visiting nurse program for the postoperative patient. Coe's participation in the American Academy of Pediatrics (AAP) and his eventual role in the development of the Academy's Surgical Section may be his most important legacy (see Surgical Section of the American Academy of Pediatrics below). He was joined in Seattle by Alexander Bill in 1948 following the latter's Boston training.

## Oswald S. Wyatt (1896-1957)

Born in Canada, Dr Wyatt (Fig. 1-3) was both an undergraduate and a medical school student of the University of Minnesota. After graduating as the first general surgery resident in 1918 from the Hennepin County General Hospital, he served in the US Army. Dr Wyatt then opened a general surgery practice in Minneapolis. At the urging of Coe, Wyatt took a leave of absence in 1927 and spent time at Washington University, St Louis, and Children's Memorial Hospital, Chicago; at the latter he learned clinical pediatrics from Dr Joseph Brennemann and clinical pediatric surgery from Dr Edwin Miller. On returning to Minneapolis he confined his practice to the surgical care of children, with a special interest in myelomeningocele. He continued over the next 30 years as a practicing pediatric surgeon with a clinical appointment at the University of Minnesota. He was joined in 1946 by Boston-trained Dr Tague Chisholm. This union formed the foundation for the largest private practice group of pediatric surgeons in the United States, a group that has continued its successful practice until now.

## Sir Denis Browne (1892-1967)

Denis Browne was a native Australian who became the father of pediatric surgery in both Australia and England. Confining his practice to the surgery of child maldevelopment, he emigrated to England after World War II, never to return to his native Australia. His contributions were many, and his colleagues felt that his recognition might have been still greater had not his personality been described as brilliant and bold, yet simultaneously confrontational. In addition to

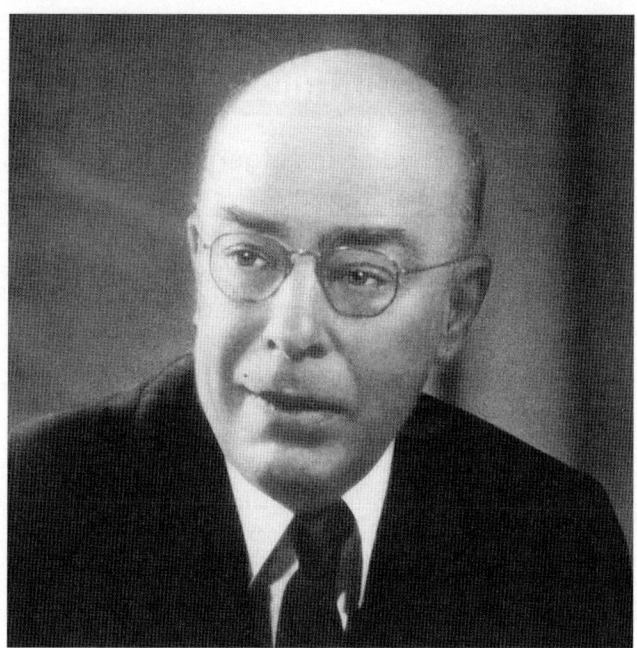

**FIGURE 1-3** Oswald S. Wyatt (1896-1957).

his contributions in a variety of pediatric specialties including orthopedics, urology, and otolaryngology, the focus of his pediatric surgery interests was on esophageal maladies. He most notably led pediatric surgery to its due recognition as an independent specialty by gaining the certification for Australian pediatric surgeons as Fellows in the Royal College of Surgeons, Pediatric Surgery, in 1967, 8 years before similar certification recognition in the United States.

## Max Grob (1901-1976)

Grob was a native of Switzerland and he was known as the father of pediatric surgery in his country. He trained in Zurich and under Monnier was appointed to the resident staff of the children's hospital in Zurich. After additional experience in Paris, he became the Swiss example of Gross, focusing his talent on a variety of pediatric surgical maldevelopment diseases including cleft deformity and Hirschsprung disease. However, his major contributions may have been his correction of congenital heart defects where he pioneered the use of both hypothermia and the heart–lung machine in children. He eventually succeeded Monnier as Chief of Surgery, Zurich Children's Hospital.

## THE BOSTON SCHOOL OF PEDIATRIC SURGERY

William E. Ladd was named Surgeon-in-Chief of Boston Children's Hospital to succeed James S. Stone, MD, in 1927. Thomas H. Lanman joined Ladd as an associate in pediatric surgery that same year, and he particularly focused on the correction of esophageal atresia (EA) and pulmonary pathology. Not until 10 years later, in 1937, when Ladd had become full time at Boston Children's Hospital, did the training program officially begin; in the interim George Cutler, Henry Hudson,

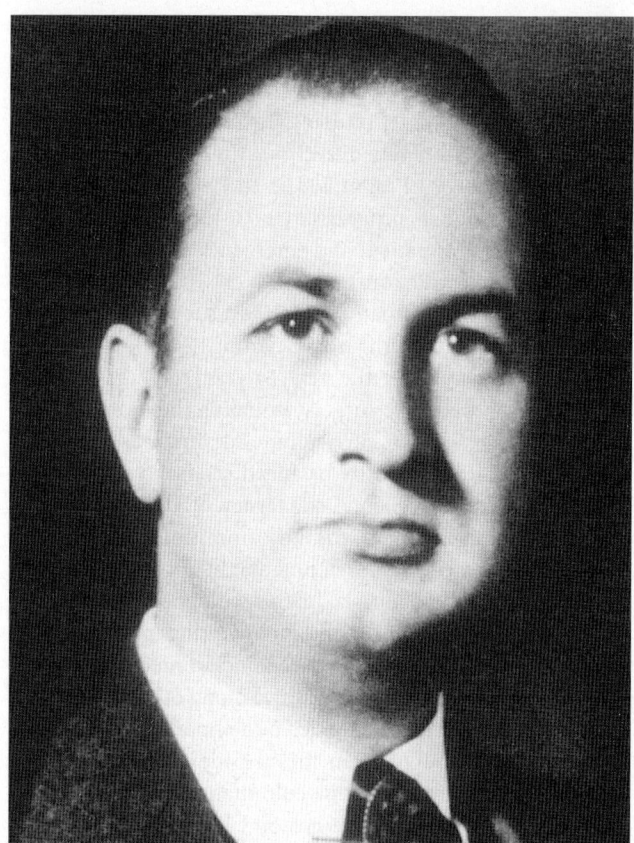

**FIGURE 1-4** Robert E. Gross (1905-1988).

Patrick Mahoney, and John Chamberlain each spent time with Ladd. The training program under Ladd included such notable trainees as Robert E. Gross, Jesus Lozoya-Solis, Orvar Swenson, and Alexander Bill. At Ladd's retirement in 1945, he was succeeded, after a contested selection, by Robert E. Gross, who almost single-handedly trained the future leaders of the field.

Gross (Fig. 1-4) was born in Baltimore in 1905, the son of a piano maker. Many of Gross's formative years were spent in Minnesota, where he graduated from Carleton College. He subsequently graduated from the Harvard Medical School in 1931. As chief surgical resident in 1938 at age 33, when Ladd was out of town, Gross is credited with initiating the field of congenital heart surgery when he successfully divided a patent ductus arteriosus in a 7-year-old girl. In cardiac surgery Gross also demonstrated resection of aortic coarctation and the use of homografts for aortic replacement. In 1940, with Ladd, Gross coauthored the text *Abdominal Surgery in Infants and Children*; then in 1952, Gross wrote *The Surgery of Infancy and Childhood*. These textbooks codified the then contemporary field of pediatric surgery. In 1970, he authored the *Atlas of Children's Surgery*. The commitment to excellence in technical surgery was legendary for Gross, and even now his sign hangs in the Boston Children's Hospital operating room, declaring "If an Operation Is Difficult, You Are Not Doing It Properly." Gross subsequently died in 1988.

Most importantly, in his 23 years (1945-1968) as training director, no fewer than 69 surgeons had the opportunity to train with Gross, many of whom became subsequent leaders in training programs in pediatric surgery throughout the United States. He also altered the format of the training program to a 3-year pyramid requiring the 6 selected residents to have previous training. The 3-tiered system included a 1st year junior residency, a 2nd year senior residency, and a following year as chief resident. To avoid a complete turnover of residents on July 1 each year, Gross started a new junior resident every 2 months. The 2nd year senior residents advanced through a progression of 6-month rotations on general surgery, outpatient and emergency department, plastic surgery, and cardiac surgery.

In 1968, Judah Folkman (1933-2008) succeeded Dr Gross as Surgeon-in-Chief, with Gross devoting his time exclusively to cardiac surgery. Over the next 14 years, Folkman trained 21 residents in pediatric surgery, initiating the more conventional 2-year residency curriculum. As much as the Gross years were characterized by balanced scientific surgery and clinical–technical excellence, the legacy of Dr Folkman was his creative thinking and striking commitment to scientific inquiry. He defined the developmental biology of blood vessel formation, "angiogenesis," along with the application of angiogenesis inhibitors for the putative therapy of diseases characterized by neovascularization, including cancer, vascular malformations, and retinopathy, among others. The Folkman years were also characterized by a remarkable dedication to provocative thought from the bedside during "professor rounds" to the operating room, culminating in a massive surgical research program at the Boston Children's Hospital.

With Folkman's return to a near full-time pursuit of research in vascular biology in 1982, Boston Children's Hospital recruited W. Hardy Hendren, a previous Gross trainee, from the Massachusetts General Hospital to assume the position of Chairman, Department of Surgery. In the subsequent 16 years under Hendren's leadership, 16 additional pediatric surgeons were trained. Remarkably, 7 of those 16 subsequently assumed faculty positions at Boston Children's Hospital. It was during this time that the productive research laboratory of Judah Folkman in angiogenesis and Jay Vacanti in tissue engineering was complemented by Dr Hendren's clinical excellence in complex cloacal deformity reconstructive surgery. Dr Hendren also enjoyed the honor of being named the first Robert E. Gross Professor of Surgery at the Harvard Medical School.

In 1998, Moritz M. Ziegler was selected to succeed Dr Hendren. A trainee of Dr Koop's Children's Hospital of Philadelphia program, he arrived from Cincinnati, where he had served for 9 years as Surgeon-in-Chief, succeeding Lester Martin, a Gross trainee, who had founded the Cincinnati program. Dr Ziegler assumed the position of Chairman, Department of Surgery, as well as Surgeon-in-Chief, and he succeeded Hendren as Robert E. Gross Professor of Surgery. Robert Shamberger, MD, succeeded Ziegler as Department of Surgery Chairman in 2002, and he continues in that position today.

The Boston School of Pediatric Surgery provided a remarkable formative legacy to the evolution of this specialty—the father, Ladd; the mentor, Gross; the scientist, Folkman; the clinician, Hendren; the educator, Ziegler; and the clinical oncologic surgeon, Shamberger; and from this heritage more than 100 pediatric surgeons were trained, more than 20 of whom had by 2012 risen to the position of pediatric surgical program director.

## THE EVOLUTION OF ORGANIZED AMERICAN PEDIATRIC SURGERY

### Certification in Pediatric Surgery, American Board of Surgery

Although the Surgical Section of the AAP was the first organization of pediatric surgeons, the alignment was with pediatricians, and a membership requirement included certification by the American Board of Surgery (ABS). The first formal effort at pediatric surgical board certification was initiated in 1955, when C. Everett Koop petitioned the ABS for certification of special proficiency in pediatric surgery. The request was formally denied in 1957, apparently because pediatric surgery crossed many existing specialties, and such certification would foster more specialty boards. A second effort was initiated in 1960 by E. H. Christopherson, Executive Director of the AAP, a request denied in 1961 by the ABS when a definition for pediatric surgery was incompletely formulated, and the ABS instead suggested that pediatric surgeons seek Surgical Section AAP membership as their home for recognition. A third effort began in 1965 and culminated in a direct petition to the ABS by Mark Ravitch, seeking an affiliate board for pediatric surgery. The ABS agreed to study the problem. A fourth effort was launched in 1967, seeking reapplication for an affiliate board status. In the final analysis, the ABS Committee chaired by John Kirklin of Alabama recommended against such an affiliate board status. Next, in 1971, Harvey Beardmore of Montreal, with support from the AAP, the Canadian Association of Pediatric Surgery, and the American Board of Pediatrics, was invited to present to the ABS. An ABS Committee of Drs Reemstma, Nardi, and Drapanis was appointed to liaison with a pediatric surgical committee of Beardmore, Gross, Holder, Kiesewetter, Cloud, Clatworthy, and Koop. Negotiations continued, and despite a moratorium on new requests for subspecialty certificates by the American Board of Medical Specialties, the ABS under new chairman David Sabiston unanimously approved certification in pediatric surgery in 1972. "Special Certification in Pediatric Surgery" under the aegis of the ABS was officially and finally approved at the American Board of Medical Specialties meeting in April 1973. The first examination for "special competence in pediatric surgery" occurred in April 1975, in Darado Beach, Puerto Rico, an exam written by Harvey Beardmore, Judson Randolph, and Marc Rowe and administered to all qualifying pediatric surgeons, no "grandfathering" being done.

The relationship between pediatric surgery and the ABS continued to mature, and in 2000 a so-called pediatric surgery "sub-board" of the ABS was developed that consisted of 6 pediatric surgical members, 1 of whom as sub-board leader also served on the parent ABS. Over time as the ABS assumed in-training examination responsibility for resident trainees that complemented their written qualifying and oral certifying exam responsibilities, they turned to the sub-board for their leadership in exam question writing, curricular reform, and an assessment of competency and maintenance of certification.

In the final analysis, this quest for specialty certification took a remarkably long 18 years, and it required the efforts and commitment of many. Pediatric surgeons Ladd, Koop, Gross, Pickett, Swenson, Bill, Potts, Clatworthy, Ravitch, Bishop, Snyder, Izant, Beardmore, Smith, Cloud, Holder, and Kiesewetter, multiple general and thoracic surgeon members of the ABS, and, in the end, support from urologists as well as pediatricians were critical to accomplishing this milestone.

## Surgical Section of the American Academy of Pediatrics

The AAP itself was founded in 1930, and in 1934, Dr Herbert Coe of Seattle led a Round Table Discussion on the Acute Abdomen of Childhood, the first discussion of a surgical topic at the AAP. Coe subsequently in 1946 wrote to request of AAP President Joseph Wall, MD, that a section on surgical conditions in infants be included in the Academy program. Thereafter, Coe expanded his request to include consideration of a surgical fellowship affiliate member category to be established at the AAP for physicians not certified in pediatrics but who specialized in surgery and treated children exclusively. Coe was subsequently appointed to chair an academy committee to explore an enlarged scope of membership to physicians in allied branches of medicine who confined their work to the pediatric age group. In December 1947, the AAP Board established a new class of membership known as "Affiliate Fellows" who were surgeons, pathologists, psychiatrists, allergists, and others devoting most or all of their time to the care of children. This was more formally expanded to form new AAP Sections of Allergy, Mental Growth and Development, and Surgery in June 1948.

The first meeting of the Surgical Section occurred on November 21, 1948, at the 17th Annual Meeting of the AAP in Atlantic City (Fig. 1-5). Coe was directed to choose a steering committee of 5, which he chaired: O. S. Wyatt, Robert E. Gross, Jesus Lozoya, William E. Ladd, and Henry Swan. Of the 20 charter members, those present at the first meeting were Ladd, Coe, Wyatt, Bowman, Ingraham, Koop, Lanman, Lozoya, Potts, and Swan. The other 10 approved charter members were Bill, Cachof, Chisholm, Gross, Moore, Mustard, MacCollum, Serinanan, Swenson, and Wilkinson. Requirements for membership for these 20 charter members included their practice of not less than 90% children's surgery. The first meeting was devoted to a discussion of interesting cases, a review of training needs, as well as a strategy for the development of a Board of Pediatric Surgery.

The Surgical Section evolved its governance to an elected Executive Committee whose members would eventually each succeed to the office of committee chairperson. The Section also developed a series of awards. The William E. Ladd Medal awarded by the AAP is the highest recognition an American pediatric surgeon can receive. The first medal was awarded in 1954 to Thomas Lanman, Ladd's protégé, and during the first 50 years of the Section, 23 such medals were awarded, 4 recognizing nonpediatric surgeons whose contributions in EA, urology, nutrition, and transplantation each had a remarkable impact on the surgical care of children. The Section also has hosted overseas guests as a part of its annual meeting, and in 1997 that award was renamed the Stephen Gans Overseas Lecturer in honor of the late Dr Gans. The annual meeting also came to evolve an annual resident papers competition, and following the death in 1987 of Jens Rosenkrantz, the Section's 1977 Chairperson, the Rosenkrantz Fund was established at the AAP to support this resident competition. Finally, in 1997, following the death of Dr Arnold Salzberg of Richmond, Virginia, the Arnold Salzberg Mentorship Award

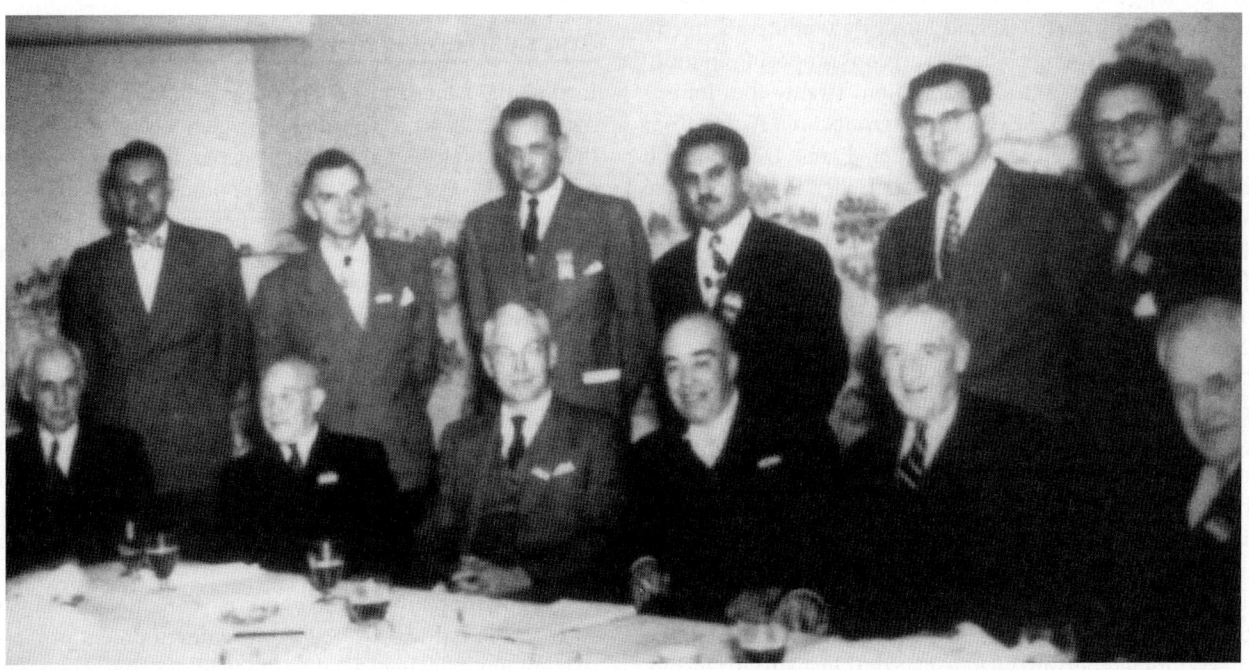

**FIGURE 1-5** First charter meeting of the Surgical Section, American Academy of Pediatrics, Atlantic City, November 21, 1948. Standing (*left to right*): Henry Swan Jr, J. Robert Bowman, Willis Potts, Jesus Lozoya-Solis, C. Everett Koop, and Professor Fontana. Seated (*left to right*): William E. Ladd, Herbert E. Coe, Franc Ingraham, Oswald S. Wyatt, Thomas H. Lanman, and Clifford Sweet.

was established by the Section to recognize that pediatric surgeon most known for contributing in a role as mentor to future pediatric surgeons.

For its 50th anniversary year, 1998, the Surgical Section was recognized for its leadership in American surgery and pediatrics. After beginning as a quite exclusive organization, it has evolved into a more inclusive role, counting among its 500-plus members either certified pediatric surgeons or those devoting a minimum of 50% of their activity to the surgical care of the pediatric age group.

In the last decade the AAP has further codified its relationship to the surgical specialties with the formation of the Surgical Advisory Panel (SAP), a group with representation from the multiple children's surgical specialties whose broad agenda has included advocacy for patient safety and quality, enhancement of trauma care systems, relevant review of Academy policies and procedures, and surgeon-specific coding and compensation issues.

## American Pediatric Surgical Association

The concept of an independent surgical organization for pediatric surgeons was felt to resolve one of the perceived barriers to becoming a recognized specialty; the others included the lack of certification, lack of training standards, and previous professional affiliation with another specialty, namely, pediatrics. Young members of the field particularly desired to have a professional identification with fellow pediatric surgeons rather than with pediatricians.

In October 1968, at the American College of Surgery meeting in Atlantic City, a group of pediatric surgeons—C. Everett Koop, Keith Ashcraft, John Campbell, Dale Johnson, and Lucian Leape—discussed the advisability of securing an identity by standing alone as a group of surgeons. Koop advised that because of strong ties to the AAP, it would be up to the younger surgeons to carry this initiative. Two months later Leape and Tom Boles resolved to act by sending a letter in April 1969 to 18 young pediatric surgeons proposing an independent pediatric surgical organization. Twenty-four founding members formed the organizing group: Fred Arcari, Tom Boles, Jack Campbell, Al Delorimier, Frank DeLuca, Bob Filler, Rick Fonkalsrud, Ed Free, Alex Haller, Bob Izant, Dale Johnson, Peter Kottmeier, Lucean Leape, Jules Lister, Lester Martin, John Raffensperger, Jud Randolph, Jim Rosenkrantz, Marc Rowe, Bill Sieber, Ide Smith, Bob Soper, Jim Talbert, and Ed Tank. Over the next 12 months a series of meetings occurred addressing the various needs: to raise standards of the specialty, to credential/approve residency training programs, to define requirements for residency training, to require for membership a 100% restriction to the practice of pediatric surgery, and to develop the mechanics of electing officers. The group sought and received endorsement from most of the leaders of pediatric surgery, and in January 1970, an invitation for charter membership in the American Pediatric Surgical Association (APSA) was mailed to 200 of the then 300 current members of the Surgical Section of the AAP. The criteria for membership included US or Canadian citizenship, practice confined to the surgery of infants and children, certification by the ABS or fellowship in the Royal Canadian College of Surgeons, and at least 2 years' experience in practice

after completion of the residency. The first official meeting of the new organization was held on April 17, 1970, at Pheasant Run, Illinois. Harvey Beardmore called the meeting to order, E. Thomas Boles Jr was nominated as temporary chairman, and Lucian Leape as temporary secretary. Robert Gross was elected President, and C. Everett Koop president-elect. At the suggestion of Robert Soper, Program Committee Chair, the *Journal of Pediatric Surgery* was to become the official journal of the new society, as was a requirement that papers presented at the annual meeting be submitted for publication in that journal. Furthermore, the subscription to the *Journal* would be included in the annual APSA membership fee. Robert Izant had drafted both bylaws and articles of incorporation. Half of the paid 191 charter members attended the meeting and approved the founding resolution:

> Be it resolved that a new society, The American Pediatric Surgical Association, now be formed to encourage specialization in the field of pediatric surgery, to promote and maintain the quality of education in pediatric surgery, to raise the standards of the specialty by fostering and encouraging research in pediatric surgery, to establish standards of excellence in the surgical care of infants and children, and to provide a forum for the dissemination of information with regard to pediatric surgery.

APSA has thrived well in its first 42 years. It hosts a highly successful annual spring meeting, and its committees monitor multiple clinical parameters and subspecialty programs, pediatric surgical manpower, continuing education requirements as well as an online method of continuing medical education (CME) accreditation, ethical issues in pediatric surgery, as well as practice management parameters. In 1998, the APSA Foundation was formed, with a mission to raise philanthropic dollars, largely from APSA membership, to support 2 or more annual competitive seed grants for those young pediatric surgeons beginning a research career.

## American College of Surgeons

In 1967 the American College of Surgeons (ACS) began listing "pediatric" as a legitimate category of surgery. In 1969 the ACS established an Advisory Council for Pediatric Surgery, and C. Everett Koop was appointed as the first Advisory Council Chairman. This Council was recognized for the specialty of pediatric surgery, a group of surgeons who at the time lacked independent specialty recognition or board certification. After a long history of being included in the annual postgraduate course offerings of the ACS as well as on the forum for presentation of "What's New," pediatric surgery achieved the status of having its own Surgical Forum in 1988, the 44th issue of that publication. Finally, the ACS not only included pediatric surgery in its activities of surgical education, standards, and ethics but, since 1985, has also represented pediatric surgery in both political and socioeconomic advocacy areas.

Perhaps most important is the partnership role that the ACS has played with APSA by their development of 2 areas that are mutually beneficial to the field of surgery as a whole and the role that the ACS plays in it as well as to the specific benefit of the pediatric surgeon. In 2008, the Pediatric Surgical Case Log Registry was developed at the ACS to serve as a repository of electronic data of clinical case procedures along with a limited notation of operative outcome assessed and entered by the individual surgeon. This voluntary registry has become a valuable tool for those surgeons contemplating recertification.

A second venture is the formation, under the aegis of the ACS but in partnership with APSA, of the National Surgical Quality Improvement Program, Pediatric (NSQIP-P). It began as a model based on the original NSQIP developed in the Veteran's Administration Hospitals. Thereafter, it was successfully modeled for both private and academic health system models of adult care, but it had not previously been applied to the pediatric surgical specialties. After several years in development, a multispecialty program (excluded were ophthalmology and cardiovascular surgery) was developed designed to employ at participating hospitals a trained nurse specialist to review more than 120 variables in real time on a predetermined inpatient case type and frequency, assessing morbidity and mortality up to 30 days postoperatively. This then would permit the calculation by regression analysis of best practice "low outliers" and worst practice "high outliers." Data-driven process improvement would follow, and the hope for a favorable outcome similar to that occurring in adult hospital participants was the ultimate outcome target. In 2009, a proof of principle was realized when an alpha phase of 4 hospitals (Yale New Haven Children's Hospital, A.I. DuPont Children's Hospital, Children's Hospital of Wisconsin, and the Children's Hospital, Denver) reported a review of more than 3000 patients. A year later the beta phase report from more than 40 participating hospitals and 37,000 patients reinforced the proof of principle and, after calculating observed/expected ratios (O/E), opened the way for high outliers to influence low outliers in process improvement. This first ever risk-adjusted multispecialty assessment of children's surgical quality and safety holds great promise for the future.

## Association of Pediatric Surgical Training Program Directors

After the development of the Boston School of Pediatric Surgery, trainees dispersed from the Ladd and Gross training milieu to establish training programs at a variety of American children's hospitals and university hospitals. Around 1950 such pediatric surgical training programs were "self-declared" and were approved by the Conference Committee on Graduate Training in Surgery, sponsored jointly by the American Medical Association (AMA) and ABS. Over the next 30 years the name of this review group and its constituency changed several times: Conference Committee on Graduate Education in Surgery (1950), Liaison Committee on Graduate Medical Education (1974), and the Accreditation Council on Graduate Medical Education (ACGME) in 1981, the latter sponsoring the Residency Review Committees (RRCs). These training programs varied in length (1-4 years) as well as their emphasis on neonatal surgery, urology, and cardiac surgery. Dr Herbert Coe, as Chairman of the Surgical Section, AAP, had as early as 1952 appointed a review committee to oversee the then-approved programs. In 1966, the Surgical Section of the AAP published a booklet listing 18 US and 2 Canadian fellowships plus 17 US and 4 Canadian

residency positions in pediatric surgery. A Surgical Section Committee on Postgraduate Education and Residency Training was appointed to develop standards. H. William Clatworthy Jr was committee chair, and members included Drs Chisholm, Ferguson, Haller, Kiesewetter, and Randolph. They published the *Special Requirements for Residency Training in General Pediatric Surgery* in September 1967. This document was also studied by the American Board of Medical Specialties, and a revised "Essentials" was formatted. The revised form was subsequently sent to the AMA Council on Medical Education and its Liaison Committee for Specialty Boards. By spring 1970, the "Clatworthy Committee" had completed 25 program site surveys, and they recommended approval of 12 US programs, provisional approval of 4 Canadian training programs, and nonapproval for 8 programs; 1 program was "tabled."

As the Clatworthy Committee continued its activity during the time that APSA was founded, between 1970 and 1972, the function was assumed by the APSA Education Committee. Recognition of "index cases" and their importance to training came to the forefront, and the Surgical Section's Post-graduate Education Committee wrote a new document entitled *Special Requirements for Residency Training in General Pediatric Surgery*. Thereafter, the APSA Education Committee under Jud Randolph, Committee Chair, continued to evaluate training programs and recommend them for approval to the ABS until 1977. However, before the first examination to award the "Certificate of Special Competence in Pediatric Surgery" in 1975, the approval of programs by the RRC and ABS was indeterminate, and in August 1976, an invitation to reapply for approval was tendered by the ACGME to the training directors. The RRC assumed control of the approval process of training programs by 1977, it developed the "Essentials" on listing the series of requirements to be met to gain approval, and the list of approved programs was reported in the Directory of Graduate Medical Education published by the AMA. The RRC approved the following numbers of US programs: 1977, 5; 1978, 10; 1979, 1; 1980, 1; 1982 to 1991, 5; 1992 to 1994, 5; by 2008 there were 33 American and 7 approved Canadian training programs; and by 2011 this number, respectively, had increased to 39 and 9, a total of 48 programs.

In the mid-1970s, the selection process of residents for training in pediatric surgery moved from the apprentice model of random interviews and selection to a formalized matching process organized within pediatric surgery by ad hoc members of the APSA Education Committee. Also, by the early 1980s, the training program directors themselves formed the Association of Pediatric Surgical Training Program Directors to develop a structured training curriculum for pediatric surgical trainees as well as to oversee the selection process. This organization, under the guidance of J. L. Grosfeld and D. R. Cooney, was formally incorporated in 1989. In the meantime, the APSA Education Committee formally adopted a new focus of defining training requirements in pediatric surgery for residents in general surgery as well as defining CME requirements. By 1990 the training program directors turned over the matching function to the National Resident Matching Program. Since that time there have been refinement of the program requirements that include case numbers and case quality, careful scrutiny of the surgeon's role in primary management of the critically ill newborn and pediatric patient while in his or her intensive care unit setting, development of a standardized in-service exam for resident trainees, and a contemporaneous scrutiny of North American manpower needs for this specialty field.

## Pediatric Surgical Publication

After publication of *The Surgery of Childhood, Including Orthopaedic Surgery* by Deforest Willard in 1910, a more major modern compilation awaited the assimilation of the Boston Children's Hospital experience. This was tabulated by publication of *Abdominal Surgery of Infancy and Childhood* in 1941 by William E. Ladd and Robert E. Gross. Eleven years thereafter, Gross's classic *The Surgery of Infancy and Childhood* was published. The early 1960s brought publication of the 2-volume *Pediatric Surgery*, a multiauthored text project spearheaded by Dr Welch and including Benson, Mustard, Ravitch, and Snyder as coeditors. An additional series of American pediatric surgeons have followed as editors or authors of texts dealing with a variety of pediatric surgical topics.

Publication of articles in journals devoted to pediatric surgery began when Drs Owen Wangensteen and Alton Ochsner, editors of *Surgery*, invited Mark Ravitch to serve as section editor of a section on pediatric surgery in 1958.

As chairman of the Surgical Section's Publication Committee in 1964, Stephen L. Gans, MD (Fig. 1-6), observed that few papers presented at the annual meeting were in fact

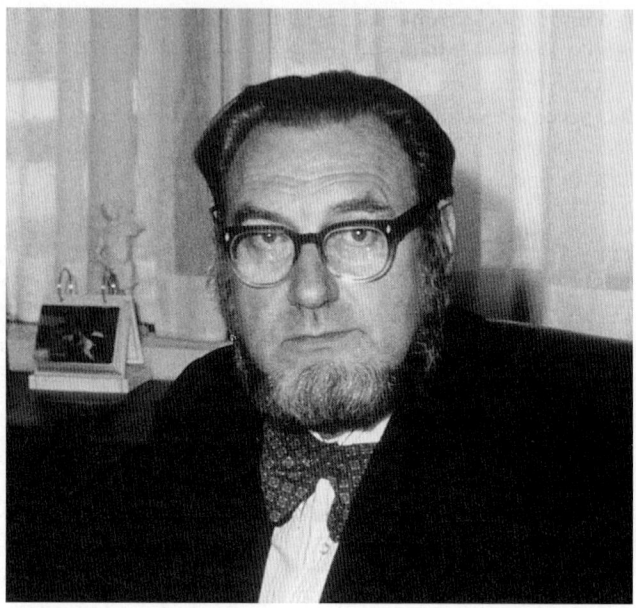

**FIGURE 1-7** C. Everett Koop (1916–2013).

being published. He perceived that as a specialty needing to secure appropriate recognition, it would be necessary to have a journal unique to the specialty. Gans enlisted and received positive feedback to that effect from 20 prominent pediatric surgeons from the United States and Canada, a group that eventually constituted an "Advisory and Editorial Board." To add an international audience, Gans met that same year with the Council of the British Association of Pediatric Surgeons. In February 1966, the *Journal of Pediatric Surgery* was founded after Dr Henry Stratton, president of Grune & Stratton in 1965, agreed to publish this journal. In that same year both the British Association of Pediatric Surgeons and the Surgical Section of the AAP approved it as their official organ. Stratton and Gans also asked C. Everett Koop, MD (Fig. 1-7), to serve as the first Editor-in-Chief of the *Journal*. In the inaugural issue, I. S. Ravdin, MD, John Rhea Barton Professor of Surgery at the University of Pennsylvania School of Medicine, wrote an introductory editorial, and in the subsequent issue the editor outlined the goals of the *Journal*: "to publish clinical experience, pertinent laboratory and clinical investigation, case reports, and an abstract section of the world's literature."

In 1967, the first supplement to the *Journal* was published, a *Conference on the Biology of Neuroblastoma*. In 1971, the newly formed APSA also had chosen the *Journal of Pediatric Surgery* as its official publication. A second supplement entitled *Advances in Endoscopy of Infants and Children* was published in 1971. In 1977, Stephen Gans assumed the role as Editor-in-Chief, prompting a letter from Dr Gross in which he stated: "I think the *Journal* has done more to advance children's surgery, not only here but around the world, above *anything* else in the last couple of decades." In 1979 the *Journal* announced its association with the Canadian Association of Pediatric Surgeons. A third supplement was published in 1981 dedicated to C. Everett Koop, MD, on his retirement from the Children's Hospital of Philadelphia. In 1984 Peter Rickman retired as Editor for Europe, and he was replaced by

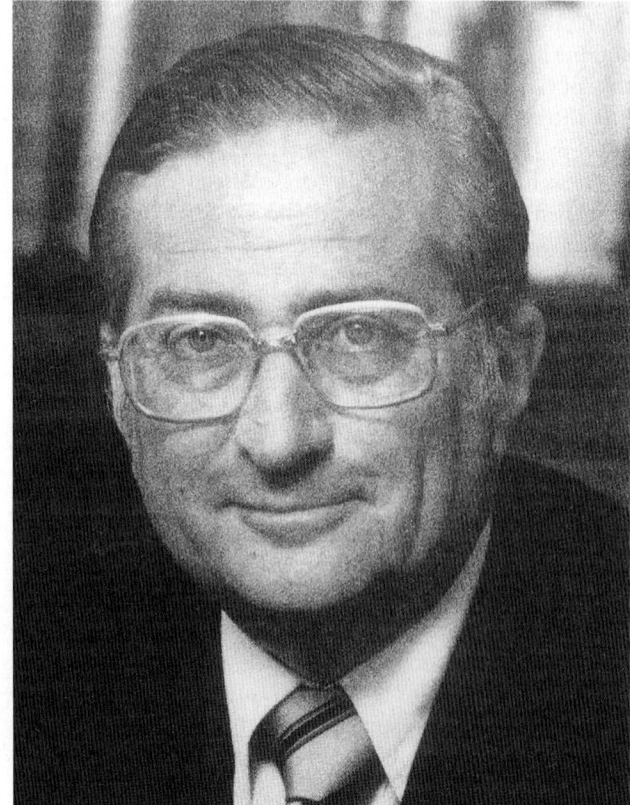

**FIGURE 1-6** Stephen L. Gans (1920-1994).

John Scott (United Kingdom) and Michel Carcassonne (Continental Europe). In 1985 the *Journal* grew from a bimonthly to a monthly publication. In 1988, the Pacific Association of Pediatric Surgeons announced its affiliation with the *Journal*. Also that same year Dan Young became Editor for the British Isles, and in 1990 Jan Molenaar was appointed Editor for Europe. In 1994 Takeshi Miyano was appointed Editor for Asia. Following the death of Dr Gans, Dr J. L. Grosfeld became the third Editor-in-Chief of the *Journal* in 1995.

In 1992 the second American journal devoted to pediatric surgery appeared with publication of *Seminars in Pediatric Surgery*, J. L. Grosfeld serving as Editor-in-Chief. Four issues were published annually. In 1997, the third journal, *Pediatric Endosurgery and Innovative Techniques*, was published with Thom E. Lobe, MD, as Editor-in-Chief. *Pediatric Surgery International* with coeditors Puri and Coran from Europe and the United States is still another publication with increasing success and impact factor for pediatric surgical publication.

## THE TIMELINE OF CONTRIBUTIONS TO DISEASE MANAGEMENT

See Table 1-1.

### Esophageal Atresia

Although this entity had been recognized since the mid-17th century, the first American description of EA was by Thomas Hill in 1840. McKenzie in 1880, Plass in 1919, and Rosenthal in 1931 each reported series of cases defining associated anomalies and the relative frequency of each entity. The first unsuccessful attempt at repair of pure EA occurred in Europe in 1888 and in the United States at Chicago by H. M. Richter in 1913. The mortality remained 100% even after a rekindled effort by Sampson in 1939, Shaw in 1939, and Lanman in 1940 for the primary repair of EA-tracheoesophageal fistula (TEF). The first survivor of pure EA was treated by staged repair in 1935 by Humphreys and Ferrer, and for EA-TEF, the staged-repair approach was also successfully used in 1940 by Logan Leven in Minneapolis and William Ladd in Boston, esophageal continuity eventually being achieved by the creation of an anterior chest wall subcutaneous skin-lined "neoesophagus." Cameron Haight, a thoracic surgeon at the University of Michigan, after several unsuccessful attempts, completed the first successful primary repair of EA-TEF in 1941. Since that time the only modifications have been operative approach variations including the application of thoracoscopic techniques and a variety of strategies for "long gap" EA, and there have been variations in esophageal replacement for patients with pure EA.

Outcomes for patients with EA have continued to improve, and risk factors analyzing such outcomes have been defined by a variety of classification systems.

### Diaphragmatic Hernia

The first description of a diaphragmatic hernia (DH) was in a term infant in 1752 by McCauley and Hunter, who dissected the body of the infant who died after 1.5 hours of life. This description included recognition of mediastinal shift along with a compressed development of the ipsilateral lung. The 19th century saw further clinical descriptions, but not until 1925 did Hedblom report survival of newborns treated in the United States with DH. In 1940, Ladd and Gross reported that 9 of 16 infants survived neonatal repair, and the first survivor less than 24 hours of age was not reported until 1946 by Gross.

From the 1940s to the 1980s, the approach to DH treatment focused on minor operative technical variations, and because little progress was being made in disease outcomes, risk factors and "predictive" prognostic factors were sought in an effort to triage or stratify patients for predicting survival with the emergent repair techniques. Finally, after describing the adverse influence of operation on respiratory compliance and gas exchange, Nakayama and coworkers in 1991 defined an advantage to preoperative stabilization, a finding confirmed by Breaux and West. These series reported survivors, in whom extracorporeal membrane oxygenation (ECMO), first used in DH infants in 1981, was utilized, serving as a bridge to repair. The overall patient survival was perhaps slightly improved but certainly not worsened by this delayed-repair technique. A more aggressive application of ECMO was reserved for the high-risk neonate where an EXIT procedure was coupled with immediate ECMO therapy as a mechanism to protect the lungs from adverse ventilator effects while early maturation occurs. The outcome of this strategy applied to the highest-risk newborn group requires definition.

Additional progress in critical care, ventilation strategies, and pharmacologic manipulation in the 1990s produced transient enthusiasm but little sustained efficacy for the DH patient. Fetal repair, touted experimentally in the 1980s and clinically applied in the 1990s by Harrison, Adzick, and others, has been disappointing in improving outcomes. Wilson's work on tracheal occlusion to enhance pulmonary development was first reported in 1993 and has now undergone fetal surgical application, especially in Europe where extreme-risk patients are managed with that adjunct (PLUG: plug the lung until it grows). The application of perfluorocarbon liquid ventilation has been reported by Hirschl to have potential benefit in enhancing lung development and tissue oxygenation while the infant is also receiving ECMO support.

### Abdominal Wall Defects

The first description of an omphalocele was Pare's report in 1634, and documented gastroschisis was first described in 1733. The early 1800s saw the first successful repair of an omphalocele in Europe, with the first American successes not coming until the early 20th century. The first successful repair of a gastroschisis did not occur until 1943. Escharotic treatment was promoted extensively in the 20th century for omphalocele, as was the development of skin flaps, the latter following Gross's successes in closing giant omphaloceles reported in 1948. Such flaps were used for gastroschisis in 1952. Izant reported the value of abdominal wall manual stretching in 1966, and in 1967 Schuster described

| TABLE 1-1 | Historical Timeline: Pediatric Surgery |
|---|---|

<table>
<tr><td colspan="2">1600</td><td>1938</td><td>Congenital heart surgery begins with successful ligation of a patent ductus arteriosus by Robert E. Gross</td></tr>
<tr><td>1634</td><td>Pare describes omphalocele</td><td>1941</td><td>Cameron Haight performs first successful primary repair of esophageal atresia</td></tr>
<tr><td colspan="2">1700</td><td>1941</td><td>Ladd and Gross publish Abdominal Surgery in Infancy and Childhood</td></tr>
<tr><td>1733</td><td>Gastroschisis described</td><td>1945</td><td>First gastroschisis repair</td></tr>
<tr><td colspan="2">1750</td><td>1946</td><td>Rhoads performs first successful abdominoperineal pull-through for imperforate anus</td></tr>
<tr><td>1752</td><td>McCauley/Hunter describe neonate with a diaphragmatic hernia</td><td>1946</td><td>Ehrenpreis and Whitehouse and Kernahan (in 1948) describe the distal aganglionic segment of Hirschsprung disease</td></tr>
<tr><td colspan="2">1800</td><td>1948</td><td>Swenson and Bill perform first successful abdominoperineal pull-through for Hirschsprung disease; Duhamel (in 1956) and Soave (in 1964) procedures described</td></tr>
<tr><td>1840</td><td>Thomas Hill describes esophageal atresia</td><td rowspan="2">1948</td><td rowspan="2">Hiatt describes meconium ileus patient salvage from 100% mortality with an ostomy and luminal irrigation</td></tr>
<tr><td></td><td>First omphalocele repair</td></tr>
<tr><td colspan="2">1850</td><td colspan="2">1950</td></tr>
<tr><td>1852</td><td>London Hospital for Sick Children founded</td><td>1953</td><td>Salk vaccine slows polio epidemic; first successful human kidney transplant, Murray</td></tr>
<tr><td>1855</td><td>Children's Hospital of Philadelphia founded as nations first</td><td rowspan="2">1953</td><td>Miculicz and Bishop/Koop and 1966, Santulli enterostomies; and 1970, O'Neill tube</td></tr>
<tr><td>1860</td><td>Edinburgh Royal Hospital for Sick Children founded</td><td>Enterostomy with irrigation applied to meconium ileus and becomes care standard</td></tr>
<tr><td>1886</td><td>Danish pediatrician Harold Hirschsprung describes megacolon</td><td rowspan="2">1953</td><td rowspan="2">Stephens describes pelvic floor levator mechanism in relationship to the management of imperforate anus; Barnard and Louw define in utero vascular occlusion mechanism for intestinal atresia</td></tr>
<tr><td>1888</td><td>First unsuccessful attempt at esophageal atresia repair</td></tr>
<tr><td>1898</td><td>Description of the embryology of intestinal malrotation from Johns Hopkins</td><td colspan="2">1960</td></tr>
<tr><td colspan="2">1900</td><td>1963</td><td>First human liver transplant, Starzl, Denver; first survivor of a liver transplant, Starzl, 1967. Both patients were children</td></tr>
<tr><td>1908</td><td>Fredet describes first pyloromyotomy in Paris</td><td>1965</td><td>Bill/Dobbins apply rectal suction biopsy to diagnose Hirschsprung disease</td></tr>
<tr><td>1914</td><td>Dr William Ladd, Boston, attends to injured children in Halifax Harbor explosion. Ladd devotes career to the surgical care of children as do Coe (Seattle) and Wyatt (Minneapolis)</td><td>1968</td><td>Dudrick, Wilmore, Vars, and Rhoads describe normal growth of infant with short bowel syndrome secondary to intestinal atresia when fed exclusively by vein</td></tr>
<tr><td>1925</td><td>Hedbloom performs first successful repair of neonatal diaphragmatic hernia</td><td>1968</td><td>First successful human heart transplant, Barnard, South Africa</td></tr>
<tr><td>1928</td><td>Penicillin discovered in Britain</td><td rowspan="3">1969</td><td rowspan="3">Noblett successfully applies gastrografin as a meconium solubilizing agent as well as a diagnostic contrast agent for distal bowel obstruction</td></tr>
<tr><td>1930</td><td>Rice/Wagenstein describe "invertogram" radiograph to aid in leveling imperforate anus to high/low</td></tr>
<tr><td>1930</td><td>Formalized pediatric surgical resident training begins at Boston Children's Hospital</td></tr>
<tr><td>1935</td><td>Ferrer/Humphries perform successful esophageal atresia staged repair</td></tr>
<tr><td>1936</td><td>Ladd procedure for intestinal malrotation described by Ladd and Gross</td></tr>
<tr><td>1938</td><td>Anderson and Farber (in 1944) describe linkage of meconium ileus, pancreatic insufficiency, and lung disease</td></tr>
</table>

*(Continued)*

TABLE 1-1    **Historical Timeline: Pediatric Surgery** *(Continued)*

| 1970 | |
|---|---|
| 1970 | Martin modifies Duhamel procedure to manage total colon aganglionosis |
| 1972 | Simpson describes role of the UGI radiograph for the diagnosis of malrotation |
| 1973 | First description of laparoscopic peritoneoscopy in neonates by Stephen Gans |
| 1975 | American surgeons Lilly and Altman demonstrate success with Kasai operation for biliary atresia |

| 1980 | |
|---|---|
| 1981 | First application of ECMO for a neonate with diaphragmatic hernia |
| 1982 | Pena and de Vries describe midline posterior sagittal anorectoplasty as a therapy for imperforate anus |
| 1987 | First description of a laparoscopic appendectomy for acute appendicitis |

| 1990 | |
|---|---|
| 1990 | Harrison reports attempt at fetal in utero congenital diaphragmatic hernia repair |
| 1991 | Nakyama reports success after initial patient stabilization/delayed repair for diaphragmatic hernia |
| | De La Torre Mondragon applies one-stage transanal pull-through to manage Hirschsprung disease; Georgeson applies laparoscopic techniques |
| 2000 | Langer describes diagnostic laparoscopy application for malrotation determining who will benefit from a Ladd procedure |
| | Relationship forged between American Pediatric Surgical Association and American College of Surgeons to develop National Surgical Quality Improvement Program Pediatric, a real-time, risk-adjusted data set designed to permit the comparison of hospital quality/safety performance outcomes leading to process improvement with the adoption of best practice standards; alpha phase (2010) and beta phase (2012) published |

the application of a prosthetic "silo" to temporarily hold the extruded abdominal viscera during a staged repair. In 1969 Allen and Wrenn modified the material to the more pliable Silon (silastic-coated Dacron) and the technique to gradual bedside closure of the silo without the need for skin wound closure at each reduction step. The University of Pennsylvania nutrition team—Rhoads, Dudrick, Vars, and Wilmore—first applied total parenteral nutrition (TPN) to an infant with short-bowel syndrome in 1966-1967. A few years later, Filler and others began applying TPN to a variety of catastrophic neonatal conditions that precluded enteral nutrition, and newborns with gastroschisis or ruptured omphalocele received considerable benefit from this maneuver. In addition, Shaw proposed in 1975 that omphalocele and gastroschisis were of common developmental origin. This unifying theory is an important contribution to our understanding of the development of abdominal wall defects.

## The Newborn Intestinal Obstructions

### Intestinal Atresia

The principle of failure of vacuolization and reabsorption as the etiology of atresia was first recognized in Europe at the turn of the 20th century, and it was not challenged until the vascular accident theory was suggested by South Africa's Louw and Barnard in the 1950s. Early American reports of atresia by Davis and Poynter and Webb and Wangensteen only emphasized poor outcomes, a survival of less than 10% extending even up until the 1950s. The last half of the 20th century demonstrated improved suture technique, suture material, and better metabolic support with TPN during the prolonged postoperative period of intestinal recovery. Additionally, the classification of atresia was refined, and

associated anomalies were cataloged. In fact, the association of trisomy 21 with duodenal atresia became a focal point for the debate of who should receive nutritional support and operative intervention, a debate in the 1980s that crystallized our current ethical approach of support for such children.

## Malrotation and Volvulus

The first embryologic description of malrotation occurred at Johns Hopkins University in 1898, an observation confirmed in 1915. A number of authors subsequently described the association of malrotation with volvulus, but the classic paper is that of Ladd and Gross from 1936 in which 21 cases were described along with the treatment of counterclockwise detorsion, division of the bands over the duodenum, and placement of the cecum into the left upper quadrant, the so-called Ladd operation. The major contribution since that time is the improved management of short-bowel syndrome along with an enhanced diagnostic sensitivity of the contrast upper gastrointestinal radiograph as described by Simpson in 1972. Langer reported the minimally invasive approach to malrotation, including the definition of how to recognize when the narrowness of the mesenteric pedicle defines those at risk for volvulus who require a formal Ladd operation.

## Meconium Ileus

Europeans first described in the early part of this century the linkage of meconium bowel obstruction and pancreatic insufficiency as well as the linkage of pancreatic disease to chronic pulmonary disease. However, Anderson in 1938 and Farber in 1944 first described meconium ileus, linking it to cystic fibrosis and lesions in the pancreas. The entity was uniformly fatal until the 1948 report of Hiatt describing therapeutic success with enterotomy and saline irrigation. Thereafter, a variety of surgical techniques were developed for this diagnosis: the Mikulicz ileostomy by Gross in 1953, the resection with proximal-to-distal end-to-side enterostomy by Bishop and Koop in 1953, a modification with proximal-to-distal side-to-end enterostomy reported by Santulli in 1961, resection with primary anastomosis by Swenson in 1962, and tube enterostomy with irrigation by O'Neill in 1970. Nonoperative management was recommended by Noblett's 1969 application of gastrografin enema administration. When nonoperative irrigation therapies fail, at least enterotomy–irrigation with gastrografin or enzymes (Viokase), sparing the need for a stoma, is almost always successful. Initially reported by Kalayoglu in 1971, this technique has withstood the test of time and today in uncomplicated meconium ileus, outcomes approach 100% survival.

Finally, the recognition of the genetics of cystic fibrosis in the mid-1980s and improved critical care have advanced not only diagnosis but also the outcomes of treatment of this disease.

## Hirschsprung Disease

The Danish pediatrician Harold Hirschsprung first described the clinical entity that bears his name in 1886, and although distal aganglionosis was described in 1901 in Europe, the pathophysiology was misunderstood until the work of Ehrenpreis in 1946 and the Americans Whitehouse and Kernahan and Zuelzer and Wilson in 1948. They described the absence of ganglion cells in the myenteric plexus of the distal bowel of patients with Hirschsprung disease. In that same year the pioneering efforts of Swenson and Bill at Boston Children's Hospital described the first successful operative treatment for Hirschsprung Disease. These last 50 years have seen refinements of 3 procedures, Swenson's pull-through and the Soave and Duhamel pull-throughs from Europe. Additionally, the refinement of diagnosis occurred with Swenson's full-thickness rectal biopsy in 1959, Bodian's submucosal biopsy in 1960, and the rectal suction biopsy technique reported by Dobbins and Bill in 1965. Martin modified the Duhamel side-to-side procedure by application of the endostapling device to eliminate the common wall in its entirety in 1962, and, thereafter, his modification was also applied to total colonic aganglionosis in 1972. Similarly, Coran and others modified the Soave procedure and also applied it to the management of total colonic aganglionosis in 1969. Extended small-bowel aganglionosis as a complex entity had its management facilitated by preservation of salt and water resorptive capacities of the distal ileum and colon reported by both Kottmeier and Velcek in 1981, Kimura in 1988, and Stringel in 1986. Ziegler in 1987 also defined a role for small-bowel myectomy in the treatment of extensive aganglionic diseases involving most of the gastrointestinal tract, a technique, if not obstruction relieving, probably at least serving as a bridge to transplantation.

Although more recent contributions have focused on the definition of the disease pathophysiology and other physiologic motility mediators, the most relevant contemporary contributions have changed what was once a 3-stage treatment of colostomy–pull-through–colostomy closure to a 2-stage plan of leveling colostomy–pull-through and finally

to the current application of single-stage primary pull-through. More recently the latter operation has been facilitated by the application of a minimally invasive laparoscopic surgical technique as initially advocated by Georgeson and others.

## Imperforate Anus

The earliest American contribution for this condition was the Wangensteen and Rice report in 1930 describing the invertogram radiographic technique as a method to define the location of the distal rectum relative to the perineum. This distance dictated a classification of low or high lesions treated by perineal anoplasty versus colostomy with delayed pull-through procedure, respectively. Jonathan Rhoads at the University of Pennsylvania reported the first case of a single-stage abdominoperineal pull-through for high imperforate anus, a technique confirmed by a report a year later by Norris. Douglas Stephens of Australia, in 1953, described the critical importance of pelvic floor muscles in determining fecal continence, and his operative procedure emphasized the need to incorporate the pull-through rectum within the puborectalis sling. Over the next 30 years this remained the standard approach to imperforate anus, and additional contributions instead emphasized associated anomalies especially related to the sacrum and spinal cord (Carson in 1984; Karrer in 1988) and urinary tract (McLorie in 1987). The landmark report by de Vries and Friedland in 1974 detailed the embryologic development of the human anus and rectum and led to a new improved therapeutic approach, the posterior sagittal anorectoplasty, reported by de Vries and Pena in 1982. This operation, a variation of a procedure described in France almost 150 years earlier, has become the procedure of choice in most centers. It has totally changed our understanding of the functional physiology and anatomy of the pelvic floor and enlightened our understanding of an anorectal "sphincter complex." As an operative procedure this approach has been of particular benefit for the treatment of complex cloacal malformations.

## Surgical Research/Investigation

In his presidential address to the APSA in May 1991, Robert Filler of Toronto categorized both the major contributions and the importance of areas of pediatric surgical research. Although his analysis limited contributions to those reported in the APSA meeting venue, the category of "impact areas" is likely relevant. They include treatment of DH, ECMO support, and critical care, total parenteral as well as surgical enteral nutrition, fetal surgery, treatment of imperforate anus and fecal continence, liver and biliary tract surgery, gastroesophageal reflux, inflammatory bowel disease including the diagnosis and treatment of necrotizing enterocolitis, and large-bowel surgery. The 10 papers achieving the highest "citation-index" score dealt with the following: *Pathophysiology of Necrotizing Enterocolitis* by Barlow in 1974, *Conservative Management of Splenic Trauma* by Douglas in 1971, *Percutaneous Endoscopic Gastrostomy* by Gauderer in 1980, *Outcomes from Diaphragmatic Hernia* by Dibbins in 1974, *Splenorrhaphy* by Ratner in 1977, *Patent Ductus Arteriosus Ligation in Prematures* by Gay in 1973, *Survival Prediction for Congenital Diaphragmatic Hernia* by Raphaely in 1973, *Necrotizing Enterocolitis* by Bell in 1973, *Esophageal Corrosive Burns* by Haller in 1971, and *Fetal Repair of Diaphragmatic Hernia* by Harrison in 1981.

Pediatric surgeons have also contributed to our understanding of entire fields of basic biology. Donahoe, in a series of experiments, defined the role of Müllerian-inhibiting substance (MIS) in the molecular determination of human sexual development. Similarly, Folkman has defined the entire field of vascular biology and angiogenesis both as it dictates the developmental biology of organs and organ systems and as it provides rate-limiting influences in a variety of pathologic (retinopathy, nephropathy, etc), neoplastic (tumor angiogenesis), and normal developmental processes (liver regeneration, gut adaptation, myocardial revascularization).

Perhaps most relevant to clinical pediatric surgery has been the translation of basic research in such entities as necrotizing enterocolitis by Ford and coworkers to clinical outcomes of treatment such as the randomized trial led by Moss et al that defined the role of operation versus drainage in perforative NEC. In like manner the critical randomized trial of fetal intervention for congenital myelomeningocele led by Adzick has refined the most appropriate algorithm of treatment for that entity.

## SELECTED READINGS

Amoury RA. "Matchmaker–matchmaker." The evolution of pediatric surgical training programs and the selection of candidates for pediatric surgical training through the first quarter century of the American Pediatric Surgical Association. *J Pediatr Surg* 1995;30:143–157.

Fonkalstrud EW. Pediatric surgery—a specialty come of age. *J Pediatr Surg* 1991;26:239–247.

Gans SL. Editorial: the "*Journal of Pediatric Surgery*": in recognition of its first 25 years. *J Pediatr Surg* 1996;26:1–3.

Goldbloom RB. Halifax and the precipitate birth of pediatric surgery. Pediatrics 1986;77:764.

Hendren WH. Pediatric surgery, then and now. *Arch Surg* 1994;129:345–352.

Johnson DG. Presidential address: excellence in search of recognition. *J Pediatr Surg* 1986;21:1019–1031.

Koop CE. Editorial: the birth of a journal. *J Pediatr Surg* 1981;16:3.

Koop CE. Pediatric surgery: the newest specialty for the youngest patient. *Trans Stud Coll Physicians Phila* 1981;3:195–208.

Koop CE. Pediatric surgery: the long road to recognition. *Pediatrics* 1993;92:618–621.

Lanman TH. William E. Ladd, MD—an appreciation. *Pediatrics* 1954;14: 668–672.

Leape LI. A brief account of the founding of the American Pediatric Surgical Association. *J Pediatr Surg* 1996;31:12–18.

Nance MI. The Halifax disaster of 1917 and the birth of North American pediatric surgery. *J Pediatr Surg* 2001;36:405–408.

Randolph U. The first of the best. *J Pediatr Surg* 1985;20:580–591.

Zwicky J. A brief history of the origins of the surgery section of the American Academy of Pediatrics. *Arch Am Acad Pediatr* [unpublished data].

# Ethical Considerations in Pediatric Surgery

# CHAPTER 2

*Donna A. Caniano*

## KEY POINTS

1. The primary duty of the pediatric surgeon as healer is one of promoting good and acting with beneficence, while keeping the patient at the center of all decisions.

2. The pediatric surgical informed consent process includes the elements of providing information that includes risks, benefits, outcomes, and alternate therapies; assessment of the ability of patient/guardian to make decisions; and the ability of the patient/guardian to make decisions free of coercion.

3. A clinical team's common moral framework is essential to address concerns of ethical conflict.

4. The pediatric surgeon has the responsibility to inform patients and families about medical error and adverse events. Failure to do so is a breach of professional and ethical norms.

5. When innovating a new operative therapy, the early development of a formalized research protocol will help to define risks, benefits, and outcomes. The informed consent process for innovative procedures needs to be done to a higher standard.

Pediatric surgical ethics came into existence with the convergence of several interrelated factors: technological advances in medicine after World War II, activism of the 1960s, and recognition that the traditional paternalistic approach to patient care contradicted contemporary notions of individual rights. In October 1971 an audience attending The Joseph P. Kennedy Jr. Foundation International Symposium on Human Rights, Retardation and Research was shown a documentary film from The Johns Hopkins Hospital about a newborn infant with trisomy 21 whose parents refused to give permission for lifesaving surgical care to repair a congenital intestinal obstruction. For the first time the public was permitted inside the "secret sanctum" of pediatric medical decision making, a place historically reserved for parents and physicians. Subsequently, in 1973 Duff and Campbell reported in *The New England Journal of Medicine* that 43 of 299 consecutive deaths (14%) in the neonatal intensive care unit at the

Yale-New Haven Hospital resulted from decisions to withdraw or withhold lifesaving treatment. This article caused a furor in the lay press, as the American public raised concerns over the morality and legality of allowing certain infants to die without treatment. In 1977 when Shaw et al published a survey of the attitudes of pediatric surgeons and pediatricians about difficult choices in treating and not treating infants with a variety of congenital anomalies, the centrality of ethics was firmly situated in pediatric surgical decision making.

In this chapter the moral dimensions of pediatric surgical health care will be considered as they relate to care decisions for individual patients, in addition to the larger context of societal interests in pediatric surgical practice. Since this textbook focuses on operative pediatric surgery, specific issues in pediatric surgical ethics will be discussed: informed consent, decision making for infants and children with uncertain prognosis, disclosure of surgical error, and professional responsibilities for surgical innovation and research.

The ethical responsibilities of the pediatric surgeon are shaped by the unique relationship of the 3 parties: the infant or child patient, the parents, and the pediatric surgeon. Medical ethicists have characterized the primary duty of the surgeon, as healer, as one of promoting good and acting with beneficence, while keeping the patient at the center of all decisions. The ethical duty of beneficence requires pediatric surgeons to: (1) honor their fiduciary role as experts in the benefits, risks, and expected outcomes for proposed treatments; (2) accept the vulnerability of their pediatric patients and parents; and (3) place the interests of their patients over personal or third-party interests. Furthermore, pediatric surgeons are obliged to provide care for their infant patients with major congenital anomalies over an extended period of time, often well into adulthood.

## INFORMED CONSENT

The doctrine of informed consent rests with the widely accepted concept in western societies, and increasingly among many cultures, that competent persons or their designated surrogates (ie, parents for their minor children) have the ethical and legal right/responsibility to make their own medical and surgical decisions, and to choose which course of treatment is preferable. Medical decisions include consideration of the patient's goals and values, based on cultural, religious, social, and other relevant norms. In *The Virtues in Medical Practice*, Pellegrino and Thomasma broadened informed consent to include the fiduciary responsibility of the physician in safeguarding patient integrity within a relationship governed by the promotion of healing, honesty, and compassion. Thus, informed consent respects patient autonomy (in pediatrics, the child and parents), and requires physicians to provide the information necessary to make reasoned decisions. Informed consent implies that the ethical principles of beneficence, nonmaleficence, and justice are upheld, along with the patient's autonomous right to decision making.

Given the ever-increasing diversity of contemporary society, pediatric surgeons may encounter children and parents from diverse and heterogeneous cultures. In the context of surgical decision making, culture implies a common and accepted way that a group of individuals think, feel, and act when faced with choices. As a cultural group they are characterized by generally shared beliefs, values, attitudes, behaviors, and notions of what is meant by certain actions. For example, most people from western cultures consider disease to be a disruption in biological processes, while individuals from other cultures may consider disease as having spiritual or metaphysical causes. While most people from progressive western countries embrace advanced technological life-preserving treatments, individuals from other cultures may employ a holistic approach to the use of life-extending therapy. For example, parents may question how prolongation of life for an imperiled infant would affect the well-being of their family and extended community. When persons from a minority culture immigrate to another country, they may adopt the prevailing attitudes of the majority population, adhere strictly to their native beliefs, or adopt a mixture of western attitudes and their native cultural mores. During the process of informed consent, the pediatric surgeon should seek ways to reduce cultural barriers by asking questions about patient/parental values, actively listening to their answers, indicating that their views are important, giving ample time to the discussion, and, when necessary, seeking assistance from experts who better understand the prevailing cultural beliefs.

Four elements comprise the essential components of the informed consent process:

1. The provision of information, in clear and understandable language, about the nature of the surgical disorder, the recommended plan for diagnosis and treatment, the potential benefits and risks of the proposed operation, anticipated outcome, and long-term prognosis. The range of possible alternative treatments should be presented, including the option of no treatment.

2. An assessment by the pediatric surgeon of the patient's/parents' understanding of the information.

3. An assessment by the pediatric surgeon of the patient's/parents' competence to make these decisions.

4. The ability of the patient and parents to make decisions free of coercion or manipulation by the pediatric surgeon or others.

In the United States and in most countries parents have the legal and ethical responsibility to be the surrogate decision makers for their minor children, until the adolescent reaches 18 years of age and she/he can give legal consent for surgical treatment. Certain exceptions to parental surrogacy for consent include the ability of minor children to seek treatment for sexually transmitted diseases and care of pregnancy-related matters and contraception. Pediatric patients with chronic illnesses, such as cystic fibrosis, sickle cell disease, muscular dystrophy, and end-stage liver or renal disease, may be given "mature minor" legal designation so that they can make their own medical decisions. In these cases it must be determined that the patient has sufficient maturity to understand the disease, its chronic and potentially terminal nature, and the benefits/risks of life-extending therapies.

The American Academy of Pediatrics recognizes that older children and adolescents should be involved in discussions and decisions about their health care and that their assent should be obtained prior to embarking on treatment. The process of assent is similar to informed consent and is characterized by:

1. The use of developmentally appropriate language to help the child/adolescent become aware of the nature of the medical/surgical condition

2. Explaining what the patient can expect with the proposed diagnostic tests and treatments, including how pain will be monitored and controlled

3. Active solicitation of the patient's understanding and willingness to accept the proposed treatment and/or operation.

Seeking assent from an older child or adolescent may be challenging when the proposed surgical procedure involves an alteration of bodily image or function, even if temporary in duration. In these situations it may be helpful to invoke assistance from patient support groups and other patients with similar health challenges. Another concern rests with the adolescent's overly optimistic view of the anticipated postoperative result, in terms of either improved bodily image or "perfect" function.

An example of a unique challenge for pediatric surgeons is the informed consent process for weight reduction surgery in morbidly obese adolescents. While objective evidence indicates that pediatric morbid obesity is associated with serious metabolic derangements and a lower quality of life, the optimal surgical intervention remains to be defined by multi-institutional prospective clinical trials. Specific issues about bariatric surgery that should be considered during the informed consent process with adolescent patients and their parents include the following:

1. Ability of the adolescent and parents to retain information about the proposed bariatric intervention and its risk/benefit profile. A study of adult patients who underwent gastric bypass surgery indicated that two thirds were unable to correctly recall information about the risks of the operation in the immediate postoperative period.

2. Adolescent patients may have a limited understanding of the irreversibility of certain bariatric operations, such as the gastric bypass. They may not fully realize that the new anatomic arrangement will be permanent and may include potentially unpleasant lifelong side effects.

3. The long-term consequences of bariatric surgery performed during adolescence are unknown in terms of unanticipated and unforeseen problems. While reduction of associated metabolic derangements and reasonable weight loss are achieved in the early postoperative period, it is unknown whether these benefits are maintained over several years and into adult maturity.

4. As a result of media publicity showing former morbidly obese individuals transformed into svelte and highly attractive persons after bariatric surgery, adolescent patients and their parents may have an overly optimistic view of the postoperative outcome in terms of physical appearance and overall well-being.

5. The pediatric surgeon is obligated to disclose her/his postoperative results following each type of bariatric operation, including complications and durable weight loss.

Pediatric surgeons who embark on weight reduction procedures for adolescents should be working within a hospital environment that supports a comprehensive screening program for associated comorbidities, psychosocial assessment and counseling for the patient and parents, preoperative attempts at weight loss, and postoperative long-term follow-up. Bariatric adolescent patients and their parents should also be made aware of how care will be transitioned on reaching adulthood.

## DECISION MAKING FOR INFANTS AND CHILDREN WITH UNCERTAIN PROGNOSIS

The American historian and philosopher Lewis Mumford observed, "In so far as ethics provides a sound guide for living, it must have life's own attributes, its pliability, its adaptiveness to the occasion." It is in the neonatal intensive care unit that pediatric surgeons are most likely to encounter substantive moral dilemmas, and where holding to rigid moral and ethical absolutes may lead to conflict between parents and well-intentioned caregivers. For example, situations that involve extremely premature infants with substantial intestinal loss or infants with multiple congenital anomalies affecting several organ systems may invoke uncertainty regarding their overall prognosis and the benefits of surgical intervention and continued utilization of life-sustaining therapies. Making decisions to proceed with operative treatment brings into conflict the ethical principles of beneficence (acting with the best interests of the infant) and autonomy (the parents' decision-making authority for their infant).

A cross-cultural study of parental involvement in decision making for extremely premature infants with severe intraventricular hemorrhages evaluated 2 similar academic neonatal intensive care units in the United States and France. The investigator, a sociologist, observed 2 interesting aspects of the decision-making process: (1) the physician's degree of medical certainty about the infant's clinical status and prognosis determined whether parents were allowed to make a choice to continue or discontinue treatment, and (2) parents were more likely to be involved in end-of-life decisions when the physicians deemed either the prognosis to be dismal for neurologic recovery or the infant to be clearly in a terminal situation. This study points out the degree of control that physicians have in determining whether a given infant's prognosis is categorized as being uncertain, and, therefore, open to significant parental involvement in continuation of treatment.

Since contemporary surgical health care is a team endeavor and, in most pediatric hospitals, seeks a patient- and family-centered approach, a common moral framework should be developed to address situations of ethical conflict. The team members should: (1) be familiar with how to articulate their views and feelings about a given moral issue; (2) understand how to clarify their values relative to considerations of withdrawal or withholding life-sustaining treatment; and (3) have an agreed-upon method for all members to use in moral decision making.

Baylis and Caniano proposed guidelines for resolution of a moral problem in situations where there is conflict or uncertainty. These guidelines include identification of the decision makers (ie, parents); outline of all medical information; definition of available treatment options; explanation of how each treatment option offers cure, amelioration, prospect for functional status, and relief of pain or suffering; clarity around the values of the parents; and arrival at a consensus resolution. An outcome that all parties can agree on requires mutual respect and support of all team members and parents. It is helpful to acknowledge at the outset that there is no one right "answer" or resolution, and that in severe illness, decisions are rarely happy and are usually painful. Finally, the health care team members should recognize that in situations of prognostic uncertainty, parental values, as well as their religious and cultural beliefs, may exert considerable influence on whether to continue or withdraw life-sustaining treatment.

Recognition that physicians benefit from review of complex patient scenarios centered on difficult ethical decision making has resulted in the institution of regular "ethics rounds" by several medical and surgical journals. Since decisions about whether to operate on extremely premature infants with necrotizing enterocolitis remain one of the most challenging areas for pediatric surgeons and their colleagues, 2 recent journals profiled similar clinical situations. In the case outlined by Yamada et al the authors concluded that the pediatric surgeons would be justified to refuse further operative intervention for an extremely premature infant with significant associated morbidity and extensive bowel loss, despite parental request for aggressive treatment. Meadow et al present the case of an extremely premature infant with an intraventricular hemorrhage, lung disease, and probable extensive necrotizing enterocolitis. The parents, practicing Jehovah's Witnesses, refused abdominal surgery unless the pediatric surgeons agreed to use no blood products intraoperatively. At an emergency ethics committee meeting, the physicians presented the various options, including that surgery would almost definitely require administration of blood products. The parents were also told about the infant's poor prognosis for survival given his deteriorating clinical condition. The parents were asked about their preferences for treatment and they reiterated love for their infant and wishes that he not suffer, but were adamant that he not be given blood products. The ethics committee members then met without parental presence and decided that the preferences of the parents for comfort care should be followed, given the infant's poor prognosis for survival. Five commentators (no pediatric surgeons) discussed the case in terms of its process for decision making, parental involvement, and outcome. It is obvious that the ethics committee members were influenced by the pediatric surgeon's explanation to the parents that, even with surgical intervention and the administration of blood products, the infant had a low chance for survival. It is possible that if the pediatric surgeon had given the parents a better prognosis for survival with operation and blood product administration, the ethics committee members may have recommended seeking a court order to proceed with aggressive treatment measures, including emergency surgical intervention.

## SURGICAL ERROR

In 1999 the Institute of Medicine's report *To Err Is Human* estimated that nearly 100,000 patients die annually in the United States as a direct result of medical error, while many more patients suffer serious harm from an error that causes unnecessary morbidity, prolongs hospitalization, and increases the cost of care. Since this report most hospitals have embarked on improving "systems of care" and reducing or eliminating preventable harm to patients. Some examples of these efforts include standardized protocols for central venous catheter insertion (elimination of catheter-associated infection), preoperative surgical site marking (prevention of wrong site surgery), and surgical checklists (review of all relevant details before commencement of the operation). Despite these efforts a pediatric surgeon may commit an error as a result of an incorrect diagnosis, intraoperative injury to a vital structure, failure to recognize a complication, or delay in instituting treatment in a timely manner. Surgical morbidity and mortality conference is the professional setting for open disclosure of mistakes and complications, at which peers discuss errors for the purpose of improvement in performance and identification of system problems.

What are the ethical obligations of surgeons to disclose an error to a patient? The Code of Professional Conduct, adopted by the American College of Surgeons in 2003, listed several responsibilities of its fellows in rendering care to surgical patients. Among these was the duty to "fully disclose adverse events and medical errors." In addition, hospitals in the United States, as mandated by the Joint Commission on Accreditation of Healthcare Organizations, require that patients and their families be informed about medical errors and adverse events, and failure of the physician to do so is considered a breach of professional and ethical norms. While surgeons-in-training usually receive education in how to deliver "bad news" to patients, they often receive little, if any, direction in how to communicate medical error. When an error is committed by the pediatric surgeon, particularly an intraoperative mistake that has adverse consequences, the emotions of shame, guilt, and fear of legal liability can easily overwhelm even the most experienced clinician. Moral courage, including self-recognition that "I made a mistake," and honesty of purpose should guide the pediatric surgeon's conversation with the parents.

The pediatric surgeon should (1) inform the parents (and patient, if appropriate) in clear language that an error occurred; (2) assume responsibility for the error; (3) explain how the mistake was corrected; (4) discuss how the patient will be treated henceforth; (5) share any predictable adverse sequelae; and (6) explain how the pediatric surgeon and institution will prevent a future error. Finally, the pediatric surgeon should communicate regret and humility for having caused harm, and be clear that all resources of the hospital will be available for future treatment related to the error.

Following a surgical error, the pediatric surgeon should endeavor to preserve the patient and parents' trust, the underlying principle in the patient–physician relationship. The offering of an apology by the pediatric surgeon is the optimal way for both parties to acknowledge, recover, and heal after a surgical error. For the pediatric surgeon, who is the power holder, it expresses vulnerability and thereby permits the patient and parents to feel less vulnerable and more in control of a difficult situation. Effective language in the apology includes "I am sorry," "I am responsible," and "I am available to review and answer your questions now and in the future." A genuine apology for surgical error requires honesty, generosity, humility, commitment, and courage on the part of both the pediatric surgeon and the patient/parents.

## INNOVATION AND RESEARCH IN PEDIATRIC SURGERY

Contemporary western societies place high value on medical technology and on progress achieved through innovation. The history of pediatric surgery is filled with the successful introduction of operations to correct a myriad of congenital and acquired conditions. While the Federal Food and Drug Administration (FDA) requires clinical studies before approval of new drugs, surgeons have great latitude in developing new operations. Traditionally, there has been minimal or no oversight of surgical innovation, giving surgeons freedom to develop new operations, modify existing procedures, and introduce new treatment. Most "new" operations are performed at a single academic center, the results of the institutional series are presented at a professional meeting, and 1 or more papers detailing the clinical outcomes are published in surgical peer-reviewed journals. Surgeons then adopt the "new" operation, several clinical series in multiple institutions are evaluated, and a more realistic assessment of its benefits, risks, and outcomes can be determined over an extended period of time. Proponents of surgical progress applaud the freedom to create and innovate, while others caution that lack of oversight carries risks of injuring patients or not helping them with new operations. The historical record of surgery contains now-abandoned operations that caused harm (the jejunal-ileal bypass for morbid obesity, gastric freezing for ulcer disease) and procedures that were not beneficial (internal mammary ligation for angina, sympathectomy for Hirschsprung disease).

Clinical innovation and clinical research are distinct entities that remain linked in the practice of modern medicine. Innovation is the introduction of something new (new treatment, new operation, or new device). The innovator's goal is to benefit a patient or group of patients with a given condition (eg, rectosigmoidectomy and pull-through introduced by Ovar Swenson for Hirschsprung disease; minimally invasive repair of pectus excavatum introduced by Donald Nuss). Clinical research involves formal testing of a hypothesis in adequate patient volumes to arrive at new knowledge that will benefit humans (with or without benefit to study participants). In most clinical research studies 1 or more treatments or operations are evaluated/compared, with the highest validation accorded to prospective, randomized clinical trials (RCTs) in multi-institutional settings.

While surgical innovation is not inherently problematic, given its intended goal of patient benefit by an operation that is safer, more effective, or less likely to cause morbidity, lack of organized oversight and ability to protect patients from overzealous innovation is cause for concern. Since new operations or innovative techniques are often accompanied by the belief (by both patients and surgeons) that they are better than the traditional approach, it is helpful to consider them as nonvalidated until they are proven to be safe and/or superior. Recently, the Society of University Surgeons published guidelines for the responsible introduction of surgical innovation. An innovation was defined as a new or modified surgical procedure that differs from currently accepted local practice, with outcomes yet to be described, and which may carry risk to the patient. In addition, if the surgical innovation is planned and the surgeon seeks to test a hunch, theory, or hypothesis about the innovation, the surgeon is obliged to obtain specific and additional patient consent. The guidelines recommend a process that safeguards patient interests: review of the planned surgical innovation by a local surgical innovations committee, submission to the national innovations registry, and additional informed consent that outlines the experimental nature of the proposed innovation. During the course of a commonly accepted operation, surgeons are often required to make unanticipated modifications based on unique patient anatomy and other circumstances. These situations, often considered tinkering, do not rise to the level of surgical innovation, but do warrant full disclosure to the patient and family postoperatively.

The dangers of unregulated research came to light in the years following World War II, when the Nazi medical and surgical experiments were revealed during the Nuremberg war crimes tribunal. In 1966 Dr Henry Beecher, a respected medical researcher, published an article in *The New England Journal of Medicine* about research on humans that he considered to be risky and performed without appropriate patient consent. As a consequence of these events, the federal government of the United States required that all research on humans funded by public monies be subject to local institutional review to assure ethical acceptability. In 1974 the US Congress established a National Commission for the Protection of Human Subjects of Biomedical and Behavioral Research, a multidisciplinary group of prominent scientists, physicians, ethicists, lawyers, and religious leaders, who met for 3 years to develop guidelines about the ethical conduct of human experimentation. Their final report culminated in the Belmont Report, published in 1979, which serves as the ethical foundation for all human research conducted in the United States. Two areas of comment in that report have special significance for pediatric surgeons: (1) the development of new operations, intended to have immediate patient benefit rather than the generation of new knowledge, should be made part of a formal research effort at the early stages to determine their benefit, safety, and outcomes; and (2) the informed consent standards for research need to be higher than those for clinical practice because of the presumption that participation may not necessarily benefit the subject. The pediatric community was singled out as a group that must take special care in conducting human research because of the vulnerable nature of its potential research subjects.

One of the best examples of clinical research in pediatrics involves the treatment of childhood cancer, which is characterized by ongoing prospective randomized investigation directed by the collaboration of multiple specialists from surgery, pediatric oncology, radiation therapy, and pathology. Since 1969 the treatment of Wilms tumor has achieved steady improvement in survival because of ongoing clinical trials that seek to lessen treatment morbidity, reduce long-term adverse sequelae, and understand the unique biological and genetic characteristics of this malignancy. That nearly all children with newly diagnosed Wilms tumor have been enrolled in these studies and that they can anticipate a survival above 90% speak to the merits of clinical investigation. Given this degree of success, it is surprising that pediatric surgeons are involved in so few other clinical trials, outside of the realm of childhood cancer. One reason that pediatric surgeons may be reluctant to participate in RCTs is a perceived lack of clinical equipoise, or the uncertainty about which treatment or operation provides the best outcome, given 2 or more alternatives. Pediatric surgeons often tend to hold firm in the belief that a "favorite" operation (one that she/he has performed with good results) is better than other procedures, despite lack of substantiated evidence from published reports that a specific operation has superior outcomes when compared with other operations for the same condition. A more nuanced concept of clinical equipoise, proposed by Freedman, holds that community equipoise is a state of uncertainty within a professional specialty regarding the relative merits of competing procedures or treatments. This interpretation of clinical equipoise allows the individual pediatric surgeon to have strong preference for a given operation, yet acknowledge that there is reasonable uncertainty within the profession (and supported by the published literature) about the best operation or treatment.

Should pediatric surgeons have an ethical and professional obligation to participate in clinical research? We may look to the principles of medical ethics outlined for the members of the American Pediatric Surgical Association, which lists 7 distinct obligations, including:

> *Members shall strive to maintain existing skills and to develop or acquire new medical and surgical knowledge through continuing practice in order to benefit patients…Members shall recognize a responsibility to participate in activities benefitting the community.*

Pediatric surgeons are uniquely positioned to engage in clinical research through cooperative prospective investigation. Many of the common congenital anomalies are relatively uniform in their anatomic derangements and pathophysiology, such as Hirschsprung disease and gastroschisis. Significant variability exists in the management of common pediatric surgical conditions, such as appendicitis. If prospective multi-institutional clinical research were to indicate optimal treatment for common pediatric surgical diseases, patients would benefit, surgeons would gain knowledge, care could be standardized, and health care costs could be potentially reduced for any given condition.

As found in the childhood cancer trials, the findings of each clinical study refine and reset standards of treatment, develop new questions for investigation, and lead to ongoing prospective research. When multiple centers enroll a large number of patients in prospective clinical study, the emergence of unintended consequences (ie, unanticipated early morbidity) may come to light far sooner than studies performed by single institutions with small numbers of patients.

## SELECTED READINGS

Baylis F, Caniano DA. Medical ethics and the pediatric surgeon. In: Oldham KT, Colombani PM, Foglia RP, et al, eds. *Principles and Practice of Pediatric Surgery*. Philadelphia, PA: Lippincott Williams & Wilkins; 2005:349–356.

Biffl WL, Spain DA, Reitsma MA, et al. Responsible development and application of surgical innovations: a position statement of the Society of University Surgeons. *J Am Coll Surg* 2008;206(3):1204–1209.

Bylaws of the American Pediatric Surgical Association. Principles of medical ethics. http://www.eapsa.org.

Caniano DA. Ethical issues in pediatric bariatric surgery. *Semin Pediatr Surg* 2009;18:186–192.

Duff RS, Campbell AGM. Moral and ethical dilemmas in the special-care nursery. *N Engl J Med* 1973;289:890–894.

Ells C. Culture, ethics and pediatric surgery. *Semin Pediatr Surg* 2001;10: 186–191.

Freedman B. Equipoise and the ethics of clinical research. *N Engl J Med* 1987; 317(3):141–145.

Kohn L, Corrigan J, Donaldson M, eds. *To Err Is Human: Building a Safer Health System*. Washington, DC: National Academic Press; 2000.

Maean A, Tichansky DA. Patients postoperatively forget aspects of preoperative patient education. *Obes Surg* 2005;15:1066–1069.

Meadow W, Feudtner C, Antommaria AHM, et al. A premature infant with necrotizing enterocolitis whose parents are Jehovah's Witnesses. *Pediatrics* 2010;126:151–155.

Orfali K. Parental role in medical decision-making: fact or fiction? A comparative study of ethical dilemmas in French and American neonatal intensive care units. *Soc Sci Med* 2004;58:2009–2022.

Pellegrino ED, Thomasma DC. *The Virtues in Medical Practice*. New York, NY: Oxford University Press; 1993.

Shaw A, Randolph JG, Manard B. Ethical issues in pediatric surgery: a national survey of pediatricians and pediatric surgeons. *Pediatrics* 1977;60:588–599.

The American College of Surgeons. Code of Professional Conduct. Chicago, IL. http://www.facs.org/memberservices/codeofconduct.html. Accessed August 4, 2010.

Weiss PM, Miranda R. Transparency, apology, and disclosure of adverse outcomes. *Obstet Gynecol Clin North Am* 2008;35:53–62.

Yamada NK, Kodner IJ, Brown DE. When operating is considered futile: difficult decision in the neonatal intensive care unit. *Surgery* 2009;146:122–125.

# Fetal Surgery, Diagnosis, and Intervention

## CHAPTER 3

*Jesse D. Vrecenak and Alan W. Flake*

## KEY POINTS

1. Fetal surgery has the potential to alter the natural history of congenital disease.

2. Patient selection requires detailed understanding of disease pathophysiology.

3. Potential benefits of prenatal intervention must offset the significant risks for both mother and fetus.

4. Improvements in imaging technology permit more detailed diagnosis of congenital anomalies and provide better prognostic information.

5. A multidisciplinary approach is necessary for patient selection and counseling.

6. Prevention of preterm labor is a focus of preoperative, intraoperative, and perioperative management.

## DEVELOPMENT OF FETAL SURGERY

Fetal surgery is a specialty born of clinical necessity. Pediatric physicians and surgeons had long observed that certain congenital anomalies could cause irreversible organ damage before birth, leading to fetal or neonatal death despite all efforts at treatment. As new imaging technologies emerged, our ability to prenatally diagnose anatomic anomalies and to understand the correlation between their prenatal pathophysiology and postnatal outcomes improved. In specific conditions, progressive organ destruction occurred in utero, raising a compelling rationale for fetal surgery. It was the logical progression of thought to consider whether repair of the defect in utero might reverse the pathophysiology, restore normal development, and lead to good quality of life with survival.

Fetal surgery requires several unique considerations, including maternal–fetal monitoring, anesthesia, tocolysis, and methods of hysterotomy and uterine closure, in addition to the technical aspects of each individual procedure. Animal models have played a key role in the development of techniques to allow the mother and fetus to undergo operation safely and successfully. Since its inception, fetal surgery has developed rapidly, driving improvements in prenatal diagnosis, technical innovations, and better understanding of the pathophysiology and natural history of candidate disorders, as well as the unique physiology of the fetus and pregnant mother. The fetus is, in essence, a patient within a patient, protected by layers of maternal abdominal wall, uterine wall, and chorioamniotic membranes, and management of obstetric complications remains critical to the success of fetal interventions.

The first report of successful therapeutic intervention on the fetal patient was the transfusion of a hydropic fetus for Rh disease by Sir A. W. Liley, which remains the treatment for Rh disease today. This transfusion was guided by radiographs and contrast instillation and represents the first acknowledgment of the fetus as a patient. Following a few attempts at open fetal exchange transfusion during the 1960s, modern fetal surgery was conceived and developed by Michael Harrison and colleagues at the University of California, San Francisco (UCSF) during the late 1970s and 1980s. There, the concept of a multidisciplinary fetal treatment program was developed, along with experimental models of fetal disease in sheep and monkeys, which allowed study of the pathophysiologic rationale and technical feasibility of human open fetal surgery. The fetal lamb model allowed evaluation of the pathophysiology of specific fetal defects, while researchers used the primate model to develop the anesthetic, tocolytic, and technical methods required to conduct fetal interventions in humans. In the early 1980s, this research allowed the first systematic clinical application of open fetal surgery by Harrison and colleagues.

Although the prerequisites for fetal surgery formulated during this early work continue to apply with only minor modifications (Table 3-1), both our understanding of fetal disease processes and our ability to make accurate diagnoses and prognoses have drastically improved since the advent of the field. Rapid advances in imaging technologies, including high-resolution ultrasound, ultrafast MRI, and fetal echocardiography, now allow precise definition of anatomic detail and characterization of structural abnormalities. Furthermore, fetal karyotyping, molecular diagnosis, and maternal serum screening allow far greater accuracy in identifying genetic diagnoses or syndromes. The clinical and research experience accumulated over the past 30 years has allowed better understanding of the natural history of prenatally

| TABLE 3-1 | Prerequisites for Fetal Surgery |
| --- | --- |

1. Accurate diagnosis and staging possible
2. Absence of associated anomalies
3. Natural history, pathophysiology, and prognosis of the disease are understood
4. No effective postnatal therapy
5. Feasibility and ability of in utero surgery to reverse disease pathology documented in animal models
6. Procedures performed in specialized multidisciplinary fetal treatment centers, adhering to strict protocols and with the informed consent of the mother or parents

diagnosed disease, and provided a metric by which to gauge the success of fetal intervention.

Randomized controlled trials (RCTs) provide the ultimate test of the efficacy of fetal surgery, although the design and execution of such trials remains challenging due to the rarity of appropriate subjects, ethical challenges, and the resources required for organization, financing, and impartial evaluation of results obtained. The first RCT to evaluate open fetal surgery for correction of an anatomic defect was the recently completed Management of Myelomeningocele Study (MOMS). The MOMS trial was a large multicenter RCT that demonstrated efficacy for prenatal repair of myelomeningocele (MMC) compared with postnatal repair, providing the first evidence-based justification for open fetal surgery. Although fetal surgery was originally felt to be appropriate only for lethal anomalies, the success of this trial may allow application of these techniques for other nonlethal conditions in which prenatal intervention might alter the course of irreversible organ damage or decrease morbidity that impacts quality of life. A RCT of fetoscopic laser separation versus amnioreduction of monochorionic (MC) twins with twin-to-twin transfusion syndrome (TTTS) performed in Europe has also demonstrated efficacy for fetal intervention. Other trials are either under development or underway including fetoscopic tracheal occlusion for congenital diaphragmatic hernia (CDH). The future of fetal intervention depends on developing evidence-based support for fetal interventional procedures, which will be a major focus in coming years.

In this chapter, we discuss the pathophysiology, diagnosis, selection criteria, and operative management of the fetal patient, with specific focus on several disorders representing the spectrum of fetal surgery, that is, CDH, congenital cystic lung lesions (congenital cystic adenomatoid malformation [CCAM]/bronchopulmonary sequestration [BPS]), sacrococcygeal teratoma (SCT), TTTS, and MMC.

## PATHOPHYSIOLOGY OF FETAL SURGICAL DISEASE

### Congenital Diaphragmatic Hernia

CDH is generally a unilateral defect in the left (90%) or right (10%) hemidiaphragm due to failure of closure of the foramen of Bochdalek between 8 and 10 weeks of gestation,

resulting in herniation of abdominal viscera into the thoracic cavity with or without herniation of the liver. CDH occurs in 1 out of every 2500 to 5000 live births and is most often sporadic, although familial cases have been reported. It may occur as part of a syndrome, and associated abnormalities have been observed in 25% to 57% of cases, including 95% of stillborn cases. Such abnormalities may include congenital heart defects, hydronephrosis, renal agenesis, intestinal atresia, extralobar sequestrations, and neurologic defects such as hydrocephalus, anencephaly, and spina bifida. CDH may be associated with chromosomal abnormalities including trisomy 21, 18, and 13 in 10% to 20% of prenatally diagnosed cases.

A majority of the morbidity observed in CDH can be related to the pulmonary hypoplasia and resulting pulmonary hypertension. Pulmonary hypoplasia, which likely occurs as a result of compression of the lung by herniated viscera during the branching phase of pulmonary morphogenesis, affects the lung at both gross and cellular levels and represents a fixed component of CDH pathophysiology. Not only are a decrease in overall lung weight and fewer bronchial divisions, bronchioles, and alveoli observed, but the hypoplastic pulmonary vascular bed leads to an increase in pulmonary vascular resistance as well as a decreased area for gas exchange. Increased vasoreactivity represents a reversible defect resulting from increased muscularization of arterioles and extension of the muscle into the distal acinar unit. Pulmonary hypertension leads to persistence of the fetal circulation with shunting through the ductus arteriosus or foramen ovale, causing hypoxemia and acidosis. The pulmonary vasculature becomes extremely sensitive to hypoxemia, acidosis, and other stimuli, and the consequent pulmonary vasospasm can lead to an inability to ventilate using conventional protocols. Because of these developmental effects, the pathophysiology of prenatally diagnosed CDH is significantly related to the timing of herniation and the volume occupied by the herniated abdominal viscera within the thoracic cavity. If herniation occurs after the majority of lung development is complete, the manifestations of the defect are far less severe, and a much better outcome is observed. Thus, CDH incorporates a spectrum of diseases ranging from mildly affected infants with relatively normal lung development and vascular reactivity to those with such severe hypoplasia that they are unable to survive postnatally.

However, improvements in postnatal management, including novel ventilation strategies, have significantly changed the natural history of the disease in recent years. Liver position has historically been the most important factor predictive of poor outcome, and lung volume measurements have not been proven to provide additional prognostic information, although they can confirm disease severity. Recently, the observed to expected lung area to head circumference ratio (O/E LHR) measured by ultrasound or MRI has been used preferentially to predict morbidity and mortality. However, while valuable for prenatal counseling, none of these measurements have proven highly predictive of mortality in a given fetus in the modern era of "gentilation"-based care. These improvements in postnatal management likely contributed to the failure of the first fetal surgical RCT of fetoscopic tracheal occlusion to demonstrate benefit for prenatal intervention, as the control group had a survival rate much higher than that predicted on the basis of historical data. As a result, the indications for fetal intervention are a matter of continued debate and further studies are underway.

## Congenital Cystic Lung Lesions

Congenital cystic lung lesions are space-occupying echo-dense and/or solid thoracic masses and represent a spectrum of diseases ranging from congenital CCAM to BPS, with an intermediate category of "hybrid" lesions exhibiting characteristics of both types. CCAM is a benign multicystic lung mass, which generally involves only 1 lobe of the lung without right or left predominance and derives its blood supply from the pulmonary circulation. Such lesions may be macrocystic (cysts 2-10 cm) or microcystic, are characterized histologically by an overgrowth of terminal respiratory bronchioles forming cystic structures, and may result from a failure of bronchiolar maturation or focal pulmonary dysplasia during the fifth or sixth week of gestation. Although this tissue is nonfunctional for normal gas exchange, connections do exist between the cyst and the tracheobronchial tree, which can lead to air trapping. The incidence of such lesions is unknown, and there are no known associated anomalies.

BPS, by contrast, is a mass of nonfunctioning lung tissue derived from the developing foregut that has systemic arterial supply, most commonly from the thoracic aorta. Both extralobar (25%) and intralobar (75%) forms are observed, with the extralobar form distinguished by the presence of its own pleura, without communication to the native tracheobronchial tree. Intralobar forms result from early ectopic lung budding, may be found within the normal lung tissue, and may or may not have connections to the tracheobronchial tree. Venous drainage is most commonly to the pulmonary veins for intralobar BPS, and to the subdiaphragmatic veins for extralobar lesions. The incidence of BPS is estimated at 1 in every 1000 live births without gender specificity for intralobar forms, but there is a 4 to 1 female predominance for extralobar lesions. Approximately 10% of fetuses with intralobar BPS have associated anomalies including CDH, tracheoesophageal fistula, congenital heart defects, aneuploidy, and/or foregut duplication, and the presence of such anomalies increases to 50% in fetuses with extralobar BPS.

CCAM and BPS lesions may be small and of minimal prenatal clinical significance or may grow to cause physiologic derangement via rapid growth and mediastinal compression, which may result in polyhydramnios, cardiac failure, and fetal hydrops via mass effect or tension hydrothorax resulting from lymphatic secretion from BPS masses. Fetal hydrops and placentomegaly can also cause the development of the maternal mirror syndrome, in which the mother develops progressive preecclamptic symptoms, which "mirror" fetal pathophysiology and may result from the release of placental vasoactive factors. Because 15% to 20% of prenatally diagnosed CCAM lesions and nearly two thirds of BPS lesions will shrink in size substantially before birth, frequent surveillance is required to determine the natural history of a given lesion and development of fetal hydrops is currently considered to be the only indication for fetal intervention.

## Sacrococcygeal Teratoma

SCT refers to a presacral neoplasm containing tissue derived from all 3 germ layers and lacking organ specificity. Four types have been identified, with Type I lesions being completely external, Type II lesions having both external and small internal pelvic components, Type III lesions having both an external component and a larger internal pelvic component extending into the abdomen, and Type IV being completely internal. The incidence of SCT is estimated at 1 in 20,000 to 1 in 40,000 live births, with 3:1 female predominance. Associated malformations have been observed in 10% to 40% of affected fetuses.

These tumors are highly vascular, and due to the often very large tumor mass, significant arteriovenous (AV) shunting can occur. This vascular steal can lead to high-output cardiac failure, placentomegaly, and fetal hydrops, with other complications including tumor rupture, fetal anemia, and urologic obstruction. The pathophysiology of prenatally diagnosed SCT is far more severe than that of postnatally diagnosed lesions with an estimated mortality of 30% to 50%. Neonatal death may occur as a result of obstetric complications, including hemorrhage from tumor rupture, as well as from preterm labor incited by polyhydramnios or uterine distention from tumor mass, which can also cause dystocia. Three subsets have been identified: Group A represents those fetuses with a tumor diameter ≤10 cm, absent or mild vascularity, and slow growth, Group B has a tumor diameter of 10 cm or greater, pronounced vascularity, and rapid growth, while Group C has a tumor diameter of 10 cm or greater, a predominantly cystic lesion with absent or mild vascularity, and slow growth. Both Groups A and C are associated with good maternal and fetal outcomes, while the rapid growth observed in Group B presents a far greater risk of perinatal mortality and preterm delivery. Fetal mortality approaches 100% once fetal hydrops and placentomegaly develop, which are frequently preceded by a rapid phase of tumor growth. If left untreated, maternal mirror syndrome can be observed. Rarely, SCTs can undergo malignant degeneration.

## Twin-to-twin Transfusion Syndrome

TTTS refers to the unbalanced exchange of circulation between interplacental communications of MC twins. Such unbalanced flow occurs in 10% to 15% of MC twin gestations, creating the potential for TTTS. The overall prevalence of TTTS is approximately 1 in 2000 pregnancies and usually occurs during the second trimester. The involved vascular anastomoses are most commonly AV, allowing unidirectional flow. In TTTS, the donor twin becomes hypovolemic and oliguric, while the recipient becomes hypervolemic and polyuric, leading to physiologic hormonal alterations in each. The renin–angiotensin system becomes activated in the donor twin in the effort to preserve intravascular volume, resulting in hypertension, reduced placental perfusion, and growth retardation, while the recipient increases renal perfusion and urine output to counter this volume overload and may be exposed to renin–angiotensin upregulation via transfer of effectors through placental shunts. Common cardiac abnormalities in the recipient include myocardial hypertrophy,

AV valvular regurgitation, and increased velocities of pulmonic and aortic outflow, as well as pulmonic stenosis and right ventricular outflow tract obstruction, which may reflect increased cardiac afterload due to systemic hypertension. The natural progression of TTTS is highly variable and unpredictable, occurring at any time during gestation. If untreated, however, TTTS is associated with a nearly 90% mortality rate in both fetuses, and the far lower mortality rates following selective laser ablation thus represent an unequivocal success for fetal intervention.

## Myelomeningocele

MMC, commonly referred to as open spina bifida, represents the first application of fetal surgery to a nonlethal disorder, and is defined as a defect in the vertebral arches allowing protrusion of meninges and neural elements with devastating neurologic consequences. Despite wide appreciation that folic acid can reduce the rate of MMC, MMC continues to occur in approximately 1 in every 2000 live births, and the true incidence is even higher as many MMC fetuses are aborted.

The development and validation of the "2-hit" hypothesis was a critical step in the consideration of MMC as a target of fetal therapy despite its nonlethal nature. This hypothesis suggests that neurologic damage occurs not only as the result of the first "hit" of failed neurulation but also from the second "hit" due to exposure of the spinal cord to the amniotic fluid and mechanical effects within the intrauterine environment. Evidence suggests that a significant component of neural damage is acquired by this mechanism, providing a compelling rationale for fetal intervention. As a result of the loss of CSF through the open spinal defect, MMC fetuses also have an Arnold-Chiari II malformation, with hindbrain herniation, low-lying venous sinuses, a small posterior fossa, and secondary brain stem compression. This secondary effect may cause a significant component of the morbidity and mortality associated with MMC.

Current postnatal treatment yields a mortality rate of 14% by age 5 in all MMC neonates, which rises to 35% in cases of symptomatic brain stem compression from the Arnold-Chiari malformation. Significant neurologic morbidity is observed, including paralysis and both bowel and bladder dysfunction. The neurologic deficits acquired in utero are irreversible; hydrocephalus occurs in 85% of cases and requires placement of a shunt in at least 80%, with associated shunt-related complications creating yet another source of morbidity. Although 70% of patients have an IQ higher than 80, only half are ultimately able to live independently, underscoring the considerable effect of MMC on quality of life.

## DIAGNOSTIC PRINCIPLES OF FETAL DISEASE

### Fetal Imaging Modalities

Novel imaging modalities have been a critical part of many advances in fetal surgery, allowing diagnosis and definition of complex anatomic abnormalities early in gestation. 3D ultrasound has become a standard of care, allowing more rapid examination of surface anatomy and more sensitive detection of neural tube defects than conventional 2D ultrasound. Before ultrafast T2-weighted MRI techniques, fetal movement often degraded the study due to the length of time necessary to acquire MRI images using a low-strength magnet. Ultrafast MRI represents a significant advance in fetal imaging. Although originally used primarily for CNS imaging, we now use MRI in the evaluation of many other organ systems. Such static images can provide extremely detailed information and more sensitive identification of primary pathology and associated anomalies. Furthermore, MRI may allow better prediction of neurologic function and thus provides valuable guidance for parental counseling.

## Congenital Diaphragmatic Hernia

CDH is often found incidentally on screening anatomic ultrasound, although polyhydramnios may prompt a dedicated study. Diagnostic findings include the presence of viscera in either the right or left hemithorax above the level of the diaphragm, or at the level of the 4-chambered heart view. The fluid-filled abdominal viscera can be easily distinguished from the surrounding lung based on its hypoechoic signal. Determination of liver position is the most important prognostic indicator but can be more difficult due to its similar echodensity to the surrounding lung. However, hepatic vasculature can be identified by ultrasound and MRI techniques, allowing excellent discrimination (Fig. 3-1A). In right-sided CDH, the liver may be the only organ herniated into the chest, making this diagnosis more challenging. Other common findings include a small or invisible lung, an ipsilateral diaphragmatic defect, or mediastinal shift. Differential diagnosis of such findings includes type I CCAM, bronchogenic cyst, neurenteric cysts, and cystic mediastinal teratoma, all of which can appear hypoechoic and be confused with herniated bowel. The presence of peristalsis in herniated bowel loops may help to distinguish true CDH, and the location of the gallbladder may provide further guidance, as it may be displaced medially, located in the left upper quadrant, or herniated into the right chest.

Liver position is the most reproducible independent prognostic factor in CDH, and can be assessed by either ultrasound or MRI, with herniation predictive of poorer outcome. The ratio between right lung area (measured at the level of the 4-chambered heart view) and head circumference (LHR) can be measured by ultrasound. It has been validated both prospectively and retrospectively as a prognostic indicator when measured in the 22- to 24-week gestation window. Controversy exists, however, regarding the clinical utility of LHR measurements that likely relates to variable skill and experience of sonographers taking the measurements. Although this measurement does not provide additional independent predictive information beyond liver position, it can provide confirmation of disease severity. Measurement of LHR is somewhat subjective, and intraobserver variability may yield differences of 0.2 to 0.3. Due to its subjective nature, the predictive value of LHR may vary by center, and may only be able to be validated within a single center over time. Other authors have suggested that the O/E LHR may be a more widely useful

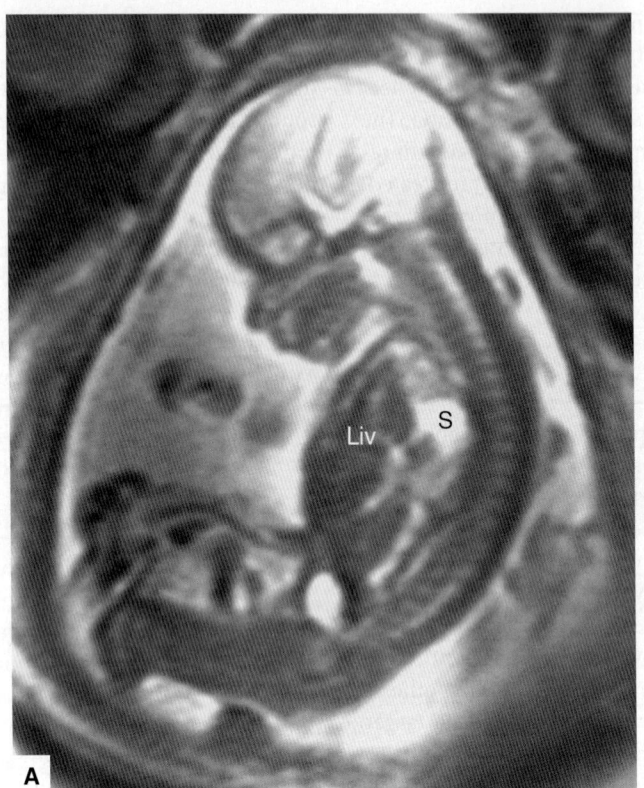

A

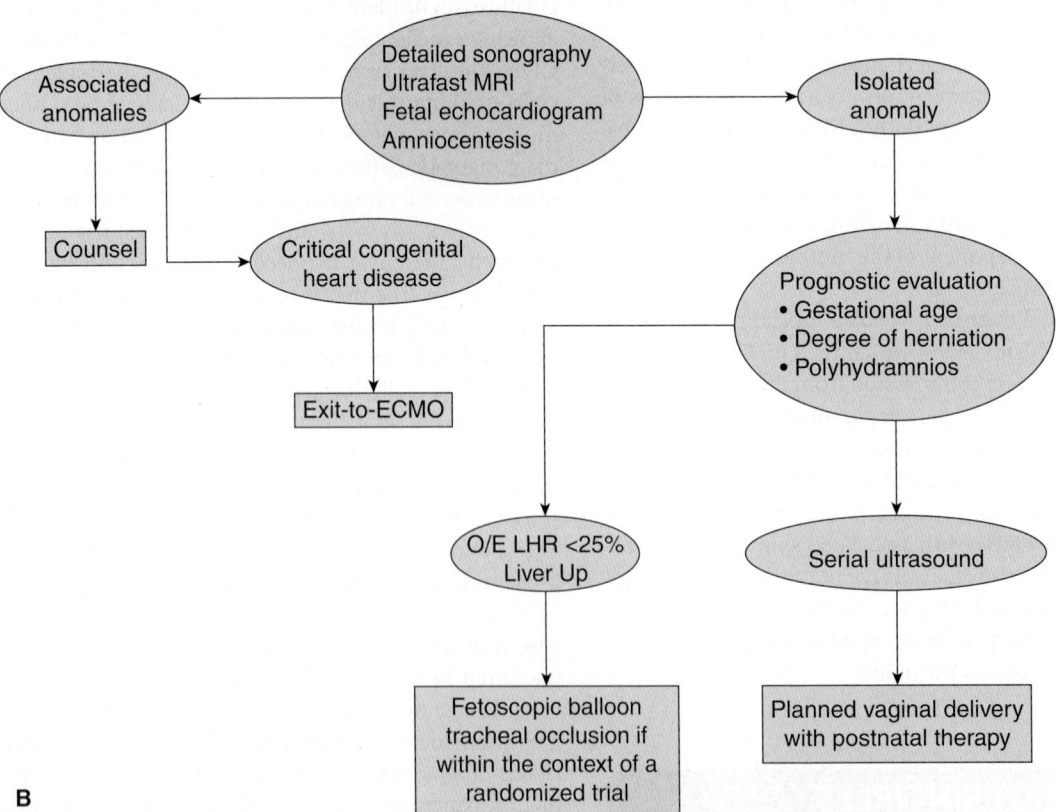

B

**FIGURE 3-1 A.** Sagittal section of fetal MRI demonstrating liver (Liv) herniated above the diaphragm. The stomach (S) is also seen in the thorax posterior to the liver. **B.** Algorithm for the management of fetal CDH.

parameter because it is predictive of mortality independent of gestational age. Importantly, advances in postnatal management have improved survival rates over the past several years, requiring contemporaneous controls for any study of fetal intervention. Our current algorithm for the management of fetuses with CDH is shown in Fig. 3-1B. Although some centers advocate the use of ex utero intrapartum treatment (EXIT)-to-extracorporeal membrane oxygenation (ECMO) for severe CDH, this strategy is currently reserved for fetuses with coincident severe cardiac disease at the Children's Hospital of Philadelphia (CHOP) due to maternal morbidity and concerns about quick and potentially inaccurate judgments regarding need for ECMO. In addition, fetoscopic balloon tracheal occlusion is an experimental treatment for the most severe subset of CDH patients that should only be offered within the context of a randomized clinical trial.

## Congenital Cystic Lung Lesions

Prenatal diagnosis of cystic lung lesions generally relies on the identification of an echogenic mass in the fetal chest (Fig. 3-2A). Because these lesions represent a spectrum of diseases, this mass may be solid, cystic, or mixed. Doppler ultrasound generally reveals evidence of either pulmonary (CCAM) or systemic (BPS) arterial supply, except in the case of hybrid lesions, which may have both. The differential diagnosis includes bronchogenic or neurenteric cysts, CDH, congenital lobar emphysema, and peripheral bronchial atresias or stenoses. CCAMs may be microcystic or macrocystic, and ultrasound may reveal mediastinal shift away from large lesions or polyhydramnios from esophageal compression. Severely affected fetuses may ultimately become hydropic, and usually die before or shortly after birth if managed expectantly. BPS presents as a uniformly echogenic lesion, often triangular, and Doppler ultrasound should reveal evidence of systemic blood supply arising from the thoracic or infradiaphragmatic aorta. Such lesions may be associated with pleural effusion, which may cause tension hydrothorax. Predominantly microcystic CCAMs typically grow slowly and plateau around 28 weeks, while macrocystic CCAMs have a less predictable growth pattern and rapid growth may occur after 28 weeks, requiring closer surveillance. CCAM size can be monitored via measurement of the ratio between CCAM volume and head circumference (CVR). A CVR greater than 1.6 on presentation has been associated with an 80% chance of developing hydrops, requiring close surveillance 2 to 3 times per week, whereas a CVR less than 1.6 portends a lower likelihood of hydrops and such fetuses can be monitored weekly (<1.2) or twice weekly (1.2–1.6) through 28 weeks. The presence of hydrops or mediastinal shift portends a poor prognosis if untreated, whereas the survival rate is greater than 95% for microcystic CCAM in the absence of hydrops. In hydropic fetuses, management depends on gestational age, as shown in Fig. 3-2B.

## Sacrococcygeal Teratoma

SCT usually presents as a caudal and/or intrapelvic mass identified on screening anatomic ultrasound or on a study indicated for uterine size too large for dates. Due to the heterogeneous nature of these tumors, SCTs exhibit a disorganized appearance by ultrasound and may be cystic, solid, or mixed. They may exhibit irregular echogenicity as a result of tumor necrosis, cystic degeneration, internal hemorrhage, or calcifications, and are very vascular. Other tumor characteristics that can be assessed by ultrasound include evidence of bladder obstruction, hydronephrosis, ureteral dilation, and evidence of tumor rupture. Once this complex mass is identified by ultrasound, MRI can provide valuable anatomic definition and help to distinguish any intrapelvic component (Fig. 3-3A). Doppler ultrasound can demonstrate reversal of diastolic blood flow in the umbilical arteries due to vascular steal by the tumor. Because of the very poor prognosis once hydrops has developed, frequent monitoring by ultrasound and fetal echocardiography is critical if fetal intervention is to be successful.

Due to the presacral location of these tumors, the differential diagnosis includes MMC, meconium pseudocyst, and obstructive uropathy, making detailed examination of the kidneys and spine critical to the evaluation of such a lesion. Following confirmation of an SCT, fetal echocardiogram is a critical part of the workup, given the prevalence of a steal syndrome and hydrops among affected fetuses. Echocardiographic parameters include IVC diameter (≥6 mm may indicate early cardiac failure), fractional shortening index, combined ventricular output (≥600 mL/kg may be consistent with early heart failure), and descending aortic flow velocity. Growth rates are an important prognostic indicator, and serial assessment of tumor size is critical in determining eligibility for fetal intervention. As in other states contributing to fetal heart failure, poor prognostic signs include signs such as cardiomegaly, hydrops characterized by ascites and skin edema, and increased preload indices. Again, decisions regarding fetal therapy depend on both physiology and gestational age, as shown in Fig. 3-3B.

## Twin-to-twin Transfusion Syndrome

Ultrasound represents the primary method of detecting TTTS, and all MC, diamniotic twin gestations should be screened frequently starting in the second trimester. Both a >65% difference in maximum vertical amniotic fluid pocket (MVP) size and a >25% discordance in estimated fetal weight have been shown to be associated with a higher risk and shorter time to the development of TTTS. Usually, the syndrome is recognized following observation of oliguric oligohydramnios in 1 twin and polyuric polyhydramnios in the other (poly/oli) (Fig. 3-4A). Other ultrasound features include concordant fetal gender and Doppler changes within the fetal vasculature. The presence or absence of a visible bladder provides important staging information, and should be assessed. Quintero staging describes several ultrasound features (Table 3-2) but does not include cardiovascular indices that are important in pathophysiology and prognosis. The CHOP cardiovascular scoring system described by Rychik et al (Table 3-3) can help in assessing disease severity and choosing co-twins for fetal treatment. In suspected cases, further evaluation of at least the recipient twin with echocardiography is necessary to determine

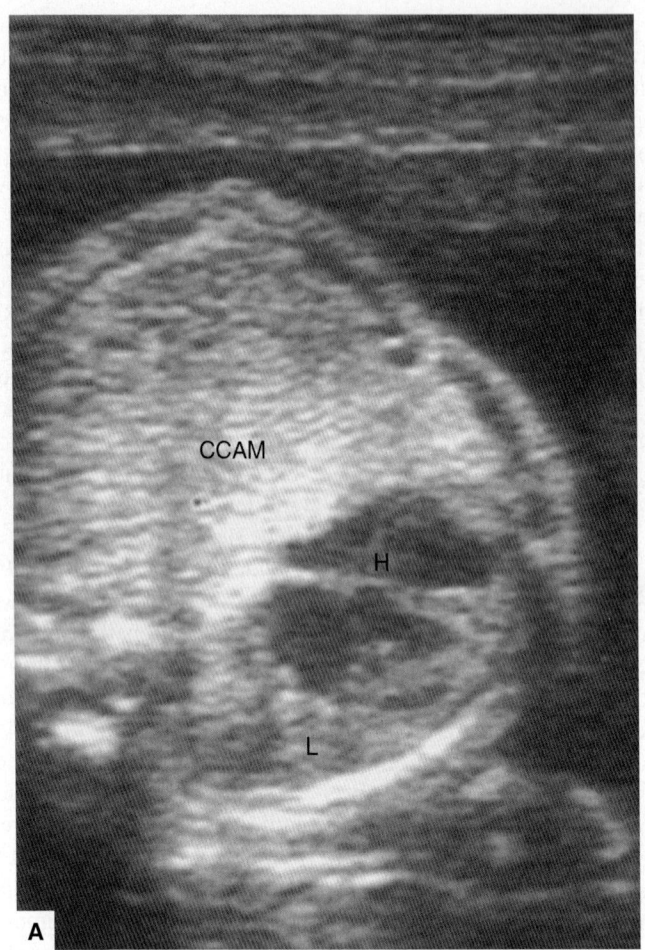

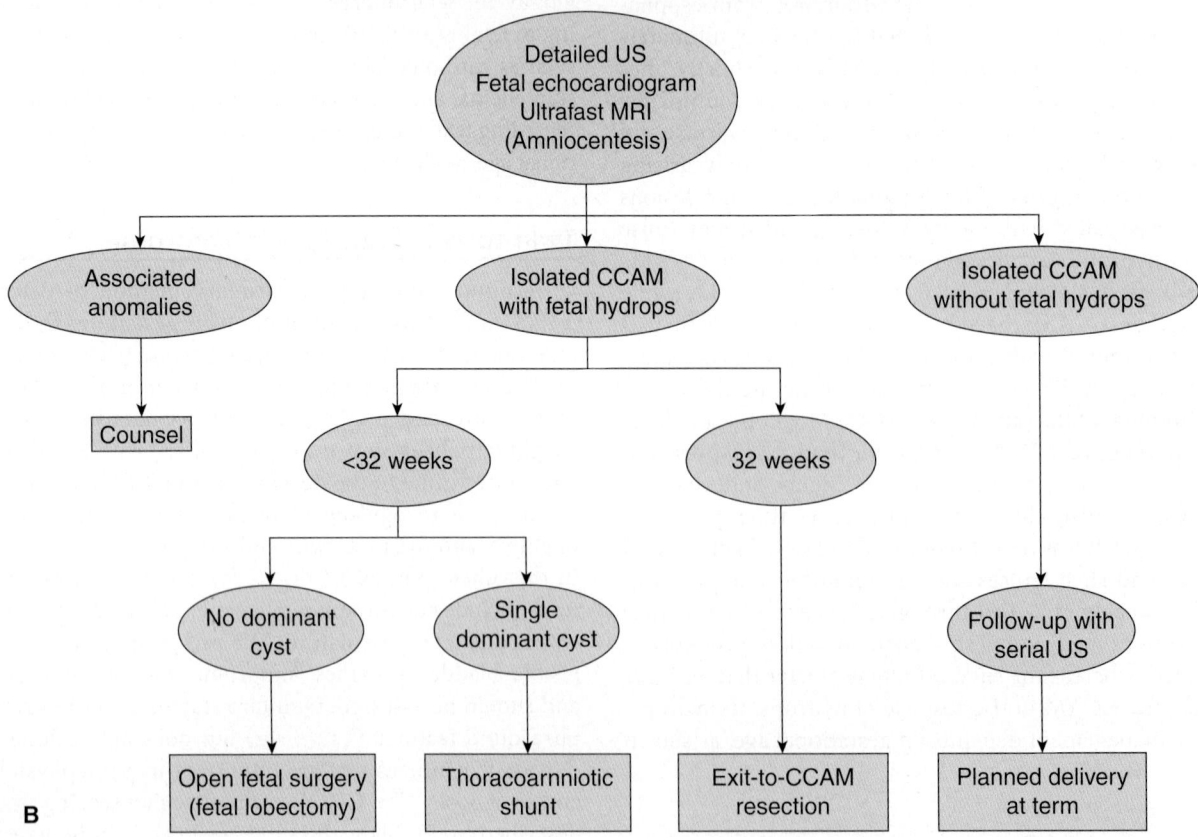

**FIGURE 3-2** **A.** Fetal ultrasound demonstrating echogenic microcystic CCAM (CCAM). The compressed contralateral lung is seen (L) as is the marked shift of the mediastinum and heart (H). There is evidence of early hydrops with skin edema. **B.** Algorithm for the management of fetal CCAM.

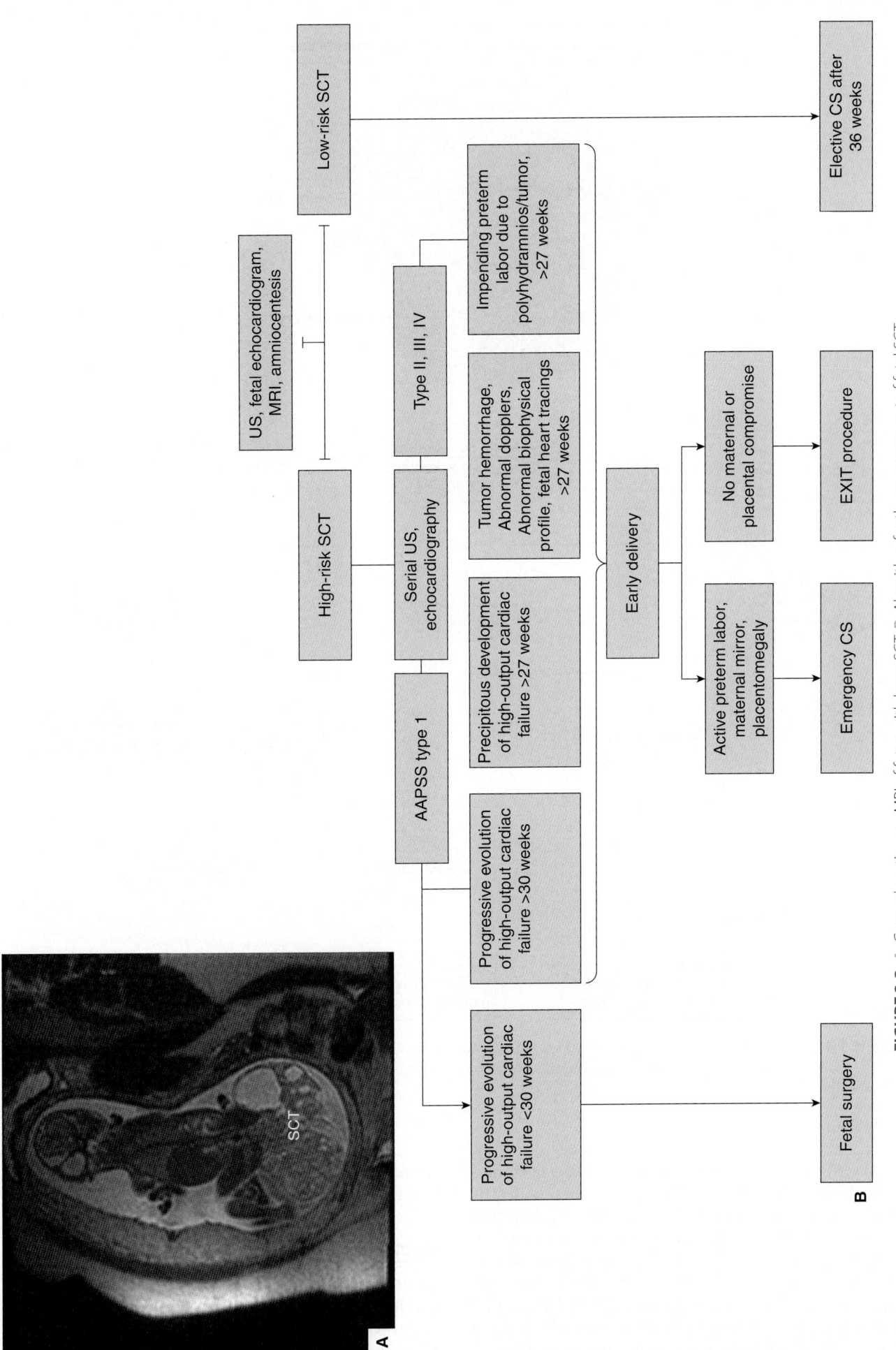

**FIGURE 3-3** A. Coronal section on MRI of fetus with large SCT. B. Algorithm for the management of fetal SCT.

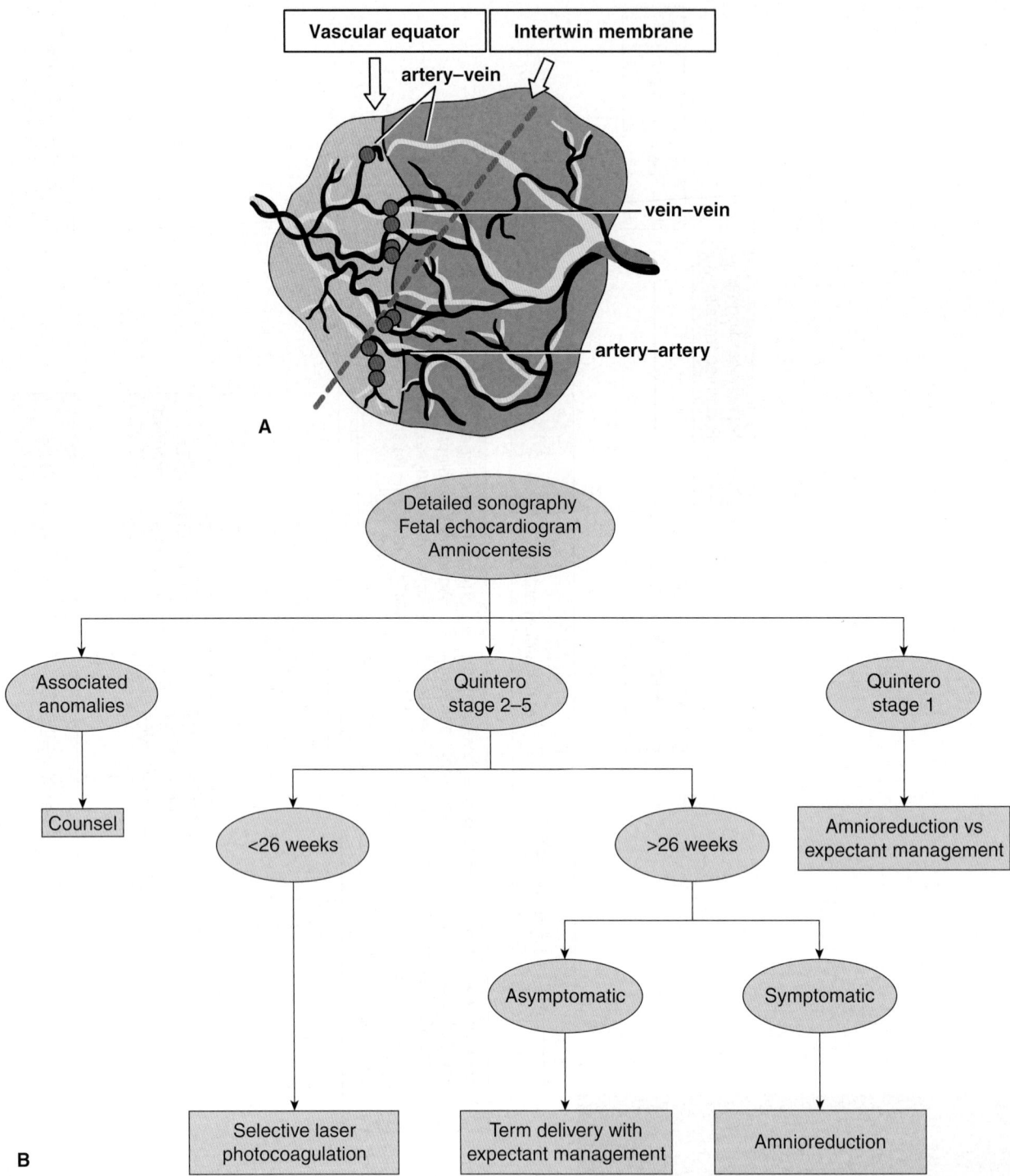

**FIGURE 3-4** **A.** Schematic representation of the types of vascular communications in TTTS and the concept of the placental/vascular equator. The circles represent the laser ablation sites required to completely separate the placental circulation. **B.** Algorithm for the management of fetal TTTS.

the severity of the physiologic alteration. Signs of cardiomyopathy associated with TTTS may include cardiomegaly or hypertrophy, atrioventricular regurgitation, decreased systolic function, and ductus venosus abnormalities on Doppler examination. In 5% of cases, significant RV outflow tract stenosis may be present. A full anatomic scan should be performed to eliminate coincident defects, ascites, hydrops, or preexisting brain damage, as well as assessment of maternal cervical length to determine whether

cerclage might be indicated. Our current treatment algorithm for TTTS is shown in Fig. 3-4B.

## Myelomeningocele

Ultrasound demonstration of the open spinal cord defect remains a mainstay of MMC detection, but MRI has become of particular importance in documenting CNS anatomy and pathology. Serial imaging via ultrasound was critical in

**TABLE 3-2    Quintero Staging of TTTS**

| Stage | Findings |
| --- | --- |
| 1 | Polyhydramnios in recipient sac (MVP >8 cm) and oligohydramnios in the donor sac (MVP <2 cm) |
| 2 | No visible bladder in donor twin |
| 3 | Doppler abnormality consisting of absent or reversed flow in the umbilical artery, reversed flow in the ductus venosus, or pulsatile flow in the umbilical vein |
| 4 | Ascites or hydrops in either fetus |
| 5 | Demise of either fetus |

the development of the 2-hit hypothesis, as affected fetuses were observed to lose movement in the lower limbs and to develop worsening hydrocephalus and hindbrain herniation over the course of gestation. In fact, early gestation fetuses may not show evidence of the Arnold-Chiari II malformation at all, while later gestational fetuses almost uniformly demonstrate these changes. In addition to identification of the defect and level, ultrasound is very important in assessing limb movement, which remains a selection criterion for fetal intervention.

MRI, however, can provide additional anatomic detail and elucidate sac contents, particularly in cases with oligohydramnios, low-lying fetal head, maternal obesity, or posterior spine position. Additionally, MRI is far more sensitive at detecting associated CNS malformations, and it is better able to assess the degree of hindbrain herniation and hydrocephalus (Fig. 3-5A). Evaluation for hydrocephalus is an important part of MMC monitoring, as shunts are commonly required postnatally to prevent further neurologic insult. The current treatment algorithm for MMC reflects the recent success of the MOMS trial, as shown in Fig. 3-5C.

# TREATMENT OPTIONS FOR FETAL SURGICAL ANOMALIES

## Ethical Considerations and Preoperative Management

Fetal surgery is unique in its involvement of a healthy patient who undertakes considerable surgical risk without expectation of direct benefit, creating a unique subset of ethical concerns. Such concerns have been explored and an ethical framework has been well established. In general, the fetus achieves independent moral status as a patient once he/she reaches the point of viability. The previable fetus, then, is a patient only when the pregnant woman chooses to continue her pregnancy and presents for treatment on behalf of her fetus. For the eligible fetus, the risks of such a procedure are clearly offset by the considerable benefit of salvage, but the fetus cannot be considered to be an independent or autonomous decision maker, and the beneficence-based obligation to the fetus must be balanced with both beneficence- and autonomy-based obligations to the mother. Thus, the fetus is

not a separate patient, and maternal safety is a primary concern in considering fetal intervention.

Furthermore, the mother is under no obligation to present her fetus for treatment, and she must be provided all necessary information for truly informed consent. The treatment team has a responsibility to consider the risks to the mother in the context of the likelihood of fetal loss or severe, irreversible disability. For this reason, both fetal and maternal factors can be contraindications to open fetal surgery, including chromosomal abnormalities, significant anatomic abnormalities, maternal obesity, heavy smoking history, or other medical conditions. Patient selection should take place through multidisciplinary evaluation following a screening process including detailed ultrasonographic examination for characterization of the defect and any other abnormalities, ultrafast fetal MRI for anatomic definition, fetal echocardiogram to assess heart function and detect any cardiac abnormality, and karyotyping. Following this evaluation, cases should be reviewed by a multidisciplinary team of fetal surgeons, obstetricians, anesthesiologists, radiologists, a nurse coordinator, sonographers, and social workers.

Eligible families must undergo extensive counseling to discuss the proposed surgical procedure, and postoperative and postnatal care. A team meeting provides an appropriate forum for the family to learn about the procedure and its risks, benefits, and alternatives. Depending on gestational age, all appropriate options should be discussed in a nondirective manner, including termination, expectant management with palliative or best available postnatal treatment, and prenatal therapy. Parents must understand the likely outcomes of all possibilities, as well as the risks involved. For any fetal surgery, complications may include preterm labor, premature rupture of membranes, chorioamnionitis, uterine rupture, medication side effects, risk of fetal demise, as well as surgical complications and future reproductive issues. The mother must be counseled regarding the need for cesarean section in this and all future pregnancies, and care must be taken to "allow" families to opt for nonsurgical management.

## Invasive Procedures

The spectrum of fetal interventions includes not only open fetal surgery but also minimally invasive fetal operations such as shunting or fetoscopic procedures, as well as the EXIT procedure.

Fetoscopy first became available in the 1970s, and was initially used primarily as a diagnostic tool. With the development of more sophisticated camera equipment and specialized endoscopic tools, minimally invasive interventions have become not only feasible but also widely applied. Procedures performed in this manner range from laser coagulation of placental anastomoses in TTTS to balloon tracheal occlusion for CDH. Complications of these procedures may include bleeding, separation or rupture of fetal membranes, chorioamnionitis, or preterm delivery. Most fetoscopic procedures can be performed entirely percutaneously and without carbon dioxide insufflation, minimizing maternal and fetal risks. Such cases usually require only local anesthesia, while procedures that could cause fetal pain generally involve intramuscular administration of an opioid and a paralytic

| TABLE 3-3 | CHOP Cardiovascular Staging of TTTS (Rychik et al) | | |
|---|---|---|---|
| **Variable** | **Parameter** | **Finding** | **Score** |
| Donor | Umbilical artery | Normal | 0 |
| | | Decreased diastolic blood flow | 1 |
| | | Absent/reversed diastolic blood flow | 2 |
| Recipient | Ventricular hypertrophy | None | 0 |
| | | Present | 1 |
| | Cardiac dilation | None | 0 |
| | | Mild | 1 |
| | | More than mild | 2 |
| | Ventricular dysfunction | None | 0 |
| | | Mild | 1 |
| | | More than mild | 2 |
| | Tricuspid regurgitation | None | 0 |
| | | Mild | 1 |
| | | More than mild | 2 |
| | Mitral regurgitation | None | 0 |
| | | Mild | 1 |
| | | More than mild | 2 |
| | Tricuspid inflow | Double peak | 0 |
| | | Single peak | 1 |
| | Mitral inflow | Double peak | 0 |
| | | Single peak | 1 |
| | Ductus venosus | All antegrade | 0 |
| | | Absent diastolic blood flow | 1 |
| | | Reverse diastolic blood flow | 2 |
| | Umbilical vein | No pulsations | 0 |
| | | Pulsations | 1 |
| | Right-sided outflow tract | Pulmonary artery > aorta | 0 |
| | | Pulmonary artery = aorta | 1 |
| | | Pulmonary artery < aorta | 2 |
| | Pulmonary regurgitation | None | 0 |
| | | Present | 1 |

| | |
|---|---|
| **Cardiovascular Grade 1** | **Score = 0–5** |
| **Cardiovascular Grade 2** | **Score = 6–10** |
| **Cardiovascular Grade 3** | **Score = 11–15** |
| **Cardiovascular Grade 4** | **Score = 16–20** |

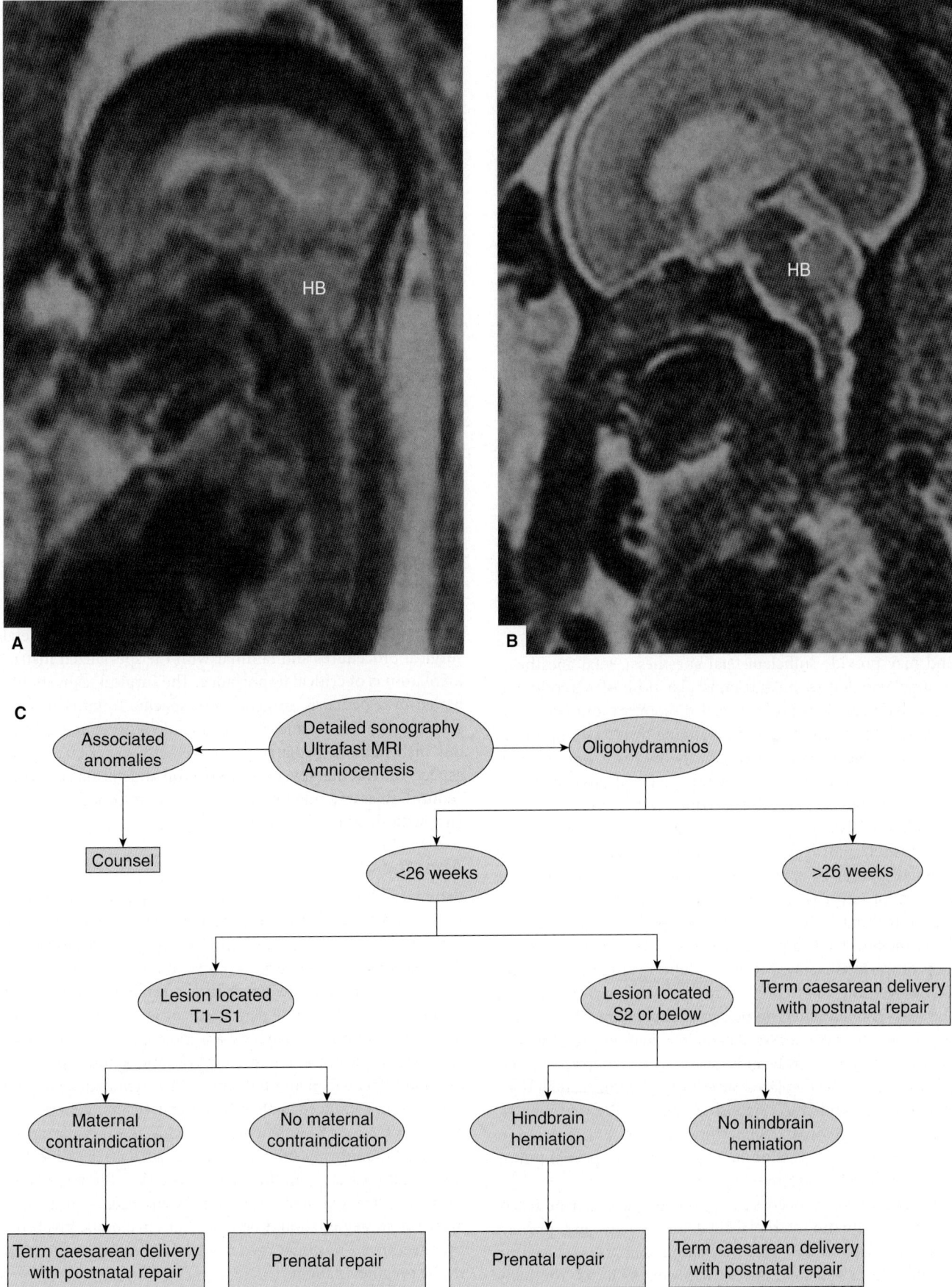

**FIGURE 3-5 A.** MRI appearance of hindbrain herniation in Arnold-Chiari II malformation. **B.** Reversal of hindbrain herniation 3 weeks after fetal repair of MMC. Fluid spaces in the cisterna magna are uniformly restored after fetal repair. **C.** Algorithm for management of fetal MMC.

agent. Similarly, the lack of a hysterotomy obviates the need for extensive tocolysis, and most procedures are performed with only a single dose of indomethacin or nifedipine. RCTs have demonstrated benefit for fetoscopic laser ablation in TTTS and are currently being conducted for fetoscopic tracheal occlusion for CDH. In the case of tracheal occlusion, it is hoped that the lower rates of preterm delivery in fetoscopically treated cases will allow demonstration of benefit that may have been obscured by such obstetric complications in the earlier trial of open surgery.

The EXIT procedure was originally used to remove tracheal clips that had been placed during an earlier procedure to promote lung growth in CDH, but it was subsequently applied to difficult airway cases such as large anterior neck masses. The indications for the procedure have now expanded, and it should be considered in any case in which difficulty obtaining an airway or ventilating a patient due to a large obstructing mass is anticipated. Examples include giant anterior neck masses (cervical teratomas), congenital high airway obstruction syndrome (CHAOS), hypoplastic craniofacial syndrome, thoracic masses (large CCAMs), mediastinal tumors, or as a bridge to ECMO in severe CDH or other cyanotic lesion, with the intent to minimize the risk of hypoxemia and acidosis.

During an EXIT procedure, the mother is positioned supine with a left lateral tilt to maximize venous return and maximize blood supply to the uterus and placenta. A deep inhalational general anesthetic is maintained to achieve uterine relaxation. Although inhaled agents cross the placenta and may provide sufficient fetal anesthesia, fetal anesthesia is supplemented by an intramuscular dose of narcotic and a paralytic agent to prevent fetal discomfort and breathing during the procedure. Careful mapping by ultrasound of the placental edges is performed and the uterus is opened with the same absorbable stapler used in open fetal surgery to control blood loss during the procedure. A peripheral intravenous line is always established for fluid resuscitation, blood transfusion, and drug administration if necessary. A pulse oximeter should be applied to the exposed fetal hand in order to monitor oxygenation during the procedure, and continuous transthoracic fetal echocardiography provides constant assessment of fetal cardiac function and volume status. Infusion of warmed lactated Ringer solution is used to maintain uterine volume and to prevent spasm of the cord vessels, and the fetus is maintained on placental circulation while an airway is established. In cases of giant fetal neck masses, tracheal anatomy may be significantly distorted or compressed, and the carina may be displaced superiorly, yielding a small window through which to establish an airway. Rigid bronchoscopy and/or operative tracheostomy may be sufficient, but in some cases decompression of a cystic mass or partial tumor resection may be required.

Success of this procedure rests on adequate uterine relaxation to maintain uteroplacental blood flow and prevent placental separation. This relaxation can cause bleeding complications postoperatively, and oxytocin is routinely administered immediately following division of the fetal cord. Maternal risks inherent to this procedure include hemorrhage, scar dehiscence or uterine rupture in a subsequent pregnancy (due often to classical cesarean incision required to avoid the placenta or atraumatically deliver a large tumor),

and wound infection. Generally, the fetus is felt to be able to be maintained on placental circulation for around 60 minutes, although procedures as long as 2.5 hours have been performed successfully. Fetal risks of this procedure include bradycardia, hypoxic/anoxic brain injury, hemorrhage, and death. These complications may occur due to cord compression, placental abruption, or loss of myometrial relaxation, all of which result in inadequate uteroplacental gas exchange.

## General Principles of Open Fetal Surgery

### Personnel and Equipment

Care of the fetal surgery patient requires a multidisciplinary team with clearly defined roles, as well as highly specialized equipment. Because the mother and fetus have separated, although there are codependent anesthetic concerns, both an obstetric anesthesiologist and a pediatric anesthesiologist are necessary. A sonographer and an echocardiographer should be an integral part of the surgery team, and a high-resolution ultrasound machine with color Doppler should be used to identify fetal and placental anatomy and to assess for potential hazards such as velamentous cord insertion. Ultrasound images before and after maternal incision are used to select the optimal site for hysterotomy. During the procedure, continuous echocardiography should be used in combination with pulse oximetry to monitor fetal heart rate, cardiac function, and volume status. An OR nursing team trained in fetal surgical procedures and familiar with the specialized instrumentation is of critical importance. The surgical team should be led by a pediatric surgeon with specific training in fetal surgical techniques, and should include a perinatologist. In our institution, 2 pediatric surgeons with experience in all aspects of fetal therapy are scrubbed on all fetal surgical procedures, to assure maximal expertise and to broaden experience with these uncommon procedures.

### Anesthesia

Patients should be admitted prior to the planned procedure for monitoring and initiation of tocolysis with indomethacin. Antibiotics should also be administered preoperatively to decrease the risk of maternal complications and chorioamnionitis. At the time of the procedure, anesthetic management should be initiated with placement of an epidural catheter to assist in both intraoperative and postoperative pain management. Typically, a fentanyl/bupivacaine mixture provides optimal pain control and reduces uterine irritability. General anesthesia is induced with inhalational agents, generally at a MAC of 2 to 2.5, sufficient to provide uterine relaxation. Maternal monitoring should include a radial arterial line, frequent cuff pressures, multiple large-bore IV catheters, a Foley catheter, pulse oximetry, and continuous EKG. Fluid management strategies should be aimed at euvolemia, given the predilection to postoperative noncardiac pulmonary edema in the pregnant patient.

### Positioning and Draping

Patients should be positioned supine with a left lateral tilt provided by a roll under the right side, in order to maximize venous return due to decreased caval compression by the uterus. Skin prep should include mid-thorax to mid-thigh, and the operative field can be squared with sterile towels and covered with a fenestrated and pocketed drape.

## Incision and Exposure

In general, the uterus is exposed through a low transverse abdominal incision. Placental position guides the fascial incision; if posterior, the fascia may be divided in the midline from the umbilicus to the symphysis pubis, while an anterior placenta dictates that muscle and fascia be divided transversely to allow anterior rotation of the uterus and a posterior hysterotomy. A ring retractor can then be positioned for the abdominal wall.

## Opening the Gravid Uterus

Prior to hysterotomy, the uterus is palpated to determine whether sufficient relaxation has been achieved. Transuterine ultrasound is used to confirm fetal and placental position prior to hysterotomy. Under ultrasound guidance, electrocautery is used to map the placental margins on the surface of the uterus and a safe site for hysterotomy is determined, avoiding uterine vasculature. Unlike a standard cesarean section, the lower segment of the uterus is avoided due to increased risk of amniotic fluid leak, chorioamnionitis, and preterm labor.

Once a site is chosen, opposing 0 PDS traction sutures are placed through the uterine wall and fetal membranes under ultrasound guidance (Fig. 3-6A and B). Using electrocautery, a 2-cm incision is made in the myometrium between the sutures and the membranes are visualized. A sharp trocar placed over the anvil of a specialized uterine stapler is then placed through the fetal membranes and the stapler is fired once in either direction (Fig. 3-6C). It is important to use a uterine stapler intended for fetal surgery, as it compresses the myometrium and controls the membranes to minimize blood loss during hysterotomy while maintaining membrane integrity for closure. Absorbable staples are used to avoid subsequent fertility issues. Using a Level I rapid infuser, warmed lactated Ringer's solution is infused into the amniotic space via a catheter to maintain amniotic fluid volumes and fetal temperature, while preventing cord compression. A fetal peripheral intravenous line is then placed for infusion of fluids, blood, or medications.

## Closure of the Gravid Uterus

Proper uterine closure is critically important, as the fetus must be returned to the amniotic space in such a way as to allow gestation to continue as normally as possible. The closure must have adequate strength to prevent uterine rupture, must be watertight to prevent amniotic fluid leaks, and must not contribute to preterm labor or future infertility. A 2-layer closure should be performed, using double-armed full thickness 0 PDS stay sutures approximately 2 cm apart and 2 cm back from the staple line and a running 2-0 PDS suture through myometrium and membranes (Fig. 3-6D). Prior to completing the running layer, approximately 400 cm$^3$ of warmed lactated Ringer's solution containing 500 mg of oxacillin should be instilled into the amniotic cavity and adequate amniotic fluid volumes should be confirmed by ultrasound. An omental flap should be used to buttress the uterine closure, and the

maternal laparotomy should be closed in layers. Skin closure should be performed with an absorbable subcuticular layer, and dressings should consist only of a transparent Tegaderm, in order to allow continued fetal monitoring by ultrasound postoperatively.

## Tocolysis and Postoperative Care

Preterm labor can compromise even the most carefully conducted intervention, and adequate tocolysis is of paramount importance to the success of any open fetal surgical procedure. Preoperative placement of an epidural catheter provides analgesia once the uterine relaxing effects of inhaled anesthesia have worn off, preventing a maternal stress response and uterine irritability. Placement of an indomethacin suppository preoperatively begins the process, and a loading dose of 6 g IV magnesium sulfate is administered during hysterotomy closure. A maintenance infusion of magnesium sulfate is continued at 2 to 4 g/h for 18 to 24 hours postoperatively, and indomethacin suppositories are placed every 6 hours postoperatively to 24 hours. Patients must be closely monitored for signs of magnesium toxicity, and serum magnesium levels should be checked frequently during this period. In addition, daily fetal echocardiography is required to detect any signs of indomethacin toxicity, which can manifest as ductal constriction, oligohydramnios, or tricuspid regurgitation. Uterine activity is monitored by tocodynamometer, and fetal heart rate is followed for any signs of distress. Daily ultrasound performed during the inpatient hospitalization assesses for fetal movement, amniotic fluid and membrane status, and serial anatomic evaluation.

During the postoperative period, fluid status must be carefully managed. Both the physiology of pregnancy and the magnesium sulfate regimen predispose the patient to noncardiogenic pulmonary edema, one of the most serious complications observed in otherwise healthy mothers. Empiric furosemide diuresis can be added if signs of pulmonary edema develop. After 48 hours, patients begin a tocolytic regimen of 10 to 20 mg oral nifedipine every 6 hours, which is continued through delivery. Patients can usually be discharged by postoperative day 4, but should be required to remain on modified bed rest for the first 2 weeks after discharge. In the absence of uterine irritability, patients can then be allowed moderate activity, although they should remain nearby and return for twice-weekly ultrasounds with obstetric assessment. Once the fetus reaches 36 weeks' gestation, lung maturity is assessed by amniocentesis, and cesarean section is performed once the lungs are mature.

## DETAILED PROCEDURES FOR INDIVIDUAL ANOMALIES

Specific procedures to be discussed include those supported by evidence or commonly performed, including lobar resection for CCAM, debulking procedure for SCT, laser ablation of placental anastomoses in TTTS, and fetal MMC repair.

Prenatal repair using a 2-step method in liver-down CDH fetuses failed to demonstrate any improvement in outcome, while the prenatal reduction of the liver in cases involving

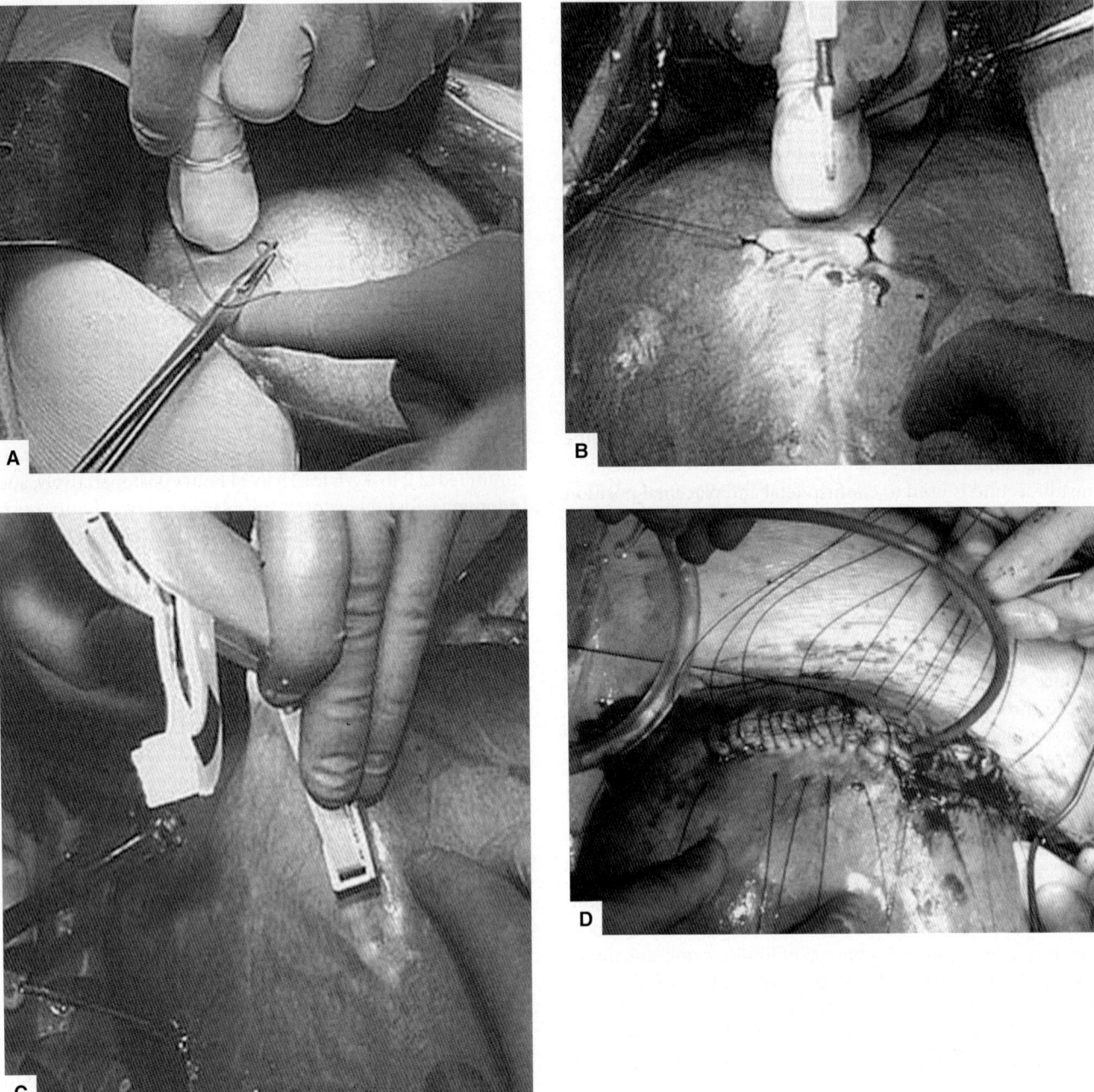

**FIGURE 3-6** **A.** Illustration of traction suture placement. Ultrasound imaging reveals the position of the fetus and the margins of the placenta so that the hysterotomy can be performed safely in a region that will provide the optimal exposure of the fetus. In this illustration, the ultrasound probe is placed against the exposed uterus and is seen guiding the safe placement of the first traction suture in the center of the planned hysterotomy. **B.** Illustration of division of the myometrium and membranes between traction sutures using the electrocautery. **C.** Enlarging the hysterotomy using a specialized surgical stapler. Through a window in the uterus created by electrocautery, a surgical stapler with absorbable staples is inserted. The myometrium and membranes are then divided and fused together with a single firing of this stapler. With minimal effort, this technique facilitates control of the fragile chorionic and amniotic membranes while providing reliable hemostasis. **D.** Illustration of uterine closure near completion with catheter instillation of antibiotics. In this illustration, the hysterotomy is approximated with 2 layers of absorbable suture. Before completion of the closure, the amniotic fluid volume is restored with warmed Ringer lactate solution infused through a catheter. The final 100 cm³ of volume is an antibiotic solution.

liver herniation acutely kinks the umbilical venous return and is incompatible with survival. Tracheal occlusion was conceived as a surrogate method of improving lung development, but a randomized trial failed to show benefit, perhaps due to higher-than-expected survival in the control group. Although tracheal occlusion is again under study for treatment of CDH using fetoscopic methods, there is currently no basis of evidence for its application by open or minimally invasive techniques outside of a randomized trial. The technique for fetoscopic tracheal occlusion has been described in detail elsewhere and will not be described here.

## Lobar Resection for CCAM

### Rationale

Large CCAM lesions can increase central venous pressure due to mediastinal shift and cardiac compression. In addition to pulmonary hypoplasia secondary to lung compression, studies simulating CCAM in the fetal lamb with gradual inflation of an intrathoracic balloon have demonstrated a temporal relation between this increase in venous pressure and the development of hydrops, which resolves following deflation of the balloon. Other studies have shown significant compensatory lung growth following fetal resection. Due to the nearly 100% mortality following the development of hydrops, these results support fetal lobar resection for a select group of fetuses. Because growth arrest of these tumors has been observed with steroid administration, CCAMs at risk for the development of hydrops (CVR >1.4) or in early stages thereof are empirically treated with a course of betamethasone. Fetal lobar resection is recommended for those fetuses without a dominant cyst in whom hydrops persists or progresses prior to 32 weeks' gestation. After that point, EXIT delivery is indicated, with resection of the mass.

### Fetal Thoracotomy and CCAM Resection

The hysterotomy site is chosen to easily access the affected side of the chest. A fetal hand and arm are grasped, and the fetus is rotated into the hysterotomy to expose the chest wall, leaving the head and remainder of the body within the amniotic sac. A pulse oximeter is secured to the fetal hand and a fetal IV is placed. Prior to the fetal thoracotomy, the fetus is pretreated with atropine and fluid volume to counter the reactive bradycardia and fetal cardiac collapse that can occur with abrupt removal of cardiac compression following removal of the mass.

A large posterolateral thoracotomy is performed at the sixth intercostal space using electrocautery, and the lesion generally bulges through the wound due to the increased intrathoracic pressure. Using a small rib retractor, the lobe containing the CCAM is exteriorized, and its attachments to surrounding lung tissue are divided. The lobar pulmonary artery is taken first to prevent further congestion of the lobe. The bronchus can then be ligated and the pulmonary vein is taken last (Fig. 3-7). Residual fusion of pulmonary parenchyma can be taken with the stapler if extensive. The thoracotomy is then closed and the ribs reapproximated using pericostal monofilament absorbable sutures. Running monofilament absorbable suture is used to reapproximate the muscle layers anatomically and subcutaneous tissues, and continuous absorbable suture is used to close the skin.

### Specific Postoperative Considerations

Daily ultrasounds should be performed following the procedure to document resolution of hydrops, which should occur within 1 to 2 weeks. After that, twice-weekly ultrasounds can be used to monitor lung growth and mediastinal position.

### Planned Delivery

Timing for delivery should be dictated by obstetric considerations and should be planned as late as possible to minimize

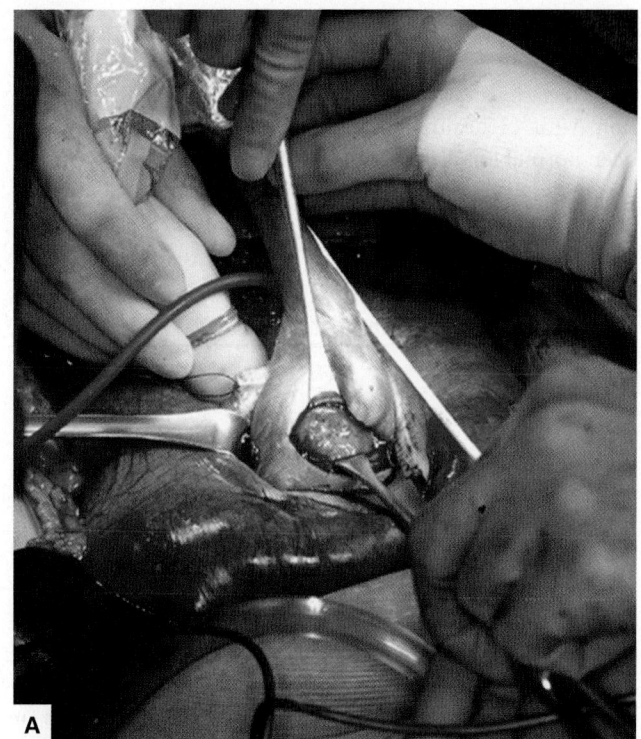

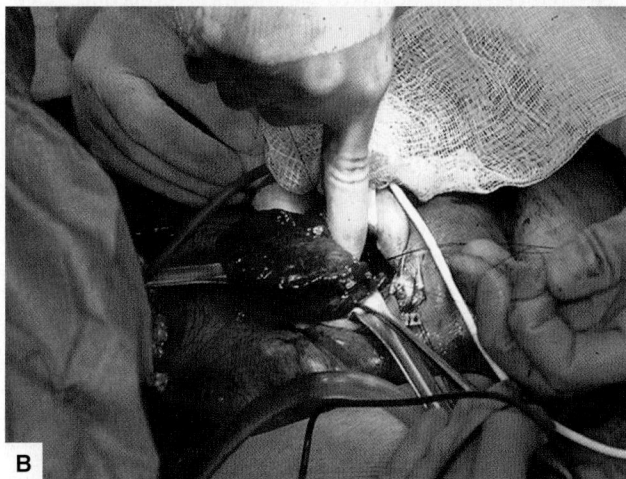

**FIGURE 3-7 A.** Resection of a fetal CCAM. The picture illustrates the fetal position with the arm and chest wall exposed and the head within the uterus. Continuous echocardiographic monitoring is performed during the procedure, and an IV and a pulse oximeter are placed on the exposed hand. A thoracotomy has been performed and the tumor can be seen bulging out of the incision. **B.** A hilar dissection is performed. Here the pulmonary artery and bronchus have already been divided and the pulmonary vein is being ligated prior to removal of the tumor.

complications related to prematurity. Because the airway is not compromised and respiratory function at the time of delivery should not be compromised once the mass has been resected, fetuses can be delivered by cesarean section via the fetal surgical incision rather than via the EXIT procedure. The hysterotomy is often very thin and occasionally limited uterine dehiscence is encountered. The edges of the hysterotomy should be freshened back to healthy tissue and closed in layers.

## Outcomes

In the CHOP experience with microcystic CCAM, 24 resections have been attempted between 21 and 31 weeks' gestation, with 13 healthy survivors. Developmental testing has been normal for all survivors. In macrocystic CCAM, associated with a predominant, thoracoamniotic shunt, a survival rate of approximately 75% and good quality-of-life indicators are expected.

## Debulking Procedure for SCT

### Rationale

Rapid tumor growth in SCT can lead to fetal death via high-output cardiac failure due to vascular steal. Serial Doppler assessment of human fetuses with large SCTs has demonstrated the evolution of fetal hydrops and placentomegaly in association with high-output physiology during periods of rapid tumor growth. Debulking eliminates the pathway for vascular steal and should reverse those physiologic changes. Because the development of hydrops is uniformly fatal in these fetuses, the rationale for fetal debulking is compelling prior to 28 weeks' gestation for Type I SCT. If hydrops or placentomegaly develops after 28 weeks, the fetus should be delivered early and debulked via the EXIT procedure. Debulking procedures should be performed early in the evolution of hydrops, as the presence of the maternal mirror syndrome is a contraindication to fetal surgery.

### Debulking of the Fetal SCT

The hysterotomy site is chosen to allow exteriorization of the tumor mass and the caudal end of the fetus. Because of the proximity of the umbilical cord to the rim of the hysterotomy,

the fetus should be closely monitored for signs of cord compression. Apart from the tumor and the caudal end, care should be taken that the remainder of the fetus remains within the amniotic sac (Fig. 3-8A). With the extreme volume reduction that would result from inadvertent delivery of the entire fetus, uterine contraction could lead to preterm labor.

Following exposure of the tumor, a Hegar dilator should be placed in the rectum and the skin incised around the anorectal sphincter complex. Fetal skin is then incised around the base of the tumor taking care to avoid the large subcutaneous veins, and a tourniquet applied around the tumor where the skin has been incised to restrict blood flow. Division of the base is best performed using the handheld harmonic scalpel combined with suture ligation of larger vessels prior to and during release of the tourniquet. A 90-mm thick tissue stapler can be used to debulk the tumor externally if the pedicle is narrow enough (Fig. 3-8B). No attempt should be made to dissect any intrapelvic component or to remove the coccyx. If fetal blood loss is excessive, intravenous boluses of crystalloid and warm blood can be given. If severe bradycardia or cardiac arrest occurs, then code medications can be given and cardiopulmonary resuscitation can be performed. Following closure of the fetal sacral wound, the fetus can be returned to the amniotic cavity.

### Specific Postoperative Considerations

Because of the risk of maternal mirror syndrome, maternal fluid balance must be closely monitored until the hydrops and placentomegaly improve. Fetal echocardiography should be performed frequently to assess ventricular diameters, combined ventricular output, descending aortic flow, umbilical vein flow, and IVC diameter. If fetal high-output physiology fails to resolve, umbilical blood sampling can be performed to

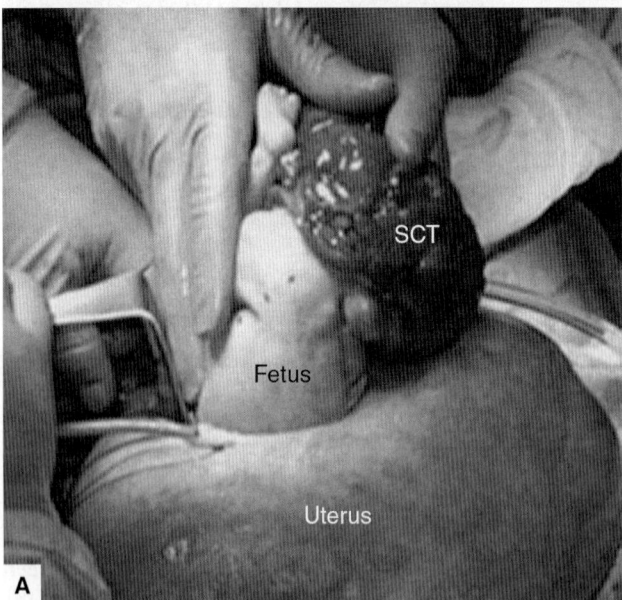
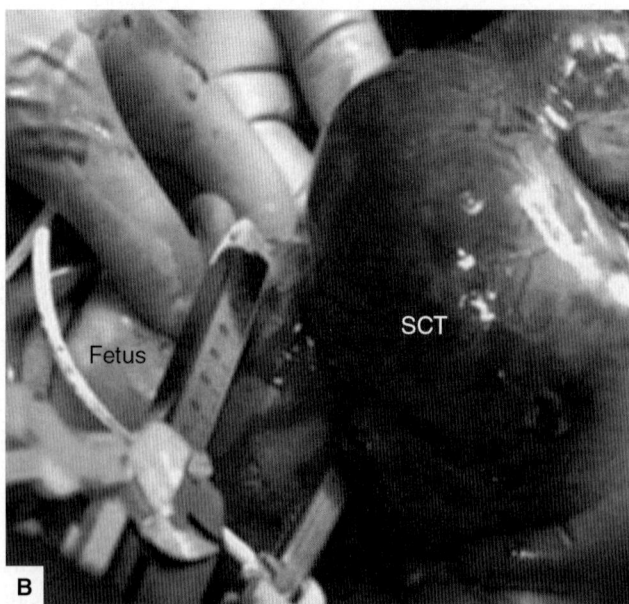

**FIGURE 3-8** **A.** Exposure of SCT during open fetal surgery for resection. In this photograph, the surgeon has delivered the caudal end of the fetus and the teratoma from the hysterotomy while leaving the fetal head and upper torso in the amniotic cavity. **B.** Division of the vascular pedicle of an SCT using a surgical stapler. The skin surrounding the base of the tumor has been incised, and a tourniquet applied. The vascular pedicle has been skeletonized by harmonic dissection and major vessels have been suture ligated. The remaining pedicle is now being divided with a vascular stapler.

check for fetal anemia, as fetal blood transfusion may reverse this pathophysiology in these cases. Once hydrops resolves, the fetus can be delivered via standard cesarean section, with timing dictated by obstetric considerations. Definitive resection of residual tumor and the coccyx must be undertaken after birth due to the risk of malignant degeneration.

## Outcomes

Since 1995, the CHOP experience includes 5 debulking procedures with 4 survivors. Of these, 1 required postnatal treatment of pulmonary metastases associated with a germ cell tumor, but has no evidence of disease at 11 years of age. Another survivor had significant morbidity likely related to emboli at the time of tumor resection.

## Fetoscopic Laser Coagulation for TTTS

### Rationale

Because TTTS occurs due to an imbalance of flow through a MC placenta, fetoscopic laser coagulation targets the anastomoses in which this imbalance exists. In essence, the goal of the therapy is to mimic a dichorionic state, preventing the oliguria and hypovolemia in the donor, and the coincident polyuria and volume overload in the recipient. The rationale for this treatment is based on the concept that all placental communicating vessels are accessible on the surface along the placental equator, and that coagulation of these anomalous anastomoses should prevent fetal blood exchange. This theory was tested in a RCT, which showed that laser coagulation increased survival by 25% and led to less premature delivery (33 weeks vs 29 weeks) as compared with amniodrainage when both procedures were performed between 16 and 26 weeks. Because many Quintero Stage I patients do not progress, most fetal centers use laser to treat only Stage II and above, although a trial of selective laser coagulation for Stage I disease is currently underway in Europe.

### Laser Coagulation

Although initially conceived as a procedure performed through a minilaparotomy, laser coagulation is usually now performed percutaneously. The procedure is most often performed under local anesthesia, although general or regional anesthesia can be used depending on surgeon and patient preferences.

A 2 to 3 mm fetoscope is inserted either with or without a trocar under ultrasound guidance. Placental vasculature is extensively mapped using direct visualization and Doppler ultrasound to identify anastomoses between the twin circulations and define the placental equator. All anastomoses between the placental circulations are targeted for ablation with a Diode laser system (30-50 W). Amnioreduction may be performed at the end of the procedure to relieve intrauterine pressure.

### Specific Postoperative Considerations

Although rates of neurologic morbidity are low (approximately 7% at 3 years of age), ultrasound examination can be used to detect CNS pathology postoperatively or during the first week of life, particularly in infants delivered prematurely.

## Outcomes

Because the procedure is now performed percutaneously, the risk of placental abruption is low (1%), and preterm premature rupture of membranes (PPROM) is the most frequent complication of the procedure. PPROM occurs in 28% of cases, and most often occurs within 3 to 4 weeks. The use of selective coagulation has improved survival rates of at least 1 twin to 65% to 85%, and 35% to 50% for both twins.

## Technique of Fetal MMC Repair

### Rationale

Serial ultrasonographic images of human fetuses with MMC demonstrate an apparent loss of function over the course of gestation, leading to the "2-hit" hypothesis of acquired intrauterine damage. The rationale for prenatal MMC repair rests on the potential to prevent significant and irreversible neurologic disability by minimizing the contact between exposed neural elements and amniotic fluid.

Recently, this theory was tested in a large, multicenter RCT (MOMS), which compared prenatal and postnatal repair in singleton pregnancies between 19 and 26 weeks at randomization, with evidence of an isolated MMC with an upper boundary between T1 and S1 and hindbrain herniation. Selection bias was minimized by the agreement of all other fetal treatment centers in the United States not to perform prenatal MMC repair during the trial. Enrollment was planned to be 200 patients (100 in each group), but the trial was terminated early (after randomization of 183 patients) for efficacy of prenatal surgery.

The MOMS trial is of particular importance as it provides the first evidence to support the use of fetal surgery for a nonlethal condition, and demonstrates that prenatal intervention can alter the natural history of MMC. Although the prenatal group had more severe disease and preterm delivery occurred more often, this group showed significant improvement in rates of shunt placement (40% vs 82%), degree and presence of hindbrain herniation, as well as functional neurologic outcomes, including the ability to walk without orthotics (42% vs 21%). In the postnatal group, 98% of patients met the primary end point of death or shunt placement by 12 months, whereas only 68% of the prenatally treated group did so. Although prenatal surgery conferred a significant advantage over postnatal treatment overall, not all fetuses benefited, and these potential benefits must be weighed against the maternal and fetal risks, including intraoperative complications, risk of wound problems and/or uterine rupture, preterm rupture of membranes, oligohydramnios, and prematurity, with its associated issues. These collective factors underscore the need for careful patient selection.

### Fetal MMC Repair

The abdominal incision should be in a low transverse position for most patients, although a vertical incision may be required in those patients with BMI >30 or with a previous vertical scar. The hysterotomy site is chosen in order to avoid the placenta and place the MMC defect in the middle of the incision. Fetal anesthesia is provided by the maternal inhalational anesthetic, and an intramuscular dose of a narcotic and paralysis agent. The neural placode is then sharply dissected

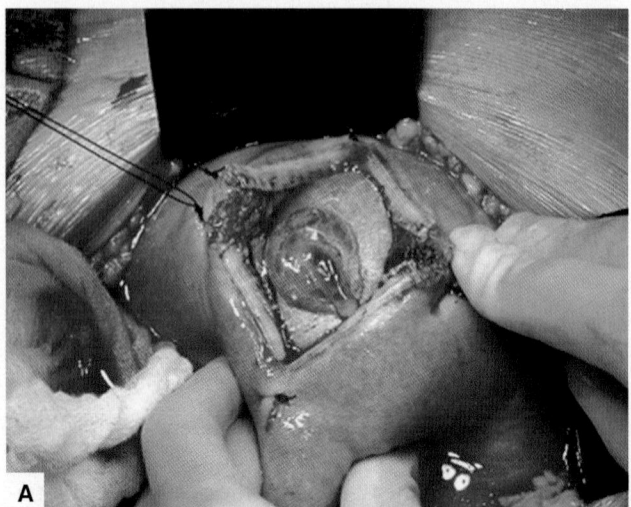

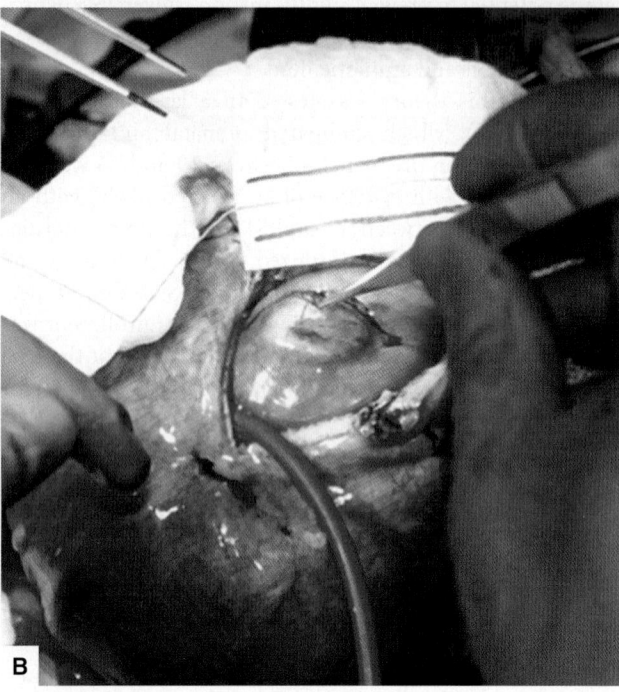

**FIGURE 3-9 A.** Exposure of the MMC during open fetal surgery for prenatal repair. **B.** Excising the MMC sac prior to the 3-layer closure.

from surrounding tissue and drops back into more anatomic position (Fig. 3-9). The dura is reflected over the defect and closed with a running suture. The paravertebral muscle fascia is mobilized and closed over the defect in the midline. The skin can then be closed, although in some cases AlloDerm may be required. Monofilament absorbable suture of small caliber should be used for closure of all layers.

## Specific Postoperative Considerations

Daily echocardiography should be performed during the period of initial tocolysis to assess ductus arteriosus constriction. Weekly targeted ultrasound should monitor for oligohydramnios and membrane status. A biophysical profile should be obtained at every visit after 25 weeks, and a comprehensive ultrasound should be performed monthly to monitor fetal growth.

## Outcomes

The risk of preterm labor is a major source of morbidity following the procedure. In the MOMS trial, fetuses treated prenatally delivered at an average gestational age of 34.1 weeks, as compared with 37.3 weeks in the postnatal surgery group. In the prenatal surgery group, 13% of fetuses delivered prior to 30 weeks. Rates of the respiratory distress syndrome were higher in the prenatal surgery group (21% vs 6%), likely related to prematurity. Maternal complications also occur more commonly in cases treated prenatally, including scarring or dehiscence of the uterine closure, oligohydramnios, chorioamniotic separation, placental abruption, and premature rupture of membranes. However, to balance this risk, prenatally treated patients clearly experience more normal neurologic development and a less severe phenotype than would be predicted by anatomic level in a majority of cases. Hindbrain herniation has been observed to improve or resolve completely after fetal intervention, improving brain stem function and avoiding the need for shunting (Fig. 3-5B).

## Maternal Morbidity

Fortunately, no maternal deaths have been reported related to fetal surgery, although significant short-term morbidity has been observed. Premature labor, PPROM, and chorioamniotic membrane separation occur frequently. Pulmonary edema is a common complication, although judicious fluid management during the postoperative period can minimize its incidence and severity. Transfusion has been occasionally required.

In general, reported reproductive outcomes for future pregnancies have been good, with fertility rates similar to background. The risk of uterine dehiscence/rupture appears to be similar to that reported for classical cesarean section (14%/14%). This risk may be compounded by the occurrence of preterm labor, which occurs at a rate similar to background. The miscarriage rate for subsequent pregnancies has been reported to be 18%, which is likely not increased over background when adjusted for age (normal range: 12% for women under 20 to 26% in women over 40). Perinatal loss other than that related to uterine rupture has not been observed, although this has been reported to occur more frequently following cesarean delivery. No increase in infertility has been observed.

## Efficacy and Future of Fetal Surgery

The anomalies discussed in this chapter represent the full spectrum of efficacy. In some cases, fetal surgery has clearly altered the natural history of the disease and improved outcomes (CCAM, SCT, TTTS, MMC). For CDH, fetal intervention remains controversial as interventions have not yet shown benefit, and selection of a patient cohort appropriate for fetal therapy has become increasingly difficult as improvements in postnatal management have increased survival rates even in severely affected fetuses.

Dramatic progress has been made in imaging and diagnosis of fetal anomalies, and technical development continues to allow more minimally invasive forms of therapy.

As imaging modalities become more sophisticated, our capabilities for image-guided intervention will move to ever earlier gestational time points. In doing so, preterm labor and premature delivery can likely be decreased, although improvements in tocolysis should be a priority to optimize patient outcomes. In the near future, RCTs must be conducted to establish clear benefit to patients, allowing fetal surgery to transition from experimental therapy to standard of care.

## SELECTED READINGS

Abraham RJ, Sau A, Maxwell D. A review of the EXIT (ex utero intrapartum treatment) procedure. *J Obstet Gynaecol* 2010;30(1):1–5.

Adzick NS. Fetal myelomeningocele: natural history, pathophysiology and in-utero intervention. *Semin Fetal Neonatal Med* 2010;15(1):9–14.

Adzick NS. Open fetal surgery for life-threatening anomalies. *Semin Fetal Neonatal Med* 2010;15(1):1–8.

Adzick NS, Thom EA, Spong CY, et al. A randomized trial of prenatal versus postnatal repair of myelomeningocele. *N Engl J Med* 2011;364:993–1004 [Epub ahead of print].

Bebbington M. Twin-to-twin transfusion syndrome: current understanding of pathophysiology, in-utero therapy and impact for future development. *Semin Fetal Neonatal Med* 2010;15(1):15–20.

Bouchard S, Johnson MP, Flake AW, et al. The EXIT procedure: experience and outcomes in 31 cases. *J Pediatr Surg* 2002;37:418–426.

Cavoretto P, Molina F, Poggi S, et al. Prenatal diagnosis and outcome of echogenic fetal lung lesions. *Ultrasound Obstet Gynecol* 2008;32(6):769–783.

Chervenak FA, McCollough LB. Ethics of maternal–fetal surgery. *Semin Fetal Neonatal Med* 2007;12(6):426–431.

Deprest JA, Flake AW, Gratacos E. The making of fetal surgery. *Prenat Diagn* 2010;30:653–667.

Golombeck K, Ball RH, Lee H, et al. Maternal morbidity after maternal–fetal surgery. *Am J Obstet Gynecol* 2006;194(3):834–839.

Harrison MR, Adzick NS, Bullard KM, et al. Correction of congenital diaphragmatic hernia in utero VII: a prospective trial. *J Pediatr Surg* 1997;32:1637–1642.

Hedrick HL. Management of prenatally diagnosed congenital diaphragmatic hernia. *Semin Fetal Neonatal Med* 2010;15(1):21–27.

Senat MV, Deprest J, Boulvain M, et al. Endoscopic laser surgery versus serial amnioreduction for severe twin-to-twin transfusion syndrome. *N Engl J Med* 2004;351:136–144.

Watanabe M, Flake AW. Fetal surgery: progress and perspectives. *Adv Pediatr* 2010;57(1):353–372.

Wilson RW, Hedrick HL, Liechty KW, et al. Cystic adenomatoid malformation of the lung: review of genetics, prenatal diagnosis and in utero treatment. *Am J Med Genet A* 2006;140(2):151–155.

Wilson RD, Johnson MP, Flake AW, et al. Reproductive outcomes after pregnancy complicated by maternal–fetal surgery. *Am J Obstet Gynecol* 2004;191(4):1430–1436.

Wilson RD, Lemerand K, Johnson MP, et al. Reproductive outcomes in subsequent pregnancies after a pregnancy complicated by open maternal–fetal surgery (1996–2007). *Am J Obstet Gynecol* 2010;203(3):209.e1–209.e6.

# Gastrointestinal, Pulmonary, Cardiac, and Neurologic Developmental Physiology of the Premature and Term Newborn

# CHAPTER 4

*Brian T. Bucher and Brad W. Warner*

## KEY POINTS

1. The morphologic and immunologic development of the gastrointestinal system progresses rapidly during the third trimester, and therefore is immature in preterm neonates.

2. Human breast milk is ideally adapted to match the digestive capacities of the newborn infant and contains several factors for the protection and development of the neonatal gastrointestinal tract.

3. Respiratory distress syndrome is highly prevalent in preterm infants and may lead to bronchopulmonary dysplasia and chronic lung disease in older children.

4. Several circulatory changes occur immediately after birth to switch from the parallel fetal circulation to the serial circulation of the newborn infant.

5. The preterm neonate is at high risk for intraventricular hemorrhage (IVH) and those infants with IVH have a higher risk of mortality.

# GASTROINTESTINAL SYSTEM

## Embryology of the Gastrointestinal System

### The Hollow Organs

The entire respiratory and gastrointestinal system is derived from the endoderm after cephalocaudal and lateral folding of the yolk sac of the embryo. After folding, the primitive gut can be divided into three sections: the foregut, the midgut, and the hindgut. These sections can be distinguished not only by their morphologic pattern, but also by their gene expression patterns that give rise to a variety of organs of the gastrointestinal tract. The foregut extends from the oropharynx to the liver outgrowth and gives rise to the thyroid, esophagus, respiratory epithelium, stomach, liver, biliary tree, pancreas, and the proximal part of the duodenum. The midgut continues past the liver outgrowth to the transverse colon and develops into the small intestine and proximal colon. The hindgut extends from the transverse colon to the cloacal membrane and forms the remainder of the colon and rectum as well as the urogenital tract.

The respiratory epithelium appears as a bud of the esophagus around the fourth week of gestation and a tracheoesophageal septum develops to separate the foregut into ventral tracheal epithelium and dorsal esophageal epithelium. Failure of development of this tracheoesophageal septum leads to the formation of a spectrum of tracheoesophageal clefts and fistulae. The esophagus is initially short, but lengthens to its final extent by 7 weeks. After the esophageal lengthening is complete, the cuboidal epithelium is gradually replaced with squamous epithelium.

The stomach begins as a dilatation of the foregut at 5 weeks of gestation. Over the next several weeks, the stomach undergoes a variety of longitudinal and anterior–posterior axis rotations until it assumes its final position at 22 weeks. The gastric fundus is formed between 12 and 16 weeks of gestation followed by formation of the antrum and pylorus by 20 weeks gestation. Neural crest cell and vagal innervation begins at 7 weeks and continues until birth. The development of gastric glands begins around 10 weeks of gestation and continues until they reach an adult form by 17 weeks gestation. Parietal and chief cells appear between 11 and 12 weeks of gestation.

The duodenum is formed from the terminal portion of the foregut and the proximal portion of the midgut. Around 5 weeks of gestation, the duodenum lumen is obliterated by the rapid proliferation of epithelial cells. The lumen is recanalized by 8 weeks of development, and over next 4 weeks, the epithelium forms the characteristic duodenal Brunner's glands.

The small intestine and colon undergo a rapid elongation beginning at 5 weeks of gestation. Due to this rapid growth, the developing small intestine herniates out of the abdominal cavity at 6 weeks of gestation and returns to the abdominal cavity beginning at 10 weeks of gestation. During their return, the small intestine and colon go through a 270° counterclockwise rotation so that, upon its return, the proximal jejunum (ligament of Treitz) lies on the left side of the spine at or above the level of the gastric antrum. The cecum ultimately becomes fixed to the right lower quadrant of the abdomen. Similar to the duodenum, the crypts and villi of the small intestine and colon develop around 14 weeks of gestation.

The colon is formed from a combination of the distal midgut and the proximal hindgut. The midgut contributes the cecum to the distal two thirds of the transverse colon. The hindgut gives rise to the distal third of the transverse colon through the upper part of the anal canal. The goblet and epithelial cells are present in the colon by 11 weeks gestation. From 13 to 17 weeks the colon crypt and villi begin to develop. Around 20 weeks gestation the colon villi begin to disappear and the diameter of the colon begins to increase beyond that of the small intestine.

## Intestinal Mucosa and Immunologic Development

The surface area of the gut presents a large surface area for the interaction of the preterm neonate and the microbial community. Establishment of the intestinal microflora occurs immediately after birth, and therefore the gut must have innate mechanisms to distinguish beneficial microbes and microbial products from harmful ones. These innate mechanisms include breast milk ingestion, gastric acid secretion, intestinal mucus production, intestinal motility, and a submucosal immune system. Breast milk contains maternal immunoglobulins and various types of white blood cells that are thought to be protective to the newborn gastrointestinal tract. Gastric acid secretion creates an inhibitory environment for intestinal microorganisms. Intestinal mucous production protects the intestinal wall and contains many antimicrobial immunoglobulins and glycoproteins. In addition, it serves as a natural defensive layer isolating the enterocytes from any potentially pathogenic bacteria. As mentioned below, intestinal motility serves to propel luminal contents caudally and serves to increase or decrease the luminal contact time with the intestinal epithelium. Finally Peyer patches, aggregation of submucosal lymphoid tissue, serve as coordinators of the local immune response with the production of various cytokines, immunoglobulins, and other humoral mediators after interaction with pathogenic bacteria.

While the majority of the above-mentioned systems are fully functioning in the newborn infants, the preterm infant lacks many of these protective mechanisms. Preterm infants with respiratory failure may not tolerate enteral feedings with breast milk. In addition, many preterm infants in the neonatal intensive care unit (NICU) are started on acid-suppressive medication, such as antihistamines or proton pump inhibitors, thus ablating the protective effect of gastric acid secretion. As discussed in detail below, intestinal motility is not fully developed in preterm infants leading to stasis of luminal contents and bacterial overgrowth. Peyer patches develop around 19 weeks gestation; however, they increase in number late in gestation. Therefore, the local immune response may be suppressed in preterm infants compared to those born at full term. The combination of all the above risk factors predisposes the preterm infant to bacterial overgrowth and invasion resulting in necrotizing enterocolitis (NEC).

## Enteric Nervous System and Intestinal Motility

The enteric nervous system (ENS) is derived from neural crest cells, a population of migratory cells originating from the neural ectoderm. These cells migrate along the gut in a craniocaudal direction and exist along the entire length of the gut by 7 weeks of gestation. After migration, these cells differentiate to form the myenteric and submucosal plexus of the ENS. Following the formation of the ENS, the visceral mesoderm differentiates into the muscle layers of the gut along a similar craniocaudal pattern. By 14 weeks of gestation, the circular and longitudinal smooth muscle layers of the gut are fully developed along its entire length.

Fetal swallowing is identifiable at 11 weeks of gestation. Therefore, during the majority of gestation, intestinal contents are propagated distally. This may serve to deliver hormones and growth factors to the developing intestinal epithelium. The sucking reflex is present by 23 weeks gestation; however, no effective negative pressure is generated before 32 weeks of gestation. From 32 to 36 weeks, swallowing is not associated with the episodes of sucking. Coordinated sucking, swallowing, and breathing are not mature until 36 weeks gestation.

The esophagus possesses an unsynchronized pattern of peristalsis after development, which propels contents either cranially or caudally. This process becomes more coordinated as gestation progresses and is fully mature by term. The lower esophageal sphincter is immature in preterm infants with a resting pressure of approximately 4 mm Hg. Therefore, gastroesophageal reflux disease (GERD) can be a significant problem with premature infants and lead to apneic episodes, bradycardia, and aspiration pneumonia. By term, however, the lower esophageal sphincter has matured with a resting pressure of 18 mm Hg.

The stomach also undergoes significant motor development during the final months of gestation. Vagally mediated gastric emptying is determined by a response to gastric volume that is not fully developed in the premature infant. Gastric motility increases and becomes more forceful during the early postnatal period. In addition, the pylorus function is delayed in a preterm infant. The ultimate result is that, despite small stomach volumes, gastric emptying is longer in preterm infants compared to term infants.

The motility of the small bowel and colon also develops with time. Rhythmic activity can be noted in the small bowel by 6 to 7 weeks of age, and at 4 months, peristaltic waves can be seen. There is an ordered progression of increasing peristaltic frequency, amplitude, and duration as gestation progresses. After birth, meconium is passed within 24 hours; however in premature infants, this may be delayed up to 1 week after birth. After feeding is initiated in premature infants, there are bands of unrelated rhythmic contractions rather than organized peristaltic waves. Mature migratory motor complexes develop within 3 weeks of feeding premature infants.

## Development of the Intestinal Microflora

The human intestine contains more microflora than any other part of the body. In addition, the interaction of the intestine with the resident microorganisms is becoming increasingly recognized as having a crucial impact on the development of disease. The fetal gut is sterile and only becomes colonized after birth. The organisms populating the neonatal intestine range from beneficial (*Lactobacillus* and *Bifidobacterium* species) to potentially harmful or opportunistic (*Escherichia coli*, *Pseudomonas aeruginosa*, *Clostridia*, Staphylococcus species) organisms. The initial organisms colonizing the neonatal gut depend on a variety of factors including the delivery method (vaginal vs cesarean section), type of initial feeding (breast vs formula fed), and gestation age. Infants delivered via the cesarean section or are formula fed have been shown to have a delay in the gut colonization by beneficial organisms such as *Lactobacillus* or *Bifidobacterium*. In addition, the presence of other neonatal comorbidities has been shown to be a risk factor for the increased presence of opportunistic or virulent pathogens such as *P. aeruginosa*.

The presence of beneficial bacteria in the neonatal gut has led to the hypothesis that certain neonatal diseases, particularly NEC, could result from an imbalance of beneficial versus harmful bacteria. It has been suggested that optimizing the bacterial flora of the neonatal gut can have beneficial health effect and prevent the occurrence of certain diseases. This optimization is accomplished through the administration of probiotics such as *Lactobacillus* and *Bifidobacterium*. Several prospective randomized controlled trials have documented a reduction in the incidence of late-onset sepsis in very-low birthweight infants (less than 1500 g). However, there currently is not enough evidence to support the routine use of prophylactic probiotics in the prevention of NEC in preterm infants.

## Liver and Biliary Tree

The liver develops as an outgrowth of the distal foregut around the third week of gestation. This outgrowth is initially composed of rapidly growing cells, and by the 10th week of development the weight of the liver is approximately 10% of the developing fetus. During this initial period the liver serves as the primary production source of red and white blood cells, a function that gradually declines during the final 8 weeks of gestation. The connection between the liver and the foregut becomes the common bile duct and gallbladder beginning around the seventh week of gestation.

Around 12 weeks of gestation, bile begins to form in the hepatic cells and is excreted into the biliary system. However, the bile acid pool size is decreased in premature infants, and the duodenal bile acid concentrations are below the critical micelle concentrations. An immature enterohepatic circulation also contributes the low bile acid concentration in premature infants. In addition, fetal bile acids are very different from adult bile acids. In fetal and preterm infant's bile, taurine conjugates predominate, whereas in older infants, glycine conjugates predominate. At term the luminal bile acid concentration increase to 50% of adults and conjugation also switched to the more soluble monoglucuronide and diglucuronide pigments.

The cytochrome P450 biotransformation system develops at variable rates for different activities. Those systems that depend on nicotinamide adenine dinucleotide phosphate (NADPH) for electron transfer are relatively inactive in the fetus and newborn because NADPH is not available in significant amounts until after birth. The fetal level of alcohol dehydrogenase is 30% of the adult level and 50% during the first year of life. Quantitatively, glucuronidation is the one of the most important reactions for eliminating compounds, and development varies depending on the substrate. Compounds excreted as glucuronides are subject to reabsorption in the intestine. In the fetus these compounds cannot be removed from the body, as there is no stooling; and without intestinal microflora, they are not hydrolyzed except in small part by intestinal glucuronidases.

Bilirubin is the end product of heme degradation. Once bilirubin is made in the reticuloendothelial system or the hepatocytes, it passes into the blood by diffusion and is bound to albumin. The ability of the liver to remove bilirubin from circulation is limited in the fetus and preterm infant and the major route of bilirubin excretion is via the placenta. The activity of the uridine diphosphoglucuronosyl transferase is only 1% of the adult at term and increased exponentially after birth. At birth there is a rapid rise in bilirubin (peak serum level of 5- 6 mg/dL at 3-5 days of life) with the removal of the placenta.

## Pancreas

The pancreas is formed a dorsal and ventral but originating from the endoderm of the duodenum at 5 weeks of gestation. During the duodenal C-loop formation around the seventh week of gestation the ventral bud rotates caudal and dorsal to the dorsal bud to form the uncinate process of the pancreas. The ventral pancreatic duct joins part of the dorsal duct to form the main pancreatic duct. Smaller ducts from the dorsal bud can persist as an accessory pancreatic duct. Failure of fusion of the ventral and dorsal pancreatic ducts results in pancreas divisum. This may be clinically apparent with recurrent bouts of pancreatitis due to the majority of the gland draining through the small, accessory ampulla. By 9 and 12 weeks of gestation, endocrine and exocrine cells can be identified, respectively. Microscopically, primitive acini and zymogen granules are visible by 16 weeks. By 20 weeks, the pancreas looks mature and can secrete more than 20 enzymes, the most significant of which are a-amylase, chymotrypsin, trypsin, and lipase. Islet cells appear at 12 weeks, and by 16 weeks, insulin can be detected in β cells.

Amylase, lipase, and proteases are all important for digestion of nutrients in the newborn infant. Amylase may or may not be present in the fetus, but lipase and proteases appear at 14 weeks of gestation. The amounts of these enzymes and their secretion in response to stimuli such as secretin are lower at birth and increase slowly. Salivary amylase, breast milk a-amylase, and intestinal brush border glucoamylase also aid in fat and carbohydrate digestion in the newborn. Thus, complex carbohydrate and high-fat diets may cause diarrhea and at the same time may induce amylase and lipase production. Soy formulas stimulate production of lipase and trypsin as compared to cow's milk-based formulas.

Pancreatic proteases (trypsin and chymotrypsin) are produced in relatively low amounts in preterm and newborn infants. In addition, peptic proteolytic activity is diminished in the newborn stomach, perhaps because of the lower gastric acid output. Breast milk also contains protease inhibitors that affect trypsin and chymotrypsin. Gastric pH increases with food intake, as does the activity of proteases over the first few days of life. Infants have more food antibodies than adults, indicating that food proteins are more likely to be absorbed intact without digestion.

## Digestion and Absorption

Human breast milk is ideally adapted to match the digestive capacities of the newborn infant. The gastrointestinal system of a newborn is not able to digest and absorb complex nutrients; therefore, breast milk can provide the total nutritional requirement of the newborn for at least the first 6 months of life.

The digestion of fat in the neonate starts with the secretion of lipases by the oral or gastric mucosa. These lipases are primarily responsible for the digestion of medium chain fatty acids present in breast milk. The advantage of medium chain fatty acids is that they do not require the presence of bile salts for absorption, which are found in decreased concentrations in preterm and term infants. Therefore, medium chain fatty acids can be directly absorbed into the blood stream. In contrast long chain fatty acids, digested primarily by a lipase present in breast milk, require bile salts for absorption, and must be processed by the liver before absorption into the blood stream. Preterm infants have a reduced bile acid pool and therefore have a decrease in fat absorption capacity. This also can lead to decreased absorption of fat-soluble vitamins.

Protein digestion also starts in the stomach. The presence of stomach acid converts pepsinogen to pepsin, which starts the digestion of dietary protein. Pancreatic proteases in the duodenum such as trypsin, chymotrypsin, and carboxypeptidases A and B accelerate this digestive process. The degraded proteins are then absorbed as primary amino acids or dipeptides by the small intestine epithelium.

Carbohydrates in breast milk exist primarily as lactose and are digested lactase into glucose and galactose. Lactase, present in the proximal small bowel, increases in concentration up to 10 months of age, then decreases to adult concentrations. A deficiency of lactase is present in premature infants, jaundiced infants treated with phototherapy, and in certain disease states such as gastroenteritis, neonatal surgery, cystic fibrosis, immune deficiencies, prolonged diarrhea, and malnutrition. The ability of preterm and term infants to digest more complex carbohydrates is limited by a deficiency in pancreatic amylase compared to adults. By 4 months of age, however, the production of pancreatic amylase is such that the infants diet can be expanded to include these macronutrients.

## Gastroesophageal Reflux Disease

Gastroesophageal reflux disease is extremely common among preterm and term infants. Immature esophageal peristalsis and a weak lower esophageal sphincter in preterm infants contribute to the propensity for reflux of gastric contents.

The presenting symptoms of GERD in premature and term infants can be highly variable. Reflux may present as spitting up small quantities after feeding. It may also present as aspiration symptoms with bradycardia and apnea. Prolonged reflux can lead to food aversion, and failure to thrive.

The diagnosis of GERD begins with the exclusion of secondary causes of proximal gastrointestinal obstruction, such as pyloric stenosis, annular pancreas, or duodenal web. A radiographic upper gastrointestinal series can be used to identify such causes of GERD. A frequent study used to identify GERD is 24-hour esophageal pH monitoring. Several scoring systems are available to determine the severity of GERD based on parameters measured on during the pH monitoring (total duration of pH <4, number of episodes of pH <4, duration of longest episode, etc).

Treatment of GERD usually begins with positional changes during and after feeding. This is usually in addition to a modified prone position such as an elevated head-of-bed while sleeping. Dietary maneuvers such as thickening feeds with cereal or more frequent, smaller feeding volumes may be beneficial. Pharmacologic inhibition of gastric acid secretion with antacids, histamine-2 receptor antagonists, or proton pump inhibitors can be used for infants who are refractory to position maneuvers. Severe or life-threatening GERD may be amenable to surgical intervention with a fundoplication, which can be performed as either an open or a laparoscopic procedure.

## Neonatal Jaundice

Neonatal jaundice is one of the most common medical disorders of the newborn infant. Jaundice results when the liver fails to sufficiently clear bilirubin from the plasma. This occurs when there is excessive bilirubin formation, impaired bilirubin uptake or conjugation by the liver, or impaired bilirubin excretion. There are multiple causes of neonatal jaundice: idiopathic, infectious, cardiovascular, metabolic, toxic, genetic, endocrine, anatomic, and extrahepatic.

The majority of newborn infants will have some transient elevation of their bilirubin level termed physiologic jaundice. This temporary elevation results from a number of factors including relative increases in bilirubin load on the liver and relative decreases in hepatic uptake, metabolism, and excretion of bilirubin. There is no formal level of total serum bilirubin that marks physiologic jaundice, rather the temporal pattern of total serum bilirubin is the hallmark of this disorder.

The normal serum bilirubin levels for healthy infants vary according to region, race, gender, and gestational age (GA). Recent population studies have documented a total serum bilirubin level of 17.5 mg/dL as the upper limit of normal infants with physiologic jaundice. Uncontrolled neonatal hyperbilirubinemia can lead to acute bilirubin encephalopathy, which, if left unchecked, can develop into kernicterus or chronic bilirubin encephalopathy. Acute bilirubin encephalopathy (ABE) is an acute progress of decreased mental status and tone in newborns with hyperbilirubinemia. Kernicterus is final sequelae of this process with the development of extrapyramidal disturbances, auditory abnormalities, gaze palsies, and dental dysplasia. While there is no total serum bilirubin level that defines ABE or kernicterus, the majority of cases occur when the total serum bilirubin level is greater than 30 mg/dL.

Treatment of neonatal hyperbilirubinemia begins with identification of the infants at risk for hyperbilirubinemia. The decision to initialize treatment is based on a number of factors including the infant's race, GA, birthweight, comorbidities, total serum bilirubin level, and bilirubin-to-albumin ratio. Once hyperbilirubinemia is identified there are several treatment strategies available. By far the most common treatment of hyperbilirubinemia is phototherapy. The primary event in phototherapy is the photochemical conversion and isomerization of bilirubin by the absorption of a photon by bilirubin. Photochemical conversion with structural isomerization to lumirubin produces a more water-soluble molecule that can be excreted in the urine. Other treatment options include an exchange transfusion to remove bilirubin mechanically or pharmacologic modification of the bilirubin metabolic pathway to increase bilirubin clearance.

# RESPIRATORY SYSTEM

## Embryology of the Respiratory System

The development of the respiratory system begins at approximately 25 days of gestation and is divided into 5 stages. The embryonic stage begins with the formation of a lung bud on the ventral surface of the esophagus. This process is regulated by retinoic acid signaling within the esophageal endoderm. The lung bud and all epithelial derivatives are therefore of endodermal origin. As the lung bud expands, tracheoesophageal ridges develop to separate the lung from the underlying esophagus to ultimately form the tracheoesophageal septum. The lung bud continues to expand to form the larynx and trachea. The bud then begins to under morphologic branching to begin the formation of the distal airways beginning around the fifth week.

The second stage, the pseudoglandular stage, begins around the sixth week after the formation of the right and left main stem bronchi and ends around the 17th week of gestation. This stage is characterized by progressive branching of the distal airways for 15 to 20 generations. In addition, the pulmonary vasculature begins to develop within the mesenchyme surrounding the branching lung bud. By the end of the pseudoglandular stage the gross lung morphology is identical to that of an adult.

The third stage, the canalicular stage, begins around the 17th week. It is characterized by the development of acini at the terminal bronchiole. In addition, airway epithelial cells and pulmonary capillaries fuse to form a surface for gas exchange. Finally selected epithelial cells differentiate into type II pneumocytes and begin surfactant production. The canalicular stage ends around the 20th week of gestation.

The fourth stage, the saccular stage, is characterized by further development of the acini into respiratory bronchioles. The process increases the surface area for gas exchange in the lung and lasts between 26 and 36 weeks of gestation. This stage is present in the majority of premature infants at birth.

The final alveolar stage occurs between 32 and 36 weeks gestation. The respiratory bronchioles septate and expand to form the alveoli. The rate of alveolar formation is maximal at 36 weeks gestation and continues until approximately 2 years of age.

Surfactant is a complex mixture of phospholipids, proteins, and cholesterol. By weight, phospholipids make up the majority of surfactant. In particular, saturated phosphatidylcholine comprises approximately 50% of surfactant. There are a variety of proteins in surfactant that are responsible for surfactant processing and host defense. Surfactant is produced by Type II epithelial cells of the distal airways. Lung maturity in the fetus can be predicted by the lecithin phosphatidyl/sphingomyelin (L/S) ratio in amniotic fluid, which is a marker for surfactant. An increase in this ratio of 2:1 is considered indicative of fetal lung maturity. Surfactant production and other aspects of lung maturation can be accelerated in utero by exogenous glucocorticoid administration.

## Respiratory Changes at Birth

In order for efficient gas exchange at birth, the pulmonary fluid must be removed from the lung. This process is aided by a variety of mechanisms occurring during labor and after birth. A surge in catecholamines during active labor induces a change in sodium ion transport of the lung epithelium from that of excretion to absorption. This process is regulated by epinephrine levels during labor. After birth, intravascular Starling forces occurring during respiration also aid in the resorption of pulmonary fluid. Any process that prevents or attenuates the normal evacuation of pulmonary fluid can lead to development of postnatal respiratory distress.

After birth the first mechanical breath is aided by a small amount of fluid present in the postnatal lung. This fluid aids to decrease the surface tension of the alveoli and lowers the opening pressure of the alveoli. In addition a large amount of surfactant produced during labor functions to lower the alveoli opening pressure. Surfactant also allows the creation of the functional residual capacity (FRC) by preventing all the air from leaving the lung during expiration. Any relative surfactant deficiency at birth causes a decrease in FRC and high opening pressures during respiration. This process can contribute to respiratory distress.

At birth there is a drop in pulmonary vascular resistance due to ventilation of the lungs which mechanically tends to open the pulmonary capillaries. Further, changes in the oxygen tension within the pulmonary vascular bed cause vasodilatation. The net result is a significant drop of the pulmonary vascular resistance and a reversal of the right to left shunt present in the fetal circulation.

Fetal breathing is continuous in early gestation and becomes episodic during late gestation. The regulation of breathing in the fetus involves an interaction of oxygen, carbon dioxide, and a variety of neurochemicals. An increase in either oxygen or carbon dioxide tension will stimulate fetal breathing in experimental models. In addition, a variety of neurochemicals including muscimol, prostaglandin $E_2$, and g-aminobutyric acid act to regulate fetal breathing.

The transition from fetal breathing to continuous breathing at birth involves a complex series of neurochemical changes that are only recently discovered. It had been thought that transient hypoxia stimulates the infant into continuous breathing. However, several recent studies have indicated that the separation of the infant from the placenta is a possible stimulus for continuous breathing. Indeed, several lines of laboratory evidence support the notion that placental-produced prostaglandins act to inhibit fetal continuous breathing. Abrupt cessation of prostaglandin stimulation when the umbilical cord is clamped may facilitate the switch from fetal to continuous breathing.

The respiratory rate of a newborn helps to minimize the external work of breathing. In addition, chest wall compliance of an infant is at least 5 times greater than the lung compliance, as opposed to the adult where the two are equal. Respiratory muscle fiber types (especially diaphragmatic) change during development so that during the newborn period there are more oxidative fibers, which are less likely to fatigue. As in adults, diaphragmatic muscle function is impaired by accumulation of lactate and decreasing intracellular pH. However, the blood supply of the diaphragm appears to be preserved during hypoxia and hypotension as compared to skeletal muscle.

## Apnea of Prematurity

Apnea is loosely defined as a cessation of breathing for greater than 10 seconds in the absence of airway obstruction. There are multiple identifiable causes of apnea in newborn infants including central nervous system (CNS), respiratory and cardiovascular, gastrointestinal, and metabolic causes. However, the majority of premature infants will have idiopathic apnea of prematurity. It is estimated that 80% of infants less than 1500 grams will have 1 documented episode of apnea while in the neonatal intensive care unit. Current evidence supports the notion that idiopathic apnea of prematurity is due to immature brain stem respiratory control centers present in premature infants.

The diagnosis of apnea of prematurity is based on the clinical observation of an apneic episode. Significant episodes can be defined as any apneic period lasting greater than 10 seconds, accompanied bradycardia (<100 beats per minute) or arterial hypoxemia. There is no consensus on how many apneic episodes are necessary for the diagnosis of apnea of prematurity. However, a single documented episode should prompt a medical workup for possible reversible causes.

The therapy for apnea of prematurity begins with the identification and treatment of reversible medical causes. Any electrolyte abnormalities, hypoxemia, hypoglycemia, or anemia should be corrected. Once reversible causes have been excluded, treatment with continuous positive airway pressure (CPAP) and/or methylxanthines such as caffeine or aminophylline should be initiated. These agents most likely act within the CNS to increase the sensitivity of the respiratory control center to carbon dioxide. Multiple randomized control trials have documented the ability of these compounds to reduce the incidence of apneic episodes in premature infants. There is no consensus on the duration of therapy with methylxanthines. However, by 36 weeks postconceptual age, the respiratory control centers in the brainstem should be fully developed and weaning trial of methylxanthines may begin.

## Respiratory Distress Syndrome

Respiratory distress syndrome (RDS) is a constellation of disorders that ultimately lead to clinical signs of respiratory distress. Previously termed hyaline membrane disease, this is a disease of the premature infant with an increase in prevalence occurring with decreasing GA. It is estimated that approximately 50% of newborns between 26 and 28 weeks gestation will be diagnosed with RDS, compared to less than 20% of infants greater than 31 weeks gestation.

The pathologic hallmark of RDS is a relative deficiency in surfactant production in the lung of premature infants. The lack of surfactant increases the opening pressure of the alveoli leading to progressive atelectasis and loss of FRC. The loss of FRC causes ventilation/perfusion mismatching, which can lead to hypoxemia and a reflexive increase in pulmonary vascular resistance. This increase in pulmonary vascular resistance further exacerbates the arterial hypoxemia.

Treatment of infants with RDS begins with prompt recognition of respiratory distress. Adequate oxygenation and ventilation via oxygen therapy or positive pressure ventilation must be initiated without delay to prevent hypoxemia, which can worsen RDS. Surfactant replacement therapy is initiated at doses of approximately 100 to 150 mg of phospholipid per 1 kg of body weight via the endotracheal tube. Attention to adequacy of ventilation, as assessed by $Po_2$, $Pco_2$, pH, and oxygen saturation, is necessary on a continuous basis to adjust to the rapid changes in respiratory status occurring in these critically ill infants.

## Bronchopulmonary Dysplasia

Bronchopulmonary dysplasia (BPD) is end result of long-term positive pressure ventilation and oxygen therapy in newborns treated for a respiratory disorder. A National Institute of Child Health and Human Development/National Heart, Lung, and Blood Institute Workshop proposed a severity-based definition of BPD for infants <32 weeks' GA. Mild BPD was defined as a need for supplemental oxygen ($O_2$) for ≥28 days but not at 36 weeks' postmenstrual age (PMA) or discharge, moderate BPD as $O_2$ for ≥28 days plus treatment with <30% $O_2$ at 36 weeks' PMA, and severe BPD as $O_2$ for ≥28 days plus ≥30% $O_2$ and/or positive pressure at 36 weeks' PMA. The underlying pathophysiology of BPD is multifactorial. Barotrauma and oxygen therapy related to the need for positive pressure ventilation have been indicated in the development of BPD. Indeed several strategies of gentile ventilation with permissive hypercapnea have reduced the incidence of BPD in premature and term newborns. Inflammation, infection, and poor nutritional intake have also all been linked to the development of BPD.

The treatment of BPD involved a multidisciplinary approach to minimize the risk factors and maximize the supportive care of premature infants. As mentioned above, gentile ventilation strategies with permissive hypercarbia and low tidal volume to minimize the barotrauma are a key strategy in the treatment of BPD. Administration of oxygen to maintain oxygen saturation between 90% and 95% should keep the goal $PaO_2$ less than 100 mm Hg. Any possible infection, including pneumonia, should be identified at treated.

Adequate nutritional therapy should be initiated to meet the metabolic demands of the critical ill infant. The use of pharmacologic agents such as bronchodilators, diuretics, and corticosteroids have not been adequately studied in large trials and should be used as the patient's clinical situation dictates.

# CARDIOVASCULAR SYSTEM

## Embryology of the Cardiovascular System

The events leading to the development of the cardiovascular system begin on the 15th day of life when the cardiac progenitor cells migrate to the lateral plate mesoderm from the primitive streak. At the same time blood islands appear in the mesoderm to begin the formation of red blood cells and vascular system. In the cardiogenic area of the mesoderm these blood islands converge to form a straight heart tube by the 20th day of life. Around the 23rd day of life the heart tube begins to bend to form the cardiac loop, normally to the right (D-loop formation). The looping process signals the atrial portion of the heart tube, the bulbus cordis, the truncus arteriosus, and the primitive ventricle to form the morphologic common atrium, right ventricle, outflow track, and the left ventricle, respectively. This process is completed by the 28th day of gestation and cardiac contraction with subsequent circulation is begun. Beginning on the 27th day of gestation, septation begins on the endocardial surface through the development of soft tissue masses called endocardial cushions. Septation is finished by the 37th day with the formation of atrial and ventricular septa, atrioventricular canals, heart valves, and the aortic and pulmonary channels.

The aortic arches develop from the distal part of the truncus arteriosus. During the fourth and fifth week of life these arches become associated with the pharyngeal arches to form 5 pairs of arteries: I, II, III, IV, and VI. The fifth arch is only present in a third of embryos, and completely regresses. The first and second aortic arches regress to form the maxillary artery and hyoid and stapedial arteries, respectively. The third arch forms the common, internal, and external carotid arteries. The fourth aortic arch forms the subclavian artery on the right and the aortic arch on the left. The sixth aortic arch becomes the left and right pulmonary arteries and the ductus arteriosus, which persists during fetal circulation.

## Physiology of the Fetal and Neonatal Cardiovascular System

In the fetus, after embryogenesis is complete, the circulation is converted from a serial circulation into two parallel circulations that will exist until gestation. A schematic diagram of fetal circulation is shown in Fig. 4-1. Blood returns to the fetus from the placenta via the umbilical vein. After entering the abdomen, the blood in the umbilical vein supplies the liver then joins the portal vein via the ductus venosus. A sphincter present at the junction of the umbilical vein and the ductus venosus regulates umbilical vein blood flow. Only 40% to 60% of the placental blood enters the ductus venous, and the remainder is shunted to the hepatic vasculature via the hepato-portal venous system.

The ductus venosus joins the retrohepatic vena cava near the junction of the hepatic veins. However, due to several valves in the inferior vena cava, the 2 streams of blood are not well mixed. These valves separate the vena cava blood flow into a high velocity, posterior and leftward stream of blood originating from ductus venosus, and a low velocity, anterior and rightward stream of blood originating from the inferior vena cava. After entering the right atrium, blood from the ductus venosus is preferentially directed into the left atrium via the foramen ovale due to the cephalad portion of conduit of the foramen termed the crista dividens. Therefore, the highly oxygenated blood originating from the placenta is directed to the left atrium and subsequent systemic circulation. The crista dividens directs blood returning from the inferior vena cave directly into the right ventricle via the tricuspid valve. Blood returning from the superior vena cava is also preferentially directed into the right ventricle by another valve situated in the right atrium, the crista interveniens.

In the fetus, due to the parallel circulation of blood, the cardiac output consists of both right and left ventricle output. In addition, the various shunts in the circulatory system allow differential output from each ventricle. The right ventricle's stroke volume is responsible for approximately 65% of the total cardiac output, approximately 300 mL/kg/min. Of the blood ejected through the right ventricle, less than 10% is directed through the lungs and the remainder enters the descending thoracic aorta via the ductus arteriosus. The majority blood from the left ventricle (35% of cardiac output) enters the ascending thoracic aorta to supply the developing brain.

The differences in cardiac output from the left and right ventricles do not parallel oxygen delivery to the upper and lower body. As mentioned above, the highly oxygenated blood returning from the placenta is directed via a series of valves toward the foramen ovale and into the left atrium. This allows the blood from the left ventricle to have a higher oxygen concentration than blood from the right ventricle. The net result is that the highly oxygenated blood is directed toward the head and upper extremities, and the poorly oxygenated blood is directed down the descending aorta toward the placenta for reoxygenation.

Fetal hemoglobin allows more oxygen to be carried in fetal blood than in maternal blood because the dissociation curve is shifted left and is steeper (higher affinity for oxygen). The fetus also has less need of oxygen with no thermoregulation work and no respiratory work, which is roughly 30% of normal term newborn oxygen consumption. In fact, although fetal oxygen delivery (22 mL $O_2$/kg/min) is less than that in the newborn (60 mL $O_2$/kg/min), oxygen consumption is also decreased (7 mL $O_2$/kg/min compared to 18 mL $O_2$/kg/min). Thus, the oxygen extraction fraction is constant at 30%.

The regulation of fetal cardiac output and blood is controlled by a complex network of local, regional, and neural regulatory mechanisms. Similar to adult circulation as global oxygen concentrations fall, blood flow to both the brain and myocardium increase to preserve oxygen delivery to these vital organs. Baroreceptor and chemoreceptors are present in the carotid arteries and aortic arch during gestation. These receptors trigger reflex bradycardia with acute increases in arterial blood pressure.

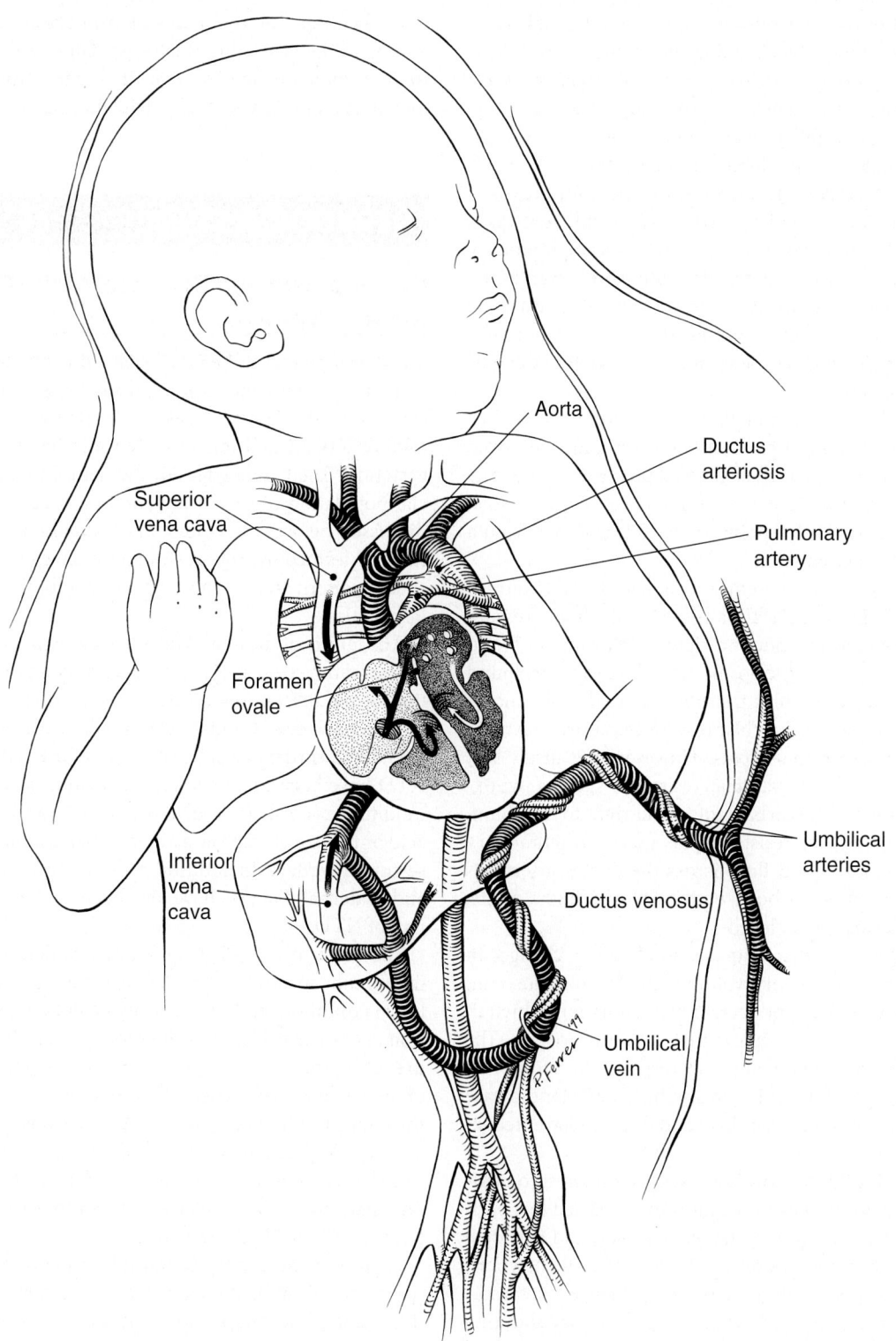

**FIGURE 4-1** Schematic diagram of fetal circulation.

Autonomic innervation to the heart and cardiovascular system is not fully developed until gestation. However, circulating catecholamines also participate in regulation of the circulation before the development of the autonomic nervous system of the heart. Alpha-adrenergic stimulation increases arterial blood pressure, decreases cardiac output, and increases in blood flow to the lung. Beta-adrenergic stimulation causes an increase in heart rate without a change in arterial blood pressure and cardiac output. Cholinergic stimulation decreases blood pressure and heart rate and increases pulmonary blood flow.

## Circulatory Changes at Birth

A profound series of changes occur at birth as the newborn is removed from placental circulation. These changes begin with the onset of spontaneous respiration and the exclusions of placental blood flow by clamping the umbilical cord. Respiration increases oxygen delivery to the pulmonary alveoli and causes physical distension of the lungs. Gas exchange across the alveolar–capillary membrane causes an increase in pulmonary capillary hemoglobin oxygen content.

Pulmonary blood flow increases due to a mechanical expansion from distended alveoli and from oxygen-initiated vasodilatation of the pulmonary arteries. The drop in pulmonary resistance decreases right ventricular output and reverses the flow in the ductus arteriosus to left to right. Whereas only 10% of the right ventricular output during gestation; after birth, 90% of right ventricle blood flow is directed to the pulmonary circulation.

As both pulmonary blood flow and pulmonary venous return increase, left atrial pressure increases and right atrial pressure decreases. When the left atrial pressure exceeds the pressure in the right atrium, the foramen ovale closes against the crista dividens. At this point the fetus transitions from a parallel to a serial circulation.

The ductus arteriosus can remain patent for several hours to days after birth. During gestation the relatively high pressure in the pulmonary artery causes a right to left shunt of blood flow across the ductus arteriosus. After birth the profound drop in pulmonary vascular resistance as well as a concurrent increase in systemic vascular resistance causes a decrease of blood flow across the ductus. However, any insult that increases the pulmonary vascular resistance such as hypoxemia or acidosis can exacerbate this small right to left shunt. Once systemic vascular resistance has exceeded pulmonary vascular resistance, blood flow across the ductus arteriosus reverses. In a healthy newborn, within 10 to 15 hours of life, the ductus arteriosus has closed.

In the newborn, cardiac output is modified by changes in heart rate rather than stroke volume. Hypoxemia causes an increase in heart rate by inducing hyperventilation, which in turn stimulates stretch receptors that act on heart rate. The ability to increase stroke volume in response to hypoxemia increases with age. Older children also have a greater increase in afterload for a given volume load and thus will have steeper Frank–Starling curves.

Gastrointestinal blood flow is of particular interest to pediatric surgeons. Blood flow to the intestine is related to 4 variables: cardiac output, local metabolic changes, and neuronal and hormonal control reflexes. As in the adult, the newborn gut blood flow is particularly sensitive to changes in cardiac output. Systemic hypotension causes preferential shunting of blood from the splanchnic circulation toward the cerebral and myocardial circulation. In addition, any disease of the descending aorta (ie, coarctation) will decrease blood flow to the intestine. Compared to the dormant fetal intestine, the initiation of feedings for the newborn infant causes a profound series of local metabolic changes that act to decrease intestinal vascular resistance and increase blood flow. Increased metabolic demand may lead to hypoxia with the release of vasodilators including $K^+$, $Mg^{++}$, histamine, bradykinin, vasoactive intestinal peptide (VIP), etc.

Several systemic neural and humoral factors also regulate intestinal blood flow. Alpha-adrenergic stimulation constricts vessels to intestine, and beta-adrenergic stimulation causes vasodilatation. The renin–angiotensin system also constricts vessels to the gastrointestinal tract. Glucagon and cholecystokinin increase flow to intestines and pancreas. Gastrin increases blood flow to the gastric mucosa.

## NERVOUS SYSTEM

### Development and Disorders of the Central Nervous System

The development of the CNS begins during the second week of gestation with the formation of the neural plate by the ectoderm. The lateral edges of the neural plate undergo a folding process and form the neural tube around day 20 of gestation. The lateral edges of the neural fold contain a special population of cells, the neural crest cells, which will be discussed below. The cranial and caudal ends of the neural tube are termed neuropores and undergo closure in a rostral–caudal pattern around the 25th (cranial) or 28th (caudal) day of gestation.

Any failure of the neural tube to close will result in a variety of neural tube defects (NTD), depending on the specific location of the defect. Rostral defects will result in anencephaly or encephalocele. Caudal defects will lead to spina bifida or a related disorder. Several risk factors for the development of NTD have been identified. These include several potentially modifiable risk factors such as poor maternal intake of folic acid or the use of valproic acid or carbamazepine for maternal seizure disorders. In addition, a family history of both NTD and maternal diabetes have also been shown to increase the risk of NTD.

The most severe NTD is of complete failure of the rostral neural tube to close leading to anencephaly. Anencephaly is a lethal condition, and the majority of infants with this condition are either stillborn or die shortly after birth. Partial failure of the anterior neural tube to close leads to the formation of an encephalocele where the intracranial contents herniate through a midline skull defect. These lesions typically exist as part of a Mendelian genetic disorder such as Dandy–Walker syndrome, Joubert syndrome, or median cleft face syndrome. The majority of these defects will require surgical correction to prevent lethal hydrocephalus.

Failure of the caudal neural tube to close will result in a spectrum of spina bifida defects that have a wide range in severity. The mildest form of the disease is spina bifida occulta in which the posterior components of the vertebral column fail to close, but there is no involvement of the spinal cord or meninges. These children are often asymptomatic. A meningocele results from a defect that involves the meninges of the spinal cord, but the neural tissue is preserved. These children are often asymptomatic, but elective repair is usually performed to protect the nerve roots. The most severe form of caudal NTD is termed a myelomeningocele. This defect involves all layers of the neural tube (spinal cord, meninges, and vertebral bodies). These children usually exhibit a variety of neurologic defects depending on the level and severity of the myelomeningocele. Meningoceles or myelomeningoceles can result in downward traction of the CNS with subsequent herniation of the brainstem and cerebellum through the foramen magnum. This process results in a variety of Chiari malformations depending on the severity of the displacement. These infants will often require either surgical decompression or cerebrospinal fluid (CSF) shunting to prevent the development of hydrocephalus.

The neural tube undergoes anterior–posterior segmentation, termed dorsal induction, between 5 and 6 weeks of gestation to form the basal plate, containing the motor-related parts of the CNS, and the alar plate, containing the sensory portion of the CNS. Abnormalities in the formation of these divisions will give rise to holoprosencephaly. CNS defects include a marked reduction in the neocortex, absent olfactory bulbs and tracts, and hypertelorism with abnormalities of the nose and face. Several genetic defects associated with holoprosencephaly have been identified: Trisomy 13 or 18, Pallister–Hall syndrome, and Rubinstein–Taybi syndrome. Prognosis is dependent on the severity of the neurologic defects.

After closure, the neural tube undergoes neurulation, a segmentation and division process between 5 and 6 weeks of gestation, to form 3 primitive brain vesicles: the prosencephalon, the mesencephalon, and the rhombencephalon. The prosencephalon ultimately develops into the cerebral hemispheres, pituitary gland, thalamus, hypothalamus, and epiphysis. The mesencephalon develops several neuron groups that control eye movement and hearing. In addition, the basilar portion of the mesencephalon forms the crus cerebri, which serves as a link between the cerebral cortex and the spinal cord. The rhombencephalon gives rise to the medulla oblongata, cerebellum, and pons. Any failure of formation of the above segments can lead to a variety of disorders including schizencephaly, aprosencephaly, agenesis of the corpus callosum, and seto-optic dysplasia.

Neurons and glia proliferate in the cerebral cortex from 6 to 12 weeks gestation. At this time, the full adult complement is reached with no further formation of neurons, although glial proliferation continues throughout life. Disorders of neuronal proliferation include microcephaly or megalencephaly, in which the brain is small or large, respectively, but otherwise is normally developed. Microcephaly is usually clinically defined as infants with an occipitofrontal circumference of less than 2 standard deviations for age and gender. Infants may have no neurologic signs initially, but later develop mental retardation. There is a genetic cause in 60% of the infants and an association with maternal radiation, alcohol, phenylketonuria, anticonvulsants, organic mercurials, excessive vitamin A, and rubella. Infants with megalencephaly may have normal function or severe mental retardation with epilepsy and have associated neurocutaneous syndromes such as tuberous sclerosis, neurofibromatosis, and Sturge–Weber syndrome.

The normal development of the cerebral cortex involves migration of neurons from the ventricular zone, where they are generated, to the outer surface of the neural tube (the cortex) starting around 10 to 20 weeks of gestation. Cerebellar neurons are generated from the epithelial lining of the rostral half of the fourth ventricle and then migrate out radially interacting with the granule cells, Purkinje cells, and glial cells. Disorders of neuronal or glial migration include

lissencephaly, cobblestone malformation syndrome, or periventricular nodular heterotopia. Similar to the disorders of neuronal proliferation above, these children typically appear to be normal in the newborn period. However, they typically develop seizures around 3 to 6 months of life and progress to infantile spasms. Mental retardation can develop later in life. Management of these disorders includes suppression of seizures and infantile spasms. The majority of these infants will require a gastrostomy for feeding.

Myelination occurs as oligodendrocytes arise in the ventricular zone and migrate out along axons, forming their myelin sheaths. One oligodendrocyte can produce myelin for up to 50 axons. Deficiencies in myelination have been identified in cerebral and cerebellar atrophy syndromes such as Pelizaeus–Merzbacher disease and Alexander disease. These diseases are characterized by a slow and progressive onset of hypotonia, seizures, and mental retardation. Death usually occurs in the adolescent years. Defects in myelination have also been seen in disorders of amino acid metabolism and malnutrition.

## Development and Disorders of the Neuromuscular System

Motor neurons arise from the basal plate of the spinal cord around 4 weeks of gestation. These neurons ultimately form the ventral horn of the spinal cord. Unlike the CNS, myelination of the peripheral neurons occurs from the actions of Schwann cells, which can only produce myelin for 1 axon. The corticospinal (or pyramidal) tracts are the only direct anatomic pathway from the motor cortex to the spinal cord. Its impulses are modulated by the cerebellum and the extrapyramidal system. Motor neurons in the spinal cord develop rostrocaudally beginning at 10 to 12 weeks. The speed of a neural signal depends on myelination of the axon, which is most rapid in the first 6 months of life and occurs in a caudal cephalic direction. Development of fetal tone also occurs in this direction.

Muscle development begins in the mesoderm with the formation of segmental somites arranges longitudinally along the developing embryo. Specific cell populations, termed dermatomyotomes, located in the somites give rise to the axial and limb musculature. The basic morphology of the adult musculature is present by 7 weeks of gestation and spontaneous contraction begins around 8 weeks. Combined movements of the limb, trunk, and head occur at 12 to 16 weeks. By 16 weeks the mother can recognize lower limb and trunk movements (quickening). After 35 weeks movement is decreased, and more time is spent in fixed postures.

Muscle fibers can be divided into type groups, type I and type II. Type I fibers, typically referred to as slow-twitch fibers, primarily use oxidative metabolism and are fatigue resistant. Type II fibers are divided into type IIa and IIb subtypes. These fast-twitch fibers primarily use anaerobic metabolism and are not fatigue resistant. Primitive muscle fibers, typed as IIc fibers, are believed to be precursors to both type I and II fibers. Type I fibers appear at about 18 weeks of gestation and are smaller than type II fibers until after birth. Most muscle fibers in the 20- to 26-week-old fetus are type IIc fibers. Type IIa and IIb fibers appear during the last month of gestation.

The presence of major clinical reflex patterns is dependent on GA. Tactile reflexes such as grasping are evident around 28 weeks. The tonic reflex (turning of the head to one side with extension of the contralateral arm and flexion of the ipsilateral arm) appears around 35 weeks gestation. Sucking and rooting reflexed develop around 30 weeks but do not become vigorous until 35 weeks. The Moro or startle reflex (extension and abduction of the upper extremities with opening of the hands and an audible cry) starts to develop around 30 weeks gestation but is not complete until 38 weeks.

Of the disorders of the neuromuscular system, cerebral palsy (CP) is one of the most common. CP is characterized by disordered motor function present in infancy and accompanied by changes in muscle tone (typically spasticity or rigidity), muscle weakness, involuntary movements, ataxia, or a combination of these abnormalities. The etiology of CP is likely multifactorial with several known risk factors such as peri- and postnatal brain injury, brain injury related to prematurity, and other developmental abnormalities. Cerebral palsy is classified by the predominant type of motor abnormality (spastic, hypotonic, ataxic, or mixed) in addition to the distribution of limb involvement (hemiplegia, quadriplegia, or diplegia). The prognosis of an infant with CP is related to several factors including the clinical type of cerebral palsy, the degree of delay in meeting milestones noted at subsequent evaluations, the pathologic reflexes present, and the degree of associated deficits in intelligence and sensation.

## Metabolism and Metabolic Disorders of the Nervous System

The primary fuel of the brain, regardless of gestation age, is glucose, which is metabolized through aerobic and anaerobic glycolysis to form adenosine triphosphate (ATP). The neonatal glycolytic rate is one tenth of the adult rate; however, the tolerance of perinatal infants for hypoxemia is greater. This tolerance cannot be explained by increased ability for anaerobic metabolism but by a decreased demand for energy as the immature brain performs less work than the mature brain. Even though the oxidative metabolism decreases, anaerobic metabolism alone cannot support it. Alternate substances for energy include lactate, ketone bodies, free fatty acids, and amino acids. Transport mechanisms for ketone bodies are 10-fold faster in the immature infant, resulting in more efficient use of alternative fuels. When newborns are hypoglycemic, lactate is used and can support up to 58% of energy needs.

Hypoglycemia is one of the most common correctable metabolic disorders in preterm and term infants. The definition of clinically important hypoglycemia is controversial, but most neonatologists agree that a blood glucose of less than 2.5 mmol/L (46 mg/dL) is a threshold that should prompt further evaluation and treatment. The causes of neonatal hypoglycemia can be grouped into 4 categories: poor adaptation to extrauterine life, hyperinsulinism, increased metabolic demands due to other illness, and inborn errors of metabolism. The signs of neonatal hypoglycemia are dependent on the duration and severity of hypoglycemia. Early signs of hypoglycemia include tachycardia, irritability, and diaphoresis. Late signs include depressed consciousness and neonatal seizures. Treatment of neonatal hypoglycemia begins with prompt repletion of blood glucose with intravenous dextrose. After stabilization of the infant, a prompt search for the underlying cause must be undertaken.

## Intracranial Pressure and Cerebral Blood Flow

The normal intracranial pressure in newborns is about 6 mm Hg. The normal cerebral perfusion pressure (difference between mean arterial pressure and intracranial pressure) varies between 20 mm Hg in preterm infants at birth and 80 mm Hg at 12 months, which corresponds to a cerebral blood flow rate in newborns of about 40 mL/100 g/min. Monroe-Kellie doctrine states that the skull is a rigid cavity and has a fixed volume consisting of the brain parenchyma, intravascular blood, and CSF. However, this doctrine is not applicable to infants and young children as for the first 3 years of life, subacute or chronically elevated ICP leads to the separation of cranial sutures, followed by cranial enlargement.

Autoregulation of cerebral blood flow has been demonstrated in both premature and full-term infants. The cerebral vasculature is responsive to changes in arterial oxygen and carbon dioxide tension. There is an inverse relationship between cerebral blood flow and oxygen tension below 50 mm Hg. Elevated $PaCO_2$ dilates cerebral blood vessels and will increase cerebral blood flow. Higher levels of hypercarbia abolish autoregulation, as the vessels are maximally dilated. Other mediators of metabolic autoregulation are changes in tissue pH, potassium, and calcium ions. Systemic alkalization as a means to diminish pulmonary hypertension and improve oxygenation will impair cerebral blood flow. This becomes a limiting factor for this type of therapy.

## Intraventricular Hemorrhage

Intraventricular hemorrhage (IVH) is defined as bleeding into the germinal matrix tissues of the developing brain and is a frequent cause of significant morbidity and mortality in preterm infants. Approximately 25% of all preterm infants less than 1500 g will suffer an IVH, and half of these will occur in the first 8 hours of life. In addition, the majority (95%) of IVHs will occur in the first 5 days of life.

The pathophysiology of IVH has been attributed to fluctuations in cerebral blood flow to the immature germinal matrix. In the developing brain, the germinal matrix is the site of proliferation of neuronal and glial precursors. In the fetus and preterm infant the germinal matrix requires a rich blood supply, but its vessels are poorly supported with large diameters and few supporting structures. Therefore, severe alterations in systemic blood pressure can lead to abnormal stress on these fragile structures resulting in IVH. Indeed, abrupt changes in blood pressure that occur with RDS, rapid volume reexpansion, tracheal suctioning, pneumothorax, hypoxemia, hypercapnea, acidosis, low hematocrit, pneumothorax, abdominal examination, and seizures can all contribute toward the development of IVH.

Two conditions associated with IVH include periventricular hemorrhagic infarction and periventricular leukomalacia. Periventricular hemorrhagic infarction is an infarction that is followed by bleeding. This is secondary to decreased cerebral blood flow because the blood vessels serving the periventricular white matter have limited ability to vasodilate. After the infarction, hemorrhage occurs with reperfusion. Venous hemorrhagic infarction occurs with increased venous pressure because of obstruction of venous outflow caused by a large germinal matrix hemorrhage or an acutely distended lateral ventricle from an IVH. Abrupt changes in right atrial pressure associated with pneumothorax, suctioning, and high ventilator pressures may also lead to venous hemorrhage. Clinical features of infarction are hypotonia in the newborn period leading to hemiparesis or quadriparesis later on in life.

Periventricular leukomalacia is symmetrical, nonhemorrhagic, ischemic insult to the periventricular white matter. These watershed zones are particularity sensitive to hypoxic insults. It is difficult to see on ultrasound when hemorrhage is present. Clinical features include hypotonia in the lower extremities in the newborn period and spastic diplegia in older children.

Clinical signs of IVH are often nonspecific and often go unrecognized. These include apneic and bradycardic spells, hyperglycemia, and persistent metabolic acidosis. Infants with large IVH may have an acute drop in hematocrit, new-onset seizures, and depressed level of consciousness. Due to the subtle clinical signs, many NICUs routinely screen high-risk infants for IVH with bedside cranial ultrasonography. A grading system for IVH had become well adopted. A grade 1 IVH describes blood in the germinal matrix only. A grade 2 IVFH is blood filling the lateral ventricles without distention, while a grade 3 is blood filling and acutely distending the ventricular system. A grade 4 describes hemorrhage within the brain parenchyma.

The most effective means of preventing IVH is to avoid preterm birth. Antenatal steroids have been shown to decrease the risk of subsequent IVH development, likely through the prevention of RDS. Postnatal abrupt changes in blood pressure by volume reexpansion or pharmacologic means should be avoided. In addition, indomethacin, an inhibitor of the cyclooxygenase pathway of prostaglandin synthesis, has been found to decrease the incidence and severity of IVH in very-low-birth-weight preterm infants. Current recommendation is that all preterm infant less than 1250 g receive prophylactic indomethacin for the first 48 hours of life.

The mortality rate for infants with IVH is higher compared with their GA-matched peers without hemorrhage. However, infants with IVH are more likely to die from underlying disease predisposing to IVH such as NEC and BPD. In the neonatal period, infants with IVH are at risk for the development of seizures and posthemorrhagic hydrocephalus. Preterm infants surviving the neonatal period with parenchymal involvement by IVH are believed to be at particular risk for cognitive disability. For infants with grade I and II hemorrhages, there are no developmental sequelae, as compared to infants of comparable prematurity without an IVH.

## SELECTED READINGS

Anderson RH, Backer EJ, Penny DJ, Redington AN, Rigby ML, Wernovsky G. *Pediatric Cardiology*. 3rd ed. Philadelphia, PA: Churchill Livingstone/Elsevier; 2010.

Creasy RK, Resnick R, Iams JD. *Creasy and Resnik's Maternal-Fetal Medicine: Principles and Practice*. 6th ed. Philadelphia, PA: Saunders/Elsevier; 2009.

MacDonald MG, Seshia MMK, Mullett MD. *Avery's Neonatology: Pathophysiology and Management of the Newborn*. 6th ed. Philadelphia, PA: Lippincott Williams & Wilkins; 2005.

Sadler TW. *Langman's Medical Embryology*. 11th ed. Philadelphia, PA: Lippincott Williams & Wilkins; 2010.

Swaiman KF, Ashwal S, Ferriero DM. *Pediatric Neurology: Principles and Practice*. 4th ed. Philadelphia, PA: Mosby Elsevier; 2006.

# CHAPTER 5

# Renal Developmental Physiology and Pediatric Fluid and Electrolyte Management

*Scott J. Keckler and David W. Tuggle*

## KEY POINTS

1. Fetal urine production begins at 10 to 13 weeks gestation, and although urine production increases thereafter throughout pregnancy, glomerular filtration rate (GFR) is always lower in preterm infants.

2. Renal function changes quickly in the fetus and newborn with an increasing GFR and tubular maturity leading to enhanced concentrating ability.

3. Calculation of maintenance fluid requirements is size dependent; however, practically, calculations are more typically based on body weight rather than body surface area.

4. Premature infant fluid requirements are different from term infant requirements in both total fluid volumes and electrolyte content.

5. To avoid serious neurologic injury, sodium abnormalities should not be corrected quickly.

## RENAL EMBRYOLOGY

The development of the human kidney is a complex process that requires precise timing. Three sets of excretory organs develop: pronephros, mesonephros, and metanephros. During the fourth week of gestation the pronephros appears and rapidly regresses but the ductal structures are utilized by the mesonephros that consists of tubules and glomeruli, which are a simple version of those seen later. The metanephros, the permanent kidney, develops in the sixth week of gestation after regression of the former 2 primitive kidneys. As this appearance and regression process occurs, the collecting system and tubules contact each other leading to the final functional unit or nephron. Upon final formation, the fetal kidney begins to produce urine by 10 to 13 weeks of gestation, and the number of nephrons continues to increase to approximately 1 million by 36 weeks of gestation. Initially, the fetal kidneys are in close approximation in the pelvis with the hilum facing ventrally. During fetal elongation, the kidneys ascend in the abdomen and rotate 90° medially, and by the ninth week, they are in the normal anatomic position. The blood supply to the developing kidneys is initially from surrounding vessels but during the cranial ascent regress, and formation of the renal vessels is seen by the ninth week as well. The complex interaction required for normal kidney development and position allows for a large number of malformations to occur.

## RENAL FUNCTION

Urine produced by the fetal kidney is excreted into the amniotic fluid, and by 20 weeks, it becomes the major portion of the overall amniotic fluid volume. Fetal urine production is initially brisk at 5 mL/h, reaching 40 mL/h by term. As a consequence, fetal anuria/oliguria manifests with oligohydramnios by approximately 24 weeks. While the fetal kidney does excrete urine, the majority of electrolyte balance is regulated by the placenta. During the first postnatal days, the kidney begins the transition from fetal to neonatal function. When compared to adults, the neonatal kidney has decreased renal function owing to the low mean arterial pressure and high vascular resistance, and this is the primary reason for the decreased glomerular filtration rate (GFR) of neonates. The initial GFR in term infants is approximately 20 mL/min $\times$ 1.73 $m^2$ and doubles within the first 2 weeks. In comparison, preterm infants have a significantly decreased GFR. Measurement of GFR using serum creatinine is rapid and easy to perform; however, results should be interpreted with caution as initial values represent maternal serum creatinine. Neonatal creatinine values take 1 to 2 weeks to approach a reliable steady state. In preterm infants, normal values may not be seen until 4 weeks of age and initial values may remain unchanged or even increase early on. While the initial GFR is decreased, a rapid diuresis of nonconcentrated urine typically occurs in the first few days of life with an average loss of 5% of birth weight. The combination of decreased GFR and overall tubular immaturity leads to an inefficient concentrating ability of the kidney. While adults are able to concentrate urine to 1200 mOsm/L, term infants typically concentrate to 800 mOsm/L and preterm infants are further limited to 550 mOsm/L. Subsequent to overall renal immaturity, fluid losses and replacement must be monitored closely, especially with preterm infants.

## NORMAL FLUID PHYSIOLOGY

The distribution of body fluids varies widely among newborns, infants, children, and adolescents. An understanding of these differences is important for pediatric surgeons who care for critically ill patients with varying fluid shifts secondary to surgical pathology. Total body fluids are divided into 2 components; intracellular and extracellular, which are further divided into interstitial fluid and plasma. As children age, the portion of total body water (TBW) in the extracellular space decreases as the amount of skeletal muscle and connective tissue increases, shifting TBW into the intracellular compartment.

The ratio of intracellular to extracellular fluid and TBW varies with age and weight. Lean individuals have a greater proportion of water compared to body weight. The converse is seen in patients with higher amounts of adipose tissue, which contains little water. Clinically, this principle is seen in extremely premature neonates (28 weeks) whose TBW-to-weight ratio is 80%. In term infants, this approaches 70%, and pubertal children are much like adults with 50% to 60% of TBW-to-weight ratio. In healthy patients, obligatory fluid losses occur and are divided into sensible and insensible. Sensible fluid losses are measurable and include urine or stool output, but will also occur with drainage tubes in either the gastrointestinal tract or pleural cavity. The majority of insensible fluid losses are from the skin (75%) and the remainder is from the respiratory tract. Water losses from the lungs are used to humidify inspired air and are subsequently exhaled. Fluid loss from the skin is difficult to measure but occurs from convective and conductive effects in the environment. At birth sweat glands are immature, but by 2 weeks of age, visible sweat can be seen in term neonates. However, the volume is negligible in the calculation of daily maintenance fluids. Overall insensible water losses account for approximately 40% to 50% of calculated maintenance fluids for an infant in a stable environment. The patient in an unstable environment, combined with an intensive care setting, poses a challenge concerning optimal fluid balance and management. In this situation, insensible losses become a major source of water loss, and slight changes in ambient room temperature, humidity, or a radiant warmer can have profound effects on overall fluid balance. In addition to external forces, internal metabolic changes may increase insensible water losses such as fever or hypermetabolic states. These effects are summarized in Table 5-1.

| TABLE 5-1 | Conditions that Alter the Estimate of Insensible Fluid Loss |
|---|---|
| **Condition** | **Adjustment** |
| Caloric expenditure change | |
| Fever | 12.5%/1°C temperature change |
| Hypermetabolic conditions | Increase estimate by 25%–75% |
| Hypothermia | Decrease by 12%/1°C temperature change |
| Hypometabolic states | Reduced by 10%–25% |
| Environmental change | |
| Humidified inspired air | Reduced insensible loss |
| Plastic covering in isolette | Reduced insensible loss |
| Uncovered nursing in isolette | Increased insensible loss |
| Decreased room humidity | Increased insensible loss |

## FLUID REPLACEMENT

Maintenance fluid therapy is designed to replace both water and electrolytes under normal metabolic conditions. Initially, maintenance fluid therapy was calculated based on caloric energy expenditure. Over the ensuing years, multiple modifications have led to the common "100, 50, 20" rule, which is widely used today (see Table 5-2).

## NORMAL ELECTROLYTE PHYSIOLOGY

Electrolytes are an integral component of maintenance fluids in children and are required for homeostasis. When one considers the short-term replenishment of fluids, the most commonly added electrolytes are sodium, chloride, and potassium. The precise daily replacement of these essential ions is difficult to determine based on the available literature and daily fluctuations in fluid balance.

| TABLE 5-2 | Fluid Requirements for Children of Different Weights (The Two Most Commonly Used Formulas) |
|---|---|
| **Body Weight (kg)** | **Maintenance Fluids** |
| 1-10 | 100 mL/ kg/day |
| 11-20 | 1000 mL/day + 50 mL/kg/day over 10 kg |
| 21 and up | 1500 mL/day + 20 mL/kg/day over 20 kg |
| 1-10 | 4 mL/kg/h |
| 11-20 | 2 mL/kg/h |
| 21 and up | 1 mL/kg/h |

## Sodium

Term infants have a decreased capacity to excrete the daily sodium load when compared to adults, and the tubules will reabsorb sodium even when faced with hypernatremia. The resulting effect is a dilute urine and continued sodium excess. Fortunately, after 2 weeks this situation tends to correct itself with maturation of the kidney. The proper amount of sodium has been estimated to be 2 to 3 mEq/kg/day for term infants, 3 mEq/kg/day for infants <32 weeks, and increases to 4 to 5 mEq/kg/day for very premature infants and the critically ill. Normal saline contains 154 mEq/L, so a saline solution containing approximately one fifth of the normal amount will provide the 2 to 3 mEq/kg/day required for term infants who are otherwise healthy. As children age and renal function matures, the amount of sodium required per day increases.

## Chloride

Historically, chloride has not played a significant role in electrolyte management, but the effects of chloride should not be discounted. The daily requirement for chloride is essentially the same for sodium, 2 to 3 mEq/kg/day. Chloride is the major anion undergoing transport in the loop of Henle, with bicarbonate playing a lesser role. Subsequently, disorders in chloride transport may result in acid–base alterations. For instance, with an excess of chloride in the serum, bicarbonate is not reabsorbed in the kidney, with a resulting hyperchloremic metabolic acidosis. Alkalotic states may be seen with deficits in serum levels of chloride. Alterations in chloride and the acid–base abnormalities may be iatrogenic, so judicious use of chloride-containing fluids is warranted.

## Potassium

The usual recommended daily potassium requirement for newborns is 2 mEq/kg/day and, traditionally, replacement is not started until documentation of urine output. The potential for potassium excess exists in renal-impaired patients or those undergoing cardiac surgery, and frequent monitoring is paramount. When potassium replacement is required, it is frequently given with chloride, although preparations containing phosphate or acetate are available.

## ABNORMAL FLUID AND ELECTROLYTE PHYSIOLOGY

Pediatric surgeons frequently encounter pathologic conditions that lead to shifts in fluid balance and derangements in electrolytes. The previously mentioned guidelines for maintenance fluid need to be tailored to the clinical situation, with additional fluid given according to ongoing losses and/or fluid shifts.

Traumatic soft tissue injuries, severe burns, peritonitis, or extensive surgical procedures are all associated with a redistribution of fluid from the intravascular space to the extravascular space. These "third space losses" have been attributed to osmotic and hydrostatic forces as well as cytokine production from injured tissues. The clinical situation will dictate the amount and type of fluid necessary for adequate fluid balance. Bowel obstructions are a classic example of major fluid shifts at work. Both the intestinal lumen and associated soft tissues see an increase in fluids and this can be difficult to measure; therefore, an accurate measurement of intake and output is necessary. A related scenario frequently seen is the association of systemic sepsis, which will further increase the amount of fluid shifted into the abdomen. With severe sepsis, the entire "third space" of the body may see large shifts of fluid. Pancreatitis with severe sepsis is a frequently seen clinical scenario that illustrates the above point, and the amount of replacement necessary can be massive. The composition of "third space losses" has been extensively studied with transmembrane potentials and radioisotopes, providing a guide for the type of fluid necessary for replacement. Based on the data, a balanced salt solution with other additives as needed is an appropriate choice for fluid replacement. Some surgeons would prefer Lactated Ringer's solution because it provides a close approximation of the fluid losses. However, some clinicians may prefer to avoid the lactate administration. The actual fluid chosen is not as important as an understanding of the clinical situation and an accurate measurement of fluid intake and output. The renal compensation in otherwise healthy children will usually take care of any minor excess or deficits.

Another source of fluid loss that complicates fluid and electrolyte replacement is external loss from body cavities or the gastrointestinal tract. An accurate measurement of the ongoing loss will provide an idea for the amount of fluid needed and the composition of electrolytes lost depending on the source (Table 5-3). When calculating the volume and type of replacement, a standard maintenance fluid calculation should be used with additional replacement based on the amount lost from the source, with a milliliter per milliliter regimen. To most accurately replace the lost electrolytes, the output fluid should be sent for analysis; however, this may become tedious and not cost-effective, so rough approximations of electrolytes allow the surgeon to begin an appropriate fluid replacement strategy.

| TABLE 5-3 | Composition of Gastrointestinal Secretions | | | |
|---|---|---|---|---|
| Type | Na (mEq/L) | K (mEq/L) | Cl (mEq/L) | $HCO_3$ (mEq/L) |
| Salivary | 10 | 25 | 10 | 30 |
| Stomach | 60 | 10 | 130 | |
| Duodenum | 140 | 5 | 80 | |
| Ileum | 140 | 5 | 104 | 30 |
| Colon | 60 | 30 | 40 | |
| Pancreas | 140 | 5 | 75 | 115 |
| Bile | 145 | 5 | 100 | 35 |

One of the most common clinical scenarios encountered by pediatric surgeons requiring extensive fluid shifts and management is peritonitis, which can range from simple appendicitis in a 10-year-old to necrotizing enterocolitis in a premature neonate. The initial fluid management may require an estimation of the physiologic insult, but often a "guess" based on experience is utilized at the beginning. To better estimate the degree of fluid requirement, Filston advocated one method of calculating a "guess" at the volume needed to replace fluid loss from intraabdominal pathology: (1) divide the abdomen into 4 quadrants (4 quadrants = 1 maintenance fluid volume); (2) estimate the effects of peritonitis (maximum of 4 quadrants of 100% of the maintenance volume) and surgical manipulation (maximum of 4 quadrants or 100% of the maintenance volume); and (3) add this volume to the maintenance fluids plus any losses measured and then given back as maintenance fluid for the calculated maintenance and the remainder as Ringer lactate solution. The above strategy can be cumbersome to use, so the most commonly utilized indicator of adequate fluid resuscitation is urine output. Sepsis may compound peritonitis and greatly increase the amount of fluid required. Insensible fluid losses are exaggerated, and obligatory isotonic volume loss occurs in both the bowel and soft tissues. These fluid losses must be replaced prior to any use of ionotropic agents to increase cardiac output or renal perfusion pressure. The typical pediatric fluid mix is too hypotonic in this situation. Therefore, a balanced salt solution, such as Ringer lactate solution, provides a better source of volume resuscitation. Care must be taken to avoid volume excess. It has been shown that hypervolemia, especially in preterm infants, has been implicated in the reopening of a previously closed ductus arteriosus when more than 170 cc/kg/24 h is given.

Another common problem encountered by pediatric surgeons is pyloric stenosis, which is a classic example of derangements in both fluids and electrolytes. The excessive vomiting seen in these infants leads to an overall loss of volume as well as a loss of chloride. A hypochloremic, hypokalemic metabolic alkalosis with associated volume depletion quickly develops. Renal compensation for the chloride loss involves retaining bicarbonate to maintain electroneutrality, with a resulting paradoxical aciduria. Normal saline should be used initially for resuscitation. After urine output is documented, potassium should be added as these infants typically have a deficit in total body potassium. After adequate volume and electrolyte replacement, a general anesthetic can be safely given for operative correction.

## Disorders of sodium

Hypernatremia is defined as a serum sodium concentration greater than 145 mEq/L and it is most often seen in older pediatric patients associated with dehydration. The clinical signs of dehydration may not be as apparent when compared to isotonic dehydration secondary to osmosis and a relative preservation of the extracellular fluid space. Neurologic symptoms including irritability, weakness, or lethargy are the most common clinical manifestation of hypernatremia. When evaluating a patient with hypernatremia it is important to measure serum and urine osmolarity, as well as the sodium content and specific gravity of the urine. Initially patients should be treated with isotonic fluids and, as volume expansion occurs, hypotonic fluids may then be given. Rapid correction of sodium may lead to cerebral edema and permanent neurologic deficits; slowly correcting the sodium over 48 to 72 hours is recommended.

Hyponatremia, defined as a serum sodium concentration less than 135 mEq/L, is more frequently seen in the pediatric population. While hypernatremia is most commonly seen with dehydration, hyponatremia may be seen in hypo-, hyper-, or euvolemic states, and proper treatment depends on recognizing the corresponding fluid state. Symptoms of hyponatremia are rarely seen until the sodium decreases below 120 mEq/L. Nausea and vomiting may be seen as well as neurologic symptoms, which can range from confusion to seizures or coma. The brain is particularly sensitive to changes in serum osmolarity that are associated with hyponatremia, and rapid correction may lead to central pontine myelinolysis, secondary to fluid shifts out of neural tissue. An algorithm for the diagnosis of hyponatremia is presented in Fig. 5-1. With chronic hyponatremia, brain injury can usually be avoided by limiting correction to <18 mmol/L in 48 hours. There is some evidence to suggest that correcting acute or postsurgical hyponatremia by less than 4 mmol/L may be associated with an excess mortality. Therefore, to attempt to avoid secondary injury, correction of hyponatremia should probably take place over 48 hours and with more than 4 mmol/L/24 h but less than 18 mmol/L/48 h correction rates. Postsurgical patients or those undergoing volume resuscitation for severe trauma, sepsis, or burns frequently develop hypervolemic or euvolemic hyponatremia secondary to excessive administration of hypotonic fluids. In the presence of normal renal function, simple fluid restriction will correct most cases. Other causes of hyponatremia include congestive heart failure, cirrhosis, and the nephrotic syndrome. These are associated with an increase in total body sodium and water; fluid restriction is initiated but diuretics may need to be added. The syndrome of inappropriate antidiuretic hormone (SIADH) may also cause a low serum sodium in a euvolemic state, and urine concentrations of sodium are increased. Initial therapy for SIADH includes water and sodium restriction. Rarely, cerebral salt wasting may also cause hyponatremia in children with neurologic injury or disease. Treatment for hyponatremia is summarized in Table 5-4.

## Disorders of Potassium

Potassium is the primary intracellular cation and plays an important role in regulating the cellular transmembrane potential. Disorders of potassium are frequently seen in the hospitalized pediatric population, and symptoms range from cardiac dysrhythmias to muscle weakness. Hyperkalemia is defined as a serum level greater than 5.5 mEq/L in children and 6 mEq/L in newborns. When compared to adults, children better tolerate hyperkalemia. The most common cause of hyperkalemia is hemolysis of the drawn lab specimen and an analysis should be repeated to rule this out. Other causes include renal failure or iatrogenic ones

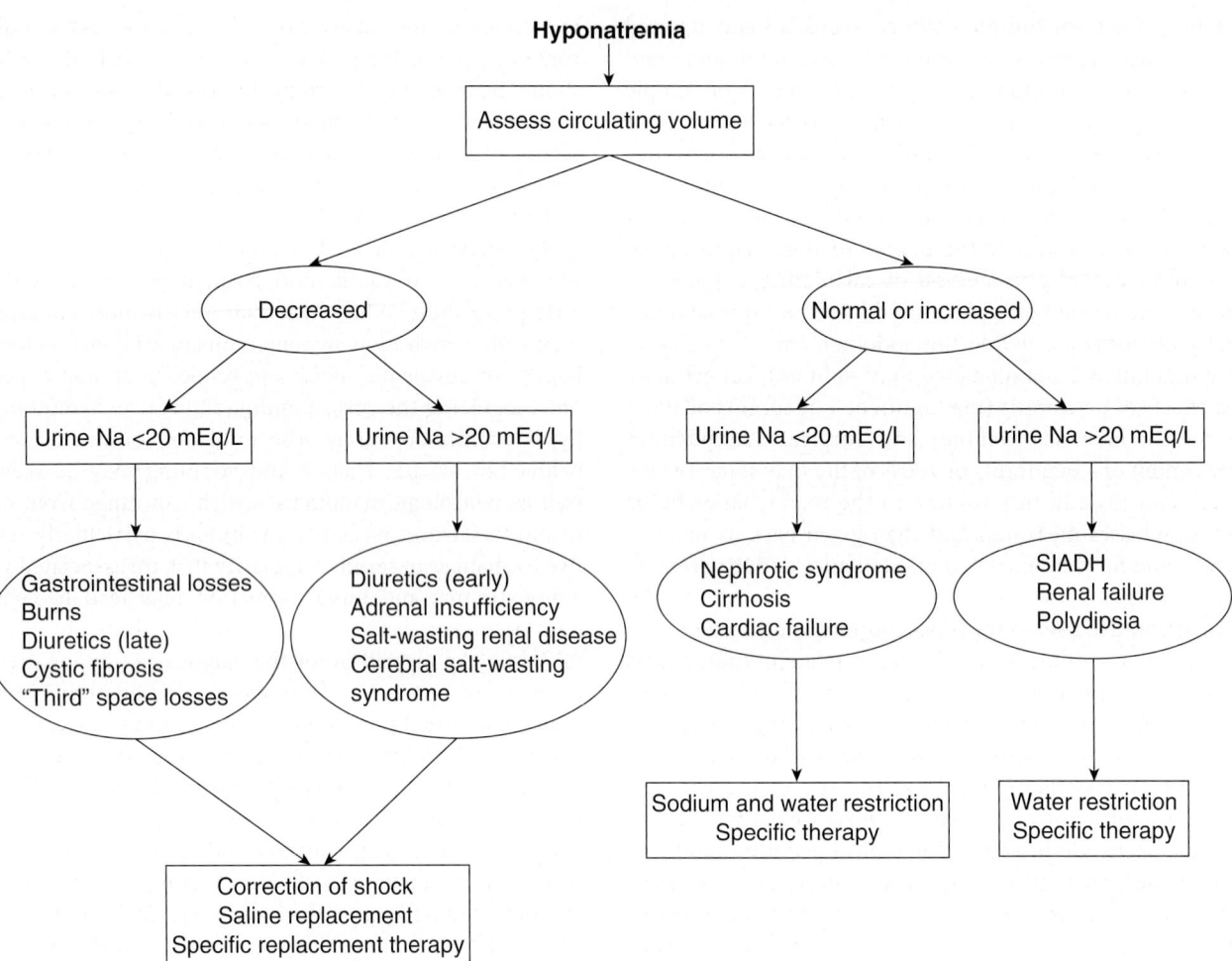

**FIGURE 5-1** Algorithm for the assessment of hyponatremia. From Perkins RM, Levin DL. *Pediatr Clin North Am* 1980;27(3):567, with permission.

secondary to parenteral nutrition or potassium-containing fluids. Hyperkalemia will be demonstrated on an electrocardiogram (ECG) as peaked T waves followed by widening of the QRS complex. When serum levels approach 9 mEq/L, ventricular fibrillation is seen but may occur with any elevated level. Table 5-5 lists an approach to symptomatic hyperkalemia.

Hypokalemia (serum K concentration <3mEq/L) has multiple causes, which include decreased intake or increased excretion in the urine or gastrointestinal tract. Severe diarrhea or administration of loop diuretics is a frequent cause seen in hospitalized patients. Asymptomatic mild hypokalemia may not require treatment except in the patient receiving digitalis. Symptomatic patients should be first treated

with oral supplementation if possible with a dose ranging from 0.5 to 1 mEq/kg. If intravenous replacement of large concentrations of potassium is necessary, continuous cardiac monitoring in an ICU setting is recommended. In addition, frequent monitoring of serum potassium levels is recommended during oral or intravenous replacement to avoid hyperkalemia. Difficulty replacing potassium should prompt a reevaluation of ongoing losses or evaluating the serum concentration of magnesium.

| TABLE 5-4 | Treatment of Symptomatic Hyponatremia |
|---|---|

Calculate Na+ deficit needed to bring serum Na+ to 125 mEq/L
(125 − observed Na+) × weight (kg) × 0.6 = mEq/L

Administer 2 mL of 3% NaCl/mEq required, as calculated above, over 5-30 min, based on acuteness of situation

Closely follow serum Na+ level and potential for fluid overload

| TABLE 5-5 | Treatment of Hyperkalemia |
|---|---|

1. Stop potassium administration
2. Give 50 mg/kg calcium gluconate IV over 5-15 min with ECG monitoring; watch for bradycardia
3. Give 1-2 mEq/kg NaHCO$_3$ IV over 5 min
4. Give 4 mL/kg glucose insulin as bolus, then IV at 4-8 mL/kg/h (4 units regular insulin/100 mL of D$_{25}$); may increase to 6 units/100 mL D$_{25}$ if hyperglycemia develops
5. Sodium polystyrene sulfonate 1 g/kg via rectum in sorbitol
6. Dialysis
7. Loop diuretics may be effective with adequate renal response
8. Monitor K+ frequently

## SELECTED READINGS

Bell EF, Warburton D, Stonestreet BS, Oh W. Effect of fluid administration on the development of symptomatic patent ductus arteriosus and congestive heart failure in premature infants. *N Engl J Med* 1980;302(11):598–604.

Friedman AL. Pediatric hydration therapy: historical review and a new approach. *Kidney Int* 2005;67(1):380–388.

Kelly LK, Seri I. Renal developmental physiology: relevance to clinical care. *NeoReviews* 2008;9;e150–e161.

Letton RW Jr. Electrolyte disorders. In Mattei P, ed. *Surgical Directives: Pediatric Surgery*. Philadelphia, PA: Lippincott Williams & Wilkins; 2003.

Snyder CL, Spilde TL, Rice H. *Fluid Management for the Pediatric Surgical Patient*. http://emedicine.medscape.com/article/936511-overview; 2010. Accessed 30.08.2010.

Verbalis JG, Goldsmith SR, Greenberg A, Schrier RW, Sterns RH. Hyponatremia treatment guidelines 2007: expert panel recommendations. *Am J Med* 2007;120(11 suppl 1):S1–S21.

# Metabolic Response to Illness and Operation

# CHAPTER 6

*Tom Jaksic, Stephen B. Shew, and*
*Ivan M. Gutierrez*

## KEY POINTS

1. Children have reduced metabolic reserves and are particularly susceptible to the adverse effects associated with the catabolic response to critical illness.

2. The metabolic response to injury is proportional to the degree of stress.

3. Both protein degradation and protein synthesis increase during illness; however, quantitatively the former predominates. Hence, net negative protein balance ensues.

4. Adequate supplementation of protein is the most important nutritional intervention in children during illness.

5. In illness the breakdown of existing skeletal muscle stores and consequent release of amino acids is driven by increased requirements. These needs include amino acids to synthesize new proteins and the conversion of these amino acids to form glucose through the process of gluconeogenesis. During the metabolic stress state, this catabolic process is refractory to inhibition by the supplementation of dietary glucose.

6. Energy expenditure can be measured either directly or indirectly. Direct calorimetry is very precise but not practical as a method to use in sick children. Indirect calorimetry requires a leak-free system, which can be difficult to achieve in children with uncuffed endotracheal tubes or not breathing calmly. Other indirect methods include deuterated water and $^{13}$C-labeled bicarbonate, which have been shown to correlate with indirect calorimetry.

7. In neonates and children, the increase in resting energy expenditure associated with surgery is very brief and is measured in hours.

8. Free fatty acids are the primary source of energy in stressed patients. In neonates, with limited stores, this makes them more susceptible to develop essential fatty acid deficiency. The quantity of lipid necessary to obviate fatty acid deficiency is relatively limited. Newer experimental data support the use of lipid-limited omega-3 formulas, in highly selected patients with cholestasis and a long-term requirement for parenteral nutrition.

9. During illness neural pathways, hormones, and inflammatory mediators mediate the prolonged metabolic response. The ability to effectively modulate these responses could result in an amelioration of the net negative protein balance that exists during stress states. Neural pathway modulation is achieved with adequate sedation and analgesia and has been shown to decrease the hypercatabolic state in ill neonates. Hormonal and inflammatory mediator modulation remains experimental at this time.

## INTRODUCTION

Surgery, trauma, and sepsis are accompanied by a constellation of metabolic aberrations that tend to be profound and predictable. Sir David P. Cuthbertson described the fundamental aspects of this metabolic response to injury in the adult over 50 years ago. By observing patients with long-bone fractures and utilizing complementary animal models, he determined that the excessive output of nitrogen following the stress of injury was a result of the catabolism of whole-body protein rather than merely the loss of muscle mass surrounding the site of injury. Diet, particularly protein intake, affected the degree of catabolism. Regardless of the etiology of the injury, the metabolic response seemed to be stereotypic and was characterized by a short "ebb" phase marked by relative hypometabolism followed by a subsequent prolonged rise in metabolic activity termed the "flow" phase. The mechanisms for these changes, however, remained largely obscure until Francis D. Moore carefully elucidated the hormonal and substrate response to surgery. In the early 1980s, a class of short peptide mediators called cytokines were isolated from human white blood cells, and it became evident that neural and endocrine changes accompanying injury along with the release of these peptides were responsible for the unified metabolic response to injury. Recent research has demonstrated that the metabolic sequelae of illness and operation in the neonate and child qualitatively resemble those in the adult, although profound quantitative differences exist. Overall, it is necessary to understand these metabolic alterations in order to design improved therapies to augment the short-term benefits of the pediatric metabolic stress response while obviating its long-term harmful effects.

## METABOLIC RESERVES

Children and adults rely on the metabolism of carbohydrates, lipids, and proteins to meet the catabolic demands of injury. Table 6-1 outlines the macronutrient metabolic reserves of reference neonates, children, and adults in terms of percentage of total body weight. Carbohydrate stores remain constant and do not afford significant reserves at any time during maturation. Lipid stores are low at birth and increase somewhat through development, with premature infants having even greater proportionately reduced reserves. The most striking difference in body composition between a healthy adult and a child or neonate is the quantity of protein available in times of injury. Adults have triple the protein stores that neonates possess, and even the elderly have proportionately twice the quantity of protein present in the neonate.

Not only do neonates and children have reduced stores, they have much higher baseline requirements. The resting energy expenditure for adults is one third that reported for growing premature neonates when standardized for weight. This inverse relationship of higher energy expenditure with decreased body weight also holds between mammalian species and is partially related to body surface area. Another obvious etiology for the increased demand is the need for growth itself. The quantity of energy and protein required to obtain optimal growth rates in term neonates and children compared to the requirement for weight and protein balance in adults is listed in Table 6-2. The protein requirements of the full-term neonate are about 3 times those of the adult, with the 10-year-old child more closely resembling the adult. Congruent with this trend, stable premature neonates minimally require 2.8 g/kg/day of protein in order to maintain growth rates approximating that in utero, which is 3.5 times the requirement for protein balance in the adult.

Thus, the child, and particularly the neonate, is potentially much more susceptible to the deleterious effects of protracted catabolic stress imposed by injury because of the presence of reduced stores and markedly increased baseline metabolic demands.

| TABLE 6-1 | Body Composition of Humans at Birth, Childhood, and as Nonobese Adults (Percent Total Body Weight) | | |
|---|---|---|---|
| | % Fat | % Protein | % Carbohydrate |
| Birth | 14 | 11 | 0.4 |
| 10 years | 17 | 15 | 0.4 |
| Adult | 19 | 34 | 0.4 |

| TABLE 6-2 | Recommended Energy and Protein Requirements in Healthy Humans | |
|---|---|---|
| Age | Protein Requirement (g/kg/day) | Energy Requirement (kcal/kg/day) |
| Birth | 2.2 | 120 |
| 10 years | 1 | 70 |
| Adult | 0.8 | 35 |

## NUTRIENT METABOLISM

The pediatric response to illness and operation has predictable effects on protein, energy, carbohydrate, and lipid metabolism. Increased intracellular utilization and enhanced interorgan transport are its hallmarks. Alterations in vitamin and trace mineral nutrition appear less pronounced, although much additional research is needed to accurately assess requirements. An understanding of these changes in nutrient metabolism allows for the provision of metabolic support to facilitate growth and recovery in even the most severely ill child (Table 6-1).

### Protein Metabolism

Amino acids are the key building blocks required for growth and tissue repair. The majority of amino acids (98%) reside in proteins, with the remainder being in the free amino acid pool. Proteins themselves are not static, as they are continually degraded and synthesized in a process termed protein turnover. The reutilization of amino acids released from protein breakdown is extensive, as is evidenced by the fact that protein turnover is more than 2 times protein intake. Newborns have a protein turnover of 6.7 g/kg/day, whereas adults have a protein turnover of approximately 3.5 g/kg/day. A salient advantage of having high protein turnover is that a continual flow of amino acids is available for new protein synthesis; hence, maximal adaptability is present in times of injury. This process does, however, consume energy and is partially responsible for the elevated resting energy expenditure evident in traumatized patients.

In significantly stressed patients such as those with severe burn injury or with pulmonary insufficiency requiring extracorporeal membrane oxygenation, protein turnover is twice that in normal subjects (Table 6-2). Generally, there is a redistribution of amino acids away from skeletal muscle to the wound, tissues involved in the inflammatory response, and the liver. Acutely needed enzymes, serum proteins, and glucose are thus synthesized. There is also a marked rise in the circulation of hepatically derived acute-phase proteins (ie, fibrinogen, haptoglobin, $\alpha^1$-antitrypsin, transferrin $\alpha^1$-acid glycoprotein, and C-reactive protein) and a concomitant decrease in hepatically derived nutrient transport proteins such as albumin and retinol-binding protein. Although an increase in both whole-body protein synthesis and whole-body protein degradation exists in illness, it is the latter that predominates. Thus, patients after illness manifest net negative protein balance, which clinically may be noted by weight loss, negative nitrogen balance, and skeletal muscle wasting.

One of the driving forces for the catabolism of muscle is the unbridled production of glucose from amino acids (gluconeogenesis). Glucose is the preferred substrate for the brain, red blood cells, and the renal medulla as well as being the most versatile fuel for energy production elsewhere in the body. Interestingly, the provision of dietary glucose alone is relatively ineffective in quelling endogenous glucose production in stressed states. Gluconeogenesis is evident in illness, from adults to premature neonates, and actually appears, on a per-kilogram basis, to be accentuated in low-body-weight patients (presumably because the brain, a glucose-requiring organ, is proportionately larger in this cohort).

In fasting subjects, alanine and glutamine are readily synthesized by muscle and account for over 60% of the total amino acids released from this tissue, and in ill and injured patients, alanine and glutamine transport from muscle is further accentuated. Alanine, by deamination to pyruvate, contributes 3 carbon units to the liver for glucose production, and glutamine serves a dual role as an intestinal energy source and gluconeogenic precursor. Glutamine given intravenously (or enterally) promotes mammalian intestinal growth and development; however, it is not a classically essential nutrient in that it is readily synthesized in adults and neonates. Whether glutamine supplementation may be of benefit in maintaining intestinal integrity in stressed states remains unclear. One study has suggested a decreased incidence of systemic sepsis, although not necrotizing enterocolitis, in enterally fed very low-birth-weight infants when glutamine supplementation was given. The study unfortunately lacked an isonitrogenous control group. About one-half of the glutamine liberated from the muscle is converted to alanine in the intestine and then transported, via the portal vein, to the liver. Hepatic glucose is then produced and released to the bloodstream to become an available energy source for the brain, wound, and even muscle. This interchange between muscle and liver is termed the glucose–alanine cycle. Two further important substrate cycles are present within the liver. Because hepatic gluconeogenesis utilizes the carbon skeletons produced by the deamination of amino acids, the ammonia moiety released must be detoxified by the liver through the urea cycle, which generates urea as a soluble end product. The urea is then able to be safely excreted from the body in the urine. Glycolysis is often activated as a mode of energy production because of the anaerobic environment of some injured tissues. Although this process is less than 10% as efficient as the aerobic oxidation of glucose, its 3-carbon product lactate may be reutilized by the liver by reduction to pyruvate and subsequent resynthesis of glucose. This process is termed the Cori cycle. Figure 6-1 summarizes the effects on endogenous substrate utilization imposed by illness or surgery.

Although the catabolism of skeletal muscle to generate glucose is an excellent short-term adaptation in children, it is limited in duration because of the reduced stores available. Without elimination of the inciting stress for catabolism, the progressive loss of diaphragmatic and intercostal muscle leads to respiratory compromise while the loss of cardiac muscle may lead to fatal arrhythmia after approximately one third of the lean body mass dissipates. Fortunately, amino acid nutritional supplementation does improve protein balance, and the mechanism for this change in ill premature neonates appears to be an increase in protein synthesis while protein degradation rates remain constant. The quantity of protein administration required to optimally enhance protein accretion is higher in unwell than in stable children. Infants demonstrate 25% higher protein degradation after surgery, 100% increase in urinary nitrogen excretion with bacterial sepsis, and 100% increase in protein breakdown if they are ill enough to require extracorporeal membrane oxygenation. Children under treatment for cancer also demonstrate increased net protein breakdown.

The quality, or precise amino acid composition, of formulas that best increase whole-body protein balance has yet to be determined, although stable isotope techniques now exist to address this issue. Neonates have immature biosynthetic pathways that alter their capacity for the synthesis of specific amino acids. A conditional essentiality for the amino acid histidine is present until about 6 months of age, and current data suggest that the biosynthetic pathways for cysteine, taurine, and proline may be of limited capacity in the premature neonate. There is little doubt that specific disease states may further accentuate certain amino acid requirements as exemplified by the increased proline demands noted in severe burn injury.

The provision of adequate dietary protein required to maximize protein synthesis, facilitate wound healing and the inflammatory response, as well as preserve skeletal muscle protein mass is the single most important nutritional intervention in ill or postoperative children. The quantity of protein (or amino acid solution) administered should be 3 to 4 g/kg/day for low-birth-weight infants, 2 to 3 g/kg/day for term neonates, and 1.5 g/kg/day for older children. Certain severely stressed states may require additional protein supplementation; hence, growth rates must be monitored closely. Nitrogen balance determination is also clinically useful but has an inherent bias toward apparent protein accrual when none actually exists. Excessive protein administration should be avoided, as toxicity to protein allotments of 6 g/kg/day in neonates has been reported and includes azotemia, pyrexia, a higher incidence of strabismus, and somewhat lower IQ.

## Energy Metabolism

Increases in energy requirement during acute illness and following surgery closely parallel the elevated protein needs. Protein retention is augmented by an adequate energy allotment, and this is particularly evident when protein intake is marginal. A careful appraisal of energy requirements in stressed states is required, as both underestimates and overestimates of energy needs are associated with potentially deleterious consequences.

The energy requisites of ill children and neonates are dependent on their resting metabolic rate, degree of illness, physical activity, and need for growth. Formally, resting energy expenditure encompasses the basal metabolic rate plus diet-induced thermogenesis (the heat generated by the consumption of food); however, the latter is quantitatively small even in neonates. Resting energy requirements may be

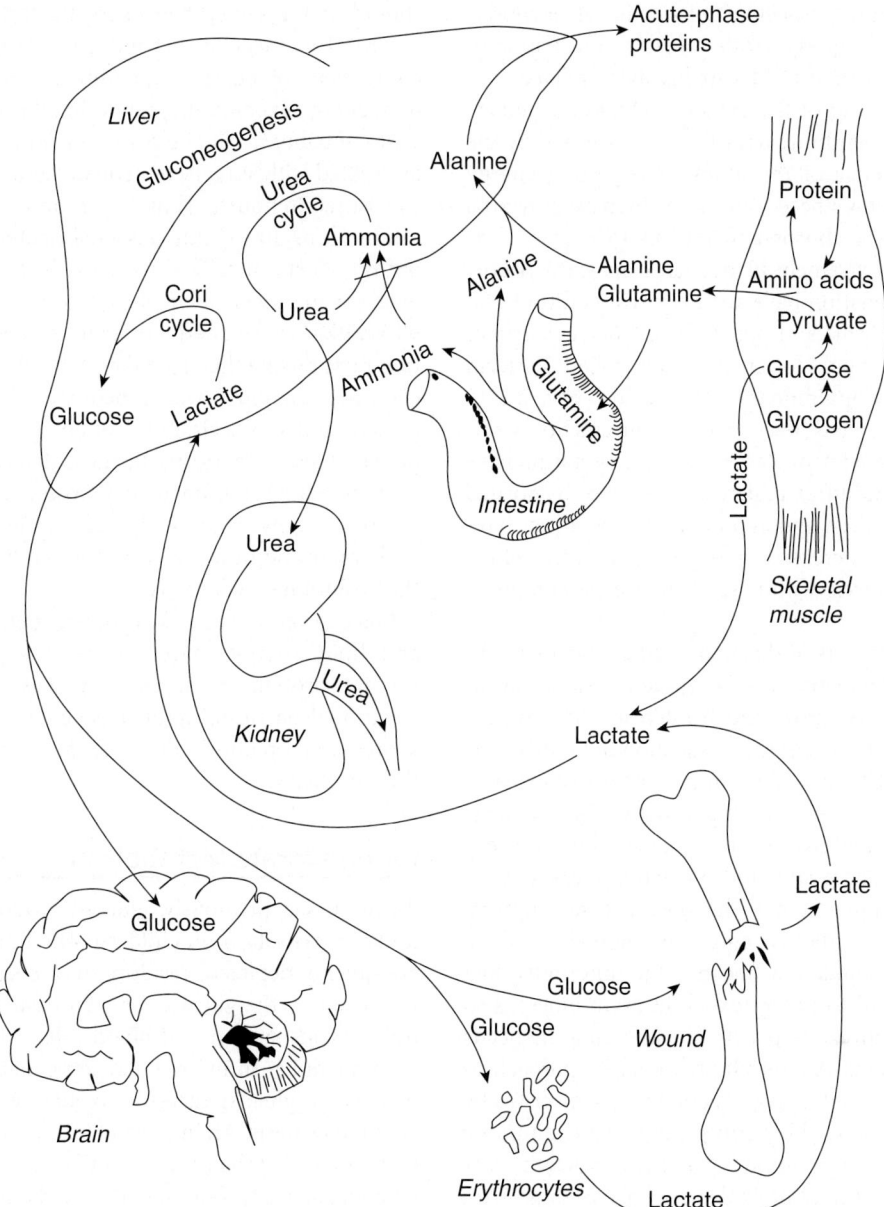

**FIGURE 6-1** Diagrammatic representation of the metabolic response to illness or operation. The endogenous utilization of substrates after injury is characterized by the release of alanine and glutamine from protein breakdown in skeletal muscle and the gastrointestinal tract for subsequent conversion to glucose and acute-phase proteins in the liver. The newly generated glucose can be utilized by those tissues of the body that are glucose-obligate, such as the wound and central nervous system. The by-products of anaerobic metabolism (ie, lactic acid) are then transferred to the liver for reconversion into glucose via the Cori cycle.

determined directly or indirectly. The direct method measures the heat released by a subject at rest and is based on the principle that all energy is eventually converted to heat. In practice, a subject is placed in a thermally isolated chamber, and the heat dissipated is accurately measured for a prolonged period. Although extremely precise, this technology is not easily applicable to pediatric patients. The indirect methods all rely on the estimation of energy production based on the quantities of $O_2$ consumed and/or $CO_2$ produced by the whole body during a specific time interval. Indirect calorimetry, the most venerable technique, relies on the measurement of $VO_2$ (the volume of oxygen consumed) and $VCO_2$ (the volume

of $CO_2$ produced) and usually a correction factor based on urinary nitrogen excretion to calculate the energy production rate. In practice, this involves the creation of a leak-free system, the use of a microcomputer-controlled gas exchange measurement device, termed a metabolic cart, and a 24-hour urinary nitrogen collection. Intubated patients with uncuffed endotracheal tubes and those who are not breathing calmly or regularly pose difficulties. Two newer stable isotope techniques with the advantage of not requiring a leak-free system, doubly labeled water ($^2H_2^{18}O$), and $^{13}C$-labeled bicarbonate, have also been used successfully in pediatric surgical patients to assess total energy expenditure over a period of several days and several hours, respectively. For clinical purposes, all of the indirect techniques provide valuable information in pediatric patients, and their results are highly correlated.

The extent and timing of the evident increase in pediatric resting energy expenditure appear to be governed by the severity and persistence of the illness. The resting energy expenditure in the flow phase of injury is increased by 50% in children with severe burns and returns to normal during convalescence. Extremely ill neonates on extracorporeal membrane oxygenation have an energy expenditure that exceeds published norms and persists after the cessation of extracorporeal life support for an extended period. Preterm neonates with bronchopulmonary dysplasia also have a 25% increase in energy needs over basal requirements. Conversely, stable extubated neonates 5 days after operation have resting energy expenditures that resemble those of normal infants. In fact, newborns undergoing major operations have only a transient 20% increase in energy expenditure, which returns to baseline levels within 12 hours unless complications ensue.

The quantitative aspects of this increased energy expenditure, particularly in patients who continue to remain ill for extended periods, have drawn much interest. The prospective evaluation of a linear regression equation to predict resting energy expenditure in stable surgical neonates explains approximately 80% of the variability noted. The generation of predictive equations in critical illness, however, has been markedly less successful, and the actual measurement of energy expenditure remains the only accurate option. Although standard predictive equations can come close to approximating population means, the interindividual variability with regard to energy expenditure in illness is so high that these equations do poorly in estimating the needs for a particular patient. A clinically reasonable approach to determine precisely total energy requirements in critically ill children is to measure the resting energy expenditure by metabolic cart and then multiply by a stress or activity factor to compensate for the additional energy needs for growth, wound healing, and physical activity. In convalescent pediatric burn patients, this factor appears to be 1.2. A clinical surgical stress score for surgical neonates has been evolved but has not been correlated directly with actual substrate requirements. Neonatal serum levels of C-reactive protein have also been only qualitatively correlated with energy expenditure in surgical neonates.

In clinical practice, the pediatric surgeon rarely has the benefit of measured resting energy expenditure or the use of a validated conversion factor. Fortunately, good reference data exist in children of various ages to allow for a safe and adequate energy allotment in most patients provided that a few basic principles are borne in mind. In healthy children, resting energy expenditures is approximately 65% to 70% of the total energy expenditure, with the remainder of energy needs made up of energy used for physical activity, growth, and diet-induced thermogenesis. After an initial very short ebb phase, the resting energy expenditures of ill patients tend to be higher than those of comparable controls, but their activity levels (which usually make up 25%-30% of total energy expenditure) tend to be proportionately lower. Because the growth rates for healthy and ill children ideally

should be the same, their energetic costs are similar in this regard. The effect of diet-induced thermogenesis, the final component of energy expenditure, comprises only 5% of total energy expenditure, rendering this a relatively insignificant contributor. The increase in resting energy expenditure associated with surgery in neonates and children is very brief (measured in hours). Thus, the recommended dietary caloric intake for healthy children is a reasonable starting point in all but the most critically ill patients. Postoperative parenterally fed neonates given adequate amino acid intake require 85 to 90 kcal/kg/day of energy to achieve adequate protein accretion rates during the first 3 days following surgery. Ventilated extremely low-birth-weight neonates receiving 3 g/kg/day of protein and 105 kcal/kg/day of energy subjected to surgical patent ductus arteriosus ligation demonstrate marked net protein synthesis immediately postoperatively. Overfeeding calories is, however, of no benefit to the maintenance of lean body mass and only results in the synthesis of excess fat and the evolution of a fatty liver.

Once protein needs have been met, both carbohydrate and lipid energy sources have similar beneficial effects on net protein synthesis in pediatric surgical patients. A rational partitioning of these energy-yielding substrates is predicted on knowledge of carbohydrate and lipid utilization in illness.

## Carbohydrate Metabolism

As discussed previously, glucose production and availability are a priority in ill children. The limited glycogen stores are quickly depleted, resulting in a need for gluconeogenesis to supply the glucose for vital tissues including the central nervous system, red blood cells, white blood cells, and renal medulla. In injured and septic adults, there is a 3-fold increase in glucose turnover, oxidation, and an elevation in gluconeogenesis. An important feature of the metabolic stress response is that the provision of dietary glucose does not halt gluconeogenesis; consequently, the catabolism of muscle proteins continues. It is clear, however, that a combination of glucose and amino acids effectively improves protein balance in illness, even in premature neonates with respiratory distress during the first week of life, primarily by augmenting protein synthesis.

In early nutritional support regimens for surgical patients, glucose and amino acid formulations with minimal lipids (only to obviate fatty acid deficiency) were often utilized. A further tendency existed to provide energy allotments well over requirements. As may be predicted, the excess glucose was synthesized to fat, resulting in a net generation of carbon dioxide. The synthesis of fat from glucose has a respiratory quotient (RQ), defined as the ratio of $CO_2$ produced to $O_2$ consumed, of about 8.7. In clinical situations, this high RQ is not attained, as glucose is never purely used for fatty acid synthesis. Nonetheless, the provision of excess glucose will result in an elevated RQ and thus increase the ventilatory burden on the child. The mean RQ in postsurgical neonates fed a high-glucose diet was approximately 1, while comparable neonates fed with less glucose, and lipids at 4 g/kg/day, had an RQ of 0.83. In contrast to glucose metabolism, excess lipids are merely stored as triglycerides and do not result in an augmentation of $CO_2$ production. Utilizing high-glucose total parenteral nutrition, hypermetabolic adult patients fed excess caloric allotments had a 30% increase in $O_2$ consumption, a 57% increase in $CO_2$ production, and 71% elevation in minute ventilation. Thus, avoidance of overfeeding and the utilization of a mixed fuel system of nutrition employing both glucose and lipids to yield energy theoretically and practically of utility in stressed patients, many of whom also have respiratory failure. Such an approach also often obviates problems with hyperglycemia in the relatively insulin-resistant ill patient.

## Lipid Metabolism

Lipid metabolism, analogously to protein and carbohydrate metabolism, is generally accelerated by illness and trauma. Initially during the brief ebb phase following trauma or in early septic shock, lipid utilization is compromised, and triglyceride levels rise with an attendant decrease in the metabolism of intravenously administered lipids. In the predominant flow phase of injury, however, adult patients demonstrate lipid turnover rates 2- to 4-fold higher than in comparable controls, and they are proportional to the degree of injury. Conceptually similar to the increased protein turnover noted in illness, this process involves the recycling of free fatty acids and glycerol into, and hydrolysis from, triglycerides. Both metabolic processes result in a continual flow of substrates through the plasma pool, although at an energetic cost, which is reflected by an elevation in the resting metabolic rate. Approximately 30% to 40% of the released fatty acids are oxidized for energy, and the RQ values postinjury are in the vicinity of 0.8. Thus, this suggests that free fatty acids are, in fact, the prime source of energy in stressed patients. When subjected to uncomplicated abdominal surgery, infants and children have a quantitatively small but statistically significant reduction in RQ, implying an increased oxidation of free fatty acids. Neonatal surgical patients demonstrate a decline in plasma triglycerides, also consistent with an increased use of free fatty acids for energy production. The glycerol, released along with free fatty acids from triglycerides, can be converted to pyruvate, which then, in turn, may be utilized as a gluconeogenic precursor. As with other catabolic processes in illness and trauma, the provision of dietary glucose does not decrease glycerol clearance or diminish lipid recycling.

Normal ketone body metabolism is markedly altered by severe illness. The product of incomplete fatty acid and pyruvate oxidation is acetyl-CoA, which, through a condensation reaction within the hepatocyte, forms the ketone bodies acetoacetate and β-hydroxybutyrate. In starved healthy subjects, a major adaptation to help preserve skeletal muscle mass is the use of ketone bodies generated by the liver as an energy source for the brain (which cannot directly oxidize free fatty acids). However, in the 3-day period following trauma, there is a negligible elevation in serum ketone body levels as compared to healthy fasting controls. This observation may be understood in light of serum insulin levels, as ketogenesis is inhibited by even low concentrations of the hormone, a fact clearly evident to physicians by the absence of ketotic problems in type II diabetes. Hence, the high insulin concentrations seen in severe injury and after major operations ablate the ketotic adaptation of starvation.

The energy needs of the injured patient are met largely by the mobilization and oxidation of free fatty acids. In conjunction with these increased demands, ill neonates have limited lipid stores. Hence, they evolve biochemical essential fatty acid deficiency within 1 week if administered a fat-free diet. In infants, linoleic and linolenic acid, are considered essential, with arachidonic acid and docosahexaenoic acid (DHA) deemed as possibly conditionally essential. When there is a lack of dietary linoleic acid, the formation of arachidonic acid (a tetraene) by desaturation and chain elongation cannot occur, and the same pathway entrains available oleic acid to form 5,8,11-eicosatrienoic acid (a triene). Empirically, a triene-to-tetraene ratio greater than 0.4 is characteristic of essential fatty acid deficiency. The clinical syndrome consists of dermatitis, alopecia, thrombocytopenia, increased susceptibility to bacterial infection, and failure to thrive. To obviate essential fatty acid deficiency in injured infants, the prompt allotment of linoleic acid and linolenic acid is recommended at 4.5% and 0.5% of total calories, respectively.

The provision of commercially available lipid solutions to parenterally fed surgical neonates obviates the risk of essential fatty acid deficiency, results in improved protein utilization, and does not significantly increase carbon dioxide production or metabolic rate. These advantages, however, are balanced by some potential risks. The administration of lipids in excess of the patient's ability to metabolize them can result in hypertriglyceridemia and increased plasma concentrations of free fatty acids. The free fatty acids displace unconjugated bilirubin from albumin and can result in kernicterus. In very low-birth-weight infants, lipid infusion rates restricted to 2 to 3 g/kg/day minimize this problem. The administration of fat emulsions has also been associated with an inhibition of polymorphonuclear leukocyte function and with an interference of pulmonary diffusing capacity, resulting in hypoxemia. A neonatal intensive care unit case–control study has shown that neonates with coagulase-negative staphylococcal bacteremia were 5.8 times as likely as controls to have received intravenous fat emulsions before the onset of the infection. A prospective randomized trial of intravenous fat infusion in adult trauma patients noted an increased incidence of pneumonia and length of hospital stay in patients receiving lipids. The latter report unfortunately did not employ isocaloric controls, so it is unclear if the excess calories or the lipids per se may have been deleterious. Although the evidence is far from conclusive, at present the possible adverse effects of lipid administration have resulted in most centers starting lipid supplementation in ill neonates and children at 0.5 g/kg/day and advancing over a period of days to 2 to 4 g/kg/day while closely monitoring triglyceride levels. Lipid administration is usually restricted to a maximum of 30% to 40% of total calories, although this practice has not been validated by clinical trials. Newer experimental data support the use of omega-3 intravenous lipid formulations at 1 g/kg/day, in highly selected patients with cholestasis and a long-term requirement for parenteral nutrition.

## Vitamin and Trace Mineral Metabolism

Vitamin and trace mineral metabolism in ill and postoperative pediatric patients has not been well studied. For the neonate and child, the fat-soluble vitamins A, D, E, and K, as well as the water-soluble vitamins, ascorbic acid, thiamine, riboflavin, pyridoxine, niacin, pantothenate, biotin, folate, and vitamin $B_{12}$, are all required and are routinely administered. Because vitamins are not stoichiometrically consumed in biochemical reactions but rather act as catalysts, the administration of a large supplement of vitamins in stressed states is not logical from a nutritional standpoint. The trace minerals that are required for normal development are zinc, iron, copper, selenium, manganese, iodide, molybdenum, and chromium. Trace minerals are usually used in the synthesis of the active sites of a ubiquitous and extraordinarily important class of enzymes called metalloenzymes. There are over 200 zinc metalloenzymes alone, and both DNA and RNA polymerases are included in this group. As with vitamins, the role of metalloenzymes is to act as catalysts; hence, unless there are excessive losses such as enhanced zinc loss with severe diarrhea, large nutritional requirements would not be anticipated in illness. The Recommended Dietary Allowances in the United States are reviewed periodically and are set to meet the vitamin and trace mineral needs of practically all healthy individuals. These levels have been used in stressed children, and at present little evidence exists that they are nutritionally inadequate. In children with severe hepatic failure, copper and manganese accumulation occurs. Therefore, parenteral trace mineral supplementation is limited to once per week in these patients.

The pharmacologic use of vitamins and trace minerals in pediatric illness is controversial. Reviews of both vitamin and trace mineral toxicity demonstrate that excessive dosage is clearly a health risk. The use of vitamin A supplementation to facilitate the orderly regeneration of airways in premature neonates (a group that appears be relatively vitamin A deficient) has been perhaps the best-studied model. A randomized, blinded, controlled clinical trial has shown that preterm neonates supplemented with a liberal, although far from toxic, amount of vitamin A for 4 weeks developed less bronchopulmonary dysplasia than did controls. Further corroborative studies are necessary to substantiate this finding.

## Summary of Nutrient Metabolism

The pediatric metabolic response to injury and operation is proportional to the degree of stress and causes an increase in the turnover of proteins, fats, and carbohydrates, thus making needed substrates readily available for the immune response and wound healing. Because this process requires energy, the resting energy expenditure of ill patients increases. Whole-body protein degradation rates are elevated out of proportion to synthetic rates, and negative protein balance also ensues. The catabolism of limited skeletal muscle stores is driven by the increased need for new proteins and by gluconeogenesis, which is refractory to inhibition by glucose in the diet. Glucose remains the major energy source for the brain, and in contradistinction to starvation, ketone body synthesis is not elevated. Free fatty acid oxidation is activated and continues as the primary fuel for most of the body. An appropriately designed mixed fuel system of nutritional support replete in protein does not quell this metabolic response, but can result in anabolism and continued growth in ill children.

## METABOLIC RESPONSE MECHANISMS

Although the provision of substrates can usually support the pediatric surgical patient until the illness is resolved, much interest is currently being paid to avoiding the initiation and ameliorating the consequences of a prolonged metabolic response to injury. In order to do so, a consideration of the mechanisms engendering this adaptation is necessary. Three integrated systems are involved: neural pathways, hormones, and inflammatory mediators.

### Neural Pathways

Injury with its attendant pain perception through afferent sensory nerve fibers results in a rapid and direct initiation of the metabolic response to stress. During gestation, cutaneous sensory receptors start to develop at 7 weeks, begin to synapse with the dorsal horn cells before 14 weeks, and are integrated by the thalamus and connected to the cerebrum by 24 weeks. Functional maturity of the neonatal cerebral cortex as suggested by electroencephalographic patterns of sleep and wakefulness may be seen before 30 weeks, and bursts of activity are present bilaterally in the cerebral hemispheres by 20 weeks. Both substance P, a neurotransmitter thought to be associated with pain perception, and opioid receptors are found in the fetus. The in vitro stimulation of 20-week fetal pituitary cells results in the release of endorphins.

The functional nature of this system is implied by the significant increases in blood pressure and heart rate that are evident in premature and full-term unanesthetized neonates subjected to heel sticks and circumcision. A randomized controlled trial of preterm neonates undergoing patent ductus arteriosus ligation with and without the addition of 10 µg/kg of fentanyl to an anesthetic regimen of nitrous oxide and d-tubocurarine demonstrated significantly less hyperglycemia, lower initial levels of gluconeogenic substrates, and, at 2 and 3 days postoperatively, a lower 3-methylhistidine/creatinine ratio (an index of protein catabolism) in the fentanyl group. This study clearly demonstrated that the metabolic response caused by surgery could be blunted by adequate anesthesia in the premature neonate. The magnitude of the metabolic stress response has been related to morbidity and mortality in adult patients; hence, optimal anesthesia and analgesia may improve outcomes after major surgery. Such a view is also supported by data in neonates, who are potentially even more at risk because of reduced stores of skeletal muscle and adipose tissue. Although satisfactory general anesthesia appears to be beneficial in decreasing the catabolism induced by surgery, it has its own primary metabolic effects, which vary according to the specific anesthetic used. For example, isoflurane anesthesia in endotracheally intubated dogs is associated with a rapid decrease in lipolysis, peripheral glucose utilization, and, perhaps most importantly, protein synthesis.

The reduction of protein synthesis is markedly greater than a concurrent modest decrease in protein degradation; thus, net protein catabolism is elevated. Halothane–nitrous oxide anesthesia also results in increased protein losses, suggesting that, from a metabolic standpoint, extended courses of general anesthesia may be harmful.

The neuroendocrine response to injury has been relatively well defined. Once the nociceptive response to injury occurs, the neural impulses are relayed to the brainstem and hypothalamus, thus activating the neuroendocrine axis. Catecholamines are released from the adrenal medulla by the sympathetic nervous system while the secretion of adrenocorticotropic hormone from the anterior pituitary results in a systemic increase in cortisol. Growth hormone release from the anterior pituitary and antidiuretic hormone secretion by the posterior pituitary are also stimulated. Head-injured patients demonstrate marked increases in resting energy expenditure and protein degradation, which are associated with a profound elevation in circulating catecholamines. Sedation markedly reduces this hypercatabolism, and brain death eliminates it.

## Hormones

The hormonal stress response of neonates, children, and adults shares many common features. After injury, an increase occurs in catecholamines, growth hormone, glucagon, cortisol, and aldosterone, which is accompanied by a brief initial suppression in insulin concentration followed by a rapid rise in insulin levels. Overall, the hormonal changes in neonates and children appear to be of greater magnitude but of shorter duration than those in older children and adults. In premature neonates studied after undergoing patent ductus arteriosus ligation with nitrous oxide anesthesia and paralytic agents, glucocorticoid and epinephrine concentrations reached a peak by 6 hours, aldosterone levels returned to normal in 12 hours, and insulin-to-glucagon ratios remained elevated at 24 hours. Although the primary hormonal response appears relatively brief, elevated levels of protein breakdown as reflected by 3-methylhistidine excretion were present at 2 and 3 days after surgery. In full-term neonates undergoing repair of complex congenital heart defects, a similar pattern of hormonal changes is evident, with insulin levels remaining elevated at 24 hours. The effect of age on the pediatric hormonal response to operation appears limited. Patients ranging in age from 2 to 20 years who were subjected to elective surgery under general anesthesia had similar postoperative elevations of cortisol and prolactin. The rise in insulin concentrations following surgery in a group of children ranging in age from 1 month to 10 years was found to be related to the severity of the surgical stress but not to age.

Because survival rates in major injuries, such as burns, are inversely related to lean body mass, persistent protein loss in illness is a major clinical concern. An explanation of this change in intermediary metabolism based solely on currently known hormonal concentrations becomes somewhat of an exercise in rationalization. The catecholamines, glucagon, and cortisol are catabolic hormones; hence, the mobilization of amino acids from skeletal muscle, increased hepatic gluconeogenesis, and lipolysis can be understood on this basis. The relative hyperglycemia that is often present, especially when

dietary glucose is administered, also may be related to these hormones. The persistent increase in net protein degradation is, however, not entirely consistent with the levels of the anabolic hormone insulin found in the serum. Injury in neonates and children results in a very brief initial drop in insulin concentrations followed by an increase in insulin levels over baseline. Although it is known that in healthy subjects even low concentrations of insulin can formidably decrease protein breakdown, this does not seem to be the case in injury. Hence, persistent protein degradation has been postulated to be the result of a postreceptor defect in insulin action. This is partially supported by the finding that burn patients do not demonstrate the same degree of inhibition of protein breakdown as do normal controls when subjected to hyperinsulinemic euglycemic conditions. A randomized prospective study has shown modest improvements in protein balance for children on extracorporeal membrane oxygenation placed on a euglycemic hyperinsulinemic clamp.

Stringent euglycemic control, through the use of insulin infusions, remains highly controversial in the pediatric intensive care unit. The potential benefits include a reduction in infection rates, preservation of lean body mass, and improved survival. The clear danger is the induction of hypoglycemia and associated morbidity and mortality. Continuous glucose monitoring is now feasible in critically ill children and an National Institutes of Health (NIH)-sponsored randomized prospective trial of tight glucose control in pediatric postcardiac bypass patients is ongoing.

Growth hormone is another anabolic hormone elevated in operative or accidental trauma. The administration of modest amounts of recombinant growth hormone to normal subjects while insulin and insulin-like growth factor (IGF-1) concentrations are kept constant resulted in an enhancement of lipolysis and increased protein synthesis in the whole body but not in skeletal muscle. Although the increased fat mobilization is consistent with what is seem in trauma, it must be surmised that the elevations of growth hormone noted in the ill patient are still insufficient to result in net protein synthesis. A confounding feature of examining the effect of growth hormone is that it stimulates the synthesis and release of IGF-1 by the liver. The administration of recombinant IGF-1 alone in humans is associated with lipolysis, increased fatty acid oxidation, increased energy expenditure, and decreased protein oxidation. The injection of 0.2 mg/kg of recombinant growth hormone in children after severe burn injury resulted in increased concentrations of IGF-1 and insulin as well as the catabolic hormones, glucagon, and the catecholamines. Because in clinical studies it is very difficult to control for the concomitant alteration in other hormones induced by recombinant growth hormone, it is rarely possible to say if the effects noted are primary or secondary.

A uniform finding in neonates, children, and adults, after the provision of recombinant human growth hormone, regardless of mode of injury, is an enhancement of fatty acid utilization. Other effects noted in burn patients have been decreased hospital stay, accelerated donor site split-thickness skin graft healing, and stimulated whole-body and leg protein synthesis. The enhancement of leg protein synthesis is presumably a secondary effect. Augmented whole-body protein synthesis has been corroborated by body composition studies, nitrogen balance assessment, and stable isotopic investigations. The major side effect of growth hormone given in the short term has been hyperglycemia, although the mechanism remains to be fully defined. In contrast, IGF-1 seems to act by increasing insulin sensitivity and thus induces hypoglycemia. In extremely ill patients, the modulation of the hormonal response to injury may be of utility in augmenting protein preservation. Currently, the administration of recombinant growth hormone and IGF-1, either individually or in concert, is being explored, and their untoward metabolic side effects are being studied. At present, the hormonal manipulation of the pediatric patient during illness and after trauma remains an experimental technique. The metabolic effects of manipulations such as cardiac bypass and extracorporeal membrane oxygenation that are associated with significant hormonal dilution are also unknown.

## Inflammatory Mediators

The presence of inflammatory mediators, or cytokines, may be found in the circulation within hours of elective surgery or trauma. This group of peptides is secreted by the white blood cells, and they engender some of the prototypic metabolic and inflammatory responses to injury. For the most part, the neonatal cytokine response does not differ significantly from that of older children and adults. The first cytokine to be characterized was interleukin-1 (IL-1), of which IL-1B was found to be the most active isoform. IL-1 is secreted by activated macrophages in response to injury, and it results in the mobilization of leukocytes, the liberation of endorphins, a rise in core body temperature, and anorexia. Although IL-1 was thought initially to be a key stimulant of net protein degradation, more accurate assays have recently brought this concept into question. There, in fact, seems to be no detectable difference in IL-1 levels before and after surgery in the neonate, child, and adult. Studies of IL-1B in sepsis have yielded conflicting data with both an elevation and depression in concentrations being reported in infected infants and children. Interleukin-6 (IL-6) appears to be a markedly more metabolically active cytokine. It is released from activated macrophages and T cells and is found in increased concentrations in the serum of children within 2 hours of surgery, remaining elevated up to 24 to 48 hours postoperatively. IL-6 levels are directly correlated with increased protein turnover, greater protein catabolism, the incidence of postoperative complications, and subsequent mortality. Neonates with sepsis or necrotizing enterocolitis also demonstrate elevations in IL-6 concentrations, which are positively correlated with severity of illness and mortality. Another effect of IL-6 is the reprioritization of hepatic protein synthesis, in times of injury, away from the transport proteins albumin and transferrin to the acute-phase proteins.

Tumor necrosis factor (TNF) is also released by activated macrophages during stress. It is thought to act in cooperation with other major cytokines, such as IL-1B, in activating the release of prostaglandins, which, in turn, produce the hypotension associated with septic shock. In neonates and children with sepsis or necrotizing enterocolitis, TNF serum levels have been consistently elevated. However, this association has not been demonstrated in response to operative stress. The release of interleukin-2, interleukin-8, γ-interferon, and

many growth factors is also known to augment the immunologic and hormonal response to injury, but their precise effect on metabolism remains unclear.

At present, no effective in vivo experimental modulation of cytokine action exists to ameliorate the negative nitrogen balance accompanying injury. In vitro, the administration of cyclooxygenase inhibitors does decrease cytokine-mediated prostaglandin $E_2$ synthesis and consequent protein breakdown.

## CONCLUSION

Injury and operation in the pediatric population result in a series of predictable metabolic changes characterized by increased protein, carbohydrate, and lipid utilization with consequent negative protein balance and increased resting energy expenditure. All of these alterations are proportional to the magnitude of the stress imposed. A summary of the metabolic changes accompanying injury and operation as contrasted to the adaptive response to starvation is outlined in Table 6-3. Neonates and children are particularly susceptible to the loss of lean body mass and its attendant increased morbidity and mortality because they have an intrinsic lack of endogenous stores and greater baseline requirements. Therapeutic nihilism is, however, unwarranted, as the judicious administration of carbohydrates, lipids, vitamins, trace minerals, and particularly protein can promote growth and wound healing in even the very ill child. Although the exact profile of substrate allotment remains to be perfected, the

| TABLE 6-3 | Summary of Hormone and Substrate Responses to Illness and Operation Compared to Starvation | |
|---|---|---|
| | **Starvation** | **Illness/ Operation** |
| Glucagon | ↑ | ↑ |
| Insulin | ↓ | ↓ then ↑ |
| Catecholamines | ↓ | ↑ |
| Cortisol | ↓ | ↑ |
| Protein turnover | ↓ | ↑↑ |
| Skeletal protein breakdown | ↑ then nl or ↓ | ↑↑ |
| Amino acid oxidation | ↑ then nl or ↓ | ↑↑ |
| Skeletal protein synthesis | ↓↓ | ↑ |
| Protein balance | ↓ | ↓–↓↓ |
| Glucose turnover | ↓ | ↑ |
| Fatty acid turnover | ↓ | ↑ |
| Ketone body synthesis | ↑ | ↓ |

nl, normal.

deleterious consequences of a prolonged catabolic response can often be reduced or even eliminated. In addition, the utilization of adequate analgesia and anesthesia is a readily available and proven means of reducing the magnitude of the catabolism associated with operation and injury. Finally, as hormonal and cytokine-mediated metabolic alterations are better understood, therapeutic interventions may become available to directly modulate the metabolic response to illness, thus potentially further improving clinical outcome in pediatric surgical patients.

## SELECTED READINGS

Agus MS, Javid PJ, Piper HG, et al. The effect of insulin infusion upon protein metabolism in neonates on extracorporeal life support. *Ann Surg* 2006;244:536–544.

Agus MS, Jaksic T. Critically low hormone and catecholamine concentrations in the primed extracorporeal life support circuit. *ASIAO J* 2004; 50:65–67.

Anand KJ, Aynsley-Green A. Measuring the severity of surgical stress in newborn infants. *J Pediatr Surg* 1988;23:297–305.

Anand KJS, Brown MJ, Bloom SR, Aynsley-Green A. Studies on the hormonal regulation of fuel metabolism in the human newborn infant undergoing anaesthesia and surgery. *Horm Res* 1985;22:115–128.

Cuthbertson DP. The metabolic response to injury and its nutritional implications: retrospect and prospect. *J Parent Ent Nutr* 1979;3:108–109.

Freeman J, Goldmann DA, Smith NE, et al. Association of intravenous lipid emulsion and coagulase-negative staphyloccocal bacteremia in neonatal intensive care units. *N Engl J Med* 1990;323:301–308.

Goran MI, Peters EJ, Herndon DN, Wolfe RR. Total energy expenditure in burned children using the doubly labeled water technique. *Am J Physiol* 1990;259:E576–E585.

Hunter DC, Jaksic T, Lewis D, et al. Resting energy expenditure in the critically ill: estimations versus measurement. *Br J Surg* 1988;75:875–878.

Jaksic T, Shew SB, Keshen TH, Dzakovic A, Jahoor F. Do critically ill surgical neonates have increased energy expenditure? *J Pediatr Surg* 2001;36:63–67.

Jones MO, Pierro A, Garlick PJ, McNurlan MA, Donnell SC, Lloyd DA. Protein metabolism kinetics in neonates: effect of intravenous carbohydrate and fat. *J Pediatr Surg* 1995;30:458–462.

Jones MO, Pierro A, Hashim IA, et al. Postoperative changes in resting energy expenditure and interleukin 6 level in infants. *Br J Surg* 1994; 81:536–538.

Keshen T, Miller R, Jahoor F, et al. Glucose production and gluconeogenesis are negatively related to body weight in mechanically ventilated, very low birthweight neonates. *Pediatr Res* 1997;41:132–138.

Meis SJ, Dove EL, Bell EF, et al. A gradient layer calorimeter for measurement of energy expenditure of infants. *Am J Physiol* 1994;266: R1052–R1062.

Miller RG, Keshen TH, Jahoor F, Shew SB, Jaksic T. Compartmentation of endogenously synthesized amino acids in neonates. *J Surg Res* 1996;63:199–203.

Piper HG, Alexander JL, Shukla A, et al. Real-time continuous glucose monitoring in pediatric patients during and after cardiac surgery. *Pediatrics* 2006;118:1176–1184.

Powis MR, Smith K, Rennie M, et al. Effect of major abdominal operations on energy and protein metabolism in infants and children. *J Pediatr Surg* 1998;33:49–53.

Puder M, Valim C, Meisel JA, et al. Parenteral fish oil improves outcomes in patients with parenteral nutrition-associated liver injury. *Ann Surg* 2009;250:395–402.

Shew SB, Beckett PR, Keshen TH, Jahoor F, Jaksic T. Validation of a [13C] bicarbonate tracer technique to measure neonatal energy expenditure. *Pediatr Res* 2000;47:787–791.

Shew SB, Keshen TH, Glass NL, Jahoor F, Jaksic T. Ligation of a patent ductus arteriosus under fentanyl anesthesia improves protein metabolism in premature neonates. *J Pediatr Surg* 2000;35:1277–1281.

Sullivan JS, Kilpatrick L, Costarino AT, et al. Correlation of plasma cytokine elevations with mortality rate in children with sepsis. *J Pediatr* 1992; 120:510–515.

van Lingen RA, van Goudoever JB, Luijendijk IHT, et al. Effects of early amino acid administration during total parenteral nutrition on protein metabolism in pre-term infants. *Clin Sci* 1992;82:199–203.

Ward Platt M, Tarbit, MJ, Aynsley-Green A. The effects of anesthesia and surgery on metabolic homeostasis in infancy and childhood. *J Pediatr Surg* 1990;25:472–478.

# Pediatric Surgical Critical Care:
## Cardiopulmonary Monitoring[1], Advanced Hemodynamic Monitoring[2], Acute Cardiopulmonary Resuscitation[1], Pharmacology[3], Respiratory Failure, and ECMO[4]

# CHAPTER 7

*Ronald B. Hirschl[1],*
*Steven L. Moulton, Jane Mulligan, and Victor A. Convertino[2],*
*Pamela D. Reiter and Steven L. Moulton[3],*
*Artur Chernoguz and Jason S. Frischer[4]*

## Conventional Cardiopulmonary Monitoring

### KEY POINTS

1. Pulse oximetry provides a measure of oxygen saturation as well as information on heart rate and perfusion. The end-tidal carbon dioxide ($etCO_2$) helps document effective ventilation; and in patients with healthy lungs, the maximal $etCO_2$ assayed over minutes provides an approximation of the $Paco_2$.

2. The $SvO_2$ level serves as a measure of oxygen dynamics, assessing the adequacy of oxygen delivery as well as consumption.

3. Assessment of central venous pressure should be performed at end-expiration; central venous oxygen saturation ($ScvO_2$) may be used to guide treatment in patients with sepsis.

Monitoring is integral to the management of the critically ill patient and is one of the essential services provided by the intensive care unit (ICU). Whether by invasive or non-invasive means, the overall goal is to maintain cardiovascular and respiratory stability. In this chapter, we discuss monitoring and management of the critically ill patient with particular emphasis on the use of such monitoring to maintain optimal oxygen delivery and perfusion and to interpret and treat cardiovascular and respiratory derangement and pathophysiology.

## TRADITIONAL NONINVASIVE MONITORING

Although monitors are an essential part of modern critical care, they are designed to supplement rather than replace clinical judgment. The physical examination is an important component in the assessment of perfusion and intravascular volume status. Warmth and color of extremities, capillary refill, assessment of oral and ocular mucous membranes, axillary moistness, urinary output measurement in the patient without renal insufficiency, and the fullness of the anterior fontanel in the newborn and infant may be integrated with data gained via invasive and noninvasive monitoring to assess the cardiopulmonary status. Cool, mottled extremity skin, capillary refill greater than 2 seconds, urinary output less than 0.5 mL/kg, orthostatic change with a fall in pressure of 20 mm Hg or a rise in pulse of 20 beats per minute with elevation of the head of the bed, a flat fontanelle, and dry mucous membranes are all clinical parameters that indicate inadequate cardiac output and/or perfusion.

One of the most basic of noninvasive monitoring procedures is that of electrocardiographic monitoring (ECG). Typically, ECG leads are placed on the right upper chest, the left upper chest, and the left lower chest in the anterior axillary line such that data from leads I, II, and $V_1$ are provided. ECG monitoring should be used routinely in all critically ill patients to assess heart rate and evidence for dysrhythmias, metabolic abnormalities, and myocardial ischemia. However, once routine monitoring raises suspicion of an abnormality, the 12-lead ECG is a much more specific and complete means of evaluation.

Core temperature monitoring is crucial in the critically ill child. Because of the relatively high surface area-to-mass ratio, children are at increased risk for hypothermia when compared to adults. In neonates, skin temperature probes reflect core body temperature accurately and may be used to servo-regulate over-bed warmers; whereas in infants and children beyond the neonatal period, rectal, esophageal, bladder, or intravascular probes are effective means for continuous temperature monitoring. Additional means for warming, such as under- and over-body warming blankets, warming of the ventilating gas, warming of administered fluids and blood products, as well as warming ambient temperature should all be considered in the pediatric patient at risk for hypothermia.

Blood pressure should be measured in all critically ill patients using sphygmomanometry even when more invasive means of blood pressure monitoring are in use. The width of the cuff should be 40% of the extremity circumference at the midpoint of the limb, and the length should be twice the recommended width. The approximate systolic blood pressure is first identified during cuff deflation, after which the cuff should be reinflated to a point just above this level. Subsequent slow deflation of the cuff is performed as the systolic pressure is identified at the point where the first of the 5 phases of Korotkoff sounds are audible. The diastolic pressure is noted as the point where those sounds disappear or are abruptly muffled (phase IV or V). A Doppler probe may be useful to ascertain systolic blood pressure in the settings of hypotension, elevated peripheral vascular resistance, and/or poor perfusion by identifying return of pulsatile arterial flow distal to a deflating proximal extremity blood pressure cuff. Automatic blood pressure devices may be programmed to accurately and automatically measure blood pressure at various intervals. The deflating cuff identifies the presence of minute alterations in cuff pressure, which are associated with the appearance and disappearance of the Korotkoff sounds and the mean blood pressure at the point of maximum amplitude of such changes.

## RECENT ADVANCES IN NONINVASIVE MONITORING

### Pulse Oximetry

Pulse oximeters provide more than just oxygen saturation: they also provide information on heart rate and perfusion. As such, the pulse oximeter is one of the most important noninvasive monitoring tools in the ICU. The pulse oximeter probe is usually placed on the fingers or toes. If the probes fail to function appropriately at those sites, more central locations such as the ears, lips, and nose may be used. These devices function by emitting light at 2 wavelengths, usually 660 nm (red) and 940 nm (near infrared), which is transmitted through the tissues to a photodetector. The transmitted light is differentially absorbed by reduced hemoglobin and oxyhemoglobin, which allows estimation of hemoglobin saturation. In addition, the transmission of light changes with each pulsation as a function of the volume of blood in the tissues (Fig. 7-1). This pulsatile change of light absorbency allows determination of the pulse rate. In the setting of poor peripheral perfusion because of low cardiac output, hypothermia,

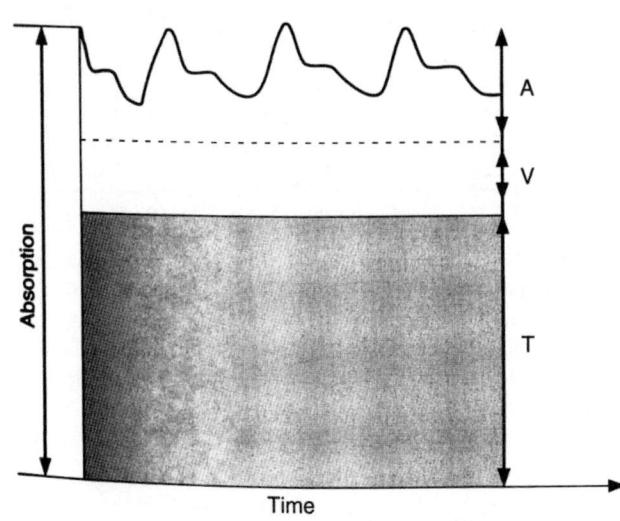

**FIGURE 7-1** The absorption of light for assessment of hemoglobin saturation by a pulse oximeter is illustrated. Light is absorbed by tissue (T), venous blood (V), and arterial blood (A) with the variation in light absorption resulting from alterations in arterial blood volume with each pulsation.

increased vascular resistance, or vascular compromise, device failure should suggest the presence of physiologic compromise at the site of the oximeter. For example, pulse oximeters can be placed on extremities with questionable arterial perfusion in order to provide continuous localized monitoring.

Frequently, with reduced perfusion, patient motion artifact, or methemoglobinemia, the "default" saturation of the device is 85%. It is important to realize, therefore, that if the hemoglobin saturation abruptly decreases to 85%, the patient and device should be assessed for pulse oximeter artifact by noting whether a valid heart rate is displayed by the pulse oximeter. Other sources of error in pulse oximeter analysis include the presence of venous blood pulsation (AV fistula), the presence of nail polish or similar materials on the skin, ambient room light that affects the photodetector, and high levels of carbon monoxide, in which case the oximeter cannot differentiate between carboxyhemoglobin and oxyhemoglobin and overestimates the true hemoglobin oxygen saturation. The presence of fetal hemoglobin does not affect the oxygen saturation reading because hemoglobin F has a similar absorbency to hemoglobin A. The accuracy of the pulse oximeter-derived oxygen saturation may be limited at levels less than 70% to 80%. Intravascular administration of methylene blue or fluorescein induces a falsely low reading because of absorption of light at the particular wavelengths used.

### Carbon Dioxide Monitoring

etCO$_2$ monitoring has been used routinely in the operating room and is now becoming more commonplace in the ICU. Such devices function by assessing the absorption of infrared light as it passes through expired gas. Two techniques are used: sidestream monitoring, in which a sample of expired gas is continuously aspirated and assessed, or mainstream monitoring, which evaluates gas as it is exhaled. A disadvantage

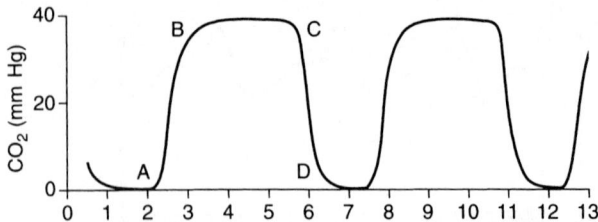

**FIGURE 7-2** The waveform generated by a $CO_2$ analyzer during tidal breathing is shown. The partial pressure of $CO_2$ is 0 mm Hg at the beginning of expiration (**A**) because of the dead space in the conducting airways. The (**B,C**) interval represents the alveolar $P_{CO_2}$. The end-tidal $P_{CO_2}$ is at point C. The $P_{CO_2}$ then decreases during inspiration (**C,D**) before the cycle is repeated.

of the sidestream technique is that tidal volume and minute ventilation measurements may be inaccurate. A disadvantage of the mainstream method is that it requires additional dead space in the ventilating circuit. The techniques are equivalent with regard to accuracy.

The $etCO_2$ helps one to document that ventilation is effectively being performed following endotracheal tube placement and at any time when the endotracheal tube position is in question. Single-use $etCO_2$ detectors may be used to document the same. In addition, in patients with healthy lungs, the maximal $etCO_2$ assayed over a few minutes provides a good approximation of the $Paco_2$ (Fig. 7-2). As such, the $etCO_2$ may be used to follow the effect of ventilator manipulation on $CO_2$ elimination. Unfortunately, ventilation/perfusion mismatch in the setting of respiratory insufficiency often results in a decrease in $etCO_2$ relative to $Paco_2$. In this situation the $etCO_2$ may be useful only for trend analysis. Moreover, the arterial $Pco_2$–$etCO_2$ gradient and the arterial $Pco_2$/$etCO_2$ ratio reflect the degree of ventilation/perfusion mismatch and are useful to monitor therapy.

### Transcutaneous Blood Gas Monitoring

Transcutaneous $Po_2$ ($tcPo_2$) and $Pco_2$ ($tcPco_2$) electrodes assess the diffusion rates of oxygen and carbon dioxide through the skin. The $Po_2$ at the skin is substantially lower (approximately 53 mm Hg) than arterial $Po_2$. To counteract this diffusion-induced reduction in $Po_2$, the electrode and skin are heated to 44°C, which increases capillary $Po_2$ approximately 45 mm Hg, causing the measured $tcPo_2$ and $Pao_2$ to be approximately equal. This puts the skin at risk for burns unless the position of the heated electrode is changed every 6 hours. It is important to recognize that if the hemoglobin–oxygen dissociation curve is shifted, the standardized heating procedure produces inaccurate estimations of $Pao_2$. Both the $tcPo_2$ and $tcPco_2$ are unreliable in patients in shock with low cardiac output and poor perfusion. Because central perfusion is less often compromised than that in the periphery, the electrode is optimally placed on the trunk, avoiding areas of thick skin or hair. The $tcPo_2$ accurately reflects the $Pao_2$ in children and young adults, especially at $Pao_2$ levels less than 60 mm Hg. Because production of $CO_2$ by the skin is enhanced during heating, the $tcPco_2$ measurement may be 20 to 30 mm Hg higher than the $Paco_2$.

Trends in $Pao_2$ and $Paco_2$ can still be followed even though the $tcPo_2$ and $tcPco_2$ values may be inaccurate.

## Cardiac Output

A number of ways to determine cardiac output noninvasively have been investigated, including the following: (1) thoracic electrical bioimpedance, (2) suprasternal Doppler ultrasound, and (3) transesophageal/transtracheal Doppler ultrasound. With transthoracic electrical bioimpedence (TEI), 2 electrodes are placed on either side of the cervical and the lower chest region followed by passage of small currents between each pair of electrodes. Thoracic resistance is a function of the pulsatile change in the fluid volume of the thoracic cavity with each cardiac cycle. An equation based on patient characteristics of height, weight, sex, and deviation from ideal body weight can be utilized to convert measured changes in impedance to cardiac output. Although little interest has been paid to this technique in the past because of low reliability under a variety of circumstances, recent technical advances have provided a more reproducible and accurate method of estimating cardiac output. The feasibility and validity of this technique in the pediatric population has been demonstrated and may offer one practical means for measuring cardiac output in neonates.

Doppler ultrasound may be utilized to assess the velocity of blood flow within the aorta via probes placed at the suprasternal notch, esophagus, or trachea. The cross-sectional area of the aorta is determined either via ultrasound measurement or through a nomogram based on age, sex, height, and weight. Once velocity of blood flow and aortic cross-sectional area are known, cardiac output may be calculated. Although the accuracy and reliability of Doppler-determined cardiac output vary, overall validity appears to be improved when (1) direct measurement of the aortic diameter is used instead of a nomogram, and (2) transesophageal or transtracheal ultrasound is utilized. The Doppler technique cannot be used in patients with aortic stenosis or insufficiency. This technique requires experience in manipulation of the Doppler signal before accurate results can be obtained.

## Echocardiography

Echocardiography is becoming a standard tool in the ICU to assess the cardiovascular status of the patient in shock. While determination of detailed congenital heart anatomy is in the domain of the cardiologist, evaluation of general cardiac function, left ventricular filling, and presence of pericardial effusion and/or cardiac tamponade require little training and can provide substantial information in the newborn, infant, and child with cardiovascular compromise.

## INVASIVE MONITORING

### Systemic Arterial Catheters

Arterial catheter placement is indicated in those patients who require frequent blood pressure monitoring and in those who require more than 2 or 3 blood gas samples per day. The

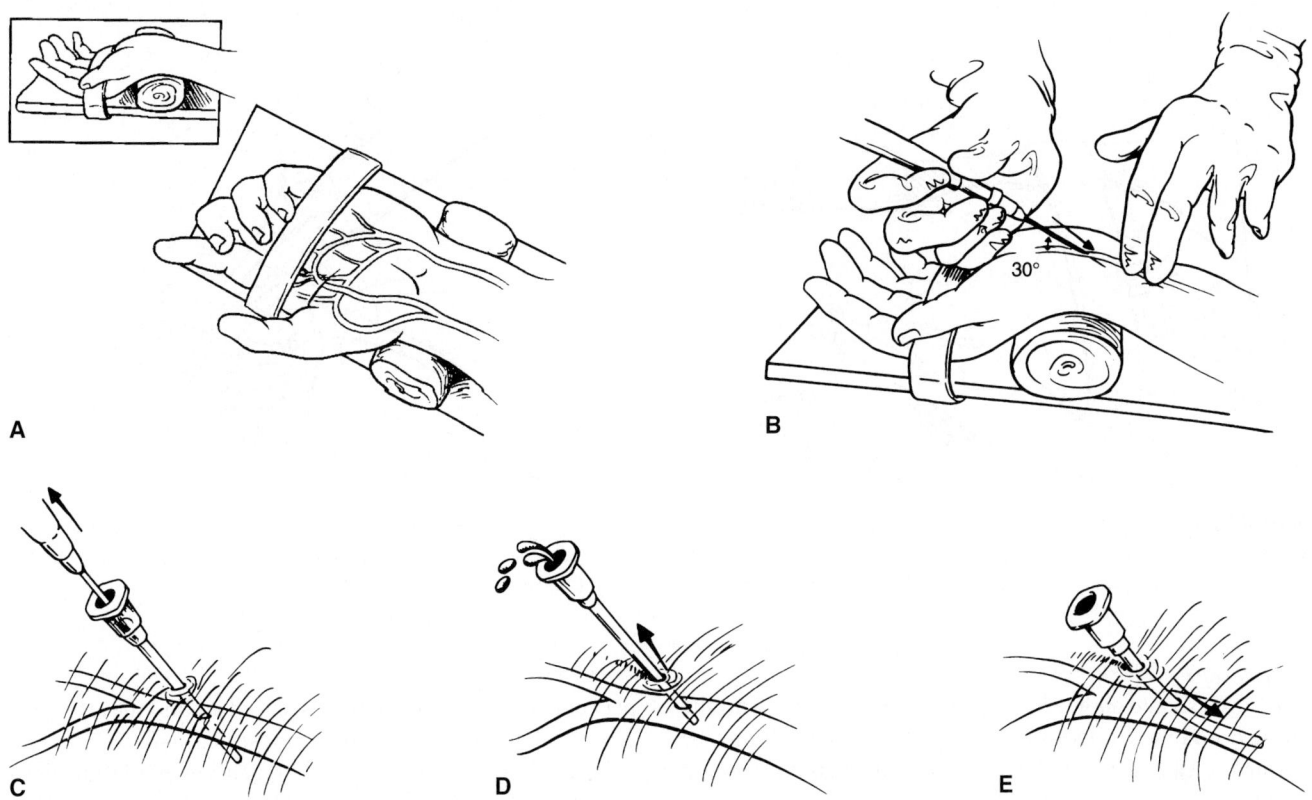

**FIGURE 7-3** Percutaneous insertion of a catheter into the radial artery. The hand is taped securely to an arm board with a roll placed under the wrist (A). The radial pulse is palpated, and the needle/catheter guided at approximately a 30° angle through the artery (B). As the needle/catheter is withdrawn and passes into the artery, blood may be observed to flow into the hub. The needle/catheter is then advanced a second time, the needle removed (C), the catheter withdrawn until blood return is observed (D), and the catheter advanced down the lumen of the artery (E).

most common arterial access site utilized in non-neonates is the radial artery (70%), followed by the posterior tibial and femoral artery. Peripheral arteries are best used because of the low complication rate should thrombosis occur. However, the femoral artery has frequently been cannulated using the Seldinger technique in children, with few complications. The superficial temporal artery is easily identified and cannulated in neonates. However, because of concern for retrograde flow of air or debris into the carotid artery circulation, it should be used only if extreme care is taken during flushing of the catheter.

Arterial cannulations in children are performed via either the percutaneous or cutdown methods. Percutaneous insertion should be attempted primarily in most cases. Typical catheter sizes for arterial cannulation include 24- or 22-gauge in neonates, 22-gauge in large infants and children, and 20-gauge in older children and adolescents. Two methods of percutaneous cannulation are commonly used: (1) the direct cannulation method and (2) the transfixion technique. I prefer the transfixion technique in which the catheter and needle are advanced through the artery as the pulse is palpated (Fig. 7-3). The needle frequently abuts the head of the radius, which is directly under the artery. Withdrawal of the catheter and needle may demonstrate a flash of blood, at which point the needle and catheter are advanced once again. The needle is then removed, the catheter withdrawn until blood return is visualized, and the catheter advanced down the lumen of

the artery. The catheter is sutured in place and secured with tape as a sterile dressing is placed over the cannulation site. At times a wire, such as a 0.0015-inch diameter wire, which fits through a 24-French catheter, may be used to advance the catheter into the artery when difficulties are encountered with placement.

The technique of arterial cut-down of the radial or posterior tibial artery is most often utilized in neonates and infants. A 6- to 8-mm transverse incision is performed over the arterial site, and blunt dissection is used to identify the artery (Fig. 7-4). The radial artery is often located deeper than one might expect, frequently lying directly on the head of the radius. It is unusual to observe or palpate pulsations in the artery. An appropriately sized over-the-needle catheter is introduced directly down the lumen of the artery. The needle is removed. The catheter is advanced into the artery only if blood flow returns from the catheter. Otherwise, the catheter is slowly removed until blood flow return is noted, at which point the catheter is advanced. It is rare that artery ligation is required.

The umbilical artery provides an excellent site for arterial access in neonates who are less than 10 days of age, with umbilical artery catheters being placed in up to 30% of neonates who are admitted to the neonatal ICU. Umbilical tape or a heavy suture may be placed around the base of the umbilical cord to reduce bleeding. An incision on the inferior aspect of the umbilicus, approximately 1 to 2 cm above

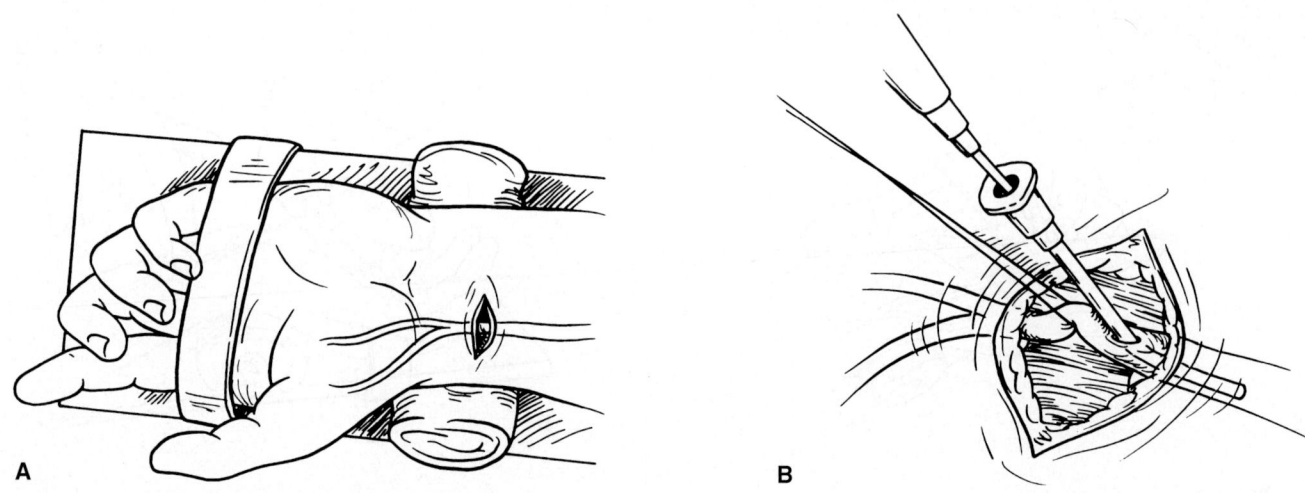

**FIGURE 7-4** Insertion of a catheter into the radial artery by the cut-down technique. A 1-cm incision is performed over the area of the radial artery just proximal to the wrist (**A**). The artery is identified on the head of the radius and retracted distally with a suture as a needle/catheter is advanced into the lumen of the artery (**B**). Ligation of the artery is usually not necessary.

skin level, should allow identification of one of the 2 ventrally located umbilical arteries (Fig. 7-5). If the artery cannot be located or cannulated in the umbilical stump, another option is to perform an infraumbilical curvilinear incision with identification of the umbilical artery in the space of Retzius, which exists posterior to the linea alba and anterior to the peritoneum. After a 4-0 suture is placed around the artery for retraction, the artery is partially transected, and a 3.5-French (preterm or small neonate) or 5-French catheter is advanced into the artery after being flushed with heparinized saline. The catheter is advanced gently, as resistance is often met at a point approximately 5 to 6 cm from the umbilicus as the

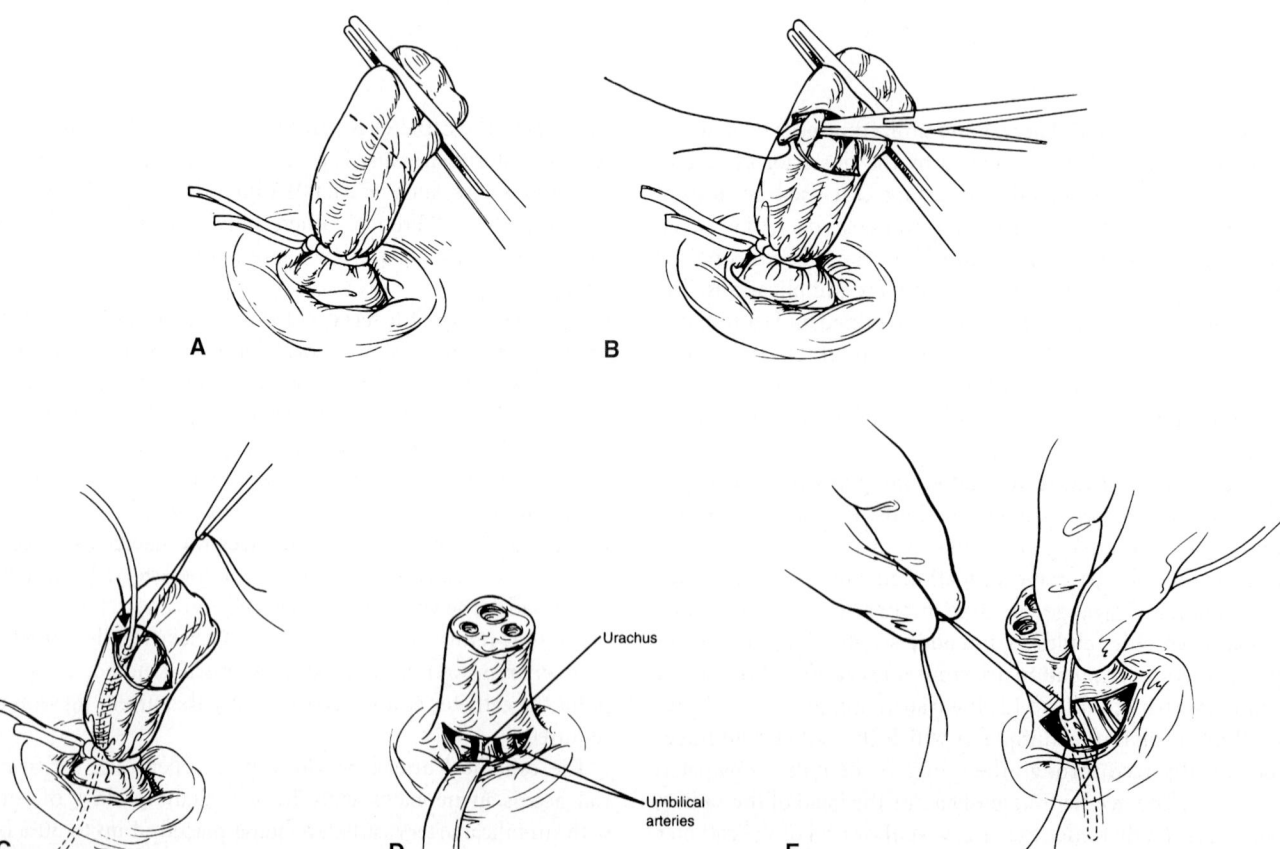

**FIGURE 7-5** Insertion of a catheter into the umbilical artery. An incision is performed on the inferior aspect of the umbilicus 1 to 2 cm above the base (**A**). One of the 2 arteries is identified, surrounded with a suture (**B**), incised, and cannulated (**C**). If an artery cannot be identified in the umbilical cord, an infraumbilical incision will allow access to (**D**) and cannulation of (**E**) an umbilical artery in the space of Retzius.

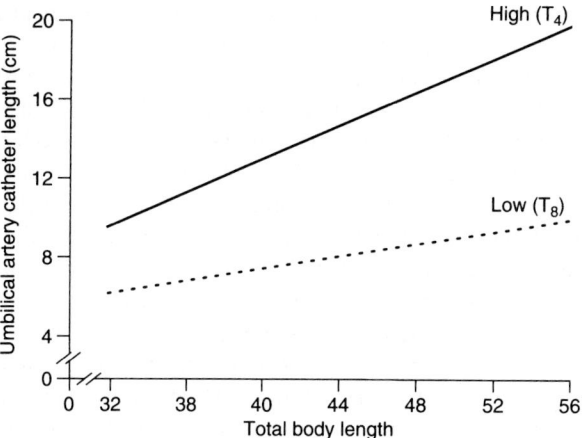

**FIGURE 7-6** Umbilical artery catheter insertion length as a function of patient total body length. (Adapted from *Klaus MH, Fanodroff AA. Case of the High-Risk Neonate, 4th ed. Philadelphia: W.B. Sanders; 1993.*)

catheter passes from the hypogastric artery into the femoral artery. The final catheter position should be either above the mesenteric vessels (T-9 to T-11) or below the renal vessels (L-4). The data from Fig. 7-6 may be used to determine the insertion length of the umbilical artery catheter. Advancing the catheter a length equivalent to 0.65 times the distance between the umbilicus and the shoulder plus the length of the umbilical stump will place the catheter in the L-4 vertebral region. A radiograph should be performed to document catheter position following placement.

A transducer is connected to the arterial catheter via noncompliant tubing, and a continuous-flow system is used to provide flushing of the catheter with heparinized saline or dextrose water. At no time should the catheter be flushed in a bolus fashion because large amounts of fluid may be incidentally introduced. Studies have demonstrated that flush may appear in the carotid artery distribution after injection of only 0.3 to 0.75 mL of flush into the radial artery of a neonate. Care should be taken to minimize blood waste, especially in small neonates. Systems that provide on-line information with regard to $PaO_2$, $Paco_2$, and pH have been developed and are becoming more reliable. Other devices avoid blood waste by aspirating the blood into proximal tubing for later reinfusion after sample withdrawal.

Systolic and diastolic blood pressures may be artificially elevated as a result of catheter whip in a large artery and artificially decreased if dampening of the signal occurs from air or clot in the connecting tubing or if the tubing is too narrow, too long, too compliant, or kinked. Systolic and diastolic arterial pressure data obtained from a peripheral systemic arterial catheter often are greater and less, respectively, than those measured in the aorta. The mean arterial pressure, however, is the same in both. The mean arterial pressure may be estimated by adding the diastolic blood pressure plus one-third of the difference between the systolic and diastolic blood pressure and is the most reliable parameter of blood pressure.

Complications of arterial catheter placement are surprisingly low. Distal embolization or ischemia is rare, and tissue loss even more so. Thrombosis of the vessel most frequently occurs in the radial artery in small newborns and infants after prolonged catheterization. Follow-up ultrasound evaluation has demonstrated that the majority of obstructed arteries recanalize following catheter removal. If the pulse is lost in an extremity following attempted or successful arterial catheter placement, the catheter should be removed, and systemic anticoagulation considered. If the limb is nonviable, then surgical exploration should be entertained. Although acute vascular injury may lead to chronic ischemia and limb length discrepancy, arterial exploration is technically difficult and often unrewarding in neonates and infants. In those cases, consideration for heparin anticoagulation, administration of streptokinase or urokinase, and observation will often result in improvement in limb perfusion.

The incidence of clinically significant aortic thrombus formation in patients with umbilical artery catheters is between 3% and 6%. The incidence of adverse thromboembolic events appears to be greater in those patients with a low (L-4 or lower) abdominal umbilical artery catheter. Overt aortoiliac thrombosis accompanied by decreased lower extremity blood flow, and hypertension may be managed with supportive care and antihypertensive therapy. More severe sequelae should be treated with systemic heparinization and/or fibrinolytic therapy with surgical thrombectomy performed if limb-threatening ischemia, renal failure, visceral compromise, or systemic acidosis is present. If unilateral lower extremity ischemia occurs in a patient with an umbilical artery catheter in place, consideration should be given to angiography and/or thrombolytic therapy via the catheter before it is removed.

Sepsis related to arterial catheters occurs in fewer than 1% and in 2% to 5% of cases with radial and umbilical artery catheters, respectively. No medications, except for heparin and papavarin, should be administered via any arterial line.

## Central Venous Catheters

The central venous pressure (CVP, right atrial pressure) serves as an excellent monitor of volume status, especially in children. In the pediatric population, the central venous pressure is as reliable as pulmonary artery or pulmonary capillary wedge pressure assessment in patients who have normal cardiac function and in whom high positive end-expiratory pressures (PEEP) are not being applied.

Central venous access may be obtained by cut-down or by percutaneous means (see Chapter 9: Vascular Access Procedures). Most commonly, access by cut-down is obtained via the external jugular vein, the common facial vein, or the saphenous vein at the saphenofemoral junction with placement of either a tunneled broviac silastic or a standard polyurethane catheter. The external jugular vein has a more direct, straight path to the superior vena cava (SVC) in neonates and infants than in children and adolescents. The common facial vein should be traced back to the internal jugular vein before cannulation to ensure proper identification. The femoral vein may be cannulated via the saphenous vein, which is easily identified in the anteromedial subcutaneous tissues of the upper thigh/groin. In newborns, the umbilical vein may be used to gain access to the central venous circulation. A 5- or 8-French catheter may be advanced via the umbilical vein to the left portal vein through the ductus venosus and into the right atrium. Difficulty with incidental passage into the portal venous system is frequent and may be recognized by the development of resistance before the predicted catheter insertion length. When this problem is encountered, the catheter should be removed a short distance, twisted, and gently reinserted. The catheter should be removed if radiography demonstrates placement in the portal venous system.

Percutaneous access to the central veins is most commonly performed via the subclavian, internal jugular, or femoral veins. In children, a 21-gauge needle is used to access the subclavian vein. The patient should be placed in the Trendelenburg position, and a roll placed under the back. Placement can be done "blindly" following anatomical landmarks, or the assistance of bedside fluoroscopy or ultrasound guidance may be a useful adjunct. The needle is advanced at a point approximately 5 mm below the clavicle in the area of the midclavicular line until the clavicle is encountered. The needle is then walked down and advanced underneath the clavicle just lateral to the point where the first rib and the clavicle come into approximation. The hub of the needle is then brought in an inferior and lateral direction. The needle is advanced in a superior and medial direction under the clavicle toward the sternal notch as the vein is encountered. Once the needle is within the lumen of the vein, as evidenced by free return of blood during aspiration, a "J"-wire is passed through the needle, the needle is removed, and the catheter is placed over the wire into the central venous position in the SVC or right atrium.

The internal jugular vein is most frequently accessed from a point one fingerbreadth above the clavicle between the heads of the sternocleidomastoid muscle (SCM). The needle is oriented toward the ipsilateral nipple and enters the vein at a 45° angle. An alternative approach is posterior to the sternocleidomastoid with the needle entering the skin at the junction of the lower and middle thirds of the posterior margin of the SCM while the needle is oriented toward the sternal notch. The femoral vein is located medial to the artery in the groin. The vein may be identified by aspiration with a 21-gauge needle at a 45° angle approximately one fingerbreadth medial to the palpated femoral artery pulse and 1 to 2 fingerbreadths below the inguinal ligament. Ultrasound guidance is advised during central venous access, especially during internal jugular cannulation.

Assessment of central venous pressure should be performed at end-expiration because it is at this point that the CVP is least affected by the patient's ventilatory status. Pressure measurements should be performed using a transducer placed at the level of the right atrium. Variation in central venous pressure with the cardiac cycle should be documented. Normal right atrial pressure is 5 to 10 mm Hg.

The central venous oxygen saturation ($ScvO_2$), as determined via a central venous pressure catheter, may be used to guide treatment in patients with sepsis. Such goal-directed therapy may decrease the mortality of adult patients with severe sepsis and septic shock.

The most common complication of central venous catheter placement is sepsis, which occurs with an incidence of from 5% to 10%. Sepsis is most often managed with antibiotic therapy and catheter removal or replacement, although in the pediatric population central venous catheter sepsis may, if necessary, be treated successfully with antibiotics and maintenance of the catheter in situ. Vascular thrombus formation likely occurs in all patients with central venous catheters. However, these thromboses are clinically significant in only 5% to 10% of patients. Catheter-induced superior vena caval occlusion may result in hydrocephalus, pulmonary lymphangiectasia, and chylothorax, with the majority of such cases occurring in patients under 1 year of age. Other complications associated with placement and maintenance of a central venous catheter include catheter breakage, catheter dislodgment and embolization, pneumothorax in 6% of cases, hydrothorax following malposition of the catheter into the thoracic cavity, subclavian artery puncture leading to hemorrhage, brachial plexus injury, and thoracic duct injury when a left subclavian or internal jugular vein catheterization is attempted. Wire breakage with embolization may occur if the wire is withdrawn inappropriately through the introducing needle.

## Measurement of Abdominal Pressure

Recognition of elevated intraabdominal pressure (IAP) is important in ICU patients with shock. The abdominal physical examination provides general assessment of whether the abdomen is distended and taut and thus concerning for abdominal compartment syndrome (ACS). Other signs of ACS include decreased urine output or anuria, reduced venous return, cyanosis of the lower extremities, high ventilator pressure requirements, and development of metabolic acidosis. Cardiac output may be reduced by as much as 30% due to compression of the diaphragm and heart. While pathologic IAP has not been well-defined in pediatric patients, any pressure greater than 20 mm Hg is considered to be consistent with ACS and potentially physiologically compromising in adult patients. IAP is most effectively assessed via a liquid-filled bladder catheter with a manometer placed through the access port of the bladder catheter drainage system. Emergent decompression of the abdomen via exploratory laparotomy should be performed following recognition of ACS. The abdomen should be decompressed by enlargement of the abdominal wall by placement of a synthetic mesh or through use of a silo or by open abdominal wall packing. Placement of such a pressure-monitoring balloon catheter via the oral or nasal route into the stomach has also been used for such measurements.

## Pulmonary Arterial Catheters

The use of pulmonary artery (PA) catheters has been largely replaced by central venous pressure monitoring since, as mentioned previously, CVP assessment is accurate in most infants and children. In addition, prospective, randomized, controlled trials in adults have shown that mortality is increased in patients in whom a pulmonary artery catheter is used for central pressure monitoring. Thus, the rate of use of PA catheters in the ICU has decreased dramatically. Even so, there are times when right atrial catheter assessment of cardiopulmonary status may be inadequate in patients with pulmonary, renal, or cardiac insufficiency, those who remain hypotensive or hypoperfused despite apparently adequate volume resuscitation, and those who require pharmacologic intervention to enhance cardiac output. Such patients may benefit from the additional information provided by a pulmonary arterial catheter. A 5-French catheter is appropriate for

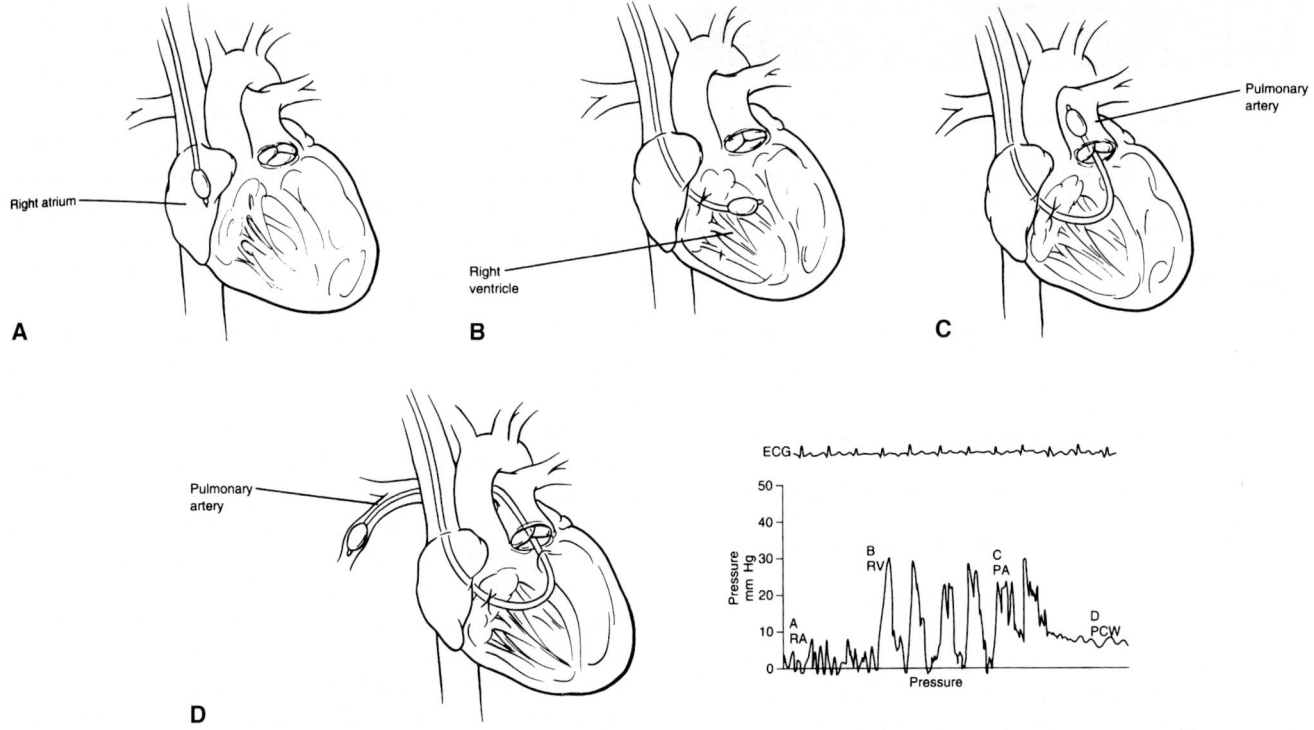

**FIGURE 7-7** Pulmonary artery catheter placement is illustrated. Vascular pressure waveforms may be used to monitor passage of the catheter through the right atrium (**A**), right ventricle (**B**), the pulmonary artery (**C**), and into the wedged position in the pulmonary artery (**D**). (Pulmonary capillary occlusion pressure = PAOP and reflects left atrial filling pressure.)

patients approximately 25 to 30 kg in weight, and a 7-French catheter is appropriate for older patients. Most catheters have 5 lumina: (1) a port for injection of either 0.5 or 1.5 mL of air into an inflatable balloon at the tip of the catheter; (2) a thermistor probe near the tip, which allows determination of core body temperature and thermodilution cardiac output; (3) a fiberoptic bundle for determination of pulmonary arterial mixed venous oxygen saturation; (4) a port distal to the inflatable balloon that allows assessment of pulmonary arterial pressures when the balloon is deflated and left atrial pressures when inflated; and (5) 1 or 2 additional proximal infusion/pressure-monitoring ports usually placed in the right ventricle and/or right atrium.

Pulmonary arterial catheters are most often placed via a subclavian or internal jugular approach. In young children (less than 2 years old), the femoral venous approach may make transcardiac passage of the catheter easier. Once venous access is established, an introducer catheter is placed; the balloon is inflated and tested; and all monitoring infusion ports are flushed and zeroed. The balloon is inflated as the catheter is gently advanced: right atrial, right ventricular, pulmonary arterial, and, finally, pulmonary wedge waveforms should be observed (Fig. 7-7). The pulmonary arterial catheter may curl in the right heart, or the tip may impinge in the trabeculae of the right ventricle. Catheter placement may be especially difficult in those patients with right ventricular hypertrophy or dysfunction. Counterclockwise rotation while advancing the catheter, placing the patient in the left decubitus position, and raising or lowering the head of the bed may all aid in catheter placement. Occasionally, fluoroscopy or echocardiography

may help to guide insertion. The balloon should "wedge" or occlude the pulmonary artery at the end of the 1.5-mL insufflation with rapid return of a pulmonary artery pressure waveform on deflation. The ability to wedge the balloon with <1.0 mL of air may indicate that placement of the catheter is too distal in the pulmonary artery. Chest radiographs should be obtained to document correct placement.

The balloon should remain inflated during passage of the catheter through the right heart in order to reduce the incidence of arrhythmias. Treatment of arrhythmias is rarely required, and lidocaine should be administered only if sustained ventricular tachycardia is induced at the time of placement.

Rupture of the pulmonary artery is a rare but lethal complication. Hemoptysis and/or cardiopulmonary collapse may follow balloon inflation during a wedge pressure measurement. Those patients with pulmonary arterial hypertension and coagulation deficiencies are at highest risk. This complication may be avoided by maintaining the tip of the catheter <2 cm lateral to the spine on chest radiograph; inflating the balloon with the minimal volume necessary to achieve a wedge tracing; and minimizing the frequency of wedge pressure assessment.

The distal port of the catheter should be continuously monitored for permanent wedging, which can lead to pulmonary infarction. If permanent wedging is observed, the catheter should be withdrawn until appropriate pulmonary arterial and wedge tracings are observed during deflation and inflation of the balloon, respectively. A number of other complications of pulmonary artery catheter placement are

| TABLE 7-1 | Complications of Pulmonary Artery Catheter Placement |
|---|---|
| Pulmonary artery thrombus formation/embolus | |
| Pulmonary infarction | |
| Ventricular arrhythmias | |
| Right bundle branch block | |
| Sepsis | |
| Perforation of the right ventricle | |
| Pulmonary artery rupture | |
| Cardiac valvular damage | |
| Knotting of catheter in right ventricle | |

summarized in Table 7-1. Valvular damage may occur during withdrawal of the catheter with an inflated balloon. Knotting of the catheter in the right ventricle may require manipulation under fluoroscopy.

## Measurement of Pulmonary Artery Pressure

The right atrial pressure may fail to represent the left ventricular preload in the setting of sepsis, acquired respiratory distress syndrome (ARDS) with application of high ventilator pressures, pulmonary hypertension, pulmonary embolus, pulmonary fibrosis, and cardiac dysfunction. In such cases, assessment of the left atrial pressure (LAP), as an approximation of left ventricular end-diastolic volume (LVEDV), may be accomplished during inflation of the pulmonary arterial catheter balloon. A static column of blood, without intervening valves, is then interposed between the distal catheter pressure monitoring site and the left atrium. This pulmonary artery occlusion pressure (PAOP) provides an estimate of LAP and, therefore, pulmonary capillary pressure, which is a determinant of the hydrostatic forces resulting in pulmonary edema. A PAOP greater than 25 mm Hg in normal lungs and greater than 18 mm Hg in the setting of sepsis and ARDS will frequently result in the development of pulmonary edema. The PAOP may also be used to assess LVEDV in order to optimize cardiac contractility. Unless cardiac compliance is altered (sepsis, restrictive pericarditis, cardiomyopathy) or mitral valve disease is present, the PAOP will accurately reflect LVEDV. Accurate assessment of LVEDV is also dependent on the location of the pulmonary arterial catheter tip: unless the tip is posterior to the level of the left atrium in the supine patient, alveolar pressures may exceed those of venous and/or arterial pulmonary vascular pressures, resulting in occlusion of the venous and/or arterial vasculature distal to the pulmonary artery catheter during a variable period of the respiratory cycle. This will preclude accurate assessment of LAP. Fortunately, the flow-directed pulmonary arterial catheter inserts most frequently at or below the left atrium because a predominance of blood flow is distributed to the dependent regions of the lungs.

PAOP should be assessed at end-expiration because the effects of ventilation on intrathoracic pressures and, therefore, PAOP may be significant. It is at this point that intrathoracic pressures are closest to atmospheric pressure. Application of PEEP may result in overestimation of the LAP by the PAOP. This effect is less significant in the injured, noncompliant lung. Under such circumstances, PAOP will exceed the LAP by only 1 mm Hg for every 5 cm $H_2O$ increase in applied PEEP. For this reason, and because of the potential for alveolar collapse and deterioration in gas exchange that may accompany even transient periods of ventilator disconnect in the patient with severe respiratory insufficiency, PAOP should be measured and reported without any attempt to reduce the effect of PEEP in such patients. All central pressures should be obtained from a paper tracing, rather than a digital output, so that end-expiratory pressures may be specifically identified and recorded.

## Measurement of Cardiac Output

Invasive cardiac output assessment is frequently performed in the ICU using the temperature indicator dilution technique. An indicator of iced or room-temperature saline is injected into any central venous port. It is important to inject the bolus rapidly and at the same point in the respiratory cycle. Room temperature injectate-determined cardiac outputs are no less accurate than those assessed using iced-saline injections. In general, 5-mL injectate volumes are used, except in infants and small children in whom 1-mL iced saline injections are preferred. After mixing of the bolus with blood in the right ventricle, the blood temperature is assessed by a thermistor located at the tip of the pulmonary artery catheter (Fig. 7-8). Once the initial blood temperature, the volume of injectate,

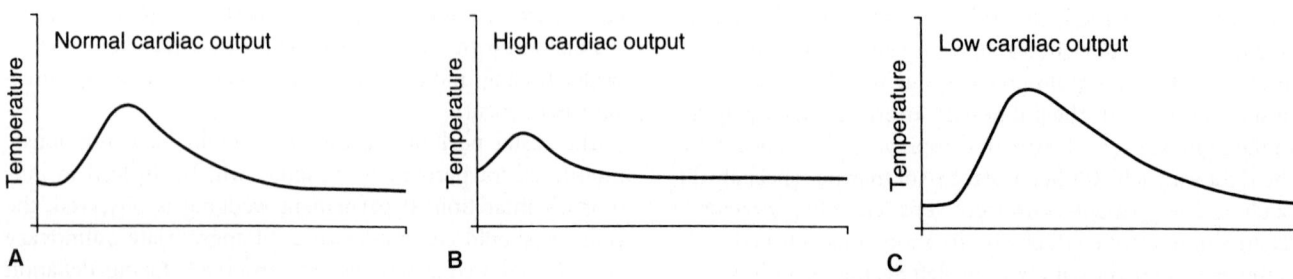

**FIGURE 7-8** This figure illustrates thermodilution cardiac output determination during periods of normal (**A**), high (**B**), and low (**C**) cardiac output. The magnitude and duration of the change in temperature are inversely proportional to the cardiac output.

the injectate temperature, and the change in blood temperature as a function of time are known, cardiac output can be determined.

The accuracy of cardiac output assessment is improved by performance of measurements in triplicate. Any irregular curves or assessments that deviate by more than 10% are discarded. The mean of the remaining 3 individual measurements has an overall accuracy of ±10%.

The Fick equation may also be applied to invasively determine cardiac output

$$\text{Cardiac output} = \frac{(SaO_2 - SvO_2) \times Hgb \times 1.36 \times 10}{VO_2}$$

Calculation of the Fick-determined cardiac output requires assessment of the mixed-venous oxygen saturation via a pulmonary arterial catheter, arterial oxygen saturation, and airway oxygen consumption ($VO_2$). Because of the inherent error present in each of the variables incorporated into the calculation, the Fick cardiac output has an overall error of approximately ±5%. In addition, the Fick-calculated cardiac output overestimates the thermodilution cardiac output by approximately 5% to 10%. A number of studies have demonstrated the feasibility of on-line Fick calculation of cardiac output through assimilation of data obtained from continuous oxygen consumption monitoring, arterial pulse oximetry, and mixed-venous oximetry.

## Mixed Venous Oximetry Monitoring

The oxygen hemoglobin saturation in mixed venous pulmonary artery blood is referred to as the $SvO_2$. As oxygen delivery ($DO_2$) increases or oxygen consumption ($VO_2$) decreases,

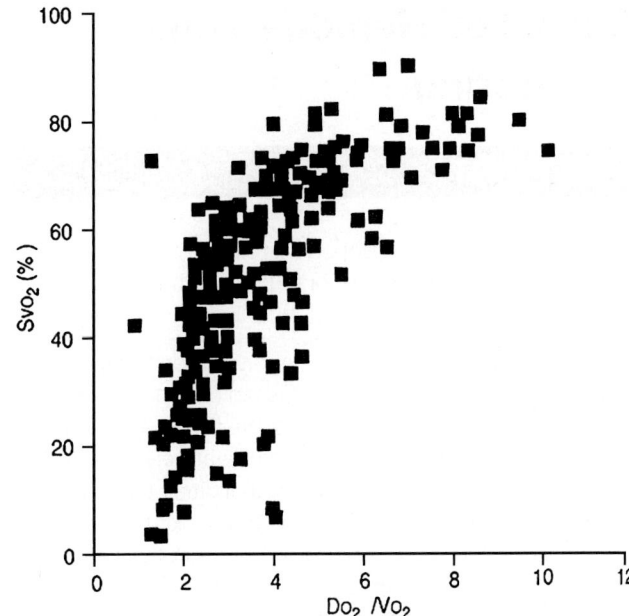

**FIGURE 7-10** The relationship of the mixed venous oxygen saturation ($SvO_2$) and the ratio of oxygen delivery to oxygen consumption ($DO_2/VO_2$) in normal eumetabolic, hypermetabolic septic, and hypermetabolic exercising canines. (Reprinted with permission from *Hirschl RB, Heiss K. Cardiopulmonary critical care and shock. In: Oldham KT, Calambani PM, Foglia RP, eds. Surgery of Infants and Children. Scientific Principles and Practice. Philadelphia: Lippincott-Raven; 1997:149–182.*)

more oxygen remains in the venous blood. The result is an increase in $SvO_2$ (Fig. 7-9). In contrast, if $DO_2$ decreases or $VO_2$ increases, relatively more oxygen is extracted from the blood, and, therefore, less oxygen remains in the venous blood. A decrease in $SvO_2$ is the result. The $SvO_2$ serves as an excellent monitor of oxygen kinetics because it specifically assesses the adequacy of oxygen delivery in relation to oxygen consumption ($DO_2/VO_2$ ratio Fig. 7-10).

Many pulmonary arterial catheters contain fiberoptic bundles that provide continuous mixed-venous oximetry data. Emitted light is reflected from circulating red blood cells and transmitted via the receiving fiberoptic bundle to an analyzer, where the data on the reflected light at 3 wavelengths are assessed to provide accurate determination of hemoglobin oxygen saturation. Continuous $SvO_2$ monitoring provides a means for assessing the adequacy of oxygen delivery, early identification of cardiopulmonary instability, rapid assessment of the response to therapy, and cost savings in critically ill patients because of a diminished need for other data such as sequential blood gas monitoring. A decrease in $SvO_2$ to less than 65% or a change in $SvO_2$ over 5% to 10% should be investigated by assessing the factors that determine the $SvO_2$ cardiac output, $SaO_2$, and hemoglobin level with consideration for variables that might result in an increase in oxygen consumption. The accuracy of $SvO_2$ monitoring may be diminished under certain circumstances where arteriovenous shunting occurs such as in the occasional patient with cirrhosis or sepsis. Importantly, this means that in situations where vasoregulation is altered, the $SvO_2$ may be normal even though the oxygen delivery at the tissue level is inadequate.

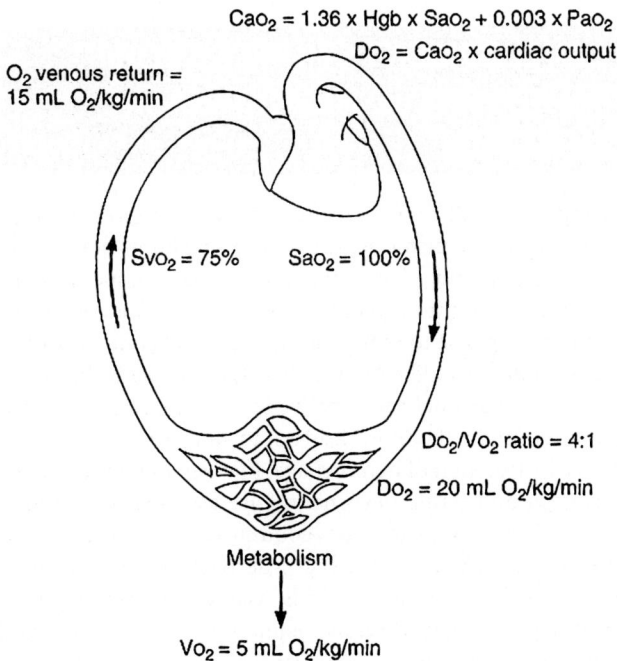

**FIGURE 7-9** Oxygen consumption ($VO_2$) and delivery ($DO_2$) relationships. (Reprinted with permission from *Hirschl RB. Oxygen delivery in the pediatric surgical patient. Can Opin Pediatr 19946:341.*)

# Advanced Hemodynamic Monitoring

## KEY POINTS

1. Algorithms can be developed that noninvasively can predict hemorrhage prior to the initiation of shock.

2. The components integral to integrated monitoring systems include: a ventilator; 3/5-lead ECG; pulse oximeter; noninvasive blood pressure (NIBP); end-tidal carbon dioxide (etCO$_2$); patient temperature; invasive arterial and intracranial pressure capabilities; Ethernet communications; closed-loop control of oxygenation, ventilation, and IV fluid control; an integrated electronic medical record (data storage/export); alarming, intravenous (IV) pumps along with smart help, connected by powered USB ports. The system should support several external IV pumps and other yet to be developed noninvasive monitors, all connected via powered-USB ports. Other potential modules that could be included are an oxygen concentrator, patient warming, and an anesthesia control module.

Continuous patient monitoring started in the 1960s, when the technology for monitoring astronauts' vital signs was transferred to the bedside. Over the past 50 years patient monitoring systems have incorporated a variety of invasive and noninvasive sensor technologies to derive and display clinically important parameters. Patient monitoring systems are set to evolve once again as new sensing technologies merge with rapid advances in computing technology. Within this context, the application of advanced modeling techniques to standard physiological waveform data is leading to the discovery of several, previously unknown, hemodynamic relationships. The next generation of patient monitoring systems will be noninvasive functional tools that are able to estimate hemodynamic states in real-time, predict physiological reserve, and optimize care of the patient.

The goal of this chapter section is to familiarize the reader with several existing and a number of new sensor technologies for advanced hemodynamic patient monitoring in the setting of acute injury, specifically hemorrhage. The setting of acute blood loss has been chosen because the physiology of hemorrhage is typically rapid and compensatory, without the confounding effects of an insidious medical illness. The application of these new sensing and machine-based technologies will be transferable to many other areas of disease detection and monitoring. By improving our ability to recognize early changes in the pathophysiology of illness or injury we hope to limit disease progression, guide early therapy, and promote rapid recovery, thereby improving patient outcomes.

## BACKGROUND

Trauma causes more than 5 million deaths worldwide each year (see also Section VIII, Trauma). It is the leading cause of death during the first 3 decades of life in the United States and the fourth leading cause of overall mortality, with over 170,000 trauma-related deaths in the United States each year. One third of these deaths are due to hemorrhage, which is the most common cause of "potentially survivable" traumatic death. The majority of these "potentially survivable" deaths are due to torso injuries and noncompressible hemorrhage, injuries that are difficult to identify early, hard to clinically monitor, and nearly impossible to effectively treat, outside of early operation. Unrecognized or poorly controlled hemorrhage leads to tissue hypoperfusion, organ ischemia, and tissue acidosis. The latter develops whenever cellular oxygen demand exceeds tissue oxygen supply, mandating an increase in anaerobic metabolism and an accelerated production of lactic acid. If the respiratory rate does not rise to adequately reverse the state of acidosis, and if hemorrhage to resuscitation volumes are inadequate, tissue and blood pH will continue to decline and the situation will evolve into an "irreversible" phase of hemorrhagic shock.

Humans can lose as much as 40% to 50% of their central blood volume without exhibiting clinically meaningful changes in mental status, pulse rate and character, systolic and mean blood pressures, arterial oxygen saturation, etCO$_2$, and respiratory rate. However, the lack of specificity associated with these "traditional" vital signs compromises their usefulness in the early detection and monitoring of acute blood loss. The resulting challenge is that shock is easily diagnosed in its latter stages, when therapy is less effective and more difficult to control. New sensors and new methods are needed to identify early physiological responses to acute blood loss.

## DEVELOPMENT STRATEGY FOR AN ADVANCED HEMODYNAMIC MONITOR

Changes in tissue perfusion and tissue oxygenation are compensatory mechanisms by which the body shunts blood away from the periphery (eg, skin, subcutaneous tissue, muscle, gastrointestinal tract) to other, more vital organs (eg, heart, brain) in response to reductions in systemic blood flow (cardiac output). An algorithm that includes some indicator of systemic oxygen delivery relative to consumption at the tissue level might therefore lead to an improved method for the early detection of hemorrhage. In current practice, tissue perfusion and tissue oxygenation are assessed by standard measurements of heart rate, blood pressure, central venous pressure, cardiac output, oxygen-derived variables, urinary output, and blood lactate levels. Gathering these types of physiological data currently requires several invasive and noninvasive techniques, some of which are discontinuous, expensive, and time-consuming to apply. The ideal solution should utilize a minimum number of sensors that provide the practitioner with continuous physiological observations and predictions.

We began with a comprehensive review of currently available noninvasive hemodynamic measurements that would linearly correlate with hemorrhage. Using advanced signal processing and waveform analysis techniques to discover linear and nonlinear relationships within the waveform data that correlated with hemorrhage, we sought to develop algorithms capable of processing real-time noninvasive hemodynamic data to quickly and reliably estimate blood loss and predict hemodynamic decompensation. A more detailed discussion of the depths of this technology is beyond the scope of this text.

## NONINVASIVE HEMODYNAMIC MONITORING

A wide variety of standard and advanced hemodynamic measurements have been shown to linearly correlate with hemorrhage, observations that can be extended by applying advanced computing techniques to noninvasive waveform data. State-of-the-art feature extraction and machine learning techniques can be leveraged to uncover linear and nonlinear relationships within the waveform data and determine whether or not these relationships could be exploited in the context of building and evaluating models for estimating blood loss and predicting hemodynamic decompensation.

Our goal is to develop algorithms that can quickly and reliably estimate hypovolemia using easily applied noninvasive physiological sensors.

## AN ADVANCED HEMODYNAMIC MONITOR

The feature extraction and machine learning methods were used to analyze complex physiological waveform data generated in a human model of severe, acute hemorrhage. This model uses lower body negative pressure (LBNP) as a method for investigating cardiovascular changes under conditions of controlled, experimentally induced hypovolemic hypotension. For every 15 mm Hg of negative pressure that is applied to an experimental subject's lower body, approximately 500 cc's of blood are pulled away from the head and torso to be redistributed to the pelvis and lower extremities. LBNP, as a surrogate for acute blood loss, reduces central blood volume and cardiac output, eventually leading to severe hypotension and decompensation. A model to safely and noninvasively induce hemodynamic decompensation in human subjects to identify early compensatory responses associated with hemorrhage has been developed at the United States Army Institute of Surgical Research (USAISR). The model uses LBNP to redistribute blood away from the head and torso to the pelvis and lower extremities, to cause experimentally induced hypovolemic hypotension (see Fig. 7-11). Victor

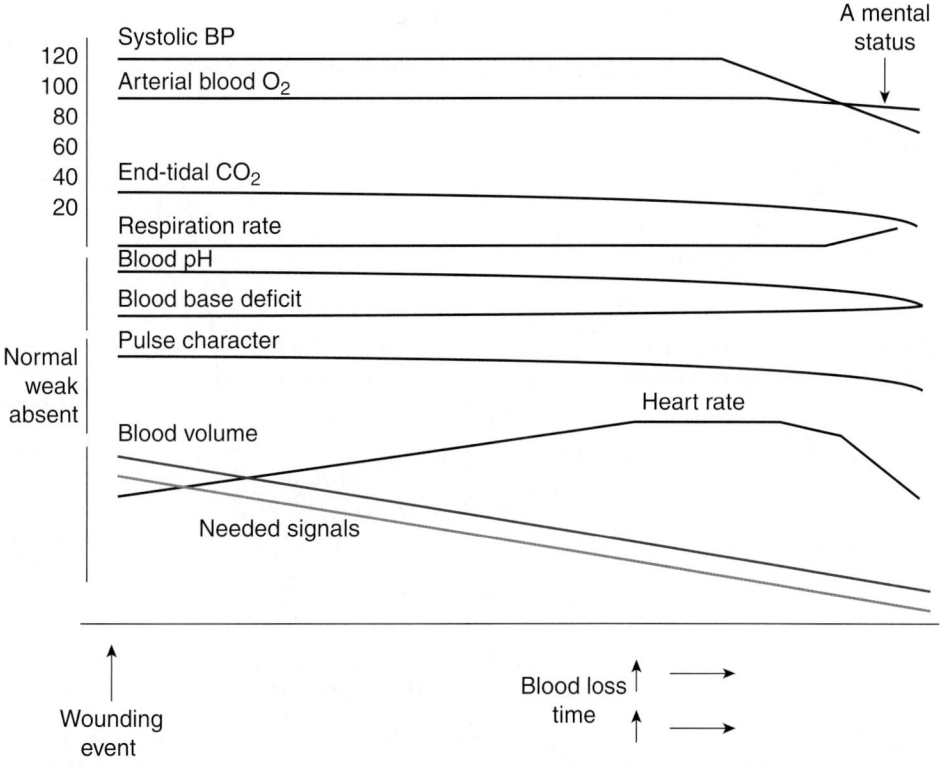

**FIGURE 7-11** The time course of standard vital signs measured on current medical monitors (*black lines*) during the dynamic compensatory phase of progressively reduced central blood volume (*red line*) simulated by LBNP. Green line indicates signals required to track blood loss.

Convertino and his colleagues have demonstrated that LBNP applied to humans mimics the hemodynamic and compensatory responses observed during hemorrhage of anesthetized animal models without attenuating peripheral vasoconstriction. Related experiments in humans have further demonstrated that reductions in central venous pressure and stroke volume, along with elevations in muscle sympathetic nerve activity caused by hemorrhage of 400 to 550 mL in humans, can be reproduced by approximately 20 mm Hg LBNP. LBNP is therefore an experimental surrogate for hemorrhage. Progressive LBNP reduces central blood volume and cardiac output, increases sympathetic nerve activity, reduces tissue oxygen content and pH, and eventually leads to severe hypotension and decompensation.

Application of LBNP provides a method of investigating continuous and simultaneous physiological responses under conditions of controlled, experimentally induced central hypovolemia. By defining hemodynamic decompensation as the primary outcome variable, investigators at the USAISR have studied the dynamics (time course) of standard vital signs. Their experiments have verified data reported in the trauma literature that during the early compensatory phase of hemorrhage, there are no clinically meaningful changes in what have been termed traditional or "legacy" vital signs. These vital signs and their failure to meaningfully change with the loss of as much as 40% to 50% of central blood volume are illustrated in Fig. 7-11. This figure illustrates the need for a device that reliably detects and estimates the level of blood loss in real-time (the red line in Fig. 7-11). It further describes our inability to tease apart the dynamically complex mechanisms (signals) that underlie the compensatory phase of hemorrhage (the green line in Fig. 7-11).

Continuous, noninvasively measured physiological signals from more than 120 human LBNP experiments have been analyzed by Grudic and Mulligan using feature extraction and advanced statistical methods to build predictive models of acute blood loss and hemodynamic decompensation. The resulting algorithms use continuous, NIBP waveform data. Statistically unbiased accuracy estimates on all subjects showed a correlation of 0.95 for: (1) estimated LBNP level (or volume of blood loss in cc's), and (2) predicted level at which the test subject will experience hemodynamic decompensation, or cardiovascular collapse.

This technology quickly, accurately, and noninvasively predicts LBNP, which correlates with how much central blood volume has been redistributed to the pelvis and lower extremities; that is, how much blood a patient has "lost" (see Fig. 7-12, *red dots*). More importantly, it provides real-time information on the predicted level of "blood loss" (LBNP) that will cause hemodynamic decompensation for that specific individual (Fig. 7-12, *blue dots*). Humans who are exposed to LBNP will collapse at different times and at different levels of LBNP. The early identification of trauma patients who are more likely to

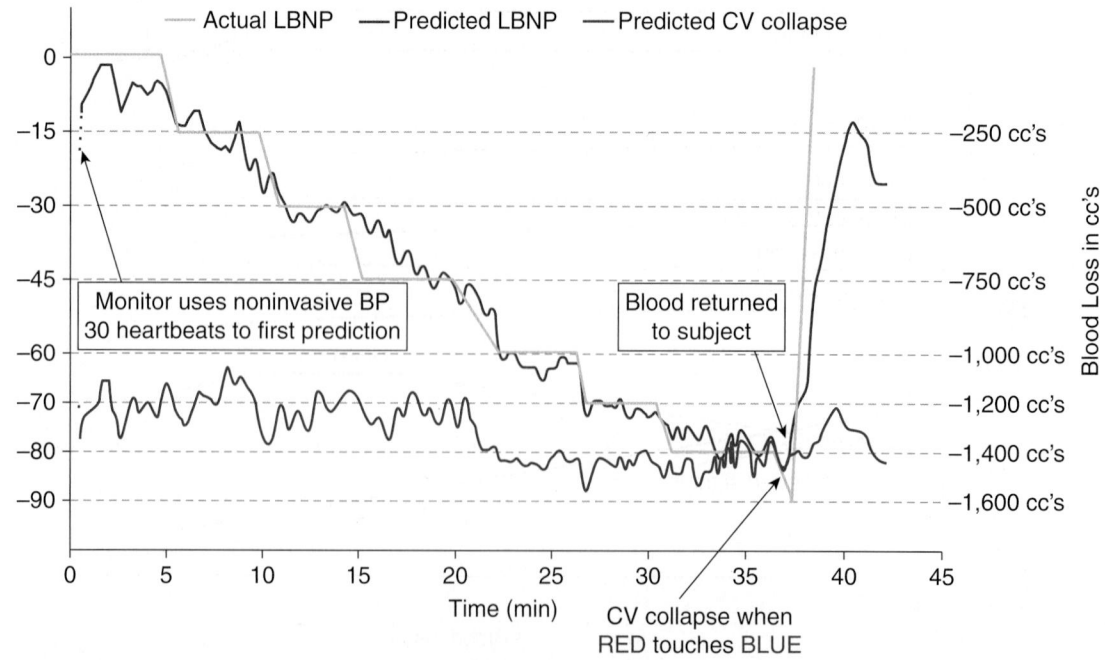

FIGURE 7-12  Live LBNP experiment. CipherSensor (Flashback Technologies, Inc., Longmont, CO) is a prototype noninvasive device designed to provide real-time information on blood loss volume (*red line*) and predict the amount of bleeding that will cause hemodynamic collapse (*blue line*). Stepwise drops in LBNP are marked by the *green line*. If the *red* and *blue* waveforms continue to converge, bleeding is ongoing. If the red waveform flattens, blood loss has stopped or IV fluid therapy is keeping up with blood loss. If the *red* and *blue* waveforms are diverging, then IV fluid resuscitation efforts are replenishing intravascular volume.

experience hemodynamic decompensation with less blood loss could prove critical to early intervention, establishing a triage order and better outcomes, since these patients are at greatest risk for rapid development of hemorrhage shock.

The physiological mechanisms that underlie greater tolerance to LBNP are under investigation. Preliminary results indicate that high tolerant (HT) individuals have a significantly greater elevation in heart rate than low tolerant subjects. The greater heart rate response of HT individuals may be due to greater cardiac vagal withdrawal and higher sympathetic nerve activity, the latter enhancing vasoconstriction to support blood pressure. Additionally, HT subjects have significantly greater oscillations in cerebral blood flow velocity and arterial blood pressure than low tolerant subjects. These are metrics that no human can detect or decipher in a beat-to-beat fashion. Their incorporation into future algorithms may, however, allow greater precision in the prediction of hemodynamic decompensation and the early identification of patients at greatest risk for CV collapse.

## EMERGING MONITORING PLATFORMS

To develop and evaluate models and algorithms for intelligent patient monitoring, we must have real patient data and a way to reconstruct the clinical context under which these data are generated. In other words, we need to obtain physiological measurements or signals from the patient's monitor; a well-annotated dataset that contains both physiological data and clinical annotations is key to the development of intelligent patient monitoring systems.

The ideal solution will be an integrated platform composed of physiological monitoring and therapeutic hardware devices, linked by a suite of software applications. The components integral to the next generation of tightly integrated monitoring systems include: a ventilator; 3/5-lead ECG; pulse oximeter; NIBP; etCO$_2$; patient temperature; invasive arterial and intracranial pressure capabilities; Ethernet communications; closed-loop control of oxygenation, ventilation and IV fluid control; an integrated electronic medical record (data storage/export); and alarming and smart help. The system should support several external IV pumps and other yet to be developed noninvasive monitors, all connected via powered-USB ports. Other potential modules that could be included are an oxygen concentrator, patient warming, and an anesthesia control module.

## DECISION SUPPORT

Noninvasive monitoring of cardiac, pulmonary, and tissue perfusion functions may be combined with an information system that predicts hospital outcome and provides therapeutic decision support. The lack of effective data integration and knowledge representation in patient monitoring limits its utility to clinicians. Intelligent alarm algorithms that use artificial intelligence techniques have the potential to reduce false alarm rates and to improve data integration and knowledge representation. Crucial to the development of such algorithms is a well-annotated data set. In previous studies, clinical events were either unavailable or annotated without accurate time synchronization with physiological signals, generating uncertainties during both the development and evaluation of intelligent alarm algorithms.

## SUMMARY

The combination of new noninvasive sensing and new state-of-the-art mathematical tools for waveform data analysis are giving rise to a new generation of tightly integrated "intelligent" patient monitoring systems. These systems will collect and synchronize exponentially growing amounts of vital sign data with electronic patient care information. They will enable the development of closed loop control and real-time clinical decision support, able to provide timelier, more cost-effective, assistive and autonomous patient care.

# Acute Cardiopulmonary Resuscitation

## KEY POINTS

1. For neonatal and pediatric patients, in the majority of circumstances hypoperfusion is secondary to low cardiac output caused by hypovolemia and preload reduction.

2. Patients with hypotension and reduced systemic vascular resistance are managed best initially via a continuous IV infusion of dopamine.

3. Variables that enhance the oxygen delivery/consumption dynamic include cardiac output, arterial oxygen concentration, hemoglobin concentration, and oxygen consumption.

## OPTIMIZING CARDIAC OUTPUT

The goal of the cardiopulmonary system is to deliver oxygen to and to remove metabolic waste and carbon dioxide from the peripheral tissues. Shock indicates a failure of the system to adequately perfuse the tissues. Shock is usually accompanied by either a reduction in cardiac output with an increase in systemic vascular resistance (eg, hypovolemic, obstructive, or cardiogenic shock) or an increase in cardiac output with a reduction in blood pressure secondary to a decrease in systemic vascular resistance (eg, anaphylactic, neurogenic, endocrinologic, and septic shock) (Fig. 7-13).

Minimum monitoring in the setting of impaired perfusion would include serial blood pressures and vital signs in addition to continuous ECG monitoring. Important physical

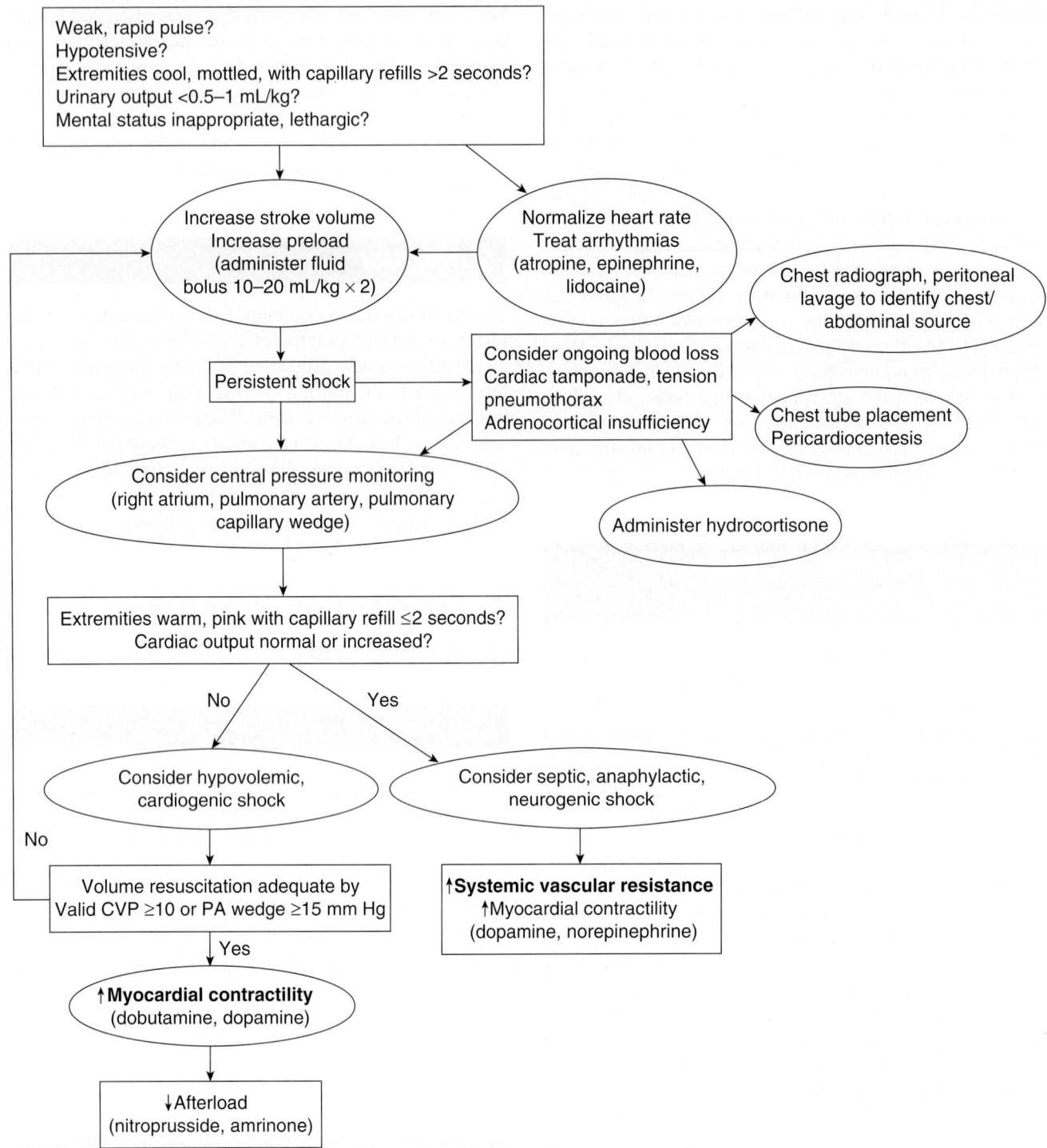

**FIGURE 7-13** An approach to the diagnosis and treatment of shock. (Reprinted with permission from *Hirschl RB, Heiss K. Cardiopulmonary critical care and shock. In: Oldham KT, Calambani PM, Foglia RP, eds. Surgery of Infants and Children. Scientific Principles and Practice. Philadelphia: Lippincott-Raven; 1997:149–182.*)

findings indicating poor perfusion or hypovolemia include poor skin turgor, cool extremities with pale color, a flat anterior fontanelle, dry mucous membranes, and capillary refill >2 seconds. Collapsed peripheral veins; a rapid, weak pulse; tachypneic, shallow breaths; cool extremities; and a reduction in glomerular filtration rate and renal blood flow as manifested by a reduction in urine output are more serious indicators of hypoperfusion. A change in the level of consciousness of the patient such as restlessness, anxiety, agitation, or unresponsiveness suggests greatly impaired oxygen delivery. It is important to recognize that hypoperfusion in children is often accompanied by a normal blood pressure until the point has been reached where complete hemodynamic collapse supervenes. The lower limit of normal systolic blood pressure in children may be approximated by the formula 80 + (2 × age in years).

In the majority of instances in neonatal and pediatric patients, hypoperfusion is secondary to low cardiac

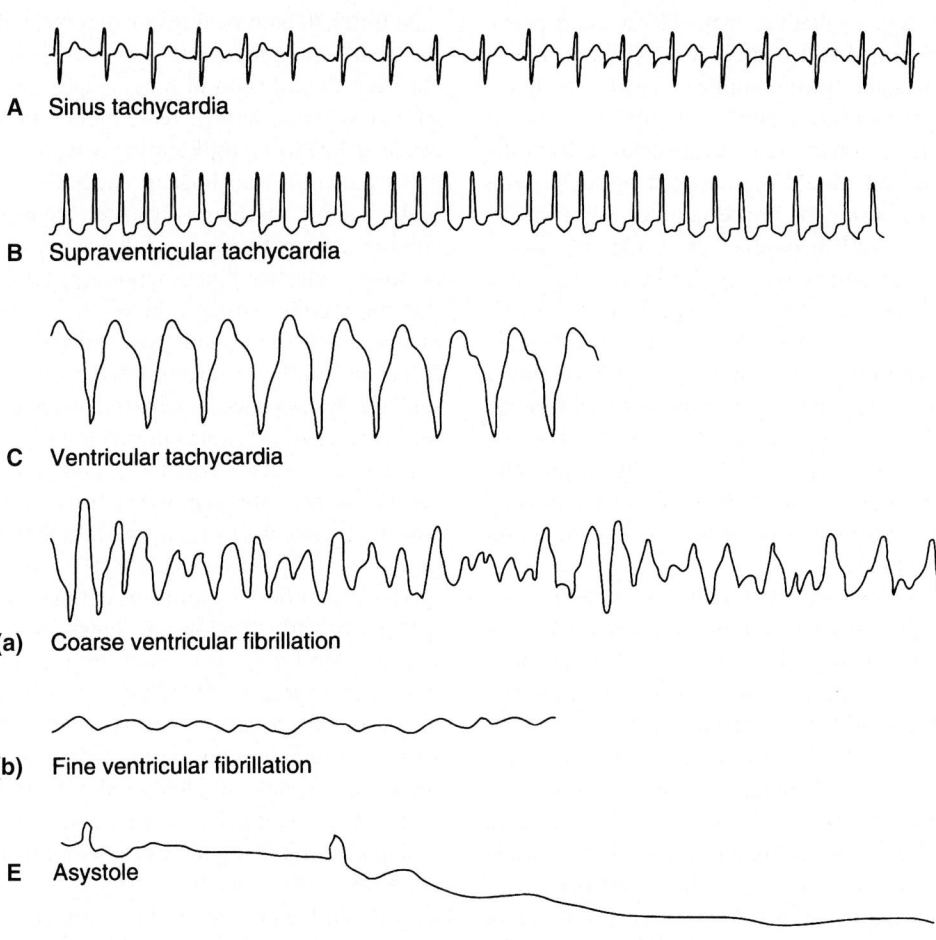

**FIGURE 7-14** Electrocardiographic findings demonstrating (**A**) the regular rhythm and P, QRS, and T sequence of sinus tachycardia at 180 beats/min, (**B**) the rapid, regular rhythm of supraventricular tachycardia at 320 beats/ min, (**C**) the wide QRS complex of ventricular tachycardia, (**D**) the disorganized depolarizations of coarse (a) and fine (b) ventricular fibrillation, and (**E**) the flat-line ECG of asystole. (Adapted from *Chameides L. Textbook of Pediatric Advance & Life Support. Dallas: American Heart Association; 1994.*)

output caused by hypovolemia and preload reduction. Volume resuscitation should be initiated with administration of repeated 10 mL/kg doses of crystalloid or 5% albumin over 15- to 20-minute time periods until hypotension and hypoperfusion resolve. It is not unusual for the hypovolemic, hypoperfused patient to require 40 to 60 mL/kg of crystalloid before resuscitation is adequate. Transfusion may be required to enhance oxygen-carrying capacity when the hemoglobin is <10 g/dL in neonates and <7 g/dL in older infants and children in whom a normal cardiac output and $SaO_2$ can be achieved. A hemoglobin >13 g/dL may be necessary in those patients with compromise in $SaO_2$ or cardiac output to optimize oxygen delivery.

A central venous pressure >10 to 15 mm Hg is usually associated with sufficient volume repletion. Persistent shock despite volume administration should lead one to suspect ongoing blood loss or additional causes of hypotension such as cardiac tamponade, tension pneumothorax, adrenocortical insufficiency, sepsis, neurogenic shock, or anaphylaxis. The presence of additional organ system failure and/or persistence of hypoperfusion despite adequate resuscitation may be an indication for pulmonary arterial catheter placement

for purposes of pulmonary arterial and left atrial pressure, mixed-venous oxygen saturation, and cardiac output assessment. Such invasive information may be critical to establishing the contribution of alterations in cardiac output or vascular tone to the shock state and the need for pharmacologic intervention. In patients who are too young for pulmonary arterial pressure monitoring or in whom the etiology of cardiac insufficiency remains unclear, echocardiography is a safe and noninvasive method for assessing cardiac function, ventricular filling, and for the presence of congenital heart disease or pericardial effusion/cardiac tamponade.

Arrhythmias contributing to the hypoperfused state should be treated. Arrhythmias can be classified into those that are too fast, too slow, or disorganized/absent and into those that are atrial or ventricular in origin (Fig. 7-14). Tachyarrhythmias may be caused by stimulation by catecholamines, digitalis, hypoxemia, electrical irritability, or other causes. For all of these arrhythmias, therefore, the patient should be evaluated for evidence of hypoxia, acidosis, electrolyte imbalance, or specific medication toxicity. Atrial tachyarrhythmias typically result from either sinus tachycardia or supraventricular tachycardia. Sinus tachycardia is associated with an underlying cause (fever, agitation, hypovolemia, and pain), which must be identified and treated. Most children maintain hemodynamic stability with supraventricular tachycardia, which, therefore, can be treated with adenosine on an emergent, rather than urgent, basis. Ventricular tachycardia is more hazardous and should be managed promptly with IV adenosine, amiodarone, or procainamide. Any tachyarrhythmias associated with hemodynamic instability should be immediately attended to be synchronized cardioversion at a dose of 0.5 to 1 J/kg, increasing to 2 J/kg if required. Bradyarrhythmias are often secondary to inadequate ventilation and oxygenation. Less often, slow rhythms may be secondary to vagal stimulation, sinus node abnormalities, heart block, hypercalcemia, or hypermagnesemia. Administration of IV atropine 0.02 mg/kg, isoproterenol 0.1 to 1.0 µg/kg/min, and epinephrine 0.01 mg/kg of 1:10,000 IV bolus, or an infusion of 0.1 to 1.0 µg/kg/min may increase heart rate, conduction velocity, and contractility.

Patients with hypotension and reduced systemic vascular resistance are managed best initially via a continuous IV infusion of dopamine. Dopamine is an endogenous catecholamine that results in enhancement of renal and splanchnic blood flow at doses between 1 and 5 µg/kg/min. β-Adrenergic receptor effects become apparent between 5 and 10 µg/kg/min, and α-adrenergic receptor-induced vasoconstriction develops at doses between 10 and 20 µg/kg/min. Therefore, dopamine provides enhancement of myocardial contractility at lower doses but splanchnic and peripheral vasoconstriction at higher infusion rates. Complications of dopamine administration are relatively few. These include the induction of arrhythmias, peripheral ischemia at high infusion rates, and skin loss following extravasation. Total body oxygen consumption and carbon dioxide production increase between 15% and 30% with the use of dopamine, epinephrine, and norepinephrine in normal adults. Most patients benefit from monitoring of the mixed-venous blood oxygen saturation during periods of pressor support to ensure that the advantages of an increase in oxygen delivery outweigh the costs of increased oxygen utilization (Table 7-2).

At times, dopamine infusion may be inadequate to produce the desired hemodynamic response. Such patients may benefit from the infusion of norepinephrine to further enhance vasoconstriction and increase blood pressure. Doses in the range of 0.05 to 1.0 µg/kg/min are typical.

For patients in cardiogenic shock (low cardiac output and high systemic vascular resistance), appropriate intravascular volume resuscitation is best followed by administration of the synthetic, selective β-adrenergic agent dobutamine. Myocardial contractility, stroke volume, and cardiac output typically increase, and the pulmonary capillary wedge pressure falls. Infusions are titrated from initial doses of 2 to 5 µg/kg/min until the desired effect is achieved or a maximum of 20 µg/kg/min is reached. Minimal alteration in heart rate or systemic vascular resistance is noted with dobutamine, although myocardial oxygen consumption is usually increased. Epinephrine at doses of 0.1 to 1.0 µg/kg/min may be used to provide potent α- and β-adrenergic effects in patients who are unresponsive to either dopamine or dobutamine infusions.

Patients with cardiogenic shock and elevated systemic vascular resistance may benefit from simultaneous administration of a systemic vasodilator to reduce cardiac afterload resistance, decrease myocardial stroke work, and increase stroke volume. In addition to cardiac output, the associated reductions in right and left atrial pressures may enhance gas exchange if myocardial dysfunction is associated with pulmonary edema. Systemic vasodilators such as sodium nitroprusside (initial dose 0.2-0.5 µg/kg/min; maximum 10 µg/kg/min) and phentolamine (1-20 µg/kg/min) may be utilized in conjunction with pressors to enhance myocardial function and cardiac output. Amrinone is a phosphodiesterase inhibitor that effectively enhances cardiac contractility while inducing systemic arterial vasodilation. An increase in oxygen consumption is not observed during the administration of amrinone. The loading dose of amrinone is 0.75 mg/kg over 5 to 10 minutes followed by a continuous infusion (CI) between 5 and 10 µg/kg/min.

Lactic acidosis is often observed in the setting of shock as the glycolytic pathway production of adenosine triphosphate predominates. Because of the untoward effect of metabolic acidosis on myocardial function and the efficacy of administered inotropes, a pH <7.20 should be corrected by hyperventilation if the $Paco_2$ > 40 mm Hg and/or by administration of IV sodium bicarbonate 1 to 2 mEq/kg. The total bicarbonate deficit may be calculated by the following:

$$\text{Total HCO}_3 \text{ deficit (mEq)} = \text{Base deficit (mEq/L)} \times \text{Weight (kg)} \times 0.3$$

One-half of this dose may be given over 1 to 2 hours followed by administration of the remainder over the ensuing 24 to 48 hours if indicated. Administration of sodium bicarbonate in the setting of hypoventilation may result in hypercarbia from production of $CO_2$. Therefore, in patients in whom hypercarbia may be of concern, *tris*-hydroxymethylaminomethane (THAM) may serve as an effective buffer in the setting of metabolic acidosis. A 3.6% solution of THAM (tromethamine) may be administered at a dose of 6 to 8 mL/kg over 20 minutes. The total dose over 24 hours should not exceed 40 mL/kg. Adverse effects may include hypoglycemia as well as hyperkalemia, hypervolumia, and

| TABLE 7-2 | Agents Commonly Administered in the Setting of Cardiac Insufficiency | |
|---|---|---|
| Drug | Dose (µg/kg/min) | Effect |
| Dopamine | 2-20 | Renal and splanchnic vasodilation at low dose; inotrope; vasoconstrictor |
| Dobutamine | 2-20 | Predominant inotrope |
| Epinephrine | 0.1-1 | Inotrope; vasoconstrictor |
| Nitroprusside | 0.2-10 | Vasodilator |
| Amrinone | 5-10 | Inotrope; vasodilator |
| Isoproterenol | 0.1-1 | Inotrope; chronotrope |
| Norepinephrine | 0.05-1 | Inotrope; vasoconstrictor |

hypernatremia, and, for this reason, THAM should be utilized with caution in patients with renal insufficiency

## OPTIMIZING OXYGEN DELIVERY/ CONSUMPTION (DO₂/VO₂) RELATIONSHIPS

Enhancement in cardiac output is associated with improvement in the SvO₂ and the DO₂/VO₂ ratio. SvO₂ and DO₂/VO₂ ratio are, however, dependent on 3 additional factors: arterial blood oxygenation, hemoglobin concentration, and oxygen consumption. The SaO₂ can often be enhanced through application of supplemental oxygen or positive-pressure ventilation. The uses of PEEP and positive-pressure ventilation are limited by their effects on cardiac output, the incidence of barotrauma, and the risk for ventilator-induced lung injury with application of peak inspiratory pressures (PIPs) >30 cm $H_2O$ and/or tidal volumes > 6 mL/kg. Assessment of the "best PEEP," which identifies the level of PEEP at which oxygen delivery and SvO₂ are optimal, should be performed in any patient requiring an FiO₂ > 0.60. The FiO₂ should be adjusted to maintain the SaO₂ greater than 85%. Additional interventions such as high-frequency oscillation, prone positioning, inverse-ratio ventilation, nitric oxide (NO) administration, and surfactant administration may enhance SaO₂. Likewise, the effects of transfusion or other ventilator manipulation on oxygen kinetics may be assessed.

One of the most efficient ways to enhance oxygen delivery is to increase the oxygen-carrying capacity of the blood. For instance, an increase in hemoglobin from 7.5 to 15 g/dL will be associated with a 2-fold increase in oxygen delivery at constant cardiac output (Fig. 7-15). Blood viscosity is increased with blood transfusion, which may result in a reduction in cardiac output. However, a number of studies have now demonstrated that the hematocrit overshadows the viscosity in the final determination of oxygen delivery.

Oxygen consumption may be elevated because of sepsis, burns, agitation, seizures, hyperthermia, hyperthyroidism, and increased catecholamine production or infusion. A number of interventions may be applied to reduce oxygen consumption, such as sedation and mechanical ventilation. Paralysis may enhance the effectiveness of mechanical ventilation while simultaneously reducing oxygen consumption. In the appropriate setting, hypothermia may be induced with an associated reduction of 7% in VO₂ with each 1°C decrease in core temperature.

Continuous mixed-venous oxygen saturation monitoring may enhance the practitioner's ability to optimize oxygen consumption and delivery relationships. For instance, the "best PEEP" may be determined by continuous monitoring of the SvO₂ as the PEEP is sequentially increased from 5 to 15 cm $H_2O$ over a short-time period. The point where the SvO₂ is maximal indicates the PEEP at which oxygen delivery is optimal. The result of various interventions designed to increase cardiac output, such as volume administration, infusion of inotropic agents, administration of afterload-reducing drugs, and correction of acid–base abnormalities, may be assessed by the effect on the SvO₂.

## CARDIOPULMONARY RESUSCITATION

The response to an unplanned in-hospital cardiac arrest begins with institution of the ABCs of cardiopulmonary resuscitation (CPR). Unresponsiveness and breathlessness should be confirmed. If carotid or brachial artery pulses are absent, external cardiac massage is instituted. The priority should be to start CPR with chest compressions immediately,

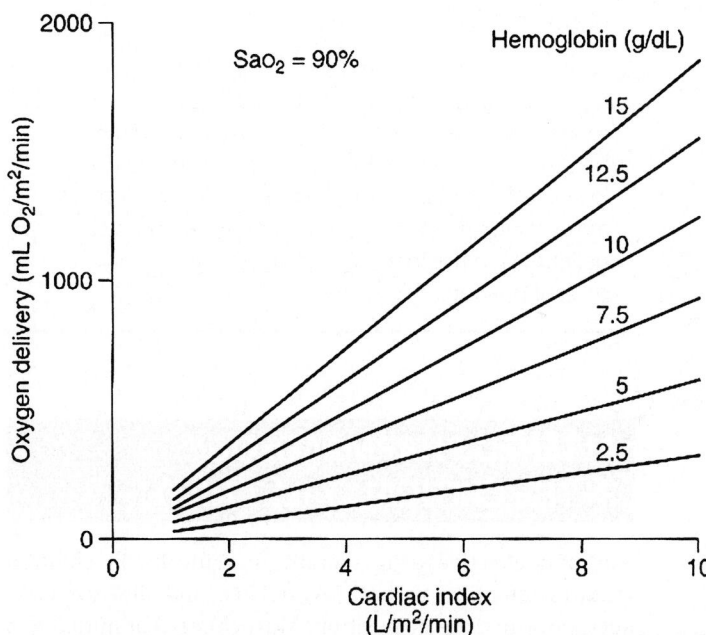

**FIGURE 7-15** The relationship of hemoglobin concentration and cardiac index to oxygen delivery at a constant SaO₂ = 90%. Note the strong influence of hemoglobin concentration on DO₂. (Adapted from *Hirschl RB, Heiss K. Cardiopulmonary critical care and shock. In: Oldham KT, Calambani PM, Foglia RP, eds. Surgery of Infants and Children. Scientific Principles and Practice. Philadelphia: Lippincott-Raven; 1997:149–182.*)

while a second rescuer prepares to provide ventilations. As soon as possible, the airway is cleared, endotracheal intubation is performed, and breathing is instituted at a rate of 1 breath every 6 to 8 seconds. The compression rate should be at least 100 compressions per minute at a depth of at least one third of the anteroposterior (AP) diameter of the chest or approximately 1½ inches in infants and approximately 2 inches in children. Those performing CPR should avoid long interruptions to secure the airway, check the heart rhythm, or move the patient. If IV access is not available, resuscitation medications such as atropine, epinephrine, and lidocaine may be administered via the endotracheal tube. In that case, medications should be diluted in 1 to 2 mL of normal saline and injected into the endotracheal tube to be followed by application of positive-pressure ventilation. All cardiac arrest medications except for bicarbonate may be administered via the endotracheal tube. During cardiac arrest, IV fluids should be administered to correct hypovolemia; positive-pressure ventilation and oxygen should be provided to correct hypoxemia; and sodium bicarbonate should be administered in an initial dose of 1 mEq/kg or as directed by blood gas analysis to correct metabolic acidosis. Other medications of use in cardiac arrest include atropine to accelerate the cardiac rate; epinephrine to increase systemic vascular resistance, blood pressure, and myocardial contractility and automaticity; and amiodarone for the child with ventricular tachycardia or ventricular fibrillation. Suggested doses and frequency of dosing during cardiac arrest are shown in Table 7-3. If ventricular fibrillation is present, external defibrillation should be performed with an initial setting of 2 J/kg. If unsuccessful, this should be repeated immediately with 4 J/kg. Higher energy levels may be considered in the setting of refractory ventricular fibrillation, not to exceed 10 J/kg or the adult maximum dose. It is critical that the underlying etiology of the cardiac arrest be identified: hypoventilation, hypoxia, hypo/hyperkalemia, and hypovolemia are among the most frequent causes of cardiac arrest in children. Pulseless electrical activity (PEA), indicated by the presence of organized electrical activity on ECG with ineffective myocardial contractions, is relatively frequently observed during cardiac arrest. Possible etiologies include tension pneumothorax, cardiac tamponade, hypovolemia, and hypocalcemia. Algorithms for the management of specific cardiac rhythm disturbances and general cardiopulmonary support during CPR are shown in Figs. 7-16 to 7-19.

# Pharmacologic Support for Acute Pediatric Illness

## KEY POINTS

1. Critical illness is associated with changes in drug disposition; dosage adjustments may be required to prevent drug toxicity and/or treatment failure.

2. IV fluid resuscitation is common in the pediatric ICU; isotonic fluids are recommended as first-line therapy, while colloid solutions are reserved for refractory cases.

3. Prophylactic antibiotics have little value beyond the first 24 hours following a surgical procedure.

4. Venous thromboembolism (VTE) is uncommon in children. Strategies to further reduce VTE include risk screening on admission, lower extremity sequential compression devices and, for high risk children, pharmacologic agents.

5. Provision of adequate analgesia and sedation is a fundamental practice in the PICU. Assessment tools (including validated scoring systems) should be used to guide therapy. Strategies to identify the lowest effective dose of opioids and benzodiazepines are encouraged in an effort to reduce dependence, delirium, and risk for drug withdrawal upon discontinuation.

| TABLE 7-3 | Medications Used During Management of Cardiac Arrest |
|---|---|
| **Drug** | **Dose and Instruction** |
| Atropine | IV/IM/ET IO/IN (0.02 mg/kg; minimum 0.1 mg, maximum 0.5 mg infant/child and 1 mg adult; may repeat × 1) |
| Sodium bicarbonate | IV (1 mEq/kg) give slowly based on blood gas analysis |
| Epinephrine | First dose:<br>0.01 mg/kg (0.1 mL/kg of 1:10,000) IV/IO/ET<br>0.1 mg/kg (0.1 mg/kg of 1:1000) ET<br>Subsequent doses:<br>0.1 mg/kg (0.1 mL/kg of 1:1000) q 3-5 min IV/IO/ET |
| Lidocaine | 1 mg/kg IV/ET/IM slowly, repeat q 5 min PRN; then begin IV infusion |
| Bretylium | Initial dose: IV<br>5 mg/kg<br>Subsequent doses:<br>10 mg/kg |

IV, intravenous; IM, intramuscular; ET, endotracheal tube instillation; IO, intraosseous; IN, intranasal.

## ALTERED PHARMACOLOGY IN THE CRITICALLY ILL CHILD

Safe and effective drug therapy in critically ill children requires attention to both age-related and illness-related alterations in drug disposition. Most children admitted to a

## Asystole

Check 2 leads
Intubate/IV access
EPI 0.1 mL/kg of 1:10,000 IV
▽
Atropine 0.02 mg/kg IV
(min 0.1 mg; max 1 mg)
▽
EPI 0.1 mL/kg of 1:1000 IV
q 3–5 min
▽
Consider EPI drip

*Consider hypoxia, ↑K+, ↓K+, acidosis, overdose, hypothermia*

## Pulseless Electrical Activity (PEA/EMD)

CPR
Intubate/IV access
EPI 0.1 mL/kg of 1:10,000 IV
▽
EPI 0.1 mL/kg of 1:1000 IV
q 3–5 min

Consider EPI drip

Assess for:
1. Hypovolemia
2. Tamponade
3. Tension PTX
4. Hypothermia
5. Hypoxia/acidosis

## Symptomatic Bradycardia
(poor perfusion, hypotension, resp distress)

Airway/IV access
▽
EPI 0.1 mL/kg of 1:10,000 IV
▽
Atropine 0.02 mg/kg IV
repeat × 1 q 5 min
▽
EPI 0.1 mL/kg of 1:10,000 IV
repeat q 3–5 min
▽
Consider EPI drip

## V FIB/Pulseless VT

Asynch shock 2 J/kg
▽
Asynch shock 4 J/kg × 2
▽
CPR
Intubate/IV access
EPI per asystole protocol
q 3–5 min
Asynch shock 4 J/kg
▽
Lidocaine 1 mg/kg IV
Asynch shock 4 J/kg
▽
Bretylium 5 mg/kg IV
Asynch shock 4 J/kg
▽
Bretylium 10 mg/kg IV
Asynch shock 4 J/kg
▽
Repeat Lido or Bret,
then shock again 4 J/kg

*(Repeat EPI every 3–5 min)*

## V TACH

**Unstable:**
IV access (defibrillate immediately if critically unstable)
Otherwise, consider sedation
Cardiovert (synch) 1 J/kg
▽
Cardiovert (synch) 2 J/kg
▽
Cardiovert (synch) 4 J/kg × 2
▽
If recurs add lidocaine
and cardiovert

**Stable:**
Lidocaine 1 mg/kg IV
▽
Lidocaine drip
Sedate
▽
Cardiovert (synch)
0.5–2 J/kg
▽
Bretylium 5 mg/kg IV
▽
Bretylium 10 mg/kg IV
▽
Overdrive pacing

## SVT

**Unstable:**
Cardiovert (synch)
0.5–1 J/kg
▽
Cardiovert (synch)
2 J/kg
▽
Cardiovert (synch)
4 J/kg

**Stable:**
1. Vagal maneuvers
2. Adenosine
3. Dig/β-blocker
4. Verapamil *(avoid if <1 yr)*

▽ = Assess pt, continue if no response

**FIGURE 7-16** Algorithm of stepwise procedures in the resuscitation of the pediatric patient in acute cardiorespiratory arrest.

pediatric intensive care unit (PICU) have multisystem organ involvement that will cause significant changes to the pharmacokinetic and pharmacodynamic profiles of medications. Additionally, since critically ill children are often exposed to more than 20 different medications during their illness, special attention must also be given to drug–drug interactions. Lastly, the influence of body composition and weight on drug dosing in a population that relies on milligram per kilogram (mg/kg) dosing must be considered. The prevalence of obesity in childhood is increasing and may require calculation of ideal and adjusted body weight to deliver the most appropriate dose to a child. In general, the highest dose recommend for a child is the maximum dose approved for adults. All of these factors make the management of drug therapy in the critically ill infant and child a distinct challenge.

Drug disposition is represented by 4 major domains: absorption, distribution, metabolism, and elimination. The critically ill child may experience dramatic alterations in all 4 domains during the acute and convalescence

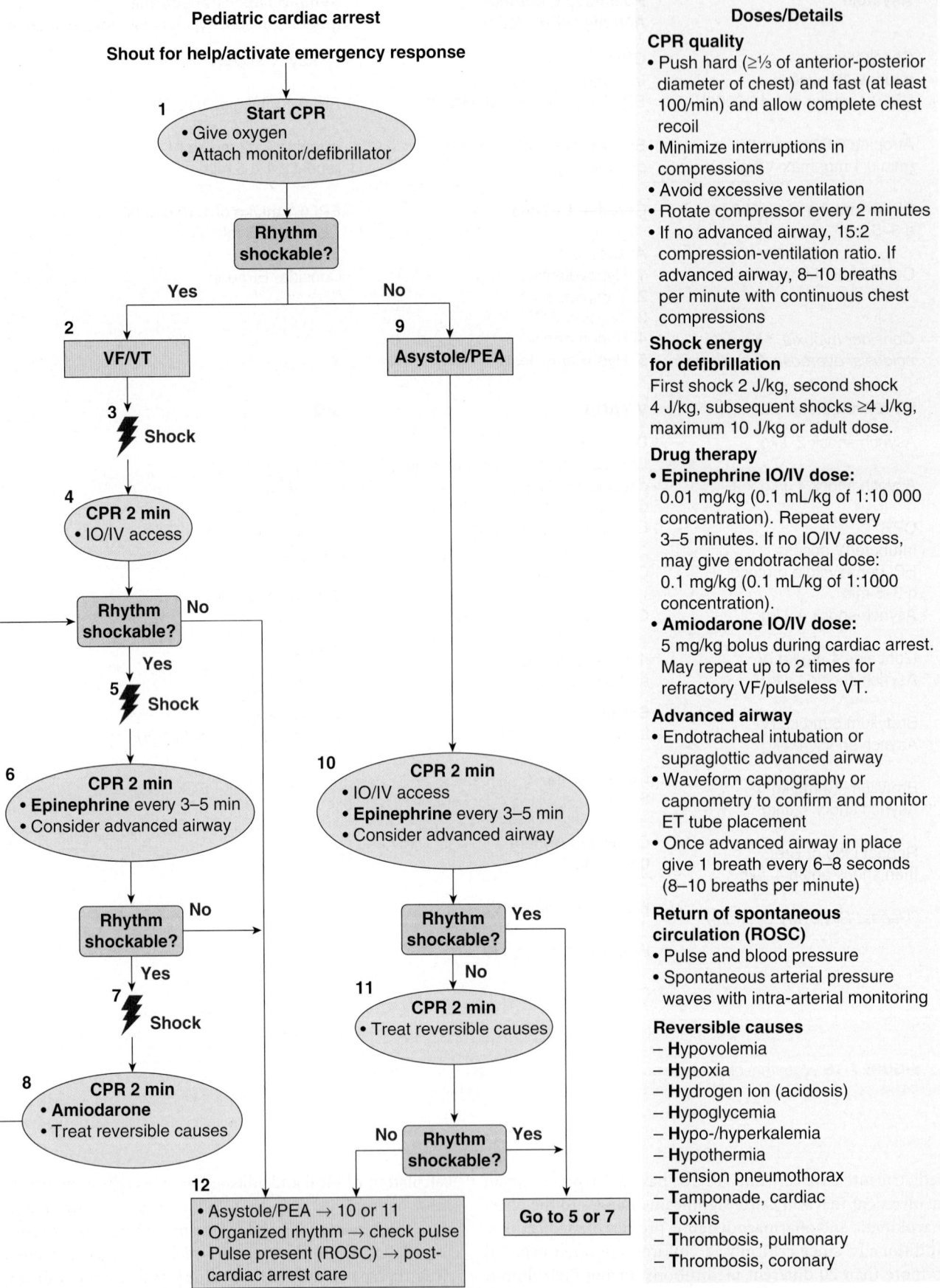

**Pediatric cardiac arrest**

**Shout for help/activate emergency response**

**1 Start CPR**
- Give oxygen
- Attach monitor/defibrillator

**Rhythm shockable?**

Yes → **2 VF/VT**

No → **9 Asystole/PEA**

**3 Shock**

**4 CPR 2 min**
- IO/IV access

**Rhythm shockable?** No

Yes

**5 Shock**

**6 CPR 2 min**
- **Epinephrine** every 3–5 min
- Consider advanced airway

**Rhythm shockable?** No

Yes

**7 Shock**

**8 CPR 2 min**
- **Amiodarone**
- Treat reversible causes

**10 CPR 2 min**
- IO/IV access
- **Epinephrine** every 3–5 min
- Consider advanced airway

**Rhythm shockable?** Yes

No

**11 CPR 2 min**
- Treat reversible causes

**Rhythm shockable?** No / Yes

**12**
- Asystole/PEA → 10 or 11
- Organized rhythm → check pulse
- Pulse present (ROSC) → post-cardiac arrest care

**Go to 5 or 7**

**Doses/Details**

**CPR quality**
- Push hard (≥⅓ of anterior-posterior diameter of chest) and fast (at least 100/min) and allow complete chest recoil
- Minimize interruptions in compressions
- Avoid excessive ventilation
- Rotate compressor every 2 minutes
- If no advanced airway, 15:2 compression-ventilation ratio. If advanced airway, 8–10 breaths per minute with continuous chest compressions

**Shock energy for defibrillation**
First shock 2 J/kg, second shock 4 J/kg, subsequent shocks ≥4 J/kg, maximum 10 J/kg or adult dose.

**Drug therapy**
- **Epinephrine IO/IV dose:**
  0.01 mg/kg (0.1 mL/kg of 1:10 000 concentration). Repeat every 3–5 minutes. If no IO/IV access, may give endotracheal dose: 0.1 mg/kg (0.1 mL/kg of 1:1000 concentration).
- **Amiodarone IO/IV dose:**
  5 mg/kg bolus during cardiac arrest. May repeat up to 2 times for refractory VF/pulseless VT.

**Advanced airway**
- Endotracheal intubation or supraglottic advanced airway
- Waveform capnography or capnometry to confirm and monitor ET tube placement
- Once advanced airway in place give 1 breath every 6–8 seconds (8–10 breaths per minute)

**Return of spontaneous circulation (ROSC)**
- Pulse and blood pressure
- Spontaneous arterial pressure waves with intra-arterial monitoring

**Reversible causes**
- **H**ypovolemia
- **H**ypoxia
- **H**ydrogen ion (acidosis)
- **H**ypoglycemia
- **H**ypo-/hyperkalemia
- **H**ypothermia
- **T**ension pneumothorax
- **T**amponade, cardiac
- **T**oxins
- **T**hrombosis, pulmonary
- **T**hrombosis, coronary

**FIGURE 7-17** Resuscitation algorithm for the pediatric patient in acute cardiopulmonary arrest. Reprinted with permission from *Kleinman ME, Chameides L, Schexnayder SM, et al. 2010 American Heart Association Guidelines for Cardiopulmonary Resuscitation and Emergency Cardiovascular Care Science; Part 14: pediatric advanced life support. Circulation 2010;122:S876–S908.*

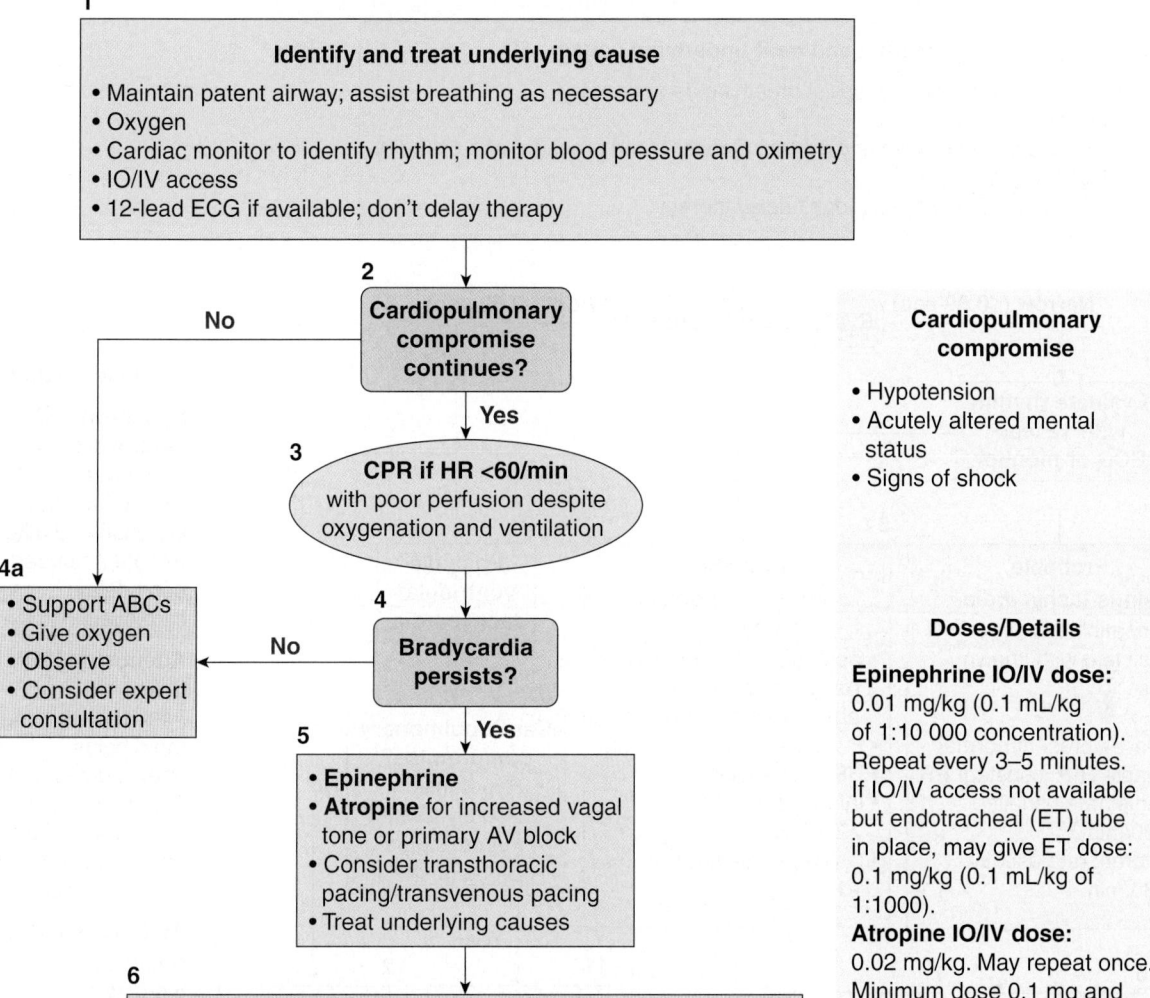

**Pediatric bradycardia**
with a pulse and poor perfusion

**1**

**Identify and treat underlying cause**

- Maintain patent airway; assist breathing as necessary
- Oxygen
- Cardiac monitor to identify rhythm; monitor blood pressure and oximetry
- IO/IV access
- 12-lead ECG if available; don't delay therapy

**2**

No — **Cardiopulmonary compromise continues?**

Yes

**3**

**CPR if HR <60/min** with poor perfusion despite oxygenation and ventilation

**4a**
- Support ABCs
- Give oxygen
- Observe
- Consider expert consultation

**4**

No — **Bradycardia persists?**

Yes

**5**

- **Epinephrine**
- **Atropine** for increased vagal tone or primary AV block
- Consider transthoracic pacing/transvenous pacing
- Treat underlying causes

**6**

**If pulseless arrest develops, go to cardiac arrest algorithm**

**Cardiopulmonary compromise**

- Hypotension
- Acutely altered mental status
- Signs of shock

**Doses/Details**

**Epinephrine IO/IV dose:**
0.01 mg/kg (0.1 mL/kg of 1:10 000 concentration). Repeat every 3–5 minutes. If IO/IV access not available but endotracheal (ET) tube in place, may give ET dose: 0.1 mg/kg (0.1 mL/kg of 1:1000).
**Atropine IO/IV dose:**
0.02 mg/kg. May repeat once. Minimum dose 0.1 mg and maximum single dose 0.5 mg.

**FIGURE 7-18** Diagnosis and treatment algorithm for the pediatric patient with acute severe bradycardia. Reprinted with permission from *Kleinman ME, Chameides L, Schexnayder SM, et al. 2010 American Heart Association Guidelines for Cardiopulmonary Resuscitation and Emergency Cardiovascular Care Science; Part 14: pediatric advanced life support. Circulation 2010;122:S876–S908.*

phases of their illness because of changes in cardiac output, vascular tone, membrane integrity, end-organ perfusion, metabolic capacity, and endogenous production of plasma proteins. Inattention to these changes can lead to drug toxicity and/or treatment failure. Equally important is the fact that these alterations are not static. As a child's illness/injury improves, it follows that drug disposition will again change and require a change in the drug therapy plan.

Many drug disposition alterations can be anticipated and adjustments in drug therapy can be performed prospectively. Knowing which medications require dosing adjustments will depend on the characteristics of the patient as well as the drug (Table 7-4). Protein binding sensitivity, metabolic dependence on blood flow or enzyme capacity, and degree of renal clearance all influence the decision to modify drug therapy.

## ABSORPTION AND DISTRIBUTION

Oral absorption of drug therapy will be compromised during critical illness due to reduced blood flow to the gastrointestinal tract, decreased transporter proteins across biologic membranes, and impaired gut motility. The IV route is the preferred route of drug administration as it provides the highest and most reliable bioavailability of drug. Drug distribution (the movement of drug throughout the body) will be affected by changes in the integrity of cellular membranes, plasma protein production, extra- and intracellular fluid volumes, and body composition. Critical illness often results in a shift away from plasma protein production (namely albumin), and toward acute-phase reactant production ($\alpha_1$ glycoprotein and C-reactive protein). In fact, trauma and acute stress can result

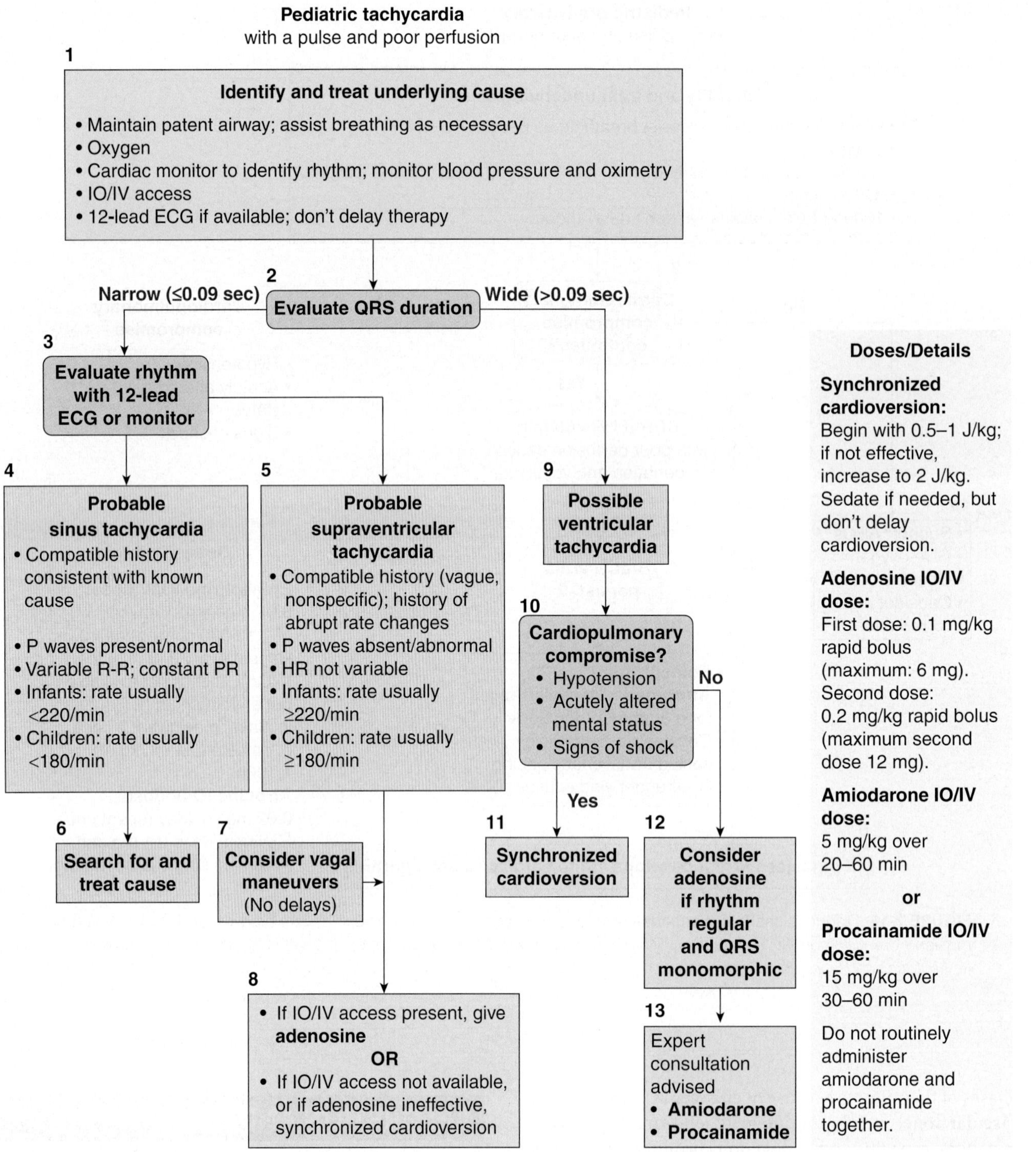

**Pediatric tachycardia**
with a pulse and poor perfusion

**1**

**Identify and treat underlying cause**

- Maintain patent airway; assist breathing as necessary
- Oxygen
- Cardiac monitor to identify rhythm; monitor blood pressure and oximetry
- IO/IV access
- 12-lead ECG if available; don't delay therapy

**2**

Narrow (≤0.09 sec) **Evaluate QRS duration** Wide (>0.09 sec)

**3**

**Evaluate rhythm with 12-lead ECG or monitor**

**4**

**Probable sinus tachycardia**

- Compatible history consistent with known cause

- P waves present/normal
- Variable R-R; constant PR
- Infants: rate usually <220/min
- Children: rate usually <180/min

**5**

**Probable supraventricular tachycardia**

- Compatible history (vague, nonspecific); history of abrupt rate changes
- P waves absent/abnormal
- HR not variable
- Infants: rate usually ≥220/min
- Children: rate usually ≥180/min

**9**

**Possible ventricular tachycardia**

**10**

**Cardiopulmonary compromise?**

- Hypotension
- Acutely altered mental status
- Signs of shock

No

Yes

**6**

**Search for and treat cause**

**7**

**Consider vagal maneuvers**
(No delays)

**8**

- If IO/IV access present, give **adenosine**

**OR**

- If IO/IV access not available, or if adenosine ineffective, synchronized cardioversion

**11**

**Synchronized cardioversion**

**12**

**Consider adenosine if rhythm regular and QRS monomorphic**

**13**

Expert consultation advised
- **Amiodarone**
- **Procainamide**

**Doses/Details**

**Synchronized cardioversion:**
Begin with 0.5–1 J/kg; if not effective, increase to 2 J/kg. Sedate if needed, but don't delay cardioversion.

**Adenosine IO/IV dose:**
First dose: 0.1 mg/kg rapid bolus (maximum: 6 mg). Second dose: 0.2 mg/kg rapid bolus (maximum second dose 12 mg).

**Amiodarone IO/IV dose:**
5 mg/kg over 20–60 min

or

**Procainamide IO/IV dose:**
15 mg/kg over 30–60 min

Do not routinely administer amiodarone and procainamide together.

**FIGURE 7-19** Diagnosis and treatment algorithm for the pediatric patient with tachycardia. Reprinted with permission from *Kleinman ME, Chameides L, Schexnayder SM, et al. 2010 American Heart Association Guidelines for Cardiopulmonary Resuscitation and Emergency Cardiovascular Care Science; Part 14: pediatric advanced life support. Circulation 2010;122:S876–S908.*

in a 50% reduction in serum albumin concentrations. Medications that are highly protein bound to albumin (eg, many anticonvulsants) will experience a higher free fraction and since the free drug is the pharmacologically active drug, have a more profound clinical effect, and increased risk of toxicity. Conversely, medications bound to $\alpha_1$ glycoprotein (eg, morphine, clindamycin) can experience a reduced physiologic response because free concentrations of these drugs actually

decrease during acute pathologic stress. When a drug normally exhibits more than 80% protein binding, even a small change in the bound fraction of that medication can have a significant influence on pharmacologic outcome.

As serum concentrations of albumin fall, fluid will shift from intra- to extravascular compartments. This fluid shift can be further complicated by administration of fluid to the surgical patient to optimize perfusion. These fluid shifts

| TABLE 7-4 | Summary of Pharmacokinetic Alterations During Various Phases of Critical Illness | |
|---|---|---|
| Physiologic State | Typical Pharmacokinetic Alterations | Anticipated Changes in Drug Therapy |
| Early acute stress | Reduced serum albumin, reduced CYP450 metabolism | Reduction in dose of highly protein (albumin) bound medications; reduction in dose and/or interval of medications metabolized by CYP450 system |
| Early postoperative phase with fluid shifts | Increased $V_d$ of water-soluble medications | Increased dose of water-soluble medication |
| Renal dysfunction | Reduced GFR | Prolonged dosing interval of renally eliminated medications, especially when CrCl falls below 50 mg/m² |
| Hepatic dysfunction | Lower serum albumin production, reduced enzymatic metabolism capacity | Reduction in dose of highly protein bound medications and prolongation of dosing interval for medications with capacity-limited characteristics |
| Shock | Reduced blood flow to kidney and liver | Reduction in dose and/or prolongation of dosing interval for medications with flow-limited characteristics |

together with changes in cellular membrane integrity (capillary leak syndrome) may result in marked changes in compartment volumes (volume of distribution, $V_d$). The $V_d$ is an important variable in determining loading doses of medications and dose adjustments may be required. In general, the initial dose(s) of water-soluble and ionic charged medications (eg, aminoglycosides and β-lactams) will need to be increased to achieve target serum concentrations in the patient experiencing volume overload. However, because only free drug is available for clearance, over time the clearance of drug affected by reduced protein binding also increases, making the net effect on the patient more difficult to predict. In general, drug dosing of highly protein-bound drugs may need to be acutely reduced, but should return to normal as the child clinically improves and drug clearance approaches baseline values. Moreover, when the serum albumin falls below 2.5 g/dL, medications with high-protein binding characteristics will likely need to be acutely adjusted because there will be a substantially higher free fraction of drug available for pharmacologic activity.

## METABOLISM AND ELIMINATION

Critical illness is associated with alterations in metabolic rate. Aerobic conditions are maintained during the hyperdynamic state of early illness, when blood flow and oxygen delivery to the organs (including the liver) may be increased. Medications that are considered flow-dependent will experience an increase in drug clearance. As illness persists, however, and oxygen demand exceeds oxygen supply, the patient begins to transition to anaerobic metabolism and a decrease in drug clearance. Changes in drug clearance due to altered hepatic blood flow can be predicted by monitoring changes in the hemodynamic variables of the individual. Changes in hepatic function can alter drug activity due to influence on drug metabolism, transportation, and presentation of the drug molecule to hepatocyte and isoenzyme capacity.

Drug clearance is further determined by the amount of metabolic enzyme production available—this is termed capacity-limited clearance. Medications that follow capacity-limited clearance depend heavily on hepatic enzyme activity. Dosage adjustments during acute illness are often required because the liver is preoccupied with the production of acute phase reactants rather than the production of enzymes responsible for drug biotransformation. Additionally, the metabolic activity of many enzyme systems can be inhibited by proinflammatory cytokines. The most dramatic change occurs in the cytochrome P-450 isoenzyme (CYP) system. This system is responsible for most drug–drug interactions and oxidation reactions. Understanding which isoenzymes are responsible for drug metabolism is useful in predicting a patient's clinical response to drug therapy during critical illness. Variability in CYP activity is influenced not only by critical illness and age, but also by genetic composition. Genetic polymorphisms in the CYP family have been identified and can account for interpatient variability in drug response. Polymorphisms have also been identified in drug transporter as well as drug target genes. The influence of genetic variability on drug dosing in the PICU is a new area of study that is gaining interest.

After the metabolic fate of a drug has been determined, most medications will require renal clearance for drug removal. Renal elimination of drug involves both filtration and secretion. Drug filtration occurs within the glomerulus while drug secretion occurs along the nephron. During periods of ischemia and hypoperfusion, cardiac output directed toward the renal bed is decreased and drug clearance is hindered. In clinical practice, the glomerular filtration rate can be estimated using the child's serum creatinine concentration, age, and height. Many medications will require dose or interval changes when calculated creatinine clearance falls below 50 mL/m². For children with renal failure necessitating renal replacement therapy (hemodialysis, peritoneal dialysis, continuous renal replacement therapy with or without filtration), it is essential to know the extent of drug removal by the specific renal therapy. Properties of the drug (hydrophilicity, molecular weight, plasma protein binding, $V_d$) will help distinguish which drugs are dialyzable. In general, drugs with low molecular weight, low protein binding, and high water-solubility will be dialyzed. Drugs with extensive tissue distribution and high lipophilicity will be less affected (or cleared) by dialysis.

The application of therapeutic drug monitoring (collection and interpretation of serum drug concentrations) for those medications with a narrow therapeutic index is a valuable tool in calculating the best drug regimen. Measuring serum drug concentrations is helpful in children with drug disposition variability, especially those who are critically ill. This drug-dosing approach optimizes drug therapy, while minimizing drug toxicity. It has been shown to improve patient outcomes while maintaining cost-effectiveness. Close consultation with clinical pharmacy services can aid in the proper dosing of medications during all phases of critical illness.

## CLINICAL USE OF PLASMA EXPANDERS

Critically ill and postoperative patients may require IV fluid resuscitation due to intravascular volume loss from trauma, surgery, drainage, and third spacing. Low volume status and hypovolemic shock can be managed with crystalloid and/or colloid solutions. The choice between crystalloid and colloid for fluid resuscitation continues to be debated with the use of human albumin at the center of this debate. While the use of albumin may have advantages in certain patient populations, it does warrant scrutiny due to its potential risks and higher cost when compared to crystalloids.

Colloids (eg, albumin, dextran-70, hetastarch 6%) have large molecular weights and as such are thought to remain in the intravascular space for prolonged periods of time after administration. Those who support the use of colloids argue that colloids improve microcirculation better than crystalloids. With the exception of 25% albumin, the provision of colloid results in equal volumes of intravascular volume expansion. Twenty-five percent (25%) albumin maintains an oncotic pressure approximately 5 times greater than normal plasma, and can expand much greater volumes (Table 7-5). Crystalloids (0.9% saline, lactated ringers) cross into the interstitial space more freely, resulting in only a quarter of the volume remaining in the intravascular space. Despite the theoretical volume expansion advantage of colloids, they have not been shown to be superior to crystalloids in most patient populations. This lack of superiority may be due to the physiological changes present in the critically ill, including endothelial cell injury with resulting capillary leak. This leak allows intravascular fluid to escape into the interstitial space with little regard for molecular weight. Additionally, colloid molecules may leak into the interstitial space, resulting in an oncotic pressure gradient favoring more tissue swelling.

There have been many randomized trials in critically ill adults comparing crystalloid and protein-based plasma volume expanders. Those studies designed to compare normal saline to lactated ringers found that saline was associated with a greater degree of progressive hyperchloremic metabolic acidosis, elevated serum creatinine, and reduced urine output. A meta-analysis published by the Cochrane Injuries Group Reviewers compared 0.9% saline to 5% albumin. They concluded no difference between the 2 therapies. However, a separate meta-analysis (which included pediatric trials) suggested that albumin may actually increase the risk of mortality. Acknowledging the limitations of these meta-analyses (namely, heterogeneity of methods and selection criteria) and new concerns regarding the safety of albumin, researchers were prompted to study fluid resuscitation in distinct patient populations using well-planned controlled and randomized methods. The Saline Versus Albumin Fluid Evaluation (SAFE) Study randomly assigned 6997 patients to receive either saline or 4% albumin for fluid resuscitation. No difference in 28-day mortality, incidence of organ failure, ICU length of stay, duration of mechanical ventilation, or renal replacement therapy was detected between the 2 study groups. However, further evaluation of the 6 predefined subgroups demonstrated differences in patient outcomes between albumin- and saline-treated groups. The use of albumin was favored in patients with sepsis and septic shock, but was associated with increased mortality in trauma patients.

| TABLE 7-5 | Comparison of Intravascular Volume Expanders | | | | |
|---|---|---|---|---|---|
| Fluid Classification | Infused Volume (mL) | Equivalent Intravascular Volume Expansion (mL) | Oncotic Pressure (mm Hg) | Calculated Osmolarity (mOsm/L) | Sodium (mmol/L) |
| Normal saline (0.9%) | 1000 | 250 | 0 | 308 | 154 |
| Lactated ringers | 1000 | 250 | 0 | 274 | 130 |
| Dextrose 5% in water | 1000 | 100 | 0 | 252 | 0 |
| Dextran-70, 6% | 500 | 500 | 193 | 0.3 | 154 |
| Albumin 5% | 500 | 500 | 20-30 | 290-310 | 140-160 |
| Albumin 25% | 100 | 500 | 120-150 | 310 | 140-160 |
| Hydroxyethyl starch (Hetastarch) 6% | 500 | 500 | 312 | 310 | 154 |

While the SAFE trial helped reduce fears about the short-term safety of 4% albumin, it did not answer any questions about 25% albumin.

Most pediatric trials have predominately focused on the evaluation of fluid resuscitation in the setting of septic shock or congenital heart repair. In these trails, the use of colloid and crystalloid resulted in similar outcomes, yet total volume infused (mL/kg) tended to be lower in the colloid group. In clinical practice, crystalloid is used as first line therapy for volume expansion, especially in trauma patients. Doses of 20 mL/kg, repeated as needed up to 60 mL/kg, are infused to achieve outcomes such as improved cardiac filling, increased central venous pressure, increased urine output, and reduction in acidosis. When crystalloids fail to sustain plasma volume for extended periods, then colloid is considered. Albumin 5% is the preferred colloid because hetastarch and dextran can reduce factor VIII:C and vWF levels. Hespan, a particular brand of hetastarch, can reduce glycoprotein IIb/IIIa availability and interfere with platelet adhesion and clot formation. Lastly, dextran has been associated with anaphylactoid reactions and nephrotoxicity.

## APPROPRIATE USE OF ANTIMICROBIALS

Children admitted to the ICU after a traumatic injury or surgical procedure are at high risk of developing a hospital-acquired infection. Consequently, antibiotics are among the most commonly prescribed medications in the ICU. Selection of the most appropriate antimicrobial regimen can avoid treatment failures and reduce unnecessary exposure to excessive antimicrobials, which has been associated with the emergence and spread of resistance.

## PHARMACODYNAMICS OF ANTIMICROBIALS

Antimicrobials can be classified by their spectrum of activity or killing technique. Some agents are considered "static" (inhibit growth and replication) while others are "cidal" (cause bacterial cell death). The inhibition or killing of bacteria by an antibiotic will depend on the ability of the antimicrobial to attain and sometimes sustain a concentration that exceeds the minimum inhibitory concentration (MIC) of the organism.

Concentration-dependent killing antibiotics (fluoroquinolones, aminoglycosides, macrolides, ketolides, metronidazole, and daptomycin) will kill bacteria when their concentrations are well above the MIC—and the killing will be further enhanced as the concentration of antibiotic at the site of infection is increased. The maximum concentration ($C_{max}$) of an antibiotic-to-MIC ratio has been used to predict clinical outcomes. A ratio of 10:1 at the site of infection is often used as the clinical target. The concentration-dependent killing antibiotics also exhibit a postantibiotic effect (PAE). This effect allows for the concentration of an antibiotic to fall below the MIC (even undetectable) yet remain effective at inhibiting microbial growth. A long PAE allows for a longer drug dosing interval. The duration of PAE is both drug- and species-dependent. The most well-known classes of drugs with a significant PAE include the aminoglycosides and fluquinolones.

Time-dependent killing antibiotics are effective only when the concentration of the antimicrobial is higher than the MIC of the organism. Generally, maximum killing will occur at 3 to 4 times the MIC and further increases in drug concentration will not lead to greater killing. If the concentration of the antimicrobial falls below the MIC, then proliferation of the organism occurs. Time-dependent antimicrobials include the penicillins, cephalosporins, aztreonam, vancomycin, carbapenems, linezolid, tigecycline, doxycycline, and clindamycin. Here, the time above MIC has been used to predict clinical outcomes. This pharmacodynamic characteristic has prompted some researchers to study CIs of these antibiotics. The results of these CI studies have revealed conflicting conclusions, but this administration technique offers an alternative to patients who may experience treatment failure due to inadequate time above the MIC.

## SELECTION AND DURATION OF ANTIMICROBIALS

Selection (or implementation) of empiric antimicrobial therapy should be based on the child's history (drug allergies, age, and concomitant drug therapy), physical exam (including presence of any organ dysfunction), knowledge of suspected pathogens for the site of infection, and local susceptibility patterns. Central-line infections and VAP are 2 of the most common infections observed in the PICU. According to the Surviving Sepsis Campaign, prompt recognition and investigation of potential infectious sources are paramount. Delays in initiation of appropriate antimicrobials beyond 1 hour are associated with worse clinical outcomes. Ideally, antimicrobials should be started within 1 hour of recognition (or earlier)—using the basic principles outlined in Fig. 7-20. Traditionally, combinations of drugs active against gram-positive and gram-negative organisms are used—with the addition of anaerobic coverage in certain clinical situations (Table 7-6). Important trends in antibiotic resistance (multidrug resistant gram-positive organisms and resistant gram-negative bacilli) must be considered when choosing antibiotics. For example, an increase in methicillin-resistant *Staphylococcus aureus* (MRSA) resulted in heavy use of vancomycin, which in turn resulted in an increase in vancomycin-resistant enterococci. Resistance rates are generally much higher in ICU settings than non-ICU settings. Narrowing the spectrum of activity by using the fewest number of antibiotics is encouraged as a way to reduce resistance rates. Choosing the correct dosing strategy, based on known killing pharmacodynamics, is also important in minimizing drug resistance. Low antibiotic dosing may fail to clear an infection and predispose the patient to harboring resistant pathogens. While the duration of antimicrobial coverage is continually debated, the optimal duration of treatment will depend on the site of infection and pathogen

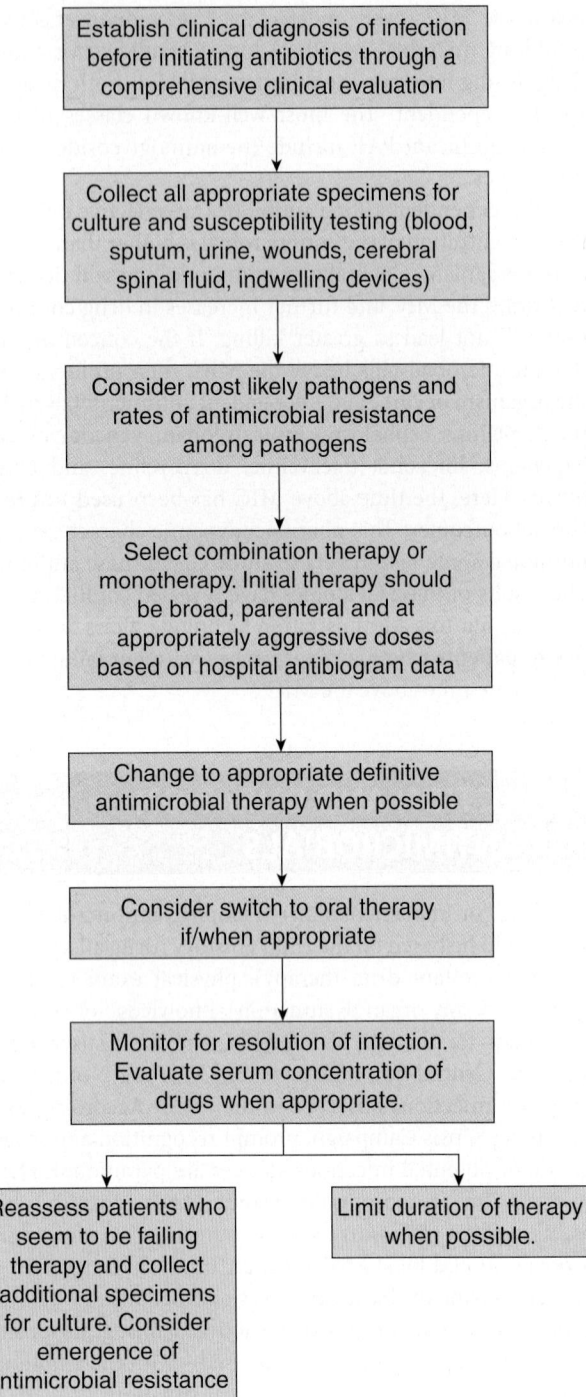

Establish clinical diagnosis of infection before initiating antibiotics through a comprehensive clinical evaluation

↓

Collect all appropriate specimens for culture and susceptibility testing (blood, sputum, urine, wounds, cerebral spinal fluid, indwelling devices)

↓

Consider most likely pathogens and rates of antimicrobial resistance among pathogens

↓

Select combination therapy or monotherapy. Initial therapy should be broad, parenteral and at appropriately aggressive doses based on hospital antibiogram data

↓

Change to appropriate definitive antimicrobial therapy when possible

↓

Consider switch to oral therapy if/when appropriate

↓

Monitor for resolution of infection. Evaluate serum concentration of drugs when appropriate.

Reassess patients who seem to be failing therapy and collect additional specimens for culture. Consider emergence of antimicrobial resistance

Limit duration of therapy when possible.

**FIGURE 7-20** Basic principles of antimicrobial use in the critically ill child.

isolated. Today, there is a trend toward limiting treatment duration, yet some infections are particularly hard to treat given the difficulty of antibiotic penetration into the tissues involved. Examples include endocarditis, osteomyelitis, undrained abscesses, and meningitis. When the presence of one of these infections is certain, prolonged antibiotic courses are usually necessary and accepted. For most other hospital-acquired and surgical infections, however, shorter treatment durations are preferable.

Risk of infection during the perioperative period can be reduced through proper preparation of the operative site and use of prophylactic antibiotic administration. To be effective, the appropriate antibiotic(s) must be administered within 1 hour before the operation so that tissue levels are high at incision time. Antibiotic coverage should be continued throughout the operative procedure; indeed, some antibiotics may need to be re-dosed for extended (more than 4 hours) surgical procedures. The spectrum of antimicrobial coverage can be limited to skin flora unless there is violation of hollow viscus mucosa. In general, cefazolin alone is adequate for coverage of skin flora contamination. Cephalosporins with anaerobic coverage (cefoxitin or cefotetan) should be used for procedures involving the appendix and for some gynecologic procedures. Vancomycin may be considered prior to placement of external ventricular drains and intraventricular shunts. Prophylactic antibiotics have no value beyond the first 24 hours following surgery. Their continued use puts patients at risk for antibiotic-associated infections, drug resistance, and the emergence of fungal infections.

New antimicrobials for use in the ICU are in various phases of research and development. Fifth-generation cephalosporins with a broad range of activity (including MRSA) are in phase III clinical trials. Investigational glycopeptides and lipoglycopeptides have shown promising results against a variety of multidrug-resistant strains of *Staphylococcus* and *Enterococcus* species. The ultimate fate of these and other new antimicrobials has yet to be determined.

## VENOUS THROMBOEMBOLISM: PROPHYLAXIS AND TREATMENT

Hospital-acquired venous thromboembolism (VTE), which includes deep vein thrombosis (DVT) and pulmonary embolism (PE), is a well-known and recognized complication in medical and postsurgical *adult* patients. VTE can be life-threatening, may prolong hospital stay, require invasive treatment, and result in chronic disability. Risk assessment and thromboprophylaxis decisions in adults have been well studied and recommendations are based on solid principles and scientific evidence. Conversely, VTE in critically ill children is poorly studied. The lack of data regarding the clinical approach to VTE risk in children is further complicated by the changing balance between pro- and anticoagulant factors that occurs throughout infancy and childhood. There appears to be a bimodal distribution of VTE prevalence in children, with peaks at birth, 1 year, and again at 12 to 14 years. Although the risk of VTE in children is certainly lower compared to adults, recent reports suggest that the incidence of VTE in children is increasing. Data from Canadian and Dutch registries report an annual incidence of pediatric DVT and PE between 0.07 and 0.14 per 10,000 children (or 5.3 per 10,000 hospital admissions) in children aged 1 month to 18 years, with a peak incidence in infants younger than 1 year of age and a mortality rate of 2.2%. Recent US registry and multicenter trial data report rates as high as 28.8 to 58 per 10,000 pediatric hospital admissions, with mortality rates ranging between 18% and 21%. Admittedly, the increase in pediatric VTE incidence may be the result of increased awareness;

| Suspected Site of Infection | Likely Pathogens | Empiric Therapy | Comment | Duration of Therapy After Negative Culture Achieved |
|---|---|---|---|---|
| Unknown | *Staphylococcus, Streptococcus, Pseudomonas, Enterococci, Enterobacter* | Cefotaxime or ceftazidime plus vancomycin | Consider double coverage with meropenem if pseudomonas is highly suspect | 10-14 days |
| Central nervous system (related to trauma or shunt) | *Staphylococcus, Pseudomonas,* gram-negative enterics (distal shunt contamination) | Vancomycin plus ceftriaxone, ceftazidime, or meropenem | Must maximize dose to achieve antibiotic penetration | Minimum of 2 weeks |
| Intraabdominal | Primary bacterial peritonitis may be caused by a single organism (Group A *Streptococcus, E. coli, S. pneumococcus, B. fragilis*) while secondary peritonitis is typically polymicrobial (enteric aerobes and anaerobes) | Ampicillin–sulbactam, piperacillin–tazobactam, carbapenem or cefotaxime plus metronidazole | For suspected *C. difficile*, consider oral metronidazole, vancomycin, or rifaximin | 5-14 days, depending on the site. Shorter courses are appropriate for appendicitis while longer course are required for severe peritonitis |
| Catheter-related (intravascular central lines) | *Staphylococcus* sp. | Vancomycin | Consider catheter removal if treatment fails | 10 days |
| Respiratory tract (including ventilator-associated pneumonia) | *Klebsiella, Serratia, Staphylococcus, Pneumococcus, Pseudomonas, Acinetobacter,* and *Stenotrophomonas* | Ceftazidime, cefepime, or antipseudomonal fluoroquinolone ± aminoglycoside | Ampicillin–sulbactam is adequate for suspected aspiration pneumonia | 7-14 days |
| Urinary tract | *E. coli, Enterobacter, Enterococci* | Fluoroquinolone (except moxifloxacin), trimethoprime–sulfamethoxazole, aminoglycoside | | 3-7 days (simple) 14 days (complex) |

All regimens should be reassessed after 48-72 hours based on clinical and microbiological data and therapy should be narrowed when possible.

nevertheless, it does raise important surveillance and recognition issues that most PICUs are not addressing.

In the critical care setting, the risk of VTE is generally increased due to immobility (with decreased blood flow), damage to blood vessel walls from trauma and/or line insertion, and a tendency to be hypercoagulable secondary to inflammatory conditions. Specific VTE risk factors identified in children include the presence of a central venous catheter, immobility, sepsis, orthopedic surgery, major trauma, history of VTE in the patient or a family member, malignancy, elevated estrogen, burns greater than 30% body surface area, acquired or inherited thrombophilia, age less than 1 year old or older than 14 years, obesity, and hypercoagulable states (eg, disseminated intravascular coagulation, lupus, diabetic ketoacidosis, nephrotic syndrome, or hemolytic uremic syndrome).

Criteria for initiating VTE prophylaxis in pediatric patients remain variable, due to the lack of consensus guidelines. One approach is to consider therapy when 3 or more of the above risk factors have been identified. Options for prophylaxis of VTE in children include mechanical and medicinal. Most children admitted to the PICU will not require any form of prophylaxis. Compression stockings or intermittent compression devices are excellent options for older children. Unfractionated heparin (UFH) or low-molecular-weight heparin (LMWH) should be considered for those who do not fit or cannot tolerate mechanical therapy. Laboratory monitoring of UFH or LMWH is not considered necessary with lower prophylactic doses. Duration of prophylaxis generally does not exceed the length of ICU stay.

In children with a documented VTE, conventional anticoagulant therapies can be used (Table 7-7). The decision to use thrombolytic therapy, in addition to anticoagulant therapy, should be made in consultation with the hematology service. In most critically ill children with VTE, UFH is the preferred agent during the acute phase of treatment because it has a shorter half-life compared to LMWH and the anticoagulant effect can be reduced sooner if needed. Regardless of agent selected, close monitoring of anti-Xa serum concentrations is needed to guide safe and effective therapy. An example of a standardized treatment protocol for anticoagulation therapy

| TABLE 7-7 | Overview of Conventional Anticoagulation Therapy for Documented Venous Thrombolembolism in Children | | |
|---|---|---|---|
| Episode | Initial (Acute Phase) Treatment: Target Anti-Xa Activity | Extended (Subacute Phase) Treatment: Target Anticoagulant Activity | Duration of Therapy |
| First | Unfractionated heparin: 0.3-0.7 units/mL<br>Low-molecular-weight heparin: 0.5-1.0 units/mL | Warfarin: INR 2.0-3.0<br>Low-molecular-weight heparin: 0.5-1.0 units/mL | 3-6 months or 6-12 months if VTE is idiopathic<br>12 months lifetime if risk factors persist |
| Recurrent | Unfractionated heparin: 0.3-0.7 units/mL<br>Low-molecular-weight heparin: 0.5-1.0 units/mL | Warfarin: INR 2.0-3.0<br>Low-molecular-weight heparin: 0.5-1.0 units/mL | 6-12 months with an underlying risk factor that has resolved<br>12 months lifetime if idiopathic and risk factors persist |

is illustrated in Fig. 7-21. The recommended duration of UFH in the critically ill child is 5 to 10 days, with transition to LMWH as soon as possible. Extended anticoagulation therapy in children is achieved with either LMWH or warfarin. Fixed tablet sizes of warfarin make this choice less flexible than LMWH in children, but avoid frequent subcutaneous injections. The international normalized ratio (INR) should be assessed after 5 days of warfarin therapy and whenever there is evidence of clinical bleeding. Other antithrombotic agents (fondaparinux, IV direct thrombin inhibitors) have been used in children when conventional therapy has failed. Oral direct thrombin inhibitors are a new class of agents that have been studied in adults after knee and hip replacement surgery. Pediatric data are lacking and their role in children remains unknown.

## PROPHYLAXIS OF STRESS-RELATED MUCOSAL DAMAGE

Children admitted to the PICU are at risk for stress-related mucosal damage (SRMD). Morbidity due to SRMD can prolong the length of ICU stay and mortality is substantially higher in patients with bleeding due to SRMD, compared to those without. The prevalence of SRMD in children depends largely on the definition and presence of underlying disease states. Early endoscopic evidence of mucosal damage is apparent in many children admitted to the ICU; however, the prevalence of overt bleeding (gross blood, hematemesis, coffee ground nasogastric aspirate, hematochezia, or melena) and clinically important bleeding (overt bleeding resulting in adverse hemodynamic outcome or a fall in hemoglobin) ranges from 5% to 51% and 1.6% to 10%, respectively. More recent studies have reported even lower rates of GI bleeding, perhaps due to widespread use of prophylactic therapy and to improved monitoring and attention toward the child's hemodynamic status. Despite the reduced prevalence of SRMD with overt bleeding, prophylaxis remains a key therapy in critically ill children.

The pathophysiology of SRMD is multifactorial and involves an imbalance between mucosal protective defenses and hostile physiologic factors. During stress, splanchnic perfusion is impaired, resulting in decreased oxygen delivery, impaired gastric mucosa integrity, and reduced bicarbonate secretion. At the same time, there is hypersecretion of gastric acid and pepsin, and an elevation in free radical production. As the permeability of the gastric mucosa is compromised, influx of hydrogen ion occurs and the circular process of further damage to the gastric mucosa continues. Since most lesions caused by stress occur in the acid-producing area of the stomach (fundus and upper body), it follows that acid-blocking therapies have the potential to reduce damage.

Risk factors for SRMD in children include mechanical ventilation, coagulopathy, Pediatric Risk of Mortality score (PRISM) ≥10, low intragastric pH, renal/hepatic failure, trauma, pneumonia, shock, severe head injury, major surgery, and high-dose corticosteroids. Additional risk factors identified in adults include burns greater than 35% total body surface area and head/spinal cord injuries. Prevention of SRMD has been achieved using antacids, sucralfate, histamine type-2 receptor antagonists (H2RA), and proton pump inhibitors (PPI). The frequent dose administration requirements with antacids (every 3 hours) and the potential for drug–drug interference with both antacids and sucralfate result in the infrequent use of these agents in pediatrics. The 2 most common regimens for SRMD prophylaxis include H2RAs or PPIs. These agents have been shown to be superior to placebo in preventing SRMD by reducing overt and clinically important bleeding. Comparative trials between H2RAs and PPIs have however failed to show a superior agent. Therapeutic goals of these antisecretory agents include the achievement of a gastric pH above 4 to prevent stress-related mucosal lesions or a gastric pH above 6 to maintain a clot if bleeding has occurred.

H2RAs are considered first-line therapy for the prevention of SRMD, primarily due to their pharmacoeconomic advantage. They reduce gastric acid through competitive (and reversible) inhibition of histamine-stimulated acid secretion. H2RAs are generally well tolerated, but thrombocytopenia has been associated with their use. The most widely used H2RAs are ranitidine and famotidine, due to their lower risk of drug–drug interactions. Tolerance to acid inhibition by H2RAs may occur as early as 3 days—a phenomenon which cannot be overcome by increasing the dose. The second most common regimen for SRMD prevention includes a PPI. These agents are more potent than H2RAs and reduce acid

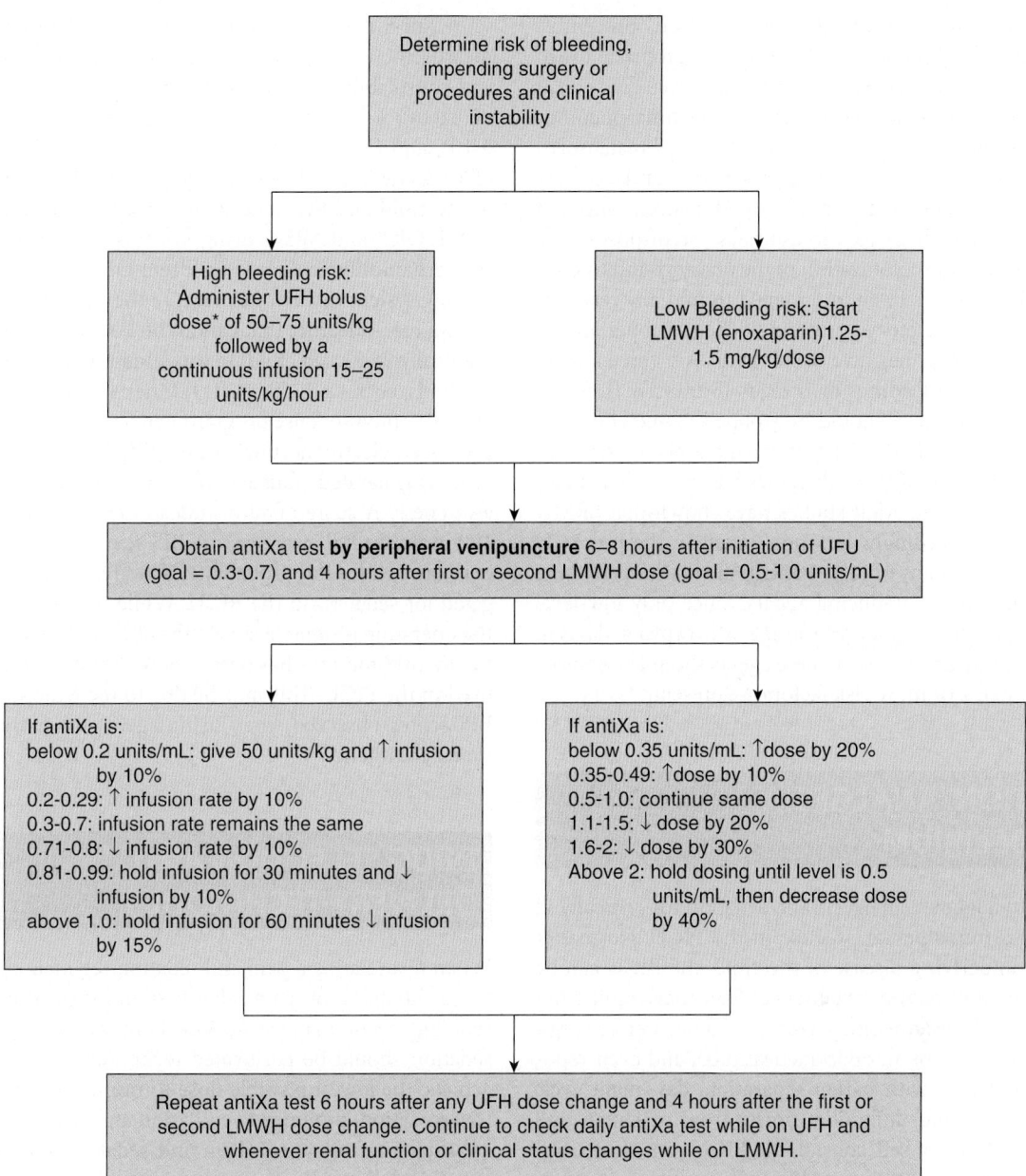

**FIGURE 7-21** Anticoagulant treatment algorithm in children with documented venous thromboembolism. May use total body weight for dosing, unless child is obese. For obese children, please consult pharmacy for calculation of an appropriate "dosing weight". *Bolus heparin is contraindicated in children with a recent cerebrovascular accident, active bleeding, severe thrombocytopenia, or cardiac mechanical prosthesis. UFU, unfractionated heparin.

through irreversible inhibition of the hydrogen–potassium ATPase pump—the final step in acid production. Unlike H2RAs, PPIs inhibit gastric acid secretion mediated by histamine, sympathomimetic, muscarinic, and vagal pathways. PPIs only inhibit actively secreting proton pumps; therefore, it can take 2 days to achieve full acid inhibition. Tolerance does not seem to develop with PPIs; however, they may precipitate rebound hypersecretion of acid production upon discontinuation. PPIs are metabolized via the CYP 450 system, so caution should be exercised regarding drug–drug interaction potential and interpatient variability due to genetic polymorphisms in the CYP2C19 gene.

The decision to start SRMD prophylaxis should be made only after surveying the child's risks. The simple act of admission to the PICU does not warrant routine SRMD prophylaxis. One study has suggested that risk of clinically important GI bleeding in children is directly related to the number of risk factors present. The presence of a single risk factor does not merit prophylaxis, but, when 2 or more risk factors are present, then the risk:benefit ratio favors prophylaxis. Many centers use mechanical ventilation, coagulopathy, or major trauma coupled with one additional risk factor as triggers to initiate SRMD prevention.

Once risk factors for SRMD have resolved, preventive therapy should be discontinued. Chronic inappropriate use of acid reduction therapy is expensive and may place the child at increased risk for adverse events, such as nosocomial pneumonia, *Clostridium difficile*-associated diarrhea, and malabsorption of nutrients. Adult data have shown that antisecretory agents are associated with an increased concentration of gram-negative bacilli in gastric aspirates, predisposing the patient to retrograde colonization of the pharynx and trachea and VAP. Two studies in children failed to find any relationship between antisecretory agents, incidence of upper airway colonization of gram-negative bacilli and VAP. Once a child is tolerating enteral feedings or is ready to transfer from the ICU, SRMD prevention should be stopped. Some clinicians feel that the benefit of SRMD prophylaxis has been overstated and that routine use of these therapies has led to their inappropriate use. Indeed, adult studies have shown that SRMD prophylaxis is exceedingly common—even in the non-ICU setting—and that many of these patients are discharged home unnecessarily on acid-reducing agents. Since only low-level evidence is available to support routine SRMD prophylaxis in critically ill children, the use of these agents should be considered only when 2 or more risk factors are present.

## SEDATION, ANALGESIA, AND DELIRIUM

Provision of adequate analgesia and sedation for critically ill children is a fundamental practice in the PICU. No matter the age or underlying disease of the child, the PICU can be a frightening and painful experience. Pain may result from invasive procedures, dressing changes, trauma, a prior surgical event, presence of an endotracheal tube, and even repositioning. Together with parent separation, day–night cycle disruption, loud and unfamiliar noises from machines and monitors, and loss of self-control, the PICU can cause emotional distress and anxiety. Although nonpharmacologic interventions such as verbal reassurance, parent presence, and psychological maneuvers may help, the use of pharmacologic intervention is often necessary. Choosing the correct agent and dosing regimen can facilitate patient-ventilator synchrony, improve oxygenation, reduce catecholamine surges, and provide patient comfort. The clinical approach to analgesia and sedation in the PICU has evolved over the past decade and clinicians are now implementing thoughtful, evidence-based, patient-targeted approaches to drug selection. This method can provide the most appropriate balance of analgesia and sedation while avoiding the pitfalls of over sedation.

Tools to help measure a child's response to analgesia and/or sedative therapy utilize subjective and objective indicators. Current assessment tools in the PICU are based predominately on validated scoring systems performed at regular intervals. These scoring systems use self-reported indicators of pain in the communicative child, while physiologic markers and observations of a patient's response to a standardized intervention are used in the noncommunicative child. Pain and sedation assessment tools include (1) the COMFORT score (an 8-item score based on behavioral and physiologic measurements); (2) the FLACC score (face, legs, activity, cry, and consolability); (3) the Oucher (self-report of pain based on faces); a Numerical score (a self-reported verbal score 0-10), and (5) the State Behavioral Score (SBS). The choice of assessment tool depends largely on the developmental age of the child and the underlying severity of illness. Both the COMFORT and SBS scoring systems have been validated in mechanically ventilated children. One drawback to these scoring systems is that they require the patient to respond to a stimulus—a feature that cannot be assessed properly in the medically paralyzed child. In this situation, brain monitoring methods, such as the Bispectral Index (BIS), may be considered. BIS monitors use programmed algorithms to evaluate a processed electroencephalogram (EEG) pattern. A numeric value is generated (range: 0-100) and provides a measure of awareness. A score of zero indicates coma while a score of 100 indicates full awareness. A BIS score below 60 generally correlates with a low probability of awareness and is often targeted for sedation in the PICU. While frequently applied in the operating room to evaluate the effects of general anesthesia, the BIS monitor has been met with some criticism when used in the PICU. This may be due to the wide variability in BIS scores observed when using agents other than inhalational anesthetics.

## DRUG SELECTION AND DELIVERY TECHNIQUES

When formulating a pain and sedation regimen, the primary focus should be on pain relief first and then, if necessary, a sedating agent may be added. Titration of analgesia and sedation should be performed using defined end-points to achieve the lowest possible dose to minimize adverse events (oversedation, prolonged ventilation and ICU stay, delirium, constipation, tolerance). Pain and sedation goals should be assessed daily and therapeutic targets should change as the child recovers from illness. Nurse-directed algorithms and protocols, based on patient-specific goals, are one way to titrate analgesia and sedation while minimizing the cumulative exposure to opioids and benzodiazepines (BZDs). A second technique, termed "daily interruption", has been used successfully in older children and adults. This technique uses a sedation holiday, whereby continuous analgesia and sedation infusions are turned off until the patient awakens and begins to demonstrate agitation. Infusions are then restarted at 50% of the previous dose. Data in adults have shown that daily interruption can decrease the duration of mechanical ventilation and length of stay in the ICU. Sedation vacations, however, are not without risk and have not been well studied in young children.

A small percentage of children admitted to the PICU may be suitable candidates for intermittent pain and sedation therapy. Mild–moderate pain can be controlled with nonsteroidal agents such as acetaminophen, ketorolac, and ibuprofen or intermittent opioid administration. Ketorolac has been associated with serious gastrointestinal side effects and, as a result, many centers limit its duration to 2 to 5 days.

Some postoperative children older than 6 years of age, who are developmentally appropriate, can benefit from patient-controlled analgesia (PCA). This technique of drug administration allows the child to self-administer a preset dose of IV opioid via a pump. The pump is programmed with limits to avoid excessive drug delivery. PCA yields better pain control with higher patient satisfaction compared to traditional intermittent nurse-administered dosing. The choice of agent will depend on body composition, historical tolerance, organ function, and hemodynamic stability of the patient.

## OPIOIDS

Opioids relive pain through stimulation of 6 major opioid receptors: mu (μ), kappa (κ), delta (δ), nociceptin, epsilon (ε), and sigma (σ). These receptors are located in the central nervous system and peripheral tissues. Morphine, fentanyl, and hydromorphone represent the most commonly used IV opioids in the PICU. Important differences exist between these agents and include lipophilicity, duration of action, active metabolites, and opioid receptor affinity (Table 7-8). Some opioids exhibit a context-sensitive half-life, where the observed half-life is dependent on the duration of drug administration. Both fentanyl and morphine exhibit clinically relevant context-sensitive half-lives, making these agents intermediate to long acting with prolonged administration. This phenomenon does not appear evident with remifentanil, which retains its short half-life irrespective of administration duration. When opioids are administered as a CI, patients can quickly develop tolerance. Fentanyl and remifentanil lead to tolerance the fastest because of their strong affinity for the opioid receptor. One strategy to minimize the impact of opioid tolerance is to rotate opioids when tolerance is suspected.

Morphine is the most hydrophilic of the opioids. It is hepatic metabolized via glucuronidation into morphine-3-glucoronide (inactive) and morphine-6-glucoronide (potent active metabolite). Both metabolites are renal cleared and can accumulate in the presence of renal insufficiency. Morphine is considered the preferred agent in obese children because it is least likely to deposit into fatty tissue. Fentanyl has a rapid onset of action and is remarkably fat soluble, posing a higher risk of drug accumulation and delayed recovery after discontinuation, particularly in obese children. Hydromorphone is a semisynthetic opioid with a slight potency advantage over morphine with perhaps less pruritus. Remifentanil is an ultra-short-acting synthetic opioid with many unique features, including its independence of hepatic metabolism and lack of drug–drug interactions. Remifentanil is generally reserved for intraoperative use, but some studies have reviewed its use in the PICU. A notable feature of remifentanil in the ICU is the rapid development of tolerance and requirement for escalating doses after only 1 to 3 hours. Meperidine is not recommended for routine use due to its low potency, propensity to cause nausea and vomiting, drug–drug interactions, and accumulation of its active metabolite (normeperidine) in patients with renal insufficiency. Normeperidine has neuroexcititory effects including tremor, delirium, and seizures. Methadone is an opioid with both μ-receptor activity and N-methyl-D-aspartate (NMDA) receptor antagonistic activity, making it useful in chronic pain and opioid-tolerant states.

## BENZODIAZEPINES

Midazolam and lorazepam are the most commonly used BZDs used in the PICU. Diazepam was one of the first BZDs to be used in the PICU for sedation, but active metabolites with half-lives that far exceed the parent drug have limited its routine use. Diazepam, however, retains its important role in the management of seizures and muscles spasms. All BZDs provide anxiolytic, sedative, and hypnotic effects by binding to the α-subunit of the γ-aminobutyric acid (GABA) receptor. This binding causes chloride movement across the neuronal membrane, resulting in hyperpolarization.

| TABLE 7-8 | Comparison of Commonly Used Opioids and Benzodiazepines in the PICU | | | | | |
|---|---|---|---|---|---|---|
| | Receptor Activation | Onset of Action (min) | Metabolism | Active Metabolite | Relevant Context-Sensitive Half-Life | Lipophilicity |
| Morphine | μ weak κ, δ | 2-10 | Hepatic glucuronidation | Yes | Yes | + |
| Fentanyl | μ | 1-3 | Hepatic CYP3A4 | No | Yes | ++++ |
| Hydromorphone | μ | 2-5 | Hepatic conjugation | No | Unknown | ++ |
| Remifentanil | μ | <1 | Nonspecific plasma esterases | No | No | +++ |
| Midazolam | GABA | 2-5 | Hepatic CYP3A5 | Yes | Yes | ++ |
| Lorazepam | GABA | 10-15 | Hepatic glucuronidation | No | Yes | ++ |

GABA, γ-Aminobutyric acid.

Midazolam is the shortest acting of the commonly used BZDs. It is water-soluble and undergoes extensive biotransformation via the CYP3A5 isoenzyme to a renal eliminated active metabolite. Genetic polymorphisms in the CYP3A5 isoenzyme have resulted in discernible over sedation in patients with known enzyme variants. Midazolam is prone to drug accumulation and increased sedation with renal insufficiency due to its renal eliminated active metabolite. A large amount of pediatric data has demonstrated its clinical efficacy as a CI in doses ranging from 0.05 to 0.2 mg/kg/h. Lorazepam is a longer-acting BZD metabolized by hepatic glucuronidation (phase II enzyme system) to inactive metabolites. The pharmacokinetics of lorazepam are less influenced by critical illness, drug interactions, and liver disease. IV lorazepam, however, contains propylene glycol which can cause hyperosmolar metabolic acidosis, acute tubular necrosis, and renal failure. This toxicity has limited its use as a CI for prolonged periods in the PICU. An osmolar gap that exceeds 10 to 15 reflects significant propylene glycol accumulation and warrants discontinuation of lorazepam. The best use of lorazepam is as an intermittent IV or oral agent for acute agitation, or as part of a withdrawal prevention strategy (discussed below).

## KETAMINE

Ketamine is classified as an anesthetic agent that imparts both amnesia and analgesia. It acts as an agonist at opioid receptors and as an antagonist at N-methyl-D-aspartic acid NMDA receptors. Metabolism of ketamine is via methylation to an active metabolite (norketamine), which undergoes further hydroxylation with subsequent renal elimination. Children with significant hepatic or renal disease may require lower doses of ketamine. Properties of ketamine that make it an attractive agent in the PICU include its relative hemodynamic stability profile and limited effects on the respiratory system. While ketamine can be administered as a CI, its predominate role in the PICU is as an intermittent adjunct during procedures, especially in the spontaneously breathing child. Ketamine administration usually results in an increase in heart rate and blood pressure due to the release of endogenous catecholamines. This action explains the bronchodilator effects of ketamine. There are a number of controversies surrounding the use of ketamine, including its effects on intracranial pressure (ICP), pulmonary vascular resistance (PVR), and the central nervous system (CNS). Early reports suggested that ketamine was associated with an increase in ICP, making it contraindicated in children with head trauma. More recent investigations have not supported this finding and instead suggest that ketamine's effect on transmembrane calcium may be of benefit in head trauma. Ketamine, through NMDA antagonism, can block the influx of calcium that occurs after the release of neuroexcititory neurotransmitters following head trauma. This reduction in intracellular calcium may reduce the effects of delayed neuronal necrosis. The effect of ketamine on PVR has also been debated. Some studies report an increase in PVR following ketamine administration and advise caution in children with congenital heart defects. Other studies using ketamine, including those evaluating its use during cardiac catheterization procedures, have reported excellent safety profiles with short recovery times. One last concern with ketamine is its effect on the CNS. Many children experience hallucinations as they recover from ketamine. This has been termed an emergence reaction and can be easily managed and minimized with the coadministration of midazolam or lorazepam.

## ETOMIDATE

Etomidate is an IV anesthetic agent used for induction of anesthesia and rapid sequence intubation. Etomidate potentiates GABA and causes a rapid loss of consciousness. It has limited effects on the cardiovascular system and can reduce ICP while improving cerebral perfusion pressure. A disadvantage of etomidate is its adverse effect on endogenous corticosteroid production. A single dose of etomidate alone can inhibit 11-β-hydroxylase, the enzyme necessary for production of cortisol. Etomidate has also been associated with increased infectious complications in patients receiving prolonged infusions. Lastly, etomidate contains 35% propylene glycol and this can accumulate and cause toxicities. In summary, etomidate should be used clinically in the PICU for intermittent procedural sedation only; prolonged infusions should be avoided due to multiple safety concerns.

## DEXMEDETOMIDINE

Dexmedetomidine is the newest agent to be used in the PICU. Dexmedetomidine is a potent α-2-adrenergic agonist that imparts sedative, analgesic, and anxiolytic effects without causing respiratory depression. It is highly protein bound and is metabolized into inactive methyl and glucoronide conjugates. It was originally approved for short-term use in adults, but has now been studied as a CI (0.3-0.7 mcg/kg/h) in mechanically ventilated infants and children requiring escalating doses of opioids and BZDs. It is especially useful for sedation in those children close to extubation in whom less respiratory depression is desirable. Dexmedetomidine has also been used as intermittent therapy for procedural sedation for the spontaneously breathing child. An additional role for dexmedetomidine is with opioid and BZD withdrawal to reduce the signs and symptom of withdrawal.

Current experience with dexmedetomidine in children is promising, but limited. There is a paucity of data in children with head trauma, and thus it cannot be recommended in this patient group until further studied. Prolonged administration of dexmedetomidine infusions remains an area of research. Although dexmedetomidine is generally well tolerated, recent reports have highlighted the observation of reduced heart rate, particularly with therapy initiation. This vagotonic effect may be potentiated with coadministration of fentanyl or propofol. Close hemodynamic monitoring is recommended with this agent and bradycardia may limit its generalized use.

## PROPOFOL

Propofol is a sedative/amnestic agent with no analgesic properties. It is formulated in an oil-in-water emulsion and should be counted as a caloric source (1.1 kcal/mL). Propofol facilitates the binding of GABA to its receptor, but in a distinctly different manner than BZDs. It is metabolized by the liver via CYP2B6 and glucuronidation into inactive metabolites. Propofol is a negative inotrope and can reduce mean arterial blood pressure; care should be taken when using propofol in a hemodynamically unstable child. Propofol has the benefit of a quick onset of action with rapid and predictable recovery. It has been studied in children as an induction agent and for procedural sedation. Despite the many advantages of short-term propofol, it is considered contraindicated for longer periods due to a constellation of symptoms termed the "propofol-related infusion syndrome" or PRIS. These symptoms include metabolic acidosis, dysrhythmias, rhabdomyolysis, and fatal cardiac failure. The mechanism of PRIS is related to mitochondrial disruption and long-chain fatty acid transportation, and is correlated to both dose and duration of infusion. For this reason, propofol dosing should not exceed 4 mg/kg/h or extend beyond 24 hours. If PRIS is suspected, immediate discontinuation of propofol is advised and administration of IV carnitine is suggested.

## DELIRIUM

Delirium is defined as a disturbance of consciousness and cognition that develops over a short period of time. Other terms to describe this phenomenon include ICU psychosis, ICU syndrome, and acute "confusional" state. Delirium has been well described in adult ICU patients with prevalence rates between 20% and 80%. Rates observed in children are much lower (less than 5%), but may be due to developmental changes that make diagnostic criteria difficult to assess. Three categories of delirium have been described: hypoactive (decreased responsiveness, withdrawal and apathy); hyperactive (agitation and emotional lability); and mixed. Hyperactive delirium is associated with high plasma concentrations of dopamine, while hypoactive and mixed forms are associated with normal or low dopamine concentrations. The presence of delirium is associated with prolonged hospital stay, worse functional outcome, and higher mortality. There is mounting evidence to suggest that the dose of BZD, especially lorazepam, may contribute to the development of delirium. This increased risk may be due, in part, to the altered levels of neurotransmitters such as serotonin, dopamine, norepinephrine, and glutamate secondary to GABA activation. Recent studies have shown reduced rates of delirium when dexmedetomidine is used in place of lorazepam.

When an episode of acute delirium is suspected, management includes typical antipsychotics (haloperidol) and atypical antipsychotics (risperidone). Haloperidol is preferred in hyperactive delirium because it is specific to the dopamine-2 receptor. Risperidone with its broad affinity for dopamine-2, serotonin, $\alpha_1$, and histamine-1 receptors is more effective for hypoactive and mixed subtypes of delirium. Therapy is typically provided on an as needed basis. Other atypical antipsychotics (olanzapine, quetiapine, and ziprasidone) have been used with some success and offer an alternative to haloperidol.

## PREVENTION AND MANAGEMENT OF DRUG WITHDRAWAL

Prolonged administration of opioids and BZDs are often necessary to provide pain relief and sedation in the PICU setting. Drawbacks to their use include the development of physiologic dependence, and, if abruptly discontinued, symptoms of withdrawal. Features of drug withdrawal include neurologic excitability, gastrointestinal dysfunction, and autonomic dysfunction (Table 7-9). Risk factors for the development of withdrawal are cumulative dose and duration of exposure. Children considered at high-risk for withdrawal include those who have received CIs of opioids and/or BZDs for periods exceeding 7 days. Management strategies used to control withdrawal range from a gradual tapering of the drug to substitution of another agent to control symptoms. The most widely accepted physiologic-based technique involves a methodical reduction in dose with an eventual transition to an oral intermittent agent. The process of discontinuing an opioid used for prolonged periods begins with a reduction in dose (10-20%) every 12 to 24 hours. If the child exhibits signs and symptoms associated with withdrawal, then the taper can be slowed. When transition to an oral agent is desired, methadone (in doses of 0.1-0.2 mg/kg every 6 hours) can be initiated. This dose is not an equipotent conversion, but rather represents a low supportive regimen thought to deflect withdrawal. Methadone has a half-life that can exceed 24 hours, so after 1 to 2 days of every 6 hours dosing, the CI of opioid should be discontinued and the methadone interval should be lengthened to every 12 hours and eventually to every 24 hours. A similar process can be applied to discontinuation of CIs of BZDs, with a gradual reduction in dose and then a transition to intermittent lorazepam (0.1-0.2 mg/kg every 6 hours). Since the half-life of lorazepam is shorter

| TABLE 7-9 | Features of Opioid and Benzodiazepine Withdrawal | |
|---|---|---|
| **CNS Irritability** | **GI Dysfunction** | **Autonomic Dysfunction** |
| Poor sleep pattern | Diarrhea | Sweating |
| Agitation | Vomiting | Yawning |
| Irritability (crying/inconsolable) | Abdominal pain | Sneezing |
| | Poor feeding | Fever |
| Tachypnea | | Tachycardia |
| Uncoordinated suck | | Hypertension |
| Tremors | | Pupillary dilatation |
| Convulsions | | |
| Fever | | |
| Myoclonic jerking | | |

CNS, central nervous system; GI, gastrointestinal.

than methadone, it is not necessary to "load" the patient with 1 to 2 days of intermittent therapy before discontinuation of the infusion of BZDs. A typical transition would be to start intermittent lorazepam and begin the taper of the infusion at the same time, with discontinuation of the infusion after 3 to 5 doses of scheduled lorazepam. The tapering and transition process of opioids and BZDs can take 7 to 14 days to complete, but is often necessary to avoid complications. Repeated assessment of the child during this process is required. Scoring systems are available to evaluate a child's progress (Withdrawal Assessment Tool-1). When a child exhibits breakthrough symptoms of withdrawal, the taper can be slowed or rescue doses of a short-acting agent (fentanyl or midazolam) can be administered. Children requiring short-term (less than 7 days of) opioid or BZD infusion therapy can be weaned quickly over 24 to 48 hours, with the dose being reduced initially by 50%, then by 25% every 6 hours.

## DELIVERY OF EVIDENCED-BASED CARE THROUGH "BUNDLES"

Care bundles are defined as a set of processes that individually have been shown to improve patient outcomes and, if used together, can have an even greater positive impact on patient care. In general, a care bundle represents at least 3 or 4 individual elements of care that are intended to improve clinical outcomes in a select patient population. These evidence-based interventions are designed to target a cohort of patients with a common disease or procedure. By "bundling" these elements into one general practice, we can consistently deliver quality care. Examples of care bundles used in the critical care setting include central-line insertion bundles, prevention of VAP bundles, surgical site infection bundles, urinary catheter care bundles, severe sepsis and septic shock bundles, and prevention of catheter-related bloodstream infection bundles. Bundles should be expected to evolve over time as new evidence enters the literature. While care bundles can improve the provision of evidence-based care, they are not intended to represent a comprehensive list of interventions. Additionally, there will be situations in which certain elements of a bundle may be contraindicated in an individual patient. Nevertheless, bundles are intended to be used on all patients for a given disease/clinical situation at all times. The power of a care bundle is truly recognized when all elements are consistently implemented.

# Acute Respiratory Failure and Ecmo

## KEY POINTS

1. Respiratory failure in premature infants occurs in up to 1% of all live births. Respiratory distress syndrome (RDS) affects 10% of premature births.

2. Treatment strategies to minimize chronic bronchopulmonary dysplasia (BPD) as a consequence of respiratory failure include surfactant administration, use of continuous positive airway pressure (CPAP), judicious use of oxygen, bronchodilators, corticosteroids, pulmonary vasodilators, sildenafil, prostanoids, and diuretics.

3. In mechanical ventilator support, barotrauma is likely caused by volumetric overexpansion of the lung rather than the pressure peak of the respiratory cycle. Therefore, as lung compliance changes with progression or regression of disease, the PIP must be changed accordingly.

4. ECMO outcomes are directly influenced by days of pre-ECMO ventilator support, patient age >10 years, cancer, renal and liver failure, and a history of a pre-ECMO cardiac arrest.

Respiratory failure in the neonatal and pediatric population represents a unique challenge from the standpoint of diagnosis, as well as therapy. A number of causes, including congenital, developmental, infectious, and metabolic defects commonly precipitate rapid respiratory collapse, leading to significant morbidity, and, in some cases, death. A number of pharmacologic, ventilator, and surgical interventions successfully improved survival rates in a variety of causes, while others remain lethal despite the most aggressive efforts. Improved survival, however, increased the incidence of secondary morbidities. These often result in the need for chronic pulmonary support, with its own host of complications. The following section discusses common and most severe pathophysiologic respiratory issues occurring in neonatal and pediatric patients. Current therapeutic interventions as well as the evolving role of extracorporeal life support measures are specifically addressed.

## PATHOPHYSIOLOGY OF RESPIRATORY FAILURE

### Lung Development

Fetal lung development begins in the fourth week of gestation with formation of the tracheoesophageal septum, effectively separating the primitive respiratory system (the laryngotracheal diverticulum) from the proximal alimentary tract (esophagus). The lungs then normally progress through 5 stages of intrauterine development: the embryonic, psuedoglandular, canalicular, saccular, and alveolar periods. This is followed by several years of maturation during childhood. However, aberrations at any point in this process may result in congenital anomalies whose clinical features may be traced back to that period of intrauterine development (Table 7-10). For instance, failure of separation of the pleuroperitoneal canal into the thoracic and peritoneal cavities by formation of the diaphragm during the seventh week may result in herniation of the primitive gut into the thorax. The compressive effect of the intrathoracic

| TABLE 7-10 | Pulmonary Development | | |
|---|---|---|---|
| Post Conception Time (Weeks) | Stage | Developmental Events | Associated Congenital Anomalies |
| 4-6 | Embryonic | | |
| | | Formation of tracheoesophageal septum | Tracheoesophageal fistula |
| | | First division airway branching | Pulmonary agenesis |
| | | Neural tube closes | Vascular ring |
| | | Mesonephric tubules form | Renal and pulmonary agenesis (Potter syndrome) |
| | | Formation of aorta and pulmonary arteries | |
| 7-16 | Pseudoglandular | | |
| | | Transverse septum divides primitive thoracic and peritoneal cavities | Diaphragmatic hernia |
| | | Branching of pulmonary vasculature | Congenital lymphangiectasia |
| | | Appearance of lymphatics | Ectopic lobes |
| | | Formation of precious blood vessels | Congenital pulmonary cysts |
| | | | Lung hypoplasia |
| 17-28 | Canalicular | | |
| | | Saccules develop | Lung hypoplasia |
| | | Capillaries penetrate primitive saccules | Respiratory insufficiencies of newborn |
| | | Epithelium attenuates forming septae | |
| 29-35 | Saccular | | |
| | | Type II pneumocyte proliferation with surfactant production | Apnea of prematurity |
| 36-40 | Alveolar | | |
| | | Alveolar proliferation | Lobar emphysema |
| | | | Cystic fibrosis |

Data from *Langston C, Thurlbeck W. Conditions altering normal lung growth and development. In: Thibeault DW, Gregory GA. ed. Neonatal Pulmonary Care. Norwalk, CT: Appleton-Century-Crofts, 1986:1–27.*

intestines during the pseudoglandular period of lung development is felt to inhibit the normal branching of primitive bronchi. Likewise, the continued effect of compression of fetal lungs during the cannalicular and saccular periods prevent normal acinar development and functional vascular ingrowth with formation of gas-exchange units. The result is that infants with congenital diaphragmatic hernia (CDH) may have hypoplastic lungs characterized by both decreased bronchial branching and deficient arborization and vascularization of the terminal acinus. Repair of the diaphragmatic defect may be successful, but postnatal branching does not occur, and the hypoplasia is irreversible, accounting for the poor prognosis in these patients. Table 7-10 outlines several other congenital pulmonary anomalies and their proposed stages of maldevelopment.

## Pulmonary Hypoplasia

The compressive effect of an intrathoracic space-occupying mass (eg, intestines in CDH) is one cause of lung hypoplasia; however, several other intrauterine factors have also been linked to this developmental problem. Abnormalities of

amniotic and lung fluid volume have been found to adversely affect normal lung development. Both experimental animal models and human studies have found that deficiencies of lung fluid, whether by inadequate urine production, chronic leak of amniotic fluid, or tracheal drainage, are associated with lungs that are hypoplastic. Similarly, studies of tracheal ligation causing increased intrapulmonary fluid in animal models have demonstrated enlarged lungs with increased alveolar development. While promising initially, clinical trials conducted at the turn of the century failed to demonstrate improved morbidity or mortality in CDH patients treated with tracheal occlusion. Despite these results, modifications to the occlusion techniques and management are currently under investigation and approach randomized testing.

## Respiratory Failure of Prematurity

Respiratory failure in premature infants is one of the most common reasons for admission to the neonatal ICU, occurring in up to 1% of all live births. RDS is, overwhelmingly, a disease of prematurity, affecting 10% of premature births, while being exceptionally rare in term infants. It manifests itself with tachypnea, increased work of breathing, and increased oxygen requirement. Lungs of patients with RDS are structurally immature and do not produce sufficient amounts of surfactant, leading to the progressive and unrelenting development of intrapulmonary shunting, hypoventilation, hypoperfusion, hypoxemia, hypercarbia, and acidosis. The risk of developing RDS is directly proportional to the degree of prematurity. A number of maternal risk factors have been identified, including history of prior preterm births and socioeconomic status. Infant risk factors for developing RDS include male sex, Caucasian race, maternal diabetes, and delivery via the cesarean section. However, drastic racial disparities in the incidence and mortality have been identified.

Latest respiratory support measures have substantially decreased the mortality of RDS (17/100,000 live births in 2007). Survivors, especially the extremely low birth weight infants, are at significant risk (85%) of developing BPD, or chronic scarring of the lung parenchyma from prolonged mechanical ventilation and oxygen toxicity. While the mortality from RDS has markedly improved, the incidence has been increasing due to the rising rates of premature births.

Patients usually present within the first day of life with tachypnea, grunting, nasal flaring, and retractions accompanied by decreased pulmonary compliance, hypoxemia, and hypercarbia secondary to ventilation–perfusion mismatch. Acidosis results from both hypercarbia and inadequate tissue oxygenation with anaerobic metabolism. Findings on chest x-ray include a homogeneous ground-glass appearance and air bronchograms in cases of significant hyaline membrane formation and atelectasis.

The underlying pathology of RDS is the deficiency or inadequacy of surfactant, a phospholipoprotein secreted by Type II pneumocytes to assist in alveolar expansion via reduction of the air/fluid interface. The resulting increase in alveolar surface tension reduces alveolar compliance, which causes massive atelectasis and pulmonary collapse, requiring mechanical ventilation. Histologically, RDS lungs are characterized by insufficient alveolar growth, a wide separation of alveolus from the vasculature, and accumulation of intraalveolar fibrin. Biochemical evidence of surfactant deficiency may be obtained by measuring lecithin/sphingomyelin ratios in the tracheal aspirate or gastric aspirate of neonates less than 1 hour old. A ratio of less than 2 is suggestive of a surfactant abnormality. Long-term effects of severe cases of RDS include persistent pulmonary function abnormalities, increased susceptibility to pulmonary infections, reactive airway disease, and BPD.

The benefits of exogenous surfactant administration as a treatment or prevention of RDS in newborns have been convincingly demonstrated and guide current medical practice. Early administration of animal-derived surfactant appears to hold the greatest benefit by reducing morbidity and mortality due to RDS. The presence of the protein fraction is a key attribute of this benefit over synthetic compositions. The physiologic effects of exogenous surfactant administration are to increase lung volume, improve dynamic lung compliance, and increase the arterial–alveolar oxygen ratio. These effects are brought about by maintaining lower alveolar opening pressure and thereby minimizing atelectasis. Surfactant administration has been found in multiple studies to produce an approximately 56% reduction in mortality, a finding that holds true for all patient profiles except very low-birth-weight infants (<700 g). In addition, almost all studies have found a significantly decreased rate of pulmonary leaks in patients treated with surfactant, and a meta-analysis of selected series demonstrated a significantly decreased rate of intraventricular hemorrhage and BPD. High-risk infants have been treated both prophylactically before the diagnosis of RDS is made and as rescue therapy for patients with established disease. In both instances, exogenous surfactant has produced improvements in survival; however, according to one study, prophylactic administration resulted in significantly lower mortality than rescue therapy. These results have been confirmed by others. Despite its overwhelming success, surfactant administration may have a limited benefit in specific subpopulations. Response to surfactant is decreased in the setting of congenital infections and birth asphyxia and is thought to be related to inflammation-mediated inactivation of surfactant in the lung.

Administration of corticosteroids to the mother at high risk of preterm delivery at 24 to 34 weeks of gestation significantly reduces the morbidity and mortality in preterm infants. Mori et al (2011) recently showed an improved survival in extremely preterm infants, as early as 22 to 23 weeks. In addition to reduction in RDS, prenatal corticosteroids have been associated with significant decrease in intraventricular hemorrhage and necrotizing enterocolitis.

## Persistent Pulmonary Hypertension

Persistent pulmonary hypertension of the newborn (PPHN) results in a shunting of pulmonary blood flow away from the high resistance pulmonary vasculature, interfering with adequate gas exchange. It occurs in 1 to 2/1000 births and is a cause of mortality in up to 20% of these patients. Severe respiratory distress, hypoxemia, acidosis, and hypercarbia increase pulmonary vascular tone, further exacerbating the illness.

Causes of PPHN can generally be subdivided into abnormalities in the development of the vasculature, or inadequate conversion from fetal to postnatal circulatory physiology. Pulmonary hypoplasia, for any reason, including CDH, renal agenesis, and urogenital obstruction, leads to substantial reduction in the pulmonary vascular cross-sectional area and an increase in vascular resistance. Abnormal proliferation of the pulmonary smooth muscle represents a barrier to gas exchange and is one of the causes of PPHN. This phenomenon is not well understood, but may be seen in the setting of meconium aspiration and postterm delivery. It has been suggested that hyperperfusion of the fetal lung, caused by maternal use of nonsteroidal antiinflammatory (NSAID) and SSRIs may contribute to the development of PPHN. Finally, infectious and parenchymal diseases can interfere with the normal postdelivery conversion to postnatal circulation, which may cause PPHN.

Medications and supportive therapy aimed at reversing this cycle are frequently employed and include, in addition to surfactant, bicarbonate, indomethacin to assist ductus arteriosus closure, pulmonary vasodilators, NO, prostanoids, and even extracorporeal life support (see below).

## Response of the Lung to Injury

### Mediators

Although many different stimuli can induce acute lung injury, the immunologic response, the histologic changes, and the pattern of respiratory failure are similar for all. The extent of pulmonary injury may vary greatly, manifesting clinically as a transient, minor oxygen requirement at its least to catastrophic respiratory failure requiring all the mechanical and pharmacologic resources of an ICU as in the case of ARDS. This latter event is a significant cause of neonatal and pediatric morbidity and mortality, accounting for 8% of all ICU patient days in one study and having an overall mortality of 52% to 70%. The major clinical causes of ARDS in the pediatric population include shock, sepsis, and drowning, although trauma, burns with or without smoke inhalation, and fat embolism are also associated conditions. In all of these settings the lung may function as both a target and a generator of the immunologic cascade that develops. The overall injury pattern is characterized by endothelial permeability with fluid and protein accumulation in the interstitium and subsequently the alveoli. Without reversal of the cascade by homeostatic mechanisms, the ongoing inflammation may lead to parenchymal fibrosis, chronic persistent lung disease, and/or the demise of the patient.

The mechanical effect of this inflammatory state in the lungs of patients with ARDS or any acute lung injury is to raise the opening pressure of many of the gas-exchanging units to the extent that alveoli remain collapsed and cannot take part in gas exchange. This is exhibited clinically by reduced lung volume, decreased compliance, and perhaps most importantly by decreased functional residual capacity (FRC). FRC is the volume at the point of end-expiration, which defines the balance between the alveolar tendency to collapse and the opposing drive of the chest wall to expand. A low FRC is associated with an increase in the shunt fraction and is the cause of hypoxemia in these patients. Increasing shunt fraction represents the accumulation of blood flow that does not undergo effective gas exchange. Mechanical ventilation with high PEEP is aimed at counteracting the loss of FRC and maintenance of recruitment of more alveoli for gas exchange at end-expiration. Similarly, with the loss of lung compliance, much higher transpulmonary pressures are required to produce the same lung volumes as a normal lung (Fig. 7-22). The normal exponential rise in volume for a given unit of pressure above FRC is concave until the closing pressure is exceeded. In addition to this mechanical effect on alveolar opening, an alveolus filled with the proteinaceous hyaline membranes of ARDS will not have normal gas exchange, exacerbating hypoxemia and arterial hypercarbia.

## MEDICAL THERAPY

### Nonpharmacologic Respiratory Care

The treatment of patients with respiratory failure is aimed at decreasing the work of breathing, improving lung compliance, and minimizing atelectasis, with the ultimate goal of promoting gas exchange. A number of simple measures can be utilized to promote these goals before institution of pharmacologic or mechanical support. Attention to patient position and postural drainage, chest physiotherapy, and appropriate suctioning and positive-pressure techniques are important aspects of pediatric respiratory care.

### Continuous Positive Airway Pressure

Recent improvements in the care for premature infants resulted in an increasing number of survivors. However, these patients often progress to the development of chronic lung disease, which can be traced to the insult from mechanical ventilation. In an effort to reduce the damaging effects of volutrauma and barotrauma in infants, alternative ventilation measures are considered more seriously. First referred to as "continuous distending pressure" when it was introduced in the 1930s, CPAP was repopularized by Gregory in the 1960s for RDS. Since then the application of this respiratory support method has expanded to include a wide range of respiratory problems including pneumonia, bronchiolitis, chemical or aspiration pneumonitis, pulmonary edema, obstructive sleep apnea, apnea of prematurity, and weaning from mechanical ventilation. CPAP provides pressure throughout the respiratory cycle to maintain airway pressure above ambient pressure and maintain patency of small airways and alveoli. In this way, it decreases the work of breathing, increases the FRC, decreases ventilation–perfusion mismatch, and improves oxygenation.

CPAP is considered by most clinicians to be a safer modality of respiratory support than mechanical ventilation. This does not, however, mean that it is without some inherent risks. Air trapping and over distension of the lungs can occur and are associated with worsening ventilation–perfusion mismatch, adversely elevated intrapulmonary pressures, and decreased right heart filling. In cases of pulmonary hypertension with already reduced pulmonary blood flow, impeding

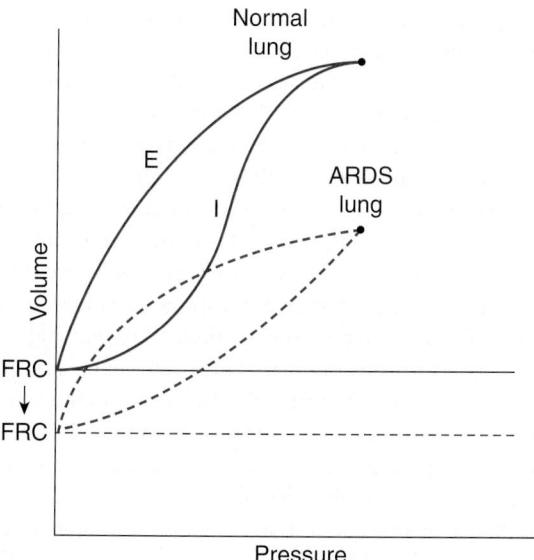

**FIGURE 7-22** Changes in FRC and compliance seen with ARDS. Greater pressures are required in patients with ARDS to produce the same lung volumes. In normal lungs changes in volume are exponential with changes in pressure, but this relationship is lost in the lungs of patients with ARDS. E, expiration, I, inspiration.

of further blood flow from elevated intrapulmonary pressures may worsen hypoxia. In addition, blood return from the head from lung over distension or excessively tight straps around the neck may occasionally be associated with increased ICP or intracranial hemorrhage in neonates. Another serious complication of CPAP is mucous plugging or kinking of the device, both of which may not be detected by the manometer but will be associated with decreased air flow to the patient. Continuous pulse oximetry and bradycardia monitors are therefore essential monitoring equipment during CPAP use. Infants displaying increased apneic episodes during CPAP administration should alert the clinician to the possibility of mucous plugging. Other hazards of this type of respiratory support include gastric distension and reflux aspiration, an event that may be difficult to detect when a face mask is obscuring visualization of the infant's mouth. For this reason, most clinicians advocate the routine use of a gastric tube for decompression.

Local skin irritation and airway mucosal breakdown from the delivery system may also occur, but are rare when properly fitting devices are applied by experienced personnel. Despite this long list of possible complications, CPAP remains an exceedingly safe system of respiratory support when instituted by properly trained persons and provides a less invasive, highly effective means of supporting patients with respiratory failure of multiple etiologies. CPAP use has become more popular as a part of a hybrid ventilation therapy known as INSURE (Intubation SURfactant Extubation). This modality involves a brief intubation period for the purposes of administration of surfactant, followed by extubation to noninvasive ventilator support, such as CPAP. This therapy avoids all mechanical ventilation and appears to significantly reduce the need for mechanical ventilation, requirement of additional surfactant administration, and incidence of BPD compared to mechanical ventilation strategies.

Derivative modalities, such as nasal intermittent mandatory ventilation (NIMV), are also gaining popularity. This approach is designed to deliver ventilator-generated breaths via nasal prongs to augment alveolar recruitment. Early data on its benefits over conventional nasally administered CPAP are not sufficient to make strong recommendations. Overall, the popularity of noninvasive ventilator approaches is growing, suggesting the trend toward a reduction in intubation of premature infants.

## PHARMACOLOGIC THERAPY

### Oxygen Therapy

Perhaps the most common respiratory therapy in the pediatric patient is the provision of oxygen. There are a variety of delivery systems available for oxygen, each having advantages depending on the degree of oxygen support necessary. It is important that any gas directed into the upper or lower airways be warmed and humidified as impairments in ciliary function, damage to mucous glands, ulceration of airways, impaired surfactant activity, and atelectasis may result from cold dry air in the bronchial tree. Low-flow oxygen may be given by nasal cannulas at flow rates of 0.1 to 6.0 L/min. Oxygen is directed posteriorly to the turbinates such that even the mouth-breathing patient will acquire an $FiO_2$ of 25% to 50% oxygen through entrainment of the nasopharygeal gas. Although the greatest advantage of the nasal cannulas is ease of administration, the largest disadvantage is that it is difficult to estimate exactly what $FiO_2$ is being delivered. A simple face mask is another low-flow oxygen delivery system that can give 6 to 10 L/min. Gas from the oxygen source is mixed with atmospheric gas entering around the mask or through its ports. Typically face masks provide an $FiO_2$ of 35% to 55%. Nonrebreathing face masks incorporate a reservoir of 100% oxygen with a one-way valve such that all inspired gas is oxygen, whereas exhalation occurs through a one-way port on the mask, preventing entrainment of gas during inspiration. These masks must be tight-fitting, and all the ports in place, to ensure that 100% oxygen is being given. Another alternative for providing higher concentrations of oxygen is the oxygen tent. Humidified gas flows into a clear plastic hood that encloses the patients head. Although some regional variation of oxygen may occur in the hood, an $FiO_2$ of 80% to 100% can be administered while access to the body of the patient is maintained.

### Oxygen Toxicity

As with any drug, there are significant toxicities associated with high-dose oxygen. Pulmonary physiologic abnormalities resulting from prolonged exposure to an $FiO_2$ of 100% include decreased ciliary function and mucous clearance, atelectasis from lack of inert gases, capillary leak with protein transudation, and type II pneumocyte injury with impaired surfactant production and function. Endothelial and alveolar epithelial injury are believed to be mediated by the increased production of free radicals including superoxide, hydrogen peroxide, and the hydroxyl free radical, all of which are upregulated by the provision of their excess substrate, oxygen. Also implicated in the etiology of hyperoxic lung injury are the arachidonic metabolites of the lipoxygenase and cyclooxygenase pathways, and their inhibition has been shown in some animal studies to lessen the injurious effects of high-dose oxygen. The direct toxic effect of these free radicals damages endothelial cells resulting in protein leakage and interstitial edema followed by alveolar edema. Activation of neutrophils and macrophages induces increased cytokine response, which in turn recruits more leukocyte infiltration with perpetuation of the injury. Oxygen may also be harmful for patients with chronic lung diseases, such as BPD, cystic fibrosis, or chronic obstructive pulmonary disease. These patients may require a slight degree of hypoxia to promote respiratory drive. The administration of oxygen alleviates this drive, effectively depressing ventilation and exacerbating hypercarbia and respiratory failure. In addition to the direct toxic pulmonary effect of oxygen, high-dose oxygen has also been found to cause retrolental fibroplasia or retinopathy of prematurity (ROP), direct central nervous system injury manifest as seizures or paralysis, and depression of erythropoiesis. The safe dose of oxygen for neonates is unknown; however, an $FiO_2$ less than 50% to 60% in children and adults appears to be well tolerated on a long-term basis. Total oxygen delivered, duration of therapy, and underlying pulmonary and systemic disease should all be considered in the pediatric patient requiring oxygen. While the role of oxygen in development of ROP has been known for several decades, safe oxygen saturation targets are still lacking. Since the acceptance of the 2-stage model of development of ROP, which involves the sequence of hyperoxic and hypoxic insults to the retina, the movement toward lower and narrower oxygen saturation goals has grown. Recent meta-analysis has revealed that lower oxygen saturations (70%-96%) in the early weeks of life, followed by higher saturations (94%-99%) later on, were associated with reduced risks of severe ROP. Typically, the oxygenation goals are inversely proportional to the gestational age; however, this strategy may interfere with the supportive therapies necessary in the setting of poor pulmonary development. In fact, evidence suggests that lower oxygenation targets may result in an overall increase in mortality.

## Bronchodilators

Because bronchospasm may be a central or exacerbating factor in the respiratory failure of pediatric patients, selective and nonselective bronchodilators are useful tools in the management of these patients. Stimulation of the $\beta_2$ receptor on bronchial and vascular smooth muscle results in bronchial relaxation and vasodilation, whereas $\beta_1$-receptor activation in cardiac tissue causes inotropic and chronotropic effects. For this reason, selective $\beta_2$ agonists such as albuterol and terbutaline, usually given in aerosolized form, are the first line of therapy in patients with bronchospasm. These drugs enable the beneficial effects of bronchodilation while minimizing the tachycardia of nonselective medications and may also enhance the mucociliary clearance of the bronchial tree.

## Corticosteroids

Although the beneficial effect of steroids in the treatment of the asthmatic patient is clear, their use in cases of RDS is more controversial. It is believed that the inflammation in the early postnatal period interferes with effective alveolar arborization and vascularization, leading to chronic pulmonary consequences, such as BPD. The theoretical advantage of steroids in patients with RDS is to ameliorate the lung damage and fibrosis associated with this inflammatory response. Glucocorticoid treatment inhibits the inflammatory response via multiple mechanisms, including inhibition of prostaglandins and leukotrienes, blocking the release of arachidonic acid, and via suppression of cyclooxygenases. Indeed, an uncontrolled study by Meduri and Chinn of adult patients with ARDS found an 86% survival rate in patients who responded to steroids. Neonatal respiratory failure has been shown to respond to steroids in selected circumstances. Although the beneficial effects of steroids in the treatment of pediatric patients with RDS have not been fully elucidated, the deleterious side effects of this class of drugs are plain. Prolonged steroid use in children is associated with growth retardation and impaired neurologic development, and much shorter courses are known to cause hyperglycemia, hypertension, fluid retention, mental status changes, peptic ulcer disease, immunosuppression, and suppression of the pituitary–adrenal axis. These harmful effects must be balanced with potential positive effects in the patient with severe respiratory failure. There is no consensus on the optimal dosage, duration, or potency of glucocorticoid utilized. In a recent move, the American Academy of Pediatrics has recommended against high dose dexamethasone for the treatment or prophylaxis of chronic lung disease in preterm infants. Currently, the recommendations for the lower doses are not backed by sufficient benefit, but this therapy appears to have fewer systemic side effects. It appears that the greatest benefit from systemic steroids may be derived by the patients with the higher than average risk of BPD. The optimal timing of the administration is also in question, but appears to trend toward late administration (>1 week).

## Pulmonary Vasodilators

Pulmonary vasodilators have been used to try to reverse the cycle of hypoxemia, acidosis, hypercarbia, and persistent pulmonary hypertension seen in infants with respiratory failure. Medications such as nitroprusside, nitroglycerin, and the calcium channel blockers as well as tolazoline have been employed with mediocre results. The limiting factor with all these drugs is that they are associated with a decrease in systemic vascular resistance in addition to pulmonary vascular resistance. The result, more often than not, is systemic hypotension with decreased peripheral perfusion and persistent right-to-left shunting. This may lead to further acidosis and perpetuation of the pulmonary hypertension.

## Nitric Oxide

NO or endothelium-derived relaxing factor, by virtue of its exceedingly short serum half-life, has the advantage of being a selective pulmonary vasodilator when delivered as an inhalational agent. By gaining access to the vasculature of those areas of the lung that are better ventilated, it can also decrease ventilation–perfusion mismatch. It was in 1987 that Palmer et al discovered that the substance responsible for vascular smooth muscle relaxation was the endothelium-derived relaxing factor called NO. Since that time intense scientific research has implicated NO in a variety of basic regulatory functions and demonstrated its ubiquitous nature in a host of mammalian systems. NO is a colorless gas resulting from the cleavage of the guanidine nitrogen group from l-arginine to form citrulline (Fig. 7-23). This reaction is catalyzed by several isoforms of nitric oxide synthase (NOS), is dependent on the presence of cofactors such as NADPH, and may be blocked by a number of l-arginine analogues. Endothelial cell-liberated NO rapidly diffuses to the subjacent smooth muscle and activates guanylate cyclase to increase cGMP, lowering intracellular calcium concentration and inducing smooth muscle relaxation. NO reaching the vascular space is rapidly bound by the heme unit of hemoglobin, inactivating it, ultimately forming methemoglobin, and preventing it from having systemic vasodilatory effects. However, increased formation of methemoglobin reduces the blood's oxygen-carrying capacity, requiring close monitoring. Physiologic levels of methemoglobin are less than 1%, but the maximum safe level of methemoglobin is not known, especially in premature infants. It is, however, known that prolonged iNO therapy at high concentrations may lead to the accumulation of this toxic metabolite. Recent evidence suggests that acute administration of high concentration iNO, combined with high oxygen concentration therapy, may be associated with higher concentrations of methemoglobin. In severe cases, the therapy may need to be withdrawn to eliminate this potentially critical side effect.

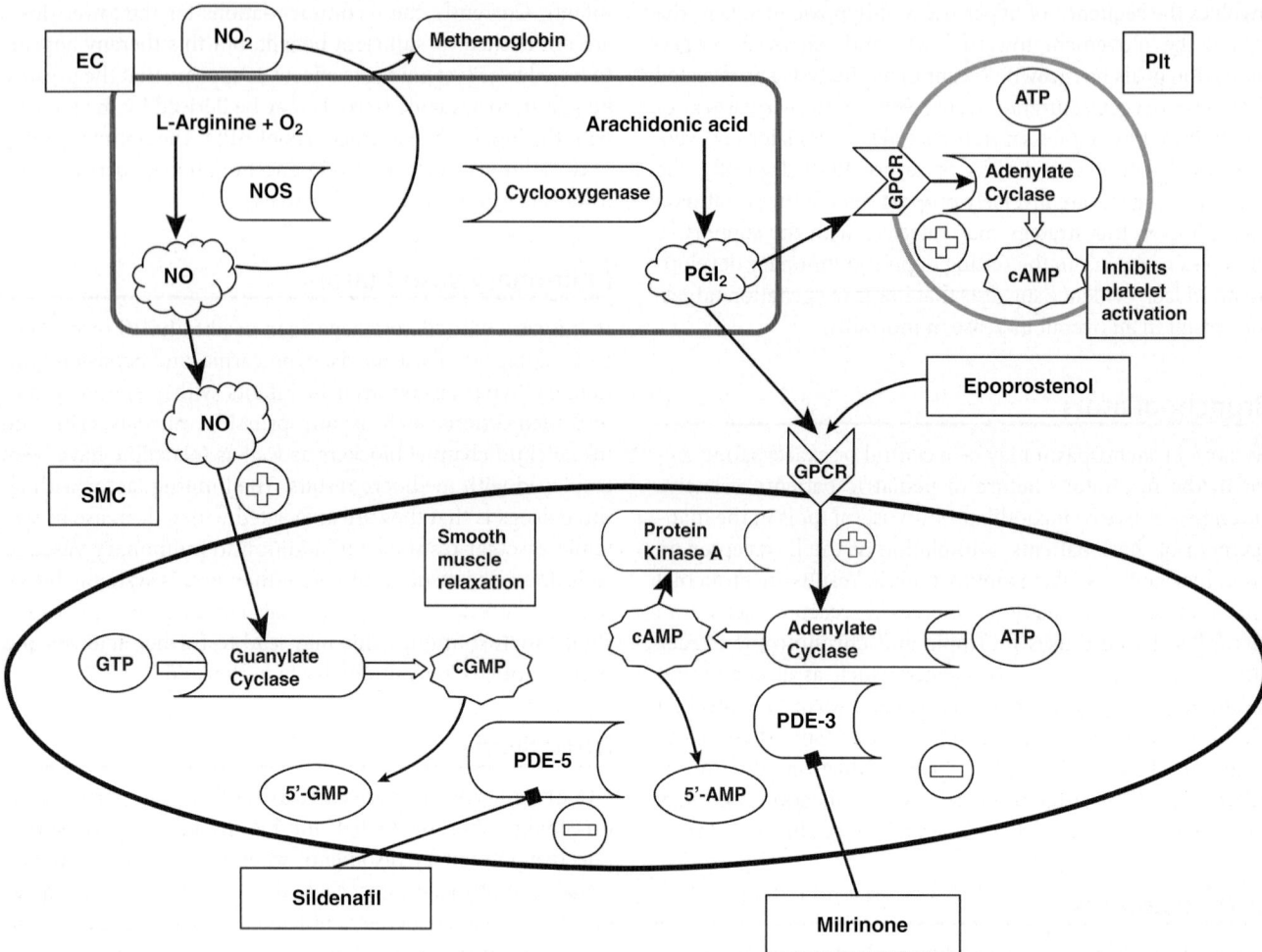

**FIGURE 7-23** Biochemical pathways of the vascular smooth muscle relaxation. EC, endothelial cell; Plt, platelet; SMC, vascular smooth muscle; NO, nitric oxide; NOS, nitric oxide synthase; $NO_2$, nitrous oxide; ATP, adenosine triphosphate; cAMP, cyclic adenosine monophosphate; GTP, guanosine triphosphate; cGMP, cyclic guanosine monophosphate; PDE 3,5, phosphodiesterase 3,5; GPCR, G-protein-couple receptor; $PGI_2$, prostacyclin I2.

Premature animal model studies with inhaled nitric oxide (iNO) demonstrated a reduction in pulmonary inflammation and alveolar development, laying the groundwork for its use in humans. iNO therapy is a useful adjunct in the preterm and term neonates with PPHN and has been demonstrated to improve oxygenation in multiple studies. It is evident, however, that the improved oxygenation resulting from iNO administration decreases the need for ECMO in infants. Neurodevelopmental deficits are important sequelae in critically ill patients with PPHN, often resulting in behavioral, cognitive, and neurosensory defects. Interestingly, iNO use in these patients is not associated with an increase in adverse neurologic outcomes. It can also be argued that by preventing the need for ECMO and its associated complications, in some patients, use of iNO may actually be even more beneficial. Unfortunately, up to 40% of infants with pulmonary hypertension do not respond to inhaled NO therapy, requiring alternative therapeutic interventions. In fact, despite acknowledging the long-term benefit in pulmonary disease, the NIH, in a recent consensus statement, has stated that there is a lack of evidence for routine use of iNO therapy in premature infants. The panel specifically pointed to the infants <34 weeks gestation or <1000 g birth weight to be particularly resistant to this modality. Newer studies are targeting the specific populations which may derive the greatest benefit from the iNO therapy.

## Sildenafil

NO activity in pulmonary smooth muscle is mediated by the generation of cGMP, leading to relaxation and reduction of the pulmonary vascular tone. The short half-life of NO is related to the action of phosphodiesterase-5 (PDE-5), an enzyme inactivating cGMP (Fig. 7-23). Sildenafil is a selective PDE-5 inhibitor and has recently become a commonly used treatment of PPHN. Sildenafil has been shown to improve exercise capacity in adults with pulmonary hypertension. In one trial, Namachivayam et al demonstrated that a single dose of sildenafil was protective from the rebound pulmonary hypertension resulting from iNO weaning. In addition, sildenafil was associated with reduced ventilator time after withdrawal of iNO and may be associated with improved oxygenation and survival. The utility of sildenafil as a stand-alone therapy is questionable at this time, but may provide substantial benefit, especially in situations when other supportive measures are unavailable.

## Prostanoids

Prostanoids such as epoprostenol are increasingly used for the treatment of pulmonary hypertension. Prostanoids exert a potent vasodilatory effect via a different mechanism from NO and sildenafil. Epoprostenol binds a G-protein–coupled receptor and signals adenylate cyclase to convert ATP to cAMP (Fig. 7-23). cAMP activates protein kinase A, which inhibits myosin light chain kinase, relaxing vascular smooth muscle. In addition to vasodilatory effects, epoprostenol also blocks vascular proliferation and platelet aggregation. Due to its short half-life (2-3 minutes), epoprostenol is typically delivered in a continuous fashion. While initial studies focused on the IV delivery of epoprostenol, its propensity to cause systemic hypotension and worsen the ventilation-perfusion mismatch has shifted the interest to inhaled delivery. One study has demonstrated an improvement in oxygenation index in neonates with persistent pulmonary hypertension who have failed iNO therapy. Precise indications and optimal method of delivery for the use of this therapy have not been clearly established.

## Surfactant

Multiple prospective randomized trials have demonstrated a decrease in mortality with the use of surfactant in neonatal respiratory failure. Please see "Respiratory Failure of Prematurity" (above) for further discussion.

## Diuretics

Acute lung injury of any cause is characterized by increased endothelial permeability with increased interstitial fluid accumulation (edema) and impaired oxygen exchange. Diuretics can be used in these patients to decrease intravascular volume, thereby minimizing hydrostatic forces across the endothelium and decreasing the interstitial fluid content. Although maintaining a low intravascular volume is beneficial for oxygenation in acute lung injury, overuse of diuretics may be detrimental if intravascular volume is compromised to the point of a decrease in cardiac output and end-organ perfusion. Frequently in patients with RDS and leaky capillary syndrome, anasarca is present, indicative of total body fluid overload, although intravascular volume is low. These patients usually require further fluid resuscitation to preserve renal and peripheral tissue perfusion until the capillary leak stops and normal mobilization of fluid occurs. Diuretic use may then help augment the normal diuretic process. A recent Cochrane review did not find sufficient evidence to recommend the routine use of furosemide in preterm infants with RDS. The authors cited that the transient improvement in the pulmonary function did not outweigh the risks of a patent ductus arteriosus (PDA) and hemodynamic instability.

## Caffeine

The use of caffeine in neonates as a preventive measure for the development of BPD has been questioned. Nevertheless, limited data suggest that caffeine may have a small, but significant long term pulmonary and neurological protective effect. Precise timing and dosages, as well as specific patient groups benefiting from this therapy have yet to be determined.

# MECHANICAL VENTILATION

Mechanical ventilation is indicated for persistent inadequate pulmonary gas exchange secondary to a range of pathophysiologic processes or as a prophylactic maneuver for impending respiratory compromise. The decision to intubate and place a patient on ventilatory support is a complex one and dependent on the nature and time course of respiratory failure as well as the failure of the multitude of less invasive supportive techniques discussed above. Although absolute criteria for mechanical ventilation on the basis of arterial blood gas measurements cannot be applied universally, infants with a $PaO_2$ less than 50 mm Hg and children with a $PaO_2$ less than 60 mm Hg generally require intubation and ventilatory support. Similarly, hypoventilation with acute rises in $Paco_2$ greater than 55 mm Hg and associated acidosis usually requires mechanical ventilation. Once an airway has been successfully obtained, however, strict adherence to a preset $Paco_2$ is unnecessary as long as severe acidosis (pH < 7.20-7.25) is not present. Allowing $Paco_2$ to rise in order to minimize barotrauma of mechanical ventilation is an increasingly common strategy of ventilator management (see "Permissive Hypercapnia" below). Mechanical ventilation may also be necessary in patients with acceptable $PaO_2$ and $Paco_2$ but with increased work of breathing. In this setting, or in any patient with severely compromised compliance and FRC, early mechanical ventilation enables control of oxygenation before respiratory collapse. Another indication for mechanical ventilation is to hyperventilate patients to treat head injury. Hyperventilation with concomitant hypocapnia has been used successfully in patients with brain swelling from closed head injury or near drowning by incurring temporary cerebral vasoconstriction, which decreases brain swelling and minimizes ICP.

# CONVENTIONAL MECHANICAL VENTILATION

## Pressure-Controlled or Pressure-Limited Ventilation

Mechanical ventilation has developed along 2 distinct modes for supplying oxygenated gas; pressure-controlled and volume-controlled. Pressure-controlled ventilators are used almost exclusively in mechanical ventilation of neonates and infants less than 10 kg. They supply a given continuous flow of gas until a preset pressure pop-off is met, at which point the PIP is maintained at a plateau level for the remainder of the predetermined inspiratory time. An exhalation valve then releases, and the continuous flow of the circuit and natural recoil of the chest cavity carry the exhaled gas out (Fig. 7-24). The tidal volume delivered may be altered by increasing the inspiratory time, increasing the flow of gas, or increasing the occlusion of the inspiratory valve, thereby increasing the PIP. Tidal volume is also significantly affected by patient variables such as lung and chest wall compliance as well as airway resistance and leak around the endotracheal tube. Initial settings for ventilation of a neonate may be determined by

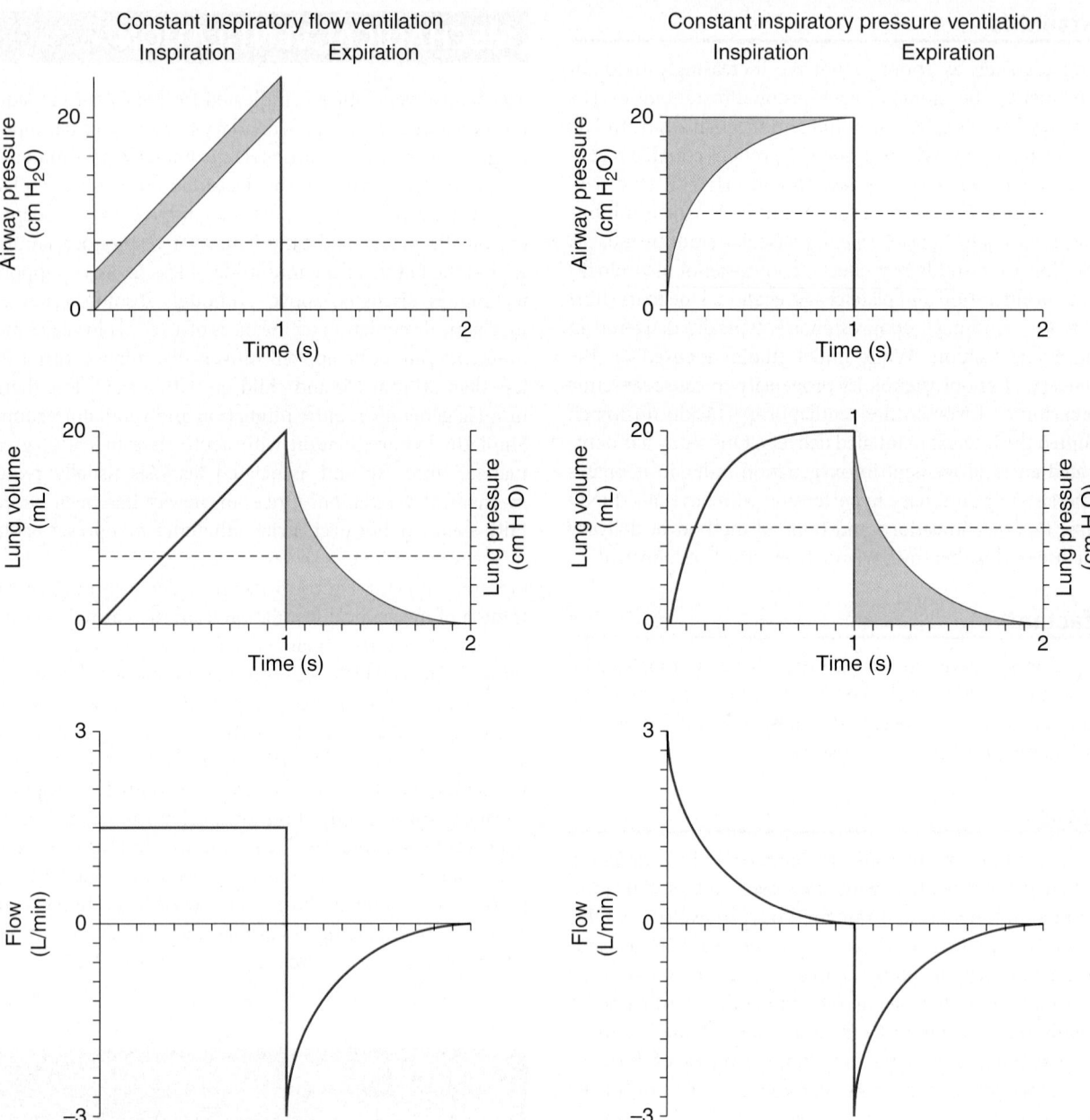

**FIGURE 7-24** Mechanical ventilation: idealized pressure, volume, and flow relationships. A 20-mL tidal volume is delivered during a 1-second inspiratory time. On the *left* is depicted volume-controlled ventilation, where an initial rise in airway pressure is needed to overcome airway resistance. Thereafter, airway pressure, lung volume, and lung pressure are defined by lung compliance. On the *right* is depicted pressure-controlled ventilation, where lung volume, lung pressure, and flow are exponential functions of time. Peak airway inspiratory pressure is higher, and mean airway pressure is lower, in volume ventilation compared with pressure ventilation; lung peak pressure is the same. *Shaded areas* represent the pressure required to overcome flow resistance; *unshaded areas* represent pressure required to overcome lung elastic properties. (Adapted from *Chatburn RL: Principles and practice of neonatal and pediatric mechanical ventilation. Respir Care 1991;36:569–595.*)

hand ventilating to see what PIP is required for normal chest excursion and good air movement by auscultation. A PIP more than 20 to 25 PIP unit as cm $H_2O$ should be avoided, as some studies have implied an increase in barotrauma associated with higher levels.

Once the PIP is determined, the frequency or rate may be selected, typically in the range of 30 to 40 breaths per minute, to maintain the desired $Paco_2$. Slower rates may be necessary in patients with restrictive airway disease, so as to avoid air trapping and over-inflation. Rates as high as 150 breaths per minute have been used successfully in patients with PPHN to induce a respiratory alkalosis. At high frequencies, inspiratory time will be sacrificed, equilibrium of gases cannot occur in terminal airways, and oxygenation may be decreased. Conversely, increasing the inspiratory time (with a slower rate) may maximize oxygenation. In patients with severe restrictive disease, inversion of the inspiratory/expiratory ratio (I/E ratio) will promote $CO_2$ elimination. The flow rate of gas may also be manipulated to change the time at which the PIP is achieved and alter the length of the plateau phase of pressure-controlled ventilation. Flow rates of 8 to 12 L/min are typical for neonates and allow for spontaneous breathing between ventilator breaths with minimal resistance. Higher flow rates are required when ventilation is at higher PIPs, whereas flow rates that are too high create turbulence, sacrificing tidal volume. The PEEP can also be altered to improve oxygenation. PEEP prevents the collapse of alveoli at end-expiration and therefore improves FRC and ventilation–perfusion mismatch. Commonly used PEEP values of 4 to 7 cm $H_2O$ are well tolerated, and increases to 10 cm $H_2O$ may significantly improve oxygenation. Higher PEEPs are associated with an increased risk of barotrauma and may impede venous return, compromising cardiac output. Last, $FiO_2$ should be adjusted so that the lowest level possible is used and the risk of oxygen toxicity (as discussed above) is minimized.

More modern pressure-controlled ventilators also supply demand flow so that the patient's inspiratory effort is sensed by microprocessors, a valve is opened, and an increased flow of gas is provided above the basal level of gas. This enables the ventilator to be synchronized with the patient's breathing pattern, theoretically decreasing the degree to which the patient is "fighting" the ventilator with his or her breathing cycle. Because detection of the small changes of pressure generated by infant breathing is difficult, pressure-controlled ventilators may also be equipped with a variety of devices that more accurately detect infant respiratory effort, including an abdominal pressure transducer for sensing diaphragmatic movement, a monitor of chest wall impedance connected to the ECG leads, and a flow-sensing device in the patient's airway to detect spontaneous breaths (pneumotachograph). Whether these devices, designed to better synchronize ventilatory breaths with infant breathing, will actually reduce the work of breathing and have clinical benefit remains to be seen.

In their most basic form, pressure-controlled ventilators provide a simple, easy-to-use, inexpensive, and effective mode of ventilating neonates and infants. Because high PIPs are felt by some to be responsible for the barotrauma of ventilators, pressure-controlled ventilators have the theoretical advantage of reducing the risk of this complication. This is true; however, only if the PIP is set lower so that the volumetric expansion of the lung is limited. Barotrauma is likely actually caused by volumetric overexpansion of the lung rather than simply the pressure peak of the respiratory cycle. This emphasizes one of the important aspects of pressure-controlled ventilator management. As lung compliance changes with progression or regression of disease, the PIP must be changed accordingly. Marked improvements in the patient's compliance must be accompanied by decreases in the PIP so as to avoid volumetric overexpansion and barotrauma. Because actual tidal volume is not known in older ventilators and may vary depending on air leaking around the noncuffed endotracheal tube, constant vigilance for changes in clinical parameters must be maintained. Similarly, endotracheal tube occlusion or kinking with a dramatic drop in tidal volume delivered may not affect functioning of the ventilator and may go undetected.

## Volume-Controlled Mechanical Ventilation

Pediatric patients weighing more than 10 kg are usually ventilated by means of a volume-controlled ventilator. This mode of ventilation delivers a constant flow of gas up to a preset volume during the inspiratory phase. As opposed to pressure-controlled ventilation, in which the PIP is attained immediately, volume-controlled ventilators slowly build pressure according to the compliance of the patient's lungs and chest wall. The mechanism for inspiratory flow delivery of volume-controlled ventilators is variable such that different waveforms of pressure may be administered. The ventilatory rate and tidal volume delivered are chosen to approximate that of a normally respiring person: 10 to 20 breaths per minute and a 5- to 6-mL/kg tidal volume. Higher tidal volumes approaching 10 to 15 mL/kg may be used and are not harmful in normal lungs but do not offer perceptible advantages. In spontaneously breathing patients, pressure support (PS) may be provided, which delivers high flows of gas at low pressures throughout the inspiratory cycle, decreasing the force necessary for the patient to pull air through the endotracheal tube. Although the relatively low sensitivity of the trigger for PS causes a delay in its onset compared to initiation of a patient breath, it can significantly decrease the work of breathing.

As in pressure-controlled ventilation, PEEP is routinely set at a low level (2–4 cm $H_2O$) so as to promote FRC and prevent atelectasis. In patients with severely compromised compliance, as in the case of ARDS, PEEP may be increased to 10 cm $H_2O$. If oxygenation needs are still not met, or very high concentrations of $O_2$ are still required, a trial of pressure-controlled ventilation should be attempted so as to lower $FiO_2$ to reasonable levels (<0.60). The beneficial effects of PEEP to keep alveoli and terminal airways open and recruit previously unventilated lung segments must be balanced with its negative effect on venous return and cardiac output. Right ventricular afterload is also increased with PEEP, most likely secondary to elevation of pulmonary vascular resistance. This inhibition of cardiac output by PEEP may be counterbalanced to some degree with inotropes and by increasing intravascular volume; however, the margin of error is small, as too much intravascular volume will eventually inhibit oxygenation. Impeding venous return with PEEP can also adversely increase ICP and lead to decreased cerebral perfusion. Auto-PEEP is a phenomenon in which alveolar pressure remains higher than airway pressure at end-expiration. When airway resistance is high, the time constant for expiration is several times that of inspiration, and air trapping occurs. Tidal volume is exchanged at near-total lung capacity, and the possibility for lung over distension is high.

As mentioned above, pressure- and volume-controlled ventilation may be used in any one of 4 different cycling modes: assist-control (A/C), intermittent mandatory ventilation (IMV), synchronized intermittent mandatory ventilation (SIMV), or pressure-support ventilation (PSV). In A/C mode, the preset tidal volume is delivered whenever the patient initiates a breath. If the spontaneous rate is less than the machine backup rate, the ventilator will initiate a breath. The minute ventilation is therefore determined by the preset tidal volume, the patient respiratory rate, and/or the backup rate. Problems are encountered with the use of A/C when the machine cannot detect the small pressure changes of infant breathing. In addition, although breaths are considered synchronized, there may be no synchrony with inspiratory mechanics. Inspiratory flow and the length of inspiration of the ventilator may not coincide with the patient's. Patient agitation and tachypnea may occur, resulting in excessive machine breaths, hypocapnia, and respiratory alkalosis. In patients with obstructive disease, air trapping occurs.

In the IMV mode, the ventilator delivers a set-time cycled breath without regard to the patient's respiratory efforts; however, it also delivers gas flow between breaths, enabling the patient to have some spontaneous breaths. This is an appropriate mode that provides consistent ventilation in a patient who is apneic or paralyzed. IMV has been used successfully in the neonatal population as well. However, in the older, conscious patient, work of breathing may be significantly increased as the patient struggles to breathe at his or her own rate while the ventilator cycles independently.

In the SIMV mode, the ventilator waits a preset time to sense patient initiation of a breath and then delivers the full tidal volume like an assist-control breath. The patient is able to breathe spontaneously between breaths with the support of gas flow only and no increased pressure. This enables patients to continue to exercise respiratory muscles and assume the work of breathing gradually. For this reason, SIMV has been used in older patients as a means of weaning, but with less success in infants.

Pressure-support ventilation allows the patient to control breathing to a much greater extent in that the initiation of a breath triggers the ventilator to increase the pressure to a preset limit and maintain it there until the patient finishes inspiration. The patient controls the length of both inspiration and expiration, and the degree of work done by the patient can be adjusted by changing the level of pressure. PSV has been used successfully for weaning in a variety of patient populations. Its disadvantages lie in that it depends on patient respiration such that apneic patients will not be actively ventilated. Once again, small infants may not generate large enough pressure changes to trigger the ventilator, and the inspiratory flow pattern of PSV is also not well tolerated by some patients.

## High-Frequency Ventilation

High-frequency ventilation delivers very small volumes at a supraphysiological high rate and relies on convection current and laminar versus turbulent air flow in the small airways to promote gas exchange. Whereas conventional ventilation incurs large volume changes during standard inspiration and expiration, with expansion and collapse of alveoli during the respiratory cycle, high-frequency ventilation provides continuous alveolar expansion with gas exchange occurring throughout the ventilatory cycle. Although the exact mechanism by which these ventilators promote gas exchange has not been elucidated, it is likely that the exchange occurs secondary to a combination of gas diffusion principles: asymmetric velocity profiles, Taylor dispersion, pendelluft, or molecular diffusion (Fig. 7-25). Pendelluft refers to the peripheral mixing of gas in alveolar units with variable time constants. In disease states, where time constants are extremely variable in the same lung area, this effect is amplified so that those with a short time constant are emptying into those units with a longer time constant. Taylor dispersion refers to the gas dispersion that occurs as a result of the relationship of axial air flow to the radial diffusion of gases in a tube, an effect that is enhanced with the turbulent flow at airway branch points. Asymmetric velocity profiles describe the net gas flow that

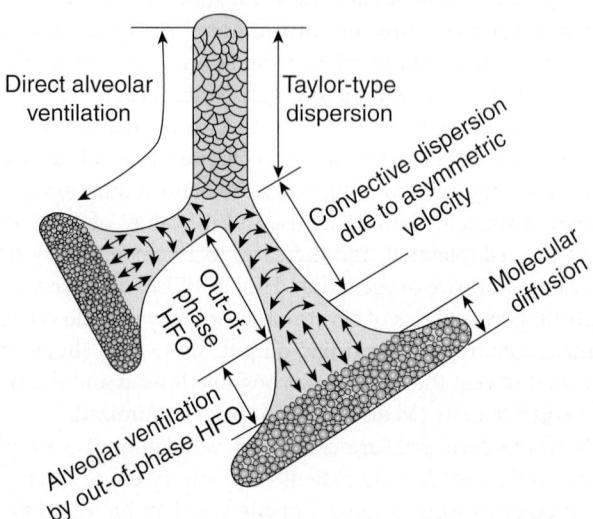

**High-frequency ventilation**

**FIGURE 7-25** Modes of gas transport during high-frequency ventilation. These mechanisms may interact and are not mutually exclusive. HFO, high-frequency oscillation. (Adapted from *Chang HK. Mechanisms of gas transport during ventilation by high-frequency oscillation. J Appl Physiol 1984;56:553.*)

occurs because inspiration has a parabolic velocity profile, whereas in expiration the velocity profile is flat. The result is that high-frequency ventilation can provide equivalent gas exchange at lower peak inspiratory pressures, a theoretical advantage in terms of volutrauma and barotrauma.

The 2 forms of high-frequency ventilation that have been used most commonly in pediatric patients are the high-frequency jet ventilator (HFJV) and the high-frequency oscillatory ventilator (HFOV). HFJV utilizes a small-bore cannula extending to the tip of the endotracheal tube for infusion of gas, and surrounding gases are entrained or pulled into the stream of injected gas. Large tidal volumes may be administered by HFJV; however, volumes less than anatomic dead space often result in normal oxygenation and carbon dioxide elimination. High flow rates without significant back pressure are determined by alterations in frequency of flow, PEEP, inspiratory time, and patient characteristics. Minute ventilation is very difficult to assess with these ventilators, and adjustments in the ventilator parameters must be dictated by clinical assessment. Frequencies in the range of 150 to 600 may be employed, with a resulting triangular-shaped pressure waveform. Expiration is completely passive. HFJV has been associated with earlier resolution of pulmonary interstitial emphysema, decreased bronchopleural fistula output, and ventilation that may be effective to the point of respiratory alkalosis. One of the major difficulties associated with HFJV is humidification and heating of gas. Inadequate humidification has resulted in several reports of necrotizing tracheobronchitis. Air trapping may also be a problem. Compared to conventional ventilation, prospective trials in patients with RDS have not shown a benefit to HFJV, so its use is mainly as salvage therapy.

HFOV uses a rapidly cycling piston pump or an acoustic speaker to generate very high-frequency small-tidal-volume breaths. This oscillating energy source is augmented by variable gas flow, providing an undercurrent of gas flow as well, and enables active rather than passive expiration. Similar to HFJV, tidal volume is unknown, and adjustments in ventilator parameters are based strictly on clinical parameters. Although initial clinical studies found no improvement in respiratory status associated with HFOV, and in fact noted an increase in complications, optimal parameters of ventilation had not been maintained, and patient's poor outcomes may have been secondary to excessive conventional ventilation before entrance into the study. Since then, several reports have found much more encouraging results. Kohelet et al found that 37 of 41 infants with PPHN responded to HFOV with improved gas exchange by 1 hour after initiation of treatment, and 34 patients survived. In one other study, HFOV was also been found to supplant ECMO in the treatment of neonatal respiratory failure. Schwendeman et al ventilated 94 neonates eligible for ECMO by standard criteria and found that HFOV avoided ECMO in 48 of these patients. Although those patients who developed chronic lung disease (20/84 survivors) were more likely to have undergone ECMO, they were also more likely to have hypoplastic lung syndromes and have had longer conventional ventilation courses. Similarly, in a comparative study of HFOV versus conventional mechanical ventilation in patients who were eligible for ECMO, Clark et al showed a decreased incidence of chronic lung disease in patients treated with HFOV.

More recent prospective randomized studies have confirmed the efficacy of HFOV in improving oxygenation, decreasing the length of time on the ventilator, decreasing the chronic lung disease in these patients, and lowering hospital costs, compared to conventional mechanical ventilation. HFOV has also been successful when combined with NO in the treatment of PPHN. In a prospective crossover study comparing HFOV to NO alone versus HFOV and NO in combination, Kinsella et al found that of 125 patients failing either NO or HFOV ventilation alone, 32% responded to the combination of the 2. With the advent of multiple new therapies for respiratory failure, determining which single or combination treatment will be most efficacious for a particular infant will be difficult. In an interesting study by de Lemos et al, the authors identified several echocardiographic findings of decreased ventricular function in respiratory failure patients that reliably predicted which patients would not respond to HFOV and would ultimately require ECMO. This finding is congruent with the fact that elevated mean airway pressure is necessary for HFOV, and patients who cannot tolerate this from a cardiac standpoint will have a fall in cardiac output and not respond to HFOV. From these data, it may be possible to predict which patients will benefit from HFOV and which will require immediate triage to ECMO.

## ADVERSE EFFECTS OF MECHANICAL VENTILATION

### Barotrauma

The major deleterious effect of mechanical ventilation is barotrauma. This may appear as one of any of the air-leak syndromes, including pneumothorax, bronchopleural fistula, pneumomediastinum, subcutaneous emphysema, pulmonary interstitial emphysema (PIE), pneumopericardium, and even pneumoperitoneum. Infants at highest risk are those with hypoplastic lungs and premature infants; however, manual ventilation, RDS, meconium aspiration, and vigorous resuscitation are also risk factors. All of these air-leak syndromes are the result of over-expansion of the lung with alveolar damage and either free rupture of the alveolus into the pleural space or more limited dissection of air into the peribronchial and perivascular connective tissues and then around adjacent structures. Pulmonary interstitial emphysema, a common finding in preterm infants on mechanical ventilation, may be seen as tubular collections of air that do not change with alterations in patient position. Continued accumulation of air in the interstitium may result in airway collapse and a requirement for greater ventilatory support because of worsening V/Q mismatch. The treatment of less severe forms of air leak such as pulmonary interstitial emphysema is to decrease ventilatory pressures or to change to high-frequency ventilation and serial x-ray follow-up. In cases of pneumothorax in patients on positive-pressure ventilation, immediate chest tube placement is essential to prevent progression to a potentially fatal complication, tension pneumothorax. Self-limited pneumopericardium likewise may be followed but, in cases of hemodynamic compromise, urgent pericardiocentesis is required.

### Bronchopulmonary Dysplasia

Chronic lung damage from prolonged mechanical ventilation and high oxygen concentration was first described by Northway et al in 1967. On pathologic examination of these lungs, mucosal hyperplasia in small airways is seen impinging on the lumen and causing atelectasis. Interstitial edema, fibrosis, and thickening of the basement membrane and vascular wall are also seen and certainly contribute to the poor gas exchange found in these patients. BPD is defined clinically as oxygen dependence present for more than 28 days after mechanical ventilation and in association with an abnormal chest x-ray. BPD is a disease common to premature infants but may occur in any pediatric patients. The 2 factors universally associated with its development are prolonged positive-pressure ventilation and high oxygen concentration. Free radical formation has been implicated as an etiologic agent, implying a therapeutic role for antioxidants such as vitamin E and superoxide dismutase; however, no studies have proven this efficacy. The implications of lifelong pulmonary compromise with its incalculable cost to patients and society require that clinicians work toward minimizing the exposure of their patients to this complication.

### Permissive Hypercapnia

Historically, the goal of respiratory therapy in the compromised patient has been to maintain near-normal levels of blood oxygen and carbon dioxide. Although this goal remains for control of blood oxygen levels, it has been found more recently that strict $Paco_2$ control is unnecessary. In fact, in light of the above discussion of the many deleterious effects of pressure and volume during mechanical ventilation, maintenance of normal carbon dioxide levels may have significant costs. In pathologic states of respiratory failure with diffuse airway collapse and reduction in FRC, the normal lung segments must be overinflated to result in enough ventilation for normocarbia. Subsequently, the normal lung segments may be damaged by trying to compensate for collapsed airways elsewhere. The precise levels of $Paco_2$ that are acceptable without significant risk of neurologic impairment are not clear and are likely highly dependent on the gestational age, birth weight, as well as comorbidities of the infant. Levels $Paco_2$ 45 to 55 mm Hg appear to be beneficial, provided that pH >7.20 can be maintained. In the awake, spontaneously breathing patient, hypercapnia is associated with acidemia, headache, narcosis, respiratory depression, and ultimately hypoxia. However, in the ventilated patient whose oxygenation is preserved, it is well tolerated. Gradual rises in $Paco_2$ are accompanied by renal accumulation of bicarbonate with a compensatory metabolic alkalosis and near-normal pH.

With proper patient selection and incremental increases in $Paco_2$, permissive hypercapnia is a useful technique in the management of patients with respiratory failure to minimize the damage imposed from mechanical ventilation. Guidelines for management of adults with respiratory failure have included maintaining oxygen saturations greater than 90%, keeping PIP less than 35 cm $H_2O$, and lowering the tidal volume to allow a slow rise in $Paco_2$. Although further application and controlled studies have yet to be performed in the neonatal and pediatric population, permissive hypercapnia could be a valuable strategy in the management of these patients.

## LIQUID VENTILATION

Another promising therapy in assisted ventilation of pediatric patients with respiratory compromise is liquid ventilation by means of perfluorocarbons. Perfluorocarbons are uniquely suited for use in ventilation as they are biologically inert substances with extremely high respiratory gas solubility, low viscosity, and relatively low surface tension. They are nonabsorbable, immiscible, and chemically nonreactive substances that are eliminated by aerosolization through the lung. Liquid ventilation using perfluorocarbon has several theoretical advantages. They can reduce lung distending pressure, facilitate homogeneous lung expansion, maintain FRC, and act as a lavage for debris and infectious materials in the airways. There are presently 2 means of liquid ventilation being extensively studied as alternative therapies: total (tidal) liquid ventilation, in which full tidal volumes are instilled through the endotrocheal tube (ET), and perfluorocarbon-assisted gas exchange (PAGE) in which an amount of perfluorocarbon equal to the FRC is instilled, and then the patient is ventilated with respiratory gas in the conventional manner.

Extensive animal studies of liquid ventilation have demonstrated it to be a safe and effective mode of respiratory support. Wolfson et al studied surfactant-deficient premature lambs and found that, compared to conventional ventilation, lambs ventilated with total liquid ventilation demonstrated improved hemodynamic stability, better gas exchange, improved respiratory compliance, decreased barotrauma, and improved survival. Whereas histologic sections of the gas-ventilated animals showed thick hyaline membrane formation, those from the liquid-ventilated lambs showed thin septa and no alveolar exudate or hyaline membranes. In fact, no study has found histologic abnormalities associated with liquid ventilation. In a similar model using partial liquid ventilation compared to conventional mechanical ventilation, dramatic improvements in oxygenation and survival have been seen. Because of the higher airway resistance associated with ventilating with a liquid and the heaviness of perfluorocarbons, concerns have arisen that liquid ventilation could compromise pulmonary vascular resistance and adversely affect cardiac output. Several animal studies have demonstrated preserved cardiac output and no change in $VO_2$, carbon dioxide production, or respiratory quotient.

Few human clinical studies of liquid ventilation have been reported; however, Greenspan et al found that 3 premature infants with severe hyaline membrane disease who had failed conventional therapy responded to short courses of liquid ventilation with increased respiratory compliance and improved and persistent oxygenation. Liquid ventilation was administered to a group of 19 neonatal, pediatric, and adult patients on ECLS at the University of Michigan, and it resulted in improved pulmonary compliance (0.18-0.29 mL cm $H_2O^{-1}$ $kg^{-1}$), decreased A-a gradient (590-471 mm Hg), and an overall survival of 58%. In a recent study by Leach et al, 10 premature infants underwent PAGE for 24 to 72 hours and demonstrated improved arterial oxygen tension by 138%, increased dynamic compliance by 61%, and a decrease in the oxygenation index from 49 to 17. No adverse effects of the perflubron ventilation were seen. Clearly further studies are warranted to establish efficacy of this promising new treatment modality.

# ECMO

Extracorporeal membrane oxygenation (ECMO) is an invasive supportive modality aimed to provide adequate gas exchange and perfusion to a patient with acute cardiopulmonary failure. ECMO provides time for the recovery of cardiac function and restoration of sufficient pulmonary activity by maintaining necessary perfusion, oxygenation, and ventilation. More importantly, it potentially obviates the need for aggressive vasopressor and inotropic administration, and protects the lungs from excessive baro-/volutrauma, and toxic oxygen concentrations. The role of ECMO in the resuscitative efforts in children and adults has been evolving since its first successful use more than 3 decades ago. Careful assessment of risks and benefits continues to redefine the groups of patients who will draw the greatest benefits from extracorporeal support. ECMO requires a significant allocation of resources in the form of renewable supplies, sophisticated monitoring equipment, and, most importantly, specially trained dedicated experienced teams of healthcare professionals. ECMO can last anywhere from several days to several weeks, depending on the clinical course and goals of treatment. Nevertheless, the key principle of ECMO remains that it is a supportive measure rather than a therapeutic modality. Thus, while precise indications and contraindications for this therapy may be debated, the overarching principle is that the patient's condition must be reversible, provided that appropriate treatment can be administered within a reasonable amount of time.

## ECMO INDICATIONS

Specific indications for ECMO are difficult to define, and appropriately evolve to accommodate new information from the modern diagnostic techniques and beneficial effects of improved therapeutic modalities. Therefore, most clinicians are instructed to follow more general guidelines. Extracorporeal life support is indicated whenever the expected patient-specific mortality is 80% or higher. Estimation of this criterion is quite difficult to achieve, aside from cases of specific anatomic defects that are amenable to repair, but are clearly lethal otherwise. Patient population-specific considerations may include more objective parameters. Neonates are stratified using the oxygenation index (OI). OI = Mean airway pressure $\times$ 100 $\times$ $FiO_2/PaO_2$. OI > 30 to 40 on arterial blood gas measurements over a 2- to 6-hour period is generally considered an indication for ECMO. Contraindications in neonates include the presence of a fatal genetic abnormality, severe brain damage, significant intraventricular hemorrhage, major organ damage not amenable to transplantation. Most centers recognize the birth weight <2 kg and gestational age <34 weeks as relative contraindications, but these parameters are subject to change as therapeutic and monitoring techniques improve. Pediatric respiratory and cardiac patient populations lack specific indications, aside from the general mortality considerations mentioned earlier. However, it has been noted that the patients subjected to prolonged mechanical ventilation (>3 weeks) and high oxygen concentrations sustain irreversible pulmonary damage, precluding successful withdrawal of ECMO therapy. Finally, due to the necessity of continuous anticoagulation, patients whose conditions are immediately related to significant bleeding risks are typically not considered candidates for ECMO. Recently, some centers have been moving toward extending the selection criteria to include infants born after just 32 weeks gestation and those weighing 1.7 kg.

Neonates with respiratory distress without underlying anatomic cardiac abnormalities are generally regarded to draw the greatest benefit from ECMO. Patients with severe cases of persistent pulmonary hypertension (PPHN), meconium aspiration syndrome (MAS), and congenital diaphragmatic hernia (CDH) are routinely considered for ECMO. Pediatric patients with bacterial or viral pneumonia, as well as acute respiratory distress syndrome (ARDS) represent typical ECMO candidates. Neonates and pediatric patients with correctable cardiac anomalies (ie, shunting septal defects) are also usual candidates for extracorporeal support, as well as those needing a bridge to visceral transplant.

## ECMO PHYSIOLOGY/CIRCUIT DESIGN

Although the specific components of the ECMO circuit have evolved to address various technical limitations and evolving needs, the basic design has remained virtually intact. The 3 main components of the circuit are the engine (roller or centrifugal pump), the membrane oxygenator, and the heat exchanger (Fig. 7-26). After the establishment of dedicated

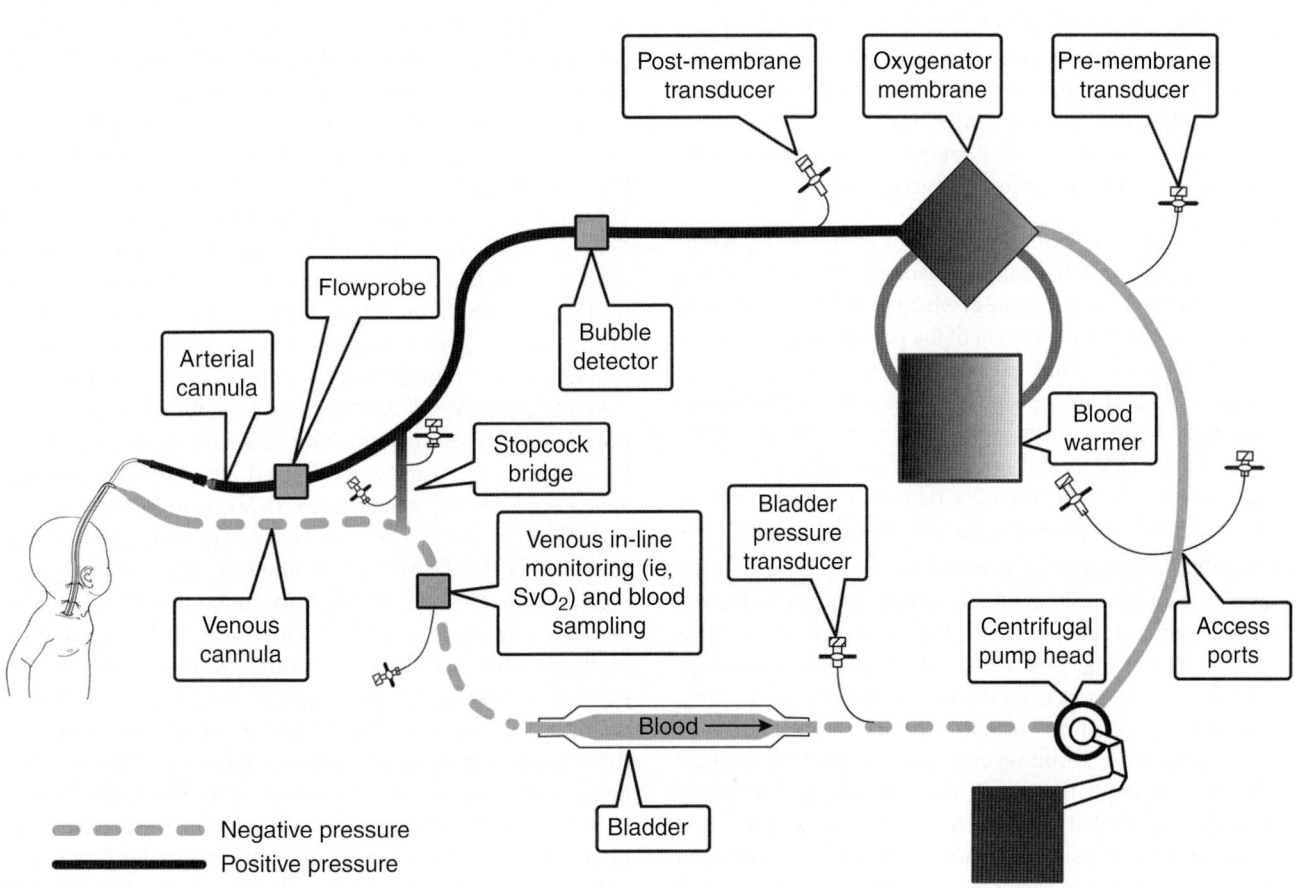

**FIGURE 7-26** Diagram of a venoarterial extracorporeal life-support circuit.

venous and if necessary, arterial access points, venous blood is shunted from the patient, along a series of flexible tubes with the help of gravity and the pump via negative pressure. Pump design involves either a mechanical cam or roller, sequentially squeezing the tubing and moving the blood forward, or a magnetic field-based rotating platform. The flow rate through the entire system is adjustable and is typically titrated based on the perfusion needs. Servoregulation is an important part of this fragment of the circuit and is accomplished using a mechanical bladder system. Since excessive negative pressure in the drainage limb of the ECMO circuit may result in significant hemolysis and damage to the vena cava and right atrial walls, the bladder serves to alert the perfusionist to the generation of significant negative pressures and can be set to interrupt the flow before irreversible damage occurs. Drained blood is then directed to the membrane oxygenator. This device interfaces the bloodstream and the flow of sweep gas in a countercurrent manner. This allows the oxygenation of the blood and removal of carbon dioxide. The partial pressures of oxygen and carbon dioxide in the sweep gas can, and are routinely adjusted to address the dynamic metabolic scenario. The size of the oxygenator is directly proportional to the surface area of the membrane interface and is estimated based on the size of the patient and the expected level of support. Following the oxygenator the blood is rewarmed and directed to the designated arterial access point in the patient. Technical advances have allowed the integration of a number of monitoring and therapeutic devices into the ECMO circuitry. These allow not only real-time monitoring of the acid/base, electrolyte, hematologic, and coagulation status of the bloodstream, but also the incorporation of fluid removal and renal replacement machinery into the circuit, if necessary. A functional circuit also allows a customizable, but virtually any number of necessary access points used for blood sampling and necessary infusions.

Caring for a patient on ECMO requires that several important considerations are consistently accounted for:

1. While the amount of flow generated by the ECMO machinery often exceeds what can be reasonably necessary, often, the limiting factor is the rate at which blood can be shunted away from the venous system of the patient into the circuit. Therefore, careful fluid balance must be maintained at all times, especially in the setting of systemic inflammatory response. Additional flow limitation is created by the size of the oxygenator, as well as the access cannulas. It is important to remember that attempts to increase the flow rate are associated with increased shear stress and hemolysis.

2. Despite the advances in material design and coating, the exposure of blood to synthetic materials, such as ECMO tubing initiates massive deposition of protein and activation of the clotting system. This not only depletes the coagulation factors, increasing the risk of pathologic bleeding, but also perpetuates unstable circuit- and system-wide thrombogenesis. Resulting clot can interfere with the flow of blood through the circuit and efficient gas exchange. In order to combat this problem, active anticoagulation, typically with heparin, and normalization of coagulation factor concentrations are required. This is a complex and dynamic process, necessitating frequent monitoring and prompt reactive transfusions of factor concentrates and blood products.

3. Despite the attempts to normalize the coagulation status and the laminar flow through ECMO circuitry, continuous consumption of blood cells, especially erythrocytes is inevitable. Therefore, careful monitoring and frequent transfusions may be required to maintain adequate oxygen-carrying capacity of the blood while on extracorporeal support.

## METHODS OF ECMO AND CANNULATION TECHNIQUES

Application of ECMO requires that appropriate vascular access is established in the patient either prior to or at the time of cannulation. Central cannulation is most often used when intraoperatively the patient cannot be weaned off cardiopulmonary bypass, in the immediate postoperative period, or due to constraints of peripheral vascular anatomy. In cases of central cannulation, the cannulas are placed directly into the right atrium or the vena cava for venous drainage and into the ascending aorta for arterial return. While this approach has several advantages, including providing optimal flow, postoperative bleeding is a major drawback. Therefore, in most cases, a peripheral approach is preferred. Vascular access can be obtained percutaneously, via an open Seldinger technique, or, in nonemergent conditions, via a cut-down. A variety of ECMO cannulas with a wide range of sizes and flow characteristics are commercially available for use with different circuit designs. As discussed above, the decision on the optimal size of the cannula depends largely on the specific patient characteristics. In addition, the goals of the specific ECMO support must be considered when choosing the cannula and access technique. The ideal cannula is short in length and has the widest lumen possible, which maximizes the amount of laminar flow through the system with the lowest resistance. However, limitations due to the anatomy and the size of the patients dictate the choice of the cannula. Cannula sizes are reported based on the outer diameter, which does not account for the thickness of the tubing wall and results in a variability of internal diameters. ECMO cannula walls are often wire-reinforced to minimize kinking and obstruction to flow.

While a number of variations and combinations of access points can be used to attain sufficient flow of blood through the circuitry, they can be subdivided into 3 main categories: venoarterial (VA), venovenous (VV), and double lumen venovenous (DLVV). Several factors are considered in the selection of the ECMO access method. VA cannulation is indicated in cases of respiratory dysfunction with an accompanying underlying cardiac deficit. This is the more common method, since significant pulmonary dysfunction, such as persistent pulmonary hypertension, evokes secondary cardiac stress. In neonates, VA ECMO is usually established via the internal jugular vein (cannula draining the right atrium) and common carotid artery (with the flow directed at the aortic arch). A right-sided cannulation is preferred due to a more direct course of the vasculature to the target locations. The cannulated vessels may be distally ligated and the majority may not be repaired following decannulation. Neurological outcomes are a natural concern in these cases and there have been attempts to establish whether this practice leads to any significant neurological sequelae, but to date the studies have resulted in contradictory findings. It is still unclear whether the ligation or repair of the neck vessels in neonates is detrimental in the long term. Other disadvantages of the VA neck cannulation include the risk of particulate embolization, reduction in pulmonary perfusion, potential reduction in cardiac output, and the loss of pulsatile systemic flow. Larger patients are candidates for groin cannulation, allowing the use of the common femoral vessels in establishing either primary, or additional ECMO access. There is no consensus on the appropriate or acceptable ages or weights that are deemed safe cut-offs for the use of this technique. However, most clinicians do not use the femoral vessels for ECMO cannulation in children weighing less than 15 to 20 kg or those who cannot walk.

Venovenous ECMO is established by the cannulation of 2 larger veins, typically using internal jugular and femoral venous vessels. Typically, the cannula placed in the internal jugular vein is well positioned to drain the right atrium and oxygenated blood is returned to the circulation via the femoral venous cannula. The converse design can also be utilized, so that blood is removed from the femoral vessel and returned to the right atrium. Alternative to this design is the placement of a double lumen cannula into the right atrium through the internal jugular vein, which allows both the drainage and reperfusion within the right atrium. One major limitation of either the VV or the DLVV system is the potential for re-circulation secondary to the close positioning of the drainage and the reperfusion cannulas. This phenomenon is especially critical at high flow rates, increasing the fraction of the oxygenated blood pool that re-enters the drainage cannula without circulating through the system. Nevertheless, VV or DLVV is an acceptable ECMO modality in patients without cardiac dysfunction. It's major

While a number of variations and combinations of access points can be used to attain sufficient flow of blood through the circuitry, they can be subdivided into 3 main categories: venoarterial (VA), venovenous (VV), and double lumen venovenous (DLVV). Several factors are considered in the selection of the ECMO access method. VA cannulation is indicated in cases of respiratory dysfunction with an accompanying underlying cardiac deficit. This is the more common method, since significant pulmonary dysfunction, such as persistent pulmonary hypertension, evokes secondary cardiac stress. In neonates, VA ECMO is usually established via the internal jugular vein (cannula draining the right atrium) and common carotid artery (with the flow directed at the aortic arch). A right-sided cannulation is preferred due to a more direct of the vasculature to the target locations. The cannulated vessels may be distally ligated and the majority may not be repaired following decannulation. Neurological outcomes are a natural concern in these cases and there have been attempts to establish whether this practice leads to any significant neurological sequelae, but to date the studies have resulted in contradictory findings. It is still unclear whether the ligation or repair of the neck vessels in neonates is detrimental in the long term. Other disadvantages of the VA neck cannulation

include the risk of particulate embolization, reduction in pulmonary perfusion, potential reduction in cardiac output, and the loss of pulsatile systemic flow. Larger patients are candidates for groin cannulation, allowing the use of the common femoral vessels in establishing either primary, or additional ECMO access. There is no consensus on the appropriate or acceptable ages or weights that are deemed safe cut-offs for the use of this technique. However, most clinicians do not use the femoral vessels for ECMO cannulation in children weighing less than 15 to 20 kg or those who cannot walk.

Venovenous ECMO is established by the cannulation of 2 larger veins, typically using internal jugular and femoral venous vessels. Typically, the cannula placed in the internal jugular vein is well positioned to drain the right atrium and oxygenated blood is returned to the circulation via the femoral venous cannula. The converse design can also be utilized, so that blood is removed from the femoral vessel and returned to the right atrium. Alternative to this design is the placement of a double lumen cannula into the right atrium through the internal jugular vein, which allows both the drainage and reperfusion within the right atrium. One major limitation of either the VV or the DLVV system is the potential for re-circulation secondary to the close positioning of the drainage and the reperfusion cannulas. This phenomenon is especially critical at high flow rates, increasing the fraction of the oxygenated blood pool that re-enters the drainage cannula without circulating through the system. Nevertheless, VV or DLVV is an acceptable ECMO modality in patients without cardiac dysfunction. Its major advantage is that it avoids the involvement and subsequent ligation or injury of the carotid artery. This technique is being used more frequently in the centers that initiate support for all noncardiac patients via the VV route, converting to VA if the need arises.

A number of cannulation techniques can be utilized and possess unique advantages and limitations under certain clinical conditions. If possible, direct visualization and adequate control is preferred to avoid excessive injury to the vessels and allow easier repositioning than the percutaneous technique. The following describes the usual approach to cervical ECMO cannulation. Anesthesia can be administered locally to the site of the incision, but a general anesthetic is indicated in many situations. It is critical to administer a paralytic for the procedure to prevent spontaneous respiration in a patient. Failure to do so may put the patient at risk for an air embolism. The child is positioned supine at the edge of the bed and his neck is hyperextended over a transverse shoulder roll. The head is turned to the left to assist in exposure of the right neck vessels. A 2- to 3-cm transverse incision is made along the anterior edge of the SCM, one finger's breadth cephalad to the right clavicle (Fig. 7-27A). The platysma is divided with electrocautery and retractors can be placed to assist further dissection. The dissection can be carried through the fibers of the sternocleidomastoid, or the muscle can be retracted anteriorly or posteriorly, depending on the relative size and location of the incision. The carotid sheath is identified and incised to reveal the carotid artery, internal jugular vein, and the vagus nerve. The vein is gently dissected and encircled with proximal and distal ligature ties. The inferior thyroid vein may be encountered and should be

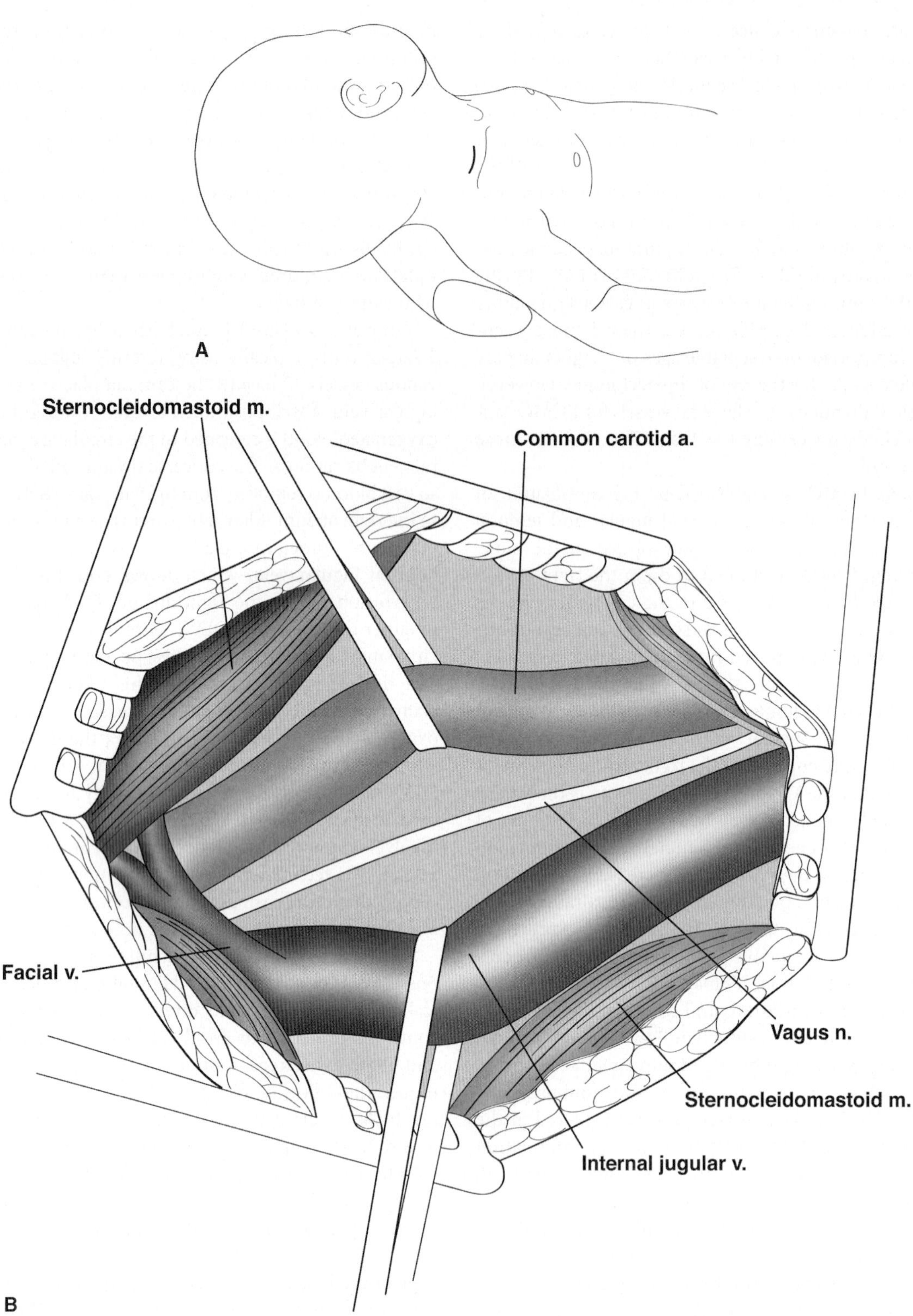

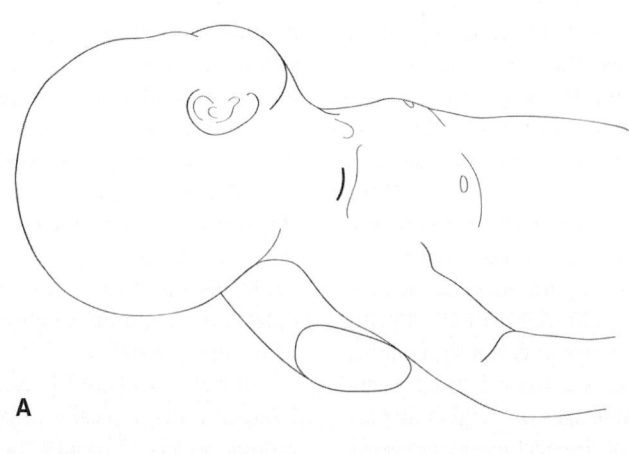

**A**

Sternocleidomastoid m.

Common carotid a.

Facial v.

Vagus n.

Sternocleidomastoid m.

Internal jugular v.

**B**

**FIGURE 7-27** **A.** Proposed position and incision site for cervical cannulation. **B.** Exposure of the internal jugular vein and carotid artery.

ligated. The carotid artery is mobilized and controlled with ligature ties in a similar fashion. It should be noted that no arterial branches should be encountered at this level. The vagus nerve should be identified and protected from dissection (Fig. 7-27B). Once the vessels are dissected free and mobilized sufficiently, a bolus of heparin (typically 100 units/kg) should be administered and circulated for 3 to 5 minutes

before proceeding. This dosage should be adjusted for coagulopathic patients. This usually raises activated clotting times (ACT), a rapid anticoagulation measurement, above 300 seconds, which, if possible, should be verified. The carotid artery is then distally ligated, proximal control is established, and a transverse arteriotomy is made. Fine prolene sutures are placed at the arteriotomy to prevent intimal dissection and

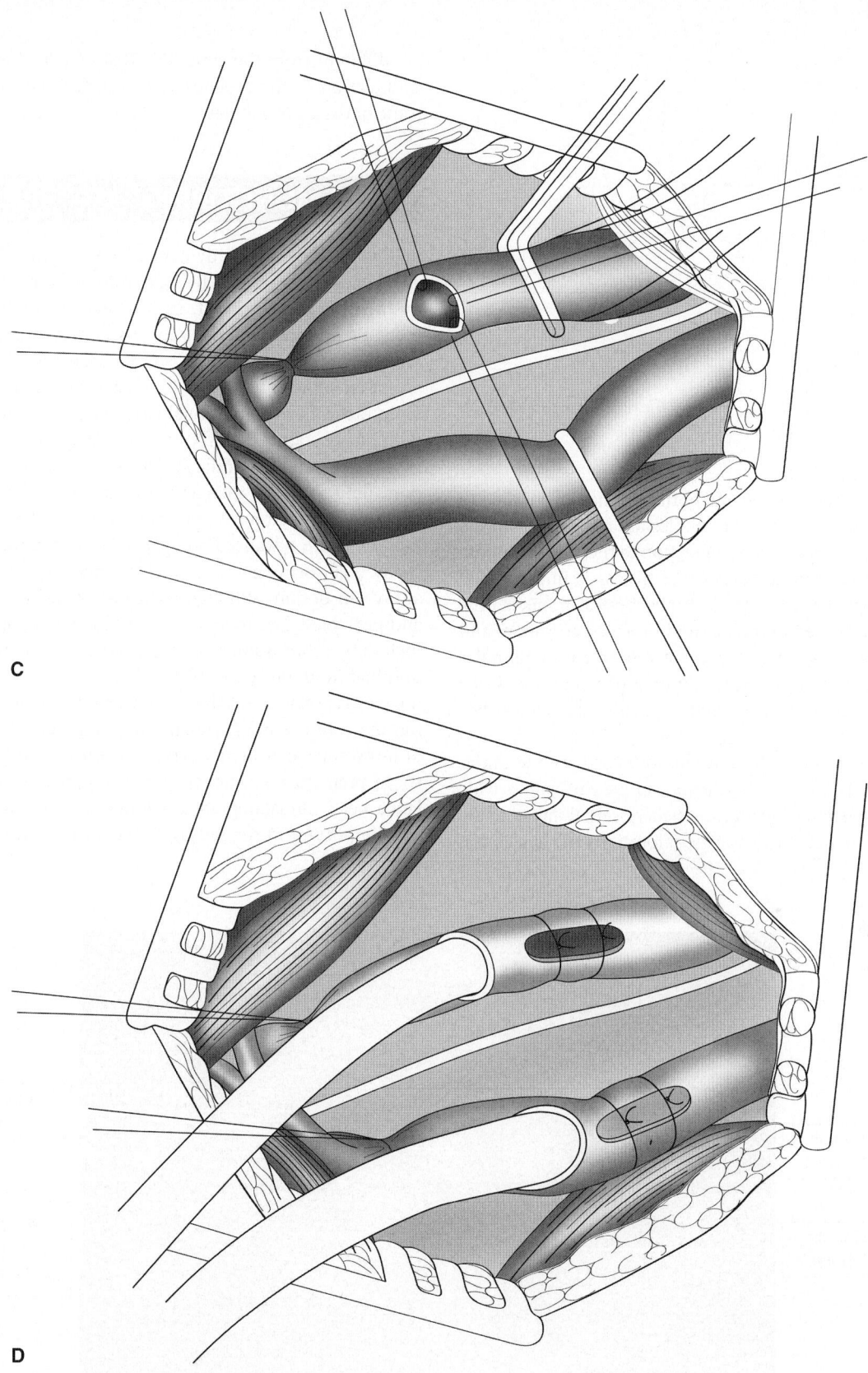

C

D

**FIGURE 7-27** *(Continued)* **C.** Carotid arteriotomy prepared for arterial cannulation. **D.** Arterial and venous cannulas secured within the vessels.

assist in retraction during cannulation (Fig. 7-27C) The arterial cannula is placed within the vessel at a predetermined distance (usually 2.5-3 cm in a neonate) and secured with 2 silk ligatures tied over a soft plastic bumper placed on the anterior surface of the vessel. The venous cannula is then placed in a similar fashion and secured at the 6- to 8-cm mark in a newborn (Fig. 7-27D). In the case of DLVV, the cannula should be placed such that the reinfusion orifice faces the tricuspid valve. This maneuver minimizes the recirculation of the blood within the right atrium. Once the ECMO circuit

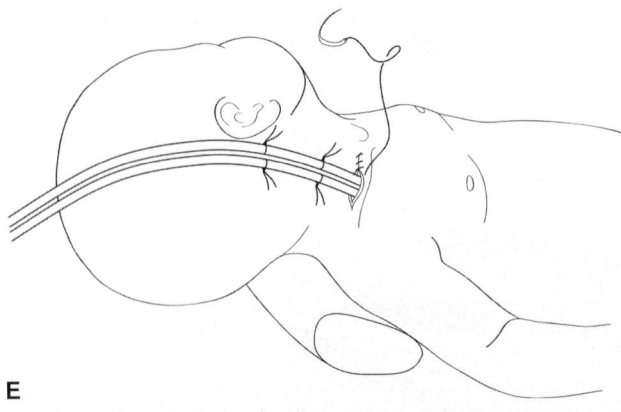

**E**

**FIGURE 7-27** *(Continued)* **E.** Closure of the neck incision and securing of the external ECMO tubing to the patient.

is prepared for cannulation and both cannulas are verified to be in proper position, the air bubbles are removed from the cannulas in preparation for connection to the ECMO circuit. After unclamping the cannulas, the bypass is initiated and support slowly advanced to goal over several minutes. The cannulas are secured to the mastoid process periosteum and scalp with heavy sutures to prevent movement of cannulas (Fig. 7-27E). The intrathoracic cannula positions should be confirmed with chest x-ray and transthoracic echocardiogram (Fig. 7-28).

Anatomic considerations must be addressed prior to initiation of cannulation. CDH patients can present with a wide variation of anatomical patterns. Their vessels, tethered to the intrathorcaic structures, may exist at locations and angles that are different from the expected. This may lead to abnormal cannulation of the azygous vein, which is an unacceptable route of drainage and new vascular access must be sought.

## ECMO MONITORING

ECMO physiology is dynamic, and at times unpredictable. Measures should be taken to prevent catastrophic dysfunction of the circuit, and to prepare for the management of multiple potential complications. Imaging studies are an inevitable part of ECMO management. Chest x-rays are often sufficient to verify the placement of the cannulas, endotracheal tube, additional vascular access catheters, and pulmonary status. Chest x-rays may need to be performed more frequently if significant changes to the ventilator support, fluid shifts, or changes in cannula position occur. Due to the difficulty in moving or repositioning of the patient on ECMO, more advanced studies, such as computed tomography (CT) or magnetic resonance imaging (MRI), are not always an option, although transport on ECMO is possible and portable CT scanners are available. Sonographic studies including echocardiograms are used to assess the intraabdominal fluid, position of cannulas, direction of the ECMO flow, and cardiac status throughout the run, assisting in steering the care toward successful decannulation. Elevated risk of intraventricular hemorrhage in neonates, and, even more so, in premature newborns often prompts frequent surveillance head ultrasonographic studies. This point is particularly important in the setting of therapeutic anticoagulation

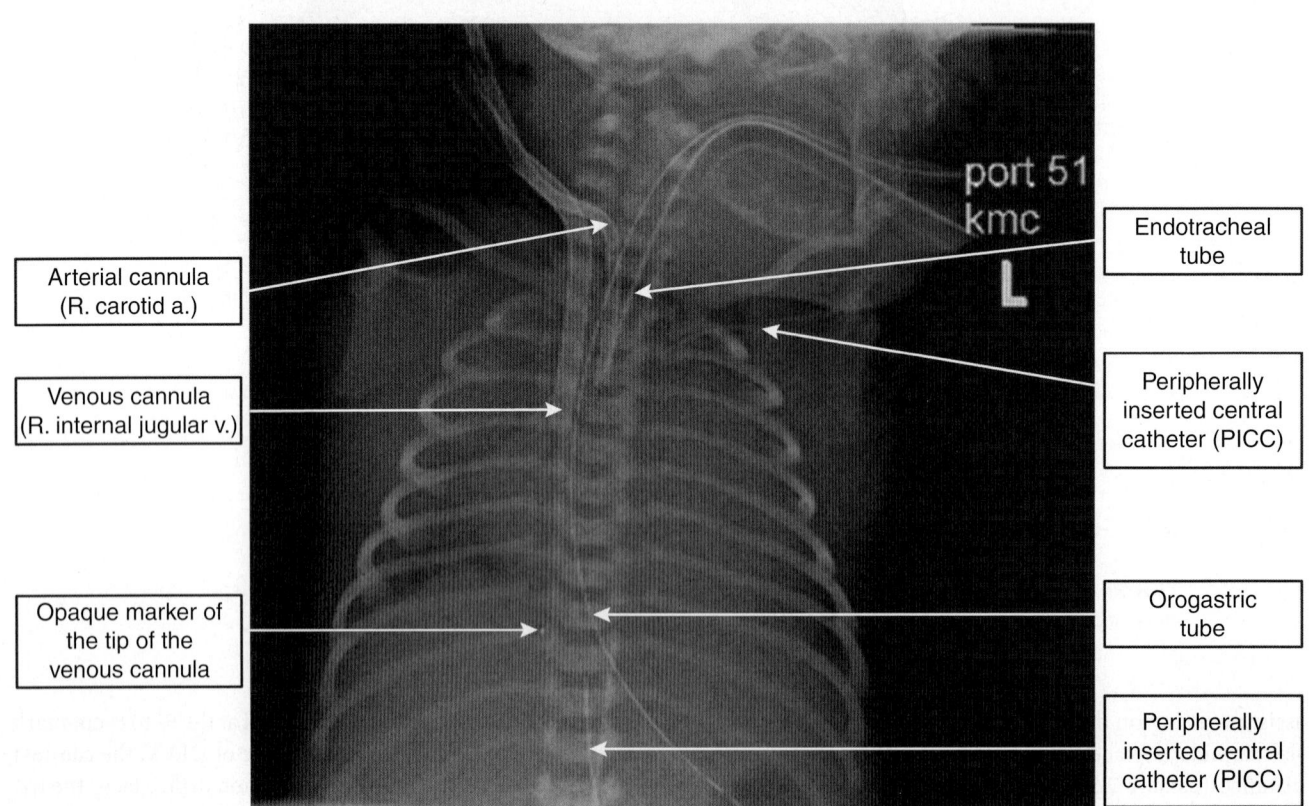

Arterial cannula (R. carotid a.)

Venous cannula (R. internal jugular v.)

Opaque marker of the tip of the venous cannula

Endotracheal tube

Peripherally inserted central catheter (PICC)

Orogastric tube

Peripherally inserted central catheter (PICC)

**FIGURE 7-28** Key landmarks after trans-cervical arteriovenous ECMO cannulation.

**GENERAL PRINCIPLES**

and relatively rapid platelet consumption that exists while on ECMO. Frequent blood sampling to assess the evolving coagulopathy, acid/base, electrolyte, and metabolic abnormalities allow careful management of these parameters. Electrolytes often require aggressive replacement to maintain normal physiologic concentrations despite an altered metabolism while on extracorporeal support. Since the patient on ECMO is anticoagulated with a continuous heparin infusion, careful monitoring of the coagulation pathways is essential using combinations of the quantitative and functional coagulation panels. Acid/base abnormalities are common in patients requiring ECMO. Once support is initiated, care must be taken to gently, but purposefully normalize the respiratory and metabolic abnormalities underlying the acid/base disturbances. One should be careful not to correct hypercapnea or acidosis too rapidly, due to their influence on cerebral perfusion and potential risks of ischemia or hemorrhage. By maintaining adequate organ perfusion, titrating the rates of gas exchange, re-establishing near-physiologic fluid status, and administering necessary medications, the clinician should be able to maintain a normal physiologic acid/base balance.

## NUTRITION ON ECMO

Patients on ECMO are often not candidates for enteral nutrition and must rely on parenteral feeding. Despite sedation and maintenance of some of the physiologic function by an external support device, the neonatal and pediatric patients are under significant catabolic stress. Their nutritional requirements may seem excessive, but careful adherence to the suggested guidelines is essential. Jaksic et al recently summarized these recommendations to include the following key points.

1. Neonates on ECMO require up to 3 mg/kg/day protein intake. This recommendation addresses the marked negative nitrogen balance on ECMO. Nevertheless, this recommendation must be carefully weighed against the existing or evolving hepatic and renal dysfunction.

2. Energy requirements in neonates on ECMO are similar to healthy neonates. Excess caloric intake may exacerbate the respiratory status.

3. Enteral feeding may benefit patients stable on ECMO. However, limited data call for additional caution in the neonatal population.

## ECMO COMPLICATIONS

While ECMO is a life-saving technology, it comes at a price of increased risks of a number of minor and devastating complications. Aggressive measures are routinely taken to minimize the risks and they merit a discussion.

## INTRACRANIAL HEMORRHAGE

The reported incidence of neurologic complications attributed to ECMO in children and infants ranges from approximately 10% to 17%. They contribute significantly to the overall morbidity of ECMO and must not be overlooked. Cranial imaging is recommended as a part of the precannulation workup to help determine the candidacy for ECMO. The risk of intracranial hemorrhage (ICH) is inversely proportional to the gestational age and neonates less than 34 weeks gestational age are at a particularly high risk. Prior to initiation of ECMO, critically ill neonates are often stressed by severe hypoxic injury, which has been linked to aberrant cerebral vasomotor regulation. In the setting of wide variation in cerebral perfusion secondary to the initiation of ECMO, administration of epinephrine, requirement for CPR, and massive fluid shifts, the risk of ischemic or hemorrhagic events is elevated. In an environment of therapeutic anticoagulation, ECMO patients are at an even higher risk of significant ICH. The incidence of ICH has been reported to up to 8% and was substantially higher in neonates and has been shown to significantly impact survival in ECMO patients. Neurologic surveillance in the ECMO population is challenging due to the frequent need for continuous sedation and the inability, in many cases, to move the head of the patient. Neuroimaging is a critical component of ECMO management and utilizes several modalities. Cranial ultrasounds can be performed in infants and are useful in assessing for intracranial hemorrhage while the fontanels are open. CT and MRI imaging can be performed in older children, but consideration has to be given to the risk of transporting these critically ill patients. This concern may be alleviated as portable imaging modalities are becoming more available. Imaging protocols differ among institutions and vary from daily, to imaging as dictated by clinical suspicion. One study found that nearly all instances of bleeding were seen in the first 5 days of ECMO initiation. This lead the authors to recommend surveillance imaging on "as needed" basis following that period.

In cases of VA ECMO, the flow through the right carotid artery is interrupted, as is the venous drainage via the internal jugular vein. The latter is thought to contribute to the risk of intracranial hemorrhage by increasing cerebral venous pressure, but convincing evidence for this is lacking. A number of short-term changes and long-term adaptations in cerebral circulation associated with the ligation of the carotid artery have been described, but the clinical significance of these is unclear. After discontinuation of VA ECMO, cerebral circulation is never restored to its original condition. Attempts to repair the carotid artery were thought to assist in restoring cerebral flow and avoiding potential neurological complications in the future. However, longer follow-up determined that this maneuver may be associated with significant vascular stenosis or occlusion. While these changes may not be linked to neurological defects, the benefit of the reconstruction remains doubtful.

## AIR EMBOLISM

The incidence of air in the circuit is variable and has been reported in nearly 5% of neonatal and pediatric respiratory ECMO patients. This potentially fatal complication can result from a number of maneuvers involved in the cannulation and routine maintenance of the circuit. Meticulous technique must be observed during the cannulation and decannulation to maintain a seal of the open vessels, particularly the veins. All air bubbles noted in the cannulas and tubing must be expunged. The patient should be paralyzed in order to prevent spontaneous respiration and generation of negative pressures within the venous system during the brief moments when the vessel is open. The ECMO circuit is repeatedly accessed throughout the run, primarily to collect blood and infuse medications. Each event must be accompanied by vigilant and careful monitoring for potential air entry into the system, especially at the negative pressure (prepump) segment of the circuit. If air entry is detected, the patient must be immediately isolated from the circuit flow and effort must be made to aspirate or recirculate the air to the venous side of the circuitry for expulsion via the membrane. If the air is noted to enter the patient's circulation, the circuit should be stopped and the patient placed in the Trendelenburg position to prevent entry into the cerebral circulation. Immediate identification and correction of the underlying cause of the occurrence of air in the circuit is vital to the successful return to ECMO.

## MEMBRANE DYSFUNCTION

Oxygenator membrane, the "lung" of the ECMO circuit is subject to continuous flow, and, therefore, to wear and tear. One of the most common causes of the failure of the membrane is the progressive formation of clot within the membrane, resulting in the inability to efficiently oxygenate and ventilate the passing blood. Accumulation of water condensation may also contribute to the failure, but is being addressed by the design alterations allowing appropriate drainage of vapor. Membrane failure is typically manifested by gradual increases in premembrane pressures, a corresponding transmembrane pressure gradient, along with increases in consumption of coagulation factors, fibrinogen, and platelets. On occasion, a clot can embolize from a proximal part of the circuit and cause an acute occlusion of the membrane. The associated abrupt cessation of ECMO support may require aggressive resuscitative efforts while the entire ECMO circuit, or the membrane, are prepared for replacement. Alternative designs of the ECMO circuitry allow the diversion of flow through an emergency shunt around the membrane to allow continued flow while the membrane is replaced.

## RACEWAY TUBING RUPTURE

This potentially devastating event results from the wear of the roller pump on the tubing and may lead to substantial bleeding and interruption of ECMO support. This complication has become exceedingly rare (<1% in neonatal and pediatric respiratory ECMO) with improvements in tubing materials. In addition, this technical consideration is not relevant in the centrifugal pump design circuits, since the flow is not generated via mechanical pressures exerted onto the circuit. In case of a raceway rupture, the circuit must be stopped to prevent further bleeding and new tubing has to be integrated into the circuit to resume ECMO support as rapidly as possible.

## ACCIDENTAL DECANNULATION AND CANNULATION SITE BLEEDING

One of the most dreaded complications of ECMO is the mechanical dislodgement of the cannulas from the vessels. Cannula positions should be routinely and meticulously tracked using external length measurements and radiographic imaging. Undue tension or tethering that may contribute to accidental decannulation should be eliminated. Efforts must be made to secure the cannulas at several points to the patient using sutures. If dislodgement occurs, the cannulation site is treated as an open wound, requiring temporary control with manual pressure and an emergent surgical exploration. The patient should be maintained using aggressive ventilator and cardiac resuscitation measures.

Cannulation site bleeding has been reported in up to 7% of neonates and over 16% of pediatric respiratory ECMO patients. This event is typically a result of the interaction of anticoagulated blood with a foreign surface. The bleeding is usually self-limiting, but should not be overlooked, as it may reflect a severe coagulopathy, or impending cannula dislodgement.

## LIMB ISCHEMIA

While cannulation using the common femoral artery has a benefit of preserving cerebral circulation, it exposes the patient to the development of critical limb ischemia and, potentially, limb loss. The occlusion of the distal flow by the ECMO catheter has been reported to occur in approximately half of the patients cannulated through the groin, but is thought to be underestimated as some patients do not survive long enough to develop ischemia. A recent study from Columbia University has not detected any significant patient or technical factors that may predict the development of ischemia. The use of distal perfusion catheters aimed to re-perfuse the threatened limb by directing a portion of the arterial return antegrade may provide relief to this situation (Fig. 7-29). However, while this technique appears to restore partial flow to the limb, it is not without complications. Cases of distal ischemia and compartment syndrome have been described and warrant caution. Nevertheless, the authors suggest that due to the lack of specific predictors, distal perfusion catheters in common femoral cannulation patients should be considered.

## INFECTION/SEPSIS

Infectious complications are a natural concern in ECMO patients, exposed to significant metabolic stress with indwelling intravascular catheters. ELSO registry data

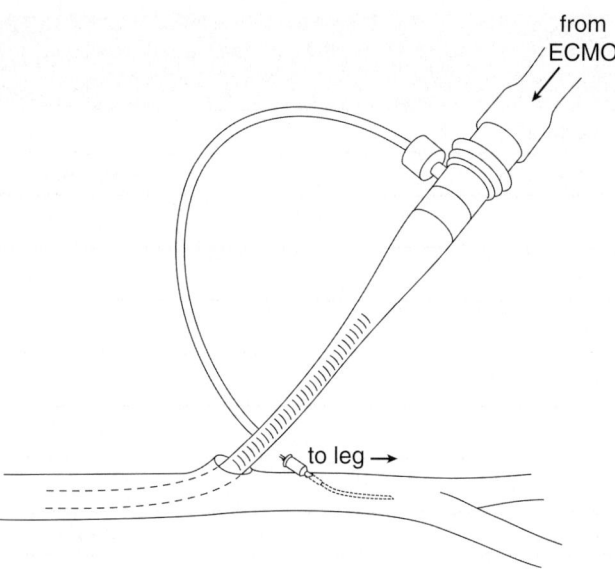

**FIGURE 7-29** Femoral artery cannulation with antegrade distal perfusion catheter.

report that 6% of neonates and more than 18% of pediatric patients on respiratory ECMO are diagnosed with infections, but other reports cite an almost 30% incidence (O'Neill, 2001). Search for the risk factors revealed that a prolonged course of ECMO is the greatest risk factor in the development of infection, although, naturally, there is some disagreement on the "safe" duration. Some reports advocate routine surveillance cultures after the 10-day mark of the ECMO run for early identification and treatment of infection. Similar duration has been recently demonstrated in the adult ECMO literature. Other risk factors include length of hospitalization and surgical procedures on ECMO. Cardiac ECMO patients appear to be at increased risk of infection than those requiring bypass for respiratory reasons. Well-tested antibiotic or care protocols, however, are lacking. It remains to be seen how the development of multidrug resistant infectious agents will affect the incidence and morbidity of ECMO population.

## RENAL FAILURE

Massive fluid shifts are a reality of ECMO and must be handled carefully to prevent significant fluid overload, while maintaining sufficient intravascular volume to sustain ECMO function. Renal perfusion is a key element of this process and is constantly changing with the fluid status and inflammation-mediated capillary leak. ECMO acts as a double-edged sword with respect to renal function, since it causes a reduction of pulsatile flow, while allowing relatively easy incorporation of renal replacement therapy. In addition, integration of hemofiltration devices into the ECMO circuit can allow for a dynamic removal of fluid and solutes without significantly affecting protein and cellular fractions. While fluid removal options are multiple, it is imperative to retain renal perfusion and near-physiologic urine output throughout the ECMO run. Askenazi et al recently determined that acute renal injury and need for renal replacement therapy independently predicted mortality in neonates and children on ECMO.

## ECMO CPR

Over the last several decades, the indications of ECMO have evolved to exclude certain patient groups, as their illnesses were deemed irreversible, obviating the long-term benefit of ECMO. On the other hand, this therapy has acquired other indications. A clear example is the apparent benefit of ECMO as a measure in CPR. Its utility in aiding the resuscitative efforts in patients with both respiratory and cardiac diseases has led to the recommendation of ECMO CPR (E-CPR) in cases of pediatric cardiac arrest due to reversible conditions, or those amenable to transplantation. While progressive, such recommendations are made in the setting of broad range of resources and practice protocols among different institutions. Due to the inherent urgency of E-CPR, the personnel involved must be readily aware of the needs and capabilities of this therapy. Recent data demonstrate that use of E-CPR in patients who failed conventional CPR measures resulted in survival of almost 40% of the patients. The authors outlined the potential groups that draw the greatest benefit from this therapy in pediatric cardiac patients and newborns with respiratory problems. Another consideration is the degree of clinical deterioration of the candidate patients, as the survival rates were substantially affected by the presence of severe metabolic acidosis. This potentially reflects the severity of the condition prior to and during CPR, as well as the incidence of serious neurological damage and other system dysfunction. The effectiveness of the administered CPR is critical to the survival of the E-CPR patient. Several considerations must be made prior to the entry of E-CPR into mainstream usage. First, the logistic and resource allocation parameters must be adjusted to ensure that a trained E-CPR team is committed and available. Diagnostic measures must be streamlined in order to rapidly recognize the patients who are candidates for E-CPR and allow prompt access to therapy. Finally, in addition to confirming the survival benefits of E-CPR, long-term outcomes must be closely examined, focusing specifically on the effect of the complications inherent to ECMO therapy, such as neurological deficits.

## ECMO BRIDGE TO TRANSPLANT

The role of ECMO as a bridge to transplant has undergone significant changes. While its utility in lung transplant patients is becoming more popular, it is an extremely useful modality in cardiac patients awaiting heart transplants. It has been generally understood that the greatest benefit of ECMO comes within the first 10 to 14 days, after which the mortality rates and the risk of complications rise sharply, disqualifying the patients from the transplant. Therefore, ECMO support as a bridge to transplant is considered a short-term modality. Recent emergence of miniaturized mechanical ventricular assist device (VAD) as a bridge to transplant in the pediatric population is currently under investigation, but the preliminary results indicate that ECMO may serve as a "bridge-to-bridge" technology for the VAD. Up to one third of patients studied received short-term ECMO support prior to transitioning to the VAD and its use was not associated with the overall mortality. Long-term results are yet to be examined, but it appears that ECMO continues to be useful in the patients awaiting cardiac transplants.

## ECMO OUTCOMES

The role of ECMO in the arsenal of neonatal and pediatric therapy is continuously evolving. Its use has risen with improvements in materials and better understanding of its benefits. On the other hand, improvements in medical therapy, such as the development of vasodilatory medications and improved techniques in ventilation, have obviated the need for ECMO in many patients. Better understanding of the risks and complications lead to more specific indications for ECMO. Survival outcomes for neonates and pediatric patients requiring respiratory and cardiac ECMO for the most common diagnoses, as listed in the ECLS Registry Report from January 2012 (Extracorporeal Life Support Organization International Summary) are listed in Table 7-11. Generally, the ideal candidate for ECMO has a high risk of mortality due to a reversible pulmonary or cardiac condition. Several other factors may come into consideration when evaluating the patient for ECMO. In a recent review of the ELSO registry, Zabrocki et al found that children 10 to 18 years old had a slightly, but significantly lower survival rate than younger patients (50% vs 55%-61%). Patients that required mechanical ventilation pre-ECMO longer than 14 days had a significantly lower survival (38%), compared to those on the ventilator for less than 2 weeks, although no differences in survival among ventilation strategies were identified. In addition to the duration of pre-ECMO ventilator support duration, patient age >10 years, cancer, renal failure, liver failure, and history of cardiac arrest all were predictors of mortality.

## SECOND COURSE ECMO

Re-institution of ECMO support may be technically challenging, but feasible in many cases. However, the benefits and the criteria for repeat ECMO are still unclear. Since the criteria for institution and the withdrawal of ECMO, specific endpoints, age, and weight criteria are not always well-defined, and practice varies among centers. Overall, up to 5% of the patients may undergo a second run of ECMO with short-term survival rates similar to single-run ECMO patients. It has been suggested that longer initial ECMO runs, renal failure, and age >3 years are negative prognostic factors for second course ECMO. However, in a recent publication, Bohuta et al cautioned against reinstitution of ECMO citing the significant decrease in survival after 1 year (15.4%) in second-run EMCO patients. Furthermore, the authors identified a substantially high rate of significant neurologic complications

| TABLE 7-11 | Survival Outcomes for Neonates and Pediatric Patients Requiring Respiratory and Cardiac ECMO |
|---|---|
| **Neonatal** | |
| **Respiratory** | **% Survival** |
| Overall | 75 |
| CDH | 51 |
| MAS | 94 |
| PPHN | 77 |
| RDS | 84 |
| Sepsis | 75 |
| **Cardiac** | **% Survival** |
| Overall | 39 |
| Congenital defect (0-30 days) | 38 |
| Congenital defect (31 days-1 year) | 45 |
| Pediatric | |
| **Respiratory** | **% Survival** |
| Overall | 56 |
| Viral pneumonia | 63 |
| Bacterial pneumonia | 58 |
| ARDS (Postop/trauma) | 59 |
| ARDS (non-Postop/trauma) | 52 |
| **Cardiac** | **% Survival** |
| Overall | 48 |
| Congenital defect (1-16 years) | 46 |

Data from *ECLS Registry Report International Summary. Extracorporeal Life Support Organization. January 2012. http://www.elsonet.org/.*

in the few survivals. The emotional toll of this action on the family must also be carefully considered.

## NEUROLOGIC SEQUELAE

Concern for future neurologic deficits after ECMO is significant. A number of defects have been reported, including transient auditory deficits (>25%), seizures (20%-70%), mild cerebral palsy (20%), to incapacitating cerebral palsy (5%). The rates of these complications are comparable to other critically ill patients not treated with ECMO. However, the rates of complications may differ among patient groups. Follow-up of cardiac ECMO patients has determined that greater than 25% of the patients develop significant neurodevelopmental deficits. Further research is necessary to determine which groups may be more susceptible to serious developmental complications and require additional surveillance. It is essential to realize that the neurologic deficits are, in large part, due to the severity of the underlying illness necessitating extracorporeal support, rather than the ECMO itself.

# GROWTH RESTRICTION

Up to one third of the neonates have feeding difficulties following ECMO. The problems may stem from the generalized neurological deficits, as well as the localized pain and discomfort at the cannula sites. Underlying mechanisms for these difficulties include uncoordinated suck and swallow, gastroesophageal reflux, slowed transit, and delayed gastric emptying. CDH patients are particularly prone to these challenges, due to underlying foregut dysmotility. Up to 50% of CDH patients require gastrostomy tubes for feeding and 42% require Nissen fundoplication following their ECMO course, exposing them to additional surgical interventions and complications. Persistent respiratory difficulties and feeding problems contribute to the higher incidence of growth restriction in these patients.

# RESPIRATORY SEQUELAE

Respiratory complications after ECMO are common and likely stem from the underlying pulmonary disease. Following ECMO, the children are more likely to require prolonged supplemental oxygen therapy (15% at 4 weeks) and develop serious pulmonary infections (25%). CDH patients may be even more susceptible to long-term pulmonary deficits, which most likely are a reflection of the severity of the underlying disease.

## SELECTED READINGS

### Conventional Monitoring and Cardiac Resuscitation

Bartlett RH. Critical Care Physiology. Boston: Little-Brown; 1995.

Kleinman M, Chameides L, Schexnayder SM, et al. Pediatric Advanced Life Support: 2010 American Heart Association Guidelines for Cardiopulmonary Resuscitation and Emergency Cardiovascular Care. Pediatrics 2010;126(5):e1361–e1399.

Cilley RE. Arterial access in infants and children. Semin Pediatr Surg 1992;1(3):174–180.

Hudson I, Houston A, Aitchison T, et al. Reproducibility of measurements of cardiac output in newborn infants by Doppler ultrasound. Arch Dis Child 1990;65(1 spec no):15–19.

Landers S, Moise AA, Fraley JK, et al. Factors associated with umbilical catheter-related sepsis in neonates. Am J Dis Child 1991;145(6):675–680.

Maar S. Searching for the holy grail: a review of markers of tissue perfusion in pediatric critical care. Pediatr Emerg Care 2008;24:883–887.

Pearson EG, Rollins MD, Vogler SA, et al. Decompressive laparotomy for abdominal compartment syndrome in children: before it is too late. J Pediatr Surg 2010;45(6):1324–1329.

Poets CF, Southall DP. Noninvasive monitoring of oxygenation in infants and children: practical considerations and areas of concern. Pediatrics 1994;93(5):737–746.

Tobias JD. Transcutaneous carbon dioxide monitoring in infants and children. Pediatr Anesth 2009;19:434–444.

Knirsch W, Kretschmar O, Tomaske M, et al. Cardiac output measurement in children: comparison of the ultrasound cardiac output monitor with thermodilution cardiac output measurement. Intensive Care Med 2008;34:1060–1064.

### Advanced Monitoring

Awad AA, Ghobashy MA, Stout RG, Silverman DG, Shelley KH. How does the plethysmogram derived from the pulse oximeter relate to arterial blood pressure in coronary artery bypass graft patients? Anesth Analg 2001;93:1466–1471.

Awad AA, Stout RG, Ghobashy M, et al. Analysis of the ear pulse oximeter waveform. J Clin Monit Comput 2006;20(3):175–184.

Lima A, Beelen P, Bakker J. Use of peripheral perfusion index derived from the pulse oximetry signal as a noninvasive indicator of perfusion. Crit Care Med 2002;30(6):1210–1213.

Keller G, Cassar E, Desebbe O, Lehot JJ, Cannesson M. Ability of pleth variability index to detect hemodynamic changes induced by passive leg raising in spontaneously breathing volunteers. Crit Care 2008;12(2):R37.

Cannesson M, Desebbe O, Rosamel P, et al. Pleth variability index to monitor the respiratory variations in the pulse oximeter plethysmographic waveform amplitude and predict fluid responsiveness in the operating theatre. Br J Anaesth 2008;101(8):200–206.

Wesseling K, Settels J, De Wit B. The measurement of continuous finger arterial pressure noninvasively in stationary subjects. In: Schmidt T, Dembrot T, Blumchen G, eds. Biological and Psychological Factors in Cardiovascular Disease. Springer-Verlag: Berlin; 1986:335–376.

Leonetti P, Audat F, Girard A, Laude D, Lefrère F, Elghozi J. Stroke volume monitored by modeling flow from finger arterial pressure waves mirrors blood volume withdrawn by phlebotomy. Clin Auton Res 2004;14(3):176–181.

Scalea TM, Holman M, Fuortes M, et al. Central venous blood oxygen saturation: an early, accurate measurement of volume during hemorrhage. J Trauma 1988;28(6):725–732.

Grudic G, Mulligan J. Outdoor path labeling using polynomial mahalanobis distance. In: Robotics: Science and Systems Conference, 2006.

Soller BR, Yang Y, Soyemi OO, et al. Noninvasively determined muscle oxygen saturation is an early indicator of central hypovolemia in humans. J Appl Physiol 2007;104:475–481.

### Pharmacology

Anand KJ, Wilson DF, Berger J, et al. Tolerance and withdrawal from prolonged opioid use in critically ill children. Pediatrics 2010;125:e1208–1225.

Devlin JW, Roberts RJ. Pharmacology of commonly used analgesics and sedatives in the ICU: benzodiazepines, propofol, and opioids. Crit Care Clin 2009;25:431–449.

Goldenberd NA, Bernard TJ. Venous thromboembolism in children. Hematol Oncol Clin N Am 2010;24:151–166.

Reveiz L, Guerrero-Lozano R, Camacho A, et al. Stress ulcer, gastritis and gastrointestinal bleeding prophylaxis in critically ill children: a systematic review. Pediatr Crit Care 2010;11:124–132.

Scaglione F, Paraboni L. Pharmacokinetics/pharmacodynamics of antibacterials in the intensive care unit: setting appropriate dosing regimens. Int J Antimicrob Agents 2008;32(4):294–301.

The SAFE Study Investigators. A Comparison of albumin and saline for fluid resuscitation in the intensive care unit. N Engl J Med 2004;350:2247–2256.

Zagli G, Tarantini F, Bonizzoli M, et al. Altered pharmacology in the intensive care unit patient. Fundament Clin Pharmacol 2008;22:493–501.

### Respiratory Failure and ECMO

Askenazi DJ, Ambalavanan N, Hamilton K, et al. Acute kidney injury and renal replacement therapy independently predict mortality in neonatal and pediatric noncardiac patients on extracorporeal membrane oxygenation. Pediatr Crit Care Med 2011;12:e1–6.

Brown KL, Goldman AP. Neonatal extra-corporeal life support: indications and limitations. Early Hum Dev 2008;84:143–148.

Corbet A. Clinical trials of synthetic surfactant in the respiratory distress syndrome of premature infants. Clin Perinatol 1993;20:737–760.

Gerstmann DR, Minton SD, Stoddard RA, et al. The Provo multicenter early high-frequency oscillatory ventilation trial: improved pulmonary and clinical outcome in respiratory distress syndrome. Pediatrics 1996;98:1044–1057.

HIFI Study Group. High-frequency oscillatory ventilation compared with conventional mechanical ventilation in the treatment of respiratory failure in preterm infants. N Engl J Med 1989;320:88.

Jobe A. Pulmonary surfactant therapy. *N Engl J Med* 1993;328:861–868.

Kinsella JP, Truog WE, Walsh WF, et al. Randomized multicenter trial of inhaled nitric oxide and high-frequency oscillatory ventilation in severe, persistent pulmonary hypertension of the newborn. *Pediatrics* 1997;131:55–62.

Kugelman A, Durand M. A comprehensive approach to the prevention of bronchopulmonary dysplasia. *Pediatr Pulmonol* 2011;46:1153–1165.

Mori R, Kusuda S, Fujimura M. Antenatal corticosteroids promote survival of extremely preterm infants born at 22 to 23 weeks of gestation. *J Pediatr* 2011;159:110–114e1.

Roberts JD, Polaner DM, Lang P, et al. Inhaled nitric oxide in persistent pulmonary hypertension of the newborn. *Lancet* 1992;340:818.

Stayer SA, Liu Y. Pulmonary hypertension of the newborn. *Best Pract Res Clin Anaesthesiol* 2010;24:375–386.

Wirbelauer J, Speer CP. The role of surfactant treatment in preterm infants and term newborns with acute respiratory distress syndrome. *J Perinatol* 2009;29(Suppl 2):S18–S22.

Zabrocki LA, Brogan TV, Statler KD, Poss WB, Rollins MD, Bratton SL. Extracorporeal membrane oxygenation for pediatric respiratory failure: survival and predictors of mortality. *Crit Care Med* 2011;39:364–370.

# CHAPTER 8

# Nutritional Supplementation in Pediatric Surgery

*Walter J. Chwals*

## KEY POINTS

1. Although optimal growth of the neonate can be insured with a caloric intake from 100 to 150 kcal/kg/D, during acute metabolic stress (injury) states, characterized by increased C-reactive protein and decreased prealbumin serum concentrations, daily energy repletion should be based on either measured energy expenditure values or basal metabolic rate.

2. The metabolic rate increases 10% to 13% per degree centigrade elevation and 7.2% per degree Fahrenheit elevation.

3. The nutritional caloric regimen for the metabolic impact of acute injury in infants does not require the replacement of calories allotted for growth.

4. Glycemic control during the resuscitative and stabilization phase of acute illness may provide a favorable impact on patient morbidity and mortality.

5. Indirect calorimetry is a useful energy assessment tool. During critical illness, changes in daily energy repletion are dependent on the magnitude and duration of the acute metabolic stress response, but do *not* include energy required for growth, insensible losses, or activity.

6. Both enteral and parenteral nutrition are effective in reducing the hypermetabolic response to injury as well as reducing protein catabolism.

## OVERVIEW

Optimal nutritional therapy is an essential requirement in the postoperative care of pediatric surgical patients, especially infants and children in the intensive care setting. Growth velocity during early infancy is higher than at any other time during childhood and is exceeded only by intrauterine growth rates. Daily energy needs range from 100 kcal/kg/day in term infants to 150 kcal/kg/day in very premature babies. Although these energy needs decrease in older children, growth and activity requirements still exceed those of normal adults. In the surgical population, particularly in critically ill patients, metabolic status is significantly altered. Perioperative acute tissue injury markedly *reduces* these energy needs, due to the injury-related induction of catabolic metabolism (which inhibits growth), sedation (which inhibits activity), and environmental temperature control (which reduces insensible heat loss). In concert, these factors result in a substantial *decrease* in energy needs, especially in the mechanically ventilated child. To account for these alterations in energy metabolism, caloric amounts equal to measured energy expenditure (MEE) values or basal energy requirements should be provided to prevent overfeeding (ie, the provision of calories and/or nutritional substrates in excess of the energy required to maintain the metabolic homeostasis). Overfeeding can create or prolong the requirement for mechanical ventilation (increased ventilatory workload), impair liver function (induced hepatic steatosis and cholestasis), and increase injury-induced hyperglycemia (increased risk of infection). Nutritional assessment of critically ill pediatric patients can be quantitatively accomplished by measuring the visceral protein pool (ie, serum C-reactive protein [CRP]), the acute-phase protein pool (ie, serum prealbumin), and energy expenditure. Serum prealbumin levels decrease and CRP levels increase with a magnitude and duration proportional to injury severity, and the values return to normal as the acute injury response resolves. Serum CRP concentrations have been shown to correlate well with MEE; however, predictive equations for energy expenditure are inaccurate. A substantial percent of preterm infants are dependent on total parenteral nutrition (TPN) to prevent hypoglycemia and provide a sufficient energy intake due to inadequate bowel absorptive function. However, diminished tolerance for parenteral glucose delivered at high rates frequently provokes hyperglycemia in this patient population. Hyperglycemia is further increased in the presence of infection, which impairs hepatic glucose uptake and enhances insulin resistance. Hyperglycemia can cause immunocompromise and is associated with an increased risk of infection-related morbidity and increased mortality in both adult and pediatric intensive care populations. To avoid overfeeding during acute injury states, critically ill infant and pediatric patients should be administered basal energy requirements until serial serum CRP concentrations decrease in association with *increasing* serum prealbumin concentrations, at which time caloric intake can be safely advanced. While enteral nutritional delivery is generally preferred, parenteral nutrition is often necessary due to intestinal dysfunction.

## ENERGY REQUIREMENTS

The assessment of energy expenditure has been widely used to characterize alterations in metabolism and to determine daily caloric requirements accompanying a variety of clinical states in both health and disease. Energy can be partitioned into (1) maintenance metabolic needs (BMR, activity, and heat loss to the environment) and (2) energy required for growth. Energy requirements are age-related and are 3 to 4 times higher for infants than for adults.

In healthy, term babies, the BMR is about 40 to 45 kcal/kg/day in the neonate, increases to about 60 kcal/kg/day by approximately the fourth to fifth month of life, and then gradually declines to about 20 to 25 kcal/kg/day during adolescence, largely due to a relative decrease in the growth of parenchymal organs with high oxygen consumption rates (brain, liver, kidney, and heart) and an increase in muscle mass (with relatively low oxygen consumption) and fat. Total daily energy requirements for healthy, uninjured children decrease progressively with age, from 90 to 120 kcal/kg/day (with 2.5-4 g/kg/day protein) during the first year of life gradually down to 30 to 60 kcal/kg/day (with 1.5 g/kg/day protein) during the adolescent and teenage years. However, estimates of energy requirements in the postsurgical setting are often unreliable, especially in critically ill pediatric patients, due to a high degree of interpatient variability. An accurate measure of energy expenditure can provide information necessary for appropriate nutritional repletion, including the type and amount of macronutrient substrates needed. In disease states, especially during critical illness, these considerations may substantially aid in improving mortality and morbidity outcomes following acute injury states, particularly by allowing for crucial metabolic resuscitation while avoiding the administration of calories in great excess of actual energy requirements. While a variety of assessment techniques have been described, indirect calorimetry is the method most frequently employed. Indirect calorimetry can be carried out at the patient's bedside using a metabolic cart to measure energy expenditure on the basis of oxygen consumption and carbon dioxide production. If indirect calorimetry is unavailable, BMR values should be used as a guide for daily caloric administration until the acute injury response resolves (see Nutritional Assessment and Resuscitation in the Postinjury Setting below).

## PROTEIN REQUIREMENTS

Growth can be expressed in terms of protein accretion, which is the amount of protein generated as new tissue. Nitrogen accounts for approximately 2% of total body weight at birth in contrast to just about 3% in the adult. Most of this difference is made up in the first year of life because of rapid somatic growth. During this first year, the infant' body length and body weight increase by 2-fold and 3-fold, respectively. Parenchymal growth is particularly accelerated during this period. For instance, the brain mass grows to 60% of its normal adult size during the first year of life. However, energy needs to take metabolic precedence, so that protein will be preferentially used as an energy source (even if protein delivery is low) if nonprotein substrate delivery is inadequate to meet energy needs.

In the healthy infant, protein as a function of body weight is highest in the neonate (0.93 g/kg/day) and decreases progressively from that point. Protein accretion is 0.5 g/kg/day during the second and third months of life, 0.26 g/kg/day during the fifth and sixth months of life, 0.18 g/kg/day from 9 to 12 months of age, and 0.08 g/kg/day between 2 and 3 years of age. Protein accretion is dependent on the amount of protein actually absorbed (metabolizable protein), the efficiency of conversion of various dietary proteins into tissue protein (estimated at 90% for breast milk but only 70% for soy protein found in infant formulae), and the protein lost during breakdown.

Protein lost because of incomplete enteral absorption and breakdown can be estimated by measuring stool, urine, and skin nitrogen content and the loss is calculated to be approximately 0.95 g/kg/day of protein during the first year of life. Taking these factors into account and allowing for the interpatient variability, the estimated enteral protein requirement is approximately 2.6 g/kg/day during the neonatal period, 2 g/kg/day at 2 to 3 months of age, and 1.3 g/kg/day at 1 year of life. Values may be somewhat less for parenteral delivery because of decreased absorptive losses.

In the premature or small-for-gestational-age (SGA) child, protein needs are proportionately higher (ranging to 3.5 g/kg/day) owing to substantially increased urinary nitrogen losses and increased catch-up growth requirements (~20% higher than the 3 g/kg/day needed to support intrauterine growth rates).

During the acute injury period in children (see Acute Metabolic Stress Response below), it is particularly important to meet daily protein requirements. Current recommendations include 3 to 4 g/kg/day in neonates, 2.5 to 3 g/kg/day in infants, 2 g/kg/day in children and adolescents, and 1.5 g/kg/day in teenagers. Early adequate protein administration increases synthetic rates in tissue with rapid turnover (eg, bone marrow, intestinal endothelium, etc) and promotes endogenous protein sparing during the injury-induced catabolic phase.

## NONPROTEIN CALORIC REQUIREMENTS

Most infant formulas provide a relatively balanced delivery of nonprotein calories, in the range of 45% of total calorie intake each for carbohydrate and fat. In the postnatal period, infant metabolism is characterized by a greater dependence on lipid substrate in addition to carbohydrate substrate for energy needs. There is substantial evidence that premature infants, because of impaired fat absorption by immature gut, may benefit from increased concentrations of medium-chain triglycerides (MCTs) in enteral formulas. Carbohydrates remain important as a source of energy for children and are optimally provided in the form of starches, such as those found in cereals. Generally, standard balanced dietary distribution recommendations include 15% protein, 35% fat, and 50% carbohydrate caloric intake daily.

## FACTORS MODIFYING ENERGY METABOLISM AND ENERGY REQUIREMENTS

Factors known to influence metabolic demand include age, gender, the type, amount, and route of macronutrient substrate administration, ambient temperature, body temperature, activity level, and acute metabolic stress. The metabolic rate increases in direct proportion to endogenous (body) temperature. The metabolic rate is dependent on body temperature and has been shown to increase 10% to 13% for each degree centigrade (or 7.2% for each degree Fahrenheit) of body temperature elevation. Tissue injury elicits an acute metabolic stress response, which can have complex and profound effects on energy requirements in children, particularly during infancy. The consideration of critically ill subjects introduces additional variables that include the effects of disease type (ie, trauma vs sepsis) and severity (magnitude and duration) on the extent of the inflammatory response. In addition, the ability of the host to respond to the metabolic injury challenge is effected by conditions that deplete the endogenous metabolic substrate reserve (eg, malnutrition, cancer cachexia, etc) and, thus, further alters energy expenditure. In order to understand how this occurs, the mechanisms of the response, how energy metabolism is affected, how this condition predisposes to excess caloric delivery in critically ill infants, and how to avoid overfeeding are discussed below.

## ACUTE METABOLIC STRESS RESPONSE

In response to a variety of local or systemic injury stimuli (such as trauma, sepsis, and acute inflammatory conditions), a series of metabolic changes occur that characterize the acute injury response state. Among the early features of the injury response is the release of cytokines, followed rapidly by important alterations in the hormonal environment. Increased counter-regulatory hormone concentrations are associated with insulin and growth hormone resistance. As a result of this response, a sequence of metabolic events is initiated that includes the catabolism of endogenous stores of protein, carbohydrate, and fat to provide essential substrate intermediates and energy necessary to fuel the ongoing response process. Amino acids from catabolized proteins flow to the liver, where they provide substrate for the synthesis of acute-phase proteins and glucose (gluconeogenesis). Therefore, the acute metabolic stress response to injury represents a hypermetabolic, hypercatabolic state that results in the loss of endogenous tissue. Growth, which is an anabolic process, is inhibited during periods of acute metabolic stress.

As the acute metabolic stress response resolves, adaptive anabolic metabolism ensues to restore catabolic losses. In children, this phase is characterized by the resumption of somatic growth.

Insulin is a potent anabolic hormone responsible for glycogen synthesis and the storage of carbohydrate, lipogenesis and the storage of fat, and new protein synthesis. Insulin and insulin-like growth factor 1 (IGF-1) are essential hormones for somatic growth in infants and children. Acute metabolic stress is characterized by substantial increases in serum concentrations of catecholamines, glucagon, and cortisol, which are referred to as counterregulatory hormones because they oppose the anabolic effects of insulin. Serum concentrations of these metabolic stress-related hormones increase as a result of cytokine release.

The predominant effect of counterregulatory hormones is to mediate the catabolism of endogenous macromolecular reserves as part of the acute metabolic stress (inflammatory) response to injury. Glucagon induces glycolysis and gluconeogenesis, resulting in increased serum lactate and alanine concentrations and, thus, provides the substrate necessary for the endogenous regeneration of glucose (the Cori cycle and alanine cycle). These cycles are major contributors to altered carbohydrate metabolism during acute metabolic stress. Cortisol induces muscle proteolysis and promotes gluconeogenesis. Glucocorticoids cause the muscle proteolysis associated with cytokine release, and they have been shown to be a predictor of protein breakdown and hypermetabolism in acutely stressed adults. The major amino acid sources for gluconeogenesis are alanine and glutamine from skeletal muscle and gut, respectively. Hepatic uptake of these amino acids is accelerated during acute metabolic stress. Catecholamines cause hyperglycemia by promoting hepatic glycogenolysis, by causing conversions of skeletal muscle glycogen to lactate (which is then transported to the liver for conversion to glucose through the Cori cycle), and by suppressing the pancreatic secretion of insulin. Catecholamines also induce lipolysis, which results in the mobilization of free fatty acids. Finally, catecholamines, in addition to glucagon and cortisol, induce hypermetabolism, which is associated with an increase in the BMR.

Surgical trauma per se may not produce a particularly severe injury insult. In general, the predominant metabolic stress (injury) insult associated with operative procedures in children derives from the underlying disease process that necessitates the operation rather than the procedure itself.

## ANABOLIC HORMONE RESISTANCE DURING ACUTE METABOLIC STRESS

Insulin and growth hormone act to promote somatic growth. During acute metabolic stress states, in response to tissue injury (eg, sepsis, inflammation, and trauma), these anabolic functions are inhibited by counterregulatory hormones to facilitate catabolism (anabolic hormone resistance). Insulin resistance is characterized by increased glucose production, lipolysis, fatty acid oxidation, and proteolysis as well as decreased glucose uptake and storage despite high serum glucose, amino acid, and insulin concentrations. Acute injury states, therefore, are typically associated with high serum glucose concentrations (hyperglycemia) in direct proportion to the magnitude and duration of the injury insult. Randomized prospective evaluation of the use of insulin to reduce injury-induced hyperglycemia have demonstrated decreased morbidity and mortality in critically ill adults in the absence of excess caloric delivery, likely due to decreased hyperglycemia-induced immunosuppression. Because insulin is known to promote protein anabolism, primarily by decreasing proteolysis, the protein breakdown observed in acute metabolic stress states has been ascribed to insulin resistance.

In health, the major actions of growth hormone are to decrease protein catabolism and promote protein synthesis, to promote fat mobilization and the conversion of free fatty acids to acetyl coenzyme A, and to decrease glucose oxidation while increasing glycogen deposition. However, the anabolic effects of growth hormone, particularly as they relate to protein metabolism, are mediated principally by IGF-1. During acute metabolic stress, IGF-1 concentrations decrease and IGF-1 inhibitory binding protein concentrations increase. In this state, the substrate-mobilizing effects of growth hormone prevail and result in increased lipolysis and free fatty acid oxidation. However, there is relative growth hormone resistance as the anabolic effects mediated by IGF-1 are inhibited due to the actions of counterregulatory hormones.

## OVERFEEDING

Overfeeding occurs when the administration of calories or specific substrate exceeds the requirements to maintain metabolic homeostasis. These requirements, which vary according to the patient's age, state of health, and underlying nutritional status, are substantially altered during periods of injury-induced acute metabolic stress. Excess nutritional delivery during this period can further increase the metabolic demands of an acute injury and place an added burden on the lungs and liver. The result is not only to exacerbate pulmonary and hepatic pathophysiologic processes, but also to increase the risk of mortality. Stress metabolism cannot be reversed by overfeeding during critical illness. Instead, overfeeding further increases the negative impact of metabolic stress by increasing hyperglycemia-associated risks associated with it and by augmenting the pulmonary and hepatic workload. Excess caloric delivery has been shown to increase injury-associated morbidity and mortality in both animal and human investigations. Younger pediatric patients are particularly vulnerable in this regard. It is important, therefore, to ensure that calorie intake does not exceed demand during the period of acute metabolic response in critically ill infants and children.

Excess caloric delivery, particularly excess carbohydrate administration, causes lipogenesis. Lipogenesis is the biosynthesis of fat from excess carbohydrate and results in increased carbon dioxide production. Glucose administered in excess of maximum oxidation rates undergoes fat biosynthesis (lipogenesis), resulting in substantial increases in carbon dioxide production. Since fatty acid oxidation is the predominant energy-generating pathway during the acute injury response, excess lipid administration also promotes lipogenesis by reducing carbohydrate oxidation. Pulmonary functional compromise results from the increased work of breathing due to excess carbon dioxide production. This effect is harmful in critically ill postoperative children and can induce or prolong the requirement for mechanical ventilation and intensive care length of stay. Preterm infants are especially vulnerable to the respiratory effects of overfeeding because of their immature pulmonary development and limited respiratory reserve. Furthermore, excess protein delivery has been shown to increase respiratory sensitivity to carbon dioxide.

Overfeeding also negatively affects hepatic morphology and function. Acute metabolic stress increases lipolysis and free fatty acid oxidation relative to glucose oxidation, owing to counterregulatory hormone-induced insulin resistance. These endocrine effects reduce the efficiency with which exogenous carbohydrate is metabolized. With excessive carbohydrate delivery, serum insulin, glucose, glucose oxidation, and fatty acid oxidation increase, and lipogenesis remains high. These metabolic events increase the hepatic workload and further predispose the liver to hepatic cellular injury, resulting in hepatic dysfunction. Lipid overfeeding with long-chain triglyceride (LCT) formulations can inhibit the ability of the reticuloendothelial system of the liver to clear bacteria during acute injury states. Decreased hepatic bacterial clearance is associated with increased bacterial sequestration in the lung, resulting in increased pulmonary neutrophil activation and the release of inflammatory mediators. Enteral replacement of LCT with MCT, which is absorbed directly into the blood from the gut, preserves liver reticuloendothelial system function and reduces lung bacterial sequestration. Parenteral lipid overfeeding heightens risk of induced hepatic dysfunction because standard lipid emulsions (eg, intralipid) contain high concentrations of linoleic acid, a omega-6 fatty acid and arachidonic acid precursor that selectively stimulates the synthetic pathways of prostaglandins with high inflammatory activity, thus, increasing inflammatory changes (steatosis, cholestasis, and fibrosis) within the liver parenchyma. In contrast, the use of lipid emulsions with omega-3 fatty acid (fish oil), which stimulates arachidonic acid pathways with lesser inflammatory activity, has been suggested as a strategy to improve or reverse parenteral nutrition associated liver disease (PNALD). This strategy may be particularly important in critically ill infants and children requiring long-term parenteral nutrition (eg, with necrotizing enterocolitis, gastroschisis, short gut syndrome, etc). In these patient populations especially, the use of intralipid should not exceed 1 g/kg/day. Furthermore, the administration of even minimal amounts of enteral feedings can stimulate intestinal trophic hormone secretion, thus reducing the inflammatory effects of bacterial translocation and decreasing PNALD.

Another negative effect of overfeeding is the exacerbation of injury-induced hyperglycemia. As discussed previously, the response to acute injury can itself result in hyperglycemia. Tissue injury results in the increased secretion of cytokines followed by counterregulatory hormones and growth hormone. Cytokine-induced counterregulatory hormones increase hepatic glucose production (glycogenolysis due primarily to epinephrine and glucagon) and decrease peripheral glucose uptake (primarily due to insulin resistance). Growth hormone increases peripheral lipolysis and fatty acid oxygenation, which amplifies hyperglycemia by decreasing the necessity for serum glucose utilization as an energy fuel. Thus, the degree of stress-related hyperglycemia is directly related to the magnitude of the acute injury insult and the availability of substrate that can be mobilized.

Progressively severe immunosuppression, as well as an array of toxic cellular effects, is known to be associated with increasing hyperglycemia. Deficiencies in white blood cell activation and function, including impaired granulocyte adhesion, chemotaxis and phagocytosis, decreased respiratory burst, and impaired intracellular killing, as well as decreased immunoglobulin function and complement fixation, have all been demonstrated in vitro in direct association with hyperglycemia and have been shown to improve with glucose control. Functional leukocyte abnormalities have been associated with sustained blood glucose levels greater than 120 mg/dL and become more severe as serum levels increase.

Hyperglycemia can also result from excess caloric delivery from either parenteral or enteral routes. Parenteral nutrition is more typically associated with overfeeding-related hyperglycemia, in part due to the absence of natural physiologic mechanisms such as ileus and malabsorption resulting in vomiting and diarrhea, which can help to protect the body against excessive caloric nutrition administered enterally. Overfeeding can be particularly harmful in critically ill patients during acute injury (catabolic) states where, in contrast to anabolic states, excess calories cannot be effectively stored in glycogen, adipose tissue, and muscle. Thus, excess caloric delivery in this patient population can further increase injury-related hyperglycemia.

Numerous studies have associated hyperglycemia with increased mortality and morbidity in critically ill adult and pediatric patient populations. Furthermore, studies in adult and pediatric intensive care populations using insulin therapy have demonstrated significantly improved mortality and morbidity associated with tight glycemic control (blood glucose, 80-110 mg/dL). This therapy has also resulted in a higher rate of transient hypoglycemia, substantially greater in enterally versus parenterally fed patients. Therapeutic glycemic target adjustment (<150 vs <110 mg/dL), more accurate monitoring (point-of-care), parenteral nutrition, and appropriately applied algorithms have been shown to reduce insulin-induced hypoglycemia.

## NUTRITIONAL ASSESSMENT AND RESUSCITATION IN THE POSTINJURY SETTING

Alterations in the energy requirement of pediatric patients in response to an acute metabolic stress can be dramatic. Growth velocity during early infancy is higher than at any other time during childhood and is exceeded only by intrauterine growth rates. These additional growth requirements must be met by age and weight-appropriate increases in protein-calorie delivery in the metabolically unstressed (anabolic) pediatric patient.

However, acute injury markedly alters energy needs. First, acute injury induces a catabolic response that is proportional to the magnitude, nature, and duration of the injury. Increased serum counterregulatory hormone concentrations induce insulin and growth hormone resistance. This results in the catabolism of endogenous stores of protein, carbohydrate, and fat to provide essential substrate intermediates and energy necessary to support the metabolic stress response. Approximately 30% to 35% of predicted energy requirements for healthy infants are needed for growth. These requirements diminish during childhood to approximately 10% for adolescents, finally approaching normal adult maintenance requirements in the late teenage period. Growth-related requirements are inversely proportional to gestational age and approach 50% in very low birth weight babies. During the injury-induced catabolic response period, however, somatic growth cannot occur. Therefore, the caloric allotment for growth, which is substantial during infancy and early childhood, should *not* be administered. Second, children treated in the intensive care setting are frequently sedated, and their activity level is markedly reduced, further lowering energy needs. Third, the intensive care environment is temperature-controlled and insensible energy losses are substantially reduced. This is especially true for children who are mechanically ventilated because, in addition to reduced energy needs for the work of breathing, these patients are ventilated with heated, humidified air. This practice alone can reduce insensible losses by one third. In concert, these factors result in substantial decreases in energy needs. Although increments in energy expenditure associated with the magnitude and duration of injury response per se have been documented, these positive values are substantially less than the reduction in daily needs due to inhibited growth, decreased activity, and decreased insensible heat losses. Therefore, if calorie repletion based on the predicted requirements for healthy infants and children is administered during the acute phase of metabolic stress in critically ill infants, clinically significant overfeeding is likely.

To account for these alterations in energy metabolism, caloric amounts equal to MEE values or basal energy requirements should be provided. The significance of this therapeutic strategy is to avoid the provision of calories and/or nutritional substrates in excess of the energy required to maintain the metabolic homeostasis of the injury response. Gender-based basal energy expenditure data are available in the publications of Fritz Talbot and/or Schofield for infants and children up to 18 years of age.

The value of indirect calorimetry in the intensive care setting lies in the fact that estimations of energy expenditure based on equations derived from other clinical criteria are notoriously inaccurate. Although average MEE values in large series of patients tend to differentiate various degrees of injury, individual subjects can respond to similar injury states with widely diverse MEE values. The actual MEE is frequently much less than predicted values based on the clinical grounds. For this reason, predictive equations, even those specifically derived from pediatric populations, are significantly inaccurate (in approximately 75% of critically ill children) and most frequently overestimate the daily energy expenditure leading to excess caloric administration, especially if an arbitrary incremental amount is added to account for metabolic stress. During the course of the metabolic stress response, energy expenditure may change substantially in response to alterations in the injury insult (magnitude, duration, second injury insult, etc). For this reason, it is important to measure energy needs daily during the acute injury response period. Measurements can be carried out at bedside within 30 minutes or less, dependent on patient stability.

Infant energy expenditure after complication-free surgical procedures does not increase substantially above measured baseline values. The characteristics of injury metabolism will be present only during the acute stress response period. For surgical stress alone, this period is relatively short, generally less than 48 hours. For this reason, studies that attempt to evaluate surgically related acute stress changes during later postoperative periods are potentially flawed and may introduce misleading conclusions. The magnitude of the stress response becomes much more difficult to predict if a substantial portion of the injury insult results from an additional, nonsurgical factor, such as burn trauma or sepsis. In a study of infants with a wide variety of stress insults, there was substantial interpatient variability in MEE relative to the predicted BMR. This variability, in large part, may be attributable to substantial differences in the acute metabolic demands imposed by the underlying disease process (eg, trauma, burns, sepsis, etc) and the ability of the host to meet these demands (size and recruitability of host endogenous metabolic reserves).

Nutrition assessment of critically ill infants must account for the acute metabolic impact due to injury severity and can be best accomplished clinically by serial measurement of (1) the visceral (or constitutive) protein pool and (2) the acute-phase protein pool in addition to (3) energy expenditure (see above). The variations of the injury response can thus be established on the basis of serial changes (response pattern) in the serum concentrations of CRP, an acute phase protein pool marker, and prealbumin, a visceral protein pool marker. Serum CRP and prealbumin concentrations are readily measured in most hospital clinical laboratories. Albumin should not be used because acute catabolic and anabolic changes, which occur in association with the evolving metabolic response to injury, have a smaller impact on overall serum levels of this visceral protein due to its substantially larger pool size and much longer endogenous serum half-life. Within 12 to 24 hours following injury, serum prealbumin levels fall, reflecting catabolic metabolism, and CRP levels rise because of hepatic reprioritization of protein synthesis in response to injury. During this acute metabolic injury response state, calories should be administered to match only MEE-established needs. If indirect calorimetry is unavailable, only basal metabolic needs should be administered. Serum prealbumin and CRP levels are inversely related (ie, serum prealbumin levels decrease and CRP levels increase with a magnitude proportional to injury severity, and then return to normal as the acute metabolic response to injury resolves), and should be measured serially to establish the injury response pattern. Acute phase protein changes have been shown to correlate well with glycemic response changes. Serum blood glucose, prealbumin, and

CRP concentrations have also been shown to be useful in predicting clinical outcome in critically ill infants. Furthermore, serum CRP concentrations have been shown to correlate well with MEE in this patient population. Decreases in serum CRP values in conjunction with increases in serum prealbumin indicate resolution of the postinjury inflammatory (metabolic stress) response and cessation of catabolic metabolism. In this regard, increasing serum prealbumin levels are particularly important, signifying the resumption of somatic growth (adaptive anabolic phase) at which time calories can be advanced to promote growth recovery. This method provides a potentially useful guide to advance calories delivery and optimize growth recovery without overfeeding infants during the acute phase of the metabolic response to injury.

## Nutritional Delivery

The protein-energy reserves in healthy, well-nourished children are adequate to serve as an endogenous nutritional resource for up to 5 days with minimal exogenous support. In critically ill children with severe preoperative injury necessitating surgical intervention, especially in malnourished patients and preterm infants, nutritional administration should be started within the first 24 to 48 hours postoperatively. Malnutrition ranges from approximately 25% to 50% among critically ill children.

## Enteral Nutrition

Enteral nutritional delivery is generally the optimal route of nutritional support provided that intestinal function is adequate to absorb the nutrients provided. Oral intake is preferred but should be monitored on a 24-hour basis to ensure that daily protein caloric goals are met. When oral feeding is insufficient, short-term enteral administration may be achieved via nasogastric, nasoduodenal, or nasojejunal feeding tubes. Nasoduodenal tubes may be useful in decreasing gastroesophageal reflux and subsequent aspiration, and thus facilitate improved enteral feeding tolerance, but are more easily dislodged. Nasojejunal tubes are better in this regard but are more difficult to position properly.

Enteral motility and absorption is often compromised in association with severe acute metabolic stress (tissue injury). In this circumstance, elemental formulations (predigested) may be useful. Elemental formulas generally consist of proteins in the form of amino acids and polypeptides, carbohydrates in the form of mono-/disaccharides and limit dextrans, and fat predominantly in the form of MCTs (absorbed directly into the blood rather than via lacteals). In the absence of normal brush border function, these nutrients can still be absorbed in the small bowel. Furthermore, enteral preparations pass little (if any) residual into the large bowel. It is important to note that the entire 24-hour caloric budget need not initially be provided enterally and that, in circumstances of even substantial bowel functional compromise, small amounts of enteral delivery, in conjunction with parenteral nutrition, can be well tolerated while offering the additional advantage of supporting the intestinal barrier.

Feeding intolerance is not only a manifestation of inadequate intestinal function but also represents a physiologic mechanism against overfeeding. Suggestive signs and symptoms include increasing abdominal distention with vomiting and/or diarrhea, often associated with crampy abdominal pain. High formula osmolarity, excessively rapid rate advancement, and early bolus feeding are frequently associated with these symptoms. Increased reducing substances (>0.5%) and fat (>10% of ingested fat in a 3-day collection sample) in the stool confirm carbohydrate and fat malabsorption, respectively. Fat malabsorption usually accompanies carbohydrate malabsorption. Initial use of diluted formula mixtures and continuous-drip feeding regimens reduce feeding intolerance.

Other complications associated with enteral delivery are sinusitis, gastritis, bowel perforation, tracheal intubation, pneumatosis intestinalis, and aspiration pneumonia.

## Parenteral Nutrition

Although the preferred route of nutritional support is enteral, parenteral nutrient delivery is often necessary in critically ill children, especially infants, due to gastrointestinal dysfunction. Since the body has no physiologic defense against excess parenteral caloric delivery, overfeeding is common using this modality, particularly in the intensive care setting. Hepatic, respiratory, and immunologic complications associated with excessive, inappropriate, and long-term parenteral nutrient administration have been discussed above. In addition, catheter-related risks include increased infection rates, venous thrombosis, vascular perforation, endocarditis, and embolism. Catheter tip placement into the right atrium about 1 cm with infants in particular allows for better dilution of hyperosmolar infusates, thus reducing the risk of superior or inferior vena cava infusate-induced endothelial injury with secondary thrombotic occlusion. Failure to appropriately monitor and adjust fluid and electrolyte balance can lead to a wide variety of metabolic disturbances. Complications involving catheter placement include, but are not limited to, pneumothorax, arterial perforation, hemothorax, and cardiac tamponade.

## Parenteral Versus Enteral Nutrition

The value of early (within 48 hours) versus late (≥5 days) has been suggested to be beneficial in patients with depleted endogenous reserves (eg, malnutrition, cancer cachexia, repeated injury insult, etc). Both enteral and parenteral nutrition have been shown to reduce the hypermetabolic response to injury and reduce protein catabolism in comparison with unfed patients. Enteral nutrition is preferred to parenteral nutrition, assuming adequate intestinal absorptive function and peristalsis are present. However, the gut mucosal barrier can be supported with a small fraction of the total daily energy requirement, even if gut function is partially compromised. The visceral protein response is significantly greater and occurs earlier with enteral nutrition versus parenteral nutrition after severe injury. A number of studies have demonstrated a significant benefit of enteral nutrition over parenteral nutrition in appropriately matched, critically ill adults. However, a recent critical review of numerous human studies involving critically ill patients receiving TPN determined that the predominant cause of stress-associated hyperglycemia in these study populations, in addition to the intense counterregulatory hormone and cytokine response to injury, was due to an excessive intravenous administration of dextrose. This observation is important because hyperglycemia can increase the risk of sepsis, wound infection, and abscess formation, all of which have been associated in greater frequency with parenteral in contrast to enteral nutritional administration in various clinical trials. While iatrogenic hyperglycemia due to intravenous carbohydrate overfeeding has been associated with significant increases in mortality and morbidity due to infectious complications in a substantial number of studies involving critically ill patients receiving TPN, it is important to note that many children, particularly infants in the intensive care setting, will initially require a large (if not total) portion of their daily caloric requirement to be administered parenterally. It is, therefore, obligatory that practitioners to ensure that caloric delivery is optimized and appropriately suited to the metabolic status of the critically ill child so that the true benefits of nutritional support in the postoperative setting can be achieved without increasing the associated risks of morbidity and mortality, particularly with respect to overfeeding.

## SELECTED READINGS

Alaedeen DI, Walsh MC, Chwals WJ. Total parenteral nutrition-associated hyperglycemia correlates with prolonged mechanical ventilation and hospital stay in septic infants. *J Pediatr Surg* 2006;41(1):239–244; discussion 239–244.

Alaedeen DI, Queen AL, Leung E, et al. C-reactive protein-determined injury severity: length of stay predictor in surgical infants. *J Pediatr Surg* 2004;39(12):1832–1834.

Botrán M, López-Herce J, Mencía S, et al. Enteral nutrition in the critically ill child: comparison of standard and protein-enriched diets. *J Pediatr* 2011;159(1):27–32.

Brunengraber LN, Robinson AV, Chwals WJ. Relationship of serum C-reactive protein and blood glucose levels with injury severity and patient morbidity in a pediatric trauma population. *J Pediatr Surg* 2009;44(5):992–996.

Burke PA, Young LS, Bistrian BR. Metabolic vs nutrition support: a hypothesis. *JPEN J Parenter Enteral Nutr* 2010;34(5):546–548.

Chwals WJ, Fernandez ME, Jamie AC, et al. Relationship of metabolic indexes to postoperative mortality in surgical infants. *J Pediatr Surg* 1993;28(6):819–822.

Chwals WJ, Fernandez ME, Jamie AC, et al. Detection of postoperative sepsis in infants with the use of metabolic stress monitoring. *Arch Surg* 1994;129(4):437–442.

De Wit B, Meyer R, Desai A, et al. Challenge of predicting resting energy expenditure in children undergoing surgery for congenital heart disease. *Pediatr Crit Care Med* 2010;11(4):496–501.

Druyan ME, Compher C, Boullata JI, et al. Clinical guidelines for the use of parenteral and enteral nutrition in adult and pediatric patients: applying the GRADE system to development of A.S.P.E.N. clinical guidelines. *JPEN J Parenter Enteral Nutr* 2012;36(1):77–80.

Rangel SJ, Calkins CM, Cowles RA, et al. Parenteral nutrition-associated cholestasis: an American Pediatric Surgical Association Outcomes and Clinical Trials Committee systematic review. *J Pediatr Surg* 2012; 47(1):225–240.

Ho MY, Yen YH, Hsieh MC, et al. Early versus late nutrition support in premature neonates with respiratory distress syndrome. *Nutrition* 2003; 19(3):257–260.

Hofer N, Zacharias E, Müller W, et al. An update on the use of C-reactive protein in early-onset neonatal sepsis: current insights and new tasks. *Neonatology* 2012;102(1):25–36.

Kudsk KA. Beneficial effect of enteral feeding. *Gastrointest Endosc Clin N Am* 2007;17(4):647–662.

Letton RW, Chwals WJ, Jamie A, et al. Early postoperative alterations in infant energy use increase the risk of overfeeding. *J Pediatr Surg* 1995; 30(7):988–992; discussion 992–993.

Lucas A, Bloom SR, Aynsley-Green A. Gut hormones and 'minimalenteral feeding'. *Acta Paediatr Scand* 1986;75(5):719–723.

Mehta NM, Bechard LJ, Dolan M, et al. Energy imbalance and the risk of overfeeding in critically ill children. *Pediatr Crit Care Med* 2011; 12(4):398–405.

Mehta NM, Compher C. A.S.P.E.N. Clinical Guidelines: nutrition support of the critically ill child. *JPEN J Parenter Enteral Nutr* 2009;33(3): 260–276.

Moghazy AM, Adly OA, Abbas AH, et al. Assessment of the relation between prealbumin serum level and healing of skin-grafted burn wounds. *Burns* 2010;36(4):495–500.

Pons Leite H, Gilberto Henriques Vieira J, Brunow De Carvalho W, et al. The role of insulin-like growth factor I, growth hormone, and plasma proteins in surgical outcome of children with congenital heart disease. *Pediatr Crit Care Med* 2001;2(1):29–35.

Preissig CM, Rigby MR. Pediatric critical illness hyperglycemia: risk factors associated with development and severity of hyperglycemia in critically ill children. *J Pediatr* 2009;155(5):734–739.

Puder M, Valim C, Meisel JA, et al. Parenteral fish oil improves outcomes in patients with parenteral nutrition-associated liver injury. *Ann Surg* 2009;250(3):395–402.

Rangel SJ, Calkins CM, Cowles RA, et al. Parenteral nutrition-associated cholestasis: an American Pediatric Surgical Association Outcomes and Clinical Trials Committee systematic review. *J Pediatr Surg* 2012;47(1):225–240.

Rosmarin DK, Wardlaw GM, Mirtallo J. Hyperglycemia associated with high, continuous infusion rates of total parenteral nutrition dextrose. *Nutr Clin Pract* 1996;11(4):151–156.

Tueting JL, Byerley LO, Chwals WJ. Anabolic recovery relative to degree of prematurity after acute injury in neonates. *J Pediatr Surg* 1999;34(1): 13–16; discussion 16–17.

Vlasselaers D, Milants I, Desmet L, et al. Intensive insulin therapy for patients in paediatric intensive care: a prospective, randomised controlled study. *Lancet* 2009;373(9663):547–556.

Yu X, Larsen B, Urschel S, et al. The profile of inflammatory and metabolic response in children undergoing heart transplantation. *Clin Transplant* 2012;26(2):E137–E142.

GENERAL PRINCIPLES

# CHAPTER 9

# Vascular Access Procedures

*Kristen A. Zeller and John K. Petty*

## KEY POINTS

1. Prevention of central line associated bloodstream infections (CLABSI) begins with prevention of the need for central lines. Excellence with placement of peripheral intravenous lines is foundational to prevention of such infections.

2. The intraosseous (IO) route provides rapid vascular access in a crisis. This route may be used effectively in older patients (adolescents and young adults) and in different locations (femur, humerus, radius, both malleoli, and even sternum) than had been traditionally thought to be ideal for this approach.

3. Although the pediatric surgeon commonly performs central venous catheterization, an understanding of the spectrum of approaches and anatomic options will help with the most difficult cases of vascular access.

4. When placing a central venous catheter (CVC), the use of central line insertion checklists and bundles can minimize the risk of CLABSI.

5. Children with long-term indwelling catheters who develop CLABSI present a challenging problem. A systematic approach to this problem will prioritize the health of the child and still preserve vascular access sites.

6. Whether using the guidance of anatomic landmarks or ultrasound imaging, meticulous technique and knowledge of anatomy are imperative for achieving safe central venous access. Ultrasound guidance can be particularly helpful with catheterization of the internal jugular vein.

Vascular access is a key that unlocks the door of acute pediatric care. Although the access itself is not therapy, it enables therapy in nearly every realm of pediatric care. Contemporary neonatology, oncology, critical care, infectious disease, anesthesia, and trauma care depend heavily on reliable vascular access for diagnosis, monitoring, and treatment.

Pediatric vascular access can challenge the person on both ends of the catheter. For so many children, "the needle" creates more anxiety than any other component of acute health care. Children at varying developmental levels do not understand their need for vascular access. Even children who do understand will typically subjugate an emotional response in order to cooperate. The family and the care provider do well to ensure appropriate comfort, environment, and analgesia to the child who needs vascular access. The care provider confronts additional challenges when pursuing vascular access in the pediatric patient and must consider the following: the acuity of the situation, the size of the child, the nature of the access needed, the anatomy of the child, and the duration of need for vascular access. The skill of vascular access is much more than the technique.

The pediatric surgeon is the provider of vascular access sometimes as first choice and sometimes as last resort. Because of the breadth of application and the challenges of these procedures in children, the pediatric surgeon is often asked to help these children. In many child healthcare institutions, vascular access procedures comprise the most common pediatric surgical intervention, and children stand to benefit greatly from a surgeon who is skilled in these procedures.

## PERIPHERAL INTRAVENOUS ACCESS

The peripheral intravenous catheter (PIV) is the most ubiquitous form of vascular access. Healthcare providers with varied training are capable of placing these catheters, from the prehospital setting to the intensive care unit. It can generally be placed rapidly and used immediately. Placement of a PIV involves very low morbidity, and modern catheters, made from materials such as Teflon® or polyurethane, are more flexible, more resistant to infection, less thrombogenic, and more conducive to very small veins than previous generations of catheters. Catheter sizes range from 14 to 26 gauge and vary in length from 3/4 to 2 inches. These short catheters have very good flow characteristics, as the flow of fluid through a cylinder is inversely proportional to the length of the cylinder. The PIV is the preferred method for rapid infusion of intravenous (IV) fluids and blood products in the setting of acute trauma, burns, or shock. Compared with vascular access through a long, thin CVC, the PIV may be preferred for infusion of more viscous fluids such as packed red blood cells and platelets, as the catheter may be less likely to thrombose. The PIV will support infusion of nearly all fluids and medications, but it should be avoided for vesicant chemotherapy, fluids containing a high concentration of dextrose (greater than 12.5%), calcium chloride, and high dose vasopressors. Infiltration with such solutions can cause tissue damage, necrosis, and sloughing.

Selection of a site for placement of a PIV is a function of the age and the anatomy of the child. Frequent sites include the dorsum of the hand, the cephalic and basilic veins in the forearm, the median cubital vein in the antecubital fossa, and the greater saphenous vein at the ankle. In infants, PIVs may be placed in scalp veins, such as the superficial temporal vein or the posterior auricular vein. In addition, infants tolerate placement of a PIV in the dorsum of the foot better than older children. The external jugular vein is a better site for placement of a PIV in older children than it is in infants. This site can be difficult to access in infants, and a PIV may more easily become dislodged here, due to the mobility of the surrounding tissue. The external jugular vein is a better option for percutaneous or cutdown central venous access in an infant than it is for peripheral venous access. If traditional sites for access are not available, suitable veins on the torso may be identified for placement of a PIV.

Although PIVs are frequently placed by other healthcare providers, the pediatric surgeon should be familiar with their insertion. In an awake child placement of a PIV may be facilitated by applying a local anesthetic cream to the anticipated site of catheter placement, if the urgency of the need for the PIV permits. Antisepsis should be observed in the placement of these catheters, including hand hygiene, clean gloves, and use of a skin antiseptic such as chlorhexidine, iodine, or alcohol. The seemingly simple technique of PIV placement involves a complex interaction of vision, touch, and motion. A tourniquet is applied as appropriate. The vein is located by sight and by palpation. The catheter and needle are inserted through the skin peripheral to the target vein. The catheter and needle are advanced toward the middle of the vein at a superficial angle. When a flash of blood is returned in the catheter, the needle is immobilized and the catheter is steadily advanced over the needle. Tubing is attached to the catheter, and the catheter is flushed to confirm intravascular placement. The catheter is secured with tape or an adhesive dressing.

A successfully placed PIV should be watched closely for signs of phlebitis, infection, or infiltration. The great disadvantage of the PIV is longevity. A PIV should generally be changed or removed within 96 hours to reduce the risk of phlebitis or bacterial colonization, although in many children, these catheters may be safely left in place for longer periods of time, as long as they are monitored closely. Given recent attention to the prevention of CLABSI, it bears mentioning that perhaps the most effective way to prevent CLABSI is to obviate the need for a central line at all. In this respect, expertise with PIV is an essential component of infection control.

Innovative approaches to the PIV may increase success at identification of veins and placement of these catheters. Experienced nurses and dedicated IV nurse specialists increase successful PIV placement, particularly on the first attempt. Although placement of a PIV should be a broadly acquired skill, there should be an effort to concentrate this skill among specialized providers. This is particularly true for children with difficult IV access due to age, weight, previous PIVs, and cooperativeness. Additional techniques that may be useful to identify veins include transillumination of an extremity with a traditional light source, which may help identify subcutaneous veins in infants and very small children. Side transillumination with the Veinlite (Translite, Sugar Land, TX) can identify subcutaneous veins in larger children. Used increasingly for central venous access, two-dimensional (2D) ultrasound can also be used to identify peripheral veins and guide catheter placement. Projection of near-infrared light with the VeinViewer (Christie Medical Holdings, Memphis, TN) identifies veins that may not be otherwise visible. The Vein Entry Indicator Device (Vascular Technologies, Nes Ziona, Israel) uses a pressure sensor to identify the change in pressure when the needle enters a vein and emits an audible signal to the practitioner to allow advancement of the catheter while the needle is in the vein. Although these technologies are not standard for placement of PIVs, they may become increasingly useful for difficult PIV placement or placement of PIVs in nontraditional locations.

Despite dedicated efforts to establish a PIV, it is not always possible. Alternatives to peripheral IV access include peripheral vein cutdown catheter placement, IO needle placement, and central venous catheterization. These alternative forms of access should be considered particularly in cases of trauma or shock, in which placement of a PIV may be ultimately achievable, but may take a longer period of time to establish.

## PERIPHERAL VEIN CUTDOWN

In the era of improved percutaneous central venous access and expanded use of IO needles, the need for cutdown peripheral IV access is less common than perhaps it once was. However, a peripheral vein cutdown is an invaluable approach for the placement of a peripherally inserted central catheter (PICC). Although the choice of catheter may vary, the approach to the peripheral veins is similar.

The greater saphenous vein at the ankle is a good choice for vascular access in a crisis, when other options have failed. Because it is located far from the head, neck, and chest, it allows an individual or a team to concentrate on obtaining venous access without interfering with other potential simultaneous procedures, such as endotracheal intubation, chest compressions, or thoracostomy. After application of a tourniquet below the knee, a transverse skin incision is created medial and cephalad to the medial malleolus. Subcutaneous dissection with a fine hemostat exposes the vein. The vein is dissected circumferentially and encircled with a fine ligature. After selection of an appropriately sized catheter, the vein can be entered with direct venipuncture through the incision. Alternatively, the catheter can be passed percutaneously through a skin puncture site inferior to the incision and then directed through the vein under direct vision in the incision. The catheter is secured and the incision is closed.

Veins of the forearm can also be used for cutdown. The basilic and the cephalic veins cross the antecubital fossa in a superficial location. A median cubital vein runs obliquely between the two and provides collateral venous drainage. Their location, size, and patency should be confirmed with placement of a tourniquet and palpation or with ultrasound. In most children, an incision in the antecubital crease overlying the brachial pulse will allow access to both the basilic vein and the median cubital vein. For placement of a PICC line, we find it is generally easier to advance the tip of the catheter into the central venous circulation through the basilic or median antecubital veins, due to the angle at which the basilic vein joins the subclavian vein. The cephalic vein lies to the radial side of the antecubital fossa and serves as another option for cutdown access, but manipulation of the arm may be required to advance the tip of a PICC line into the subclavian vein.

## INTRAOSSEOUS ACCESS

The IO route provides rapid access to the systemic venous circulation. The medullary cavity is rich in sinusoids that drain into a central venous canal and then enter the venous circulation through emissary veins. The marrow space does not collapse and is of sufficient size to provide a sufficient target even in very small patients. For all of these reasons, the IO route is the first choice for vascular access in cases of shock or trauma when peripheral IV access is unsuccessful. Compared with urgent central venous access, it is more rapid and does not involve the same risk of acute complications.

Because of the resistance of the medullary cavity and the size of the needles used, IO access is not ideal for rapid volume infusions. A 15-gauge IO needle will generally support flows equivalent to a 20-gauge IV. IO infusions should be delivered with a pump rather than by gravity flow alone. Medications administered IO are rapidly absorbed comparable to IV medications, with no need to adjust the dosage.

IO access in children is most frequently obtained on the anteromedial surface of the tibia. A point 1 to 2 cm inferior and medial to the tibial tuberosity is selected for access (Fig. 9-1). A local anesthetic is infiltrated into the skin, soft

tissue, and periosteum in awake patients. The IO needle and stylet are advanced perpendicular to the tibia with a slight angulation toward the toes, away from the growth plate. The needle is rotated as it is advanced. Once a loss of resistance is appreciated, the stylet is removed. If a syringe placed on the needle will aspirate blood or marrow, this confirms placement in the medullary space. Laboratory studies may be obtained through an IO needle. If blood cannot be aspirated from the IO needle, it does not necessarily mean that the needle is incorrectly placed. Crystalloid should be infused through the needle by gravity or by gentle flush. As this infusion is started, the site must be inspected and the calf muscles must be palpated for signs of extravasation. Ease of infusion without swelling around the site further confirms intramedullary placement. The needle is secured to the extremity, and a dressing is applied.

Although the proximal tibia is the most commonly selected site of IO access, other sites lend themselves to IO placement as well. The distal femur, proximal humerus, distal radius, medial or lateral malleolus, sternum, and iliac crest provide additional options for IO access. An IO should not be used in children with underlying bone disease, such as osteogenesis imperfecta or osteopenia. Nor should an IO be placed in a bone with a known fracture or at the site of a previously failed IO attempt, because of the risk of extravasation and compartment syndrome. It was previously thought that IO needles should only be placed into medullary spaces with red marrow, thus restricting the use of IO access to young children. As experience has grown, it has become clear that medullary spaces with yellow marrow (quiescent marrow that has been replaced by fat) are acceptable for IO infusions. Thus, IO access has become an option for rapid vascular access in older children, adolescents, and adults.

Specialized needles for IO access are sized 16 or 18 gauge and have a stylet to prevent obstruction of the needle with bone spicules. Spinal needles and bone marrow needles may also be used for IO access. These needles are manually inserted and may be more challenging to place in larger patients. Recently developed devices may simplify IO placement beyond traditional manually placed needles. The EZ-IO (Vidacare, San Antonio, TX) uses a handheld driver, much like a drill, to advance the needle through the cortex of the bone into the marrow space. This device can place IO needles of differing sizes, depending on the anatomic location chosen and the size of the patient. The Bone Injection Gun (WaisMed, Kansas City, MO) is held against the skin and a spring-loaded mechanism advances the needle through the cortex. This device is also capable of placing IO needles of different sizes.

Complications of IO access are uncommon. The most common complication is IO needle malposition or dislodgement, resulting in fluid extravasation into the adjacent soft tissues. If this is promptly recognized, alternative vascular access should be secured. If this is not promptly recognized, the patient can develop soft tissue damage and even compartment syndrome. Osteomyelitis is an extremely rare, but potentially serious complication related to placement technique, duration of infusion, and infusion of hypertonic fluids. Thus, IO needles should be removed within the first 24 hours, once more durable vascular access has been obtained. Placement

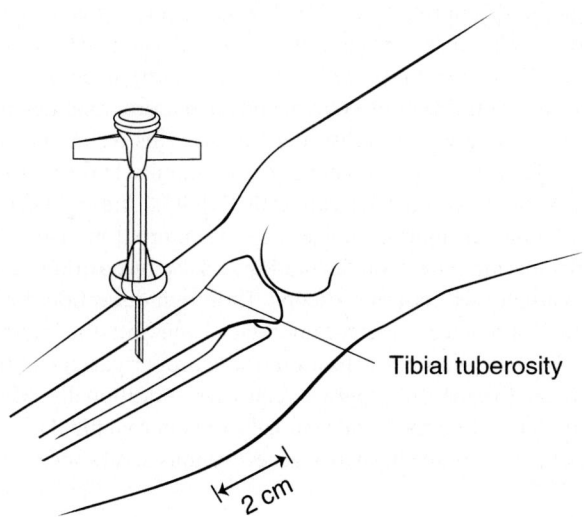

**FIGURE 9-1** Intraosseous access. At 1 to 2 cm below the tibial tuberosity, a needle is introduced into the bone marrow at an angle of 45° to 60° away from the growth plate.

Tibial tuberosity

2 cm

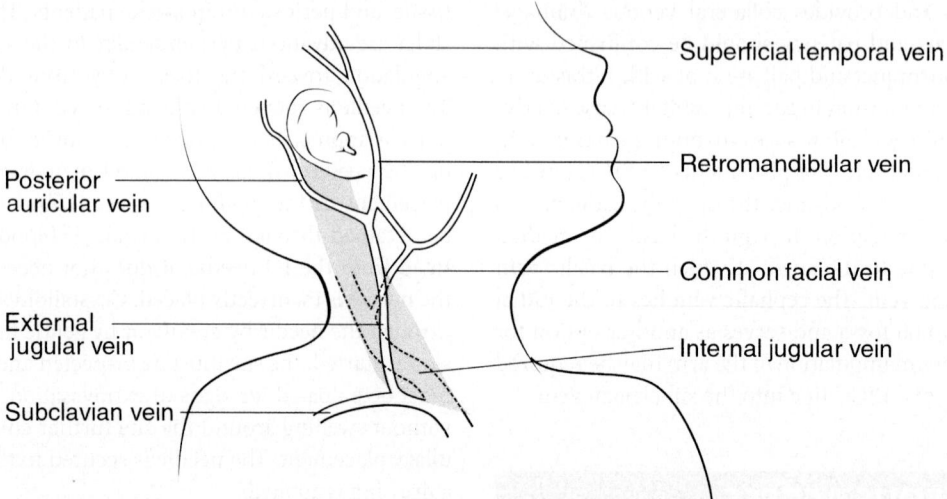

**FIGURE 9-2** The external jugular vein is formed by the union of retromandibular and posterior auricular veins. The common facial vein is joined by the anterior division of the retromandibular vein and drains into the internal jugular vein behind the sternocleidomastoid muscle. An incision at the midpoint between the inferior border of the ear and the sternal notch allows dissection of external jugular and common facial veins.

extremity veins are difficult to locate. This vein can also allow easy access into the central venous system by either percutaneous or cutdown methods and is associated with virtually no risk of pneumothorax, hemothorax, or pericardial tamponade. The external jugular vein begins just behind the angle of the mandible by the union of the posterior auricular vein with the posterior division of the retromandibular vein. It descends obliquely across the sternocleidomastoid muscle and pierces the deep cervical fascia just above the clavicle to drain into the subclavian vein (Fig. 9-2). Despite its superficial location, the advancement of catheters can occasionally be difficult because of excess mobility of the vein, angulation of the juncture point with the subclavian vein, as well as the presence of many tributaries. In surgically exposing this particular vein, the midpoint between the mandible and the clavicular head, directly over the anterior border of the sternocleidomastoid muscle, is selected as a landmark. This landmark not only provides consistent access to the external jugular veins, but also serves as a focus of dissection for the internal jugular or common facial veins when necessary.

Upon identification of the superficial external jugular vein, a small transverse neck incision is made. Once isolated, the external jugular vein is ligated cephalad with a fine ligature. A small transverse venotomy is made, and the cannula is advanced into the superior vena cava. The transverse cervical vein, supraclavicular vein, and anterior jugular vein can alter the direction of advancement of the catheter away from the subclavian vein; when available, fluoroscopy can facilitate the proper catheter placement into a central vein.

## Common Facial Vein

The facial vein is joined by the anterior division of the retromandibular vein and drains directly into the internal jugular vein (Fig. 9-2). Because of this direct drainage, catheters can be advanced into the central venous system more reliably. The patient is usually positioned with the neck in full extension and the head turned slightly away from the intended site of the dissection. A small transverse skin incision is made at the midpoint between the inferior tip of the ear and sternal notch at the anterior border of the sternocleidomastoid muscle. Using this landmark will avoid dissecting in close proximity to the mandibular branch of the facial nerve near the mandible. Blunt dissection with a fine hemostat can accomplish dissection through the superficial cervical fascia. When it is difficult to directly locate the common facial vein, the internal jugular vein should be identified first before proceeding to the point at which the facial vein joins the internal jugular vein. After proximal and distal control of the vein has been established, a subcutaneous tunnel to the anterior chest can be made using either a Frazier suction tip or a small chest tube (8 Fr chest tubes will accommodate Broviac catheters 4.2 Fr or smaller). After the catheter length is measured to approximately the nipple line, it is cut with a scissor at an angle. At this point, the common facial vein is ligated distally, and a small transverse venotomy is created using a #11 scalpel blade. The catheter is passed through the internal jugular vein into the central venous system, and then a proximal ligature is placed gently to establish hemostasis. This technique can be performed, even in small premature infants, at the bedside in the neonatal intensive care unit (NICU). The right facial vein allows straight drainage into the internal jugular vein and superior vena cava, facilitating consistent positioning of the catheter without fluoroscopy. Thorough dissection down to the confluence of the common facial vein into the internal jugular vein allows visualization of the proper passage of the catheter toward the superior vena cava. Additionally, when cannulation into the facial vein fails, the internal jugular vein may be used as an alternative access venous access site.

## Internal Jugular Vein

If the common facial vein dissection has been carried close to the internal jugular vein, one can easily complete the internal

of an IO needle can cause a fracture, and follow-up radiographs should be obtained in any child in whom such a fracture is suspected. Injuries to the growth plate are hypothetically possible, but demonstrable cases of limb growth disturbances have not been reported. Fat embolization could hypothetically occur in patients whose red marrow has been replaced with yellow marrow, such as adolescents and adults. However, clinically significant fat embolism from IO placement has not been documented.

## CENTRAL VENOUS ACCESS

Central venous catheter placement is a mainstay of the pediatric surgeon's armamentarium, and also a common source of frustration. Despite the frequency with which central access is performed, even the most seasoned and experienced surgeon can be humbled by a difficult access case. A variety of factors make central venous access procedures a frequent occurrence for the pediatric surgeon: small patients with precarious peripheral access, necessity for long-term parenteral nutrition, and chronic disease processes such as malignancy or cystic fibrosis. Product advances in catheters have also led to more widespread applications for central lines. CVC placement, even in small premature infants, has become accepted as routine. Central veins are accessed in infants and children either by cutdown or by a percutaneous method. External or internal jugular, facial, femoral, and subclavian veins are the preferred sites for central venous access. Despite advances in access techniques and devices, catheter-related infection, venous thrombosis, and technical placement misadventures remain the most frequently encountered complications of central venous access.

## AVAILABLE DEVICES

Several devices are available for either temporary (percutaneous) or permanent (tunneled) access. The proper catheter selection depends on the needs and the condition of the patient. For a short-term central venous access (less than 2 weeks), percutaneous polyvinyl catheters are frequently used. Although younger patients usually require general anesthesia, this type of access can be performed at the bedside in older patients. These catheters are available in various catheter diameters, lumen sizes, and lengths. These nontunneled catheters are not recommended for chronic use because of higher infection and thrombosis rates. Some newer percutaneous central venous lines are now available as Silastic® catheters, potentially increasing the safety profile.

When long-term central venous access is anticipated, tunneled Silastic® central venous lines are preferred. Catheters comprised of Silastic® (Dow Corning, Midland, MI) are the device of choice for long-term venous access because it is less thrombogenic and also less traumatic to veins than polyvinyl material. Broviac®, Hickman®, and Groshong® catheters (Bard Access Systems, Salt Lake City, UT) feature a cuff that provides mechanical stability and reduces infection rates. Broviac® catheters are the most commonly used tunneled CVC for pediatric patients.

Another type of tunneled central venous device is the totally implantable reservoir. Similar in design, the added subcutaneous ports are available in titanium or plastic. Because these devices do not have an external catheter, they allow easier care and are more readily accepted by active pediatric or adolescent patients. This also makes them ideal for patients in need of intermittent therapies. Despite some speculation of decreased complication rates, recent studies have demonstrated no significant differences when internal reservoirs are compared to externalized, tunneled catheters. These implantable ports, which are available in single or double lumen, have been extensively used in pediatric oncology patients as well as patients with cystic fibrosis, who frequently require long-term, but often intermittent, IV treatments.

PICC have become increasingly popular as an alternative for patients needing long-term venous access. Through a suitable peripheral vein, usually at the antecubital fossa, a small-caliber (2-4 Fr) Silastic catheter is inserted to the desired length into the proximal central vein. PICC lines are used in a wide variety of patients, and bedside placement may reduce overall cost. Although the risks of infection and thrombosis of PICC lines do not differ significantly from traditional CVCs, the obvious potential catheter-related thoracic "placement" complications at the time of catheterization are virtually eliminated. The overall incidence of infection or thrombosis is low, and phlebitis is reported in fewer than 10% of cases. The PICC line is often used in infants needing central access for intermediate duration, and its use has contributed to minimizing the frequency of tunneled catheter placements in this patient population. Large series of successful experiences with PICC lines, even in very small premature infants, have now been reported. In infants, other common access sites include saphenous veins and even scalp veins. A combined concept of peripherally inserted CVCs with completely implanted small subcutaneous ports exists with the P.A.S. PORT® (Smiths Medical, Dublin, OH) device. The P.A.S. PORT is a brachial vein inserted titanium system. The polysulfone catheter has a sensor wire that permits nonfluoroscopically guided catheter tip placement with a cath finder instrument. Although this device possesses certain advantages, no large experience in pediatric patients has been reported.

For patients who have an anticipated need for intermittent cross-sectional imaging, whether by CT or by MRI, a variety of central access catheters have been designed to withstand the power injections needed for contrast infusion. These catheters are available as percutaneous central lines, PICCs, and port-a-caths (PowerLine® CVC, PowerPICC®, PowerPort®, Bard Access Systems). Additionally, radiolucent port-a-caths are available, which minimize scatter artifact from the device itself.

## CENTRAL VENOUS ACCESS BY CUTDOWN

### External Jugular Vein

The external jugular vein is easily visible, and it can be percutaneously accessed using angiocatheters. It provides an alternative peripheral venous access site, especially when

jugular vein dissection without creating another neck incision. Alternatively, the internal jugular vein can be dissected above the clavicle and between the two heads of the sternocleidomastoid muscle. Although a unilateral internal jugular vein can be sacrificed to accommodate the venous catheter without significant morbidity, ligation of the internal jugular vein should be avoided whenever possible, particularly in premature infants. In older patients, placement of a purse-string suture on the anterior wall of the vein before venotomy results in secure positioning of the catheter as well as complete hemostasis. Alternatively, after temporary proximal and distal control of the internal jugular vein has been achieved, tension can be placed on the encircling loosely placed silk ties, and a 20-gauge angiocatheter can be used to perforate the anterior vein wall. Through this opening, silicone catheters (2.7 or 4.2 Fr) can be placed easily into the central venous system without ligating the internal jugular vein.

### Saphenofemoral Vein

The greater saphenous vein, which drains into the femoral vein at the infrainguinal area, is consistent in its location. During an emergency situation, particularly in small infants, a cutdown technique can rapidly expose the greater saphenous vein at the groin. This vein is able to accommodate larger CVCs for rapid infusion of fluid, blood products, and medications. Long-term CVCs are also frequently placed via this particular vein with subcutaneous tunnels to the anterior abdominal wall or distal thigh in infants without significant morbidity (Fig. 9-3). The femoral vein lies just medial to the femoral artery. A transverse skin incision is made just below the inguinal ligament, medial to the femoral pulsation. Dissection is accomplished with a fine hemostat, and the saphenous vein is usually identified in the subcutaneous plane, superficial to the femoral fascia. When a temporary catheter is being placed, this vein can then be accessed using either J-wire–directed Seldinger technique or direct cannulation via a small venotomy. When chronic

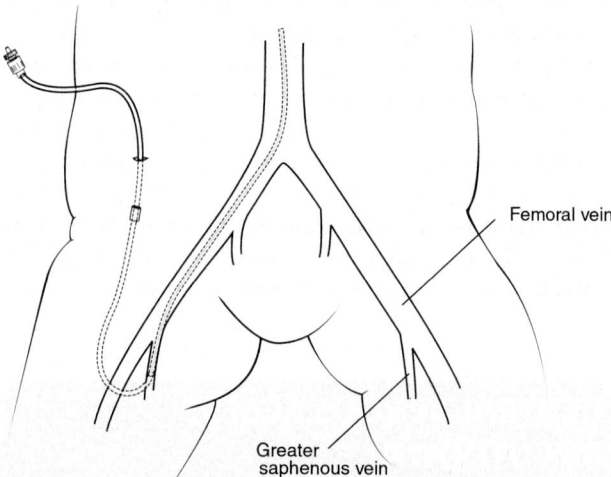

**FIGURE 9-3** A saphenofemoral vein at the inguinal region can be accessed to place tunneled catheters. Subcutaneous tunnel can be created on either the anterior abdominal wall or the distal thigh. This vein is also an ideal alternative site for temporary central venous catheter access by the cutdown method.

central venous access is desired, a subcutaneous tunnel to the appropriate site is made, and the appropriately trimmed length of catheter can be advanced into the iliac vein or inferior vena cava. Despite some concerns for catheter-related infections because of the close proximity to the perineum, access from this site eliminates the risk of thoracic complications and is well tolerated without an increase in morbidity. Inferior vena cava thrombosis remains a concern with any lower extremity catheter, and therefore, it is optimal to locate catheter tip away from renal vein orifices.

## PERCUTANEOUS CENTRAL VENOUS ACCESS

A Swedish radiologist revolutionized vascular access in 1952 when he had a "severe attack of common sense" and developed the now universally used method employing three simple tools: a needle, a wire, and a catheter. The Sven-Ivar Seldinger technique is ubiquitously employed for vascular access. The Seldinger technique makes it possible to safely access central veins percutaneously, thereby avoiding the more belabored cutdown approach. Patients in need of chronic central venous access, whether for nutritional support, administration of chemotherapeutic agents, or other IV therapies, may require periodic replacement of central lines. Percutaneous access allows repeated use of the same vein for multiple catheter placements. However, percutaneous central venous access has its limitations. The most obvious is the potential for injury due to a blind approach. Bleeding risk is greater, and correction of coagulopathy and thrombocytopenia must be addressed prior to initiating the procedure. Arterial puncture and pneumothorax are well-documented complications, the frequency of which can be minimized, but not eliminated, by meticulous technique and knowledge of anatomic landmarks.

### Femoral Vein

The femoral vein has a consistent relationship medial to the femoral artery. With the patient's legs in slight abduction, a percutaneous needle is introduced medial to the arterial pulsation, well below the inguinal crease. Gentle aspiration of the syringe is maintained during the advancement of the needle. When blood is aspirated, the position of the needle is stabilized, and the guidewire is introduced through the needle's hub. The needle is then withdrawn, and the puncture site is enlarged with a #11 scalpel blade. After the dilation is introduced over the wire, the percutaneous CVC can be placed over the wire. Catheter tip position can be confirmed either in the iliac vein or inferior vena cava by radiograph. This technique carries a low complication rate, and the potential infection rate can be kept to a minimum with diligent care of the insertion site.

### Internal Jugular Vein

The internal jugular vein begins at the jugular foramen at the skull base as a continuation of the sigmoid sinus. It descends through the neck in the carotid sheath lateral to the carotid artery and crosses the triangle formed by the sternal and

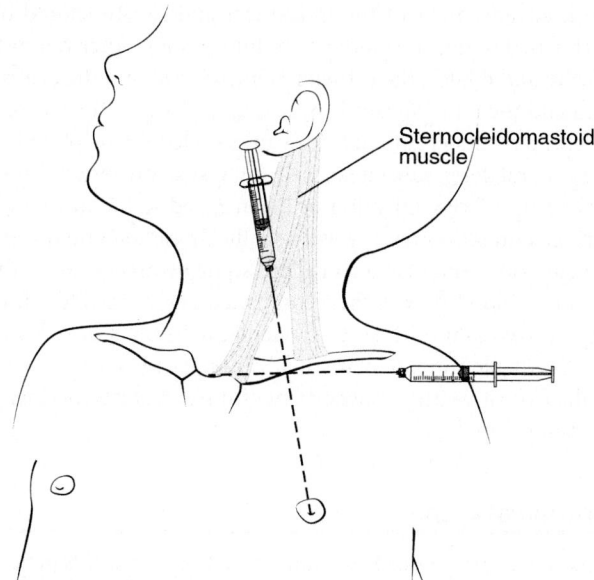

**FIGURE 9-4** Percutaneous access for central venous catheter can be performed safely even in small infants. For internal jugular vein access, a needle is introduced at the apex of the triangle formed by the two heads of the sternocleidomastoid muscles and aimed toward the ipsilateral nipple. The subclavian vein can be located by introducing the needle horizontally at the mid-clavicle and advancing it toward the sternal notch.

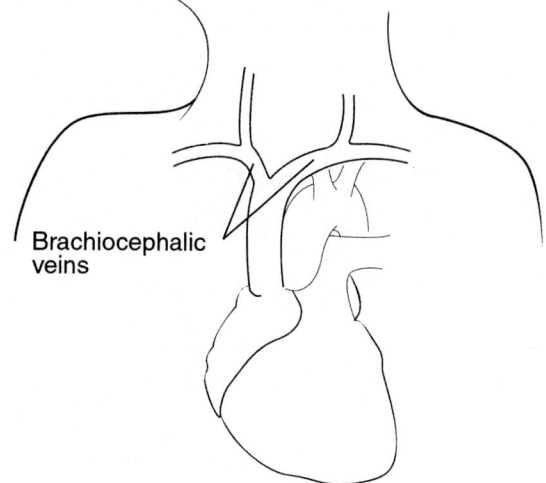

**FIGURE 9-5** Central venous anatomy. The angle at which the subclavian vein joins the internal jugular vein to become the brachiocephalic vein is more acute on the right side. Because of this anatomy, access to the left subclavian vein is often easier. In infants, this difference of central venous anatomy is even more prominent.

clavicular heads of the sternocleidomastoid muscle and clavicle. It then joins the subclavian vein behind the medial end of the clavicle to form the brachiocephalic vein. After a shoulder roll is placed to hyperextend the neck, the patient is positioned in Trendelenburg with the head turned slightly away from the insertion site. The carotid pulse is palpated, usually at the level of the cricoid cartilage, and the needle is introduced at the apex of the triangle formed by the two heads of the sternocleidomastoid muscle and clavicle. The internal jugular vein lies lateral to the carotid pulse. By keeping the finger gently on the carotid artery, one can avoid arterial puncture and maintain an accurate landmark for proper percutaneous access. The needle is advanced toward the ipsilateral nipple (Fig. 9-4). After aspiration of venous blood, the guidewire is introduced, and the catheter can be subsequently placed using the standard Seldinger technique.

The right internal jugular vein is preferentially used because it has a straighter, more direct drainage into the brachiocephalic vein. Although the left internal jugular vein can also be accessed using the same technique, potential injury to the thoracic duct along with the presence of a higher positioned pleura and a more acute angle where it joins the subclavian vein makes this access more difficult. The advantage of internal jugular vein cannulation is a low associated risk of thoracic complications; however, the discomfort of the catheter in the neck does not make it an ideal choice for long-term use, especially in children.

## Subclavian Vein

This is our preferred method and site to establish central venous access, even in infants as small as 2 kg. It has a

relatively reliable landmark, and the subsequent chest wall catheter location is much more comfortable for patients. The subclavian vein begins at the outer border of the first rib as a continuation of the axillary vein. It courses behind the medial third of clavicle and joins the internal jugular vein at the scalenus anterior muscle. The angle at which the subclavian joins the internal jugular vein to form the brachiocephalic vein is much more acute on the right side (Fig. 9-5). Additionally, this angle is more acute in young infants less than 1 year of age.

With the patient in the Trendelenburg position, a small shoulder roll is placed to separate the clavicle and the first rib space, allowing easier access to the subclavian vein. A saline-filled 3- or 5-mL syringe with attached needle is inserted 1 to 2 cm below the clavicle at its midpoint and is then directed toward the sternal notch (Fig. 9-4). The more acute angle of the subclavian vein insertion into the brachiocephalic vein in small infants requires advancement of the needle toward the contralateral shoulder. Brief hesitation of ventilation by an anesthesiologist at this time can minimize the risk of potential pneumothorax. Use of a larger syringe may create too much negative pressure and cause the vein to collapse. After blood returns, the needle position is secured, the syringe detached, and the guidewire is introduced. The wire tip position must then be confirmed by fluoroscopy in the superior vena cava. Occasionally the wire does not travel down toward the superior vena cava despite repeated manipulation under fluoroscopy. In this case, reintroducing the J-wire over a shorter 18-gauge angiocatheter can often properly redirect the wire toward the superior vena cava. (Note: It is always imperative to insert the flimsy "J" end of the wire and not its stiffer straight end to avoid any penetrating venous or cardiac injury.) For temporary percutaneous catheters, an introducer can be placed over a wire, and CVCs of various sizes and luminal diameters can be eventually placed. For tunneled chronic venous access, a small incision is made at the wire

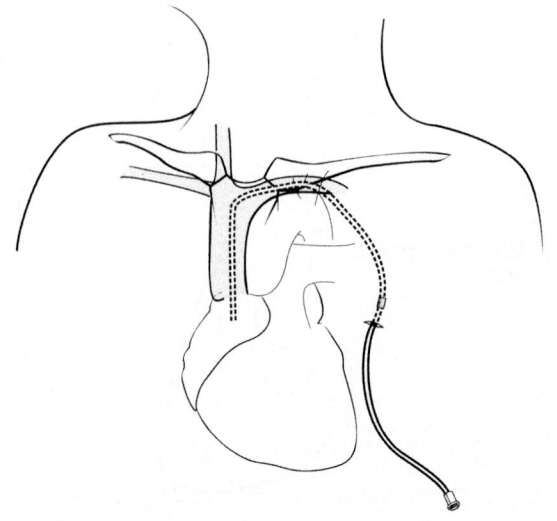

**FIGURE 9-6** Tunneled central venous catheter. The catheter tip is lined up at the nipple line to position the catheter tips at the junction of the superior vena cava and right atrium. Subcutaneous tunnel along with a cuff minimizes catheter dislodgement as well as potential infectious complications.

insertion site. A subcutaneous tunnel is made to the anterior medial chest using a tunneling device. In girls, potential injury to breast tissue must be avoided during the creation of the subcutaneous tunnel or pocket. After positioning of the Dacron cuff 2 to 3 cm proximal to the catheter exit site, the catheter length is prepared by measuring it to the nipple line. This usually ensures a final catheter tip position at the distal superior vena cava and right atrial junction (Fig. 9-6).

The vein dilator and peel-away sheath are threaded over the wire. The advancement of the dilator should be limited to the level of the superior vena cava to avoid any potential cardiac injury. Particularly, when larger introducers (10 or 13 Fr) are

used, advancement of the introducer and sheath should be performed under the guidance of fluoroscopy. After removal of wire and dilator, the catheter is introduced into the central vein and the outer sheath is peeled away. Despite the use of a careful technique, catheter tips can occasionally be placed in the contralateral subclavian vein or ipsilateral internal jugular vein. A brisk injection of heparinized saline in a 3-mL syringe under fluoroscopy will usually flip catheter tip toward the superior vena cava a so-called "squiggle maneuver." Bidirectional blood flow is then confirmed before instillation of heparinized saline. The infraclavicular incision is closed with an absorbable subcuticular stitch, and the catheter is secured at the exit site with nonabsorbable suture. A sterile occlusive dressing is applied.

## Umbilical Vein

This vein can provide immediate central venous access in neonates for administration of fluid, medication, and transfusion of blood products. In some instances, an umbilical venous cannula can also be used to administer parenteral nutrition. Cannulation of the umbilical vein is possible up to several days after birth. The patient is kept in a stable position, and the umbilical area is sterilely prepared. A piece of umbilical tape is tied around the base of the umbilicus. Next, the distal portion of the umbilical cord is cut with a scalpel or scissors, leaving a stump 1 cm in length. The thin-walled umbilical vein is located close to the periphery of the stump, on the cephalad side. The vein is then suspended using forceps, and a catheter (3 or 5 Fr) is introduced (Fig. 9-7). Occasionally, dilatation of the vein is required. A simple method to gauge the proper position of the catheter is to measure the length from the xiphoid to the umbilicus and add 1 cm; however, this catheter tip position should be confirmed by a radiograph, tip location optimally to be 1 cm above the diaphragm. Occasionally, a catheter may enter the portal vein, and this

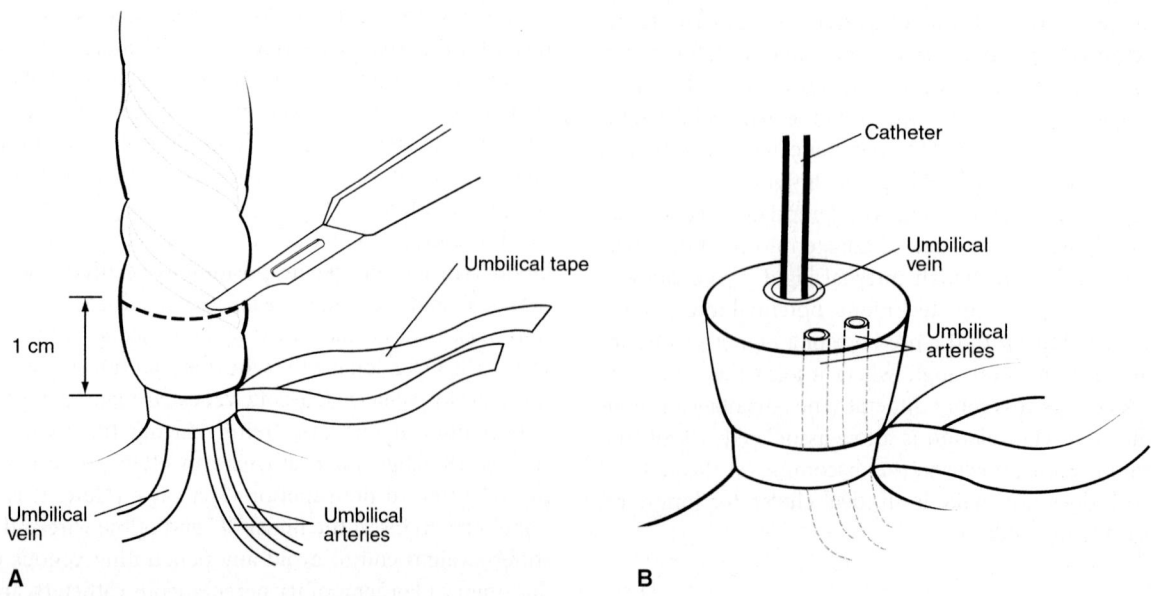

**A**                                                    **B**

**FIGURE 9-7 A.** Umbilical vessel catheterization. An umbilical tape is tied around the base of the cord, and the distal portion is cut with a scalpel, leaving a stump 1 cm in length. **B.** The umbilical vein is located at the cephalad aspect of the stump, and the two umbilical arteries are identified at the caudal aspect of the cord on either side of the urachal remnant.

should be repositioned to prevent thrombosis. Although the long-term use of an umbilical catheter is discouraged because of potential concerns of necrotizing enterocolitis, sepsis, perforation, and thrombosis, these catheters have been used for an extended period with caution, especially in extremely low-birth-weight infants.

## ULTRASOUND GUIDANCE

Improvements in ultrasound technology and expansion of it applications throughout medicine have introduced an element of "sight" to the previously blind approach to percutaneous central venous access. Although operator dependent, ultrasound is a helpful tool for access procedures due to its portability and ease of use. Proponents cite its safety benefits, reporting fewer complications and decreased time to achieve access. Controversy surrounds whether or not ultrasound guidance should be the standard for all access procedures, yet few will argue against its benefit as an adjunct for difficult cases. One area in which data supporting its use are strongest is vascular access for children. Ultrasound is most often used for placement of internal jugular catheters, but there is a growing experience with its use in subclavian line placement as well. Two-dimensional ultrasound (B-scan) is the preferred modality due to its ability to create an anatomic depiction of the subcutaneous tissues. Color-flow Doppler may be used to enhance the image further. Sterile probe covers allow for preservation of the sterile field when incorporating ultrasound guidance. With both the carotid artery and internal jugular vein in view, inadvertent arterial puncture may be avoided (Fig. 9-8). The artery and vein are differentiated by the artery's pulsatility and the vein's compressibility

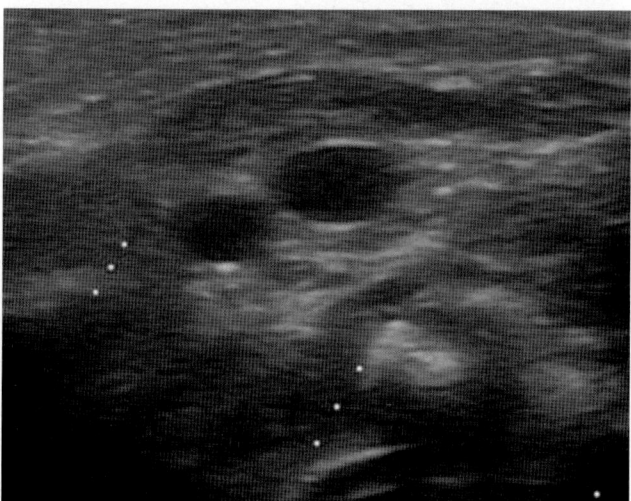

**FIGURE 9-8** Ultrasound-guided central venous access. At the bedside or in the operating room, ultrasound can be used to guide the placement of an internal jugular vein catheter. In the transverse plane, the right carotid artery and right internal jugular vein can be identified, demonstrating the location of the artery medial (*left*) to the vein (*right*). With downward compression of the ultrasound probe against the skin, the vein collapses while the artery remains patent.

with slight downward pressure of the probe against the tissue. The probe may be oriented transversely or longitudinally along the targeted vessel, and the vein accessed under ultrasound guidance by viewing the needle's signal in real time as it enters the vein. Aspiration of venous blood confirms access, and a guidewire is inserted. Catheter placement proceeds in the standard fashion.

## COMPLICATIONS OF CENTRAL VENOUS ACCESS

### Infection

The incidence of catheter-related infection can be quite variable depending on the type of catheter, area of placement, and the patient population. Infection is the most common complication of CVC access, and the incidence has been reported to range from 3% to 60%. Numerous clinical factors, including patient age, influence the risk of catheter infection. The highest incidence of catheter infection has been reported in the neonatal population. Others have demonstrated greater risk of catheter infection in pediatric patients with clinical conditions such as short-bowel syndrome, neutropenia, and other chronic illnesses. Catheter infections generally are categorized into three types: exit site infection, subcutaneous tunnel or pocket infection, and CLABSI.

Catheter exit site infections involve only the skin surrounding the catheter and most commonly are caused by skin flora, particularly *Staphylococcus epidermidis*. Such infections are reported to occur in 11% to 34% of all central venous access catheters. The location of the catheter and the exit-site care may have a direct effect on the incidence of infection. Although there are implications of increased infection rates in femoral venous catheters, several reports have supported the use of the femoral site for central venous access for chronic use without a significant incidence of infection or other complications. Difference in technique regarding site care has also been related to site infection rates; however, no single method has proven to be consistently better in regard to lowering the overall complication rate. Such infections are usually minor in severity, and they may be treated with local wound care and antibiotics with an excellent response. Infection cure without catheter removal can be accomplished in the majority of patients. Although the subcutaneous implantable infusion port eliminates this type of infection due to its internalized access site, it does carry the disadvantage of a potential pocket infection.

Significant tenderness, induration, erythema, and occasionally expressible purulent drainage at the exit site or at the port incision site represent a catheter tunnel or pocket infection. These infections result from a local process in the subcutaneous tissue plane that has extended proximally from the skin wound to the site of catheter entry into the central vein. This type of infection usually requires removal of the venous access device in addition to IV antibiotic therapy. Although there are several reports of successful treatment with antibiotic therapy alone, the majority of reports note difficulty in achieving cure of extensive subcutaneous infections without catheter removal because of poor antibiotic penetration, the foreign material that makes up the vascular access device, and a lack of adequate wound drainage. Regardless of the specific treatment applied, it is imperative that such infections be promptly treated to prevent progression to systemic sepsis.

The third and the most significant type of infection associated with venous access is CLABSI. Patients generally experience a variable degree of systemic signs and symptoms of bacteremia or fungemia when no other source for infection is identified. Frequently, patients do not demonstrate obvious local signs of catheter infection, nor do they demonstrate consistent microbiologic culture results. Several studies have indicated that the introduction and migration of bacteria from the skin exit site into the central venous circulation results directly in sepsis. There are a variety of protocols established to accurately diagnose and identify offending organisms. Such protocols usually include blood cultures from both peripheral and central sites along with direct and indirect sampling of the device itself. Quantitative analysis of blood cultures can also enhance the probability of accurate diagnosis. Coagulase-negative *Staphylococcus* is the most frequently identified organism responsible for CVC-related sepsis; however, various other gram-positive and gram-negative bacteria as well as fungi may be the offending organisms.

The initial therapy for CLABSI in the absence of an associated tunnel or pocket infection begins with empiric IV antibiotic therapy as soon as the appropriate cultures have been obtained. Antibiotics should be administered through the catheter, but if the patient's condition deteriorates, or if positive blood cultures persist, the catheter must be removed. Nevertheless, when a patient presents with problems that necessitate the need for repeated and chronic central venous access, the limited availability of other possible venous access sites should be carefully considered before the catheter is removed (Fig. 9-9).

Recognizing a strong correlation between skin flora and organisms causing catheter-related sepsis, researchers have focused much attention on reducing skin colonization to prevent venous access device infection. Prophylactic antibiotic therapy once was proposed to deter subsequent catheter sepsis. However, several studies have demonstrated that there is no improvement in the rate of line sepsis with such prophylactic antibiotics. Another area of study to reduce the incidence of line infection involves manipulation of the biomaterial of the catheter. The presence of a cuff on the tunneled catheter may create a mechanical barrier against the migration of skin organisms along the catheter. Antimicrobial material has been used in subcutaneous cuffs and topical disks to dress the exit site: VitaCuff® (Bard Access Systems, Salt Lake City, UT), BIOPATCH® (Ethicon, Somerville, NJ), and SILVASORB® (Medline Industries, Mundelein, IL). Additionally, antiseptic and antimicrobial impregnated devices may provide more than just a mechanical barrier to infection. They have been shown to be beneficial for adult patients, but their use in children is not yet approved in the United States. Preliminary reports suggest they are safe and may be useful, particularly in pediatric intensive care patients. More recently, the use of

70% ethanol locks for patients requiring long-term access has been proposed as a means of reducing catheter-related infections. At this time, data are limited to a small number of case series, and prospective randomized trials are forthcoming.

The greatest improvement in rates of CLABSI has been seen with the implementation of a central line "bundle." Bundles are groupings of best practices and evidence-based interventions that, when applied together, result in substantially greater improvement than when implemented individually. The key components of the central line bundle are proper hand hygiene, maximal barrier precautions upon insertion, chlorhexidine skin antisepsis, optimal catheter site selection, and daily review of line necessity with prompt removal of unnecessary lines. A central line insertion checklist will also provide a systematic approach to ensure that all processes related to central line placement are performed routinely.

## Thrombosis

Venous thrombosis is occasionally seen as a complication of chronic central venous access. It occurs at variable rates and presents a variety of clinical conditions. Pathologic findings range from a small fibrin sheath within or around a catheter to a large venous thrombosis causing obstruction of venous return from the involved area, even to the extent of superior vena caval occlusion. Several etiologic factors have been identified. Catheter type, size, location, and the underlying condition of the patient have all been implicated as potential factors producing thrombus formation. The increased disturbance of blood flow and the larger surface areas in multiple-lumen catheters have also been suggested to be etiologic factors. Furthermore, several studies have demonstrated an association between thrombosis and infection, and numerous protocols exist for use of various thrombolytic agents to manage systemic line sepsis effectively.

## TECHNICAL COMPLICATIONS

Several complications can occur at the time of catheter placement. Bleeding, arrhythmia, nerve injury, and malposition of the catheter represent the majority of potential problems during the cutdown access procedure, making percutaneous access of the subclavian vein preferable. However, potential complications of this technique include arterial puncture, pneumothorax, hemothorax, thoracic duct injury, nerve injury, and even pericardial tamponade. The incidence of pneumothorax is most common and has been reported at approximately 4%. However, any thoracic complication can potentially lead to life-threatening conditions. Thorough preoperative evaluation should include a detailed history and physical exam, particularly focusing on the type and location of previous CVCs. Patients should be screened for significant thrombocytopenia or other coagulopathy that would preclude a safe percutaneous puncture of a central vein. Early recognition of these conditions may prevent unexpected bleeding problems during the procedure. In addition, in those patients having had multiple previous central lines, preoperative

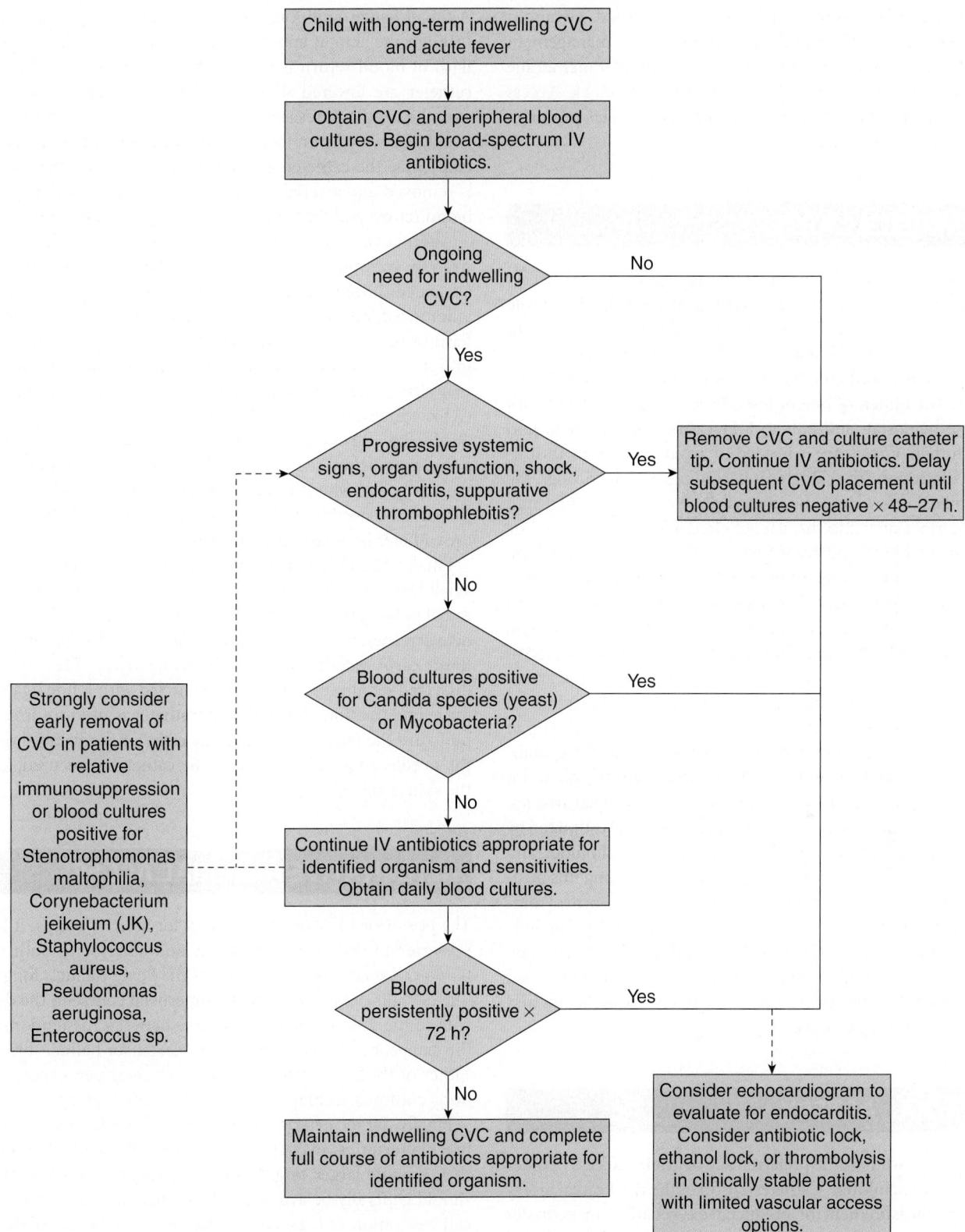

**FIGURE 9-9** Treatment algorithm for central line associated bloodstream infection (CLABSI) in the patient with a long-term indwelling central venous catheter (CVC), emphasizing effective treatment of the infection and preservation of vascular access.

venous duplex ultrasonography may be quite useful to more accurately assess the degree of patency of a particular central vein. Intraoperative ultrasound and fluoroscopy may guide safer catheter placement. Most of all, detailed attention to the insertion technique can often prevent these serious potential complications.

## ARTERIAL ACCESS

Arterial catheters facilitate care of the most critically ill children. They permit continuous monitoring of blood pressure, serial blood gas measurement, and access for blood sampling.

They are most useful for patients who need advanced mechanical ventilation, infusions of inotropes, management of elevated intracranial pressures, extracorporeal membrane oxygenation (ECMO), and resuscitation from shock. Access is most commonly obtained at the umbilical, radial, posterior tibial, or femoral arteries.

## UMBILICAL ARTERY

Neonates less than 10 days old may have arterial access through one of the paired umbilical arteries. Under sterile conditions, the umbilical stump is divided 0.5 to 1 cm from the skin. The umbilical arteries are located along the inferior aspect of the cord on either side of the midline urachal remnant. The lumen of one of the arteries is gently dilated with a fine hemostat, and a 3- to 5-Fr catheter is advanced into the lumen. Great care is needed to avoid creation of an intimal dissection. The catheter is passed retrograde through the umbilical artery, into the internal iliac artery, and then into the aorta. Entry into the arterial circulation is recognized by return of blood and transduction of an arterial waveform. The catheter is sutured in place, and a radiograph is obtained to confirm placement. If placement in one of the umbilical arteries is unsuccessful, placement in the other artery should be attempted. If the umbilical artery is unable to be dilated in the umbilical cord, it may be preferable to access the artery through an infraumbilical skin incision and dissection in the space of Retzius. A low umbilical artery catheter (tip at L3-L5) is estimated by 60% of the distance from the umbilicus to the shoulder, and has a hypothetical advantage of not interfering with perfusion of the mesenteric or renal arteries. A high umbilical artery catheter (tip at T6-T9) is estimated by 110% of the distance from the umbilicus to the shoulder, and has a lower incidence of arterial vasospasm, making this position preferable for the smallest premature newborns. Complications of umbilical artery catheters are rare, but include infection, thrombosis, hemorrhage, and distal embolization. Neonates with high umbilical artery catheters should be fed cautiously because of concerns of mesenteric ischemia and necrotizing enterocolitis.

## RADIAL ARTERY

The radial artery is the preferred site of arterial access in older infants and children. Catheterization of the right radial artery allows measurement of preductal oxygenation in neonates with significant flow across a patent ductus arteriosus. Radial artery catheters are placed percutaneously in larger infants or children or by cutdown in smaller infants. The radial pulse is palpable at the wrist between the styloid process of the radius and the flexor carpi radialis muscle tendon. An Allen test is performed to be certain that the ulnar artery supplies the deep palmar arch, and thus the hand should remain perfused with a catheter in the radial artery. The hand is then secured with a roll behind the wrist, creating 45° of dorsiflexion.

For percutaneous insertion, the surgeon palpates the radial pulse proximal to the anticipated point of insertion.

A small-gauge angiocatheter (24 or 22 gauge) is inserted through the skin at approximately 30° to 45° angle. When a flash of blood return is seen in the catheter, the needle and catheter are lowered slightly, and the catheter is advanced over the needle. If resistance is encountered, the catheter and needle are withdrawn together, to avoid shearing of the catheter. Once the catheter is advanced in the artery, the needle is removed and arterial placement is confirmed with arterial blood return and transduction of an arterial waveform.

Alternative techniques for placement include the transfixation technique, whereby the catheter and needle are advanced through-and-through the radial artery. The needle is removed, and the catheter is withdrawn gradually until a flash of blood returns. The catheter is then gently advanced into the lumen of the artery. A modified Seldinger technique may also be used, either with a needle-wire-catheter assembly (Arrow International, Reading, PA), or with a small butterfly needle (having cut away the phlebotomy tubing) followed by a fine guidewire. The needle is advanced into the lumen of the artery, and when blood returns, the guidewire is advanced through the needle. With the wire in the lumen of the artery, the catheter is advanced over the wire.

Finally, the radial artery may be accessed by cutdown. A small transverse incision is made in a skin fold overlying the radial pulse at the wrist. Blunt dissection with a fine hemostat between the tendons of the abductor pollicis longus and the flexor carpi radialis identifies the radial artery. The artery is dissected circumferentially and encircled with a fine ligature for gentle traction. A small angiocatheter is used to directly puncture the radial artery, and the catheter is advanced over the needle under direct vision. The catheter is secured, and the skin is closed.

## ALTERNATIVE ARTERIAL ACCESS

The posterior tibial artery is useful for arterial access. It lies posterior to the medial malleolus and anterior to both the tendo calcaneus and the tendon of the flexor hallucis longus. The dorsalis pedis artery runs a superficial course in the dorsum of the foot. Its pulse is palpable between the tendons of the extensor hallucis longus and the extensor hallucis brevis. Either of these two arteries may be accessed percutaneously or by cutdown, as may be done for the radial artery.

Finally, larger arteries, such as the femoral, axillary, and brachial arteries, may be used for arterial access. Although they provide larger targets for percutaneous insertion, they should generally be avoided unless other sites have failed, as catheterization of these larger arteries carries a risk of distal embolization.

### SELECTED READINGS

Abboud PA, Kendall JL. Ultrasound guidance for vascular access. *Emerg Med Clin North Am* 2004;22(3):749–773.

Bonventre EV, Lally KP, Chwals WJ, Hardin WD, Atkinson JB. Percutaneous insertion of subclavian venous catheters in infants and children. *Surg Gynecol Obstet* 1989;169:203–205.

Broviac JW, Cole JJ, Scribner BH. A silicone rubber atrial catheter for prolonged parenteral alimentation. *Surg Gynecol Obstet* 1973;136(4): 602–606.

Cilley RE. Arterial access in infants and children. *Semin Pediatr Surg* 1992; 1(3):174–180.

Cobb LM, Vinocur CD, Wagner CW, Weintraub WH. The central venous anatomy in infants. *Surg Gynecol Obstet* 1987;165:230–234.

Filston HC, Grant JP. A safer system for percutaneous subclavian venous catheterization in newborn infants. *J Pediatr Surg* 1979;14:564.

Hind D, Calvert N, McWilliams R, et al. Ultrasonic locating devices for central venous cannulation: meta-analysis. *BMJ* 2003;327:361–367.

La Quaglia MP, Caldwell C, Lucas A, et al. A prospective randomized double-blind trial of bolus urokinase in the treatment of established Hickman catheter sepsis in children. *J Pediatr Surg* 1994;29(6):742–745.

Loughran SC, Borzatta M. Peripherally inserted central catheters: a report of 2506 catheter days. *J Parent Ent Nutr* 1995;19:133–136.

Maecken T, Grau T. Ultrasound imaging in vascular access. *Crit Care Med* 2007;35(5 suppl):S178–S185.

Marschall J, Mermel LA, Classen D, et al. Strategies to prevent central line-associated bloodsteam infections in acute care hospitals [published erratum in *Infect Control Hosp Epidemiol* 2009 Aug;30(8):815]. *Infect Control Hosp Epidemiol* 2008;29(suppl 1):S22–S30.

Mermel LA, Allon M, Bouza E, et al. Clinical practice guidelines for the diagnosis and management of intravascular catheter-related infection: 2009 Update by the Infectious Diseases Society of America [published erratum appears in *Clin Infect Dis* 2010;50(3):457 and *Clin Infect Dis* 2010;50(7):1079]. *Clin Infect Dis* 2009;49(1):1–45.

Seldinger SI. Catheter replacement of the needle in percutaneous arteriography; a new technique. *Acta Radiol* 1953;39(5):368–376.

Silvestre ME, Abecasis F, Veiga-Pires JA, eds. *Pioneers in Angiography*. New York: Elsevier Science Publishers (Biomedical Division); 1987.

Statter MB. Peripheral and central venous access. *Semin Pediatr Surg* 1992;1(3):181–187.

Tobias JD, Ross AK. Intraosseous infusions: a review for the anesthesiologist with a focus on pediatric use. *Anesth Analg* 2010;110(2):391–401.

Verghese ST, McGill WA, Patel RI, et al. Ultrasound-guided internal jugular venous cannulation in infants. *Anesthesiology* 1999;91:71–77.

Whitman ED. Complications associated with the use of central venous access devices. *Curr Prob Surg* 1996;33(4):309–388.

Wiener ES. Catheter sepsis: the central venous line Achilles' heel. *Semin Pediatr Surg* 1995;4(4):207–214.

# Pediatric Anesthesia and Analgesia

# CHAPTER 10

*Alan Bielsky and David M. Polaner*

## KEY POINTS

1. Analgesic dosing is administered to perioperative children based on age-specific pain assessment scoring.

2. Analgesics available to children include all dosage routes, specific drug concentrations, and dosing frequencies based on pediatric age-specific drug distribution and utilization differences.

3. Regional anesthetic techniques can often be combined with perioperative analgesics, assuring continued pain control well into the postoperative period.

4. Use of the patient-controlled analgesia (PCA) is both effective and safe in pediatric pain control.

5. Clear fluids administered PO in healthy infants and children 3 to 4 hours before the induction of general anesthesia is safe.

6. The uptake of inhalational anesthetics occurs more rapidly in children than in adults.

## GOALS OF PEDIATRIC ANESTHESIA

The goals of pediatric anesthesia are to maintain physiological homeostasis, providing analgesia (elimination of the sensation of pain), amnesia (loss of memory), and akinesia (absence of movement) during the operative procedure.

## ANESTHETIC RISKS

Complications associated with anesthesia in children are numerous. They can include sore throat, dental damage, nausea and vomiting, aspiration, drug reactions or anaphylaxis, dysrhythmias, and unanticipated intraoperative crises (eg, airway, bleeding) that could cause further morbidity and even death.

The American Society of Anesthesiologist (ASA) Physical Status Classification provides a means to describe and stratify the patient's preoperative physical condition. It is not a risk assessment system and has never been validated as such, but rather is designed to concisely describe the health status of the patient prior to the induction of anesthesia. There are 6 categories within this classification system: I, healthy patient; II, mild systemic disease with no functional limitations; III, severe systemic disease with definite functional limitation; IV, severe systemic disease that is a constant threat to life; V, moribund patient who is not expected to survive 24 hours with or without surgery; and VI, brain-dead patient who is an organ donor. A classification of "E" is added to any of the above categories if the surgical procedure is emergent. The rate of complications may increase with ASA scores III and above and the number and nature of coexisting diseases. There may also be an increased rate of complications for emergency procedures, and when the duration of preoperative fasting was less than 8 hours.

A study beginning in 1954 and reflecting more than 150,000 patients from 0 to 20 years of age indicated a mortality of 1.8/10,000 in the 0- to 10-year age range from 1954 to 1966 and decreasing to 0.8/10,000 in the same age range from 1966 to 1978. From 1966 to 1978, the mortality was 0.6/10,000 in the 10- to 20-year age range. In the current era, anesthetic mortality in adults has been estimated to have decreased an additional order of magnitude, but good pediatric data are still lacking. Although studies have placed the perioperative mortality risk at 0.2 to 1.8/10,000, these numbers reflect the unstratified increased risk, including infants with congenital heart disease, pulmonary hypertension, and various congenital anomalies, and do not accurately reflect anesthetic-specific mortality. It is evident from the data that age less than 30 days or the presence of congenital heart disease may significantly increase risk of perioperative cardiac arrest and other complications. The risks associated with regional anesthetics in children appear to be very small, even though these blocks are generally placed when children are under general anesthesia. Data from the 2 Association of French Speaking Paediatric Anaesthetists (ADARPEF) studies in France, the Association of Paediatric Anaesthetists of Great Britain and Ireland audit of epidural anesthesia, and the Pediatric Regional Anesthesia Network in the United States demonstrate that long-term complications are extremely rare (<1:10,000). The risk of anesthesia for infants less than 1 year old in the hands of pediatric anesthesiologists is decreased toward that of adults. Overall, their rate of cardiac arrest for infants less than 1 year old is significantly less than that of nonpediatric anesthesiologists. There is a higher incidence of respiratory complications in preterm and former preterm infants (ie, apnea, atelectasis, aspiration, and postextubation stridor) in the perianesthetic period than among full-term infants. The causes and treatment of these respiratory complications are discussed in the section on postanesthetic care and postoperative follow-up.

## Malignant Hyperthermia

Malignant hyperthermia (MH) is an inherited muscle disorder unmasked by exposure to volatile anesthetics and succinylcholine that results in a hypermetabolic state due to sustained muscle contraction. Normally, a reduction in myoplasmic concentration of calcium initiates muscle relaxation. In MH, because the RyR1 channels remain in a mostly open state, intramyoplasmic calcium accumulates at an accelerated rate and calcium removal pumps are overwhelmed. The resulting accelerated metabolism leads to increased oxygen consumption and increased carbon dioxide and heat production.

MH events occur in 1 in 15,000 children and 1 in 40,000 adults. It is seen most commonly between the ages of 3 and 30 years. When trauma cases are eliminated, there is an equal male-to-female ratio.

The genetic transmission of MH was initially thought to be autosomal dominant. However, because there is a variable clinical expression of this disease state, heterogeneity is more likely. There are now 3 recognized modes of inheritance (autosomal dominant, autosomal recessive, and multifactorial). Chromosome 19 has been linked to MH. A child with a first-degree relative with a history of MH should be treated as susceptible, and should receive a nontriggering anesthetic.

The clinical presentation of MH is variable, but often the earliest clues are signs of increased metabolism, most evident by an unexplained rise in exhaled carbon dioxide, or masseter muscle spasm (trismus) following the use of a depolarizing muscle relaxant (ie, succinylcholine). Estimates of the progression from masseter spasm to true MH crisis range from 30% to 50%. In a full triggering episode, tachypnea, tachycardia, unstable blood pressure, cyanotic, mottled, and/or diaphoretic skin, and generalized muscle rigidity soon ensue. The precipitous elevation of temperature, for which the condition is named and which can easily exceed 43°C, is frequently not the initial finding. In addition, rhabdomyolysis and subsequent myoglobinuria occur, and can produce renal injury if not anticipated and promptly treated. This hypermetabolic state leads to hypoxia, hypercarbia, and a concomitant respiratory and metabolic acidosis. Ventricular arrhythmias and electrolyte abnormalities may follow.

A second type of clinical presentation similar to MH involves sudden generalized muscle rigidity and cardiac arrest and/or a volatile anesthetic agent. There is an immediate increase in serum potassium with concomitant rhabdomyolysis and myoglobinuria. Recent research has now classified this as anesthesia-associated rhabdomyolysis, and is found typically in patients with preexisting myopathies.

Late complications of MH included renal failure, hepatic failure, pulmonary edema, disseminated intravascular coagulation, and neurologic damage ranging from seizures to coma to even death.

MH can occur after exposure to any of the volatile anesthetic agents (ie, sevoflurane, isoflurane, and desflurane) with or without the concomitant use of succinylcholine. Recrudescences can occur after successful initial treatment. Laboratory evaluation may reveal hyperkalemia, hypoxemia, hypercarbia, respiratory and metabolic acidosis, myoglobinuria, and increased creatine phosphokinase (CPK). A preoperative elevation of CPK can be seen in approximately one third of MH susceptible patients.

Treatment for the patient with a suspected MH episode is multifaceted. The first step is to discontinue all potential triggering agents (depolarizing muscle relaxants, volatile anesthetic agents) and call for help. The patient should be hyperventilated with 100% oxygen, and the surgical procedure should be concluded as soon as possible.

Dantrolene is the only drug effective for the treatment of MH. Dantrolene dissociates the excitation–contraction coupling of actin and myosin in muscle by inhibiting the release of calcium from the sarcoplasmic reticulum. It acts specifically on skeletal muscle without any clinical effect on cardiac or smooth muscle. Dantrolene is given intravenously as a 2.5 mg/kg bolus, followed by 1 to 2 mg/kg until the patient's symptoms are controlled. The dose is repeated every 6 hours and tapered over the next 24 to 72 hours.

The patient should be observed in the intensive care unit. Acid–base imbalance can be corrected with sodium bicarbonate. Hyperkalemia can be corrected with insulin and glucose, calcium, sodium polystyrene sulfonate, sodium bicarbonate, and furosemide. Temperature control methods include chilled intravenous fluids, surface cooling, stomach, bladder, rectal, and/or surgical wound lavage. Furosemide and mannitol can be used to increase urine output in an effort to prevent renal failure, which can be precipitated by myoglobinuria. Dysrhythmias are ultimately controlled by decreasing serum potassium levels, but can also be treated with lidocaine or procainamide.

An arterial line should be placed to monitor beat-to-beat variations in blood pressure as well as to sample blood for pH, $Paco_2$, $Pao_2$, electrolytes, CPK, and a coagulation profile. A urinary catheter provides a means to measure urine output, to detect myoglobinuria, and to assist in central cooling (via lavage) when necessary.

If a MH-susceptible patient is to be anesthetized, a nontriggering anesthetic technique (ie, no volatile anesthetics or succinylcholine) must be used. An anesthesia machine should have its vaporizers removed or disabled. The machine should be flushed with high-flow oxygen for 15 minutes to eliminate the possibility of any residual volatile agents, or filters containing a resin that removes residual vapor should be placed on both inspiratory and expiratory limbs of the breathing circuit.

In addition to patients with a known history of MH, patients with known muscle diseases such as Becker muscular dystrophy, central core disease, King-Denborough syndrome, myotonia congenita, Schwartz-Jampel syndrome, and other muscular dystrophies are susceptible to a hyperkalemic response to succinylcholine that can mimic MH.

The Malignant Hyperthermia Association of the United States (MHAUS) can provide counseling via a 24-hour-a-day hotline.

## Latex Sensitivity

Latex sensitivity involves an IgE-mediated anaphylactic reaction in latex-sensitized patients on exposure to latex antigen. Typical contact points involve the skin or mucous membranes such as the mouth, eyes, genitals, bladder, or rectum.

There are numerous risk factors for developing latex sensitivity. These include coexisting atopy and/or multiple allergies, associated allergies to kiwi, banana, avocado, and other fruits, prolonged or frequent exposure to latex products (ie, healthcare workers with glove exposure, patients status post-multiple surgical procedures). In pediatrics, latex sensitivity is most commonly seen in patients with neural tube defects (ie, myelomeningocele, spina bifida), and patients with congenital urologic abnormalities (who require recurrent instrumentation of the genitourinary tract) or a history of balloon or glove intolerance. Diagnostic testing is not necessary for patients with a positive history.

Most children's hospitals have removed latex-containing products from their inventories, and this practice is highly advisable. Gloves, catheters, tourniquets, elastic bandages, ace wraps, intravenous tubing injection ports, medication stopper vials, adhesive tape, bandaids, syringe plungers, rubber bands, Penrose drains, instrument mats, rubber-shod clamps, vascular tags, and bulb syringes for irrigation all may contain latex, but latex-free alternatives are readily available.

Perioperatively, latex anaphylaxis may have numerous signs and symptoms. Onset is usually 20 to 60 minutes after exposure to antigen. Signs and symptoms may include urticaria, flushing, diaphoresis, hypotension, tachycardia, perioral edema, periorbital edema, and bronchospasm. Initial treatment involves the discontinuation of all latex product use. The presence of powder in gloves may help to transmit the latex antigen. After all latex-containing products are removed from the patient's immediate environment, the patient should be given 100% oxygen. All anesthetic agents should be discontinued, and the patient's intravascular volume should be maintained. Epinephrine can be given as needed in doses of 0.5 to 2 µg/kg/dose. Secondary treatment involves the use of corticosteroids (Solu-Medrol, 1-2 mg/kg), antihistamines (diphenhydramine, 0.5-1.0 mg/kg), catecholamine infusions (epinephrine, 0.05-0.1 µm/kg/min), aminophylline infusion or albuterol nebulizer, ranitidine (1 mg/kg), and/or sodium bicarbonate (0.5-1 mEq/kg).

## PREOPERATIVE EVALUATION

### Patient History

The pediatric history should begin with a birth history to determine whether the child was full-term or premature (less than 37 weeks postconceptual age) and whether there were any perinatal complications. Postconceptual age at the time of the planned operation should be determined. A history of apnea of prematurity, bronchopulmonary dysplasia, mechanical ventilation and intubation, and/or intraventricular hemorrhage is especially important to elicit. Infants born prematurely have an increased risk of apnea following exposure to general anesthetics of any type, even if there was no prior history of apnea of prematurity. The etiology is postulated to be due to immaturity of central ventilatory control. The risk is estimated to be between 10% and 20% for children less than 60 weeks postconceptual age, and thus these children should be admitted overnight for apnea monitoring. Anemia (hemoglobin <10 g/dL) has been reported to increase the risk of postanesthetic apnea. The use of spinal anesthesia for these children has been reported to reduce the risk of apnea, but carefully controlled studies are lacking. Caffeine (10 mg/kg before surgery and continued for 24 hours afterward) has also been demonstrated to reduce the incidence of postanesthetic apnea in ex-premature infants by acting as a central ventilator stimulant, the same mechanism by which it reduces apnea of prematurity. There are no data at all in term infants; many centers admit term infants less than 4 weeks of age for monitoring, although these practices are not evidence-based. Elective operations in ex-premature infants are best postponed, if possible, until after the child reaches 60 weeks postconceptual age. As always, a thorough history of prior hospitalizations and surgical procedures should be obtained in an effort to determine whether there were any anesthetic problems, and a review of prior anesthetic records is very informative.

Data in the last decade from animal experiments and some retrospective data in humans have raised concerns that exposure to general anesthetics in infancy might lead to neurodevelopmental problems in later childhood. At this time, the findings are somewhat in conflict and several long-term, prospective randomized trials are underway to try and elicit more conclusive information. While these data are concerning and suggest that elective procedures requiring general anesthesia might best be postponed until at least past infancy, it is certainly prudent to make the decision about surgery primarily based on the need and optimal timing of the operation.

Effects of anesthesia can include decreased respiratory muscle activity, depressed ciliary clearance, depression of the central respiratory response to hypoxia and hypercarbia, and decreased lung volumes and increased intrapulmonary shunting. Therefore, the presence of any respiratory diseases (ie, asthma, bronchopulmonary dysplasia, chest wall deformities) can increase the risk of anesthetic complications. Obstructive sleep apnea and sleep-disordered breathing are increasing in incidence, and can affect the responses to opioids as well as general anesthetics and sedatives.

Concurrent medical illnesses must be determined before surgery. Active upper respiratory infection might demand postponement of elective surgery, but this is dependent on the severity and time course of the illness, the presence or absence of underlying conditions of the patient, and the nature of the operation and anesthetic. If the patient is afebrile and nontoxic, and the illness is mild, then the child should be considered for elective surgery, although increased risks of laryngospasm, desaturation, and prolonged postoperative oxygen requirement may still exist. The laryngeal mask airway has been shown to produce less airway stimulation than an endotracheal tube, and may be preferable in this situation if it can be used safely for the operation.

The pediatric preoperative history must also elicit the presence or absence of conditions such as diabetes, a history of seizures, gastroesophageal reflux, heart disease (ie, history of a murmur, cyanosis, and/or surgery), and/or sickle cell disease or other hematological abnormalities. These conditions necessitate that the patient be medically optimized before elective surgery. Anatomic anomalies can complicate airway management, and may preclude the use of regional anesthetics.

To complete the pediatric patient history, allergies to known drugs and/or latex, current medications the patient is taking, and NPO status should be listed in the patient's chart.

## Family History

Preoperative evaluation of the pediatric patient must also include a pertinent family history. Unusual reactions to surgery or anesthesia in blood relatives of the patient should be listed. If a family history of MH is elicited, then the patient's family should be queried as to how the diagnosis was made (ie, muscle biopsy). Parents with sickle cell disease or trait or thalassemia should explain the extent of their disease and whether or not their child has been tested. Atypical pseudocholinesterase, a rare inherited trait, will cause prolonged paralysis after the administration of succinylcholine or mivacurium for neuromuscular blockade. Any neuromuscular disorders in parents or blood relatives may alter the anesthetic plan for the pediatric patient. In particular, a history of muscular dystrophy, myopathic disease, or unexplained death of a male child in infancy should preclude the use of succinylcholine.

## Physical Exam

The physical examination of the pediatric patient before surgery includes a focused evaluation of the airway, dentition, cardiovascular and respiratory systems, potential block sites, and the patient's neurological status and deficits.

Loose or missing teeth should be noted before instrumentation of the patient's airway. Anatomic abnormalities, including limited range of motion of the neck and jaw, may make airway instrumentation difficult or call for special techniques such as fiberoptic intubation. The presence of wheezing, rales, and/or rhonchi may increase the risk of anesthetic complications.

If cardiac auscultation reveals a murmur, its etiology must be determined. Innocent or functional murmurs are audible in nearly 25% of children at one time or another. These murmurs are soft blowing systolic ejection murmurs of less than 3/6 intensity with normal first and second heart sounds, and are heard in children with normal exercise tolerance who are acyanotic, and growing normally. However, the presence of an abnormal murmur, cyanosis, decreased exercise tolerance, poor weight gain, diaphoresis with feeding, decreased femoral pulses, or a precordial heave necessitates a preoperative evaluation by a pediatric cardiologist.

## Laboratory Evaluation

Unless a physical exam or history suggests otherwise, routine preoperative laboratory evaluation is not necessary for most pediatric patients. Laboratory evaluation of the pediatric patient scheduled for surgery should only be done to detect targeted significant physiological abnormalities that may impact the child in the perioperative period.

The incidence of previously undetected anemia in children presenting for elective surgery is extremely low (0.29%). A hemoglobin level of 10 g/dL is a safe level for the performance of major surgery in the otherwise healthy patient. There is no documented minimum hemoglobin level that provides for the safe administration of anesthesia.

Patients who are at risk for severe and/or physiologically debilitating anemia should be tested. These patients include premature infants, patients with chronic disease who demonstrate any signs or symptoms suggestive of anemia, children whose surgery may result in any considerable blood loss, and patients with hemoglobinopathies (ie, thalassemia, sickle cell disease).

There is an increasing rate of sexual activity among younger adolescents. Anesthetic medications can increase the incidence of spontaneous abortion and are potential teratogens. The female adolescent patient should be queried as to her sexual activity as well as whether or not she has begun her menses. Given all these factors, preoperative urine pregnancy tests are performed routinely for all postmenarchal girls at many centers. If this is not standard policy, it should be considered after the patient and family have been informed of the potential risks if the test is positive.

## NPO Status

Prolonged fasting is not necessary for the normal healthy child. Clear fluid ingestion on the day of surgery improves the child's preoperative experience and behavior and decreases the child's thirst and hunger. Clear fluids consumed 2 hours before the induction of anesthesia have no adverse effect on residual gastric fluid volume in healthy children and therefore do not increase the risk of pulmonary aspiration. Prolonged fasting may be detrimental in allowing continued undiluted secretion of gastric acid. Clear fluids may therefore dilute gastric acid secretions and, by stimulating gastric emptying, provide a beneficial effect.

Preoperative feeding instructions should begin with the cessation of all food 8 hours before induction of anesthesia. This includes solid food, candy, chewing gum, milk, milk products, formula, orange juice, and orange juice containing pulp. Breast-feeding may continue up to 4 hours prior to the scheduled surgery time. Breast milk passes from the stomach faster than formula but slower than clear liquids. Cow's milk and soy-based infant formulas empty somewhat faster than solids, and can be offered up to 6 hours prior to anesthetic induction.

All patients presenting for emergency surgery must be assumed to have a full stomach regardless of the NPO status. The anesthetic management should proceed as if the child has a full stomach. Other patients at risk for aspiration of gastric contents during general anesthesia include pregnant patients, obese patients, patients with esophageal disease, patients with GI obstruction, and those with a history of emesis during induction of anesthesia. In addition, children with increased intracranial pressure, premature infants, and those who are heavily sedated or have preexisting gastroesophageal reflux are also at increased risk for aspiration.

# PREOPERATIVE PREPARATION

## Premedication Goals

There are often multiple reasons for the administration of preoperative medications to the pediatric patient. Anxiety should be reduced in the child, which often leads to a reduction in parental anxiety. This will help to facilitate the separation of the child from the parents and can also aid in the acceptance of a face mask for the induction of anesthesia or an intravenous cannula for induction. Preoperative analgesics can help to decrease the pain from an injury or disease and/or ease the transition from the stretcher to the operating bed. Blockade of detrimental autonomic (vagal) reflexes and a decrease in airway secretions can be provided by preoperative medications, but is not routinely required. A decrease in the volume and acidity of gastric contents (aspiration prophylaxis) and subacute bacterial endocarditis prophylaxis can also be part of the patient's preoperative preparation.

## Premedications for Sedation

The ideal premedicant should have a rapid onset, short duration, painless administration, reliable sedation, and be associated with little or no respiratory compromise. Premedications to decrease separation anxiety are usually unnecessary in healthy infants less than 8 months old. Sedative premedications should also be avoided or used at reduced dosage in children with central nervous system disease (ie, abnormal central ventilatory control mechanisms, hypoventilation, and increased intracranial pressure) or airway abnormalities. Sedative premedications can be administered via multiple routes.

## Oral

Midazolam is the most commonly administered oral premedication for children. It is a short-acting benzodiazepine with an oral dose of 0.25 to 0.5 mg/kg PO, with a maximum dose of 15 mg. If the commercial oral preparation is not available, the intravenous solution can be used for oral administration but contains the preservative benzyl alcohol, which has a bitter taste. It must therefore be mixed with a flavored syrup or with acetaminophen to mask the taste. The drug produces a calm, cooperative child who will accept a mask induction. After oral administration, sedation usually occurs within 10 to 15 minutes and lasts approximately 30 minutes. Respiratory depression can occur when midazolam is given concurrently with narcotics, but is uncommon when used as a sole agent in the aforementioned doses.

Diazepam, another benzodiazepine, can also be given orally in doses of 0.1 to 0.3 mg/kg PO. Its main disadvantage is its long duration of action. It is similar to midazolam in its ability to cause respiratory depression when given with narcotics.

Ketamine is a phencyclidine derivative that provides amnesia and intense analgesia. It has a reliable and fast onset, usually within 5 to 10 minutes, producing a dissociative state in which the eyes remain open but the patient is noncommunicative. Oral dose is typically 5 mg/kg. Ketamine is a sympathetic nervous system stimulant and can cause an increase in both heart rate and blood pressure. Cerebral metabolic rate for oxygen, intracranial pressure, and intraocular pressure can also be increased. Copious secretions can occur with its use, and concomitant use of an antisialagogue is suggested. Its use is contraindicated in children with an active upper respiratory infection because it may add further to an irritable airway and lead to laryngospasm. Emergence delirium consisting of vivid dreams and hallucinations after ketamine use can be prevented by the addition of a benzodiazepine at the time of the ketamine administration. Ketamine is not commonly used, and is generally reserved for the most combative and uncooperative children.

## Nasal

The nasal route is less traumatic than intramuscular. The intravenous preparation of midazolam can be given by the nasal route in doses of 0.25 to 0.5 mg/kg. Although the onset may be more rapid than the oral route, it produces significant burning on administration, thus the oral route is usually preferred.

Ketamine is also effective intranasally in doses of 1 to 5 mg/kg. Its nasal administration is better tolerated than that of midazolam.

## Intramuscular

Intramuscular premedications should be used as the last resort, only after other routes are found to be unavailable or contraindicated. Their use is generally limited to combative or otherwise uncooperative children. Opioids, benzodiazepines, and ketamine can be given intramuscularly, with the latter 2 most commonly used in combination. The child must be monitored closely for any evidence of respiratory depression after administration.

Ketamine is administered intramuscularly at a dose of 3 to 5 mg/kg, using the most concentrated preparation available. Midazolam (0.05 mg/kg) and glycopyrrolate (1-2 mcg/kg) can be mixed in the same syringe and administered simultaneously.

## Parental Presence in the Induction Area

The induction of anesthesia can be stressful for the child. Parental presence in the induction area during induction for children greater than a year of age may provide some benefits. These include avoiding separation distress and possibly decreasing long-term behavior problems after surgery and minimizing the need for preoperative premedication, as well as a significant increase in parental satisfaction with the perioperative experience. However, not all parents, especially those who are highly anxious themselves, are able to calm an anxious child in this situation, and in very rare circumstances they may be disruptive. In order for this intervention to be most effective, the parent must be instructed in what to expect, how to best aid their child (distraction, singing, and telling stories are much more effective than simple comforting talk), and that they will be escorted from the induction area as soon as the child loses consciousness or if any complications develop.

Neonates and children who are critically ill during the induction of anesthesia require great vigilance and rapid responses to their changing clinical course. Therefore, parental presence during induction is not recommended.

## ANESTHETIC MANAGEMENT

### Mask Induction

Mask induction is performed for most elective pediatric operations in the United States. This avoids the trauma of starting an intravenous line and, in addition, produces vasodilation, making intravenous cannula placement easier. Mask induction is also of benefit in the patient with a difficult airway because it is easier to maintain spontaneous ventilation.

Inhalational anesthetics consist of the potent inhalational anesthetics (volatile agents) and nitrous oxide. The volatile agents are in a liquid state at room temperature and require an agent-specific vaporizer for delivery. These agents are capable of providing amnesia, analgesia, and some muscle relaxation. All the inhalational agents will depress ventilation in a dose-dependent manner. Tidal volume decreases with some increase in respiratory rate. In addition, the patient's ventilatory response to hypoxemia is depressed by the inhalational anesthetics.

In general, the uptake of inhalational anesthetics occurs more rapidly in children than in adults because of increased respiratory rates and cardiac index and a greater proportional distribution of cardiac output to vessel-rich organs.

Sevoflurane produces a smooth and rapid mask induction. Its pleasant odor is tolerated without associated coughing and/or laryngospasm. It can be used for both induction and maintenance of anesthesia; however, it has been associated with a higher incidence of emergence agitation than other volatile agents. Sevoflurane does decrease the activity of respiratory muscles, although spontaneous ventilation is usually well preserved.

Nitrous oxide is a weak inhalation anesthetic with a very low blood gas solubility, which provides for a rapid onset and elimination. It is nearly odorless and does not irritate the airways. After approximately 3 to 5 minutes of inhalation with 70% nitrous oxide, most children become somewhat sedated and euphoric, and will better tolerate the introduction of a volatile agent, although dysphoria and activation can occasionally be seen. Nitrous oxide has analgesic properties, and may be used to facilitate the placement of an intravenous cannula with local anesthesia in a child in whom a full inhalation induction is contraindicated or not desired. Nitrous oxide has minimal myocardial or respiratory depression but may increase pulmonary artery pressure. Because it is typically delivered in concentrations of 60% to 70%, it is contraindicated in those patients with a need for high inspired oxygen concentration. It is also contraindicated in the presence of air contained in closed body spaces (ie, pneumothorax, bowel obstruction) because it is capable of rapidly diffusing into air spaces and causing expansion.

### Intravenous Induction

Intravenous induction is fast, reliable, and safe. It is used less often than other methods because most children are fearful of receiving a "shot" (intravenous catheter placement).

Propofol provides a more rapid awakening with less postoperative side effects than other intravenous induction agents, and, due to its antiemetic properties, is also associated with less postoperative nausea and vomiting (PONV). Its high first-pass hepatic degradation provides for a rapid return to consciousness. A decrease in blood pressure can be seen as a result of its ability to decrease both cardiac output and systemic vascular resistance. Propofol can be used as a continuous infusion in combination with opioids with or without nitrous oxide as a total intravenous anesthetic, but it has no analgesic properties on its own. In addition, it is useful for brief and repeated anesthetics needed for radiotherapy. A continuous infusion is also a useful technique for anesthetizing children undergoing radiologic procedures. Propofol is painful on injection when given through a peripheral vein. This can be diminished by using a larger antecubital vein or by infusing lidocaine prior to the induction dose.

Thiopental is infrequently used in the United States, due to both its very long elimination half-life and limited availability. It is a highly lipid-soluble barbiturate that is capable of crossing the blood–brain barrier quickly and inducing unconsciousness within 30 seconds. Its rapid redistribution provides for early awakening after a single dose. Thiopental can decrease both cardiac output and systemic vascular resistance, leading to a fall in blood pressure with induction. It is contraindicated in patients who are hypovolemic or those with depressed cardiac function. Like all barbiturates, it has no analgesic effects.

Etomidate is a desirable intravenous induction agent when hemodynamic stability is essential. It has a relative lack of cardiovascular side effects producing little or no change in stroke volume, cardiac output, or contractility. Sympathetic nervous system tone is also preserved, so there is little effect on systemic vascular resistance. Etomidate may be a useful intravenous induction agent for the head-injured patient because it causes a decrease in intracranial pressure by decreasing cerebral blood flow and metabolic rate without decreasing cerebral perfusion pressure. It has no analgesic activity. Intravenous induction is associated with pain on injection and myoclonic movements. Etomidate has the ability to transiently suppress adrenal function for 4 to 8 hours after an induction dose, and although this has not been shown to increase morbidity and mortality repeated dosing is not recommended.

Ketamine is a phencyclidine derivative that causes central dissociation while providing analgesia and amnesia. It can provide analgesia for insertion of invasive monitoring devices before induction of anesthesia (ie, cardiac surgery) or in patients having limited intravenous access. It is often the drug of choice in children who are hypovolemic or hemodynamically unstable. Adrenergic stimulation produced by ketamine can raise the blood pressure and heart rate by releasing endogenous catecholamines, a side effect that can be used to advantage in the hemodynamically unstable child or the child with asthma, but the drug itself has negative inotropic properties. Thus, if the patient is already exhibiting maximal adrenergic drive, ketamine may produce a fall in blood pressure, and should be used with caution in the hypovolemic patient. Ketamine is contraindicated in patients with increased intracranial pressure because it is a cerebral vasodilator and also increases cerebral metabolic rate.

Emergence delirium can occur after the use of ketamine. This may consist of visual, auditory, and/or proprioceptive hallucinations, which are typically seen within 24 hours after the use of ketamine. Premedicating the patient with a benzodiazepine such as midazolam can decrease the incidence of this side effect.

## Maintenance of Anesthesia

Both inhalation and intravenous anesthetics are commonly utilized for maintenance of anesthesia, often in combination as a "balanced" anesthetic technique. While sevoflurane is often used for maintenance as well as induction, both isoflurane and desflurane have advantages that make them suitable as maintenance agents as well. Isoflurane, although not suitable for mask induction because of its irritating odor and potential for causing coughing and/or laryngospasm on induction by mask, is commonly used for anesthetic maintenance. Its primary advantages are low cost and smooth emergence. Desflurane is used after induction for maintenance of anesthesia. The main advantage of desflurane is its low solubility in blood and tissues, which permits rapid changes in anesthetic depth and rapid emergence. The low tissue solubility also is advantageous during long cases, where this characteristic results in less accumulation of the agent in the vessel-rich tissue beds. Its very pungent odor is associated with a very high incidence of coughing and laryngospasm, and it therefore should not be used for inhalational induction. The rapid emergence associated with this drug has not been shown to speed the discharge of outpatients. A wide variety of opioids are used as adjuncts to maintenance, including both long-acting agents such as morphine, hydromorphone, and methadone, and short-acting opioids such as fentanyl, sufentanil, and remifentanil. Assuming that the patient is expected to be extubated at the end of the procedure, it is important to titrate the drug to effect to avoid overdosage and permit spontaneous ventilation to resume prior to extubation.

The use of muscle relaxants ("paralyzing agents") is much less common in pediatric anesthesia than in adults, especially as an adjunct to intubation. Most infants and children can easily and safely be intubated "deep" and many operations do not require muscle relaxation. For intraabdominal and intrathoracic procedures, however, muscle relaxation often can improve operating conditions for the surgeon. In these situations, nondepolarizing relaxants are used much as they are in adult anesthesia, and similarly require reversal at the end of the case if any residual neuromuscular blockade is present. The use of a nerve stimulator to aid in dosing and to measure of adequacy of reversal is mandatory.

## Monitoring: Routine and Special

Monitoring during anesthesia and surgery is a critical and central function of the anesthesiologist. Careful and vigilant monitoring can provide early warnings of impending adverse events so that intervention can be implemented prior to catastrophic incidents. Standard monitors include a precordial or esophageal stethoscope, noninvasive automated blood pressure cuff, electrocardiogram, pulse oximeter, inspiratory and expiratory gas analyzer, and temperature. While in older children monitors are generally placed before the induction of anesthesia, in young uncooperative infants and children

it is common to begin with just a pulse oximeter and precordial stethoscope, and place the other monitors as consciousness is lost. This requires a high level of vigilance and careful observation.

Intraarterial or central venous catheters are reserved mainly for operations associated with large fluid shifts, significant blood loss, or potential for hemodynamic instability. An arterial line is also indicated for constant blood pressure monitoring in operations requiring controlled hypotension to decrease blood loss. The arterial line can also be used for frequent blood sampling, and analysis of respiratory variation in the pressure waveform has been demonstrated to be a highly reliable dynamic index of fluid responsiveness, and thus can be used to guide fluid replacement. A central venous line also provides a reliable means of administering fluids and vasoactive drugs.

## Fluid Management

The goal of perioperative fluid management is to maintain fluid homeostasis with normal organ perfusion and normal glucose and electrolyte balance. Preoperative deficits, maintenance fluids, and ongoing intraoperative third space loss and blood losses must be replaced. The endpoint of therapy is sustained normal blood pressure and heart rate, adequate tissue perfusion, and urine output of 0.5 to 1 mL/kg/h.

Preoperative fluid deficits result from fasting and can be calculated by multiplying the patient's normal fluid maintenance rate by the number of hours fasted. This calculated fluid deficit is usually replaced over the first 3 hours of surgery, with half given in the first hour. The normal fluid maintenance rate is derived from the patient's daily fluid requirement, which depends directly on metabolic demand. Specifically, 100 mL of water is required for each 100 calories of expended energy. Related to weight: 0 to 10 kg = 4 mL/kg/h, 11 to 20 kg = 40 mL/h + 2 mL/kg/h, and >20 kg = 60 mL/h + 1 mL/kg/h. It is common to give 10 mL/kg rapidly in the fasted infant or child once intravenous access is established to counteract the hemodynamic effects of anesthetic induction.

Glucose-containing solutions are not routinely used for intraoperative fluid replacement. Anesthesia decreases glucose requirements because of a decrease in the patient's metabolic rate and the stress response to surgery and anesthesia simultaneously produces an increase in serum glucose levels. Hypoglycemia is rare even in fasting children. Neonates in the first few days of life, premature infants with low glycogen stores, and those patients previously receiving parenteral nutrition are exceptions, but the glucose load should be titrated to the patient's needs and measured glucose levels.

Fluid lost during the surgical procedure can be from transudation into the interstitial space or evaporation from exposed tissues as well as from actual blood loss. The amount of fluid lost depends on the amount of tissue exposed and the degree of surgical manipulation. Fluid losses are highest in infants undergoing intestinal surgery. Suggested replacement volumes are 1 to 2 cc/kg/h for inguinal herniorrhaphy, 3 to 5 cc/kg/h for thoracic surgery, and 10 to 20 cc/kg/h for intraabdominal procedures. It is best, however, to guide replacement with a measurement of fluid deficit and responsiveness, which can be done if an arterial cannula is present and the patient is receiving positive pressure ventilation.

Blood loss may be replaced with isotonic crystalloid solutions in a ratio of 1:3 (for every 1 mL of blood loss, 3 mL of crystalloid is given). This is because all balanced salt solutions will redistribute to all active fluid compartments. Alternatively, blood loss may be replaced in a 1:1 ratio with a colloid such as albumin or blood. The maximum allowable blood loss is calculated as estimated blood volume × (starting hematocrit − target hematocrit)/(starting hematocrit). Estimated blood volumes are 100 to 120 cc/kg premature infant, 90 cc/kg full-term infant, 80 cc/kg 3 to 12 months old, and 70 cc/kg for children greater than 1 year old. Hypotonic crystalloids should not be used in the perioperative period because they promote hyponatremia, due to the increased endogenous secretion of antidiuretic hormone (ADH). Excessive use of normal saline, as opposed to balanced salt solutions, may lead to a hyperchloremic metabolic acidosis.

# POSTANESTHETIC CARE/ POSTOPERATIVE FOLLOW-UP

## Monitoring

Monitoring in the postoperative period should consist of assurance of a patent airway, adequacy of ventilation and oxygenation, and hemodynamic stability. Initial evaluation consists of obtaining the patient's heart rate and respiratory rate via auscultation. A noninvasive blood pressure cuff can be used to obtain information regarding the patient's hemodynamic status. Like in the operating room, pulse oximetry has become one of the most important monitors in the postanesthetic care unit.

## Postextubation Croup and Stridor

Postextubation croup is now relatively uncommon. Previously, it was thought that the trachea in infants and children is funnel-shaped rather than cylindrical, with the narrowest portion at the cricoid cartilage. Recent data suggest this is not so, and that the vocal cords are the narrowest point. Nevertheless, excessively tight-fitting endotracheal tubes are the cause of significant morbidity in small children. The thin mucosal and submucosal layers in the subglottis are surrounded by the cricoid ring, making this region particularly susceptible to ischemic injury from endotracheal tube compression. Transmural pressures corresponding to leak pressures of greater than 25 to 30 cm $H_2O$ can produce edema and tracheal mucosal injury, which can lead to croup and stridor in the short term, and subgottic stenosis in extreme cases in the long term.

The small diameter of the airways in infants and children increases resistance to flow. Because airway resistance is inversely proportional to the radius raised to the fourth power, a small amount of edema in a small infant airway produces a great increase in resistance and a change from laminar to turbulent flow. It is important to properly size endotracheal tubes, and if a cuffed tube is used, to choose a design specifically engineered for pediatric patients and carefully position the cuff in the mid trachea.

## Postoperative Nausea and Vomiting

PONV is one of the most common causes of delayed discharge from the postanesthesia care unit and the most common cause of unanticipated admission following out-patient surgery. The reported incidence varies very widely, in large part due to dissimilarities in study methodology. Patients undergoing strabismus surgery, middle ear surgery, intraabdominal and laparoscopic procedures, and orchidopexy have an increased risk.

Treatments include ondansetron (0.1 mg/kg IV) and dexamethasone (0.1 mg/kg IV). These are best administered prophylactically. For children especially susceptible, a total intravenous anesthetic with propofol and remifentanil may be less emetogenic than an inhalation anesthetic. The use of neural blockade for analgesia can reduce the need for opioids, which are known to increase the incidence of PONV.

# PAIN CONTROL

## Introduction

Management of acute postoperative pain management in infants and children continues to grow in both sophistication and efficacy. Improved surgical techniques have been coupled with better understanding of pharmacology, new drugs and routes of administration, and increased use of both central neuraxial and peripheral nerve blocks to improve postoperative comfort and function, and speed recovery. In the past 2 decades there has been increased recognition of analgesic needs in children, as well as an increased emphasis on the treatment of pediatric pain. Along with the obvious benefits of improved postoperative pain control, however, has come an increased risk of complications and adverse outcomes. These rare but potentially catastrophic events clearly point to the necessity of expert and judicious assessment and management of medications, sophisticated understanding of the patient's underlying conditions and developmental physiology, and coordination of care and management with the acute pain service and anesthesiologists. With this information we can provide effective and compassionate analgesic care while minimizing the risk of adverse outcomes.

## Physiologic Effects of Pain

Despite the increased emphasis on recognition and assessment of pain in children, both inadequate analgesia and inappropriate use of analgesic modalities persist even in children's hospitals. The "fifth vital sign" mandate from the Joint Commission (JCAHO), while increasing the use of pain scoring, has not necessarily improved the use of appropriate interventions to treat pain, and on a busy postoperative unit has the unintended potential to encourage the perfunctory assignment of pain scores without careful assessment of the patient. Thus, the proper use of age and cognitively appropriate scores and the assessment of the results of analgesic therapy are the cornerstones of effective analgesic treatment. A frank preoperative discussion with the child's parents and a developmentally appropriate conversation with the patient are also important to set reasonable expectations for analgesic needs, plans, and outcomes.

Inadequate analgesia has been shown to have adverse effects on multiple organ systems. Cortisol and other stress hormone levels are increased in the face of inadequate analgesia. In the postoperative patient, the catabolic state induced by these stress hormones may have an adverse effect on wound healing. A child must have adequate pain control before he can be discharged home, so inadequate analgesia can prolong the length of stay, and it can also limit or prevent the ability to participate in activities necessary for rehabilitation, such as ambulation, pulmonary toilet, and return to preoperative levels of function. Regional analgesia is reported to be most effective at blunting the stress response to surgery, but systemic opioids and clonidine have both been shown to diminish the catecholamine and the cortisol response to surgical and postsurgical stress in infants and children.

## Risks of Over- and Under-treatment

Like all therapeutic modalities, analgesics are not without their risk. Oversedation and ileus can result from excessive opioid dosing in situations where either multimodal treatment or alternative therapies are better choices. Children with obstructive sleep apnea have been shown to have increased sensitivity to opioids. This is not only due to their blunted ventilatory responses to hypercarbia and hypoxia; children with chronic intermittent hypoxemia have increased analgesic sensitivity to opioids as well, and need lower doses to achieve equipotent analgesic effects. At the opposite end of the spectrum, children who have been on long-term opioid therapy will be tolerant, and children with partial or full thickness burns over greater than 20% of their surface area will have upregulation of opioid receptors and require even more opioid than the increased doses expected due to tolerance alone. Using standard dosing schemes will likely result in under-treatment of their pain. Thus it is important to have a thorough understanding of the individual patient's underlying medical condition before prescribing an analgesic regimen so that neither over- nor underdosing occurs.

The provision of postoperative analgesia for children is most effective when it is planned and delivered as a collaborative effort between surgeon and anesthesiologist. The surgeon and anesthesiologist optimally should discuss the anticipated postoperative analgesic needs before the operation so that the anesthetic can be optimized for the postoperative analgesic plan. For example, timing of block placement (before or after the completion of the surgical procedure) can dramatically change the intraoperative anesthetic requirement. Coordination of the intraoperative and postoperative plans can result in better analgesic outcomes.

## Monitoring Postoperative Analgesia

### Pain Scales and Assessment

Assessment of pain in infants and children, and of the efficacy of analgesic management, can be more difficult than in adults.

Subjective assessment by an observer, which relies on the limitations of interpretation of behavior and vital signs, is never as accurate as a self-assessment tool, but it is an obvious necessity due to the constraints imposed by the developmental and communication limitations of preverbal or developmentally delayed children. Whenever observational pain scales are used there is a risk of misinterpreting hunger, irritability, or disorientation as pain. Thus, it is important to use pain assessment tools that are validated for a particular age and developmental state, and are designed to limit the influence of confounding factors on the pain score. In addition, it is important to actually score each parameter in the scale and not to give a "gestalt" total score based on the observer's general impression.

### Infants

Several scales are available to score pain in infants. One should note that these scoring systems rely on critical observation of behavior and facial expression, and not vital signs, which can be altered by other factors, although signs of autonomic activation, such as blood pressure and heart rate, may influence clinical decision making. The FLACC scale is an acronym for *Facial expression, Legs, Activity state, Crying, and Consolability*, and was developed for the assessment of postoperative patients; but it has also been used and validated in other settings. One assigns a score of 0 to 2 for each parameter, and sums the individual ratings to give a total score. The scale descriptors are shown in Table 10-1. The revised FLACC scale has been validated from ages 2 months to 18 years, so it can be used for older nonverbal children with developmental disabilities (see below). Once users are trained in making the observations, scoring is fairly simple and quick, making it a particularly useful tool in the clinical setting. Other observational scales such as the CHEOPS (Children's Hospital of Eastern Ontario Pain Scale) have been developed and validated for both postoperative and procedural pain, but they have somewhat more complex scoring systems and thus require both more training and time to use. The CHEOPS is often used in research studies where greater precision may be desired, but it is used by many clinicians as well and has been validated in children from 1 to 7 years of age.

### School-Aged Children

Several observational and self-reporting scales have been developed for use in younger children. In most circumstances the use of a self-reporting scale is preferable to an observational one, since pain is by definition a subjective experience, and observational measurements are, in many ways, surrogates for the patient's own assessment of their feelings and condition. If the clinician is not sure that the self-report is accurate, it can be modified with an observational score.

In addition to the CHEOPS, a modified version of the FLACC is available for use in older children. Several variations of the faces scale are available, but we prefer the modified Bieri scale because it has been best validated to correspond to the 10-point verbal numeric and visual analog scales. The child is asked to point to the face that best reflects how they feel. It is important to note that the scale is not intended to be used as an observational scale; that is, the faces are not meant to reflect the child's own facial expression. We use this scale

| TABLE 10-1 | Suggested Doses and Pharmacokinetic Data for Nonopioid Analgesics | | | |
|---|---|---|---|---|
| Drug | Route | Dosage Guidelines | Half-life | Duration |
| Acetaminophen | IV | 10 mg/kg/dose every 4 h or 15 mg/kg every 6 h, maximum dose 3000 mg/day | Neonates: 7 h[a] Children and adolescents: 3 h Adults: 2.4 h | 4-6 h |
| | PO | 10-15 mg/kg/dose every 4-6 h, maximum dose 3000 mg/day | Neonates: 2-5 h Adults: 2-3 h | 4 h |
| | PR | 40 mg/kg loading dose, followed by 20 mg/kg/dose every 6 h | | |
| Ibuprofen | PO | 4-10 mg/kg/dose every 6-8 h, maximum dose 40 mg/kg/day, no greater than 2400 mg/day | Children: 1-7 years: 1-2 h Adults: 2-4 h | 6-8 h |
| Ketorolac | IV | 0.5 mg/kg/dose every 6 h, maximum of 30 mg/dose, maximum course of 8 doses | Children: ~6 h Adults: ~5 h | 4-6 h |

[a]Currently not FDA labeled for children under 2 years of age.

in preschool- and school-aged children, especially those who have trouble giving accurate or consistent verbal numerical scores. There are some younger school-aged children who may use the verbal numerical score better in reverse (ie, 10 = no pain, 0 = worst pain imaginable) because they associate higher scores with better performance on school tests, and thus a higher score reflects feeling better. This strategy is worth trying if a child seems to have trouble reporting accurate scores with the verbal numeric scale, although there are no published data to support this tactic.

## Teenagers

Teenagers and older school-aged children can effectively use any of the adult pain scales. The most common ones are the verbal numeric scale (0 = no pain, 10 = worst pain imaginable) and the visual analog scale (a 100-mm line labeled "no pain" on the left and "worst possible pain" on the right; the patient marks the line in a spot corresponding to their level of pain).

## Developmentally Delayed Older Children

Older developmentally delayed children with cognitive impairment and an inability to express their needs present an increased challenge for assessment. An observational pain scale is necessary, and the revised FLACC has been best validated for this patient population. The revised FLACC has additional definitions that are specific to developmentally delayed children. One should remember that the child's parent can be sensitive to the subtleties of a developmentally impaired child's expressions and behavior, and they can often (but not always) provide valuable aid in making these assessments.

## Drug Research in Children

Until the last 10 years very little was known about specific drug metabolism and distribution of the majority of analgesics used in pediatric patients. In fact, it is well recognized that pediatric patients have been understudied and neglected in drug research. In the FDA's *The Pediatric Exclusivity Provision January 2001 Status Report to Congress* it was noted that Children

are subject to many of the same diseases as adults, and by necessity, are often treated with the same drugs. According to the American Academy of Pediatrics only a small fraction of all drugs marketed in the United States has been studied in pediatric patients, and a majority of marketed drugs are not labeled, or are insufficiently labeled, for use in pediatric patients. Safety and effectiveness information for the youngest pediatric age groups is particularly difficult to find in product labeling.

The absence of pediatric testing and labeling poses significant risks for children. Inadequate dosing information exposes pediatric patients to the risk of adverse reactions that could be avoided if such information were provided in product labeling. The absence of pediatric testing and labeling may also expose pediatric patients to ineffective treatment through underdosing, or may deny pediatric patients the ability to benefit from therapeutic advances because physicians choose to prescribe existing, less effective medications in the face of insufficient pediatric information about a new medication. The failure to produce drugs in dosage forms that can be used by young children (eg, liquids or chewable tablets) can also deny them access to important medications.

The drug industry has recently expanded its research in pediatric analgesics to meet FDA requirements and much of the drug information found here is based on these recent studies. However, it is important to recognize that many of the recommendations and information contained in this chapter on specific drugs are for unlabeled use. This is particularly true for preterm and term neonates and infants where there is very little information on any drugs.

## GENERAL PRINCIPLES ON USE OF PAIN MEDICATION IN CHILDREN

### Pharmacology

The safe and effective use of analgesic medications in children relies on an understanding of both modes of action of the medication, physiology of the patient, ability of the

| TABLE 10-2 | Suggested Doses of Oral Opioids in Infants and Children | | |
|---|---|---|---|
| Opioid Drug | Dosage Guidelines | Onset | Duration |
| Codeine | 0.1 mg/kg/dose every 4-6 h for 2-3 doses, then every 6-12 h | 30-60 min | 6-8 h (22-48 h after repeated doses) |
| Morphine | Immediate release: 0.2-0.5 mg/kg/dose every 4-6 h | 15-60 min | 3-5 h |
| | Sustained release: 0.3-0.6 mg/kg/dose every 12 h | 1-2 h | 8-12 h |
| Hydromorphone | Children: 0.03-0.1 mg/kg/dose every 4-6 h | 15-30 min | 4-5 h |
| | Adolescents: 1-4 mg every 3-4 h | | |
| Hydrocodone (in Violin, Lortab elixir) | Children: 0.15-0.2 mg/kg/dose every 4-6 h | 10-20 min | 3-6 h |
| | Adolescents: 1-2 tabs q 4-6 h (limited due to acetaminophen content; see acetaminophen recommendations in the text) | | |
| Oxycodone | Immediate release: 0.1-0.2 mg/kg/dose every 4-6 h | | |
| | Sustained release: 0.2-0.4 mg/kg/dose every 12 h | | |

patient to metabolize and clear drugs, and differences in genetically determined responses from patient to patient. *Pharmacokinetics* refers to the process by which a medication is absorbed, distributes into tissue compartments, is metabolized by different organs, and then eliminated. *Pharmacodynamics* refers to the actions and effects of medications on target sites throughout the body.

Pertinent pharmacokinetic considerations in children can be illustrated with the concept of "volume of distribution," which refers to the amount of drug administered in a theoretical volume of tissue in order to achieve a specified tissue or fluid concentration. In children, high body water content in the first year of life, as well as low relative protein composition can significantly alter blood levels of medications depending on the drug's specific characteristics. The concept of clearance also demonstrates the pharmacokinetic variation seen in children. Clearance is defined as the volume of a theoretical body compartment from which a specified drug is entirely eliminated over a period of time. Clearance can be affected by liver metabolism, plasma enzymatic degradation, and urinary clearance.

There are 3 pharmacokinetic parameters to understand for the safe and effective use of analgesic drugs: half-life, context-sensitive half-life, and peak onset. Half-life refers to the time required for the measured tissue or fluid level to decrease by 50%. Context-sensitive half-life is a variation of this concept used to describe the effect of continuous infusion of a medication on the half-life of the medication when the infusion is stopped. Peak onset is a measure of the time required to see maximum effect of the administered drug. As such, it is more accurately a pharmacodynamic measurement.

Used together, pharmacokinetic and pharmacodynamic characteristics can be matched to level and duration of pain and individual patient characteristics to achieve continuous effective analgesia.

## Nonopioid Analgesics

For outpatient care acetaminophen and nonsteroidal antiinflammatory drugs (NSAIDs) are the mainstay of treatment

either as single agents or in combination with oral opioids (see Table 10-2). Around the clock administration appears to produce better analgesia than PRN dosing for both minor pain and when administered as an adjunctive therapy for major pain.

## Acetaminophen

As a first-line therapy, acetaminophen is the most commonly used oral analgesic for mild to moderate pain. Acetaminophen is administered via the intravenous, oral, or rectal route. Acetaminophen is more predictable in its effects when given intravenously or orally than rectally due to its erratic absorption from the latter route. If given per rectum, dosing must be altered to take the pharmacokinetic differences into account. The toxicity of acetaminophen is very low at clinically recommended doses. However, the use of acetaminophen combined with other over-the-counter and prescription combination products (ie, acetaminophen/codeine, multisymptom cold medications) has been a frequent cause of significant toxicity. Liver damage or failure can occur with doses exceeding 200 mg/kg/day. Thus it is important to carefully avoid coadministration of acetaminophen and acetaminophen/opioid combination products. Also, there have been recent reports of toxicity in patients who received prolonged administration, only minimally more than the recommended daily dosing limits. Thus the daily limit is now suggested to be 50 mg/kg/day or a maximum of 3 g/day.

## Nonsteroidal Antiinflammatory Drugs

Ibuprofen is the prototypic oral NSAID. Naproxen is also available in suspension, and either can be used in synergy with acetaminophen for effective, nonsedating postoperative analgesia by alternating their administration schedule (eg, acetaminophen at 8:00 and 12:00, ibuprofen at 10:00 and 14:00). NSAIDs can affect platelet function via inhibition of the cyclooxygenase pathway, so they should be used with caution in patients at risk for postoperative bleeding. They are also gastric irritants, so administration with food is often desirable. Because they may reduce renal blood flow, they should be used with caution in children with renal impairment. COX2 drugs, such as celicoxib, can be used in children with fewer concerns for platelet function inhibition or renal effects.

## Oral Opioids

When pain is more severe, oral opioids can be added for short-term use. The most commonly used oral opioids are oxycodone and hydrocodone (Table 10-2). These drugs are available as single agent preparations and are also commonly formulated in fixed combination with acetaminophen, that is, as oxycodone/acetaminophen (Percocet®) and hydrocodone/acetaminophen (Loratab®). When using these combination drugs, the dose is based on the opioid component. Other concomitantly administered similar NSAIDs must be discontinued.

Although codeine is another common oral opioid, its use is strongly discouraged because of pharmacogenomic concerns. Codeine is metabolized to morphine via the cytochrome P-450 2D4 isoenzyme. One to ten percent of people (Asians 1%-2%, African Americans 1%-3%, and Caucasians 5%-10%) are poor metabolizers as a result of a genetic polymorphism. Thus, patients with this defect get no effect from this drug. A very small percentage of patients (primarily from East Africa) are ultra-rapid metabolizers. These patients convert 10 to 15 times the amount of parent drug to the active compound, producing clinical toxicity. The other oral opioids are superior drugs from all standpoints and should be used instead.

Morphine, oxycodone, and hydrocodone are available as suspensions, are active as administered, and are metabolized by multiple routes. Practical considerations include the controlled substance class, as hydrocodone is a Schedule III controlled substance while morphine and oxycodone are both Schedule II.

When dealing with more protracted pain, it becomes prudent to utilize medications that are longer acting. These can provide a baseline of pain relief, and allow for concomitant use of short-acting analgesic medicines for breakthrough pain. Available longer-acting opiates include extended release morphine (MS Contin®), oxycodone extended release (Oxycontin®), and methadone. Methadone is both a μ-opioid receptor agonist and an NMDA receptor antagonist, resulting in multimodal analgesic action. Although it is an excellent drug for patients with prolonged analgesic needs, it has a very long elimination half-life and slow onset of action, and doses must be titrated upward to effect (see below).

## Intravenous Analgesics

For severe pain not amenable to oral analgesics, an intravenous opioid can be titrated to effect; options for pain relief are dependent on severity and location of pain and age. Intravenous opioids administered intermittently via continuous infusion and as part of a PCA infusion have a long track record of both safe and efficacious use in children. This is confirmed by a recent large multicenter prospective study of opioid infusions in children. Morphine continues to be the mainstay of intravenous opiate therapy. With a typical onset of 3 to 5 minutes and a half-life of roughly 3 to 4 hours, it can be given as a one-time dose or as a part of PCA. Side effects specific to morphine include histamine release that can cause venodilation and, if hypovolemia is present, hypotension, as well as pruritus in many patients. Additionally, as morphine is metabolized by glucuronidation into morphine-3-glucuronide and morphine-6-glucuronide, the potential for accumulation of these metabolites exists in patients with impaired renal function. These metabolites are still active at opioid receptors and can produce symptoms of opioid overdose. Although infants have low activity in pathways of glucuronidation, they have more active sulfation pathways, and are able to metabolize morphine at similar rates to older children once they are more than 1 month of age.

Hydromorphone is a semisynthetic opiate with 5 times the potency of morphine. It has a peak onset of approximately 15 minutes and a half-life of 2.5 to 3 hours. It can be used as a single-time bolus or as part of a PCA regimen. Specific advantages of hydromorphone over morphine are that hydromorphone causes less histamine release, and does not have active metabolites that could accumulate in a patient with renal insufficiency. Although the half-life is shorter than morphine's, the duration of analgesia is roughly the same.

Fentanyl is the prototypical short-acting synthetic opiate agonist. Due to its lipophilicity, it can be administered via intravenous, intramuscular, neuraxial, transdermal, intrabuccal, and intranasal delivery. With a peak onset of 6 minutes, one-time dosing results in a half-life of 3 to 4 hours, although with a considerably shorter duration of analgesia of approximately 45 minutes. The context-sensitive half-life of the drug, however, can lead to accumulation when multiple doses are administered. Fentanyl is metabolized by the liver to nonactive metabolites, and can be used in patients with renal failure. Fentanyl is available in a transdermal-delivery system that offers continuous release up to 72 hours, but this application is reserved for chronic pain and is not recommended for acute usage. Fentanyl's best indication in acute postoperative pain management is for severe pain of intermittent short duration that requires rapid treatment, or via infusion in patients unable to tolerate morphine or hydromorphone. It's hemodynamic stability has made it popular for use in neonates, although it must be used with considerable caution in those who are not mechanically ventilated. Because of it's very potent μ-receptor avidity, tolerance can develop more rapidly than with morphine or hydromorphone. Additionally, chest wall rigidity is more common, especially when higher doses are administered as an intermittent bolus.

The advent of ultra-short-acting synthetic opiates warrants mention due to their demonstration of pharmacokinetic unsuitability for postoperative analgesia. Alfentanil and remifentanil provide the anesthesiologist with the ability to use powerful opiates during a procedure while maintaining the ability to discontinue administration and have quick offset of opiate effects. While these medicines can be useful for

| TABLE 10-3 | Suggested Doses of Intravenous Opioids for Infants and Children | | | |
|---|---|---|---|---|
| Drug | Dose (Intermittent) | Peak Effect | Effective Duration of Action | Starting Rate for Continuous Infusion |
| Fentanyl | 0.5-1 mcg/kg/dose (best for intermittent short duration analgesia; titrate to effect) | 1-3 min | 30-60 min | 0.5-1 mcg/kg/h |
| Hydromorphone | Children: 0.015 mg/kg/dose every 3-6 h<br>Adolescent: 1-4 mg every 3-6 h | 15 min | 4-5 h | 5-10 mcg/kg/h |
| Morphine | 0.05-0.1 mg/kg/dose every 2-4 h | 10-15 min | 2-4 h | 10-20 mcg/kg/h |
| Methadone | 0.1 mg/kg/dose every 4 h for 2 doses, then every 6-12 h | 10-20 min | 6-8 h (22-48 h after repeated doses)<br>Same | n/a |

sedation or as adjuncts during general anesthesia, they have no role in postoperative analgesia.

Methadone warrants its own category, as it is a long-acting synthetic opiate with unique qualities. It can be delivered by intravenous and oral routes, and it has, in addition to opiate receptor agonism, NMDA receptor antagonism that makes it useful in opioid-resistant pain states. It is metabolized in the liver and excreted in feces, making it suitable for use in patients with renal insufficiency. Methadone's analgesic duration is at least 4 to 8 hours, while its elimination half-life is up to 150 hours. This unique pharmacokinetic quality requires careful dosing (see Table 10-2) as initiation of therapy can induce enzymatic degradation for 5 to 7 days leading to initially low blood levels, and rebound elevated blood levels after this if the dose is quickly escalated. We suggest consultation with the pain service to aid in its initial prescription. A specific contraindication to methadone is QT prolongation, as methadone may induce torsades de pointes in patients with QT prolongation due to congenital or acquired causes (hypokalemia, hypomagnesemia).

## Delivery Systems of Opiate Therapy

Oral administration of medicines remains the most used route and is most acceptable to children of all ages. However, consideration must be given to potential causes of reduced effectiveness of oral delivery, specifically gastrointestinal processes inhibiting gastric motility and absorption. If gastrointestinal pathology prohibits oral administration and intravenous access is not available, consideration could be given to transbuccal or sublingual administration. An alternative is rectal administration, which is usually acceptable in younger patients. With rectal administration of medicine, however, there is considerable variation of pharmacokinetics due to the differing uptake in various parts of the colon.

Intramuscular or subcutaneous administration is mentioned only to be strongly discouraged. Although these injections provide quick drug uptake, it results in variable pharmacokinetic parameters, and more importantly is greatly feared by children. This route should be utilized only as a last resort, and avoided entirely in patients with poor perfusion conditions such as shock and hypovolemia, as uptake is greatly reduced in these states.

Intravenous administration of opiate medications remains the most reliable route of delivery. This method can be utilized with single time dosage or continuous infusion (Table 10-3). PCA is widely accepted in pediatrics. PCA utilizes timed and measured intravenous administration of opiate medications (Table 10-4). The patient is granted autonomy in determining the need for on-demand analgesia, while the inherent safeguard of self-titration

| TABLE 10-4 | PCA Dosing Recommendations | | |
|---|---|---|---|
| | Morphine | Fentanyl | Hydromorphone |
| Solution | 1 mg/mL | 10 mcg/mL | 0.1 mg/mL or 1 mg/mL |
| Bolus dose | 15-20 mcg/kg (max 1.5 mg) | 0.25 mcg/kg | 3-4 mcg/kg (max 0.3 mg) |
| Lockout time | 8-10 min | 5 min | 8-10 min |
| Basal infusion | 0-20 mcg/kg/h | 0-1 mcg/kg/h | 0- 4 mcg/kg/h |
| Maximum starting dose (for nonopioid tolerant patients) | 30 mcg/kg/h | 1-2 mcg/kg/h | 5 mcg/kg/h |

is ensured, as an over-sedated patient will not administer more boluses. A lockout interval, during which additional demand doses are blocked, ensures that the previous demand dose reaches peak effect before another can be initiated, preventing "stacking" of doses. A bolus or "rescue" dose can also be set that can be administered by the nurse if analgesia is inadequate with the PCA settings. Continuous basal infusions, administered at modest doses (5-10 mcg/kg/min), are used much more commonly than in adults, and are thought to maintain more even analgesic levels with less need for demand activation, especially during sleep. Although there is a potential increase in the risk of associated respiratory depression, data from the UK audit attest to their safety when used cautiously in appropriate pediatric patient populations. Basal rates are contraindicated when concomitant central neuraxial opioids have been administered.

Inherent to the safe use of PCA is a patient able to comprehend its use, and parental understanding of the absolute prohibition of the parent pushing dose-administration buttons. Continuous pulse-oximetry and cardiopulmonary monitoring is necessary for patients receiving PCA. The software of PCA pumps allows the practitioner to determine the number of demands for dosage as compared with actual doses delivered, aiding the clinician in assessing the adequacy of the PCA settings. These should be reviewed daily and appropriate modifications to the setting made as needed.

Variants of the PCA model used in infants and patients unable to understand or operate a PCA pump include nurse-controlled analgesia and parent-controlled analgesia. Strict guidelines and education by a dedicated pain service are critical for the safe and effective use of these modalities.

## Adjuncts to Opiate Therapy

### Ketorolac

Ketorolac is the only currently available parenteral NSAID. It is commonly used as an adjunct to opioids for severe pain, or when opioids are contraindicated or not tolerated. It is administered intravenously at 0.5 mg/kg q6 h. Like other NSAIDs, it can reduce renal blood flow, and cause gastric irritability and prolonged bleeding times by decreasing platelet adhesion. Caution is warranted when using ketorolac in patients with renal insufficiency or the potential for unacceptable microvascular bleeding. It is advisable to check renal function if a course of therapy must exceed 48 to 72 hours.

### Gabapentinoids

The introduction of gabapentinoid drugs such as gabapentin and pregabalin has provided an excellent nonopioid adjuvant to acute pain management. These medications bind to the $\alpha 2\delta$ subunit of voltage-gated calcium channels, thereby stabilizing excitable sensory neurons. While not a rescue therapy, these medicines can act as a well-tolerated adjunct to opiate therapy, presenting few drug interactions, and no increased risk of respiratory depression. Their onset of action is quite slow, so these agents should be started preoperatively.

### Tramadol

Tramadol is a synthetic opioid analog with weak µ-receptor antagonism. It has an additional action of inhibiting norepinephrine and serotonin uptake, which can provide an alternative analgesic target for neuropathic pain. Tramadol can decrease the seizure threshold, so it should be used with caution in patients with seizure disorders and in those receiving antidepressant therapy, such as has been reported with the serotonin syndrome.

### Ketamine

Ketamine is a racemic NMDA receptor antagonist. In low doses it can be used as an analgesic; as the dose is escalated it has increasingly potent dissociative sedative properties and can be used as an anesthetic induction agent. It can be given orally, intramuscularly (for sedation of an uncooperative patient), and intravenously. To provide analgesia while maintaining an awake state requires low infusion rates of 0.1 to 0.3 mg/kg/h, a range that also helps minimize the dysphoria that is associated with higher doses. Caution should be used in patients with elevated intracranial or intraocular pressure and congestive heart failure. Ketamine is not a "routine" analgesic and is generally used in consultation with the pain service.

### Benzodiazepines

Benzodiazepines act on the GABA receptors of the central nervous system and can be used as both sedatives and muscle relaxants. Although they are not analgesics themselves, they are commonly used adjuncts in children who have muscle spasms, particularly following orthopedic surgery of the extremities. They are also occasionally indicated in children with excessive anxiety. For the former purpose, a long-acting benzodiazepine such as diazepam is most commonly prescribed at a dose of 0.05 to 0.1 mg/kg q4 to 6 h. One must be aware of the synergy between opioids and benzodiazepines that can increase the risk of respiratory depression.

## Regional Analgesia Techniques

Although available since the early 20th century, regional anesthesia techniques have enjoyed a renaissance with both the advent of ample evidence of clinical benefit and the development of new techniques and technology to facilitate nerve blockade. Specific goals of regional anesthetic techniques are to provide alternatives to opiate analgesia, thereby reducing the potential opiate side effects such as respiratory depression, sedation, pruritis, decreased gut motility, and dysphoria. Other specific benefits of regional anesthesia include the ability to provide continuous infusions, the limited nature of clinically significant tachyphylaxis and tolerance, and the synergistic coadministration with opiate therapy. Regional anesthesia is also readily used as a part of multimodal analgesia, where multiple agents are used in smaller doses in order to minimize dose-related side effects of individual therapy modalities. Repeated safety audits of regional anesthesia techniques have all revealed acceptable safety profiles with few untoward events.

Regional anesthesia can be divided broadly into *neuraxial* and *peripheral* nerve blocks. Neuraxial nerve blocks utilize the accessibility of spinal nerves as they pass from the intrathecal space, through the epidural space, through plexuses, and on to peripheral nerves. The decision to use either a neuraxial or peripheral nerve block is related to the nature of the surgery, presence of coagulopathy, ability of the patient to tolerate hemodynamic changes, and the need for continuous ambulatory analgesia.

## Local Anesthetics

Local anesthetic medicines are classified as amino esters or amino amides. The amino esters, comprised of procaine, chlorprocaine, and tetracaine, are metabolized by plasma pseudocholinesterase. The amino amides lidocaine, bupivacaine, and ropivacaine are metabolized be the liver cytochrome P450 enzymes. Local anesthetics inactivate voltage-gated sodium channels and thereby block the propagation of neuronal impulses. As such, increasing concentrations will result in a progression from predominantly sensory block to sensory and motor blockade.

Special consideration must be given to toxicity in the pediatric setting. While just as effective on neural structures in infants and children, pharmacokinetic differences in infants and children can result in increased susceptibility to local anesthetic toxicity. Uptake of local anesthetics is faster in the pediatric setting due to higher relative cardiac output and increased regional blood flow. Serum proteins, specifically human serum albumin and $\alpha_1$-acid glycoprotein, are lower in infants, thereby decreasing protein binding and increasing effective serum concentrations. Finally, hepatic cytochrome immaturity can lead to decreased breakdown of the local anesthetics. These factors combined with an apparent increased susceptibility to cardiac toxicity warrant extra vigilance in infants and children.

## Local Anesthetic Toxicity

Local anesthetic toxicity syndrome (LATS) is a result of either overdosage and excessive systemic absorption of local anesthetic or inadvertent intravascular injection of these drugs (see Table 10-5 for suggested maximum doses). It is particularly important to remember that a given dose of local anesthetic in infants under 6 months of age will produce higher systemic levels of free drug than in older children, due to decreased protein binding. Infants thus must have the total dose of administered local anesthetic reduced by about 25% to avoid toxicity.

LATS is initially manifested by central nervous system hyperexcitability that appears as tremor and tinnitus, and can progress to seizures. As local anesthetics are often administered to a sedated or anesthetized child, these initial CNS signs are often masked, and the first sign of LATS may indeed be cardiac in nature. The cardiac manifestations of LATS are widening of the QRS complex with T wave elevation, bradycardia and bradydysrhythmias, torsades de pointe, ventricular fibrillation, and asystole.

## Treatment of Local Anesthetic Toxicity

Once LATS is recognized, immediate treatment is essential to prevent total cardiovascular collapse. Once identified by

| TABLE 10-5 | Maximum Doses of Local Anesthetics (Except for 2-Chloroprocaine, Infusion Rates Should Be Decreased by 25% in Infants Less Than 6 Months of Age) | |
|---|---|---|
| Local Anesthetic | Dose (mg/kg) | Maximum Infusion Rate (mg/kg/h) |
| Bupivacaine (with or without epinephrine) | 2.5 | 0.4 |
| Ropivacaine and Levobupivacaine | 3.0 | 0.5 |
| Lidocaine with epinephrine | 7 | |
| Lidocaine without epinephrine | 4.5 | |
| Mepivacaine with epinephrine | 7 | |
| Mepivacaine without epinephrine | 5 | |
| Tetracaine | 1.5 | |
| 2-Chloroprocaine | 20 | 12 |

cardiac or neurologic symptoms, the injection of any local anesthetic should be immediately discontinued. It is essential to utilize anesthesia services in these crises, as they have intimate knowledge of both the pharmacologic and pathophysiologic nuances of these emergencies. Airway management should proceed in order to both ensure delivery of 100% oxygen and avoid respiratory acidosis (which can potentiate local anesthetic toxicity). Basic and advanced cardiac life support algorithms should be followed. Drugs specifically to avoid include vasopressin, calcium channel blockers, β-blockers, and lidocaine, as they can worsen the cardiac effects of local anesthetics.

Once the above resuscitation measures have begun, it is prudent to begin "lipid rescue therapy," which is a recently developed modality of effectively altering toxic tissue concentrations of local anesthetics. 20% lipid emulsion is bolused intravenously (1.5 mL/kg) over 1 minute, and then followed with a continuous infusion of 0.25 mL/kg/min. Up to 2 additional boluses may be given for refractory cardiovascular collapse, and the infusion can be raised to 0.5 mL/kg/min for refractory hypotension. The lipid emulsion infusion should be continued for at least 10 minutes after successful resuscitation, and the patient should be monitored for an extended period of time in an appropriate location. More information on lipid rescue therapy is available at www.lipidrescue.org.

## Neuraxial Blocks

### Subarachnoid Blockade

The subarachnoid block caries multiple monikers, namely a "spinal" block or an "intrathecal" block. While the names differ, the technique does not vary. A spinal needle, typically with a "pencil point" to reduce risk of postdural-puncture headache, is utilized to pass through subcutaneous tissue and fascia in the lumbar level below the termination of the spinal cord. Local anesthetic can be administered for surgical anesthesia, with the potential addition of preservative free opiate for postoperative analgesia. Advantages of the subarachnoid block include the speed of onset, and the low doses of medicines needed to accomplish a clinical effect. Disadvantages include the potential for "high spinal" in which cardiopulmonary centers are affected, inability to both titrate to effect and leave a catheter in place for continuous infusion, and the possibility of blood pressure swings and postdural puncture headache. Intrathecal opiates also pose the risk of postoperative respiratory depression, and as such, require both continuous postoperative cardiopulmonary and pulse-oximetry monitoring and caution when using additional opiates.

## Epidural Blockade

The epidural block is a neuraxial technique that can be placed at multiple points along the neuraxis corresponding to the location of surgery, and is typically named by the access point such as caudal, lumbar, or thoracic (Figs. 10-1 and 10-2). Although older children and adolescents can experience hypotension with higher levels of epidural blockade, hemodynamic stability is the rule in infants and young children. This block is amenable to single injection dosing or catheter placement for continuous postoperative infusion. Continuous neural blockade requires care by a pain service for safety and optimal management.

The "caudal" block is an epidural nerve block starting at the level of the sacral hiatus in which a needle is passed though the sacrococcygeal ligament into the epidural space located between the sacrum and coccyx. This space is easily accessible in children, is amenable to catheter placement, and is frequently utilized in the pediatric setting for both lower extremity and genitourinary procedures. It is used less frequently in older patients as significant calcification of the sacrococcygeal ligament makes placement of the block more difficult.

Lumbar epidurals are block performed typically at the L4-5 or L3-4 interspace, are amenable to catheter placement, and utilized in lower extremity procedures, as well as some lower abdominal or urologic operations. Because the needle is placed below the conus medullaris there is no risk of direct injury to the cord. Accidental dural puncture, which although uncommon, can occur with epidural placement at any level, can result in headache. Like any continuous block utilizing a catheter, infection is a risk, although with proper care this can be recognized early when only skin inflammation is present, thus permitting intervention before deep infection ensues.

Thoracic epidurals are blocks performed most frequently at the T7-8 interspace and are utilized for both surgical procedures of the abdomen and chest. Specific risks inherent to thoracic epidural block, albeit exceedingly rare (<1:10,000), are pneumothorax and injury to the spinal cord. Regardless, the ability to treat abdominal and chest pain, specifically in the presence of the need for deep breathing, makes thoracic epidural catheters an essential component of the analgesic armamentarium.

## Paravertebral Blockade

Moving distally from the neuraxium, the paravertebral space provides an access point for unilateral blockade of multiple spinal intercostal nerves (Fig. 10-3). The wedge-shaped thoracic paravertebral space is bounded posteriorly by the transverse process and rib heads, medially by the vertebral body and intervertebral disks, and anterolaterally by the parietal pleura. In the paravertebral space, local anesthesia targets the spinal intercostal nerve, the dorsal rami, the anterior and posterior rami communicantes, and the sympathetic chain. There is also clinical and radiographic evidence of communication between multiple intercostal levels. The space is accessed by a variety of techniques including landmark-based, ultrasound-guided, and loss-of-resistance techniques.

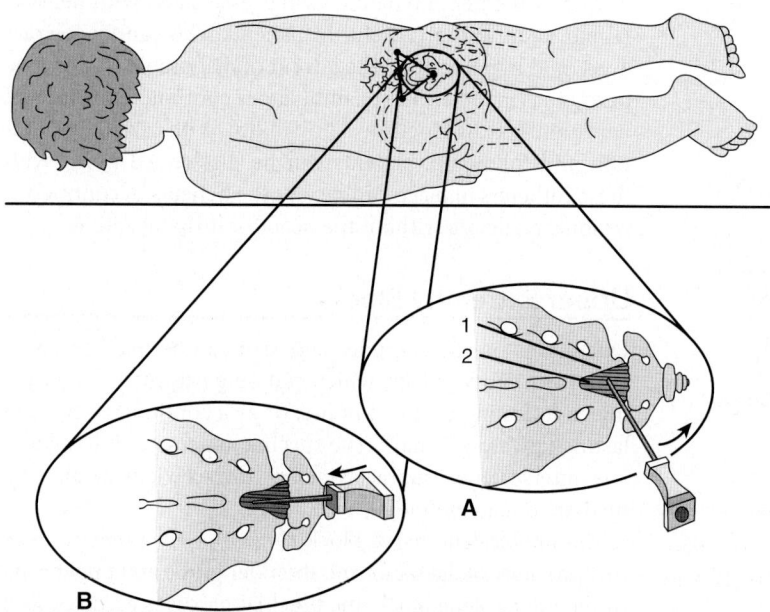

**FIGURE 10-1** Caudal block. The landmarks of the sacral cornua and coccyx are palpated. The needle (A) is inserted through the sacrococcygeal membrane at a right angle to the skin. The needle (B) is then depressed and redirected in a cephalad direction and advanced a short distance.

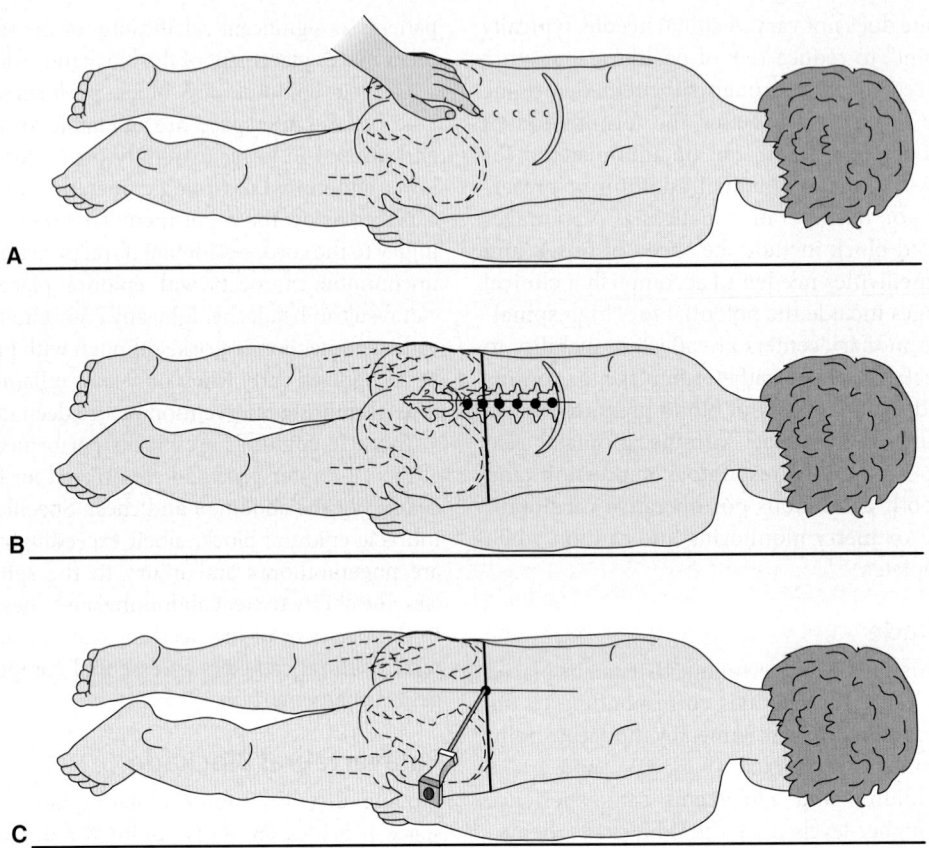

**FIGURE 10-2** Lateral position for epidural anesthesia. The lumbar spine is palpated (**A**). The intersection of the spine with a line across the top of the iliac crest marks the L4-5 interspace (**B**). The needle is inserted (**C**).

The paravertebral block is useful in the setting of somatic chest pain, specifically that of chest wall and breast procedures, rib fractures, and chest tubes. Contraindications to paravertebral blockade include sepsis, infection at the injection site, local anesthetic allergy, and empyema. Anticoagulation is a relative contraindication, as current evidence is not sufficient to obviate or encourage this modality as an alternative to neuraxial block in the setting of coagulopathy or platelet-inhibiting medicines.

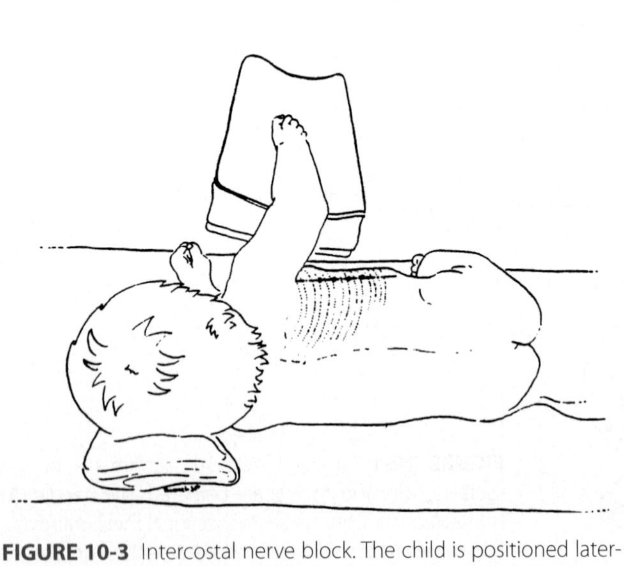

## Peripheral Nerve Blockade

Peripheral nerve blockade can selectively target both nerve plexi and individual nerves. They can be used in a variety of extremity and body wall operations, and can provide surgical anesthesia and postoperative analgesia. These blocks are devoid of the hemodynamic swings associated with neuraxial blockade, and are useful in patients who cannot tolerate even mild hypotension. The advent of disposable elastomeric pumps has made the use of ambulatory continuous peripheral nerve and plexus blockade a possibility. With careful instruction and follow-up, patients can be discharged home with these catheters in place and receive the benefits of continuous regional analgesia without the need for hospitalization.

## Upper Extremity Blocks

Operations on the shoulder and arm can be managed with upper extremity blocks, which can be performed as a single injection lasting up to 24 hours, or as a continuous infusion lasting upward of 3 days. The specific upper extremity blocks are interscalene, supraclavicular, infraclavicular, axillary, median, ulnar, and radial.

The interscalene nerve block (Fig. 10-4) is a plexus block that provides analgesia for the shoulder girdle and upper arm. In the interscalene block, the brachial plexus is accessed as it

**FIGURE 10-3** Intercostal nerve block. The child is positioned laterally or semiprone, and the midaxillary line is identified. Injection is made below the border of sequential ribs.

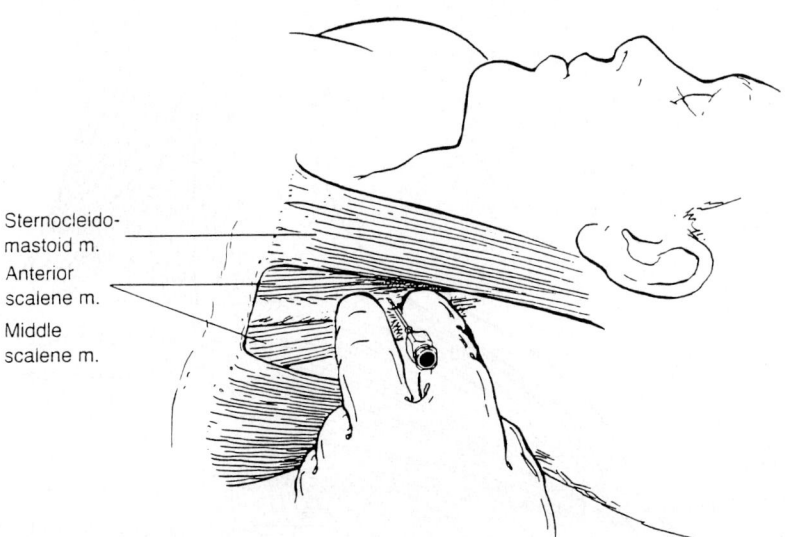

**FIGURE 10-4** The interscalene approach. With the patient supine and the head turned away from the examiner, the groove between the anterior and middle scalene muscles is palpated behind the sternocleidomastoid muscle. The needle is inserted and directed both posteriorly and caudad.

exits the neuraxium between the anterior and middle scalene muscle at the approximate C-6 level. Potential complications include intravascular injection, intrathecal injection, and extremely rarely, spinal cord damage. Common and acceptable side effects can include ptosis, meiosis, and mild voice changes. Of note, this block can also cause transient phrenic

block, and as such, should be used with caution in patients with pulmonary disease, and should not be performed bilaterally.

The supraclavicular block (Fig. 10-5) is utilized for surgical procedures of the upper and lower arm, and its aim is to block the brachial plexus before it dives underneath the clavicle. As such, potential complications include intravascular injection,

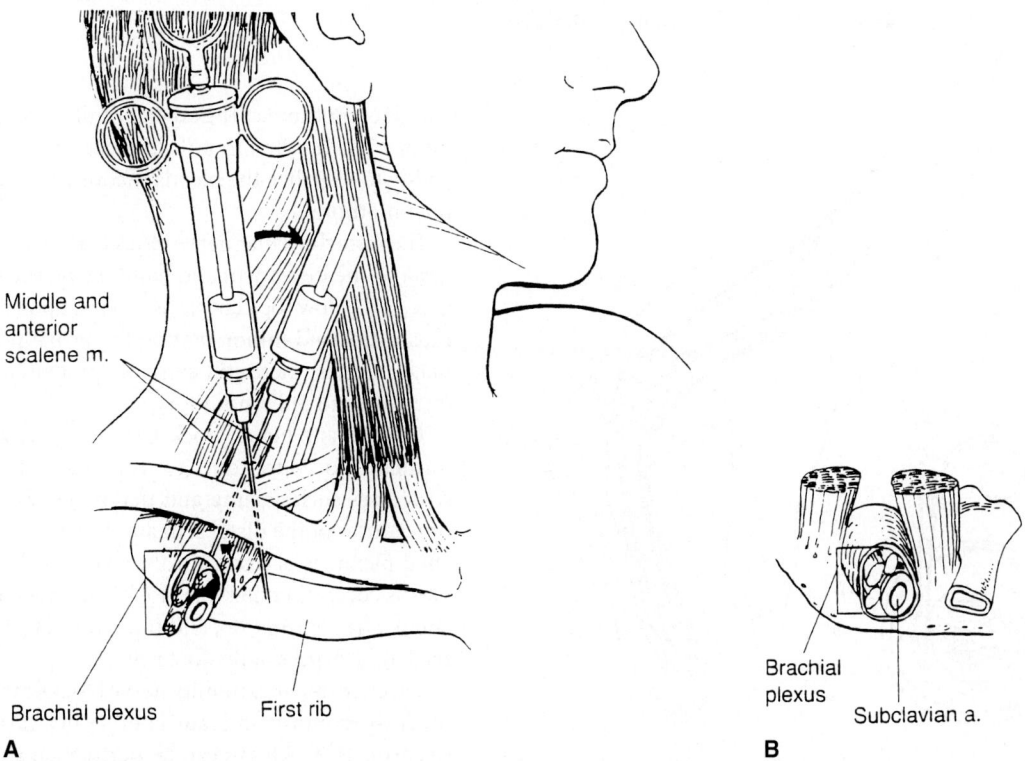

**A**   **B**

**FIGURE 10-5** Brachial plexus block, supraclavicular approach. (**A, B**) The plexus is formed by ventral rami from C5-T1, and it is enveloped by a continuous fascial sheath. The plexus via this approach is accessed behind the clavicle, between the heads of the anterior and middle scalene muscles. The needle is walked along the first rib until the plexus is located just behind the subclavian artery crossing the rib.

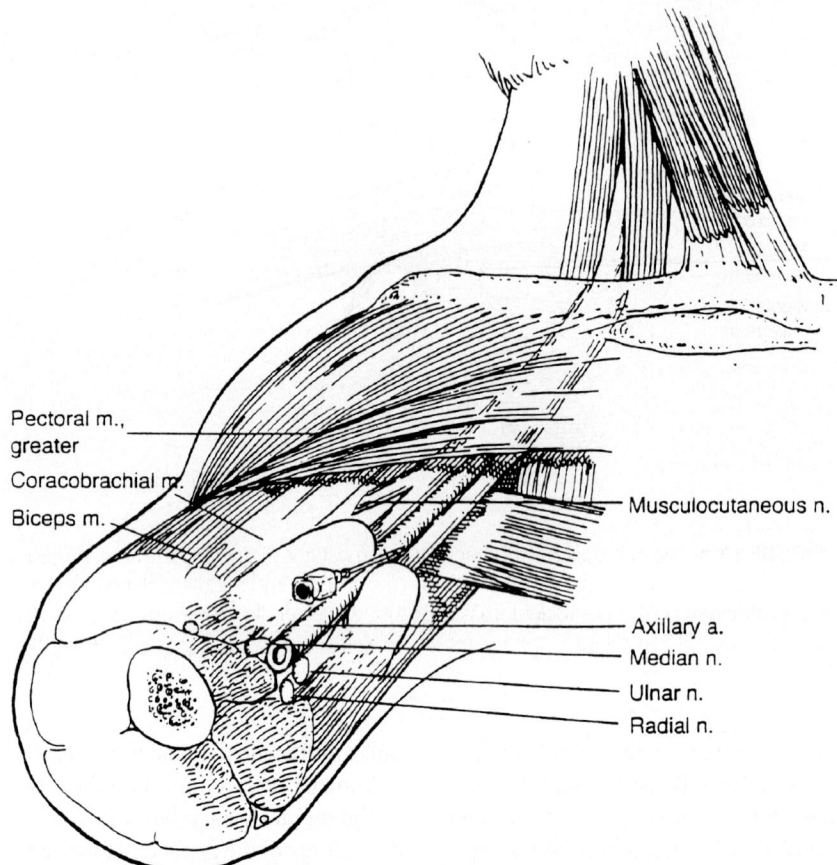

Pectoral m., greater

Coracobrachial m.

Biceps m.

Musculocutaneous n.

Axillary a.

Median n.

Ulnar n.

Radial n.

**FIGURE 10-6** The axillary block. The patient is positioned supine with the arm abducted 90° from the body. Along the medial aspect of the upper arm, just above the crossing of the inserting pectoral muscles, the axillary arterial pulse is palpated. At this point the median, ulnar, and radial nerves as well as the musculocutaneous nerve are organized as individual trunks in immediate proximity to the artery.

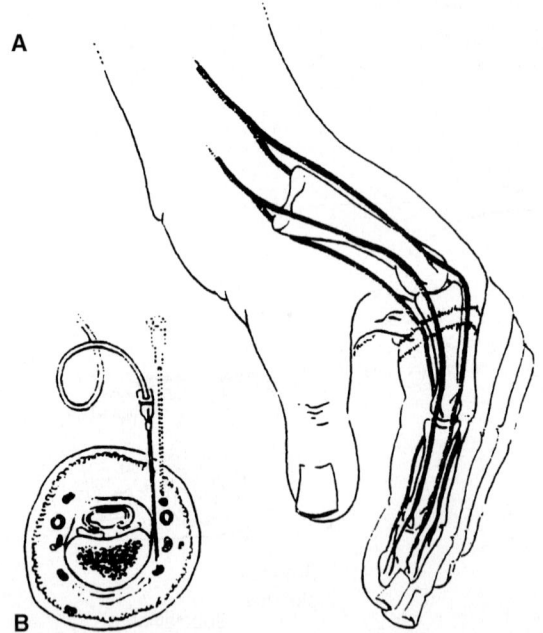

A

B

**FIGURE 10-7** Digital nerve block. The base of the selected digit should be stabilized with one hand, and a syringe with a fine needle should be guided along either side of the proximal phalanx or the distal metacarpal or metatarsal. After aspiration, a small volume of epinephrine-free local anesthetic is injected.

and pneumothorax. The advent of ultrasound guidance technology has resulted in a resurgence of this technique, as the ability to visualize the plexus theoretically reduces the risk of pneumothorax.

The infraclavicular nerve block can be used to provide analgesia to the lower arm and hand. Here, the brachial plexus is accessed below the clavicle as it passes posterior to the pectoralis major and minor. Noting the proximity to the lung and major vessels, there still exists the potential for intravascular injection and pneumothorax.

The axillary nerve block (Fig. 10-6) is a commonly performed procedure due to the ease of avoiding critical structures such as lung and major vessels. It can be used in procedures of the distal arm and hand. In this block, the brachial plexus is accessed in the axilla at the level of brachial plexus cords. Of note, this block does not cover the musculocutaneous distribution, and thus will not provide blockade to the lateral aspect of the forearm.

Selective upper extremity nerve blocks can be performed on the median, ulnar, and radial nerves in a variety of areas along the arm. These blocks can be performed with small doses of local anesthetic while allowing the patient to maintain control of the upper arm (Fig. 10-7). These blocks, however, are not typically amenable to continuous catheter placement, and are more often supplanted by plexus blocks.

## Lower Extremity Blocks

Analgesia for procedures of the hip, leg, ankle, and foot can be managed with the use of lower extremity nerve blocks. These blocks typically affect motor function of the leg, so caution must be used with postoperative ambulation. The lower extremity nerve blocks include the lumbar plexus, fascia iliaca, femoral, and sciatic nerve blocks.

The lumbar plexus nerve block aims to anesthetize the L1-L4 plexus as it forms within the psoas muscle, thereby blocking the femoral, obturator, and lateral femoral cutaneous nerves. It is utilized in operations of the hip and upper leg. As this is a deep, noncompressible area, caution is warranted as the potential for retroperitoneal bleeding and injury to the kidney exists.

The fascia iliaca block aims to anesthetize both the femoral and lateral femoral cutaneous, and often obdurator, nerves in the suprainguinal region as they pass through the fascia iliaca compartment bordered posteriorly by the iliacus muscle, anteriorly by the fascia iliaca, and inferiorly by the inguinal ligament. While useful in surgical procedures of the upper leg, there can be considerable variability in the degree of nerve blockade for each individual nerve.

The femoral nerve block (Fig. 10-8) is achieved by identifying the infrainguinal portion of the femoral nerve before

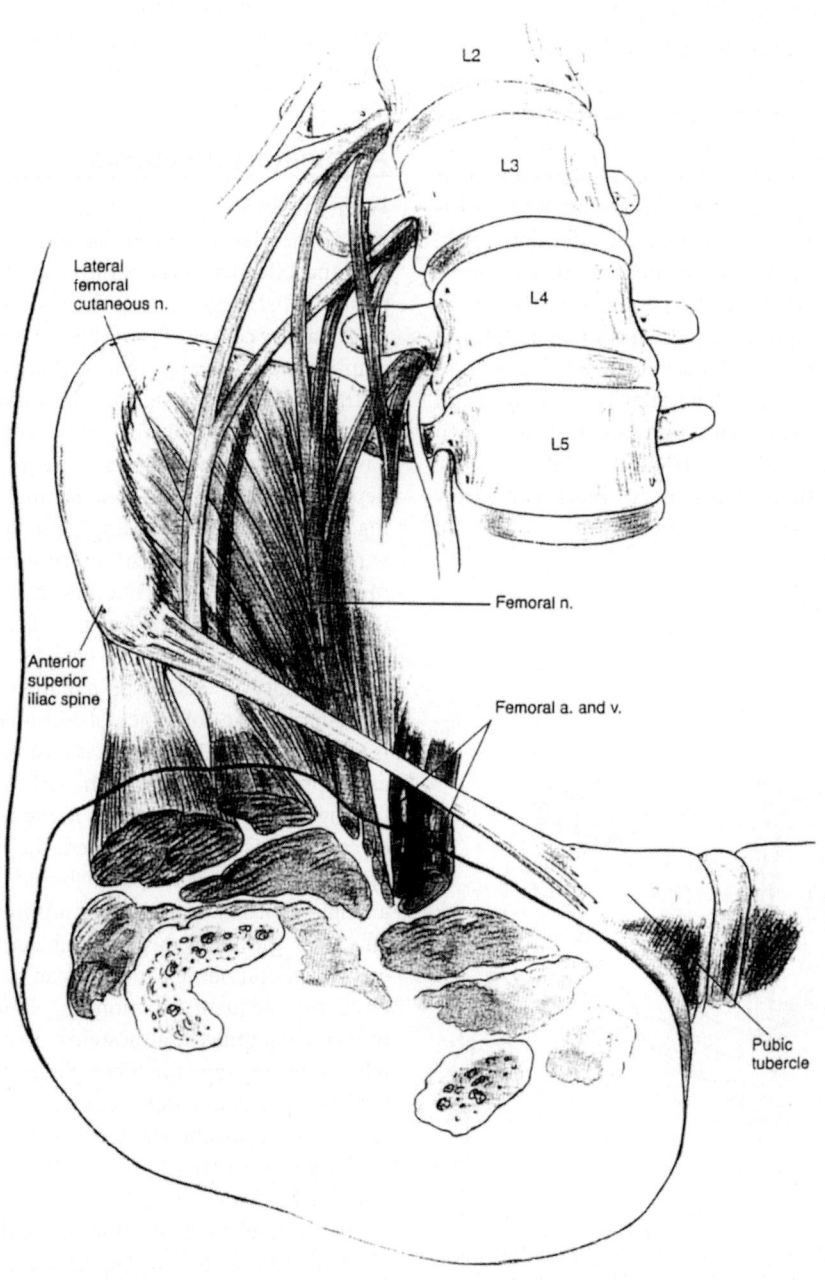

**FIGURE 10-8** Femoral nerve block. The femoral nerve is located just below the inguinal ligament lateral to the femoral artery pulse. The needle is inserted 1 cm below the inguinal ligament and directed cephalad. During injection and for several minutes thereafter, distal compression is maintained in an effort to distribute the anesthetic cephalad along the nerve sheath.

it branches into anterior and posterior segments. A successful block will provide sensory block to the anterior thigh and knee, and will also result in quadriceps weakness.

The sciatic nerve block can be performed at a myriad of points along the posterior leg, although the branching of the sciatic nerve into the common peroneal and anterior tibial nerves is localized at the popliteal fossa. Sciatic nerve blockade results in sensory block to the lower leg, ankle, and foot, although it spares the posteromedial portion of the calf and foot as this is innervated by the saphenous nerve.

## Body Wall Blocks

### Ilioinguinal–Iliohypogastric Block

The iliohypogastric nerve originates from L1, and emerges from the transverse abdominus muscle to provide sensory innervation to the posterior lateral gluteal region and the skin of the lower abdomen above the pubis (Fig. 10-9). The ilio-inguinal nerve also originates from L1 and follows a similar course with the iliohypogastric nerve, but eventually emerges from the internal oblique to run with the spermatic cord through the inguinal ring into the inguinal canal. This nerve provides sensory innervation to the penile root, the upper and inner aspect of the thigh, the upper scrotum in males, and mons pubis and lateral portion of labia in females. The nerves can be blocked along the abdominal wall with both blind and ultrasound-guided techniques, although evidence has shown that ultrasound-guided techniques result in greater success. The potential complications of this nerve block can rarely include injury to bowel, hematoma, and transient femoral nerve blockade.

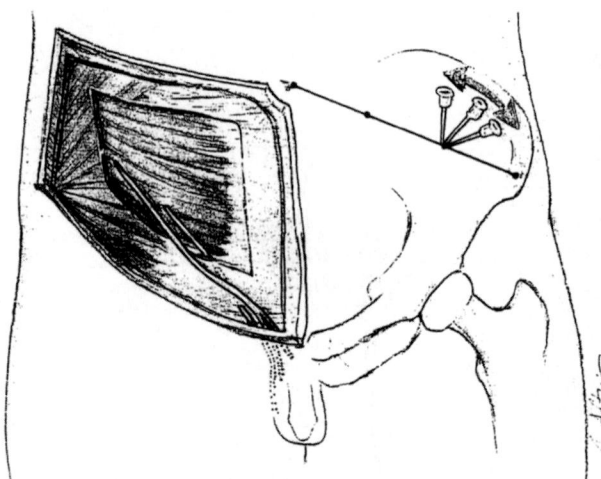

**FIGURE 10-9** Ilioinguinal and iliohypogastric nerve block. These nerves can be blocked by direct inspection and perineural infiltration of an agent at inguinal exploration. An equally efficacious approach is to insert a needle just medial to the anterior superior iliac spine. The iliohypogastric nerve is blocked by injecting anesthetic as the needle is directed laterally toward the inside of the ilium, whereas the ilioinguinal nerve is blocked when the needle is directed along the inguinal canal.

## Transverse Abdominis Plane Block

The transverse abdominis plane block (TAP block) aims to anesthetize terminal intercostal portions of the T8-L1 somatic afferents. This block can provide sensory analgesia for the abdominal wall skin, muscle, fascia, and parietal peritoneum. As such, it is a supplemental block for intraperitoneal procedures as it does not cover visceral pain from intraabdominal sources, but can be used effectively to reduce opiate and NSAID medication dosages and improve pain control. The TAP block can be performed as a blind or ultrasound-guided technique, although the ease and success of ultrasound guidance have been readily demonstrated. The block aims to deposit local anesthetic in the interconnected plexus of terminal sensory afferents located between the internal oblique and transverse abdominus muscle. This block results in multidermatome spread of local anesthetic yet with controlled minimal serum concentrations of local anesthetic.

## Ambulatory Analgesia

With the increased prevalence of ambulatory procedures comes the elevated need for techniques that provide both safe and effective postoperative analgesia and the ability to be safely discharged home. As postoperative pain and nausea are 2 leading causes of postoperative admission, effective preemptive measures and treatment are needed.

The perfect analgesic for ambulatory surgical procedures would be effective against both somatic and visceral pain, have no emitogenic effects, have no associated respiratory depression, and be both long lasting and amenable to redosing. As such, no perfect single medicine exists. Therefore, it is most effective to utilize multimodal and targeted therapy in order to achieve the maximum and synergistic benefit of multiple drugs at low doses in order to minimize their side effects.

The ability to discharge a patient home after operation relies heavily on tolerance of PO medications. If the patient is taking oral medications, it is wise to utilize an NSAID such as ibuprofen in combination with an acetaminophen containing opiate medicine. If a nerve block, either single-shot or continuous, has been placed, these medicines can still be utilized for rescue pain, and should also be prescribed after a single-shot nerve block and administered as the analgesic effects of the block begin to abate. Patients with continuous peripheral nerve catheters can be discharged home after ensuring adequate functioning of both the block and the infusion equipment, although it is critical to have 24-hour telephone coverage for these patients in order to both troubleshoot problems and recognize potential local anesthetic toxicity. It is not the standard of care and it is unacceptable to discharge a patient home with an indwelling continuous neuraxial block.

The same elastomeric pumps used for continuous plexus blockade can be used to deliver local anesthetic into a fascial plane or into a wound bed to provide continuous field blockade to a large incision. They require the same conscientious and meticulous follow-up as the plexus blocks. Infusion rates must be calculated to not exceed the toxic levels of the local anesthetic on a per kilogram per hour basis.

## Antiemetic Agents

Any anesthetic and opiate exposure carries the risk of associated nausea and vomiting. While seemingly innocuous, these symptoms are a considerable cause for hospital admission of ambulatory surgical patients as well as patient dissatisfaction. Accordingly, multimodal therapy is warranted in the treatment of post-operative nausea and vomiting (PONV).

Ondansetron is a 5HT serotonin receptor antagonist commonly used in prophylaxis of and treatment for PONV. It is a well-tolerated medicine available via intravenous, intramuscular, oral, and sublingual routes. Its half-life in children is 2.5 to 3 hours, and multiple "rescue doses" have not been shown to be effective. Caution should be used in patients taking selective serotonin reuptake inhibitors, and for patients with long QT syndrome or other bradyarrhythmias.

Dexamethasone has also been proven as effective anti-nausea prophylaxis. While the mechanism remains unclear, dexamethasone used in combination with other antiemetic medicines provides excellent PONV prophylaxis with minimal side effects, and no clinically significant impact on post-operative wound infection. Caution, however, should be used in patients with diabetes and with cancer patients receiving chemotherapy as their regimen may include carefully calculated doses of steroids. A single 0.1 mg/kg dose administered after induction is effective.

Metoclopramide is a dopamine receptor antagonist useful in treatment of PONV. It can be used with other antiemetic medications. The medicine must be administered slowly to avoid dysphoria and extrapyramidal symptoms. Caution should be used in patients receiving antipsychotics, patients with movement disorders, and small bowel obstructions. Sedation is a notable side effect and thus it should be used with caution in patients with decreased mental status and in conjunction with other sedating drugs.

Scopolamine is an anticholinergic medication available in a transdermal formulation. It is useful in the ambulatory setting due to its long duration of 72 hours when a patch is placed. Because it is available only in 1.5 mg patches its use is limited to children weighing more than 40 kg. While it may take up to 3 hours to reach peak effect, the placement of a scopolamine transdermal patch is an excellent "baseline" of nausea prophylaxis that can be supplemented with the aforementioned medications. It is prudent, however, to inform the patient to remove the patch for excessive sedation, double vision, and dry mouth. It is also important to instruct the remover of the patch to wash his or her hands after handling a scopolamine patch as significant transfer of the drug can occur with patch manipulation.

## SELECTED READINGS

Badner J, Pei D, Boyett JM, Cook E Jr, Ratain MJ. A pharmacogenetic study of uridine diphosphate-glucuronosyltransferase 2B7 in patients receiving morphine. *Clin Pharmacol Ther* 2003;73:566–574.

Bailey A, McNaull P, Jooste E. Perioperative crystalloid and colloid fluid management in children: where are we and how did we get here? *Anesth Analg* 2010;110:375–390.

Berde CB, Sethna NF. Analgesics for the treatment of pain in children. *N Engl J Med* 2002;347:1094–1103.

Bortone L, Ingelmo P, Grossi S, et al. Emergence agitation in preschool children: double-blind, randomized, controlled trial comparing sevoflurane and isoflurane anesthesia. *Pediatr Anesth* 2004;16:1138–1143.

Brown KA, Laferriere A, Lakheeram I, Moss IR. Recurrent hypoxemia in children is associated with increased analgesic sensitivity to opiates. *Anesthesiology* 2006;105:665–669.

Coller JK, Barratt DT, Dahlen K, Loennechen MH, Somogyi AA. ABCB1 genetic variability and methadone dosage requirements in opioid-dependent individuals. *Clin Pharmacol Ther* 2006;80:682–690.

Davidson A. Anesthesia and neurotoxicity to the developing brain: the clinical relevance. *Pediatr Anesth* 2011;21:716–721.

Eccofey C. Safety in pediatric regional anesthesia. *Paediatr Anesth* 2012;22(1):25–30.

Fitzgerald M, Walker SM. Infant pain management: a developmental neuro-biological approach. *Nat Clin Pract Neurol* 2009;5:35–50.

Hancock DL. Latex allergy prevention and treatment. *Anesthesiol Rev* 1994;21(5):153–163.

Hicks CL, von Baeyer CL, Spafford PA, van Korlaar I, Goodenough B. The Faces Pain Scale-Revised: toward a common metric in pediatric pain measurement. *Pain* 2001;93:173–183.

Kain ZN, Caldwell-Andrews AA, Mayes LC, et al. Family-centered preparation for surgery improves perioperative outcomes in children: a randomized controlled trial. *Anesthesiology* 2007;106:65–74.

Kokinsky E, Thornberg E. Postoperative pain control in children: a guide to drug choice. *Paediatr Drugs* 2003;5:751–762.

Landau R, Kern C, Columb MO, Smiley RM, Blouin JL. Genetic variability of the mu-opioid receptor influences intrathecal fentanyl analgesia requirements in laboring women. *Pain* 2008;139:5–14.

Lonnqvist PA, Morton NS. Postoperative analgesia in infants and children. *Br J Anaesth* 2005;95:59–68.

Madadi P, Ross C, Hayden M, et al. Pharmacogenetics of neonatal opioid toxicity following maternal use of codeine during breastfeeding: a case-control study. *Clin Pharmacol Ther* 2009;85:31–35.

Mauch J, Martin Jurado O, Spielmann N, Bettschart-Wolfensberger R, Weiss M. Resuscitation strategies from bupivacaine-induced cardiac arrest. *Paediatr Anaesth* 2012;22(2):124–129.

Morton NS, Errera A. APA national audit of pediatric opioid infusions. *Paediatr Anaesth* 2010;20:119–125.

Murat I. Perioperative fluid therapy in pediatrics. *Pediatr Anesth* 2008;18:363–370.

Pizov R, Eden A, Bystritski D, Kalina E, Tamir A, Gelman S. Arterial and plethysmographic waveform analysis in anesthetized patients with hypovolemia. *Anesthesiology* 2010;113:83–91.

Rosenbaum A, Kain ZN, Larsson P, Lönnqvist PA, Wolf AR. The place of premedication in pediatric practice. *Pediatr Anesth* 2009;19:817–828.

Ross JR, Rutter D, Welsh K, et al. Clinical response to morphine in cancer patients and genetic variation in candidate genes. *Pharmacogenomics J* 2005;5:324–336.

Sia AT, Lim Y, Lim EC, et al. A118G single nucleotide polymorphism of human mu-opioid receptor gene influences pain perception and patient-controlled intravenous morphine consumption after intrathecal morphine for postcesarean analgesia. *Anesthesiology* 2008;109:520–526.

Stoddard FJ, Sheridan RL, Saxe GN, et al. Treatment of pain in acutely burned children. *J Burn Care Rehabil* 2002;23:135–156.

Sun L. Early childhood general anaesthesia exposure and neurocognitive development. *Br J Anaesth* 2010;105:i61–i68.

Taylor EM, Boyer K, Campbell FA. Pain in hospitalized children: a prospective cross-sectional survey of pain prevalence, intensity, assessment and management in a Canadian pediatric teaching hospital. *Pain Res Manag* 2008;13:25–32.

Trescot AM, Datta S, Lee M, Hansen H. Opioid pharmacology. *Pain Physician* 2008;11:S133–S153.

von Ungern-Sternberg BS, Boda K, Chambers NA, et al. Risk assessment for respiratory complications in paediatric anaesthesia: a prospective cohort study. *Lancet* 2010;376:773–783.

Wilder RT, Flick RP, Sprung J, et al. Early exposure to anesthesia and learning disabilities in a population-based birth cohort. *Anesthesiology* 2009;110:796–804.

# Transfusion Medicine and Coagulation Disorders

# CHAPTER 11

*Gregory T. Banever*

Hematologic abnormalities are frequently encountered in the ill pediatric patient. Many excellent reviews of the physiology and pathophysiology of blood disorders and coagulation are currently available. This chapter is designed to complement rather than replace them. The goal is to provide a practical guide for the practicing surgeon and to aid in the formulation of diagnostic and treatment algorithms for the care of actual patients.

## ANEMIA

In the strictest sense, anemia is defined as a hemoglobin value or hematocrit level that is below 2 standard deviations from the mean for a given patient's age and sex. This definition, however, does not serve to identify those patients with clinically significant reductions in RBC mass, which is usually defined as the level at which tissue oxygenation is compromised. In fact, most decisions to transfuse RBCs are based on clinical judgment, currently available clinical and experimental data, accepted clinical guidelines, and personal experience.

The range of "normal" hematocrit levels for a particular age group can be rather broad. Likewise, the acceptable minimum hematocrit for any given patient is variable. In general, red cell transfusion is not considered in an otherwise healthy *asymptomatic* child until the hematocrit is less than approximately 21% (hemoglobin <7.0 g/dL). Even this is not an absolute indication for transfusion, as we have seen healthy children tolerate levels less than this with minimal physiologic embarrassment. Furthermore, in stable critically ill children, a recent randomized controlled trial demonstrated that a hemoglobin level of 7 g/dL is feasible as a transfusion threshold without affecting outcome. Some children with chronic anemia (eg, chronic renal insufficiency) have established compensatory mechanisms to such a degree that they can tolerate hematocrit levels much lower than those stated above. On the other hand, children with a hematocrit value higher than a minimally acceptable standard but who are clinically compromised may require transfusion regardless of the absolute hematocrit.

Newborns have a hematocrit value that normally varies between 47% and 60% but gradually decreases to a "physiological nadir" at approximately 2 to 3 months of age. This value can be as low as 28% in healthy infants. This nadir also coincides with the normal replacement of fetal hemoglobin (HbF), the predominant form in neonates, with the adult type. HbF has a higher affinity for oxygen and demonstrates a relative left shift of the oxygen–hemoglobin dissociation curve. Congenital hemoglobinopathies affecting the adult form of hemoglobin (eg, sickle cell anemia, thalassemia, etc) typically become clinically apparent after 2 to 3 months, when most of the unaffected HbF has been replaced with the defective adult form. Healthy newborns are not transfused unless they are clinically compromised by a low hematocrit. Critically ill neonates, especially premature infants, are often empirically transfused to hematocrit levels of 30% or higher depending on the clinical scenario.

There are accepted indications for empiric blood transfusion in the setting of acute blood loss typically encountered in the trauma bay or operating room. Most protocols suggest transfusion for acute losses that result in hypotension or mental status changes. In some truly emergent circumstances, it may be necessary to transfuse type-specific or type O blood because of the time required to properly cross-match units of blood.

There is no universally accepted standard for an "optimal" hematocrit level for a given patient about to undergo elective surgery. The decision regarding preoperative transfusion is thus often made jointly by the surgeon and anesthetist, who consider the age and cardiorespiratory status of the patient, the nature of the procedure, anticipated blood loss, and the patient's baseline hematocrit. In general, a preoperative hematocrit value of approximately 30% would be considered a safe and adequate level for major procedures in most patients.

Blood volume varies according to age from approximately 70 mL/kg in adults to 80 mL/kg in newborns and up to 90 mL/kg in premature infants. We use 80 mL/kg as a convenient estimate for newborns and children up to 30 kg. A typical blood transfusion volume in children is between 10 and 15 mL/kg of packed RBCs, depending on the indication. The expected change in hematocrit for a given volume of transfusion can be estimated by the formula: (volume transfused × hematocrit of transfused blood)/blood volume. Because the hematocrit of packed RBCs is approximately 50% to 60%, one should expect in the absence of ongoing bleeding a rise in hematocrit of approximately 6 to 8 points for every 10 mL/kg of packed RBCs transfused. Patients who have less than the calculated expected rise should be evaluated for ongoing bleeding or hemolysis.

Efforts to minimize transfusions for elective adult surgery have led to several strategies that are being tested in the pediatric surgical population. First, acute normovolemic hemodilution typically involves pre- or intraoperative removal of whole blood and replacement with a crystalloid solution. With subsequent intraoperative bleeding, the hemodiluted patient will thus lose less hemoglobin per milliliter of blood lost. The previously removed whole blood can be transfused back as needed. Next, devices that process and return blood lost during surgery are in developmental and experimental stages for infants and children. Also, preoperative administration of erythropoietin and the use of deliberate hypotension are being employed in selected circumstances. It is believed that a combination of some or all of these techniques will help minimize or even eliminate the need for allogenic transfusions in the future.

## SICKLE CELL DISEASE

Normal adult hemoglobin is composed of two pairs of globin subunits, each in turn made up of an α chain and a β chain. The common hemoglobinopathies consist of defective β-chain subunits in which the normal β chains (hemoglobin A) are replaced by one or more of sickle cell, hemoglobin C, or β-thalassemia β chains. Patients with SCD include those who are homozygous for sickle cell (hemoglobin SS disease) as well as those who are doubly heterozygous for sickle cell and hemoglobin C disease (hemoglobin SC disease) or β-thalassemia (hemoglobin Sβ disease).

Persons with the heterozygous sickle cell trait are generally asymptomatic while those with homozygous disease generally have severe alterations of RBC function. These result in increased cell rigidity and adherence, with the potential for conversion to an elongated "sickle" shape due to polymerization of the abnormal hemoglobin. Sickling is induced by hypoxia, acidosis, dehydration, or hyperosmolarity. This

is clinically manifest by vasoocclusive "crises," which are extremely painful and can result in tissue injury and organ dysfunction.

Crises can occur anywhere in the body and are frequently recurrent and characteristic in a given individual. Painful abdominal crises can pose a diagnostic dilemma, as they often mimic acute surgical processes. Most patients with an acute abdominal crisis will have had similar episodes in the past, which can help avoid unnecessary surgery. Nevertheless, these patients must be observed very closely for signs of a true abdominal catastrophe.

Acute splenic sequestration typically causes a rapid fall in the hemoglobin level and platelet count. Complications include hypovolemic shock and death. Recurrent episodes of sequestration are an indication for splenectomy.

Patients with SCD who undergo elective surgical procedures usually require preoperative preparation to avoid complications of the disease during and after operation. This typically involves transfusion therapy to decrease the relative amount of sickle hemoglobin. Recommendations have varied, but an aggressive approach involving decreasing the level of hemoglobin S to less than 30% has been used for years in many centers. However, data from a large multicenter trial suggest that patients treated with a more conservative approach, involving transfusion to a hemoglobin level of 10 g/dL, have a similar incidence of SCD-related complications and fewer transfusion-related complications. During and after the procedure, it is important to avoid conditions that are known to be conducive to sickling. This often requires careful monitoring in an intensive care setting and early consultation with hematologists and intensivists. Atelectasis and hypoxia require aggressive management to avoid the acute chest syndrome. This potentially lethal complication is characterized by severe chest pain, tachypnea, fever, and pulmonary infiltrates on chest radiograph. The treatment is aggressive and includes intensive respiratory support and exchange transfusion. Other perioperative complications include sepsis, painful crises, and cerebrovascular accidents.

## HEREDITARY SPHEROCYTOSIS

Hereditary spherocytosis is an inherited defect in a red cell membrane protein that results in increased red cell fragility and hemolytic anemia. Splenectomy relieves the hemolysis and is essentially curative. Affected children should undergo splenectomy after the age of 5 years to minimize the risk of postsplenectomy sepsis. If gallstones are detected by preoperative ultrasound, patients typically undergo cholecystectomy. By use of current minimally invasive techniques, cholecystectomy and splenectomy can be combined in a single laparoscopic procedure with very little morbidity.

## THROMBOCYTOPENIA

A normal platelet count is between 150,000 and 400,000/mm³. In general, adequate hemostasis for most surgical procedures requires a platelet count of at least 50,000/mm³, and spontaneous bleeding typically occurs when the platelet count falls below 10,000/mm³. Although there are several known congenital syndromes that include thrombocytopenia as one of their features, most patients encountered in pediatric surgery have an acquired form of thrombocytopenia.

Sepsis is a common cause of thrombocytopenia in neonates. Platelet consumption is felt to play a large role, although bone marrow suppression seems likely to be involved as well. This is of special concern in patients who have had an operation and in premature infants, who are at significant risk of intraventricular hemorrhage. Autoimmune platelet destruction can also occur in newborns as a result of maternal antibodies directed at inherited paternal platelet antigens. Known as neonatal isoimmune thrombocytopenia, it is difficult to treat with random donor platelets because of the prevalence of the PL^A1 antigen, which is usually the target antigen. Maternal platelets can be used when necessary.

Recommendations vary according to individual preferences, but in general, platelet transfusion is recommended for neonates who have any degree of thrombocytopenia and who are actively bleeding, and for those with a platelet count less than 20,000/mm³. It is common practice to transfuse critically ill newborns for platelet counts less than 50,000/mm³. The usual replacement dose is 10 mL/kg of standard random donor platelet concentrates.

Idiopathic thrombocytopenic purpura (ITP) most commonly occurs in preschool-age children, but can occur in all age groups. Thought to be caused by an autoimmune process, the disease typically occurs in the setting of a viral illness. Most patients recover within 1 month, and almost all recover within 6 months of the diagnosis. Those with severe thrombocytopenia can be treated with corticosteroids or intravenous (IV) immune globulin (IgG), with good temporary results. Transfused platelets are destroyed rapidly. Splenectomy provides effective relief in most patients but is rarely necessary except in cases of life-threatening hemorrhage or refractory thrombocytopenia.

Thrombocytopenia can also be caused by certain classes of drugs such as sulfa antibiotics, phenothiazines, and antiseizure medications. This usually responds to withdrawal of the offending drug. Thrombocytopenia also commonly occurs in the setting of hematologic malignancy, caused by either the primary disease process (eg, leukemia) or its treatment. From the pediatric surgical standpoint, this becomes a problem when a surgical procedure is required. Central line placement is a common example and in general is felt to be safe with a platelet count of 50,000/mm³ or more. There are some patients, however, whose platelet counts cannot be raised significantly with random donor platelet transfusions. These patients may benefit from single-donor platelet transfusions or by having platelets transfused continuously during the procedure.

## DISORDERS OF PLATELET FUNCTION

Aspirin and nonsteroidal antiinflammatory drugs cause an inhibition of platelet aggregation by inhibiting platelet cyclooxygenase and thus reducing levels of thromboxane $A_2$. The effect of these drugs is permanent for a given population of exposed platelets. The effect can last for up to 2 weeks, as the half-life for platelets in the circulation is 7 to 10 days. The effect can be reversed in cases of severe hemorrhage with platelet transfusion, assuming that a significant serum level of the drug is not present.

Other antiplatelet agents include glycoprotein IIb/IIIa inhibitors and theinopyridines. The former class of drugs prevents thrombin from binding to platelet receptors, interfering with platelet aggregation. The latter inhibits both aggregation and secretion via the ADP/P2Y12 receptor.

There are rare congenital causes of platelet dysfunction such as Glanzmann thrombasthenia and the Bernard–Soulier syndrome. These are characterized by a prolonged bleeding time and can be treated temporarily in cases of severe bleeding with platelet transfusion. Platelet dysfunction also occurs in the setting of significant uremia. Hemodialysis can help, but in the emergent setting cryoprecipitate or desmopressin can be used. Patients who have excessive bleeding during or immediately after hemodialysis may have received an excessive heparin dosage and should be considered for empiric protamine administration (1 mg of protamine sulfate for every 100 units of heparin).

The most common inherited disorder of hemostasis is von Willebrand disease with a prevalence of approximately 1% in the general population. Clinically significant disease affects only approximately 0.1%, and the severe form of the disease is extremely rare. Several subtypes have been described, most of which are inherited as autosomal dominant traits. The disorder is caused by a quantitative and qualitative defect in von Willebrand factor (vWF), which mediates platelet adhesion and aggregation and acts as a carrier for plasma coagulation factor VIII. It is characterized by a family history of bleeding, a prolonged bleeding time, and a prolonged activated partial thromboplastin time (aPTT). The diagnosis can be confirmed by several in vitro tests. Patients with clinically mild forms of the disease who undergo minor surgical procedures may need no specific treatment. Desmopressin (DDAVP) improves bleeding times in certain patients with von Willebrand disease by causing a release of factor VIII from hepatic stores and vWF from endothelial cells. It is useful only for very minor operations and some dental procedures. Patients with more severe forms of von Willebrand disease and those who are to undergo major operative procedures can be treated with cryoprecipitate or vWF concentrates.

## COAGULATION DISORDERS

Screening children for disorders of hemostasis should include a careful clinical and family history, which will identify the vast majority of patients with potential coagulation problems. Although it is common for parents to report a history of "easy bruising," specific questions should address a history of petechiae, large hematomas (eg, into joints or after minor trauma), or excessive bleeding during minor surgical procedures such as circumcision and dental procedures. In adolescents, a history of excessive menstrual flow or prolonged bleeding after shaving is important. A history of renal or hepatic dysfunction should be sought. A medication history including over-the-counter medications is also important. A family history of excessive bleeding should be specifically addressed as well. On physical examination, petechiae, ecchymoses, and evidence of renal or hepatic dysfunction should be documented.

Otherwise healthy children without evidence of a bleeding disorder by history or physical examination generally do not require screening laboratory studies in anticipation of most operative procedures. Those considered at risk for a bleeding disorder should undergo further studies. The first series of tests typically includes a complete blood count, an aPTT, a prothrombin time (PT), and a fibrinogen level. Most patients should also have a bleeding time. Prolonged clotting studies should be evaluated with further studies including individual factor assays, a thrombin time, plasma mixing studies, and von Willebrand testing.

## INHERITED DISORDERS OF COAGULATION

The most common inherited coagulation factor deficiency is hemophilia, an X-linked recessive disorder that occurs at a rate of 1 in 5000 births in the United States. Two third of cases have factor VIII deficiency or hemophilia A. The severity of bleeding in hemophilia A varies substantially and correlates with factor VIII levels. Those with a level more than 30% of normal have essentially normal hemostasis and a normal aPTT. Levels less than 5% are associated with spontaneous hemorrhage into joints and soft tissues. Affected individuals with levels between 5% and 30% may have relatively normal hemostasis except during surgery or major trauma.

Patients with hemophilia A can be treated with cryoprecipitate or factor VIII concentrate. Human recombinant factor VIII preparations are available, which minimize the risk of infectious complications. For major elective surgery, the goal is to achieve a level of factor VIII that is at least 80% of normal during the procedure and sustain minimum levels of 30% to 50% for 1 to 2 weeks after surgery. The half-life of circulating factor VIII is 8 to 12 hours. Levels should be checked often, and replacements given as needed.

The second most commonly inherited coagulation factor deficiency is factor IX deficiency, or hemophilia B, which is clinically indistinguishable from hemophilia A. Purified or recombinant factor IX is used to maintain similar perioperative levels as described above. The half-life of factor IX is 18 to 30 hours.

Deficiencies of most other coagulation factors have been reported but are much less prevalent than the hemophilias and are generally associated with less severe bleeding.

## ACQUIRED DISORDERS OF COAGULATION

Profound coagulopathy that is difficult to correct occurs in the setting of severe hepatic dysfunction. Most coagulation factors (I, II, V, VII, IX, X, XI, XII, and XIII) are synthesized in the liver and are diminished with severe liver disease. Temporary improvement can occur after the infusion of FFP or cryoprecipitate, but full correction is rarely possible, and therapy should generally be directed at the underlying liver disease.

Vitamin K is a fat-soluble cofactor that is required for the production of factors II (prothrombin), VII, IX, and X by the liver. It is also required for the production of the endogenous anticoagulants protein C and protein S. Vitamin K deficiency results in a deficiency of these factors and subsequent prolongation of the PT.

Newborns are naturally vitamin K deficient and can have severe bleeding complications if replacement is not given shortly after birth, a practice that has become a standard of care in neonatal nurseries. Vitamin K deficiency can also occur in the setting of disease states that result in poor intestinal absorption or be caused coincidentally by medications such as certain broad-spectrum antibiotics. Vitamin K can be administered intramuscularly or intravenously. In newborns 0.5 to 1.0 mg is administered intramuscularly. In older children and adults, dosages up to 25 mg can be administered by either route. Results are typically seen in several hours, although full correction can take up to 24 hours. In the emergent setting, rapid correction of coagulopathy can be achieved with the administration of FFP or cryoprecipitate.

Disseminated intravascular coagulation (DIC) results in a profound coagulopathic state caused by the unchecked activation of the coagulation cascade and subsequent consumption of coagulation factors, fibrinogen, and platelets. In pediatric surgery, the most common clinical scenarios are severe sepsis or a critically injured child. The diagnosis can usually be made on clinical grounds but is confirmed by laboratory evidence of a consumptive coagulopathy and elevated levels of fibrin degradation products (fibrin monomer, D-dimer levels). Treatment is directed at the underlying cause and includes general supportive measures and replacement of coagulation products with FFP, cryoprecipitate, and platelets as indicated. Use of heparin, antithrombin, and protein C concentrate have been described for refractory cases, but must be used with caution until more evidence is available.

Another cause of coagulopathy seen in pediatric surgery is that encountered in trauma victims with extensive brain injury. This is thought to be related to release of tissue factor into the circulation and is associated with severe brain parenchymal injury and a poor prognosis. FFP or cryoprecipitate may be required if bleeding occurs. Profound hypothermia, especially in the setting of trauma or a major operation, can result in an acquired coagulopathy that is usually reversible by active rewarming. Last, large-volume transfusions of RBCs can result in coagulopathy because of citrate toxicity, hypocalcemia, dilution of coagulation factors, thrombocytopenia, or hypothermia.

## DISORDERS OF THROMBOSIS

Clinically significant deep venous thrombosis (DVT) is relatively uncommon in children when compared with adults. The vast majority of thrombotic events in children are associated with serious underlying disorders or other predisposing factors, such as the presence of a central line. The incidence of embolic events or other serious complications is smaller still. Perhaps the exceptions are central lines, which are associated with a significant incidence of venous thrombosis, and disorders of endogenous anticoagulation, which can cause recurrent and potentially serious thrombotic events. Nevertheless, DVT prophylaxis with subcutaneous heparin or sequential compression devices are rarely indicated in pediatric patients, although judgment should be exercised in patients who are at higher risk (history of thrombotic event, malignancy, orthopedic procedures, obesity, paralysis, immobility, pubertal, or adolescent patients).

Protein C is a vitamin K-dependent circulating anticoagulant that inhibits activated factors V and VIII. There are 2 basic groups of patients with congenital protein C deficiency, one in which the disorder is inherited as an autosomal dominant trait with variable penetrance (incidence of 1 in 20,000) and another that behaves clinically as an autosomal recessive trait with a prevalence of approximately 1 in 200 to 300 individuals. Patients who are homozygous for the latter trait present in the newborn period with purpura fulminans, retinal thrombosis with detachment of the retina and blindness, and other severe thrombotic complications. The diagnosis is confirmed by one of several assays for protein C activity. The treatment depends on the type of deficiency present and the clinical setting. Neonates with purpura fulminans or other serious thrombotic complications should be treated with FFP or protein C concentrate, if available. Older patients with acute thrombosis are treated with heparin. FFP or protein C concentrate can be used prophylactically in these patients as well. Chronic warfarin therapy is used to prevent thrombotic events in affected patients, but it typically needs to be started in the setting of full heparinization to prevent thrombotic complications.

Protein S is another vitamin K-dependent component of the natural anticoagulation system, which acts as a cofactor for protein C. The clinical manifestations and treatment are essentially the same.

Most common of the anticoagulant protein defects, Factor V Leiden is caused by a point mutation in factor V at the protein C binding site. Otherwise known as activated protein C resistance, this condition prevents the typical proteolysis that helps maintain the balance of the coagulation system. Most patients do not develop thrombosis until after puberty, and the condition can be diagnosed with a functional assay.

Lupus anticoagulant and anticardiolipin antibodies are antiphospholipid antibodies that are strongly associated with a high risk of thrombosis and thrombocytopenia. Specific therapy is not available, but patients with unexplained thrombotic events such as DVT should be evaluated for the presence of a lupus anticoagulant or anticardiolipin antibody and treated with chronic anticoagulant therapy. Specific immunologic assays are available for detection.

Antithrombin III (ATIII) is a circulating anticoagulant synthesized in the liver that inhibits the action of thrombin and activated factor X. This inhibition is potentiated greatly by heparin, and ATIII is an essential cofactor for the action of heparin as an anticoagulant. Individuals with an inherited deficiency of ATIII typically develop thrombotic complications such as DVT in adolescence and early adulthood and are at higher risk for thrombotic complications in the perioperative period and in the settings of trauma or pregnancy. The diagnosis is confirmed by one of several available assays for ATIII activity. Chronic therapy is with an oral anticoagulant such as warfarin. Purified ATIII preparations can be used in the setting of acute thrombosis or in the perioperative period.

There are several technical considerations that deserve mention. One is cardiac surgery, which can result in a significant risk for thrombotic events. Care of these patients, especially in the critical care setting, often involves striking a careful balance between hemostasis and the tendency for thrombosis. This is also true for organ transplantation, particularly in very small children in whom anastomoses and vascular conduits are at high risk for thrombosis. Anticoagulation is not a good option in some cases such as liver transplantation, but here an intentional "undercorrection" of the patient's coagulopathy (eg, avoiding platelet transfusion in the absence of significant bleeding) is often used. The incidence of asymptomatic vascular thrombosis is also quite high in children who have long-standing central venous catheters. Although complications are rare, these patients are at risk for postphlebitic syndrome and difficulty with central venous access should it become necessary again. Several well-known thrombotic syndromes have been associated with central venous catheters, including renal vein thrombosis from indwelling catheters in the inferior vena cava placed via a femoral approach; portal vein thrombosis caused by umbilical vein catheters and resulting in portal hypertension; and superior vena cava syndrome, which after central line placement results in severe head and arm edema, chylothorax, and potentially death, especially in neonates. Anticoagulation and fibrinolytic therapies should be considered in the acute setting but are associated with significant risks. All patients should also undergo a workup for inherited disorders of coagulation.

Thrombocytosis is defined as a platelet count above 500,000/mm$^3$ and can be classified as primary or secondary. Primary thrombocytosis is caused by a stem cell defect and occurs in the setting of myeloproliferative diseases or as an idiopathic phenomenon. It is extremely rare in the pediatric population. Secondary thrombocytosis is caused by splenectomy, sepsis, or the physiological response to the stress of surgery or trauma. It is also associated in rare cases with hypoxemia, epinephrine injection, and iron-deficiency anemia. Actual thrombotic events are extremely rare in cases of thrombocytosis in children regardless of the cause or the degree of thrombocytosis, with the possible exception of iron-deficiency anemia, which has been associated with thrombotic complications in published anecdotal case reports. Prophylactic therapy is almost never indicated except in the rare case of thrombocytosis associated with iron-deficiency anemia, in patients with a history of thrombosis, and in those felt to be at significant risk for thrombosis.

## ANTICOAGULATION THERAPY

Heparin exerts its effects on coagulation by inducing a conformational change in the naturally circulating anticoagulant ATIII protein, which markedly increases its inhibitory effect on thrombin and activated factor X. The most common indication for heparin therapy in children is acute thrombosis such as DVT. It is also indicated as prophylaxis for procedures that are considered high risk for thrombosis, and during fibrinolytic therapy. In its most commonly used form, after an initial bolus the unfractionated drug is given as a continuous IV infusion. The dosage used varies according to institutional and individual preferences but is typically in the range of 50 to 100 units/kg as an IV bolus followed by 10 to 25 units/kg/h as a continuous infusion. Therapy is monitored by maintaining aPTT levels at 1.5 to 2.5 times the control value. The effective half-life of heparin is variable between 60 and 90 minutes; therefore, repeat aPTT values should be done 4 to 6 hours after a bolus or a change in the infusion rate. Emergent reversal of the effect of heparin can be brought about by the IV administration of protamine.

Heparin therapy can be complicated by recurrent thrombosis with inadequate anticoagulation or, less frequently, by bleeding. Heparin can also cause thrombocytopenia in some patients. A drop in platelet count below 100,000/mm³ typically occurs approximately 5 to 7 days after initiation of therapy but can occur more quickly in a presensitized patient. The syndrome is characterized by thrombosis rather than bleeding, and although most affected patients are asymptomatic and require only cessation of heparin, the rare patient develops a significant acute vascular occlusion referred to as the *white clot syndrome*. In patients who still require anticoagulation, oral warfarin, low-molecular-weight heparin (LMWH), or porcine-derived heparin can be utilized.

Sodium warfarin (warfarin, Coumadin®) is an oral agent that exerts its anticoagulant effect by inhibiting the vitamin K-dependent posttranscriptional modification of factors II (prothrombin), VII, IX, and X as well as anticoagulant proteins C and S. The effect of the drug is not seen for 2 to 4 days. Therapy is monitored by measuring the international normalized ratio (INR). The effect of warfarin can be reversed by administration of vitamin K, which takes up to 24 hours, or by administration of FFP, which replaces the defective factors immediately.

Patients receiving chronic anticoagulant therapy with warfarin require a carefully monitored withdrawal of therapy before elective surgery. Regardless of the indication for anticoagulation therapy, the risk of an acute thrombotic event during the several days that the agents are withheld is very small and in most cases does not outweigh the risk of major bleeding if therapy were to be continued through the operative period. The goal is to allow the INR to fall to 1.5 or less during the operation, which can usually be achieved by withholding 5 doses of warfarin. The INR should be checked the day before operation, and if it is higher than 1.5, a small subcutaneous dose of vitamin K can be administered (0.02 mg/kg). For patients on warfarin with atrial fibrillation, mechanical heart valves, or previous venous thromboembolism, the following recommendations are made based upon thrombosis risk. High-risk patients should receive therapeutic dose LMWH, but IV heparin is acceptable. Those with low risk should be given low-dose LMWH or no bridging medication. Continuous heparin infusions should be stopped 4 hours prior to surgery and restarted 12 to 48 hours postoperatively depending on hemostasis and the risk of postoperative bleeding. Patients on LMWH should receive their last preoperative dose the day before surgery, at 50% of the usual dose, and generally can be restarted the day after the procedure assuming the bleeding risk is low. These are recommendations extrapolated from extensive data in studies on adults; however, these recommendations provide reasonable guidelines for the management of children on oral anticoagulation therapy.

## TRANSFUSION MEDICINE

Modern blood storage techniques have resulted in a shelf life of RBC products stored at 4°C of up to 42 days. Whole blood is collected and mixed immediately with a citrate–phosphate–dextrose solution as an anticoagulant. One of several commercially available nutrient solutions is typically added, which extends the viability of the RBCs to 6 weeks. Despite these techniques stored blood products undergo a progressive change in milieu as a result of continued anaerobic metabolism by the RBCs. There is a decline in 2,3-DPG (2,3-Disphosphoglycerate) levels, a drop in pH, and a decreasing posttransfusion viability of the RBCs themselves. These and other issues related to storage have been generating debate with regards to blood product age and possible impact on clinical outcomes.

The availability of whole blood is limited in most pediatric centers because of the demand for more specialized blood components and the limited indications for whole blood. Thus, the most commonly used RBC replacement product is packed RBCs. These are units of blood in which the cells have been separated from the plasma. One adult unit typically has a volume of 250 to 300 mL and a hematocrit between 50% and 60%. The usual transfusion volume in newborns and children is 10 to 15 mL/kg given over 1 to 4 hours, or more quickly in emergent situations. Because the volume load associated with a blood transfusion can be significant in small children, and especially newborns, a diuretic such as furosemide may be given during or after the transfusion.

For most patients no further processing of the packed RBCs beyond a type and cross-match is required. Packed RBC units that have not been further processed will have residual donor plasma and leukocytes. In the immune-competent host, these residual components are generally not a concern, but in certain immune-incompetent patients they can pose potentially serious risks. The risks include infectious disease transmission, graft-versus-host (GVH) disease, and transfusion reactions. Patients with a history of febrile nonhemolytic or urticarial transfusion reactions should receive washed RBCs when transfusion is required. These are units that have been processed by extensive washing with normal saline to remove nearly all traces of plasma. These patients may also require leukocyte-depleted RBCs. High-grade leukocyte depletion can be accomplished by specialized filtering systems and is also indicated for selected severely immune-compromised patients. Lastly, irradiation of blood products will further decrease the likelihood of GVH disease; and this technique is used routinely in most centers for immune-compromised patients.

Transfusions in neonates pose multiple potential concerns. Neonates are typically transfused with 10 to 20 mL/kg of packed RBCs at a time. For babies less than 4 months old and whose initial antibody screen is negative, it is unnecessary to routinely cross-match blood before transfusion. The blood is routinely CMV-negative and should also be screened for hemoglobin S. Babies less than 1000 g should receive irradiated blood because of the risk of GVH disease. The lower pH and higher potassium levels in stored blood pose a potential hazard, so fresh blood (less than 72 hours old) or washed RBCs should be used. Although packed RBCs have relatively low levels of citrate compared to whole blood, a large transfusion in a newborn can precipitate hypocalcemia from citrate toxicity.

Random donor platelets are isolated from fresh whole blood by a multistep centrifugation process that results in a unit of platelet concentrate ($5\text{-}7 \times 10^{10}$ platelets) suspended in 50 to 70 mL of plasma per unit of whole blood. Single-donor platelets can be prepared by apheresis, which yields 3 to $4 \times 10^{11}$ platelets, usually suspended in 250 mL of plasma. Platelets are filtered to remove microaggregates but are not routinely depleted of RBCs and leukocytes. They can also be washed, irradiated, or volume-reduced if indicated. Cross-matching is not necessary for platelets, and ABO compatibility is routinely practiced in many blood banks but is not strictly necessary for most patients. Because of the concern of Rh-alloimmunization, platelets from an Rh-positive donor should not be given to an Rh-negative individual.

The volume transfused is usually 5 to 10 mL/kg, which should result in a "bump" in platelet count, conventionally measured at 1 hour after transfusion, of 40,000 to 50,000/mm$^3$. Patients who have hypersplenism, bleeding, or sepsis, and those who are consuming platelets for another reason may not have a significant increase in platelet count after transfusion. In patients who have had multiple platelet transfusions and have less than the expected rise in platelet count after transfusion, the possibility of immune-mediated destruction of platelets should be considered. These patients may benefit from single-donor platelet transfusions rather than random donor platelets. Alternatives such as leukocyte depletion and human leukocyte antigen (HLA) class I matching may be necessary in some patients.

## MASSIVE TRANSFUSION

A common definition of massive blood loss is one circulating blood volume in 24 hours. Uncontrolled bleeding is a major source of preventable mortality in both the operating room and the trauma bay. Massive transfusion protocols (MTPs) have been developed to both streamline the process from a logistical standpoint and provide guidelines for the appropriate usage of blood products. Most current MTPs have been developed for adults, and are frequently initiated when a patient has or is expected to require 10 units or more of RBCs in 24 hours. Pediatric protocols are being developed, and typically extrapolate from adult MTPs. An example is provided in Fig. 11-1. Data from both civilian and military investigations have led to the general recommendation of a 1:1:1 ratio of PRBC:FFP:platelet units for damage control resuscitation scenarios. This is a departure from previous practices that

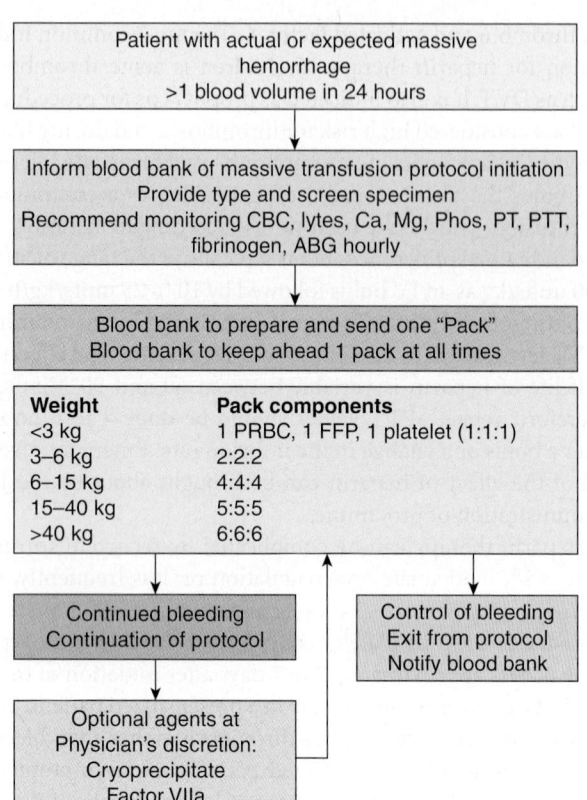

**FIGURE 11-1** Example of a massive transfusion protocol for pediatric patients.

utilized less nonerythrocyte products and administered them later in the course of treatment. Also, due to the degradation of blood product quality over time, many protocols call for units that are less than 2 weeks old.

Significant hemorrhage has been successfully controlled with recombinant factor VIIa in both adults and children. The supporting data for this "off-label" use are limited in the pediatric age group. Factor VIIa predominantly interacts with tissue factor at the site of injury to activate factor X to Xa, thereby stimulating clot formation via thrombin and then fibrin. The incidence of thromboembolic complications is quite low, but it still remains an investigational adjunct.

## TRANSFUSION REACTIONS

Transfusion reactions generally take one of 3 forms: hemolytic reactions caused by blood group antigen incompatibility, febrile nonhemolytic reactions caused by transfused leukocyte cytokines, and urticarial reactions caused by plasma protein antigens. The most worrisome of the 3, the hemolytic reactions, are also the least common. ABO incompatibility is the most common cause and is usually the result of a clerical error. The response is typically immediate, with widespread intravascular hemolysis being caused by activation of the complement system. Symptoms include fever, chills, hemoglobinuria, abdominal pain, and back pain. The reaction may progress to include tachycardia, hypotension, and shock. Complications include severe anemia, renal failure, and DIC.

Treatment involves general supportive measures and immediate cessation of the transfusion. Mannitol, alkalization of the urine, and corticosteroids are often used as well. Confirmation of a suspected transfusion reaction can be made through laboratory testing.

Febrile nonhemolytic reactions are more common. Patients present with fever and chills during a transfusion, and these reactions occur in patients who have a history of prior transfusion or pregnancy. Therapy is directed at the symptoms (antipyretics, analgesics); however, corticosteroids may be required in severe or refractory cases. Future transfusions should be with leukocyte-depleted and washed RBCs.

The most common transfusion reactions are urticarial and can be localized to the transfusion site or instead be generalized. The target antigen is presumed to be a plasma protein. Therapy is with antihistamines, although occasionally corticosteroids are required. Washed cells or medical pretreatment should be used for future transfusions.

Transfusion-related GVH disease has been mentioned as a risk for immune-compromised patients. GVH may also be encountered when biological relatives donate blood for a pediatric patient. The transmitted lymphocytes may not be recognized as foreign due to haplotype similarities, and lymphocyte proliferation with host tissue destruction could ensue. GVH typically occurs within 2 weeks of the transfusion and is manifest by pancytopenia, hepatitis, a characteristic maculopapular rash, and diarrhea. Mortality can be high, depending on the degree of reaction severity. Treatment is generally nonspecific and has disappointing results. The risk is minimized by using irradiated blood products.

Infectious complications can occur with any blood product, but the overall incidence has improved over time. CMV is transmitted by leukocytes, and infection can be prevented in susceptible individuals by using blood from seronegative donors or by using washed or leukocyte-depleted blood products. The incidence of infection by the human immunodeficiency virus (HIV) has been lowered to approximately 0.14 to 1.1 per million units of blood products by screening programs. Most estimates of hepatitis C transmission rates have fallen to below 2 per million units transfused. Transfusion-related hepatitis B infection is uncommon because of screening programs and the routine immunization of children against hepatitis B, but it still carries an approximate rate of up to 1 in 100,000 per unit. Other potentially transmitted agents include hepatitis A, West Nile virus, and several parasites and bacteria. Because of these and the risk of other as yet unknown infectious hazards, the use of blood transfusion should be limited to those with clear-cut indications and to situations in which risk–benefit considerations are in favor of transfusion.

## SELECTED READINGS

Barcelona SL, Thompson AA, Coté CJ. Intraoperative pediatric blood transfusion therapy: a review of common issues. Part I: hematologic and physiologic differences from adults; metabolic and infectious risks. *Paediatr Anaesth* 2005;15(9):716–726.

Barcelona SL, Thompson AA, Coté CJ. Intraoperative pediatric blood transfusion therapy: a review of common issues. Part II: transfusion therapy, special considerations, and reduction of allogenic blood transfusions. *Paediatr Anaesth* 2005;15(10):814–830.

Bihl F, Castelli D, Marincola F, Dodd RY, Brander C. Transfusion-transmitted infections. *J Transl Med* 2007;5:25.

D'Alessandro A, Liumbruno G, Grazzini G, Zolla L. Red blood cell storage: the story so far. *Blood Transfus* 2010;8(2):82–88.

Douketis JD, Berger PB, Dunn AS, et al. The perioperative management of antithrombotic therapy: American College of Chest Physicians Evidence-Based Clinical Practice Guidelines (8th edition). *Chest* 2008;133(6 suppl):299S–339S.

Goldenberg NA, Manco-Johnson MJ. Pediatric hemostasis and use of plasma components. *Best Pract Res Clin Haematol* 2006;19(1):143–155.

Greer SE, Rhynhart KK, Gupta R, Corwin HL. New developments in massive transfusion in trauma. *Curr Opin Anaesthesiol* 2010;23(2):246–250.

Hermans C, Altisent C, Batorova A, et al. Replacement therapy for invasive procedures in patients with haemophilia: literature review, European survey and recommendations. *Haemophilia* 2009;15(3):639–658.

Israels SJ, Michelson AD. Antiplatelet therapy in children. *Thromb Res* 2006;118(1):75–83.

Lacroix J, Hébert PC, Hutchison JS, et al. Transfusion strategies for patients in pediatric intensive care units. *N Engl J Med* 2007;356(16):1609–1619.

Marchant WA, Walker I. Anaesthetic management of the child with sickle cell disease. *Paediatr Anaesth* 2003;13(6):473–489.

Prabhakar H, Haywood C Jr, Molokie R. Sickle cell disease in the United States: looking back and forward at 100 years of progress in management and survival. *Am J Hematol* 2010;85(5):346–353.

Sarkar S, Rosenkrantz TS. Neonatal polycythemia and hyperviscosity. *Semin Fetal Neonatal Med* 2008;13(4):248–255.

Segel GB, Francis CA. Anticoagulant proteins in childhood venous and arterial thrombosis: a review. *Blood Cells Mol Dis* 2000;26(5):540–560.

Vichinsky EP, Haberkern CM, Neumayr L, et al. A comparison of conservative and aggressive transfusion regimens in the perioperative management of sickle cell disease. *N Engl J Med* 1995;333(4):206–213.

Weldon BC. Blood conservation in pediatric anesthesia. *Anesthesiol Clin North Am* 2005;23(2):347–361, vii.

# Wound Healing

# CHAPTER 12

*Stig Sømme*

## KEY POINTS

1. Wound healing, like the body's response to injury, undergoes the three phases of inflammation, proliferation, and remodeling.

2. Inflammatory cell infiltration is a key step in wound healing, stimulated in part by endothelial cells, monocytes and cytokines.

3. The wound's fibrin plug brings collagen synthesizing fibroblasts to the wound, the cells that also stimulate the production of mucopolysaccharides.

4. "Scarless" fetal wound healing may relate to an altered inflammatory response, collagen composition and hyaluronic acid composition when compared to adult wound healing and scar formation.

5. Negative pressure is an important therapeutic adjunct for the treatment of delayed healing wounds.

## INTRODUCTION

Wound healing is a fundamental part of recovery from surgery. After tissue damage, the body responds in a predictable manner to repair and restore function. Wound healing involves blood clotting factors, inflammatory mediators, connective tissue formation, and remodeling processes. In the fetus some wounds will heal without a scar, but after birth scar formation is expected. Individuals respond to wound healing differently, resulting in differences in scar formation. Some chronic (eg, diabetes, malnutrition) and genetic (eg, Ehlers–Danlos) conditions negatively affect the healing of a wound.

## RESPONSE TO INJURY

The repair process after tissue injury from trauma or surgically created wounds has been divided into 3 phases: inflammation, proliferation, and remodeling (Fig. 12-1). These 3 phases overlap, but each has identifiable characteristics that will be discussed in more detail. Wound healing is the tissue's ability to restore function after injury. There is an urgency to restore function, minimize loss of fluid, and avoid infection. This may explain why perfect repair, or regeneration, is not possible. Regeneration is a term used for restoration of the tissue without a scar or signs of previous injury. It is found to take place only in fetal tissue and in certain organs such as liver and bone.

## WOUND HEALING PHASES

All wounds undergo the same 3 steps (inflammatory, proliferative, and remodeling phases) progressing toward repair and restoration of function. Acute wounds heal in a predictable fashion, progressing through these 3 phases. Chronic wounds do not proceed past the inflammatory phase.

### Inflammatory Phase

The inflammatory phase starts immediately after injury or incision and lasts for approximately 6 days. This phase represents the body's attempt to limit blood loss by creating a seal over the wound and is followed by removal of necrotic tissue and debris. During the inflammatory phase there is an increase in vascular permeability. Cells migrate into the tissue stimulated by chemotaxis. These cells release several cytokines and growth factors which activate migrating cells (Fig. 12-2).

### Hemostasis, Inflammation, and Increased Vascular Permeability

Hemostasis is triggered by the exposure of subendothelial collagen to platelets; this is mediated by Von Willebrand factor. Platelet adhesion to the endothelium is facilitated by integrin receptor GPIIb-IIIa. This results in aggregation of platelets, vasoconstriction, and activation of the coagulation cascade. The binding of platelets results in the release of biologically active proteins from the platelets' α granules and dense bodies (eg, platelet-derived growth factor [PDGF], transforming growth factor β [TGF-β], insulin-like growth factor type I [IGF-I], fibronectin, fibrinogen, thrombospondin, Von Willebrand factor, and vasoactive amines). The increased vascular permeability observed is a result of the release of these biologically active proteins by platelets and

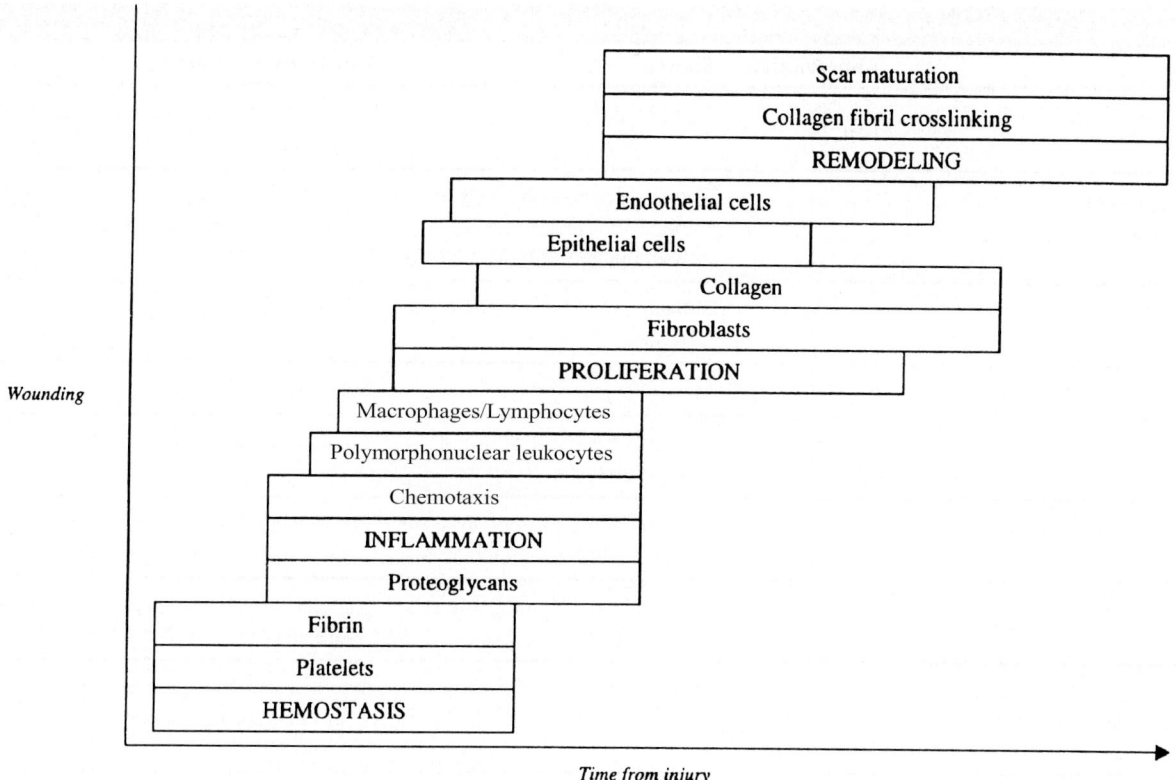

**FIGURE 12-1** Schematic timeline of the events involved in wound healing.

mast cells. The most important mediators are histamine and serotonin. Prostaglandin and thromboxane A2 are released from the breakdown of cell membranes and assist in platelet aggregation and vasoconstriction.

Both the intrinsic and extrinsic clotting pathways are activated. Thrombin activates platelets and triggers fibrin formation from fibrinogen. The resulting fibrin strands trap erythrocytes and other cells in the blood to form a blood clot (Fig. 12-3). Ultimately, this results in the formation of a scaffold for inflammatory cells, fibroblasts, and endothelial cells, allowing hemostasis and the wound healing process.

Macrophages and neutrophils are the predominant cell types to migrate into tissue in response to injury. Neutrophils (polymorphonuclear cells or PMNs) appear first, followed

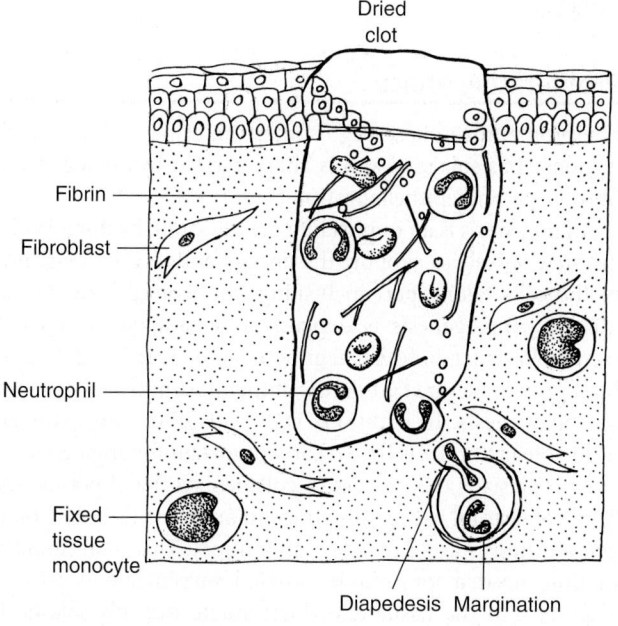

**FIGURE 12-2** The inflammatory phase of wound healing with neutrophil cellular infiltration.

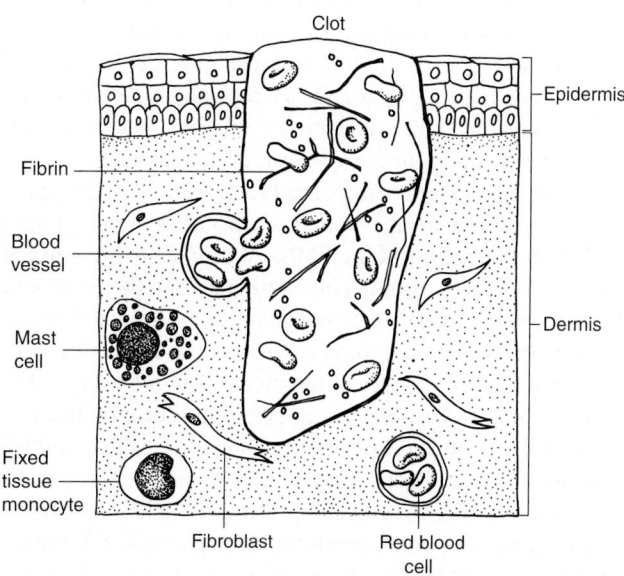

**FIGURE 12-3** Hemostasis at the wound site with deposition of a fibrin clot.

| TABLE 12-1 | Cytokines and Growth Factors Implicated in Tissue Repair | | |
|---|---|---|---|
| **Factor** | **Abbreviation** | **Source** | **Functions Regulated** |
| Platelet-derived growth factor | PDGF | Platelets and macrophages | Fibroblast proliferation, chemotaxis, and collagenase production |
| Transforming growth factor β | TGF-β | Platelets, polymorphonuclear neutrophil leukocytes, T lymphocytes, and macrophages | Fibroblast proliferation, chemotaxis, collagen metabolism, and the action of other growth factors |
| Transforming growth factor α | TGF-α | Activated macrophages and many tissues | Similar to EGF functions |
| Interleukin-1 | IL-1 | Macrophages | Fibroblast proliferation |
| Tumor necrosis factor | TNF | Macrophages, mast cells, and T lymphocytes | Fibroblast proliferation |
| Fibroblast growth factor | FGF | Brain, pituitary, macrophages, and many other tissues and cells | Fibroblast proliferation, stimulates collagen deposition and angiogenesis |
| Epidermal growth factor | EGF | Saliva, urine, milk, and plasma | Stimulates epithelial cell proliferation and granulation tissue formation |
| Insulin-like growth factor | IGF | Liver, plasma, and fibroblasts | Stimulates synthesis of sulfated proteoglycans, collagen, and cell proliferation |
| Human growth factor | HGF | Pituitary and thus plasma | Anabolism |
| Connective tissue growth factor | CTGF | Fibroblasts | Mesenchymal cell to fibroblast differentiation |
| Hypoxia-inducible factor 1-α | HIF-1α | | Angiogenesis |
| Vascular endothelial growth factor | VEGF | | Angiogenesis |

by macrophages. Integrin molecules, a family of cell surface receptors, are important for the migration and activation of neutrophils and macrophages.

Monocytes and endothelial cells increase the migration of PMNs into the injured tissue through the release of interleukin-1 (IL-1) and tumor necrosis factor-α (TNF-α). The PMNs release lysosomes, elastase, and other proteases, promoting further migration of PMNs and facilitating the breakdown of damaged tissue. PMNs and macrophages are phagocytes, which have the ability to remove damaged tissue and dead cells in preparation for the synthesis of new tissue.

Macrophages are very important to the wound healing process. They appear in the wound when PMNs are dwindling and induce apoptosis of the PMNs. Within 24 to 48 hours of injury, monocytes from the blood migrate into the tissue and become macrophages. Chemotactic agents from the initial response to the wound (complement c5a, thrombin, fibronectin, collagen, TGF-β) recruit monocytes into the wound. The process of transforming monocytes into macrophages is facilitated by specific integrins in the tissue, which control adhesion-mediated gene induction in monocytes. The macrophages release matrix metalloproteinases, collagenases, and other enzymes to break down the damaged tissue in preparation for regeneration. In addition, macrophages release numerous cytokines and growth factors important for the wound healing process (see Table 12-1).

After about 5 days, T lymphocytes appear in the wound. They stimulate other cells (primarily macrophages) and process the antigens presented by macrophages. These antigens include foreign material from bacteria, viruses, and other pathogens.

## Proliferative Phase

The proliferative phase begins after the initial inflammatory response has subsided and is characterized by angiogenesis, fibroplasia, and epithelialization (Fig. 12-4).

Angiogenesis is an important part of wound healing. Without new vessels to support the energy and oxygen demands of the cells taking part in healing, the wound cannot heal quickly. Angiogenesis is dependent on angiogenic growth factors. Vascular endothelial growth factor (VEGF) and fibroblast growth factor (FGF) are 2 of the most potent stimulants of angiogenesis. In addition, TGF-β, TGF-α, and hypoxia-inducible factor-1α (HIF-1α) are important for angiogenesis.

Fibroplasia is the process of collagen synthesis performed by fibroblasts for use in the extracellular matrix (ECM). Collagen synthesis starts 3 to 5 days after injury. This is the amount of time needed for undifferentiated mesenchymal cells to migrate into the tissue and differentiate into fibroblasts. It appears that the initial proliferation of fibroblasts comes from tissue-derived mesenchymal cells capable of differentiation.

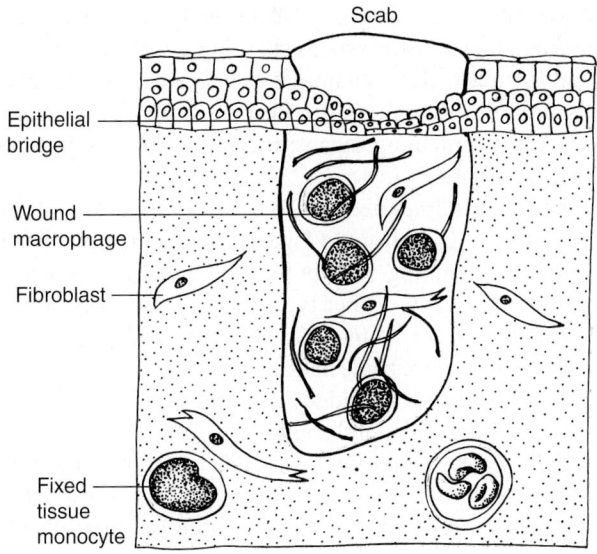

**FIGURE 12-4** Fibroblasts infiltrate the wound site in response to signaling from wound macrophages.

| TABLE 12-2 | Extracellular Matrix Components | |
|---|---|---|
| **Component** | **Structure** | **Function** |
| Collagen | Triple helical glycoprotein molecules rich in proline, hydroxyproline, and glycine | Strength, support, and structure for all tissues and organs |
| Elastin | Stretchable hydrophobic protein interacting with glycosylated microfibrils | Allows tissues and structures to expand and contract |
| Fibronectin | Specialized adhesive glycoprotein | Mediates cell matrix adhesion |
| Laminin | Large, complex, adhesive glycoprotein | Binds cells to type IV collagen and heparan sulfate |
| Proteoglycans | Heterogeneous, long glycosaminoglycan chains covalently linked to a core protein | Moisture stores, shock absorption, sequestration of cytokines |
| Hyaluronic acid | Very large, specialized, nonsulfated glycosaminoglycan | Provides a fluid environment for cell movement and differentiation and binds to cytokines |

These cells are not as pluripotent as the mesenchymal cells found in bone marrow. The bone marrow-derived mesenchymal cells respond later.

The factors involved in the differentiation of mesenchymal cells to fibroblasts are not well characterized, but most likely involve connective tissue growth factor (CTGF). Interestingly, TGF-β and CTGF differentiate fibroblasts into the myofibroblasts responsible for wound contraction. The presence of a large number of myofibroblasts can lead to hypertrophic scars and keloids.

Epithelialization takes place very soon after an injury to the skin and replaces the clot that initially protects the wound (Fig. 12-4). Epidermal cells migrate from the basal layer of the residual epidermis or the epithelium-lined dermal appendages to form a fine layer over the wound. The migrating epidermal cells are guided by dermal integrins, allowing them to migrate between the fibrinous eschar and the underlying dermal tissue. The migrating epidermal cells use phagocytosis to remove debris as they migrate.

## Extracellular Matrix

The ECM consists of a framework of (1) glycosaminoglycans (GAG) primarily proteoglycans (eg, hyaluronic acid); and (2) fibrous proteins such as collagen, elastin, fibronectin, and laminin. The ECM provides a lattice network for cells to migrate and differentiate. Early in wound healing a fibrin plug forms the wound matrix; this plug consists of fibrin, fibrinogen, fibronectin, and vitronectin. GAGs and proteoglycans are then synthesized, and finally collagen is synthesized by fibroblasts. GAGs form a hydrated gel that occupies a large volume and provides a matrix optimized for cell migration and collagen deposition (Table 12-2).

## Collagen Formation

There are at least 16 types of collagen identified; each differs in its polypeptide composition. Glycine, proline, and a third amino acid, often hydroxyproline, form a tripeptide. Glycine plays an important role in the structure of collagen because of its small size, which makes it critical for the formation of the triple helix (Fig. 12-5). Integrins help direct fibroblasts and thus are important in collagen synthesis. Reconstructing the ECM is a dynamic process with degradation and synthesis happening at the same time.

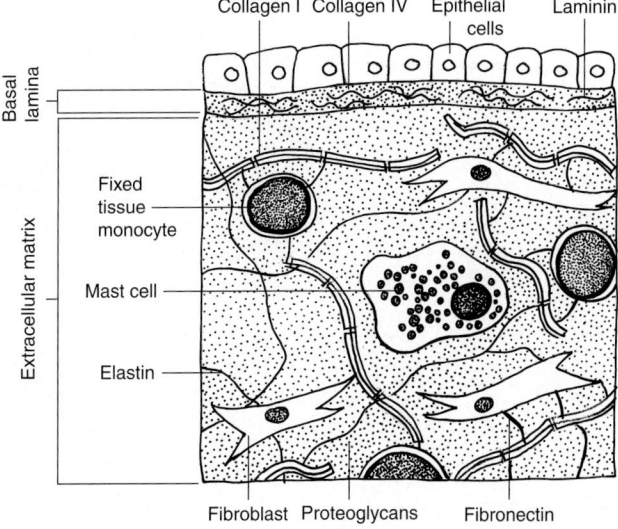

**FIGURE 12-5** The triple helical conformation of the type I procollagen molecule.

| TABLE 12-3 | Molecular Structure of Collagen Types I Through VI | |
|---|---|---|
| Type | Molecular Configuration[a] | Distribution |
| I | $[\alpha1(I)]_2\alpha2(1)$ | All connective tissues except cartilage and basement membranes |
| II | $[\alpha1(II)]_3$ | Cartilages and vitreous humor |
| III | $[\alpha1(III)]_3$ | Distensible connective tissues (eg, fetal skin, blood vessels, and uterus) |
| IV | $[\alpha1(IV)]_2\alpha2 (IV)$ | Basement membranes |
| V | $[\alpha1(V)]_2\alpha2 (V)$ | Essentially all tissues |
| VI | $[\alpha1(VI), \alpha2 (VI), \alpha3 (VI)]$ | Essentially all tissues |

[a]γ-Chains are composed of about 1000 amino acids and are rich in glycine, proline, and hydroxyproline. Most collagens contain 3 α chains interacting in a helical structure.

In adult scars, type III collagen is first produced, followed largely by type I. In fetal and newborn tissue, type III collagen remains the dominant type of collagen. Collagen is synthesized in fibroblasts and secreted into the ECM in a triple helix configuration called procollagen. Procollagen has propeptides attached to the carboxy and amino terminals. Specific proteases cleave the propeptides resulting in the formation of a collagen monomer. These monomers self-assemble into collagen fibrils in the ECM. Vitamin C is important for the hydroxylation of proline and the formation of stable triple helices. Vitamin C deficiency is called scurvy, a condition in which collagen becomes frail. Scurvy affects all collagen containing organs, including skin, teeth, capillaries, and bones.

Osteogenesis imperfecta (OI) is a disorder of collagen type I. In type I OI, 1 out of 2 genes producing procollagen is defective, resulting in only half the quantity of collagen type I pro-$\alpha_1$ chains. Other types of OI involve gene mutations that alter the amino acid sequence and prohibit the formation of mature triple helices. This leads to brittle bones and is important to consider in a child with multiple fractures consistent with child abuse.

Ehlers–Danlos syndrome is another condition that leads to defective collagen production. It can affect collagen type I, III, V, and other parts of collagen synthesis. Ehlers–Danlos results in unusually elastic skin and joints, and can also lead to fragile blood vessels and otosclerosis (Table 12-3).

## Glycosaminoglycans

GAG are also known as mucopolysaccharides. They are produced by fibroblasts or cells in the fibroblast family (eg, chondroblasts, osteoblasts). The addition of a protein moiety to a GAG is called a proteoglycan (Fig. 12-6). Proteoglycans have negatively charged side chains because of their sulfate or carboxyl groups. $Na^+$ is bound to the side chains and is followed by water. The large amount of water incorporated into the ECM provides tissue turgor and the ability to withstand pressure. Proteoglycans play an important role in controlling migration of cells, nutrients, hormones,

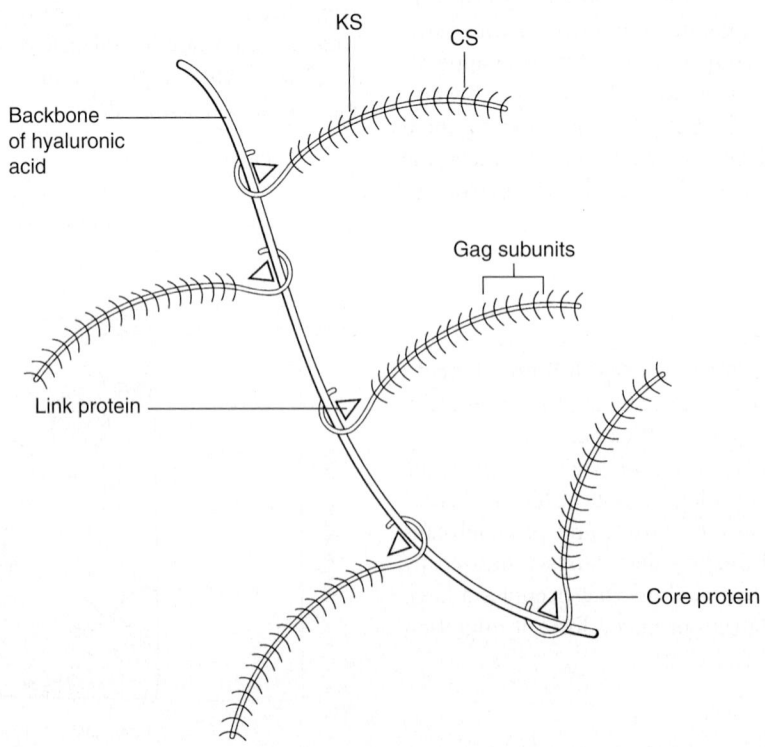

**FIGURE 12-6** The structure of a representative proteoglycan (KS, keratan sulfate; CS, chondroitin sulfate) demonstrating the "bottle-brush" architecture.

## TABLE 12-4  Glycosaminoglycans and Their Tissue Distributions

**Repeating Disaccharide (A-B)**

| Glycosaminoglycan | Molecular Weight (Da) | Monosaccharide A | Monosaccharide B | Linked to Protein | Tissue Distribution |
|---|---|---|---|---|---|
| Hyaluronic acid | $4000 - 8 \times 10^8$ | D-Glucuronic acid | N-Acetyl-D-glucosamine | − | Most connective tissues, skin, cartilage, and synovial fluid |
| Chondroitin sulfate | 5000-50,000 | D-Glucuronic acid | N-Acetyl-D-galactosamine | + | Cartilage, bone, and skin |
| Dermatan nitrate | 15,000-40,000 | D-Glucuronic acid or L-iduronic acid | N-Acetyl-D-galactosamine | + | Skin and blood vessels |
| Heparan sulfate | 5000-12,000 | D-Glucuronic acid or L-iduronic acid | N-Acetyl-D-glucosamine | + | Lungs, arteries, and cell surfaces |
| Heparin | 6000-25,000 | D-Glucuronic acid or L-iduronic acid | N-Acetyl-D-glucosamine | + | Skin, lungs, liver, and mast cells |
| Keratan sulfate | 4000-19,000 | D-Galactose | N-Acetyl-D-glucosamine | + | Cartilage and intervertebral disc |

and metabolites. Because of their many different side chains and core proteins, they have the ability to alter the ECM environment.

As previously mentioned, the GAG, hyaluronic acid, is predominant in fetal tissue and appears to facilitate a perfect deposition of collagen. Hyaluronic acid is composed of nonsulfated disaccharide units, and does not have an attached protein moiety. It provides an ideal environment for cell migration into the wound. In adult tissue where sulfated GAGs predominate, a denser scar is formed (Table 12-4).

### Remodeling Phase

Collagen is synthesized by fibroblasts as part of the healing process. There is a dynamic balance between breakdown and synthesis. The balance is weighted heavily toward synthesis in the beginning stages of healing. As part of the maturation of the wound, excessive collagen is broken down by collagenases and the scar becomes less prominent.

The wound also contracts and becomes slightly smaller and less visible. Myofibroblasts are specialized fibroblasts responsible for wound contraction. They are present between 1 and 4 weeks after the injury but peak around 2 weeks. In acute wounds, they undergo apoptosis and then disappear after they have completed the wound contraction.

Research has shown that TGF-β and CTGF help to differentiate the fibroblast into a myofibroblast. When hypertrophic scars form, myofibroblasts are present beyond the usual time period or are present in excessive amounts. This may be related to ongoing autocrine TGF-β stimulation.

The wound strength increases rapidly between 1 and 6 weeks after injury. At 3 weeks, the breaking strength increases as a result of cross-linking of collagen. The wound reaches close to its final strength after 2 months. At a year, the wound strength plateaus and is approximately 70% that of normal skin.

## TYPES OF WOUND REPAIR

### Primary

After most operations the wound is repaired by primary closure. The edges of the wound are approximated using sutures, glue (eg, Dermabond), paper tape strips, or staples. Following approximation, the wound follows the usual steps of healing (Fig. 12-7).

### Secondary

Contaminated wounds have a high risk of wound infection (>30%). Thus, it is not advised to close the skin and subcutaneous tissue of contaminated wounds. The wound can be packed with saline-soaked gauze daily up to several times daily. This will minimize contamination in the wound, allow granulation tissue formation, and ultimately results in healing and contraction of the wound. Some contaminated wounds, for example, ileostomy closures, can be closed with a purse-string suture and left partially open. This has been shown to significantly reduce wound infection rates, but also provides a favorable scar (Fig. 12-8).

### Delayed Primary

Some surgeons advocate leaving contaminated, or potentially contaminated, wounds open for 3 to 5 days and then closing the wound after a bed of granulation tissue has formed. Closure of the wound can usually take place at the bedside. Sutures are often left in place, but untied, at the time of operation (Fig. 12-9).

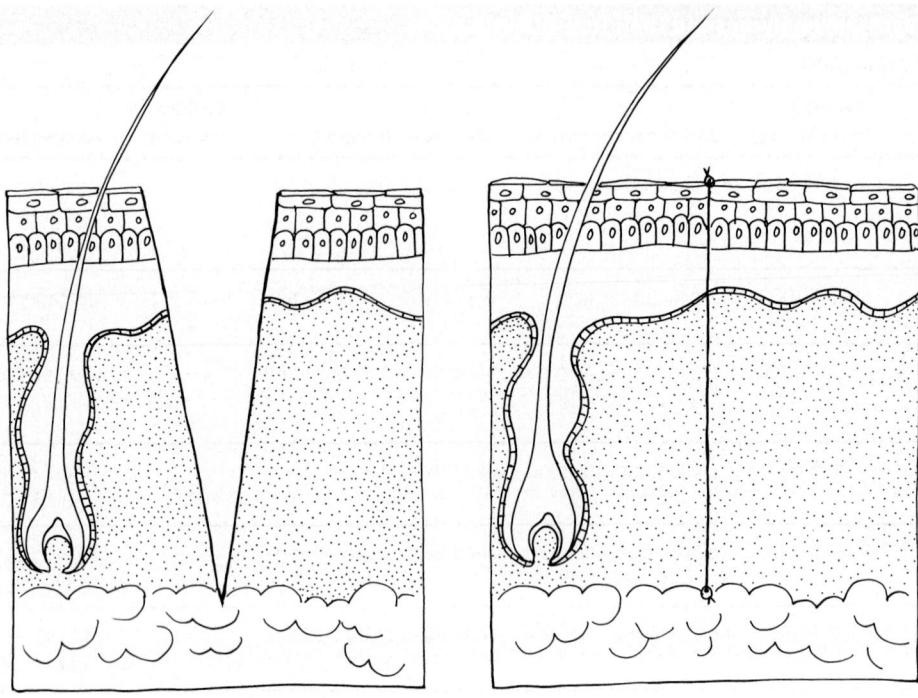

**FIGURE 12-7** Schematic depiction of primary wound healing.

## PEDIATRIC WOUNDS

In general, pediatric wounds are treated according to the same principles as adult surgical wounds. However, there are subtle differences. Children rarely have chronic conditions that impair wound healing and lead to complications (eg, type 2 diabetes, atherosclerosis, and obesity). Children also have a lesser amount of subcutaneous fat, resulting in decreased dead space. This may allow for the closure of wounds that would be considered contaminated and only amenable to closure by secondary intention in adults. Contaminated wounds such as wounds from stoma closure and the laparoscopic incisions for appendectomy in perforated appendicitis can be closed primarily. In addition, the trauma of dressing changes and suture removal make primary closure of most wounds the preferred option in children.

Laparoscopic surgery has been shown to decrease the frequency of superficial surgical site infections. Laparoscopy has been widely adopted among pediatric surgeons because

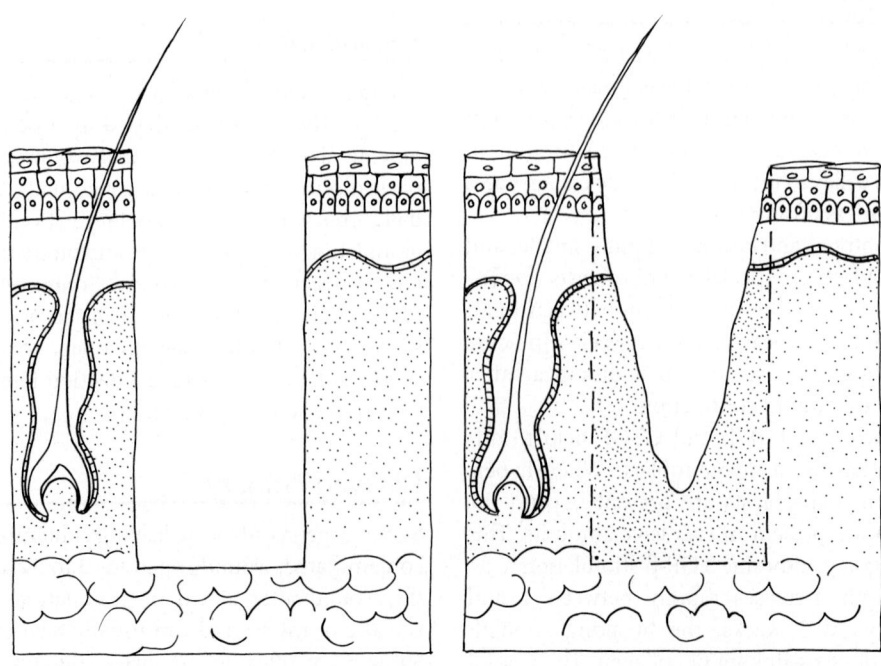

**FIGURE 12-8** Schematic depiction of secondary wound healing.

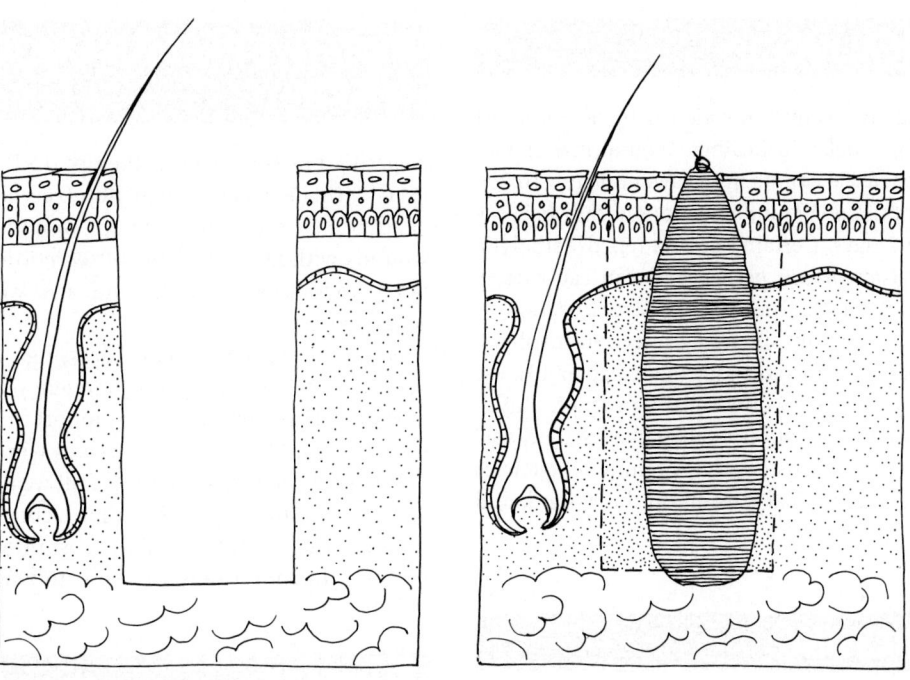

**FIGURE 12-9** Schematic drawing depicting delayed primary wound healing.

of the benefits of smaller wounds, less pain, and less risk of wound infection.

## EXCESSIVE SCARRING

Some patients will develop scars out of proportion to what one would expect. There are 2 types of excessive scarring: hypertrophic scars and keloids. Both types share in common the deposition of excessive amounts of collagen as a response to wound healing.

Hypertrophic scars have boundaries within the original wound and become less prominent over time. In addition, these scars usually do not cause functional impairment of joints. Rarely is the removal of a hypertrophic scar indicated.

Keloids typically extend beyond the borders of the original wound and can lead to functional impairment. Occasionally, keloids contain histamine-releasing mast cells and as a result are very pruritic. The treatment of keloids is difficult and often involves a combination of scar revision with triamcinolone injections intra- and postoperatively. Unfortunately, the long-term outcome is often not satisfactory, as keloids can recur.

Burn wounds can cause problems with contractures over joints and cosmetically displeasing results. The topic of burns is covered elsewhere in this text (see Chapter 83).

## FETAL WOUND REPAIR

Pediatric surgeons have noticed how well infants and young children heal after surgical procedures. The scar formation is significantly less than in adults, and children return to normal function and activity much more rapidly than adults. Fetal wound healing has received focused research since Somasundaram and Prathap demonstrated repair without scar formation in fetal rabbits in 1969.

Several differences in the dermal tissue repair of fetus and adult have been described: (1) fetal wounds have less inflammation than adults; (2) more hyaluronic acid is present in the fetal wound; (3) fetal wounds exhibit less collagen deposition, despite high rates of production; (4) fetal wounds have fine and reticular collagen deposits and a greater ratio of type III to I collagen; and (5) T lymphocytes predominate in fetal wounds.

Fetal wound healing and scar formation are not uniform throughout all organs or throughout gestation. Anecdotal reports have described children who underwent in utero diaphragmatic hernia repair having a dense scar of the diaphragm in addition to adherent intestine and stomach on subsequent postnatal operations. Longaker has confirmed this observation in fetal lambs, demonstrating that diaphragmatic incisions heal with scar formation whether or not they were exposed to amniotic fluid. In contrast, facial musculature in full-thickness lip wounds has been shown to heal without scar formation in a model for cleft lip repair.

There are multiple questions related to fetal wound healing that still need to be answered. Does the fetal wound healing response represent a different response to injury or are the observed results the effect of an immature response and the growth characteristics of developing tissue? When does the fetus acquire the ability to respond to wounds, and when does this response become prone to scar formation? Finally, what alterations in the genetic response to injury are necessary to create a scar-less repair or is the lack of scarring a response to the environment in which the fetus is located?

## DELAYED HEALING

In the pediatric patient, wound infection is by far the most common reason for a delay in healing. Wound infection is present when the bacterial counts in the awound are >10,000 bacteria per gram of tissue. Wound infections usually become apparent after 5 to 7 days. Certain bacteria (eg, β-hemolytic streptococcus and *Clostridium perfringens*) can cause early infections (before 5 days). The most severe infection is necrotizing fasciitis, a rapidly spreading infection involving the deep fascia and subcutaneous tissue (see Chapter 13).

Other reasons for delayed wound healing include radiation, chemotherapy, malnutrition, connective tissue disorders, medications (eg, corticosteroids), vitamin deficiencies (vitamin C and A), mechanical tension on the wound, and ischemia.

## WOUND DRESSING

Pediatric surgical wounds are most often dressed with only steri-strips. The more complicated wounds (eg, gastroschisis closure wounds and G-tube sites) often require additional wound care and may benefit from specialized dressings. We have seen benefits from using a silicone-based dressing in neonates with gastroschisis or other complex wounds as these dressings are less traumatizing to the skin and require less frequent changes.

It has been shown that leaving an occlusive dressing on for several days speeds up epithelialization. The slightly acidic environment and low oxygen tension on the wound surface appears to be an ideal setting for granulation tissue formation. In contaminated wounds and wounds with a lot of secretions, an absorptive dressing is necessary and more frequent dressing changes are performed to reduce the bacterial counts.

Currently, several biological skin coverage options are available (see below). These materials can be very expensive compared to a traditional dressing; however, they may provide improved healing in children with complicated wounds or wounds without adequate coverage.

MatriStem®: Decellularized and sterilized ECM from porcine bladder.

AlloDerm®: Decellularized and sterilized human donor skin ECM without epidermis.

Apligraf®: A living cell hybrid product consisting of bovine type 1 collagen, human fibroblasts, and matrix proteins. In addition, there is an upper epidermal layer of human keratinocytes. Unlike human skin, Apligraf does not contain melanocytes, Langerhans cells, macrophages, and lymphocytes, or other structures such as blood vessels, hair follicles, or sweat glands.

Surgisis®: Biologic grafts harvested from porcine small intestinal submucosa. Surgisis is extracted from the intestine in a manner that removes all cells, but leaves the ECM intact.

Permacol™: Consists of acellular porcine dermis.

## NEGATIVE PRESSURE WOUND THERAPY

Negative pressure wound therapy (NPWT) is now being used with increasing frequency (see also Chapter 13). It is advocated for many different wounds, but in particular wounds with large amounts of secretions, chronic wounds, open abdominal wounds, and any wound left open or reopened.

Negative pressure wound dressings can be left on for several days decreasing the frequency of painful dressing changes. There are data to support improved neovascularization and blood flow to tissues with the use of NPWT. Scientific evidence, however, is still weak. In several studies and a Cochrane review clear improvements in outcome have not been demonstrated. Taking cost into consideration, it is possible that physicians are over-utilizing NPWT.

## SUMMARY

Wound healing is a field with tremendous potential for ongoing research both to facilitate healing and to improve cosmetic results. Many of the principles of wound care have not changed since sterile surgical techniques were introduced. Substantial progress, however, has been made in alternative biological materials used in complex wound closures. The ongoing research into fetal wound healing will hopefully bring results that will benefit patients in the near future.

### SELECTED READINGS

Burnweit C, Bilik R, Shandling B. Primary closure of contaminated wounds in perforated appendicitis. *J Pediatr Surg* 1991;26:1362–1365.

Dabiri G, et al. Hic 5 promotes the hypertrophic scar myofibroblast phenotype by regulating the TGF-beta 1 autocrine loop. *J Invest Dermatol* 2008;128:2518–2525.

Ethridge R, Leong M, Phillips L. Wound healing. In: Sabiston DC, ed. *Textbook of Surgery*. 18th ed. Philadelphia, PA: WB Saunders Co.; 2007.

Longaker M, Adzick N, Jackson L, et al. Studies in fetal wound healing. VII. Fetal wound healing may be modulated by hyaluronic acid stimulating activity in amniotic fluid. *J Pediatr Surg* 1990;25:430–433.

Sauerland S, Jaschinski T, Neugebauer EAM. Laparoscopic versus open surgery for suspected appendicitis. *Cochrane Database Syst Rev* 2010; 10: CD001546. doi: 10.1002/14651858.CD001546.pub3.

Somasundaram K, Prathap K. Intra-uterine healing of skin wounds in rabbits foetuses. *J Pathol* 1970;100:81–86.

Ubbink DT, Westerbos SJ, Evans D, Land L, Vermeulen H. Topical negative pressure for treating chronic wounds. *Cochrane Database Syst Rev* 2008; 3:CD001898. doi: 10.1002/14651858.CD001898.pub2.

Whitby DJ, Longaker MT, Harrison MR, et al. Rapid epithelialisation of fetal wounds is associated with the early deposition of tenascin. *J Cell Sci* 1991;99:583–586.

# CHAPTER 13

# Surgical Infection: Classification, Diagnosis, Treatment, and Prevention

*John R. Gosche and Samuel Smith*

## KEY POINTS

1. Findings on physical examination often suggest the origin and likely causative organisms in patients with infections involving the skin and subcutaneous tissues.

2. When planning operative intervention for lymphadenitis, it is important to preoperatively plan either incision and drainage for abscess formation or lymphadenectomy for suspected mycobacterial infection.

3. A high index of suspicion of necrotizing fasciitis and early surgical intervention are keys to optimizing patient outcomes.

4. Laboratory and imaging studies are important adjuncts for the diagnosis of body cavity infections.

We live in a hostile environment. Since the beginning of life on earth, all living organisms have been under attack by would-be invaders seeking to use the nutrients within living tissues for their own survival, often to the detriment of the host. To combat the constant threat of invasion, all living organisms have developed measures to resist microbial invasion. In higher organisms, the mechanisms to resist microbial invasion have become quite complex and are usually extremely effective. However, occasionally resistance to invasion is overcome, due either to a break in host defenses or to a microbial adaptation that creates a more effective invader. When host invasion occurs, the resulting infection will frequently require medical treatment. In some cases, effective treatment also includes surgical intervention.

Unfortunately, many of the disease conditions that require surgical treatment, as well as the nature of the surgical intervention itself, alter host defense mechanisms and thus create further opportunities for microbial invasion. It is not surprising therefore that postoperative infection is the most common complication associated with many surgical procedures. Thus, instituting measures to decrease the risk of postoperative wound infections, in addition to early recognition and expeditious treatment of surgical site infections (SSIs) when they do occur, are essential aspects of optimal surgical care.

## HOST DEFENSES

### Epithelial Barriers

In higher organisms, all exposed body surfaces (external and internal) are covered by a layer of epithelial cells that serve as a mechanical barrier against microbial invasion, while invasion between cells is inhibited by close apposition of the cellular membranes of adjacent epithelial cells. Besides creating a mechanical impediment to microbial invasion, most epithelial surfaces also have specialized adaptations that limit bacterial attachment and invasion. For example, the epidermis of the skin is composed of multiple layers of cells, the outer layers of which are inanimate, keratinized cells creating a dry, acidic inhospitable environment. Continuous cell shedding facilitates removal of attached organisms, while glandular secretions contain free fatty acids, lysozymes, and β-defensins that inhibit microbial growth. In the respiratory tract, a continuous layer of mucous covers the epithelial surface, trapping inhaled pathogens, which are then swept toward the pharynx by the continuous movement of cilia on the luminal surface of the epithelial cells. In addition, glandular secretions contain defensins and immunoglobulins that inhibit bacterial growth and attachment to epithelial surfaces. The urinary tract maintains sterility via a continuous flow of urine which has bacteriostatic properties due to its low pH, high ammonia and urea content, and high osmolality. In the gastrointestinal system, the epithelial defense mechanisms vary at different levels of the digestive tract. The saliva is rich in antibacterial agents including lysozyme and phospholipase A2. In the stomach, low pH and proteases kill most ingested microorganisms. Beyond the pylorus, a continuous mucous layer covers the epithelial surface, trapping organisms and inhibiting contact with the epithelial cell surface. In addition, secreted immunoglobulins coat microbial surfaces thereby inhibiting attachment, while continuous peristalsis propels unattached microorganisms distally for elimination.

### The Immune Response

Destruction of microorganisms that breach epithelial barriers and enter the body is dependent on the immune system. The human immune system is often considered as 2 separate components, the innate immune response and the adaptive (acquired) immune response. However, there are multiple interactions and effector mechanisms that are shared between these 2 arms. The immune response in humans is very complex, and therefore a complete discussion is beyond the scope of this chapter.

## Innate Immunity

Innate immunity is the more ancient of the immune responses and is present in all multicellular organisms. The components of the innate immune response are preformed and functional, allowing immediate recognition and destruction of invading microorganisms. Components of innate immunity include several of the epithelial adaptations noted previously (ie, defensins, lysozyme), plus cellular effectors (macrophages, dendritic cells, neutrophils, and natural killer [NK] cells) and humoral components (complement, interferons). Innate immune responses rely on detection of carbohydrates, lipids, or other cellular components (eg, double-stranded RNA) that are unique to microorganisms (ie, pathogen-associated molecular patterns or PAMPs) by pattern-recognition receptors (PRRs). Examples of PRRs include: the Toll-like receptors (TLRs), a family of intracellular and cell surface receptors that activate downstream adapter proteins resulting in induction or suppression of genes that help to orchestrate the immune response; mannan-binding lectins (MBLs), a serum protein that binds to a unique polysaccharide on the surface of many bacteria and yeasts (mannan) thereby facilitating phagocytosis and activation of the complement system; and nucleotide-binding oligomerization domain (NOD)-like receptors (a.k.a., nucleotide-binding domain, leucine-rich repeat containing proteins or nucleotide leucine rich receptors [NLR]), a family of cytoplasmic receptors that recognize microbial and stress-induced molecules causing activation of caspases that cleave and activate inflammatory cytokines, and activate NF-κB, a transcription factor for genes involved in the immune response.

The innate immune response has several important roles, one of which is to activate the adaptive immune response as discussed in the section that follows. Other critical functions include the elaboration of signals that trigger inflammation and the killing of invading microorganisms. Both cellular and humoral components of the innate immune system contribute to microbial destruction. The cellular mediators include phagocytic cells (eg, neutrophils, macrophages, and dendritic cells) that are capable of recognizing and ingesting foreign material. Once ingested, the resulting phagosome containing the microbe fuses with a lysosome that contains acid hydrolases and enzymes (eg, nitric oxide synthase, NAPH oxidase, superoxide dismutase, and myeloperoxidase) capable of producing reactive oxygen intermediates. These enzymatic processes cause microbial destruction, and in macrophages and dendritic cells allow partial digestion of microbial proteins for presentation on the surface of the phagocyte. Another cellular mediator of microbial killing is the NK cell. NK cells are lymphocytes that possess some, but not all T-cell surface markers. Unlike other cellular killers, NK cells are not phagocytic. Instead, NK cells kill by releasing perforins (pore forming proteins) and proteases (granzymes) in close proximity to target cells resulting in cell death by apoptosis or osmotic cell lysis. NK cells are activated by interferons and macrophage-derived cytokines but are inhibited by surface receptors that recognize major histocompatibility complex (MHC) class I alleles (thus preventing killing of host cells). MHC class 1 alleles frequently are downregulated on the surface of virus infected and tumor cells, which facilitates attack by NK cells.

Humoral mediators of microbial killing include defensins, lysozyme, LPS-binding protein, pentraxins (eg, C-reactive protein, serum amyloid protein), collectins (eg, MBL, surfactant proteins A and D), and the complement system. Several of these humoral factors directly attack invading microorganisms (eg, lysozyme hydrolyzes peptoglycans in the cell wall of bacteria, defensins form pore-like membrane defects), while others contribute to phagocytosis by opsonization or activation of the complement system. The complement system consists of approximately 30 known serum and membrane-bound proteins and protein regulators that are synthesized mainly in the liver. Once activated, the complement system has 3 main roles: lysis of cells, generation or inflammatory and chemotactic mediators, and facilitation of phagocytosis by opsonization through attachment to foreign material. There are 3 known pathways for activation of the complement system, all of which ultimately lead to activation of C3 (Fig. 13-1). Once activated, C3 binds and activates additional proteins leading to cell lysis and generation of inflammatory signals and opsonins. The "classical pathway" is activated when IgG or IgM antibodies bind an antigen allowing activation of C1q by the antibody's Fc fragment. Activated C1q autoactivates 2 associated proteins (C1s, C1r) leading to recruitment and activation of additional proteins (C4, C2) generating C3 convertase. The "alternative pathway" is activated when cell surface molecules (eg, lipopolysaccharides) directly bind C3 causing a conformational change leading to hydrolysis and activation of C3 and binding of factor B. Once bound, factor B is cleaved by a serine protease and the resultant complex (hydrated C3 + Bb) functions as the C3 convertase of the alternative pathway. Finally, the "lectin pathway" is activated when MBL binds mannan on the surface of a microbe. MBL is structurally similar to C1q and is associated

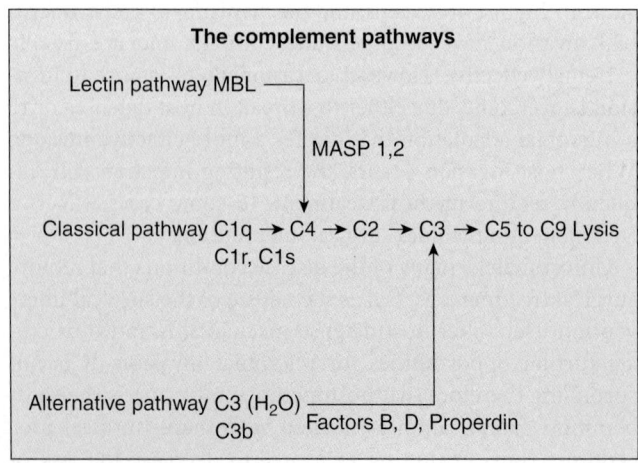

FIGURE 13-1 Three pathways for activation of the complement system. (Reprinted with permission from *Frank MM. Complement disorders and hereditary angioedema. J Allergy Clin Immunol 2010;125(2):S262–S271.*)

with mannose-binding lectin-associated serine proteases (MASPs). Binding of MBL to mannan causes activation of MASP, which like C1r and C1s bind and activate C4 and C2 resulting in generation of C3 convertase. C3 convertases cleave C3 into a and b fragments. The C3b binds with the C3 convertase creating C5 convertase, which in turn cleaves C5 into a and b fragments. The complement cascade continues as C5b complexes with C6 and C7, which in turn interact with C8 and C9 to create a pore-forming complex that penetrates the cell membrane causing loss of osmotic equilibrium and cell lysis. Besides cell lysis, some small fragments generated during the complement cascade also serve other important functions including chemotaxis and anaphylaxis (C3a, C4a, and C5a) as well as opsonization (C3b).

## Adaptive Immunity

The adaptive immune system is evolutionarily a relative newcomer being present only in vertebrates. Like innate immunity, the adaptive immune system has both cellular and humoral components. However, unlike the innate immune system, most of the response elements for the adaptive immune response are not preformed, but rather are generated and/or amplified following exposure to a pathogen. Thus there is a lag time between exposure to a pathogen and maximal activation of the adaptive immune response. Also, unlike the innate immune system which responds to common PAMPs, the individual components of the adaptive immune system recognize and respond to very specific antigens. Finally, unlike innate immune responses, prior exposure to a pathogen results in "immunologic memory." Thus, subsequent invasion of the same or a similar pathogen are met by a more rapid and robust immune response.

Cellular elements of the adaptive immune system include the T (a.k.a., thymus-derived) and B (a.k.a., bursa of Fabricius or bone marrow-derived) lymphocytes. Both begin as lymphoid progenitors in the bone marrow or fetal liver and must undergo a series of maturation steps to become fully functional. One step, common to both T and B lymphocytes, is a series of genomic rearrangements that culminate in the generation of a unique surface protein receptor (T-cell receptor [TCR] in T-cells, immunoglobulins in B-cells) that accounts for the lymphocyte's antigen binding specificity. During maturation, T and B cells also acquire additional surface receptors that dictate function and are necessary for interaction with other immunologically active cells or pathogens. In addition, lymphocytes that express receptors that react with "self" proteins or fail to recognize self MHC proteins are identified and destroyed by apoptosis.

Activation of the adaptive immune response to most pathogens begins with the innate immune system. Initially invading microorganisms are ingested by antigen presenting cells (APCs) (dendritic cells, macrophages, B-cells, and basophils) and are partially digested. Inside the APC, microbial antigens are reprocessed and presented on the surface of the APC in conjunction with "self" MHC proteins. APCs are present in large numbers in the skin and mucosa. Engulfment of foreign material induces migration of the APC to regional lymph nodes where interaction with T cells can occur. T-cell activation is initiated when the TCR recognizes

a peptide/MHC complex on the surface of an APC, which results in clustering of other membrane-associated molecules (CD3 and CD4 or CD8) at the interface between the T cell and the APC. This APC–T cell interface is further stabilized by the interaction of adhesion molecules (LFA-1 on T-cells to ICAM-1 on APCs). T-cell activation also requires costimulatory signals (eg, B7 protein on the APC must interact with CD28 on the helper T cell). Failure of this secondary signaling results in a state of anergy specific to that antigen. Activated T cells produce cytokines that induce activation of downstream effectors. One of these cytokines, interleukin-2 (IL-2) produces a positive-feedback effect by inducing T-cell activation and clonal expansion of antigen-specific helper T cells. This positive feedback effect is inhibited by a different protein called cytotoxic T lymphocyte antigen-4 (CTLA-4), which also binds B7 and blocks IL-2 synthesis. CTLA-4 synthesis occurs in activated T cells and is important for inducing quiescence and generating memory cells.

T cells perform important functions which are determined by the expression of surface proteins (CD4 and CD8). Most CD4+ lymphocytes perform "helper" functions, of which there are 2 subpopulations, Th-1 cells and Th-2 cells. CD4+ cells are activated when TCRs interact with an antigen–MHC class II complex. Activated CD4+ helper cells produce cytokines that stimulate specific effector responses. Th-1 helper cells produce IL-2 and gamma interferon that activate cytotoxic T-cells and macrophages (cell-mediated responses); while Th-2 helper cells produce IL-4, IL-5, IL-6, and IL-10 which stimulate B cells (antibody-mediated response). The balance of Th-1 to Th-2 cells is regulated by IL-12, which increases the number of Th-1 cells, and gamma interferon, which inhibits the proliferation of Th-2 cells. Cytotoxic T-lymphocytes (CTLs) are CD8+ lymphocytes and are primarily involved in killing virus-infected and tumor cells. CD8+ cells recognize antigens associated with MHC class I molecules on the surface of infected cells. CTLs kill by inserting perforins and releasing degradative enzymes called granzymes into infected cells. CTLs also induce apoptosis by surface expression of Fas ligand which engages the Fas receptor (CD95) on the surface of the target cell.

Another class of T lymphocytes is the regulatory T cell. Regulatory T cells account for only 5% to 10% of CD4+ lymphocytes. They express CD4, CD25 (IL-2 receptor α chain), and CTLA-4 on their surface and produce the immunosuppressive cytokines (TGFβ and IL-10), but not IL-2. Activated regulatory T cells suppress proliferation and cytokine production of CD4+ and CD8+ T cells and thus downregulate the immune responses to foreign antigens. Regulatory T cells induce tolerance and are important for preventing autoimmune responses.

The humoral arm of the adaptive immune response requires activation of B lymphocytes which results in the production of antibodies (immunoglobulins) by plasma cells. Immunoglobulins serve a number of important functions including neutralization of toxins and viruses, opsonization of microbes to facilitate phagocytosis, complement activation, and blocking attachment of microbes to mucosal surfaces. B cells recirculate through secondary lymphoid organs (lymph nodes, spleen, and mucosal-associated lymphoid organs) where contact with foreign antigens is most likely to occur. In lymph nodes, B cells are concentrated in the cortex in contact with follicular dendritic cells. Foreign antigens may enter B-cell rich regions of the lymph node by diffusion or by being carried on the surface of macrophages, follicular dendritic cells, or other B cells. In addition, B-cell activation can occur via T-cell dependent or independent pathways, although most antibody responses require the participation of T cells. T-independent antigens include protein or polysaccharide molecules with repeating molecular patterns that are capable of cross-linking multiple immunoglobulin receptors on the surface of the B lymphocyte. T-cell dependent B-cell activation begins with binding of antigen by the immunoglobulin (IgM or IgD) component of the B-cell receptor (BCR). B-cell activation requires cross-linking of BCRs, phosphorylation of BCR-associated proteins, and the assembly of an intracellular signaling complex (signalosome). The signalosome leads to internalization of the antigen, which is then processed, loaded onto MHC proteins, and presented on the surface of the B cell for recruitment and activation of CD4+ Th-2 helper cells. Once activated, B cells may become short-lived plasma cells that release large amounts of IgM, or they may undergo further maturation. B-cell maturation includes class-switching (ie, change in antibody production from IgM or IgD to IgG, IgA, or IgE), and affinity maturation (a.k.a., somatic hypermutation) via a series of nucleotide substitutions in the heavy and light chain variable regions resulting in the generation of antibodies with higher affinity. B-cell maturation processes occur in response to cytokine signals. Ultimately, some activated lymphocytes become quiescent long-lived memory T and B cells, which are capable of being rapidly reactivated during subsequent exposures to an antigen. Thus, subsequent exposures to a pathogen are met by the more rapid appearance of high affinity IgG, IgA, or IgE immunoglobulins (secondary response), while first encounters with a pathogen (primary response) initially generate lower affinity IgM antibodies and require a lag time of 2 weeks or more to generate high affinity IgG, IgA, or IgE antibodies.

## Immunity in Infants and Children

Globally, more than 2 million children die annually due to infectious diseases. Multiple developmental deficiencies in the immune system contribute to the increased risk of death due to infection in infants and children. In the neonate, the skin is fragile at birth and more susceptible to trauma. Tracheal secretions at birth are devoid of IgA and antimicrobial peptides including β-defensins increase with gestational age. In the gastrointestinal tract, gastric pH of the neonate is higher and intestinal peristalsis is less efficient. The neonate, however, does have some unique epithelial defense adaptations. These include the vernix caseosa, which limits desiccation of the skin, lowers surface pH, and contains a number of antimicrobial substances (lysozyme, α-defensins, ubiquitin, psoriasin, and free fatty acids). In addition, human breast milk contains antimicrobial peptides including lactoferrin and lysozyme. Human breast milk also contains factors that modulate TLR signaling, which are thought to support the establishment of beneficial bacteria as part of the intestinal microflora.

At birth many components of the innate immune system are deficient. Serum levels of most of the complement system proteins (C1q, C2, C3, C4, C5, factor B, and properdin) are significantly lower in neonates than in adults. C3 levels decrease initially after birth, but recover by 3 weeks of age and reach adult levels by about 6 months of age. Levels of several of the acute phase proteins (MBL, C-reactive protein [CRP], and lipopolysaccharide binding protein [LBP]) are also low at birth, but rise during the first weeks of life. Circulating neutrophil counts are higher in newborns than in adults, but neonates have decreased numbers of granulocyte and monocyte precursors. As a result, neonates frequently have an inadequate pool of neutrophils to respond to infection. Furthermore, the neutrophils in neonates exhibit functional impairments in chemotaxis, rolling adhesion, transmigration and lamellipodia formation (due to decreased expression of complement receptor 3 and L-selectin), and microbial killing (due to a decrease in granule content of antimicrobial peptides and impaired oxidase activity). APC function in the neonate is also impaired due to decreased surface expression of MHC class II molecules and decreased numbers of resident dendritic cells in secondary lymphoid organs. The latter alteration contributes to inefficient antigen presentation. Finally, the production of some cytokines by APCs in the neonate is decreased (eg, IFNγ, TNF, and IL-12p70), while the production of other cytokines (eg, IL-6, IL-10, and IL-23) exceeds that of adults.

The adaptive immune system of the neonate is naïve. Thus, responses to foreign antigens have the characteristics of a "primary responses." In addition, T-helper cell function in the neonate is generally depressed and altered production of cytokines by neonatal APCs results in a bias toward Th-2 responses and against Th-1 responses. Diminished Th-1 responsiveness contributes to greater vulnerability to certain microbial infections, while increased Th-2 responsiveness is believed to increase susceptibility to allergic reactions. Th-1 mediated responses are also impaired by regulatory T-cells, which are relatively more abundant and more potent in the fetus and in the newborn.

Antibody responses to both thymus-dependent and thymus-independent antigens are also impaired in neonates and infants. In part this is due to the architectural immaturity of the secondary lymphoid structures where foreign antigens are processed. Specifically, lymph node germinal centers do not appear until around 4 months after birth, and marginal zone B-cell numbers in the spleen do not reach adult levels until around 2 years of age. Absence of lymphoid germinal centers, alterations in the function of APCs, and decreased expression of the costimulatory molecules by neonatal B-cells all contribute to decreased responses to thymus-dependent antigens. Decreased numbers of marginal-zone B cells in the spleen and low serum levels of the complement protein C3, coupled with decreased expression of the corresponding receptor (CD21) on the surface of neonatal B cells, contribute to impaired responses to T-cell independent antigens. Even after activation, B cells in neonates and infants generate fewer antibody secreting plasma cells, which accounts for decreased antibody titers of shorter duration. In addition, impaired antibody maturation results in the production of lower affinity antibodies and limited expression of certain classes of immunoglobulins. Thus, serum levels of IgM reach adult levels at approximately 1 year of age, while adult levels of IgG are not attained until approximately 5 to 7 years of age and serum IgA levels do not reach adult levels until 10 to 14 years of age (although salivary levels of IgA reach adult levels by around 2 months of age). The IgG2 subclass of immunoglobulin is known to be particularly effective at recognizing polysaccharide antigens. Low levels of IgG2 combined with impaired responses to T-cell independent antigens are believed to contribute to the increased susceptibility of infants and neonates to infections caused by encapsulated bacteria.

## RISK FACTORS FOR INFECTION

### Microbial Virulence

The virulence of a microbial pathogen is generally defined as the ability of the organism to cause disease. The virulence of a given microbial pathogen is reliant in part on the relative susceptibility of the host. Virulence can be thought of as the gene products of an organism that facilitate colonization, growth, and survival within the host organism and allow spread to a new host. The key steps are initial colonization and attachment, multiplication and nutrition, evasion of host defenses (in some cases this also includes invasion of cells involved in the immune response), and lastly exit to spread to a new host. Microbial examples include the PapG P-pili of uropathogenic *Escherichia coli*, which allows attachment and colonization of the kidney and subsequent pyelonephritis. Another example is the Type III secretion system (TTSS) of *Pseudomonas aeruginosa*, which mediates the delivery of toxins directly into host eukaryotic cells and allows invasion and subsequent serious infections such as pneumonia. Bacterial capsules have long been recognized as important virulence factors. For example, *E. coli* that express the K5 capsule are not associated with significant infections in neonates while K1 capsule *E. coli* are associated with meningitis and disseminated sepsis. The K1 capsule camouflages the bacteria because of similarity with host tissues. Group B streptococcus (GBS) capsule is the most well-defined virulence factor of GBS. The capsule protects GBS from opsonization by C3 through inhibition of the alternative complement pathway in the absence of type-specific antibodies to capsular antigens. However, GBS may also express other factors that allow it to resist opsonophagocytosis and cause life-threatening neonatal bacterial infection.

### Immunodeficiencies

Defects in immune function can be classified as primary immunodeficiencies (ie, a defect in immune function not attributable to another illness) and secondary immunodeficiencies (ie, immunodeficiency arising in a previously normal individual attributable to an associated condition). Secondary immunodeficiencies are much more common than primary immunodeficiencies. In fact most serious or prolonged illnesses have a suppressive effect on immune function.

The primary immunodeficiencies comprise more than 130 different disorders. Most are rare with prevalence rates of approximately 1:10,000 births. Many primary immunodeficiencies are due to a defect in a single gene; however,

variations in penetrance and interactions between genetic and environmental factors can result in wide phenotypic variability. Commonly applied classification systems divide these conditions into: combined T- and B-cell deficiencies; predominantly antibody deficiencies; immune dysregulation; defects of phagocyte number, function, or both; defects in innate immunity; autoinflammatory disorders; and complement deficiencies. All primary immunodeficiencies are characterized by increased susceptibility to recurrent or severe infections caused by specific pathogens. Responsible pathogens and types of infectious complications will depend on the nature of the immune defect.

Secondary deficiencies in immune function can result from a multitude of preexisting conditions. Common etiologies include severe burns and trauma, severe malnutrition, specific viral infections (eg, cytomegalovirus [CMV], Epstein-Barr virus [EBV], and human immunodeficiency virus [HIV]), neoplasias (eg, leukemias, lymphomas), medical therapies (eg, immunosuppressive or chemotherapeutic drugs, irradiation), and chronic disease states (eg, renal failure, diabetes mellitus). Extremes of age, including newborn and premature infants, are also associated with alterations in immune function as described previously. While some of these etiologic agents are known to affect the function of specific cellular components of the immune system (eg, HIV infects CD4+ T helper cells, EBV encodes an IL-10 like protein [BRCF-1] that inhibits Th1 responses), most cause global deficiencies due to impairment of cellular division and/or maturation of 1 or more elements of the immune response. Affected patients are at increased risk of developing infections due to opportunistic organisms, or may experience increased frequency or severe complications associated with infections caused by common pathogens.

An underlying immune deficiency should be considered in any patient with a history of chronic or recurrent infections or a history of infections due to unusual pathogens. A record of the types, locations and frequency of infections, as well as the causative organisms should be sought. Recurrent gastrointestinal or respiratory symptoms or a history of growth failure or chronic weight loss may suggest a primary etiology or may be attributable to recurrent infections. A history of chronic medical illnesses as well as any history of recent or current drug exposures or medical treatments may suggest a possible etiology. A family history of frequent or recurrent infectious complications in an ancestor might suggest a primary immunodeficiency; however, it is important to remember that most patients have no family history since many of these conditions arise from de novo mutations or they may be the first occurrence of an autosomal recessive disease. Finally, findings on physical examination (eg, absent tonsils, partial albinism, telangiectasias, petechiae, and microcephaly) may also suggest a primary immunodeficiency.

While the laboratory evaluation of a patient with a suspected immunodeficiency can become quite complex, the initial studies should include at least a complete blood count (CBC), with differential, skin tests to check for cellular immune responses to common antigens and viral serologies (ie, HIV). Additional studies including measurements of total and specific antibody or complement component titers and tests of lymphocyte and granulocyte function may be indicated depending on the patient's history and results of preliminary laboratory studies.

Treatment for patients with primary immunodeficiencies includes antibiotic prophylaxis to decrease the risk of infections caused by common and opportunistic organisms, replacement of specific deficiencies (ie, immunoglobulins) where available, and possible gene therapy or bone marrow transplantation depending on the diagnosis. The treatment for secondary immunodeficiencies is primarily directed at identifying and correcting the underlying etiology. However, patients often receive antibiotic prophylaxis and may benefit from specific replacement therapy (eg, intravenous immunoglobulin infusions) or cytokine treatment (eg, granulocyte-macrophage colony stimulating factor) to stimulate production of immune cells until normal immune function is restored.

## Colonization of the Newborn

The human body comprises 10 times more microbial cells than human cells due to the large number of microbes that inhabit the gastrointestinal tract. In the first year of life, the infant intestinal tract progresses from sterility to an adult-like colonization of $10^{12}$ microbes per milliliter in the colon. The gastrointestinal microflora of an infant is initially composed of organisms from environmental exposures such as maternal vaginal, fecal, or skin microbiota. The rate at which the gastrointestinal tract of the newborn infant is colonized and the types of organisms in the newborn infant's intestinal microflora are influenced by the route of delivery, diet, maternal flora, and the neonatal environment.

Newborns delivered vaginally are colonized by anaerobic bacteria, predominantly *Bacteroides*, within 1 week of age. In infants delivered by C-section, anaerobic colonization is delayed, and the infant's microflora is initially more reflective of the hospital's flora than that of their mother. Beginning approximately 1 week postnatally, mode of feeding becomes the most important determinant of gastrointestinal flora in otherwise healthy neonates. In breast-fed infants lactobacilli and bifidobacteria outnumber *Enterobacteriaceae* in the gastrointestinal tract by nearly 1000-fold. In contrast, *Enterobacteriaceae* predominate in formula-fed infants. However, a complex bacterial microflora is established more rapidly in formula-fed infants than in breast-fed infants, possibly due to the iron content of infant formulas which fosters bacterial growth. The introduction of formula feedings in breast-fed infants causes a change in the bacterial profile to one that is more typical of formula-fed infants. Ultimately, the transformation of the intestinal microbial flora to a pattern that is adult-like is associated with the transition from a milk-based diet to the typical toddler diet. This transition is marked by a decrease in the relative numbers of *E. coli* and *Clostridium* spp., and an increase in *Bacteroides* and gram-positive anaerobic cocci.

Normal commensal bacteria have a number of positive effects on gastrointestinal physiology and immune function. The presence of bacteria in the gastrointestinal tract improves mucosal barrier function by activating genes responsible for epithelial cell turnover and mucus secretion resulting in the growth of intestinal villi and crypts and an overall increase in gut mass. Some intestinal microbes also synthesize essential vitamins and generate short-chain fatty acids that are absorbed and metabolized by the colonic epithelium. Commensal organisms also contribute to development of the neonatal immune system by releasing antigens that induce a low-grade inflammatory response that stimulates the growth and maturation of mucosa associated lymphoid tissues (Peyer patches and lymphoid follicles) in the neonatal intestine. The presence of normal microbial flora in the gut also inhibits the growth of enteric pathogens by competing for nutrients, secreting antibacterial substances, and interfering with adherence to mucosal surfaces. Finally, the resident microflora may also provide a protective effect by degrading bacterial toxins. Paucity of immune stimulation in infancy associated with alterations in the normal neonatal intestinal microbial flora has proposed as an etiology for the increasing prevalence of allergies and autoimmune disorders in many western countries. However, this association has not been proven.

The development of gastrointestinal microflora in preterm neonates is frequently disrupted by multiple environmental influences in the neonatal intensive care unit (ICU). Some of these factors include frequent exposure to broad-spectrum antibiotics, gavage feeding, formula feeding, and alterations in intestinal motility. The hostile environment of the neonatal ICU increases the likelihood that the intestinal tract will become colonized with: (1) gram-negative enteric pathogens such as *E. coli*, *Enterobacter*, and *Klebsiella*, (2) coagulase-negative *Staphylococcus*, and (3) *Candida* species. Recently there has been an increasing interest in the use of nonpathogenic commensal bacteria (probiotics) to promote colonization of the gut with beneficial organisms in an attempt to improve the maturity and function of the gut mucosal barrier. A recent meta-analysis of 11 previous studies that used probiotics for prevention of necrotizing enterocolitis (NEC) in preterm neonates reported significant decreases in death and the development of NEC, with a 30% reduction in NEC overall. Multiple strains of probiotics have been studied including: *Bifidobacterium breve*, *Lactobacillus GG*, *Saccharomyces boulardii*, *Bifidobacterium bifidus*, *Lactobacillus BB-L*, *Streptococcus thermophilus*, *Bifidobacterium infantis*, *Lactococcus acidophilus*, *Bifidobacterium lactis*, and *Bifidobacterium longum*. Additional randomized studies are required to determine the most efficacious bacterial agent(s), as well as optimal timing, dosage, and contraindications. Identifying the environmental and genetic factors that determine the characteristics of our gut microflora and how this microflora influences our physiology and health are promising areas for future research.

## Inflammatory Responses and Their Definitions

Mediators produced as part of the immune response, as well as toxins released by bacteria result in a constellation of symptoms that clinicians recognize as an inflammation. Inflammatory responses reflect the body's response to injury and are necessary for controlling the causative agent and for initiating wound repair. However, inflammation is not necessarily synonymous with infection, since inflammatory responses can be induced by injurious agents other than invading microbial pathogens.

Inflammatory responses may be acute or chronic, local, regional, or systemic. Inflammation progresses from local to systemic via a stepwise progression depending on the magnitude and persistence of the inciting event. Stage 1 or local inflammatory responses result when chemical mediators including histamine, prostaglandins, leukotrienes, and bradykinin are released by resident tissue cells (histiocytes, macrophages, dendritic cells, and mast cells). These mediators result in the 4 classical signs of inflammation: rubor (redness due to vasodilation), calor (warmth due to vasodilation), dolor (pain due to nerve stimulation), and tumor (swelling due to local tissue edema). These initial mediators also induce an influx of humoral and cellular response elements. Subsequently, a regional response (stage II) develops when cytokines and products of complement system activation (C3a and C5a) are released into the local circulation and recruit cellular elements of the immune system to the site of injury. Early responders include macrophages and neutrophils which kill invading microorganisms and eliminate injured tissue. Early responders also release cytokines, enzymes, and nitric oxide that further contribute to local signs of inflammation. If the initial response is able to contain and eradicate the stimulus, the local production of proinflammatory stimuli decreases and endogenous antagonists are released causing a downregulation of the inflammatory response. However, if the injurious agent exceeds local control, inflammatory cytokines (eg, IL-1, IL-6, IL-8, interferon-$\gamma$, and TNF-$\alpha$) and bacterial toxins enter the central circulation resulting in systemic signs of inflammation (stage III). Unfortunately, if systemic inflammation persists serious negative consequences will result leading due end-organ dysfunction as a result of effects on metabolism, circulatory integrity, and hemostasis.

In 1991, the American College of Chest Physicians and the Society of Critical Care Medicine proposed specific definitions for clinical syndromes of systemic inflammation and organ failure that were applicable to adults. While an update of these criteria published in 2003 noted criteria that were excluded in children and refined hemodynamic definitions, these criteria were still not consistently applicable to the pediatric age group. However, in 2005 the International Pediatric Sepsis Concensus Conference proposed new definitions for syndromes of inflammation in pediatric patients. Thus, "systemic inflammatory response syndrome" (SIRS) was defined as the presence of 2 or more of the following criteria: temperature >38.5°C or <36°C; tachycardia (ie, >2 SD above normal for age in the absence of external stimuli or persistent elevation for >0.5 to 4 hours) or bradycardia in children <1 year of age (ie, <10th percentile for age in the absence of external stimuli or drugs for >0.5 hours); respiratory rate >2 SD above normal for age or requirement for mechanical ventilation for an acute process; or leukocyte count elevated or depressed for age or 10% immature neutrophils. Other definitions proposed by this group include "infection" (ie, suspected or proven infection caused by any pathogen or a clinical syndrome associated with a high probability of infection), "sepsis" (ie, SIRS as a result of a suspected or proven infection), "severe sepsis" (ie, sepsis plus cardiovascular dysfunction, acute respiratory distress syndrome, or 2 or more other organ dysfunctions), and "septic shock" (ie, sepsis with cardiovascular organ dysfunction). The panel also has proposed specific criteria for definitions for organ dysfunction in pediatric patients. While the primary goal for establishing these definitions was "to facilitate the performance of successful clinical studies in children with sepsis," these syndromes also are useful clinically since they have prognostic implications.

# SKIN AND SUBCUTANEOUS TISSUE INFECTIONS

Infections of the skin and subcutaneous tissue are relatively common. Most are attributable to opportunistic invasion by commensal organisms associated either with a minor break in skin integrity and/or obstruction of or damage to cutaneous glands and hair follicles. Bacteria including gram-positive cocci such as *Staphycoccal* and *Steptococcal* spp. are most frequently responsible. However, infections involving subumbilical or intertriginous regions of the body are sometimes due to gram-negative bacterial and fungal organisms. Infections due to resistant organisms, such as methicillin-resistant *Staphylococcus aureus* (MRSA), should be suspected in patients with a history of recurrent skin and soft tissue infections in either the patient or their kindred, or when an infection does not respond to appropriate empiric antibiotic therapy. Infections due to resistant organisms were previously primarily associated with exposure to a hospital environment; however, multiple recent reports have shown an increase in the prevalence of antibiotic-resistant organisms as causative agents of community-acquired infections.

Most infections affecting the skin and subcutaneous tissues do not require surgical intervention and respond well to local treatment measures (eg, warm compresses, antibiotic ointments, or creams) and antibiotic therapy directed at eradicating the most likely causative organisms. Occasionally, surgical consultation is requested due to disease chronicity or when an invasive infection or abscess is suspected. Important aspects of the medical history include the time course of the present infection, trauma to the affected site that preceded the onset of infection, prior episodes of skin or subcutaneous infections in the patient or other recent contacts, therapeutic interventions for the current or prior infections, and the responses to those treatments. In addition, any history of skin conditions (eg, atopic dermatitis, eczema, and acne) or systemic illnesses (eg, diabetes, known immunodeficiencies) that might increase the risk of skin infections and/or complications should be sought.

Physical examination should include a visual assessment of location, extent, and appearance (ie, erythema, pustule formation, and skin discoloration) of the primary site of infection, as well as skin abnormalities affecting other areas of the body. The primary site should be gently palpated to assess for tenderness, tissue induration, fluid collections, or retained foreign bodies. The clinician should also note evidence of a systemic response to infection including tachycardia, pyrexia, or generalized malaise as these may suggest a more serious, invasive infection that might require immediate, aggressive surgical treatment.

Diagnostic imaging is seldom required as part of the assessment of skin and soft tissue infections. However, plain radiographs may be useful to identify retained radioopaque foreign bodies when there is a prior history of penetrating trauma. Ultrasound examination may allow identification of retained radiolucent foreign bodies or subcutaneous collections (seromas, hematomas, and abscesses) that may be difficult to identify on physical examination due to surrounding tissue edema. Ultrasound examination can also be useful for assessing extent of subcutaneous tissue involvement, as well as depth of invasion of the inflammatory process as evidenced by altered appearance of subcutaneous fat and fascial planes associated with accumulation of tissue fluid. While axial imaging including computed tomography (CT) or magnetic resonance imaging (MRI) is primarily obtained when a deep tissue infection is suspected, these studies will also allow assessment of the extent of skin and subcutaneous tissue infections and will demonstrate subcutaneous fluid collections.

The primary indication for surgical treatment of skin and subcutaneous skin infections is to drain an abscess. The benefits of abscess drainage include a decrease in the bacterial inoculum, as well as a change in the local tissue environment (ie, improved perfusion, improved oxygen delivery, and normalization of pH) that allows increased bacterial killing by inflammatory cells and improved antibiotic penetration and effectiveness. Thus, an important aspect of abscess drainage is to assure that the cavity has been adequately and completely drained. Occasionally, nonloculated localized abscesses can be managed with needle aspiration in conjunction with antibiotic therapy; however, these patients must be followed closely to assure adequate clinical response. Another option for managing deeper infections is to perform percutaneous drainage with placement of a drain. The benefit of this approach is the potential for improved cosmesis, while still allowing for long-term drainage. However, for this approach to be successful all parts of the abscess cavity must communicate freely. Incision and drainage is most appropriate for large or loculated abscesses. At the time of drainage, the surgeon must confirm that all loculated collections are opened to allow complete drainage of the abscess cavity. The cavity should be inspected for evidence of foreign or necrotic material, which should be removed. For localized abscesses, the surgical site is covered with a dry gauze dressing. However, placement of a drain or gauze packing may be more appropriate for deep or extensive cavities in order to prevent reaccumulation of fluid and recurrence of the abscess. Patients commonly receive antibiotic therapy at the time of incision and drainage, but these can usually be discontinued postoperatively when cellulitis has resolved. Studies suggest that results of gram stains and cultures of fluid obtained from abscess cavities at the time of incision and drainage seldom affect treatment decisions, and thus are probably not indicated. However, this recommendation may not apply to patients with extensive cellulitis, systemic manifestations, multiple or recurrent lesions, cutaneous gangrene, or in patients with impaired host defenses, as these infections may be polymicrobial or due to virulent or resistant organisms.

## Hidradenitis Suppurativa

Hidradenitis suppurativa is a chronic skin disease associated with recurrent infections involving the apocrine glands. The condition most commonly affects the axillae and inguino-femoral regions. Other common sites of involvement include the perineum and buttocks. In women, it may also affect the infra- or intermammary skin. The etiology of hidradenitis suppurativa is unknown. It is frequently attributed to clogging or plugging of the apocrine glands. Factors that have been proposed as contributors to apocrine gland obstruction include hormonal stimuli (androgen excess), smoking, obesity, and genetic predisposition (a positive family history increases the risk of developing the disease). Females are more commonly affected than males and this condition is seldom seen in prepubescent individuals.

Patients initially present with 1 or more localize areas of erythema and tenderness involving the axilla, perineum, or inguinal region. Over time these tender nodules may spontaneously rupture or coalesce forming painful deep dermal abscesses. Ultimately the inflammatory process leads to fibrosis and dermal scarring. Persistent or recurrent lesions may lead to skin contractures and the formation of sinus tracts. In many patients, the disease is characterized by an indolent but slowly progressive course with patients experiencing periods of relative quiescence interspersed with flares of increased disease activity. Disease flare-ups are associated with stress, increased perspiration (heat, humidity), hormonal changes (monthly cycles in women), and friction (tight-fitting clothes).

The diagnosis of hidradenitis suppurativa is made clinically as there is no confirmatory test. The differential diagnosis includes multiple other acute and chronic skin infections and autoimmune diseases (ie, Crohn disease) with cutaneous involvement. However, the presence of multiple simultaneous lesions, recurrent lesions in the same or new locations, and bilateral lesions primarily located in the milk line are considered diagnostic of hidradenitis suppurative. When the diagnosis is uncertain, biopsies and cultures may suggest an alternative etiology. Figure 13-2 presents a proposed diagnostic algorithm.

Treatment of early hidradenitis suppurativa is primarily medical. The mainstay of initial management is antibiotic therapy either by topical or systemic routes. Clindamycin 1% topical solution twice daily has been shown to be similar in efficacy to tetracycline 500 mg twice daily. Other antibiotic regimens that have been studied include combination therapy with oral clindamycin and rifampin, and monotherapy with dapsone. Besides its antibacterial effects, dapsone provides antiinflammatory and immunomodulatory benefits through inhibition of myeloperoxidase. Other therapeutic options that are not as well established include retinoids, antiandrogen therapy, immunosuppressive, and antiinflammatory agents. In addition, botulinum toxin injections, radiotherapy, cryosurgery, carbon dioxide laser treatments, and photodynamic therapy have been attempted with variable success. Besides medical therapy, patients should be advised to lose weight, stop smoking, and to avoid tight fitting clothes as these may decrease the incidence of disease flare-ups. Also, avoidance of deodorants, depilation products, and shaving are frequently recommended although their association with hidradenitis suppurativa is controversial.

Surgical therapy is primarily indicated in acute disease for drainage of abscess cavities. However, incision and drainage alone was associated with a 100% recurrence rate after a median of 3 months in 1 study. For intractable disease, surgery is widely considered the most effective treatment. Unfortunately, even aggressive, wide local excision of areas of scarred and inflamed tissues as well as surrounding apocrine

## Evaluation algorithm

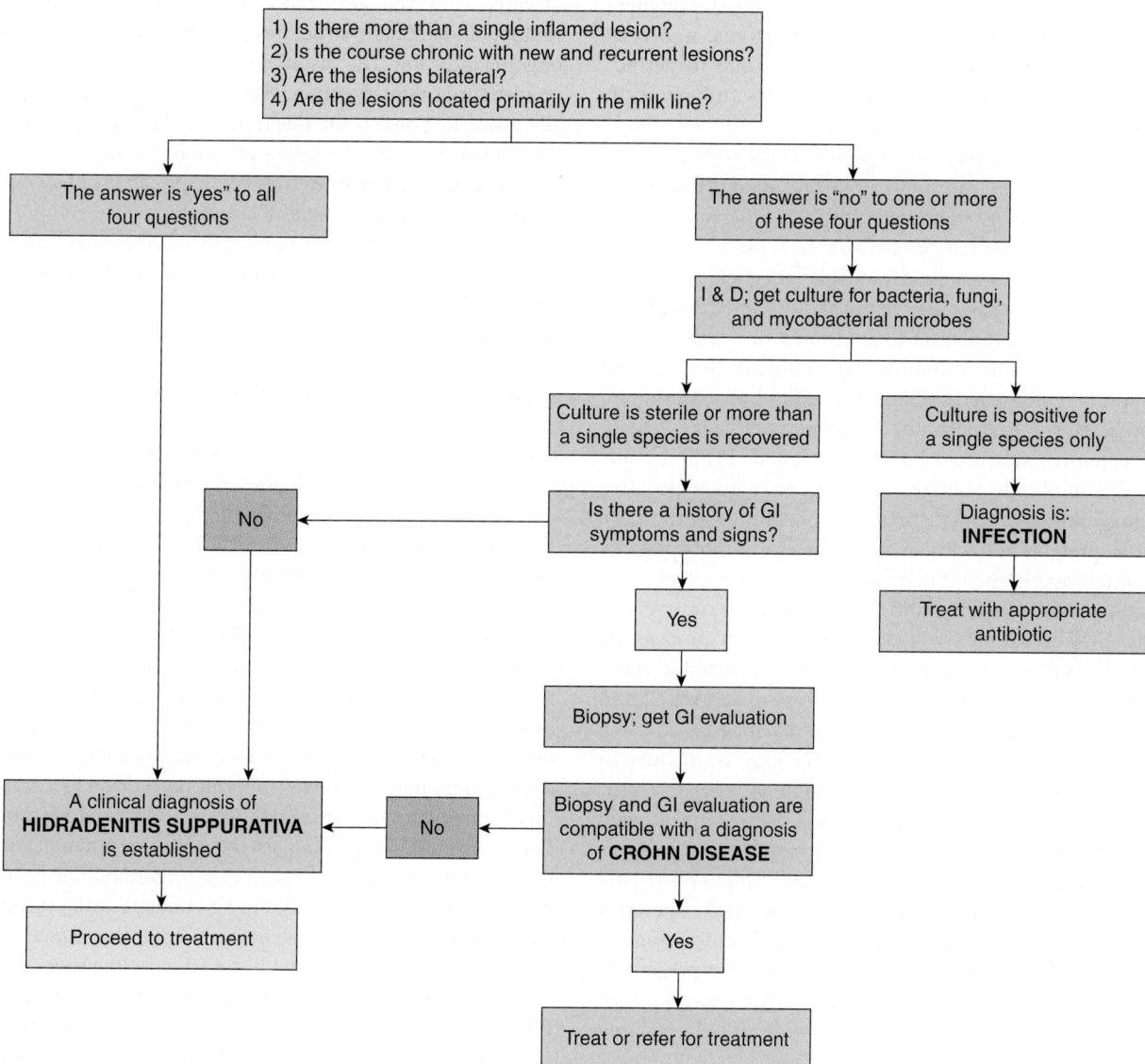

**FIGURE 13-2** Proposed algorithm for evaluation of a patient with suspected hidradenitis. (Reprinted with permission from *Alikhan A, Lynch PJ, Eisen DB. Hidradenitis suppurativa: a comprehensive review. J Am Acad Dermatol 2009;60(4):539–561.*)

gland containing skin is associated with significant recurrence rates. In one study recurrence rates of 37% and 50% were observed following radical excision of inframammary and inguinoperineal areas, respectively, with lower rates of recurrence observed following radical excision of disease involving the perineum (0%) and axillary area (3%). In addition, wide excision with either skin graft or flap closure has been associated with lower recurrence rates than excision and primary closure (PC) likely reflecting less extensive tissue removal with the latter approach.

## Pilonidal Abscess

Pilonidal disease is similar to hidradenitis suppurativa in that it is a disease of postpubertal teenagers, frequently has a chronic, indolent course with intermittent exacerbations resulting in the development of chronic cysts and sinuses, and is more commonly observed in obese and hirsute individuals.

Unlike hidradenitis however, pilonidal disease occurs more commonly in males than in females (ratio of between 2 and 4:1), and of course pilonidal disease affects the intergluteal cleft. The incidence is highest in Caucasians and lower among Asians and individuals of African descent.

Given the similarities between the 2 conditions, it is not surprising that one proposed etiology of pilonidal disease is similar to that of hidradenitis suppurative (ie, obstruction of hair follicles allowing secondary infection with abscess and skin sinus formation). Other proposed etiologies include a foreign body reaction to hairs embedded in the skin, and a congenital anomaly associated with congenital pilonidal dimples.

The diagnosis of pilonidal disease is based on clinical presentation. Patients may present acutely with pain, induration, and erythema or frank abscess formation with fluctuance involving the sacrococcygeal region. Alternatively, patients may also present with 1 or more skin sinuses at or near the midline in the sacrococcygeal region, or with a chronic nonhealing wound of the gluteal cleft, with or without purulent or blood-stained drainage. The differential diagnosis includes dermoid cyst, sacrococcygeal teratoma, anorectal fistula, sacral osteomyelitis, and infections due to actinomycosis or chronic granulomatous infections (tuberculosis, syphilis).

More than 50% of patients present initially with an acute abscess requiring incision and drainage. In most patients, incision and drainage can be performed under local anesthesia in an outpatient setting. However, some patients may require general anesthesia to enable adequate drainage. At the time of drainage, the cavity should be irrigated and hair, debris, and granulation tissue should be debrided. Ideally, midline incisions should be avoided since they tend to heal poorly. Following drainage, the wound may simply be left open, closed over a drain, or packed with gauze if there is an extensive subcutaneous cavity present. While broad-spectrum antibiotic therapy covering both gram-negative and anaerobic organisms is frequently instituted at the time of initial presentation with an acute abscess, in most patients antibiotics can be discontinued once erythema resolves.

Unfortunately, incision and drainage is not curative and nearly 50% of patients will develop recurrent disease. At the time of follow-up patients should be instructed to thoroughly clean the area at least daily with soap and water, and to perform regular hair removal either by shaving or using depilatory creams. Since local trauma may contribute to the development of ingrown hairs, some surgeons recommend avoiding activities such as bicycle riding or prolonged sitting. In patients with chronic or recurrent infections and drainage, excision of the chronically inflamed tissues and sinus tracts should be considered. Multiple operative approaches have been described to treat chronic pilonidal disease. It is beyond the scope of this chapter to present all or even most of these operative procedures; however, they all incorporate varying degrees of excision of inflamed and infected tissues and differ primarily in regards to placement of incisions and closure techniques. Unfortunately, all surgical procedures for chronic pilonidal disease carry some risk of recurrence.

One unusual complication of long-standing pilonidal disease is the potential for malignant degeneration, affecting approximately 1% of patients usually with chronic disease for 2 or more decades. The most frequent secondary tumor is a well-differentiated squamous cell carcinoma.

## Perianal Infections

See Chapter 54: Anorectal Prolapse, Abscess and Fissure.

## Breast Abscess

See Chapter 16: Breast Disease.

## Lymphatic Infections

The lymphatic system transports interstitial fluid and lymphatic structures are intimately involved in the immune response. Therefore, it is not surprising that the lymphatic system is frequently affected by invasive infections. In many cases, involvement of the lymphatic system is transient and reflects the spread of invading pathogens along lymphatic channels from the point of entry. However, sometimes invading microorganisms will multiply in lymphatic structures and establish an active site of ongoing infection. The vast majority of these infections do not require surgical intervention. However, surgeons are occasionally asked to assist in the diagnosis and treatment of patients who either are not responding to initial therapy or in whom chronicity or other features suggest the possibility of an opportunistic infection or a neoplastic process.

Lymphatic infections can generally be categorized as acute or chronic. Acute infections of lymphatic channels (lymphangitis) and lymph nodes (lymphadenitis) persist for up to 2 weeks and are usually associated with invasion by either a viral or bacterial pathogen. Chronic lymphadenitis, lasting more than 6 weeks, is most commonly attributable to infections by opportunistic organisms such as fungi, bacteria of low virulence, and occasionally even parasites. Infections lasting between 2 and 6 weeks (subacute infections) have a much broader range of possible etiologies.

Besides chronicity, other clinical features provide important clues to the likely etiology of a lymphatic infection. Lymphatic drainage follows well-defined patterns. Therefore, location is a good indicator of a likely site of entry and should elicit a focused history and physical in search of symptoms and signs of recent or ongoing infections involving the sites drained by the involved lymph nodes. Involvement of multiple nodal basins suggests invasion through deep structures having more than 1 pathway for lymphatic drainage, or nodal involvement by a systemic infection or inflammatory process. Other physical findings can also be useful. Erythema, tenderness, and fluctuance that involves a single node or group of nodes are usually attributable to an acute bacterial infection, while erythema and tenderness without fluctuance, often involving more than 1 nodal basin (due to invasion through deep structures), is more consistent with a viral etiology. Finally, the appearance of the overlying skin or draining material in patients with chronic lymphadenitis may suggest invasion by a specific microorganism.

Laboratory tests are seldom of value when treating patients with acute infections, but may be helpful for identifying the etiology of a chronic lymphatic infection. Leukocyte counts and markers of inflammation (C-reactive protein, erythrocyte sedimentation rates) are usually abnormal but are nonspecific. A leukocyte differential with an increase in immature white blood cells suggests a bacterial origin, but this etiology is frequently suggested by findings on clinical examination. Cultures from a likely site of invasion may suggest a pathogen; however, these results may not correlate with the organisms isolated from an associated infected lymph node. Serologic testing on patients with chronic lymphatic infections may reveal evidence of active infection by *Bartonella henselae*, syphilis (venereal disease research laboratory test [VDRL]), toxoplasmosis, CMV, histoplasmosis, or coccidiomycosis. Serologic testing from HIV should be considered in any patient with diffuse lymphadenitis or a history of recurrent infections caused by opportunistic organisms. Finally, a strongly positive intradermal tuberculin skin test is consistent with an infection due to *Mycobacterium tuberculosis*, while lesser reactions are commonly associated with infections due to a nontuberculous mycobacterium. Figure 13-3 presents a

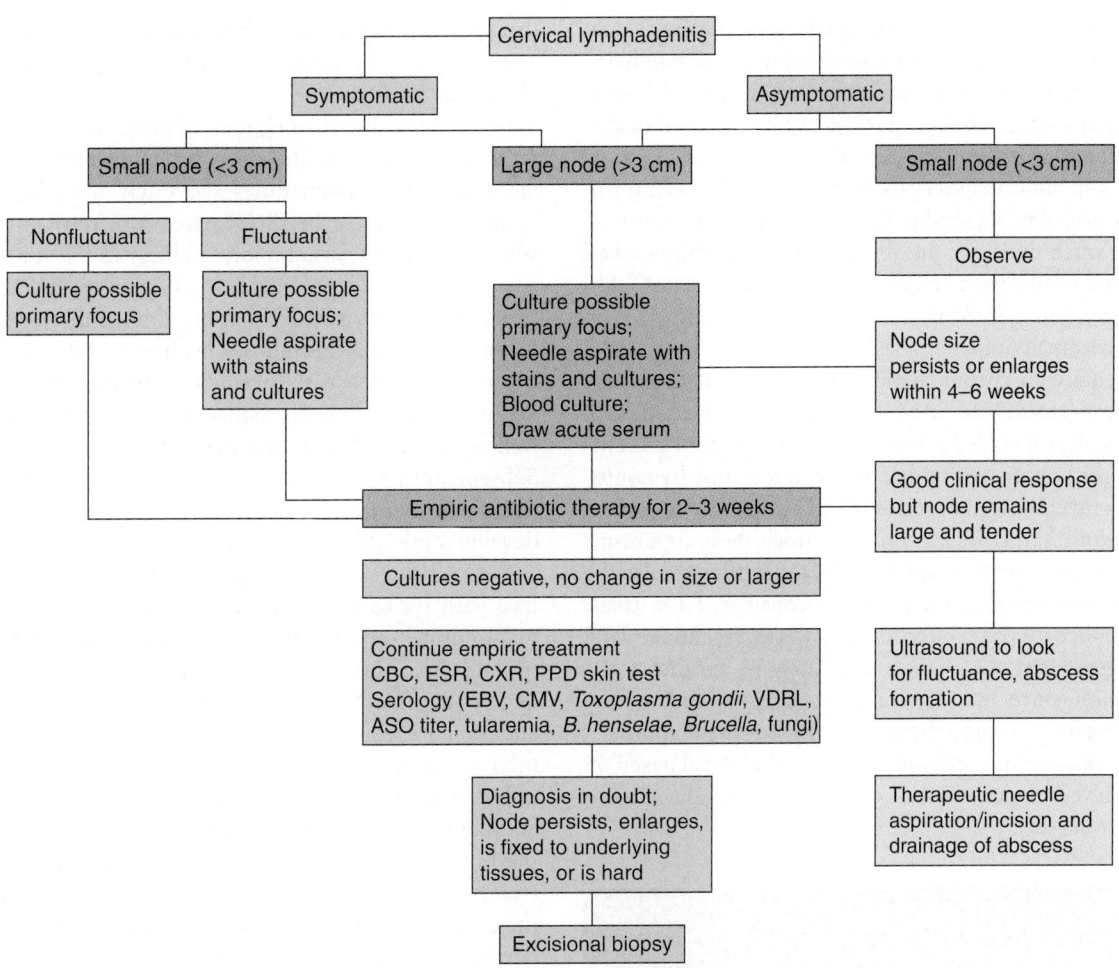

**FIGURE 13-3** Diagnostic and treatment algorithm for cervical lymphadenitis. (Reprinted with permission from *Darville T, Jacobs RF. Chapter 51: Lymphadenopathy, lymphadenitis and lymphangitis. In: Jenson HB, Baltimore RS, eds. Pediatric Infectious Diseases: Principles and Practice. Philadelphia, PA: W.B. Saunders Co.; 2002:610–629.*)

proposed diagnostic algorithm for infections involving the cervical lymph nodes.

Ultrasonography (US) is the most frequently employed and useful diagnostic study for evaluating patients with infections of the lymphatic system. US is noninvasive, avoids exposure to ionizing radiation, and can be performed in most patients without sedation. High-resolution US allows assessment of nodal size and architecture, and can also provide useful information about involvement of nearby nodes or surrounding structures that may not be readily apparent on clinical examination. In the acute setting, US can be used to confirm that a cervical swelling is nodal in origin, to identify fluid collections that may require drainage and to both direct and assess the adequacy of percutaneous drainage procedures. In the patients with subacute or chronic lymphatic infections, serial US examinations can provide an objective measure of nodal size thus allowing assessment of response to treatment. US may also demonstrate features that suggest a specific etiology. Findings in patients with chronic nodal enlargement that suggest an inflammatory etiology by gray-scale US include a ratio of the long axis to the short axis of involved lymph nodes of greater than 2, central irregular hyperechogenicity, blurred margins, and central necrosis. Findings by color Doppler examination that are consistent with inflammation

include hilar vascularity with a low pulsatility index. US findings, however, are not definitive for ruling out neoplasia, since none of the features alone or in combination will consistently distinguish between benign and malignant etiologies. Finally, while cross-sectional imaging (CT and MRI) is seldom required in patients with nodal infections, these studies may provide important anatomical information in patients with suspected atypical mycobacterial infections that require nodal excision.

Surgical treatment of lymphatic infections primarily includes drainage of abscesses in patients with acute infections and excision of involved nodes in patients with chronic lymphadenitis. Abscess development is usually heralded by the development of fluctuance, and is commonly associated with gram-positive coccal, *Staphylococci*, and *Streptococci* infections. Treatment options include simple needle aspiration or more formal wide surgical drainage. Needle aspirations can frequently be performed at the bedside or in the clinic under local anesthesia, with or without sedation, and have the potential of avoiding a postoperative scar. However, 2 or more aspirations may be required to treat recurrent fluctuance. More formal surgical drainage is preferred in patients who are unable to tolerate needle aspirations under local anesthesia and in patients with loculated fluid collections. The goal of either approach is to evacuate necrotic and infected material as completely as possible in order to facilitate antibacterial killing of any remaining viable organisms. Frequently, aspirated or drained fluid is sent for gram stain, cultures, and special stains as indicated by the clinical situation. These studies may not alter initial management, but can be very useful for redirecting therapy in patients who fail to respond to the initial course of treatment. Following open drainage, the abscess cavity is usually packed with gauze to assist with hemostasis and to prevent early skin closure. This gauze packing can be removed over a period of several days on an outpatient basis.

In patients with chronic lymphadenitis, biopsies are most commonly performed to rule out neoplasia. However, surgical debridement of involved nodes may be required for patients with chronic lymphadenitis due to infections cause by nontuberculous mycobacterial species (most commonly *Mycobacterium avium-intracellulare* complex) since these organisms often respond poorly to antimycobacterial therapy. In the past, complete surgical excision was considered the treatment of choice for these infections. However, recently several series suggest that observation alone may be another treatment option since many infections resolve spontaneously within 6 months. At present, the optimal treatment approach remains controversial, and should be individualized based on extent of involvement, clinical course, and parental wishes.

# INFECTIONS INVOLVING DEEP TISSUES AND BODY CAVITIES

## Necrotizing Fasciitis

Necrotizing infections involving the fascia and deeper tissues are uncommon in children but may be life-threatening and are frequently associated with significant morbidity. There are an estimated 500 to 1500 cases of necrotizing fasciitis in the United States annually, with reported incidence rates of 0.8 to 3.2 per million children per year.

Necrotizing infections of the fascia are classified into 2 types based on whether they are polymicrobial (Type I) or monomicrobial (Type II) in origin. In the pediatric age group, monomicrobial infections occur more commonly than polymicrobial infections. Organisms isolated from polymicrobial necrotizing infections nearly always include a combination of a anaerobic microorganism (most commonly *Bacteroides* or *Peptostreptococcus*) with 1 or more facultative anaerobic species such as streptococci (other than group A) or members of the *Enterobacteriaceae* (*E. coli, Enterobacter, Klebsiella*, and *Proteus*). Type II infections are most commonly caused by invasive group A β-hemolytic streptococci (GABHS). Over the past decade, type II infections due to MRSA have been increasing in frequency.

Unlike adults, most pediatric patients that develop type II necrotizing fasciitis are previously healthy, the most common predisposing condition being a recent varicella infection. In contrast, more than half of type I infections occur in children with preexisting medical conditions including trauma, recent surgery, chronic illness (eg, diabetes mellitus), malnutrition, obesity, immunosuppression, or intravenous

drug use. In the neonate, type I necrotizing fasciitis may be associated with omphalitis, circumcision, placement of scalp electrodes, and NEC.

Necrotizing fascial infections develop when virulent bacteria gain entry into the deep subcutaneous tissues either via a disruption (sometimes seemingly innocuous) of the epithelial barrier or by direct extension from a contiguous site. Causative bacteria rapidly multiply in the subcutaneous tissues and produce enzymes (collagenases, hyaluronidase, lipase, and streptokinase) that breakdown tissue planes and cause small vessel thromboses leading to tissue necrosis. As thrombosis and necrosis expands to involve perforating cutaneous vessels and nerves, bullae, ulceration, and necrosis, as well as numbness and anesthesia affect the overlying skin. Subsequently, with release of toxins and breakdown products from tissue necrosis into the circulation, patients may develop septic shock and multi-organ failure.

Necrotizing fasciitis is a rapidly progressive disease. Therefore, early recognition and aggressive treatment are necessary to minimize morbidity and mortality. Unfortunately, early in the course of the disease, it may be difficult to distinguish necrotizing fasciitis from cellulitis or other less serious skin and subcutaneous tissue infections. Symptoms that should increase suspicion include high fevers, tachycardia out of proportion to fever, altered mental status, systemic toxicity, and pain that seems out of proportion to or extends beyond the border of skin findings. As the disease progresses, skin changes include progressive discoloration, induration, anesthesia, and frank gangrene. In addition, crepitus on palpation develops in approximately one third of patients with type I necrotizing infections. Drainage, if present, is frequently thin and watery ("murky dishwater").

Diagnostic studies can help to identify changes suggestive of the diagnosis and to determine the extent of soft tissue involvement, but should not delay intervention when there is a high degree of suspicion. Plain radiographs demonstrate gas in the soft tissue in more than 50% of patients with type I necrotizing fasciitis. Both MRI and CT will delineate the extent of disease and identify gas in the soft tissues. MRI is more sensitive than CT for differentiating healthy from necrotic tissue but may overestimate the extent of fascial involvement. Finally, US can also help to establish the diagnosis by demonstrating irregular thickening of the deep fascia and fluid or gas collections along fascial planes.

Effective treatment requires concomitant aggressive surgical debridement and empiric antibiotic therapy. Patients with suspected group A β-hemolytic streptococcal infections should be started on high-dose intravenous penicillin plus clindamycin. Clindamycin not only serves as an antimicrobial agent, but also reduces the synthesis of exotoxins due to its antiribosomal effect. Patients with suspected type I necrotizing infections should be started on broad-spectrum antibiotics effective against both aerobes and anaerobes (eg, clindamycin plus a third-generation cephalosporin, or ampicillin, gentamicin, and metronidazole).

Surgical exploration is indicated when the index of suspicion is high. If the diagnosis is uncertain, exploration can begin with a "finger test" during which a small incision is made and the surgeon introduces a finger to the level of the deep fascia. Positive findings include a lack of bleeding, the return of foul smelling, dishwater-like thin pus, and minimal resistance to finger dissection. Operative management requires aggressive debridement of all devitalized tissue until obviously viable freely bleeding tissue is encountered. Often sequential debridements are required and wounds should be reexamined (preferably in the operating room) on a daily basis until only viable tissue is encountered. Initially after debridement the wound is packed open. Wound closure should not be undertaken until the patient is clinically doing well. Options for managing the resultant soft-tissue defect include vacuum-assisted wound closure, skin grafts, or flap closure with or without fascial reconstruction.

While the morbidity associated with necrotizing fasciitis in children is considerable, the mortality rate in the pediatric age group is lower than in adults (≈5% overall, ≈0% in patients with type II disease). The majority of deaths associated with necrotizing fasciitis occur in patients with preexisting comorbidities and in patients at the extremes of age.

## Muscle Compartment Infections

Infections of skeletal muscle (infectious myositis) are uncommon but may be due to invasion by a wide range of microorganisms including viruses, bacteria, fungi, or parasites. Infectious myositis can affect a single muscle group or multiple muscle groups (polymyositis). Polymyositis typically is due to a systemic viral or parasitic infection, and other than the infrequent need to obtain a biopsy to help identify an etiology, seldom requires surgical intervention. However, localized myositis, which is more commonly associated with bacterial invasion, frequently comes to the attention of surgeons due to questions about whether symptoms or signs are attributable to another surgical disease or due to the requirement for surgical drainage and debridement.

Initially, myositis may present with only fever, chills and malaise, and relatively few local symptoms. Physical examination may reveal only minimal tenderness and swelling, and the diagnosis can be easily overlooked. However, as the condition progresses, patients develop increasingly severe localizing pain and swelling that conforms to the shape of the involved muscle. The overlying skin may be warm to touch but erythema is usually absent. Aspiration of the affected muscle belly at this stage will often return pus (pyomyositis). Subsequently, systemic manifestations of sepsis and shock may develop if the condition is not recognized and appropriately treated.

Bacterial invasion of skeletal muscle can occur via local spread from contiguous sites of infection or by hematogenous spread from a distant focus. Up to 50% of patients have a recent history of blunt or penetrating trauma or vigorous exercise. Other predisposing conditions include immunodeficiencies, rhabdomyolysis, and diabetes mellitus. While multiple different types of bacteria have been associated with pyomyositis, S. aureus is the responsible etiologic agent in more than two thirds of cases. Invasion by group A Streptococci account for only 1% to 5% of cases but can have a fulminant course resulting in myonecrosis. Similarly, invasion by Clostridial organisms can cause a rapidly progressive, life-threatening disease associated with gas gangrene. Myositis due to fungi and parasites are typically seen only in immunosuppressed patients.

Diagnostic imaging studies can help narrow the differential diagnosis and identify the extent of disease. Plain radiographs may reveal soft tissue swelling or gas in the soft tissue plains and may identify other causes of musculoskeletal pain. Ultrasound examination will typically show only muscle swelling early in the disease, but can localize focal abscesses once suppuration has developed. Finally, cross-sectional imaging techniques (CT and MRI) provide better anatomic detail and demonstrate enlargement of the involved muscles as well as abscess formation and changes in contrast enhancement consistent with inflammation.

Treatment consists of early surgical drainage of abscesses and debridement of necrotic tissue. Purulent material should be sent for immediate gram stain and aerobic and anaerobic, as well as fungal cultures. Initial empiric antibiotic therapy typically includes a β-lactamase–resistant penicillin to cover S. aureus. Antibiotic coverage for MRSA should also be considered in patients with chronic illnesses or recent hospitalizations and in centers where there is a high incidence of community-acquired MRSA. Empiric treatment for presumed group A streptococcal infections based on gram stain results typically includes high-dose penicillin G and clindamycin. Persistent fever and pain should prompt reassessment to rule out incompletely drained abscesses or a previously unrecognized site of infection. Pyomyositis can progress to compartment syndrome, so open surgical drainage including possible fasciotomy should be considered in patients who progress or fail to improve following initial limited percutaneous drainage.

## Osteomyelitis

While infections of the bone or bone marrow are not commonly treated by pediatric surgeons, patients with osteomyelitis can present with symptoms that raise concern for other conditions that are managed by pediatric surgeons. Infections spread to the bone or joints via 3 primary routes: hematogenous, direct contamination (ie, through penetrating injuries), or direct extension from a nearby infection. In children, osteomyelitis most commonly arises from hematogenous spread and the most common causative organism is S. aureus. Group A Streptococci, Streptococcus pneumoniae, and Kingella kingae are also commonly seen in infants and children, while in neonates group B Streptococci and gram-negative enteric are important etiologic pathogens. Osteomyelitis associated with penetrating injuries or due to spread from contiguous soft tissue infections is frequently polymicrobial. In almost half of children, a bacterial pathogen is never isolated.

Infections of the bone in children characteristically involve the metaphysis of long bones. In neonates, the cartilaginous epiphyses receive their blood supply via metaphyseal blood vessels which accounts for the higher incidence of concomitant joint involvement. Common presenting symptoms include pain, fever, and swelling around the site of infection. Older children will also frequently present with decreased mobility or a limp. In neonates, the presenting symptoms may be nonspecific and include irritability or poor feeding. Laboratory evaluation typically demonstrates leukocytosis and elevated markers of inflammation (eg, erythrocyte sedimentation rate and C-reactive protein). Blood cultures may identify a causative organism since bacteremia is more common in children than in adults.

Plain radiographs of the involved bones during the early stages of osteomyelitis will usually demonstrate only soft tissue swelling and obliteration of tissue planes. Periosteal elevation and lytic lesions are not typically seen until 10 to 14 days after the onset of clinical symptoms. Plain radiographs are also useful for identifying fractures or changes suggestive of malignant lesions. Technetium ($^{99m}$Tc)-labeled bone scans are nearly 90% sensitive for detecting osteomyelitis, and are particularly useful for identifying multifocal involvement and for identifying the site of involvement in patients with poorly localized disease. Ultrasound findings in patients with acute osteomyelitis include deep soft tissue swelling, elevation of the periosteum, subperiosteal collections, and cortical erosion. MRI allows definition of the extent of bone marrow and soft tissue involvement, and is particularly useful for excluding extradural collections in patients with involvement of the spine. However, findings on MRI may overestimate the extent of bony involvement since reactive inflammation causes a signal pattern that is similar to active infection.

Empiric treatment for patients with acute osteomyelitis should include antimicrobial agents active against *S. aureus*. In communities where the rate of MRSA isolates exceeds 10%, antimicrobial agents effective against these organisms (eg, vancomycin or clindamycin) should be administered. Surgical treatment is indicated for drainage of subperiosteal or intraosseous abscesses in patients with acute osteomyelitis, for debridement or drainage of associated contiguous infections and for debridement of devascularized bone in patients with chronic osteomyelitis. Patients with an associated acute septic arthritis should undergo urgent drainage to relieve vascular compression that may result in avascular necrosis of the affected epiphysis.

## Body Cavity Infections

### Peritoneal Cavity Infections: Peritonitis

Intraabdominal infections are common in infants and children but comprise a heterogeneous group. Infections arising within the abdomen should be conceptualized as 2-compartment infections since the intraabdominal focus of infection interacts with the dense microbial flora of the intestine with subsequent possible changes in gut wall permeability or ileus with bacterial overgrowth. Primary intraabdominal infections are those that arise in the absence of an identifiable anatomic breakdown. The classic example is primary peritonitis.

### Primary Peritonitis

Primary peritonitis (spontaneous bacterial peritonitis) is an infection of the peritoneum in the absence of an obvious source. It is frequently seen in patients with nephrotic syndrome, ascites, or intraabdominal fluid that becomes infected from hematogenous spread of bacteria from a distant focus. Infection can develop in girls as a result of bacterial contamination through the fallopian tubes. Primary peritonitis is a monomicrobial infection with the usual causative organisms being gram-positive cocci, particularly *Streptococcus*. Other common organisms are *E. coli*, *Klebsiella pneumoniae*, and *Staphylococcus*.

Clinically these children present with the signs and symptoms of peritonitis with fever and abdominal pain. Many patients will undergo exploration for presumed appendicitis, at which time the diagnosis will be made. If the diagnosis is suspected before exploration, it can be confirmed by performing paracentesis and sending a fluid sample for cell count, differential, gram stain, and culture. A polymorphonuclear leukocytes (PMN) count >250 cell/mm3 suggest the diagnosis. Culture of the peritoneal fluid sample increases the positivity from 50% to ~80% if the fluid is directly inoculated into blood cultures bottles at the bedside. Unless definitive identification of the responsible organism has occurred, initial therapy is empiric and is chosen to provide adequate gram-positive and gram-negative coverage. Clinical improvement should be seen within 48 hours.

## Peritoneal Dialysis-Associated Peritonitis

Chronic peritoneal dialysis is well established as a treatment of choice for pediatric end-stage renal disease. The development of peritonitis is the most common complication associated with peritoneal dialysis. Peritoneal contamination arises primarily by intraluminal contamination of the dialysis catheter during bag and tubing changes. The primary pathogens are: gram-positive cocci (50%-75%), enteric gram-negative bacteria (30%), and fungi (10%). The diagnosis is suspected when cloudy dialysate is noted along with abdominal pain. A cell count on the dialysate >100 WBC/mm$^3$ and a differential >50% polymorphonuclear leukocytes support the diagnosis. Most cases can be successfully managed with intraperitoneal administration of cephalosporin or vancomycin combined with an aminoglycoside. Intermittent versus continuous dosing of intraperitoneal antibiotics are equally effective. Catheter removal is indicated in the absence of response within 4 to 5 days. Fungal peritonitis is associated with a high failure rate without removal of the infected peritoneal dialysis catheter.

## Secondary Peritonitis

Secondary peritonitis results from gastrointestinal contamination of the peritoneal cavity, either localized or diffuse. Most frequently this is the result of NEC in preterm neonates and appendicitis in children. Secondary peritonitis is commonly polymicrobial with enteric gram-negative rods (*Enterobacteriaceae*) and anaerobes (*Bacteroides*, *Clostridia*). Bacterial synergism plays a significant role in the pathophysiology. Clinical presentation is characterized by systemic manifestations of the septic response. These vary particularly in the neonate, and include fever/temperature instability, bradycardia/tachycardia, tachypnea, and hypotension. Nausea and vomiting and/or feeding intolerance are common. Physical findings are critical and include abdominal distension, tenderness, guarding, and rebound. Abdominal radiographs can demonstrate ileus, pneumoperitoneum, pneumatosis, mass effect, and/or an appendicolith.

Management initially includes resuscitation along with broad-spectrum antibiotics that cover gram-negative and anaerobic bacteria. The primary treatment is operative with the goal of eliminating ongoing contamination and reducing the bacterial load. Once the goals of operative intervention have been achieved, systemic antibiotics are continued until the patient demonstrates clinical improvement with resumption of diet, normal white count, and resolution of fevers. Continued lack of improvement after 5 to 7 days should prompt a search for a source of ongoing infection.

Intraabdominal abscesses arise as a consequence of peritonitis. The location is related to the primary infection, the peritoneal circulation, and the gravity. Common locations include subphrenic spaces, the pericolic gutters, and the pelvis. Responsible organisms mirror those recovered from secondary peritonitis. Intraabdominal abscesses generally present as a recurrent or persistent infection following treatment of secondary peritonitis but can be the primary presentation of secondary peritonitis. Fever and leukocytosis are present frequently with anorexia. The diagnosis is confirmed with ultrasound or CT scan. Management includes appropriate antimicrobials and drainage. Antibiotic coverage is altered based on clinical response and the results of culture obtained at the time of drainage. Drainage can frequently be performed percutaneously using ultrasound or CT guidance. Open drainage is typically reserved for multiple or poorly localized abscesses. Drainage and antibiotics are maintained until temperature and leukocyte counts have normalized and catheter drainage is minimal.

## PLEURAL CAVITY INFECTIONS— EMPYEMA

See Chapter 30: Lung Infections: Lung Biopsy, Lung Abscess, Bronchiectasis, and Empyema.

## PERIOPERATIVE (SURGICAL SITE) INFECTIONS

### Prevalence and Cost

Based on the CDC National Nosocomial Infection Surveillance (NNIS) system reports, SSIs are the third most frequently reported nosocomial infection, accounting for 14% to 16% of all nosocomial infections among hospitalized patients. Among surgical patients, SSIs were the most common nosocomial infection, accounting for 38% of all such infections. Of these SSIs, two thirds were confined to the incision, and one third involve organs or spaces accessed during the operation. A 1992 analysis showed that each SSI resulted in 7 additional postoperative hospital days, adding $3,152 in extra charges. The additional cost attributable to SSI for cardiac or orthopedic cases can exceed $30,000.

### Definitions

Table 13-1 lists proposed criteria for diagnosing SSIs.

### Incidence

The incidence of SSIs in adults has been extensively studied but only a few reports have looked at incidence of SSIs in pediatric surgical patients. It is generally assumed that the incidence of SSI is lower in pediatric patients, but the incidence has varied from 2.5% to 13.6%. A recent series from the Netherlands reported an overall infection rate of 6.6%. In this series, clean sites had a SSI rate of 2.8% while the rate for dirty sites increased to 30%. Emergency procedures likewise had a higher infection rate (14.8%) compared with elective cases (4%). Not surprisingly most of the dirty cases were performed emergently. Ninety-four percent of the infections appeared within 3 weeks of the procedure. Duration of the surgical procedure greater than 1 hour and inpatient procedures were associated with significantly higher infections rates. These data suggest that similar strategies to those recommended in the adult literature should help decrease the incidence of SSIs in pediatric patients.

## PREVENTION OF SSIs

### Antimicrobial Prophylaxis

Since the 1960s the effectiveness of antimicrobials administered shortly before skin incision has been repeatedly demonstrated. Despite this substantial demonstration and publication of guidelines, prophylactic antibiotic usage remains frequently suboptimal. This is due to inappropriate timing of administration and/or excess duration of administration, along with inappropriate selection of the antimicrobial agents. The baseline results from the National Surgical Infection Prevention Project suggested substantial opportunity for improvement in prophylactic antimicrobial usage with only 56% of patients receiving the initial antimicrobial dose within 1 hour before the incision. Discontinuation of antimicrobial prophylaxis within 24 hours of the surgery end-time occurred only 41% of the time. On the positive side, 93% of the patients received appropriate antimicrobial agents based on published guidelines.

The current recommended guidelines for parenteral antimicrobial prophylaxis include: (1) initiation of prophylaxis within 1 hour before the incision (2 hours for vancomycin); (2) redosing of the antibiotic for cases that are prolonged (eg, readministration of cefazolin within 240 minutes for cases lasting longer than 4 hours); and (3) discontinuation of antibiotics within 24 hours following completion of the procedure.

### Preoperative and Intraoperative Management

Preexisting medical conditions are a major risk factor for SSI. Some of these conditions including obesity or prolonged hospitalization are not readily amenable to timely intervention. Other risk factors can be fairly easily optimized including: (1) lowering hemoglobin A1C concentrations in patients with diabetes; (2) discontinuing smoking at least 30 days prior to an elective procedure; and (3) treating concomitant infections preoperatively. However, data are limited regarding the success of these interventions in preventing SSI.

There are better data to support the value of specific perioperative approaches as a means to decrease the risk of SSIs. Preoperative hair removal by shaving has been consistently shown to *increase* SSI rates. It is currently recommended that

## TABLE 13-1 Criteria for Defining a Surgical Site Infection (SSI)

### Superficial Incisional SSI

*Infection occurs within 30 days after the operation and infection involves only skin or subcutaneous tissue of the incision and at least one of the following:*

1. Purulent drainage, with or without laboratory confirmation, from the superficial incision
2. Organisms isolated from an aseptically obtained culture of fluid or tissue from the superficial incision
3. At least one of the following signs or symptoms of infection: pain or tenderness, localized swelling, redness, or heat and superficial incision is deliberately opened by surgeon, unless incision is culture-negative
4. Diagnosis of superficial incisional SSI by the surgeon or attending physician

*Do not report the following conditions as SSI:*

1. Stitch abscess (minimal inflammation and discharge confined to the points of suture penetration)
2. Infection of an episiotomy or newborn circumcision site
3. Infected burn wound
4. Incisional SSI that extends into the fascial and muscle layers (see "Deep Incisional SSI" below)

*Note:* Specific criteria are used for identifying infected episiotomy and circumcision sites and burn wounds.

### Deep Incisional SSI

*Infection occurs within 30 days after the operation if no implant[a] is left in place or within 1 year if implant is in place and the infection appears to be related to the operation and infection involves deep soft tissues (eg, fascial and muscle layers) of the incision and at least one of the following:*

1. Purulent drainage from the deep incision but not from the organ/space component of the surgical site.
2. A deep incision spontaneously dehisces or is deliberately opened by a surgeon when the patient has at least one of the following signs or symptoms: fever (>38°C), localized pain, or tenderness, unless the site is culture-negative
3. An abscess or other evidence of infection involving the deep incision is found on direct examination, during reoperation, or by histopathologic or radiologic examination
4. Diagnosis of a deep incisional SSI by a surgeon or attending physician

*Notes:*

1. Report infection that involves both superficial and deep incision sites as deep incisional SSI
2. Report an organ/space SSI that drains through the incision as a deep incisional SSI

### Organ/space SSI

Infection occurs within 30 days after the operation if no implant[a] is left in place or within 1 year if implant is in place and the infection appears to be related to the operation and infection involves any part of the anatomy (eg, organs or spaces), other than the incision that was opened or manipulated during an operation and at least one of the following:

1. Purulent drainage from a drain that is placed through a stab wound[b] into the organ/space
2. Organisms isolated from an aseptically obtained culture of fluid or tissue in the organ/space
3. An abscess or other evidence of infection involving the organ/space that is found on direct examination, during reoperation, or by histopathologic or radiologic examination
4. Diagnosis of an organ/space SSI by a surgeon or attending physician

[a]National Nosocomial Infection Surveillance definition: a nonhuman-derived implantable foreign body (eg, prosthetic heart valve, nonhuman vascular graft, mechanical heart, or hip prosthesis) that is permanently placed in a patient during surgery.
[b]If the area around a stab wound becomes infected, it is not an SSI. It is considered a skin or soft tissue infection, depending on its depth.
Reprinted with permission from *Horan TC, Gaynes RP, Martone WJ, et al. CDC definitions of nosocomial surgical site infections, 1992: a modification of CDC definitions of surgical wound infections. Infect Control Hosp Epidemiol 1992;13(10):606–608.*

hair be removed by clipping immediately before the procedure or not at all. Preoperative showering with chlorhexidine has *not* been shown to be helpful in decreasing SSI rates. Skin preparation with an antiseptic agent is an established effective measure to decrease the incidence of SSI; however, the available data have not conclusively demonstrated superiority of chlorhexidine over iodophors. Similarly, there are currently no conclusive data regarding any specific antiseptic agent for preparation of surgical team members' hands and forearms.

The conduct of the operation is another potential but unproven area in which the risk of SSI may be altered. While the use of drains without clear indications has been clearly associated with an increase in the risk of SSI, the value of gentle handling of tissue, thorough irrigation of contamination, complete removal of devitalized tissue, and avoidance of dead space have not been conclusively proven. Similarly, studies of various approaches to managing closed wounds with wound dressings and ointments have also yielded little data that supports a specific technique.

PC of infected or dirty wounds would seem to be a significant risk factor for developing SSI. However, published data have not consistently proven this to be true. Previous randomized prospective studies over the past 3 decades have shown no decrease in the risk of wound infections associated with delayed primary closure (DPC) in patients with complicated appendicitis. In contrast, a more recent randomized trial demonstrated that PC of dirty wounds due to perforated appendicitis, other perforated viscus, traumatic wounds more than 4 hours old, or intraabdominal abscesses in adult patients was associated with a 4 times higher incidence of wound infections as compared with DPC (48% vs 12%, respectively). However, this study enrolled only 51 patients of which 2 were withdrawn due to early mortality. In addition, nearly half of the patients in the DPC group were judged unsuitable for closure on evaluation at 72 hours after surgery, suggesting that the patients treated by DPC may represent a subset of the patients randomized to this treatment arm. Furthermore, overall length of stay and costs of care did not differ between treatment groups or in patients that developed wound infections.

Several reports suggest that laparoscopic surgery may be associated with a decrease in the incidence of SSIs in adults. A recent meta-analysis that compared laparoscopic versus open appendectomy for treating adults with complicated appendicitis reported that laparoscopic appendectomy was associated with a decrease in the rate of SSIs without a significant difference in the incidence of intraabdominal abscesses. However, the quality of the available data was considered moderate to poor. Similarly, a recent retrospective analysis of a large database that compared the incidence of SSI associated with open versus laparoscopic appendectomy, cholecystectomy, antireflux surgery, or gastric bypass reported that patients treated with laparoscopy were 72% less likely to experience a SSI. Multiple other nonrandomized, mostly retrospective studies, have also shown an advantage to laparoscopic surgery in reducing the incidence of SSI in adult patients. To date there appear to be no published reports comparing the incidence of SSI associated with laparoscopic versus open surgery in the pediatric age group.

The effects of avoidance of hypothermia, maintenance of higher tissue oxygen concentrations, and management of hyperglycemia on SSIs have all been reported in the adult surgical literature. The importance of maintaining normal intraoperative and postoperative core temperature in adult surgical patients is now fairly well-accepted. A prospective trial reported that preventing hypothermia by maintaining a core temperature of 36.6°C in adult colorectal patients resulted in a 3-fold decrease in the rate of SSIs (Kurz et al., 1996). The value of using increased inspired oxygen concentrations (80% vs 30%) in the intraoperative and immediate postoperative periods in adult patients has been more controversial. However, a meta-analysis of 4 trials comparing different inspired oxygen concentrations in the perioperative period concluded that the data overall favored the use of higher oxygen concentrations (Chura et al., 2007). Avoidance of significant hyperglycemia in the intraoperative and postoperative period has also been shown to decrease the incidence of deep SSI and mediastinitis in adult patients undergoing cardiac surgical procedures. Avoidance of elevated blood glucose levels (>200 mg/dL) at 6:00 AM on postoperative days 1 and 2 after cardiac surgery is now one of the adult performance measures aimed at decreasing the incidence of SSI.

Maintenance of normal core temperature during surgical procedures has been common practice in pediatric surgery for many years. However, its effect on SSI in the pediatric age group has not been adequately studied. Interestingly, hypothermia during surgery appeared to protect against SSI by univariate analysis in a group of pediatric patients undergoing posterior spinal fusion. Finally, the roles of higher concentrations of inspired oxygen and tighter serum glucose control as measures to decrease the incidence of SSI in pediatric surgical patients remain unknown.

## Probiotics

Despite close adherence to antimicrobial guidelines, nosocomial infection remains a significant cause of morbidity and mortality in surgical patients. Recently there has been increasing interest in the use of supplemental nonpathogenic bacteria (probiotics) as a means to decrease colonization by pathogenic organisms and thus decrease the risk of SSI. There have been multiple trials of probiotics but the use of multiple different agents, differences in patient populations studied and differing end points have made it difficult to develop a clear sense of their usefulness in the clinical setting. A recent paper reported a randomized placebo-controlled trial of Lactobacillus *rhamnosus* strain GG (Culturelle, ConAgra Foods) on the incidence of nosocomial infection in a pediatric ICU. The *L. rhamnosus* strain GG was not shown to be effective in decreasing infection during interim analysis and the study was terminated due to safety concerns related to case reports of proven sepsis with this particular agent. However, multiple clinical trials of probiotics in the treatment of acute viral diarrheal disorders, *Clostridium difficile* colitis, bacterial overgrowth in short bowel patient, and NEC have demonstrated significant benefits.

Another strategy, referred to as synbiotic therapy, is to administer beneficial bacteria (probiotic) in combination with a poorly digestible dietary fiber (prebiotic). Prebiotics are nondigestible food ingredients that stimulate the growth and/or activity of beneficial bacteria. The results to date with synbiotic therapy have been mixed. Some studies have failed to show an effect on postoperative wound infections in patients undergoing mixed abdominal or colorectal procedures. Proposed explanations for the lack of effect include the relatively short duration of administration, oral instead of jejunal administration, and a relatively high percentage of low-risk operations resulting in low overall infection rates. Other studies, however, have noted significant decreases in rates of infection, decreased ICU lengths of stay and decreased days on mechanical ventilation with synbiotic therapy in patients with a various surgical conditions known to be associated with rates of infection and morbidity.

Available data suggest that probiotics and synbiotics may ultimately prove to be useful adjunctive treatments to decrease the incidence of SSIs. Additional research is required to identify the most effective and safest prebiotic and/or probiotic agents, as well as the optimal treatment regimens and the patients and diseases that are most likely to benefit from this therapy.

## Treatment of Surgical Site Infections

Probably the most important detail for postoperative care is to monitor the surgical incision for development of a SSI. Early identification and treatment of a superficial SSI may prevent spread of the infection and avoid major subsequent complications. When a SSI is suspected, the incision should be opened. Purulent material should be sent for cultures to confirm the diagnosis and to provide information that may help direct antimicrobial therapy. The wound should be irrigated and any foreign material or necrotic tissue should be debrided. While many wounds can be opened at the bedside or in the clinic, adequate local wound care may require general anesthesia in the operating room. For extensive or deep infections, a systemic antibiotic regimen that covers the likely causative organisms (taking into account local resistance patterns) should also be instituted.

Traditionally opened wounds have been managed with wet-to-dry dressings which are associated with significant pain and anxiety on the part of the patient and family. Recently, negative pressure wound therapy (a.k.a., vacuum assisted closure or VAC) has been increasingly applied to children and neonates with complicated open wounds. Wound VAC therapy promotes wound healing by approximating wound margins, reducing tissue edema, removing tissue exudate and infectious material, increasing tissue perfusion, and promoting granulation tissue growth. Patients treated with VAC therapy typically require dressing changes every 2 to 3 days instead of the 2 to 3 times per day often required for wet-to-dry dressings. In very young patients, it has been noted that higher rates of granulation tissue formation can result in ingrowth and plugging of the pores in polyurethane foam. Therefore, the use of polyvinyl alcohol foam and more frequent dressing changes may be necessary in young children. At present there is limited data regarding optimal negative pressure settings that should be applied to wounds in pediatric patients. Negative pressures of 125 mm Hg, which are commonly used in adult patients, are based on animal models that showed this amount of negative pressure was associated with the highest rate of granulation tissue formation. However, concerns about the risks of using this amount of negative pressure in small children, particularly in neonates, have been raised. Published retrospective data suggest that adequate wound healing can be achieved using lower negative pressures (100 mm Hg) in children younger than 4 years of age. Another author proposed using negative pressures of between 50 and 75 mm Hg in children less than 2 years of age, and between 75 and 125 mm Hg in children more than 2 years old based on consensus of an expert panel; however, the authors note that these recommendations may not be appropriate for use in all circumstances.

## SELECTED READINGS

Alikhan A, Lynch PJ, Elsen DB. Hidradenitis suppurativa: a comprehensive review. *J Am Acad Dermatol* 2009;60(4):539–561.

Baharestani M, Amjad I, Bookout K, et al. V.A.C. therapy in the management of pediatric wounds: clinical review and experience. *Int Wound J* 2009;6(suppl 1):1–26.

Bone RC, Balk RA, Cerra FB, et al. Definitions for sepsis and organ failure and guidelines for the use of innovative therapies in sepsis. The ACCP/SCCM consensus conference committee. American College of Chest Physicians/Society of Critical Care Medicine. *Chest* 1992;101(6):1644–1655.

Bonilla FA, Oettgen HC. Adaptive immunity. *J Allergy Clin Immunol* 2010;125(2):S33–S40.

Chuang SC, Lee KT, Wang SN, et al. Risk factors for wound infection after cholecystectomy. *J Formos Med Assoc* 2004;103(8):607–612.

Chura JC, Boyd A, Argenta PA. Surgical site infections and supplemental perioperative oxygen in colorectal surgery patients: a systematic review. *Surg Infect (Larchmt)* 2007;8(4):455–461.

Cohn SM, Giannotti G, Ong AW, et al. Prospective randomized trial of two wound management strategies for dirty abdominal wounds. *Ann Surg* 2001;233(3):409–413.

Deshpande G, Rao S, Patole S, et al. Updated meta-analysis of probiotics for preventing necrotizing enterocolitis in preterm neonates. *Pediatrics* 2010;125(5):921–930.

Goldstein B, Giroir B, Randolph A, et al. International pediatric sepsis consensus conference: Definitions for sepsis and organ dysfunction in pediatrics. *Pediatric Crit Care Med* 2005;6(1):2–8.

Honeycutt TC, El Khashab M, Wardrop RM, et al. Probiotic administration and the incidence of nosocomial infection in pediatric intensive care: a randomized placebo-controlled trial. *Pediatr Crit Care Med* 2007;8(5):452–458.

Horan TC, Vegas AA, Jodra VM, Garcia ML. Nosocomial infection in surgery wards: a controlled study of increased duration of hospital stays and direct cost of hospitalization. *Eur J Epidemiol* 1993;9(5): 504–510.

Howard DP, Datta G, Cunnick G, et al. Surgical site infection rate is lower in laparoscopic than open colorectal surgery. *Colorectal Dis* 2010;12(5):423–427.

Imai E, Ueda M, Kanao T, et al. Surgical site infection risk factors identified by multivariate analysis for patient undergoing laparoscopic, open colon, and gastric surgery. *Am J Infect Control* 2008;36(10):727–731.

Kurz A, Sessler DI, Lenhardt R. Perioperative normothermia to reduce the incidence of surgical-wound infection and shorten hospitalization. *N Engl J Med* 1996;334(19):1209–1215.

Levy MM, Fink MP, Marshall JC, et al. 2001 SCCM/ESICM/ACCP/ ATS/SIS international sepsis definitions conference. *Crit Care Med* 2003;31(4):1250–1256.

Linam WM, Margolis PA, Staat MA, et al. Risk factors associated with surgical site infection after pediatric posterior spinal fusion procedure. *Infect Control Hosp Epidemiol* 2009;30(2):109–116.

Markides G, Subar D, Riyad K. Laparoscopic versus open appendectomy in adults with complicated appendicitis: systematic review and meta-analysis. *World J Surg* 2010;34(9):2026–2040.

McCord SS, Naik-Mathuria BJ, Murphy KM, et al. Negative pressure therapy is effective to manage a variety of wounds in infants and children. *Wound Repair Regen* 2007;15(3):296–301.

Pettigrew R. Delayed primary wound closure in gangrenous and perforated appendicitis. *Br J Surg* 1981;68(9):635–638.

Rayes N, Seehofer D, Neuhaus P. Prebiotics, probiotics, synbiotics in surgery—are they only trendy, truly effective or even dangerous? *Langenbecks Arch Surg* 2009;394:547–555.

Richards C, Edwards J, Culver D, et al. Does using a laparoscopic approach to cholecystectomy decrease the risk of surgical site infection? *Ann Surg* 2003;237(3):358–362.

Romy S., Eisenring MC, Bettschart V, et al. Laparoscope use and surgical site infections in digestive surgery. *Ann Surg* 2008;247(4):627–632.

Stevens DL, Bisno AL, Chambers HF, et al. Practice guidelines for the diagnosis and management of skin and soft-tissue infections. *Clin Infect Dis* 2005;41:1373–1406.

Uludag O, Rieu P, Niessen M, Voss A. Incidence of surgical site infections in pediatric patients: a 3-month prospective study in an academic pediatric surgical unit. *Pediatr Surg Int* 2000;15(5–6):417–420.

Zerr KJ, Furnary AP, Grunkemeier GL, et al. Glucose control lowers the risk of wound infection in diabetics after open heart operations. *Ann Thorac Surg* 1997;63(2):356–361.

# CHAPTER 14

# Office-Based Ambulatory Surgery

*Wallace W. Neblett III and Joshua B. Glenn*

## KEY POINTS

1. Procedural analgesia and sedation are both safe and applicable to office setting surgical procedures in children as long as support personnel are appropriately trained and monitoring and resuscitation equipment is available.

2. Emergent and scheduled surgical procedures are both amenable to an office location site. Incision and drainage of a superficial abscess is a common such procedure.

3. Infection drainage is best accompanied with enteral antibiotic therapy in the face of local cellulitis and even lymphangitis; however, when proximal lymphadenitis is present, parenteral antibiotics are indicated.

4. In the presence of a truncal or extremity penetrating/puncture wound in a child, a retained foreign body should be suspected and excluded.

## INTRODUCTION

Many commonly encountered minor pediatric surgical problems can be diagnosed and treated in the pediatric surgeon's office. The office setting is ideal for the management of such problems and there has been substantial growth of office-based surgery in recent years. The reasons for this include patient satisfaction, surgeon convenience, and cost savings. Certain preparations are required to facilitate office procedures, including training of office staff, making available appropriate surgical instruments, and provision of suitable analgesia.

## SEDATION AND ANALGESIA IN THE OFFICE SETTING

Provision of safe and effective anxiolysis and pain control during procedures for children in the ambulatory setting is a challenge for the surgeon, which may effectively limit the spectrum of procedures that can be provided in the surgical clinic. A variety of methods should be considered as possible solutions.

## Topical Anesthesia

Clinical experience with a variety of local anesthetic agents applied topically to reduce discomfort during painful procedures in children has demonstrated efficacy during venipuncture and intravenous (IV) cannulation. In our clinic, we have noted a substantial reduction in discomfort when topical anesthetics are used prior to tissue infiltration with local anesthetics. Topical application of 2.5% lidocaine and 2.5% prilocaine cream (EMLA cream) has been used in clinical practice for more than 25 years. Efficacy is enhanced by application of a thick layer of cream for 60 to 90 minutes prior to the procedure, and this is facilitated by use of small occlusive dressing. Parents can be instructed to apply the medication to the anticipated wound site for up to 1 hour in advance of the procedure in infants up to 3 months and for up to 4 hours for older infants and children.

Other topical anesthetic agents, including tetracaine (4%) gel and liposomal lidocaine (4%), have a more rapid onset of action, so, application time required is only 30 to 60 minutes.

Other needle-free strategies for local anesthetic administration include a lidocaine/tetracaine topical patch with an integrated heating component, which accelerates penetration of local anesthetic agents through the stratum corneum. Iontophoresis allows an ionic form of a local anesthetic to be accelerated into the subcutaneous or submucosal tissue under the influence of low-voltage direct electrical current. De Cou and co-workers described successful utilization of iontophoresis to administer lidocaine and epinephrine for a series of pediatric surgery office procedures with satisfactory results.

## Local Anesthesia

Infiltration of local anesthetic into tissue at the site of surgical procedures is the most basic method to provide analgesia. Local anesthetics such as lidocaine and bupivacaine are useful in office procedures, although each has important differences in rate of onset, duration of blockage, and safe dosage limits (Table 14-1). Signs and symptoms of toxicity range from tinnitus, lightheadedness, and nausea to seizures, arrhythmias, and cardiovascular collapse. Local anesthetics must be administered with strict attention to dosage limitations to avoid serious complications.

| TABLE 14-1 | Local Anesthetic Maximum Dosages for Tissue Infiltration[a] | |
|---|---|---|
| **Local Anesthetic** | **Maximum Dose** | **Onset/Duration of Action** |
| 1% Lidocaine plain (no epinephrine) | 4.5 mg/kg (0.45 mL/kg) (not to exceed 300 mg) | Rapid/60-120 min |
| 1% Lidocaine with epinephrine | 7 mg/kg (0.7 mL/kg) (not to exceed 300 mg) | Rapid: 60-120 min |
| 0.25% Bupivicaine plain (no epinephrine) | 2 mg/kg (0.8 mL/kg) (not to exceed 175 mg) | Slow: 240-480 min |
| 0.25% Bupivicaine with epinephrine | 3 mg/kg (1.2 mL/kg) (not to exceed 225 mg) | Slow: 20-480 min |

[a]For patients older than 3 months. Reduce dosage by 20% in newborn and infants under 3 months.

## Digital Block

The block is performed by injecting the local anesthetic with a small-bore needle into the web space along each lateral surface of the selected digit (Fig. 14-1). Epinephrine-containing anesthetics are best avoided because of the risk of tissue ischemia due to vasoconstriction of the digital arteries.

## Penile Block

A penile block can be used for circumcision or other penile procedures. This block is performed by infiltrating around the dorsal penile nerves at the level of the pubic bone using an epinephrine-free local anesthetic. A ring block can be used, as well, with good efficacy.

## Procedural Sedation

Provision of analgesia, immobilization, and anxiolysis in the clinic setting has long been a challenge for the pediatric surgeon. However, for many surgical clinics associated with a children's medical center, a balance of patient comfort and safety is currently possible due to improvements in monitoring due to routine availability of pulse oximetry, development of new pharmacologic agents of shorter duration but greater potency, evolution of procedural sedation safety guidelines, and the development of hospital-based procedural sedation services devoted to provision of moderate to deep sedation at sites outside the operating room.

Ketamine has been long used for painful procedures as a sedative/hypnotic with analgesic properties. This medication produces a dissociative state that allows painful procedures to be performed with tolerable patient movement. Patients usually maintain a stable airway with spontaneous respiration, but at times, may experience apnea, hypotension, laryngospasm, and postprocedural hallucinations and nightmares.

Benzodiazepine or propofol, in combination with a narcotic, may be used to achieve moderate sedation. Patients receiving these combinations of sedatives and analgesics require continuous monitoring and supplemental oxygen during the procedure along with postanesthesia recovery unit-like care following the procedure.

Low concentration (<50%) nitrous oxide inhalation appears to be an efficacious technique to achieve procedural analgesia and sedation while maintaining protective laryngeal reflexes. This agent has a rapid onset, is short-acting, and has a

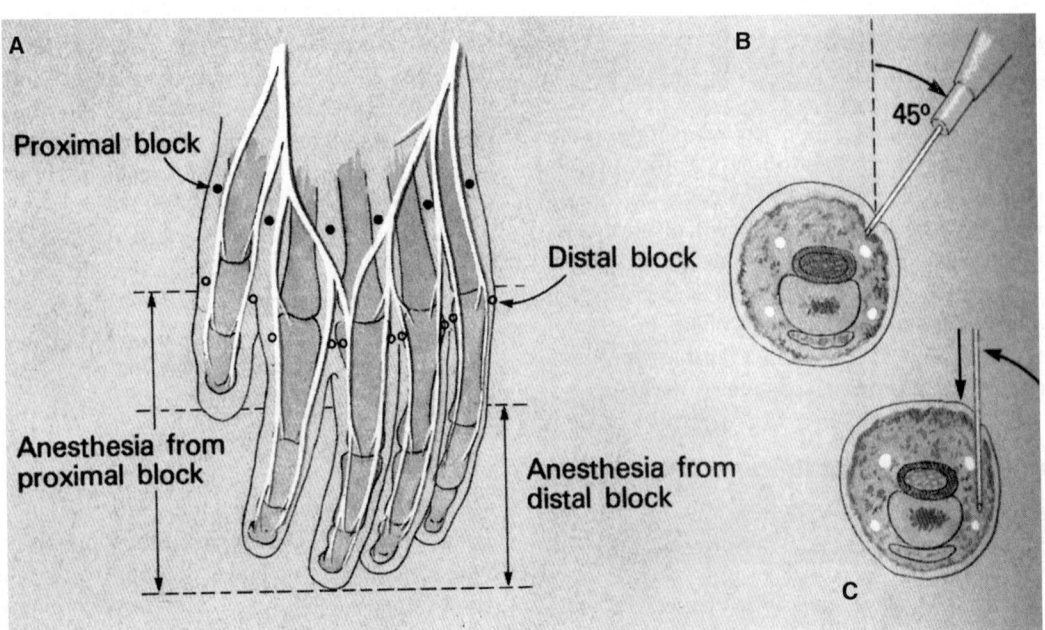

**FIGURE 14-1** Anatomy and technique of administering a digital nerve block anesthetic. The block can be administered proximally or distally on the lateral aspect of the digit using small volumes of agent (**A**) and the infiltration should be completed with additional injection along flexion and extension surfaces (**B, C**).

well-documented safety record. Reported advantages of using this modality include excellent pain control, minimal need for advance preparation of the patient, low complication rate, and lack of need for postoperative monitoring. Early experience with this technique in a pediatric surgical clinic practice indicates it to be a cost-effective and safe alternative to conscious sedation or general anesthesia for minor pediatric surgical procedures.

## SUPERFICIAL INFECTIONS

Superficial infections are a common problem among pediatric patients. Suppuration occurs frequently and often requires surgical drainage. Infection of a variety of congenital lesions may lead to abscess formation, including thyroglossal cyst, branchial cleft cyst, and preauricular cyst and sinus. Conservative incision and drainage with packing may be required to clear the acute infection. Definitive resection of the predisposing lesion will be required once the acute infection has resolved.

### *Staphylococcal aureus* Skin and Soft Tissue Infections

During the last decade, there has been a dramatic worldwide increase in community-associated methicillin-resistant *Staphylococcus aureus* (CA-MRSA) skin and soft tissue infections (SSTI). CA-MRSA now accounts for more than 75% of community-acquired infections.

Surgical drainage of abscesses is an essential component of treatment for these patients. Traditionally, the procedure involved an adequate incision to allow evacuation of pus and necrotic tissue, hemostat disruption of loculated pockets, irrigation of the abscess cavity, and insertion of a small penrose drain or gauze wick packing. A culture should be performed to clarify antibiotic sensitivities.

Several recent reports have described a minimally invasive technique of abscess drainage involving placement of a silastic vessel loop or one-fourth inch penrose drain introduced through a central stab incision into the abscess cavity and exteriorized through a second peripheral incision made at the cavity margin. The results reported in 2 small retrospective reviews suggest that this technique is safe and equivalent in outcome to standard incision and drainage, although one study reported a need for additional drainage procedures in 5% of patients.

### Paronychia

Paronychia is the most common infection of the hand and occurs as a result of any process that disrupts the nail fold/ nail plate junction, such as penetrating trauma, nail biting, or hangnails. The infection begins as an infection of the lateral nail fold but can process to involve the eponychium and opposite nail fold, creating a *runaround* infection. As infection progresses, pus can accumulate along the nail bed, causing elevation of the nail plate.

Early paronychia can be treated with oral antibiotics, warm soaks, and splinting for comfort. Surgical drainage is required when the infection progresses to an abscess. In that case, the affected portion of the nail plate should be elevated from the nail bed and removed to achieve effective drainage (Fig. 14-2). This can be readily accomplished using a digital block to provide analgesia.

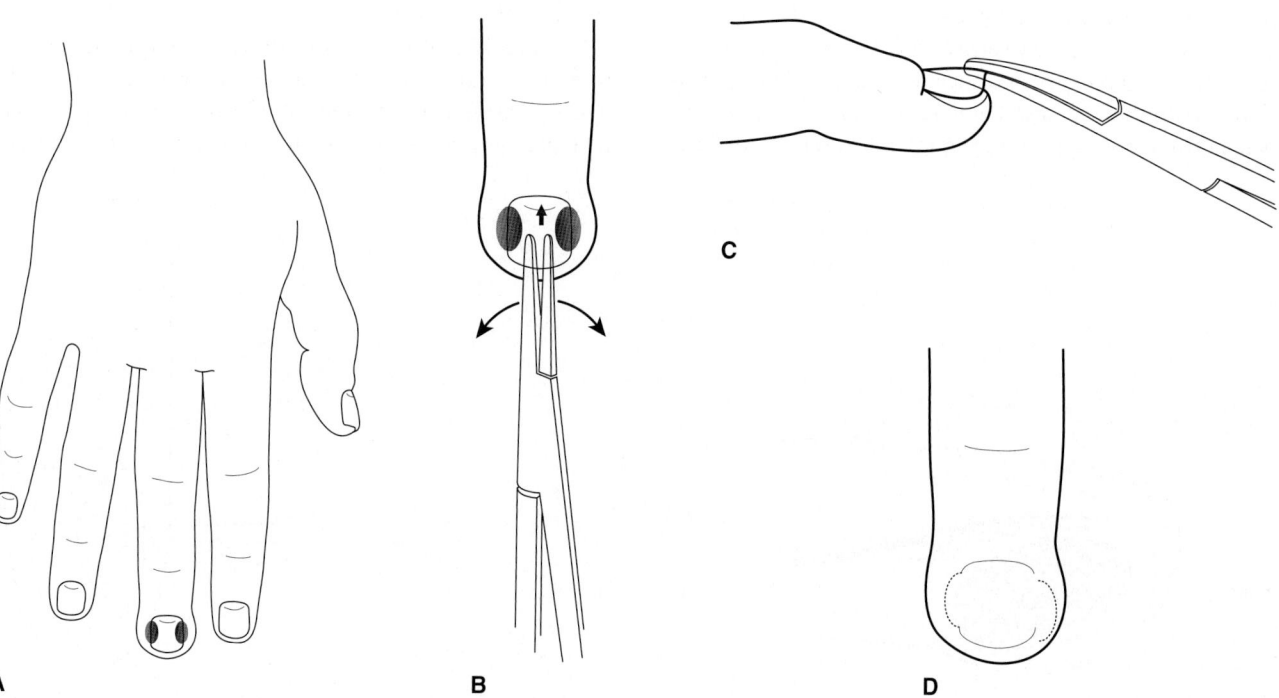

**FIGURE 14-2** Management of acute paronychia (A). A hemostat is used to separate the nail from its bed all the way to the nail root (B). The elevated nail can then be gently extended and pulled out from beneath the overlying proximal eponychia (C). Any residual granulation tissue should be debrided (D).

## Felon

A felon occurs as a result of infection within the closed space formed by the multiple vertical septae that originate along the periosteum of the distal phalanx and insert into the skin. Patients experience throbbing pain and rapid onset of swelling of the entire pulp of the distal phalanx. Drainage may be performed through the classic midaxial hockey stick incision carried down to the periosteum followed by blunt division of the vertical septae from their periosteal attachments to allow drainage of all the septal compartments (Fig. 14-3A and B). The incision should be placed on the noncontact side of the digit (radial side of thumb and ulnar side of the fingers) and should not extend around the tip of the digit.

Drainage may also be performed through a central vertical incision extending from the distal flexion crease to the fingertip. This incision avoids the neurovascular bundle, provides effective drainage, and heals well.

## Ingrown Toenails

Onchocryptosis or ingrown toenails (IGTN) is a common problem in the general population and in children, and occurs most frequently in adolescents. The great toes are exclusively affected with the lateral edge more frequent than medial.

The disorder is characterized by the abnormal extension of the lateral margin of the nail plate into the nail groove with resultant erosion into the dermis along the skin fold. This results in local pain, edema, and tenderness with pressure and commonly progresses to the development of cellulitis, granulation tissue, and nail fold hypertrophy. Debilitating pain may impede wearing normal footwear and participation in daily activities. The primary physician has often prescribed antibiotics to treat the local inflammation prior to referral to the pediatric surgeon for treatment.

For patients in an early stage of IGTN, conservative measures may be successful and include nail care, proper trimming, hydrotherapy, and antibiotics. More advanced cases benefit from more aggressive surgical intervention, which can

be usually performed in the clinic setting. Treatment options include:

1. Avulsion of the entire nail, with or without chemical destruction of the nail bed
2. Wedge excision of the nail edge
3. Wedge excision with surgical matrixectomy targeted to destroy the lateral horns of the matrix and hence to prevent regrowth of the lateral nail plate into the skin fold
4. Wedge excision of nail edge with chemical destruction of the lateral matrix using concentrated phenol (88%) or NaOH (10%)

Several studies have demonstrated an unacceptably high recurrence rate for nail plate avulsion without matrixectomy. Complete segmental matrixectomy, in theory, should prevent recurrence by achieving permanent removal of the offending lateral edge of the nail plate; however, surgeon experience with this procedure may affect success rates. Several authors have demonstrated a lower incidence of symptomatic IGTN recurrence by using topical phenol to accomplish chemodestruction of the matrix, but at the cost of increased postoperative infection rate and prolonged wound healing. Experience with NaOH chemical matrixectomy in adults and children indicates outcomes comparable to using phenol with a better side effect profile.

Children with IGTN in advanced stages are best managed with a surgical approach, which can be carried out in the surgical clinic in the majority of patients (approximately 75%). Initial topical anesthesia, accomplished by application of EMLA cream along the base of the toe for 40 to 60 minutes, improves tolerance of subsequent injections. Digital block using 1% plain xylocaine followed by infiltration along the edge and at the base of the ingrown segment provides effective and complete anesthesia for the procedures in those children able to cooperate.

Bleeding is controlled using a rubber band or small penrose drain tourniquet. We prefer to perform avulsion of the ingrown portion of the toenail, sharp excision of the nail fold plus any associated granulation tissue and including

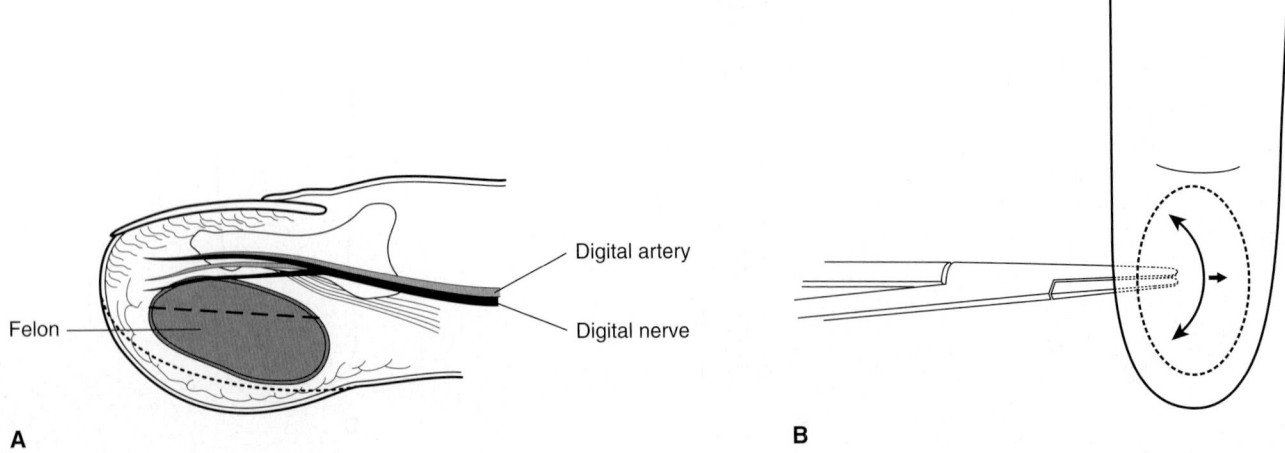

**A**

Felon —

Digital artery

Digital nerve

**B**

**FIGURE 14-3** Management of an acute felon. A distal digit ulnar surface incision is made into the infected soft tissue (A). A hemostat is then inserted and infectious loculations are bluntly separated (B).

the germinal matrix at the base of the ingrown nail segment. Curettage can be used for any remaining matrix. Complete removal of the germinal matrix is essential, and failure to accomplish this will lead to recurrence of a troublesome nail spicule along that edge. There is a definite learning curve in performing this part of the otherwise simple procedure.

Chemical matrixectomy may be performed in lieu of surgical matrixectomy by using an application of 10% NaOH to the germinal matrix followed by curettage and then neutralization of the base with glacial acetic acid. This approach may be technically simpler and has a lower reported recurrence rate: surgical matrixectomy 20% and chemical matrixectomy 12%.

Following completion of the procedure, a compressive circumferential gauze wrap is applied prior to removal of the tourniquet. No sutures are needed as the dressing compresses the skin edge against the normal remnant nail bed and achieves excellent tissue approximation. The dressing should be tight enough to prevent bleeding, but elastic dressing material that might cause tissue ischemia should be avoided. The dressing can be removed by the family at home 3 days postoperatively, after a brief warm water soak. Thereafter, care includes application of topical antibiotic ointment, a dry band-aid, and comfortable footwear.

## Perianal Abscess

Perianal abscess (PA) occurs commonly in infants, presenting usually within the first year. Affected babies are usually otherwise healthy and there is no need to search for an underlying condition in infants. There is a strong male predominance (>90%). Older children are more likely to have an underlying cause, including immunodeficiency, immune suppression, diabetes, and inflammatory bowel disease (most commonly Crohn disease).

Patients present with an indurated or fluctuant tender area of perianal swelling, which is usually discovered by the parent during bathing or diaper change. The babies are usually fretful and may have a low-grade fever. This disorder may occasionally be confused with staphylococcal SSTI, which commonly occurs on the nearby buttock or perineum. Proximity within 1 to 2 cm of the anus should alert the clinician to the actual diagnosis.

PA probably arises as a result of infection within an obstructed crypt of Morgagni at the dentate line, which then necessitates into the adjacent perianal space. Some authors have proposed a congenital defect to explain the frequent occurrence in infancy. Others have proposed a role of androgens affecting the anal glands to explain the striking male predominance. The frequent coincidence of fistula-in-ano (FIA) is testimony to the crypt's role in the pathogenesis of PA.

Surgical drainage is the mainstay in treatment of PA, although there are dissenting opinions. Simple needle aspiration with or without antibiotics was reported to achieve cure in 62% of a group of 47 infants with PA. Another report characterizes PA as a self-limited process and encourages supportive care only in the absence of severe symptoms.

In our clinic, simple incision and drainage is the recommended treatment in an infant with a symptomatic PA. This can usually be accomplished in the clinic procedure room without

general anesthesia by using topical EMLA cream supplemented by local infiltration of 1% xylocaine with epinephrine. A limited radial incision centered over the inflammatory mass is used to evacuate the abscess. The incision should be oriented to allow subsequent incorporation into a fistulotomy incision for the 40% to 50% of patients who develop recurrent suppuration associated with persistent FIA. The fistula virtually always arises in the crypt closest to the abscess. The abscess cavity is packed lightly with a small gauze wick, which will be removed the following day at the time of initiation of warm baths.

There is controversy regarding the utility of performing the initial drainage procedure in the operating room under anesthesia in order to allow a search for a FIA and, if found, a fistulotomy to be performed as part of that same operative procedure. We feel the high resolution rate after simple incision and drainage of the abscess warrants a more conservative approach and favors a delayed treatment for the child with persistent symptoms due to FIA.

## MINOR TRAUMA

### Superficial Lacerations

A wide variety of minor surgical problems may be encountered in the office that result from minor trauma. As with any traumatic wound, the status of tetanus immunization should be assessed and addressed. Although a detailed discussion of the management of minor lacerations in the pediatric age group is beyond the scope of this chapter, many superficial lacerations lend themselves to being managed in the surgeon's office if the office is appropriately staffed and supplied.

### Fingertip Injuries

#### Fingertip Avulsions

Laceration of the fingertips is among the most common injuries, although major fingertip trauma, including partial amputation and extensive fractures, obviously require the support of specialized equipment and other advanced technologies. More simple lacerations and partial avulsion of the fingertip or nail bed are amenable to treatment in the office. In young children, satisfactory healing of the wound, as well as a functional sensate fingertip, is usually achieved using digital block, cleansing and closure of the wound with or without sutures (Steri-Strips, Dermabond), and the application of antibiotic ointment. An appropriate nonadhesive dressing is also indicated.

#### Nail Bed Injuries

Partial nail avulsions with firm adherence of the nail plate to the bed are best treated conservatively and not explored. Complete or near-complete avulsions require removal of the nail and inspection of the nail bed for lacerations. Nail bed lacerations require repair with a 6-0 or smaller absorbable suture, and minimal to no debridement of the nail bed should be performed. Digital block is the preferred method of anesthesia and a penrose tourniquet provides a bloodless field. A small hole is made in the nail for drainage then the nail is secured back into the nail fold with either suture or tissue adhesive (Dermabond). The nail then serves as a splint to keep the nail fold open for new nail growth and provides a cover for the nail bed. The finger should be dressed with an appropriate nonadherent dressing and splinted.

## Subungual Hematoma

A subungual hematoma, whether occurring on a toe or a finger, is a painful, acute problem frequently encountered in the surgeon's office. The traumatic event leading to development of the hematoma is generally a direct blow to the nail. It may be associated with a distal phalanx fracture or nail bed laceration. Regardless of the etiology, an acutely painful hematoma can be managed by evacuation directly through the surface of the nail, which usually does not require anesthesia. Traditionally, this procedure has been simply carried out by heating the tip of a paper clip in an open flame and then applying it to the surface of the nail at its midportion, burrowing through the nail into the hematoma with the evacuation of blood through the puncture site (Fig. 14-4). A somewhat more sophisticated method of accomplishing trephination involves the use of a handheld, battery-powered cauterizing unit. The heating element of this unit easily penetrates the nail, producing similar results (Fig. 14-4). If associated with distal phalanx fracture, antibiotics are advised, as well as splinting and close follow-up.

## Subcutaneous Foreign Bodies

A patient with a foreign body embedded in the hand or foot often presents to the surgeon for treatment in the office. The type of foreign body may vary from fragments of wood and metal to needles, toothpicks, and graphite fragments from lead pencil stab wounds. On many occasions, because a retained foreign body in the subcutaneous tissue is suspected, a radiograph or sonogram of region is obtained. If the object is radiopaque and relatively superficial, it can be quite inviting to attempt to remove it using a local anesthetic in the office. A word of caution is needed at this point because on a radiograph many of these objects appear to be deceptively easy to access. In contrast, many of these cases require the benefits of a general anesthetic and dynamic radiographic guidance for removal in the operating room. However, should the foreign body appear superficial or be palpable, consideration for office removal is appropriate. In order to dislodge foreign bodies wedged between the nail and the nail bed, partial or total removal of the nail may be required.

## Puncture Wounds

Puncture wounds of the foot may also fall into the category of retained foreign body materials. Contaminated material may have been inserted into the plantar aspect of the foot as a result of the puncture wound. Patients may visit the surgeon's office after being treated with antibiotics, but persistent pain, erythema, and swelling may indicate persistent infection. A radiograph of the foot is appropriate to establish a baseline for bony structures, as well as to search for possible retained portions of radiopaque material. A few of those puncture wounds may require incision and drainage of a plantar abscess followed by a short course of outpatient antibiotic therapy. A small number of patients with persistent infection require specific gram-negative antimicrobial therapy; and a still smaller number progress to osteomyelitis and require long-term IV antibiotic therapy. Patients with cellulitis or lymphangitis may be appropriately treated with oral antibiotics, but those with regional lymphadenitis, persistent cellulitis, or bony changes suggesting osteomyelitis require parenteral antibiotics.

## Hair Tourniquet

A somewhat less common entity seen in the office that requires diligent surgical intervention is strangulation of a digit with an embedded circumferential hair (Fig. 14-5). This problem

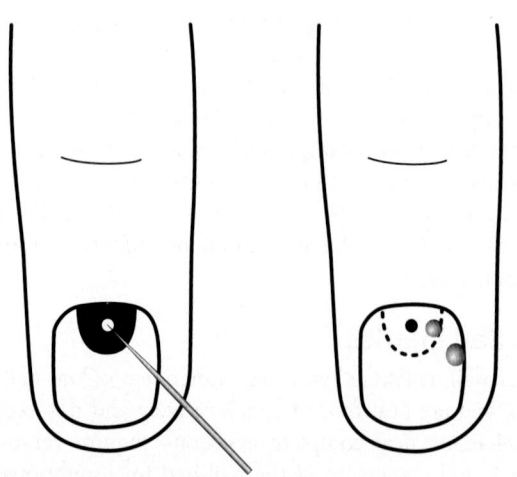

FIGURE 14-4 A subungual hematoma is drained with either an electrocautery or a heated pin, and a hole is "burned" through the nail directly over the painful hematoma effecting drainage and relieving the pressure.

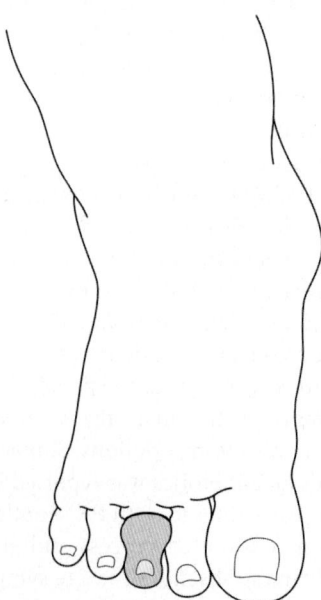

FIGURE 14-5 A circumferential enwrapping hair foreign body has produced a proximal crevice and distal swelling of the digit.

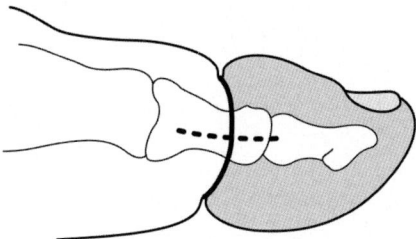

**FIGURE 14-6** Bilateral longitudinal incisions are made at the level of the foreign body crevice to ensure division of the constricting band when the foreign body itself cannot be identified and removed.

occurs most frequently in neonates and young children. They appear with an obvious constriction ring around the digit with distal edema and a proximal crevice secondary to a constricting foreign body, usually a hair. Generally, removal of the constricting hair or other foreign material successfully preserves the digit. With the use of magnification and persistence, these strangulating hairs can easily be removed, not uncommonly in segments. This problem may also occur in male children as a constricting band around the base or shaft of the penis. When the foreign body is hidden by secondary edema, an alternate therapy is controlled lateral and medial longitudinal incision in to the soft tissue (and through the encircling foreign body), parallel to the long axis of the digit (Fig. 14-6).

## Minor Scald and Contact Burns

Minor burns and scald injuries less than 10% body surface area can safely be treated in the office. Cool the burn area with towels moistened with saline and carefully cleanse with mild soap and water. Bullae should be debrided and all necrotic tissue removed. An antibiotic ointment is then applied—Silvadene for extremities and trunk and Bacitracin for facial burns. Digits should be wrapped individually with fluffed gauze separating them in order to prevent maceration and adherence. Tetanus immunization status must be checked and tetanus immunization administered as appropriate. Prophylactic oral antibiotics are not indicated, but appropriate pain management is essential.

## MISCELLANEOUS SURGICAL PROBLEMS

Although a detailed discussion of the numerous benign lesions of the integument presenting for surgical resection is beyond the scope of this chapter, many of these lend

themselves to removal in the office under local anesthesia with or without sedation. Consideration might be given to office excision of various pigmented nevi because of concerning features or change, family history of melanoma, or other indicators of malignant risk (eg, dysplastic nevus syndrome) depending on specific individual factors. Other benign neoplasms or lesions appropriate for excision or biopsy in an ambulatory setting include epidermoid and dermoid cyst, pilomatrixoma, lipoma, pseudorheumatoid nodule, granuloma annulare, and pyogenic granuloma.

Infants requiring circumcision may have that procedure performed in the clinic using a penile block and a papoose board for passive restraint. Labial adhesions may be separated as an office procedure using topical anesthesia and/or sedation. Following blunt dissection or manual separation of the filmy labial adhesions, the parents should be instructed to apply estrogen cream to the labia for 10 to 14 days, postprocedure. This enhances cornification of the labial epithelium, which aids in preventing recurrence of the condition.

## SUMMARY

Although the majority of a pediatric surgeon's office practice involves consultation, counseling, preoperative evaluation, and postoperative care, a wide variety of minor surgical problems can be treated on an ambulatory basis in the surgical clinic. Outfitting the clinic with appropriate surgical instruments, insuring adequate training of office personnel, and selection of suitable methods of local anesthesia/procedural sedation will expand the spectrum of care that can be provided in a cost-effective and time-efficient office-based ambulatory setting.

## SELECTED READINGS

Burnweit C, Diana-Zerpo JA, Nahmad MH, et al. Nitrous oxide analgesia for minor pediatric surgical procedures: an effective alternative to conscious sedation? *J Pediatr Surg* 2004;39:495–499.

De Cou JM, Abrams RS, Hammond JH, et al. Iontophoresis: a needle free electrical system of local anesthesia delivery for pediatric surgical office procedures. *J Pediatr Surg* 1999;34:946–949.

Ladd AP, Levy MS, Quilty J. Minimally invasive technique in treatment of complex subcutaneous abscesses in children. *J Pediatr Surg* 2010;45:1562–1566.

Odell CA. Community-associated methicillin-resistant *Staphylococcus aureus* (CA-MRSA) skin infections. *Curr Opin Pediatr* 2010;22:273–277.

Ross AK, Eck JB. Office-based anesthesia for children. *Anesthesiol Clin North Am* 2002;20:195–210.

Yang G, Yanchar NL, Lo AYS, et al. Treatment of ingrown toenails in the pediatric population. *J Pediatr Surg* 2008;43:931–935.

# PART II

## THE HEAD AND NECK

# CHAPTER 15

## Head and Neck Lesions

*Richard G. Azizkhan*

### KEY POINTS

1. To successfully manage patients with branchial cleft anomalies, surgeons must have a thorough understanding of the embryology, anatomy, and clinical presentation of these lesions.

2. To minimize recurrence and injury to critical structures related to the larynx, surgeons must have in-depth knowledge of normal and pathological neck anatomy in the context of congenital and acquired lesions (ie, thyroglossal duct cysts, dermoid cysts, and other midline lesions).

3. Torticollis is a common acquired condition related to scarring and atrophy of the sternocleidomastoid muscle and adjacent cervical muscles. Most patients can be treated nonoperatively; however, rarely, patients require surgical intervention to prevent complications such as facial hemihypoplasia and life-long craniofacial asymmetry.

4. Vascular lesions are the most common benign neoplasms affecting the salivary glands in children. Pleomorphic adenoma is the most common benign epithelial tumor. The high rate of local recurrence of this tumor is problematic.

5. Malignant neoplasms of the salivary glands (mucoepidermoid carcinomas and acinous cell carcinomas) are uncommon, and most lesions can be managed with surgical excision. High-grade malignancies are extremely rare and tend to occur in younger patients.

6. Cervical lymphadenitis can be either acute or chronic, caused by a spectrum of etiologies, including viral, bacterial (aerobic, anaerobic, and mycobacterial), fungal, and protozoan infections. Understanding the spectrum and presentation of diseases is essential to selecting appropriate pharmacological and surgical management approaches.

## INTRODUCTION

Head and neck lesions in children are extremely common and can be subdivided by etiology into lesions that are congenital and those that are acquired. Most congenital lesions, such as anomalies of the second branchial apparatus and thyroglossal duct cysts, are of embryonic origin. They are usually easily diagnosed on physical examination and seldom require an additional workup. Some of these lesions, however, may not be easily recognized or may not cause clinical problems until adolescence or adulthood. Knowledge of their embryologic origin and their relationship to normal neck structures is essential to successful management. This chapter therefore focuses on the embryology, pathobiology, and surgical management of congenital head and neck lesions. We also present an overview of neonatal torticollis, salivary gland lesions, and acquired lesions caused by neoplasms and inflammatory processes.

## LESIONS OF EMBRYONIC ORIGIN

### Anomalies of the Branchial Apparatus

Branchial apparatus anomalies comprise a heterogeneous group of congenital malformations stemming from incomplete in utero resorption of pharyngeal clefts and pouches. Fistulae, cysts, sinus tracts, and cartilaginous remnants are all clinical manifestations arising from these embryonic events. Although all of these lesions are present at birth, many do not become clinically apparent for months or years. In many cases infection is the initial manifestation. Cysts developing from branchial structures usually appear later in childhood than sinuses, fistulae, and cartilaginous remnants, which are observed in infancy. Complete fistulae are more common than external sinuses, and during childhood both are more common than branchial cleft cysts. The incidence of these anomalies in adults is quite different, with cysts occurring more frequently than either sinuses or fistulae.

### History

The term *branchial* is derived from the Greek word *brankhia*, meaning gills. The first description of a cervical fistula is credited to Hunczowski in 1789. In 1832, Von Ascherson described the embryonic origin of fistulae arising from the branchial apparatus. A more in-depth understanding of these lesions has been derived from studies conducted by of a number of renowned embryologists of the 19th and early 20th centuries (Proctor, Wilson, Lyall, Stahl, and Frazer).

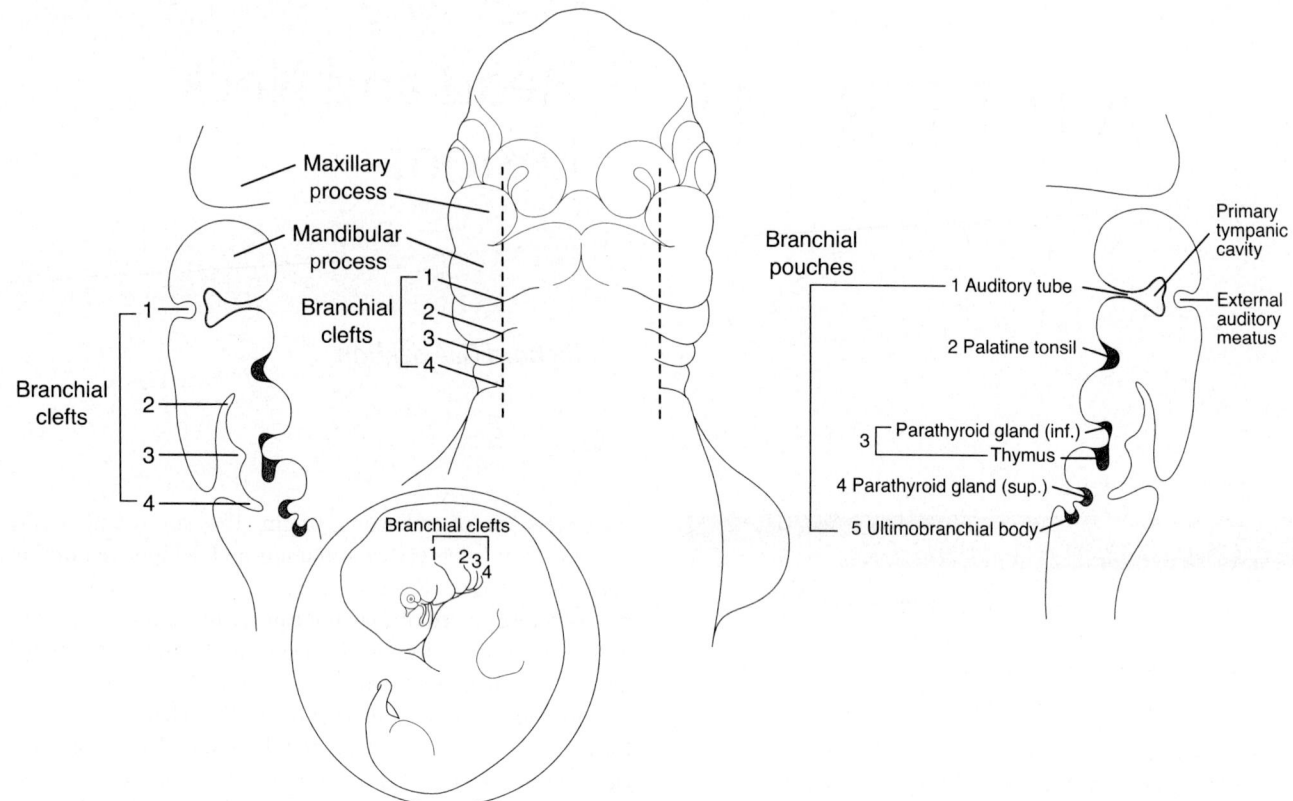

**FIGURE 15-1** Five-millimeter human embryo at the fifth week of gestation (*inset*). Schematic representation of the head and neck region demonstrating the branchial clefts and pouches at the 5-mm embryo stage. Sagittal sections taken through the branchial apparatus depict the location of the external clefts and the internal pouches. The embryonic derivation of important head and neck structures within this region is noted.

## Embryology

Four pairs of branchial arches, clefts, and pharyngeal pouches appear in the head and neck region during the fourth to eighth weeks of gestation (Fig. 15-1). At this early stage of development, the clefts are external ectodermal infoldings (resembling the gills of a fish) between the arches and are matched internally by pharyngeal endodermal pouches. This branchial apparatus develops into many of the structures of the lower face and neck.

As the embryo grows, the arches coalesce and obliterate all of the clefts except for a portion of the first, which becomes the eustachian tube and the auditory canal (Fig. 15-1). The first branchial arch forms the mandible and contributes to the maxillary process of the upper jaw. Abnormal development of this arch results in a wide range of facial deformities, including cleft lip and palate, an abnormal shape or contour of the external ear, and malformed internal ossicles; these deformities comprise 8% of branchial cleft anomalies. The second branchial arch forms the palatine tonsil, the tonsillar fossa, and the hyoid bone. Ninety percent of branchial abnormalities arise from the second cleft. These abnormalities are thought to be due to incomplete obliteration as the first arch overgrows the second, third, and fourth clefts and fuses with the lateral branchial wall. The third arch gives rise to the inferior parathyroid glands and the thymus (Fig. 15-1). The fourth branchial arch stops higher in the neck to form the superior parathyroid glands.

The ventral portion of this arch also forms the ultimobranchial body, which is responsible for the development of the thyrocalcitonin-producing parafollicular cells of the thyroid gland. Anomalies of the third and fourth clefts and pouches occur but are rare.

## Anatomy and Pathologic Variants

**Anomalies of the Branchial Clefts.** First branchial cleft remnants occur along a line extending from the external auditory canal to a point just below the midportion of the mandible. If external openings are present, they are generally found below the mandible and above the hyoid bone (Fig. 15-2). The fistula courses upward to a connection with the external auditory canal. First branchial cleft anomalies include sinuses opening onto the skin or into the pharynx; fistulae with communications between the skin and the pharynx; and cysts without extension to either surface.

Second branchial cleft lesions most commonly appear as cysts or external openings along the anterior border of the sternocleidomastoid muscle, usually near the junction of the caudal and middle third of the muscle (Fig. 15-2). Those with an external opening typically have a history of drainage of clear mucus. The fistula courses upward along the carotid sheath, between the external and internal carotid arteries, in front of the hypoglossal nerve, and ends in the tonsillar fossa. A fistulagram can demonstrate the course of the tract but is generally not essential for future operative planning.

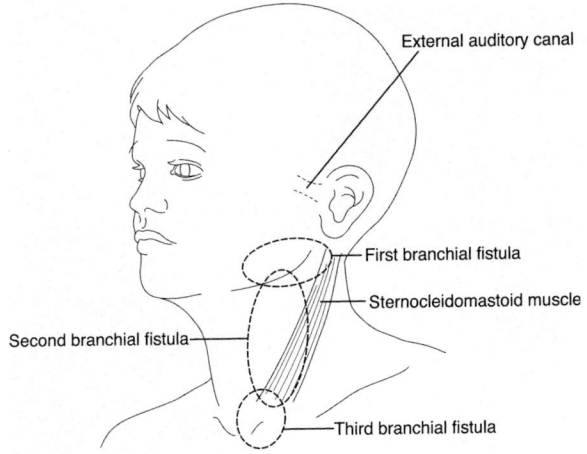

**FIGURE 15-2** Regions of the neck where first, second, and third branchial cleft fistulae or cysts are most commonly seen.

A third branchial cleft fistula is very uncommon. It generally is seen as an external opening along the anterior border of the clavicular head of the sternocleidomastoid muscle; it may occur in the same areas as lesions of the second cleft but ascends posteriorly to the carotid artery rather than through the bifurcation (Fig. 15-2). The fistula pierces the thyrohyoid membrane and enters the pyriform sinus. Related but distinct embryonic pyriform sinus lesions are also thought to be derived from the third or fourth branchial pouch and will be discussed in more detail in a following section of this chapter.

While a definitive case of a complete fourth branchial cleft fistula has not been documented, based on our understanding of human embryology, such a fistula would course from a low anterior cervical external opening into the chest. Here it would encircle either the subclavian artery on the right or the aortic arch on the left and would then ascend to a connection with the cervical esophagus or pyriform sinus.

**Anomalies of the Branchial Pouches.** Although significant anomalies of the first pouch are rare, minor anomalies are common in association with first branchial arch aberrations. The second branchial pouch is involved in the development of the palatine tonsils, and it sometimes persists as an internal sinus. This structure is a blind tract of varying depth within or close to the palatine tonsil, which might be a factor in recurrent tonsillitis. Failure of development of the third and fourth branchial pouches results in the absence of the thymus and parathyroid glands (DiGeorge syndrome), which is involved in neonatal tetany and impaired cellular immunity. An infection might first arise as an inflammatory mass on the anterior lower neck and then fistulize through a tract that runs directly from the skin to the pyriform sinus. The external exit is generally in the lower neck in the region of the thyroid gland. The differential diagnosis of recurrent abscesses of the anterior neck must thus consider a persistent third branchial pouch. Other anomalies arising from the third and fourth branchial pouches may appear as cystic structures in the neck. Cervical thymic cysts (discussed later in this chapter) are generally found on the left side of the neck but may be seen anywhere along the migratory path of

descent of the thymus and the pharynx to the anterior mediastinum. Parathyroid cysts can be located anywhere around the thyroid gland or in the mediastinum.

**Anomalies of the Branchial Arch Remnants (Cartilages).** Most branchial arch remnants disappear, with the exception of those that contribute to bony structures or ligaments. Occasionally, however, remnants persist as small, triangular masses deep in the skin along the anterior border of the sternocleidomastoid muscle. They present cosmetic problems only and are easily removed.

## Clinical Presentation and Evaluation

Most branchial cleft lesions can be diagnosed from a medical history and by performing a physical examination. When a sinus is present, lesions are diagnosed in the first decade of life. However, when there is no external sinus, the diagnosis may not be made until the patient is well into adolescence or adulthood.

Branchial cleft sinuses and fistulae are bilateral in 20% of cases and have a slight female preponderance. An external sinus or fistula is manifested by intermittent clear mucoid drainage from a skin ostium located in the midneck along the anterior border of the sternocleidomastoid muscle (Fig. 15-3A and B). In some cases, the tract itself may be palpable. Preoperative probing of the tract or injecting it with a colored dye or water-soluble contrast should be avoided because it may lead to infection, thus making excision more difficult and recurrence more likely. Familiarity with the cited embryology should help one to identify the branchial cleft origin and its likely associated tract. The diagnosis is often apparent on examination, rendering further radiographic evaluation unnecessary. Internal sinuses drain into the tonsillar fossa and appear as a mass or an inclusion cyst when the draining tract becomes obstructed.

Branchial cleft cysts appear after infancy. They are located higher in the neck than the external ostia of sinuses and fistulae, and can be identified as a palpable mass at the level of the carotid bifurcation (Fig. 15-4A and B). They may be more difficult to diagnose, as they tend to lie deep to the anterior border of the sternocleidomastoid muscle in its upper third. These cysts can occur when the cutaneous opening of a sinus tract becomes occluded. It is not unusual for a branchial cleft cyst or sinus tract to become secondarily infected, and it may be the infection that initially alerts the physician to the lesion. Branchial cleft cysts can be confused with and should be distinguished from macrocystic lymphatic malformations (formerly called cystic hygromas), hemangiomas, lymphadenopathy, and particularly, lymphatic or metastatic tumors.

## Diagnosis

When the diagnosis is uncertain, ultrasonography can be extremely useful in identifying deep cysts and characterizing their contents, as well as in differentiating solid and cystic masses. Additionally, real-time ultrasonography with Doppler imaging can identify associated vascular structures. The extensive differential diagnosis of a mass at the angle of the jaw includes adenopathy, macrocystic lymphatic malformations, dermoids, and parotid lesions, as well as primary and

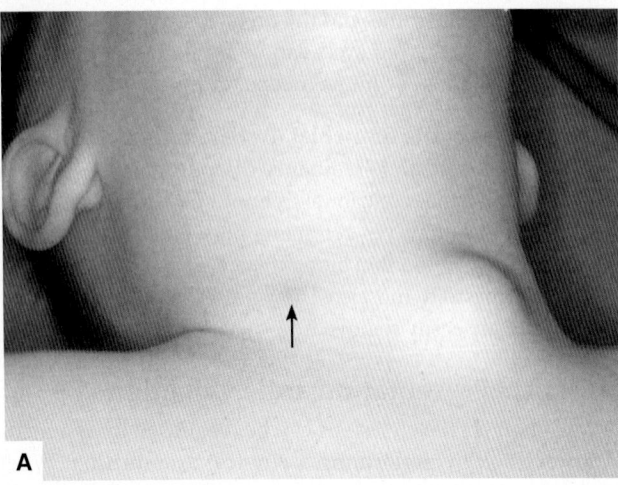

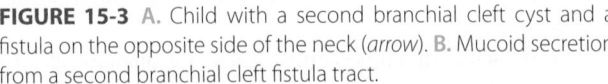

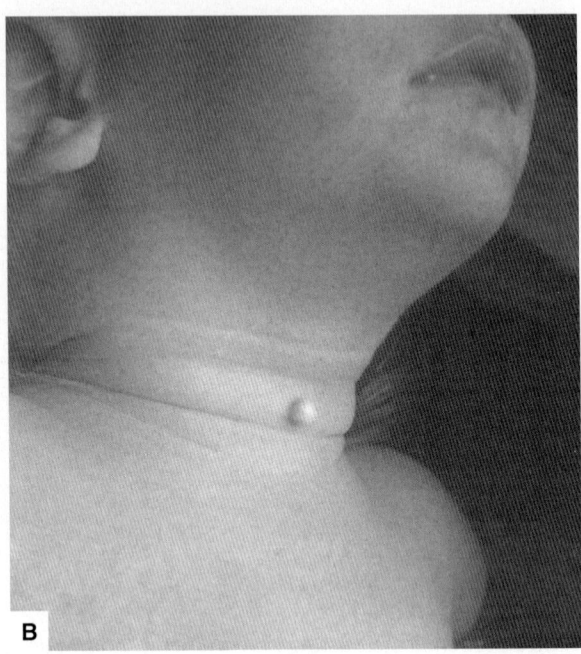

**FIGURE 15-3 A.** Child with a second branchial cleft cyst and a fistula on the opposite side of the neck (*arrow*). **B.** Mucoid secretion from a second branchial cleft fistula tract.

metastatic neoplasms of lymphatic origin. Further diagnostic studies with computed tomography, magnetic resonance imaging, or fine-needle aspiration biopsy may be indicated, particularly for solid masses. Determination of the specific etiology of the mass, however, often requires surgical exploration. Incision and drainage are sometimes necessary. In such cases, it is important to keep in mind that branchial cleft anomalies are anatomically related to nerves and vessels that are vulnerable to injury during drainage procedures.

## Treatment

Because of the likelihood of infection developing in any of the branchial lesions, complete excision of the cyst and sinus tract is generally recommended at the time of diagnosis in a noninfected lesion. Surgery in infants is delayed until 3 to 6 months of age to minimize the risks of anesthesia associated with neonatal surgery. In older children, surgical procedures

are scheduled conveniently to minimize the risk of intervening infection. Infected cysts and sinus tracts should be treated with appropriate antibiotics and warm soaks. If they are fluctuant, needle aspiration or incision and drainage should be performed and definitive resection deferred until the infection has completely resolved. Attempts at complete excision during active infection significantly increase the risk of injury to major vessels and nerves. Excision of the entire tract is of paramount importance because recurrence and infection are common with an incomplete excision. With a complete excision, the recurrence rate in most series is less than 7%.

## Surgical Procedures

**First Branchial Cleft Fistulae.** A first branchial cleft fistula generally requires an extensive procedure due to its proximity to the parotid gland and facial nerve. The procedure is carried out with a general anesthetic. The patient is

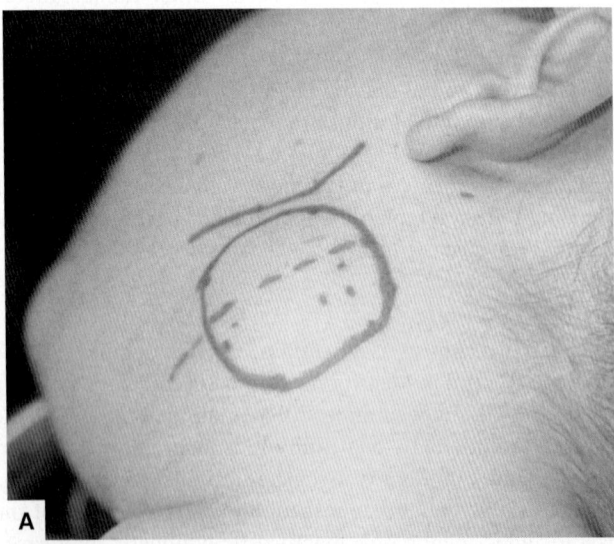

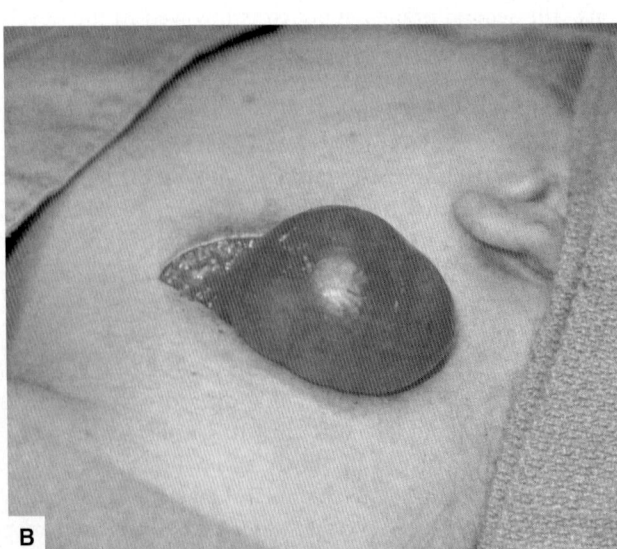

**FIGURE 15-4 A.** Child with a second branchial cleft cyst. **B.** The cyst is exposed at surgery.

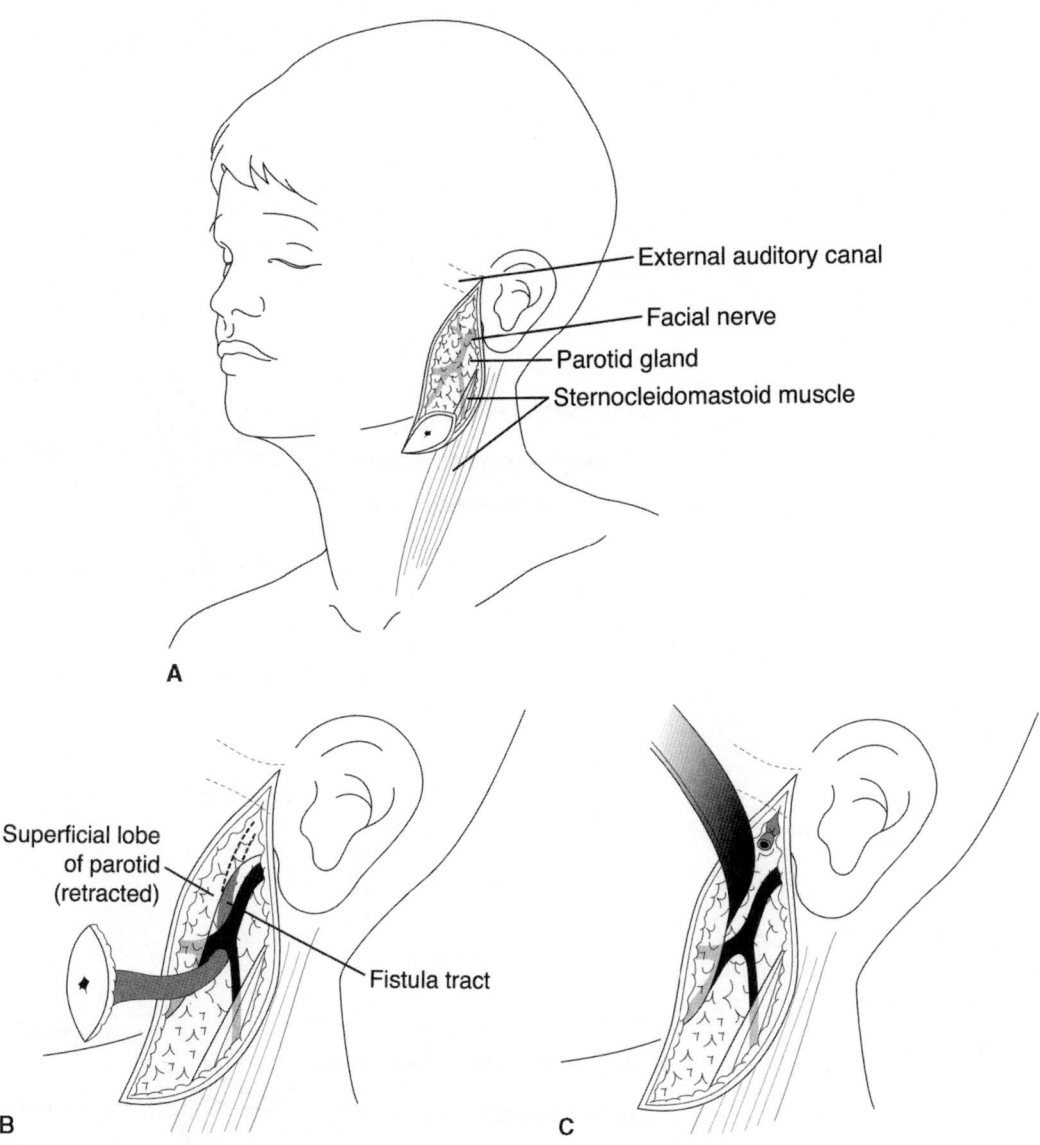

**FIGURE 15-5** Exposure of a first branchial cleft fistula. **A.** The fistula has been circumscribed with an elliptical incision carried superiorly just anterior to the ear. The superficial lobe of the parotid is identified. **B.** The superficial lobe of the parotid gland is reflected medially to expose the branches of the facial nerve and the fistula tract. **C.** The fistula is ligated as it enters the cartilage of the external auditory canal.

positioned supine with a transverse roll beneath the shoulders and the head turned slightly away from the side of the lesion. The incision should be carried from an ellipse around the external opening up over the mandible and in front of the ear, in order to expose the superficial lobe of the parotid and the nerve (Fig. 15-5A). A nerve stimulator is useful in identifying the facial nerve. The fistula tract can then be safely dissected away from the nerve (Fig. 15-5B). The tract is suture ligated and divided at its connection with the external auditory canal (Fig. 15-5C).

**Second Branchial Cleft Sinuses or Fistulae.** Excision of a second branchial cleft sinus or fistula is the most common operation performed in this group of branchial lesions. The procedure is carried out with a general anesthetic, and the patient is positioned as described for a first cleft fistula excision. When a skin opening is present, some surgeons place a fine lacrimal duct probe to help facilitate dissection;

this is a delicate maneuver, however, requiring care to avoid puncturing the tract wall. A transverse elliptical incision, in a skin crease if possible, is made around the external opening (Fig. 15-6A). If a cyst is present with no opening, a transverse incision is made. Sharp dissection of the tract and cyst, if present, is performed with fine scissors. To avoid injury to surrounding structures, the dissection remains right on the wall of the tract. After dissection is initiated, the course of the fistula can be determined by placing it on gentle traction and palpating more superiorly in the neck. In most cases, a transverse counter incision is made 3 to 4 cm above the first to safely and completely excise the tract (Fig. 15-6B). The dissection is carried deeper in the neck via the second incision up to the tonsillar fossa, where the tract is ligated with an absorbable suture and divided (Fig. 15-6B, *inset*). The incisions are irrigated with saline and suctioned dry. The platysma, subcutaneous tissue, and skin are closed in layers with absorbable sutures.

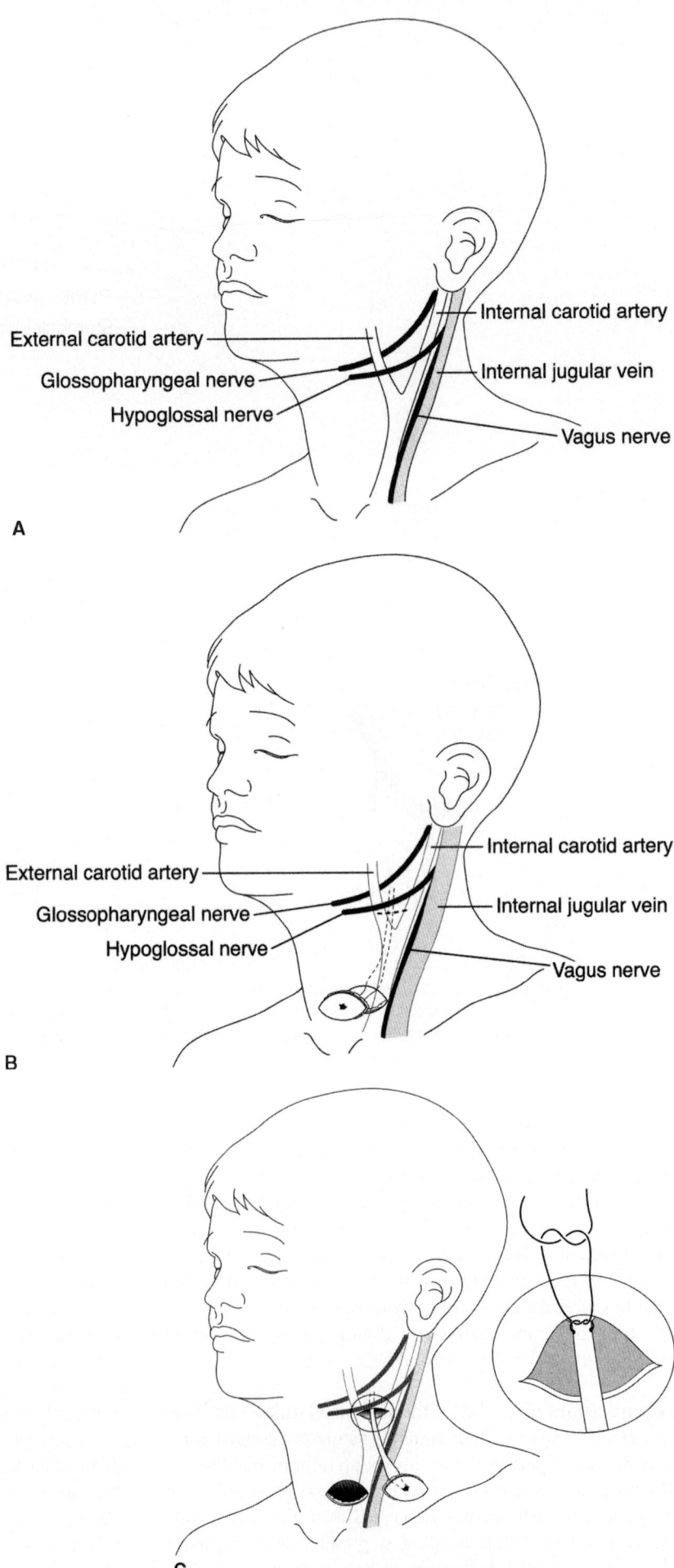

External carotid artery

Internal carotid artery

Glossopharyngeal nerve

Internal jugular vein

Hypoglossal nerve

Vagus nerve

A

External carotid artery

Internal carotid artery

Glossopharyngeal nerve

Internal jugular vein

Hypoglossal nerve

Vagus nerve

B

C

**FIGURE 15-6** **A.** Anatomy of the neck in relation to a second branchial cleft fistula. **B.** The fistula opening is circumscribed by an incision. The tract is carefully dissected away from surrounding neck structures by staying on the fistula wall. The tract courses cephalad between the external and internal carotid arteries. A counter incision (*dotted line*) may be required to complete the dissection. **C.** The tract is ligated as it enters the pharynx (*inset*) and the incisions are closed in layers with absorbable sutures.

**Third and Fourth Branchial Cleft Anomalies.** The principles of excision of third and fourth branchial cleft anomalies are the same as those for first and second branchial cleft anomalies.

## Complications and Recurrence

Morbidity is caused by injury to the nerves and vessels near the tract at the time of surgery, whereas recurrence is caused by incomplete excision. The likelihood of these complications increases when inflammation occurs adjacent to the anomaly prior to or at the time of surgical excision. In the absence of infection, recurrence is rare. However, when infection precedes excision, recurrence exceeds 20%. In light of these facts, excision is indicated at diagnosis. Although rare, squamous cell carcinoma has been reported with branchial cleft cysts, this complication does not appear until adulthood.

## Pyriform Sinuses and Cysts

Pyriform sinus lesions are rare lesions of the branchial apparatus and, as mentioned earlier, are thought to be third or fourth branchial derivatives. They usually appear as an abscess or mass in the left neck, specifically the thyroid lobe, and commonly communicate with the left pyriform sinus; as such, they may have an air–fluid level. In infants, a cyst may be asymptomatic or cause respiratory distress. Children may have a history of repeated upper respiratory infections and

sore throats, as well as tenderness of the thyroid, with or without suppuration. Like other branchial anomalies, pyriform sinuses and cysts are often infected at presentation. Acute suppurative thyroiditis as a result of an internal fistula is the most common presentation. The diagnosis is based on the finding of left lower neck pain and swelling, demonstrated by a barium swallow (Fig. 15-7A) or endoscopy of the pyriform sinus fistula, or findings at surgery. When active infection and inflammation are present, a barium swallow may fail to show a tract. Once the inflammation subsides, however, the tract can be readily demonstrated. Complete excision is necessary to prevent a recurrence, and anatomy requires excision of the involved portion of left thyroid lobe in the process of tracing the fistula to the pyriform sinus (Fig. 15-7B). During dissection of the pyriform sinus cyst via a transverse neck incision, placement of an endoscope or a guidewire into the pyriform sinus has been found to be helpful in delineating the extent of the cyst.

## Cervical Thymic Cysts

The thymus arises as a pair of primordia from the third branchial pouch. The paired glands normally descend from the pharynx and fuse as they reach the aortic arch during the eighth week of gestation. The development of a congenital thymic cyst is thought to be due to persistence of the thymopharyngeal duct, which normally is obliterated.

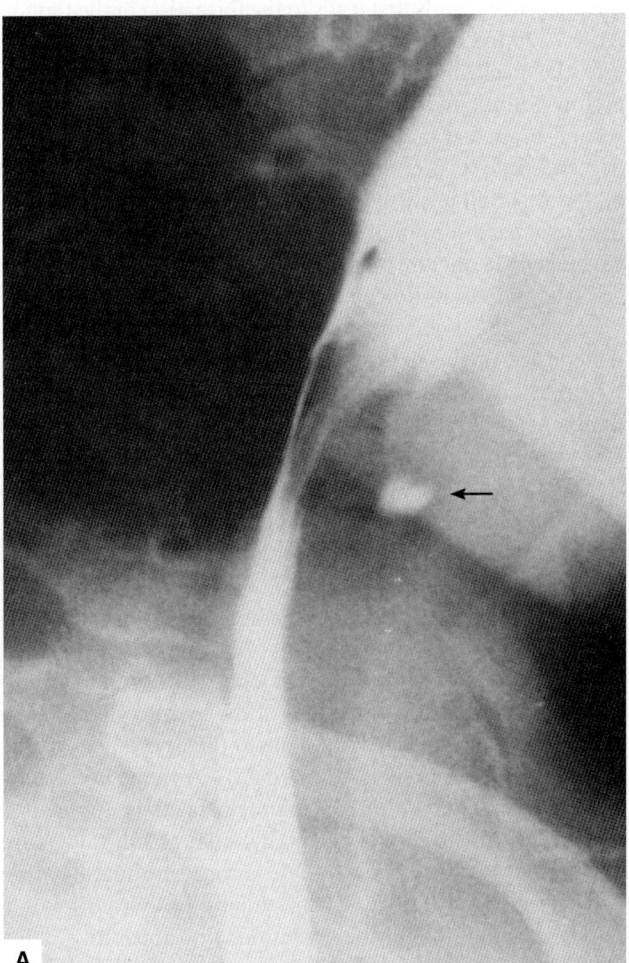

**A**

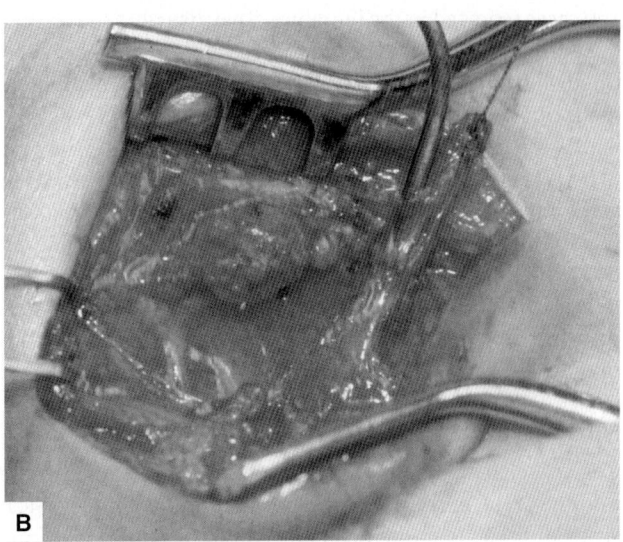

**B**

**FIGURE 15-7 A.** Contrast study demonstrating a left pyriform sinus tract (*arrow*). **B.** At operation, the pyriform sinus tract involves an abscessed left lobe of the thyroid. The sinus tract has a metal flexible probe inserted into the tract. A left thyroid lobectomy encompassing the sinus tract was required.

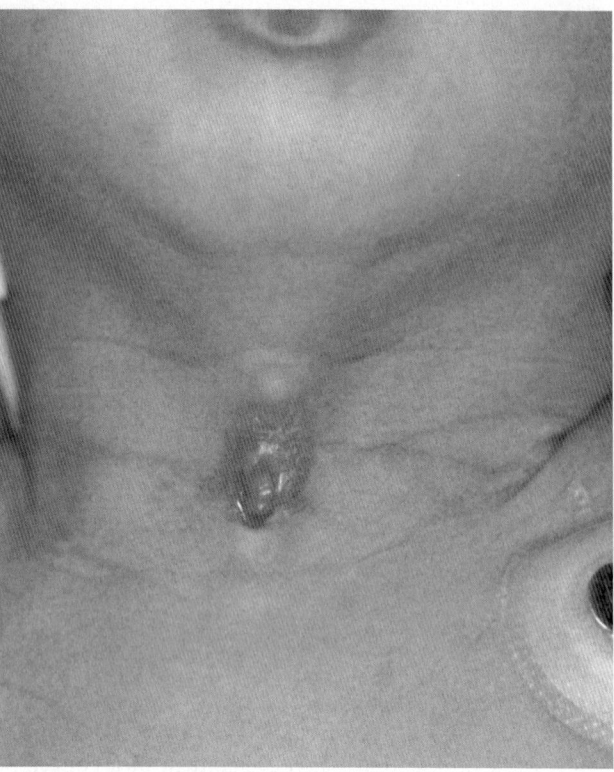

**FIGURE 15-8** Unrepaired midline cleft in an infant.

Cervical thymic cysts are extremely rare, with less than 100 cases reported in the literature. They usually arise as solitary, unilateral neck masses and are clinically difficult to distinguish from branchial cleft cysts or macrocystic lymphatic malformations. Excision is performed by sharp dissection, with a transverse skin crease incision over the cyst. The cystic mass is typically found adjacent to the carotid sheath. In some cases, the cyst extends into the mediastinum, requiring splitting of the upper sternum. The pathologic finding of the thymic tissue in the cyst wall confirms the diagnosis. Because of the common embryonic origin of the thymus and parathyroid, parathyroid tissue is frequently found within thymic cysts.

## Midline Cervical Clefts

Cervical clefts are a rare anomaly of newborns found in the midline of the neck. They appear as raw, protuberant, vertical strips of tissue that often contain skin tags, sinuses, and cartilaginous remnants (Fig. 15-8). These lesions are attributed to abnormal midline fusion of branchial arch pairs during the third and fourth weeks of gestation. Excision is indicated mainly for cosmesis, and therefore is usually delayed for several months. The cleft is excised via a series of Z-plasty incisions to prevent skin contractures that would form following a simple vertical elliptical incision.

## Thyroglossal Duct Cysts

Thyroglossal duct cysts are one of the most common lesions in the midline of the neck. Although they are embryonic in origin, they rarely manifest in neonates. They are more commonly seen in preschool-aged children (25%) and in children up to 10 years old (40%). Frequently, however, these lesions are not identified until after the age of 20 (33%).

### History

First described by Vater in 1723, the thyroglossal duct became known as the canal of His following studies by His in 1885 and 1891. In 1893, Schlange proposed that in addition to cyst resection, resection of the middle of the hyoid bone was also important. A manuscript authored by Sistrunk and published in the *Annals of Surgery* in 1920 earned him the distinction of being the first to fully understand surgical anatomy. Sistrunk was the first to realize that the duct traverses the hyoid bone up to the foramen cecum. He maintained that complete surgical excision of a thyroglossal duct cyst requires that the central portion of the hyoid bone and the duct, up to the base of the tongue, had to be resected in continuity with the cyst. This has remained the basic principle of the operation, which is known as the Sistrunk procedure.

### Embryology

Thyroglossal duct cysts are ectodermal remnants that may produce midline masses along the line of descent of the thyroid gland in the neck, from the base of the tongue to the pyramidal lobe of the thyroid gland. The embryogenesis of the thyroglossal duct is intimately associated with that of the thyroid gland, the hyoid bone, and the tongue. During the fourth to seventh weeks of gestation, the foramen cecum is the site of the development of the thyroid diverticulum; this structure arises caudal to the central tuberculum impar, which is one of the pharyngeal buds that leads to the formation of the tongue. As the tongue develops, the thyroid diverticulum descends into the neck, maintaining its connection to the foramen cecum. Simultaneously, the hyoid bone develops from the second branchial arch, and the thyroid gland develops and descends into its pretracheal position in the neck. As a result of these simultaneously occurring events, the thyroglossal duct may pass in front of, behind, or through the hyoid bone. Normally, the duct involutes and is resorbed once the thyroid gland completes its descent in the anterior neck.

Because the embryologic thyroglossal tract never reaches the surface of the neck, thyroglossal duct cysts never have a primary external opening. Secretion by epithelium-lined remnants of the duct can, however, lead to thyroglossal duct cyst formation anywhere along the course of the thyroglossal tract in the neck if the duct does not disappear. The stimulus for secretion by these remnants can occur at any time, thus accounting for the delayed appearance of these cysts in older children, adolescents, and adults.

Errors in thyroid descent or persistence of the thyroglossal duct can lead to the formation of lingual or other ectopic thyroid tissue, a pyramidal thyroid lobe, or a thyroglossal duct cyst. Complete failure of descent of the thyroid gland results in a lingual thyroid, which develops at the base of the tongue. In such instances, there is no thyroid tissue in the neck. Ectopic thyroid tissue within the thyroglossal duct remnant is reported in 20% to 45% of cases. Thyroid function studies are, however, not required unless there is concern about hypo- or hyperthyroidism. If a significant amount of thyroid tissue is removed at the time of the operation, a postoperative radionuclide scan should be obtained to make certain that sufficient residual thyroid tissue remains. Furthermore, for patients with large lingual thyroid gland and no normal thyroid tissue in the neck, clinical treatment should begin with the administration of thyroid hormone to decrease the size of the mass.

## Clinical Presentation and Evaluation

Thyroglossal cysts are typically found in the anterior midline of the neck at or immediately adjacent to the hyoid bone but may occasionally be suprasternal (7%) or sublingual (3%). They are characteristically smooth, soft, and nontender, and are generally apparent on physical examination. Because of the attachment of the thyroglossal duct cyst to the hyoid bone, a typically positioned mass moves with swallowing. Nevertheless, this condition can be difficult to evaluate in young children and may also occur with other lesions located near the hyoid bone. If the diagnosis is not apparent on physical examination because of atypical features or location of the mass, inflammation, or additional neck pathology, studies such as ultrasonography, computed tomography, and magnetic resonance imaging can be invaluable in differentiating possible lesions. The differential diagnosis includes ectopic thyroid tissue, thyroid neoplasm, dermoid cyst, sebaceous cyst, lipoma, and submental lymphadenitis. Owing to communication with the base of the tongue at the foramen cecum, thyroglossal cysts commonly become infected, and patients may report infection as the first manifestation. This infection may spontaneously drain or require surgical incision and drainage prior to excision.

## Treatment

A thyroglossal duct cyst is treated by complete excision of the cyst and its tract up to the base of the tongue and including the central portion of the hyoid bone (Sistrunk procedure). This technique has reduced the incidence of recurrence to less than 10% from the 25% recurrence rate for cystectomy alone. An operation should be performed as early as possible to avoid the morbidity of intervening infection. If infection does occur, a course of antibiotics should be administered and the operation deferred until the inflammatory process is fully resolved. In some cases, incision and drainage are indicated prior to cyst resection. Complete surgical excision during active infection is inadvisable because of both the difficulty of the operation when infection is present and the risk of injury to the surrounding structures, which results in a higher incidence of recurrence.

Although papillary adenocarcinoma in thyroglossal duct specimens is not seen in children, it is reported in up to 10% of patients undergoing the Sistrunk procedure in adulthood. This observation lends further support to the cited rationale for early and complete excision.

## Surgical Procedure

The operation is performed with a general anesthetic with the patient in a supine position and the neck extended (Fig. 15-9A-F). A 3- to 4-cm transverse curvilinear incision is marked in a skin crease overlying the cyst and taken down through the platysma muscle. The cyst is usually found just beneath this layer. Dissection of the cyst and the thyroglossal duct follows the principle of Sistrunk, removing the

midportion of the hyoid bone and the duct up to the base of the tongue. The cyst is dissected mostly by sharp dissection. Care is taken to avoid rupturing it during the procedure. When previous infection has occurred, a somewhat wider resection may be required to remove all portions of the cyst distorted by the inflammatory process. On dissection, a short duct is usually found in a cephaloposterior position. It is then traced to the area of the hyoid bone.

The hyoid bone is transected on either side of the duct, leaving a 1- to 1.5-cm defect in the hyoid (Fig. 15-9D). When the cyst is suprasternal, a counterincision overlying the hyoid bone may be necessary. The strap muscles firmly attached to the hyoid are easily dissected with electrocautery. The duct is identified on the undersurface of the hyoid and is dissected up to the base of the tongue, where it is ligated with an absorbable suture and divided. It is sometimes helpful to place a finger at the base of the tongue, pushing ventrally to facilitate ligation of the duct at the foramen cecum (Fig. 15-9G and H). If necessary, bleeding from the cut surfaces of the hyoid is controlled with bone wax. No attempt is made to approximate the hyoid in the midline. Following an extensive dissection, a drain is occasionally necessary. The incision is closed in layers with absorbable sutures.

## Complications and Recurrence

An uncommon but potentially dangerous postoperative complication is wound hemorrhage with resultant airway compression. Avoiding this situation requires careful hemostasis rather than routine drainage. Because of anatomic distortion or variability in neck anatomy, mistaking thyroid cartilage for the hyoid bone has been reported; this may result in severe injuries to the larynx. Wound infections are infrequent and respond to antibiotic therapy.

The recurrence rate following the primary resection of a previously uninfected thyroglossal duct cyst is 5%, and recurrence generally happens within 1 year of the procedure. It is usually attributed to incomplete excision of part of the cyst or its tract but can, however, be caused by distortion of the tissues due to inflammation or inadequate resection of the hyoid bone or the central stalk leading to the foramen cecum. Additionally, the presence of multiple tracts or rupture of the cyst at the time of excision can lead to recurrent disease.

Recurrence typically manifests with infection in the upper neck. A course of antibiotics is administered until the inflammation has resolved, and a second operation is then performed through the same incision. Reexcision of persistent cysts is associated with recurrence rates as high as 25% to 35%.

## Preauricular Sinuses, Pits, and Cysts

### Embryology

Although preauricular sinuses, pits, and cysts are sometimes classified with first branchial cleft anomalies, they are not of true branchial cleft origin. Rather, they represent ectodermal inclusions related to aberrant development of the auditory tubercles. Sinuses and pits are thought to occur when the ectoderm is enfolded during the development and merging of the 6 hillocks of the ear. The sinuses are often short and end

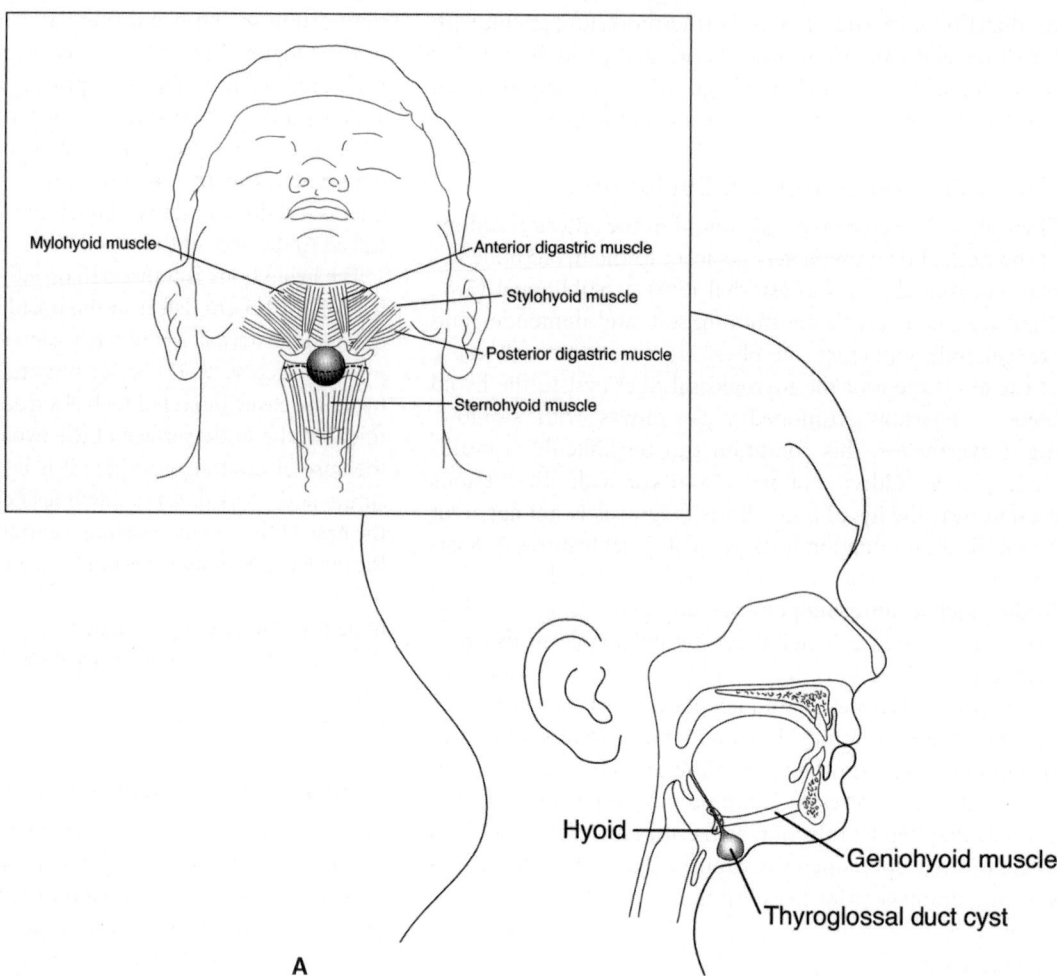

A

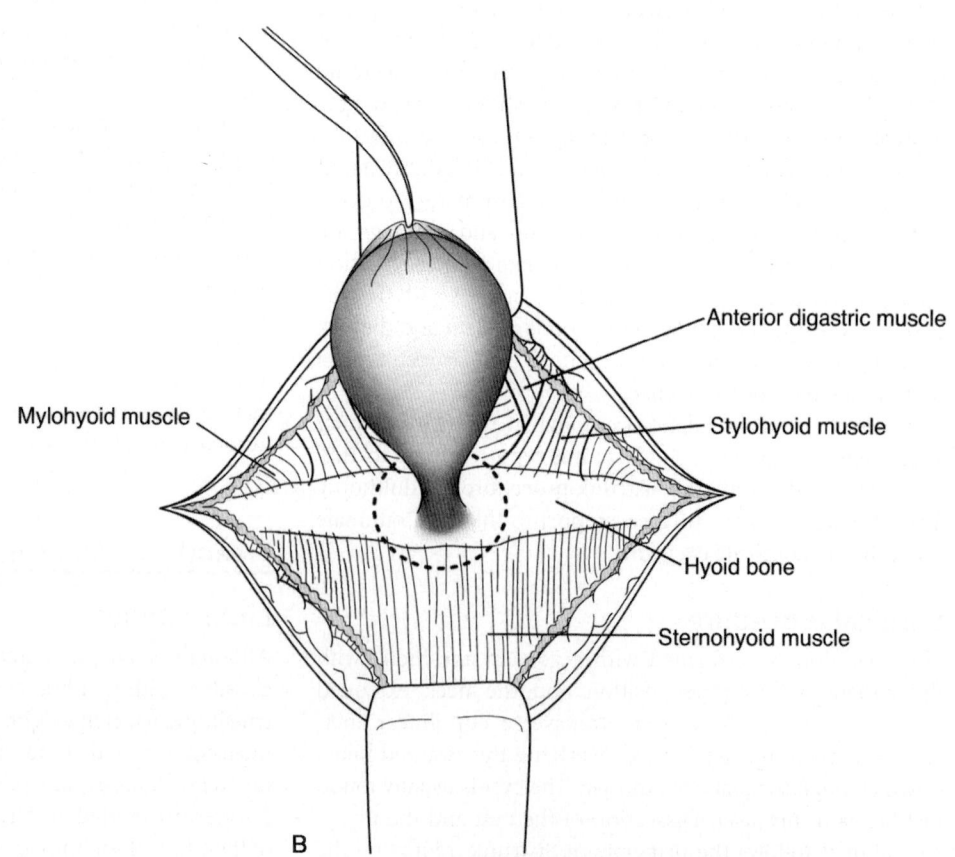

B

**FIGURE 15-9** **A.** Anterior neck anatomy and a thyroglossal duct cyst extending through the hyoid bone. Lateral view and anterior frontal view (*inset*). The incision is represented by the *dotted line*. **B.** The platysma has been opened and the cyst dissected free, exposing the hyoid and deep anterior cervical muscles. The *dotted line* marks the area that will be incised with electrocautery. **C.** The hyoid bone is transected on both sides of the thyroglossal duct. **D.** The thyroglossal duct is then dissected to the foramen caecum. **E.** The appearance of a typical midline thyroglossal duct cyst in an 8-year-old male. **F.** At operation, the cyst and the resected central hyoid bone as well as the remaining tract attached to the base of the tongue can be readily seen. **G.** Pushing the base of the tongue anteriorly with a finger placed in the mouth of the patient facilitates visualization, dissection, and ligation of the tract. **H.** Once the thyroglossal duct cyst has been removed, the platysma, subcutaneous tissue, and skin are closed in layers using absorbable sutures.

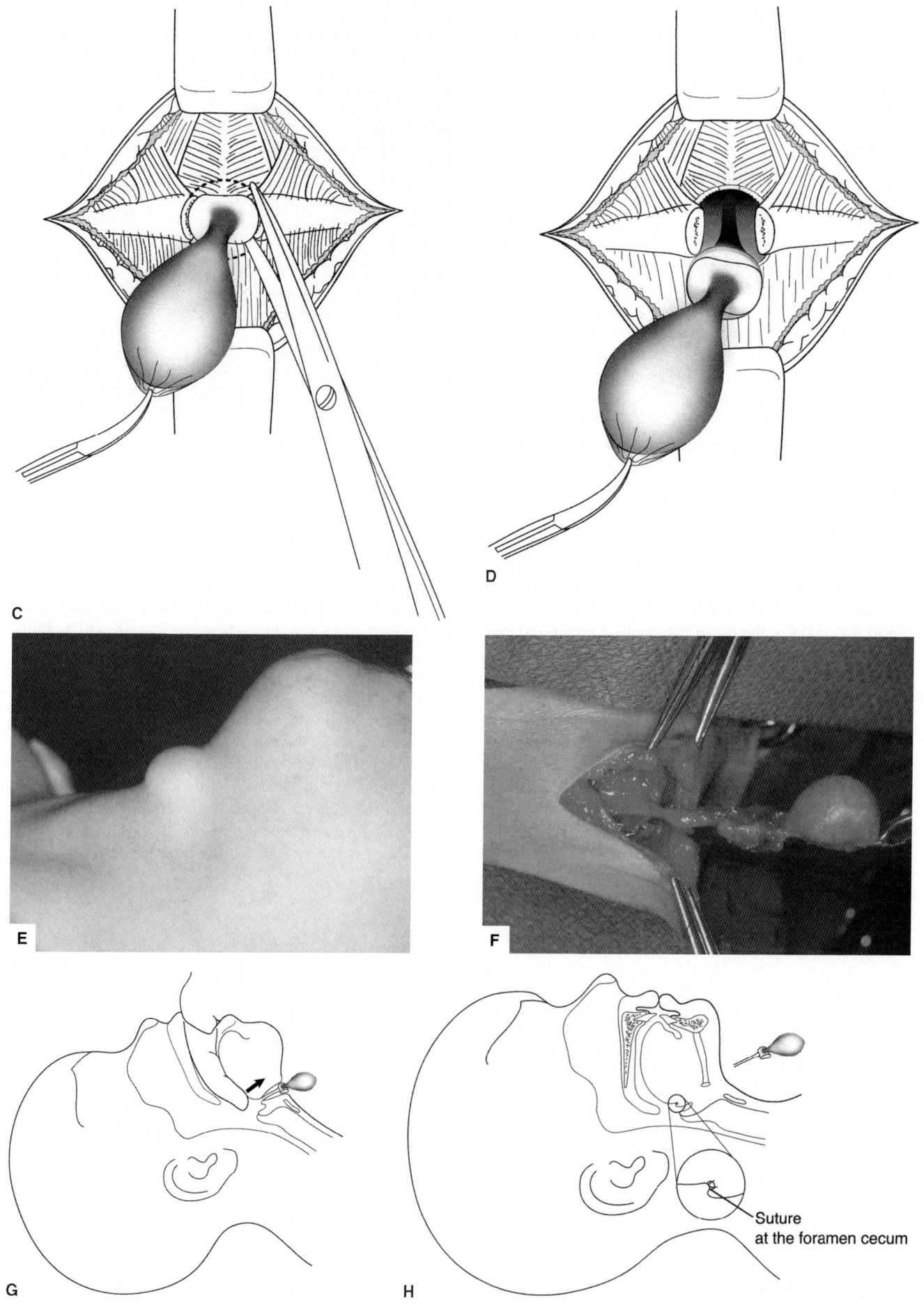

C

D

E

F

G

H                                                                                  Suture
                                                                                   at the foramen cecum

**FIGURE 15-9** *(Continued)*     **227**

blindly. They occasionally connect internally to the external auditory canal. The sinus tracts extend from the skin through the subcutaneous tissue close to the superficial temporal artery and characteristically terminate in the cartilage of the external auditory canal.

## Incidence

Preauricular anomalies are much more common than first branchial cleft anomalies, with an incidence ranging from 15.5 to 43.7 per 10,000 births in various populations. These anomalies more commonly appear in people of Asian and African-American descent and are slightly more common in females than in males (3:2). Preauricular sinuses may be associated with other congenital anomalies such as deafness. They also have an increased incidence of concomitant renal anomalies (eg, branchio-oto-renal [BOR] syndrome).

Preauricular sinuses can be either inherited or sporadic. When inherited, these lesions show an incomplete autosomal dominant pattern with reduced penetrance and variable expression. The appearance of bilateral preauricular sinuses is associated with an increased likelihood of being inherited.

## Clinical Aspects

Most preauricular cysts are bilateral. When unilateral, they more commonly arise on the right side. These anomalies are commonly observed at birth, and are typically located superior to the tragus of the ear in the cymba conchae and subcutaneous tissue superficial to the parotid fascia (Fig. 15-10). The tract of sinuses and cysts is lined with stratified squamous epithelium.

Most sinuses and cysts are asymptomatic; however, parents often report sebum intermittently draining from the sinuses. The sinuses extend down to the temporalis fascia and may be juxtaposed to the perichondrium of the helix. Occasionally, these patients develop infections that result in an abscess. In this setting, a thorough examination will reveal a preauricular lesion as opposed to a first branchial anomaly.

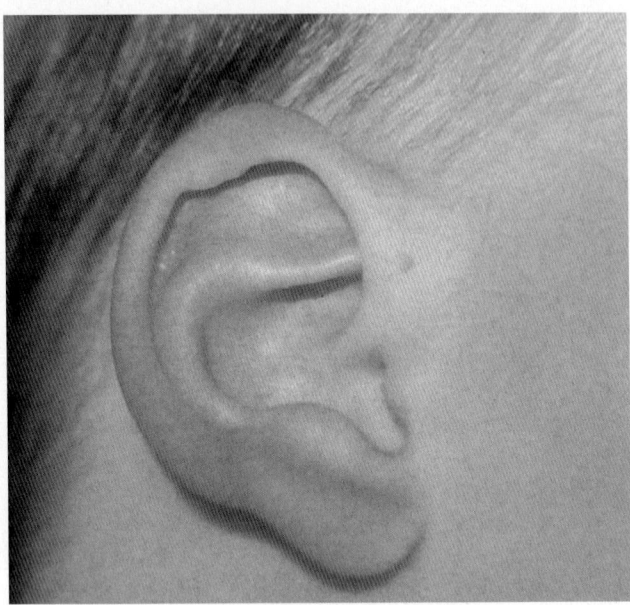

**FIGURE 15-10** A preauricular sinus.

## Treatment

Excision is recommended for lesions that form a palpable mass or drain sebaceous material because they are the most likely to become infected (Fig. 15-11). Complete surgical excision of the subcutaneous cyst and sinus tract down to the level including the cartilage of the external auditory canal is the treatment of choice for the uninfected draining sinus. Care should be taken to avoid rupture of the sinus and to perform a complete excision. If infection is present, excision should be delayed because it makes dissection more difficult and increases the risk of incomplete excision and hence recurrence. Infection, which is most commonly staphylococcal, should be treated with antibiotics and warm soaks to encourage drainage and control surrounding inflammation. In some patients, needle aspiration or incision and drainage is required to control the infection. Once the infection

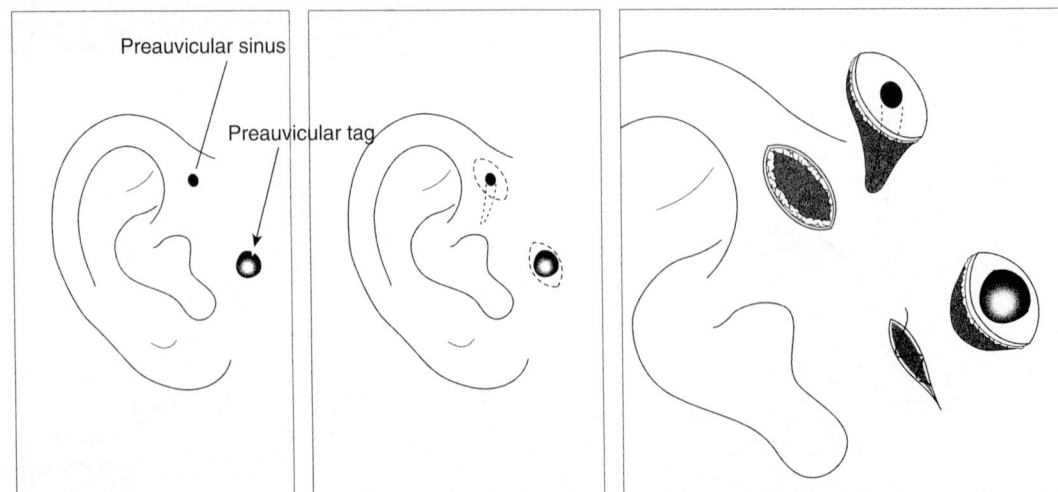

**FIGURE 15-11** Operative technique used to excise a preauricular sinus or skin tag. An elliptical incision is placed around the sinus and dissection of the skin and a block of subcutaneous tissue is carried to the temporalis muscle fascia or to the perichondrium of the helix.

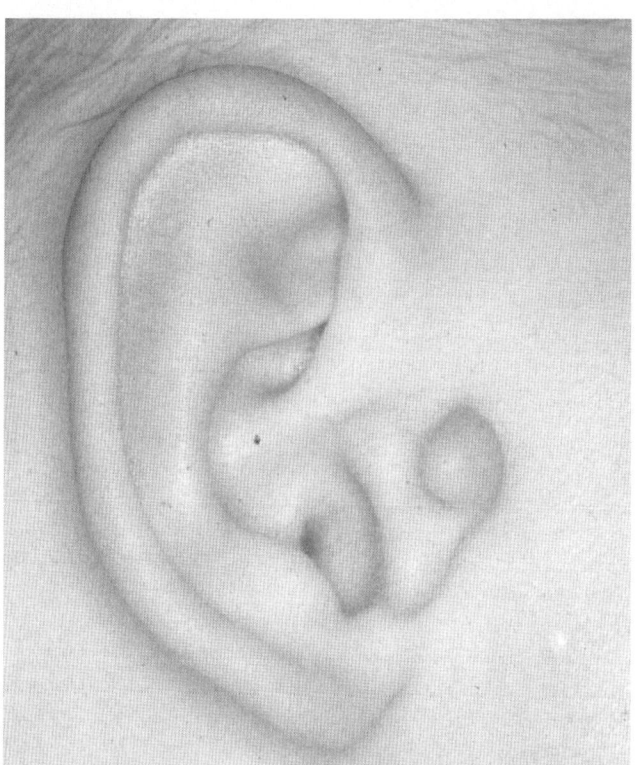

**FIGURE 15-12** Photograph of a preauricular skin tag with a cartilaginous component at its base.

is completely resolved, definitive excision is performed. When the cyst or sinus has only simple single tract involvement, recurrence is uncommon. By contrast, when the sinus has multiple branches, recurrence is as high as 42%. Because postoperative wound infection is common, all patients should undergo a course of antibiotics.

## Skin Tags

Preauricular skin tags (Fig. 15-12) are common embryological remnants that may include cartilage and are located just medial to the external ear canal. These lesions reflect minor incomplete or aberrant migration of the ear anlage. Most children with these lesions are otherwise normal, and surgical excision is performed primarily because of aesthetic concerns (Fig. 15-11). Children with preauricular tags that occur in conjunction with other more complex ear malformations frequently have significant hearing impairment.

## Dermoid and Epidermoid Cysts

### Embryology

Dermoid cysts are derived from ectodermal elements that were either buried beneath the skin and superficial muscles (eg, the platysma and orbicularis oculi) or failed to separate from the neural tube. They form along the lines of embryonic fusion in the anterior neck and are differentiated from superficial epidermoid cysts histologically by the accessory glandular structures they possess, including sebaceous glands, hair follicles, connective tissues, and papillae. Both dermoid and epidermoid cysts contain sebaceous material within the cyst cavity.

## Pathology

Dermoid and epidermoid cysts are generally unilocular and are seen at birth. They gradually expand with age because of secretions from the entrapped glands and the accumulation of epithelial material.

The lining of a dermoid cyst is thicker than that of an epidermoid cyst and may contain dystrophic calcification. The lipid material in dermoids is from the sebaceous glands. This material resembles the texture of cheese and contains cholesterol crystals in addition to glandular secretions.

The dermoid cavity is lined with a thick stratified squamous keratinized epithelium surrounded by dermal appendages such as hair follicles and sebaceous, eccrine, and apocrine glands.

## Clinical Presentation

Dermoid cysts are most commonly found along the supraorbital palpebral ridge, and commonly appear as a swelling in the corner of the eyebrow (Fig. 15-13). Although they are attached to the underlying bony periosteum, they are usually minimally mobile and nontender. In this setting, most patients do not require preoperative imaging. However, when lesions on other parts of the face or skull are immobile, patients should undergo a skull radiograph to assess whether there is bony defect in the skull (Fig. 15-14). Midline dermoid cysts of the skull, including the nasal bridge, may occasionally penetrate the calvarium, forming a dumbbell-shaped mass with dermoid elements on either side of the bone (Fig. 15-15). Patients with midline lesions should undergo a computed tomography scan or a magnetic resonance imaging scan to ensure that there is no intracranial extension.

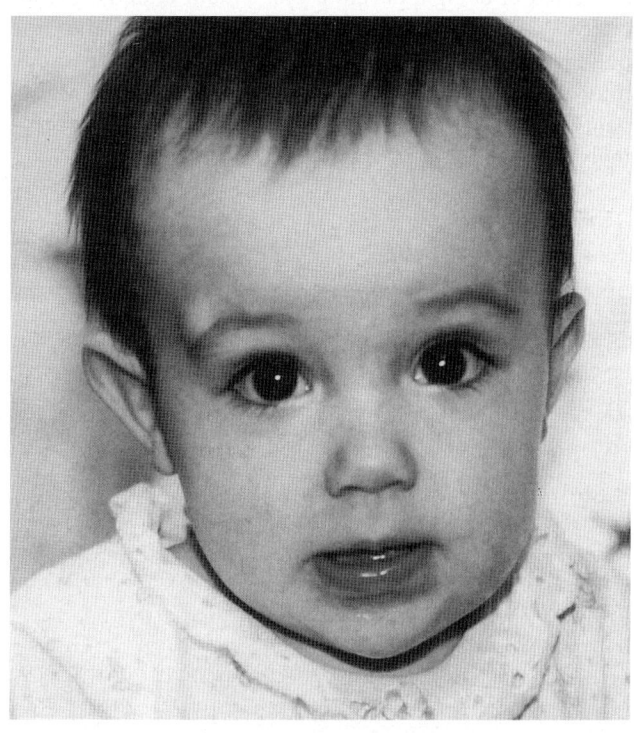

**FIGURE 15-13** Right lateral eyebrow soft tissue nodule. This is the classic location for an angular dermoid cyst.

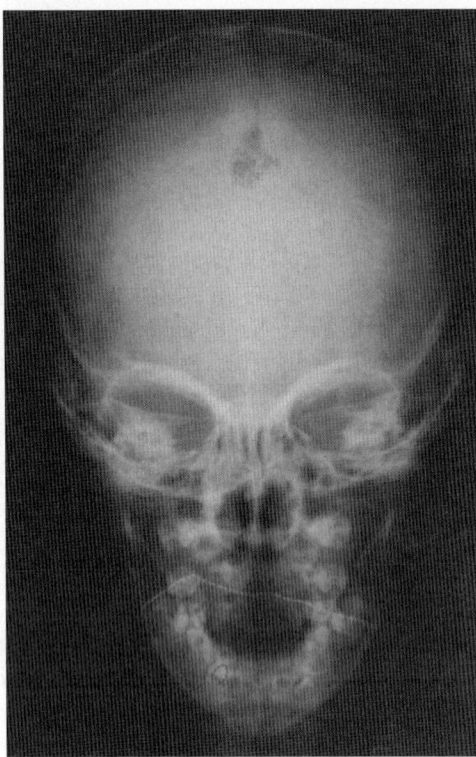

**FIGURE 15-14** Skull radiograph depicting a cranial bone defect beneath a scalp soft-tissue nodule.

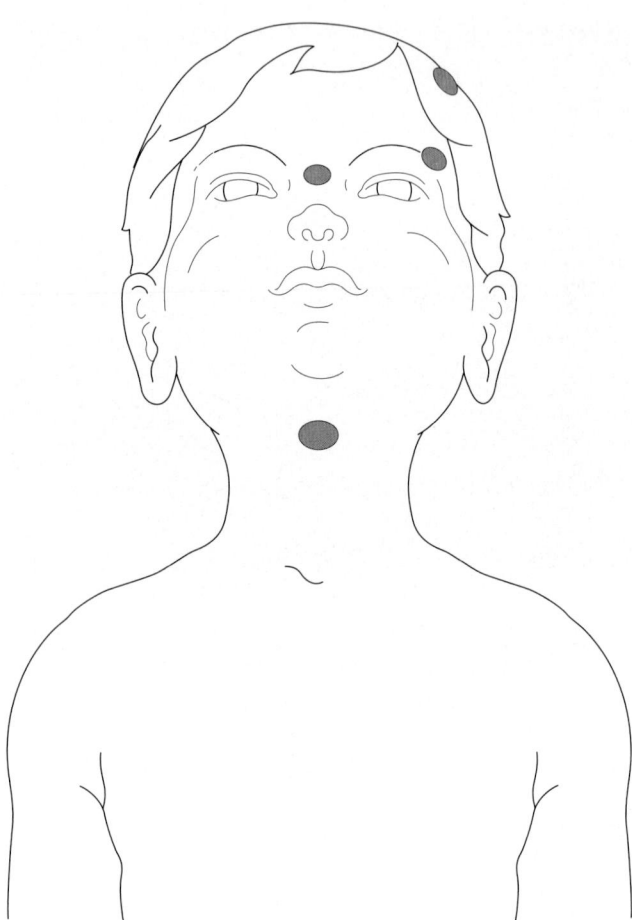

**FIGURE 15-16** Diagram of the typical locations for dermoid cysts of the head and neck: the extended angular dermoid, the internal angular (nasal bridge) dermoid, and the midline neck dermoid.

Dermoid cysts can also be found in the midline of the neck overlying the hyoid bone and, as such, are frequently confused with midline thyroglossal duct cysts (Fig. 15-16). They are, however, more superficial and lack connections to the hyoid bone and the tongue. Any midline scalp lesion suspected of being a dermoid cyst should undergo preoperative evaluation with magnetic resonance imaging to rule out intracranial extension. Expanding lesions can erode into adjacent bone; however, this rarely occurs. Malignant degeneration of dermoids is also possible but exceedingly rare.

## Treatment

Complete surgical excision is the treatment of choice for all dermoid and epidermoid cysts; this confirms the diagnosis, prevents infection, and ensures aesthetic outcomes. If dermoid cysts are seen during the neonatal period, the operation can be postponed until the child is 6 to 12 months old. Complete removal of the capsule is of utmost importance in decreasing the risk of recurrence. Aspirating or opening these cysts may result in spillage of cyst contents, which in turn may lead to infection or recurrence.

Excision should be performed with a general anesthetic and with meticulous technique. Attention should be paid to the important nerves such as the branches of the facial nerves supplying the forehead and the supraorbital nerves. Injury to the supraorbital branches of facial nerve can be avoided if the incision is made at the hairline of the eyebrow with minimal lateral and medial dissection, staying on the cyst wall. The cyst is usually deep into the muscles and may be adherent to the periosteum. When there is neurapraxia or stretching of the superior branch of the facial nerve, there may be a postoperative inability to elevate the eyebrow. This inability diminishes over several months. Transection or the use of electrocautery can, however, result in permanent injury to the nerves.

Rarely, the cyst may extend into the orbit. In this setting, care should be taken not to injure the eye and the

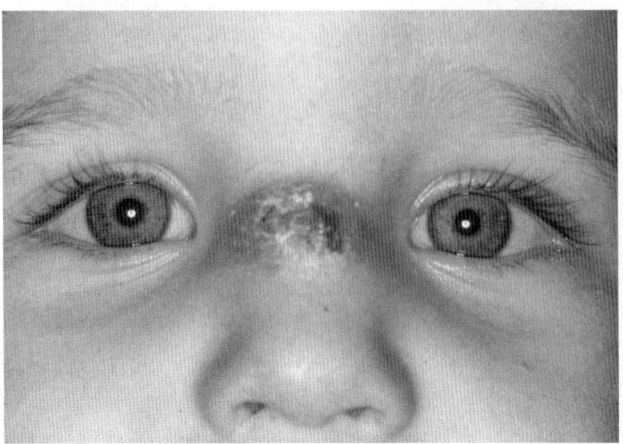

**FIGURE 15-15** A midline nasal bridge dermoid cyst that is connected to an intracranial component through the cribriform plate.

surrounding muscles and nerves. A midline cyst should be approached with caution, and preparations made for a possible craniotomy.

## ACQUIRED LESIONS

### Torticollis

#### History

The term *torticollis* is derived from the Latin *tortus*, meaning twisted, and *collum*, meaning neck. Interestingly, this deformity is said to have affected Alexander the Great (third century BC). Although Antyllus may have performed tenotomies in the fourth century, the sternocleidomastoid was not divided in the treatment of torticollis until 1641. This procedure took place in Amsterdam and is credited to Minnius. Heusinger first described a sternocleidomastoid tumor in 1826.

#### Pathophysiology

Although torticollis in infants can be caused by a number of conditions (eg, cervical hemivertebrae, adenitis, fasciitis, and an ocular muscle imbalance), the most common cause seen in pediatric surgical practice is fibrosis and shortening of the sternocleidomastoid muscle, which pulls the head and neck to the side of the lesion. Pathologically, the basic abnormality is due to the deposition of collagen and fibroblasts around individual atrophied muscle fibers. The severity and distribution of fibrosis differ widely among patients, and in rare cases (2%-8%), fibrosis occurs bilaterally. The maturity of the fibrous tissue in neonates suggests that the condition begins during fetal life and may be related to abnormal fetal positioning. Support for this hypothesis comes from the association of torticollis with congenital dislocation of the hip and tibial torsion. Also, the reported incidence of breech deliveries is about 20% to 30%, which is much higher than the normal incidence. However, because a history of obstetrical difficulties is present in close to two thirds of patients, the etiology of torticollis remains controversial.

#### Diagnostic Principles

The patient's medical history and a physical examination usually confirm the diagnosis of sternocleidomastoid torticollis. The condition first becomes apparent between 2 and 8 weeks of age, with infants demonstrating the characteristic posture of the face and chin tilted away from the affected side and the head tilted toward the ipsilateral shoulder. A 1- to 3-cm fibrotic mass within the middle or lower third of the sternocleidomastoid muscle is also commonly, but not always, seen. Without appropriate intervention, marked facial and cranial asymmetry usually develop by 6 months of age. Although rarely necessary, ultrasonography may be useful in distinguishing torticollis from other lesions. For patients older than 6 months of age or those with advanced lesions, an evaluation of potential craniofacial asymmetry (eg, plagiocephaly or facial hemihypoplasia) should be carried out either by standardized photography with the head in a cephalostat or by computerized tomography. Older children with torticollis should be evaluated for cervical rotary subluxation,

ocular torticollis, and midbrain lesions. In rare circumstances, pathologic gastroesophageal reflux that resolves with effective antireflux therapy may accompany torticollis (Sandifer syndrome).

#### Treatment

The natural history of untreated torticollis is complete resolution in 50% to 70% of cases by 6 months of age. In about 10% of cases, the lesion and sternomastoid shortening persist beyond 12 months. Because the outcome is difficult to predict, we advocate that parents perform range-of-motion and stretching exercises under the guidance of a physiotherapist or physician. Active exercises may involve having the child look toward a toy or some other object away from the involved side. Passive rotation of the neck toward the lesion with flexion away from the lesion may help to stretch the muscle and reduce the size of the mass. These exercises should be integrated into play activities and performed several times a day. For more advanced lesions or for lesions that do not respond to nonoperative treatment, surgery is indicated. The development of facial hemihypoplasia is the major criterion for surgical intervention (Fig. 15-17).

#### Surgical Procedure

After the administration of a general anesthetic, the patient is placed in a supine position with a roll beneath the shoulders. The neck is extended and the head is turned slightly away from the lesion. The field is draped to allow rotation of the head during the procedure. A transverse skin-crease curvilinear incision over the width of the affected

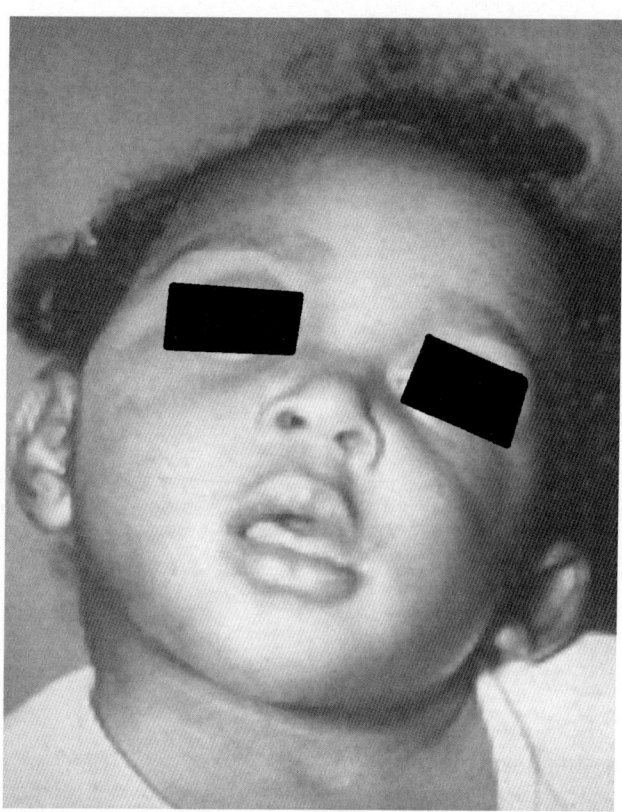

**FIGURE 15-17** Torticollis in a 20-month-old child with hemifacial distortion and plagiocephaly.

sternocleidomastoid muscle is made 3 to 4 cm above the clavicle. The dissection is taken down through the platysma to the sternocleidomastoid muscle. The external jugular vein is doubly ligated and divided if necessary. The muscle is dissected circumferentially at the level of the convergence of the sternal and clavicular heads, which should be 1 to 1.5 cm caudad to the spinal accessory nerve (Fig. 15-18A and B). The muscle is divided at this level with electrocautery. The divided ends of the muscle are then elevated from the underlying carotid sheath, taking care to avoid injury to the spinal accessory nerve. While the head is turned from side to side, the depth of the wound is palpated to identify any tight bands. Occasionally, the deep cervical fascia lateral to the sternocleidomastoid muscle requires release. In severe cases, the fascia around the omohyoid muscle and the carotid sheath requires release. A layered closure is performed with absorbable sutures.

An alternative technique that has been used successfully entails dividing the involved sternocleidomastoid muscle in a stepwise manner and reattaching the most caudal superior and most cephalic inferior end of this muscle together (Fig. 15-18C and D). Theoretically, this leaves the child with an elongated sternocleidomastoid muscle that is less likely to contract in the cephalic-caudal dimension.

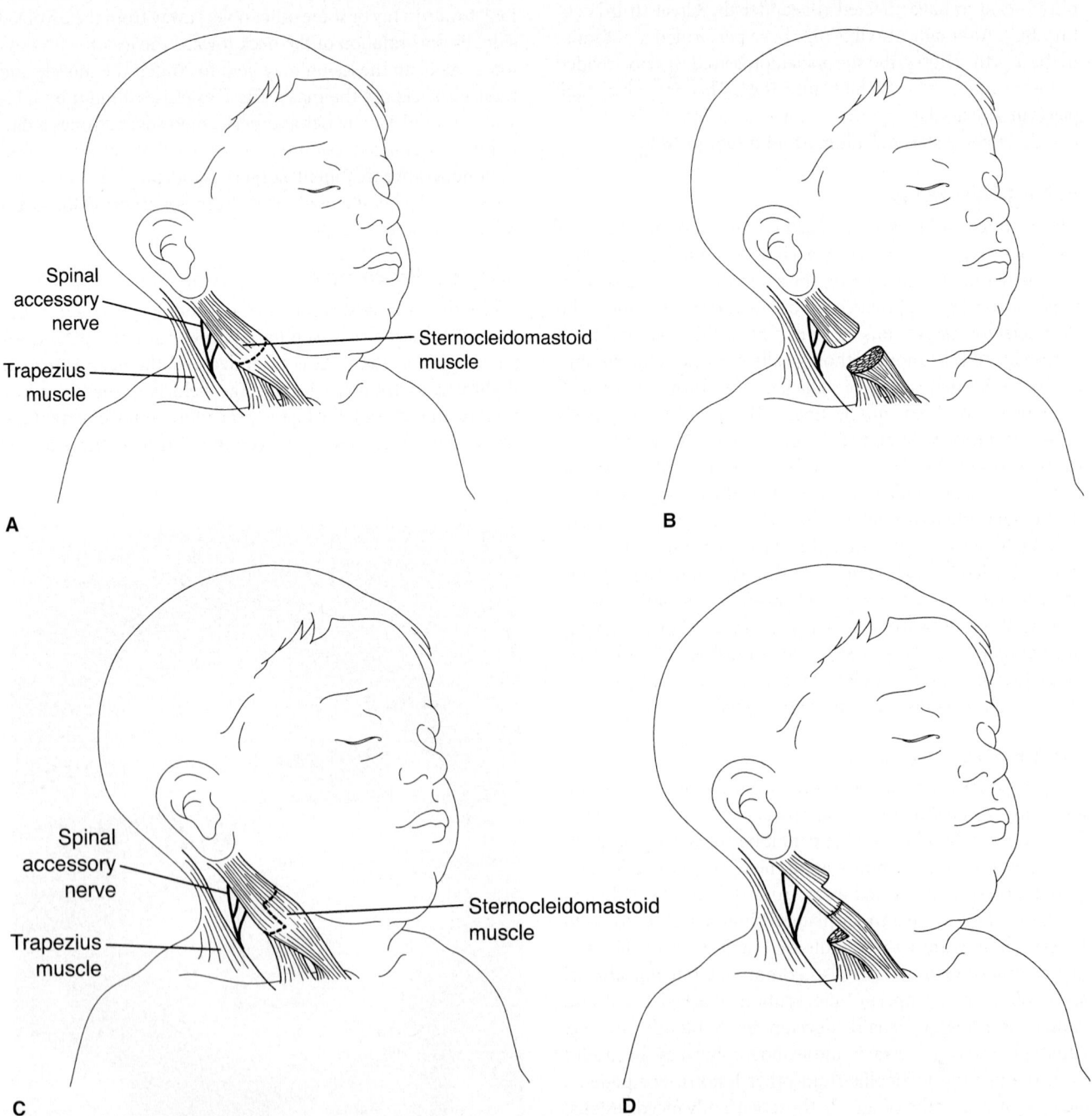

**FIGURE 15-18** Surgical treatment of torticollis. **A.** The transverse cervical incision is extended through the platysma. **B.** The sternocleidomastoid muscle is then divided in the area of fibrosis cephalad to the sternal and clavicular heads but caudal to the spinal accessory nerve. This technique generally provides an excellent release, and the 2 cut ends of the muscle retract. **C.** An alternative procedure is to lengthen the sternocleidomastoid muscle using a stair-step incision in the muscle. **D.** The long ends of the sternocleidomastoid muscle are approximated together. This procedure recreates the normal anterior cervical contour.

Postoperatively, the patient is placed in a supine 30° position with the head up and without a pillow for 48 hours. Physical therapy is then started, with a goal of achieving full range of motion within 7 to 10 days after surgery. Over the subsequent 3 to 6 months, older children must be retrained in front of a mirror to eliminate their previous postural habits. The resolution of facial and cranial asymmetry is gradual and may take several months or even years to occur.

## Outcomes and Complications

Although the vast majority of patients can be treated nonoperatively, close follow-up is necessary to ensure a full range of motion of the neck and resolution of the sternocleidomastoid fibrosis or mass. When surgery is required, the best results are obtained if it is performed between the first and second year of life. It is generally successful only when followed up with adequate postoperative physical therapy. The reported recurrence rate following surgery is less than 3%.

A wound hematoma is the most common surgical complication. The muscle may reunite or become attached to fascia as the wound heals, and the need for a second operation has been reported.

## Salivary Gland Lesions

The salivary glands comprise many minor glands found throughout the oral cavity, pharynx, and paranasal sinuses and 3 major glands—the parotid, submandibular (submaxillary), and sublingual. In the pediatric population the parotid is the most frequently involved salivary gland, whereas in adults the submandibular and minor salivary glands are more often involved. Submandibular and minor salivary gland lesions are also more likely to be malignant than parotid neoplasms.

Clinically, salivary gland tumors fall into 3 histologic groups: benign, low-grade malignant tumors, and high-grade malignant tumors (Table 15-1). Low-grade malignancies are associated with a 15% risk of recurrence and a low mortality rate, while high-grade malignancies have a 50% risk of recurrence and a high mortality rate.

## Benign Lesions

The most common benign neoplasms affecting the major salivary glands in children are vascular lesions such as hemangiomas, hemangioendotheliomas, and lymphatic malformations (Chapter 75). Pleomorphic adenoma (mixed tumor) is the most common benign epithelial tumor; all other benign lesions are rare. This tumor usually arises in the lateral portion of the parotid gland, grows slowly, and is painless; it peaks at ages 10 to 13. The mass is usually less than 3 cm in diameter and is firm and freely mobile. The high rate of local recurrence of this tumor is problematic, and is often seen following enucleation. Surgical treatment consists of a superficial or total parotidectomy that includes a margin of normal tissue in all directions around the tumor, with dissection and preservation of the facial nerve. (This procedure is described later in the chapter.)

Other benign epithelial lesions such as Warthin tumors and cystadenomas are treated similarly. Because patients with Warthin tumors may develop bilateral disease, they must be followed to observe the contralateral gland.

| TABLE 15-1 | Salivary Gland Lesions in Children | |
|---|---|---|
| | **Malignant** | |
| **Benign** | **Low-grade** | **High-grade** |
| Hemangioma | Mucoepidermoid carcinoma | Undifferentiated carcinoma |
| Lymphatic malformation | Acinous cell carcinoma | Undifferentiated sarcoma |
| Hemangioendothelioma | | Carcinoma from mixed tumor |
| Pleomorphic adenoma (mixed tumor) | | Adenocarcinoma |
| Cystadenoma | | Adenoid cystic carcinoma |
| Warthin tumor | | Squamous cell carcinoma |
| Lymphoepithelial tumor | | Mesenchymal sarcoma |
| | | Rhabdomyosarcoma |
| | | Lymphoma |
| | | Malignant epithelial tumor |

## Low-Grade Malignancies

Two low-grade malignant neoplasms occasionally appear in children: mucoepidermoid carcinomas and acinous cell carcinomas (acinic cell carcinomas). In most cases, both of these lesions have a benign course. However, because they occasionally exhibit malignant behavior, it is inappropriate to classify them either as completely benign or completely malignant. Both lesions tend to be clinically similar to a mixed tumor, being firm, mobile, slow growing, and painless. The parotid (most commonly) and submandibular glands are the major sites.

## High-Grade Malignancies

Although there are a large number of cell types in this group (Table 15-1), they are all extremely rare. High-grade malignancies tend to occur at a younger age (average 5.3 years) than benign and low-grade tumors (average 9.7 and 9.5 years, respectively). Also, their rate of growth and the severity of local symptoms are generally more pronounced than in benign and low-grade malignant tumors. Most of these lesions show aggressive biologic behavior. The classic physical findings of malignant parotid tumors are facial nerve paralysis and fixation. In the submandibular gland, fixation and involvement of the lingual, hypoglossal, or marginal mandibular branch of the facial nerve indicate advanced disease.

## Diagnosis and Surgical Treatment

Ultrasonography can be helpful in evaluating infants with hemangiomas, hemangioendotheliomas, and lymphatic malformations. Computed tomography and magnetic resonance imaging enhance our ability to differentiate various salivary gland lesions and determine the extent of nodal and other involvement. For some nonvascular tumors, fine-needle aspiration cytology may also be useful in helping to establish a preoperative diagnosis and in treatment planning. Depending on the clinical situation, an excisional biopsy or a glandectomy is preferable to reduce the risk of recurrence. When a complete excision is not feasible, an incisional biopsy can establish the diagnosis and facilitate the development of postoperative treatment planning. Minor salivary gland lesions require complete excision.

### Parotidectomy

In cases of parotid involvement, treatment generally consists of either a superficial lobectomy or a total parotidectomy with sparing of the facial nerve unless it is invaded by tumor. There does not appear to be a role for routinely performing modified neck dissection in children with low-grade lesions, but it may be beneficial for those with high-grade lesions.

A parotidectomy is performed without muscle relaxants and with the nerve stimulator available. The patient is placed in a supine position with the neck extended and the head turned away from the lesion. A sterile transparent adhesive drape is useful in order to view the entire distribution of the facial nerve. This nerve runs between the 2 anatomic lobes of the parotid gland and should be preserved unless involved by the tumor. The incision is carried from in front of the ear to just below the angle of the mandible. To improve exposure, it is occasionally extended behind the ear (Fig. 15-19A). The digastric muscle is exposed, and the main trunk of the facial nerve is identified between the digastric muscle and the external auditory canal. When the tumor involves the superficial lobe, that portion of the parotid is carefully resected, preserving the underlying branches of the facial nerve (Fig. 15-19B and C). If the tumor is in the deep lobe, the facial nerve branches are carefully retracted and the underlying lobe is resected (Fig. 15-19D and E). When a malignant tumor encases the nerve or a major branch, sacrifice of the nerve with immediate sural nerve grafting is recommended. The facial nerve has the highest success rate (about 90%) in peripheral nerve grafting. Following this procedure it may take 6 months or more for function to be restored.

### Resection of the Submandibular Gland

Submandibular gland resection is performed through a submandibular incision (Fig. 15-20A and B). The subcutaneous tissue and platysma are traversed and the mandibular branch of cranial nerve VII must be identified and preserved; this nerve controls the ability to raise the commissure of the lip on the ipsilateral side. Because damage to the lingual nerve (deep to the submandibular gland) and its branch, the chorda tympani, results in a loss of taste, it too must be identified before dividing the deep blood supply to the gland. Although the hypoglossal nerve is also deep to the submandibular gland, it is usually not seen during excision and is unlikely to be damaged during resection.

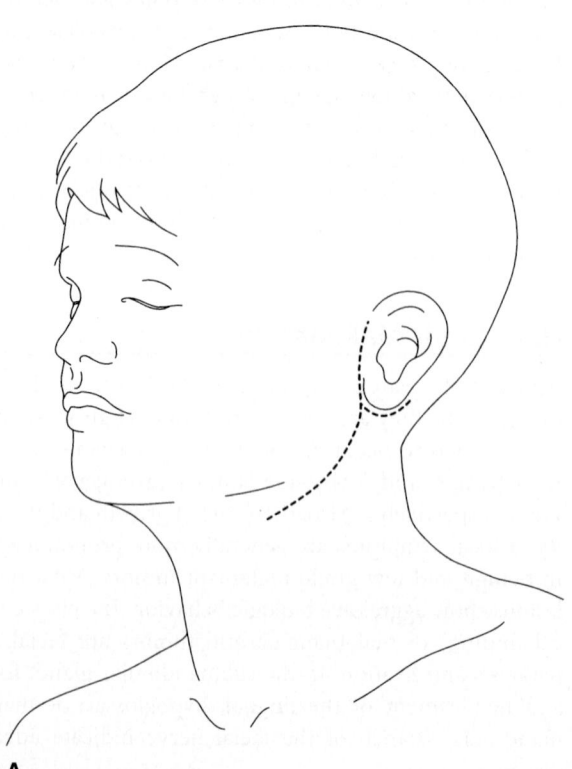

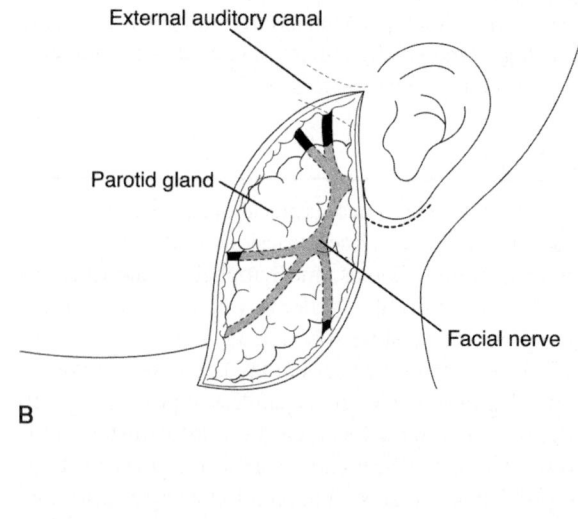

**FIGURE 15-19** A. Preauricular and superior neck incision (*dotted line*) for a parotid gland resection. B. The superficial lobe of the parotid gland is exposed through the incision.

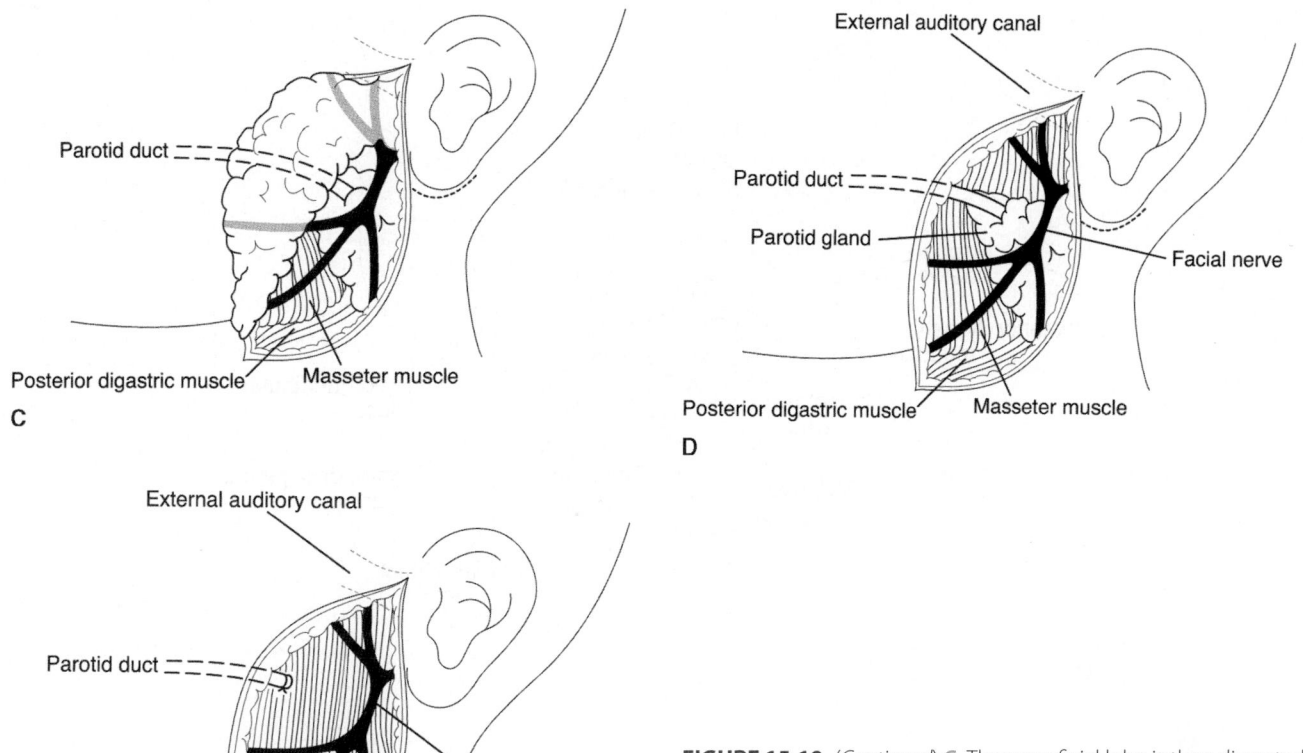

C

D

E

**FIGURE 15-19** (*Continued*) **C.** The superficial lobe is then dissected from the deeper lobe, preserving the facial nerve and its branches. **D.** When removing the deep lobe of the parotid gland, the facial nerve usually can be preserved except when the tumor involves the nerve. **E.** The facial muscles, including the masseter muscle, and facial nerve after resection of the entire parotid gland.

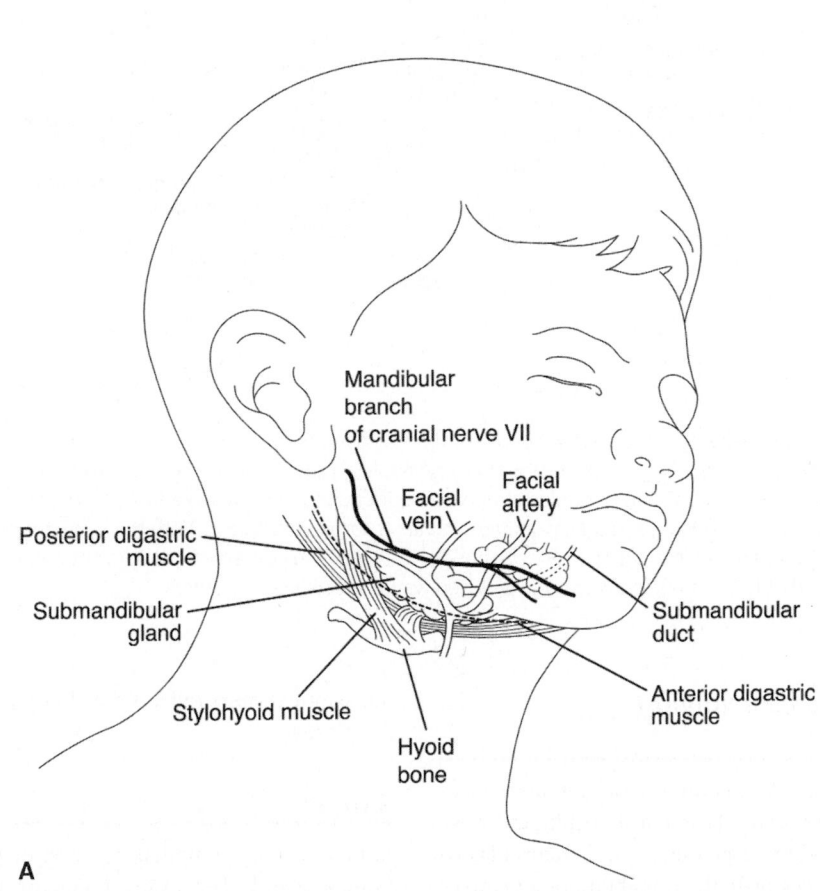

A

**FIGURE 15-20** Excision of the submandibular gland. **A.** Anatomy of the submandibular region with a curvilinear incision identified with a dotted line.

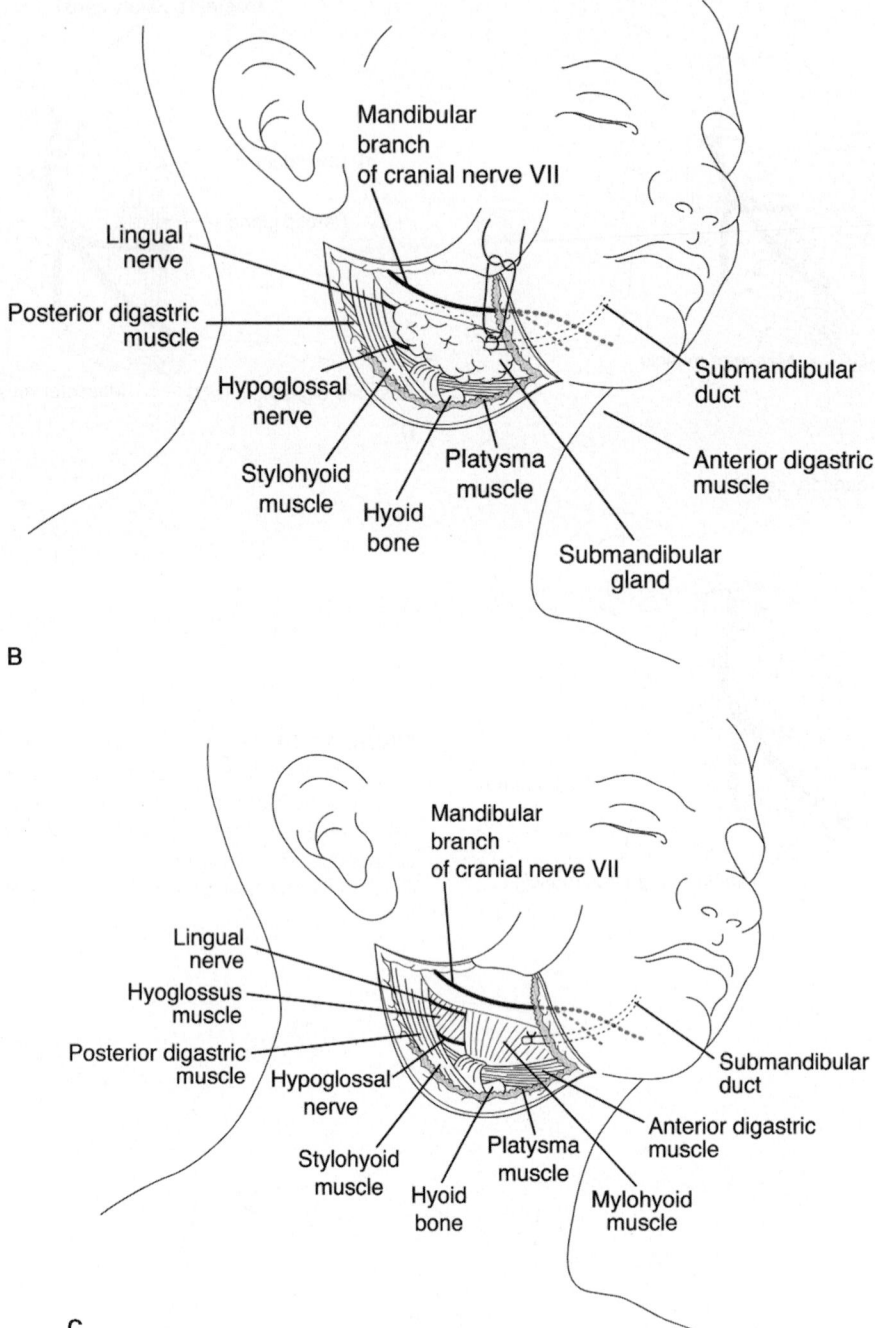

B

C

**FIGURE 15-20** (*Continued*) **B.** Exposure of the submandibular gland after traversing the platysma. Branches of the facial vein and artery involving the gland are divided. The marginal mandibular, lingual, and hypoglossal nerves are identified and preserved during dissection. The submandibular gland duct is ligated with an absorbable suture. **C.** With the submandibular gland excised, the anterior cervical muscles are seen. The platysma is reapproximated with absorbable fine sutures, and wound is closed with a subcuticular closure.

## Metastatic Neoplasms Involving the Parotid Gland

Because the parotid gland is a common site for metastases of primary lesions of the scalp, face, cheek, orbit, and nose (eg, lymphomas, rhabdomyosarcomas, and neuroblastomas), clinicians must investigate the possibility of a primary lesion outside the gland in all cases of suspected malignancy. It is important to keep in mind that the clinical behavior of metastatic tumors reflects the biologic features of the primary neoplasm.

## Ranula

*Ranula* is a term applied to a cyst or pseudocyst of the sublingual gland. The cystic form, or simple ranula, has an epithelial lining and is due to partial ductal obstruction. It arises as a cystic swelling in the oral cavity on the floor of

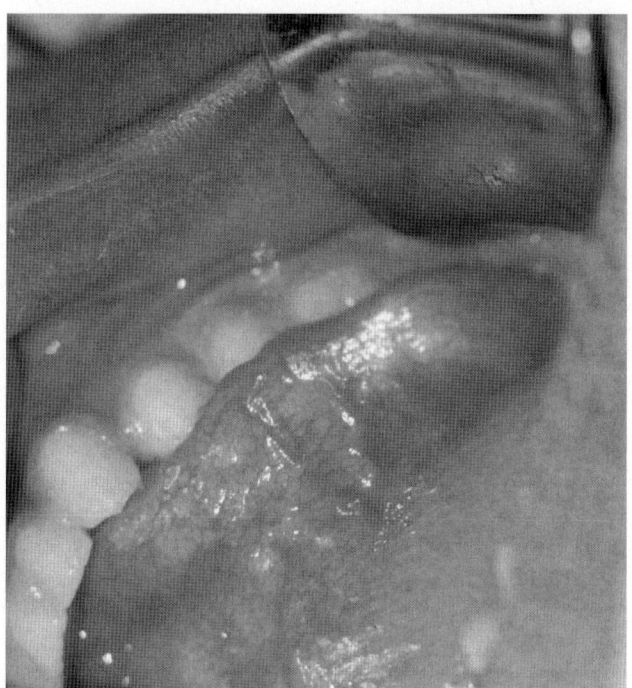

**FIGURE 15-21** Ranula in the floor of the mouth in an adolescent male.

the mouth (Fig. 15-21). Rupture of the duct due to complete ductal occlusion may result in extravasation or dissection of amylase-containing secretions between the anterior neck muscles, forming a pseudocyst. This lesion, which is called a plunging ranula, is unlike a simple ranula in that it lacks an epithelial lining.

Treatment of a simple ranula consists of unroofing the cyst and marsupializing the cut edge of the cyst wall to the oral mucosa, with a running, locked absorbable suture (Fig. 15-22A and B). This approach is effective in two thirds of patients. In cases of recurrence, resection of the sublingual salivary gland may be required. A plunging ranula requires resection of the involved sublingual gland in continuity with the pseudocyst wall. This operation is performed either with a transoral approach or with a combination of oral and cervical incisions, depending on the size of the lesion. Care must

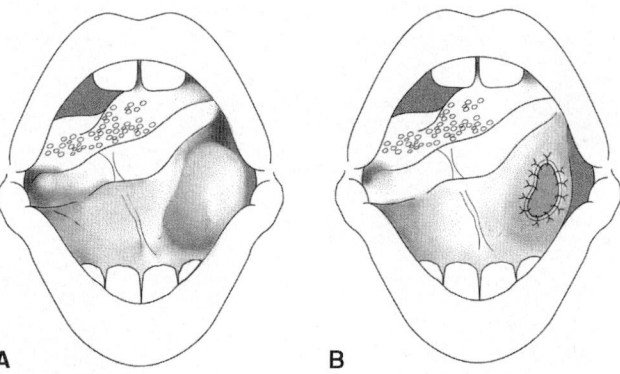

**A**          **B**

**FIGURE 15-22** Ranula marsupialization. **A.** The position of a simple ranula in the floor of the mouth. **B.** Marsupialization of the ranula is accomplished through a transoral excision of the roof of the cyst with suturing of the cyst lining to the sublingual mucosa.

be taken during this dissection to preserve the hypoglossal and lingual nerves, which may become entrapped in the mass.

# INFLAMMATORY LESIONS

Because the head contains a number of structures through which bacteria or viruses can enter the body, the cervical lymph nodes frequently become involved in infections and inflammatory diseases. In this section, we will describe the most common acute and chronic lesions of the cervical lymph nodes.

## Acute Cervical Lymphadenitis

Enlarged cervical lymph nodes are the most common neck masses in childhood. When their etiology is viral, lesions are often bilateral, relatively short in duration, rarely suppurative, and generally resolve spontaneously. Acute suppurative cervical lymphadenitis is, however, the most common cause of cervical lymph node enlargement in children requiring treatment (Fig. 15-23A and B). It generally originates from a bacterial infection arising in the upper respiratory tract or oropharynx. Although the 2 most common etiologic organisms are penicillin-resistant *Staphylococcus aureus* and *Streptococcus hemolyticus*, anaerobes have also been cultured.

The diagnosis of bacterial suppurative cervical lymphadenitis is generally apparent; there is rapid, unilateral enlargement of one or more cervical lymph nodes and marked tenderness, warmth, and erythema. The fever is usually mild and is often accompanied by irritability and malaise. Also, leukocytosis with a high band count is commonly seen. Affected nodes often enlarge and become abscessed. In many cases there may be associated cellulitis and thinning of the overlying skin, leading to spontaneous drainage of purulent material. If fluctuance is identified, drainage is mandatory. Needle aspiration can be both diagnostic and therapeutic. Purulent fluid aspirated from the fluctuant node should be cultured for both aerobic and anaerobic bacteria. Warm soaks and treatment with appropriate antibiotics should be initiated. Repeated aspirations may occasionally be necessary. If the child appears to be ill or is quite young, hospital admission for the administration of intravenous antibiotics and close observation is indicated. Needle aspiration combined with antibiotic therapy usually effects a complete resolution. If, however, the abscess is large or fluctuance persists or recurs after needle aspiration, incision and drainage should be performed with a general anesthetic. The placement of a small Penrose drain may facilitate irrigation and dressing changes performed by parents. Some surgeons prefer to place a light packing that is changed daily in the abscess cavity. Following abscess drainage, complete healing generally occurs within 2 weeks.

## Subacute or Chronic Lesions

### Chronic Cervical Lymphadenitis

Children occasionally develop impressively enlarged lymph nodes that are mildly inflamed, minimally tender, and

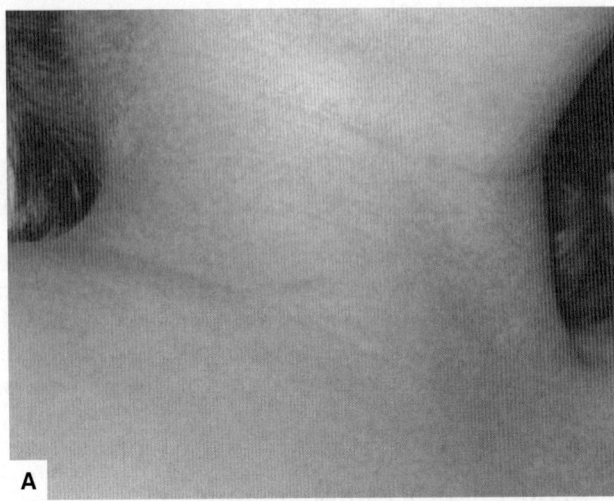 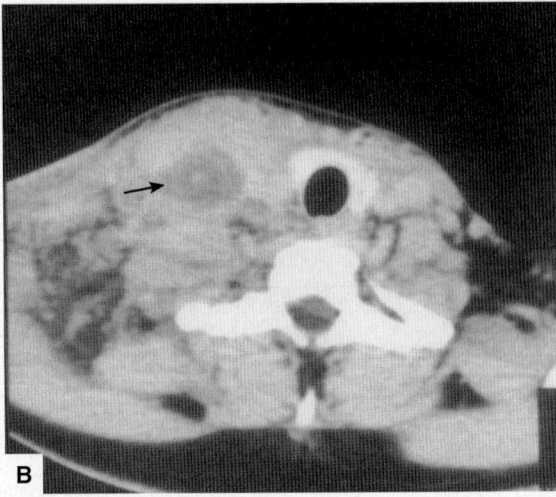

**FIGURE 15-23** Acute suppurative lymphadenitis. **A.** Deep cervical lymphadenitis in a young teenager with severe anterior cervical tenderness and erythema. This patient had no palpable fluctuance in the neck. **B.** The cervical abscess (*arrow*) is seen on computed tomography.

nonfluctuant. Node enlargement may appear suddenly or slowly over a period of days to weeks and, in contrast to acute suppurative cervical lymphadenitis, there are no obvious associated prodromal or systemic symptoms. In such cases, the differential diagnosis may encompass a wide range of clinical entities, including a reactive response to a nonspecific viral or bacterial infection, an atypical mycobacterial infection, a *Mycobacterium tuberculosis* infection, cat scratch disease, and infectious mononucleosis. Rarer entities such as toxoplasmosis, cytomegalovirus, human immunodeficiency virus, sarcoidosis, histoplasmosis, actinomycosis, and a malignancy must also be considered in the differential diagnosis.

A complete medical history must be obtained, and a thorough physical examination must be performed. A complete blood cell count and diagnostic tests that may rule out conditions considered in the differential diagnosis are also necessary. A chest radiograph may also be useful to exclude mediastinal adenopathy or pulmonary infiltrates. After an initial evaluation, most children should receive a full course of an antistaphylococcal antibiotic and undergo frequent reexamination by the same physician to assess the response to therapy. The persistence of a single dominant lymph node for longer than 6 to 8 weeks mandates an excisional biopsy to exclude the diagnosis of neoplasm. Nodes present in the supraclavicular space and posterior triangle tend to be more of a concern in regard to malignancy than those found in the submandibular or anterior triangle.

## Mycobacterial Lymphadenitis

Mycobacterial infections comprise 7% to 8% of cases of chronic lymphadenitis in children. Of these cases, 18% to 34% involve the head and neck region. Most mycobacterial lymphadenitis in the United States is caused by the atypical mycobacteria of the *Mycobacterium avium-intracellulare scrofulaceum* (MAIS) complex (Fig. 15-24), a group of 10 to 15 mycobacteria that produce a specific, localized form of lymphadenitis. Infection occurs predominantly in children 1 to 5 years of age, and the breakdown of the mucosal barrier

with the eruption of teeth during this time may permit entry of atypical mycobacterial pathogens. Infection is rarely seen after age 12. The portal of entry is primarily through the mucous membranes of the oropharynx and tonsils. These infections typically involve the submandibular nodes unilaterally, with overlying skin involvement and sinus tract formation. The nodes are generally minimally tender, dull red, and of a rubbery consistency. Atypical mycobacterial lymphadenitis is thought to be a local process, without associated intrathoracic or systemic disease, unless the child is immunocompromised. Purified protein derivative skin testing in children with atypical mycobacterial infection is either negative or weakly positive. Because these organisms grow very slowly, cultures may take as long as 1 month before organisms are identifiable. The treatment of choice is resection in continuity of grossly involved nodes and overlying skin and sinus tracts. Care must be taken to avoid injury to the mandibular branch of the facial nerve during resection of these nodes. Adjuvant antibiotic therapy with

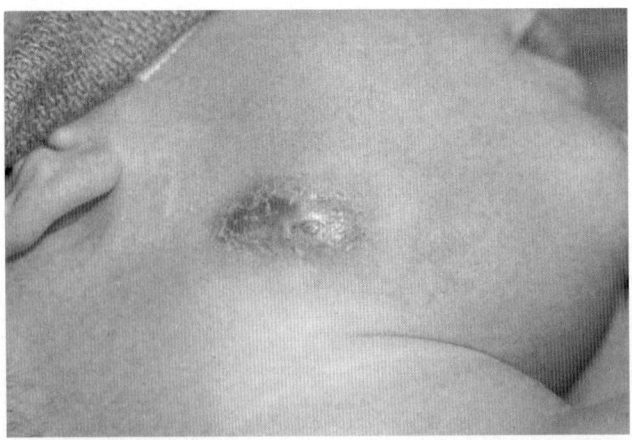

**FIGURE 15-24** Atypical mycobacterial infection involving the left submandibular nodes.

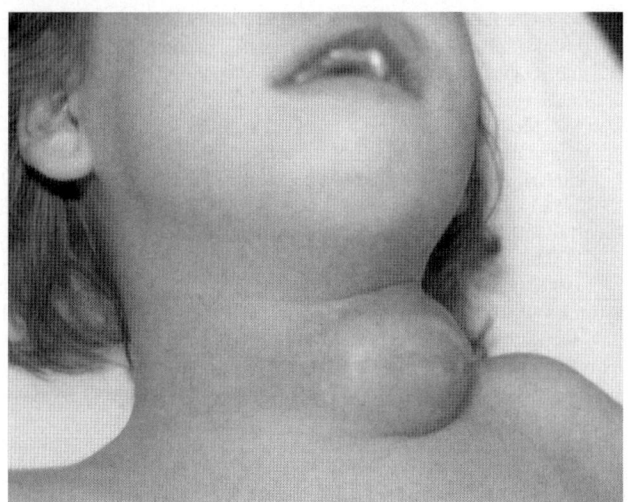

**FIGURE 15-25** Scrofula in the left neck of a 5-year-old girl. (*Courtesy of Lester Martin, MD, Cincinnati Children's Hospital Medical Center, Cincinnati, OH.*)

Biaxin® (clarithromycin) is carried out for several days preoperatively and 3 weeks postoperatively. Antibiotic therapy without surgery is ineffective.

In underdeveloped countries, tuberculous cervical lymphadenitis, also known as scrofula, is almost exclusively due to *Mycobacterium tuberculosis* (Fig. 15-25). It is thought to be an extension of a primary pulmonary infection and usually involves the supraclavicular nodes. In contrast to MAIS, it is generally accompanied by the systemic manifestations of tuberculosis, and so a history of the patient's exposure to tuberculosis should be obtained. Purified protein derivative skin testing, a chest x-ray, lymph node needle aspiration cytology, or an excisional biopsy with culture provides the diagnosis. Because lymphadenitis is thought to be the manifestation of a systemic disease, it is treated pharmacologically with a 2-year course of antituberculous chemotherapy. Most children respond well, with resolution of the lesion within 3 months of the initiation of therapy.

## Cat Scratch Disease

Cat scratch disease is a common cause of lymphadenopathy in childhood. The disease begins as a minor infection or pustule that forms 3 to 5 days after the infliction of a superficial wound, usually by a cat. The child typically develops tender regional lymphadenopathy in 2 to 4 weeks. The site of inoculation is generally an extremity, resulting in inguinal, epitrochlear, or axillary adenopathy. However, scratches in the area of the head and neck may result in significant cervical lymphadenopathy, which may be accompanied by mild systemic symptoms of fever and malaise early in the course of the disease. Generally, only 1 or 2 nodes are involved. In addition to lymphadenitis, complications such as encephalitis, retinitis, and osteomyelitis have been reported in a small number of patients. *Rochalimaea henselae*, a pleomorphic gram-negative bacillus, has been identified as the infectious agent. This organism can be detected on Warthin–Starry silver impregnation stains of both affected lymph nodes and inoculum sites.

Although not done routinely, in most cases a skin test antigen prepared from the aspirate of an involved node can confirm diagnosis. Cat scratch disease is usually self-limiting, with the resolution of regional adenopathy within 6 to 8 weeks. Antibiotics are not generally effective despite in vitro sensitivities. Occasionally, suppuration requires drainage. Persistent adenopathy, especially in older children and adolescents, should prompt an excisional biopsy to exclude a malignancy.

## Other Causes of Cervical Lymphadenopathy

Other infectious diseases associated with cervical lymphadenitis include: actinomycosis, toxoplasmosis, tularemia, infectious mononucleosis, *Yersinia* infection, nocardiasis, blastomycosis, and acquired immunodeficiency syndrome. Kawasaki disease, an acute vasculitis seen in children, also is frequently accompanied by unilateral cervical lymphadenitis. A nodal biopsy may be required to establish the diagnosis.

When cervical lymphadenopathy persists for several weeks in older children and adolescents, it is worrisome due to the possibility of Hodgkin and non-Hodgkin lymphomas. Cervical node enlargement is often the first sign of lymphoma, and the pediatric surgeon should be consulted for a lymph node biopsy. A chest radiograph is mandatory prior to the biopsy to exclude a mediastinal mass. If undetected, such a mass could cause airway collapse on induction of anesthesia.

## NEOPLASTIC LESIONS

Neoplasms involving the head and neck account for 5% of all malignancies in children. More than 50% of these malignancies are lymphomas or soft tissue sarcomas. Lymphoid tumors tend to predominate, and Hodgkin and non-Hodgkin lymphomas (Chapter 95) occur with almost equal frequency in the head and neck region in children. Rhabdomyosarcomas (Chapter 91) are the most frequent solid tumors, accounting for about 10% of all malignant childhood tumors in this region. Other head and neck tumors that occur in the pediatric population include thyroid carcinomas, neuroblastomas (Chapter 89), salivary gland carcinomas, nasopharyngeal carcinomas, and melanomas.

Age is a factor in the type of head and neck tumor encountered. Neuroblastoma is the most frequent diagnosis in children younger than 6 years. In this age group the next most common malignant tumors are non-Hodgkin lymphomas, followed by rhabdomyosarcomas, and Hodgkin lymphomas. Children from 7 to 13 years of age, however, have an equal risk for either Hodgkin or non-Hodgkin lymphoma, followed by thyroid carcinoma and rhabdomyosarcoma. In contrast, adolescents are most commonly diagnosed with Hodgkin lymphoma.

A high index of suspicion is critical to facilitate the early diagnosis and treatment of all malignant lesions, and treatment must be individualized according to the type of tumor. In all patients, this necessitates a multidisciplinary approach involving close collaboration of the primary care pediatrician, oncologist, surgeon, and radiologist.

# SELECTED READINGS

Altman RP, Hechtman DH. Congenital lesions: thyroglossal duct cysts and branchial cleft anomalies. In: Baker RJ, Fischer JE, eds. *Mastery of Surgery*. Vol 1. 4th ed. Philadelphia: Lippincott Williams & Wilkins; 2001:382–388.

Altman RP, Margeleth AM. Cervical lymphadenopathy from atypical mycobacteria: diagnosis and surgical treatment. *J Pediatr Surg* 1975;10:419–422.

Berger C, Pfyffer GE, Nadal D. Treatment of nontuberculous mycobacterial lymphadenitis with clarithromycin plus rifabutin. *J Pediatr* 1996;128:383–386.

Fallat ME. Neck. In: Oldham KT, Colombani PM, Foglia RP, eds. *Surgery of Infants and Children: Scientific Principles and Practice*. Philadelphia: Lippincott-Raven; 1997:835–855.

Filston HC. Common lumps and bumps of the head and neck in infants and children. *Pediatr Ann* 1989;18:180–186.

Healy G. Malignant tumors of the head and neck in children: diagnosis and treatment. *Otolaryngol Clin North Am* 1980;13:483–488.

Lawrence WT, Azizkhan RG. Congenital muscular torticollis: a spectrum of pathology. *Ann Plast Surg* 1989;23:523–529.

Miller D, Hill JL, Sun CC, et al. The diagnosis and management of pyriform sinus fistulae in infants and young children. *J Pediatr Surg* 1983;18:377–381.

Pinder SE, Colville A. Mycobacterial cervical lymphadenitis in children: can histological assessment help differentiate infections caused by nontuberculous mycobacteria from *Mycobacterium tuberculosis*? *Histopathology* 1993;22:59–64.

Scott MA, McCurley TL, Vnencak-Jones CL, et al. Cat scratch disease; detection of *Bartonella henselae* DNA in archival biopsies from patients with clinically, serologically, and histologically defined disease. *Am J Pathol* 1996;149:2161–2167.

Seibert RW. Diseases of the salivary glands. In: Bluestone CD, Stool SE, eds. Pediatric Otolaryngology. 2nd ed. Philadelphia: WB Saunders Co; 1990:948–960.

Sistrunk WE. Technique of removal of cyst and sinuses of the thyroglossal duct. *Surg Gynecol Obstetr* 1928;46:109–112.

Spiro RH. The parotid gland. In: Baker RJ, Fischer JE, eds. *Mastery of Surgery*. Vol. 1. 4th ed. Philadelphia: Lippincott Williams & Wilkins; 2001:320–327.

Telander RL, Filston HC. Review of head and neck lesions in infancy and childhood. *Surg Clin North Am* 1992;72:1429–1447.

Waldhausen JHT, Tapper D. Head and neck sinuses and masses. In: Ashcraft KW, Murphy KP, Sharp RJ, Sigalet DL, Snyder CL, eds. *Pediatric Surgery*. 3rd ed. Philadelphia: WB Saunders Co; 2000: 987–999.

THE HEAD AND NECK

# PART III

## CHEST WALL AND THORACIC DISEASE

# CHAPTER 16 | Breast Disease

*Leslie Ann Taylor and Richard G. Azizkhan*

## KEY POINTS

1. Breast conditions apparent at birth include athelia and polythelia. Newborns should be examined for polythelia because of the conditions that can be associated with it, including renal agenesis, supernumerary kidneys, renal cell carcinoma, congenital cardiac defects, pyloric stenosis, epilepsy, and ear abnormalities.

2. The 2 main conditions of the breast that can appear in the first few weeks of life are neonatal gynecomastia, with or without galactorrhea, and neonatal mastitis.

3. Premature thelarche can occur with no other signs of puberty or be the first indication of precocious puberty. Girls with premature maturation should be followed carefully to determine the true cause so that surgically treatable lesions can be managed early.

4. Prepubertal gynecomastia in boys is rare and usually found with sexual precocity, although some cases are caused by tumors.

5. Virginal or juvenile hypertrophy, usually beginning at the onset of puberty, can lead to skin ulceration of the breast and psychosocial consequences. Medical treatment with danazol is possible, but may cause permanently suppress ovulation and cyclic bleeding. Surgical options include total mastectomy with an implant or reduction mammoplasty.

6. Bilateral deficiency of breast growth related to delayed thelarche or puberty in adolescent girls requires endocrine evaluation and karyotyping.

7. Fibroadenomata are the most common discrete solid masses found in the adolescent breast and large masses should be excised to preserve normal breast tissue and rule out the very small chance of cancer.

8. Most cystosarcoma phylloides are benign and should be locally excised. Subcutaneous mastectomy is appropriate if they are malignant.

9. Juvenile secretory carcinoma is a slow-growing tumor that can recur locally and metastasizes to the axillary lymph nodes. This tumor is not hormone-dependent and can occur in both girls and boys, with a mean age of occurrence is 9 years. A simple mastectomy with axillary node sampling is indicated.

10. Other causes of breast masses in pubertal girls include lesions of the rib, skin, or chest wall, which can be differentiated with a plain chest x-ray or a computed tomography scan.

11. Metastatic breast masses include rhabdomyosarcoma, Ewing sarcoma, lymphoma, neuroblastoma, ovarian dysgerminoma, and acute leukemia.

12. The most common disorder of the breast in adolescent boys is gynecomastia. Only 1% of boys find the condition troublesome enough to undergo surgery.

---

Breast disorders in children encompass a wide range of causes and include developmental anomalies, tumors, infections, hormonal imbalances, and, rarely, trauma. The vast majority of breast conditions in children of all ages are benign. Most breast conditions are age specific. In this chapter, the chronologic presentation of breast conditions will be emphasized (Tables 16-1 and 16-2).

## EMBRYOLOGY AND NORMAL DEVELOPMENT

During the sixth week of fetal life, epidermal cells migrate in the underlying mesenchymal layer to produce a thickened ridge. This primitive mammary ridge is known as the milk line. The mesenchyme becomes the fibrous and fatty tissue of the breast stroma. In normal human development, the multiple breast structures extending from the axilla to the groin regress during the ninth week of gestation, except at the level of the pectoralis muscle. Up to the fifth month of fetal life, there is further differentiation of the breast structure, with the nipple, areola, and lactiferous ducts taking form.

The Tanner stages of pubertal maturity are the 5 stages of female breast development. Stage 1 is the preadolescent stage with elevation of the nipple only. Stage 2 is the breast bud stage that occurs at about 11 years with elevation of the breast

**TABLE 16-1 Breast Conditions in Girls**

| Age (years) | Lesion | Diagnosis | Treatment |
|---|---|---|---|
| 0–1 | Developmental | Neonatal gynecomastia | Observation |
| | Infectious | Neonatal mastitis | Antibiotics, drainage |
| 1–4 | Developmental | Premature thelarche | H&P, bone age endocrine evaluation |
| | Mass | Galactocele | Excision |
| | | Metastatic nodule | Excision |
| 4–10 | Developmental | Precocious puberty | H&P, bone age endocrine evaluation |
| | Mass | Metastatic nodule | Excision |
| 10–18 | Developmental | Pubertal growth | H&P, observation |
| | | Virginal hypertrophy | Reduction mammoplasty Mastectomy |
| | | Macromastia | Reduction mammoplasty |
| | Infectious | Lactation mastitis | Antibiotics, drainage |
| | Mass | Fibroadenoma | Serial exam, excision |
| | | Metastatic nodule | Excision |

and nipple as a small mound with enlargement and darkening of the areola. In Stage 3, further enlargement of both the breast and the areola occur. Most girls reach Stage 4 by age 12 years, with the areola and nipple projecting to form a secondary mound above the level of the breast. Stage 5 is the mature breast in which there is projection of the nipple only, as the areola becomes recessed. Montgomery glands, which provide lubrication to the areola, form (Fig. 16-1).

# BREAST CONDITIONS APPRARENT AT BIRTH

Breast conditions apparent at birth in males and females include congenital absence of nipple, termed athelia. True amastia, which is complete absence of the breast, will not be recognized until puberty. Polythelia, the persistence of

**TABLE 16-2 Breast Conditions in Boys**

| Age (years) | Lesion | Diagnosis | Treatment |
|---|---|---|---|
| 0–1 | Developmental | Neonatal gynecomastia | Observation |
| | Infectious | Neonatal mastitis | Antibiotics, drainage |
| | Mass | Galactocele | Observation, excision |
| 1–10 | Developmental | Prepubertal gynecomastia | H&P, endocrine evaluation |
| | Mass | Galactocele | Observation, excision |
| 10–18 | Developmental | Pubertal gynecomastia | H&P, weight reduction Subcutaneous mastectomy |
| | Mass | Metastatic nodule | Excision |
| | | Other | Endocrine evaluation |

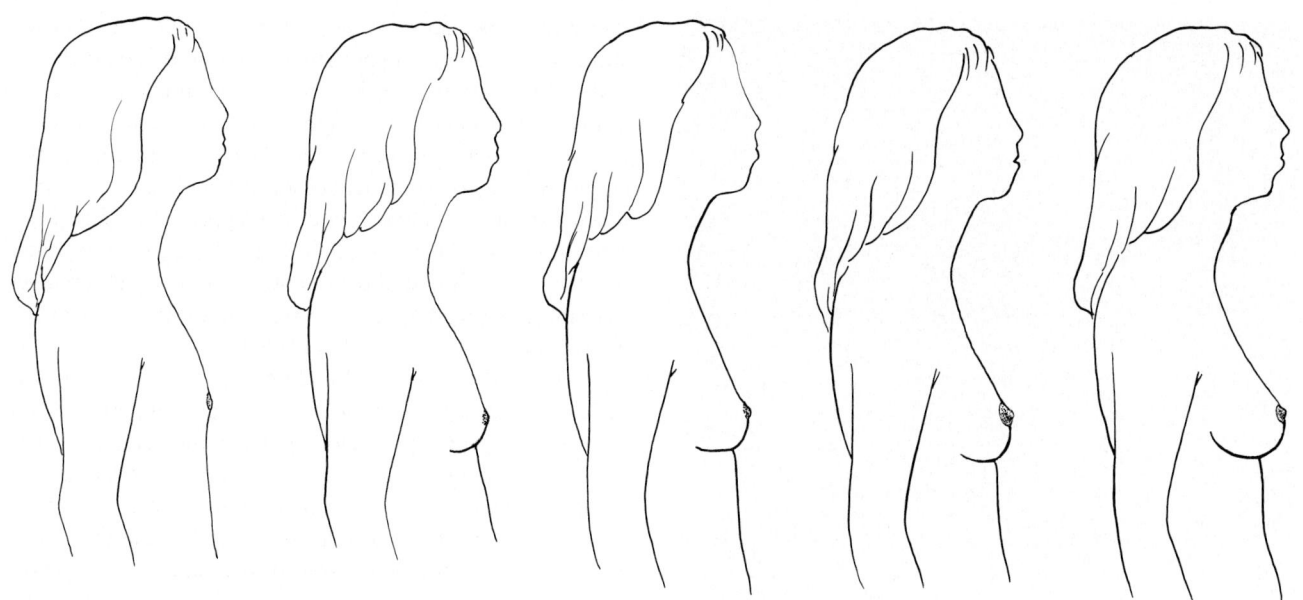

**FIGURE 16-1** Tanner stages of breast development in pubertal girls, stage 1 to 5.

multiple nipples along the milk line due to failure of regression of the cephalad or caudad extent of the mammary ridge, may be either unilateral or bilateral. Polythelia occurs in about 2% of the population. The appearance of these supernumerary nipples ranges from pigmented macula to fully developed nipples. Rarely nipple development can occur distant to the milk line. Newborns should be examined for polythelia because several conditions that can be associated with polythelia require further investigation, including renal agenesis, supernumerary kidneys, and renal cell carcinoma. Also, congenital cardiac defects, pyloric stenosis, epilepsy, and ear abnormalities have been associated with polythelia.

Polythelia forecasts polymastia, the development of supernumerary breast tissue that is subject to the same pathologic conditions as normal breast tissue, including pubertal enlargement, premenstrual swelling, lactation, and carcinoma. Polymastia may not be recognized until puberty if no nipple complex is present. The tissue mass may be mistaken for a lipoma or another soft tissue tumor. If the cosmetic defect is prominent, simple excision can be performed. Bilateral breast absence occurs in ectodermal dysplasia. This disorder includes dystrophic nails, reduced body hair, dental abnormalities, the absence of eccrine sweat glands, and hyperkeratotic palmar and plantar skin.

Poland syndrome is a congenital disorder characterized by absent chest wall structures that may include ribs, clavicles and pectoralis muscle, as well as digital anomalies. In some cases, lack of breast development is seen only at puberty. Management of this defect will be discussed under the section "Developmental Anomalies of the Adolescent Female Breast". Widely spaced nipples should prompt investigation for Turner syndrome with ovarian agenesis or dysgenesis, and Fleisher syndrome with bilateral renal hypoplasia.

## BREAST CONDITIONS IN THE FIRST FEW WEEKS OF LIFE

In either gender, there are 2 main conditions of the breast that can appear in the first few weeks of life including neonatal gynecomastia, with or without galactorrhea, and neonatal mastitis. Neonatal gynecomastia is breast enlargement caused by maternal estrogens that have crossed the placenta. Both newborn girls and boys have estrogen receptors in the breast. Girls may also have copious vaginal secretions due to this estrogen stimulation. Galactorrhea may be seen in both genders. The colostrums-like fluid has been colloquially called "witch's milk" (Fig. 16-2). Boys tend to have less breast enlargement and 1 study noted a correlation between breast

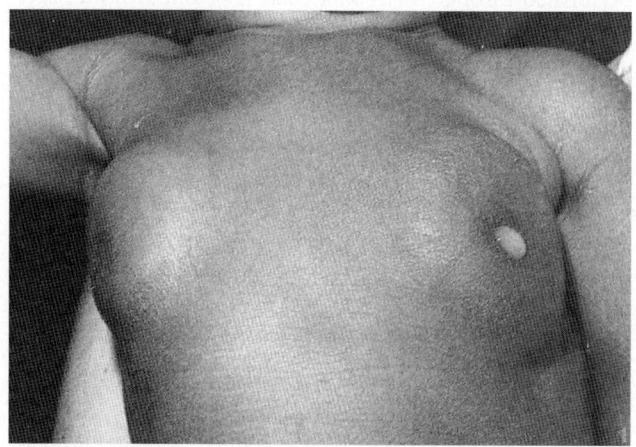

**FIGURE 16-2** Neonatal gynecomastia with galactorrhea ("witch's milk") exuding from the left nipple. (From *Liebert P. Color Atlas of Pediatric Surgery. New York: Elsevier Science Publishers; 1989:52.*)

245

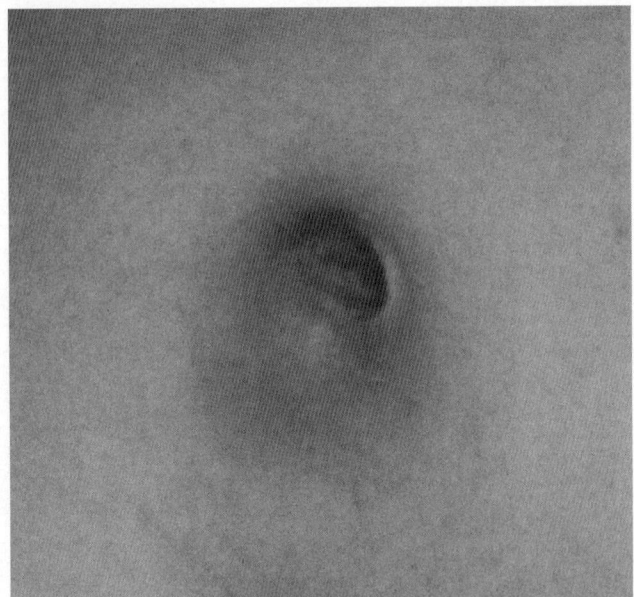

**FIGURE 16-3** Neonatal mastitis.

size in newborn males and the level of testosterone in umbilical cord blood as the only factor accounting for the difference in breast size in boys and girls. There was no difference in the levels of other hormones known to be involved, such as estradiol, progesterone, thyrotropin, and prolactin. Spontaneous regression of the gynecomastia occurs over several weeks. Manipulation of the infant's breast should be discouraged as it may lead to infection.

A second disorder specific to newborn breast tissue is neonatal mastitis, which usually occurs at 2 to 4 weeks of age. A swollen, tender, erythematous breast bud is a presenting symptom (Fig. 16-3). The cause is not easily documented, but the bacteriology has been well studied. *Staphylococcus aureus*, including methicillin-resistant *Staphylococcus*, is the predominant cause. Gram-negative and mycobacterial pathogens have also been documented. The treatment consists of antibiotics and warm compresses to encourage spontaneous drainage. If fluctuance develops, incision and drainage should be performed through a circumareolar incision, avoiding excision of the breast bud.

Children of either gender can develop a galactocele, although this is a rare condition. Ultrasound may confirm its cystic nature. Excision is the recommended treatment, with preservation of the subareolar disk of breast tissue.

## BREAST CONDITIONS IN PREPUBERTAL GIRLS

Normal puberty occurs between the ages of 8 and 14 years. Thelarche usually precedes menstruation and the growth of pubic hair. Premature thelarche is defined as bilateral breast development in girls younger than 8 years with no other signs of puberty. When this occurs at about the age of 2 years, it is usually transient and benign. Thelarche beginning between the ages of 6 and 8 years usually progresses into a normal

thelarche. The cause of premature thelarche is transient stimulation of the hypothalamic–pituitary–gonadal axis with follicle-stimulating hormone predominating. There is ultrasound evidence for a high incidence of follicular cysts. Precocious puberty can be distinguished from premature thelarche by menstruation, ovulation, and pregnancy. As during normal thelarche, 1 breast bud may appear and enlarge significantly earlier than the other. Careful examination should distinguish this breast bud from other types of breast masses. Excision of or damage to the breast bud leads to iatrogenic breast absence and should be avoided.

Precocious puberty has 3 main categories: true precocious puberty, pseudo precocious puberty, and idiopathic precocious puberty. True precocious puberty indicates early activation of the hypothalamic–pituitary axis. Menstruation and ovulation are present. Pseudo precocious puberty has several causes. Stimulation can be related to ingestion of medications such as corticosteroids, contraceptives, digoxin, anticonvulsants, and estrogen. Tumors of the ovary or the adrenal or hypothalamic area can act as an endogenous source of hormones. Pseudo precocity can also occur in McCune–Albright syndrome (polyostotic fibrous dysplasia) and primary hypothyroidism. Precocious puberty may also be idiopathic. A girl presenting with premature maturation should be followed carefully to determine the true cause so that surgically treatable lesions can be managed early.

Premature thelarche may be the first indication of precocious puberty. Bone age and assessment of estrogenization by measuring the vaginal maturation index and serum estradiol levels help in this differentiation. Hypothyroidism should also be ruled out. Other rare causes of breast enlargement or mass in prepubertal girls include tumors metastatic to the breast.

## BREAST CONDITIONS IN PREPUBERTAL BOYS

Prepubertal gynecomastia in boys is extremely rare and usually found with sexual precocity. A feminizing tumor of adrenal, testicular, or hepatic origin may be discovered after vigilant evaluation. Other rare causes of breast enlargement in prepubertal boys include metastatic tumors. A thorough endocrine evaluation should precede any attempt at surgical intervention.

## BREAST CONDITIONS IN PUBERTAL GIRLS

As previously described, normal puberty occurs between the ages of 8 and 14 years with thelarche preceding menstruation and the growth of pubic hair. Hormones participating in normal breast development include estrogen, progesterone, prolactin, growth hormone, and corticotropin. Syndromes of breast overgrowth and breast deficiency will be discussed, as well as breast tumors and masses found in pubertal girls.

## Developmental Anomalies of the Adolescent Female Breast

Virginal or juvenile hypertrophy is a developmental abnormality characterized by a rapid, painful, enormous increase in the connective fibrous tissue of the breast. It usually begins at the onset of normal pubertal development and may be unilateral or bilateral. It may be asymmetric. Virginal hypertrophy must be differentiated from unilateral giant fibrosarcoma and gravid hypertrophy, for which treatment is different. Virginal hypertrophy must also be differentiated from drug-induced breast gigantism like that caused by D-penicillamine. In virginal hypertrophy, no specific hormonal abnormality has been identified except a possible oversensitivity to estrogen that usually regresses in 1 to 3 years. The development of other secondary sexual characteristics is normal.

Virginal hypertrophy is not a premalignant condition nor is it related to other tumors. Its morbidity comes mostly from the great weight of the breasts, which can lead to skin ulceration and breakdown, and from the psychosocial consequences of this obvious deformity. Medical treatment with danazol is possible. The mechanism of action of danazol is thought to be the suppression of the pituitary–ovarian axis through the alteration of the sex steroid metabolism, and the interaction of danazol with sex hormone receptors. Side effects include suppression ovulation and cyclic bleeding, and mild androgenic effects that may be permanent. For these reasons, its indications for use should be carefully evaluated before it is used.

Surgical options for correcting virginal hypertrophy include total mastectomy with an implant or reduction mammoplasty. Both procedures have drawbacks. The safety of silicone breast implant after a total mastectomy has been questioned. Unless all hypersensitive breast tissue is excised, a recurrence should be expected with a need for secondary reduction mammoplasty. Patients must be informed that breast sensitivity and the ability to breast-feed will be lost with mastectomy or mammoplasty.

Virginal hypertrophy must also be differentiated from macromastia, another condition of breast enlargement, in which the histology is normal. Patients with macromastia usually complain of back and shoulder pain and posture problems. Reduction mammoplasty is usually curative, but should be delayed until full skeletal maturity is achieved (Figs. 16-4 and 16-5).

There are several causes for a deficiency of breast growth in adolescent girls. The tuberous breast anomaly occurs when the breast itself has a very small base, but a large nipple area, with the appearance that the breast tissue has prolapsed in the nipple. Treatment involves mammoplasty to broaden the base and reposition the nipple. Another type of bilateral breast deficiency occurs with atrophy secondary to chronic illness or primary weight loss. In eating disorders such as anorexia nervosa where there is hypothalamic suppression, hypoestrogenism contributes to breast atrophy. The breast tissue normalizes when nutrition is improved.

A bilateral breast deficiency can also occur with delayed thelarche or delayed puberty, with no secondary sexual characteristics present by age 14 years. Endocrine evaluation and

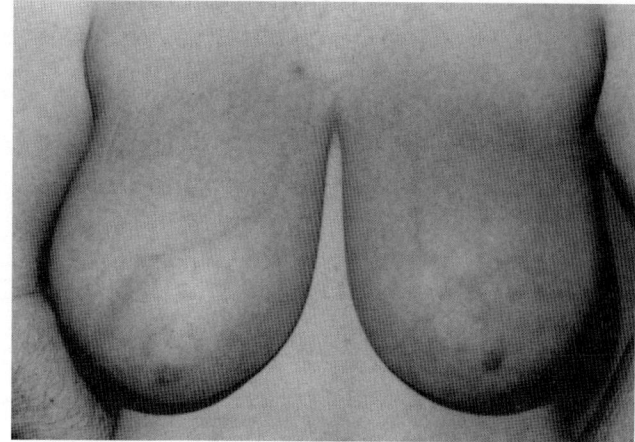

**FIGURE 16-4** Adolescent girl with debilitating macromastia.

karyotyping are necessary. The differential diagnosis includes adrenal hyperplasia, gonadal dysgenesis, pituitary hypogonadism, and hermaphroditism.

Unilateral breast deficiency occurs in Poland syndrome with unilateral deficiency of the pectoralis muscle, ribs, and costal cartilage. The musculoskeletal defects are apparent at birth, but adequacy of breast development cannot be determined until puberty. The cosmetic deformity, rather than any physical limitation, is the major problem (Figs. 16-6 and 16-7). An asymmetric pectus excavatum can also cause a unilateral breast deficiency. Chest wall and breast reconstruction can be staged or performed simultaneously in treating either of these conditions. It is usually best to wait until the normal breast has fully developed before proceeding with breast reconstruction. For Poland syndrome, latissimus dorsi muscle transposition with a simultaneous submuscular mammary prosthesis, or a mammary prosthesis alone, is used in the mild form. A contralateral breast procedure may be required for symmetry.

Other causes of unilateral breast deficiency include iatrogenic excision of 1 breast bud and chest wall radiation. An anterolateral thoracotomy in infancy or childhood has been associated with maldevelopment of the breast and pectoral muscle. Some authors recommend the avoidance of incision above the seventh or eighth intercostal space, or division of the pectoralis muscle. Another iatrogenic cause of breast

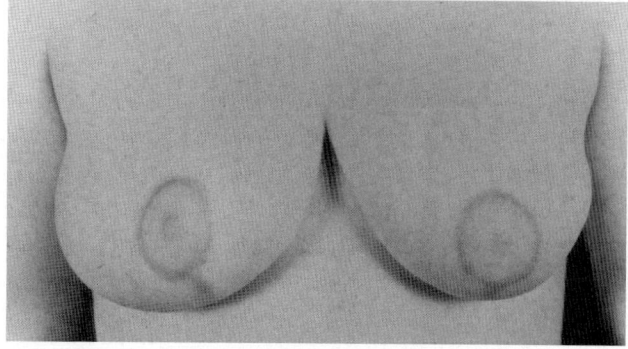

**FIGURE 16-5** Reduction mammoplasty for macromastia.

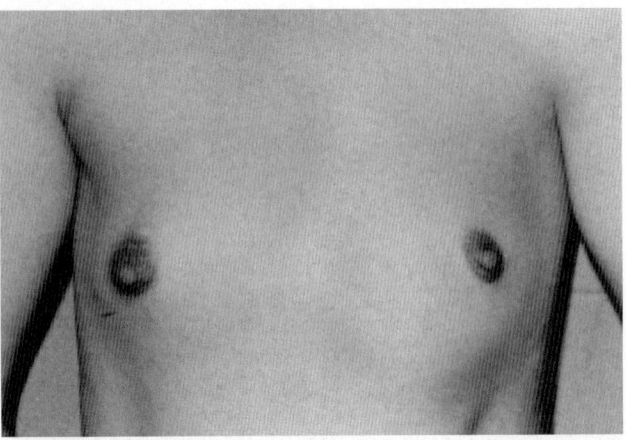

**FIGURE 16-6** Mild Poland syndrome with absent left pectoralis muscle.

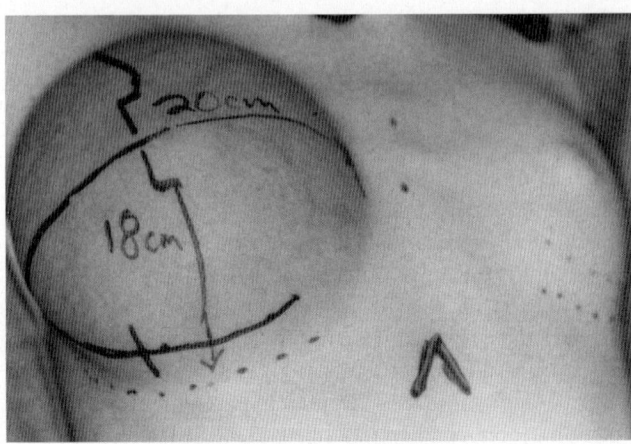

**FIGURE 16-8** Extremely large fibroadenoma.

deficiency is improper placement or positioning of a chest tube or tunneled central venous catheter that causes injury to the breast bud.

## Neoplastic Diseases of the Adolescent Female Breast

Single or discrete masses can be found in the breast on self-exam, or during the physician's examination. The differential diagnosis is similar to that in older women, but fortunately, breast cancer is rare in teenagers. Less than 0.1% of all breast cancer occurs in women younger than 20 years. Fibrocystic disease may be associated with tenderness to palpation before the menstrual period. Reassurance is indicated. The girl should be reexamined over the course of 2 menstrual cycles, and aspiration should be attempted for any cystic masses that persist. If a mass cannot be aspirated, excision may be indicated. A bloody nipple discharge can also occur in teenagers, and may represent an intraductal papilloma or papillomatosis. Treatment is the same as for adults.

Fibroadenomata are the most common discrete solid masses found in the adolescent breast, occurring most frequently in African American teenagers, with a peak at ages 14 and 15. These are firm, smooth, encapsulated, nontender, and mobile. They may involve a large part of the breast (Figs. 16-8 to 16-10). They develop slowly and are asymptomatic and noted incidentally. Some may enlarge rapidly enough to become uncomfortable and cause breast deformity. A clinical diagnosis is usually sufficient, and mammography is rarely useful in examining the adolescent breast because of its dense fibrous structure. Ultrasound can distinguish cystic from solid masses, and may obviate the need for needle aspiration. On ultrasound, a fibroadenoma is well-circumscribed, hyperechoic, and homogeneous. If the fibroadenoma is large, it should be excised to preserve normal breast tissue and rule out the very small chance of cancer. It is rare that a breast implant is needed after excision of large fibroadenoma, as the breast architecture usually reforms. Local recurrence is rare; however, other areas of fibroadenoma may develop in the ipsilateral or contralateral breast. Multiple giant fibroadenomata may require a simple mastectomy with reconstruction because of deformity of the breast.

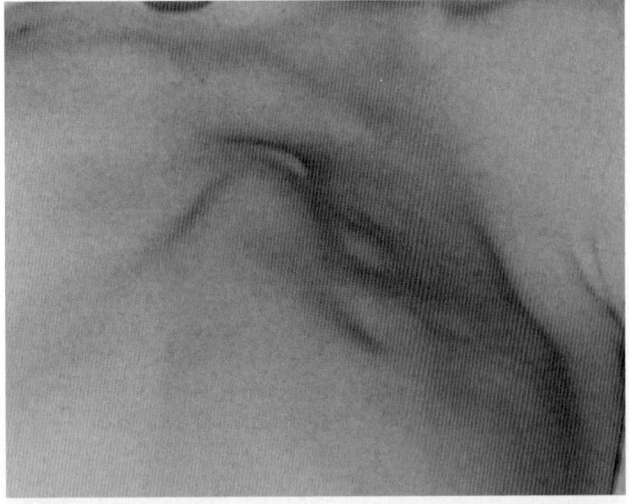

**FIGURE 16-7** Severe Poland syndrome with absent left pectoralis muscle and sternal and costal deformity.

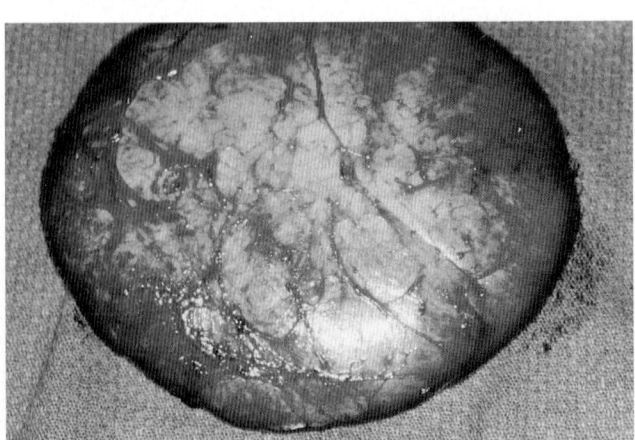

**FIGURE 16-9** Specimen of extremely large fibroadenoma.

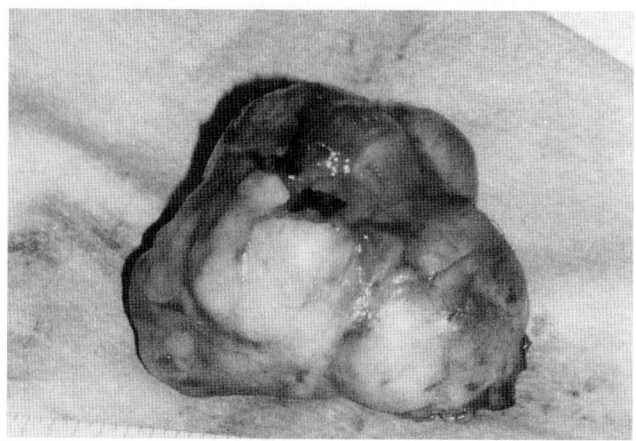

**FIGURE 16-10** Typical fibroadenoma specimen with encapsulated borders.

Cystosarcoma phylloides is another mass seen in the adolescent breast. It can grow rapidly and is distinguished histologically from fibroadenoma by a greater amount of hypertrophy and greater cellularity of the stroma. Seventy-five percent are benign. Those that are malignant rarely metastasize. Local excision is indicated if they are benign. Subcutaneous mastectomy is appropriate if they are malignant.

Juvenile secretory carcinoma is a slow-growing tumor that can recur locally and metastasizes to the axillary lymph nodes. This tumor can occur in both girls and boys, and the mean age of occurrence is 9 years. It is not a hormone-dependent tumor. A simple mastectomy with axillary node sampling is indicated. Other pathological types of breast cancer are rare.

Infiltrating ductal carcinoma is rare in adolescents, but has been reported. Conditions predisposing to its development include previous chest wall irradiation or a family history of breast cancer. Breast carcinoma in the postpubertal female responds to the treatment used in adult women and should be managed accordingly. Both lymphatic and systemic metastases follow a course similar to that in adults. Mammography is not recommended in adolescent girls, as interpretation is difficult because of the fibrous nature of the breast tissue at this age and the risk of radiation exposure.

Other causes of breast masses in pubertal girls include lesions of the rib, skin, or chest wall that can be differentiated with a plain chest x-ray or a computed tomography scan. Metastatic breast masses are well described and include rhabdomyosarcoma, Ewing sarcoma, lymphoma, neuroblastoma, ovarian dysgerminoma, and acute leukemia.

## Infections of the Adolescent Female Breast

Infectious breast conditions specific to adolescents include mastitis or an abscess in the lactating breast. Erythema and fluctuance with significant tenderness may occur and can be managed as they would be in an older female, with antibiotics, warm compresses, and drainage of clearly fluctuant areas. Mastalgia or mastodynia can also occur in adolescents and should be treated with breast support and analgesics.

# BREAST CONDTIONS IN PUBERTAL BOYS

The most common disorder of the breast in adolescent boys is gynecomastia. This is a discrete disk of glandular tissue, and is not the same as lipomastia, the breast enlargement found in obese boys, nor is it overdevelopment of the pectoralis muscle. The cause of pubertal gynecomastia is thought to be an increase in conversion of androgens to estrogens at tissue sites like those in the breast at a time in development when daytime secretion of testosterone is low. It is a common condition, and 60% of boys develop it after 1 to 2 years of puberty. Ninety percent of boys with gynecomastia have bilateral involvement, although development may be asynchronous.

In only about 2% to 3% of boys with gynecomastia is a major endocrine disturbance or other entity the cause. These include ingestion of drugs, including use of marijuana and other street drugs, and Klinefelter syndrome, which can be confirmed if the testicles are small (Table 16-3). A thorough

| TABLE 16-3 | Causes of Gynecomastia |
|---|---|
| Normal pubertal development | |
| Drug effect | |
|   Estrogens, testosterone | |
|   Isoniazid | |
|   Phenothiazine | |
|   Meprobamate | |
|   Hydroxyzine | |
|   Reserpine | |
|   Spironolactone | |
|   Digoxin | |
|   Marijuana, amphetamines, heroin | |
| Excessive estrogen production | |
|   Feminizing tumors, usually adrenal | |
| Insufficient androgen production | |
|   Klinefelter syndrome | |
|   Testicular failure | |
|   Luteinizing hormone deficiency | |
| Thyroid disease | |
| Chronic liver disease | |
| Pulmonary disease | |
|   Tuberculosis | |
|   Bronchiectasis | |

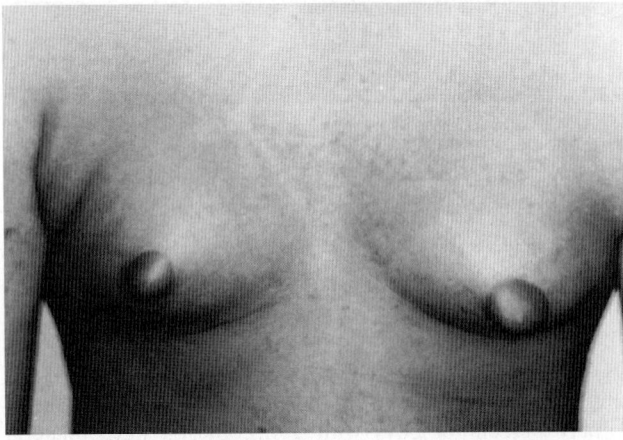

**FIGURE 16-11** Grade 1 male pubertal gynecomastia with breast tissue disk, frontal view.

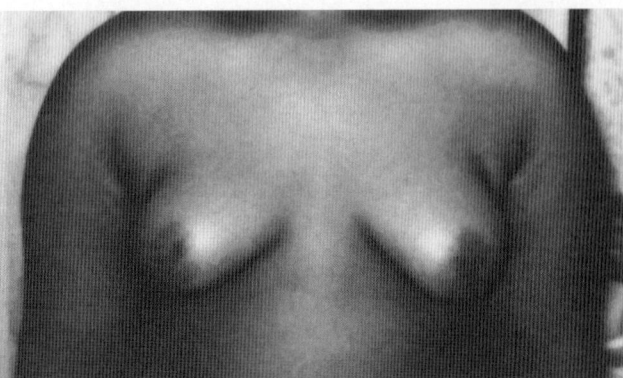

**FIGURE 16-13** Grade 2 male pubertal gynecomastia with enlarged breast tissue and significant fatty involvement of the chest wall, frontal view.

history and physical examination can aid in distinguishing pubertal gynecomastia from other conditions. Both mammography and ultrasound can be useful in differentiating gynecomastia from fatty enlargement. A grading system has been developed to describe pubertal gynecomastia. Grade 1 is a localized disk of breast tissue with little additional fatty tissue (Figs. 16-11 and 16-12). Grade 2 is diffuse enlargement of the breast on a fatty chest where the edges of the breast tissue and the fat are difficult to distinguish (Figs. 16-13 and 16-14). Grade 3 is diffuse enlargement with significant excessive fatty tissue. Many boys who come for surgical evaluation of gynecomastia are overweight, and weight loss should be encouraged before surgery is recommended.

Only 1% of boys with pubertal gynecomastia find the condition troublesome enough either physically or socially to undergo surgery. Both submammary and circumareolar incisions have been described. A circumareolar incision may give limited exposure, but provides a superior cosmetic result. After submammary incision, a flap is raised and the breast tissue excised down to the pectoralis fascia. All mammary tissue must be excised, including the axillary tail. The use of liposuction to taper the edges of the resection to reduce dishing deformity has been described. Drains may be needed

to ensure adequate closure of the flap (Fig. 16-15). There is rarely a need for excision of the excessive skin, as it shrinks with time, and some authors recommend skin excision only as a secondary procedure.

Neurofibroma of the chest wall and breast may resemble gynecomastia, but can be distinguished histologically by diffuse replacement of the breast stroma by a benign neurofibromatous proliferation. There are rare reports of breast cancer in pubertal boys, and as with girls, other tumors can metastasize to the breast.

## BREAST CONDITIONS IN CHILDREN UNRELATED TO AGE

Breast conditions that can occur at any age include hemangioma, with a characteristic vascular pattern, lymphangioma, and soft tissue tumors such as lipoma and granular

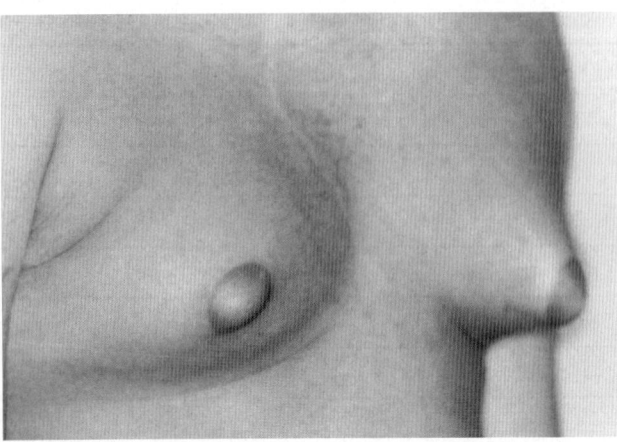

**FIGURE 16-12** Grade 1 male pubertal gynecomastia, lateral view.

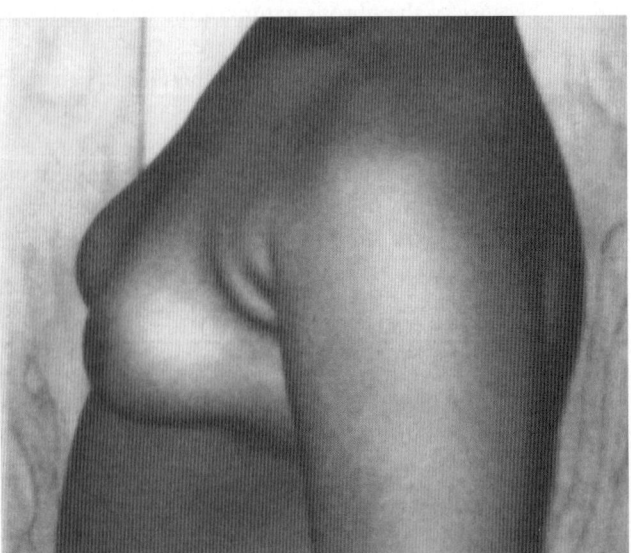

**FIGURE 16-14** Grade 2 male pubertal gynecomastia, lateral view.

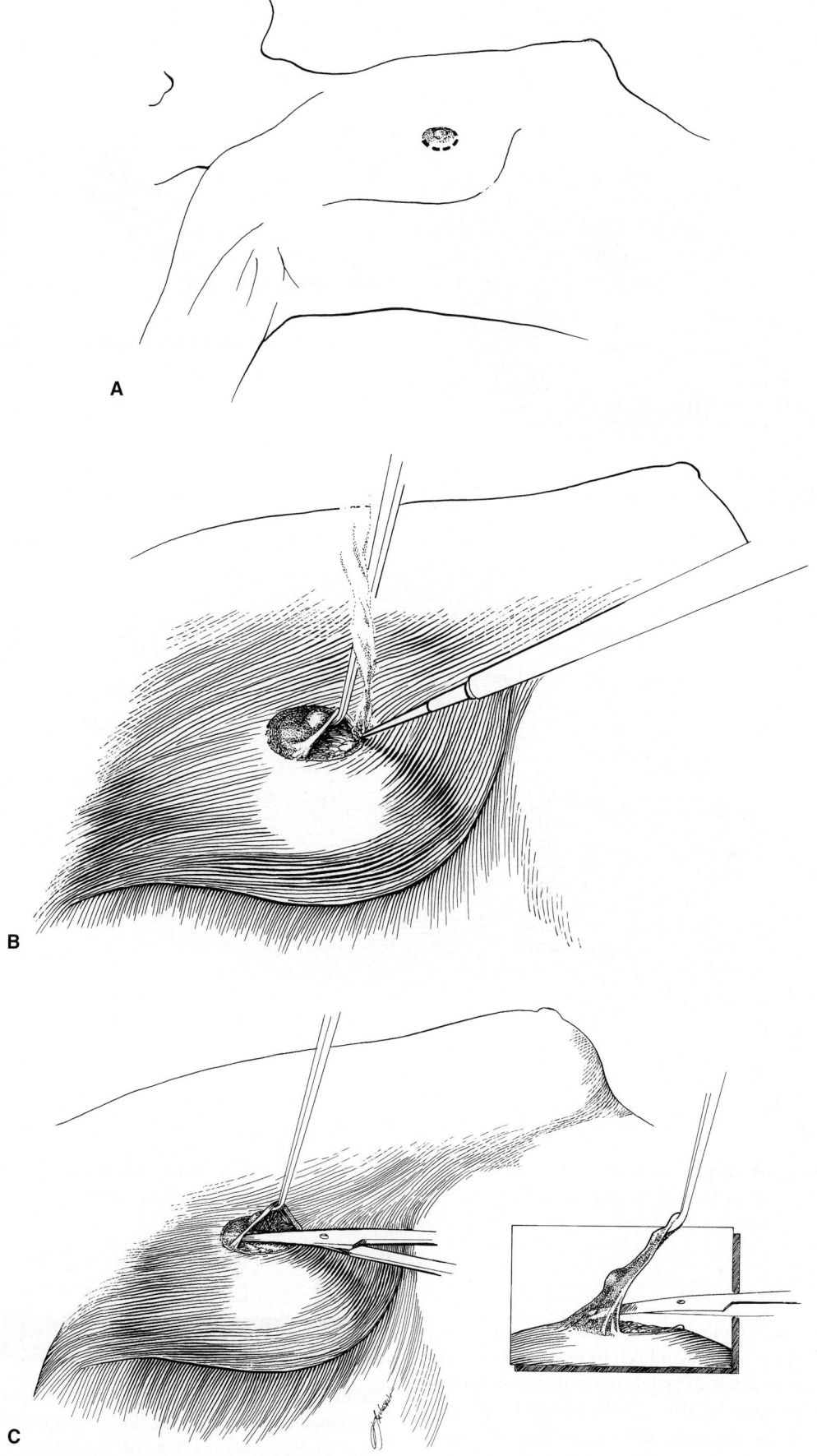

A

B

C

**FIGURE 16-15** Operative technique for subcutaneous mastectomy for male pubertal gynecomastia. **A.** A circumareolar incision is made extending approximately 50% around the nipple. **B, C.** The nipple is elevated off of the underlying breast tissue with sharp dissection and electrocautery for hemostasis.

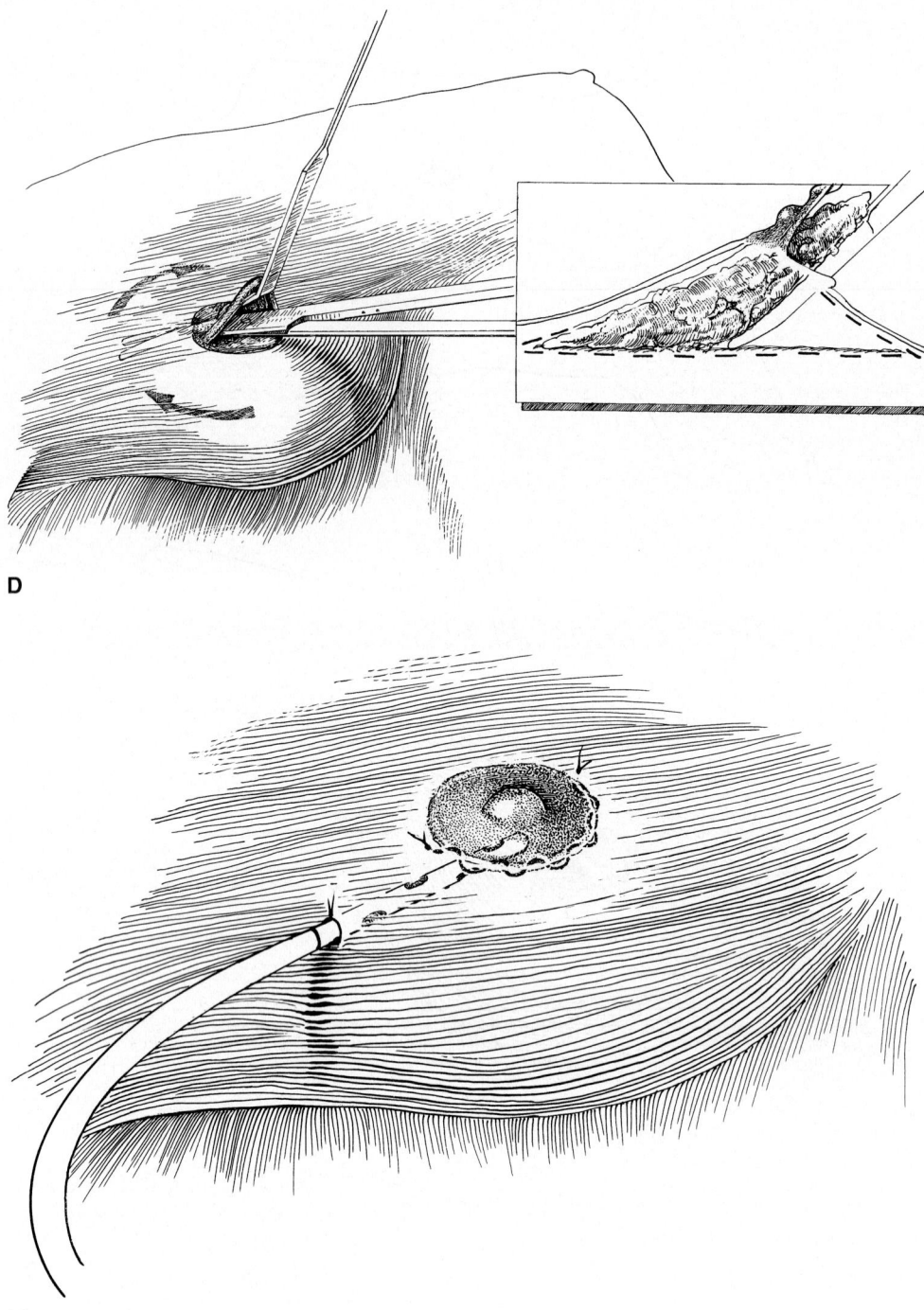

**D**

**E**

**FIGURE 16-15** (*Continued*) **D.** The glandular and adipose tissue are resected down to the pectoralis fascia. The peripheral margins of the dissection are tailored to provide a smooth contour of the anterior chest wall. **E.** A small, closed suction drain is placed to prevent seroma collection.

cell myoblastoma. Simple cysts and galactocele are easily distinguished by ultrasound and can be excised. Care must be taken during excision to avoid injury to the subareolar breast bud, especially in girls. A circumareolar incision should be used. Fat necrosis may occur after an unrecognized trauma, and may appear as a discrete mass, but because there is less fat in the breast of children and adolescents, compared with those of adult women, this is an uncommon problem.

## CONCLUSION

Knowledge of the embryology and development of the breast facilitates the diagnosis of breast conditions in children in most cases. A vast majority of breast lesions are benign. For most children, observation of the breast and reassurance of the parents is all that are required. In prepubertal patients who require surgery, attention to anatomy and future function must be kept foremost in mind.

## SELECTED READINGS

Bauer BS, Jones KM, Talbot CW. Mammary masses in the adolescent female. *Surg Gynecol* 1987;165:63–65.

Bland KI, Copeland EM, eds. *The Breast: Comprehensive Management of Benign and Malignant Disease*. Philadelphia: WB Saunders Co; 1991.

Bond SJ, Buchino JJ, Nagaraj HS, McMasters KM. Sentinel lymph node biopsy in juvenile secretory carcinoma. *J Pediatr Surg* 2004;39:120–121.

Brook I. The aerobic and anaerobic microbiology of neonatal breast abscess. *Pediatr Infect Dis J* 1990;10:785.

Clune JE, Kozakewich HP, VanBeek CA. Nipple adenoma in infancy. *J Pediatr Surg* 2009;44:2219–2222.

Coen P, Kulin H, Ballantine T, et al. An aromatase-producing sex cord tumor resulting in prepubertal gynecomastia. *N Eng J Med* 1991;324:317.

Conter V, D'Angelo P, Rovelli A, et al. Isolated breast relapse after allogenic bone marrow transplantation for childhood acute lymphoblastic leukemia. *Med Pediatr Oncol* 1992;20:165.

Corpron CA, Black CT, Singletary SE, et al. Breast Cancer in adolescent females. *J Pediatr Surg* 1995;30:322–324.

Dehner LP. *Pediatric Surgical Pathology*. Baltimore: Williams & Wilkins; 1987.

El-Tamer MB, Song M, Wait RB. Breast masses in African American teenage girls. *J Pediatr Surg* 1999;34:1401–1404.

Ferguson T, McCarty K, Filston H. Juvenile secretory carcinoma and juvenile papillomatosis: diagnosis and treatment. *J Pediatr Surg* 1987;22:637–639.

Francis G, Hoffman WH, Gala RR, et al. A relationship between neonatal breast size and cord blood testosterone level. *Ann Clin Lab Sci* 1990;201:239–244.

Gobbi D, Dall'lgna P, Alaggio R, et al. Giant fibroadenoma of the breast in adolescents: report of 2 cases. *J Pediatr Surg* 2009;44:e39–e41.

Halper S, Rubenstein D. Aplasia cutis congenital associated with syndactaly and supernumerary nipples: report of a second family with similar clinic findings. *Pediatr Dermatol* 1991;8:32–34.

Herrera LJ, Lugo-Vincente H. Primary embryonal rhabdomyosarcoma of the breast in an adolescent female: a case report. *J Pediatr Surg* 1988;33:1582–1584.

Kangesu T. Cystic hygroma of the breast in childhood. *Br J Clin Pract* 1990;44:787–788.

Karnak I, Kotiloglu E, Tanyel FC, et al. Axillary breast tissue in an adolescent girl. *J Pediatr Surg* 1995;30:1369.

Kattan J, Droz JP, Charpentier P, et al. Ovarian dysgerminoma metastatic to the breast. *Gynecol Oncol* 1992;46:104–106.

Kithara S, Wakabayashi M, Shiba T, et al. Mammary duct ectasia in children presenting bloody nipple discharge: a case in a pubertal girl. *J Pediatr Surg* 2001;36:E2.

Koltuksuz U, Aydin E. Supernumerary breast tissue: a case of pseudomamma on the face. *J Pediatr Surg* 1997;32:1377–1378.

Kupfer D, Dingman D, Broadbent R. Juvenile breast hypertrophy: report of a familial pattern and review of the literature. *Plast Reconstruct Surg* 1991;2:233–236.

Laituri CA, Garey CL, Ostile DJ, et al. Treatment of adolescent gynecomastia. *J Pediatr Surg* 2010;45:650–654.

Le-Merrer M, Renier D, Briard ML. Scalp defect, nipple absence and ear abnormalities, another case of Finlay syndrome. *Genet Couns* 1991;2:233–236.

Martino A, Zamparelli M, Santinelli, et al. Unusual clinical presentation of a rare case of phylloides tumor of the rest in an adolescent girl. *J Pediatr Surg* 2001;36:941–943.

Meggorini ML, Labi FL, Nusiner MP, et al. An overview of adolescent breast disorders. *Clin Exp Obstet Gynecol* 1991;18:265.

Miliauskas JR, Leong AS. Adenoid cystic carcinoma in a juvenile male breast. *Pathology* 1991;23:298–301.

Moore RL, Mungara A, Shayan K, et al. Bilaterally symmetric juvenile fibroadenoma and tubular breast deformity in a prepubescent girl. *J Pediatr Surg* 2007;42:1133–1136.

Murphy JJ, Morzaria S, Gow KW, et al. Breast cancer in a six year old child. *J Pediatr Surg* 2000;35:765–767.

Nakamarua M, Okabe I, Shimizumi H, et al. Ultrasonography of ovary, uterus and breast in premature thelarche. *Acta Paediatr Jpn* 1991;33:645–648.

Olcay I, Gokoz A. Infantile gynecomastia with bloody nipple discharge. *J Pediatr Surg* 1992;27:103–104.

Palnaes-Hansen C, Fahkenkrug L, Hastrup N. Tubular adenoma of the breast in a pregnant girl: report of a case. *Eur J Pediatr Surg* 1991;1:364–365.

Rissanen TJ, Makarainen HP, Kallioinen MJ, et al. Radiology of the male breast in gynecomastia. *Acta Radiol* 1992;33:110–114.

Roger DA, Lobe TE, Rao BN, et al. Breast malignancy in children. *J Pediatr Surg* 1994;29:48–51.

Sadove AM, van Aalst JA. Congenital and acquired pediatric breast anomalies: a review of 20 year's experience. *Plast Reconstr Surg* 2005;115:1039–1050.

Samuelove R, Siplovich L. Juvenile gigantomastia. *J Pediatr Surg* 1988;23:1014–1015.

Serour F, Gilad A, Kopolovic J, et al. Secretory breast cancer in childhood and adolescence: report of a case and review of the literature. *Med Pediatr Oncol* 1992;20:341–344.

Shamberger RC, Welch KJ, Upton J. Surgical treatment of thoracic deformity in Poland's syndrome. *J Pediatr Surg* 1989;24:760–765.

Simmons PS. Diagnostic considerations in breast disorders of children and adolescents. *Obstet Gynecol Clin North Am* 1992;19:91–102.

Simmons RM, Cance WG, Iacicca MV. A giant juvenile fibroadenoma in a 12-year-old girl: a case for breast conservation. *Breast J* 2000;6:418.

Singh O, Singh Gupta S, Upadhyaya VD, et al. Cystic lymphangioma of the breast in a 6-year-old boy. *J Pediatr Surg* 2009;44:2015–2018.

Soto L, Jie T, Saltzman DA. Giant cell fibroblastoma of the breast in a child—a case report and review of the literature. *J Pediatr Surg* 2004;39:229–230.

Vergier B, Torjani M, de-Mascarel I, et al. Metastases to the breast: differential diagnosis from primary breast carcinoma. *J Surg Oncol* 1991;48:112–116.

Wadie GM, Banever GT, Moriarty KP, et al. Ductal carcinoma in situ in a 16 year old adolescent boy with gynecomastia: a case report. *J Pediatr Surg* 2005;40:1349–1353.

West KW, Rescorla FJ, Sherer LR, et al. Diagnosis and treatment of symptomatic breast masses in the pediatric population. *J Pediatr Surg* 1995;30:182–186.

# Pectus Excavatum

# CHAPTER 17

*Frazier W. Frantz, Michael J. Goretsky, and
Robert C. Shamberger*

## KEY POINTS

1. Surgical repair of pectus excavatum is indicated for patients with a severe pectus deformity and associated physiologic impairment.

2. Cardiorespiratory impairment associated with severe pectus excavatum has been characterized and measured by pulmonary function testing, morphologic and functional echocardiographic assessment, cardiovascular magnetic resonance imaging (CMR), and incremental exercise testing.

3. Relief of cardiac compression after pectus repair is associated with increased stroke volumes and subsequent improvements in exercise capacity and cardiovascular performance.

4. The optimal timing for pectus excavatum repair appears to be 10 to 14 years of age, when the chest wall is still malleable. Repairs done in this age range are associated with a low incidence of recurrent pectus excavatum.

5. The Nuss procedure is now used for the majority of primary pectus excavatum repairs.

6. Open repair is used primarily for patients with severe asymmetry of the chest wall, mixed pectus deformities, or if there are objections to having a substernal bar in place for 2 to 3 years.

7. Both the Nuss procedure and open repair methods provide excellent results with low complication and recurrence rates.

## INTRODUCTION

Pectus excavatum is a depression of the sternum and lower costal cartilages. The depression can appear quite deep and the condition is commonly referred to as "funnel chest." The most common deformity of the anterior chest wall, pectus excavatum is estimated to occur in 1 in 500 to 1000 children and is much more common in males. While pectus excavatum is usually noted at birth or within the first year of life, it often worsens during the growth spurts that occur during late childhood or adolescence.

## PATHOPHYSIOLOGY

The etiology of pectus excavatum remains unknown. Early investigators attributed its development to an abnormality of the diaphragm, but there has been little evidence to support this theory except for the reported occurrence of pectus excavatum in patients with a congenital diaphragmatic hernia. The higher prevalence of pectus excavatum in patients with conditions such as Marfan syndrome has focused attention on defects in collagen formation as a potential etiology. In addition, the incidence of pectus deformities among members of the same family has been reported as high as 40%, suggesting a potential genetic link. Scoliosis has been identified in 26% of patients recently diagnosed with pectus excavatum.

As a structural abnormality of the chest wall, pectus excavatum potentially has a negative impact on the normal mechanics of the respiratory muscles and can limit complete expansion of the heart and lungs by compressing these structures in the thoracic cavity. If it does, this functional impairment could manifest as symptoms of cardiorespiratory insufficiency.

Infants and young children with pectus excavatum rarely have symptoms, but many older children do develop symptoms, particularly in association with exercise. Exercise intolerance is the most common symptom and is considered to result from the inability to increase minute ventilation and/or the inability to increase cardiac output in the setting of increased metabolic demands. Other symptoms include chest pain at the site of the deformity, shortness of breath, palpitations, and, rarely, syncope.

Some authors have stated that pectus excavatum does not cause cardiovascular or pulmonary impairment, relegating cardiopulmonary symptoms to psychological effects associated with the deformity. This opinion contrasts, however, with the general clinical impression that many patients have increased stamina following surgical repair. A multitude of clinical studies investigating pulmonary and cardiac function in patients with pectus excavatum have been undertaken to identify and quantify potential physiologic impairment in affected patients. Historically, these studies have produced inconsistent results.

More recently, the use of meta-analysis has facilitated statistical analysis of data from original series that were difficult to interpret individually due to small sample size and large variances within each study. The increase in referrals for pectus excavatum repair since the introduction of the Nuss procedure has provided larger patient series for analysis. In addition, newer technologies have made possible more objective and precise characterization of the cardiovascular structure and function in this patient population. The combination of these factors has helped to better define the potential physiologic impairment present in patients with pectus excavatum and to appreciate the improvements in cardiovascular function that can occur because of pectus repair.

In general, abnormalities in pulmonary function produced by pectus excavatum are difficult to demonstrate because of the wide range of normal pulmonary function parameters, which heavily depend on both physical training and body habitus. Studies of pulmonary function at rest in patients with pectus excavatum, using plethysmography to measure lung volumes and spirometry to measure airway function, have demonstrated varied patterns of obstructive and/or restrictive impairment in almost half of the patients studied. Analysis of pulmonary function studies in over 800 patients with pectus excavatum who have presented for surgical repair to the Children's Hospital of The King's Daughters in Norfolk, VA, demonstrated mean decreases of 15% below predicted values for forced vital capacity (FVC), forced expiratory volume at 1 second of expiration ($FEV_1$), and forced expiratory flow, midexpiratory phase ($FEF_{25\%-75\%}$). Similar results were observed in 327 patients, aged 8 to 21 years, enrolled in a multicenter study of pectus excavatum. Studies from Lawson, Kelly, and Sigalet and associates comparing pulmonary function tests before Nuss repair and after bar removal in pectus patients have demonstrated small but significant improvements in pulmonary function. The body of literature on postoperative pulmonary function studies, however, has shown variable results, ranging from mild improvement to deterioration in measured parameters. This inability to document consistent improvement after surgical repair in pulmonary function among patients observed to have enhanced exercise capacity has focused attention on cardiovascular changes brought about by pectus repair as the principal contributors to enhanced cardiorespiratory function.

Cardiac impairment from pectus excavatum has been extensively evaluated. Early studies utilizing right heart catheterization in patients with pectus excavatum demonstrated decreased stroke volumes and cardiac outputs compared to normal subjects, as well as limited increases in stroke volume during transition from rest to exercise. More recent cardiac evaluations have employed noninvasive testing with computed tomography (CT) scanning, electrocardiography, and echocardiography. Patients evaluated with these modalities for surgical repair at Children's Hospital of The King's Daughters have been found to have a 17% incidence of mitral valve prolapse (vs 1% in the normal pediatric population) and a 16% incidence of dysrhythmias, including first-degree heart block and right bundle branch block. Utilizing transthoracic echocardiography to calculate ventricular volumes, Kowaleski and associates demonstrated significant increases in right ventricular (RV) systolic, diastolic, and stroke volumes, presumably due to the relief of sternal compression, after open pectus repair in 60 patients. Left ventricular stroke volumes were also significantly increased, but only in the patient subset with severe deformities. To overcome the potential shortcomings of transthoracic echocardiography associated with the abnormal anatomy of the anterior chest wall in pectus excavatum, Krueger and associates prospectively studied end-diastolic RV dimensions and left ventricular ejection fraction (LVEF) using intraoperative transesophageal echocardiography (TEE) before and after open surgical correction of pectus excavatum in 17 adults. As evidence of significantly improved cardiovascular function after pectus repair, significant increases were noted in RV end-diastolic diameter, area, and volume, as well as in LVEF. Similar findings have been reported by Huang and associates using intraoperative TEE in 10 patients undergoing Nuss repair to quantitate morphological and functional changes in the RV during retrosternal dissection and turning of the pectus bar (to elevate the sternum). Significant increases were demonstrated in RV volumes, as measured by maximum RV short-axis distance, and in RV systolic function, as represented by RV tricuspid annular plane systolic distance.

Most recently, Saleh and associates used CMR to compare cardiothoracic structure and function in 30 patients with pectus excavatum and 25 healthy control subjects. The CMR protocol included cardiac cine images, pulmonary artery flow quantification, time-resolved 3-dimensional (3D) contrast-enhanced MR angiography (CEMRA), and high spatial resolution CEMRA. LV (LVEF) and RV ejection fractions (RVEF), ventricular long and short dimensions, midventricle myocardial shortening, pulmonary-systemic circulation time, and pulmonary artery flow were quantified. The patients with pectus excavatum had significant reductions in the RV short axis diameter at both end-diastole and systole and an associated significant increase in RV long axis diameter at end-diastole, reflecting geometric distortion of the RV due to sternal compression. This abnormal pattern of myocardial shortening due to compression-induced changes in RV anatomy was associated with a statistically significant reduction in resting RVEF of approximately 6% (mean ± SD in pectus excavatum patients 53.9% ± 9.6% vs 60.5% ± 9.5% in controls, $P = 0.013$) in patients with pectus excavatum relative to controls, potentially mimicking restrictive RV physiology. No significant differences between patients with pectus excavatum and controls were found in LVEF, LV myocardial shortening, pulmonary-systemic circulation time, or pulmonary flow indices.

Reports of enhanced exercise performance and improved cardiovascular function after pectus repair are, perhaps, the most impressive in realizing the beneficial physiologic effects of pectus repair. Most of these have focused on the relief of cardiac compression by the sternal deformity with subsequent increase in stroke volume. Beiser and colleagues used cardiac catheterization in 6 patients and demonstrated a 38% increase in cardiac index during intense upright exercise after open pectus repair. Current evaluation techniques employ noninvasive incremental exercise testing with cycle ergometer or treadmill to a predetermined threshold and continuously measure expired fractional concentrations of oxygen and carbon dioxide ($CO_2$). Pulmonary function testing can be incorporated into this protocol. From these data, pertinent cardiorespiratory parameters, such as oxygen uptake (a measure of the amount of oxygen that can be delivered to the tissues with exercise), $CO_2$ output, and oxygen pulse (an indirect measure of stroke volume) can be calculated. Using this methodology, Malek and associates characterized the cardiovascular impairment in 21 patients with pectus excavatum, demonstrating, in comparison to reference values, significantly lower maximum oxygen uptake (76% predicted) and oxygen pulse (86% predicted) during maximal exercise testing. Haller and associates tested 15 patients with pectus excavatum before and 6 months after open pectus repair, along with 6 healthy control subjects, and observed increased exercise tolerance in 66% of patients and significantly higher oxygen pulse during exercise. Similarly, Sigalet and associates conducted exercise testing in 26 patients with pectus excavatum before and at least 3 months after Nuss bar removal and noted significant improvements in oxygen pulse (82.5% vs 77.1% predicted) and maximum oxygen uptake (76.6% vs 70.8% predicted). Using meta-analysis, Malek and associates reviewed quantitative measures of preoperative and postoperative cardiovascular function compiled from 169 pectus excavatum patients in 8 studies that met predetermined inclusion criteria. The principal finding was that average cardiovascular function increased by greater than one-half standard deviation following the surgical repair of pectus excavatum.

## PREOPERATIVE ASSESSMENT

Among the many published methods of scoring the severity of the sternal depression, those of Haller have received the greatest acceptance. Using measurements obtained from CT (Fig. 17-1), Haller calculated an index by dividing the transverse breadth of the chest by the narrowest sternovertebral distance. An index greater than 3.25 generally is considered severe. The measurements for the index can also be reliably obtained from a routine chest radiograph.

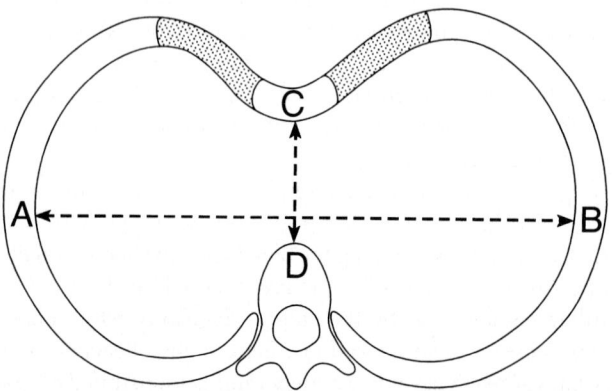

**FIGURE 17-1** Schematic depiction of a computed tomography image of the chest demonstrates the method of obtaining measurements for the Haller index. (A, B) The breadth of the chest is divided by the narrowest sternovertebral distance (C, D) to obtain the index (A-B/C-D). Ratios of >3.25 are considered to represent a significant depression.

While the Haller index provides a basis for defining the severity of the deformity, clinical evidence of physiologic impairment combined with the results of CT imaging and cardiopulmonary testing often provides a more comprehensive assessment for decisions regarding surgical intervention. A proposed evaluation and treatment algorithm is depicted in Fig. 17-2. In addition to static pulmonary function testing and plethysmography, it is often useful to obtain workload evaluations to define the degree of impairment in cardiopulmonary output in a child being assessed for surgical repair.

## SURGICAL REPAIR

Numerous methods of surgical repair have been proposed and used. The continued use of multiple techniques bespeaks the failure to achieve uniformly superior results by any one method. All techniques have some risk of recurrence. Selection of an approach must be based not only on the ultimate results and long-term recurrence rates, but also on the potential complications intrinsic to the procedure. A technique that achieves safe, satisfactory correction of pectus excavatum with total preservation of the perichondrial sheaths of the costal cartilage, preservation of the intercostal muscle bundles, and anterior fixation of the sternum was reported by Baronofsky in 1957 and by Welch in 1958. This technique has been used in more than 700 cases at Children's Hospital Boston over the past 3 decades.

In 1997, Nuss described minimally invasive pectus excavatum repair by placing a convex steel bar beneath the sternum and anterior to the heart through lateral thoracic incisions to elevate the sternum. Since this initial report, the Nuss procedure has been performed in more than 1400 patients at Children's Hospital of The King's Daughters alone. Numerous modifications have optimized the safety and effectiveness of the technique. These improvements include (1) routine use of thoracoscopy with $CO_2$ insufflation for better visualization and safety and (2) pectus bar stabilization and fixation using both an attached metal stabilizer on the lateral bar and pericostal suturing around the bar and the underlying ribs medially to minimize postoperative bar displacement.

Two other types of repair should be mentioned. Haller and associates use a 3-point "tripod" fixation by placing an osteotomy and creating oblique chondrotomies of the upper costal cartilages angled from anteromedial to posterolateral. The medial portion of the costal cartilage attached to the sternum can then be laid on the lateral portion of the cartilage attached to the rib to help support the sternum anteriorly.

A "sternal turnover" technique was proposed by Judet and by Jung in the French literature. This technique has been employed primarily by Wada, who reported a large series from Japan. The "sternal turnover" technique essentially uses a "free graft" of the sternum that is rotated 180° and secured to the costal cartilages. This technique is a radical approach for children with pectus excavatum, considering the major complications reported when infection occurs and the generally successful alternatives available.

The majority of repairs now rely on the Nuss technique. Open repair is used primarily for patients with severe

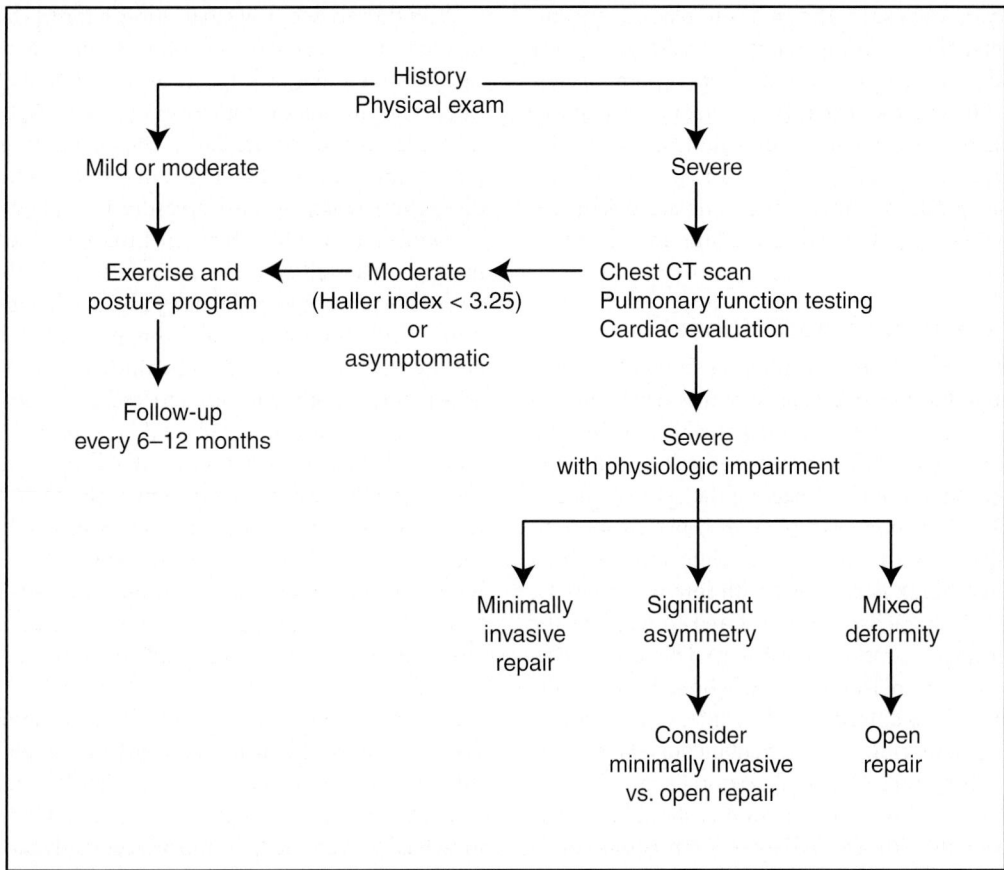

**FIGURE 17-2** Evaluation and treatment algorithm for primary repair of pectus excavatum.

asymmetry of the chest wall (particularly when it involves the lower "floating" ribs), mixed pectus deformities (elements of both excavatum and carinatum), or for individuals who do not wish to have the bar in place for 2 to 3 years. These approaches are described in depth in this chapter.

## Nuss Procedure

Minimally invasive pectus repair is indicated for patients with a severe pectus excavatum deformity and associated physiologic impairment. Specific inclusion criteria include 2 or more of the following:

1. CT index greater than 3.25 with associated cardiac or pulmonary compression;

2. pulmonary function studies demonstrating restrictive and/or obstructive impairment;

3. cardiology evaluation demonstrating cardiac compression, displacement, mitral valve prolapse, murmurs, or conduction abnormalities; and

4. documentation of progression of the deformity with advancing age in association with development of or worsening of physiologic symptoms (ie, shortness of breath, lack of endurance, exercise intolerance, palpitations, and chest pain).

The optimal timing for minimally invasive repair appears to be 10 to 14 years of age while the chest wall is still malleable. Surgery in these children is associated with a shorter recovery and ensures that support from the pectus bar is provided during the adolescent growth spurt. Repair at a younger age is certainly appropriate in the setting of severe cardiac or pulmonary compression with associated clinical signs of physiologic impairment. Bars placed in children at younger ages are typically left in situ for longer periods of time as these children grow. Repair in postpubertal patients in characterized by a higher likelihood of requiring placement of multiple bars due to increased chest wall stiffness, but is generally well tolerated.

Prior to surgery, the patient's anterior chest wall circumference (from right to left midaxillary lines) at the level of the deepest sternal depression should be measured to approximate appropriate pectus bar length. The length selected is typically 1 to 1.5 inches shorter than this outer circumference. Any patient with a history of eczema or atopy should be skin tested for metal allergy. Those patients with positive skin tests or history of nickel allergy should have titanium bars placed. These titanium bars must be specially ordered and will arrive prebent from the manufacturer (Biomet Microfixation, Jacksonville, FL) based on measurements from the patient's chest wall and chest CT scan.

## Surgical Technique

The patient is placed in the supine position with both arms abducted to expose the lateral chest wall on each side. A single dose of cefazolin is administered. After prepping, important landmarks to identify on the anterior chest wall include the deepest point of the sternal deformity and the lateral ridge of the deformity on each side. The goal is to place the pectus bar in a horizontal plane encompassing the intercostal spaces at the pectus ridge on each side and the deepest point of sternal depression. Bilateral thoracic incisions are planned at this level. If multiple bar placement is planned, it may be necessary to make separate thoracic incisions for each bar placed. In female patients, inframammary incisions are performed because they provide good access to the anterior chest wall and enhanced cosmesis.

## Creation of the Transthoracic Tunnel

The first step of the repair process entails creation of a tunnel extending through the subcutaneous/submuscular tissues on one side of the chest, beneath the medial ribs and sternum in the intrathoracic and mediastinal spaces, and out through the subcutaneous/submuscular tissues on the opposite side of the chest (Fig. 17-3). A thoracoscopic port is placed approximately 2 interspaces below the planned right thoracic incision, and pneumothorax is achieved with low-pressure $CO_2$ insufflation. A 30° thoracoscope is inserted to confirm the internal anatomy in preparation for substernal dissection. Lateral transverse thoracic incisions are made on each side of the chest wall from mid- to anterior-axillary lines and advanced medially to the pectus ridge in a subcutaneous plane using blunt and sharp dissection. If there is pectoralis muscle present at the level of this dissection, the tunnel should be made beneath it. In patients with sternal depression predominantly involving the upper chest, care should be taken not to create the tunnel too high on the chest wall because bar placement at this site could interfere with the nerves and vessels of the axilla and/or cause chronic pain.

With thoracoscopic visualization, a tonsil clamp is inserted through the subcutaneous tunnel on the right side and into the pleural space to create a soft tissue defect in the intercostal muscles (thoracostomy). It is important that this defect is positioned medial to the pectus ridge because bar placement lateral to this ridge can result in intercostal muscle disruption when upward pressure is applied by the pectus introducer, and subsequent bar instability. The pectus introducer is inserted into the tunnel through this defect and, with thoracoscopic guidance, advanced beneath the sternum. While upward pressure is applied by the introducer to elevate the sternum, the blunt tip dissects the pericardium and pleura off the sternum to create a substernal tunnel. The tip of the introducer should be kept in view during the entire substernal dissection to avoid injury to the heart. If the sternal depression is too deep or the chest wall is too stiff to allow visualization of the introducer tip during this dissection, external elevation of the sternum can be achieved with mechanical retraction introduced via a subxiphoid incision. The surgeon's finger can be inserted into the subxiphoid space and used to manually guide the introducer tip beneath the sternum.

Bilateral thoracoscopy should be considered to optimize visualization of the displaced heart in the left chest. During this process, the EKG monitor is closely watched to detect evidence of arrhythmia or injury pattern. Once the mediastinum has been crossed, the introducer is advanced through the intercostal muscles of the left chest medial to the pectus ridge and into the subcutaneous/submuscular tunnel on that side. The edges of the introducer are then grasped by the surgeon and assistant and elevated to correct the sternal depression.

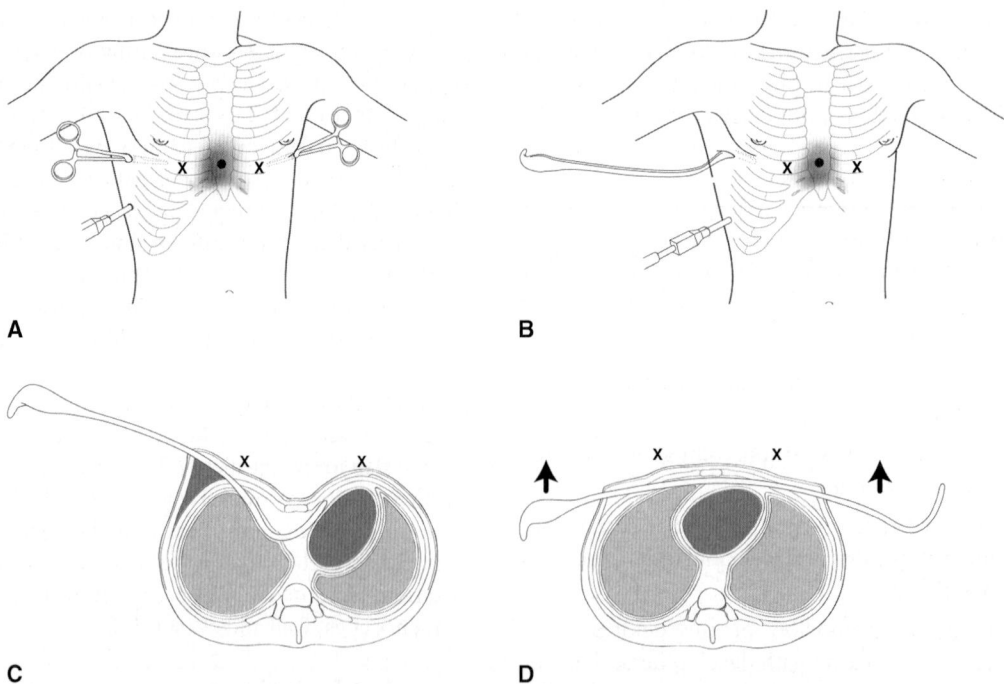

**FIGURE 17-3** Nuss procedure, creation of the transthoracic tunnel. **A.** Bilateral subcutaneous tunnels are created to pectus ridge (X) on each side in the horizontal plane of deepest sternal depression (•). With thoracoscopic visualization, a tonsil clamp is inserted through intercostal space medial to pectus ridge and into right pleural space. **B.** The pectus introducer is advanced through the tunnel and right intercostal defect. **C.** Creation of substernal tunnel with the pectus introducer. **D.** Introducer is advanced through intercostal space medial to the left pectus ridge. Upward traction is placed on the introducer to stretch intercostal muscles.

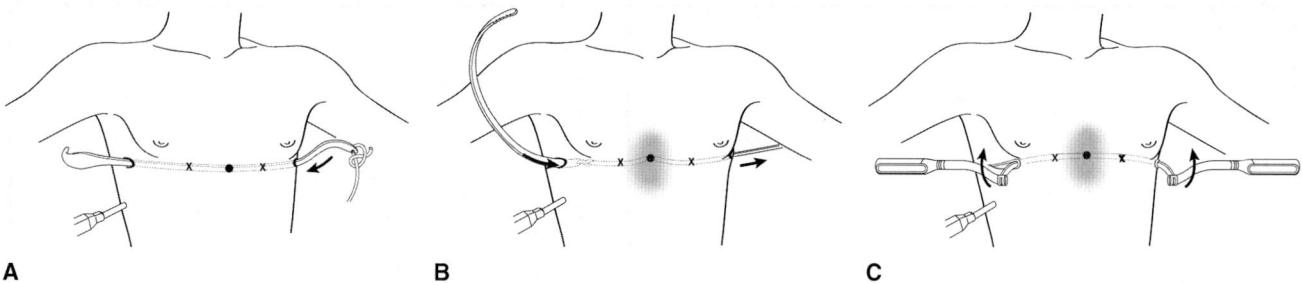

**FIGURE 17-4** Pectus bar insertion. **A.** Umbilical tape is advanced into the transthoracic tunnel via withdrawal of the introducer. **B.** The bent pectus bar is secured to the umbilical tape and pulled through the tunnel with the convexity oriented posteriorly. **C.** The pectus bar is rotated 180° with bar flippers.

Once the introducer is in place in the transthoracic tunnel, the effectiveness of single bar placement can be judged visually and is indicated by complete correction of the pectus excavatum deformity on the chest wall and complete flattening of the sternum visualized thoracoscopically. If residual depression remains, creation of a second transthoracic tunnel in preparation for multiple bar placement can be undertaken at this time. Alternatively, the surgeon can proceed with pectus bar placement, and creation of a second tunnel, if necessary, can proceed after the first bar is in place. When it is obvious preoperatively that multiple bar placement will be necessary due to the nature or severity of the pectus deformity, the more cephalad transthoracic tunnel, which is usually less depressed, should be created first. The upper introducer can then be left in place to provide sternal elevation and facilitate safer dissection of the lower tunnel at the deepest point of sternal depression.

### Pectus Bar Insertion

Once complete correction of the pectus deformity has been visualized with the introducer in place, preparations are made for pectus bar insertion (Fig. 17-4). A bar of appropriate length is bent into an optimal configuration to match the patient's chest wall contour. A semicircular shape with a relatively short, flat central apex (to support the sternum) flanked by gentle, convex curves on each side is used most commonly. Bars bent on the ends only with a rectangular configuration should be avoided because they typically result in undercorrection of the deformity.

An umbilical tape is secured through the eyelet at the tip of the introducer. Under thoracoscopic visualization, the introducer is withdrawn, and the umbilical tape is deposited in the tunnel and then secured to the pectus bar. Using thoracoscopic guidance and gentle traction on the tape, the bar is pulled into the right pleural space and through the tunnel in a convex configuration. The umbilical tape is removed, and the bar is rotated 180° using bar flippers applied on each side of the bar. With the bar in place, the sides of the pectus bar should rest comfortably against the lateral ribs and chest wall musculature. If adjustments to the bar configuration are necessary, the bar can be reflipped 180°, remodeled, and returned to final configuration without removing the bar from the tunnel.

Immediate correction of the pectus deformity should be observed after bar insertion. If there is evidence of residual sternal depression on the external chest wall or thoracoscopic visualization, placement of a second substernal bar should be undertaken.

Single bar placement inferior to the body of the sternum should be avoided. Even if this is the deepest point of depression and results in immediate correction of the deformity after bar placement, this location is unstable and carries a higher risk of bar displacement. A bar placed inferior to the sternal body (ie, subxiphoid) in combination with a second bar placed under the bony sternum is a much more stable configuration.

### Bar Stabilization and Fixation

The final step of repair is bar stabilization and fixation to the chest wall to minimize the risk of bar displacement (Fig. 17-5). The current technique favored by the authors utilizes 3-point fixation, with lateral fixation provided by securing a metal rectangular stabilizer to one end of the bar (usually on the left) and placing multiple interrupted absorbable sutures through the holes in the stabilizer and bar on both sides for attachment to the underlying fascia and periosteum. Medial fixation involves attachment of the bar to underlying ribs using pericostal polydioxanone sutures (PDS) placed with the Endoclose® needle (Covidien, Norwalk, CT) through the lateral thoracic incision under thoracoscopic guidance. When multiple bars are placed, the stabilizers are typically placed on opposite sides of the chest wall to avoid overlap of the hardware on one side. Single stabilizer placement is preferred to prevent "pinching" of the ribs during future chest wall growth.

Once the pericostal sutures have been placed around the pectus bar and underlying ribs, there is no further need for thoracoscopy, and attention can be focused to evacuation of the pneumothorax. This is accomplished by cutting the insufflation tubing and placing the end of the tube under water seal. The evacuation of $CO_2$ is facilitated by placing the patient in the Trendelenburg position with the right side elevated and administering a series of large positive pressure breaths. As the soft tissues and skin incisions are closed, progressive decrease and eventual cessation of bubbling through the tubing should be observed. The trocar can then be removed, and a chest x-ray is obtained to exclude the presence of residual pneumothorax. If bubbling persists, a chest tube should be inserted and secured in place.

### Postoperative Care

The central focus of postoperative care after minimally invasive pectus repair is pain control and pulmonary toilet.

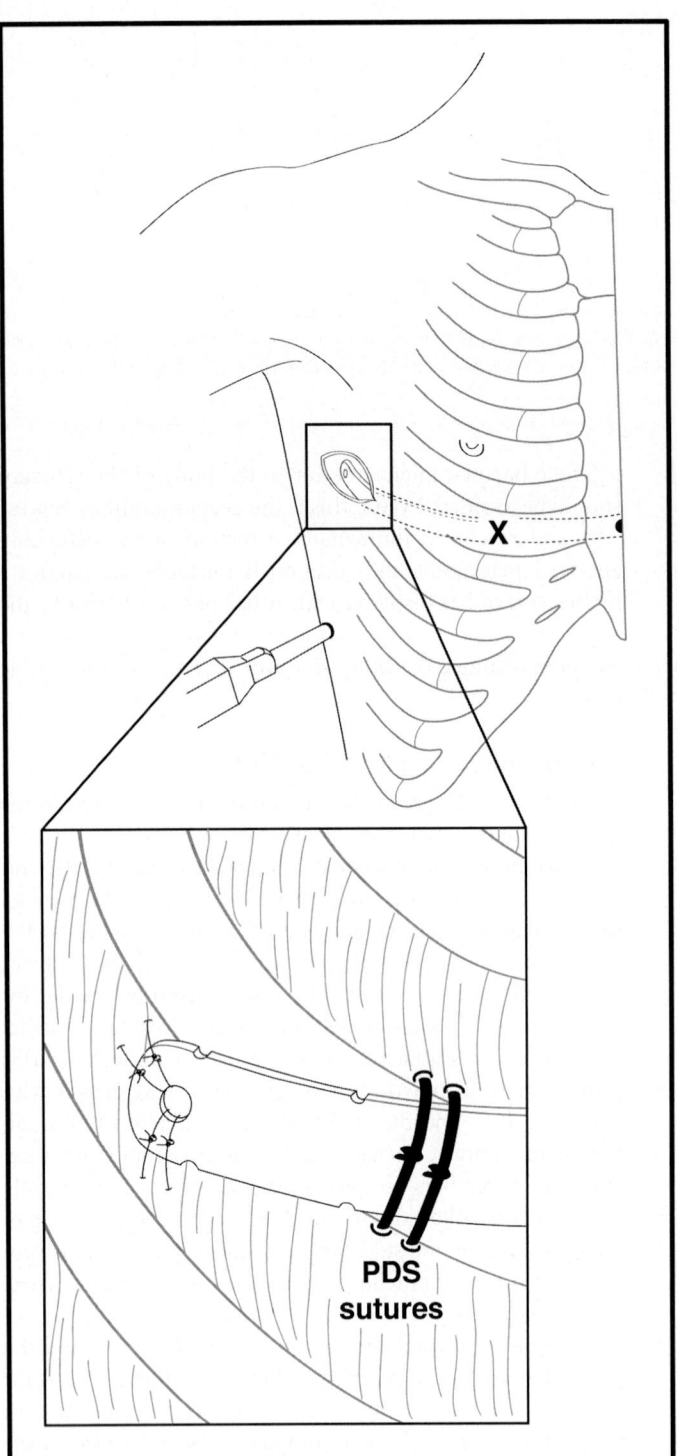
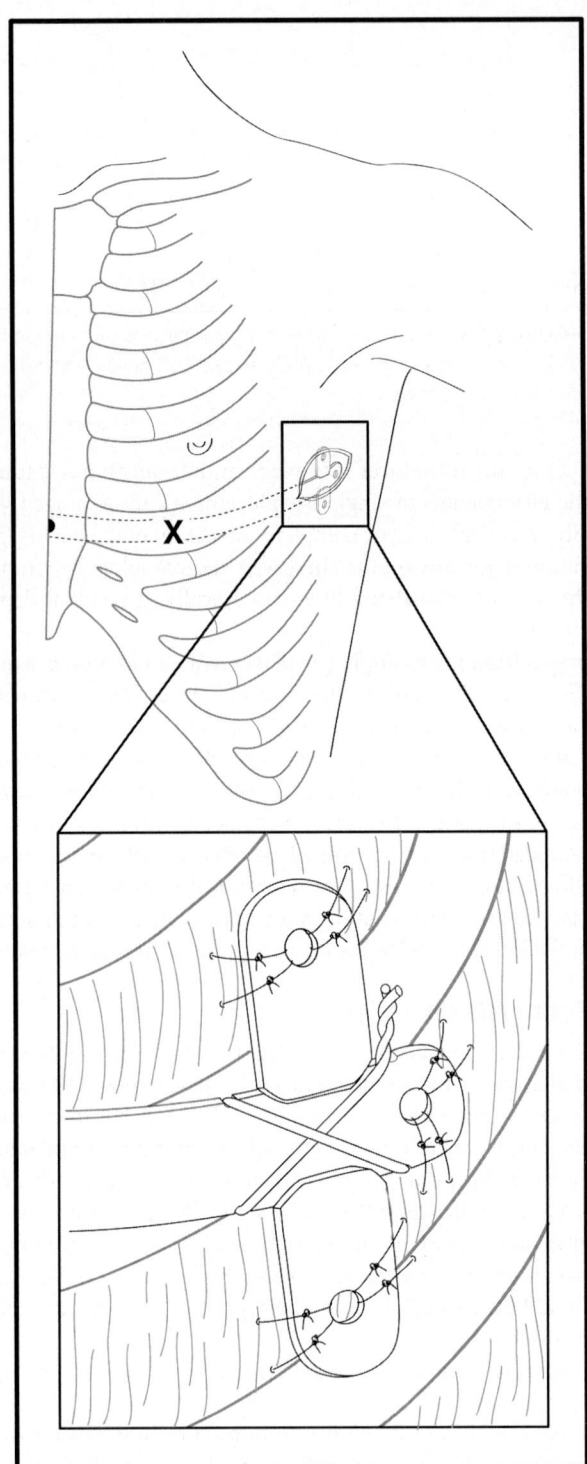

**FIGURE 17-5** Bar stabilization and fixation. The left-sided stabilizer is secured to the bar with # 3 surgical steel wire. The right side of the bar is secured with pericostal sutures of 0 or 1 polydioxanone sutures (PDS). The lateral bar is secured with absorbable sutures placed through holes in the bar and stabilizer.

The authors' current pain management regimen includes a combination of patient-controlled analgesia (PCA) with narcotic drugs, intravenous ketorolac, and muscle relaxants. Most recently, local anesthetic infusion has been continuously administered in a regional manner via bilateral thoracic On-Q® catheters (I-Flow Corporation, Lake Forest, CA). These catheters are typically placed intraoperatively and loaded prior to the initiation of pectus repair. They will infuse for 4 days postoperatively. Perioperative antibiotics are continued for 24 hours. Over the typical 4- to 5-day in-hospital postoperative recovery, patients are transitioned from intravenous to oral medications, with the expectation that they will require narcotics for an additional 2 weeks.

Physical activity is restricted after repair to minimize the risk of bar displacement. Patients are able to resume aerobic activities at 6 weeks and competitive sports at 3 months postrepair. Most patients who attend school can return in 2 to 3 weeks.

## Bar Removal

The pectus bars should remain in the chest for 2 to 4 years after repair to ensure permanent remodeling of the chest wall (Fig. 17-6). The far end of this range is appropriate for younger patients and those actively undergoing pubertal growth.

Bar removal is typically undertaken as an outpatient procedure. After induction of general anesthesia, the patient is positioned supine with both arms abducted to expose the lateral chest wall. Ideally, the previously placed hardware is palpable. If it is not, and particularly if the patient has grown considerably since bar placement, it is helpful to have fluoroscopy available to help localize the position of the bar. Positive pressure ventilation with positive end-expiratory pressure (PEEP) is maintained throughout the procedure to minimize the chance of developing a pneumothorax during the exposure and removal of the bar. Incisions through previous incision sites are preferred, and both sides of the bar should be exposed and mobilized. In some cases, heterotopic calcifications will have formed around the bar and may require dissection with osteotomes to free the bar from this encasement. The wire attaching the stabilizer and bar should be cut and removed. Both ends of the bar should be straightened using the bar flippers or Malti bender. The stabilizer can be disengaged from the bar at this point. The bar is then slowly removed with traction, using a bone hook inserted through the hole in the lateral bar. Close attention is paid to the EKG

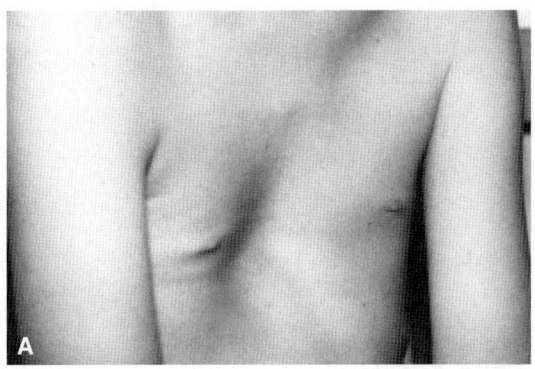

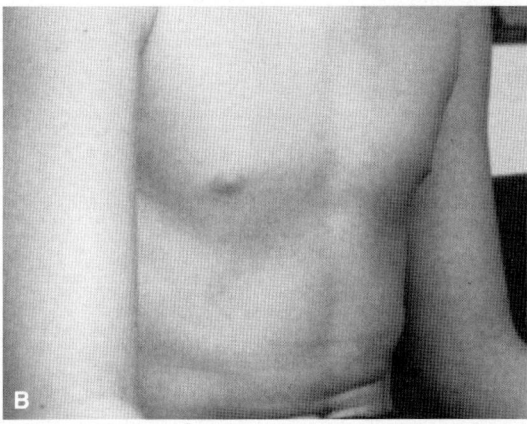

**FIGURE 17-6** **A.** A preoperative photograph of a 7-year-old-boy prior to pectus excavatum repair at age 9 years. **B.** A postoperative photograph obtained 4 years after the surgery and 1 year after removal of the bar. (Reproduced with permission from *Donald Nuss, Children's Hospital of The King's Daughters, Norfolk, VA*.)

monitor during this process. Ideally, the bar is removed via the right chest incision to minimize the bar length that must pass anterior to the heart during removal. After wound closure, a chest x-ray is typically obtained in the recovery room.

## Open Surgical Repair

One dose of cefazolin is administered immediately prior to surgery. A transverse incision is made below and well within the nipple lines. In females, particular attention is taken to place the incision within the projected inframammary crease, thus avoiding the potential complication of a breast deformity. Skin flaps are mobilized using electrocautery, primarily in the midline to the angle of Louis superiorly and to the xiphoid inferiorly (Fig. 17-7). Pectoral muscle flaps are elevated off the sternum and costal cartilages, preserving the entire pectoralis major and portions of the pectoralis minor muscle in the flap. This plane is defined by identifying the areolar plane just anterior to the costal cartilages and lateral to their junction with the sternum. An empty knife handle is used to develop this plane, and the muscle flap is then retracted anteriorly with a small right-angle retractor. Muscle dissection and elevation is carried to the costochondral junctions of the third to fifth ribs. Particular attention is paid to avoid injury to the intercostal bundles, which would result in significant bleeding.

Subperichondrial resection of the costal cartilages with specially designed Welch perichondrial elevators is performed by removing the third, fourth, and fifth cartilages but preserving the costochondral junctions. Occasionally the second costal cartilages are involved, particularly in older patients. Segments of the sixth and seventh costal cartilages are resected to the point where they flatten to join the costal arch, which is generally equal in length to the fourth and fifth cartilages. Familiarity with the cross-sectional shape of the medial ends of the costal cartilages facilitates their removal. The second and third cartilages are broad and flat, the fourth and fifth are circular, and the sixth and seventh are narrow and deep at their junction with the sternum.

Two parallel transverse sternal osteotomies, extending through the anterior cortex, are created using a Hall air drill (Zimmer USA, Inc, Warsaw, IN). These are placed 2 to 4 mm apart at the point where the sternum is displaced posteriorly. A short segment of the anterior cortex is then removed along with the underlying cancellous bone. This allows the sternum to be brought forward. The posterior table of the sternum is fractured behind the osteotomy by anterior elevation of the sternum. The osteotomy must be of adequate size to allow the sternum to come forward easily.

Welch would divide the rectus muscle from the tip of the sternum with electrocautery. The authors currently avoid this division because an unsightly depression at the tip of the sternum can result. If strut fixation is used, division of the rectus muscle is generally not required unless the xiphoid is protruding acutely forward. Welch would then close the sternal osteotomy with nonabsorbable sutures intentionally overcorrecting the position of the sternum 30° to 35°. While this is successful in younger children, the extent of correction is limited in older patients, leading the authors to routinely use strut fixation in these cases.

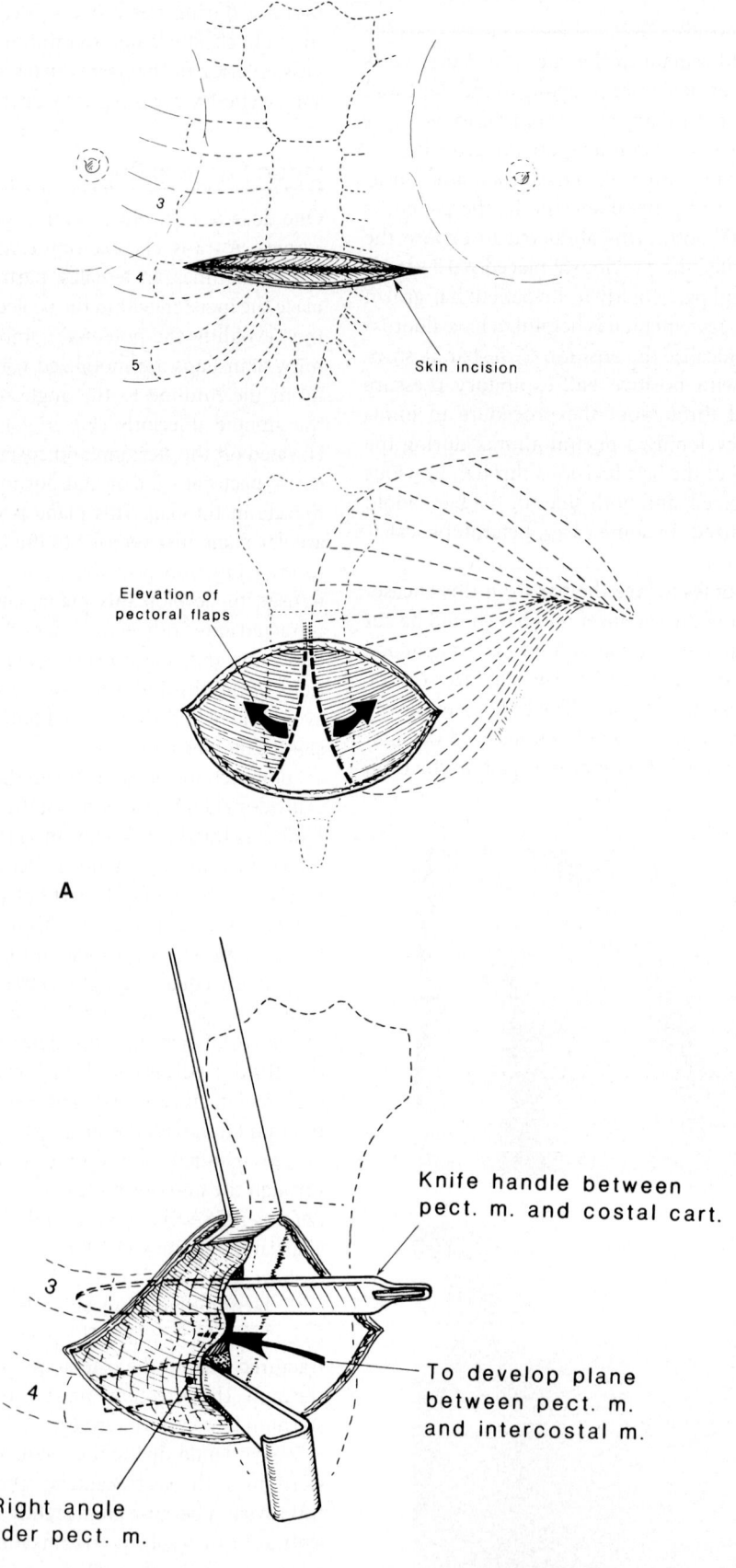

**FIGURE 17-7** "Open" pectus excavation repair. **A.** A transverse incision is placed below and well within the nipple lines at the site of the future inframammary crease. The pectoralis major muscle is elevated from the sternum along with portions of the pectoralis minor and serratus anterior bundles. **B.** The correct plane of dissection of the pectoral muscle flap is defined by passing an empty knife handle directly anterior to a costal cartilage after the medial aspect of the muscle is elevated with electrocautery. The knife handle is then replaced with a right-angled retractor, which is pulled anteriorly. The process is then repeated anterior to an adjoining costal cartilage. Anterior distraction of the muscles during the dissection facilitates identification of the avascular areolar plane and avoids entry into the intercostal muscle bundles.

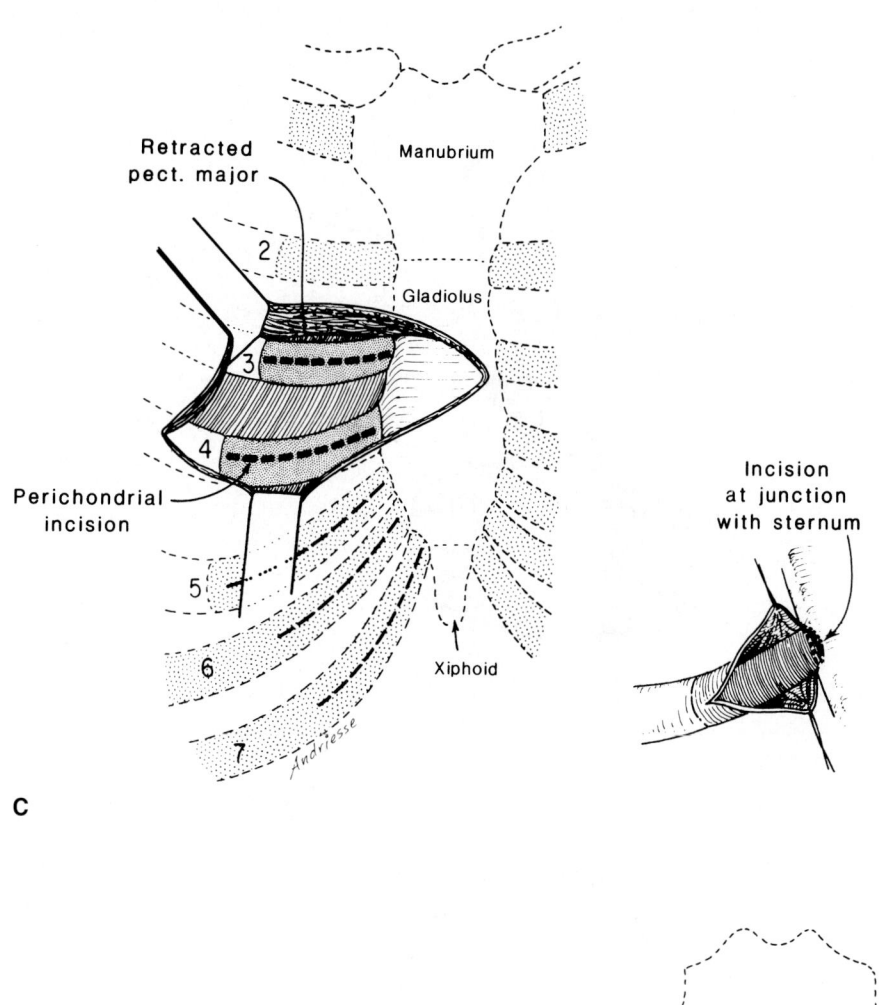

C

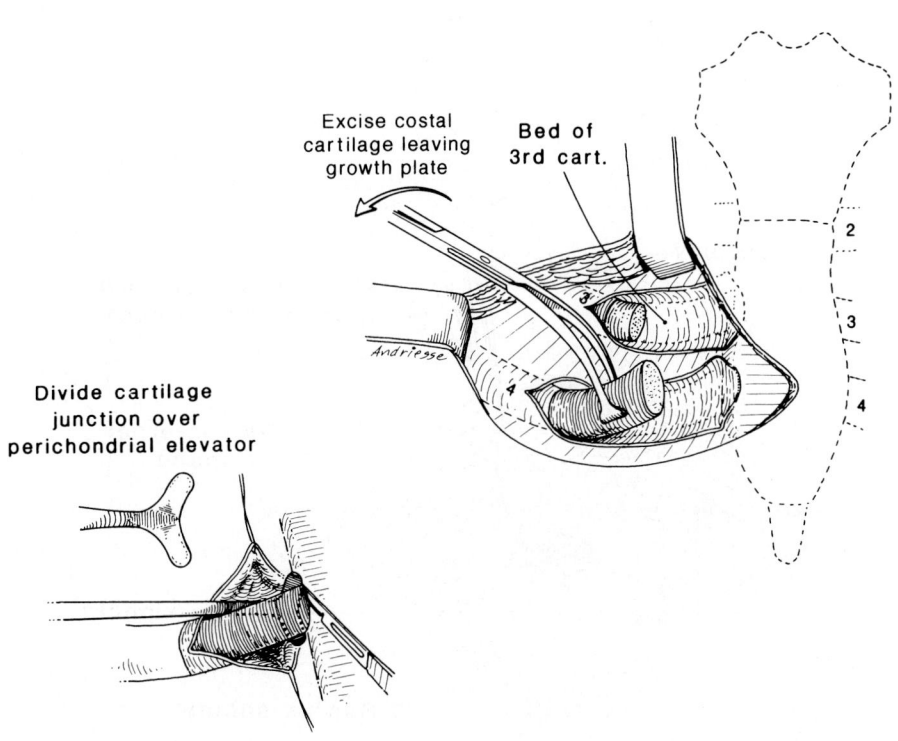

D

**FIGURE 17-7** (*Continued*) **C.** Subperichondrial resection of the costal cartilages is achieved by incising the perichondrium anteriorly. It is then dissected away from the costal cartilages in the bloodless plane between the perichondrium and the costal cartilage. Cutting back the perichondrium 90° in each direction at its junction with the sternum (*inset*) facilitates visualization of the back wall of the costal cartilage. **D.** The cartilages are divided at the junction of the sternum with a knife with a Welch perichondrial elevator held posteriorly to elevate the cartilage and protect the mediastinum (*inset*). The divided cartilage can then be held with an Allis clamp, elevated, and divided laterally, preserving the costochondral junction with a segment of costal cartilage.

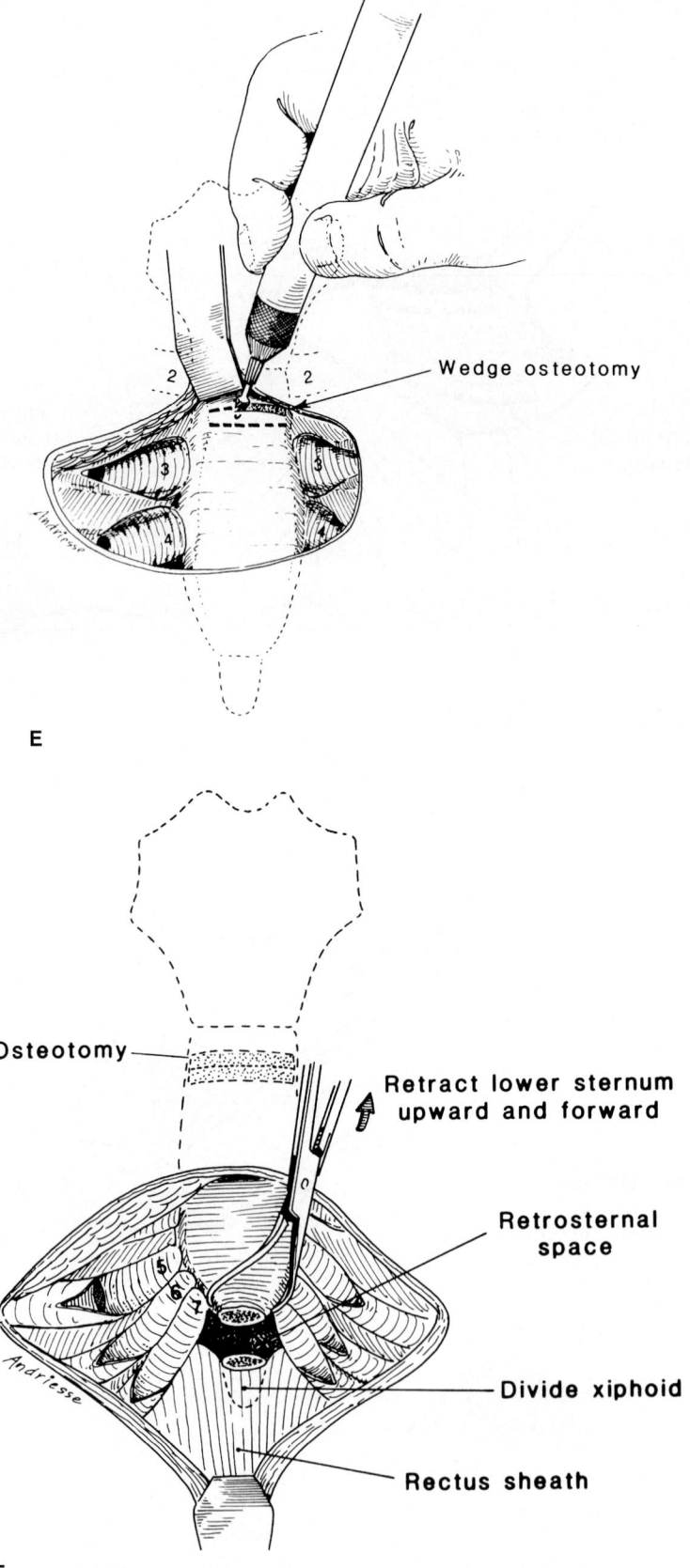

E

F

**FIGURE 17-7** (*Continued*) **E.** A sternal osteotomy is created above the level of the last deformed cartilage and the posterior angulation of the sternum, generally the third cartilage but occasionally the second. Two transverse sternal osteotomies are created through the anterior cortex with a Hall air drill 2 to 4 mm apart. **F.** The base of the sternum and the rectus muscle flap are elevated with 2 towel clips, and the xiphoid is divided from the sternum with electrocautery. This procedure allows entry into the retrosternal space. This step is not necessary when a retrosternal strut is used. Preservation of the attachment of the perichondrial sheaths and xiphoid avoids an unsightly depression that can occur below the sternum.

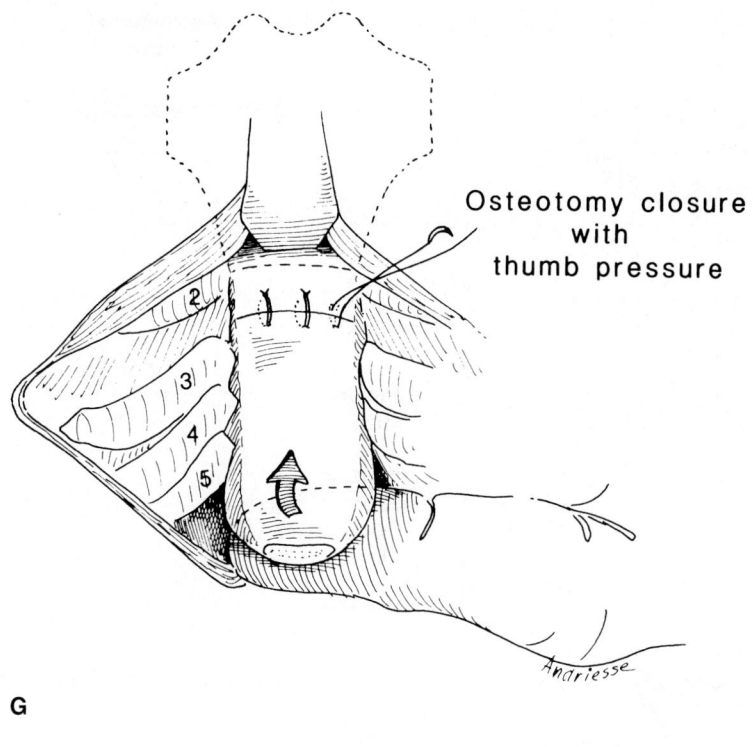

Osteotomy closure
with
thumb pressure

G

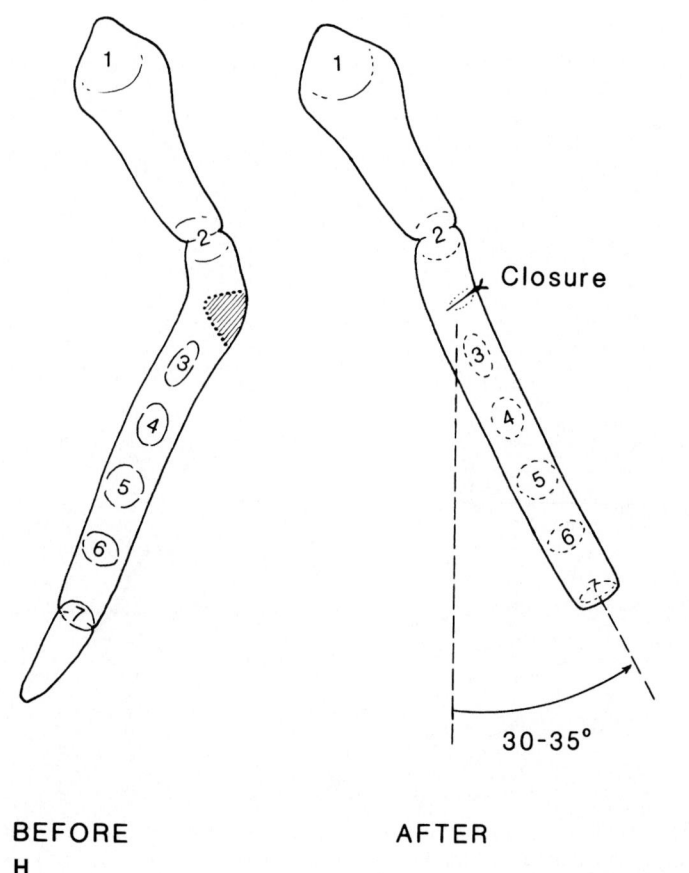

Closure

30-35°

BEFORE                    AFTER
H

**FIGURE 17-7** (*Continued*) **G.** With the nonstrut method the osteotomy is closed with several heavy, nonabsorbable sutures as the sternum is elevated by the assistant. **H.** Correction of the abnormal position of the sternum is achieved by the creation of a wedge-shaped osteotomy that is then closed, bringing the sternum anteriorly into an overcorrected position.

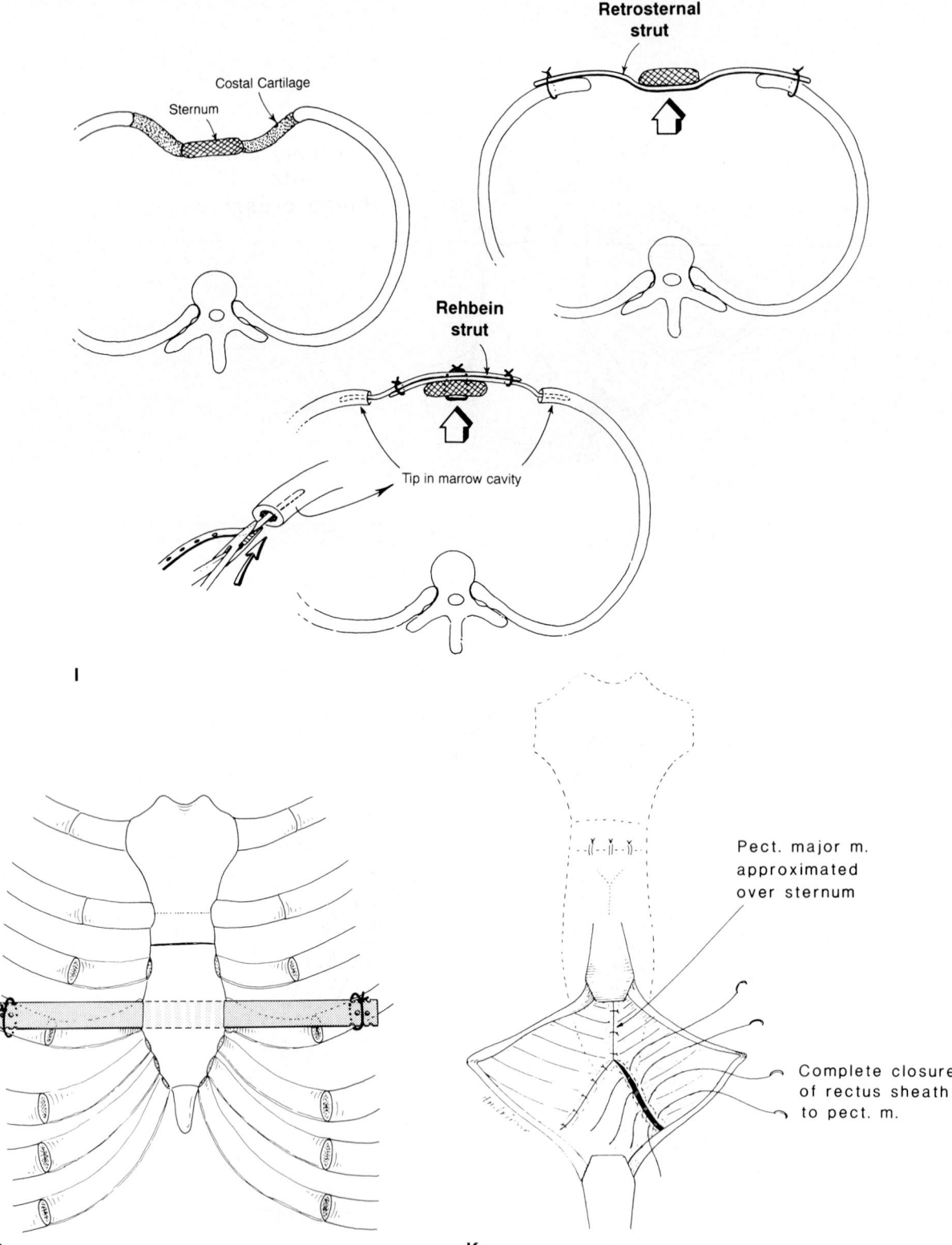

**FIGURE 17-7** (*Continued*) **I.** The use of both retrosternal struts and Rehbein struts (David Scott Company, Framingham, MA). The Rehbein struts are inserted into the marrow cavity (*inset*) of the third or fourth rib and are then joined to each other medially to create a metal arch anterior to the sternum. The sternum is sewn to the arch to secure it in its new forward position. The retrosternal strut (V. Mueller, Baxter Operating Room Division, McGraw Park, IL) is placed behind the sternum and is secured to the rib ends laterally to prevent migration. **J.** Anterior depiction of the retrosternal struts. The perichondrial sheath to either the third or fourth rib is divided from its junction with the sternum, and the retrosternal space is bluntly dissected to allow passage of the strut behind the sternum. It is secured with 2 pericostal sutures laterally to prevent migration. Division of the perichondrial sheath immediately adjacent to the sternum avoids injury to the internal mammary vessels, which are more lateral. **K.** The pectoral muscle flaps are secured to the midline of the sternum, advancing the flaps to obtain coverage of the entire sternum. The rectus muscle flap is then joined to the pectoral muscle flaps. (A–H and K reproduced with permission from *Shamberger RC, Welch KJ. J Pediatr Surg 1988;23:615–622.* I and J reproduced with permission from *Shamberger RC. In: Shields TW, ed. General Thoracic Surgery. 4th ed. Baltimore: Williams & Wilkins; 1994:538.*)

Struts can be used to hold the sternum securely forward. They are especially helpful in correcting extensive sternal rotation or severe depression. Fixation with struts is also required in all patients with Marfan syndrome or other connective tissue disorders where risk of recurrence is high. Strut fixation also avoids the need to divide the lowest 1 or 2 sets of intercostal bundles, which is required to produce adequate sternal mobility with suture fixation. Division of the intercostal bundles also contributes to the unsightly hollow at the distal end of the sternum.

Two methods of strut fixation are available. The first, employing a set of Rehbein struts, is shown in Fig. 17-7(I). The struts are placed in the marrow cavity of a rib to each side of the sternum. The arch of the struts is created anterior to the sternum and secured with stainless steel wire. The sternum is then secured to the Rehbein strut. The second technique uses a retrosternal approach as described by Adkins and Blades, and later by Jensen and colleagues. Critical to this technique is safe dissection from the 2 sides of the sternum of a path for the strut to traverse posterior to the sternum and anterior to the pericardium. It is helpful to employ a Kittner dissector to create this plane. This technique is treacherous in patients who have had prior cardiac surgery.

At the conclusion of the procedure, the wound is flooded with warm saline to remove clots. A single medium Hemovac drain (Snyder Laboratories, Inc, New Philadelphia, OH) is brought through the inferior skin flap, with the suction ports in a parasternal position to the level of the highest costal cartilage resected. The pectoralis muscle flaps are sutured to the sternum, advancing the muscles medially and inferiorly to cover the underlying sternum with muscle. The rectus muscles, if divided, are then reattached to the lower sternum medially and to the pectoralis muscles laterally. A postoperative chest radiograph is obtained in the recovery room. Perioperative antibiotics are continued with 3 postoperative doses of cefazolin. In patients of all ages, blood loss generally is well below the transfusion requirement.

The correction of pectus excavatum is technically most easily performed on young children, but recent reports have described major abnormalities of chest wall growth in children who have undergone repair at an early age. In 1990, Martinez first described a deficiency in thoracic growth in children following the repair of pectus excavatum. This was most noticeable in children operated on early in the preschool years. More recently, Haller and colleagues reported on 12 children in their teens who presented with apparent limited growth of the ribs and who had resection of the costal cartilages at an early age that had caused a bandlike narrowing of the midchest (Fig. 17-8). In some cases, the first and second ribs in which the costal cartilages have not been resected show apparent relative overgrowth, producing an anterior protrusion of the upper sternum. This occurrence has been attributed by Haller to injury during surgical repair of the costochondral junctions, which are the longitudinal growth centers for the ribs, and to decreased growth of the sternum resulting from injury to its growth centers or vascular supply. Weber and Kurkchubasche reported severe impairment of respiratory function with a restrictive defect in a 14-year-old boy after a standard repair of pectus excavatum at 4 years of age. The impairment was so severe that a sternotomy with

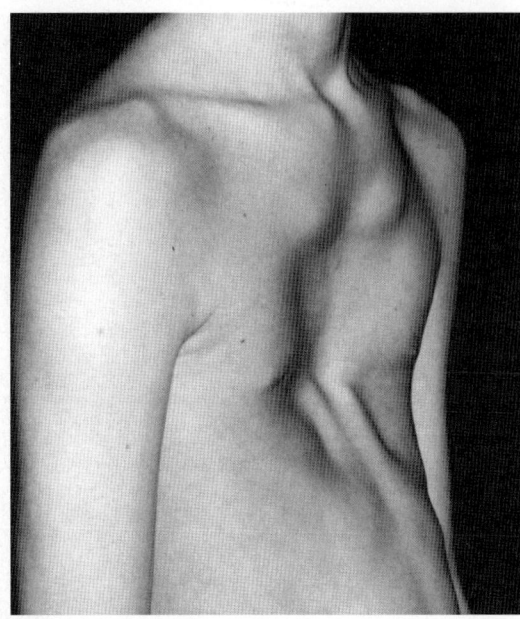

**FIGURE 17-8** A photograph of a 13-year-old boy who underwent pectus excavatum repair when he was 4 years old, demonstrating undergrowth of the resected costal cartilages and relative overgrowth of the upper ribs and manubrium.

separation of the sternal halves was performed to increase the thoracic volume and relieve symptoms.

Perichondrial sheaths, bone, or prosthetic material that cannot grow will form a bandlike stricture across the chest and should not be joined posterior to the sternum in a growing child. This complication of delayed thoracic growth has been described primarily in children who underwent repair in early childhood and can be avoided by delaying surgery until children are older. The complication is unique to open repair, as the Nuss procedure does not involve resection of the costal cartilages.

Preservation of the costochondral junction, leaving a segment of the cartilage on the osseous portion of the rib (Fig. 17-7D), may also minimize growth impairment. The authors delay use of the open procedure until a child is at least 10 to 12 years of age, when the chest has less remaining growth, to both minimize the risk of abnormal thoracic growth and to limit the opportunity for recurrence of the pectus excavatum.

The open surgical technique achieves excellent results in most patients (Fig. 17-9), with few and limited complications. Appropriate patient selection and timing of the procedure are critical to obtaining optimum results.

## COMPLICATIONS OF PECTUS EXCAVATUM REPAIR

Complications of pectus excavatum repair should be few and minor. A multi-institutional report of the Nuss and open procedures has demonstrated that complications are similar in both procedures. If the pleura is entered during open repair, the opening should be made large enough to prevent development of a tension pneumothorax intraoperatively. At the

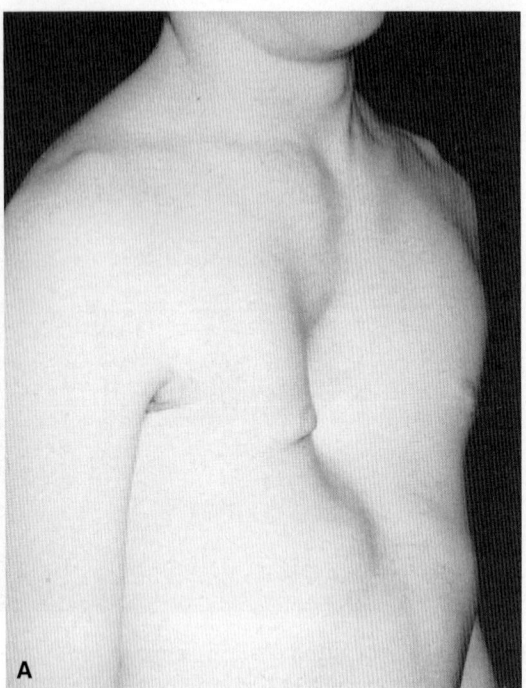 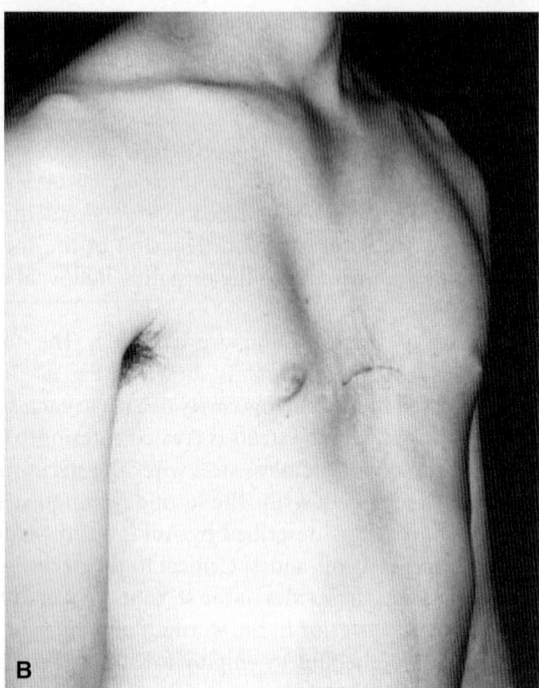

**FIGURE 17-9** **A.** A preoperative photograph of a 15-year-old boy with symmetric pectus excavatum. **B.** Eighteen-month follow-up after the correction of pectus excavatum with Rehbein struts.

conclusion of the procedure, pleural air is aspirated through a catheter that is withdrawn when the defect is covered by the pectoralis muscle closure.

In a series of open procedures, 2% of patients had a limited pneumothorax requiring aspiration or observation. In a series of more than 700 open repairs, only 4 patients needed tube thoracostomy, which generally has not been required in the last decade. Wound infection was rare with the use of perioperative antibiotic coverage. The most distressing complication following surgical correction of pectus excavatum is major recurrence of the deformity after the original repair. This occurred in 17 of 704 open repairs reported. It is difficult to predict which patients will have a major recurrence, but they often have an asthenic or "Marfanoid" habitus with poor muscular development and a narrow anterior–posterior chest wall diameter. The incidence of recurrence after primary Nuss repair in the series from Children's Hospital of The King's Daughters is approximately 1%.

A late postoperative complication unique to the Nuss repair, bar displacement, has decreased in incidence from 12% when the procedure was first use to 2% following implementation of 3-point bar fixation with wired stabilizers and PDS pericostal sutures. Approximately half of the patients who have experienced bar displacement required surgery to reposition the bar.

## RECURRENT PECTUS EXCAVATUM

Correction of recurrent pectus excavatum is generally a formidable task, although results can be very good. Sanger and associates reported their experience with secondary correction. They resected the regenerated fibrocartilage plate, repeated the osteotomy, and closed the pectoral muscles behind the sternum. Ten patients had very good results.

Although recurrences often appear symmetric, they are in fact frequently right-sided with a deep right parasternal "gutter" and sternal obliquity. Recurrence often progresses, particularly during the period of rapid growth at puberty. The Nuss procedure has been used successfully to treat recurrent pectus excavatum after failed primary Nuss, Ravitch, and Leonard repairs. In general, recurrences after initial Nuss repair tend to occur within months of surgery and are due to malpositioned or displaced bars. Recurrences after initial Ravitch repairs tend to occur in patients repaired at a young age who then develop gradual recurrences that accelerate during pubertal growth. When considering minimally invasive repair for recurrence after initial Ravitch repair, keep in mind that diffuse osteochondrodystrophy with excessive calcification and rigidity of the chest wall is not remediable by substernal bar placement.

From a technical standpoint, the challenge of redoing a Nuss repair lies in the pleural and pericardial adhesions that often obstruct visualization of the sternum and compressed mediastinal structures. Thoracoscopy is particularly useful to facilitate necessary lysis of adhesions. The vascular nature of these adhesions renders the Harmonic scalpel particularly useful. In comparison to a primary repair, a redo Nuss repair is more likely to require multiple bar placement and have more frequent and serious complications, particularly with regard to the necessity for tube thoracostomy for air leak, hemothorax, and pleural effusions. Despite these drawbacks, redo Nuss repair has achieved very favorable patient satisfaction and clinical results, deemed excellent in 66%, good in 30%, and fair in 2% of patients with recurrence.

# SELECTED READINGS

Baronofsky ID. Technique for the correction of pectus excavatum. *Surgery* 1957;42:884–890.

Beiser GD, Epstein SE, Stampfer M, et al. Impairment of cardiac function in patients with pectus excavatum, with improvement after operative correction. *N Engl J Med* 1972;287:267–272.

Haller JA Jr. Severe chest wall constriction from growth retardation after too extensive and too early (<4 years) pectus excavatum repair: an alert. *Ann Thorac Surg* 1995;60:1857–1864.

Haller JA Jr, Loughlin GM. Cardiorespiratory function is significantly improved following corrective surgery for severe pectus excavatum. *J Cardiovasc Surg* 2004;41:125–130.

Haller JA Jr, Kramer SS, Lietman SA. Use of CT scans in selection of patients for pectus excavatum surgery: a preliminary report. *J Pediatr Surg* 1987;22:904–906.

Huang PM, Liu CM, Cheng YJ, et al. Evaluation of intraoperative cardiovascular responses to closed repair for pectus excavatum. *Thorac Cardiovasc Surg* 2008;56:353–358.

Kelly RE Jr, Goretsky MJ, Obermeyer R, et al. Twenty-one years of experience with minimally invasive repair of pectus excavatum by the Nuss procedure in 1215 patients. *Ann Surg* 2010;252:1072–1081.

Kelly RE Jr, Shamberger RC, Mellins RB, et al. Prospective multicenter study of surgical correction of pectus excavatum: design, perioperative complications, pain and baseline pulmonary function facilitated by internet-based data collection. *J Am Coll Surg* 2007;205:205–216.

Koumbourlis AC. Pectus excavatum: pathophysiology and clinical characteristics. *Pediatr Respir Rev* 2009;10:3–6.

Kowalewski J, Brocki M, Dryjanski T, et al. Pectus excavatum: increase of right ventricular systolic, diastolic, and stroke volumes after surgical repair. *J Thorac Cardiovasc Surg* 1999;118:87–93.

Krueger T, Chassot PG, Christodoulou M, et al. Cardiac function assessed by transesophageal echocardiography during pectus excavatum repair. *Ann Thorac Surg* 2010;89:240–244.

Lawson ML, Mellins RB, Tabangin M, et al. Impact of pectus excavatum on pulmonary function before and after repair with the Nuss procedure. *J Pediatr Surg* 2005;40:174–180.

Malek MH, Berger DE, Housh TJ, et al. Cardiovascular function following surgical repair of pectus excavatum. *Chest* 2006;130:506–516.

Malek MH, Fonkalsrud EW, Cooper CB. Ventilatory and cardiovascular responses to exercise in patients with pectus excavatum. *Chest* 2003;124:870–882.

Nuss D, Kelly RE Jr. Indications and technique of Nuss procedure for pectus excavatum. *Thorac Surg Clin* 2010;20:583–597.

Nuss D, Kelly RE Jr, Croitoru DP, Katz ME. A 10-year review of a minimally invasive technique for the correction of pectus excavatum. *J Pediatr Surg* 1998;33:545–552.

Redlinger RE Jr, Kelly RE Jr, Nuss D, et al. One hundred patients with recurrent pectus excavatum patients repaired via the minimally invasive Nuss technique—effective in most regardless of initial operative approach. *J Pediatr Surg* 2011;46:1177–1181.

Saleh RS, Finn JP, Fenchel M, et al. Cardiovascular magnetic resonance in patients with pectus excavatum compared with normal controls. *J Cardiovasc Magn Reson* 2010;12:73.

Shamberger RC, Welch KJ. Cardiopulmonary function in pectus excavatum. *Surg Gynecol Obstet* 1988;166:383.

Shamberger RC, Welch KJ. Surgical repair of pectus excavatum. *J Pediatr Surg* 1988;23:615.

Sigalet DL, Montgomery M, Harder J, et al. Long-term cardiopulmonary effects of closed repair of pectus excavatum. *Pediatr Surg Int* 2007;23:493–497.

Torre M, Varela P, Asquasciati C, et al. Bilateral Endoclose approach for the stabilization of the bar in pectus repair. *J Laparoendosc Adv Surg Tech* 2009;19:S227–S228.

Weber TR, Kurkchubasche AG. Operative management of asphyxiating thoracic dystrophy after pectus repair. *J Pediatr Surg* 1998;33:262–265.

Welch KJ. Satisfactory surgical correction of pectus excavatum deformity in childhood; a limited opportunity. *J Thorac Surg* 1958;36:697–713.

*Jennifer Bruny*

1. The main indications for medical intervention for children with pectus carinatum are severity of symptoms and the degree to which the deformity interferes with activities. This is a subjective decision-making process that requires the input of the surgeon, parent, and adolescent.

2. Surgical repair and bracing can be effective treatments of pectus carinatum.

3. Newer approaches include minimizing the extent of cartilage resection and thoracoscopic and subpectoral cartilage resection using minimally invasive techniques.

4. Surgical intervention on the chest is indicated for patients with Poland syndrome and functional impairment, mainly those with aplastic ribs. In less severe cases, surgical repair to the chest is mainly for cosmesis.

5. Several surgical approaches have been used to address the thoracic insufficiency associated with thoracic deformity syndromes, but the outcomes are generally poor. More promising are recent reports of procedures using vertical expandable prosthetic titanium ribs.

## PECTUS CARINATUM

### Introduction

Pectus carinatum is a chest wall deformity caused by an overgrowth of the costal cartilages. This causes anterior protrusion of the sternum with narrowing of the sides of the chest wall, resulting in a bowed appearance often referred to as "pigeon chest." This deformity can occur in patients with connective tissue disorders, in association with scoliosis, in families, or sporadically in patients without any other abnormalities.

Pectus carinatum occurs in 1 of 300 births. It is more common in males by a 4:1 ratio. It is often apparent at birth, but becomes more noticeable and more severe during periods of rapid growth, such as puberty.

### Etiology

The varied patient population affected by pectus carinatum has led to different theories about its etiology. Most of these theories focus on an abnormality in the cartilage. Damage to the growth plates in the costochondral junction, leading to the overgrowth of the costal cartilages, is thought to be the cause among the sporadic patient population. Efforts to identify a cause in genetically linked patients have led to more intensive study of collagen synthesis and structure. Studies of skin and cartilage collagen have focused on the ratios of collagen types and the stability of collagen I and II. The consistent finding of collagen with unstabilized end terminals suggests a specific mutation, but the exact mutation has not been determined.

### Associated Defects and Syndromes

Approximately 20% of patients have associated anomalies. These include numerous conditions such as cardiac defects, microcapnia, bilateral clubfeet, hemifacial microsomia, microphthalmia, tracheoesophageal fistulae, congenital laryngeal stridor, a dolichocephalic skull, scoliosis, and other musculoskeletal anomalies. The family history is positive for a chest wall deformity in approximately 25% of cases.

The incidence of pectus carinatum is higher in patients with Poland syndrome and Marfan syndrome. Any suspicion of Marfan stature should prompt a genetic work-up and evaluation of the aortic root. The Currarino-Silverman syndrome is associated with an abnormally short, U-shaped, unsegmented sternum and a high carinatum deformity. Individuals with the sporadic, genetic King syndrome have short stature, low-set ears, malar hypoplasia, micrognathia, kyphoscoliosis, cryptorchidism, slowly progressive myopathy with contractures, proptosis, and downslanted palpebral fissures. The singular event that leads to identification may be an episode of malignant hyperthermia, usually with a fatal outcome. To avoid this outcome, the syndrome must be identified preoperatively. Although many of the features of these syndromes are well known and, thus, intuitive, any abnormal facies or other worrisome features mandate genetic evaluation.

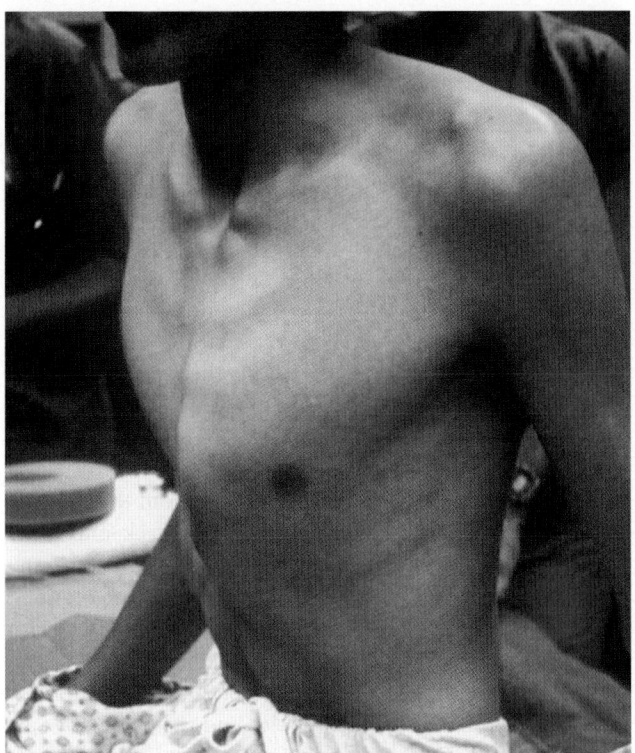

**FIGURE 18-1** An adolescent male with an asymmetric chondrogladiolar pectus carinatum deformity.

## Clinical Presentation

### Classification and Descriptions of Deformities

Pectus carinatum deformities have been categorized by descriptive terms referring to the structures involved or classified as type I, II, or III. Two common descriptive categories are chondrogladiolar and chondromanubrial (Figs. 18-1 to 18-3). The chondrogladiolar type is more common and involves the inferior costal cartilages and the gladiolus. The sternum is protuberant and has parallel incurvings of the adjoining costal cartilages, which intensifies the appearance of the sternum.

The chondromanubrial type affects the superior costal cartilages and the manubrium. Either type can be symmetric or asymmetric.

An alternative classification system refers to the defects as type I, II, or III. Type I, also known as keel chest, has a symmetric appearance. The maximal apex of the protrusion is inferior as described for chondrogladiolar. Type II is a symmetric chondromanubrial deformity also known as the Pouter deformity. Type III is an asymmetric or lateral protrusion, which can be associated with a depression on the opposite side.

### Symptoms

While pectus carinatum patients do not complain of respiratory limitations as frequently as pectus excavatum patients do, functional limitations are sometimes found. There is some evidence of incomplete exhalation with pectus carinatum. This can lead to decreased stamina, exercise-induced wheezing, or shortness of breath. There is not strong evidence to support major cardiac or pulmonary abnormalities in these patients. Improvement in exercise stamina has sometimes been reported following surgical repair, but physiologic data are lacking.

More commonly, patients present complaining of pain. This can be due to pressures in the chest wall that develop from the cartilage overgrowth. The pain is often localized over the cartilage, and may be manifested as discomfort while lying on the sternum. Alternatively, patients may complain of neuropathic pain that is related to compression of intercostal nerves. This pain is often sharp and associated with rotational motion.

Psychological and social impacts of pectus carinatum can be quite significant. In the emotionally at-risk adolescent population, the impact of the physical appearance can manifest as poor self-image and self-esteem. This can contribute to anxiety and poor motivation, and ultimately alter peer relationships and performance in activities. The parental reaction to the deformity will often shape the child's attitude. A parent who draws great attention to the deformity can heighten the child's anxiety.

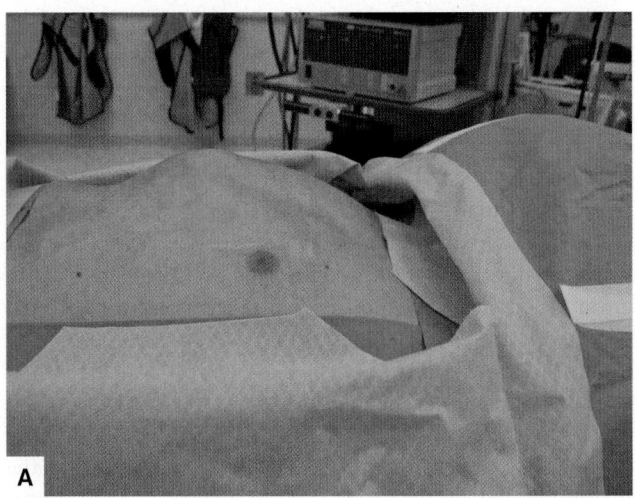
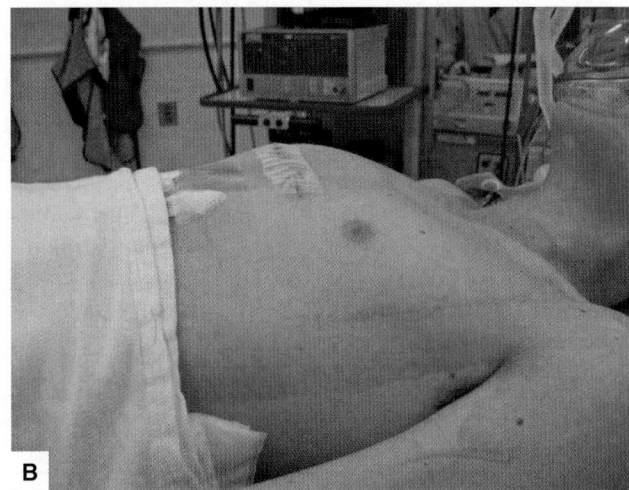

**FIGURE 18-2** A 16-year-old male with a chondrogladiolar pectus carinatum deformity (**A**) before and (**B**) after surgical repair.

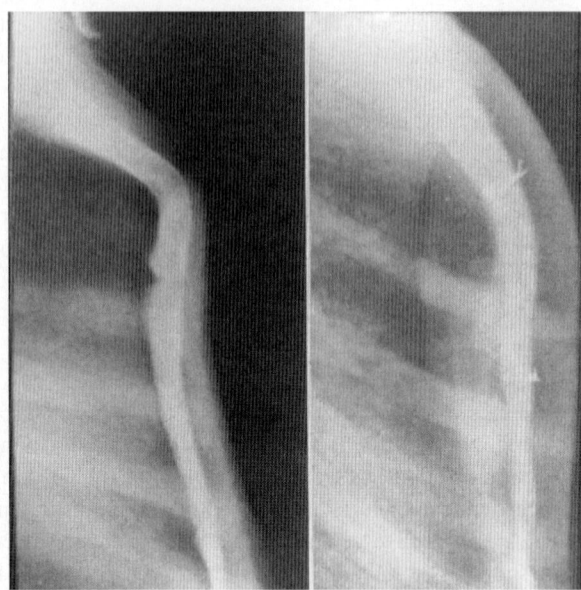

**FIGURE 18-3** Radiographs of a child with a chondromanubrial pectus carinatum deformity before and after surgical repair.

## Diagnostic Evaluation and Indications for Intervention

Consideration of intervention for pectus carinatum first requires a thorough history and physical examination by a pediatric surgeon. Any suspicion of an underlying congenital or syndromic issue (particularly suspicion of Marfan syndrome) should prompt referral to a geneticist or cardiologist.

While radiographs are not required, they can be useful in quantifying the severity of the deformity. In patients with a chest wall deformity, a pelvimeter can be used to compare measurements of the sagittal thoracic diameters in a vertical position. The standard points of measurement are the upper manubrial margin (diameter T1), the sternal angle (diameter T2), and the costal arch intersection (diameter T3). The T1/T2 ratio is the most valuable index, by direct or radiographic measurement of the deformity. While this ratio is approximately 0.75 in a normal population, the ratio is lower—approximately 0.65—in children with pectus carinatum. A single-plane chest radiograph at the level of maximum deformity is sufficient to identify the internal bony landmarks for computerized tomography (CT) and also can be used to document correction.

Unlike pectus excavatum, pectus carinatum has no ratio value that serves as a threshold to indicate intervention may be necessary. Consideration of intervention is mainly based on the patient's symptoms and the degree to which the deformity interferes with activities. This is a very subjective decision-making process that requires the input of the surgeon, parent, and adolescent.

## Management

### Operative

Ravitch first performed surgical repair of chondromanubrial deformities in 1946 and chondrogladiolar deformities in 1960. There have been many reports of alternatives and modifications since that time. The most common surgical procedure currently performed for pectus carinatum was named for Ravitch, although there are now several variations.

A transverse incision is made just below the nipple line. In females, this incision is curved downward bilaterally to fall in the projected inframammary crease. Skin flaps are raised from the angle of the manubrium to the xiphoid. The pectoralis muscles are then raised as flaps off the sternum and the costal cartilages out to the costochondral junctions. The rectus muscle is detached from the sternum and the lower costal cartilages. Cartilage resection is then performed with preservation of the perichondrium (Fig. 18-4A to C). Electrocautery is used to score the perichondrium transversely with vertical crosshatches at either end. A periosteal elevator is used to separate the perichondrium from the cartilage circumferentially. The sternum is brought back into a flat position by reefing the perichondrium, performing an osteotomy, or both. An anterior transverse sternal osteotomy is very effective for correcting a symmetric chondrogladiolar deformity. In the case of asymmetric deformities with sternal twisting, an oblique wedge osteotomy can be performed (Fig. 18-4D). The pectoralis muscles and rectus muscles are reapproximated with absorbable suture. A drain is left in the bed of the flaps.

The length of each cartilage to be removed and the number of cartilage levels removed have been areas of variation and debate. Most authors recommend unilateral limited resection in only mild, focal deformities. Longer unilateral deformities often require bilateral cartilage resection to achieve a good result. More recently, there have been several reports of minimizing the extent of cartilage resection. In 2009, Fonkalsrud reported a 38-year experience of changing trends in surgical repair. Almost all of the last 303 patients, about one third of the total patients in the study, had only short segments of cartilage excised with suture reattachment. Similarly, there have been descriptions of both thoracoscopic and subpectoral cartilage resection using minimally invasive techniques. The thoracoscopic patients wore chest binders for 1 year after the surgery.

In 2009, Abramson described 5 years of experience with implantable stainless steel bars. This technique drew from the principles of the Nuss minimally invasive repair for pectus excavatum. This procedure was carried out on patients with malleable chest walls that could be manually compressed into a corrected position by the surgeon's hands. A subcutaneous bar (now modified to a submuscular bar) is tunneled over the area of maximal deformity, and fixation plates are attached to the ribs laterally. Manual pressure is applied over the chest wall to achieve correction, and then the bar and fixation plates are attached to one another. The short-term results have been good, without recurrences after the bar was removed. Long-term results and comparative data are not yet available.

Chondromanubrial deformities are approached through a high transverse incision. A wedge-shaped osteotomy is performed at the point of maximal protrusion. Closure of the osteotomy corrects both the posterior depression of the lower sternum and the anterior angulation of the manubrium. The second costal cartilage may also need to be removed to prevent buckling (Fig. 18-3).

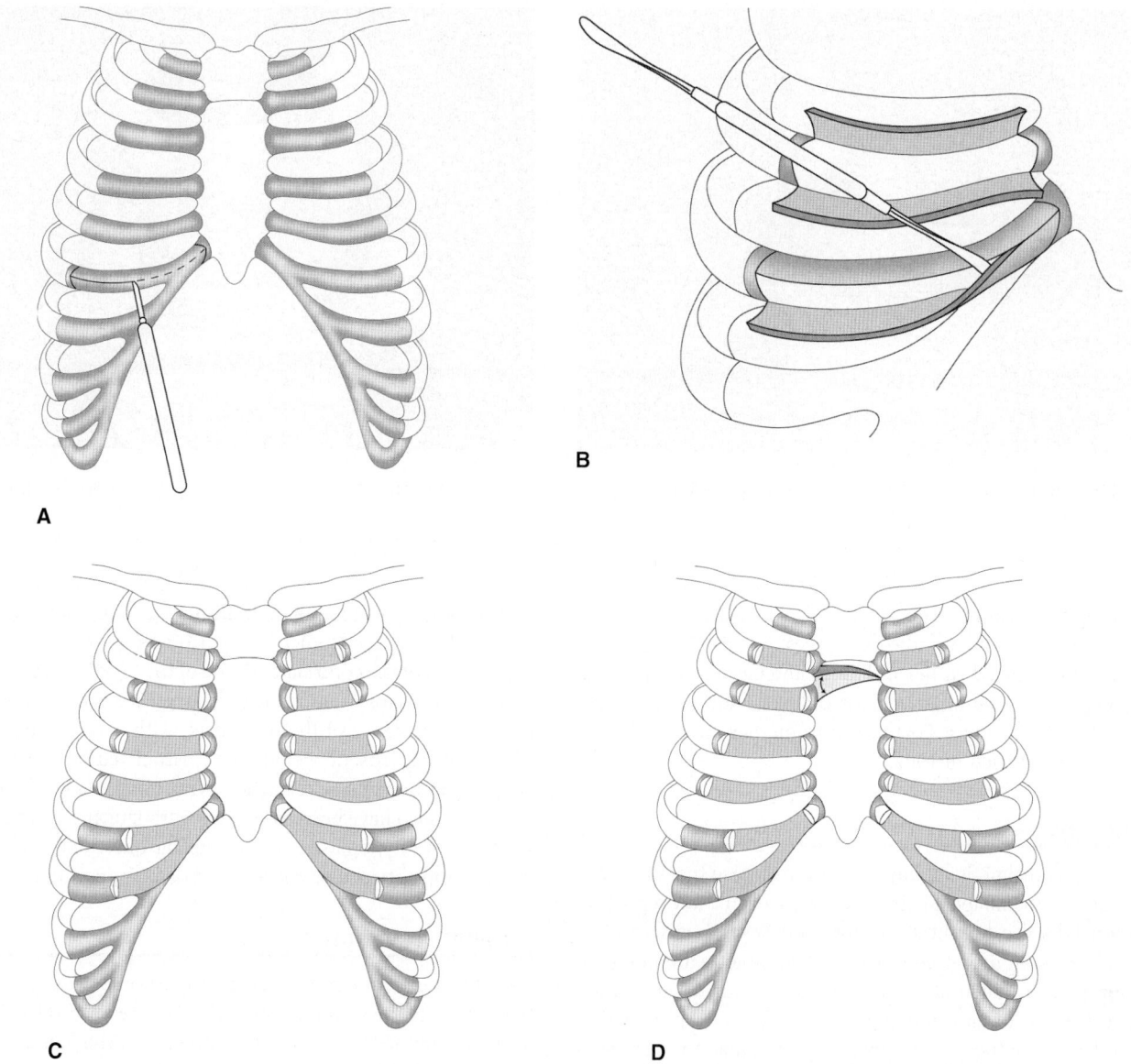

**FIGURE 18-4** Exposure for open repair of pectus carinatum including subperichondrial cartilage excision. **A.** Electrocautery scores the perichondrium with a V-shaped incision delineating the medial aspect of the dissection. **B.** A freer elevator dissects subperichondrially to free the cartilage. **C.** Following resection of the second to seventh cartilages on each side. **D.** The sternal twist of the mixed deformity is corrected by a wedge osteotomy of the anterior sternal cortex with the widest aspect on the posterior depressed sternal border.

## Nonoperative

Nonoperative therapy has mainly been applied to chondrogladiolar type deformities. Early descriptions in the 1970s reported that casting to remodel the chest wall achieved minimal success. The initiation of bracing in Brazil in the early 1990s was followed by several reports with more encouraging results using custom-fit orthotic bracing devices. This approach has gained increasing popularity over the past 2 decades.

Bracing is based on Wolff law stating that bone and surrounding tissue growth are influenced by external pressures placed on them. This is the same concept that Nuss and Abramson relied on and can also be applicable when the force is completely external to the patient. Pressure placed on the prominent area of the chest wall will theoretically remodel the growing tissues. The brace is prescribed for between 12 and 24 hours a day (Fig. 18-5A and B). The recent

literature generally concludes bracing is effective. Many authors consider bracing to be most effective at younger ages (around 12 years old), and less effective when the chest wall is less malleable (16 years and older). Major limitations of bracing often involve patient compliance and patient education is necessary for optimal compliance. Many centers are using bracing as first-line therapy and then using surgery in the case of brace failures.

## POLAND SYNDROME

### Introduction

In 1841, Poland, with the help of a fellow medical student, reported a case of a deficiency of the pectoralis major and minor muscles discovered during the autopsy of a man

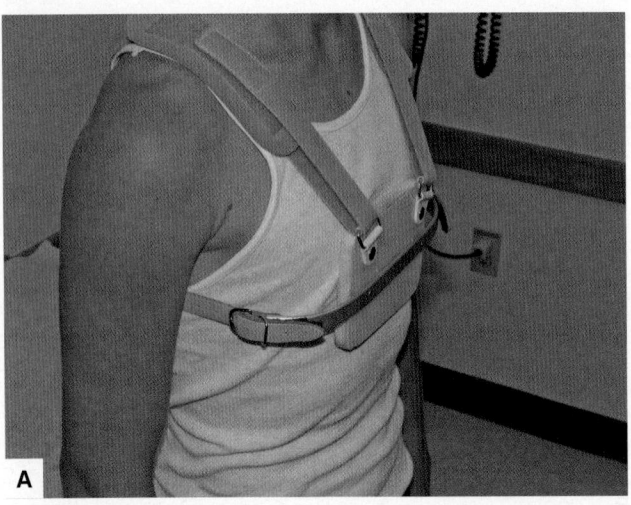
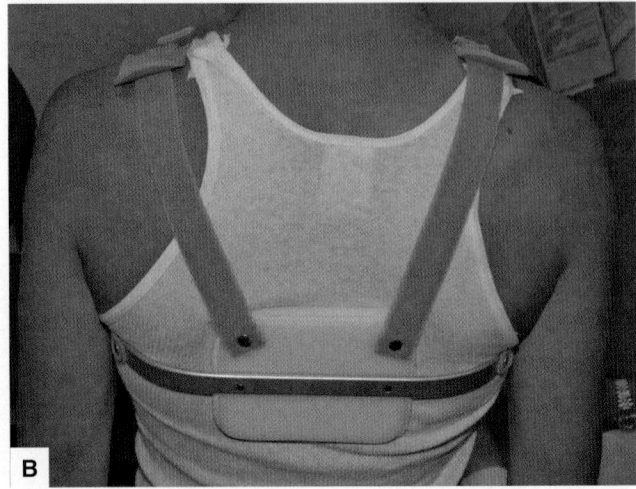

**FIGURE 18-5** Pectus carinatum orthotic compression brace. **A.** Oblique view of the patient wearing the brace with anterior compression plate visible. **B.** Posterior compression plate view of the brace.

hanged for stealing. The subject also had syndactyly with an absence of the middle phalanges. Similar descriptions had been reported earlier in France and Germany. Although Thompson first summarized the full spectrum of anomalies in 1895, the eponym Poland syndrome has stuck since the term was first used in 1962.

## Etiology

Poland syndrome is mainly a sporadic disease that occurs in about 1 in 30,000 live births. There have been a few reports of familial disease, but these are quite rare. Several causative factors have been proposed. These include potential teratogens, injuries from failed abortion attempts, abnormal migration of embryonic tissues, and hypoplasia of the subclavian artery. This later hypothesis is supported by examination of the subclavian artery of affected individuals. A study of 8 children with Poland syndrome showed these children had markedly reduced velocity in the arterial volume of the affected upper extremity during systole, as measured by real-time echo Doppler duplex scanning. Arteriography of affected individuals has revealed arterial stenoses. However, the arterial hypoplasia might result from, rather than be causative of, the hypoplasia of the arm and upper chest.

The pectoralis major is the most common area that fails to develop in children with Poland syndrome. The right side is affected more commonly (66%) than the left. In a series of 75 patients, the pectoralis minor and the costal portion of the pectoralis major were absent in all patients. In addition, hand anomalies were present in 50 patients, athelia or amastia in 37, and abnormalities of the chest wall cartilage in 10 patients. In all the series compiled, 70% of children with Poland syndrome were male.

## Associated Defects and Syndromes

Moebius syndrome, consisting of neonatally recognized facial paralysis and palsy of the sixth cranial nerve (and occasionally of cranial nerves III, V, IX, and/or XII), has been associated with Poland syndrome. Other syndromes associated with Poland syndrome include Bonnevie–Ullrich syndrome, Adams–Oliver syndrome, Parry–Romberg skin syndrome (depression of the contralateral side of the forehead and chin), and morning glory syndrome (unilateral congenital developmental disturbance of the optic disk, with severely impaired or completely absent vision often associated with nasoencephalocele and Duane retraction syndrome). Cases of Poland syndrome also have been associated with leukemia and carcinoma of the hypoplastic breast, raising questions about the relationship between developmental defects and tumors.

## Clinical Presentation

By definition, children with Poland syndrome have aplasia or hypoplasia of the sternocostal portion of the pectoralis major. This is combined with 1 additional lesion of the hand, breast, or chest wall. The degree of each abnormality can be quite variable.

Associated trunk anomalies include an absence of the pectoralis minor, serratus anterior, rectus abdominis, and latissimus dorsi. There may also be an absence or hypoplasia of the nipple, elevation of the nipple, or hypoplasia of the breast. Poland syndrome accounts for 1 out of 6 patients with breast hypoplasia or aplasia. Chest cavity abnormalities can include a small thoracic cage, scoliosis, and kyphosis. Deficient axillary hair as well as alopecia of the mammary region are also observed. The subcutaneous fat over the pectoralis is sometimes deficient. In more severe cases, there is a rotational abnormality of the sternum that requires correction. In extreme instances, there can be absence of intercostal muscles, the costal cartilage, and the anterior portions of 2 or 3 ribs. The lung may herniate through the chest wall in the area of rib aplasia, but this is rare, occurring only in 8% of patients. There is a report describing a child with Poland syndrome with the absence of the right hemidiaphragm and the ipsilateral lung. Except in extreme instances, compensatory actions negate the loss of muscle, and the arm does not exhibit a functional deficit.

The most common hand anomalies are symbrachydactyly (80%), an absence of phalanges (60%), and hypoplasia of the entire hand (33%). Other hand anomalies include an absence of digits, carpal hypoplasia, carpal coalition syndrome, nail agenesis, ectrodactyly and camptodactyly, a simian crease, a delta phalanx, an absence of extensor tendons, metacarpal phalangeal dislocation, interphalangeal dislocation, a congenital constriction band, and polydactyly. The syndactyly is usually incomplete and simple. The forefingers are affected more often than the thumb. The middle phalanges are hypoplastic or absent and there is only 1 interphalangeal joint.

The extent of the involvement of the upper extremity tends to be proportional to the extent of hypoplasia of the hand syndactyly. Upper limb anomalies that are occasionally part of Poland syndrome include the Sprengel deformity, radial-ulnar synostosis, axillary webs, and skin dimpling. All components of the upper extremity and the ipsilateral side may be smaller than on the contralateral side. The ipsilateral side may be hypopigmented. One third of patients have hypoplasia of the forearm and 15% of patients have hypoplasia of the full arm. The entire forearm can be absent. A child may hold the affected shoulder higher than its counterpart.

## Management

Surgical intervention on the chest is indicated for functional reasons, mainly in patients with aplastic ribs. The skin and pleura are in close proximity and the loss of chest wall stability may be significant. Paradoxical respiratory motion may occur. In less severe cases, surgical repair to the chest is mainly for cosmesis. Preoperative CT scan can assess the configuration of the chest wall and the quality of the latissimus dorsi muscle. A muscle with hypoplasia would not make a suitable flap.

Replacement of aplastic ribs can be accomplished with autologous rib grafts or Marlex mesh. In cases of hypoplastic ribs with significant depression of the affected side, cartilage resection very much like a carinatum repair is necessary. Contralateral cartilage resection is often required as well to correct the abnormal position and rotation of the sternum.

Coverage of the muscular defect can be achieved with a muscular graft. Using the latissimus dorsi muscle can result in an improved appearance, but the loss of strength in that added to a deficit from the absence of the pectoralis major muscle might be unacceptable in an athletic adolescent. Effective alternatives include a free transposition flap with a neurovascular bundle or the use of a rectus flap. The rectus flap has the disadvantage of creating abdominal wall laxity or weakness.

Breast reconstruction is best achieved after puberty. This allows for better balance with the normally developed contralateral breast. A breast prosthesis can be combined with a muscle flap to achieve optimal results. The most prominent part of treatment of hand anomalies is separating syndactyly. Operations on the hand should be initiated by age 1 year.

# THORACIC DEFORMITY SYNDROMES

## Jarcho–Levin Syndrome: Spondylothoracic Dysplasia

In 1938, Jarcho and Levin detailed an autosomal recessive deformity found most often in Puerto Ricans. Multiple rib and vertebral anomalies cause respiratory failure in early infancy. Hemivertebrae of the thoracic and lumbar spine, posterior rib fusion, and a shortened chest cage result in a crab-like radiographic appearance. Also associated with Jarcho–Levin syndrome are heart and kidney problems, camptodactyly, syndactyly, long digits, a prominent occiput, a broad forehead, a wide nasal bridge, anteverted nares, and upslanted palpebral fissures. The shortened vertebral height creates the small chest, limiting surgical options and usually resulting in death before age 18 months.

## Cerebrocostomandibular Syndrome

In 1966, Smith and associates reported an association among micrognathia, costal anomalies, and mental retardation. The ribs are aplastic just lateral to the posterior rib angles. The rib involvement varies in extent and number. The aplastic portion contains cartilage, fibrous tissue, and skeletal muscle. The poorly supported thoracic cage causes ineffective flail-like respiration with an early lethal course because of respiratory insufficiency. Associated defects include abnormal tracheal cartilages, low birth weight, glossoptosis, a cleft soft palate, vertebral anomalies, and elbow hypoplasia. The underlying cause and inheritance pattern remain unknown.

## Jeune Syndrome: Asphyxiating Thoracic Dystrophy

In 1954, Jeune described a newborn with a narrow rigid chest and cartilage anomalies. This form of osteochondrodystrophy is inherited in an autosomal recessive model and has variable skeletal involvement. The chest is narrow and cylindrical with clavicles that are more transverse and higher than usual. The anterior–posterior and transverse diameters, as well as the circumference, are reduced. The ribs are broad, short, and horizontal and terminate in the lateral chest. The costochondral junctions have disorganized endochondral calcification and are prominent, as in a rachitic rosary. The narrow, rigid, small-volume thoracic cage causes respiration to depend on diaphragmatic excursion. The abdomen is protuberant. Associated skeletal anomalies include shortened extremities with short, wide bones. Small, square iliac bones form the hypoplastic pelvis. Some patients have renal disease and a few have hepatic failure.

Progressive respiratory problems make management of this disorder difficult. A spectrum of pulmonary hypoplasia has been reported. Thus, many children with Jeune syndrome die of respiratory distress.

## Treatment of Thoracic Deformity Syndromes

Several surgical approaches have been tried to address the thoracic insufficiency caused by these skeletal abnormalities. These approaches have typically involved a median sternotomy with rib interposition grafts and outcomes have been generally poor. More promising have been recent reports of procedures using vertical expandable prosthetic titanium ribs. The device was originally intended for use with patients with scoliosis and most of the studies have involved these patients. The device has now been applied to patients with Jeune

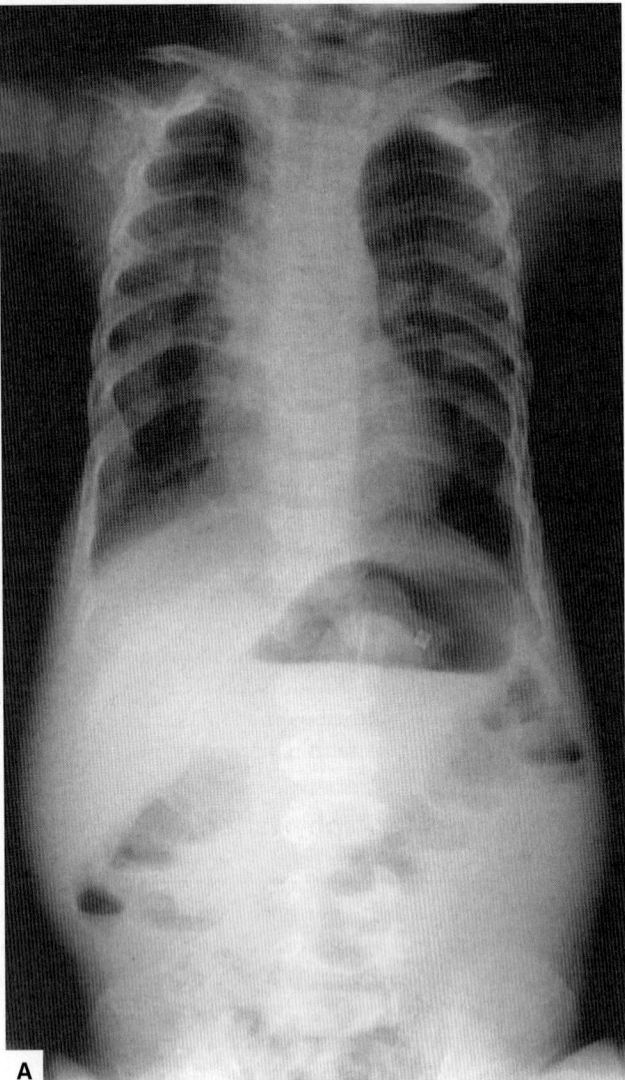
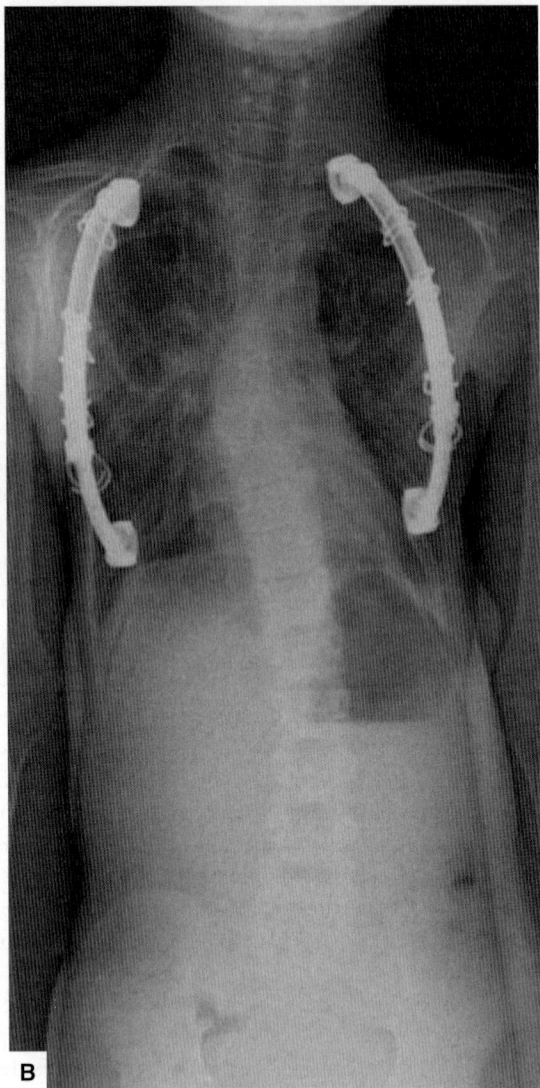

**FIGURE 18-6** Radiographs of a child with Jeune syndrome (**A**) before surgical repair at 12 months of age and (**B**) 9 years postoperative at 10 years of age.

syndrome and other types of spondylocostal dysplasia. Early experience showed very young patients on ventilators could achieve enough improvement in lung function to be weaned off respiratory support. The clinical and radiographic changes over time can be quite remarkable (Fig. 18-6). Measurable changes in pulmonary function have not been reliably proven.

## SELECTED READINGS

Abramson H, D'Agostino J, Wuscovi S. A 5-year experience with a minimally invasive technique for pectus carinatum repair. *J Pediatr Surg* 2009;44:118–124.

Bouvet JP, Leveque D, Bernetieres F, Gross JJ. Vascular origin of Poland syndrome? A comparative rheographic study of the vascularisation of the arms in eight patients. *Eur J Pediatr* 1978;128:17–26.

Fonkalsrud EW. 912 open pectus excavatum repairs: changing trends, lessons learned: one surgeon's experience. *World J Surg* 2009;2:180–190.

Fonkalsrud EW, Mendoza J. Open repair of pectus excavatum and carinatum deformities with minimal cartilage resection. *Am J Surg* 2006;191:779–784.

Frey AS, Garcia VF, Brown RL, et al. Nonoperative management of pectus carinatum. *J Pediatr Surg* 2006;41:40–45.

Haje SA, Bowen, JR. Preliminary results of orthotic treatment of pectus deformities in children and adolescents. *J Pediatr Orthop* 1992;12:795–800.

Jeune M, Carron R, Beraud C, et al. Polychondrodystrophie avec blocage thoracique d'evolution fatale. *Pediatr* 1954;9:390–392.

Ravitch MM. The operative treatment of pectus excavatum. *Ann Surg* 1949;129:429.

Ravitch MM. Operative correction of pectus carinatum (pigeon breast). *Ann Surg* 1960;5:705–714.

Smith DW, Thileller K, Schachenmann G. Rib-gap defect with micrognathia, malformed tracheal cartilages, and redundant skin: a new pattern of defective development. *J Pediatr* 1966;69:799–803.

Waldhausen JHT, Redding GJ, Song KM. Vertical expandable prosthetic titanium rib for thoracic insufficiency syndrome. A new method to treat an old problem. *J Pediatr Surg* 2007;42:76–80.

# CHAPTER 19

## Ectopia Cordis and Sternal Defects

*Jonathan I. Groner*

## KEY POINTS

1. The nomenclature for ectopia cordis is confusing and inaccurate; only a few survivors of "true" ectopia cordis have ever been reported.

2. Thoracic ectopia cordis or "true" ectopia cordis is an extremely rare condition in which the bare heart beats outside the body on the newborn's chest, and is frequently tilted so that the apex is near the patient's chin.

3. Thoracoabdominal ectopia cordis is an omphalocele variant involving major deficiencies of the abdominal wall (superior to and including the umbilicus), diaphragm, and lower sternum. Although the heart may protrude (and may be visible), it is typically covered with attenuated pericardium or skin, and is properly oriented.

4. Sternal cleft is a condition in which there is a deficit in the superior sternum. In some patients with large clefts, the heart appears to protrude out of the chest when the patient performs a Valsalva maneuver.

5. Patients with ectopia cordis often have structural abnormalities of the heart, whereas patients with sternal clefts usually have normal hearts.

6. Sternal clefts can usually be repaired in a single stage with primary closure or autologous tissues. In contrast, repairs of ectopia cordis generally require staged operations and the use of prosthetic materials.

## INTRODUCTION

Ectopia cordis refers to a rare congenital anomaly, sometimes considered bizarre or even horrifying, in which the heart is located outside the thoracic cavity. The exposed heart is frequently tilted so that the apex of the heart is near the patient's chin. Sternal clefts, however, can range in severity from relatively minor defects in the sternum to large sternal deficiencies through which the heart, although covered by pericardium and skin, herniates out of the chest with crying or straining. This condition is so dramatic and it has at times mistakenly

been called "partial ectopia cordis" or "thoracocervical ectopia cordis" (because the protruding heart appears to rise through the sternal cleft into the neck), even though the heart is structurally normal and in the anatomically correct position.

The first reported case of ectopia cordis is attributed to Niels Stensen in 1671 ("the sternum was split, and the heart, liver, and spleen, most of the intestines and right kidney have passed out through the slit being thus uncovered..."). Others, however, credit Haller or Martinez, who both reported cases in 1706. Operative repair was first described in 1925 by Cutler and Wilens, who attempted unsuccessfully to create a subcutaneous pocket over the left chest to cover the exposed heart. The infant died 11 hours after surgery. An early and celebrated case of a sternal cleft involved E. A. Groux of Hamburg, who, in the 1850s, exhibited himself at many universities and claimed that more than 2000 physicians had examined his heart through the V-shaped defect in his sternum. When Groux performed a Valsalva maneuver, his heart thrust forward, allowing direct palpation of its activity. Investigators made numerous studies on Groux and were able to determine, for example, that contraction of his heart preceded palpation of his radial pulse.

The history of ectopia cordis and its variations is colorful, and the terminology is often confusing. Antiquated texts have reported some extremely bizarre cases. These include a still-born infant with a heart that hung like a medallion on his neck and a Napoleonic soldier who was discovered on autopsy to have his heart located in his left renal fossa (in place of the kidney). This chapter will be limited to the management of sternal clefts and thoracic and thoracoabdominal ectopia cordis, which a pediatric surgeon has a reasonable chance of encountering during a career.

## EMBRYOLOGY OF STERNAL CLEFTS AND ECTOPIA CORDIS

The embryology of midline thoracic defects has been debated since they were first described. Sternal clefts (sternal defects without displacement of the heart) may be caused by the absence of sternal elements or the failure of sternal fusion. The sternum and the pectoral muscles are derived from the mesoderm. During the sixth week of gestation, lateral

| TABLE 19-1 | Some Thoracic and Cardiac Anomalies Associated with Ectopia Cordis |
|---|---|
| **Thoracic** | |
| Cleft sternum | |
| Deficient/absent pericardium | |
| Diaphragmatic hernia | |
| Pulmonary hypoplasia | |
| Absent lung (rare) | |
| **Cardiac** | |
| Tetralogy of Fallot | |
| Pulmonary artery stenosis | |
| Ventricular septal defect | |
| Atrial septal defect | |
| Transposition of the great vessels | |
| Hypoplastic left ventricle | |
| Left ventricular diverticulum | |
| Double outlet right ventricle | |

| TABLE 19-2 | Extrathoracic Anomalies Associated with Ectopia Cordis |
|---|---|
| **Head and neck** | |
| Anophthalmia[a] | |
| Cleft lip[a] | |
| Cleft palate[a] | |
| Cleft tongue[a] | |
| Cranial defects including encephalocele and anencephaly[a] | |
| **Abdomen** | |
| Omphalocele[a] | |
| Diastasis recti | |
| Fibrous midline bands or scars[a] | |
| Cloacal exstrophy[a] | |
| **Extremities** | |
| Digital amputations[a] | |
| Digital fusions[a] | |

[a]A feature strongly suggestive of mechanical teratogenesis following rupture of the chorion or yolk sac.

mesodermal plates move ventrally creating 2 parallel strips of mesenchyme, and during the seventh through tenth week, these strips merge craniocaudally to form the sternum and part of the manubrium. The cartilaginous sternum then develops multiple ossification centers proceeding in a craniocaudal sequence. Sternal clefts occur from the failure of superior sternal fusion, resulting in a V-shaped or U-shaped defect of the sternum. This defect is also called a congenital bifid sternum. In extreme cases, the entire sternum may be absent.

In the third week of embryonic life, the intraembryonic and extraembryonic celom are demarcated by the folding of the embryo. An early theory suggested that ectopia cordis results when the ventral body walls "catch the heart outside their place of convergence rather than inside," resulting in the heart being positioned on the anterior chest wall. This complicated mechanism does not provide an adequate explanation for thoracoabdominal defects, nor does it explain the numerous intracardiac lesions seen in these patients (Table 19-1).

Cantrell's classic work attributed defects in the upper torso to a developmental failure of the mesodermal components of the sternum and upper abdomen. This defect occurs during days 14 to 18 of embryonic life—immediately after differentiation of the primitive embryonic mesoderm into its splanchnic and somatic layers. The diaphragmatic and pericardial defects result from failure of the transverse septum to develop. Cantrell blamed the complex cardiac lesions on "faulty development of the epimyocardium which is derived from the splanchnic mesoderm corresponding to that portion of the somatic mesoderm from which the pericardium is derived."

The preceding theories all suffer from a failure to account for the numerous malformations identified in these infants *exclusive of the torso* (Table 19-2). In 1985, Kaplan and others advanced a concept that explains not only ectopia cordis and a cleft sternum but also the associated anomalies: mechanical teratogenesis (band disruptions) following rupture of the chorion or yolk sac. The association between ectopia cordis and band disruption anomalies is based on the observation that infants with thoracoabdominal and thoracic defects

(including a cleft sternum) frequently have extrathoracic stigmata of band disruptions, such as an encephalocele, a cleft of the calvaria or face, oblique fibrous bands, anophthalmia, or digital malformations. The compression that results from rupture of the chorion and/or yolk sac at the time of cardiac descent (21 days) would affect the thorax (hindering development of the lungs), prevent midline fusion of the developing chest wall, and fix the heart's position outside the chest with a cranially pointing apex. An early rupture would also explain the multiple clefts and deformities seen in these patients. Thoracoabdominal ectopia cordis is thought to result from a combination of mechanical compression of the thorax and tethering of the heart to the umbilical region by a band. Photographic evidence of such fibrous bands ("gubernaculum cordis") can be found in case reports.

An amniotic rupture later in gestation, but before sternal fusion is complete at 6 weeks, could result in a cleft sternum, a normal heart location, and fewer extrathoracic defects. According to the mechanical teratogenesis theory, intracardiac lesions are the result of "deformational strains on the developing great vessels and cardiac septa" due to "the early aberrant location of the heart."

Numerous contemporary photographs of patients with ectopia cordis or a cleft sternum demonstrate evidence of congenital bands. A case report of a congenital bifid sternum, for example, shows an infant with "a 4-mm wide raised midline raphe extending from the xiphoid to the umbilicus" that is most likely a congenital fibrous band.

## PATHOPHYSIOLOGY OF STERNAL CLEFTS AND ECTOPIA CORDIS

Sternal clefts can be dramatic at birth, but because of the normal cardiac anatomy and normal position of the heart, these clefts are not life-threatening. Thoracic ectopia cordis, on the other hand, often requires urgent surgical intervention because the exposed heart will rapidly become desiccated if it is not covered with tissue. The most serious threat is the combination of decreased oxygenation (due to pulmonary hypoplasia) and decreased oxygen delivery (due to intrinsic cardiac defects) that can rapidly cause tissue hypoxia and acidosis. Hypothermia results from exposure of the viscera. In thoracoabdominal ectopia cordis, the amnion-covered abdominal cavity compounds heat and fluid loss. Particularly in thoracic cases, the aberrant position of the heart causes the great vessels to have an unusual orientation. Attempts to reposition the heart into the mediastinum will kink the great vessels and cause cardiac arrest. Attempts to cover the heart in an extrathoracic position (with local tissue) may lead to severe cardiac tamponade with the same end result.

## DIAGNOSIS OF ECTOPIA CORDIS

### Modern Classification System

The vast majority of midline thoracic defects can be classified into 3 major groups: cleft sternum, thoracic or true ectopia cordis, and thoracoabdominal ectopia cordis (Table 19-3).

### Simple Sternal Clefts

Simple sternal clefts range from V-shaped or U-shaped clefts in the upper sternum to absence of the entire sternum (Fig. 19-1). A diagnosis is made by physical examination. Although the heart is in the anatomically correct position, cardiac pulsation is plainly visible, and when the patient cries or strains, the heart protrudes through the cleft and may appear to rise above the clavicles. The misnomer *partial ectopia cordis* has been applied in the past, but in patients with sternal clefts, the heart is always covered by both pericardium and skin, although in some cases, the skin has an attenuated or scarred area in the middle of the defect. The edges of the bony defect are plainly palpable, and a raphe or fibrous band may extend down to the umbilicus. When the defect is large, paradoxical motion of the mediastinal structures may be noted with respiration.

### Thoracoabdominal Ectopia Cordis

In thoracoabdominal ectopia cordis, the midline defect usually extends from the midsternum to the umbilicus. The thoracoabdominal group includes a diverse spectrum of lesions, ranging from giant omphaloceles and diaphragmatic defects, with the heart prolapsed almost entirely out of the thorax, to a skin-covered omphalocele discovered at the time of operation to have a diaphragmatic defect through which the heart is visible in the pericardium (Fig. 19-2). Virtually all these patients have cardiac lesions, and the incidence of left ventricular diverticula is unexpectedly high. Although the displaced heart may be plainly visible on physical examination, it is essentially always covered by a membrane of pericardium or thin, pigmented skin.

| TABLE 19-3 | Classification of Midline Defects of the Upper Torso | | |
|---|---|---|---|
| | **Sternal Cleft** | **Thoracoabdominal Ectopia Cordis** | **Thoracic Ectopia Cordis** |
| Other names | Bifid sternum, partial ectopia cordis and, rarely, thoracocervical ectopia cordis (both misnomers) | Cantrell pentalogy (most, but not all cases in this category meet Cantrell criteria) | Ectopia cordis extrathoracica nuda, ectopia cordis cum sterni fissura, complete ectopia cordis, true ectopia cordis |
| Relative frequency | Rare | Although rare, possibly the most common of the 3 conditions | Very rare |
| Associated cardiac anomalies | Rare | Very common | Very common |
| Heart covering | Present (skin, soft tissue, and pericardium); in some cases, the skin is scarred or attenuated in the middle of the defect | Heart is usually covered: pericardium; thin, pigmented skin or sometimes normal skin | Always absent (naked heart) |
| Heart position | Normal anatomic location and orientation; may protrude superiorly and anteriorly with crying or straining | Normal orientation and relatively normal relationship to liver and lungs; often partially prolapsed below the diaphragm | Extremely abnormal: heart outside thoracic cavity, cardiac apex pointed toward chin, atrial appendages often visible |
| Abdominal wall | Generally intact but may have diastasis recti or midline fibrous raphe | Significant midline abdominal wall and anterior diaphragmatic defects always present—usually a moderate-sized omphalocele (sometimes with prolapsed abdominal contents), cloacal exstrophy (rare) | Usually associated with abdominal wall defects: diastasis recti, attenuated midline skin, small omphalocele; rarely associated with giant omphalocele |
| Survival | Excellent | Fair | Poor |

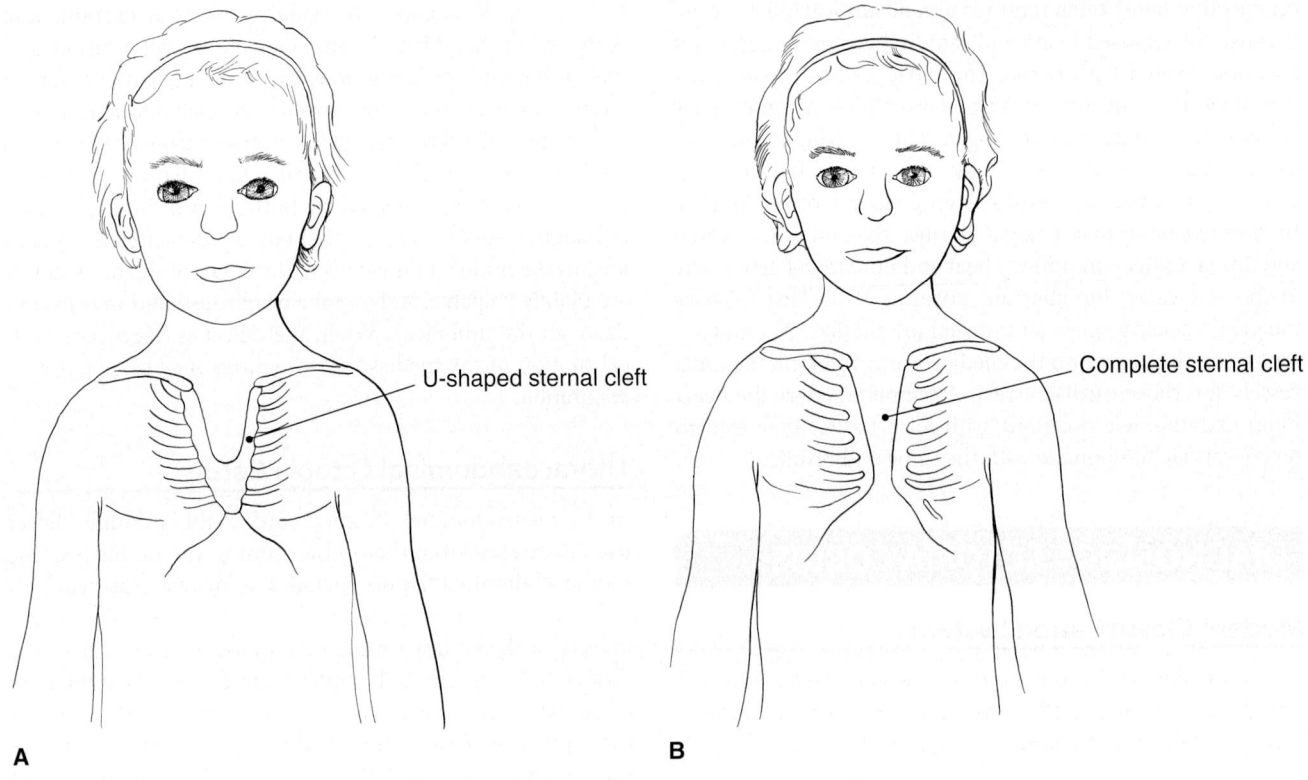

**FIGURE 19-1** **A.** Partial sternal cleft. **B.** Complete sternal cleft.

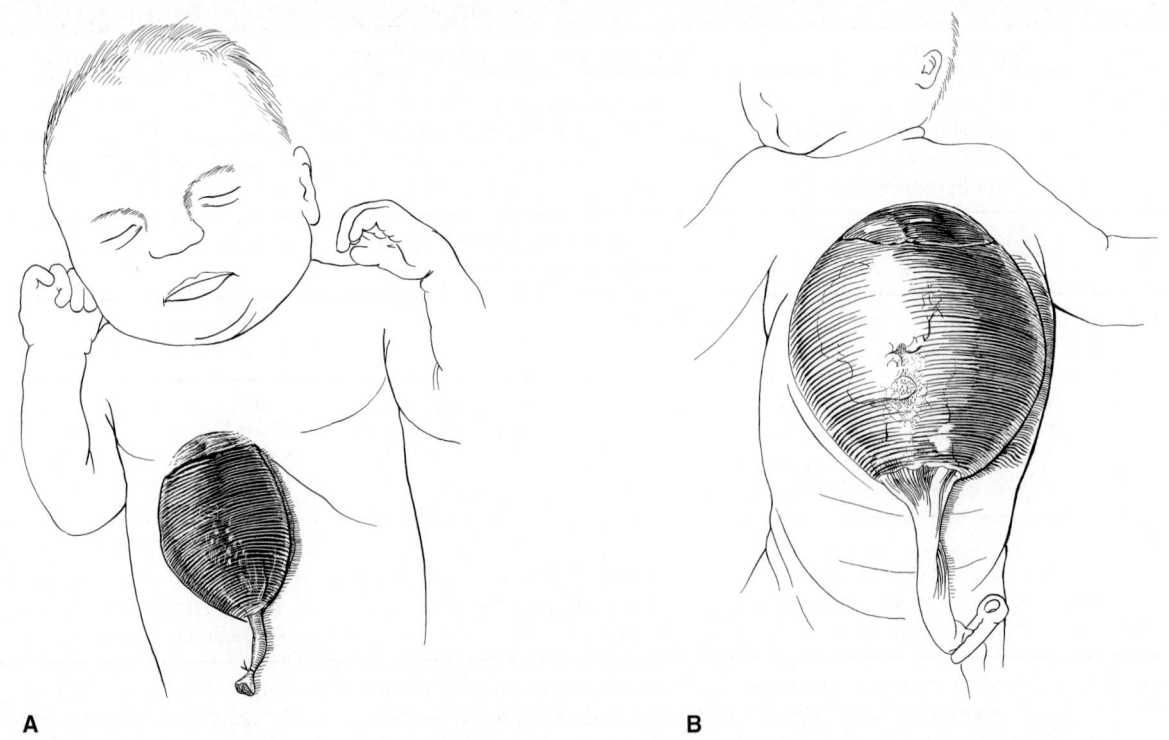

**FIGURE 19-2** **A.** Thoracoabdominal ectopia cordis with an omphalocele. **B.** Severe thoracoabdominal ectopia with a very large associated omphalocele.

Within this group is a large subset with the syndrome of defects known as the pentalogy of Cantrell. This pentalogy consists of (1) a midline supraumbilical abdominal wall defect, (2) a defect of the lower sternum, (3) a deficiency of the anterior diaphragm, (4) a defect in the diaphragmatic pericardium, and (5) congenital intracardiac defects. Not all thoracoabdominal cases appear to fit into the Cantrell syndrome. Exceptions include thoracoabdominal ectopia cordis with a complete sternal cleft and rare cases in which the abdominal wall defect extends below the umbilicus (ie, cloacal exstrophy).

## Thoracic or True Ectopia

Thoracic or true ectopia cordis is also called ectopia cordis extrathoracica nuda because the heart is not only outside the chest but also devoid of any covering. This lesion is always associated with a cleft sternum, and some form of midline abdominal wall abnormality is usually present as well. Classically, the heart sits on the anterior chest wall with the apex pointed toward, and sometime touching, the chin (Fig. 19-3). The atrial appendages are often visible, positioned on the anterior chest wall. The great vessels pass through the sternal cleft into the mediastinum. A severe intracardiac defect is almost always present. If an infant with thoracic ectopia cordis does not have a severe cardiac anomaly, he may present to the surgeon appearing pink and vigorous with his cardiac apex bouncing on his chin—an extremely rare and dramatic sight.

There is controversy in the literature about whether a patient with a "naked" upturned heart, who also has a large (or even giant) abdominal wall defect, belongs to the thoracic (ie, thoracic ectopia cordis with omphalocele) or the thoracoabdominal (ie, thoracoabdominal defect with true ectopia cordis) category. It should be noted that, in almost all well-documented cases of thoracic ectopia cordis, *an abdominal wall defect* (such as a small omphalocele or diastasis recti with thin, pigmented supraumbilical skin) *is also present.* Therefore, regardless of the size of the abdominal wall defect, any patient with a completely bare, vertically rotated, extrathoracic heart belongs to the thoracic category. This is the lesion that represents the greatest surgical challenge—and the highest risk for mortality.

## Prenatal Diagnosis of Midline Thoracic Defects

The increased use of fetal ultrasonography has permitted prenatal diagnosis of midline thoracic wall defects. A complete sternal cleft was diagnosed at 21 weeks' gestation in an infant who underwent surgical repair at age 26 days. In another case, ultrasonogram revealed ectopia cordis, tetralogy of Fallot, and an omphalocele in a 33-week fetus. The infant was delivered by elective cesarean section at 38 weeks but expired the next day despite an attempt at surgical repair. The authors commented that "termination of pregnancy is probably justified after a very early diagnosis." Although termination has been described in several cases after ultrasound diagnosis of ectopia cordis, the incidence of elective terminations is unknown. In cases in which a pregnancy is carried to term following an ultrasound diagnosis of ectopia cordis, cesarean section (performed in a children's hospital or in close proximity to one) is recommended to avoid injury to the exposed heart.

## Preoperative Evaluation

Preoperative evaluation of infants with ectopia cordis must be combined with their initial assessment and stabilization. After a thorough examination and documentation of

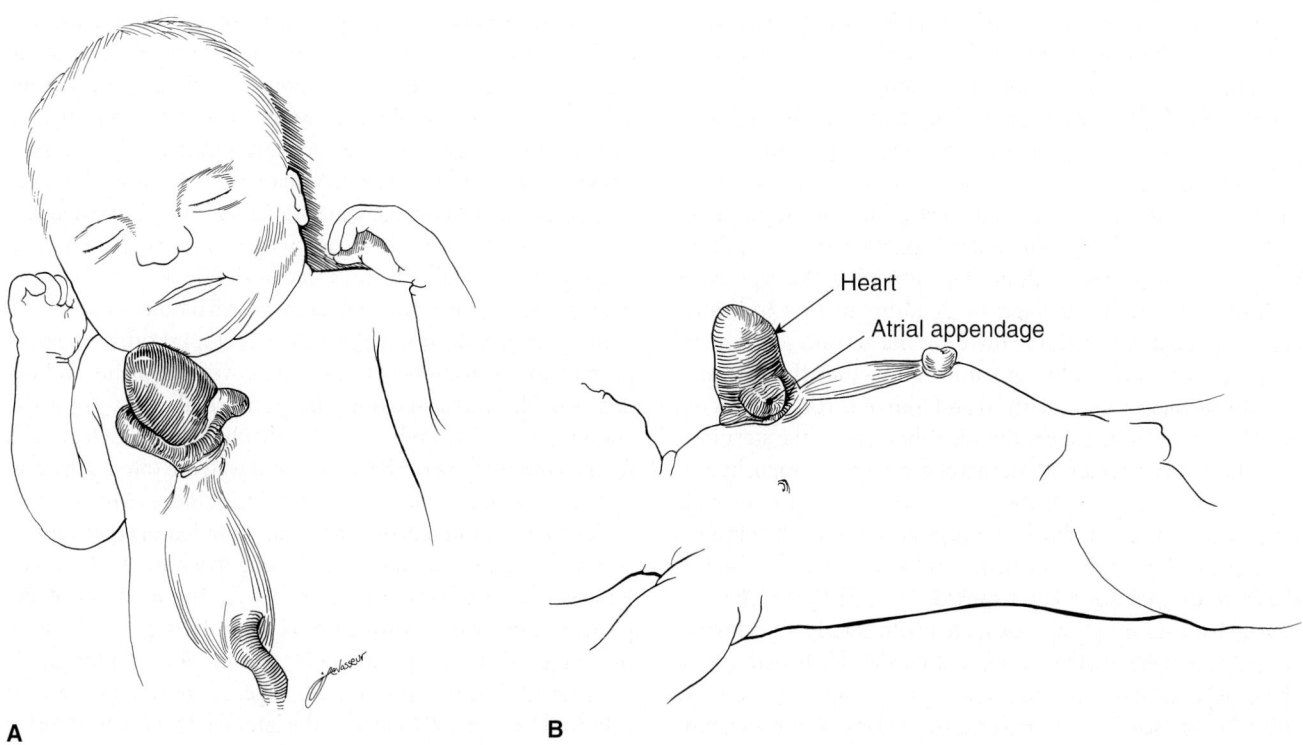

A          B

**FIGURE 19-3** A, B. True ectopia cordis or ectopia cordis extra thoracica nuda, the naked heart.

all abnormalities (particularly those outside the chest), all infants should have a plain chest radiograph and routine laboratory tests. An intravenous line, an umbilical artery catheter, and a bladder catheter should be placed, and frequently an endotracheal tube as well. An echocardiogram is essential for diagnosing the extent of the intracardiac lesions. If the heart is exposed, this procedure can be performed using a sterile cover over the transducer. An ultrasonogram of the head should be used to evaluate severe intracranial lesions, such as intraventricular hemorrhaging or severe hydrocephalus.

## SURGICAL TREATMENT OF A CLEFT STERNUM

Sternal clefts are rare, representing only 0.15% of all chest wall defects. While sternal clefts do not require emergency evaluation and infants are often referred for surgical consultation on an elective or outpatient basis, repair of the primary condition during the infant's first month allows the surgeon to take advantage of the highly compliant thorax of the neonate. The goals of surgical repair are to provide bony protection of the mediastinal structures and eliminate a significant cosmetic deformity. Repair also eliminates the paradoxical motion of the thoracic structures, although the physiologic significance of this effect is uncertain. If other conditions need to be stabilized first or the infant is not able to tolerate repair during the first month, repair can be delayed until the child is older.

In the past, synthetic materials were recommended for repairing sternal clefts: Marlex mesh, wire mesh, Teflon, or an acrylic patch. Because of the risk of infection, however, these techniques have been abandoned in favor of autogenous tissue. In older patients (including adolescents), repair is performed through a transverse inframammary incision. The anterior periosteum of the sternal bars can be divided laterally and folded over medially to bridge the gap in the sternum. This area is then reinforced with rib grafts to create a bony sternum without compressing the intrathoracic contents.

Other methods of cleft repair "lengthen" the cartilaginous portions of the ribs to bridge the midline gap. The Sabiston technique uses oblique incisions in the costal cartilages to create sliding chondrotomies that allow the sternal bars to be moved medially and sutured together in the midline (Fig. 19-4). Another method of lengthening the ribs is to transpose the costal cartilages by dividing the first and third cartilages near the midline, dividing the second and fourth cartilages laterally, and then suturing together the first and second cartilages, and the third and fourth cartilages, to create 2 long ribs from 4 short ribs on either side of the sternum.

In the neonate, repair of a sternal cleft can be accomplished by suture closure (Fig. 19-5). The procedure is performed through a vertical midline incision. The pericardium and diaphragm are separated from the subcutaneous tissues, and the edges of the cleft are mobilized and exposed. For complete clefts, the sternal bars are simply approximated with stainless steel wires or heavy, nonabsorbable sutures. For partial (U-shaped) clefts, the fused area of the sternum (often the cartilaginous xiphoid) must be excised before bringing the halves of the sternum together. The hemodynamic status must be carefully monitored to ensure that there is no cardiac compression before the

sternal sutures are tied. The pectoralis muscles are then closed over the sternum, and the skin is closed. No drains are used.

Although all of the above techniques have been used with success, long-term follow-up (over many years) is difficult to document. There appear to be no reports describing failures with any of these methods.

## MANAGEMENT OF ECTOPIA CORDIS

The management of ectopia cordis begins immediately after birth. The exposed heart and viscera should be covered with warm, moist saline pads, and the entire upper torso covered with clear plastic wrap to prevent heat loss and desiccation. Many infants require urgent endotracheal intubation for ventilatory support, and inotropic support may be needed in patients with a low cardiac output.

A preoperative echocardiogram is essential not only for prognosis but also to aid in the hemodynamic treatment of patients with severe cardiac disease. A recent review of 10 ectopia cordis cases (2 thoracic, 8 thoracoabdominal), all involving conotruncal defects and all managed at a single institution, demonstrated survival beyond infancy in 5 patients (1 thoracic and 4 thoracoabdominal). All these patients had cardiac surgery delayed until repair of the ectopia cordis had been completed. Interestingly, 2 of these patients underwent an aortopexy for treatment of aortic compression of the trachea or left main stem bronchus. Three children underwent total repair at 9 months, 2.6 years, and 3.3 years of age (the latter 2 had initially been treated in other countries). The other survivors had undergone single-ventricle palliation as toddlers. The previous ectopia cordis repair did not alter the surgical course of these patients. One infant, however, underwent delayed closure of his midline defect 1 day after his definitive cardiac repair.

All patients with thoracic ectopia cordis and many patients with thoracoabdominal ectopia cordis should be taken to the operating room within a few hours of delivery. The anesthetic technique for a newborn with ectopia cordis uses intravenous fentanyl and pancuronium. Intraoperative ventilation with a high inspired oxygen concentration is recommended to improve tissue oxygenation because these patients may have a low cardiac output and ischemia. Inhalational agents are avoided not only because they can cause gaseous distention of the intestine, making closure difficult in thoracoabdominal cases, but also because these agents can depress myocardial function.

In patients with thoracoabdominal ectopia cordis, the purpose of the operation is to provide coverage of the midline defect of the torso, separate the pericardial cavity from the abdominal cavity, and close the diaphragmatic defect. The fascial components of the abdominal wall are often deficient, and creative maneuvers are required to achieve closure.

Cantrell's original article provides detailed descriptions of several patients, ranging in age from newborn to 16 years. His technique is as follows (Fig. 19-6). The junction of the pericardium and peritoneum is sharply separated along the edge of the diaphragmatic defect. The diaphragm is then sutured to the anterior rib cage. Abdominal closure is achieved by vertically incising the lateral edges of the anterior rectus sheaths to create relaxing incisions so that the rectus abdominis muscles meet in the midline. For larger defects,

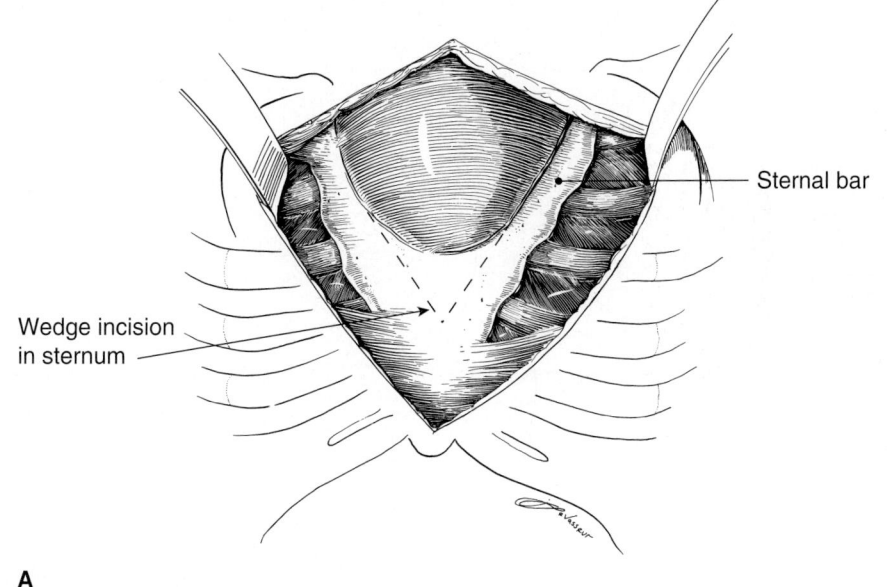

Sternal bar

Wedge incision
in sternum

**A**

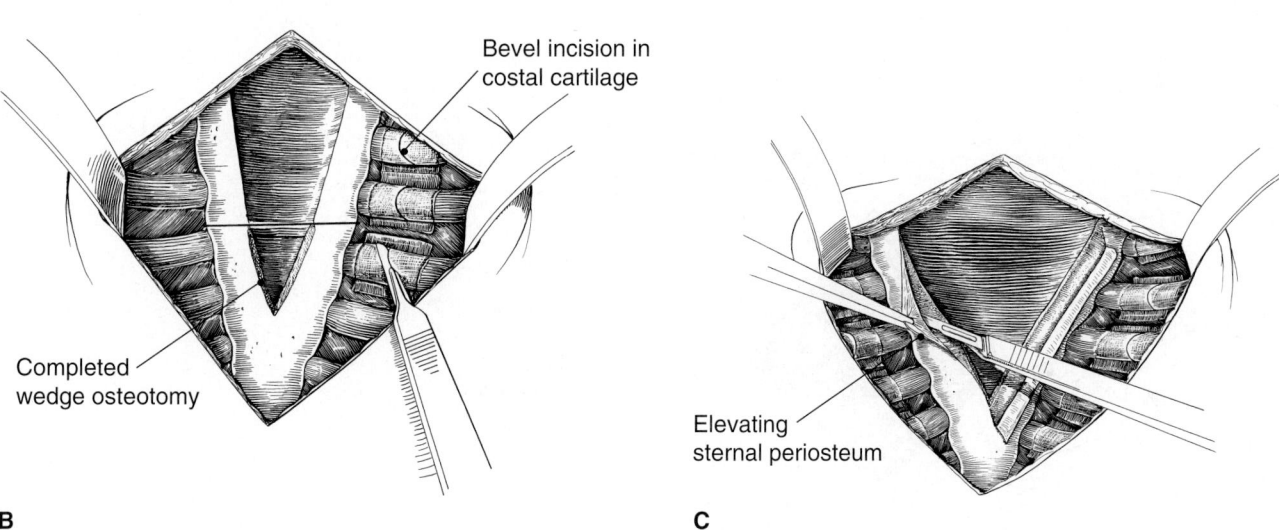

Bevel incision in
costal cartilage

Completed
wedge osteotomy

**B**

Elevating
sternal periosteum

**C**

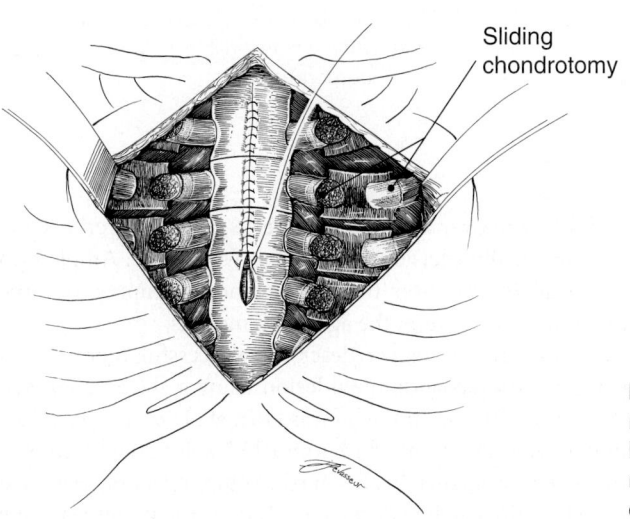

Sliding
chondrotomy

**D**

**FIGURE 19-4** The Sabiston technique for sternal cleft repair. **A.** Pectoral muscles have been reflected and a wedge incision has been created in the lower sternum. **B.** After reflecting the perichondrium, a beveled incision is made through each costal cartilage. **C.** A periosteal flap is then made for each sternal bar. **D.** Sternal bar approximation is facilitated by the sliding chondrotomies and the position is held; the periosteum is then closed.

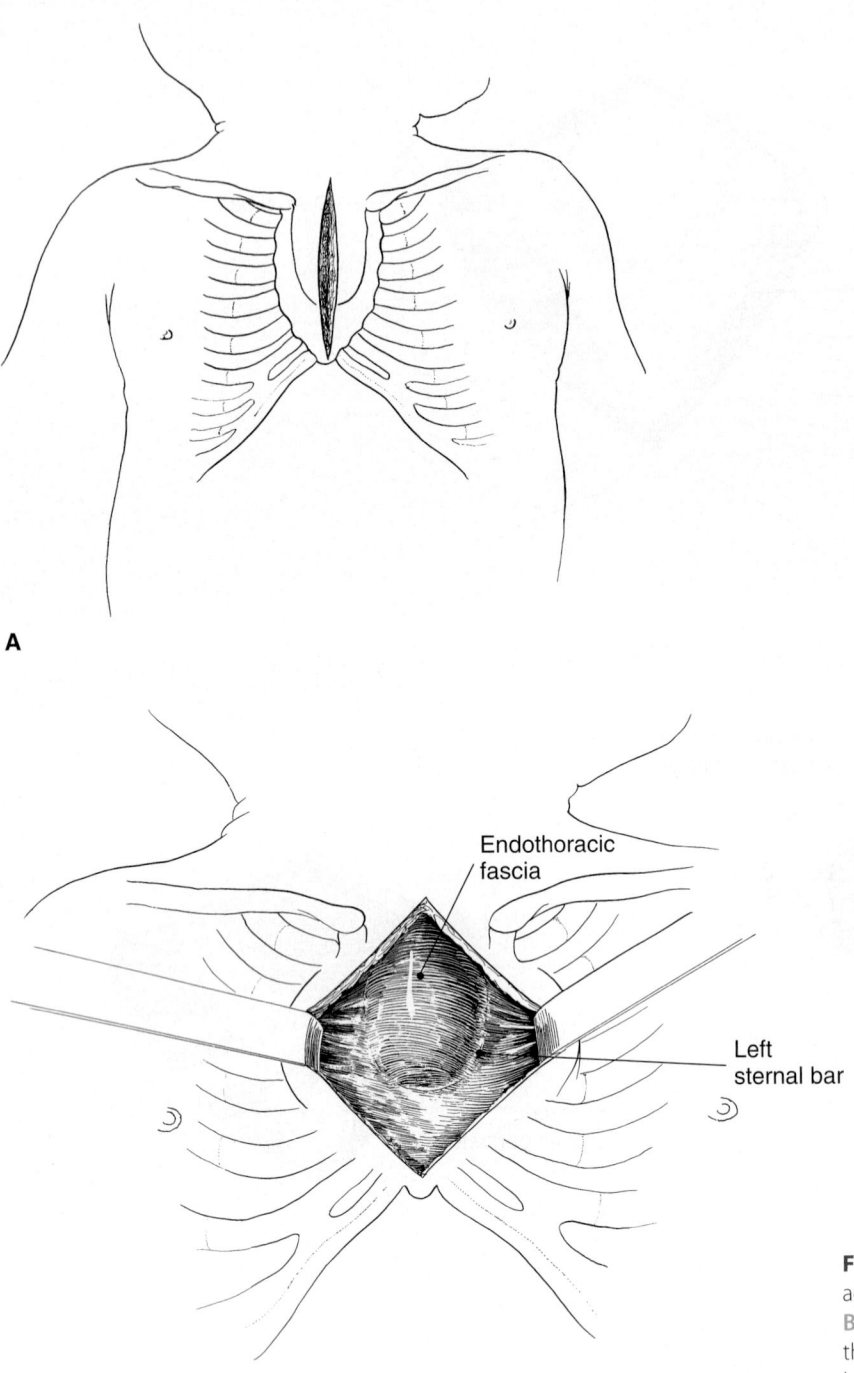

**A**

**B**

Endothoracic
fascia

Left
sternal bar

**FIGURE 19-5** Sternal cleft repair in the newborn age group. **A.** A vertical midline incision is made. **B.** The sternal bars are visualized on either side of the cleft where mediastinal structures are covered by the endothoracic fascia.

Cantrell used autologous fascia lata to reinforce flaps of anterior rectus sheath rotated to meet in the midline. A commercial bioprosthetic patch, such as polytetrafluoroethylene (PTFE), might be a better choice today (Fig. 19-7). Where the diaphragmatic defect was larger and the heart was quite prominent within the abdominal cavity, Cantrell described dissection of the heart and pericardium from the surrounding structures to allow the heart to partially retract within the thoracic cavity.

The use of tissue expanders in the repair of thoracoabdominal ectopia cordis was reported in 1987. Bilateral subpectoral tissue expanders were placed 3 days after a silastic silo was sutured over the defect. The expanders were inflated to 150 mL each over a period of 2 weeks, and then removed at the time of silo excision and a definitive closure. Ample skin was available to cover the heart without compression. The infant died of sepsis at the age of 3.5 months.

A more recent report described successful repair of an extensive thoracoabdominal lesion using a staged approach (Fig. 19-8). This infant, who was born at 38 weeks' gestation, underwent placement of a 2-mm PTFE soft tissue patch over the defect immediately after birth. Suture plication was used to reduce the patch over the next 2 days. The infant was then returned to the operating room where tissue coverage was achieved (over the plicated patch) with bilateral, bipedicled pectoralis major and rectus abdominis myocutaneous flaps.

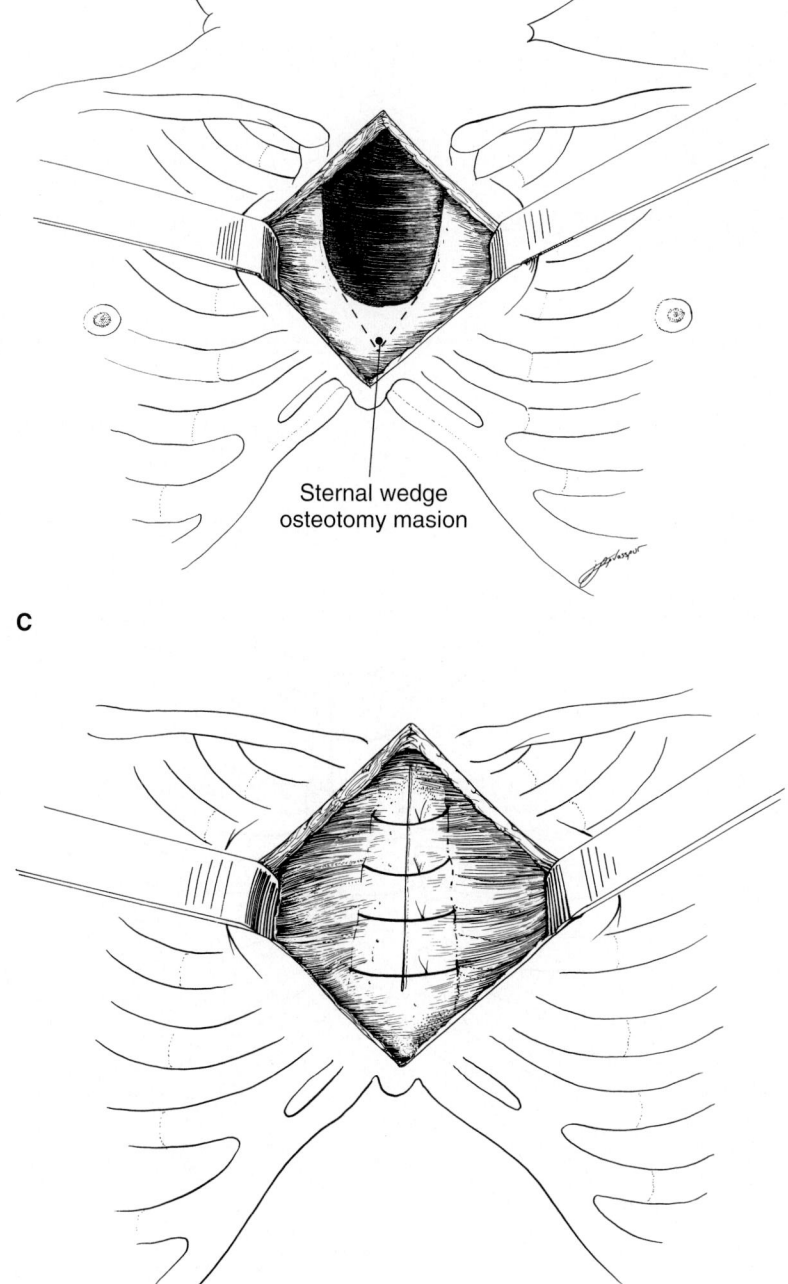

Sternal wedge
osteotomy masion

**C**

**D**

**FIGURE** 19-5 (*Continued*) **C.** A distal wedge of the sternum is removed and the sternal bars are undermined, permitting safe placement of nonabsorbable sutures. **D.** Approximation of the sternal bars with stainless steel wire or heavy, nonabsorbable sutures placed around the sternum.

Prior to closure, intraoperative tissue expansion was performed with saline inflation of 2 large Foley catheters placed under the abdominal portion of the flaps. The abdomen was then closed without cardiac compression. Donor sites in the anterior axillary lines healed by secondary intention. No mention was made of the diaphragmatic defect or its repair. This infant was operated on again at the age of 7 months because of extrusion of the PTFE patch. It was excised, and the bilateral, bipedicled flaps were remobilized for coverage. At 3-year follow-up, the infant was clinically stable, but had a sternal cleft and unrepaired congenital cardiac disease (double-outlet right ventricle, ventricular septal defect, and subpulmonic stenosis).

Surgical repair of thoracic ectopia cordis is one of the most difficult challenges a pediatric surgeon can face because the heart can be oriented in an almost upside-down position. Tilting the apex away from the chin and back toward the diaphragm occludes the great vessels and causes immediate arrest. The strategy, therefore, is to attempt to bring the heart partially into the mediastinum and cover the exposed portion with skin, without radically changing the orientation of the apex. The goals of surgical therapy are to (1) cover the heart to protect it from desiccation and trauma, (2) preserve cardiac output by preventing vessel kinking, (3) repair the associated abdominal wall defect, and (4) stabilize the thoracic cavity so that spontaneous ventilation will be effective.

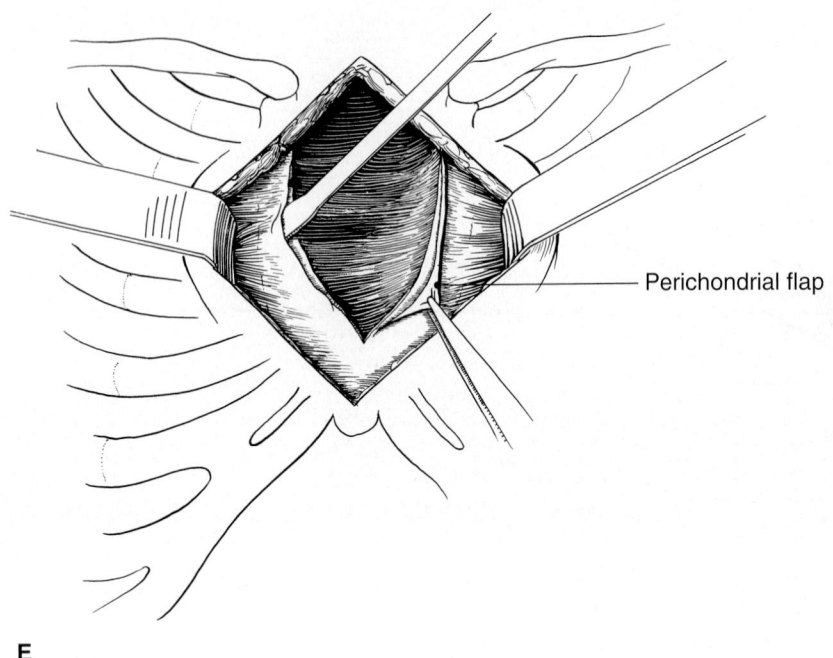

Perichondrial flap

E

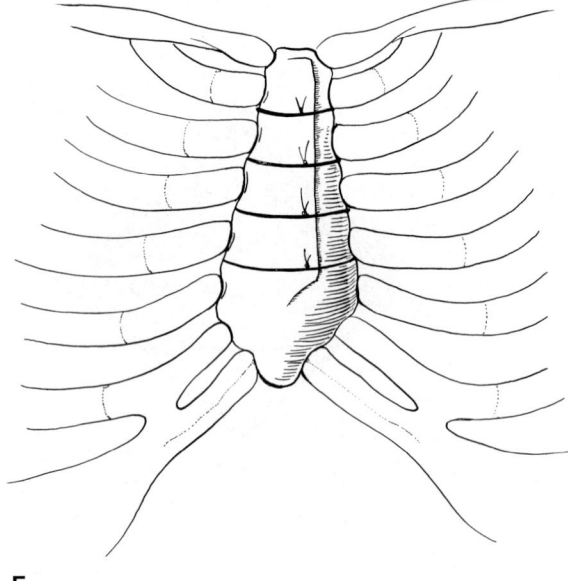

F

**FIGURE 19-5** (*Continued*) **E.** For a more U-shaped cleft, an extensive wedge must be excised from the xiphoid end of the sternum to permit approximation. A flap of perichondrium is raised. **F.** Peristernal sutures are placed, and the perichondrium flap is imbricated to tighten and hold the approximation.

## Documented Historical Cases of Ectopia Cordis Repair

### 1975

A 3-kg term male infant was pink and active on arrival at the children's hospital. The heart protruded completely outside the chest cavity and was uncovered. The sternum was cleft except at the manubrium, and the upper abdominal midline was covered by shiny, attenuated skin to the umbilicus. No other abnormalities were apparent except for hypertelorism. The initial evaluation consisted of a chest radiograph, which revealed normal-appearing lung fields.

The patient's first operation was performed at 7 hours of life, and involved taking down the anterior attachment of the diaphragm and mobilizing the great vessels from the heart into the mediastinum in an attempt to create space for the heart within the chest. After reattachment of the diaphragm

at a lower level, attempts were made to close the widely split sternum directly or with a Dacron patch, but tamponade occurred. Skin flaps were then mobilized to the anterior axillary line, and the skin was closed directly over the heart with interrupted sutures. The midline abdominal wall defect was similarly closed.

The infant recovered from this operation but remained ventilator-dependent and eventually required a tracheostomy. Cardiac catheterization revealed a small ventricular septal defect with a left-to-right shunt. After 6 months of mechanical ventilation, an attempt was made to stabilize the flail chest and enlarge the thorax by placing an acrylic patch in the manubrial area. The gap in the sternal halves was bridged by a piece of Dacron reinforced (on its external surface) with Marlex. Skin flap ischemia developed, and after 2 revisions the prosthesis was removed because of infection. A second attempt to stabilize the chest with a prosthesis again failed because of infection and was removed.

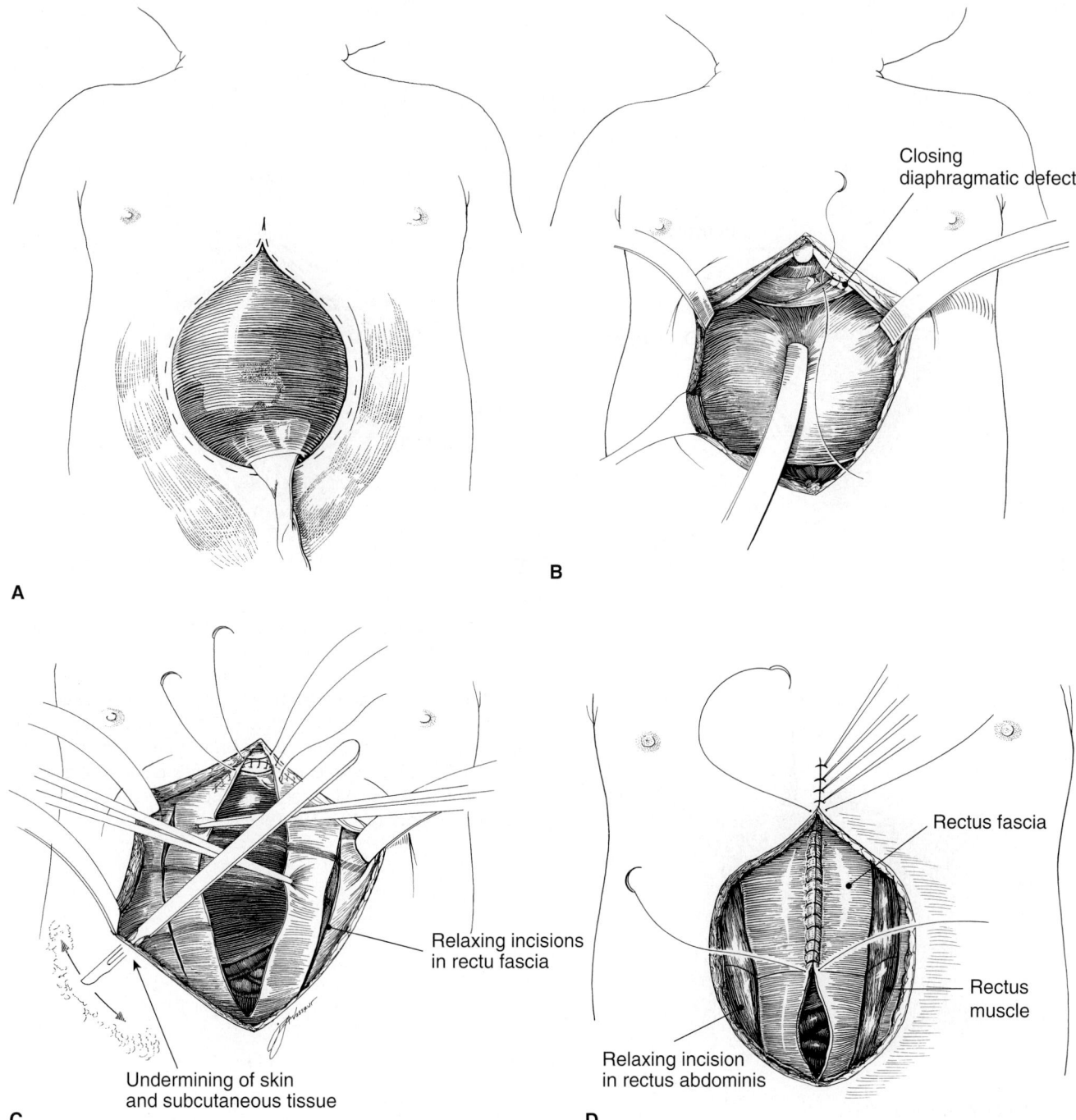

**FIGURE 19-6** Steps in repairing a pentalogy of Cantrell. **A.** An incision is made around the omphalocele. **B.** The junction of the pericardium and peritoneum is sharply incised along the edge of the midline anterior diaphragmatic defect and then the diaphragmatic remnants are sutured to the anterior rib cage. This procedure functionally creates a new pericardium and separates the heart above from the abdominal contents below. **C.** After sharply undermining the skin and subcutaneous tissue, lateral relaxing incisions are made in the anterior abdominal wall fascia to relieve tension and facilitate a primary midline closure. **D.** Midline skin closure completes the abdominal wall reconstruction.

The child remained ventilator-dependent and was eventually discharged home where he received ventilator support. At age 4, the patient was weaned to nocturnal ventilator support. At the age of 6, a bone graft was performed (using iliac crest) between the manubrial remnants. Within 3 months of this operation, the patient was independent of the ventilator, and his tracheostomy was removed a short time later.

At age 12, the patient participated in a full range of activities, including swimming and baseball, while wearing a plastic shield to protect his heart. When the shield was removed, the subcutaneous heart was plainly visible. The patient is now an adult and has occasionally appeared on television to tell his story.

### 1982

A male infant was born with an absent sternum and a bare heart but no cardiac disease. The initial repair consisted of skin coverage with widely mobilized skin flaps. At the age of 19 months, the patient underwent a second operation, in

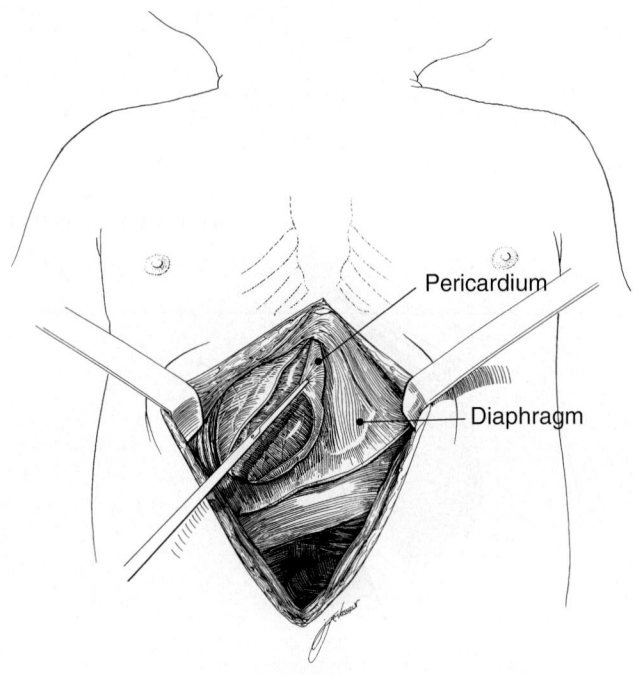

Pericardium

Diaphragm

A

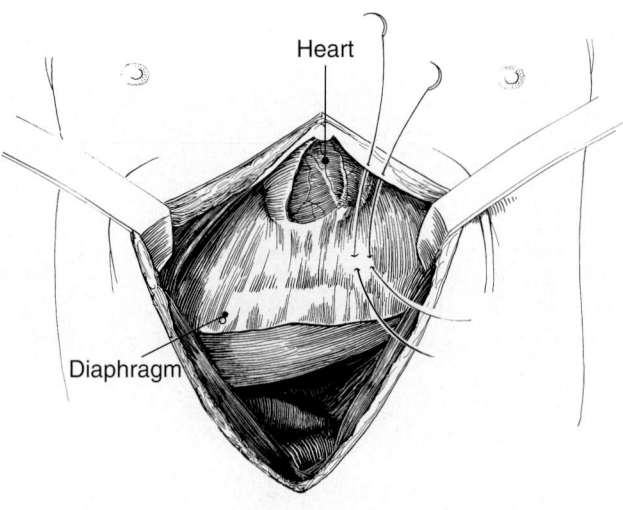

Heart

Diaphragm

B

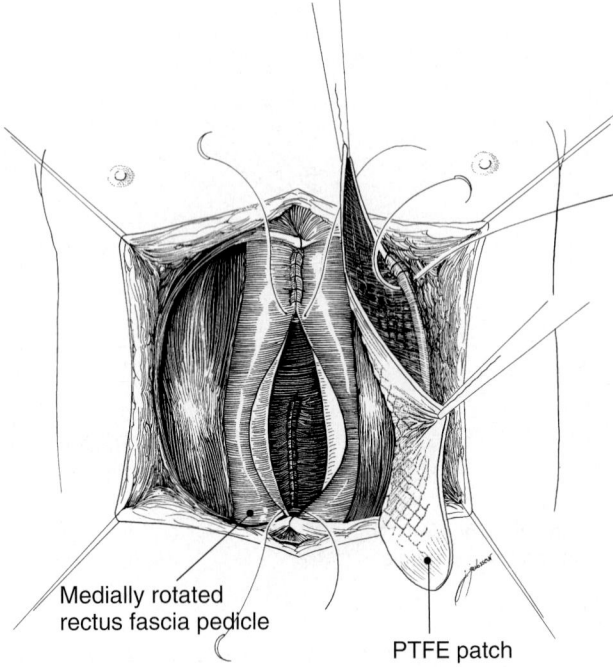

Medially rotated
rectus fascia pedicle

PTFE patch

C

**FIGURE 19-7** Repair techniques for larger thoracoabdominal defects. **A.** The heart and pericardium are dissected free to facilitate the retraction of the heart within the thoracic cavity. **B.** The heart is isolated from the abdomen by a series of stitches between the diaphragm and anterior costal margin. **C.** Relaxing incisions permit approximation of the anterior rectus sheath in the midline. A prosthetic polytetrafluoroethylene (PTFE) patch is placed externally to augment the attenuated abdominal musculature. **D.** The PTFE graft is located external to the rotated anterior rectus sheath.

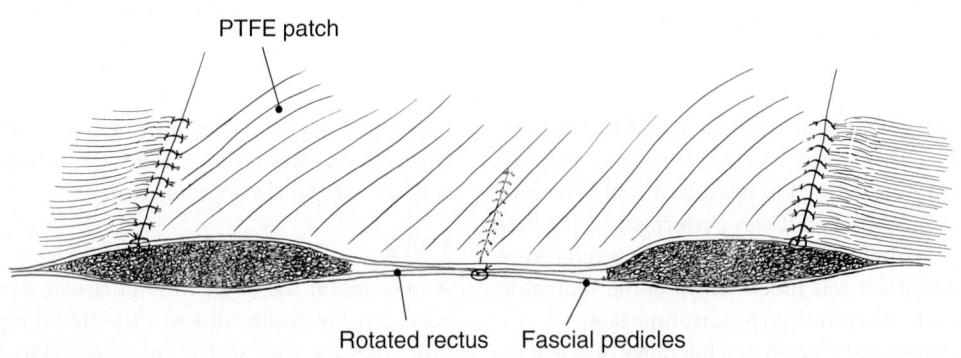

PTFE patch

Rotated rectus    Fascial pedicles

D

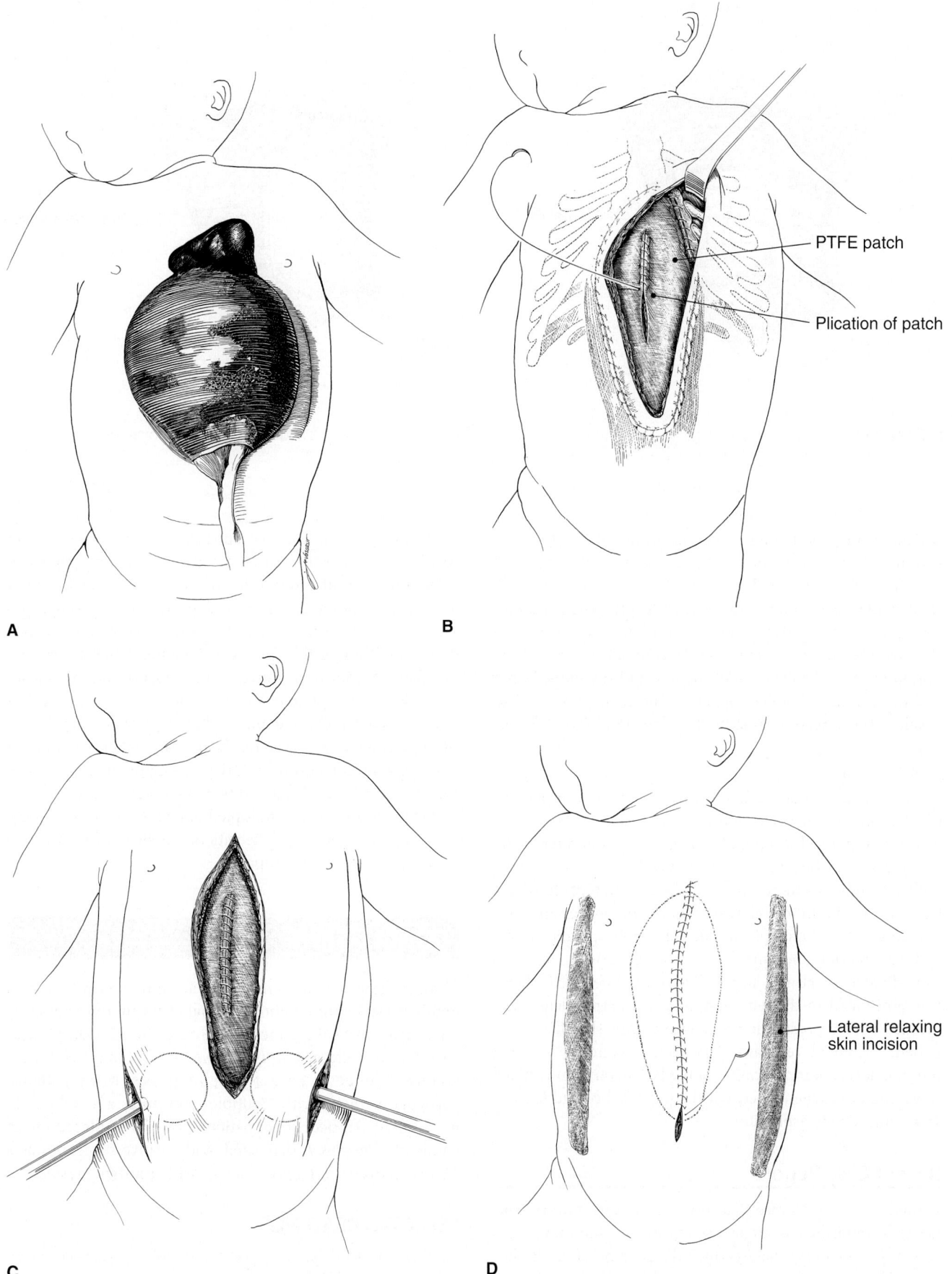

**A**

PTFE patch

Plication of patch

**B**

**C**

Lateral relaxing
skin incision

**D**

**FIGURE 19-8** Staged repair for extensive thoracoabdominal ectopia cordis. **A.** Large membrane-covered defect. **B.** A PTFE patch is sutured circumferentially to the musculofascial margins of the defect. Over several days, plication of the prosthetic patch reduces content into the chest and abdomen. **C.** Tissue expansion over the abdominal portion of the defect facilitates myocutaneous closure using bipedicle and pectoralis major and rectus abdominis flaps. **D.** Lateral relaxing incisions facilitate midline skin closure.

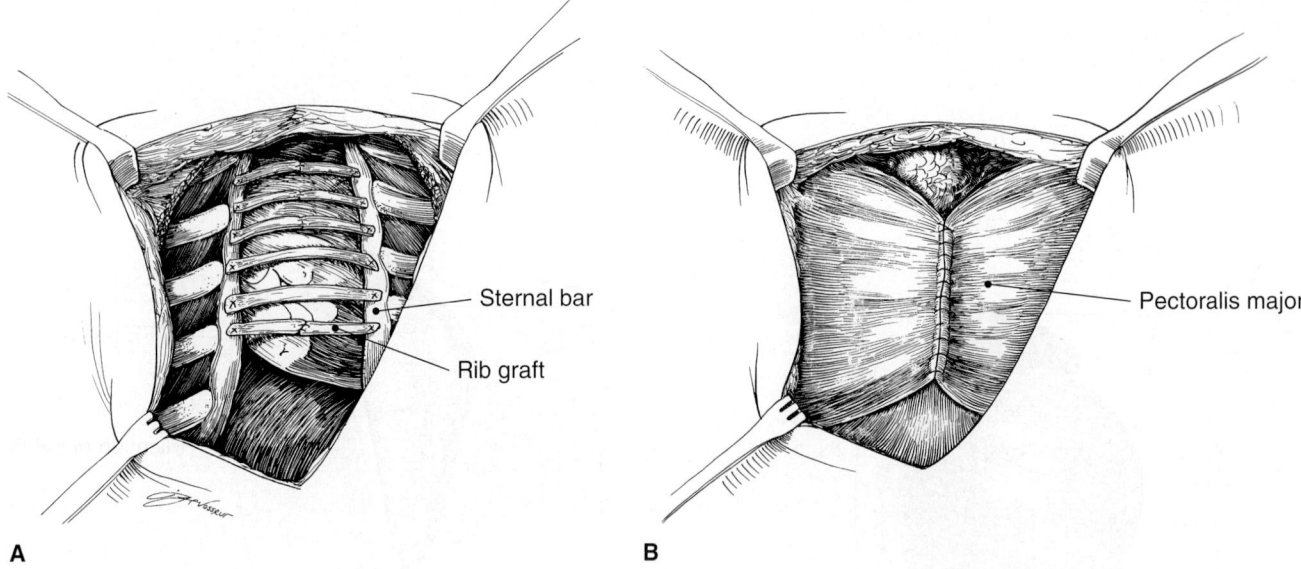

**A**

**B**

**FIGURE 19-9** Second-stage thoracic ectopia cordis repair. **A.** Free rib grafts positioned over the midline defect. **B.** Pectoralis muscles approximated in the midline on top of the rib graft.

which, the mediastinum was enlarged by mobilizing the pericardium. This allowed the heart to recede partially back into the chest. The anterior defect was then bridged with 6 rib strut grafts, each more than 6 cm in length. The pectoralis muscles were then advanced to the midline to cover most of the ribs. The skin flaps were closed to complete the operation. The infant was extubated immediately and discharged after 6 days. At 2-month follow-up, only 3 of the 6 rib struts had ossified. The others remained soft and malleable (Fig. 19-9).

### 1988

A 2.6-kg female infant was born with thoracic ectopia cordis, a small omphalocele, and no intracardiac lesions on an echocardiogram. The operation began 2 hours after birth. The pleural cavities were entered, and the thymus was partially excised to make room for the heart. Attempts to return the heart to the thorax caused severe hypotension and bradycardia. After repair of an anterior diaphragmatic hernia and an anterior abdominal wall, the left costal cartilages were divided, creating a larger cavity for the heart. The heart was positioned in the left chest, and the sternal defect was bridged with a prosthetic and covered with skin flaps. The patient remained ventilator-dependent secondary to a left phrenic nerve injury. Plication of the left diaphragm resulted in ventilator independence, but the patient died suddenly at 10 months due to aspiration.

### Recent Case Report

Ectopia cordis is so rare that most of the literature continues to be published as single case reports. Furthermore, each case requires careful analysis (including examination of photographs) because there continues to be confusion between "true" ectopia cordis (naked heart beating outside the chest) and thoracoabdominal ectopia cordis (covered, partially protruding heart associated with abdominal wall defect) and even large sternal clefts.

The only recent case that appears to meet the criteria of "true" ectopia cordis was reported in 2 separate papers in 2010. The fetal ultrasound demonstrated an upturned heart outside the thoracic cavity, and postpartum photographs appear to demonstrate that the heart is completely extra-thoracic (although the apex is not pointed toward the chin, as other authors have noted). Furthermore, no significant omphalocele component was described. This patient underwent a staged repair. At birth, skin flaps over a prosthetic sheet were used to cover the heart. The patient required a tracheostomy for chronic ventilator support at 1 month of age. At age 18 months, a complex reconstruction using craniofacial hardware and multiple bone grafts was performed. Following this operation, the patient was successfully weaned from chronic ventilator support.

## CONCLUSION

Midline thoracic defects may have a common etiology, but a highly variable presentation. Sternal clefts are rare, but early repair and survival are the general rule. Thoracic and thoracoabdominal ectopia cordis are also rare, but in general these lesions continue to have a poor prognosis. Many patients, particularly those with multiple congenital anomalies, do not survive. An occasional patient, however, if placed in the hands of a prepared, dedicated, and creative surgeon, has a chance of overcoming great odds—with gratifying results.

## SELECTED READINGS

Acastello E, Majluf R, Garrido P, et al. Sternal cleft: a surgical opportunity. *J Pediatr Surg* 2003;38:178–183.

Amato JJ, Zelen J, Talwalkar NG. Single-stage repair of thoracic ectopia cordis. *Ann Thorac Surg* 1995;59:518–520.

Cantrell JR, Haller JA, Ravitch MM. A syndrome of congenital defects involving the abdominal wall, sternum, diaphragm, pericardium, and heart. *Surg Gynecol Obstet* 1958;107:602–614.

Diaz JH. Perioperative management of neonatal ectopia cordis: report of three cases. *Anesth Analg* 1992;75:833–837.

Greenberg BM, Becker JM, Pletcher BA. Congenital bifid sternum: repair in early infancy and literature review. *Plast Reconstr Surg* 1991;88:886–889.

Hochberg J, Ardenghy MF, Gustafson RA, et al. Repair of thoracoabdominal ectopia cordis with myocutaneous flaps and intraoperative tissue expansion. *Plast Reconstr Surg* 1995;95:148–151.

Hornberger LK, Colan SD, Lock JE, et al. Outcome of patients with ectopia cordis and significant intracardiac defects. *Circulation* 1996;94 (suppl II):II32–II37.

Kaplan LC, Matsouka R, Gilbert EF, et al. Ectopia cordis and cleft sternum: evidence for mechanical teratogenesis following rupture of the chorion or yolk sac. *Am J Med Genet* 1985;21:187–202.

Mohan R, Peralta M, Perez R, et al. Chest wall reconstruction in a pediatric patient with ectopia cordis. *Ann Plast Surg* 2010;65:211–213.

Ravitch MM. *Congenital Deformities of the Chest Wall and Their Operative Correction.* Philadelphia: WB Saunders Co; 1977:19–20.

Ravitch MM. *Sternal Clefts. Congenital Deformities of the Chest Wall and Their Operative Correction.* Philadelphia: WB Saunders Co; 1977:1–68.

Shamberger RC, Welch KJ. Sternal defects. *Pediatr Surg Int* 1990;5:156–164.

Skandalakis JE, Gray SW, Ricketts R, Skandalakis LJ. The anterior body wall. In: Skandalakis JE, Gray SW, eds. *Embryology for Surgeons.* 2nd ed. Philadelphia: WB Saunders Co; 1977:551–559.

Van Allen MI, Myhre S. Ectopia cordis thoracalis with craniofacial defects resulting from early amnion rupture. *Teratology* 1985;32:19–24.

# Airway Endoscopy and Pathology, and Tracheotomy

# CHAPTER 20

*Alexandros Georgolios, Charles Johnson III,
and Charles Bagwell*

## KEY POINTS

1. A child's airway is shorter and smaller in caliber than the adult's, the larynx is placed more anterior, and the structures are more collapsible. Prior to ages 8 to 10 years, the smallest portion of the airway is the subglottic trachea.

2. Stridor merits immediate investigation and is nearly always an indication for airway endoscopy.

3. The principal advantage of rigid over flexible bronchoscopy involves better control of the airway, but also allows access to instruments, removal of foreign bodies, or more effective suctioning capability.

4. Rigid and flexible bronchoscopy are complementary techniques used in various circumstances to assess airway anatomy and function, in some cases concurrently.

5. In the rare urgent case when establishment of an airway is critical and endotracheal intubation fails, the treatment of choice in children is needle access of the trachea with a large-bore angiocath.

6. Retention sutures are placed parallel to the proposed site for a pediatric tracheotomy incision in mid-trachea. These can provide exposure of the trachea and allow replacement in the case of accidental tracheal dislodgement in the early postoperative period.

7. There are various and numerous challenging issues for the parents after the patient is discharged home with a new tracheostomy. These may include skin and stoma care, suctioning, humidification and routine changes of the tracheostomy ties and the tracheostomy tube itself, and education for emergent situations.

## AIRWAY ENDOSCOPY AND PATHOLOGY

### History of Airway Endoscopy

Curiosity regarding the mysteries of respiratory function and the need to remove airway foreign bodies have long evoked an interest in airway inspection. Early writings describe Hippocrates' recommendation that a tube be inserted into the upper airway to allow a suffocating patient to breathe. However, it was not until 1807 that the first device for showing the inner cavities of the upper airway was demonstrated by Phillip Bozzini. This primitive instrument, called a *Lichtleiter* (light conductor), consisted of a candle and a series of mirrors contained within a tin and leather housing. A crude laryngoscopic device introduced by Benjamin Babington in 1829 comprised a set of polished mirrors that could reflect sunlight and allowed a view of the upper larynx. In the 1850s, another instrument designed to allow visualization of vocal cord and laryngeal function was constructed from connected mirrors and demonstrated before the Royal Society by a London voice teacher. The term *endoscopy* was coined by Antonin Jean Desormeaux, a French neurologist who produced a similar instrument in 1853. His device used a lens and an attached light source fueled by an alcohol–turpentine mixture.

Despite the demonstration of such devices, their insufficiencies in directing illumination into the airway prevented their use in medical practice. With Edison's invention of the light bulb in 1878, this major obstacle was overcome. In the 1890s, Gustav Killian developed the first electric headlight, and in 1897, he also became the first practitioner to remove a foreign body from the distal airway by endoscopic means. His expertise in this newly developing field, which he named bronchoscopy, was widely acknowledged. Under his leadership the University of Freiburg (Germany) became the center of endoscopic airway evaluation.

The modern era of endoscopic practice began in 1915 with development of the rigid bronchoscope by Chevalier Jackson. This device consisted of a hollow metallic tube connected to a light source at the distal end, which can be inserted into the patient's airway via the mouth. Although it allowed a look into airways previously unseen, it did not provide the desirable illumination or range of vision. The introduction of rigid fiber-optic instruments came in 1968 with the invention of the Storz ventilating bronchoscopic system for pediatric use (Fig. 20-1). This bronchoscope replaced earlier hollow-tube devices with a glass-filled telescope that fit into the open channel of the bronchoscope itself. Opposing convex–concave surfaces in the telescope created lenses, allowing excellent light transmission with little refractive error and

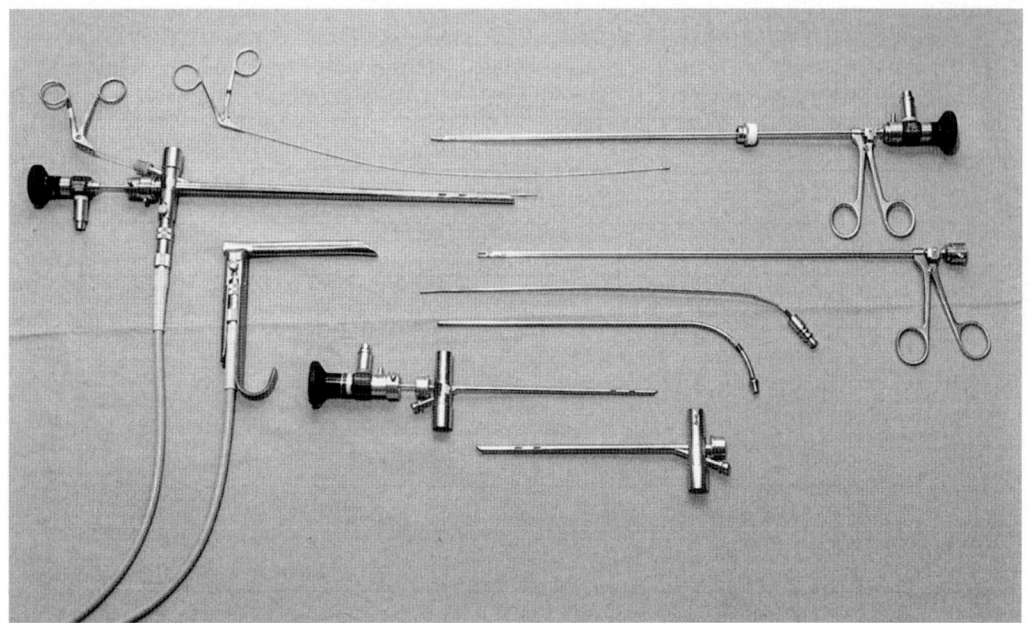

**FIGURE 20-1** Instrumentation for rigid bronchoscopy in children. Note the diminutive size of Storz bronchoscopes, from the 2.5-mm, 20-cm bronchoscope applicable for use in premature infants to the 6-mm, 30-cm bronchoscopes for older children. An anterior commissure laryngoscope is shown along with a variety of instruments that can be passed through the bronchoscope instrument channel for biopsy or suction purposes. Storz foreign body instruments are also shown with their attached housing to accommodate a rod-lens telescope; this unit can be advanced through the bronchoscopic tube for removal of a wide variety of foreign bodies.

high resolution. This arrangement resulted in high-quality magnified images and a controlled ventilation system suitable for use even in neonates. It paved the way for advancements in instrumentation, foreign body removal, suctioning, and laser capacity. Today this same instrumentation is combined with video recording devices that enable archiving, documentation, and teaching.

In 1966, the first flexible fiber-optic bronchoscope was developed by Shigeto Ikeda. This advance made the distal tracheobronchial tree visible. In 1978, Wood and Fink demonstrated a prototype flexible bronchoscope for pediatric use with a 3.5 mm outer diameter. Subsequent miniaturization of flexible bronchoscopes to 2.2 mm has allowed passage through small endotracheal or tracheostomy tubes or the nares, while maintaining effective gas exchange (Fig. 20-2). Newer small-diameter bronchoscopes with suction channels now allow physicians to visualize the airways of premature infants and children without a need for general anesthesia and without significantly altering the anatomy and normal physiology of the upper airway during instrumentation.

It is clear that ongoing improvements in instrumentation will continue to enhance and expand the usefulness of airway endoscopy in the future, for both diagnosis and treatment.

## Airway Anatomy

Compared to that in older patients, a child's airway is shorter and smaller in caliber, the larynx more anterior, and the structures more collapsible. Prior to ages 8 to 10 years, the smallest portion of the airway is the subglottic trachea, an area defined by the underlying cricoid cartilage, the only circumferential

cartilaginous tracheal ring. In contrast, in older children the glottic orifice represents the smallest cross-sectional area. Because of this unique subglottic anatomy, care is required with endotracheal intubation and airway procedures to minimize trauma to this region. Endotracheal tubes that are too large may produce circumferential scarring at the level of the cricoid cartilage from mucosal or submucosal injury. This can be significant since a 50% reduction in cross-sectional area results for every millimeter of airway edema or narrowing of the lumen of an infant's airway. Tables 20-1 and 20-2 list rigid

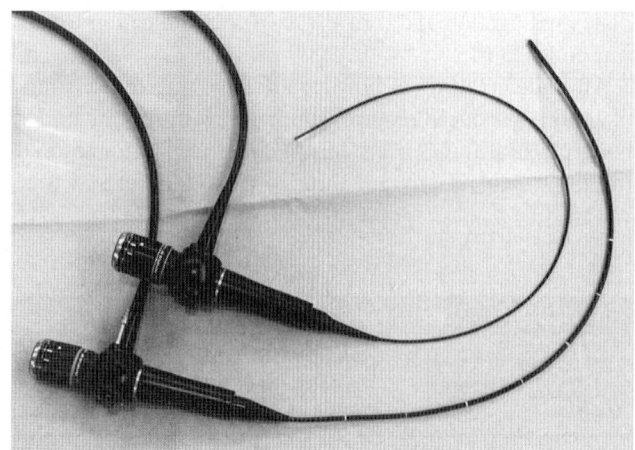

**FIGURE 20-2** Flexible pediatric bronchoscopes. The larger model has an outer diameter of 3.6 mm, with channels for suction and passage of (fine) instruments. The thinner version has an outer diameter of 2.2 mm with no suction channel.

| TABLE 20-1 | Sizes of Rigid Storz Bronchoscopes | | | |
|---|---|---|---|---|
| Sheath Size | Length (cm) | Insertable Length (cm) | Maximum Outer Diameter (mm) | Maximum Inner Diameter (mm) |
| 2.5 | 20 | 16 | 4.1 | 2.8 |
| 3.0 | 20 | 16 | 5.2 | 3.5 |
| 3.5 | 20 | 16 | 5.9 | 4.5 |
| 3.0 | 26 | 23 | 5.2 | 3.5 |
| 3.5 | 26 | 23 | 5.9 | 4.4 |
| 3.7 | 26 | 23 | 6.3 | 4.9 |
| 4.0 | 26 | 23 | 7.5 | 5.1 |
| 3.5 | 30 | 27 | 6.0 | 4.4 |
| 3.7 | 30 | 27 | 6.3 | 4.8 |
| 4.0 | 30 | 27 | 7.5 | 5.0 |

and flexible bronchoscope sizes for correlation with the size of the tracheal lumen in children of various ages. The correct fit of the child's uncuffed endotracheal tube can be calculated as follows.

$$4 + \frac{\text{years of age}}{4} = \text{tube size (mm)}$$

In determining the correct fit of an endotracheal tube, it is prudent to have an air leak at less than 18 to 25 cm of water pressure. This is particularly important in patients with conditions such as Down syndrome, in which airway caliber is typically reduced.

## Pathophysiology

Stridor is a physical sign best characterized as the harsh sound produced by turbulent airflow through a partial obstruction. As discussed later in this chapter, severe stridor merits immediate investigation and is nearly always an indication for airway endoscopy.

An understanding of how a pathologic respiratory sound like this is produced requires familiarity with specific underlying physical forces. Certain principles of physics apply to the movement of any gas through a partially closed tube.

In a static system, pressure exerted by a gas is equal in all directions. However, when there is linear movement of gas, additional pressure is created in the forward vector with a corresponding fall in the lateral pressure. This phenomenon is referred to as the Venturi principle.

As a result of Venturi forces, the flexible airway of a child may narrow momentarily (or even close) during either inspiration or expiration, obstructing the airflow. Once the pressure drops, the lumen can reopen. This pattern of intermittent flow creates vibrations of the lumen that are often strong enough to result in the audible respiratory sounds referred to as stridor.

Viewing the respiratory tree as 3 distinct regions helps in determining the possible pathologic causes of stridor. These regions include (1) a supraglottic and supralaryngeal region (including the pharynx), (2) an extrathoracic tracheal region (including both the glottis and the subglottis), and (3) an intrathoracic tracheal region (including primary and secondary bronchi). Supraglottic lesions often cause stridor during inspiration, whereas lesions of the intrathoracic trachea or bronchi are aggravated during expiration. This is best explained as follows: as air passes through a narrowed supraglottis, the Venturi forces and pharyngeal pressures combine to constrict the airway. In this first region stridor is generally inspiratory. Expiration has the opposite effect on the supraglottic regions, forcing the airway open. A patient with a pattern of inspiratory stridor should be carefully investigated for upper airway lesions such as choanal atresia, expanding lesions in the tongue (such as dermoid cyst or internal thyroglossal duct cyst), or lack of structural airway support as seen in Pierre-Robin syndrome from mandibular hypoplasia or in Beckwith–Wiedemann syndrome from macroglossia.

The second region, the extrathoracic trachea, is a neutral region affected equally by both inspiration and expiration. Both the vocal ligament and the subglottis are independent

| TABLE 20-2 | Sizes of Olympus Flexible Bronchoscopes | | |
|---|---|---|---|
| Model | Size (Outer Diameter in mm) | Minimum Size of Endotracheal Tube for Passage (mm) | Size of Suction Channel (mm) |
| BF-P20 | 5.0 | 7.5 | 2.2 |
| BF-3C30 | 3.6 | 4.5 | 1.2 |
| BF-N20 | 2.2 | 3.0 | None |

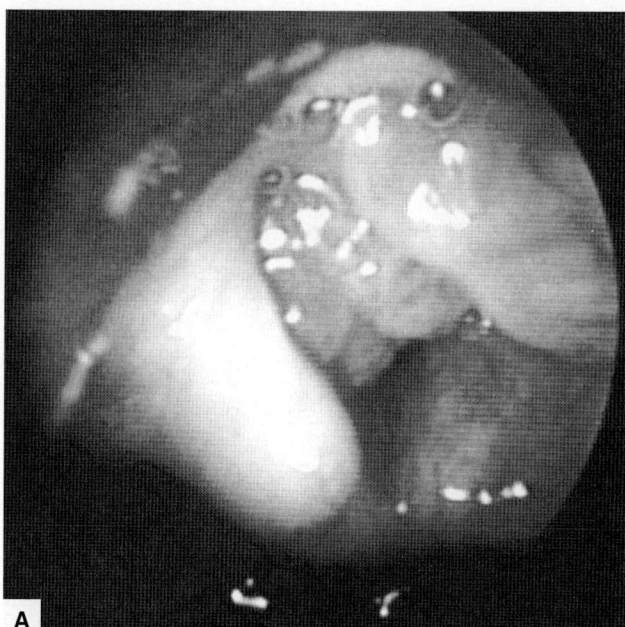 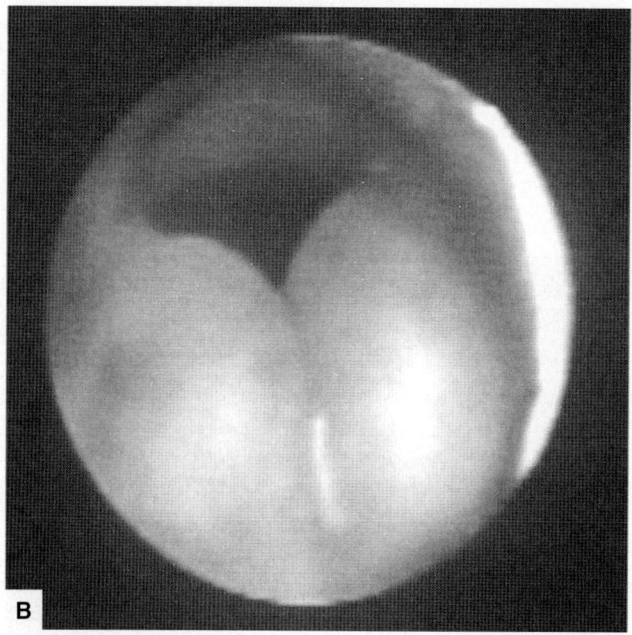

**FIGURE 20-3** Lesions of the larynx and upper airway. **A.** Laryngeal papilloma. A toddler presented with progressive stridor and a confusing history suggesting a laryngeal foreign body. The diagnosis of airway papillomata was established endoscopically and confirmed with a biopsy. A $CO_2$ laser resection produced initial good results; long-term results are unknown. **B.** Laryngeal cysts. An infant presented at a few months of age with rapidly progressive stridor. Cysts demonstrated in the glottic region were amenable to $CO_2$ laser resection with an immediate resolution of symptoms.

of fluid dynamics like the Venturi principle. Because airflow depends on absolute lumen size, the airway cannot contract or expand dynamically. When stridor develops in this region, the glottic and subglottic lumens have reached a critically small size (Fig. 20-3). Since stridor is heard during both inspiration and expiration, it is called biphasic. Breathing requires tremendous effort through a critically narrowed opening, and biphasic stridor often heralds respiratory collapse. Accordingly, this physical finding may represent a medical emergency likely to require intubation or a tracheotomy.

In the third airway (intrathoracic) bronchial region, the positive pressure from expiratory forces within the chest narrow the bronchial lumen, even in normal children. As air moves during expiration, the Venturi principle again adds a constricting force. The intrathoracic forces and the Venturi forces act jointly to close the lumen against a foreign body or another lesion. The resultant sound is expiratory in phase, manifest as stridor best described as "wheezing."

## Patient Assessment and Diagnostic Guidelines

Physical examination of a patient with airway distress must be prompt, thorough, and organized. The clinician should look for tachypnea and signs of fatigue that may signal respiratory collapse. These include flaring of the nasal alae, the use of accessory neck or chest muscles, drooling (when tachypnea prohibits swallowing secretions), or an upright "tripod" posture with the neck hyperextended in an attempt to improve airflow. If the child appears in respiratory distress, examination of the airway should not be undertaken in a nonsecure setting at risk of precipitating respiratory arrest.

Rather, the patient should quickly be moved to a setting with ready access to emergency airway intervention by a medical team experienced in pediatric airway management.

In a well-oxygenated, stable child, an additional examination can proceed. A thorough assessment should include information regarding the child's prior health, as well as any conditions that may have a bearing on the developing respiratory system, including prematurity, endotracheal intubation, or known pediatric syndromes. The duration of symptoms and their progression over time may offer clues regarding the nature of an underlying process; a slowly decreasing airway lumen may be caused by a gradually enlarging subglottic hemangioma, whereas the rapid onset of symptoms may indicate laryngotracheitis (croup). Since the airway and upper gastrointestinal tracts are in juxtaposition, abnormalities in eating or swallowing may suggest vascular rings, mediastinal masses, or a wide range of other lesions, including foreign bodies in the esophagus (Fig. 20-4). The concern for foreign body aspiration in the young child should prompt questions regarding witnessed episodes of choking, coughing, or cyanotic spells, especially if food or objects were in the mouth at the time (Fig. 20-5). Physical examination should also include careful examination of the head, neck, and chest. Clues to an airway lesion may be present elsewhere on the body, as in the case of airway hemangiomas; 50% of children with these lesions also have visible hemangiomas elsewhere on the body.

In addition to obtaining a careful history and performing a thorough physical examination of the stable child, an appropriate roentgenographic evaluation is indicated. The physician should request plain views of the soft tissues of the neck and chest in the anteroposterior and lateral planes. In the

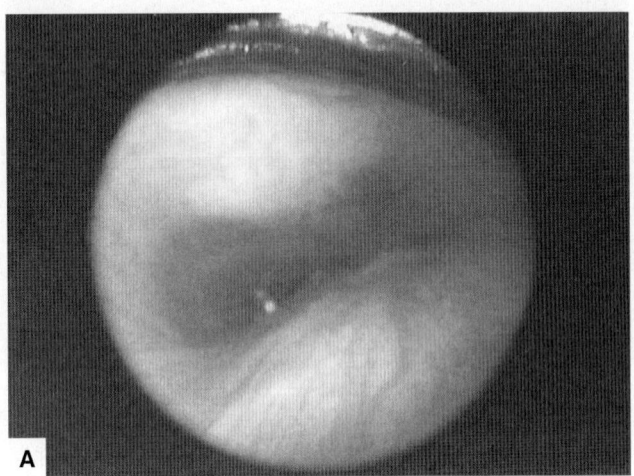

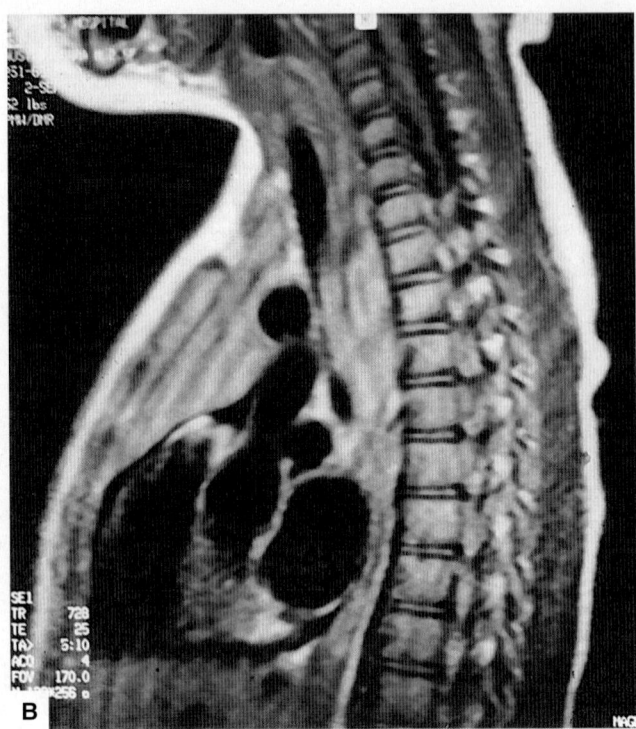

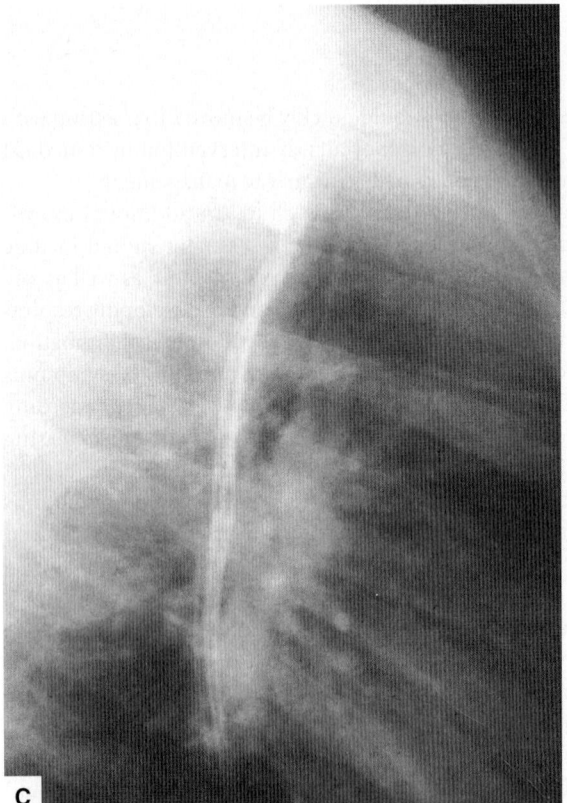

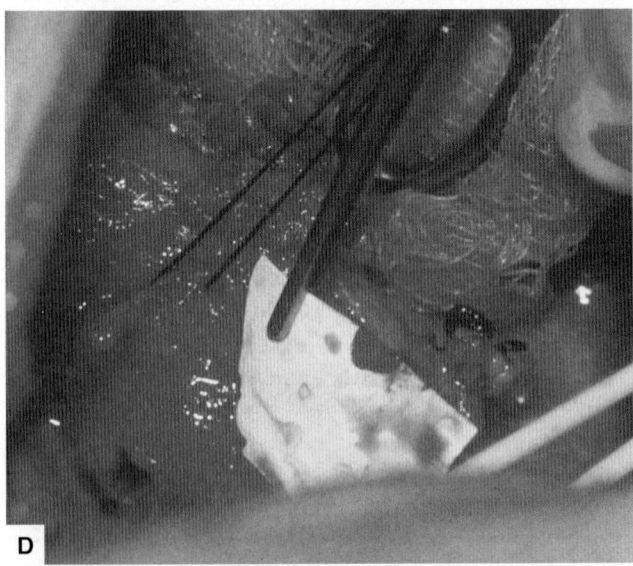

**FIGURE 20-4** A 3-year-old child presented to a local practitioner with increasing stridor and was found to have distal airway collapse on bronchoscopic evaluation (**A**). A subsequent magnetic resonance image showed a posterior mediastinal mass (**B**), initially thought to represent a hemangioma. Lack of response to systemic steroids prompted a repeat scan and a subsequent barium swallow that demonstrated a region of esophageal irregularity (**C**). A thoracotomy revealed a dense, inflammatory mass encasing the upper esophagus; an irregular plastic fragment was found embedded in the muscular wall of the esophagus (**D**) without communication with the esophageal lumen from which it had eroded. The child's recovery was uneventful, with complete resolution of her stridor.

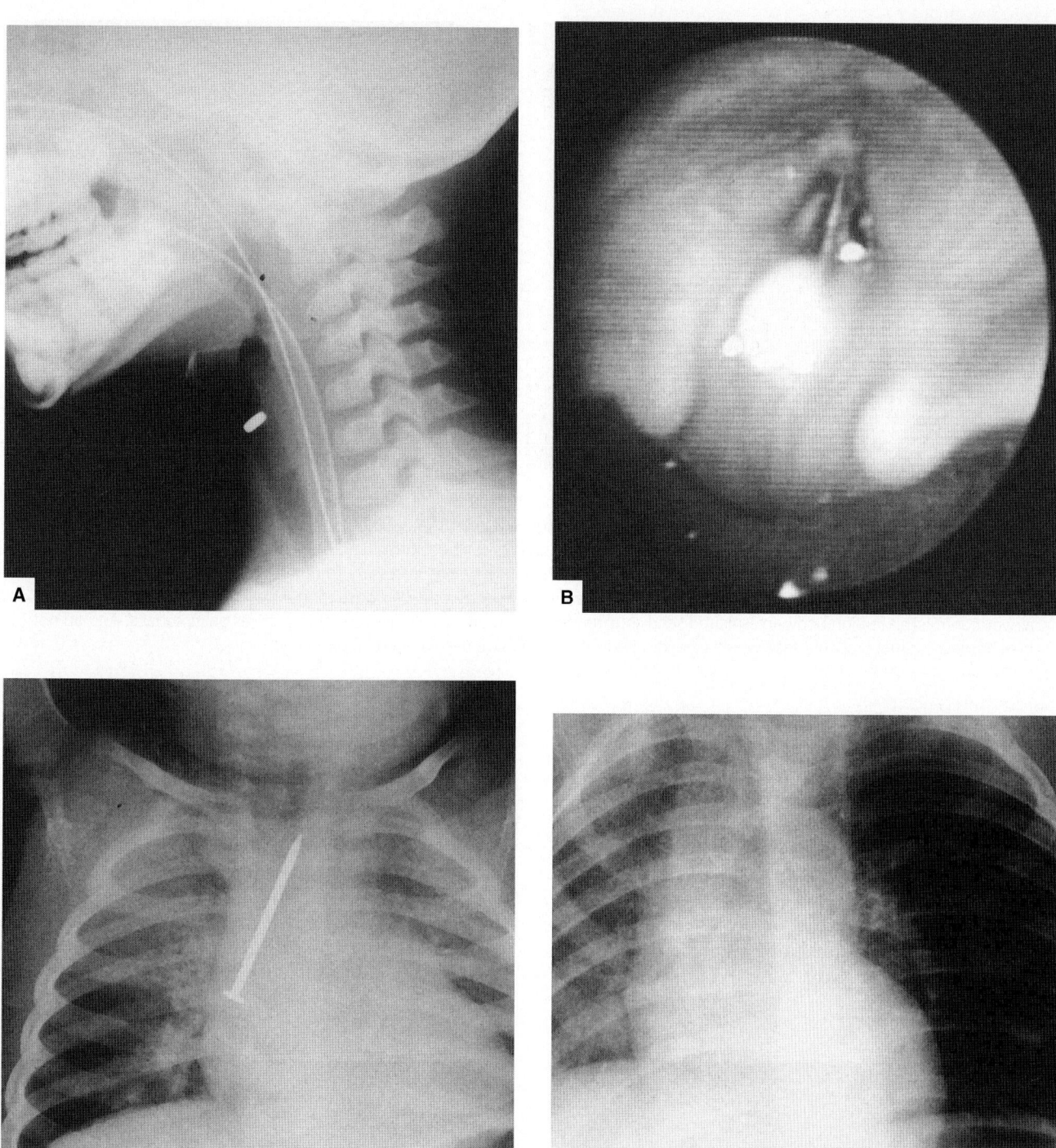

**FIGURE 20-5** Foreign bodies in the airway. **A.** A youngster arrived at the emergency room *in extremis*, having fallen while chasing a sibling. This lateral neck film demonstrates a radiopaque foreign body in the larynx. At the autopsy, the coroner reported a plastic chess piece tightly impacted in the glottic orifice, completely obstructing the lumen. **B.** A toddler presented in late January with a history of stridor and a voice change of 6 weeks' duration. On bronchoscopic evaluation, a foreign body was visible in the glottic orifice, a piece of plastic from a home-made Christmas ornament that had been aspirated as an unwitnessed event. The symptoms resolved after its removal. **C.** The nail shown on this chest radiograph was aspirated by a toddler who presented with mild respiratory symptoms. An attempt to remove it with a flexible bronchoscope resulted in a disastrous outcome. Removal of a foreign body should be attempted only by those with pediatric experience and proper equipment for secure airway control and foreign body extraction. **D.** An infant presented with obstructive emphysema, as seen on a chest radiograph, caused by a popcorn kernel impacted in the left main stem bronchus. This radiographic image should prompt rigid bronchoscopy to exclude airway foreign bodies.

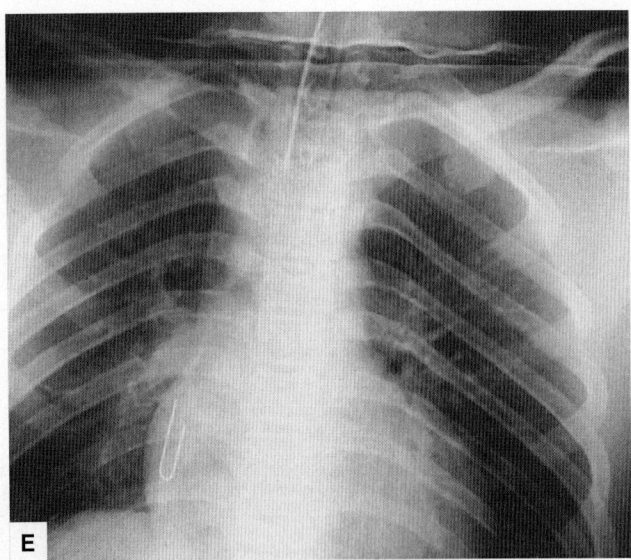

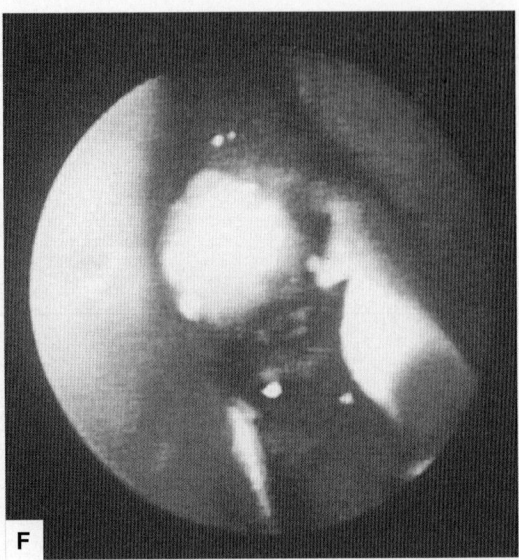

**FIGURE 20-5** (*Continued*) **E.** A teenager presented to a local practitioner having aspirated a broken paper clip at school. Multiple attempts were made to remove the proximal foreign body using flexible instrumentation, resulting in displacement of the foreign body distally and prompting referral. Although the paper clip could be visualized with a rigid bronchoscope, it could not be removed endoscopically as it tended to hook into the tracheal wall. A thoracotomy was necessary to remove it. **F.** Removal of an aspirated foreign body with Storz foreign body instruments through a rigid bronchoscope, demonstrating excellent visualization with secure airway control. This foreign body, an aspirated sand spur, tended to migrate distally because of tiny spikes on its surface. If it had not been retrieved, distal bronchiectasis would have resulted, which may have necessitated lung resection.

anteroposterior view, the tracheal air column is enhanced with the use of a high-kilovoltage technique and should reveal a normal right lateral deviation just below the thoracic inlet caused by the presence of the aortic arch. Distortion of the air column to the left or into the midline suggests a right-sided aortic arch or mediastinal mass.

It is particularly important to obtain roentgenograms during both inspiration and expiration because mobile pharyngeal tissues bulge outward during expiration, mimicking a retropharyngeal abscess or mass. Persistent pulmonary hyperaeration during expiration is indirect evidence of the bronchial obstruction seen when a foreign body is present. If a roentgenogram cannot be obtained in true expiration or inspiration, fluoroscopy may be indicated to ascertain respiratory effort and segmental ventilation.

Computed tomography with enhancement has improved radiographic evaluation, allowing the analysis of both hard and soft tissue structures (eg, airway structures, adjacent masses or lesions, and lung parenchyma) to within millimeters of size and also location (Fig. 20-6).

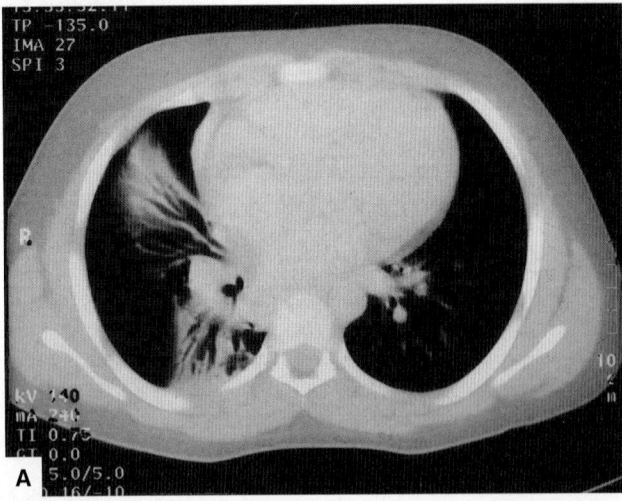

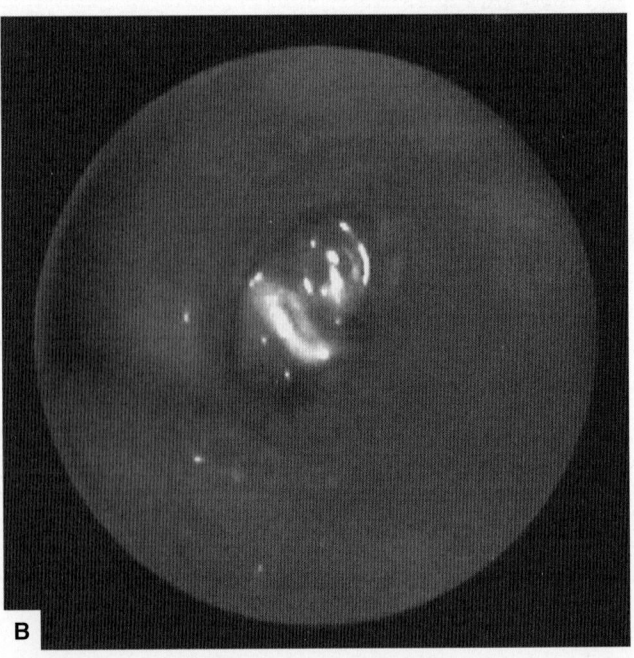

**FIGURE 20-6** Advanced bilobar bronchiectasis seen on a computed tomogram (**A**) due to a foreign body (a sunflower seed) lodged in the bronchus intermedius (**B**). The radiograph was normal 3 weeks after an uneventful foreign body removal.

# INDICATIONS FOR LARYNGOBRONCHOSCOPY

A worsening airway obstruction or an overall worsening condition of the child's respirations indicates the need for laryngobronchoscopy. In a stable patient in the office setting, direct laryngoscopy with flexible instrumentation can be performed under topical anesthesia. In a stable patient who requires a more thorough evaluation, laryngoscopy should be performed in the operating room as part of any airway endoscopic examination. These procedures enable a diagnosis to be made and assist in the planning of further treatment. If indicated, samples for bacteriological culture can be taken, and definitive treatment of an obstructing lesion can be performed under the same anesthetic.

For a child who has signs of respiratory distress, urgent endoscopic evaluation is mandatory. Early intervention in the setting of worsening stridor may avoid more extreme measures such as endotracheal intubation or a tracheostomy under critical conditions. It should be noted that once an endotracheal tube has been passed, the opportunity for diagnosis is greatly compromised.

If poor weight gain and difficulty in feeding are present in addition to concerns regarding airway compromise, endoscopy may be revealing of chronic conditions such as laryngomalacia or reflux-related irritation/inflammation.

Additionally, if imaging techniques such as computed tomography or echocardiography suggest an abnormality such as a vascular ring, endoscopy may confirm the diagnosis (Fig. 20-7).

## Endoscopic Evaluation

Careful inspection of the pharynx, larynx, trachea, and bronchi provides critical information on lumen size, vocal cord mobility, and the presence of dynamic compression, inflammation, or infection. Cooperation and teamwork between the surgeon and the anesthesiologist is absolutely imperative, as well as a surgical nurse/assistant who is familiar with the endoscopic equipment material. The preparation for airway endoscopy should include a discussion of an overall strategy and the resources required to handle all possible contingencies. The attending pulmonologist should also be available, especially when the patient has a history of pulmonary dysfunction or previous bronchoscopic procedures. The possible need for urgent airway access by cannula or a tracheostomy should be kept in mind for any airway procedure, and the appropriate instruments should be available in the operating room. A surgical cricothyrotomy is rarely advisable in young children; emergency airway access can be achieved faster and with less risk through the use of a large-bore angiocatheter (12- or 14-gauge) by direct, percutaneous tracheal puncture. Oxygenation can be performed through this intratracheal cannula using the hub of a 3-mm endotracheal tube connector attached to the bag valve mask or anesthesia circuit, until intubation or formal tracheotomy can be performed.

## Utility and Limitations of Rigid and Flexible Bronchoscopy

Rigid and flexible bronchoscopy are complementary techniques used in various circumstances to assess airway anatomy and function, in some cases concurrently. Bronchoscopy may be diagnostic or therapeutic. Sometimes the diagnosis is already known, other times, there may be unexplained symptoms or undiagnosed disease that can be clarified only by direct examination of the airway. It is within the setting of airway obstruction or compromise that most difficulties occur. While both rigid and flexible bronchoscopy have advantages as well as disadvantages, both require an understanding of the unique anatomy of infants and children, and the potential risks involved in any attempt to visualize anatomical structures of the airway. Regardless of which endoscopic procedure is used, the importance of gentle technique cannot be overemphasized.

Rigid bronchoscopy has a more invasive character and is best utilized to visualize the oropharynx, larynx, vocal cords, and proximal tracheal bronchial tree. The procedure may be performed in an endoscopy suite with available anesthesia, but for most children it is more appropriately performed in the operating room under general anesthesia; it may be combined with flexible bronchoscopy for better distal airway visualization and suctioning.

The indications for rigid bronchoscopy usually involve severe or progressive airway obstruction, suspected foreign body aspiration, or a variety of surgical interventions, such as airway stent placement or dilation of tracheal or bronchial stenosis. The overall benefits to be gained from rigid bronchoscopy in children are shown in a large-scale study conducted by Wiseman over a 15-year period where the use of rigid bronchoscopy contributed to the final diagnosis in almost 90% of patients, with no mortality and a morbidity rate of only 3.5%.

The principal advantage of rigid over flexible bronchoscopy involves better control of the airway, but also allows access to instruments, removal of foreign bodies, or more effective suctioning capability.

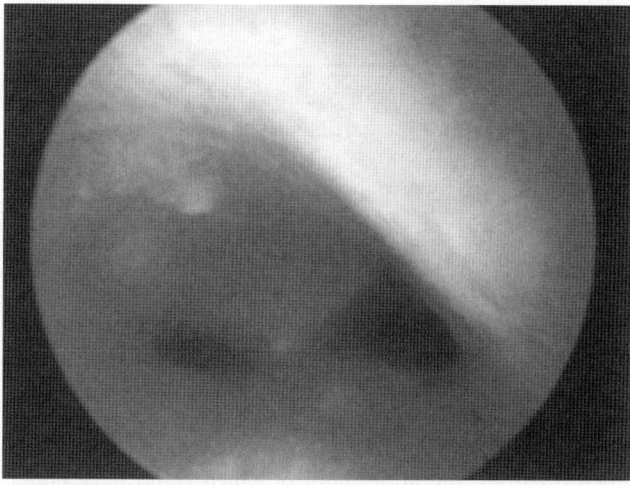

**FIGURE 20-7** A vascular ring is demonstrated on bronchoscopy in a young child with intermittent airway symptoms; these symptoms resolved after division of the ring and a concomitant aortopexy.

Since the rigid bronchoscope can be placed only through the mouth, proper positioning requires neck hyperextension, usually upon a gently folded towel placed just below the occiput. This entails some risk for children with physical conditions that limit wide opening of the mouth or limited neck mobility, as seen in patients with Down syndrome or Arnold–Chiari malformation.

Unlike rigid bronchoscopy, flexible fiber-optic bronchoscopy can be carried out under topical anesthesia with or without intravenous sedation. Its use extends to settings beyond a hospital operating room, such as an intensive care unit. In addition, since flexible bronchoscopes can be passed through mouth or naris, this technique may be useful in evaluating children with anatomic anomalies or maxillofacial trauma that make passage of a rigid scope difficult. Since the airway of patients who undergo flexible bronchoscopy through an endotracheal tube can be obstructed during the endoscopic examination, careful attention must be paid to oxygen saturation and carbon dioxide levels during the procedure in order to ensure physiological stability.

The standard pediatric flexible bronchoscope has a 3.5 to 3.7 mm outside diameter and a 1.2-mm suction channel. This instrument can be used in infants weighing as little as 700 g, and most term newborns can breathe around it spontaneously for short periods. To minimize the risk of hypoxia, small infants can undergo bronchoscopy through a face mask adapter, either breathing spontaneously or being manually ventilated by an anesthesiologist. Examination of the distal airways in intubated infants usually requires extubation, use of a rigid bronchoscope, or possible use of a very small flexible bronchoscope.

Ultrathin flexible bronchoscopes offer many advantages for examination of the lower airways of infants and small children. The most important of these is the ability to pass through small endotracheal or tracheostomy tubes while maintaining effective gas exchange. Ultrathin flexible bronchoscopes can be used for other purposes as well, including in situ evaluation of (the placement of) tracheostomy tubes and the dynamics of the posterior trachea near the tip of tracheostomy tubes, and for retrograde direct laryngoscopy in infants with tracheostomies. They have also been used to direct the placement of balloon catheters for dilation of bronchial stenoses, to examine peripheral airways beyond the subsegmental bronchi in infants, and for intraoperative assessment of bronchial patency during pulmonary resection. Despite this wide array of possible uses, ultrathin flexible bronchoscopes provide only limited working channels and limited suction capability.

While visualization of airway patency and management of obstructive lesions are best accomplished using a rigid bronchoscope with the patient under general anesthesia, the use of a flexible bronchoscope with the patient under sedation and local anesthesia allows a more dynamic view of the airway. Although tracheoesophageal fistulae are best identified and their location is assessed by rigid endoscopy (Fig. 20-8), other conditions such as tracheomalacia are best assessed in a dynamic state. When rigid endoscopy is used to assess dynamics of airway motion, anesthesia must be lightened to allow for spontaneous respiration and assess collapse from tracheomalacia.

The widespread use of flexible bronchoscopy by nonsurgeons may lead to confusion regarding its value or role in diagnosis or management. Wood reported the use of flexible

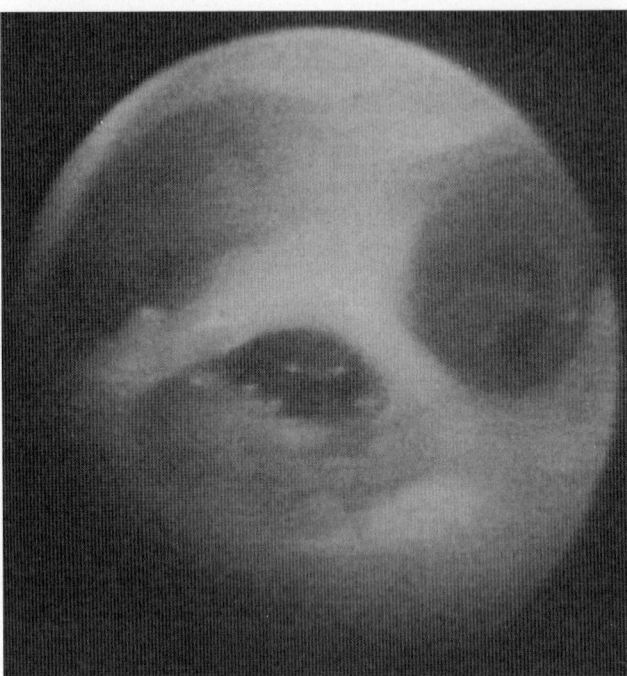

**FIGURE 20-8** A newborn with esophageal atresia demonstrated a distal tracheoesophageal fistula at the level of the carina. A routine bronchoscopic evaluation prior to a thoracotomy provided important information, revealing the presence of a proximal fistula and providing an estimation of the distal esophageal length.

bronchoscopy in 1000 children undergoing laryngoscopy or bronchoscopic procedures over a 5-year period. He found endoscopic information of direct relevance to the suspected diagnosis in 75% of patients and demonstrated other unsuspected abnormalities in 15%; normal findings were encountered in only 9% of the patients studied. As in the Wiseman study cited earlier, Wood reported no mortality and a morbidity rate of only 3%, the major complications being abscess formation, laryngospasm, and pneumothorax. Accordingly, when used by well-trained individuals familiar with pediatric airway issues, both flexible and rigid bronchoscopic techniques have unique advantages and specific limitations.

## Airway Foreign Bodies

Sudden onset of respiratory distress is highly suggestive of foreign body aspiration, particularly in toddlers and younger children. The average age for fatal events from aspiration is only 15 months; 75% of aspiration events occur in children younger than 4 years. Endoscopy for evaluation and management of airway foreign bodies should be performed only in the operating room setting with surgical and anesthesia teams in attendance (Fig. 20-9). If foreign body aspiration is suspected, general anesthesia should be induced in a manner that minimizes the effects on spontaneous ventilation. Should assisted ventilation be necessary, avoiding positive airway pressure may reduce the chance of foreign body dislodgement or distal migration, both of which could have potentially disastrous results.

When removing large or dangerous foreign bodies that might result in occlusion of the airway or injury to delicate

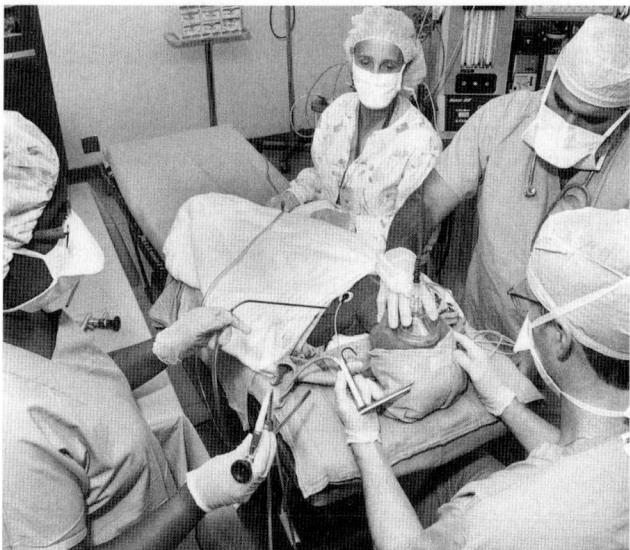

**FIGURE 20-9** Layout for rigid bronchoscopy. Layout for rigid bronchoscopy in a pediatric patient is demonstrated. Note that the patient is positioned with the neck slightly hyperextended on a folded towel, the eyes taped and protected, and the chest exposed for visualization. Induction of anesthetic can usually be performed without intubation, allowing the surgeon a first look at most noncritical airways. An anterior commissure laryngoscope, which provides excellent visualization in difficult pediatric airway cases, is shown. Nursing personnel skilled in equipment use and in the performance of this procedure are necessary. Organization of the entire team to review the proposed "game plan" prior to such procedures is essential, especially in cases of anticipated difficult airway access.

tissues, conversion to a tracheostomy may need to be considered. Thoracotomy should be reserved for the rare complications of endoscopic removal (eg, airway perforation or a major injury to the trachea or bronchus) or cases where the foreign body cannot be removed by endoscopic techniques and must be extracted by bronchotomy or through lung parenchyma. A lobectomy may be required in rare cases when a foreign body has caused a pulmonary abscess, the destruction of parenchyma, or chronic bronchiectasis.

The significant risks involved in removing foreign bodies without secure airway control and less than optimum instrumentation mandate against attempts to use any technique other than rigid endoscopy in an operating room setting. As noted by Kelly and Mantor, if occult foreign bodies are found during flexible bronchoscopy, conversion to rigid instrumentation should be carried out before attempting foreign body removal. It is important to note that foreign body aspiration can masquerade as other pediatric respiratory illness, as illustrated by a study conducted by Wood and Gauderer showing foreign bodies in 1% of all patients undergoing flexible endoscopy for a wide variety of reasons.

We have found flexible and rigid bronchoscopy to be complementary instruments in the operating room setting for occasional foreign bodies that are so distally located that then cannot be reached by flexible bronchoscopy alone. In such a case, the removal of demonstrable foreign bodies can occur under rigid instrumentation under the same general anesthetic. When used in conjunction with rigid bronchoscopes, flexible scopes assist not only in the diagnosis for borderline cases but also in the removal of difficult or fragmented objects from those distal airways.

## Treatment with Laser Therapy

Lasers can be useful for resection or fulguration of a number of airway lesions (Fig. 20-10). Although a carbon dioxide laser provides a superficial depth of penetration making it safe for routine airway use, the laser beam cannot be passed through a fiber-optic cable; special laser bronchoscopic tubes are required to focus the beam directly on the target tissue

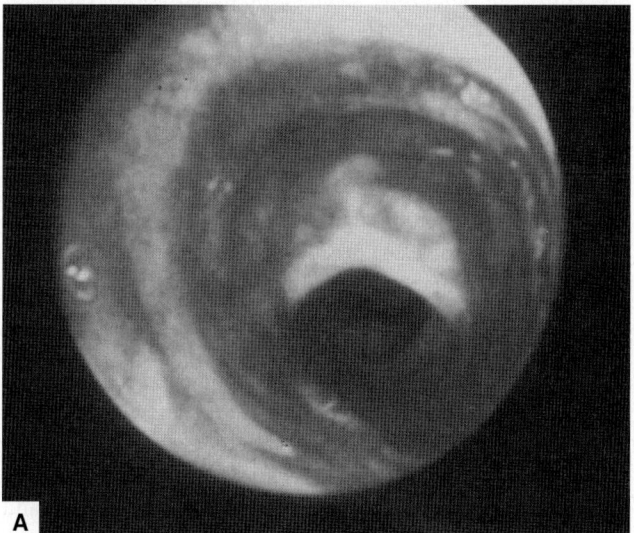

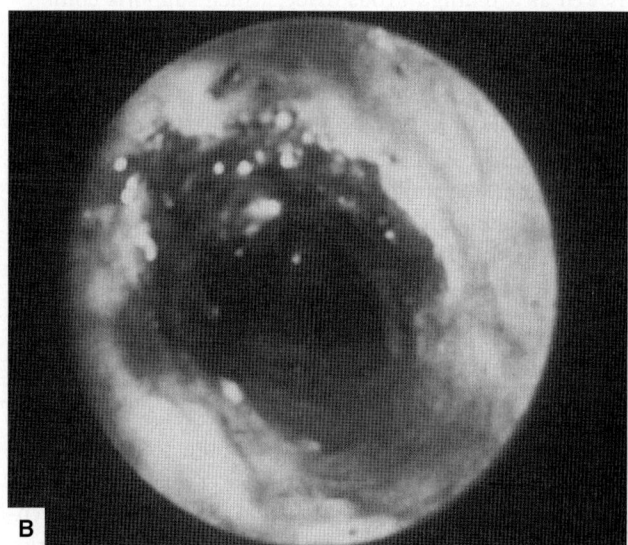

**FIGURE 20-10** An adolescent presented with a long history of airway difficulties dating to infancy when a tracheostomy was done because of respiratory distress. Subsequent decannulation was also performed. Over subsequent childhood years he did well, although he demonstrated severe dyspnea on exertion. A bronchoscopic evaluation showed a thick web in the distal trachea (**A**), presumably from the distal tracheostomy cannula, leaving a tracheal lumen of only a 4- to 5-mm diameter. Resection of this dense web was accomplished with a YAG laser; there was significant enlargement of the tracheal lumen (**B**) and complete resolution of symptoms.

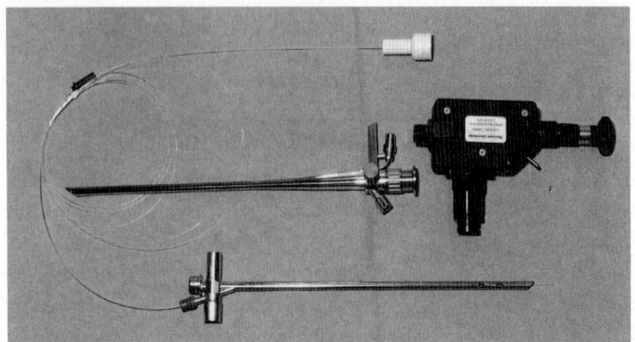

**FIGURE 20-11** Laser bronchoscopy. Equipment for laser bronchoscopy includes a carbon dioxide laser bronchoscope and housing, shown in the center. Because a carbon dioxide laser beam cannot be passed down a fiber-optic cable, it must be transmitted directly through the special bronchoscope by a series of mirrors; manipulation of the joystick moves the laser beam. As shown, fiber-optic cables can be passed down the instrument channel of a Storz bronchoscope to allow the use of a KTP or YAG laser.

(Fig. 20-11). This is a major drawback since the smallest such bronchoscopic tube is 7 mm in diameter, too large for most infants. In contrast, the YAG laser beam can pass through a fiber-optic cable and is easily inserted via the instrument channel of rigid bronchoscopes. However, its depth of penetration is significantly greater, thus increasing the risk of tracheal penetration or deep tissue injury. Its use should involve the minimal effective power setting with a short duration of laser burst. The KTP laser incorporates elements of both the carbon dioxide and YAG lasers with lesser tissue penetration, while allowing beam transmission via a fiber-optic cable.

Concerns pertaining to anesthesia during laser surgery on airway include minimizing thermal injury and using the lowest possible inspired oxygen concentration (preferably less than 30%) compatible with adequate oxygen saturation as well as avoiding nitrous oxide, which supports combustion. Flammable items in the airway such as endotracheal tubes or stents must be shielded from exposure to the laser beam to prevent laser fire from ignition. The safest techniques involve the use of metal airways, the use of a laser through the rigid bronchoscope, or the use of insufflation anesthesia or jet ventilation with a suspension laryngoscopy apparatus, although laser ignition of normal tissue can still occur with prolonged periods of lasering, especially on high energy settings.

## Conclusions

Children with airway lesions, including foreign bodies, may present with symptoms ranging from subtle to dramatic and with varying indications for endoscopic evaluation and treatment. Familiarity with basic tenets of bronchoscopic techniques and equipment for use in children is mandatory prior to undertaking airway evaluation of any child. Once anesthesia has been induced, surgeons are dependent on their own skills and the assistance of the anesthesiologist and nursing staff in attendance to ensure a successful outcome and avoid potentially disastrous complications.

# TRACHEOTOMY

## Relevant Surgical History

Tracheotomy dates back to surgical reports from as early as 124 BC. The invention of metal tracheotomy tubes, replaced in the late 1950s with relatively atraumatic plastic tubes designed at the Hospital for Sick Children in London, created an era in which tracheotomy was a frequently performed procedure. Since then, improvements in endotracheal tube design (eg, high-volume, low-pressure balloons), coupled with the receptance of nasotracheal intubation for long-term ventilatory support, have led to diminished enthusiasm for tracheotomy along with a deliberative process of patient selection.

## Disease Pathophysiology

While in the past, tracheotomies were frequently performed in an emergency setting, either in combination with another surgical procedure or after a short period of assisted ventilation, their use is now much more circumscribed. The basic disease processes that may require or benefit from a tracheotomy are listed in Fig. 20-12.

Although this list is quite extensive, the overall indications are straightforward: either the airway is anatomically compromised or long-term ventilator support is anticipated.

## Diagnostic Principles

The diagnostic procedures required to determine the need for tracheotomy should demonstrate either an anatomic obstruction or a functional impairment of airway patency. Such diagnostic procedures fall into 3 broad categories: (1) endoscopic (rigid or flexible), (2) anatomic (computed tomography or magnetic resonance imaging), or (3) functional (cineradiography). For lesions that cause airway obstruction (congenital anomalies, masses or tumors, trauma), a diagnostic procedure for anatomic detail (computed tomography or magnetic resonance imaging) is usually done first, followed by rigid endoscopy under a general anesthetic to evaluate the oropharynx, larynx, and trachea. With proper preoperative counseling of the parents, the definitive procedure can be performed under the same anesthetic once findings are confined endoscopically.

Functional obstructions may be visualized by cineradiography of the upper aerodigestive tract. Swallowing studies that demonstrate esophageal motility and upper airway protective mechanisms may be the most useful, although endoscopic evaluation may still be necessary to further define the problem (eg, visualization of vocal cord movement with spontaneous respiration).

Evaluation for tracheotomy for indications of excessive secretions or assisted ventilation should require more deliberation. The severity, frequency, and degree of damage caused by recurrent lung infections may determine the need for, and timing of tracheotomy. Inability to wean from a ventilator, coupled with respiratory function testing, lung compliance, and chronic carbon dioxide retention, may help to quantify the degree of damage and accordingly need for long-term ventilation assistance. Central nervous system impairment, respiratory failure, and thoracic dystrophy requiring a

| AIRWAY OBSTRUCTION | SECRETIONS | ASSISTED VENTILATION |
|---|---|---|

- Congenital anomalies:
  Choanal atresia
  Micrognathia
  Laryngo or tracheal:
    Atresias/stenosis
    Webs/malacia

- Masses or tumors:
  Hemangiomas
  Teratomas
  Lymphangiomas
  Neurofibroma

- Trauma:
  Maxillofacial
  Cervical
  Iatrogenic:
    Intubation injury/
    Acute or chronic

- Functional:
  Vocal cord paralysis
  Cricoarytenoid fixation

- Preliminary procedure:
  Craniofacial reconstruction
  Laryngotracheal reconstruction

- Infections:
  Acute epiglottis
  Chronic and/or recurrent
    Pneumonias
  Laryngotracheobronchitis

- Tracheal toilet

- CNS impairment:
  Oropharyngeal function
  Central apnea
  Chronic aspiration
  Coma

- Respiratory failure:
  Chronic and/or recurrent

- Thoracic dystrophy

**FIGURE 20-12** Indications for a tracheotomy.

permanent tracheostomy may present ethical as well as medical decision-making challenges. Such treatments may likely be determined more by the family's wishes and the long-term prognosis than by specific diagnostic criteria.

## Treatment Options

Establishing a surgical airway may be clinically urgent or elective. In the rare urgent case when establishment of an airway is critical and endotracheal intubation fails, the treatment of choice is needle access of the trachea with a large-bore angiocath. This can be quickly performed, even in a combative hypoxic child, in seconds.

## Tracheotomy

In preparation for elective tracheotomy (see Figs. 20-13 to 20-17), the child is anesthetized via endotracheal intubation or through a ventilating rigid bronchoscope, if necessary for airway security. The neck should be fully extended over a rolled towel or sandbag with the occiput just resting on the table surface. This position straightens the cervical trachea and elevates it to the skin surface.

The thyroid cartilage can usually be palpated; in many children, the tracheal rings can be also felt. The neck incision should be placed transversely in the midcervical region approximately 1 fingerbreadth above the sternal notch and is only 2 to 3 cm long. With proper retraction, a larger incision should not be necessary (Fig. 20-13). Small subcutaneous cervical veins are ligated or cauterized, as a bloodless

field is crucial. With gentle retraction, strap muscles can be bloodlessly separated in the midline and retracted laterally. At this point, dissection of overlying soft tissue should expose the underlying trachea allowing cricoid cartilage and some

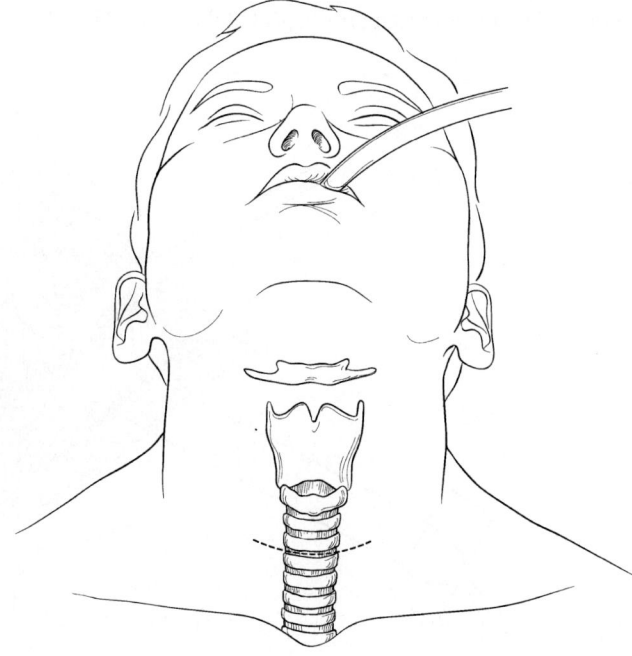

**FIGURE 20-13** With an endotracheal tube in place, a roll horizontally beneath the shoulders, and the neck extended, a tracheotomy skin incision is made horizontally to the midline approximately one finger breadth above the sternal notch.

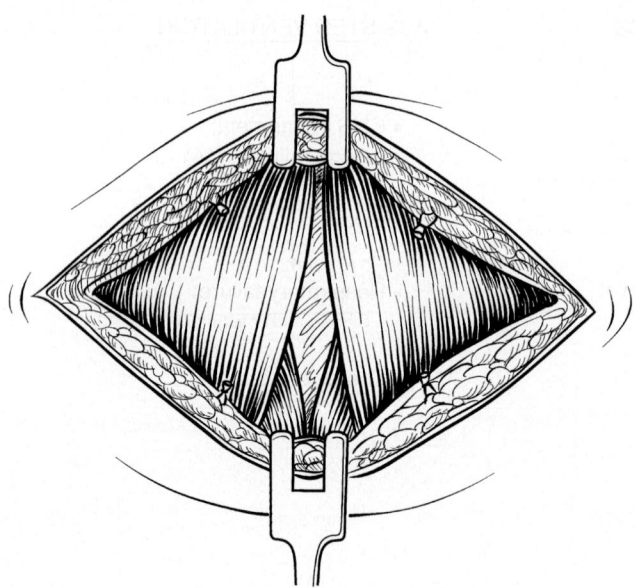

**FIGURE 20-14** After dividing the skin and subcutaneous tissue, the strap muscles are exposed with gentle cephalocaudal retraction, and the midline raphe of the neck is visualized and subsequently incised.

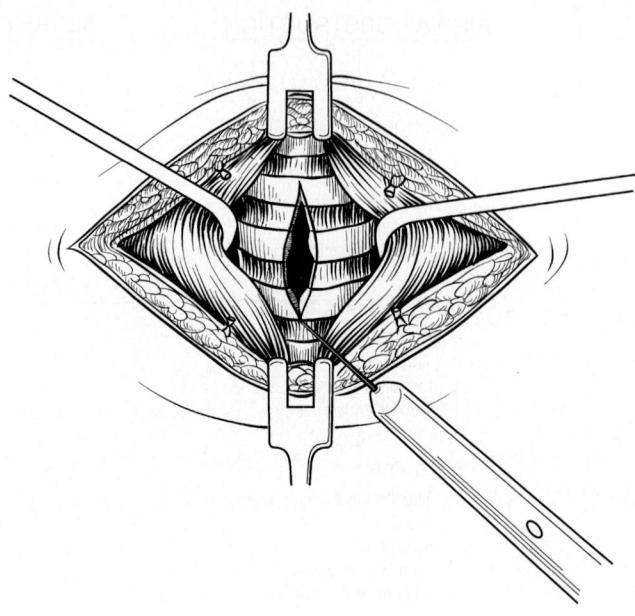

**FIGURE 20-15** With cephalocaudal retraction of the skin and subcutaneous tissue and lateral retraction of the strap muscle, the top 3 or 4 cartilaginous rings are exposed and identified. With a fine-tip electrocautery, an anterior midline tracheotomy is performed usually across rings 2 and 3 with the opening sized to accommodate the selected tracheotomy tube.

tracheal rings to be palpated. While the optimum position for tracheotomy is through tracheal rings 2 through 4, this region is usually obscured by the overlying thyroid isthmus. Once this is divided (in the midline) with the cautery, tracheal rings are easily exposed (Fig. 20-14).

Retention sutures of 3-0 Prolene or 2-0 Silk are placed parallel to the proposed site for incision in mid-trachea. These are secured to the chest for gentle lateral traction, to provide exposure of the trachea and to allow replacement in the case of accidental tracheal dislodgement in the early postoperative period before the tract is formed.

The anesthesiologist slowly withdraws the endotracheal tube until it is just above the superior aspect of the tracheal incision.

Maintaining gentle traction on the retention sutures to spread the tracheal incision open, the surgeon rotates the tracheotomy tube in position. It is imperative to have selected the range of tracheotomy tubes prior to the procedure. The size can be estimated from the endotracheal tube size used, although a useful formula to predict the tracheotomy tube size is

$$\text{Internal diameter (ID)} = (\text{age yr})/3 + 3.5$$

Of note, the neonatal tracheotomy tubes are shorter than the pediatric ones of the same diameter.

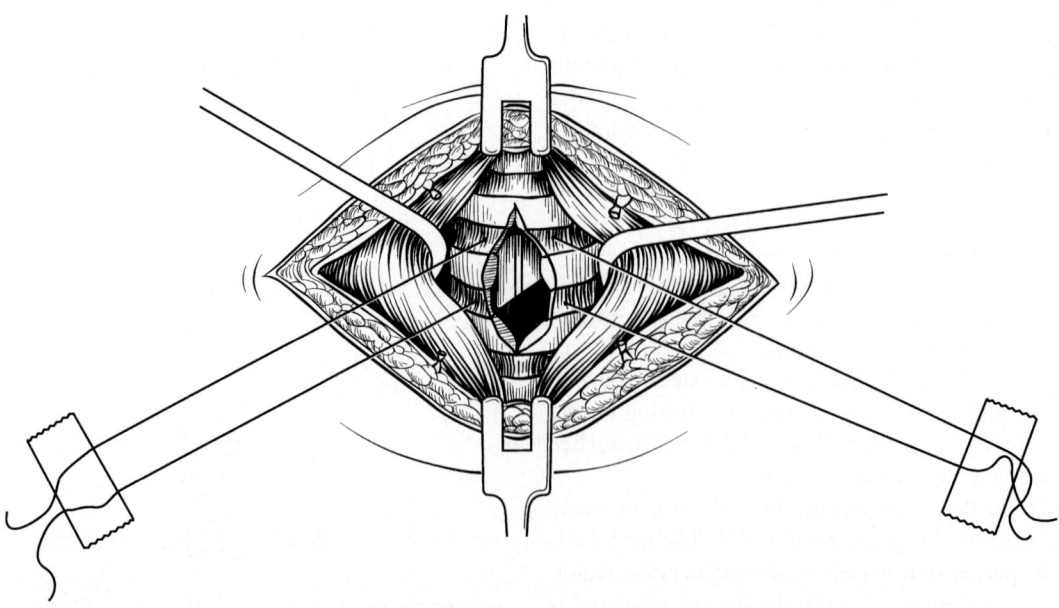

**FIGURE 20-16** The endotracheal tube is visualized beneath the tracheotomy, and on either side of the incision in the tracheal wall a stay suture of 3-0 Prolene is placed to permit retraction of the opening during the procedure and to secure rapid access to the tracheotomy opening after the procedure should the tube become inadvertently displaced.

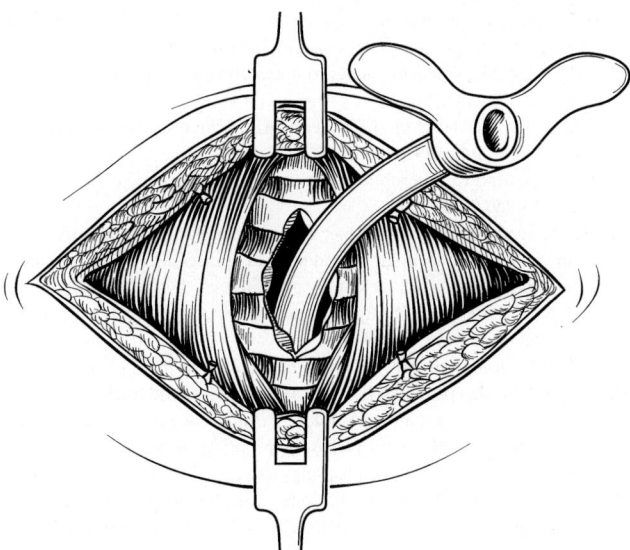

**FIGURE 20-17** With traction laterally on the stay suture and after withdrawal of the endotracheal tube tip proximal to the tracheotomy opening, the curved tracheotomy tube is gently inserted under direct vision.

Once the tracheotomy tube is inserted, the placement is verified by auscultation *of* the lung fields for equal breath sounds bilaterally, ensuring that the tracheotomy tube sits above the carina (Fig. 20-18). Right main stem positioning is not unusual if the tube is too long. A chest radiograph is obtained postoperatively to further confirm the position and to check for a rare pneumothorax. Because such a small incision is made, the skin and soft tissue usually surround the tracheotomy tube and no suturing of the skin is required.

Prior to securing the tracheotomy tube, the patient's neck should be flexed and the positioning towel removed when the appropriate tracheotomy tapes are secure in place. They should be snug, not to allow more than 2 fingers under the tape. A piece of slit gauze may be placed under the tracheotomy tube to prevent skin irritation.

The morbidity of pediatric tracheotomy is significant including increased rate of infections and risk of occlusion from tenacious secretions (especially in cold weather months with indoor heating which results in low humidity). Moreover, there is a need for specialized nursing care and equipment as well as family education and support for the difficult socialization issues that result from decreased social acceptance of children with tracheotomy.

## Treatment Effectiveness and Patient Outcomes

Although reports in the literature are sparse, the overall tracheotomy rate for a children's hospital neonatal intensive care unit (NICU) was 0.7% from Sidman et al, in a review of 10,428 NICU admissions. Since the use of tracheotomies is low and has greatly decreased over the past 15 years, long-term outcomes are less defined. Except for patients receiving tracheotomies for airway access during another surgical procedure, children who undergo tracheotomies are currently younger, smaller, more frequently neurologically impaired, and more likely to have these surgically created airways be permanent than in earlier reports.

The early complication rate (<30 days) of 10% to 15% includes inadvertent dislodgment, tube blockage, or air entrainment in the neck or mediastinum. Late complications are reported in upward of 50% of patients, with episodes of obstruction from mucous secretions, granulation formation, infection, and bleeding all frequently observed. Although children with tracheostomies have reported overall mortality rates of 25% to 30%, this is principally from coexisting morbid conditions. The mortality rate directly attributable to the tracheotomy itself rarely exceeds 1% to 3% in most large series.

Home care and detailed long-term medical evaluations are critical issues to children with tracheostomies. Chronic ventilator-dependent patients and/or patients with tracheostomy alone are now routinely cared for at home. Centers with sufficient patient volumes usually have a tracheotomy team composed of a surgeon, a nurse, a speech therapist, a social worker, and a respiratory therapist.

After detailed and thorough teaching, the bulk of this care can be provided by the parents or other caregivers at home. Visiting nurses and respiratory therapists (for those on home ventilators) provide continued teaching and ongoing evaluation. This has revolutionized the care of these children and has allowed them to benefit from the nuturing environment of family life at home. Many attend school in special education classes or are fully integrated into mainstream programs.

There are various and numerous challenging issues for the parents after the patient is discharged home with a new tracheostomy. These may include skin and stoma care, suctioning, humidification, and routine changes of the tracheostomy ties and the tracheostomy tube itself. Parents are also instructed to monitor the amount of liquid intake that the young patient takes on a daily basis, and to encourage a copious fluid intake to keep respiratory secretions thin. Normal saline instillation ("salt water squirts") to the tracheostomy

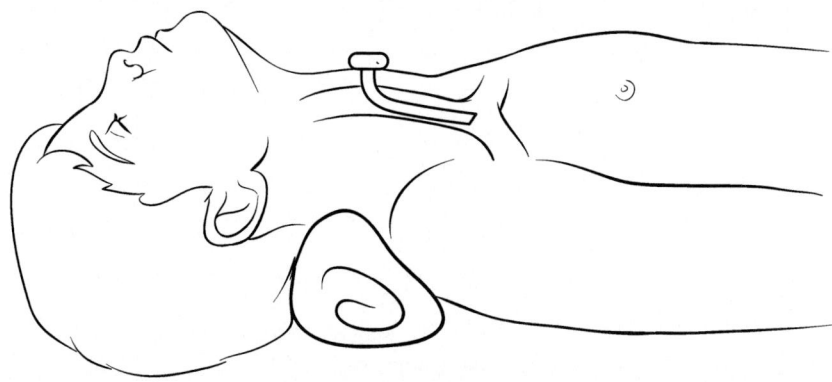

**FIGURE 20-18** Lateral depiction of proper placement of a tracheotomy tube with the tube tip brought to lie just above the carina.

with subsequent suctioning can also decrease the viscosity of the respiratory secretions. Parents must be educated on chest physical therapy to mobilize the secretions and facilitate coughing and expectoration. Tracheostomy emergencies are the most frightening occurrences that a parent can face. Special education on CPR principles and self-inflating bag ventilation are essential to cope with these situations.

When the tracheostomy is no longer deemed necessary and removal is contemplated, the entire trachea is evaluated for stenosis, granulation formation, infection, polyps, tracheomalacia, or other conditions that could preclude or complicate the decannulation process. After this evaluation, and treatment (if required), the process leading to decannulation may proceed. Over several days to several weeks, depending on the patient and family's level of comfort, the tracheostomy tube may sequentially be downsized. As the tracheal lumen becomes progressively less occluded by the downsized tube, the child should be noted to breathe and phonate around it. When a sufficiently small tube remains in place, it may be blocked temporarily or capped. If this procedure is well tolerated, decannulation can be performed preferably in an operating room setting, after bronchoscopic evaluation to confirm airway patency. After decannulation, the child should be admitted to the hospital for close observation in a monitored setting, as the development of recurring respiratory difficulties may necessitate urgent tracheostomy replacement. After decannulation, an adhesive Vaseline gauze bandage may be applied; the tracheotomy site usually seals spontaneously over several days. If a persistent fistula occurs, operative excision and primary closure can be performed at a later date on an elective setting.

## SELECTED READINGS

Bagwell CE. CO: laser excision of pediatric airway lesions. *J Pediatr Surg* 1990;25:1152–1156.

Bagwell CE. Surgical lesions of pediatric airways and lungs. In: Koff PB, Eitzman DV, Neu J, eds. *Neonatal and Pediatric Respiratory Care.* St. Louis, MO: CV Mosby Co; 1993:128.

Bailey B. Laryngoscopy and laryngoscopes—who's first?: the forefathers/four fathers of laryngoscopy. *Laryngoscope* 1996;106:939–943.

Bank DE, Krug SE. New approaches to upper airway disease. *Pediatr Emerg* 1995;13:473–487.

Boyd AD. Chevalier Jackson: the father of American bronchoesophagology. *Ann Thorac Surg* 1994;57:502–505.

Finer NN, Etches PC. Fiberoptic bronchoscopy in the neonate. *Pediatr Pulmonol* 1989;7:116–120.

Godfrey S, Springer C, Maayan C, et al. Is there a place for rigid bronchoscopy in the management of pediatric lung disease? *Pediatr Pulmonol* 1987;3:179–184.

Helmers RA, Sanderson DR. Rigid bronchoscopy—the forgotten art. *Intervent Pulmonol* 1995;16:393–399.

Kelly SM, Marsh BR. Airway foreign bodies. *Thorac Endosc* 1996;6:253–276.

Manning PB, Wesley JR, Polley TZ Jr, et al. Esophageal and tracheobronchial foreign bodies in infants and children. *Pediatr Surg Int* 1987;2:346–351.

Mantor PC, Tuggle DW, Tunell WP. An appropriate negative bronchoscopy rate in suspected foreign body aspiration. *Am J Surg* 1989;158:622–624.

Marks SC, Marsh BR, Dudgeon DL. Indications for open surgical removal of airway foreign bodies. *Ann Otol Rhinol Laryngol* 1993;102:690–694.

Marsh BR. The historic development of bronchoesophagology. *Otolaryngol Head Neck Surg* 1996;114:689–716.

Martinet A, Closset M, Marquette CH, et al. Indications for flexible versus rigid bronchoscopy in children with suspected foreign body aspiration. *Am J Respir Crit Care Med* 1997;155:1676–1679.

Othersen HB Jr. Trachea, lungs and pleural cavity. In: Welch KJ, ed. *Complications of Pediatric Surgery.* Philadelphia: WB Saunders Co; 1982:184–198.

Palmer PM, Dutton JM, McCulloch TM, Smith RJ. Trends in the use of tracheotomy in the pediatric patient: the Iowa experience. *Head Neck* 1995;17:328–333.

Reiliey IS. Airway foreign bodies: update and analysis. *Int Anesthesiol Clin* 1992;30:49–55.

Rimell PL, Shapiro AM, Mitskavich MT, et al. Pediatric fiberoptic laser rigid bronchoscopy. *Otolaryngol Head Neck Surg* 1996;114:413–417.

Wiseman NE, Sanchez I, Powell RE. Rigid bronchoscopy in the pediatric age group: diagnostic effectiveness. *J Pediatr Surg* 1992;27:1294–1297.

Wood RE. The diagnostic effectiveness of the flexible bronchoscope in children. *Pediatr Pulmonol* 1985;1:188–192.

Wood RE, Gauderer MW. Flexible fiberoptic bronchoscopy in the management of tracheobronchial foreign bodies in children: the value of a combined approach with open tube bronchoscopy. *J Pediatr Surg* 1984;19:693–698.

# CHAPTER 21

## Posterior Laryngeal Cleft

*Michael J. Rutter and Richard G. Azizkhan*

## KEY POINTS

1. Most type 1 and type II clefts can be repaired endoscopically.

2. When open cleft repair is required, a transtracheal approach with a layered closure is recommended.

3. When there is a higher risk of repair breakdown, an interposition graft is recommended.

4. Before embarking on cleft repair, consideration should be given to: (a) placement of a gastrostomy tube; (b) fundoplication; and (c) performing a tracheotomy.

5. Type IV clefts that involve the carina require a highly individualized approach.

6. Even in the presence of optimal intervention, morbidity and mortality rates remain high.

## HISTORY

Posterior laryngeal cleft is a rare congenital anomaly resulting from embryologic failure of the laryngotracheal groove to fuse. This condition was first described by Richter in 1792 in reference to a baby with multiple congenital anomalies. No further reports occurred until 1949, when Finlay reported a posterior laryngeal cleft progressing to the level of the mid-cricoid found on autopsy in a child with longstanding stridor. In 1955, Petterson performed the first successful repair of a posterior laryngeal cleft using a lateral pharyngotomy approach. However, it was not until 1982 that Donahoe performed the first successful repair of a posterior laryngeal cleft extending to the carina. At that time, the survival rate of children with posterior laryngeal clefts of any severity was less than 60%. Over the past 3 decades, transtracheal and translaryngeal repair of longer laryngeal clefts has replaced the laryngeal pharyngotomy approach, while over the past decade, endoscopic repair of shorter clefts has been enthusiastically adopted. Although overall survival rates have steadily increased, the mortality rate of children with long type IV clefts still exceeds 90%.

## EMBRYOLOGY

The laryngotracheal groove appears at day 25 of normal embryonic development, with lateral indentations fusing to form a tracheoesophageal septum. This fusion commences distally and progresses proximally, reaching the first tracheal ring by day 34. The 2 lateral chondrification centers of the cricoid fuse ventrally at 40 to 42 days and dorsally at 46 to 48 days. Disruption of normal development often results in a variety of anomalies, including those associated with the spectrum of tracheoesophageal fistulae and esophageal atresia. Approximately 20% of patients with posterior laryngeal clefts also have a concurrent tracheoesophageal fistula (TEF).

## CLASSIFICATION SYSTEM

The most useful classification system is that proposed by Benjamin and Inglis. It is an anatomic classification that divides posterior laryngeal clefts into the following 4 subtypes:

▶ Type I: A supraglottic interarytenoid cleft present to, but not below, the level of the true vocal cords. This cleft could be considered a deep interarytenoid notch.

▶ Type II: A partial cricoid cleft that extends into, but not through, the posterior cricoid cartilage.

▶ Type III*: A total cricoid cleft with or without extension of the cleft into the cervical trachea.

▶ Type IV*: A cleft extending to the thoracic trachea.

While this is an anatomical classification system, it has some predictive values in that the outcomes of type III and IV clefts are worse than those for type I or II cleft. Although there is also some correlation with presenting symptoms, this correlation is not strong. It is important to note that these symptoms are not indicative of the severity of the cleft, for there is a great deal of symptom overlap between the types of cleft.

---

*When the cleft extends below the level of the cricoid cartilage, it may be termed a laryngotracheoesophageal cleft.

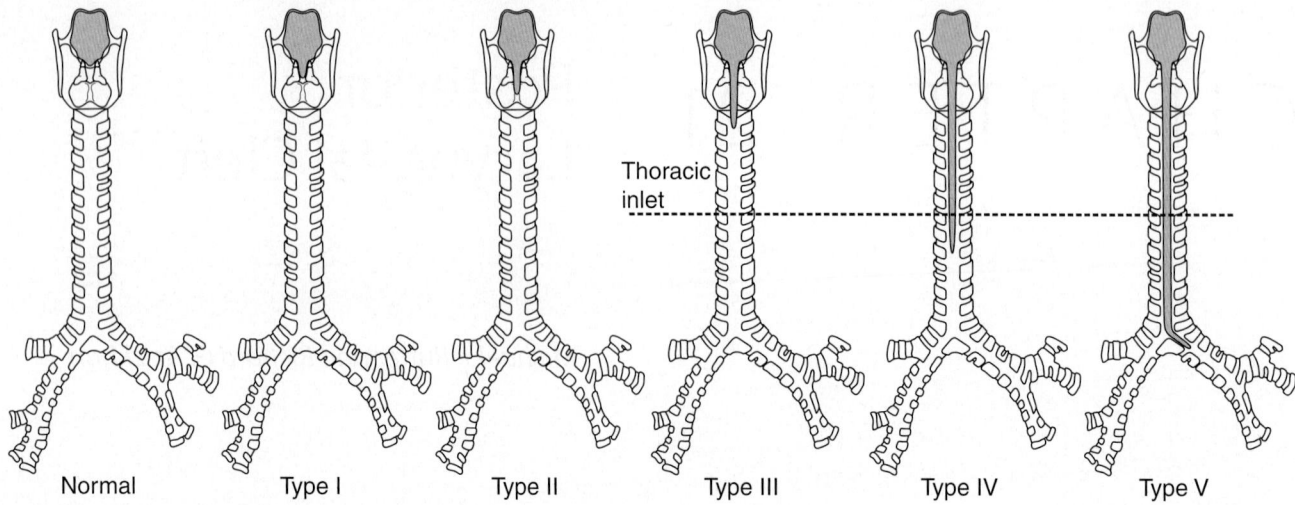

Normal    Type I    Type II    Type III    Type IV    Type V

Thoracic inlet

**FIGURE 21-1** Posterior laryngeal cleft classification. (Modified from Benjamin B, Inglis A. *Ann Otol Rhinol Laryngol* 1989;98:417–420.)

Based on our experience, a modification to the classification system would include mention of the submucous cleft cricoid. This may involve either a child without a mucosal cleft in whom the cricoid cartilage has a posterior defect or a child with a type I or type II mucosal cleft with a longer submucosal cleft (ie, the absence of the posterior plate of the cricoid cartilage). The relevance of these conditions is that they are likely to be associated with subglottic stenosis, particularly an elliptical cricoid with prominent subglottic lateral shelves. Management of these children is especially challenging because not only is repair of the posterior cleft required, but expansion of the subglottic lumen is also desirable.

A further modification to this classification system that allows for differing severities of type IV clefts is provided in Fig. 21-1. A short type IV cleft can be adequately repaired with a cervical approach, whereas a cleft that approaches the carina usually requires a transthoracic/transcervical approach. A long type IV cleft presents a greater anesthetic challenge and has a poorer prognosis. A rare variant of the type IV cleft is a cleft that extends into a bronchus. Infants with long type IV cleft are particularly challenging to manage, as they usually have associated microgastria and severe gastroesophageal reflux disease. These children frequently have other congenital anomalies, including cartilaginous anomalies of the tracheobronchial tree.

## PRESENTATION AND DIAGNOSIS

Both the incidence and significance of type I clefts are controversial. In most large series of posterior laryngeal clefts, the relative proportions of type II, III, and IV clefts are reasonably constant, whereas the relative proportion of type I clefts varies greatly. This discrepancy implies a variation in diagnostic techniques. Although the type I cleft is defined as a mucosal deficiency down to the level of the vocal fold, the enthusiasm with which the interarytenoid notch is probed may influence the interpretation of the depth of the interarytenoid notch and whether it approaches the level of the vocal fold. The

authors' view is that a type I cleft and a deep interarytenoid notch are demarcated more so by symptomatology than by anatomy. Whether the interarytenoid cleft is anatomically viewed as a deep notch or a cleft is irrelevant; the relevance lies in whether the defect is symptomatic. If a child aspirates through the posterior mucosal defect, dietary modification or surgical repair is required.

Type II and some type III clefts are diagnostically challenging in that patients may present with vague symptoms such as chronic coughing and repeated chest infections, often due to chronic aspiration. However, these symptoms vary greatly. Because they can be subtle and may mimic other common disorders, a clinician may be blinded by the child's more overt anomalies. Children with type IV clefts usually present with severe aspiration that may be clinically indistinguishable from the symptoms of a TEF with distal esophageal atresia. In all cases, a high index of suspicion is thus essential. All children with a TEF should be evaluated to rule out the presence of a laryngeal cleft, as this anomaly coexists in a small, although not insignificant, percentage of patients with a TEF.

In symptomatic cases, early presentation is with feeding problems, choking, chronic coughing, wheezing, cyanotic spells, and apnea. Aspiration pneumonia may result. There may be associated stridor due either to redundant mucosa on the edge of the cleft or to a small or elliptical cricoid ring. Severe tracheomalacia may significantly compromise the airway, especially in children with an associated TEF.

Although diagnostic tools include flexible nasopharyngoscopy, fiberoptic endoscopic evaluation of swallowing, video fluoroscopy–barium swallow, and flexible bronchoscopy, the gold standard for diagnosing a cleft and for excluding other airway pathology remains rigid bronchoscopy and esophagoscopy (Figs. 21-2 and 21-3). Nevertheless, it is common for a laryngeal cleft to be undiagnosed or misdiagnosed on initial evaluation with flexible or rigid bronchoscopy. The cleft is often hidden by redundant mucosa in the posterior glottis, and it may be useful to place an endotracheal tube through the glottis and carefully inspect the postcricoid region with a rigid endoscope. If there is any suspicion that a cleft is present, the interarytenoid area should be probed with a right-angled

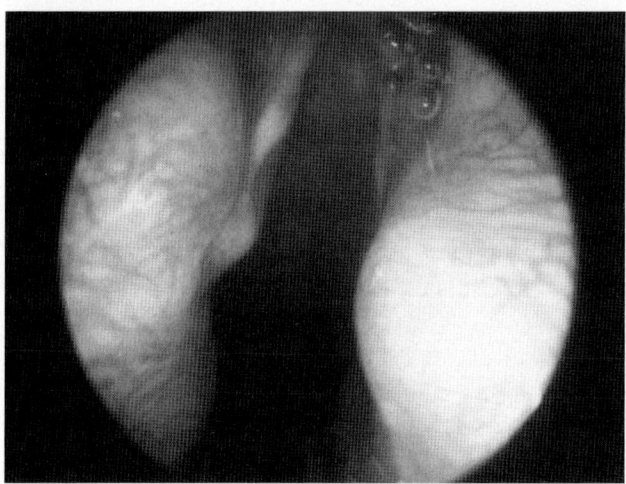

FIGURE 21-2 Endoscopic view of a type III cleft in a 2-month-old infant—glottic level type III posterior laryngeal cleft repair—anterior laryngotomy and tracheotomy.

probe. The presence of redundant mucosa between the vocal cords should always raise suspicion of a posterior laryngeal cleft. Although flexible bronchoscopy provides a superb view of the anterior commissure, the view of the posterior glottis is inadequate.

Other relevant investigations include the assessment of pulmonary function and the evaluation of other congenital anomalies. The presence of another congenital anomaly warrants a genetic evaluation.

## COEXISTENT ANOMALIES

Most children with a posterior laryngeal cleft have other congenital anomalies, which may be grouped into those that compromise the airway and those that do not. Anomalies

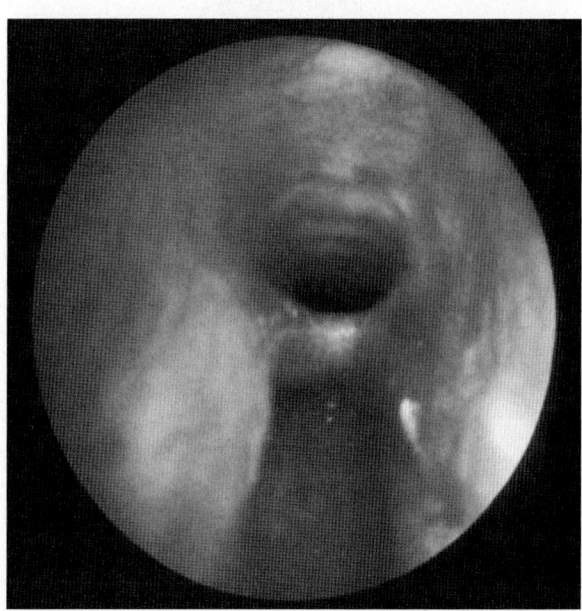

FIGURE 21-3 Endoscopic view of a type III cleft in a 2-month-old infant—tracheoesophageal level.

compromising the airway include tracheomalacia (always present in varying severity), laryngomalacia, vocal cord paralysis, subglottic stenosis, TEF, and innominate artery compression. Anomalies that do not affect the airway include esophageal atresia, gastroesophageal reflux, other gastrointestinal anomalies (particularly an imperforate anus), a cleft lip and palate, congenital heart defects, hypertelorism, and hypospadias. Opitz-Frias syndrome comprises several of these anomalies and is seen in at least 10% of children with a posterior laryngeal cleft. Gastroesophageal reflux is present and significant in most children with posterior laryngeal clefts. Frequently, it is sufficiently severe to cause pathologic consequences; when this occurs, it is better termed as gastroesophageal reflux disease.

## OPERATIVE INTERVENTION

### Presurgical Considerations

In the absence of other more severe anomalies, a posterior laryngeal cleft should be repaired as soon as possible in order to prevent chronic microaspiration with consequent long-term pulmonary compromise. In some children, however, there may be minimal symptomatology, and in selected cases it may be justifiable to delay the repair. For many children, there may be other medical problems that take precedence over the laryngeal cleft repair. The most common problem is the need for repair of a TEF and esophageal atresia. The complex nature of these disorders requires an interdisciplinary approach.

Prior to the repair, consideration needs to be given to whether a tracheotomy, a gastrostomy tube, a fundoplication, or a combination of all these is needed. A tracheotomy is often warranted in the presence of significant stridor or airway compromise due to vocal cord paralysis, subglottic stenosis, or, most commonly, severe tracheobronchomalacia. An advantage of a tracheotomy is that there is no pressure on the suture line of the repair from an endotracheal tube, as may occur with a single-stage repair. In certain cases, however, a tracheotomy may have negative consequences. If a tracheotomy is performed in a child with moderate-to-severe tracheomalacia but relatively few airway symptoms, the child may not be able to be decannulated for months or years.

A gastrostomy has the advantage of eliminating the need for oral feeding, hence limiting the potential for aspiration. In a single-stage procedure, it also has the advantage that the repair site will not lie between a nasogastric tube and an endotracheal tube. However, a gastrostomy tube does not prevent aspiration of saliva and gastroesophageal reflux. A gastrostomy may only be required for a few weeks after a successful cleft repair. Prolonged gastrostomy use without oral stimulation ultimately leads to oral aversions and other feeding problems.

Gastroesophageal reflux disease is usually present, and the refluxate may adversely affect the healing of a fresh repair site. Possible solutions include acid suppression, a gastrojejunal tube, or a jejunal tube. However, a fundoplication remains the most definitive intervention.

## SURGICAL PROCEDURES

As cited earlier, type I clefts are uncommon and may be over-diagnosed. They do not necessarily require operative intervention, but surgery is warranted when associated symptoms are present. Repair may be either endoscopic or open. In our experience, type III and IV clefts require open repair. In most cases, surgical intervention reveals that a cleft is more extensive than previously suspected on endoscopy. Although a lateral pharyngotomy was the mainstay of operative intervention for many years, it carried significant risks to the recurrent laryngeal nerves. In addition, access is suboptimal with a longer cleft.

### Open Repair

We recommend a transtracheal approach for repair of type III, IV, and some type II clefts. Figures 21-4 to 21-13 illustrate a type III cleft repair. Anesthetic is provided through a shortened oral RAE endotracheal tube placed through the tracheal stoma in a child with a preexisting tracheotomy. In a single-stage procedure, after induction with an oral or nasal endotracheal tube, a temporary low tracheotomy can be placed and a shortened oral RAE tube introduced through the low tracheotomy to maintain anesthesia. An esophageal bougie is then placed. With the patient's neck well extended, a transverse neck incision is made in a skin crease close to the level of the cricoid cartilage. Subplatysmal skin flaps are raised, and the strap muscles and thyroid isthmus divided and carried laterally. This exposes the anterior trachea. A beaver blade is used to enter the airway, and great care is

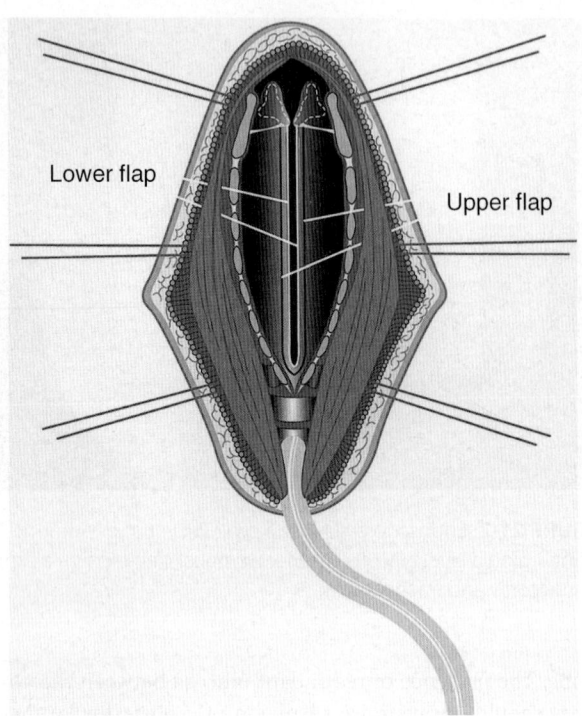

**FIGURE 21-5** Type III posterior laryngeal cleft repair—developing a plane between the tracheal and esophageal mucosal layers of the cleft.

taken to stay strictly in the midline. The anterior trachea is opened from the second or third tracheal ring up through the cricoid cartilage and cricothyroid membrane. The airway is held retracted with Prolene stay sutures, and the extent of the posterior cleft is ascertained. In children with a long

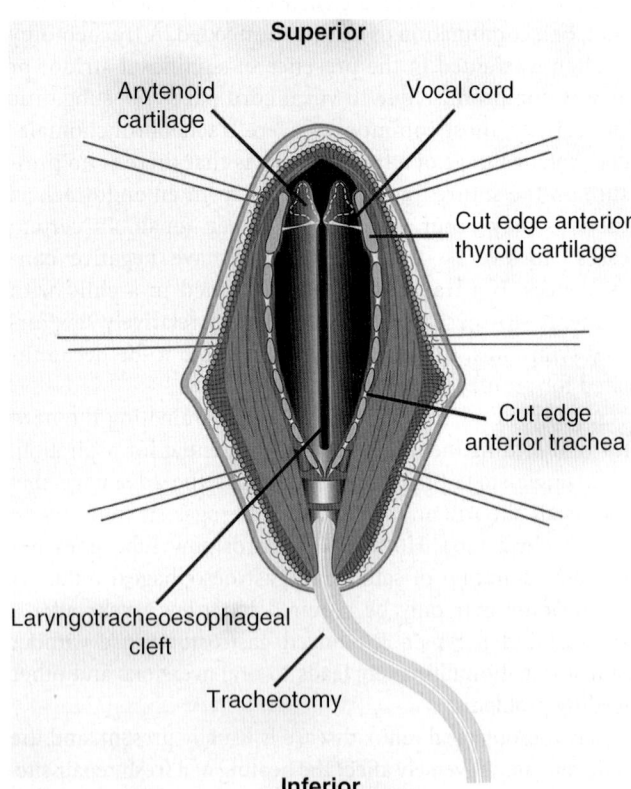

**FIGURE 21-4** Type III posterior laryngeal cleft repair—an anterior laryngotomy and a tracheotomy.

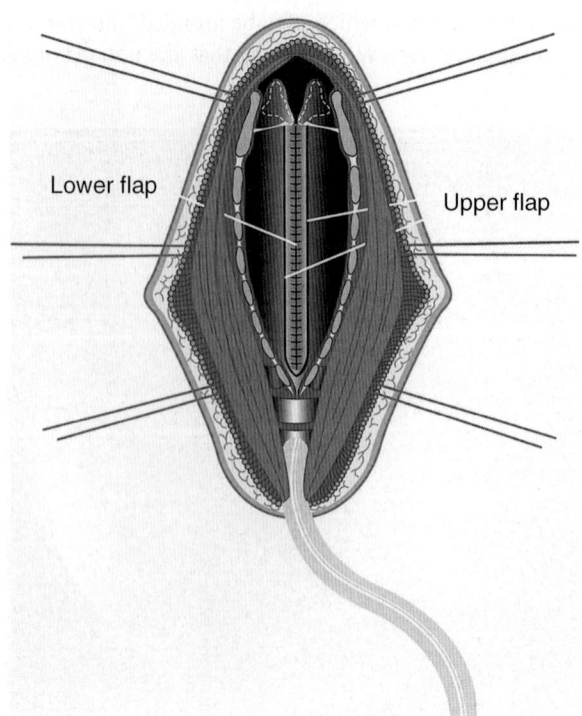

**FIGURE 21-6** Type III posterior laryngeal cleft repair—esophageal mucosal layer.

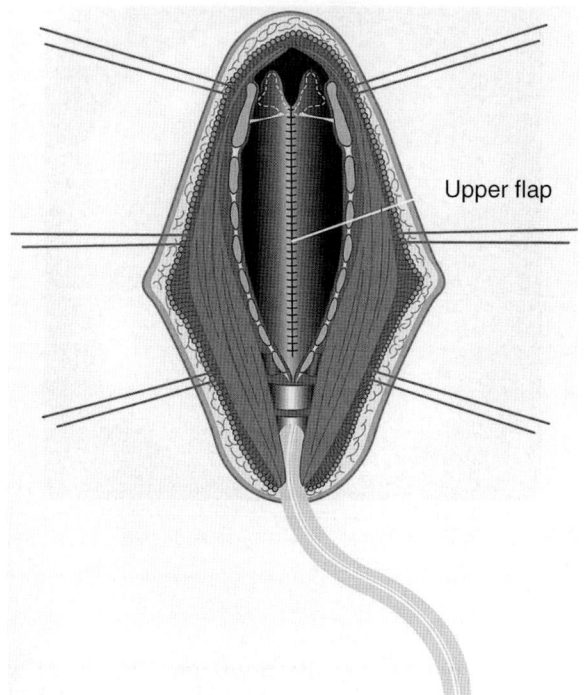

Upper flap

**FIGURE 21-7** Type III posterior laryngeal cleft repair—tracheal mucosal layer.

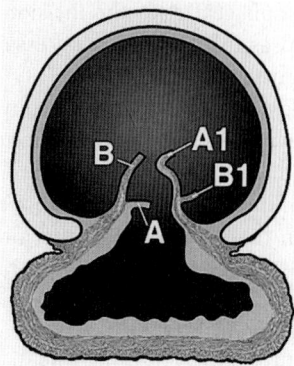

**FIGURE 21-10** Posterior laryngeal cleft—developing a dissection plane between the esophageal and tracheal mucosal layers.

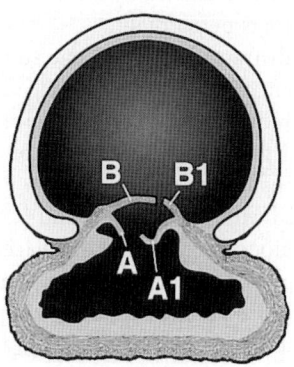

**FIGURE 21-11** Posterior laryngeal cleft—aligning mucosal flaps.

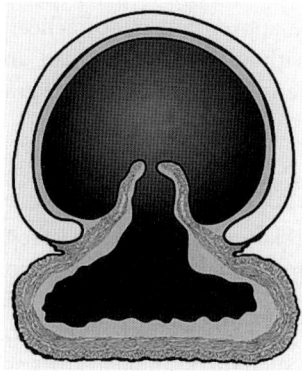

**FIGURE 21-8** Posterior laryngeal cleft—axial view.

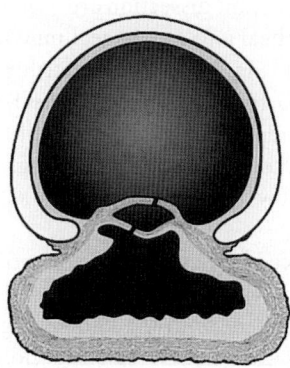

**FIGURE 21-12** Posterior laryngeal cleft—closure with noncontiguous suture lines.

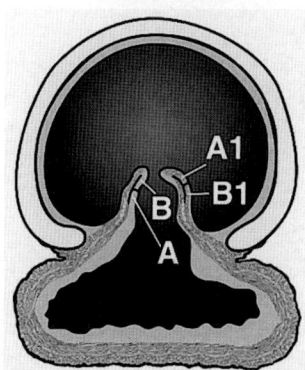

**FIGURE 21-9** Posterior laryngeal cleft—planned mucosal incisions in edges of the cleft. **A**. Short esophageal flap; (**A1**) long esophageal flap; (**B**) long tracheal flap; (**B1**) short tracheal flap.

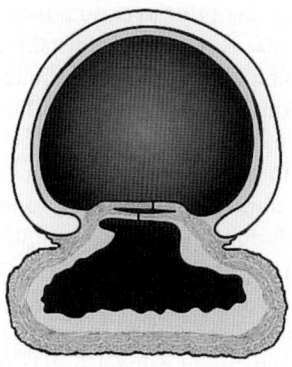

**FIGURE 21-13** Posterior laryngeal cleft—view immediately following repair.

311

laryngotracheoesophageal cleft, the incision in the anterior trachea is carried as inferiorly as is necessary to gain good exposure to the posterior cleft.

The larynx must then be split. To avoid damage to the vocal cords, this procedure should be done exactly in the midline, through the anterior commissure. In young children, the level of the anterior commissure lies one third of the way between the superior and inferior notches of the thyroid cartilage, closer to its inferior border. This procedure is most accurately performed with an assistant providing a televised view of the glottis with a rigid 30 Hopkins rod telescope. This endoscopic view enables the surgeon to place a pair of Jake forceps between the true vocal cords (from below). Opening these forceps distracts the cords, allowing an excellent view of the anterior commissure. A beaver blade is then visualized by the endoscope as an anterior laryngofissure is performed.

The larynx is distracted with Prolene sutures and the full extent of the cleft can be observed (Fig. 21-4). A significant amount of redundant mucosa is typically present. This requires removal to prevent airway compromise while still maintaining a tension-free 2-layer repair. The edges of the cleft are infiltrated with 1% lidocaine and 1:100,000 epinephrine, and 3-0 Monocryl stay sutures are placed along the edge of the cleft to provide traction. The mucosa along the edge of the cleft is then incised or excised, depending on the amount of redundant mucosa present. Particular care should be taken at the apex of the cleft distally and over the arytenoid cartilages proximally. The aim is to repair the cleft 3 to 4 mm above the level of the true vocal folds.

Both sharp and blunt dissection are used to create a plane between the tracheal and esophageal mucosal layers of the edges of the cleft (Fig. 21-5). This procedure should ideally be performed so that additional tracheal mucosa is preserved on one side of the cleft and additional esophageal mucosa is preserved on the other side (Figs. 21-8 to 21-13). This method allows for noncontiguous suture lines upon 2-layer closure.

Once this procedure has been performed, the esophageal mucosa is closed with interrupted 4-0 or 5-0 sutures over the esophageal bougie, with the knots lying in the esophageal lumen (Figs. 21-6 and 21-12). This closure commences distally, and the suture at the apex of the cleft should be tied like a purse string. Each suture can act as a retractor to allow placement of the following suture before being cut. After the esophageal mucosa is closed, we place a thin layer of fibrin glue on the suture line prior to closing the tracheal mucosa. The tracheal mucosa is then closed distally to proximally in an identical fashion to the esophageal mucosa. Sutures are placed with the knots lying in the tracheal lumen (Figs. 21-7 and 21-12), and particular care is taken over the most distal and proximal sutures. This layer is further reinforced with a very thin film of fibrin glue. Figures 21-14 to 21-19 illustrate this operative technique in a 1-year-old child.

In a single-stage procedure (ie, without a tracheotomy), the patient is then nasally intubated. The tip of the tracheotomy tube should lie distal to the repair site. The anterior trachea is then closed using 4-0 PDS (polydioxanone) sutures through the tracheal rings and cricoid and 5-0 Vicryl sutures in the cricothyroid membrane if required

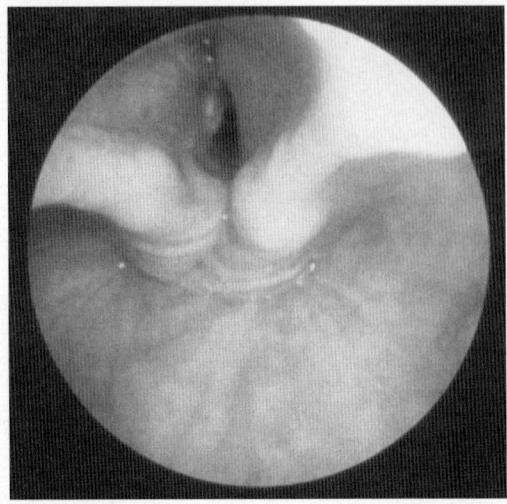

**FIGURE 21-14** Endoscopic view of a type III cleft—preoperative glottic level.

(Figs. 21-20 and 21-21). The larynx must be closed with particular care so as not to overlap the vocal cords at the anterior commissure. This technique is best performed with figure-of-8 or mattress sutures at the level of the anterior commissure and further figure-of-8 or mattress sutures above and below the anterior commissure. This suture line is also reinforced with fibrin glue, and the neck is then closed in layers over a Penrose drain. If closure of the cricoid over an age-appropriate endotracheal tube cannot be accomplished without tension, a small anterior cartilage graft will allow tension-free closure. The graft may be costal cartilage or thyroid alar cartilage.

## Endoscopic Repair

Type I and type II laryngeal clefts are best repaired endoscopically, as this approach does not require a complete laryngofissure and therefore does not place the vocal cords or voice at risk. However, if laryngeal exposure is inadequate, access may be a problem; in such cases, an open approach may therefore

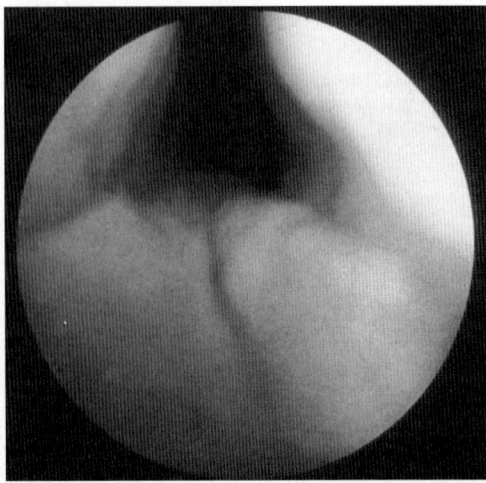

**FIGURE 21-15** Endoscopic view of a type III cleft—preoperative posterior glottis.

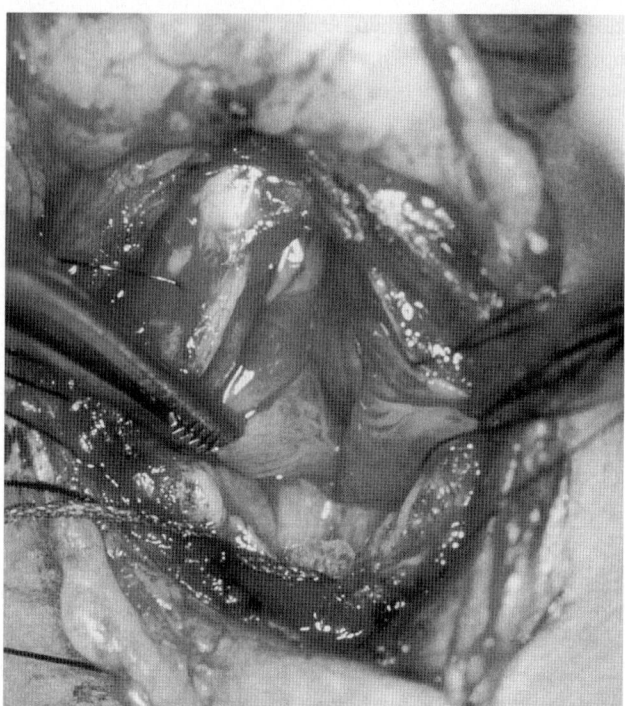

**FIGURE 21-16** Intraoperative view of a type III cleft. Open trachea with redundant mucosa.

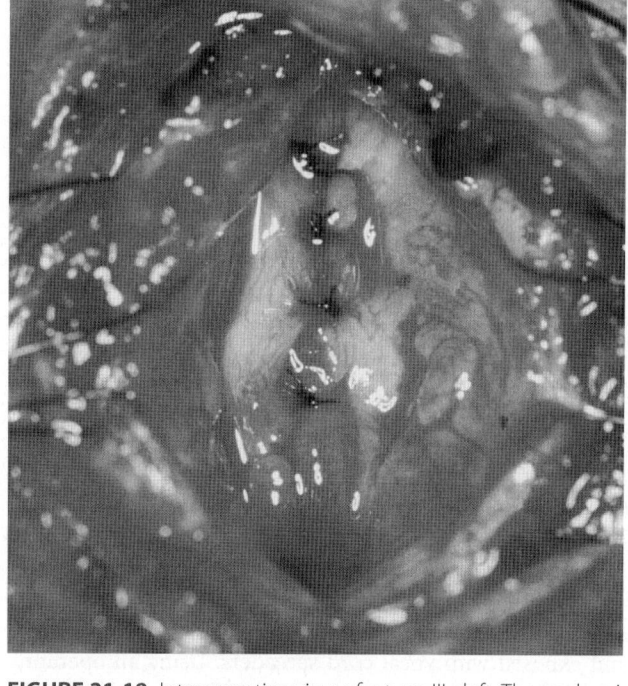

**FIGURE 21-18** Intraoperative view of a type III cleft. The trachea is open, and the cleft has been repaired.

be required. Similarly, an open approach may be preferable in children with an associated subglottic stenosis, as this allows both lesions to be addressed concurrently.

The original descriptions of endoscopic laryngeal cleft repairs involve creating tracheal and esophageal mucosal flaps and performing a painstaking 2-layer closure with very fine (6-0) PDS sutures on a BV-1 needle. This is a technically challenging procedure with a significant risk of repair breakdown. In recent years, we have changed our philosophy regarding endoscopic cleft repairs, and now prefer a 1-layer mass closure technique with only 1 or 2 heavy sutures placed in a mattress fashion. Our rationale is that an endoscopic repair is most likely to break down starting at the proximal aspect of the repair, and that a heavy proximal suture lessens the risk of dehiscence. The most proximal suture should pass through the cuneiform cartilage bilaterally, as this further lessens the risk of dehiscence.

Our technique is to position the patient with the larynx suspended on a suitable laryngoscope (eg, medium Lindholme)

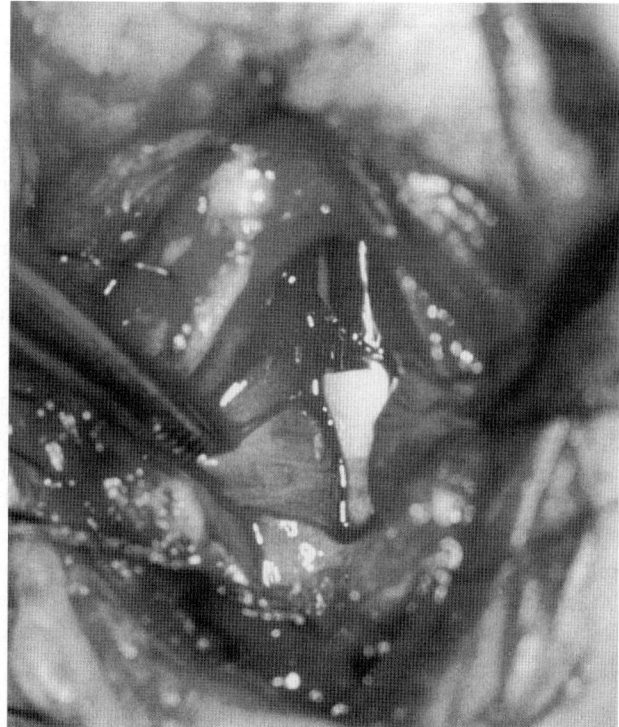

**FIGURE 21-17** Intraoperative view of a type III cleft. The trachea is open, and an esophageal bougie is displayed.

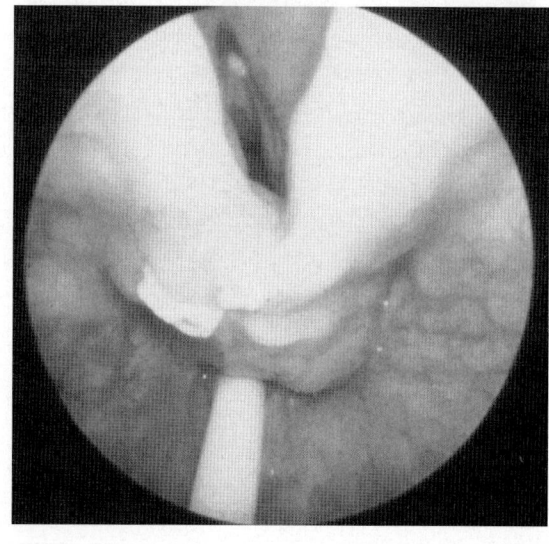

**FIGURE 21-19** Endoscopic view of a repaired type III cleft 10 days postoperatively.

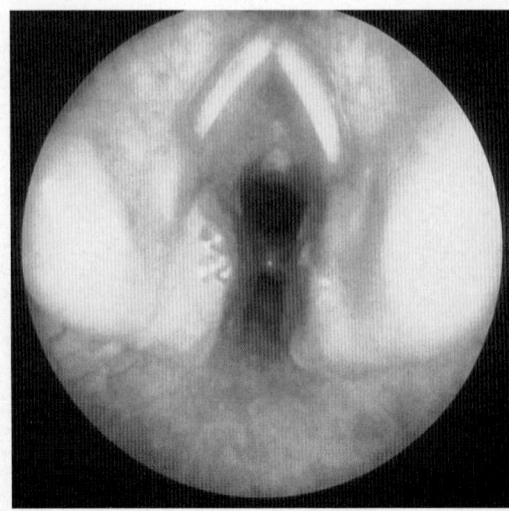

**FIGURE 21-20** Endoscopic preoperative view of a type III cleft in a 1-month-old infant.

and exposed with vocal cord spreaders. Using an operating microscope and microlaryngeal instruments, we denude the mucosa of the inner aspect of the cleft, with particular attention to the apex of the cleft. Rather than removing a narrow strip of mucosa, the mucosal excision is more aggressive in order to maximize the demucosalized surface area on either side of the cleft. The raw surfaces are opposed by the placement of 4-0 PDS sutures on a taper needle. These sutures are placed in a horizontal mattress fashion. The first throw of the distal suture commences at the mucosal edge of the esophageal side and exits at the mucosal edge of the tracheal aspect on the same side of the larynx, with the suture having incorporated a large "bite" of tissue. The second throw of the needle is on the opposite side of the larynx from close to the mucosal edge on the tracheal side, exiting close to the mucosal edge on the esophageal side. The suture may be tied down with at least 6 throws, as PDS is notoriously slippery. If required,

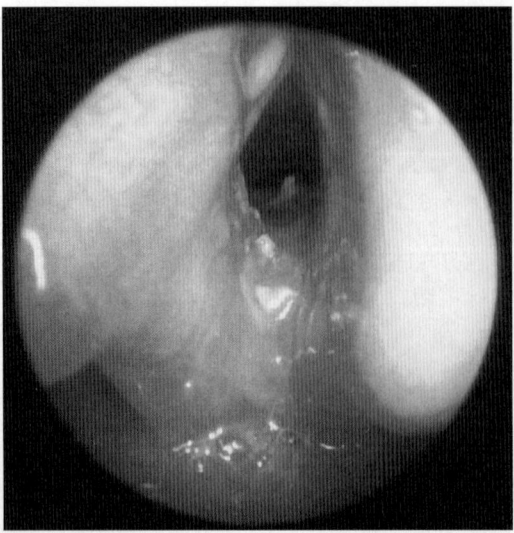

**FIGURE 21-21** Endoscopic view of a type III cleft in a 1-month-old infant 1 week postoperatively (single stage).

additional sutures are then placed more proximally, with the most proximal suture involving the cuneiform cartilage if possible to minimize the risk of the suture pulling through.

## Interposition Grafts

The use of interposition grafts is reserved for cases in which the risk of failure is either higher or potentially catastrophic. The relative risk of failure is higher in revision cases, children with a history of TEF repair, and children with Opitz-Frias syndrome. Failure is potentially catastrophic in children with type IV clefts. In all of these cases, consideration should be given to the use of interposition grafts. Suggested graft material includes temporal fascia and tibial periosteum, both of which are used as free grafts. However, in our institution, if a small graft is needed, clavicular periosteum is easily harvested from within the surgical field. If a larger graft is desired, sternal periosteum may also be obtained from the surgical field and is abundant. Periosteum is robust, but exceedingly difficult to place sutures through; thus, once the esophagus is repaired, the periosteum is laid over the esophageal suture line and stabilized with a small amount of fibrin glue. Tracheal mucosa is then closed over the top of the periosteum.

## Revisions

Laryngeal cleft repairs have a recognized failure rate. The repair is at the greatest risk of breakdown either at the distal end of the repair with TEF formation, or at the proximal end with cleft recurrence. Laryngeal cleft failures usually occur within weeks of the initial repair; however, late occurrences have been described several years after a successful initial repair.

## Type IV (Long) Clefts

Infants born with a long type IV cleft are challenging to manage for a variety of reasons. Severe aspiration is inevitable. Airway maintenance may be problematic, as an endotracheal tube may reside in the esophagus or trachea, with the "tracheoesophagus" being a common cavity. Other congenital anomalies are common and the closer the cleft is to the carina, the greater the likelihood of other major congenital anomalies; these may be classified as airway and nonairway anomalies. Airway anomalies associated with long laryngeal clefts include bronchial stenosis and bronchomalacia, which is usually left-sided. Cartilage abnormalities of the laryngotracheal complex are common and may include areas of cartilage aplasia and conjoined tracheal rings.

Nonairway anomalies include microgastria, polysplenia, and annular pancreas. Microgastria may result in uncontrollable gastroesophageal reflux, and is not amenable to a fundoplication. Prior to embarking on surgical repair of the laryngeal cleft, a decision must be made as to whether the child is salvageable.

In a child who has a highly abnormal left bronchus and associated tracheal cartilage abnormalities or in a child who has a sustained significant anoxic brain injury, the prospects of an acceptable long-term outcome are remote. If a child is deemed worth salvaging, controlling gastroesophageal reflux is highly desirable. Although an esophagogastric separation with a Roux-en-Y approach is attractive, subsequent cleft repair is more prone to dehiscence, possibly due to a compromise of the esophageal blood supply. Our current approach in a child with microgastria who cannot undergo a fundoplication is to cross-staple the stomach with a vented gastrostomy tube proximal to the staple line and a feeding gastrostomy tube distal to the staple line.

There are many methods to repair a type IV cleft, primarily because none of the approaches is ideal. The dilemmas fundamentally relate to issues of access and issues of oxygenation. Access may be through a lateral thoracotomy approach, a transsternal approach, or a cervical approach, either transtracheally or from an extended lateral pharyngotomy. Oxygenation may be achieved with the use of intubation, extracorporeal membrane oxygenation, or cardiopulmonary bypass. Having had experience with all of these methods, our current preference is to perform a transcervical repair whereby the upper trachea is exposed and transected at the lower border of the cricoid cartilage. The trachea distal to the transection is then "peeled up" off the esophagus. This is achieved by dividing the mucosa on either side of the cleft at the apex of the tracheoesophageal mucosal junction. The dissection is continued down to the apex of the cleft and, ideally, is continued a few millimeters into the tracheoesophageal groove distal to the apex of the cleft. In most children with a long laryngeal cleft, the trachea is relatively short, and this can therefore be achieved through a transcervical approach. However, if access is cramped, a limited sternotomy improves access. During this procedure, oxygenation may be obtained by an endotracheal tube placed in the trachea with the tip of the tube lying in the right mainstem bronchus. The left lung is partially ventilated through the Murphy eye of the endotracheal tube, which should lie at the carinal level. The proximal aspect of the laryngeal cleft can then be dissected, commencing at the lower border of the cricoid and progressing proximally to the arytenoids. Performing a complete laryngofissure is an option to improve access if required. The esophageal aspect of the cleft is then repaired with interrupted sutures, with the knots placed in the esophageal lumen. At this point, an interposition graft may be placed from beyond the carina up to the arytenoids; we recommend sternal periosteum as an ideal graft material because it is abundant and readily available. The posterior trachea may then be repaired in a distal to proximal fashion, with the repair being performed from the posterior aspect of the trachea. This approach permits oxygenation, as the endotracheal tube remains in position while the posterior trachea is repaired. Once the distal trachea has been repaired, the proximal tracheal mucosa may be repaired from the lower border of the cricoid cartilage to the arytenoids. The transected trachea may then be reconnected to the cricoid cartilage. The problem with this approach is that the posterior tracheal mucosa will have a 4-point anastomosis at the lower border of the cricoid, and is therefore at a higher risk of dehiscence. However, if the interposition graft and the esophageal mucosa are intact, the tracheal dehiscence eventually heals. In the event that a TEF redevelops at this site, it is easier to manage and repair than a dehiscence close to the carina.

To minimize the pressure on the suture line, we recommend managing the postoperative airway with a transnasal endotracheal tube. Although placement of a tracheotomy tube is inevitable, if this can be delayed for 2 or 3 weeks following surgery, the tip of the tracheotomy tube will not be as great a threat to the integrity of the distal repair. A stormy postoperative course is routine in these children.

## OUTCOMES

Success rates for posterior laryngeal cleft repair vary between 50% and 90%. Breakdown of the repair usually occurs within a month of surgery, but a late breakdown (even years later) may also occur. The success of an operative repair is negatively influenced by several factors. The more severe the cleft, the higher the incidence of breakdown or fistula formation through the repair. The type of operation chosen influences outcome, and a transtracheal repair remains superior to a lateral pharyngotomy or an endoscopic repair because of the excellent exposure provided by this approach. Similarly, a 2-layer repair is superior to a single-layer closure. Because of problems with intractable reflux, microgastria is also associated with repair breakdown. Revision surgery, whether for a recurrent cleft or a secondary H-type TEF, is less successful than primary surgery. An adequate primary procedure offers the best chance of success. However, the most influential factor compromising successful cleft repair is the presence of a coexistent congenital TEF (repaired or otherwise), although the reasons for this are unclear.

The most common site of breakdown is the most distal end of the cleft repair, usually seen as a persisting TEF—and these acquired H-type fistulae are notoriously difficult to find. Success may also be compromised by excessive redundant mucosa obstructing the airway, which may require trimming with a carbon dioxide laser. Patients with a coexisting subglottic stenosis should have it repaired at the time of the cleft repair. Other significant complications seen after cleft repair include vocal cord paralysis (especially after a lateral pharyngotomy) and a collapsing larynx caused by an inadequate posterior cricoid.

Historically, the mortality rate of children born with a posterior laryngeal cleft approached over 90%. Although the current mortality rate is unknown, it is presumed to be less than 10%. Certainly, mortality and morbidity rates rise with the severity of the cleft. The greatest influence on survival, however, is often not the cleft itself or the associated aspiration but other coexisting congenital anomalies, especially neurologic or cardiac lesions.

## SELECTED READINGS

Bakthavachalam S, Schroecer JW Jr, Holinger LD. Diagnosis and management of type 1 posterior laryngeal clefts. *Ann Otol Rhinol Laryngol* 2010;119(4):239–248.

Benjamin B, Inglis A. Minor congenital laryngeal clefts: diagnosis and classification. *Ann Otol Rhinol Laryngol* 1989;98(6):417–420.

Bent JP III, Bauman NM, Smith RJ. Endoscopic repair of type 1A laryngeal clefts. *Laryngoscope* 1997;107(2):282–286.

Berkovits RN, Bax NM, van der Schans EJ. Surgical treatment of congenital laryngotracheo-oesophageal cleft. *Prog Pediatr Surg* 1987;21:36–46.

Donahoe PK, Gee PE. Complete laryngotracheoesophageal cleft: management and repair. *J Pediatr Surg* 1984;19(2):143–148.

Evans KL, Courtney-Harris R, Bailey CM, Evans JNG, Parsons DS. Management of posterior laryngeal and laryngotracheoesophageal clefts. *Arch Otolaryngol Head Neck Surg* 1995;121:1380–1385.

Parsons DS, Stivers FE, Giovanetto DR, Phillips SE. Type I posterior laryngeal clefts. *Laryngoscope* 1998;108(3):403–410.

Rahbar R, Chen JL, Rosen RL, et al. Endoscopic repair of laryngeal cleft type I and type II: when and why? *Laryngoscope* 2009;119(9):1797–1802.

Robie DK, Pearl RH, Gonsales C, Restuccia RD, Hoffman MA. Operative strategy for recurrent laryngeal cleft: a case report and review of the literature. *J Pediatr Surg* 1991;26(8):971–973; discussion 973–974.

Ryan DP, Muehrcke DD, Doody DP, Kim SH, Donahoe PK. Laryngotracheoesophageal cleft (type IV): management and repair of lesions beyond the carina. *J Pediatr Surg* 1991;26(8);962–969; discussion 969–970.

Schraff SA, Zur KB, Jacobs I, Darrow DH, Cott RT, Rutter MJ. The clinical relevance of the submucosal cricoid cleft. *Int J Pediatr Otorhinolaryngol* 2007;71(7)1099–1104.

Walner DL, Stern Y, Collins M, Cotton RT, Myer CM III. Does the presence of a tracheoesophageal fistula predict the outcome of laryngeal cleft repair? *Arch Otolaryngol Head Neck Surg* 1999;125(7):782–784.

# CHAPTER 22

# Tracheal Stenosis and Tracheomalacia

*Patricio Herrera, Priscilla P. L. Chiu, and Peter C. W. Kim*

## KEY POINTS

1. Tracheal narrowing due to fixed (ie, complete tracheal rings) and/or dynamic (eg, tracheomalacia) airway obstruction can cause life-threatening respiratory distress in infants and children.

2. Expedient investigations for tracheal stenosis must include echocardiography, cross-sectional imaging by computed tomography (CT) or magnetic resonance imaging (MRI), and bronchoscopy to determine the cause and define the extent of airway compromise.

3. Optimal management of tracheal obstruction requires a multidisciplinary and yet individualized approach. Conservative management without surgical intervention may be warranted in select patients depending on severity of symptoms and extent of narrowing as the airway caliber in congenital tracheal stenosis (CTS) and tracheomalacia will improve with patient growth in many cases.

## INTRODUCTION

Airway obstruction of the infant or pediatric trachea can precipitate acute and life-threatening respiratory compromise. While infections and foreign bodies are the most common causes of airway compromise in children, intrinsic airway narrowing due to CTS caused by complete tracheal rings or airway compression caused by anomalous cardiovascular anatomy and/or tracheomalacia represent the more challenging conditions for the pediatric surgeon to manage, especially in the setting of acute respiratory distress. Moreover, these 2 conditions may coexist in the same patient, presenting a complex clinical condition that requires thorough and systematic evaluation. This chapter will present the pathophysiology of airway obstruction, the diagnostic paradigm, and the surgical options for the treatment of tracheal stenosis and tracheomalacia.

## DISEASE PATHOPHYSIOLOGY

### "Fixed" Tracheal Obstruction: Congenital Tracheal Stenosis

Congenital tracheal stenosis is a rare condition defined as the congenital reduction in tracheal diameter due to the presence of abnormal and complete cartilaginous rings replacing the normal compliant C-shaped tracheal cartilages. It has been estimated that the incidence of CTS is approximately 1 in 65,000 live births. In addition to fixed narrowing due to small complete cartilaginous tracheal rings and a reduced mural compliance during respiration, there is hypertrophy of submucosal glands and connective tissue, further narrowing the tracheal cylinder in the affected segment. This malformation of the airway can be associated with a number of other congenital anomalies, including vascular or cardiac malformations in 25% to 70% of cases. Lung hypoplasia and total lung agenesis are also frequently associated with CTS, suggesting that lung and airway malformations may arise from a common developmental defect. Several classifications of CTS have been described including the morphologic classification by Cantrell and the functional classification by Anton-Pacheco being the most commonly used. According to the Cantrell classification, there are 3 morphologic types of the stenosis: diffuse hypoplasia, funnel type, and segmental stenosis (Fig. 22-1). This classification is particularly useful for determining the technique for reconstruction of the airway. The functional classification stratifies patients into mild, moderate, and severe categories according to presenting symptoms and age of presentation that could further help in defining prognosis and need for surgery. Interestingly, our experience representing more of a population-based patient cohort demonstrated that segmental narrowing is uncommon while longer segment narrowing involving more than 50% of tracheal length is the most common phenotype.

Typically, patients with CTS present in 2 distinct periods in infancy: in the early neonatal period and in the second half of the first year of life when physical activity level escalates with mobility, with respiratory distress often

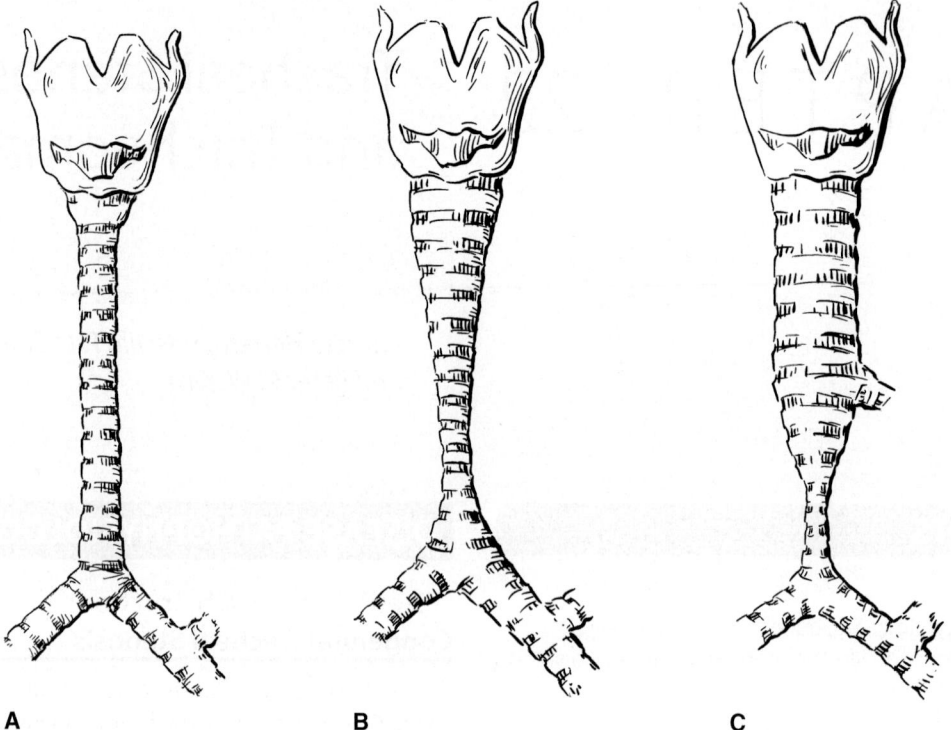

**FIGURE 22-1** The 3 most common types of tracheal stenosis. **A.** Full-length stenosis. **B.** Funnel-shape stenosis. **C.** Segmental stenosis, usually associated with a tracheal bronchus.

precipitated by an acute episode of respiratory tract infection. In our series, males and females were equally affected. Five of 13 patients were premature at birth (ie, gestational age <36 weeks) with a mean gestational age of 31 weeks. The mean age at diagnosis was 3.8 months with 4 patients diagnosed under age 2 months. Ten patients presented with cardiac arrests or "near death" spells and 6 had initial arterial pH less than 7.2. Nine of 13 patients were intubated and ventilated prior to their eventual repair. Five of 9 patients were supported with high-frequency oscillatory ventilation preoperatively, indicating the challenge in maintaining adequate ventilation in these patients. In summary, many CTS patients presenting acutely in the early neonatal period are critically ill and warrant emergent management of an obstructed airway including any associated cardiac and great vessel anomalies.

In contrast, some of the older CTS patients present with less acute signs and symptoms, often having been treated for asthma or "chronic wheezing" before they are finally investigated. These patients can often be minimally symptomatic unless exercising where they generally experience poor exercise tolerance following exertion compared to their age-matched peers, presenting with shortness of breath or "windedness" associated with biphasic stridor. Many of these late-presenting patients can be observed without surgical intervention as they appear to have a "self-selected" treatment option for their airway narrowing. In contrast, those presenting in early or late infancy require careful evaluation, and clinical experience and judgment with regard to optimal treatment option will need to be individualized depending on the severity of symptoms and anomalies.

## "Dynamic" Tracheal Obstruction: Vascular Compression and Tracheomalacia

Dynamic airway narrowing results from 2 distinct pathophysiologies: tracheal compression by adjacent vascular structures due to anomalous anatomy (eg, vascular rings [VRs]) or from intrinsic airway weakness known as tracheomalacia.

### Vascular Compression

Tracheal narrowing may result from anomalous cardiovascular anatomy such as VRs, including pulmonary artery sling, double aortic arch, and aberrant right subclavian artery. In such cases, tracheal narrowing may be secondary to direct mechanical tracheal compression by the vessel or VR with associated tracheomalacia, a condition also known as vascular tracheobronchial compression syndrome. However, 50% to 65% of VR patients also have CTS from complete tracheal rings resulting in primary tracheal obstruction, making this condition more complex in its diagnosis and management. Symptomatic patients often present with airway and/or esophageal obstructive symptoms such as dysphagia, stridor, and respiratory distress. Radiological investigations including CT typically reveal the anomalous vascular anatomy with the associated airway narrowing. Bronchoscopy remains the gold standard in visualization of the airway, with identification of the pulsatile narrowing in the tracheal lumen due to VR as well as any intrinsic airway obstruction from associated complete tracheal rings. Once the diagnosis is made, surgical intervention is required to relieve the obstructive symptoms.

The complexity of VR and associated CTS has raised debate over the optimal treatment of this distinct population of CTS patients. Some reports have advocated surgical correction of VR alone, as translocation or reimplantation of the anomalous vessel may relieve airway compression and significantly improve symptoms. However, others have promoted combined CTS and VR repair, as VR associated with long-segment CTS due to complete tracheal rings may require definitive tracheal repair. In such cases, unrepaired CTS from complete tracheal rings may result in the persistence of airway obstructive symptoms following VR repair alone. Therefore, the indications for selective VR repair or combined VR and CTS repairs are unclear, requiring adequate preoperative assessments of both cardiovascular and tracheal anatomies to define the nature of airway obstruction and the management options.

## Tracheomalacia

Tracheomalacia, either primary or secondary, is characterized by the abnormal compliance (structural resistance) of the tracheobronchial tree resulting in occlusion of the airway lumen. Symptoms range from a brassy cough and expiratory stridor to the more serious "dying spells," which often occur during or within 10 minutes of feeding. With tracheomalacia, the pathophysiology is quite different from CTS since there is no rigid or fixed reduction in airway caliber, but a dynamic obstruction that only manifests in moments of higher respiratory demand. This creates higher airflow and extramural mechanical compression to the abnormally compliant airway lacking structural rigidity. This dynamic stress causes collapse of large and intermediate-sized airways. However,

if the small peripheral bronchi are affected, it will mimic obstructive bronchial disease with air trapping due to muscle spasm, but will only respond to sedation and positive pressure ventilation and not to β-blockers or inhaled steroid therapy. When more proximal trachea or bronchi are involved, dynamic compromise is evident at the moment of extubation from surgery or mechanical ventilation following respiratory infection, where extubation fails due to poor respiratory mechanics.

Tracheomalacia is often associated with other congenital lesions, the most common being esophageal atresia with or without tracheoesophageal fistula (EA/TEF). The classic barking cough of the tracheomalacia patient should be an indication for close observation during feeding for EA/TEF patients. Most children with tracheomalacia will improve spontaneously, usually by 1 year of age, and can be managed symptomatically, with humidified air and chest physiotherapy. However, patients with "dying spells," recurrent pneumonia, or those who cannot be extubated, will require more aggressive interventions.

## DIAGNOSTIC PRINCIPLES

A thorough clinical examination of the pediatric patient presenting with respiratory distress is imperative, as other causes such as foreign bodies as well as infectious and inflammatory conditions of the lungs and airway must be first ruled out (Fig. 22-2). Once that has been accomplished, diagnostic

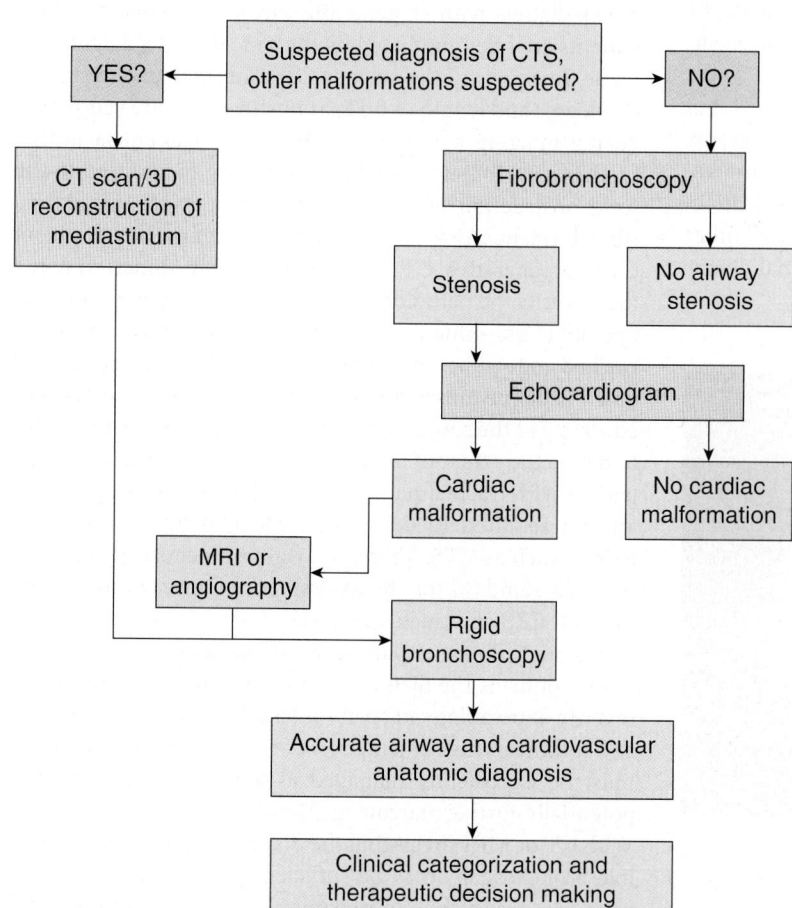

**FIGURE 22-2** Diagnostic evaluation of a child with suspected tracheal obstruction. Evaluation is based on the severity of symptoms, the age of the patient, and the clinical presentation. There are several options available for establishing the diagnosis of the tracheal obstruction—usually not all of them are required. Bronchoscopy is the definitive diagnostic method. Comprehensive examination is very important, because associated aerodigestive and cardiovascular anomalies are frequent in such patients. (From Herrera P, Caldarone C, Forte V, et al. The current state of congenital tracheal stenosis. *Pediatr Surg Int* 2007;23:1033–1044.)

tests focused on the airway must be performed. Multiple yet complementary imaging modalities are required to fully investigate the patient presenting with the signs and symptoms of airway obstruction. Although direct visualization of airway narrowing using an endoscope is considered the gold standard, recent progress in real-time and dynamic imaging technology including CT and MRI has made these noninvasive technologies a critical requisite and determinant in both diagnosis and surgical planning, particularly in small infants with critically narrowed airways where even simple diagnostic instrumentation may potentially exacerbate further airway narrowing.

The following is a summary of the investigative tools and the recommended approach to the investigation of the patient presenting with airway obstruction.

## Radiological Imaging

A thorough preoperative assessment of patients, including cardiac evaluation, is imperative in the preparation of CTS patients prior to operative repair. In our experience, CT of the neck and chest with intravenous contrast provides excellent imaging of the aerodigestive tract in addition to definition of cardiovascular anomalies (Fig. 22-3). The use of CT is favored over MRI as the speed of imaging by CT without the need for general anesthesia results in less invasive and more rapid imaging of the often precarious and unstable airway patient. The clinical symptoms of airway or esophageal obstruction should be initially investigated with imaging studies including CT scan of the chest to determine the cardiac and aerodigestive tract anatomies. CT cross-sectional imaging enhanced with 3-dimensional reconstruction provides further details of the anatomic relationship between these vital structures to facilitate operative approach and planning.

MRI for airway imaging has little advantage over CT but does provide the favored imaging for cardiovascular anatomy with dynamic imaging that may capture airway compression not revealed by CT. Therefore, the addition of MRI in the investigation of the airway patient can supplement other functional studies and provide important mediastinal details without radiation exposure to the patient.

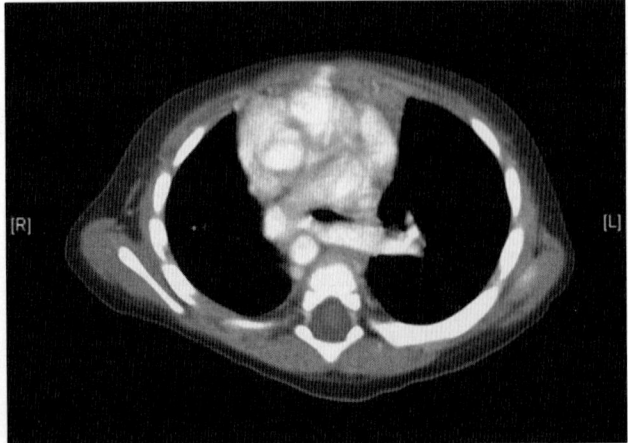

**FIGURE 22-3** CT imaging of the tracheal obstruction associated with anomalies vascular anatomy. The image shows cross-sectional details of a compressed trachea due to anomalous vascular anatomy.

## Echocardiogram

Preoperative echocardiogram is essential for identifying intracardiac defects and the potential presence of pulmonary hypertension. Children with coexisting CTS and intracardiac anomalies represent a high-risk group for morbidity and mortality following CTS repair. Although some centers have reported success in simultaneous surgical correction of CTS and the cardiac defects usually in the older age group and excluding PDA and VRs, our data suggested that these 2 conditions posed a significant operative morbidity and mortality risk. This was particularly compounded in infants less than 1 month of age. Moreover, the development of refractory pulmonary hypertension can result in postrepair cardiac failure, especially in patients with endocardial cushion defects. Other congenital anomalies coincident with CTS in the presence or absence of cardiac anomalies further contribute to patient morbidity and outcomes. Although echocardiogram is necessary and precise in assessing cardiac anatomy and function, echocardiogram information on adjacent great vessels must be interpreted with caution and in conjunction with CT or MRI, especially for formulating surgical plans.

## Bronchoscopy

Patients with CTS often present with acute respiratory failure and respiratory acidosis, especially when precipitated by concomitant pulmonary infection. Some CTS patients remain asymptomatic until an acute infectious episode exacerbates the underlying airway obstruction, precipitating acute respiratory distress with an acute life-threatening episode. These patients are often intubated by the time the CTS diagnosis is made. Imaging studies such as CT scans may underestimate the degree and length of CTS, as positive pressure ventilation during imaging may mask underlying tracheomalacia that further contributes to tracheal narrowing in addition to the fixed obstruction of CTS. When patients were imaged via rigid bronchoscopy and CT scans to define the extent of CTS, preoperative CT imaging invariably underestimated the severity of pathology compared to bronchoscopy and operative assessment. The presence of endotracheal or tracheostomy tubes often contributed significant artifact and failed to define the extent of CTS as well. Furthermore, bronchoscopy of the spontaneously breathing patient is necessary to define the extent of the dynamic airway obstruction in the patient with tracheomalacia, while spontaneous respirations are not required to define the extent of fixed obstructive lesions such as CTS. Therefore, rigid bronchoscopy remains the gold standard for the assessment of airway obstruction for both CTS and tracheomalacia.

Although direct visualization of the airway by an endoscope confirms the diagnosis and often aids in assessing the severity of pathology in terms of length and diameter in CTS, any additional instrumentation of critically narrowed airway must be expediently managed as any manipulation could potentially further narrow an already compromised airway. With CT or MRI suggesting the diagnosis, confirmatory flexible bronchoscopy may be sufficient particularly in affected neonates and infants. In dynamic airway compromise, rigid bronchoscopy is necessary both for diagnosis and during surgical intervention to optimally calibrate the suspended airway. Patency of the airway following an induced Valsalva maneuver confirms effectiveness of the suspension.

## ANESTHETIC CONSIDERATION

Close and careful consultation among cardiac, anesthetic, otolaryngology, critical care, and general and thoracic surgical teams is necessary and critical in surgical planning particularly in the treatment of CTS. Although a number of case series have reported successful repair without the need for cardiopulmonary support, the need of cardiopulmonary support in the form of either ECMO or full bypass especially in cases where combined cardiac and tracheal repair is planned is invaluable and safe. In most affected neonates and infants, carefully planned use of appropriate cardiopulmonary support must be anticipated in our experience.

The placement and positioning of an endotracheal tube particularly following slide repair require discussion with the anesthetic team. Although planned, on-table extubations following repair can be accomplished in select patients, most patients require the placement and maintenance of the endotracheal tube in place for several days until intraluminal swelling is subsided to allow leakage of airway around the endotracheal tube for possible extubation.

## TREATMENT OPTIONS: RESULTS/OUTCOMES

### Fixed Obstruction

Historically, CTS and attempts to repair the underlying tracheal lesions have been associated with significant morbidity and mortality. However, recent reports suggest that surgical intervention has resulted in significant improvement in survival. Some children with less severe forms of CTS may be asymptomatic in early infancy only to present later with acute respiratory distress. Although immediate control of the airway may be required including early intubation or possible tracheostomy, the best management strategy is not to manipulate the already compromised airway until an efficient work-up can be completed and definitive treatment plans are made. Definitive interventions are indicated when patients experience significant respiratory compromise from CTS and/or fail to wean from ventilatory support. The variability in the severity of CTS warrants careful investigation in each patient and thoughtful planning before proceeding to surgery. In general, commonly used surgical procedures for the treatment of CTS consist of tracheal resection with end-to-end anastomosis, patch tracheoplasty, and slide tracheoplasty. Given the rarity of these lesions, few centers have had extensive experience with the management of CTS. It is clear from a review of the literature that CTS patients represent a heterogeneous group depending on the severity of pathology, symptoms, and associated anomalies. Surgical teams must be prepared to provide the whole spectrum of treatment options ranging from extubation and observation, to resection, to combined cardiac and tracheal repair. Today, there is a general trend toward using slide tracheoplasty as a preferred and versatile technique for CTS repair in many centers. In our center, our approach is first to assess whether a simple observation alone would suffice safely depending on patient history, severity of symptoms, and pathology. If surgical repair is warranted, the following treatment options may be considered.

### Tracheal Resection

As experience with the surgical treatment of segmental tracheal stenosis has accumulated, tracheal sleeve resection with end-to-end anastomosis has proved to be an effective and reliable method of treatment (Fig. 22-4). Grillo reported the results of this operation in 901 patients with an operative mortality of 1% and only 4% failures mainly in adult patients (Wright and Grillo, 2004). Although only a few of his patients were children, the basic operative principles are the same in the pediatric population. The technique of segmental resection can be used with the same rate of success in neonates as well as in older children. As indicated by Grillo, complications can be minimized if the following principles are observed:

▶ The preoperative diagnosis should be anatomically and functionally accurate.

▶ The surgical approach should be made carefully in a stepwise fashion, and no irrevocable move should be made until the surgeon is able to proceed to resection.

▶ The surgical technique should be meticulous and great attention should be paid to avoid tracheal devascularization or anastomotic tension.

▶ The tracheal surgeon should have access to expert help in radiology and anesthesiology, an experienced special nursing unit, and the help and advice of consultants, especially otolaryngologists.

It is generally accepted that up to a third of the length of the affected trachea can be resected safely while resection up to 50% of the length with additional proximal and distal release procedures to reduce tension along trachea has been reported. A short segment involving 2 to 5 rings can be readily resected primarily. However, in CTS, the length of affected segment is often underestimated and one has to be cautious in choosing this approach as the definitive technique in the correction of CTS.

### Tracheoplasty

The general principle in tracheal reconstruction for CTS is not to make the airway diameter anatomically normal, but approximate newly reconstructed airway as wide as possible. Repair of CTS by tracheoplasty can be categorized into 2 main approaches: patch or slide technique. Various materials have been used for patch including native trachea, cartilage (either costochondral or thyroid), pericardial, and anterior wall of esophagus. The patch technique at best enlarges compromised tracheal diameter by 30% to 40% depending on the size and shape of the patch while having a minimal effect on the length of narrowed trachea.

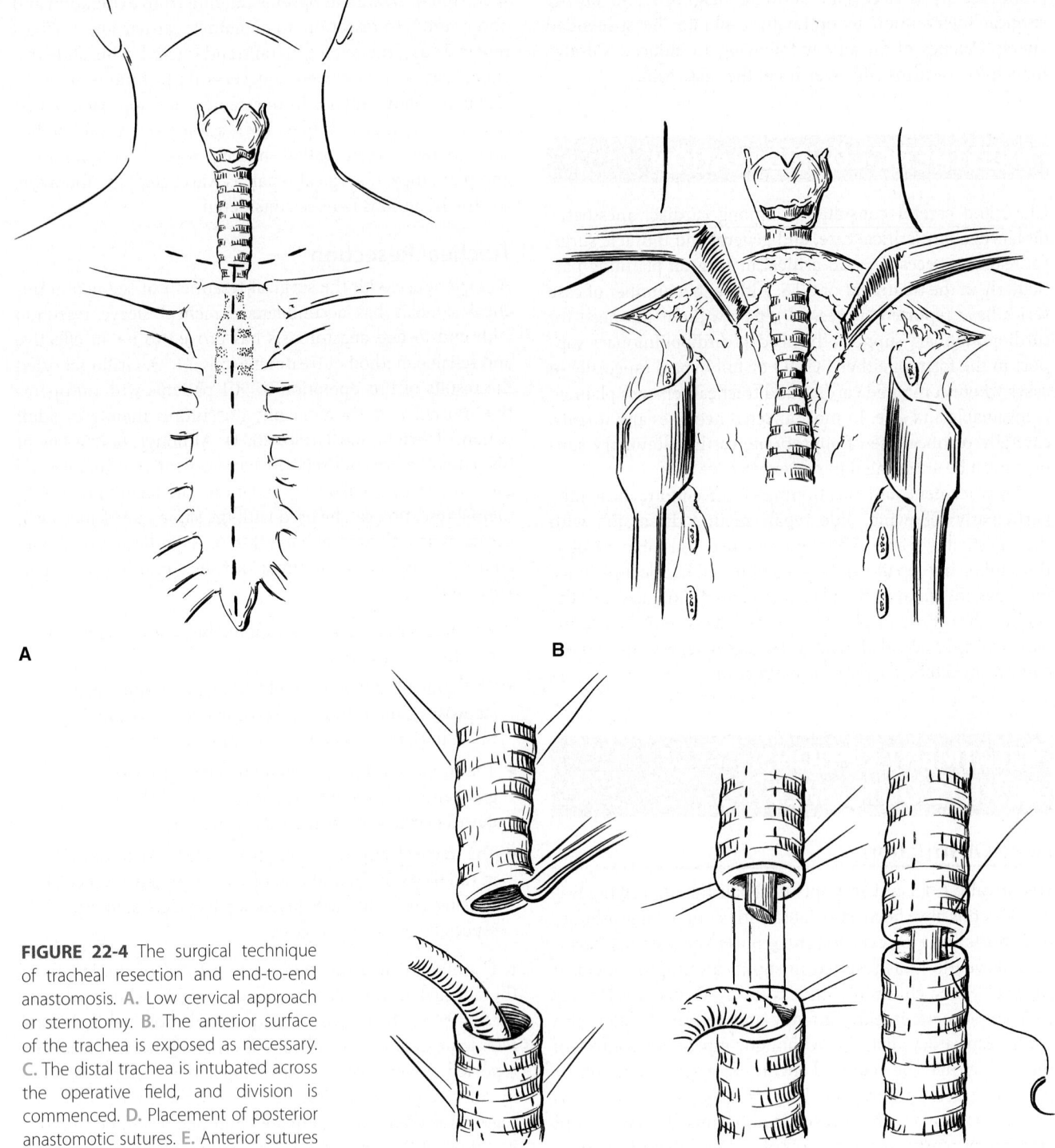

**FIGURE 22-4** The surgical technique of tracheal resection and end-to-end anastomosis. **A.** Low cervical approach or sternotomy. **B.** The anterior surface of the trachea is exposed as necessary. **C.** The distal trachea is intubated across the operative field, and division is commenced. **D.** Placement of posterior anastomotic sutures. **E.** Anterior sutures with transanastomotic intubation.

The largest series and most extensive experience in the use of autologous pericardial patch tracheoplasty comes from Backer's group at the Children's Memorial Hospital in Chicago, IL, that, since 1982, has operated on 23 children with long-segment tracheal stenosis—all with complete tracheal rings (Fig. 22-5). They employed cardiopulmonary bypass (CPB) in all of the patients. There were 2 early deaths for an operative survival of 92%. The first death occurred in an 8-day-old child who had associated agenesis of the right lung; the second occurred as a result of patch dehiscence. There were 3 late deaths: 5, 7, and 13 months after the operation, all from airway complications. The major disadvantages

of patch tracheoplasty are the need for postoperative intubation for stenting and ventilatory support and the development of granulation tissue and restenosis.

Slide tracheoplasty has now become the procedure of choice in repairing CTS in many centers including ours. The slide technique initially described by Tsang et al. and popularized by Grillo doubles tracheal diameter of the affected segment while shortening the length approximately by a third to half, further reducing airway resistance. Slide tracheoplasty is most appropriate when a long segment of trachea is narrowed. Briefly, this procedure uses only autologous tracheal tissue and is performed by transecting the

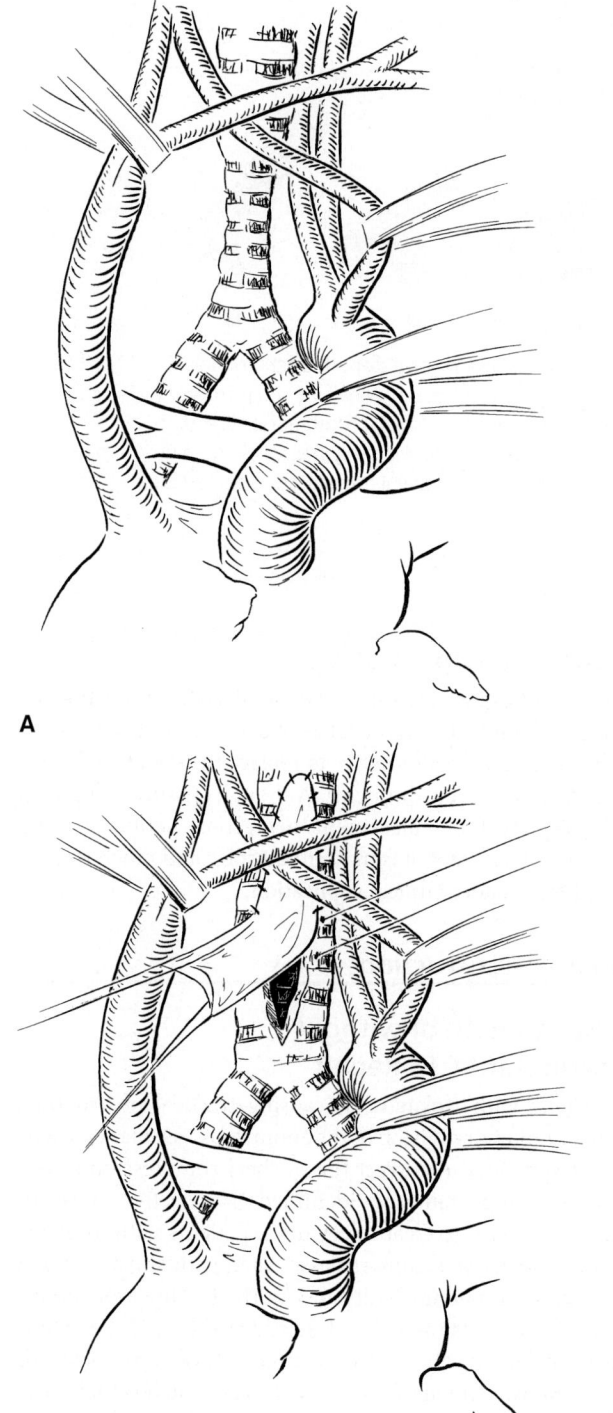

A

B

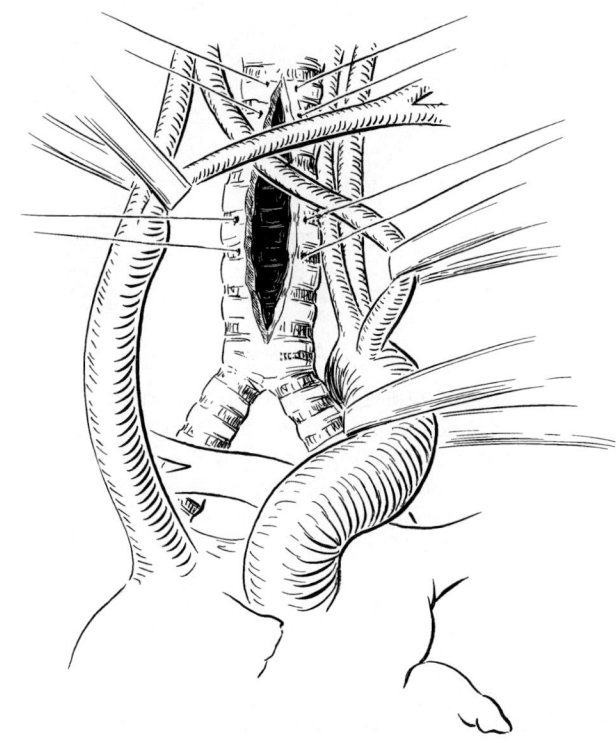

C

**FIGURE 22-5** The surgical technique of pericardial patch tracheoplasty. **A.** The trachea is exposed through an anterior sternotomy. **B.** The trachea is incised along the entire length of the stenosis. **C.** A pericardial patch is sutured to the edges of the tracheal cut. The correction is carried out using a CPB or distal intubation or by advancing the laryngeal endotracheal tube after opening the narrow tracheal lumen.

trachea into 2 equal segments (Fig. 22-6). The anterior wall of the lower half of the trachea and the posterior wall of the upper trachea are incised. These segments are then slid over each other and anastomosed with absorbable monofilament suture. Patient survival rates greater than 90% using this technique are now reported, and complications including granulation tissue following repair have been considerably less while allowing continued tracheal growth. Although restenosis requiring bronchoscopic dilatation or reoperation has been reported, the incidence of this complication appeared to be lower with slide technique, and in our cohort of 45 patients, only 1 patient developed granulation tissue

requiring bronchoscopic dilatation. The most recent review of our experience further affirms the effectiveness of the slide technique demonstrating no early or late mortality following slide tracheoplasty.

With the success of the slide technique, confounding comorbidity of these CTS patients has become the most critical prognostic determinant of surgical outcomes. We have previously identified 3 significant variables: patients less than 1 month of age at repair, associated chromosomal anomalies, and associated significant cardiac anomalies. In our multicenter review, 19 CTS patients were diagnosed with comorbid intracardiac anomalies. Of these, 10 died following CTS

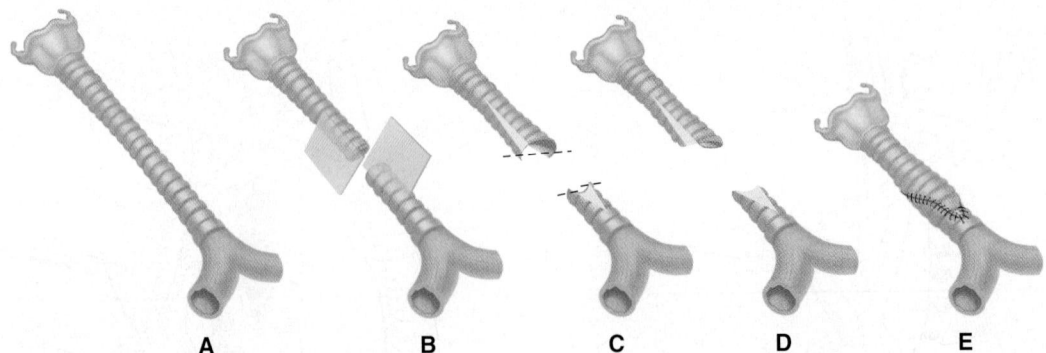

**FIGURE 22-6** Surgical technique for slide tracheoplasty. **A.** This diagram shows a native stenotic trachea involving the whole length of the trachea. **B.** The stenotic segment is divided into 2 with the upper half incised posteriorly and lower half incised anteriorly. **C, D.** The edges of the 2 halves are trimmed to allow smooth apposition with anastomosis of the slide tracheoplasty. **E.** The final representation of the shorter and wider trachea following slide tracheoplasty. (From Herrera P, Caldarone C, Forte V, et al. The current state of congenital tracheal stenosis. *Pediatr Surg Int* 2007;23:1033–1044.)

repair (53% mortality). Only 9 of 49 CTS patients without intracardiac anomalies died, representing the most favorable survival rate in all centers (18% mortality). CPB was utilized for 54 of the 68 repairs (79% of cases), including all cases in which the cardiac anomalies were simultaneously repaired at the time of CTS repair. There was no difference detected in the surgical treatment of CTS patients with associated intracardiac lesions and those repaired at age less than 1 month as both groups represented very high mortality risk for CTS repair.

### CTS Repair Associated with VR

There are few reports in the literature describing the long-term outcomes of patients treated for airway obstruction due to VR alone or combined VR and CTS. The combination of VR with CTS has consistently resulted in higher surgical mortality following combined VR and CTS repairs compared to isolated VR repair. The main concern has been that VR repair alone without simultaneous or staged CTS repair would result in persistent airway obstruction, resulting in a second and more morbid sternotomy following the primary VR repair procedure. Therefore, the approach to the CTS patient with co-diagnosed VR represents a challenge for clinical decision making.

In our experience, the selective correction of VR alone without CTS repair can be offered based on the patient's bronchoscopically determined airway obstructive disease if the fixed obstructive component from CTS is minimal (see VR Repair with or without Concomitant CTS Repair below). However, it is requisite that concurrent bronchoscopic evaluation of the airway be performed immediately after the VR is corrected to ensure that critical airway narrowing is relieved without residual significant CTS lesion. Simultaneous repair of the underlying CTS lesion may be required if the fixed obstruction involves a long segment of the trachea as determined preoperatively or intraoperatively. In such cases, the surgical team should be prepared to perform the combined repair rather than doing the repairs in a more morbid staged approach.

### Tracheal Transplantation

Recently, an allograft from cadaveric decellularized trachea seeded with cultured epithelial cells derived from the patient has been used as an alternative to replace the complete length of trachea or even bronchi. Although tissue-engineered tracheal graft for replacement or reconstruction appears promising in concept, it is in its infant stage and much work is needed for broader clinical application.

## Dynamic Obstruction

### VR Repair with or without Concomitant CTS Repair

In patients with isolated VR causing tracheal obstruction, reimplantation or division of the anomalous vascular anatomy may be sufficient to correct the tracheal compression symptoms. More importantly, we identified that selective VR repair may be sufficient to treat selected VR patients with localized airway obstructive symptoms associated with short-segment CTS with minimal morbidity and mortality. However, almost half of the patients treated with selective VR repair had some persistent airway obstructive symptoms postrepair secondary to extensive tracheobronchomalacia or the residual unrepaired complete tracheal rings. Surprisingly, most of these patients did not require subsequent surgical repair of residual airway obstruction, indicating that conservative treatment in some cases of CTS may be appropriate. Together, these data suggest that VR repair alone may be sufficient treatment of focal vascular tracheobronchial compression with or without associated short-segment CTS but not for those VR patients with extensive, long-segment CTS, or tracheomalacia.

### Aortopexy

Tracheomalacia can be treated by several surgical techniques. Aortopexy, the suspension of the aorta to the posterior aspect of the sternum, is the gold standard for surgical management of tracheomalacia (Fig. 22-7). Aortopexy must be preceded by bronchoscopy to confirm the diagnosis of tracheomalacia,

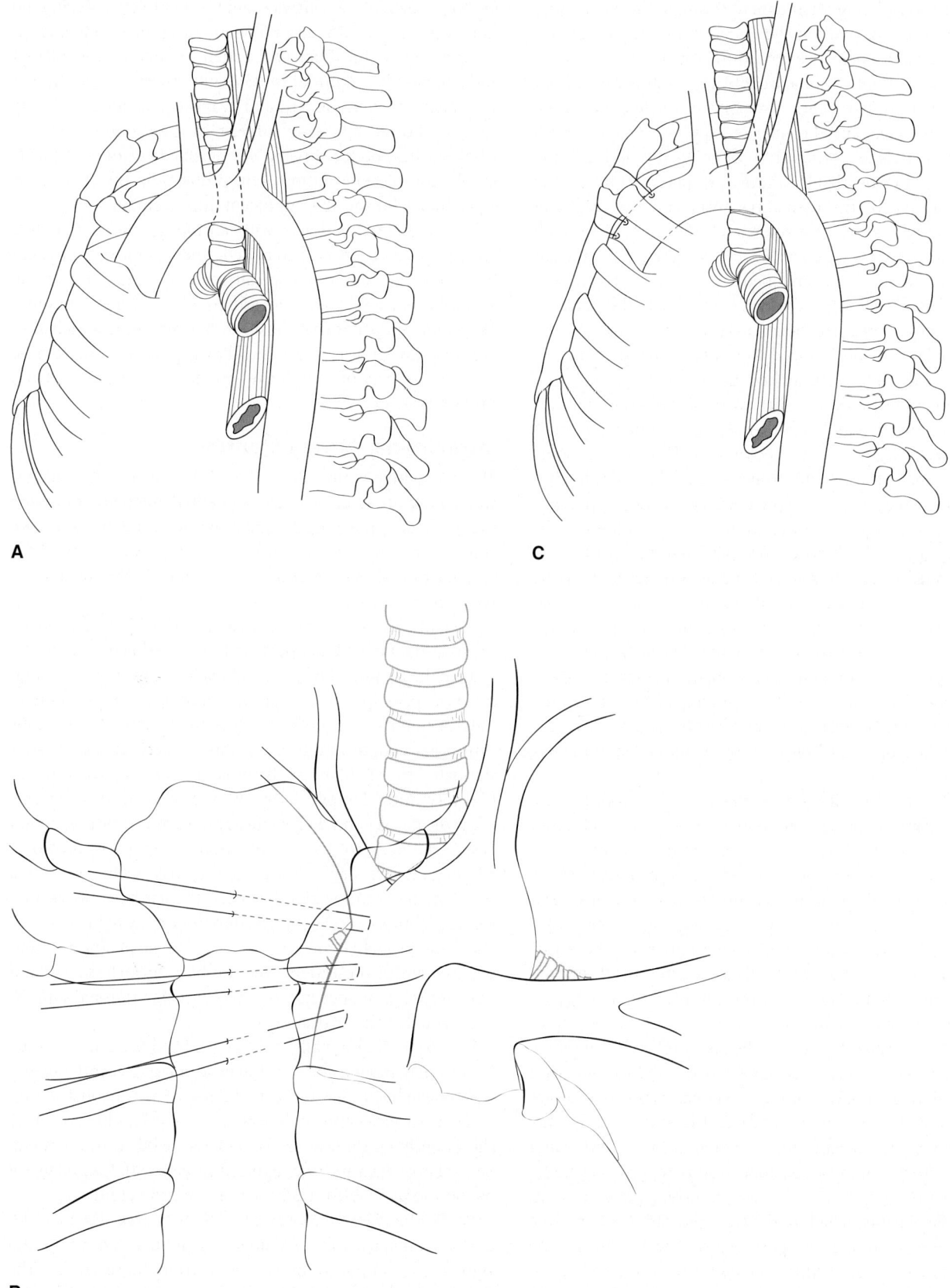

**A**

**C**

**B**

**FIGURE 22-7** Surgical procedure of aortopexy. **A.** Left anterior thoracotomy. The aorta is exposed by opening the pericardium transversely just below its reflection on the arch of the aorta. Sutures are placed through the adventitia and wall of the ascending aorta and through the origin of the innominate vessel. The sutures are then passed through the sternum, and traction is applied evenly to all the sutures to bring the aorta to the sternum. The degree of correction is assessed bronchoscopically. **B, C.** The position of the aorta before and after surgical correction of tracheomalacia by aortopexy.

with anesthesia being maintained through the ventilating bronchoscope. This method allows continuous intraoperative monitoring of the corrective procedure. An anterior thoracotomy or more recently thoracoscopic approach is carried out through the third left anterior interspace. The left lobe of the thymus is resected, and the anterior aspect of the aortic arch and great vessels are exposed by opening the pericardium. Interrupted nonabsorbable sutures are placed through the adventitial wall of the ascending aorta and the origin of the innominate vessel. The sutures are then passed through the sternum to a subcutaneous plane, along the anterior surface of the sternum, and tied in sequence. Traction is applied evenly to all sutures to bring the aorta to the sternum, while the degree of correction is assessed bronchoscopically. Cough reflex can be induced to confirm the adequacy of airway patency of now suspended malacic trachea.

Our experience indicates that aortic suspension by aortopexy is an effective and safe method of treatment for most patients with segmental tracheomalacia. However, in some patients, usually those with involvement of the entire trachea or tracheal collapse at or below the level of the carina, aortopexy alone may not sufficient and airway stenting may be used. The rationale behind an aortopexy assumes that the trachea is pulled anteriorly, suspended from the sternum, taking off the extra weight from the anterior wall of the tracheomalacic airway, when the baby is lying supine. This changes the configuration of the cross-section of the malacic trachea from a flat ellipse to almost a circle and prevents contact between its anterior and posterior walls, improving airflow dynamics. In addition, anterior displacement of the trachea creates more room for the esophageal bolus to move without disturbing tracheal diameter.

The results of treating tracheomalacia by aortopexy have been the subject of several reports. Filler and colleagues reviewed their experience with the surgical treatment of 32 children with severe tracheomalacia associated with EA. In 29, an aortopexy alone eliminated airway collapse, relieving all symptoms of airway obstruction. Splinting was also necessary in 2 of the 32 patients at the initial operation, when the aortopexy failed to prevent tracheal collapse. Currently, 29 children are well (mean follow-up 6.6 years), 2 have a tracheostomy in place, and 1 died at home of unknown causes. In a group of 7 patients described by Rode, substantial relief of symptoms was achieved following an aortopexy over a follow-up period of more than 24 months. In the 28 neonates and children we have operated on for tracheomalacia, the indication for surgery was inability to extubate the patient in 14 (all underwent surgery with the endotracheal tube in situ), recurrent cyanotic episodes (dying spells) in 12, and recurrent pneumonia in 6 cases. Four patients had more than 1 indication. There were no operative or immediate postoperative deaths. In the late postoperative course, 3 children died for reasons unrelated to the original operation.

Postoperative complications included paresis of the left diaphragm due to phrenic nerve injury in 1 patient, and wound infection in 2 patients. Operative results in relation to the original indication for surgery showed that of the 14 patients operated on with the endotracheal tube, 13 could be extubated, although 2 required tracheal splinting. Intraoperative bronchoscopy showed that tracheomalacia persisted in those 2 patients. An airway splint was employed during the same operation, with an autologous rib graft in one and an internal stent in the other. One patient could not be extubated and eventually required subsequent tracheostomy. In the 12 patients treated for repeated cyanotic episodes, all of the episodes ceased following surgery. In the group of patients whose indication for surgery was repeated episodes of pneumonia, complete resolution of the problem occurred in all but 4 patients, who showed significant improvement.

The surgical experience with aortopexy shows that this operation has been well tolerated, and operative complications have been minimal in all reports. Evaluation of the aortic suspension by an echocardiogram in a limited number of patients indicates that the aorta has remained attached to the sternum for at least 1 year following surgery. There have been no reports of long-term vascular complications from the aortopexy.

## Intraluminal Airway Stenting

The alternative approach to the treatment of tracheomalacia requires that the airway be stented open to overcome the tracheal narrowing. Tracheotomy with positive pressure ventilation can serve to both stent the airway to maintain patency as well as serve as an access route for clearing airway secretions.

Recently, balloon-expandable stents, initially developed for the treatment of vascular obstructions, have been successfully used in the treatment of tracheomalacia in children. Although the basic principle of intraluminal stenting is simple enough, the placement of foreign body in the lumen of trachea remains somewhat counterintuitive and this concern is further substantiated by debilitating inflammatory and reactive granulation formation. Despite early enthusiasm, clinical criteria for the indications and relative efficacy of each procedure are not clearly defined. To date, no prospective comparison of outcomes between stents and aortopexy has been performed. A more recent innovation has been the use of endovascular stents (Palmaz stents) deployed into the airway to provide tracheal and bronchial integrity (Fig. 22-8). The positioning and deployment of these stents require both bronchoscopic and fluoroscopic guidance in order to ensure that luminal support is provided in the critical regions.

Self-expanding metallic stents have been used successfully for vascular, biliary, and urethral procedures. Recently, airway stents have been used to treat adults with airway obstruction when a surgical approach was not possible, due to either the underlying disease or the general health of the patient. Several investigators have reported success with limited use of balloon-expandable metallic airway stents in children.

While the use of endovascular stents to treat severe cases of tracheomalacia of the infant airway is an attractive option, significant complications can arise from these stents. The Achilles heel with the use of balloon-expandable stents is the formation of granulation tissue. Foreign body reaction against the metal grid can result in granulation tissue formation resulting in airway obstruction and hemoptysis. Long-term stent use can be associated with stent migration or erosion into adjacent structures, the most significant of which are the pulmonary vessels resulting in life-threatening bleeds.

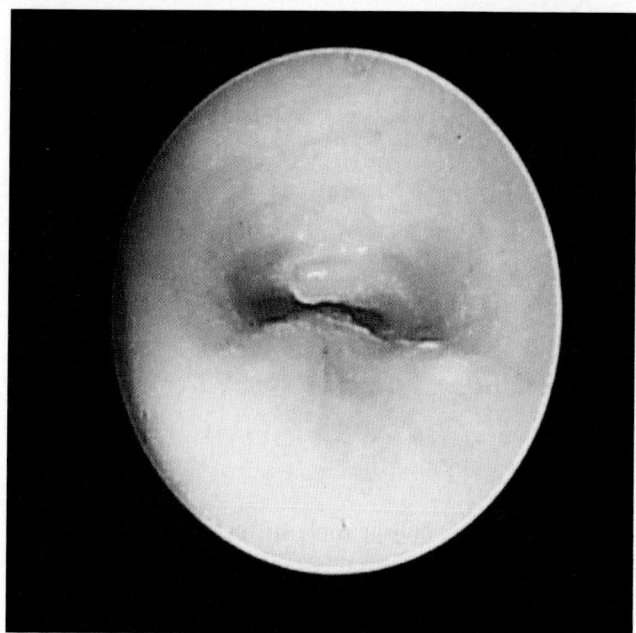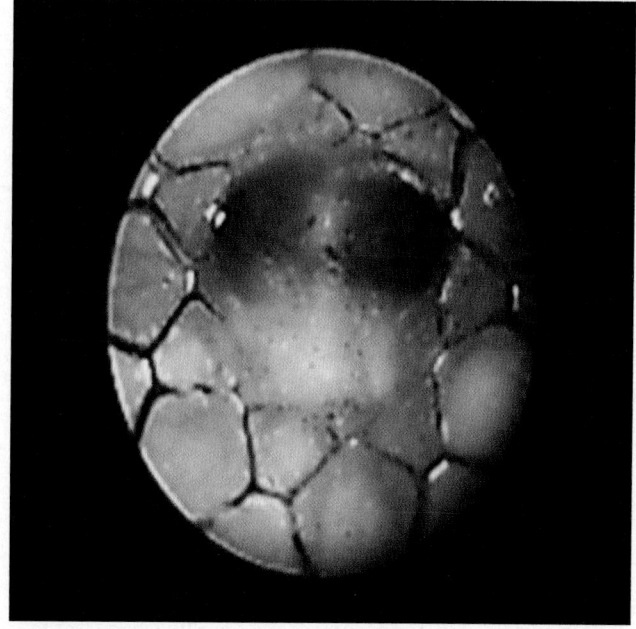

**FIGURE 22-8** Insertion of intratracheal expandable metallic stent for tracheomalacia. The obstructed airway in tracheomalacia (*left*) as seen via bronchoscopy with the collapse of the anterior and posterior tracheal wall. The insertion of the metallic stent (*right*) splints the airway to maintain patency.

The long-term effect of stenting on airway growth remains unanswered. In the largest reported series using balloon-expandable stents, no child had the stent in situ for more than 2 years. The risk of airway obstruction was considered minimal as the stents could be further expanded with balloon dilation to accommodate growth. Our data suggest that this is not the case. Balloon-expandable stents, such as other metallic stents, have the disadvantage of being difficult to reposition or to remove. Two patients in this series had tracheal stents in place for longer than 2 years, and both of these patients experienced significant airway obstruction due to the formation of granulation tissue. Of the 9 patients who underwent stent removal in our series, 7 had successful extractions without any significant complications. Two patients who had stents in place for more than 2 years experienced severe airway obstruction secondary to stent collapse. One child died and the second required emergent tracheal resection and reconstruction. Although efforts are being made to improve the mechanics of stent design and impregnation using bioactive molecules to reduce granulation tissue formation, the use of intraluminal stent for dynamic airway obstruction today, however, remains as application of exclusion and palliation.

## SELECTED READINGS

Anton-Pacheco J, Cano I, Garcia A, Martinez A, Cuadros J, Berchi F. Patterns of management of congenital tracheal stenosis. *J Pediatr Surg* 2003;28(10):1452–1458.

Cantrell JR, Guild HG. Congenital stenosis of the trachea. *Am J Surg* 1964;108(2):297–305.

Cheng W, Manson DE, Forte V, et al. The role of conservative management in congenital tracheal stenosis: an evidence-based long-term follow-up study. *J Pediatr Surg* 2006;41(7):1203–1207.

Chiu P, Kim P. Prognostic factors in the surgical treatment of congenital tracheal stenosis. *J Pediatr Surg* 2006;41(1):221–225.

Filler RM, Forte V, Fragatu JC, Matute J. The use of expandable metallic airway stents for tracheobronchial obstruction in children. *J Pediatr Surg* 1995;30:1050–1056.

Filler RM, Rossello PJ, Lebowitz RL. Life-threatening anoxic spells caused by tracheal compression after repair of oesophageal atresia, correction by surgery. *J Pediatr Surg* 1976;11:739–748.

Forsen JWJ, Lusk RP, Huddleston CB. Costal cartilage tracheoplasty for congenital long-segment tracheal stenosis. *Arch Otolaryngol Head Neck Surg* 2002;128(10):1165–1171.

Grillo HC. Slide tracheoplasty for long-segment congenital tracheal stenosis. *Ann Thorac Surg* 1994;58:613–621.

Grillo HC, Zannini P. Management of obstructive tracheal disease in children. *J Pediatr Surg* 1984;19:414–416.

Herrera P, Caldarone C, Forte V, et al. The current state of congenital tracheal stenosis. *Pediatr Surg Int* 2007;23(11):1033–1044.

Jacobs JP, Elliott MJ, Haw MP, Bailey CM, Herberhold C. Pediatric tracheal homograft reconstruction: a novel approach to complex tracheal stenosis in children. *J Thorac Cardiovasc Surg* 1996;112:1549–15610.

Jaquiss RDB, Lusk RP, Spray TL, Huddleston CB. Repair of long-segment tracheal stenosis in infancy. *J Thorac Cardiovasc Surg* 1995;110:1504–1512.

Johnson DG. Tracheal stenosis. In: Fallis JL, Filler RM, Lemcine G, eds. *Pediatric Thoracic Surgery.* New York, NY: Elsevier Science Publishers; 1991.

Kamata S, Usui N, Ishikawa S, et al. Experience in tracheobronchial reconstruction with a costal cartilage graft for congenital tracheal stenosis. *J Pediatr Surg* 1997;32(1):54–57.

Katz M, Konen E, Rozenman J, Szeinberg A, Itzchak Y. Spiral CT and 3D image reconstruction of vascular rings and associated tracheobronchial anomalies. *J Comput Assist Tomogr* 1995;19:564–568.

Rutter M, Willging J, Cotton R. Nonoperative management of complete tracheal rings. *Arch Otolaryngol Head Neck Surg* 2004;130(4):450–452.

Tsang V, Murday A, Gilbe C, Goldstraw P. Slide tracheoplasty for congenital funnel shaped tracheal stenosis. *Ann Thorac Surg* 1989;48(5):632–635.

Valerie E, Durrant A, Forte V, Wales P, Chait P, Kim P. A decade of using intraluminal tracheal/bronchial stents in the management of tracheomalacia and/or bronchomalacia: is it better than aortopexy? *J Pediatr Surg* 2005;40(6):904–907.

Wright CD, Grillo HC, Wain JC, et al. Anastomotic complications after tracheal resection: prognostic factors and management. *J Thorac Cardiovasc Surg.* 2004;128(5):731–739.

# Gastrointestinal Endoscopy, Caustic Ingestions, and Foreign Bodies

# CHAPTER 23

*Robert A. Cina and Andre Hebra*

## KEY POINTS

1. Pediatric surgeons should be trained to conduct both rigid and flexible endoscopy of the aerodigestive tract to maximize outcomes for children who have aspirated or ingested a foreign body or toxic substance.

2. The sequelae of ingestion are usually minimal, but the risk of complications arising from ingestion of even the most benign foreign body, a coin, approaches 5% in children requiring treatment in a hospital.

3. Ingestion of lithium button batteries should be considered a true emergency, since serious injury to the esophagus can occur in less than 2 hours.

4. Given the marked variability of symptoms seen with foreign bodies in the aerodigestive tract, ranging from mild dysphagia to perforation with sepsis and shock, the best axiom to follow is always be suspicious and prepared to deal with multiple outcomes.

5. Treatment options for removal of esophageal foreign bodies depend on the type of foreign body and include (1) rigid esophagoscopy, (2) flexible esophagoscopy, (3) awake bougienage, and (4) balloon extraction.

6. A wide variety of household chemicals may damage the esophagus, but the most serious injuries are caused by strong alkali products with a pH of >12.

7. Children with a suspected corrosive esophageal exposure should be given intravenous fluids and antibiotics immediately.

8. The most reliable method of imaging and determining extent of injury from caustic ingestion is upper endoscopy, ideally performed within the first 24 to 48 hours.

9. Dilation remains central for managing esophageal strictures following caustic injury.

## INTRODUCTION

Endoscopy, initially scorned as a curiosity by the Vienna Medical Society following Phillip Bozinni's introduction of the *Lichtleiter* (light conductor) in 1806, has gained widespread acceptance and is indispensible in the modern practice of pediatric surgery. The invention of an electrically generated light source offered the most drastic improvement for the field, and recent technologic advancements in fiber optics and digital imaging have vastly improved its functionality.

While there were several "early adopters" of this technology, Chevalier Jackson is considered by many as the father of modern bronchoesophagology. His innovative efforts led directly to the development of diagnostic instruments and tools for the removal of foreign bodies. This ultimately decreased the mortality rate for foreign bodies in the aerodigestive tract from 24% to 2%. In Jackson's time, endoscopists were an elite group of subspecialists who tried to limit the widespread use of these techniques, but the drastic improvement in outcome ultimately led to the widespread adoption of endoscopy. To this day, endoscopy remains a vital component of a pediatric surgeon's armamentarium in the treatment of a child or infant who has aspirated or ingested a foreign body or toxic substance. Pediatric surgeons should be trained to conduct both rigid and flexible endoscopy of the aerodigestive tract in order to maximize outcomes and minimize complications.

This chapter will focus on current diagnostic and treatment modalities for esophageal foreign bodies and caustic ingestions. The preferred intervention for these challenges varies widely and is usually institutionally driven. Several management strategies will be discussed.

## FOREIGN BODIES

### Disease Pathophysiology

While a 4-hour-old neonate is the youngest reported patient with an esophageal foreign body, these objects are most commonly found in children between the ages of 9 months and 3 years. Poison centers reported 4163 pediatric coin ingestions in 2008, with 3304 of the incidents occurring in children less than 6 years of age. The sequelae of ingestion are usually minimal; however, the risk of moderate to major complications arising from ingestion of even the most benign foreign body, a coin, approaches 5% in those children who require treatment in a hospital.

Children are particularly prone to foreign body ingestion given their natural curiosity of the world around them

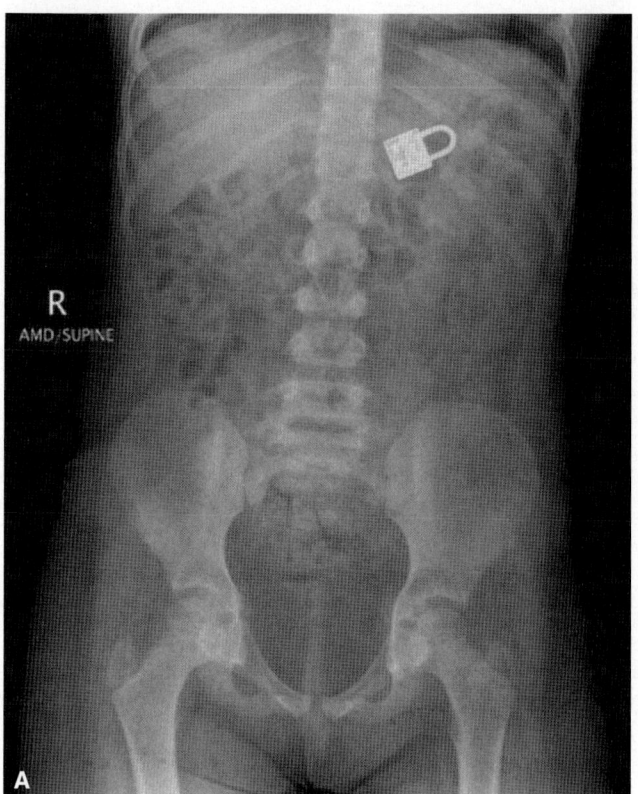
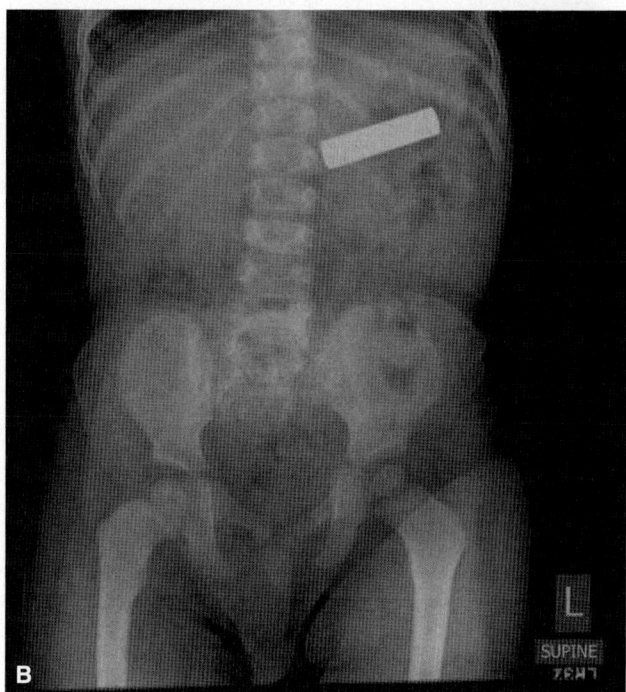

**FIGURE 23-1** Chest radiograph demonstrating (A) a lock and (B) a AAA battery in the stomach.

and their propensity to explore the world with their mouth (Fig. 23-1). While over 80% of all foreign body ingestions occur among children, only 50% of the incidents are witnessed. These foreign bodies commonly become lodged in the esophagus at 4 principal sites of physiologic narrowing. The most common site of impaction is the proximal esophagus at the level of the thoracic inlet (69%), while less common areas include the midesophagus (21%) at the levels of the aortic arch and mainstem left bronchus, and just proximal to the lower esophageal sphincter (10%). Impaction of a blunt foreign body at a site other than those listed above should raise concern about a previously unknown esophageal abnormality or an unreported prior surgical repair of the esophagus, such as repair of a tracheoesophageal fistula.

Common types of foreign bodies are listed in Table 23-1. Impacted esophageal foreign bodies can be classified as food bolus impactions or true foreign bodies that were not intended for ingestion. Food bolus impactions tend to afflict older children, and are more likely to arise in the presence of underlying esophageal pathology (Fig. 23-2). When these occur, it is necessary to rule out either an anatomic narrowing, such as a stricture or Schatzki ring, or an underlying motility disorder. Eosinophilic esophagitis most frequently presents as food impaction, and an esophageal mucosa biopsy is warranted in any patient with this history. Diagnosis and treatment may be aided by skin testing, and pharmacotherapy should be initiated if eosinophilic esophagitis is confirmed. Foreign body ingestion is likely to be significantly underreported since many accidental ingestions pass spontaneously with no ill effect. Small, blunt objects will usually pass spontaneously without the need for endoscopic intervention, while larger, irregularly shaped objects have a higher likelihood of becoming impacted. Complications following foreign body ingestion of any type are proportionally related to the time until diagnosis, and, in some instances, can include severe injury and even death. Prompt diagnosis and appropriate intervention are important to minimize morbidity and mortality.

## Button Battery Ingestion

Button battery ingestion deserves special attention since the increasing spread of electronic devices has led to an explosion in the number of these ingestions within the last 25 years.

| TABLE 23-1 | Types of Foreign Bodies in the Aerodigestive Tract[a] | | |
|---|---|---|---|
| **Airways** | **Percent** | **Esophagus** | **Percent** |
| Bones and meat | 27 | Coins | 58 |
| Nuts and vegetables | 22 | Food | 20 |
| Coins and disks | 17 | Metal | 8 |
| Metal objects | 14 | Plastic parts | 4 |
| Safety pins | 9 | Bones | 3 |
| Plastic parts | 8 | Safety pins | 3 |
| Batteries | 3 | Batteries | 2 |

[a]It is believed that the incidence of ingestion or aspiration of button batteries is increasing because of the increased availability of these devices. Note that the percentages illustrate the average obtained from reviewing the recent literature on the subject.

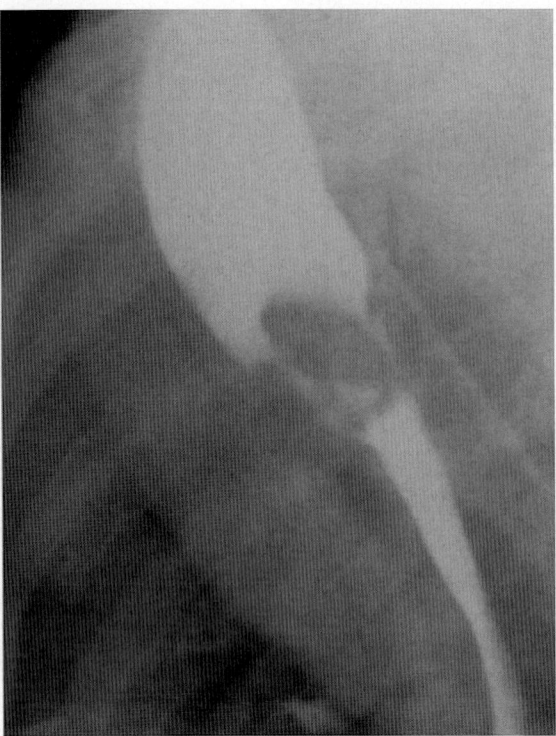

**FIGURE 23-2** Radiograph of a nonopaque esophageal foreign body (prune pit) in a 9-year-old patient with esophageal atresia repaired at birth. The mild stricture at the anastomotic site was responsible for the retention of this foreign body. Note the size discrepancy between the proximal and distal esophagus.

This number has gradually increased every year, reaching 2476 button battery ingestions in children in 2008, a 10-fold increase from the 1983 incidence of 243. This drastic rise in button battery ingestions and the consequent risks have resulted in revision of treatment guidelines for patients suspected of ingestion.

Litovitz et al recently reported a comprehensive analysis of button battery ingestion over the past 25 years. While the overall rate of clinically significant complications in this analysis was only 1.3%, the percentage of cases with clinically significant outcomes increased 4.4-fold from the first 3 to the last 3 years of the analysis. Furthermore, the rate of major or fatal outcomes increased 6.7-fold between those same time points (1985 to 1987 and 2007 to 2009). In cases in which mortality was reported and the battery diameter was known, 94% involved a diameter >20 mm. In contrast, no clinically significant outcomes were observed with batteries 15 to 18 mm in diameter.

The higher risk of esophageal injury due to lithium-based batteries appear to be related to their increased availability, larger size, greater capacitance and energy density, and long shelf life. Lithium batteries are designated with a 2-letter prefix, which designates the type of electrochemical system used and the form, and a number, which indicates diameter in millimeter followed by height. For example, the CR 2032 battery uses a manganese dioxide (C) electrical system, is (R)ound, and measures 20 mm in diameter, and 3.2 mm in height.

Battery-induced local injury to the esophageal wall is thought to be caused by (1) the generation of an external electrolytic current that causes tissue hydrolysis and produces hydroxide at the negative pole of the battery, (2) leakage of alkaline hydroxide, and (3) physical pressure on the tissue. While lithium batteries do not contain hydroxide, they typically have increased capacitance and twice the voltage potential of other button batteries and generate more hydroxide than other batteries. Clinically, injury occurs from the narrow end of the battery (the negative pole) and causes necrosis. This injury can cause serious burns in less than 2 hours. Given the rapidity of injury, all battery ingestions known to be located in the esophageal region should be considered true emergencies and endoscopically extracted immediately. Figure 23-3 illustrates the National Battery Ingestion Hotline treatment algorithm for button battery ingestion. (Updates to the algorithm can be found on their website at *http://www.poison.org/battery/guideline.asp.*)

## Clinical Presentation

There is marked variability in the manifestation of symptoms seen with foreign bodies in the aerodigestive tract, ranging from mild dysphagia to perforation with sepsis and shock. Given this variability, the best axiom to follow when dealing with a possible foreign body ingestion or aspiration is always be suspicious and be prepared to deal with multiple outcomes.

Up to 50% of children can be asymptomatic despite a radiographically confirmed impaction. Symptomatic patients will generally present with dysphagia, odynophagia, poor feeding, vomiting, and occasionally chest discomfort (Table 23-2). Hypersalivation occurs reflexively secondary to obstruction, and as a consequence of being unable to swallow any liquid including their own saliva, patients will drool. Up to one third of patients, particularly those who are younger, have respiratory symptoms that manifest as coughing and stridor (Fig. 23-4). While gagging is rare, a brief coughing spell frequently occurs immediately following the ingestion. Patients with prolonged impactions are more likely to present with respiratory symptoms, weight loss, failure to thrive, and stridor. Rarely, unexplained sepsis is caused by perforation.

## Diagnostic Principles

### History and Physical Exam

Most patients receiving medical attention for ingestions do so after the ingestion was reported by the child or observed or strongly suspected by one of the child's caregivers. A complete history should be elicited from the child and the parents or other caregiver present at the time. The history should include the time when the suspected ingestion took place, the type of object thought to be ingested, and the severity and duration of symptoms (Fig. 23-5).

Physical examination is a focal point of the workup, although it is only abnormal in roughly 10% of patients. Important aspects to note on the exam are the presence of drooling, the absence or presence of wheezing, unilateral hyperinflation, crepitance, and fever on examination. While the presence of wheezing would indicate possible aspiration, crepitance and fever are suggestive of perforation and require expeditious management. Examination of the abdomen

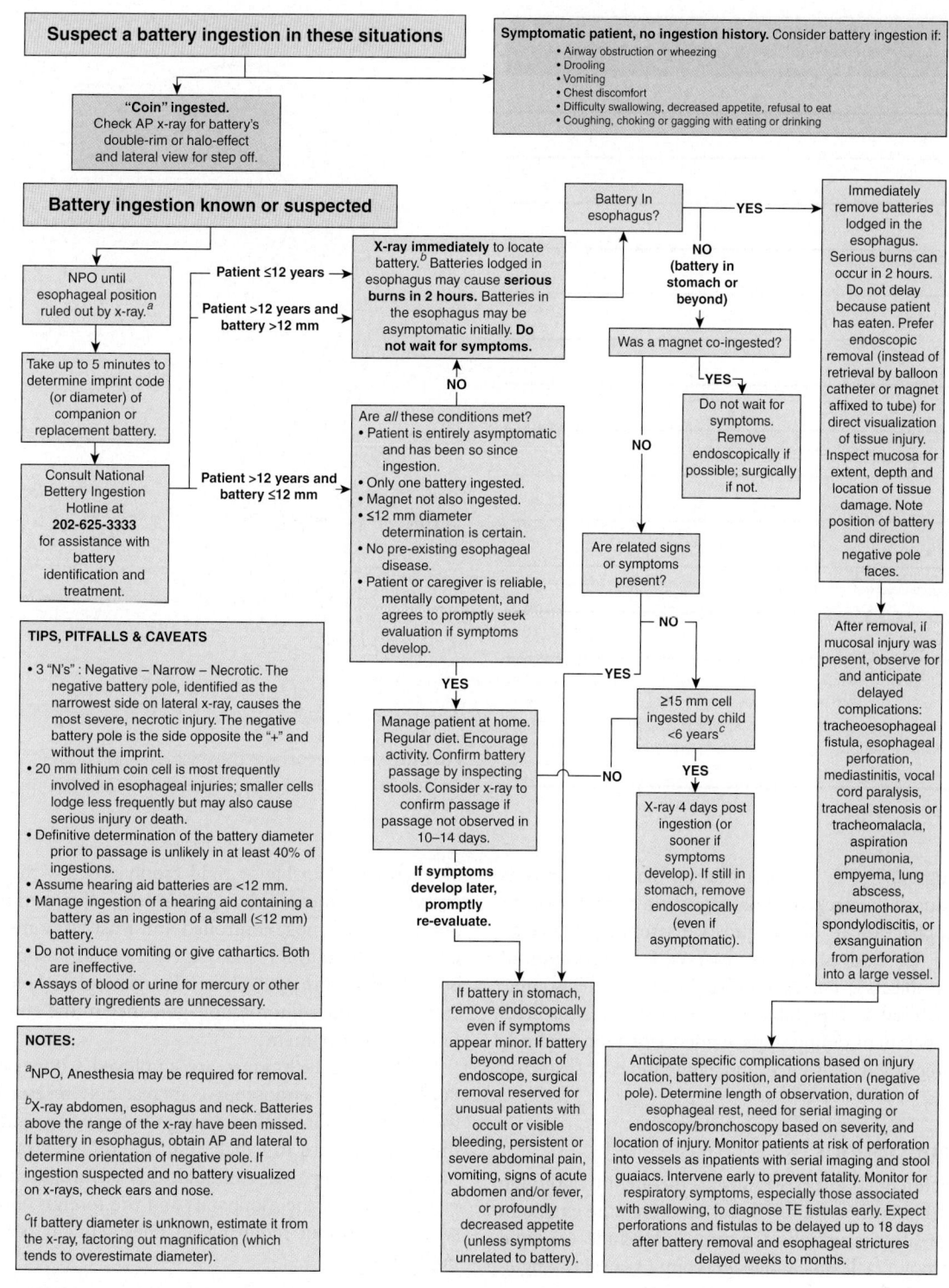

**FIGURE 23-3** National Button Battery Treatment Guidelines from the National Capital Poison Center. (Reprinted from National Capital Poison Center. http://www.poison.org/battery/guideline.asp.)

should focus on the presence of peritonitis, guarding, bowel sounds, and distension, as these may indicate either small bowel obstruction or perforation.

## Radiographic Evaluation

The best initial radiographic study is a posterior–anterior and lateral chest x-ray, including the soft tissues and spine of the neck (Fig. 23-6). These are very useful in distinguishing whether the foreign body is located in the esophagus or trachea. The orientation of the object, especially a flat object such as a coin or button battery, can also help distinguish location. Typically, coins that are located in the trachea will be oriented on the sagittal plane, with the narrowest dimension in the anterior–posterior direction, since successful negotiation of the vocal cords requires this. Coins located in the esophagus also are best visualized on the anterior–posterior view, but are typically lying in the coronal plane. Button batteries characteristically will have a "halo" appearance on

| TABLE 23-2 | Clinical Symptoms Caused by Esophageal Foreign Bodies[a] |
|---|---|
| Symptoms | Percent |
| Vomiting | 43 |
| Odynophagia | 38 |
| Dysphagia | 35 |
| Salivation | 29 |
| Gagging/choking | 25 |
| Coughing | 24 |
| Anorexia | 17 |
| Dyspnea | 8 |
| Stridor | 8 |
| Asymptomatic | 6 |
| Hematemesis | 2 |
| Hemoptysis | 0.5 |

[a]Reported in a review of 484 cases (Crysdale et al. *Ann Otol Rhinol Laryngol* 1991;100:320–324). Curiously, asymptomatic cases were unusual, which is different from our own series of 123 cases in which 20% were asymptomatic. Note that respiratory symptoms were quite common (coughing, dyspnea, and stridor).

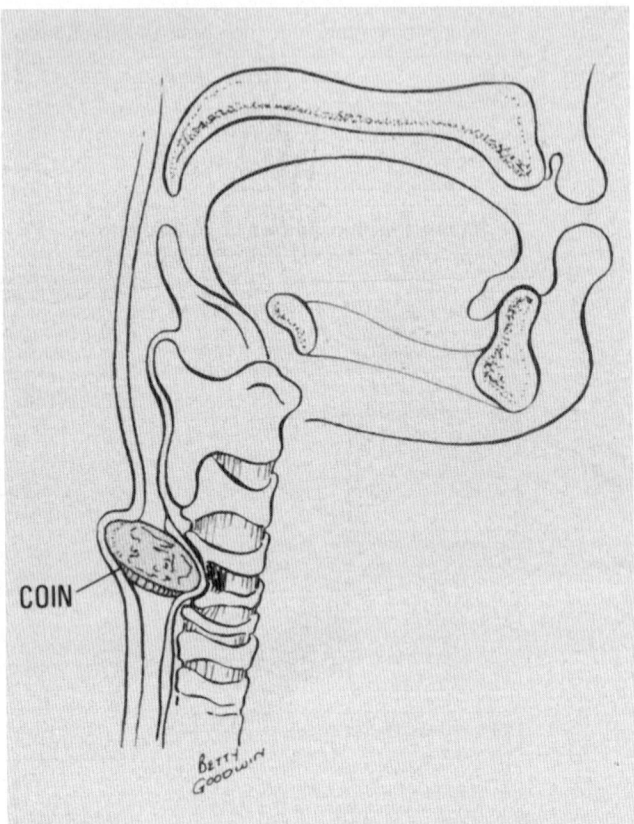

COIN

**FIGURE 23-4** Mechanism by which a foreign body (coin) lodged in the proximal esophagus can cause airway compromise.

chest radiographs (Fig. 23-7), a finding that very rarely is also reproduced by stacked coins. There is a limited role for barium esophagram in the diagnosis of esophageal foreign bodies, and this study should be reserved for localization of radiolucent objects if necessary (Fig. 23-2). A water-soluble contrast material is preferable if perforation is suspected. Failure to document radiographic evidence of a foreign body does not preclude its existence, and a high index of suspicion is necessary.

## Treatment Options

Esophageal foreign bodies are rarely life threatening, although certain objects, such as button batteries, do require emergent removal. Treatment options for removal include (1) rigid esophagoscopy, (2) flexible esophagoscopy, (3) awake bougienage, and (4) balloon extraction. Each of these techniques is advocated strongly by varying pediatric subspecialties. While surgeons and gastroenterologists generally advocate for endoscopic removal, emergency medicine and radiology literature supports bougienage or balloon extraction. There are no significant differences in the success or complication rates of each removal option, although nonendoscopic removal is usually reserved only for the most straightforward cases that meet strict criteria and thus is not universally applicable. For these straightforward cases, there does not appear to be a statistical difference in the complication rates associated with any of these procedures, but important cost considerations are evident. As a rule, bougienage in the emergency room is the least expensive, but also the least controlled method

of treatment. Flexible or rigid esophagoscopy may increase costs by a factor of 10 when performed in the operating room, but is also the most controlled and least risky method. The intermediate option, less expensive than esophagoscopy, but offering more control than bougienage, is Foley catheter extraction under fluoroscopic guidance in the emergency or radiology department.

While these techniques are employed with growing frequency, surgical endoscopy is increasingly reserved for only the most difficult cases involving foreign bodies and remains the gold standard to which all of the other extraction techniques are compared. Although this technique offers direct visualization of the esophagus and the foreign body, it does so at the cost of requiring an anesthetic in the pediatric population.

## Esophagoscopy

Widely available, high-quality flexible endoscopes are well suited for most pediatric foreign body removal procedures; however, a rigid endoscope can be indispensable in certain situations. Thus, familiarity with each is essential. Flexible fiber-optic scopes suitable for pediatric use are available from many manufacturers, including Olympus, Pentax, and Fuji. Advances in optics and image processing continue to improve image quality. Pediatric-sized endoscopes with usable ports are typically no smaller than 8 to 9 mm in diameter. The working port allows for the use of a variety of tools, including biopsy and foreign body forceps, graspers, snares,

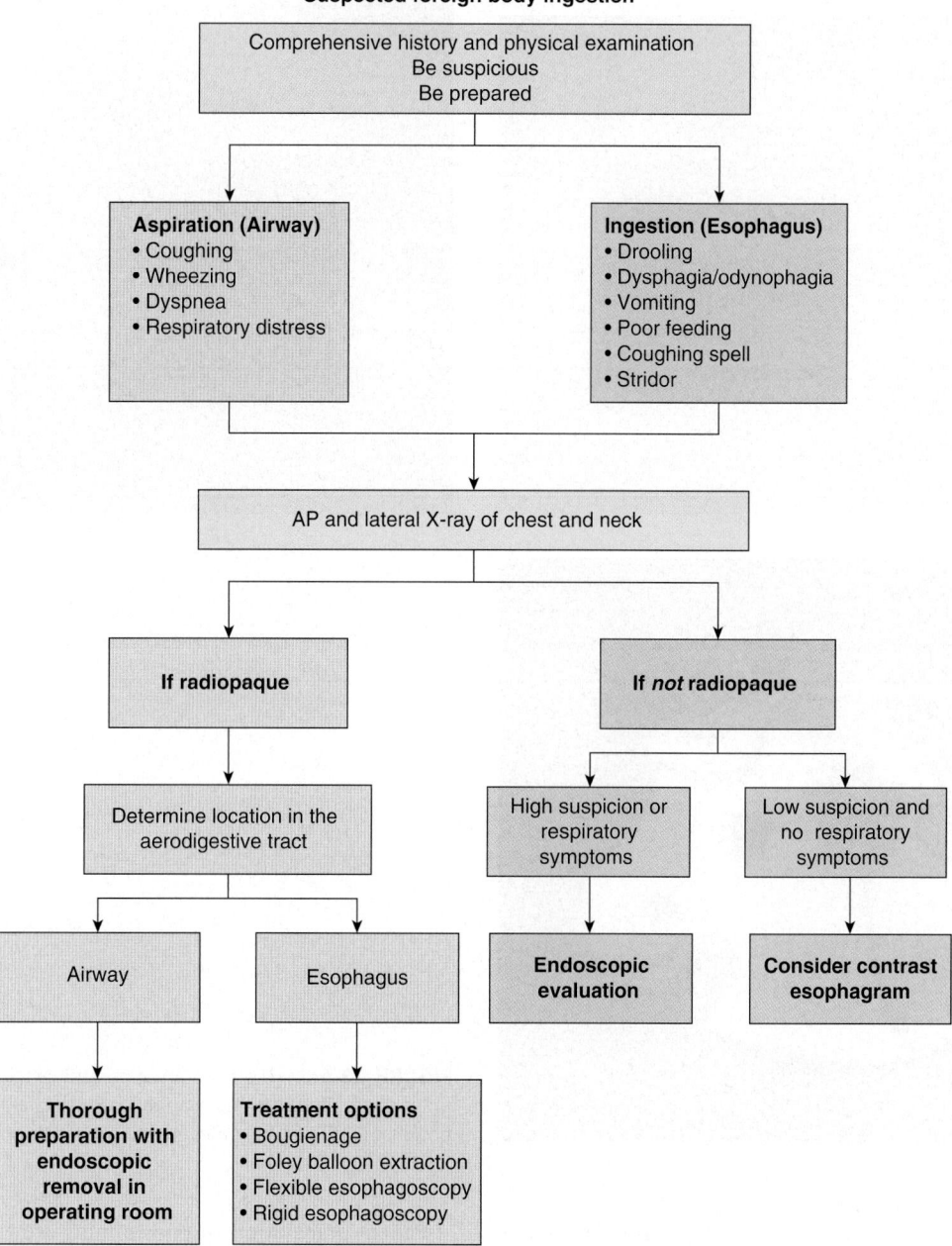

**Suspected foreign body ingestion**

Comprehensive history and physical examination
Be suspicious
Be prepared

**Aspiration (Airway)**
• Coughing
• Wheezing
• Dyspnea
• Respiratory distress

**Ingestion (Esophagus)**
• Drooling
• Dysphagia/odynophagia
• Vomiting
• Poor feeding
• Coughing spell
• Stridor

AP and lateral X-ray of chest and neck

**If radiopaque**

**If *not* radiopaque**

Determine location in the aerodigestive tract

High suspicion or respiratory symptoms

Low suspicion and no respiratory symptoms

Airway

Esophagus

**Endoscopic evaluation**

**Consider contrast esophagram**

**Thorough preparation with endoscopic removal in operating room**

**Treatment options**
• Bougienage
• Foley balloon extraction
• Flexible esophagoscopy
• Rigid esophagoscopy

**FIGURE 23-5** Suggested management and assessment of aerodigestive foreign bodies.

baskets, injectors, and cautery devices. Flexible fiber-optic scopes offer a better view of the esophageal mucosa, provide aspiration and suction capability without the need to switch out instruments, and have multiple instruments that can be used to deliver therapy such as band ligation, and sclerotherapy injection devices.

Rigid esophagoscopes also come in a variety of sizes. The authors frequently use optical rigid esophagoscopes by Karl-Storz Endoscopy, which are 30 cm in length, combined with the use of optical forceps. While the authors do not routinely use these scopes for foreign body extraction, they can offer advantages in difficult cases, especially when used in combination with a flexible scope. Repeated esophageal intubation can be avoided with rigid esophagoscopy, offering advantages over flexible esophagoscopy for the removal of organic foreign body matter from the esophagus.

## Flexible Esophagoscopy

For flexible esophagoscopy, the patient is brought to the operating room where a general endotracheal tube anesthetic is induced and the tube taped to the right side of the patient's mouth. The neck is extended slightly to facilitate passage of the endoscope into the esophagus. With the scope unlocked and manipulated to have a gentle curve, it is introduced into the mouth and into the esophagus. Lifting the trachea upward (toward the ceiling) aids in easy passage of the scope. Visualization of the esophageal mucosa is often facilitated by intermittent distension of the esophagus with the judicious application of air. When a foreign body is visualized, the state of the esophageal mucosa should be noted, along with the presence of ulceration, and the type of foreign body. Blunt foreign bodies may be grasped with a coin grasper or similar device. Manipulation of the tip of the scope is best

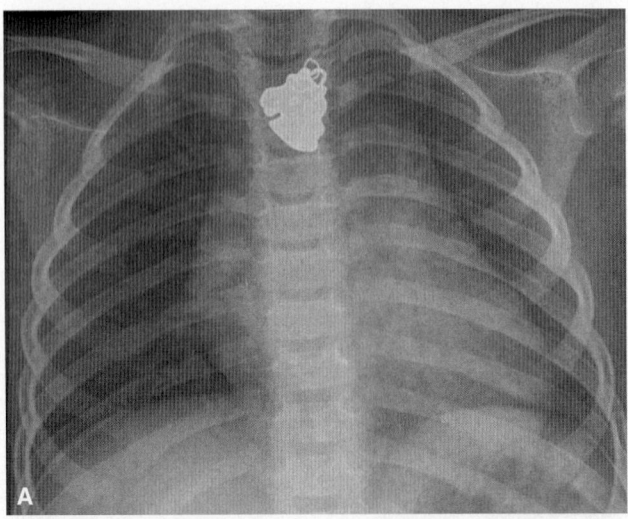

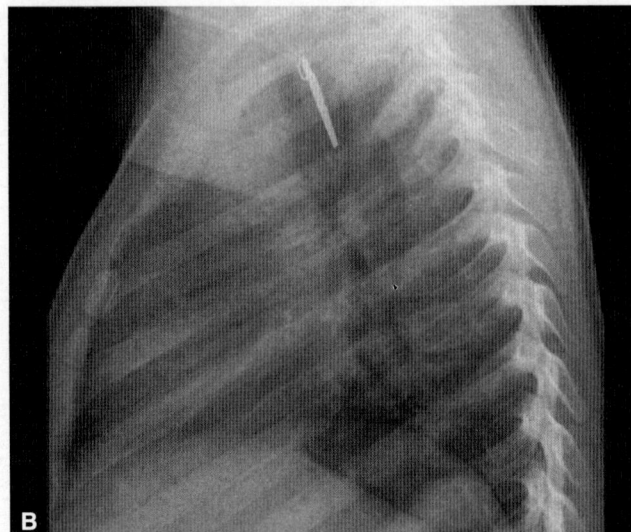

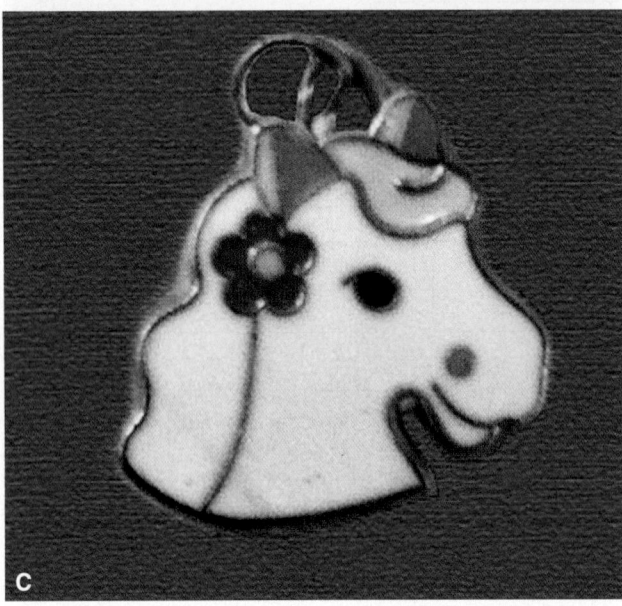

**FIGURE 23-6** **A.** Posterior–anterior and **(B)** lateral chest radiographs help discern either esophageal or tracheal location of foreign bodies. **C.** Depicts the retrieved foreign body.

achieved using one hand to twist and position the scope near the patient's mouth, with the other hand manipulating the controls of the scope. Sharp foreign bodies, such as open safety pins facing upward, represent a greater challenge. If these are positioned so that they can be advanced without causing damage to the esophageal mucosa, they can be grasped by the spring, passed into the stomach without difficulty, flipped 180°, and extracted with the scope. Other oddly shaped foreign bodies or those without graspable edges can be extracted with a Roth retrieval net, polypectomy snare, endoscopic baskets, or improvised baskets fashioned from a condom.

## Rigid Endoscopy

A rigid open-channel esophagoscope, alone or in combination with an optical telescope, is used by many for the routine management of foreign bodies. The operating room environment, with a general anesthetic, provides for complete airway control, increases the safety of manipulating the scope, and makes endoscopy a more comfortable experience for both the patient and surgeon.

Patient preparation and positioning are vital to the proper use of esophagoscopes. The patient should be positioned on a generous shoulder roll with the neck extended in the "sniffing position" (Fig. 23-8). A tooth guard is recommended to avoid injury to the patient's teeth. The esophagoscope should be then advanced along the right side of the tongue, which can be retracted to gain better visualization. A Macintosh laryngoscope can also be used to help aid in the initial positioning of the scope. Under direct vision, the scope is introduced into the back of the pharynx with the lip of the beveled portion anterior, which allows for the elevation of the laryngeal opening of the cricopharyngeus. The patient's mandible and maxilla are supported with the surgeon's left hand, using the thumb and index finger to guide the scope and protect the teeth. The right hand is used to firmly grasp and manipulate the scope. While performing this maneuver, it is vital to advance the scope only when the lumen of the pharynx or esophagus is clearly visualized. If the cricopharyngeus does not open with elevation of the lip of the scope against the posterior portion of the larynx, the esophageal lumen should be identified by passing a soft red rubber catheter as

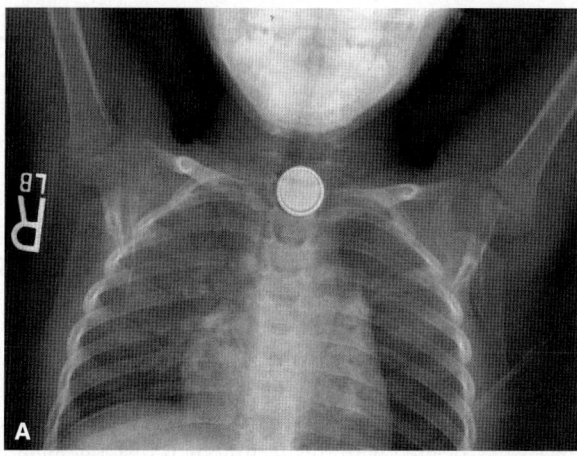 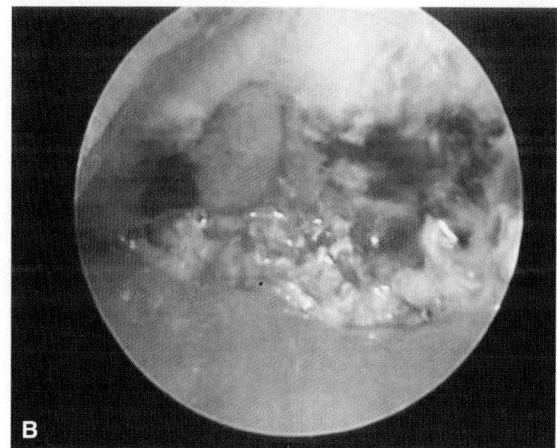

**FIGURE 23-7** **A.** Radiograph of a button battery in the esophagus and (**B**) findings at endoscopy.

a lumen finder. The scope can then be passed over this, acting as a guide, into the esophageal lumen under direct vision. The scope should never be advanced with force, or blindly when a lumen is not seen. The optical forceps make removing graspable foreign bodies straightforward. Additionally, since the scope has a larger working channel than the flexible endoscope, sharp objects can be pulled into the sheath before removal, making for a safer extraction.

Removal of organic foreign material from the esophagus is easier with a rigid esophagoscope. The larger working channel allows for repeated piecemeal passes at the material before extraction and, because larger graspers can fit through the channel, facilitates the removal of larger pieces. Moreover, since the esophagoscope does not require removal when each of the pieces of material is extracted, less esophageal trauma results from frequent intubations.

## Bougienage

Awake bougienage is advocated by many pediatric emergency physicians as a safe, readily available, highly effective, and inexpensive treatment for blunt esophageal foreign bodies. An observational case series reported by Arms et al in 2008 reported their experience with this technique over a 12-year period. Eligibility criteria included a witnessed coin ingestion occurring less than 24 hours before presentation, which could be radiographically determined to be in the esophageal lumen, in a patient with no prior history of esophageal foreign body, esophageal surgery, or other disease. Of 620 patients identified with esophageal coins, 461 met the inclusion criteria for bougienage, although 89 of these patients underwent endoscopy due to patient, parent, or physician preference. The total number of patients undergoing endoscopy was 248 and the coin was successfully removed in all but 1 of these patients. Bougienage was attempted in 372 patients and successful in 355 (95%), with only 17 patients failing bougienage therapy. The average length of stay for patients undergoing bougienage was 2.2 hours, compared to 6.1 hours for patients undergoing endoscopy.

Bougienage has been employed in the authors' own pediatric emergency department and with the very strict criteria used in its application (Table 23-3), is a reasonably safe, effective, and inexpensive first-line treatment modality for the minority of patients who qualify (Fig. 23-9). Prior to the procedure, written informed consent is obtained from the parents. Then the length of bougie necessary to reach the stomach is estimated

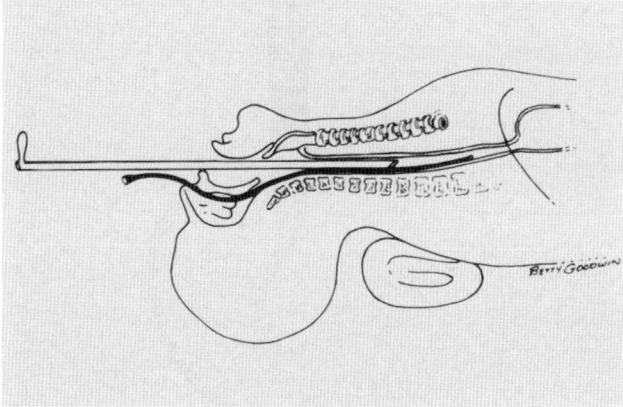

**FIGURE 23-8** Technique for the insertion of a rigid endoscope into the esophagus. A "red" soft nasogastric tube passed through the nose into the esophagus helps guide the placement of the endoscope into the esophageal lumen.

| TABLE 23-3 | Criteria for Application of Bougienage |
| --- | --- |

*Criteria for esophageal bougienage:*

1. Single coin ingested
2. Coin radiographically located in the esophagus
3. Witnessed ingestion of <24 h duration
4. No prior history of esophageal foreign body, esophageal disease (GE reflux, esophagitis, stricture, or hiatal hernia) or esophageal surgery
5. No known GI tract anomalies or surgery that would prevent the spontaneous passage of the coin from the stomach and through the intestinal tract
6. No acute respiratory distress (tachypnea, stridor, or wheezing)
7. Physician performing procedure has received in-service education from physician experienced in the bougienage technique for coin advancement.

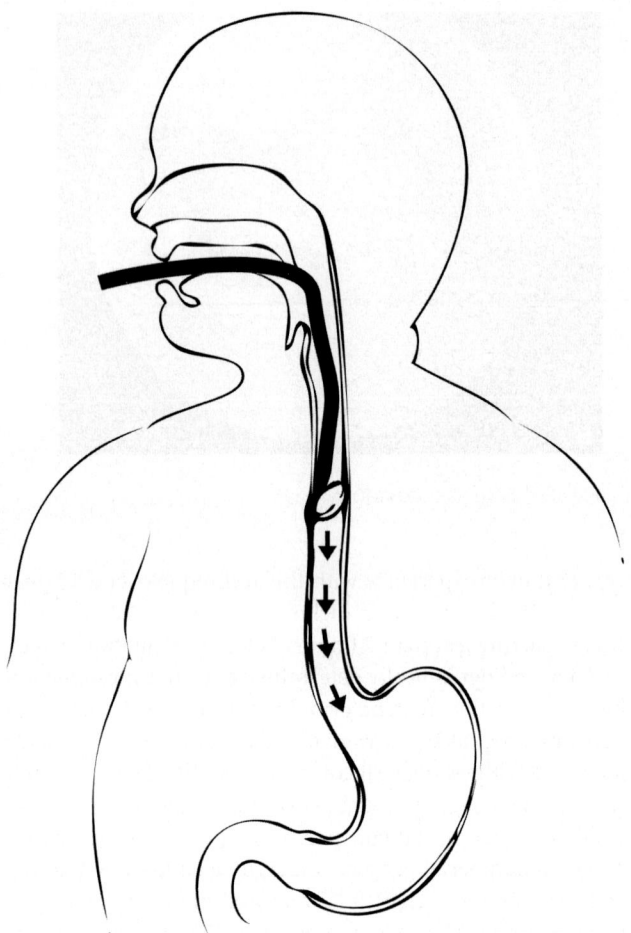

**FIGURE 23-9** Technique for pushing a coin into the stomach using a mercury-weighted bougie.

by measuring the distance from the nares to the ears and epigastrium. This distance is marked with a piece of circumferential tape on the bougie. Bougie size is determined by the patient's age (Table 23-4).

The patient is seated in the upright position, arms wrapped at the side by a cloth sheet and restrained from behind by an assistant. A stack of tongue depressors is used to induce a gag and act as a bite block, after which the bougie is gently advanced into the oropharynx, esophagus, and stomach to the depth marked previously on the bougie. Repeat radiography is obtained to ascertain the displacement of the coin into the stomach.

| TABLE 23-4 | Bougie Size as Determined by Patient's Age | |
|---|---|---|
| **Patient Age (Years)** | | **Bougie Size** |
| 1-2 | | 28F |
| 2-3 | | 32F |
| 3-4 | | 36F |
| 4-5 | | 38F |
| 5 and above | | 40F |

## Balloon-Tipped Catheter

The extraction of smooth esophageal foreign bodies using a Foley balloon catheter was initially reported by Bigler over 55 years ago. Initially, catheters were used to push coins down into the esophagus, but catheters currently are used for coin extraction (Fig. 23-10). This technique has gained acceptance in several disciplines, particularly radiology and emergency medicine, but has achieved limited acceptance among surgeons. Nonetheless, several larger studies have demonstrated safety and efficacy. A large survey of the North American Pediatric Radiologists involving 2500 blunt esophageal foreign body extractions since the 1970s documented a 95% success rate with 1 major complication. While rare, a potential hazard associated with this technique is dislodgement of the coin from the esophagus into the airway during extraction.

In 2006, Little et al reported the retrospective institutional experience at Children's Mercy Hospital in Kansas City, MO. Over a 16-year period, the attending pediatric surgeon or the pediatric surgery fellow on call performed procedures on 555 patients with esophageal foreign bodies. Balloon extraction was attempted in 478 children and was successful 88% of the time, demonstrating an overall success rate of 75% for all presenting patients. The highest failure rate, 25%, occurred among children less than 1 year of age. The patient charges were significantly less with balloon extraction, averaging

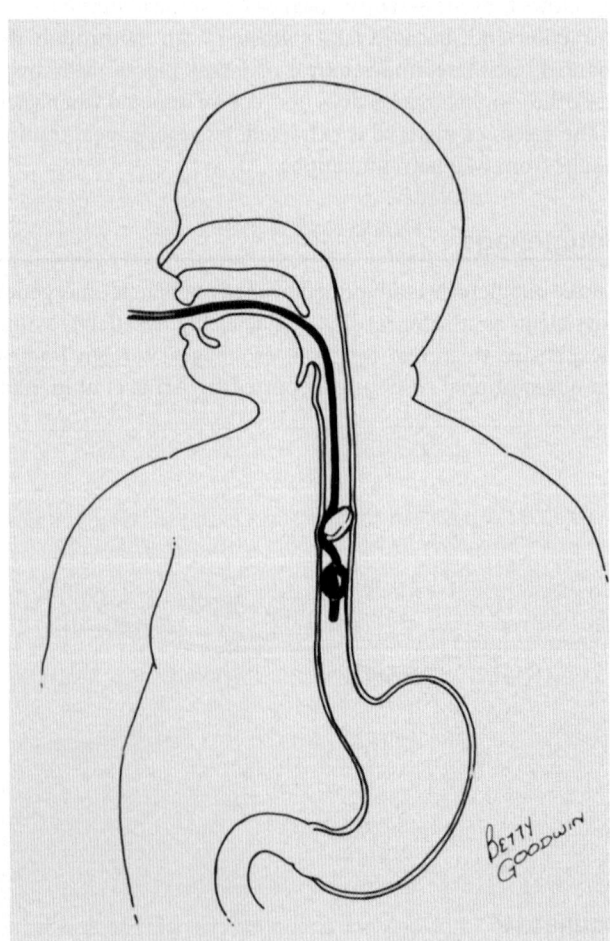

**FIGURE 23-10** Technique for extracting a coin from the esophagus using a balloon-tipped catheter.

$955, while operating room and recovery room costs averaged $2440. Exclusion criteria for balloon extraction listed in this study include impaction for more than 7 days, a sharp object, radiographic evidence of esophageal or airway perforation, and an underlying structural abnormality of the esophagus. The advantage of this technique is that it can be performed in the pediatric emergency room or radiology suite, resulting in a lower overall patient cost. The lack of airway protection during the procedure remains its biggest disadvantage, and although balloon extraction is less costly than endoscopy, bougienage is more economical. Nonetheless, Little's report demonstrates that balloon-tipped catheter extraction is a generally safe technique that avoids general anesthesia.

## Authors' Preferred Operative Procedure

At the Medical University of South Carolina, esophageal foreign bodies are managed in collaboration between the surgeons and emergency medicine colleagues. Esophageal foreign bodies that meet criteria to allow for bougienage are dislodged in the emergency department. The majority of foreign bodies are managed with either flexible or rigid esophagoscopy with removal accomplished by using a coin grasper, as described above. A number of endoscopic devices are available to aid in removal of oddly shaped objects. The authors have found endoscopic snares and the Roth Net retriever to be the most useful in removal of objects that do not have a graspable edge.

## Outcomes and Complications

The success rates for removal of esophageal foreign bodies by endoscopy, bougienage, or Foley extraction are excellent. Endoscopy has the highest success rate for all patients, given the strict inclusion criteria required for alternate techniques. Complications caused by retained esophageal foreign bodies are primarily related to injury of the esophagus from pressure or electrically induced necrosis causing stricture or possibly perforation. Perforation is the most advanced form of this injury and typically manifests as mediastinitis causing fever, tachycardia, chest pain, odynophagia, and dyspnea. Perforation can also result in tracheoesophageal fistula, esophago-aortic fistulas, extraluminal migration of the foreign body, and the development of false esophageal diverticula.

## CAUSTIC INJURY OF THE ESOPHAGUS

Exposure to both acids and alkalis is significant source of morbidity within the pediatric population in the United States. The groups at risk represent a bimodal age distribution, with children aged less than 6 years at greatest risk for accidental ingestion, and adolescents 13 and older at greatest risk for deliberate self-inflicted injury.

In 2008, there were 1,204,673 cases of reported single agent ingestion of nonpharmacologic substances in the United States. Ingestion accounted for 79.3% of toxic exposure, was implicated in 77% of fatalities, was unintentional 82% of the time, and occurred in the home 9 times out of 10. Children younger than 6 made up for nearly half of all human exposures, with children less than 3 years of age involved in 38.7% of cases. A male predominance was found in children younger than 13; however, this gender bias was reversed in teenagers. In 2008, 134,422 children ingested cleaning products, with 5215 suffering moderate-to-severe injuries, and 14 fatal injuries, not including children who ingested noncleaning alkali and acid substances. Most ingestions by children are accidental with trivial amounts ingested and account for a small fraction of fatal exposures across the population. The rate of esophageal caustic injury is difficult to discern given the current method of data reporting, although it suggests that these injuries occur most often in children less than 6 years, and commonly within 12 months to 3 years of life. These children have been ambulatory, have access to cabinets or areas where caustic chemicals are kept, and have suboptimal supervision.

The pattern of injury seen following caustic ingestion varies with the pH (acid or base), the concentration of the ingestant and its pH level, and viscosity. A wide variety of household chemicals may damage the esophagus, but the most serious injuries are caused by strong alkali products with a pH of >12. While injury to the lips, oropharynx, and upper airway can occur with many caustic agents, esophageal injury accounts for not only the most serious injuries, but also those with the majority of long-term complications. These burns commonly arise from household cleaning products such as strong lyes that contain sodium and potassium hydroxides, drain cleaners, and laundry detergents and cleaning agents with sodium phosphate, sodium carbonate, and ammonia.

Although the ingestion of cosmetics and hair relaxer is common, this type of exposure is generally of minor significance. Ahsan and Haupert examined this issue in a large retrospective study examining 163 charts of patients with possible caustic ingestion. Of the 59 patients who ingested hair relaxer, only 3 were found by endoscopy to have mild esophagitis, the most severe injury found. Although clinical data should ultimately drive the decision to perform endoscopy in patients with this particular ingestion, the data would suggest that severe injury with these agents is extremely rare, and as a rule these patients do not require routine endoscopy.

Public education efforts, federally mandated legislation imposing stricter packaging standards, and safer products have diminished the rate and severity of caustic ingestion injury in the United States, compared with other countries, where unintentional injuries are more severe. Other less industrialized countries, however, have adopted novel strategies adapted to local culture and standards and these efforts are having an impact on caustic ingestion injuries worldwide.

## Pathophysiology

Haller delineated the mechanisms of esophageal caustic burns in his seminal papers published in 1964 and 1971. Exposure to strong alkalis causes injuries that penetrate deeply as a consequence of liquefaction necrosis and can cause local thrombosis of blood vessels, further potentiating the damage. This type of injury is usually limited to the esophagus, although the stomach is sometimes affected. Alkalis become soluble once they form soaps with fat, further causing an edematous loosening of the tissue that allows for even deeper penetration.

Neutralization of the substance occurs only by the tissues themselves, which is required for the reactions to cease. These agents cause injury very quickly and as little as 1 mL of a 30% solution of sodium hydroxide (NaOH) can cause transmural injury and necrosis within 1 second of contact. Although injury typically affects the esophagus, injury of the stomach can occur less frequently following exposure.

Acids and corrosives with a pH <7 cause coagulation necrosis and generally are less injurious than their alkali counterparts. The coagulum, which forms following injury on the mucosal surface, limits deeper penetration of the caustic substance. Combined with the naturally present protective mechanisms of the normally alkaline pH and squamous epithelium of the esophagus, this coagulum limits the severity of esophageal injury from acids. Acidic injury of the esophagus is responsible for only 10% to 20% of esophageal burns. Gastric injury, however, is more severe and localized to the prepyloric area as a consequence of antral pooling and spasm.

Following the initial insult, second and third degree burns result in additional destruction, which takes place over the first week as a consequence of inflammation and vascular thrombosis. Granulation tissue and weakening of the esophageal wall are seen starting at about 10 days postinjury. Increased fibrogenesis resulting in stricture and dysmotility is typically observed at 3 to 4 weeks following exposure. Stricture formation occurs in approximately 20% to 30% of third degree burns and is a direct consequence of both the depth and circumferential involvement of the injury.

## Management

### Caustic Esophageal Injury—Acute Phase

Early signs and symptoms following caustic ingestion may not correlate with the severity of tissue injury. When present, dysphagia is the most common symptom, followed by drooling, excessive salivation, vomiting, and the inability or refusal to drink. While clear signs of perforation, including crepitance and mediastinitis, are indicative of caustic esophageal injury, the presence or absence of milder symptoms cannot accurately predict the occurrence or severity of the esophageal lesion. Children with a suspected corrosive esophageal exposure should receive intravenous hydration immediately to assuage the effects of a potential third-space fluid volume loss secondary to damaged tissue (Fig. 23-11). Intravenous antibiotics should be instituted immediately to protect against oropharyngeal flora. While considered "standard of care" in the past, systemic administration of corticosteroids has been shown to be of no benefit, and may be harmful due to its effects as an immunosuppressant. Attempts to neutralize the corrosive agent by making the child drink should be discouraged as they can lead to emesis and repeat exposure of the esophageal mucosa to the ingestant. Neutralization agents (acetic acid for lye, sodium bicarbonate for acid) should also be avoided, as these can cause additional thermal injury from the strongly exothermic reaction resulting from the neutralization process.

Documentation of the injury following symptomatic ingestion should always be performed as it is the only way to determine the extent of injury. Radiologic evaluation does not reliably detect or grade acute injury. The most reliable method of imaging is upper endoscopy (Fig. 23-12), ideally performed within the first 24 to 48 hours. Earlier endoscopy may not show the full extent of the injury, while later endoscopy increases the risk of perforation. The surgeon should note the presence or absence of esophageal or gastric lesions, and determine the severity of involvement.

Flexible endoscopy can be safely performed in all but the most severe injuries. This allows passage of the scope through the area of injury so that both the esophagus and stomach can be visualized. Although rigid esophagoscopy is still commonly used, the scope should only be advanced up to the injury, given a higher risk of perforation if the scope is advanced aggressively. Endoscopy should be performed under general anesthesia with a protected airway, especially in the presence of signs or symptoms of upper airway involvement. Endoscopy is contraindicated in patients who are hemodynamically unstable, in respiratory distress, have clinical evidence of perforation, or have severe oropharyngeal edema. In the presence of mediastinitis, pleural effusion, or perforation, esophagoscopy is unlikely to yield additional benefit, and a thoracotomy is indicated.

Injuries are commonly encountered at the level of the inferior constrictor muscle, at the aortic arch, or in the area of the lower esophagus. Acute burns appear as edematous mucosa covered with a grayish exudate in an area of luminal narrowing (Fig. 23-12). Use of a grading scale, that proposed by Estretta or Hawkins, is useful as a prognostic indicator. If circumferential burns are noted, every attempt should be made to place a nasogastric tube across the area of injury under endoscopic vision. The purposes of this are 2-fold. First, it allows a means to access the distal gastrointestinal (GI) tract for the institution of enteral feeds. Second, having access through the stricture is important if future dilation or esophageal stenting becomes necessary. If this is impossible, a gastrostomy is indicated.

In patients with even the mildest of burns, a strict nil per os status should be maintained until the patients are able to swallow their own secretions. Patients with grade II and III burns should undergo a barium esophagram to ensure esophageal patency prior to the resumption of oral feeds.

### Caustic Esophageal Injury—Recovery Phase and Management of Chronic Strictures

Early clinical signs and symptoms of esophageal obstruction warrant radiographic evaluation during the recovery period to assess the development of stricture formation. If there is evidence of increasing luminal occlusion, treatment options include placement of a nasogastric tube under vision or a gastrostomy to assist in the placement of a transesophageal string for continuous loop dilation.

### Dilation

Several options are available for the management of esophageal strictures following injury. Dilation remains central. The authors prefer to delay initial bougienage until three to 3 to 4 weeks postinjury. While early prophylactic bougienage has been advocated by others, there are no data supporting a reduced rate of stricture formation, and bougienage carries a theoretical increased risk of perforation.

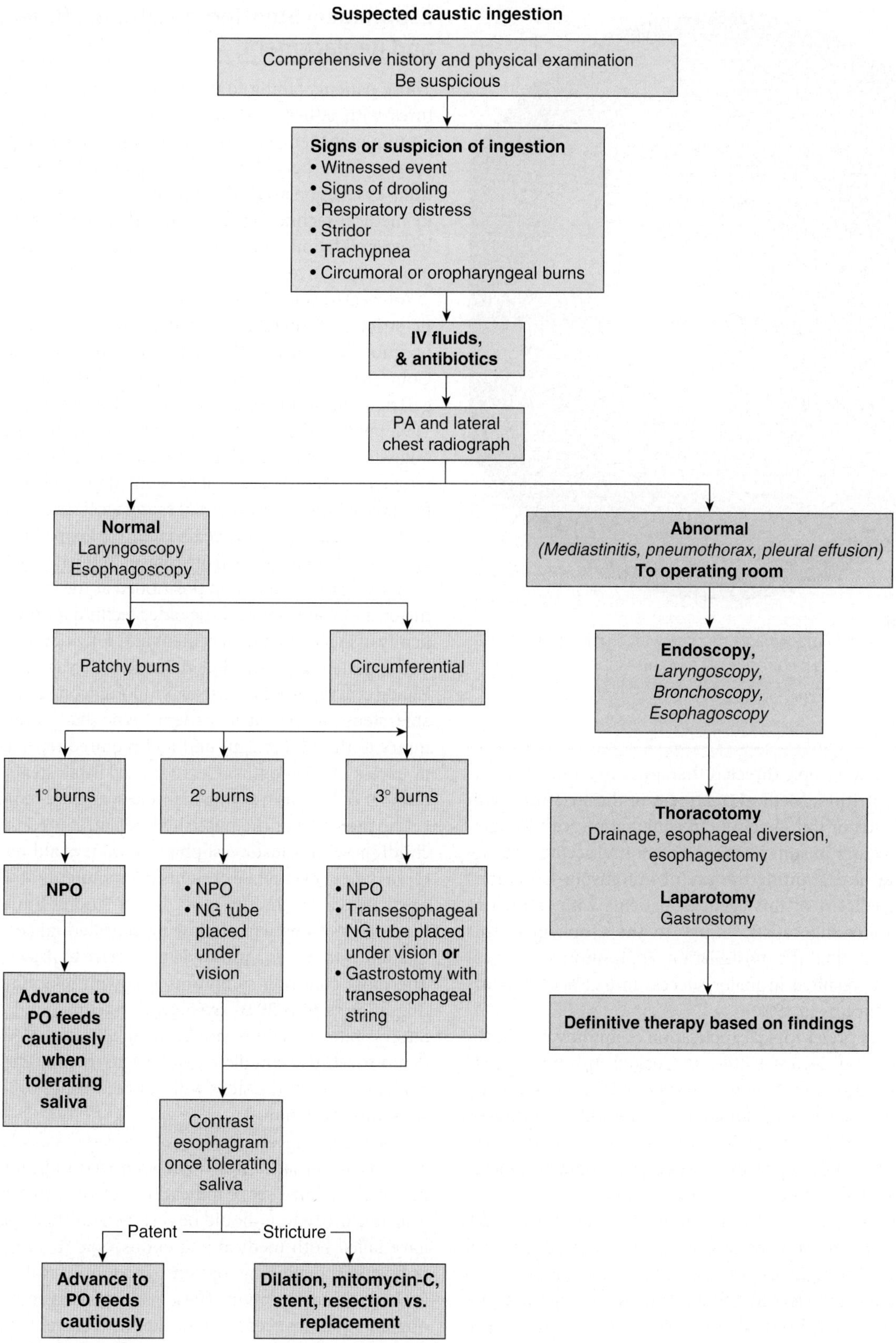

**Suspected caustic ingestion**

Comprehensive history and physical examination
Be suspicious

**Signs or suspicion of ingestion**
• Witnessed event
• Signs of drooling
• Respiratory distress
• Stridor
• Trachypnea
• Circumoral or oropharyngeal burns

**IV fluids,
& antibiotics**

PA and lateral
chest radiograph

**Normal**
Laryngoscopy
Esophagoscopy

**Abnormal**
*(Mediastinitis, pneumothorax, pleural effusion)*
**To operating room**

Patchy burns

Circumferential

**Endoscopy,**
*Laryngoscopy,
Bronchoscopy,
Esophagoscopy*

1° burns

2° burns

3° burns

**Thoracotomy**
Drainage, esophageal diversion,
esophagectomy

**Laparotomy**
Gastrostomy

**NPO**

• NPO
• NG tube
placed
under
vision

• NPO
• Transesophageal
NG tube placed
under vision **or**
• Gastrostomy with
transesophageal
string

**Definitive therapy based on findings**

**Advance to
PO feeds
cautiously
when
tolerating
saliva**

Contrast
esophagram
once tolerating
saliva

— Patent — Stricture —

**Advance to
PO feeds
cautiously**

**Dilation, mitomycin-C,
stent, resection vs.
replacement**

**FIGURE 23-11** Suggested management and assessment in patients suspected of having ingested a caustic substance.

Several methods of dilation are available, including weighted Maloney dilators, wire-guided Savary dilators, continuous loop Tucker dilators passed antegrade or prograde, balloon dilators, and endoscopically placed stents. The choice of these dilators is governed by the anatomic configuration of the stricture. Fluoroscopic guidance is recommended to help decrease the risk of esophageal perforation, which has been reported to be as high as 0.8%. Short strictures are most amenable to dilation, while long, tight, eccentric strictures are the most prone to perforation.

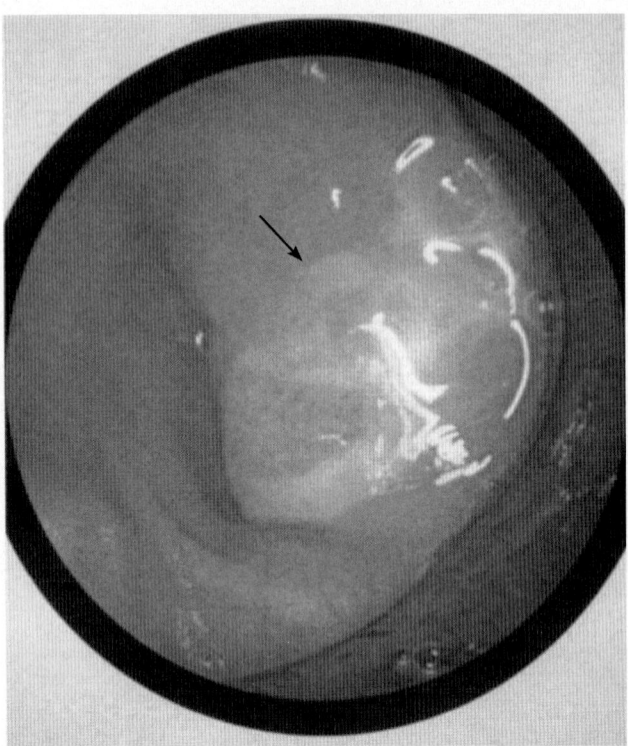

**FIGURE 23-12** Inflamed, friable mucosa with a gray covering exudate (*arrow*) following a corrosive burn of the esophagus.

## Mitomycin-C

The goal of endoscopic directed therapy is to allow for complete oral nutrition. Medical treatment of the strictures with corticosteroids or mitomycin-C in conjunction with bougienage is necessary in some cases. A recent multicenter trial by Rosseneu et al examining the use of mitomycin-C demonstrated the efficacy of this agent in patients with refractory strictures following caustic injury to the esophagus. This study showed that the postdilation application of topical mitomycin-C resulted in major success in 62.5% of patients and partial success in 19%.

The authors prefer topical application of mitomycin-C over steroid injection. Neuro Patties are soaked in mitomycin-C at a concentration of 0.1 mg/mL and placed on the overlying mucosa of the stricture postdilation for a period of 5 minutes. The tissues of the proximal esophagus and oropharynx are protected from the drug by the use of either a rigid esophagoscope or flexible endoscope with an overtube.

The authors utilize the 8.6 to 10 mm OD Guardus overtube (US endoscopy) for this application, due to the larger channel size compared to rigid scopes. The mitomycin-soaked Neuro Patty is placed at the level of the stricture by passing the scope through the well-lubricated fully assembled overtube. The scope is then placed into the esophagus in a standard fashion and the overtube advanced over, but not past, the scope. Once in proper position, which can be confirmed both by fluoroscopy and endoscopy, the scope and the inner tube can be removed. A snare through the working port of the scope is used to grasp the string of a mitomycin-C soaked Neuro Patty, which is then directly applied to the stricture through the overtube. The authors generally apply the drug so that mucosal contact time is at least 5 minutes.

## Esophageal Stenting, Segmental Resection, and Replacement

Those patients failing to experience resolution of their strictures with either medical or endoscopic therapy represent a unique challenge. Until recently, the remaining treatment options have been limited to segmental esophageal resection, esophagoplasty, or esophageal replacement. Advances in medical technology have introduced a treatment option between dilation and these more invasive and complication-prone alternatives.

Advocated initially in 1966 as a measure to prevent caustic stricture formation following injury, esophageal stenting was not described in the pediatric population until 1986 by Coln and Chang. These early reports primarily used nasogastric tubes to maintain patency of the esophagus. Mutaf in 1996 published a report of a large series of pediatric patients following caustic ingestion who had a modified polytetrafluorethylene (PTFE) nasogastric stent deployed for prolonged periods of time as treatment of esophageal strictures refractory to dilation therapy. Two years later, De Peppo et al described customized stents made from Silastic tubing, which was fitted over nasogastric tubes and positioned at the stricture site. The major disadvantages of these older techniques involve the difficulty associated with placement and retention of the stent, as well as patient support while the stent is in place. Most recently, Zhang et al reported the use of Nitinol silicone covered retrievable stents in pediatric patients who had suffered caustic injury to their esophagus and had required repeated dilations in excess of 12 months. Currently available stents come in a number of lengths, varying diameters, and are removable.

The mainstay of the published pediatric literature involves children with caustic esophageal injury, although several reports describe the use of stents in strictures following esophageal atresia repair. The most recent studies limit the use of these stents to patients following repeated failed attempts at dilation, and not as a prophylactic device to prevent stricture. The most common symptoms following placement include migration (up to 29%) dysphagia, retching, and chest pain. Success rates are good, with between 50% and 85% of patients demonstrating a complete response to therapy, defined as the ability to remove the stent without recurrence or the need for subsequent dilation.

Since esophageal stenting of "benign" caustic strictures remains an off-label, non-FDA-approved indication, there is no clearly defined set of indications for the procedure. Therefore, this procedure should be reserved for those patients who have failed both medical and endoscopic treatment, and the only other remaining options are esophageal replacement and segmental resection. These patients will generally have an ongoing dilation requirement due to recurrent symptoms of dysphagia, food impaction, and feeding difficulties. The decision to stent should be based on a number of factors, including patient size and the nature, location, and length of the stricture. Strictures present within 2 cm of either the upper esophageal or lower esophageal sphincter are not ideally treated with stent placement. Stent interference with the upper esophageal sphincter results in a high incidence of dysphagia and retching, while severe reflux and aspiration can complicate stent placement through the lower esophageal sphincter.

Chronic strictures, which fail to respond to dilation and stenting, require esophagoplasty, segmental resection, or esophageal replacement. A comprehensive review of these techniques is discussed in Chapter 25.

## SELECTED READINGS

Aggarwal SK, Gupta R. Esophageal foreign body mimicking esophageal atresia. *Indian Pediatr* 2005;42:392–393.

Ahsan S, Haupert M. Absence of esophageal injury in pediatric patients after hair relaxer ingestion. *Arch Otolaryngol Head Neck Surg* 1999;125:953–955.

Anderson KD, Rouse TM, Randolph JG. A controlled trial of corticosteroids in children with corrosive injury of the esophagus. *N Engl J Med* 1990;323:637–640.

Arms JL, Mackenberg-Mohn MD, Bowen MV, et al. Safety and efficacy of a protocol using bougienage or endoscopy for the management of coins acutely lodged in the esophagus: a large case study. *Ann Emerg Med* 2008;51:367–372.

Bigler FC. The use of a Foley catheter for removal of blunt foreign bodies from the esophagus. *J Thorac Cardiovasc Surg* 1966;51:759–760.

Bronstein AC, Spyker DA, Cantilena LR Jr, et al. 2008 Annual Report of the American Association of Poison Control Centers' National Poison Data System (NPDS): 26th Annual Report. *Clin Toxicol (Phila)* 2009;47:911–1084.

Coln D, Chang JH. Experience with esophageal stenting for caustic burns in children. *J Pediatr Surg* 1986;21:588–591.

De Peppo FD, Zaccara A, Dall'Oglio L, et al. Stenting for caustic strictures: esophageal replacement replaced. *J Pediatr Surg* 1998;33:54–57.

Gaudreault P, Parent M, McGuigan MA, et al. Predictability of esophageal injury from signs and symptoms: a study of caustic ingestion in 378 children. *Pediatrics* 1983;71:767–770.

Gilchrist BF, Valerie EP, Nguyen M, et al. Pearls and perils in the management of prolonged, peculiar, penetrating esophageal foreign bodies in children. *J Pediatr Surg* 1997;32:1429–1431.

Haller JA, Bachman K. The comparative effect of current therapy on experimental caustic burns of the esophagus. *Pediatrics* 1964;34:236–245.

Haller JA Jr, Andrews HG, White JJ, Tamer MA, Cleveland WW. Pathophysiology and management of acute corrosive burns of the esophagus: results of treatment in 285 children. *J Pediatr Surg* 1971;6:578–584.

Kramer RE, Quiros JA. Esophageal stents for severe strictures in young children: experience, benefits, and risk. *Curr Gastroenterol Rep* 2010;12:203–210.

Litovitz T, Whitaker N, Clark L, et al. Emerging battery-ingestion hazard: clinical implications. *Pediatrics* 2010;125:1168–1177.

Little DC, Shah SR, St Peter SD, et al. Esophageal foreign bodies in the pediatric population: our first 500 cases. *J Pediatr Surg* 2006;41:914–918.

Macpherson RI, Hill JG, Othersen HB, et al. Esophageal foreign bodies in children: diagnosis, treatment, and complications. *AJR Am J Roentgenol* 1996;166:919–924.

Mutaf O. Treatment of corrosive esophageal strictures by long-term stenting. *J Pediatr Surg* 1996;31:681–685.

Rosseneu S, Afzal N, Yerushalmi B, et al. Topical application of mitomycin-C in oesophageal strictures. *J Pediatr Gastroenterol Nutr* 2007;44:336–341.

Yalcin S, Karnak I, Ciftci AO, et al. Foreign body ingestion in children: an analysis of pediatric surgical practice. *Pediatr Surg Int* 2007;23:755–761.

Zhang C, Yu JM, Fan GP, et al. The use of a retrievable self-expanding stent in treating childhood benign esophageal strictures. *J Pediatr Surg* 2005;40:501–504.

# Esophageal Atresia

# CHAPTER 24

*Paolo De Coppi and Agostino Pierro*

## KEY POINTS

1. Most cases of esophageal atresia and tracheoesophageal fistula (EA/TEF) occur sporadically. In 50% to 80% of cases, there are associated anomalies, most frequently musculoskeletal malformations, followed by cardiovascular, genitourinary, gastrointestinal, and chromosomal anomalies.

2. Unlike other congenital malformations, EA is infrequently diagnosed prenatally.

3. Polyhydramnios is present in 95% of patients with isolated EA without TEF, and in 35% of cases with distal TEF.

4. All infants with EA should have an echocardiogram before operative repair because of the high incidence of congenital cardiac anomalies.

5. In neonates with EA/TEF, the diagnosis can be confirmed by tracheobronchoscopy and/or esophagoscopy.

6. Surgical repair should be done soon after birth. It is not an emergency procedure, but neonates requiring mechanical ventilation should be operated on promptly to avoid gastric distension and possible perforation.

7. Physiological stable neonates with EA and TEF can be managed with a single operation to divide the distal fistula and perform the esophageal anastomosis.

8. In 10% of neonates with EA and TEF who are very premature or physiological unstable, ligation of the TEF is performed first and the esophageal anastomosis is done as a secondary stage repair when the baby is stable.

9. Thoracoscopic repair offers a scarless repair with faster recovery and less postoperative pain and may also potentially protect from later problems such as winged scapula and thoracic asymmetry.

## INTRODUCTION

Esophageal atresia and tracheoesophageal fistula (EA/TEF) constitute a relatively rare malformation, affecting approximately 1 in 2500 to 4500 live births with a slight preponderance of males in the ratio of 3:2. It was first described in 1670 by Durston in a set of conjoined twins. This was followed by a report of EA with TEF by Thomas Gibson in his landmark treatise, *The Anatomy of Human Bodies Epitomized*, published in 1684.

In 1913, Richter proposed a plan of management that involved dividing the TEF, feeding the neonate via a gastrostomy, and performing a delayed esophageal anastomosis when difficulties had been overcome. In 1939, William Ladd and N. Logan Leven were independently the first to achieve long-term survival for children with EA/TEF, but only by a staged approach. The first successful primary repair of an EA was performed by Cameron Haight on March 15, 1941, at the University of Michigan. This was accomplished through a left thoracotomy, which is now used only if a right-sided aortic arch is found on preoperative echocardiography. Haight's success was soon followed by others and survival increased, reaching approximately 75% in late 1960 and almost 100% today in children with no severe associated anomalies.

## EMBRYOLOGY

The pathogenesis of EA remains unknown, and because most cases of EA occur sporadically, it is highly unlikely that a simple, inheritable genetic mechanism is responsible. The parallel development of both teratogenic and genetic models of EA/TEF has demonstrated that the fundamental developmental aberration appears to be the disturbance of the process of separating the foregut into a respiratory (ventral) and a gastrointestinal (dorsal) component. The study of the genetic models shows that factors that are expressed in a well-defined dorsoventral pattern within the anterior foregut at the time of separation are fundamental to this process and that loss of the dorsoventral boundary of expression domains disrupts the physical separation of the foregut. This has been demonstrated for both respiratory and gastrointestinal markers (Nkx2.1 and Sox2), as well as for factors with more dynamic expression patterns (Sonic hedgehog [Shh] and Nog). In the animal model of the disease, exposure to a teratogenic agent such as doxorubicin disturbs this precisely regulated dorsoventral expression of Shh, leading to failed separation of trachea and esophagus. This finding provides a unique insight into how a nongenetic factor can disrupt a specific developmental process.

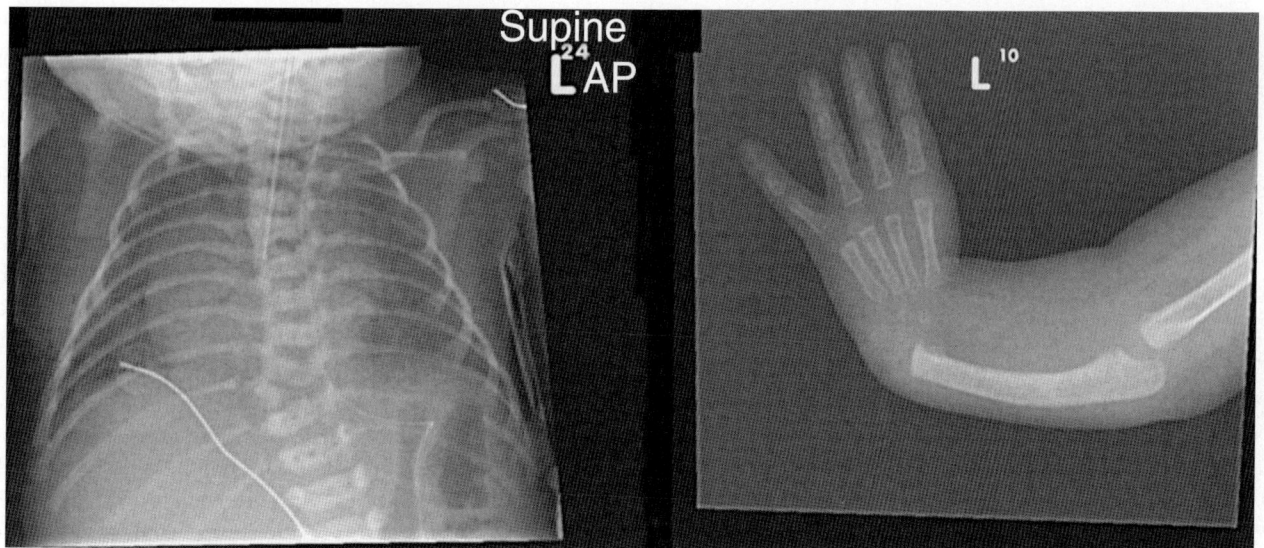

**FIGURE 24-1** Chest radiograph in a baby with EA and vertebral anomalies, radial hypoplasia, and club hand.

Although the precise etiology of the majority of human EA/TEF cases remains elusive, understanding of the interplay between molecular and morphogenetic events may in the future provide targets for modulation therapy. This could lead to possible prevention of EA/TEF, perhaps similar to the prevention of neural tube defects by the administration of folic acid.

## ASSOCIATED MALFORMATIONS

Most cases of EA/TEF occur sporadically, and in 50% to 80% of cases, there are associated malformations (Fig. 24-1). The most frequent associated anomalies are musculoskeletal malformations (20%-70%), followed by cardiovascular (atrial septal defect, tetralogy of Fallot, coarctation, and right-descending aorta, 20%-50%), genitourinary (15%-25%), gastrointestinal (anorectal atresia, duodenal atresia, and malrotation; 15%-25%), and chromosomal anomalies (5%-10%), including trisomies 13, 18, and 21. Well-recognized associations include CHARGE (Coloboma, Heart defect, Atresia of the choana, Retardation, Genital hypoplasia, and Ear deformities) and VACTERL (Vertebral anomaly, Anal atresia, Cardiac anomaly, Tracheoesophageal fistula, Esophageal atresia, Renal anomaly, and Limb malformation).

## CLASSIFICATION

Various classifications have been used to describe the anatomic types of EA. In 1953, Gross took into consideration the presence and the position of the fistula to develop the following classification: Type A, EA without fistula (8.5%); Type B, EA with proximal fistula (1%); Type C, EA with distal fistula (85%); Type D, EA with proximal and distal fistula (1.5%); Type E, H-type fistula without atresia (4%). In 1962, Waterston proposed criteria for survival that are no longer

relevant. More recently, Spitz in 1994 described a classification that correlates survival with birth weight and presence or absence of major cardiac anomaly: Group I, birth weight >1500 g and no major cardiac anomaly (97% survival); Group II, birth weight <1500 g or major cardiac anomaly (59% survival); and Group III, birth weight <1500 g plus major cardiac anomaly (22% survival).

## DIAGNOSIS

Unlike other congenital malformations, EA is infrequently diagnosed prenatally. Polyhydramnios is present in 95% of patients with isolated EA without TEF, and in 35% of cases with distal TEF. Serial fetal ultrasound scans indicating absent or small stomach bubble and maternal polyhydramnios are predictive of EA without TEF only in up to 40% of cases. Neonates with EA present at birth with excessive salivation and inability to clear secretions from the mouth, and require repeated suctioning. Feeding should not be attempted since it could result in aspiration, regurgitation, choking, coughing, and cyanotic episodes. A wide-bore (10-12F) catheter should be passed through the mouth, and in neonates with EA, it will stop at 9 to 10 cm from the lower alveolar ridge. A plain x-ray of the chest and abdomen will show the tip of the catheter arrested in the superior mediastinum (T2-T4).

The presence of gas in the stomach and beyond signifies the presence of a distal TEF (Fig. 24-2). The absence of intestinal air suggests the diagnosis of a pure EA without distal fistula. A contrast study of the upper pouch is performed only in infants with pure EA to exclude the presence of a proximal TEF. All infants with EA should have an echocardiogram before operative repair because of the high incidence of congenital cardiac anomalies. This may also help to define the position of the aortic arch and therefore to determine the side of the thoracic repair, which is done on the side opposite the aortic arch (Fig. 24-3).

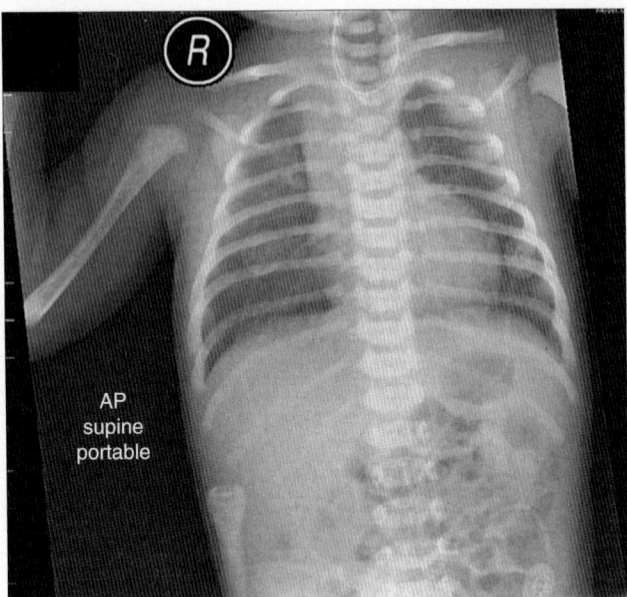

**FIGURE 24-2** Radiograph in a newborn with EA and a distal TEF, with gas seen in the gastrointestinal tract beyond the duodenal bulb.

## Bronchoscopy or Esophagoscopy

In neonates with EA/TEF, the diagnosis can be confirmed by tracheobronchoscopy and/or esophagoscopy. Tracheobronchoscopy using a rigid 3.5-mm endoscope can be performed before the repair to visualize the distal TEF and exclude the presence of an upper pouch fistula. The latter can be difficult to visualize and the dorsal membranous region of the trachea can be gently probed with the tip of a 3F ureteric catheter to avoid missing a small upper pouch fistula. Alternatively, a rigid esophagoscopy can be performed to confirm the diagnosis.

## TREATMENT

Once the diagnosis has been established, the upper pouch is continuously aspirated using a Replogle tube attached to low-pressure suction to remove secretions and prevent

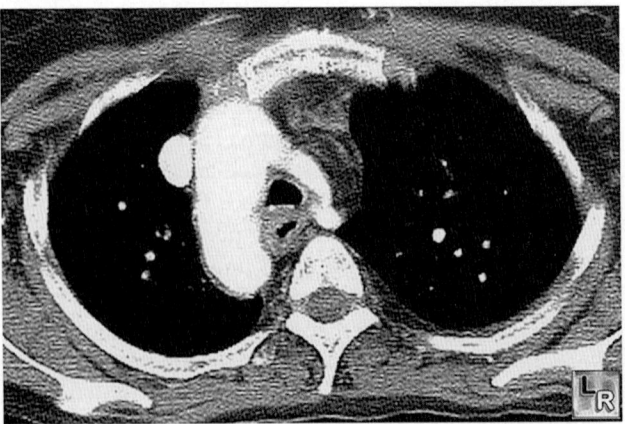

**FIGURE 24-3** A CT scan of a baby with EA and right-sided aortic arch.

aspiration. Dextrose and saline intravenous fluids are administered (usually 10% dextrose and one fourth of the normal percentage saline solution). Surgical repair should be done soon after birth. It is not an emergency procedure, but neonates requiring mechanical ventilation should be operated on promptly to avoid gastric distension and possible perforation.

Most neonates with EA and TEF can be managed with a single operation to divide the distal fistula and perform the esophageal anastomosis. Gastrostomy should be avoided except in patients with pure EA and no TEF. Preterm infants with severe respiratory distress syndrome needing ventilator support require an emergency transpleural ligation of the TEF. In these infants, the esophageal anastomosis should be performed when the infants are physiologically stable. In neonates with EA and TEF with bronchial or distal carina, a long gap between the upper and lower esophageal pouches is common. These babies are usually treated initially with a feeding gastrostomy and continuous suction of the upper pouch by the Replogle tube.

The alternatives for definitive treatment are various and include (1) delaying primary anastomosis, usually to several weeks from birth, with the optimal time based on the assessment of the gap; (2) cervical esophagostomy and subsequent esophageal replacement; and (3) elongation of esophageal pouches by traction (Foker technique) and subsequent esophageal anastomosis.

## Thoracotomy

In the more usual scenario of a left-sided aortic arch, a right posterolateral thoracotomy is generally employed. The infant is placed in the lateral position with the right arm raised over the head to facilitate the thoracic approach. A transverse incision is done posteriorly just below the inferior angle of the scapula. The chest is entered through the fourth intercostal space and the pleura swept off the chest wall, ideally maintaining an extrapleural approach. The azygos vein is ligated with absorbable sutures and divided.

The lower esophagus and TEF are identified and a vessel loop can be passed around the fistula to help in the dissection (Fig. 24-4). TEF is divided and the tracheal side is closed with 5-0 nonabsorbable suture (Fig. 24-5). The anaesthetist can push on the Replogle tube to help identify the upper esophageal segment. A stay suture may assist in its mobilization and avoids unnecessary handling of the proximal pouch during mobilization. Particular care should be taken in its dissection because of the close adherence to the trachea.

The esophageal ends can be anastomosed in a single layer using small-caliber absorbable or nonabsorbable sutures (5-0 or 6-0) to achieve continuity (Fig. 24-6). Multiple sutures can be placed on the posterior wall of the esophagus and pulled together before tying to allow more distribution of the tension. A transanastomotic tube can be passed to allow postoperative early feeding. The anastomosis is completed on the anterior wall, with special care taken to ensure that the mucosa layer is included in the anastomosis (Fig. 24-7).

A chest drain is normally not required and the chest wall can be closed by approximation of the ribs with an absorbable suture and closure of muscle and skin layers.

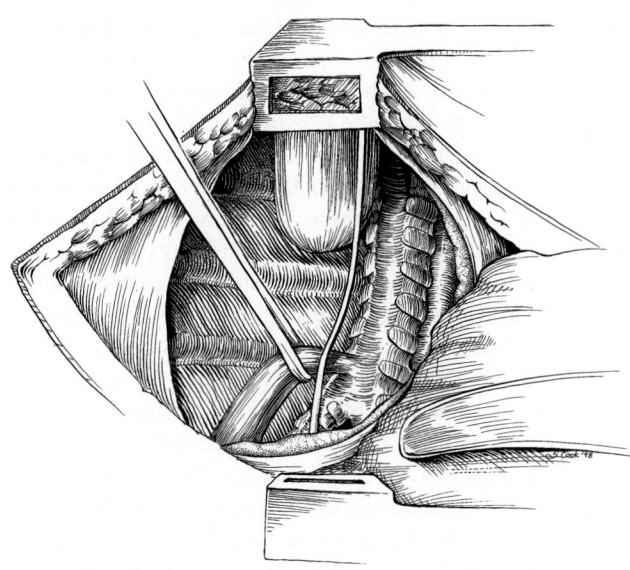

FIGURE 24-4 Initial dissection of a TEF. The distal esophagus is controlled with an umbilical tape, and the vagus nerve is identified and preserved.

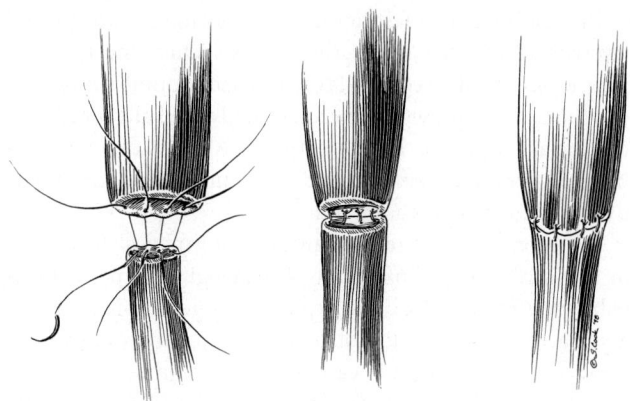

FIGURE 24-6 A single-layer esophageal anastomosis is constructed with 5-0 silk sutures. An 8-Fr feeding tube is placed across the anastomosis just before placement of the last anterior sutures.

Foker recently described a technique of esophageal growth induced by traction of esophageal pouches. Following progressive traction, a primary anastomosis is performed. This technique can be used in long-gap EA with distal TEF and pure EA. The long-term results of this procedure are unclear.

## Thoracoscopy

Greater experience with minimally invasive techniques in infants and children has led to the use of thoracoscopy in neonates with EA. The first thoracoscopic repair was performed on a 2-month-old infant with isolated EA at the International Pediatric Surgical Endoscopy (IPEG) meeting in Berlin in 1999 by Steven Rothenberg, MD, and Thom Lobe, MD.

Thoracoscopy is usually performed with both lungs ventilated, although a bronchial blocker is sometimes used to achieve single lung ventilation. The neonate is positioned semiprone and a 3- or 5-mm Hasson cannula is inserted below the tip of the scapula. The chest is insufflated to a pressure of 5 to 8 mm Hg using $CO_2$ at a flow rate of 1 to 4 L/min and the lung gradually collapses. Once collapsed, a maximum pressure of 6 mm Hg is recommended. A 30° telescope is used and 2 additional 3- or 5-mm ports are inserted, 1 up in the axilla and the other more posteriorly to achieve a good triangulation with the other ports. An additional instrument is usually helpful for lung retraction. For better visualization, the azygos vein usually is divided between ligatures or coagulated closed with monopolar or bipolar hook diathermy. In favorable cases, the esophageal ends may be in proximity and the azygos vein may not need to be divided. The TEF is transfixed and ligated with a nonabsorbable suture (polypropylene 4-0). Visualization of the upper pouch can be facilitated by the anaesthetist gently pushing on the Replogle tube.

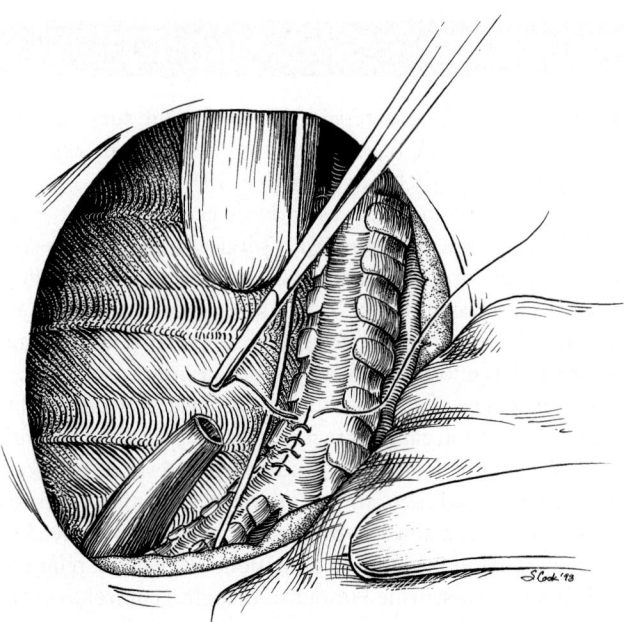

FIGURE 24-5 The fistula is divided, leaving a 1-mm cuff of esophagus on the trachea. The cuff is oversewn with interrupted fine silk sutures.

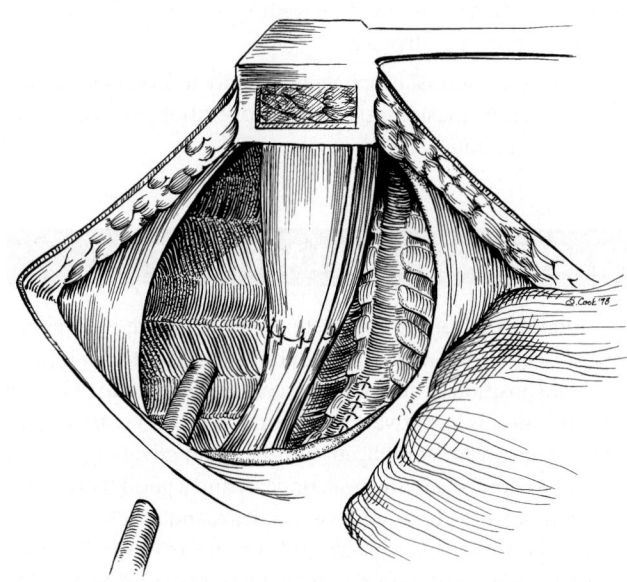

FIGURE 24-7 The completed repair.

The esophageal anastomosis is performed with several interrupted stitches as described above. Once the first few sutures are positioned, a Silastic transanastomotic nasogastric tube can be passed by the anaesthetist and advanced into the distal esophagus by the surgeon. A chest drain is also inserted via the lowest port site since immediate postoperative pneumothorax is common.

The thoracoscopic repair can be performed at birth and in low-birth-weight infants. It is challenging to perform in babies less than 1.5 kg body weight. Early gestational age and associated anomalies do not represent a contraindication to thoracoscopy, although in early series, anastomotic leaks and recurrent fistula have been described. In addition, anastomotic stricture requiring balloon dilatations seems to occur more frequently. Finally, preliminary studies suggest that thoracoscopic repair of EA/TEF may be associated with acidosis, hypercapnia, and decreased cerebral oxygen saturation. The effects of these phenomena on future brain development are unknown. Thoracoscopic repair offers a scarless repair with faster recovery and less postoperative pain and may also potentially protect from later problems such as winged scapula and thoracic asymmetry.

## POSTOPERATIVE TREATMENT

Postoperatively, the neonates are monitored in the intensive care unit. The authors prefer to follow the guidelines:

1. Restrict intravenous fluid for 24 hours at 75% maintenance.

2. Administer intravenous antibiotics for 48 hours.

3. Do not perform routine mechanical ventilation.

4. Administration of systemic paralytic and analgesic agents and mechanical ventilation are recommended for the first 5 postoperative days in patients with anastomosis performed under tension. This should prevent movements and further tension on the anastomosis, and reduce the risk of an anastomotic leak and subsequent stricture formation.

5. Administer proton pump inhibitors for 2 weeks.

6. Start transanastomotic tube feeding or oral feeding on the second postoperative day.

7. Perform a contrast esophagogram only if there is a clinical suspicion of anastomotic leakage (pneumothorax) or stricture formation.

## ESOPHAGEAL REPLACEMENT

In situations of failure to anastomose the native esophagus, the most common alternative conduits include stomach (gastric transposition or gastric tube), colon, and jejunum. Gastric transposition is a relatively simple operation and is associated with fewer severe complications. The main advantages are a single anastomosis in the neck or chest and a good blood supply with decreased risk of ischemia, leak, and stricture.

Spitz performed 138 gastric pull-ups for EA over 21 years. There were no graft failures, but a 4.6% mortality and a 12% leak rate. A total of 20% of the patients needed anastomotic dilation for stricture. Good function has been maintained long-term. This operation can now be performed with minimally invasive techniques and faster recovery for the patients. A gastric tube can be constructed as either a reversed or isoperistaltic tube from the greater curvature of the stomach. The blood supply is generally excellent, and it tends to retain its tubular shape. It does, however, reduce the stomach capacity, and peptic ulcerations may occur because of acid production. Complications such as anastomotic leak in 50% of cases and stricture formation in 66% of cases seem significant, but the long-term outcome was reasonable in terms of swallowing. Colonic transposition is widely used because it is relatively simple, but it is associated with short- and long-term complications, with increased risk of leakage and anastomotic strictures. Moreover, with time the colonic graft becomes redundant causing swallowing problems and food impactions. Redundancy may require redo surgery and it is unclear whether there is a risk of malignant degeneration in the colonic mucosa that is exposed to gastric acid. A very large series from Egypt reported 775 colon interpositions over a 30-year period (mostly for caustic strictures) with excellent results. Only 10% of the upper anastomoses leaked; the proximal stricture rate was 5% and overall mortality 1%. Jejunal interposition by pedicled or free grafts has been used by a few pediatric surgeons to repair a long-gap EA with some success. Significant complications, however, such as graft necrosis, ischemia, and strictures, occur on a frequent basis.

Finally, due to recent advances in biomaterial science and cellular biology, it is possible that in the near future esophageal tissue engineering could represent a valid alternative. Numerous attempts to shape a neoesophagus in vitro have been described in the last decade and in the near future will likely have clinical application similar to what has happened for the bladder, urethra, trachea, and large vessels.

## OUTCOME

Since the first successful repair of EA by Haight, survival rates for infants with EA have steadily improved from approximately 50% in the 1940s to more than 90% today.

Complications can arise as early or late events. The early complications are associated with surgical techniques as well as certain patient factors that in turn may compound the effect of surgical techniques (Fig. 24-8). These complications include anastomotic leaks, anastomotic stricture, recurrent TEF, and esophageal dysmotility with an associated risk of aspiration.

The incidence of anastomotic stricture varies widely and is the most common cause of recurrent surgery in children with EA and TEF. The majority of studies report a stricture rate of between 37% and 52%. In our experience, routine contrasts are not necessary, since only symptomatic strictures need to be treated. Balloon multiple dilatations are usually required and should be performed under radiological control to avoid esophageal perforation (Fig. 24-9).

Recurrent TEF occurs in 3% to 15% of cases, usually following an anastomotic leak. The majority of recurrent TEFs present early, but some can occur months and even years after

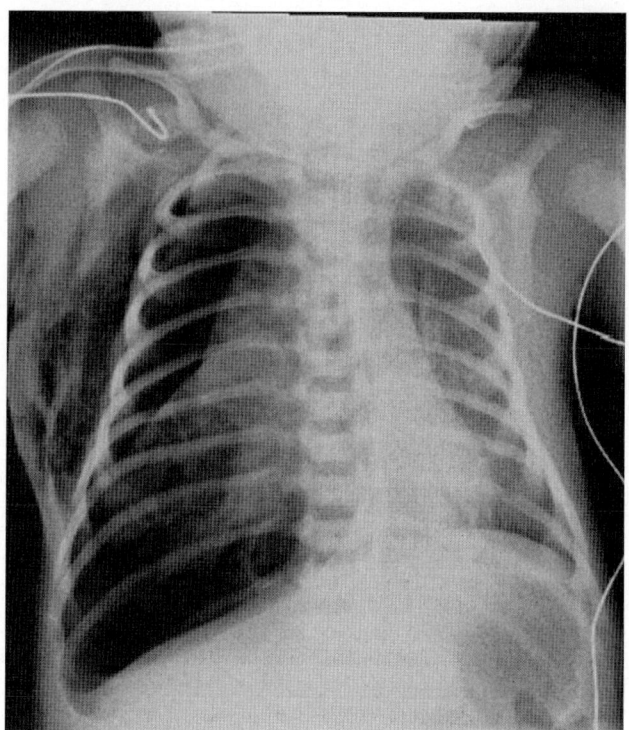

**FIGURE 24-8** Postoperative chest radiograph after thoracoscopic EA repair. Right pneumothorax, mediastinal shift, and subcutaneous emphysema may occur and postoperative drainage is recommended.

the initial repair. The presenting symptoms usually involve coughing, choking, cyanosis with feeding, and/or recurrent chest infections. The diagnosis is made either by tube esophagogram or by direct visualization of the fistula during bronchoscopy.

Tracheomalacia is a common finding among neonates with EA and often manifests itself as a typical barking cough. Tracheomalacia is defined as generalized or localized weakness of the trachea that allows the anterior and posterior tracheal wall to come together during expiration or coughing. Tracheomalacia can cause life-threatening events or deaths during the first few months of life. In general, however, tracheomalacia improves with age and becomes significant in only 10% to 20% of infants, with even fewer requiring surgical intervention.

Bronchoscopy during spontaneous ventilation is the gold standard for diagnosis. Surgery is reserved to infants with severe tracheomalacia having life-threatening events. The operation of choice is an aortopexy that can be performed via a left anterior thoracotomy or via thoracoscopy. The ascending aorta is sutured to the posterior surface of the sternum, lifting the aorta forward and opening the tracheal lumen.

Gastroesophageal reflux disease (GERD) can affect up to 60% of babies following EA repair. Although the majority of these patients can be treated medically with proton-pump inhibitors, about 28% will require surgical correction of their reflux. The Nissen fundoplication, which is usually performed laparoscopically, is the procedure of choice, but is associated with a high failure rate (40%) partly due to the inherent dysmotility of the esophagus. Long-term follow-up studies in patients with EA with endoscopic surveillance are warranted, since continuing reflux of gastric content in the esophagus is a risk factor for the development of intestinal metaplasia and esophageal cancer.

Chest wall and spinal deformities are more common in patients who have had a thoracotomy, especially if portions of the serratus anterior and latissimus dorsi muscle groups and their nerve supply had to be divided. These procedures can be associated with the development of scoliosis later in childhood.

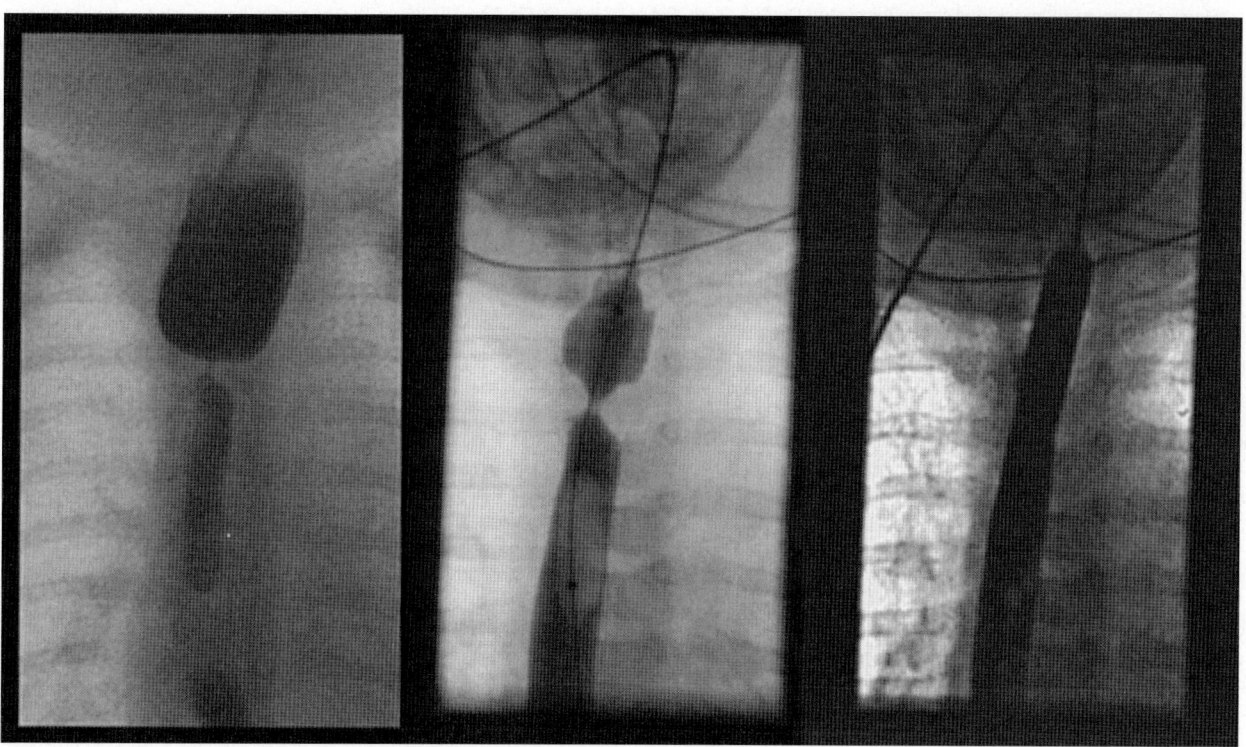

**FIGURE 24-9** Anastomotic stricture and balloon dilatation under fluoroscopic control.

In a long-term follow-up extending into adulthood, Sistonen et al have found significant esophageal morbidity associated with EA. Symptomatic gastroesophageal reflux, dysphagia, and esophageal motility disturbances, as well as columnar epithelial metaplasia, are common in adults with repaired EA. Surgical complications, patient age, and impaired esophageal motility were significant predictors of development of epithelial metaplasia, suggesting that a tight primary esophageal anastomosis and reoperations due to surgical complications further impair esophageal motility and predispose to epithelial metaplasia later. In conclusion, it is important to follow children operated on for EA and/or TEF for many years and arrange for continuing monitoring of these patients into adulthood.

## SELECTED READINGS

Ashcraft KW, Goodwin C, Amoury RA, et al. Early recognition and aggressive treatment of gastroesophageal reflux following repair of esophageal atresia. *J Pediatr Surg* 1977;12:317–321.

Bax KM. Jejunum for bridging long-gap esophageal atresia. *Semin Pediatr Surg* 2009;18(1):34–39.

Bishay M, Giacomello L, Retrosi G, et al. Decreased cerebral oxygen saturation during thoracoscopic repair of congenital diaphragmatic hernia and esophageal atresia in infants. *J Pediatr Surg* 2011;46(1):47–51.

Boyle EM Jr, Irwin ED, Foker JE. Primary repair of ultra-long-gap esophageal atresia: results without a lengthening procedure. *Ann Thorac Surg* 1994;57:576–579.

Chetcuti P, Phelan PD. Gastrointestinal morbidity and growth after repair of oesophageal atresia and tracheo-oesophageal fistula. *Arch Dis Child* 1993;68:163–166.

Chittmittrapap S, Spitz L, Kiely EM, et al. Anastomotic stricture following repair of esophageal atresia. *J Pediatr Surg* 1990;25:508–511.

Delius RE, Wheatley MJ, Coran AG. Etiology and management of respiratory complications after repair of esophageal atresia with tracheoesophageal fistula. *Surgery* 1992;112:527–532.

Durston W. A narrative of a monstrous birth in Plymouth, October 22, 1670; together with the anatomical observations taken thereupon by William Durston, Doctor in Physick, and communicated to Dr. Tim Clerk. *Philos Trans R Soc B Biol Sci* 1670;5:2096–2098.

Ein SH, Shandling B. Pure esophageal atresia: a 50-year review. *J Pediatr Surg* 1994;29:1208–1211.

Engum SA, Grosfeld JL, West KW, et al. Analysis of morbidity and mortality in 227 cases of esophageal atresia and/or tracheoesophageal fistula over two decades. *Arch Surg* 1995;130:502–508.

Filler RM, Messineo A, Vinograd I. Severe tracheomalacia associated with esophageal atresia: results of surgical treatment. *J Pediatr Surg* 1992;27:1136–1141.

Filston H. Esophageal atresia and tracheoesophageal fistula. In: Ashcraft KW, Sharp RJ, Murphy JP, Snyder CL, Sigalet DL, eds. *Pediatric Surgery*. 3rd ed. Philadelphia: WB Saunders Co; 1999 [chapter 27].

Foker JE, Kendall Krosch TC, Catton K, Munro F, Khan KM. Long-gap esophageal atresia treated by growth induction: the biological potential and early follow-up results. *Semin Pediatr Surg* 2009;18(1):23–29.

Gross RE. *The Surgery of Infancy and Childhood*. Philadelphia and London: WB Saunders Co; 1953.

Haight C, Towsley HA. Congenital atresia of the esophagus with tracheo-esophageal fistula: extrapleural ligation of fistula and end-to-end anastomosis of esophageal segments. *Surg Gynecol Obstet* 1943;76:672.

Hamza AF. Colonic replacement in cases of esophageal atresia. *Semin Pediatr Surg* 2009;18(1):40–43.

Holder TM, Ashcraft KW. Esophageal atresia and tracheoesophageal fistula. *Curr Prob Surg* 1966;38:1–65.

Holland AJ, Ron O, Pierro A, et al. Surgical outcomes of esophageal atresia without fistula for 24 years at a single institution. *J Pediatr Surg* 2009;44(10):1928–1932.

Ioannides AS, Copp AJ. Embryology of esophageal atresia. *Semin Pediatr Surg* 2009;18(1):2–11.

Kluth D. Atlas of esophageal atresia. *J Pediatr Surg* 1976;11:901.

Kosloske AM, Jewell PF, Cartwright KC. Crucial bronchoscopic findings in esophageal atresia and tracheoesophageal fistula. *J Pediatr Surg* 1988;23:466–470.

Ladd WE. The surgical treatment of esophageal atresia and tracheoesophageal fistulas. *N Engl J Med* 1944;230:625.

Lai JY, Sheu JC, Chang PY. Experience with distal circular myotomy for long-gap esophageal atresia. *J Pediatr Surg* 1996;31:1503–1508.

Leven NL. Congenital atresia of the esophagus with tracheoesophageal fistula: report of successful extrapleural ligation of fistulous communication and cervical esophagostomy. *J Thorac Surg* 1940;10:648.

MacKinlay GA. Esophageal atresia surgery in the 21st century. *Semin Pediatr Surg* 2009;18(1):20–22.

Manning PB, Morgan RA, Coran AR, et al. Fifty years' experience with esophageal atresia and tracheoesophageal fistula. *Ann Surg* 1986;204:446–453.

McKinnon LJ, Kosloske AM. Prediction and prevention of anastomotic complications of esophageal atresia and tracheoesophageal fistula. *J Pediatr Surg* 1990;25:778–781.

Moriarty KP, Jacir NN, Harris BH, et al. Transanastomotic feeding tubes in repair of esophageal atresia. *J Pediatr Surg* 1996;31:53–55.

Mortell AE, Azizkhan RG. Esophageal atresia repair with thoracotomy: the Cincinnati contemporary experience. *Semin Pediatr Surg* 2009;18(1):12–19.

Othersen HB Jr, Parker EF, Chandler J, et al. Save the child's esophagus, part II: colic patch repair. *J Pediatr Surg* 1997;32:328–333.

Pedersen JC, Klein RL, Andrews DA. Gastric tube as the primary procedure for pure esophageal atresia. *J Pediatr Surg* 1996;31:1233–1235.

Poenaru D, Laberge JM, Neilson IR, et al. A new prognostic classification for esophageal atresia. *Surgery* 1993;113:426–432.

Pretorius DH, Drose JA, Dennis MA, et al. Tracheoesophageal fistula in utero: twenty-two cases. *J Ultrasound Med* 1987;6:509–513.

Puri P, Ninan GK, Blake NS, et al. Delayed primary anastomosis for esophageal atresia: 18 months' to 1 years' follow-up. *J Pediatr Surg* 1992;27:1127–1130.

Raffensperger JG, Luck SR, Reynolds M, et al. Intestinal bypass of the esophagus. *J Pediatr Surg* 1996;31:38–47.

Rintala RJ, Sistonen S, Pakarinen MP. Outcome of esophageal atresia beyond childhood. *Semin Pediatr Surg* 2009;18(1):50–56.

Robertson DF, Mobaireek K, Davis GM, et al. Late pulmonary function following repair of tracheoesophageal fistula or esophageal atresia. *Pediatr Pulmonol* 1995;20:21–26.

Ron O, De Coppi P, Pierro A. The surgical approach to esophageal atresia repair and the management of long-gap atresia: results of a survey. *Semin Pediatr Surg* 2009;18(1):44–49.

Sistonen SJ, Koivusalo A, Nieminen U, et al. Esophageal morbidity and function in adults with repaired esophageal atresia with tracheoesophageal fistula: a population-based long-term follow-up. *Ann Surg* 2010;251(6):1167–1173.

Spitz L. Gastric transposition in children. *Semin Pediatr Surg* 2009;18(1):30–33.

Spitz L, Kiely E, Bereton RJ. Esophageal atresia: five year experience with 148 cases. *J Pediatr Surg* 1987;22:103–108.

Spitz L, Kiely EM, Morecroft JA, et al. Esophageal atresia: at-risk groups for the 1990s. *J Pediatr Surg* 1994;29:723–725.

Stanwell J, Drake D, Pierro A, Kiely E, Curry J. Pediatric laparoscopic-assisted gastric transposition: early experience and outcomes. *J Laparoendosc Adv Surg Tech A* 2010;20(2):1771–1781.

Stringer MD, McKenna KM, Goldstein RB, et al. Prenatal diagnosis of esophageal atresia. *J Pediatr Surg* 1995;30:1258–1263.

Waterston DJ, Bonham-Carter RE, Aberdeen E. Oesophageal atresia—tracheoesophageal fistula: a study of survival in 218 infants. *Lancet* 1962;1:819–822.

Weber TR, Smith W, Grosfeld JL. Surgical experience in infants with the VATER association. *J Pediatr Surg* 1980;15:849–854.

Wheatley MJ, Coran AR, Wesley JR. Efficacy of the Nissen fundoplication in the management of gastroesophageal reflux following esophageal atresia repair. *J Pediatr Surg* 1993;28:53–55.

Zani A, Pierro A, Elvassore N, De Coppi P. Tissue engineering: an option for esophageal replacement? *Semin Pediatr Surg* 2009;18(1):57–62.

# CHAPTER 25

# Esophageal Replacement

*Richard G. Azizkhan*

## KEY POINTS

1. When native esophagus is not available, there are a number of esophageal replacement techniques that are effective in restoring the continuity of the gastrointestinal tract.

2. Selection of the appropriate technique depends on the anatomy and function of the stomach, the availability of the colon, and the experience and preference of the surgeon.

3. The 2 dominant replacement procedures are colon interposition and gastric pull-up. The overall outcomes of these 2 procedures are comparable, although both have strong proponents.

## HISTORICAL OVERVIEW

The decision to replace the esophagus of a child is one of the most difficult decisions a pediatric surgeon must make. Although most surgeons attempt to preserve the native esophagus, there is sometimes no alternative but to consider esophageal replacement. Fortunately, the need for this procedure has decreased in recent years because of public health initiatives concerning the avoidance of caustic ingestion and because of the increased success pediatric surgeons have had in lengthening the upper pouch of patients with long-gap esophageal atresia by performing myotomies. Esophageal replacement is, however, used in the management of a number of conditions, including congenital absence of the stomach, long-gap esophageal atresia, severe injury to the esophagus from caustic ingestion, prolonged gastroesophageal reflux disease, trauma, and inflammatory and infectious conditions.

In 1894, Bircher first devised a neoesophagus by creating an antethoracic skin tube that was constructed to traverse the gap between the proximal esophagus and the stomach. While this procedure allowed patients to eat as normally as possible, the frequency of fistulae and strictures was high.

Subsequently, 4 operative replacement techniques, all of which were developed for adults following resection of esophageal carcinoma, were adapted for use in children. In the most widely used technique (colon interposition), the right or left colon is used as an esophageal substitute. First reported by Lundblad in 1921, this technique was adapted to children in 1955 by Dale and Sherman. They used a retrosternal isoperistaltic colon graft based on the middle colic artery for esophageal replacement. In 1957 Sherman and Waterston modified this technique, creating a transthoracic interposition graft. In 1982 Freeman and Case modified the technique by using a posterior route through the esophageal hiatus.

The stomach is also used as an esophageal substitute either by creating a gastric tube (gastric tube interposition) or by transposing the entire stomach to traverse the gap between the cervical esophagus and the abdomen (gastric interposition). Described by both Gavriliu and Heimlich in the mid-1950s, the reversed gastric tube approach was later adapted to children by Burrington, Anderson, and Randolph. The key proponents in the use of the entire stomach for esophageal replacement have been Spitz and Coran.

The fourth esophageal replacement technique, jejunal interposition, was performed by Roux in 1907 and Herzen in 1908, and adapted for use in children by Leven and Varco in 1950s. Although Ring, Varco, and a number of other authors have advocated its benefits, the popularity of this technique has not grown. It is now seldom used unless other approaches fail. A technical distinction between jejunal interposition and the other more commonly used procedures is that the former is multistage and more complicated. Jejunal interposition may require a microvascular anastomoses and has an early risk of infarction of the entire graft; in contrast, replacement with colon or stomach can generally be accomplished at an early age in 1 operation.

The aim of all of these replacement techniques is to restore continuity of the gastrointestinal tract with a conduit that provides the best overall function and the fewest complications. To this end, as much proximal native esophagus as possible should be preserved, particularly the cricopharyngeus, and when possible, the lower esophageal sphincter. In addition, the conduit should bridge the defect through a course that is straight and short and encourages dependent drainage.

Before considering esophageal replacement, surgeons should weigh all options for preserving the native esophagus, for while each of the replacement techniques has advantages

**TABLE 25-1    Advantages and Disadvantages of Various Methods of Esophageal Replacement**

| Type of Replacement | Advantages | Disadvantages |
| --- | --- | --- |
| Colonic interposition | Can usually attain adequate length<br>Versatility of the conduit for many esophageal problems | Potentially precarious blood supply<br>Leaks (25%–35%)<br>Strictures (15%–30%)<br>Redundancy of colonic loop, kinks<br>Slow transit time |
| Gastric tube interposition | Good blood supply<br>Adequate length<br>Rapid transit | Long suture line<br>Leaks from cervical anastomosis (50%)<br>Strictures (25%–30%)<br>Gastroesophageal reflux |
| Gastric transposition | Good blood supply<br>Adequate length<br>Ease of procedure | Respiratory problems<br>Poor gastric emptying<br>Gastroesophageal reflux |
| Jejunal interposition | Size of intestine appropriate<br>Good peristaltic activity | Vascular supply precarious<br>Adequate length difficult to attain<br>Gastroesophageal reflux |
| Free jejunal graft | Size of intestine appropriate<br>Good peristaltic activity | Microvascular anastomosis required<br>Prolonged operating time<br>High incidence of graft necrosis<br>Gastroesophageal reflux |

and disadvantages (Table 25-1), none is entirely free of short- or long-term complications.

## GENERAL CONSIDERATIONS

Surgeons must consider the possibility of the eventual need for esophageal replacement in any child with a difficult esophageal problem. Should replacement become necessary, attention to detail and planning ahead permits more flexibility for choosing the appropriate organ for substitution. Coexisting conditions and concurrent or anticipated surgical procedures must be carefully considered should replacement become necessary. For example, if the creation of a reversed gastric tube is a possibility, then placement of a gastrostomy on the lesser curve of the stomach is mandatory to avoid compromising construction of the tube at a later date. Because some children with esophageal atresia have the VACTERL association (vertebral, anal, cardiac, tracheoesophageal, renal, and limb abnormalities) with anorectal anomalies, the selection of the colostomy site for imperforate anus affects the availability of the colon for later use. A right transverse colostomy or proximal sigmoid colostomy provides versatility for the colonic pull-through and the coloesophageal conduit. Placement of an esophagostomy on the left side in the neck makes eventual anastomosis of the cervical esophagus and the replacement conduit easier and safer.

Occasionally, anatomic considerations dictate the choice of substitute. If the infant has a symptomatic short colon (ie, severe diarrhea), the use of a portion of the colon as an esophageal substitute is likely to further exacerbate intestinal problems. If a baby has a congenitally small stomach, it may be impossible to create a gastric tube with any stomach left as a reservoir; in this situation, colon interposition would be appropriate.

Prior to any replacement procedure, thorough radiologic evaluation of the stomach and gastrointestinal tract is essential.

## COLON INTERPOSITION

Colon interposition is ideal for situations in which the distal esophagus can be retained with the lower esophageal sphincter intact, but can also be used to provide a direct conduit to the stomach. Both subcutaneous and intrathoracic colonic interposition grafts using right transverse and descending colon, as well as ileocolic segments, have been described. Intrathoracic colon interposition can be performed through the anterior (retrosternal) or posterior (left retrohilar) mediastinum. We prefer a single-stage isoperistaltic descending colon graft placed in the left retrohilar position. This approach generally provides adequate length and vascular supply from the left colic artery.

### Preoperative Management

A mechanical bowel preparation and an oral antibiotic are administered the night before surgery. An intravenous antibiotic (cefoxitin) is given preoperatively, and the patient is placed supine in a 45° right lateral decubitus position. This positioning is optimal for the cervical, abdominal, and thoracic approaches.

## Surgical Technique

There are several possible surgical techniques for colonic grafts used as esophageal substitutes (Fig. 25-1). The portion of the colon to be used for esophageal replacement depends largely on the length required. The most common approach, which employs a segment composed of a portion of the transverse and descending colon placed in the left hemithorax in the retrohilar position, is particularly suited for patients with long-gap atresia. The transverse and distal colonic graft

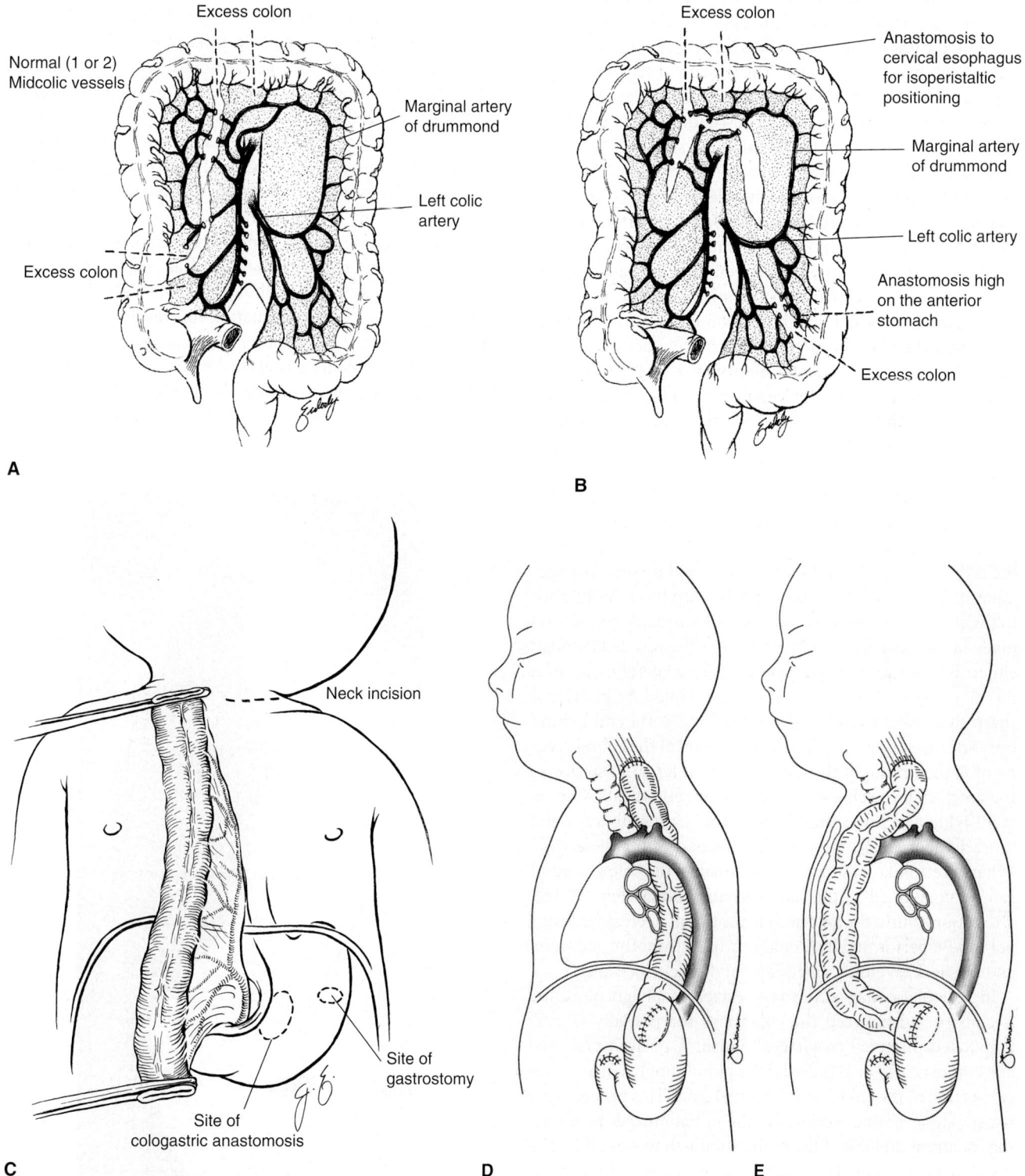

**FIGURE 25-1** Isoperistaltic retrohilar descending colon interposition. **A.** Isolation of an ascending colonic segment based on the middle colic artery and vein. **B.** Isolation of a transverse descending colonic segment based on the superior branch of the left colic artery and vein and the marginal artery of Drummond. **C.** The colon segment is brought behind the stomach through the gastrohepatic ligament, taking care not to torse the vascular pedicle. **D.** Lateral view showing the retrohilar position of the colon conduit with completed esophageal and gastric anastomoses. Note the completed pyloroplasty. **E.** Lateral view demonstrating an alternative approach with the colon conduit placed in the retrosternal position.

is vascularized from the left colic artery, and the transverse colon segment remains viable through a collateral blood supply from the marginal artery of Drummond (Fig. 25-1A). Alternatively, the ascending and/or transverse colon can also be used as an esophageal conduit (Fig. 25-1B). The ascending colon conduit is based on the right colic artery, while the transverse colon graft is based on the middle colic vessel.

After exploration through an upper midline abdominal incision, the gastrocolic ligament is incised, freeing the transverse colon from the stomach. The left lateral segment of the liver is mobilized by dividing the left triangular ligament, and the peritoneum lateral to the descending colon is incised from the splenic flexure to the proximal sigmoid. Next, the peritoneum of the transverse colon and left colon is incised, dividing the left branch of the middle colic artery and preserving the marginal arcade and the left colic artery and its arcades. The phrenoesophageal ligament is incised, expanding the esophageal hiatus, and dissection of the gastroesophageal junction is carried into the mediastinum along the esophagus. A sufficient length of colon is measured to allow the proximal end of the colonic segment to reach the area of the anticipated esophagocolic anastomosis (Fig. 25-1C). On division of the colon, back bleeding should be noted at both the proximal and distal ends of the segment, indicating an adequate blood supply. A colocolic anastomosis reestablishes intestinal continuity.

When the retrohilar approach is used, a left lateral thoracotomy is performed by dividing the latissimus dorsi muscle and preserving the serratus muscles. The chest is entered at the fifth or sixth intercostal space. To avoid torsion, the segment of colon and its vascular pedicle are brought anterior to the pancreas behind the stomach and through an incision made in the gastrohepatic ligament. It is then passed through either the expanded esophageal hiatus or a lateral incision in the diaphragm. A retrohilar tunnel is created by blunt and sharp dissection lateral to the descending aorta and behind the aortic arch (Fig. 25-1D). The upper end of the colonic segment is then brought through the Sibson fascia posterior to the subclavian vessels and lateral to the carotid sheath. Care in identifying and protecting the recurrent laryngeal nerve and thoracic duct is necessary during this part of the dissection. When a retrohilar approach is not feasible, the colon conduit can be positioned in the retrosternal position (Fig. 25-1E). Dissection within the anterior mediastinum to create the tunnel can be performed by a dual approach from the abdomen and the neck, avoiding an additional thoracic incision.

In cases of esophageal atresia, a cervical esophagocolostomy is constructed between the colon and the partially (1 cm) amputated proximal esophageal pouch. A delayed proximal anastomosis may be required if the blood supply to the cervical portion of the colon conduit is marginal. This procedure is usually done several weeks after the initial procedure, allowing for strengthening of the blood supply to the conduit. The distal anastomosis is made between the colon and the distal esophageal remnant. Both anastomoses are created with a single layer of 5-0 monofilament absorbable sutures. When the entire esophagus is replaced, a cervical esophagocolostomy or a pharyngocolostomy and a cologastrostomy (along the lesser curve) can be constructed. We routinely perform a Heineke–Mikulicz pyloroplasty and place a gastrostomy. We also place

a Penrose drain in the cervical wound below the platysma and a dependently positioned chest tube in the left chest.

## Postoperative Management and Outcomes

All patients are closely monitored in the intensive care unit or a step-down unit until their respiratory status is stable. A water-soluble contrast study (Fig. 25-2) is obtained on the seventh postoperative day; if no leakage is present, the cervical drain and chest tube are removed. The patient is first given clear liquids and then advanced as tolerated. If a cervical leak is noted, the patient is observed *nil per os* (NPO) for an additional 2 weeks. We often continue to provide enteral tube feedings through one of several approaches, including a gastrojejunal, nasojejunal, or nasogastric jejunal feeding tube. The contrast study is then repeated.

The success rate of this procedure is approximately 82% and the mortality is 1% to 2%. Most leaks occur at the coloesophageal anastomosis. Although they usually close spontaneously, 50% require dilatation of resulting strictures. Leaks of either the proximal or distal anastomosis occur in 25% to 35% of patients. Vocal cord paralysis caused by injury to the recurrent nerve during dismantling of the cervical esophagostomy occurs in 3% to 5% of patients. Long-term

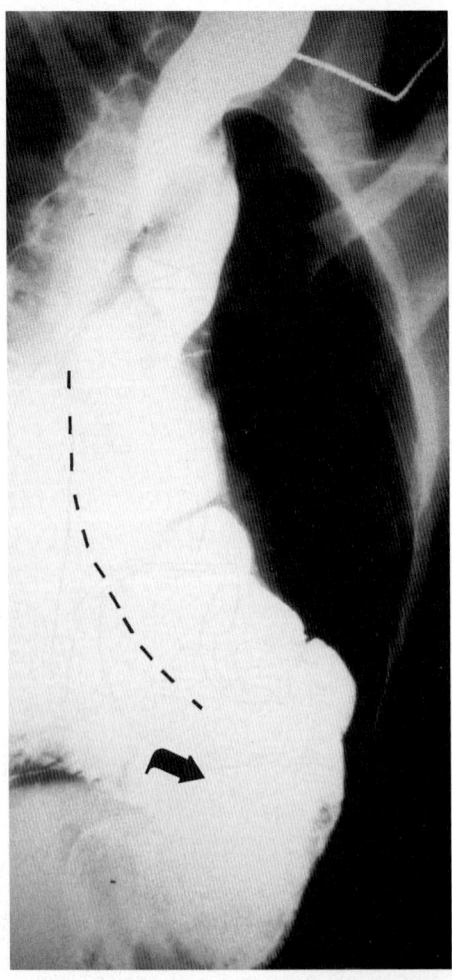

**FIGURE 25-2** Postoperative contrast study of a retrohilar colon interposition in a 16-year-old male 14 years after surgery. The *dotted line* marks the mediastinal border. The *curved arrow* points to the stomach.

follow-up indicates that severe redundancy of the colon conduit (Fig. 25-3A) occurs in 15% to 20% of patients and may require operative revision because of severe stasis or obstruction (Fig. 25-3B). Long-term outcomes are comparable to outcomes achieved with gastric pull-ups, and both approaches should be included in the surgical armamentarium.

Gastroesophageal reflux continues to be an unpredictable and daunting problem with colon interposition as well as with all other methods of esophageal replacement. If reflux esophagitis or aspiration becomes problematic after colon interposition, we perform a partial wrap fundoplication.

## GASTRIC TUBE INTERPOSITION

Gastric tube placement has an advantage over colon substitution in that the neoesophagus is lined entirely with gastric mucosa, which decreases the likelihood of peptic ulceration. It also has the advantages of ease of construction and long, straight length, which appeal to surgeons who must bridge long gaps in small children. Either an isoperistaltic tube based at the antrum or a reversed tube based at the fundus can be placed in the retrosternal or left retrohilar spaces. A limitation is gastric size. If the stomach is small or inflexible, this approach is unfeasible.

### Preoperative Management

When gastric tube replacement is planned, we obtain a preoperative upper gastrointestinal contrast study to document gastric volume. This study is particularly important in patients with esophageal atresia, many of whom have very small stomachs. A gastric reservoir of at least 200 to 250 mL is optimal to maintain adequate gastric capacity after tube construction. Should a gastric tube interposition be unfeasible, a mechanical bowel preparation and oral antibiotics are administered to prepare the colon for a possible colon interposition. An intravenous antibiotic is given preoperatively, and the patient is placed supine in a 45° right lateral decubitus position on the operating table.

### Surgical Technique

Surgery begins with an abdominal exploration. Particular attention is paid to the stomach and to the location of a previously placed gastrostomy. The gastrostomy is dismantled and closed. The stomach and gastroesophageal junction are mobilized, and care is taken to preserve the blood supply and avoid injury to the spleen. If a native esophageal stump remains, as in esophageal atresia, it is resected. Failure to do this may create unwanted torque on the tube as it is drawn into the chest. If the native esophagus is still present, as in a corrosive injury, it is resected to prevent the development of carcinoma in the burned segment. The duodenum is mobilized with an extensive Kocher maneuver to enhance mobilization upward into the chest and to facilitate pyloroplasty.

The cervical esophagus or a previously placed cervical esophagostomy is then dissected out at the site for anastomosis. The distance between the cervical and distal esophagus must correlate with the eventual length of the gastric tube. We next assess blood supply and measure the greater curvature of the stomach and determine whether a tube of adequate length can be constructed (Fig. 25-4A). If there is insufficient length or if the blood supply of the stomach and the gastroepiploic circulation is inadequate, a colon interposition becomes necessary. The dimensions of the tube along

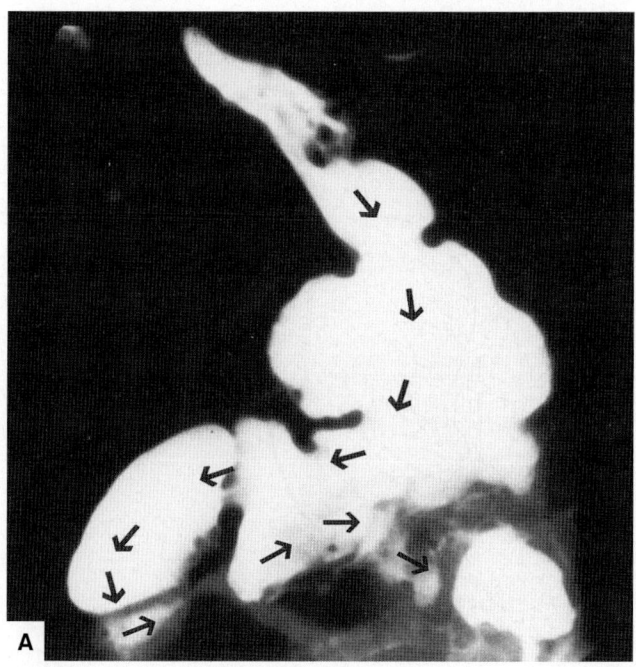
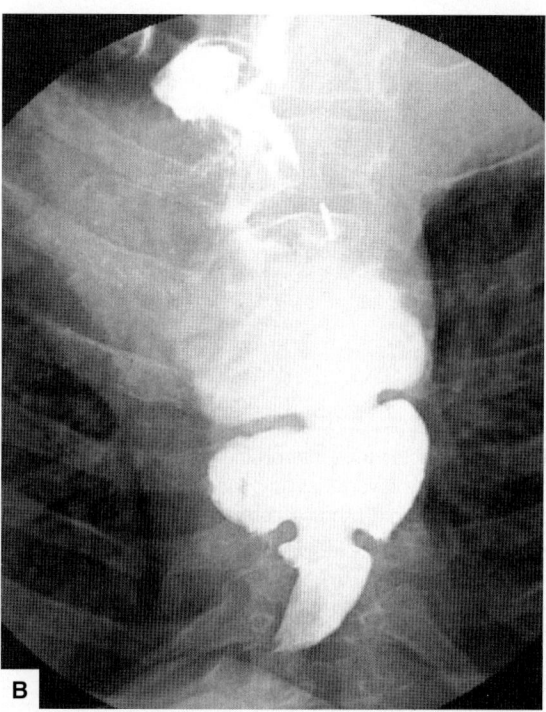

**FIGURE 25-3  A.** Postoperative contrast study of a colon interposition demonstrating severe redundancy in a 3-year-old girl who had long-gap esophageal atresia. The *arrows* follow the tortuous course of the retrosternal conduit. This patient had significant obstruction with severe stasis. **B.** Following partial resection the conduit is now straight and empties into the small stomach promptly.

the greater curvature of the stomach are then marked out. Although an antrally based tube can be considered, in most cases a reversed gastric tube based at the fundus is required to gain adequate length to the neck. The gastric tube should begin at least 2 cm from the pylorus so that gastric emptying through the pyloric channel is not compromised.

The stomach is then opened along the greater curve at the site of the eventual proximal end of the tube. A 20- to 24-Fr round chest tube is inserted and passed along the greater curve to the fundus, which helps to define the circumference

of the gastric tube. The gastric tube is then created using a gastrointestinal anastomosis (GIA) stapler along the superior border of the chest tube (Fig. 25-4B). Many surgeons reinforce the staple line with hand-sewn seromuscular stitches (Fig. 25-4C). It is important to ensure that the fundal end of the gastric tube is not too narrow, particularly because this angle becomes critical as this tube is drawn into the chest. We then divide the short gastric vessels while preserving the gastroepiploic arcade. We do not routinely perform a splenectomy.

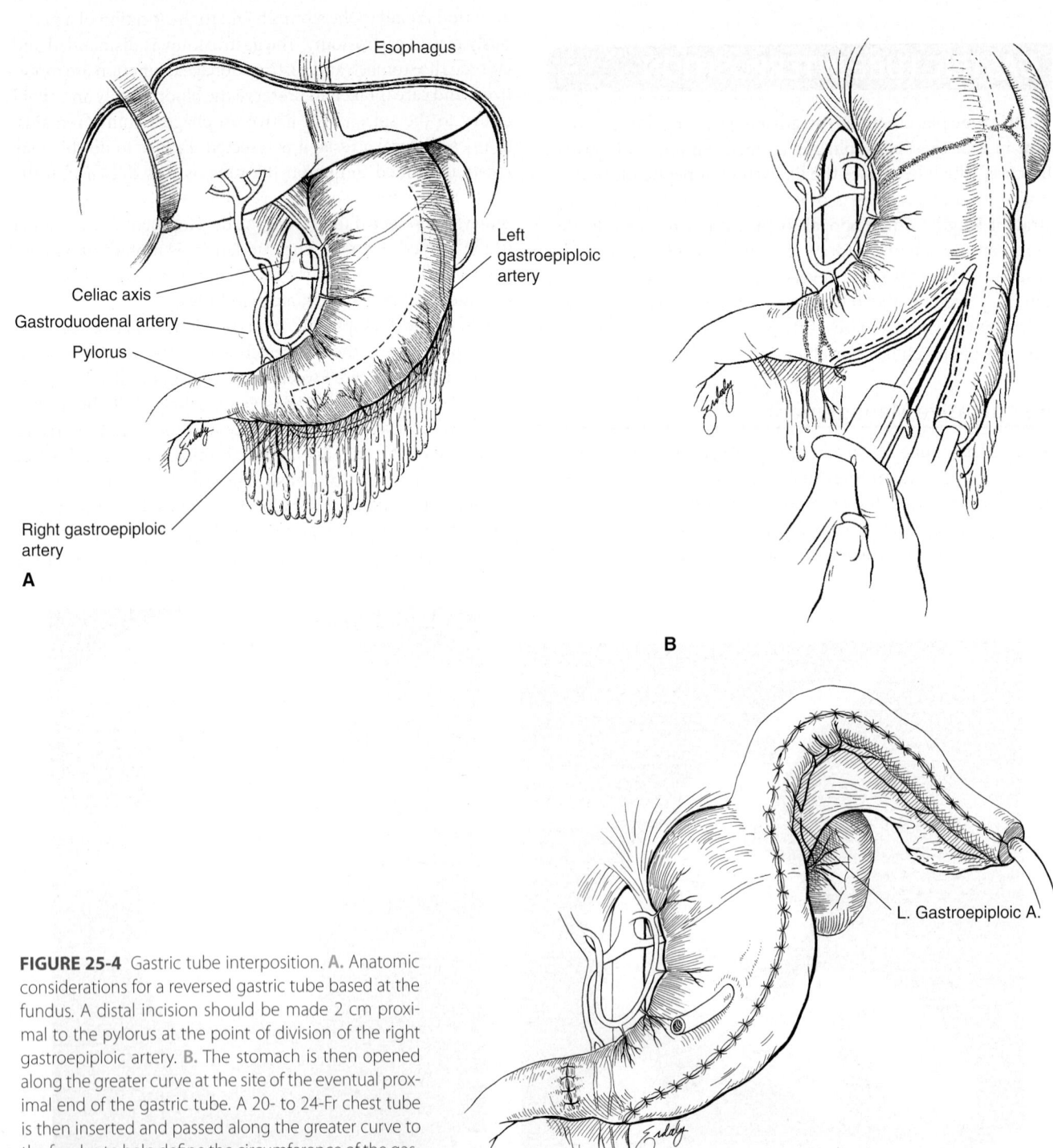

**FIGURE 25-4** Gastric tube interposition. **A.** Anatomic considerations for a reversed gastric tube based at the fundus. A distal incision should be made 2 cm proximal to the pylorus at the point of division of the right gastroepiploic artery. **B.** The stomach is then opened along the greater curve at the site of the eventual proximal end of the gastric tube. A 20- to 24-Fr chest tube is then inserted and passed along the greater curve to the fundus to help define the circumference of the gastric tube. The tube is then created using multiple firings of a GIA stapler along the superior border of the chest tube. **C.** Completed reversed gastric tube, gastrostomy, and pyloroplasty.

Once the gastric tube is created, the next step is to choose the anatomic route to the neck. Although the posterior mediastinum along the location of the native esophagus is the most logical route, it is frequently unavailable because of inflammation or infection. In addition, mediastinal dissection for this route risks injury to the recurrent laryngeal nerves. An alternative is to create a retrosternal tunnel. Although this method is easier to perform, the conduit has the disadvantage of being longer and more tortuous.

We prefer the retrohilar approach, which may require enlargement of the esophageal hiatus. The graft can also be placed in a retrosternal position via an opening anterior to the diaphragm below the xiphoid. A left thoracotomy is required to place the gastric tube behind the left lung. To complete the dissection, a space is created through the thoracic inlet into the neck. Careful identification and dissection prevent injury to the subclavian vessels, thoracic duct, and recurrent nerve. The gastric tube must be drawn into the neck under direct visualization in order to prevent torsion of the graft and its blood supply. An incision in the sternal fascia or removal of the clavicular head is sometimes required to create adequate space for the tube at the suprasternal notch.

Once the gastric tube is brought into the neck, the fundal angle and the vascular supply along the length of the tube are reassessed. A pyloroplasty is performed to improve gastric emptying, and a gastrostomy is recreated to facilitate postoperative drainage and feeding. Performing the pyloroplasty and gastrostomy at this stage permits additional time to elapse so that any ischemia of the proximal end of the gastric tube becomes evident.

Next, any redundancy of the tube is trimmed off (the cut edge should bleed briskly), and a single-layered anastomosis of the tube with the cervical esophagus is performed. Some surgeons advocate a double-layered anastomosis. Our experience, however, shows that this does not decrease the incidence of leaks and may in fact increase the incidence of stricture. If the gastroepiploic blood supply to the cervical anastomosis is in question, we stage the procedure by oversewing the proximal end of the gastric tube and tacking it to the sternocleidomastoid muscle, leaving a cervical esophagostomy. We perform a delayed cervicogastric anastomosis 2 to 4 weeks later.

## Postoperative Management and Outcomes

As with colon interposition, patients are carefully monitored in the intensive care unit or a step-down unit until their respiratory status is stable. A water-soluble contrast study assessing the graft for leaks is obtained on the seventh postoperative day; if no leakage is present, the cervical drain and chest tube are removed. The patient is observed after ingesting clear liquids and advanced as tolerated. If a cervical leak is noted, the patient is managed NPO for an additional 2 weeks; the contrast study is then repeated. Leaks of the cervical anastomosis occur in up to 50% of cases, resulting in a stricture rate of 30%.

A 70% success rate with this technique has been reported and, as with other techniques, the mortality rate is low (3%-5%). However, the long suture line required and its potential for leakage are disadvantages. Although shorter tubes with shorter suture lines can be used, these necessitate anastomosis

within the chest and present the risk of a leak with consequent mediastinitis. Another disadvantage is the diminution of stomach size. Gradual compensation with growth of the stomach can, however, be expected over several years.

While many solutions have been proposed to solve the problem of GER into and up the tube (eg, partial wraps), it remains a problem. Although leaks are common, because the cervical anastomosis is typically well vascularized, healing usually occurs without further surgical intervention.

## GASTRIC TRANSPOSITION

The advantages of a whole stomach transposition include its simplicity, having a single anastomosis, and having a long, well-vascularized conduit without long suture lines. Since the stomach has a rich blood supply, this procedure ensures esophagogastric anastomosis healing, thus avoiding multiple-stage operations. A low incidence of anastomotic leaks and strictures is another advantage of this technique.

### Preoperative Management

We use the same preoperative preparation for gastric transposition as for colon interposition and gastric tube replacement. Positioning for surgery is also the same.

### Surgical Technique

Whether gastric transposition is performed using an open or endoscopic approach, the fundamentals remain the same. The procedure begins with abdominal exploration and mobilization of the stomach and duodenum. A previously placed gastrostomy is dismantled and closed. The left gastric and short gastric arteries are divided, leaving the stomach dependent on the gastroepiploic and right gastric arteries for its blood supply (Fig. 25-5A). The greater omentum is separated from the stomach, taking care to preserve the gastroepiploic vessels. The gastroesophageal junction and lower 5 cm of the distal esophagus are dissected and mobilized. The esophagogastric junction is then divided with a GIA stapler, and the cardia is oversewn. A generous Kocher maneuver is performed to gain optimal length of the mobilized stomach. Adequate length of the mobilized gastric transposition is verified when the apex of the gastric fundus can reach past the clavicles and the pylorus overlies the xiphoid process (Fig. 25-5B).

The bed of the intrathoracic esophagus is used as the channel for the gastric transposition (unless this is precluded by extensive fibrosis from previous surgery or inflammation), for it is the shortest route to the cervical esophagus (Fig. 25-5C and D). In addition, this route provides a straight course, avoids potential compression at the thoracic inlet, and may prevent gastric dilatation within the mediastinum. Once blunt dissection of distal esophageal bed has reached the level of the carina, a low anterior cervical incision is made and dissection is carried out through the platysma; the carotid sheath and sternocleidomastoid muscle are retracted laterally, and the larynx and trachea are retracted medially (Fig. 25-5C). The esophagus is identified, mobilized, and encircled with a

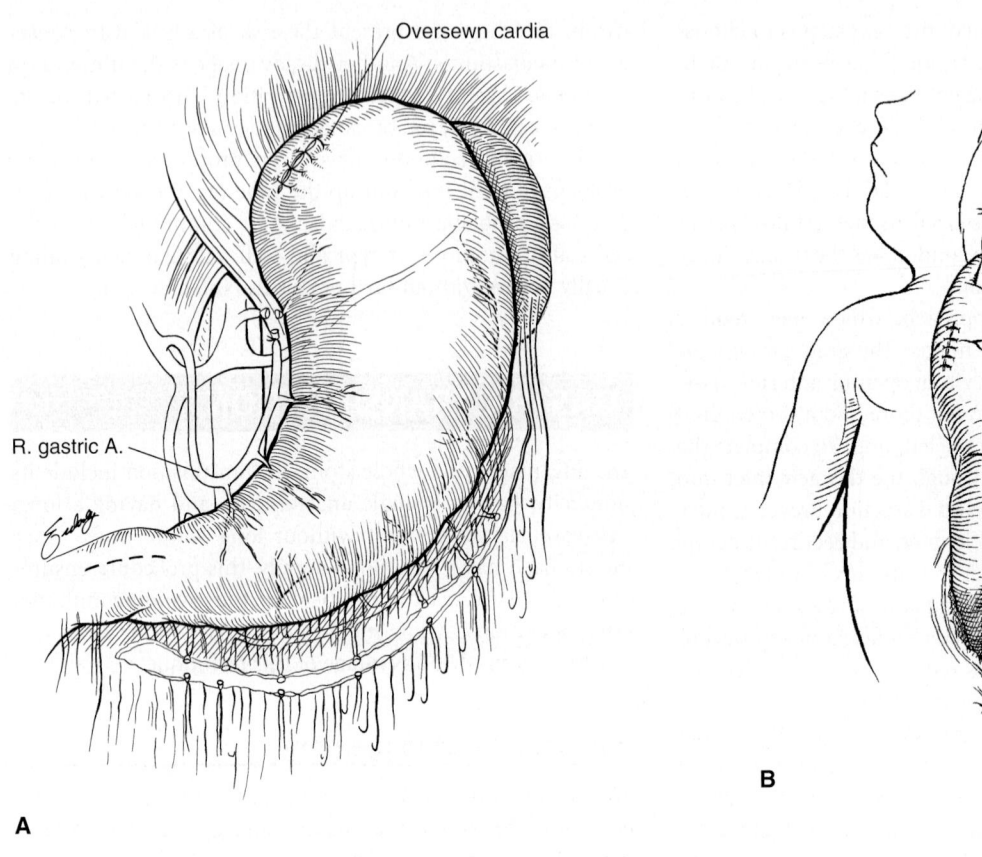

Oversewn cardia

R. gastric A.

A

B

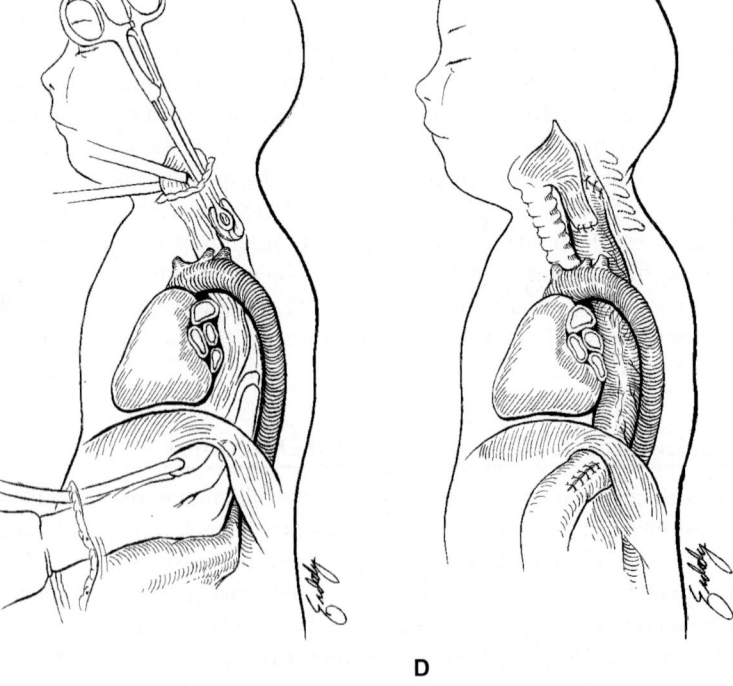

C

D

**FIGURE 25-5** Gastric transposition. **A.** Mobilization of the stomach for whole gastric interposition. The right gastric and gastroepiploic vessels are preserved. A wide Kocher maneuver is performed to facilitate gastric mobilization. The gastroesophageal remnant is divided, stapled, and oversewn at the cardia. **B.** Assessing the cephalad "reach" of the stomach after division of the left gastric vessels. Note the position of the apex of the gastric fundus over the clavicles. **C.** Developing the mediastinal tunnel using a combined transabdominal and transcervical approach. **D.** Final position of the whole gastric interposition graft with completed esophagogastric anastomosis and pyloroplasty.

Penrose drain, taking care to identify and protect the recurrent laryngeal nerve. Blunt midline dissection along the anterior border of the esophagus is carried down to the level of the carina. In cases of lye stricture, an esophagectomy is performed when possible to avoid mucocele formation or malignancy. In some cases, a left lateral thoracotomy is required to place the transposed stomach in the retrohilar position within the chest, as was previously described in the colon conduit procedure.

To minimize the intraabdominal portion of the stomach, the gastric conduit is pulled all the way into the chest through the hiatus. The pylorus lies just below the diaphragm. The upper anastomosis can be performed at the original gastroesophageal junction or this can be oversewn and a fresh opening and anastomosis can be performed at the fundus. When an endoscopic approach is used, it is important to ensure that there is no twisting or angulation of the gastric fundus as it is brought into the mediastinum. Otherwise, there is a risk of gastric outlet obstruction. A pyloroplasty is then done, a cervical closed suction drain is inserted, and a left chest tube is placed.

## Postoperative Management and Outcomes

Postoperative management follows the same guidelines as those in the previously described replacement techniques.

Anastomotic leaks and strictures occur with a frequency of 12%. Many surgeons avoid this type of reconstruction because of the risk of peptic esophagitis, particularly with an intrathoracic anastomosis. This complication is lowered by higher anastomosis with the cervical esophagus. Some surgeons point out that transposing the stomach in infants and small children may lead to pulmonary compromise or growth failure. However, this claim has not been substantiated in long-term studies conducted by Spitz and other investigators. Although the success rate of this technique is approximately 88%, the mortality rate of 7% is higher than those for the previously described techniques.

Coran has described a partial gastric transposition performed through the right chest for primary treatment of long-gap esophageal atresia in neonates; this approach may allow the advantage of performing a single-stage procedure. To reduce the risk of GER, he completes the procedure with a partial fundoplication.

## JEJUNAL INTERPOSITION

While the small bowel is rarely used for primary esophageal substitution in children, it is sometimes required as a secondary strategy when other approaches have failed or when neither the colon nor the stomach is available for esophageal reconstruction. With this technique, the entire esophagus can be replaced in a multiple-stage procedure. Additionally, jejunal pedicle grafts are particularly useful in the replacement of short segments of the distal esophagus. Free jejunal grafts with microvascular anastomoses are also used in the cervical region.

### Preoperative Management

We follow the same preoperative preparation as outlined in the previously cited procedures.

### Surgical Technique

Initially, a cervical esophagostomy and a gastrostomy are done. The jejunal interposition is then created; this procedure usually takes place when the patient is at least 1 year old. The Roux-en-Y limb of the proximal jejunum is created in the standard fashion, using an upper midline incision because it facilitates the passage of the jejunum along the antethoracic route. The first major jejunal artery and vein distal to the ligament of Treitz are preserved to ensure adequate vascularity of the remaining proximal jejunum. Once the first major vessel has been

identified, the next 2 or 3 major vessels of the primary arcade are located (Fig. 25-6A). Adequacy of the remaining blood supply can be tested with the aid of atraumatic neurosurgical aneurysm clips placed prior to division of vessels. With this blood supply ensured, the vessels are taken and the bowel is divided approximately 6 to 12 cm distal to the ligament of Treitz (Fig. 25-6B). Next, the bowel is tested for length by placing it on the chest. Although a suitable length of bowel is present, at this stage it usually falls short of the neck because it is confined by the mesentery. This confinement results from both the peritoneal covering and the radial origin of the mesenteric vessels. The peritoneum and accompanying lymphatic tissue and autonomic fibers that invest the vessels must be carefully dissected free—this being the most delicate and tedious part of the operation. The peritoneum is incised radially into the secondary arcade at several points along the jejunal limb, which contributes to lengthening. The second and most effective way of gaining length is by opening up 1 or more of the secondary arcades. Not only does division at 2 or 3 points gain length, but the redundancy of the bowel also is effectively reduced as the disparity between intestinal and mesenteric lengths is decreased. Before one divides any point of the arcade, however, it is important to ensure that the blood supply after division will be adequate. These divisions are carried out until sufficient length is achieved. This technique reliably provides enough jejunum to reach as high as necessary. The blood supply to the cervical end is the most susceptible to ischemia.

It is the venous drainage rather than the arterial supply that seems to be most critical to the viability of the graft. Among the factors that can contribute to venous obstruction, compression within the mediastinal and diaphragmatic hiatus may be the most important. The jejunal isoperistaltic graft is positioned in the retrohilar thorax, and the end of the jejunum is brought out through the cervical opening; a cervical jejunostomy is thus created. This procedure is usually performed with 6-0 interrupted absorbable suture. When the jejunal graft is viable, a jejunogastrostomy is performed. Distal intestinal continuity is then restored with a jejunojejunostomy. A gastrostomy is also performed.

Six to 8 weeks later, the second stage of the interposition operation is done. This consists of performing the cervical anastomosis between the jejunum and the cervical esophagus. The anastomosis is fashioned after the distal end of the cervical esophagus and the jejunal limb are mobilized (Fig. 25-6C).

### Free Jejunal Grafts

When free jejunal grafts are used, an appropriate length of jejunum is harvested, providing primary vessels for arterial and venous anastomoses. The primary arterial vessel is flushed with a cold solid organ preservation solution (ie, University of Wisconsin solution), and the graft is kept on the iced solution until the neck vessels are prepared for anastomosis. Usually, the facial vein and the external carotid artery are used to perform the microvascular anastomosis. The jejunal conduit is placed in the retrosternal or retrohilar position and the vascular anastomosis is then performed. If there is good flow and viability of the conduit, a cervical esophagojejunostomy and gastrojejunostomy are completed.

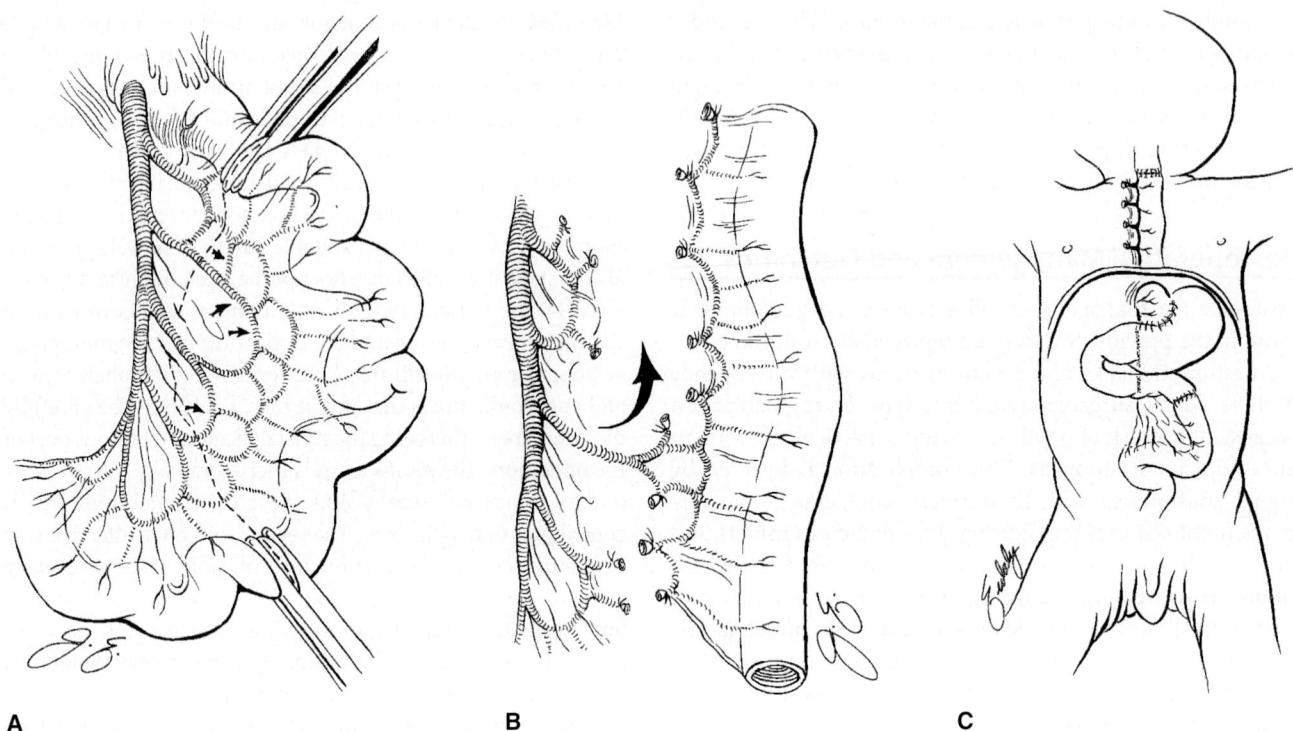

A                                     B                                    C

**FIGURE 25-6** Free jejunal graft. **A.** The jejunum is divided just beyond the first vasa recta artery. **B.** Preservation of the critical vascular pedicle to maintain a viable graft. In patients who receive a free graft, these vessels are used for microvascular anastomoses to the neck recipient vessels. **C.** The graft is brought into the chest via the esophageal hiatus and can be placed in either the retrosternal or intrathoracic position.

## Postoperative Management and Outcomes

Postoperative management follows the same general guidelines as described earlier for other replacement techniques.

The use of the jejunum as an esophageal substitute has an initial advantage in terms of adequacy of length and absence of graft failures. Moreover, these advantages increase with time. Continued active peristalsis and the absence of intrinsic disease of the jejunum make it an attractive long-term substitute. Nevertheless, the technical difficulty of this procedure as well as the requirement of several stages is an obvious drawback. Other disadvantages are that the relatively short length of the mesenteric vessels feeding the jejunum limits the use of a transposed jejunal segment and that the long lengths of an esophageal gap cannot be traversed without risking ischemia.

The success rate of jejunal interposition is approximately 75%; the mortality rate is approximately 5%. As with other esophageal replacement techniques, gastroesophageal reflux is sometimes problematic.

## SELECTED READINGS

Ahmad SA, Sylvester KG, Hebra A, et al. Esophageal replacement using the colon: is it a good choice? *J Pediatr Surg* 1996;31:1026–1030; discussion 1030–1031.

Anderson KD, Randolph JG. The gastric tube for esophageal replacement in children. *J Thorac Cardiovasc Surg* 1973;66:333–342.

Anderson KD, Noblett H, Belsey R, Randolph JG. Long-term follow-up of children with colon and gastric tube interposition for esophageal atresia. *Surgery* 1992;111:131–136.

Azar H, Chrispin AR, Waterston DJ. Esophageal replacement with transverse colon in infants and children. *J Pediatr Surg* 1971;6:3–9.

Burgos L, Barrena S, Andrés AM, et al. Colonic interposition for esophageal replacement in children remains a good choice: 33-year median follow-up of 65 patients. *J Pediatr Surg* 2010;45:341–345.

Choi RS, Lillehei CW, Lund DP, et al. Esophageal replacement in children who have caustic pharyngoesophageal strictures. *J Pediatr Surg* 1997;32:1083–1087; discussion 1087–1088.

Dunn JC, Fonkalsrud EW, Applebaum H, et al. Reoperation after esophageal replacement in childhood. *J Pediatr Surg* 1999;34:1630–1632.

Gross RE, Firestone FN. Colonic reconstruction of the esophagus in infants and children. *Surgery* 1967;61:955–964.

Hamza AF, Abdelhay S, Sherif H, et al. Caustic esophageal strictures in children: 30 years' experience. *J Pediatr Surg* 2003;38:828–833.

Marujo WC, Tannuri U, Maksoud JG. Total gastric transposition: an alternative to esophageal replacement in children. *J Pediatr Surg* 1991;26:676–681.

Pedersen JC, Klein RL, Andrews DA. Gastric tube as the primary procedure for pure esophageal atresia. *J Pediatr Surg* 1996;31:1233–1235.

Reinberg O, Genton N. Esophageal replacement in children: evaluation of the one-stage procedure with colic transplants. *Eur J Pediatr Surg* 1997;7:216–220.

Ring WS, Varco RL, L'Heureux PR, Foker JE. Esophageal replacement with jejunum in children; an 18 to 33 year follow-up. *J Thorac Cardiovasc Surg* 1982;83:918–927.

Spitz L. Gastric transposition in children. *Semin Pediatr Surg* 2009;18:30–33.

Stanwell J, Drake D, Pierro A, Kiely E, Curry J. Pediatric laparoscopic-assisted gastric transposition: early experience and outcomes. *J Laparoendosc Adv Surg Tech* 2010;20:177–181.

Tannuri U, Tannuri ACA, Gonçalves MEP, Cardoso SR. Total gastric transposition is better than partial gastric tube esophagoplasty for esophageal replacement in children. *Dis Esophagus* 2008;21:73–77.

Touloukian RJ, Tellides G. Retrosternal ileocolic esophageal replacement in children revisited. Antireflux role of the ileocecal valve. *J Thorac Cardiovasc Surg* 1994;107:1067–1072.

# CHAPTER 26

# Achalasia

*Philip K. Frykman and Richard G. Azizkhan*

## KEY POINTS

1. Esophageal achalasia has profound impact on a child's growth and development with many children presenting with failure to thrive.

2. Symptoms include dysphagia, regurgitation of undigested food, and nocturnal wheezing in older children; and respiratory difficulties such as wheezing, chronic coughing, bronchitis, pneumonitis, and recurrent pneumonia in younger children.

3. Classic radiographic findings of a barium esophagogram are dilated esophagus with a "bird's beak" narrowing of the lower esophageal sphincter (LES).

4. Esophageal manometry is the gold standard study to confirm the diagnosis of achalasia. The hallmark manometric findings are increased LES resting pressure, absence of peristalsis, and failure of LES to relax to swallowing.

5. The primary treatment of choice for children with achalasia is surgical, specifically the modified Heller esophagomyotomy (EM).

6. Either a laparoscopic or thoracoscopic approach can be used with similar success. Currently, the preferred approach is a laparoscopic Heller EM with concomitant fundoplication.

7. Long-term outcomes show around 90% relief of dysphagia with rapid resumption of normal diet and growth with diminution of respiratory symptoms.

## INTRODUCTION

Achalasia is an esophageal motility disorder characterized by the absence of peristalsis and failure of the lower esophageal sphincter (LES) to relax in response to swallowing. Its incidence in the United States and Europe is 0.2 to 1 per 100,000 per year, with children comprising only 5% of the patient population. The impact of achalasia on the growth and development of children is, however, profound.

## PATHOPHYSIOLOGY

Swallowing is a complex coordinated set of neuronal impulses originating in the swallowing center of the medulla. These impulses first act on the striated pharyngeal musculature, propelling a food bolus into the upper esophagus; a peristaltic wave then moves it down the esophagus. The LES, which is a high-pressure zone at the gastroesophageal junction, acts as a valve to prevent the reflux of gastric contents into the esophagus. It relaxes when reached by the peristaltic wave transporting the food bolus into the stomach. In contrast to this normal process, achalasia is characterized by obstruction at the gastroesophageal junction and abnormal peristalsis in the body of the esophagus. Manometric techniques have clearly defined a combination of hypertensive sphincter resting pressures and incomplete relaxation in response to a swallow. Additionally, contractions in the lower two thirds of the body of the esophagus are irregular or absent.

Although peristalsis appears to be under vagal control, the innervation of the esophagus is not well understood. The LES has intrinsic myogenic tone, which is modulated by neural and hormonal mechanisms. The vagus nerve sends both excitatory and inhibitory nerve fibers to the LES. However, their degree of influence on LES tone is unclear. Interestingly, the LES continues to relax on swallowing, suggesting a degree of autonomy. Hormones and gut peptides found to increase LES pressure are gastrin, motilin, substance P, and bombesin; those that decrease this pressure are secretin, gastric inhibitory peptide, neuropeptide Y, and vasoactive intestinal peptide.

Electron microscopic studies of the dorsal motor nuclei and vagus nerves of some patients with achalasia reveal fewer ganglion cells and neurodegenerative changes. Induced lesions of dorsal motor nuclei in animal models produce a picture that mimics achalasia. Immunohistochemical studies of distal esophagi show reduced levels of vasoactive intestinal peptide and nitric oxide, both of which are mediators of smooth muscle relaxation. Physiologic investigations have shown a hypersensitivity of LES contractions to cholinergic agonists. This particular finding forms the basis on which botulinum toxin, a potent inhibitor of acetylcholine release from presynaptic nerve terminals, has been used therapeutically albeit with limited efficacy and durability.

The protozoan *Trypanosoma cruzi* destroys the esophageal myenteric ganglia, causing an achalasia-like disorder called Chagas disease (found in South America). An increased incidence of varicella zoster virus antibodies has been detected in the myenteric ganglia in patients with achalasia. Thus, a number of diseases in which damage to these myenteric ganglia occurs have been implicated as causes of achalasia. There is also a higher incidence of achalasia in patients with Sjögren syndrome (an immune disorder). These patients have histocompatibility DQw1 and histologic findings suggestive of T-cell-mediated destruction of myenteric ganglia. In patients with achalasia who have had esophageal resections, the characteristic neuropathic finding is a reduction in or absence of myenteric ganglion cells, often associated with a variable degree of chronic inflammation within the myenteric plexus. In sum, these observations and findings suggest that neuropathic abnormalities may be acquired as the result of a variety of processes.

In children, achalasia has been associated with glucocorticoid deficiency, microcephaly, and neuropathies, suggesting a more generalized disease process. While very rare, Allgrove syndrome, also known as "AAA syndrome" for the triad of adrenal hypoplasia, achalasia, and alacrimia, is the most commonly cited of these disorders. Cases of familial achalasia have predominantly been found in families with consanguinity, suggesting an autosomal recessive mode of inheritance. Because of the small number of familial cases reported, however, this association is unclear.

## DIAGNOSIS

A cardinal feature of children with achalasia is profound weight loss and/or growth retardation as a result of inadequate nutrition. Their weight often falls below the fifth percentile for their age. Respiratory complaints and dysphagia are also common. Younger children frequently present with respiratory difficulties caused by recurrent aspiration, such as wheezing, chronic coughing, bronchitis, pneumonitis, recurrent pneumonia, and bronchiectasis. Dysphagia, which is found more commonly in older children, may be accompanied by nocturnal coughing and regurgitation of undigested food. Because of the broad range of symptoms, differential diagnosis is sometimes difficult.

The diagnostic workup begins with a plain chest roentgenogram, which may reveal nonspecific findings such as mediastinal widening, an airfluid level in the midesophagus, or abnormal pulmonary markings due to chronic aspiration (Fig. 26-1A). A barium swallow is generally then performed and typically reveals a dilated upper esophagus with smooth tapering to the classic "bird's beak" appearance of the LES (Fig. 26-1B). Manometry is the gold standard for confirming the diagnosis of achalasia, generally indicating a resting LES pressure 15 to 20 mm Hg, incomplete LES relaxation on swallowing, and the absence of peristalsis in the entire esophagus. Endoscopy is performed to rule out the possibility of an organic obstruction or infection in the distal esophagus, and although an esophageal emptying scan with a semisolid radionuclide meal is not required to establish the diagnosis, it can be used to assess esophageal motility when manometry cannot be performed.

## TREATMENT

### Overview

The 2 primary therapeutic modalities used to treat achalasia are pneumatic dilation (PD) and esophagomyotomy (EM) (Fig. 26-1C). Although there have historically been proponents of each of these procedures, numerous reports have been published that document clinical improvement in adult patients ranging from 65% to 85% with either modality. Moreover, a comparative evaluation is difficult to make in that criteria for classifying results differ from one study to another and follow-up studies are often inadequate. Despite the controversy, in many cases of adult achalasia, PD is frequently performed as the initial treatment modality; it has low morbidity and fair clinical success and involves a short hospital stay with a rapid return to normal activity. There is also general agreement that if 1 or 2 attempts at nonoperative treatment fail to provide satisfactory long-term relief of dysphagia, surgical treatment is then initiated. An esophagectomy should be considered for patients who have a tortuous or severely dilated esophagus and for those in whom symptoms are not relieved by an EM; however, this is rarely seen in children.

### Childhood Achalasia

While the pediatric experience with achalasia is much more limited, outcomes differ from those in the adult population. Several studies have revealed an age-related correlation with successful treatment. In a study conducted by Azizkhan et al, only 25% of children showed significant improvement with PD alone, and no child under age 9 responded to this treatment. In general, the younger the patient, the less the success achieved by one or multiple dilations. However, a recent study by Lee et al found that all of the children treated with PD as the initial mode of therapy had recurrent symptoms and 93% required additional intervention. This group was compared with 53% of patients receiving EM as initial treatment that developed recurrent symptoms and 40% required additional intervention. The study also showed that 47% of children initially treated PD went on to have EM performed. The authors concluded that patients treated with EM had a statistically significant longer symptom-free duration, fewer hospital admissions with similar complication rates compared with the PD treated patients. Two case series of laparoscopic Heller myotomy and Dor fundoplication in children with achalasia (Patti et al and Mattioli et al) showed greater than 90% relief of dysphagia with low complication rates. In light of multiple studies and the authors' experience, we recommend that EM should be the initial therapy for achalasia in children of all ages. PD should be reserved for children who may not tolerate an operation or for EM patients who developed recurrent dysphagia. Additionally, endoscopic botulinum toxin injection of the LES has been shown to have only transient relief of symptoms, and therefore has essentially no role in treatment of children.

While the modified Heller EM is the standard surgical treatment for achalasia, controversy exists over whether this is best performed through a laparoscopic versus a thoracoscopic approach. While both approaches show similar

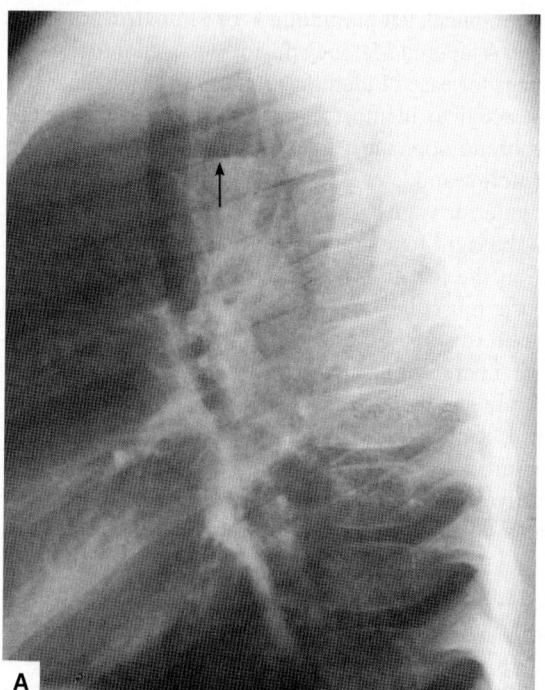 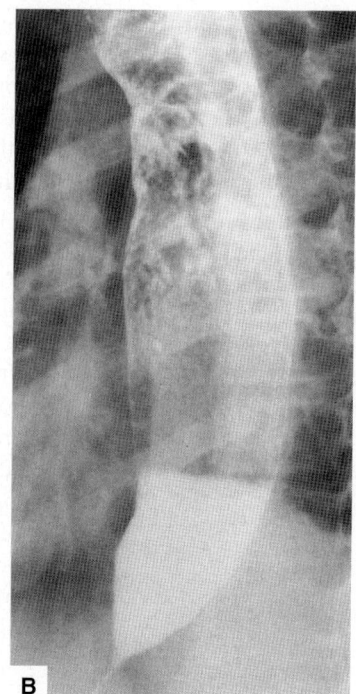 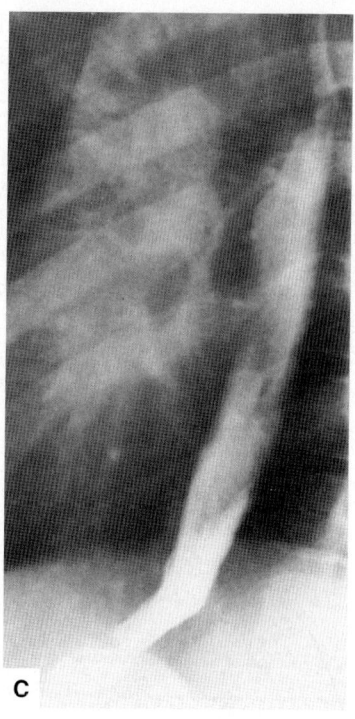

**FIGURE 26-1 A.** Lateral chest radiograph in a 12-year-old male with achalasia. Note the airfluid level in the dilated esophagus (*black arrow*). **B.** Barium esophagogram in the same patient showing a dilated esophagus with a bird beak LES. **C.** Following a transthoracic modified Heller procedure, the esophagus empties promptly as seen on the esophagogram.

overall effectiveness and rates of complications, the complication profiles differ somewhat. The initial minimally invasive approach was a left thoracoscopic approach, based on the traditional left thoractomy used to perform the modified Heller EM. The thoracoscopic approach has limited hiatal access with suboptimal visualization of the gastric cardia leading to an elevated rate of incomplete myotomy and recurrent dysphagia. Currently, the laparoscopic approach is preferred because of the lower rate of incomplete myotomy owing to easy gastric access, but a higher incidence of postmyotomy GERD from extension of the myotomy onto the cardia. Consequently, most pediatric surgeons performing the laparoscopic approach also perform a fundoplication as well. Debate continues regarding whether a fundoplication should be performed at the time of the EM, and if so, which type of fundoplication should be performed. Regardless of which approach is used, after the operative procedure, respiratory symptoms diminish and there is a rapid resumption of normal diet, normal growth, and normal activity.

## Complications

Both PD and EM entail potentially serious risks to patients. The reported incidence of esophageal perforation after forceful dilation is between 1% and 5%, and treatment for perforation generally necessitates surgical intervention. Gastroesophageal reflux (GER) and peptic esophagitis are significant problems with the modified Heller EM, occurring in approximately 10% to 30% of pediatric patients. These disorders are also difficult to treat medically. It appears that the absence or very low incidence of postdilation reflux is related to the fact that it is difficult to disrupt the oblique fibers of the gastroesophageal junction with a dilator.

Regardless of the type of treatment, all patients require close long-term follow-up. Although the initial results may be good or even excellent, symptoms often reappear. Moreover, achalasia is associated with a slightly increased risk of esophageal cancer.

## Pneumatic Dilation in Children

The aim of treatment with PD is relief of obstruction by successfully reducing LES tone while maintaining an effective barrier to GER. This procedure is performed under intravenous sedation or general anesthesia. Fluoroscopy facilitates the placement of a pneumatic dilator in the distal esophagus. Air or contrast is forced into the balloon until the pressure reaches the desired amount. Although the technique of PD is similar in all patients, the number of dilations and the maximal diameter of the dilating balloon are individually determined according to clinical, radiologic, and especially manometric criteria. The patient is held NPO for a 24-hour period, with frequent checks of vital signs. A barium swallow is subsequently performed to rule out the possibility of esophageal perforation and evaluate relief of obstruction. If there are no complications, a soft diet is begun the next morning and the patient is discharged.

## Laparoscopic Heller Myotomy with Dor Fundoplication

### Preoperative Preparation

The patient is positioned in the lithotomy position with the table tilted in reverse Trendelenburg. The patient is prepared by emptying the esophagus and stomach with an orogastric tube. Flexible esophagoscopy may be required to confirm that there is no retained food material in the esophagus.

## Operative Technique

A 5-port technique employing 4- and 5-mm trocars as shown in Fig. 26-2. A pneumoperitoneum is established with a Veress needle, and standard $CO_2$ insufflation. A 5-mm trocar is placed through the umbilicus; a right upper quadrant trocar 4 or 5 mm is placed for the articulated liver retractor secured to a holder; a 4- or 5-mm trocar is placed at the left costal margin as the right hand working port; a 4- or 5-mm trocar in the epigastrium right of midline for the left-hand working port; supraumbilical, left of midline 4- or 5-mm trocar for the laparoscope. A tapered Maloney dilator is passed into the distal esophagus for ease of identification of the esophagus. The liver is retracted to identify the gastroesophageal junction, next the phrenoesophageal ligament is divided mobilizing only the anterior and lateral crural attachments (Fig. 26-3A). Next, the anterior vagus is identified, gently mobilized, and pushed to the right to avoid injury. A longitudinal myotomy is started on the left anterior aspect using hook cautery to coagulate the muscular layer (Fig. 26-3B). A Maryland dissector is used to spread the longitudinal muscle fibers; once the circular fibers are encountered, these are elevated with the hook cautery and divided. Once the submucosal layer is identified, it protrudes through the myotomy. Great care should be taken to avoid bleeding and mucosal perforation. Intraoperative esophagoscopy can be helpful to reduce the risk of mucosal perforation, especially in patients who have had previous esophageal dilatations. The edges of the myotomy are grasped with the each hand and gently pulled apart to widen the myotomy and facilitate submucosal herniation (Fig. 26-3C). The myotomy is extended proximally well onto the dilated esophagus and distally onto the cardia to the transverse esophageal vessels. The esophageal muscle is separated from the mucosa for at least one third of the circumference of the esophagus. To check for mucosal perforation, air is insufflated into the esophagus using a nasogastric tube. If a mucosal perforation occurs, this can be closed with fine suture and covered with an anterior fundoplication (Dor or Thal).

Although controversial, an antireflux procedure is often added to minimize the risk of postoperative reflux. If an antireflux procedure is added, the general consensus is that a partial wrap (Dor or Toupet procedure) should be performed. We routinely perform a 180° anterior Dor fundoplication to cover the exposed submucosa and to mitigate risk of GERD. The fundus is sutured to the left and right edges of the myotomy with nonabsorbable 3-0 sutures (Fig. 26-4A and B). This can be accomplished by either intracorporeal or extracorporeal knot tying.

## Postoperative Management

Most patients have the nasogastric tube removed prior to emergence from anesthesia and are kept NPO on the day of the operation. A liquid diet is started the day after surgery, and, if tolerated, can be advanced to a soft diet for 2 weeks. If there is any concern regarding mucosal perforation, an esophagram with water-soluble contrast should be performed prior to starting a diet. Pain control with acetaminophen and low dose morphine sulfate is usually adequate. Most patients are discharged on the first or second postoperative day.

## Thoracoscopic Heller Myotomy

### Operative Technique

The preoperative preparation is essentially identical to that described above for the laparoscopic procedure. During this procedure, the anesthetized patient is secured in the Trendelenburg position with the left side up. Four ports are needed (Fig. 26-5). One 5-mm port for the thoracoscope is placed in the superior portion of the midclavicular line; two 4- or

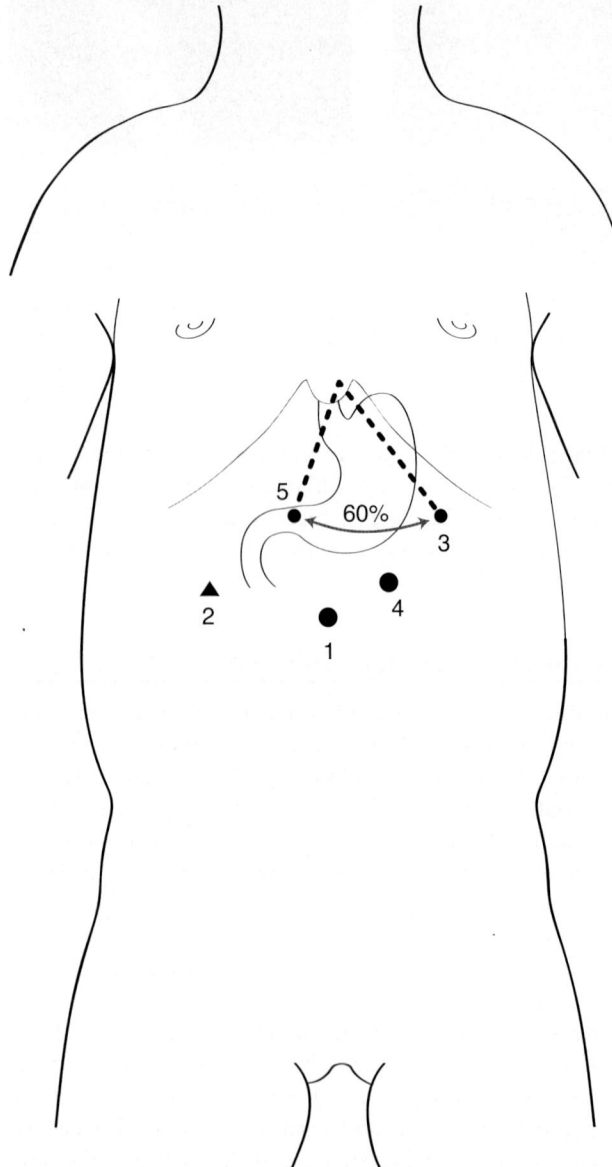

**FIGURE 26-2** The location of the 5 trocars in order of placement. A 5-mm port is placed in the umbilicus using an open technique (*1*). A second port is placed near the liver edge and in the right midclavicular line for the liver retractor (*2*). The third trocar is placed at the left costal margin in the anterior axillary line (*3*). The fourth trocar is placed in the supraumbilical region, left of midline (*4*); and the fifth trocar is placed in the epigastrium to the right of midline (*5*). Ports 3 and 5 (left and right hands, respectively) should be placed approximately 60° apart in relation to the hiatus, as this provides an optimal working angle.

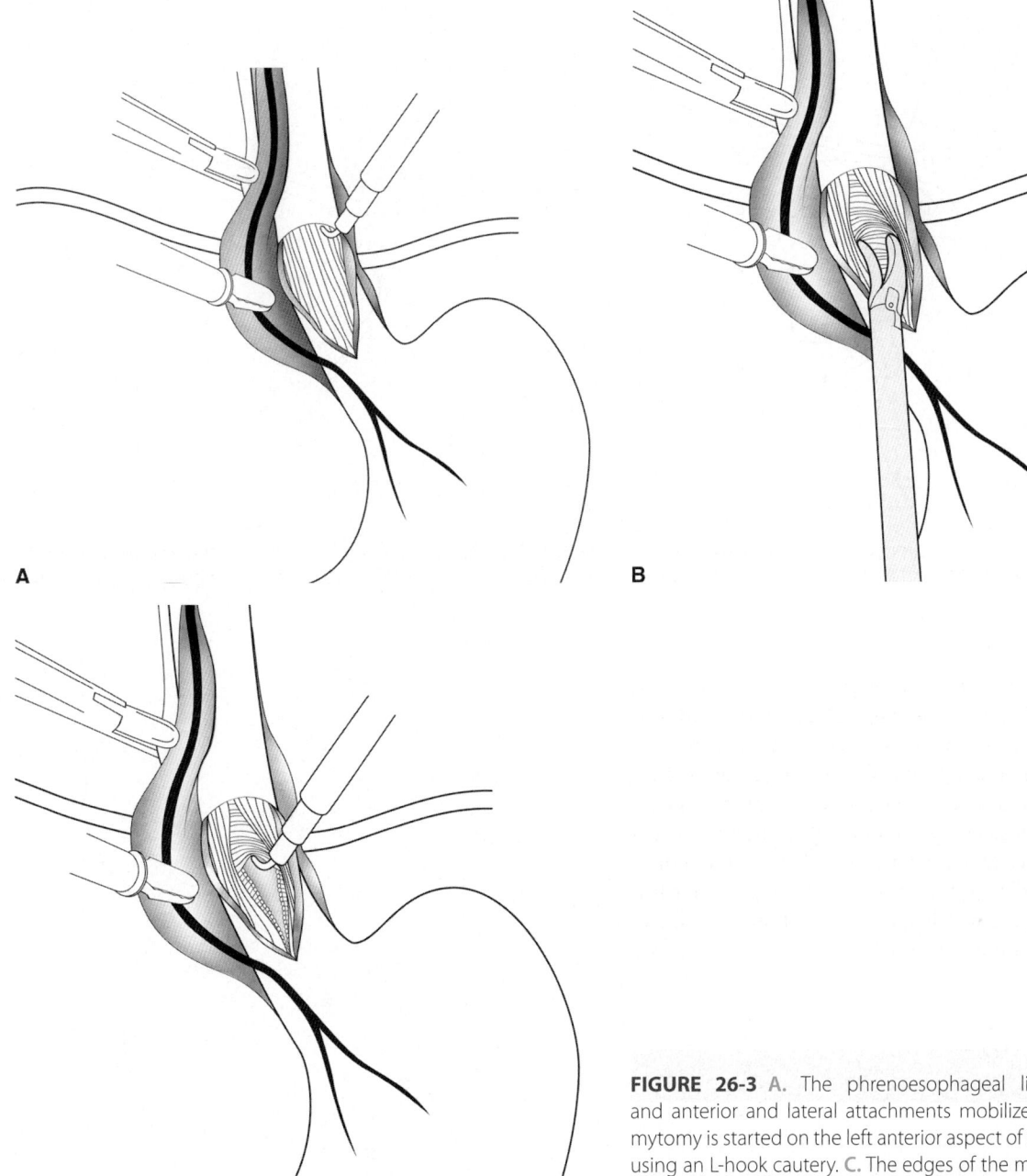

**A**

**B**

**C**

**FIGURE 26-3 A.** The phrenoesophageal ligament is divided and anterior and lateral attachments mobilized. **B.** A longitudinal myotomy is started on the left anterior aspect of the distal esophagus using an L-hook cautery. **C.** The edges of the myotomy are grasped and gently pulled apart to widen the myotomy.

5-mm ports for the dissector and grasper are placed 1 to 2 interspaces below the thoracoscope anteriorly and posteriorly to the midclavicular line; and one 5-mm port for the cautery and scissors used to divide the esophageal muscle and free it from the underlying mucosa is placed close to the diaphragm. A tapered Maloney dilator is passed into the distal esophagus for ease of identification and mobilization from the mediastinum. Some surgeons have found that a flexible endoscope placed transorally into the distal esophagus permits easy identification with transillumination of the esophagus.

The pleura is incised overlying the esophagus, and dissection is carried both superiorly and inferiorly to free it from the posterior mediastinum. The esophagus must be mobilized superiorly to the level of the inferior pulmonary vein and inferiorly to the hiatus of the diaphragm; this mobilization step is best accomplished using blunt dissection. Umbilical tape

is then wrapped around the esophagus for retraction. The esophagus is vertically incised using the laparoscopic shears, and the esophageal muscle is dissected from the underlying mucosa on the distal third of the esophagus inferiorly to the cardioesophageal junction (Fig. 26-6A). Graspers are used to hold the cut muscle edges, and the mucosa is pushed away from the muscle using a Kittner dissector (Fig. 26-6B). The muscle should be stripped away from the mucosa approximately one third of the circumference of the esophagus, with half of this circumference on either side of the incision. Esophagoscopy is also helpful at this stage to gauge the distal extent of the obstruction and when the EM has been anatomically successful.

The most significant risk at the time of myotomy is perforation through the mucosa. Repairing the small hole with fine absorbable sutures and buttressing the repair site with

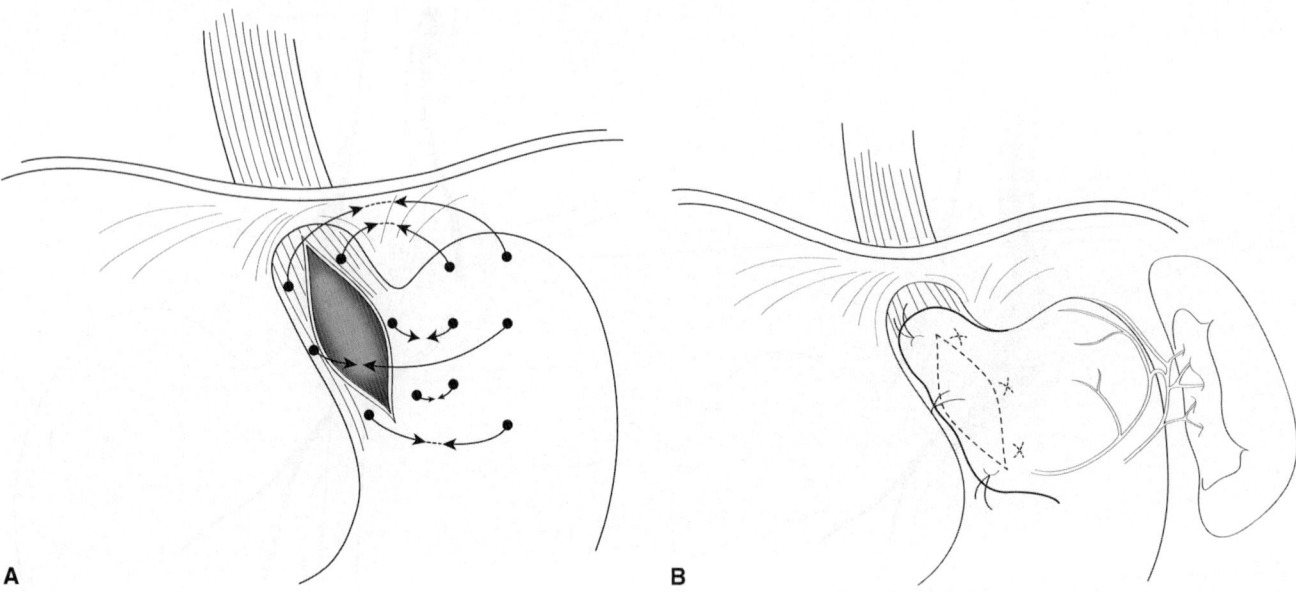

**A**    **B**

**FIGURE 26-4** **A.** Completed myotomy extending down just beyond the gastroesophageal junction. The numbers show suture placement for 180° anterior Dor fundoplication. **B.** Two nonabsorbable sutures are placed to secure the anterior stomach to each edge of the myotomy.

a vascularized tissue pedicle of pleura is usually all that is required. A thoracostomy tube is placed and positioned near the myotomy at closing, and usually removed on postoperative day 1 or 2 once a diet is resumed. The postoperative management is the same as that for the laparoscopic technique.

The minimally invasive procedures offer the advantages of smaller incisions, less postoperative pain, and a shorter hospital stay than the open approaches. The decision regarding appropriateness of which approach to choose should, of course, be based on the individual patient and the surgeon's skill set.

## OUTCOME

The vast majority of patients have immediate and lasting relief of symptoms following an EM. It is prudent to perform postoperative manometry once the patient has recovered to document the level of LES pressure following the myotomy. Most children have postoperative LES pressures between 7 and 10 mm Hg. Patti et al and Mattioli et al reported case series of laparoscopic Heller myotomy and Dor fundoplication in children with achalasia showed greater than 90% relief of dysphagia medium (mean 24 months) and long-term follow-up (mean 45 months), respectively. Neither series reported GERD based on symptoms (Patti et al) nor by pH probe monitoring (Mattioli et al) using this approach.

Residual dysphagia within a year occurs in approximately 5% to 10% of patients after a thoracoscopic EM. It is usually caused by an inadequate EM. Making sure the myotomy extends onto the cardia reduces the risk of this complication. Rarely, a second myotomy must be performed if symptoms remain severe.

A study in which children were followed up for an average of 8 years after a myotomy, a higher incidence of recurrent dysphagia was noted, especially in adolescent girls. Some of

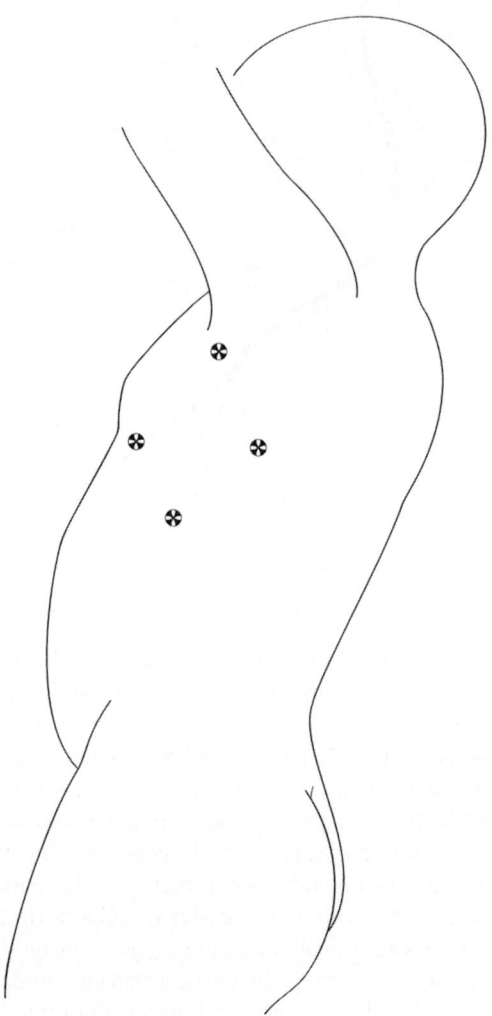

**FIGURE 26-5** The location of the 4 trocar sites on the left lateral chest wall for a thoracoscopic EM. The camera is usually held at the most cephalad site for optimal viewing of the procedure, which is performed near the diaphragm.

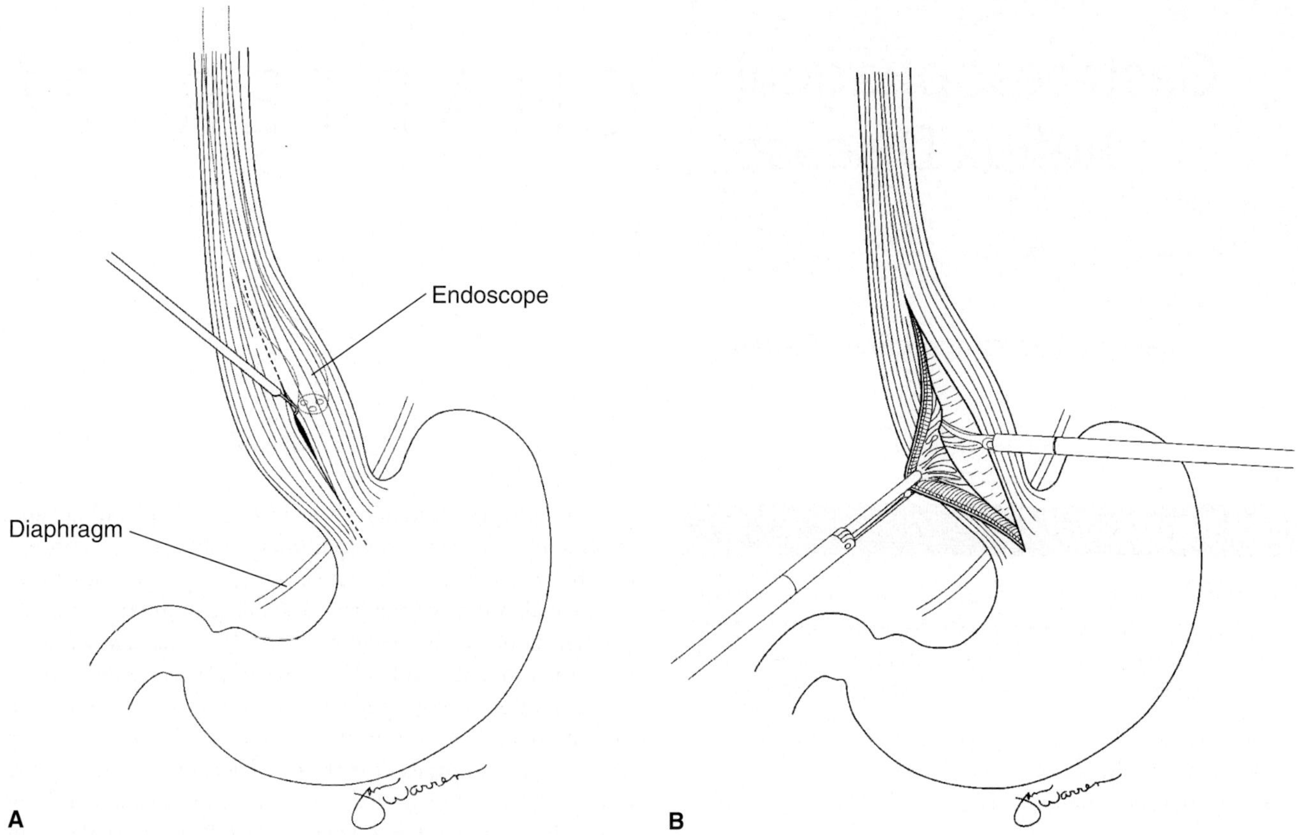


**FIGURE 26-6** A. After the parietal pleura has been opened, the myotomy is begun in the distal third of the esophagus with an endoscopic J hook connected to electrocautery. A large dilator or esophagoscope is prepositioned in the distal esophagus to facilitate the myotomy. B. The muscle is elevated on either side of the myotomy with graspers to anchor the edge of the muscle, while the endoscopic scissors are used to dissect the muscle from the underlying mucosa.

these patients appeared to have significant but transient dysmotility associated with pregnancy, and symptoms improved after delivery. More than 85% of the patients have had long-term relief of symptoms and resumption of appropriate growth.

## SELECTED READINGS


Azizkhan RG, Tapper D, Eraklis A. Achalasia in childhood: a 20-year experience. *J Pediatr Surg* 1980;15:452–456.

Boyle JT, Cohen S, Watkins JB. Successful treatment of achalasia in childhood by pneumatic dilatation. *J Pediatr* 1981;99:35–40.

Holcomb GW, Richards WO, Riedel BD. Laparoscopic esophagomyotomy for achalasia in children. *J Pediatr Surg* 1996;31:716–718.

Hunter JG, Trus TL, Branum GD, Waring JP. Laparoscopic Heller myotomy and fundoplication for achalasia. *Ann Surg* 1997;225:655–665.

Lee CW, Kays DW, Chen MK, Islam S. Outcomes of treatment of childhood achalasia. *J Pediatr Surg* 2010;45(6):1173–1177.

Lemmer JH, Coran AG, Wesley JR, Polley TZ Jr, Byrne WJ. Achalasia in children: treatment by anterior esophageal myotomy (modified Heller operation). *J Pediatr Surg* 1985;20:333–338.

Marlais M, Fishman JR, Fell JM, Haddad MJ, Rawat DJ. UK incidence of achalasia: an 11-year national epidemiological study. *Arch Dis Child* 2011;96(2):192–194.

Mattioli G, Esposito C, Pini Prato A, et al. Results of the laparoscopic Heller-Dor procedure for pediatric esophageal achalasia. *Surg Endosc* 2003;17(10):1650–1652.

Mehra M, Bahar RJ, Ament ME, et al. Laparoscopic and thoracoscopic esophagomyotomy for children with achalasia. *J Pediatr Gastroenterol Nutr* 2001;33(4):466–471.

Monnig PJ. Familial achalasia in children. *Ann Thorac Surg* 1990;49:1019–1022.

Morris-Stiff G, Khan R, Foster ME, Lari J. Long-term results of surgery for childhood achalasia. *Ann R Coll Surg Engl* 1997;79:432–434.

Myers NA, Jolley SG, Taylor R. Achalasia of the cardia in children: a worldwide survey. *J Pediatr Surg* 1994;29:1375–1379.

Nihoul-Fekete C, Bawab F, Lortat-Jacob S, Arhan P. Achalasia of the esophagus in childhood. Surgical treatment in 35 cases, with special reference to familial cases and glucocorticoid deficiency association. *Hepatogastroenterology* 1991;38(6):510–513.

Patti MG, Albanese CT, Holcomb GW 3rd, et al. Laparoscopic Heller myotomy and Dor fundoplication for esophageal achalasia in children. *J Pediatr Surg* 2001;36(8):1248–1251.

Tryhus MR, Davis M, Griffith JK, Ablin DS, Gogel HK. Familial achalasia in two siblings: significance of possible hereditary role. *J Pediatr Surg* 1989;24:292–295.

Vane DW, Cosby K, West K, Grosfeld JL. Late results following esophagomyotomy in children with achalasia. *J Pediatr Surg* 1988;23:515–519.

Woltman TA, Pellegrini CA, Oelschlager BK. Achalasia. *Surg Clin North Am* 2005;85(3):483–493.

# Gastroesophageal Reflux Disease

# CHAPTER 27

*Stephen G. Jolley and J. Brent Roaten*

## KEY POINTS

1. Understanding the historical perceptions and experience with gastroesophageal reflux disease (GERD) in infants and children allows the clinician to evaluate the efficacy and reasonableness of proposed treatment modalities.

2. The presence of GERD in children can be suspected by clinical history, but confirmation requires quantitative testing, which is often invasive.

3. The most reliable test to confirm the presence or absence of GERD in children is extended esophageal pH monitoring. This test can also give important information about the probability of spontaneous resolution of GERD with time, and the probability that respiratory symptoms associated with the risk for sudden infant death are caused by GERD.

4. Medical therapy of childhood GERD is often successful in controlling symptoms, but may not eliminate the GERD over time.

5. Antireflux operations in children with GERD can be performed safely with good long-term control of GERD and minimal morbidity and mortality. More than 1 approach and type of antireflux operation can be used in children to maximize the advantages and minimize the side effects.

6. The same quantitative evaluation used preoperatively to confirm GERD in children should be used for postoperative evaluation when there is a question about whether GERD is still present or has been eliminated.

7. Asymptomatic children may have GERD and be at risk for serious complications of GERD, particularly infants with congenital anomalies associated with a high prevalence of GERD.

## INTRODUCTION

A simplified definition of gastroesophageal reflux disease (GERD) is the adverse effects of excessive movement of gastric contents into the esophagus due to a defective gastroesophageal junction. The key to understanding and treating this disease entity in humans is an accurate concept of what constitutes a defective gastroesophageal junction. Normal functions of the gastroesophageal junction include (1) relaxation with swallowing to allow passage of food from the esophagus into the stomach, (2) relaxation to permit eructation or vomiting when necessary to relieve gastric distention, and (3) intermittent relaxation that permits only physiological episodes of gastroesophageal reflux during the initial 2 hours after meals, primarily while awake and only rarely during sleep. Contrasting with GERD is achalasia, in which there is inadequate relaxation with swallowing and impaired esophageal emptying.

Descriptions of childhood GERD have been recorded as early as 1828 in Paris, where children who succumbed to malnutrition with repeated emesis were found to have esophageal ulcers at autopsy. Over a century later GERD was recognized as a disease entity in children, mainly due to the descriptions of "chalasia" by Berenberg and Neuhauser in Boston and partial thoracic stomach by Astley and Carre in Belfast. These investigators noted that symptoms associated with GERD in treated children would usually disappear by 2 years of age with postural therapy and weaning to solid food. It is for this reason that GERD has been considered to be self-limiting in infants and children.

Surgical intervention for childhood GERD was not generally considered until the 1950s because the experience with antireflux operations in children was limited and because medical antireflux therapy was felt to be uniformly successful. Since then, many infants and children with GERD have been identified as having complications severe enough to warrant an antireflux operation. Some older children with severe complications of GERD even presented to clinicians without prior symptoms of GERD or with symptoms of GERD that had resolved during infancy.

The major complications of childhood GERD that may require surgical intervention include recurrent regurgitation of feedings with or without growth retardation, intractable pain or irritability associated with esophageal mucosal injury, esophageal stricture or columnar cell metaplasia (Barrett) of the esophageal mucosa, and life-threatening respiratory symptoms. The antireflux operation is currently the third most commonly performed operation on most pediatric surgical services.

# DIAGNOSIS OF GASTROESOPHAGEAL REFLUX DISEASE IN CHILDREN

## Clinical History and Physical Examination

The clinical history is the initial screening tool used to identify children who may have GERD. A common indicator of childhood GERD is recurrent, effortless emesis without bile. This regurgitation of feedings may or may not result in poor growth. Many children with GERD are identified because of life-threatening respiratory symptoms or disease. These respiratory complaints include apnea, choking, respiratory arrest, an apparent life-threatening event (ALTE), recurrent aspiration pneumonia, chronic coughing or stridor, recurrent wheezing, and chronic lung disease. Advanced esophagitis, seen in approximately 10% to 20% of children with GERD referred for surgical intervention, is usually associated with pain, dysphagia, hematemesis, irritability, or esophageal stricture. Unusual neurological symptoms or breathholding may result from esophagitis in a small number of children with GERD.

Unfortunately, the clinical history of affected children is usually not specific for GERD. For example, infants with emesis, even effortless emesis, may not have GERD. Obstructive lesions of the alimentary tract, swallowing disorders, impaired esophageal emptying, disorders of gastric emptying, small bowel motility disorders, infections, food allergies, increased intracranial pressure, and metabolic disorders can produce recurrent emesis in children. Furthermore, respiratory symptoms or disease from GERD in infancy are similar to those associated with sepsis, central nervous system (CNS) trauma or malformation, seizure disorders, central apnea or increased periodic breathing, congenital heart disease, allergies, primary lung disease, or Munchausen by proxy. In most children who have only GERD, the physical examination is usually unremarkable.

## Diagnostic Studies

Radiographs taken during a liquid barium meal are used primarily to exclude obstructive lesions of the esophagus, stomach, or duodenum. Occasionally, other congenital lesions that may produce symptoms that mimic GERD (eg, swallowing disorders, tracheoesophageal fistula) can also be detected during the barium meal. The entire swallowing sequence—esophagus, stomach, and duodenum—must be visualized to exclude anatomic lesions that may produce symptoms resembling those of GERD.

Many clinicians still use the presence of reflux episodes during the barium meal to confirm or exclude GERD in children. This practice is associated with frequent diagnostic errors, such as high false-positive or false-negative rates, even in institutions where an attempt is made to quantitate or grade the severity of reflux episodes. The presence of a large hiatal hernia detected during the barium meal is usually indicative of GERD, but not all hiatal hernias (eg, paraesophageal or type II hiatal hernia) are associated with a defective gastroesophageal junction. An examination of the chest area with radiographs during the barium meal is helpful if a child has congenital heart disease, unsuspected mediastinal mass, or chronic lung disease.

A *radionuclide scan* of the upper alimentary tract performed with ingested technetium-labeled sulfur colloid offers no advantage over the barium meal, except for the quantitation of gastric emptying and the potential for quantitation of esophageal emptying. Gastric emptying in children has been studied more extensively than esophageal emptying and is important to measure when considering GERD. The percentage of gastric emptying at 30 and 60 minutes, corrected for the delay in emptying produced by postcibal reflux episodes (corrected gastric emptying), can give an estimate of effective gastric emptying. Even though gastric emptying abnormalities do not cause GERD, they may be seen in association with GERD or may produce symptoms that are similar to those caused by GERD, such as vomiting. A distribution of gastric emptying abnormalities seen in children with symptoms of GERD is shown in Table 27-1.

*Gastroesophageal manometry* has limited usefulness in the identification of GERD in children. Most manometric studies of the esophagus have focused on static measurements of lower esophageal sphincter pressure (LESP). In children with GERD, however, the LESP may be increased, normal, or decreased. Gastroesophageal reflux episodes can result

| TABLE 27-1 | Distribution of Findings from Extended Esophageal pH Monitoring and Radionuclide Liquid Gastric Emptying Studies in Infants with Gastroesophageal Reflux Disease | | | |
|---|---|---|---|---|
| | | Incidence of Corrected Gastric Emptying[a] | | |
| Reflux Pattern | ZMD[b] | Slow (%) | Control (%) | Rapid (%) |
| Type I | + | 7.7 | 9.4 | 13.2 |
| | − | 8.4 | 10.1 | 14.4 |
| | | | | Total = 63.2% |
| Type II | + | 3.9 | 2.7 | 6.1 |
| | − | 4.1 | 3.0 | 6.5 |
| | | | | Total = 26.3% |
| Type III | + | 0.7 | 2.2 | 3.6 |
| | − | 0.5 | 1.3 | 2.2 |
| | | | | Total = 10.5% |
| All patterns | + | 12.3 | 14.3 | 22.9 |
| | − | 13.0 | 14.3 | 23.2 |
| Total | | 25.3% | 28.6% | 46.1% |

[a]Expected percent gastric emptying of apple juice at 30 min if no postcibal reflux episodes occur.
[b]ZMD indicates mean duration of reflux episodes during sleep: (+) = prolonged; (−) = normal.

from a persistently decreased basal LESP or an inappropriate relaxation of LESP with a rise in gastric pressure. Therefore, prolonged monitoring of dynamic LESP changes is probably more important in the identification of GERD using manometric methods, although this technique has been used infrequently in children. Current manometric evaluation of the esophagus in children includes measurement of upper esophageal sphincter pressure and relaxation, measurement of LESP and relaxation with swallowing, and a profile of propagated or nonpropagated peristaltic waves in the esophageal body. Children with suspected primary or secondary esophageal motility disorders benefit most from gastroesophageal manometry.

Endoscopic evaluation of the esophageal mucosa by *esophagogastroscopy* is attempted to identify mucosal injury as a consequence of GERD. This evaluation is accomplished by both visualization and biopsy of the mucosa. No other diagnostic study can define mucosal abnormalities better than endoscopy. Visual inspection of the esophageal mucosa can identify erosive esophagitis, peptic ulceration, or stricture, but may miss the presence of Barrett esophagus. Esophageal mucosal biopsy 2 cm or more cephalad from the gastroesophageal junction is necessary to detect the presence of Barrett esophagus, for which most evidence favors chronic mucosal metaplasia from GERD as the likely cause. Histological types of Barrett esophagus include specialized columnar epithelium, fundic-type epithelium, and junctional epithelium, although some clinicians consider only the specialized columnar epithelium to represent Barrett esophagus. The incidence of Barrett esophagus detected in children during endoscopy has been reported to be as high as 12.5%.

Esophageal mucosal biopsy may be used to detect lesser degrees of esophageal mucosal injury from GERD, but there is not universal agreement on a system specific for GERD. (Other diseases alone or diseases that produce vomiting can be associated with injury to the esophageal mucosa). Histologic findings associated with the presence of esophagitis include basal cell hyperplasia, shortened rete pegs, increased neutrophils, and the presence microscopically of increased eosinophils. Chronic forms of esophagitis usually do not have a prominent neutrophil presence in mucosal specimens.

The most accurate study currently used to identify GERD in children is *extended esophageal pH monitoring* for 18 to 24 hours. It was devised to measure the frequency and duration of acid reflux episodes over time, so it is necessary to document the presence of gastric acid (pH 2 or less) prior to initiating esophageal pH monitoring. The methodologies used for the performance and analysis of this study vary in accuracy. Table 27-2 shows the relative accuracy of each method in the same population of children.

The principal methods and analysis for esophageal pH monitoring used in infants and children are the Johnson–DeMeester method (composite pH score, reflux index—percentage of total time esophageal pH <4) and the Jolley–Johnson method (<2 hour and >2 hour postcibal pH scores). The Johnson–DeMeester method has been subsequently modified by Boix-Ochoa and by Vandenplas for children. Methods of esophageal pH monitoring for which there are no reported normal values in children should be avoided in the routine evaluation and care of children with GERD.

| TABLE 27-2 | Comparison of the Accuracy for Methods of Extended Esophageal pH Monitoring in a Single Population of Infants and Children | | |
|---|---|---|---|
| **Methods of Esophageal pH Analysis** | False (+) | False (−) | Percentage of Accuracy |
| **Johnson–DeMeester** | | | |
| pH score (normal ≤18) | 3% | 50% | 81% |
| Reflux index (total % of time pH <4) | | | |
| If normal: ≤5% | 33% | 42% | 64% |
| ≤9% | 3% | 50% | 81% |
| **Euler pH score (normal ≤50)** | 13% | 42% | 81% |
| **Jolley–Johnson pH score** | | | |
| <2 h postcibal (normal ≤64) | | | |
| Apple juice | 3% | 83% | 69% |
| Milk formula | 3% | 58% | 78% |
| Combined | 3% | 75% | 72% |
| >2 h postcibal (normal ≤64) | 3% | 3% | 97% |

The calculations necessary to derive the >2 hour postcibal esophageal pH score can be done manually or by computer. Even though the widespread acceptance of the >2 hour postcibal esophageal pH score has been hindered by the cumbersome calculations with the strict protocol and nursing participation needed for the performance of the 18- to 24-hour esophageal study, the improved accuracy is worth the extra effort. A normal range for this esophageal pH score is ≤64 and is independent of patient age. Esophageal pH measurements obtained for normal children >2 hour postcibal are comparable to the normal values reported for adults >2 hour postcibal. Abnormal regurgitation of duodenal contents into the esophagus has been suggested by some investigators to be a significant factor in GERD, but is very difficult to document using pH monitoring of the esophagus or stomach. Special probes that may detect bilirubin have been employed in adults to detect refluxed duodenal contents in the stomach and esophagus.

## Patterns of Reflux Episodes

In children with GERD, there are at least 3 detectable patterns of reflux episodes on the esophageal pH record (Fig. 27-1). The type I reflux pattern is characterized by a continuously high frequency of reflux episodes into the third and fourth hours after drinking apple juice. In contrast, the type II reflux pattern is characterized by a high frequency of reflux episodes for 30 to 45 minutes longer than the 2 hours seen in normal children fed apple juice. The type III reflux pattern is a mixture of the type I and type II reflux patterns, but behaves clinically like the type I reflux pattern. Each reflux pattern

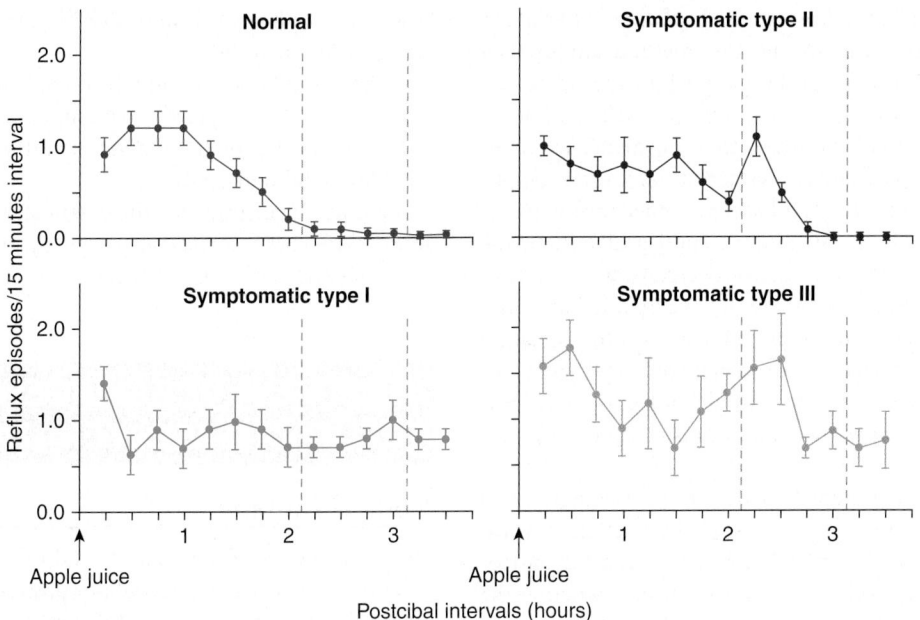

**FIGURE 27-1** Patterns of gastroesophageal reflux episodes following apple juice feedings in normal children and symptomatic children with GERD. *Bars* represent the standard error of the mean. (From Jolley SG, Johnson DG, Herbst JJ, et al. The significance of gastroesophagel reflux patterns in children. *J Pediatr Surg* 1981;16:859–865.)

has prognostic importance and associated clinical findings, which are detailed in Table 27-3.

Another parameter found in the esophageal pH record is the mean duration of acid reflux episodes that occur during sleep and after the first 2 hours postcibal (ZMD). The normal value for the ZMD is 3.8 minutes or less. A prolonged ZMD correlates with the presence of reflux-induced respiratory symptoms in children with GERD; a normal ZMD with the absence of such symptoms. The accuracy of ZMD in a large group of infants and older children with respiratory symptoms or disease thought to be caused by GERD was 97%, with a 6% false-negative rate and no reported false-positive values. The prolonged ZMD is significantly less likely to be detected prior to 39 weeks rather than after 39 weeks postconceptual age in children who are ultimately found to have a prolonged ZMD. Postterm infants with apnea or choking episodes have the highest prevalence of a prolonged ZMD in the first 6 months, whereas children with recurrent aspiration pneumonia, chronic coughing, or chronic wheezing have the highest prevalence of a prolonged ZMD in the first year of life.

A prolonged ZMD in combination with the type I or type III reflux pattern carries an approximately 10% risk for sudden death due to GERD if the GERD is not controlled completely. The risk of sudden infant death due to GERD in infants with the type II reflux pattern and a prolonged ZMD is approximately 2%. All other combinations seen on prolonged esophageal pH monitoring do not appear to be associated with a risk for sudden infant death from GERD. Studying the high-risk combination of a prolonged ZMD and the type I or type III reflux pattern in almost 500 young infants over a 10-year period confirmed GERD as a cause for some sudden infant death syndrome (SIDS) deaths. In infants with a type I reflux pattern and a prolonged ZMD, the risk for SIDS from GERD is 6.8% (34 times the risk for SIDS reported in normal healthy infants at the time the study was published in 1991).

The incidence of the 3 reflux patterns and a prolonged ZMD can vary according to the population studied. Examples of the possible combinations of findings and their incidence are presented in Table 27-1.

## Impedance Plethysmography of the Esophagus

A more recent procedure proposed to confirm the diagnosis of GERD in children is *impedance plethysmography of the*

| TABLE 27-3 | Clinical Findings Associated with Abnormal Patterns of Gastroesophageal Reflux Episodes in Infants | | |
|---|---|---|---|
| | | Spontaneous Resolution | |
| Pattern Type | Associated Conditions[a] | By 1 Year of Age (%) | Reproducibility (%) |
| I | Decreased or normal LESP, large hiatal hernia | 10 | 90 |
| II | Increased LESP, antral or pylorospasm, diarrhea | 70-80 | 70 |
| III | Decreased or normal LESP, large hiatal hernia, change to type I pattern after 10 months of age | 13 | 60 |

[a]LESP, lower esophageal sphincter pressure.

369

*esophagus*, also called *intraluminal esophageal impedance.* Like esophageal pH monitoring, this method employs an intraluminal small-caliber probe placed into the nares and positioned in the esophagus. The probe is usually combined with a pH sensor along with the 4 to 6 impedance channels (1-2 cm apart) that measure electrical resistance in the esophageal lumen. There is always a baseline impedance between the esophageal walls. In an empty esophageal lumen, the impedance is high. The impedance decreases as a bolus of fluid passes in the lumen, but increases as a bolus of air passes in the lumen. It is generally assumed that a gastroesophageal reflux episode is indicated by a drop in impedance that begins at the most distal channel, and a swallowing episode is indicated by a drop in impedance that begins at the most proximal channel.

The technique is designed to detect the frequency and duration of all episodes of gastroesophageal reflux, not just acidic gastroesophageal reflux. It can detect nonacid gastroesophageal reflux episodes, as well as determine whether the episodes are liquid, gas, or a mixture of both. The major problem with this technique is the lack of evidence for a significant role of nonacid gastroesophageal reflux episodes in the pathogenesis of GERD in children. This is not the case with the measurement of acid gastroesophageal reflux episodes with a pH probe.

Other issues concern an arbitrary threshold to define the detection and clearance of gastroesophageal reflux episodes with impedance technology, the inclusion of events less than 15 seconds in duration as gastroesophageal reflux episodes, and the assumption that all retrograde flow in the esophagus is gastroesophageal reflux. (Retrograde flow of contrast material in the esophagus can be seen without gastroesophageal reflux and with a closed gastroesophageal junction during a barium meal.) The thresholds for the definition of a gastroesophageal reflux episode during esophageal pH monitoring are not arbitrary. A level of pH <4 is used to determine the occurrence and duration of a gastroesophageal reflux episode, as described in work published in the 1940s by Hollander, which defined the activation of pepsin (from pepsinogen) as beginning at pH 4 and ending below pH 1, a reason why esophagitis is considered a form of "acid-peptic" disease. The 15-second minimum length of a confirmed gastroesophageal reflux episode was obtained from the minimum length of time necessary to detect a drop in esophageal pH below 4 and then a return to a pH above 4 with an interval between the drop and rise. Such a definition was necessary to distinguish a gastroesophageal reflux episode from movement artifact on an esophageal pH recording moving at a speed of 20 cm (8 in) per hour.

Since a pH sensor is included with the esophageal impedance probe, useful information is not lost when the combined probe is used for prolonged esophageal monitoring in children. Impedance data do have promise for detecting gastroesophageal reflux episodes in patients who do not make sufficient gastric acid for an esophageal pH probe to detect, such as those on acid-suppression medication or those rare patients with congenital achlorhydria. It can also be a useful investigative tool for the immediate postprandial period if the gastric acid is buffered by nonacidic feedings, and may be useful to detect retrograde esophageal flow and esophageal dysmotility in patients with esophageal motility disorders.

At the current time, the authors do not consider impedance monitoring of the esophagus to be superior to pH monitoring of the esophagus for the diagnosis and evaluation of treatment for childhood GERD.

Suggested algorithms for the diagnostic workup of infants and children with GERD suspected by clinical history and physical examination are shown in Figs. 27-2 to 27-4.

## TREATMENT OF GASTROESOPHAGEAL REFLUX DISEASE IN CHILDREN

### Medical Therapy

The cornerstones of treatment for GERD in children are the strict maintenance of the upright or prone-elevated (30°-45°) posture at all times and the thickening of feedings. Small frequent feedings, nasogastric or nasojejunal feedings, and total parenteral nutrition may be used temporarily to provide nutritional support in GERD with severe complications until antireflux medications can be administered (Table 27-4) or an operation can be performed.

The medications used for childhood GERD include antacids, cytoprotective gels (sucralfate, alginic acid), histamine-receptor blockers (cimetidine, ranitidine, and famotidine), proton pump inhibitors (omeprazole, lansoprazole), cholinergic agonists (bethanechol), and dopamine antagonists (metoclopramide, domperidone, cisapride). Antacids, histamine-receptor blockers, and proton pump inhibiters are designed to reduce acid in the refluxed gastric material. Cytoprotective gels cover the esophageal mucosa to provide a shield to acid injury and promote healing. Some cytoprotective gels, such as alginic acid, also provide thickening of gastric contents. Cholinergic agonist and dopamine antagonists have been used to improve competence of the diseased gastroesophageal junction. The desired additional effects may also include an improvement in esophageal and gastric emptying.

Unfortunately, not all of the medications used for GERD in children have been approved by the US Food and Drug Administration for such purposes. Domperidone is not available in the United States, and cisapride has been limited by the manufacturer to restricted use because of rare cardiovascular side effects. Furthermore, the long-term effects and side effects of the newer medications, such as the proton pump inhibitors and the dopamine antagonists, are unknown in children.

### Operative Therapy

The major antireflux operations in children may be classified as either a fundoplication or a gastropexy (Fig. 27-5). Newer endoscopic antireflux procedures with a stapling device or a radiofrequency probe or injection device attempt to control GERD by closing the angle of His with a partial fundoplication or by thickening the wall of the distal esophagus, respectively. The authors have no experience with these newer endoscopic approaches to control GERD,

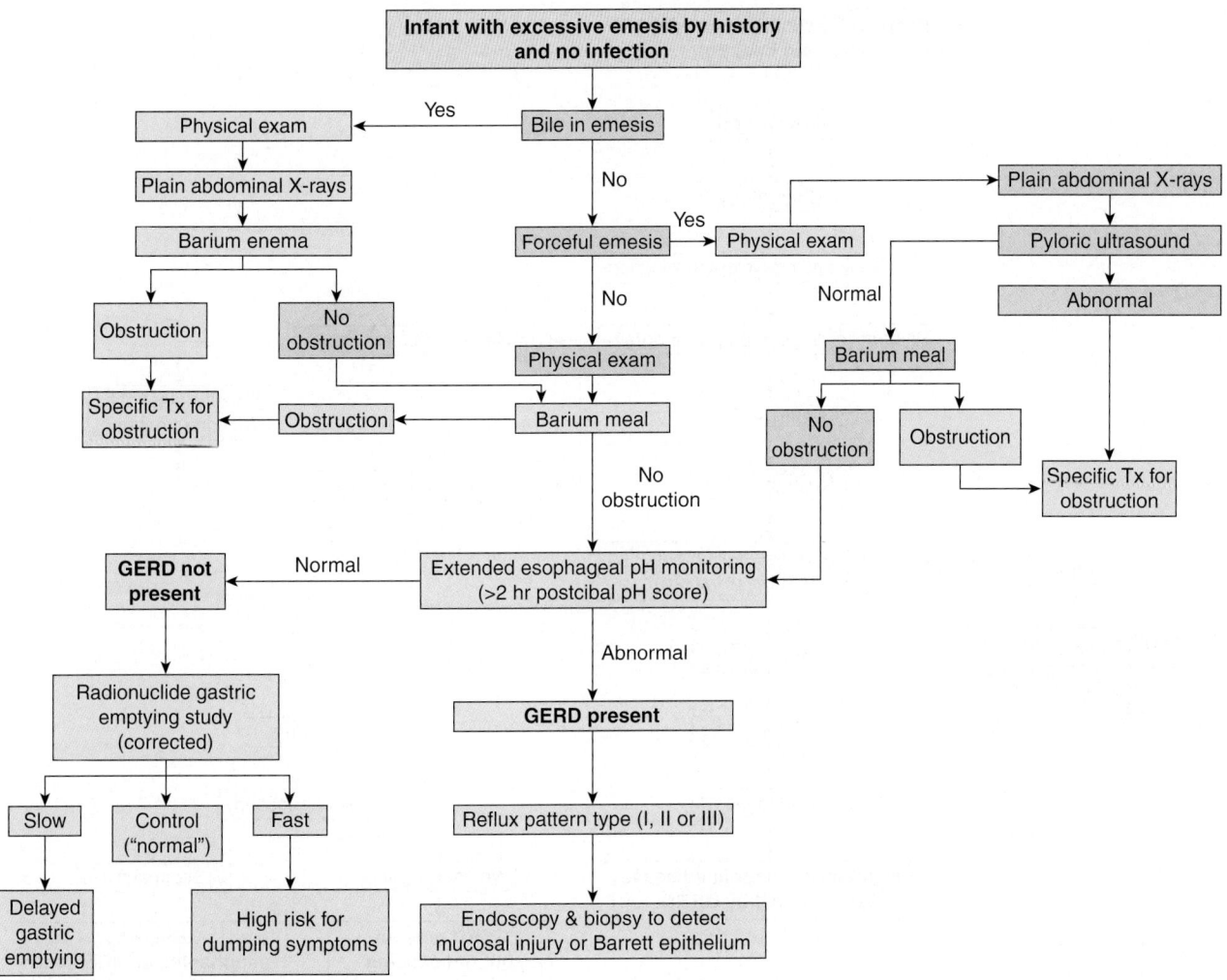

**FIGURE 27-2** Suggested sequence for the diagnostic workup of infants and children with suspected GERD and excessive emesis. (From Jolley SG. In: Giuli R, Tygat GNJ, DeMeester TR, Galmiche JP, eds. *Esophageal Mucosa. Amsterdam: Elsevier Science*; 1994:735–740 with permission.)

but have extensive experience performing fundoplication and gastropexy in children.

Both the fundoplication and gastropexy can be performed by the open or the minimally invasive (laparoscopic) approach. Two major types of fundoplication have been well studied in children: the 360° fundic wrap (Nissen) and the 230° to 270° anterior fundic wrap (Thal). Both work by a nipple valve effect and eliminate most physiological as well as pathological episodes of acid reflux early in the postoperative period. Although fundoplication usually results in a normal or increased resting LESP, the surgeon does not need to achieve an increase in resting LESP over preoperative values to control GERD. Early postoperative extended esophageal pH monitoring can be used to document the effective control of GERD. Side effects and complications of these fundoplications are shown in Table 27-5.

The main gastropexy used for GERD in children was described by Boerema. The apparent effect of this anterior gastropexy on the diseased gastroesophageal junction is to improve competence by "tightening" the gastric sling muscle fibers and increasing the intraabdominal esophageal length. The "tightening" is achieved by the proper spatial orientation of the gastric sling fibers around the angle of His and by producing the proper tension on the gastric sling fibers

as the lesser gastric curvature is approximated to the right subhepatic anterior abdominal wall. Intraoperative esophageal manometry may be a necessary adjunct to assure the proper performance of the gastropexy by those surgeons having limited experience with the Boerema gastropexy. The effect of gastropexy on physiological reflux episodes is usually not as pronounced as following a fundoplication. Early postoperative extended esophageal pH monitoring used to document the effective control of GERD shows more normal acid reflux episodes following feedings than seen with fundoplication. Complications and side effects associated with the Boerema gastropexy are also shown in Table 27-5.

## Open Versus Minimally Invasive Approach

Major antireflux operations in children can be performed with a standard laparotomy (open technique) or laparoscopically (minimally invasive technique). Indications for both approaches in children are identical, but the type of approach may be limited by previous laparotomies or anatomic deformity (eg, severe scoliosis). For example, patients with complex cardiac anomalies that cannot tolerate pneuomoperitoneum may not be good candidates for laparoscopy

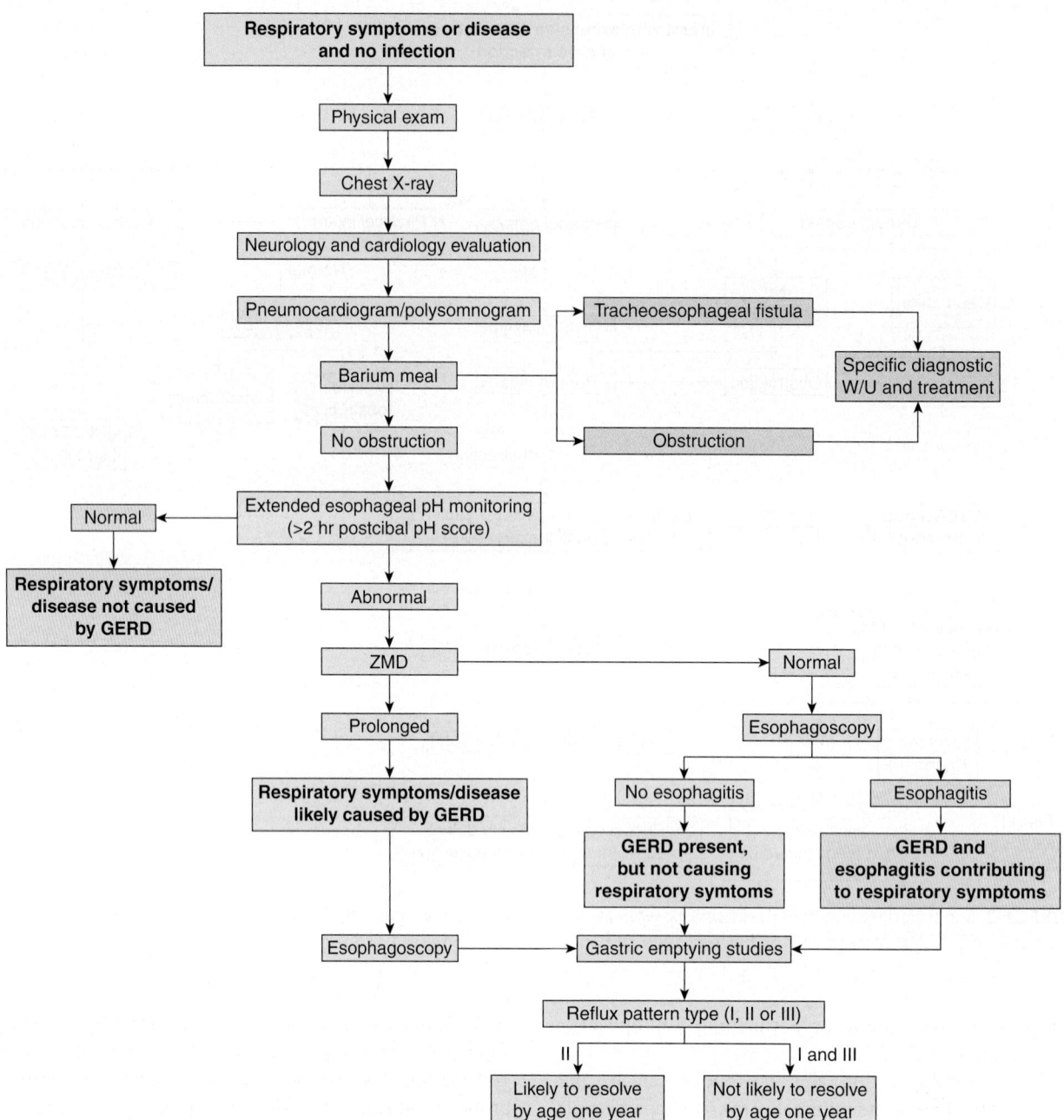

**FIGURE 27-3** Suggested sequence for the diagnostic work-up of infants and children with respiratory symptoms or disease suspected to be caused by GERD. ZMD, mean duration of reflux episodes during sleep; W/U, workup.

and the family should be advised of the possible need for conversion to an open procedure. The fundoplications are the most commonly performed antireflux operations by both approaches, but the minimally invasive technique is still evolving. The authors perform both types of antireflux operations and use both the standard laparotomy and minimally invasive approaches.

Potential advantages of the minimally invasive approach include faster postoperative recovery with resumption of full feedings and normal activity, decreased physiological stress, less pain, and a lower incidence of adhesive small bowel obstruction. Another minimally invasive laparoscopic approach using robotic techniques has been described in children, but the authors have no experience with that method.

There is a distinct learning curve for the performance of the minimally invasive antireflux operation in children, and the long-term control of GERD with this approach so far appears to be inferior to the open approach. This may be due to a steep learning curve, which the senior author finds to be a significant issue in producing an antireflux operation with the minimally invasive technique that is comparable to the same operation performed by the author using the open technique. The short-term (<2 years) control of clinical symptoms and the complication rate of minimally invasive fundoplication in children appear to be similar to the open approach once the surgeon has arrived at the flat portion of the learning curve. However, quantitative postoperative studies with extended esophageal pH monitoring are notably lacking in most series of minimally invasive fundoplications reported in

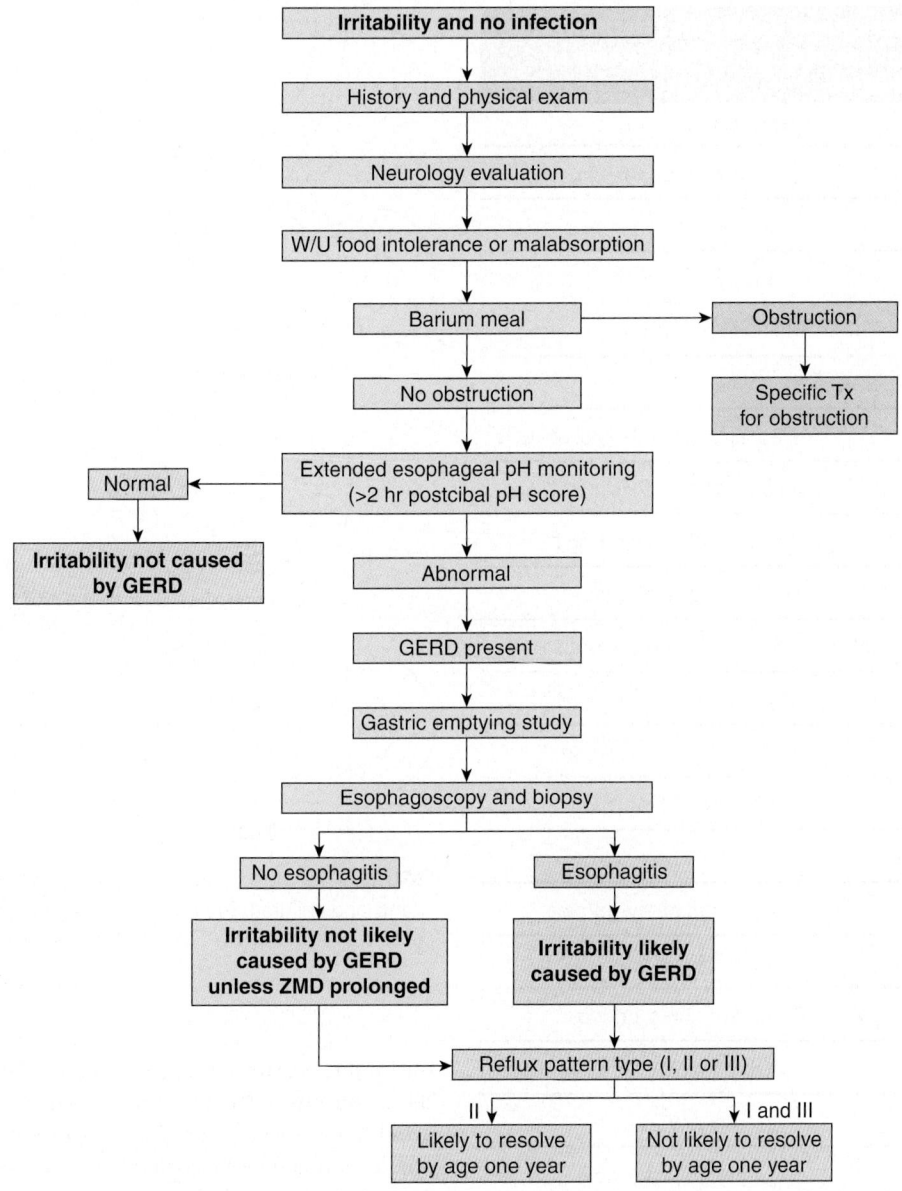

**FIGURE 27-4** Suggested sequence for the diagnostic workup in infants and children with irritability suspected to be caused by GERD. ZMD, mean duration of reflux episodes during sleep; Tx, treatment; W/U, workup.

children. In the few series of children reported with postoperative esophageal pH studies using the Johnson–DeMeester or reflux index method of pH analysis, which have a low false-positive rate and a very high false-negative rate (Table 27-2), the recurrence of GERD during the first 2 years is 10% to 20%. This rate of recurrence for GERD is similar to the senior author's experience, and is currently higher than for the same operation performed by standard laparotomy (Table 27-5). The above information should be disclosed to the child's family or legal guardian during the informed consent process when a surgeon proposes an antireflux operation for a child with GERD.

## Operative Techniques

The preoperative preparation for an antireflux operation is virtually identical to any other nonemergent abdominal operation in a child. Perioperative antibiotics are used

routinely. All patients receive a balanced general anesthetic after being placed in a supine position. If the open approach is used, a transverse upper abdominal incision is performed to access the peritoneal cavity (Fig. 27-6). For the Boerema gastropexy, the open laparotomy incision intersects the midline abdomen three fourths of the distance from the upper xiphoid toward the umbilicus. When the minimally invasive approach is used, at least 4 ports of 5 mm are placed in the abdominal wall to access the peritoneal cavity. The size of the patient determines the position of the ports (Fig. 27-6). The smaller patient, 2 to 10 kg, is turned perpendicular to the bed, while the larger patient is placed in pediatric or adult stirrups, depending on size. All organs in the peritoneal cavity are inspected routinely by vision and palpation (open approach) or by vision alone (minimally invasive approach), but an incidental appendectomy is not performed.

Following exploration of the peritoneal cavity, attention is focused on the stomach and esophageal hiatus in the

| TABLE 27-4 | Medications Used in the Treatment of Gastroesophageal Reflux Disease in Children |
|---|---|
| **Medication** | **Oral Dosage** |
| Antacids | 5-15 mL/dose, q3-6 h |
| Cytoprotective gels | |
| Alginic acid | 5-30 mL/dose, q6 h |
| Sulcralfate | 40-80 mg/kg/d, q6 h |
| Histamine-receptor blockers | |
| Cimetidine | Neonate: 5-20 mg/kg/d, q6-12 h |
| | Infant: 10-20 mg/kg/d, q6-12 h |
| | Child: 20-40 mg/kg/d, q6 h |
| Ranitidine | 5-10 mg/kg/d, q6-12 h |
| Famotidine | Neonate: 0.5-1 mg/kg/dose, qd |
| | Infant: 0.5 mg/kg/dose, q12 h |
| | Child: 1-2 mg/kg/d, q12 h |
| | Adolescent: 20 mg, bid |
| Proton pump inhibitors | |
| Omeprazole | 0.2-3.5 mg/kg/day, qd-bid |
| Lansoprazole | <10 kg: 7.5 mg, qd |
| | 11-30 kg: 15 mg, qd-bid |
| | >30 kg: 30 mg, qd-bid |
| Cholinergic agonists | |
| Bethanechol | 0.4-0.8 mg/kg/day, q6 h |
| Dopamine antagonists | |
| Metoclopramide | 0.4-0.5 mg/kg/day, q6 h |
| Cisapride | 0.2-0.3 mg/kg/dose, tid-qid |
| Domperidone | 1.2-2.4 mg/kg/day, q6 h |

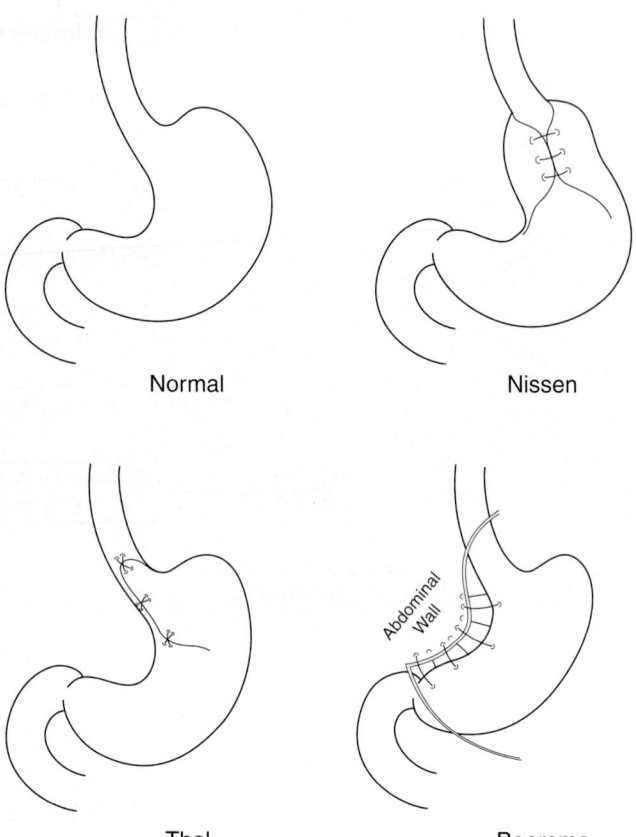

**FIGURE 27-5** Three antireflux operations used by the author in infants and children. The normal stomach is also depicted for comparison. (From Jolley SG. *Surg Clin North Am* 1992;72:1365–1391.)

diaphragm. The phrenoesophageal attachments are divided completely around the entire circumference of the lower esophagus, with care taken to minimize trauma to both the anterior and posterior vagal nerve trunks, as well as their branches. Both vagal nerve trunks are kept with the esophagus as it is mobilized from the lower mediastinum. At least 3 cm of lower esophagus are mobilized. The crus of the diaphragm is then approximated behind the esophagus with a figure-of-8 suturing technique using 2-0 nonabsorbable sutures. A curved hemostat tip should pass easily between the closed crus and the esophagus containing a nasogastric tube.

From this point onward, the 3 antireflux operations used in children differ. For the *Nissen fundoplication* (Fig. 27-7), 3 or more of the upper short gastric vessels are divided to mobilize the fundus. The posterior gastric fundus is then passed behind the esophagus in a manner described by Tunell and Smith to avoid "corkscrewing" or twisting of the fundus. A 360° fundoplication is then performed around the esophagus, which contains a weighted Hurst esophageal bougie large enough to efface the esophagus. The bougies used generally depend on the child's size, and are usually 20F to 34F in infants and 32F to 50F in older children. Three interrupted 2-0 nonabsorbable sutures are used to attach the fundus to the anterior esophageal muscularis and complete the fundoplication with a length of 2 to 3 cm. The loose nature of the fundoplication is demonstrated by being able to pass easily a right-angled clamp between the wrapped fundus and the esophagus containing the bougie. With the bougie in place, the diaphragm is sutured with nonabsorbable sutures to the esophagus at 3 points around the esophageal hiatus. This portion of the operation can be performed either before or after the fundic wrap, but is easier if done before performing the fundic wrap.

For the laparoscopic approach, the surgeon stands at the child's feet, with an assistant on either side. After a standard skin prep and draping, the umbilicus is anesthetized with local anesthetic and a transumbilical incision, large enough to accommodate a 5-mm trocar, is made directly into the cicatrix. The abdomen is then insufflated to 12 to 15 mm Hg of mercury, depending on the size of the patient. Lower pressures may be required in the neonate to allow adequate ventilation and this must be carefully monitored by the

| TABLE 27-5 | Common Side Effects and Complications of Antireflux Operations[a] | | | | | |
|---|---|---|---|---|---|---|
| | **Nissen** | | **Thal** | | **Boerema** | |
| Side Effect/Complication | Laparotomy | Laparoscopy (%) | Laparotomy (%) | Laparoscopy (%) | Laparotomy (%) | Laparoscopy (%) |
| *Recurrent GERD*[b] | | | | | | |
| Immediate[c] | 1.1% | 25% | 1.2% | 33% | 2.4% | 0% |
| Short-term[d] | 1.7% | 25% | 1.6% | 33% | 4.3% | |
| Intermediate-term[e] | 2.9% | 25% | 2% | | 4.3% | |
| Long-term[f] | 3-5% | | 3%-5% | | 4%-5% | |
| Paraesophageal hernia | 5% | 12.5% | 5% | 0% | <1% | 0% |
| Reoperation within 5 years[g] | 10.3% | 25% | 3.1% | | 4.3% | |
| | **Nissen** | | **Thal** | | **Boerema** | |
| Inability to burp or vomit | 1-2 years | | 2-3 months | | <1 month | |
| **Gas-bloat: Preoperative gastric emptying**[h] | | | | | | |
| Slow | 15%[i] | | 15% | | 15% | |
| Control | <1% | | <1% | | <1% | |
| Fast | 10% | | 10% | | 10% | |
| **Gas-bloat: Postoperative gastric emptying** | | | | | | |
| Slow | 30% | | 30% | | 30% | |
| Control | 0% | | 0% | | 0% | |
| Fast | 0% | | 0% | | 0% | |
| **Dumping syndrome: Preoperative gastric emptying**[h] | | | | | | |
| Slow | 0%[i] | | 0% | | 0% | |
| Control | <1% | | <1% | | <1% | |
| Fast | 20% | | 20% | | 20% | |
| **Dumping syndrome: Postoperative gastric emptying** | | | | | | |
| Slow | 0% | | 0% | | 0% | |
| Control | 0% | | 0% | | 0% | |
| Fast | 45% | | 45% | | 45% | |
| Small-bowel obstruction | 5% | | 1% | | 1% | |
| Esophageal obstruction | <1% | | Rare | | Rare | |
| Chronic abdominal pain unrelated to gas-bloat, obstruction, or paraesophageal hernia | Unusual | | Unusual | | 9% | |

[a]Represents the senior author's experience with the Nissen fundoplication, Thal fundoplication, and Boerema gastropexy, performed by laparotomy and laparoscopy and used for the treatment of GERD in infants and children.
[b]Defined by abnormal 18 to 24 hours esophageal pH monitoring (*N* = 502 patients studied postoperatively: Nissen = 159, laparoscopic Nissen = 24, Thal = 248, laparoscopic Thal = 9, Boerema = 58, laparoscopic Boerema = 4).
[c]Less than 3 months postoperatively.
[d]Three months to 5 years postoperatively.
[e]Five to 10 years postoperatively.
[f]More than 10 years postoperatively.
[g]Reoperation for recurrent GERD, paraesophageal hernia, or small-bowel obstruction.
[h]Corrected for postcibal gastroesophageal reflux episodes.
[i]Percentage of patients with findings who develop gas-bloat or dumping syndrome.

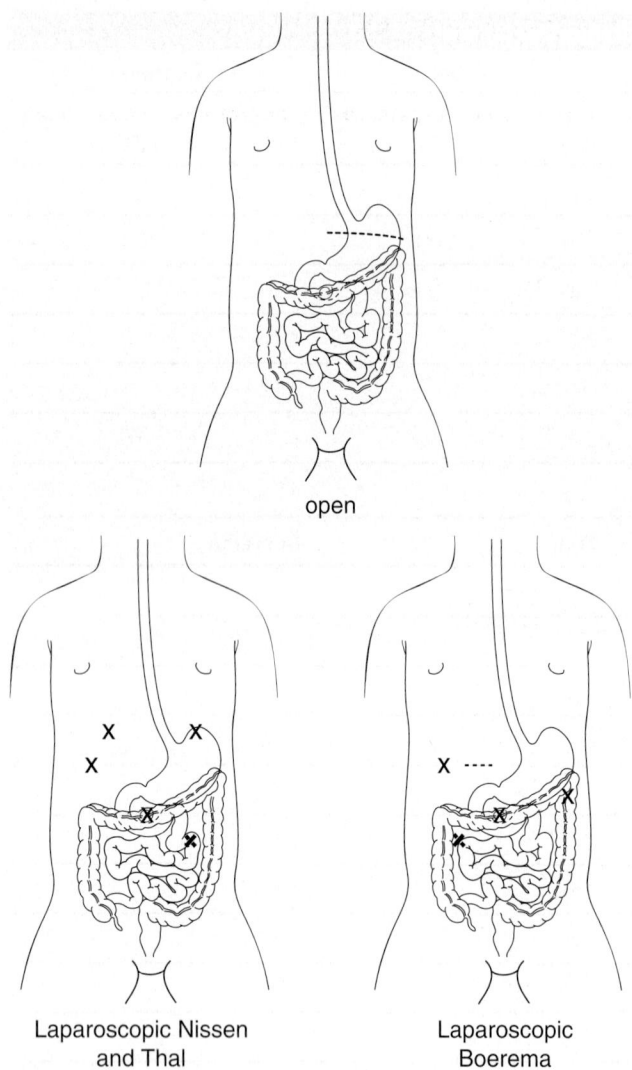

open

Laparoscopic Nissen
and Thal

Laparoscopic
Boerema

**FIGURE 27-6** The location of incision for open laparotomy and port sites (**X**) for laparoscopy used to approach antireflux operations in children. **A.** Open laparotomy, (**B**) laparoscopic Nissen and Thal fundoplication, and (**C**) laparoscopic Boerema gastropexy. *Dotted lines* or ports on laparoscopic approach indicate optional access sites.

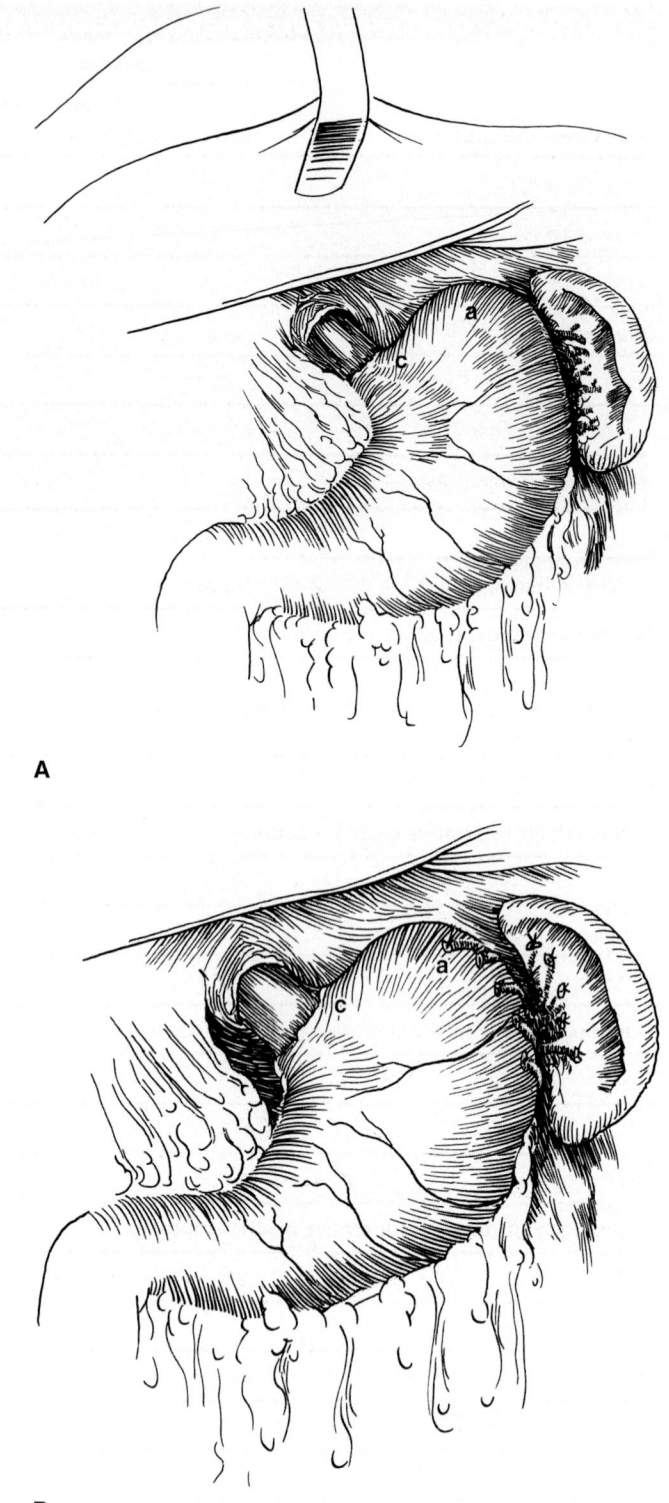

A

B

**FIGURE 27-7** Steps used to perform the Nissen fundoplication in children include (**A**) exposure of the anatomy prior to dissection, (**B**) division of the short gastric vessels,

anesthesiologist. The patient is then placed in reverse Trendelenburg position and the monitor placed directly over the patient's head. A 5-mm scope with a 30° lens is then placed through the umbilical port and, under direct visualization, a 5-mm right subcostal port is placed. A 5-mm fan-type retractor is then introduced and used to retract the left lobe of the liver to reveal the gastroesophageal junction. Subsequently, 2 working ports are placed, the first in the right midepigastrium and the second in the optimal location for a gastrostomy tube (if needed). Finally, a fifth port is placed in the left lower quadrant for retraction (Fig. 27-6).

A harmonic scalpel device is then used to divide the short gastric vessels along the greater curvature of the stomach. Once this is completed, the retroesophageal dissection is begun from the left exposing the left crura of the esophageal hiatus. Attention is then directed to the gastrohepatic ligament, which is opened using the harmonic scalpel. The retroesophageal dissection is completed using both blunt

dissection and sharp dissection with the aid of the harmonic scalpel. An appropriately sized Hurst bougie is passed into the stomach and an umbilical tape is passed posterior to the esophagus. The tape is then used to elevate the esophagus to expose and facilitate the crural closure. Next, the crura are approximated with 2 to 3 interrupted 2-0 nonabsorbable sutures. The fundus is grasped through the retroesophageal

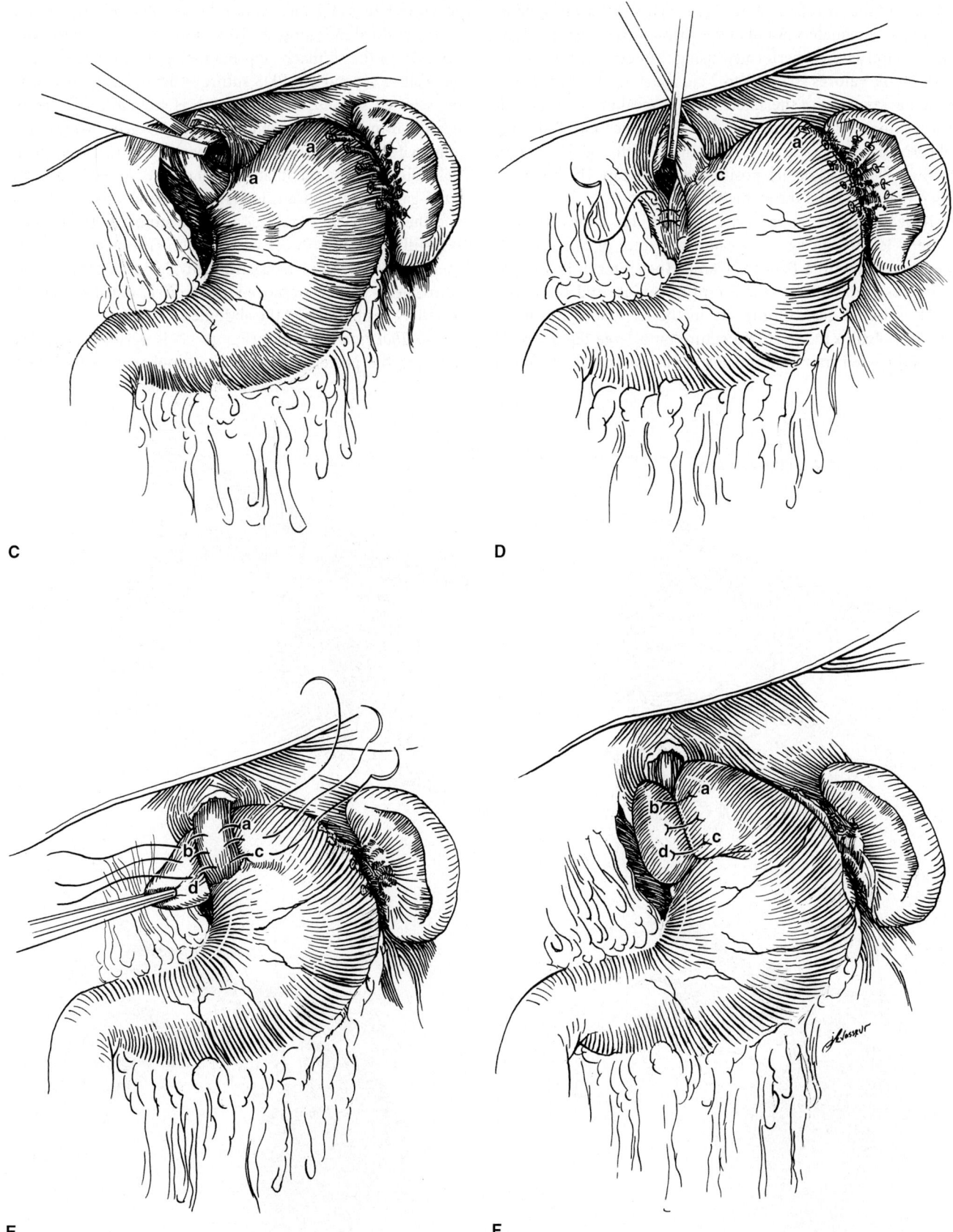

C

D

E

F

**FIGURE 27-7** (*Continued*) (**C**) mobilization of the distal esophagus, (**D**) closure of the diaphragmatic crus, (**E**) passage of the posterior gastric fundus around the esophagus with subsequent suturing of the fundus to the esophagus, and (**F**) completed fundoplication. Here **a** indicates anterior fundus; **b** posterior fundus; **c** anterior angle of His; and **d** posterior angle of His.

space and the so-called "shoe-shine" maneuver performed to ensure an adequate amount of stomach for the wrap. The fundoplication is then performed using 3 interrupted 2-0 nonabsorbable sutures spaced 1 to 2 cm apart, with care taken to include a portion of the anterior esophageal muscularis with each suture. After completing the fundoplication, 3-0 nonabsorbable sutures are used to fix the wrap to the diaphragm at the 3, 9, and 12 o'clock positions of the wrap. The bougie is then removed from the stomach.

If required, an appropriate location for a gastrostomy tube is located along the greater curvature of the stomach and grasped with a Babcock clamp. The stomach is brought into close proximity to the 5-mm trocar site and the previously selected gastrostomy site in the left upper quadrant. A 2-0 polydioxanone (PDS) suture on a large taper needle is then passed transabdominally above the trocar site and a generous bite is taken just above the selected gastrostomy site on the body of the stomach. This suture is then used to place traction on the stomach, approximating it with the abdominal wall. A second 2-0 PDS suture is then placed inferior to the selected site. Once the stomach is secured in this manner, the 5-mm trocar is removed and a 14-gauge needle and guidewire are placed into the stomach. The tract is sequentially dilated using the dilator kit of choice. An appropriately sized gastrostomy button is placed over the smallest dilator and the wire used to guide it into the stomach. The balloon is insufflated under direct visualization. The stay sutures are then loosely tied over the gastrostomy device. All trocars and instruments are then removed under direct visualization, followed by desufflation of the abdomen.

The *Thal fundoplication* (Fig. 27-8) is performed by first suturing the posterior wall of the esophagus to the crural

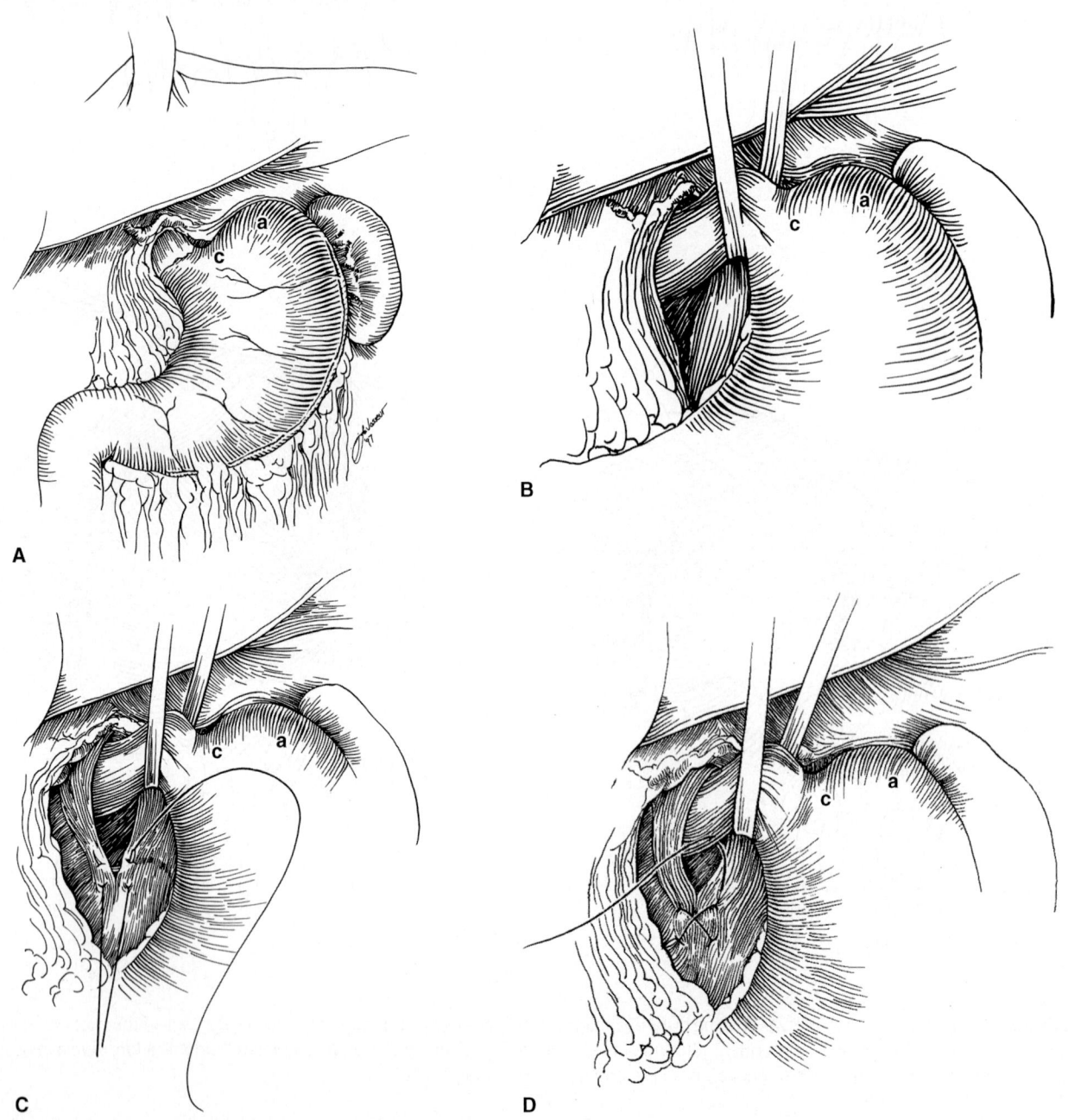

**FIGURE 27-8** Steps used to perform a Thal fundoplication in children include (**A**) exposure of the anatomy prior to dissection, (**B**) dissection of the distal esophagus, (**C**) closure of the diaphragmatic crus, (**D**) suture fixation of the posterior esophagus to the crural closure,

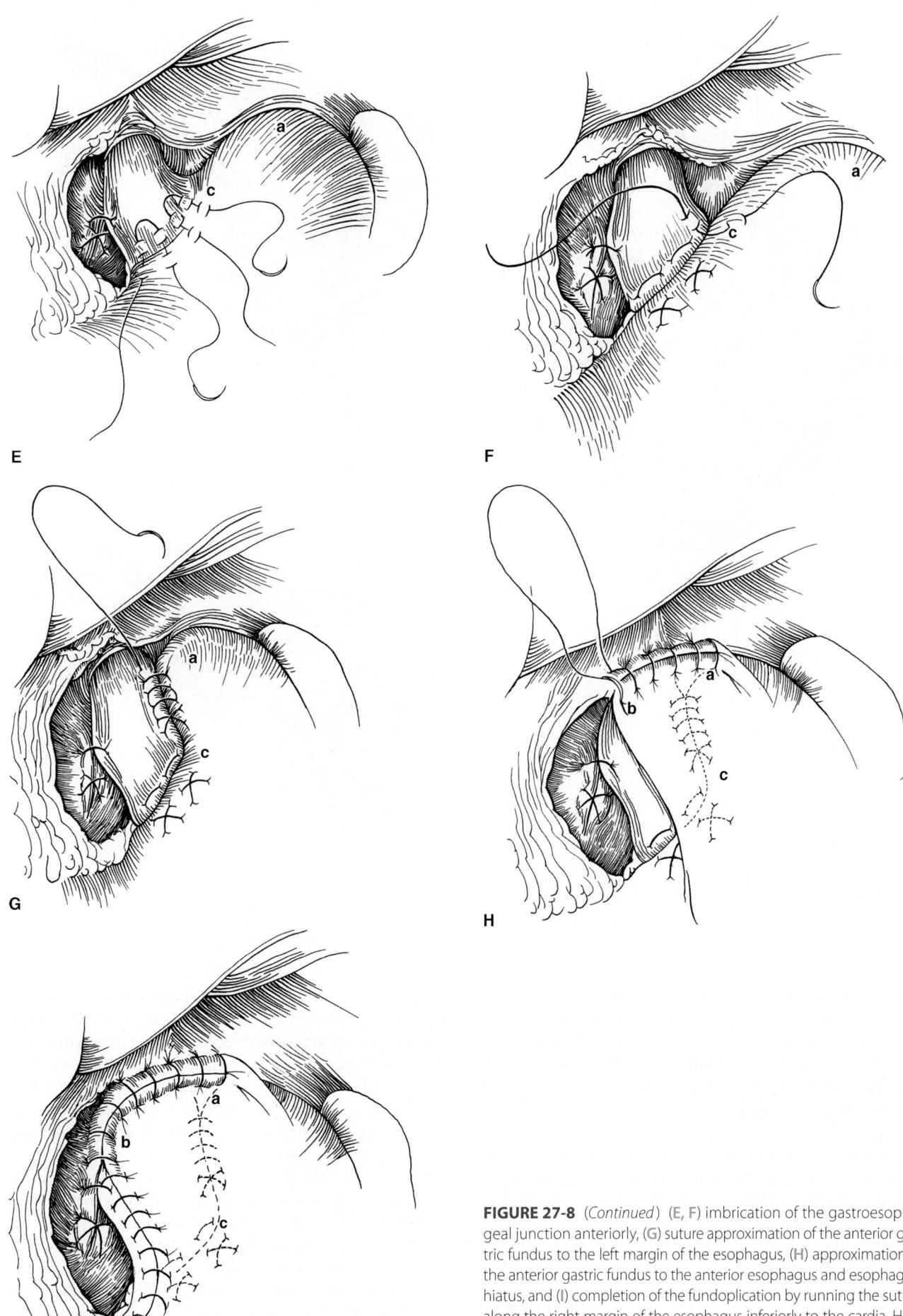

E

F

G

H

I

**FIGURE 27-8** (*Continued*) (**E, F**) imbrication of the gastroesophageal junction anteriorly, (**G**) suture approximation of the anterior gastric fundus to the left margin of the esophagus, (**H**) approximation of
the anterior gastric fundus to the anterior esophagus and esophageal
hiatus, and (**I**) completion of the fundoplication by running the suture
along the right margin of the esophagus inferiorly to the cardia. Here
**a** indicates anterior fundus; **b** posterior fundus; and **c** anterior angle
of His.

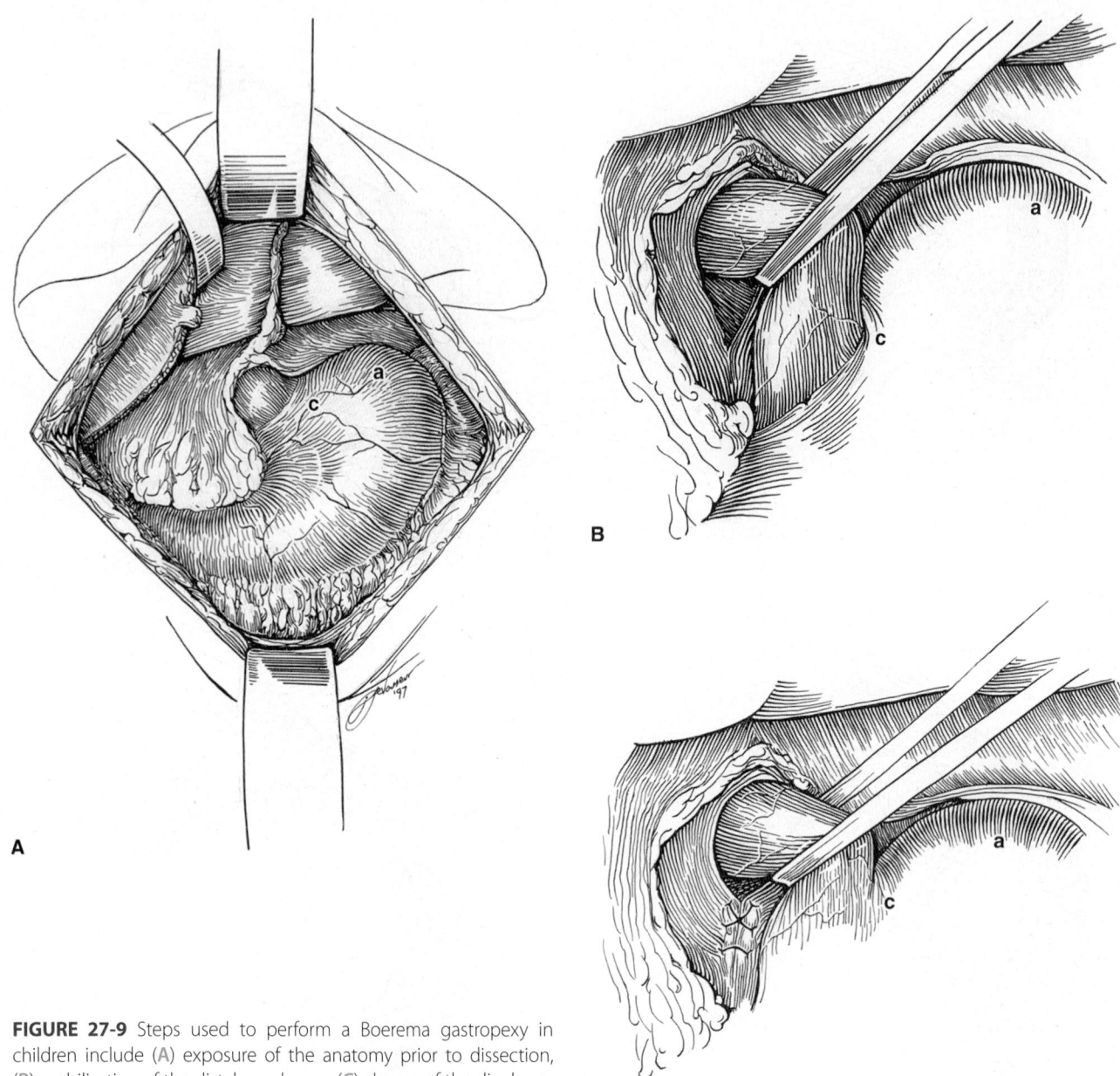

**FIGURE 27-9** Steps used to perform a Boerema gastropexy in children include (**A**) exposure of the anatomy prior to dissection, (**B**) mobilization of the distal esophagus, (**C**) closure of the diaphragmatic crus,

closure with nonabsorbable sutures to assure at least 2.5 cm of intraabdominal esophagus posteriorly. Anteriorly, the gastroesophageal junction is imbricated using interrupted nonabsorbable 3-0 sutures. At approximately 230° to 270° from the lesser curvature portion of the gastroesophageal junction and anteriorly around the angle of His, the imbrication is carried out with a CV-4 Gortex suture (WL Gore & Associates, Inc, Phoenix, AZ). This same suture is then used, in a running fashion, to approximate a rectangle of anterior gastric fundus to the anterior intraabdominal esophagus to complete the 230° to 270° anterior fundoplication. The suture is run up the left portion of intraabdominal esophagus to the esophageal hiatus, and then across the esophageal hiatus in the diaphragm to the right portion of the intraabdominal esophagus. Completion of the fundoplication is accomplished by running the Gortex suture down the right margin of the esophagus to the cardia, where the suture is tied to itself. Interrupted

nonabsorbable 2-0 sutures can be used to perform the fundoplication in place of the running Gortex suture, if desired. The fundoplication is performed with only a nasogastric tube in the esophagus. When performed by laparoscopy, the Thal fundoplication utilizes the same laparoscopic approach and port locations as used for the Nissen fundoplication. The intraabdominal portion of the operation is otherwise identical to the open approach.

The *Boerema gastropexy* (Fig. 27-9) is performed in the open approach by dissecting the skin and subcutaneous fat away from the anterior rectus sheath to the right of the ligamentum teres hepatis. This step is not needed, however, for the minimally invasive approach. At least 4 nonabsorbable 2-0 sutures are then placed through the full thickness of muscle and fascia of the right subhepatic abdominal wall to the right of the ligamentum teres hepatis and 1 to 2 cm cephalad to the incision for the open approach, or

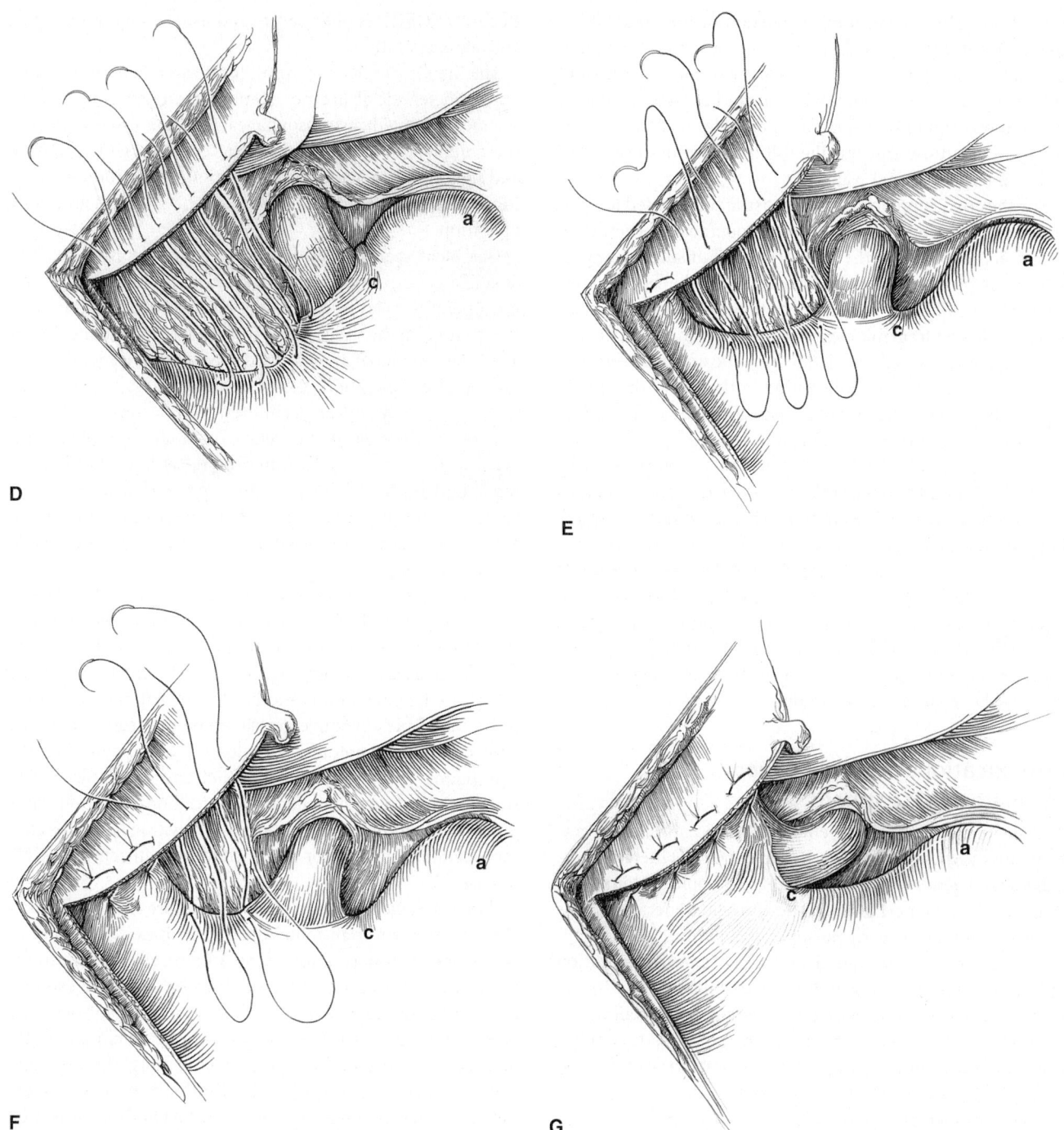

D

E

F

G

**FIGURE 27-9** (*Continued*) (D) placement of the sutures for fixation of the lesser gastric curvature to the right subhepatic anterior abdominal wall, and (E-G) sequential tying of the fixation sutures from distal to proximal to achieve the appropriate tension on the gastric sling fibers to tighten the gastroesophageal junction and increase the length of intraabdominal esophagus. Here **a** indicates anterior fundus, **c** anterior angle of His.

to an imagined transverse upper abdominal incision in the same spot for the minimally invasive approach. Each suture placed though the abdominal wall is passed also through the muscle sling fibers along the lesser curvature portion of the stomach in 1-cm intervals. The most laterally placed suture in the abdominal wall is the most distally placed suture in the stomach, and the most medially placed suture is at the ligamentum teres hepatis in the abdominal wall and the lesser curvature portion of the gastroesophageal

junction in the stomach. Prior to tying each suture and approximating the lesser curvature of the stomach to the posterior rectus fascia and peritoneum of the right subhepatic abdominal wall, the tension on the esophagus is checked and the bowel is kept away from the area. The sutures are tied sequentially from lateral to medial (distal to proximal on the stomach) to complete the gastropexy.

When the Boerema gastropexy is performed by laparoscopy, the port sites differ from those used in the fundoplications

GASTROESOPHAGEAL REFLUX DISEASE

381

(Fig. 27-6). The intraabdominal portion of the operation is the same as for the open approach. One variation is that fixation of the lesser curvature portion of the stomach to the right subhepatic anterior abdominal wall can be via a small skin incision or a right lower quadrant port (Fig. 27-6), as long as the fixation sutures traverse the full thickness of muscle and fascia in the abdominal wall.

For the open approach, the nasogastric tube is used for gastric decompression for 1 to 3 days postoperatively. Thereafter, a diet appropriate for the patient's age is instituted gradually as the postoperative ileus resolves. For the laparoscopic approach, a child only undergoing a fundoplication or gastropexy is allowed to drink clear liquids early on postoperative day 1 and is advanced as tolerated to a postoperative antireflux surgery diet prior to discharge. If the infant or child is also undergoing placement of a gastrostomy tube, the tube is left to gravity drainage overnight and elevated for use early on postoperative day 1. Feeds are initiated in a continuous fashion for the first 24 hours and then converted to bolus feedings on postoperative day 2. Prior to discharge from the hospital, but after the first 24 to 48 hours and full feedings have been tolerated, a postoperative extended esophageal pH study is recommended to document the control of GERD with the operation. The stay sutures are removed prior to discharge, but not before day 2 or 3. Follow-up extended esophageal pH monitoring is recommended at 5- to 10-year intervals postoperatively, regardless of symptoms.

## Complications and Side Effects of Operative Treatment

The complications and side effects of the 3 antireflux operations are shown in Table 27-5. Recurrent GERD literally indicates a recurrence of the defective gastroesophageal junction that was documented prior to the antireflux operation. This is uncommon in the early postoperative period. Since symptoms similar to those caused by GERD (emesis, aspiration episodes or respiratory symptoms, irritability, refusal to eat, or poor growth) can be caused by infection, poor swallowing, impaired esophageal emptying, slow or rapid gastric emptying, and overfeeding, a complete evaluation of the child with suspected recurrent GERD is warranted.

The consumer-driven trend for less invasive operations has been accompanied by a trend for less invasive or abbreviated testing for GERD. Until there is a clearly proven equivalent and less invasive test for GERD, it is a serious mistake to omit critical evaluation techniques for GERD that are invasive, such as extended esophageal pH monitoring, in both the preoperative and postoperative evaluations. At a minimum, the postoperative reevaluation should include a barium meal, extended esophageal pH monitoring (Jolley–Johnson method), and a radionuclide gastric emptying study. Repeat endoscopy may be needed to evaluate for persistent mucosal injury.

If extended esophageal pH monitoring is normal, then recurrent GERD is unlikely. If a repeat operation is needed, it should be directed at correcting the abnormality producing the child's symptoms. When both the patient and the type of antireflux operation are selected properly, the long-term (>10 years) development of recurrent GERD is less than 5%.

Recurrent GERD is often severe and usually requires a repeat antireflux operation.

The inability to burp or vomit for a variable period of time is a characteristic of all types of antireflux operations. Because the reconstructed gastroesophageal junction usually restricts the complete evacuation of gastric contents with vomiting and may result in acute gastric dilation, induction of vomiting should be avoided in children who have had an antireflux operation.

Gas-bloat seems to be related to a preoperative delay in effective gastric emptying (corrected gastric emptying) or a postoperative delay in gastric emptying related to intraoperative trauma to the vagal nerve trunks. In most infants under age 1, any gas-bloat symptoms resolve within 6 months after an antireflux operation. Unfortunately, the gas-bloat symptoms may not disappear in children with persistent CNS disease or severe vagal nerve injury, or in children older than age 1 at the time of operation. The delay in gastric emptying found postoperatively in these patients usually can be reversed with prokinetic agents (eg, metoclopramide or cisapride) or a gastric drainage procedure (eg, pyloroplasty or pyloromyotomy).

Dumping symptoms can occur with any antireflux operation postoperatively. The main factor in the development of the dumping symptoms postoperatively is a rapid preoperative effective gastric emptying. A reduction in gastric volume related to the operation is another factor that may contribute to the rapid postoperative gastric emptying seen in children with dumping symptoms. Symptoms may be controlled by eliminating disaccharides in the diet and by administering small-volume frequent or continuous feedings. In most infants under age 1, dumping symptoms resolve within 6 months after the operation, except for some children with chronic CNS disease.

Paraesophageal hiatal hernia is far more likely following a fundoplication than following a gastropexy. The cause of paraesophageal hernia following an antireflux operation is unknown, but important factors may be excessive esophageal dissection, an inadequate closure of the diaphragmatic crus, poor nutrition, chronic gagging or retching, severe delayed gastric emptying, or chronic lung disease with hyperaeration of the lungs. The fundoplication is usually intact in paraesophageal hernia associated with Nissen fundoplication. Simple operative reduction of the paraesophageal hernia and intact Nissen fundoplication is all that is needed to treat children with large paraesophageal hernias or children with symptoms and signs of mechanical obstruction of the herniated stomach, such as epigastric pain, refusal to eat, postcibal vomiting, gastric bleeding, proximal gastric ulcer, or gastric volvulus. The same is true for paraesophageal hiatal hernia associated with an intact Boerema gastropexy. Recurrent GERD with paraesophageal hernia in association with Nissen fundoplication or Boerema gastropexy requires a redo antireflux operation. A large paraesophageal hiatal hernia associated with the Thal fundoplication often indicates a failed operation with recurrent GERD, requiring reoperation with repeat fundoplication to repair the paraesophageal hernia.

Postoperative small-bowel obstruction can occur following any antireflux operation (Table 27-5), but occurs more often following Nissen fundoplication. Most postoperative small-bowel obstructions are caused by adhesions and appear within 2 years following an antireflux operation. Some postoperative small-bowel obstructions are caused by ileoileal intussusceptions and appear within the first week after an operation. Reoperation is usually needed to relieve the obstruction. An obstruction of the distal esophagus from antireflux operations in children is rare following the Thal fundoplication and Boerema gastropexy, but is more likely to occur following Nissen fundoplication due to a "tight" wrap or severe associated dysmotility of the esophageal body with impaired esophageal emptying preoperatively. Reoperation and redo fundoplication may require a distal esophagocardiomyotomy to relieve the esophageal obstruction.

Chronic abdominal pain may be seen following Boerema gastropexy at the site of suture fixation of the stomach to the anterior abdominal wall, and is unrelated to small-bowel obstruction, paraesophageal hiatal hernia, or gas-bloat. Children experiencing chronic abdominal pain may require reoperation with conversion of the gastropexy to a fundoplication to control the pain. Wound infection occurs in 2% to 3% of patients, but major infection resulting from gastric or esophageal leak is rare. It is also rare for an infant or child who has only GERD to die as a result of complications from an antireflux operation. The operative mortality is less than 5% in children with life-threatening associated diseases, and less than 1% in children with no associated diseases. Reoperation in the first 5 years postoperatively is more likely with the Nissen fundoplication than with the Thal fundoplication or Boerema gastropexy (Table 27-5).

## Selection of Antireflux Operation

Successful antireflux operations in children depend on both patient selection and selection of operation. The selection of an antireflux operation for children is based both on the ability of the operation to control the GERD long-term and on the potential side effects and complications from the operation (Fig. 27-10). In children who have antireflux operations due to recurrent emesis secondary to GERD, the presence of associated CNS disease, advanced esophagitis, and a prolonged ZMD are important. For children with CNS disease and repeated emesis, the Nissen fundoplication with gastrostomy is performed. Often, these children do not take oral feedings well even after the GERD has been controlled. If a gastrostomy was not placed during the initial operative procedure, a subsequent gastrostomy is usually needed for supplemental feedings. The Nissen fundoplication has fared better than the Thal fundoplication or Boerema gastropexy in children who have CNS disease or require a feeding gastrostomy.

When no CNS disease is present, the presence of advanced esophagitis or a prolonged ZMD must be considered. Children with advanced esophagitis have better long-term control of the esophagitis with the Nissen fundoplication than with the Thal fundoplication or Boerema gastropexy. In children without advanced esophagitis who have a prolonged ZMD, the Thal fundoplication provides good long-term control of emesis equivalent to the Nissen fundoplication and with a lower incidence of postoperative small-bowel obstruction.

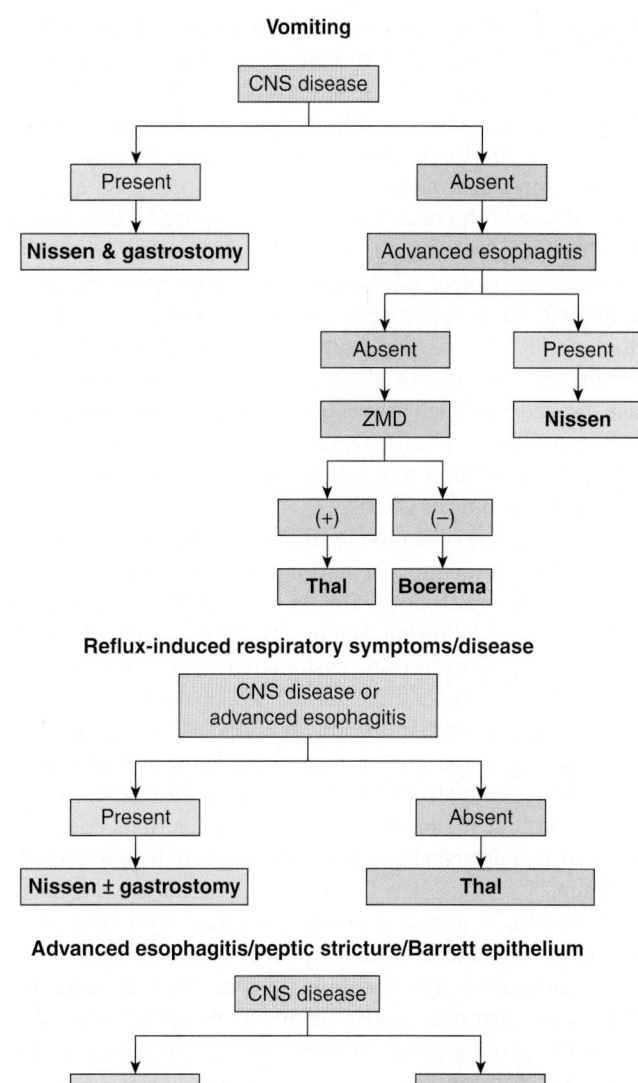

**FIGURE 27-10** General algorithm for the selection of an antireflux operation in infants and children based on the complication of GERD, associated CNS disease, and the prolonged (+) or normal (–) value for the mean duration of acid reflux episodes during sleep (ZMD) derived from extended esophageal pH monitoring. (From Jolley SG. *Surg Clin North Am* 1992;72:1365–1391.)

Although the most physiologic of the antireflux operations discussed, the Boerema gastropexy is unsuitable for children with a prolonged ZMD. The angulation of the esophagus produced by the Boerema gastropexy can actually prolong the ZMD further by impeding the esophageal clearance of acid reflux episodes, even though the frequency of acid reflux episodes has been decreased to a normal level. This can lead to postoperative respiratory symptoms from acid reflux episodes that are not cleared from the esophagus. However, the Boerema gastropexy is the procedure of choice in neurologically normal children with recurrent emesis, a normal ZMD, and no advanced esophagitis.

A Thal fundoplication is the antireflux operation of choice for infants and children with reflux-induced respiratory symptoms and no evidence of CNS disease or advanced esophagitis. When CNS disease or advanced esophagitis are also present, the Nissen fundoplication is the procedure of choice, with or without gastrostomy, respectively. The Nissen fundoplication is the procedure of choice for peptic esophageal stricture or Barrett esophagus, except for children with coexistent primary esophageal dysmotility. For these children, the Thal fundoplication provides adequate control of GERD without impeding esophageal emptying, as is sometimes found following Nissen fundoplication. When esophagitis has progressed to severe esophageal stricture or shortening, more complex operative procedures such as segmental esophageal resection, with anastomosis or esophageal replacement, or Collis gastroplasty in addition to fundoplication, may be required to control symptoms of GERD.

As a protective operation for feeding gastrostomy, the Nissen fundoplication fares better than the Thal fundoplication and Boerema gastropexy. This is because the normal acid reflux episodes following feedings may not be well tolerated by children with swallowing dysfunction and the Nissen fundoplication eliminates these normal postcibal reflux episodes for a longer period than the Thal fundoplication or Boerema gastropexy. A lesser curvature gastrostomy with a Boerema gastropexy may prevent GERD associated with gastrostomy placement, but it cannot eliminate the deleterious effect of even normal postcibal acid reflux episodes in these impaired children.

Performing a gastric drainage procedure with antireflux operation in children is controversial. Several factors must be considered in this decision: (1) Only 15% of children with slow corrected gastric emptying preoperatively subsequently develop gas-bloat symptoms. (2) In most infants with gas-bloat symptoms and slow corrected gastric emptying, the symptoms resolve within 6 months after an antireflux operation. (3) Slow corrected gastric emptying in children older than age 1 or with chronic CNS disease is more likely to produce gas-bloat symptoms and less likely to resolve following antireflux operation. (4) Gastric drainage procedures predispose the child to long-term serious side effects such as dumping symptoms and bile reflux gastritis. Currently, a concomitant pyloroplasty is performed only in children who are older than age 1 and have demonstrated slow corrected gastric emptying preoperatively.

## Treatment According to Complications of Childhood GERD

The goal of antireflux therapy in children is to provide the best long-term control of GERD with the lowest risk for death or other side effects directly related to therapy.

### Recurrent Emesis

In infants with recurrent emesis caused by GERD and without advanced mucosal injury, the first consideration is the presence or absence of growth retardation (Fig. 27-11). Infants with growth retardation are initially treated with upright positioning, thickened feedings, and medication (histamine-receptor blocker plus metoclopramide) for at least 6 weeks. For a child with the type I or type III reflux pattern and a

prolonged ZMD, the option of a repeat extended esophageal pH study on medication is discussed with the child's family or legal guardian. If repeat esophageal pH indicates that the medication is controlling the GERD, then the child may be treated with the aggressive medical antireflux regimen described and the addition of home apnea monitoring. If, however, repeat esophageal pH monitoring on medication indicates that the GERD is not controlled, then an antireflux operation is recommended (Fig. 27-10). The other option to be considered by the family or legal guardian of an infant with recurrent emesis, growth retardation, a prolonged ZMD, and the type I or type III reflux pattern is to proceed directly to an antireflux operation because of the high risk for sudden death from this kind of GERD. All patients treated nonoperatively have their progress reevaluated after 6 weeks of therapy. If there has been improvement in weight gain, resolution of emesis, and no significant apnea or bradycardia, the nonoperative therapy is continued at least until the child is 10 to 12 months of age, when another extended esophageal pH study should be repeated with the child off medications for 48 hours. A child with persistent poor weight gain, persistent emesis, or significant apnea or bradycardia, should have an antireflux operation (Fig. 27-10).

For patients with a normal ZMD, the aggressive medical antireflux regimen described should be tried, and the patient reevaluated after 6 weeks. An antireflux operation should be recommended for patients who continue to lose weight during the trial of medical therapy or who continue to have poor weight gain at the time of reevaluation. Patients with improved weight gain on nonoperative therapy should have their therapy continued with follow-up extended esophageal pH monitoring off medications at 10 to 12 months of age. Infants with the type II reflux pattern can be treated the same as those with the type I or type III reflux pattern, except that nonoperative antireflux therapy is *always* preferred in those infants who continue to improve and have no significant apnea or bradycardia (even with a prolonged ZMD).

In infants with no growth impairment from recurrent emesis, nonoperative antireflux therapy is usually best. Initially, the nonoperative therapy consists of postural treatment and thickened feedings for at least 6 weeks in infants with a normal ZMD. This regimen is followed by the addition of medications (histamine-receptor blocker plus metoclopramide) if the child's emesis has not improved (Fig. 27-11). In contrast, in infants with no growth impairment from recurrent emesis but with a prolonged ZMD, antireflux medications are used initially and the treatment scheme is similar to that for infants with growth retardation from emesis and a prolonged ZMD. An antireflux operation is usually reserved for infants with no improvement in emesis after extensive medical antireflux therapy, or for infants with a prolonged ZMD and the type I or type III reflux pattern who are at risk for sudden death from the GERD.

In children treated nonoperatively and followed with repeated extended esophageal pH monitoring off medication at 10 to 12 months of age, a normal study means that all antireflux treatment and home monitor for apnea can be discontinued. If the child still has GERD on follow-up, repeat endoscopy should be performed and an antireflux operation

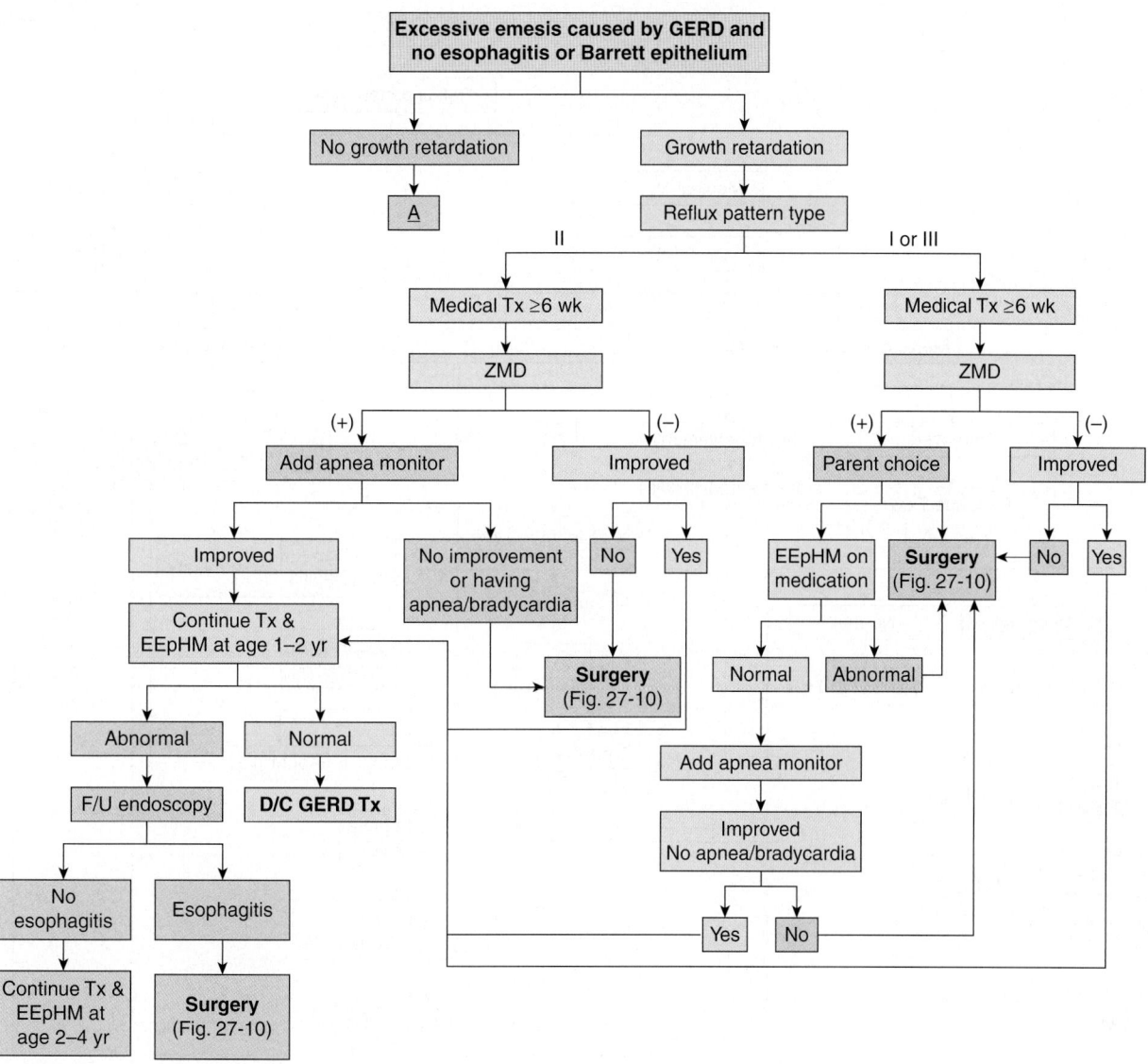

**FIGURE 27-11** Suggested treatment sequence for infants with excessive emesis caused by GERD. EEpHM, extended esophageal pH monitoring; ZMD, mean duration of reflux episodes during sleep; Tx, treatment; F/U, follow-up; D/C, discontinue.

considered if esophagitis is present. When there is no evidence of mucosal injury, then antireflux medication may be continued and the same follow-up evaluation repeated at 2 to 4 years of age. In general, children over 1 year of age with continued emesis and GERD are unlikely to have the GERD resolve spontaneously. An antireflux operation should be strongly considered in these children because their only other alternative is lifelong antireflux medication.

Infants with reflux-induced respiratory symptoms or esophagitis found during their initial evaluation for GERD should be treated according to the algorithms for respiratory symptoms (Fig. 27-12) and esophagitis (Fig. 27-13) instead of the algorithm for recurrent emesis from GERD.

## Respiratory Symptoms or Disease

Infants with respiratory symptoms or disease caused by GERD, and no advanced esophagitis, always require the use of home apnea monitors as an adjunct when nonoperative antireflux treatment is appropriate (Fig. 27-12). The decision between operative and nonoperative antireflux

therapy is determined initially by the pattern of reflux and not by the severity of the respiratory event precipitating an evaluation for GERD. Infants with the type II reflux pattern usually can be treated safely with the upright posture, thickened feedings, and medication (histamine-receptor blocker plus metoclopramide). If respiratory or GERD symptoms persist after 6 weeks, or if there are significant apneic or bradycardic events while on nonoperative therapy, then an antireflux operation (Fig. 27-10) should be recommended. Nonoperative antireflux therapy should be continued as long as the child remains asymptomatic. Follow-up extended esophageal pH monitoring should be performed off medication after the child is 10 to 12 months of age.

In infants with the type I or type III reflux pattern, an antireflux operation is recommended because these patients are at the highest risk for sudden death from GERD during infancy. Since increased periodic breathing or central apnea can coexist in patients with reflux-induced respiratory symptoms or disease, a postoperative sleep evaluation for

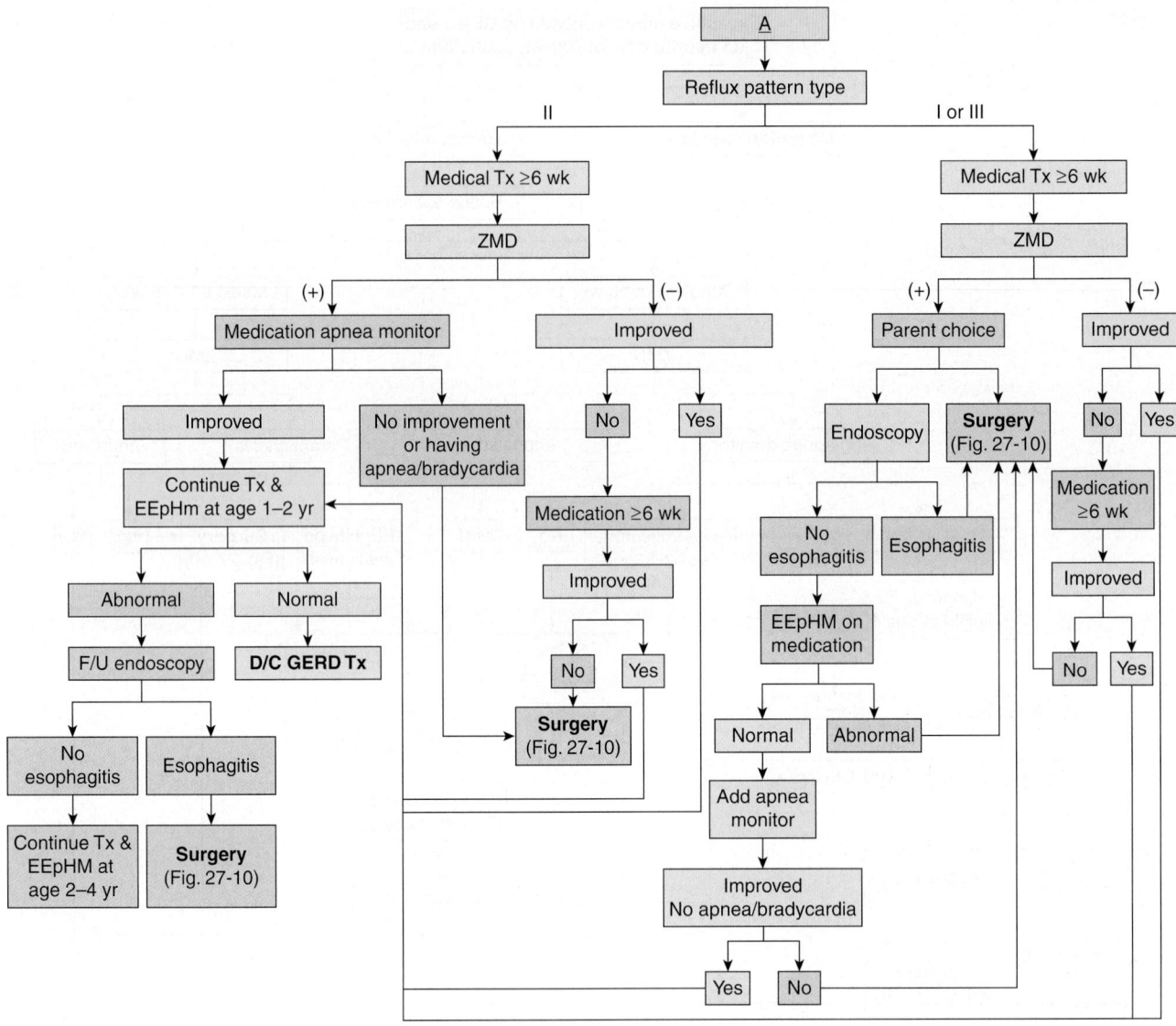

**FIGURE 27-11** (*Continued*)

breathing may indicate the need for home apnea monitoring even though the GERD has been controlled. A reasonable alternative to an antireflux operation that can be discussed with the family or legal guardian of the infant with the type I or type III reflux pattern is the aggressive medical antireflux regimen stated above and repeated extended esophageal pH monitoring while the infant is on the prescribed medications. No improvement on the esophageal pH study performed with the child on medication indicates a need for an antireflux operation. Demonstrated control of the GERD with the antireflux medication permits the infant to continue nonoperative therapy while on home apnea monitors as long as respiratory symptoms and other reflux symptoms disappear and there are no significant apnea or bradycardia events. Follow-up extended esophageal pH monitoring should be performed in these infants off medication after they reach 10 to 12 months of age.

For children who are treated nonoperatively and have a normal follow-up esophageal pH study off medication, all antireflux treatment and home apnea monitoring can be discontinued. Children with persistent GERD may have home apnea monitors discontinued if the ZMD becomes normal. Endoscopy should be repeated in children with persistent GERD to determine the presence or absence of esophageal mucosal injury. An antireflux operation is warranted in children found to have esophagitis. Antireflux medication may be continued in children with no esophageal mucosal injury, with the same follow-up evaluation repeated at 2 to 4 years of age. In general, children over 1 year of age with continued respiratory symptoms from GERD are unlikely to have the GERD resolve spontaneously. An antireflux operation is a logical choice for these children.

## Advanced Esophagitis, Peptic Esophageal Stricture, and Barrett Epithelium

In most children, advanced esophagitis without esophageal stricture or Barrett epithelium usually requires an antireflux operation (Fig. 27-13). When a normal ZMD is present, a trial of nonoperative treatment with the upright position,

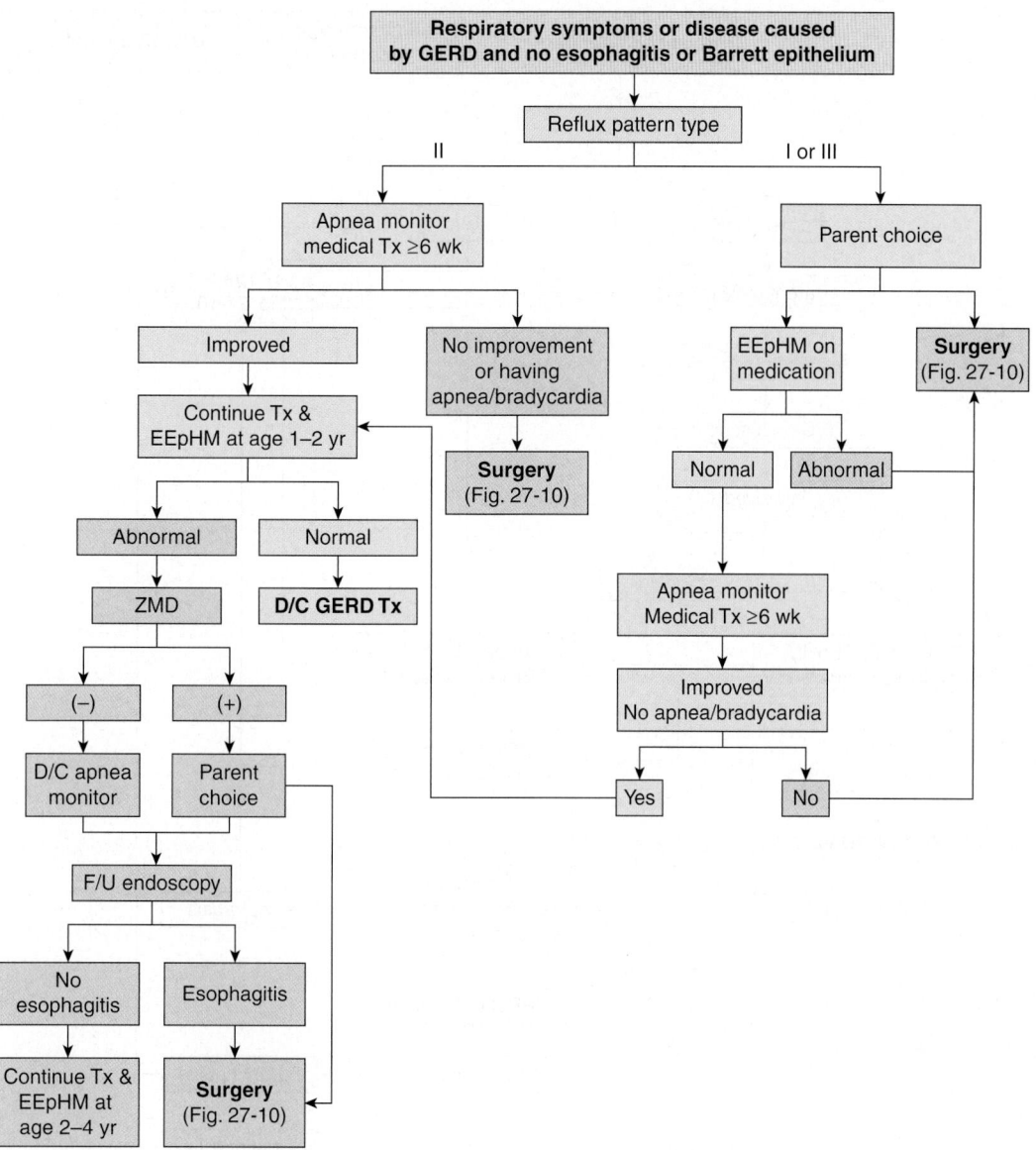

**FIGURE 27-12** Suggested treatment sequence for infants with respiratory symptoms or disease caused by GERD. EEpHM, extended esophageal pH monitoring; ZMD, mean duration of reflux episodes during sleep; Tx, treatment; F/U, follow-up; D/C, discontinue.

thickened feedings, cytoprotective gels, and antiacids or medication (histamine-receptor blocker or proton pump inhibiter, and metoclopramide) can be used for at least 6 weeks with close follow-up and repeated endoscopy. No improvement in the esophagitis on follow-up endoscopy would be an indication that an antireflux operation is needed to control the GERD. However, documented improvement in the mucosal injury while on antireflux medications would encourage continued nonoperative antireflux therapy with repeated extended esophageal pH monitoring off medication *and* endoscopy when the child is 10 to 12 months of age. A complete resolution of the GERD and esophagitis would indicate that all medications could be discontinued. In children with persistent GERD and resolved esophagitis on follow-up, antireflux medication should be continued with repeated extended esophageal pH monitoring and endoscopy at 2 to 4 years of age. The persistence of esophagitis and

GERD on follow-up at 10 to 12 months or 2 to 4 years of age is an indication that an antireflux operation is needed to control GERD. The presence of a peptic esophageal stricture or Barrett epithelium at any age is an indication for an antireflux operation.

The main long-term problem associated with Barrett esophagus is the increased risk for developing adenocarcinoma of the esophagus. Adenocarcinoma of the esophagus is more likely with the specialized columnar type of epithelium and has a rising incidence in humans. Adenocarcinoma of the esophagus related to Barrett esophagus has been reported rarely in childhood. Although Barrett esophagus has been unlikely to regress following aggressive medical or operative antireflux therapy in adults, the authors have seen substantial and complete regression of the Barrett epithelium in children treated with an antireflux operation and no evidence of GERD on follow-up studies.

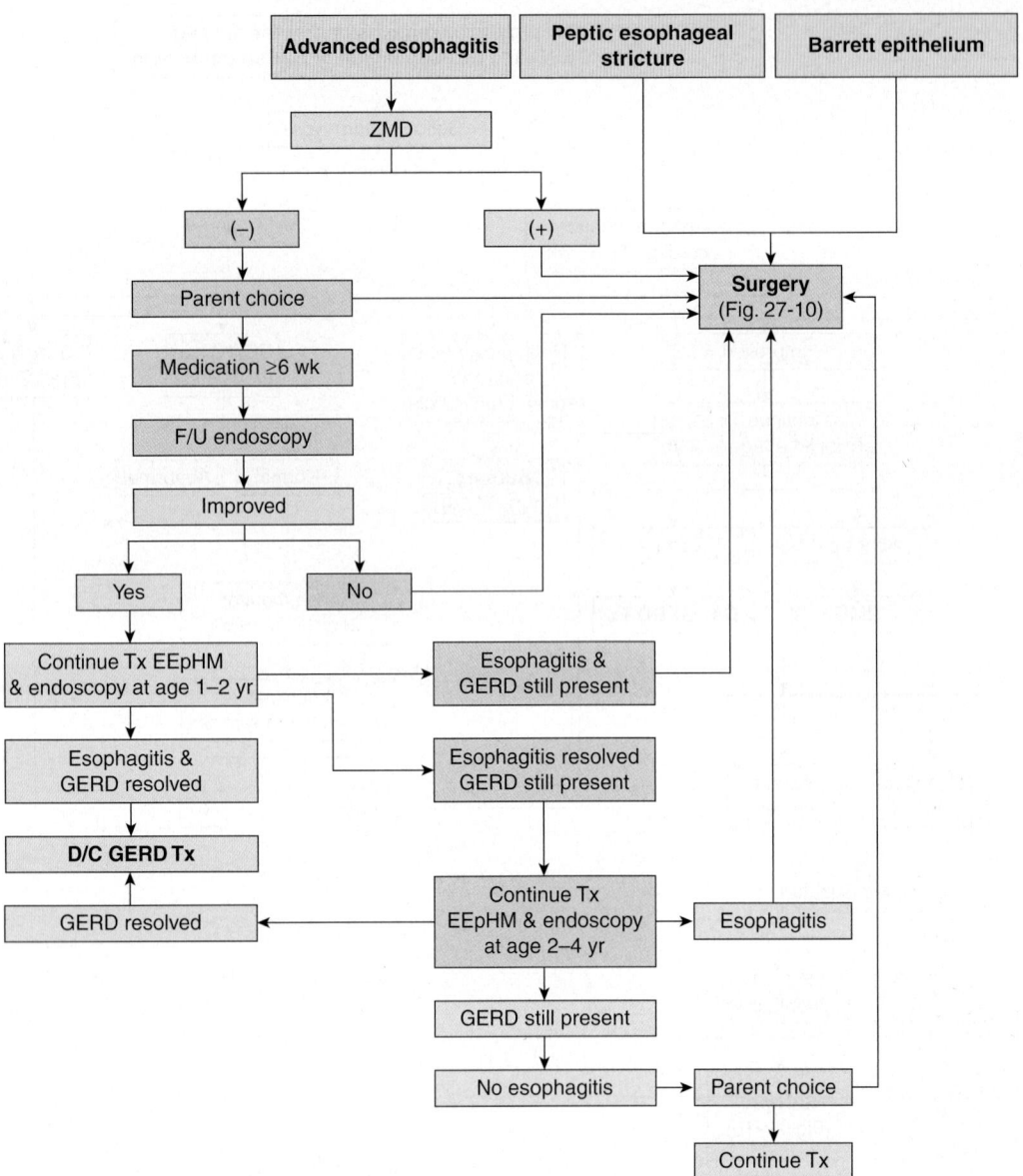

**FIGURE 27-13** Suggested treatment sequence for infants and children with advanced esophagitis, peptic esophageal stricture, and Barrett epithelium caused by GERD. EEpHM, extended esophageal pH monitoring; ZMD, mean duration of reflux episodes during sleep; Tx, treatment; F/U, follow-up; D/C, discontinue.

An antireflux operation in children with Barrett esophagus is an attempt to control symptoms of GERD and to halt the progression of columnar metaplasia by reducing additional esophageal mucosal injury. Because of the increased risk for adenocarcinoma, children with Barrett esophagus should have esophagoscopy with an esophageal mucosal biopsy performed at several levels annually for at least the first 5 years to detect any early signs of dysplasia. The best interval for surveillance endoscopy thereafter is not known, but can probably be as long as every 4 to 5 years in children who have no signs of progression (histologic type or extent of mucosal area involved) or dysplasia. As in the adult experience, total esophagectomy and esophageal substitution may provide the best chance for curing adenocarcinoma of the esophagus associated with Barrett esophagus in children when severe dysplasia appears on

esophageal biopsy. The risk for developing adenocarcinoma of the esophagus in children with Barrett esophagus is probably higher than for adults due to the longer life expectancy for children.

## Feeding Gastrostomy and Operations in Neurologically Impaired Children

Infants and children referred for feeding gastrostomy usually require a protective antireflux operation. Most patients already have GERD even if they are asymptomatic. In more than two thirds of the patients who do not have GERD initially, GERD will be induced acutely following placement of a feeding gastrostomy operatively or endoscopically. The specific concerns in these children with GERD include: (1) GERD may be present without symptoms and these patients can die suddenly from the "asymptomatic" GERD or develop long-term problems from the GERD. (2) Patients without GERD prior to gastrostomy may develop GERD in the long term from the progression of their CNS disease instead of from the feeding gastrostomy. (3) With time, the GERD resulting from feeding gastrostomy may resolve as the stomach pulls away from its attachment to the anterior abdominal wall and if CNS disease is either not present or improves in the patient. (4) Caretakers for children with feeding gastrostomy often do not administer gastrostomy feedings in a physiologic manner or as instructed, thereby resulting in the regurgitation of gastrostomy feedings even in the absence of GERD. A protective antireflux operation is performed in infants and children referred for placement of a feeding gastrostomy because most patients have GERD by extended esophageal pH monitoring following gastrostomy placement and one cannot predict which patients will further develop GERD due to their underlying disease process or have GERD resolve in the long term. It is reasonable to place a feeding gastrostomy tube without an antireflux operation in a child as long as the risk of GERD is discussed with the child's family or legal guardian and as long as follow-up extended esophageal pH monitoring is performed after gastrostomy placement to document the presence or absence of GERD. If GERD is present, then follow-up evaluation for GERD is needed until the GERD has resolved, as determined by extended esophageal pH monitoring.

It is well known that children with CNS disease are at high risk for GERD. An understanding of the potential alimentary tract motility disorders associated with GERD in these patients is necessary for a realistic assessment of expectations by the surgeon, the primary care physician, and the patient's family or legal guardian. Nearly all neurologically impaired infants and children have some element of swallowing dysfunction, which may lead to oropharyngeal aspiration. These patients can aspirate refluxed gastric contents in addition to saliva and food taken orally. Unless the gag reflex is absent, most children have episodes of gagging and choking with frequent episodes of aspiration pneumonia. Even when GERD has been contributing to respiratory symptoms or disease, it is unlikely that all symptoms will be "cured" by an antireflux operation. The best chance to improve respiratory symptoms or disease often means the avoidance of oral feedings (ie, a feeding gastrostomy) as well as an antireflux operation.

Esophageal peristalsis and clearance of refluxed gastric acid also may be disordered in children with CNS disease. This disorder results in chronic respiratory symptoms or disease from aspiration similar to the complications associated with swallowing dysfunction. As mentioned previously, esophageal obstruction may occur following fundoplication if esophageal clearance is severely impaired preoperatively. Gastric emptying in neurologically impaired children is more likely to be uncoordinated, with values that are slow or rapid. As a result, these patients are more likely to have gagging and retching associated with gas-bloat or dumping symptoms following an antireflux operation. In children older than age 1, these symptoms are not likely to improve, whereas the symptoms usually improve in infants whose CNS disease is not progressive. A gastric drainage procedure may reduce the occurrence of gagging and retching caused by gas-bloat symptoms.

**TABLE 27-6    Prevalence of Gastroesophageal Reflux Disease in Infants with Repaired Congenital Anomalies[a]**

| Congenital Anomaly | N | % With GERD | % of Patients With GERD Reflux Pattern Type | | | % With Risk for Sudden Infant Death from GERD |
|---|---|---|---|---|---|---|
| | | | I | II | III | |
| Intestinal malrotation | 65 | 83.1% | 72% | 17% | 11% | Low[b] = 6.2% |
| | | | | | | High[c] = 26.1% |
| | | | | | | Total = 32.3% |
| Abdominal wall defect (gastroschisis/omphalocele) | 70 | 80% | 59% | 29% | 12% | Low = 12.9% |
| | | | | | | High = 20.0% |
| | | | | | | Total = 32.9% |
| Bochdalek diaphragmatic hernia (left side) | 20 | 65% | 92% | 8% | 0% | Low = 0% |
| | | | | | | High = 10.0% |
| | | | | | | Total = 10.0% |
| Esophageal atresia with tracheoesophageal fistula (Gross type C) | 37 | 70% | 85% | 11% | 4% | Low = 0% |
| | | | | | | High = 32.4% |
| | | | | | | Total = 32.4% |

[a]The prevalence of GERD was determined by extended esophageal pH monitoring in 180 infants with repaired congenital anomalies suspected to have a high association with GERD. All infants were asymptomatic at the time of initial study.
[b]Type II pattern of reflux in combination with a prolonged mean duration of sleep reflux (ZMD).
[c]Types I and III patterns of reflux in combination with a prolonged ZMD.

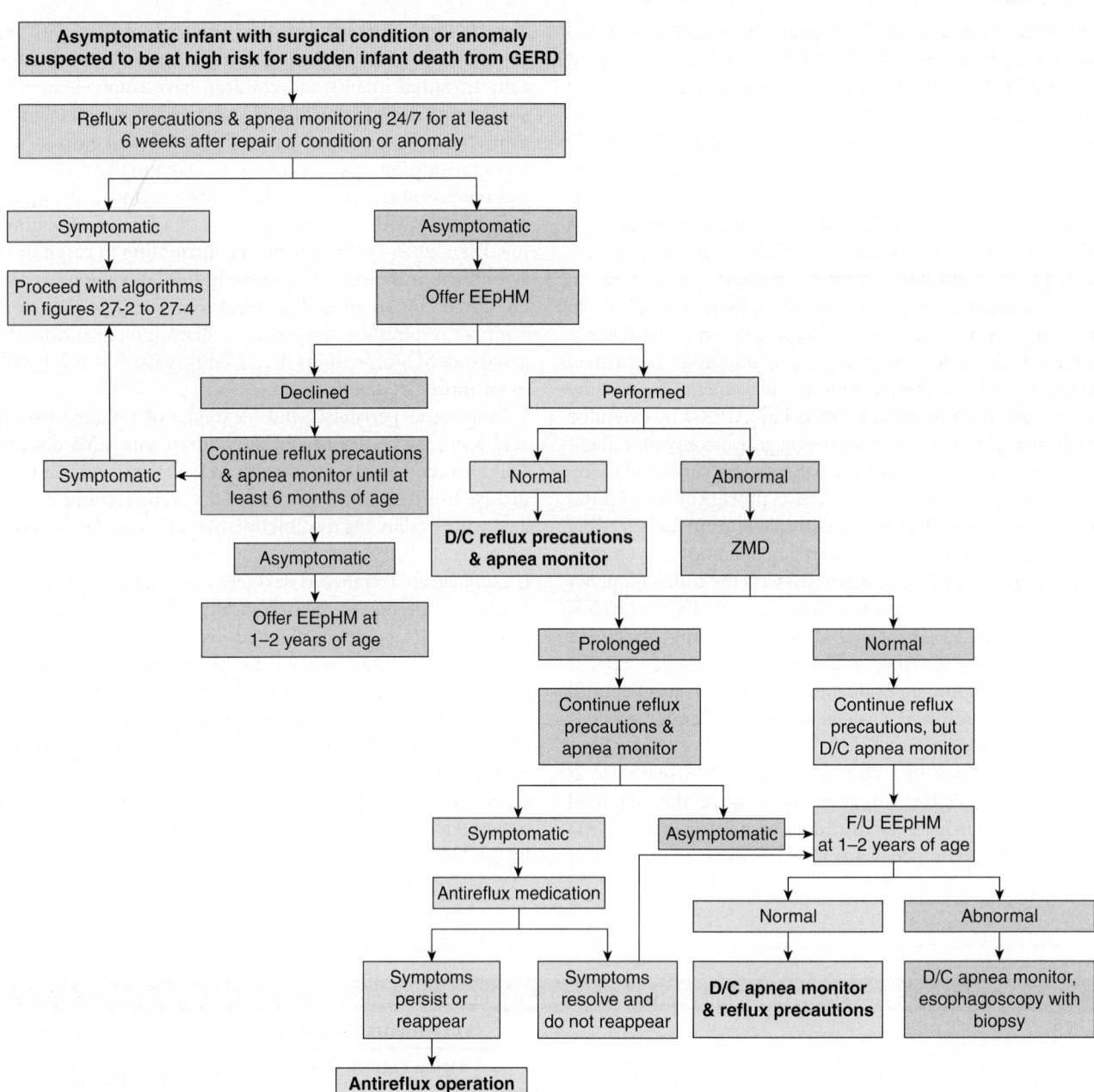

**FIGURE 27-14** Evaluation and treatment algorithm for asymptomatic infant with a surgical condition or anomaly suspected to be at significant risk for sudden infant death from GERD. EEpHM, extended esophageal pH monitoring; ZMD, mean duration of reflux episodes during sleep; Tx, treatment; F/U, follow-up; D/C, discontinue.

The occurrence of symptoms following an antireflux operation in neurologically impaired infants and children appears to be related directly to the progression or persistence of alimentary tract motility disorders associated with CNS disease, of which GERD is only one component. Chronic gagging and retching related to alimentary tract motility disorders from CNS disease in childhood are likely causes for the reported increased incidence of complications such as recurrent GERD and paraesophageal hernia following an antireflux operation. A frank discussion about the problems associated with CNS disease in children and the expectations of an antireflux operation in controlling those problems usually helps the child's family or caregiver avoid unrealistic expectations.

## Asymptomatic Children with GERD

Over time, more children are being identified with GERD but without symptoms suggestive of GERD. This observation has occurred because of an increased awareness of GERD in children, and the sophisticated technology (eg, esophageal pH monitoring) that is available to examine the function of the gastroesophageal junction. The clinical groups of children who provide evidence for the existence of "asymptomatic" GERD include (1) older children with peptic esophageal stricture who either had no symptoms of GERD previously or had symptoms of GERD that resolved after infancy, (2) infants with the type I reflux pattern documented by extended esophageal pH monitoring who continue to have GERD after age

1 even though all symptoms have disappeared, and (3) infants with the type I reflux pattern and a prolonged ZMD who die suddenly from GERD even though no symptoms referable to GERD occurred.

Some of the information on asymptomatic GERD was derived from studies of repaired congenital anomalies, such as esophageal atresia, diaphragmatic hernia, intestinal malrotation, and abdominal wall defects, which were considered clinically to be risk factors for the presence of GERD (Table 27-6). Although presumed to be similar to infants and children with symptoms of GERD, the natural course of infants and children with asymptomatic GERD may be quite different. The treatment of asymptomatic children with severe mucosal injury or Barrett epithelium secondary to GERD should be the same as for symptomatic children. On the other hand, asymptomatic infants with GERD and a normal ZMD should be treated only with the upright posture, and follow-up extended esophageal pH monitoring performed after 10 to 12 months of age as long as the infant remains asymptomatic. If symptoms of GERD develop, then aggressive treatment of the GERD with medication, or possibly an antireflux operation, may be warranted according to the algorithms outlined previously for symptomatic patients. In asymptomatic infants with GERD and a prolonged ZMD, home apnea monitors should be used in addition to upright positioning of the infant. More aggressive treatment of GERD is reserved for the infant who develops symptoms of GERD or unexplained episodes of apnea, bradycardia, or ALTEs. An algorithm for the treatment of an asymptomatic infant with the risk for sudden infant death from GERD is shown in Fig. 27-14.

## SUMMARY

In summary, a working knowledge of 18- to 24-hour esophageal pH monitoring and the motility disorders of the esophagus and stomach that may be associated with GERD is necessary to understand GERD in infants and children. The results of surgical therapy for childhood GERD cannot be assessed accurately without this knowledge. To a large degree, antireflux operations can be tailored to the child's situation, which includes a combination of clinical symptoms and findings on objective tests for GERD and associated alimentary tract motility disorders. The presence of severe complications from GERD in "asymptomatic" infants and children is an area that requires further study and may play a key role in understanding the overall contribution of GERD in human disease and adaptation to the environment.

## SELECTED READINGS

Ashcraft KW, Holder TM, Amoury RA, et al. The Thal fundoplication for gastroesophageal reflux. *J Pediatr Surg* 1984;19:480–483.

Astley R, Carre IJ. Gastro-oesophageal incompetence in children. With special reference to minor degrees of partial thoracic stomach. *Radiology* 1954;62:351–361.

Avansino JR, Lorenz ML, Hendrickson M, et al. Characterization and management of paraesophageal hernias in children after antireflux operation. *J Pediatr Surg* 1999;34:1610–1614.

Barrett NR. Chronic peptic ulcer of the oesophagus and "oesophagitis." *Br J Surg* 1950;38:175–182.

Berenberg W, Neuhauser EBD. Cardio-oesophageal relaxation (chalasia) as a cause of vomiting in infants. *Pediatrics* 1950;5:414–420.

Billard C. Traites des maladies des enfans nouveaux-nes et a la mamelle. In: Billard MC ed. *Atlas D'anatomie Pathologique pour server A L'histoire des Maladies des Enfans*. Paris, France: Imprimerie de H Balzac; 1828:271–295.

Blot WJ, Devesa SS, Kneller RW, et al. Rising incidence of adenocarcinoma of the esophagus and gastric cardia. *JAMA* 1991;265:1287–1289.

Boerema I. Hiatus hernia: repair by right-sided, subhepatic, anterior gastropexy. *Surgery* 1969;65:884–893.

Carre IJ, Astley R. The fate of the partial thoracic stomach (hiatus hernia) in children. *Arch Dis Child* 1960;35:484–486.

Celik A, Loux TJ, Harmon CM, et al. Revision Nissen fundoplication can be completed laparoscopically with a low rate of complications: a single-institution experience with 72 children. *J Pediatr Surg* 2006;41:2081–2085.

Euler AR, Byrne WJ. Twenty-four-hour esophageal intraluminal pH probe testing: a comparative analysis. *Gastroenterology* 1981;80:957–961.

Forshall I. The cardio-oesophageal syndrome in childhood. *Arch Dis Child* 1955;30:46–54.

Grunow JE, Al-Hafida AS, Tunell WP. Gastroesophageal reflux following percutaneous endoscopic gastrostomy in children. *J Pediatr Surg* 1989;24:42–45.

Halpern LM, Jolley SG, Tunell WP, et al. The mean duration of gastroesophageal reflux during sleep as an indicator of respiratory symptoms from gastroesophageal reflux in children. *J Pediatr Surg* 1991;26:686–690.

Herbst JJ, Book LS, Johnson DG, et al. The lower esophageal sphincter in gastroesophageal reflux in children. *J Clin Gastroenterol* 1979;1:119–123.

Hoeffel JC, Nihoul-Fekete C, Schmitt M. Esophageal adenocarcinoma after gastroesophageal reflux in children. *J Pediatr* 1989;115:259–261.

Hollander F. What is pH? An explanation of the various measures of acidity employed in gastroenterology. *Gastroenterology* 1945;4:497–508.

Johnson LF, DeMeester TR. Twenty-four-hour pH monitoring of the distal esophagus. A quantitative measure of gastroesophageal reflux. *Am J Gastroenterol* 1974;62:325–332.

Jolley SG. Gastroesophageal reflux disease as a cause for emesis in infants. *Semin Pediatr Surg* 1995;4:176–189.

Jolley SG, Halpern LM, Tunell WP, et al. The risk of sudden infant death from gastroesophageal reflux. *J Pediatr Surg* 1991;26:691–696.

Jolley SG, Herbst JJ, Johnson DG, et al. Patterns of postcibal gastroesophageal reflux in symptomatic infants. *Am J Surg* 1979;138:946–950.

Jolley SG, Johnson DG, Herbst JJ, et al. An assessment of gastroesophageal reflux in children by extended pH monitoring of the distal esophagus. *Surgery* 1978;84:16–23.

Jolley SG, Johnson DG, Herbst JJ, et al. The significance of gastroesophagel reflux patterns in children. *J Pediatr Surg* 1981;16:859–865.

Jolley SG, Leonard JC, Tunell WP. Gastric emptying in children with gastroesophageal reflux. I. An estimate of effective gastric emptying. *J Pediatr Surg* 1987;22:923–926.

Jolley SG, Smith EI, Tunell WP. Protective antireflux operation with feeding gastrostomy. Experience with children. *Ann Surg* 1985;201:736–740.

Jolley SG, Tunell WP, Leonard JC, et al. Gastric emptying in children with gastroesophageal reflux. II. The relationship to retching symptoms following antireflux surgery. *J Pediatr Surg* 1987;22:927–930.

Lopez M, Kalfa N, Forgues D, et al. Laparoscopic redo fundoplication in children: failure causes and feasibility. *J Pediatr Surg* 2008;43:1885–1890.

Meehan JJ, Georgeson KE. The learning curve associated with laparoscopic antireflux surgery in infants and children. *J Pediatr Surg* 1997;32:426–429.

Sterling CE, Jolley SG, Besser AS, et al. Nursing responsibility in the diagnosis, care and treatment of the child with gastroesophageal reflux. *J Pediatr Nurs* 1991;6:435–440.

Tovar JA, Olivares P, Diaz M, et al. Functional results of laparoscopic fundoplication in children. *J Pediatr Gastroenterol Nutr* 1998;26: 429–431.

Tunell WP, Smith EI. Suture alignment for cuff creation in Nissen fundoplication. *Surg Gynecol Obstetr* 1981;152:347–349.

Vandenplas Y, Goyvaerts H, Helven R, et al. Gastroesophageal reflux, as measured by 24-hour pH monitoring, in 509 healthy infants screened for risk of sudden infant death syndrome. *Pediatrics* 1991;88: 834–840.

Wenzl TG, Moroder C, Trachterna M, et al. Esophageal pH monitoring and impedence measurement: a comparison of two diagnostic tests for gastroesophageal reflux. *J Pediatr Gastroenterol Nutr* 2002;34:519–523.

Werlin SL, Dodds WJ, Hogan WJ, et al. Mechanisms of gastroesophageal reflux in children. *J Pediatr* 1980;97:244–249.

# CHAPTER 28

## Mediastinal Cysts, Tumors, and Myasthenia Gravis

*Steven Teich, Jennifer H. Aldrink, and Jonathan I. Groner*

## KEY POINTS

1. Robotic surgery offers advantages for the resection of selected solid mediastinal chest masses.

2. A calcified mass in the posterior mediastinum is most commonly of neural cell origin.

3. Neuroblastomas that arise in the mediastinum usually have a more favorable prognosis than those in other locations.

4. A careful and thorough evaluation for potential airway obstruction is required prior to biopsy for patients with a large anterior mediastinal mass. Alternative sites of biopsy should be investigated if general anesthesia is of considerable risk.

5. A calcified mass located within the anterior mediastinum is typically a teratoma.

6. Complete surgical resection is the goal for mediastinal germ cell tumors.

7. Mediastinal hemangiomas are rare causes of respiratory distress or feeding difficulties in infants. Propranolol may help shrink these lesions, but it has not been prospectively studied.

8. Lymphatic malformations (cystic hygromas) are benign lesions that may envelop vital structures. Interventional radiology techniques offer highly effective treatment of macrocystic mediastinal lesions.

9. The role of thymectomy for myasthenia gravis (MG) is controversial, and there is a lack of prospective studies documenting efficacy.

## ANATOMY

The mediastinum is the portion of the thoracic cavity that lies between the 2 pleural sacs. It is bounded superiorly by the thoracic inlet, inferiorly by the diaphragm, anteriorly by the sternum, and posteriorly by the vertebral bodies and costovertebral sulci. Classic anatomic definitions of the mediastinum in adults may fail to convey a clear, precise understanding of the surgical anatomy in childhood. In the pediatric population, it is preferable to divide the mediastinum into 3, rather than 4, compartments. The *anterior mediastinum* is defined as the area between the sternum and the pericardial sac including the cephalad portion of the mediastinum. The *middle mediastinum* remains bounded by the anterior and posterior surfaces of the pericardium. The *posterior mediastinum* encompasses the area from the posterior aspect of the pericardium to the vertebral bodies and their costovertebral sulci, including the cephalad portion of the mediastinum.

These definitions provide clinicians with descriptive terminology that is more consistent with the surgical anatomy in the pediatric age group. For instance, a neurogenic tumor arising from the third sympathetic ganglion should be considered a superior mediastinal mass, but in order to formulate an accurate differential diagnosis, the posterior position of the lesion is the most important information to be imparted. The visceral contents of these 3 redefined mediastinal compartments are listed in Table 28-1.

## INTRODUCTION

Mediastinal masses are not common in the pediatric age group, but a wide variety of both benign and malignant lesions do arise in the mediastinum. While each patient represents a unique treatment opportunity, it is important to recall the 4 basic principles that form the foundation for clinical decision making regarding lesions in this region: (1) The morbidity and mortality associated with mediastinal cysts and tumors (both benign and malignant) are well documented. (2) The majority of mediastinal masses in children are malignant. (3) Although an infrequent complication in patients with benign disease, death may occur precipitously as a result of loss of airway control. (4) Virtually all mediastinal masses (both benign and malignant) require surgical intervention either for an initial diagnostic biopsy or as definitive therapy.

The treatment priorities for children with mediastinal masses that are a natural extension of these basic principles include (1) securing the airway, (2) providing a prompt, accurate diagnostic evaluation, and (3) achieving complete excision (or an appropriate biopsy) of the index lesion with minimal morbidity.

| TABLE 28-1 | Visceral Contents of the Mediastinal Compartments as Redefined for the Pediatric Population | | |
|---|---|---|---|
| **Anterior** | **Middle** | **Posterior** |
| Thymus | Pericardium | Esophagus |
| Ascending aorta | Heart | Vagus nerves |
| Aortic arch | Trachea (distal) | Descending aorta |
| Brachiocephalic vessels | Hilar structures | Thoracic duct |
| Trachea (proximal) | Lymph nodes | Lymph nodes |
| Lymph nodes | | Sympathetic nerves |

| TABLE 28-2 | Mediastinal Masses: Incidence Data (Summary of 7 Series From 1970 to 2003) | |
|---|---|---|
| **Type of Mass** | **Total** | **Percentage** |
| Benign | | |
| Thymus | 43 | 14.6 |
| Teratoma | 44 | 15 |
| Cystic hygroma | 24 | 8.2 |
| Hemangioma | 11 | 3.7 |
| Granuloma | 4 | 1.4 |
| Bronchogenic cyst | 32 | 10.9 |
| Enterogenous cyst | 22 | 7.5 |
| Neurofibroma | 25 | 8.5 |
| Ganglioneuroma | 69 | 23.5 |
| Other | 20 | 6.8 |
| | 294 | 39% |
| Malignant | | |
| Thymoma | 15 | 3.2 |
| Lymphoma | 237 | 51.2 |
| Germ cell | 16 | 3.5 |
| Sarcoma | 23 | 5 |
| Neuroblastoma | 167 | 36.1 |
| Other | 5 | 1.1 |
| | 463 | 61% |

## INCIDENCE

Table 28-2 summarizes the pediatric data reported by 7 American medical centers from 1970 to 2003. Of the 757 children reviewed, 39% had benign conditions. Forty percent of the benign lesions were in the anterior portion of the mediastinum, and another 40% were observed in the posterior compartment. Thymic cysts or hyperplasia (14.6%), teratomas (15%), and vascular tumors (11.9%) accounted for the overwhelming majority of benign anterior mediastinal masses. Tumors of neural origin (32%) and enteric duplications (7.5%) represented virtually all of the posterior lesions. Bronchogenic cysts (10.9%) and granulomatous infections (1.4%) were the only conditions that consistently occurred in the middle segment of the mediastinum.

Among children with mediastinal tumors reported in this data set, 463 (61%) had a malignancy. More than 50% of these patients had lymphoma, which was typically seen in the anterior compartment of the mediastinum. Other lesions observed anteriorly included malignant thymomas (3.2%) and germ cell tumors (3.5%). Neuroblastomas accounted for 36.1% of malignant lesions, and this was the only type of cancer that arose in the posterior aspect of the mediastinum. Sarcomas were relatively uncommon (5%) and frequently extended beyond the borders of any single anatomic area.

## DIAGNOSTIC EVALUATION

The evaluation of children with mediastinal tumors has changed significantly during the last decade as diagnostic imaging techniques continue to evolve. A vast array of studies is available to help assess patients with mediastinal masses and define the nature of their lesions, but the diagnostic armamentarium should be used judiciously in an attempt to control costs. Specific questions to be answered preoperatively include: (1) What is the anatomic location and extent of the lesion? (2) What is the consistency—cystic, solid, or complex? (3) Is it likely to be benign or malignant? (4) Is there evidence of vascular, gastrointestinal, or neurologic involvement? Once these questions have been answered, the clinician has the information necessary to proceed with safe, effective surgical intervention.

The following recommendations are presented as suggested guidelines for use of the various diagnostic techniques.

▶ Chest radiographs (posteroanterior and lateral) are appropriate for the initial study of all patients with mediastinal cysts and tumors.

▶ Computed tomography (CT) scans of the chest are a logical second test in the vast majority of children due to excellent resolution, especially for anterior or middle mediastinal compartment masses. CT can assess the nature, size, location, and involvement of other organs by mediastinal masses with a high degree of accuracy.

▶ Magnetic resonance imaging (MRI) is an important diagnostic imaging modality because of its superior soft tissue characterization, but should not be used routinely because of the relatively high cost, image artifact caused by cardiac and respiratory motion, and the need for sedation in infants and young children. MRI is particularly helpful in defining the extent of disease in patients with suspected intraspinal or vascular involvement as well as the evaluation of foregut duplication cysts.

- Positron emission tomography (PET) is not indicated as an initial imaging modality for evaluating nonvascular mediastinal masses, but it appears extremely useful for staging of lymphomas, assessing response to treatment, and evaluating lymphomas when other imaging modalities have limited diagnostic capabilities, such as discriminating between fibrous scar and necrotic tissue in a posttreatment residual mass.
- Ultrasound is the most precise method of defining the cystic nature of lesions that are indeterminate on CT scan, and can also define the intrinsic characteristics and anatomic borders of the thymus. Ultrasound is also routinely used as a guide for invasive diagnostic studies such as needle biopsies and cyst aspirations.
- Esophagoscopy is indicated for the assessment of intrinsic lesions of the esophagus.
- Bronchoscopy is infrequently required, but is used occasionally to obtain culture material in patients with suspected infectious lesions.
- Anatomic considerations limit the few indications for mediastinoscopy in pediatric patients, but the procedure is very useful in the assessment of adolescents with isolated anterior mediastinal lymphadenopathy.

## VIDEO-ASSISTED THORACOSCOPIC SURGERY AND ROBOTIC SURGERY

Since 1990 and the refinement of laparoscopic surgical techniques and equipment, video-assisted thoracoscopic surgery (VATS) has evolved into the preferred technique for the surgical evaluation of mediastinal masses in children. Although the technique may be more cumbersome and time-consuming than a traditional thoracotomy, its main advantages are minimal morbidity, less postoperative pain, and a shorter recovery time. The anterior and posterior surfaces of the mediastinum are easily accessible, and the pulmonary hila can be well visualized. The only location difficult to assess is the posterior mediastinum at the level of the inferior pulmonary vein because exposure in this area requires division of the inferior pulmonary ligament.

Single-lung ventilation with a complete ipsilateral pneumothorax is crucial to the success of this procedure. In children more than 6 or 7 years old, a double-lumen endotracheal tube can be used, but double-lumen tubes are not available for younger children, and the only way to achieve single-lung ventilation is by selective intubation of the main stem bronchus. Many infants and small children do not tolerate single-lung ventilation well, so thoracoscopy may not be as useful a technique in the preschool age group.

The use of thoracoscopy in the diagnosis of mediastinal lymphadenopathy is controversial. Although fine-needle aspiration and percutaneous needle biopsies of mediastinal nodes are accurate for the identification of metastatic carcinoma, the success rate for the definitive diagnosis of lymphoma and thymoma is between 20% and 40%. Studies in both children and adults report a diagnostic accuracy of 80% to 90% for VATS for a wide variety of nonmetastatic mediastinal malignancies, including Hodgkin and non-Hodgkin and acute lymphocytic leukemia. Although mediastinoscopy and a parasternal mediastinotomy both provide access for the biopsy of anterior mediastinal masses, VATS has the advantage of allowing visualization of the entire pleural cavity and access to many more nodal areas for sampling.

The use of VATS for resection of benign cystic mediastinal masses is well accepted. The cysts are usually aspirated and then excised with a combination of sharp and blunt dissection. Cystic lesions of the anterior and middle mediastinum are amenable to resection, but the use of thoracoscopy for excision of posterior mediastinal tumors, most of which are solid and neurogenic in origin, is controversial. Robotic surgery has been gaining acceptance in pediatric surgery over the past 5 years and appears to be well suited for the resection of selected solid mediastinal masses because the articulating instruments are capable of moving around a rigid mass. Dissecting around mediastinal structures such as the azygous vein, superior vena cava, and phrenic nerve are facilitated by the 3D visualization that the robot provides.

In summary, thoracoscopy is a minimally invasive procedure with a low morbidity and mortality that is useful for the biopsy of selected malignant mediastinal tumors and excision of some cystic lesions. VATS is not appropriate for resection of solid or complex tumors that have a high risk of malignancy. Robotic surgery appears to offer advantages for the resection of selected solid mediastinal chest masses.

## NEURAL TUMORS

Lesions of neural origin are the most common type of tumor arising in the mediastinum. In the 7 series of mediastinal masses reviewed, 34% of tumors were of neural origin. Sixty-four percent of these lesions were malignant neuroblastomas. The benign lesions were ganglioneuromas or neurofibromas. Most of these neural tumors arise in the paravertebral position and may appear on a lateral chest radiograph in the posterior mediastinum, although others may not be visible by plain radiographs (Fig. 28-1). The anatomic position of neurofibromas is much more variable, as these lesions arise from the sympathetic, parasympathetic, and/or intercostal nerves and frequently extend beyond the borders of any single compartment within the mediastinum.

## NEUROBLASTOMAS

All 167 of the malignant neural tumors collated in the 7 series reviewed were neuroblastomas. Approximately 25% of all neuroblastomas arise in the chest, representing the most common cause of a mediastinal mass in children younger than 2 years. In the largest study of thoracic neuroblastoma patients to date, the Pediatric Oncology Group (POG) noted that patients with mediastinal neuroblastomas are younger than their counterparts with extrathoracic primary tumors (0.9 vs 1.8 years). In this study, 50% of the patients with mediastinal neuroblastomas were asymptomatic at the time of presentation, 20% had mild upper respiratory complaints,

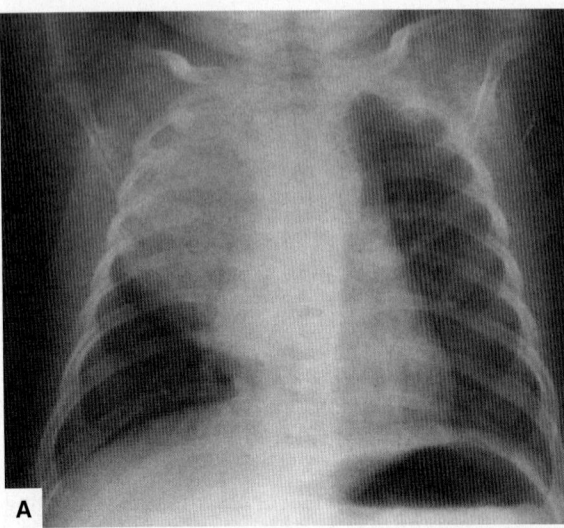

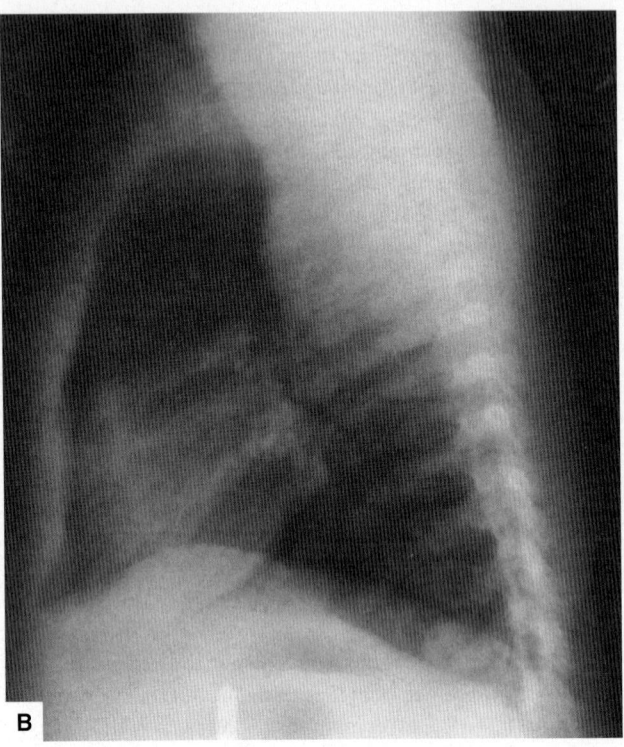

**FIGURE 28-1 A.** Opacification of the right upper hemithorax is apparent on a posteroanterior chest radiograph of a 2-month-old child with respiratory distress. The ribs appear to be eroded and splayed apart, indicating that the lesion is arising in the posterior of the mediastinum. **B.** On a lateral view the characteristic posterior position of the tumor is confirmed.

14% had severe respiratory distress, and 16% had neurologic symptoms including spinal cord compression (9%), opsoclonus (4%), or Horner syndrome (3%). Dumbbell tumors with an extradural extension through the neural foramina into the spinal canal were observed in 16 patients (17%).

In comparison to patients with abdominal neuroblastomas, children with primary neuroblastomas originating in the thorax have an excellent prognosis, with survival rates of 75% or higher. This may be related to the fact that they present at a younger age and have lower-stage tumors, although this improved survival rate holds true independent of other clinical and biological variables. More than 66% of the children with a thoracic neuroblastoma enrolled in the POG protocols had well-localized lesions without evidence of lymph node metastases, while only 18% had evidence of disseminated disease at diagnosis. In stark contrast, 66% of patients with extrathoracic neuroblastoma presented with distant metastases.

The actuarial survival of the patients included in the POG study was 88% at 4 years. As expected, the best outcome (100% survival) was for the children who underwent complete excision of their primary tumors. The results achieved in those who underwent a biopsy alone or incomplete resection followed by chemotherapy were quite satisfactory, however, and appeared to be closely related to age and to the extent of disease at presentation. Overall, 27 of the 30 children (90%) who had an incomplete excision of their tumor survived. Of the 52 children who were younger than 1 year at diagnosis, 50 survived. The presence of residual tumor extending into the intervertebral foramen was not associated with a poor prognosis. It is important to note that radiation therapy was utilized in only 2 of the 96 patients in this study.

Based on this experience, complete surgical resection at the time of diagnosis remains the primary goal for children with thoracic neuroblastoma as long as morbidity and mortality can be minimized. An initial biopsy or an incomplete resection followed by chemotherapy and delayed excision may be considered appropriate in order to avoid radical surgical procedures and their attendant increased risk of postoperative complications. A standard posterolateral thoracotomy through the fourth or fifth intercostal space is recommended for children with thoracic neuroblastoma. This provides appropriate access for virtually all apical tumors and the majority of those at the midthoracic level. Low-lying lesions can be difficult to deal with through a standard thoracotomy incision because the proximity of the diaphragm may prevent good visualization of tumor margins. For bulky lesions low in the thorax, a thoracoabdominal approach is recommended. The improved exposure facilitated by circumferential detachment of the diaphragm greatly enhances the opportunity for complete tumor resection in this anatomic area. Thoracoscopic approaches to resection have also been well described, and complete gross resection of thoracic neuroblastomas has been safely achieved in several series.

## GANGLIONEUROMAS

In the series reported by the 7 medical centers, 69 children had benign tumors arising from the sympathetic chain. Ganglioneuromas account for approximately 24% of all the intrathoracic neural tumors, and are typically asymptomatic lesions identified incidentally on radiographs in children older than 2 years of age. This is in contrast to neuroblastoma, which usually presents as a symptomatic tumor in a child younger than 2 years. There are no characteristics on diagnostic imaging that reliably define ganglioneuromas as benign, so all suspected ganglioneuromas should be approached in a similar fashion to neuroblastomas and resected as completely as possible.

The benign nature of ganglioneuromas may be suspected intraoperatively because ganglioneuromas are quite firm, fibrous, and avascular in comparison to their malignant counterparts. Intervertebral involvement may be observed, and complete excision is recommended as long as this can be achieved safely and without significant risk to the spinal cord. Gentle dissection using a blunt-tipped atherosclerotic plaque elevator usually frees the tissue extending into the intervertebral foramina. If the resection results in significant bleeding from the foramina, gentle packing with thrombin-soaked oxycellulose or the application of fibrin glue usually suffices to control the hemorrhage. Vigorous packing or excessive use of electrocautery in this area must be avoided in order to prevent the development of an expanding extradural hematoma or direct damage to the spinal cord.

## LYMPHOMA

Lymphoma is the third most common type of malignancy reported in childhood, accounting for 16% of pediatric cancers, and the most frequently observed malignant condition in the mediastinum (Table 28-2). In the reported series, 237 children (51.2%) with malignant mediastinal lesions were diagnosed as having either Hodgkin disease (35%) or non-Hodgkin lymphoma (65%). Since surgery is of little or no therapeutic value in patients with lymphoma, the role of the surgeon is to achieve an accurate histologic diagnosis with minimal morbidity.

Although most children with mediastinal lymphoma have enlarged nodes in the supraclavicular or cervical areas that are accessible for biopsy, a direct approach to the mediastinum is required occasionally. Data from adult patients suggest that ultrasound or CT-guided percutaneous needle biopsies are 80% to 90% accurate in defining the presence of metastatic carcinoma in the anterior compartment of the mediastinum,

but the results achieved in patients with lymphoma are much less reliable. In order to prescribe the most appropriate chemotherapy protocol, it is absolutely critical to be able to differentiate Hodgkin disease from non-Hodgkin lymphoma, and lymphoblastic from nonlymphoblastic histology. Needle biopsies of children with suspected lymphoma may not provide a reliable definition of these issues and as such are not recommended. Immunophenotyping is frequently used to confirm the histologic diagnosis. This technique may be particularly helpful in situations where adequate biopsy material is difficult to obtain. Unfortunately, most antibodies used for immunohistochemical characterization of lymphatic tissue are not completely specific. In the majority of cases, the definitive diagnosis of lymphoma should not be established on the basis of immunostaining alone.

Thoracoscopy represents a safe and minimally invasive method for the biopsy of mediastinal tumors. This method provides excellent visualization of the mediastinum. A chest tube is usually left in place for 1 to 2 days for lung reexpansion. Following removal of the chest tube, the patient may be discharged or may begin chemotherapy. If a direct approach to the anterior mediastinum is required, the favored method is the Chamberlain procedure with resection of the third or fourth costal cartilage (Fig. 28-2A). With this incision, it is usually possible to remain in an extrapleural plane, and once direct visualization of the underlying tissue is attained, an open biopsy with secure hemostasis is easily achieved (Fig. 28-2B). A chest tube is not required, and postoperative discomfort is minimal. Patients treated in this fashion are typically ready for discharge or initiation of chemotherapy on the first or second postoperative day.

Unfortunately, a significant percentage of children with lymphoma present with evidence of bulky disease in the anterior mediastinum (Fig. 28-3). This condition represents a major anesthetic risk because of the propensity to produce a life-threatening airway compromise. The airway problems associated with pediatric mediastinal tumors have been well

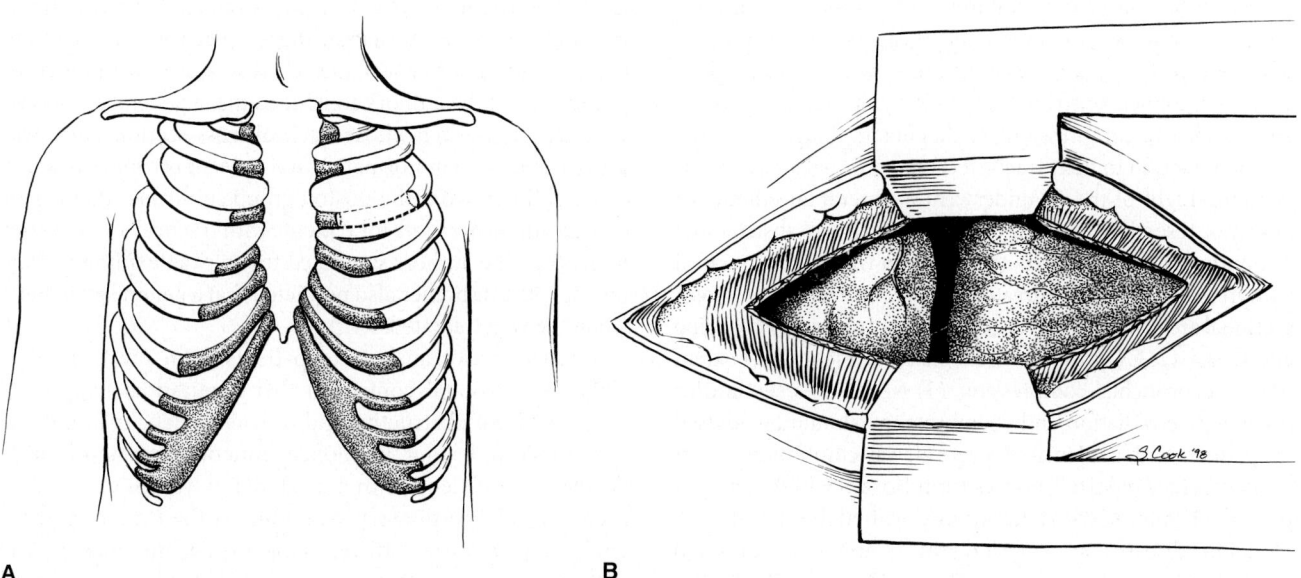

A          B

**FIGURE 28-2** Chamberlain procedure. This anterior–parasternal approach to the mediastinum is used in the biopsy of bulky anterior mediastinal tumors. **A.** Typically, a transverse incision is made and the third or fourth costal cartilage is resected. This provides exposure to the underlying mediastinum. **B.** The internal mammary vessels are divided.

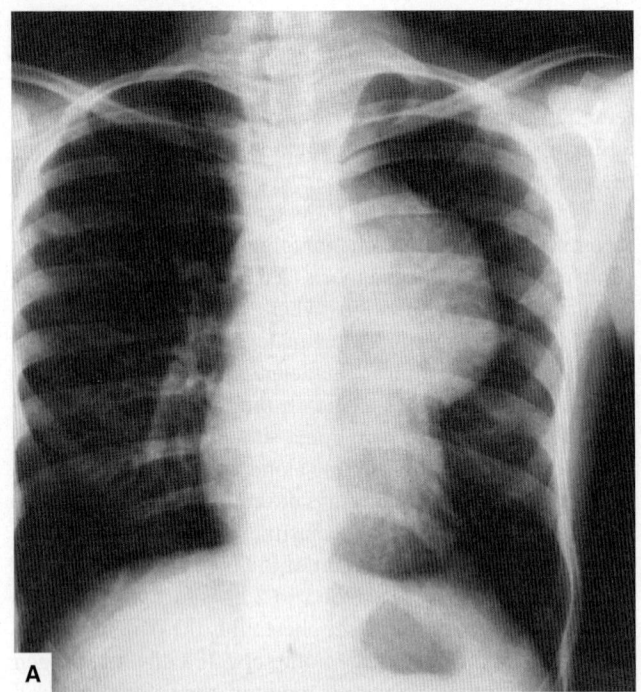

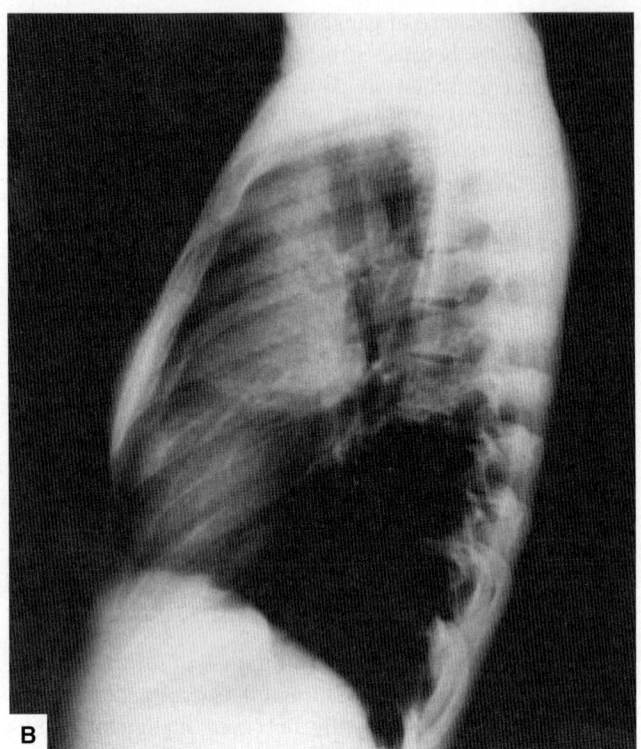

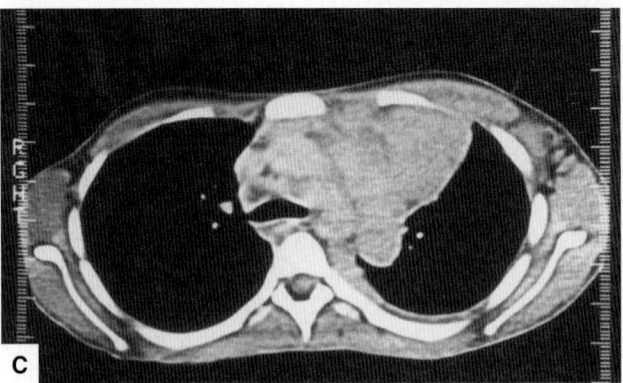

**FIGURE 28-3 A.** Anteroposterior chest radiograph obtained to evaluate an adolescent female with orthopnea. A large mass obliterating the left cardiomediastinal silhouette is noted. **B.** A lateral chest radiograph confirms the anterior position of the tumor. **C.** Computed tomography demonstrates complete occlusion of the left main stem bronchus when the patient is supine.

documented. Azizkhan reviewed the Johns Hopkins experience with 50 consecutive children with mediastinal tumors: 30 had respiratory symptoms at diagnosis, and 9 had evidence of a life-threatening airway compromise with either dyspnea at rest, orthopnea, or stridor. Of the 30 symptomatic children, 13 had airway compression on diagnostic imaging studies, with a reduction in their tracheal cross-sectional areas of 35% or more. Eight of the 13 underwent a general anesthetic for biopsy or resection, and 5 developed total airway obstruction. The authors concluded that: (1) Children with severe tracheal compression (defined as greater than a 33% decrease in cross-sectional area) were at grave risk for airway obstruction during anesthesia. (2) CT provided a reliable assessment of the extent of tracheobronchial compression. (3) Needle biopsies and/or preoperative radiation and chemotherapy should be advised for patients with evidence of severe airway compromise.

Shamberger reported a series from Boston Children's Hospital of 42 children with anterior mediastinal tumors, 40 with Hodgkin disease or non-Hodgkin lymphoma. Although respiratory symptoms were present in 21 cases (50%), with the exception of orthopnea, symptoms could not be correlated with the degree of tracheal narrowing. The cross-sectional area of the trachea was moderately compromised

(less than 75% of expected area) in 23 patients and severely narrowed (less than 50% of expected area) in 7. In 29 patients with mild-to-moderate narrowing (between 50% and 100% of normal), an endotracheal anesthetic was used without complication, and the authors concluded that a general anesthetic was safe for children whose tracheal cross-sectional area was greater than 50% of normal. A more recent prospective study on 31 children from the Boston group confirmed that a general anesthetic was safe for patients with tracheal areas greater than 50%. The authors suggested that a peak expiratory flow rate of >50% or higher also predicted that a general anesthetic would be well tolerated.

A retrospective analysis of patients from the Columbus Children's Hospital confirmed that mediastinal lymphoma produced both obstructive and restrictive deficits in pulmonary function testing. Pulmonary function was significantly decreased in patients with non-Hodgkin lymphoma, in children who had respiratory symptoms at the time of presentation, and in those with very large mediastinal masses. The authors' current protocol at Nationwide Children's Hospital in Columbus, OH, for the preoperative evaluation of children with bulky mediastinal tumors includes: (1) an assessment of symptoms with particular interest to the presence of dyspnea, orthopnea, or stridor; (2) standard posteroanterior and lateral chest radiographs; (3) CT to evaluate the magnitude of tracheal narrowing; (4) echocardiography to rule out the presence of pericardial effusion or cardiac compromise; (5) pulmonary function studies with inspiratory and expiratory flow loops in both upright and supine positions; and (6) room air oxygen saturation at rest. Asymptomatic patients with normal flow loops and children with no significant tracheal narrowing (>50% of normal) are considered appropriate candidates for general endotracheal anesthesia. Those with evidence of severe anatomic or physiologic impairment who require surgical intervention for a definitive diagnosis of lymphoma are treated with a general anesthetic with the patient breathing spontaneously in the sitting position or with a local anesthetic with or without adequate sedation. If the patient is so unstable that a biopsy cannot be obtained safely, the authors recommend the use of radiotherapy or chemotherapy to reduce the size of the mediastinal tumor. If radiotherapy is used, a portion of the lesion in an accessible area should be shielded in order to preserve a segment of untreated tissue for a subsequent biopsy. This technique usually provides an accurate assessment of the histopathology of the primary tumor. Alternatively, pleural fluid, if present, may be obtained for cytologic evaluation, avoiding the risk of a general anesthetic in these symptomatic patients.

## GERM CELL TUMORS

The mediastinum is the second most common extragonadal site for germ cell tumors. Sixty of the 757 patients (8%) in the reported review had tumors of germ cell origin. Benign lesions were observed in 44 of these 60 patients (73%), and 16 others had malignant tumors (Table 28-2). Lesions of germ cell origin accounted for 15% of all of the benign tumors reported and 3.5% of the malignancies.

Germ cells arise in the caudal portion of the yolk sac between the fourth and sixth weeks of embryonic life and migrate to the primordial gonad developing in the urogenital ridge. If this migration is not completed properly, these pluripotential cells may remain in extragonadal sites adjacent to the midline, giving rise to germ cell tumors. Germ cells have the potential to develop into a wide variety of mature tissues, forming a teratoma, or they can differentiate into frankly malignant lesions with embryonic elements, as in embryonal carcinoma, or extraembryonic tissue, as in choriocarcinoma. Germ cells can also remain undifferentiated and be classified as a seminoma or dysgerminoma. Germ cell tumors of the mediastinum usually arise during the teenage years. Klinefelter syndrome may be observed in up to 20% of these patients.

Cancer of germ cell origin is uncommon, accounting for less than 3% of all the malignant tumors in childhood. Alpha fetoprotein (half-life 5 days) and the β-subunit of human chorionic gonadotropin (half-life 16 hours) have proven to be sensitive serum markers of residual and/or recurrent disease in patients with malignant germ cell tumors. Although Norris's classification of teratomas as either mature or immature is well accepted, the accuracy and applicability of the germ cell tumor staging systems presently used in adults have not been verified in children. The current Children's Oncology Group (COG) protocol includes the following clinical/pathologic staging system for patients with malignant extragonadal germ cell tumors:

▶ Stage I: Localized disease, with complete resection, negative tumor margins, tumor markers positive or negative

▶ Stage II: Microscopic residual disease, capsular invasion, lymph nodes negative, tumor markers positive or negative

▶ Stage III: Gross residual disease or biopsy only, gross lymph node involvement, cytologic evidence of tumor cells in ascites or pleural fluid, tumor markers positive or negative

▶ Stage IV: Distant metastases

The completed Pediatric Oncology Group/Children's Oncology Group (POG/COG) intergroup study of high-risk mediastinal germ cell tumors was reported by Billmire. The study reviewed 36 children with primary malignant germ cell tumors arising in the mediastinum. The tumor arose in the anterior mediastinum in 34 cases, while 2 infants had intrapericardial tumors. Mean tumor diameter was 13.3 cm for children less than age 5 years and 13.9 cm for children 5 years or older. There were 8 stage I/II tumors, 19 stage III tumors, and 9 stage IV tumors. Fourteen patients underwent prechemotherapy resection and 18 patients received neoadjuvant therapy followed by resection after at least 4 cycles of chemotherapy. Four patients underwent tumor biopsy alone without additional surgery. In this series, 26 patients survived with a 4-year survival rate of 71% and 4-year event-free survival of 69%. The tumor was the cause of death for 5 patients, all males with stage III or IV tumors.

Complete resection of the primary tumor at diagnosis, if possible, clearly offers the best prognosis for children with both benign and malignant lesions. If complete resection is not feasible at initial presentation, then biopsy, neoadjuvant chemotherapy, and delayed resection is appropriate and does not appear to adversely affect outcome. Although total excision is sufficient for the vast majority of patients with both mature and immature benign tumors, long-term follow-up is recommended because a small percentage of these patients will develop either a benign recurrence or malignant transformation. Children with malignant lesions should receive multiagent chemotherapy with a combination of cisplatin, bleomycin, and etoposide. Serial measurement of serum alpha-fetoprotein and/or beta-human chorionic gonadotropin levels is recommended because this may well provide evidence of recurrent or residual tumor before a lesion is apparent on physical examination or diagnostic imaging.

## VASCULAR LESIONS

Hemangiomas and lymphatic malformations (cystic hygromas) are vascular anomalies that represent approximately 12% of all benign mediastinal lesions. These lesions may be present at birth but not become evident until later in life. The principles of management for lesions in the mediastinum are similar to those recommended for their counterparts in extrathoracic locations.

Hemangiomas are the most common tumors of infancy. Also referred to as "infantile hemangiomas," they affect approximately 5% to 10% of Caucasian infants but are less common in other infants. These tumors are usually not identified at birth but during the first to third week of life. They are usually insignificant lesions that increase in size during the first 6 to 12 months of life, but typically undergo gradual spontaneous involution thereafter, a process that takes many years.

Hemangiomas are neoplastic proliferations of blood vessels composed of variable but generally thin and uniform fibromuscular walls lined by a single layer of benign endothelial cells. The majority of mediastinal hemangiomas are capillary lesions, which may produce life-threatening airway obstruction as they grow. Other types of benign vascular neoplasms observed in the mediastinum include arteriovenous malformations, angiofibromas, angiolipomas, glomus tumors, and hemangiopericytomas.

Mediastinal hemangiomas are uncommon in childhood. Only about 50 cases were reported by the early 1990s. Pediatric patients with mediastinal hemangiomas are typically brought to medical attention during the first few months of life for an evaluation of fullness in the neck, feeding difficulties, or respiratory symptoms ranging from mild wheezing to severe respiratory distress. Bronchoscopy usually demonstrates external compression of the tracheal lumen. A solid mass in the anterior or middle portion of the mediastinum can be observed on a CT scan. MRI can be helpful in differentiating vascular tumors consistent with hemangiomas. Although these imaging studies are useful for defining the anatomic boundaries of the tumor, there are no unique characteristics on diagnostic imaging that can definitively identify the lesion as a hemangioma and a mediastinal hemangioma is seldom diagnosed definitively by noninvasive means.

Treatment modalities for most hemangiomas include observation, propranolol, steroids, and rarely arterial ligation or embolization or resection (either partial or complete). Observation usually suffices. Despite the striking appearance and occasional rapid growth of hemangiomas, spontaneous regression almost always occurs with minimal residual scarring. Observation is contraindicated, however, when the hemangioma is located in the mediastinum and produces symptoms of airway obstruction.

The treatment of mediastinal lymphatic malformations requires a multimodal approach and may include both operative resection and image-guided percutaneous sclerotherapy. Patients require multiple treatments, and both short-term and long-term follow-up with imaging studies. (see Chapter 75). Given the rarity of mediastinal lymphatic malformations and the complexity of their treatment, consideration should be given to referral to a specialty center with substantial experience and technical expertise.

## THYMUS CYSTS AND NEOPLASMS

Among the children in the series from the 7 medical centers, 58 (7.7%) had lesions of the thymus. Forty-three of the 58 patients had benign conditions (75%), and 15 had a

malignancy. The benign lesions included 11 thymic cysts, 12 benign thymomas, 14 hyperplastic glands, and 6 other less common problems. These 43 thymic lesions accounted for 14.6% of all benign mediastinal masses and approximately one half of the benign tumors observed in the anterior compartment of the mediastinum. The 15 children with cancer of the thymus represented only 3.2% of all of the malignant conditions reported and 5.6% of the malignant tumors that in the anterior mediastinum (Table 28-2).

## Thymic Embryology

Thymic epithelium appears in the sixth week of development from the third and often fourth branchial clefts and pharyngeal pouches. By the eighth week, the 2 thymic anlages unite in the midline and begin descending into the chest. On occasion, the thymus fails to descend into the chest and can be found in the neck (Fig. 28-4). By the tenth week, T cells are present in the gland. Ectopic thymic tissue can be found anywhere between the posterior pharynx and the diaphragm. At birth, the thymus usually weighs approximately 30 to 40 g.

## Thymic Anatomy and Function

The thymus is the central organ of the immune system. It lies in the anterior superior mediastinum with the lower border reaching the level of the fourth costal cartilages. The vascular supply is derived from branches of the internal thoracic and

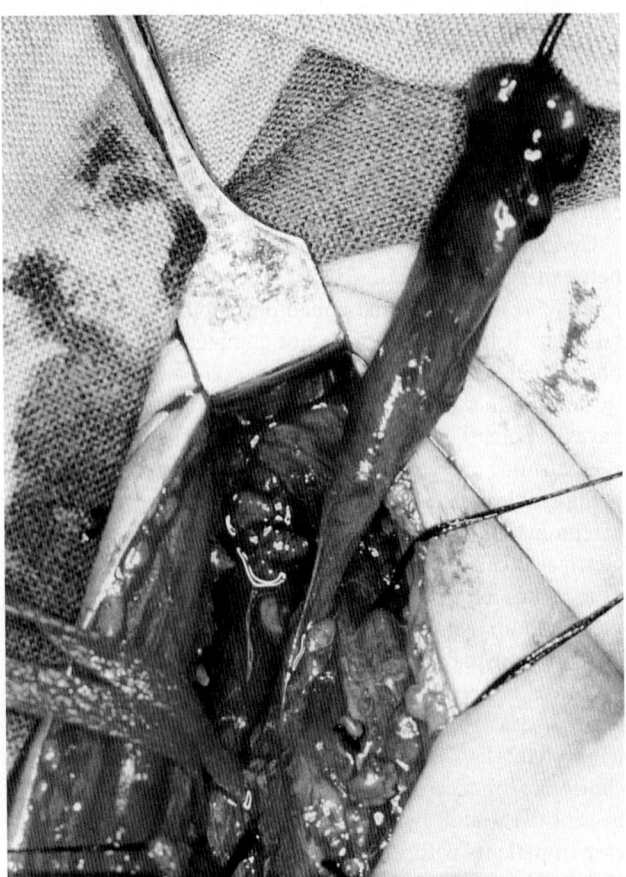

**FIGURE 28-4** Cervical thymus found in the neck of a newborn when exploration was performed for an esophageal perforation.

inferior thyroid arteries. The gland drains into the brachiocephalic, internal thoracic, and inferior thyroid veins. The thymus undergoes involution with age, decreasing to one third of its original size in adults.

Histologically, the thymus is divided into lobules with cortical and medullary compartments. The cortex contains the immunologically incompetent thymocytes. T-cell differentiation takes place in the cortex, and mature T cells reside in the medulla.

The thymus remains quite prominent on standard chest radiographs during the first year of life, and differentiating a normal but large gland from a benign or malignant tumor may be difficult. Indeed, 14 of the 41 benign lesions collated in the data review were described as hyperplastic glands. With the recent advances in diagnostic imaging, this dilemma should no longer represent a common clinical problem. There are now well-established criteria for ultrasound, CT, and MRI that should provide clear differentiation of a hyperplastic thymus from a benign or malignant thymoma.

Involution of the thymus in response to physiologic stress and sepsis is a well-known phenomenon, but rebound thymic hyperplasia, which has been described much less frequently, may represent a diagnostic dilemma. This condition has been reported to occur following recovery from cardiac surgery and major burns and after chemotherapy for a variety of malignant conditions. Idiopathic thymic hyperplasia can also be seen in association with Graves disease, Addison disease, acromegaly, and during therapy for hypothyroidism.

Thymic cysts are uncommon lesions that appear with equal frequency in both the neck and anterior mediastinum. These cysts are usually unilocular, thin-walled spaces lined with squamous epithelium. Abundant lymphocytes are observed in the cyst wall. The presence of thymic tissue containing Hassall corpuscles differentiates these lesions from lymphatic malformations. Unilocular thymic cysts should be resected because they are prone to developing intralesional bleeding and infection and may undergo rapid expansion with a potential for airway obstruction.

Multilocular thymic cysts are uncommon lesions usually observed in patients with systemic immune-mediated conditions (eg, Sjögren disease) or certain tumors (eg, Hodgkin disease). The lesions are inflammatory and have visible septations on ultrasound and contrast-enhanced CT. Gallium-67 uptake has also been reported. Multilocular thymic cysts occur in both children and adults with human immunodeficiency virus (HIV) infections. Although these lesions do not resolve spontaneously with antiretroviral therapy, some authors have advised observation rather than resection because the majority of patients reported to date have remained asymptomatic.

Thymomas are uncommon, but when they do occur are almost equally likely to be benign or malignant (Fig. 28-5). In the collated series, 47% of all of the thymic masses reported were thymomas. There are very little data available on the treatment of these tumors in childhood, and recent advances in management of these tumors rely on experience with adult patients.

The current clinicopathologic staging system for thymoma is presented in Table 28-3. Stage I lesions that demonstrate no histologic evidence of invasion are considered benign, and complete resection is curative. None of the 45 stage I

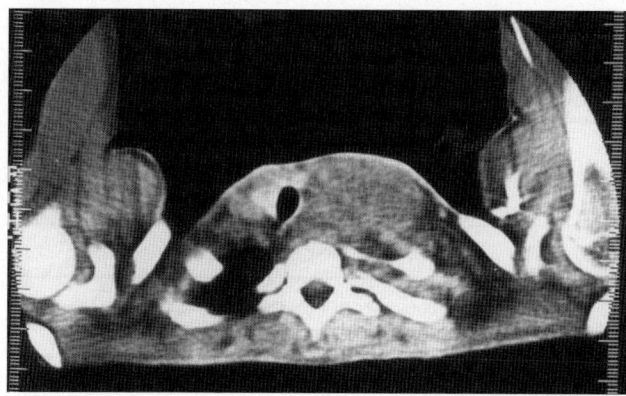

**FIGURE 28-5** Computed tomography scan demonstrating a malignant thymoma that produced significant tracheal displacement and distortion.

patients reported by Wilkins from Massachusetts General Hospital developed recurrence. Stage II, III, and IV thymomas are defined as malignant lesions, and their treatment is less well standardized. Without doubt, the most important therapeutic modality for patients with malignant thymoma is surgery. Patients with resectable lesions have an excellent prognosis, particularly when adjuvant radiotherapy is used. Nakahara reported 48 stage III patients, all of whom received radiotherapy following resection of their thymoma, with survival rates of 100% at 5 years and 95% at 10 years. Multiagent chemotherapy (cisplatin–doxorubicin–cyclophosphamide) has been employed with very limited success in patients with disseminated disease.

## MYASTHENIA GRAVIS

Clinical features of MG include weakness and fatigability of skeletal muscles, which worsen with repeated activity and improve with rest. Ptosis and diplopia occur early in most patients. Physical findings include motor weakness with preservation of sensation, coordination, and deep tendon reflexes. A scale for measuring the severity of symptoms was designed by Osserman (Table 28-4).

Children account for 10% of all MG cases. Three forms of MG occur during childhood: transient neonatal, genetic or congenital, and juvenile. Transient neonatal MG occurs in infants born to mothers with MG. The disease lasts from a few hours to several weeks with complete recovery. Congenital

| TABLE 28-3 | Staging of Thymomas |
|---|---|
| **Stage** | **Description** |
| I | An encapsulated lesion with no gross or microscopic invasion of adjacent tissues |
| II | Microscopic invasion of the capsule or adjacent pleura |
| III | Macroscopic invasion of surrounding tissues (ie, lung, pericardium, vena cava, and aorta) |
| IV | Disseminated disease that is intrathoracic or extrathoracic |

| TABLE 28-4 | Osserman Classification of Myasthenia Gravis |
|---|---|
| Group | Muscle Involvement |
| I | Focal disease (ocular muscle) |
| IIA | Generalized disease (mild) |
| IIB | Generalized disease (moderate) |
| III | Severe generalized disease |
| IV | Myasthenic crisis |

MG occurs in infants whose mothers do not suffer from MG. Symptoms are usually confined to ptosis with little or no generalized weakness. Juvenile MG is similar, both clinically and etiologically, to adult-onset MG. Approximately 75% of juvenile MG cases occur after age 10. Juvenile MG occurs more frequently in females. Initial symptoms are usually ptosis and diplopia, but up to 40% of patients may develop respiratory compromise.

The cellular pathophysiology of MG was initially theorized by Dale. After determining that acetylcholine (ACh) was released at motor nerve terminals, Dale suggested that weakness from MG was related to altered motor end plate function. The weakness of muscles after repetitive nerve stimulation led Harvey and Masland to propose that MG was due to a deficiency of ACh synthesis, a block of the ACh receptor, or an excess of cholinesterase (ChE) at the motor end plate. In some patients, a lack of ACh receptors at the neuromuscular junction was subsequently determined by further biochemical analysis.

An autoimmune etiology for the decrease in ACh receptors was suggested by Simpson. Anti-ACh receptor antibodies have subsequently been identified in 85% of MG patients. In addition, thymic abnormalities have been found in nearly all MG patients. T cells have a major role in the autoantibody response of MG. What triggers the autoimmune response remains unknown.

## Treatment of Myasthenia Gravis

Since there is no cure for MG, the main treatment goal is to achieve remission. The 4 methods of treatment for MG include enhancing neuromuscular transmission with ChE inhibitors, immunosuppression, short-term immunotherapies, and a surgical thymectomy. ChE inhibitors are the first line of treatment for MG. The purpose of using ChE inhibitors is to treat the symptoms by increasing ACh at the neuromuscular junction. These inhibitors have no effect on the pathologic basis of MG. Patients with MG usually benefit from taking ChE inhibitors, but improvement may be partial or may decrease over time.

The addition of an immunosuppressive agent is indicated when ChE inhibitors fail to alleviate weakness. Corticosteroids are the most commonly used second-line agents. The mechanism of action for immunosuppressive agents includes decreasing both the cellular and humoral responses to autoimmunity. Improvement can be seen in 70% of patients

taking corticosteroids. High-dose treatments are used to treat exacerbations of symptoms, and the amount is tapered to the lowest level possible to maintain remission. Azathioprine, cyclosporine, and cyclophosphamide have also been used to treat MG. Azathioprine is used when steroids and ChE inhibitors are not adequate or to avoid the side effects of steroids. Cyclosporine and cyclophosphamide are alternative agents used in the setting of refractory MG or intolerance of other immunosuppressive agents.

Short-term immunotherapies include plasma exchange and intravenous immunoglobulin. Using plasmapheresis to remove the antibodies from the circulation has resulted in short-term clinical improvement. This technique is used for patients in myasthenic crisis (respiratory compromise) or perioperatively for patients undergoing a thymectomy. Improvement following plasmapheresis lasts only a few weeks as antibody levels are reestablished. Immunoglobulin is indicated for the same patient population as plasmapheresis. The mechanism of action of immunoglobulin is unknown.

The role of thymic excision for the treatment of MG remains controversial. The guidelines from the American Academy of Neurology for the treatment of MG (published in 2000) recommend thymectomy only "as an option" to increase the chance of remission. While nonrandomized case series claim improvement in 60% to 100% of MG patients undergoing thymectomy, prospective randomized studies comparing thymectomy to medical management are lacking. Current indications for a thymectomy include resection of a thymoma and inducing MG regression. A thymectomy should be recommended for all children with generalized MG who have increased medication requirements for symptom control. Surgical resection is an elective procedure and should be performed only when the patient is strong and stable. Patients may have worsening symptoms after surgery, and the time required to reach maximal recovery varies. Thymectomies performed within 12 months of onset have better remission rates. Buckingham's computer-matched series of patients comparing early thymectomy to medical treatment is a compelling argument for surgery at diagnosis.

Treatment options for the 3 types of childhood MG are outlined in Table 28-5. Transient neonatal MG may or may not require intervention. Treatment with a ChE inhibitor may be needed for a few days or longer. Congenital MG symptoms can be treated successfully with ChE inhibitors. Juvenile MG treatment options are the same as the treatment for adult-onset MG. Drug therapy initially with ChE inhibitors is recommended. An exacerbation of symptoms or an insufficient response to ChE inhibitors requires that corticosteroids be added.

A thymectomy can be performed by a transcervical, transsternal, or thoracoscopic method. The authors prefer a transcervical approach. Preoperative evaluation consists of a routine chest radiograph to rule out the presence of thymoma, and pulmonary function tests as a baseline evaluation of respiratory muscle strength. The patient is given the usual dose of anticholinergic medication orally on the morning of surgery. A collar incision is made approximately 1 cm above the sternal notch (Fig. 28-6A and B). The pretracheal strap muscles are split in the midline and retracted laterally. The cervical thymus is grasped by clamps, and traction is applied

| TABLE 28-5 | Treatments for Childhood Myasthenia Gravis |
|---|---|
| **Type** | **Treatment** |
| Transient neonatal | Supportive |
| | Cholinesterase inhibitors—short-term |
| | corticosteroids |
| Congenital | Cholinesterase inhibitors |
| | Corticosteroids |
| Juvenile | Cholinesterase inhibitors |
| | Corticosteroids |
| | Immunosuppressive drugs |
| | Intravenous immune globulin |
| | Plasmapheresis |
| | Thymectomy |

superiorly to mobilize the thymus. The gland is dissected from surrounding structures and from the innominate vein that lies deep to it in the upper chest. Traction is applied with serially positioned clamps, and by blunt dissection, the thymus is mobilized from within the chest (Fig. 28-6C-I). Vascular structures are ligated with hemoclips. The lowest clip is usually noted at the level of the pulmonary artery on the postoperative chest radiograph (Fig. 28-7). The wound is closed with a soft suction drain left in place for 24 hours.

Unlike patients who undergo surgery using a transsternal approach, those who undergo surgery using a cervical approach are frequently extubated in the operating room or recovery room when spirometry indicates that they are at preoperative levels of pulmonary function. Anticholinergic agents may have increased efficacy and are given in incremental doses as indicated by bedside spirometry during the postoperative period. Discharge times are shorter after surgery with the transcervical approach than with the transsternal approach.

The success of a thymectomy in inducing remission in MG varies from 24% to 90%. Remission may be complete or partial and is defined as a reduction in medication dosage needed. Variables that improve postoperative remission include early surgical intervention, the presence of bulbar symptoms, the presence of other immune diseases, and the onset of symptoms between ages 12 and 16 years. Rodriquez found that 80% of patients with juvenile MG were estimated to be alive at 40 years of age compared to 90% in the general population.

## BRONCHOGENIC AND ENTERIC CYSTS

Bronchogenic and enteric cysts, which are commonly located in the middle or posterior mediastinum, represented 7.1% of all of the mediastinal masses in the reported review and accounted for 18.4% of the benign lesions. Although

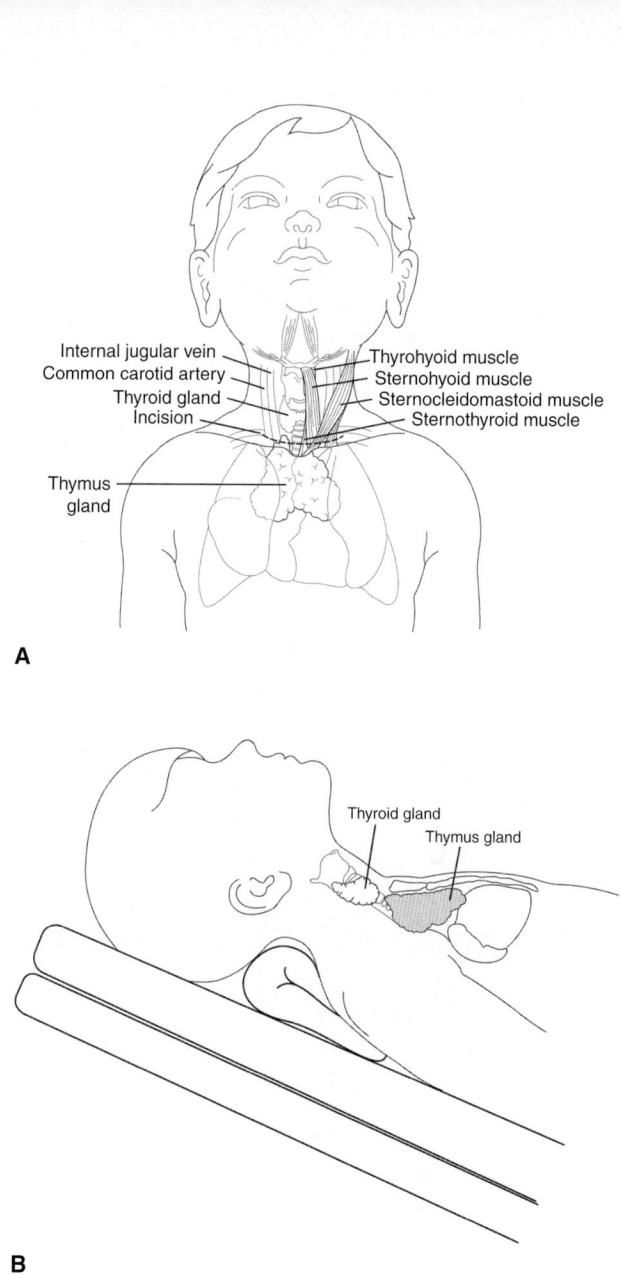

A

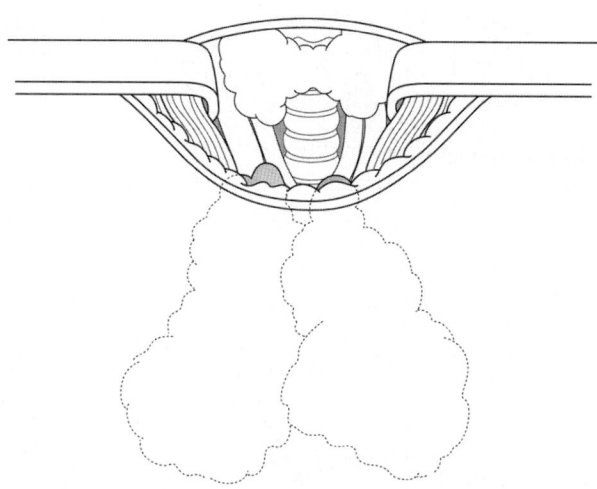

B

C

**FIGURE 28-6** **A.** Anatomy of the superior mediastinum and neck. The collar incision is depicted by the *dotted line*. **B.** A lateral anatomic view demonstrates the positioning of the patient with the neck moderately extended. **C.** Strap muscles are separated in the midline and they are mobilized for lateral retraction.

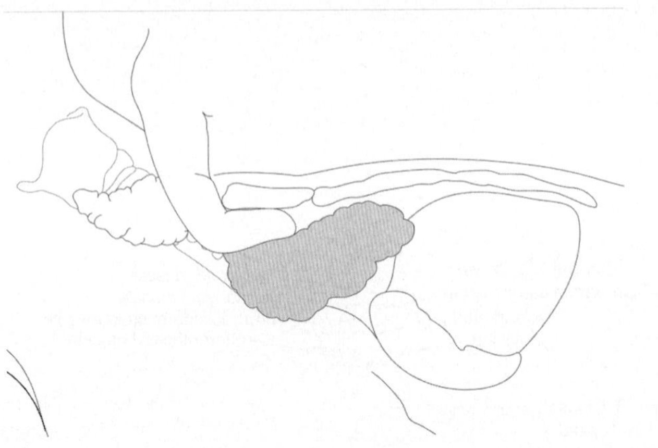

**D**

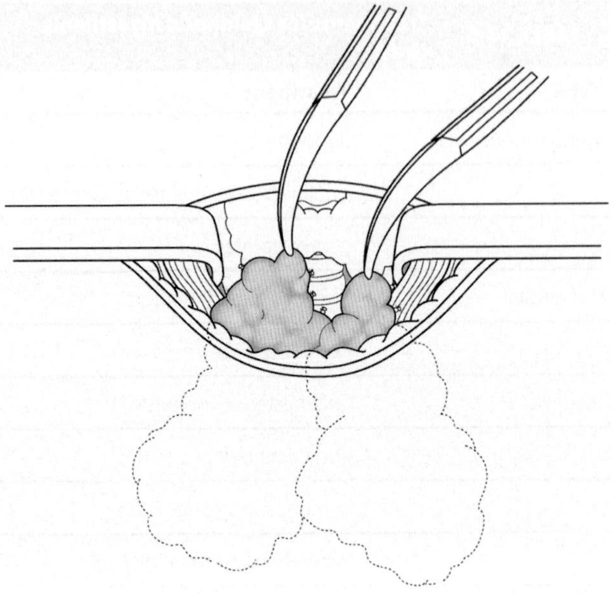

**E**

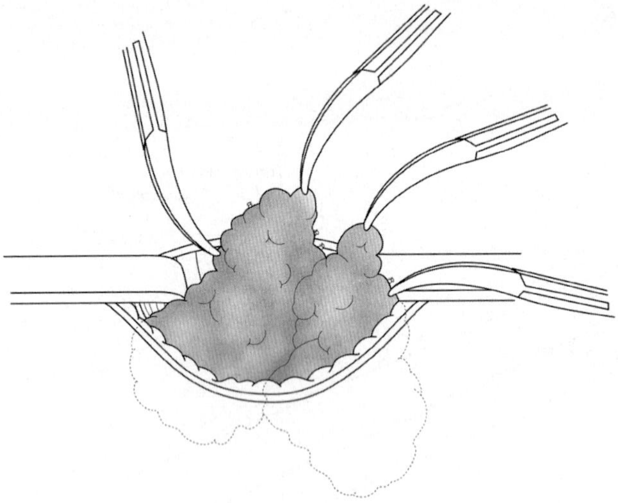

**F**

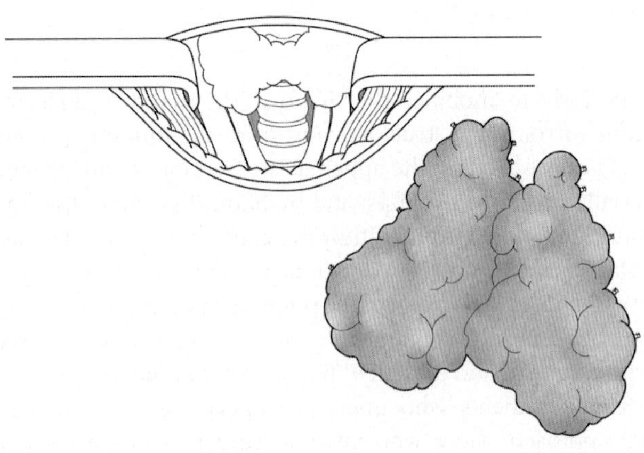

**G**

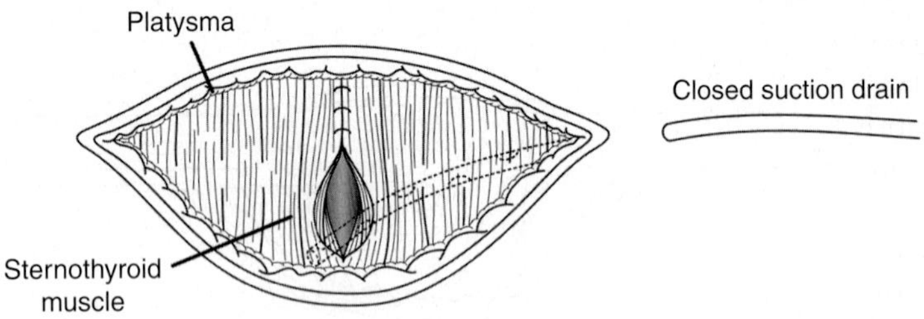

Platysma

Sternothyroid
muscle

Closed suction drain

**H**

Sternothyroid
muscle

Platysma

Closed suction
drain

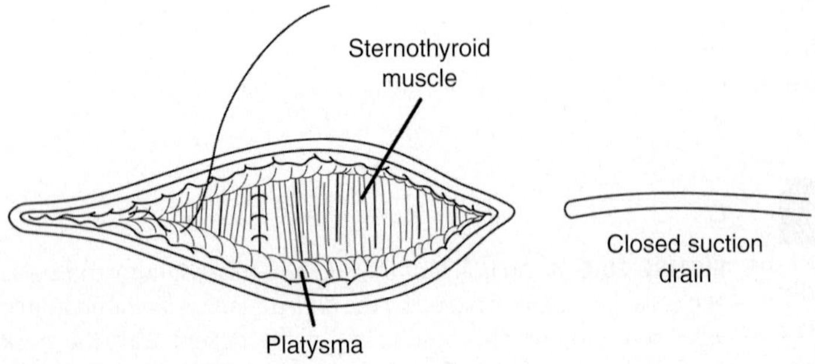

**I**

**FIGURE 28-6** (*Continued*) **D.** The dissection into the superior mediastinum is facilitated by blunt finger dissection between the posterior surface of the sternum and the thymus. **E.** The thymus is grasped and cephalad traction is applied by serially positioning clamps. **F.** The thymus is mobilized by segmental dissection while maintaining cephalic traction. Vascular clips or ligatures are used to ligate vessels. **G.** The thymus is delivered from the superior mediastinum. **H.** A soft suction drain is placed for 24 hours in the retrosternal space through a separated stab wound in the neck. The strap muscles are approximated in the midline. **I.** Final wound closure.

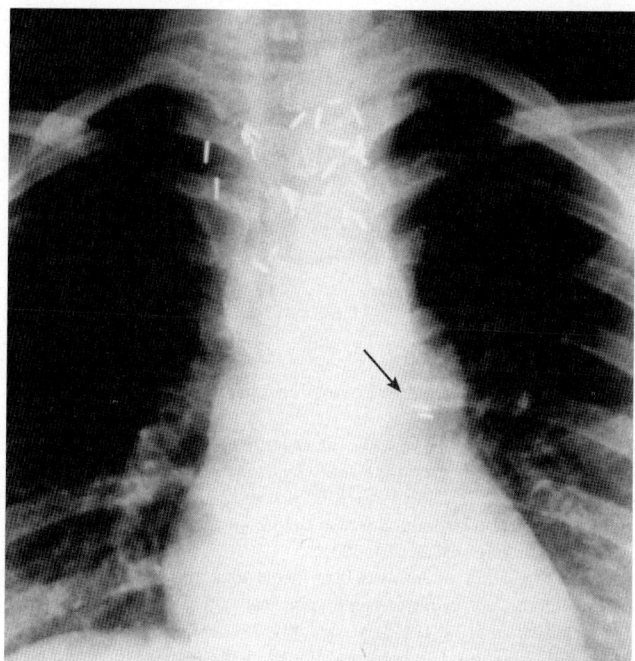

**FIGURE 28-7** Postoperative chest radiograph. Note metallic clips at the level of the pulmonary arteries (*arrow*).

malignant thymoma, germ cell tumors, and Hodgkin disease may all have cystic components, the majority of cystic mediastinal tumors are benign lesions that are congenital in origin. In the reported review, gastroenteric duplications (22) were less common than bronchogenic cysts (32).

Congenital mediastinal cysts generally arise from the foregut as a result of anomalous budding of the primordia of the esophagus or tracheobronchial tree. Each of the 3 types of foregut cysts (bronchogenic cysts, enteric duplications, and the rare neuroenteric cysts) has characteristic histologic and anatomic features. Occasionally, the pathologic characteristics of both enteric duplications and bronchogenic cysts coexist, and these composite structures are referred to as bronchopulmonary foregut malformations.

On a CT scan, a foregut cyst usually appears as a smooth, rounded cystic mass with homogeneous attenuation. The lesion typically has a thin wall and is commonly located in the carinal, paratracheal, or paraesophageal region. The cyst contents generally have attenuation values similar to those of water, but higher levels can be observed if the lesion contains mucus, blood, or debris. Bronchogenic and enteric cysts are not enhanced in the presence of intravenous contrast.

## Bronchogenic Cysts

The respiratory tract develops as a ventral bud off of the primitive foregut on about the 22nd day of gestation, and division into left and right main stem bronchi is usually complete by day 26. Abnormal budding from the tracheobronchial tree is believed to result in bronchogenic cysts. These lesions may be completely encapsulated, or they can communicate with the airway. Although most bronchogenic cysts arise in the mediastinum, they also occur in the pulmonary hilum, the lung parenchyma, or the neck, and can even be found below the diaphragm. Bronchogenic cysts are usually lined with ciliated columnar or cuboidal epithelium and have a fibromuscular wall that may contain both cartilage and bronchial mucous glands.

Bronchogenic cysts are a well-recognized cause of respiratory distress in newborns and these cysts can also produce recurrent pulmonary infections in older infants and children. In a review of 20 patients with bronchogenic cysts, the most common presenting symptom was fever, followed by recurrent pneumonia, a cervical mass, and respiratory distress. On standard chest radiographs, bronchogenic cysts usually appear as radiolucent spherical lesions that are variable in size and may cause a mediastinal shift (Fig. 28-8A and B). On CT scanning, bronchogenic cysts appear as well-defined, spherical, nonenhancing masses. If the cyst is infected or filled with secretions, it may be radiodense. If there is communication with the tracheobronchial tree, an air-fluid level will frequently be observed.

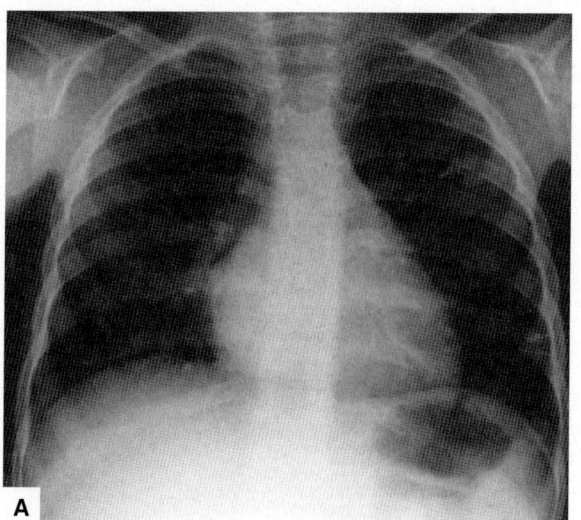

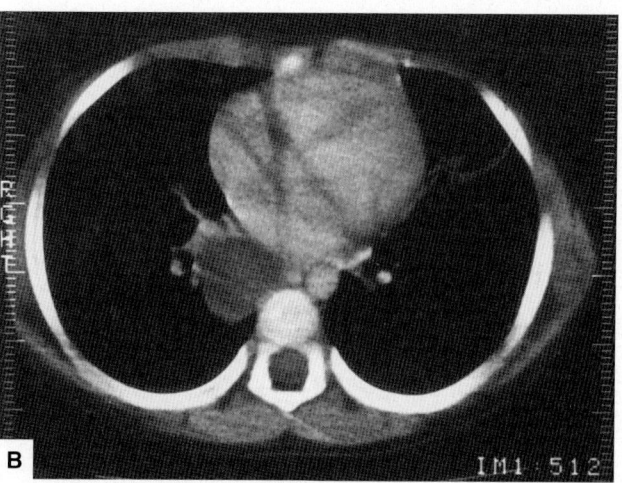

**FIGURE 28-8** **A.** Posteroanterior chest radiograph obtained for the evaluation of persistent wheezing that failed to respond to bronchodilator therapy. A retrocardiac mass is noted on the right. **B.** With computed tomography a thin-walled apparently cystic lesion is observed adjacent to the left lower lobe bronchus.

Bronchogenic cysts should be resected. A thoracoscopic approach can be used for easily accessible lesions. If a thoracotomy is elected, a muscle-sparing technique is most appropriate. If a complete resection is difficult because a portion of the cyst wall is densely adherent to the bronchus, esophagus, or trachea, the mucosa should be stripped and a segment of the cyst wall left behind.

## Enteric and Neuroenteric Cysts

Enteric cysts, also called enterogenous cysts and enteric duplications, have somewhat thicker muscular walls and are typically spherical or tubular in configuration. Because these lesions are lined with mucus-producing epithelium, they gradually enlarge and usually produce symptoms in infancy or early childhood resulting from the compression of adjacent organs.

Esophageal duplications, a subset of enteric cysts, constitute 15% of all gastrointestinal duplications. These lesions may contain cartilage and respiratory epithelium similar to bronchogenic cysts, and they tend to occur in older children. Esophageal duplications typically have well-developed muscular walls lined with gastric or intestinal mucosa.

Neuroenteric cysts are the least common type of congenital mediastinal cyst. They communicate with the meninges through a defect in the neurospinal axis and may be suspected on a chest radiograph because of the associated vertebral anomalies. A neuroenteric cyst has thin, fibrous walls lined with simple or pseudostratified epithelium. These lesions may produce neurologic symptoms if spinal cord compression occurs, and meningitis is a real threat, particularly if there is open communication with the gastrointestinal tract. Surgical management may require the assistance of colleagues in both neurosurgery and orthopedics in order to ensure proper closure of the dural membrane and stabilization of the vertebral column.

## SELECTED READINGS

Adams GA, Schochat SJ, Smith EI, Shuster JJ, Jashi VV, Altshuler G. Thoracic neuroblastoma: a POG study. *J Pediatr Surg* 1993;28:372–378.

Azizkhan RG, Dudgeon DL, Buck JR, Colombani PM, Yaster M, Nichols D. Life-threatening airway obstruction as a complication to the management of mediastinal masses in children. *J Pediatr Surg* 1985;20:816–822.

Billmire DF, Grosfeld JL. Teratomas in childhood: analysis of 142 cases. *J Pediatr Surg* 1986;21:548–551.

Billmire D, Vinocur C, Rescorla F, et al. Malignant mediastinal germ cell tumors: an intergroup study. *J Pediatr Surg* 2001;36:18–24.

Boardman SJ, Cochrane LA, Roebuck D, Elliott MJ, Hartley BE. Multimodality treatment of pediatric lymphatic malformations of the head and neck using surgery and sclerotherapy. *Arch Otolaryngol Head Neck Surg* 2010;136:270–276.

Childress ME, Baker CP, Samson PC. Lymphangioma of the mediastinum: report of a case with review of the literature. *J Thorac Surg* 1956;31:338–348.

DeCou J, Schlatter M, Mitchell D, Abrams R. Primary thoracoscopic gross total resection of neuroblastoma. *J Laparoendosc Adv Surg Tech* 2005;15:470–473.

Evoli A. Acquired myasthenia gravis in childhood. *Curr Opin Neurol* 2010;23:536–540.

Hack HA, Wright NB, Wynn RF. The anaesthetic management of children with anterior mediastinal masses. *Anaesthesia* 2008;63:837–846.

King DR, Patrick LE, Ginn-Pease ME, McCay KS, Klopfenstein K. Pulmonary function is compromised in children with mediastinal lymphoma. *J Pediatr Surg* 1997;32:294–300.

Lee EY. Evaluation of non-vascular mediastinal masses in infants and children: an evidence-based practical approach. *Pediatr Radiol* 2009;39(suppl 2):S184–S190.

Meehan JJ, Sandler AD. Robotic resection of mediastinal masses in children. *J Laparoendosc Adv Surg Tech* 2008;18:114–119.

Nakahara K, Ohno K, Hashimoto J, et al. Thymoma: results with complete resection and adjuvant postoperative irradiation in 141 consecutive patients. *J Thorac Cardiovasc Surg* 1988;95:1041–1047.

Noi M, Nakamura M, Yoshida S, Ishii T, Amae S, Hayashi Y. Thoracic removal of neurogenic mediastinal tumors in children. *J Laparoendosc Adv Surg Tech* 2005;15:80–84.

Perkins JA, Manning SC, Tempero RM, et al. Lymphatic malformations: review of current treatment. *Otolaryngol Head Neck Surg* 2010; 142:795–803.

Rodriquez M, Gomez MR, Howard FM Jr, Taylor WF. Myasthenia gravis in children: long term follow-up. *Ann Neurol* 1983;13:504–510.

Shamberger RC, Holzman RS, Griscom NT, Tarbell NJ, Weinstein HJ, Wohl ME. Prospective evaluation by computed tomography and pulmonary function tests of children with mediastinal masses. *Surgery* 1995;118:468–471.

Shiels WE 2nd, Kang DR, Murakami JW, Hogan MJ, Wiet GJ. Percutaneous treatment of lymphatic malformations. *Otolaryngol Head Neck Surg* 2009;141:219–224.

Simpson JA, Behan PO, Dick HM. Studies on the nature of autoimmunity in myasthenia gravis: evidence for an immunodeficiency type. *Ann NY Acad Sci* 1976;274:382–389.

Truong MT, Perkins JA, Messner AH, Chang KW. Propranolol for the treatment of airway hemangiomas: a case series and treatment algorithm. *Int J Pediatr Otorhinolaryngol* 2010;74:1043–1048.

Wilkens EW Jr, Castleman B. Thymoma: a continuing survey at the Massachusetts General Hospital. *Ann Thorac Surg* 1979;3:252–256.

# CHAPTER 29

## Congenital Lung Malformations:
CPAM, Bronchopulmonary Sequestration, Congenital Lobar Emphysema, and Bronchogenic Cyst

*Steven Rothenberg and
Timothy M. Crombleholme*

## KEY POINTS

1. Treatment of bronchopulmonary malformations may vary somewhat depending on the time of diagnosis and the presentation, but in most cases, complete resection is the desired therapy.

2. New minimally invasive techniques allow treatment with much less pain and morbidity and long-term consequence for the infant or child.

3. Bronchopulmonary sequestration (BPS) lesions may be asymptomatic, but postnatal resection should be considered because of the risks of infection, hemorrhage, and malignant transformation.

4. The surgical approach to BPS is straightforward, with the exception of the management of anomalous blood supply. Intraoperative death due to hemorrhage from unrecognized anomalous vessels has been reported.

5. Congenital pulmonary airway malformation (CPAM) is increasingly being diagnosed by routine prenatal ultrasound, allowing for prenatal consultation and planning. The need for fetal intervention is rare and limited to cases with severe hydrops and a predicted mortality of near 100%.

6. The treatment of choice in infants with CPAM is complete resection of the CPAM, usually by lobectomy.

7. The treatment for patients with symptomatic congenital lobar emphysema (CLE) is surgical resection; in most cases, a complete lobectomy.

8. The operative approach to resecting bronchogenic cysts depends on their location and involvement of adjacent structures, such as the trachea or mainstem bronchi, which may require repair.

## INTRODUCTION

There is a broad spectrum of bronchopulmonary malformations that present in early infancy and childhood. These include bronchopulmonary sequestrations (BPS), congenital pulmonary airway malformation (CPAM), congenital lobar emphysema (CLE), and bronchogenic cysts. These lesions may be detected by prenatal diagnosis, present as acute respiratory distress in the newborn period, or may remain undiagnosed and asymptomatic until late in life. Treatment may vary somewhat depending on the time of diagnosis and the presentation, but in most cases, complete resection is the desired therapy. New minimally invasive techniques now allow this to be done with much less pain, morbidity, and long-term consequences for the infant or child.

## BRONCHOPULMONARY SEQUESTRATION

Bronchopulmonary sequestration is a rare congenital malformation of the lower respiratory tract. It consists of a nonfunctioning mass of lung tissue that lacks normal communication with the tracheobronchial tree and receives its arterial blood supply from the systemic circulation. There appears to be a spectrum of sequestration with, at one extreme, an abnormal vessel supplying a nonsequestered lung and, at the other extreme, abnormal pulmonary tissue but without anomalous vascular supply.

The majority of sequestrations fall into 2 categories: intralobar sequestration (ILS) and extralobar sequestration (ELS). ILS, defined as a lesion that lies within the normal lobe and lacks its own visceral pleura, accounts for 75% of BPS in infants and children. ELS is a mass located outside the normal lung and has its own visceral pleura. ELS accounts for 25% of cases in infants and children and may be either intrathoracic or subdiaphragmatic (Savic et al 1979; Collins et al 1987).

Terminology has become increasingly complicated. The term "malinosculation" describes the spectrum of congenital lung anomalies with an abnormal connection of 1 or more of the 4 major components of the lung tissue (Clements and Warner 1987). Congenital bronchopulmonary foregut malformation (CBPFM) refers to intralobar or extralobar BPS associated with a communication with the gastrointestinal tract. The spectrum of CBPFM includes ILS, ELS, congenital cystic adenomatoid malformation (CCAM), bronchogenic cyst, Scimitar syndrome, and duplication cyst. While much emphasis has been placed in the past in differentiating between BPS and CPAM, it is now clear that features of both can coexist in the same lesion, referred to as a hybrid lesion.

The majority of sequestrations occur in the lower lobes, but they can occur anywhere in the chest, as well as below the diaphragm and in the retroperitoneal space (Fig. 29-1A and B). Approximately 20% of ELS are located below the diaphragm. Approximately 60% of ILSs involve the left lower lobe, the majority in the posterior basal segment. CBPFM is more common on the right side. Communication with the foregut is much more common with ELS than with ILS. The systemic vascular supply for both ILS and ELS generally arises from the lower thoracic or upper abdominal aorta (Fig. 29-1C and D). The majority of cases have a single arterial feeder, but up to a third may have multiple vessels. The venous drainage is usually normal to the left atrium, but abnormal drainage to the right atrium, vena cava, or azygos vein has been documented. ELS and ILS have been reported together in the same patient.

ELS and CPAM type II (described later in this chapter) coexisting together has been reported in 25% to 50% of ELS cases (Conran et al 1999). The exact embryologic basis for the development of BPS of the lower respiratory tract is unclear. The lesion likely occurs early in embryologic development prior to the separation of the aortic and pulmonary circulations. One explanation is that there is an abnormality in lung bud formation. This might result in not only BPS, but also a

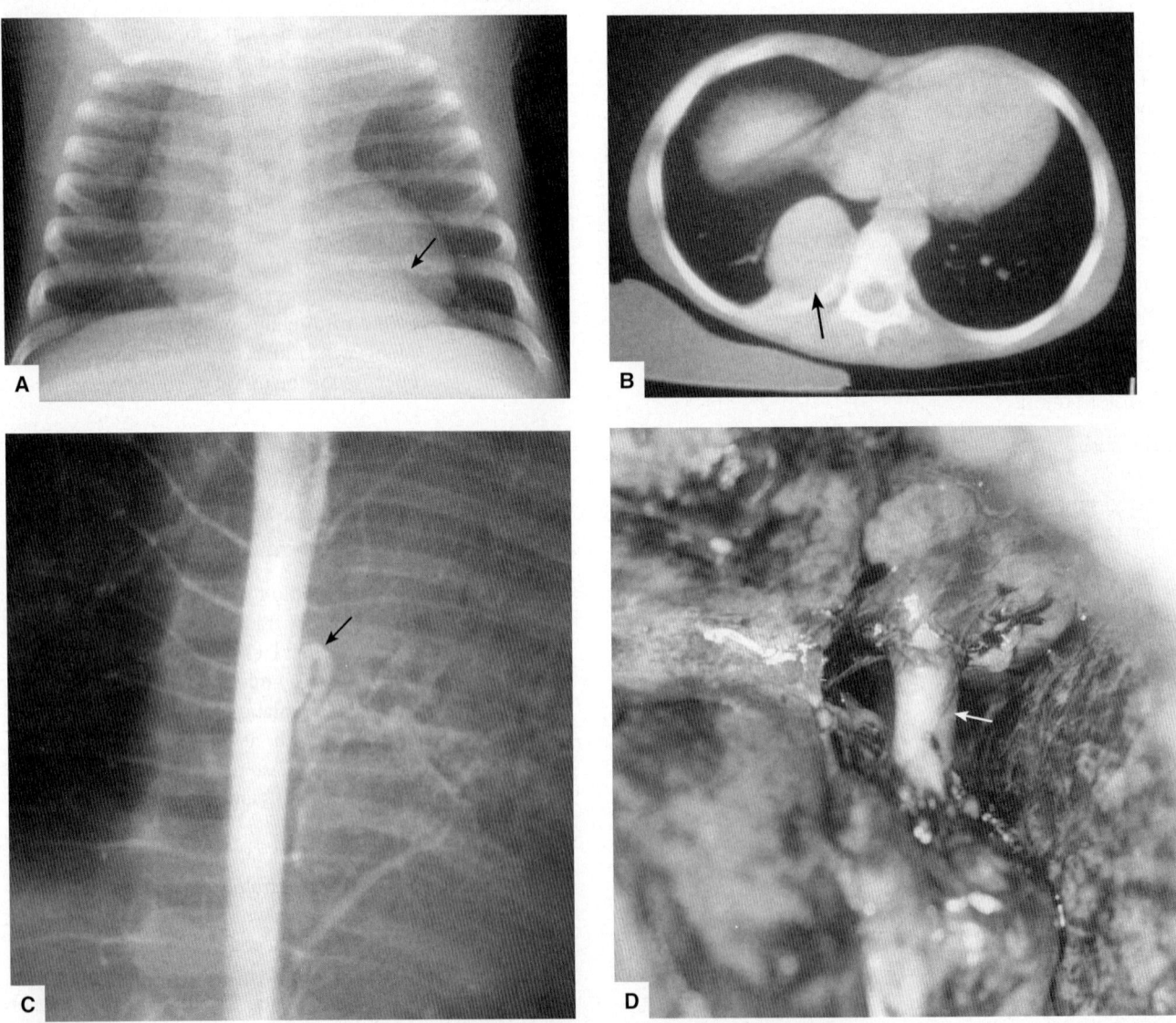

**FIGURE 29-1 A.** Plain chest radiograph of a female infant demonstrating extralobar sequestration (*arrow*) at left posteromedial base. **B.** Extralobar sequestration (*arrow*) right lower lobe of lung demonstrated by CT. **C.** Thoracic aortogram demonstrating a systemic artery (*arrow*) coursing directly to the pulmonary sequestration. **D.** The systemic artery (*arrow*) to an intralobar sequestration after dissection from its inferior pulmonary ligament location.

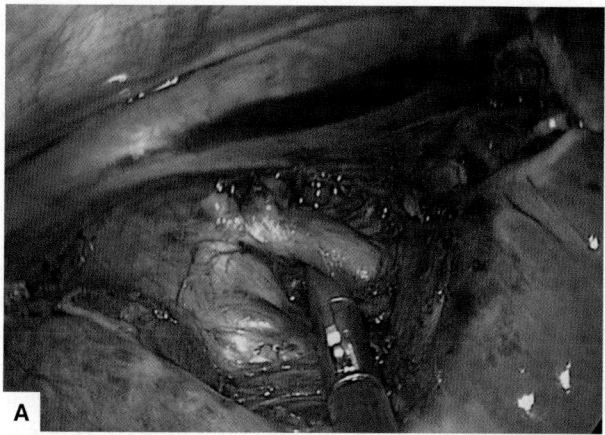 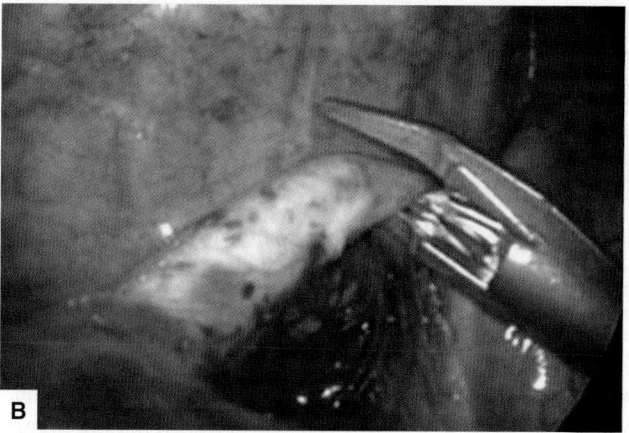

**FIGURE 29-2** **A.** The systemic artery to an extralobar bronchopulmonary sequestration is dissected out using a thoracoscopic approach. **B.** The artery is being clipped with a 5-mm clip applier.

spectrum of anomalies, including CPAM, bronchogenic cyst, foregut duplication, and even CLE. Another explanation is that a portion of the developing lung bud is mechanically separated from the rest of the lung by compression from cardiovascular structures, traction by aberrant systemic vessels, or inadequate pulmonary blood flow. Whatever the etiology, it is clear that there is a spectrum that exists between BPS, CPAM, and other bronchopulmonary malformations, and all need to be considered in the diagnosis when one of these lesions is encountered.

The newborn with intraabdominal BPS usually has no respiratory compromise and can undergo elective resection. The treatment of the newborn with an intrathoracic BPS is determined by the severity of associated pulmonary hypoplasia. Therapeutic needs may vary from minimal (not requiring ventilatory support) to severe (requiring ventilatory and vasopressor support, high-frequency oscillatory ventilation, and/or extracorporeal membrane oxygenation [ECMO]). Large pleural effusions should be treated immediately by tube thoracostomy. In the infant with pulmonary hypoplasia secondary to BPS, thoracotomy should be deferred until it is clear the infant has stabilized (Hazebrock et al 1989; Langer et al 1989). The infant's condition may deteriorate after surgery because of changes in chest wall compliance, pulmonary vascular resistance, and pulmonary hypertension superimposed on pulmonary hypoplasia.

The surgical approach to BPS is straightforward, with the exception of the management of anomalous blood supply. Despite exposure to systemic blood pressure, arteries are often large, thin-walled, and elastic, rather than muscular (Fig. 29-2A and B). In 20% of cases, these vessels are subdiaphragmatic in origin; in 15%, more than 1 vessel is present (Carter 1959). Subdiaphragmatic origin of anomalous vessels is more common with right-sided lesions (Gottrup and Lund 1978). These vessels can retract into the mediastinum or diaphragm and continue to bleed.

Intraoperative death due to hemorrhage from unrecognized anomalous vessels has been reported (Harris and Lewis 1940). Of note, one series reported that 60% of right-sided intralobar sequestrations had anomalous venous return compatible with the Scimitar syndrome (Collin et al 1987). Scimitar syndrome is characterized by anomalous pulmonary venous return from the right lung. This anomalous return may be total or partial.

The syndrome derived its name from the curvilinear pattern, similar to the shape of a scimitar (a curved sword), seen on chest radiograph with partial anomalous venous return to the inferior vena cava (Kramer et al 2003).

The importance of preoperative assessment of venous drainage, as well as arterial supply, is underscored by the reports of postoperative deaths due to ligation of anomalous veins that constituted the sole or major venous drainage of the entire ipsilateral lung (O'Mara et al 1978; Thilenius et al 1983).

Even though these lesions may be asymptomatic, postnatal resection should be considered because of the risks of infection, hemorrhage, and malignant transformation (Elias and Aufses 1960; Juettner et al 1987). When cardiac decompensation is the result of BPS, embolization of the feeding vessels may be considered. The long-term outcome of intrathoracic BPS is determined by the extent of pulmonary hypoplasia. In extralobar BPS, resection results in no loss of pulmonary parenchyma. Resection of intralobar BPS often requires at least some resection of normal lung parenchyma, if not a segmentectomy or lobectomy, and the loss of pulmonary tissue may compound the underlying pulmonary hypoplasia in the short term (Fig. 29-3). In the long term, removal of the BPS will provide room for compensatory lung growth in the remaining pulmonary parenchyma.

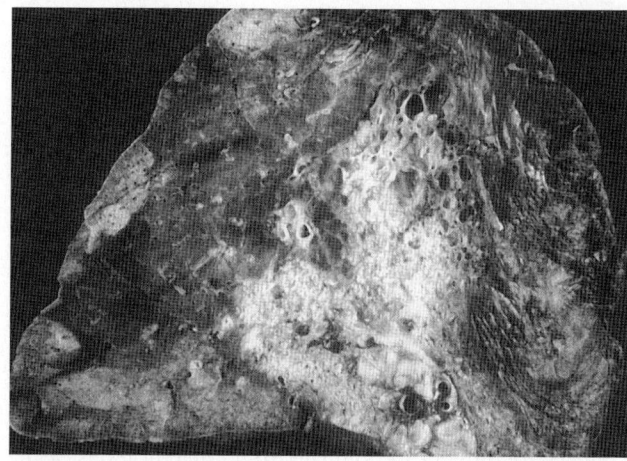

**FIGURE 29-3** Intralobar pulmonary sequestration identified in a lobectomy specimen.

# CONGENITAL CYSTIC ADENOMATOID MALFORMATION/CONGENITAL PULMONARY AIRWAY MALFORMATION

Congenital cystic adenomatoid malformation (CCAM) or congenital pulmonary airway malformation (CPAM), the newer term suggested by Stocker to replace CCAM, is a rare developmental anomaly of the lower respiratory tract. These terms encompasses a spectrum of conditions with debatable origins. Affected patients may be completely asymptomatic or present with severe respiratory distress in the newborn period. Some patients become symptomatic later in life with acute respiratory distress, acute infection, or other manifestations.

CPAMs are relatively uncommon, with the reported incidence being between 1/25,000 and 1/35,000. Many cases that previously would not have been detected until complications arose later in life are now detected by routine prenatal ultrasound. Thus the role of the pediatric surgeons has changed from simply dealing with a patient with acute respiratory issues to often providing prenatal consultation for the expectant parents.

CPAM is slightly more common in males and may affect any lobe of the lung (Hernanz-Schulman 1993) and the lesions are equally distributed between the right and the left side. The lesion is unilobar in 80% to 95% of cases and bilateral in fewer than 2% (Stocker et al 1977). Rare cases have been reported of multilobar involvement of 1 lung or bilateral lesions (Rempen et al 1987).

Unlike BPS, CPAMs have a communication with the tracheobronchial tree, albeit via a minute, tortuous passage. In contrast to BPS, CPAMs usually derive their arterial blood supply and venous drainage from normal pulmonary circulation, but anomalous arterial and venous drainage of CPAM has been reported (Rashad et al 1988), as well as so-called "hybrid" CPAMs that have a systemic blood supply (Cass et al 1997).

CPAM is a lesion characterized histologically by a multicystic mass of pulmonary tissue with a proliferation of bronchial structures (Stocker et al 1977; Miller et al 1980). This may represent a failure of bronchiolar structures to mature, which normally occurs at approximately the fifth or sixth week of gestation during the pseudoglandular stage of lung development (Stocker et al 1977; Miller et al 1980; Shanji et al 1988). Alternatively, it may represent focal pulmonary dysplasia, since skeletal muscle has been identified within the cyst walls (Leninger and Haight 1973). Others have suggested that it may be the result of airway obstruction (Moerman et al 1992; Langston 2003). The gestational age and location of the airway obstruction may determine whether CPAM, BPS, or lobar emphysema results (Keswani et al 2005; Kunisaki et al 2006).

The pathogenesis is uncertain, but appears to result from an abnormality of the branching morphogenesis of the lung and represents a maturational defect. The different types of CPAMS are thought to originate from different levels of the tracheobronchial tree and at different stages of lung development. CPAM is distinguished from other lesions and

normal lung by 5 main criteria: (1) polypoid projections of the mucosa, (2) an increase in smooth muscle and elastic tissue within the cyst walls, (3) an absence of cartilage in the cystic parenchyma, (4) the presence of mucous secreting cells, and (5) the absence of inflammation. While the CPAM portion of the lung does not participate in normal gas exchange, there are connections to the tracheobronchial tree that can lead to air-trapping and respiratory distress in the newborn period.

The exact mechanism resulting in CPAM is unknown, but is thought to include an imbalance between cell proliferation and apoptosis (increased cell proliferation and decreased apoptosis as compared to gestational controls). CPAMs are hamartomatous lesions that comprise both cystic and adenomatous overgrowth of the terminal bronchioles. If large cysts develop in utero, they can compress and compromise the growth of normal surrounding tissue.

In 1977, Stocker et al originally subdivided CCAMs into 3 types: I, II, and III, based on pathologic characteristics (Fig. 29-1). Stocker later revised this classification to CPAM type 0 to IV (Stocker et al 1994). The 5 types were intended to represent the spectrum of malformations of 5 successive groups of airways. Type 0, a condition previously described as acinar dysplasia (Davidson et al 1998), is described as bronchial; type I as bronchial/bronchiolar; type II as bronchiolar; type III as bronchiolar/alveolar duct; and type IV as peripheral. Because of the broad spectrum of malformations covered by this expanded classification system, Stocker (1994) suggested the term CPAM was more appropriate, but CCAM and CPAM are both in common usage. Reported prevalence rates for postnatal cases vary and range from <1% for type 0 lesions, 50% to 65% for type I, 10% to 40% for type II, 5% to 10% for type III, and 10% to 15% for type IV.

Type I lesions consist of single or multiple cysts lined by ciliated pseudostratified epithelium. These cysts are usually quite large (3-10 cm) and few in number (1-4). Type I lesions are usually associated with a favorable outcome. Type II lesions are more numerous cysts and smaller (usually less than 1 cm in diameter) and are lined by ciliated, cuboidal, or columnar epithelium. Respiratory bronchioles and distended alveoli may be present between these cysts. There is a high frequency of associated congenital anomalies with type II lesions and the prognosis often depends on the severity of associated anomalies. The most commonly associated anomalies are: genitourinary, such as renal agenesis or dysgenesis; cardiac, including truncus arteriosus and tetralogy of Fallot; jejunal atresia; diaphragmatic hernia; hydrocephalus; and skeletal anomalies (Stocker et al 1977). The type III lesions are usually large homogeneous microcystic masses that cause mediastinal shift. These lesions have bronchiole-like structures lined by ciliated cuboidal epithelium, separated by masses of alveolar-sized structures lined by nonciliated cuboidal epithelium. The prognosis in type III CPAMs is variable but can, in severe cases, present with nonimmune hydrops in utero and cardiorespiratory compromise in the newborn (Adzick et al 1985; Harrison et al 1990). Type IV CPAMs are characterized by very large cysts up to 10 cm lined by flattened epithelium resting on loose mesenchyme. These lesions can have areas of focal stromal hypercellularity with histologic overlap of cystic pleuropulmonary blastoma, which may be clinically indistinguishable (McSweeney et al 2003; Hill and Dehner 2004).

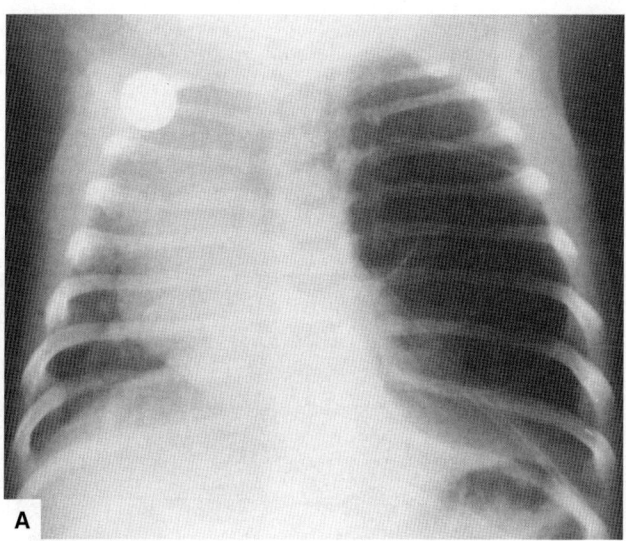
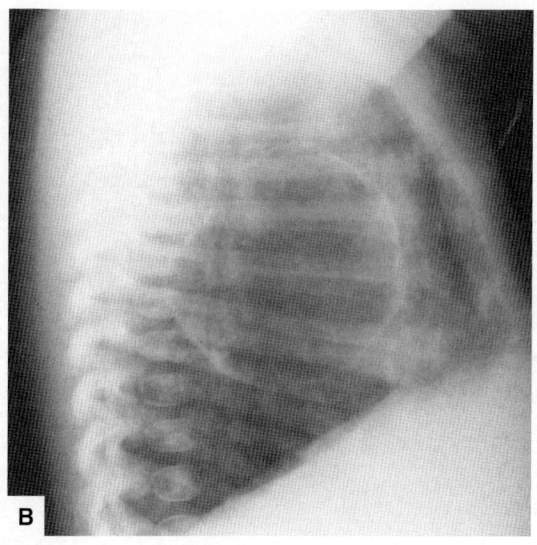

**FIGURE 29-4** Antero-postero (**A**) and lateral (**B**) views of CCAM in left upper lobe of a 1-month-old male with respiratory distress.

The presentation of CPAM is quite variable and can extend from the early prenatal period to late in adult life. The spectrum runs from an incidental finding on a routine chest x-ray in a completely asymptomatic patient, to severe respiratory distress in the newborn period (Fig. 29-4). More and more of these lesions are now picked up in the prenatal period on routine screening ultrasound, allowing for prenatal consultation and planning. Prenatal diagnosis by ultrasonography is generally classified as either microcystic lesions with cysts <5 mm, which appear echogenic and solid, or macrocystic lesions of 1 or more cysts >5 mm, and includes massive pulmonary involvement with the development of hydrops. Hydrops can develop in up to 40% of cases and regression of the lesion is seen in up to 60% during the course of gestation. The need for fetal intervention is rare and limited to those cases with severe hydrops with a predicted mortality of near 100%. MRI is being used more frequently to examine the fetus and can help differentiate CPAM from other thoracic lesions, such as congenital diaphragmatic hernia, foregut duplications, and others (Fig. 29-5).

The differential diagnosis of CPAM includes other cystic diseases of the lung including BPS, bronchogenic cyst, and CLE. The primary differentiation between CPAM and BPS is based on 2 anatomic points. BPS has no connection to the tracheobronchial tree and is supplied by an anomalous systemic artery. CPAM is usually not. However, the difference between the 2 lesions is not as discreet as once thought and it is more likely that the 2 are variants of the same abnormal developmental pathway.

In the neonatal period, the diagnosis is usually suspected based on clinical presentation and the initial chest x-ray. A computed tomography (CT) scan is usually definitive, although the exact diagnosis may not be made until surgical exploration is performed (Fig. 29-6). Diagnosis later in life is usually dependent on late symptoms or, in some cases, an incidental finding on a routine chest x-ray. CT scan is still the gold standard.

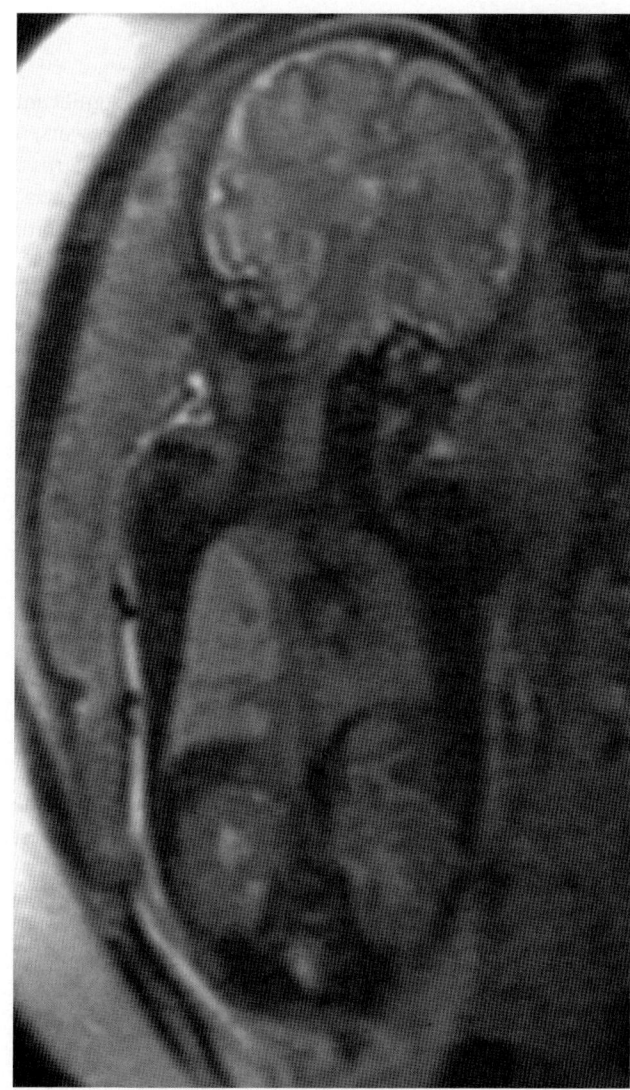

**FIGURE 29-5** MRI of fetus with CPAM diagnosed in utero. The involved fetal lung is lighter due to the fluid within the cystic structures in the lung parenchyma.

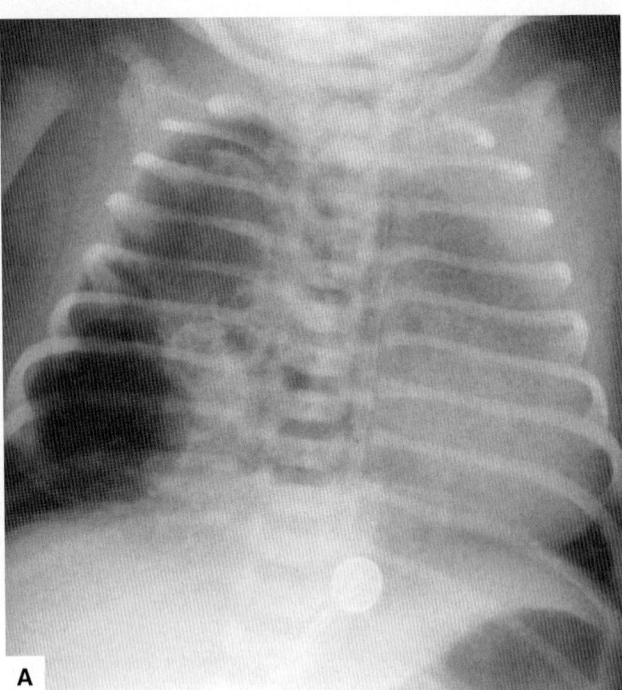

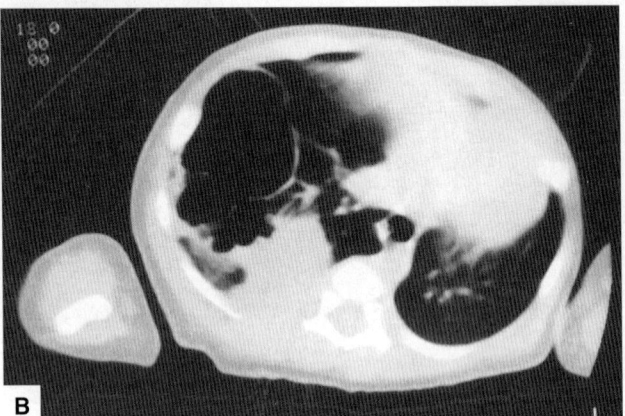

**FIGURE 29-6** Chest radiograph (**A**) and corresponding CT (**B**) of a 2-day-old tachypneic male showing right lower lobe CPAM.

The infant with type I, II, or IV CPAM may be at significant risk for air trapping in the CPAM, which may acutely worsen the respiratory status (Stocker et al 1977; Bailey et al 1990). In cases of unilateral CPAM, selective intubation of the contralateral bronchus may be a useful temporizing measure until resection of the CPAM can be accomplished. Pneumothorax is an additional concern in CPAM, especially in the type I or II lesions, and may require tube thoracostomy (Bentur et al 1991). The treatment of choice in CPAM is complete resection of the CPAM, usually by lobectomy (Fig. 29-7A-C). In rare cases of extensive involvement of nearly the entire lung, resection of multiple lobes or pneumonectomy may be necessary. There are several reports, however, detailing potentially lethal problems associated with pneumonectomy in newborns resulting from mediastinal shift with vascular compression of the trachea and remaining bronchus (Szarnicki et al 1978). Because of these risks, some groups advocate a nonanatomic resection to preserve as much pulmonary parenchyma as possible to allow postoperative compensatory growth and avoid postpneumonectomy complications (Mentzer et al 1992).

The newborn with a CPAM detected antenatally that subsequently regresses also needs careful postnatal evaluation (MacGillivray et al 1993; Adzick et al 1998). Often subtle abnormalities will be evident on chest radiography, but chest CT scanning may be necessary to detect residual CPAM tissue. Several authors have recommended that as long as these lesions are asymptomatic, they may be observed closely and managed without resection (Adzick et al 1993; MacGillivray et al 1993; Aziz et al 2004; Hsieh et al 2005). The argument against this approach includes the reported cases of myxosarcoma, embryonal rhabdomyosarcoma, pleuropulmonary blastoma, and bronchoalveolar carcinoma arising in CPAMs or indistinguishable from them (Stephanopoulos and Catsaros 1963; Wecla et al 1977; Benjamin and Cahill 1991; d'Agostino et al 1997).

Primary lung tumors are rare during the first 2 decades of life, but 4% of those reported were associated with congenital cystic lesions of the lung, including CPAM (Benjamin and Cahill 1991). While CPAM-associated malignancies often arise only after decades, the youngest patient reported with a malignancy was only 13 months of age (Ozcan et al 2001). Because there is an anomalous connection to the tracheobronchial tree, infection is an additional potential complication (Stephanopoulos and Catsaros 1963; Benjamin and Cahill 1991; Ozcan et al 2001; Hasiotou et al 2004; Galadzas et al 2005; Poi et al 2005).

Some have argued that asymptomatic CPAMs should be followed expectantly, and that the risks of surgery in infancy outweigh the potential benefits (Aziz et al 2004). However, the continued presence of CPAM represents a lifelong risk of both infection and malignant transformation. In centers with significant experience in lung resection in infants, CPAMs can be safely resected with virtually no morbidity and mortality (Tsai et al 2007). The authors' approach is to obtain a postnatal CT scan and perform a muscle-sparing thoracotomy or thoracoscopic lobectomy or lung resection when possible to retain normal lung tissue. An added benefit to resection over observation is that the remaining lung undergoes significant compensatory growth within months of the surgery. This does not occur if the CPAM is left in situ. The long-term outcome of infants with CPAM following resection is excellent. If residual CPAM is left behind or the mass is not resected, the child will remain at risk for infectious and potentially malignant complications. The authors recommend prophylaxis against respiratory syncytial virus (RSV) in infancy in those with significant associated pulmonary hypoplasia, pulmonary hypertension, or chronic lung disease. Children who survived open fetal surgery for CPAMs associated with hydrops appear to be still doing well from 1 to 7 years postoperatively.

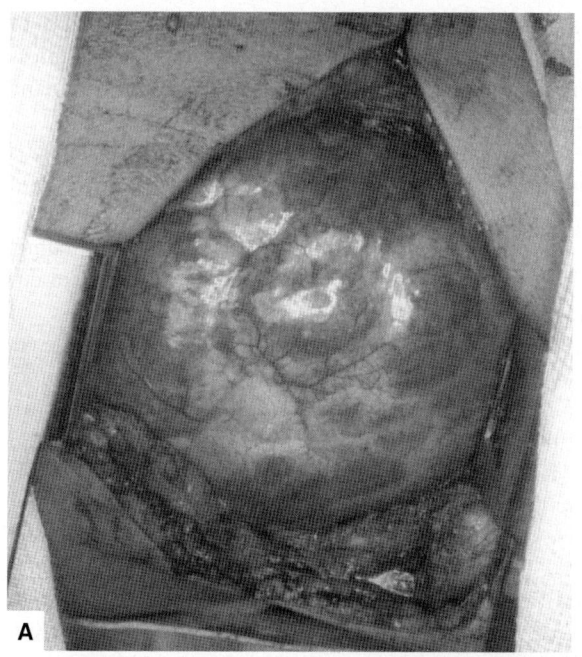

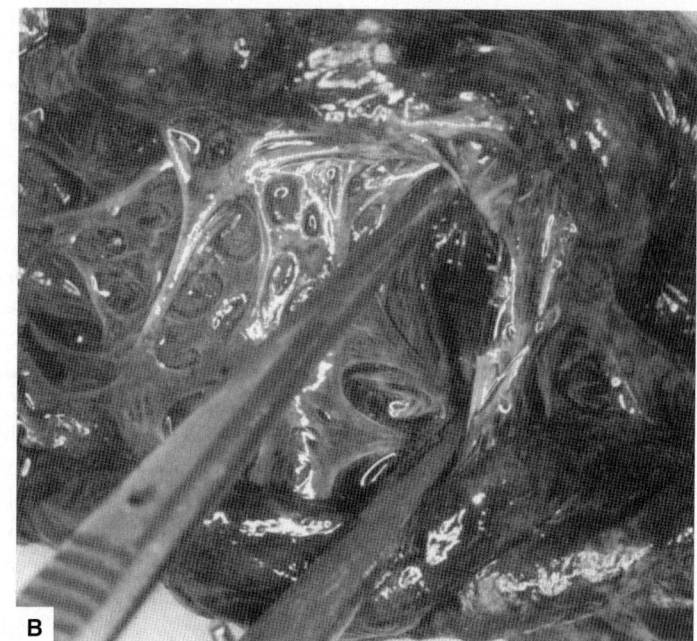

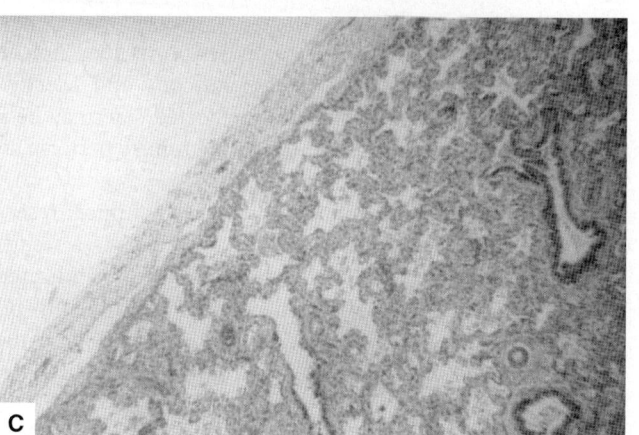

**FIGURE 29-7** **A.** Transthoracic inspection of a lobar CPAM at operation. **B.** Cut section of the operative specimen demonstrating cystic and solid components of the CPAM. **C.** Histology of a solid CPAM in which the section demonstrates the microcystic disease.

## CONGENITAL LOBAR EMPHYSEMA

CLE is a rare anomaly of lung development that often presents in the neonatal period with hyperinflation of 1 or more pulmonary lobes. Other terms for this entity include congenital lobar overinflation and infantile lobar emphysema. CLE is characterized by overinflation, either by retained fluid produced in the lobe or segment prenatally, or by air trapped in the lobe or segment postnatally (Clements 1999). CLE is thought to be a consequence of inappropriate bronchial valvular mechanism caused by localized malformations, deficiencies of bronchial cartilage mucosal folds, or extrinsic bronchial compression (Clements 1999). Overinflation may be due to an increase in the number of normally expanded alveoli, called a polyalveolar lobe (Hislop and Reid 1970; Mani et al 2004). The most frequently documented cause of CLE is obstruction of the developing airway, which occurs in approximately 25% of cases. Airway obstruction can either be intrinsic or extrinsic, although intrinsic is the most common. This results in a ball-valve type obstruction, which causes air

trapping and histologic changes of alveolar distension without structural anomaly.

The upper lobes tend to be the most frequently involved with the left side more common (40%-50%) than the right (20%). Almost half of all cases involve the left upper lobe (Eber 2007), and the right middle lobe is the next most often affected. The middle lobe is involved in 25% to 30% of cases and lower lobe disease is extremely rare, 2% to 5%.

CLE lesions rarely contain cysts and appear homogeneous by prenatal ultrasound and MRI. Some authors have suggested that both CLE and polyalveolar lobe may be 2 outcomes of a similar inciting lesion during lung development (Mani et al 2004). The timing of development of this lesion during lung development may account for different anatomical and functional bronchial abnormalities (Mani et al 2004). Prenatally, lobar emphysema appears as a homogeneously enlarged lobe or segment that may be impossible to distinguish from a type III CPAM. Lobar emphysema tends to follow a different prenatal history from type III CPAM, however, and can continue to enlarge slowly throughout gestation with resulting mediastinal shift and compression. Postnatally, the neonate may also present with a radioopaque mass on chest x-ray due to delayed clearance of lung fluid of the affected lobe. The differential diagnosis must include the other types of congenital cystic lung disease, as previously mentioned.

CLE is a relatively rare, occurring in 1/20,000 to 1/30,000 infants. The male-to-female ratio is 3:1. Progressive hyperinflation is the end result of a number of variations of disruption of bronchopulmonary development. These disturbances may cause a change in the number of airways or alveoli and alveolar size. Up to a third of CLE cases are found to have a polyalveolar lobe in which there is a 3- to 5-fold increase in the number of alveoli but a normal number of bronchial branches. In the past, this was thought to be a distinct entity from CLE, but it is more likely that this is the normal response of the lung parenchyma distal to a complete bronchial obstruction in utero.

More than half of patients with CLE develop symptoms within the first few days of life, while others do not become symptomatic until 1 to 4 months of age. Symptomatic neonates may develop rapidly progressive respiratory failure, with 10% to 15% requiring emergency thoracotomy. The typical findings in CLE in an infant will be noticeable shift in apical cardiac impulse to the contralateral side, decreased breath sounds over the affected hemothorax, and hyperresonance to percussion. Plain chest radiograph is usually diagnostic with lobar hyperinflation, mediastinal and tracheal shift, compression and collapse of ipsilateral unaffected lobe or lobes, and flattening or inversion of the ipsilated diaphragm (Fig. 29-8A and B). The differential diagnosis includes pneumothorax, giant type I CPAM, large pneumatocele, and complete collapse of a lobe or lobes with compensatory overinflation of the remaining lobe. The most important radiographic differential diagnosis is tension pneumothorax, which can easily be mistaken for CLE and vice versa. The complete collapse of the entire lung in tension pneumothorax versus the compression of adjacent lobes in CLE should be apparent on plane radiographs.

CT scan of the chest, if the infant is sufficiently stable, is helpful in delineating the anatomy of the involved lobe and more importantly extrinsic cases of CLE such as bronchogenic cyst. Similarly, echocardiography should be obtained prior to surgery to exclude potential associated cardiovascular anomalies.

Treatment of the asymptomatic patient is controversial, since the lung parenchyma in the affected lobe is normal and, if CLE is due to cartilaginous weakness in the lobar bronchus, may resolve over time. Flexible bronchoscopy is helpful to identify potentially reversible causes of endobronchial obstruction either from mucous plugs, granulation tissue, or extrinsic compression from a bronchogenic cyst or vascular anomaly. Lobar emphysema from inspissated mucous plugs or viral bronchiolitis does not require resection. Similarly, CLE secondary to extrinsic compression from a bronchogenic cyst may respond to excision of the cyst with preservation of the affected lobe.

It is important to note that some newborns may not be stable enough for either CT or bronchoscopy, and selective intubation of the bronchus of the unaffected side may be a life-saving temporizing measure, allowing time to perform an emergency thoracotomy and lobectomy.

Treatment for the symptomatic patient is surgical resection. In most cases, a complete lobectomy versus a wedge or segmentectomy of the involved lobe is indicated (Fig. 29-9A-D). This is favored because of the difficulty, on a macroscopic level, of determining which portion of the lung is involved and which is not. The increased difficulty

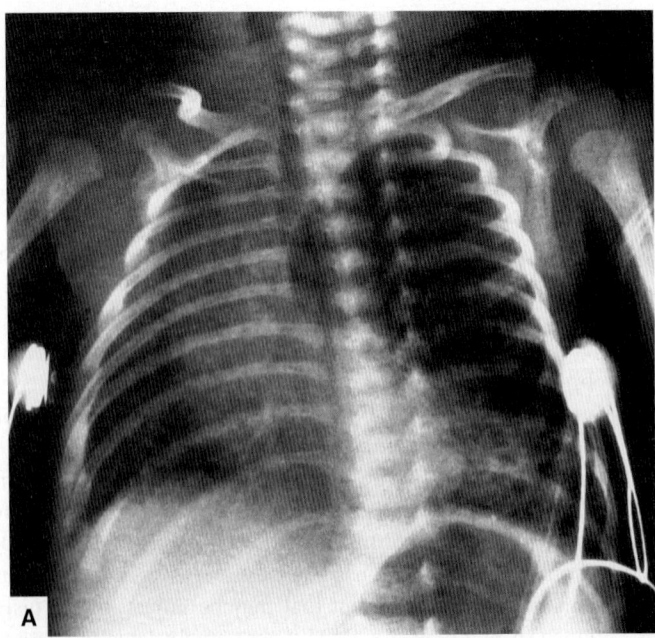
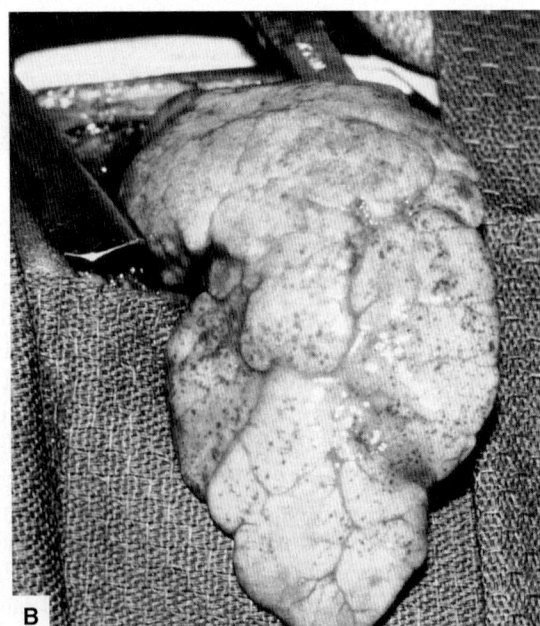

**FIGURE 29-8** **A.** Chest radiograph in an infant with CLE. Note the hyperlucent lung, the compressed atelectatic normal lung, and the shift of the mediastinum. **B.** Intraoperative photograph of child with CLE. The involved segment "pops out" when opening the chest. When the positive pressure is removed, the emphysematous lobe remains distended while the normal lobes collapse.

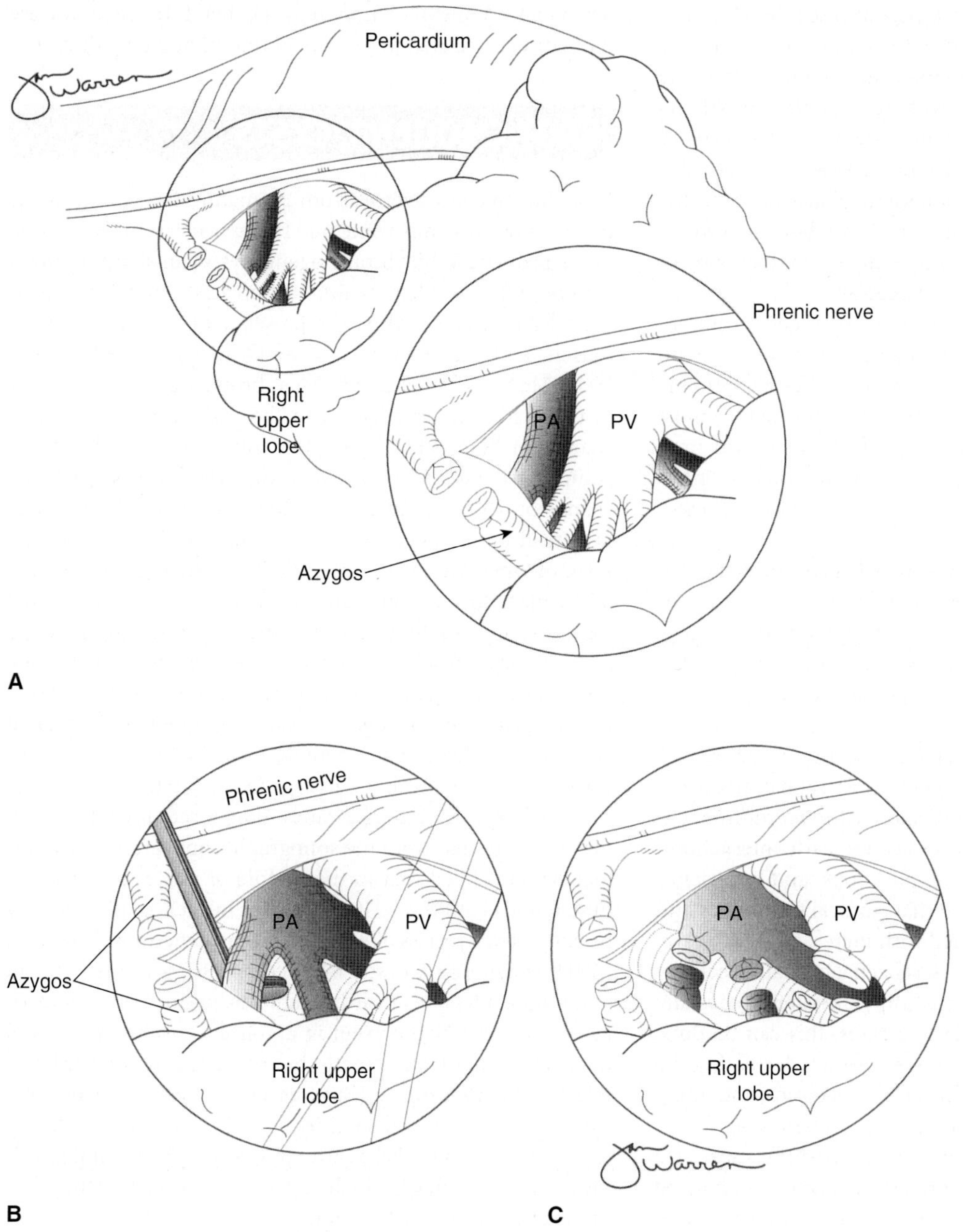

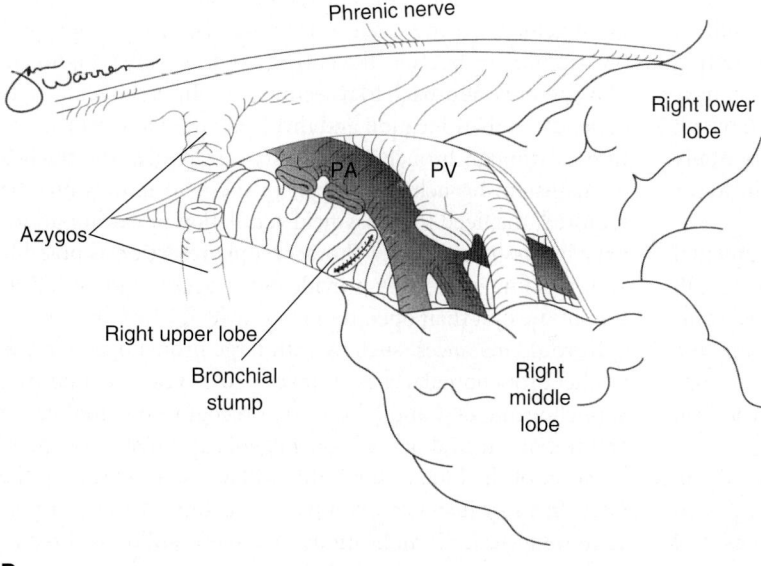

**A**

Pericardium

Right upper lobe

Phrenic nerve

PA  PV

Azygos

**B**

Phrenic nerve

Azygos

PA  PV

Right upper lobe

**C**

PA  PV

Right upper lobe

**D**

Phrenic nerve

Right lower lobe

PA  PV

Azygos

Right upper lobe

Bronchial stump

Right middle lobe

**FIGURE 29-9** Details of a right upper lobectomy. **A.** With the upper lobe retracted caudally and laterally, the azygos vein is ligated and divided. The mediastinal pleura overlying the hilum is opened, exposing the pulmonary vasculature. The inset is enlarged for clarity. **B.** The right upper lobe lobar and segmental branches of the PA and PV are sequentially dissected, ligated, and divided. **C.** View of the right pulmonary hilum after the upper lobe vessels have been divided. **D.** View of the hilar region after suture ligation and division of the right upper lobe bronchus.

415

and morbidity associated with a partial resection does not warrant the limited benefits of preserving a portion of the lung. Since lobar bronchial abnormality is most often the cause of CLE, only lobectomy will address the underlying problem. There are cases where more than 1 lobe appears to be involved or there may be bilateral disease. There are also cases where there are no clear anatomic planes between the upper and lower lobe lobes, and segments of both are grossly involved. In these cases, segmentectomy or another type of lung preserving surgery becomes necessary.

The symptomatic neonate needs to be operated on immediately. In extreme cases, an emergency thoracotomy with decompression of the chest cavity can be a life-saving intervention and an emergency lobectomy is performed. In most neonatal cases, however, especially with the increased incidence of prenatal diagnosis, the baby is asymptomatic or has only mild-to-moderate symptoms and a semi-elective resection can be performed.

The timing of surgery remains somewhat controversial, but there is little evidence to suggest that delayed resection benefits the child in any significant way. In fact, delayed surgery may increase the risk of infection or respiratory compromise. Early resection maximizes the compensatory lung growth of the remaining lobe(s).

Many centers have recommended resection at between 1 and 6 months of age to allow for some growth and decrease the risk of the anesthetic, but data to support this recommendation are limited. The authors have favored early intervention to minimize the risk of later complications, and experience in our centers has demonstrated that surgical techniques and anesthetic care are not associated with increased risk in early resection. The standard therapy has been a formal lobectomy through a posterolateral thoracotomy incision, especially in emergent cases. In more elective cases, this can be done using a muscle-sparing approach (see below), decreasing the morbidity associated with a formal thoracotomy, including scoliosis, shoulder girdle weakness, and chest wall deformity, all well documented in infants. Due to the sheer size of the emphysematous lobe, thoracoscopic resection may be exceedingly challenging and a sizable incision will be needed to remove the lobe even if it can be safely resected.

There is also an acquired form of lobar emphysema (ALE), which typically develops in preterm infants as a result of lung injury from positive-pressure ventilation in the setting of bronchopulmonary dysplasia (BPD). Barotrauma, oxygen toxicity, lung immaturity, and suction trauma have all been suggested as contributing factors. ALE more commonly affects the lower lobes than does CLE, with the right lower lobe most often affected.

Bronchoscopy may be helpful in diagnosing segmental bronchial collapse during exhalation. This can result in "ball valve" air trapping in the affected lobe and may be compounded by problems with increased mucus production, inadequate ciliary clearance from bronchial metaplasia, bronchial mucosal hyperplasia, and peribronchial fibroplasia seen in BPD.

Most mild or only moderately severe cases of ALE can be managed nonoperatively with ventilatory strategies to minimize air-trapping and lung injury. In severe cases of ALE unresponsive to medical treatment, lobectomy can be beneficial. While resection may be helpful, outcomes are more directly related to severity of underlying lung disease.

## BRONCHOGENIC CYSTS

Bronchogenic cysts result from premature foregut remnants that originate in embryonic bud tissue prior to the formation of the bronchi. While bronchogenic cysts can share common features with esophageal duplication cysts, they are histologically characterized by the presence of cartilage, smooth muscle, and glands in the cyst wall (Stocker 2001; Langston 2003; McAdams et al 2000). Most bronchogenic cysts occur in the mediastinum adjacent to the distal trachea or mainstem bronchi (Stocker 2002; McAdams et al 2000). Bronchogenic cysts can also be found within the lung parenchyma (Langston 2003; McAdams et al 2000), although this is a controversial point, since some have considered these lesions a form of type I CPAM (Stocker 2002). Bronchogenic cysts are unilocular, do not communicate with the tracheobronchial tree, and are usually filled with mucus. Bronchogenic cysts can enlarge to produce airway compression and may ulcerate the cyst wall lining due to ectopic gastric mucosa (Eber 2007). Histologically, bronchogenic cysts are lined with ciliated columnar epithelium and contain bronchial mucous glands, elastic tissue, and hyaline cartilage (Maier 1948).

Bronchogenic cysts are rarely diagnosed prenatally, but may be suspected from the sonographic appearance of a unilocular fluid-filled cyst in the middle or posterior mediastinum (Avni et al 1986). Alternatively, a bronchogenic cyst may be suggested by mass effect on adjacent structures. Patel et al (2004) diagnosed a cystic mass compressing the left atrium at the time a fetal echocardiogram was performed. Bronchogenic cysts can also present in atypical locations, such as in the neck or subdiaphragmatic, but retain the unilocular fluid-filled cystic appearance (Bagolan et al 1999). Bronchogenic cysts may be best evaluated by bronchoscopy and chest CT (Fig. 29-10A and B). Echocardiography may be helpful in ruling out other etiologies, such as pericardial cyst, and the effect of the cyst on cardiac function.

Surgical resection of cystic thoracic lesions is indicated due to risk of infection, cyst enlargement, airway compromise, impingement on the trachea or bronchus, heart, esophageal obstruction, or because the etiology of the cyst is unknown. The operative approach to resecting these bronchogenic cysts depends on their location and involvement of adjacent structures. Although bronchogenic cysts can involve the trachea or mainstem bronchi and repair of these structures may be required, the need for cross-field ventilation or cardiopulmonary bypass is very rare. Thoracoscopic resection is possible and, in some cases, may provide better access and visualization of the cyst than open thoracotomy (Fig. 29-11).

In some instances, such as with large bronchogenic cysts, tracheobronchomalacia may take 1 to 2 years to improve. Bronchogenic cyst and CLE form a recognized combination and initial removal of the bronchogenic cyst may allow preservation of the lobe to see if this will allow resolution of the CLE. In most instances, complete resection of the cyst prevents long-term complications and these children do very well on long-term follow-up.

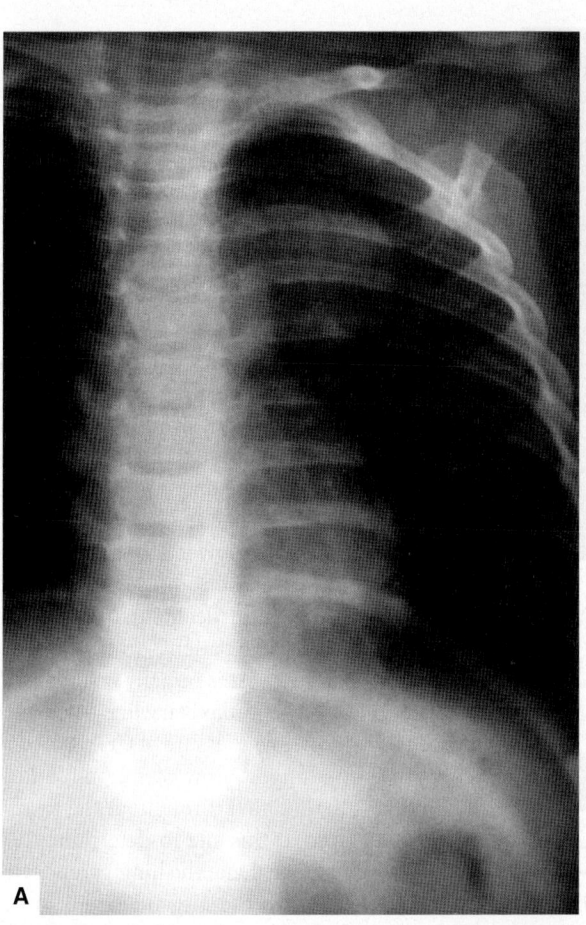

FIGURE 29-10 Mediastinal bronchogenic cyst. **A.** Chest radiograph depicting a left mediastinal mass. **B.** Chest CT
scan depicting a left posterior mediastinal paravertebral mass with a cyst.

A

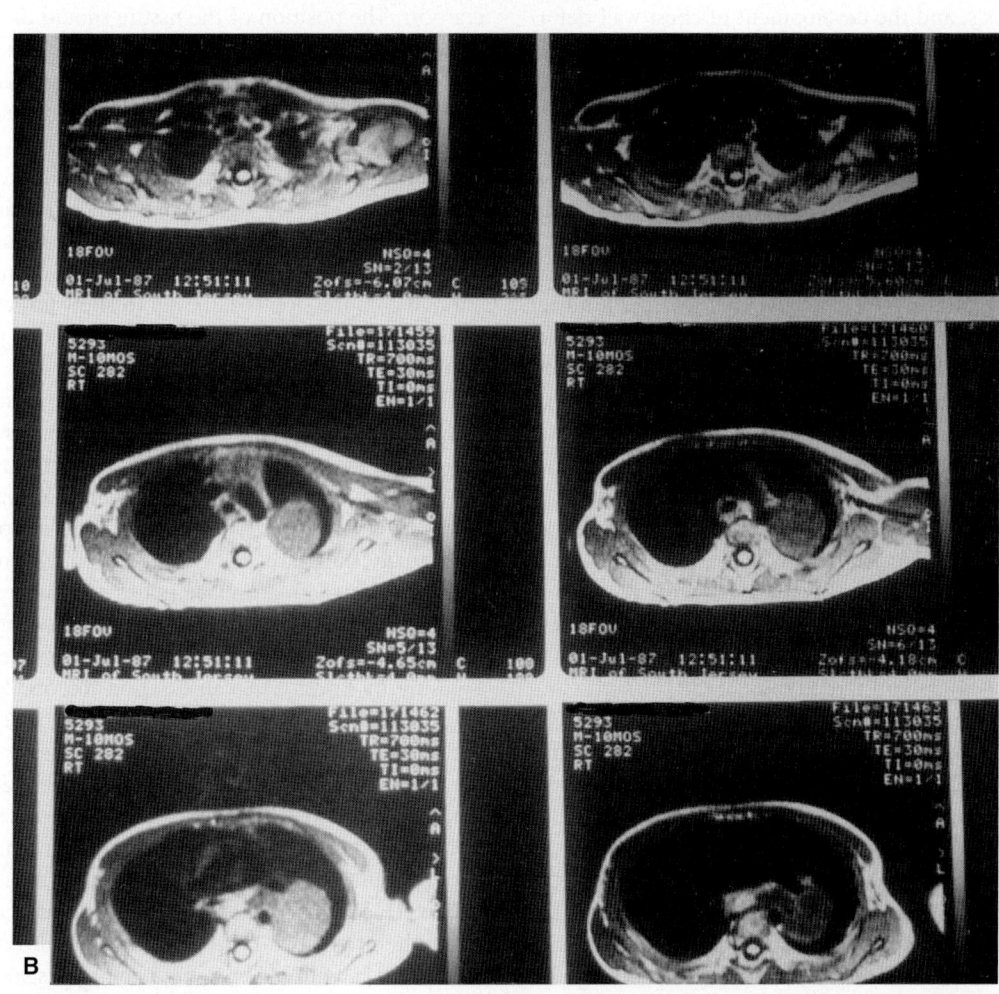

B

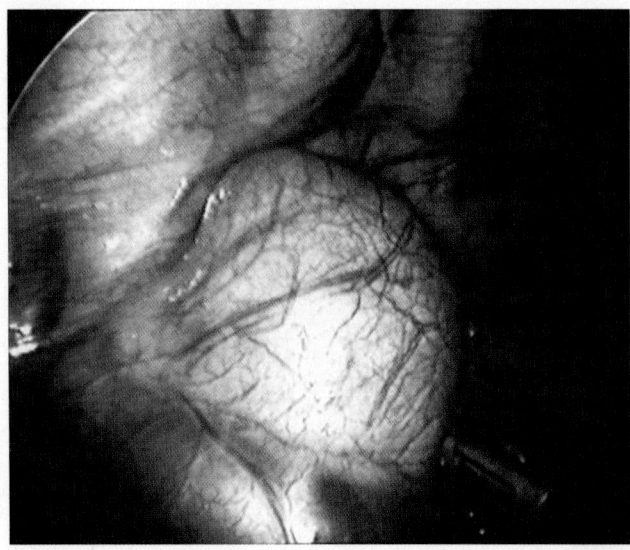

**FIGURE 29-11** Thoracoscopic visualization of a bronchogenic cyst surrounded by lung parenchyma.

# MINIMALLY INVASIVE TECHNIQUE

## Muscle-Sparing Thoracotomy

A formal posterolateral thoracotomy in neonates and infants can have unintended morbidity related to decreased shoulder mobility, scoliosis, and the development of chest wall deformities on long-term follow-up. As a consequence, minimally invasive techniques, such as muscle-sparing thoracotomy or thoracoscopic techniques, have become the preferred approaches in neonates and children.

The technique for a muscle-sparing thoracotomy involves 4- to 5-cm transverse incision in the midaxilla at about the level of the nipple. Skin and subcutaneous flaps are raised 6 to 10 cm circumferentially, freeing the anterior surface of the latissimus dorsi and serratus anterior muscles. The anterior border of the latissimus dorsi is identified and the areolar tissue between it and the serratus anterior is divided, pulling the latissimus posteriorly and the serratus anteriorly and exposing the ribs. This level skin incision easily accommodates entry into the chest from as low as the seventh intercostal space to as high as the third intercostal space. The intercostal muscles and parietal pleura are incised as for a standard thoracotomy. Two Finichetto chest wall retractors are placed at 90° to each other. One spreads the ribs, while the second retracts the latissimus posteriorly and serratus anteriorly. Patience is required with the use of this technique as initial exposure will be limited until relaxation of the latissimus and serratus occurs with time. Overly aggressive retraction with the Finichetto retractor can result in rib fractures, especially in neonates, but this can be avoided by simply allowing time for muscular relaxation.

The procedure for a lobectomy or segmental resection is then the same as for standard thoracotomy (Fig. 29-9A-D). The closure of a muscle-sparing thoracotomy uses standard pericostal sutures to reapproximate the ribs. In addition to a standard chest tube, if indicated, a small closed suction drain is left above and below the raised muscle flaps to evacuate dead space and prevent accumulation of air or serous fluid. The TLS drain is placed to vacutainer suction every 4 to 8 hours and is usually ready for removal, along with the chest tube, if placed, on postoperative day 1.

## Thoracoscopic Lobectomy

For the past decade, the authors have preferred to use minimally invasive techniques to perform lobectomies in all infants with congenital cystic lesions. The benefits of avoiding a formal thoracotomy and the morbidity associated with it greatly outweigh the disadvantages of the increased technical difficulty and operative time. In fact, with experience, the operative times have equaled or are faster than with a standard thoracotomy.

The technique of a lower lobectomy is detailed here for discussion purposes. The room setup is organized so that the patient is in the lateral decubitus position and the surgeon and assistant are at the patient's front with the monitor at the patient's back. The chest is initially insufflated through a Veres needle placed in the midaxillary line at the fifth or sixth interspace. A low flow, low pressure of $CO_2$ is used to help complete collapse of the lung. A flow of 1 L/min and pressure of 4 to 6 mm Hg is maintained throughout the case. The first port (a 5 mm) is placed at this site to determine the position of the major fissure and evaluate the lung parenchyma. Using a 4- or 5-mm 30° lens allows the surgeon to look directly down on the fissure and the instruments. In general, this will be the camera port. The position of the fissure should dictate the placement of the other ports, as the most difficult dissection occurs in this plane. The working ports (3 or 5 mm) are then placed in the anterior axillary line between the fifth, eighth, or ninth interspace.

Entering the chest, the anatomy is often difficult to identify because the cysts are occupying so much space. To free up space and improve visualization, the cysts are involuted using the Ligasure device. The cysts are grasped and sealed until enough compression is achieved to allow for identification of all anatomic structures. The compressed lobe is much easier to manipulate with laparoscopic instruments.

The first step is mobilization of the inferior pulmonary ligament. Care should be taken to look for a systemic artery coming off the aorta in case this is a misdiagnosed sequestration or one of the hybrid lesions. The inferior pulmonary vein (PV) is dissected out, but not ligated at this point. Ligation prior to division of the PV can lead to congestion in the lower lobe, which can create space issues especially in the smaller child and infant. The fissure is then approached going from anterior to posterior. In cases of an incomplete fissure, the Ligasure or Endo-GIA can be used to complete the fissure (Fig. 29-12A and B). Gradually the pulmonary artery (PA) to the lower lobe is isolated. Often it is necessary to dissect into the parenchyma of the lower lobe to gain extra exposure and length. If possible, the artery can be ligated at its main trunk to the lower lobe as it passes through the fissure, but is often easier to dissect out the vessel after the first or second bifurcation. This also provides a longer segment of artery to work with. The bronchus to the lower lobe lies directly behind the artery and can often be palpated before it is seen.

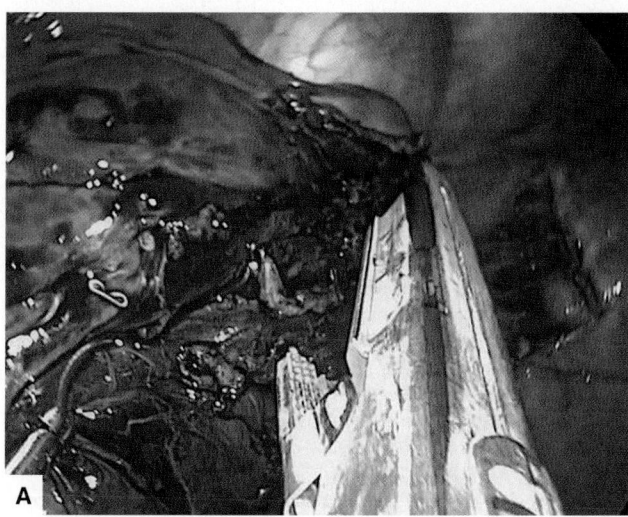
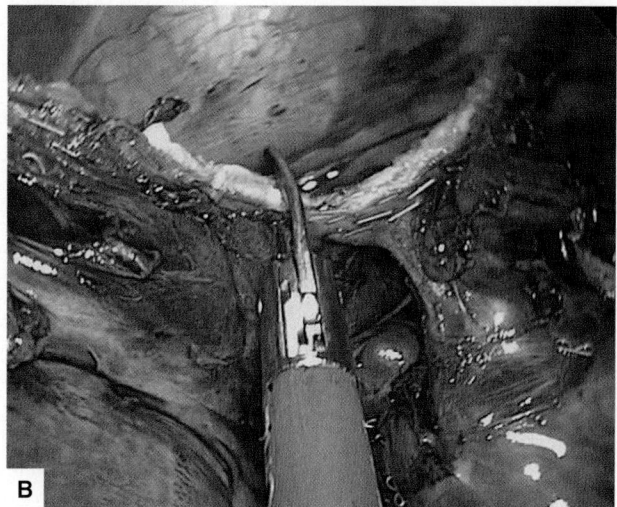

**FIGURE 29-12** Thoracoscopic division of incomplete lobar fissure in process of performing a lobectomy. **A.** After identifying the plane for dissection the Endo-GIA being applied to divide lung parenchyma. **B.** Final division of incomplete fissure to expose the underlying vascular structures and bronchus to be ligated.

Once the artery is divided, the improved exposure facilitates complete dissection of the vein. The vein can also be ligated in assorted ways depending on the size of the vessel. Prior to isolation and ligation of the vein, it is helpful to divide the pleura along the posterior border of the lobe to complete its mobilization. The inferior PV is then divided and the bronchus to the lower lobe isolated. The bronchus is divided with the Endo-GIA in larger children or cut sharply and closed with 3-0 polydioxanone sutures (PDS) in smaller patients. In infants and patients under 5 kg, it is possible to seal the bronchus with Endo-clips (Fig. 29-13). The specimen is then brought out through the lower anterior axillary line trocar site, which is slightly enlarged if necessary, either whole or piecemeal with a ring forceps. If more than 1 lobe is involved on the same side, a lung-sparing procedure should

be performed. (An example of this is a case where the CPAM appeared on the CT scan to involve just the left lower lobe.)

The authors have performed over 200 thoracoscopic lobectomies for congenital lung lesions. The average length of hospital stay is now under 48 hours, and complications have been almost nonexistent. The authors highly recommend this approach, as well as early intervention, since the surgery becomes much more difficult if a significant pulmonary infection occurs before resection.

## SELECTED READINGS

Adzick NS, Harrison MR. Management of the fetus with a cystic adenomatoid malformation. *World J Surg* 1993;17:342–349.

Adzick NS, Harrison MR, Crombleholme TM. Fetal lung lesions: management and outcome. *Am J Obstet Gynecol* 1998;179:884–889.

Adzick NS, Harrison MR, Glick PL, Globus MS, Anderson RL, Mahony BS. Fetal cystic adenomatoid malformation: prenatal diagnosis and natural history. *J Pediatr Surg* 1985;20:483–488.

Bailey PV, Tracy T Jr, Connors RH, et al. Congenital bronchopulmonary malformations: diagnostic and therapeutic considerations. *J Thorac Cardiovasc Surg* 1990;99:597–603.

Benjamin DR, Cahill JL. Bronchioloalveolar carcinoma of the lung and congenital cystic adenomatoid malformation. *Am J Clin Pathol* 1991;95:889–892.

Bentur L, Canny G, Thoener P, et al. Spontaneous pneumothorax in cystic adenomatoid malformation: unusual clinical and histologic features. *Chest* 1991;99:1292–1293.

Bezzuti RT, Isler RJ. Antenatal ultrasound detection of cystic adenomatoid malformation of lung: report of a case and review of the recent literature. *Clin Ultrasound* 1983;11:342–346.

Boulot P, Pages A, Deschamps F, et al. Early prenatal diagnosis of congenital cystic adenomatoid malformation of the lung (Stocker's type I): a case report. *Eur J Obstet Gynecol Reprod Biol* 1991;41:159–162.

Carter R. Pulmonary sequestration. *Ann Thorac Surg* 1969;7:68–88.

Cass DL, Crombleholme TM, Howello LJ, et al. Cystic lung lesions with systemic arterial blood supply: a hybrid of congenital cystic adenomatoid malformation and bronchopulmonary sequestration. *J Pediatr Surg* 1997;32:986–990.

Chinn DH, Filly RA, Callen PW, et al. Congenital diaphragmatic hernia diagnosed prenatally by ultrasound. *Radiology* 1983;148:119–123.

Clements BS. Congenital malformations of the lungs and airways. In: Tausig LM, Landau LI, eds. *Pediatr Respiratory Medicine*. St Louis: Mosby; 1999:1106–1122.

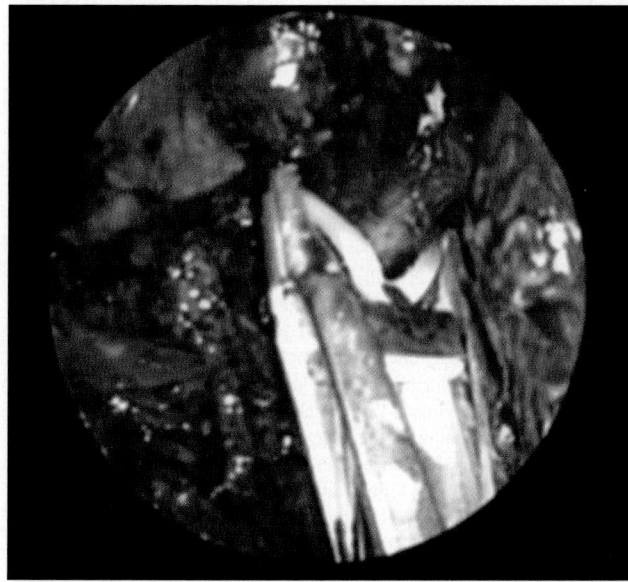

**FIGURE 29-13** Thoracoscopic application of a locking Endo-clip to occlude the proximal bronchus just prior to division.

Clements BS, Warner JO. Pulmonary sequestration and related congenital bronchopulmonary-vascular malformations: nomenclature and classification based on anatomical and embryological considerations. *Thorax* 1987;42:401–408.

Cochia R, Sobonya RE. Congenital cystic adenomatoid malformation of the lung and bronchial atresia. *Hum Pathol* 1981;12:947–950.

Collin P, Desjardins JG, Khan AH. Pulmonary sequestration. *J Pediatr Surg* 1987;22:750–753.

Cone APD, Adam AE. Cystic adenomatoid malformation of the lung (Stocker type III) found on antenatal ultrasound examination. *Br J Radiol* 1984;57:176–178.

Coran RM, Stocker JT. Extralobar sequestration with frequently associated congenital cystic adenomatoid malformation, type 2: a report of 50 cases. *Pediatr Dev Pathol* 1999;2:454–462.

Crombleholme TM, Leichtly KW, Howell LJ, et al. Cystic adenomatoid malformation volume ratio predicts outcome in prenatally diagnosed cystic adenomatoid malformation of the lung. *J Pediatr Surg* 2002;37:331–338.

Dan SM, Martin JN, White SJ. Antenatal ultrasound findings in cystic adenomatoid malformation. *Pediatr Radiol* 1981;10:180–182.

Davidson LA, Batman P, Fagan DG. Congenital acinar dysplasia: a rare cause of pulmonary hypoplasia. *Histopathology* 1998;32:57–59.

Deacon CS, Smart PJ, Rimmer S. The antenatal diagnosis of congenital cystic adenomatoid malformation of the lung. *Br J Radiol* 1990;63:968–970.

Deluca FG, Wesselhoelft CW. Surgically treatable cause of neonatal respiratory lung distress. *Clin Perinatol* 1978;5:37–47.

Demos NJ, Teresi A. Congenital lung malformations: a unified concept and a case report. *J Thorac Cardiovasc Surg* 1975;70:260–264.

DeParedes CG, Pierce WS, Johnson DG, Waldenhausen JA. Pulmonary sequestration in infants and children; a 20-year experience and review of the literature. *J Pediatr Surg* 1970;5:136–141.

De Santis M, Masini L, Noia G, et al. Congenital cystic malformation of the lung: antenatal ultrasound findings and fetal-neonatal outcome. Fifteen years' experience. *Fetal Diagn Ther* 2001;15:246–248.

Diwan RV, Brennan JN, Phillipson EH, et al. Ultrasonic prenatal diagnosis of Type III congenital cystic adenomatoid malformation of lung. *J Clin Ultrasound* 1983;11:218–221.

Dolkhart L, Reimer F, Helmuth W, et al. Antenatal diagnosis of pulmonary sequestration: a review. *Obstet Gynecol Surg* 1992;47:515–520.

Duncombe GJ, Dickeson JE, Kikiros CS. Prenatal diagnosis and management of congenital cystic adenomatoid malformation of the lung. *Am J Obstet Gyn* 2002;187:950–954.

Elias K, Aufses AH. Squamous cell carcinoma occurring in an intralobar pulmonary sequestration. *Exp Med Surg* 1960;18:36–46.

Gerle RD, Jaretski A, Ashley CA, et al. Congenital broncho-pulmonary foregut malformation: pulmonary sequestration communicating with the gastrointestinal tract. *N Engl J Med* 1968;278:1413–1419.

Gonzalez-Cuezzi F, Boggs JD, Raffensperger JG. Brain heterotopia in the lungs: a rare case of respiratory disease in the newborn. *Am J Clin Pathol* 1980;73:281–285.

Gottrup F, Lund C. Intralobar pulmonary sequestration: a report of 12 cases. *Scand J Respir Dis* 1978;59:21–29.

Harrison MR, Adzick NS, Jennings RW, et al. Antenatal intervention for congenital cystic adenomatoid cystic malformation. *Lancet* 1990;336:965–967.

Hazebrock FWJ, Pattenier JW, Tibboel D, et al. Congenital diaphragmatic hernia: the impact of preoperative stabilization. *J Pediatr Surg* 1989;24:678–684.

Heithoff KB, Sane SM, Williams HJ, et al. Bronchopulmonary foregut malformations. a unifying etiological concept. *Am J Roentgenol* 1976;126:46–55.

Hernanz-Schulman M. Cysts and cystlike lesions of the lung. *Radiol Clin North Am* 1993;31:631–649.

Hernanz-Schulman M, Stein IM, Neblett WW, et al. Pulmonary sequestration: diagnosis with color flow sonography and a new theory of associated hydrothorax. *Radiology* 1991;180:817–821.

Hobbins JC, Grannum PAT, Berkowitz RL, et al. Ultrasound in the diagnosis of congenital anomalies. *Am J Obstet Gynecol* 1979;134:331–345.

Hubbard AM, Crombleholme TM. Prenatal and neonatal lung lesions. *Semin Roentgenol* 1998;33:117–125.

Johnson JA, Rumack CM, Johnson ML, et al. Cystic adenomatoid malformation: antenatal demonstration. *Am J Roentgenol* 1984;142:483–484.

Juettner FM, Pinter HH, Hammer G, et al. Bilateral intralobar pulmonary sequestrations: therapeutic implications. *Ann Thorac Surg* 1987;43:660–662.

Keswani SG, Crombleholme TM, Pawel BR, et al. Prenatal diagnosis and management of mainstem bronchial atresia. *Fetal Diagn Ther* 2005;20:74–78.

Kravitz RM. Congenital malformations of the lung. *Clin North Am* 1994;41:453–472.

Kunisaki SM, Fauza DO, Nemes LP, et al. Bronchial atresia: the hidden pathology within a spectrum of prenatally diagnosed lung masses. *J Pediatr Surg* 2006;41:61–65.

Laberge JM, Flageole H, Pugash D, et al. Outcome of the prenatally diagnosed congenital cystic adenomatoid lung malformation: a Canadian experience. *Fetal Diagn Ther* 2001;16:178–186.

Landing BH, Dixon LG. Congenital malformations and genetic disorders of the respiratory tract. *Am Rev Respir Dis* 1979;120:151–158.

Langer JC, Filler RM, Bohn DJ, et al. Timing of surgery for congenital diaphragmatic hernia: is emergency operation necessary? *J Pediatr Surg* 1989;23:731–738.

Langston C. New concepts in the pathology of congenital lung malformations. *Semin Pediatr Surg* 2003;12:17–37.

Leninger BJ, Haight C. Congenital cystic adenomatoid malformation of the left lobe lower lobe with compression of remaining lung. *Clin Pediatr* 1973;12:182–186.

MacGillivray TE, Adzick NS, Harrison MR, et al. Disappearing fetal lung lesions. *J Pediatr Surg* 1993;28:1321–1325.

Marcus SF, Lobb MO. The antenatal diagnosis by ultrasonography of type III congenital cystic adenomatoid malformation of the lung: case report. *Br J Obstet Gynaecol* 1986;93:1002–1005.

May DA, Barth RA, Yeager S, et al. Perinatal and postnatal chest sonography. *Radiol Clin North Am* 1993;31:499–516.

Mendoza A, Wolf P, Edwards DK, et al. Prenatal ultrasonographic diagnosis of congenital adenomatoid malformation of the lung. *Arch Pathol Lab Med* 1986;110:402–404.

Mentzer SJ, Filler RM, Phillips J. Limited pulmonary resections for congenital cystic adenomatoid malformation of the lung. *J Pediatr Surg* 1992;27:1410–1413.

Miller JA, Corteville JE, Langer JC. Congenital cystic adenomatoid malformation in the fetus: natural history and predictors of outcome. *J Pediatr Surg* 1996;31:805–808.

Miller RK, Sieber WK, Yunis EJ. Congenital cystic adenomatoid malformation of the lung: a report of 17 cases and review of the literature. *Pathol Annu* 1980;1:387–407.

Moerman P, Fryns JP, Vandenberghe K, et al. Pathogenesis of congenital cystic adenomatoid malformation of the lung. *Histopathology* 1992;21:315–321.

Morin C, Fillatrault P, Russo P. Pulmonary sequestration with histologic changes of cystic adenomatoid malformation. *Pediatr Radiol* 1989;19:130–133.

Morin L, Crombleholme TM, Lewis F, et al. Bronchopulmonary sequestration: prenatal diagnosis with clinicopathologic correlation. *Curr Opin Obstet Gynecol* 1994;6:479–481.

Moulik D, Robinson L, Daily DK, et al. Perinatal sonographic depiction of intralobar pulmonary sequestration. *J Ultrasound Med* 1987;6:703–706.

Nicolaides KH, Blatt AJ, Greenough A. Chronic drainage of fetal pulmonary cysts. *Lancet* 1987;1:618–619.

O'Mara CS, Baker RR, Jeyasingham K. Pulmonary sequestration. *Surg Gynecol Obstet* 1978;147:609–616.

Ozcan C, Celik A, Ural Z, et al. Primary pulmonary rhabdomyosarcoma arising within cystic adenomatoid malformation: a case report and review of the literature. *J Pediatr Surg* 2001;36:1062–1065.

Rashad F, Gaisoni E, Gaglione S. Aberrant arterial supply in congenital cystic adenomatoid malformation of the lung. *J Pediatr Surg* 1988;23:107–108.

Rempen A, Feige A, Wiinsch P. Prenatal diagnosis of bilateral cystic adenomatoid malformation of the lung. *J Clin Ultrasound* 1987;15:3–8.

Romero R, Chernenak FA, Katzen J, et al. Antenatal sonographic findings of extralobar pulmonary sequestration. *J Ultrasound Med* 1982;1:131–132.

Savic B, Birtel FJ, Thalen W, et al. Lung sequestration: report of seven cases and review of 540 published cases. *Thorax* 1979;34:96.

Shanji FM, Sachs JH, Perkins DG. Cystic diseases of the lungs. *Surg Clin North Am* 1988;68:581–618.

Stephanopoulos C, Catsaros H. Myxosarcoma complicating a cystic hamartoma. *Thorax* 1963;18:144–145.

Stocker JT, Madewell JER, Drake RM. Congenital cystic adenomatoid malformation of the lung: classification and morphologic spectrum. *Hum Pathol* 1977;8:155–171.

Stocker JT, Drake RM, Madwell JE. Cystic and congenital lung disease in the newborn. *Perspect Pediatr Pathol* 1978;4:93–98.

Szarnicki R, Maurseth K, deLoval M, et al. Tracheal compression by the aortic arch following right pneumonectomy. *Ann Thorac Surg* 1978;25:321–324.

Taguchi T, Suita S, Yamanouchi T, et al. Antenatal diagnosis and surgical management of congenital cystic adenomatoid malformation of the lung. *Fetal Diagn Ther* 1995;10:400–405.

Takeda S, Miyoshi S, Inoue M, et al. Clinical spectrum of congenital cystic disease of the lung in children. *Eur J Cardiothorac Surg* 1999;15:11–18.

Tander B, Yalcin M, Yilmaz B. Congenital Lobar emphysema: a clinicopathologic evaluation of 14 cases. *Eur J Pediatr Surg* 2003;13:108–111.

Thakral CL, Maji DC, Sajwani MJ. Congenital lobar emphysema: experience with 21 cases. *Pediatr Surg Intl* 2001;17:88–93.

Thilenius OG, Ruschhaupt DG, Replogh RL, et al. Spectrum of pulmonary sequestration: association with anomalous pulmonary venous drainage in infants. *Pediatr Cardiol* 1983;4:97–100.

Walker J, Cudmore RE. Respiratory problems and cystic adenomatoid malformation of the lung. *Arch Dis Child* 1990;65:649–659.

Warner CL, Britt RL, Riley HD Jr. Bronchopulmonary sequestration in infancy or childhood. *J Pediatr* 1958;53:521–528.

Wecla K, Grippo R, Unger R, et al. Rhabdomyosarcoma of lung arising in a congenital cystic adenomatoid malformation. *Cancer* 1977;40:383–388.

# Lung Infections: Lung Biopsy, Lung Abscess, Bronchiectasis, and Empyema

# CHAPTER 30

*Harsh Grewal and Barry Evans*

## LUNG INFECTIONS

The incidence of community-acquired pneumonia is estimated to be almost 200 per 100,000 population and complications of community-acquired pneumonia lead to hospitalization in less than 10% of these cases. The majority of children hospitalized for community-acquired pneumonia have empyema, which will often require surgical consultation and possible surgery. Other reasons for surgical intervention include necrotizing lung infection resulting in abscess formation, lung infection in the immunocompromised child, and lung infection associated with bronchiectasis.

## THORACOSCOPIC LUNG BIOPSY

### Essentials of Diagnosis

▶ Undiagnosed interstitial infiltrates in the immunocompromised child and possible diffuse interstitial lung disease in the immunocompetent child are the most common indications for lung biopsy.

▶ Lung biopsy is safe and effective for evaluating the immunocompromised child with suspected infection not responding to empiric antibiotic, antifungal or antiviral therapy, and if serology, high-resolution computerized tomography (HRCT), and broncho-alveolar lavage (BAL) are not diagnostic.

▶ Video-assisted thoracoscopic surgery (VATS) is indicated if the child can tolerate single lung ventilation and transbronchial lung biopsy cannot be performed for technical reasons.

### Indications

Jacobaeus first described thoracoscopy in 1910, when he used it to facilitate collapse therapy for pulmonary tuberculosis. He also used it to perform pleural biopsies. Although the use of thoracoscopy in children was reported in 1971, it was popularized for use in children in 1976 by Rodgers. Today there are fewer indications for lung biopsy than in the past, due to improved diagnostic evaluation using a combination of BAL specimens, HRCT, and genetic testing. Indications for thoracoscopic lung biopsy are listed in Table 30-1. Most children with primary interstitial lung disease have the diagnoses made with the other diagnostic modalities, obviating the need for a biopsy in every patient.

In the immunocompromised patient, however, the appearance of a nodule or a localized or diffuse pulmonary infiltrate presents a diagnostic dilemma and lung biopsy frequently proves invaluable. Since the abnormal finding could be neoplastic, infectious, or a noninfectious inflammatory process, or even possibly a genetically mediated lung disorder, and the therapy could be potentially toxic, a tissue diagnosis becomes crucial. Transbronchial lung biopsy in these infants and children is technically difficult

| TABLE 30-1 | Indications for Lung Biopsy Using Video-Assisted Thoracoscopic Surgery |
|---|---|

**HIV/AIDS (only if BAL is not diagnostic)**

Interstitial infiltrates

    Pneumocystis carnii pneumonia (PCP)

    Lymphoid interstitial pneumonitis (LIP)

    Pulmonary lymphoid hyperplasia (PLH)

    Miliary tuberculosis

**Immunosuppressed following chemotherapy/bone marrow transplant (only if BAL is not diagnostic)**

Interstitial infiltrates

    PCP

    CMV pneumonia

    Mycoplasma pneumonia

    RSV pneumonitis

    Fungal

Nodular infiltrates

    Malignant neoplasm (primary or metastatic)

    Lymphoma or lymphoproliferative disorder

    Fungal

**Diffuse interstitial lung disease (only if all other modalities are not diagnostic)**

Nonspecific or usual interstitial pneumonitis

Desquamative interstitial pneumonitis

LIP/PLH

Others

    Bronchiolitis obliterans

    Sarcoidosis

    Pulmonary hemosiderosis

AIDS, acquired immune deficiency syndrome; BAL, broncho-alveolar lavage; CMV, cytomegalovirus; RSV, respiratory syncytial virus.

and associated with a higher complication rate than in adult patients.

## Diagnostic Algorithm

The child with pulmonary symptoms and an abnormal chest radiograph (CXR) who may require a lung biopsy can be categorized in 1 of 2 ways: as an immunocompetent child with possible diffuse interstitial lung disease or as an immunocompromised child with interstitial infiltrates.

The immunocompromised child with an abnormal CXR should have a sputum examination, CBC, and appropriate serologies. If an infection is suspected and the patient is neutropenic, empiric antibiotics are the usual first step. If the child fails to show clinical improvement despite the addition of antifungal or antiviral therapy, HRCT and bronchoscopy with BAL are the usual next steps to obtain a diagnosis. If these are not diagnostic, transbronchial lung biopsy, if technically feasible, is indicated. An alternative to transbronchial or open lung biopsy in the child who can tolerate single lung ventilation is thoracoscopic lung biopsy to obtain tissue for diagnosis. If the patient is not neutropenic or infection is not highly suspect,

bronchoscopy with BAL may be a satisfactory first step. In children with diffuse or interstitial lung disease with a workup that has not resulted in a diagnosis, or children with suspected malignant pulmonary infiltrate, HRCT followed by lung biopsy with video-assisted thoracoscopic surgery (VATS) is usually indicated. Although BAL may provide a diagnosis, HRCT followed by VATS lung biopsy is the more commonly used approach, has a higher diagnostic accuracy, and is safer. Alternatives include transbronchial lung biopsy or image-guided percutaneous needle biopsy. HRCT is useful to diagnose as well as localize interstitial disease for biopsy preoperatively. An algorithm outlining this approach is shown in Fig. 30-1.

## Operative Procedure

General anesthesia is preferable and should be done with a double lumen endotracheal tube, selective bronchial intubation, or use of a bronchial blocker as appropriate for the weight and size of the child. The child is positioned in the lateral decubitus position. Anterior or posterior rotation may be necessary depending on the site of the lesion (Fig. 30-2).

Trocar placement is dictated by the location of the lesion to be biopsied. A valved trocar, which allows carbon dioxide insufflation if the lung does not collapse, is usually used for the telescope and this is placed in the sixth intercostal space in the mid or posterior axillary line. A 5-mm, 0°- or 30°-telescope is used in almost all patients. A 2-mm scope is now available, but the authors have not used it for thoracoscopic lung biopsy. Two additional ports are placed: a 5 mm for a grasper or retractor and a 12 mm for an endoscopic stapler in larger children. The lung to be biopsied is grasped and resected with the endoscopic linear stapler (Fig. 30-3A). In smaller children in whom a 12-mm stapler cannot be accommodated, 2 endoloops can be used to snare a tongue of lung tissue that can then be cut with endoscopic scissors (Fig. 30-3B).

Following biopsy, the lung is inspected for hemostasis and "aerostasis." It is important to ensure that there is no air leak in these sick, and often ventilated children. A chest tube is placed in all ventilated patients through 1 of the port sites. In nonventilated patients with compliant lungs, a chest tube may be avoided by using a catheter to aspirate the hemithorax. The anesthesiologist expands the lung as the catheter is withdrawn from the hemithorax while applying suction through the catheter. A postoperative CXR confirms lung expansion. Lung biopsy specimens should be sent fresh to the pathologist, and if interstitial lung disease is suspected, the specimens need to be inflated just prior to fixation.

## Outcome

The diagnostic yield of HRCT is low in acquired diffuse pulmonary disease and is relatively low in acquired focal lung diseases. It is much higher, however, for genetically mediated diffuse interstitial lung disorders. The diagnostic accuracy of lung biopsy in children is high, around 95% and the results significantly alter therapy in most patients. Thoracoscopic (VATS) lung biopsy is safe, with minimal air leaks in children who tolerate single lung ventilation, and less than 1% of patients require transfusion for bleeding.

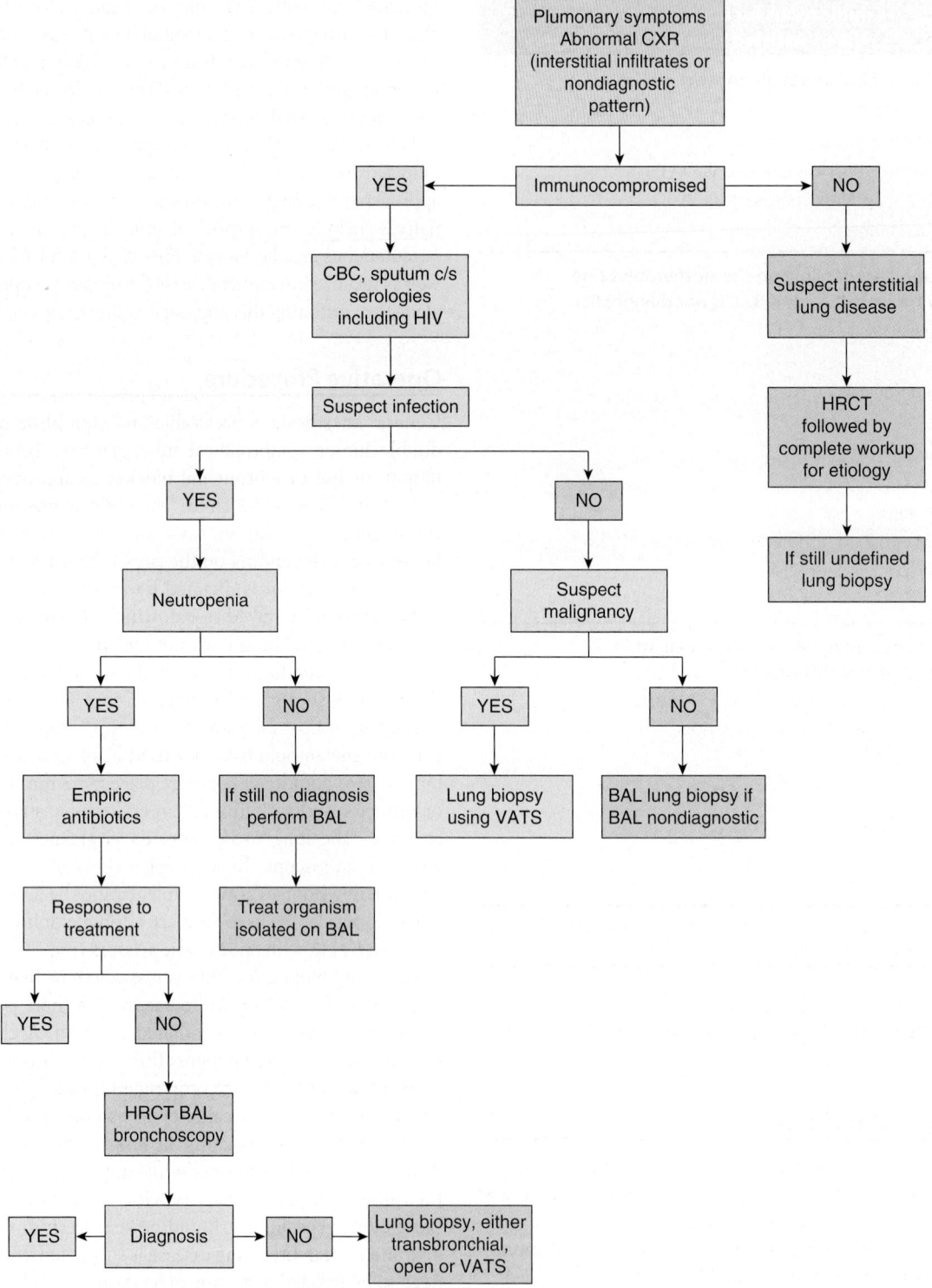

**FIGURE 30-1** Algorithm outlining an approach for lung biopsy in children.

## EMPYEMA

### Essentials of Diagnosis

► Childhood empyema is the most common local complication of community-acquired pneumonia requiring hospitalization in children 18 years or younger.

► The diagnosis of empyema should be considered in all children with fever, cough, respiratory distress, and parapneumonic effusion on CXRs.

► Ultrasound or computed tomography (CT) may be useful in defining the nature and extent of the effusion, and especially the presence of loculations.

► If thoracentesis is performed, a diagnosis of empyema is made if there is frank pus, positive gram stain, or culture of pleural fluid. Additional diagnostic criteria are pleural fluid pH <7.0, pleural fluid glucose <40 mg/dL, and pleural fluid LDH >1000 IU/dL.

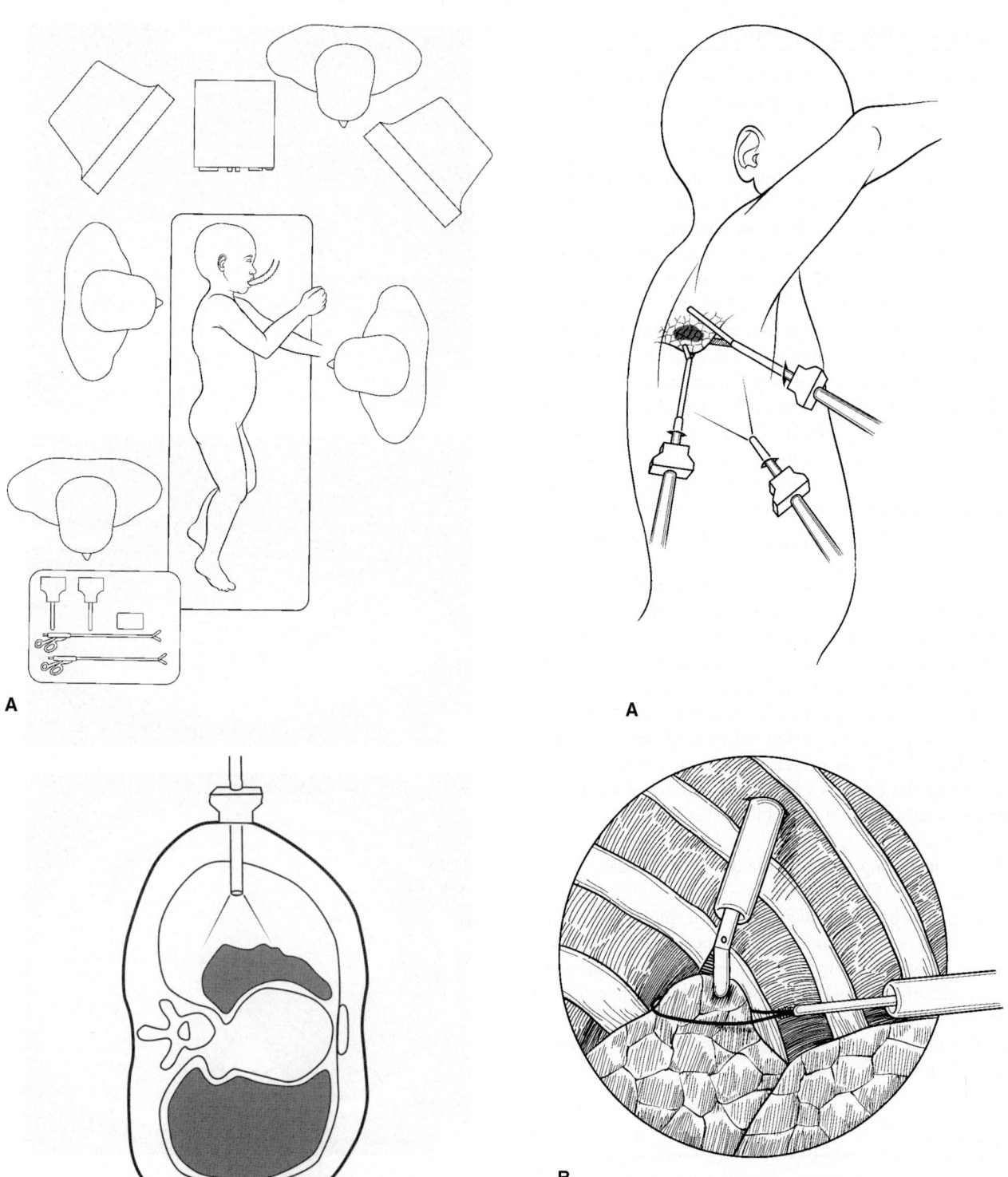

**FIGURE 30-2** Thoracoscopic lung biopsy. **A.** Authors' preferred room setup with patient in the lateral decubitus position. **B.** Lateral decubitus position is followed by insertion of a trocar in the sixth intercostal space in the mid to posterior axillary line. Lung collapse may be assured by use of a double-lumen tube, selective intubation, use of a bronchial blocker, or by $CO_2$ insufflation.

**FIGURE 30-3** Lung biopsy using a thoracoscopic technique. **A.** The lung to be biopsied is put under tension and a linear stapler is fired to secure hemostasis and control air leak. **B.** An endoloop is effective in smaller children as an adjunct to control the cut lung surface.

## Etiology and Pathophysiology

The first description of empyema as pus in the pleural space is attributed to Hippocrates, around the fourth century BC. Closed drainage of empyema with a chest tube was introduced following the report of the Empyema Commission in 1918 by Evart Graham, who showed that open drainage to atmospheric pressure was associated with high mortality.

Childhood empyema is the most common local complication of community-acquired pneumonia requiring hospitalization in children 18 years or younger. It is estimated that approximately 9 to 10 per 100,000 children are hospitalized for empyema complicating community-acquired pneumonias. Direct infection of a parapneumonic effusion is the most common cause of empyema, although it may also result from spread of infection to the pleural space from an abdominal infection, esophageal perforation, retropharyngeal or prevertebral infections, or introduction of infection by trauma or surgery. Children with immune deficiencies, hypogammaglobulinemia, Down syndrome, congenital heart disease, and cerebral palsy may be predisposed to develop empyema.

*Streptococcus pneumoniae*, *Haemophilus influenzae*, and *Staphylococcus aureus* are the most common pathogens cultured from empyema, but often no organism is isolated on culture of pleural fluid. Anaerobic bacteria may be cultured in patients with aspiration pneumonia or lung abscess complicated by empyema. The highest incidence of empyema is in the 1- to 5-year age group, followed by the ≤1-year age group. The introduction of heptavalent pneumococcal conjugate vaccine does not appear to have reduced rates of local complications such as empyema in children; in fact the rates seem to be increasing.

Traditionally, empyemas are divided into 3 stages: (1) the exudative stage—characterized by a thin, sterile, pleural exudate; (2) the fibrinopurulent stage—the fluid is now turbid and loculated, with a fibrinous, pleural peel; and (3) the organizing stage—with a thick exudate and an organized, pleural peel encasing the lung and rendering it immobile. Simple exudative effusions can progress to complicated effusions, including empyema in as little as 24 to 48 hours, but more commonly take 3 to 5 days.

## Diagnosis

The diagnosis of empyema should be considered in all children with fever, cough, respiratory distress, and parapneumonic effusion on CXRs (Fig. 30-4A). Ultrasound (Fig. 30-4B) or CT (Fig. 30-4C) may be useful in defining the nature and extent of the effusion. The authors recommend initial chest ultrasound rather than CT to image the pleural cavity for the presence or absence of loculations. Ultrasound is more accurate in imaging loculated fluid, is portable and cheaper, and there is no radiation exposure. The authors also recommend using a diagnostic and management algorithm based on early ultrasound in suspected empyema (Fig. 30-5). If thoracentesis is performed, a diagnosis of empyema is made if there is frank pus, positive gram stain, or culture of pleural fluid. Additional diagnostic criteria are pleural fluid pH <7.0, pleural fluid glucose <40 mg/dL, and

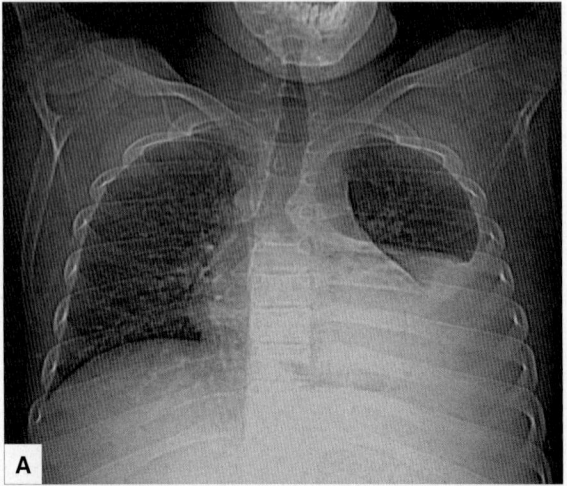

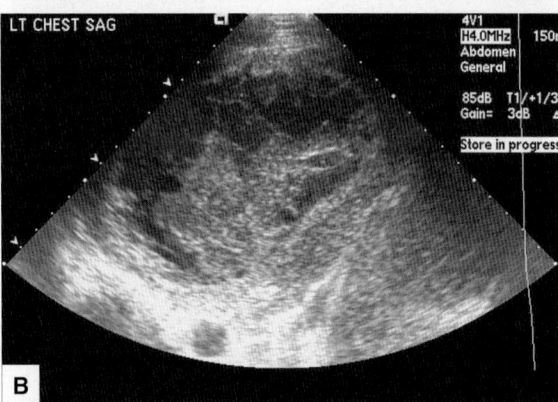

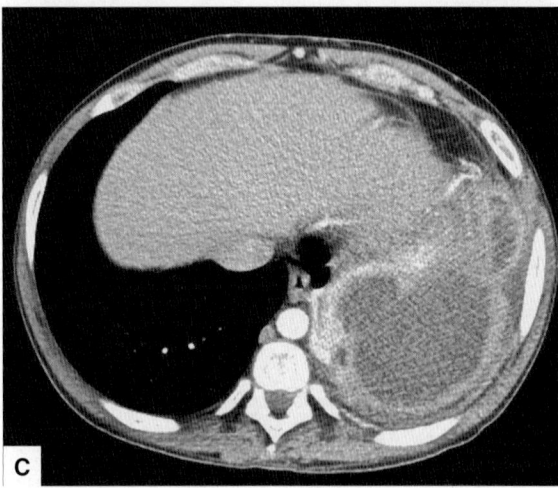

**FIGURE 30-4** **A.** Chest radiograph showing a parapneumonic effusion that suggests an empyema. **B.** Ultrasound examination revealing a complex fluid collection in the chest, typical of a loculated empyema. **C.** Computerized tomographic (CT) scan of an empyema demonstrating a complex mass in the pleural space.

pleural fluid LDH >1000 IU/dL. An alternative management algorithm derives from the position paper of the American Pediatric Surgical Association New Technology Committee and includes the use of fibrinolytic therapy for parapneumonic effusions and empyema (Fig. 30-6). The decision to use image-guided catheter placement and fibrinolytic therapy is dependent on local expertise and experience.

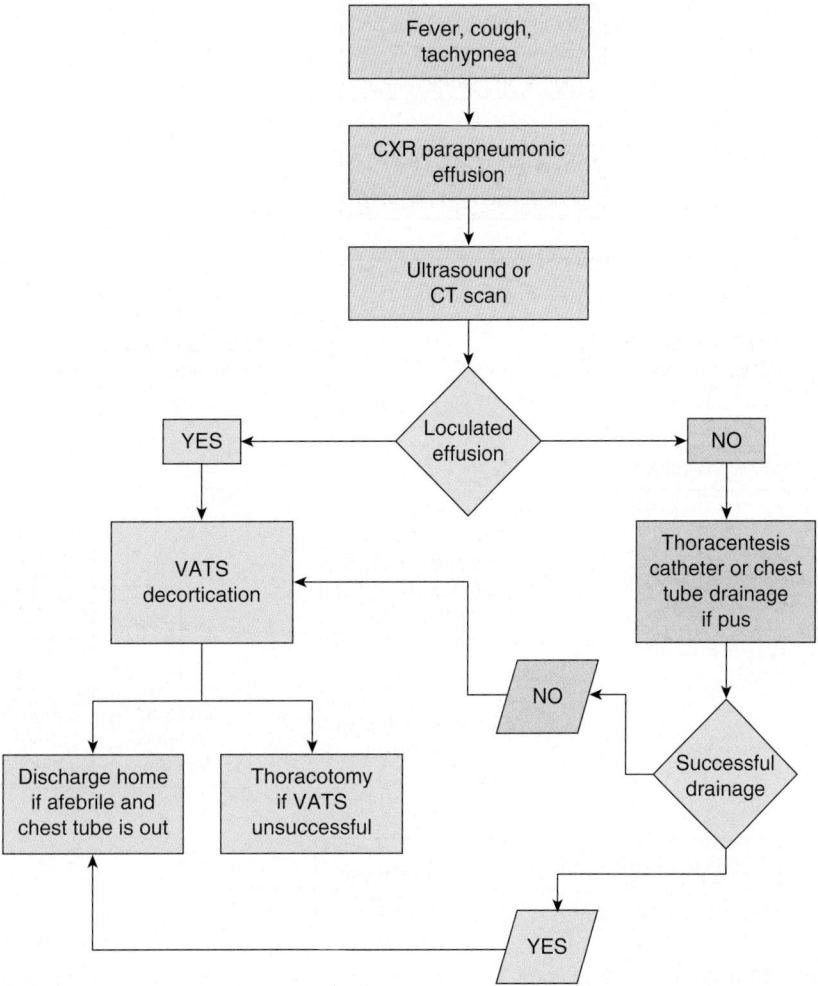

**FIGURE 30-5** Algorithm outlining diagnostic and therapeutic approach for a child with an empyema.

## Management

Initial antibiotic treatment alone may successfully treat an empyema, especially in the early stages, prior to becoming thick and loculated. In the child with a persistent empyema, in addition to using antibiotics to sterilize the pleural cavity, the goals of treatment are to drain and obliterate the pleural space, thus, allowing the lung to expand and function normally. The timing and method of attaining these goals are controversial. During the initial exudative stage, the fluid is thin and free flowing and its removal by thoracentesis or chest tube drainage may result in a cure. Most patients, however, are treated initially by their primary care physicians with antibiotics, and by the time these patients are admitted to the hospital (usually 3-5 days later), the empyema has often progressed to the loculated, fibrinopurulent, or organizing stage.

Although chest tube drainage may be successful in some patients in the fibrinopurulent or loculated stage, this stage usually results in prolonged hospital stay. Fibrinolysis has been advocated as an alternative to surgical therapy for the management of empyema, but there is conflicting evidence regarding the economic benefit, morbidity, and length of hospital stay for fibrinolysis compared to VATS. Fibrinolysis is an alternative to early VATS for the treatment of loculated effusions not responding to antibiotics (Fig. 30-6). In practice, the authors perform early ultrasound, as soon as the patient is suspected to have an empyema, and if there are loculations on imaging, proceed directly to VATS, as outlined in the treatment algorithm depicted in Fig. 30-5. Thoracentesis or chest tube placement is not required prior to VATS.

## Operative Management

VATS is performed using general anesthesia. A single lumen endotracheal tube is used in the majority of patients, with selective bronchial intubation if possible. Arterial or central lines are not routinely used. The patient is positioned in the lateral decubitus position with the involved side up. Trocar placement is dictated by the location of the loculated empyema. Usually 1 valved trocar, which allows $CO_2$ insufflation if the lung does not collapse, is used for the telescope and this is placed in the sixth intercostal space in the mid or posterior axillary line (Fig. 30-7). A 5- or 10-mm, 0°- or 30°-telescope is used.

Prior to insufflation, pleural fluid or pus should be aspirated with a large bore suction aspirator. After pneumothorax

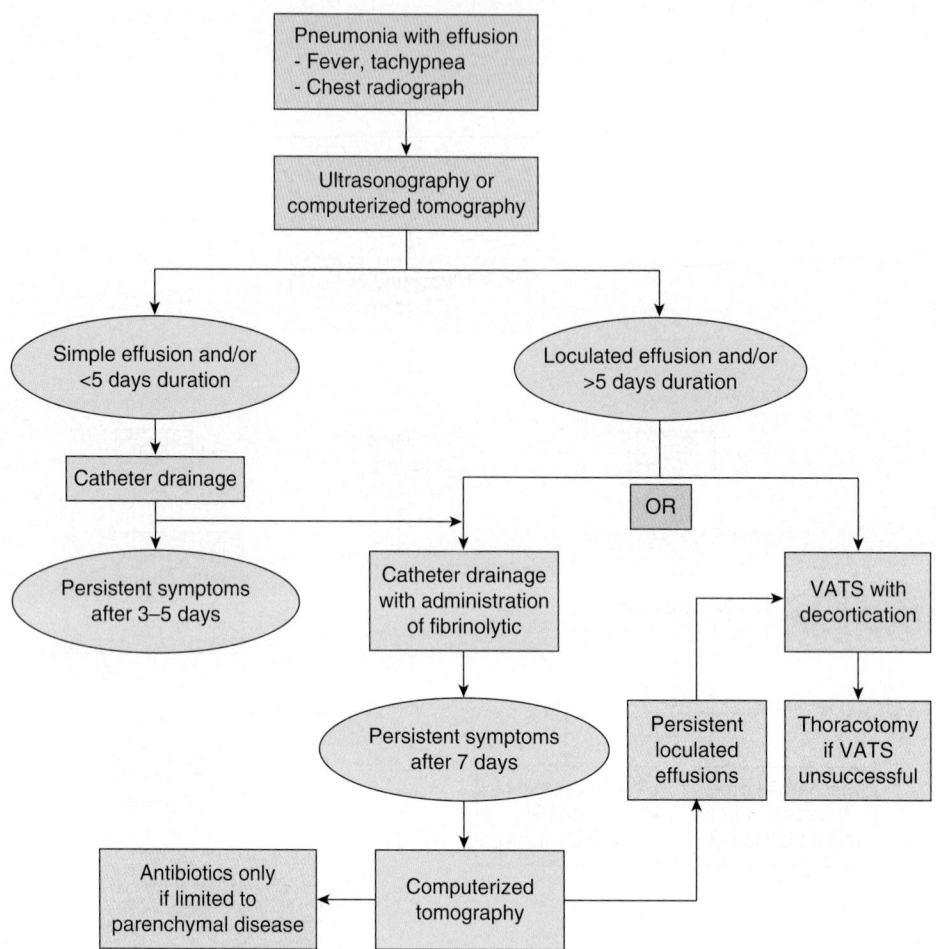

**FIGURE 30-6** Alternate algorithm for the treatment of children with pneumonia and parapneumonic effusions or empyema. (Used with permission from Kokoska ER, Chen MK; New Technology Committee. Position paper on video-assisted thoracoscopic surgery as treatment of pediatric empyema. *J Pediatr Surg* 2009;44:289–293.)

is induced and the lung is collapsed, additional incisions in the intercostal space are made under thoracoscopic visualization to allow instruments to be introduced directly into the thoracic cavity. These skin incisions should be placed so that they can be incorporated into a formal thoracotomy incision, if needed. A variety of curved and straight, ring, stone, and dressing forceps can then be used (Fig. 30-8). The pleural cavity is debrided of all fibrinous and purulent material (Fig. 30-9). All adhesions are lysed and the lung is inspected.

If the lung is encased and does not expand, the lung must be decorticated. A plane is developed between the lung and the encasing "peel" using a sponge or Kittner dissector and decortication is performed. If there is excessive bleeding and visualization is inadequate, VATS should be converted into a minithoracotomy. After irrigation and hemostasis, either 1 or 2 chest tubes are placed through the trocar incisions (Fig. 30-10).

Postoperative recovery usually occurs in the pediatric surgery ward unless a child requires postoperative ventilation. Chest tubes are removed when they stop draining or drainage is <50 mL/day and CXR confirms lung expansion. Intravenous antibiotics are usually continued until the patient is afebrile (temperature ≤38.5°C). Patients are

discharged from the hospital on oral antibiotics when they are afebrile.

## Outcome

Historically, the mortality for childhood empyema ranges from 0% to 10%, with thoracotomy and decortication rates of up to 50%. Compared to nonsurgical approaches, surgical approaches using thoracotomy or VATS show advantages in reductions in complications, failures, and hospital stays. The smaller incisions needed for VATS have the additional advantages of reducing morbidity and patient discomfort (Table 30-2).

# BRONCHIECTASIS

## Essentials of Diagnosis

▶ Bronchiectasis is a descriptive term for abnormally thickened and irreversibly dilated bronchi, usually associated with chronic suppuration.

▶ The diagnosis of bronchiectasis should be considered in a child with recurrent or chronic cough with sputum

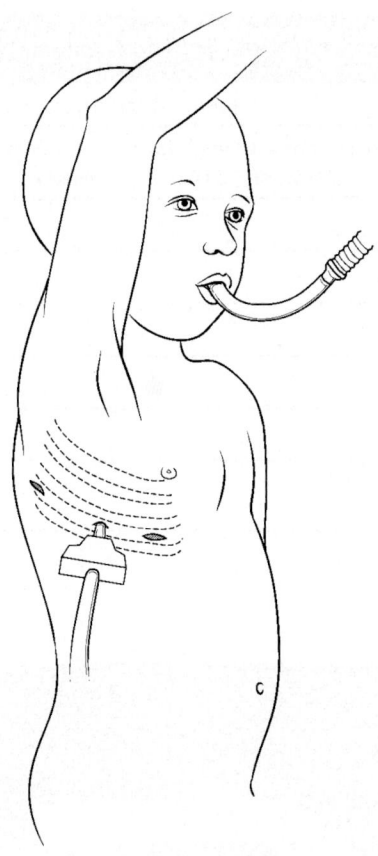

**FIGURE 30-7** Position and port access sites for video-assisted thoracoscopic management of an empyema.

production, or with hemoptysis associated with recurrent or localized pulmonary suppuration.

▶ Bronchiectasis is most commonly associated with cystic fibrosis, although noncystic fibrosis bronchiectasis, a heterogenous group of diseases, is not as uncommon as previously thought.

▶ Bronchiectasis may be suspected on CXR, but diagnosis requires HRCT.

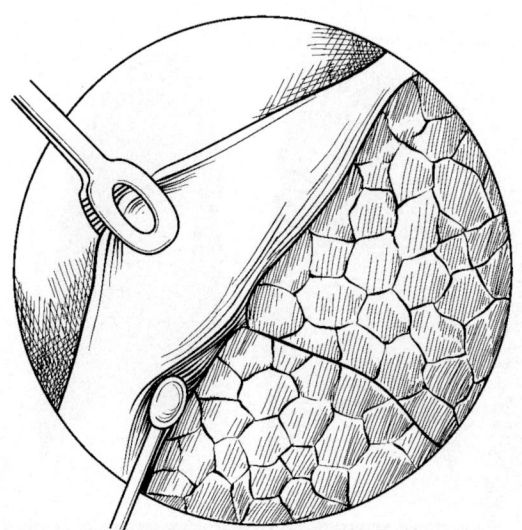

**FIGURE 30-8** Thoracoscopic dissection of the encircling peel from off of the lung surface.

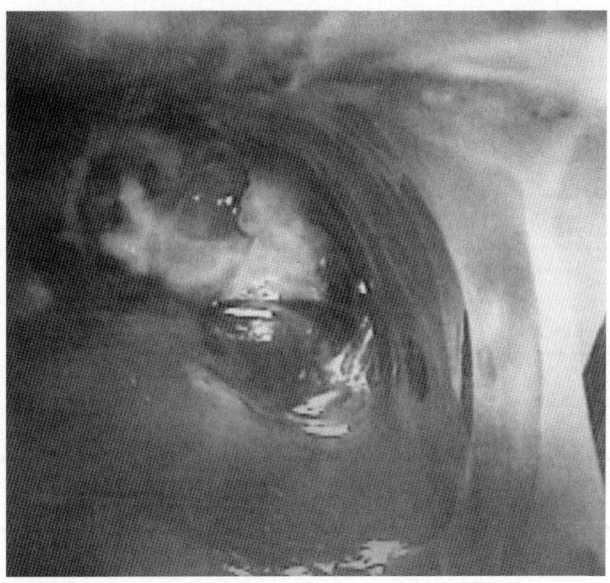

**FIGURE 30-9** Thoracoscopic debridement and decortication of the lung and pleural space.

## Etiology and Pathophysiology

Bronchiectasis, a descriptive term for abnormally thickened and irreversibly dilated bronchi, usually associated with chronic suppuration, was initially used by Laennec in 1819. Osler recognized the role of bronchial inflammation and bronchial obstruction in his textbook published in 1892. The introduction of effective antibiotics for childhood pneumonia, immunization against pertussis and measles, aggressive

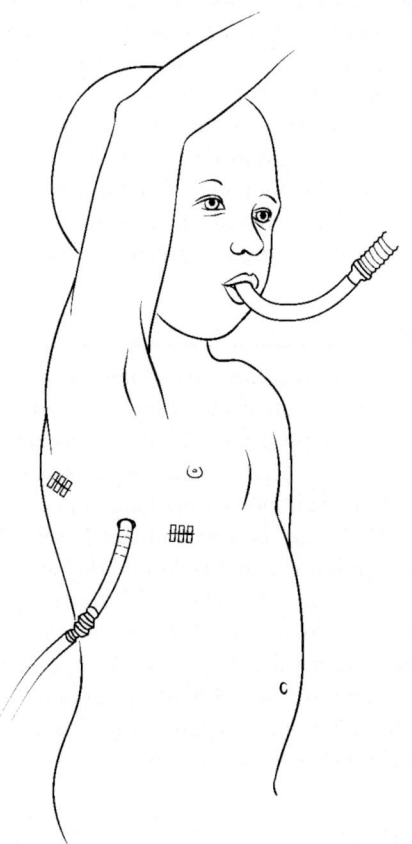

**FIGURE 30-10** Port and chest tube sites following VATS treatment of an empyema.

| TABLE 30-2 | Outcomes for Treatment of Empyema Using Operative Therapy with Video-Assisted Thoracoscopic Surgery, Thoracotomy, or Nonoperative Therapy | | | |
|---|---|---|---|---|
| | Operative Therapy | | Nonoperative Therapy | |
| | VATS (Number = 176) | Thoracotomy (Number = 175) | Chest Tube and Antibiotics (Number = 3183) | Primary Fibrinolytic Therapy (Number = 64) |
| Age (years) | 5.1 | 6.7 | 5 | 4.1 |
| Mortality (%) | 0 | 0 | 3.3 | 0 |
| Failure (%) | 2.8 | 3.1 | 23.6 | 9.4 |
| Complication rate (%) | 5.4 | 5.2 | 5.6 | 12.5 |
| Length of hospital stay (day) | 11.2 | 10.6 | 20 | 10.7 |

Adapted from Avansino JR, Goldman B, Sawin RS, Flum DR. Primary operative versus nonoperative therapy for pediatric empyema: a meta-analysis. *Pediatrics* 2005;115:1652–1659.

treatment of cystic fibrosis, and prompt removal of foreign bodies causing airway obstruction have made bronchiectasis a rare problem. Due to this rarity, there may be a significant delay in diagnosis of bronchiectasis, especially in the noncystic fibrosis group.

Bronchiectasis develops as a result of inflammatory destruction of the bronchial epithelial lining, as well as progressive damage to the bronchial and peribronchial supporting connective tissue. The loss of mucociliary transport mechanisms and functional obstruction of the bronchial lumen result in ongoing inflammation, suppuration, and permanent tissue damage. In the past, postinfectious or postobstructive bronchiectasis was common. Today the exact etiology is often unknown. The most common classification systems consider cystic fibrosis as the major cause of bronchiectasis in children. The other cases are classified into a group described as noncystic fibrosis-related causes, including those related to immune deficiency states, primary ciliary dyskinesia syndrome, post-lung transplantation, and allergic bronchopulmonary aspergillosis.

## Diagnosis

The diagnosis of bronchiectasis should be considered in a child with recurrent or chronic cough with sputum production, or with hemoptysis associated with recurrent or localized pulmonary suppuration. CXR may be suggestive; usually showing increased pulmonary markings, honeycombing, and atelectasis. There may be predominant lower lobe involvement, although lingular and right middle lobes may also be involved. Bronchiectasis in cystic fibrosis may preferentially involve the upper lobes. In the past, bronchography was recommended to make the diagnosis. However, HRCT of the lung is the diagnostic modality of choice today (Fig. 30-11). An algorithm outlining an approach to diagnosis and management of bronchiectasis is shown in Fig. 30-12.

## Management

The preferred treatment for bronchiectasis is medical management including intravenous, oral, and inhaled antibiotics,

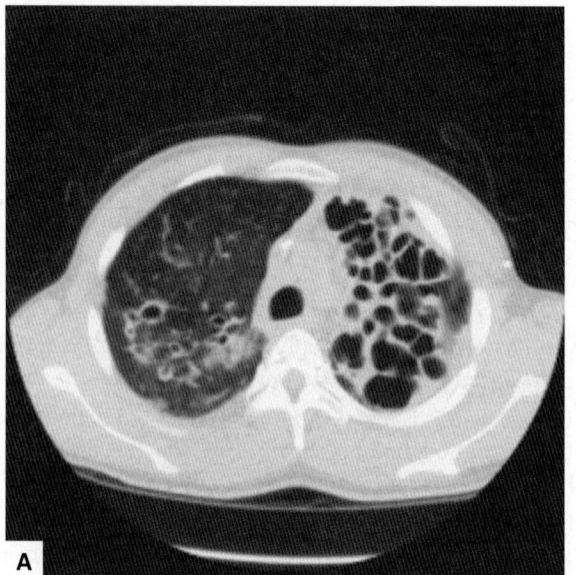

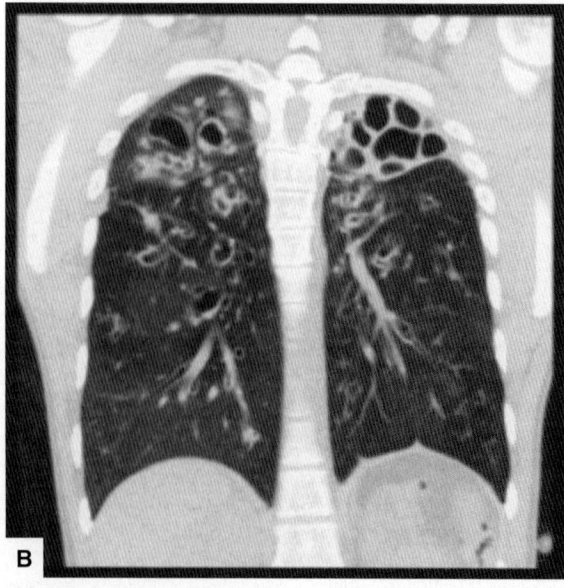

**FIGURE 30-11 A.** Axial image and (**B**) coronal image of HRCT demonstrating bronchiectasis in a child with cystic fibrosis.

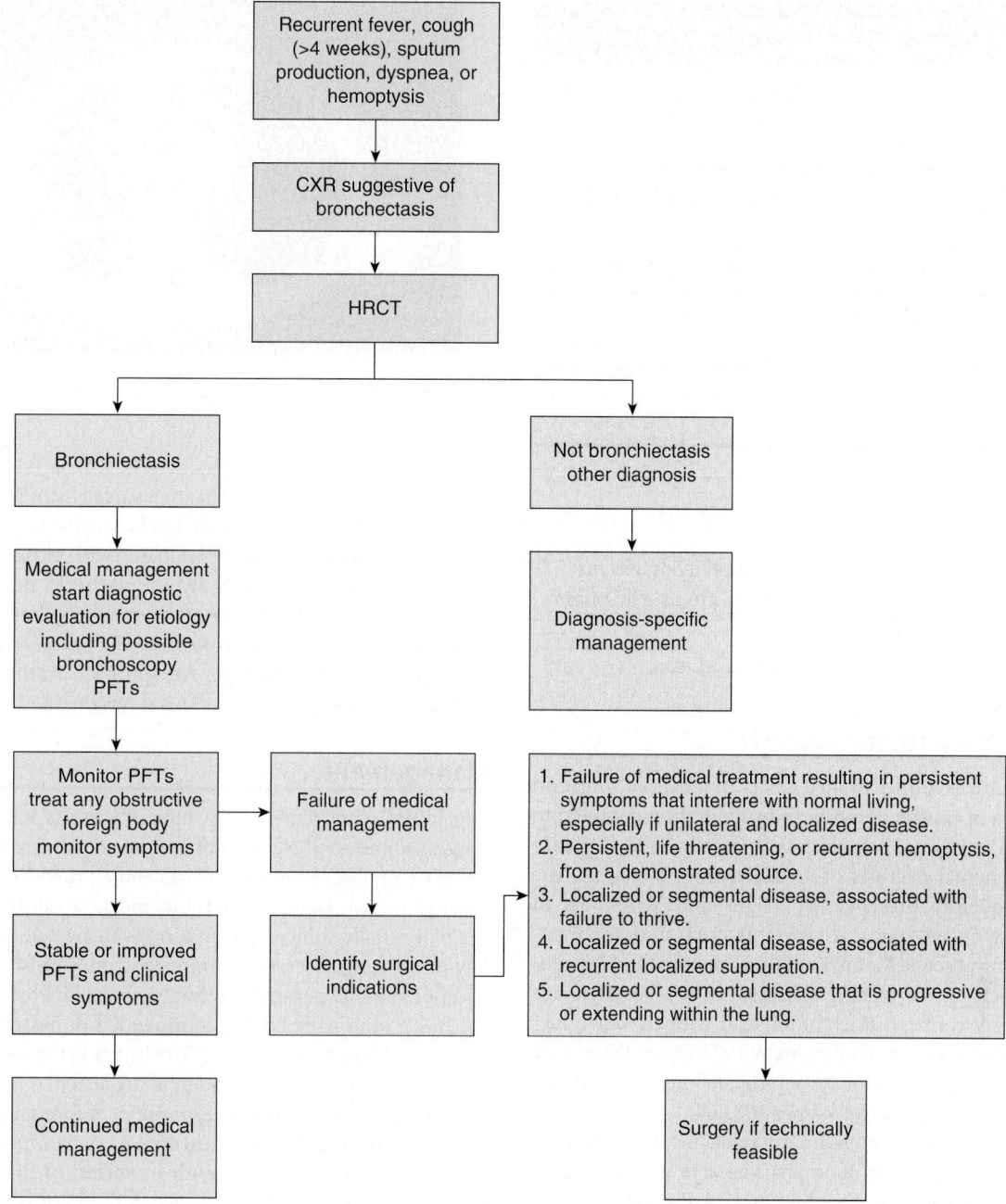

**FIGURE 30-12** Algorithm for the diagnosis and management of bronchiectasis.

The boxes in the figure read:

- Recurrent fever, cough (>4 weeks), sputum production, dyspnea, or hemoptysis
- CXR suggestive of bronchectasis
- HRCT
- Bronchiectasis
- Not bronchiectasis other diagnosis
- Medical management start diagnostic evaluation for etiology including possible bronchoscopy PFTs
- Diagnosis-specific management
- Monitor PFTs treat any obstructive foreign body monitor symptoms
- Failure of medical management
- Stable or improved PFTs and clinical symptoms
- Identify surgical indications
- Continued medical management
- Surgery if technically feasible

1. Failure of medical treatment resulting in persistent symptoms that interfere with normal living, especially if unilateral and localized disease.
2. Persistent, life threatening, or recurrent hemoptysis, from a demonstrated source.
3. Localized or segmental disease, associated with failure to thrive.
4. Localized or segmental disease, associated with recurrent localized suppuration.
5. Localized or segmental disease that is progressive or extending within the lung.

along with a program of postural drainage, chest physiotherapy, and mucolytic agents. This is especially true for patients with cystic fibrosis and primary ciliary dyskinesia.

Indications for surgery are listed in Table 30-3. Preoperative management includes intensive medical management, pulmonary function testing, and localization by HRCT of the diseased segment to be removed. Segmental or lobar resection with conservation of the functioning lung is the operation of choice. On occasion, it may be necessary to perform resection of the lingular lobe along with the left lower lobe, or right middle lobe with right lower lobectomy, since there may be concurrent involvement of these neighboring lobes or segments. The lung resection may be performed by thoracotomy or VATS, depending on the extent of intrathoracic adhesions and the surgeon's expertise with thoracoscopy.

## Outcome

Results are good in 75% to 90% of patients receiving surgical treatment for localized bronchiectasis. Serious complications are uncommon, although empyema and bronchopleural fistulas have been reported in up to 15% of operated patients. Mortality is less than 1% in reported series.

## LUNG ABSCESS

### Essentials of Diagnosis

▶ Rarely a cause of lung infection in children, a lung abscess is a thick-walled cavity of localized infection with an area of central necrosis and suppuration confined to the lung parenchyma.

| TABLE 30-3 | Indications for Surgery in Children with Bronchiectasis |
|---|---|
| 1. | Failure of medical treatment resulting in persistent symptoms that interfere with normal living, especially if unilateral and localized disease |
| 2. | Persistent, life-threatening, or recurrent hemoptysis from a demonstrated source |
| 3. | Localized or segmental disease associated with failure to thrive |
| 4. | Localized or segmental disease associated with recurrent localized suppuration |
| 5. | Localized or segmental disease that is progressive or extending within the lung |

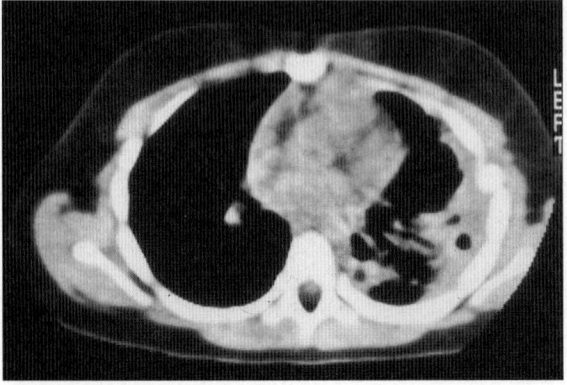

**FIGURE 30-13** CT scan demonstrating a lung abscess.

- ► The presence on CXR of a fluid-filled cavity or a cavity with an air fluid level that measures >2 cm usually raises suspicion of a lung abscess.

- ► CT scan of the chest confirms the diagnosis.

## Etiology and Pathophysiology

A lung abscess is a thick-walled cavity of localized infection with an area of central necrosis and suppuration confined to the lung parenchyma. The abscess is usually a consequence of a parenchymal necrosis of an active lung infection. The patient frequently presents with signs and symptoms of cough, fever, and dyspnea. An early description of the treatment for lung abscesses is attributed to Bonet in the 17th century. The occurrence of lung abscesses in the pediatric age group has always been uncommon and with the introduction of antibiotics has become rare. A 1934 report listed lung abscesses as responsible for 33 per 100,000 pediatric admissions, while today the rate is <1 per 100,000.

There are 4 common routes for microbial invasion: (1) postpneumonic, (2) aspiration of oropharyngeal or gastrointestinal contents, (3) hematogenous seeding, and (4) direct spread from the abdomen or from trauma and surgery. Lung abscesses have been classified as primary when they occur in a previously healthy child and secondary when they occur with a preexisting condition. Secondary abscesses are often multiple. Common risk factors in children are altered mental states with swallowing dysfunction, hematologic and oncologic disorders resulting in immunodeficiency states, primary immunodeficiencies, and bronchial obstructive conditions. *S. aureus*, *Streptococcus* species, and anaerobes are the most common bacterial pathogens isolated. Multiple organisms are often cultured from lung abscesses in children.

## Diagnosis

Fever, cough, purulent sputum, and dyspnea in a child should make one suspect a lung abscess. Like most other respiratory infections in children, lung abscesses are usually first discovered on CXR. Along with CXR, sputum examination with cultures should be done. The presence of a fluid-filled cavity or a

cavity with an air-fluid level that measures >2 cm is characteristic of lung abscess. If this is pleural based, the possibility of a loculated empyema should be evaluated with ultrasonography or CT (Fig. 30-13). CT may also be useful in documenting multiple abscesses, differentiating them from other congenital or acquired lung cysts, and possibly as part of treatment to guide percutaneous drainage. An approach to the diagnosis and management of lung abscesses is outlined in Fig. 30-14.

## Management

The initial management of a lung abscess is with intravenous antibiotics. The choice of antibiotic will depend on the presence or absence of risk factors and culture results. In the absence of risk factors, anaerobic and gram-positive coverage will usually suffice. If aspiration is suspected as the etiology or for lung abscesses in immunocompromised children, additional gram-negative coverage is needed. Postural drainage has traditionally been recommended to hasten recovery. The total duration of antibiotic treatment is not well defined, but 2 to 3 weeks at the minimum is suggested.

In the absence of clinical response or if foreign body aspiration is suspected, bronchoscopy is recommended. This is, however, risky and can result in spread of infection and even fatal aspiration. If bronchoscopy does not help or is not performed, CT-guided drainage may be possible in managing chronic lung abscess, especially if the abscess is peripherally located and if there is evidence of pleural symphysis between the lung and pleura adjacent to the abscess cavity. Another option is VATS drainage of abscesses that are superficial. While rare, surgical resection of the abscess cavity and necrotic lung may be performed as a formal thoracotomy and lobectomy, or it may be done using VATS with a linear endoscopic stapler. Single lung anesthesia using either a double lumen endotracheal tube or a bronchial blocker placed bronchoscopically is advantageous in preventing spillage and complications in the contralateral lung. The authors' approach to managing lung abscesses is included in Fig. 30-14.

## Outcome

Children with primary lung abscesses have a good prognosis for cure, with resolution of abscess cavities in more than 70% of children by 3 months. The mortality is usually less than

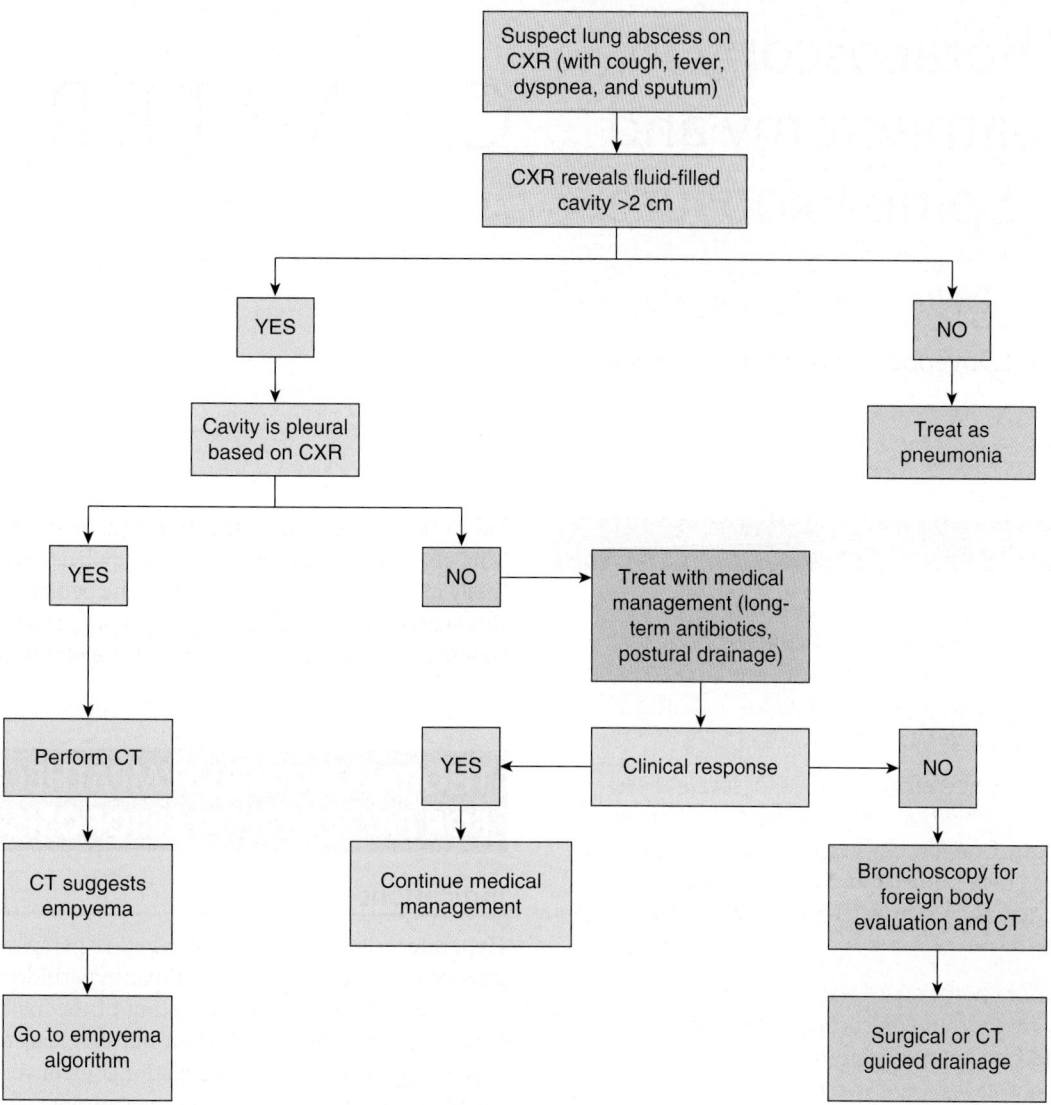

**FIGURE 30-14** Algorithm for the diagnosis and management of lung abscess.

5%. In children with secondary lung abscesses, mortality is higher, ranging from 10% to 30%, with the underlying disease being more important in determining outcome.

## SELECTED READINGS

Avansino JR, Goldman B, Sawin RS, Flum DR. Primary operative versus nonoperative therapy for pediatric empyema: a meta-analysis. *Pediatrics* 2005;115:165–1659.

Chang AB, Redding GJ. Bronchiectasis. In: Chernick V, Boat TF, Wilmott RW, Bush A, eds. *Kendig's Disorders of the Respiratory Tract in Children*. Philadelphia: Saunders Elsevier; 2006:463–477.

Glüer S, Schwerk N, Reismann M, et al. Thoracoscopic biopsy in children with diffuse parenchymal lung disease. *Pediatr Pulmonol* 2008;43:992–996.

Gow KW, Chen MK, New Technology Committee. American Pediatric Surgical Association New Technology Committee review on video-assisted thoracoscopic surgery for childhood cancer. *J Pediatr Surg* 2010;45:2227–2233.

Grewal H, Jackson RJ, Wagner CW, Smith SD. Early video assisted thoracic surgery (VATS) in the management of empyema in children. *Pediatrics* 1999;103:e63.

Kokoska ER, Chen MK, New Technology Committee. Position paper on video-assisted thoracoscopic surgery as treatment of pediatric empyema. *J Pediatr Surg* 2009;44:289–293.

Laberge J-M. Infections of the lung and airway. In: O'Neil JA, Grosfeld JL, Fonkalsrud EW, et al, eds. *Principles of Pediatric Surgery*. 2nd ed. St. Louis: Mosby; 2003:357.

Nagasawa KK, Johnson SM. Thoracoscopic treatment of pediatric lung abscesses. *J Pediatr Surg* 2010;45:574–578.

Puligandla PS, Laberge JM. Respiratory infections: pneumonia, lung abscess, and empyema. *Semin Pediatr Surg* 2008;17:42–52.

Rodgers BM, Talbert JL. Thoracoscopy for diagnosis of intrathoracic lesions in children. *J Pediatr Surg* 1976;11:703–708.

Rothenberg SS, Kuenzler KA, Middlesworth W. Thoracoscopic lobectomy for severe bronchiectasis in children. *J Laparoendosc Adv Surg Tech A* 2009;19:555–557.

Sirmali M, Karasu S, Türüt H, et al. Surgical management of bronchiectasis in childhood. *Eur J Cardiothorac Surg* 2007;31:120–123.

Stafler P, Carr SB. Non-cystic fibrosis bronchiectasis: its diagnosis and management. *Arch Dis Child Educ Pract Ed* 2010;95:73–82.

Wilson S, Grundy R, Vyas H. Investigation and management of a child who is immunocompromised and neutropenic with pulmonary infiltrates. *Arch Dis Child Educ Pract Ed* 2009;94:129–137.

# Thoracoscopy for Sympathectomy and Spine Exposure

# CHAPTER 31

*Katherine P. Davenport and Timothy D. Kane*

## KEY POINTS

1. For thoracoscopic sympathectomy for primary hyperhidrosis and thoracoscopic spine exposure for release of thoracic scoliosis, video-assisted thoracoscopic surgery (VATS) offers several advantages, including shorter hospital stay for patients and lower morbidity.

2. Surgical treatment is recommended for severe cases of primary hyperhidrosis or those refractory to medical management. Upper thoracic sympathectomy interrupts transmission of impulses from the sympathetic ganglia to the sweat glands and can offer immediate and permanent relief.

3. Compensatory sweating (CS) occurring in the back, chest, and thighs is the most common side effect of thoracoscopic sympathectomy, but the reported incidence and severity are lower than in adults and very few adolescent patients express regret for having undergone thoracoscopic sympathectomy.

4. The initial access for thoracoscopic spine exposure should be just above the level of the central-most portion of the proposed release.

5. At each level, the intervertebral space is entered by using electrocautery to incise the pleura and overlying fascia between the segmental vessels superior and inferior to the line of incision and standard curets and other extraction devices are used to remove the disk.

6. When all the selected disks have been removed, the bone graft that has been harvested from the iliac crest and morcellated can be packed into each intervertebral space.

## INTRODUCTION

The use of thoracoscopic methods to perform surgical procedures in infants and children has burgeoned over the several years. Familiarity with approaches and instrumentation along with the more widespread use of these techniques has led to the routine use of thoracoscopy in some institutions. This chapter focuses on 2 growing applications for a minimally invasive thoracic approach in the pediatric population: thoracoscopic sympathectomy for primary hyperhidrosis and thoracoscopic spine exposure for release of thoracic scoliosis.

## THORACOSCOPIC SYMPATHECTOMY FOR PALMAR HYPERHIDROSIS

### Indications

Hyperhidrosis is a condition of excessive perspiration beyond physiological needs. Primary palmar hyperhidrosis (PHH) is part of a triad of excessive sweating of the axillae, feet, and hands. The etiology is unknown but can lead to significant psychological, social, and occupational inconvenience. Conservative management with antiperspirants, iontophoresis, botox injections, and systemic medications such as anticholinergics are temporary, but may be effective for mild forms of hyperhidrosis. Surgical treatment is recommended for severe cases or those refractory to medical management. Upper thoracic sympathectomy interrupts transmission of impulses from the sympathetic ganglia to the sweat glands and can offer immediate and permanent relief. Although rarely performed via an open approach, the video-assisted thoracoscopic technique offers the benefit of high visibility of the surgical field, low morbidity, short hospital stay, and excellent cosmetic results.

Most hyperhidrosis series involve adult populations who have had longstanding symptoms since childhood and have undergone sympathectomy 10 to 15 years after the onset of symptom onset. Others have reported improved outcomes for children compared to adults with regard to long-term satisfaction as well as decreased severity and incidence of compensatory sweating (CS). These reports advocate earlier intervention for children. While not as common in the United States, increased palmar sweating is frequently seen in children and adolescents living in warmer climates, such as the area around the Negev Desert in Israel, where the largest pediatric experience has been reported. Dedicated pediatric series report good postoperative results with considerable improvement in social settings and scholastic achievement.

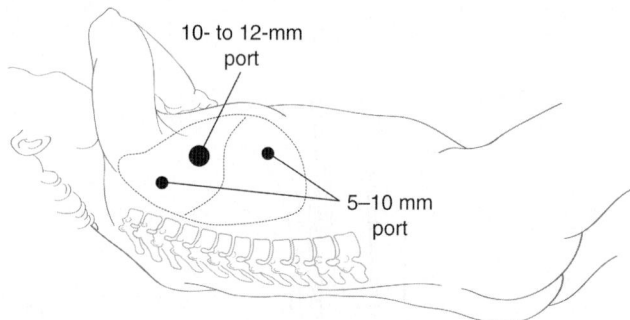

**FIGURE 31-1** Patient positioning for a thoracoscopic sympathectomy. The shoulders are elevated on a block, and both arms are extended and abducted.

## Operative Approach

The goal of surgery is to interrupt the sympathetic supply to the palms through destruction of the relevant ganglions in the upper thoracic sympathetic chain. For palmar hyperhidrosis, it is generally accepted that a sympathectomy (removing or ablating the ganglia) or sympathotomy (transecting the chain between ganglia) at the T2 and T3 level is the most effective. Since this condition tends to be bilateral, the procedure is usually carried out on both sides. Cohen and his colleagues described elevating the anesthetized patient on a shoulder roll and extending both arms, allowing access to both axillae. A reversed Trendelenburg position is also helpful. The procedure is relatively short (20-30 minutes per side) and is performed in the apex of the hemithorax. Therefore, lung isolation techniques are not necessary for thoracoscopic sympathectomy. Some surgeons use a single 10- to 11-mm incision to accommodate an operating thoracoscope, which has a 5-mm channel to accept a Maryland-style dissector or an L-hook electrocautery probe alongside the 5-mm scope (Fig. 31-1). The authors use similar patient positioning but prefer to use a 5-mm trocar and thoracoscope as depicted in Fig. 31-2. A 5-mm electrocautery hook instrument is then introduced through a second stab incision (with or without a trocar) to perform the sympathectomy. These patients are typically adolescents although the authors have performed this procedure in a couple of children less than 10 years of age. The operating thoracoscope has a large diameter and is

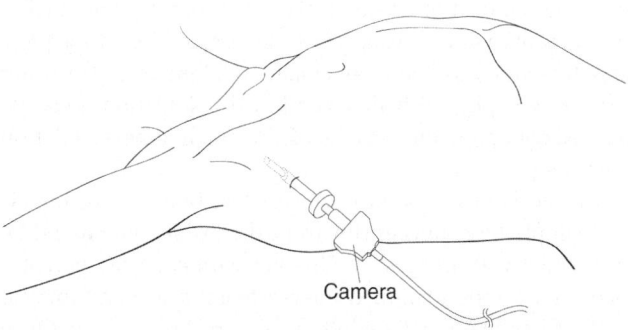

**FIGURE 31-2** Patient positioning with a smaller 5-mm access trocar and 5-mm telescope. A second access incision will be placed medially, adjacent, and 1 interspace lower (with or without an additional trocar) for electrocautery probe device use.

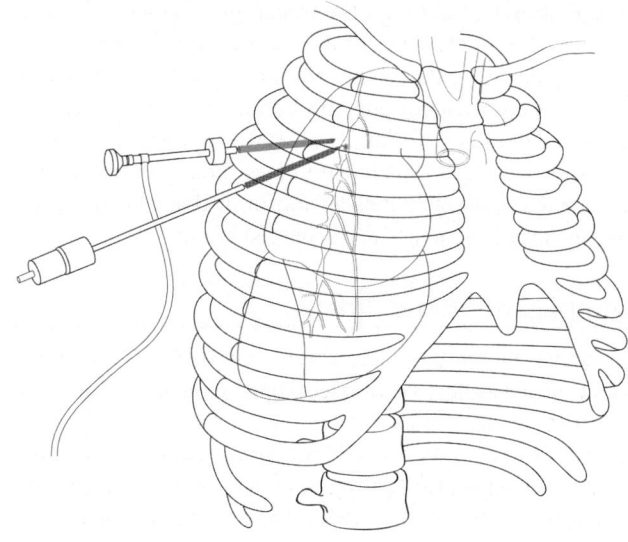

**FIGURE 31-3** Internal view of the technique for sympathectomy. The area between the second and third ganglion is selected and entering and exiting fibers are destroyed by electrocautery.

thus more difficult to negotiate through the tighter rib interspaces in smaller patients (Fig. 31-3).

After access is achieved, the operating table is tilted about 30° to 40° toward the opposite side so that the combination of gravity and 4 to 6 mm Hg $CO_2$ insufflation act to push the lung inferiorly to expose the superior sympathetic ganglion chain. The area between the second and third ganglia is selected, and all connecting fibers are destroyed with the cautery device. Once the chain is exposed, the hook is used to divide the chain and/or ablate the ganglia.

Preoperatively, temperature probes are placed on both palms and connected to the anesthesia monitor. The palmar temperature should be noted prior to sympathectomy and the adequacy of the procedure assessed by observing a slight increase in temperature of the palmar surface immediately following division of the sympathetic chain. The temperature change is typically only 0.2°C to 0.4°C and after the patient has emerged from anesthesia, their hands will be flushed, dry, and warm.

Methods of dividing the sympathetic chain vary among surgeons and range from clipping the chain (without division) between T2 and T3 to completely resecting the T2 and or T3 ganglia. Clipping the chain has been advocated by some to retain the potential of reversibility if intolerable CS occurs. This is also the reason cited for staged operations, with the first procedure involving thoracoscopic injection of the sympathetic chain with local anesthetic (lidocaine or bupivicaine) to assess the effects of temporary sympathectomy over the course of a couple of days and observe if the amount of CS would preclude the recommendation to proceed with definitive sympathectomy. This staged approach has not been described in children, where CS seems to be less of an issue. Resection of the ganglia at T2 and T3 and/or multiple levels (T4) has led to a greater amount of CS in adults. The authors' preference is to use electrocautery to divide the chain completely between the ganglia, along with associated nerve fibers traveling out along the accompanying rib heads. Post-procedural pneumothoraces are evacuated by a combination of aspirating $CO_2$ through the trocar and maintaining positive pressure on the lungs to force any air out of the chest as the surgeon closes the wound and no chest tubes are placed. If there is any residual pneumothorax on the postoperative chest radiograph, inhalation of 100% oxygen for several hours or overnight usually eliminates the problem. As long as the pneumothorax is smaller and/or unchanged on the following day, the patients are discharged home.

## Complications and Pitfalls

CS occurring in the back, chest, and thighs is the most common side effect of thoracoscopic sympathectomy. The reported frequency ranges from 45% to 90% in adult series, and varies in severity and subsequent patient dissatisfaction. Most series report that despite residual CS, patients still prefer the elimination of their PHH. The reported incidence and severity of compensatory hyperhidrosis in adolescents have not been as high or as bothersome and very few express regret for having undergone thoracoscopic sympathectomy.

Horner syndrome can occur in up to 6% of cases and be temporary or permanent. The incidence of Horner syndrome is increased with the inclusion of T1 ganglion in the resection, and for this reason such inclusion is not advised. Other complications of thoracoscopic sympathectomy are infrequent and include wound infection, pneumonia, pneumothorax, and hemothorax requiring tube thoracostomy. With the exception of CS, long-term morbidity associated with thoracoscopic sympathectomy is relatively low.

## THORACOSCOPIC SPINE EXPOSURE

### Indications

Pediatric surgeons are being asked with increasing frequency to provide thoracoscopic exposure for thoracoscopic scoliosis surgery. The traditional approach to the anterior thoracic spine has been by posterolateral thoracotomy. With continued advances in endoscopic instrumentation, video-assisted thoracoscopic surgery (VATS) has become a viable surgical option and is associated with shorter operative time, decreased blood loss, less postoperative pain, and shorter hospital stay when compared to an open approach.

### Operative Approach

The authors use single lung anesthesia either with a double-lumen endotracheal tube for older patients or a Fogarty balloon catheter as a bronchial blocker (Fig. 31-4). The patient is placed in a lateral decubitus position, as would be the case for an open thoracotomy, and the table can be rotated to displace the patient anteriorly as necessary to facilitate exposure of the spine.

The initial access for the telescope should be in a neutral position just anterior to the anterior axillary line, at or just above the level of the central-most portion of the proposed release. For instance if the release is to include levels from T7 through T10, the telescope should be placed at the level of about T8 or T9 (Fig. 31-5).

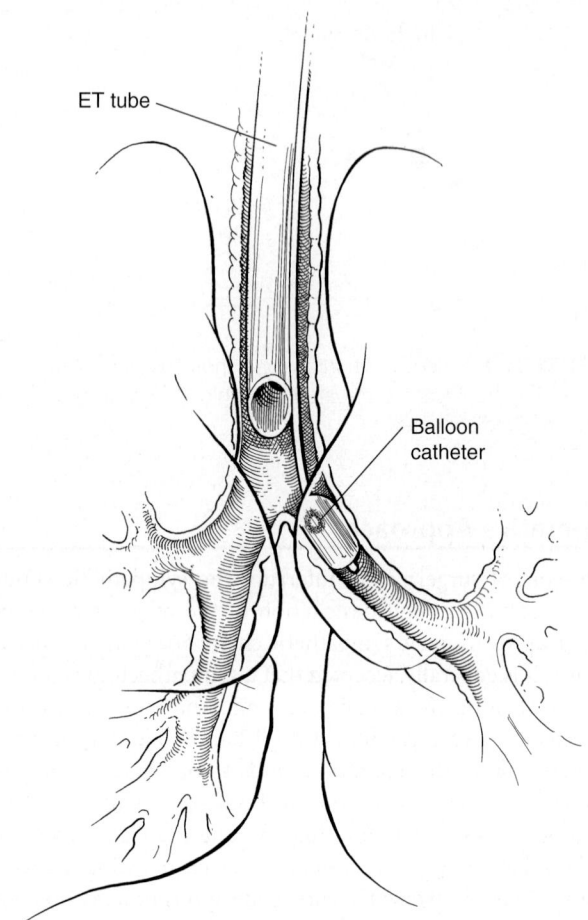

**FIGURE 31-4** Bronchial blocker used in a small infant to occlude ventilation of the left lung. The noncuffed endotracheal tube can be directed into the right main stem bronchus to ventilate the right lung. A Fogarty catheter is directed down the left main stem bronchus and is inflated to occlude its orifice. A flexible bronchoscope passed through the endotracheal tube is used to properly position these 2 devices and thus allow the left lung to remain deflated throughout the procedure.

Since conventional sized orthopedic instruments are used to perform the diskectomies, the authors use Thoracoport® trocars (Covidien, Norwalk, CT), which are shorter than conventional trocars and have grooved sides to prevent slippage from the rib interspaces. The ports have removable rubber caps that can be taken on and off either to accommodate the removal of tissue or placement of larger or smaller instruments without leakage of gas. Use of $CO_2$ to a pressure of about 6 to 8 mm Hg enables the lung to collapse and expose the spine. Whether continued insufflation is necessary depends on the success of the single-lung ventilation technique.

The level of the central-most vertebral body can be identified simply by counting ribs from the inside, but should be confirmed with images. A Kirchner wire is placed percutaneously into the identified intervertebral space and imaged with either plain radiographs or C-arm fluoroscopy. Once the appropriate levels are identified, the release can be carried out. Additional access ports are provided at appropriate levels (approximately 90° perpendicular to the disk space) to permit direct access to the selected disk space. These ports

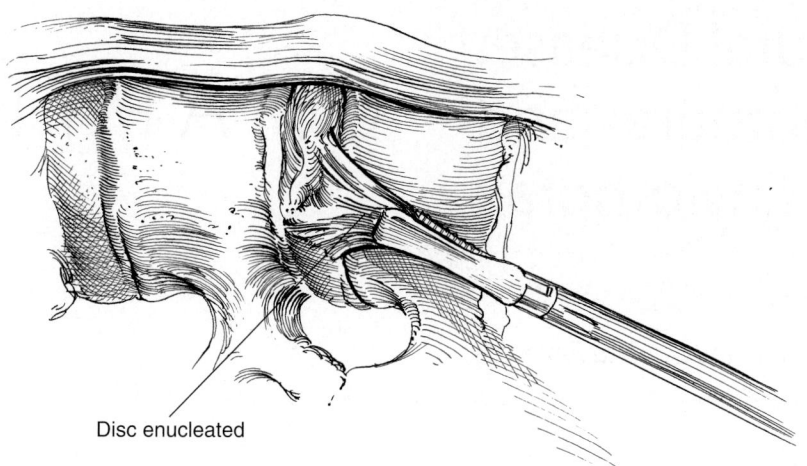

Disc enucleated

**FIGURE 31-5** Technique of diskectomy.

can also be used for repositioning the telescope so that the intervertebral space can be seen from all angles as is necessary to clean out the disk and establish hemostasis.

At each level, the intervertebral space is entered by using electrocautery to incise the pleura and overlying fascia between the segmental vessels superior and inferior to the line of incision. Standard curets and other extraction devices are used to remove the disk, and the remaining space is packed temporarily with a plug made of Gelfoam (Upjohn Company, Kalamazoo, MI) to maintain hemostasis until all the selected disks have been removed (Fig. 31-6). The bone graft that has been harvested from the iliac crest and morcellated is then introduced and packed into each intervertebral space. At the end of the procedure, the patient's lung is allowed to reexpand, and a chest tube is introduced into the most inferior port site for drainage as necessary.

While the patient still must endure the discomfort of the orthopedic procedure and posterior fixation if required, in appropriately selected patients, the morbidity and added

discomfort of a large thoracotomy incision are eliminated with this approach.

## Complications and Pitfalls

As previously mentioned, the thoracoscopic technique for spine exposure can significantly minimize the perioperative and postoperative morbidity found with the open approach. Single lung ventilation is necessary in order to collapse the ipsilateral lung and provide adequate visualization of the field. Single lung ventilation often requires double lumen endotracheal tube placement, which is not always feasible for smaller patients. In such cases, other options to achieve single lung ventilation may be necessary. Pediatric patients treated by the authors have had no postoperative hemorrhaging or other significant problems requiring reoperation after thoracoscopic-assisted spine exposure and release.

## SELECTED READINGS

Cohen Z, Shinar D, Levi I, et al. Thoracoscopic upper thoracic sympathectomy for primary palmar hyperhidrosis in children and adolescents. *J Pediatr Surg* 1995;30:471–473.

Holcomb GW, Mencio GA, Green NE. Video-assisted thoracoscopic diskectomy and fusion. *J Pediatr Surg* 1997;32:1120–1122.

Huang EY, Acosta JM, Gardocki RJ, et al. Thoracoscopic anterior spinal release and fusion: evolution of a faster, improved approach. *J Pediatr Surg* 2002;37:1732–1735.

Li PY, Gu HH, Liang WM. Sequential one-lung ventilation using one Arndt endobronchial blocker in a pediatric patient undergoing bilateral, video-assisted thoracoscopic surgery (VATS). *J Clin Anesth* 2009;21:464.

Mares AJ, Steiner Z, Cohen Z, et al. Transaxillary upper thoracic sympathectomy for primary palmar hyperhidrosis in children and adolescents. *J Pediatr Surg* 1994;29:382–386.

Rodgers B, Moazam F, Talbert J. Thoracoscopy in children. *Ann Surg* 1979;189:176–180.

Steiner Z, Cohen Z, Kleiner O, et al. Do children tolerate thoracoscopic sympathectomy better than adults? *Pediatr Surg Int* 2008;24:343–347.

Steiner Z, Kleiner O, Hershkovitz Y, et al. Compensatory sweating after thoracoscopic sympathectomy: an acceptable trade-off. *J Pediatr Surg* 2007;42:1238–1242.

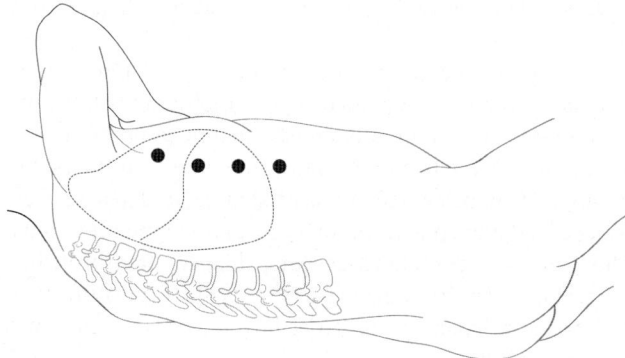

**FIGURE 31-6** Patient positioning for thoracoscopic spinal exposure and release. In the left lateral decubitus position, ports are placed in or anterior to the midaxillary line. Ports are in line and the telescope can be exchanged as successive levels are released.

# Pleural Disease: Pneumothorax and Chylothorax

# CHAPTER 32

*Anthony C. Chin and Marleta Reynolds*

## Pneumothorax

### KEY POINTS

1. A pneumothorax results from a tear in the visceral or parietal pleura with the introduction and/or accumulation of air in the pleural space.

2. A pneumothorax may be spontaneous or, more frequently, acquired.

3. A patient with a pneumothorax may present with respiratory complaints and chest pain, but with minimal lung collapse, the breath sounds may be normal.

4. An upright anterior-to-posterior chest radiograph, upon expiration when feasible, is the standard diagnostic test used to identify a pneumothorax.

5. Treatment may include observation, needle aspiration, placement of an intercostal catheter or tube, or surgical intervention. This may include invasive thoracoscopy or thoracotomy with pleurodesis or pleurectomy, and possibly resection of underlying bullae, cysts, or abnormalities thought to be responsible for the pneumothorax.

6. Surgical treatment using video-assisted thoracoscopic techniques (VATS) or open thoracotomy is indicated when an air leak continues for more than 3 to 5 days or in a pneumothorax that recurs within 48 hours following adequate treatment.

### INTRODUCTION

A pneumothorax results from a tear in the visceral or parietal pleura with the introduction and/or accumulation of air in the pleural space. Although known for centuries to occur from penetrating chest injuries, the danger of air in the chest was not appreciated until the late 18th century. During the 19th century, when a pneumothorax was commonly due to tuberculosis, John B. Murphy popularized collapse therapy for treating tuberculosis. In 1932, Kjaergaard described the rupture of a subpleural bleb as the most common cause of pneumothorax.

### ETIOLOGY

A pneumothorax may be spontaneous or acquired. A spontaneous pneumothorax is classified as primary or secondary. The most common cause of a primary spontaneous pneumothorax is rupture of an apical subpleural bleb. While this seldom affects prepubescent children, it is more likely to occur in young, tall, thin males, especially those who smoke. It is hypothesized that a rapid increase in the vertical growth compared to the horizontal growth of the thorax increases the negative pressure in the apex of the lung causing the formation of subpleural blebs.

Secondary spontaneous pneumothorax results from a complication of underlying lung disease. The most common causes of secondary spontaneous pneumothorax in children are asthma and cystic fibrosis. A neonate being treated for hyaline membrane disease, meconium aspiration, or other acute pulmonary condition may develop secondary spontaneous pneumothorax from a combination of the disease and treatment with positive pressure ventilation. In older children, cystic fibrosis and *Pneumocystis carinii* infection associated with immunosuppression are relatively common causes of secondary pneumothorax. Asthma, pneumonia with lung abscess, Marfan syndrome, esophageal rupture, and metastatic cancer can also be associated with secondary pneumothorax.

An acquired pneumothorax is encountered much more frequently than a spontaneous pneumothorax. Blunt and penetrating chest trauma often lead to a pneumothorax and are discussed in Chapter 80. Iatrogenic injury to the pleura or lung from placement of central lines and pacemakers using a percutaneous technique can cause a pneumothorax. Thoracentesis, percutaneous lung biopsy, transbronchial lung biopsy, barotrauma created by positive pressure ventilation, and laparoscopic procedure may also result in a pneumothorax.

### PRESENTATION AND DIAGNOSIS

A patient with a pneumothorax may present with respiratory complaints and chest pain. Physical findings associated with a pneumothorax may be misleading. With minimal lung

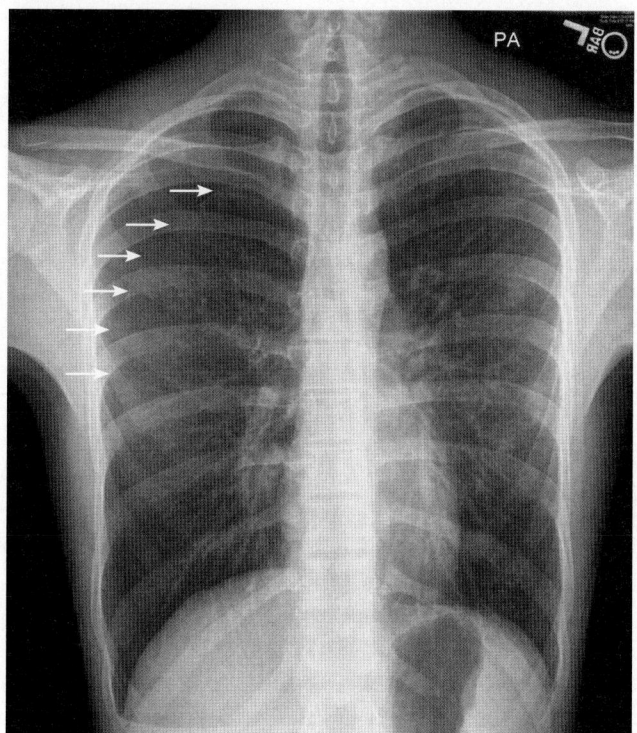

**FIGURE 32-1** Chest radiograph depicting a right partial pneumothorax. *Small white arrows* illustrate the visceral pleura.

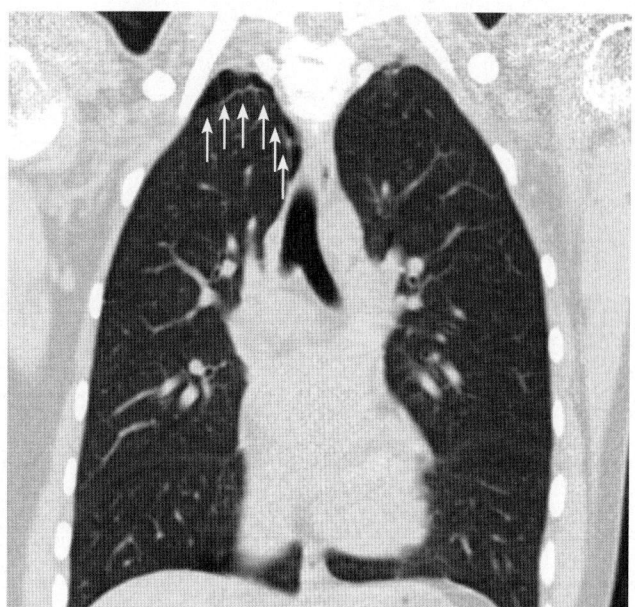

**FIGURE 32-2** CT scan depicting numerous apical subpleural bullae (indicated by *small white arrows*).

collapse, the breath sounds may be normal. Decreased breath sounds and hyperresonance to percussion will be found on the ipsilateral chest when more of the lung collapses. A pneumothorax under tension results in a mediastinal shift to the contralateral side of the chest with tracheal deviation, jugular venous distension, and decreased cardiac preload with tachycardia, sweating, pallor, and hypotension. Cardiovascular collapse will ensue if needle aspiration or emergency tube thoracostomy is not performed.

An upright anterior-to-posterior chest radiograph, upon expiration when feasible, is the standard diagnostic test used to identify a pneumothorax. The radiograph reveals partial to complete collapse of the lung. A thin line outlines the visceral pleura (Fig. 32-1) and there is no evidence of lung markings beyond the line of visceral pleura. An estimation of the volume of collapsed lung can be made using a formula and monogram (Paape and Fry). The authors find it easier to describe the pneumothorax by measuring the distance from the apex of the lung to the top of the chest cavity.

To prevent unnecessary exposure to radiation, a CT scan is not recommended for most patients. However, a CT scan can reveal bullae, which have been reported in upward of 45% of patients with spontaneous pneumothorax and are highly prevalent in patients with recurrent pneumothorax (Fig. 32-2). A CT scan can also be very useful in evaluating patients with a pneumothorax in the setting of complex cystic lung disease. The scan can identify sites of adhesions and the exact location and size of a pneumothorax, and can help differentiate between a lung cyst and a pneumothorax. The scan may also reveal underlying pathology or contralateral disease and identify patients who would benefit from early intervention.

## TREATMENT

The aim of treatment for a pneumothorax is to evacuate the air from the pleural space to allow the pleural disruption to heal and to establish fusion of the visceral and parietal pleura to prevent recurrence. Treatment depends on the size and cause of the pneumothorax and may include observation, needle aspiration, or placement of an intercostal catheter or tube. Surgical intervention may include invasive thoracoscopy or thoracotomy with pleurodesis or pleurectomy. It may also include resection of underlying bullae, cysts, or abnormalities thought to be responsible for the pneumothorax (Fig. 32-3).

## OBSERVATION OR NEEDLE ASPIRATION

A small primary spontaneous pneumothorax (<20% of the hemithorax) in an otherwise healthy and clinically stable child may be treated with observation on an outpatient basis. Air is reabsorbed at a rate of 1.25% per day, which for a small pneumothorax <20% would mean a reduction of 5% per day. Serial radiographs are then used to monitor resolution. A patient with a small primary or acquired pneumothorax who cannot be safely managed as an outpatient will require inpatient observation. Under these circumstances, oxygen therapy may speed resolution. For patients with simple pneumothoraces limited to less than 20% to 30% of chest size, intercostal needle aspiration may be considered. In one large series, catheter aspiration for simple pneumothorax was successful in 69% of patients. The treatment was more successful in a small pneumothorax as compared with a large pneumothorax (87% vs 61%). Complications including hemothorax and retained catheter tips occurred in 2.3% of the cases.

**439**

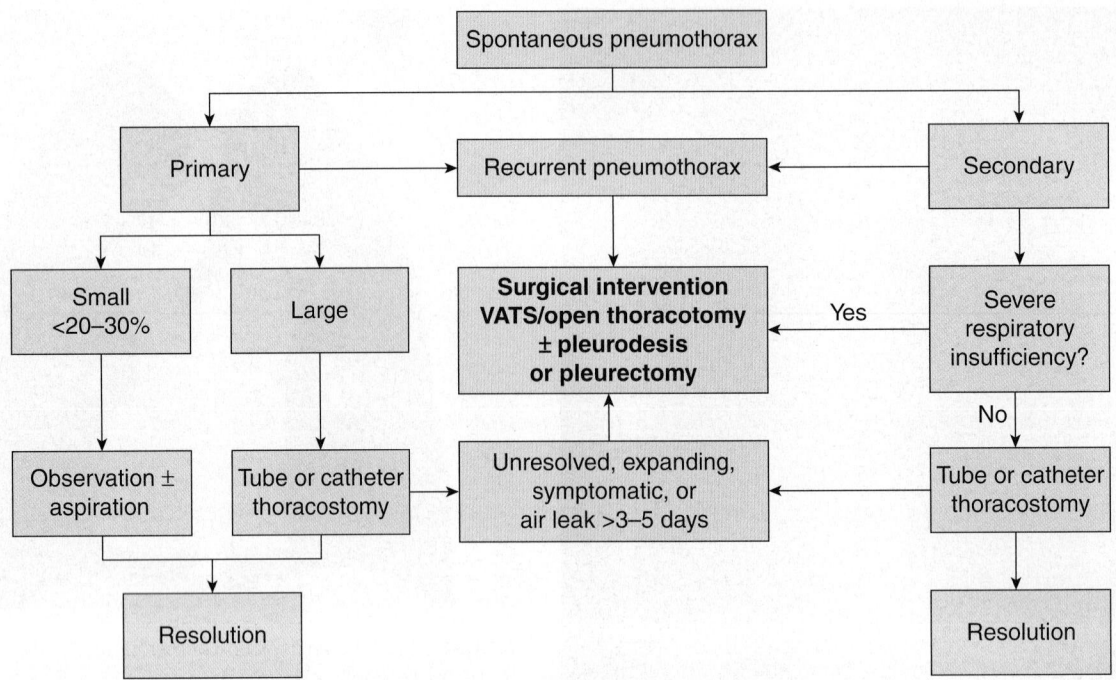

**FIGURE 32-3** Proposed treatment algorithm for the management of a spontaneous pneumothorax.

## TUBE OR CATHETER THORACOSTOMY

A tube or catheter thoracostomy is recommended for the patient with a large primary pneumothorax or secondary spontaneous pneumothorax. Tube size will depend on the size of the child. Neonates can be treated with a 10- or 12-Fr tube. Tubes 16 Fr and larger can be used for children older than 3 years of age. A larger tube (20-40 Fr) will be needed if fluid is present in the chest and might easily occlude a smaller tube. Conscious sedation and local or general anesthesia may be used to facilitate tube placement. Atropine may be useful to avoid a vasovagal response.

The patient is placed in the lateral position and an area of skin surrounding the second to fourth intercostal space in the anterior axillary line is prepped and draped. The skin, subcutaneous tissue, and intercostal muscle are anesthetized with a local anesthetic. An intercostal nerve block is used at the level of tube or catheter insertion and at 1 rib above and below. A transverse incision is made approximately 1 rib below the chosen intercostal space and a subcutaneous tunnel created. If necessary, a curved clamp or scissors is used to create the tunnel. The pleura is penetrated with a blunt instrument above the rib to avoid the intercostal vessels and nerve, and air should escape. A tube is placed through the subcutaneous tunnel and into the chest. The tube is advanced anteriorly to the apex. The tube is then sutured to the skin and a sterile occlusive dressing applied.

The tube may be attached to a water seal or Pleur-Evac drainage system. A Heimlich valve can be used for ease in transport or for outpatient management. Gentle suction of 15 to 20 cm $H_2O$ may be applied if the lung is not immediately expanded. Reexpansion pulmonary edema can develop if the lung is expanded too rapidly, regardless of method used to reexpand the lung. The tube can be removed when the lung is completely expanded and the air leak has disappeared for at least 24 hours.

The risk of recurrent pneumothorax following nonsurgical therapy is upward of 50% to 60% in the pediatric population and is more common in children older than 9 years of age. For this reason, surgery has been recommended following the first recurrence in children older than 9 years. In younger patients, surgery may not be recommended until after the second recurrence. When an air leak persists for more than 72 hours, surgical intervention should be considered. Whenever a primary or secondary spontaneous pneumothorax recurs, surgical treatment is indicated. Some have suggested that surgical intervention be considered in patients with a first episode of secondary spontaneous pneumothorax with severe respiratory insufficiency, since this may restore pulmonary function and minimize risk of developing a tension pneumothorax.

## CHEMICAL PLEURODESIS

Pleural symphysis can be accomplished chemically with instillation of caustic agents into the chest via a tube or catheter thoracostomy. It should be considered for patients with a primary pneumothorax that does not resolve with observation or aspiration. Talc is the most effective agent but can be associated with acute respiratory failure following instillation. Tetracycline was used extensively prior to its removal from the market in 1991. Doxycycline and other tetracycline derivatives are successful in inducing pleural symphysis in 75% to 84% of patients. Instillation may be imprecise unless performed with VATS or open thoracotomy. Pleural sclerosing agents cause pain and fever and will not be effective in a patient with a persistent air leak or an incompletely expanded lung. Chemical pleurodesis may also seriously complicate future reoperation in the thorax and should not be used in potential lung transplant patients.

## SURGICAL INTERVENTION

Surgical treatment using video-assisted thoracoscopic techniques (VATS) or open thoracotomy is indicated when an air leak continues for more than 3 to 5 days or in a pneumothorax that recurs within 48 hours following adequate treatment. Apical blebectomy and pleurodesis using open thoracostomy or VATS yields recurrence rates of 0% to 5%. The goal of surgical therapy is to prevent recurrent pneumothorax with excision of the ruptured bleb and to chemically/mechanically abrade the pleura or perform an apical pleurectomy to induce adhesions between the visceral and parietal pleura.

### Video-Assisted Thoracoscopy

VATS is considered by most the modality of choice for management of recurrent or persistent pneumothorax, with potentially lower complications for most patients. Compared to open thoracotomy, VATS is associated with better surgical outcomes, shorter hospital stays, and better cosmetic results. In most published series, the effectiveness and recurrence rate are similar to that of open surgery, although in some series there may be a minimally higher recurrence rate with thoracoscopy.

A double-lumen endotracheal tube can greatly facilitate VATS and should be used whenever possible. The patient is placed in the lateral position. A 5-mm, 30° thoracoscope is placed into the fourth to sixth intercostal space in the midaxillary line through an appropriately sized introducer. When the lung is collapsed upon slow insufflation and visualization is obtained, the insufflation may be lowered or turned off. This will improve venous return to the heart during the procedure. The lung is examined for bullae with the most likely location in the apex of the upper lobe (Fig. 32-4). The anesthesiologist

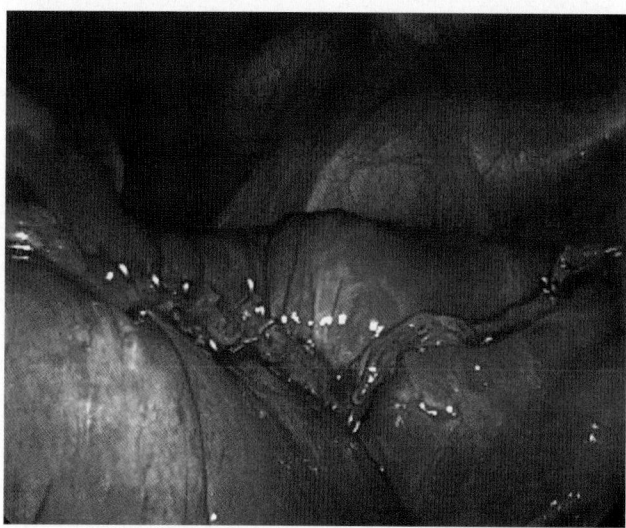

**FIGURE 32-5** Staple line following wedge resection of apical bullae.

may be able to assist in identifying the site of the air leak. It is important to note that bullae may be noted in the lower lobes during 12.5% of VATS procedures and found along the superior edges of the major and minor fissures.

Under direct vision, additional working ports may be placed anterior and posterior to the camera port and triangulated toward the apex. A 12-mm port is necessary to accommodate an Endo-GIA when a stapled wedge resection is to be performed (Fig. 32-5). In smaller children or when a small lesion is recognized, an alternative approach would be placing an endoloop through a much smaller port may also accomplish a similar goal. The suture line is inspected and fibrin glue may be injected over the staple line. Bullectomy with subsequent mechanical and chemical pleurodesis are both associated with acceptable outcomes.

Bialas et al reported that blebectomy plus chemical pleurodesis appears to have less risk of ipsilateral recurrence, but longer postoperative stay and chest drainage. A chemical pleurodesis may be performed as described earlier. The authors prefer an apical mechanical pleurodesis, since one can never be certain of the need to perform a thoracotomy in the future. A bovie scraper or similar abrasive device is inserted through a port site to perform a mechanical pleurodesis on the parietal and visceral pleura (Fig. 32-6). An alternative is to perform an apical pleurectomy. A chest tube is inserted through 1 port site and connected to a Pleur-Evac drainage system. A "U" stitch is placed around the tube site to facilitate tube removal and prevent post-pull pneumothorax.

### Open Thoracotomy

When open thoracotomy is indicated, the routine prep and drape is performed and an incision made over the fourth rib. The latissimus dorsi muscle is incised and the serratus anterior muscle is spared and retracted. The incision is continued through the intercostal muscle and into the chest. When the area of leak is identified, it is resected and treated in a similar fashion as with VATS. A chest tube is brought out through a separate incision, positioned in the apex, and attached to a Pleur-Evac drainage system.

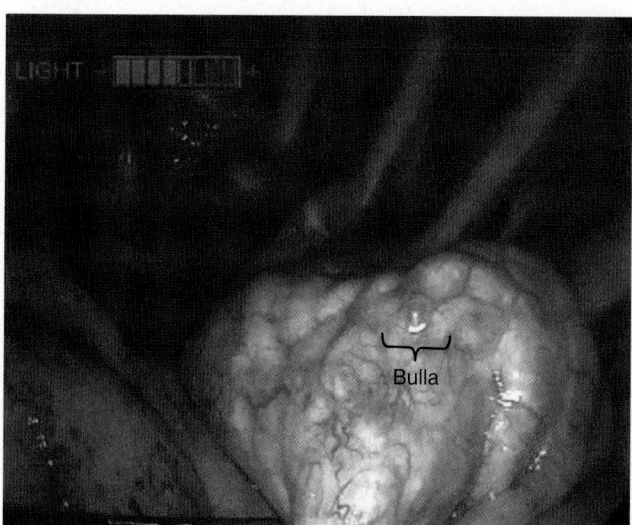

**FIGURE 32-4** Video-assisted thoracoscopic view of an apical bulla.

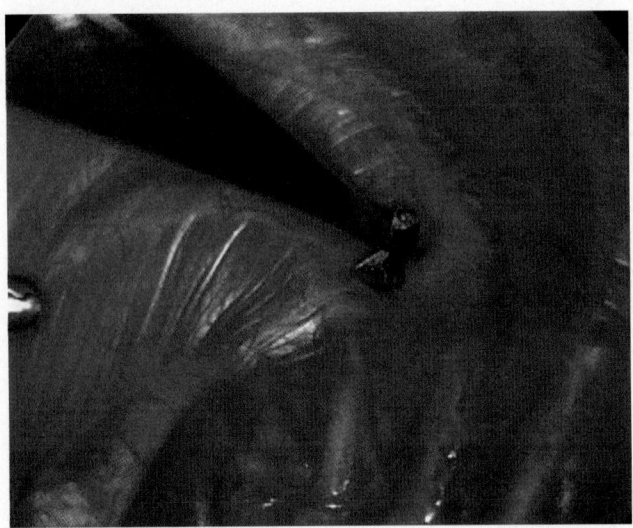

**FIGURE 32-6** Video-assisted thoracoscopic mechanical pleurodesis with a bovie scraper.

# Chylothorax

1. Chylothorax is a potentially life-threatening disorder with respiratory, nutritional, and immunological consequences due to the accumulation of lymphatic fluid in the pleural space.

2. Nontraumatic causes of chylothorax are generally obstructive and associated with congenital abnormalities.

3. Traumatic causes of chylothorax result from thoracic duct rupture or injury with a subsequent lymphatic leak from the duct.

4. Clinical presentation is that of a pleural effusion and includes respiratory compromise, cyanosis, diminished breath sounds, and dullness to percussion on the affected side.

5. A suspected diagnosis of chylothorax is confirmed with cytologic and biochemical analysis of the effusion.

6. The primary modes of treatment include evacuation of the pleural space, use of medium-chain triglycerides (MCT) enteral feeds, or enteric rest with parenteral nutrition.

7. When medical therapy fails surgical management is used.

8. During therapy it is important to prevent significant ongoing chyle loss, if possible, and to treat the potential complications from the ongoing loss of chyle.

## INTRODUCTION

Chylothorax is a potentially life-threatening disorder with respiratory, nutritional, and immunological consequences due to the accumulation of lymphatic fluid in the pleural

space. Therapeutic drainage leads to loss of fluid and nutritional depletion of proteins, lipids, and electrolytes. Lymphocytopenia of T cells leads to immunodeficiency.

Chylothorax was first described by Virchow in 1856. Mortality secondary to chylothorax historically has exceeded 50%, and although much improved, mortality (at approximately 10%) and morbidity remain significant.

## ANATOMY AND PHYSIOLOGY

The lymphatic system transports lipids and lipid-soluble vitamins (A, D, E, and K), collects protein-rich interstitial fluid from the interstitial spaces, and forms an integral part of the immune system by returning lymphocytes into circulation.

Chyle is primarily produced in the intestinal lacteal system. In the mucosal cell, long chain fatty acids (>12 carbon atoms) are esterified into triglycerides and pass into the lymphatic system as chylomicrons. The turbid and milky appearance of chyle is attributed to chylomicrons. The medium-chain fatty acids (<10 carbon atoms) do not become esterified and pass directly into the portal venous blood as free fatty acids bound to albumin.

The thoracic duct transports chyle produced from the intestinal tract to the venous system. It is reported to transport between 1.5 and 2.5 L/day at a rate of 1.4 mL/kg/h and may increase depending on meals and water absorption. The anatomic course of the thoracic duct provides understanding of the etiology and management of chylothorax (Fig. 32-7). Chyle is collected in the cysterna chyli from which the thoracic duct arises at approximately the level of the first to second lumbar vertebrae in the midline. There is a rich collateral network of lymphatics; however, it is usually described as a singular structure. The duct enters the thorax through the aortic hiatus into the posterior mediastinum. It follows a course in the right chest between the aorta and azygous vein and behind the esophagus to the level of

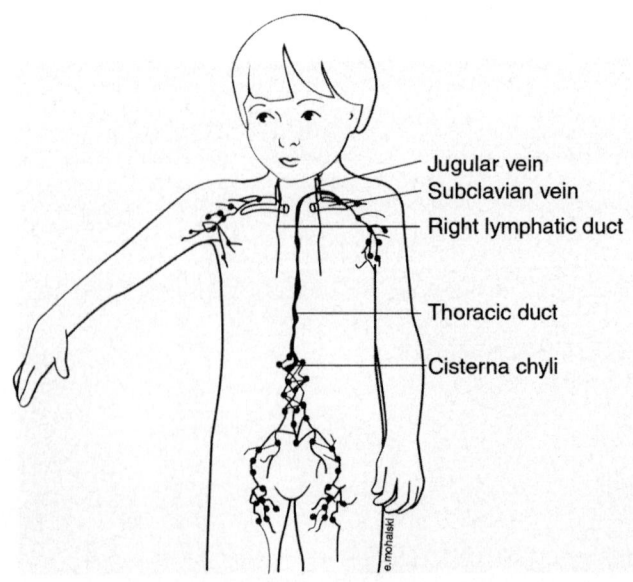

**FIGURE 32-7** Schema of lymphatic drainage.

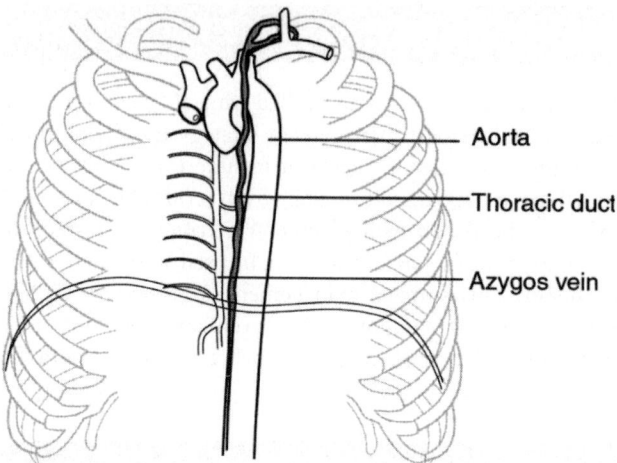

**FIGURE 32-8** Anatomical illustration of the pathway of the thoracic duct.

the fourth to sixth thoracic vertebrae. At this level, the duct crosses to the left mediastinum and travels, extrapleural, behind the aorta along the left subclavian artery into the junction of the left internal jugular vein and subclavian vein (Fig. 32-8). Lymph from the right side of the head, neck, thorax, lung, chest wall, and arm drain into the right lymphatic duct entering the right jugulo-subclavian vein. There may be duplicated ducts with drainage into either the subclavian vein, the jugular vein, or combinations. Variations of this drainage may be the rule. Injury or disruption of the thoracic duct below the fifth thoracic vertebra generally produces a right chylothorax, while injury or disruption of the thoracic duct above the fifth thoracic vertebra generally produces a left chylothorax.

## ETIOLOGY

Nontraumatic causes of chylothorax are generally obstructive and associated with congenital abnormalities. These include generalized lymphatic malformations, atresia, or absence of the thoracic duct. Patients with Turner, Noonan, or Down syndrome may have chylothorax with an associated vascular or lymphatic malformation. Obstruction of thoracic duct drainage may also arise from malignancies, inflammation, fibrosis, infections, and superior vena cava thrombosis.

Traumatic causes result from thoracic duct rupture or injury with a subsequent lymphatic leak from the duct. This may be due to hyperextension of the vertebral column during exercise or birth, penetrating trauma, central line placement, or situations where increased thoracic pressure results in thoracic duct disruption. The most common cause of a chylothorax in a tertiary pediatric hospital is postcardiac surgery with direct injury to the thoracic duct, central venous thrombosis, and/or high venous pressure. With an increase in the performance of complex cardiothoracic procedures in children, the incidence of chylothorax has increased from between 0.9% and 1.5% to upward of 6.6%.

## PRESENTATION AND DIAGNOSIS

Clinical presentation is that of a pleural effusion. Patients may present with respiratory compromise, cyanosis, diminished breath sounds, and dullness to percussion on the affected side. A chylothorax is the most common cause of pleural effusion in the first few days of life; however, other causes need to be excluded. Chylothorax also should be suspected when there is an extensive pleural effusion following cardiothoracic or mediastinal surgery. A chest radiograph reveals haziness of the affected side with blunting of the costovertebral angles (Fig. 32-9). Layering of the free fluid may be appreciated on lateral decubitus view and ultrasound may assist in discriminating an effusion from parenchymal consolidation and loculated empyemas. Lymphoscintagraphy, via subcutaneous or intradermal injection, and lymphangiography, via direct injection into a lymphatic vessel, are 2 specific lymphatic imaging modalities. Filtered 99m-technium is the most common radionuclide used. There are, however, significant limitations for its use in children due to pain and difficulty in cannulation of a lymphatic vessel. A CT scan may assist in defining lymphatic and vascular anatomy and abnormalities.

Ultimately, diagnosis is established with cytologic and biochemical analysis of the effusion (Table 32-1). Characteristically, the fluid is described as milky-white in appearance

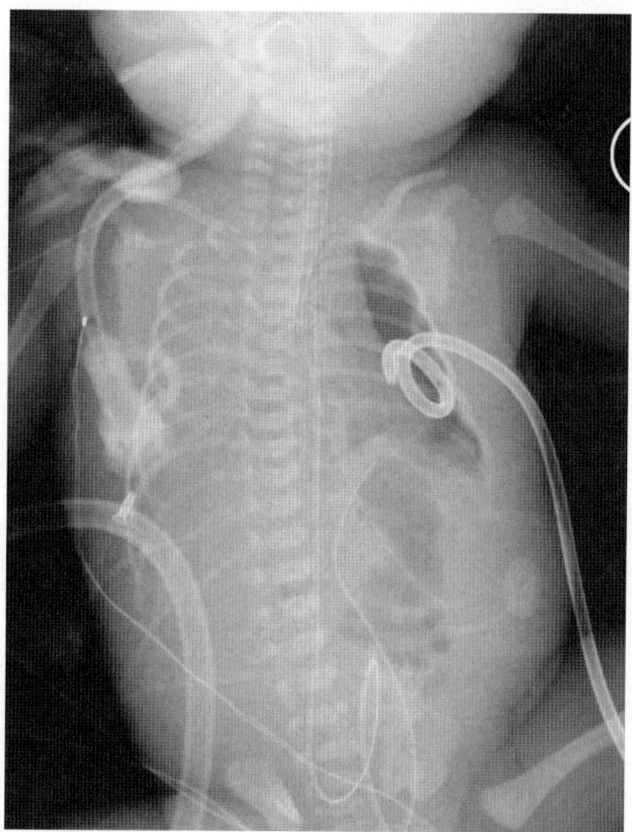

**FIGURE 32-9** Chest radiograph of an infant with bilateral chylothorax. The left chest is drained with a pig-tailed catheter.

| TABLE 32-1 | Diagnostic Characteristics of Chyle |
|---|---|
| pH | 7.4-7.8 |
| Milky or turbid appearance<br>▸ Enterally fed patient<br>▸ Presence of chylomicrons | + Sudan III test |
| Sterile | |
| Bacteriostatic | |
| Triglyceride level | >1.1 mmol/L, >100 mg/dL |
| Absolute cell count<br>▸ Lymphocyte predominant | >1000 cells/μL<br>>70%-80% |

in a nonfasting patient. This is attributed to the presence of long-chain fatty acids transported by chylomicrons that stain with Sudan III. The fluid is sterile, does not clot, and is bacteriostatic. The triglyceride and protein content is elevated in relationship to serum. The diagnosis of a pseudochylothorax is made when there is a high presence of cholesterol and the absence of triglycerides or chylomicrons. Cellular analyses reveal an absolute cell count >1000 cells/μL with a lymphocyte fraction greater than 70% to 80%.

## MANAGEMENT

There are no randomized controlled clinical trials to provide evidence for the best management strategy for chylothorax. The primary modes of treatment include evacuation of the pleural space, use of medium-chain triglyceride (MCT) enteral feeds, or enteric rest with parenteral nutrition. In refractory cases octreotide or somatostatin can be used, and when medical therapy fails surgical management is used (Fig. 32-10). During therapy, it is important to prevent and treat the potential complications from the loss of chyle due to chylothorax.

## MEDICAL MANAGEMENT

The use of enteral low-fat or MCT feeds is based on the theory that enterocytes directly absorb the medium-chain fatty acids into the circulation, thus reducing flow through the thoracic duct and allowing spontaneous healing. Enteral feeding with MCT provides nutritional support while maintaining gut-barrier protection. In a large series, 71% of children with postoperative chylothorax had complete resolution of their drainage with changes to enteral nutrition only. If the chylous drainage persists and does not improve, the therapy may be to exclude all enteral feeding and provide nutrition

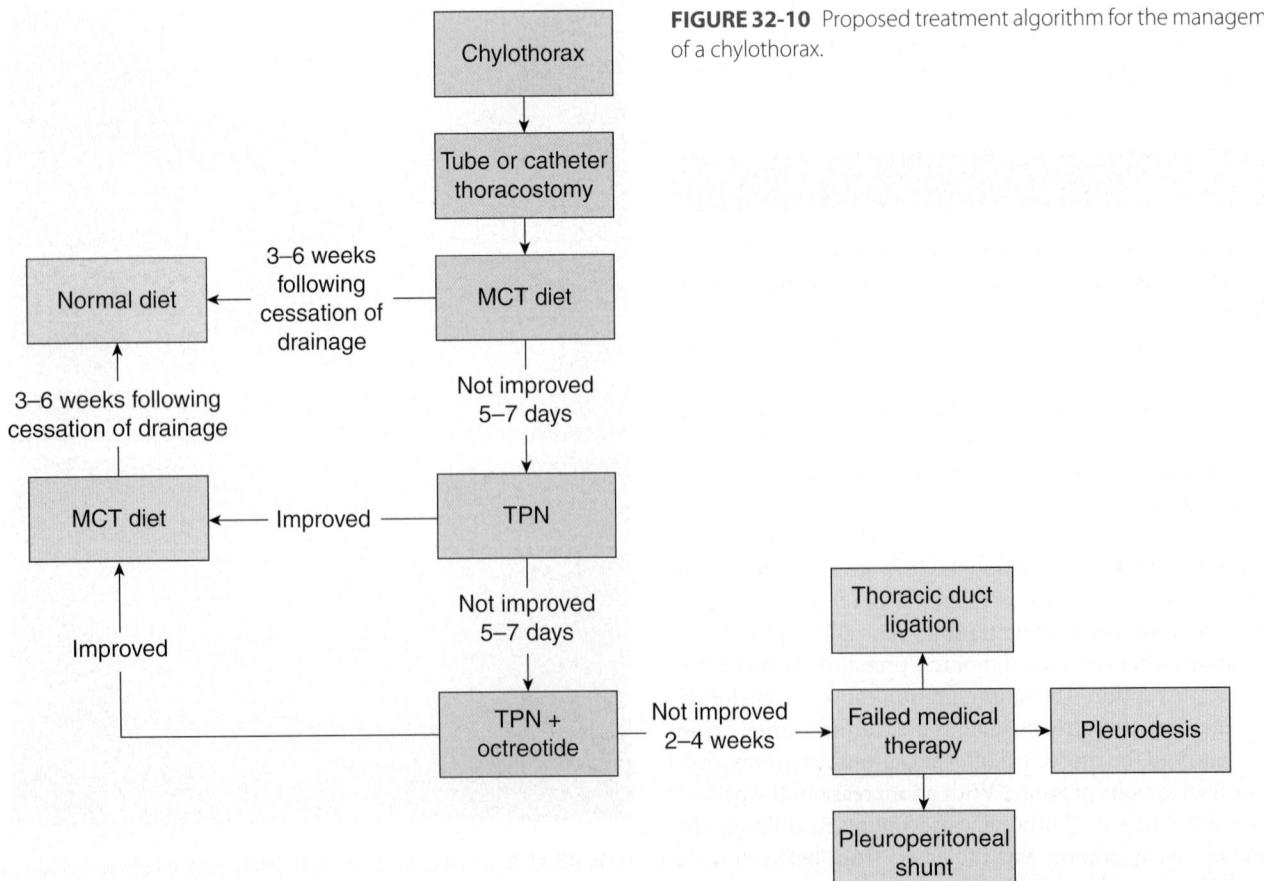

**FIGURE 32-10** Proposed treatment algorithm for the management of a chylothorax.

parenterally. Adjuvant therapy may be necessary, including antithrombotic cardiac medication that lowers central venous pressure, albumin, electrolytes repletion, and the addition of lipid-soluble vitamins and essential fatty acids (omega 3 and omega 6). Patients with chylothorax have been treated with intravenous immunoglobulin (IVIG) to maintain IgG levels in the normal range. The clinical benefit is unclear.

Somatostatin and its synthetic analog, octreotide, have been successfully used in the management of chylothorax. The mechanism of action is not clearly understood, but it is hypothesized that these agents may reduce leak via contraction of the lymphatic vessel or reduction of intestinal blood flow. There may also be somatostatin receptors on lymphatic vessels that respond by reducing lymphatic production or triglyceride absorption from the gut. The recommended continuous dosage is titrated in a stepwise fashion from 0.5 µg/kg/h to 10-15 µg/kg/h. In patients with limited IV access, a dosage of 5 µg/kg/dose every 8 hours is increased every 24 hours by 5 µg/kg/dose, to a maximum of 40 µg/kg/day. Potential complications include cutaneous flushing, abdominal distension, hypothyroidism, hypo/hyperglycemia, liver impairment, renal dysfunction, ileus, and necrotizing enterocolitis.

Success has been reported with the use of corticosteroids in postoperative patients and in medical conditions such as Noonan syndrome and Behcet disease. The presence of venous thrombosis may require anticoagulation, thrombolytic therapy, or intervention to remove the obstruction. Patients with high central venous pressure or right atrial failure may require agents to lower this pressure and improve diastolic function. There are case reports of successful management of chylothorax with nitric oxide, high positive-end expiratory pressure ventilation, and Etilefrine, a sympathomimetic drug that causes smooth muscle contraction.

The literature includes varying definitions of what constitutes improvement of a chylothorax and how long a mode of therapy should be attempted. Some define improvement as drainage that is <2 mL/kg/day, while others specify <5 mL/kg/day. Many authors base their therapeutic approach on 10 mL/kg/day for improvement and >10 mL/kg/day as failure. Most series performed in children recommend attempting medical management for 2 to 4 weeks before a surgical procedure is considered. Nonoperative management of chylothorax in children appears to be successful in more than 80% of reported cases.

## SURGICAL MANAGEMENT

Timing of surgery is not well defined. Some advocate that persistence of an effusion for more than 2 weeks or drainage >100 mL/year of age/day indicates failure of medical therapy and need for surgery. Patients with elevated central venous pressure, thrombosis, or a cavopulmonary anastomosis may fail medical management and require more aggressive therapy sooner.

Chemical pleurodesis has been described as a treatment of choice. Many agents have been described, including the use of fibrin glue, talc, bleomycin, OK 432, doxycycline, and povidone-iodine. These agents may be instilled through a chest tube or with the assistance of VATS.

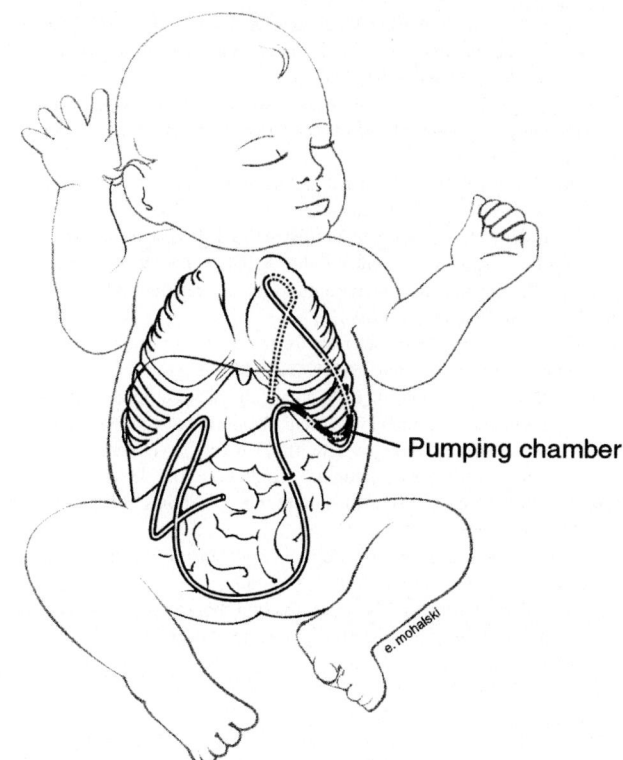

**FIGURE 32-11** Position of the pleuroperitoneal shunt.

Mechanical pleurodesis and thoracic duct ligation may be performed via open thoracotomy or via VATS. The site of disruption may be identified with lymphoscintigraphy or lymphangiography. The use of 1% Evans blue dye subcutaneously in the thigh or enterally fed milk/cream prior to surgical intervention may also assist in identifying the site of rupture, which allows for direct surgical ligation of the leak. If the site of rupture cannot be identified, mass ligation or identification of the thoracic duct proximal to the disruption is necessary. The inferior pulmonary ligament is divided in the right thorax and the thoracic duct is identified as it enters the chest between the aorta and azygous vein just posterior to the esophagus.

Pleuroperitoneal shunts have been used in the management of chylothorax (Fig. 32-11). These shunts are useful in patients who cannot tolerate a major procedure or when thoracotomy or pleurodesis is contraindicated. The shunts have a pump and 1-way valve that move chyle from the pleural space into the abdomen to be absorbed by the peritoneum. This technique may have the advantage of limiting nutritional and fluid losses. The presence of vena cava thrombosis or instances of elevated central venous pressure may limit the effectiveness of these shunts. They are prone to clotting, are labor-intensive, and initially require frequent pumping. The pump may be exteriorized to facilitate pumping and for added patient comfort.

## SELECTED READINGS

### Pneumothorax

Baumann MH, Strange C. Treatment of spontaneous pneumothorax: a more aggressive approach? *Chest* 1997;112:789–804.
Bertrand PC, Regnard JF, Spaggiari L, et al. Immediate and long term results after surgical treatment of primary spontaneous pneumothorax by VATS. *Ann Thorac Surg* 1996;61:164–165.

Bialas R, Weiner TM, Phillips JD. Video-assisted thoracic surgery for primary spontaneous pneumothorax in children: is there an optimal technique? *J Pediatr Surg* 2008;43:2151–2155.

Chung P, Wong K, Lan L, et al. Thoracoscopic bullectomy for primary spontaneous pneumothorax in pediatric patients. *Pediatr Surg Int* 2009;25:763–766.

Delius RE, Obeid FN, Horst M, et al. Catheter aspiration for simple pneumothorax. *Arch Surg* 1989;124:833–836.

Gossot D, Galetta D, Stern JB, et al. Results of thoracoscopic pleural abrasion for primary spontaneous pneumothorax. *Surg Endosc* 2004;18:466–471.

Kjaergaard H. Spontaneous pneumothorax in the apparently health. *Acta Med Scand* 1932;(suppl 43):1–159.

Light RW, Vargas FS. Pleural sclerosis for the treatment of pneumothorax and pleural effusion. *Lung* 1997;175:213–223.

O'Lone E, Elphick HE, Robinson PJ. Spontaneous pneumothorax in children: when is invasive treatment indicated? *Pediatr Pulmonol* 2008;43:41–46.

Ozcan C, McGahren ED, Rodgers BM. Thoracoscopic treatment of spontaneous pneumothorax in children. *J Pediatr Surg* 2003;38:1459–1464.

Paape K, Fry WA. Spontaneous pneumothorax. *Chest Surg Clin North Am* 1994;4:517–538.

Poenaru D, Yazbeck S, Murphy S. Primary spontaneous pneumothorax in children. *J Pediatr Surg* 1994;29:1183–1185.

Waller DA, Forty J, Morritt GN. Video-assisted thoracoscopic surgery versus thoracotomy for spontaneous pneumothorax. *Ann Thorac Surg* 1994;58:372–377.

## Chylothorax

Allen EM, van Heeckeren DW, Spector ML, et al. Management of nutritional and infectious complications of postoperative chylothorax in children. *J Pediatr Surg* 1991;26:1169–1174.

Azizkhan RG, Canfield J, Alford BA, et al. Pleuroperitoneal shunts in the management of neonatal chylothorax. *J Pediatr Surg* 1983;18:842–850.

Beghetti M, La Scala G, Belli D, et al. Etiology and management of pediatric chylothorax. *J Pediatr* 2000;136:653–658.

Buttiker V, Fanconi S, Burger R. Chylothorax in children: guidelines for diagnosis and management. *Chest* 1999;116:682–687.

Chan EH, Russell JL, Williams WG, et al. Postoperative chylothorax after cardiothoracic surgery in children. *Ann Thorac Surg* 2005;80:1864–1871.

Christodoulou M, Ris HB, Pezzetta E. Video-assisted right supradiaphragmatic thoracic duct ligation for non-traumatic recurrent chylothorax. *Eur J Cardiothorac Surg* 2006;29:810–814.

Cummings SP, Wyatt DA, Baker JW, et al. Successful treatment of postoperative chylothorax using an external pleuroperitoneal shunt. *Ann Thorac Surg* 1992;54:276–278.

Epaud R, Dubern B, Larroquet M, et al. Therapeutic strategies for idiopathic chylothorax. *J Pediatr Surg* 2008;43:461–465.

Graham DD, McGahren ED, Tribble CG, et al. Use of video-assisted thoracic surgery in the treatment of chylothorax. *Ann Thorac Surg* 1994;57:1507–1512.

Kosloske AM, Martin LW, Schubert WK. Management of chylothorax in children by thoracentesis and medium-chain triglyceride feedings. *J Pediatr Surg* 1974;9:365–371.

Le Coultre C, Oberhansli I, Mossaz A, et al. Posoperative chylothorax in children: differences between vascular and traumatic origin. *J Pediatr Surg* 1991;26:519–523.

Marts BC, Naunheim KS, Fiore AC, et al. Conservative versus surgical management of chylothorax. *Am J Surg* 1992;164:532–535.

Panthongviriyakul C, Bines J. Post-operative chylothorax in children: an evidence-based management algorithm. *J Pediatr Child Health* 2008;44:716–721.

Rheuban KS, Kron IL, Carpenter MA, et al. Pleuroperitoneal shunts for refractory chylothorax after operation for congenital heart disease. *Ann Thorac Surg* 1992;53:85–87.

Soto-Martinez M, Massie J. Chylothorax: diagnosis and management in children. *Pediatr Resp Rev* 2009;10:199–207.

# CHAPTER 33

# Diaphragmatic Hernias and Eventration

*Thomas Tracy Jr and Francois I. Luks*

## KEY POINTS

1. The 2 most critical elements of congenital diaphragmatic hernia (CDH) are pulmonary hypertension and hypoplasia.

2. While a diagnosis of diaphragmatic hernia is theoretically possible from the 12th week on, in reality, the earliest CDH can be detected with current ultrasonographic equipment is 14 to 15 weeks, or late in the first and early in the second trimester.

3. Left-sided CDH is found in 80% to 85% of cases; right-sided defects in 10% to 15% of patients in different series. Rarely are the defects bilateral.

4. Most infants with a diaphragmatic hernia will present at birth or shortly after with varying degrees of respiratory distress.

5. Antenatal intervention for severe CDH is an appropriate therapeutic option in very few patients.

6. The first line of treatment of a newborn with suspected or documented diaphragmatic hernia is respiratory support.

7. The key to a successful CDH repair rests in the security of the sutures and the freedom from tension on the repair.

8. Innovative approaches to endoscopic and even laparoscopic efforts at repair now are considered routine for 25% to 45% of newborns with CDH.

9. For infants in immediate distress in the delivery room or intensive care unit, extracorporeal membrane oxygenation (ECMO) may be lifesaving and is considered by many as mandatory for supporting infants with CDH and in managing high-risk deliveries of fetuses with known CDH.

10. Major institutions in the United States have reported survival outcomes for patients with CDH that range from 70% to 85%.

11. For patients with diaphragmatic herniation through the foramen of Morgagni, operative reduction and repair is generally easily accomplished through the abdomen using open or minimally invasive techniques.

12. Traumatic hernias may be repaired through an abdominal approach during exploration following blunt or penetrating trauma. If recognition of the trauma has been delayed, a transthoracic incision or thoracoscopic approach might be preferable.

13. Congenital or acquired abnormalities of the diaphragm and phrenic nerve can lead to unilateral or bilateral diaphragmatic eventration that can be repaired through abdominal and thoracic open approaches and minimally invasive surgery.

## INTRODUCTION

The 2 most critical elements of congenital diaphragmatic hernia (CDH) are pulmonary hypertension and hypoplasia. Pulmonary hypertension was first demonstrated in CDH patients in 1971 by Rowe and Uribe. The associated morphologic finding of increased arteriolar muscularization is the foundation for the persistent pulmonary hypertension of the newborn (PPHN), leading to persistent fetal circulation (PFC). Morphometric examinations of the lungs of infants who have died with CDH, as well as of experimental animals with CDH, demonstrate uniform loss of pulmonary mass and decreased bronchial branching as well as alveolar:arteriolar ratios. Pulmonary hypoplasia resulting from the arrest of alveolar development at the midcanalicular stage is a central factor in mortality, long-term morbidity, and restrictions on the quality of outcomes with CDH.

The present and future medical and surgical management of CDH has been one of the central focal points of pediatric surgery for the past 25 years. Several large and small animal models of CDH have been developed to yield extensive information about significant alterations in fetal physiology that accompany CDH in utero. These models have been central to the identification of specific defects in the disordered lung architecture and function that result from absent or abnormal fetal diaphragmatic development. These models have also served as the foundation for the first attempts at surgical intervention and pharmacologic modulation of CDH in utero.

This period of research and discovery about CDH has yielded many widely accepted clinical best practices. Continuing studies are looking at several approaches, including fetal interventions and postnatal pulmonary growth augmentation. Inconsistent outcomes and the disparity of outcomes in different centers and nations are realities that must be addressed.

## CLASSIFICATION

Diaphragmatic hernias are categorized by the location of herniation or by their etiology. The 4 classes are:

1. Posterolateral hernias through the foramen of Bochdalek
2. Anterior subcostal hernias through the foramen of Morgagni
3. Central, paraesophageal hernias
4. Acquired traumatic hernias

## EMBRYOLOGY

Embryologic hypotheses for CDH remain focused on the formation of the diaphragm, which takes place during the fourth through the eighth weeks of gestation. The completed diaphragm is derived from the following essential fetal components: (1) the septum transversum, which forms the central tendon; (2) bilateral pleuroperitoneal membranes or folds that are reinforced by striated muscle components; and (3) the mesentery of the esophagus that forms crural and dorsal structures. Long-standing hypotheses propose that incomplete or absent fusion of the pleuroperitoneal folds is responsible for the posterolateral diaphragmatic defect and subsequent development or migration of the liver, spleen, stomach, and variable lengths of intestine in the hemithorax.

The embryologic sequence of events through the 4-week period of diaphragmatic development begins with formation of the septum transversum as mesoderm between the developing heart and liver. Its fusion ventrally leaves bilateral pleuroperitoneal canals that result from the remaining posterolateral defects. It has been assumed that the early fusion of the septum transversum ventrally and the large posterolateral defects is necessary for lung development. Lung expansion burrows into the surrounding mesenchyme to form bilateral folds that subsequently fuse with septum transversum to form the pleuroperitoneal membrane. Myoblasts and eventually associated nerves from cervical segments penetrate these membranes to form the neuromuscular component. Final diaphragmatic formation and remodeling requires that the esophageal mesentery contributes to the development of the crura as the most dorsal portion of the diaphragm.

Failures of these boundary structures have been the focus of most theories of CDH. Alternatively, it is interesting to speculate on what would happen to the diaphragmatic development process if the lungs failed to develop. This same question has been recently posed in teratogenic experiments using nitrofen to induce primary pulmonary hypoplasia. The resultant diaphragmatic defect duplicates the posterolateral defects seen with CDH. The mechanism for either nitrofen-induced hypoplasia or the formation of defects may result from a disturbance in the retinoic acid pathway inferred from vitamin A deficiency and CDH formation in rats. A decreased incidence of CDH has been found for vitamin A-supplemented, nitrofen-treated animals. No human corollary for retinoic acid deficiencies or receptor expression has been found.

In a similar fashion, some embryologists have proposed that failure of myoblast migration from cervical segments 3, 4, and 5 may be a contributing factor to diaphragmatic agenesis, leaving the unmuscularized membrane as the "sac" that is occasionally seen. In either case, a total failure of the development of the lung cavity does not adequately explain agenesis of the diaphragm.

The formation of a diaphragmatic defect in the 9th or 10th week will easily allow transit of abdominal organs into the chest. The intestinal contents are returning to the abdomen at this stage of development. An intriguing area of study is the identification of the signals responsible for malposition of the liver or the relative cardiac hypoplasia that can occur with both small and large defects, even with adequate fusion of the septum transversum between the heart and liver. Genetic studies have identified that genes essential for organ development such as Sonic Hedgehog (Shh), Gli2, Gli3, Wt1, platelet-derived growth factor receptor $\alpha$, Fog2, Gata4, and Gata6, are all candidates whose expression or mutation have demonstrated effects on heart, lung, and diaphragmatic development. Wt1 null mice, Gli2-, and Gli3-null mice demonstrate specific diaphragmatic defects. A finding in one study of pulmonary hypoplasia with or without a CDH linked to a mutation in Fog2, led to several major proposals to utilize high throughput analysis based on mutagenesis. The magnitude of interest in genetic studies to understand the genotypic and phenotypic manifestation of CDH is evidenced by the formation of more than 23 mouse knockout models and the identification of approximately 50 known genes associated with pulmonary or diaphragmatic development or defects. New subgenomic sequencing will play a pivotal role in determining the significance of these genes in multipatient analysis.

Embryologic interactions between the components of diaphragmatic development and the cellular and molecular processes of pulmonary parenchymal growth are likely to occur at many levels and gestational time points. Understanding the fetal development of the lung in conjunction with diaphragmatic defects is essential as a foundation for any attempts at early or late fetal intervention. The roles and mechanisms of growth factors such as epimorphin as it contributes to bronchial branching must be defined along with epithelial scatter factors and their receptors. These and other signals and signaling mechanisms may offer the earliest targets for embryologic and fetal intervention for the growing number of investigators focused on abnormal lung development as the inciting factor or the result of CDH.

The ontogeny and differentiation of important pulmonary parenchymal cell populations, such as type II pneumocytes and stretch sensitive pulmonary fibroblasts, will need to be defined to further understand qualitative and quantitative alterations that have been demonstrated in surfactant and matrix proteins experimentally and postnatally. Late gestational amniotic fluid and fetal lung fluid contribute to the induced parenchymal cellular proliferation found after fetal bronchial ligation in vivo and in similarly obstructed in vitro lung explants. This growth occurs without excessive sustained fluid-dependent increases in intrabronchial luminal pressure. There have been no extraordinary increases observed in currently identified growth factors following tracheal occlusion. Promoters for stretch-dependent cell cycle gene transcription and proliferation have been described in the pulmonary and vascular systems. They may be the basis for observed growth of lungs with fetal tracheal obstruction, as well as observed postnatal compensatory growth with density-dependent distention of hypoplastic lungs of infants with CDH.

Embryologically associated anomalies have been defined through fetal and postnatal autopsy series. A more dynamic understanding of the associated defects has been gleaned from intensive fetal screening and ultrasonography. The incidence of associated defects ranges from 20% to nearly 60%, depending on whether it is based on autopsy or ultrasound data. Karyotypic abnormalities are usually trisomy 13 or trisomy 18. The majority of neural defects include anencephaly, encephalocele, hydrocephalus, and myelomeningocele. The majority of nonneural tube defects are commonly found in the cardiovascular system as ventricular septal defects, vascular rings, and congenital aortic coarctation. Associated extralobar pulmonary sequestrations have been described, as has esophageal atresia and omphalocele. More recently reported is foregut dysmotility far beyond what would be associated with long-standing esophagogastric compression and obstruction. Embryologic connections between CDH defects and the neuromuscular changes in the esophagus and the stomach have not yet been as clearly defined. Critical tracheomalacia associated with structurally abnormal tracheal cartilage has been problematic for survivors following protracted and intensive newborn treatment for severe CDH.

## BOCHDALEK HERNIAS

### History of Surgical Management and Operative Repair

Perhaps the most notable historical event for operative management of diaphragmatic hernia was the success of delayed operative repair that followed the prolonged survival of infants and children who surprisingly escaped without any apparent respiratory compromise. In the original reports by Gross and Ladd in 1934, only the fittest to survive arrived for surgical consideration. Excellent operative results were reported and their textbooks gave directions for management designed to achieve greater than 90% survival in those infants and children who were fortunate to make it beyond the newborn period. Over 7 decades later, the best current series show that in some centers we have achieved up to 90% survival for all infants. The main milestones along the way and their published contributors are listed in Table 33-1.

The "age of enlightenment" that followed the accomplishments of Ladd and Gross can be roughly divided into the following periods:

1. Immediate operation and attempted repair

2. Immediate operation followed by extracorporeal membrane oxygenation (ECMO)

3. Delayed operation after ventilatory or ECMO stabilization

4. Fetal intervention

| TABLE 33-1 | The History of Congenital Diaphragmatic Hernia | |
| --- | --- | --- |
| Year | Author | Milestone |
| 1754 | McCauley | First anatomic description of CDH from postmortem |
| 1848 | Bochdalek | Defined posterolateral defect responsible for hernia |
| 1888 | Nauman | First unsuccessful surgical attempts at repair |
| 1901 | Aue | First successful adult repair |
| 1931 | Hedblom | 75% of patients died before the end of the first month |
| 1940 | Ladd and Gross | 31 repairs in the first year of life reviewed with 17 survivors; 9 of 16 survive CDH in Boston Children's series |
| 1946 | Gross | First reported survival of infant less than 24 hours old |
| 1953 | Gross | Immediate operation will yield 95% survival |

*(Continued)*

| TABLE 33-1 | The History of Congenital Diaphragmatic Hernia *(Continued)* | |
| --- | --- | --- |
| **Year** | **Author** | **Milestone** |
| 1960s | | First newborn mechanical ventilators |
| 1971 | Rowe and Uribe | Persistent pulmonary hypertension associated with CDH |
| 1977 | Collins | Description of the "honeymoon period" |
| 1977 | German | First report of support of CDH with ECMO following successful use for cardiopulmonary support in infants (1971, White; 1976, Bartlett) |
| 1984 | Reynolds | Era of emergent repair reviewed and reevaluated |
| 1984 | Hazebroek | First efforts at preoperative stabilization and emergent surgery questioned (1984, Langer) |
| 1986 | ELSO | ELSO–ECMO registry formed and the search for predictors of survival begins (Adzick, Bohn, Bartlett, Krummel, Stolar, Bailey, Tracy) |
| 1986 | Sawyer | First institutional improvements with ECMO (1987, Weber) |
| 1987 | Langham | First registry review of 93 CDH infants treated with ECMO for assumed >95% mortality finding 42% survival |
| 1990 | Connors | First report of repairs during ECMO stabilization |
| 1990 | Harrison | First report of successful in utero repair; followed by clinical trials with dismal results reported in 1993 and prospective trial completed without benefit in 1997 |
| 1992 | Glick | First experimental evidence of surfactant deficiency and clinical application |
| 1992 | Kinsella | Nitric oxide administered for pulmonary hypertension to newborns with no effect (reported in 1997) |
| 1993 | Wilson | First experimental fetal tracheal obstruction reverses hypoplasia |
| 1994 | Wilson | Antenatal diagnosis not predictive |
| 1994 | Van Meurs | First patient to receive a lobar lung transplant for CDH |
| 1995 | Sigalet | First trial of high frequency oscillatory ventilation; without subsequent benefit in multicenter trial (1997, Kinsella) |
| 1995 | Hirschl | First use of perfluorochemical liquid ventilation in CDH |
| 1995 | Wung and Stolar | Permissive hypercapnia, low pressure ventilation and delayed surgery |
| 1996 | | The first multi-institutional and multidisciplinary CDH registry is formed with its first report (Lally) delivered 1997 |
| 1998 | Harrison and Adzick | First clinical experience with fetal tracheal ligation reported |
| 1999 | Kays | Detrimental effects of standard medical therapy in congenital diaphragmatic hernia described; approach 90% survival for inborn patients |
| 2000 | Adzick | Fetal tracheal occlusion results in 33% survival with 15 patients |
| 2001 | Stolar | 76% survival for 120 patients with postnatal diagnosis |
| 2001-2005 | | First demonstrations and series of thoracoscopic repairs |
| 2009 | Lansdale | Endoscopic repair of CDH has greater recurrence rates and operative times but similar survival and patch usage compared with open surgery |

ECMO, extracorporeal membrane oxygenation; ELSO, Extracorporeal Life Support Organization.

## Presentation and Diagnosis

### Antenatal

The diaphragm is completely formed by 10 to 11 weeks of gestation (Fig. 33-1). A diagnosis of diaphragmatic hernia is therefore theoretically possible from the 12th week on. In reality, the earliest CDH can be detected with current ultrasonographic equipment is 14 to 15 weeks, or late in the first and early in the second trimester. At that gestational age, the diagnosis is based on the presence of cystic or heterogeneous ultrasound shadows in the fetal thorax. Even with optimal resolution, the differential diagnosis includes any space-occupying lesion in the chest, such as cystic adenomatoid malformation (CCAM), sequestration, or foregut duplication. By 18 weeks, the diaphragm can often be seen as an uninterrupted hypoechoic line, separating thorax and abdomen. The combination of heterogeneous echoes in the thoracic cavity and the inability to visualize the entire diaphragm on the ipsilateral side is suggestive of a diaphragmatic hernia. Left-sided CDH is found in 80% to 85% of cases; right-sided defects in 10% to 15% of patients in different series. Rarely are the defects bilateral.

A diagnosis of diaphragmatic hernia before 24 to 25 weeks of gestation has been linked to a poor prognosis in several series. While it appears logical that long-standing herniation would be particularly detrimental to pulmonary development, other intrathoracic processes, such as CCAM, are not always associated with pulmonary hypoplasia, even if the lesion is present early in the second trimester. This lends some credence to the possibility of primary fetal pulmonary hypoplasia as the cause rather than the result of CDH. Conversely, a late diagnosis of diaphragmatic hernia does not rule out early onset of the condition. Therefore, neither gestational age at diagnosis, nor any of the other criteria of severity currently in use is infallible in predicting outcome of children with diaphragmatic hernia.

Other diagnostic criteria, in addition to direct sonographic visualization of the diaphragmatic hernia and herniated intestinal loops, include the presence of the gastric bubble above the diaphragm (Fig. 33-2). This is observed in the same transverse plane as the 4-chamber cardiac view. Additionally, an abdominal circumference far below the normal for gestational age suggests that a large portion of the abdominal viscera (including the liver) have herniated into the chest. The latter criteria are helpful in differentiating a diaphragmatic hernia from isolated intrathoracic lesions. Mediastinal shift (to the right in a left-sided hernia) and displacement of the heart can often be seen as well, but are

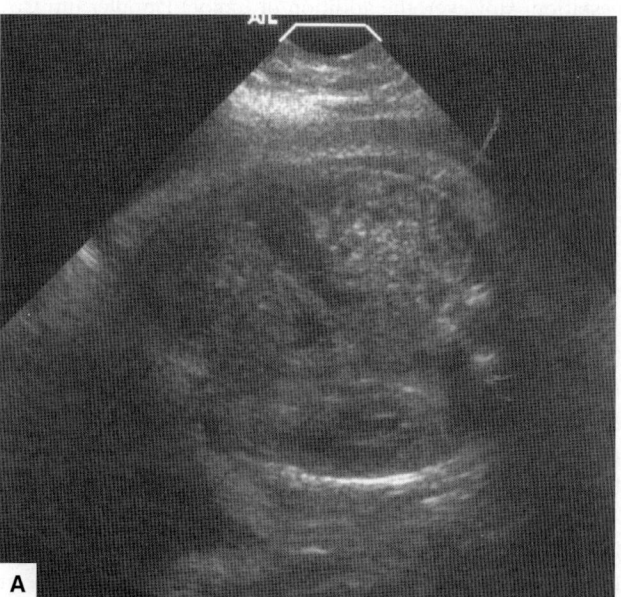

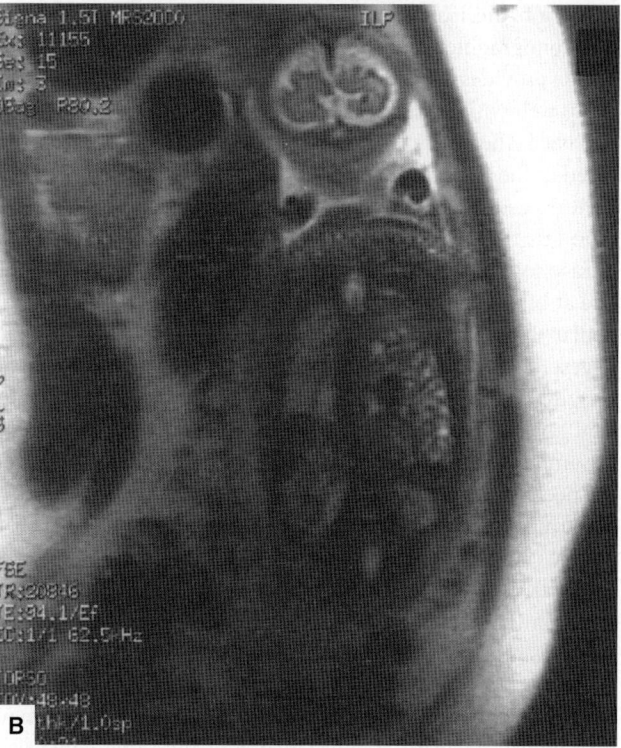

**FIGURE 33-2** Fetal ultrasound (A) and MRI depicting (B) a left diaphragmatic hernia in utero with liver, bowel, and stomach in the left chest.

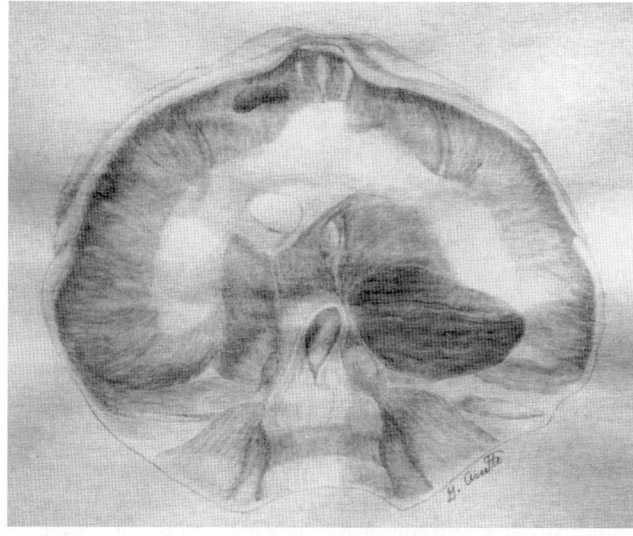

**FIGURE 33-1** Embryologic anatomy of the diaphragm. A posterolateral defect provides the basis for a foramen of Bochdalek hernia. An anterior paramedian defect provides the basis for a foramen of Morgagni hernia.

common to any intrathoracic space-occupying lesion, including CCAM. Extreme mediastinal shift may be associated with fetal hydrops. This occurs presumably by compression of the inferior vena cava and impairment of venous return, causing heart failure in the fetus. While this is a known complication of a CCAM, it is highly unusual for a fetus with diaphragmatic hernia to become hydropic.

In severe forms of diaphragmatic hernia, the liver is partially intrathoracic. This may be suggested antenatally by a smaller than expected abdominal circumference, or more directly by visualizing its location above the diaphragm. Practically, this is difficult to do by plain ultrasonography, as the lungs have an echodensity similar to that of the liver in early gestation. However, the addition of (color) Doppler ultrasonography may demonstrate flow through the ductus venosus and the junction with the vena cava and the right atrium. An abnormally long and tortuous ductus, with a course toward the left of the midline and reaching the level of the heart, is suggestive of intrathoracic herniation of the left lobe of the liver.

Polyhydramnios is a common, very nonspecific sign of severe diaphragmatic hernia. The presumed mechanism for this is kinking and obstruction of the upper gastrointestinal tract (esophagogastric junction and/or gastric outlet) caused by herniation of the stomach into the chest cavity. The fetus is thus unable to swallow the amniotic fluid, which interrupts the normal cycle of amniotic fluid secretion/excretion and reabsorption. Polyhydramnios usually presents late in fetal life, and is considered an ominous sign.

By the 18th week, lung tissue can normally be identified by ultrasonography. In diaphragmatic hernia, as well as with other intrathoracic processes, the amount of lung tissue seen may be dramatically reduced, and in severe forms, totally absent on the ipsilateral side. In the plane of a 4-chamber ultrasonographic view, the lung-to-head circumference ratio (LHR) provides a reproducible parameter that appears to correlate well with severity and survival. The best predictor for survival is the ratio of the right lung 2-dimensional area, measured at the level of the right atrium, to head circumference. LHR exceeding 1.5 correlates with 100% survival, whereas a ratio less than 0.6 is uniformly fatal. Early second trimester ultrasonography is notoriously inaccurate in predicting lung size at birth, and regressing thoracic lesions (CCAM in particular) have allowed seemingly absent lungs to develop later in gestation. Recently, the use of ultrafast magnetic resonance imaging (MRI) has been described to accurately visualize the fetal lungs, and this modality may prove useful in predicting the amount of pulmonary hypoplasia at birth, and, therefore, the need for antenatal intervention.

Cardiac anomalies have been described in up to 10% of patients with diaphragmatic hernia. A contralateral shift of the heart is seen in the 4-chamber view, along with a rotational shift of the pulmonary artery and the pulmonary veins, if they can be visualized. Left-sided CDH is characterized by left ventricular hypoplasia. Although the etiology of this is not clear, direct compression by the herniated viscera may be a culprit or again, a consequence of the same constellation of potential genetic alterations. This situation can be reproduced in both surgical and teratogenic animal models of CDH. The dual hit hypothesis may apply, similar to that offered for pulmonary hypoplasia that results from a primary developmental defect followed by loss of domain or adjacent organ pressure. Further support for a causative relationship between left ventricular mass deficit and intrathoracic mass effect is offered by the fact that "classic" experimental fetal surgery, with reduction of viscera in the abdomen, reverses the effect on the heart. This is in contrast to experimental tracheal obstruction to cause lung hyperplasia. With the latter technique, the hyperplastic lungs, rather than abdominal viscera, compress the heart as the end result.

Apart from the left-sided hypoplasia, the most common anatomic congenital heart defect is an atrial septal defect. Other accompanying anomalies in spontaneous CDH include malrotation of the intestine, patent ductus arteriosus, patent foramen ovale, tricuspid or mitral valve regurgitation, undescended testes, and accessory spleen.

## Neonatal Period

Most infants with a diaphragmatic hernia present at birth or shortly after with varying degrees of respiratory distress. This may be the result of primary pulmonary hypoplasia. The most severe form is seen with aplasia of the diaphragm. The ipsilateral lung is virtually nonexistent and the contralateral lung is severely hypoplastic. Due to the primary insufficiency of any remaining lung tissue to provide gas exchange after birth, this condition is usually not compatible with life.

More commonly, the lack of respiratory tissue is not the basis of the refractory hypoxia. Rather, there will be a short period of relatively adequate ventilation and oxygenation (honeymoon period), followed by rapidly progressing hypoxia. This refractory hypoxia is most often caused by severe pulmonary hypertension (PPHN), whereby the newborn reverts to an antenatal pattern of blood circulation with a resultant bypass of the pulmonary bed. This PFC is characterized by severe vasoconstriction of the pulmonary arteries, and there is a progressive and often extreme right-to-left shunt with resultant ventilation/perfusion mismatch. Although hypoxia, hypercarbia, acidosis, and a variety of vasoconstricting agents are known to worsen pulmonary hypertension, the initial stimulus for PFC is unknown. It is likely that the immaturity of the pulmonary vasculature and, to a lesser degree, the surfactant system renders the infant prone to this condition.

Even in the absence of PFC, progressive hypoxia may occur due to worsening lung compression by intrathoracic viscera. As the neonate swallows air, the stomach and intestinal loops become distended, further compressing the thoracic cavity and the mediastinum. Clinical examination of a baby with diaphragmatic hernia may then reveal absent or decreased breath sounds on the ipsilateral side, evidence of dextrocardia (in left-sided hernia) and, rarely, intrathoracic bowel sounds. Massive herniation of distended viscera in the thorax may be clinically visible as a barrel chest, while the abdomen is typically scaphoid.

The diagnosis is usually confirmed with a chest radiograph, demonstrating intrathoracic intestinal loops, a nasogastric tube curled up in the chest, absence of a diaphragmatic shadow on the affected side, mediastinal and cardiac shift to the contralateral side, and occasionally intrathoracic location of the left lobe of the liver (Fig. 33-3).

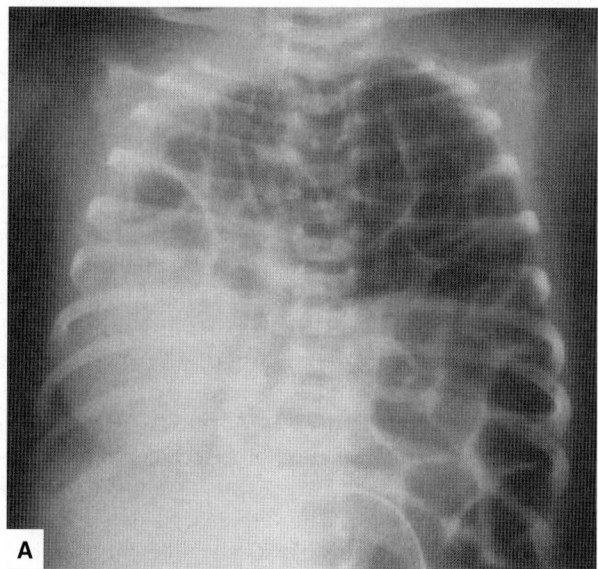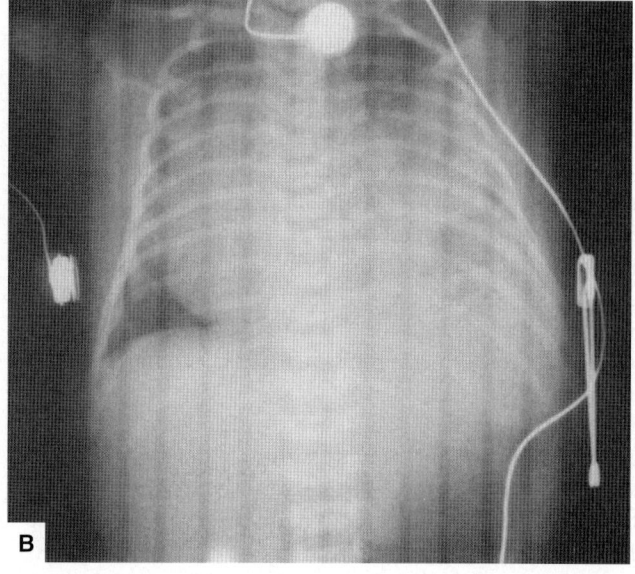

**FIGURE 33-3** Chest radiographic diagnosis of a diaphragmatic hernia. **A.** Profound filling of small bowel loops with gas. Loops are herniated into the left chest, and with increasing distention and contralateral lung hypoplasia they appear to herniate across the midline producing a profound mediastinal shift to the right. **B.** A cystic and solid mass effect in the left lower chest cavity is compatible with either herniated bowel and solid organ (spleen or liver) or even a cystic adenomatoid malformation of the lung.

## Infancy and Childhood

Occasionally, diaphragmatic hernia is not diagnosed until later in infancy, or even in early childhood. A routine chest radiograph may reveal many of the features described above, albeit in a less severe form. Rarely, the child may present with evidence not of respiratory distress, but of incarceration, intrathoracic sigmoid volvulus, or even acute or ruptured appendicitis. Less dramatic presentations of dyspnea on exertion, mild reactive airway disease, or viral or bacterial respiratory infection should prompt investigations that lead to the delayed diagnosis of CDH.

## Management of Bochdalek Hernias

### Antenatal

If the presence of a CDH is strongly suspected antenatally, minimum management should include consultation with a pediatric surgeon and a neonatologist and counseling for the parents. More institutions have recently formalized the evaluation and fetal management of CDH through combinations of perinatologists, geneticists, neonatologists, pediatric surgical subspecialists, and counselors or social workers. As for fetal management for other congenital anomalies, a consensus of options for further diagnostic and therapeutic steps is identified. The parents can then make informed decisions about therapy. They should also be prepared for the often urgent events that can occur at term.

Ten percent of fetuses with CDH have a chromosomal anomaly. Karyotypic investigation should therefore routinely be performed before fetal management is considered. If the prognosis is dismal (chromosomal anomalies, lethal syndrome), the parents may opt for termination of the pregnancy. If not, the optimal therapeutic course needs to be chosen. Antenatal intervention for severe CDH has been extensively studied experimentally throughout the last 2 decades, but is appropriate as an actual therapeutic option in very few patients.

Fetal surgical options were developed after years of animal experiments in several models. These studies improved the understanding of the pathophysiology and helped determine the limits and technical requirements for in utero or ex utero intervention. Fetal surgery for CDH has been characterized as physiologically sound and technically feasible using methods of "open" (via hysterotomy) and "closed" (endoscopic) fetal manipulation. Operative reduction of the viscera to the abdomen and closure of the diaphragmatic defect using a polytetrafluoroethylene patch has been shown to reverse pulmonary hypoplasia in animal models (sheep and nonhuman primates) as well as in few reported clinical cases. Open fetal surgery for diaphragmatic hernia, however, has sometimes included laparotomy, thoracotomy, and even partial liver resection, which has proven to be excessively invasive, with associated morbidity and mortality. The Fetal Treatment Center at the University of California, San Francisco, the first group with more than anecdotal experience with open fetal surgery, determined that CDH repair via an open hysterotomy should not be used in fetuses with CDH if the liver was herniated. In patients without an intrathoracic liver, the outcome of fetal repair showed no advantage over postnatal management. These patients are clearly best treated after birth.

Despite the dismal results of conventional open fetal surgery, new theoretic and technical developments continued to make fetal surgery a viable option. The finding that tracheal occlusion causes fetal lung growth allowed its application to the treatment of CDH-associated pulmonary hypoplasia. The use of minimally invasive techniques, developed in animal models, allowed tracheal occlusion to be performed endoscopically, with the fetus left in utero, minimizing the effects of surgery on the gravid uterus. Early clinical results were mixed. Fetal tracheal occlusion led to variable degrees of lung hyperplasia and hypertrophy, as well as detrimental effects on lung development and maturation. It appears that prolonged tracheal occlusion causes a disappearance of the surfactant-producing type II pneumocyte population. Furthermore, uncontrolled lung growth after tracheal obstruction led to fetal hydrops by mediastinal compression in several cases.

Methods of tracheal occlusion have included clips applied (endoscopically or not) after dissection of the fetal neck and exposure of the trachea. A second procedure was required at birth, with the fetus on placental support, to release the obstruction. The risks of this technique to the trachea (damage to tracheal rings, tracheomalacia, tracheomegaly, recurrent laryngeal nerve injury) were significant, and further development of the lungs (both before and after birth) was mixed. The latest iteration of fetal tracheal occlusion uses a completely endoscopic (tracheoscopic) method of balloon occlusion. Clinical trials of these methods have followed technical developments (Table 33-2). Methods of "open" fetal tracheal occlusion have uniformly fallen short of the marked improvement in postnatal survival of controls or of methods of management discussed later. There is limited proof that endotracheal occlusion with a detachable balloon can be a viable option in cases where there is prenatal evidence that survival would otherwise be dismal. Despite its disadvantages, fetal tracheal obstruction may still be designed and applied in such a way to achieve sufficient "catch-up" lung growth and molecular and cellular maturation to allow for postnatal survival. If risks are deemed reasonable, this approach may become a viable option for the fetus with severe diaphragmatic hernia. International organization and Food and Drug Administration (FDA)-monitored trials may determine the patient selection and safety parameters to allow for a structured application of this late antenatal treatment.

## Special Considerations for Fetal Diagnosis and Management

One of the major hopes for the treatment of CDH was that reliable antenatal predictors of severity and survival would emerge, leading to improved prenatal diagnostic accuracy. As shown in Table 33-3, the predictive value of the simple prenatal diagnosis of CDH is in apparent sharp contrast to the specificity of more technically advanced predictors of outcomes and survival, such as measured fetal LHRs. Many studies have attempted to correlate prenatal diagnosis of CDH and the timing of diagnosis with survival. The wide variability in perinatal management, however, has had a great impact on survival. Kays et al reported a survival rate of 20 of 22 prenatally diagnosed infants, whereas other centers have rates as low as 53%. Other studies have consistently found that prenatal diagnosis does not correlate with adverse outcome. None of these survival figures are statistically different from overall survival following postnatal diagnosis in each respective center. Most recently, however, a group that was previously skeptical of the validity of any prenatal predictor of survival has shown in its own series, that LHR <0.8 was associated with 100% mortality.

Anatomic and ultrasonographic or physiologic/biochemical factors in prenatal studies have been analyzed to determine their ability to predict mortality. The refinement in sonographic demonstration of fetal anomalies in addition to the diaphragmatic defect has allowed for a greater set of fetal variables that can be used to evaluate postnatal outcome. The current range of fetal features subjected to analysis (Table 33-3) now includes gestational age at the time of diagnosis, side of diaphragmatic hernia, degree of polyhydramnios, presence of liver and/or stomach herniation, lung fluid content as measured by MRI, opposite lung 2-dimensional area at the level of the heart, simultaneous head circumference, and left ventricular mass by an area–length method. The only major human fetal physiologic parameter to be reported is the characteristic of fetal breathing-related fluid flow in the trachea of fetuses with CDH. Using color Doppler, fluid displacement can be measured and spectral Doppler used to assess fluid flow velocity waveforms. Low-volume

| TABLE 33-2 | Reported Results of Fetal Management of Congenital Diaphragmatic Hernia | | | |
|---|---|---|---|---|
| Procedure | Date | N | Survival (%) | Comment |
| Open fetal surgery ("classic" repair) | 1993/1997 | 18 | 7 (39%) | 1 late neonatal death |
| Open fetal surgery (tracheal clip) | | | | |
| San Francisco | 1998 | 28 | 6 (21%) | 1 died in infancy |
| Philadelphia | 2000 | 15 | 5 (33%) | |
| Endoscopic tracheal clip | 1998 | 16 | 11 (69%) | 3 vocal cords damaged |
| Clip or balloon | 2004 | 11 | 8 (73%) | For LHR <1.4; no difference in postnatal survival/morbidity |
| Detachable balloon (Eurofoetus) | 2009 | 207 | 192 (93%) | 49% survival at discharge |

**TABLE 33-3    Proposed Predictors of Outcome and Survival for Children with Congenital Diaphragmatic**

**Fetal**

Prenatal ultrasound diagnosis of CDH

Gestational age at diagnosis of CDH

Side of CDH

Polyhydramnios

Associated anomalies diagnosed by fetal ultrasound

Abdominal circumference at umbilicus position

Mediastinal shift

Thoracic position of stomach

Thoracic position of liver and liver volume

Right lung 2-dimensional area

Transverse/sagittal thoracic diameter

Lung area to head circumference ratio (contralateral lung) (LHR)

Observed/expected lung-to-head ratio (O/E LHR)

Lung fluid content by magnetic resonance imaging (MRI)

Head/thorax circumference ratio

Observed/expected lung volume (3-dimensional ultrasound or MRI)

Lung/thorax transverse area ratio

Tracheal fluid volume and flow

Left ventricular mass

Size of ventricular aorta and pulmonary artery

Cardioventricular index (LV/RVsize)

Cardiovascular index (aortic/pulmonary artery [Ao/PA] size)

Left/right ventricular width

Left ventricular volume

Amniotic fluid lecithin/sphingomyelin ratio (experimental)

Amniotic fluid phosphatdylglycerol (experimental)

**Postnatal**

Gestational age gender race at delivery

Birth weight

1 + 5-min Apgar

Side of CDH

Association anomalies

Thoracic position of liver

Thoracic position of stomach

Percentage aerated ipsilateral/contralateral lung on chest x-ray

Measured mediastinal shift on chest x-ray

Presence of immediate respiratory distress

Requirement for cardiopulmonary resuscitation

"Honeymoon period"

Physiologic parameters

Preductal $P_{AO_2}$ <100

Postductal $P_{AO_2}$ <50

$a\text{-}A_{DO_2}$

**Ventilatory**

Tidal volume

Status/dynamic compliance

Functional residual capacity

Ventilatory index

(Peak inspiratory pressure [PIP] × respiratory rate [RR] × $CO_2$/1000)

Oxygenated index

(Mean arterial pressure [MAP] × $FiO_2$/$PaO_2$)

**Cardiac**

Left ventricular volume

Cardiac arrest

**Infancy**

Time of mechanical ventilation

Oxygen dependence

Extracorporeal membrane oxygenation (ECMO) mechanical/patient complications

Neurodevelopmental outcome

**Postmortem**

Lung weight/body weight ratio

Radial alveolar count

flow was identified in fetuses with lethal CDH. Survivors had flow values that approached normal with increasing flow during gestation and progressive lung growth similar to infants without CDH.

Specific anatomic findings associated with CDH have attracted attention because of their apparent significance during early attempts at open fetal repair of CDH. Albanese et al have carefully analyzed the finding of liver herniation into the fetal chest. Herniation of a major portion of the liver indicated a greater need for postnatal ECMO (53% vs 19% in patients with CDH without liver herniation). Survival for this small group of ECMO-treated infants was surprisingly only 43%, less than the 58% for all ECMO-treated newborns, according to the Extracorporeal Life Support Organization (ELSO) registry, which encompasses more than 2000 infants treated since 1986.

The liver had herniated into the chest in 27 of 53 patients (51%) reported by the group at the University of Florida at Gainesville (Kays et al), with 77% of patients since 1992 presenting with liver and/or stomach in the chest. This finding was not significantly different from previous periods of study at that institution. In contrast to the series reported by Albanese et al, survival for those patients with greater than 50% of liver mass in the chest was 79%, and reached 85% for those with any amount of liver and/or stomach in the chest. The discrepancy in outcome may indeed be due to the prognostic implications of fetal liver position and intrathoracic volume. Other factors to be considered are the percentage of patients with a right-sided CDH in any study, and the fact that these are often small neonates with poor cardiac function and severe cardiopulmonary hypoplasia.

A focus on the hypothetical association of cardiac hypoplasia has been attempted experimentally and clinically. Ten echocardiographic variables in 12 fetuses demonstrated that left heart dimensions and volume were below the expected range. However, they did not predict postnatal outcome in a series of patients with a globally poor outcome. In a separate study of left ventricular mass based on postnatal echocardiographic data, all patients with a left-sided CDH had significantly lower indexed left ventricular mass than did control infants with pulmonary hypertension not related to CDH.

## Lung-to-Head Ratio

Prospective evaluation of pulmonary hypoplasia relative to overall fetal development has been reported in several series. Using an axial view of the fetal chest at the level of the heart (4-chamber view), the long axis of the contralateral lung is obtained and a perpendicular line is drawn. The product of these 2 axes is divided by the head circumference, giving a LHR. This ratio normalizes lung size for gestational age, with head circumference as its surrogate.

The LHR and its correlation with survival were initially reported in a small series of 32 fetuses, but 17 could not be evaluated due to termination, exclusion of patients, or withdrawal of support for severe pulmonary insufficiency. Survival was only 47% for the group and no other prenatal variables were reported to correlate with outcome. This and subsequent attempts to establish the validity of LHR have been hampered by historical and variable postnatal

treatment modalities, the retrospective nature of most studies, and unclear measurement methods of LHR. Consequently, survival of infants with CDH and an LHR of 1.0 to 1.4 has ranged from 30% to 70%, and that of infants with an LHR <1.0 has ranged from 0% to 50%. Most recently, Aspelund et al reported 100% mortality for LHR <0.8, which can be characterized as extreme pulmonary hypoplasia. Furthermore, LHR is not as constant as was previously thought. More recently, the Eurofoetus group has advocated the use of observed/expected LHR (O/E LHR) as a more reliable and gestational-independent, factor.

## Role of Prenatal Therapy

While open surgical repair of the diaphragm and endoscopic surgical clipping of the fetal trachea no longer find supporters, fetoscopic tracheal occlusion (FETO) using an endotracheally deployed detachable balloon has been shown to be a feasible technique. It carries a relatively low morbidity for the fetus, can often be performed percutaneously, and has shown to generate accelerated fetal lung growth. The timing and duration of tracheal occlusion appear to be critical. The occlusion is typically performed between 28 and 30 weeks and is removed 4 to 6 weeks later. In a recent series of more than 200 patients, LHR increased from a preoperative average of 0.7 to 1.7 after occlusion, and mean gestational age at delivery was 35 weeks.

The place of FETO in the overall treatment of CDH remains controversial. Following a randomized controlled trial in 2004 by Harrison et al, prenatal treatment is generally no longer recommended for LHR >1.0. In patients with an LHR >1.0 (or O/E <25%), survival at birth was greater than 90%. Only 50% of patients, however, survived to be discharged. It can be argued that this "true" survival rate is not significantly better than many postnatal series that include severe CDH. If the recent report that LHR <0.8 is associated with 100% mortality is confirmed, FETO may have a role in cases of extremely severe CDH with nonsurvivable pulmonary hypoplasia. Even so, widespread acceptance awaits carefully conducted trials currently under way. In the United States, these trials are occurring under the auspices of the FDA.

## Postnatal Management

The first line of treatment of a newborn with suspected or documented diaphragmatic hernia is respiratory support. The recommended flow of management steps is depicted in Fig. 33-4. Most babies will require endotracheal intubation. Ventilation with 100% oxygen, even if the baby is not acutely hypoxic, may help decompress intestinal loops that are already distended with nitrogen-rich room air. A nasogastric tube is necessary for the same reason.

Assisted ventilation aims at providing optimal oxygenation and minimal barotrauma, to avoid ipsilateral alveolar damage that would worsen alveolar-capillary gas diffusion and contralateral tension pneumothorax. Although adequate ventilation and carbon dioxide elimination is ideal, hyperventilation is contraindicated. Moderate permissive hypercapnia is clearly preferable to hypocapnia. Monitoring should, at minimum, include systemic arterial pressure measurement

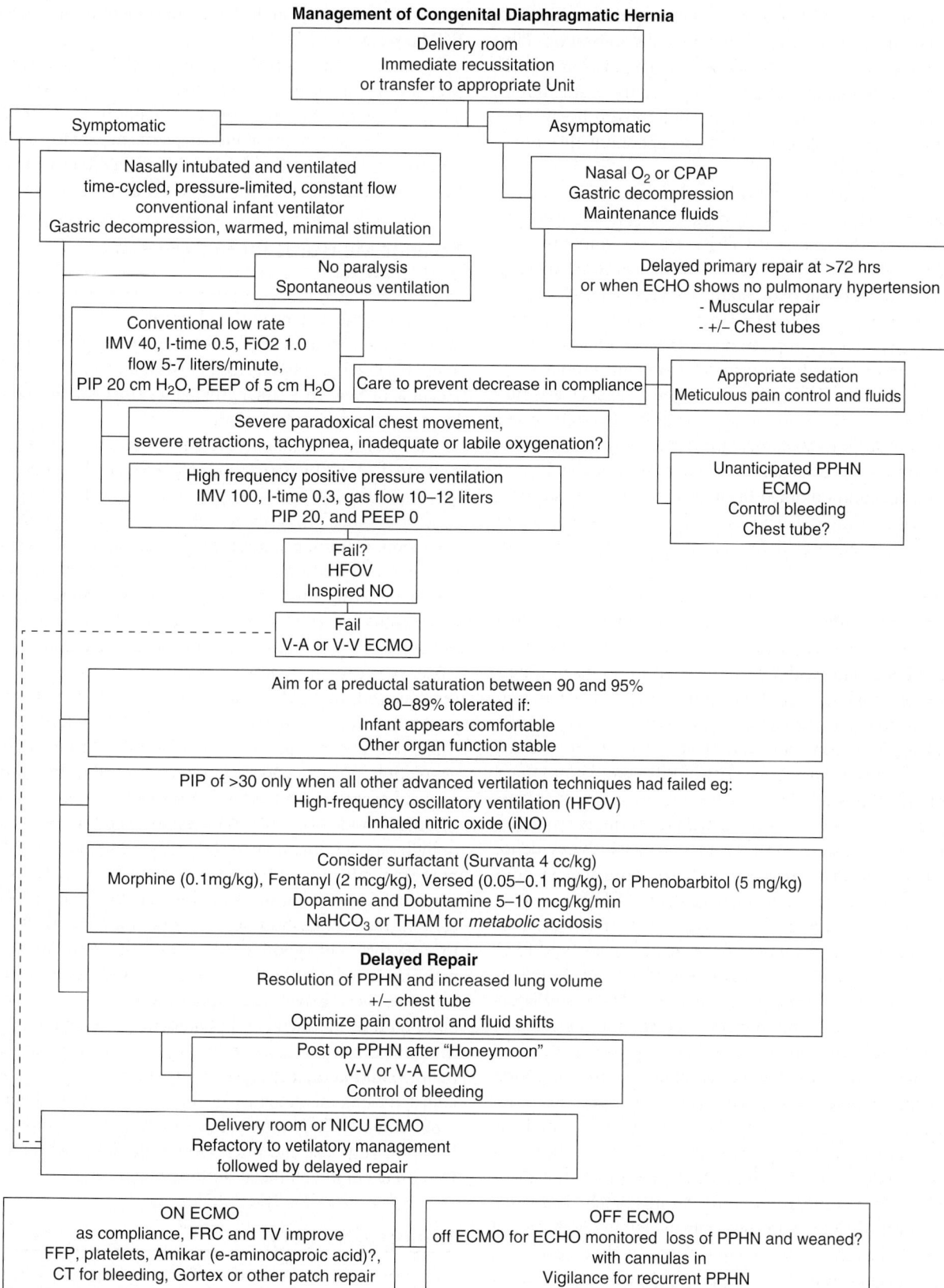

**Management of Congenital Diaphragmatic Hernia**

Delivery room
Immediate recussitation
or transfer to appropriate Unit

Symptomatic

Asymptomatic

Nasally intubated and ventilated
time-cycled, pressure-limited, constant flow
conventional infant ventilator
Gastric decompression, warmed, minimal stimulation

Nasal O₂ or CPAP
Gastric decompression
Maintenance fluids

No paralysis
Spontaneous ventilation

Delayed primary repair at >72 hrs
or when ECHO shows no pulmonary hypertension
- Muscular repair
- +/– Chest tubes

Conventional low rate
IMV 40, I-time 0.5, FiO2 1.0
flow 5-7 liters/minute,
PIP 20 cm H₂O, PEEP of 5 cm H₂O

Care to prevent decrease in compliance

Appropriate sedation
Meticulous pain control and fluids

Severe paradoxical chest movement,
severe retractions, tachypnea, inadequate or labile oxygenation?

Unanticipated PPHN
ECMO
Control bleeding
Chest tube?

High frequency positive pressure ventilation
IMV 100, I-time 0.3, gas flow 10–12 liters
PIP 20, and PEEP 0

Fail?
HFOV
Inspired NO

Fail
V-A or V-V ECMO

Aim for a preductal saturation between 90 and 95%
80–89% tolerated if:
Infant appears comfortable
Other organ function stable

PIP of >30 only when all other advanced vertilation techniques had failed eg:
High-frequency oscillatory ventilation (HFOV)
Inhaled nitric oxide (iNO)

Consider surfactant (Survanta 4 cc/kg)
Morphine (0.1mg/kg), Fentanyl (2 mcg/kg), Versed (0.05–0.1 mg/kg), or Phenobarbitol (5 mg/kg)
Dopamine and Dobutamine 5–10 mcg/kg/min
NaHCO₃ or THAM for *metabolic* acidosis

**Delayed Repair**
Resolution of PPHN and increased lung volume
+/– chest tube
Optimize pain control and fluid shifts

Post op PPHN after "Honeymoon"
V-V or V-A ECMO
Control of bleeding

Delivery room or NICU ECMO
Refactory to vetilatory management
followed by delayed repair

ON ECMO
as compliance, FRC and TV improve
FFP, platelets, Amikar (e-aminocaproic acid)?,
CT for bleeding, Gortex or other patch repair

OFF ECMO
off ECMO for ECHO monitored loss of PPHN and weaned?
with cannulas in
Vigilance for recurrent PPHN

**FIGURE 33-4** Algorithm depicting the preferred management schemes for diaphragmatic hernia.

via an umbilical artery catheter, urine output, and preductal and postductal pulse oximetry. Preductal oxygen saturation (right arm) is an indicator of optimal oxygenation, whereas postductal oxygen saturation reflects the amount of right-to-left shunt (ie, the degree of ventilation/perfusion mismatch due to pulmonary hypertension). Some controversy exists whether the measurement of preductal or postductal PO₂ provides an accurate uniform prediction of survival. Many studies have shown no correlation with postductal blood gas measurement because the degree of ductal or foraminal shunting is highly variable and may be temporary due to the degree and quality of the resuscitation and stabilization. Liberal use of echocardiography allows the diagnosis of associated cardiac anomalies and, more importantly, evaluation of right and left ventricular function, pulmonary artery flow (and pressure), and degree of right-to-left shunt through a patent ductus arteriosus.

Based on the extensive evidence of structural immaturity determined in morphologic studies, several investigators have hypothesized that CDH lungs are immature and surfactant deficient. Surfactant has been measured in lung tissue of CDH nonsurvivors and in several animal models with variable results. The fetal lamb model has yielded data regarding deficiencies in pulmonary surfactant and the beneficial effects of immediate postnatal treatment, although not delayed treatment. The significance of the deficiency was further underscored by information gained from ECMO-treated infants who, despite exogenous surfactant treatment, demonstrated continued surfactant deficiencies in bronchoalveolar lavage (BAL) fluid obtained during the course of treatment. On the basis of the deficiencies noted, several management protocols have advocated immediate treatment with exogenous surfactant.

This suggestive biochemical abnormality has been contradicted by other human fetal and animal studies. In the first careful prospective evaluation of surfactant composition in BAL fluid of infants with CDH, the concentrations of different phospholipids are similar to those of age-matched controls. This study has even greater significance as BAL samples were taken from conventionally treated and ECMO-treated infants covering a range of severity of PPHN and pulmonary hypoplasia. This study in a relatively small group of infants challenges the data that suggest a primary pulmonary surfactant deficiency exists in CDH. There is no conclusive evidence to accept or refute the immediate or delayed use of exogenous pulmonary surfactant in the management of CDH.

In addition to optimization of oxygenation, treatment aims at preventing or reducing pulmonary hypertension and PFC. A tendency toward alkalosis may be beneficial, but hyperventilation and hypocapnia are unwarranted. Most vasodilators are not specific to the pulmonary circulation and are therefore rarely recommended. Tolazoline is probably the best known agent and if used at all will often require correction of systemic hypotension, usually with dopamine. Recently, inhaled nitric oxide (iNO) has been introduced in patients with refractory pulmonary hypertension. As NO only affects capillaries associated with alveoli that are ventilated, it theoretically reduces ventilation/perfusion mismatch. The vasodilator effect of NO is only local, since it is rapidly degraded once it reaches the systemic circulation. In short-term use, at doses varying from 20 to 80 ppm, NO does not appear to have major side effects. Unfortunately, its efficacy is erratic and tachyphylaxis often occurs. While initial case reports suggested that iNO improved oxygenation in some infants, large randomized, controlled trials demonstrated that early administration of iNO did not reduce deaths or ECMO use in patients with CDH. Anecdotal and experimental reports indicate that with prolonged survival, the pulmonary vasculature may become not only less reactive, but also more responsive to the direct effects of NO. Therefore, there may

be a basis for a trial late in the management of prolonged or ECMO refractory PPHN.

If conventional ventilatory support at less than extreme pressures is unable to maintain adequate oxygenation, use of a high frequency jet ventilator or oscillator may be necessary. In cases of persistent instability, hypoxia, hypercarbia, and/or pulmonary hypertension, ECMO is indicated, provided that the child meets the inclusion criteria (Fig. 33-4).

## Specific Measures for Preoperative Stabilization

The management steps outlined in this section are based on survival data from several centers and designed to follow similar guidelines popularized at Morgan Stanley Children's Hospital of New York (formerly Babies Hospital) and adapted by many centers internationally.

The majority of infants are intubated and mechanically ventilated. A nasogastric tube is placed to decompress the gastrointestinal tract. The pressure- or volume-regulated ventilator is set primarily to achieve adequate, gentle chest excursion. Commonly, good chest excursion and acceptable oxygenation (preductal $PaO_2$ >50 torr) becomes possible with ventilator settings that ranged from an intermittent mandatory ventilation (IMV) of 15 to 40 breaths per minute and pressures of 20/5 to 25/5 cm $H_2O$. If oxygenation is unsatisfactory, peak inspiratory pressure is not increased further. Instead, the IMV is raised immediately to 100 breaths per minute and pressures reduced to 18/0 to 20/0 cm $H_2O$ (high-rate positive pressure ventilation). During high-rate ventilation, positive end-expiratory pressure is discontinued to avoid excessive inadvertent air trapping.

Once a mode of ventilation is established (ie, conventional or high rate) it is maintained. Adjustments to mechanical support are made only in response to changes in preductal oxygenation. Little attention is paid to the regulation of $PaCO_2$ early in the stabilization period. Should the $PaCO_2$ decrease to <40 torr with good oxygenation, the peak inspiratory pressure is reduced or the IMV is lowered. As oxygenation improves, permissive hypercapnia allows the $PaCO_2$ to rise to 50 to 60 torr. Preductal and postductal pulse oximetry assist in monitoring right to left shunting and in adjusting the ventilator. Fluid and electrolyte management must be carefully adjusted using maintenance or slightly less than maintenance requirements. These infants have an exaggerated antidiuretic hormone response and often require fluid restriction to prevent excess fluid volume and extracellular water.

## Timing of Surgery

This decision will remain one of continuing controversy and debate, as a current meta-analysis has failed to define a benefit for an immediate or delayed approach. Proponents of urgent surgery remain convinced that intrathoracic viscera are able to exert negative influences on the mediastinum through progressive venous obstruction and intraluminal air if not reduced. Both sides point to measured and deleterious compliance changes from organ displacement (the need to repair early) or the resuscitation and diminished chest wall dynamics during urgent repair. Whether ECMO is applied early for stabilization or late for rescue, there remain clinicians that do not feel that ECMO provides any survival advantage over their particular medical management strategy and there is international evidence to support poorer ECMO outcome than seen consistently in US centers. Further, there are also those groups that feel that, without resolution of PPHN and evidence of adequate pulmonary ventilation, repair is absolutely not indicated.

In the absence of any definite prenatal or postnatal predictors, the current standard of care will follow the following sequence:

1. Immediate resuscitation of all infants with CDH.

2. Initiation of pressure-limited maximal ventilatory support allowing for permissive hypercapnia.

3. Operative repair after progressive and monitored (ECHO) resolution of PPHN and shunt over a period generally >72 hours.

4. ECMO support for progressive PPHN, hypoxia, falling cardiac output, or $O_2$ delivery.

5. ECMO support following operative repair resulting in the onset or recurrence of PPHN.

6. Operative repair: (a) following a course of ECMO stabilization and resolution of PPHN, (b) during a course of ECMO stabilization with evidence of deteriorating or fixed, unimproved pulmonary compliance.

## Surgical Repair of Bochdalek Hernias

### Elective Repair of a Left CDH Without ECMO Support or Prior to ECMO Anesthetic Management

The anesthetic management for operative reduction of the hernia and repair of the defect has become more established with a clear understanding of the benefits of appropriate postnatal resuscitation and improved ventilation nodes. The major priorities are for preservation of minute ventilation and cardiac output. For those infants with adequate spontaneous ventilation, the challenge to not drive $PaCO_2$ down following induced paralysis can be met by an adequate period of preoperative evaluation and observation. Just as desired during the initial resuscitation phases, the avoidance of exaggerated chest excursions is necessary. Appropriate narcotic levels must be achieved in order to ablate the stress response. Doses of fentanyl reaching 25 µg/kg/h are required. Pancuronium is used as a muscle relaxant and isoflurane is an appropriate inhalation agent. As before, there is no need for mask or laryngeal ventilation regardless of the how stable the infant is. With even the slightest gastric distention, the entire clinical picture can be reversed. A rapid sequence intubation must be accomplished if the baby is not already intubated.

### Surgical Procedure for Open Transabdominal Repair

The core principles and maneuvers for adequate and rapid transabdominal repair provide the foundation for

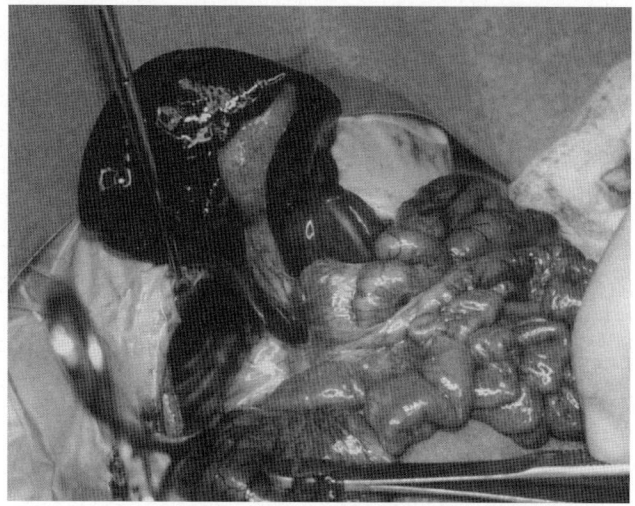

**FIGURE 33-5** Right-sided diaphragmatic hernia visualized after abdominal incision and visceral reduction. A clamp marks the anterior diaphragmatic rim.

minimally invasive approaches and the current advances in minimally invasive surgery (MIS). As discussed later, thoracoscopic techniques may be suitable for a growing number of infants. Expeditious patch repair may be best achieved through open abdominal or thoracoscopic procedures. There are still technical and anatomic structural hurdles that contribute to a high rate of hernia recurrence in open cases. There is not yet adequate follow-up of MIS cases to validate whether there is a higher rate of recurrence in MIS versus open cases.

The infant is placed on the operating table or positioned supine on the infant radiant warmer (Figs. 33-5 to 33-7). There is no specific need to move the baby from the bed/platform especially if there is ongoing oscillatory or other specialized ventilation or iNO delivery. A small bump made up of 1- or 2-folded small towels or diapers is placed under the left flank. Arterial blood pressure and blood gases should ideally be monitored from a right radial arterial line for preductal determinations. Postductal monitoring can be performed via umbilical artery lines. Central venous pressure is preferentially measured from an internal jugular or subclavian line, although femoral lines through the inferior vena cava or umbilical venous lines to the right atrium are also possible. A Foley catheter is placed with a stopcock for intraabdominal pressure monitoring; the same provision is made for the naso- or orogastric tube. Both of these sites are useful to judge the degree of pressure that develops with abdominal wall closure.

Following positioning and skin preparation, the application of drapes should be accomplished to allow access to both sides of the chest. Sudden deterioration might be the result of a contralateral pneumothorax requiring an immediate tube thoracostomy. The left chest must be exposed either for placement of a chest tube or for the very rare necessity of performing a mini thoracotomy to release adhesions in the most apical portions of the chest or to allow for the occasional bimanual reduction of a herniated liver, spleen, or kidney.

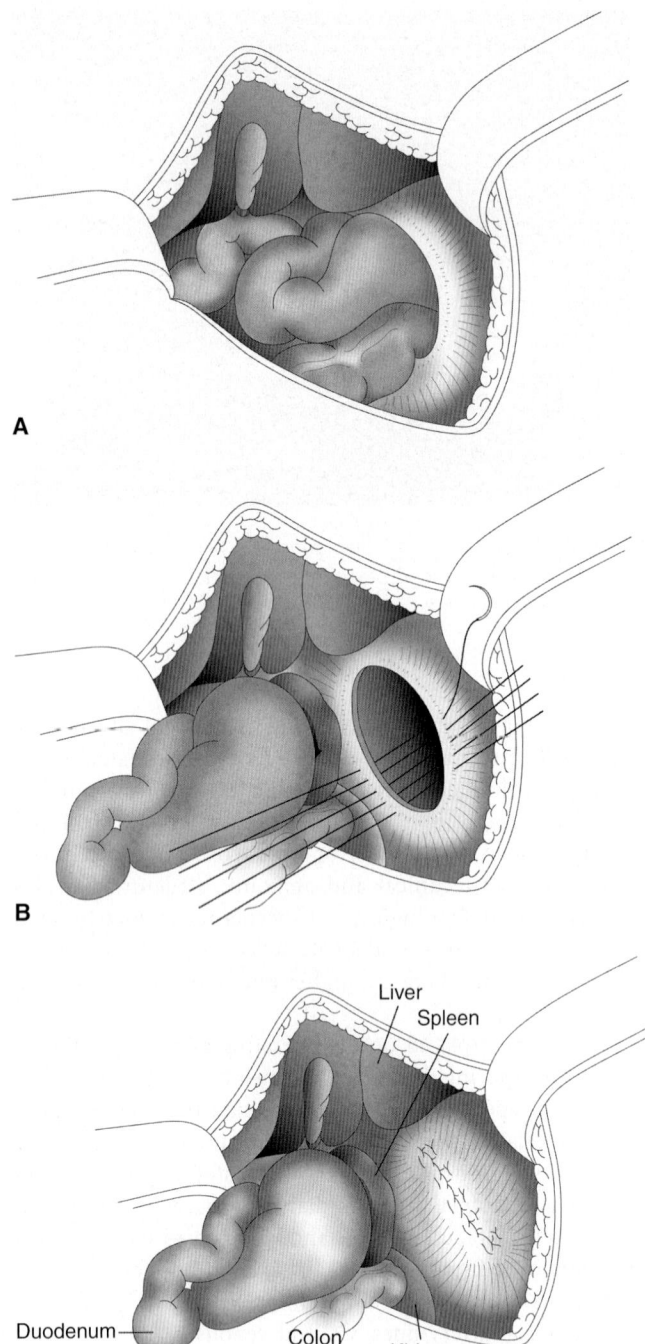

**A**

**B**

Liver
Spleen

Duodenum
Colon
Kidney
**C**

**FIGURE 33-6** Primary transabdominal repair of a diaphragmatic hernia. **A.** The viscera are reduced; a maneuver facilitated by retraction or placement of a trans-defect tube to relieve the vacuum. **B.** The edges of the diaphragm are mobilized. The posterior edge may be deficient and may be best exposed by sharply incising the overlying peritoneum. **C.** Simple or mattress sutures are placed and tied, obliterating the defect.

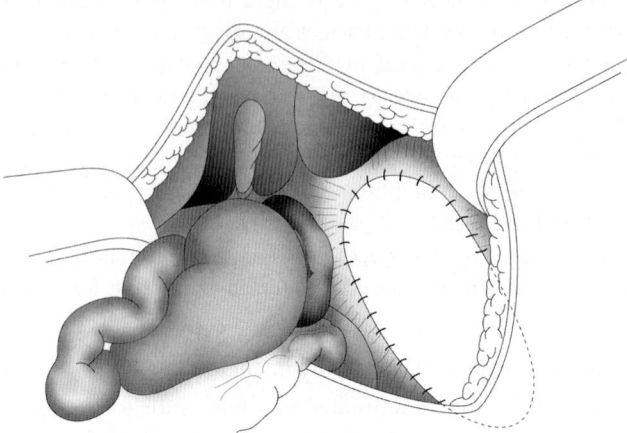

**FIGURE 33-7** Prosthetic repair of a diaphragmatic hernia. A measured prosthetic (Gortex®) patch is positioned, allowing for some redundant tenting, and it is circumferentially secured with interrupted suture technique.

has been adequate resolution of pulmonary hypertension at the time of the elective repair, postoperative or delayed PPHN may require the use of ECMO.

Once the peritoneum is opened, the incision must be generous enough to allow for evisceration of the nonherniated small and large bowel. Small Richardson retractors are placed on the costal border of the incision. Gentle downward retraction of the abdominal contents will reveal the diaphragmatic defect and an estimation of the degree of solid organ herniation. A large defect will allow the almost immediate reduction of intestinal contents by gentle traction using fine ring forceps. The mesentery of the bowel should flow with the intestine from the defect. The formation of mesenteric or subserosal hematomas should be avoided at all costs.

Segments of small bowel and large bowel usually can be reduced simultaneously. Once the jejunum and duodenum have been identified, special attention must be directed to a gentle reduction of the stomach due to the fragile connection of the short gastric vessels to the herniated spleen. If the spleen does not freely return through the diaphragmatic defect at the time of intestinal traction, gentle finger reduction should be applied to the spleen, liver, and left kidney in that order. The reduction of each herniated organ may require the gentle placement of laparotomy pads and/or small malleable retractors on each organ to maintain its intraabdominal position during the manual reduction process and diaphragmatic hernia repair.

Small defects often pose a challenge for the reduction of the spleen and occasionally the kidney. Exposure of the defect is the same and the introduction of air through the defect will negate the small but perceptible influence of negative intrathoracic pressure. This is best performed by manual distraction of the superior edge of the diaphragmatic defect or by retraction of the defect by a vein retractor. When the "suction" is relieved, the reduction proceeds as previously described with great care to enable the reduction of a large spleen through a small defect.

Once the reduction is complete, the borders and extent of the muscular defect must be identified. In some infants, the

The operative procedure is begun with a left subcostal incision 2 finger breadths below the costal margin. Abdominal wall muscle flaps are no longer used because they diminish the all-important compliance of the chest wall when compared to the current prosthetic patch repair. Hemostasis is critical when dividing the rectus muscles medially and the oblique muscles laterally. Although it is assumed that there

medial edge may demonstrate a normal hiatus and crura. The largest defects, including agenesis of the diaphragm, may have almost no medial muscle, thus, exposing the distal esophagus and aorta. When there is adequate medial muscle present, the posterior border should be traced laterally to expose the entire muscle leaf, which may appear rolled on itself in the retroperitoneum and covered by a thin peritoneal adhesion. Once this adhesion is divided with electrocautery, the posterior portion of the diaphragm can be unfurled from medial to lateral. A residual hernia sac or an associated extralobar pulmonary sequestration often attached to the edge of the diaphragm may be readily apparent or require a search. Both should be resected and hemostasis achieved by cautery and ligature of any larger vessels. The anterior diaphragm is usually well developed when present. Once the anterior and posterior edges are freed and absolute hemostasis accomplished, each edge should be simultaneously grasped with forceps or baby Allis clamps to determine if they can be approximated. The goal is a tension-free closure to prevent further decreases in compliance. If the edges are easily approximated, 2-0 silk or other nonabsorbable sutures are placed without tension in an interrupted fashion from medial to lateral. The use of pledgets is time-consuming for the surgeon and operating room staff and it invites the use of excess tension in the repair without any proven advantage.

Prior to closure, a 10- or 12-Fr chest tube may be placed in the left chest to water seal for drainage. Some surgeons contend that this tube is unnecessary and its presence prevents the lung from full expansion. In the authors' opinion, however, that contention is difficult to understand, considering the compensating rate of lung growth that will occur months and years later. Chylous effusions and hemo- and hydrothoraces that may occur are for the most part limited by chest drainage from causing potentially serious consequences of mediastinal pressure and shift, especially in anticoagulated newborns.

Cases of large diaphragmatic defects or agenesis require prosthetic replacement. An adequate diaphragmatic border or alternatively anterior and posterior ribs must be identified to anchor the prosthetic patches. Gortex® (Gore Association, Tucson, AZ) patches have been used, while anticipating future materials that will provide better fusion with native tissue at its borders. Currently, there is an unacceptable high rate of recurrence of the hernia with prosthetic repairs. Lyophilized dura, Marlex, and Vicryl mesh, Dacron-reinforced Silastic, porcine small intestinal submucosa (SIS), and alloderm, among other regenerative matrices, have all been reported as diaphragmatic substitutes in the literature.

Primary repair of these defects requires minimal or almost no dissection following visceral reduction. A prosthesis is cut larger than the defect, only to be trimmed after the patch is inset and contoured to a convex shape. The prosthesis is fixed in position with interrupted nonabsorbable sutures. Again, interrupted sutures without pledgets are expeditious and effective and 3-0 Prolene is used due to its ease of control and tying. A small Allis clamp is used to grasp and elevate the 10th rib posteriorly to facilitate sutures placement around the rib and into the patch. Anteriorly, a vein retractor or Allis clamp can elevate the costal margin and isolate the 8th rib to place sutures around it. The posterior half is tied first and a chest tube is placed. The anterior sutures are then tied.

It is uncommon and surprising to find no anchoring structures medially. The only option in this situation is to place several tacking sutures to the crural remnant directly adjacent to the gastroesophageal junction. The left lobe of the liver is allowed to rest against the medial prosthetic edge to partition off the medial abdominal compartment. These maneuvers are required in only the severest cases. No attempts to suture to aortic adventitia or to the esophagus should be made.

In the performance of CDH repairs with or without prosthetic material, no soft tissue flaps are used. Procedures to repair malrotation associated with CDH are unnecessary at this juncture and are meddlesome. No appendectomy is performed and it is not necessary to manually manipulate the colon to extrude meconium through the anus in preparation for closure of the abdomen. Throughout the procedure, the surgeon must remain aware that extralobar pulmonary sequestrations can be associated with CDH. These are found with their systemic blood supply on either the thoracic or abdominal sides of the repair. Although these are felt to be the least consequential of all bronchopulmonary malformations, they should be resected at the time of repair.

The key to a successful repair rests in the security of the sutures and the freedom from tension on the repair. Apart from setting the stage for recurrence, the most important immediate consequence of tension is in its effect on pulmonary compliance. Alterations in the pressure–volume curves are indicative of tension. Likewise the same pressure effects will become apparent if the abdomen is closed under tension. The fundamental closure of the abdomen in the era of emergent repair was a skin only closure after generous elevations of skin flaps. Obviously some repairs allowed for a layered closure and the goal of such a closure can be accomplished in most cases. Interrupted absorbable sutures are appropriate. Monitoring of the intraabdominal pressure can prove helpful, as pressures greater than 8 to 10 mm $H_2O$ will begin to translate into decreased compliance. This is the time for the greatest judgment. For those infants with long-term stability after resolution of PPHN, and clear evidence of excess pulmonary reserve and tidal volume, the changes in compliance will be well tolerated. The performance of bedside compliance and tidal volume measurements are extremely helpful in this regard as an ongoing analysis of pulmonary function during the course of preoperative management.

If the abdominal wall cannot be primarily closed without undue tension, a Gortex prosthesis or preferably Vicryl mesh is used under a skin closure. Gortex has significant extrusion problems, as shown by experience in omphalocele and gastroschisis. The acceptance of a ventral hernia for an unstable or precarious infant is a small price to improve survival and can be easily rectified later. The occasional infant will require the placement of a silastic silo to house the viscera to allow gradual and progressive reduction of the abdominal contents prior to closure.

Postoperative management should proceed as it had prior to the procedure. Pain control with continuous fentanyl or morphine is essential to eliminate postoperative stress. The single chest drain or tube, if placed, must not be placed on suction; water seal is sufficient.

## Video-Assisted Thoracoscopic Repair of CDH

For many centers, CDH repair has evolved into advanced endoscopic approaches and video-assisted thoracoscopic surgery (VATS), used not only for the visual clarity and precision they provide, but also because of concerns about minimal interference on chest wall compliance. As with all minimally invasive procedures, there are also aspirations for better pain management, wound healing, and cosmesis. Outcome measures would be shorter periods of ventilatory/$O_2$ support, shorter hospital stay, and fewer recurrences or other complications. No study has been large enough or designed with enough power to assure the benefit of endoscopic approaches. What can be determined is that these procedures can be successfully accomplished as a technical extension of current thoracoscopic procedures in newborns.

Experienced teams caution that patients should be carefully selected based on accumulated experience. The anatomy is important and sicker newborns will have the liver herniated into the chest with an almost certain significant defect. A prolonged procedure using $CO_2$ insufflation has the potential for hypoxia, hypercarbia, acidosis, and hypothermia, all of which can trigger for pulmonary hypertension. Three well-written initial series (in Boston, Seattle, and Ann Arbor, Michigan) all point to the concern for complete resolution of PPHN prior to consideration of an endoscopic approach. Common characteristics in a group of 33 patients at Milwaukee Children's Hospital who underwent successful thoracoscopic repair included absence of congenital heart defects, no need for ECMO, ventilatory peak inspiratory pressure of less than 26 cm $H_2O$, and oxygenation index less than 5 on the day of planned surgery. Intraoperative acidosis was demonstrated in some of the patients in these series and reversed with the cessation of insufflation. Patch closure was a strong relative indication for conversion to open surgery. Suture techniques are still being developed, extending from extracorporeal ties and anchors to internal auto sutures.

The technical details are similar to all neonatal thoracoscopic instrumentation and strategic trocar placement for triangulation. Generally, the first trocar for the thoracoscope (5 mm, 30°) is placed in the anterior axillary line in the fourth intercostal space. A clamp is used to bluntly spread through the intercostal musculature into the chest to protect against bowel injury. A radially expandable sleeve is slipped into the chest and then dilated with the trocar and dilator. Insufflation pressure is initiated at 4 to 5 mm Hg. Three to 4 ports are employed and 3 mm instrumentation is used. Pericostal sutures are arranged laterally and interrupted sutures with or without pledgets are placed after the bowel is returned to the abdomen and the posterior diaphragmatic leaf is dissected and developed.

Innovative approaches to endoscopic and even laparoscopic efforts at repair now are considered routine for 25% to 45% of newborns with CDH. Improvements in outcome have resulted from a focus on stabilization and the measured effect on pulmonary function found after a rapid procedure. Although operative times have dropped dramatically below 2.5 hours and will continue to do so, technical ability should not trump the cautions coming from centers with long-term experience in selecting infants for MIS approaches. Experienced surgeons

can guide the judgment required to recognize the prudent application of simple, rapid thoracoscopic repair. Limited outcome data may indicate a greater recurrence with MIS, but the power of any study is so insufficient that the best observation of outcome indicates equivalence across all centers.

# ECMO IN THE CDH INFANT

While there are many excellent reviews of ECMO in the immediate stabilization of oxygenation and ventilation of infants with severe PPHN and lung hypoplasia, it is beyond the scope of this chapter to review all facets of the application of ECMO in CDH. ECMO is discussed here to elucidate the basic maneuvers for those unstable infants and for those infants that become unstable after repair.

ECMO is used in the delivery room and is primarily reserved for infants failing conventional therapy or for infants who were initially stabilized or repaired and subsequently showed evidence of inadequate oxygen delivery, progressive metabolic acidosis, and organ failure despite maximal conventional therapy. Extracorporeal support is ideally instituted before inordinate ventilatory pressures are employed. An alveolar–arterial dissolved oxygen difference ($AdO_2$) >600 torr for more than 4 hours or decreased cardiac output despite inotropic support is an indication for ECMO. ECMO should not be considered without some evidence of potentially adequate lung parenchyma. However, there have been no adequate predictors uniformly demonstrated at all centers. ECMO can be instituted preoperatively for a patient who cannot be stabilized if there is a reasonable expectation of adequate lung parenchyma and a potentially reversible pulmonary hypertensive pathophysiology.

## ECMO Technique

When ECMO is necessary, most centers prefer venoarterial ECMO. The expertise to achieve predictable and stable positioning of the newer highly efficient double lumen cannulae for venovenous ECMO is not present in many programs. In addition, the occasional severe distortion and shift of the mediastinum lends itself to more dependable placement of separate venous and arterial cannulae.

The patient is heparinized with 100 units/kg in all cases. Extrathoracic cannulation is accomplished at the bedside using either an 8- or 10-Fr end hole arterial perfusion cannula and a 10- or 12-Fr multiple side hole venous drainage catheter (Elecath, Rahway, NJ). Flow is instituted slowly to prevent severe and sudden changes in cerebral blood flow and velocity associated with intracranial hemorrhage. The maintenance of pump flows sufficient to meet tissue oxygen requirements with minimal ventilator and supplemental oxygen support usually requires not more than 125 mL/kg/mm. The flow may also be dependent on the degree of cardiac dysfunction (stun) due to excessive prebypass use of high concentrations of inotropes and NO. Often there is a significant "oxygen debt" when going on bypass, especially in those infants transported over long distances and after relatively prolonged ventilatory management. $O_2$ saturation may not rise until cardiac output is restored in lieu of near total right-sided bypass. Target preductal O$_2$ saturation need not exceed 95%. Weaning from ECMO is best guided primarily by inline monitoring of mixed venous oxygen saturation, which is maintained at 65% to 70%.

## Repair of CDH During ECMO

For those infants in immediate distress in the delivery room or intensive care unit, ECMO may be lifesaving and is now considered by many as mandatory for the support of infants with CDH and in managing high risk deliveries of fetuses with known CDH. The operative considerations for ECMO in unrepaired infants must include extreme care for cannula placement. Mediastinal shift during CDH repair may require cannula adjustment during the ECMO run and after the repair. The decision to repair during the course of ECMO or following successful resolution of PPHN has not been studied. Proponents of either method focus on opposing fears of excessive bleeding following repair in heparinized infants and the exaggerated or recurrent PPHN after repair. Case reports document both occurrences without providing irrefutable data to support either method so the controversy continues. The dramatic reversal of the pathophysiology is unusual while on bypass except in the special situation of progressive mediastinal shift due to venous obstruction in herniated viscera. These infants will not only show progressive deterioration, but also may develop a metabolic acidosis and demonstrate decreased dynamic pulmonary compliance and functional residual capacity (FRC).

Repair of the CDH on ECMO follows appropriate correction of platelet counts to ≥100,000. The repair may occur late in the course of ECMO and attention to falling antithrombin III levels allow for more precise heparin regulation. Fresh frozen plasma (10-20 mL/kg) should be administered as a source of this important heparin cofactor. Trials of e-aminocaproic acid (Amicar) have been attempted in ECMO patients to prevent bleeding by inhibiting fibrinolysis. The inhibitory effects of aminocaproic acid appear to be exerted via inhibition of plasminogen activators and through antiplasmin activity. No specific controlled trials for CDH repair on ECMO have been completed.

The dissection and repair are the same when ECMO is not used. Use of electrocautery is liberal and precise. More often, these are the patients with diaphragmatic agenesis or large defects that will require prothetic patch repair. These are ideal candidates for placement of the patch with running hemostatic suture. In the repair of smaller defects, extreme care must be given to the reduction of the liver and spleen and the subsequent retraction on all organs. A capsular or serosal tear can become a life-threatening catastrophe. The use of fibrin sealants seems intuitive, but efficacy data have not been published. A chest tube is clearly necessary not to compound the sequelae of the repair by a significant hemothorax. Precise control of heparin, platelets, and fluids postoperatively is essential. The authors and others have observed that those parameters are more easily controlled early in the course of ECMO and this has served as the motivation for earlier repair.

An analysis of the Extracorporeal Life Support Organization (ELSO) ECMO registry failed to show any difference in overall outcome for CDH infants treated with venovenous (VV) versus venoarterial (VA) ECMO. More than 80% of these infants received VA ECMO and suffered more neurologic complications compared to infants receiving VV ECMO, who had a predominance of renal complications.

## OUTCOME FOR CONGENITAL DIAPHRAGMATIC HERNIA

In no other newborn condition has there been a greater opportunity for variability in outcome based on an astounding number of possible management schemes (Table 33-3 and Fig. 33-8). In addition, numerous individual variations

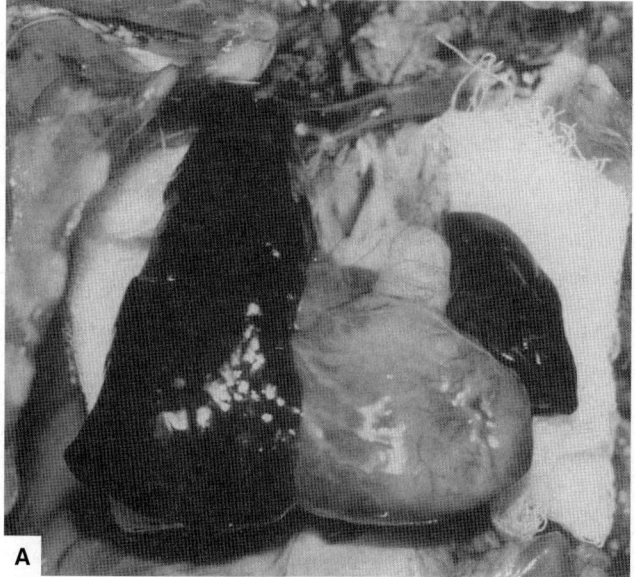 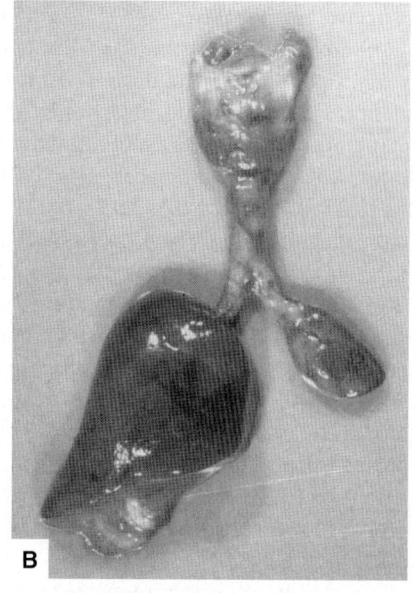

**FIGURE 33-8** Outcome limiting pulmonary hypoplasia. **A.** Autopsy specimen depicting in situ the small left lung and the mediastinal shift of the heart toward the right side. **B.** A fixed explanted specimen emphasizes the bilateral nature of the pulmonary hypoplasia.

result from the numbers and types of physician and allied caregivers involved in CDH care from the prenatal period through early childhood. The vast majority of management options are often not consistent within and among institutions. It is not a surprise that major institutions in the United States using the "best" postnatal surgical and medical management have reported survival outcomes that range from just over 35% to just under 85% for individual groups.

The poor infant survival of less than 50% of CDH cases throughout the 1980s should have been a very powerful impetus to change the wide phase and amplitude swings of postnatal management. Fetal intervention then became the potential mechanism to obviate the persistence of rugged therapeutic individualism and random uncontrolled applications of postnatal management. In other clinical areas, such as pediatric oncology, multidisciplinary consensus regimens that were thoughtfully proposed and tested resulted in dramatic improval of childhood cancer outcomes. Fortunately, out of the apparent ashes of lost opportunities of the last 3 decades of CDH management, a new gold standard for survival has arisen. The report of 92% survival for patients born at the University of Florida Medical Center in Gainesville and 89% survival for patients treated there is a landmark achievement. The true significance of this work, which was presented to the American Surgical Association, was that the authors meticulously duplicated prior work through precise, diligent, and expert imitation of previously reported best practice. Kayes et al in a study of 53 unselected infants with CDH were able to confirm the potential for excellent postnatal survival. This achievement was based on an earlier benchmark established through the innovation of Wung and Stolar. These investigators reversed the status quo of ventilatory and pharmacological management to achieve a 94% survival in a group of infants with CDH. These achievements by 2 separate groups and centers indicate that management uniformity can be achieved, translated, and transplanted into other centers.

Perhaps the most current evaluation of the broadest perspective on survival can be gleaned from the CDH Study Group. The survival rate for the entire Congenital Diaphragmatic Hernia Study Group registry was 67%, and 61% for those receiving ECMO. From data derived from an analysis of 3100 patients, the study group determined that among ECMO-treated children, survivors had a greater estimated gestational age ($38 \pm 2$ vs $37 \pm 2$ weeks; $P < 0.01$), greater birth weights ($3.2 \pm 0.5$ vs $2.9 \pm 0.5$ kg; $P < 0.001$), were less often prenatally diagnosed (53% vs 63%; $P < 0.01$), and were on ECMO for a shorter period of time ($9 \pm 5$ vs $12 \pm 5$ days; $P < 0.001$). Therapy-related variables, including the duration of ECMO, the nature of diaphragmatic repair, and the type of abdominal closure and certain comorbidities, particularly the presence of a concomitant severe cardiac abnormality, were independently associated with outcome. The overall survival reported by this large group of centers interested in the management of CDH should be a more contemporary benchmark for the lowest levels of possible survival for neonatal management of CDH.

Long-term morbidity following intensive postnatal management and rescue with ECMO is emerging as a significant concern. Table 33-2 lists the extensive complications that have been reported. Only with improved survival has the next challenge of morbidity emerged. There is no major series apart from follow-up studies of ECMO-treated infants that has even attempted to correlate prenatal variables with morbidity following survival. The general experience is that markedly improved survival with ECMO has been achieved, but with significant neurologic, pulmonary, and gastroenterologic morbidities. Late deaths are also well described. Few similar studies have been done accounting for significant variabilities in different modalities of ventilatory management.

It is no longer reasonable to assume that CDH infants will have a 50% to 60% mortality. However, 10% to 20% of fetuses surviving to term will have associated severe or lethal associated anomalies. Using the best possible combination of postnatal management, another 10% of neonates suffer mortality directly related to pulmonary hypoplasia and hypertension. Why then is the international figure for survival a further 20% lower than the best series? Ongoing arguments that all centers are equal clearly are inaccurate and unsubstantiated claims. It is reasonable to assume that in the future, a postnatal focus on care and outcome should rapidly result in the expected >75% survival. This can be achieved by duplication of best center practice through internal consolidation and standardization of management. Those centers achieving that result must continue to carefully analyze prenatal variables. Postnatal outcome relative to fetal presentation must also be analyzed with an eye to stratification of the complexity of the patients' neonatal course and functional score throughout infancy and childhood.

## DIAPHRAGMATIC HERNIATION THROUGH THE FORAMEN OF MORGAGNI

There are 3 potential sites for herniation through the sternal attachments of the diaphragm. Two short muscular bands of variable thickness extend from the anterior part of the central tendon to attach to the back of the xiphoid process. Lateral to these bands are narrow triangular openings in the diaphragm that enclose the superior epigastric arteries, veins, and the lymphatics that drain into the anterior phrenic lymph nodes. Each sternocostal hiatus also contains a variable amount of fat and areolar tissue. Occasionally, and particularly in obese individuals, the sternal attachments are also composed of fatty areolar tissue rather than muscular band.

Herniation of abdominal viscera through these potential weakened areas does occur, but is uncommon in children. It is thought that trauma may be an etiologic factor, but developmental defects can also be responsible. A peritoneal sac is invariably present. The protrusion of the sac and the extension of the defect in the diaphragm are usually located to the right because of the presence of the heart and pericardial attachments on the left side. Occasionally, the sac lies behind the sternum or even in free communication with the pericardium. Omentum is frequently present in the sac, but portions of the transverse colon, stomach, or liver may also reside in the hernia. When the entire stomach is involved, it appears in contrast studies to be "upside-down."

The symptoms of the retrosternal hernias vary from feelings of mild substernal pressure or epigastric pain to dyspnea and severe episodic vomiting. Strangulation of the contained viscera is possible, though it rarely occurs. Hematemesis may develop from mucosal congestion when the stomach is present in the hernia.

Chest x-ray is often diagnostic without the need for contrast studies. Operative reduction and repair is generally easily accomplished through the abdomen with interrupted nonabsorbable sutures using open or MIS techniques. In the MIS cases, extracorporeal traction sutures have been shown to allow for tension-free closures.

## TRAUMATIC DIAPHRAGMATIC HERNIATION

The muscular fibers of the diaphragm are arranged in a radial pattern to the top of the 12th rib, while the more medial fibers of the posterior diaphragm arise from the lumbocostal arch, the vertebrocostal trigone, forming a potential weak area. Severe abdominal trauma in infants and children may rupture this triangular space as the result of a sharp increase in the intraabdominal pressure. The thin posterolateral fibers of the diaphragm may also be disrupted. This posterolateral portion is virtually always the area that ruptures with trauma.

Other intraabdominal injuries occur in association with these traumatic posterior hernias. The hernia, however, can exist alone. It is not uncommon that the herniation of abdominal contents into the chest is delayed, occurring within 1 or 2 days, several weeks, or even months later. Since the incidence of strangulation is high in traumatic diaphragmatic hernia, early diagnosis and treatment are essential. Palpation of the posterior diaphragm should always be done in operations for abdominal trauma. Ruptures are much more common on the left side, presumably because the liver tends to diffuse intense localized pressure in the right side. Ultrasound can be used to differentiate fluid from hollow viscera in the chest of those children who are being followed nonoperatively and is therefore useful in resolving the differential diagnosis.

### Operative Repair of Traumatic Hernias

The viscera are withdrawn through an abdominal approach generally used for an exploration following blunt or penetrating trauma. The diaphragm is closed with interrupted sutures inserted at least 1 cm from the edges of the defect. Some surgeons use felt pledgets above the sutures to make the closure more secure, but this is generally unnecessary. The sutures should not be tied too tightly.

When recognition of a traumatic diaphragmatic hernia has been delayed, but the child is otherwise in good health, a transthoracic incision or thoracoscopic approach might be preferable (Fig. 33-9). The open approach should be made through the ninth interspace and permits a transcostal extension of the incision to the abdomen if reduction of the viscera is difficult from above.

In acute situations, pulmonary contusions, head injuries, avulsion of the mesenteric root, rupture of the liver or spleen, and lacerated hollow viscera are frequent concomitant injuries with traumatic diaphragmatic hernia. After such severe abdominal trauma resulting in diaphragmatic rupture, children tend to have fewer of these complicating problems if they survive to reach the hospital.

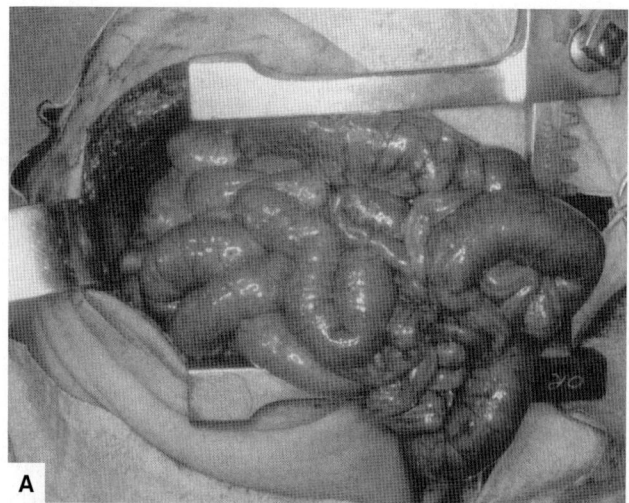

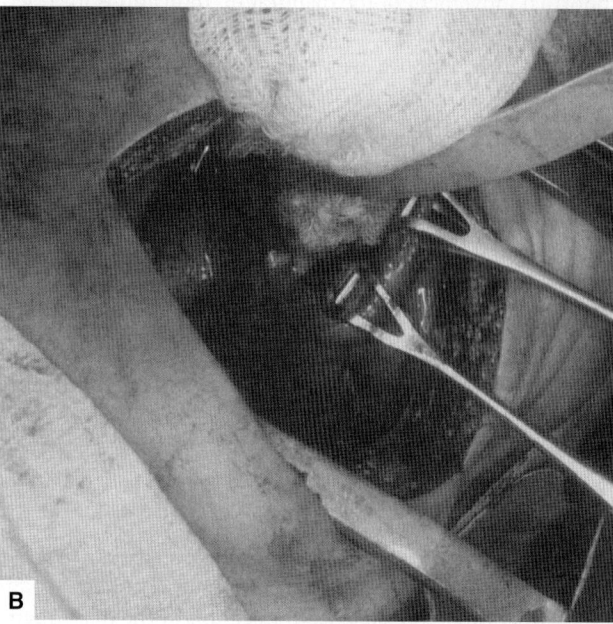

**FIGURE 33-9** Transthoracic repair of a diaphragmatic hernia. **A.** A seventh, eighth, or ninth interspace posterolateral incision is preferred and immediate inspection of herniated intestine is possible. **B.** After careful reduction of herniated viscera, the hernia "rim" is identified and the defect is then closed by a suture technique.

# DIAPHRAGMATIC EVENTRATION

Congenital or acquired abnormalities of the diaphragm and phrenic nerve lead to elevation of part or all of the hemidiaphragm. The resulting diaphragmatic eventration can be unilateral or bilateral. However, it is most commonly found on the left side. The congenital form results in marked muscular thinning of the diaphragm with areas that have poor or absent muscle development between the pleura and peritoneum. Common acquired causes are birth trauma or phrenic nerve injury during cervical or thoracic operations. Occasionally, invasion by tumors or phrenic nerve injury due to pleural or pulmonary infections may be identified as the etiology.

The elevation of the hemidiaphragm is due to increased abdominal pressure resulting in lung compression. Further respiratory difficulties occur due to paradoxical motion generated by negative intrathoracic pressure. With a very high extensive eventration, the differential diagnosis between a CDH and eventration may be impossible without selective imaging such as CT scanning or visualization at operation.

Small eventrations are generally asymptomatic and noted on postoperative or perinatal films. Severe symptoms occur with progressive lung compression and paradoxical diaphragmatic movement. Further, there may be mediastinal movement, which causes tracheal shifts resulting in wheezing or stridor on exertion. Certain gastrointestinal symptoms are occasionally noted such as dysphagia and reflux-type symptoms related to the abnormal position of stomach and esophagus with a left-sided eventration.

Plain x-rays demonstrate the diaphragmatic eventration. The symptoms prompt the diagnostic investigation that subsequently may lead to ultrasound or fluoroscopy to confirm abnormal movement of the diaphragm. Indications for operation include the presence of symptoms. Repair should also be considered for those eventrations that cause considerable lung compression that persists after phrenic nerve trauma. A paresis of the phrenic nerve may take 6 to 9 months to recover; however, recovery after a year's period of observation is usually not achievable.

There have been reports suggesting a link between maternal/fetal β-hemolytic streptococcal infection and diaphragmatic hernia and eventration. Antenatal diagnosis in 1 infant with a subsequent β-hemolytic streptococcal pulmonary infection demonstrated a diaphragmatic eventration in the perinatal period. There is no direct evidence that this infection leads to either diaphragmatic disruption or phrenic nerve damage.

## Surgical Management

Those infants with bilateral eventration may require mechanical ventilation before successful plication of the diaphragm. Other patients will be symptomatic, but not require ventilation preoperatively and most often will not require ventilation postoperatively.

The procedure is designed to fix the paralyzed or atrophic diaphragm in the low thoracic position to initially prevent paradoxical movement and shift in the mediastinum. The variability of procedures and independent preferences for

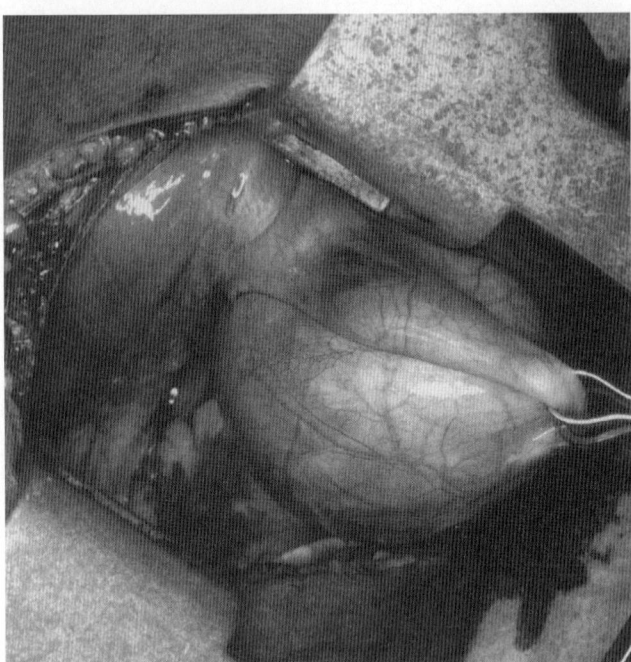

**FIGURE 33-10** Transthoracic exposure of a diaphragmatic eventration. A sixth, seventh, or eighth posterolateral thoracotomy incision is made. The tented-up diaphragm is easily visualized with corresponding lung compression and thoracic space loss secondary to intraabdominal visceral protrusion into the chest.

the methods of repair make comparisons almost impossible. Abdominal and thoracic open and MIS approaches have all been described. For the open thoracic exposure, the sixth or seventh interspace is entered, the inferior pulmonary ligament is divided, and the distribution of the branches of the phrenic nerve identified (Fig. 33-10).

Four to 6 rows of 2-0 Prolene sutures for children and 3-0 Prolene sutures for infants are placed from the antrolateral to the posterior medial position (Fig. 33-11). In the thin attenuated diaphragm, pledgeted sutures are usually not required as the bulk of tissue prevents any cutting effect from the suture material. As in the repair of the diaphragmatic hernia, achievement of the convex position is all that is required. Complete flattening of the diaphragm has led to serious complications and an increased incidence of recurrence. Once all the sutures are placed, the configuration of the repair should resemble a sail that is about to be reefed. Sutures are then tied individually and sequentially from medial to lateral. A small chest tube is placed and attached only to seal water.

Several important facets of the operation should be remembered regardless of the approach. Sutures should not be blindly placed through the diaphragm. This potentially jeopardizes infradiaphragmatic structures, which may be caught in the repair causing either hemorrhage or microperforation to elevated large or small bowel. The distribution of the phrenic nerve must be carefully identified and avoided. Additionally, removal of the attenuated diaphragmatic muscle does not always need to be performed. The need for exposure is not great, therefore just as this operation lends itself to video-assisted techniques, surgeons definitely should consider performing muscle-sparing thoracotomies.

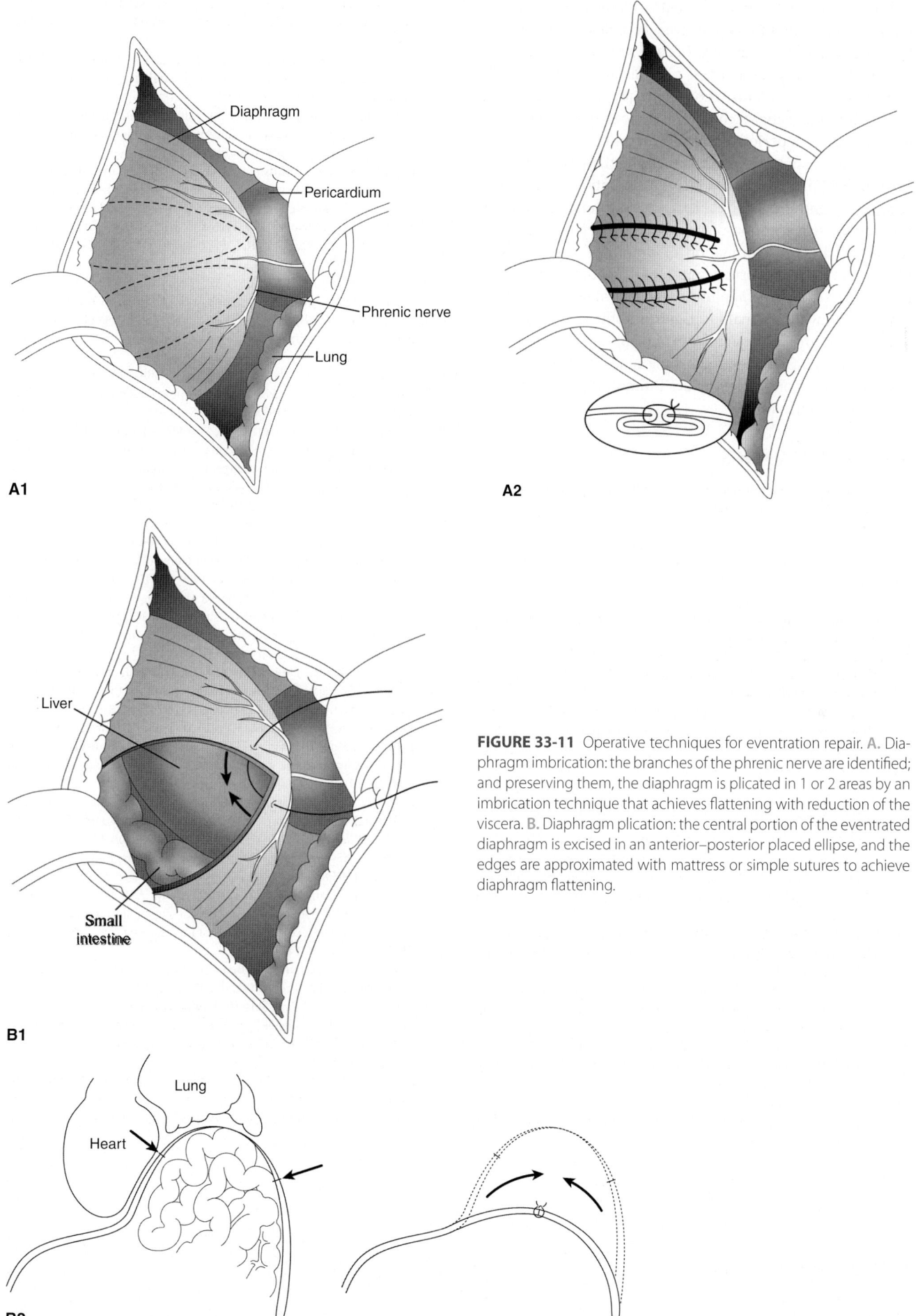

**A1**

- Diaphragm
- Pericardium
- Phrenic nerve
- Lung

**A2**

**B1**

- Liver
- Small intestine

**FIGURE 33-11** Operative techniques for eventration repair. **A.** Diaphragm imbrication: the branches of the phrenic nerve are identified; and preserving them, the diaphragm is plicated in 1 or 2 areas by an imbrication technique that achieves flattening with reduction of the viscera. **B.** Diaphragm plication: the central portion of the eventrated diaphragm is excised in an anterior–posterior placed ellipse, and the edges are approximated with mattress or simple sutures to achieve diaphragm flattening.

- Lung
- Heart

**B2**

The postoperative management is straightforward and usually results in immediate near complete expansion of the lung. Chest tube removal occurs within the next 24 to 48 hours and early discharge is possible after adequate pain control. For those infants who have required bilateral repair, a transabdominal approach may be more effective and is usually followed by a period of improved ventilation allowing for more rapid weaning from mechanical ventilation.

Complications of plication include disruption of the repair, recurrent eventration, and even rupture secondary to adjacent fibromuscular disruption or tension in the repair. Successful repair will lead to elimination of pulmonary compression with restoration of normal pulmonary volumes and functional reserve. Successful plication will eliminate paradoxical motion following normal localization of the diaphragms. In long-term studies, measurements of diaphragmatic thickness showed that plicated diaphragms maintained growth in proportion to the contralateral side. Pulmonary function tests also become normalized.

## SELECTED READINGS

Albanese CT, Lopoo J, Goldstein RB, et al. Fetal liver position and perinatal outcome for congenital diaphragmatic hernia. *Prenat Diagn* 1998;18(11):1138–1142.

Azarow K, Messineo A, Pearl R, Filler R, Barker G, Bohn D. Congenital diaphragmatic hernia—a tale of two cities: the Toronto experience. *J Pediat Surg* 1997;32(3):395–400.

Clark RH, Hardin WD Jr, Hirschl RB, et al. Current surgical management of congenital diaphragmatic hernia: a report from the Congenital Diaphragmatic Hernia Study Group. *J Pediatr Surg* 1998;33(7):1004–1009.

Fauza DO, Wilson JM. Congenital diaphragmatic hernia and associated anomalies: their incidence, identification, and impact on prognosis. *J Pediatr Surg* 1994;29(8):1113–1117.

Finer NN, Tierney A, Etches PC, Peliowski A, Ainsworth W. Congenital diaphragmatic hernia: developing a protocolized approach. *J Pediatr Surg* 1998;33(9):1331–1337.

Flake AW, Crombleholme TM, Johnson MP, Howell LJ, Adzick NS. Treatment of severe congenital diaphragmatic hernia by fetal tracheal occlusion: clinical experience with fifteen cases. *Am J Obstet Gynecol* 2000;183:1059–1066.

Geary MP, Chitty LS, Morrison JJ, Wright V, Pierro A, Rodeck CH. Perinatal outcome and prognostic factors in prenatally diagnosed congenital diaphragmatic hernia. *Ultrasound Obstet Gynecol* 1998;12(2):107–111.

Gross WE, Ladd RE. Congenital diaphragmatic hernia. *N Engl J Med* 1940;223:917.

Harrison MR, Adzick NS, Flake AW, et al. Correction of congenital diaphragmatic hernia in utero: VI. Hard-earned lessons. *J Pediatr Surg* 1993;28:1411–1417.

Harrison MR, Adzick NS, Bullard KM, et al. Correction of congenital diaphragmatic hernia in utero VII: a prospective trial. *J Pediatr Surg* 1997;32(11):1637–1642.

Harrison MR, Keller RL, Hawgood SB, et al. A randomized trial of fetal endoscopic tracheal occlusion for severe fetal congenital diaphragmatic hernia. *N Engl J Med* 2003;349(20):1916–1924.

Harrison MR, Mychaliska GB, Albanese CT, et al. Correction of congenital diaphragmatic hernia in utero IX: fetuses with poor prognosis (liver herniation and low lung-to-head ratio) can be saved by fetoscopic temporary tracheal occlusion. *J Pediatr Surg* 1998;33(7):1017–1022. Discussion 1022.

Karamanoukian HL, O'Toole SJ, Rossman JR, et al. Can cardiac weight predict lung weight in patients with congenital diaphragmatic hernia? *J Pediatr Surg* 1996;31(6):823–825.

Kays DW, Langham MR Jr, Ledbetter DJ, Talbert JL. Detrimental effects of standard medical therapy in congenital diaphragmatic hernia. *Ann Surg* 1999;230(3):340–348. Discussion 348–351.

Lipshutz GS, Albanese CT, Feldstein VA, et al. Prospective analysis of lung-to-head ratio predicts survival for patients with prenatally diagnosed congenital diaphragmatic hernia. *J Pediatr Surg* 1997;32(11):1634–1636.

Metkus AP, Filly RA, Stringer MD, Harrison MR, Adzick NS. Sonographic predictors of survival in fetal diaphragmatic hernia. *J Pediatr Surg* 1996;31(1):148–151. Discussion 151–152.

Morin L, Crombleholme TM, D'Alton ME. Prenatal diagnosis and management of fetal thoracic lesions. *Semin Perinatol* 1994;18(3):228–253.

Pfleghaar KM, Wapner RJ, Kuhlman KA, Spitzer AR. Congenital diaphragmatic hernia: prognosis and prenatal detection. *Fetal Diagn Ther* 1995;10(6):393–399.

Pusic AL, Giacomantonio M, Pippus K, Rees E, Gillis DA. Survival in neonatal congenital hernia without extracorporeal membrane oxygenation support. *J Pediatr Surg* 1995;30(8):1188–1190.

Reyes C, Chang LK, Waffarn F, Mir H, Warden MJ, Sills J. Delayed repair of congenital diaphragmatic hernia with early high-frequency oscillatory ventilation during preoperative stabilization. *J Pediatr Surg* 1998;33(7):1010–1014. Discussion 1014–1016.

Rowe MI, Uribe FL. Diaphragmatic hernia in the newborn infant: blood gas and pH considerations. *Surgery* 1971;70:758–761.

Somaschini M, Locatelli G, Salvoni L, Bellan C, Colombo A. Impact of new treatments for respiratory failure on outcome of infants with congenital diaphragmatic hernia. *Eur J Pediatr* 1999;158(10):780–784.

Steimle CN, Meric F, Hirschl RB, Bozynski M, Coran AG, Bartlett RH. Effect of extracorporeal life support on survival when applied to all patients with congenital diaphragmatic hernia. *J Pediatr Surg* 1994;29(8):997–1001.

Thebaud B, Mercier JC, Dinh-Xuan AT. Congenital diaphragmatic hernia. A cause of persistent pulmonary hypertension of the newborn which lacks an effective therapy. *Biol Neonat* 1998;74(5):323–336.

Thebaud B, Azancot A, de Lagausie P, et al. Congenital diaphragmatic hernia: antenatal prognostic factors. Does cardiac ventricular disproportion in utero predict outcome and pulmonary hypoplasia? *Intens Care Med* 1997;23(10):10062–10069.

VanderWall KJ, Kohl T, Adzick NS, Silverman NH, Hoffman JI, Harrison MR. Fetal diaphragmatic hernia: echocardiography and clinical outcome. *J Pediatr Surg* 1997;32(2):223–225. Discussion 225–226.

Vanamo K. A 45-year perspective of congenital diaphragmatic hernia. *Br J Surg* 1996;83(12):1758–1762.

vd Staak FH, de Haan AF, Geven WB, Doesburg WH, Festen C. Improving survival for patients with high-risk congenital diaphragmatic hernia by using extracorporeal membrane oxygenation. *J Pediatr Surg* 1995;30:(10):1463–1467.

Wilson JM, Fauza DO, Lund DP, Benacerraf BR, Hendren WH. Antenatal diagnosis of isolated congenital diaphragmatic hernia is not an indicator of outcome. *J Pediatr Surg* 1994;29(6):815–819.

Wilson JM, Lund DP, Lillehei CW, Vacanti JP. Congenital diaphragmatic hernia—a tale of two cities: the Boston experience. *J Pediatr Surg* 1997;32(3):401–405.

Wung JT, Sahni R, Moffitt ST, Lipsitz E, Stolar CJ. Congenital diaphragmatic hernia: survival treated with very delayed surgery, spontaneous respiration, and no chest tube. *J Pediatr Surg* 1995;30(3):406–409.

# PART IV

## ABDOMINAL DISEASE

# CHAPTER 34

# Abdominal Wall Defects: Omphalocele and Gastroschisis

*Saleem Islam*

## KEY POINTS

1. Omphalocele and gastroschisis are distinct clinical entities.

2. Associated anomalies and chromosome abnormalities are common in omphalocele, and rare in gastroschisis.

3. Prenatal diagnosis is common in both entities, which aids in planning for delivery and early postnatal care treatment.

4. Early delivery and cesarean section delivery methods are not warranted.

5. The surgical management is highly individualized for each entity, and depends on the overall condition of the newborn, associated anomalies, eviscerated organs, size of abdominal cavity, gestational age, and comorbidities among others.

6. Overall survival for infants with gastroschisis is over 90%, but is less for infants with omphalocele because of associated anomalies or chromosome abnormalities.

Abdominal wall defects represent one of the most common congenital surgical problems encountered in neonates. While often discussed as one topic, gastroschisis and omphalocele are different and distinct entities; in this chapter, we will be discussing them separately in terms of management and outcomes.

## EMBRYOLOGY

The embryologic etiology of congenital abdominal wall defects is not completely understood, and remains a controversial subject. Most authorities currently believe that gastroschisis and omphalocele are embryologically distinct.

In gastroschisis, the abdominal wall defect is usually located to the right of an intact umbilical cord. The eviscerated contents are not enclosed in a sac. Older hypotheses include rupture of the amniotic membrane at the base of the cord, abnormal regression of the right umbilical vein, and disruption of the vitelline artery resulting in ischemia at the base of the umbilicus. Currently, the ventral body folds theory that suggests failure of migration of the lateral folds (more frequent on the right side) is most accepted. This would make the gastroschisis defect occur early in gestation and prior to development of an omphalocele. Due to the increasing incidence of gastroschisis, there have been a number of possible causative factors that have been considered including tobacco, environmental exposures, lower maternal age, and low socioeconomic status, all suggested by epidemiologic studies but not proven.

Omphaloceles are not considered to occur as a failure of lateral body wall closure. As these defects will have the umbilical cord coming off the defect itself, it is thought to result from a failure of the intestinal loops to return to the abdomen following the period of physiologic herniation during the 6th to the 10th week of gestation. Etiologically, there are not many teratogens that are implicated in omphalocele causation.

## ASSOCIATED ANOMALIES

Gastroschisis has been considered to be an isolated defect with occasional presence of intestinal atresia (10%-12%). However in a recent review of the literature, a number of anomalies were noted with gastroschisis including cardiac, limb, renal, and occasional chromosomal. These were very few cases, but they suggest that in some patients there may be a genetic component to the defect.

Infants with omphalocele have a high incidence of associated conditions that can significantly impact outcome. These include isolated cardiac or renal anomalies, chromosomal defects (trisomies 13, 18, and 21), and recognizable syndromes such as prune belly, Beckwith–Wiedemann, and pentalogy of Cantrell. Patients with a pentalogy syndrome have (Fig. 34-1) an epigastric or higher position of the defect, while a hypogastric or lower defect (Fig. 34-2) occurs when an omphalocele complicates cloacal exstrophy. It is imperative to identify potentially lethal anomalies associated with omphalocele either prenatally or immediately after birth so as to anticipate perioperative complications and counsel the parents of affected infants.

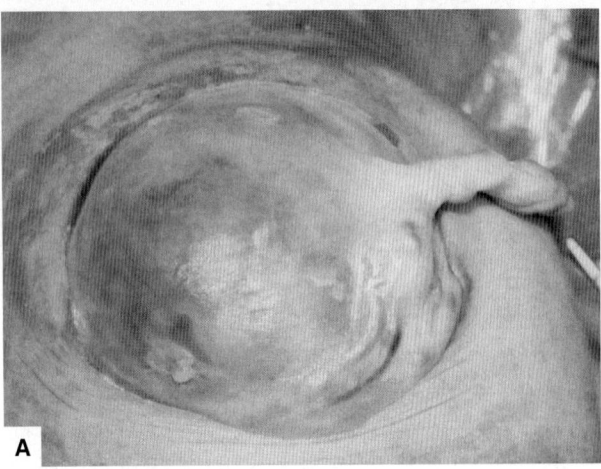

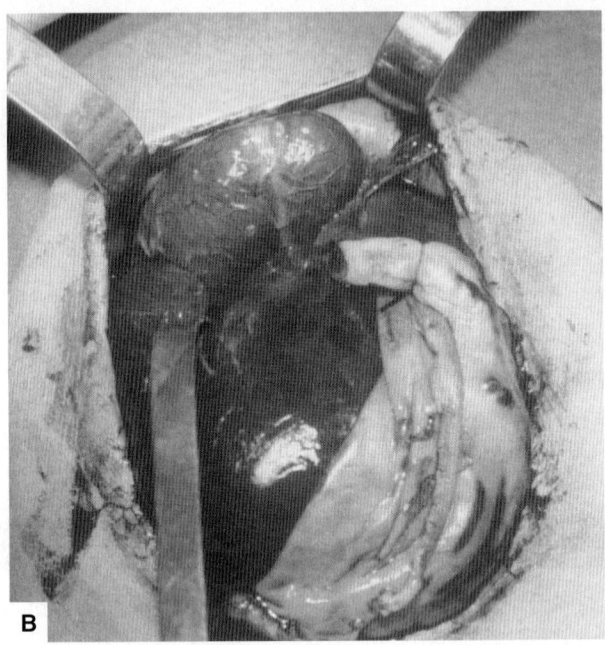

**FIGURE 34-1** **A.** An omphalocele where a prominent pulsation was present at its cephalic end. **B.** This baby had pentalogy of Cantrell with an exposed heart just beneath the omphalocele membrane.

## EPIDEMIOLOGY

The incidence of abdominal wall defects is increasing, primarily due to the rise in gastroschisis. This increase has been reported worldwide over the past few decades. In the United States, the reported rates are 3.9 to 4.6 per 10,000 births. The rates of omphalocele have declined in the recent past especially in developed nations, due to prenatal diagnosis and termination of pregnancy. This represents a significant "hidden mortality" in omphaloceles, and has been documented in multiple reports that studied the fate of prenatally diagnosed defects.

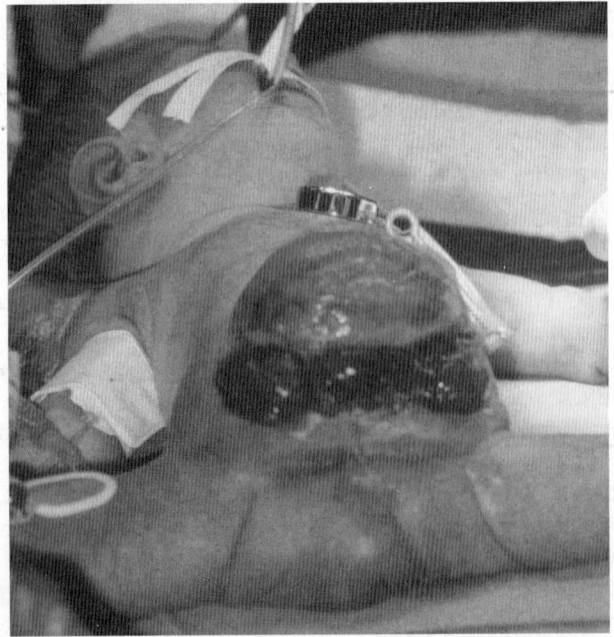

**FIGURE 34-2** An omphalocele cephalad to the exposed bowel and bladder plates of classic cloacal extrophy.

## PRENATAL DIAGNOSIS AND MANAGEMENT

### Gastroschisis

A majority of gastroschisis are now diagnosed prenatally. Suspicion for an abdominal wall defect is noted with an elevated maternal serum α-fetoprotein, which would trigger a high-level ultrasound. Current ultrasound and MRI technology allow for more accurate diagnosis and other structural defects can be noted, including renal, limb, or cardiac. After making the diagnosis of gastroschisis, more intensive follow-up ultrasounds are done, biweekly until the 30th week of gestation and then weekly until delivery. Ultrasound markers that are considered as poor prognostic indicators include gastric dilation, bowel thickening, and dilation. There is controversy over the importance of bowel dilation as a marker for intestinal damage—typically dilation of the intestine over 17 mm is considered worrisome for the development of a bowel obstruction. It is important to note that a majority of fetuses with gastroschisis will have poor growth and have evidence of Intrauterine growth retardation (IUGR). The significance of this finding is not well understood at this time. "Vanishing" gastroschisis has also been described, and is thought to represent a small defect that closes off prior to delivery with an intestinal atresia where the bowel may have suffered vascular compromise (Fig. 34-3). This may result in severe congenital short bowel syndrome.

### Omphalocele

Similar to gastroschisis, most omphaloceles are diagnosed prenatally. The prenatal management of omphaloceles is distinct from gastroschisis. This is due to the fact that there is a much higher incidence of associated anomalies and chromosomal defects. After making a diagnosis of omphalocele

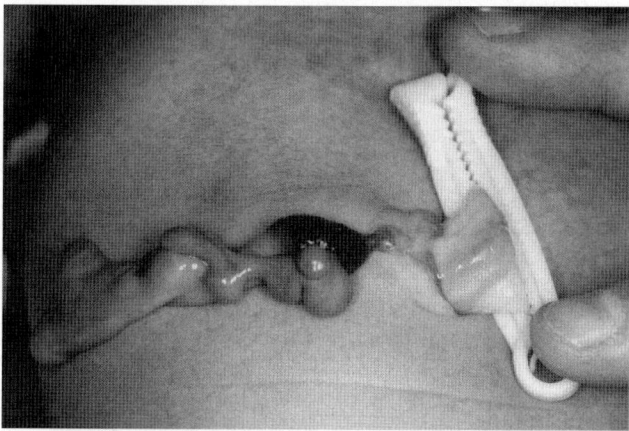

**FIGURE 34-3** The rare gastroschisis variant where the protruding bowel apparently experienced in utero ischemic necrosis. Also termed vanishing gastroschisis due to the closure of the defect in utero.

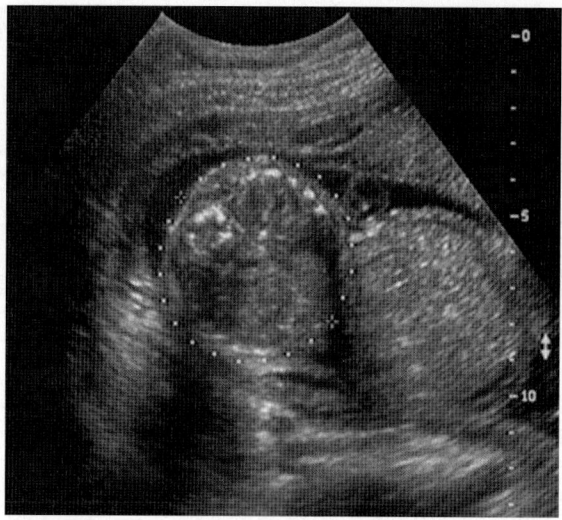

**FIGURE 34-4** Prenatal ultrasound image depicting a large omphalocele. The *white dots* are encircling the herniated contents.

(Fig. 34-4), most parents will be offered an amniocentesis to determine the chromosomes. Diagnosing severe cardiac defects with ultrasound is critical. In a study from Norway, it was noted that two thirds of patients opted for termination of pregnancy after a diagnosis of omphalocele was made, which highlights the increasing number of families who take this option. In some cases, the omphalocele defect gets smaller during gestation, which may represent an involution, becoming a hernia of the cord. A special situation is that of a ruptured omphalocele. These defects may be difficult to distinguish from a gastroschisis, but should be suspected when there is significant herniation of the liver, or associated cardiac, renal, or limb abnormalities.

## PERINATAL MANAGEMENT

### Gastroschisis

Studies have shown that it is the deleterious effects of amniotic fluid on the fetal intestine that causes the thickened and matted appearance and dysfunction. Animal studies documented an improvement by amniotic fluid exchange and preterm delivery, which prompted human trials at preterm delivery. Recent data strongly suggest that there is no benefit to preterm delivery on the intestine, and that there is a detriment in outcomes from a pulmonary standpoint. Therefore, elective preterm delivery has fallen out of favor. In the case where there is ultrasonographic evidence of gastric or intestinal dilation, preterm delivery may be recommended.

There is controversy over the route of delivery as well. Most studies would suggest that there is no benefit to the fetus with gastroschisis to have a cesarean delivery. However, a large proportion of abdominal wall defects are offered elective cesarean section deliveries. Some centers prefer a scheduled c-section to allow for more planned management of the neonate. Our recommendations are that in the absence of an obstetric indication (CP disproportion, placenta previa, etc), a term vaginal delivery be performed.

Once the neonate is delivered, standard care is performed. Routine endotracheal intubation is not required for gastroschisis. The bowel is assessed and covered with warm saline-soaked gauze, and placed into a plastic covering that covers the torso and legs. This allows safe transport to the neonatal unit, especially if that unit is at another facility, by minimizing fluid and heat losses from the uncovered bowel. If there is obvious ischemia or twisting of the intestine, this may need more urgent evaluation and correction. All neonates with gastroschisis have some intravascular volume depletion and rapid intravenous access is obtained and fluid resuscitation instituted. In addition, broad-spectrum intravenous antibiotics are started and gastric decompression performed.

### Omphalocele

The recommendation for omphalocele is a term, vaginal delivery unless otherwise indicated by fetal or obstetric indications. In cases where the defect is particularly large, or ruptured with extensive liver herniation, cesarean section may be indicated to avoid liver injury.

For patients with an intact amnion lined sac, postnatal management consists of covering the membrane with petrolatum, or saline-soaked gauze. The neonate should receive standard airway management. Urgent evaluation with echocardiogram and renal ultrasound should be obtained. If the karyotype is not obtained prenatally, or if the neonate appears to have characteristic features, chromosomal analysis should be sent. The results may have a significant impact on further management.

## SURGICAL MANAGEMENT

### Gastroschisis

Surgical options for gastroschisis repair are less complex and varied compared to omphalocele. The reason is the more uniform size of the defect and absence of liver and

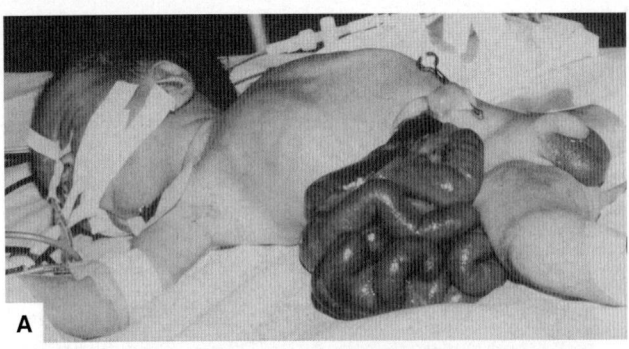

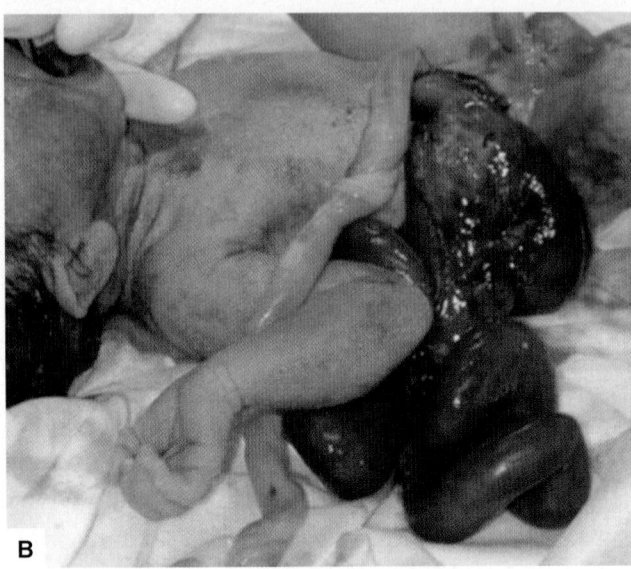

**FIGURE 34-5 A.** The right paramedian gastroschisis defect is associated with variable degrees of visceral protrusion. Thickened foreshortened bowel filled with meconium. **B.** Newborn gastroschisis with matted and ischemic bowel. The ischemia resolved with slight detorsion and suspension in a silo.

other organs involved (Fig. 34-5). In general, we divide gastroschisis into "simple" and "complex" based on the presence or absence of intestinal ischemia, bowel atresia, perforation, or significant associated anomaly. Management and outcomes vary significantly based on the defect being simple or complex. All neonates will require the use of total parenteral nutrition (TPN) for a variable length of time and will require some form of central access either a peripherally inserted central catheter (PICC) or a surgically placed line.

## Silo Placement with Staged Closure

Schuster first used a silo for gastroschisis in 1967, which involved sewing Teflon sheets to the abdominal wall with serial reduction of the contents. This was modified later by using silastic and not closing the skin over the silo. In the 1990s, the preformed silo became available that changed the treatment algorithm significantly. The use of the silo has become commonplace in most centers and preferred due to the ease of use, gentle reduction with potentially less abdominal compartment syndrome and intestinal ischemia.

The silo comes in multiple ring sizes (2-15 cm available—4-6 cm most common used sizes). The rings either have a metal spring inside them or are otherwise elastic (Fig. 34-6). After initial assessment of the newborn and establishment of IV access, the intestine is closely examined and the meconium may be gently reduced through the anus by manipulation of the colon. The size of silo is chosen based on the defect—the ring must completely fit inside the abdominal cavity. If the defect is too small or is thought to be causing

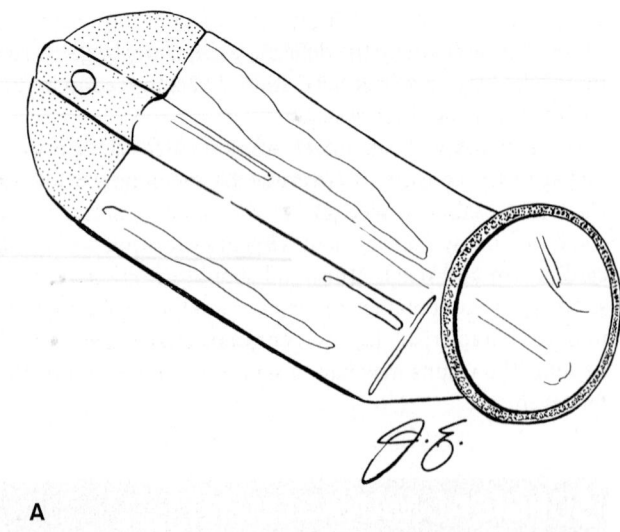

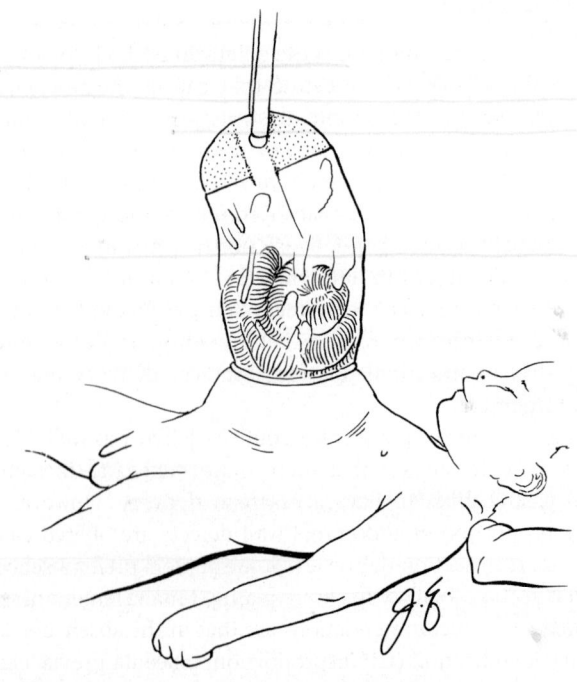

**FIGURE 34-6 A.** Pre-made silastic silo with a wire-ring covered base. **B.** Silo positioned and suspended.

intestinal ischemia, immediate enlargement of the fascial defect is indicated to remove the tourniquet effect (Fig. 34-7). After lubricating the silo with warm saline, the intestines are gently placed into the bag and the ring is bent and gradually placed into the abdomen. One must ensure that nothing is trapped between the abdominal wall and the ring. A dressing is placed at the base of the silo and the top is suspended with gentle tension. Over the course of the next 2 to 5 days, the silo is gradually reduced by twisting from the top down, taking care not to exert high pressure (Fig. 34-8). The silo placement and reduction is usually performed in the neonatal intensive care unit (NICU) under sedation, thus intubation is not required. When the contents are completely reduced, the silo is removed and the fascial defect closed, usually in the operating room. In some cases, a formal closure is not performed and a dressing with the cord remnant and adherent gauze may allow gradual spontaneous closure.

## Primary Closure

In cases deemed suitable, patients may have complete reduction of the intestines and primary fascial closure performed shortly after birth. In a multicenter, randomized trial of silo versus primary closure, no significant differences were noted in outcome; however, the study was underpowered and did not meet accrual targets. While there are some reports of bedside immediate reduction, most centers perform it in

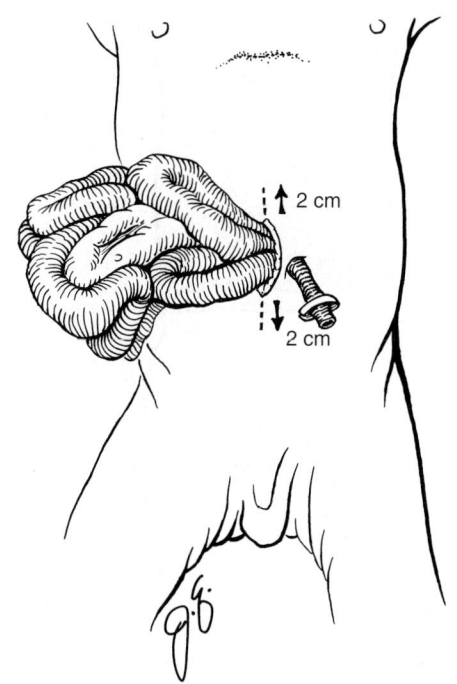

**FIGURE 34-7** Vertical incisions extended the right paramedian opening to permit stretching, reduction, and primary fascial and skin closure. In the event that primary closure proves difficult, the broadened base of the defect created by the incision(s) permits application of an appropriate silo for delaying staged closure.

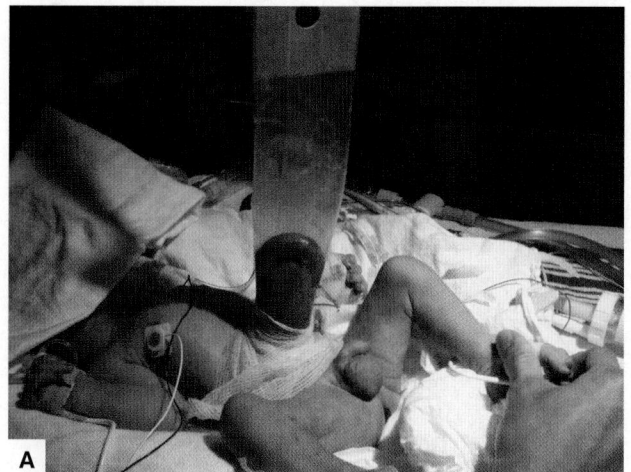

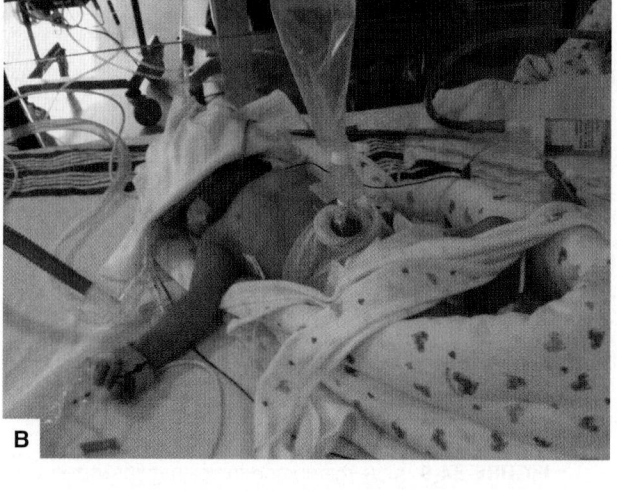

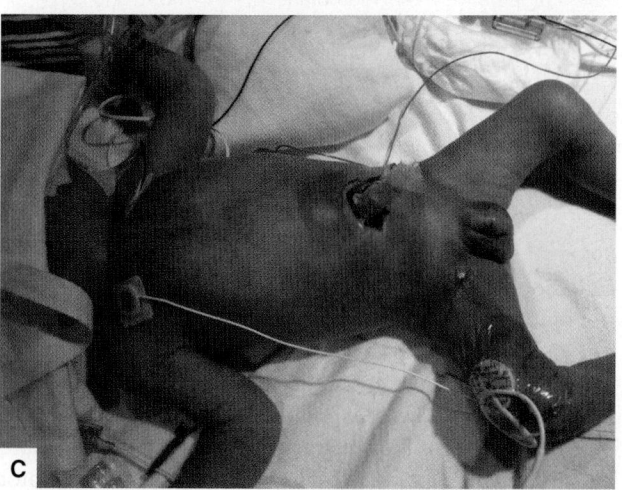

**FIGURE 34-8** **A.** Newborn with initial 5 cm silo placed at bedside. Intestines clearly visible. **B.** Same patient with silo reduction performed. Note the ties on the twisted portion of the silo and the reduction of viscera into abdominal cavity. **C.** Complete silo reduction of the viscera. The silo was removed and the defect closed primarily without any issues.

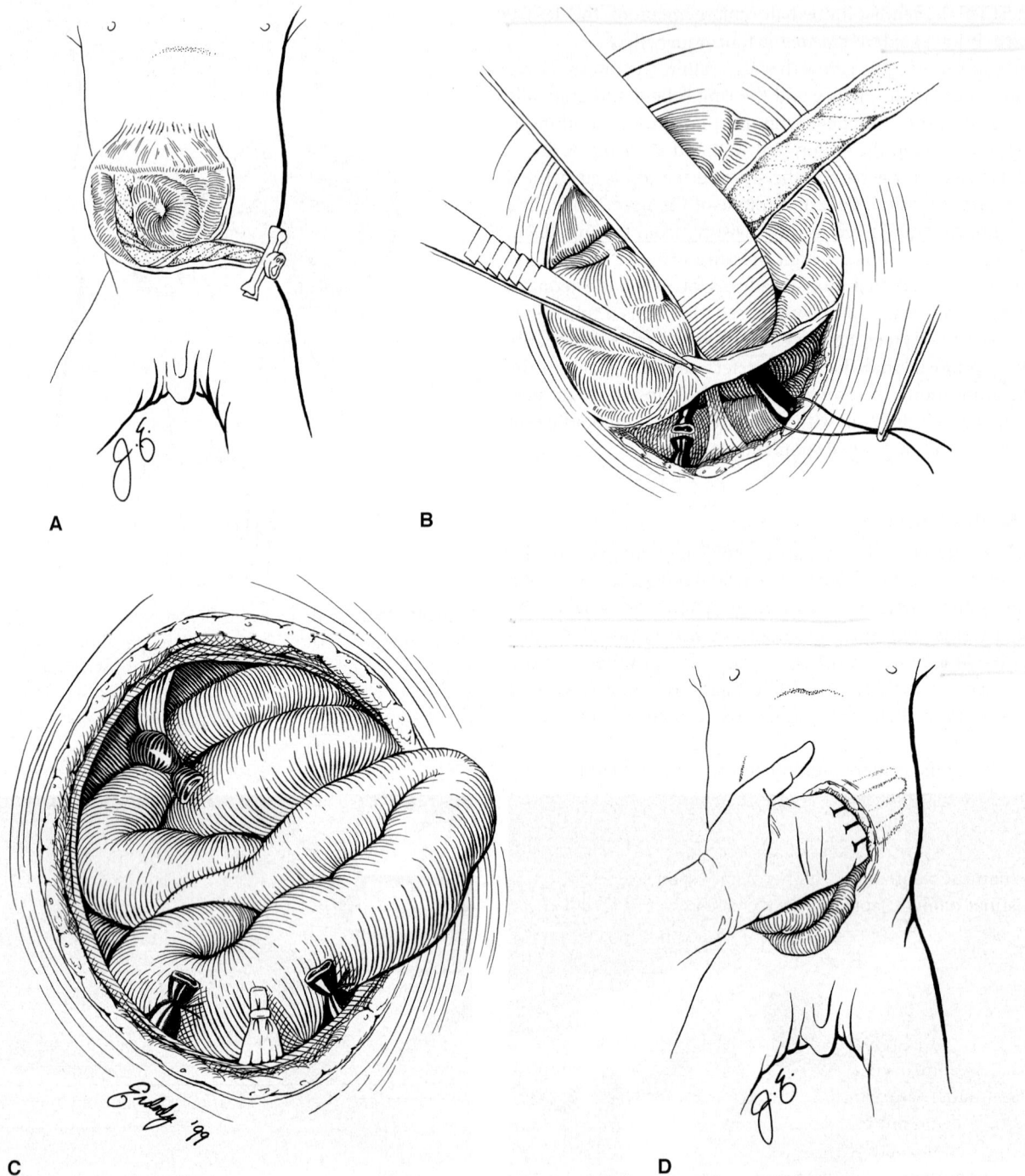

**FIGURE 34-9 A.** A membrane-intact medium-sized omphalocele. Preoperatively the membrane is kept moist and clean by warm saline-soaked gauze or by coverage of the infant's torso by a bowel bag containing warm sterile saline. **B.** The junction of the membrane with skin and fascia is incised and the umbilical arteries and umbilical vein are identified, isolated, and ligated. **C.** The membrane has been removed and the umbilical vessels ligated and divided. **D.** Manual stretching of the abdominal wall musculature is best accomplished by placing a finger from each hand into the peritoneal cavity and distracting them to stretch the muscle. This maneuver is repeated in 4 quadrants around the defect being careful to protect the liver at its ligamentous attachments.

the operating room under general anesthesia to facilitate the closure. After careful inspection of the bowel, and evacuation of meconium as described previously, the intestines are gently and gradually reduced with forceps, taking care not to cause a serosal injury, which is more likely in very matted bowels. The defect may need to be extended cephalad and caudad if it is too small to allow reduction (Fig. 34-9).

Occasionally, thickened and edematous loops of bowel may not reduce despite stretching of the peritoneum. In this event, safe closure is not feasible, and a silo should be placed for a more gradual reduction. In addition, assessment of the intraabdominal pressure should be done prior to closure by monitoring the peak inspiratory and mean airway pressures, and arterial blood gasses for the development of a respiratory

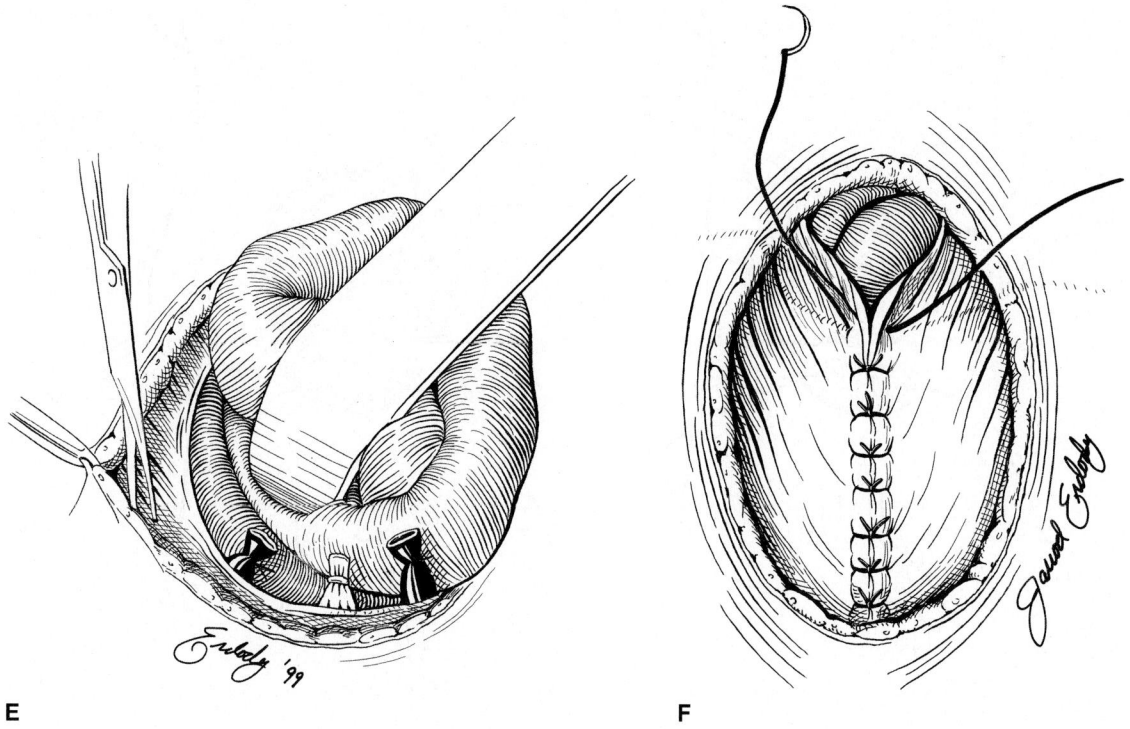

E

F

**FIGURE 34-9** *(Continued)* **E.** The skin is elevated and sharply dissected off at the underlying fascia in a circumferential fashion. **F.** The fascia is closed with interrupted sutures, and the degree of wound tension dictates suture selection.

acidosis. Some centers monitor intragastric or bladder pressures as a marker of intraabdominal pressure. If the pressure is too high, then the viscera should be extruded and a silo placed. There are a number of reports that describe prolonged mechanical ventilation, higher ventilation pressures, and intestinal damage from primary closure. However, there are also other series that have favorable outcomes from the same procedure, which indicates proper patient selection plays an important role in deciding primary versus silo closure.

The early management of infants with initially nonreducible gastroschisis plus intestinal atresia (complicated gastroschisis) is controversial. Our approach has been to support these infants with parenteral nutrition, close the abdomen after a silo, and not perform an initial ostomy. A more definitive procedure may then be undertaken 3 to 6 weeks later under more favorable conditions when the intestine is less matted. If an ostomy proves necessary, it should be located lateral to the silo. In some cases, we have been able to perform an ostomy and decompress the proximal intestine so that a complete reduction can be performed and the ostomy may be located at the umbilicus to avoid additional scars. One advantage of an initial ostomy is the possibility of instituting early enteral feeds and avoiding parenteral nutrition-induced cholestasis and limiting proximal intestinal dilation. In cases where there is an intestinal atresia, one must be cognizant of the fact that there may be associated short bowel syndrome due to loss of intestine.

## Omphalocele

A number of options exist for the surgical management of the infant with an omphalocele, based on the size of the

defect and the child's underlying clinical state. An important consideration is the size of the defect in relation to the neonate. The definition of "giant" or "large" omphaloceles is not standardized according to body weight, which leads to discrepancy in the literature and an inability to compare the treatment strategies coherently. That is why there are a multitude of different techniques described for treating the problem. The defect may be repaired immediately after birth, in a staged fashion in the neonatal period, or in a delayed fashion.

### Immediate Repair

The treatment of choice for small- to medium-sized omphaloceles is primary closure in the early neonatal period as a single operation (Fig. 34-9). After establishment of general anesthesia, the omphalocele sac is typically excised to the level of the skin and fascia. The umbilical vessels and urachus must be carefully ligated (Fig. 34-9C). The abdominal contents are thoroughly examined and the abdominal cavity manually enlarged by stretching (Fig. 34-9D). The defect may need to be extended 2 to 3 cm at its superior and inferior areas to allow for a more tension-free linear closure. Skin flaps are raised and the fascia is then closed with interrupted sutures of absorbable material (Fig. 34-9E and F). Closure of the skin may also include a formal umbilicoplasty to create a central scar.

Primary fascial closure of larger abdominal wall defects can lead to a sudden increase in intraabdominal pressure that may compromise ventilation and impair venous return from the lower limbs, intestines, and kidneys. Reported complications of early fascial closure in infants with both gastroschisis and omphalocele include hypotension, bowel ischemia,

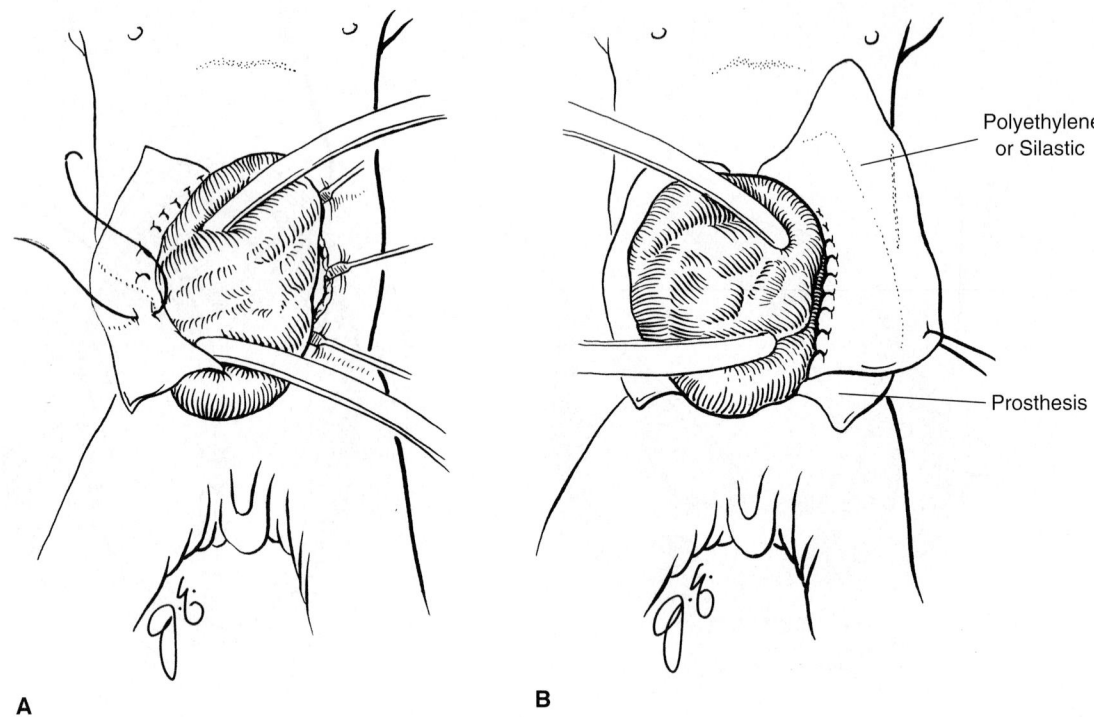

Polyethylene
or Silastic

Prosthesis

**A**

**B**

**FIGURE 34-10** **A, B.** After removal of the membrane, the skin is undermined circumferentially a short distance exposing the musculofascial margins of the defect. A sheet(s) of silicone-coated dacron is then sutured to the fascial ring with a running stitch of nonabsorbable suture.

respiratory, and renal failure. As mentioned previously, measurement of abdominal pressure may be used as a predictor of the success of primary closure. In our experience, we have closely observed both the ventilatory and hemodynamic status of the infant during closure as a means to avoid serious complications.

## Staged Neonatal Repair

In infants who do not tolerate early primary closure, or in those whom closure is not attempted, a number of options exist. Most defects can be closed during the first week of life using a modified silo technique. This procedure involves excision of the sac, possible enlargement of the incision, and the creation of minimal skin flaps. Next, a reinforced silastic sheet is sutured to the fascial margins (Fig. 34-10A and B) and to itself to create a silo (Fig. 34-10C and D). The silo is gradually reduced in size by daily compression of its contents into the abdomen until the viscera are fully reduced (Fig. 34-10E). Such incremental reduction can be performed over 7 to 10 days in the NICU without general anesthesia and with the infant's status closely monitored (Fig. 34-10F and G). Final fascial and skin closure is then accomplished in the operating room. In some cases, where the liver is not intimately attached to the sac, the preformed silos as described for gastroschisis may be used instead. Only the risk of infection and silo disruption limit the time span of this technique. The amnion inversion technique as initially described by De Lorimer involves using the existing omphalocele covering as a modified silo and gradually reducing the defect with eventual excision of the superficial part of the membrane and fascial closure. As with the silastic silo, this can usually be accomplished in the NICU and completed in 7 to 10 days of life (Fig. 34-11).

In some cases, the defect may not allow fascial closure without compromise of the abdominal contents and compartment syndrome. In those cases, a variety of prosthetic materials have been utilized to bridge the gap. Goretex has been used as a completely synthetic material that does not become incorporated, while biologic choices such as Alloderm®, Surgisys®, and Permacol® that allow vascular ingrowth have also been used. Skin closure is then performed over the patch after raising flaps. Skin breakdown and patch infection are the biggest risks from this repair.

## Delayed Repair

In some infants with a large or giant omphalocele, closure in the neonatal period is not feasible and a prolonged or multistaged repair is necessary. There may be significant cardiac lesions that preclude a major operative intervention in the neonatal period. In the classic Gross type repair that was first described in the 1950s and 1960s, a large ventral hernia is created by removing the sac and approximating mobilized skin flaps to protect the abdominal viscera (Fig. 34-12A–C). Six to 12 months later, primary closure is considered. The amnion inversion technique described in the previous section may also be used to obtain skin coverage and leave a large ventral hernia to be repaired later in life.

Complete initially nonoperative techniques are useful adjuncts to the management of large omphaloceles. Synthetic coverings such as Op-Site or antibiotics such as silver sulfadiazine, povidone–iodine, or triple antibiotic ointment can be topically applied to the sac to induce eschar formation with subsequent epithelialization from the margins of the defect. This technique may be combined with a modified pressure dressing that encourages the development of

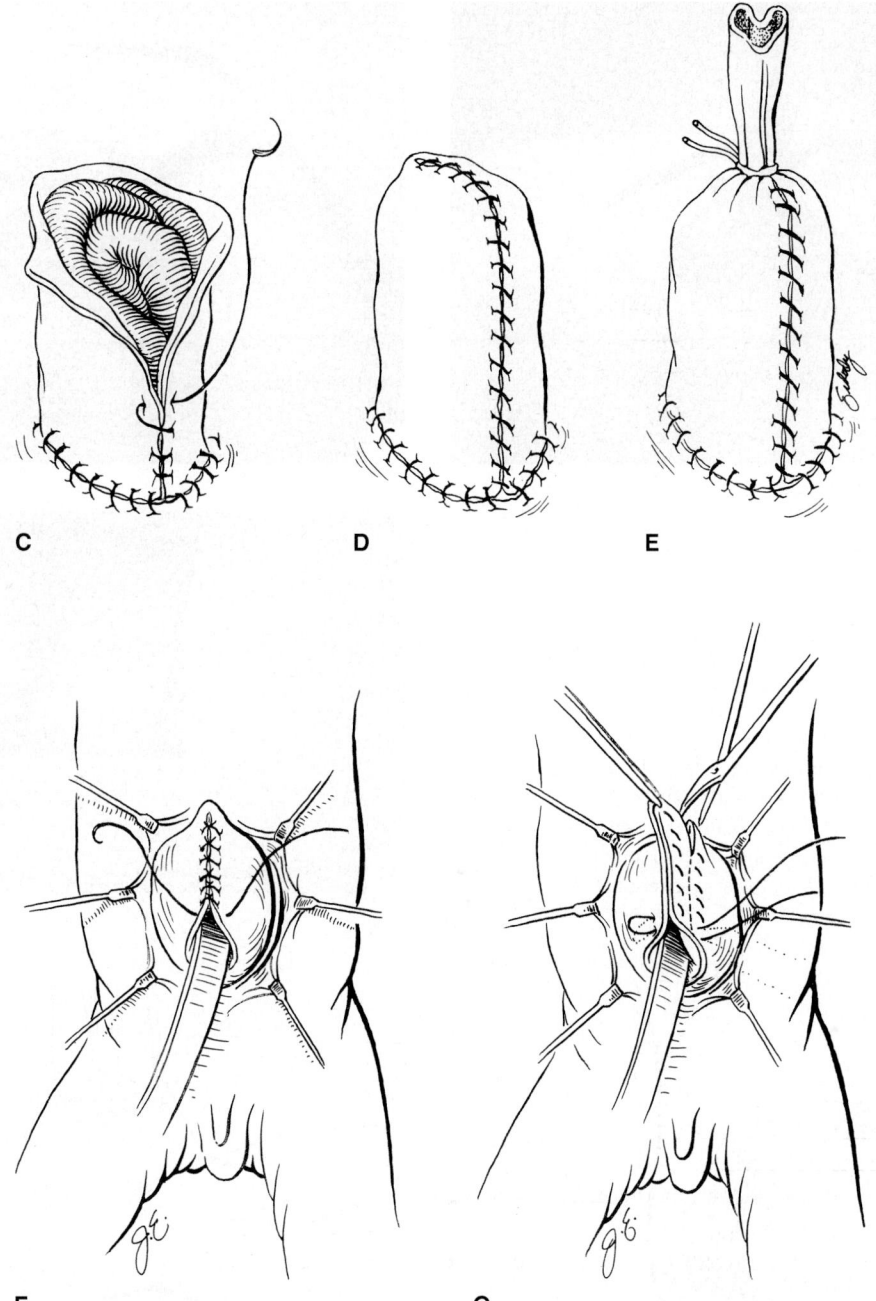

**FIGURE 34-10** (*Continued*) **C, D.** The membrane sheets are then sutured to one another to complete the silo. As the silo is fashioned, it is imperative that it be broader at its base than at the apex to facilitate eventual reduction. **E.** An alternate technique of apex silo closure is to apply an umbilical tape around the apex, which permits opening and inspection of silo content. **F, G.** The silo content is reduced at the bedside by a daily or every other day placement of imbricating sutures. In ventilated babies, the use of the neuromuscular blockade may facilitate this reduction. Eventually when the silo is flattened, intraoperative silo removal and fascial and skin closure follows.

abdominal domain and in some cases results in a remarkable partial or complete closure of the defect (Fig. 34-13A and B). In most cases, however, the result is a large ventral hernia amenable to delayed closure with acceptable results. This technique is usually reserved for those infants with giant omphalocele and severe underlying medical problems that preclude early primary closure. In some cases, abdominal domain remains problematic to achieve and alternative means such as tissue expanders have been utilized to help create space for reduction of the herniated contents at the time of final closure.

## Ruptured Omphalocele

The management of a neonate with a ruptured omphalocele presents a particularly difficult challenge for pediatric surgeons. If the defect is particularly large, the problem is compounded. Initial management consists of resuscitation and antibiotics as for gastroschisis and temporary coverage with a bowel bag. In most cases, a silo is created from silastic or other materials and sutured to the fascia. The superior midline part of the defect is often the most challenging as the liver and hepatic veins are adjacent and do not allow much room to place the sutures. The immediate goal is to obtain epithelial

479

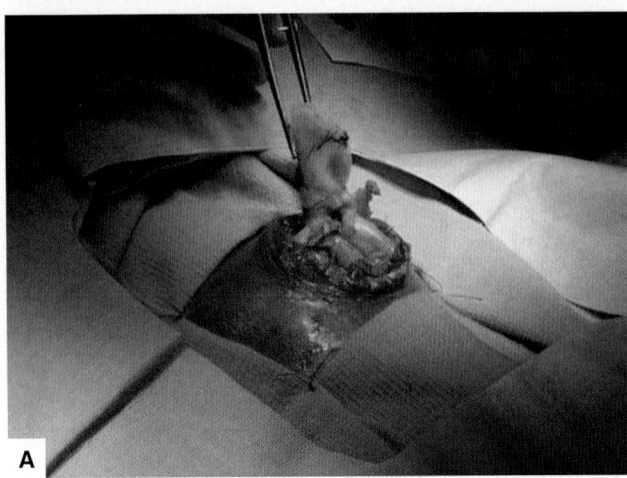

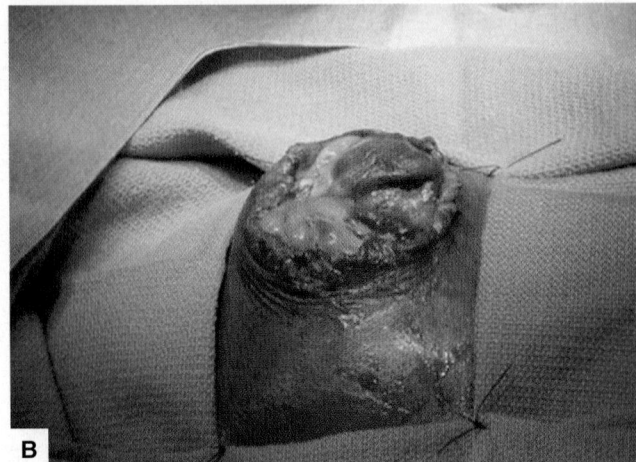

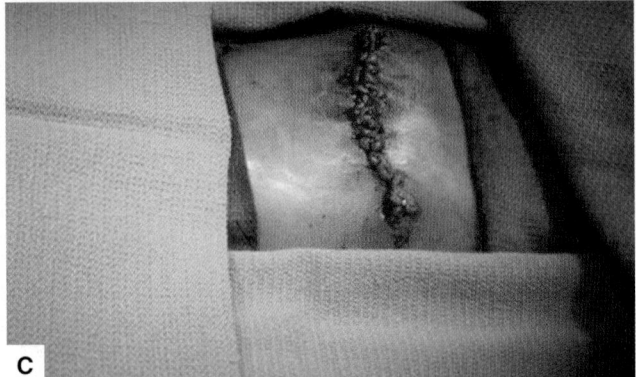

**FIGURE 34-11** **A.** Omphalocele after staged neonatal reduction with silo. The silo has already been sequentially reduced and is ready for removal and final fascial closure. **B.** After silo removal. In this case, the amnion had been left intact and inverted under the silo. **C.** The fascia and skin closed easily after the staged reduction.

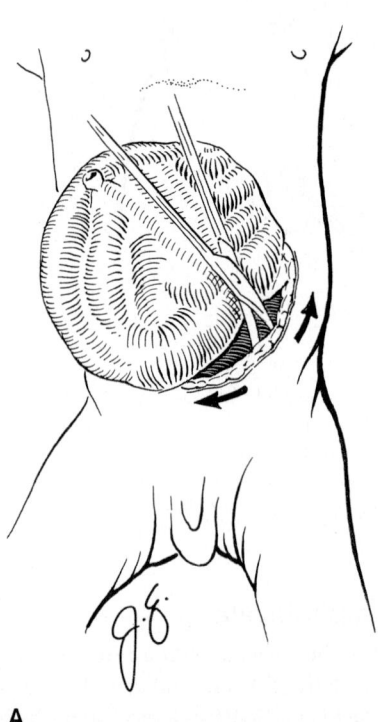

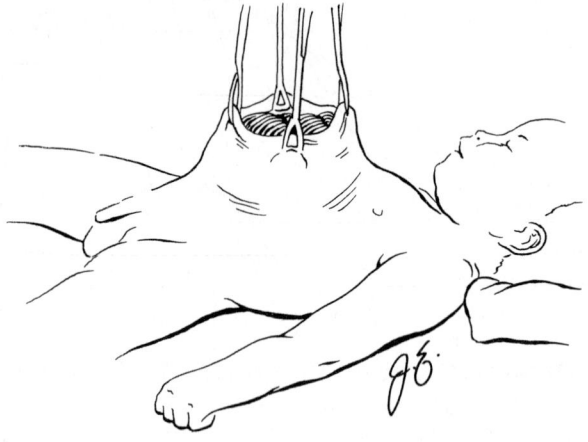

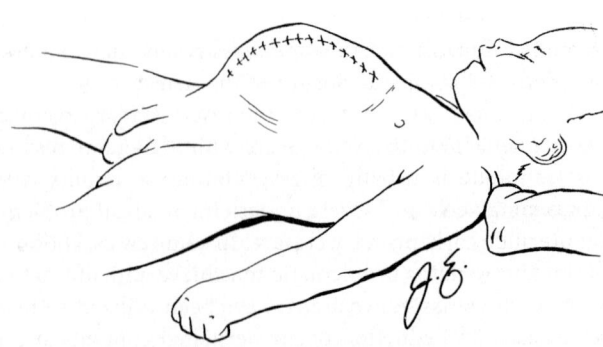

**FIGURE 34-12** Staged closure of an omphalocele. **A.** Skin flaps are elevated by significant undermining off of the anterior abdominal wall, at times extending the dissection to the midaxillary line. **B.** Either the original omphalocele membrane is left intact or it is reinforced with a synthetic patch sutured to the musculofascial margin of the defect. **C.** The skin flaps are then approximated in the midline over the defect. At a later date, the "ventral hernia" is closed.

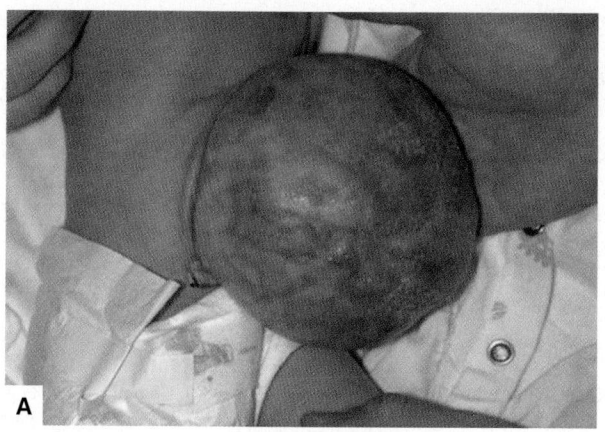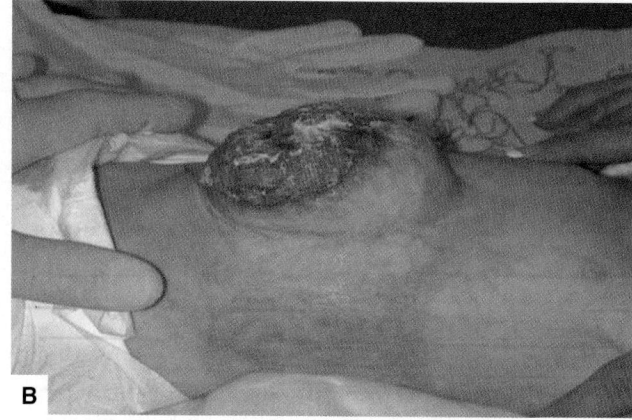

**FIGURE 34-13** **A.** Large omphalocele being managed with dressing changes using antibiotic ointment and povidone–iodine solution allowing epithelialization. **B.** Same patient after 2 months of the dressing changes and gentle pressure wrapping. Note the significant reduction. The defect flattened out and continued to close over the next 2 months.

coverage, which may require skin grafting or techniques to allow epithelialization.

## POSTOPERATIVE MANAGEMENT

### Gastroschisis

The most critical issue postoperatively in patients with gastroschisis after closure (delayed or primary) is to be cognizant that high abdominal pressures may develop and lead to complications. Abdominal compartment syndrome may cause respiratory difficulties, intestinal ischemia, and impair renal function. It is not necessary to keep these neonates intubated postoperatively, especially after a delayed closure in which there is no acute intestinal reduction. Some cases may be allowed to close by secondary intention by placing the umbilical cord stump over the defect with a sterile dressing and, thus, not require general anesthesia.

Postoperative antibiotics are continued for approximately 3 to 5 days in uncomplicated cases as prophylaxis, although this is not required. It takes a variable amount of time from the closure (2-4 weeks) for intestinal motility to improve, and during this time the neonate must be supported by parenteral nutrition. Once the oro- or nasogastric tube volume diminishes and meconium is passed, feeds may be started and gradually increased. Promotility agents are of no benefit in this period. Care must be taken to monitor liver enzymes and function for the development of cholestatic liver disease. In cases when the period of ileus or dysmotility exceeds 3 to 4 weeks, suspicion for an intestinal atresia is raised, and contrast enema followed by a small bowel follow through study may be necessary.

In about 10% of cases, there is a necrotizing enterocolitis clinical picture with sepsis, pneumatosis intestinalis, and abdominal distention. Therapy consists of bowel rest, parenteral nutrition, broad-spectrum antibiotics, and routine plain abdominal radiography to detect perforation. Most of these cases will resolve with medical management; however, those who require an operation end up with reduced bowel length and a longer hospital stay.

### Omphalocele

Postoperative management of a patient with an omphalocele is determined by the type of repair: neonatal, staged, or delayed. One must consider the impact of associated anomalies, in particular cardiac, in the postoperative care. As has been discussed for gastroschisis, in primary or staged neonatal closures, the development of an abdominal compartment syndrome is of particular concern in the first 24 to 48 hours. If a mesh closure was utilized, there is concern for an infectious complication, and antibiotics are typically continued for 3 to 7 days postoperatively as prophylaxis.

Most neonates remain intubated and on mechanical ventilation for a few days after an omphalocele repair if the defect is large, due to respiratory issues that arise from lack of proper muscle development around the defect.

Intestinal dysmotility is not a prominent feature after an intact omphalocele repair as the intestines are protected from amniotic fluid during gestation, thus allowing early enteral nutrition.

In patients with a delayed repair, dressing changes of the epithelializing defect may take a few weeks to months to complete. This may be transitioned to home during this time period with close follow-up.

## OUTCOMES

### Gastroschisis

The outlook for infants with abdominal wall defects has improved significantly in the past few decades, primarily due to improved neonatal care and the development of parenteral nutrition. Overall survival to discharge in gastroschisis exceeds 95%, and in simple gastroschisis it is 98% or higher. A subset of gastroschisis patients may demonstrate manifestations of the short bowel syndrome. This may be secondary to anatomic shortening or dysmotility. Patients with an atresia or intestinal ischemia-related issues predominate in this group, and they account for the largest number of children on the intestinal transplant list.

Most children with gastroschisis exhibit significant catch-up growth throughout the first year of life. All abdominal wall defect patients have malrotation by definition and may develop a volvulus or bowel obstruction, thus parents and caregivers need to be cautioned.

## Omphalocele

Survival in omphalocele is closely related to the associated defects and, in patients with severe cardiac or chromosomal abnormalities, the outlook remains poor. The overall mortality rate in omphalocele is approximately 34%; however, infants free of major cardiac or chromosomal defects have a 94% survival rate. Pulmonary hypoplasia and chronic lung disease can occur in these patients and those with large defects require prolonged respiratory care and have tracheostomies performed.

Gastroesophageal reflux is seen in up to 50% of survivors and is particularly severe in infants with large omphaloceles who undergo staged repair. Reoperation may be necessary for patients with postclosure abdominal wall hernias.

## SELECTED READINGS

Boutros J, Regier M, Skarsgard ED, et al. Is timing everything? The influence of gestational age, birth weight, route, and intent of delivery on outcome in gastroschisis. *J Pediatr Surg* 2009;44:912–917.

Brantberg A, Blaas HGK, Haugen SE, Eik-Nes SH. Characteristics and outcome of 90 cases of fetal omphalocele. *Ultrasound Obstet Gynecol* 2005;26:527–537.

Drewett M, Michailidis GD, Burge D. The perinatal management of gastroschisis. *Early Hum Dev* 2006;82:305–312.

Frolov P, Alali J, Klein MD. Clinical risk factors for gastroschisis and omphalocele in humans: a review of the literature. *Pediatr Surg Int* 2010;26:1135–1148.

Islam S. Clinical care outcomes in abdominal wall defects. *Curr Opin Pediatr* 2008;20:305–310.

Kidd JN, Jackson RJ, Smith SD, Wagner CW. Evolution of staged versus primary closure of gastroschisis. *Ann Surg* 2003;237:759–765.

Klein MD. Congenital defects of the abdominal wall. In: Grosfeld JL, O'Neill JA, Coran AG, et al., eds. *Pediatric Surgery*. 6th ed. Philadelphia: Mosby Elsevier; 2006:1157–1171.

Lao OB, Larison C, Garrison MM, et al. Outcomes in neonates with gastroschisis in US children's hospitals. *Am J Perinatol* 2010;27:97–101.

Minkes RK. Abdominal wall defects. In: Oldham KT, Colombani PM, Foglia RP, Skinner MA, eds. *Principles and Practice of Pediatric Surgery*. Philadelphia: Lippincott; 2005:1103–1120.

Pastor AC, Phillips JD, Fenton SJ, et al. Routine use of a silastic spring loaded silo for infants with gastroschisis: a multicenter randomized controlled trial. *J Pediatr Surg* 2008;43:1807–1812.

Puligandla PS, Janvier A, Flageole H, et al. Routine cesarean delivery does not improve the outcome of infants with gastroschisis. *J Pediatr Surg* 2004;39:742–745.

Schwartz MZ, Timmapuri SJ. Gastroschisis. In: Spitz L, Coran AG, eds. *Operative Pediatric Surgery*. 6th ed. London: Hodder Arnold; 2006:267–278.

Weber TR. Omphalocele. In: Spitz L, Coran AG, eds. *Operative Pediatric Surgery*. 6th ed. London: Hodder Arnold; 2006:257–266.

Whitehouse JS, Gourlay DM, Masonbrink AR, et al. Conservative management of giant omphalocele with topical povidone iodine and its effect on thyroid function. *J Pediatr Surg* 2010;45:1192–1197.

# CHAPTER 35

# Umbilical and Supraumbilical Disease

*Evan Kokoska and Thomas R. Weber*

## KEY POINTS

1. Umbilical hernia frequently resolves without operation.

2. When needed, persistent fascial defects ( umbilical and epigastric hernias) should be repaired before 4 to 5 years of age.

3. Urachal and vitelline remnants often present with infection, and should be excised after the infection has resolved.

Umbilical abnormalities are among the most common reasons a child is referred to the pediatric surgeon. Periumbilical disorders that might require operation include abnormal granulation tissue, fistulas, masses, or herniation. While most umbilical conditions appear relatively nonacute, proper and concise diagnosis and management are necessary to avoid potentially serious, albeit infrequent, morbidity.

## ANATOMIC CONSIDERATIONS

Basic knowledge of the anatomical basis of umbilical disease is essential. The umbilical ring forms during the fourth week of gestation as a result of infolding of the lateral folds and migration and differentiation of the muscular and fascial mesoderm. The umbilical ring represents the transition from epidermis to amnion and contains the umbilical vessels, allantois, and vitelline (omphalomesenteric) duct. Primitive gut is connected to the yolk sac via the vitelline duct. The urachus is a vestigial canal between the allantoic stalk and the superior portion of the bladder (Fig. 35-1). During normal development, epithelium from both the urachus and the vitelline duct close as a result of apoptotic cell death. The involuted urachus becomes the median umbilical ligament. Absent or incomplete apoptosis gives rise to a range of urachal or vitelline ductal abnormalities including diverticuli, sinuses, cysts, or fistulae. Thus, there exists a delicate balance between cell proliferation and apoptotic cell death during this critical stage in fetal development.

The midgut, following initial herniation through the umbilical ring (as depicted in Fig. 35-1), returns to the abdominal cavity during the 10th week of gestation. Proper closure of the umbilical ring occurs as the lateral body wall (somatopleure) folds medially around the umbilical vessels, yolk stalk, and allantoic remnants. The rudimentary rectus abdominis muscles approach one another and, with subsequent narrowing, form the linea alba. Following birth and cord separation, the obliterated umbilical arteries (medial umbilical ligaments) also contribute to umbilical ring closure as their elastic fibers serve as a sphincter mechanism allowing for slow orifice contraction.

## SPECIFIC DISORDERS

### Umbilical Hernia

The first umbilical hernia repair was mentioned by Celsus in the early first century. However, the majority of cases up to the 18th century were managed with abdominal binders. In 1890, Nota reported the first series of children undergoing hernia reduction and purse-string closure of the fascial defect. Mayo recommended transverse fascial closure in 1901 and his technique remains most frequently utilized today.

Umbilical hernia, defined as visible protrusion on straining or crying, develops as a result of incomplete ring closure and is very common in young children. The incidence ranges from 10% to 25% and is increased in girls, African American children, and low-birth-weight babies. Umbilical hernias have been associated with numerous syndromes and conditions including hypothyroidism, mucopolysaccharidosis, Down syndrome, Beckwith–Wiedemann syndrome, and exomphalos–macroglossia syndrome.

The majority of umbilical hernias close spontaneously at 3 to 4 years of age. However, there are no good long-term prospective studies that document spontaneous hernia closure rates with regard to various sized defects. Hernia straps or buttresses, in addition to potentially irritating local skin, actually delay closure by alleviating the local stress that is necessary for promoting muscular and fascial strengthening.

Bowel incarceration or strangulation is extremely rare and is the only absolute indication for urgent surgical repair. Relative surgical indications take into account the 2 factors most associated with a decreased likelihood of spontaneous closure: age greater than 3 to 5 years and fascial defect size greater than 1.5 to 2 cm. Some surgeons also promote elective repair

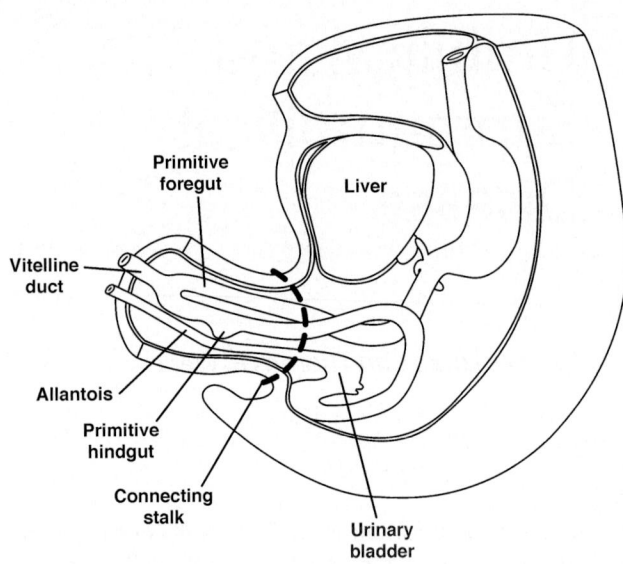

**FIGURE 35-1** Umbilicus and associated structures at 6 weeks' gestation. The embryo is attached to the developing placenta by a connecting stalk comprised of extraembryonic mesoderm through which the allantois, umbilical vessels, and vitelline duct pass.

when there is a need for general anesthesia during concurrent minor otolaryngologic, orthopedic, or other procedures.

Our surgical technique is as follows (Fig. 35-2A–F). A semicircular or "smile" incision is made along a skin crease inferior to the umbilicus. The umbilical cicatrix is raised by incising subcutaneous fat, and the underlying tissue is cleared from the defect and hernia sac. Extreme care must be taken to avoid a "button hole" injury to the skin. The management of the hernia sac is controversial. Our approach is to circumferentially incise and open the neck of the sac. Omentum is ligated and excised if necessary, and the sac is trimmed back to strong fascia. Other surgeons prefer to dissect the sac anterior to the skin and invert it unopened into the abdominal cavity.

The fascial defect is closed with interrupted stitches in a transverse fashion utilizing long-lasting absorbable suture with the knots in a buried position. It may be technically easier to place all sutures before tying them. The dermis/cicatrix below the umbilicus is sutured to fascia for cosmetic restoration using absorbable suture. Skin is closed with subcuticular suture, a liquid adhesive and steri-strips are placed, and the wound is dressed with a pressure bandage. Repair of strangulated hernia is the same as for elective cases. Complications

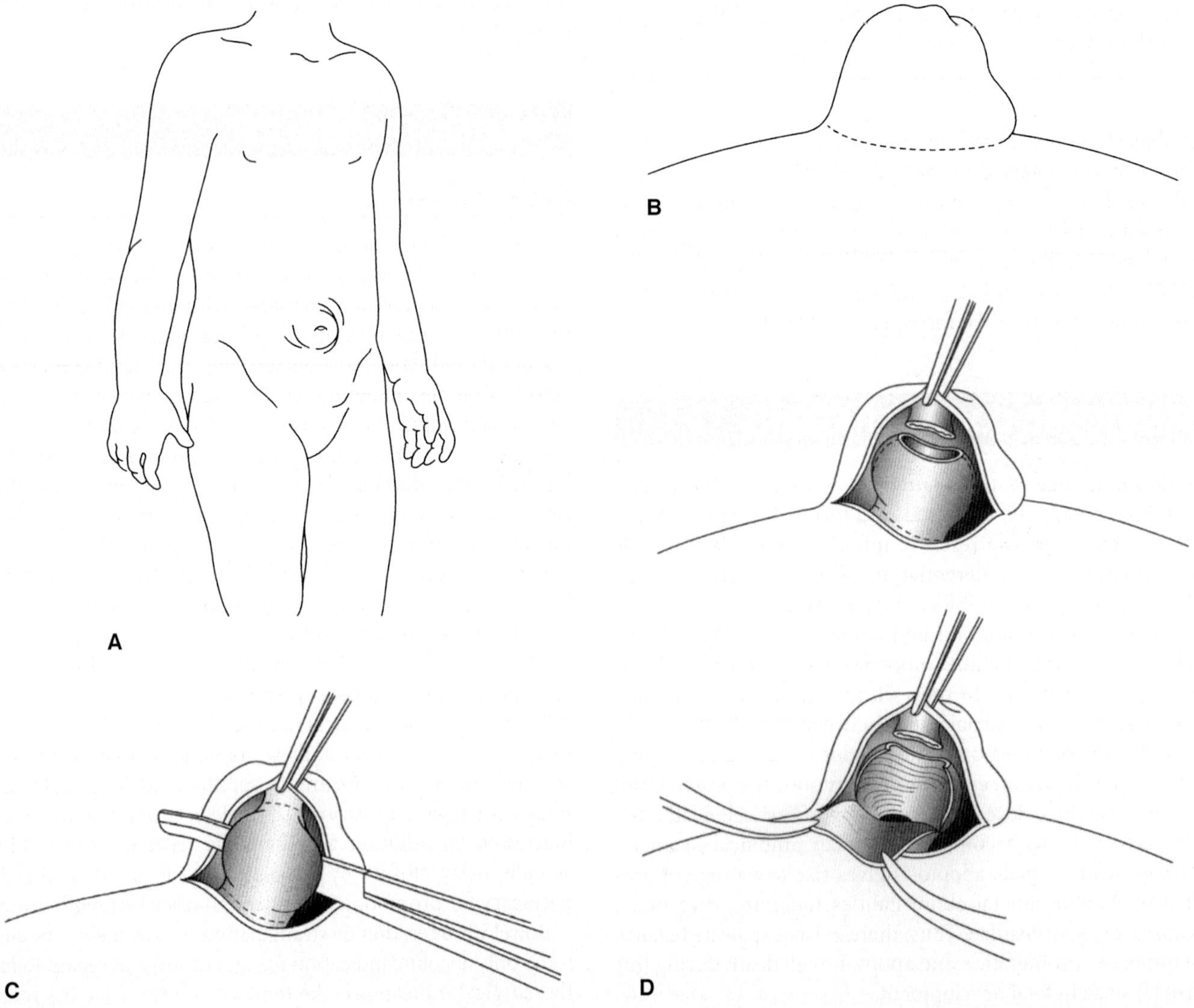

**FIGURE 35-2** Surgical repair of umbilical hernia (**A**). A semicircular or "smile" incision is made along a skin crease inferior to the umbilicus (**B**). The neck of the hernia sac is circumferentially incised and opened (**C**). Omentum is ligated and excised if necessary, and the sac is trimmed back to strong fascia (**D**). The fascial defect is closed with buried, interrupted stitches in a transverse fashion utilizing long-lasting absorbable suture.

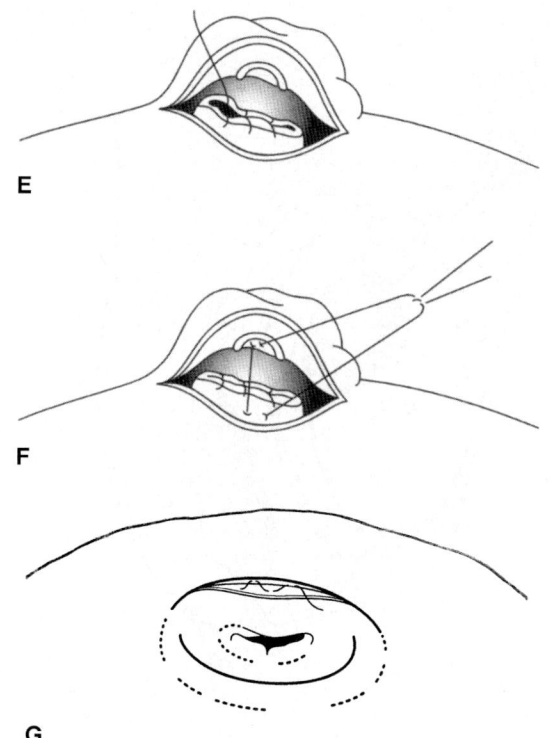

**E**

**F**

**G**

**FIGURE 35-2** (*Continued*) (**E**). The dermis/cicatrix below the umbilicus is sutured to fascia for cosmetic restoration using absorbable suture (**F**). Skin is closed with subcuticular suture (**G**), a liquid adhesive and steri-strips are applied, and the wound is dressed with a pressure bandage.

include infection (0.5%-1%), hematoma or seroma formation (uncommon), hernia recurrence (uncommon), and injury to the underlying intestine (rare). Unless postoperative concerns are present, a telephone follow-up is usually sufficient. Normal activity can generally be resumed in 2 weeks.

## Epigastric Hernia

Epigastric hernias are protrusions of abdominal contents through the interstices of decussation fibers (linea alba) of the anterior abdominal wall aponeuroses. Epigastric hernias were initially labeled as such in 1812 by Leveille. Prior to this time, epigastric hernias were considered a reflection of serious intraabdominal disease.

Sternocostal fibers from the diaphragm also attach to the abdominal wall fibers. Epigastric hernias are most common in young adults and have been generally considered as acquired defects that are a result of straining or coughing that causes tears at the site of the insertion of diaphragmatic fibers. However, epigastric hernias also occur in newborns and children, suggesting that there is a congenital component.

The overall incidence of epigastric hernia is 5%, and males are more commonly affected. Presentation may range from a small palpable mass to localized pain. Smaller hernias tend to be more painful as properitoneal fat is likely to become strangulated. Epigastric hernias are occasionally multiple and can be associated with concurrent umbilical defects.

The natural history of epigastric hernia is gradual enlargement, especially in obese children or those with chronic cough. For this reason, elective repair is generally warranted. It is important to label the site of herniation with a marker prior to anesthesia induction as the defect may be difficult to find after muscle relaxation. A transverse or midline skin incision is then made over the defect. The herniated fat is ligated and excised, and the fascia is repaired in transverse fashion with nonabsorbable suture. In the absence of confounding factors such as ascites or malnutrition, recurrence is extremely rare.

## Urachal Remnant

The incidence of patent urachus is less than 1 in 1,000 live births. Presenting symptoms include periumbilical granulation, urine excretion, pain, purulent drainage, swelling, and erythema as a result of fistulae, sinuses, or cysts (Fig. 35-3A–C). The type of lesion is determined by the stage at which normal involution is arrested.

Granulomas are common, consist of pink friable tissue that is usually associated with a local inflammatory response in the surrounding skin, and may be isolated or associated with either urachal or vitelline remnants. Initial treatment involves silver nitrate application. Granulomas with a visible stalk can also be managed in the office setting by simple ligation with an absorbable suture. Persistent lesions following several trials of silver nitrate treatment and/or ligation warrant further evaluation (Fig. 35-4). The presence of a sinus tract or fistula is at times very difficult to visualize and can be investigated with an otoscope or soft probe.

In cases with no draining sinus tract, abdominal ultrasonography can be helpful. Ultrasonography has a very high specificity and sensitivity for defining urachal duct remnants but is less helpful in the assessment of omphalomesenteric duct remnants. When a draining tract is clearly visible, fistulography with lateral radiographic views can provide a better understanding of the anatomic relationships as well as assist in differentiation from vitelline duct pathology. Contrast passage in the properitoneal space toward the bladder is suggestive of a urachal remnant. The diagnosis of a patent urachus mandates a careful search for a bladder or urethral obstruction employing either fistulography or a voiding cystourethrogram. Cystoscopy may be helpful in assessing the position of the opening.

Not unlike the vitelline duct, epithelial lines of the urachal lumen have a propensity to fill with serous or mucinous fluid and/or become infected through hematogenous or lymphatic seeding. Although rare, infected cysts have the potential to rupture into the peritoneal cavity. In addition, both benign and malignant (adenocarcinoma and yolk sac) neoplasms have been associated with urachal remnants.

Surgical therapy for urachal remnants is generally recommended to avoid infectious complications, skin breakdown, and potential malignant degeneration. Sinuses and cysts are excised through an infraumbilical approach. The best approach for fistulae is complete excision of the umbilicus, urachus, and ventral bladder cuff, as simple ligation has a high recurrence.

## Vitelline Duct Abnormalities

The in utero connection between the fetal gut and yolk sac (vitelline or omphalomesenteric duct) usually completely

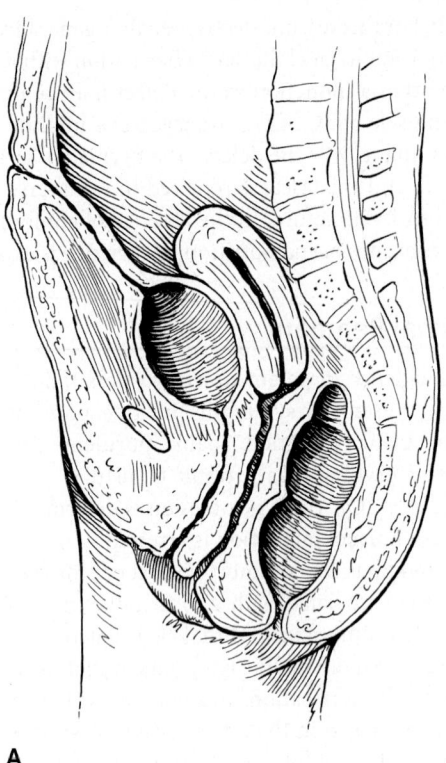

A

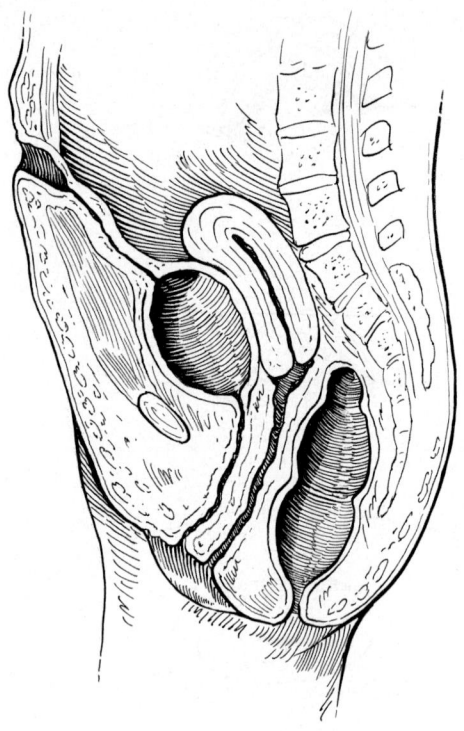

B

C

**FIGURE 35-3** Umbilical pathology associated with urachal anomalies. Absent or incomplete obliteration of the urachus can lead to various abnormalities including fistula communicating from the bladder to the umbilicus (A) and urachal sinus (B). Umbilical pathology associated with urachal anomalies. Absent or incomplete obliteration of the urachus can lead to various abnormalities including fistula communicating from the bladder to the urachal cyst (C).

involutes during the seventh to eighth week of gestation. While the patent vitelline duct is among the most frequent of the congenital malformations (2% incidence), it is also least likely to cause symptoms. Among the vitelline duct abnormalities, Meckel diverticulum is by far the most common. Umbilical disease resulting from a patent vitelline duct is less frequent and includes granluomas, enteric drainage, draining cysts and sinuses, and ileal prolapse (Fig. 35-5).

The diagnostic and therapeutic principles are similar for suspected urachal remnant and vitelline duct pathology (see Fig. 35-4). However, ultrasonography has a low sensitivity for vitelline duct pathology and is generally less helpful. During fistulography, the intraperitoneal passage of contrast dye toward bowel is suggestive of vitelline ductal abnormalities. Umbilical drainage from a patent vitelline duct is more commonly associated with a sinus rather than a fistula. Either

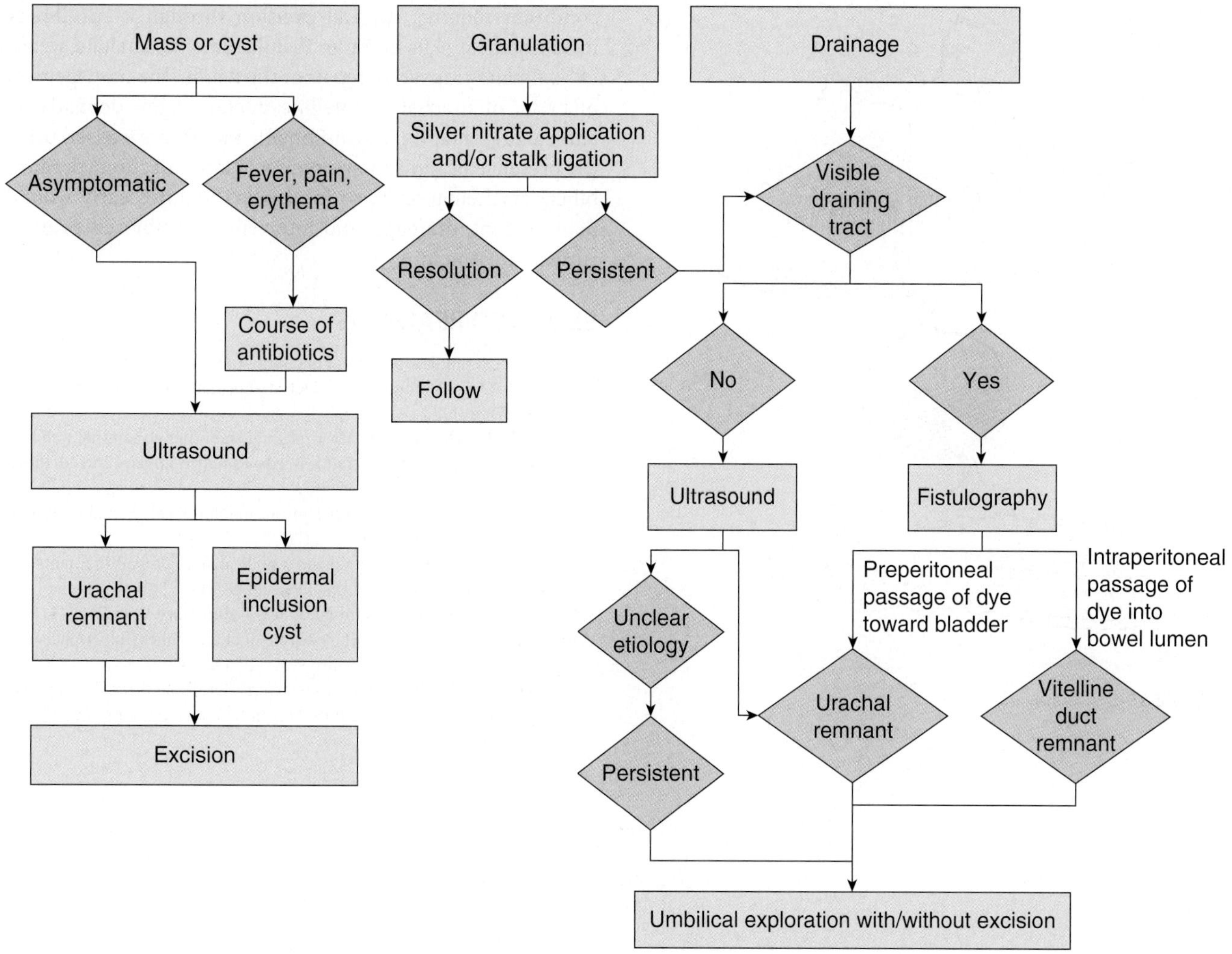

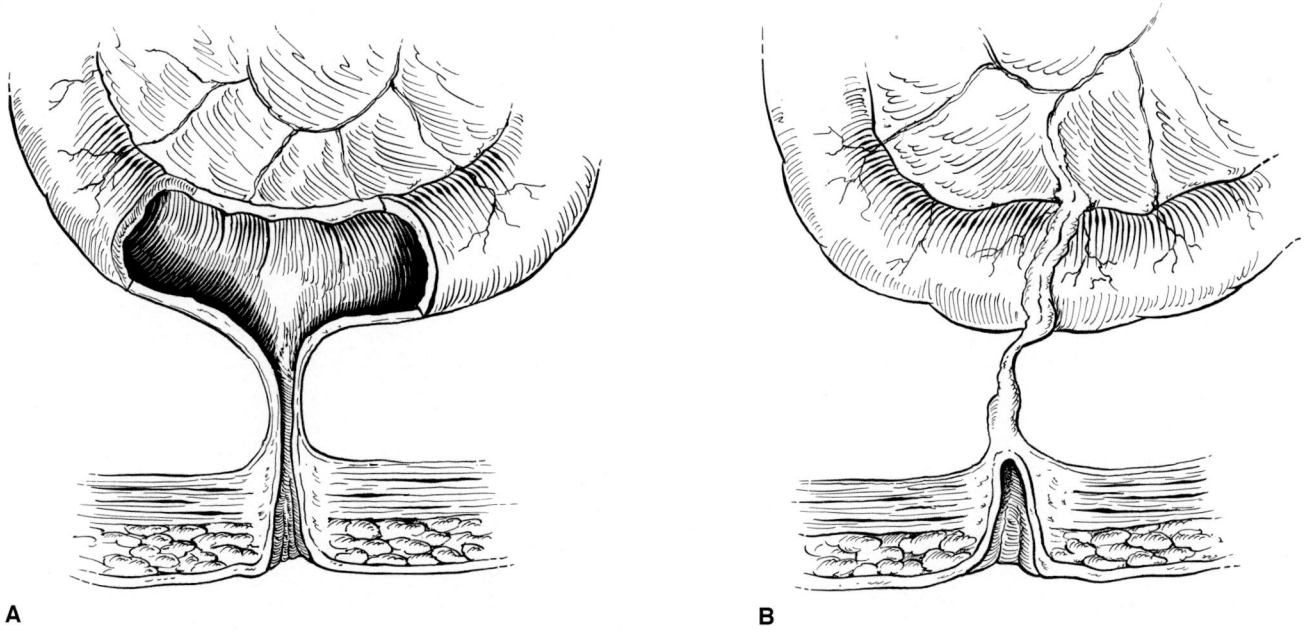

**FIGURE 35-4** Diagnostic and treatment algorithm for various umbilical disorders.

**FIGURE 35-5** Umbilical disease cause by vitelline (or omphalomesenteric) ductal abnormalities. Incomplete involution of the in utero connection between the fetal gut and yolk sac (vitelline duct) may result in enteric and/or purulent drainage as a result of an umbilico-intestinal fistula (**A**), an umbilical sinus (**B**), or rupture of a subumbilical cyst (**C**).

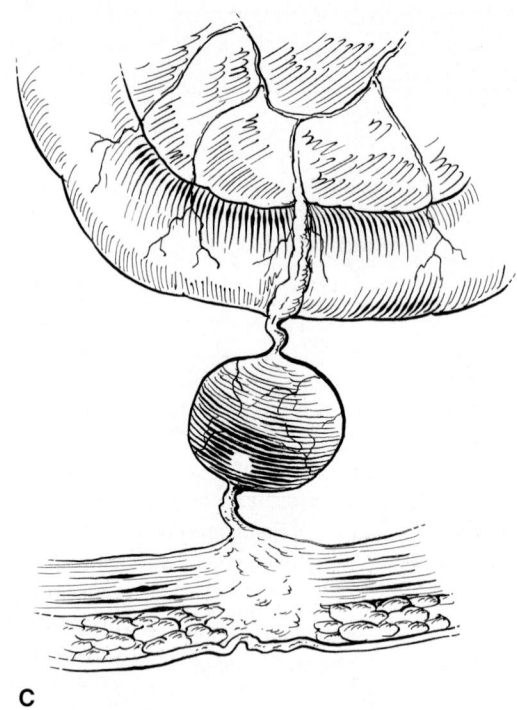

**C**

**FIGURE 35-5** (*Continued*)

condition requires surgical excision through a curvilinear infraumbilical skin incision. Fistulae may necessitate wedge excision and transverse repair of the ileum. The management of cysts, of urachal or vitelline ductal origin, depends on clinical presentation. Asymptomatic masses are excised while the presence of signs or symptoms of cyst infection (periumbilical erythema, fever, or local pain) requires early wound debridement, drainage, and intravenous antibiotics prior to surgical treatment.

## SELECTED READINGS

Blumberg NA. Infantile umbilical hernia. *Surg Gynecol Obstet* 1980;150:187–191.

Moore TC. Omphalomesenteric duct malformations. *Sem Pediatr Surg* 1996;5:116–123.

Neblett WW III, Holconb GW III. Umbilical and other abdominal wall hernias. In: Holder TM, Ashcraft KW, eds. *Pediatric Surgery.* 2nd ed. Philadelphia: WB Saunders; 1993:557.

Scherer LR III, Grosfeld JL. Inguinal hernia and umbilical anomalies. *Pediatr Clin North Am* 1993;40:1121–1126.

Skinner MA, Grosfeld JL. Inguinal and umbilical hernia repair in infants and children. *Surg Clin North Am* 1993;73:439–444.

Suita S, Nagasaki A. Urachal remnants. *Sem Pediatr Surg* 1996;5:107–115.

Vane DW, West KW, Grosfeld JL. Vitelline duct anomalies. Experience with 217 childhood cases. *Arch Surg* 1987;122:542–547.

Vermeij-Keers C, Hartwig NG, van der Werff JFA. Embryonic development of the ventral body wall and its congenital malformations. *Sem Pediatr Surg* 1996;5:82–89.

# CHAPTER 36

## Hernias of the Inguinal Region

*Michael W. L. Gauderer and Robert A. Cina*

## KEY POINTS

1. High ligation of the hernia sac by either the classic open technique or more recent laparoscopic techniques remains the standard of care for pediatric indirect inguinal hernia.

2. The issue of hernia incarceration is its frequency, especially increased in the neonatal population; the increased morbidity of operation in part related to its necessary urgency; the potential for permanent injury to the entrapped incarcerated organ; less optimal operative outcomes with potential vas and vessel injury; and treatment outcomes with greater recurrence rates.

3. The trend toward greater application of the laparoscopic technique to hernia repair seems warranted to improve the sensitivity of diagnosis, the protection of vas, vessel, and sliding hernia sac content, and the placement using magnified vision of sac closing sutures that do not jeopardize other vital structures.

4. Minimally invasive techniques may be particularly advantageous for the diagnosis and the treatment of both direct inguinal hernias as well as femoral hernias.

5. Inguinal hernia repair remains one of the most common operations for children: such hernias are most common in prematures, in boys, and on the right side.

## INDIRECT INGUINAL HERNIA

### Introduction

The management of abdominal wall hernias is a core activity of pediatric surgical practice. Salient among these is the inguinal hernia, the most frequently performed operation in the pediatric age group. Although the basic anatomy of this congenital opening has been known since antiquity, effective, sequelae-free surgical correction did not occur until the latter part of the 19th century. The advent of general anesthesia, improved equipment, aseptic surgically precise techniques, and detailed anatomical studies of the inguinal region led to the development of operations that laid the foundations of inguinal hernia repair in adults. These procedures were based on closure, with partial or total removal of the hernia sac, followed by reconstruction and reinforcement of the weakened area. It is likely that scarring resulting from these more extended dissections contributed to the decrease in recurrences.

The recognition that pediatric inguinal hernias were almost exclusively indirect and that the abdominal wall structures were intact, led early pioneers to limit the procedure to simple ligation of the hernia sac. This was initially accomplished through the external inguinal ring, a procedure that is applicable to the very young infant because in this age group the external and internal rings are almost superimposed. A more direct approach to the internal inguinal ring, by means of incising the external oblique aponeurosis, became the next step in the evolutionary process. Despite the evidence that simple ligation of the hernia sac corrected the pathology, many surgical centers continued to add a variety of reinforcing sutures. In the mid-20th century, pediatric surgical pioneers conclusively demonstrated that high ligation of the patent processus vaginalis (PPV), without excessive mobilization of the cord structures or inguinal floor reconstruction, constitutes the most effective approach to safely correct indirect inguinal hernias.

Advances in pediatric anesthesia, outpatient surgery, neonatal intensive care, material science, and surgical technique have made inguinal herniorrhaphy a well-tolerated procedure with a low complication rate. Despite this, controversies concerning the optimal management of inguinal hernias in children persist. Among these are timing of the operation (notably for hospitalized premature infants), approach to the asymptomatic contralateral side, management of incarceration (or an entrapped ovary), and, in the last 2 decades, whether the neck of the sac (at the internal ring) should be approached from below (the "open technique") or from above (employing one of several "laparoscopic" or "laparoscopic assisted techniques").

Two different approaches, which have worked well for the authors, are illustrated in this chapter. The repair of inguinal hernias in children, regardless of the technique used, can be an esthetically pleasing, highly effective, and fairly straightforward intervention. However, not infrequently, a herniorrhaphy will present the operator with significant technical

**489**

challenges. Nowhere is this more evident than in the premature neonate. A hernia repair in a very small child with an ipsilateral undescended testicle and an incarcerated bowel loop can be one of the most technically challenging procedures in pediatric surgery.

## Pathogenesis/Embryology

Indirect inguinal hernias, hydroceles, or a combination of both are related to the persistent patency of the PPV (Fig. 36-1). This outpouching (or evagination) of peritoneum is first apparent during the third month of fetal development. In boys, it is associated with the retroperitoneal migration of the testis (and its main blood supply: the spermatic vessels) from the lower pole of the kidney, across the abdominal wall (through the internal and the external inguinal rings) to the scrotum, following the path of the gubernaculum testis. This slow action, which is not fully understood, is probably an interplay involving mechanical, hormonal, and local innervation-related factors. The migration is usually complete by the seventh gestational month. The left testis reaches a final intrascrotal position before that of its right counterpart

leading to an earlier onset of the gradual obliteration of the PPV, explaining the higher incidence of right inguinal hernias. It also accounts for the increased incidence of undescended testis on the right. In girls, the gubernaculum does not have the same importance as in boys, given that the ovaries usually remain intrapelvic. The inguinal canal is narrower and the PPV (referred to as the canal of Nuck in girls) is less pronounced. Consequently, the closing of the PPV is simpler than that of boys and the incidence of hernias lower. Although the gradual obliteration of the PPV in boys begins after the descent of the testicle is completed, it continues after birth. In fact, patency rates over 80% in newborns, slightly over 50% in the 4- to 12-month age group and 20% in adulthood have been reported. As an infant grows, the inguinal canal gradually elongates and the nearly superimposed inguinal rings of the newborn age gradually migrate into their final, separate positions. The resulting longer, oblique canal (and the abdominal wall musculature) creates a valve or "shutter-like" occluding mechanism that helps prevent (but not eliminate) the entrance of intestinal loops. A PPV is a *potential* inguinal hernia, only becoming an actual, clinically detectable, symptomatic hernia when it contains an abdominal viscus. The

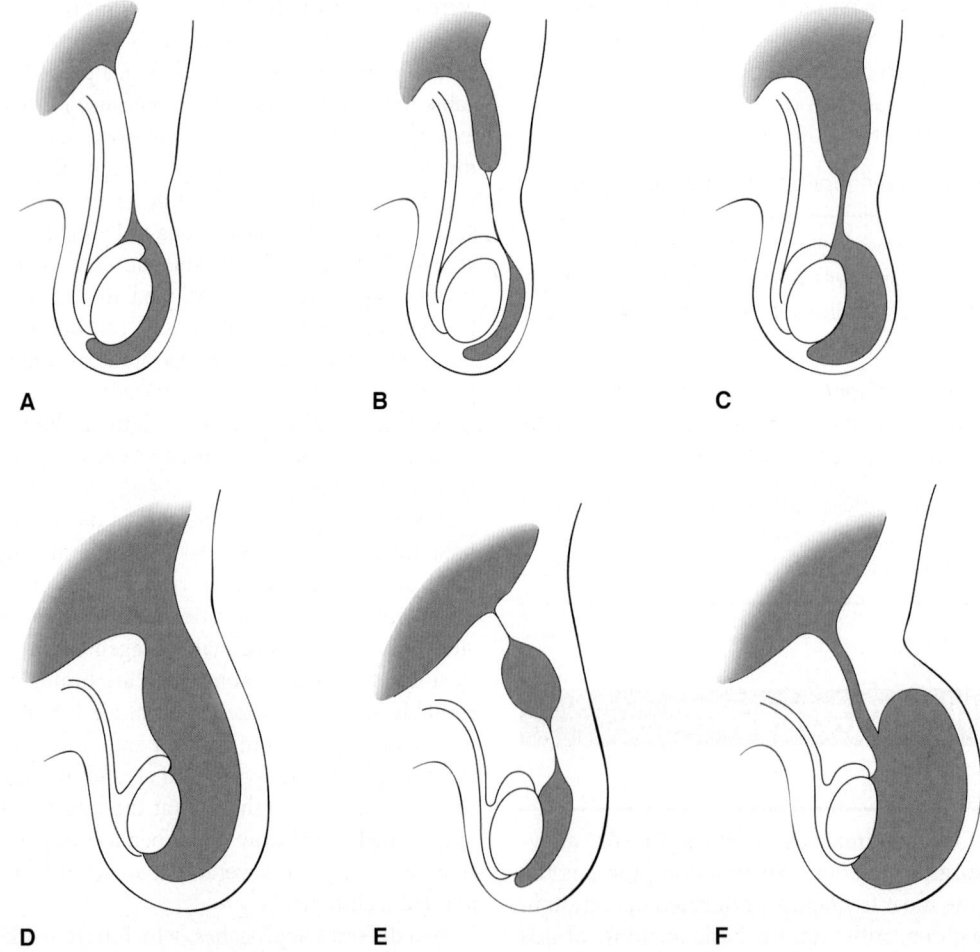

**FIGURE 36-1** Manifestations of the processus vaginalis: **A.** Normal: complete obliteration. No hernia sac. Small noncommunicating hydrocele. **B.** Complete distal obliteration: inguinal hernia sac and small noncommunicating hydrocele. **C.** Incomplete distal obliteation: inguinal hernia sac and communicating hydrocele. **D.** Total lack of obliteration: inguinoscrotal hernia sac. **E.** Incomplete proximal and complete distal obliteration: hydrocele of cord. **F.** Full-length incomplete obliteration: communicating hydrocele.

clinical significance of an asymptomatic PPV is at the center of the controversy concerning contralateral inguinal exploration, particularly if the "open" approach is used. If the PPV is thin and too narrow to admit a viscus, the patent tract may lead to a communicating hydrocele.

## Incidence and Associated Conditions

Congenital indirect inguinal hernias occur in 2% to 5% of full-term neonates. The incidence in preterm infants is substantially higher and is gestational age dependent, ranging from 9% to 11% and approaching 60% in extremely low-birth-weight infants. Inguinal hernias occur with much greater frequency in boys than in girls, with reported ratios of 5:1 to 10:1, although these differences appear to be lower in preterm infants. At clinical presentation, 60% of hernias occur on the right side (Figs. 36-2 and 36-3), 25% to 30% on the left, and 10% to 15% are bilateral. Bilateral inguinal hernias are more common in premature patients, reported to be present in 44% to 55% of children (Fig. 36-4). The clinical presentation of metachronous contralateral hernias is reported to occur in 7% to 10% of patients. A history of familial incidence is well documented as is the occurrence in twins and siblings. Race, socioeconomic status, or geographic location do not appear to influence the incidence, although, in many disadvantaged areas of the world, children may present late, with very large, difficult-to-correct hernias.

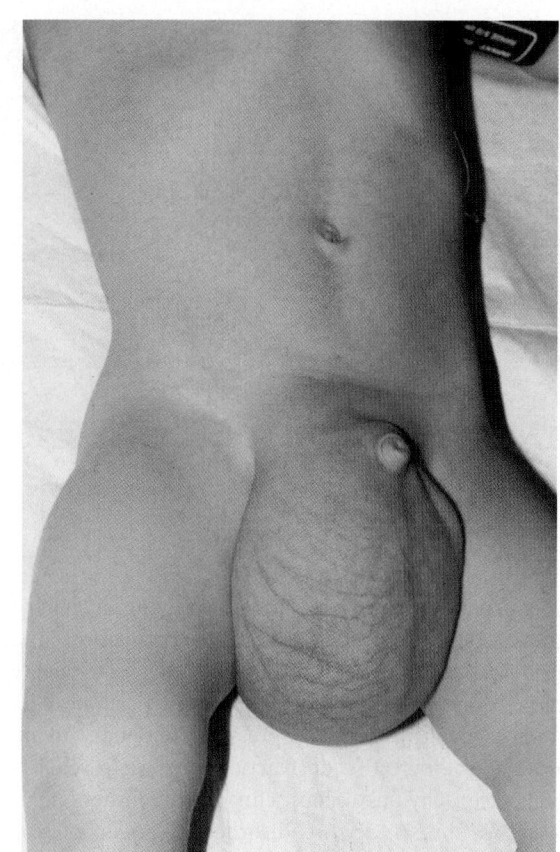

**FIGURE 36-3** Giant, unoperated right inguinal hernia in a 19-month-old former very low birth weight infant with multiple medical problems.

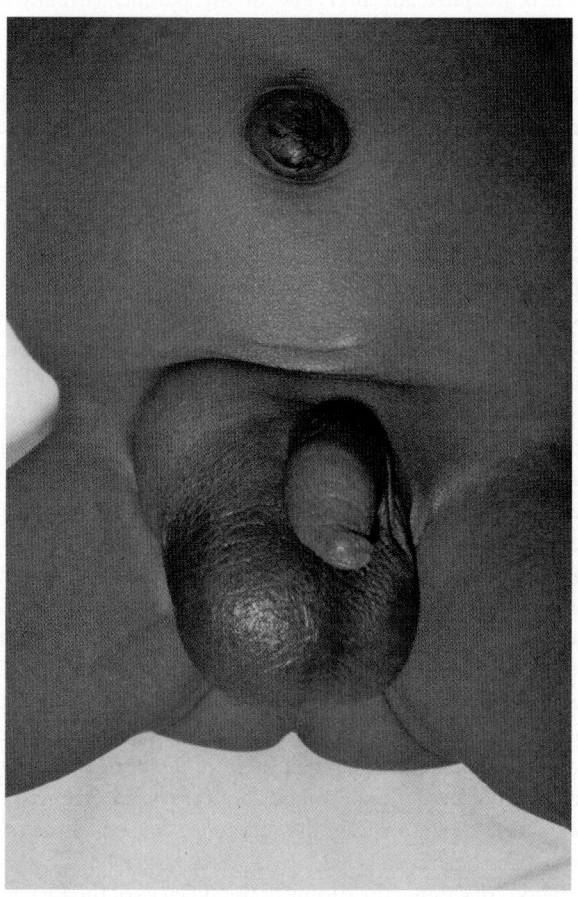

**FIGURE 36-2** Incarcerated, easily reducible, right inguinal hernia in a 2-month-old former premature infant.

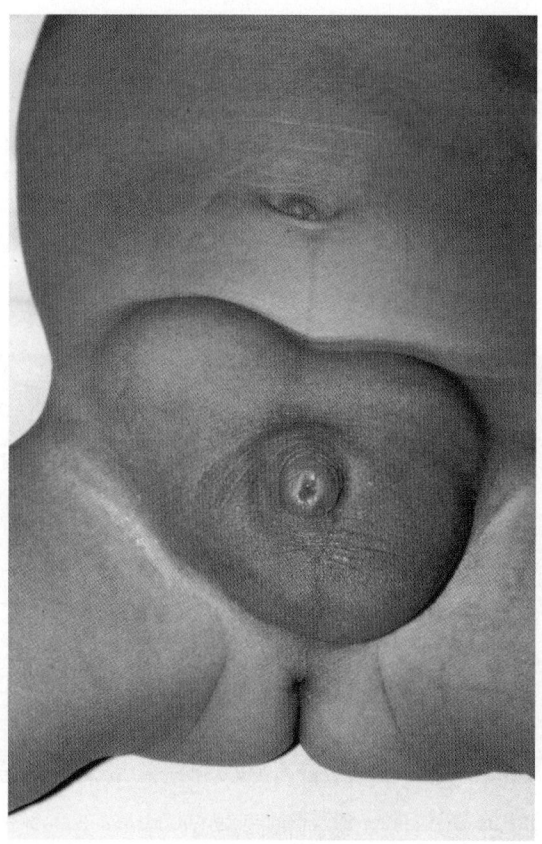

**FIGURE 36-4** Bilateral inguinal hernias and right undescended testis in a former premature infant.

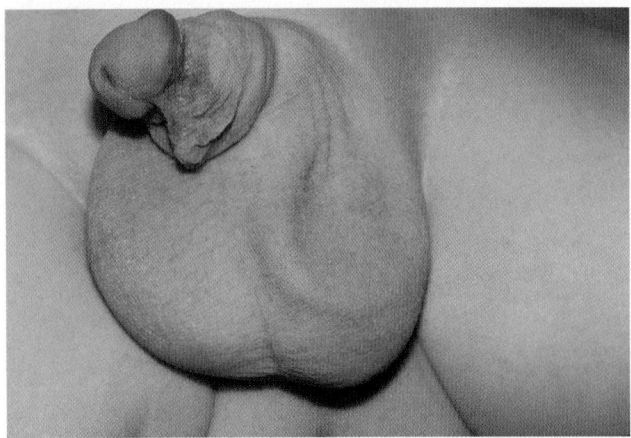

**FIGURE 36-5** Ventriculoperitoneal (VP) shunt in left inguinoscrotal hernia sac.

Several conditions are associated with inguinal hernias, the most common, particularly in the premature child, is an undescended testicle (Fig. 36-4). Others include: ventriculoperitoneal (VP) shunts (Fig. 36-5); peritoneal dialysis; increased intraabdominal pressure secondary to major abdominal wall defect reconstructions (eg, gastroschisis and omphalocele), chylous ascites, chronic coughing associated with cystic fibrosis, seizure disorders; bladder exstrophy; urologic abnormalities and intersex conditions (Fig. 36-6); as well as miscellaneous connective tissue disorders. Some strenuous physical activities in older children, such as wrestling, seem to disclose hernias, probably secondary to a previously asymptomatic PPV.

## Clinical Presentation, Diagnosis, and Differential Diagnosis

Inguinal hernias can present at any age. However, the peak incidence is during infancy and early childhood. Hospitalized premature babies are usually diagnosed in the nursery, particularly if the stay is prolonged and associated with respiratory support. Nonhospitalized children are typically brought

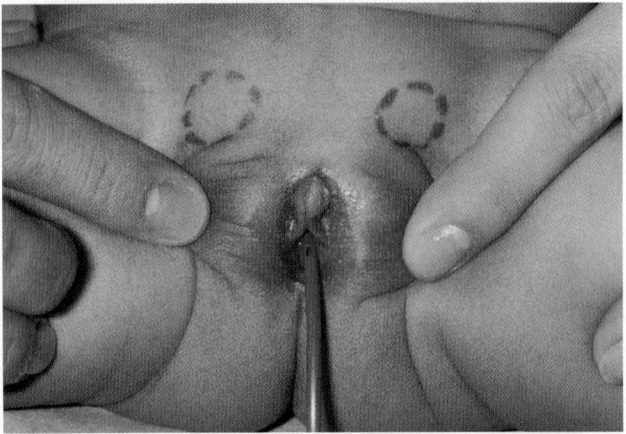

**FIGURE 36-6** Androgen insensitivity syndrome in a 2½-month-old infant. The child had bilateral inguinal hernias. The *circles* denote the position of the palpable gonads (testes) in the hernia sacs. The catheter demonstrates the short introitus and absence of vagina.

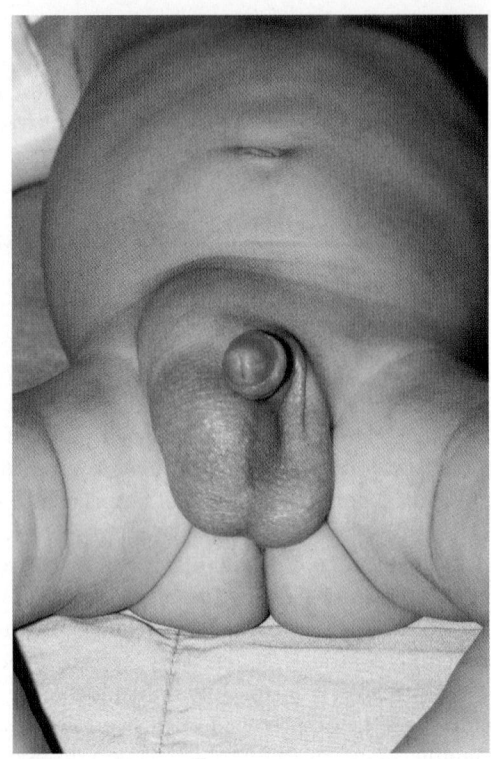

**FIGURE 36-7** Incarcerated right inguinal hernia. Notice the large inguinoscrotal swelling and the distended bowel loops visible through the abdominal wall.

to their pediatrician after one of the parents (usually the mother) noticed a bulge in the groin during diaper change or bath. The parents may also have noticed unusual "fussiness" and unexplained crying. The child is then referred to the surgeon. In 10% to 12% of children, usually those under 6 months of age, an incarceration is the first manifestation of a hernia (Fig. 36-7).

The office visit should be relaxed and reassuring. A good history is essential. It is helpful to explain what a hernia is and supplement this with a simple drawing. Using the finger of an insufflated examining glove (mimicking the hernia sac) tends to help older children understand the condition. Infants are examined on the table, with the parents or a nurse holding the child's legs. The increased intraabdominal pressure produced by struggling or crying usually makes the hernia manifest. Children who can stand unaided are best examined while standing on a small stool, between the parents and the surgeon. In most cases, the pathology is obvious. If not, coughing, blowing up a balloon or an office glove helps. In examining for a hernia in boys, it is important to determine that the ipsilateral testis is in the scrotum, because a retractile gonad can mimic a bulging hernia. In this case, the testicle is gently repositioned into the low scrotum and the exam continued. If a typical hernia is present, it is reduced and the cord examined. At this time, it is helpful to guide the index finger of the parent(s) over the spermatic cord (or round ligament) on both sides, to demonstrate the difference caused by the presence of the hernia sac (Fig. 36-8). With larger hernia sacs, a so-called "silk sign" (the sliding of the surfaces of the PPV) can be elicited. However, this sign is quite unreliable. A herniated ovary in infants presents as a smooth, mobile, well-defined

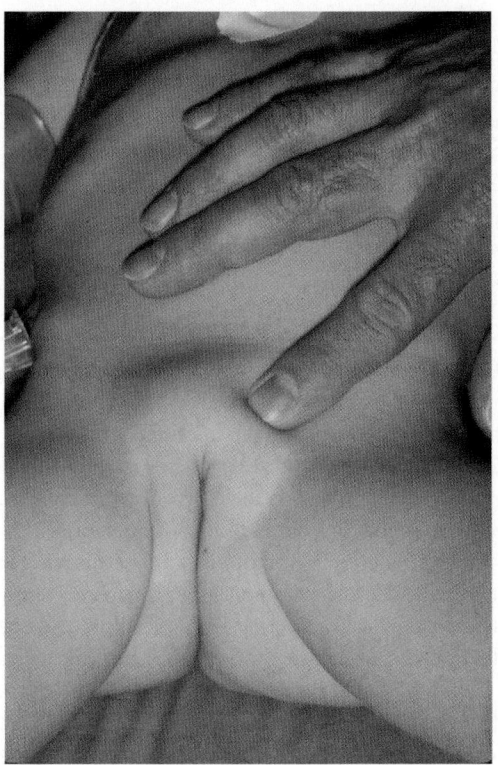

**FIGURE 36-8** Examination of the cord or, as in this case, the round ligament. Parents are encouraged to do the same to note the difference between the 2 sides. Often a "silk sign" can be elicited.

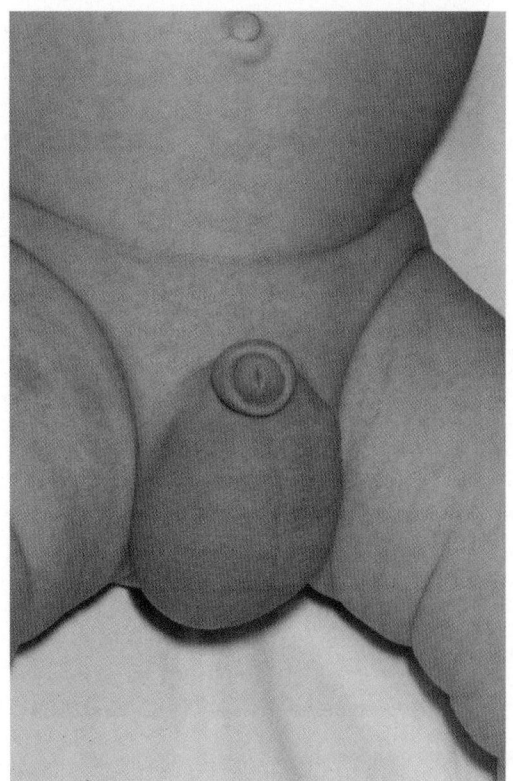

**FIGURE 36-9** Physiologic hydrocele in a 7-week-old infant. Complete spontaneous resolution followed.

swelling that can be difficult or impossible to reduce. As part of the office visit, the surgeon must address the possibility of incarceration: what it is, how to recognize it, and what steps to follow when one is suspected. This is particularly important in the youngest patients. If, during the visit, no bulge is visible and the exam is inconclusive, a simple option is to ask the parents to document the bulge using a digital camera. Although an ultrasound exam is not reliable in the diagnosis of an empty PPV, it is very helpful if the etiology of the groin mass is unclear. Other radiological examinations, such as the once advocated herniograms, do not have a place in contemporary practice.

The most common lesions in the differential diagnosis of groin masses are hydroceles (Figs. 36-9 and 36-10) and lymphadenitis (Fig. 36-11). Most hydroceles in newborns and infants are physiologic (noncommunicating). There is no history of size change; the examiner can usually determine that the bulge is below the level of the external ring, the mass is smooth and painless. Although applying a light source has been a traditional maneuver, it is unreliable in infants because thin, air-filled bowel loops will easily transilluminate. Hydroceles of the cord or the canal of Nuck can be difficult to differentiate from an incarcerated hernia. Although the mass is irreducible, the children are asymptomatic. In patients with chronic lymphadenopathy, multiple lymph nodes are commonly involved. These are smooth, mobile, and usually in or below the abdominocrural fold. However, if there is a painful, acute inflammatory process, the differential diagnosis is more difficult, particularly in girls because of the possibility of ovarian torsion with gonadal necrosis. In boys with an

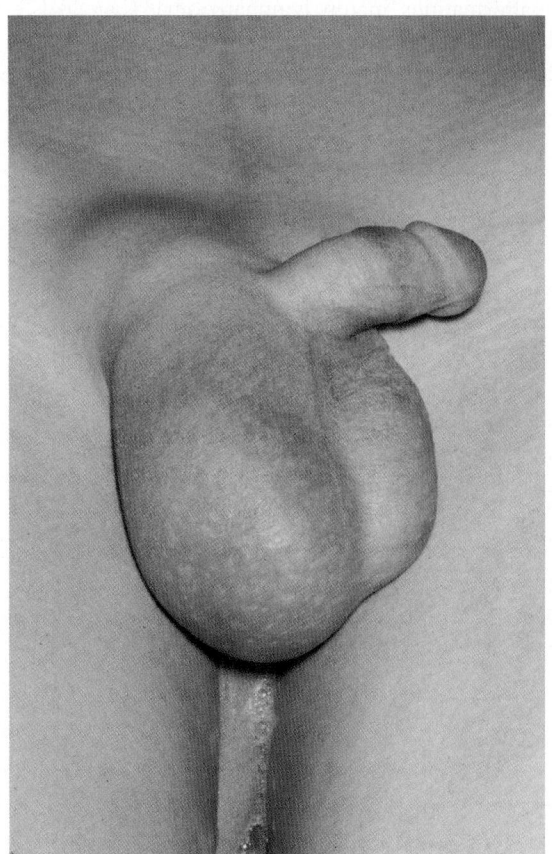

**FIGURE 36-10** Communicating hydrocele in a prepubertal boy. The painless, irreducible fluid-filled structure extended to the level of the external inguinal ring.

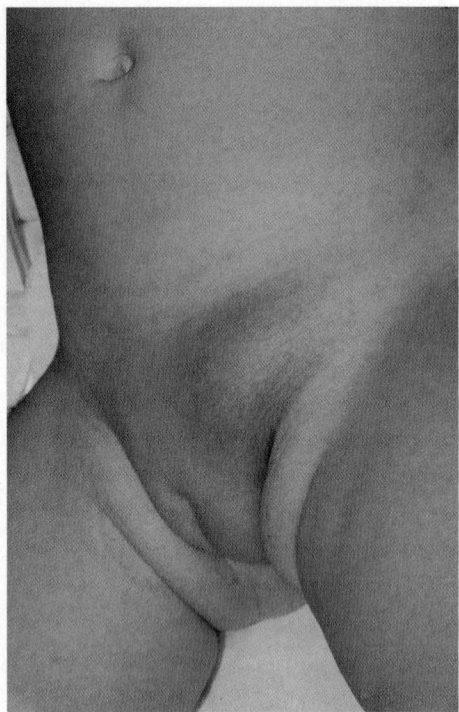

**FIGURE 36-11** Female infant with swollen, erythematous, and tender left groin. No signs of intestinal obstruction. Gonadal torsion with necrosis could not be excluded. The mass proved to be an abscess.

undescended testis (notably newborns), a painful groin bulge is likely due to gonadal torsion. Other masses include vascular malformations, mainly lymphangiomas (Fig. 36-12), and malignant lesions, such as lymphomas. A rare lesion on the patient's left side might be an engorged fragment of spleen in

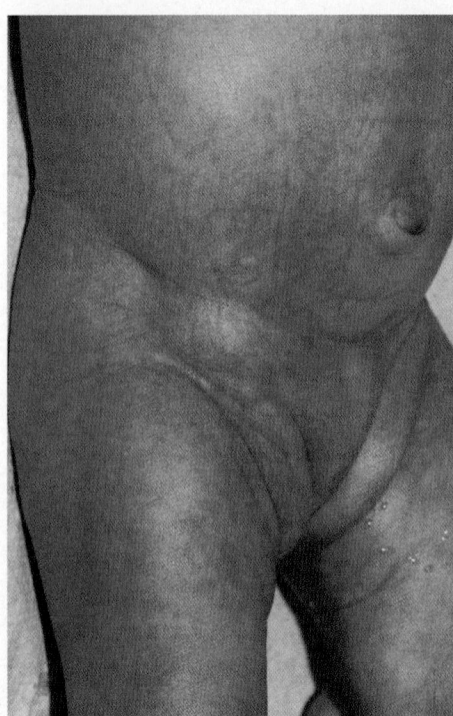

**FIGURE 36-12** Female infant with a soft, mobile, nontender right groin mass. Because of the medial and lateral extensions, a lymphangioma was suspected and confirmed operatively.

response to a viral or bacterial infection representing a remnant splenogonadal fusion from earlier development. Children with a female-appearing external genitalia and bilateral inguinal gonads need a work-up for androgen insensitivity syndrome (see also Chapter 71, Ambiguous Genitalia and Intersex Anomalies). Whether in the office or in the hospital, the importance of not missing an incarcerated hernia cannot be overstated.

## Indications and Timing of Operation

Once the diagnosis of an inguinal hernia is established, operative correction is indicated. As a general rule: the younger the child, the sooner the correction, preferably within 2 weeks. Children under 1 year, and especially those under 6 months, are most likely to develop an incarceration. There are few reasons for delay, including a diaper rash, which can be corrected in a couple of days. Infants with serious associated problems, such as congenital heart disease, should also be considered for early intervention, provided the condition is stable, because an incarceration would complicate management. Conservative measures of yesteryear, such as trusses, should never be used because they are unreliable, provide a false sense of security, and can create local skin problems. Figure 36-13 provides an algorithm for management.

Areas of controversy include the approach to the asymptomatic side, timing of correction in hospitalized newborn premature infants, and the management of the girl with an

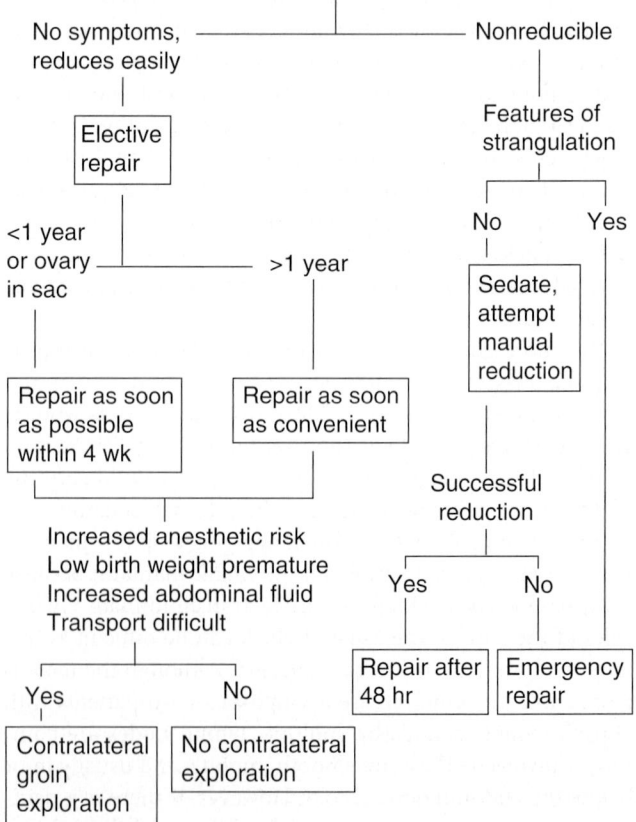

**FIGURE 36-13** Algorithm for the management of a congenital inguinal hernia.

irreducible ovary. There is a large volume of literature dealing with the question of exploration of the contralateral, asymptomatic groin when the "open" approach is used. Because the incidence of metachronous hernias is low and the incarceration rate is even lower, routine bilateral exploration is difficult to justify. Although the contralateral internal inguinal ring may be examined endoscopically by placing an endoscope through the ipsilateral open hernia sac (or through a separate trocar site) during the open approach, this method can be cumbersome and time-consuming, particularly in small patients. Exploration of the asymptomatic contralateral side is warranted, though, in patients with increased anesthetic risk, low-birth weight premature infants, those with increased intraabdominal fluid (eg, VP shunts, peritoneal dialysis), or those for whom transport, in the event of incarceration, it is difficult. If a "laparoscopic" repair is chosen, the contralateral PPV is clearly visible and, if patent, routinely closed. Concerning preterm infants in a neonatal intensive care unit, the most commonly applied practice is repair as soon as "clinically stable," or prior to discharge. Not only are these children at higher risk for incarceration, but a chronically protruding hernia can interfere with clinical progress (eg, need for respiratory support and feeding) in addition to pain. It is worth noting that the size of the hernia is usually inversely proportional to the likelihood of incarceration. It has been suggested that the girl with an irreducible ovary should be promptly operated, but most authors agree that the condition is best managed by electively placing the child on the first available slot on the operating room schedule.

## Repair Options: Conventional Open, Laparoscopic, and Laparoscopic Guided

Currently, 3 different approaches are used in clinical practice: conventional "open," through a groin incision, removing part of the hernia sac, and closing it at the internal ring from "below" or "outside" of the peritoneal cavity; fully laparoscopic "closed," occluding the internal ring with an intracorporeally placed suture from "above" or "inside," usually without excision of a part of the sac; and "laparoscopic guided/assisted," a hybrid in which the tying of the suture placed around the sac at the internal ring is done extracorporeally. There are 2 basic "open" approaches: high ligation of the sac following an incision in the external oblique aponeurosis (with or without opening the external ring), and high ligation without opening the aponeurosis or the external ring. The first, illustrated in this chapter, can be applied to all age groups. The latter (known as the Mitchell–Banks technique) is suitable for neonates whose internal and external rings are nearly superimposed. Although the pioneers in pediatric laparoscopic hernia have standardized the approach and now have very sizeable patient volumes, as well as clearly convincing results, many minor variations are published and others continue to be introduced. Laparoscopic-guided procedures aim at combining elements of the "open" method, such as the tie around the neck of the PPV, with the visualization and control provided by the endoscope.

As expected, such radically different ways to close the sac at the internal ring level have advantages and disadvantages. The pure laparoscopic and the laparoscopic-aided methods are grouped together, for simplicity, although some notable differences exist.

### Advantages of "Open" Approaches

Techniques well standardized, familiar, and applicable to a wide range of local inguinoscrotal abnormalities (including those of testicular position and different types of hydroceles); specialized endoscopic equipment not required; endotracheal intubation not necessary in all cases; use of absorbable suture material for hernia sac possible. Because of the dissection and removal of part of the sac, in addition to high ligation, the recurrence rate is very low.

### Disadvantages of "Open" Approaches

Presence of an incision and subsequent scar; dissection around vas deferens, with possible trauma and/or devascularization; inspection of contralateral deep inguinal ring cumbersome in routine cases and bowel inspection after reduction of incarceration not possible; significant postoperative edema following herniorrhaphy in small premature children, mimicking early recurrence.

### Advantages of "Laparoscopic" Approaches

Clear visualization of the anatomy (including proper anatomical identification of usual and unusual groin hernias, bowel inspection following reduction of incarceration, supplemental information in intersex conditions); defect treated at origin (PPV at the internal ring), without unnecessary additional dissection and, consequently, less local trauma; vas and vessels undisturbed; ability to recognize and treat an open contralateral PPV and unusual hernias without additional incision sites (except the "hybrid" techniques); well suited for repair of recurrences of "open" procedures; superb documentation for records, referring physician and family.

### Disadvantages of "Laparoscopic" Approaches

Limited to centers where pediatric laparoscopic skill/equipment available; endotracheal intubation required; postoperative right shoulder pain and other possible, albeit rare, complications of laparoscopy in general; permanent suture at neck of hernia sac employed by most surgeons; difficult to deal with undescended testicle (although not with sliding ovaries); not well suited for hydroceles; procedure more challenging in small infants with distended bowel loops.

Other differences continue to be subjects of debate, including *teaching of the techniques, length of operation, postoperative (local) pain, and recurrences.* For surgeons familiar with laparoscopic techniques in children, learning the laparoscopic approach should not be more difficult than mastering the open technique. An additional strength of the laparoscopic approach is that all in the operating room see the same steps as the procedure evolves. Although length of the operation initially favored the open procedures, in skilled hands the laparoscopic approach can be faster, particularly in bilateral hernias in fully endoscopic repair. Local pain does not appear to differ if fine laparoscopic instruments (3 mm diameter or less) are employed. Large series have now demonstrated that the laparoscopic closure of the hernia sac has equivalent hernia recurrence rates, compared with the open approach, although the incidence of postoperative hydrocele formation is slightly higher. Until recently, patient weight was a limiting factor in the laparoscopic repair of inguinal hernias. With the development of very fine instruments, however, premature babies with weights well below 2000 g have been successfully repaired endoscopically.

At the other end of the spectrum, a different question emerges: *when does a hernia require more than simple ligation of the sac at the internal ring?* Although the use of mesh material or reinforcing sutures is not indicated in children, select older adolescents, patients with complex hernias, and young adults benefit from one of several contemporary tension-free laparoscopic techniques, particularly the transabdominal preperitoneal (or TAPP) technique.

## Preparation and Anesthesia

Parents and children of appropriate age should be fully informed about the steps that will occur on the day of the operation. Appropriate preoperative preparation, in addition to detailed postoperative information (ie, what to expect), will reassure caregivers and decrease the number of unnecessary postprocedure telephone calls. Many outpatient facilities offer preoperative "tours" for interested parents. It should be mentioned, though, that the information must be reassuring and kept so as not to create unnecessary anxiety. Healthy patients and those not at risk for postoperative apnea are routinely operated as outpatients. The youngest age is still a matter of debate among pediatric anesthesiologists. However, in most centers a postconceptual age of 50 weeks is considered safe. Children below this age, as well as those with cardiac, chronic respiratory, or other increased risk factors, are admitted for monitored observation. Some neonatal intensive care units have their own operating room, which eliminates the need for transport.

Contemporary anesthesiologists have a large palette of options, and even the highest risk children can undergo safe general anesthesia. Intravenous access is placed in all patients. A laryngeal mask airway is commonly used for open herniorrhaphies in healthy children of appropriate age. High-risk patients, premature babies, and full-term neonates usually require endotracheal intubation. Although spinal anesthesia and sedation have been employed in some of these patients, this method can be challenging for the surgeon because it is difficult to obtain adequate abdominal wall relaxation. Endotracheal intubation is presently the standard for laparoscopic interventions. For postoperative pain control, the application of a local anesthetic is routinely employed. Most surgeons prefer the infiltration at the end of the procedure to avoid possible distortions of the anatomy or hematomas. This is supplemented with a suppository of a nonsteroidal antiinflammatory analgesic. For postdischarge pain management, a combination of nonsteroidal antiinflammatory agent plus codeine is very effective.

## Conventional or "Open" Procedure (MWLG)

The anesthetized child is reexamined. The side of the hernia, if unilateral, is confirmed. Children with long or sharp fingernails should have these clipped to avoid postoperative

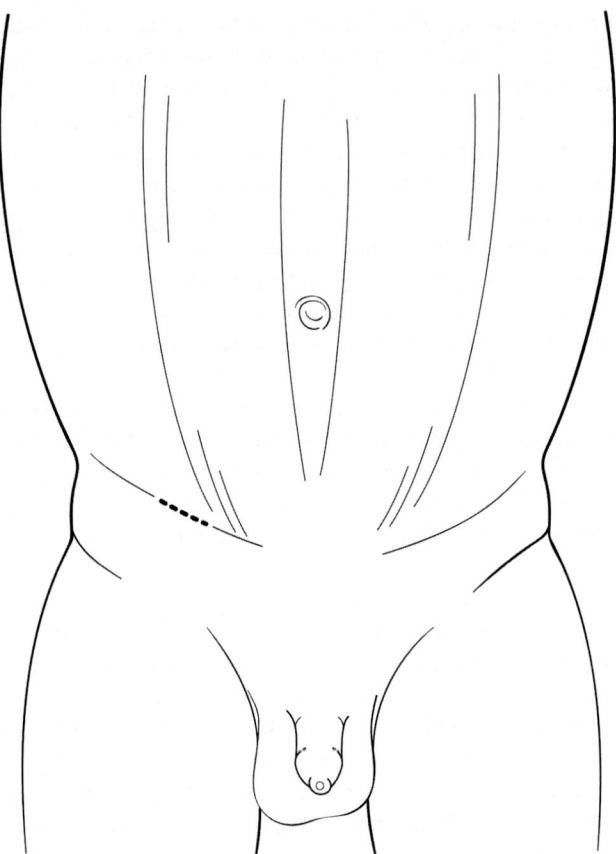

**FIGURE 36-14** Groin incision in the inguinoabdominal fold, centered over the internal ring.

wound scratching. The child's legs are lifted to enhance the visualization of the inguinoabdominal fold. The tips of a pair of forceps without teeth are used to mark the incision in the crease. These "pressure spots" obviate the use of ink, which can be removed during skin preparation. A small roll under the lower back may facilitate exposure in infants. The region is washed with an antiseptic soap solution prior to the application of the antiseptic. This is done to remove debris and oily residue of ointments. No antibiotics are administered.

Figure 36-14 shows the site of the incision, centered over the internal inguinal ring. The skin is slightly spread as the incision is made. Cautery is not used. Small bleeding vessels are temporarily clamped. The superficial epigastric vessels are retracted or tied, and the fascia superficialis (Scarpa) is incised with scissors. Blunt dissection down to the aponeurosis of the external oblique muscle follows (Fig. 36-15). Retractors are placed and the aponeurosis is exposed. To confirm the appropriate site for the incision of the aponeurosis, the inguinal ligament (Poupart) and, if necessary, the external inguinal ring may be identified. A short incision is made in the aponeurosis (solid line) and a small straight hemostat applied to each cut edge. The edges are lifted and a closed curved hemostat or scissors inserted cranially and caudally prior to extending the cut (dashed line). This is done to protect the ileoinguinal nerve from injury. In this technique the external inguinal ring is left intact, obviating the need for subsequent closure. If necessary, as in the case of an incarceration, the incision is extended caudally and the external ring opened.

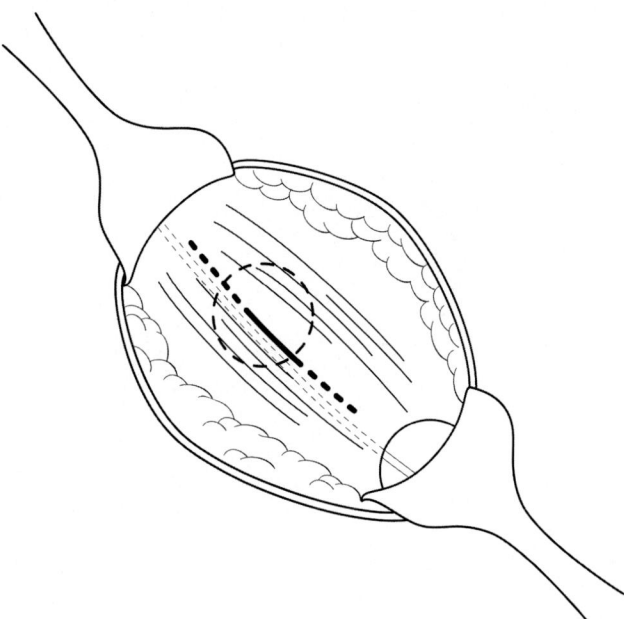

**FIGURE 36-15** Exposure of the external oblique aponeurosis. A short incision (*solid line*) is initially made, the edges are lifted, and the incision is extended proximally and distally, protecting the ilioinguinal nerve. The external ring (depicted at the distal retractor) is not routinely opened.

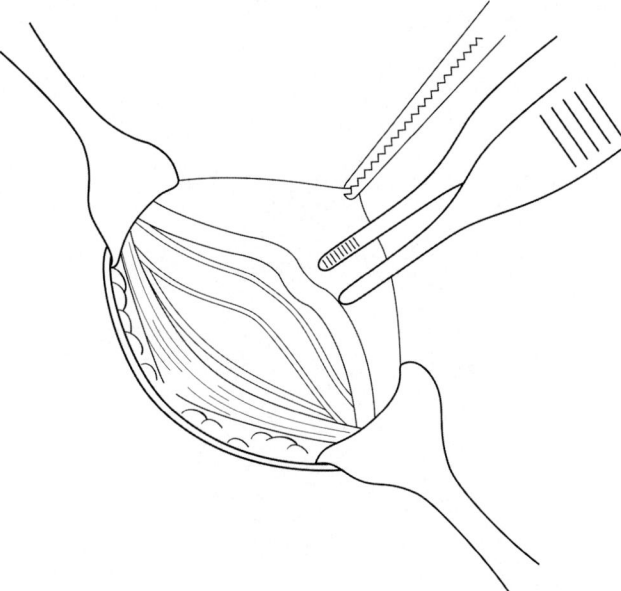

**FIGURE 36-17** The lifted anteromedially located hernia sac and the beginning of the separation of the sac from the vas and the cord vessels. The tip of a fine forceps initiates the process. Because the sac may slightly overlay the vas, special care needs to be exercised to avoid tearing it. This is particularly important in premature infants and small children.

Figure 36-16 shows the lifted, cut edges of the aponeurosis exposing the slightly bulging cremasteric fibers covering the cord. These fibers are gently split with a blunt straight hemostat (not shown). The hernia sac is in the anteromedial position of the cord and usually the first layer at the tip of the hemostat. This layer (the hernia sac) is *gently* grasped by the hemostat and lifted. The hemostat is *never* closed by clamping during this step. The edge of the sac may be clamped *after* the vas deferens and the cord vessels have been clearly identified. Figure 36-17 demonstrates the lifted sac, the vas, and the

cord vessels. "Peeling" the vessels and the vas from the sac is started with one of the prongs of a fine dissecting forceps and continued in a conventional manner. This is done very carefully to avoid tearing and entering the sac. The vas is *never* grasped with an instrument to avoid injury to its delicate wall or its blood supply. Once a safe "window" has been established between the hernia sac and the elements of the cord, the sac is cross-clamped with a straight hemostat (but not until the vas has again been clearly visualized and the absence of an intraabdominal structure in the sac, such as omentum, has been confirmed). The hernia sac is then transected and lifted. Gentle countertraction on the cord helps with the separating dissection. Should tearing of a very thin sac occur, the site is promptly secured with a hemostat. The dissection is continued cranially to the level of the internal ring. Occasionally, in thin young children, the epigastric vessels are seen through the transversalis fascia. This is the uppermost limit of dissection. It is important to avoid excessive traction on the sac in small children because the urinary bladder or a ureter can be pulled into the field and injured.

The distal portion of the sac is left undisturbed, even though it is tempting to remove it. Unnecessary dissection can endanger the vas and the vessels. If the absence of hernia sac content cannot be assured, the sac is opened and inspected (Fig. 36-18). It is then twisted and a tie of synthetic absorbable suture material (4:0 or 3:0) applied to its neck. A suture ligature of the same material follows (Fig. 36-19). This is applied distal to the regular tie to avoid tearing the sac. Excess sac is excised, allowing the stump to retract behind the lowermost fibers of the internal oblique muscle. Traction is applied to the scrotum replacing the testicle, which is often pulled up during the dissection. Alternatively a long, narrow, and smooth instrument such as a blunt periosteal elevator

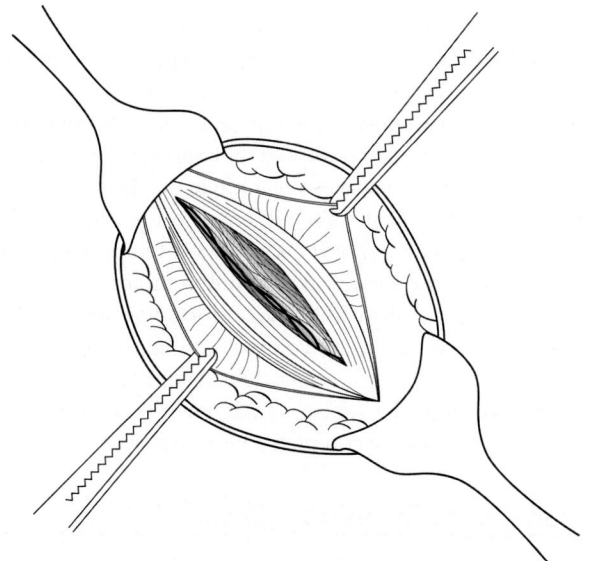

**FIGURE 36-16** The lifted edges of the external oblique aponeurosis, exposing the split cremasteric fibers and the underlying spermatic cord.

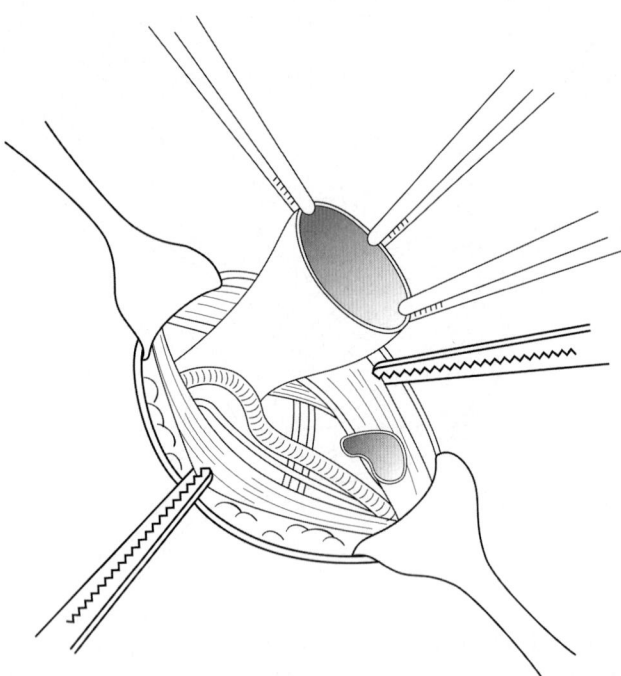

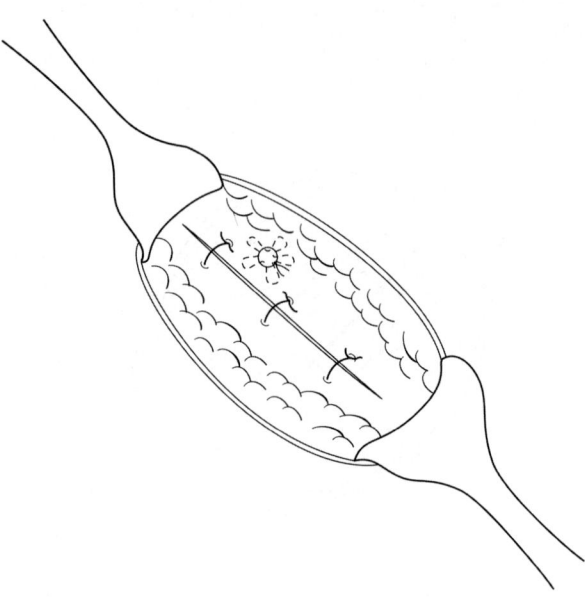

**FIGURE 36-20** The closed aponeurosis of the external oblique and the site of the closed sac.

**FIGURE 36-18** The sac has been separated from the vas and vessels of the cord, and transected. The dissection has been extended to the internal ring. The deep epigastric vessels may be seen medially, through the transversalis fascia in some thin patients. In this drawing, the sac has been opened for inspection for possible contents. The distal, collapsed sac is also seen. It is left untouched.

(or joker) can be inserted into the canal, through the incision, pushing the gonad into its scrotal position. This maneuver is useful in children in whom the surgeon wishes to avoid handling the scrotum, which may be the site of residual dermatitis. A long-lasting local anesthetic is injected in the deep and subcutaneous layers. Alternatively, the solution can be sprayed onto the exposed surfaces. The aponeurosis of the external oblique is reapproximated with a couple of stitches of synthetic absorbable material (4:0 or 3:0) (Fig. 36-20). The subcutaneous tissue is united with a couple of fine sutures of the same material (5:0 or 4:0). The skin is closed with a couple of fine subcuticular sutures (5:0). These should be "buried," slightly everting the skin, to minimize the formation of a suture reaction. Flexible collodion, if available, is applied to the incision of small infants and children. Alternatively tissue adhesive can be employed. If adhesive strips are used in infants, they must be placed in such a way that they will not lift off when the child pulls up the legs, deepening the abdominal fold. Adhesive strips are well suited for children beyond infancy. The correct position of the gonad is confirmed. Antiseptic solutions should be washed off to prevent pruritus.

Figure 36-21 demonstrates a technique that is useful in girls with a sliding Fallopian tube adherent to the inner surface of the proximal portion of the sac. This is found in approximately 20% of the girls and is more common in infancy. The sac is tied distal to the tube and a purse string suture applied to its base, carefully avoiding both tube and epigastric vessels. A thin forceps or straight hemostat invaginates the sac, returning the tube to an intraabdominal position. Figure 36-22 shows the completed hernia closure.

## Laparoscopic Technique (RAC)

Since the inception of pediatric surgery, the traditional open inguinal herniorraphy, described earlier in this chapter, continues to be the standard by which alternate repair techniques are judged. This technique requires a small incision,

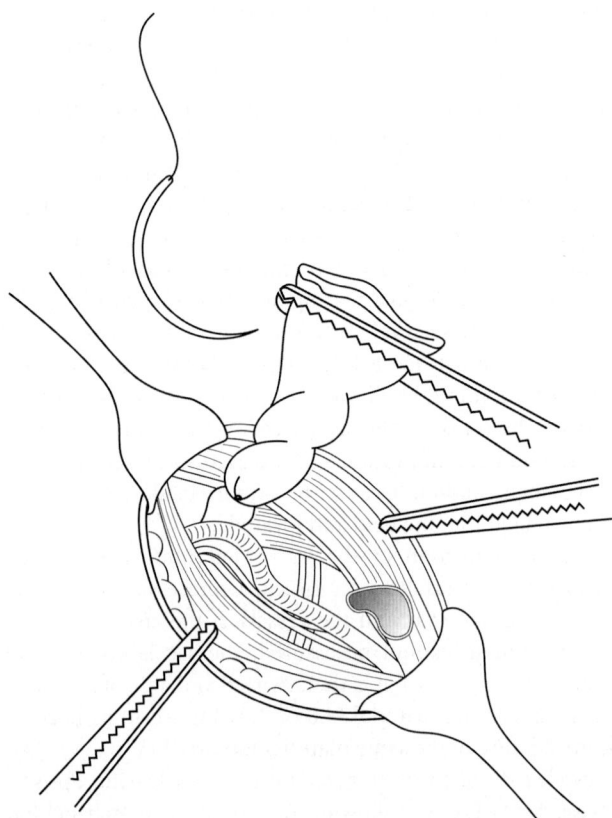

**FIGURE 36-19** The empty sac has been twisted and a ligature placed at the base that corresponds to the internal inguinal ring. A suture placed slightly above follows.

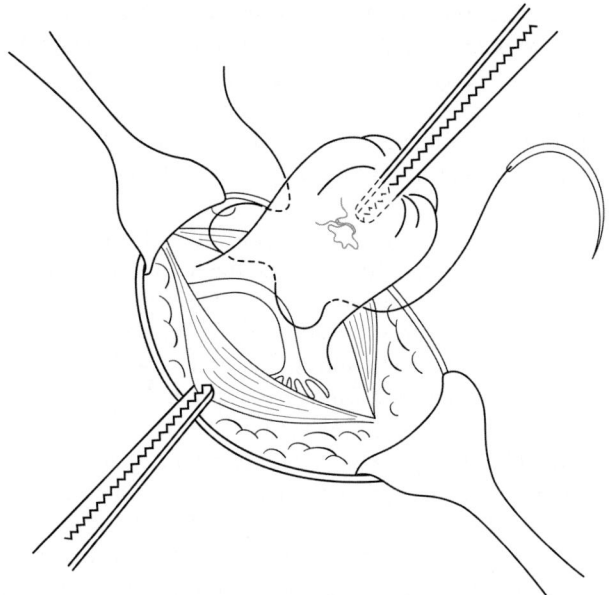

FIGURE 36-21 A technique for sliding hernias, in this case the fallopian tube. The dissected sac is tied distal to the tube. A purse-string suture is applied from the outside, carefully avoiding the tube. The beginning of the invagination process of the sac is shown.

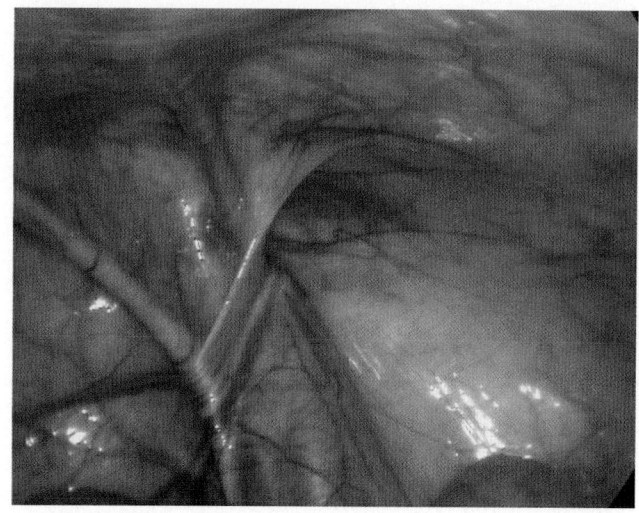

FIGURE 36-23 Laparoscopic inspection demonstrating a patent or "open" processus vaginalis, right side. The open internal ring, the vas, the testicular blood supply, the epigastric vessels, the obliterated right umbilical artery and the lateral portion of the bladder are clearly visible. (*Courtesy of Felix Schier, M.D.*)

has relatively few postoperative complications, a low recurrence rate, and is easily taught. The application of minimal access techniques to the repair of pediatric inguinal hernias in children remains controversial, yet it appears to be the trend in care of the future. Both intracorporeal and extracorporeal repair techniques have been advocated by a number of groups throughout the world. While most initial repair techniques described by pediatric surgeons involved the use of an intracorporeal suture repair (Figs. 36-23 and 36-24), refinement of the procedure has resulted in a laparoscopic-assisted

extracorporeal approach as advocated by one of the authors (RAC). The evolution of this technique has mirrored the adoption of extraperitoneal repair techniques by our adult colleagues who we must credit for being the true pioneers of laparoscopic inguinal hernia repair. Contemporary review of published repair techniques suggests that while some are clearly inferior to the traditional open repair, others appear to offer equivalent, if not superior, results. While there are several potential benefits of the laparoscopic techniques over open repair, perhaps the most striking is the ease at which it can be performed in preterm infants with equal efficacy. Furthermore, it allows for better visualization of the contralateral internal ring due to the differences in approach angles,

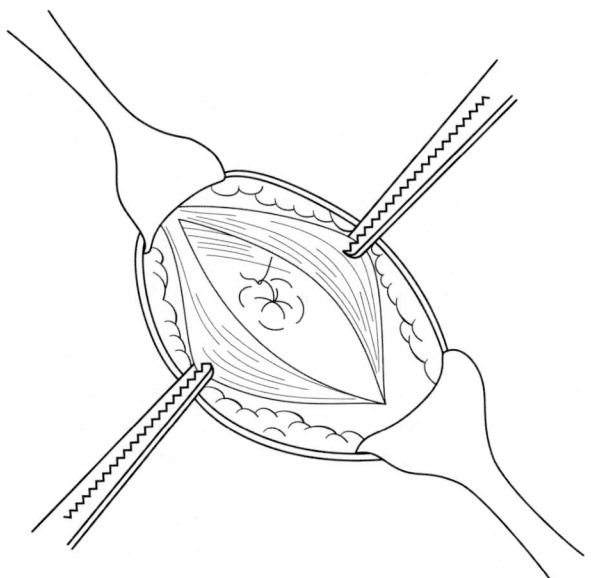

FIGURE 36-22 The sac has been invaginated and the purse-string suture tied. The sliding contents of the sac are now in a "free" intraperitoneal location.

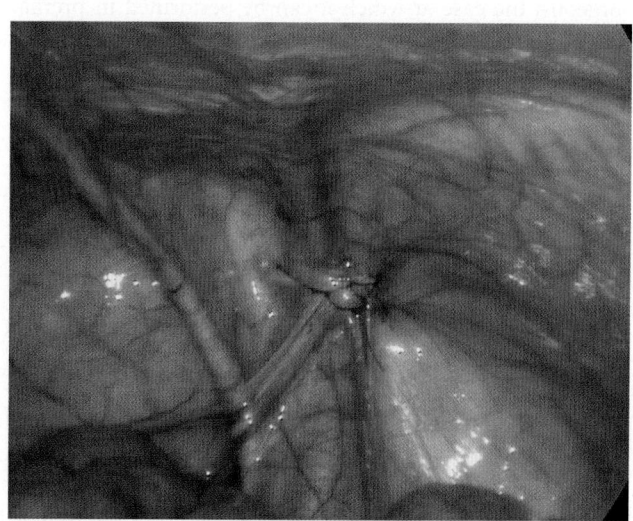

FIGURE 36-24 Fully intraperitoneal laparoscopic closure of the patent processus vaginalis at the internal ring. Notice the laparoscopically placed suture and minimal distortion of adjacent structures. (*Courtesy of Felix Schier, M.D.*)

as well as direct visualization of the vas deferens and testicular blood supply at the site of hernia ligation.

Hernia recurrence and devascularization of the testicle and the vas deferens are important factors that must be considered in the comparison of open and laparoscopic hernia repair techniques. Individual studies examining the rate of recurrence following open inguinal hernia repair during childhood indicate a rate that ranges from 0.1% to 3.8%. A recent study examining 50-year follow-up data from the Mayo Clinic demonstrated the rate is closer to the high end of that spectrum, as a recurrence rate of 2.8% in primarily nonpremature infants was found. Unfortunately, none of these reviews have collected prospective data on recurrence rate, and the actual rate is not known. Thus, a true comparison of open and laparoscopic techniques is challenging. Adding to the difficulty in comparison is the fact that while the recurrence rate of laparoscopic studies is often collected prospectively, the mean follow-up time is by historic necessity short. Grosfeld et al. reported the mean time to hernia recurrence in 71 cases to be 6 months, with 75% found at 2 years. Given these data, a 2-year follow-up is probably not sufficient to be able to evaluate laparoscopic techniques, and 5-year follow-up data are probably necessary to reliably compare laparoscopic techniques to historical controls, either untreated or treated by the conventional "open" technique.

## Operative Technique

The preferred laparoscopic technique of one of the authors (RAC) is one adapted from Patkowski and modified by our group (MUSC). The technique relies on a monofilament nonabsorbable suture to perform a high ligation of the hernia sac with full exclusion of the vas deferens and spermatic cord vessels. The technique has been reserved for those patients who are younger than 10 years of age due to data from open repair suggesting that high ligation of the sac alone may be inadequate treatment for adolescent patients. Additional benefits of this technique are the ease with which it can be taught to surgeons, the ease at which it can be performed in premature and lower-birth weight infants, and a shorter operative time resulting in decreased anesthetic time. The potential liabilities of the technique include its requirement for a general anesthetic and an unlikely need for a conversion of an extraperitoneal approach to an intraperitoneal approach. We believe that the shorter operative time offsets the first liability, while the second is purely an academic one since diagnostic laparoscopy is performed routinely on most open hernia repairs converting them to intraperitoneal procedures.

The patient is positioned supine on the bed with a small bump under the hips. After a general endotracheal tube anesthetic is induced, the abdomen and groin are prepared and draped in usual sterile fashion. A 5-mm radially expanding trocar (*Mini Step*™ Bladeless Trocar, *Autosuture*) is placed through the umbilicus using a modified open technique. This is achieved by a vertical incision placed in the base of the umbilicus that incises the skin and fascia. After a straight Jacobson microhemostatic forceps is placed through the fascial defect to ensure free entry into the abdominal cavity, the radially dilating sheath is inserted following placement

of the trocar. The abdomen is insufflated with carbon dioxide to a pressure that allows full visualization of the inguinal anatomy (8-12 cm water). Diagnostic laparoscopy ensues using a 4-mm 30° scope to both confirm the preoperative diagnosis and evaluate the contralateral internal ring. This also allows direct visualization of direct and femoral hernias if present.

An additional 3-mm stab incision is then made lateral to the umbilicus on the side opposite the hernia, and through this a 3-mm slightly curved fine-tipped (Maryland) dissector is placed. The preferred position of the surgeon is to stand on the side of the bed opposite the hernia, with a monitor setup in a straight line from the surgeon. The first step is to define the lateral and medial borders of the open internal ring by probing the area with a small 27-gauge needle. A 1-mm skin incision is then made between the lateral and medial borders of the internal ring with an 11 blade scalpel. A straight fine-tipped (Jacobson) hemostat is used to spread the superficial tissues below this incision. A 22-gauge noncutting blunt tipped (Tuohy) spinal needle is loaded with a 2-0 (or 3-0 depending on the patient's size) synthetic, monofilament, suture threaded inside the barrel and the tail pulled back along the needle. We typically use a nonabsorbable suture; however, an absorbable suture may be appropriate although our group has not studied the long-term efficacy of this. The needle and suture are inserted into the 1-mm skin incision, advanced, and passed underneath the peritoneum and the inguinal ligament, lateral to the internal inguinal ring and away from the spermatic vessels and vas. Once past the vessels, the needle is advanced through the peritoneum into the abdominal cavity and the suture is pushed through the barrel of the needle creating an internal "loop" (Fig. 36-25). The needle is then pulled out, leaving the loop of suture inside the abdomen. This loop of suture will be used to pull the other end of the suture circumferentially around the hernia sac. To accomplish this, the needle is again introduced into the 1-mm skin incision, and advanced along the anteromedial aspects of the hernia sac, over the vas, but under the peritoneum, and the needle is brought out of the previously made hole in the peritoneum through which the loop of suture is emanating. The needle is positioned so that it is going through the loop of suture. To facilitate placement of the needle during this maneuver, the vas and vessels are mobilized by grasping the adjacent peritoneum (while not touching these structures) in order to prevent injury. Hydrodissection (by injecting saline through the needle) can be used to help develop the plane between the vas/vessels and the peritoneum, although this is rarely necessary and can obscure the view.

One of the suture ends is introduced through the barrel of the empty spinal needle, and the thread is pushed through the barrel of the needle so that it passes into the loop. Finally, the loop is pulled out of the abdomen, bringing with it the caught end of suture. This last step results in the circumferential placement of suture around the internal inguinal ring, under the peritoneum but not incorporating the vas deferens and spermatic vessels. The resulting purse-string suture can be easily tied extracorporeally since the ends of the suture exit through the same 1-mm skin incision in the groin (Fig. 36-26). Prior to tying the ligature, the laparoscope

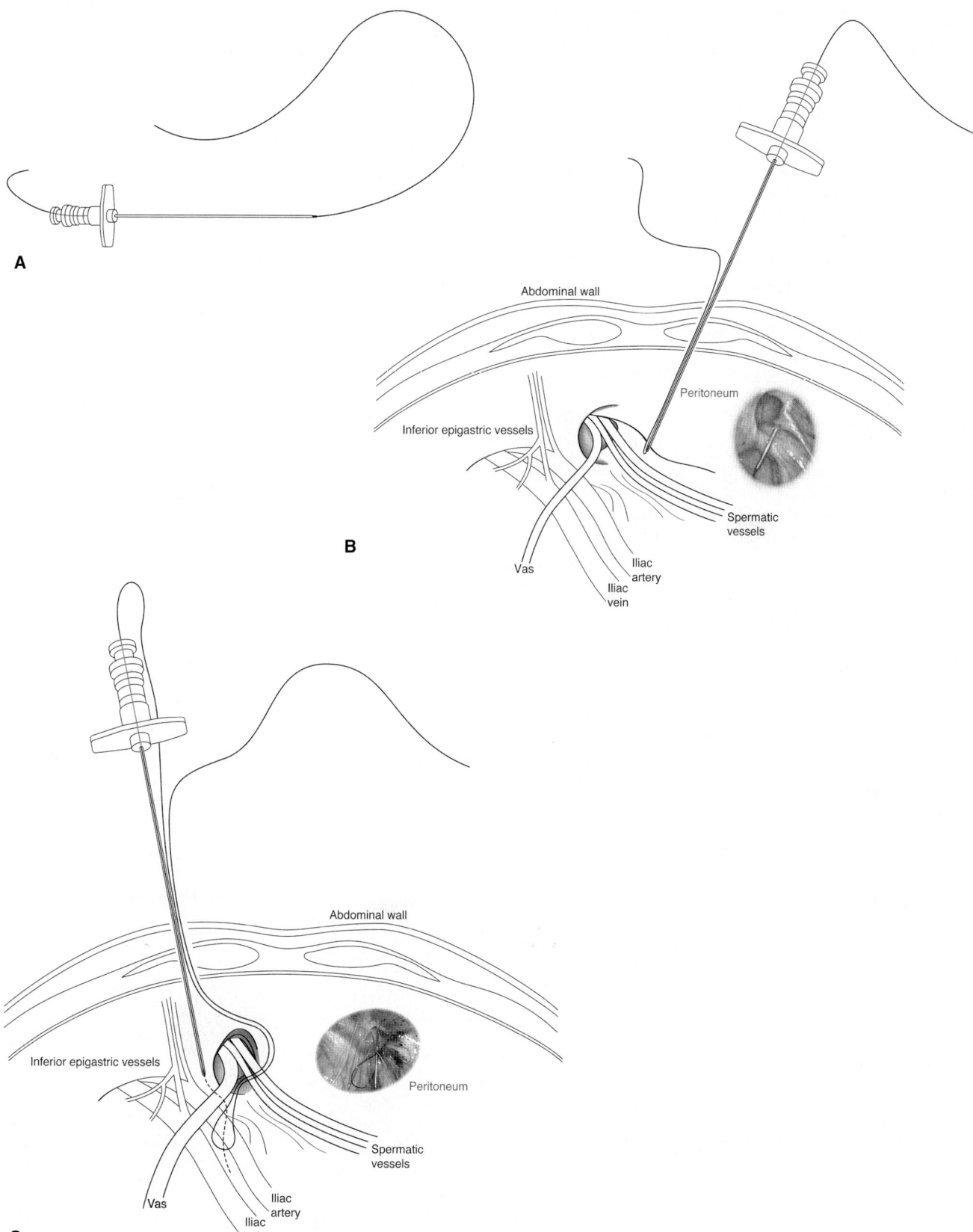

**FIGURE 36-25** **A.** The 22-guage Tuohy Spinal Needle is loaded with a 2-0 Prolene suture strand. The thread is then pulled back along the needle shaft. **B.** After a small skin incision is made over the inguinal canal, the needle is advanced along the anterolateral aspects of the hernia sac, passed the vessels, taking great care to place the needle between the peritoneum and the vessels. The needle is then pushed through the peritoneum and the internal loop remains in the abdomen as the needle is withdrawn. **C.** The needle is then advanced along the anteromedial aspects of the hernia sac, over the vas deferens, and under the peritoneum. Grasping the peritoneum near the vas (but never the vas itself) aids in the placement of this suture. The needle tip is advanced through the peritoneum and placed in the internal loop before the thread is advanced through the needle into the loop.

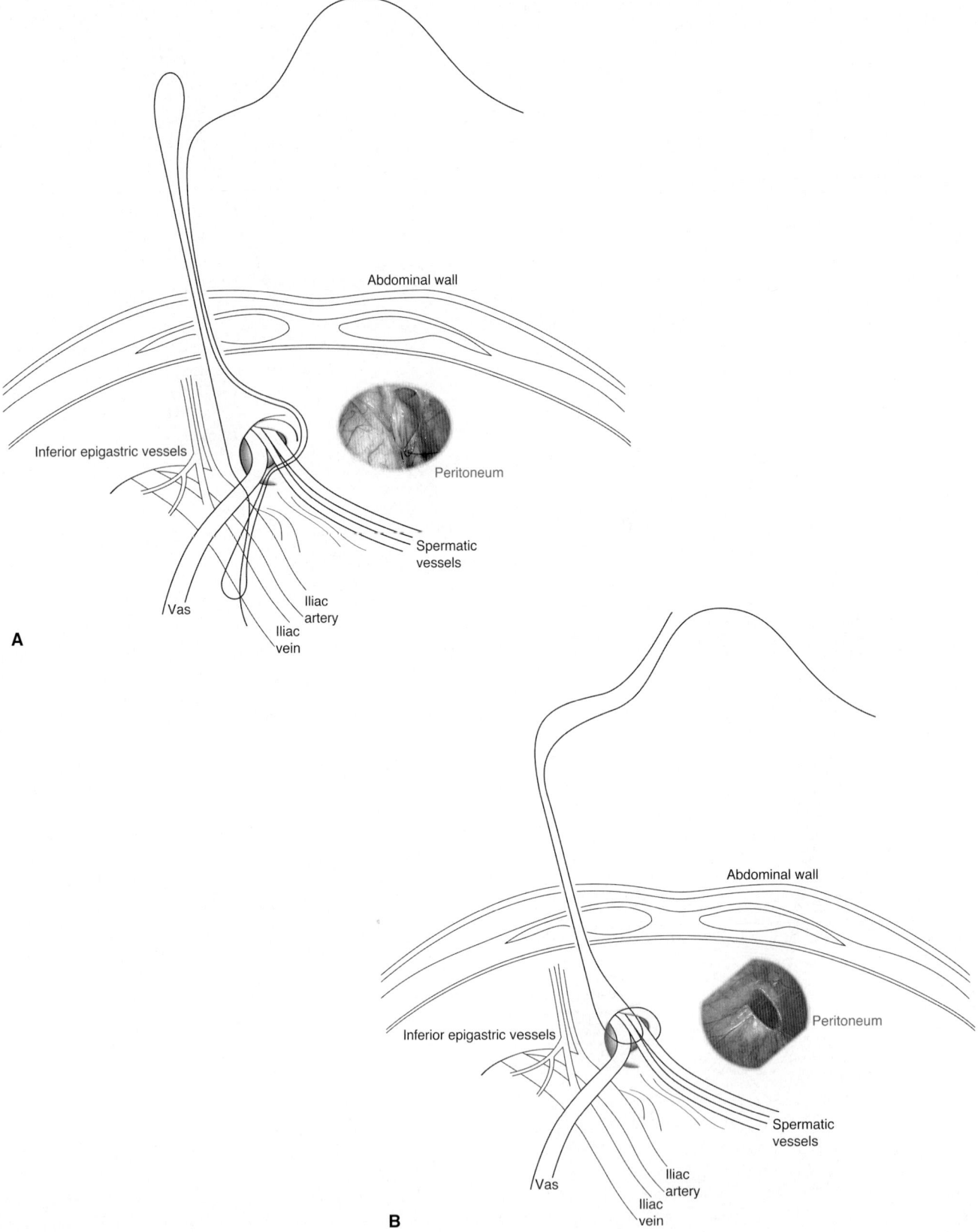

Abdominal wall

Inferior epigastric vessels

Peritoneum

Spermatic
vessels

Vas

Iliac
artery

Iliac
vein

A

Abdominal wall

Inferior epigastric vessels

Peritoneum

Spermatic
vessels

Vas

Iliac
artery

Iliac
vein

B

**FIGURE 36-26** **A.** Once an adequate length of suture is advanced through the barrel of the needle, the needle is withdrawn slightly so that only the suture and the loop are in the abdomen. It is important to have a considerable length of suture thread into the loop before the loop is withdrawn so as to ensure that the suture will be externalized. **B.** This also demonstrates the purse string suture around the hernia sac without incorporating the vas deferens or vessels. The two suture ends are elevated closing the purse string and an extracorporeal knot is tied.

is used to visualize the spermatic vessels and vas deferens, and by pulling up on the tails of the ligature, a final check can be made to ensure that these structures are not incorporated within, or damaged by the closure of the hernia sac. Once the suture is tied, the knot is buried in the subcutaneous tissue of the abdominal wall. Ilioinguinal nerve blocks are placed using the standard technique or laparoscopic guidance can be employed, to aid postoperative pain control. Following desufflation of the abdomen, the umbilical port site is closed with absorbable suture, and the skin incisions are closed with steri-strips.

This technique can be used with equal facility in both boys and girls, although we generally do modify the technique to omit the accessory instrument in performing inguinal hernia repairs in girls for obvious reasons. This technique requires a short time to learn and can be applied to both preterm and term infants, toddlers, and older children with ease. We feel that the most important technical aspects of this procedure are not only the use of nonabsorbable suture material, but also meticulous suture placement around the internal ring. The suture placement should specifically avoid skipped areas of the peritoneum through which a recurrent hernia could develop, as well as be placed so as to not interfere with the vas deferens and spermatic vessels.

## THE INCARCERATED HERNIA

An *incarceration* occurs when the contents of the sac, usually small bowel, are trapped and do not spontaneously return to the abdominal cavity. If unattended, interference with the intestinal blood supply ensues, initially occluding venous and lymphatic vessels and eventually compromising the arterial blood supply. This stage is referred to as strangulation. The swollen sac contents, pressing against the inguinal canal and its rings lead to obstruction of the blood supply to the ipsilateral gonad, jeopardizing its viability. Additionally, it has been reported that fibrous "rings" or constrictions inside the sac (believed to be attempts of the body to occlude the PPV) may contribute to incarceration in some cases (Fig. 36-27). Incarceration most commonly occurs in the first 6 months of life, when more than half of the instances are diagnosed. Infants under 3 months are particularly at risk with a reported incidence as high as 30%, falling to around 20% at 6 months and decreasing gradually thereafter.

The early manifestations of incarceration include "irritability" and unexplained crying, and occasional vomiting. Signs and symptoms of intestinal obstruction eventually follow: abdominal distention, bilious emesis, and occasionally traces of blood in the stool. On physical examination, there is a tense mass in the groin that can extend down to the scrotum. However, in heavier babies this bulge may not be initially obvious. On palpation the mass is defined, usually tender, and does not spontaneously reduce. If present beyond several hours, swelling and redness of the groin and the scrotum will be seen. The differential diagnoses include gonadal torsion and lymphadenitis. If there is doubt concerning the etiology, an ultrasonographic examination may be obtained

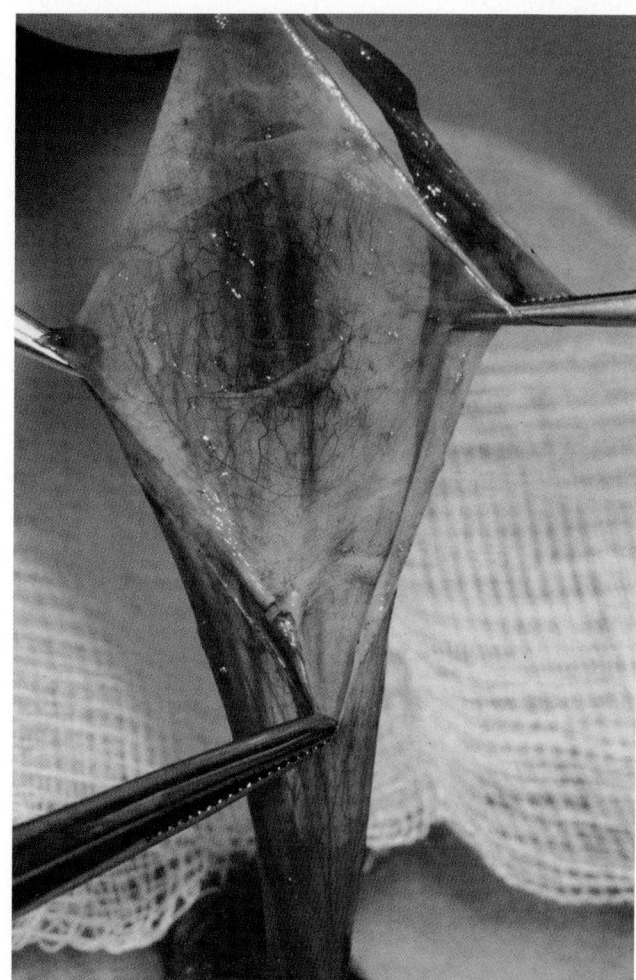

**FIGURE 36-27** Opened hernia sac demonstrating fibrous rings, believed to contribute to incarceration in some cases.

that may demonstrate peristaltic activity in the entrapped intestine. An abdominal roentgenogram will demonstrate distended loops of bowel. An air "bubble" may be visible in the affected scrotum (Fig. 36-28).

The initial approach to an incarcerated hernia, without signs of bowel compromise, is manual reduction. Figure 36-29 illustrates a commonly employed technique. One hand of the operator holds the scrotum and testis and exerts gentle distal traction following the direction of the canal. The index and thumb of the other hand apply gentle and sustained pressure downward (distally), freeing the incarceration from the edge of the external ring. If the child is too agitated or the process proves too painful, sedation and analgesia are indicated. In this case, a monitored setting is mandatory. The herniated bowel will be felt to empty gradually and then suddenly reduce. At least 80% of incarcerated hernias will reduce without an operation. Elective repair is performed 24 to 48 hours later, depending on the difficulty of reduction. The operative technique is as for an uncomplicated hernia repair. Excessive force or general anesthesia for the reduction of an incarceration is contraindicated because compromised bowel can be returned to the abdomen. This warning applies particularly to premature infants.

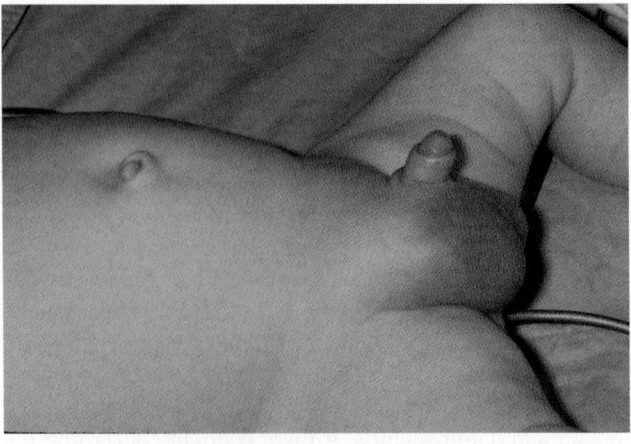

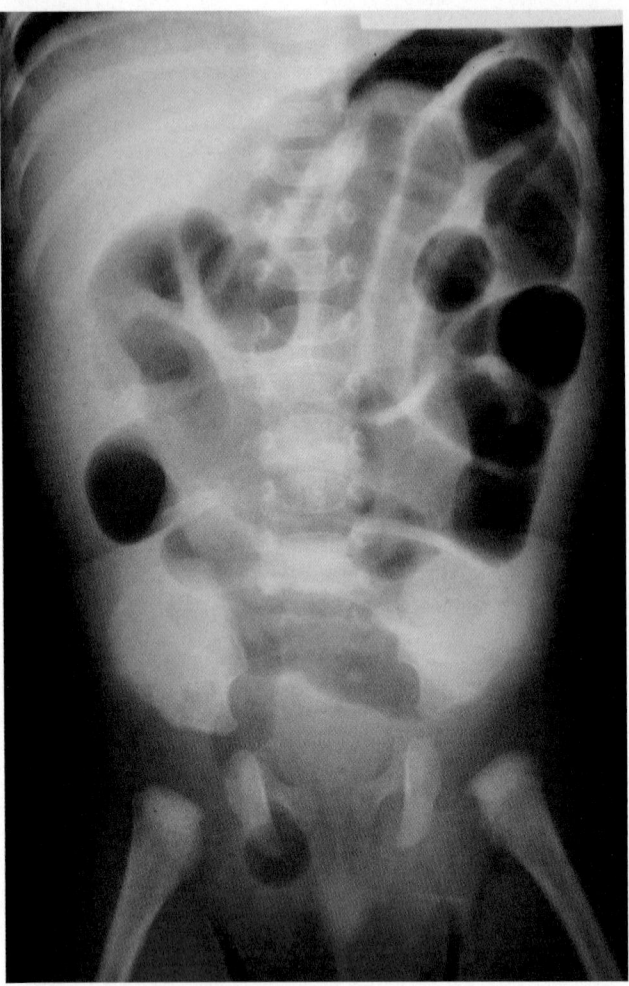

**FIGURE 36-28** Plain abdominal film of a male infant with an incarcerated right inguinal hernia. The child presented with bilious vomiting. Notice the distended loops of bowel and the air "bubble" in the right groin.

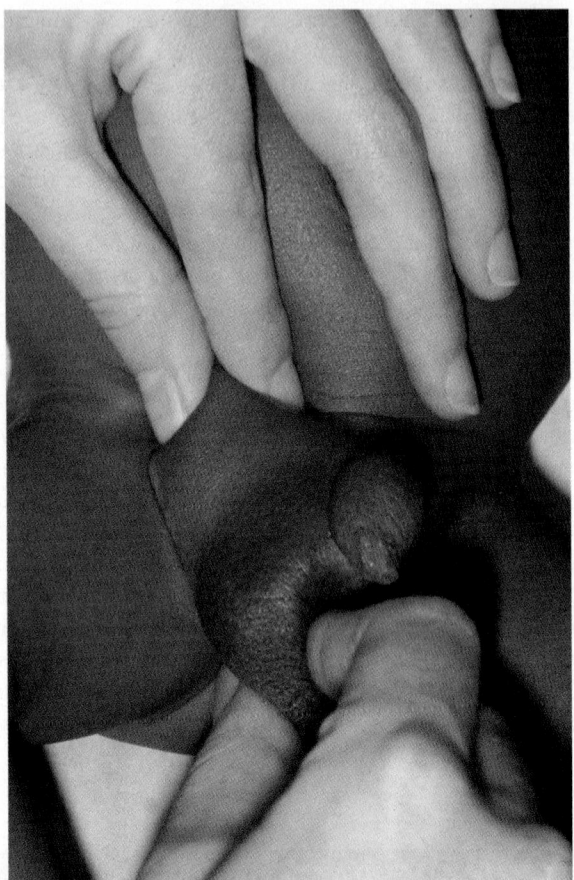

**FIGURE 36-29** Reduction maneuver for children with an incarcerated hernia. The operator's right hand places traction distally on the affected scrotum. The thumb and index finger of the other hand push the incarceration distally, away from the external ring. Slight, continuous pressure is applied until the reduction is completed.

An *emergency operation* is required when the hernia cannot be reduced (Figs. 36-30 to 36-32) or when there is evidence of strangulation (Figs. 36-33 to 36-34). The children are managed in the same manner as for any intestinal obstruction, including nasogastric decompression, intravenous hydration, and prophylactic antibiotic therapy. If the child shows signs of toxicity, the procedure is delayed until his/her condition has stabilized. A previously irreducible hernia may spontaneously reduce after the child has been anesthetized. In this case, the operation should proceed as planned. If the hernia is not reduced prior to the operation, a couple of steps differ from the previously described open procedure. The incision should be more generous, the external ring opened, and the sac grasped more distally and opened widely to permit a thorough inspection of the bowel prior to reduction. Any constricting portion of the sac is opened. If the incarcerated bowel shows signs of ischemia, it is covered with moist, warm gauze and observed for 5 to 10 minutes. Necrotic bowel can usually be resected without an additional skin incision, although an extension may be needed. A gridiron approach, through the internal oblique and transverse muscle, slightly more cranially, may be employed if additional deep exposure is required. An

adequate opening is needed for atraumatic repositioning of the anastomosed bowel. The status of the affected gonad must be assessed. Only a clearly necrotic gonad warrants removal. In addition to the conventional open techniques, laparoscopic approaches have been shown to be very successful, notably in very small children without necrotic bowel. Boys in whom

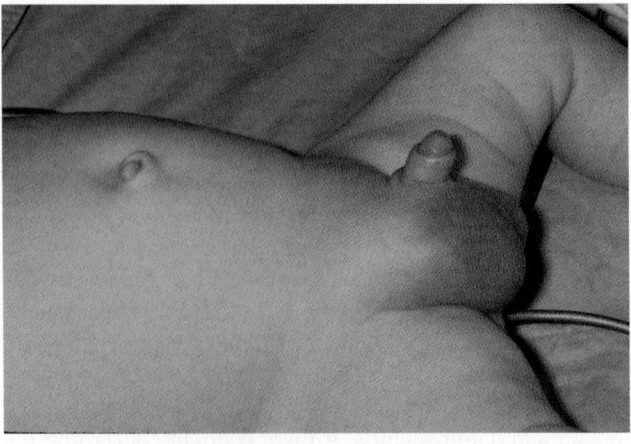

**FIGURE 36-30** Irreducible right inguinal hernia in a 6-week-old boy.

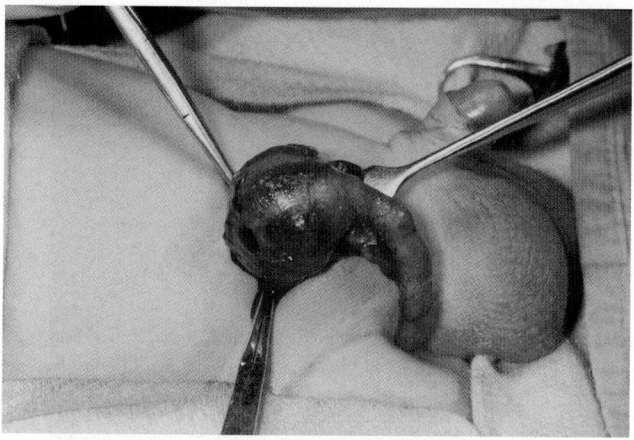

**FIGURE 36-31** Operative finding: incarcerated cecum and appendix. The appendix was removed, the cecum reduced, and the hernia repaired.

the incarceration was not easily reduced should have a long-term follow-up to assess the affected testis.

## Special Considerations

### Premature Infants

These children present the neonatologist, the anesthesiologist, and the surgeon with a set of specific problems. Concerning timing, it is generally agreed that infants in the neonatal intensive care unit should have the hernia(s) repaired prior to discharge. If operated postdischarge, they require admission and overnight monitoring because of the significant risk for postanesthesia apnea. For the surgeon the procedure can be challenging because of the small, delicate structures, the very thin sac, the often present incompletely descended testicle, and occasionally a large, "stretched" internal ring (Fig. 36-3). With the open procedure, magnification is mandatory; an undescended testicle is brought down with minimal dissection and secured to the inside surface of the scrotum, rather than being placed in the conventional neo-dartos

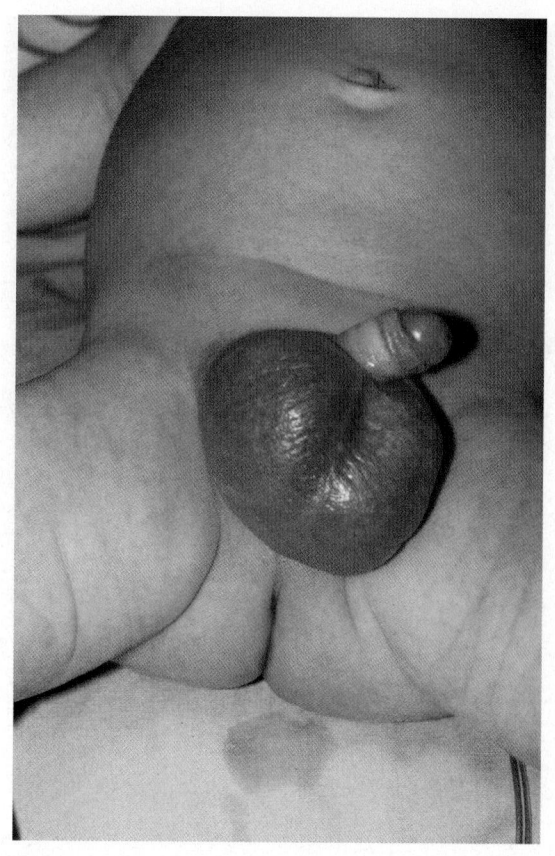

**FIGURE 36-33** Tender, swollen inguinoscrotal area in a 2½-week-old infant with intestinal obstruction. Manual reduction was not attempted.

pouch; if there is difficulty with tearing of a large sac and/or a large opening, a purse-string suture is placed *inside* the sac at the level of the internal ring.

### Undescended Testis

Incompletely descended testes are generally associated with a PPV and may be accompanied by a hernia. If the patient

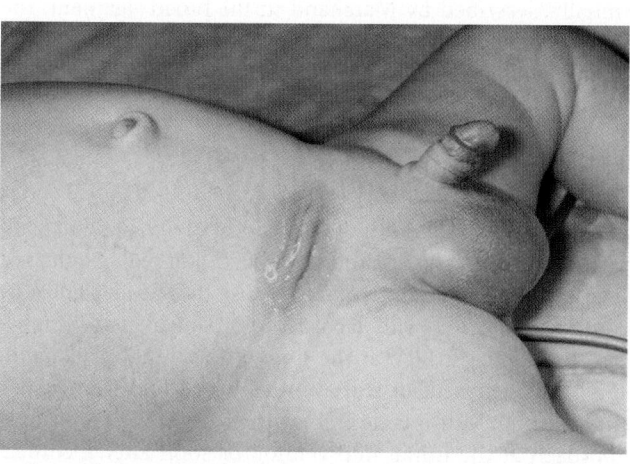

**FIGURE 36-32** Completed procedure. The incision in the inguinoabdominal fold was covered with a flexible collodion. The child recovered uneventfully and the gonad had a normal size at a 1-year follow-up.

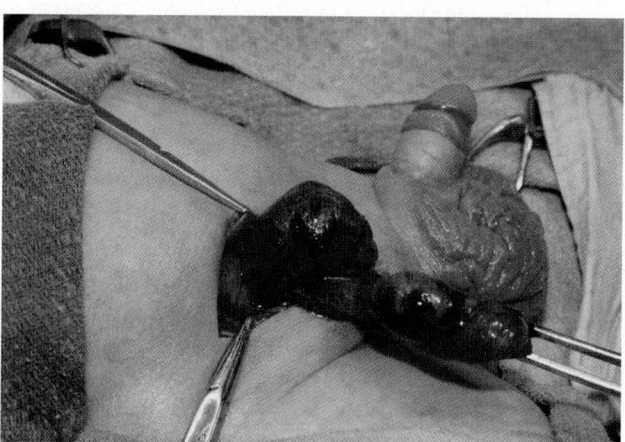

**FIGURE 36-34** Operative finding: a loop of necrotic small bowel and an equally necrotic, incompletely descended testicle. The deep layers of the incision were further opened, the necrotic segment was resected, and a primary anastomosis was performed. The testis could not be salvaged and was removed. The child made an uneventful recovery.

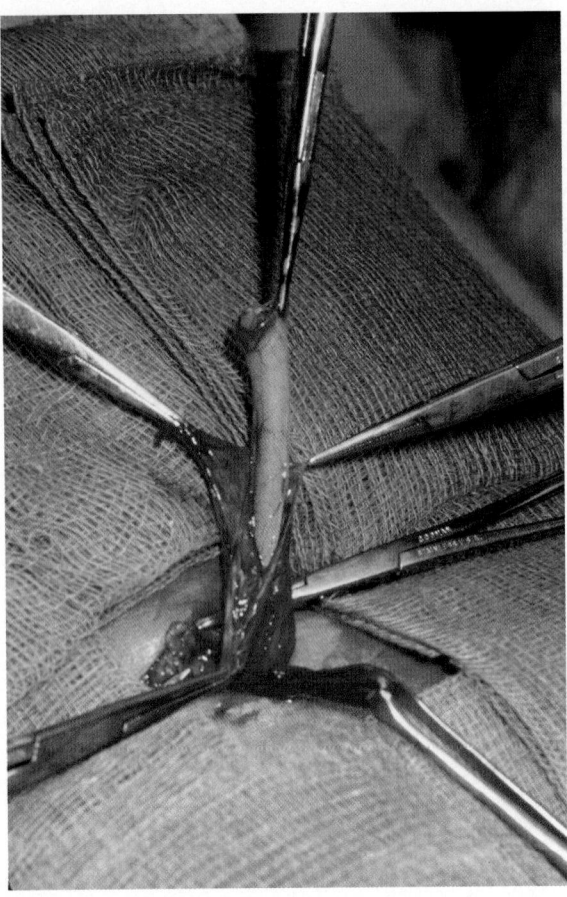

**FIGURE 36-35** An appendix adherent to a right inguinal hernia sac (Amyand hernia). The appendix was separated and removed. The hernia closure followed.

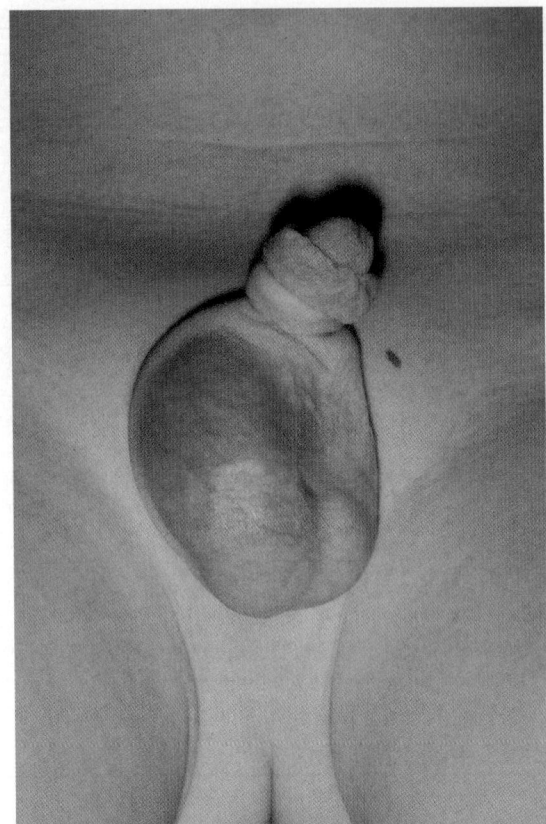

**FIGURE 36-36** Hydrocele in a young boy. Notice the bluish discoloration. Because of the rather recent manifestation and no clear history of changes in size, an ultrasound exam was obtained to rule out testicular malignancy. The testicle was normal and the child underwent a hydrocelectomy.

is a newborn or a small infant and the hernia is asymptomatic, it may be advantageous to postpone the procedure until the child is closer to 6 months or beyond. The gonad may have descended further spontaneously and the structures become easier to dissect, minimizing the danger of injury. However, the parents must be fully informed about how to recognize an incarceration and the steps to follow in such an event (Figs. 36-2, 36-35 and 36-36).

### Sliding Hernias and Unusual Intestinal Segments in Hernia Sacs

A sliding hernia is one in which an intraabdominal viscus becomes a part of the hernia sac. In a true sliding hernia, as in the case of the urinary bladder or the ureter, the structure is external to the peritoneal covering. However, other organs may be in a peritoneal fold, such as the cecum, ovary, tube, or even the uterus. Intraabdominal portions of the intestine may also be found in the sac, either freely moving or firmly adherent to its inner surface. Examples include omentum (in older children), appendix (Amyand hernia) (Fig. 36-35), and Meckel diverticulum (Littre hernia). An acutely inflamed appendix or Meckel diverticulum in a groin hernia can be difficult to distinguish from incarcerated bowel or gonadal torsion. A laparoscopic exam can clarify the anatomy before an exploration is undertaken.

### Adrenal Rests

During the testicular descent from its retroperitoneal position, small islands of adrenocortical tissue can follow and are occasionally found in the spermatic cord. These bright yellow–orange structures seldom exceed 4 to 5 mm in diameter. Although there are no reported cases of complications leaving them intact, removal through enucleation is simple. Initially described by Marchand in the broad ligament, the same eponym is often applied to these incidental findings on the cord.

### Ventriculoperitoneal (VP) Shunts and Peritoneal Dialysis

Due to the excess fluid in the peritoneal cavity, patients with VP shunts or dialysis catheters have a markedly increased incidence of inguinal hernias. Because these tubes are now routinely inserted with laparoscopic control, it is important to identify a PPV at the time of the initial placement. If a PPV is present, it will eventually lead to a hernia. For this reason, closure is desirable either using a laparoscopic approach at the initial intervention or soon after a clinical hernia manifests itself. It stands to a reason that an incarceration in these patients can significantly compound the original pathologies.

## Cystic Fibrosis

Patients with mucoviscidosis have an increased incidence of inguinal hernias, and absence of the vas deferens is a common associated finding. If, during a herniorrhaphy, a vas cannot be identified, the child should be investigated for cystic fibrosis. Additionally, specks of calcium within a hernia sac may represent calcified meconium secondary to an in utero intestinal perforation, another finding that may imply underlying cystic fibrosis with or without meconium ileus.

## Intersex

The presence of a palpable gonad in the labia of a phenotypic female, particularly if the finding is bilateral, may indicate that the child is a male with androgen insensitivity syndrome, or a hermaphrodite (see also Chapter 71, Ambiguous Genitalia and Intersex Anomalies). If an ovary is present in the hernia sac, it must be carefully examined for evidence of testicular tissue. Males with androgen insensitivity syndrome do not have fallopian tubes or a uterus. The introitus and the vaginal canal are short and the gonads tend to be small (Fig. 36-6). Hermaphrodites may have a fallopian tube in the hernia sac, and examination of the gonad will reveal an asymmetric ovotestis. In either case, the abnormal gonad should not be removed. Small wedge biopsies are taken from each pole, the gonad is replaced, and the hernia is repaired. Subsequently, appropriate investigations are carried out.

## Transverse or Crossed Testicular Ectopia

In this rare anomaly the affected gonad lies in the same canal as the normally descended testis and it is usually accompanied by an ipsilateral hernia. The contralateral scrotum is empty. The right side is affected more often. Correction depends on the anatomical findings. Because the fusion of the cords, attempts at full separation are hazardous. Following closure of the hernia, the ectopic testis is fixed to the opposite hemiscrotum.

## Postoperative Complications

The overall complication rate for inguinal herniorrhaphy, employing either the traditional open or the laparoscopic approach, is approximately 2%. However, the figure increases significantly to 15% to 20% in instances of incarceration and strangulation, particularly in premature infants.

## Edema, Hematoma, Infection, Early Suture Reaction

Inguinoscrotal edema is uncommon and almost entirely limited to premature babies and small infants. The main concern is that it can mimic an early recurrence. Wound hematomas should be rare, although scrotal discoloration can be observed after the repair of larger hernias in small children. Surgical site infection should also be rare. Fortunately, it tends to be limited to skin and subcutaneous tissue. Prompt antibiotic therapy is indicated, especially if cellulitis is noted. Occasionally, a subcutaneously placed suture will create a local reaction. Simple removal of the stitch suffices. Early and late deep or superficial suture reactions can occur with silk, and for this reason, this suture material should not be used.

## Hydrocele

A hydrocele may develop in the distal portion of the sac after several days or weeks. This usually resolves spontaneously and aspiration is rarely required.

## Iatrogenic Undescended Testis

Also known as ascending or "trapped" testicle this occurs when a previously eutopic gonad is found in an abnormally high position during the follow-up visit. This complication can be minimized by routinely repositioning the testicle into the low scrotum immediately after completing every herniorrhaphy in boys. If the gonad cannot be brought to the scrotum by simple manipulation, as in the case of a retractile testis, an orchiopexy is necessary.

## Recurrent Hernia

The reported recurrence rate following repair of an uncomplicated conventional open inguinal hernia repair is under 1%. Although early series of laparoscopic herniorrhaphies exhibited higher recurrence rates (and hydrocele formation), the contemporary series show that the recurrence rate of both methods (for straightforward hernias) is now practically similar. However, the recurrence rates rise with either method to near 20% in children who had a complex incarceration or small premature infants with large hernias and very thin sacs. Possible causes for a recurrence of an indirect inguinal hernia include an unrecognized tear of the sac, failure of the ligature, and failure to correctly identify and ligate the PPV. At times, the "recurrence" is actually a previously unrecognized direct inguinal or femoral hernia. A repeat exploration becomes necessary, being certain that the exposure is adequate. A laparoscopic approach may be advantageous because it can more easily determine the cause and site of the recurrence, followed by the appropriate repair without dissection of the cord.

## Testicular Atrophy

The exact incidence of this problem is not known. The reported incidence puts the figure at 1%, but this is probably an underestimation, particularly if the repair was prompted by an incarceration with strangulation.

## Injury to the Vas Deferens

The vulnerability of the vas deferens has been clearly demonstrated in animal models. Even gentle grasping of the vas with a nontoothed forceps can lead to wall inflammation leading to stricture. Clamping has practically the same long-term effect as transection. Accidental transection of the vas requires immediate or, if not available, delayed expert reconstruction. Although there is some circumstantial evidence linking male infertility with inguinal hernia repair, the actual risk of damage to the vas during repair of an uncomplicated hernia is not known.

## Other Complications

Chronic pain following herniorrhaphy in children is considered rare, but it may be underreported. Hypertrophic scar or keloid formation may occur if an incision is placed outside the tension lines of the skin. Silk sutures can lead to a delayed foreign body reaction, even years after a herniorrhaphy and should, therefore, not be employed.

## HYDROCELES

Three types of hydroceles are seen in the pediatric and adolescent age group: physiologic (neonates and infants), communicating (beyond the neonatal period), and (scrotal) noncommunicating (beyond infancy). The most common is the physiologic hydrocele present in many healthy male newborns and small infants. There is no communication with the abdominal cavity, and therefore no changes in size are noted. These hydroceles resolve spontaneously from a few months up to a year or beyond. Very large, tense, bilateral hydroceles are occasionally seen. Their management is controversial, but waiting is still the preferred approach. Fine needle aspiration can have palliative value.

Communicating hydroceles, which may be associated with indirect inguinal hernias, tend to occur when the children are over 1 to 2 years of age. There are clear changes in size: the scrotal swelling is barely noticeable when the child awakens in the morning and quite obvious in the evening. On examination, the scrotum exhibits a slight bluish discoloration, transilluminates, and is nontender (Fig. 36-36). Although there is usually a clear demarcation at the upper portion of the hydrocele, at times the fluid-filled sac extends to the level of the external inguinal ring. A hydrocele of the cord can be confused with an incarceration. However, the children (boys or girls) are asymptomatic. The operation for communicating hydroceles is the same as for indirect inguinal hernias. As expected, the PPV at the level of the cord is thin and can be missed. If the main, distended portion of the hydrocele cannot be easily brought into the wound, a transscrotal needle aspiration is helpful. Part of the hydrocele sac can be split or resected, although this is not usually necessary and can endanger the delicate vas deferens and vessels. Postoperative reaccumulation is uncommon and tends to resolve spontaneously. A rare manifestation of the communicating hydrocele spectrum is the abdominoscrotal hydrocele in which the fluid-filled sac has an intraabdominal extension through the inguinal canal. The intraabdominal portion may be larger than the external one and can present as an abdominal mass. An ultrasound examination is diagnostic. The surgical approach is through a groin incision. Laparoscopy may be helpful.

Noncommunicating scrotal hydroceles, mostly in older children, can have multiple causes (eg, trauma, testicular malignancy, imbalance between the fluid produced and resorbed, inflammation, infection, parasitic). A prompt ultrasound examination is indicated, particularly if the onset of the fluid accumulation is recent. The management of these hydroceles is etiology specific.

## DIRECT INGUINAL HERNIA

Direct inguinal hernias account for about 1% of all groin hernias in children. They are due to a defect in the transversalis fascia and present as a bulge medially in the groin. Usually they do not extend as distally through the inguinal canal as indirect inguinal hernias. The sac is shorter and the neck is medial to the deep epigastric vessels. These hernias are difficult or impossible to diagnose preoperatively. If, during an open herniorrhaphy, a PPV is small and short, a direct inguinal hernia must be considered, keeping in mind that in an asleep, relaxed child, the collapsed sac may be difficult to find. What is, at times, thought to be a recurrent indirect inguinal hernia may be a missed direct hernia. The open repair consists of placing interrupted sutures in the transversalis fascia between the inguinal ligament and the conjoined tendon.

With the laparoscopic approach, the surgeon has the advantage of seeing the pathology very clearly. However, the neck of the sack may be collapsed. Increasing the insufflating pressure slightly can help open the neck and identify the hernia, which is then closed with intracorporeal suturing.

## FEMORAL HERNIAS

Femoral hernias are even less common than direct inguinal hernias in children, with a reported incidence below 0.5%. However, laparoscopic examinations have disclosed higher percentages in both femoral and direct inguinal hernias. Femoral hernias present as a bulge in the groin, below the inguinal ligament, medial to the femoral pulse, protruding through the femoral canal. Because of the rarity, these hernias are often misdiagnosed preoperatively and also missed intraoperatively, when the open inguinal approach is employed. Some children have had one or more previous operations until the correct diagnosis was established and the problem corrected. There are 4 different approaches for the correction of femoral hernias in children: the femoral or infrainguinal approach, the transinguinal approach, the suprainguinal preperitoneal approach, and, more recently, the laparoscopic approach. Until the advent of the laparoscopic herniorrhaphy, the preferred operation for children with a preoperatively diagnosed femoral hernia was the infrainguinal approach through a low inguinal incision. Here the cribriform fascia is divided to expose the hernia, which is medial to the femoral vein. Cutting or cauterizing is avoided to minimize damage to the lymphatic nodes and capillaries. The sac is opened and the contents are inspected and reduced. The sac is dissected as proximally as possible, tied and suture-ligated. The stump is reduced into the pelvis. The femoral canal is closed with nonabsorbable sutures placed between the inguinal ligament and the pectineal ligament of Astley Cooper. These structures should not be drawn too tightly together in order to avoid tearing through the tissues or obstructing the femoral vein. The sutures are placed in such a manner as to produce a lattice or barrier that will obstruct and narrow the femoral canal. Scar tissue eventually completes the closing process. The wound is then closed in layers. If compromised bowel is encountered in the sac and a resection is necessary, this should be done through a separate abdominal incision. The 2 other open approaches are more complex.

Femoral hernias have been successfully repaired using laparoscopic techniques. The main advantages are clear visualization of the anatomy, precise placement of sutures at the neck of the sac, and avoidance of groin blood and lymphatic vessels. The initial results are very promising, although long-term results are not yet available.

## UNUSUAL GROIN HERNIAS

Because of the increased use of laparoscopy for examination and repair of inguinal region hernias in children, unusual types, such as combinations of indirect and direct hernias (hernia "*en pantalon*"), indirect and femoral hernias, as well as a combination of all 3 types have been documented. Although known in the adult hernia literature, the traditional open inguinal hernia repair in the pediatric age group did not permit clear identification of these unusual forms.

## CONCLUDING NOTE

The diagnosis and management of hernias of the inguinal region is a most fulfilling endeavor for every surgeon managing pediatric patients: a common pathology for which there is an effective and lasting cure. Although paradigm-shifting approaches have occurred in the last couple of decades, the basic goal is to close the neck of a congenital, low abdominal wall hernia with the least possible disturbance of vital surrounding structures. Minimally invasive procedures, such as laparoscopic repair, offer new and, hopefully, less traumatic, lasting approaches. It is possible, and quite likely, that even less invasive methods will be developed in the future. However, every surgeon who is given the privilege of caring for a child must be keenly aware of the fact that pediatric hernias comprise a broad spectrum with many variables and several remaining questions and challenges.

## SELECTED READINGS

Al-Shanafey S, Giacomantonio M. Femoral hernia in children. *J Pediatr Surg* 1999;34(7):1104–1106.

Baird R, Gholoum S, Laberge JM, et al. Prematurity, not age at operation or incarceration, impacts complication rates in inguinal hernia repair. *J Pediatr Surg* 2011;46(6):906–911.

Bittner R, Schwarz J. Inguinal hernia repair: current surgical techniques [Note: adult hernias]. *Langenbeck's Arch Surg* 2012;397(2):271–282.

DeCou JM, Gauderer MWL. Inguinal hernia in infants with very low birth weight. *Semin Pediatr Surg* 2000;9(2):84–87.

Esposito C, Turial S, Allichio T, et al. Laparoscopic repair of incarcerated inguinal hernia: a safe and effective procedure to adopt in children. *Hernia* 2012;17(2):235–239.

Grosfeld JL, Minnik K, Shedd F, et al. Inguinal hernias in children: factors affecting recurrence in 62 cases. *J Pediatr Surg* 1991;26(3):283–287.

Kaya M, Hückstedt T, Schier F. Laparoscopic approach to incarcerated inguinal hernia in children. *J Pediatr Surg* 2006;41(3):576–579.

Le Coultre C, Cuendet A, Richon J. Frequency of testicular atrophy following incarcerated hernia. *Z Kinderchir* 1983;38(suppl):39–41.

Nah SA, Giacomello L, Eaton S, et al. Surgical repair of incarcerated inguinal hernia in children: laparoscopic or open? *Eur J Pediatr Surg* 2011;21(1):8–11.

Parelkar SV, Oak S, Gupta R, et al. Laparoscopic inguinal hernia repair in the pediatric age group: experience with 437 children. *J Pediatr Surg* 2010;45(4):789–792.

Patkowski D, Czernik J, Chrzan R, et al. Percutaneous internal ring suturing: a simple minimally invasive technique for inguinal hernia repair in children. *J Laparoendosc Adv Surg Tech A* 2006;16(6):513–517.

Potts WJ, Riker WL, Lewis JE. The treatment of inguinal hernia in infants and children. *Ann Surg* 1950;132(3):566–576.

Rajput A, Gauderer MWL, Hack M. Inguinal hernia in very low birth infants: incidence and timing of repair. *J Pediatr Surg* 1992;27(10):1322–1324.

Schier F. Laparoscopic surgery of inguinal hernias in children—initial experience. *J Pediatr Surg* 2000;35(9):1331–1335.

Schier F. Laparoscopic hernia repair: an option in babies weighing 5 kg or less. *Pediatr Surg Int* 2006;22(12):1033.

Schier F, Danzer E, Bondartschuk M. Incidence of contralateral patent processus vaginalis in children with inguinal hernia. *J Pediatr Surg* 2001;36(10):1561–1563.

Schier F, Montupet P, Esposito C. Laparoscopic inguinal herniorrhaphy in children: a three-center experience with 933 repairs. *J Pediatr Surg* 2002;37(3):395–397.

Schwöbel MG, Schramm H, Glitzelmann CA. The infantile inguinal hernia—a bilateral disease? *Pediatr Surg Int* 1999;15(2):115–118.

Shandling B, Janik JS. The vulnerability of the vas deferens. *J Pediatr Surg* 1981;16(4):461–464.

Tackett LD, Breuer CK, Luks F, et al. Incidence of contralateral inguinal hernia: a prospective analysis. *J Pediatr Surg* 1999;34(5):684–687.

Tam PK, Lister J. Femoral hernia in children. *Arch Surg* 1984;119(10):1161–1164.

Vergnes P, Midy D, Bondonny JM. Anatomical basis of inguinal surgery in children. *Anat Clin* 1985;7(4):257–265.

Wiener ES, Touloukian RJ, Rogers BM, et al. Hernia survey of the Section on Surgery of the American Academy of Pediatrics. *J Pediatr Surg* 1996;31(8):1166–1169.

Zamakhshary M, To T, Guan J, et al. Risk of incarceration of inguinal hernia among infants and young children awaiting elective surgery. *CMAJ* 2008;179(10):1001–1005.

Zendejas B, Zarrouq AE, Erben YM, et al. Impact of childhood inguinal hernia repair in adulthood: 50 years of follow-up. *J Am Coll Surg* 2010;211(6):762–768.

# Stomach: Obstruction, Microgastria, Foreign Body, and Peptic Ulcer

# CHAPTER 37

*Michael G. Caty and Mauricio A. Escobar Jr*

## KEY POINTS

1. Organoaxial volvulus is the most common reported type of gastric volvulus in childhood. Children do not reliably demonstrate the triad of Borchardt (unproductive retching, localized epigastric distension, and inability to pass a nasogastric tube). Associated diaphragmatic abnormalities should be assessed.

2. Pyloric atresia (PA) is an extremely rare cause of intestinal obstruction and may occur in combination with epidermolysis bullosa.

3. A completely obstructing antral web is treated with gastrotomy and circumferential web excision with oversewing of the mucosal remnant.

4. The need for surgical therapy is dictated by the severity of microgastria. If drooling, reflux, or failure to thrive persists, gastric augmentation should be performed. The technical aspects of the procedure include creating a loop from the Roux-en-Y limb of the jejunum. This pouch is anastomosed to the side of the diminutive stomach.

5. Most gastric duplication cysts can be bluntly dissected off adjacent organs. Dissection begins in the common muscular plane between the stomach and the duplication. The duplication is peeled off the mucosa of the stomach and removed.

6. The most common type of gastric tumor in childhood is a teratoma.

7. Recommendations for button battery removal from the stomach have changed. Typically, they pass on their own. Intervention is reserved for large batteries in small children (<6 years old) or if swallowed concomitantly with a magnet. Endoscopy is preferred but laparotomy and gastrotomy for removal may be necessary.

8. Operative interventions should be considered for any persistently bleeding child with peptic ulcer disease. Some clinical indications for operative treatment are loss of 50% of the estimated blood volume in 8 hours, hemodynamic instability, and the presence of a visible vessel on endoscopy.

The majority of gastric surgery in children is either gastrostomies or antireflux procedures. The surgeon managing infants and children must be additionally aware of the many gastric lesions that result in abdominal signs and symptoms. Most of these rare lesions cause either intrinsic or extrinsic obstruction of the stomach. Other lesions result in bleeding, perforation, or mass effect on the stomach.

## OBSTRUCTIVE LESIONS

Obstructive lesions of the stomach can be divided into those causing extrinsic obstruction (volvulus) or intrinsic obstruction (pyloric atresia [PA], antral web). The majority of these entities will be diagnosed in infancy. PA, however, will be diagnosed in the immediate newborn period. The common symptom of obstructive gastric lesions is nonbilious emesis. Each of these entities will be definitely diagnosed with gastrointestinal (GI) contrast studies. Following individualized surgical repairs, they have uniformly good outcomes.

### Gastric Volvulus

Acute gastric volvulus is an uncommon surgical emergency in children. Chronic gastric volvulus is even rarer and can be very difficult to diagnose. Gastric volvulus results from an abnormal rotation of the stomach around 1 of 2 axes. Organoaxial rotation occurs about a line drawn through the gastroesophageal junction and the pylorus (Fig. 37-1A). The body of the stomach usually rotates back over the axis toward the lesser space. This is the most common reported type of volvulus in childhood. Mesentericoaxial volvulus occurs about an axis drawn through the lesser and greater curvature of the stomach (Fig. 37-1B). Combinations of these types of volvulus may occur. Gastric volvulus occurs in the setting of inadequate fixation of the stomach by absence of one or more naturally occurring points of fixation. Four "ligaments" serve to maintain the normal location of the stomach. These are the gastrosplenic, gastrocolic, gastrophrenic, and gastrohepatic. Absence or "laxity" of the gastrosplenic and gastrocolic ligaments seems to be a common factor in documented cases. Patients with gastric volvulus often have associated abnormalities of the diaphragm. Eventration of

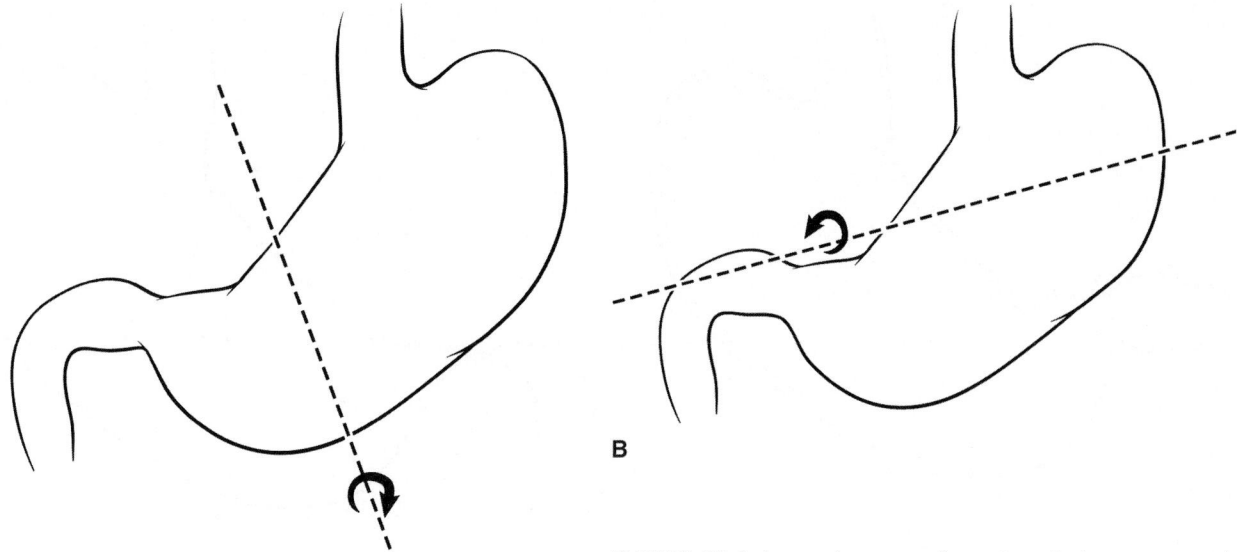

**FIGURE 37-1** Anatomic types of gastric volvulus, organoaxial volvulus (**A**), and mesentericoaxial volvulus (**B**).

the diaphragm, sliding hiatal hernia, and Bochdalek hernias have all been reported in association with gastric volvulus. Congenital asplenia, wandering spleen, and tracheoesophageal fistula have also been reported in association with gastric volvulus. Enlargement of the stomach with either air or fluid seems to contribute to volvulus in many reported series of gastric volvulus.

The majority of children with gastric volvulus present as infants. Vomiting is the most frequent presenting symptom. Children do not reliably demonstrate the triad of Borchardt (unproductive retching, localized epigastric distension, and inability to pass a nasogastric tube). Abdominal X-rays provide clues to the diagnosis as many patients have abnormal left upper quadrant gas patterns. Barium studies secure the diagnosis. Patients with mesentericoaxial volvulus will demonstrate a transverse obstruction in the middle of the stomach. Organoaxial volvulus is potentially more difficult to diagnose. The key to the diagnosis of organoaxial volvulus is the horizontal nature of the stomach. In addition, the gastroesophageal junction may be lower than normal. Associated diaphragmatic abnormalities should be assessed by examining radiographically for air or barium above the diaphragm. Howell–Jolly bodies in a peripheral blood smearing provide evidence of asplenia. In skilled hands, ultrasonography may be useful in securing a diagnosis.

Gastric volvulus should be considered a surgical emergency due to the potential for gastric necrosis. Laparoscopic approaches have been described, but exploratory laparotomy remains the gold standard therapy in children. Upon exploration, the stomach should be decompressed by a nasogastric tube if previous attempts at placement were unsuccessful. Occasionally, needle decompression is necessary.

Coexisting abnormalities should be identified and repaired. Congenital diaphragmatic hernias should be reduced and closed with nonabsorbable sutures. Hiatal hernias should be reduced and the crura closed. An antireflux procedure should be considered in the patient with clinically significant reflux. It is not clear that clinically insignificant diaphragmatic

eventration needs to be addressed acutely. In the absence of feeding difficulties, gastrostomy need not be performed, but is reasonable in the setting of a chronically distended stomach. Recurrence is prevented by anterior fixation of the stomach to 3 points on the anterior abdominal wall. Newly detected patients with asplenia should be started on penicillin prophylaxis and receive appropriate immunization. Recurrence is extremely unusual unless gastropexy is omitted, or technical failure occurs.

## Pyloric Atresia

PA is an extremely rare cause of intestinal obstruction. It has been estimated to have an incidence of 1 per million and an autosomal inheritance pattern. It may occur in combination with epidermolysis bullosa. This rare autosomal recessive disorder is characterized by a variable presentation of blistering of the skin and mucosal surfaces. The coexistence of epidermolysis bullosa and PA was once thought to have a uniformly fatal outcome; however, recent reports have described survivors. Because of this, repair of pyloric atresia should not be withheld in the patient with epidermolysis bullosa. Contemporary patients with isolated PA have uniformly good outcomes.

PA describes the total obstruction of the gastric outlet. This obstruction may result from a membrane, cord-like atresia, or gap between the stomach and pylorus (Fig. 37-2A-C). Theories of the etiology of this abnormality emphasize the failure of recanalization of the solid "cord" (epithelial plugging) state of the pylorus—a theory also used to explain duodenal atresia. In fact, PA may be associated with other intestinal atresias in a hereditary syndrome. Other authors feel that a vascular accident is involved. The coexistence of PA and epidermolysis bullosa suggests a possible role for in utero mucosal sloughing and subsequent scar formation. This theory is consistent with the observation that esophageal stricture and laryngeal stenosis occur in patients with epidermolysis bullosa.

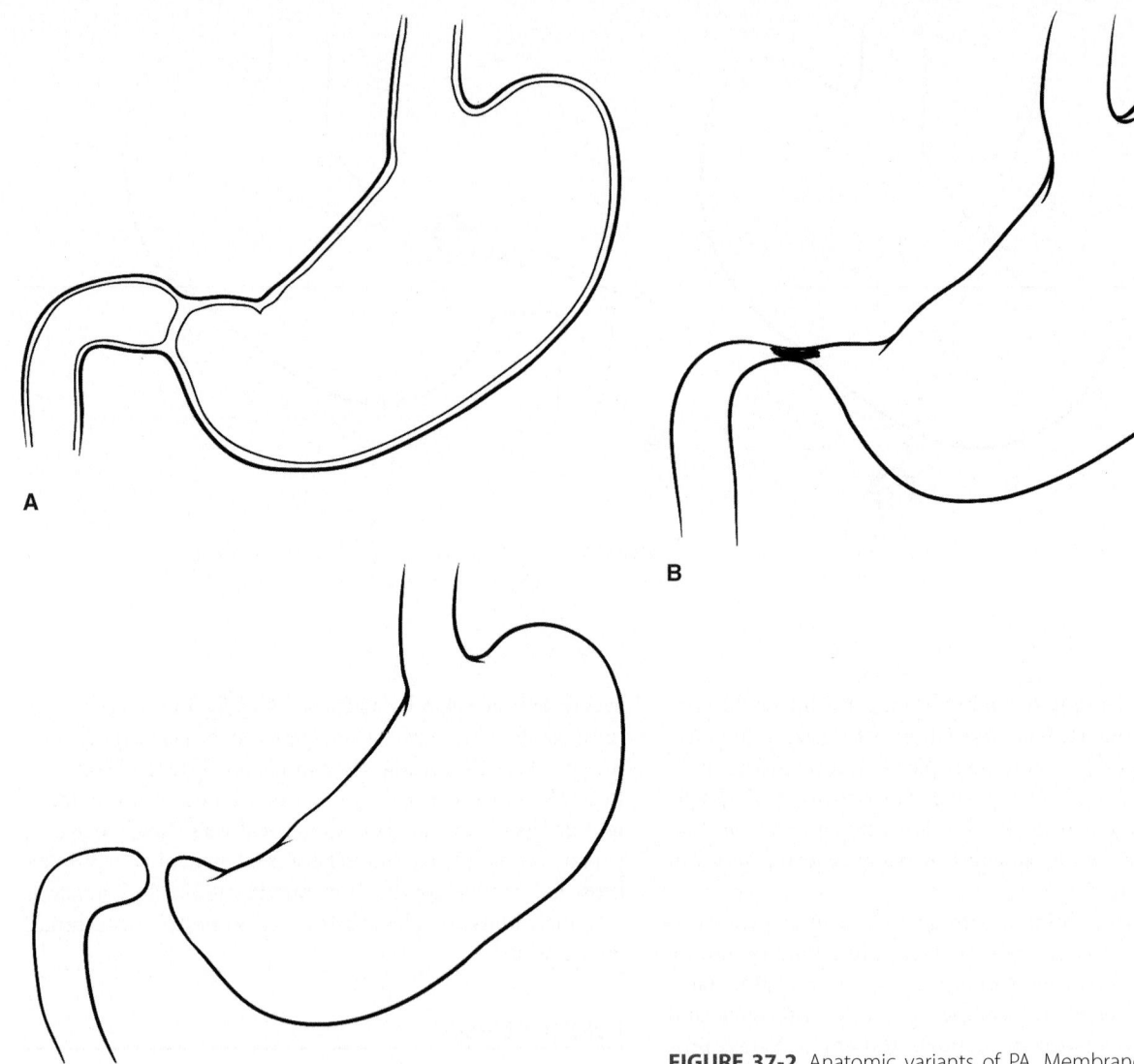

**A**

**B**

**C**

**FIGURE 37-2** Anatomic variants of PA. Membranous obstruction (**A**), cord-like atresia (**B**), and (**C**) complete disconnection.

Mothers of fetuses with PA characteristically have poly-hydramnios. Newborns with PA present with repeated non-bilious emesis. There is no abdominal distention suggestive of a distal obstruction. Plain abdominal radiographs show gastric distention and no distal air. If the diagnosis cannot be established or distinguished from duodenal obstruction due to malrotation or atresia, then a contrast study is performed.

Many patients suffer from dehydration and a hypochloremic, hypokalemic metabolic alkalosis. Fluid resuscitation should be accomplished prior to laparotomy. A nasogastric tube should be in place to decompress the distended stomach.

Technical correction of PA is adapted to the pathology discovered intraoperatively. Most newborns will have a membranous obstruction. This can be treated with a longitudinal incision over the pylorus and membrane resection. The pylorus is then closed in a Heineke-Mickulicz fashion. It is reasonable to pass a nasogastric tube through the anastomosis to facilitate early feeding and "stent" the area of edema at the anastomosis. The proximal stomach should be decompressed by a nasogastric tube. After a 7-day period, a contrast study is performed to assess the anastomosis. If the anastomosis is

patent and intact, the nasogastric tube is removed and oral feedings are started.

If there is no continuity between the distal stomach and pylorus (see Fig. 37-2C) then a gastroduodenostomy is performed. A gastrojejunostomy should be avoided to prevent the potential for the dumping syndrome, bile reflux, and marginal ulceration.

Coexistence of epidermolysis bullosa and PA makes the management more complicated. Meticulous attention to skin care is imperative. Incisions and retraction should be planned to minimize tangential trauma to the skin. Tape should not be used on endotracheal tubes, nasogastric tubes, intravenous catheters, or dressings. It may be prudent to decompress the stomach temporarily with a gastrostomy tube so that repetitive esophageal trauma from a nasogastric tube can be avoided.

## Antral Web

Gastric antral webs are another important cause of obstruction of the stomach. These occur at any age, and may be congenital or acquired. The symptoms caused by prepyloric

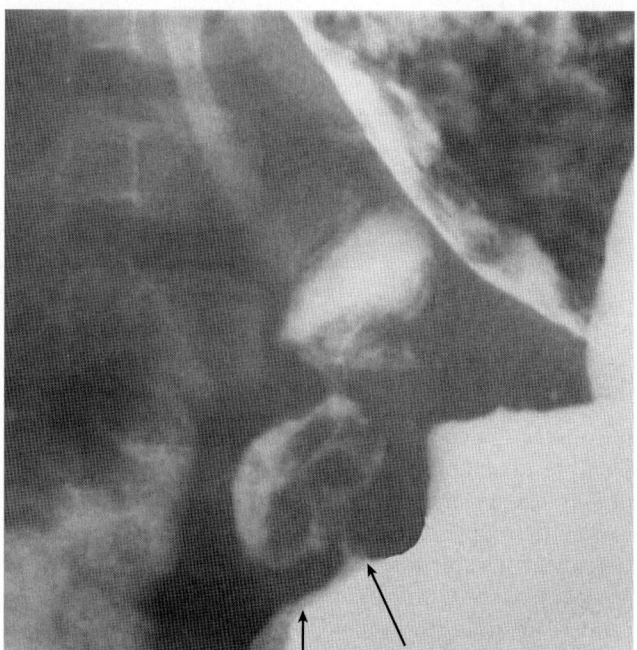

**FIGURE 37-3** Upper GI demonstrating a partially obstructing antral web (*short arrow*) immediately proximal to pyloric channel (*long arrow*). (*Courtesy of Eshan Afshani, MD.*)

membranes vary according to the degree of obstruction. Newborns with complete membranes present with nonbilious emesis and an absence of distal air on plain radiographs. Older children and adults with partial obstruction present with vomiting, epigastric discomfort, and weight loss.

The diagnosis of a complete prepyloric membrane is made with a plain abdominal radiograph or limited contrast study. The diagnosis of a partially obstructing membrane can be problematic. Often plain films are not helpful. Anterior–posterior (AP) projections of barium contrast studies may not reveal the web; therefore, oblique views should be performed in patients suspected of having a distal gastric obstruction due to an antral web (Fig. 37-3). Flexible gastroscopy may be helpful in cases in which radiographic studies are unable to reveal an etiology for distal gastric obstruction. Endoscopic criteria for the confirmation of a web include smooth mucosa on the diaphragm, a fixed opening despite peristalsis, and cessation of peristalsis at the membrane. Congenital antral webs are thought to be due to inadequate recanalization of the distal stomach. Acquired antral webs result from peptic ulcer disease and subsequent related scarring. Conversely, patients with congenital antral webs may also have associated peptic ulcer disease.

A completely obstructing antral web is treated with gastrostomy and circumferential web excision with oversewing of the mucosal remnant.

Treatment of partially obstructing webs should be individualized, as there has been some successful experience with nonoperative treatment with low residual formulas and antispasmodics. Follow-up of patients treated this way suggests the capacity for spontaneous regression of partially obstructing webs. Endoscopic dilation may be useful in partially obstructing cases, and in patients with peptic ulcer disease. Excision of the web typically resolves the ulceration.

## Congenital Microgastria

Congenital microgastria is a rare anomaly that results from the arrest of normal stomach development. The stomach develops as a fusiform dilatation of the foregut. The fetal stomach enlarges by asymmetric growth of the greater curvature. Asplenia is commonly associated with microgastria. This association suggests an event that simultaneously prevents gastric expansion and development of the spleen, which is an outgrowth of the dorsal mesogastrium. Other conditions known to coexist with microgastria are megaesophagus, situs inversus, malrotation, limb anomalies, and congenital heart disease. Associations with DiGeorge syndrome, Pierre-Robin sequence, esophageal stenosis, diaphragmatic hernia, laryngotracheoesophageal cleft, and intralobar sequestration have also been reported.

Newborns with congenital microgastria present with vomiting and aspiration pneumonia. Barium upper GI studies will demonstrate the small gastric reservoir and megaesophagus. Associated malrotation should be identified during the upper GI study.

The need for surgical therapy is dictated by the severity of the microgastria. Newborns with severe microgastria will have problematic reflux and drooling. Continuous intragastric feedings should be attempted. Some infants will adapt and ultimately gain normal reservoir function of the stomach. If drooling, reflux, or failure to thrive persists, gastric augmentation should be performed. The most widely applied technique is that of Hunt and Lawrence (Fig. 37-4). This procedure was designed to create a gastric reservoir after gastrectomy. The technical aspects of the procedure include creating a loop from a Roux-en-Y limb of jejunum. This "pouch" is anastomosed to the side of the diminutive stomach. Patients undergoing this procedure require meticulous follow-up of their nutritional status. Good quality of life but subpar growth has been reported in a patient 18 years following this procedure. If asplenia coexists, vaccination and prophylactic penicillin should be started postoperatively.

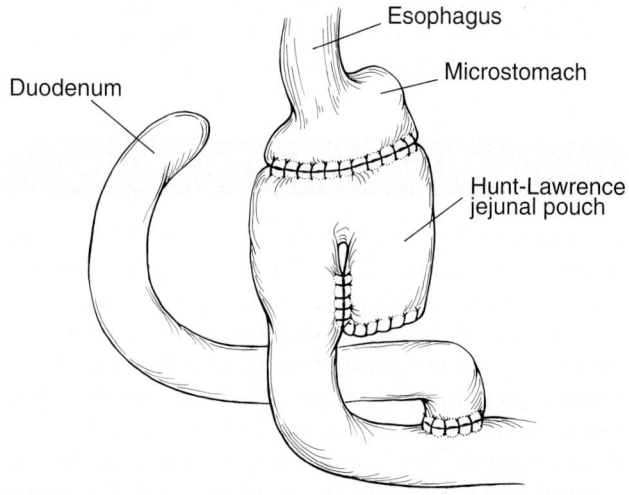

**FIGURE 37-4** Hunt–Lawrence reconstruction for gastric augmentation in congenital microgastria.

513

STOMACH: OBSTRUCTION, MICROGASTRIA, FOREIGN BODY, AND PEPTIC ULCER

# GASTRIC DUPLICATIONS

Alimentary tract duplications are mass lesions, which are congenital in origin and usually share a common wall with some part of the GI tract. They are tubular or spherical in shape and are lined with mucosa. Gastric duplications are the least common occurring alimentary tract duplication. Gastric duplications most often present in childhood. They are more common in females. Duplications of the stomach may be difficult to distinguish from other local foregut abnormalities. Criteria for the diagnosis of a gastric duplication are that the cyst be connected or in close proximity to the stomach, that it share a common muscular wall with the stomach, be lined with GI epithelium, and share a common blood supply with the stomach. A case report by Schwartz et al. challenges the concept that continuity between the duplication and the stomach wall must exist for it to be designated as a gastric duplication. Rarely, the cyst may have a communication with the pancreas.

The etiology of duplications of the stomach is speculative. One theory asserts that duplications result from persistence of diverticula that are present on the antimesenteric border of the developing fetal stomach. Other theories include abortive twinning of the stomach, fusion of longitudinal epithelial folds, coalescence of GI vacuoles, and neurenteric bands that result from endodermal-ectodermal adhesions.

Symptoms of gastric duplications include vomiting, weight loss, pain, GI bleeding, and perforation. Occasionally, duplications are asymptomatic and detected on routine upper GI study or at autopsy. Most children have a palpable mass. An upper GI study will show an extrinsic compression. Most duplications are located on the greater curvature. If diagnostic confusion exists, a computed tomography (CT) scan or abdominal ultrasound is helpful to distinguish this mass from a neoplasm, omental cyst, or pancreatic pseudocyst. Recently, the senior author diagnosed a gastric duplication with prenatal ultrasound.

The goal of operative therapy is complete excision of the cyst and preservation of gastric reservoir function. Laparoscopy is a viable option for select cases. Most cysts can be bluntly dissected off adjacent organs. Dissection begins in the common muscular plane between the stomach and the duplication. The duplication is "peeled" off the mucosa of the stomach and removed. If the duplication is large, the common septum between the stomach and duplication is excised and the cyst "marsupialized" into the stomach.

# NEWBORN GASTRIC PERFORATION

Perforation of the stomach is the least common type of GI perforation in newborns. Newborns with gastric perforation present with abdominal distension, sepsis, and respiratory impairment. Gastric bleeding may occasionally coexist. Prematurity and episodes of hypoxia are often present and degree of prematurity correlates with a high mortality. Perforation usually occurs between 2 and 8 days postpartum.

Most cases of neonatal gastric perforation are due to mechanical disruption of the stomach. Most disruptions occur as single tears on the greater curvature. This pattern of disruption was observed in experimentally overdistended stomachs of autopsied newborns. Clinical experience also suggests a "mechanical" theory of disruption as many patients prior to perforation have recently initiated positive pressure ventilation or feeding and have been noted to have gastric distension. Pathologic examination of clinical specimens supports this theory. Most specimens demonstrate little if any necrosis or inflammation if they have been obtained early in the disease process.

A minority of patients sustain perforation as a result of necrotizing gastritis due to either sepsis, obstruction secondary to duodenal atresia, "low-flow" states, or necrotizing enterocolitis.

The newborn identified to have abdominal distension and pneumoperitoneum should undergo prompt laparotomy. Fluid resuscitation, antibiotic administration, and gastric decompression should be accomplished prior to laparotomy. Needle decompression of the abdominal cavity should be considered if respiratory compromise occurs.

Most newborns will have an isolated perforation on the greater curvature. This should be closed in 2 layers. Children with extensive necrosis may require gastric resection and, in extreme cases, total gastrectomy and immediate gastric replacement or esophagoduodenostomy.

Every attempt should be made to conserve gastric reservoir function. However, evidence supports normal growth and development of children despite significant gastric resections.

# TUMORS OF THE STOMACH

## Teratomas

Gastric tumors occur rarely in children. The most common type of gastric tumor in childhood is a teratoma. Gastric teratomas predominantly occur in male infants. They usually present with upper GI bleeding. Gastric teratomas differ from most teratomas affecting children. First, teratomas at other sites (sacrococcygeal, mediastinum, gonads) are usually present in females. Teratomas of the stomach are extremely unusual in females, occurring in only 2 of 51 cases reported. Second, malignancy in a gastric teratoma has only been reported twice (endodermal sinus tumor), while the overall malignancy rate for other pediatric teratomas is approximately 20%.

Teratomas present with bleeding or mass effect. An upper abdominal mass is often present. They can be either cystic or solid. Most tumors can be resected with minimal loss of gastric reservoir function. Other reported tumors that have occurred in the stomachs of children include gastric lymphoma, leiomyoblastoma, leiomyosarcoma, polyps, lipoma, ganglioneuroblastoma, plasma cell granuloma, and carcinoma.

## Inflammatory Myofibroblastic Tumor

Recently, 2 cases of gastric inflammatory myofibroblastic tumor (IMT) have been reported in children. IMT is a rare benign neoplasm. This tumor is seen almost exclusively in children. Interestingly, it may exhibit malignant features such as local invasiveness, recurrence, distant metastasis, or malignant transformation to lymphoma. Surgical excision is required.

# GASTRIC FOREIGN BODIES

As a result of their curiosity, children swallow an assortment of foreign bodies. Many of these become lodged in the esophagus. Their removal is discussed in Chapter 22. Some pass into the stomach and are temporarily lodged there. Most objects that will pass through the esophagus will pass out of the stomach and through the entire GI tract without difficulty. Pencils, nails, and open safety pins will often have difficulty traversing the pylorus. Children with large foreign bodies should be observed for 48 hours and should undergo laparotomy and gastrotomy if they remain in the stomach.

## Button Batteries

National Battery Ingestion Hotline at the National Capital Poison Center recommendations for disc batteries are as follows. Retrieve batteries, endoscopically if possible, from the stomach or beyond if: a magnet was also ingested; the patient develops signs or symptoms that are likely related to the battery ingestion: or a large battery (≥15 mm diameter), ingested by a child younger than 6 years, remains in the stomach for 4 days or longer. Most other patients may be managed at home with a follow-up film in 2 weeks if no battery is detected in the stool. Symptomatic patients require immediate evaluation with intervention with endoscopy and possible laparotomy with gastrotomy and battery removal.

## Bezoars

Bezoars are collections of hair (trichobezoar), vegetable matter (phytobezoar), or milk (lactobezoar). Trichobezoars and phytobezoars occur most often in children and adolescents with psychiatric illness. They present with epigastric pain, distention, and vomiting. Upper GI contrast studies outline the intragastric foreign body. Large bezoars usually require gastrotomy for removal. Trichobezoars may extend through the pylorus into the duodenum and small bowel (Rapunzel syndrome). Successful laparoscopic removal has been reported in children. Lactobezoars usually occur in premature newborns and result from impaired gastric emptying. Gastric outlet obstruction due to an antral web or duodenal stenosis should be ruled out with an upper GI contrast study. Lactobezoars can usually be removed with gastric lavage and reinstitution of slow continuous feeds after resolution.

# PEPTIC ULCER DISEASE

Pediatric surgeons infrequently manage infants and children who have complications from peptic ulceration of the stomach and duodenum. Children presenting for surgical treatment invariably have serious complications such as bleeding, perforation, or chronicity. Acutely presenting ulcers are either primary or secondary in origin. Secondary ulcers usually occur in younger children who have coexisting conditions such as prematurity, burns, steroid use, immunodeficiency, and central nervous system tumors. Primary ulcers present in older children and adolescents and have a higher rate of chronicity and recurrence.

Ulcers of the stomach and duodenum result from an imbalance between acid secretion and mucosal protection. While a small number of children with ulcers are "hyper" secretors of acid, most do not have basal and maximal acid output that differ from normal. Children with ulcers secondary to Zollinger–Ellison syndrome are one exception to this generalization, as gastrin secreted by pancreatic and duodenal tumors cause excess gastric acid secretion. Additionally, consumption of nonsteroidal antiinflammatory drugs may result in peptic ulcer disease.

Pediatric patients with complicated peptic ulcer disease present with bleeding, perforation, obstruction, and chronicity. Bleeding may be manifest by either hematochezia or melena. Perforation due to peptic ulcer disease usually occurs in patients with coexisting illnesses. Obstruction is a rare complication that presents with nonbilious emesis due to pyloric scarring. Surgery for chronic ulcer symptoms has been drastically reduced due to the use of H2 antagonists, sucralfate, and proton pump inhibitors such as omeprazole. The association between the *Helicobacter pylori* infection and primary ulcer disease in children suggests a causative role. Gastric colonization and infection result in antral gastritis. This gastritis is rarely symptomatic. Its importance is in its association with duodenal ulcer disease, as they frequently coexist. Successful treatment of ulcer disease in many children requires the elimination of *H. pylori* infection and its attendant antral gastritis.

Secondary ulcer disease usually occurs in younger children with serious comorbidities such as burns, and head and other injuries. It is thought to occur by mechanisms related to breakdown of mucosal defenses and by the reduction of mucosal blood flow.

The initial treatment of ulcer disease in children is similar to that of adults. Medical management is attempted first. Agents to reduce acid production (cimetidine, ranitide, omeprazole) are combined with agents that coat or protect the mucosa (sucralfate). Continuous administration of H2-antagonists or proton pump inhibitors rather than discrete dosing twice a day seems to be superior for optimal acid suppression.

Bleeding patients should have their stomachs decompressed of retained blood and early endoscopy performed to evaluate the location of the bleeding. A number of techniques exist to arrest bleeding endoscopically. These include epinephrine injection, diathermy, and bipolar cautery. If the responsible surgeon is not performiing the endoscopy, then he or she should be in attendance so that operative strategies can be designed early.

Operative interventions should be considered for any "persistently" bleeding child. Some clinical indications for operative treatment are loss of 50% of the estimated blood volume in 8 hours, hemodynamic instability, and the presence of a "visible vessel" on endoscopy.

The choice of a particular operation for ulcer disease balances the risk of recurrence with that of the long-term sequelae. Decision regarding children is hampered by the lack of large case series comparing techniques. Nevertheless, some recommendations can be made.

Younger children with secondary ulcer disease and bleeding gastric or duodenal ulcers should have the base of the ulcers ligated through either gastrotomy or duodenotomy. This should be followed by intensive acid suppression postoperatively. Older children with secondary ulcers that are bleeding and stable should have definitive ulcer surgery performed. Options include vagotomy and pyloroplasty, proximal gastric vagotomy after vessel ligation, or vagotomy and antrectomy. Although vagotomy and antrectomy have superior rates of bleeding cessation, their use should probably be the last option in a child due to postgastrectomy sequelae.

Children with primary ulcer disease and unremitting hemorrhage should undergo ulcer and vessel ligation and definitive ulcer surgery. Options include both vagotomy and pyloroplasty or proximal gastric vagotomy.

Children with perforation of the duodenum due to ulcer disease should undergo simple closure of the duodenum with a Graham patch. Children with an ulcer predisposition may be considered for definitive ulcer surgery at the time of initial exploration.

## SELECTED READINGS

Anderson KD, Guzzetta PC. Treatment of congenital microgastria and dumping syndrome. *J Pediatr Surg* 1983;18:747–750.

Aoyama K, Tateishi K. Gastric volvulus in three children with asplenic syndrome. *J Pediatr Surg* 1986;21:307–310.

Banks PA, Woye DJ, Waitman ANI, Correll A. Mucosal diaphragm of the gastric antrum. *Gastroenterology* 1967;2:1003–1008.

Bartels RJ. Duplication of the stomach, case report and review of the literature. *Am Surg* 1967;3:747.

Bird CE, Limper MA, Mayer JM. Surgery in peptic ulceration of stomach and duodenum in infants and children. *Ann Surg* 1941;114:526–542.

Cameron AEP, Howard ER. Gastric volvulus in childhood. *J Pediatr Surg* 1987;10:944–947.

Cole C, Freitas A, Clifton MS, Durham MM. Hereditary multiple intestinal atresias: 2 new cases and review of the literature. *J Pediatr Surg* 2010;45(4):E21–E24.

Cribbs RK, Gow KW, Wulkan ML. Gastric volvulus in infants and children. *Pediatrics* 2008;122(3):e752–e762.

Haley T, Dimler M, Hollier P. Gastric teratoma with gastrointestinal bleeding. *J Pediatr Surg* 1986;21:949–950.

Hayashi AH, Galliani CA, Gillis DA. Congenital pyloric atresia and junctional epidermolysis bullosa: a report of long-term survival and a review of the literature. *J Pediatr Surg* 1991;26:1341–1345.

Holgersen LO. The etiology of spontaneous gastric perforation of the newborn: a reevaluation. *J Pediatr Surg* 1981;16:608–613.

Hunt CJ. Construction of a food pouch from a segment of jejunum as substitute for stomach in total gastrectomy. *Arch Surg* 1952;64:601–608.

Jones VS, Cohen RC. An eighteen year follow-up after surgery for congenital microgastria—case report and review of literature. *J Pediatr Surg* 2007;42(11):1957–1960.

Karnak I, Senocak ME, Ciftci AO, et al. Inflammatory myofibroblastic tumor in children: diagnosis and treatment. *J Pediatr Surg* 2001;36(6):908–912.

Lawrence W. Reservoir construction after total gastrectomy, an instructive case. *Ann Surg* 1962;155:191–198.

Lin CM, Lee HC, Kao HA, et al. Neonatal gastric perforation: report of 15 cases and review of the literature. *Pediatr Neonatal* 2008;49(3):65–70.

Litovitz T, Whitaker N. Clark L, White NC, Marsolek M. Emerging battery ingestion hazard: Clinical implications. *Pediatrics* 2010;125(6):1168–1177.

McIntyre RC, Bensard DD, Karrer FM, Hall RJ, Lilly JR. The pediatric diaphragm in acute gastric volvulus. *J Am Coll Surg* 1994;178:234–238.

Neifeld JP, Berman WF, Lawrence W Jr, Kodroff MB, Salzberg AM. Management of congenital microgastria with a jejunal reservoir pouch. *J Pediatr Surg* 1980;15:882–885.

Rosser SB, Clark CH, Elechi EN. Spontaneous neonatal gastric perforation. *J Pediatr Surg* 1982;17:390–394.

Schwartz DL, So HB, Becker JM, Schneider KM. An ectopic gastric duplication arising from the pancreas and presenting with a pneumoperitoneum. *J Pediatr Surg* 1979;14:187–188.

Tan CE, Kiely EM, Agrawal M, Brereton RJ, Spitz L. Neonatal gastrointestinal perforation. *J Pediatr Surg* 1989;24:888–892.

Touroff ASW, Sussman RM. Congenital prepyloric membranous obstruction in a premature infant. *Surgery* 1940;8:739–755.

Tunnell WP, Smith EL. Antral web in infancy. *J Pediatr Surg* 1980;15:152–155.

Velasco AL, Holcomb GW, Templeton JM, Ziegler MM. Management of congenital microgastria. *J Pediatr Surg* 1990;25:192–197.

# CHAPTER 38

## Gastrointestinal Tract Feeding Access

*Shannon Acker and David A. Partrick*

## KEY POINTS

1. Multiple techniques are in the surgeon's armamentarium for feeding access techniques in children.

2. Gastrostomy access can be achieved by a variety of technical approaches: Stamm or open gastrostomy, percutaneous endoscopic gastrostomy (PEG), laparoscopic-assisted gastrostomy, and radiologically assisted gastrostomy. The authors' preference is achieved by the visualization and inherent safety of the laparoscopic-assisted technique.

3. Gastrostomy morbidity can also be a significant feature of tube change.

4. The major morbidity of feeding enteral access tube placement relates to the need to exclude gastroesophageal reflux as a major clinical association. If present, feeding access may require a specific adjustment: gastrostomy with concomitant antireflux procedure, feeding jejunostomy being the most common alternatives available.

5. Gastrostomy remains one of the most common procedures done by pediatric surgeons.

## INTRODUCTION

Children who develop failure to thrive from a variety of clinical problems often require some type of long-term enteral access for feeds. Placement of a gastrostomy tube is indicated if oral nutrition is either not adequate or not feasible for a prolonged time interval. This can be due to an inability to swallow, inadequate caloric intake, unique feeding requirements resulting from metabolic disorders, or the practical requirement of the need for continuous enteral feeding. There are currently 5 different methods commonly used to obtain feeding access: (1) open gastrostomy (Stamm gastrostomy); (2) PEG; (3) laparoscopic gastrostomy; (4) percutaneous radiologic gastrostomy and percutaneous radiologic jejunostomy (PRG and PRJ); and (5) open jejunostomy. With the recent advances in minimally invasive treatment approaches,

PEG and laparoscopic placement are now the most common techniques utilized in children. PRG and PRJ are performed by interventional radiologists and are becoming increasingly popular at centers where this service is available.

## HISTORY

The concept of gastrostomy was first described by Egeberg in 1837. Sedillot was the first to attempt to perform the procedure, initially in dogs in 1839, and then in humans in 1846. Unfortunately his efforts were unsuccessful and all 3 of the patients died. In 1876, Verneuil performed the first successful gastrostomy. Since that time a number of modifications have been developed, the most popular of which was described by Stamm in 1894. The Stamm gastrostomy involves a purse-string suture to invaginate the serosa of the stomach around a tube. Other developments include the PEG, first described by Gauderer in 1979, the PRG described by Preshaw in 1981, and most recently, laparoscopic gastrostomy as well as single incision laparoscopic gastrostomy.

## INDICATIONS

Many conditions are potential indications for placement of some type of feeding access, including neurologic impairment with developmental delay, aspiration problems resulting in pneumonia or other respiratory complications, or congenital anatomic anomalies such as esophageal atresia. All of these problems can potentially lead to failure to thrive and the need for supplemental enteral feeds. At other times, a gastrostomy is done to secure access to the esophagus for retrograde dilation management of a stricture.

The 2 primary sites of access into the gastrointestinal (GI) tract for long-term enteral feeds are the stomach and the small bowel, specifically the jejunum. Each of the 5 procedures described below have been used in children of all ages, with similar success and complication rates. Contraindications for feeding tube placement are relatively uniform among the 5 different techniques. Absolute contraindications to gastrostomy tube placement include ascites, coagulopathy, pathology of the gastric wall, and potentially severe microgastria.

Contraindications that are specific to each procedure are described in detail below.

## TREATMENT OPTIONS

### Perioperative Management

Prior to incision, antibiotic prophylaxis is given with a cephalosporin, regardless of the chosen procedure. Following gastrostomy tube placement, the tube is typically left to gravity drainage overnight. Full-strength formula feeds are started on the first postoperative day and advanced to a goal rate as tolerated by the patient. Patients are discharged to home within 1 to 2 days, once gastrostomy teaching is complete for the family, if there are no complications or other illnesses requiring a longer hospital stay.

### Open Gastrostomy

The most common technique of open gastrostomy is Stamm gastrostomy. This is done under general anesthesia in most children, although it is possible to perform the operation under sedation and local anesthesia. Traditional gastrostomy placement has been via laparotomy incision, either midline or a left paramedian transverse incision. Upon entering the peritoneal cavity, the stomach can be directly visualized and gently grasped with a Babcock clamp. The site of gastrostomy is generally between the greater and lesser curves, and between the esophagus and pylorus on the body of the stomach. In the event the stomach is small, adjustments may need to be made; and in the circumstance where the stomach might itself be used for esophageal replacement, preserving either the lesser or greater curve should be considered. Stamm gastrostomy involves placing 2 purse-string sutures around the selected site, making a gastrotomy with either electrocautery or sharply, and placing a feeding tube into the stomach. Usually a long tube is initially placed such as Foley catheter or Malencott tube (a low-profile button device may also be chosen). The gastrostomy does not exit from the initial incision, but rather is instead brought out through a separate stab incision to the left of or above the initial incision. The stomach is secured to the abdominal wall with 4 sutures. The tube is then secured to the skin and the laparotomy incision closed. Ultimately, the gastrostomy tube is typically replaced with a gastrostomy skin-level button with a 1-way valve and a cap for closure. This exchange takes place a minimum of 3 to 4 weeks following the open gastrostomy. This requires removal of the initial tube and replacement with a button of appropriate diameter (French size) and length (abdominal wall thickness). These button devices are secured in place by either a balloon that must be inflated, or a phalange that is deformed by an obturator during tube placement. This procedure can be performed in the office setting. However, if there is concern about proper placement of the button in the stomach, a contrast study must be obtained.

Complications of open gastrostomy are similar to the complications of the other techniques discussed below. These include hemorrhage, gastric leak causing peritonitis, injury to the stomach or adjacent organs, separation of the stomach from the abdominal wall, wound infection, tube malfunction (occlusion), and tube migration leading to esophageal, gastric outlet, biliary, or small bowel obstruction. Certain strategies have been routinely employed to help decrease the risk of these complications. Preoperative prophylactic antibiotics are routinely used to prevent wound infection. Attention must be paid to the amount of tension placed at the level of the skin. It is important that the bolster that helps to secure tube position not be placed too tightly as this can lead to tissue necrosis, tube migration, and potentially separation of the stomach from the abdominal wall. However, care must also be taken to prevent the bolster from being too loose, allowing the tube to migrate distally. Other complications include persistent gastrocutaneous fistula following tube removal, gastrocolic fistula formation (more common with percutaneous techniques), erosion of the tube through adjacent organs, volvulus around a poorly positioned tube, and abscess.

A relatively common complication is tube dislodgement. This either can be a relatively simple problem to solve or can become quite complicated depending on how long after the original operative insertion the tube has been in place. If the tube is relatively new, dislodgement can lead to separation of the stomach from the abdominal wall and may require operative reinsertion. In the case of open gastrostomy, if a tube is displaced within 3 weeks of placement, it should be carefully replaced with a balloon-tipped catheter, of equal size or smaller. If a tube was placed percutaneously, this time frame should be extended to 6 weeks. Following replacement, contrast should be injected under fluoroscopic visualization to confirm placement position. If there is any difficulty in replacing the tube, the patient may need to return to the operating room. If there is evidence of contrast extravasation, peritonitis, or sepsis, immediate laparotomy is indicated.

The primary disadvantage of open gastrostomy, over other techniques presented, is the requirement for an open incision resulting in postoperative pain and scarring with increased potential for adhesion formation. The benefits, however, are well demonstrated. In children with cerebral palsy, gastrostomy tube feeding has been demonstrated in a prospective, longitudinal study to result in significant weight gain and subcutaneous fat deposition. Benefits have also been shown in patients with cystic fibrosis (CF). In a group of patients with CF and pancreatic insufficiency, although the patients had a significant decline in both height and weight for the 12 months prior to gastrostomy feeding initiation, placement of the feeding tube led to stabilization of nutritional status. Another group from the UK demonstrated similar findings in neurologically impaired children with two thirds of patients achieving catch-up growth postoperatively. However, 18% of these children experience major surgical complications. When compared with an endoscopic technique, open gastrostomy has also been associated with an increased risk of persistent gastrocutaneous fistula after tube removal. Concerns have been raised that children with severe neurologic impairment may be at risk for respiratory morbidity following gastrostomy placement due to oromotor dysfunction and aspiration. This was not found to be the case in 57 children with cerebral palsy whose number of chest infections requiring antibiotics actually decreased after gastrostomy placement. It should also be recognized that at least one half of caregivers will have an initial negative response when gastrostomy is recommended, and feeding time can be an unpleasant experience for these children and their families.

## Percutaneous Endoscopic Gastrostomy

Percutaneous endoscopic gastrostomy (PEG) is a very popular technique for gastrostomy placement and is one of the most common procedures performed in children. PEG is performed by both surgeons as well as gastroenterologists. There are multiple techniques of placing a PEG, the most popular of which is the Gauderer "pull" technique. In children, this is usually performed under general anesthesia, although it is possible to do with sedation and local anesthesia. Prior to the procedure, prophylactic antibiotics are given. An endoscope is advanced via the oropharynx into the stomach, air is insufflated, and the point of greatest transillumination and gastric indentation is marked on the anterior abdominal wall. Local anesthesia is injected at this point and a small (0.5 cm) incision is made. A trocar needle is then inserted through this incision directly into the stomach under endoscopic visualization. The needle is then removed and a guidewire is inserted via the remaining trocar that is then grasped by an endoscopic snare. The endoscope and wire are removed retrograde via the esophagus, oropharynx, and mouth as the wire advances through the abdominal wall. Then, the proximal end of the gastrostomy tube, the PEG tube itself, is connected to the wire. The wire is pulled from the skin incision, advancing the tube through the patient's mouth, esophagus, and ultimately their stomach. The endoscope is then reinserted to inspect the esophagus and stomach for mucosal injury or hemorrhage while the tube's flange is pulled to seat the tube against the interior gastric wall, which itself is advanced until it adheres to the peritoneal surface of the abdominal wall. An external bolster is placed at the skin to hold the tube in place. It is important that there is no tension on the skin. Tension is not necessary to hold the stomach at the abdominal wall; rather, it has been associated with ischemic necrosis and subsequent abdominal wall infection, tube extrusion, and separation of the stomach from the abdominal wall. Similar to open gastrostomy, the PEG tube should be replaced with a gastrostomy button approximately 4 to 8 weeks following tube placement to allow time for the stomach to firmly adhere to the abdominal wall.

Technical considerations to keep in mind in order to avoid PEG complications include both transillumination and insufflation. Inability to transilluminate is an absolute contraindication to PEG placement. Additionally, it is important to remember that the abdominal wall of children and babies is very thin, making it possible to transilluminate even when the transverse colon or small bowel lies between the abdominal wall and stomach. The primary risk of PEG placement is possible injury to hollow visceral organs during the procedure, often colon that is wedged between the stomach and abdominal wall during placement but cannot be seen due to poor visualization of the peritoneal cavity; or transverse colon that is rolled anteriorly between the stomach and skin when "over-insufflation" occurs. The risk of puncturing the colon or small bowel can be decreased by avoiding over-insufflation. This author as well as others has added laparoscopy to the PEG procedure in order to decrease the risk of injury to other intraabdominal viscera.

Benefits of PEG placement over open gastrostomy include minimal postoperative discomfort since the only abdominal wall incision is the gastrostomy tube site itself, quicker recovery with shorter procedure time, decreased length of stay, and reduction in costs. Careful consideration should be given to patient selection before proceeding with PEG placement. Although there is no consensus as to how small a child can be, it has been suggested that a placement limit be a minimum of 5 kg body weight for safe PEG insertion. Other patient factors to consider are those that would affect the ability to transilluminate the stomach including scoliosis or constipation, both common in patients with neurologic impairment. Laparoscopic-assisted PEG would likely be a better option for these patients. This may also be the preferred method in patients with a ventriculoperitoneal shunt in place in order to prevent mechanical damage to the shunt or ascending shunt infection causing meningitis. Patients with ongoing peritoneal dialysis have higher complication rates from PEG placement, including peritonitis. Open gastrostomy or laparoscopic gastrostomy with sutures holding the stomach to the abdominal wall would be preferred in this situation as well. Relative contraindications to PEG placement include previous gastric or upper abdominal surgery and severe esophageal stenosis precluding passage of an endoscope.

Despite the many advantages of PEG placement, there are a number of complications to consider as well. Authors from Norway recently reviewed 121 children who had PEG placement and found that although major complications are rare, nearly 50% of patients experienced some type of stoma-related complication. Even with these problems, 98% of families in this series would have chosen PEG insertion again due to its positive influence on their child's health. Other investigators from Australia reported that children with severe neurological dysfunction who require PEG placement have a significant long-term mortality of 39% after 13 years, a finding not directly related to the PEG itself. Additional risk comes from the fact that the gastrostomy tube alone is the only structure securing the stomach to the abdominal wall early after placement, potentially increasing the risk of a leak either intraoperatively or postoperatively if the gastrostomy tube is inadvertently removed or dislodged. A review of cases in Alberta found an increased risk of major infection compared with open gastrostomy.

The PEG tube is usually shortened down to skin level 4 to 8 weeks after operative placement when the stomach has become adherent to the anterior abdominal wall. This is typically accomplished by original tube removal and replacement with a skin-level button. However, a single-stage PEG button has now been developed and reported to be safe to place even in children weighing less than 5 kg. The single-stage PEG button involves the "push" technique with T-bar fixation, as opposed to the Gauderer "pull" technique. With this technique, following endoscopy, insufflation of the stomach, and transillumination of the anterior abdominal wall, T-bar fasteners are used to secure the stomach to the anterior abdominal wall. Next, a modified Seldinger technique is used to place a gastrostomy tube through the center of the T-bars. A review of 223 children undergoing PEG tubes and buttons revealed that children undergoing PEG button placement were more likely to spend only 1 night in the hospital versus PEG tube. Additionally, PEG buttons had fewer dislodgements.

Unfortunately, gastroesophageal reflux is a well-known complication of gastrostomy placement with a post-PEG rate of 13% to 28%. It remains difficult to predict, preoperatively, which patients might better be served by fundoplication at the time of gastrostomy tube placement. Novotny et al reviewed 863 patients who underwent PEG placement to identify preoperative factors that may require eventual fundoplication. They did this by comparing groups of patients undergoing PEG who did not require a subsequent antireflux procedure with those patients who ultimately underwent Nissen fundoplication after gastrostomy placement. Of the 863 patients reviewed, 5% of patients initially offered PEG alone, required an antireflux procedure. They found that only the diagnosis of cerebral palsy was an associated risk factor for the eventual need of an antireflux procedure. A second retrospective review of 760 patients undergoing PEG at the Johns Hopkins Children's Center found a rate of post-PEG fundoplication of 10%. Preoperative dysphagia and direct aspiration on modified barium swallow were both strongly associated with patients undergoing fundoplication following PEG.

## Laparoscopic Gastrostomy

Laparoscopic gastrostomy takes advantage of minimally invasive techniques (1-2 ports) while allowing excellent visualization of the peritoneal cavity contents to increase safety of the procedure when compared to PEG. Precise placement of the gastrostomy at the desired location in the stomach is done under the excellent magnified view provided by laparoscopy. Most surgeons utilizing this technique initially place one of the low-profile buttons with a balloon securing it within the gastric lumen, thus bypassing initial placement of a longer tube with subsequent device change making this a single-stage procedure.

Conventional laparoscopic gastrostomy is usually performed under general anesthesia. The abdomen is entered with a Veress needle and pneumoperitoneum with 8 to 12 mm Hg is created, depending on the size of the patient. This is generally performed with 2 ports, one 5-mm port for the laparoscope located at the umbilicus and a second 5-mm port in the right upper quadrant across from the previously marked gastrostomy site. The stomach can be secured to the abdominal wall with sutures to the posterior rectus fascia (through the 5-mm port site incision) or a U stitch can be placed around the gastrostomy site with excellent results. In one large series, no leaks occurred and reoperation was only necessary due to tube dislodgement in 7/461 (1.5%) children. In a second large series of 119 pediatric gastrostomy procedures from Vancouver, laparoscopic gastrostomy with primary button placement was found to be safe and easy to perform and have a significantly lower complication rate of 7.7.% compared to 14% with PEG placement. Other authors have suggested that laparoscopic gastrostomy should be the preferred method of gastrostomy placement in children. When compared to PEG placement, the advantages of laparoscopic gastrostomy include virtual feasibility in all patients,

the ability to primarily place a low-profile gastrostomy feeding device, and simplicity with the requirement of minimal laparoscopic expertise and safety. Concerns have been reported in the past about gastroesophageal reflux worsening after gastrostomy placement. Plantin et al describe a technique of laparoscopic gastrostomy where the G-button is placed on the anterior wall of the stomach near the lesser curvature (whereas most surgeons place gastrostomies near the greater curvature of the body of the stomach well away from the pylorus). They have reported that this modified laparoscopic gastrostomy placement does not aggravate gastroesophageal reflux as measured by pH probe monitoring. If indicated, laparoscopic gastrostomy is the most likely procedure for feeding access to be performed in combination with an antireflux fundoplication.

Single-site laparoscopic gastrostomy tube is the newest procedure to be added to a surgeon's armamentarium. Multiple authors have shown this to be a feasible technique with a comparable complication rate to traditional laparoscopy. The basic technique of single-site laparoscopic gastrostomy is similar to traditional laparoscopic gastrostomy. The patient is placed under general anesthesia. Local anesthesia is injected at the site of gastrostomy, midway between the umbilicus and ribs through the left rectus fascia. A 1.5-cm incision is made at this site. Dissection is carried down to the peritoneal layer and the abdomen is entered with a 3- or 5-mm trocar. A camera is placed through this trocar to visualize the anterior stomach wall. A second smaller trocar is placed through the same incision, next to the initial trocar. A grasper is introduced through the smaller trocar and is used to grasp the stomach wall. The pneumoperitoneum is evacuated and the stomach is brought out through the incision. The stomach is then sewn to the abdominal wall and a tube is placed with a similar technique to a Stamm gastrostomy. The advantages of single-site laparoscopy include the fact that the stomach is not entered blindly, preventing the risk of colon puncture, while offering the advantage of minimal postoperative pain.

## Jejunostomy

For various reasons, some children do not tolerate gastric feeds. This may be due to poor gastric emptying, gastroesophageal reflux problems not amendable to other approaches, or recurrent reflux after a previous failed antireflux procedure. These patients may require long-term enteral feeding access directly into the small intestine distal to the stomach. If a preexisting gastrostomy tube is in place, this can potentially be converted to a gastrojejunostomy tube. The gastrostomy is removed and a new feeding tube with a longer jejunal limb is placed. The jejunal limb is advanced past the pylorus and into the proximal jejunum under fluoroscopic or endoscopic guidance. Gastric decompression can simultaneously be accomplished via a second port in the gastrojejunostomy tube that opens into the stomach. The biggest problems with these "G–J" tubes are frequent dislodgement and mechanical failure. Fortunato and associates reported a mean of 2.2 replacements over a mean follow-up of 39 days. Each of these replacements has to be performed under fluoroscopy. Out of the 51 patients, 58 tube dislodgements occurred. Therefore, gastrojejunostomy tube placement and replacement may not be the best long-term option for these children. In addition, patient size may limit G–J tube placement in children less than 10 kg. An alternative, and the author's procedure of choice, is a laparoscopic-assisted jejunostomy. Laparoscopic jejunostomy is performed under general anesthesia in a similar fashion as laparoscopic gastrostomy. Two 5-mm trocars are used, the first located at the umbilicus and the second on the left side of the abdomen at the site of creation of the jejunostomy, typically through the rectus sheath. Following port placement, an atraumatic grasper is used at the left-sided port to move both the greater omentum and transverse colon superiorly, allowing identification of the first jejunal loop. The jejunum is grasped approximately 20 cm distal to the ligament of Treitz and is exteriorized through the port site. The jejunostomy is then created by fixing the loop of intestine to the abdominal wall (posterior rectus fascia), then placing a purse-string suture around the jejunum through which the feeding tube is placed. The tube is further secured by inflating its balloon. Confirmation of the tube's location within the lumen of the bowel is confirmed by visualizing the loop with the laparoscopic camera at the umbilical port. The jejunostomy is then further secured at the skin if necessary. A button can be placed initially, similar to a laparoscopic gastrostomy, obviating the need for a second procedure. Esposito et al reported their experience with 7 neurologically impaired children with gastroesophageal reflux; they had no perioperative complications with an operative time of 40 minutes and a hospital stay of 3 to 4 days. A second technique of laparoscopic jejunostomy, a laparoscopic Roux-en-Y jejunostomy, has also been described in 5 children by Neuman and offers another option that is somewhat more technically demanding. However, the advantage of this modification is the Roux-en-Y loop that avoids possible obstruction problems if the jejunostomy balloon fills or partially fills the lumen of a loop jejunostomy. In comparing a surgical jejunostomy to image-guided placement, Raval and Phillips found that of the 14 children undergoing image-guided placement, 7 (50%) eventually required surgical jejunostomy placement due to recurring tube management issues. Radiographically placed tubes required 4.6 tube adjustments per year compared to 1.5 for surgically placed jejunostomies (the majority were Roux-en-Y).

Complications of jejunostomy are similar to those of gastrostomy. The most common complication is obstruction, however as stated above, this can be avoided with Roux-en-Y jejunostomy.

Contraindications of jejunostomy vary somewhat from those of gastrostomy in general. Bowel obstruction is the only absolute contraindication. Other relative contraindications include edema of the intestinal wall, postradiation enteritis, and chronic inflammatory bowel disease such as Crohn disease or ulcerative colitis. Other contraindications have been mentioned previously including coagulopathy and ascites.

## Percutaneous Radiologic Gastrostomies and Jejunostomies

Gastrostomy tubes are traditionally placed by either surgeons or gastroenterologists. However, over the past 20 years, radiologists have begun to place both gastrostomy and gastrojejunostomy tubes under image guidance. The main benefit of PRG is that only mild sedation is required. A fluoroscopy facility is utilized, obviating the costs of either an operating room or endoscopy suite.

PRG can be performed with or without gastropexy via a gastric anchor. The basic procedure involves first distending the stomach with carbon dioxide gas via a nasogastric tube. Ultrasound is used to visualize the stomach and make sure no other organs overlie the planned puncture site. In gastrostomy, the puncture site is lateral to the rectus muscle, angled toward the fundus. In gastrojejunostomy, it is angled toward the pylorus. In order to anchor the stomach to the abdominal wall, a GI suture anchor set can be used. This consists of a gastric anchor (a short section of guidewire attached at the center by a long thread with a suture needle at the end) preloaded onto a 17-gauge puncture needle. After infiltration with local anesthetic, a 15-gauge needle with the gastric anchor preloaded is inserted into the distended stomach. Aspiration of air indicates that the needle is in the gastric lumen. Second confirmation is obtained by injecting contrast and visualizing the outline of rugal folds. The guidewire is then advanced, pushing the anchor into the gastric lumen. The needle is withdrawn, leaving the anchor in place to hold the stomach up to the abdominal wall. Next a guidewire is passed into the stomach and the tract is dilated up to the size of the desired tube. Contrast is injected into the catheter to confirm its placement in the gastric lumen. If gastrojejunostomy is desired, the catheter is advanced into the jejunum under fluoroscopic guidance. The tube is then secured to the skin by looping the string from the gastric anchor around the tube. Other authors have demonstrated success using the same technique to place jejunostomy tubes (PRJ). The jejunum is dilated with saline injection after using fluoroscopy to place an angiocatheter into an air-filled proximal loop. The jejunum is then punctured using either fluoroscopic or ultrasound guidance. One then proceeds in a fashion similar to PRG.

Complications of PRG and PRJ are similar to those of all gastrostomy tubes, described in detail above. Complications specific to radiologic placement include inadvertent puncture of the colon, small bowel, or liver at the time of tube placement or placement of a tube into the peritoneal cavity. Gastropexy is performed by some to avoid placing the tube into the peritoneum, although there is no consensus regarding the necessity of this step. A single-institution review found that radiologic percutaneous gastrostomy had a complication rate of 5.9% compared with 9.4% for endoscopic and 20% for surgical techniques. Others have reported a rate of major complication (peritonitis, bleeding, deep stomal infection, aspiration, displacement of the tube requiring a repeat procedure, and sepsis) to be less than 8% with overall risk of minor complications between 5% and 10%. The risk of wound infection is lower in PRG than in PEG because the tube is not passed through the oropharynx, avoiding contamination. For this reason, prophylactic antibiotics are not routinely given during PRG or PRJ. While the success rate of PRG approaches 100%, that of PRJ is only 85% to 95% due to the ease of collapsibility of the jejunum, high mobility making initial puncture difficult, and easy dislodgement of the punctured jejunum when trying to place the tube or anchor.

As with complications, contraindications to PRG are similar to other percutaneous techniques. This technique should not be used in patients with uncorrectable coagulopathy, portal hypertension, and varices, or in patients with interposed colon or hepatosplenomegaly making percutaneous access to the stomach difficult. Patients who have undergone previous stomach surgery certainly present a challenge; however, this is not an absolute contraindication. While massive ascites is usually a contraindication, there are some reports that preprocedural paracentesis and/or gastropexy make PRG feasible.

## PATIENT SELECTION

When the decision is made to place a tube for enteral feeding access, the choice of procedure should be made with regard to the individual patient. Before proceeding with gastrostomy or jejunostomy, the patient should first be evaluated for gastroesophageal reflux disease. There has been some debate about the necessity of an antireflux procedure concurrent with gastrostomy, particularly in children with neurologic impairment. Current recommendation is that, if there is no clinical history and no preoperative evidence of gastroesophageal reflux disease, an antireflux procedure is not indicated. There is some evidence that even in patients with abnormal pH study and symptomatic reflux disease preoperatively, an antireflux procedure is not necessary at the time of gastrostomy as reflux improves following gastrostomy. In patients with no clinical history of reflux, no further workup is required prior to gastrostomy. However, if a patient has a clinical history or signs and symptoms of reflux, they should undergo appropriate workup (contrast upper GI study and pH/impedence probe). If the workup reveals pathologic reflux, they should proceed with an antireflux procedure and laparoscopic or open gastrostomy. If there is no evidence of gastroesophageal reflux, either a percutaneous or laparoscopic gastrostomy is placed. This decision is based on patient factors such as anatomic abnormalities, comorbidities, anesthetic risks, and previous abdominal operations. The decision to proceed with either PEG or PRG depends on the availability of experienced personnel with these procedures at a given facility in addition to the above-listed patient factors that must be considered.

## SELECTED READINGS

Ackroyd R, Saincher M, Cheng S, El-Matary W. Gastrostomy tube insertion in children: the Edmonton experience. Can J Gastroenterol 2001;25:265–268.

Aprahamian CJ, Morgan TL, Harmon CM, et al. U-stitch laparoscopic gastrostomy technique has a low rate of complications and allows primary button placement: experience with 461 pediatric procedures. J Laparoendosc Adv Surg Tech A 2006;16:643–649.

Avitsland TL, Kristensen C, Emblem R, et al. Percutaneous endoscopic gastrostomy in children: a safe technique with major symptom relief and high parental satisfaction. J Pediatr Gastroenterol Nutr 2006;43:624–628.

Beres A, Bratu I. Attention to small details: big deal for gastrostomies. Semin Pediatr Surg 2009;18:87–92.

Burd RS, Price MR, Whalen TV. The role of protective antireflux procedures in neurologically impaired children: a decision analysis. J Pediatr Surg 2002;37:500–506.

Catto-Smith AG, Jimenez S. Morbidity and mortality after percutaneous endoscopic gastrostomy in children with neurological disability. J Gastroenterol Hepatol 2006;21:734–738.

Craig GM, Carr LJ, Cass H, et al. Medical, surgical, and health outcomes of gastrostomy feeding. Dev Med Child Neurol 2006;48:353–360.

Esposito C, Settimi A, Centonze A, et al. Laparoscopic-assisted jejunostomy: an effective procedure for the treatment of neurologically impaired children with feeding problems and gastroesophageal reflux. Surg Endosc 2005;19:501–504.

Fortunato JE, Troy AL, Cuffari C, et al. Outcome after percutaneous endoscopic gastrostomy in children and young adults. J Pediatr Gastroenterol Nutr 2010;50:390–393.

Gassas A, Kennedy J, Green G, et al. Risk of ventriculoperitoneal shunt infections due to gastrostomy feeding tube insertion in pediatric patients with brain tumors. Pediatr Neurosurg 2006;42:95–99.

Grant JP. Comparison of percutaneous endoscopic gastrostomy with Stamm gastrostomy. Ann Surg 1988;207:598–603.

Jones VS, La hei ER, Shun A. Laparoscopic gastrostomy: the preferred method of gastrostomy in children. Pediatr Surg Int 2007;23:1085–1089.

Kawahara H, Kubota A, Okuyama H, et al. One-trocar laparoscopy-aided gastrostomy in handicapped children. J Pediatr Surg 2006;41:2076–2080.

Neuman HB, Phillips JD. Laparoscopic Roux-en-Y feeding jejunostomy: a new minimally invasive surgical procedure for permanent feeding access in children with gastric dysfunction. J Laparoendosc Adv Surg Tech A 2005;15:71–74.

Novotny NM, Jester AL, Ladd AP. Preoperative prediction of need for fundoplication before gastrostomy tube placement in children. J Pediatr Sug 2009;44:173–177.

Novotny NM, Vegeler RC, Breckler FD, Rescoria FJ. Percutaneous endoscopic gastrostomy buttons in children. J Pediatr Surg 2009;44:1193–1196.

Plantin I, Arnbjornsson E, Larsson LT. No increase in gastroesophageal reflux after laparoscopic gastrostomy in children. Pediatr Surg Int 2006;22:581–584.

Ponsky TA, Lukish JR. Single site laparoscopic gastrostomy with a 4-mm bronchoscopic optical grasper. J Pediatr Surg 2008;43:412–414.

Raval MV, Phillips JD. Optimal enteral feeding in children with gastric dysfunction: surgical jejunostomy vs. image-guided gastrojejunal tube placement. J Pediatr Surg 2006;41:1679–1682.

Shin JH, Park AW. Updates on percutaneous radiologic gastrostomy/gastrojejunostomy and jejunostomy. Gut Liver 2010;4:S25–S31.

Sullivan PB, Juszczak E, Bachlet AM, et al. Gastrostomy tube feeding in children with cerebral palsy: a prospective, longitudinal study. Dev Med Child Neurol 2005;47:77–85.

Sullivan PB, Morrice JS, Vernon-Roberts A, et al. Does gastrostomy tube feeding in children with cerebral palsy increase the risk of respiratory morbidity? Arch Dis Child 2006;91:478–482.

Tapia J, Murguia R, Garcia G, Espinoza de los Monteros P, Onate E. Jejunostomy: techniques, indications, and complications. World J Surg 1999;23:596–602.

Terry NE, Boswell WC, Carney DE, Beck A, Lowe L, Rittmeyer C. Percutaneous endoscopic gastrostomy with T-bar fixation in children and infants. Surg Endosc 2008;22:167–170.

Truby H, Cowlishaw P, O'Neil C, Wainwright C. The long term efficacy of gastrostomy feeding in children with cystic fibrosis on anthropometric markers of nutritional status and pulmonary function. Open Respir Med J 2009;3:112–115.

van Overhagen H, Ludviksson MA, Lameris JS, et al. US and fluoroscopic-guided percutaneous jejunostomy: experience in 49 patients. J Vasc Interv Radiol 2000;11:101–106.

Wilson GJP, van der Zee DC, Bax NMA. Endoscopic gastrostomy placement in the child with gastroesophageal reflux: is concomitant antireflux surgery indicated? J Pediatr Surg 2006;41:1441–1445.

Wollman B, D'Agostino HB, Walus-Wigle JR, Easter DW, Beale A. Radiologic, endoscopic, and surgical gastrostomy: an institutional evaluation and meta-analysis of the literature. Radiology 1995;197:699–704.

Yu SC, Petty JK, Bensard DD, et al. Laparoscopic-assisted percutaneous endoscopic gastrostomy in children and adolescents. JSLS 2005;9:302–304.

Zamakhshary M, Jamal M, Blair GK, et al. Laparoscopic vs. percutaneous endoscopic gastrostomy tube insertion: a new pediatric gold standard? J Pediatr Surg 2005;40:859–862.

# CHAPTER 39

# Bariatric Surgery in Adolescents

*Mark Holterman, Allen Browne, and Ai-Xuan Holterman*

## KEY POINTS

1. The etiology of obesity is multifactorial.

2. Obesity is a chronic disease with short-term and long-term medical and psychosocial morbidity.

3. Morbid obesity may lead to shortened life expectancy.

4. No child chooses to be obese.

5. The obese child and adolescent are not the same as the obese adult.

6. Medical weight loss programs are not effective.

7. Bariatric surgery in adolescents is safe and effective.

8. Low-risk surgical options are available and effective for the majority of obese adolescents.

9. Weight management surgery is best practiced in collaboration with a multidisciplinary team.

10. Individual bariatric procedures can be chosen for the individual obese adolescent.

11. Collaborative studies are needed to advance bariatric surgery for adolescents.

---

Obesity is the most common medical condition of childhood. It is not a cosmetic issue, but a medical issue with serious, and potentially lifelong, health and psychosocial consequences.

*American Academy of Pediatrics*—June 21, 2004

Obesity is a chronic, debilitating and potentially fatal disease...
*American Society of Bariatric Physicians*—2004

## THE PROBLEM

A side effect of the advancement in technology and progress in the standard of living is the increased percentage of children and adolescents that are defined as overweight or obese. Today one third of American children are overweight or obese; an incidence that has tripled in the last 30 years. This rise in obesity is apparent across the developing world as the availability of abundant food, control of infectious disease, improved sanitation and water supplies, environmental obesity-potentiating agents (obesogens), and decreased physical activity precede an alarming rapid rise in childhood obesity. This inconvenient truth about childhood obesity is especially pertinent for pediatric surgeons who have heretofore been able to avoid the surgical care of obese children with the occasional unsettling and perhaps, guilt-ridden transfer of a severely ill morbidly obese child to an adult bariatric surgeon for a major bariatric procedure. With the alarming increase in adolescent and childhood obesity and the unique psychosocial and medical needs of children and adolescents, it has become apparent that pediatric surgeons can no longer turn their back on this problem. It is important therefore for pediatric surgeons to have a general working knowledge of the comorbidities associated with obesity and the various surgical interventions available. Of particular importance, pediatric surgeons will care for many obese children with general surgical problems. It is important to understand the particular perioperative management issues associated with the morbidly obese child.

Pediatric health care professionals all agree that the best therapy for obesity is prevention. This in itself is no small task in our "obesogenic" society. Many different programs are underway and obesity prevention will require fundamental changes in our food supply, eating habits, sedentary lifestyles, and a realization of the dangers associated with obesity. While prevention is a laudable goal, over the last decade, leaders in pediatrics have come to the realization that something needs to be done for those children and adolescents that are already morbidly obese. Ignoring their plight is irresponsible, since delayed or inadequate treatment may lead to irreparable damage to their social development and education and an increased rate of irreversible morbid conditions such as type II diabetes, hypertension, dyslipidemia and early onset of atherosclerosis, and premature death. A comprehensive multispecialty approach to the problem of the obese child is critical and can lead to weight loss and the resolution of many of the medical and psychosocial problems caused by obesity.

## OBESITY DEFINED

It is widely recognized that it is common for the average child or adolescent and their parents to have an unrealistic perception of their "weight problem" and therefore objective

523

| Height / Weight | 5-0 | 5-1 | 5-2 | 5-3 | 5-4 | 5-5 | 5-6 | 5-7 | 5-8 | 5-9 | 5-10 | 5-11 | 6-0 | 6-1 | 6-2 | 6-3 | 6-4 |
|---|---|---|---|---|---|---|---|---|---|---|---|---|---|---|---|---|---|
| 100 | 20 | 19 | 18 | 18 | 17 | 17 | 16 | 16 | 15 | 15 | 14 | 14 | 14 | 13 | 13 | 12 | 12 |
| 105 | 21 | 20 | 19 | 19 | 18 | 17 | 17 | 16 | 16 | 16 | 15 | 15 | 14 | 14 | 13 | 13 | 13 |
| 110 | 21 | 21 | 20 | 19 | 19 | 18 | 18 | 17 | 17 | 16 | 16 | 15 | 15 | 15 | 14 | 14 | 13 |
| 115 | 22 | 22 | 21 | 20 | 20 | 19 | 19 | 18 | 17 | 17 | 17 | 16 | 16 | 15 | 15 | 14 | 14 |
| 120 | 23 | 23 | 22 | 21 | 21 | 20 | 19 | 19 | 18 | 18 | 17 | 17 | 16 | 16 | 15 | 15 | 15 |
| 125 | 24 | 24 | 23 | 22 | 21 | 21 | 20 | 20 | 19 | 18 | 18 | 17 | 17 | 16 | 16 | 16 | 15 |
| 130 | 25 | 25 | 24 | 23 | 22 | 22 | 21 | 20 | 20 | 19 | 19 | 18 | 18 | 17 | 17 | 16 | 16 |
| 135 | 26 | 26 | 25 | 24 | 23 | 22 | 22 | 21 | 21 | 20 | 19 | 19 | 18 | 18 | 17 | 17 | 16 |
| 140 | 27 | 26 | 26 | 25 | 24 | 23 | 23 | 22 | 21 | 21 | 20 | 20 | 19 | 18 | 18 | 17 | 17 |
| 145 | 28 | 27 | 27 | 26 | 25 | 24 | 23 | 23 | 22 | 21 | 21 | 20 | 20 | 19 | 19 | 18 | 18 |
| 150 | 29 | 28 | 27 | 27 | 26 | 25 | 24 | 23 | 23 | 22 | 22 | 21 | 20 | 20 | 19 | 19 | 18 |
| 155 | 30 | 29 | 28 | 27 | 27 | 26 | 25 | 24 | 24 | 23 | 22 | 22 | 21 | 20 | 20 | 19 | 19 |
| 160 | 31 | 30 | 29 | 28 | 27 | 27 | 26 | 25 | 24 | 24 | 23 | 22 | 22 | 21 | 21 | 20 | 19 |
| 165 | 32 | 31 | 30 | 29 | 28 | 27 | 27 | 26 | 25 | 24 | 24 | 23 | 22 | 22 | 21 | 21 | 20 |
| 170 | 33 | 32 | 31 | 30 | 29 | 28 | 27 | 27 | 26 | 25 | 24 | 24 | 23 | 22 | 22 | 21 | 21 |
| 175 | 34 | 33 | 32 | 31 | 30 | 29 | 28 | 27 | 27 | 26 | 25 | 24 | 24 | 23 | 22 | 22 | 21 |
| 180 | 35 | 34 | 33 | 32 | 31 | 30 | 29 | 28 | 27 | 27 | 26 | 25 | 24 | 24 | 23 | 22 | 22 |
| 185 | 36 | 35 | 34 | 33 | 32 | 31 | 30 | 29 | 28 | 27 | 27 | 26 | 25 | 24 | 24 | 23 | 23 |
| 190 | 37 | 36 | 35 | 34 | 33 | 32 | 31 | 30 | 29 | 28 | 27 | 26 | 26 | 25 | 24 | 24 | 23 |
| 195 | 38 | 37 | 36 | 35 | 33 | 32 | 31 | 31 | 30 | 29 | 28 | 27 | 26 | 26 | 25 | 24 | 24 |
| 200 | 39 | 38 | 37 | 35 | 34 | 33 | 32 | 32 | 30 | 30 | 29 | 28 | 27 | 26 | 26 | 25 | 24 |
| 205 | 40 | 39 | 37 | 36 | 35 | 34 | 33 | 33 | 31 | 30 | 29 | 29 | 28 | 27 | 26 | 26 | 25 |
| 210 | 41 | 40 | 38 | 37 | 36 | 35 | 34 | 33 | 32 | 31 | 30 | 29 | 28 | 28 | 27 | 26 | 26 |
| 215 | 42 | 41 | 39 | 38 | 37 | 36 | 35 | 34 | 33 | 32 | 31 | 30 | 29 | 28 | 28 | 27 | 26 |
| 220 | 43 | 42 | 40 | 39 | 38 | 37 | 36 | 34 | 33 | 32 | 32 | 31 | 30 | 29 | 28 | 27 | 27 |
| 225 | 44 | 43 | 41 | 40 | 39 | 37 | 36 | 35 | 34 | 33 | 32 | 31 | 31 | 30 | 29 | 28 | 27 |
| 230 | 45 | 43 | 42 | 41 | 39 | 38 | 37 | 36 | 35 | 34 | 33 | 32 | 31 | 30 | 30 | 29 | 28 |
| 235 | 46 | 44 | 43 | 42 | 40 | 39 | 38 | 36 | 36 | 35 | 34 | 33 | 32 | 31 | 30 | 29 | 29 |
| 240 | 47 | 45 | 44 | 42 | 41 | 40 | 39 | 37 | 36 | 35 | 34 | 33 | 33 | 32 | 31 | 30 | 29 |
| 245 | 48 | 46 | 45 | 43 | 42 | 41 | 40 | 38 | 37 | 36 | 35 | 34 | 33 | 32 | 31 | 31 | 30 |
| 250 | 49 | 47 | 46 | 44 | 43 | 42 | 40 | 39 | 38 | 37 | 36 | 35 | 34 | 33 | 32 | 31 | 30 |

**FIGURE 39-1** BMI tabular chart expressed in pounds and feet/inches. BMI classically is defined as the individual's body mass divided by the square of their height—with the value universally being expressed in units of kg/m$^2$. The formula would then be BMI = mass (kg) divided by height in meters squared. When expressing the height and weight in feet/inches and pounds, the formula would instead be BMI = mass (lb) divided by height in inches squared times the constant 703.

measurements of body habitus are crucial. The basic metabolic index (BMI) has been the standard metric for quantifying obesity. BMI is calculated by taking the weight in kilograms divided by the height in meters squared. BMI calculations are becoming routine and should become part of the routine health status metrics collected upon initial presentation of the patient (Fig. 39-1).

It is important to remember that children have a lower normal BMI than adults and so utilizing the BMI scale to define obesity in children may be misleading. Therefore, a useful and important obesity metric in children is to compare the child's percentile BMI to the standard age and gender appropriate BMI charts. According to this system, greater than 95th percentile is considered obese and greater than 99th percentile is considered morbidly obese. These growth charts can be obtained from the Centers for Disease Control and Prevention (*http://www.cdc.gov/growthcharts/*) and online BMI calculators are readily available (eg, *http://apps.nccd.cdc.gov/dnpabmi/Calculator.aspx*). The National Institutes of Health (NIH) recommend that bariatric surgery be considered in adults with a BMI of 40 or a BMI of 35 with comorbidities (NIH, 1991). Many pediatric surgeons performing bariatric surgical procedures have adopted these standards. Others have set even more restrictive standards with the concerns for the safety of the obese adolescent contemplating those bariatric procedures with a significant risk of morbidity and mortality.

## OBESITY EPIDEMIC QUANTIFIED

Using BMI and the relevant position on the growth chart as the metric, the World Health Organization, the CDC, and the NIH have compiled alarming statistics concerning obesity in children. Childhood obesity (BMI ≥ 30) has more than tripled in the past 30 years. The prevalence of obesity among children aged 6 to 11 years increased from 6.5% in 1980 to 19.6% in 2008. The prevalence of obesity among adolescents aged 12 to 19 years increased from 5% to 18.1%. The incidence of obesity in the adult U.S. population is nearly twice this rate. The recent data suggest that the rapid rise of obesity may be leveling off but the incidence is still very troublesome. A rough calculation of the children at a BMI of ≥99% would predict a cohort of at least 300,000 U.S. children (age 12–19) with profound obesity! It is important to realize that greater than 80% of obese children become obese adults. These trends predict a serious increase in health care and societal costs.

### The Medical Comorbidities Associated with Obesity

The increased incidence and severity of obesity is accompanied by a disturbing increase in comorbid conditions. In particular, the various components of the metabolic syndrome show a profound increase in morbidly obese children including hypertension, hypercholesterolemia, and type 2 diabetes. The early appearance of atherosclerosis is a harbinger of eventual cardiovascular disease and for the first time in history the average life span is predicted to be decreased due to the obesity epidemic. Additional severe comorbidities such as nonalcoholic steatohepatitis and sleep apnea can lead to early mortality. Less severe, but still significant problems include polycystic ovary disease, focal glomerulosclerosis, orthopedic problems (Blount disease and slipped capital femoral epiphysis, low back pain, and injuries), and dermatologic problems (acanthosis nigricans, acne, and infections). Of course, it has been well established that obesity is linked to an increased incidence of colon, breast, and prostate cancer (Fig. 39-2).

### The Psychosocial Comorbidities Associated with Obesity

One must remember that every child, if given a choice, would not choose to be obese (Fig. 39-3). The medical suffering that these children endure pales in comparison to the psychosocial effects of obesity. There have been many studies documenting the lower mental health and psychological quality of life endured by obese children. They suffer from low self-esteem, depression, school phobia, bulimia and binge eating, suicide, and self-mutilation. Overweight children are teased and bullied more than their normal

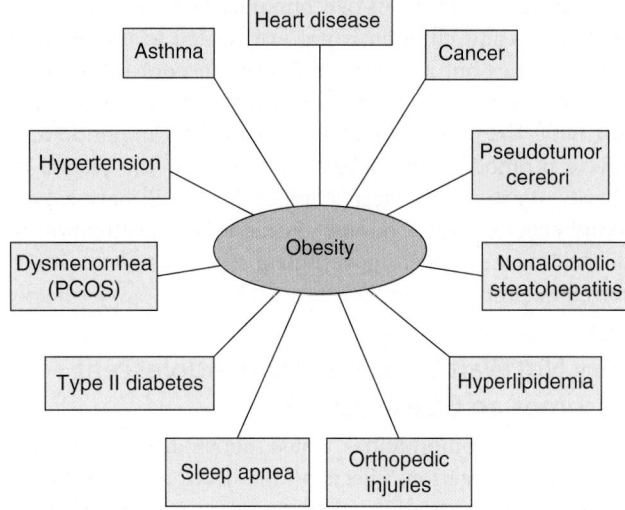

**FIGURE 39-2** Medical comorbidities associated with obesity.

weight peers. Initial studies now document a significant improvement in quality of life measurements with successful weight loss interventional therapy.

### The Societal Comorbidities Associated with Obesity

With the many medical and psychosocial comorbidities found in the obese child, it is logical to think of the economic cost to society. The costs of treating obesity-related disease are becoming an increasing portion of the health care expenditures. In addition, it has been shown that the incidence of admission of obese children with common problems and their length of stay and cost with common problems are greater than those for nonobese children.

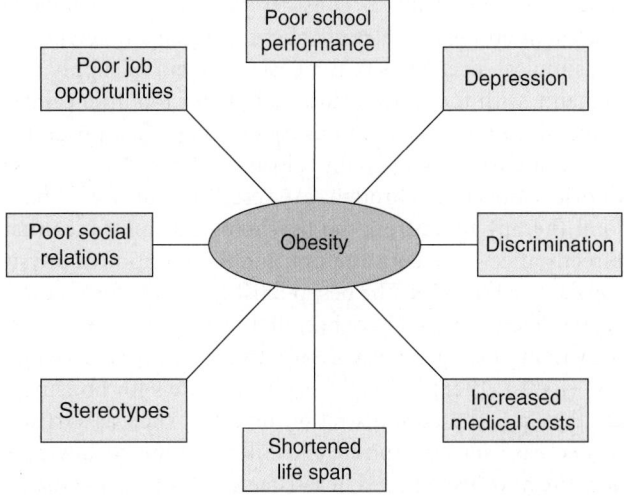

**FIGURE 39-3** The psychosocial comorbidities associated with obesity.

In addition, in calculating the cost to society, we must also consider that the loss of economic productivity in obese adolescents and children is not just related to the medical comorbidities but also manifests itself in poor school performance, low paying jobs, and decreased economic productivity. The prevalence of antiobesity discrimination also affects promotion and salary. In summary, the plague of obesity affecting adolescents and children will have a profound effect on our economy and deserves the attention of the health care workers, government officials, and parents to solve this problem.

## Why Not Wait Until the Obese Adolescent Becomes an Obese Adult?

The various comorbidities noted above have prolonged cumulative deleterious effects on the developing adolescent and child. For example, weight loss is a great cure for type II diabetes, but if weight loss is delayed for a prolonged period of time, the pancreas will not be able to recover sufficient insulin production capacity. The effect of dyslipidemia and hypertension on atherosclerosis-induced coronary artery disease, peripheral vascular disease, and stroke is cumulative over time. Earlier treatment can decrease the long-term damage. Other examples include premature death from sleep apnea, progressive liver failure secondary to nonalcoholic steatohepatitis (NASH), and the severe morbidity associated with slipped capital femoral epiphysis that often leads to joint replacement surgery.

## Treatment Options for the Morbidly Obese Adolescent

Obesity is a very complex multifactorial disease and much work is still required to sort out all of the contributory factors responsible for why some children, often in the same household, are obese and others remain normal weight. Genetic, epigenetic, behavioral, societal, and environmental factors all contribute to the development of obesity. A complete understanding of these factors may one day be understood and prevention strategies can be deployed and nonsurgical treatments implemented. Many different prevention strategies are now under evaluation. In the meantime, it is important to consider the currently available treatment options for already obese children and teens. On the simplest level, obesity is a basic problem of supply and demand, with too much caloric supply for too little caloric demand. Comprehensive nonsurgical weight loss programs encourage patients to count calories, eat healthy, increase caloric utilization through exercise, and utilize behavioral therapy to address the psychological influences that directly affect food consumption and the adoption of physically active lifestyles. The best published results for medical weight loss programs have been in the range of 10% to 20% of patients losing a meager 10% to 20% of excess weight loss (EWL). There is a high recidivism rate with nonsurgical therapy. The administration of drugs such as Orlistat to decrease fat absorption and Silbutramine to decrease appetite have also yielded unsatisfactory results and created compliance issues.

## Energy Homeostasis: The Role of the Neuroendocrine Axis and Obesity

There are important contributory factors affecting obesity that cannot be controlled through surgical approaches, including genetic predisposition, behavioral overeating, noncompliant patients, and an obesogenic society. Patients do not choose to be obese and there are many negative aspects of being obese that clearly would encourage a desire in a person to lose weight. It is clear that strong and disordered signals within the body are critical for the obesity epidemic. One particularly poorly understood concept in obesity is the notion of a set-point for a particular person's ideal BMI. In the simplest form, this concept of energy homeostasis can explain the observation that certain people have a "higher metabolism" and never gain weight, whereas other patients deposit fat as if suffering through a famine. Exposing an adolescent to a major surgical procedure with a risk for significant morbidity and mortality only to have them regain their lost weight 3 years later is a clear example of the body's set point and its desire to regain the desired amount of energy stored. Some of the neuroendocrine determinants of these feast or famine signals, as manifested by hunger or satiety, are being studied for their role in causing obesity. An eventual understanding of these central signals may result in a nonsurgical treatment option for morbid obesity. The discovery of such a treatment is not imminent and it is unlikely that one new obesity treatment will control a disease that is caused by a variety of factors, differing from patient to patient. In the meantime, an understanding of the neuroendocrine cause-and-effect relationship with obesity may prove particularly germane to bariatric surgeons. Choosing a surgical procedure with permanent irreversible anatomic rearrangement and resections could prove to have been an unnecessary risk if future discoveries lead to nonsurgical methods of altering individual patient's energy homeostasis. It is prudent to understand these signals, especially in light of the recurrence risk of morbid obesity after bariatric procedures and is particularly important to understand how the various bariatric procedures affect hormones that affect hunger and satiety.

## Weight Loss Versus Weight Gain

Homeostatic mechanisms defend strongly against weight loss through the induction of hunger and lowered metabolic rate. Weight gain is controlled less well by the body with physiologic signals attenuating fat storage. Compensatory and competing signals therefore combine to control energy homeostasis. A detailed analysis and description of the research on the role of the neuroendocrine axis is beyond the scope of this chapter. A summary of the key portions of the regulatory system for energy homeostasis will shed some important insight into the mechanism of action of the various bariatric surgical procedures. The status of body energy stores is communicated to the central nervous system (principally the arcuate nucleus of the hypothalamus) via circulating hormones, in particular leptin, insulin, and hormones released by the gut itself. Weight loss leads to a decrease in catabolic hormones and an increase in hormones that increase appetite. Release of gut hormones is mediated by food ingestion. Postsurgical changes in the basal and postprandial levels of many of these gut hormones correlate with weight loss and are different for the various weight loss procedures. Several of these hormones appear to be of particular importance and interest to the bariatric surgeon.

## Leptin

Adipocytes produce the protein leptin in direct proportion to the amount of fat stored in the body. Basic science studies have shown that mice lacking leptin or its receptor leads to the uncontrolled intake of food and profound obesity. Leptin acts on the hypothalamus to block the appetite stimulant effects of various circulating molecules. Leptin also promotes the production of α-melanocyte stimulating hormone (MSH), an appetite suppressant. This potent effect on inhibiting food intake is long term as opposed to the rapid onset but short-lived inhibition seen with cholecystokinin (CCK) and the slower suppression of hunger seen with peptide YY (PYY) (see below). Leptin resistance is proposed to be a major factor in obesity and recent animal studies report that a return of leptin sensitivity in obese diabetic mice increases exercise and helps overcome insulin resistance.

## Ghrelin

Ghrelin is a polypeptide mainly secreted by the stomach and duodenum that stimulates food ingestion through increased appetite. It acts in the CNS to increase food intake and decrease fat mobilization. It is rapidly downmodulated after food ingestion. Pharmacological blockade of ghrelin leads to decreased appetite and weight loss in animal studies. Ghrelin appears to be a significant obstacle to sustained weight loss.

## Peptide YY

PYY is a gut hormone secreted by cells in the distal gastrointestinal (GI) tract that is released in proportion to the caloric density in the lumen of the distal GI tract. PYY effectively increases satiety, decreases GI motility, and secretions. It is often expressed at lower basal levels in obese patients and this level increases after certain bariatric procedures.

## Oxyntomodulin

Oxyntomodulin (OXM), like PYY, is secreted by cells in the distal intestine in response to their exposure to nutrients. Like PYY, OXM has a direct effect on satiety. Direct infusion of OXM has been shown to acutely decrease hunger and decrease single meal calorie ingestion.

## Glucagon-like Peptide-1

Glucagon-like Peptide-1 (GLP-1) is secreted by cells in the distal intestine in response to exposure to nutrients. GLP-1 has 6 important functions that are critically important to food ingestion and homeostasis: (1) augments insulin action, (2) decreases glucagon release, (3) reduces gastric acid secretion, (4) slows gastric emptying, (5) relaxes the gastric fundus decreasing the sensation of fullness, and (6) crosses the blood–brain barrier to signal satiety to the GLP-1 receptors in the CNS. GLP-1 levels remain elevated after weight loss related to certain bariatric procedures.

## Cholecystokinin

Cholecystokinin (CCK) is released from the duodenum in response to meals and directly affects satiety through vagus nerve afferent signaling. CCK is elevated in obese patients after restrictive bariatric procedures provided the vagus nerve has not been damaged.

Upon considering the role of these gut hormones in attaining decreased hunger and weight loss, it is interesting to note that changes in these gut hormones are evident within days following bariatric surgery and that blockage of the release of these hormones with the somatostatin analog Octreotide results in increased appetite and food consumption. Even more telling is that attenuated increases in the levels of some of these gut hormones in postoperative patients correlate with poor postsurgical weight loss. Later in this chapter, we will consider the data on how the current bariatric procedures affect the release of the various gut hormones and speculate on how this information can be used to aid in the selection of the most effective weight loss operation.

## Visceral Fat

Visceral fat is an important determinant of obesity regulation and is a critical source of the atherosclerotic morbidities associated with visceral obesity. Many studies have elucidated the importance of patients with a preponderance of visceral fat as opposed to subcutaneous fat spread throughout the body. This explains the strong correlation with the waist-to-hip circumference ratio and the metabolic syndrome (dyslipidemia, hypertension, insulin resistance, prothrombotic, and proinflammatory states).

Some of the important hormones produced by the visceral fat are as follows.

*Plasminogen activator inhibitor 1 (PAI-1)* is the principal inhibitor of plasminogen activation and so promotes atherothrombosis by decreasing fibrin degradation. It is produced mainly by visceral fat tissues in the omentum and mesenteric fat. Procedures that would decrease visceral fat would theoretically directly and immediately decrease the cardiovascular risk even before significant weight loss.

*Resistin* is mainly released by abdominal fat. Resistin increases insulin resistance in peripheral tissue including muscle, heart, liver, and fat. Fat cells that are resistant to insulin cannot shut off their lipolysis and release free fatty acids directly into the portal circulation, increasing lipid abnormalities and steatohepatitis.

*Energy homeostasis and evolution* is of great importance to appreciate that the modern obesity epidemic occurred in synchrony with the advent of ready to eat high-caloric-density foods that are easily digested and rapidly absorbed. It is logical that the digestive system of *Homo sapiens* has not been able to adapt to this modern diet.

Four interesting observations are relevant: (1) The diet of our ancestors and of nonhuman primates is that of hypocaloric foods encased in fiber and cellulose. This necessitated a long small intestine to provide optimal time for calorie extraction. (2) This required primitive man to eat a large quantity of food (often quickly) to ingest enough calories. A large distensible stomach that emptied quickly enhanced food consumption capacity. (3) Once the ingested food reached the distal small intestine, further ingestion would result in calorie wasting through malabsorption and so powerful satiety signals were released. (4) Obese patients have longer small intestines than normal-weight people. In fact, intestinal length is correlated with weight not height. This series of observations helps us to understand the obesity epidemic, explains the evolutionary role of the gut hormones, and suggests methods to surgically correct patients with morbid obesity.

## Special Challenges: Adolescence and Obesity

Surviving the teenage years is a challenge for the average adolescent without a weight problem. Now consider the special challenges of being severely overweight and going through adolescence. Obese adolescents often appear quite advanced in their physical appearance but on the psychosocial side they are at various stages of maturation. This poses a special challenge in caring for these teens. It is natural to treat them like adults, when inside they function as a typical teenager with the insecurities, misunderstandings, and worldviews typical for their age group. Caring for the obese teenager therefore requires that the medical care is designed for their unique developmental phase.

Although somewhat variable between cultures and ethnic background, the age of adolescence ranges from 10 to 21. During this period, the children develop their own identity, strive for peer group acceptance, undergo sexual maturation, come to grips with their body image, and then begin to plan their future. The adolescent with a chronic illness such as obesity will struggle with all of these developmental milestones. The independence of adolescence poses special challenges for weight management programs, since teens want to be like their peers including eating like their peers. They have some degree of autonomy and can purchase their own food. They often want to rebel against their parents and weight management issues can become a huge source of friction within homes. It is important to realize that the obese adolescent suffers from 2 of our culture's greatest discriminations: being a teenager and being overweight. Supporting the patient and the family through these times is the special challenge for the various members of the weight management team.

## The Weight Management Team

Obesity is a complex disease. It is multifactorial in its etiology and in its physical, emotional, and psychosocial impact that obesity has on patient's lives. Therefore, it is logical that optimal care would be provided by a multidisciplinary weight

management team combining expertise to care for the obese patient. This is even more challenging in the care of obese children and adolescents. The ideal weight management program would include medical supervision, an experienced bariatric surgeon, dietary counselors, physical therapists/exercise instructors, social workers, and psychologists, all who have pediatric backgrounds and interest.

## SURGICAL APPROACHES TO WEIGHT LOSS

Over the years, surgical operations to achieve weight loss have been designed to decrease food consumption (restrictive procedures) or to decrease food absorption (malabsorptive procedures) or a combination thereof. The ideal surgical procedure to treat morbid obesity in adolescents would result in durable and significant weight loss (eg, >60% EWL for the remainder of the patient's life) would be safe with low operative mortality and morbidity and not lead to significant nutritional deficiencies or long-term morbidity such as liver disease or malignancy. Conceivably, in those younger children who have not reached their adult height, the ability to stop weight gain may allow them to grow into a healthier BMI. Unfortunately, a bariatric procedure that achieves all of these ideals is currently not available for adults, much less for adolescents or children. There are few reliable clinical trials directly comparing the various surgical approaches to achieve weight loss in adults. The few randomized controlled studies suffer from limited statistical power. The relevant adolescent bariatric literature, although very encouraging is nearly exclusively limited to case series reporting perioperative morbidity and mortality, EWL, long-term morbidity, and improvements in physical and psychosocial quality of life measurements. Most surgeons who currently perform bariatric procedures on adolescents are faced with the difficult decision of choosing the appropriate surgical option that balances the risk and benefits for the morbidly obese child (Fig. 39-4). There is a definite need to treat this chronically debilitating disease that will shorten the average life span of the child and cause a great deal of suffering, but on the other hand, obesity is not a life-threatening emergency that demands immediate surgical intervention. The ideal operation for obesity in children and adolescents would allow for a safe, durable attainment of a healthy BMI with minimal complications in the immediate postoperative time period and minimal long-term complications such as nutritional deficiencies, damage to the liver, or the development of malignancies in the bypassed portion of the intestine. The resolution of the associated comorbidities and not the return to ideal body weight is arguably the best measure of success.

There have been many different weight loss surgeries developed over the years. In this chapter, we will discuss in detail only those procedures that are of current use in bariatric surgery: Roux-en-Y gastric bypass (RYGB), biliopancreatic diversion with or without the duodenal switch modification (BPD or BPD/DS), the sleeve gastrectomy (SG), and the laparoscopic adjustable gastric band (LAGB) (Fig. 39-5).

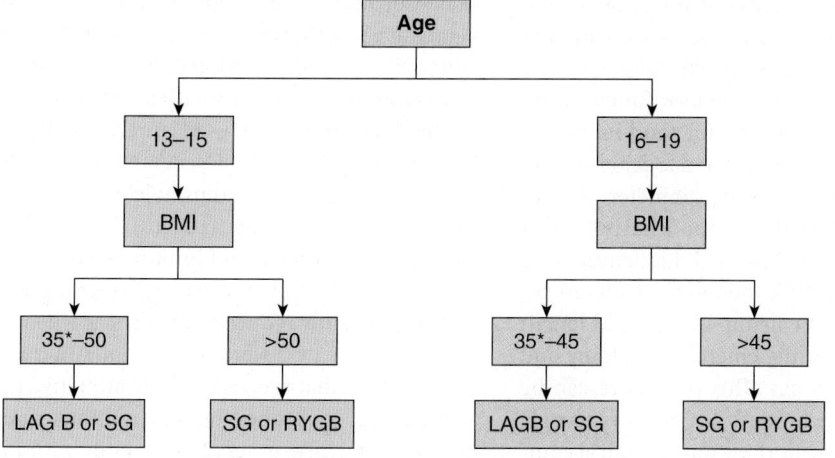

**Surgical approach to the obese teenager**

Nonresponders to the LAGB can undergo SG or RYGB
Nonresponders to SG can undergo RYGB or BPD/DS

*BMI 35–39 with obesity-related comorbidities
LAGB = Laparoscopic adjustable gastric band
SG = Sleeve gastrectomy
RYGP = Roux-en-Y gastric bypass
BPD/DS = Biliopancreatic diversion with duodenal switch
Nonresponder = Inadequate weight loss with LAGB or SG and/or persistent mechanical problems with LAGB

**FIGURE 39-4** Surgical decision protocol for bariatric surgery in adolescents.

Historically, bariatric surgery started with the introduction of purely malabsorptive procedures such as the jejunoileal bypass procedure, which resulted in profound vitamin and micronutrient deficiencies and long-term liver damage. This procedure was abandoned many years ago. A newer surgical procedure was introduced by Scopinaro and is referred to as the biliopancreatic diversion procedure (BPD). This procedure works by separating the digestive enzymes from the ingested food until a point where they are mixed in the distal GI tract. In brief, the stomach is separated from the duodenum and a long Roux limb is created between the stomach and small intestine. The biliopancreatic secretions follow their normal route and mix with the food at the point of the enteroenterostomy at the mid ileum. This creates a distal common channel in which there is limited time for digestion and absorption. The procedure has undergone modifications involving resection of a greater portion of the stomach to decrease the stomach capacity (which adds a volume restrictive component) and modifications to the length of the common channel to optimize the amount of malabsorption while minimizing vitamin and micronutrient deficiency and the dumping syndrome. BPD produces impressive weight loss but seems ill-suited for the specific needs of the morbidly obese teenager or child, in particular the high incidence of surgical complications, the irreversibility, the drastic change in anatomy, and the nutritional deficiencies such as hypocalcemia, iron deficient anemia, vitamin deficiencies, mineral deficiencies, and the unknown long-term risk of organ damage and malignancy in the excluded intestinal limb.

The duodenal switch modification to the BPD (BPD/DS) is the most effective and best studied variation of the BPD. It produces anatomy that is restrictive for caloric intake and

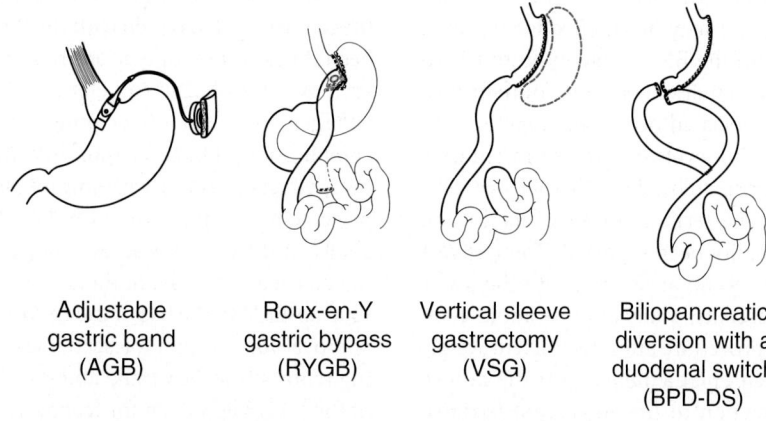

Adjustable gastric band (AGB)

Roux-en-Y gastric bypass (RYGB)

Vertical sleeve gastrectomy (VSG)

Biliopancreatic diversion with a duodenal switch (BPD-DS)

**FIGURE 39-5** Diagram of surgical options.

produces the malabsorption associated with BPD. The standard procedure begins with an aggressive resection of the greater curvature and body of the stomach and the creation of a tubularized remnant or sleeve of the stomach along the lesser curvature. This aptly named SG preserves pyloric function and results in a significantly reduced capacity for food ingestion. The second part of the procedure, called the duodenal switch, involves dividing the duodenum above the sphincter of Oddi and creating a duodenoenterostomy to the duodenal bulb. This anastomois in effect switches out the normal duodenum for a Roux limb. As with the simpler BPD, the food channel mixes with the digestive secretions in the ileum. The desired length of the common channel between the enteroenterostomy and the ileocecal valve is 100 to 150 cm. This procedure can be done with minimally invasive techniques but not surprisingly has had a higher rate of operative morbidity and surgical complications because of the complexity of the anatomical reconstruction. Of particular note, in super obese individuals, the BPD/DS is sometimes performed as a staged procedure with the SG utilized as the initial procedure to initiate weight loss. The surprising amount of weight loss seen with the SG has prompted many bariatric surgeons to offer this as a standalone bariatric procedure. There is an impressive rise in PYY, OXM, and GLP-1 after BPD, which is likely responsible for the early satiety experienced by these patients. The addition of the SG would result in a decreased amount of fasting circulating ghrelin, which would result in decreased appetite.

The SG may be of particular interest to the bariatric surgeon interested in treating morbidly obese adolescents, since it is an easily learned, relatively low-risk procedure that does not involve malabsorption and seems to yield very good weight loss. The SG can be converted later to a more aggressive procedure such as a BPD/DS or RYGB. The procedure is easily done with endoscopic staplers to divide the stomach, the LigaSure or Harmonic Scalpel to divide the short gastric vessels and removal of the resected stomach. The procedure is now gaining popularity among adult bariatric surgeons as a low-risk means of gaining calorie restriction without causing vitamin and micronutrient deficiency. The disadvantages of the procedure have been the rate of gastric leaks, gastroesophageal reflux, gastric emptying problems, and antral stenosis. Many of these problems have been minimized with the development of reinforced staple lines and modifications including the placement of an appropriate-sized transpyloric Bougie during the creation of the lesser curvature sleeve. Initial reports of the weight loss associated with the SG have been encouraging and may be an effective bariatric procedure for patients within the BMI range of 45 to 65. As mentioned, SG patients have a marked decrease in their fasting ghrelin levels and an associated decreased appetite. The effect of this change in ghrelin levels on growth in children has been questioned. Unfortunately, since the SG is a relatively new procedure, the long-term accounts of its durable effectiveness and safety have not been reported. There is very limited experience, mainly anecdotal reports, with the use of SG in morbidly obese adolescents. Many of these adolescents underwent SG as a salvage procedure after insufficient weight loss or after repeated pouch enlargements with the adjustable gastric band. The attraction to the adolescent bariatric surgeon is the ease of the operation and relative low risk of

surgical complications and long-term issues associated with malabsorption. The ability to eventually undergo a more aggressive malabsorptive procedure such as the RYGB or the BPD/DS may make starting with the SG a useful and prudent algorithm for adolescents with a BMI ≥ 45.

The most commonly used purely restrictive procedure for bariatric surgery in adolescents is the LAGB. This involves placing an inflatable adjustable silicone ring around the upper portion of the stomach just distal to the GE junction to form an upper pouch and limit food consumption. The basic physiology relies on the patient reaching a point of satiety with significantly reduced portion size when the upper pouch fills up. There are several important and distinct advantages to the LAGB that are particularly attractive to the adolescent population. The operation has minimal operative risk and can be performed in less than 1 hour with low risk of damage to internal organs, blood loss, or infection. The operative mortality rate in adults is 0.05% and there has been no report of a death in adolescents. The band itself is adjustable and so that the amount of restriction can be easily adjusted via a subcutaneous reservoir that is connected via a catheter to the band. This is particularly advantageous, since the surgical experience with an operative creation of a restricting structure (eg, vertical banded gastroplasty) has been difficult to calibrate from patient to patient and was prone to stenosing or expanding resulting in the need to reoperate. This adjustability is particularly useful in young people because their ongoing growth and maturation (both physically and mentally) can affect the amount of restriction required for adequate weight loss and then long-term management of healthy weight. Many patients after losing weight will ask for a modest loosening of the restriction, a feature that is ideal for pregnant women. Since there is no portion of the GI tract that is bypassed, the risk of malnutrition, vitamin, and micronutrient deficiency is minimal. The final advantage is the reversibility of the procedure, since the band is easily removed with a minimally invasive approach.

Unfortunately, the LAGB has not proven to be the optimal procedure for all morbidly obese adolescents. There are conflicting reports on the outcomes of the LAGB in adolescents especially when it pertains to weight loss. The biggest concern is that of a slower weight loss and lower total EWL when compared with other procedures, although several groups report similar long-term weight loss with the LAGB compared to the RYGB after 3 years or more of follow-up. Of course, the argument can be made that a slower rate of weight loss may be healthier than the rapid weight loss seen with the RYGB or BPD/DS. There has been the issue of reoperations required for hardware problems such as reservoir and catheter problems, band migration, and enlargement of the upper pouch. The historically worrisome complication of band erosion into the stomach seems to have been virtually solved with improvements in band design and placement technique over the last decade. While the adjustability of the LAGB is an advantage, it also means the adjustments need to be part of the follow-up care of the patient. The final obstacle to the use of the LAGB is the current lack of FDA approval for use in adolescents less than 18 despite convincing reports from Australia and Israel of the safety and efficacy of the LAGB approach for teenagers. FDA-approved industry-sponsored trials are underway to gather sufficient data to prove the safety and efficacy of the LAGB in the 14- to 17-year age group. There are conflicting reports in the literature, but overall, it appears that the LAGB in adolescents is most effective in adolescents with BMI less than 50 and who show a good potential for discipline when it comes to adapting to the band lifestyle. The band in these children serves as a constant reminder to not overeat and they are encouraged to choose high-protein foods with low glycemic-index carbohydrates. LAGB patients do not seem to have as significant degree of ghrelin suppression as the other surgical procedures. The LAGB procedure can be a very effective weight loss strategy for a large subset of children with the necessary intelligence, motivation and family support. It does, however, require a multispecialty approach, frequent postoperative course corrections, and band adjustments to attain maximal results. The need for frequent follow-up visits, while advantageous for maturing teenagers, can pose significant logistical problems including geographical relocation for college or work opportunities. The increasing number of surgeons throughout the country familiar with the care of LABG patients simplifies the transfer of care for these mobile young people.

## Malabsorptive and Restrictive Procedures

The most frequently performed bariatric procedure in adults is the RYGB. This is now routinely done with minimally invasive techniques and involves the separation of the majority of the stomach and anastomosing a small pouch of the upper stomach to a Roux limb of the jejunum (<150 cm). The disconnected portion of the stomach drains into the duodenum and the digestive juices mix with the food at the jejunojejunostomy. Food consumption is restricted by the creation of the small gastric pouch and the anastomosis between the stomach and the Roux limb. Similar to the BPD, malabsorption is created by the bypass of a significant portion of the absorptive surface and the delayed mixing of the food with the digestive enzymes. The amount of bypassed intestine is generally much less than that bypassed in the BPD operation. The RYGB reliably produces rapid weight loss over the first 6 to 12 months, although a significant subset of patients regain weight, which appears to be related to an adaptation process directed by the body striving to reattain its perceived ideal body weight. The weight regain can be reduced if the patient continues the other parts of their weight management program—appropriate diet, activity, and behavior. An operative mortality rate as low as 1 in 200 has been reported, but many case series report mortality rates of 1% to 3%. Mortality data on RYGB in adolescents are not available, but would be expected to be better because of the overall increased physiologic reserve of younger patients. After the RYGB, most patients have lower ghrelin levels and a higher PYY, OXM, and GLP-1 response to meals than their BMI-matched controls.

## Results of Weight Loss Procedures in Adolescents

Recommendations for the optimal bariatric surgery procedure for adolescents will certainly depend on the results of the various centers performing weight loss surgery in this age group. Unfortunately, the available data suffer the usual limitations associated with various surgeons reporting results from their respective case series. There have been no randomized controlled trials performed, for example comparing RYGB to LAGB in teens. A careful analysis of the available data is consistent with the following interpretation. The LAGB system can be very effective for 60% to 80% of patients with a BMI less than or equal to 45. They can be expected to undergo a percent excess weight loss (% EWL) of 50 to 60, which is durable but slower to achieve than the RYGP. The LAGB operation can be done very safely with low surgical morbidity rates and a shallow learning curve. There is an additional learning curve involving postoperative management and optimizing the band adjustments. There is a long-term surgical morbidity rate as high as 15% for band slippage, pouch enlargement, and mechanical problems associated with the port and catheter. Many of the patients who suffer from pouch enlargement are nonresponders to LAGB and this is correlated with a higher initial BMI. Nonresponders should be converted to a more aggressive surgical procedure such as the SG or LAGB.

RYGP in comparison is a very effective weight loss surgery that can be done with mortality rates of 0.5% by experienced surgeons. The weight loss is rapid (6-12 months) in nearly all individuals, but is associated with the risk of significant vitamin and mineral deficiencies. Weight regain has been reported in 10% to 20% of patients. Presumably, this is associated with the intestine adapting to the new anatomical configuration and the body striving to regain its misguided ideal body weight. Postoperative morbidity that requires some form of surgical intervention is less frequent than with the LAGB, but often more serious such as internal hernias, bowel obstruction, bleeding from stomal ulcers, gastric pouch enlargement, and stenosis or enlargement of the gastrojejunal anastomosis.

Compared to RYGB, the SG is a technically simple surgical procedure that has been shown to be a highly effective stand-alone weight loss procedure in adults. There are little data in adolescents. Improvements in technology have allowed the development of SG into an operation with low morbidity and mortality. It appears to be an effective salvage operation for LAGB nonresponders. The SG has been utilized for nearly 10 years, and there have been no reports of significant long-term morbidity. There have been reports of regaining weight after the SG similar to the level seen with RYGB.

BPD/DS is an extremely aggressive surgical procedure with higher complication rates and should only be done by experienced bariatric surgeons in those patients suffering from extreme morbid obesity and obesity-related comorbidities. It should rarely be used as the initial procedure for adolescents, but may be necessary if a SG or RYGP is unable to control severe obesity and obesity-related comorbidities.

## Recommended Approach for Weight Loss Surgery in Adolescents

Obtaining Class I evidence from an adequately powered randomized clinical trial comparing the various bariatric surgical procedures has proved elusive in adults, but it seems impossible to realize within teenagers. Therefore, bariatric surgeons treating adolescents must develop a practical, commonsense protocol before embarking on weight loss surgery for this age group. The overarching goal is to optimize weight loss and improve or prevent comorbidities in a safe manner for all obese adolescents and children. It seems logical that the same operation will not be the best option for every obese adolescent and child especially when one considers their varying BMI status, comorbidity burden, and stages of physical and psychological maturation. Based on the evidence available, the following surgical approach to the obese adolescent is suggested as a safe and reasonable protocol that can be tested in a prospective fashion.

A simple, low-morbidity procedure such as the LAGB is best in younger patients (15 or younger) with BMI less than or equal to 50. The SG option may also become a good choice for these patients. Adolescents (15 or younger) with BMI greater than 50 will probably do better with a SG or RYGB as their initial surgical procedure and the severity of their obesity supports the additional surgical risk. The relative technical ease of the SG makes it particularly appealing to surgeons unwilling to climb the learning curve of the RYGB.

Using these recommendations, the success rate for LAGB will be optimized with fewer complications. The use of a more judicious age and BMI selection criterion could also minimize postoperative morbidity and patient frustration with wasted time and unmet expectations as the number of LAGB nonresponders decreases. The excellent safety profile with the LAGB also begs the question as to whether younger patients (eg, age <14 years old) should be treated with the LAGB. In our experience, younger patients are more compliant with the physician and parent-directed lifestyle modifications necessary to gain optimal results with the LAGB system. The use of the LAGB in these patients could control their weight at an early age without significant risk of malabsorption of critical nutrients during the rapid pubertal growth period.

Older teenagers (16-19) with a modest BMI in the range of 35 to 45 are still good candidates for the LAGB. Those with a BMI of greater than 45 should undergo a SG or RYGB as their primary operation. The excellent safety profile and the shallow learning curve may result in the SG being the procedure of choice for these older teens with higher BMI. Just as the SG may be an excellent salvage operation for unsuccessful LAGB patients, the RYGB or BPD/DS may become the best salvage operation for unsuccessful SG patients.

It is important to remember that the morbidly obese child can have very complex medical and psychosocial problems. Therefore, the establishment of a multispecialty adolescent weight management team will result in much better patient care and better patient outcomes. At the very least, an experienced nurse practitioner can offload the myriad of problems that would otherwise be directed toward the busy pediatric general surgeon interested in devoting some of his or her valuable time to treating morbidly obese children.

## Collaborative Efforts to Address the Bariatric Surgical Care of Teenagers

The importance of the obesity epidemic is evidenced by the support offered by the NIH. For example, in 2003, the National Institute of Diabetes and Digestive and Kidney Diseases (NIDDK) formed a partnership with researchers called the Longitudinal Assessment of Bariatric Surgery, or LABS. Subsequently, to help determine if bariatric surgery

is appropriate for adolescents, NIH launched a prospective study called Teen-LABS in 2007. This multiinstitutional collaboration is collecting data on the effects of bariatric surgery in teenagers. Over a 5-year period, researchers will collect data about obesity-related medical problems, other health risk factors, and quality of life from the patients before they undergo surgery and 2 years after surgery. Researchers will then compare the adolescent outcomes to data collected from adults.

## SUMMARY

The obesity epidemic is ravaging a large percentage of our children. Prevention measures have not proven successful to date and nonsurgical weight loss interventions effectively treat only a small fraction of obese children. A nonsurgical drug, device, or treatment protocol that will have a wide ranging effect on morbid obesity does not appear imminent. A surgical protocol for weight loss in morbidly obese children must be safe, effective, and adaptive to the individual child based on his or her age, degree of obesity-linked comorbidity burden, and chance for success. The stepwise escalation to surgical procedures with increasing anatomical rearrangement and risk for complications seems prudent. We have proposed an approach to treat morbid obese teenagers that takes all of these considerations into account and should provide a rational and testable protocol as we move forward with this difficult problem.

## SELECTED READINGS

Ashrafian H, Ahmed K, Rowland SP, et al. Metabolic surgery and cancer: protective effects of bariatric procedures. *Cancer* 2011;117(9):1788–1799.

Brandt ML, Harmon CM, Helmrath MA, Inge TH, McKay SV, Michalsky MP. Morbid obesity in pediatric diabetes mellitus: surgical options and outcomes. *Nat Rev Endocrinol* 2010;6(11):637–645. Epub Sep 14, 2010. Review.

Browne AF, Inge TH. How young for bariatric surgery in children? *Semin Pediatr Surg* 2009;18(3):176–185.

Christou N, Efthimiou E. Five-year outcomes of laparoscopic adjustable gastric banding and laparoscopic Roux-en-Y gastric bypass in a comprehensive bariatric surgery program in Canada. *Pediatrics* 2010;126(4):e746–e753.

Diniz Mde F, Azeredo Passos VM, Diniz MT. Bariatric surgery and the gut-brain communication—the state of the art three years later. *Nutrition* 2010;26(10):925–931. Epub Apr 14, 2010. Review.

Dixon JB, Jones K, Dixon M. Medical versus surgical interventions for the metabolic complications of obesity in children. *Semin Pediatr Surg* 2009g;18(3):168–175.

Fielding GA, Duncombe JE. Laparoscopic adjustable gastric banding in severely obese adolescents. *Surg Obes Relat Dis* 2005;1(4):399–405.

Galvani C, Gorodner M, Moser F, et al. Laparoscopic adjustable gastric band versus laparoscopic Roux-en-Y gastric bypass: ends justify the means? *Surg Endosc* 2006;20(6):934–941.

Grün F, Blumberg B. Environmental obesogens: organotins and endocrine disruption via nuclear receptor signaling. *Endocrinology* 2006;147(6 Suppl):S50–S55.

Holterman AX, Browne A, Tussing L, et al. A prospective trial for laparoscopic adjustable gastric banding in morbidly obese adolescents: an interim report of weight loss, metabolic and quality of life outcomes. *J Pediatr Surg* 2010;45(1):74–78; discussion 78–79.

Inge TH, Zeller M, Harmon C, et al. Teen-Longitudinal Assessment of Bariatric Surgery: methodological features of the first prospective multicenter study of adolescent bariatric surgery. *J Pediatr Surg.* 2007;42(11):1969–1971.

Inge TH, Zeller MH, Lawson ML, Daniels SR. A critical appraisal of evidence supporting a bariatric surgical approach to weight management for adolescents. *J Pediatr* 2005;147:10–19.

Lawson ML, Kirk S, Mitchell T, et al. One-year outcomes of Roux-en-Y gastric bypass for morbidly obese adolescents: a multicenter study from the Pediatric Bariatric Study Group. *J Pediatr Surg* 2006;41(1): 137–143.

Lee WJ, Chong K, Ser KH, et al. Gastric bypass vs sleeve gastrectomy for type 2 diabetes mellitus: a randomized controlled trial. *Arch Surg* 2011;146(2):143–148.

Melissas J, Mouzas J, Filis D, et al. Laparoscopic gastric bypass is superior to adjustable gastric band in super morbidly obese patients: a prospective, comparative analysis. *Obes Surg* 2006;16(7):897–902.

Nadler EP, Brotman LM, Miyoshi T, Fryer GE Jr, Weitzman M. Morbidity in obese adolescents who meet the adult National Institutes of Health criteria for bariatric surgery. *J Pediatr Surg* 2009;44(10): 1869–1876.

Nadler EP, Youn HA, Ren CJ, Fielding GA. An update on 73 US obese pediatric patients treated with laparoscopic adjustable gastric banding: comorbidity resolution and compliance data. *J Pediatr Surg* 2008;43(1):141–146.

Ogden CL, Carroll MD, Curtin LR, Lamb MM, Flegal KM. Prevalence of high body mass index in US children and adolescents, 2007–2008. *JAMA* 2010;303(3):242–249.

Puhl R, Brownell KD Bias, discrimination, and obesity. *Obes Res* 2001;9(12):788–805.

Santoro S, Velhate M, Malzoni C, Milleo, F, Klajner S, Campos F. Preliminary results from digestive adaptation: a new surgical proposal for treating obesity, based on physiology and evolution. *Sao Paulo Med J* 2006;124(4):192–197.

Tucker O, Sucandy I, Szomstein S, Rosenthal RJ. Revisional surgery after failed laparoscopic adjustable gastric banding. *Surg Obes Relat Dis* 2008;4(6):740–747.

Yitzhak A, Mizrahi S, Avinoach E Laparoscopic gastric banding in adolescents. *Obes Surg* 2006;16(10):1318–1322.

# Pyloric Stenosis CHAPTER 40

Edward M. Barksdale Jr and Todd A. Ponsky

## KEY POINTS

1. Curvilinear supraumbilical incision.

2. Omental traction facilitates delivery of pylorus

3. Extraluminal muscle split from duodenum to stomach antral fibers.

4. Inspect for mucosal injury.

5. Laparoscopic approach seems to be equivalent to traditional open operation.

## HISTORY

The first clinical description of pyloric stenosis is attributed to Hildanus in 1627. Although sporadic reports of infants with gastric outlet obstructive symptoms followed his initial description, it was not until the seminal work of Harald Hirschsprung in 1888 that infantile hypertrophic pyloric stenosis (HPS) was established as a distinct clinical entity. The first successful surgery followed shortly thereafter in 1899, when Lobker performed a gastrojejunostomy to successfully treat an infant with HPS. General acceptance of this procedure was not favorable due to an attendant postoperative mortality as high as 50%. Nicoll (1906) and Fredet (1907) working independently developed a technique of extramucosal pyloroplasty that would provide the foundation for pyloromyotomy first described in 1912 by Ramstedt. Although various incisions have been used to access the pylorus, the Ramstedt procedure, as it is frequently called, has remained the surgical standard until the present. Recently, the laparoscopic approach originally described by Allain and colleagues in 1991 has gained immense popularity. Laparoscopic pyloromyotomy has supplanted the open procedure as the new standard in many pediatric centers. Currently, the morbidity and mortality of pyloromyotomy regardless of approach in experienced hands is less than 10% and 0.5%, respectively.

## PATHOPHYSIOLOGY

Pyloric stenosis is one of the most common surgical conditions of early infancy presenting in approximately 3 per 1000 live births in the United States. Despite this high prevalence, the precise etiology of the condition remains poorly understood. Family history, sex, birth order, and maternal feeding patterns have all been implicated as potential risk factors. Numerous theories for the pathogenesis of pyloric stenosis have been proposed, but none has achieved general acceptance. These theories fall into 3 principal categories: (1) compensatory work hypertrophy, (2) neurologic degeneration or immaturity, and (3) abnormal endocrine or growth factor signals. Some authors have suggested that milk curds developing in the stomach can obstruct the pyloric channel leading to redundancy in the pyloric mucosa and compensatory pyloric muscle hypertrophy. Other investigators have theorized that various neural components in the pyloric antrum may be immature or defective leading to increased muscle size. Some of these theories include the deficiency of nitric oxide synthase, decreased interstitial cells of Cajal (pacemaker cells of the gut), and diminished expression of neural cell adhesion molecule (NCAM). Other authors have implicated gastrointestinal endocrine or paracrine factors such as gastrin hypersecretion in either the infant or the mother as the stimulus toward muscle hypertrophy. The familial occurrence of this condition in some patients also implicates genetic factors in the etiology. Due to the strong evidence supporting each of these major theories, the etiology is likely multifactorial and yet to be determined.

## DIAGNOSTIC PRINCIPLES

The diagnosis is primarily made by history and physical exam. The classic clinical presentation of pyloric stenosis is projectile nonbilious vomiting in an infant 3 to 6 weeks of age. Although the disease rarely presents at birth, some infants will develop a crescendo pattern of emesis that begins in the first week of life and progresses to full presentation as late as 3 to 4 months of age. Significant metabolic alkalosis and malnutrition may occur as a consequence of prolonged symptoms. The typical physical exam findings in these patients include visible peristaltic waves in the epigastrium and the presence of a palpable mass in the upper abdomen. The mass or "olive" may be distinguished by an experienced examiner in 70% to 90% of patients. Identification of this finding often requires gastric decompression and a cooperative patient. The infant is most easily examined in the supine position with either a pacifier or bottle of sugar water given to keep him or her calm. The legs are gently elevated to relax the abdominal wall musculature and the abdomen is palpated in the subxiphoid region about one half the distance to the umbilicus. The examiner must be patient and occasionally must return to reexamine the infant in order to identify the "olive." In the absence of a palpable mass, an upper gastrointestinal (UGI) contrast study or ultrasonographic evaluation will usually make the diagnosis. In most pediatric centers, the study of choice is an abdominal ultrasound (US). The ultrasonographic criteria for pyloric stenosis include a pyloric channel length >17 mm, pyloric muscle diameter >14 mm, and pyloric muscle wall thickness >4 mm. This technique is reliable and decreases the risk of aspiration. If the US is inconclusive or there is concern for gastroesophageal reflux, malrotation, or anatomic anomalies, then an UGI series should be performed. This study will demonstrate the presence of a distended stomach with narrowing and elongation of the pyloric channel—the "string" sign or "double track" sign. Other findings seen on UGI series include "shoulders" at the proximal end of the pylorus reflecting the hypertrophied muscle bulging into the gastric lumen.

The initial physical exam should also include an assessment of the patient's overall clinical status and degree of dehydration. Most infants at presentation have had significant episodes of emesis and may be dehydrated and/or cachectic. Clinically, these patients may present with dry mucous membranes, depressed fontanels, increased skin turgor, and varying degrees of malnutrition. They characteristically have a hypochloremic, hypokalemic metabolic alkalosis with some hyponatremia. The initial intravenous (IV) fluid resuscitation is begun with 5% dextrose and normal saline for severely dehydrated infants or one half normal saline for moderately dehydrated patients given as a bolus of 20 mL/kg with 10 to 20 meq/L of potassium chloride (KCl) added when the infant has voided. Once the infant's calculated deficit is 50% corrected, the sodium content is reduced until euvolemia is achieved and then he or she is maintained on one quarter normal saline until surgery. This rehydration process may take hours to days depending on the degree of dehydration at presentation. Surgical correction of this disease is not an emergency. Failure to adequately correct the alkalosis preoperatively may result in postanesthetic apnea and respiratory arrest (Fig. 40-1).

## TREATMENT OPTIONS

The Ramstedt extramucosal longitudinal pyloromyotomy has long been the classic surgical approach to HPS. Numerous incisions have been described to gain exposure to the pylorus:

midline laparotomy (Fredet), right upper quadrant oblique right-upper quadrant transverse muscle-splitting (Robertson "gridiron") or muscle-sparing (Rickham) incision, and circumbilical or transumbilical laparoscopic incision. Minimal access approaches are increasingly the preference of many pediatric surgeons due to rapid access to the pylorus. We prefer either the circumbilical approach first advocated by Tan and Bianchi or the laparoscopic repair because of its superior cosmetic results and low perioperative morbidity (Fig. 40-2).

Following adequate preoperative hydration to correct any volume deficit and/or metabolic alkalosis, the patient is brought to the operating room. Evacuation of the stomach with an orogastric or nasogastric tube prior to the induction of general anesthesia should be performed. IV antistaphylococcal antibiotics are administered for a single preoperative dose and for 24 hours postoperatively. Betadine and alcohol are used to prepare the abdomen with meticulous attention to the umbilicus. The presence of an umbilical remnant, a "wet" umbilicus, and periumbilical erythema all contraindicate an umbilical incision. As an alternate approach, we would perform the incision above the umbilicus or use a standard right upper quadrant incision.

## Circumbilical Approach

A curvilinear incision is made in a supraumbilical skin fold following the infiltration of 0.25% bupivacaine based on the patients' weight. Through sharp dissection, the midline fascia is identified and exposed approximately one third to one half the distance from the umbilicus to the xiphoid. The linea alba is opened longitudinally and the peritoneum is entered to the right of the umbilical vein. The pylorus is identified by first mobilizing the omentum with an opened moist sponge that is gently placed into the peritoneal cavity just beneath the liver. The omentum will adhere to the sponge when removed from the peritoneum. By mobilizing the omentum, the transverse colon will be easily visualized in the wound and may be directed caudally. This maneuver brings the gastric antrum into view. The greater curvature of the stomach should be grasped with a moist sponge and the pylorus can then be delivered by a gentle rocking motion. The junction of the gastric and duodenal serosa may be identified by a white line of demarcation and the prominent vein of Mayo. Prior to myotomy, the pylorus should be immobilized with placement of the surgeon's index finger of the nondominant hand on the duodenal side of the pylorus. A perpendicular serosal incision is made on the anterosuperior aspect of the pylorus beginning approximately 1 to 2 mm proximal to the duodenum and extending well on to the nonhypertrophied antrum. This is delineated by the transverse/oblique gastric fibers of the stomach. The blunt end of the knife handle is used to initially disrupt the fibers. The circular muscle of the pylorus is then further disrupted using the Benson spreader. This maneuver is performed until the gastric muscular fibers are completely separated from the gastroduodenal junction to the oblique fibers of the stomach. The gastric submucosa will bulge into the cleft. Care should be taken to avoid too vigorous spreading in the distal pylorus because the adjacent

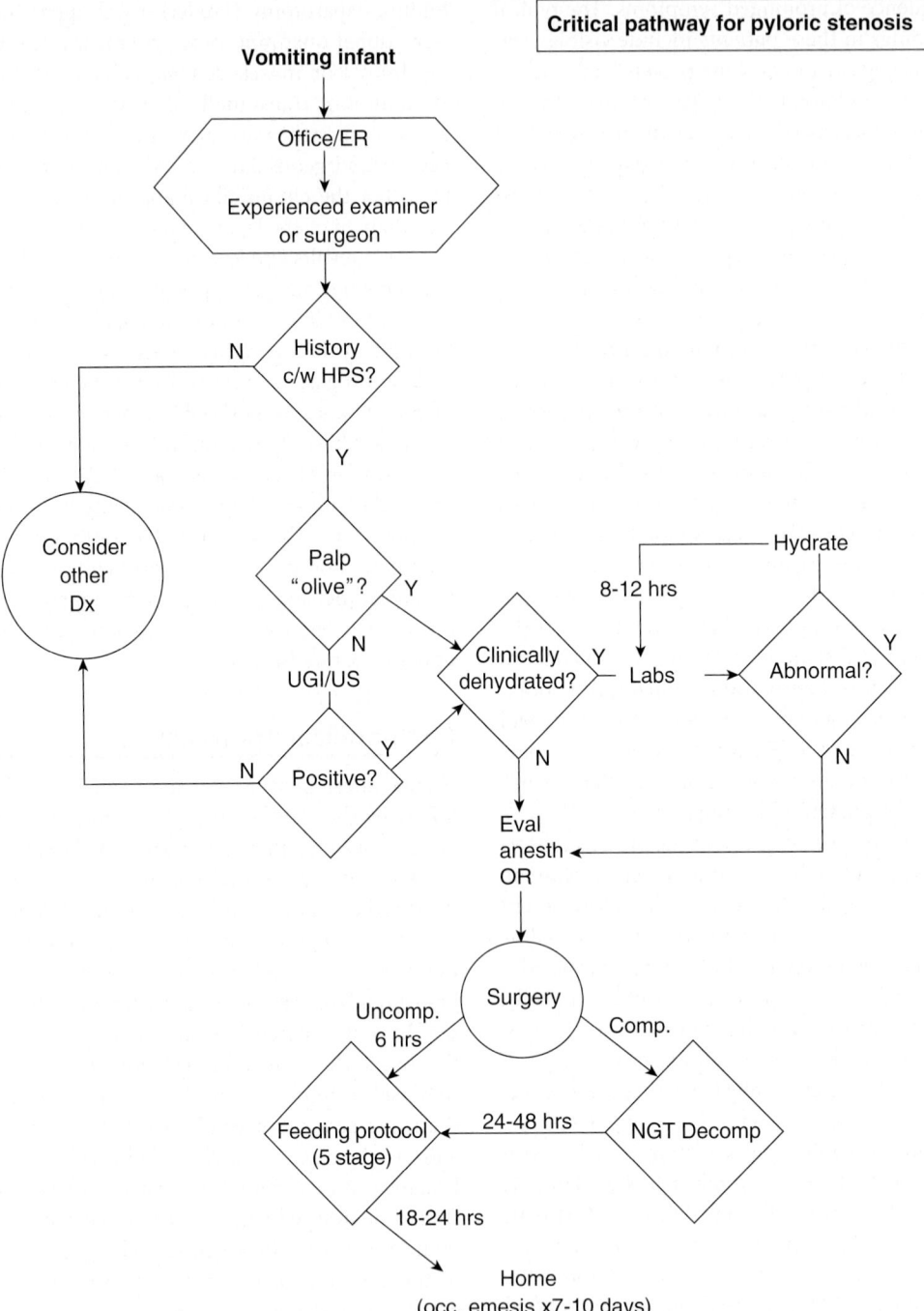

**Critical pathway for pyloric stenosis**

**FIGURE 40-1** Critical pathway for pyloric stenosis. The vomiting infant birth to 4 months of age brought to the office or emergency room (ER) for evaluation by an experienced examiner or a pediatric surgeon. Initial assessment of history and/or physical exam to assess likelihood of the diagnosis. Clear history and exam findings that are consistent with (c/w) HPS lead to an assessment of the hydration status and laboratory evaluations; electrolytes, blood urea nitrogen, creatinine, and hemoglobin/hematocrit. If hydration status is good, then the patient is referred for surgery. Equivocal history or findings necessitate either an UGI series or US. Other diagnoses (eg, gastroesophageal reflux, pylorospasm, sepsis, etc) must be considered if these studies are negative. If the study is positive, then the patient will have labs obtained and undergo rehydration and then surgery. Postoperatively, feedings are initiated per protocol at 6 hours. If surgical complications (mucosal perforation) occur, then a nasogastric tube would be left in place for 24 to 48 hours, and feedings initiated at that time per protocol. Patients are typically discharged 18 to 24 hours postinitiation of protocol. Rarely, patients will have frequent emetic episodes and require longer stays. Occasional emesis may occur for 7 to 10 days postoperatively. HPS, hypertrophic pyloric stenosis; NGT, nasogastric tube.

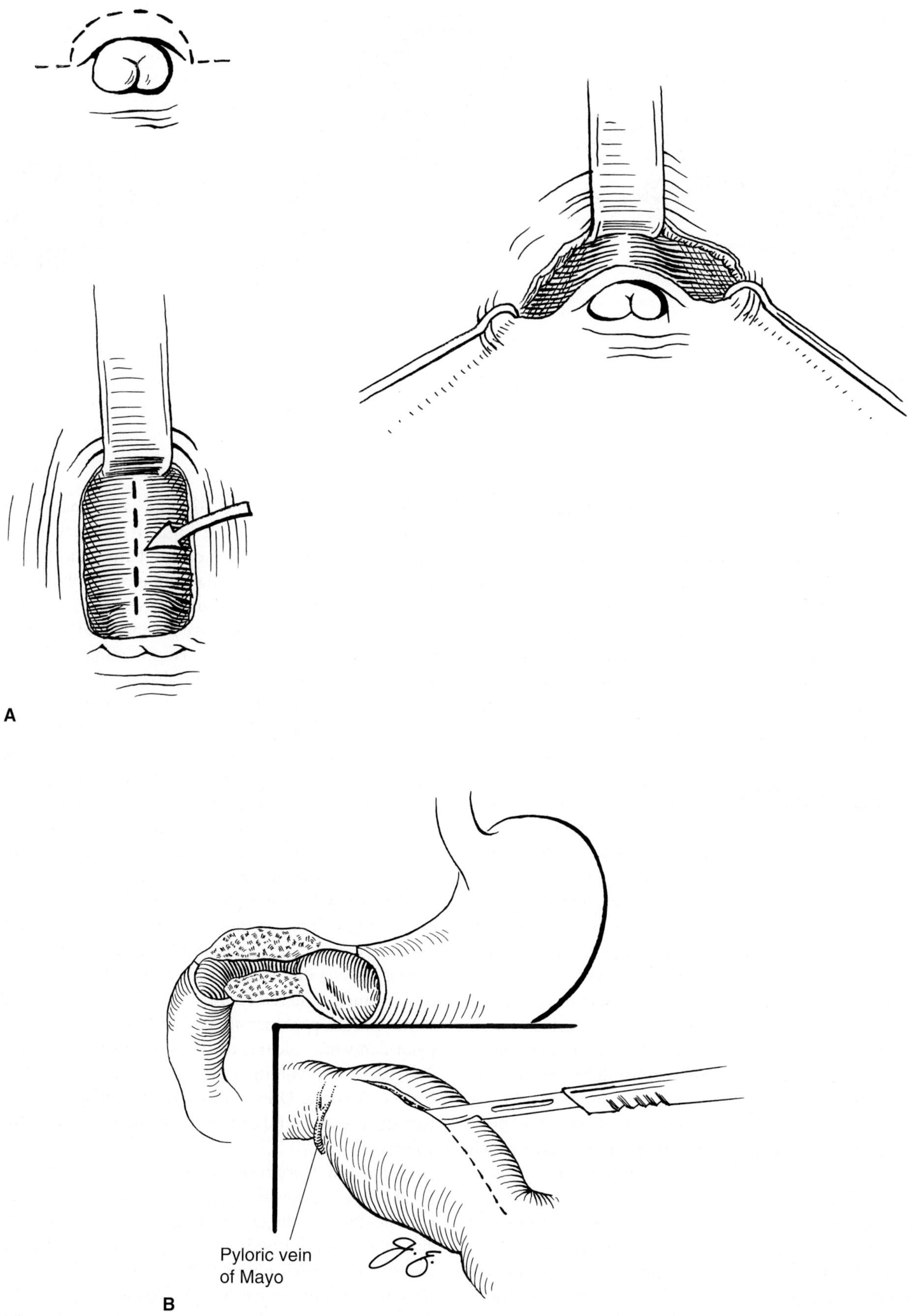

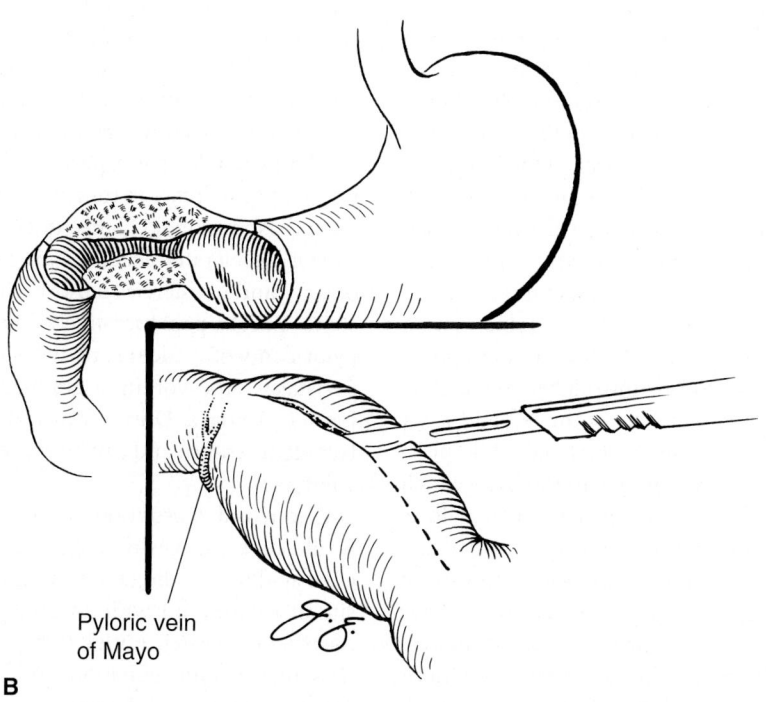

**A**

**B**

Pyloric vein
of Mayo

**FIGURE 40-2** Operative techniques for open pyloromyotomy. **A.** Curvilinear circumbilical incision approximately one half to two thirds of the distance around the umbilicus. The midline fascia is exposed and opened longitudinally. **B.** Serosal incision made into musculature of hypertrophied pylorus beginning approximately 1 to 2 mm proximal to the duodenum (vein of Mayo) and extending to the oblique fibers of the antrum.

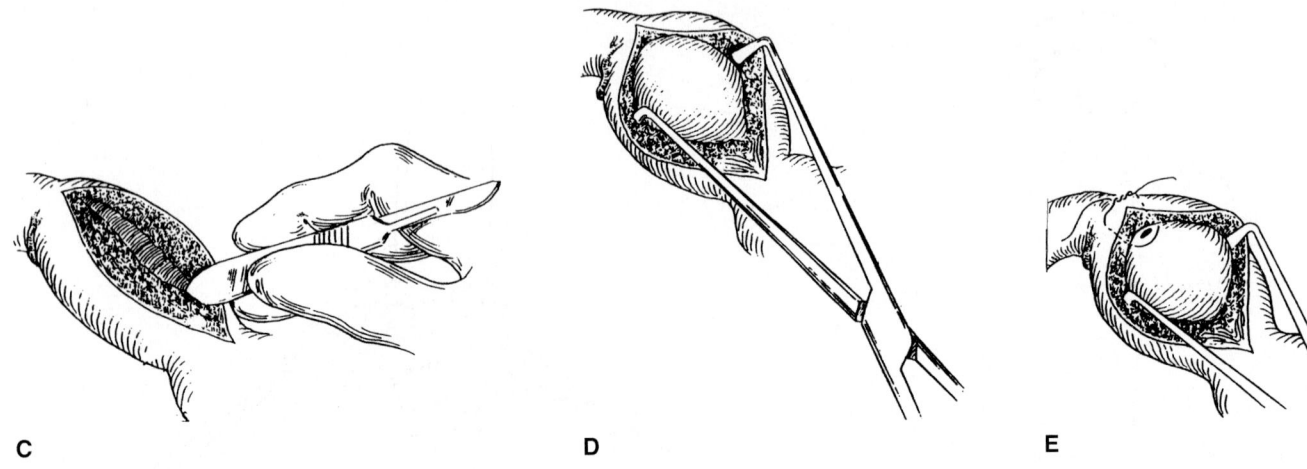

**C**　　　　　　　　　　**D**　　　　　　　　　　**E**

**FIGURE 40-2** (*Continued*) **C.** Blunt knife handle disrupts fibers. **D.** Benson spreader further separates the thickened fibers until mucosa bulges into the cleft. **E.** A perforation is closed with a mattress suture to buttress the site to the serosa.

duodenal mucosa is fragile and injury prone. Completion of the myotomy can be assessed when the 2 sides of the divided "olive" move independently. Following the completion of the myotomy, the stomach is filled with 60 to 100 cc of air, which is milked toward the antrum with gentle finger compression of the duodenum to obstruct the lumen and facilitate identification of any leaks. The presence of air bubbles or bile staining indicates a mucosal injury. Most bleeding is minor and is due to venous congestion and will stop with reduction of the pylorus into the peritoneum (Fig. 40-2).

## Laparoscopic Approach

After induction of general anesthesia, the infant is positioned transversely across the operating room table. Folded towels under the infant's head and back help to place the baby in the reverse Trendelenburg position so the intestines fall away from the upper abdomen. Following prepping and draping, 0.25% bupivacaine is injected in a subumbilical skinfold and the peritoneum is entered bluntly at the umbilicus via an open technique with a fine mosquito clamp. A 3-, 4-, or 5-mm trocar is inserted into the abdomen and a therapeutic pneumoperitoneum is established. The appropriately sized 30° angled telescope is introduced to facilitate placement of two 3-mm stab incisions in the left and right upper quadrants. Care is especially is practiced while placing the right-sided trocar to avoid injury to the liver, which may extend well below the right costal margin. A pyloric grasper is then inserted through the right upper quadrant incision to stabilize the duodenum or pylorus with care to avoid crush injury to these structures. Recently, we have used the Geiger Pyloric Immobilizer (Storz, Tutlingen, Germany) to grasp the pylorus. Although many variations to this technique exist, we place an arthroscopic blade in the left upper quadrant incision. Alternatively, electrocautery with a long tip blade is inserted through this incision and used for the myotomy. The myotomy is created from the duodenal side of the pylorus to the stomach. If cautery is used, we utilize a setting of "cut" at 8. The blunt blade of the knife or cautery is pushed into the pylorus

through the myotomy incision and is turned side-to-side to open the myotomy. The knife is then replaced with a laparoscopic pyloric spreader and the muscle is spread from the vein of Mayo to the nonhypertrophied stomach. The adequacy of the myotomy is assessed by insuring that the 2 cut edges of pylorus move independently. Air is insufflated into the stomach while compressing the duodenum to test for mucosal injury. This also insures patency of the pyloric channel and the adequate elimination of a discrete neck at the junction of the stomach and duodenum. Next, the instruments are removed and all 3 fascial incisions are closed with a 3-0 absorbable braided polyglycolic acid suture. The skin is closed with steri-strips or liquid adhesive.

In the absence of mucosal disruption, feedings are initiated at 4 to 6 hours postoperatively. Although numerous postoperative feeding regimens have been proposed, based on the principle that a period of no feeding followed by a progressive increase in tonicity and volume would limit emesis and aspiration, evidence does not support this assertion. In fact, accelerated feeding approaches show shorter length of stays and no increased morbidity. Many patients will have some emesis postoperatively likely secondary to residual pyloric mucosal edema and delay in return of normal gastric peristalsis. The vomiting gradually resolves over the ensuing 7 to 10 days. During this time, the infant has improved feeding tolerance and can be successfully advanced to higher volumes.

If mucosal disruption occurs, it must be repaired. We would repair this with a single layer of absorbable polyglycolic acid or polydioxanone suture placed transversely at the site of perforation with an omental patch. If these sutures obstruct the gastric outlet, then we would perform complete muscular reapproximation and rotate the pylorus 90° to 180°, where a second myotomy would be performed. Postoperative nasogastric decompression for 24 hours would then be indicated. A contrast study may be used prior to the initiation of feeding to insure that there is no extravasation of contrast or leak.

Although surgery is the "gold standard" therapy for HPS, nonoperative treatment strategies have been reported. Some authors have revisited the use of atropine in the management of HPS. IV atropine sulfate beginning at an initial dose of 0.4 mg/kg/day IV and advanced at increments of 0.1 mg/kg/day over an 8-day period until vomiting ceases. The infants are then maintained on oral atropine for 2 weeks. A recent study showed that 21 of 23 patients with documented pyloric stenosis recovered uneventfully without surgery. US was used to verify the normalization of the pyloric muscle postrecovery. Endoscopic and interventional radiographic guided balloon dilatation have been described, but unacceptably high rates of perforation and failure have limited the utility of these alternative techniques.

## TREATMENT EFFECTIVENESS/ PATIENT OUTCOME

The major complications following surgery include wound infection, mucosal perforation, and persistent vomiting (secondary to inadequate pyloromyotomy). The incidence of wound infections in several series has been variably reported from 1% to 5%. The relative malnourished status of these vomiting infants and the proximity of the umbilicus to the incision are likely major factors in the predisposition toward wound infection. The advent of improved antistaphylococcal antibiotics and earlier diagnosis of patients prior to severe malnutrition are likely reasons for the decline in infectious complications in more recent series. Mucosal perforation may occur in 1% to 2% of cases and, if recognized and promptly repaired, should not have significant impact on outcome but may delay the time of discharge by 24 to 48 hours. Although 30% to 90% of patients will have some degree of postoperative emesis, this typically resolves spontaneously within the first week. Persistent emesis beyond 2 weeks postoperatively should raise concern for gastroesophageal reflux (common) or inadequate myotomy (rare). The frequency of associated reflux in infants with treated HPS may be in the range of 10% to 15%. Antireflux measures and medications usually control the symptoms. Those patients who are refractory to medical therapy or have persistent projectile nonbilious emesis beyond 10 days should be suspected of having an inadequate myotomy. This is a very rare complication but tends to occur in the setting of inadequate proximal extension of the myotomy onto the gastric antrum. Diagnostic imaging studies are typically not useful because the radiographic findings of HPS may persist for many weeks to months postoperatively, despite the resolution of symptoms. Consequently, the decision to reoperate on patients with a previous myotomy should be delayed unless there is strong evidence by history that an inadequate myotomy was performed.

Considerable controversy exists in the literature over the desired access, that is, laparoscopic versus open for pyloromyotomy relative to desired outcomes such as time to full feeds, length of stay, incomplete myotomy, and cosmesis. A recent randomized controlled multicenter study from 7 institutions in North America and Europe suggests that laparoscopy has advantages over open pyloromyotomy in centers with experienced laparoscopic surgeons. In contrast, open pyloromytomy may be most feasible approach in surgeons with limited experience with the laparoscopic procedure or institutions with low volumes.

Despite several attempts to refine the technique, Ramstedt's original pyloromyotomy has been the benchmark of therapy for a century. The success and outcome of this procedure is unparalleled by alternative management approaches. In the early history of this surgery, the incidence of infectious (pneumonia/septicemia) and metabolic (shock/convulsions) complications was as high as 30% to 40% and mortality rates approached 20%. Earlier diagnosis, improved preoperative management, better anesthetic care, and an overall enhanced understanding of the pathophysiology of the disease have led to a precipitous decline in the morbidity and mortality for surgery to less than 10% and 0.5%, respectively. Currently, most uncomplicated patients may be discharged within 24 hours of surgery. Minor episodes of emesis or "wet burps" may persist for up to 2 weeks postoperatively. Most patients will have a rapid and complete resolution of vomiting by 1 week following their procedure. The hypertrophied muscle retains to normal caliber at about 3 to 4 weeks after surgery. There appear to be no major long-term residua in patients who have had surgery for HPS.

## SELECTED READINGS

Alain JL, Grousseau LD, Longis B, et al. Extramucosal pyloromyotomy by laparoscopy. *Eur J Pediatr Surg* 1996;6(1):10–12.

Aspelund G, Langer J. Current management of hypertrophic pyloric stenosis. *Semin Pediatr Surg* 2007;16:27–33.

Benson CD, Lloyd JR. Infantile pyloric stenosis a review of 1120 cases. *Am J Surg* 1964;107:429–433.

Bowen A. The vomiting infant: recent advances and unsettled issues in imaging. *Radiol Clin N Am* 1988;26(2):377–391.

Hall NJ, Pacilli M, Eaton S, et al. Recovery after open versus laparoscopic pyloromyotomy for pyloric stenosis: a double-blind multicenter randomized controlled trial. *Lancet* 2009;373(9861):390–398.

Hight DW, Benson CD, Phillippart AI, et al. Management of mucosal perforation during pyloromyotomy for infantile pyloric stenosis. *Surgery* 1981;90:85–86.

Hulka F, Harrison MW, Campbell TJ, et al. Complications of pyloromyotomy for infantile hypertrophic pyloric stenosis. *Am J Surg* 1997;173:450–452.

Nagita A, Yamaguchi J, Kanji A, et al. Management and ultrasonographic appearance of infantile hypertrophic pyloric stenosis with intravenous atropine sulfate. *J Pediatr Gastroenterol Nutr* 1996;23:172–177.

Ravitch MM. The story of pyloric stenosis. *Surgery* 1960;48:1117–1163.

Scharli A, Sieber WK, Kiesewetter WB. Hypertrophic pyloric stenosis at the Children's Hospital of Pittsburgh from 1912 to 1967. *J Pediatr Surg* 1969;4(1):108–114.

Spicer RD. Infantile hypertrophic pyloric stenosis: a review. *Br J Surg* 1982;69:128–135.

# Intestinal Rotation Abnormalities

# CHAPTER 41

*Emily Christison-Lagay and Jacob C. Langer*

## KEY POINTS

1. Normal rotation occurs early in gestation, and failure or incomplete rotation can occur.

2. Many rotation abnormalities predispose to gut volvulus.

3. The Ladd procedure, including appendectomy is the standard operative approach that can be performed open or via laparoscopy.

## INTRODUCTION

The embryology of intestinal rotation was described by Mall in 1898 and the potential surgical sequelae of anomalous intestinal rotation were described by Dott 25 years later. However, it was not until 1932 that Ladd first described 10 cases of malrotation and an operative technique for treating the condition. His account, expanded to include 21 cases by 1936, advocated the division of bands over the duodenum and placing the cecum in the left upper quadrant. Although to this day there remains some controversy regarding treatment or observation of variants of incomplete rotation, the optimal radiographic studies for diagnosis, the use of laparoscopy, and the treatment of asymptomatic rotational abnormalities in older children or children with heterotaxia syndromes (HS), the Ladd procedure remains the gold standard surgical procedure for children with intestinal malrotation who are at risk for midgut volvulus.

## EMBRYOLOGY

For a child to be born with "normal" rotation, a precisely orchestrated sequence of events must occur during the fourth through 12th weeks of gestation. The molecular mechanisms controlling the initiation and progression of left–right asymmetry are the subjects of much investigation. Transient asymmetric expression of *Nodal* around Henson node in the gastrulating embryo appears to initiate left–right specification. Subsequent asymmetric expression of *Pitx2* and *Isl1* (as a feedback loop) in the left side only of the dorsal mesentery

and *Tbx18* in the right side only appears to play a prominent role in promoting normal rotation through the differential induction of a tightly packed columnar epithelium on the left and cuboidal cells in more loosely packed mesenchymal elements on the right. This cellular architecture results in leftward "tilting" of the primitive gut tube. Misexpression of any of these elements in a murine model is associated with abnormal rotation. The macroscopic ramifications of these cellular events can be first appreciated during the fourth to fifth week postconception, when the straight tube of the primitive embryonic intestinal tract begins to elongate more rapidly than the embryo, causing it to "buckle" ventrally and force the duodenum, jejunum, ileum, ascending, and transverse colon to extend into the umbilical cord. The duodenum curves downward and to the right of the axis of the artery, initially completing a 90° counterclockwise turn. Over the next 3 weeks, the duodenum continues to rotate so that by the end of 8 weeks, it has undergone a 180° rotation. During the 10th gestational week, the intestines return precipitously back into the abdomen, led by the duodenum and jejunum and followed by the remainder of small bowel and then the colon in a left to right order. The cecum is the final portion of the intestine to return and does so by rotating superiorly and anteriorly around the superior mesenteric artery (SMA). This sequence of return causes the duodenum and proximal jejunum to be pushed to the superiorly and leftward posterior to the SMA such that they become fixed in a 270° rotation from their initial position. Fixation of the intestines in the position takes place over the fourth and fifth months of gestation. Normal rotation is summarized in Fig. 41-1.

## DEFINITIONS OF INTESTINAL ROTATION ABNORMALITIES

Variations in the sequence of herniation, rotation, and fixation are responsible for the full spectrum of intestinal rotation abnormalities and internal hernias. If the cecocolic loop returns to the abdomen prior to the return of the proximal foregut, the duodenum and jejunum are not pushed superior laterally and undergo only 180° of rotation. In this scenario, the cecum itself does not undergo proper fixation and the colon remains on the left side of the abdomen, while the midgut fills in the

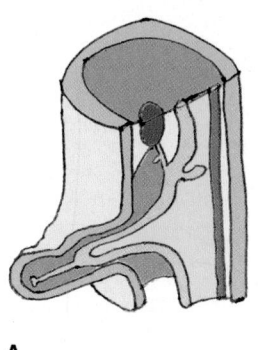
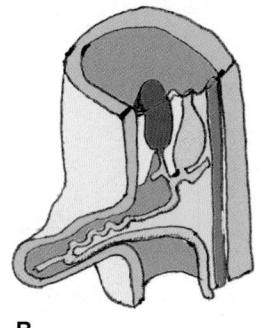
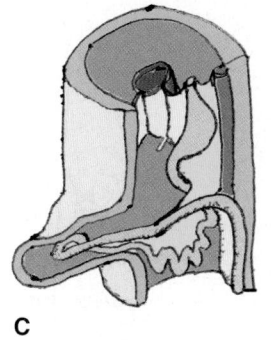
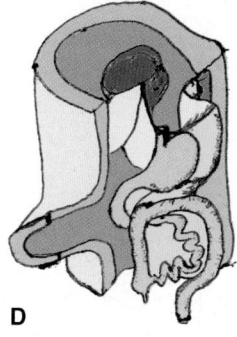

A                 B                 C                 D

**FIGURE 41-1** Normal intestinal rotation. **A.** Embryonic intestinal tube herniates into the umbilical cord. **B.** The duodenum herniates downward and undergoes a 90° counterclockwise turn. **C.** Rotation continues an additional 180°. **D.** At 10 weeks, the intestines return to the abdomen. Cecal fixation occurs postnatally.

space on the right and duodenum descends directly along the course of the SMA. This condition is classically termed "*nonrotation*," and because it is associated with a wide-based mesentery, nonrotation does not put the child at risk for midgut volvulus. Classic "*malrotation*" occurs as a result of failed extracoelomic rotation. It is also most commonly associated with the duodenal–jejunal juncture in the right upper quadrant and a midabdominal cecum fixed in place by adhesive bands to the gallbladder, duodenum, and right-sided abdominal wall ("Ladd bands"). Most importantly, classic malrotation results in a narrowed mesenteric base, which predisposes the child to potentially fatal midgut volvulus (Fig. 41-2). If the bowel makes a 90° turn clockwise, rather than counterclockwise, *reverse rotation* results. Typically in reverse rotation, the colon returns to the abdomen prior to the duodenum. As a result, the duodenum lies anterior to the SMA and the colon lies posteriorly, producing a retroarterial tunnel, which may be associated with partial mesenteric arterial, venous, and lymphatic obstruction. If the mesoderm does not fuse to the retroperitoneum over the fourth and fifth months of gestation, *paraduodenal or paracolic hernias* may form. Because of the complexity of intestinal rotation, the variations in rotational anomalies are seemingly endless. While not all variations are associated with a narrowed mesenteric base (and are thereby not all at risk for volvulus), attempts to fix the bowel to the retroperitoneum in each case can create focally obstructing bands, which require surgical division.

## EPIDEMIOLOGY

The reported incidence of rotation abnormalities varies widely, depending on the source. Autopsy series suggest that 0.5% or 1:200 people have some type of rotation abnormality. Barium enema studies in adults in the mid-1900s estimated an incidence of 1:500, but only 1:6000 present with symptoms during their lifetime. Seventy to eighty percent of these present within the first year of life, with half to three-quarters presenting within the first month. A recent population-based study estimated an incidence of about 15:1,000,000 in children less than 1 and about 10:1,000,000 in children aged 1 to 2 years. The subsequent yearly risk falls by approximately half. In the

infant group presenting with malrotation, males predominate by a factor of 2:1; this ratio disappears for older children.

Associated abnormalities are found in approximately 30% to 60% of cases and may include intestinal atresia or web (the most common associated anomaly) or, more rarely, Meckel diverticulum, intussusception, Hirschsprung disease, mesenteric cyst, and anomalies of the extrahepatic biliary system. Omphalocele, gastroschisis, and congenital diaphragmatic hernia typically present with some variation of intestinal rotation, usually nonrotation. Many children with intestinal motility disorders have associated rotation abnormalities. Finally, rotation abnormalities are commonly associated with congenital heart disease, often in the context of one of the various HS.

## CLINICAL PRESENTATION

The classic presentation of malrotation is bilious vomiting in the newborn infant. This may occur for 2 reasons: obstructive compression of the duodenum by Ladd bands or, more ominously, midgut volvulus. Midgut volvulus is due to the presence of a narrow mesenteric pedicle that acts as an axis around which the bowel may rotate, causing twisting of the SMA and superior mesenteric vein (SMV). The abdomen is not distended initially because the obstruction is very proximal. Vascular compromise may result in the passage of bloody stool; irritability, pain, abdominal distension, and peritonitis develop late in the presentation of volvulus and may portend the onset of shock. Similarly, hematemesis and abdominal wall erythema are late signs suggestive of significant bowel ischemia, which may rapidly evolve to shock and death. In older children, chronic, partial, or intermittent volvulus may present with crampy abdominal pain, intermittent vomiting, diarrhea, protein-losing enteropathy, failure to thrive, or malnutrition. Distension is frequently present, although it may be intermittent.

In the child who presents with bilious emesis, a high index of suspicion should be directed toward malrotation with volvulus. Clinical history, physical examination, hemodynamic parameters, and laboratory evidence of metabolic disarray should inform the decision to proceed with diagnostic

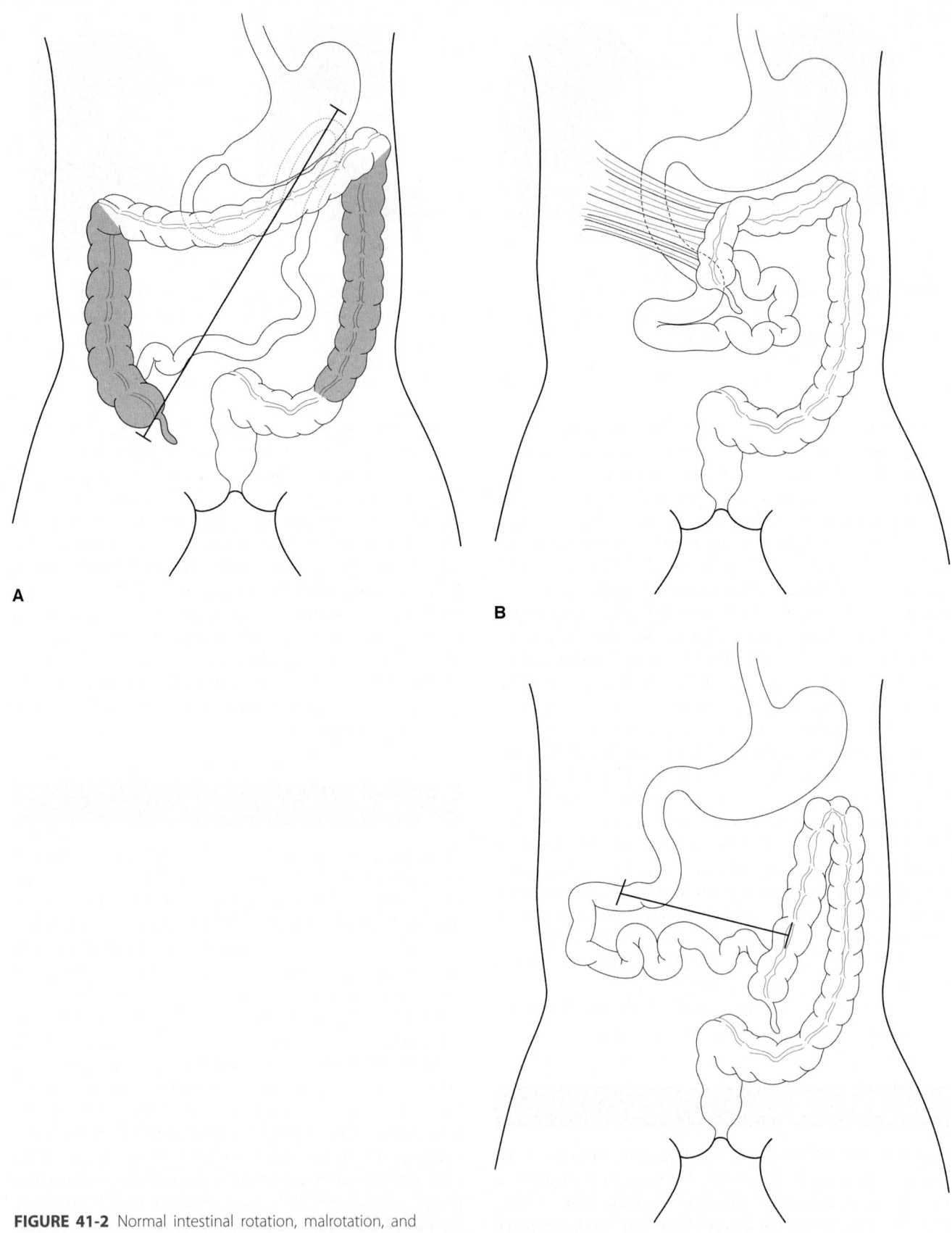

**A**

**B**

**C**

**FIGURE 41-2** Normal intestinal rotation, malrotation, and nonrotation.

imaging for evaluation or emergent operative intervention without diagnostic imaging confirmation.

Although volvulus associated with malrotation represents the condition's most acute, dramatic, and urgent presentation, duodenal obstruction from Ladd (or other congenital) bands represents a second cause of bilious emesis. Neonatal presentation of duodenal obstruction from Ladd bands may be feeding intolerance, bilious emesis, and a "double bubble" sign. Older children more commonly present with intermittent colicky abdominal pain associated with bilious emesis. An internal hernia associated with inappropriate intestinal fixation may present in a similar fashion. A recent study found that chronically symptomatic patients commonly presented with recurrent respiratory symptoms including asthma and aspiration.

## RADIOLOGIC DIAGNOSIS

The diagnosis of isolated rotational abnormality is very infrequently suggested by prenatal imaging. Sequelae of midgut volvulus: bowel dilation, meconium peritonitis, and/or fetal ascites can be detected and may increase suspicion of a rotation anomaly, although none of these signs are specific.

Plain abdominal radiography, the first exam often obtained in patients with vomiting, is nonspecific for the diagnosis of rotation abnormalities. Proximal obstruction due to congenital or Ladd bands, incomplete volvulus, or associated duodenal atresia or web may present with a large gastric or "double" bubble with a paucity of distal air. Infants with established intestinal ischemia may have pneumatosis intestinalis, which may lead to confusion with a diagnosis of necrotizing enterocolitis. Although unusual, a pattern of distal bowel obstruction consisting of multiple dilated bowel loops with air fluid levels may be seen. Most importantly, children with rotation abnormalities, including malrotation with volvulus, may initially present with a completely normal bowel gas pattern (Fig. 41-3).

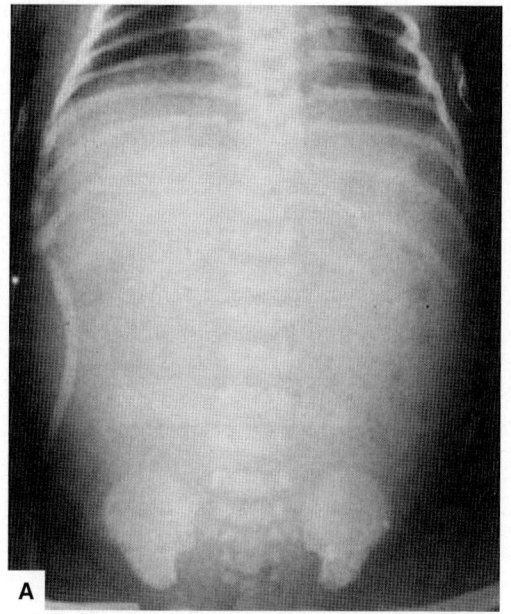
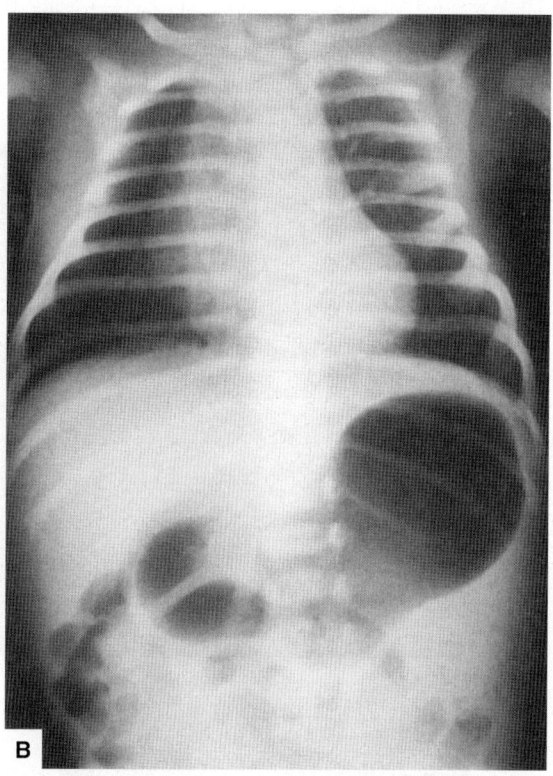
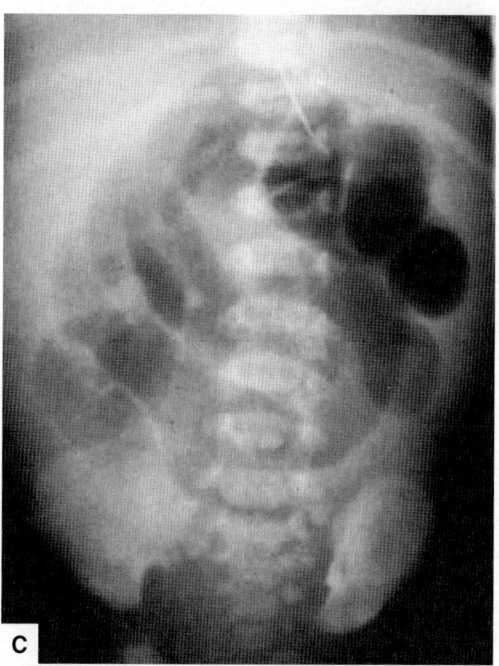
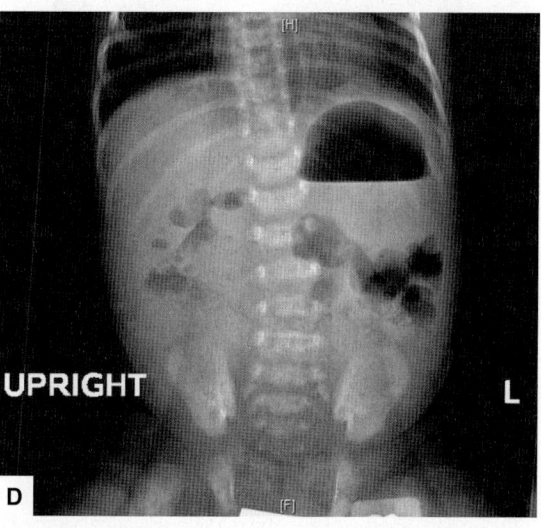

**FIGURE 41-3** The varying appearances of malrotation on plain film. **A.** Gasless abdomen; (**B**) dilated gastric bubble; (**C**) dilated small bowel suggestive of a distal obstruction; and (**D**) normal film.

The earliest reports of diagnostic imaging for the diagnosis of malrotation used barium enema to ascertain cecal position. Since the 1960s, however, upper gastrointestinal contrast radiography (UGI) to evaluate the position of the duodenal–jejunal junction (DJJ) has become the gold standard for diagnosis. However, even as the benchmark against which all other imaging modalities are measured, interpretation of the UGI series must be done with very specifically defined criteria. In order to be considered normal, the location of the DJJ must be to the left of the vertebral body at the level of the inferior margin of the duodenal bulb on an anterior-posterior (AP) projection and must travel posteriorly on the lateral projection. If the DJJ does not demonstrate these radiographic characteristics, a diagnosis of rotation abnormality should be entertained. However, it is also important to be aware that conditions such as splenomegaly, renal or retroperitoneal tumors, gastric overdistension, liver transplant, small bowel obstruction, and scoliosis may cause the DJJ to be medially or inferiorly displaced. Such findings are responsible for a false-positive rate to be as high as 15% and a false-negative rate of 3% to 6% in some studies. Often in cases in which the UGI is confusing or equivocal, radiologists move to a small bowel follow-through to the cecum or a contrast enema in the same session, in order to determine the location of the cecum and its proximity to the DJJ. A short distance between the DJJ and the cecum strongly suggests the presence of malrotation with a narrow-based mesentery, and therefore a risk of midgut volvulus. However, it should be noted that there is a wide range of variability in normal cecal positioning and fixation, especially in the neonate. Therefore, a cecum located in the right lower quadrant cannot definitively rule out malrotation, and a cecum located in the right upper quadrant or epigastrium is not diagnostic of malrotation. Examples of contrast studies in the diagnosis of intestinal rotation abnormalities are seen in Fig. 41-4.

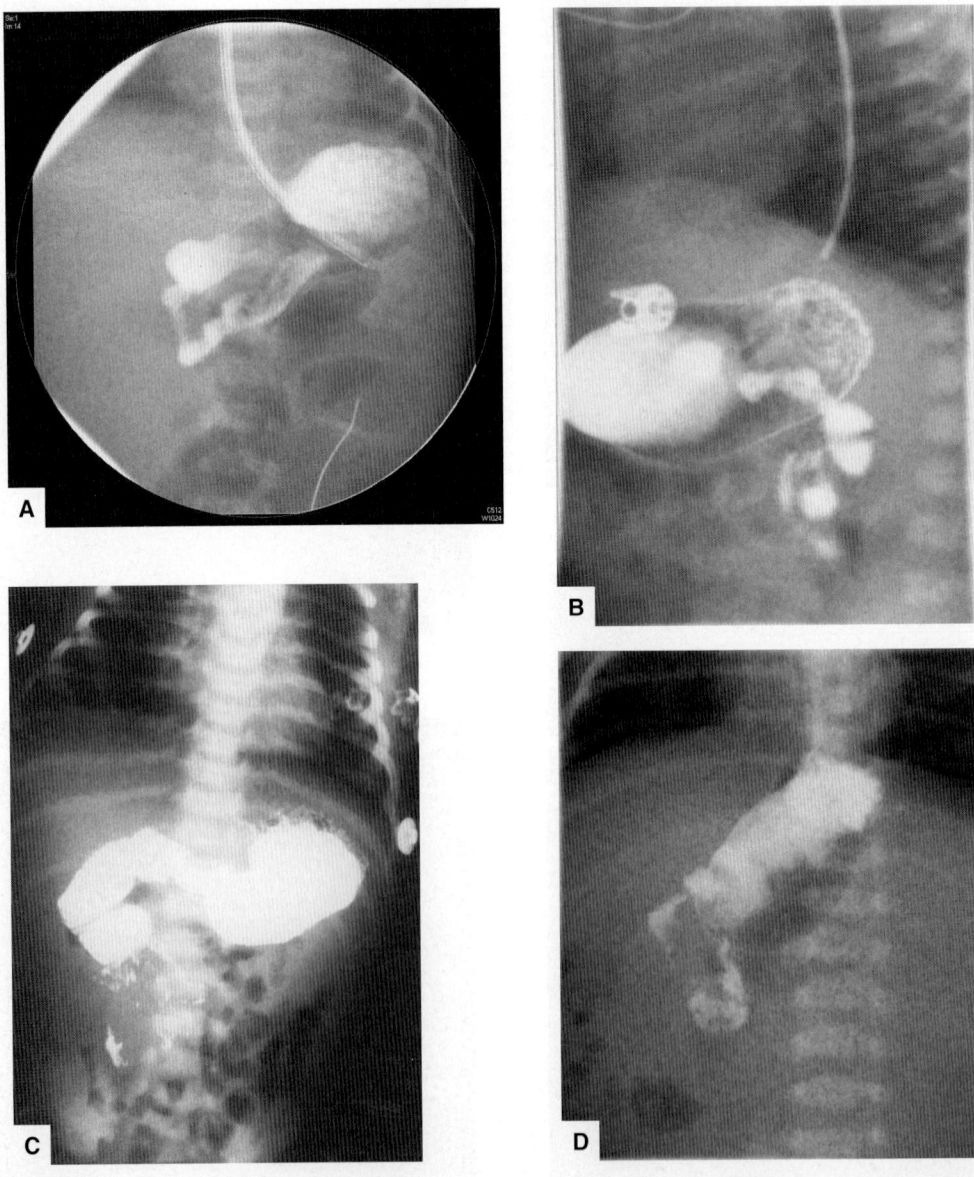

**FIGURE 41-4** Upper GI series with small bowel through. **A.** Normal contrast series showing the duodenal C-loop crossing the midline; (**B**) lateral view of malrotation, demonstrating "corkscrew" appearance of jejunum; (**C**) lateral view suggestive of duodenal obstruction secondary to Ladd bands or volvulus; and (**D**) false-positive study; DJ flexure is pushed rightward by large multicystic kidney.

More recently, ultrasound (US) has been advocated by some authors as a noninvasive screening method for malrotation. This is based on the notion that reversal of the relationship of the SMA and SMV predicts the presence of malrotation. One study correlating radiographic findings of UGI and US on the same admission found an US sensitivity of 87%, specificity of 75%, positive predictive value of 42%, and negative predictive value of 96%. This same study found that inverted orientation of the SMA/SMV axis with a "whirlpool" sign were more likely to be associated with an abnormal UGI than reversal in the anterior/posterior position. Sensitivity and specificity of a whirlpool sign to detect midgut volvulus in this study was 45% and 99%. Others have reported sensitivity as high as 92% and specificity of 100%.

While radiographic techniques are important diagnostic aids in the nonacute setting, an infant who presents in extremis with a history of bilious emesis and findings of peritonitis should be aggressively resuscitated, decompressed via a nasogastric tube, and taken for an emergent exploratory laparotomy.

## OPERATIVE TECHNIQUE

The fundamentals of operative correction of malrotation have changed little since Ladd seminal description. Most surgeons begin an open approach to a Ladd procedure via a transverse supraumbilical incision with the patient placed in the supine position. In most patients, a circumumbilical omega incision affords the same access to the midgut and mesentery with a considerable cosmetic benefit. Upon entering the abdomen, rotation and fixation of the bowel is assessed by delivering the entire midgut into the operative field. The presence of chylous ascites may indicate chronic lymphatic obstruction due to partial midgut volvulus. If volvulus is encountered, the involved loops of bowel are gently detorsed by counterclockwise rotation until the mesentery is unfurled. At this time, the bowel is assessed for viability. Reperfusion and delineating of viable from nonviable bowel may take several minutes. During this period, the bowel should be covered with a warm damp laparotomy pad or towel to help prevent evaporative losses and vasoconstriction. Following this, a Ladd procedure is performed. This operation consists of 4 discreet steps, the goal of which is to place the bowel into a position of nonrotation, with the small bowel on the right side of the abdomen and the colon on the left: (1) division of any abnormal bands (Ladd bands) fixing the bowel to the right upper quadrant retroperitoneal or intraabdominal structures; (2) mobilization and rotation of the colon toward the left, taking care not to divide the colonic mesentery in the process, so that the entire colon sits on the left side of the abdomen; (3) mobilization and straightening of the duodenum so that it heads inferiorly and all the small bowel sits on the right side of the abdomen; and (4) broadening of the base of the mesentery by dividing the congenital bands along the SMA and SMV. Many surgeons assess distal patency of the bowel by milking intraabdominal contents from the proximal duodenum through to the cecum, because of the association of duodenal atresia or web with malrotation. Most surgeons also perform an appendectomy, either by excision or using an inversion technique (Fig. 41-5).

Prior to closing the abdomen, small bowel viability should be reassessed. Any frankly necrotic sections should be resected. If the rest of the bowel is completely viable, a primary anastomosis can be performed, and if bowel viability is questionable stomas should be created. If there are large sections of bowel in which viability is still unclear, resection should not be done, and a "second-look" laparotomy should be planned for 24 to 48 hours later. More ethically problematic is the situation in which the entire midgut is clearly necrotic, and resection of the bowel will result in short bowel syndrome. Options include closing the abdomen without resection and offering palliative care, or performing a massive resection and creating intestinal failure, with long-term need for total parenteral nutrition (TPN). Although historically the prognosis for neonatal intestinal failure was dismal due to the extremely high incidence of fatal cholestatic liver failure, improvements in intestinal rehabilitation and small bowel transplantation have resulted in new management paradigms for children with extreme short bowel and, in selected cases, massive intestinal resection may be a reasonable option.

## CONTROVERSIES IN THE MANAGEMENT OF ROTATION ABNORMALITIES

Although the treatment of classic malrotation has changed little in the last 80 years, advancements in medical care and the increasing availability of diagnostic techniques have raised new questions regarding the management of rotation abnormalities.

### Role of Laparoscopy

Beginning in the mid-1990s, a laparoscopic approach to the Ladd procedure has been advocated by some surgeons. This is most commonly reserved for malrotation not associated with midgut volvulus, as the bowel in patients with volvulus can be quite friable and subject to perforation with all but the most gentle manipulation, as well as the fact that surgery must be done as quickly as possible to maximize the chance of survival.

In infants, the most commonly described technique utilizes three 3.5-mm ports, with a fourth port added to help with bowel retraction and operative exposure. In older children, 5-mm ports may be used. The operation begins with the placement of an umbilical trocar and abdominal insufflation to a pressure of 8 to 12 mm Hg, followed by the placement of 2 additional trocars in the right and left mid to low abdomen (depending on the size of the infant). Careful exploration of the abdomen is then performed and the specific anatomy of the patient delineated. Of particular importance, the presence or absence of midgut volvulus should be noted. If there is no volvulus, the next step is determination of the length of the

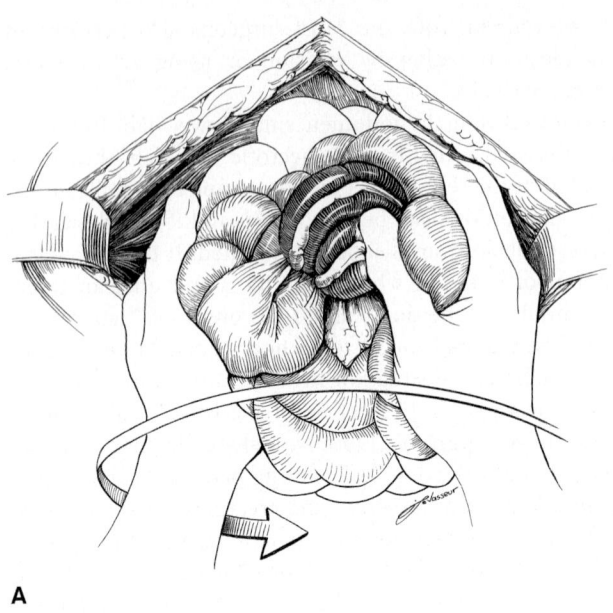

A

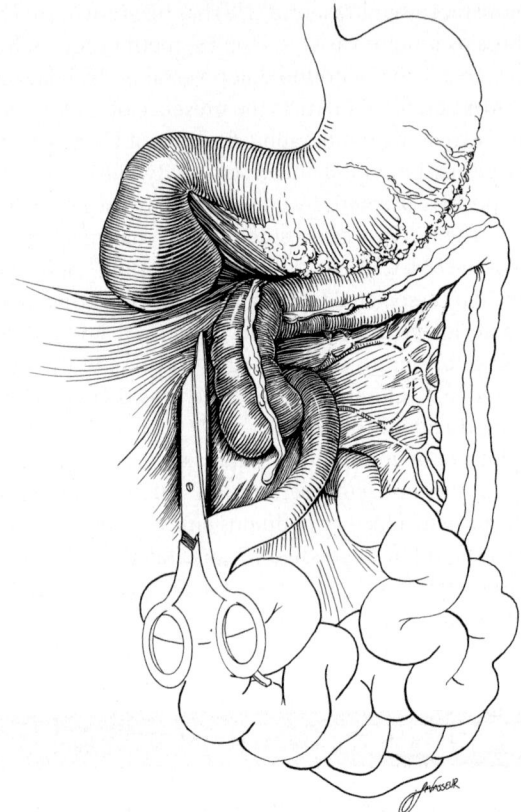

B

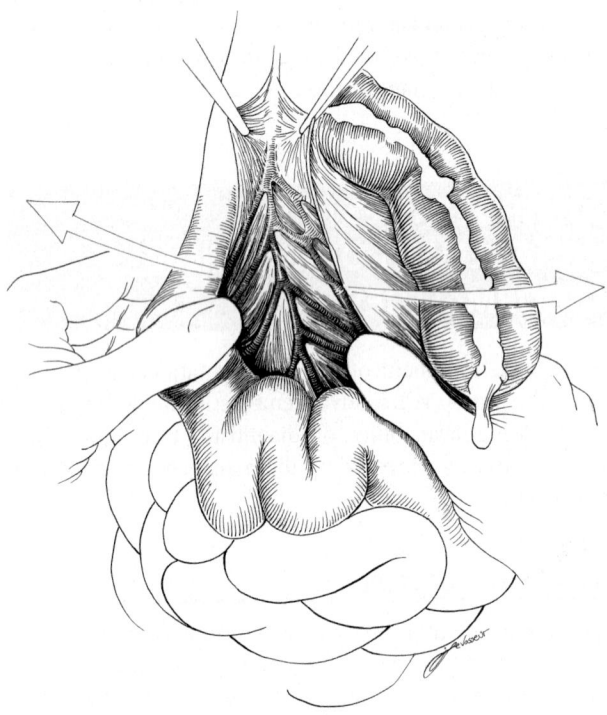

C

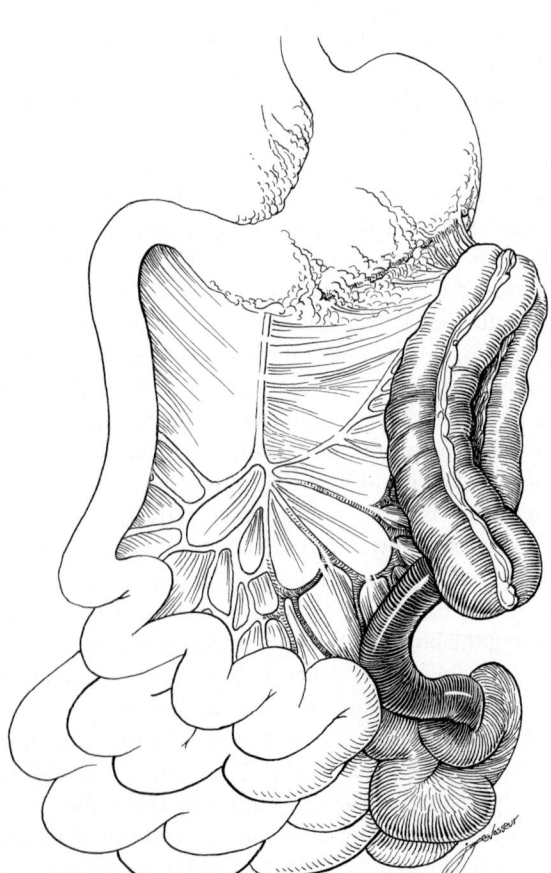

D

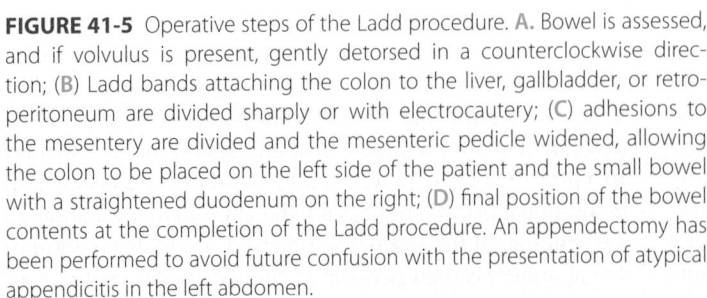

**FIGURE 41-5** Operative steps of the Ladd procedure. **A.** Bowel is assessed, and if volvulus is present, gently detorsed in a counterclockwise direction; (**B**) Ladd bands attaching the colon to the liver, gallbladder, or retroperitoneum are divided sharply or with electrocautery; (**C**) adhesions to the mesentery are divided and the mesenteric pedicle widened, allowing the colon to be placed on the left side of the patient and the small bowel with a straightened duodenum on the right; (**D**) final position of the bowel contents at the completion of the Ladd procedure. An appendectomy has been performed to avoid future confusion with the presentation of atypical appendicitis in the left abdomen.

small bowel mesentery, that is, the distance between the DJJ and the cecum. If this distance is long (in our center defined as greater than half the diameter of the abdomen), as would be seen in both near-normal rotation and in nonrotation, the patient is not considered to be at risk for midgut volvulus, and a Ladd procedure is not necessary. In this scenario, obstructing bands around the duodenum should be identified and divided, and any internal hernias should be identified and repaired. If the base of the small bowel mesentery is short, the patient should be considered to be at risk for volvulus, and a full Ladd procedure should be done. The steps are the same as for the open procedure, and dissection can be done using hook electrocautery, sharp scissors, or scissors attached to cautery. In larger children, the harmonic scalpel may also be used. If an appendectomy is performed, it can be done extracorporeally through the umbilical port site or intraabdominally with an endoloop or stapler.

Advocates of a laparoscopic approach cite decreased postoperative pain and more rapid return of bowel function (and thus shorter hospital stay) as well as an obvious cosmetic advantage. Detractors suggest that intraoperative visualization of the mesenteric pedicle is inadequate, especially in the population most commonly affected by malrotation: infants less than 1 year of age. It has also been suggested that open correction of malrotation may be more effective in preventing recurrent volvulus by facilitating the formation of intraabdominal adhesions and that the laparoscopic approach may not achieve this ancillary benefit to the same extent. Advocates of the laparoscopic approach argue that prevention of recurrent volvulus is accomplished by adequate broadening of the mesenteric base rather than by adhesions, and that adhesion formation results in a long-term risk of intestinal obstruction requiring further surgical correction. To date, there have been no large-scale studies with enough longitudinal follow-up to demonstrate this theoretical benefit.

## Atypical Radiological Findings

The group at the University of Arkansas attempted to define risk of malrotation, ischemic volvulus, and internal hernia in a group of consecutive patients undergoing operation for rotation abnormalities based on the positioning of the DJJ on initial UGI series. The rotation abnormality was described as "typical" if the DJJ was positioned to the right of the midline or if it was absent. Atypical variants of malrotation were classified as "high" if the DJJ was at or to the left of the midline but higher than the 12th thoracic vertebra and "low" if it was at or to the left of the midline below the 12th thoracic vertebra. Approximately 43% of presenting patients were classified as "typical," 32% were "high" and the remaining 25% were "low." All patients with "typical" and "low" rotation abnormalities on UGI were found to have a rotation abnormality intraoperatively, and 95% of patients with a "high" malformation on UGI were confirmed to have a rotation abnormality intraoperatively. At the time of operation, volvulus had occurred in 12 of 75 of "typical" patients versus 1 of 56 "high" and 1 of 45 "low" patients. Internal hernias were also more common in "typical" than "atypical" patients. Moreover, this group found that 11% to 13% of "atypical" patients had persistent postoperative symptoms compared to 0% of "typical"

patients. Given the cited postoperative bowel obstruction rate following Ladd procedure (8%-12%) and the relatively high incidence of continued symptomatology, the authors advocated careful discussion in patients with "atypical" radiological findings. This is a group in which a laparoscopic approach might be particularly useful.

## Asymptomatic Rotation Abnormalities

While there is general consensus that symptomatic malrotation should be addressed surgically, the role of prophylactic surgery in children with incidentally diagnosed, asymptomatic rotation abnormalities is less clear. Advocates of routine operative intervention cite reports of midgut volvulus secondary to malrotation throughout adult life and further argue that a careful history often elicits subtle symptoms of malrotation that may have been dismissed or attributed to other causes. However, population-based evidence suggests that the incidence of midgut volvulus secondary to malrotation decreases significantly after infancy and that many patients with rotation abnormalities remain asymptomatic throughout life. The only study to date that attempts to address this question used malrotation data from the Nationwide Inpatient Sample to derive a model to compare the quality-adjusted life expectancy with and without a Ladd procedure in asymptomatic patients. This group found that the greatest benefit of a Ladd procedure occurred in infants at 1 year of age and declined thereafter. By age 20, a Ladd procedure conferred more risk than nonoperative observation. These authors concluded that operative intervention should be offered to children, but not adults with asymptomatic malrotation.

Ultimately, the most important decision in an asymptomatic patient is whether there is a risk of midgut volvulus or not, that is, what is the width of the small bowel mesentery? Sometimes this can be well seen on contrast imaging, and a reasonable decision can be made regarding surgical intervention. However, contrast imaging has a clearly delineated false-positive and false-negative rate, and laparoscopy may be a safer and more definitive way of determining the need for a Ladd procedure. If at the time of laparoscopy the mesenteric base is found to be wide, the operation can be concluded, with minimal morbidity. If the mesenteric base is found to be narrow, a Ladd procedure can be done either laparoscopically or open, at the discretion of the surgeon.

## Heterotaxia Syndromes

Patients with heterotaxia syndromes (HS, defined as any arrangement of organs along the left–right body axis, which is neither situs solitus nor situs inversus) are known to have a high rate of rotation anomalies, which cover the entire spectrum from nonrotation to classic malrotation to near-normal rotation, as well as the more uncommon rotation abnormalities such as reverse rotation. The coexistence, in many cases, of congenital heart disease places these children at an increased risk of operative intervention, which has resulted in controversy around the role of generalized screening for rotation abnormalities in patients with heterotaxia, and the role of intervention in asymptomatic patients with documented rotation abnormalities. While several centers have found that the morbidity and mortality associated with a Ladd procedure in patients with HS is not increased over a control population, the procedure itself is associated with a 10% risk of postoperative bowel obstruction and overall childhood mortality in patients with HS is 23%, mainly due to cardiac disease. In our own study following 152 asymptomatic neonates with HS, only 4 developed gastrointestinal symptoms over a median follow-up of 18 months (range, 4-216), and only 1 of these 4 was found to have malrotation on UGI. Of the remaining asymptomatic patients, 43% died of cardiac disease and none developed intestinal symptoms or complications. We have therefore adopted a more conservative approach in which asymptomatic patients with HS are not screened for rotation abnormalities unless they develop symptoms. Those with documented rotation abnormalities and either mild symptoms or no symptoms are evaluated laparoscopically.

## SUMMARY

Rotation abnormalities represent a spectrum of anomalies, which may be asymptomatic or may be associated with obstruction due to bands, midgut volvulus, or associated atresia or web. The most important goal of the clinician is to determine whether the patient has midgut volvulus, in which case, an emergency laparotomy should be done. If the patient is not acutely ill, the next goal is to determine if the patient has a narrow-based small bowel mesentery, which may predispose to midgut volvulus in the future. This decision is made based on imaging studies or laparoscopy, and should be followed by the Ladd procedure if the mesenteric base is felt to be narrow. There is still controversy around the role of laparoscopy, the management of atypical and asymptomatic rotation abnormalities, and the management of rotation abnormalities in children with HS.

## SELECTED READINGS

Applegate KE, Anderson JA, Klatte E. Malrotation of the gastrointestinal tract: a problem solving approach to performing the upper GI series. *Radiographics* 2006;26:1485–1500.

Bass KD, Rothenberg SS, Chang JH. Laparoscopic Ladd's procedure in infants with malrotation. *J Pediatr Surg* 1998;33:279–281.

Chen LE, Minkes RM, Langer JC. Laparoscopic vs open surgery for malrotation without volvulus. *Pediatr Endosurg Innov Techniq* 2003;7:433–438.

Choi M, Borenstein SH, Hornberger L, Langer JC. Heterotaxia syndrome: the role of screening for intestinal rotation abnormalities. *Arch Dis Child* 2005;90:813–815.

Davis NM, Kurpios NA, Sun X, Gros J, Martin JF, Tabin CJ. The chirality of gut rotation derives from left-right asymmetric changes in the architecture of the dorsal mesentery. *Dev Cell* 2008;15:134–145.

Ladd WE. Surgical disease of the alimentary tract. *N Engl J Med* 1936;215:705–708.

Long FR, Kramer SS, Markowitz RI, Taylor GE. Radiographic patterns of intestinal malrotation in children. *Radiographics* 1996;16(3):547–556.

Malek MM, Burd RS. Surgical treatment of malrotation after infancy: a population based study. *J Pediatr Surg* 2005;40:285–289.

Malek M, Burd R. The optimal management of malrotation after infancy: a decision analysis. *Am J Surg* 2006;191:45–51.

Mazziotti MV, Strasberg SM, Langer JC. Intestinal rotation abnormalities without volvulus: the role of laparoscopy. *J Am Coll Surg* 1997;185:172–176.

Mehall JR, Chandler JC, Mehall RL, Jackson RJ, Wagner CW, Smith SD. Management of typical and atypical intestinal malrotation. *J Pediatr Surg* 2002;37:1169–1172.

Orzech N, Navarro OM, Langer JC. Is ultrasonography a good screening test for intestinal malrotation? *J Pediatr Surg* 2006;41:1005–1009.

Scoutter AD, Askew AA. Transumbilical laparotomy in infants: a novel approach for a wide variety of surgical disease. *J Pediatr Surg* 2003;38:950–952.

Weinberger E, Winters WD, Liddell RM, Rosenbaum DM, Krauter D. Sonographic diagnosis of intestinal malrotation in infants: importance of the relative positions of the superior mesenteric vein and artery. *AJR Am J Roentgenol* 1992;159:835–838.

Yu DC, Thiagarajan RR, Laussen PC, Laussen JP, Jaksic T, Weldon CB. Outcomes after the Ladd procedure in patients with heterotaxy syndrome, congenital heart disease, and intestinal malrotation. *J Pediatr Surg* 2009;44:1089–1095.

# CHAPTER 42

# Intestinal Atresia

*Eric D. Strauch and J. Laurence Hill*

## KEY POINTS

1. Intestinal atresia is a life-threatening cause of intestinal obstruction in the newborn.

2. Atresia can occur throughout the intestinal tract but is common in the small intestine.

3. The surgical goal is to establish intestinal continuity.

4. Duodenal atresia can be associated with Down syndrome, cardiac defects, and malrotation.

5. Jejunoileal atresia can be associated with cystic fibrosis, gastroschisis, and short gut syndrome.

6. Colonic atresia is uncommon, but does occur.

*Intestinal atresia* is a congenital absence of the bowel lumen, which results in obstruction. It becomes evident during prenatal ultrasonography or presents in the early neonatal period. If not corrected, the anomaly will result in death from losses of gastrointestinal (GI) fluids, pulmonary aspiration, and malnutrition. Thus, surgical creation of a continuous lumen with as much functional bowel as possible is the mainstay of management. Not until surgical technique was complemented by the ability to support the neonate through the perioperative period with nutrition and ventilation was long-term survival possible.

Atresias are classified into 3 types with variations depending on etiology and the location of the obstruction. Type I has mural continuity with a membranous luminal obstruction. In Type II atresia, a residual fibrous cord connects a dilated proximal segment to the unused smaller distal segment. Type III atresia finds a gap between the proximal and distal bowel with a mesenteric defect. The level of the obstruction is reflected in the etiology, incidence, clinical presentation, differential diagnosis, and surgical technique.

Many theories exist for the development of intestinal atresia. They can be simplified into 2 categories: an ischemic event causing necrosis and resorption of the involved bowel, or failure of the lumen to develop from the embryologic cord stage. Because of the fixation of the first and second part of the duodenum and its dual blood supply from the celiac axis and the superior mesenteric artery, it is less susceptible to vascular

accidents. Therefore, the most likely etiology for duodenal atresia is failure of luminal recanalization after the cord stage. Because of the mobility of the jejunum and ileum with the potential for compression or volvulus, and the anatomy of the arcades, these areas are more likely to suffer vascular ischemia. The presence of a mesenteric defect with Type III atresias also supports this etiology. Statistically, the more distal the atresia, the less frequent is the incidence. Realizing that the last embryonic segments to recanalize are the duodenum and the sigmoid colon, the rare occurrence of colonic atresia remains relatively discrepant and deserves further attention.

When a neonate presents with a bowel obstruction, locating the site of the lesion becomes most important in the sequence of clinical investigation and management. The approaches are quite different for the proximal lesion compared to a distal ileocolonic obstruction. A duodenal or jejunal obstruction is more likely to be atresia, and once other significant systemic anomalies are excluded, the baby is prepared more promptly for the operating room. If the obstruction is distal, then the differential diagnosis is more complex and, indeed, the assessing modality can be therapeutic (ie, meconium ileus relieved by the contrast study) and an operation may become unnecessary.

## DUODENAL OBSTRUCTION

Duodenal atresia was first described by Calder in 1733, and Ernst was credited with the first successful repair in 1914. At the beginning of the twentieth century, congenital duodenal obstruction was a lethal disease due to technical failure at operation, associated congenital anomalies, primitive neonatal care skills, and insufficient nutrition. With the advent of the operative techniques of side-to-side and subsequently the "diamond" duodenoduodenostomy accompanied by improved intensive unit care and parenteral nutrition, the survival is now 95%.

### Pathophysiology

Duodenal atresia is probably caused by failure of recanalization of the duodenum during the embryonic solid core stage. This results in either partial obstruction due to a perforate membrane or stenosis, or complete obstruction by an

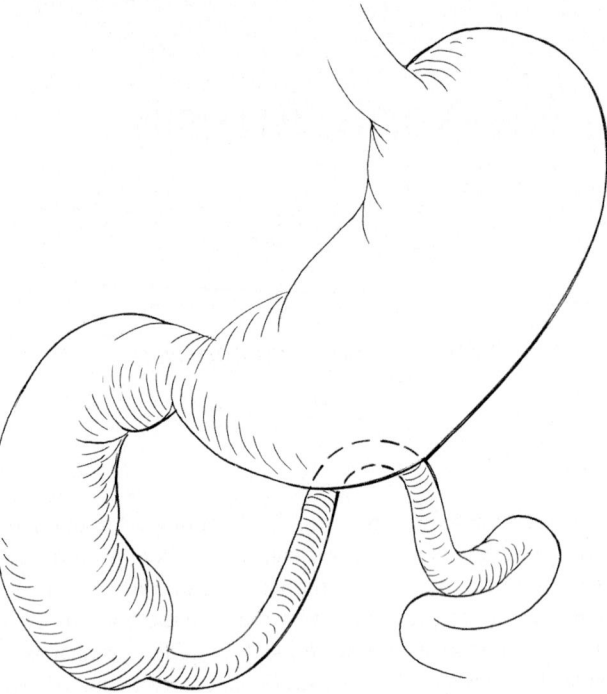

**FIGURE 42-1** Type I duodenal atresia with intact membrane causing complete obstruction.

imperforate membrane or atresia (Fig. 42-1). Failure of the pancreatic ventral anlage to rotate around the duodenum produces annular pancreas, which also has a strong association with duodenal stenosis and atresia.

These babies present with high intestinal obstruction. Polyhydramnios may be clinically evident and detected prenatally by ultrasound. The stomach and duodenum may appear dilated by fetal ultrasonography as early as 18 weeks'

gestation. Early definition is important because Down syndrome occurs in 30% of infants with duodenal atresia, and counseling of the parents for genetics as well as management options is not only indicated but is integral to the care of the baby and the family.

The intrinsic obstructive anatomy can vary among stenosis, perforate, or imperforate webs (Fig. 42-2), atresia, the compressive bands of midgut malrotation, or an in utero midgut volvulus. The anatomical variants are depicted, corresponding to the foregoing classification (Figs. 42-2A, 42-3, and 42-4). Presumably in the case of a longstanding web, elongation of the web evolves into a "windsock" shape with dilatation of the bowel well beyond the annular root of the membrane (Fig. 42-2B). This ring may not be visible on the external surface of the bowel. The externally apparent point of obstruction at the transition between the dilated and decompressed bowel is *not* the true internal origin of the web. The surgeon must always keep this variant in mind to avoid the pitfall of an unnecessary incision at the more distal transition site.

Duodenal stenosis is associated with, and probably caused by, the external compression of the anomalies of Ladd bands of midgut malrotation, annular pancreas, preduodenal portal vein, or duplications. Through the partial obstruction, swallowed air soon passes into the distal intestine and often delays the diagnosis and management. With a perforate web or stenosis, the degree of obstruction dictates the severity of proximal dilatation and generally the amount of polyhydramnios, although the latter is quite variable.

With complete obstruction, the gastric content suctioned in the delivery room can be alarming and may continue at high volume output. Usually the drainage is bile stained with the obstruction site distal to the entrance of the bile duct(s). Failure to replace this aspirate with its high concentrations of $K^+$ and $Cl^-$ rather quickly depletes the fluid compartments of the patient and leads to dehydration and hypokalemic,

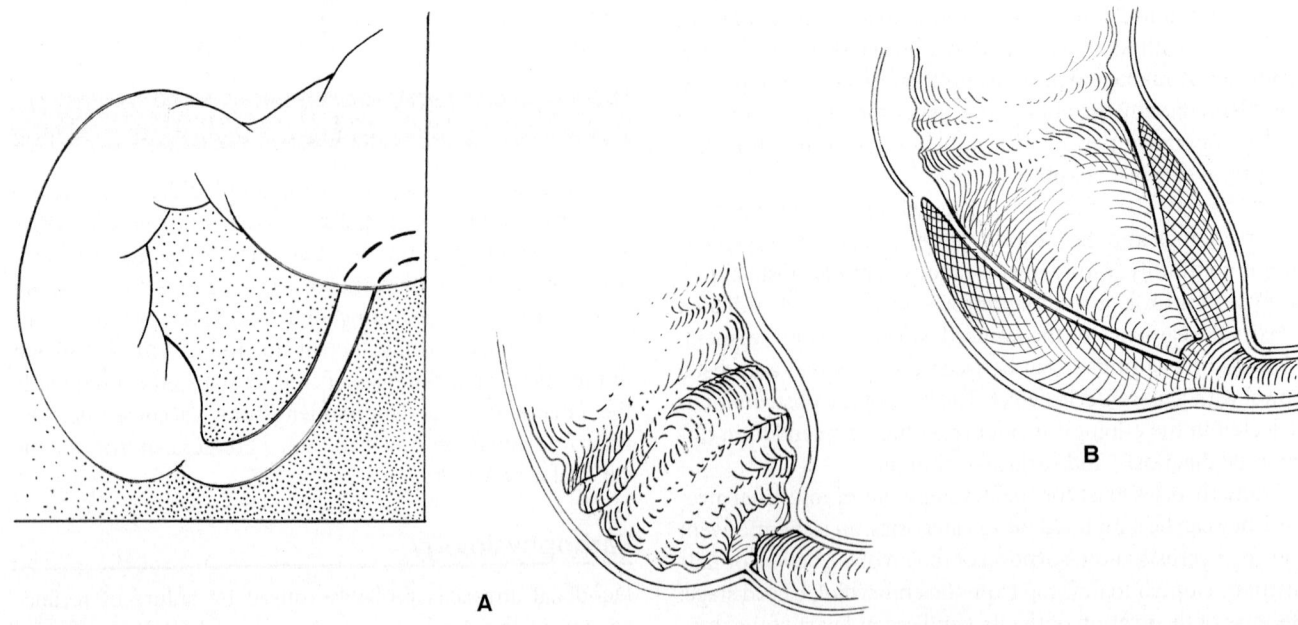

**A**

**B**

**FIGURE 42-2 A.** Type I duodenal atresia with fenestrated membrane causing near complete obstruction. **B.** Type I duodenal atresia with "windsock" diaphragm resulting in obstruction distal to the origin of the diaphragm.

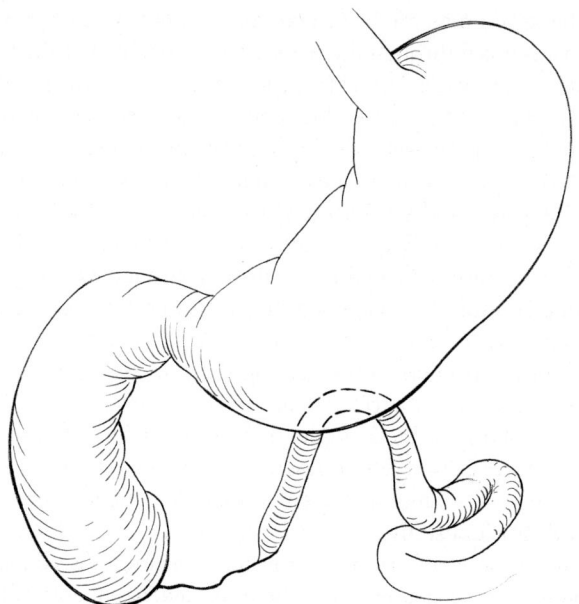

**FIGURE 42-3** Type II duodenal atresia with a complete obstruction and the proximal and distal duodenum connected by a fibrous cord.

full stomach may be visible and palpable in the epigastrium prior to decompression. If the baby has been discharged from the hospital with mother early after birth, the diagnosis may be delayed with severe emesis and dehydration.

The diagnosis can be confirmed with plain abdominal x-rays. The classic "double-bubble" sign will be seen, which is a dilated stomach and duodenal bulb layered with intraluminal air and fluid, but ordinarily no distal air pattern. If the double bubble is missing, due to the stomach and duodenum containing only fluid, then 30 to 60 mL of air can be infused via a nasogastric tube as a contrast medium. When gas is present in the distal segment, a partial obstruction due to stenosis, perforate web, or Ladd peritoneal bands can be assumed. The risk of ischemic bowel demands proceeding with urgency to avoid the catastrophy of midgut volvulus, which can be confused with duodenal atresia or stenosis. Confirmation either by a foregut contrast study or more directly by laparotomy is indicated.

Once volvulus has been excluded, the urgency to operate resolves. While resuscitation is underway by nasogastric decompression and fluid and electrolyte administration, the baby can be more fully evaluated. Echocardiography should be performed to identify a possible cardiac malformation. Ultrasonography of the head and urinary tract will assess for other anomalies of these systems, and a genetic consultation for chromosomal analysis will determine whether trisomy or Down syndrome is present.

hypochloremic alkalosis, or later to acidosis from severe hypovolemia and low cardiac output.

## Diagnosis

The diagnosis of duodenal obstruction can be determined antenatally with the findings of a dilated stomach and duodenum on ultrasound usually with polyhydramnios. After birth, the baby will present with emesis or high gastric aspirates, which are usually bilious. Because of the proximal nature of the obstruction, the baby's abdomen is scaphoid, although a

## Treatment

Prior to arrival of the baby in the operating room, overhead warming lights are secured, the warming blanket circulation is commenced, and the operating room is warmed to 24°C. After anesthesia is induced, the umbilical cord is prepped with 70% alcohol or other antiseptic agent, ligated, and divided flush with the abdominal wall. Two other techniques enhance thermal control: the drapes under the infant are not allowed to become wet during the abdominal preparation with the povidine–iodine solution and an adhesive plastic steridrape is applied to minimize heat loss and keep the baby and the drapes dry during the operation.

Traditional repair is through a transverse supraumbilical incision. In the last decade, laparoscopic techniques have been applied to repair of duodenal atresia (Fig. 42-5). A circumumbilical incision (Fig. 42-6) has also been used to improve long-term cosmesis after repair of duodenal atresia. The surgery itself despite the different approaches have the same goal of reestablishing intestinal continuity; however, there are some variations in the surgery among the different techniques.

During the traditional open repair, the abdomen is explored and inspected for fixation of the right colon and the rotation of the ligament of Treitz. If malrotation is present, the Ladd dissection begins by mobilizing the omental layers and hepatic flexure of the colon, and by exposing the duodenum by lysing the Ladd bands of the peritoneal reflections across the duodenum and pancreas. The ligament of Treitz is taken down during which time the jejunum is derotated counterclockwise under the mesenteric vessels and the terminal ileum and entire colon are rotated to the left side.

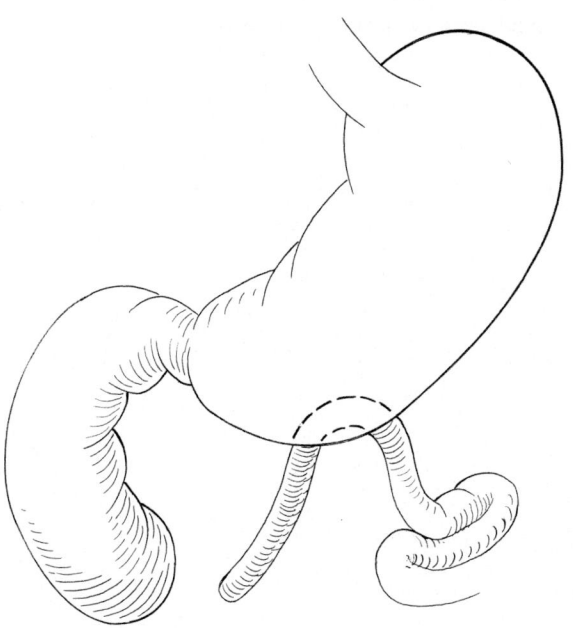

**FIGURE 42-4** Type III atresia with a gap between the proximal and distal duodenum.

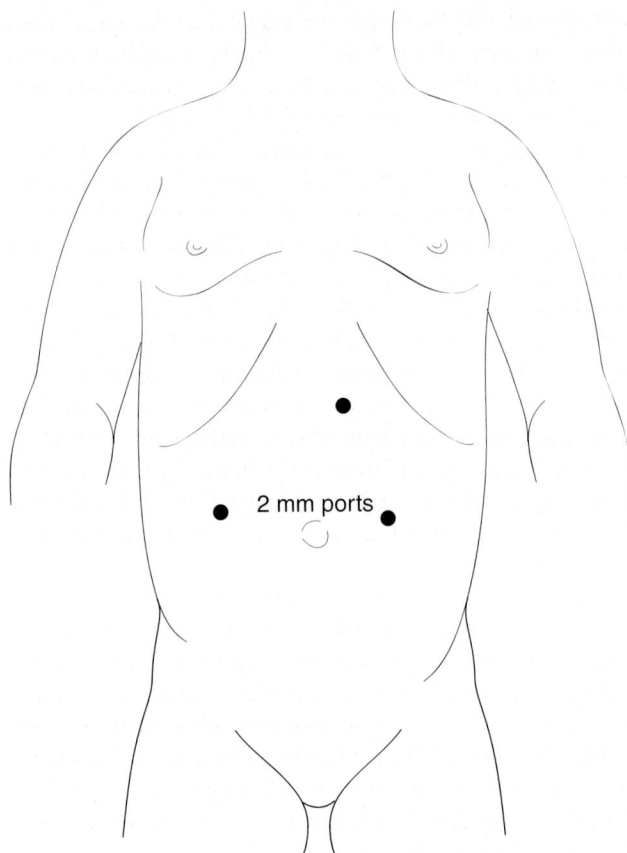

**FIGURE 42-5** Location of ports for laparoscopic duodenal atresia repair.

Otherwise a tube can be inserted per oris or via a gastrotomy and advanced through the pyloris with stretching of the web until its annular origin is evident, demarcated in the duodenal wall. A longitudinal duodenotomy is made at this origin exposing the web. The locations of the ampulla of Vater and/or ostium of the accessory duct of Santorini are identified, assisted by observing on which side of the web bile flows. The web is carefully excised preserving these ostia. A balloon catheter is inserted and directed distally through which warm saline is infused to insufflate the small intestine and detect another web, stenosis, or atretic segment. Controlled inflation of the balloon, while passing the catheter through the lumen, assures an adequate caliber at any suspect area. The duodenotomy is then closed transversely with interrupted fine sutures. If the web cannot be excised, then it is bypassed utilizing a diamond-shaped duodenoduodenostomy or duodenojejunostomy.

In the event of mural discontinuity, a transverse duodenotomy is placed at precisely the most dependent area of the dilated proximal segment (Fig. 42-7A), and a lengthy longitudinal incision is performed in the distal segment, which allows apposition without tension. The catheter is passed in both directions to assure that there is no concomitant obstruction preliminary to the anastomosis with full-thickness single layer closure. Air or saline is insufflated through the small intestine to the ileocecal valve to inspect for a second more distal atresia. The technique of Kimura (Fig. 42-7B) produces a widely patent "diamond-shaped" anastomosis. The initial orientation suture adjoins the proximal apex of the distal longitudinal duodenotomy to the midpoint of the inferior edge of the proximal transverse duodenotomy. Thus, the corners of each duodenotomy are sutured to the midpoints of the opposite duodenotomy.

This same procedure is used to bypass an annular pancreas. The pancreas should be left undisturbed. Incising or otherwise manipulating this tissue unnecessarily invites a pancreatic leak or fistula difficult to close. Also critical to anticipate is the anomaly of a preduodenal portal vein that must be identified, preserved, and similarly bypassed.

In the absence of malrotation, an extensive Kocher lysis to the mesenteric root allows examination for a duodenal obstruction as well as the anatomy of the pancreas.

If a Type I defect is present with mural continuity, then a windsock lesion must be suspected at this point. The web may be palpable or the annular origin of the web may be apparent proximal to the transitional segment of dilation.

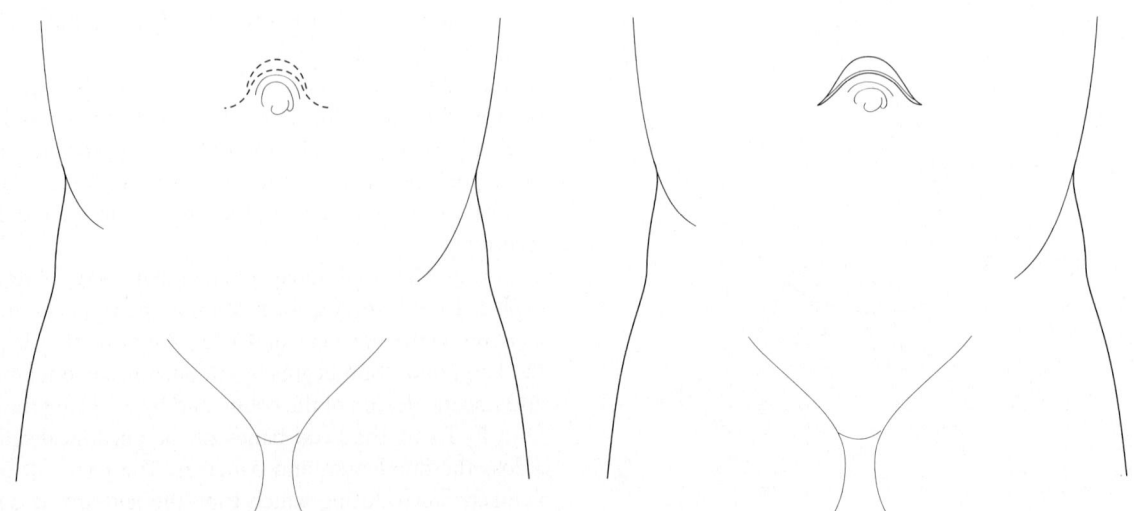

**FIGURE 42-6** Diagram of a circumumbilical incision for repair of an intestinal atresia.

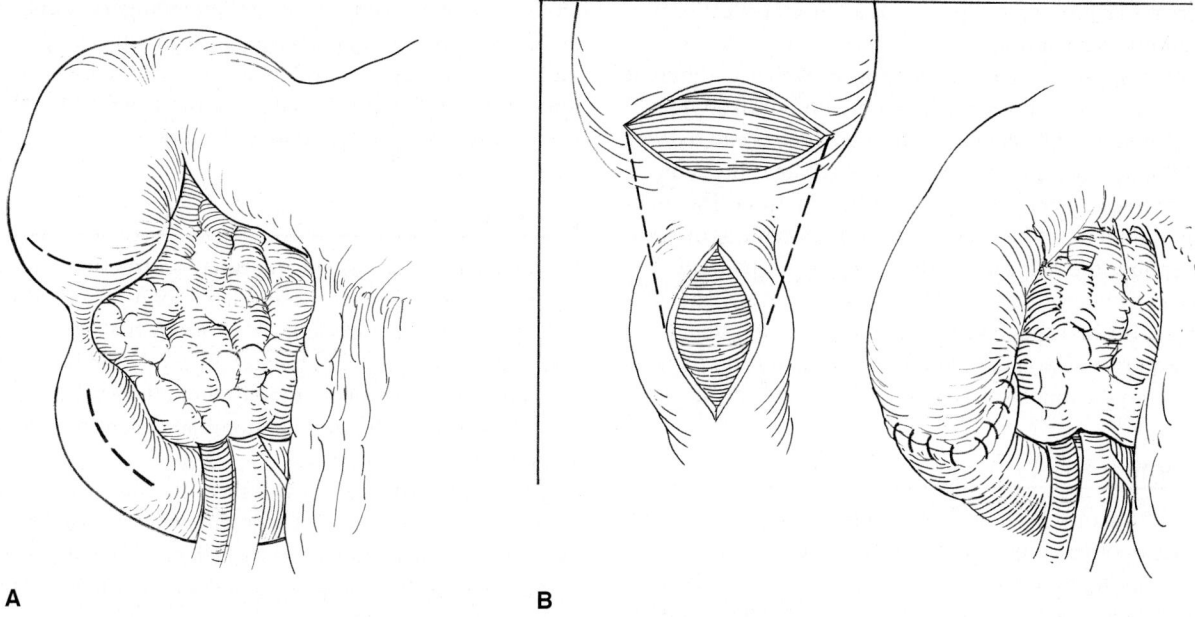

**FIGURE 42-7** **A.** To perform a diamond-shaped anastomosis, a transverse proximal duodenotomy is made 1 cm from the atresia on the lateral anterior duodenum to prevent injury to the ampulla and a longitudinal distal duodenotomy of the same length is made on the antimesenteric border. **B.** A diamond-shaped anastomosis to maintain the lumen of the duodenum.

When the proximal segment of the duodenum is excessively dilated, it has been demonstrated that the motility is both weak and has a significantly slower peristaltic frequency, which promotes stasis and bacterial overgrowth. Adhering to LaPlace law, function and long-term poor emptying can be improved by tailoring or tapering (reducing) the diameter of the dilated segment. A fold of the antimesenteric wall of the duodenum is resected along the longitudinal axis of the dilation with a catheter of appropriate caliber in the lumen, applying a GI stapler (Fig. 42-8A and B).

Duodenal atresia can be repaired through a laparoscopic approach. The patient is placed in a frog leg position. Usually

3 or 4 ports are required. The liver can be suspended with an external suture underneath the falciform ligament or a fourth port used for retraction of the liver. The anastomosis can be handsewn or completed with Nitinol U-clips. Most reports of laparoscopic repairs do not describe any tapering of the duodenum. A criticism of the laparoscopic approach is the difficulty or inability to search for a more distal atresia. A large retrospective multiinstitutional review recognized only noted 2 out of 400 cases with a second more distal atresia noted during laparoscopic repair of duodenal atresia. This study questions the need for insufflation and exploration of the distal intestine looking for a second atresia. Numerous studies

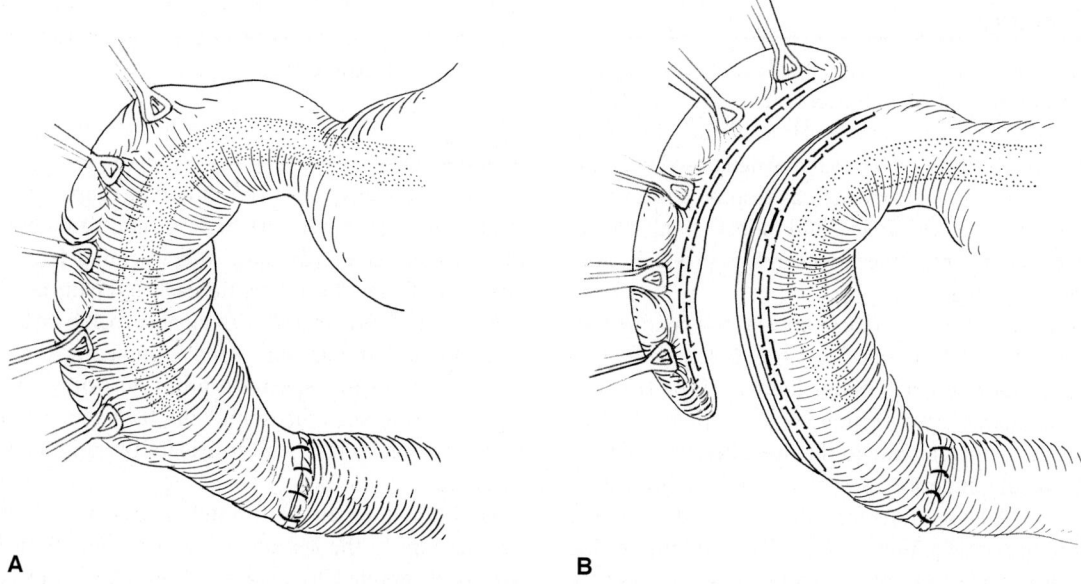

**FIGURE 42-8** **A, B.** A tapering duodenoplasty over a 20-Fr red rubber catheter performed in a massively dilated duodenum to improve contractility and emptying using a stapling device.

support the laparoscopic approach as a safe and effective way to repair duodenal atresia.

Another approach that has developed, which is different from the laparoscopic approach, is a periumbilical approach. Through a periumbilical incision the abdomen is entered and the duodenum is exposed. The surgical repair is the same as the more traditional right upper quadrant incision. The main benefit is thought to be cosmetic as a periumbilical incision heals without the scar seen in the right upper quadrant. The fascia can be opened in the midline or transversely. The incision can also be expanded in the midline as a T-shape for better exposure. Upon closure the T extension can be incorporated into the umbilical closure for improved cosmesis.

## Outcome

The mortality of this anomaly depends on the presence and influence of other congenital anomalies. Technical complications of anastomotic leak, stricture, pancreatic fistula, or a missed second atresia should rarely occur. Late complications including megaduodenum, poor motility, duodenogastric reflux, peptic ulcer, gastroesophageal reflux, and cholelithiasis are reported at a 12% to 15% incidence. As described above, megaduodenum can be effectively avoided and treated by a tapering duodenoplasty. The long-term prognosis is quite good with survival rates greater than 90% with mortality usually secondary to comorbidity.

## JEJUNOILEAL ATRESIA

Ileal atresia was first described in 1684 by Goeller, and the first successful repair was not performed until 1911 by Fockens in Rotterdam. In 1950, the overall survival was 85% to 90% but this has dramatically approached 100% during the last 45 years for numerous reasons, including the advent of intravenous (IV) nutrition in the 1960s, the improvements in ICU care, and anesthesia, as well as surgical techniques.

## Pathophysiology

In 1955, Louw and Barnard reported their canine fetal experimental observations that small bowel atresias are usually the result of an in utero mesenteric vascular accident. Tibbœl, in 1979, also showed in chick embryos that small bowel perforation can lead to atresia. Factors such as trophic and growth hormones within the amniotic fluid affect small bowel growth and development. Other mechanisms probably exist to be further elucidated.

The classification for jejunoileal atresia is expanded to 5 types, Types I to IIIa (Fig. 42-9A-C) corresponding to those described for duodenal lesions (above). Type IIIb was established to characterize separately the "apple-peel" or "Christmas tree" deformity due to the overt loss or extensive abnormality of the superior mesenteric artery blood supply (Fig. 42-9D). A large mesenteric defect extends from the atretic dilated proximal jejunum to the distal microintestine that receives its blood supply by retrograde flow from a single collateral arterial source of a residual ileocolic, right, middle, or left colic artery. The distal bowel courses as a "corkscrew"

around this single collateral vessel providing the "apple-peel" or "Christmas tree" appearance. Type IV atresia consists of multiple atretic segments often in a series of "sausage-shaped" links, or seemingly embedded in the mesentery with tiny collateral vessels supplying tenuous viability (Fig. 42-9E).

## Diagnosis

The antenatal diagnosis of intestinal obstruction with atresia should be suspected when dilated loops of intestine and polyhydramnios are evident. A newborn that presents with abdominal distention and bilious emesis should be evaluated for a bowel obstruction to establish both the level and the etiology, if feasible. The more abdominal distention, the more distal the obstruction.

A plain abdominal x-ray will show the amount and size of the dilated bowel. If a short segment of very dilated bowel is evident, proximal jejunal atresia is likely. The baby needs to be prepared for the operating room, and no further diagnostic workup is required.

In contrast, should the obstruction seem to be distal because of the degree of abdominal distention and many loops of air-filled bowel on the x-ray, then the differential diagnosis is more complicated and more information is required to differentiate ileal atresia, meconium ileus, meconium plug syndrome, Hirschsprung disease, small left colon syndrome, adynamic ileus from sepsis or drug toxicity, malrotation, or colonic atresia.

A rectal examination determines imperforate anus or stenosis, and will show if meconium or just mucus is present in the rectal vault. If the baby is stable, a water-soluble contrast enema may establish the diagnosis and be therapeutic simultaneously for meconium plug, meconium ileus, or small left colon syndrome. In ileal atresia the contrast will show a microcolon but no contrast refluxing into the dilated bowel. The baby is then prepared for the operating room.

Preparation entails nasogastric decompression, IV hydration, and electrolyte correction to replace the fluid lost from emesis, the nasogastric tube, and within the bowel lumen. Antibiotics should be administered intravenously. A careful physical exam may detect other anomalies that should be addressed before anesthesia also.

## Treatment

The operating environs itself should be prepared by warming to an ambient temperature of 24°C, and using both a warming blanket under the baby and warming lights overhead. Before or during the antiseptic wash and painting, the umbilical cord is suture ligated with an absorbable tie and cut flush with the abdominal wall. After completing the providine–iodine prep, an adhesive waterproof steri-drape is applied for 2 purposes: to keep the drapes and baby dry, which prevents evaporative heat loss, and to isolate the umbilicus from the incision.

Traditional repair is through a transverse supraumbilical incision. In the last decade laparoscopic techniques have also been applied to repair of jejunoileal atresia or, more commonly, circumumbilical incision has also been used to improve long-term cosmesis after repair of jejunoileal atresia.

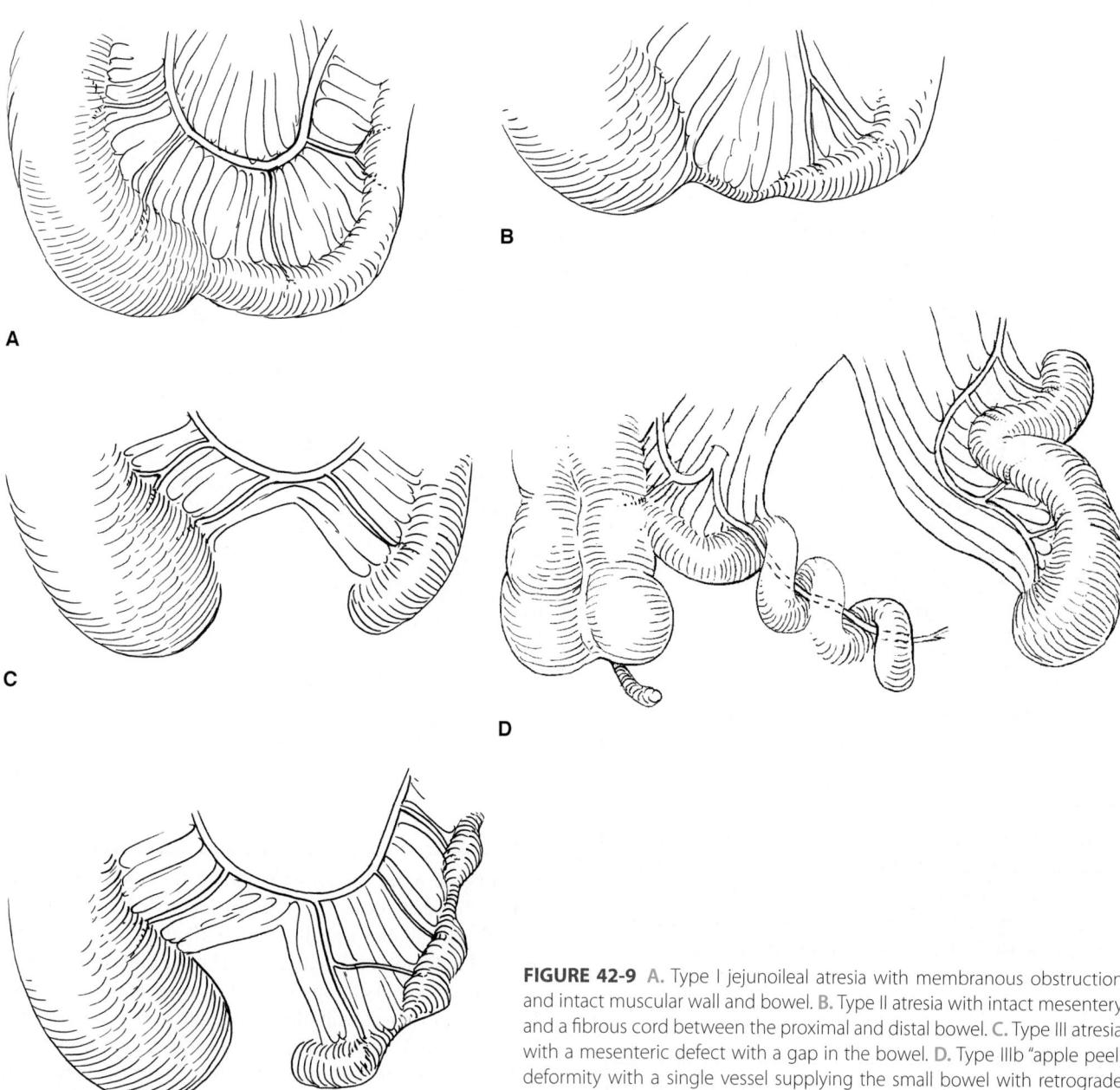

**FIGURE 42-9 A.** Type I jejunoileal atresia with membranous obstruction and intact muscular wall and bowel. **B.** Type II atresia with intact mesentery and a fibrous cord between the proximal and distal bowel. **C.** Type III atresia with a mesenteric defect with a gap in the bowel. **D.** Type IIIb "apple peel" deformity with a single vessel supplying the small bowel with retrograde flow from either the ileocolic or right colic artery. **E.** Type IV multiple jejunoileal atresias.

The surgery itself, despite the different approaches, has the same goal of reestablishing intestinal continuity.

A traditional approach is through a transverse incision 1 fingerbreadth (12-20 mm) superior to the umbilicus, is usually one half the distance from the xiphoid to the pubis, and allows exposure from the hepar to the pelvis. After transecting the rectus muscles, the peritoneum is incised and the surgeon explores first to identify the location of the cecum and ligament of Treitz to rule out midgut malrotation. The bowel will require evisceration to find the point of obstruction and assess whether additional sites of atresia coexist, which occurs in at least 10% of cases. Any site of perforation is immediately controlled to prevent further spillage of enteric content. Proximal to an atresia, the bowel is dilated and the last 10 to 15 cm is more dilated and atonic (Fig. 42-10A). It is advisable to resect this markedly dilated segment, if it is far enough from the pancreas, to enhance recovery of motility

and decrease stasis in this segment that can lead to bacterial translocation and sepsis. The remainder of the bowel proximal to the atresia will still have a diameter markedly discrepant to the distal segment. Tailoring the former by obliquely excising a longitudinal fold from the antimesenteric side of the bowel will taper the diameter and facilitate an anastomosis. With a 24-Fr catheter in the lumen and stay sutures at the ends of the segment to be tapered, a GI anastomosis stapler assists the quick excision and control of bleeding from the long cut edge of the bowel.

Before proceeding with the anastomosis, a catheter should be inserted into the excised opening of the distal segment and warm saline infused to demonstrate both patency with no secondary atresia and that flow continues into and through the colon. If a distal atretic obstruction is missed, the anastomosis is doomed to postoperative disruption, a second operation will be necessary, and the morbidity risk is increased.

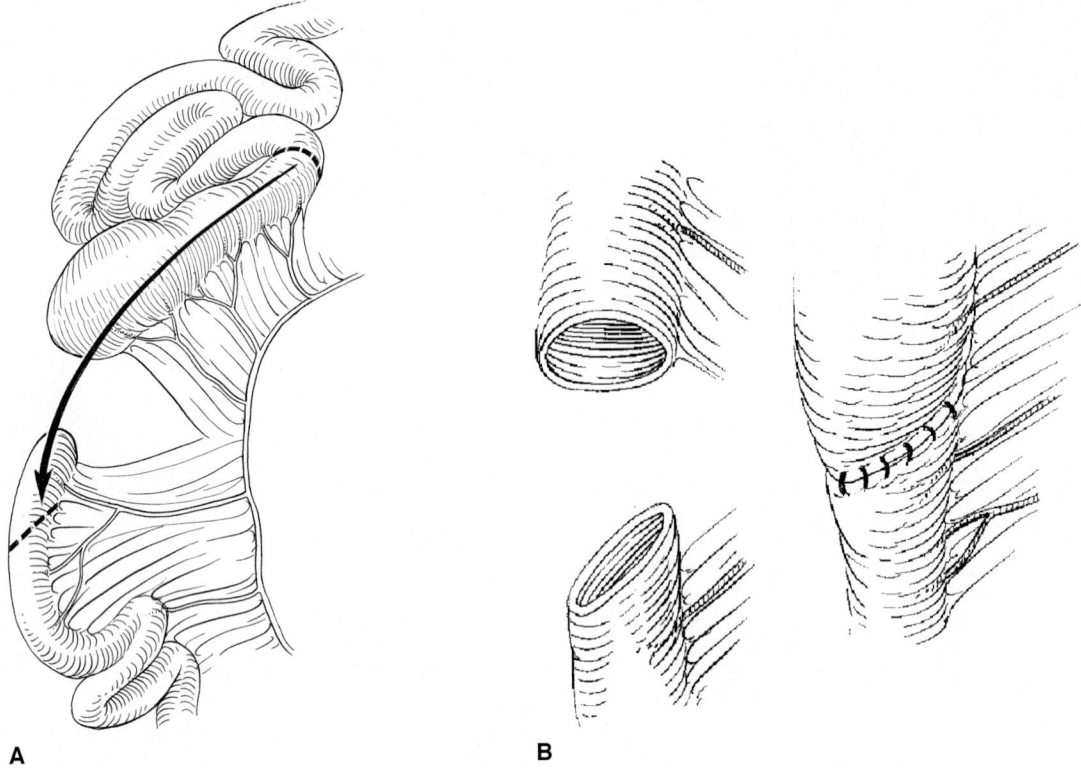

**A**

**B**

**FIGURE 42-10** **A.** Resection of the dilated bowel just proximal to the obstruction if there is adequate bowel length to allow for better contractility and avoid stasis. **B.** Completed end-to-oblique enteroenterostomy after resection.

The diameter of the anastomosis is further matched by enlarging the distal end with an incision along the antimesenteric border for a length that approximates the diameter of the proximal dilated bowel. An "end-to-oblique side" anastomosis is performed with interrupted 5-0 or 6-0 sutures (Fig. 42-10B). The mesenteric defect is closed carefully, avoiding injury to small vessels supplying blood to this anastomosis.

If the anomaly is the Type IIIb or "apple-peel" deformity, the lone blood vessel providing all the collateral blood supply must be carefully preserved. The bowel and mesentery here must not be allowed to twist when replacing the intestines into the abdominal cavity. Obstruction of this vascular source will be evident if the color becomes dusky or overtly cyanotic, and the bowel must be rearranged to reverse such an appearance before closing the abdomen.

In the presence of a perforation or concern about viability of the bowel, it may be judicious in extreme prematurity, excessive inflammation, or cardiac instability, to exteriorize the bowel by forming stomas either through the incision or separate incisions. If at all possible, stomas should be avoided and primary repair completed to prevent mucosal atrophy, enhance nutrition, avoid additional operations, and thereby reduce morbidity.

A laparoscopic or periumbilical incision can be used for repair as well. The approach for either is the same as used for duodenal atresia repair. The goals of the surgery are the same: reestablish intestinal continuity while maintaining blood supply to the intestine. Complex jejunoileal atresia that requires resection or Type IIIb or Type IV atresia can be difficult to approach laparoscopically, but are amenable to repair through a periumbilical incision.

## Outcome

The survival of a neonate with an isolated intestinal atresia should be near 100%. Overall, this success has developed dramatically in the last 40 years with the advent of total parental nutrition and neonatal ICU care. Mortality is associated with complications of prematurity, abdominal wall defects, perforation, volvulus, short gut, and cystic fibrosis. The incidence of a technical complication such as anastomotic stricture or leak is 5% to 10%. Potential long-term complications include short-bowel syndrome, adhesive bowel obstruction, renal calculi, central venous catheter sepsis, and vitamin D deficiencies. Especially in part of Types IIIb and IV anomalies, the most difficult problem to manage is the short gut syndrome. This condition requires prolonged parenteral nutrition and potentially may lead to small bowel transplantation.

## COLONIC ATRESIA

Colonic atresia is the rarest of intestinal atresias, occurring about 1 in 20,000 neonates. Potts reported the first successful repair for an infant in 1947.

## Pathophysiology

The etiology of simple colon atresia is probably an in utero compromise of the blood supply to the colon. The transverse and sigmoid colon are the most commonly affected areas.

## Diagnosis and Treatment

The baby presents with a distal bowel obstruction, failure to pass meconium, bilious emesis, and greater abdominal distention. Resuscitation and diagnosis are similar to the processes for small intestinal atresia and include fluid resuscitation, nasogastric tube decompression, abdominal radiographs, and distal contrast enema, which will show a small caliber, unused or microcolon, and a blind-ending colonic segment.

The preparation of the operating room and the baby should proceed as described above for the small intestine. A primary anastomosis is performed after the terminal 10 cm of dilated bowel is resected. Note that the unprepped colon in the newborn is sterile. The alternative option is a colostomy allowing the bowel to decompress and return to normal size. A second atretic obstruction elsewhere in the bowel must be looked for and ruled out or repaired.

## Outcome

The mortality of an isolated colonic atresia should also be low. Death is related to other infrequent malformations or perforation with peritonitis. Long-term bowel function should be normal as long as no other intestinal or systemic (ie, cystic, fibrosis, etc) bowel abnormality is present.

## SELECTED READINGS

Calder J. Two examples of children born with preternatural conformation of the guts. *Med Essays* (Edinburgh) 1733;1:203.

Doolin EJ, Ormsbee HS, Hill JL. Motility abnormality in intestinal atresia. *J Pediatr Surg* 1987;22:320–324.

Ernst NP. A case of congenital atresia of the duodenum treated successfully by operation. *Br Med J* 1916;1:644.

Evans CH. Atresias of the gastrointestinal tract. *Surg Gynecol Obstet* 1951;92:1–8.

Fockens P. Ein operativ geheilter Fall von Kongenitaler Duenndarm Atresie. *Zentralbl Chir* 1911;38:532.

Grosfeld JL. Jenjunoileal atresia and stenosis. In: Welch KJ, Randolph JG, Ravitch MM, et al., eds. *Pediatric Surgery*. Chicago: Year Book; 1986:838.

Grosfeld JL, Rescorla FJ. Duodenal atresia and stenosis: reassessment of treatment and outcome based on antenatal diagnosis, pathologic variance, and long-term followup. *World J Surg* 1993;17:301–309.

Kimura K, Mukohara N, Nishijima E, et al. Diamond shaped anastomosis for duodenal atresia: an experience with 44 patients over 15 years. *J Pediatr Surg* 1990;25:977–979.

Kimura K, Tsugawa C, Ogawa K, et al. Diamond-shaped anatomosis for congenital duodenal obstruction. *Arch Surg* 1977;112(10):1262–1263.

Louw JH. Investigations into the etiology of congenital atresia of the colon. *Dis Colon Rectum* 1964;7:471–478.

Louw JH, Barnard CN. Congenital intestinal atresia: observations on its origin. *Lancet* 1955;2:1065–1067.

Philippart AI. Atresia, stenosis, and other obstructions of the colon. In: Welch KJ, Randolph VG, et al., eds. *Pediatric Surgery*. Chicago: Year Book; 1986:984–988.

Potts WJ. Congenital atresia of the intestine and colon. *Surg Gynecol Obstet* 1947;85:14–19.

Rescorla FJ, Grosfeld JL. Intestinal atresia and stenosis: analysis of survival in 120 cases. *Surgery* 1985;98:668–676.

Spigland N, Yazbeck S. Complications associated with surgical treatment of congenital intrinsic duodenal obstruction. *J Pediatr Surg* 1990;25:1127–1130.

Stubbs TM, Horger EO. Sonographic detection of fetal duodenal atresia (Letter). *Obstet Gynecol* 1989;73:146.

Tandler J. Zur Entwicklungsgeschichte des menschlichen Duodenums. *Morphol Jb* 1902;29:187.

Tibboel D, Molenaar JC, Van Nie CJ. New perspectives in fetal surgery: the chicken embryo. *J Pediatr Surg* 1979;14:438–440.

# Meconium Ileus CHAPTER 43

*Brent E. Carlyle, Drucy S. Borowitz, and Philip L. Glick*

## KEY POINTS

1. Cystic fibrosis (CF) is an autosomal recessive disease characterized by respiratory, digestive, reproductive, and sweat gland abnormalities.

2. Meconium ileus (MI) accounts for up to 33% of neonatal intestinal obstructions and occurs in approximately 20% of newborns diagnosed with CF.

3. More than 1870 distinct mutations of the cystic fibrosis transmembrane regulator (CFTR) protein have been identified, some of which cause CF. The most common mutation is F508del, which accounts for approximately two third of all mutations in patients with CF.

4. Prenatal diagnosis of MI may be made by sonogram, most commonly showing dilated bowel or increased echogenicity within the bowel lumen. The positive predictive value of hyperechoic masses in a *high-risk* fetus is estimated to be 52%, whereas in the *low-risk* fetus the estimate is only 6.4%.

5. MI can be *simple or complicated*. In the *simple* form, thickened meconium begins to form in utero and, as it obstructs the mid ileum, proximal dilatation, bowel wall thickening, and congestion occur. In *complicated* MI volvulus, atresia, necrosis, perforation, meconium peritonitis, and pseudocyst formation may occur.

6. Nonoperative management with Gastrografin® enema is the preferred initial treatment option for simple MI. Special care should be observed to avoid hypovolemic shock with adequate prior intravenous (IV) hydration. Bowel perforation may be avoided by forgoing balloon catheter inflation and maintaining a low hydrostatic pressure during enema instillation.

7. Complicated MI and simple MI that fails enema treatment will require bowel resection with a temporary enterostomy or resection with primary anastomosis. The authors advocate a double barrel enterostomy; followed by serial irrigations of the open stomas and enteral feedings in the distal stoma to stimulate bowel growth. Bowel continuity is usually restored 6 to 12 weeks later.

8. Infants with simple MI and CF may be given breast milk or routine infant formula, enzymes, and vitamins. Those who have a complicated surgical course will require either continuous enteral feedings or total parenteral nutrition (TPN). Pancreatic enzymes must be given orally starting at 2000 to 4000 lipase units per 120 mL of full-strength formula.

9. The prognosis for patients with CF and MI is very promising; recently published studies show 1-year survival rates as high as 100%. Long-term follow-up at 13 years shows similar pulmonary function and nutritional status in CF patients with or without MI.

## INTRODUCTION

Meconium ileus (MI) is one of the most common causes of intestinal obstruction in the newborn accounting for 9% to 33% of neonatal intestinal obstructions. It is the earliest clinical manifestation of CF, occurring in approximately 20% of patients with CF.

Clinically, CF is characterized by chronic obstruction and infection of the respiratory tract, insufficiency of the exocrine pancreas, and elevated sweat chloride levels. Approximately 10% of patients with CF will remain pancreatic sufficient and tend to have a milder course. Complicated MI often results in prolonged hospital stays at great monetary and emotional cost. In the current era, prenatal diagnosis of MI with obstetrical ultrasound, coupled with improved biochemical and molecular techniques for diagnosis of CF, enable the perinatal team to counsel a family concerning the likelihood of CF in the fetus. Affected fetuses may be monitored and managed to ensure an optimal outcome. Advances in neonatal care and surgical management of infants with CF complicated by MI have greatly improved survival. Recent studies show that long-term nutritional, pulmonary, and mortality outcomes of patients with CF and MI are no worse than outcomes of CF patients without MI.

## PATHOPHYSIOLOGY OF MI

CF is an autosomal recessive disease with a heterozygote frequency estimated to be 1 in 29 in the Caucasian population. Each offspring of 2 heterozygote parents has a 1 in 4 chance of developing the illness. A family history of CF has been noted in 10% to 40% of new patients with MI. Allan, in a review of 488 families with at least 1 child with CF, reported a recurrence rate of 39% of MI in families with a previously affected sibling.

In 1989, the CF locus was localized through linkage analysis to the long arm of human chromosome 7, band q31. The disease results from mutations in the gene, which codes for a cell membrane protein termed the cystic fibrosis transmembrane (conductance) regulator. This protein has been found to be an adenosine $3',5'$-cyclic phosphate (cAMP)-induced chloride channel, which also regulates the flow of $HCO_3^-$ ions across the apical surface of epithelial cells. CFTR is 1480 amino acids long with a mass of approximately 170,000 Da. An abnormal CFTR protein results in altered electrolyte content in the environment external to the apical surface of epithelial membranes. This leads to desiccation and reduced clearance of secretions from tubular structures lined by affected epithelia. In the sweat gland, CFTR dysfunction leads to inadequate resorption of sodium, chloride, and potassium.

Over 1870 CFTR mutations have been reported to the CF Genetic Consortium as of June 2011. By far the most common mutation of the CFTR gene is a 3-base pair deletion, which results in the removal of a phenylalanine residue at amino acid position 508 of CFTR. This is called the F508del mutation, previously termed ΔF508. Globally, 66% of CF patients have at least 1 F508del mutation; however, there is wide variability within different ethnic and geographic populations. In Denmark, F508del represents 87.5% of CF mutations whereas in Tunisia, F508del only accounts for 17.9% of mutations. Worldwide, the one third of mutations not attributable to F508del are a heterogeneous group; less than 20 mutations occur at a frequency of greater than 0.1%. Certain alleles cluster with increased frequency in specific populations. For example, W1282X is common in Ashkenazi Jews, G551D is common in Celtic populations, and R553X is common in Switzerland. MI occurs most commonly in patients with the F508del and G542X mutations. Patients with 2 copies of the F508del mutation have a 24.9% chance of presenting with MI, F508del plus any "other" CF mutation confers 16.9% chance, and 2 "other" CF mutations confer a 12.5% chance of MI.

Genotype–phenotype correlation in CF is stronger for pancreatic phenotype than respiratory phenotype. In general, homozygosity of F508del nearly always confers pancreatic exocrine insufficiency. It was previously thought that pancreatic insufficiency played a central role in the pathogenesis of MI. However, work in CF mouse models suggests an alternative explanation. In the first CF mouse model (*Cftr*^*tm1UNC*^), engineered in 1992, newborn mice were noted to have severe intestinal obstruction at birth with minimal pulmonary or pancreatic involvement. This suggested the role of pancreatic insufficiency in the development of MI was minimal. Since the first mouse CFTR-knockout in 1992, 11 CF mouse models have been characterized including the 2 most common mutations, F508del and G551D. Recently, a ferret and pig model CFTR-knockout were engineered. Of note, the pig model shows 100% penetrance for MI.

Further work in the mouse models by Quinton and others has demonstrated that CF patients likely have defective $HCO_3^-$ excretion in addition to the traditionally understood $Cl^-$ excretion defect. CFTR is permeable to $HCO_3^-$ via 2 separate transport mechanisms. Intestinal fluid in patients with CF has long been known to be low in $HCO_3^-$. The defective secretion of $HCO_3^-$ leads to an altered luminal environment that is more acidic and dehydrated than seen within normal intestinal lumens. These changes lead to accumulation of mucus within the bowel lumen. In contrast, the addition of $HCO_3^-$ is known to reduce the viscosity of intraluminal fluids. $HCO_3^-$ plays an additional role as well. In the process of normal mucogenesis, mucins are excreted into the bowel lumen by the process of exocytosis. Mucins are released in a tight matrix formation around $Ca^{2+}$ ions. By chelating the $Ca^{2+}$ ions, $HCO_3^-$ helps to expand these mucins from a tight matrix into the loose, well-hydrated form that compromises normal mucus. This compacted, dehydrated mucus likely contributes to MI.

Non-CFTR genetic factors also influence MI. In a twin study, Blackman found that 82% of monozygotic twins showed concordance for MI, whereas only 22% of dizygotic and 24% of 2 affected siblings showed concordance, thus providing strong evidence for the role of modifier genes in the pathogenesis of MI. In CF, chromosomes 19q13.2 and 12p13.3 have been identified as possible modifier genes for MI. Chromosome 4q13.3 may be a modifier gene that is protective for MI. Additionally, there is some evidence for multiple loci modifier gene involvement. With the discovery of modifier genes for MI, our understanding of MI is evolving.

Abnormal intestinal motility may also contribute to the development of MI. Some patients with CF have been found to have prolonged small intestinal transit times. Non-CF diseases associated with abnormal gut motility, such as Hirschsprung disease and chronic intestinal pseudoobstruction, have been associated with MI, suggesting that decreased peristalsis may allow for increased resorption of water, thus favoring the development of MI.

## ANTENATAL DIAGNOSIS AND MANAGEMENT

Two factors should be considered when assessing the risk of MI in a fetus: ultrasound findings and the genetic risk of CF in the fetus. As of 2011, the American College of Obstetrics and Gynecology recommends that, as a routine part of obstetric care and regardless of ethnicity, all women of reproductive age should be offered preconception and prenatal CF carrier screening. Antenatal diagnosis of MI can be made in 2 different groups, a *high-risk* group and a *low-risk* group. In the *low-risk* group, the diagnosis is suspected when the sonographic

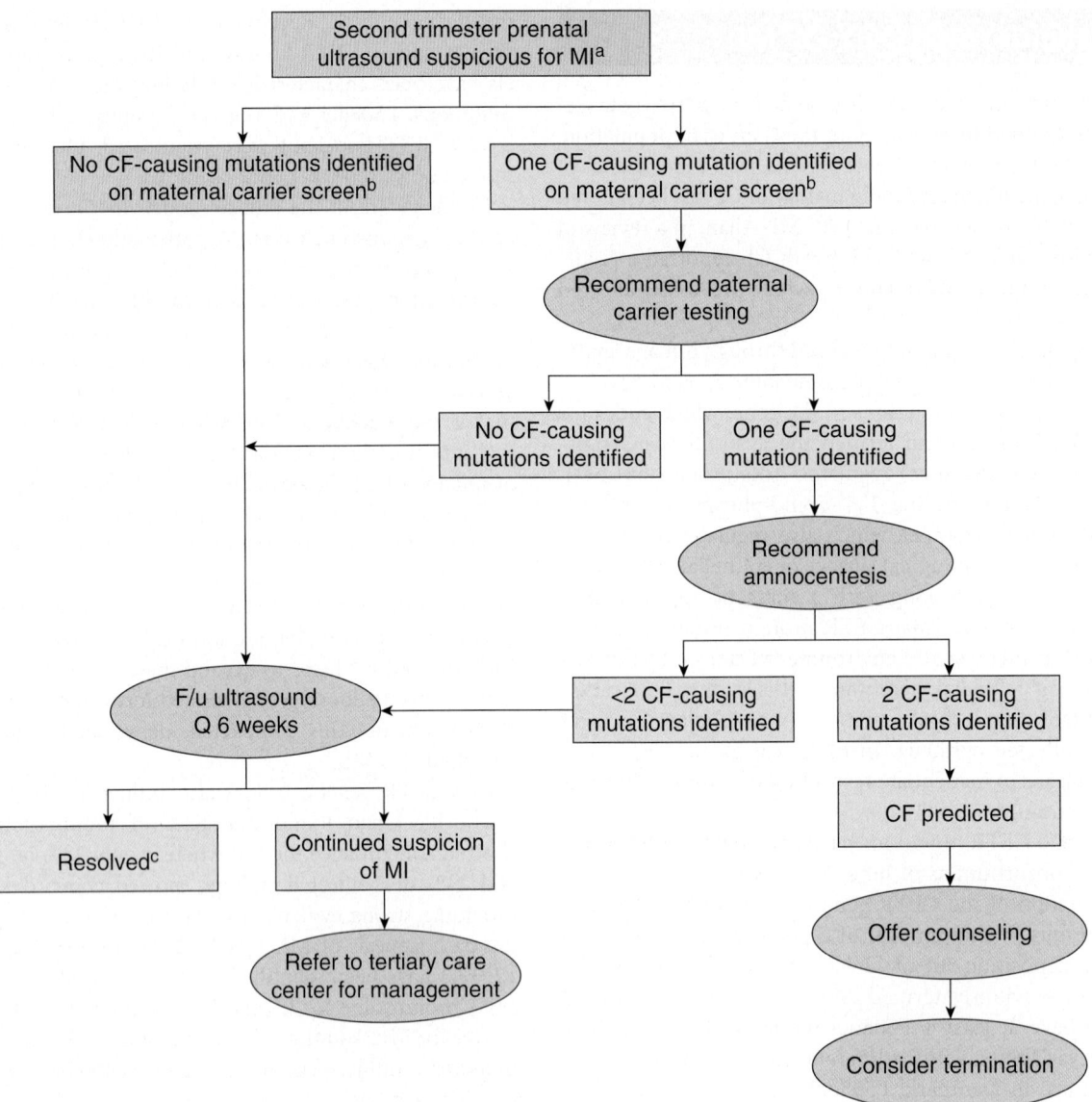

**FIGURE 43-1** Suggested algorithm for management of patients with prenatal ultrasound suspicious for MI. [a]This algorithm excludes families with a child with CF or mothers with CF, but could be adapted to those situations. [b]Maternal carrier screening is strongly recommended if it was not previously performed, but the ultrasound is suspicious for MI. [c]CF is unlikely but families and care providers should be aware that negative carrier screening cannot definitively rule out CF.

appearances of MI are found on routine prenatal ultrasound in a mother with a negative CF carrier screen. Sonographic findings consistent with MI in a fetus with parents who are known CF carriers, and all pregnancies subsequent to the birth of a CF-affected child are considered *high-risk*.

Pediatric surgeons are increasingly being consulted to evaluate fetuses suspected of having MI. We have established an algorithm that may be used in decision making and management of the fetus suspected of having MI based on prenatal ultrasound findings (Fig. 43-1).

## Sonographic Evaluation

Sonographic characteristics associated with MI include: hyperechoic masses (inspissated meconium in the terminal ileum), dilated bowel, and nonvisualization of the gallbladder on prenatal sonogram. Normal fetal meconium, when

visualized in the second and third trimesters, is usually hypoechoic or isoechoic to adjacent abdominal structures (Fig. 43-2). A hyperechoic mass has been variably defined as one with sonographic density greater than that of liver or bone. As a sonographic marker of MI, this finding is plagued by difficulties such as the subjective assessment of echogenicity, and the lengthy associated differential diagnosis. In addition to MI, hyperechoic bowel has been reported with Down syndrome, intrauterine growth retardation, prematurity, in utero cytomegalovirus infection, intestinal atresias, abruptio placenta, and fetal demise. The importance of hyperechoic fetal bowel is related to gestational age at detection with younger fetuses being at higher risk; the presence of ascites, calcification, volume of amniotic fluid, and the presence of other fetal anomalies also increase the risk of MI.

The prenatal diagnosis of MI using the sonographic feature of hyperechoic bowel must take into account the a priori

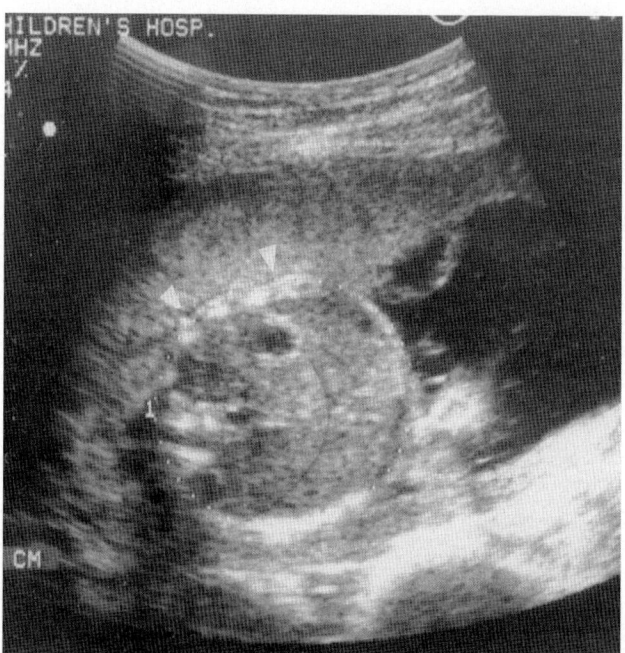

**FIGURE 43-2** Sonogram at 22 weeks' gestation demonstrating a 2 × 3-cm intraluminal (distal ileum) mass consistent with meconium inspissation (MI). (From *Irish MS, Ragi JM, Karamanoukian H, et al. Prenatal diagnosis of the fetus with cystic fibrosis and meconium ileus. Pediatr Surg Int 1997;12:434–436,* with permission.)

genetic risk of the couple. The positive predictive value of hyperechoic masses in a *high-risk* fetus is estimated to be 52%, whereas in the *low-risk* fetus the estimate is only 6.4%. Pregnancies with a 1 in 4 risk of CF show 25% to 60% association between hyperechoic bowel and CF; this association is less prevalent in the general population. In a large regional study encompassing 573,820 newborn screening sonograms, Scotet found 289 fetal cases of hyperechoic bowel. Of these, 7.6% were found to have CF, 3.7% had chromosome abnormalities and 3.7% had maternofetal infections, and a disorder of any sort was diagnosed in 32.2% of fetuses. It is crucial to note that hyperechoic bowel, in both the second and third trimesters, has been found to be a normal variant. Hyperechoic bowel, seen as an isolated event in the earlier part of the second trimester, may represent a normal variant and follow-up prenatal exams are indicated. Ruiz, in a study of 48 fetuses with hyperechoic bowel, found that 65% of cases detected by sonogram resolved with subsequent sonographic evaluation. Findings of many published studies are confounded by the use of multiple ultrasound models, numerous sonographers with unknown inter- and intraobserver reliability, and subjective assessments of hyperechogenicity. While an increase in risk of MI and CF has been associated with hyperechoic bowel, most fetuses with hyperechoic bowel do not have MI or CF.

The finding of dilated bowel on prenatal ultrasound has been reported less frequently in association with CF than hyperechoic bowel. In MI, bowel dilation is caused by obstruction by meconium, but mimics similar findings with midgut volvulus, congenital bands, bowel atresia, intestinal duplication, internal hernia, meconium plug syndrome, or Hirschsprung disease.

In addition to the findings of increased abdominal echogenicity and bowel dilation, inability to visualize the gallbladder on fetal ultrasound has been associated with CF. Combined with other sonographic features, nonvisualization of the gallbladder can be useful in the prenatal detection of the disease. However, caution should be exercised in the interpretation of a nonvisualizing gallbladder, as the differential also includes biliary atresia, omphalocele, diaphragmatic hernia, chromosomal abnormalities, and normal pregnancy.

Sonographic characteristics of fetal bowel obstruction are neither sensitive nor specific for MI. Again, the interpretation of these aforementioned sonographic findings must include consideration of the risk of the fetus of having CF. Certainly, findings suggesting MI in the *high-risk* fetus indicate a high probability of CF. In the *low-risk* fetus, suspicious ultrasound findings warrant consideration of CFTR mutation testing of both parents or, at the very least, serial follow-up examinations.

## Prenatal Testing for CF

CFTR analysis can be accomplished using a technique for recovering DNA from cells obtained from the parents by buccal brushing or directly by sampling blood. With this technique, the carrier status of parents suspected of having a fetus with CF based on sonographic findings of MI can be determined. Since the first edition of this text, commercial screening panels have become more comprehensive. Many region- and ethnic-specific panels have been developed to reflect the mutations present in a specific population. The Technical Standards and Guidelines for CFTR Mutation Testing published by the American College of Medical Genetics recommends a panethnic panel that includes 23 common mutations. This panel identifies 94% of mutations found in Ashkenazi Jews, 88% in Caucasians, 64% in African Americans, 72% in Hispanics, and 49% in Asian Americans. Thus, negative tests must still be interpreted with some caution. Even complete gene sequencing along with evaluation for duplications and deletions is not 100% accurate in finding all CFTR mutations. For example, mutations in the promoter region cannot be identified. Conversely, not all CFTR mutations cause CF. Of note, a variety of expanded screening panels are available, some of which include CFTR mutations that only variably are associated with CF. Thus, results of genetic testing need to be evaluated by someone with experience, preferably a genetic counselor.

If both parents have identified CF-causing mutations, subsequent evaluation of the fetus can be made by chorionic villus sampling or amniocentesis. If the results predict CF in the fetus, the mother should be followed at a tertiary care facility for discussion of the diagnosis and further management. Alternatively, some parents may consider termination. If either DNA analysis or amniocentesis are refused or are nondiagnostic, we recommend close sonographic follow-up at 6-week intervals.

The obvious advantage of prenatal diagnosis is that it allows the clinician to prepare for the medical and psychological needs of the parents, fetus, and newborn before, during, and after delivery and it allows the family time to adjust to the diagnosis. When an ultrasound suggests MI in a high-risk fetus, we recommend immediate referral to a tertiary care facility equipped to manage the needs of the mother, fetus, neonate, and family. At the Women and Children's Hospital of Buffalo, a multidisciplinary team of perinatologists, neonatologists, obstetricians, pediatric surgeons, and CF specialists prepares for the delivery of these high-risk neonates. Serial sonographic examinations are performed on a monthly basis until delivery. This evaluation allows the early detection of potential complications as they occur, thereby preparing the clinicians for special or urgent medical or surgical needs on delivery.

## POSTNATAL MANAGEMENT

MI is either *simple* or *complicated*. Each occurs with a frequency of approximately 50%. In the *simple* form, thickened meconium begins to form in utero and, as it obstructs the mid ileum, proximal dilatation, bowel wall thickening, and congestion occur. In *complicated* MI, thickened meconium and obstruction lead to complications such as: segmental volvulus, atresia, necrosis, perforation, meconium peritonitis (generalized), and giant meconium pseudocyst formation.

After birth, both simple and complicated MI should be managed as a newborn intestinal obstruction. Resuscitative measures including mechanical respiratory support, if necessary, and IV hydration are initiated along with gastric decompression, evaluation, and correction of any coagulation disorders and with empiric antibiotic coverage. When MI is suspected or diagnosed, immediate pediatric surgical consultation should be obtained.

### Clinical Presentation

*Simple* MI usually presents with abdominal distension at birth (Fig. 43-3). Failure to pass meconium, bilious vomiting, and progressive abdominal distention will eventually occur. Often, dilated loops of bowel become visible on exam and have a doughy character that indents on palpation. Typically, the rectum and anus are narrow, a finding which may be misinterpreted as anal stenosis.

*Complicated* MI presents more dramatically. At birth, severe abdominal distension with abdominal wall erythema and edema may be present. Abdominal distension may be so severe as to cause respiratory distress. Signs of peritonitis include tenderness, abdominal wall edema, distension, and clinical evidence of sepsis. A palpable mass may indicate pseudocyst formation. Often, the neonate needs urgent resuscitation and surgical exploration.

### Radiologic Features

Uncomplicated MI is characterized by a pattern of unevenly dilated loops of bowel on abdominal radiograph with variable presence of air-fluid levels (Fig. 43-4). As air mixes with the tenacious meconium, bubbles of gas may be seen. This soap bubble (Fig. 43-5) appearance depends on the viscosity of the meconium and is not a constant feature. However, this radiographic feature is pathognomonic and distinguishes

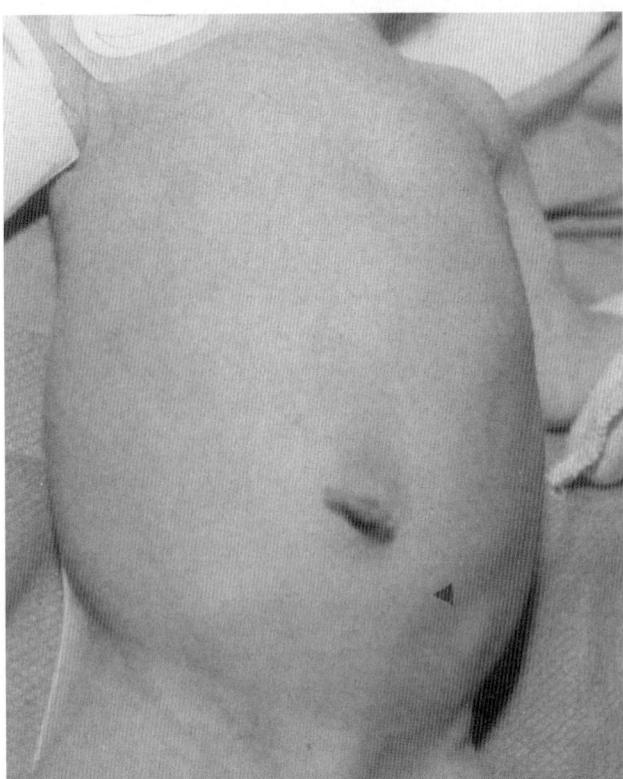

**FIGURE 43-3** Abdominal distension in an infant with MI. Note visible loops of bowel (Δ). (From *Irish MS, Gollin Y, Borowitz DS, et al. Meconium ileus: antenatal diagnosis and perinatal care. Fetal Matern Med Rev 2010;8:79–93*, with permission.)

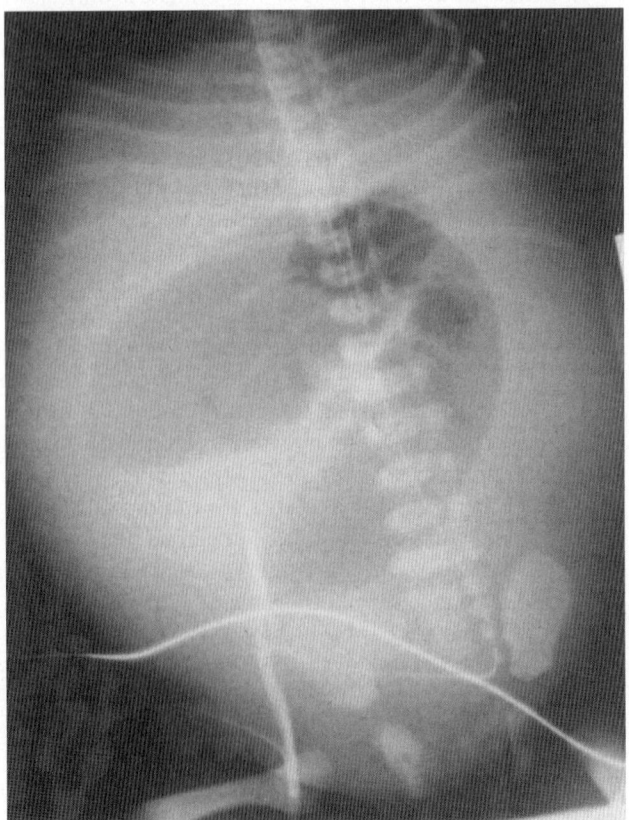

**FIGURE 43-4** Distended loop of ileum due to MI. (From *Irish MS, Gollin Y, Borowitz DS, et al. Meconium ileus: antenatal diagnosis and perinatal care. Fetal Matern Med Rev 2010;8:79–93*, with permission.)

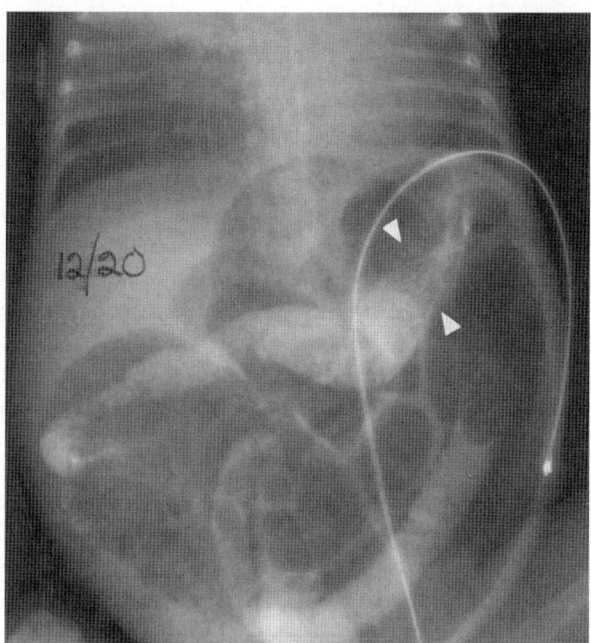

**FIGURE 43-5** "Soap bubble" appearance (Δ) of meconium mixed with water-soluble contrast material. (From *Irish MS, Gollin Y, Borowitz DS, et al. Meconium ileus: antenatal diagnosis and perinatal care. Fetal Matern Med Rev 2010;8:79–93*, with permission.)

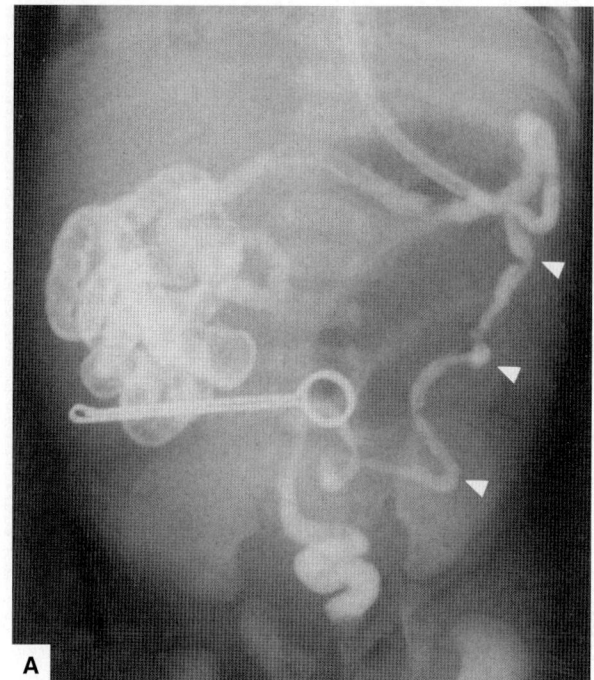

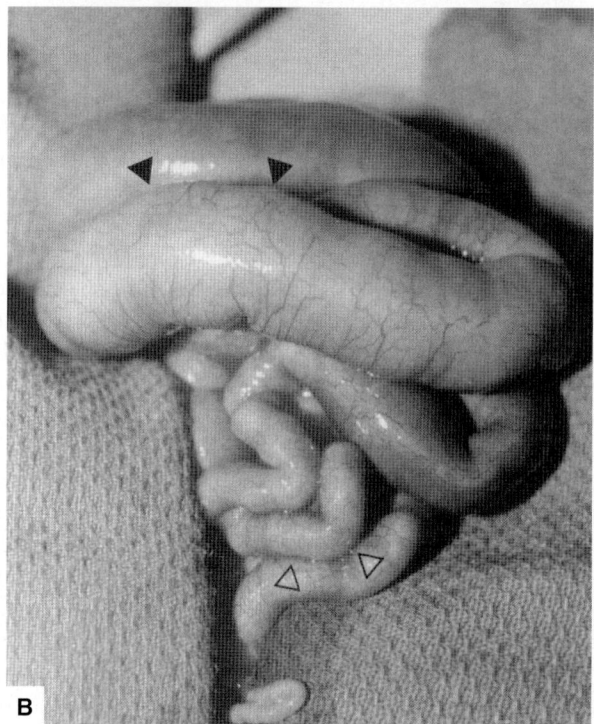

**FIGURE 43-6** "Microcolon of disuse" (Δ) (A) as seen on contrast enema radiography, and (B) at operation compared with dilated ileum (▲). (From *Irish MS, Gollin Y, Borowitz DS, et al. Meconium ileus: antenatal diagnosis and perinatal care. Fetal Matern Med Rev 2010;8:79–93*, with permission.)

MI from other causes of newborn intestinal obstruction. In a review of 58 neonates with CF and MI, Lang reported that 26% of neonates were found to have abdominal calcifications, although only half of this number were visible on plain radiograph. While each of these features alone is not diagnostic for MI, collectively, and with a family history of CF, they strongly suggest the diagnosis.

If MI is clinically and radiographically suspected, a contrast enema of barium may be performed for diagnosis, followed by a therapeutic Gastrografin® (Bracco Diagnostics Inc., Princeton, NJ) enema, if MI is likely. Some advocate water-soluble contrast initially for both diagnosis and treatment. In MI, contrast instillation is followed fluoroscopically and will demonstrate a colon of small caliber, described as the microcolon of disuse (Fig. 43-6A and B), often containing small "rabbit pellets" (scybala) of meconium (Fig. 43-7). Escobar found that 48% of neonates with CF and MI demonstrated microcolon on barium enema. Progression of the contrast proximally may also outline pellets of inspissated meconium. If contrast is successfully refluxed proximal to the obstruction, dilated loops of small bowel will be seen.

Radiologic findings in complicated MI vary with the complication. Speckled calcification seen on abdominal plain films is highly suggestive of intrauterine intestinal perforation and meconium peritonitis. A pseudocyst is suggested by radiographic findings of obstruction and a large dense mass with a rim of calcification. Historically, as many as one third of cases of complicated MI have no radiologic findings suggesting any complication. Furthermore, it is important to remember that in utero perforation (CF or non-CF related) can lead to meconium peritonitis or meconium pseudocyst formation. Therefore, in these situations, only intraoperative inspection may differentiate CF versus non-CF–related meconium peritonitis or meconium pseudocyst formation.

## Nonoperative Management

In 1969, Noblett introduced the use of enemas of Gastrografin® in treating 4 infants with MI. Gastrografin® is meglumine diatrizoate, a hyperosmolar, water-soluble, radiopaque solution

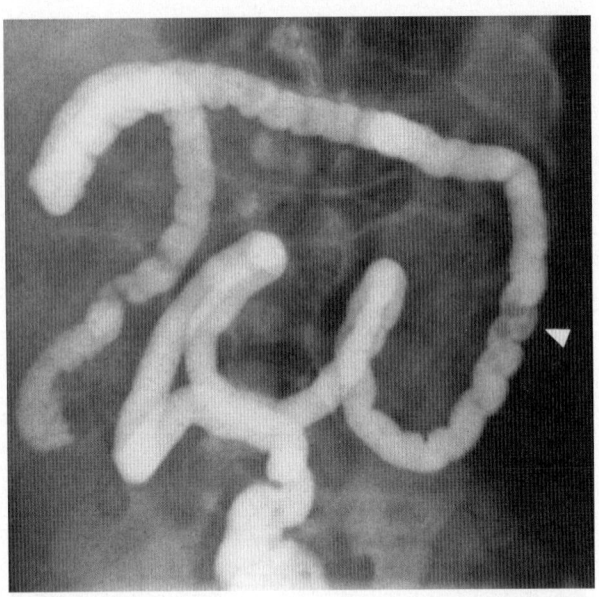

**FIGURE 43-7** "Rabbit pellets" or *scybala* (Δ). (From *Irish MS, Gollin Y, Borowitz DS, et al. Meconium ileus: antenatal diagnosis and perinatal care. Fetal Matern Med Rev 2010;8:79–93,* with permission.)

containing 0.1% polysorbate 80 (Tween 80), and 37% organically bound iodine. The osmolarity of the solution is 1900 mOsm/L. Upon instillation, fluid is drawn into the intestinal lumen, hydrating and softening the meconium mass. Both transient osmotic diarrhea and diuresis follow. Thus, adequate preenema resuscitation and hydration anticipating these fluid losses are paramount.

Under fluoroscopic control, a 25% to 50% solution of Gastrografin® is infused slowly at low hydrostatic pressure through a catheter inserted into the rectum. To minimize the risk of rectal perforation, balloon inflation is avoided. Upon completion, the catheter is withdrawn and an abdominal radiograph is obtained to rule out perforation. The infant is then returned to the neonatal care unit for intensive monitoring and fluid resuscitation. Warm saline enemas containing 4% N-acetylcysteine may be given to help complete the evacuation. Usually there is rapid passage of semi-liquid meconium, which continues in the ensuing 24 to 48 hours. Radiographs should be taken in 8 to 12 hours, or as clinically indicated, to confirm evacuation of the obstruction and to exclude late perforation. In the nonoperative management of MI, if evacuation is incomplete, or if the first attempt at Gastrografin® evacuation does not reflux contrast into dilated bowel, a second enema may be necessary. In a small study of very low birth weight infants, Shinohara concluded that reflux of the enema into the terminal ileum was essential for the bowel obstruction to be relieved. Serial Gastrografin® enemas can be performed at 12- to 24-hour intervals if necessary. However, if progressive distension, signs of peritonitis, or clinical deterioration occur, surgical exploration is indicated.

Following successful evacuation and resuscitation, we have used 5 mL of a 4% N-acetylcysteine solution be administered every 6 hours through a nasogastric (NG) tube to liquefy upper gastrointestinal (GI) secretions. Feedings, along with supplemental pancreatic enzyme replacement therapy (PERT) for those infants confirmed with CF, may be initiated

when signs of obstruction have subsided, usually within 48 hours. The success rate of patients with uncomplicated MI, treated with Gastrografin® enemas, historically range as high as 83%. Multiple contemporary studies report much lower success rates closer to 36% to 39%. Copeland and colleagues analyzed the reasons for reduced rates of success in a recent study. They hypothesized that surgeons are attempting few enemas per patient before transitioning to surgical treatment, some institutions are using enema solutions with lower osmolarity than Gastrografin® (thereby resulting in less effective meconium hydration due to decreased osmotic activity), and the enema attempts are less aggressive. Conversely, all of these help explain why the complication rates for Gastrografin® enema are decreasing.

Several potential complications exist with the use of hyperosmolar enemas in treating MI. The risk of rectal or colonic perforation can be avoided with careful placement of the catheter under fluoroscopic guidance and avoidance of inflating balloon-tipped catheters. A small study of 22 patients found a 23% perforation rate in patients when inflated balloon catheters were used. Copeland recently reported only a 2.7% perforation rate. Early perforation occurring during the administration of the enema is usually readily apparent under fluoroscopy. The risk of perforation increases with repeated enemas. Late perforation occurring between 12 and 48 hours following the enema can occur. Potential causes for late perforation include severe bowel distension by fluid osmotically drawn into the intestine or direct injury to the bowel mucosa by the contrast medium. The former appears to be the etiology in experimental models. Reports of delayed perforation associated with extensive bowel necrosis have been made. The pathogenesis of intestinal perforation associated with necrotizing enterocolitis is believed to be the ischemia produced by intestinal distension. Hypovolemic shock is a profound risk when delivering hypertonic enemas. Ischemia caused by overdistension is worsened by hypoperfusion caused by hypovolemia due to poor fluid resuscitation. Adequate fluid resuscitation (150 mL/kg/day, minimum) with anticipation of fluid losses due to osmotic diarrhea and diuresis is mandatory. Hepatotoxicity is a reported complication as well. The addition of 1% N-acetylcysteine added to the enema solution has been hypothesized to aid in dissolution of the inspissated meconium. Slow infusion carefully monitored under fluoroscopy is necessary.

## Operative Management

The prognosis for infants with MI was uniformly poor despite surgical treatment prior to 1948, when Hiatt and Wilson of Babies Hospital in New York reported the first successful surgical management of 5 infants with MI through intraoperative disimpaction of meconium with saline instilled into the bowel via a tube enterostomy (Fig. 43-8). In 1989, Fitzgerald proposed a similar technique in which an appendectomy is performed and a cecostomy catheter is placed through the appendiceal stump for insertion of irrigant and evacuation of impacted meconium (Fig. 43-9). Over the years, a number of surgical approaches in the treatment of uncomplicated MI have been proposed. Success rates with each of these methods have been variable. The approach to each infant should be

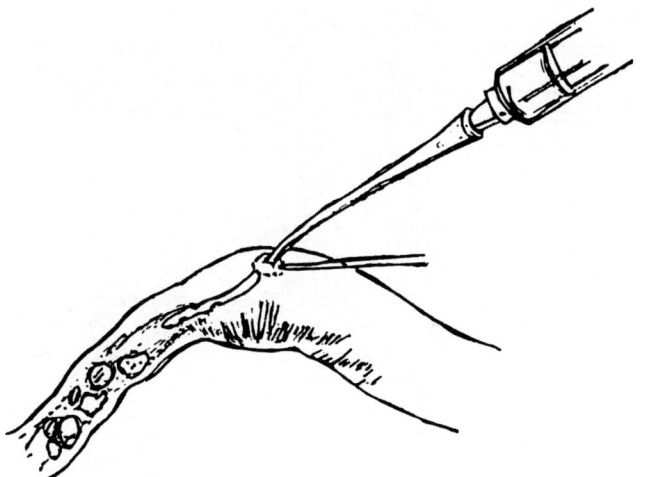

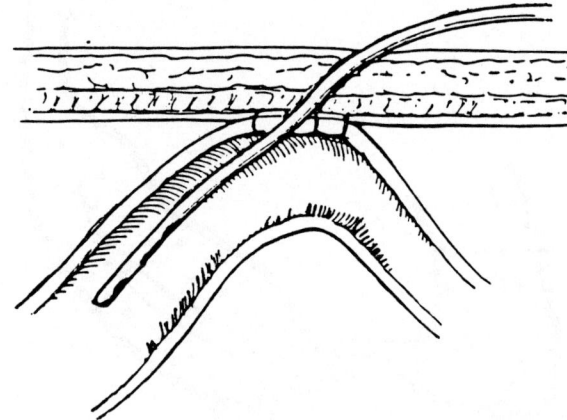

FIGURE 43-10 Technique of indwelling tube ileostomy for postoperative irrigation as described by O'Neill.

FIGURE 43-8 Technique of intraoperative irrigation of inspissated meconium via a tube enterostomy as described by Hiatt and Wilson.

individualized. The goal of operative management in simple, uncomplicated MI is evacuation of meconium from the intestine with preservation of maximal intestinal length.

Several variations upon the theme of Hiatt and Wilson's technique have involved placing indwelling ostomy tubes for purposes of postoperative bowel irrigation decompression, and/or feeding. In 1970, O'Neill described success with tube enterostomy with and without resection (Fig. 43-10). Harberg described a similar procedure in which a T-tube enterostomy is used (Fig. 43-11). The Harberg group later reported that 87% of MI resolved with T-tube placement and postoperative irrigation. In either situation, irrigations are begun on the first postoperative day and, after successful clearance of the obstruction (7-14 days), the tube may be removed and the enterocutaneous fistula allowed to spontaneously close.

Further surgical techniques have revolved around resection, anastomosis, and enterostomy through which postoperative irrigations can be delivered. The Mikulicz double-barreled

enterostomy (Fig. 43-12), first reported by Gross, has 3 distinct advantages. First, because complete evacuation of inspissated meconium is not necessary, operating and anesthetic times are reduced. Second, an intraabdominal anastomosis is avoided preventing the risk of anastomotic leakage. Third, the bowel can be opened following complete closure of the abdominal wound, thereby reducing the risk of intraperitoneal contamination. Following surgery, solubilizing agents can be given through both the proximal and distal limbs of the stoma as well as per rectum or via a NG tube. As classically described, a crushing clamp may be applied to the 2 limbs to create continuity for distal flow of intestinal fluids. Disadvantages of this and other procedures employing resection and stoma(s) are potential postoperative fluid losses through high-volume stomas, bowel shortening by resection, and the need for a second procedure to reestablish intestinal continuity.

A distal chimney enterostomy, described by Bishop and Koop (Fig. 43-13), involves resection with anastomosis between the end of the proximal segment and the side of the

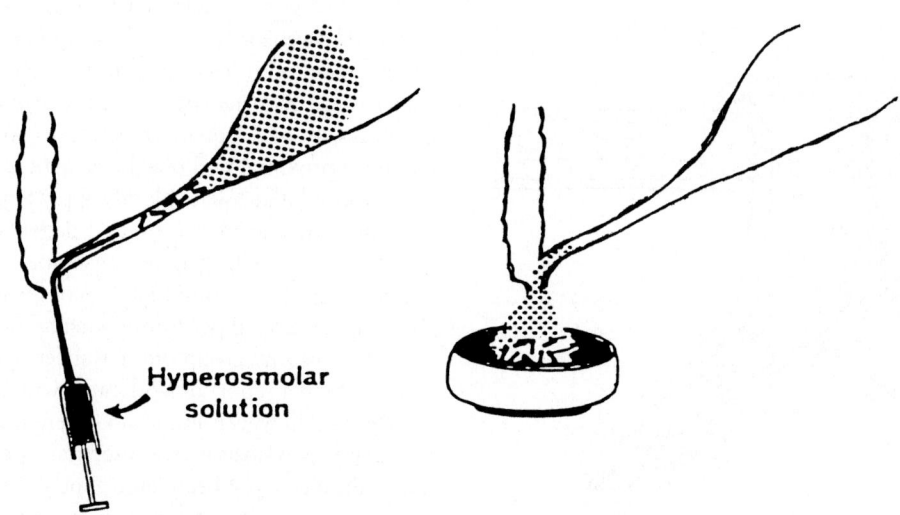

Hyperosmolar solution

FIGURE 43-9 Technique of intraoperative bowel irrigation and evacuation of meconium via the appendiceal stump as described by Fitzgerald.

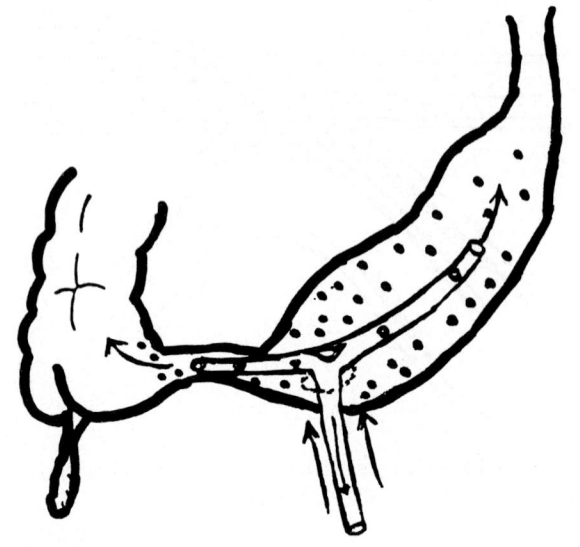

**FIGURE 43-11** Technique of indwelling T-tube ileostomy for postoperative irrigation as described by Harberg.

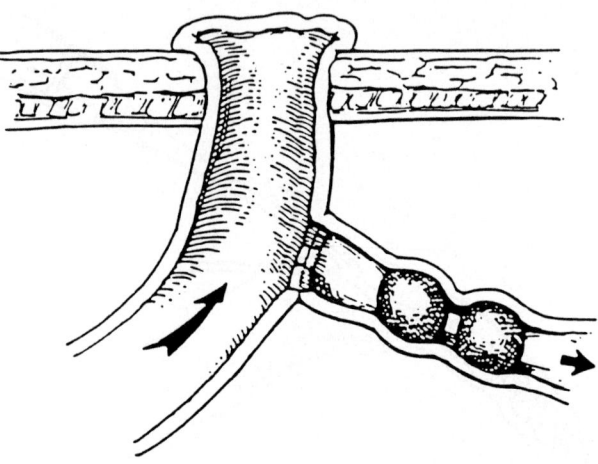

**FIGURE 43-14** Proximal enterostomy or *"reverse Bishop-Koop"* as described by Santulli.

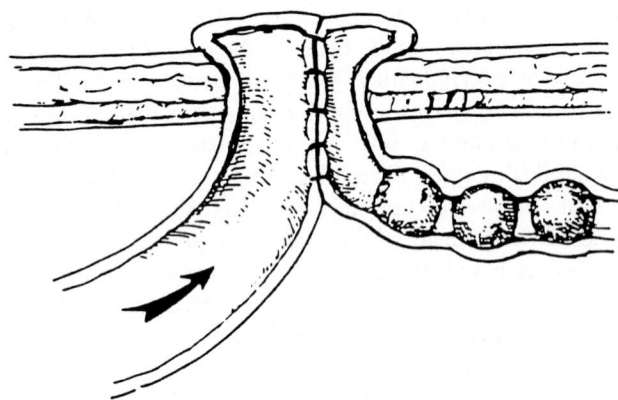

**FIGURE 43-12** The Mikulicz double-barreled enterostomy as described by Gross.

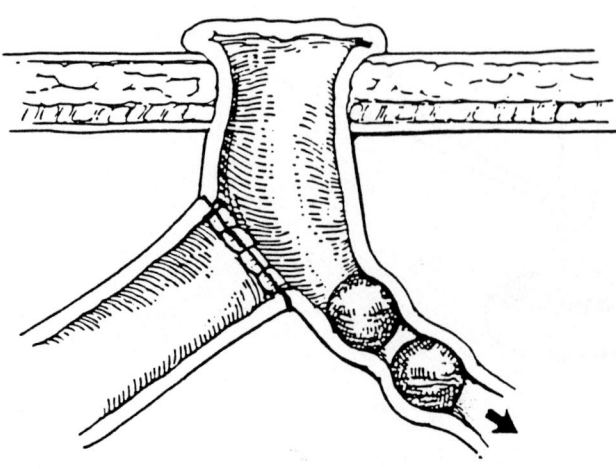

**FIGURE 43-13** The Bishop-Koop distal chimney enterostomy as described by Bishop.

distal segment of bowel approximately 4 cm from the opening of the distal segment. The open end is brought out as the ileostomy. This technique allows normal GI transit while providing a means for managing distal obstruction through the ileostomy should it occur. The reverse of the Bishop-Koop enterostomy is the proximal enterostomy described by Santulli in 1961 (Fig. 43-14). Here, following resection, the end of the distal limb is anastomosed to the side of the proximal limb. The end of the proximal limb is brought out as the enterostomy. With this arrangement, proximal irrigation and decompression is enhanced and it is not necessary to evacuate the proximal small bowel at the time of surgery. Like the distal chimney enterostomy, catheter access to the distal limb is placed, exiting through the stoma, thus providing means of irrigating the distal bowel. The apparent disadvantage with this technique is the presence of a high-output stoma and the inherent risk of dehydration. Care must be taken to replenish fluids, electrolytes, and nutrients in accordance with the stomal output. Reinstillation of stomal output from the proximal to the distal limb is often performed via the indwelling catheter.

Resection with primary anastomosis (Fig. 43-15), first suggested by Swenson in 1962, met with initial difficulty and complication with leakage from the anastomosis. Improved results were reported by later investigators that emphasize the necessity of adequate resection of compromised bowel, complete proximal and distal evacuation of meconium, and preservation of adequate blood supply to the anastomosis. In a recent study, Karimi reviewed 41 patients with MI and compared resection with primary anastomosis to resection with enterostomy. They found that 21% of the primary anastomosis group developed peritonitis whereas none of the resection with enterostomy group did. Jawaheer found a 31% complication rate in a report of MI treated with primary anastomosis. Del Pin, however, found no difference in morbidity with primary anastomosis versus resection with enterostomy. Thus far, studies have not been large enough to indisputably identify best practices for the surgical treatment of MI.

We prefer a modification of the technique originally described by Gross in 1953 in managing infants with

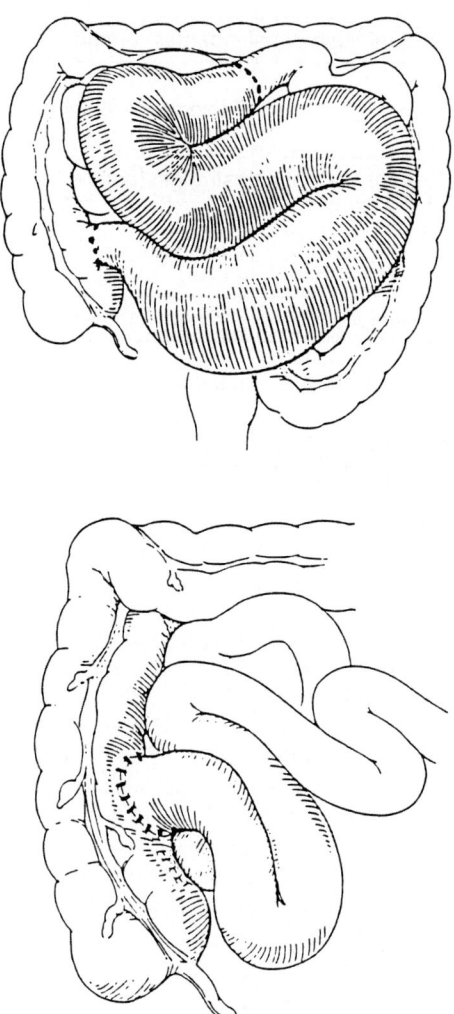

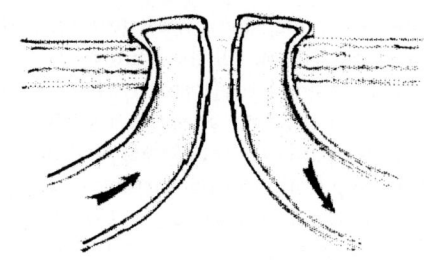

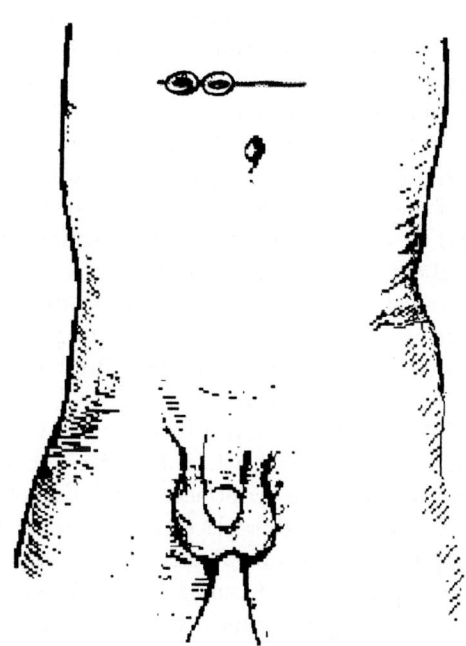

**FIGURE 43-15** Resection with primary anastomosis for meconium ileus as described by Swenson.

**FIGURE 43-16** The author's preferred method of side-by-side enterostomy when resection is necessary in the management of MI. Irrigating catheters may be inserted through either the proximal or distal stoma for irrigation, or through the distal stoma for feeding.

uncomplicated MI (Fig. 43-16). Celiotomy is performed. Upon exploration, the decision to create an enterotomy for irrigation and evacuation of the meconium, or, to resect the segment of impacted intestine, is made based on the viability and length of bowel involved. We then create side-by-side, separate enterostomies without creating a common wall (Fig. 43-16A). Stomas are placed within the abdominal incision to the right (Fig. 43-16B) and may be covered with a single ostomy collecting device. Postoperatively, each stoma may be irrigated to remove any residual meconium. Instillation of dilute enteral feedings high in glutamine, via the distal stoma, may also be performed to stimulate growth of the unused distal bowel. Intestinal continuity is generally restored within 6 to 12 weeks if bowel function has resumed, and the infant is tolerating oral feedings.

Surgery is always indicated in cases of complicated MI. Complications necessitating surgical management include persistent or worsening abdominal distension, persistent bowel obstruction, enlarging abdominal mass, intestinal atresia, volvulus, perforation, meconium cyst formation with peritonitis, and bowel necrosis. Resection is more often necessary in cases of complicated MI than with simple MI, and always requires temporary stomas.

## Postoperative Care

Initial postoperative management involves ongoing resuscitation. The fluid losses from preoperative diuresis and diarrhea, if Gastrografin® enema has been attempted, and from surgical losses must be carefully replaced. Ongoing maintenance fluids and replacement of insensible fluids, as well as GI losses (NG suction and ileostomy) must be adjusted accordingly. Instillation of 4% *N*-acetylcysteine via a NG tube or via ileostomy may help solubilize residual meconium. Stomas placed in the course of surgical management should be closed as soon as possible (6-12 weeks) to help avoid prolonged problems with fluid, electrolyte, and nutritional losses.

## POSTNATAL DIAGNOSIS OF CF

In the patient with fetal or neonatal bowel obstruction, CF must be suspected, and diagnostic tests should be performed as soon as possible. Patients should have the diagnosis of

CF confirmed or refuted by a sweat test performed using a technique, which meets all the Clinical and Laboratory Standards Institute standards (formerly NCCLS). Sweat tests may be performed any time after the first 48 hours of life, providing that the patient is not edematous. The test involves a transdermal application of pilocarpine to promote sweat gland secretion. The minimum amount of sweat needed is either 75 mg or 15 µL, depending on the technique used. This quantity may be difficult to obtain in young infants. Sweat should never be pooled from multiple sites to obtain the required quantity, since it is the rate of sweating that determines its volume and electrolyte content. A result of ≥60 mmol/L is considered diagnostic for CF, whereas results from 30 to 59 mmol/L are intermediate and ≤29 mmol/L is a negative result in a neonate. Patients with intermediate sweat test results on repeat exam and MI should be followed in a CF center. Mutation analysis, performed on buccal or blood cells, is useful in diagnosis if it yields 2 known CF-causing mutations. Patients with confirmed CF should be referred to the regional CF center or affiliate center for counseling and education about this complex, chronic disease. CF center physicians can also assist in the postoperative management of nutritional or respiratory problems. A listing of accredited centers can be obtained by calling 1-800-FIGHT CF, or from the Internet at *www.cff.org.*

Although MI is almost always associated with pancreatic insufficiency in patients with CF, a definitive test of pancreatic function should be performed. In practice, the fecal elastase (FE) test has mostly replaced the classic coefficient of fat absorption test based on a timed stool collection and measurement of fat intake. FE can be done on a small quantity of stool from a single specimen passed per rectum. Thus, patients with complex MI and an ostomy may not be able to have FE performed. Patients with CF and MI should be presumed to have pancreatic insufficiency and treatment with PERT should not be withheld while awaiting definitive evidence of PI. However, FE should be performed once bowel continuity has been restored; results are reliable even in a patient taking PERT.

## Nutritional Management

Infants with uncomplicated MI and CF may be given breast milk or routine infant formula, PERT, and vitamins. Those who have a complicated surgical course will require either continuous enteral feedings or TPN. We recommend the use of predigested infant formula (Alimentum®, Abbott Nutrition, Columbus, OH, or Pregestimil®, Mead Johnson, Glenview, IL) for enterally fed infants. Prestenotic dilation of the small bowel caused by the obstructing meconium theoretically may lead to mucosal damage, which could contribute to poor peristalsis, malabsorption, and/or bacterial overgrowth. Patients who have had complicated MI and/or sizeable bowel resection and are being fed enterally may tolerate continuous feedings better than bolus feedings. As the bowel mucosa may or may not be damaged by stasis, feedings are begun with predigested, diluted, formula, usually one half strength and at low volume (Fig. 43-17). If this is well tolerated, strength may be increased and then the volume, while observing for signs of feeding intolerance

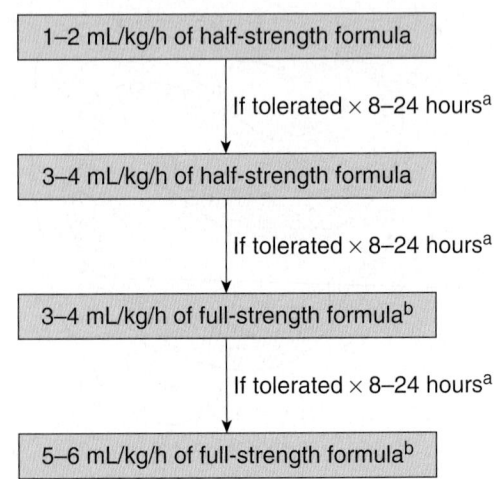

**FIGURE 43-17** One possible protocol for feeding babies s/p repair for complicated MI. [a]"Tolerated" = no abdominal distention, no heme positive stools, no emesis. [b]Once the infant is taking full-strength formula, begin pancreatic enzyme supplements. The dose of enzymes is 2000 to 5000 lipase units per 120 mL. For example, a 2.5-kg infant receiving 4 mL/kg/h formula could get one half Creon 6 capsule PO every 12 hours. Adjust the dosing interval within reason to fit in a 24-hour period. *Capsules contain enteric-coated microspheres, which should not be crushed.* The microspheres should be mixed in a tiny amount of applesauce and given orally. Even newborn infants can learn to take enzymes orally. Prescribe Desitin ointment (zinc oxide) to prevent perianal skin breakdown when starting pancreatic enzymes. Nurses should check to be sure microspheres do not remain in the mouth where they can cause mucosal breakdown.

(ie, abdominal distention, heme-positive stools, and/or increasing emesis). Once oral feedings are begun, PERT must be given orally (even with predigested formula) starting at the historical recommendation of 2000 to 4000 lipase units per 120 mL of full-strength formula. For example, a 2.5-kg infant receiving 4 mL/kg/h formula could be given one half Creon 6® capsule (6000 lipase units per capsule) PO every 12 hours. Other low-dose brands approved by the Food and Drug Administration (FDA) include Zenpep 5® and Pancreaze 4®. Capsules containing enteric-coated microspheres can be opened and the contents mixed with applesauce (Fig. 43-18). This is then given orally. The microcapsules should not be crushed, as this will expose the enzymes to the acid of the stomach where they will be inactivated. Uncrushed pancreatic enzymes should be given even with MCT-oil–containing formulas. Desitin® ointment (zinc oxide) can be applied to perianal skin to prevent skin breakdown.

Infants who have had significant bowel resection (greater than one third) may be difficult to manage, especially if the ileocecal valve has been resected. In addition, the presence of an ileostomy may lead to excessive loss of fluid and sodium. Patients with CF and an enterostomy have the double burden of excessive sweat and intestinal sodium losses and may have a total body sodium deficit. Urine sodium should be measured in infants with ileostomies especially when there is failure to grow, even if serum sodium levels are normal. Those with urinary sodium to

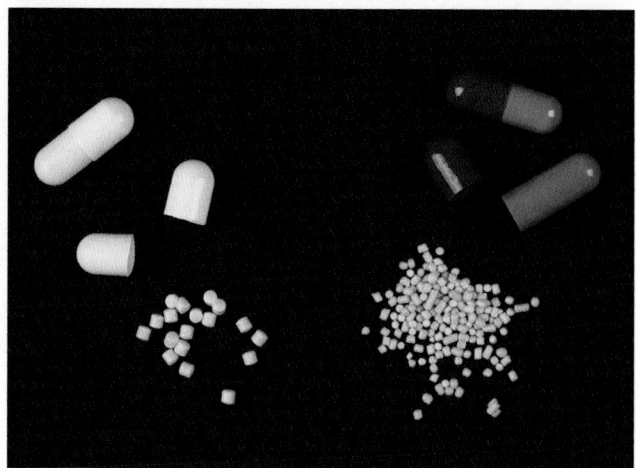

**FIGURE 43-18** Currently FDA-approved low-dose pancreatic enzyme microtablets (*left*) and microspheres (*right*).

creatinine ratio less than 17 will need sodium (and possibly bicarbonate) supplementation. Ostomies should be taken down as soon as possible. In the interim, if access to the distal, defunctionalized bowel is feasible, ostomy-drip feeds of glutamine-enriched formula may be given at low volumes to enhance bowel growth, to help prevent bacterial translocation, and to minimize TPN-associated hepatic injury. Infants with MI are at risk for cholestasis, particularly if they have had or are receiving TPN. Although neonatal cholestasis and later CF-related liver disease are different entities, Colombo found that 35% of patients with CF and MI had liver disease whereas only 12% of patients with CF *without* MI had liver disease. Alkaline phosphatase, alanine aminotransferase (ALT), aspartate aminotransferase (AST), and bilirubin should be monitored weekly.

Gastric acid hypersecretion is seen in patients who have short bowel syndrome. An acid intestinal environment inactivates pancreatic enzymes and prevents dissolution of enteric-coated microcapsules. Proton pump inhibitors or histamine-2 receptor blockers may be used as an adjunct to pancreatic enzyme therapy in patients who have had significant bowel resections. Recent work in patients without CF shows that there may be a role for growth hormone, insulin-like growth factor, epidermal growth factor, and other hormones in the treatment of short bowel syndrome.

## Pulmonary Management

Although clinical lung disease does not usually develop early, mucus plugging and atelectasis can be seen. Vigorous prophylactic pulmonary care with chest physiotherapy is initiated immediately postoperatively. The head-down position should not be used as this may increase the risk of gastroesophageal reflux and aspiration. Infants should receive inhaled albuterol twice a day followed by chest physiotherapy. Prophylactic antibiotics are not necessary and antibiotic therapy is directed on the basis of respiratory tract cultures if needed. If aminoglycosides are given, the dose is likely to be higher than in other patients (up to twice as high per dose). We recommend beginning with

gentamicin 2.5 mg/kg/dose, checking serum levels after the fourth dose, and tailoring subsequent dosage accordingly. Each increase of 1 mg/kg dose should increase peak serum levels by 1.75 mg/L.

## PROGNOSIS

Early series, subsequent to Hiatt and Wilson's report of the first survivors with MI in 1948, showed mortality rates of 50% to 67%. With the advent of improved nonoperative and operative treatments, good nutritional support, and better treatment of bacterial infection, the prognosis for infants with both complicated and simple MI has improved dramatically. Survival rates of near or at 100% have been reported. On the whole, once infants are discharged from the hospital, they do well. Long-term follow-up of patients with MI done in the modern era shows pulmonary function and nutritional status (as measured by weight and length) at age 15 years to be no different between those born with MI and those without MI.

## CONCLUSION

Advances in the perinatal diagnosis and management of both MI and CF as well as our understanding of the CFTR protein have vastly improved the outlook of affected infants. Continued success in the management of these patients will depend on prenatal diagnosis, multidisciplinary care, and innovative strategies in therapy. The goals for the future should thus include exploration of new ways to reduce perinatal complications, which add to morbidity, mortality, and the cost of medical care. With the ability to detect both MI and CF prenatally, we should begin to consider strategies that can prevent the progression of simple MI to complex MI. We have, with the creation of mouse, ferret, and pig models for CF, a unique opportunity to study the basic pathophysiology of MI. This should enable us to develop and prospectively evaluate new treatments for this disorder. In the future, prenatal interventions may even prevent MI.

### SELECTED READINGS

Anderson D. Cystic fibrosis of the pancreas and its relationship to celiac disease. *Am J Dis Child* 1938;56:344–399.

Bishop H, Koop C. Management of meconium ileus: resection, Roux-en-Y anastomosis and ileostomy irrigation with pancreatic enzymes. *Ann Surg* 1957;145(3):410–414.

Blackman SM, Deering-Brose R, McWilliams R, et al. Relative contribution of genetic and nongenetic modifiers to intestinal obstruction in cystic fibrosis. *Gastroenterology* 2006;131(4):1030–1039.

Buchanan D, Rapoport S. Chemical comparison of normal meconium and meconium from patients with meconium ileus. *Pediatrics* 1952;9(3):304–310.

Del Pin CA, Czyrko C, Ziegler MM, Scanlin TF, Bishop HC. Management and survival of meconium ileus. A 30-year review. *Ann Surg* 1992;215(2):179–185.

Donnison AB, Shwachman H, Gross RE. A review of 164 children with meconium ileus seen at the Children's Hospital Medical Center, Boston. *Pediatrics* 1966;37(5):833–850.

Escobar MA, Grosfeld JL, Burdick JJ, et al. Surgical considerations in cystic fibrosis: a 32-year evaluation of outcomes. *Surgery* 2005;138(4): 560–572.

Guilbault C, Saeed Z, Downey GP, Radzioch D. Cystic fibrosis mouse models. *Am J Respir Cell Mol Biol* 2007;36(1):1–7.

Johnson JA, Bush A, Buchdahl R. Does presenting with meconium ileus affect the prognosis of children with cystic fibrosis? *Pediatr Pulmonol* 2010;45(10):951–958.

Kerem B, Rommens JM, Buchanan JA, et al. Identification of the cystic fibrosis gene: genetic analysis. *Science* 1989;245(4922):1073–1080.

Mak GZ, Harberg FJ, Hiatt P, et al. T-tube ileostomy for meconium ileus: four decades of experience. *J Pediatr Surg* 2000;35(2):349–352.

Noblett HR. Treatment of uncomplicated meconium ileus by gastrografin enema: a preliminary report. *J Pediatr Surg* 1969;4(2):190–197.

Quinton PM. Role of epithelial $HCO_3$ transport in mucin secretion: lessons from cystic fibrosis. *Am J Physiol Cell Physiol* 2010;299(6): C1222–C1233.

Scotet V, Duquépéroux I, Audrézet MP, et al. Focus on cystic fibrosis and other disorders evidenced in fetuses with sonographic finding of echogenic bowel: 16-year report from Brittany, France. *Am J Obstet Gynecol* 2010;203(6):1–6.

# CHAPTER 44 | Hirschsprung Disease

*Daniel H. Teitelbaum, Mark L. Wulkan,*
*Keith E. Georgeson, and Jacob C. Langer*

## KEY POINTS

1. Diagnoses are typically made with suction rectal biopsy, however, when a full-thickness biopsy is needed, it is important to carefully determine your distance from the dentate line. This insures an accurate ruling in or out of Hirschsprung disease.

2. A colostomy may be needed in those with severe enterocolitis or those with a delayed diagnosis and very dilated colon. In those cases, a laparoscopic inspection of the abdomen can often facilitate the identification of the transition zone, and placement of the initial incision (see later in chapter for laparoscopic leveling biopsies).

3. The decision to perform an open versus laparoscopic-assisted or transanal pull-through probably does not affect the long-term results of the infant. Thus, the approach that the surgeon is most familiar with should be selected.

4. For total colonic Hirschsprung disease either a standard Duhamel or endorectal pull-through is acceptable, and associated with similar outcomes.

## INTRODUCTION

The first therapeutic approach to Hirschsprung disease was described by Harold Hirschsprung, himself. He performed a diverting colostomy in one of the first children he recognized with the disease itself. Over the past 100 years, tremendous advancements in the approach to this disease process have occurred. Figure 44-1 summarizes in a diagrammatic fashion some of the more commonly performed procedures in the historical development of the surgical correction of Hirschsprung disease. While many of these techniques have been retained, the dominate approach in the last decade has been the endorectal pull-through and the Duhamel approach. The chapter will thus concentrate on these operations.

## DIAGNOSIS

### Rectal Biopsy

#### Indications

The suction rectal biopsy has become the gold standard for the diagnosis of Hirschsprung disease. However, in some patients, particularly those over 4 years of age, the thick mucosal layer prevents the biopsy of sufficient submucosal tissue to make a definitive diagnosis of aganglionosis. Although it is worth attempting a suction rectal biopsy first in such patients, the diagnostic yield decreases with increased age. In other cases, a full-thickness biopsy is indicated for the child in whom there has been more than 1 indeterminate suction rectal biopsy. Although one would think that performing a full-thickness biopsy may preclude or increase the difficulty of an endorectal pull-through, the author has not found this to be the case.

#### Preoperative Preparation

No formal bowel prep is required, as this often causes excess loose stool to run into the operative field. The child's rectum is irrigated with saline at the beginning of the procedure, followed by the placement of a sponge into the proximal rectal vault to prevent stool from entering the operative field. A single dose of preoperative broad-spectrum cephalosporin is given.

#### Operative Technique

The patient is placed in the lithotomy position. The buttocks are at the very end of the bed, supported with a folded towel. The feet are placed together (plantar surfaces adjoined) with a cotton roll, and both legs are suspended on an ether screen with the lower extremities flexed at the hips (Fig. 44-2). In older patients standard stirrups are quite adequate.

Digital dilatation is followed by placement of 2 narrow anal retractors. The posterior aspect of the dentate line is identified and marked with a polyglycolic acid suture (3-0), which is used for traction. Two additional sutures are placed on the posterior wall of the rectum, at 1.5 to 2 cm and 3 cm proximal to the dentate line (Fig. 44-3). The needle should be retained on the proximal suture, and this one should be tied and kept long, as it will be used to close the defect.

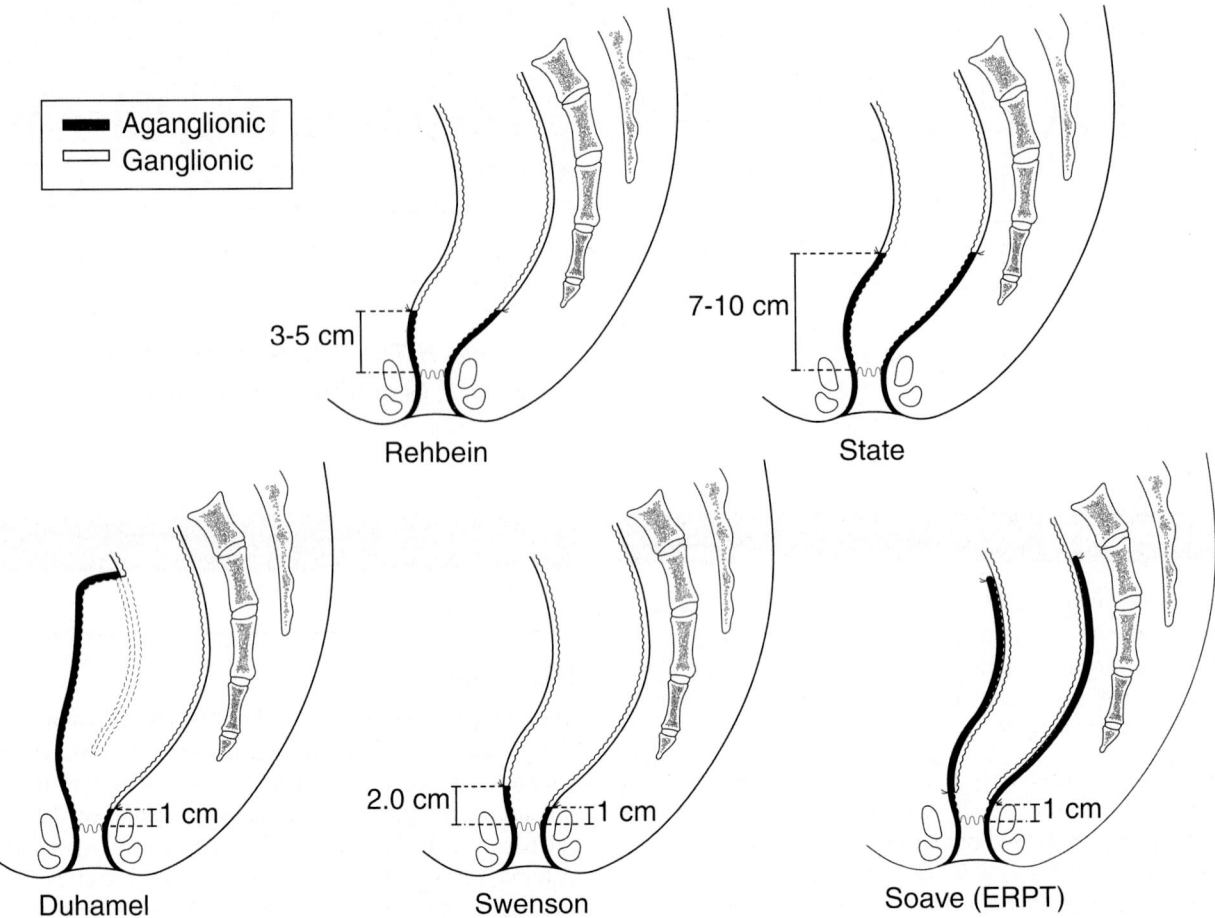

**FIGURE 44-1** Schematic illustrations of several operative pull-through techniques for the treatment of Hirschsprung disease.

The surgeon's nondominate hand holds the middle silk suture. Using a sharp curved scissors, a full-thickness incision is made on the posterior rectal wall centered on the middle suture. This can be done with 2 diagonally placed cuts around this middle traction suture, each sweeping around one half of the tissue suspended by the middle suture. Once this is done the scissors can be placed in the presacral space and gently spread. Bleeding can slightly obstruct the view at this point, however, by maintaining traction on the middle suture. The specimen is inspected and delivered off the table (Fig. 44-4).

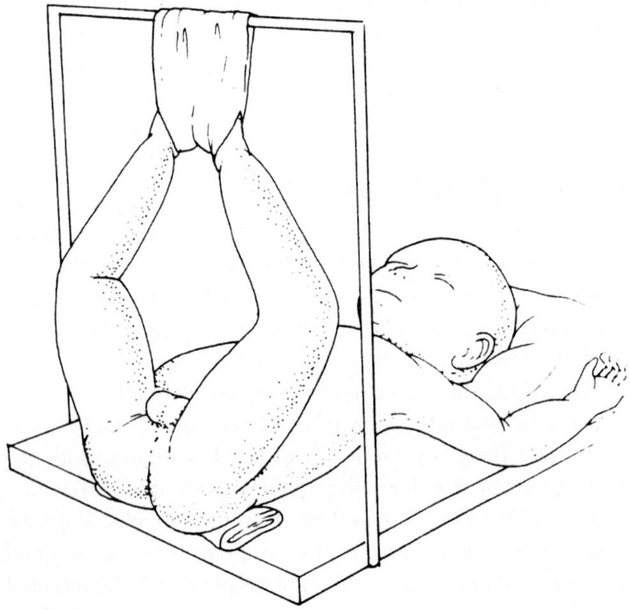

The rectal defect is closed in a running fashion using the most superiorly placed suture. Hemostasis is achieved fairly quickly once a few of these sutures have been placed. In general, this procedure can be done as an outpatient. Postoperatively, the patient is watched for bleeding and if stable may be discharged home after the procedure. It is also important to remember that the diagnosis of Hirschsprung disease can also be made by performing such a biopsy, but only carrying the incision through the submucosa and avoiding all of the muscularis propria.

## Leveling Colostomy

### Treatment Options

Although a right transverse colostomy has been advocated by some surgeons as the initial procedure, we prefer a leveling colostomy. This allows for the determination of the aganglionic level at the time of the colostomy, facilitating the subsequent pull-through. As well, placement of a leveling colostomy allows the proximal bowel to grow, which will

**FIGURE 44-2** Dorsal lithotomy "suspension" position for an infant rectal biopsy.

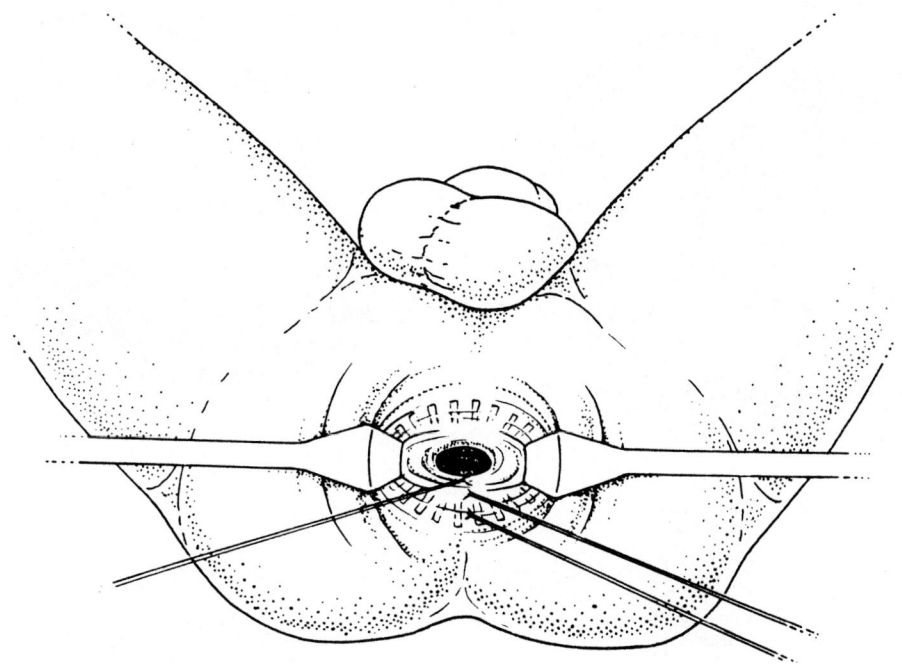

**FIGURE 44-3** Traction sutures 1 and 2 cm proximal to the dentate line.

stretch the mesentery and may simplify the subsequent pull-through. Finally, this colostomy can be closed during the pull-through avoiding a third operation. Placement of the ostomy is just proximal to the transition zone. The incision is generally an oblique one in the left lower quadrant. If the level of aganglionosis is not readily apparent, this incision can be extended, transversely, across the midline. Despite a trend toward primary pull-through in the neonatal period, a decompressing colostomy is the recommended procedure for the child with either severe enterocolitis or those patients who present in a delayed manner with markedly dilated bowel. A laparoscopic inspection of the abdomen can often facilitate the identification of the transition zone, and placement of the initial incision (see later in chapter for laparoscopic leveling biopsies).

## Preoperative Preparation

Essentially, only the diagnosis of aganglionosis is needed. The infant should receive serial rectal washouts (10 mL/kg volume for each washout) administered through a large caliber (18-20 Fr in an infant) rectal tube. The patient should be placed on broad-spectrum, intravenous antibiotics, but no formal bowel prep is required. These washouts should not be treated as enemas. The catheter for the washouts must remain in the proximal bowel, ideally above the aganglionic portion, and used to decompress the bowel.

## Operative Technique

Once the peritoneum is entered, an attempt should be made to define a transition zone. Note that the bowel proximal to the transition zone is dilated and has a diffuse hypertrophy

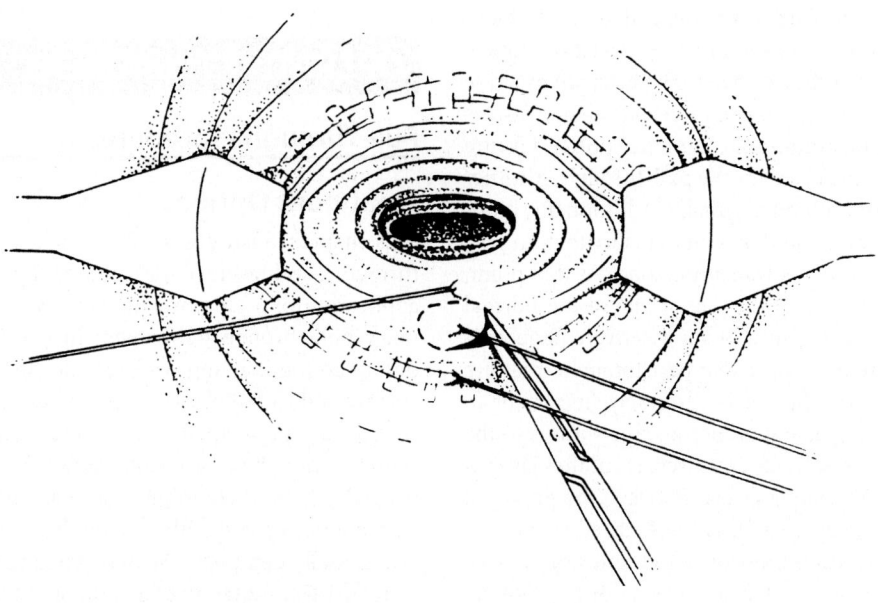

**FIGURE 44-4** Full-thickness rectal biopsy.

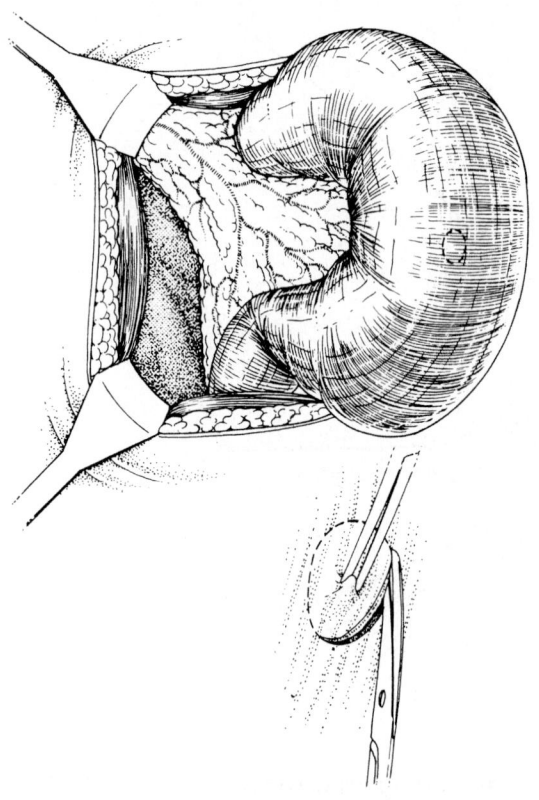

**FIGURE 44-5** "Open" seromuscular colon biopsy to level the area of ganglion cells.

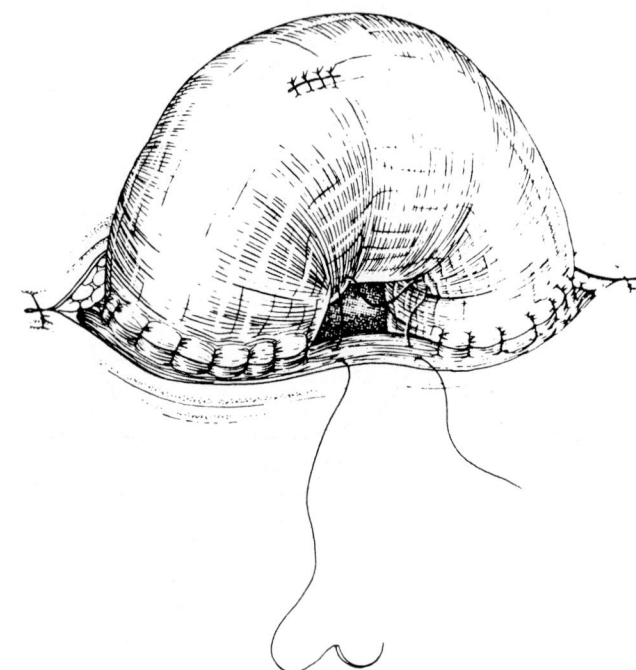

**FIGURE 44-6** Creation of a loop colostomy at the site proven to have ganglion cells.

of the muscular layer with no clearly distinguishable tinea. Occasionally in neonates, such a transition cannot be made. If this is the case, a good starting point for a seromuscular biopsy is just above the peritoneal reflection (Fig. 44-5).

A fine sharp scissors is used to make an incision only through the seromuscular layers. The muscular layer, which is fairly thick even in the aganglionic section, makes this dissection fairly easy. Blunt dissection is used to strip off the muscle. In general, a 0.5 × 0.5 cm biopsy is taken and interrupted silk sutures are placed to close the biopsy site (Fig. 44-5, *inset*).

Each biopsy is sent for frozen section, progressively moving more proximal until both ganglion cells as well as a loss of hypertrophied nerve bundles are seen. Hypertrophied nerve bundles, despite the presence of ganglion cells, demonstrates that one is still in the transition zone, and may portend future problems if this level is selected for the pull-through. Another biopsy should be taken more proximally. Additionally, biopsies from all 4 quadrants should be sent to insure that no portion of the diameter contains transition zone. At this point, a loop colostomy is created at the site of one of the normal biopsy sites (Fig. 44-6). Because of the relatively large caliber of the bowel, stomal prolapse and peristomal hernias are common complications. Thus, it is extremely important to begin the colostomy by placing numerous fine sutures to the peritoneum and transversalis fascia as well as another layer of sutures to the external oblique fascia. Between the proximal and distal loops of bowel, a stitch is then placed starting at the fascia and then to each limb of bowel and finally back to fascia; a maneuver often referred to as a "Bishop Stitch." The stomal maturation is performed by simple eversion of the

mucosa to the dermis. If no transition is found and the first few biopsies are aganglionic, it is usually beneficial to perform an appendectomy early in the course of these biopsies. Aganglionosis of the appendix indicates the presence of total colonic Hirschsprung disease.

## Postoperative Care

The stoma usually begins to work within 24 hours, and feedings can begin on the first postoperative day if there is no history of enterocolitis. It is occasionally helpful to perform intermittent dilatations of the proximal ostomy. These dilatations will prevent narrowing of the opening and allow the dilated proximal colon to return to normal size.

## OPERATIVE TREATMENT

### Pull-Through Procedures

#### Treatment Options

This chapter illustrates the Duhamel, Soave (endorectal pull-through), and Swenson procedures (Fig. 44-1), as well as the application of a laparoscopic-assisted pull-through and primary pull-through performed through the perineum without an abdominal approach. The techniques are modified to correspond to the most current manner in which these procedures are performed. Controversy arises as to which procedure yields the best results. However, long-term outcomes with all of the 3 techniques are basically similar as long as they are performed with a meticulous technique. Because an occasionally complex case may demand one modifying their standard technique, the surgeon should be familiar with all of these techniques, but use 1 technique as their primary procedure. This is the only way that one can develop consistently good results.

## Duhamel

The Duhamel technique was advanced in 1956 to avoid the tedious pelvic dissection of the Swenson procedure. The advantage of the procedure is that very little manipulation of the rectum is performed anteriorly, so that the autonomic nervous plexus to the genitourinary system is preserved. The procedure has undergone several modifications, the most important of which was the use of an automatic stapling device. The procedure is fairly straightforward and continues to be popular today. Despite the procedure's relative simplicity, several key technical points must be followed. As with other pull-through procedures, ganglionic bowel is brought down to within 1 cm above the dentate line.

### Preoperative Preparation

The child usually has a leveling colostomy, which was placed several months previously. This serves to decompress the bowel and return it to normal caliber. The operation is generally performed when the child is 6 to 12 months of age with a weight of 10 kg. More recently, a primary Duhamel pull-through has been performed with good results (see later in chapter). The child undergoes a mechanical bowel prep as well as receiving oral antibiotics. Care must be taken to give adequate rectal and colonic washouts as stool is often inspissated in the distal rectum. It is necessary to do a rectal examine on the child prior to the pull-through to insure that no residual stool is present.

### Operative Technique

A nasogastric tube is placed after induction of anesthesia. The child is placed in a supine position, the entire patient is prepped circumferentially from the abdomen to the feet. Stockinets are placed around each foot and a Foley catheter is placed after the patient has been prepped and draped. Alternatively, the child can be placed in stirrups or on skis (Fig. 44-7). Excellent exposure can be found with assistants

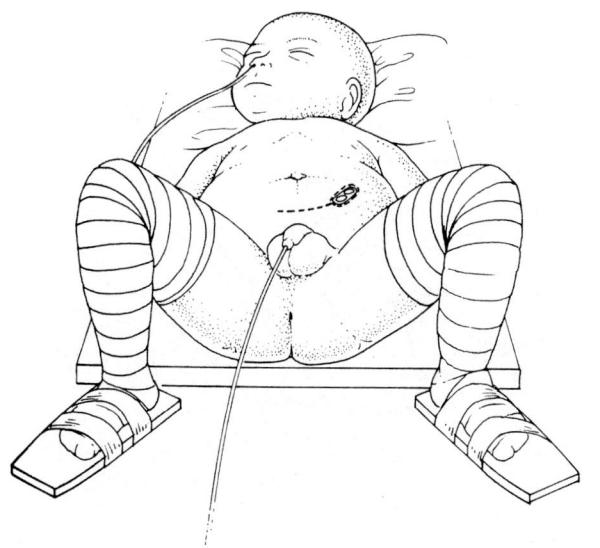

**FIGURE 44-7** Dorsal lithotomy positioning on skis.

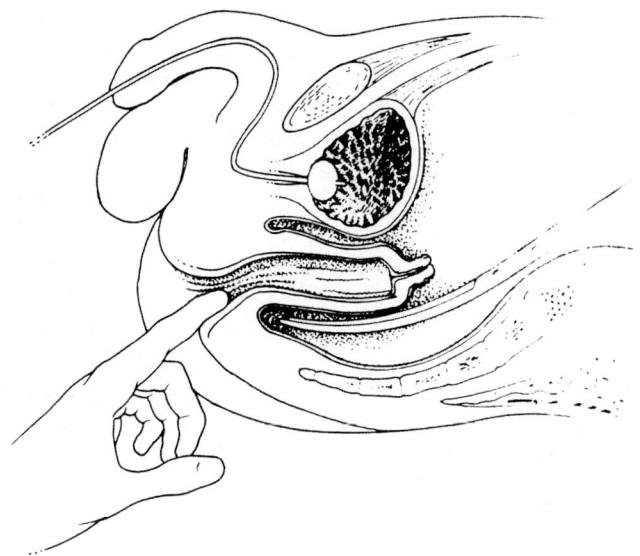

**FIGURE 44-8** Development of the retrorectal space for the Duhamel pull-through.

supporting and flexing the lower extremities at the hips during the anal anastomosis. A hockey stick or oblique incision is made incorporating the colostomy takedown. The bowel is mobilized proximal to the former colostomy and the splenic flexure is taken down, if necessary, to ensure adequate length for the pull-through. In general, the colon must reach to the level of the perineum when drawn over the child's pubis with only modest tension. Occasionally, the mesentery is foreshortened and it is necessary to ligate the inferior mesenteric artery at the aortic root. By preserving the remainder of the arcades, the bowel should maintain its viability. The ureter is carefully identified and the peritoneal reflection between the rectum and bladder is incised. The distal rectum is mobilized for approximately 4 cm below the reflection. The colostomy site is then removed.

A retrorectal space is created, with dissection carried out directly in the posterior midline. This dissection is carried down to the pelvic floor so that an assistant's finger can be felt when inserted no further than 1 to 1.5 cm into the anus. Dissection can be facilitated with a narrow towel clamp, as shown, but is usually very easily performed with the surgeon's index finger (Fig. 44-8).

Once the retrorectal dissection is done, redundant aganglionic bowel is resected down to peritoneal reflection with an automatic stapling device. Tacking sutures are placed on both left and right sides of this bowel so that it can be retracted anteriorly during the pull-through (Fig. 44-9). The ganglionic bowel is labeled mesenteric and antimesenteric with a separate undyed Vicryl suture (turns a red color as the bowel is pulled through) and silk suture, respectively. This allows the surgeon working on the pulled through segment to maintain correct orientation of the bowel as it is pulled into the anus.

At this point, the surgeon's attention is directed to the perineum. Both legs are drawn upward allowing a clear view of the anus. Narrow anal retractors are placed and held in position by 2 assistants. No separate field is created, which allows improved communication and keeps the surgeon

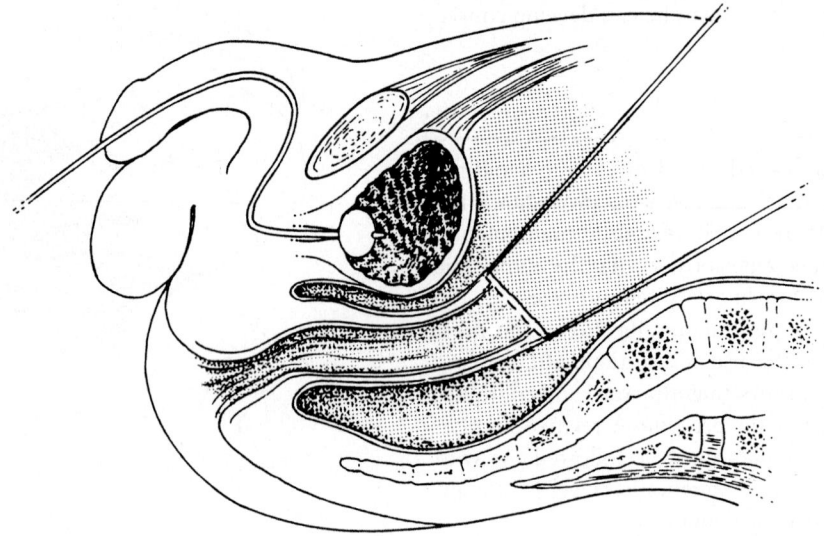

**FIGURE 44-9** Traction sutures suspend the distal rectum in preparation for the retrorectal pull-through.

and assistant within the same operative field. It is generally not found necessary to have 2 completely different set-ups. However, one should treat all of the instruments used in the perineal portion of the procedure as dirty and change gloves at the end of the anastomosis.

Using cautery, a full-thickness incision is made 1 to 1.5 cm proximal to the dentate line, posteriorly. Care is taken to maintain this distance by curving the incision as one moves laterally in each direction. Three 4-0 polyglycolic sutures are placed on the inferior aspect of this incision, 1 in the midline and 1 each on both left and right sides; needles are left on the sutures for eventual creation of an anastomosis. Sutures are directed from the mucosal side to the retrorectal space. This is done so that the suture needle can later be directed from the serosal surface of the ganglionic bowel, once it is pulled through. Three additional absorbable (4-0 polyglycolic) sutures are placed on the upper portion of this incision in similar positions. Each suture is held in position with hemostats. Use of dyed and undyed suture types prevents confusion of orientation once the ganglionic bowel is pulled through.

The surgeon operating on the anus inserts a long ring clamp into the retrorectal space toward the abdominal field (Fig. 44-10).

The 2 tacking sutures on the distal ganglionic bowel are fed into this clamp and are pulled down. The surgeon remaining in the abdominal field makes sure that the bowel does not rotate as it is brought down (Fig. 44-11).

Once the bowel is pulled through, the staple line is excised on the anterior half of the colon (Fig. 44-12) and a single-layered anastomosis is created starting with the 3 previously placed polyglycolic sutures (Figs. 44-13 and 44-14). Care is taken with each stitch so that the anterior wall of the anorectum is not incorporated into any of the sutures. Once the anterior half is anastomosed, the remainder of the staple line is excised and the anastomosis completed (Fig. 44-15).

An extra long automatic stapling device (80 mm, 3.5-mm thick staples) is placed with 1 arm in the native anal canal and

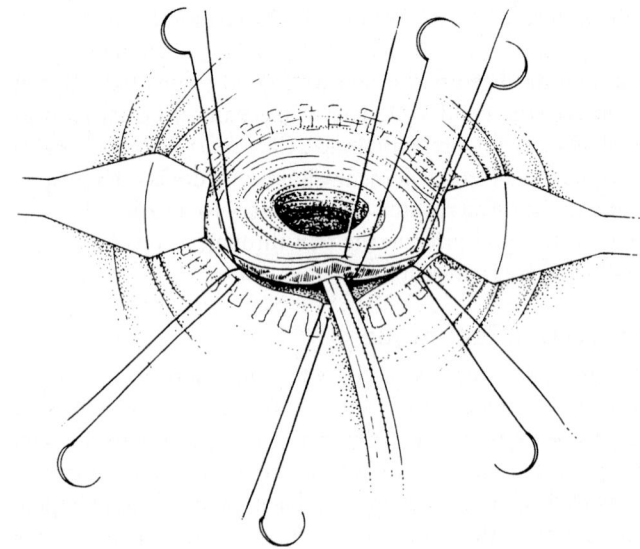

**FIGURE 44-10** A ring-clamp is inserted into the retrorectal space from below.

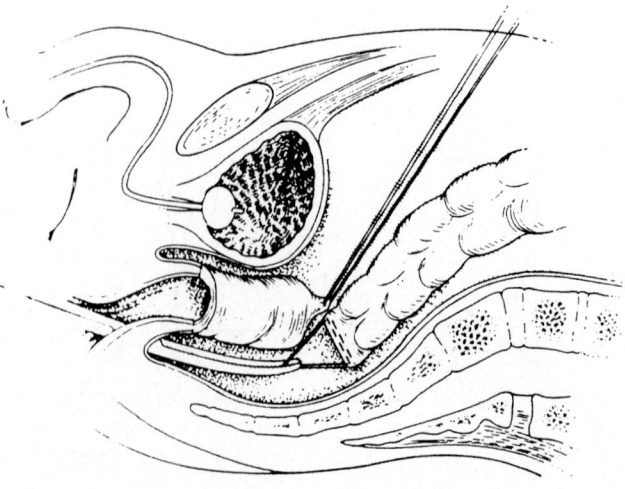

**FIGURE 44-11** The ganglionated bowel is gently pulled through the retrorectal space and angulation/twisting is prevented.

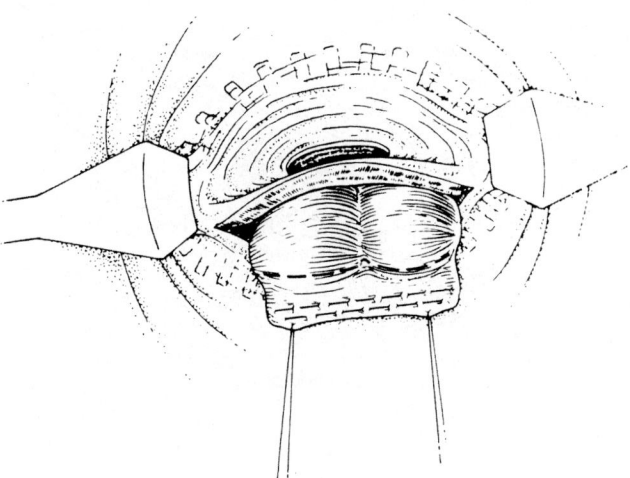

**FIGURE 44-12** An anterior wall colostomy is made just proximal to the staple line after the bowel is pulled through.

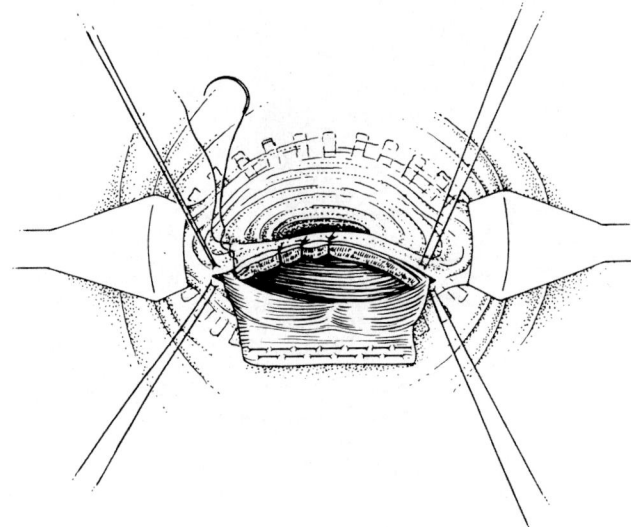

**FIGURE 44-14** A single-layer anastomosis is made from the posterior wall of the "old" rectum to the anterior wall of the pulled through rectum.

the other in the neorectum (Fig. 44-16). The stapler is fired directly in the midline. Hemostasis along the suture line is checked. The operation from below is completed at this point (Fig. 44-17).

Often, a complete anastomosis between the ganglionic and aganglionic bowel cannot be achieved with a single staple application from below, and a second firing from the abdomen is necessary (Fig. 44-18). The staple line of the remaining aganglionic rectum is opened and a small enterotomy is made in the ganglionic colon at a similar level. The abdominal surgeon places a reloaded automatic stapler between the 2 limbs of bowel to complete the anastomosis. This last step is critical. In the past, a proximal spur, left between the bowel segments, caused the eventual formation of huge fecalomas. Rarely a gastrointestinal anastomosis (GIA) device cannot approximate bowel, which is excessively thick. In this case,

the anastomosis may either be handsewn with absorbable suture or 2 large Kocher clamps may be placed in a "V"-like configuration, which will allow the bowel to anastomose over a 7- to 10-day period.

The anastomosis is completed by suturing the proximal end of the rectum to the enterostomy in the ganglionic colon in 2 layers. The neorectum is reperitonealized to prevent internal herniation of the bowel and the abdomen is closed (Fig. 44-19).

The development of a spur in the postoperative period may occasionally be seen. One generally does not need to address this from an abdominal approach. It can best be dealt with by firing a GIA stapling device through the rectum.

## Endorectal Pull-Through (Soave)

The Soave or endorectal pull-through was introduced by Franco Soave at the Institute G. Gaslini in 1955. The procedure was modified by Boley by performing a primary

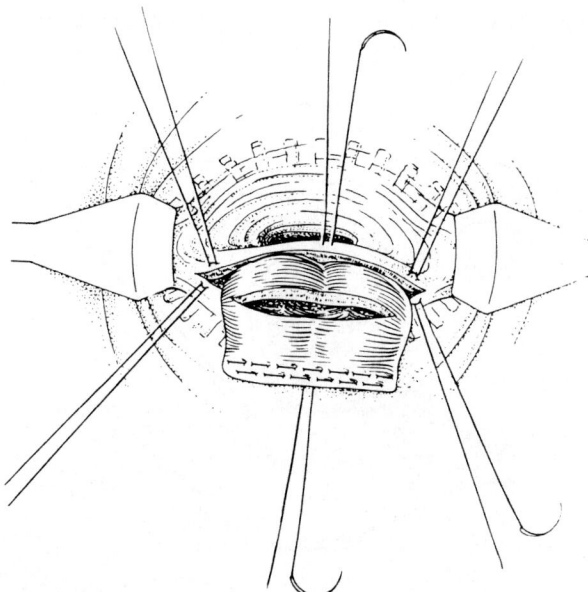

**FIGURE 44-13** A single layer anastomosis is made from the posterior wall of the "old" rectum to the anterior wall of the pulled through rectum.

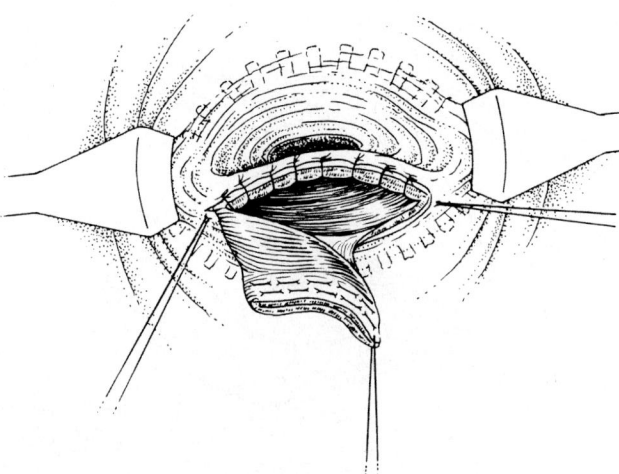

**FIGURE 44-15** The remainder of the staple line is excised and the posterior rim anastomosis of the new rectum is completed.

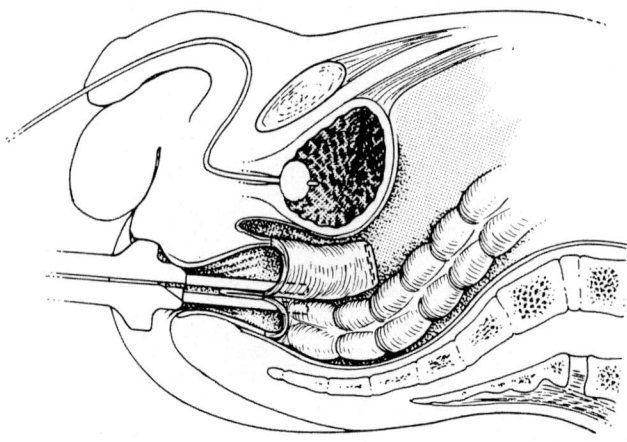

**FIGURE 44-16** A GIA stapler is placed transanally, one arm in the rectum, and one arm in the pulled-through rectum.

anastomosis at the anus and then further modified by Coran. This procedure is well suited for neonates undergoing the procedure within the first 1 to 2 weeks of life. The complication rate is identical to that seen with the standard 2-staged approach. It is actually technically easier to perform the endorectal dissection at this young age. This procedure, as is the case with the Duhamel, avoids injury to the pelvic nerves and by remaining within the muscular wall of the aganglionic segment important sensory fibers and the integrity of the internal sphincter are preserved. Although conceptually leaving behind aganglionic muscle surrounding normal bowel could lead to a high incidence of constipation, this is not observed clinically.

## Preoperative Assessment and Preparation

The operation is now typically done within the newborn period. To prepare the infant, serial rectal washouts and digital dilatations of the rectum are performed prior to beginning the pull through. The last of the rectal irrigations has 1% neomycin added to it. Intravenous antibiotics are given prior to the beginning of surgery and continued postoperatively for 2 doses after surgery.

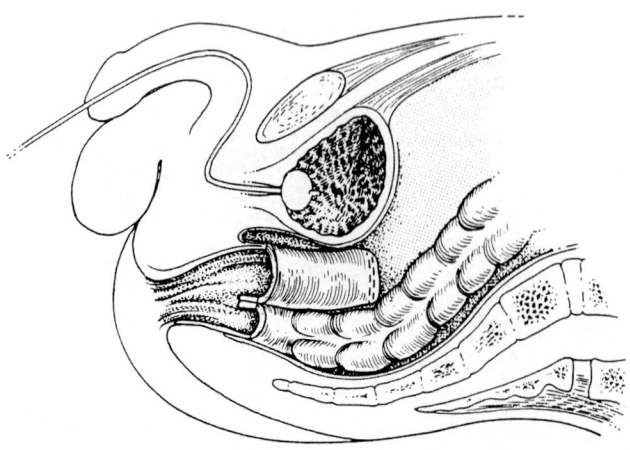

**FIGURE 44-17** The stapler has been fired, removing the common wall.

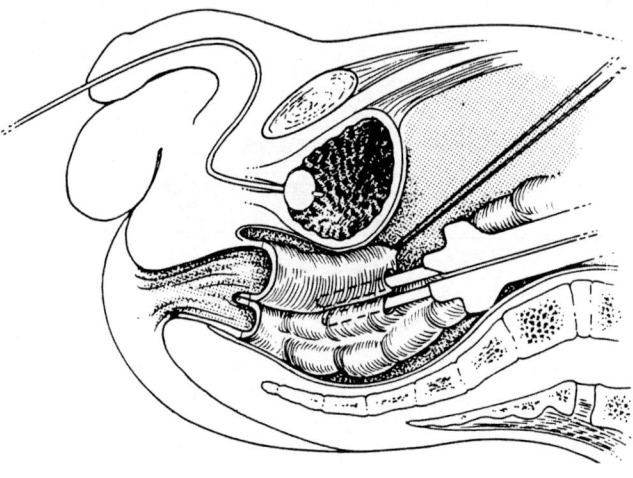

**FIGURE 44-18** To remove the common wall completely and avoid a "retained spur," the stapler is applied from the pelvic side and inserted distally, 1 arm into each lumen.

## Operative Technique

The child is placed in a supine position, with the buttocks brought to the end of the operating table, and propped slightly up with a folded towel. The legs are carefully padded and placed on wooden skis extending off the end of the table. The entire field is prepped and draped, followed by the placement of a Foley catheter. The operating table is placed in a slight Trendelenburg position. A hockey-stick incision is made incorporating the leveling colostomy. The same type of incision is made for infants undergoing a primary pull-through.

If the child was not previously leveled, the extent of aganglionosis is established with frozen section. Ganglionic bowel is mobilized proximally and is transected at the transition level with a stapling device. The distal colon is mobilized and resected to about 4 cm above the peritoneal reflection. Traction sutures are placed on either end of the distal bowel. The endorectal dissection is then started about 2 cm below the peritoneal reflection (Fig. 44-20). We have progressively

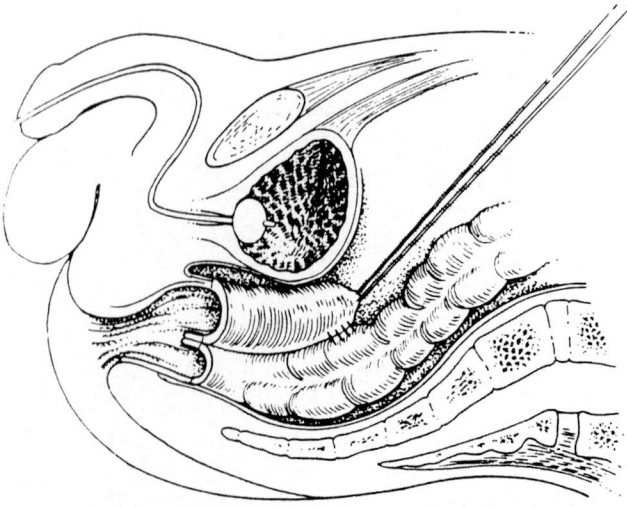

**FIGURE 44-19** The proximal colostomy is closed and the neorectum is reperitonealized.

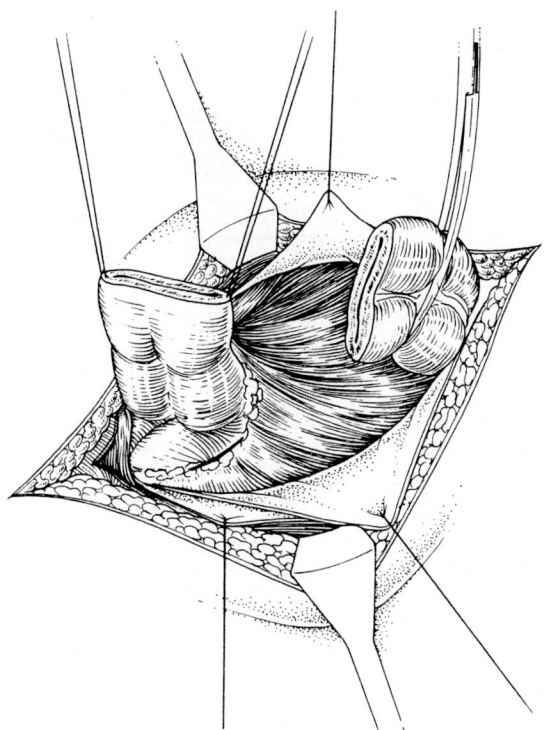

**FIGURE 44-20** The distal rectum is divided and the dissection is carried below the peritoneal reflection.

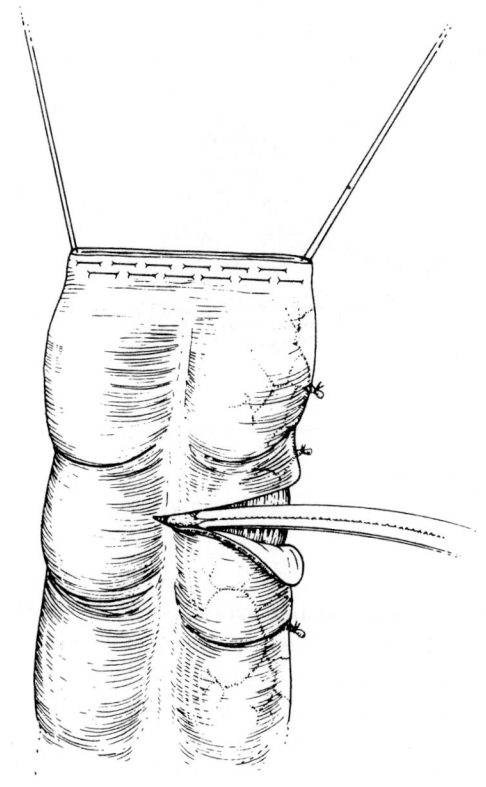

**FIGURE 44-21** Developing the plane between the submucosal and muscular layers in a circumferential fashion.

shortened the length of our endorectal dissection, because longer lengths of a muscular cuff may lead to increased bouts of constipation and enterocolitis.

The endorectal dissection usually begins by completely clearing the serosa, mesentery, and fat over a 2 cm length of bowel. The seromuscular layer is lightly incised with either sharp dissection or Bovie cautery. Once the submucosal layer is reached, the seromuscular layer is divided circumferentially using blunt dissection with a fine hemostat (Fig. 44-21).

After the plane is established, dissection is continued distally and is facilitated by an assistant pulling upward on the already dissected mucosal–submucosal tube for countertraction. In the newborn period, a cotton tip applicator is the most effective tool for this dissection. As the muscular cuff begins to develop, traction sutures are also placed in the muscle, 1 in each quadrant. Larger communicating vessels are coagulated; however, the majority of these are not cauterized during the dissection without significant blood loss, particularly in the newborn period. Dissection is carried down to within 1.5 cm of the anal opening in older children and less than 1 cm in a newborn (Fig. 44-22).

Some have advocated performing the distal part of the endorectal dissection from the transanal approach. However, once the endorectal dissection from above is started, it can proceed in a straightforward fashion. With appropriate traction and countertraction, one can perform the entire dissection in almost any sized child. Dissection from the anus requires additional time to set up and perform this portion of the procedure and delays the overall case.

One of the operating surgeons then moves to the foot of the table. Narrow retractors (Phrenic or Army-Navy) are placed at the anal–mucocutaneous junction and a ring or Kelly clamp is inserted into the rectum. An assistant at the abdominal field places the end of the mucosal–submucosal tube into the clamp. The segment is then everted onto the perineum. The end of the everted tube is placed in a clamp and held on traction by an assistant to facilitate the anastomosis (Fig. 44-23). At this point, the posterior wall of the muscular cuff is split with cautery down to just above the anal sphincters.

The submucosal/mucosal tube is incised on the anterior half, 1 cm above the dentate line for a 1-year-old and 0.5 to 0.7 cm above in a neonate (Fig. 44-24).

A Kelly clamp is inserted into this opening and the ganglionic bowel is brought down to this point by grasping the

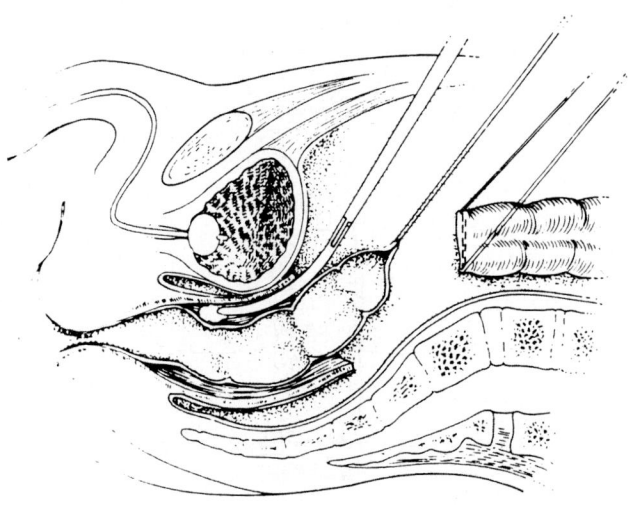

**FIGURE 44-22** The endorectal dissection is carried distally to within 1 to 1.5 cm from the anal opening.

579

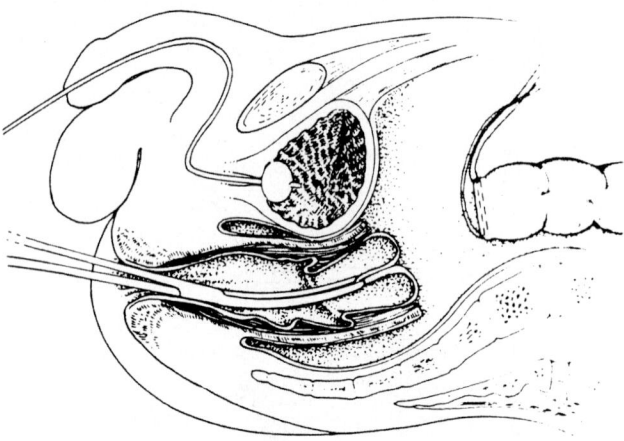

**FIGURE 44-23** The mucosal tube is grasped with a transanal inserted clamp and everted out of the rectal canal.

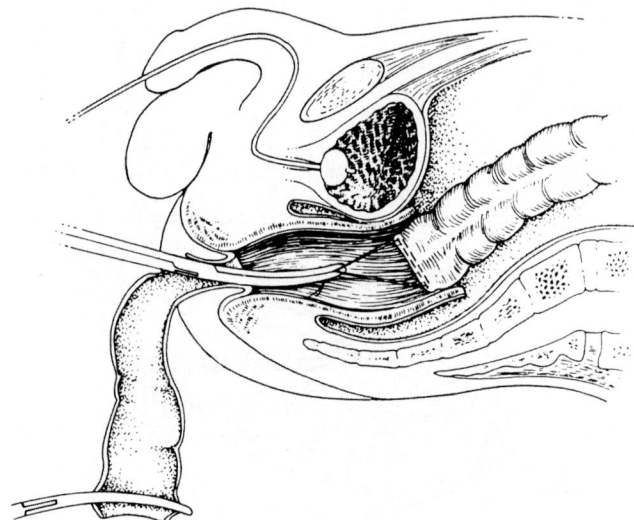

**FIGURE 44-25** The proximal ganglionated bowel is pulled under direct vision through the residual muscular sleeve.

2 previously placed traction sutures. Great care is taken not to twist the bowel as it is brought through the muscular cuff. If there is any question, the bowel should be brought back into the abdomen and rechecked. As with the Duhamel, different colored sutures on each side of the bowel are quite helpful in maintaining orientation (Fig. 44-25). Additional attention needs to be taken with long segment disease, as the greatest chance of a twist occurring is seen by pulling through the right colon.

The anterior half of the ganglionic colon is incised and is anastomosed to the anterior half of the anus with 4-0 Vicryl suture. The first sutures are placed at each corner and in the midline. Interrupted sutures are then placed in-between (Fig. 44-26). This is facilitated by the assistant pulling caudally on the midline and lateral sutures, which nicely exposes the 2 layers of the bowel.

One quarter of the remaining ganglionic colon is opened as is one quarter of the everted tube. A suture is placed in the

posterior midline and this quarter of the anastomosis is completed. Countertraction applied by an assistant on the everted tube will help with the exposure (Fig. 44-27).

After completion of the anastomosis, the colon is pulled slightly upward, which will invert the neorectum back into its correct position. Rectal exam at this point should show a well-formed anastomosis 1.5 to 2 cm above the anodermal junction. Gloves are then changed and attention is then directed to the abdominal field.

## Swenson

This technique was originally described by Swenson and Bill in 1948 and was the first successful treatment of children with Hirschsprung disease. They based their technique on the principle that the diseased portion of the bowel was the aganglionic

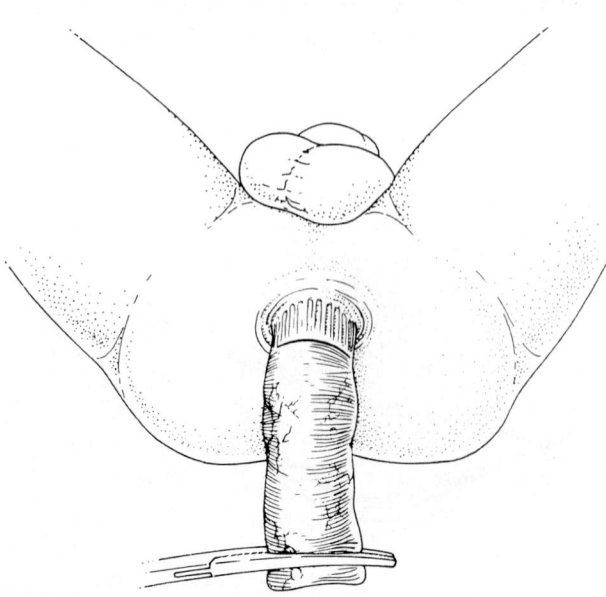

**FIGURE 44-24** With traction on the mucosal tube, incision is made 0.5 to 0.7 cm above the dentate line anteriorly.

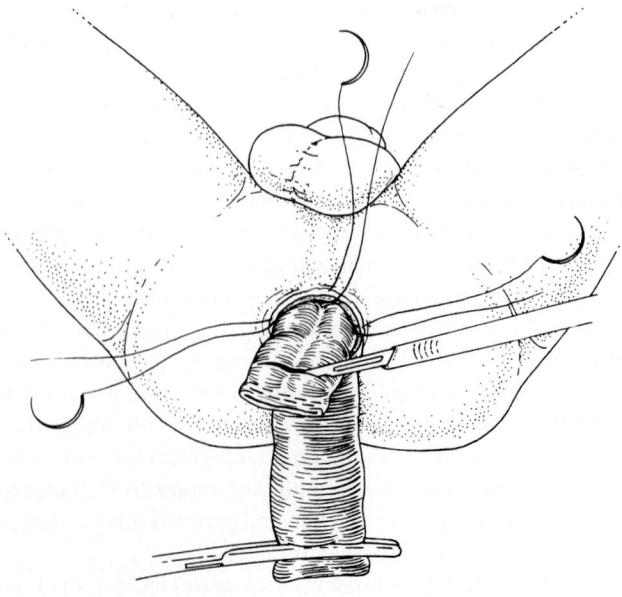

**FIGURE 44-26** The anterior wall anastomosis is completed between the distal anterior rectal wall just above the dentate line to the pulled-through rectum.

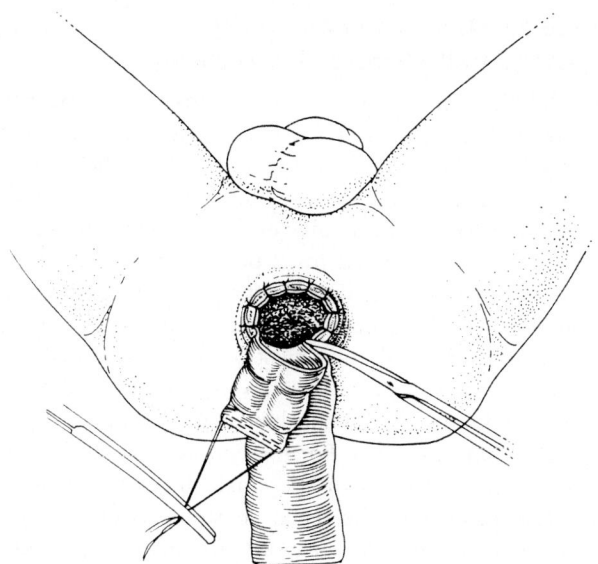

**FIGURE 44-27** The circumferential anastomosis is complete as the bowel is excised.

distal rectum, and that removal of this segment was necessary to allow for normal stooling. The initial incidence of postoperative enterocolitis was fairly high (early 16% and late 27%); and this was attributed to leaving too much aganglionic rectum. The procedure has since been modified by resecting virtually all of the posterior rectal wall (and the very topmost aspect of the internal sphincter). The technique demands meticulous dissection of the rectum down to within 2 cm of the anodermal junction. If the dissection moves off of the rectal wall, a significant incidence of injury to genitourinary innervation may occur. Properly performed, the results with this procedure are quite good; however, because of the technical difficulties of the dissection, it is not as commonly performed.

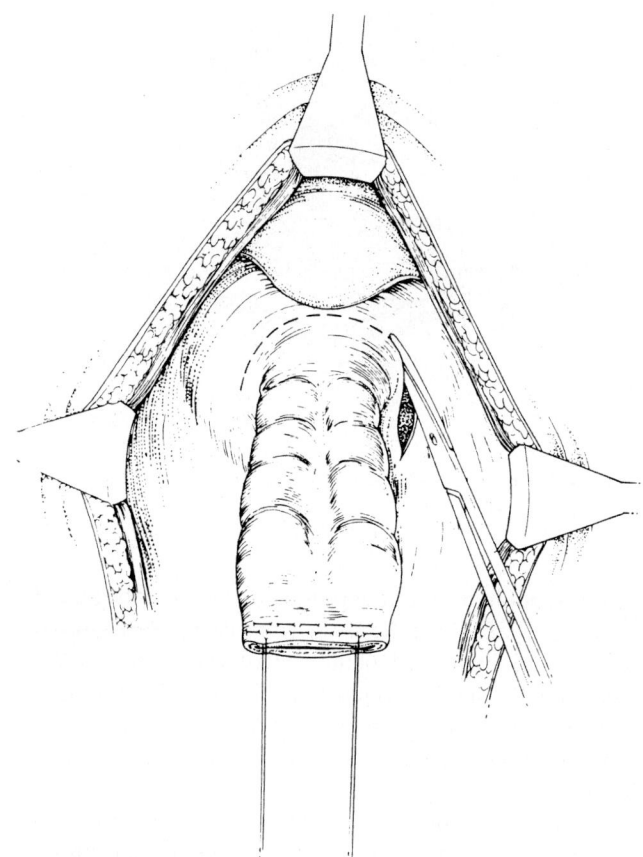

**FIGURE 44-28** The peritoneal reflection is incised anteriorly.

## Preoperative Assessment and Preparation

The child is admitted the day prior to surgery for a routine bowel prep. Assessment and preparation are similar to the other pull-throughs.

## Operative Technique

The child is positioned in a similar fashion as for an endorectal pull-through. The incision was classically described as a left paramedian incision with takedown of the colostomy; however, the modified hockey stick incision will work equally well.

The redundant aganglionic rectum is excised and proximal ganglionated colon mobilized, as needed. At this point, the peritoneal reflection over the rectum is incised (Fig. 44-28).

Following this, the operating surgeon dissects the full-thickness rectum caudally. This is a critical dissection, which demands the surgeon to stay directly on the bowel wall. Dissection is facilitated by the first assistant applying upward traction on the end of the aganglionic rectum. Multiple blood vessels enter directly into the bowel wall, each must be dissected out and can usually be coagulated. Dissection is carried down to within 2 cm of the anal verge. Dissection is not carried as far anteriorly in order to avoid autonomic nerve injury (Fig. 44-29).

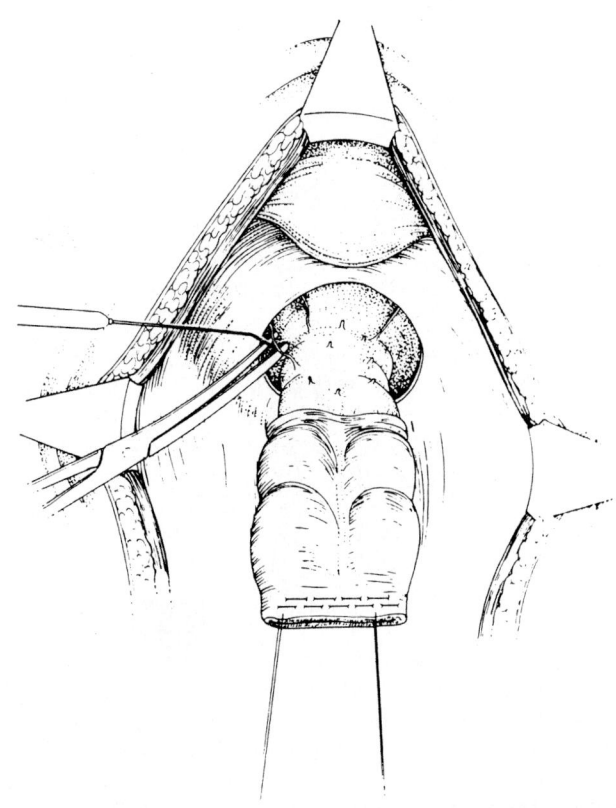

**FIGURE 44-29** Dissection continues along the outer rectal wall, taking care to proceed less aggressively anteriorly, to within 2 cm of the verge.

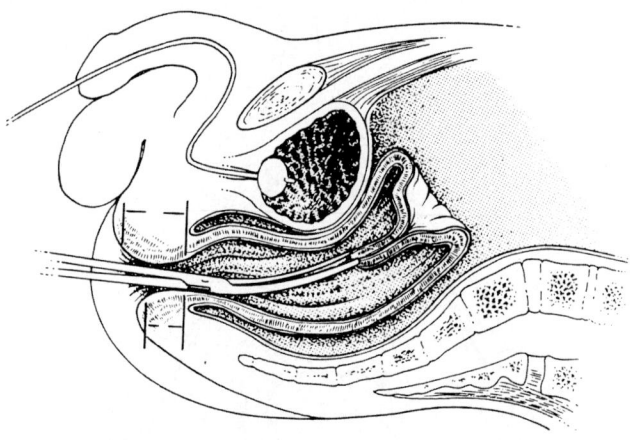

**FIGURE 44-30** The full-thickness mobilized rectum is everted out of the anal canal.

At this point, the perineal portion of the case is begun. The rectum is everted with the use of a long clamp placed into the rectum. The anterior half of the everted rectal wall is cut 2 cm away from the anodermal junction. The posterior wall will be no longer than 1 to 1.5 cm in length, so a gently curved incision, which is shorter posteriorly, is created along the anterior half of the bowel (Fig. 44-30).

The ganglionic colon is pulled through and the anastomosis is virtually identical to that for the endorectal pull-through. Classically, silk sutures have been used, but we have utilized Vicryl sutures with good results (Fig. 44-31).

The anastomosis is allowed to recede and is gently pulled upward from the perineum. Closure is essentially the same as for the previous procedures.

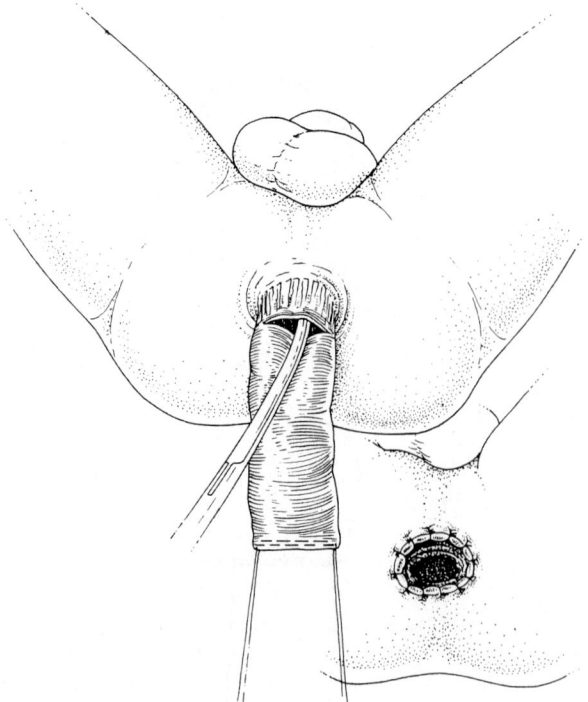

**FIGURE 44-31** The anterior half of the everted bowel is incised, the ganglionated proximal colon is advanced through the pelvic space, and the extrapelvic end-to-end anastomosis is completed with interrupted sutures.

## Postoperative Care Following all of the Pull-Through Procedures

The child has the nasogastric tube removed once gastrointestinal activity returns. The Foley catheter can usually be removed on the second postoperative day following the endorectal and Duhamel pull-through because bladder innervation has not been affected by the pelvic dissection. Antibiotics are continued for 2 postoperative days. Great attention is placed on examining the perineal region for the development of erythema or cellulitis, as this is an early sign of an anastomotic leak. Investigation of a leak consists of a contrast enema study or a CT scan with contrast. Although fairly uncommon, should a leak be demonstrated, a diverting colostomy is needed. For the endorectal pull-through, a gentle rectal exam with the small finger is performed to ensure patency of the rectal anastomosis prior to discharge. For neonates, because of their small size, a cotton tip applicator is passed instead of a finger. Parents are given thorough instructions on perineal care and the potential development of enterocolitis. To avoid perineal excoriation, we generally have the parents apply a thick coat of a zinc oxide based ointment with each diaper change. If a significant diaper rash develops, more intensified applications are used. Digital dilatations are performed in the office starting on the third week after surgery. Again, with a neonatal pull-through a 6 to 7 Hegar dilator is initially used and this is slowly advanced with subsequent clinic visits. These dilations with each clinic visit are usually enough to prevent anastomotic stricturing. It is not, however, uncommon to encounter infants and older children who develop stooling problems and enterocolitis in the post-pull–through period. Marty et al have reported a statistically lower incidence of post-pull–through enterocolitis in those individuals who undergo routine rectal washouts postoperatively for a 3-month period. Based on this, our own group has adopted this practice in many of its patients. Stool frequency is generally quite high (7-12 bowel movements per day) immediately after the pull-through. The frequency slowly decreases and is generally normal by 12 months.

## Total Colonic Hirschsprung Disease

### Treatment Options

Total colonic aganglionosis accounts for approximately 3% to 12% of infants with Hirschsprung disease. Complications associated with total colonic aganglionosis are numerous and considerably higher than for standard length Hirschsprung disease. Many infants with total colonic Hirschsprung disease will also require parenteral nutrition, making catheter sepsis, failure to thrive, stomal dysfunction, electrolyte imbalance, and dehydration commonly encountered complications. Treatment for total colonic aganglionosis generally begins with the creation of a properly formed enterostomy. Fluids and electrolytes are watched closely. Nutrition is usually initiated parenterally and slowly converted to the enteral route. Failure to thrive is common and attention to sodium and bicarbonate replacement may prevent this.

## Procedures

Despite numerous procedures suggested for this disorder, either a standard Duhamel or endorectal pull-through is acceptable, and associated with similar outcomes.

## Anal/Rectal Myotomy and Myectomy

### Treatment Options

A child with very short segment Hirschsprung disease may be a candidate for an anal/rectal myectomy. The advantage of this procedure is that it avoids an abdominal operation. The procedure must be confined to very short segment Hirschsprung disease. One must be certain that they have extended the myectomy beyond the level of aganglionosis. Because performing an inadequate myectomy may adversely affect the outcome of a subsequent pull-through, if there is any uncertainty as to the level of disease, a myectomy should be avoided. A more common use of this procedure is to alleviate a child who suffers from internal sphincter spasm and repeated bouts of enterocolitis following a pull-through procedure. Several authors have described their performance of an internal sphincterotomy on patients with persistent enterocolitis in the post-pull–through period. Overall results of these internal sphincterotomies are quite good; however, a significant period of conservative therapy should be given first, since most patients with post-pull–through enterocolitis will improve over time.

### Preoperative Assessment and Preparation

Preparation is similar to that of the other pull-through procedures.

### Operative Technique

**Transanal Approach.** The child is placed in an identical position as for the full-thickness rectal biopsy. Digital dilatation is performed and 2 narrow anal retractors are inserted and held by assistants. The posterior aspect of the dentate line is identified. A curvilinear incision through the mucosa and submucosa of the posterior wall is made starting 1 cm above the dentate line. Following this, a submucosal dissection is carried upward for several centimeters. The mucosal flap is held up with multiple silk sutures and can be extended proximally with vertical incisions on either side (Fig. 44-32).

Following this, a myotomy is performed by sharply incising the full-thickness of the muscle layer and then advanced cranially using Bovie cautery. For a myectomy, a 0.5- to 1-cm wide muscle strip is created centered around the midline. The initial strip removed should be at least 5 cm in length (Fig. 44-33). Prior to transecting this strip, 2 silk sutures are placed proximal to the point of transection, so that should further dissection be necessary, the proximal muscle will not retract beyond the reach of the surgeon. The strip should be mounted on a tongue depressor with mounting pins or suture; proximal and distal orientation must be clearly depicted (Fig. 44-33, *inset*). A frozen section confirming ganglion cells at the proximal margin must be obtained before the procedure can be terminated. The dissection can be carried out in this manner for approximately 8 cm. If the surgeon suspects

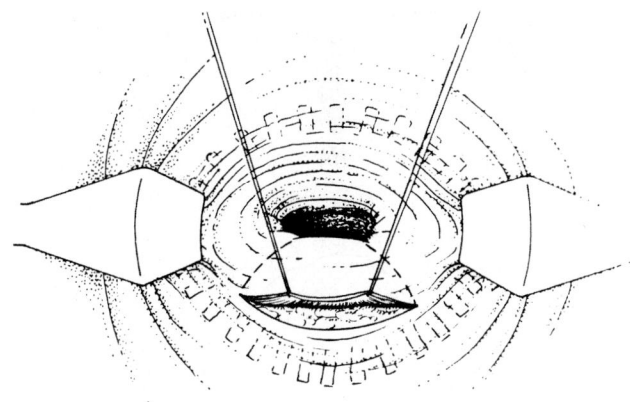

**FIGURE 44-32** A transanal mucosal flap is elevated beginning 1 cm above the dentate line.

that the level of aganglionosis is longer than this, it is advisable to forgo this approach.

Once a sufficient length of muscle has been removed, hemostasis is achieved with cautery. The wound is irrigated and closed with fine interrupted absorbable sutures approximating the mucosa/submucosal dissection.

**Transsacral Approach.** A transsacral approach can also be used for the myectomy. A vertical transsacral incision is made from the coccyx to within 1 cm of the anus and carried down to the levator muscles complex (Fig. 44-34).

The levator muscles are retracted caudally with a retractor (Fig. 44-35). With a finger in the rectum, the posterior rectal wall is exposed and a strip of rectal muscle, 1 cm wide, is removed from the dentate line proximally. The mucosa and submucosa are not incised and the rectal lumen is not entered. This approach gives an excellent exposure of the posterior rectal wall.

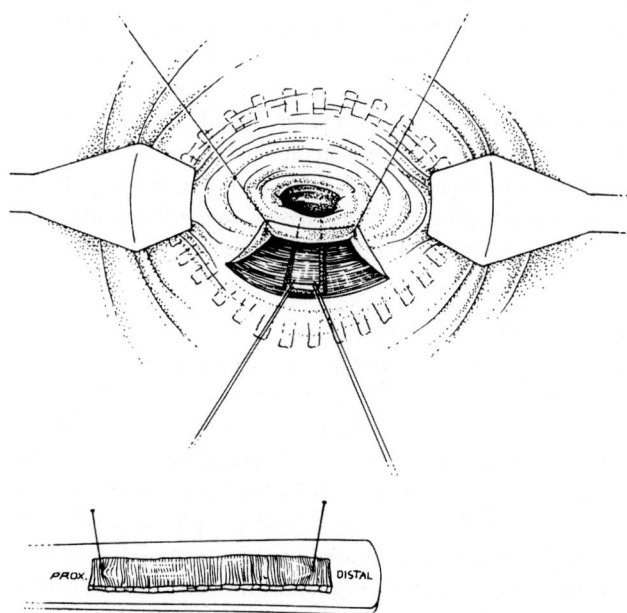

**FIGURE 44-33** A full-thickness muscular strip of 1 cm width and at least 5 cm in length should be excised and sent for frozen section diagnosis after appropriate mounting and labeling.

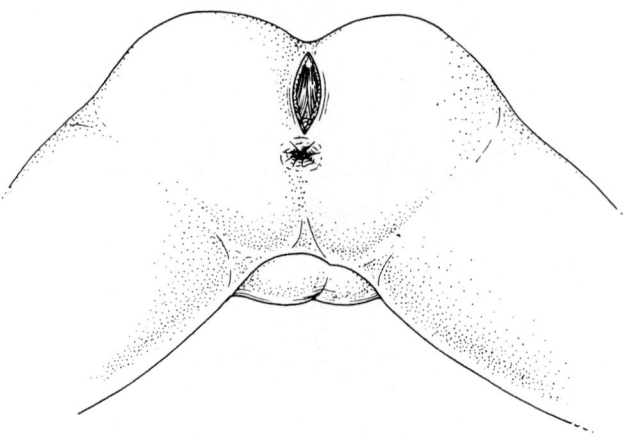

**FIGURE 44-34** Posterior midline transsacral approach for an anorectal myectomy.

## Chronic Problems Encountered with Hirschsprung Disease

### Constipation and other Stooling Issues

Not uncommonly children develop a variety of stooling abnormalities after any number of pull-through procedures. These include intermittent bouts of constipation, occasional soiling, and at times enterocolitis. Most problems with constipation or soiling can be managed with changes in diet or laxatives. Occasionally, an enema regimen will be required. Episodes of enterocolitis can often be managed with oral metronidazole. Severe cases, however, will necessitate admission, intravenous antibiotics, and rectal washouts. In the child with persistent constipation or enterocolitis, one should do a careful exam to exclude the development of a stricture or fissure, which may be the source of these symptoms. Additionally, one should consider performing a repeat rectal biopsy to confirm ganglionic bowel is present at the level of the anastomosis. Rarely, if episodes of enterocolitis or constipation are quite severe and recurrent, additional surgical therapy may be needed (ie, rectal myotomy, see above). Incontinence after a pull-through procedure may be seen in 5% or more of patients, and warrants long-term follow-up of patients for this issue. Such patients will need to be engaged into a bowel management program. In some cases, stooling disorders are so severe that consideration of a redo-pull–through should be considered.

### Second Pull-Through

This is an uncommon option and should be performed in only very select cases. The most common reason for a second procedure is when aganglionic bowel has been pulled through. Should this be the case, a second pull-through may be necessary. Another consideration would be the performance of a myectomy, if the level of aganglionosis is known to be fairly short (approximately 5 cm or less). Because of its relative ease, a Duhamel is generally the procedure of choice, no matter which original pull-through was used. We have, however, performed both an endorectal and Swenson pull-through as a second procedure. If the child has already undergone a Duhamel, one would generally resort to a Swenson

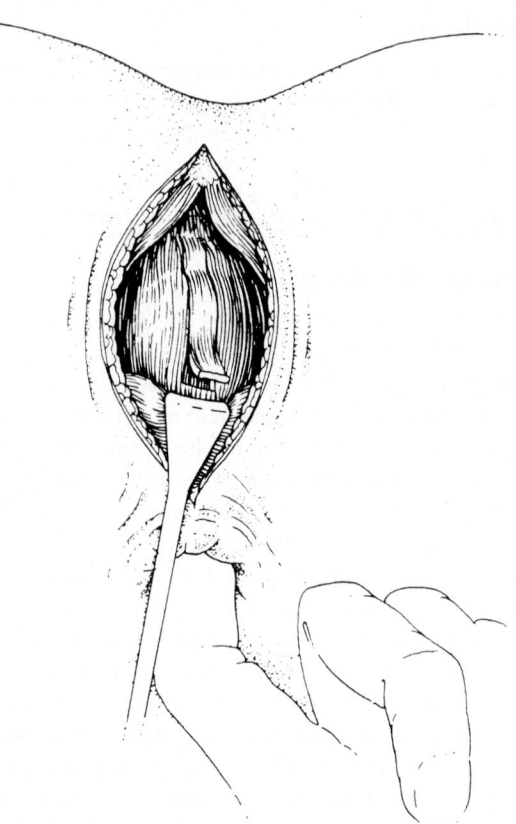

**FIGURE 44-35** With the levators retracted caudally and a transanal finger as a guide, an extramucosal strip of muscle is excised and sent for pathologic exam.

procedure. For the child with debilitating incontinence, a detailed history and exam should be performed to rule out encopresis and to assess the degree of anorectal tone. Anal manometry is particularly helpful is this group, as a lack of normal muscular control is generally felt to be a poor indicator of a successful outcome for a redo-pull–through. Some children in this latter group may best be served with a diverting colostomy, or bowel management program.

This chapter offers 2 distinct views on the laparoscopic versus transanal approach to treating Hirschsprung disease. Taken together, the sections offer a unique insight to the advantages and disadvantages to each of these approaches.

# Laparoscopic-Assisted Pull-Through for Hirschsprung Disease

*Mark L. Wulkan and Keith E. Georgeson*

## HISTORICAL BACKGROUND

Contemporary surgical management of Hirschsprung disease has progressed from 3 stages of reconstruction to a single procedure early in life. Many centers have reported their experience with primary colon pull-through using open and laparoscopic techniques. Potential advantages of a single-stage procedure over multistaged procedures include decreased morbidity, decreased hospital stay, and no need for colostomy. Delayed intestinal continuity may also retard development of anorectal continence. The use of advanced laparoscopic techniques further refines the technique of primary pull-through, decreasing perioperative morbidity and shortening full recovery from the operation. Primary laparoscopic endorectal pull-through can be performed as soon as the diagnosis is confirmed in neonates, children, and adults.

## OPERATIVE TECHNIQUE

In most children with Hirschsprung disease with a rectosigmoid or left colon transition zone, a laparoscopic-assisted endorectal pull-through is performed. If the transition zone is in the right colon, or if the patient has total colonic disease, a laparoscopic-assisted Duhamel pull-through may be performed.

### Endorectal Pull-Through

Once the diagnosis is confirmed, the patient is prepped for surgery. All patients receive preoperative antibiotics. Infants are bowel prepped with rectal irrigations alone. Older children are prepped with rectal irrigations and enteric lavage. Intravenous antibiotics are used perioperatively.

Smaller children and infants are positioned transversely at the end of the operating table and prepped circumferentially. Older children and adults are positioned in stirrups in the lithotomy position. The first trocar is placed in the right upper quadrant using a Veress needle or open technique. Two more trocars are placed in the right and left lower quadrant using visual surveillance. A forth trocar may be placed in the suprapubic position for placing traction on the colon (Fig. 44-36). In older children, the initial trocar may be placed in the standard umbilical position.

It is essential to establish the level of the transition zone at the beginning of the procedure. A seromuscular biopsy is procured grasping the serosa with a fine instrument and cutting out the specimen with fine scissors. If there is perforation or bleeding, the site may be closed with a suture.

Dissection is begun by establishing a plane at the rectosigmoid junction 5 to 10 cm above the peritoneal reflection adjacent to the colon. Mesenteric vessels are divided proximal to the level of the transition zone using an ultrasonic scalpel, electrocautery (including impedance feedback bipolar devices), and/or clips. Several techniques may be used to gain adequate length for the pull-through. The inferior mesenteric artery can be divided below the level of the vascular arcades to gain length for the pull-through. The fusion fascia of the left colon can be divided bluntly or sharply. The lienocolic ligament can also be divided for patients with a transition zone in the descending colon. The marginal artery should be carefully preserved (Fig. 44-37). Adequate mobility of the colon pedicle can be determined by grasping the colon 10 to 20 cm

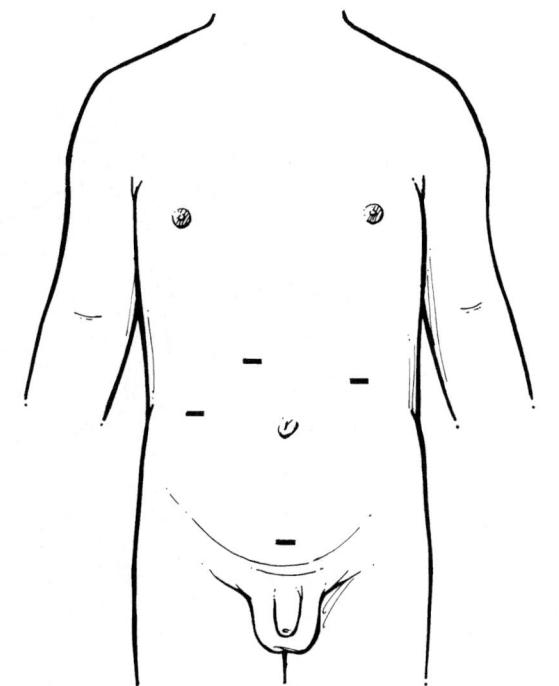

**FIGURE 44-36** Four 3.5- to 5-mm trocars are placed through the abdominal wall. Working ports are sited on either side of the optic port. The suprapubic trocar is used for retraction of the retrosigmoid colon.

above the transition zone and pushing this portion of colon deep into the pelvis. Tethering bands are divided after being identified with this maneuver.

The rectum is then circumferentially dissected to the level of the prostate or cervix anteriorly and the coccyx posteriorly. The exact level of this dissection is not critical. In general, the lower the dissection, the easier the endorectal dissection from below. Care is taken to keep the dissection close to the rectal wall to minimize the risk of injury to pelvic structures such as the ureter, vas deferens, or seminal vesicles (Fig. 44-38). This dissection can be performed with a hook cautery, fine-tipped grasper, electrocautery, or an ultrasonic scalpel.

Attention is now directed to the perineum. Traction sutures are placed at the dentate line to expose the anorectum. A mucosal incision is made one half to 1 cm above the dentate line with electrocautery. Once the plane between the submucosa and muscularis is identified, multiple fine sutures are placed in the proximal mucosal sleeve for traction. The proctectomy is continued in the submucosal plane using fine scissors, cautery, and blunt dissection (Fig. 44-39). When the level of the intracorporeal dissection is reached, the rectum will begin to prolapse through the anus. A marked decrease in bleeding in the submucosal plane is also noted. These features identify the level of the intracorporeal dissection. The muscular wall is divided circumferentially at this level and the colon is pulled through the rectal cuff (Fig. 44-40). The cuff is split posteriorly to provide room for a neorectal reservoir (Fig. 44-41). More colonic mesentery may be divided transanally if necessary. The rectum is amputated approximately 10 to 20 cm

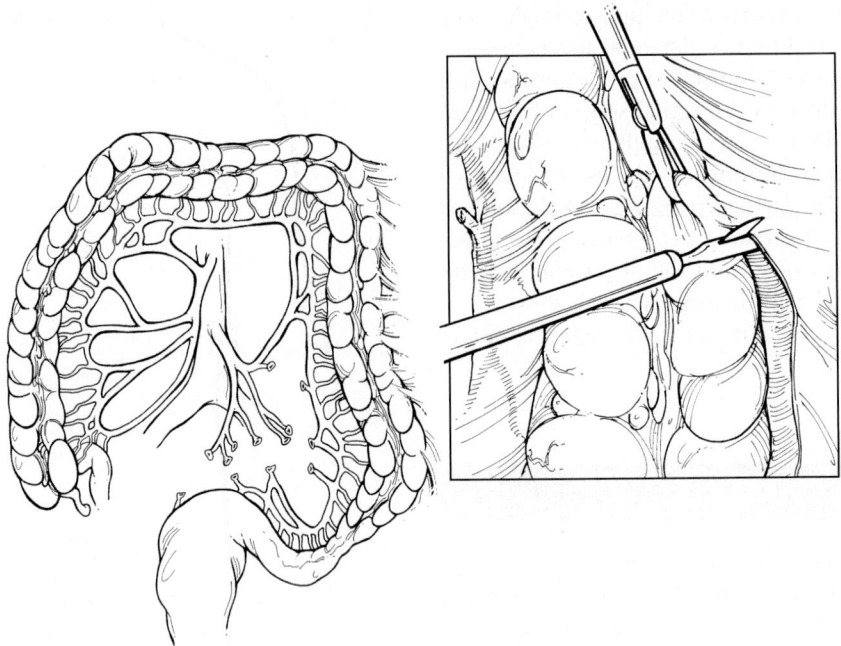

**FIGURE 44-37** Mesenteric vessels are divided proximal to the marginal artery. The left fusion fascia is divided in patients where mobilization of a longer pedicle is needed (*inset*).

above the transition zone (Fig. 44-42) and an anastomosis is performed with absorbable sutures (Fig. 44-43). The anastomosis should be watertight as there is no protective colostomy.

## Duhamel Pull-Through

A Duhamel pull-through is performed on patients with a right colon transition zone or total colonic aganglionosis. The trocars are placed as for the endorectal pull-through. Attention is first directed to determining the transition

zone. Biopsies are performed as previously described just above the suspected transition zone. If necessary, the appendix may be removed to establish total colonic aganglionosis. The gastrocolic ligament is divided using electrocautery or an ultrasonic scalpel. The mesentery is then divided to the transition zone.

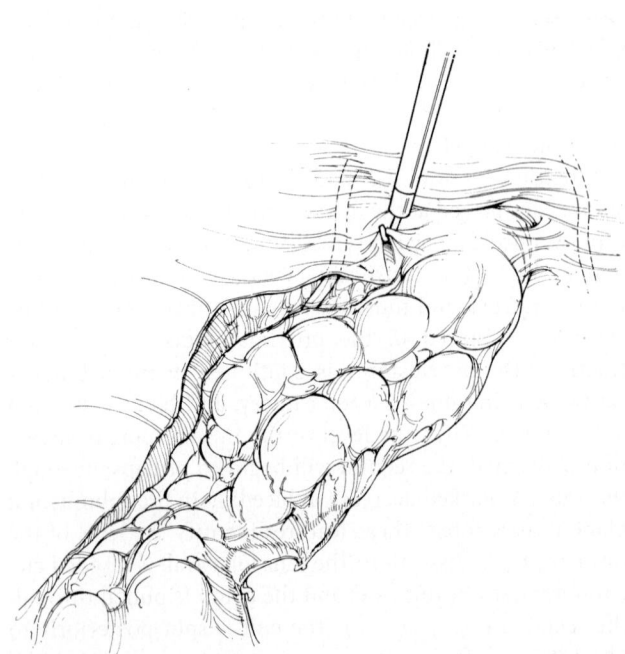

**FIGURE 44-38** Rectal dissection is performed circumferentially as close to the rectum as possible.

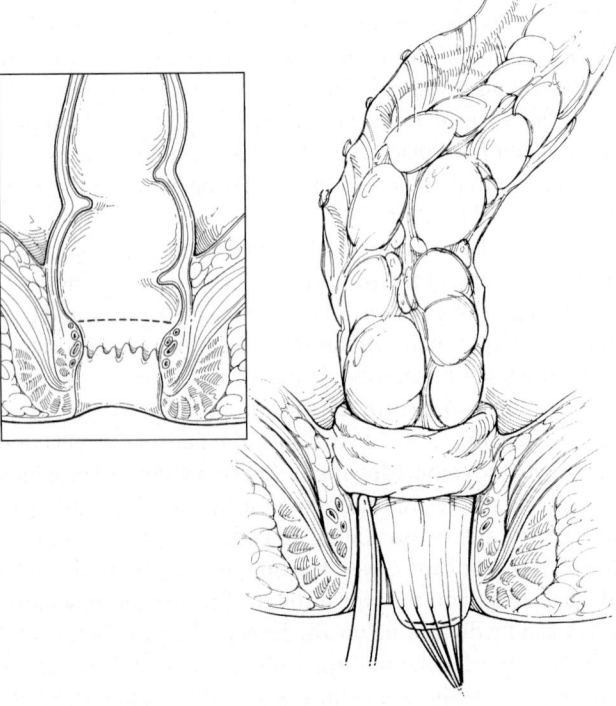

**FIGURE 44-39** Transanal mucosectomy is begun 5- to 10-mm above the dentate line. Fine traction sutures are placed in the proximal mucosal margin, and the mucosa is separated circumferentially from the muscular layer.

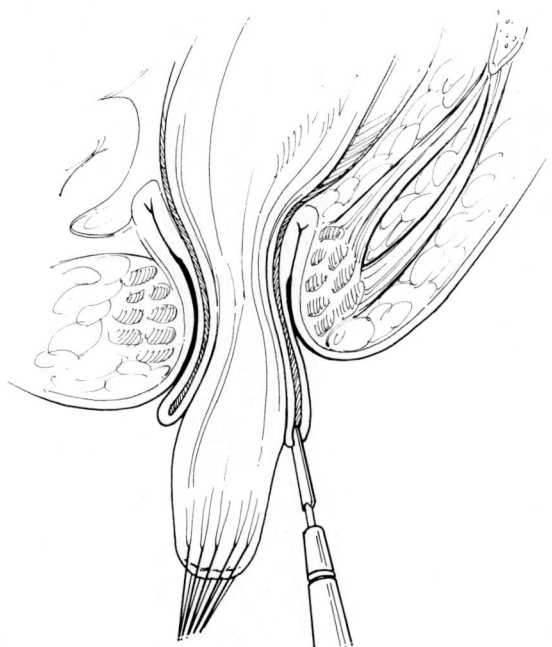

**FIGURE 44-40** The mucosectomy is extended until the laparoscopically mobilized rectosigmoid colon prolapses easily through the anus. The muscular cuff is opened and the laparoscopic and transanal planes are joined circumferentially.

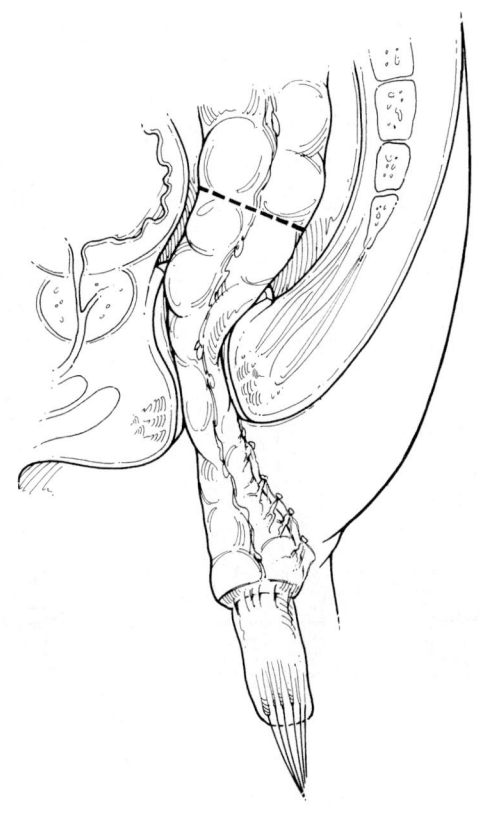

**FIGURE 44-42** The mobilized colon is pulled up through the anus to a level proximal to the transition zone.

The presacral space is dissected using a hook cautery and blunt dissection. The bowel is divided with an endoscopic stapler leaving a rectal stump length of 5 to 10 cm. One or 2 graspers are wedged deep in the pelvis and a transanal incision is made in the posterior rectum 1 cm above the dentate line onto the wedged graspers (Fig. 44-44A). The bowel is brought down through the presacral space, through the defect

in the posterior rectal wall, and through the anus (Fig. 44-44B). The bowel is amputated 10 to 20 cm above the transition zone. An anastomosis of the neorectum to the anorectal mucosa is performed transanally with interrupted, absorbable sutures. The endoscopic stapler is inserted and from below to obliterate the septum between the rectum and ganglionated bowel

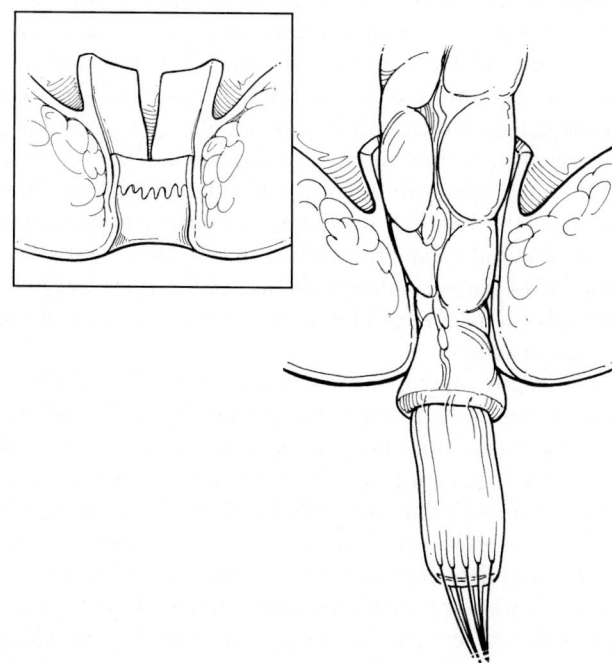

**FIGURE 44-41** The rectal cuff is split posteriorly to a level of 3 cm proximal to the dentate line.

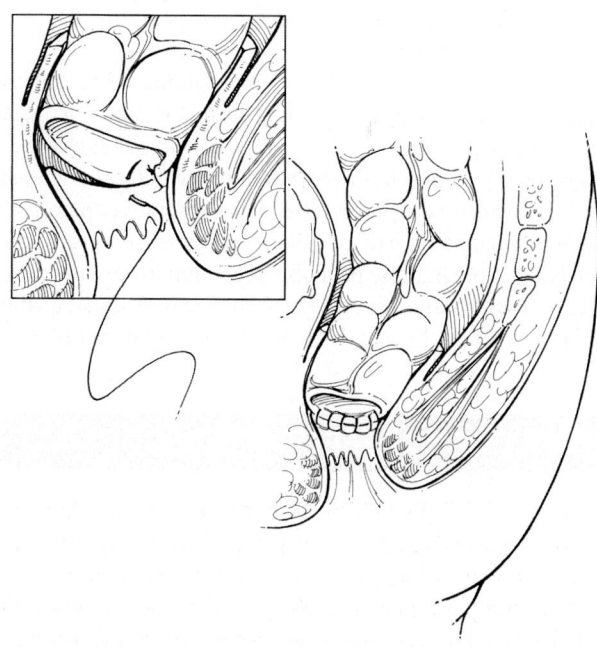

**FIGURE 44-43** The ganglionated end of the proximal colon is secured to the distal rectal mucosa with interrupted absorbable sutures.

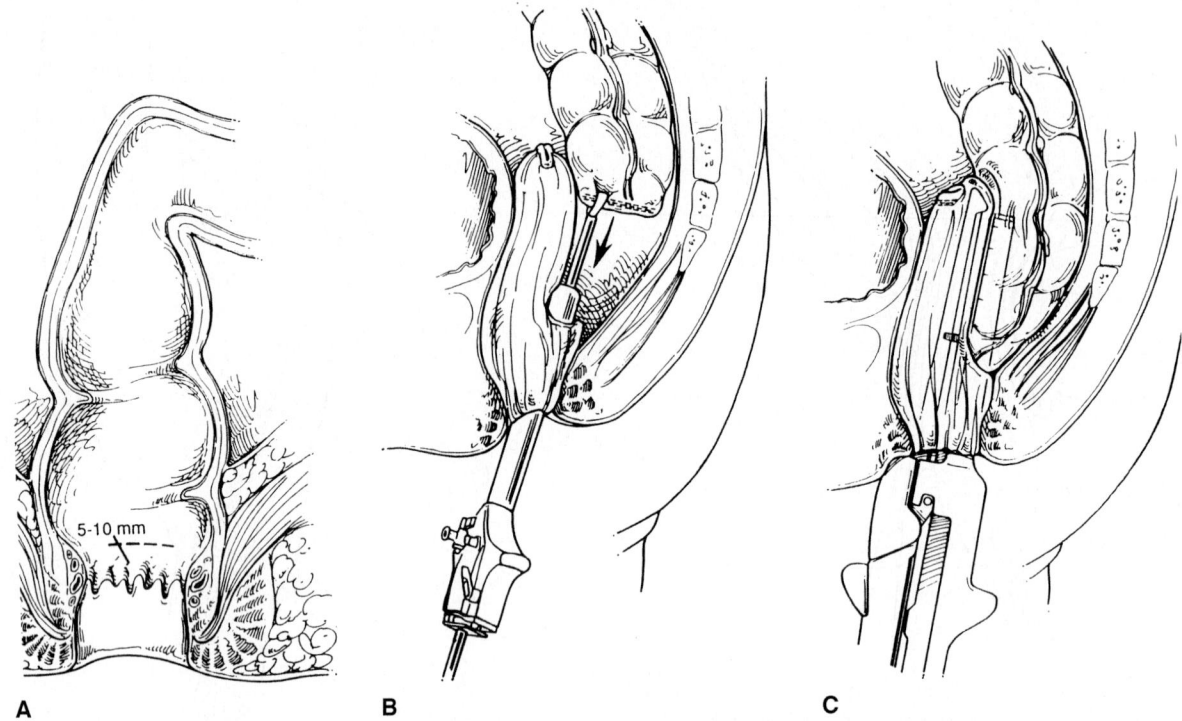

A                                    B                                    C

**FIGURE 44-44** **A.** An incision is made in the posterior rectum 1 cm above the dentate line. **B.** A 12-mm trocar is passed through the tract behind the rectum and the proximal rectal staple line grasped. **C.** The neorectal spur is obliterated using a GIA stapler.

(Fig. 44-44C). Any redividing in the rectal pouch is removed with an endoscopic GIA stapler.

## SURGICAL OUTCOMES

In the senior author's series of 25 laparoscopic primary laparoscopic pull-through procedures for Hirschsprung disease the age range was 3 days to 6 years. Average length of stay was 3½ days. Feedings were initiated on postoperative day 1 in almost all of the patients.

There were 2 perioperative complications. One patient required a transfusion for bleeding from the superior rectal artery and 1 patient had an anastomotic leak necessitating a diverting colostomy. Both patients are currently doing well. There have been no clear episodes of postoperative enterocolitis. Two patients have had mild diarrhea that responded to anorectal dilatation. In those patients old enough to develop bowel control (8/8), continence appears to be at least of equal quality to those patients who have been operated by open techniques.

## TREATMENT EFFECTIVENESS

A laparoscopic approach to the treatment of Hirschsprung disease is safe and effective. This approach appears to decrease hospital stay, less morbidity, and reduce costs compared to open techniques. Laparoscopy provides clear delineation of pelvic anatomical structures, especially in the neonate. Laparoscopy appears to reduce the formation of adhesions compared to open surgery and is associated with less postoperative pain.

Transanal dissection alone (the perineal portion of the procedure) without laparoscopy for short segment Hirschsprung disease is another minimally invasive technique used by others. However, for most infants and children with Hirschsprung disease, we prefer a combined endoscopic and transanal dissection to mobilize and remove the frequently dilated and dysfunctional colon proximal to the aganglionic segment. A significant disadvantage of the transanal technique is the lack of biopsy confirmation of the transition zone prior to the rectal mucosectomy. Additionally, some patients with Hirschsprung disease have associated intestinal dysmotility proximal to the aganglionic segment, making resection of up to 20 cm colon proximal to the ganglionic transition zone an attractive technique. Transanal dissection alone also appears to be associated with longer operative times and may lead to greater dilatation of the internal anal sphincter during mobilization of the sigmoid colon. The authors of this subsection of the chapter do not recommend the use of the transanal pull-through due to the inability to confirm the location of the transition zone.

The laparoscopic Duhamel technique is easy and efficacious in the early postoperative period. We have used this technique only for long segment Hirschsprung disease because we are concerned about the reported incidence of overflow incontinence associated with the larger dysmotile rectal reservoir created by Duhamel operation. Constipation becomes especially problematic in childhood. In patients with right colon transition zones or in total colonic aganglionosis, overflow incontinence is rarely a problem. The larger rectal reservoir created by the Duhamel technique may actually lead to improved continence in patients with long-segment disease.

Primary laparoscopic colon pull-through for Hirschsprung disease is safe and efficacious. Apparent reductions in morbidity, length of hospital stay, and cost are attainable with this technique.

# Transanal 1-Stage Soave Procedure for Infants with Hirschsprung Disease

*Jacob C. Langer*

Based on the reported success of the minimally invasive approach, and our own experience with the laparoscopic pull-through, we and others developed a simpler operation in which a one-stage pull-through could be accomplished using a completely transanal approach without any dissection of the rectum in the pelvis. This procedure is associated with the advantages of short hospital stay, minimal risk of damage to pelvic structures, a low incidence of intraperitoneal bleeding and adhesion formation, and minimal abdominal incisions.

## OPERATIVE TECHNIQUE

The patient is anesthetized, and a caudal block is given. The child is placed at the end of the operating table in lithotomy position, and the rectum is irrigated until clear. A urinary catheter is optional.

The operation is started by performing an umbilical incision, and passing a Hegar dilator through the anus in order to push the sigmoid colon up to the umbilical incision. A full-thickness biopsy is done and sent for frozen section to identify the presence of ganglion cells. While waiting for the frozen section, the surgeon can divide the mesenteric vessels to the distal sigmoid colon. When confirmation of ganglion cells has been achieved, the operation moves to the perineal dissection.

Sutures are placed to evert the anus, or an anal retractor such as the Lone Star (Lone Star Medical Products, Houston, TX) can be used. An epinephrine solution can be injected into the submucosal plane if desired. The rectal mucosa is circumferentially incised using the cautery, approximately 5 mm from the dentate line, and the submucosal plane is developed (Fig. 44-45). The proximal cut edge of the mucosal cuff is tagged with multiple fine sutures, which are used for traction. The endorectal dissection is then carried proximally, staying in the submucosal plane.

When the submucosal dissection has extended proximally 2 to 3 cm, the rectal muscle is divided circumferentially (Fig. 44-46), and the full thickness of rectum and sigmoid is mobilized out through the anus. This requires division of rectal and sigmoid vessels, which can be done under direct vision using cautery or ligatures, taking care to stay on the rectal wall (Fig. 44-47).

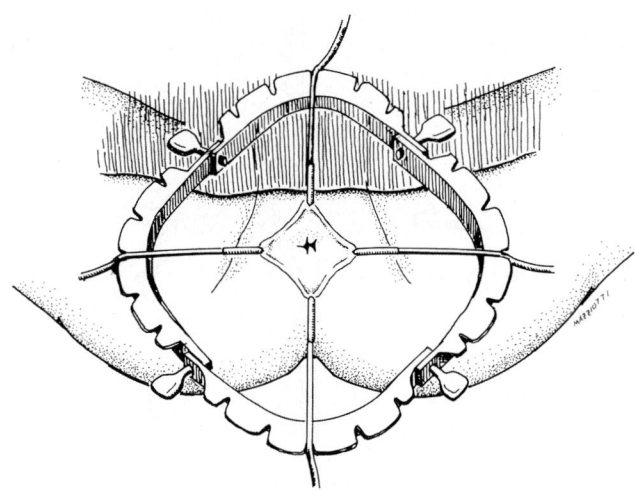

**FIGURE 44-45** Technique for transanal Soave pull-through. With an anal retractor in place, the rectal mucosa is circumferentially incised approximately 5 mm from the dentate line, and the submucosal plane is developed.

When the biopsy site containing normal ganglion cells is encountered, the colon is divided several centimeters above the biopsy (Fig. 44-48), and a standard Soave–Boley anastomosis is performed. No drains are placed. Since the mucosal dissection is very short, there is no need to divide the muscular cuff.

A digital rectal examination or calibration of the anus is done approximately 1 to 2 weeks postoperatively, and then weekly for 6 weeks. Routine daily dilatations are not done unless a stricture or cuff narrowing is detected at the weekly calibrations, or unless the child develops postoperative enterocolitis.

## SURGICAL OUTCOMES AND ONGOING CONTROVERSIES

Since the first reports of the transanal approach in the late 1990s, numerous case series involving large numbers of children have been published from virtually all continents around the world. The transanal pull-through has been shown to be effective, with both short- and long-term complication rates that are equivalent to those previously reported using a laparotomy. A number of comparative studies have also been published, comparing the transanal operation to the open approach. These studies have confirmed that the transanal pull-through is associated with shorter time to feeding, less pain, shorter hospital stay, lower cost, and improved cosmesis, as well as similar rates of incontinence, stool frequency, and obstructive symptoms on longer-term follow-up.

As the transanal pull-through has increased in popularity over the past 15 years, modifications have been introduced by various authors, which have led to a number of ongoing controversies. The first is whether a routine intraoperative biopsy should be done prior to beginning the anal dissection. Because there is approximately a 10% risk of the pathological

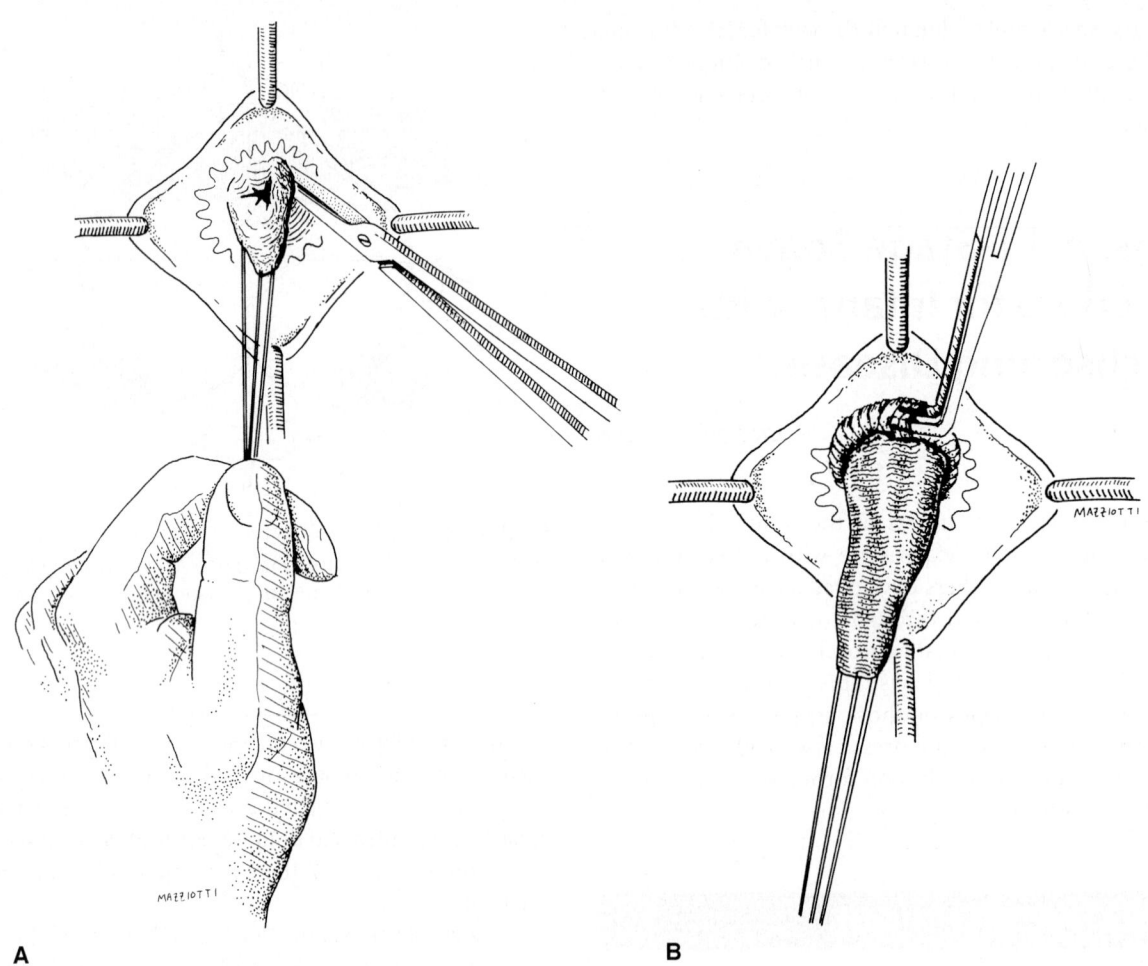

**A**

**B**

**FIGURE 44-46** Staying in the submucosal plane (**A**), the endorectal dissection is carried proximally to a point above the peritoneal reflection, where the rectal muscle is divided circumferentially (**B**).

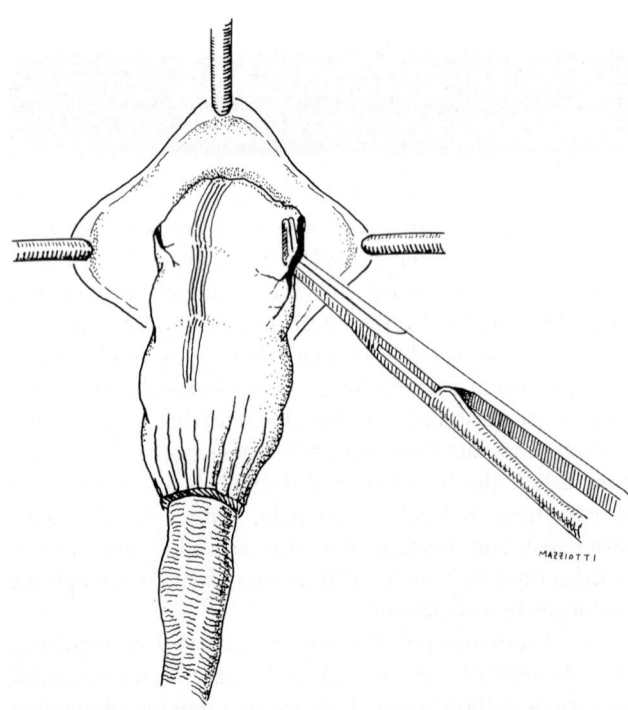

**FIGURE 44-47** The full thickness of rectum and sigmoid is mobilized out through the anus. Rectal and sigmoid vessels are divided under direct vision using cautery or ligatures.

transition zone being more proximal than the radiological transition zone, and because there is no difference in surgical outcomes in patients who undergo a preliminary biopsy, we strongly advocate this approach. The second controversy is the position in which the operation is done. Some surgeons prefer the prone position, which provides excellent visualization of the anatomy. We perform the operation in the supine position, which permits an umbilical incision or laparoscopy in order to do intraoperative biopsies or to mobilize the colon in the case of more a proximal transition zone. The third controversy is the length of the muscular cuff. We have documented a decrease in the incidence of cuff narrowing and of enterocolitis after changing our technique to a very short muscular cuff, as described above. Some authors have taken this even further and performed a Swenson procedure transanally, with no submucosal dissection at all.

No comparative studies have been published comparing the transanal pull-through to the laparoscopic pull-through. However, a recent series suggests the transabdominal versus transanal route have similar outcomes. Further, as the 2 techniques have evolved over time, they have become increasingly similar to each other, and the outcomes from reported case series are almost identical. Therefore, a direct comparison between the 2 methods has become less relevant and is unlikely to be done.

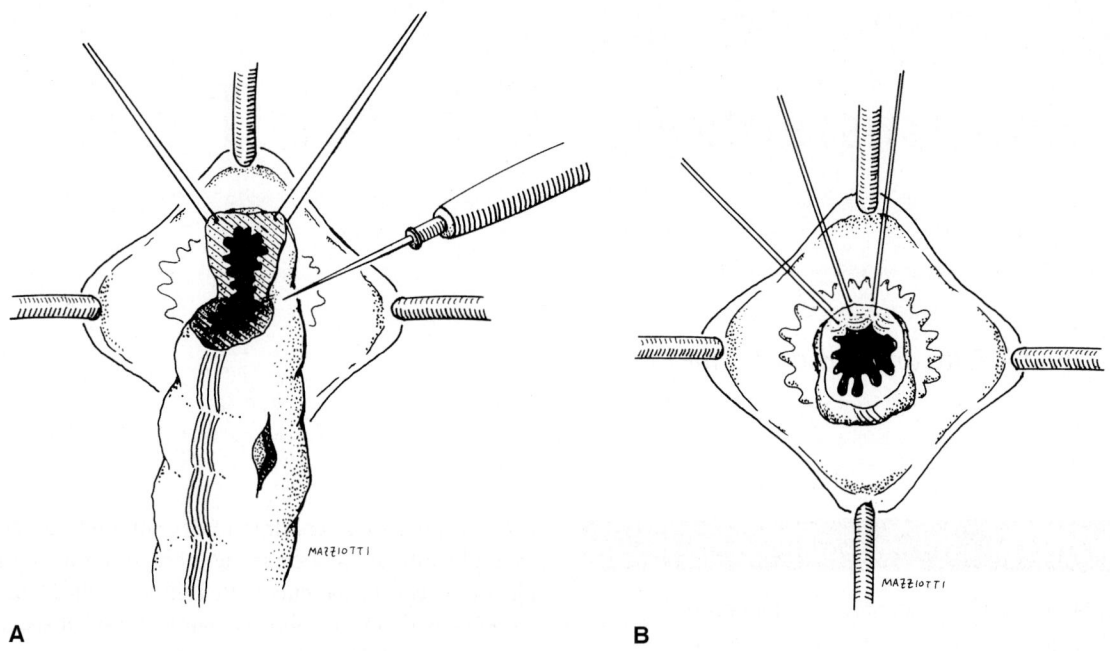

**FIGURE 44-48** After confirmation of ganglion cells by frozen section, the colon is divided several centimeters above the most proximal normal biopsy (**A**). A standard Soave–Boley anastomosis is then performed (**B**).

## SELECTED READINGS

Coran A, Weintraub W. Modification of the endorectal procedure for Hirschsprung's disease. *Surg Gynecol Obstet* 1976;143:277–282.

De La Torre L, Langer JC. Transanal endorectal pull-through for Hirschsprung disease: technique, controversies, pearls, pitfalls, and an organized approach to the management of postoperative obstructive symptoms. *Semin Pediatr Surg* 2010;19:96–106.

Escobar MA, Grosfeld JL, West KW, et al. Long-term outcomes in total colonic aganglionosis: a 32-year experience. *J Pediatr Surg* 2005;40:955–961.

Georgeson KE, Cohen RD, Hebra A, et al. Primary laparoscopic-assisted endorectal colon pull-through for Hirschsprung's disease: a new gold standard. *Ann Surg* 1999;229:678–682; discussion 682–673.

Kim AC, Langer JC, Pastor AC, et al. Endorectal pull-through for Hirschsprung's disease—a multicenter, long-term comparison of results: transanal vs transabdominal approach. *J Pediatr Surg* 2010;45:1213–1220.

Langer JC, Durrant AC, de la Torre L, et al. One-stage transanal Soave pullthrough for Hirschsprung disease: a multicenter experience with 141 children. *Ann Surg* 2003;238:569–583; discussion 583–565.

van Leeuwen K, Teitelbaum DH, Elhalaby EA, Coran AG. Long-term follow-up of redo pull-through procedures for Hirschsprung's disease: efficacy of the endorectal pull-through. *J Pediatr Surg* 2000;35:829–833; discussion 833–824.

Wildhaber B, Coran A, Teitelbaum D. Total colonic Hirschsprung's disease: a 28-year experience. *J Pediatr Surg* 2005;40(1):203–206.

Wildhaber B, Pakarinen M, Rintala R, Coran A, Teitelbaum D. Posterior myotomy/myectomy for persistent stooling problems in Hirschsprung's disease. *J Pediatr Surg* 2004;39:920–926.

Yagmurlu A, Harmon CM, Georgeson KE. Laparoscopic cecostomy button placement for the management of fecal incontinence in children with Hirschsprung's disease and anorectal anomalies. *Surg Endosc* 2006;20:624–627.

# Intussusception CHAPTER 45

Brad A. Feltis and David J. Schmeling

## ETIOLOGY AND PATHOPHYSIOLOGY

Intussusception occurs when a segment of intestine invaginates or "telescopes" into the adjacent distal bowel. Although the process can occur anywhere in the intestine, 90% of the cases in children are ileocolic (Fig. 45-1) in location. The invaginating proximal bowel is termed the intussusceptum and the receiving distal bowel segment the intussuscipiens. Intussusception can occur at any age; however, it is unusual in children younger than 3 months or older than 3 years. The peak incidence occurs between 5 and 9 months.

The majority of cases (90%) of intussusception in children are idiopathic. In these patients, viral-induced lymphoid hyperplasia has been hypothesized to account for the "lead point." Adenovirus, rotavirus, and human herpes virus 6 have all been implicated as potential causative agents.

Ten percent of children with intussusception will have an identifiable cause or "pathologic" lead point, most commonly a Meckel diverticulum. Other identifiable lead points include lymphoma and intestinal polyps (Fig. 45-2), conditions most frequently seen in older children. Certain systemic conditions can also predispose children to develop intussusception. For example, intussusception is the most common surgical complication seen in patients with Henoch–Schonlein purpura. Patients with cystic fibrosis, familial polyposis, nephrotic syndrome, and Peutz–Jeghers syndrome are also predisposed to developing intussusception.

Aggressive diagnostic workup to identify a pathologic lead point should be initiated when an intussusception is not ileocolic in location or when an intussusception occurs at an age outside the typical infant idiopathic range.

## CLINICAL PRESENTATION

Severe intermittent cramping abdominal pain occurring at intervals every 15 to 20 minutes in an infant or toddler is a hallmark of intussusception and is noted in up to 95% of children with this diagnosis. The child's abdomen is generally soft and the child may seem relatively playful and well between episodes of colic. Abdominal colic is so prevalent with intussusception that its absence should cause the clinician to be suspicious of the validity of a diagnosis of intussusception. In addition to colic, children with intussusception will frequently exhibit emesis that may become bilious, anorexia, and malaise. A picture of full-blown clinical sepsis may evolve if not diagnosed and treated in a timely way. The "classic" clinical triad for intussusception consists of abdominal pain, a palpable abdominal mass, and currant jelly stool. This triad is present in fewer than 50% of cases.

Importantly, the clinician needs to be aware that the frequency of signs and symptoms varies with age. An infant may present with only irritability or vomiting; abdominal colic becomes more common in older children—often causing the child to double over and pull his knees toward his abdomen. The physical exam finding of a palpable right upper quadrant mass is quite helpful; however, it is also quite challenging to confirm with certainty in a distressed infant or toddler. The finding of currant jelly stool is a relatively late finding and is indicative of intestinal ischemia and mucosal sloughing. The absence of currant jelly stools in the appropriate clinical setting should not delay the pursuit of a diagnosis of intussusception.

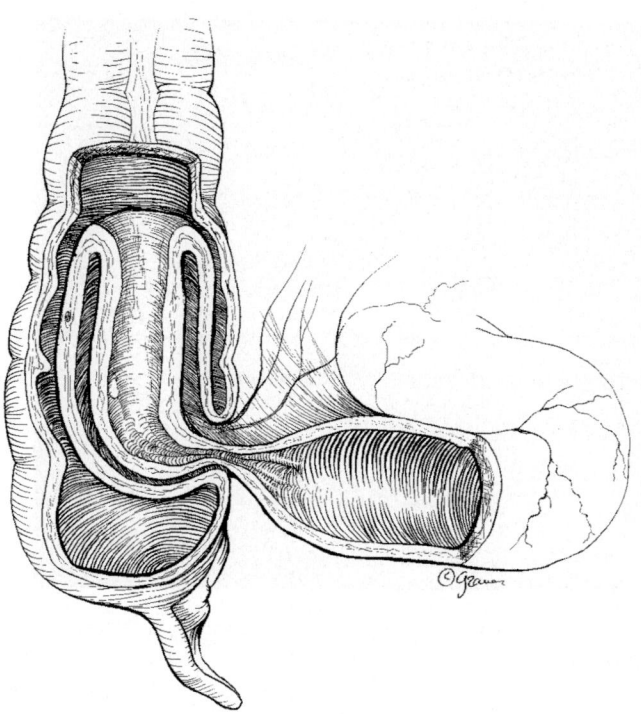

**FIGURE 45-1** Ileocolic intussusception showing how the mesenteric vessels are compressed and squeezed between the layers of the intussusceptum. Resultant edema exacerbates venous congestion leading to ischemia in the intussusceptum. Untreated, tissue pressure will exceed arterial pressure and result in necrosis.

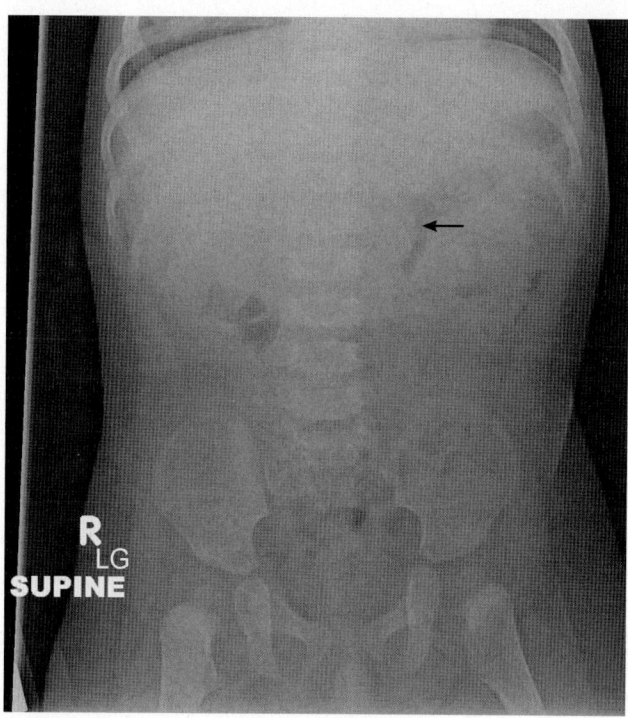

**FIGURE 45-3** Supine x-ray of a child with ileocolic intussusception. Note the characteristic paucity of gas in the right colon and iliac fossa. The lead point of the intussusceptum is in the transverse colon and is visible as a soft tissue mass in the epigastrium (*arrow*).

## EVALUATION

Radiologic studies are essential in the evaluation of intussusception. Initial studies should consist of supine frontal as well as left lateral decubitus radiographs. Although these studies are neither sensitive nor specific, they can be helpful. Bowel gas patterns are normal early in the course of intussusception, but can appear obstructive as symptoms persist. The most consistent finding is of a paucity of gas in the right iliac fossa (Fig. 45-3) in the region of the normally air containing cecum. Other helpful plain film findings include the presence of a soft tissue mass in the right upper quadrant (Fig. 45-3). Evidence of bowel obstruction is nonspecific, but

in a nonoperated infant, bowel obstruction is frequently associated with intussusception.

If the clinical findings and plain films are suggestive of intussusception, one should proceed to either air enema or positive contrast enema (water-soluble contrast in most institutions utilizing hydrostatic reduction) for confirmation and attempted reduction. If, however, the diagnosis is suspected but remains in doubt after plain films, ultrasound can be useful as a noninvasive adjunct to confirm or exclude intussusception. In experienced hands, ultrasound is both sensitive (98%) and specific (90%-100%) for intussusception. The findings of a "target" sign on transverse imaging and a "sandwich" or "pseudokidney" sign on longitudinal imaging effectively confirm the diagnosis of intussusception (Fig. 45-4). Importantly, the absence of these findings on ultrasound effectively excludes the diagnosis of intussusception. Computed tomography (CT) does not have a defined role in the evaluation of suspected pediatric intussusception. Although this imaging modality is capable of demonstrating the intussusception, exposure of the child to potentially harmful doses of radiation relegate CT use only for confounding cases.

## NONOPERATIVE MANAGEMENT

A child with intussusception is typically intravascularly volume depleted due to vomiting, decreased oral intake, and third space losses. Therefore, fluid resuscitation should be initiated in the emergency department (ED). Historically,

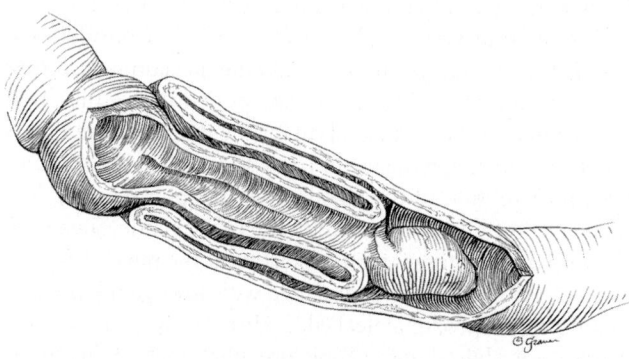

**FIGURE 45-2** Small bowel intussusception caused by polyp (the second commonest pathogenic lead point).

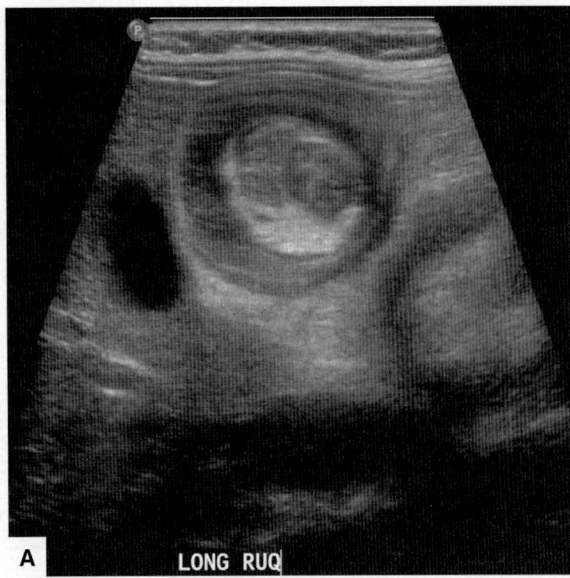
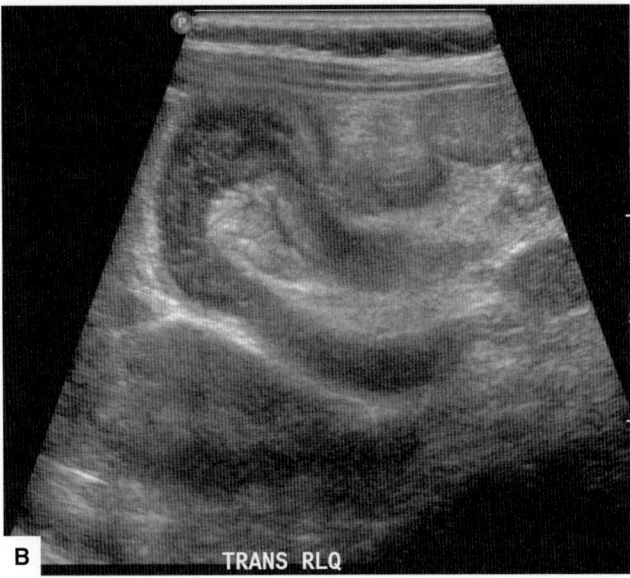

**FIGURE 45-4 A.** "Target sign": this RUQ ultrasound demonstrates a cross-sectional view of an ileocolic intussusception. **B.** "Pseudokidney sign": this RLQ ultrasound demonstrates an axial view of an ileocolic intussusception.

administration of intravenous (IV) antibiotics has been recommended prior to attempts at radiologic reduction. However, this recommendation is not well studied and many groups do not routinely provide antibiotics prior to reduction. Pediatric surgical consultation is initiated while the child is in the ED. A child with frank peritonitis or evidence of perforation is administered IV antibiotics (ie, piperacillin/tazobactam or ertapenem) and should proceed directly to surgery after volume resuscitation. The first line of therapy for all other children with intussusception is an attempt at pneumatic or hydrostatic reduction by enema performed by a pediatric radiologist.

The technique of radiologic reduction involves placing a rectal tube, usually a Foley balloon catheter. To facilitate a good seal and allow the generation and maintenance of adequate pressure, the tube is stabilized by tightly taping the buttocks. Historically, a 1 m column of barium was used as the agent of choice with a reported success rate of 70%. More recently, fluoroscopically guided pneumatic reduction (air enema, Fig. 45-5A) has gained acceptance as the procedure of choice due to greater ease of exam and a higher success rate (85%), as well as decreased risk in the event of perforation. Additionally, air enema has the advantages of lower radiation dose along with continued pressure monitoring during the procedure. The pressure of the air column is kept below 120 mm Hg. The reported perforation rate during enema reduction is 1% to 3%. Successful reduction is typically defined as resolution of the intracolonic mass associated with free reflux of air or contrast material into the terminal ileum (Fig. 45-5C). Some authors have documented successful reduction without the observation of contrast flowing into the terminal ileum. The absence of ileal reflux, attributed to a competent or edematous ileocecal valve, raises the concern for incomplete reduction and these children are best observed for resolution or recurrence of symptoms prior to discharge.

Postreduction management of these children varies. Some accumulating data suggest that children with successful enema reduction can be safely treated as outpatients. However, most admit these children for limited observation. Depending on the degree of intravascular volume depletion on admission, continued IV fluids may or may not be required. We do not administer antibiotics prior to attempted reduction and we allow the child to eat and drink as tolerated following the procedure. If the children are tolerating a diet and not having recurrent abdominal pain, we discharge them home within 23 hours of the reduction. Recurrent intussusception may occur in up to 15% of children after successful enema reduction. These children should proceed again to enema reduction. If intussusception recurs several times, a pathologic lead point needs to be strongly considered and eventual open or laparoscopic exploration may be warranted.

## OPERATIVE MANAGEMENT

Operative management of intussusception is reserved for cases of frank peritonitis, perforation, or failed enema reduction.

### Open

Open surgery has traditionally been performed via an infra-umbilical transverse right-sided incision. Consideration could also be given to an upper midline incision, which may result in better visualization or ease of delivery of the mass. Upon entering the peritoneal cavity, the intussuscepted mass is delivered through the wound. For an ileocolic intussusception, mobilization of the right colon may be necessary. The maneuver of manual reduction involves gentle squeezing ("taxis") of the intussusceptum starting at the most distal end (Fig. 45-6). This may be augmented with slow, gentle traction pulling on the proximal ileal edge. Historically, pediatric surgeons were advised not to apply proximal traction due to the risk of tearing the edematous intestine. However, accumulating experience, both open and laparoscopically, demonstrates

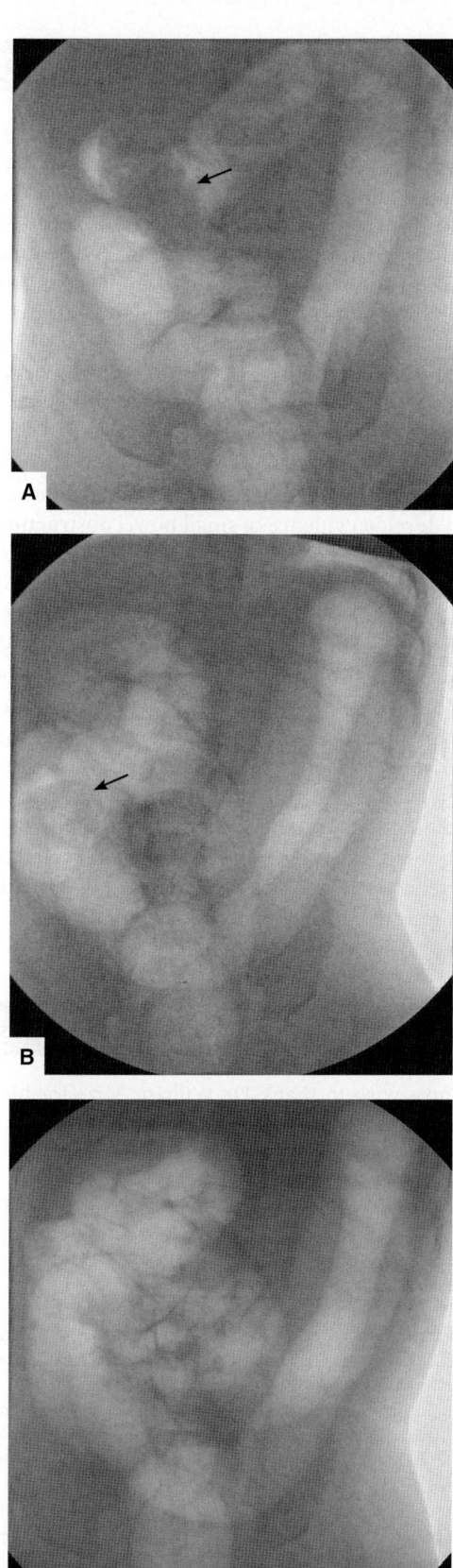

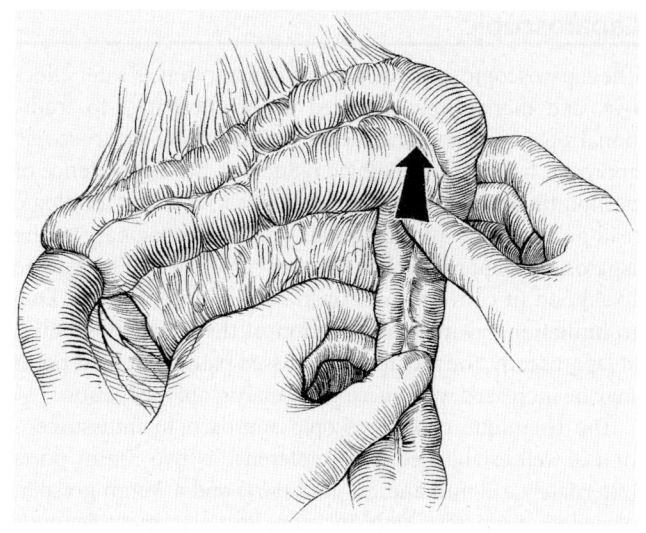

**FIGURE 45-6** The most important aspect of the manual reduction of any intussusception is the continuous squeezing of the most distal intussusceptum through the wall of the intussuscipiens. Simultaneously, an assistant gently pulls the intussusceptum out of the proximal end.

that gentle proximal traction is safe. Several minutes of continuous pressure to slowly decompress the bowel wall edema is often necessary to manually reduce the mass. Serosal tears may result during this maneuver as both the intussusceptum and intussuscipiens are quite edematous. These should be of no consequence as long as there is no full-thickness injury. It is difficult to ascertain the extent of ischemia until the bowel has been completely reduced. If manual reduction is accomplished, one must be certain that the bowel is viable and adequately perfused and the presence or absence of a pathologic lead point, most frequently a Meckel diverticulum or a polyp, is confirmed.

If, after several minutes attempting manual reduction, no progress is made, preparation should be undertaken for resection of the irreducible intussusception. For an ileocolic intussusception this will typically involve an ileocecectomy or a right hemicolectomy. This operation will be facilitated by completely mobilizing the right colon to the hepatic flexure. Our preferred approach is to perform primary end-to-end anastomosis if the resection margins are well perfused and only mildly edematous. A temporary stoma can be entertained at the discretion of the operating surgeon, but should be reserved for cases with a high likelihood of poor intestinal healing, such as poor perfusion of the resected margins, hemodynamic instability, or frank perforation with intraabdominal sepsis.

Management of the appendix remains controversial and without consensus. Historically, appendectomy was performed to eliminate confusion concerning the status of the appendix in a patient with a right-sided transverse incision. However, accumulating evidence suggests the potential of a functional immunologic role for the appendix. Additionally, the possibility exists for any patient that the appendix may have other potential uses, such as continent appendicostomy or Mitrofanoff reconstruction. Our approach is generally to leave the appendix in place if it is not included in a resection.

**FIGURE 45-5 A.** Fluoroscopic image during air enema demonstrating ileocolic intussusception with lead point in proximal transverse colon (*arrow*). Note that air is bright and bone is dark in this technique. **B.** Lead point (*arrow*) has been reduced to proximal right colon and (**C**) Intussusception completely reduced as air now opacifying multiple loops of distal small bowel.

## Laparoscopic

The laparoscopic approach to intussusception is safe, effective, and increasingly accepted as an alternative to traditional open surgery. The ideal candidate for a laparoscopic approach has failed radiologic reduction, has no evidence of peritonitis, and a duration of symptoms <1.5 days. Pathologic lead point and delayed diagnosis are not exclusionary of the laparoscopic approach, but these circumstances increase the likelihood of conversion to open surgical intervention. Due to limitations in manual palpation of the edematous bowel at laparoscopy, the incidence of missed pathologic lead point may be increased with successful laparoscopic reduction.

The technique of laparoscopic approach to intussusception is well established. Our preference is two 5-mm ports (alternately a 3-mm and a 5-mm port) and a 3-mm grasper, placed via a separate "stab" incision. Port placement depends on the location of the intussusception. The abdomen is entered via the open technique through the umbilicus. A 3- or 5-mm port is placed in this umbilical location and pneumoperitoneum is established. For ileocolic intussusception, a 5-mm port is placed in the LUQ and a 3-mm grasper is introduced through the LLQ via the stab technique. These are placed under direct telescopic vision after infiltrating the peritoneum with 0.25% bupivacaine. The goal is to reduce the intussusceptum using the atraumatic graspers. A 3-mm grasper tends to be too traumatic to the edematous bowel, because of the pressure generated over a smaller grasping surface. Some authors recommend a 10-mm grasper as the instrument of choice to assure gentle handling of the edematous bowel. The decision to upsize an existing port can be made intraoperatively. As in the open technique, the key is gentle traction just proximal and constant gentle pressure just distal to the intussusceptum. Again, due to the intestinal wall edema, several minutes of continuous pressure and traction may be required, so one should not too quickly abandon the laparoscopic technique for lack of progress. Other authors have described preoperative placement of a ballooned Foley catheter taped into the rectal vault and attached to a bag of normal saline to provide helpful intracolonic counter pressure during the attempted laparoscopic reduction. Conversion to an open technique is considered for bowel necrosis, discovery of pathologic lead point, or failure of reduction. If a decision for conversion is made, we mobilize the right colon laparoscopically and deliver the intussuscepted mass through an expanded umbilical incision.

Management of the appendix at laparoscopy is not standardized. Our practice is to leave the appendix. If appendectomy is a part of the operative strategy, it can be easily performed via an "open" technique after delivering the appendix into the umbilicus through the 5-mm port site.

Postoperative management depends on the procedure performed. Length of stay (LOS) is shorter for children requiring bowel resection treated laparoscopically (3 vs 4.5 days). If no bowel resection is performed, the patients can eat early and LOS is dictated by traditional parameters of diet and pain control, typically 1 to 2 days in an infant after successful surgical reduction.

# POSTOPERATIVE INTUSSUSCEPTION

Postoperative intussusception (POI) in children represents an uncommon but well-described phenomena. Although there is a stronger correlation with retroperitoneal dissection, POI has been observed following routine abdominal surgery as well. The precise etiology of POI is unknown. Proposed causes of an etiologic lead point include edema from bowel manipulation, adynamic ileus, suture or staple line, or postoperative adhesions. POI typically involves the small bowel and occurs within the first 2 weeks after surgery. As the incidence is less than 1%, diagnosis generally depends on maintaining a high index of suspicion in any child with a postoperative bowel obstruction. Commonly the children will fail to return normal bowel function and develop evidence of small bowel obstruction a few days postoperatively. Symptoms may include abdominal pain with distention, bilious vomiting or bilious nasogastric returns, and crampy colic. The diagnosis of POI is challenging as these symptoms are readily attributed to prolonged adynamic ileus. Routine plain films are most often not helpful for diagnosis. If POI is suspected, ultrasound is the confirmatory test of choice with a sensitivity around 80%. However, a negative ultrasound does not exclude the diagnosis of POI, and a high index of clinical suspicion with a low threshold for surgical reexploration remains key.

If diagnosed, small bowel POI requires reexploration for manual reduction. Most are easily reduced with gentle traction and resection is seldom necessary.

# ACKNOWLEDGMENTS

The authors wish to thank Dr William Mize for his excellent assistance in preparing the radiologic portion of this chapter.

## SELECTED READINGS

Applegate KE. Intussusception in children: evidence-based diagnosis and treatment. *Pediatr Radiol* 2009;39(suppl 2):S140–S143.

Bonnard A, Demarche M, Dimitriu C, et al. Indications for laparoscopy in the management of intussusception: a multicenter retrospective study conducted by the French Study Group for Pediatric Laparoscopy. *J Pediatr Surg* 2008;43(7):1249–1253.

Curtis JL, Gutierrez IM, Kirk SR, Gollin G. Failure of enema reduction for ileocolic intussusception at a referring hospital does not preclude repeat attempts at a children's hospital. *J Pediatr Surg* 2010;45(6):1178–1181.

Fraser JD, Aguayo P, Ho B, et al. Laparoscopic management of intussusception in pediatric patients. *J Laparoendosc Adv Surg Tech A* 2009;19(4):563–565.

Hryhorczuk AL, Strouse PJ. Validation of US as a first-line diagnostic test for assessment of pediatric ileocolic intussusception. *Pediatr Radiol* 2009;39(10):1075–1079.

Waseem M, Rosenberg HK. Intussusception. *Pediatr Emerg Care* 2008;24(11):793–800.

Whitehouse JS, Gourlay DM, Winthrop AL, Cassidy LD, Arca MJ. Is it safe to discharge intussusception patients after successful hydrostatic reduction? *J Pediatr Surg* 2010;45(6):1182–1186.

ABDOMINAL DISEASE

# CHAPTER 46

## Necrotizing Enterocolitis

Shannon L. Castle, Allison L. Speer,
Tracy C. Grikscheit, and Henri Ford

## KEY POINTS

1. Necrotizing enterocolitis (NEC) is the most common gastrointestinal emergency of the newborn, primarily affecting preterm infants and those with cyanotic heart disease. Up to 50% of infants who develop NEC will require surgical intervention.

2. Major risk factors for NEC include prematurity, hypoxia, bacterial infection, congenital heart disease, and initiation of enteral nutrition.

3. Infants with NEC may present with feeding intolerance, bloody stools, respiratory distress, or hypoperfusion. Clinical and radiographic criteria are summarized in the Bell grading system.

4. In an infant with suspected NEC, initial laboratory studies should include a complete blood cell count, electrolyte panel, a blood gas to determine the acid–base status of the patient, and blood cultures.

5. Infants with suspected or confirmed NEC should be treated with bowel rest, broad-spectrum antibiotics, and volume resuscitation.

6. The only absolute indication for surgical intervention is the presence of the pneumoperitoneum. Relative indications for surgery include a fixed intestinal loop on serial plain abdominal radiographs, portal venous gas on plain abdominal radiograph, abominal wall erythema, a palpable abdominal mass, a positive paracentesis, and clinical deterioration despite maximal medical therapy.

7. Based on accumulated evidence, we recommend initial peritoneal drainage (PD) only for VLBW infants who are hemodynamically unstable with respiratory embarrassment secondary to abdominal distention; however, subsequent laparotomy is warranted.

8. Definitive primary laparotomy with resection of necrotic intestine is best suited for infants weighing >1500 g or VLBW neonates who can tolerate the initial operation.

9. The standard of care for focal NEC is resection with creation of a proximal enterostomy, with or without a distal mucous fistula. Primary anastomosis may be considered in a hemodynamically stable infant with minimal peritoneal soilage.

10. Options for treatment of multifocal disease are varied, but the principal goal is resection of the obviously necrotic intestine with preservation of intestinal length to avoid short bowel syndrome.

11. Long-term complications of NEC include stricture, short bowel syndrome, and neurodevelopmental impairment.

## INTRODUCTION

Necrotizing enterocolitis (NEC) is the most common gastrointestinal emergency in the newborn. The majority of the cases occur in infants born at fewer than 36 weeks gestational age. In fact, approximately 1% to 5% of all preterm infants develop NEC. However, NEC has also been reported in term infants, particularly those with cyanotic heart disease. As a result of recent advances in the care of preterm infants, the incidence of NEC has been rising. In its most severe form, NEC is characterized by full-thickness destruction of the intestinal wall, which may lead to intestinal perforation, subsequent peritonitis, sepsis, and death. Up to 50% of infants who develop NEC will require surgical intervention. The mortality rate ranges from 10% to 50% but approaches 100% in infants with panintestinal involvement. Infants who survive may experience future morbidity such as intestinal obstruction secondary to stricture formation or adhesions, or they may develop intestinal failure characterized by intestinal dysmotility and long-term dependency on parenteral nutrition.

## PATHOGENESIS

Multiple risk factors have been implicated in the pathogenesis of NEC. These include prematurity, hypoxia, bacterial infection, congenital heart disease, and initiation of enteral nutrition. The preterm infant has an immature intestinal epithelial barrier that may facilitate the transmucosal passage of lumenal bacteria and antigens. Bacterial colonization is believed to be necessary for the development of NEC. Abnormal colonization of the intestine with pathogenic Gram negative bacteria, whether derived from the hospital environment or contaminated feedings, may predispose the preterm infant to the development of NEC. Our current hypothesis regarding the pathogenesis of NEC is that a hypoxic or ischemic insult to the intestine damages the mucosal barrier and allows indigenous bacteria from the gastrointestinal tract to invade the intestinal wall, inciting an inflammatory cascade that leads to the local release of proinflammatory mediators, which in turn exacerbate the initial epithelial injury and ultimately lead to gut barrier failure. Although no single pathogen has been consistently isolated in NEC, several bacteria, including Enterobacteriaceae, *Clostridia,* and *Staphylococcus* species, have been implicated in its development.

The intestinal epithelium serves as a selective barrier that restricts the translocation of antigens and microbes. Epithelial tight junctions, intestinal peristalsis, mucin production, and gastric acidity work synergistically to limit the number of antigens and microbes that traverse the gastrointestinal tract. In premature infants, an immature mucosal epithelial layer and immune system combined with impaired peristalsis and abnormal mucin production may predispose to increased translocation of bacteria, thereby inciting an inflammatory cascade in the epithelium and lamina propria that may contribute to the subsequent development of NEC.

Many inflammatory mediators have been implicated in the development of NEC; these include TNF-alpha, platelet activating factor, IL-1, IL-6, IL-18, endothelin-1, thomboxanes, and oxygen free radicals, to name a few. Similarly, nitric oxide, produced in high levels by inducible nitric oxide synthase during inflammation, and prostanoids, produced by the cyclooxygenase enzymes, have been shown to damage the gut barrier.

Initiation of enteral feeding is well established as a risk factor for the development of NEC, but the optimal strategy for advancing feeds in premature infants is controversial. Low volume (<24 mL/kg/day) delivery of enteral nutrition in the first 10 days of life does not appear to increase the risk of developing NEC, but according to multiple studies, rapid advancement beyond this volume significantly increases the risk of developing NEC. Feeding breast milk instead of formula lowers the incidence of NEC in both human and animal studies, but the mechanism of this protective effect of breast milk remains unclear.

## CLINICAL MANIFESTATIONS

NEC occurs most commonly in premature, low-birth-weight infants. Fewer than 10% of cases occur in full-term infants. Age at presentation is variable. NEC typically presents in the first 2 weeks of life after the onset of bacterial colonization, but it may occur later in infants born at an earlier gestational age or in very low birth weight (VLBW) infants (less than 1500 g). The incidence of NEC in preterm infants weighing between 1000 and 1500 g is approximately 4%, but approaches 10% in extremely low birth weight (ELBW) patients (less than 1000 g).

Infants with NEC may present with feeding intolerance, bloody stools, respiratory distress, or hypoperfusion. On physical exam, patients with NEC have a distended abdomen, which may be tense and erythematous. Infants with advanced NEC or intestinal perforation may demonstrate systemic signs of sepsis such as hemodynamic instability, respiratory distress, or decreased peripheral perfusion.

The Bell grading system for NEC has been widely used since its introduction in 1978 to standardize the diagnosis of NEC based on clinical and radiographic criteria. Classification based on the Bell criteria allows for uniform language in research and treatment guidelines (Table 46-1).

| TABLE 46-1 | Modified Bell's Stages of Necrotizing Enterocolitis | | | |
|---|---|---|---|---|
| **Stage Classification** | **Systemic Signs** | **Abdominal Signs** | **Radiographic Signs** | **Treatment** |
| IA suspected | Apnea<br>Bradycardia<br>Temperature instability<br>Lethargy | Mild abdominal distension<br>Emesis or high gastric residuals<br>Fecal occult blood | Normal<br>Nonspecific mild intestinal dilatation<br>Mild ileus | Bowel rest (NPO, OGT)<br>Antibiotics × 3-5 days unless symptoms progress |
| IB suspected | Same as IA | Same as IA + gross fecal blood | Same as IA + intestinal dilatation | Same as IA |
| IIA Definite<br>Mildly Ill | Same as IA | Same as IB<br>+ Absent bowel sounds<br>+/− Abdominal tenderness | Same as IB<br>+ pneumatosis intestinalis | Bowel rest<br>Antibiotics × 7-10 days |
| IIB<br>Definite<br>Moderately Ill | Same as IA + Mild metabolic acidosis<br>Mild thrombocytopenia | Same as IIA<br>+ Definite abdominal tenderness<br>+/− Abdominal cellulitis or RLQ mass | Same as IIA<br>+ Portal venous gas<br>+/− Ascites | Bowel rest<br>Antibiotics × 14 days |

*(Continued)*

**TABLE 46-1    Modified Bell's Stages of Necrotizing Enterocolitis** *(Continued)*

| Stage Classification | Systemic Signs | Abdominal Signs | Radiographic Signs | Treatment |
|---|---|---|---|---|
| IIIA<br>Advanced<br>Severely Ill<br>Bowel intact | Same as IIB +<br>Severe apnea<br>Hypotension<br>Shock<br>Respiratory acidosis<br>Metabolic acidosis<br>DIC<br>Neutropenia | Same as IIB +<br>Peritonitis<br>Marked abdominal<br>   tenderness and distension | Same as IIB + Definite<br>   ascites | Bowel rest<br>Antibiotics × 14 days<br>Fluid resuscitation<br>Inotropic support<br>Ventilator support |
| IIIB<br>Advanced<br>Severely Ill<br>Bowel perforated | Same as IIIA | Same as IIIA | Same as IIIA<br>   + Pneumoperitoneum | Same as IIIA + Surgery |

NPO, nil per os; OGT, orogastric tube; RLQ, right lower quadrant; DIC, disseminated intravascular coagulopathy.
Modified from Walsh MC, Kliegman RM. Necrotizing enterocolitis: treatment based on staging criteria. *Pediatr Clin N Am* 1986;33(1):179–201.

## DIAGNOSTIC STUDIES

### Laboratory Findings

In an infant with suspected NEC, initial laboratory studies should include a complete blood cell count, electrolyte panel, a blood gas to determine the acid–base status of the patient, and blood cultures. Laboratory abnormalities in NEC include thrombocytopenia, leukocytosis or leukopenia, metabolic acidosis, hypercapnea, and hypoxia. Leukocytosis may be present initially, but leukopenia is common, especially in severe NEC, with roughly 37% of severe cases (Bell stage III) having a WBC count less than $1.5 \times 10^3$/L. Severe thrombocytopenia ($<100 \times 10^3$/L) is associated with worse outcomes. Bacteremia is present in up to 50% of patients.

### Radiographic Studies

Plain abdominal radiographs (anterior–posterior and a left lateral decubitus) should be obtained to evaluate for signs pathognomonic for NEC (Fig. 46-1). These include intramural gas or pneumatosis intestinalis, the radiographic hallmark of NEC, portal venous gas, and, if perforation is present, free intraperitoneal air. An early, nonspecific sign is generalized dilation of the bowel. A "fixed loop," defined as a loop of bowel that remains unchanged over serial abdominal radiographs, is typically associated with transmural necrosis or distal obstruction. Portal venous gas, the result of intramural gas being absorbed by the venous system, can be seen in up to 30% of infants with NEC, and has been associated with the presence of panintestinal involvement.

Another imaging modality used to evaluate infants with proven or suspected NEC is abdominal ultrasound, which may demonstrate increased bowel wall thickness or intra-abdominal fluid collections with greater sensitivity compared to an x-ray. In the hands of an experienced ultrasonographer, ultrasound can also be used to show portal venous gas or free air, although detection of portal venous gas by ultrasound may not have the same clinical significance as detection on plain abdominal radiographs due to the high sensitivity of

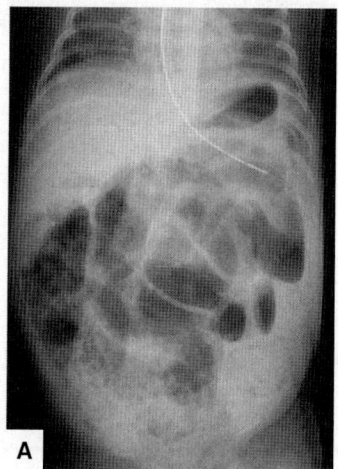 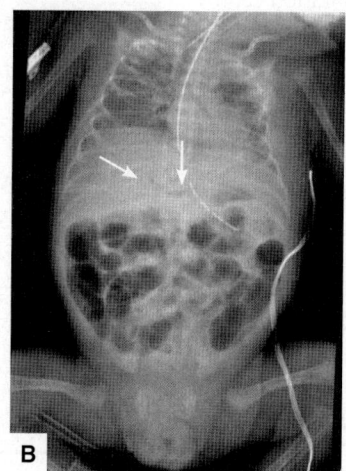 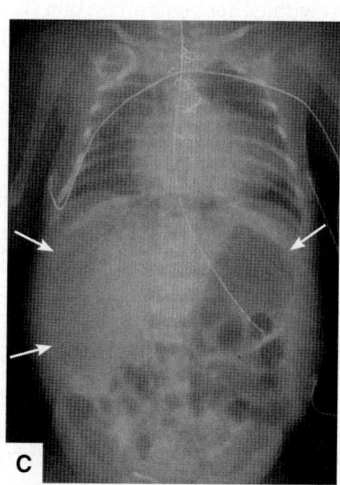

**FIGURE 46-1** Abdominal radiographs of infants with NEC showing **A.** pneumatosis intestinalis; (**B**) portal venous gas; and (**C**) free intraperitoneal air (football sign).

ultrasonography in this setting. The ultrasound is dependent on operator experience for its sensitivity, and thus should not be used as the sole imaging modality. Plain abdominal radiographs remain the standard of care.

## Differential Diagnosis

The differential diagnosis of NEC includes sepsis, ileus, bacterial or viral enterocolitis, and intestinal obstruction. Focal intestinal perforation (FIP) may present with a clinical picture similar to NEC but is truly a focal process, usually associated with a perforation in the distal ileum. FIP is more common in extremely premature (less than 26 weeks gestation) or VLBW infants. Typically it presents in the first week of life and is associated with prior treatment with cyclooxygenase inhibitors (such as indomethacin for treatment of a patent ductus arteriosus) and steroids. Patients with FIP do not always exhibit the typical clinical symptoms, laboratory results, or radiographic findings associated with NEC, but will generally have pneumoperitoneum on plain abdominal x-ray. While the surgical treatment may be similar to that for short-segment NEC, it is now recognized as a distinct clinical entity.

## MEDICAL MANAGEMENT

Infants with suspected or confirmed NEC should be treated with bowel rest, broad-spectrum antibiotics, and volume resuscitation. Oral feeding should be discontinued and an orogastric tube (OGT) should be inserted. Aggressive fluid resuscitation is vital to correct the associated hypovolemia and metabolic acidosis. Septic infants with respiratory distress may require ventilatory support as well as vasopressors to maintain adequate perfusion pressure. Infusion of blood products should be used as needed to correct thrombocytopenia or coagulopathy.

Broad-spectrum antibiotics with good activity against Gram negative and Gram positive organisms should be administered. There is little evidence to support a specific antibiotic combination or regimen, but the high rate of bacteremia seen in these infants supports the use of broad-spectrum antibiotics. Appropriate antibiotic regimens include ampicillin with either gentamicin or a third-generation cephalosporin (ie, cefotaxime), plus metronidazole or clindamycin, or piperacillin–tazobactam. Vancomycin may be added for suspected methicillin-resistant *S. aureus* or ampicillin-resistant enterococcal infection; plasma vancomycin levels should be measured to ensure that they are in the therapeutic range. Blood cultures and intraoperative cultures of surgically managed infants can then be used to further refine antibiotic coverage. If the Gram stain or intraoperative cultures indicate a fungal infection, fluconazole or amphotericin B should be added for antifungal coverage. Specific antibiotic choices should be guided by an institution-specific antibiotic nomogram. Antibiotics should be administered for 7–10 days or until the patient recovers from the septic episode as evidenced by hemodynamic stability, return of bowel function, and improvement in leukopenia. Note that the thrombocytopenia associated with NEC always trails other parameters during the recovery phase.

## SURGICAL MANAGEMENT

### Indications for Surgery

Up to 50% of infants who develop NEC may ultimately require surgical intervention. The only absolute indication for surgical intervention is the presence of pneumoperitoneum. Relative indications for surgery include a fixed intestinal loop on serial plain abdominal radiographs, which suggests the presence of a necrotic segment of the intestine, or abdominal wall erythema, which suggests the presence of a contained or walled-off perforation. Other relative indications for surgery include portal venous gas on plain abdominal radiograph, a palpable abdominal mass, a positive paracentesis, and clinical deterioration despite maximal medical therapy (Table 46-2).

Although pneumoperitoneum is the only widely accepted absolute indication for surgery, it should be noted that extensive intestinal necrosis may occur in the absence of perforation or free air on plain abdominal radiograph. Thus, surgeons must have a high index of suspicion for a gangrenous bowel and exercise good clinical judgment when managing an infant with advanced NEC without evidence of pneumoperitoneum. Most infants who require surgery will manifest indications within 24 hours from the onset of disease. The relative surgical indications for NEC are debatable, and the optimal surgical procedure remains a subject of ongoing controversy as well. Surgical approaches vary and are often determined by the extent of intestinal involvement, and the clinical stability of the child. The main goals of surgery for NEC are source control and preservation of the intestinal length. Removal of the gangrenous bowel allows for sepsis control, but massive bowel resection may result in short bowel syndrome characterized by inadequate intestinal function and malabsorption.

### The History of Primary Peritoneal Drainage

The concept of peritoneal drainage (PD) was first introduced by Ein et al in 1977. It involves placing an intraperitoneal drain, occasionally bilaterally, under local anesthesia, in an

| TABLE 46-2 | Indications for Surgery |
| --- | --- |
| Absolute | Intestinal perforation (pneumoperitoneum) |
| Relative | Fixed intestinal loop on serial plain abdominal radiographs |
| | Abdominal wall erythema |
| | Portal venous gas on plain abdominal radiograph |
| | Palpable abdominal mass |
| | Positive paracentesis[a] |
| | Failure of maximal medical therapy |
| | -Increasing respiratory support |
| | -Increasing third-space fluid losses |
| | -Persistent acidosis and thrombocytopenia |

[a]Positive paracentesis: at least 0.5 cc of free-flowing fluid that is brown or yellow-brown in color and/or has bacteria seen on Gram stain. Negative paracentesis: clear ascitic fluid and no organisms on Gram stain.

infant with NEC (or FIP) in the neonatal intensive care unit (NICU). Initially, PD was used in a series of 5 hemodynamically unstable ELBW infants with perforated NEC, who were too critically ill to tolerate laparotomy. Three of the patients survived and two did not require a subsequent operation. The investigators postulated that this approach allowed time for resuscitation, medical optimization, and stabilization by draining the intestinal perforation and relieving the increased intra-abdominal pressure. PD has steadily gained popularity over the past 3 decades and is still a subject of contemporary debate. Multiple retrospective studies have advocated PD as a definitive therapy for ELBW infants with Bell Stage III NEC. Critics argue that the majority of infants who undergo PD for NEC eventually require laparotomy. In an effort to determine whether PD or laparotomy was superior as a definitive treatment for NEC, Moss and colleagues performed a meta-analysis of 10 studies ($N = 475$). They were unable to come to a conclusion due to marked selection bias in treatment assignment in prior reports. A subsequent multi-institutional prospective nonrandomized study in Europe by Demestre et al reviewed outcomes of 44 neonates who received PD as the primary treatment for pneumoperitoneum or peritonitis from advanced NEC. The authors demonstrated that while early PD was not a definitive solution in all patients, many infants survived without the need for surgery and outcomes were comparable to historical controls who underwent primary laparotomy. In this study, 36% of neonates still required a laparotomy after PD because of progressive deterioration, and 54% of infants required delayed laparotomy for intestinal complications such as stenosis, fistula, or strictures. Sixty-four percent survived after PD only. Overall survival was 82%, and when stratified by birth weight, only 57% of ELBW neonates survived versus 95% of infants >1000 g. Demestre et al concluded that PD is the first management step for infants with pneumoperitoneum or overwhelming NEC, regardless of birth weight and gestational age. Blakely and colleagues conducted a prospective, cohort study at 16 clinical centers within the National Institute of Child Health and Human Development (NICHD) Neonatal Research Network with the goal of determining risk-adjusted outcomes among ELBW infants who underwent laparotomy versus PD for NEC or FIP. The authors suggested that infants who underwent laparotomy appeared to have better outcomes than those who underwent PD. In this study, severe NEC or FIP occurred in 156 (5.2%) of 2987 ELBW infants; 76 were treated with initial PD, and 80 underwent primary laparotomy. Survival to discharge was higher in the laparotomy cohort versus the PD cohort (57% vs 46%) as well as survival without neurodevelopmental impairment (NDI) at 18 to 22 months adjusted age (62% vs 37%). Unadjusted odds ratios (ORs) for adverse outcomes in the laparotomy group relative to the PD group were all substantially less than 1.0, favoring the laparotomy group. However, after adjustment for multiple potential confounders and restriction of the cohort by exclusion of those who were considered to be too sick for laparotomy, the adjusted OR for death at 18-22 months increased to 1.1 (95% CI: 0.41-3.21), whereas the adjusted OR for death or NDI remained low at 0.56 (95% CI: 0.19-1.69). Blakely et al recognized that while their findings suggested an important advantage of laparotomy over PD, there was still the need for a randomized trial to evaluate the relative effectiveness of these 2 surgical interventions and their outcomes.

Finally, a multi-institutional prospective randomized controlled trial in the United States and Canada was conducted comparing PD versus laparotomy in 117 preterm (<34 weeks gestational age) neonates weighing <1500 g with perforated NEC. This study demonstrated no difference in 90-day mortality (34.5% vs 35.5%) and similar secondary outcomes including dependency on parenteral nutrition and length of hospitalization. Approximately 38% of infants randomized to PD required subsequent laparotomy. Interestingly, in the nonrandomized arm of the same study, the mortality rate was only 15% for initial laparotomy versus 41% for primary PD. Therefore, one could conclude that perhaps experienced clinical judgment and careful patient selection for PD versus laparotomy can achieve better outcomes than arbitrary assignment to a particular surgical approach. In a concurrent, international multicenter randomized controlled trial, Pierro and colleagues compared PD to laparotomy as initial treatment for 69 infants with birth weight ≤1000 g and pneumoperitoneum on x-ray (NEC or FIP) and found no significant difference in mortality (51.4% vs 63.6%) but a trend toward increased survival in the primary laparotomy cohort. Seventy-four percent of neonates in the PD group required delayed laparotomy. PD as a definitive treatment was effective in only 11%. The others required remedial laparotomy or died. The investigators concluded that PD offers no real benefit in this population. This is supported by a subsequent review performed by Sola et al in 2010, which concluded that PD is associated with an excess 55% mortality compared to laparotomy based on 5 separate prospective trials.

Proponents of PD argue that it may be better suited for ELBW neonates. This claim is addressed in a follow-up study by Pierro and coworkers comparing PD and laparotomy in the same group of 69 ELBW (<1000 g) neonates with pneumoperitoneum. They found no postprocedure improvement in either group comparing heart rate, blood pressure, inotrope requirement, arterial partial pressure of oxygen/fraction of inspired oxygen ratio, and total organ failure scores. Additionally, only 4/35 infants with PD alone survived, with no difference between their pre- and postprocedure organ failure scores. The authors concluded that PD does not immediately improve the clinical status in ELBW neonates with bowel perforation. Therefore, the use of PD as a stabilizing or temporizing measure is not supported by their results. However, a retrospective study by Baird et al in 2006 showed a decrease in mortality with laparotomy, or PD followed by laparotomy, compared to PD alone in VLBW infants. In practice, we recommend initial PD for VLBW infants who are hemodynamically unstable with respiratory embarrassment secondary to abdominal distention; however, subsequent laparotomy is warranted. Definitive primary laparotomy with resection of necrotic intestine is best suited for infants weighing >1500 g or VLBW neonates who can tolerate the initial operation (Fig. 46-2).

## Peritoneal Drainage Technique

PD is usually performed in the NICU, as these infants are too unstable to be transferred to the operating room. Local

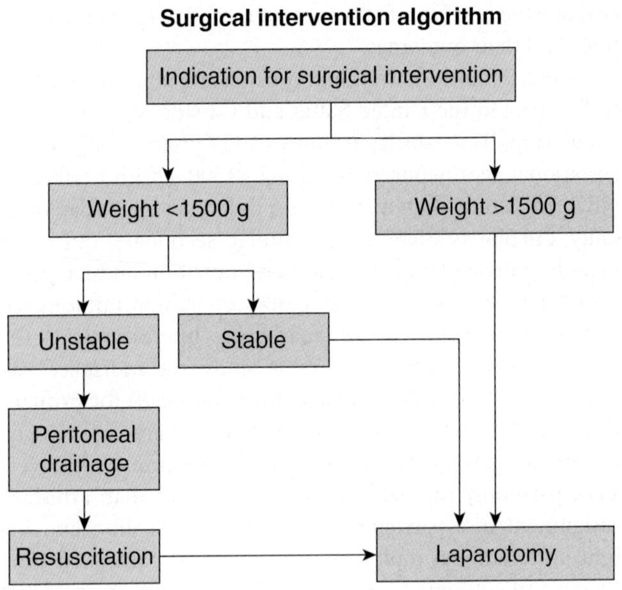

## Surgical intervention algorithm

```
        Indication for surgical intervention
                    │
          ┌─────────┴─────────┐
          ▼                   ▼
   Weight <1500 g      Weight >1500 g
          │                   │
      ┌───┴────┐              │
      ▼        ▼              │
  Unstable   Stable ──────────┤
      │                       │
      ▼                       │
  Peritoneal                  │
   drainage                   │
      │                       │
      ▼                       ▼
 Resuscitation ─────────► Laparotomy
```

**FIGURE 46-2** The algorithm outlining criteria for peritoneal drainage and laparotomy in infants with an indication for surgical intervention.

anesthesia is injected and a small incision is made in the left lower quadrant away from the liver under direct vision. It is imperative to visualize the peritoneum and open sharply to avoid iatrogenic bowel injury. A half-inch penrose is inserted with or without "side holes" that may be cut into the drain (Fig. 46-3A). The penrose is placed at the end of a hemostat and carefully advanced along the anterior abdominal wall from the left lower quadrant to the epigastrium (Fig. 46-3B). Care is taken to avoid the liver, which in premature infants is easily injured. The drain is then sutured in place to the skin. At a later date, the penrose may be gently advanced out of the abdomen over several days, if needed, to promote fistula formation.

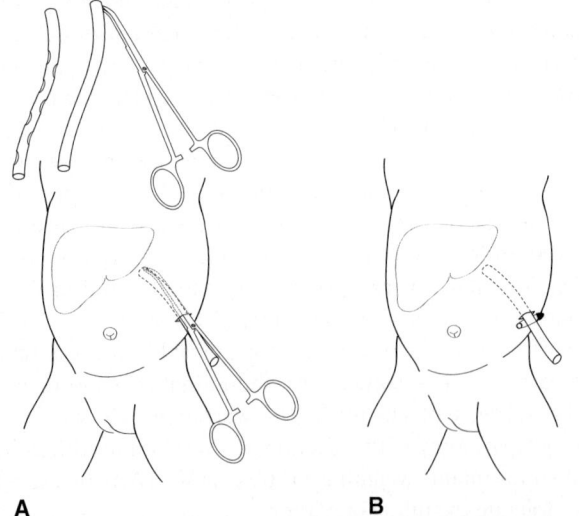

**A**                  **B**

**FIGURE 46-3 A.** A half-inch penrose with or without "side-holes" that may be cut into the drain is typically used for peritoneal drainage. **B.** The penrose is placed on the end of a snap and carefully advanced along the anterior abdominal wall from the left lower quadrant to the epigastrium. Care is taken to avoid the liver.

## Laparotomy

After optimization of the patient's condition with aggressive ventilatory support, resuscitation, administration of broad-spectrum antibiotics, OGT drainage, and correction of anemia and coagulopathy, the surgery may be begun. Preoperative correction of the patient's mean arterial pressure and intravascular volume are imperative. The surgical intervention may be performed in the NICU under appropriate conditions without an increase in complications, or the patient may be taken to the operating room if transport does not introduce any adverse risks. For laparotomy, the extent of disease may be classified as focal, multifocal (>50% viable), or panintestinal (<25% viable). Depending on the extent of NEC and the patient's condition at the time of operation, a number of different surgical options may be considered, including resection with enterostomy, proximal enterostomy, the "patch, drain, and wait" (PD&W) approach, the "clip and drop back" technique, or resection with primary anastomosis. The two fundamental principles of surgical management are removal of the gangrenous or perforated bowel while preserving bowel length.

The operation is carried out through a transverse supraumbilical incision with special care taken not to injure the liver, which may extend well below the level of the umbilicus. In an infant, this incision allows for visualization of all the intra-abdominal structures and for a 2-layer closure of the abdominal wall at the end of the procedure, thereby reducing the risk of wound dehiscence. The entire bowel is eviscerated through the incision and the intestine is carefully examined from the stomach to the rectum. Gentle fingers instead of instruments should be used when inspecting the intestine for the extent of disease and the viability of the bowel.

Precautions must be taken when evaluating the intestine adjacent to the liver, since the liver in this patient population is at risk for developing a subcapsular hematoma which, when ruptured, can lead to fatal hemorrhage. The suction tip should never touch the liver surface. Gentle fingers or silastic-coated malleable retractors may be used to carefully hold the liver out of the way during the procedure, but a no touch technique is best of all. VanderKolk et al reported that spontaneous liver hemorrhage is an important and lethal complication in very small neonates undergoing laparotomy for NEC. In their series of 68 patients, 11.8% developed this complication and only 1 patient survived. Those infants who developed liver hemorrhage had a mean gestational age of 28 weeks and a mean weight of 1262 g. The investigators reported that significant risk factors included hypotension and a large amount of fluid administration during the 24 hours preceding operation. Finally, the area of the bowel to be resected is noted and the decision whether to proceed with resection is made depending upon the length of residual intestine following the planned resection (Fig. 46-4).

## Focal Disease

If a single segment of the bowel is gangrenous or perforated, as is the case in focal NEC or FIP, only a limited resection of this area is required. When performing a resection, the mesenteric vessels are sequentially ligated on the mesenteric

**Surgical techniques algorithm**

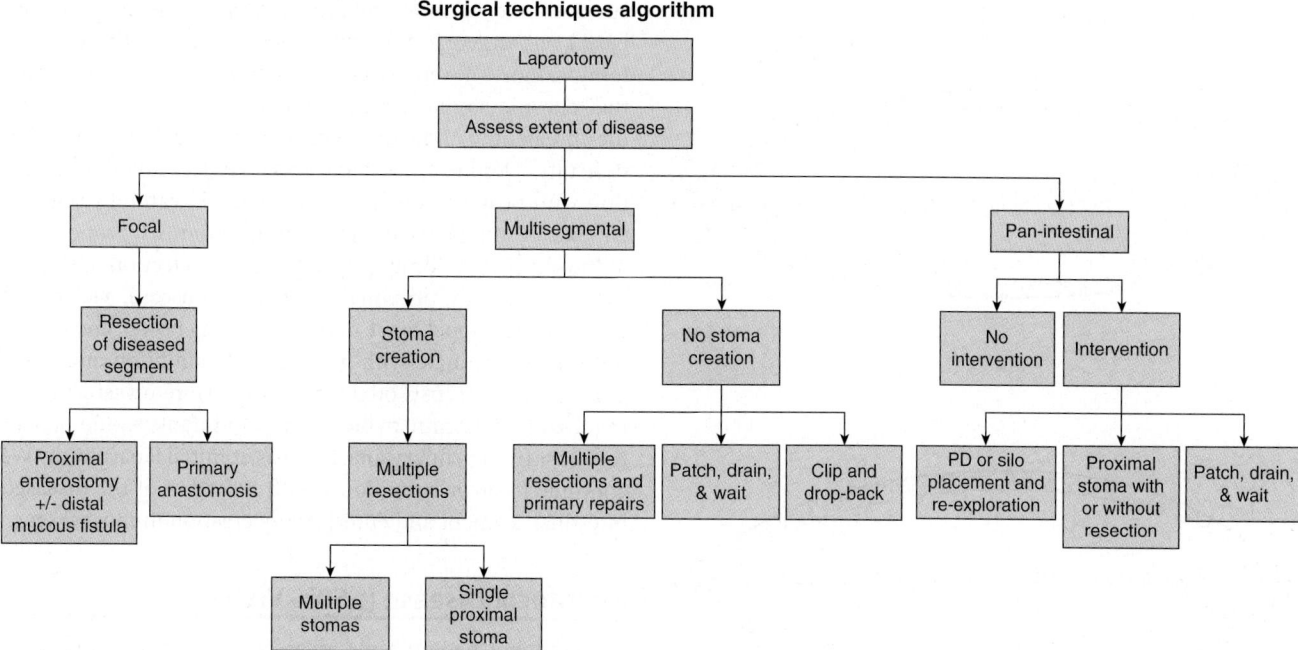

**FIGURE 46-4** The algorithm outlining available surgical techniques for the treatment of NEC depending on the extent of disease.

side. The distal ends of the mesenteric vessels adjacent to the bowel may not require ligation except for the most proximal and most distal vessel. After ligation, the vessels are divided, followed by division of the intestine proximally and distally (Fig. 46-5). In this manner, a rapid or expedient resection can be performed, which is imperative in these sick infants.

The standard of care after resection is the creation of a proximal enterostomy, with or without a distal mucous fistula. A concerted effort should be made to preserve the ileocecal valve. If only a very short segment of the terminal ileum remains after bowel resection, it can be ligated and left in the abdominal cavity as a "Hartmann" pouch. This allows for salvage of the ileocecal valve at the time of ostomy closure by avoiding the use of 2 cm of the terminal ileum required to create an enterostomy. The proximal stoma and distal mucous fistula may be exteriorized through the lateral aspect of the abdominal wound without an increased incidence of wound

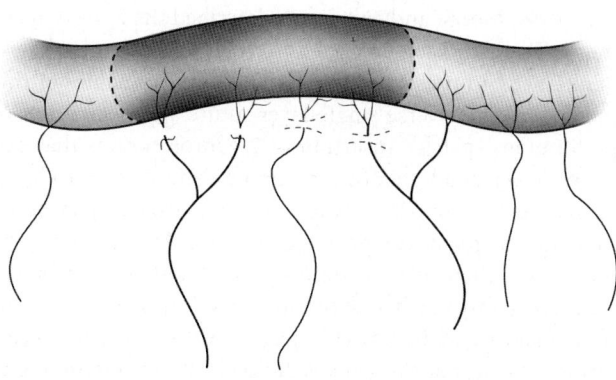

**FIGURE 46-5** When performing a resection for NEC, the mesenteric vessels are sequentially ligated on the mesenteric side. The distal ends of the mesenteric vessels adjacent to the bowel may not require ligation except for the most proximal and most distal vessel.

complications (Fig. 46-6). Prior to stoma creation, we recommend decompressing the bowel by emptying its contents; this may improve perfusion to the intestine. Interrupted fine absorbable sutures are used to approximate the seromuscular layer of the intestine to the full-thickness of the abdominal fascia in four quadrants. The surgeon should only take seromuscular bites of the intestine rather than full-thickness bites as these may lead to "side hole" fistulas. Approximately 2 cm of the intestine is left outside the abdominal wall and maturation of the end is not performed. One or more full-thickness fascial sutures are placed between the 2 ends of the bowel brought out as stomas as well as a skin bridge. This fascial and skin bridge should help to prevent prolapse and/or wound dehiscence. The remaining wound is then closed in 2 layers with continuous absorbable suture or 1 layer of interrupted absorbable suture in neonates <500 g. Historically, several types of enterostomies have been used. Although no longer practiced, 1 technique used for stoma creation was the Mikulicz enterostomy (Fig. 46-7A). The proximal and distal intestines were sewn together with continuous seromuscular fine silk suture on their anti-mesenteric borders for approximately 4 to 5 cm. A spur-crushing clamp was then used to create gradual pressure necrosis of the intervening septum between the 2 intestinal limbs. Proponents of the Mikulicz double-barrel stoma believed that this technique had a significantly lower incidence of distal intestinal strictures possibly related to early restoration of bowel continuity. Also less frequently used in NEC, or for meconium ileus from which they arose, are the Bishop–Koop technique (Fig. 46-7B) and Santulli procedure (Fig. 46-7C). The Bishop–Koop technique consists of a Roux-en-Y anastomosis between the end of the dilated proximal segment and the side of the collapsed distal segment approximately 4 cm from the distal open end, which is brought out through the skin as an ileostomy. This technique affords the opportunity for catheter placement and

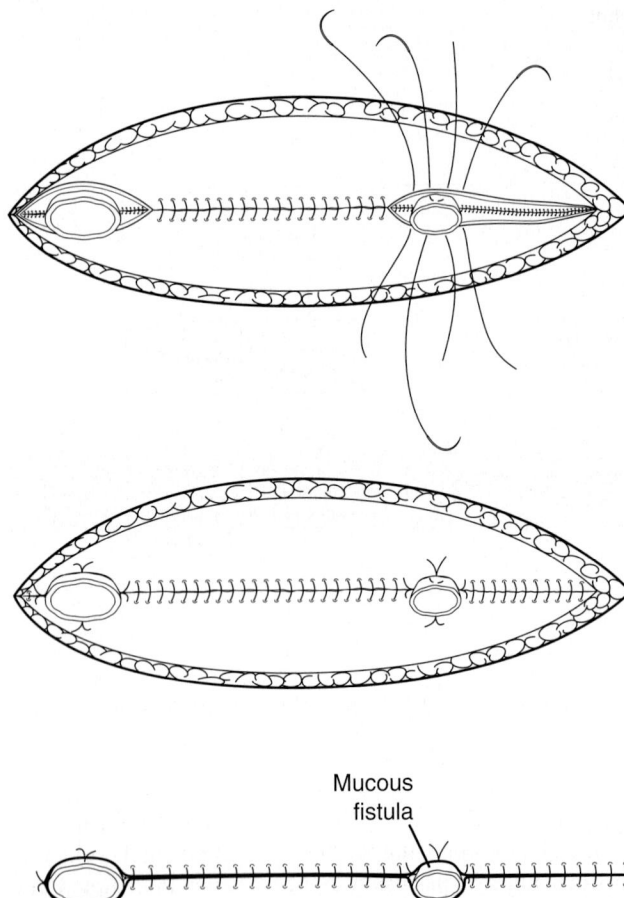

Mucous
fistula

**FIGURE 46-6** The proximal stoma and distal mucous fistula may be exteriorized through the lateral aspect of the abdominal wound without increased incidence of wound complications.

distal irrigation or feeding with either formula or proximal stoma gastrointestinal effluent. The Santulli procedure is the opposite configuration of the Bishop–Koop that connects the end of the collapsed distal segment and the side of the dilated proximal segment with exteriorization of the proximal segment. In current practice, we recommend an enterostomy of the proximal segment with or without mucous fistula creation with the distal segment. If a prolonged period is anticipated before restoration of intestinal continuity or the enterostomy is very proximal, a mucous fistula may allow for refeeding.

Although enterostomies are generally thought to be beneficial and safe, they are not without morbidity due to inadequate absorption and mechanical issues including prolapse. Proximal enterostomies may be complicated by the failure to thrive, fluid and electrolyte imbalances, challenging peristomal skin management, in addition to requiring a second operation for takedown. In a 10-year retrospective series of 73 patients who underwent laparotomy for NEC, 42% developed stoma-related morbidities. Younger gestational age and low preoperative weight were the only statistically significant predictors of stoma-related complications. Two additional studies found no difference in outcomes between laparotomy with stoma creation versus primary repair. However, other investigators have reported higher rates of sepsis, leak, and stricture formation after primary repair. In fact, Cooper et al reviewed 173 patients over 14 years and found a 48%

survival rate in those infants undergoing primary repair, based on surgeon's preference, versus 72% in the enterostomy cohort. Proponents of enterostomy creation argue that chronic stoma-related complications are almost never life-threatening and can typically be managed without great difficulty. Despite these data, some centers advocate resection with primary repair for focal NEC in carefully selected patients. Proponents of primary anastomosis propose the following criteria for appropriate patient selection: a sharply localized, usually proximal segment of disease, viable and well-perfused appearance of the remaining bowel, and a well-resuscitated neonate with good overall condition and without progressive sepsis or coagulopathy. More investigation is required to determine which cohort of infants would benefit the most from primary anastomosis at initial laparotomy. We continue to favor laparotomy with resection of the diseased intestinal segment and enterostomy creation in most cases.

## Multifocal Disease (>50% Viable)

If the patient has multiple areas of necrotic intestine separated by a viable bowel, the overall goal of the surgery should be to control sepsis and preserve intestinal length to avoid short bowel syndrome. Historically, multiple resections with multiple stomas were performed rather than a massive resection. However, this traditional approach is associated with a high morbidity and mortality rate. An alternative method is to create a single proximal enterostomy and the distal bowel is resected and reconnected with multiple primary anastomoses, thereby avoiding multiple stomas. This approach is also not without morbidity as a high jejunostomy is fraught with significant fluid and electrolyte loss as well as peristomal skin complications. Furthermore, in an unstable infant, the extra operative time for multiple anastomoses is unwise. At the time of jejunostomy closure, it is not uncommon to find anastomotic strictures. In addition, resection with primary repair has also been described for multifocal NEC. While Fasoli et al reported a higher survival rate after resection and primary anastomosis (85%) versus stoma creation (50%) in a retrospective series of 46 neonates with multifocal disease, their results should be interpreted with caution. Significant selection bias can exist in retrospective reviews. If the resection and primary anastomosis cohort were healthier to begin with, a higher postoperative survival rate would be expected.

In 1989, Moore and colleagues described the PD&W technique. This approach evolved as a result of the surgeon's desperate need to preserve bowel length. The principles of this method are transverse single-layer suture approximations of perforations (patch), insertion of 2 Penrose drains that exit in the lower quadrants (drain), and a commitment to long-term parenteral nutrition (wait), with the ultimate goal being to "resect no gut and do no enterostomies." At laparotomy, the dilated intestinal loops are decompressed, and then perforated areas are gently patched with interrupted sutures (Fig. 46-8). If the majority of the bowel is necrotic with numerous perforations, the peritoneal cavity is drained without attempting to patch unsuitable tissue. Two Penrose drains are placed from the diaphragmatic edges to the lower abdomen with loops in the pelvis, which exit via stab incisions in bilateral lower quadrants. These drains allow evacuation of fecal soilage and

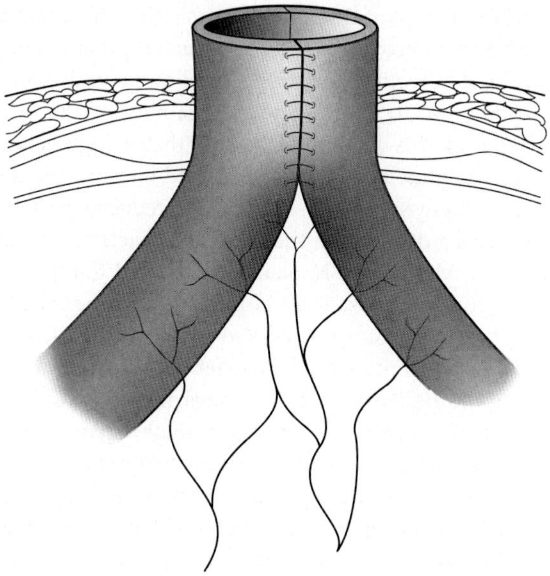

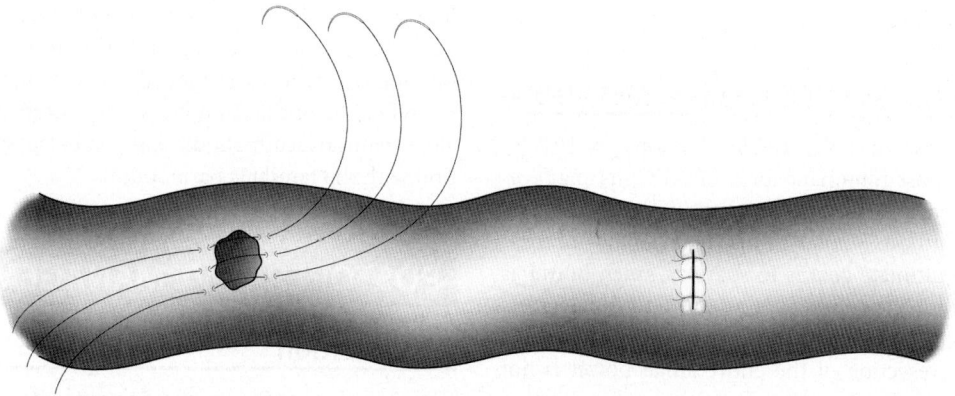

A

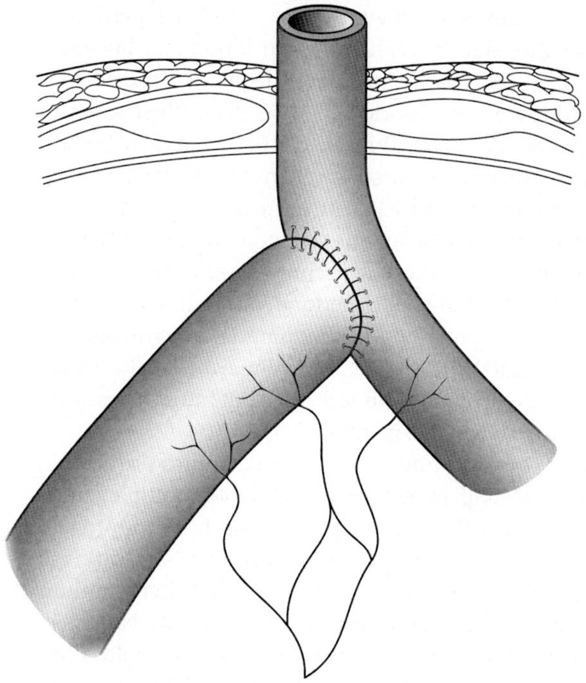

B

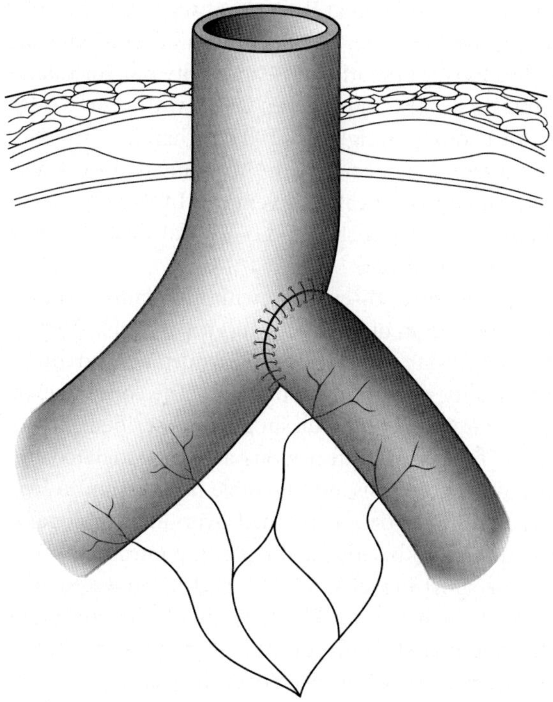

C

FIGURE 46-7 **A.** Mikulicz enterostomy. **B.** Bishop–Koop. **C.** Santulli.

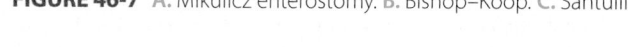

**FIGURE 46-8** After decompression of the dilated intestinal loops, perforated areas are gently patched with interrupted sutures and/or approximation to the omentum or adjacent bowel.

function essentially as enterostomies while the peritoneal cavity is obliterated by rapid adhesion formation. Finally, a gastrostomy tube is placed to ensure adequate gastric decompression. Moore et al reported good results in their series of 23 patients over 15 years. Three deaths occurred early in their experience, when gastrostomies were not performed. During their later experience, only 1 death occurred within 60 days of initial laparotomy. Critics of this technique argue that PD&W does not control sepsis, as the necrotic bowel is not resected. Additionally, the thin-walled perforated intestine often cannot support the suture and the abdominal cavity is difficult to drain adequately. Therefore, PD&W may be an alternative operative approach for multifocal NEC, but future studies are necessary to validate this method.

Another surgical option to treat multifocal NEC, described by Vaughan et al, strives to avoid multiple enterostomies and is called the "clip and drop-back" approach. At laparotomy, areas of obviously necrotic intestine are resected and the cut ends are closed with either titanium clips or stapled, leaving the bowel in discontinuity. No enterostomies or primary repairs are performed. Re-exploration to restore intestinal continuity occurs 48 to 72 hours later, after the patient is adequately resuscitated, coagulopathy is corrected, and the initial inflammatory response is controlled. The clips or staples are removed and the bowel is reanastomosed without stoma creation. In their small series of 3 patients, Vaughan and colleagues reported no anastomotic complications and a 100% survival during a follow-up period of 6 months to 7 years. In a study published in 2001 in the *Journal of Pediatric Surgery*, Molik et al utilized the clip and drop-back technique in 4 infants with 1 death and 3 requiring an enterostomy at re-exploration. In a more recent study from the United Kingdom, Ron et al reported that only half of the 13 infants with fulminant NEC who underwent the clip and drop-back technique survived to a mean of 29 months. Similar to the PD&W approach, the clip and drop-back approach is another treatment option to address multifocal NEC that requires further investigation to determine its effectiveness.

At the conclusion of the operation, the length of the remaining intestine should be noted as along with the presence of the ileocecal valve. Additionally, it is useful to place a drawing in the chart mapping out each bowel segment in order to facilitate accurate restoration of intestinal continuity at a later time, and to understand regional anatomy in case of future intestinal failure.

### Panintestinal Disease/NEC Totalis (<25% Viable)

Panintestinal disease or NEC *Totalis* develops in 19% of patients. As the most fulminant form of NEC, its management is quite challenging and controversial, with limited surgical options at best. Similar to the management of multifocal NEC, the ultimate goal is to spare as much bowel as possible. One treatment option is to resect all of the necrotic intestine and place multiple stomas or a single proximal stoma. However, resection of the entire small bowel is not usually recommended at initial exploration as the intestine with questionable viability may improve after resuscitation. Therefore, some centers advocate initial PD or silo placement

followed by re-exploration after resuscitation, if the patient and the bowel improve. Another approach is proximal diversion without resection of intestine followed by a second-look laparotomy to re-evaluate the viability of the bowel. Proponents of this technique believe that a high jejunostomy may facilitate healing of the injured intestine via distal bowel decompression with subsequent reduced metabolic demands and a decrease in the amount of bacteria and their by-products. Martin and Neblett were the first to report this approach in 1981. Luzzatto et al published in the *European Journal of Pediatric Surgery* in 1996 that proximal diversion alone allows for limitation of the extent of resection without increasing morbidity or mortality. Sugarman and Kiely later reported 80% survival after a second-look laparotomy but only 50% long-term survival. In addition to the above options, both the PD&W and the clip and drop-back techniques have been used for management of neonates with paninvolvement. Despite these surgical options, almost all of the few survivors with NEC *totalis* are left with short bowel syndrome. Gastrostomy tube placement and/or a central venous catheter placement should be considered at the time of surgery if the child will likely survive but suffer from short bowel syndrome and can tolerate a longer operation. The mortality rate for infants with panintestinal NEC approaches 100%, with nearly 100% mortality for neonates weighing <1000 g. Therefore, in select cases, the surgeon may decide with the family that treatment is futile and forego surgical intervention. In these patients, bowel should not be resected and a natural death allowed with the family at bedside.

An early, informed discussion with the family should involve an explanation of the above surgical options, postoperative morbidities such as short bowel syndrome, and finally, the high mortality rate in this population. The consequences of long-term parenteral nutrition should be described, including the need for central intravenous access, associated line infections, liver cholestasis, and possible progression to liver failure requiring liver or a combined liver–intestinal transplant. Parents should be educated regarding intestinal transplantation for short bowel syndrome and its consequences. If a transplant team is available, they should be consulted. Although patient and graft survival after intestinal transplantation has markedly improved over the past 10 years, the 1-year adjusted patient and graft survival was only 79% and 75% in 2007. In 10 years, patient and intestine survival falls to 46% and 29% for intestine-only recipients. Combined liver–intestinal transplants have an even higher mortality at both 1 and 10 years post-transplant. Given the significant morbidities and overwhelming mortality associated with panintestinal NEC, the option to not resect or surgically intervene and allow natural death should also be discussed. Communication with the family is paramount.

## POSTOPERATIVE MANAGEMENT

### Resuscitation

Postoperative management of infants after surgery for NEC is initially aimed at maintaining the hemodyamic status and supporting respiratory function. The infant with severe NEC will have significant third-spacing of fluid and aggressive fluid resuscitation and judicious use of dopamine is advised to maintain adequate blood pressure and perfusion as monitored by urine output. Infants will often be coagulopathic, thrombocytopenic; and anemic; and blood products (packed red blood cells, fresh frozen plasma, and platelets) should be used as necessary to correct to normal values. An OGT should be placed to low suction until gastric output is clear (nonbilious) and decreased in output and bowel function has resumed.

## Antibiotics

While data are conflicting on optimal duration of antibiotics after an operation for NEC, consensus guidelines state that the infant should continue to receive parenteral antibiotics for at least 7 to 10 days. Longer duration may be indicated for continued positive blood cultures.

## Feeding

Total parenteral nutrition (TPN) should be started postoperatively and enteral feeds held until the return of bowel function. Enteral feeds can then be started at trophic rates and slowly increased to the desired goal. Inability to advance nutrition may be an early sign of strictures.

## Ostomy Management and Restoration of Intestinal Continuity

Ostomy appliances should fit well to avoid spillage of enteral contents into the wound. Many surgeons delay bag placement for up to 72 hours to avoid rough handling of the wound. Jejunal and more proximal ileal ostomies will present the challenge of high output, leading to a tendency toward dehydration and electrolyte imbalances. In addition, insufficient bowel may be left proximally to allow for full nutrition to be enterally absorbed. Infants with short bowel syndrome as a result of loss of a large amount of bowel may need to be maintained on TPN indefinitely. Distal ileostomies are generally well-tolerated and surgical restoration of intestinal continuity can be done after 6 to 8 weeks to allow time for decrease in postoperative inflammation. A contrast enema should be performed prior to takedown to evaluate for the presence of any distal strictures. Any strictures identified can then be resected at the time of operation.

In patients with a proximal stoma and distal mucous fistula, nutritional needs may be met by refeeding proximal stoma output to the distal fistula once bowel function has returned but before re-anastamosis.

## PROGNOSIS

Mortality in patients with surgical NEC is 30%, compared with 7% for patients with less severe, medically treated NEC. Survival is lowest in low-birth-weight infants, with a mortality of 50% in ELBW infants.

Chronic complications include strictures, which occur in over 30% of patients with either medically treated or surgically treated NEC. Strictures are most common in the colon, but can occur anywhere in affected bowel. The possibility of strictures mandates a distal contrast study prior to ostomy closure. Any feeding difficulties in NEC survivors should prompt investigation for strictures.

Short bowel syndrome occurs as a long-term complication in approximately 10% of infants after surgically treated NEC. Short bowel syndrome occurs when the remaining intestine is insufficient to support full nutrition via enteral feeds. These infants are dependent upon TPN for all or part of their nutrition, and are thus exposed to the risks of parenteral nutrition, including line sepsis and cholestatic liver disease. Current surgical treatment for short bowel syndrome includes bowel lengthening procedures and small bowel transplant (See Chapter 50: Short Bowel Syndrome).

Major NDI is found in up to 43% of survivors of severe NEC, and 15% of survivors of mild-to-moderate NEC. The risk is highest in VLBW infants, likely impacted as well by increased comorbidities associated with prematurity in these infants.

## SELECTED READINGS

Ade-Ajayi N, Kiely E, Drake D, et al. Resection and primary anastomosis in necrotizing enterocolitis. *J R Soc Med* 1996;89:385.

Aguayo P, Fraser JD, Sharp S, et al. Stomal complications in the newborn with necrotizing enterocolitis. *J Surg Res* 2009;157(2):275–278.

Baird R, Puligandlaa PS, St Vilb D, et al. The role of laparotomy for intestinal perforation in very low birth weight infants. *J Pediatr Surg* 2006;41:1522–1525.

Blakely ML, Tyson JE, Lally KP, et al. Laparotomy versus peritoneal drainage for necrotizing enterocolitis or isolated intestinal perforation in extremely low birth weight infants: outcomes through 18 months adjusted age. *Pediatrics* 2006;117(4):e680–e687.

Cooper A, Ross AJ 3rd, O'Neill JA Jr., Schnaufer L. Resection with primary anastomosis for necrotizing enterocolitis: a contrasting view. *J Pediatr Surg* 1988;23:64–68.

Demestre X, Ginovart G, Figueras-Aloy J, et al. Peritoneal drainage as primary management in necrotizing enterocolitis: a prospective study. *J Pediatr Surg* 2002;37(11):1534–1539.

Ein SH, Marshall DG, Girvan D. Peritoneal drainage under local anesthesia for perforations from necrotizing enterocolitis. *J Pediatr Surg* 1977;12(6):963–967.

Emami CN, Petrosyan M, Giuliani S, et al. Role of the host defense system and intestinal microbial flora in the pathogenesis of necrotizing enterocolitis. *Surg Infect (Larchmt)* 2009;10(5):407–417.

Fasoli L, Turi RA, Spitz L et al. Necrotizing enterocolitis: extent of disease and surgical treatment. *J Pediatr Surg* 1999;34:1096.

Kim, SS, Albanese, CT. Necrotizing enterocolitis. In: O'Neill JA, Coran AG, Fonkalsrud E, Grosfeld JL, eds. *Pediatric Surgery*. 6th ed. Philadelphia, PA: MosbyElsevier; 2006:1427–1452.

Kosloske AM. Indications for operation in necrotizing enterocolitis revisited. *J Pediatr Surg* 1994;29:663.

Lin PW, Nasr TR, Stoll BJ. Necrotizing enterocolitis: recent scientific advances in pathophysiology and prevention. *Semin Perinatol* 2008;32(2):70–82.

Martin LW, Neblett WW. Early operation with intestinal diversion for necrotizing enterocolitis. *J Pediatr Surg* 1981;16:252.

Moore TC. Management of necrotizing enterocolitis by "patch, drain, and wait." *Pediatr Surg Int* 1989;4:110.

Moss RL, Dimmitt RA, Henry MC, et al. A meta-analysis of peritoneal drainage versus laparotomy for perforated necrotizing enterocolitis. *J Pediatr Surg* 2001;36(8):1210–1213.

Moss RL, Dimmitt RA, Barnhart DC, et al. Laparotomy versus peritoneal drainage for necrotizing enterocolitis and perforation. *N Engl J Med* 2006;354(21):2225–2234.

Petrosyan M, Guner YS, Williams M, Grishin A, Ford HR. Current concepts regarding the pathogenesis of necrotizing enterocolitis. *Pediatr Surg Int* 2009;25(4):309–318.

Rees CM, Eaton S, Khoo AK, et al. Peritoneal drainage does not stabilize extremely low birth weight infants with perforated bowel: data from the NET Trial. *J Pediatr Surg* 2010;45(2):324–328.

Rees CM, Eaton S, Kiely EM, et al. Peritoneal drainage or laparotomy in neonatal bowel perforation? A randomized controlled trial. *Ann Surg* 2008;248(1):44–51.

Sola JE, Tepas JJ 3rd, Koniaris LG. Peritoneal drainage versus laparotomy for necrotizing enterocolitis and intestinal perforation: a meta-analysis. *J Surg Res* 2010;161(1):95–100.

Sugarman ID, Kiely EM. Is there a role for high jejunostomy in the management of severe necrotizing enterocolitis? *Pediatr Surg Int.* 2001; 17:222.

VanderKolk WE, Kurz P, Daniels J, et al. Liver hemorrhage during laparotomy in patients with necrotizing enterocolitis. *J Pediatr Surg* 1996;31: 1063.

Vaughan WG, Grosfeld JL, West K, et al. Avoidance of stomas and delayed anastomosis for bowel necrosis: the 'clip and drop-back' technique. *J Pediatr Surg* 1996;31(4):542–545.

# CHAPTER 47

# Intestinal Stomas

*Thomas R. Weber*

## KEY POINTS

1. Intestinal stomas in infancy and childhood can be life-saving or can greatly improve the quality of life.

2. There are a variety of indications for both acute and chronic intestinal conditions.

3. Positioning the stoma on the abdominal wall away from bony prominences or skin depressions is important for excellent ostomy bag seal.

4. The varieties of stoma configurations (end stoma, loop stoma, end-to-side, double barreled) all have specific indications and potential complications.

5. Stoma closure is a major surgical procedure with potentially serious complications if not performed well.

The exteriorization of the intestine in a child, performed for acute or chronic intestinal conditions, can be lifesaving or can improve the quality of life if well planned and properly performed. Depending on the disorder requiring treatment, the stoma can be fashioned at any level of the gastrointestinal tract and may provide complete diversion (end stoma), partial diversion (loop stoma or vented stomas), or access to the distal bowel (mucous fistula). Each of these variations has specific indications, and knowledge of their proper use and construction is an important part of the pediatric surgeon's armamentarium. This chapter discusses the indications for enterostomas in children, some alternative methods for stoma construction, stomal complications and their management, and stoma closure.

## INDICATIONS

The indications for stomas in children can be conveniently grouped into acute (emergent) or elective and further subdivided by age group and by basic intestinal disorder (congenital or acquired). These are summarized in Table 47-1. Obviously not all of these disorders will invariably require a stoma each time they are encountered, but a stoma can be

an important alternative if primary anastomosis is felt to be unwise for a variety of reasons.

## TECHNIQUES

The various ostomy configurations are shown in Figs. 47-1 to 47-7. Each kind of ostomy has its specific indications and use, depending on the disease process, age, and body habitus of the patient, anticipated duration of ostomy need, and need for total or partial diversion.

Correct positioning of the stoma on the abdominal wall is an extremely important determinant of the quality of life experienced by the patient with a stoma. The stoma should be positioned to avoid both bony prominences (ribs, iliac crest) and skin depressions (umbilicus, scars). Exceptions include bringing the stoma directly through the umbilicus or through one end of a transverse upper abdominal incision. The latter is most useful in small infants undergoing bowel resection for necrotizing enterocolitis and where there is limited area on the abdominal wall. Otherwise, creating the stoma through a separate incision is most likely to allow an excellent immediate bag device seal. Finally, in older children, the folding point of the abdomen while seated should be avoided, as it is difficult to maintain an adequate bag seal in that location. For elective stoma construction in older children, having the ideal position of the stoma marked by an experienced enterostomal therapist before the operation is extremely helpful.

A "loop" ostomy (Fig. 47-1) is used where complete intestinal diversion is not needed. In the newborn, many surgeons use a loop colostomy in cases of Hirschsprung disease (Fig. 47-5) and loop enterostomy for a solitary small bowel perforation such as that secondary to indomethacin. In addition, multiple perforations from necrotizing enterocolitis can be managed by exteriorization of each perforation as a loop ostomy if bowel resection is not needed (Fig. 47-7). In older children, bowel injury secondary to blunt or penetrating injury can be managed by a single- or multiple-loop enterostomies if repair or resection and anastomosis are not performed. Finally, a loop enterostomy can be used to "protect" a distal anastomosis on a temporary basis.

| TABLE 47-1 | Stoma Indications |
|---|---|
| **Neonatal, congenital** | |
| Intestinal atresia | |
| Midgut volvulus | |
| Hirschsprung disease | |
| Imperforate anus | |
| Meconium ileus | |
| Meconium peritonitis | |
| Segmental absence of muscle | |
| **Neonatal, acquired** | |
| Necrotizing enterocolitis | |
| Indomethacin-associated ileal perforation | |
| **Infants and children, congenital** | |
| Midgut volvulus | |
| Hirschsprung disease | |
| **Infants and children, acquired** | |
| Traumatic bowel injury | |
| Inflammatory bowel disease | |
| Bowel obstruction | |
| Intussusception | |

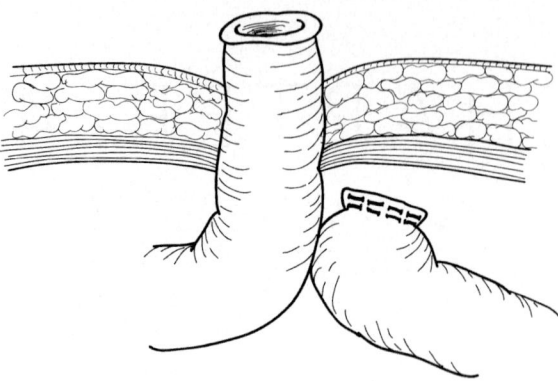

**FIGURE 47-2** An end ostomy is created by exteriorizing the proximal bowel end and oversewing the distal end, as pictured. "Tacking" the distal end so that it sits near the ostomy facilitates later ostomy closure. Maturing the ostomy with everting sutures is frequently not necessary in newborns or infants but is advisable in older children.

An end ostomy (Fig. 47-2) is used in cases in which complete enteral diversion is needed or when bowel resection is performed. Newborns with necrotizing enterocolitis, intestinal atresia, midgut volvulus, or meconium peritonitis are frequently treated with temporary end ostomy, with or without mucous fistula. In older children, end colostomy is usually used in cases of rectal injury with major contamination where repair is not possible or not completely secure.

An end-to-side ostomy with exteriorization of the distal bowel (Fig. 47-3) is extremely useful for cases of meconium ileus associated with cystic fibrosis (see Chapter 43). In this specific instance, fecal diversion with access to the distal bowel for irrigation of the thick tenacious meconium is required. Frequently, the exteriorized portion of the bowel stops draining when the distal bowel is open. In addition, this type of

ostomy can be used in cases of ileal- or right-colon atresia associated with severe microcolon, where there is a question of whether the colon can accommodate the fecal stream. This allows a gradual enlargement of the colon but still provides a means of external drainage if necessary.

Including a mucous fistula with the end ostomy is frequently done in cases of necrotizing enterocolitis because of the risk of distal stricture secondary to areas of ischemia that would result in closed-loop anatomy if the distal bowel end was closed (Fig. 47-4). A mucous fistula also allows distal bowel feeding in cases of high jejunostomy and gives access to the distal bowel for contrast x-rays before ostomy closure.

The catheterizable cutaneous cecal stoma, most often performed by appendicostomy, allows the administration of antegrade colonic enemas (ACE procedure) for children with chronic constipation or fecal incontinence. First described by Malone, this procedure has found wide application in children with refractory large bowel disorders. By creating a "valve" mechanism at the base of the appendix, where it enters the cecum, the stoma can be intermittently catheterized for

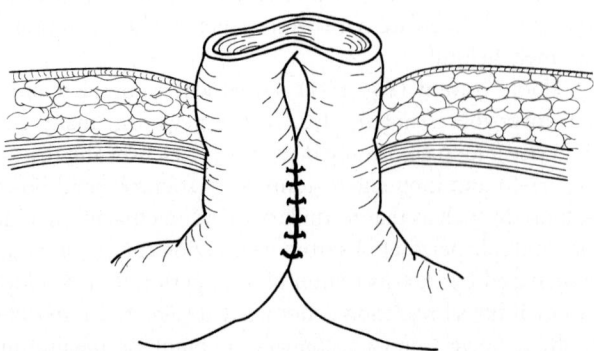

**FIGURE 47-1** Diagram of a "loop" ostomy. The bowel is left in partial continuity, with a generous opening along the antimesenteric border. In the early postoperative period, a rod or soft rubber tube can be left between the 2 limbs of the bowel to help hold it above skin level.

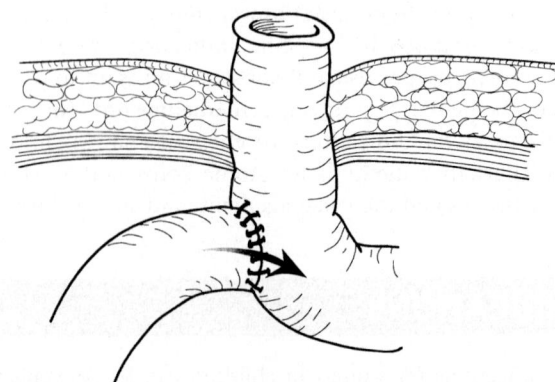

**FIGURE 47-3** An end-to-side ostomy, with exteriorization of the distal bowel end, is very useful in cases of cystic fibrosis with meconium obstruction of the distal bowel, requiring irrigation. The fecal stream will usually bypass the ostomy and progress distally if the bowel is not obstructed. This type of ostomy is also useful in cases of microcolon.

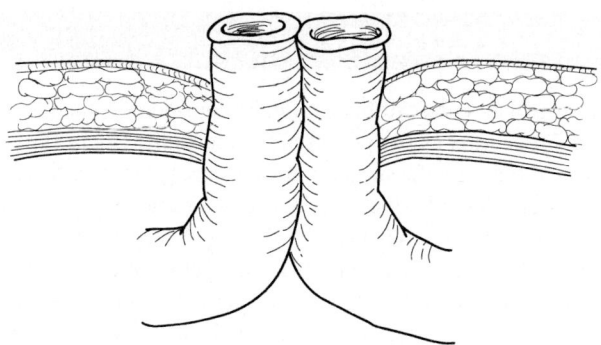

**FIGURE 47-4** An ostomy with distal exteriorization ("mucous fistula") is useful for ensuring distal bowel drainage as well as for feeding in instances of high small bowel ostomy.

the administration of enemas that can cause complete colon washout on a daily or every-other-day basis. A number of published series of large numbers of patients have demonstrated the long-term durability of this procedure and the dramatic improvement in quality of life in the majority of patients.

## COMPLICATIONS OF ENTEROSTOMIES

Although complications of stomas are unusual, they nonetheless can be serious and disabling and must be managed aggressively. The various complications are listed in Table 47-2. Stoma necrosis from insufficient blood supply should be recognizable within 24 hours after stoma formation and obviously requires operative revision. A mildly "blue" or "dusky" stoma may suffer from venous stasis only and can be safely observed for 12 to 24 hours to see if there is improvement. In cases of extensive bowel resection, such as in necrotizing enterocolitis, it is not unusual to exteriorize a stoma or mucous fistula that is marginal in viability to attempt to preserve as much bowel length as possible. It is common for these stomas to appear normal and completely viable 12 to 24 hours later with vigorous circulatory and ventilator support

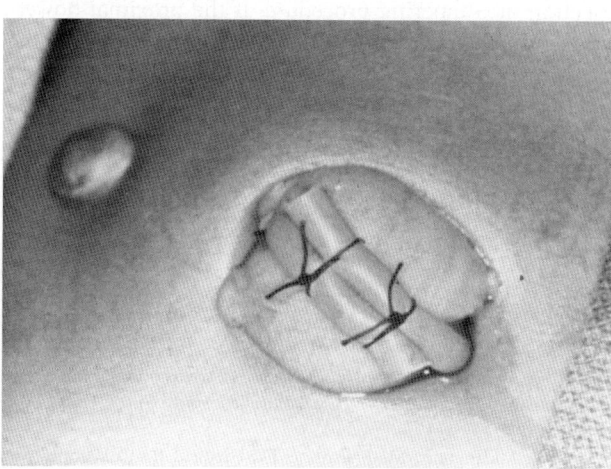

**FIGURE 47-5** Photograph of a sigmoid "loop" ostomy. A temporary soft rubber tube has been placed to help hold the stoma above the skin.

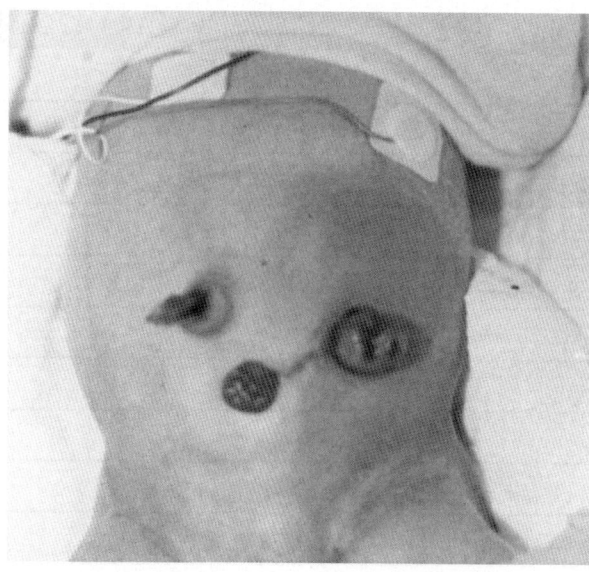

**FIGURE 47-6** End ostomy with mucous fistula placed distant from the ostomy. This form of ostomy arrangement is very useful in infants with imperforate anus, where total fecal diversion is needed as well as access to the distal bowel for radiologic studies.

and overall improvement in the patient's condition. If the appearance worsens, operative revision is mandatory.

Stricture, causing partial or complete obstruction of the stoma, can occur at either the skin or the fascia level. Mild stricture can be treated with dilatation, either digitally or with dilators. The family (or patient, if old enough) can usually be taught to perform the dilatation intermittently, if necessary. More severe or recurrent stricture must be operatively repaired, usually requiring excision of the cicatrix

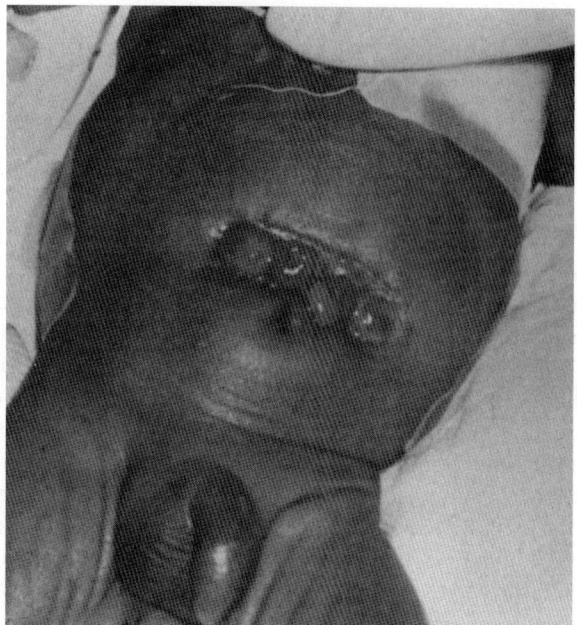

**FIGURE 47-7** Multiple ostomies in a newborn with necrotizing enterocolitis. In many of these cases, multiple bowel perforations occur, with "segments" of normal bowel. Exteriorizing multiple ostomies allows preservation of valuable bowel length. Closure can be in stages or in 1 large operation.

## TABLE 47-2    Stoma Complications

| |
|---|
| Necrosis |
| Stricture |
| Prolapse |
| Retraction |
| Wound infection |
| Skin excoriation and infection |
| Fistula |
| Appliance leakage |
| Mucosal ulceration |
| Mucosal hemorrhage |
| Variceal hemorrhage |
| Electrolyte imbalance |

at whatever level it occurs, with resuturing. Occasionally, moving the stoma to another location on the abdominal wall will be necessary.

Prolapse of an enterostomy is not unusual and requires revision only if it interferes with the function of the stoma or secure placement of the ostomy device. In the case of loop ostomies, it is generally the distal limb that prolapses. Transverse colostomies prolapse more frequently than sigmoid colostomies, and greatly dilated small or large bowel tend to prolapse at an increased rate when end ostomies are used. Ostomy prolapse can be somewhat prevented by extensive intra-abdominal suture placement, anchoring both proximal and distal limbs to the peritoneum. In addition, the use of tapering techniques, frequently with a stapling device, will allow a less dilated portion of bowel to be fashioned into a stoma that is less likely to prolapse. Finally, keeping the fascia opening small may also help prevent prolapse, although this obviously must be balanced against the possibility of stricture development at the fascia level.

Minor bleeding from a stoma is common and usually responds promptly to pressure. Occasionally caustic agents, such as silver nitrate, are required to slow or stop hemorrhage from traumatic injury or mucosal tears. Patients with an enterostomy and portal hypertension, such as infants with biliary atresia or liver abnormalities related to prolonged parenteral nutrition, can have significant, occasionally life-threatening, hemorrhage from an enterostomy. The most effective treatment for these children is closure of the ostomy at the earliest possible time, as local efforts at hemostasis are very temporary at best, and recurrent hemorrhage is the rule.

Skin problems (rash, excoriation, frank skin breakdown) are common and are best treated by consultation with an experienced enterostomal therapist. A variety of medications and protective compounds are available for local skin care. Much of the effort should be directed toward prevention of these problems by proper fitting and application of the stoma device and local skin hygiene.

# STOMA CLOSURE

Closure of an enterostomy should be considered a major surgical procedure, as the potential for morbidity is substantial. As an initial step, the surgeon must ensure patency of the distal bowel, generally through the use of contrast x-rays, either by rectal or by mucous fistula injection. Alternatively, irrigation of the distal bowel at the time of closure can be used, but this may require extensive adhesiolysis to expose all of the distal bowel and may not adequately demonstrate colonic strictures that are common in disorders such as necrotizing enterocolitis. In addition, knowledge of distal strictures may prompt the excision or repair of those lesions, with delay in closure of the ostomy until a later date. In general, having advance information regarding the anatomy and patency of the distal bowel before ostomy closure will improve the outcome of the operation.

Local incisions that encompass the ostomy (and mucous fistula, if present) are usually all that are necessary unless other procedures, such as adhesiolysis or stricturoplasty, are required. Placing the mucous fistula or oversewn distal bowel in the vicinity of the stoma facilitates this approach (Figs. 47-2 and 47-4). Adequate blood supply to each end of the bowel to be anastomosed can be assured by using sharp cutting of the bowel ends rather than electro-cautery to prepare the bowel for suture. Most surgeons prefer to hand sew the bowel anastomosis, as opposed to stapling, because the size of the bowel frequently precludes the use of staple devices. The choice of single- or two-layer and absorbable or nonabsorbable suture is strictly the surgeon's preference and is probably not as important to the outcome of the operation as are the suture placement, nutritional condition of the patient, and the blood supply to the bowel segments.

The 2 major complications of ostomy closure are leakage and stricture formation. Intraperitoneal leak must be managed promptly with reoperation. If performed early, suture repair of the leak may be possible, but more often exteriorization as an ostomy is necessary. The later complication of stricture formation can be managed by stricturoplasty or resection with another end-to-end anastomosis. Significant proximal bowel dilatation may require additional bowel resection or a tapering procedure. If the proximal bowel is sufficiently dilated, and bowel resection is not possible, then exteriorization as another ostomy with later attempted closure is advisable.

## SELECTED READINGS

Bischoff A, Levitt M, Lawal T, Pena A. Colostomy closure: how to avoid complications. *Ped Surg Int* 2010;26:1087–1092.

Chandramouli B, Srinivasan K, Jaydish S, et al. Morbidity and Mortality of colostomy and its closure in children. *J Pediatr Surg* 2004;39:596–599.

Ekenze SO, Agugua-Obyianyo NEN, Amah CC. Colostomy for large bowel anomalies in children: a case controlled study. *Int J Surg* 2007;5:273–277.

Mollitt DL, Malangoni MA, Ballantine TV, Grosfeld JL. Colostomy complications in children. An analysis of 146 cases. *Arch Surg* 1980;115:455–458.

Weber TR, Tracy TF, Silen ML. Enterostomy and its closure in newborns. *Arch Surg* 1995;130:534–537.

# CHAPTER 48  Appendicitis

*Rebeccah L. Brown*

## KEY POINTS

1. Appendicitis is a very common pediatric disorder.

2. Most cases of appendicitis are secondary to appendix lumen obstruction.

3. Appendectomy, either open or laparoscopic is the treatment of choice for non-complicated (unruptured) appendicitis.

4. Complicated (perforated) appendicitis can be treated with immediate operation, or a delayed procedure if the infection is controlled with antibiotics.

## HISTORY

Leonardo da Vinci first depicted the appendix in his anatomic drawings in 1492. Unfortunately, the drawings were not published until the eighteenth century. Consequently, Berengario Da Carpi is credited for the first description of the appendix in 1521.

Although several authors had described the pathology of the appendix, surgeon Lorenz Heister was the first to recognize in 1711 that the appendix might be the location of acute primary inflammation. In 1735, Claudius Amyand incised and drained a scrotal abscess, identified, tied off, and removed a perforated appendix through the scrotal incision. He is therefore credited with the first successful appendectomy.

In 1886, Reginald Fitz presented "Perforative Inflammation of the Vermiform Appendix with Special Reference to Its Early Diagnosis and Treatment" to the Association of American Physicians. Fitz was the first to describe "appendicitis" and suggested immediate surgical intervention (less than 3 days) for spreading peritonitis or deteriorating clinical status. Three years later, Charles McBurney published the first of his papers on appendicitis. He described the most likely location of the appendix 1.5 to 2 inches toward the umbilicus from the anterior superior iliac spine.

## PATHOPHYSIOLOGY

The association of fecalomas with perforated appendicitis had been well established since the necropsy period of the 1700s.

Consequently, the concept of appendiceal luminal obstruction leading to subsequent inflammation was not new when Wangensteen and Dennis published their "Experimental Proof of the Obstructive Origin of Appendicitis in Man" in 1939.

The etiology of appendicitis in the vast majority of patients is presumed to be based on luminal obstruction of the appendix. Intact mucosa normally secretes fluid into the lumen of the appendix. In the event of obstruction at the base of the appendix, this fluid cannot escape into the cecal lumen, and the intraluminal pressure of the appendix rises. With high pressures, venous drainage is impaired. The wall of the appendix becomes edematous, and ischemia of the mucosa ensues. Concomitant with the breakdown of the mucosal barrier is bacterial invasion of the wall of the appendix, resulting in acute appendicitis, gangrene, and ultimately perforation.

However, the sequence of events described above is not a maxim. There are other scenarios with which the surgeon needs to be acquainted. Should luminal obstruction be relieved as with extrusion of an appendicolith, there will be immediate luminal decompression with relief of symptoms. The appendix will then repair the injury. Even in the event of perforation, if the inflammatory process is well isolated from the rest of the abdomen by omentum and loops of the small bowel, the injury may be repaired in time without any detrimental effect on the patient. Significant injury to the appendix results in capillary ingrowth and the formation of granulation tissue eventually to be replaced by fibrosis. This is exactly the histopathologic picture seen in interval appendectomy specimens. Ironically, the circumferential fibrotic cicatrix compromising the appendiceal lumen may very well precipitate creation and retention of another fecaloma, resulting in appendiceal colic and/or acute appendicitis once again.

Fecalomas (fecaliths hereafter will refer to radiopaque concretions) have been documented in as many as 5% of incidental appendectomies. They are probably the most recognized cause of luminal obstruction of the appendix. Other entities may also compromise the lumen. Fibrosis, indicating remote appendicitis, has also been documented in approximately 5% of incidental appendectomies. Seeds, vegetable matter, and other foreign debris (fragments of metal, etc) may compromise the lumen. *Enterobius vermicularis* (pinworm) has been associated with appendiceal colic, although it is rarely associated with appendicitis. Finally, the lumen may be narrowed by intramural thickening secondary to a carcinoid or lymphoid hyperplasia.

Lymphoid tissue appears in the appendix shortly after birth. It is part of the secretory immune system of the gut—the gut associated lymphoid tissue (GALT). This lymphoid tissue produces secretory immunoglobulin and serves as a very effective barrier. Fortunately, the GALT located in the appendix is not indispensable. There is increased incidence of appendicitis during the influenza season, and this may be secondary to luminal narrowing due to lymphoid hyperplasia. In addition, this may explain why well-localized tenderness is often found at the McBurney point in association with mesenteric adenitis and acute gastroenteritis.

Appendiceal colic secondary to luminal compromise without associated inflammation is not unusual in children. It may be minor, of short and intermittent duration, or it may be severe and disabling. Appendiceal colic may herald the onset of acute appendicitis or may be a source of chronic, intermittent right lower quadrant pain that may pose a diagnostic dilemma for the treating physician.

## INCIDENCE

Appendicitis is the most common abdominal condition requiring surgery in the pediatric age group. The mean age of presentation is 11 to 12 years. The lifetime risk of acquiring appendicitis is 1 in 14 (7%). Appendicitis is unusual in patients less than 5 years of age and is exceptionally rare in the first year of life. In most series, males outnumber females, accounting for 55% to 65% of patients.

The incidence of perforated appendicitis in the pediatric population ranges from approximately 30% to 45%. In most instances, the appendix will perforate between 24 and 48 hours after onset of inflammation. However, 13% may perforate in less than 24 hours. The perforation rate in preschoolers ranges from 60% to 65%. Children less than 2 years of age account for 2% of pediatric appendicitis and have a perforation rate of 95%. Neonatal appendicitis is exceedingly rare, and the surgeon must be wary of other underlying conditions, such as Hirschsprung disease and necrotizing enterocolitis.

Ironically, the success rate of clinically diagnosing acute appendicitis is no better now than it was 50 years ago. A 15% to 20% negative appendectomy rate had been deemed acceptable in the past. However, with the advent of contemporary imaging strategies as well as the application of clinical practice guidelines, a 5% to 10% negative appendectomy rate is now generally considered acceptable.

## CLINICAL PRESENTATION

History and physical examination are the hallmark of diagnosing acute appendicitis, and the surgeon may expect to make the accurate diagnosis 80% to 90% of the time based on these parameters alone. In selected patients, laboratory and imaging studies may be useful adjuncts to support the diagnosis.

The time issue is important. It is highly unlikely that an inflamed appendix will perforate in the first 12 hours, when the symptomatology may not be quite as classic. Most appendices will perforate in 36 to 48 hours, and symptoms more than 72 hours are ominous for complicated appendicitis, especially in younger patients.

The paramount symptom is pain. Classically, the pain begins in the periumbilical location, but occasionally may originate in the right lower quadrant. Periumbilical pain is usually colicky secondary to stretch receptors in the appendix and mediated by visceral afferents entering the spine in the vicinity of T10. As subsequent inflammation ensues (usually within a few hours), somatic pain receptors of the parietal peritoneum become irritated, and pain localizes to the vicinity of the appendix, which usually is the McBurney point. If the appendix is located high, retrocolic, retrocecal, or in the pelvis, pain may be reported in the right upper quadrant, right flank, or suprapubic regions, respectively (Fig. 48-1). Malrotation or situs inversus may be responsible for pain in the epigastrium or left lower quadrant. An appendix lying adjacent to the bladder or right ureter may be responsible for urologic symptoms such as urgency, frequency, and dysuria.

Most patients will report anorexia. Anorexia and nausea are noted as the pressure in the appendix begins to increase. Vomiting has been reported as being important in establishing the diagnosis of appendicitis. However, some patients may perforate and never vomit. Vomiting invariably occurs after the onset of pain. As gangrene develops, or when the appendix perforates, the pain and vomiting may transiently and dramatically diminish. Subsequent spreading inflammation and secondary ileus will again exacerbate vomiting, and at this time, the emesis will usually be bilious in nature. Vomiting preceding abdominal pain is virtually never secondary to appendicitis.

Fever associated with acute appendicitis will usually hover within 1°C above normal. Fever higher than 39.4°C is usually associated with perforation or gangrene. In general, fever increases as the symptomatology progresses. High fever preceding onset of pain makes appendicitis very unlikely.

Constipation associated with appendicitis is not unusual. Diarrhea associated with appendicitis it occurs less frequently than constipation but has a more ominous significance, suggesting inflammation adjacent to the rectum. Diarrhea is more frequently associated with perforated appendicitis.

The diagnosis of appendicitis may be more difficult in children less than 5 years of age since they are less able to accurately describe their symptoms that may initially mimic other disease processes like gastroenteritis. As such, younger children are much more likely to present with perforated appendicitis.

Appendicitis is exceptionally rare in the newborn and even more difficult to diagnose. The usual presentation is vomiting, irritability, and fever followed by anorexia, diarrhea, and occasionally a stiff right hip. Diarrhea is important diagnostically and occurs in at least one-third of the younger patients with appendicitis as contrasted to older patients.

## PHYSICAL EXAMINATION

Abdominal tenderness is the most constant physical finding associated with acute appendicitis. The point of maximal tenderness is usually well localized in the right lower quadrant almost invariably at the McBurney point, located

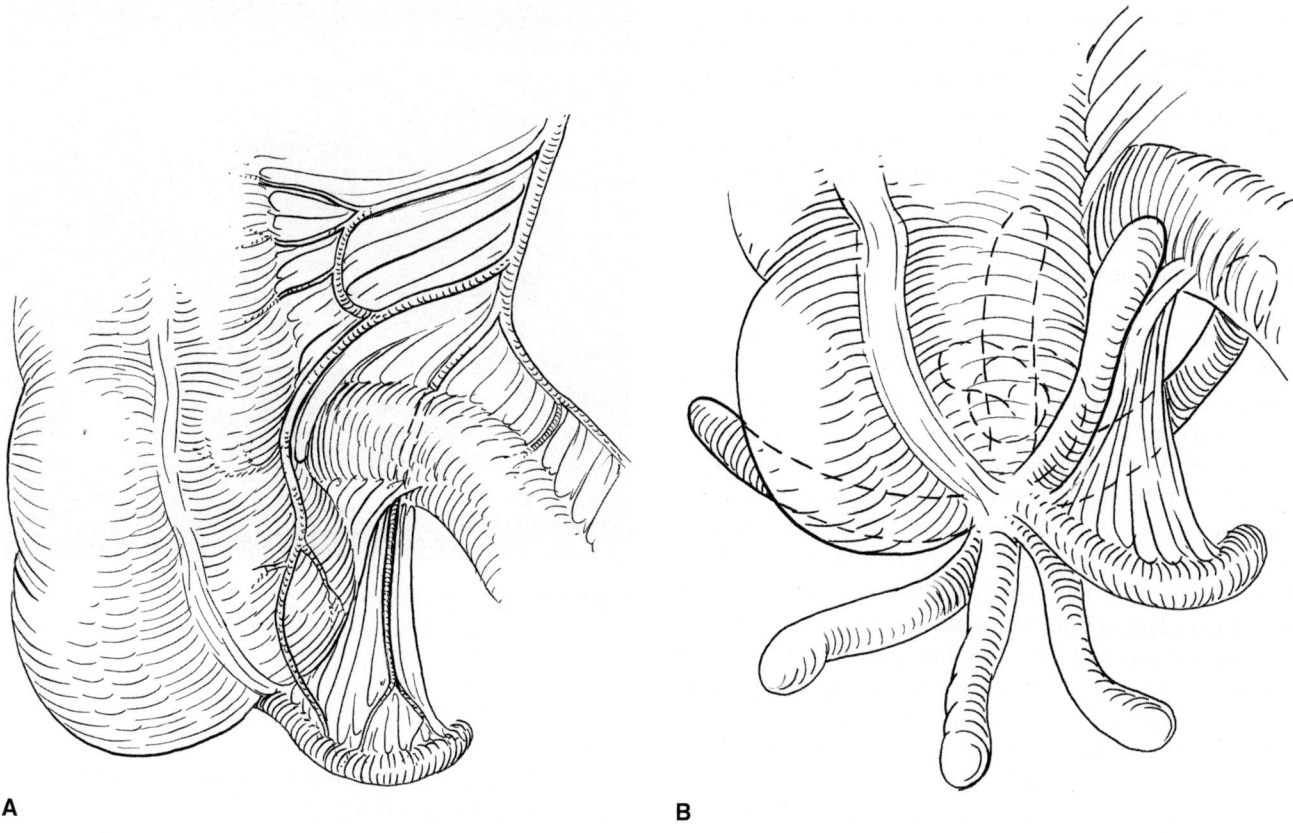

**FIGURE 48-1** Normal appendiceal anatomy. **A.** Blood supply of the appendix via the appendiceal artery. The taenia of the cecum lead to the base of the appendix. An ileocecal mesenteric fold overlays the ileocecal junction toward the base of the mesoappendix. **B.** The variety of anatomic variations in appendiceal location.

two-thirds the distance from the umbilicus to the anterior superior iliac spine.

It is valuable that the examiner be able to distinguish between the patient with appendiceal colic and the patient with acute appendicitis. The patient with appendiceal colic is obviously uncomfortable, pale, writhing, and crying with pain. He or she may experience increased pain with sudden movement and may have reflexive "dry heaves" with the pain. Patients with acute appendicitis will lie still, moan with pain, resist examination, and guard their abdomen. Both kinds of patients will have point tenderness over the appendix. The patient with acute appendicitis needs an urgent appendectomy. The patient with appendiceal colic may ultimately need an appendectomy but rarely emergently.

The second most constant physical finding is the right lower abdominal muscle spasm and involuntary guarding associated with adjacent inflammation. If intervention is delayed, rebound tenderness follows and the patient becomes quiet, resisting movement and examination. The Rovsing sign is positive when palpation in the left lower quadrant results in the patient complaining of pain in the right lower quadrant. The psoas sign is positive when the patient experiences discomfort as the right thigh is extended. The obturator sign is positive when pain is elicited with passive rotation of the flexed right thigh. As peritonitis evolves, the patient becomes increasingly febrile, tachycardic, hypotensive, and septic. The abdominal exam may be misleading if the appendix is located in a retrocolic or retrocecal position. The abdominal wall

is rather insulated from inflammation. Symptoms may be slower in onset, and physical findings may be more obscure. The patient may complain of right flank and right hip pain. Obese patients may also have more significant inflammation than appreciated upon physical exam.

A rectal examination is an important adjunct for patients with suspected appendicitis. If the appendix is located in the pelvis, anterior abdominal wall findings may be virtually absent. A large tender mass found in the pelvis without associated peritoneal findings or an inflamed pelvic appendix may be palpated rectally. In very young patients, the entire pelvis may be palpated per rectal exam. A pelvic examination should be performed in sexually active patients.

## LABORATORY STUDIES

If the history and physical exam are classic for acute appendicitis, it is unlikely that routine laboratory and imaging studies will add anything that is significant. Ordinarily, the white blood count (WBC) will range from 10,000 to 18,000. However, 20% of patients with acute appendicitis will have a normal WBC. Only 20% of patients with appendicitis will have an elevated WBC in the first 24 hours of symptoms.

A WBC greater than 20,000 suggests perforated appendicitis. Although appendicitis may occasionally be associated with a WBC greater than 25,000, one should be wary of other possible diagnoses such as pneumonia. WBCs less than 5000 may be seen with acute appendicitis, especially if a preceeding viral syndrome is responsible for this suppression. Children under 5 years of age are notorious for a slow WBC response in the face of acute appendicitis.

A left shift is probably a more significant finding than an elevated WBC. Normal values for polymorphonuclear leukocytes (PMN) are 50% up to 5 years of age, 65% from 5 to 10 years, and 75% over 10 years of age. PMN counts greater than 75% may be expected in 85% of patients with acute appendicitis.

C-reactive protein (CRP) levels may be used in conjunction with the WBC count or alone as an adjunct to the diagnosis of acute appendicitis or to guide antibiotic management for perforated appendicitis with abscess.

The urinalysis is helpful in excluding urinary tract infection and identifying patients requiring fluid resuscitation. The specific gravity and ketones may be elevated due to vomiting and dehydration. The RBC and WBC in urine may be elevated if the appendix is located adjacent to the bladder or ureter. Urinalysis cell counts greater than 15, and white cells too numerous to count or in clumps, presence of nitrites or leukocyte esterase suggest a urinary tract infection. Bactiuria is not seen with acute appendicitis, and if documented, a urine culture and possibly a urinary tract radiographic assessment should be considered.

A preoperative pregnancy test is mandatory for all pubertal female patients. An electrolyte profile is indicated for dehydrated patients.

## IMAGING

Laboratory studies and imaging rarely add significant information in cases of classic acute appendicitis, especially in boys. Imaging studies should be reserved for equivocal cases of abdominal pain when hospital observation versus discharge is anticipated, or in preparation for management of complex cases, such as perforated appendicitis with phlegmon or abscess.

Abdominal radiographs, including supine, upright, and perhaps left-lateral decubitus views, may be quite helpful if a calcified, oval, laminated fecalith is identified in the vicinity of maximal tenderness. In this setting, acute appendicitis will be documented 90% of the time. Appendicoliths may be documented in 10% to 12% of school-aged children and older with acute appendicitis. Patients under 5 years of age with acute appendicitis have a 28% incidence of appendicoliths.

Findings suggestive but not diagnostic for acute appendicitis include mildly dilated loops of the bowel with air-fluid levels in the right lower quadrant, scoliosis of the spine concave to the right, and obliteration of the lower right psoas margin. Other suggestive findings such as obliteration of the preperitoneal fat line, paucity of gas in the right lower quadrant, localized air bubbles in the right lower quadrant, and small bowel obstruction might be present.

Free air documented by abdominal radiographs in patients with acute appendicitis is extremely rare. The abdominal radiograph should include the lower chest to rule out right lower lobe pneumonia. Any patient with a cough, dyspnea or

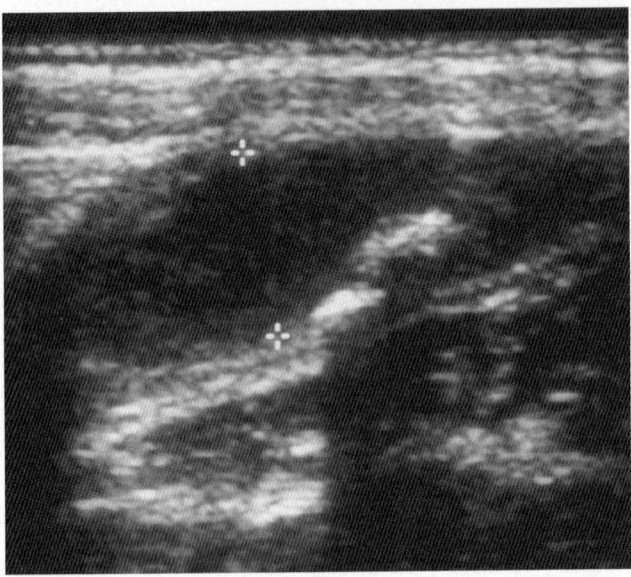

**FIGURE 48-2** Abdominal ultrasound (US) depicting acute appendicitis. The appendix is distended with increased wall thickness.

tachynea, and/or pleuritic chest pain associated with abdominal pain should have a chest x-ray.

More sophisticated imaging may be necessary to assist decision-making with patients who are difficult to evaluate, such as the obese, preschoolers, the developmentally delayed, and patients who are being observed and in whom the diagnosis remains obscure. Such imaging studies may also be helpful with immunocompromised oncology patients and those with nephritis, cardiac problems, diabetes, sickle cell disease, Henoch–Schönlein purpura, and hemolytic uremic syndrome.

Ultrasound (US) is fast, may be done portably, involves no irradiation, is inexpensive, and the results are available immediately. Diagnostic accuracy is generally greater than 90%, but it is very user-dependent. High-resolution, real-time imaging with graded compression that displaces the bowel and associated gas may document a blind-ending tubular or target-like structure that is immobile, nonperistalsing, and noncompressible. The hypoechoic wall is greater than 2 mm in thickness. The maximal diameter of the appendix must be greater than 6 mm (Fig. 48-2). The lumen is generally anechoic and the mucosa echogenic. There may be loculated adjacent fluid. If perforated with luminal decompression, the appendix may not be identifiable. Color doppler may help delineate the wall. US is especially useful to rule out gynecologic pathology or to document normal ovaries in pubescent females. One must always correlate US findings with clinical findings and exam.

In general, computerized tomography (CT) is more accurate than US, with a diagnostic accuracy of 95% to 98%. CT provides more detailed imaging of intra-abdominal and pelvic structures, and the diagnosis of appendicitis is suggested by the presence of an appendix greater than 6 mm in diameter, appendiceal wall thickening greater than 2 mm, appendicolith(s), adjacent fluid or loculated gas collections, and peri-cecal or pelvic inflammation, fat stranding,

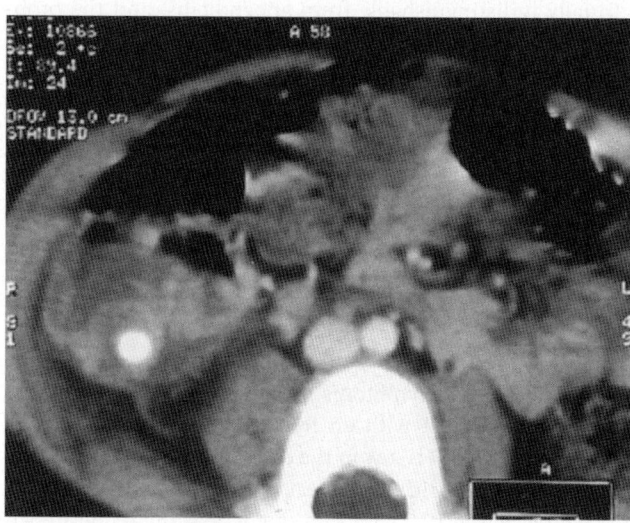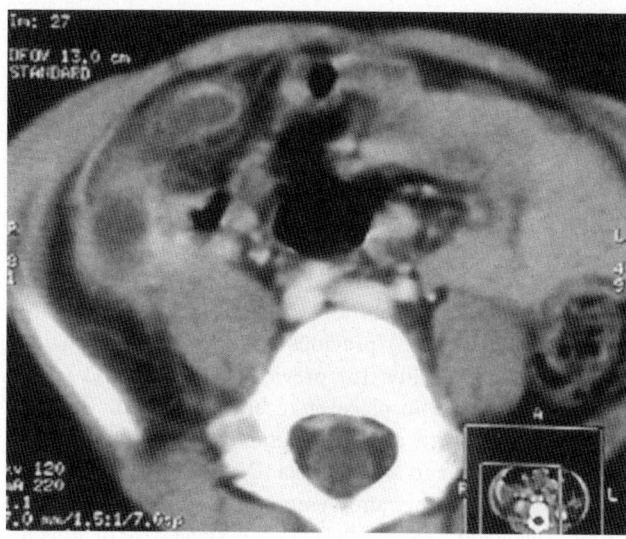

**FIGURE 48-3** Classic pelvic computerized tomography (CT) scan depicting a distended appendix with enhanced wall thickness.

phlegmon, or abscess (Fig. 48-3). The disadvantage of CT versus US is the ionizing radiation associated with CT that may predispose children to malignancy. Therefore, CT should be limited to cases in which there is still diagnostic uncertainty after US or when US is not available or reliable. Table 48-1 defines the findings of US and CT.

## DIFFERENTIAL DIAGNOSIS

### Diagnoses Virtually Indistinguishable from Appendicitis That Would not Require Operation

*Acute gastroenteritis* is a very common emergency room diagnosis for abdominal pain. Generally regarded as a viral illness, the problem presents acutely and is self-limited. Symptoms include some combination of profuse watery diarrhea, intermittent cramping, abdominal pain, fever, nausea, and vomiting. The diarrhea may persist for several days. Typically, nausea, vomiting, and diarrhea are the predominant symptoms, with abdominal pain playing a lesser role. Symptoms generally subside in 48 hours, and if they are more severe and

protracted, one should be alert for bacterial and protozoan infections.

*Mesenteric adenitis* may be diagnosed by US or CT or after a negative appendectomy. The enlarged terminal ileal mesenteric nodes are felt to be secondary to a concurrent or recently subsided upper respiratory infection. There may be fever and nausea but generally without vomiting. The pain is generally not as impressive as that with acute appendicitis, and the tenderness is more diffuse. Lymphocytosis may support the diagnosis of mesenteric adenitis. Clinically, mesenteric adenitis is frequently indistinguishable from acute appendicitis.

*Primary peritonitis* is a diffuse bacterial peritoneal infection without an apparent source. Certain disease states such as nephrotic syndrome, cirrhosis, ascites, immune deficiencies, systemic lupus erythematosus, and carcinoma are prone toward primary peritonitis. The majority of children with this problem are less than 3 years of age. The abdominal pain associated with primary peritonitis is diffuse, severe, and of unusually sudden onset. Fever is noted to be significantly higher and earlier in onset than in the case of secondary peritonitis. The WBCs may be exceptionally high (20,000-50,000). Exploratory laparotomy may reveal scant, slightly cloudy fluid, or thick, sticky fluid without an obvious source. Cultures of the fluid and all possible sources should be taken. Occasionally, peritonitis in a susceptible patient may mandate paracentesis. If Gram-positive cocci are found, then intravenous antibiotics and observation may be indicated.

*Primary omental torsion* is exceptionally rare and almost impossible to differentiate from acute appendicitis preoperatively. Intra-abdominal serosanguinous fluid is suggestive.

*Epiploic appendagitis* is also a rare cause of abdominal pain that may mimic acute appendicitis. In experienced hands, the diagnosis may be made with CT or ultrasonography. Most patients can be treated conservatively with or without anti-inflammatory medications or antibiotics. Most cases will

| TABLE 48-1 | Diagnostic Imaging for Appendicitis |
| --- | --- |
| **Ultrasound** | **Computerized Tomography** |
| Noncompressible, immobile, blind-ended structure | Thickened, tubular, structure, unopacified, greater than 6 mm |
| Thickened appendiceal wall greater than 2 mm | Appendicolith |
| Appendiceal diameter greater than 6 mm | Periappendiceal inflammation and mass effect |
| Appendicolith | Enhanced appendiceal or cecal wall |
| | Abscess, phlegmon |

resolve over a period of observation within a few days. An operation is rarely required.

## Diagnoses That Will Require Operation

*Ectopic pregnancy* must be considered in any female from menarche to menopause who complains of lower abdominal pain. Menstrual history and parity are meaningless. Since delayed passage of a fertilized egg is the problem, certain points must be kept in mind: (1) previous PID; (2) previous ectopic pregnancy; (3) previous abdominal surgery (tubal ligation); (4) infertility; (5) previous abortion; and (6) an intrauterine device in place or recently removed. The classic triad noted with ectopic pregnancy is abdominal pain, vaginal bleeding, and amenorrhea. Dizziness (hypovolemia), nausea, and vomiting, and symptoms of pregnancy, should arouse suspicion. A soft, blue cervix is suggestive of an ectopic pregnancy, and a positive pregnancy test and US are usually diagnostic.

*GI perforation* (other than the appendix) is associated with free air in 70% to 90% of cases. A gastric air-fluid level is absent in 93% of gastric perforations, and if present, a small or large bowel perforation is more likely. In the pediatric age group, 75% of patients are under 2 years of age and 50% are neonates. The decreasing order of incidence is as follows: necrotizing enterocolitis; ulcers of the duodenum, stomach, and jejunum; Hirschsprung disease; atresias; meconium ileus; and volvulus. The most likely site of perforation is the ileum, followed by the rectosigmoid, the stomach, and the duodenum.

*Gonads:* A male patient with lower abdominal pain must be examined for an empty scrotum. A scrotal testicular torsion will be obvious. However, an empty scrotum will warrant further work-up for possible intra-abdominal torsion. Females may experience lower abdominal pain secondary to hemorrhage within an ovarian cyst, rupture of an ovarian cyst, or even torsion of an adnexal structure (including ovarian cyst). Torsion in older patients is usually secondary to ovarian tumors. Gonadal torsion results in intense inflammation associated with a markedly elevated WBC. The groin needs to be examined to exclude an incarcerated or strangulated inguinal hernia.

A *small bowel obstruction* with pain in the very young suggests midgut volvulus or intussusception. If there is an abdominal scar and the obstruction has occurred more than 2 weeks postoperatively, an adhesion is the likely problem. If it has been less than 2 weeks postoperatively, one should anticipate a possible postoperative intussusception that may require operative reduction.

Tenderness in the right upper quadrant warrants an US examination that will likely demonstrate the presence of cholelithiasis with or without *cholecystitis*. The surgeon, however, must be wary of the high-riding retrocecal appendix that may well be responsible for localized right upper quadrant subcostal tenderness.

Complications of the *Meckel diverticulum* are usually encountered in patients around 2 years of age. Pain secondary to the Meckel diverticulum is unusual and may be secondary to peptic ulceration or inflammation associated with a retained foreign body (fecaloma). The presentation is virtually indistinguishable from appendicitis, and the problem is usually identified operatively.

Sixty percent of *choledochal cysts* present in patients less than 10 years of age, and females predominate 4:1. The classic presentation is right upper quadrant pain, jaundice, and a palpable mass. Infants may present with acholic stools (elevated direct bilirubin) and fever. An US is diagnostic.

## Diagnoses That May Require Operation

Pelvic inflammatory disease (PID) is more common in females who have multiple sex partners. Once contracted, the recurrence rate is 25%. Symptoms usually occur within 2 weeks after sexual contact with an infected partner. The ratio of appendicitis to PID is low in the early phase of the menstrual cycle and high during the luteal phase. The lower abdominal pain is aggravated with movement, and the tenderness is usually bilateral (6%-8% unilateral). Cervical tenderness is present in 97% of patients, followed by vaginal discharge, and adnexal enlargement. After administering appropriate antibiotics, operation may be indicated for nonresponders with a persisting or enlarging pelvic mass, a leaking abscess, intra-abdominal bleeding, or pointing abscess.

Idiopathic *intussusception* is encountered between 2 months and 5 years of age, with the peak being 4 to 10 months. While appendectomy is the most common surgical procedure for abdominal pain in patients over 2 years of age, intussusception has been responsible for the majority of surgical procedures for abdominal pain in patients under 2 years of age. The classic presentation is severe colicky abdominal pain, vomiting, and bloody stools. An abdominal mass is frequently palpable and, in time, a bowel obstruction will ensue. Intussusception beyond 3 years of age will likely be secondary to a lead point, such as the Meckel diverticulum, polyps, or other masses. A terminal ileal duplication cyst is likely in for patients less than 1 month of age. An air enema may be both diagnostic and therapeutic.

*Henoch–Schönlein purpura* results from a vasculitis secondary to allergic sensitivities in patients typically 4 to 10 years of age. The characteristic symmetrical, raised, erythematous, maculopapular rash that evolves to petechiae or purpuric lesions involves the lower extremities and buttock, and may involve the arms. Two-thirds of patients develop microscopic or gross hematuria. Two-thirds develop arthritis. Approximately 50% of patients will experience abdominal pain secondary to ischemic vasculitis. The pain may occur before the rash in 10% to 20% of patients, and vomiting may be present. Surgical lesions include intussusception and perforation in 2% to 6% of patients, but these complications rarely occur before the rash. Knee and/or ankle arthritis with abdominal pain should encourage observation for development of the rash.

Approximately 25% of all new patients with *Crohn disease* are less than 20 years of age, and 5% are less than 5 years of age. The disease is more common in Whites and those of Jewish descent. The disease is subtle in onset with anorexia, fever, malabsorption, and occasional vomiting and diarrhea. Growth failure is an important observation but may go unnoticed. The patient may present with recurrent poorly localized periumbilical pain or pain in the right lower quadrant. Ten percent may mimic acute appendicitis with an elevated WBC. Since eating exacerbates the pain, many avoid eating. More than one-third of children present with perianal disease (skin tags, fissures, fistulas). Thrush-like stomatitis and arthritis may be noted. It is important to entertain the diagnosis and inquire about a family history of Crohn disease in all patients being evaluated for right lower quadrant pain.

*Sickle cell disease* is frequently associated with cholelithiasis and its attendant morbidity. Splenic sequestration crisis usually occurs in children less than 5 years of age and is characterized by massive splenic enlargement, abdominal pain, and a rapidly falling hemoglobin. Vaso-occlusive crisis is more commonly encountered in patients greater than 4 to 5 years. Occlusion of microvasculature results in abdominal pain and even ileus simulating appendicitis. Abdominal surgical intervention in either crisis is rarely necessary.

The *hemolytic uremic syndrome* is characterized by a micro-angiopathic (renal) hemolytic anemia, acute renal failure, and thrombocytopenia. Usually seen in children less than 5 years of age, it is often preceded by a flu-like syndrome (upper respiratory infection or gastroenteritis) 1 to 2 weeks earlier. Colicky abdominal pain and abdominal tenderness with diarrhea (occult or bloody) may be noted. The surgeon must be aware of possible toxic megacolon, perforation, and intussusception. Usually, renal failure with hypertension and oliguria become evident within 2 weeks.

*Pancreatitis* may occur at any time in childhood. The pain is rather vague and midepigastric without radiation. Drugs (steroids, thiazides, L-asparaginase), systemic disease (cystic fibrosis, hyperlipidemia, lupus erythematosis), familial pancreatitis, mumps, and anatomic abnormalities (stones, ductal abnormalities) are proven associations. Serum amylase and lipase should be measured, and pancreatic US or CT scans may be useful to establish the diagnosis.

*Kawasaki disease* (mucocutaneous lymph node syndrome) is characterized by prolonged high fever, skin rashes, cervical lymphadenopathy, stomatitis, erythema, edema, desquamation of the distal extremities, and arthritis. The disease usually occurs in children less than 8 years (average 2 years). Hydrops of the gallbladder will likely result in surgical consultation. Arteritis and periarteritis lead to ischemia and possible necrosis of the GI tract, liver, adrenal gland, and urinary bladder, which in turn may necessitate surgical intervention.

## Diagnoses That Will not Require Operation

*Constipation* is a common pediatric problem and may be responsible for abdominal pain, nausea and vomiting, and even abdominal tenderness. The pain is persistent but does not progress. It is usually associated with periumbilical or poorly localized pain. Rectal examination and/or abdominal radiographs will suggest the diagnosis.

*Urinary tract infection—pyelonephritis* is suggested by chills, fever, pyuria, bacteriuria, and leukocytosis. Vomiting may be associated with surprising frequency. Dribbling, nocturnal enuresis, and daytime incontinence as well as foul-smelling urine are also suggestive.

Right lower lobe *pneumonia* may result in irritation of the lower intercostal nerves with subsequent pain, hyperesthesia,

and muscle spasm in the right lower quadrant. Cough, tachypnea, pleuritic chest pain, shallow breathing, and splinting as well as rales, dullness, decreased breath sounds, high fever, and markedly elevated WBC should suggest the diagnosis. Chest x-ray is diagnostic.

*Diabetic ketoacidosis* may be manifested by abdominal pain, tenderness, and vomiting. There will be varying degrees of fever, and the patient eventually becomes somnolent. Polyuria, polydipsia, glycosuria, and elevated serum and urine ketones associated with hyperglycemia suggest this diagnosis.

Abdominal pain (any location in the abdomen including the right lower quadrant) may be one of the earliest manifestations of *acute rheumatic fever*. Anorexia, nausea, and vomiting are associated. Fifty percent have had a preceding sore throat 1 to 5 weeks earlier. Fever, arthritis (migrating and large joints), heart murmur, skin rash (erythema marginatum), and tachycardia out of proportion to the fever suggest the diagnosis.

The *hemophiliac* presenting with abdominal pain should be imaged to rule out a possible retroperitoneal or mesenteric hematoma.

*Lead poisoning* usually occurs in patients 1 to 6 years of age who live in older at-risk dwellings. The earlier symptoms include anorexia, intermittent abdominal pain, sporadic vomiting, constipation, hyperirritability, and decreased play activity. X-rays may show broad bands of increased density of the metaphyses of the long bones.

The clinical symptoms associated with *porphyria* are rarely encountered before puberty and are usually subtle in onset. Most commonly noted is colicky abdominal pain localized in the epigastrium or right-lower quadrant. The pain may be extremely severe and is usually associated with vomiting and constipation. A cutaneous photodermatitis may be manifested as vesicles, bullae, and edema of exposed skin. The lesions may become infected and then heal with a violaceous hue. Hypertension may be present, and the classic burgundy-red urine may or may not be present.

*Ureterolithiasis* may be responsible for right-lower quadrant pain if a stone is lodged near the appendix. Pain is typically colicky in nature and the patient may be writhing in pain. Pain may be referred to the labia, scrotum, and penis. Pain and hematuria in the absence of fever and leukocytosis warrants a noncontrast CT to exclude ureterolithiasis.

## COMPLICATED APPENDICITIS

Delay in seeking medical attention is the primary reason for complicated (gangrenous or perforated) appendicitis. In addition, when significantly delayed, the presentation may be so atypical (high fever, diarrhea) that the primary practitioner may not recognize the diagnosis, leading to further delay. Currently, in most series, 30% to 45% of children with appendicitis present with perforated appendicitis. In general, the younger the patient, the greater the chance of presenting with complicated appendicitis. Although males outnumber females with acute suppurative appendicitis, the gender difference narrows with perforated appendicitis.

Perforated appendicitis may be managed in 3 ways: (1) operatively—with urgent appendectomy and drainage of associated abscesses; (2) conservatively—with intravenous antibiotics, with or without percutaneous drainage of associated abscesses, followed by interval appendectomy in 6 to 8 weeks; or (3) nonoperatively—with intravenous antibiotics, with or without percutaneous drainage of associated abscesses, and no planned interval appendectomy unless symptoms recur.

The downside to conservative management is its attendant morbidity and need for close follow-up. The patient is generally observed in-house until the infectious process is under control. There is often a period of intravenous antibiotics administered at home, drain management, subsequent convalescence, and readmission for interval appendectomy, depending on surgeon preference. There remains a possibility of exacerbation of recurrent appendicitis that could require urgent intervention, or at the very least, frequent trips to the office or emergency department to be re-assessed for recurrent symptoms. Consequently, some surgeons prefer operative intervention in all patients as soon as they are stabilized. The downside to urgent operation for perforated appendicitis is a potentially more difficult operation with increased risk for injury to adjacent structures due to the intense acute inflammatory response.

In general, if a patient with perforated appendicitis presents within 3 to 7 days and does not have a well-defined, safely-accessible abscess amenable to percutaneous drainage, the preferred management is usually urgent appendectomy after appropriate fluid resuscitation. If the patient has had prolonged symptoms greater than 1 to 3 weeks or has a well-defined, safely-accessible abscess amenable to percutaneous drainage, then a more conservative approach to management may be a safer option due to the intense peritoneal inflammatory response from the perforation, thereby increasing the difficulty and associated morbidity of an operation. An interval appendectomy after conservative management is typically performed at 6 to 8 weeks to allow the inflammatory response to subside, allowing for a safer, easier operation. However, the need for interval appendectomy after conservative treatment of perforated appendicitis has been widely debated.

## Peritonitis

Peritonitis is the most likely complication of acute appendicitis, and prompt operative intervention after a careful and thorough resuscitation is indicated. In addition, a significant number of children explored for acute suppurative appendicitis are found to have perforated appendicitis. Younger children are more likely to have diffuse peritonitis while older children are more likely to develop a walled-off abscess. This difference has been attributed to the inability of a thin omentum to effectively wall off and limit the spread of infection in younger children. If diffuse peritonitis is encountered, most surgeons would recommend evacuation of the pus and appendectomy, with or without copious saline lavage (without antibiotics). A fecalith should be sought and removed. If left behind, it may be a source of recurrent abscesses. Intra-abdominal drains are of limited value and rarely indicated.

## Abdominal Mass

Up to 10% of pediatric patients with appendicitis may present with an abdominal mass. Some masses will be palpated in the emergency department but most will be discovered in the operating room after the patient is anesthetized. The mass may be a phlegmon with a central inflamed appendix. The phlegmon will appear after 4 to 5 days from onset and accounts for 50% of appendiceal masses. One-quarter of masses will be an abscess.

An abdominal mass is best evaluated by US or contrast-enhanced CT scan, although contrast-enhanced CT provides more detail and is less user-dependent. If the patient is found to have a phlegmonous mass without a well-defined abscess and is nontoxic, he or she should be admitted for observation, serial examinations, and treated with broad-spectrum intravenous antibiotics, with adequate Gram positive, Gram negative, and anaerobic coverage. Since phlegmonous masses may evolve into well-defined abscesses over time, serial US imaging may be useful to identify potentially drainable abscesses. If a well-defined, safely-accessible abscess is identified either on presentation or on serial imaging studies, percutaneous US or CT-guided drainage may be attempted. Multiple inter-loop abscesses or a nonaccessible abscess unresponsive to antibiotics will generally require operative drainage.

## GI Obstruction

Dilated loops of the bowel in a patient with acute appendicitis may be secondary to ileus, obstruction due to adhesions, or obstruction due to an impinging mass. If the patient has dilated loops and undergoes exploration, the surgeon should take note of the terminal ileum adjacent to the ileal cecal valve. If this segment is decompressed, the ileum should be run proximally until dilatation is encountered. In this way, an adhesion may be released at the time of exploration rather than 2 or 3 weeks later when the obstruction (as opposed to ileus) becomes obvious.

# PREOPERATIVE CONSIDERATIONS

## In-House Observation

In an effort to reduce negative appendectomy rates, patients who have an equivocal presentation may be observed for several hours. Serial abdominal examinations, preferably by the same physician coupled with repeat blood counts, or US or CT imaging, should identify patients with appendicitis. Any chance of perforation while the patient is hospitalized is slight. After discharge, recurrence of focal pain coupled with fever or nausea and vomiting requires a repeat evaluation.

## Resuscitation

Any unstable patient must be thoroughly resuscitated prior to administration of a general anesthetic. This could take up to 3 to 4 hours, but it will avoid an intraoperative catastrophe. The patient must be volume-resuscitated with isotonic fluid boluses of 20 mL per kg and subsequent drip infusion.

The goal is to establish an adequate urine output of at least 1 mL per kg per hour. A nasogastric tube should be placed in order to decompress the stomach. Broad-spectrum antibiotics should be administered.

## Antibiotics

Antibiotics are administered for suspected appendicitis in order to reduce the incidence of postoperative wound infection and intra-abdominal abscess formation. Such antibiotics must be administered prior to making the skin incision.

*Escherichia coli* and *Bacteroides fragilis* are the 2 most commonly isolated micro-organisms in patients with perforated appendicitis. With this in mind, both aerobic and anaerobic coverage must be provided.

For suspected nonperforated appendicitis, a single-agent antibiotic, for example, cefoxitin or ampicillin–sulbactam, is adequate. If a patient is allergic to penicillin, clindamycin and gentamicin may be used. However, for perforated appendicitis, more broad-spectrum antibiotics may be more appropriate, and may be either single agent, for example, piperacillin–tazobactam or ertapenem; double agent (eg, ceftriaxone and flagyl); or triple agent, for example, ampicillin–gentamicin–clindamycin or ampicillin–gentamicin–metronidazole, or other variations thereof. Wound infection rates of 10% to 30% may be anticipated in acute nonperforated appendicitis when patients are not covered with antibiotics. Indeed, wound infection rates approaching 10% have been reported when normal appendices have been removed without antibiotic coverage. With preoperative antibiotics, wound infection rates of less than 3% to 4% may be anticipated for nonperforated appendicitis. There is no evidence to support the administration of further antibiotic doses in the postoperative period for uncomplicated nonperforated appendicitis. A single preoperative dose of antibiotics should suffice.

Perforated appendicitis mandates a longer course of broad spectrum antibiotic coverage, although the optimal duration of treatment is not known and varies widely among surgeons. Wound infection rates up to 80%, and intra-abdominal abscesses up to 40%, may be expected in the absence of proper antibiotic coverage. With appropriate coverage, the postoperative infection rate still approaches 20% to 30%. Traditionally, children with perforated appendicitis were treated with triple antibiotic therapy covering Gram-positive, Gram-negative, and anaerobic organisms for 10 to 14 days. More recently, single- and double-agent therapy with less frequent dosing has been shown to be equally effective to triple-agent therapy with the advantages of increased ease of administration and reduced cost. Furthermore, clinical guidelines developed by the American Pediatric Surgical Association Outcomes and Clinical Trials Committee in 2010 suggest that the length of administration of antibiotics be based not on a set time frame but rather on clinical criteria, including fever, pain, return of bowel function, and WBC count. For this management scenario, intravenous antibiotics are continued until patient is afebrile for 24 hours, pain is well controlled on oral pain medications, bowel function has returned, and WBC is normalizing. The patient may then complete the course of therapy with oral antibiotics for a total of 7 days of antibiotic therapy, including both intravenous and oral.

# APPENDECTOMY

The decision whether to do an open versus laparoscopic appendectomy for acute appendicitis is dependent upon surgeon skill and experience as well as hospital resources and training of staff. Laparoscopic appendectomy has gained widespread popularity in children and is now the preferred approach for the majority of pediatric surgeons. While studies have shown roughly equivalent outcomes for open versus laparoscopic appendectomy in children, purported advantages of the laparoscopic approach may include reduced pain, quicker recovery and return to normal activities, fewer wound infections and intra-abdominal abscesses, enhanced ability to examine the entire abdomen and pelvis when the diagnosis is unclear, and improved cosmesis. After an appropriate learning curve, operative times are similar. Cost may be slightly higher with laparoscopy, but this is thought to be balanced by a decreased length of stay, quicker return to activities, and decreased complications. Although an open appendectomy may be performed through a tiny single incision in young, thin children with similar outcomes to laparoscopy, a laparoscopic approach is preferred in older, heavier, and more muscular patients in whom a more extensive incision would be needed. It is also generally preferred for pubertal females in whom gynecologic pathology may mimic acute appendicitis or in cases in which there is diagnostic uncertainty since the entire abdomen and pelvis may be visualized. Laparoscopic appendectomy may also be associated with fewer wound complications, especially for perforated appendicitis and in obese patients due to the smaller incisions. Relative contraindications to laparoscopic appendectomy include prior abdominal or pelvic surgery in which adhesions may be prohibitive, stump appendicitis, and severe cardiac disease.

## Techniques for Open Appendectomy

A transverse skin incision is made in the right lower quadrant slightly above the anterior superior iliac spine and lateral to the rectus abdominus. The incision may be adjusted to the point of maximal tenderness. In general, the cecum is located somewhat higher in younger patients and a more cephalad incision will provide better exposure. A 1- to 2-cm incision in the direction of the fibers of the external oblique will allow insertion of the right-angle retractors. When retracted, they will expose the internal oblique. A Kelly clamp or heavy, straight Mayo scissors are used to spread in the direction of the fibers of the internal oblique and then the transversus muscle is separated further with right-angle retractors. The peritoneum is then exposed, grasped between smooth forceps, and then incised. The peritoneal incision is extended to expose the intra-abdominal region. Purulent fluid may be cultured at this time. A digital exploration is then done to locate the appendix. Babcock clamps are ideal to deliver the cecum and/or appendix into the incision. The cecum identified by taenia may be grasped with a moist gauze and rocked gently through the small incision. If the cecum is located unusually high, the sigmoid colon may occasionally be mistaken for the cecum and temporarily cause confusion.

The cecum may be difficult to extract from the iliac fossa due to its peritoneal attachments. These attachments may be incised inferior and lateral under direct vision. However, this may require lengthening the incision. With experience, the surgeon may take down these peritoneal reflections bluntly with finger dissection and avoid extending the incision. The appendix is usually located inferior and slightly posterior to the lower pole of the cecum. If it can be delivered directly into the wound, it may be possible to remove it without delivering the cecum. If the appendix is not immediately obvious, it may be located by identifying the cecal taeniae and by following them to where they converge, the base of the appendix. If the cecum is difficult to mobilize, and access to the appendix seems impossible, the incision is lengthened. It can be extended medially by dividing the internal oblique and transversus muscles into the anterior and posterior rectus sheaths, leaving the rectus muscle intact. The rectus muscle itself may easily be retracted medially. If lateral extension is required, the skin incision is lengthened "above the iliac crest." The incision in the external oblique is easily extended. The internal oblique and transversus may be divided with electrocautery. Another option is to perform a more cephalad gridiron incision through these 2 muscles. This will provide excellent exposure to the right gutter as far cephalad as the gallbladder.

A final option to remove a difficult appendix is to divide the appendix at an appropriate location near its base, and dissect the distal appendix in a retrograde fashion.

One must be very careful dissecting the base of the appendix. Occasionally the most proximal few centimeters of the appendix may be hidden under peritoneal reflections. If this "hidden" appendix is not identified, a few centimeters of proximal appendix may be left after dividing the structure, and recurrent appendicitis in the stump may be a risk.

The appendix may be removed—by one of 3 ways:

1. Simple ligation (Fig. 48-4): After the mesoappendix is divided and the cecum is clearly identified surrounding the base of the appendix, the appendiceal base is doubly ligated with 2-0 absorbable ties. The appendix is amputated and the exposed mucosa cauterized to prevent mucocele formation.

2. Purse string appendectomy (Fig. 48-5): Once the appendix is accessible, the mesoappendix is taken down between clamps and divided. Generally, 2-0, 3-0, or 4-0 absorbable suture ties are used. The mesoappendix is divided until the cecum surrounding the base of the appendix is completely exposed. The appendix is grasped with a sponge and a seromuscular purse string suture of 3-0 silk is placed in the

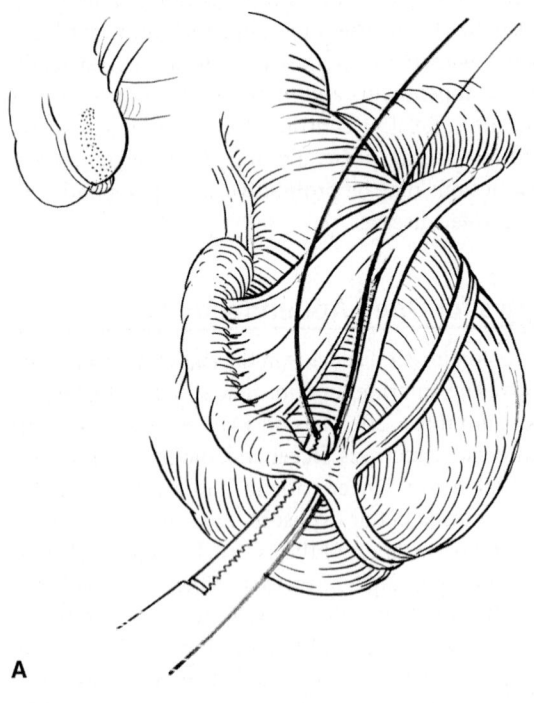

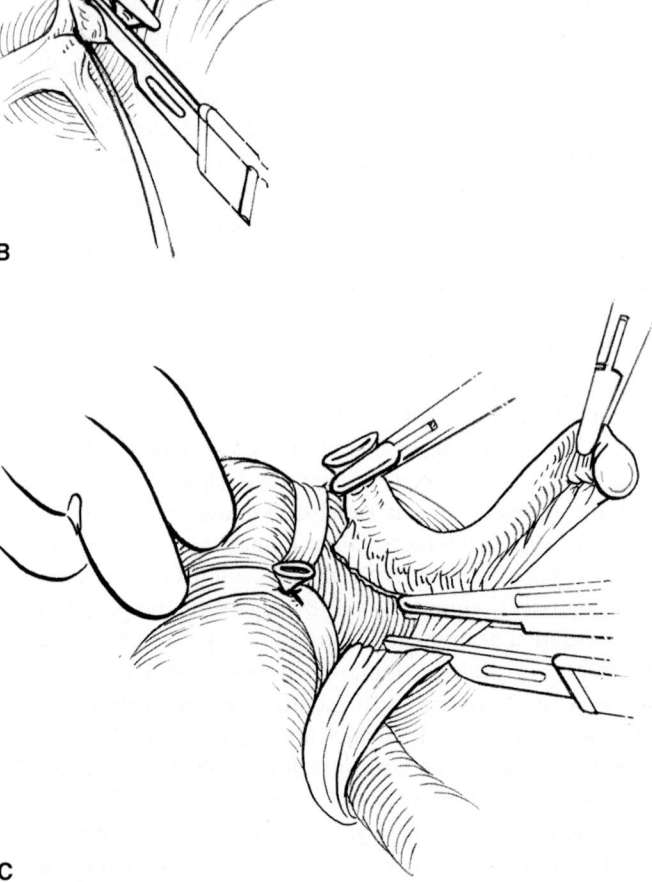

**FIGURE 48-4 A.** The appendix is visualized and delivered into the wound. **B.** The mesoappendix is carefully divided and ligated. **C.** The base of the appendix is crushed with a clamp.

A

B

C

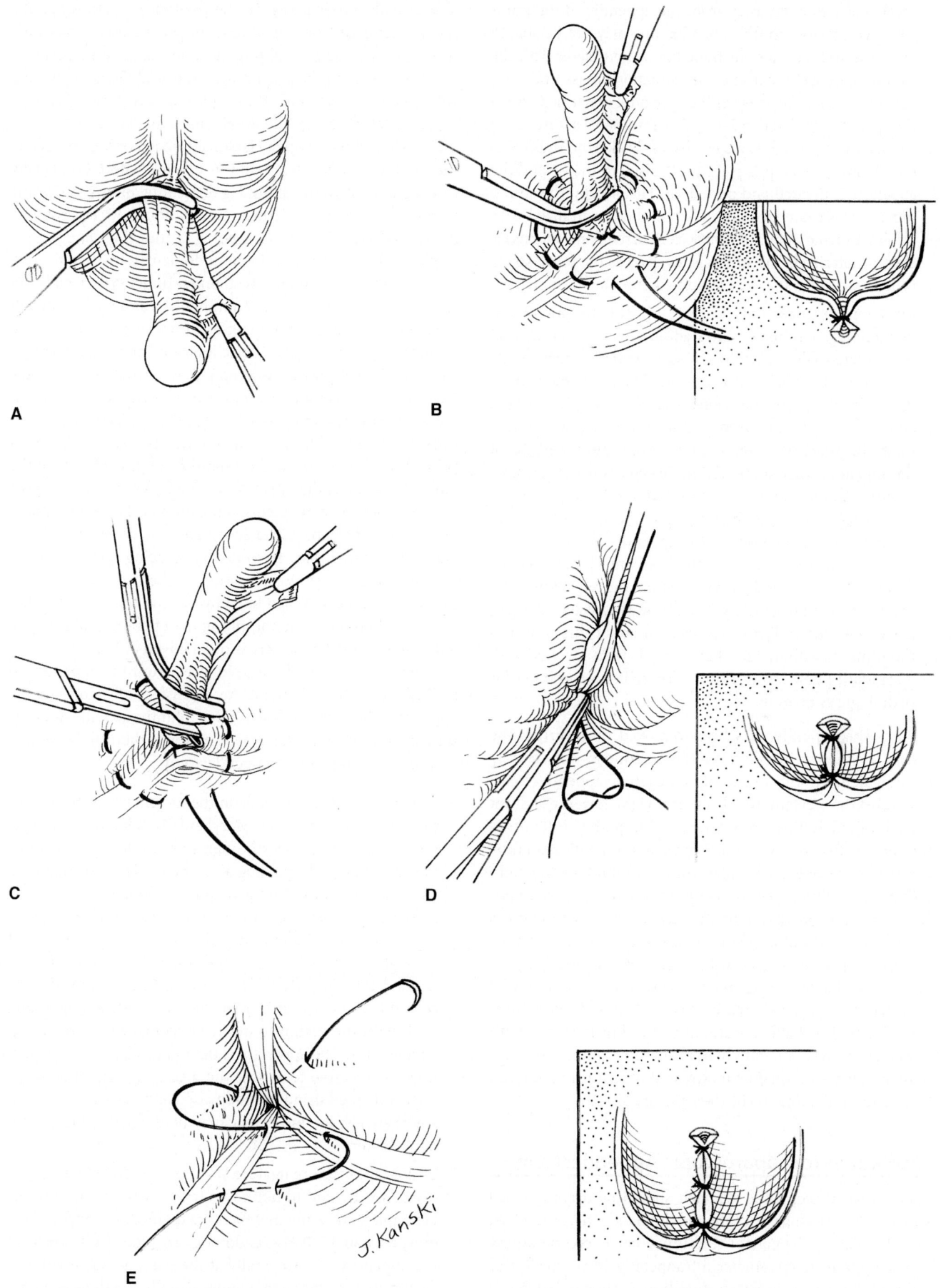

**FIGURE 48-5** **A.** The crushed base of the appendix is ligated with an absorbable suture. **B.** A seromuscular suture is placed in the cecum in a purse-string fashion approximately 1 cm away from the appendiceal base. **C.** The appendix is clamped distally and sharply amputated. **D.** The ligated stump is grasped and inverted. The purse-string suture is tied. **E.** A Z-stitch can be used to further invert the area.

cecal wall 1 to 2 cm away from the appendix. If the purse string is too close to the appendix, one may not be able to dunk the stump; if too far there may be problems with the stump (mucocele, chronic inflammation, mass effect on barium enema). The base of the appendix is crushed with a clamp and ligated with a 2-0 or 3-0 absorbable suture (used so that any enclosed localized abscess is likely to drain into the cecum). A clamp is placed just distal to the tie and the appendix is divided and passed off. Historically, the stump mucosa was cauterized with phenol, then neutralized with alcohol to avoid potential mucocele. Currently the mucosa is electrocauterized. The stump is inverted as the purse string is tied. A Z-stitch may be placed to secure the purse string.

3. Inversion appendectomy (Fig. 48-6): This technique was devised to eliminate intra-abdominal contamination encountered when cutting across an enteric structure. Its use should be confined to the incidental appendectomy. After division, the mesoappendix, still attached to the appendix, must be excised completely, including any that might be attached to the cecum surrounding the base of the appendix. This can be accomplished easily with electrocautery. A blunt tip probe is inserted into the crushed and flaccid tip of the appendix. The tip of the appendix is then pushed into (or the body of the appendix is "pulled onto" the probe) and inverted through its proximal lumen into the cecum. The inversion is continued until the reflection of the inversion is approximately 1 cm from the cecum. A tight, absorbable suture ligature is secured about this stump as the probe is withdrawn. This stump is then inverted with a standard purse string closure. There is no specimen for pathologic evaluation.

Once the appendix has been removed or inverted, the cecum is then replaced into the abdomen, which may be irrigated. In the event of a negative appendectomy, one must be certain to check for right-lower quadrant pathology including mesenteric adenopathy, inflammatory bowel disease, the Meckel diverticulum, fallopian tube or ovarian pathology, hernias, and pathology of the right kidney and gallbladder. To facilitate visual or digital exposure, the incision may be lengthened. The peritoneum is closed with a running 2-0 or 3-0 absorbable suture, and the 3 muscle layers are closed with interrupted or running 2-0 or 3-0 absorbable suture. General wound irrigation may be repeated at each level. Scarpa fascia is closed with interrupted 4-0 absorbable suture, and the skin is closed with either a running subcuticular absorbable suture, or permanent simple or vertical mattress skin sutures or staples. Steristrips and a dry sterile dressing are applied.

## Techniques for Laparoscopic Appendectomy

Prior to laparoscopy, the stomach should be decompressed with an oro- or nasogastric tube and the bladder decompressed by either having the patient void immediately preoperatively or placing a urinary catheter intraoperatively. A curvilinear infraumbilical or vertical transumbilical incision is then made to place the first port. The transumbilical approach may be more cosmetic since the umbilicus is a natural scar, and this incision is hidden within the depths of the umbilicus. It may

also provide easier access to the peritoneal cavity since the fascia is generally thinner at the center of the umbilicus where there may also be a small umbilical hernia in some patients. For the transumbilical approach, the umbilicus is everted with towel clips or toothed forceps, and a vertical incision is made directly through the umbilicus with a knife (Fig. 48-7). Then using either an open Hasson approach or Veress needle, the peritoneum is entered and insufflated with $CO_2$, usually to a pressure of 10 to 15 mm Hg depending on the size of the patient. Once there is adequate insufflation, a 30° laparoscope is inserted via a 5 to 12 mm port (12 mm if an endoscopic stapler will be used), and the abdomen is inspected. Two additional ports are then placed under direct vision, either in the left lower quadrant and suprapubic regions or in the left lower quadrant and right upper quadrant regions, depending upon surgeon preference. Single incision laparoscopy using a single umbilical port is also being performed by some pediatric surgeons. Variations on port placement are depicted in Fig. 48-8. For ergonomic reasons, I prefer to place the ports in the suprapubic and left lower quadrant regions. With both the primary and assistant surgeon standing on the left side of the table, the scope is then placed in the left lower quadrant port and the working instruments in the umbilical and suprapubic ports. It is important to clearly visualize the dome of the bladder and stay well away from it when placing the suprapubic port to avoid injury. Visualization of the right lower quadrant and appendix is facilitated by placing the patient in the Trendelenberg position and tilting the operating table to the left. The inflamed appendix is often covered with omentum. The omentum should be moved away from the appendix to facilitate exposure. If there are extensive adhesions to the appendix, they can be lysed either bluntly or with hook or scissor cautery. Once the appendix is free, there are 2 general methods to complete the appendectomy

1. Stapled: A window is made in the mesentery at the base of the appendix with a blunt Maryland dissector. Once the dissector has been passed through this window, the window may be enlarged by passing a second dissector through the window and gently pulling in opposite directions longitudinally and parallel to the mesentery (Fig. 48-9). Once there is an adequate window, an endovascular stapler is passed through the window, and the appendix is stapled and divided at the junction of the base of the appendix and the cecum (Fig. 48-10). It is important to divide the appendix flush with the cecum to avoid the complication of stump appendicitis. The appendix is then grasped in its mid-portion and elevated to expose the mesentery. The mesentery is then divided using the endovascular stapler (Fig. 48-11). Alternatively, the mesentery may be divided using careful hook cautery (Fig. 48-12).

2. Endoloop or suture ligature (Fig. 48-13): The mesentery is divided with careful hook cautery or with an endovascular stapler. Once the mesentery is divided, the appendix is grasped, and 3 2-0 PDS endoloops are placed at the base of the appendix—2 proximally at the base, as flush with the cecum as possible, and 1 more distally on the appendix. The appendix is then divided using endoscissors between the distal and proximal endoloops leaving 2 endoloops to secure the appendiceal stump. Alternatively, the appendix

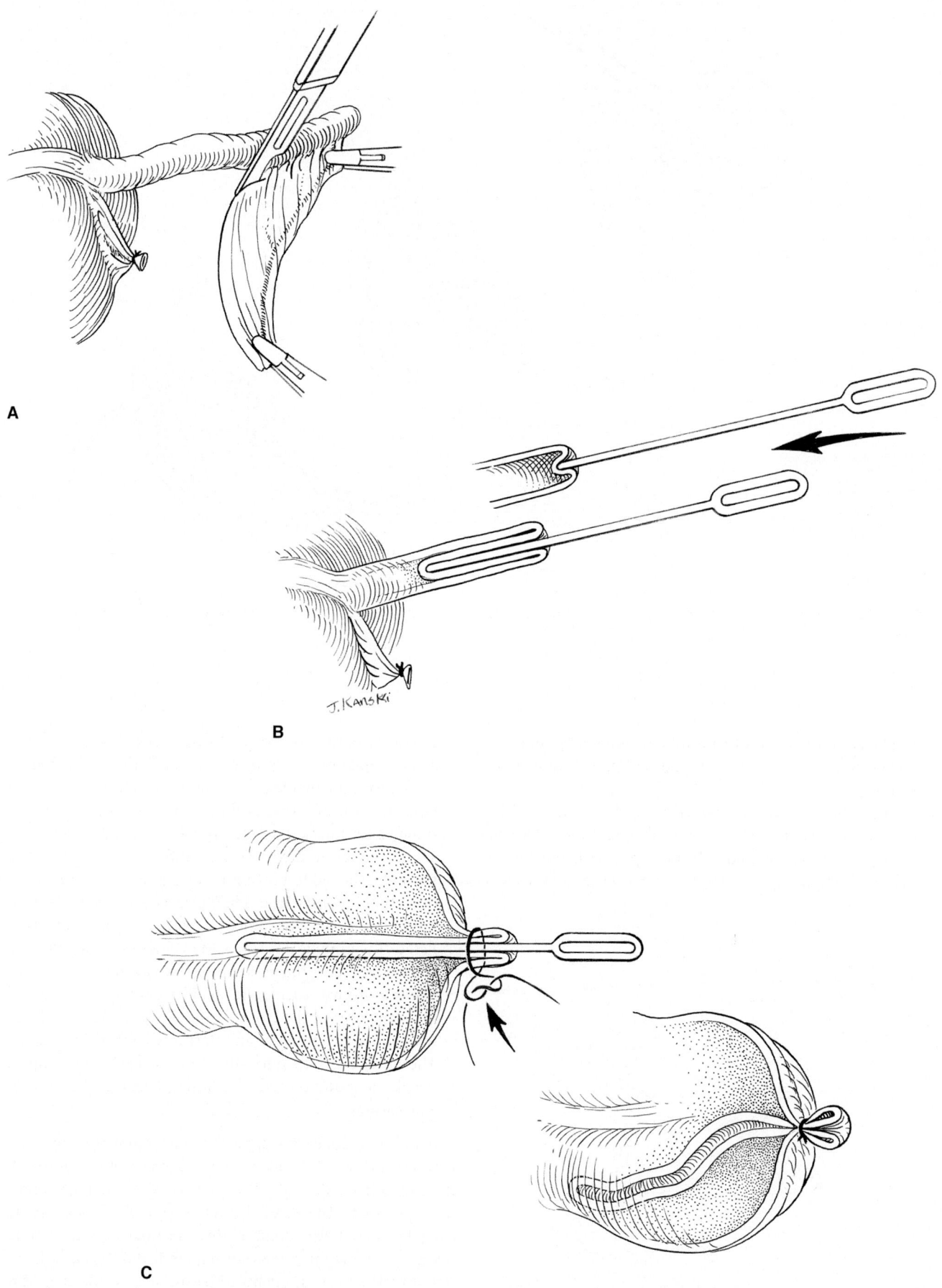

**FIGURE 48-6** Inversion-ligation appendectomy. **A.** The appendiceal mesentery after ligation is sharply excised off the appendix proper. **B.** A blunt probe is inserted at the appendiceal tip, and as the tip is gently inverted the appendix is pulled onto the probe, which is directed into the lumen of the cecum. **C.** An approximate 1-cm stump of appendix is then ligated with an absorbable suture as the probe is removed, assuring necrosis and sloughing of the inverted appendix into the lumen of the cecum.

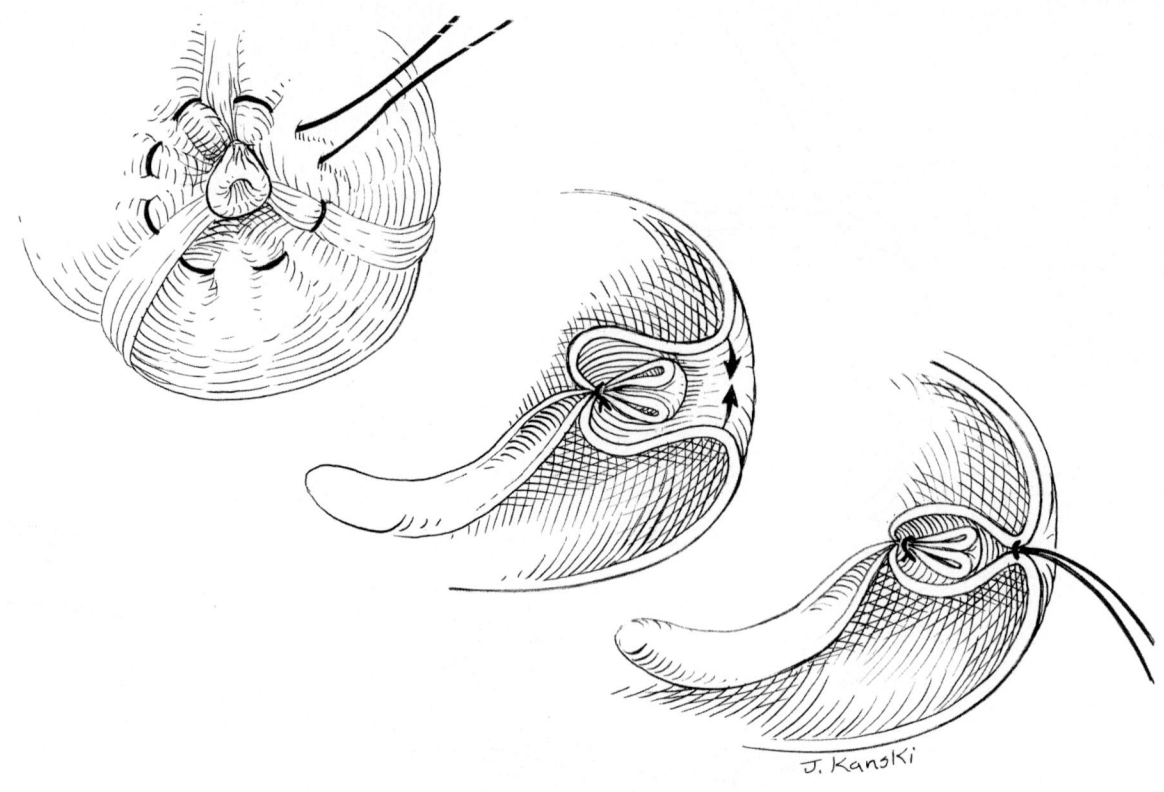

J. Kanski

**D, E**

**FIGURE 48-6** (*Continued*) **D.** A seromuscular nonabsorbable purse-string suture is placed around the ligated appendiceal stump. **E.** The purse-string is tied, further inverting the stump.

can be doubly ligated with absorbable suture as in an open appendectomy using intra- or extracorporeal knot-tying techniques.

Once the appendix is divided from the cecum and its mesentery, it is placed in an endocatch bag and retrieved through the umbilical port. If the appendix is minimally inflamed or grossly normal, it can be retrieved through the sleeve of the port without a bag. One should, however, avoid removing an appendix through the incision itself to decrease the incidence of wound infection. If there is a large amount of purulent fluid in the abdomen, it is suctioned free and the abdomen is then irrigated with normal saline until clear. If there is a fecalith, it must be searched for and removed to prevent recurrent abscesses. Once the operation is complete and hemostasis is assured, the ports are removed, and the abdomen is then completely desufflated. The umbilical fascia is then closed with a figure-of-eight heavy absorbable suture. The closure is facilitated using a groove director to avoid trapping any underlying structures in the closure. The umbilical skin is closed with either a running or an interrupted absorbable suture. The other 2 5-mm port site are closed with interrupted deeply dermally buried or running subcuticular absorbable sutures.

If a normal-appearing appendix is encountered, the abdomen must be carefully inspected to exclude other causes for the abdominal pain and associated symptoms that prompted the operation. The small bowel is carefully inspected to exclude mesenteric adenopathy, terminal ileitis, Crohn disease, tumors, intussusception, and the Meckel diverticulum. The liver and gallbladder are inspected, as are the ovaries, uterus, and fallopian tubes in females. The internal rings are inspected for patency. In most cases, the appendix is still removed to avoid further diagnostic dilemma postoperatively.

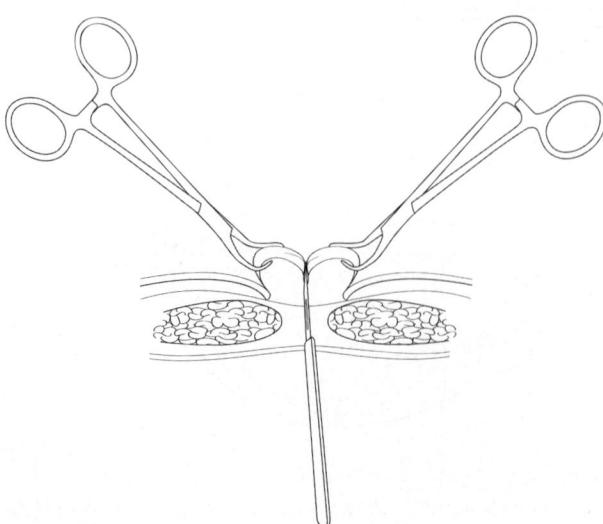

**FIGURE 48-7** The umbilicus is everted with towel clips or toothed forceps and divided in the vertical midline with a knife.

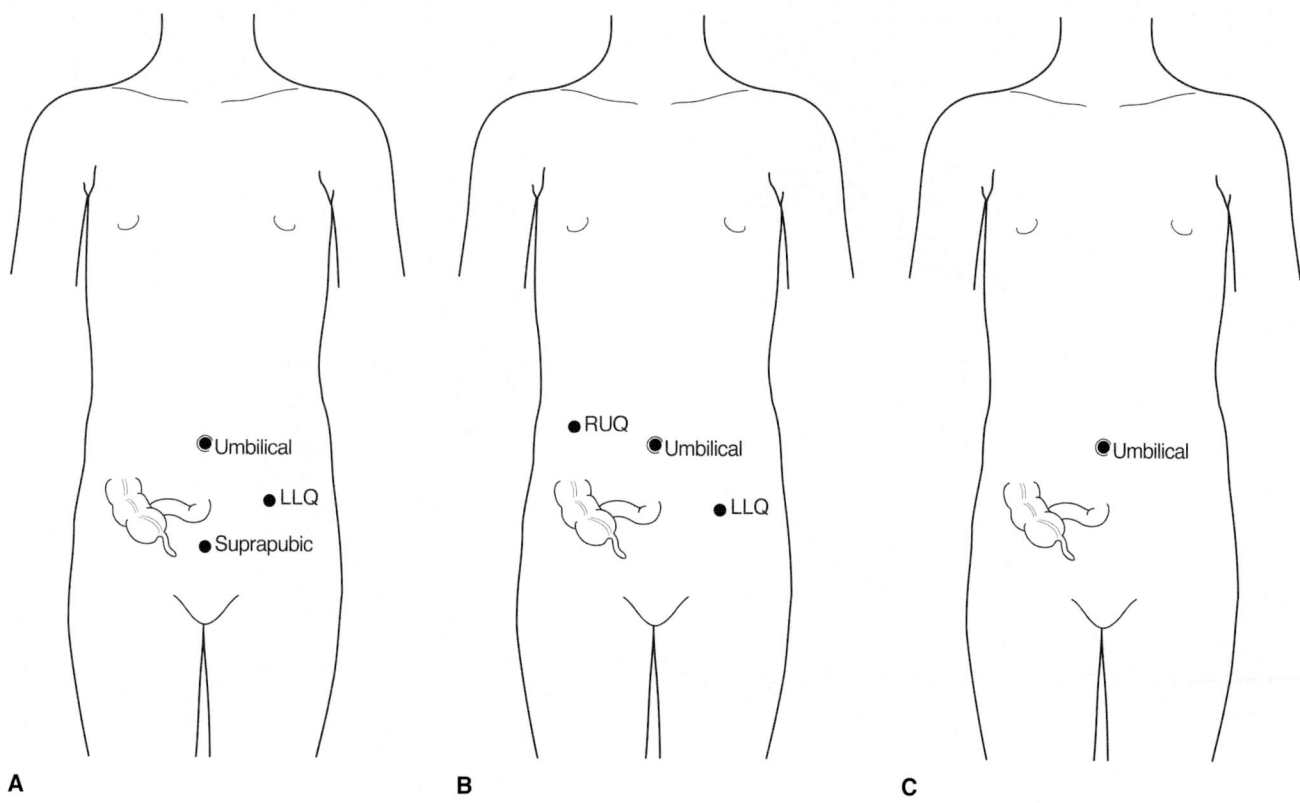

**FIGURE 48-8** Three different approaches to port placement are depicted.

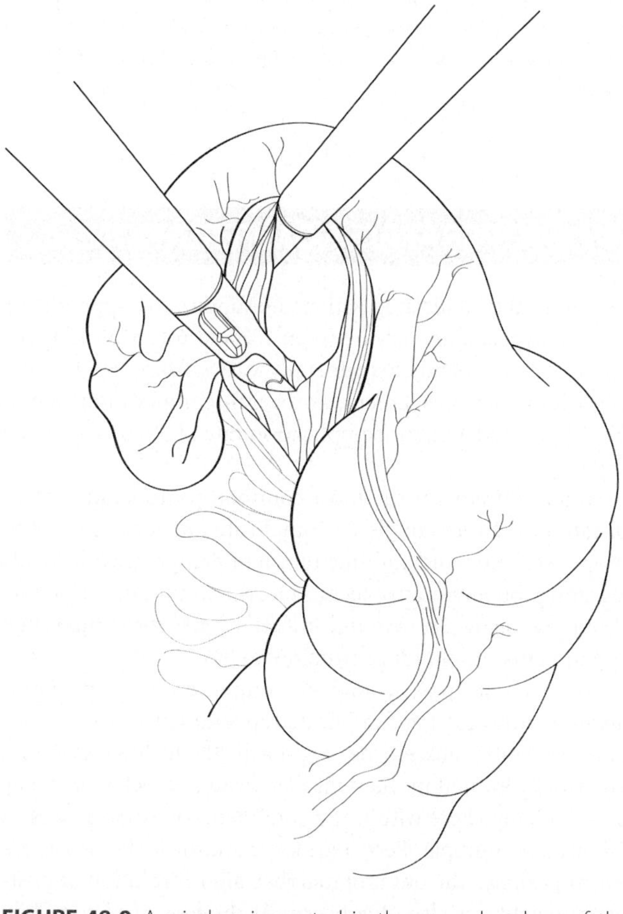

**FIGURE 48-9** A window is created in the avascular plane of the mesentery at the base of the appendix at its junction with the cecum.

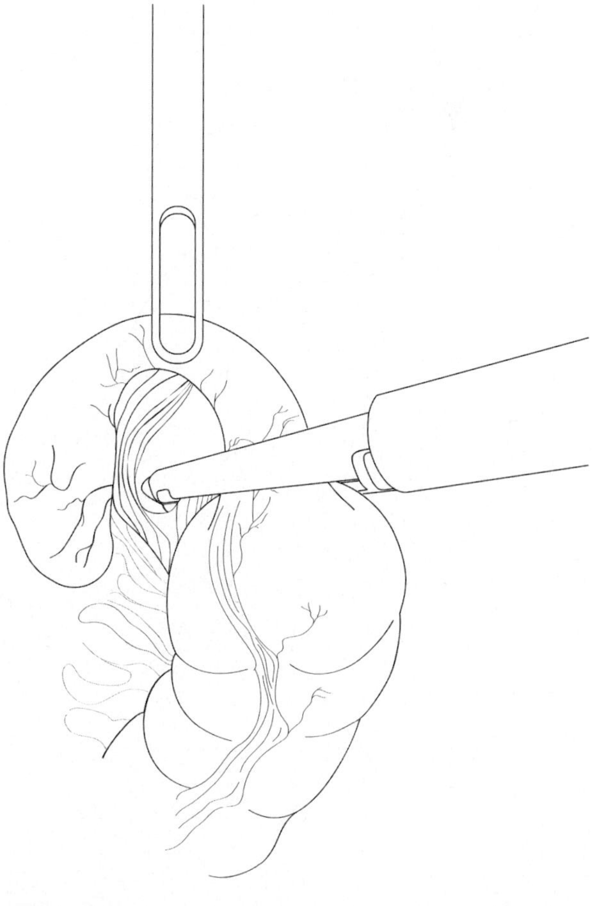

**FIGURE 48-10** An endovascular stapler is passed through the window created in the mesentery, and the appendix is divided flush with the cecum.

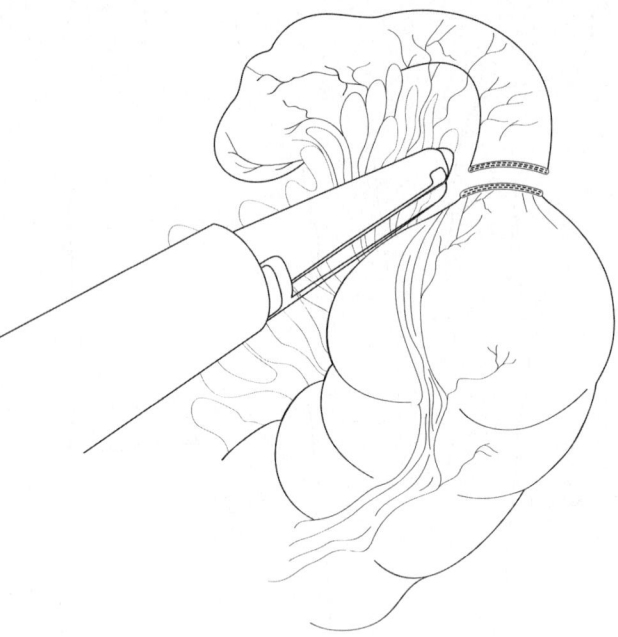

**FIGURE 48-11** The endovascular stapler is used to divide the mesoappendix.

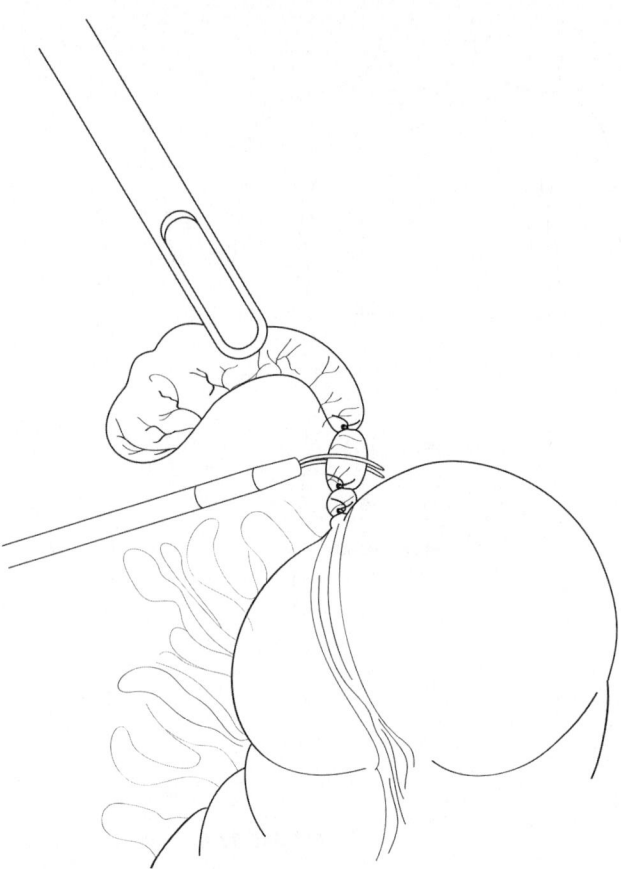

**FIGURE 48-13** Three endoloops or sutures are placed at the base of the appendix at its junction with the cecum. The appendix is then divided with endoscissors between the most distal 2 endoloops or sutures such that the appendiceal stump is doubly ligated.

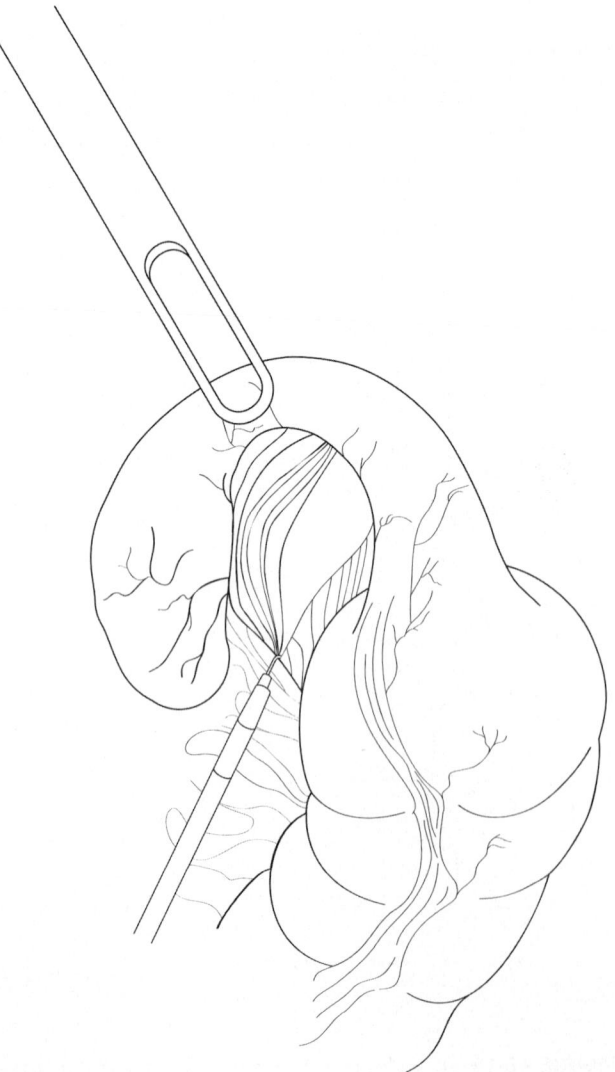

## POSTOPERATIVE COMPLICATIONS

The morbidity associated with acute suppurative appendicitis may be expected to vary between 1% and 6%. Morbidity for complicated appendicitis generally varies from 15% to 65%. With optimal management, an overall complication rate of 9% to 10% and a major complication rate of 3% to 4% can be expected.

*Wound infection* is the most common postoperative complication in either simple or complicated appendicitis. With proper selection and administration of preoperative antibiotics, and proper operative technique, the wound infection rate should be below 3%. Wound infection rates for complicated appendicitis should range from 6% to 8%.

The second most common complication is an *intra-abdominal abscess*. For complicated appendicitis, the incidence of postoperative abscess may approach 20% to 30%. Abscesses are usually located in the right iliac fossa and pelvis, but may be found anywhere within the abdomen. Interloop abscesses are usually multiple. Persistent fever and/or leukocytosis are warning signs. The onset of diarrhea after resolution of post-operative ileus is also of concern. At the first suspicion of an intra-abdominal abscess, a contrast-enhanced CT should be performed.

**FIGURE 48-12** Hook cautery is used to divide the mesoappendix.

*Small bowel obstruction* post-appendectomy is the third most common complication and has a reported incidence of 5% to 15% following complicated appendicitis. Paralytic ileus secondary to perforated appendicitis may be expected to last 3 to 5 days. Prolonged bowel dysfunction or evidence of obstruction developing after temporary recovery warrants initial conservative management with nasogastric suction, fluid replacement, and possible total parenteral nutrition. Exploration may be inevitable. Failure of conservative management and operative intervention is much more likely if the patient presents with small bowel obstruction more than 4 weeks postoperatively.

Although exceptionally rare after an appendectomy, postoperative intussusception may occur. This complication is generally encountered within 7 to 14 days (mean 8 days) of the appendectomy, and 90% present within 2 weeks of operation. In contrast, 75% of adhesive small bowel obstructions present greater than 2 weeks postoperatively. Seventy-five percent of patients have already tolerated enteral feeds before the intussusception occurs. The typical presentation is irritability, mild abdominal distention, and bilious emesis. A clue that suggests intussusception is unusually excessive nasogastric drainage associated with a rather mild to moderate partial small bowel obstruction. Contrast studies or US may be helpful. Postoperative intussusceptions are located in the small bowel and are usually short and almost always reducible at reoperation.

Other more unusual complications include a *fecal fistula*, encountered in 0.3% to 0.7% of appendectomies. This may also occur due to erroneously placed percutaneous drains. In the absence of coexisting adjacent disease (foreign body, Crohn disease) or partial distal obstruction, fecal fistulas will close. *Pylephlebitis* is an extremely rare complication resulting from septic emboli to the portal vein, and may ultimately lead to septic occlusion of the vein and liver abscesses. Chills, fever, sweats and an enlarged, tender liver in a patient who may be jaundiced suggests this complication. CT drainage is mandatory. The mortality rate may be as high as 50%.

## OTHER CONSIDERATIONS

An *incidental appendectomy* may be performed in association with another abdominal procedure. The expectation is to prevent future simple/complicated appendicitis found in 7% of the population. This is especially relevant in patients with anomalies of colon rotation where the exact eventual location of the appendix may vary. The incidence of wound infection in an otherwise clean procedure is less than 0.7%. An inversion incidental appendectomy should have no associated wound infections. Incidental appendectomies are advisable if the appendix is easily accessible, if there have been no complications with the prior procedure, and if the low risk of theoretic wound infection is acceptable. Incidental appendectomy is contraindicated in immune-suppressed patients, those with adjacent cecal Crohn disease, unstable patients, and in those who may need the appendix for a GI or urinary conduit.

The *carcinoid* is the most common neoplasm of the pediatric GI tract but is a very rare lesion. Out of the entire GI tract, the tip of the appendix is the most common site for a carcinoid followed by the midportion and the base. A carcinoid tumor may be encountered in 0.3% of pediatric appendectomies. Females outnumber males by 2 to 4:1. The tumor is very slow growing and very slow to metastasize.

At least half the children documented with carcinoids are explored because of right-lower quadrant signs and symptoms indistinguishable from appendicitis. Occasionally, there may be associated acute appendicitis, but it is rare. The association with abdominal pain is interesting, since the majority of lesions are located at the tip of the appendix and pain secondary to luminal compression would appear unlikely. If no other pathology is identified, an appendectomy will usually relieve the pain. The remainder of pediatric carcinoids are incidental findings at exploratory laparotomy or necropsy.

Pediatric carcinoids may be encountered in patients as young as 6 years of age, the mean peak age of incidence being 15 years. Although deaths from metastases have been reported in children, this is exceptionally rare. The majority of children may be managed with a simple appendectomy. The carcinoid syndrome (flushing, diarrhea, and tachycardia associated mainly with liver metastases) is virtually unheard of with pediatric appendiceal carcinoids.

Management of an appendiceal carcinoid depends on its size. An appendectomy will suffice if the lesion is less than 2 cm in size. Extension into the mesoappendix or periappendiceal fat in the resected specimen is not an issue. Lesions are less than 1 cm 70% to 90% of the time, whereas less than 25% are between 1 cm and 2 cm. Lesions greater than 2 cm are extremely unusual in children.

Current management dictates that patients with lesions greater than 2 cm in size undergo cecectomy or right hemicolectomy. It is not entirely clear that such aggressive management is warranted in children. A simple appendectomy in the pediatric patient with a carcinoid should suffice if (1) there are no pathologic nodes noted, (2) there is no lesion at the base of the appendix involving the cecum, (3) there are no large lesions involving adjacent structures, and (4) there are no implants.

*Crohn disease* may be encountered incidentally when exploring a child for presumed acute appendicitis. In fact, 15% of pediatric patients with Crohn disease present with symptoms mimicking acute appendicitis. In such patients, the normal appendix should be removed provided the adjacent cecum is grossly free of Crohn disease. Crohn disease patients who develop symptoms mimicking appendicitis may have more severe disease. Crohn disease patients who have a longer prodrome of symptoms, and who have undergone an incidental appendectomy, generally require more medication, have a higher incidence of recurrence, and have a higher potential for repeat surgical procedures.

Usually, Crohn disease involving the appendix has encroached from the cecum. However, primary Crohn disease of the appendix with no evidence of Crohn disease elsewhere in the GI tract has been rarely reported. The signs and symptoms of primary appendiceal Crohn disease are indistinguishable from those of acute appendicitis. However, the history is usually greater than 3 days, and there may have been recurrent previous episodes. Primary appendiceal Crohn disease is generally not encountered until the second and third decades. The diagnosis is established histopathologically. An appendectomy or limited cecal or ileocecal resection is advised, since the incidence of postoperative enterocutaneous fistulas in these patients is surprisingly low (3%-5%). The prognosis for patients with primary appendiceal Crohn disease is also much better (recurrence rate of 16%) than the usual patient with Crohn disease.

*Acute typhlitis* occurs in an immunocompromised patient with hematologic malignancy or following induction chemotherapy for bone marrow transplantation. Such a patient with acute cecal inflammation may present with symptoms indistinguishable from acute appendicitis. This situation presents a very critical problem in the face of profound immunodepression with an absolute neutrophil count approaching zero. If operation is done, the patient may suffer postoperative hemorrhage, wound separation, or intra-abdominal sepsis. These complications may prove to be fatal. It is suggested that sequential clinical and imaging exams be done, and every effort made to spontaneously or therapeutically correct the hematologic parameters. Mortality from a negative appendectomy in this situation may be greater than that associated with delaying the procedure until the patient is properly prepared.

*Chronic appendiceal pain* may present in one of 3 ways:

1. *Chronic appendicitis* is often used to describe any type of long-term appendiceal pain. The term "chronic appendicitis" should be reserved for the appendix infiltrated with chronic inflammatory cells such as mononuclear white cells. True chronic appendicitis is rare; probably less than 0.1%.

2. *Recurrent appendicitis* occurs when a patient develops low-grade appendicitis that resolves spontaneously before surgical intervention. When the inflammation subsides, the result is fibrosis. A reasonable incidence for remote appendicitis in the pediatric population is about 5% in incidental appendectomies.

3. *Appendiceal colic* (appendiceal cramping) is by far the most common type of chronic appendiceal pain. Complete, unrelieved obstruction of the appendiceal lumen will likely produce acute appendicitis. Partial or intermittent obstruction may result in appendiceal colic. If the material obstructing the appendiceal lumen (fecalith) is extruded, there will be immediate and complete relief of symptoms. However, if the pathology responsible for luminal narrowing remains (fibrosis), the process of entrapment of foreign material will likely be repeated.

The severity and periodicity of appendiceal colic are extremely variable. The pain may be severe and unrelenting for days. In such situations the appendix is invariably removed. The pain may also be severe but for only a brief period of time. Unless such episodes are recognized by a physician, the patient may be destined for months or years of sporadic pain until the appendix is removed. Almost as significant as the severe colic is the more mild colic that may recur sporadically every few weeks or months. This seems to concern no one except the patient and family. In time, this may have a tremendous social, academic, physical, and psychologic impact.

Appendiceal colic is episodic, of variable intensity, duration, and periodicity. The painful crises are virtually identical. Pallor is almost always evident in patients with appendiceal colic. Headaches may be reported, and if the patient is migraine-prone, the colic may precipitate a migraine. The most severe appendiceal colic may result in lightheadedness or even syncopal attacks.

Patients will frequently feel nauseated when experiencing colic. With more severe pain, reflexive vomiting ("dry heaves") occurs. Of utmost importance is the postprandial exacerbation of appendiceal colic. This usually occurs within 5 to 30 minutes after eating. In general, patients describe the discomfort as periumbilical in location. With more severe colic, the discomfort may be described as right-lower quadrant in location.

As the duration of appendiceal colic increases, the incidence of associated complaints increases. Because of the behavioral changes, the concern for possible psychological issues increases. The child may become withdrawn and depressed. There may be weight loss, since eating exacerbates the pain; therefore, the patient prefers not to eat.

If the history is classic for appendiceal colic, then the physical exam will likely confirm the diagnosis. The patient must be experiencing colic before the physical exam will be obviously positive. Pressure on an appendix that is in spasm will accentuate the pain and will also accurately identify the location of the appendix. This point of maximal tenderness will almost always be at exactly the same location from one examination to another. One needs to be alert for complaints of right flank, back, hip, and leg pain. A previously inflamed appendix that is scarred and tethered in the right gutter or iliac fossa may be responsible for such discomfort, especially when the appendix is in spasm. Patients suffering from appendiceal colic will generally be afebrile.

Laboratory studies are usually ordered to exclude other diagnoses. The WBC count is usually normal. A normal urinalysis is reassuring, and a pregnancy test, when appropriate, is mandatory.

Imaging evidence of appendiceal colic is disappointing. An abdominal radiograph is of little value unless a fecalith is documented. An abdominal–pelvic US is useful in order to exclude pathology in other organ systems (ovaries). Occasionally, barium upper- or lower-GI studies may document nonfilling, partial filling, or a filling defect of the appendix. Barium retained in the appendix for days after the study is pathologic. Delayed films 6 to 8 hours after the study may show filling of the appendix that was not seen during the study. Imaging studies utilizing CT or magnetic resonance are virtually useless.

The patient with a long history of appendiceal colic and extensive negative work-up deserves an appendectomy. The patient presenting with severe appendiceal colic, as verified by a classic history and physical exam, also deserves an expedited appendectomy. If the appendiceal colic is mild and of short duration, a 1- or 2-week period of observation is indicated. During this period one will become more confident of the diagnosis with repeated physical exams, and diagnoses such as gastroenteritis and mesenteric adenitis can be excluded. A pelvic US in a female patient is advised. Patients may present with a classic history, yet point tenderness on a physical exam has never been verified. In this situation it is incumbent upon the physician to make arrangements for patient examination when the pain is present. Finally, patients with abdominal pain may present with confusing signs and symptoms, and they are usually destined for an extensive negative work-up. Ultimately, exploratory laparoscopy or laparotomy is performed and the appendix is removed. It is recommended that in the event of chronic abdominal pain, the appendix should be removed regardless of its operative appearance. A normal external appearance of the appendix at exploration cannot assure that the lumen is not occluded.

An appendectomy in this group of patients may be expected to provide relief of pain in 70% to 95% of patients.

## PROGNOSIS

Contemporary mortality from perforated appendicitis is low. Deaths may be encountered in 0.1 to 0.2 patients per 100,000, and mortality may be expected to be less than 0.1% to 0.3% in patients with appendicitis. Mortality is generally encountered in the very young. It is usually associated with complicated appendicitis, inadequate resuscitation prior to surgery, uncontrolled sepsis, and uncontrolled intra-abdominal abscesses with secondary multiorgan system failure.

## SELECTED READINGS

Adibe OO, Amin SR, Hansen EN, et al. An evidence-based clinical protocol for diagnosis of acute appendicitis decreased the use of computed tomography in children. *J Pediatr Surg* 2011;46(1):192–196.

Aziz O, Athanasiou T, Tekkis PP, et al. Laparoscopic versus open appendectomy in children: a meta-analysis. *Ann Surg* 2006;243(1):17–27. PMCID: 1449958.

Blakely ML, Williams R, Dassinger MS, et al. Early vs interval appendectomy for children with perforated appendicitis. *Arch Surg* 2011;146(6):660–665.

Bliss D, McKee J, Cho D, et al. Discordance of the pediatric surgeon's intraoperative assessment of pediatric appendicitis with the pathologists report. *J Pediatr Surg* 2010;45(7):1398–1403.

Fisher M, Meates-Dennis M. Is interval appendectomy necessary after successful conservative treatment of appendiceal mass in children? *Arch Dis Child* 2008;93(7):631–633.

Fraser JD, Aguayo P, Leys CM, et al. A complete course of intravenous antibiotics vs a combination of intravenous and oral antibiotics for perforated appendicitis in children: a prospective, randomized trial. *J Pediatr Surg* 2010;45(6):1198–1202.

Gendel I, Gutermacher M, Buklan G, et al. Relative value of clinical, laboratory and imaging tools in diagnosing pediatric acute appendicitis. *Eur J Pediatr Surg* 2011;21(04):229–233.

Goldin A, Khanna P, Thapa M, McBroom J, Garrison M, Parisi M. Revised ultrasound criteria for appendicitis in children improve diagnostic accuracy. *Pediatr Radiol* 2011;41(8):993–999.

Gosain A, Blakely M, Boulden T, et al. Omental infarction: preoperative diagnosis and laparoscopic management in children. *J Laparoendosc Adv Surg Tech A* 2010;20(9):777–780.

Hall NJ, Jones CE, Eaton S, Stanton MP, Burge DM. Is interval appendicectomy justified after successful nonoperative treatment of an appendix mass in children? A systematic review. *J Pediatr Surg* 2011;46(4):767–771.

Kaselas C, Molinaro F, Lacreuse I, Becmeur F. Postoperative bowel obstruction after laparoscopic and open appendectomy in children: a 15-year experience. *J Pediatr Surg* 2009;44(8):1581–1585.

Kolts R, Nelson R, Park R, Heikenen J. Exploratory laparoscopy for recurrent right lower quadrant pain in a pediatric population. *Pediatr Surg Int* 2006;22(3):247–249.

Krishnamoorthi R, Ramarajan N, Wang NE, et al. Effectiveness of a staged US and CT protocol for the diagnosis of pediatric appendicitis: reducing radiation exposure in the age of ALARA. *Radiology* 2011;259(1):231–239.

Kwan KY, Nager AL. Diagnosing pediatric appendicitis: usefulness of laboratory markers. *Am J Emerg Med* 2010;28(9):1009–1015.

Lee SL, Yaghoubian A, Kaji A. Laparoscopic vs open appendectomy in children: outcomes comparison based on age, sex, and perforation status. *Arch Surg* 2011;146(10):1118–1121.

Lee SL, Islam S, Cassidy LD, Abdullah F, Arca MJ. Antibiotics and appendicitis in the pediatric population: an American Pediatric Surgical Association Outcomes and Clinical Trials Committee Systematic Review. *J Pediatr Surg* 2010;45(11):2181–2185.

Miyano G, Urao M, Lane GJ, Kato Y, Okazaki T, Yamataka A. A prospective analysis of endoloops and endostaples for closing the stump of the appendix in children. *J Laparoendosc Adv Surg Tech A* 2011;21(2):177–179.

Ostlie DJ. Single-site umbilical laparoscopic appendectomy. *Semin Pediatr Surg* 2011;20(4):196–200.

Ponsky TA, Rothenberg SS. Division of the mesoappendix with electrocautery in children is safe, effective, and cost-efficient. *J Laparoendosc Adv Surg Tech A* 2009;19(Suppl 1):S11–S13.

Schurman JV, Cushing CC, Garey CL, Laituri CA, St. Peter SD. Quality of life assessment between laparoscopic appendectomy at presentation and interval appendectomy for perforated appendicitis with abscess: analysis of a prospective randomized trial. *J Pediatr Surg* 2011;46(6):1121–1125.

Scott A, Upadhyay V. Carcinoid tumours of the appendix in children in Auckland, New Zealand: 1965-2008. *N Z Med J* 2011;124(1331):56–60.

St. Peter SD, Sharp SW, Holcomb Iii GW, Ostlie DJ. An evidence-based definition for perforated appendicitis derived from a prospective randomized trial. *J Pediatr Surg* 2008;43(12):2242–2245.

Williams RF, Blakely ML, Fischer PE, et al. Diagnosing ruptured appendicitis preoperatively in pediatric patients. *J Am Coll Surgeons* 2009;208(5):819–825.

# Inflammatory Bowel Disease

# CHAPTER 49

*D. Dean Potter and Christopher R. Moir*

## KEY POINTS

1. Inflammatory bowel disease is a serious but treatable condition in children.

2. Differentiating between Crohn disease and ulcerative colitis (UC) is extremely important.

3. In Crohn disease, surgical management should emphasize preservation of bowel length and relief of obstructing lesions.

4. Restorative proctocolectomy with colectomy is the treatment of choice for children with UC.

## INTRODUCTION

Inflammatory bowel diseases (IBD) comprise a heterogeneous group of chronic inflammatory disorders of the gastrointestinal tract. Crohn disease (CD), ulcerative colitis (UC), and indeterminate colitis (IC) are thought to develop from dysregulation of the immune system in a genetically susceptible host. Incident symptoms occur in childhood in up to one third of patients with CD and UC. Despite the fact that most pediatric patients with IBD initially respond to steroid therapy, surgical intervention is required on an average 2 years later. Establishing the correct diagnosis of CD versus UC has important implications for surgical care.

Pediatric surgeons must be aware that the majority of children present with colitis regardless of their eventual diagnosis. Epidemiologic studies suggest that up to 80% to 90% of children with CD experience colonic disease (colon only or ileocolonic), whereas only approximately 50% of adults have colonic involvement. Additionally, pediatric UC patients present more often with pancolitis as compared to adult patients who present more commonly with left-sided disease or proctitis. Adding to these disease similarities is the finding that pediatric CD presents predominantly with inflammatory and nonpenetrating phenotypes. Complicated forms of CD, such as stricturing and penetrating phenotypes, do occur in childhood; however, complicated CD more commonly results from a progressive disease despite contemporary treatment. Thus, the diagnostic dilemma of colitis in a child may not be differentiated to CD or UC until the teenage years when the adult distribution of IBD evolves. Interestingly, the incidence of CD appears to be increasing by population studies, whereas UC has remained essentially unchanged over time. To further cloud the situation, boys are at higher risk than girls for CD by a ratio of 2:1, whereas gender distribution is nearly equal in adult patients. Ultimately, the diagnosis of CD versus UC changes the indications for operation and the choice of surgical procedure.

## CLINICAL PRESENTATION

The classic presentation for CD is abdominal pain, diarrhea, poor appetite, and weight loss. Children with UC may have similar symptoms that include chronic (>2 weeks) abdominal pain, hematochezia, and tenesmus. Inflammatory extraintestinal manifestations occur in 25% to 35% of patients with either CD or UC and commonly affect the skin, joints, liver, eye, and bone. Indeed, extraintestinal manifestations of CD are more common in children with colonic disease as compared to isolated small-bowel CD involvement. Growth delay, which is commonly associated with CD, also occurs in severe UC, which is more common in pediatric patients.

A genetic predisposition has been found in pediatric patients with IBD. Population-based studies have shown that 10% to 40% of patients with IBD have a positive family history. This finding has been supported by twin studies. Concordance rates approach 50% in monozygotic twins with CD and decrease to 4% for dizygotic twins with UC. Familial cases are associated with earlier age of onset, on average 5 years younger than sporadic cases. Genetic factors not only influence disease onset but also disease phenotype and course. Ileal CD involvement is associated with *CARD15/NOD2* mutations and confers an increased incidence of operation for stricturing disease in adolescents. HLA haplotypes have long been associated with extraintestinal manifestations (B27, B35), while more recent discoveries identify HLA-DRB*0103 as being strongly associated with fulminant UC progressing to surgery. Cellular protein anomalies also play a role; polymorphisms in the NFκβ binding site of the tumor necrosis factor-alpha promoter are strongly associated with colonic disease rather than ileal or small-bowel CD involvement.

The finding that Asian immigrants to North America have an increased risk of IBD and that increased rate of disease correlates to the industrialization of Hong Kong and mainland China highlights the interplay between genetic and environmental factors. Smoking exacerbates recurrent CD but is mildly protective for UC. Similarly, appendectomy reduces the incidence of UC. Breastfeeding may confer immunity while improved sanitation and hygiene could paradoxically increase the disease by impairing functional maturity of the mucosal immune system.

## DIAGNOSIS

Once IBD has been established by ruling out infectious colitides, a standard evaluation includes contrast imaging of the small intestine, esophagogastroduodenoscopy, colonoscopy, ileoscopy, and multiple biopsies of the intestinal tract to differentiate CD from UC. Multiple imaging studies are currently available to visualize the small bowel. Standard barium small-bowel follow-through, computed tomography enterography, magnetic resonance enterography, and capsule enteroscopy all play a role in visualizing the GI tract. Indeed, a 4-way comparison of small-bowel follow-through, CT enterography, ileoscopy, and capsule enteroscopy found no statistical difference between the 4 examinations for detecting active small-bowel CD. Importantly, capsule enteroscopy should be used with caution as a first-line study due to the possibility of undetected small-bowel obstruction resulting in retained capsule. In our practice, CT enterography has been the test of choice to evaluate the small intestine due to its sensitivity and specificity to detect bowel inflammation, proximal intestinal dilation, intraperitoneal inflammatory lesions, and the extent of disease. Recently, MR enterography has become more popular due to concerns of radiation exposure during a computed tomography scan in children. Image quality and diagnostic effectiveness for MR enterography has yet to be determined as compared to CT enterography.

Upper and lower endoscopies with multiple biopsies are the mainstay of establishing the diagnosis of CD versus UC. The transmural, panintestinal inflammation of CD may be detected in up to 30% of patients during esophagogastroduodenoscopy. Visualizing the terminal ileum is extremely important. Backwash ileitis is mucosal inflammation associated with severe UC, whereas the transmural inflammation of CD results in deep linear ulcers referred to as bear claw deformity. Demonstration of nonpericryptal granulomas is a hallmark of CD on histological examination. Endoscopic findings of pseudopolyps are a result of mucosal erosion due to UC.

The classic histologic findings of UC include disruption of crypt architecture, crypt abscess formation, and infiltration of the lamina propria with leukocytes. While determining CD from UC seems straightforward; in fact, 10% to 15% of patients demonstrate findings consistent with both CD and UC. These patients have IC and require repeat evaluation in the future. The North American Society for Pediatric Gastroenterology, Hepatology, and Nutrition and the Crohn's and Colitis Foundation of America have developed recommendations to assist the clinician in differentiating CD from UC (Fig. 49-1).

Serum biomarkers have been extensively studied in both adults and children (Table 49-1). They effectively differentiate IBD from noninflammatory conditions. Distinguishing CD from UC is more problematic, but the standard findings of anti-*Saccharomyces cervisiae* antibodies (ASCA) in CD and elevated titers of perinuclear antineutrophil cytoplasmic antibody (p-ANCA) in UC remain true. Furthermore, a high ASCA titer in a patient with CD indicates a strong possibility of surgery in the near future. Unfortunately, the specificity is low for these serum biomarkers. For example, colon predominant CD is a common pediatric presentation and p-ANCA occurs in these patients. Thus, serum biomarkers are not diagnostic, but may help differentiate CD from UC when the standard evaluation is equivocal.

## CROHN DISEASE

CD is now the most prevalent form of IBD and boys are more commonly affected than girls. Incident cases occur in all ethnic groups in both urban and rural locales. A child diagnosed with CD has a 78% probability of the need for operative intervention within 20 years; those with ileocolonic disease (92%) are at highest risk. Nearly two thirds of children with small-bowel CD will require an operation, whereas approximately 60% with colonic disease require operation. Recurrence following surgical resection is nearly universal as seen by endoscopic examination, with up to 50% of these patients requiring another procedure.

## MEDICAL THERAPY

Even though the probability of operation in patients with CD is a near certainty over time, the need for early initial operation is decreasing. Improved responses to medical therapy and a general reluctance to proceed with operation in smaller children contribute to this change.

Enteral nutrition and corticosteroids are the mainstays of medical therapy for children with CD. Nutritional therapy in children helps to obviate the growth delay and osteoporotic effects of corticosteroids while maintaining a more normal lifestyle and school attendance. Improved formulas and good compliance with enteral nutrition are associated with a reduction in inflammatory mediators and healing of CD. Patient and physician noncompliance, variable insurer coverage, and frequent relapse are common reasons for the lack of widespread acceptance in the United States. Improvement has been identified in 80% to 90% of children with ileal or ileocolonic involvement versus 50% response in patients with colitis. This difference likely represents the varying genetic phenotypes and bacterial flora associated with the small intestine versus the colon.

Despite the high initial response rates to systemic corticosteroids, a recent population-based study reported 58% of children remained corticosteroid dependent or required operation by 1 year. Small-bowel disease was twice as likely to improve as compared to ileocolonic or colonic disease. Early addition of immunomodulator drugs, azathioprine or mercaptopurine, reduced the need for surgery and increased the prolonged response by 50%. Thus, early addition of immunomodulators, immunosuppressant drugs, or biologic agents

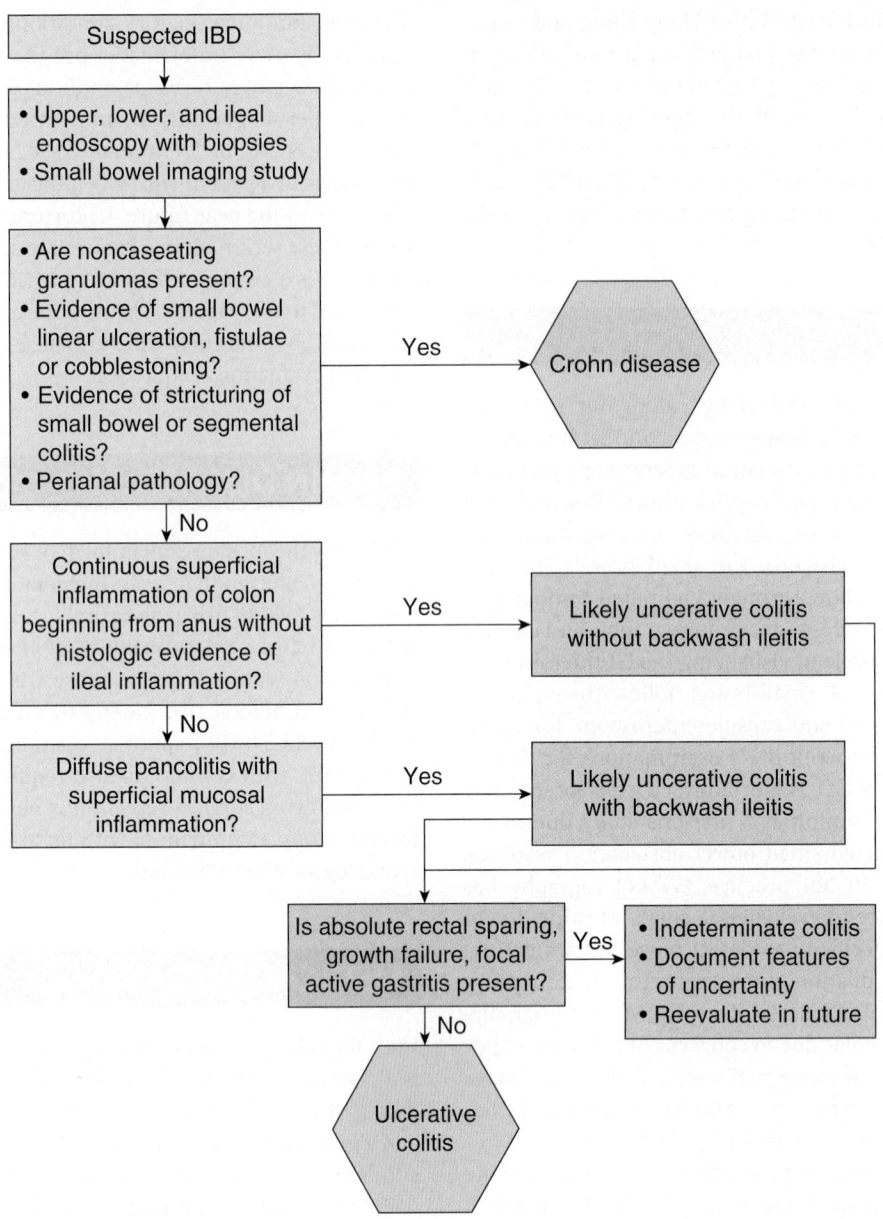

**FIGURE 49-1** Diagnostic algorithm to differentiate Crohn disease from ulcerative colitis. (Adapted from *J Pediatr Gastroenterol Nutr* 44(5):653–674.)

is commonplace. Both retrospective and population-based studies of infliximab in children have identified improved treatment benefits ranging from decreased inflammatory markers, increased height and weight, and healing of inflammatory lesion by endoscopic evaluation. However, therapy was been associated with a 30% long-term response and a nearly 50% dependence on repeated infliximab infusions. One quarter of children do not respond to infliximab therapy with nearly half of these patients having colitis.

## INDICATIONS FOR OPERATION

The decision to operate on children with CD represents a balance of medical and surgical factors designed to relieve symptoms and reduce treatment toxicity. Refractory illness

and complications of disease are the most common indications for operation in children with CD. Strictures and local perforation/penetration are most commonly identified in children who present with small-bowel and ileocolonic disease. Growth failure and symptomatic disease are more common in patients with colonic disease.

The need for early intervention has been associated with high ASCA seropositivity, *CARD15/NOD2* mutations, hypoalbuminemia, poor growth velocity, female gender, and stricturing disease. The progression to complicated CD, internal fistulae, rectovaginal fistulae, and phlegmon/abscess formation are less common indications for early operative intervention. Perforative/penetrating CD associated with intraabdominal abscess is best treated with initial percutaneous drainage of the abscess followed by operative resection.

| TABLE 49-1 | The Prevalence of Serum Biomarkers in Crohn Disease and Ulcerative Colitis | |
|---|---|---|
| Serum Biomarker | Prevalence in Crohn Disease | Prevalence in Ulcerative Colitis |
| ASCA (anti-*Saccharomyces cerevisiae* antibody) | 60%-70% | 10%-15% |
| p-ANCA (perinuclear antineutrophil cytoplasmic antibody) | 10%-15% | 60%-70% |
| I2 antibody | 55% | 10% |
| OmpC antibody | 55% | 5%-10% |
| CBir1 antibody | 55% | 10% |
| ACCA (anti-chitobioside carbohydrate antibody) | 20%-40% | <10% |
| ALCA (antilaminaribioside carbohydrate antibody) | 20%-40% | <10% |
| PAB (antipancreatic antibody) | 20%-40% | <10% |

*Note:* Data from *Current Gastroenterology Reports.* 2009;11:360–367.

## OPERATIVE PRINCIPLES

The ability of the surgeon to select an appropriate operation and reduce the recurrence risk in children with CD depends on specific disease patterns. Younger age and colonic disease

have been shown to have the lowest operative rates as compared to ileocolonic and small-bowel disease, which have the highest relative risk for operation. Three operative principles prevail: (1) preserve bowel length, (2) perform a widely patent anastomosis, and (3) complete a safe division of bowel mesentery.

Firstly, length-preserving procedures are based on known reoperative rates. The overall incidence of surgical recurrence has been reported to be 33% at 5 years and 44% at 10 years. Small-bowel and ileocolonic recurrences were more likely to need reoperation as compared to colonic disease. Short bowel syndrome is an uncommon but feared complication following operative intervention for CD. Thus, relief from the offending lesion with preservation of intestinal length is the goal of all operations for CD. Surgical margins that remove only the grossly involved bowel have been shown to be safe and do not statistically increase the risk of recurrent obstruction. The presence of nonspecific microscopic inflammation or even microscopic CD at the surgical resection margin resulted in similar recurrence rates (20%-30%) as compared to negative microscopic margins.

Stricturoplasty for active disease, as well as for fibrotic strictures, remains an excellent option for patients with multicentric activity. Preoperative imaging aides the surgeon in identifying the stenotic regions, yet intraoperative use of a balloon tipped catheter provides anatomic details as to the location of these obstructions (Fig. 49-2). The length of the stricture and noninflammatory nature of the obstruction are the two strongest factors determining success. Such length-sparing procedures are particularly attractive for children with extensive disease and skip areas. No data exist

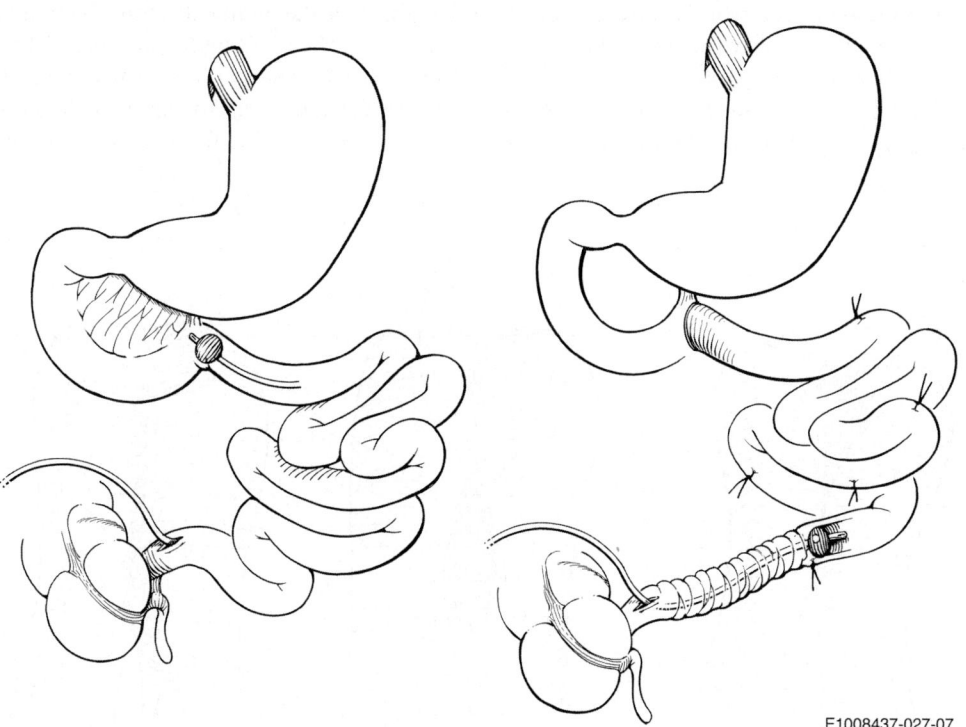

E1008437-027-07

**FIGURE 49-2** Intraoperative interrogation of the bowel lumen using a balloon tipped catheter accurately identifies multiple obstructing lesions. The balloon can be deflated to allow it to pass through the strictured bowel lumen and subsequently reinflated to identify the remaining strictures. Lesions with a luminal diameter of <2 cm require intervention. (Used with permission of Mayo Foundation for Medical Education and Research.)

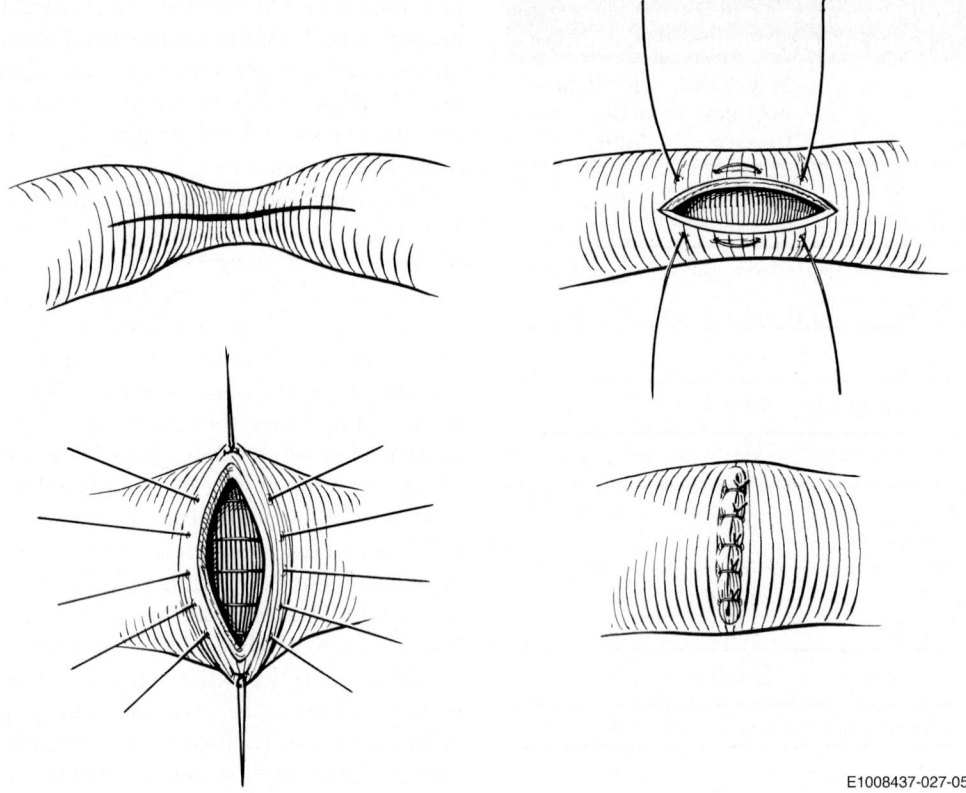

E1008437-027-05

**FIGURE 49-3** The Heineke–Mikulicz stricturoplasty involves a transverse incision through the fibrotic segment of bowel to include 1 to 2 cm of normal bowel on each side. The incision is then closed vertically to enlarge the intestinal lumen. (Used with permission of Mayo Foundation for Medical Education and Research.)

to support the relative contraindication of leaving persistent disease behind in developing children. Adverse effects on growth and the risk of malignancy have not been quantified.

The Heineke–Mikulicz stricturoplasty (Fig. 49-3) and Finney stricturoplasty (Fig. 49-4) are the two most commonly used techniques. The Heineke–Mikulicz procedure is best used for short fibrotic strictures less than 10 cm in length, while the Finney stricturoplasty can be used for strictures up to 25 cm in length. One potential drawback of a long Finney stricturoplasty is the formation of a functional bypass that results in bacterial overgrowth. Some centers advocate a side-to-side isoperistaltic stricturoplasty in these situations.

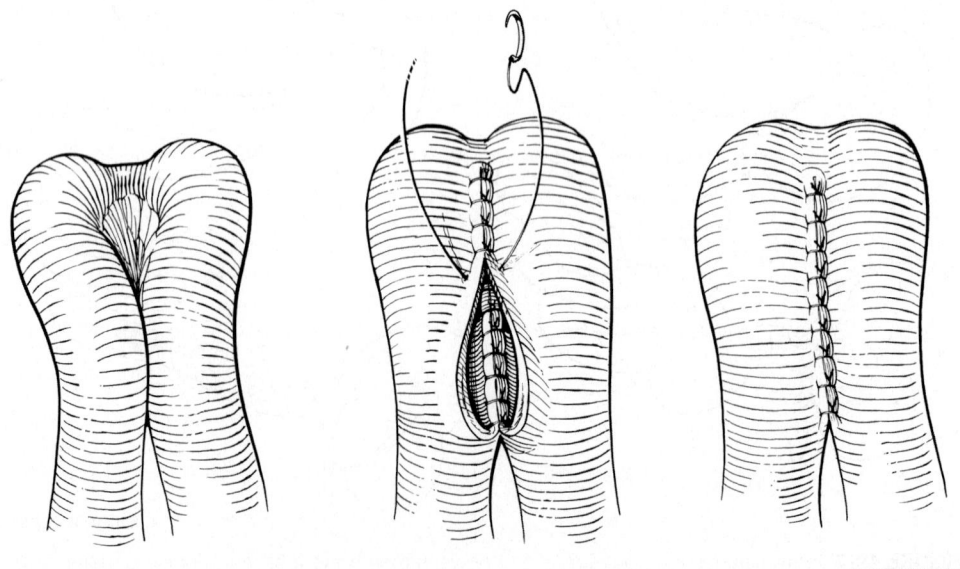

E1008437-027-06

**FIGURE 49-4** The Finney stricturoplasty is used for longer strictures up to 25 cm in length. The side-to-side stricturoplasty can be performed in 1 or 2 layers with either interrupted or running suture. (Used with permission of Mayo Foundation for Medical Education and Research.)

A meta-analysis found a leak/abscess/fistula rate of 4% and a site-specific recurrence rate of 3% for all stricturoplasty techniques. Two patients out of 1112 developed adenocarcinoma at the stricturoplasty site.

Secondly, postoperative recurrences most commonly occur at the site of anastomosis. Thus, a widely patent anastomosis is an important principle in the effort to reduce the need for reiterative surgery. Stapled side-to-side anastomosis can be twice as large as hand-sewn end-to-end techniques. Retrospective studies evaluating surgical recurrences have found the stapled anastomosis to be superior to a hand-sewn technique; however, a recent multicenter prospective trial found no difference in the endoscopic recurrence (43% vs 38% stapled vs hand-sewn) and symptomatic recurrence (22% vs 23%) for CD at 12 months postoperatively. The use of maintenance azathioprine was associated with decreased recurrences in this trial. The stapled technique lends itself well to ileocolonic anastomoses; however, consideration for this technique should be given to other small-bowel anastomoses and colonic resections. Currently, we use either a 60- or 100-mm stapler depending on the size and age of the child.

Thirdly, safe division of the bowel mesentery can be challenging when dealing with a markedly thickened and inflamed bowel. The presence of a fistula, phlegmon, or abscess adds to the complexity of the process. Resection of mesenteric lymph nodes does not improve outcomes for CD, thus division of the mesentery close to the intestinal wall preserves the vascular arcades and potentially reduces the risk of ischemic resection margins. Isolating and individually ligating mesenteric blood vessels is difficult if not impossible in these situations. Alternative energy sources such as bipolar vessel sealing devices or ultrasonic shears can assist with safe division, yet hemorrhage from markedly thickened mesentery is not uncommon with these devices. For open or laparoscopic-assisted procedures, overlapping clamps using suture ligation afford excellent control of the mesenteric blood vessels. Postoperative hemoperitoneum is exceedingly rare using these techniques.

## ILEOCOLONIC DISEASE

Ileocecal resections are the most commonly performed procedures for CD by pediatric surgeons. Limited disease allows for negative margins and anastomosis of healthy bowel. Postoperative complications are uncommon in this patient population. Postoperative recurrence rates are favorable (30%-40%) at 4 years unless extensive ileal disease is encountered. The need for a stoma is uncommon except in the situation of perforation or abscess. Limited ileocecal disease lends itself well to laparoscopic, laparoscopic-assisted, or single-incision laparoscopic procedures.

## UPPER INTESTINAL AND SMALL-BOWEL DISEASE

Gastroduodenal involvement of CD is rare in children (<5%) and is invariably associated with multicentric disease. Patients may present with nausea, vomiting, and dysphagia.

Symptomatic treatment with acid blockade and medical therapy is successful in mild-to-moderate disease. Fibrostenotic disease of the duodenum has been classically treated with gastrojejunostomy. This procedure may be complicated by anastomotic stricture and marginal ulceration in addition to poor emptying of the stomach. Heineke–Mikulicz stricturoplasty of the first, second, and third portions of the duodenum is feasible, but recurrence rates appear to be slightly higher than bypass procedures. Surgical judgment is paramount when caring for these children.

Minimally invasive techniques are applicable to limited small-bowel CD. However, up to 20% of children present with multiple small intestinal strictures. Palpation of the bowel and interrogation with a balloon-tipped catheter allow the surgeon to accurately identify all sites of obstruction. Intervention is recommended for all strictures with a luminal diameter of less than 2 cm; however, surgical judgment should prevail, since lesser strictures may progress over time. Surgeons should be aware that children presenting with significant diarrhea and small-bowel disease may have a fistula to the sigmoid colon. Flexible sigmoidoscopy would be indicted and intraoperative lithotomy positioning provides access to the lower GI tract. Combined small-bowel and sigmoid resection may be required (Fig. 49-5).

## COLONIC DISEASE

Crohn colitis represents the highest risk for a permanent ileostomy. The 20-year risk of needing a stoma ranges from 14% to 44%. This risk increases in children with significant rectal and perianal inflammation, high pediatric CD activity index scores, and female gender.

Segmental colonic resections involving the right and left colon can be safely performed laparoscopically with primary ileocolostomy or colocolostomy. High recurrence rates with permanent ileostomy rates approaching 50% have caused these procedures to fall out of favor; however, postoperative prophylaxis may decrease the current recurrence rates and need for ileostomy.

Total colectomy is an excellent alternative for the child with refractory illness. Ileostomy and a Hartmann pouch are required when severe rectal disease is present; a secondary ileorectostomy is an option once the rectal stump has healed by proctoscopic evaluation. A primary ileorectostomy can be safely performed when normal sphincter tone and rectal distensibility with insufflation is present. Fewer than 20% of patients with mild-to-moderate rectal disease progress to completion proctocolectomy.

Proctocolectomy with end ileostomy is rarely performed for children with CD, but this procedure carries the lowest rate of surgical recurrence in patients with Crohn colitis. Patients with extensive rectal and perianal disease have a poor outcome with limited segmental resections or total abdominal colectomy, yet new therapies including biologic agents hold promise to help these children avoid a permanent ileostomy. When removal of the rectal stump is required, a standard intersphincteric proctectomy is performed with tight closure of the perineum. Placement of a vascularized graft, such as

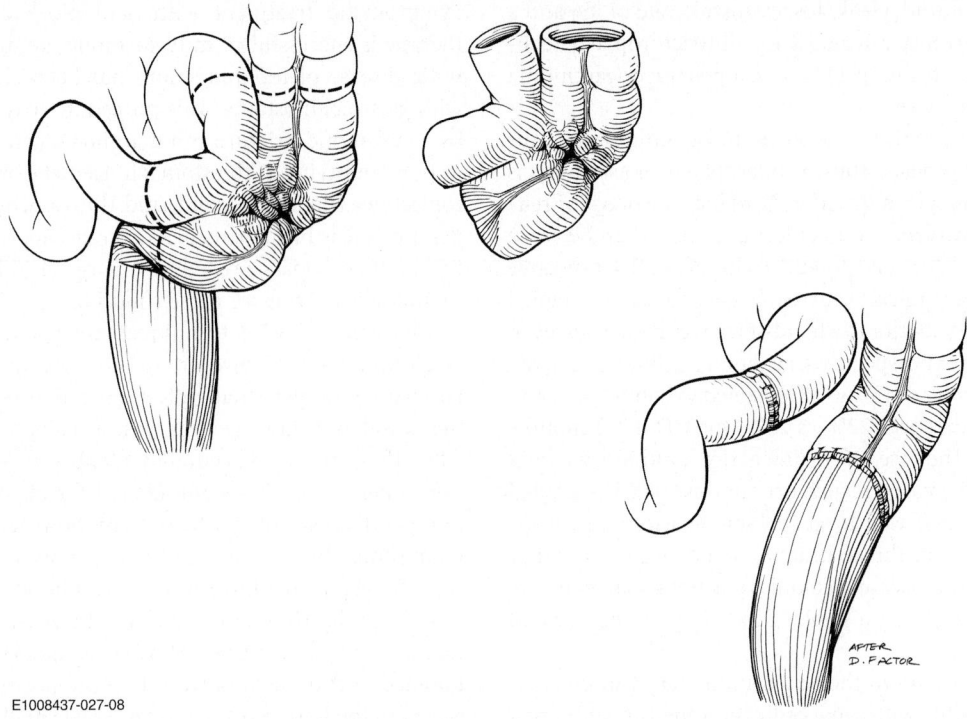

E1008437-027-08

**FIGURE 49-5** Ileal CD with sigmoid fistula. Combined ileal and sigmoid colon resection may be required. Lithotomy position allows access to the lower GI tract for flexible endoscopy and surgical staplers in this situation. (Used with permission of Mayo Foundation for Medical Education and Research.)

omentum, into the pelvis with reperitonealization following reconstruction helps avoid the chronic nonhealing wound and bowel obstructions associated with this procedure.

## PERIANAL DISEASE

Nearly 60% of patients with CD develop perianal complications; 5% to 10% have severe disease. Perianal disease can be the first sign of CD in up to one quarter of children. The most common conditions are fistula-in-ano, anal fissures, hypertrophy of the perianal skin, and stenosis. These lesions can be painful, drain purulent material, and bleed. The most common indication of surgical intervention is abscess. Examination in the office is usually very painful and may complicate the prolonged care required to heal these lesions. Thus, examination under anesthesia allows for excellent visualization of the anal canal. Endoscopy of the distal rectum is helpful. When there is concern for more extensive disease, magnetic resonance fistulography is the test of choice. It is highly sensitive (97%) and specific (100%) for the detection of fistulae.

Less is more when dealing with perianal CD. The goal of any surgical procedure for perianal CD is to treat infection with limited incision and drainage procedures and placement of draining seton sutures (Fig. 49-6). For larger abscess cavities, a mushroom catheter may be placed initially and exchanged to a seton after several weeks. The combination of surgical infection control and biologic agents has resulted in partial or complete healing of perianal CD in nearly 90% of patients.

Persistent fistulae have been treated with moderate success using fibrin glue or "plugs." Fistulotomy is the definitive

procedure for a persistent anal fistula with healing occurring in up to 80% of patients. The risk of incontinence and poor wound healing is high in patients with transsphincteric or complex fistula. Rectal mucosal flaps provide healing in 60% to 70% of patients with transsphincteric disease once a good response to

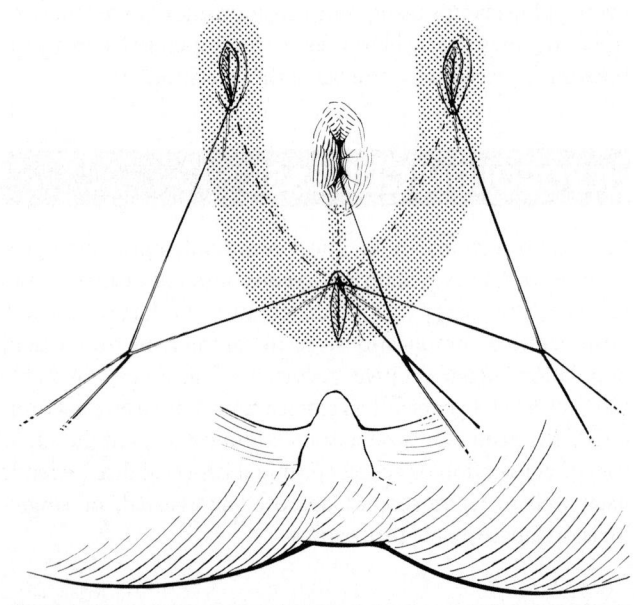

E1008437-027-14

**FIGURE 49-6** Draining setons for perianal CD. Soft vessel loops are tied loosely through fistulae or complex abscesses to allow adequate drainage of infected material. Limited manipulation and small incisions promote more rapid healing with the use of biologic agents. (Used with permission of Mayo Foundation for Medical Education and Research.)

medical therapy has been achieved. A protective ileostomy may improve the rate of healing after rectal mucosal flaps.

Rectovaginal fistulas present a complex problem to the pediatric surgeon. Following fecal diversion and optimal medical therapy, rectal mucosal flaps, vaginal mucosal flaps, and/or cutaneous advancement flaps have a success rate of 60% to 70%. Healing rates as high as 90% have been reported with well-controlled disease.

## CHRONIC ULCERATIVE COLITIS

The surgical options for children with UC are well studied, and the expectation for disease eradication is high. Optimal surgical management of pediatric patients includes restoration of normal bowel function after removal of all disease in the colon and rectum. Segmental resection of the most involved portion of the colon in an attempt to preserve function is not recommended. Limited forms of UC respond well to medical therapy and will not require surgery during childhood. Conversely, those with refractory pancolitis require restorative proctocolectomy.

## INDICATIONS FOR OPERATION

Refractory disease, defined as treatment resistance or the inability to wean from corticosteroids, is the most common indication for operation. Children are particularly sensitive to long-term corticosteroid therapy. Not only are there implications for growth and development, but bone mineralization and the risk of fracture are important considerations for the active child. Middle and high school adolescents are acutely aware of the severe side effects of medial therapy on their social opportunities and look to surgery to restore a more normal life. Preoperative discussions center on the expected quality of life and psychosocial issues associated with long-term bowel function.

Fulminant colitis with bleeding or obstruction and toxic megacolon with the potential for perforation of the colon is a presentation more common in children and adolescents as compared to adults. Many of these desperately ill children require subtotal colectomy with end ileostomy. Evaluation of the number of bloody bowel movements per day, presence of fever, anemia, hypoalbuminemia, and elevated sedimentation rate or C-reactive protein help the surgeon determine the appropriate number of stages to complete restorative proctocolectomy. Simple correction of mild abnormalities should not preclude complete reconstruction, but patients with recurring fevers, multiple bloody bowel movements, significant anemia or hypoalbuminemia, and elevated inflammatory markers are best staged with colectomy and end ileostomy. Once these children have been weaned from their corticosteroids and have regained their usual state of health, completion proctectomy with ileal-pouch anal anastomosis is completed. This may take up to 6 months of recovery for the sickest of patients. Recent data from adult studies suggest a deleterious effect of infliximab on pouch healing with increased rates of pouch leak and serious infectious complications. Currently, we delay construction of the pouch for 2 months following the administration of infliximab.

## CHOICE OF OPERATION

The proctocolectomy may be performed laparoscopically, be laparoscopic-assisted, or be open. Recently, advancements in instrumentation have allowed us to accomplish resection of the colon and rectum using single-incision laparoscopic-assisted techniques. The reconstruction can occur in 1, 2, or 3 stages. A variety of pouches that are stapled or hand-sewn to the anus have been advocated. Knowledge of each technique is required to tailor the operative approach to individual patients.

Preoperative preparation depends on the condition of the child. In general, bowel preparation is no longer used and healthy children can be admitted to the hospital on the day of their procedure. Rectal irrigation is completed prior to sterile preparation in the operating suite. The optimal site for ileostomy is marked by an enterostomal therapist. Stress dose steroids are required in steroid-dependent patients and are weaned over weeks or months. Broad-spectrum antibiotics are administered within 60 minutes of incision. Prophylaxis for venous thromboembolism is appropriate due to an acquired hypercoagulable state in patients with IBD. Positioning is supine for a subtotal colectomy with end ileostomy; however, lithotomy position is required for pouch construction (Fig. 49-7).

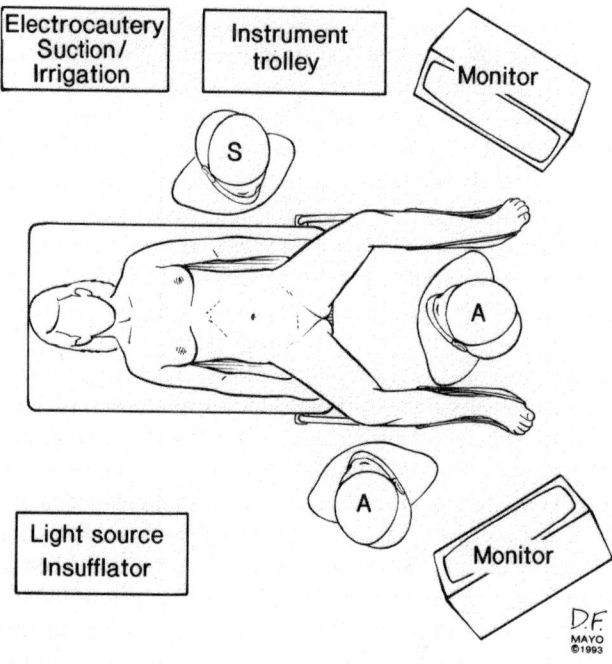

**FIGURE 49-7** The lithotomy position ensures access to the perineum for ileal-pouch anal anastomosis. This illustrates the positioning for laparoscopic rectal dissection for a right-handed surgeon. The legs must be well padded with the weight centered on the heels of the feet. Accessible stirrups allow for extension of the hips during laparoscopic colectomy and proctectomy preventing instrument collision with the legs and hip flexion during transanal mucosectomy or stapled anastomosis. (Used with permission of Mayo Foundation for Medical Education and Research.)

# LAPAROSCOPIC TECHNIQUE

For children with fulminant colitis or toxic megacolon, total abdominal colectomy with end ileostomy is appropriate. Laparoscopic or single-incision laparoscopic techniques are safe alternatives. For laparoscopic procedures, a 5-mm port is placed in the umbilicus for optical access and a 12-mm port is placed in the ileostomy site. Two other 5-mm ports are usually required and can be fashioned in the line of a future Pfannenstiel incision. The left and right lateral peritoneal attachments of the colon are mobilized. The omentum may be preserved by entering the lesser sac and freeing the anterior attachments from the transverse colon. Alternatively, the omentum may be resected by dividing its blood supply using a bipolar vessel sealing device just distal to the right gastroepiploic arcade. This may reduce the incidence of postoperative bowel obstructions. Currently, we prefer to divide the mesentery using the LigaSure device. This technique reduces the amount of mobilization required for stapling and ligates larger vessels as compared to the ultrasonic shears. Once the colon has been mobilized and the rectum has been securely divided with a stapler, the abdominal colon can be removed by slightly enlarging the ileostomy site. For single-incision laparoscopic techniques, a single-incision access device is placed in the ileostomy site. The skin incision is kept to 1.5 to 2 cm and the fasciotomy is approximately 4 cm. An accessory 5-mm umbilical port may be used to help manipulate an inflamed or edematous colon. This umbilical incision is invisible after complete healing. Resecting the omentum speeds the operation.

Proctectomy can be completed laparoscopically or by single-incision laparoscopic techniques following resection of the abdominal colon as a part of a simultaneous or staged restorative proctocolectomy. Injury to the ureters and nervi erigentes is avoided by dividing the rectal mesentery close to the bowel wall. Visualization of the ureters is usually straightforward in a child and the presacral nerves can be identified at the pelvic brim. Dissection close to the rectal wall also prevents injury to the bladder, seminal vesicles, and prostate in boys and the vagina in a girl. Adequate visualization is provided by the laparoscope and by placing the tissues on tension. In larger children, the rectum can be divided intracorporeally at the level of the levator ani muscles using a laparoscopic deflectable stapler. In smaller children, the pelvis will not accept insertion of a laparoscopic stapler to the level of the levator complex. The rectum can be divided at a level that accepts the laparoscopic stapler and the dissection continues distally to the pelvic floor. The rectum can then be everted through the anus and divided extracorporeally taking care to identify the sphincteric complex. The surgeon should be aware that for the double-stapled anastomosis, the EEA stapler will resect at least an additional centimeter of rectum to complete the anastomosis (Fig. 49-8). In small children, a stapled anastomosis may not be possible necessitating a hand-sewn technique (Fig. 49-9). This eliminates the short segment of the involved mucosa left by the stapled technique that requires surveillance; however, there are concerns for retained islands of mucosa following mucosectomy that may lead to the development of cuff adenocarcinoma.

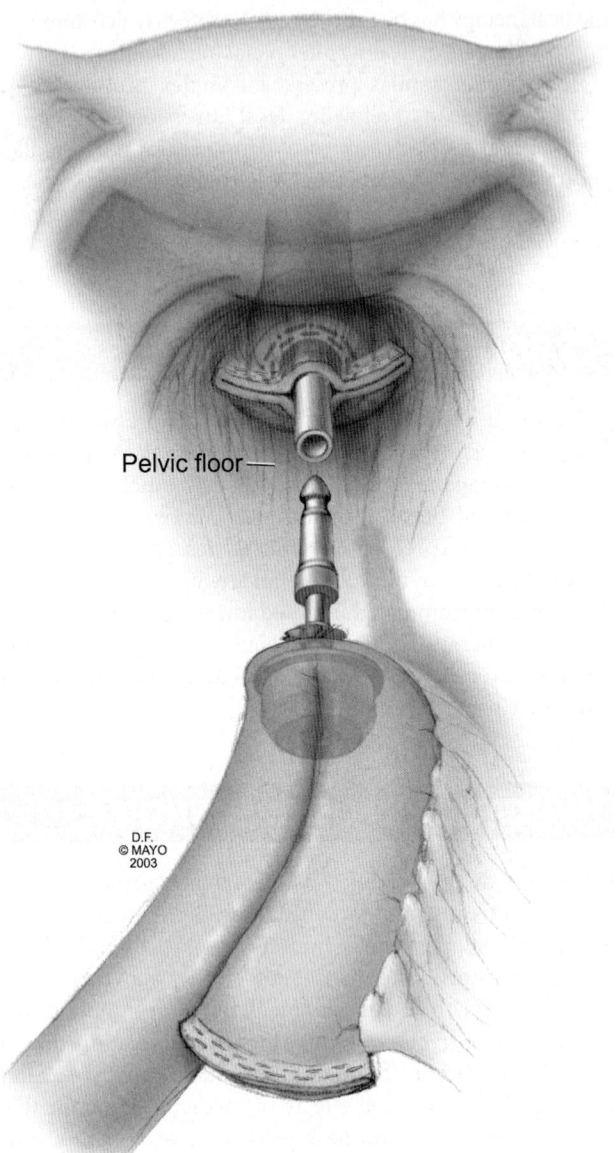

Pelvic floor—

D.F.
© MAYO
2003

E1129399-003-0

**FIGURE 49-8** Intracorporeal view of the double-stapled anal anastomosis. An EEA stapler is inserted through the short rectal stump and connected to an anvil that has been secured in the ileal pouch. The surgeon must recognize that the EEA stapler will resect approximately 1 cm of the rectal stump. (Used with permission of Mayo Foundation for Medical Education and Research.)

Pediatric surgeons have an extensive experience with mucosectomy and anal anastomosis by caring for children with Hirschsprung disease. It is expected that this experience will potentially avoid this risk in children.

A diverting ileostomy is commonly used following construction of an ileal pouch and is reversed in 6 to 8 weeks after a contrast study of the pouch demonstrates normal healing. The stoma is fashioned in an area of the ileum that easily reaches to the ileostomy site, which is approximately 20 cm from the pouch. Ileal pouch anal anastomosis can be performed without a protective ileostomy; however, this occurs in a highly selected patient group. Children who have been weaned from corticosteroids, have normal nutritional parameters, and underwent technically perfect operations without tension on the pouch are candidates. These patients

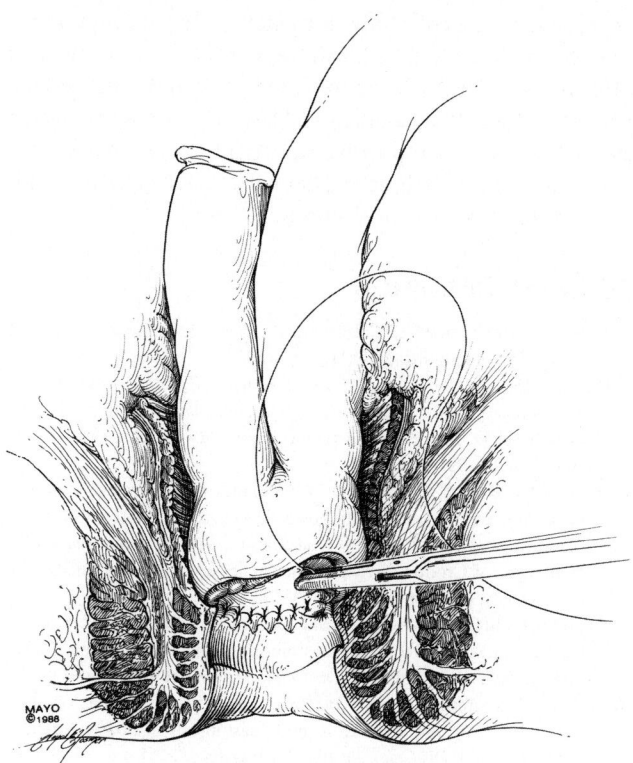

**FIGURE 49-9** Rectal mucosectomy with hand-sewn anastomosis. The mucosectomy begins approximately 5 mm above the dentate line and continues proximally to complete the pelvic dissection. The pouch is then pulled through the muscular cuff and anastomosed to the muscle complex and anal mucosa with interrupted suture. (Used with permission of Mayo Foundation for Medical Education and Research.)

are rare because an anastomotic leak and pelvic sepsis are too high a risk for poor long-term pouch function in children.

## SMALL-BOWEL MOBILIZATION

Adequate mobilization of the small bowel is mandatory to provide sufficient reach of the ileal pouch to the anus. This can be especially problematic in obese patients, patients with previous intestinal resections, or patients with shortened mesentery from steroid therapy. The first step is to completely mobilize the mesenteric attachments to the retroperitoneum as far as the third portion of the duodenum. Mobilization of the superior mesenteric artery as it crosses the inferior border of the pancreas can be helpful and is easily visualized laparoscopically. The ileum can then be drawn into the pelvis to determine its length. It should easily reach the pelvic reflection without tension. If tension remains, the ileocolic artery and vein may be divided at the origin of the superior mesenteric artery. The peritoneum over the superior mesenteric artery should be mobilized both anteriorly and posteriorly taking care not to injure the vessels. If the ileum still does not reach the pelvis without tension, consideration should be given to performing an ileostomy to allow the mesentery to lengthen over 3 to 6 months before removing the rectum. Alternatively, a formal Kocher maneuver and resection of all

the tissue to the right of the superior mesenteric artery may provide an additional 2 cm of mobility. Consideration of the pouch at this time is important, since the S-pouch will reach deeper into the pelvic as compared to a J-pouch. Attention to the length of the spout of the S-pouch is key so that emptying is not impaired. Mucosectomy with hand-sewn anastomosis requires more mobility, thus if there is significant tension, a stapled anastomosis may be more appropriate. Finally, a straight ileoanal procedure can provide the necessary length. Nearly equivalent stool frequencies with fewer episodes of pouchitis are reported; however, the postoperative time required to achieve these stool frequencies is significantly longer than in children with pouch construction.

## POUCH DESIGN

Several pouch designs have been used to restore bowel function in children. The J-, S-, W-, and lateral pouches, in addition to the straight pull-through, have all been utilized at leading pediatric centers. The functional result of each pouch appears to be comparable to the other. The S-pouch does provide an extra 2 cm of reach into the pelvis, whereas the J-pouch is easiest to construct. A J-pouch can be constructed laparoscopically, but we prefer to exteriorize the ileum and create a 15-cm pouch using linear staplers. A small pouch will not function well as a reservoir and a larger pouch may have ineffective evacuation. The capacity of the pouch does increase over the next year. The blind end of the J-pouch is obliterated by suturing the open end of the pouch to the pre-pouch ileum. A wound protector allows easier return of the pouch into the abdomen.

## POSTOPERATIVE COURSE

Most patients that have undergone minimally invasive restorative proctocolectomy do not require nasogastric decompression postoperatively. Liquid diet may be started the morning following the procedure and advanced as tolerated. This rapid progression is well tolerated and helps thicken ileostomy effluent.

Perioperative complications are commonplace following restorative proctocolectomy (30%-66%). Bowel obstruction (12%-20%), intraabdominal abscess (2%-7%), wound infection (4%-20%), and ileostomy complications predominate; however, anastomotic leak (2%-5%) and fistula (0%-10%) are the most feared complications that frequently require diverting ileostomy.

Long-term complications center on pouchitis. Pouchitis is a nonspecific mucosal inflammation that presents with fever, watery diarrhea, malaise, and worsening extraintestinal manifestations. The estimated incidence of pouchitis ranges from 23% to 46% within the first year after ileostomy closure. Nearly 50% of patients experience at least 1 episode of pouchitis following restorative proctocolectomy over their lifetime. Risk factors associated with an increased incidence of pouchitis include extensive UC, presence of backwash ileitis, preoperative thrombocytosis, concurrent primary sclerosing cholangitis, arthralgia/arthropathy, seropositive pANCA, seropositive anti-CBir1 flagellin, being a nonsmoker, and use of nonsteroidal anti-inflammatory medications. Treatment is initiated with oral ciprofloxacin or metronidazole with improvement in symptoms within 24 to 48 hours. Patients with persistent or recurrent symptoms require investigation for anastomotic strictures, retained rectal segment (cuffitis), small-volume pouch, medication-induced irritability, and CD. Chronic pouchitis is managed with daily low-dose antibiotics that are cycled weekly or monthly. Probiotics, immunosuppressants, and biologic agents have been used with moderate success. Five to 10% of ileal pouch procedures fail due to chronic pouchitis with the eventual diagnosis of CD predominating in these unfortunate patients.

## FUNCTIONAL OUTCOME

Overall, the vast majority of pediatric patients have an excellent result from restorative proctocolectomy. They have a very low rate of incontinence and less frequent stooling when compared to adult counterparts. Indeed, the stool frequency at 6 months ranges from 4 to 8 movements per day and this persists for years to come. Nighttime stooling ranges from 1 to 2 movements; however, it is not uncommon for children to sleep all night without accidents. Quality of life is similar to healthy children following restorative proctocolectomy with only the presence of pouchitis and nighttime stooling correlating to lower quality of life scores. Urinary complaints and impotence in boys are very rare, yet the incidence of retrograde ejaculation is not well-studied. Pregnancy in females is reportedly decreased following restorative proctocolectomy; however, assisted fertility has been highly successful in these patients. The potentially fewer adhesions from minimally invasive procedures may improve the fecundity rates. Pregnancy and vaginal delivery are possible following pouch procedures without increased risk of serious pouch or anastomotic complications. The mode of delivery should be determined by the patient and her obstetrician.

## INDETERMINATE COLITIS

A firm diagnosis of UC or CD cannot be established in 5% to 15% of children who require an operation for IBD. This presents a therapeutic challenge to the pediatric surgeon because of a higher rate of postoperative complications compared to patients with UC. The long-term success of restorative proctocolectomy for patients with IC approaches 85% as compared to 89% for those with UC, thus proceeding directly to a pouch procedure is tempting and justified. Yet, patients with IC that resembles CD, such as younger children and patients with seropositive ASCA antibodies, may benefit from a 6- to 12-month delay after colectomy before proceeding to restorative proctocolectomy.

## SELECTED READINGS

Abraham BP, Thirumurthi S. Clinical significance of inflammatory markers. *Curr Gastroenterol Rep* 2009;11:360–367.

Baldassano RN, Han PD, Jeshion WC, et al. Pediatric Crohn's disease: risk factors for postoperative recurrence. *Am J Gastroenterol* 2001;96:2169–2176.

Cooney R, Jewell D. The genetic basis of inflammatory bowel disease. *Dig Dis* 2009;27:428–442.

Diamond IR, Gerstle JT, Kim PCW, et al. Outcomes after laparoscopic surgery in children with inflammatory bowel disease. *Surg Endosc* 2010;4:epub.

Fazio VW, Marchetti F, Church M, et al. Effect of resection margins on the recurrence of Crohn's disease in the small bowel. A randomized controlled trial. *Ann Surg* 1996;224:563–571.

McLeod RS, Wolff BG, Ross S, et al. Recurrence of Crohn's disease after ileocolic resection is not affected by anastomotic type: results of a multicenter, randomized, controlled trial. *Dis Colon Rectum* 2009;52:919–927.

Muñoz-Juárez M, Yamamoto T, Wolff BG, et al. Wide-lumen stapled anastomosis vs. conventional end-to-end anastomosis in the treatment of Crohn's disease. *Dis Colon Rectum* 2001;44:20–25.

Ruemmele FM. Pediatric inflammatory bowel disease: coming of age. *Curr Opin Gastroenterol* 2010;26:332–336.

Saur CG, Kugathasan S. Pediatric inflammatory bowel disease: highlighting pediatric differences in IBD. *Med Clin N Am* 2010;94:35–52.

Sawczenko A, Sandu B. Presenting features of inflammatory bowel disease in children. *Arch Dis Child* 2003;88:995–1000.

Seetharamaiah R, West BT, Ignash SJ, et al. Outcomes in pediatric patients undergoing straight vs J pouch ileoanal anastomosis: a multicenter analysis. *J Pediatr Surg* 2009;44:1410–1417.

Solem CA, Loftus EV, Fletcher JG, et al. Small-bowel imaging in Crohn's disease: a prospective, blinded, 4-way comparison trial. *Gastrointest Endosc* 2008;68:255–266.

Stavlo PL, Libsch KD, Rodeberg DA, et al. Pediatric ileal pouch-anal anastomosis: functional outcomes and quality of life. *J Pediatr Surg* 2003;38:935–939.

Topstad DR, Panaccione R, Heine JA, et al. Combined seton placement, infliximab infusion, and maintenance immunosuppressives improve healing rate in fistulizing anorectal Crohn's disease: a single center experience. *Dis Colon Rectum* 2003;46:577–583.

Tung J, Loftus EV, Freese DK, et al. A population-based study of the frequency of corticosteroid resistance and dependence in pediatric patients with Crohn's disease and ulcerative colitis. *Inflamm Bowel Dis* 2006;12:1093–1100.

Working group of the North American Society of Pediatric Gastroenterology, Hepatology, and Nutrition and the Crohn's and Colitis Foundation of America. Differentiating ulcerative colitis from Crohn disease in children and young adults. *J Pediatr Gastroenterol Nutr* 2007;44:653–674.

Yamamoto T, Fazio VW, Tekkis PP. Safety and efficacy of strictureplasty for Crohn's disease: a systematic review and meta-analysis. *Dis Colon Rectum* 2007;50:1968–1986.

# CHAPTER 50

# Short Bowel Syndrome

*Megan K. Fuller, Jeffrey J. Dehmer,
and Michael A. Helmrath*

## KEY POINTS

1. Due to the repair and growth capacity of the bowel, it is crucial to minimize the length of bowel resected at initial and subsequent operations.

2. Early and consistent administration of enteral nutrition, utilizing enteral feeding access if necessary, helps maximize intestinal adaptation.

3. Careful consideration of the location of stomas and mucous fistulae can minimize the length of the operation to reestablish intestinal continuity.

4. Distal refeeding through a mucous fistula is a useful technique for maintaining enteral nutrition despite the presence of a very proximal stoma.

5. Intestinal failure associated liver disease and catheter-related septic complications may be reduced with application of liver-protective feeding strategies and ethanol lock devices.

6. Autologous intestinal reconstruction surgery should only be considered after sufficient time has passed to allow for maximal adaptation of the remnant bowel.

7. Formal multidisciplinary intestinal failure teams can improve patient outcomes.

## INTRODUCTION

Short bowel syndrome (SBS) is the most common cause of intestinal failure and can be the result of congenital disorders, extensive surgical resection, or both. In addition, primary defects in absorption or in peristalsis can contribute to this disorder. The end result is a remaining bowel of insufficient length and/or functional capacity to meet the fluid and/or nutritional needs of the patient without parenteral nutrition (PN) support. The causes of SBS in the pediatric population have changed over the years and are myriad. The most common is necrotizing enterocolitis (NEC), comprising some 35% of cases. Other causes include intestinal atresias, abdominal wall defects (mainly gastroschisis), intestinal volvulus, complicated

meconium ileus, and the long-segment Hirschprung disease, as shown in Fig. 50-1. Apart from primary intestinal pathology, mesenteric vascular occlusion necessitating resection may occur from invasive monitoring devices and reduced perfusion states secondary to shock, as well as the use of vasoconstrictive inotropic agents that can result in an ischemic or necrotic bowel.

Neonatal cases comprise 80% of all pediatric SBS. Surprisingly, data on the incidence and mortality related to SBS are incomplete. The published incidences of SBS in very low and extremely low birth weight neonates at 16 tertiary centers in the United States are 0.7% and 1.1%, respectively, although this excluded cases in term infants. There is a bimodal mortality distribution in this population. The first peak corresponds mainly to infants who undergo massive initial bowel resections and the later peak represents deaths due to complications of SBS, namely central venous catheter (CVC) sepsis and intestinal failure associated liver disease. The survival rate for children with SBS has been quoted as 73% to 89% with lower rates in patients requiring chronic PN.

## GENERAL PRINCIPLES

SBS is a complex clinical problem and as such, many institutions have developed formal multidisciplinary teams specifically designed to care for these difficult patients. This approach is associated with reduced morbidity and mortality. Although each patient requires an individualized approach, several management principles should be considered in each case. The third trimester through the first year of life is a period of rapid intestinal growth. Therefore, even short segments of the bowel have the potential for significant increased growth. This concept is of utmost importance when considering resection of bowel with questionable viability at an initial operation. As the intestine has a remarkable ability to heal after ischemia, it is often impossible to predict the fate of the bowel without the benefit of time, supporting the liberal use of second-look operations prior to committing to resection. In conditions such as NEC, procedures such as the "clip-and-drop" approach have demonstrated that sections of bowel initially deemed nonviable will survive and can function in the future. This further emphasizes the point that the bowel has a

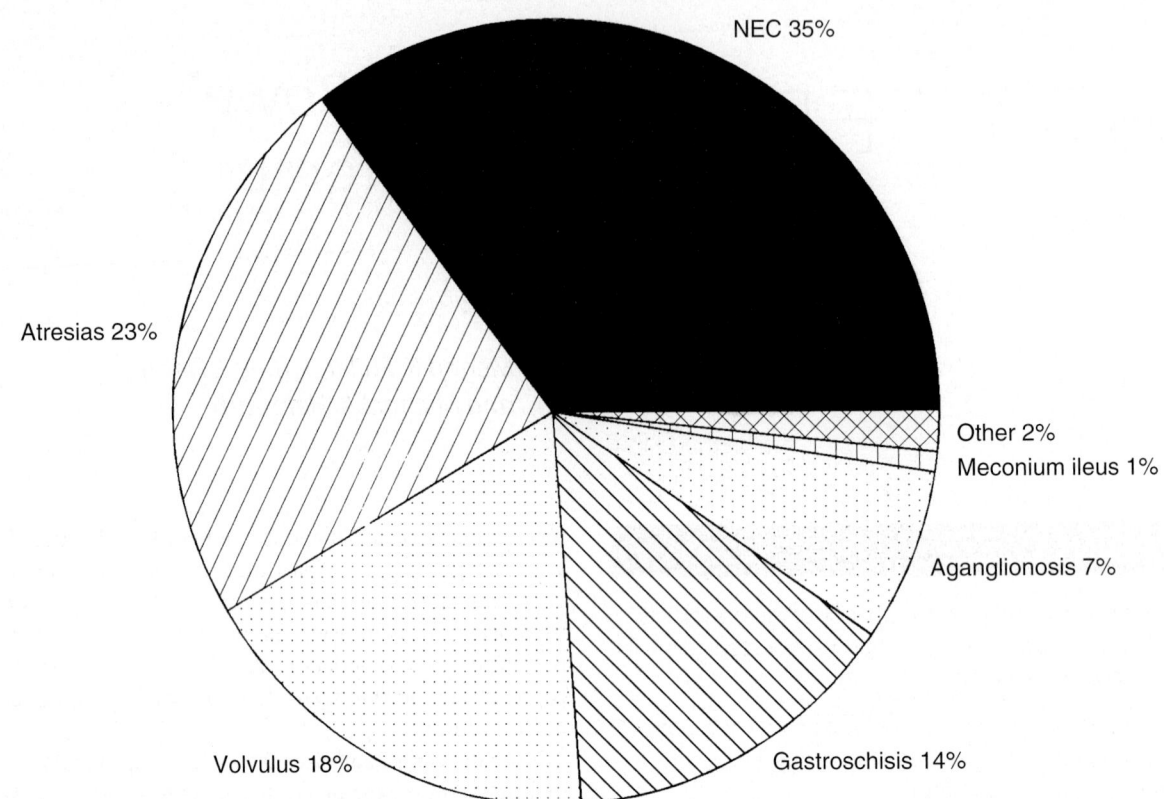

NEC 35%

Atresias 23%

Other 2%

Meconium ileus 1%

Aganglionosis 7%

Volvulus 18%

Gastroschisis 14%

**FIGURE 50-1** The causes of short bowel syndrome.

remarkable ability to heal. Based on this principle, resections of the intestine in patients with NEC should be directed to avoid excessive loss of bowel length.

Enteral nutrition is the most potent driver of intestinal adaptation and initial operative plans should consider options for early initiation of feeds. Careful placement of intestinal stomas and distal mucous fistulas obviates the need for an extensive laparotomy in the future when reestablishing intestinal continuity. This approach helps avoid potential complications that may result in long postoperative periods without enteral nutrition. It also allows early restoration of intestinal continuity, which, in turn, augments the adaptive response. Furthermore, it minimizes complications including PN-associated liver disease and CVC infections. Although there can be technical difficulties with regards to wound complications and application of the ostomy appliance with 2 stomas in close proximity, this is outweighed by the potential avoidance of additional intestinal injury during extensive operative mobilization.

## NUTRITIONAL CONSIDERATIONS

The ultimate goal of all nutritional strategies is to maintain appropriate growth, maximize bowel adaptation, and minimize complications. A multidisciplinary approach has been shown to improve long-term outcomes for these children. To achieve these goals, the surgeon's role centers on performing an appropriate initial operation and considering the need for secure, long-term vascular and enteral access.

PN is essential to initially support the nutritional needs of these children; however, up to 60% of children on long-term PN develop hepatic dysfunction. In addition to the risk for development of cirrhosis, liver disease has been associated with hindered bowel adaptation. A lipid-reduction protocol that limits the amount of fat to less than 1 g/kg/day at our institution has shown a dramatic decrease in the incidence of elevated directed bilirubin and liver enzymes. Another strategy for patients with continued elevation of liver function tests is the use of omega-3 fatty acids (Omegaven®—Fresenius Kabi AG, Bad Homburg, Germany), which have shown benefit in 1 study. New prospective studies are underway to examine these strategies more closely and establish appropriate evidence-based usage guidelines. Finally, aggressive prevention of sepsis is essential to any liver-protective nutritional approach.

Sepsis is generally secondary to catheter-related infections (CRI) and rates are significantly higher in children with SBS (7.8 vs 1.3 per 1000 catheter days). In addition, enteric organisms are much more frequently obtained in cultures compared to infections in children without intestinal failure (62% vs 12%). Strict antiseptic technique should always be employed at the time of catheter placement and upon access. Preferably, all CVCs placed should be cuffed and tunneled, as they have longer lives and decreased infection, migration, and dislodgement in comparison to simple CVCs or peripherally inserted central catheters (PICCs). Each central line site should be carefully documented as well as any CRI and their causative organisms, if identified. Strategies for catheter salvage and diagnosis of bloodstream infections are outlined by the Infectious Disease Society of America. However, as noted in the guidelines, pediatric patients and specifically neonates pose difficulties in proving CRI by culture criteria. In this case, suspected catheter infections should be treated with catheter salvage unless there is clinical decline or recurrence of infection after treatment, in which case the catheter should be removed. On removal of infected catheters, the tip should be sent for culture.

Prevention and treatment of CRI may include antibiotic and 70% ethanol locks. These strategies function by attacking the biofilm lining the catheter and both have studies demonstrating efficacy and drawbacks. Antibiotic locks are recommended in treatment strategies for catheter salvage, but their use for prevention of infection can promote bacterial resistance and requires heparin to maintain patency. Ethanol locks have shown reduction of CRIs. Despite reports suggesting that polyurethane catheter degradation occurs, a study of prolonged exposure to ethanol demonstrated no appreciable changes in catheter integrity of either polyurethane or silicone catheters, however these treated catheters may be susceptible to increased thrombosis. Side effects of ethanol intoxication include dizziness, nausea, and dyspnea; however, with a dwell time of 3 to 4 hours and withdrawal of ethanol prior to usage, there were no reports of adverse events.

In addition to the provision of PN to support growth, it is vital to begin enteral feeds early to promote bowel adaptation and gut barrier function while decreasing incidence of PN-related liver disease. A meta-analysis looked at feeding recommendations in the literature and found the best evidence for initiation of enteral feeds early to promote adaptation. In addition, consensus based on clinical data recommends administering enteral nutrition in a continuous fashion. To accomplish these goals, the surgeon must consider methods of secure enteral access.

Initially feeds may be started via oro/nasogastric (NG) or oro/nasojejenal (NJ) routes; however, in 1 study, up to 59% of feeding tubes placed in neonates were malpositioned or accidently removed, making them impractical in the long term. Thus, placement of gastrostomy tubes (GT) is indicated in this population. In general, if a patient tolerates NG feeds, he or she will tolerate GT feeds. If there is difficulty with high residuals or poor gastric emptying, a NJ tube may be tried to evaluate the ability of the bowel to tolerate enteral nutrition. NJ tubes can then be converted to gastrojejunal (GJ) tubes for long-term feeding. One study examined outcomes for antireflux surgery versus GJ tubes in neurologically impaired patients with reflux. Among this patient population, only 8% of children failed management with a GJ tube and 14% transitioned to oral or gastric feeds by the end of the follow-up period. Numerous studies have demonstrated safety and efficacy of antireflux procedures, but we typically first attempt to feed via GJ or NJ tubes in our neonatal patients with reflux and SBS to avoid potential complications that limit the ability to provide enteral nutrition.

Several GT techniques have been described as safe including open, laparoscopic, and percutaneous. No consensus has been reached regarding radiographic or endoscopic placement of feeding tubes as there are conflicting data. Surgically placed tubes are also safe, but the open technique has been supplanted by more minimally invasive methods at several centers. In one study of PEG versus laparoscopic placement, PEG tubes had a higher incidence of significant complications. Some surgeons utilize laparoscopy to guide PEG placement to prevent colonic injury or peritoneal placement. After initial placement, conversion to low-profile devices is preferred in the pediatric population (eg, MIC-KEY© or BardButton©).

Initiation of enteral feeds should be in a low-volume, continuous manner and should be started as soon as physiologically possible depending on the underlying disease process and surgical procedure. Breast milk (either donor or maternal) feedings have demonstrated decreased days of PN, reduction in cholestasis. This effect may be secondary to the presence of high levels of IgA, long-chain fats, growth factors, and free amino acids, specifically glutamine, within the milk. In patients with protein allergies, or in older patients, an elemental amino-acid-based formula is advised.

Feeds should be advanced in a systematic fashion based on the lack of emesis, abdominal distension, and skin breakdown and considering the amount and consistency of stool output. Fluid losses via stomas, decompressing tubes, and stool should be carefully replaced mL for mL with an appropriate electrolyte solution. If there is evidence of feeding intolerance, we recommend decreasing the volume of enteral feed rather than discontinuation. Frequent starts and stops will make it difficult to determine the amount of feeds the patient will tolerate and will lead to a lack of enteral stimulation to promote bowel adaptation. However, in cases of systemic illness or sepsis, we would halt feeds until resolution. Electrolytes should be carefully monitored in these children, especially as stool output approaches 40 to 50 mL/kg/day. In these children, consider addition of antidiarrheal or antisecretory medications or the addition of fiber in the form of 3% pectin. Pectin has been demonstrated to improve gut adaptation in some animal studies. In children at or exceeding 40 to 50 mL/kg/day of stool output, feeds should be decreased in instances of persistent fluid or electrolyte derangements, specifically when $CO_2$ levels fall below 20 on serum chemistries. Another instance to hold or limit feeds is significant skin breakdown. Skin breakdown can be a significant and difficult problem in this patient population. Skin care should be initiated prior to any sign of breakdown and an established wound care program utilized at the first signs of breakdown. Reducing substance levels have not been clinically beneficial in our practice and are not utilized.

As enteral feeds are increased slowly to goal, PN should be concomitantly decreased and growth measures should be closely followed during this time. If enteral volume has been maximized with unmet caloric needs, concentrating feeds can be attempted. If intestinal continuity has not been reestablished, we opt for continued PN and improved growth until after surgery. Aggressive occupational and physical therapy should be provided during this period to help establish oral motor skills for eventual transition to oral feeds. Initiating oral feeds is generally begun once or twice daily by holding 1 hour of continuous feed then offering that amount orally. This should be advanced at the clinician's discretion, but if the child is not yet at full enteral feeds, use of oral feeds should be minimal. If children are 4 to 6 months of age, solids may also be offered. Children with long-term SBS even if weaned off PN should be closely monitored for appropriate growth and pubertal development. Adolescence in particular is a time of rapid growth and may require increased nutritional supplementation. Micronutrient deficiencies are also common, particularly $B_{12}$, iron, zinc, vitamin D, and calcium. Of note, normal levels of calcium, vitamin D, and phosphorus did not ensure good bone mineral density in adolescents and DEXA scans have been recommended to determine appropriate bone growth.

## FEEDING ADJUNCTS

Careful consideration regarding stoma placement with relationship to the distal bowel (mucous fistula) and abdominal incision greatly influences the high incidence of complications. Regardless of the pathology necessitating creation of an intestinal stoma, complications occur in up to 38% of patients in 1 retrospective review and as high as 68% in premature infants with NEC. The most common complications that occur include stricture, prolapse, necrosis, skin excoration, and retraction with an overall rate increased to 43% in premature infants.

Based on these data, one must consider the duration of diversion required prior to stoma reversal, as the definitive management to many of these stomal complications is reanastomosis. Certainly there are pros and cons in any decision to take a child back to the operating room to reestablish intestinal continuity, but a few principles can be used to assist in management. A common clinical scenario that supports the decision to take down stomas earlier is recurrent episodes of dehydration and electrolyte imbalance, which may occur particularly if the stoma is very proximal. Several studies do promote early reversal in these instances, citing the benefits of avoiding systemic complications associated with high stomal output.

In lieu of withholding enteral feeds, which is relatively counterproductive unless clinically necessary, or proceeding directly to reanastomosis, one option to manage stomal output is refeeding enteral output through the distal mucous fistula. The rationale for distal refeeding is relatively straightforward and it has benefits beyond simply increasing the percentage of daily calories obtained through the enteral route.

Described as early as 1985, refeeding distal mucous fistulas can result in improved overall enteral nutrient absorption, maintenance of distal bowel mucosal integrity, and stimulation of mucosal growth, and improved aboral peristalsis. In cases where there is a proximal jejunal stoma, distal feeding will also permit enterohepatic circulation to persist as long the terminal ileum remains intact, decreasing the risk of hepatic complications. Overall, clinically, this can improve weight gain and reduce some of the requirements for PN in SBS patients. In a case report, even a minimal amount of rectal tube feeding has been suggested to be beneficial with regard to the aforementioned parameters. Distal refeeding also provides an environment conducive to adaptation of the remnant bowel, which occurs via early increases in crypt depth, villus height, and crypt fission as well as permanent increases in the number of crypts and bowel caliber. Although the mechanisms by which this occurs are still being elucidated, enteral nutrition provides growth factors, immunologic stimuli, and vital nutrients to the bowel during this period. Despite the readily apparent theoretical advantages of feeding the distal bowel, there are still no definitive prospective data to support utilizing this therapy routinely. In 2006, a review could only identify 30 patients in 5 appropriate studies over a 10-year period. The results of their analysis concluded that this clinical technique is safe, can potentially reduce PN-related complications in SBS patients, and all studies reported significant weight gain in the included patients. Providing enteral content in one form or another is particularly important if the colon remains intact but out of intestinal continuity, as it plays a critical role in sodium reabsorption from the lumen. Practical aspects of refeeding include collection of proximal stoma effluent every 4 to 6 hours and feeding distally via a syringe pump with barrier cream application to prevent peristomal skin irritation. The most commonly employed catheter is 8-French (red rubber, Foley, or NG). We do not recommend refeeding if accessing the distal mucous fistula is difficult and cannot be done as part of routine care.

Although there are no concrete data to suggest the optimal time of stoma reversal in all patients, there is some evidence to suggest that always performing reanastomosis as early as possible is not necessarily better and that those early patients may have a higher rate of postoperative complications than those whose intestinal continuity is reestablished later. In particular, among infants undergoing early (<10 weeks after initial operation) stoma reversal, these authors found a longer requirement for mechanical ventilation and for postreversal PN. Intuitively, it makes sense that in children without compelling reasons to proceed with early reoperation to reverse stomas, a later approach allows time for natural weight gain and for resolution of any other medical issues that may arise during the complicated hospitalization period for these children.

With modern pediatric surgical techniques, early closure can be accomplished safely even in small patients, with no strict weight limit required in our opinion. Regardless of the initial pathology necessitating intestinal resection, if a stoma is to be created, it is beneficial to plan the operation such that any subsequent attempt at establishing intestinal continuity can be done via a local incision and without requiring full adhesiolysis and mobilization of the bowel. This avoids taking down adhesions that are providing systemic blood supply to the healing intestine and may increase injury or time for return of gastrointestinal function.

In summary, the decision to create stomas during an initial abdominal operation is typically driven by the underlying disease process. The management of the stomas should be driven by the overall clinical status of the patient. Unless there is a compelling reason to proceed with early anastomosis, waiting and allowing for some growth and adaptation of the remnant bowel is clinically prudent. Distal mucous fistula refeeding is a viable option to delay stoma reversal if tolerated by the patient and appropriate given their overall medical and social situation. When planning stomas during an initial surgical intervention, placement to allow subsequent reversal through a smaller incision rather than a full laparotomy may have beneficial effects through preservation of new vasculature to the at-risk segments of bowel.

# AUTOLOGOUS INTESTINAL RECONSTRUCTION SURGERY

Despite our best efforts for the medical management of the SBS and its complications, some patients will have a persistent requirement for PN. Small bowel series images demonstrate that intestinal failure can result in a dilated bowel without other pathology, such as a distal stricture. In select patients with a significantly dilated bowel who continue to have PN requirements or other complications, surgical reconstruction may augment the functional capacity of the remnant intestine. Description of a variety of novel surgical techniques to address SBS such as reversed intestinal segments and colonic interposition grafts can be found in several small case series. None of these historical techniques stood the test of time until Bianchi published a procedure to lengthen the bowel in a porcine model in 1980. The procedure was originally referred to as intestinal loop lengthening, but is now more commonly called LILT (longitudinal intestinal lengthening and tailoring). As the Bianchi procedure is technically challenging, it was primarily performed in centers with experience caring for patients with intestinal failure. Twenty-three years later, a new novel procedure was described that autologously reconstructed loops of the dilated bowel by serially alternating partial division of the intestine with a linear stapler. The procedure was named "serial transverse enteroplasty," or STEP, and was quickly adopted as it is technically less challenging than the LILT, resulting in an increase in surgical procedures available to patients with short bowel syndrome. The LILT and STEP procedures represent the bulk of autologous intestinal reconstructive surgery performed today.

A visual representation of the components of LILT is shown in Fig. 50-2. LILT involves dividing the mesentery of the small bowel into 2 leaflets (Fig. 50-2A). Most surgeons use a stapler to divide the bowel into 2 segments (Fig. 50-2B), each half of the original diameter and supplied by one of the mesenteric leaflets. The leaflets are separated (Fig. 50-2C) and isoperistaltic anastomoses are created and the length of the bowel is effectively doubled (Fig. 50-2D). Several modifications to this procedure have been published. Bianchi described the use of electrocautery to divide the bowel rather that a stapler, followed by Lembert sutures to form the new bowel loops and preserve additional intestinal mass. Georgeson et al described the formation of a nipple valve distally to promote proximal small bowel dilation sufficient to perform a Bianchi procedure. Oblique division of the dilated bowel can reduce the number of anastomoses performed during a LILT procedure.

Several studies describe results of LILT as shown in Table 50-1. Waag et al reported no intraoperative deaths and 17 of 18 survivors were completely weaned from PN by 10 months postoperatively in their series of 25 patients over 15 years. The following year, Thompson et al identified 16 patients from their institution and describe 46% to be completely weaning from PN at 1 year and the remaining independent for 5 years. Of the 5 patients followed for 10 years, 3 remained on enteral nutrition alone. They confirm that results are influenced by remnant length, liver status, PN requirement, and age, indicating the importance of patient selection. Hosie et al included important concepts in their review about patient selection—dependence on PN, inability to achieve at least 50% of nutritional requirements enterally, and at least 6 months of nonsurgical therapy. Their age range was 4 months to 12 years with a mean of 25 months. Weaning from PN was achieved in 39% at an average of 9.1 months postoperatively. Perhaps most importantly, they highlight key considerations for surgical therapy: all bowel segments must be in continuity, a bowel diameter of 5 cm, intrinsic adaptation must be stimulated over a "sufficient time interval," although this is not explicitly defined. The most recent description of outcome in these patients gives similar results with 36 of 53 patients weaning from PN in the short-term follow-up and 23 of 29 remaining free with long-term follow-up. They did not find any significance of the presence of the ileocecal valve in terms of mortality, although the patients with an entire colon or only a small right colon resection did better. In their study, a high mortality rate in children with severe liver disease has led to that becoming an exclusion criteria for LILT.

Although within individual studies, analysis may vary, evaluation of patients that benefit from LILT identifies several common factors, including initial bowel length greater than 40 cm (particularly with a retained ileocecal valve) and the lack of liver disease. Patients with preexisting liver disease universally do worse, and it was suggested that patients with more mild hepatic dysfunction are self-selected for better outcomes after surgery. Furthermore, it is noted that in the Bianchi operative series, survivors underwent surgery at an average of 83 weeks of age compared with 10.9 weeks in nonsurvivors. This suggests that age at the time of surgery is an important factor, perhaps due to the higher degree of innate adaptation that has taken place prior to surgery.

The STEP procedure was first described in 2003 with the first human application later that year. The STEP procedure involves making alternating staple lines in the mesenteric and antimesenteric portions of the bowel perpendicular to its long axis. As with LILT, this does require that the bowel be dilated prior to operative intervention. As shown in Fig. 50-3, sequential STEP procedures have been successfully performed as the bowel can redilate postoperatively. Several additional indications for STEP have been described including atresia with a dilated proximal bowel and recalcitrant D-lactic acidosis.

Several short series of STEP results have been published; however, an international database has been created (http://www.stepoperation.org) with the first results published in 2007. In analyzing 38 patients across 19 centers in 3 countries with 12.6 months of median follow-up, significantly increased mean intestinal length was reported to be associated with an increase in enteral feed tolerance among those patients with SBS. Complications included staple line leak, bowel obstruction, intraabdominal abscess, progression of disease requiring transplantation, and 3 deaths (7.9%).

Although there are much more long-term data with LILT, based on existing data, the results of LILT and STEP appear comparable, with both procedures resulting in increased enteral nutrition tolerance, decreased PN-related complications, and potential avoidance of intestinal transplantation. Although both procedures did result in similar rates of weaning from PN, there was a trend toward more rapid weaning after STEP than LILT. Significant early and late complications did not differ. Of note, this analysis does include 14 adult

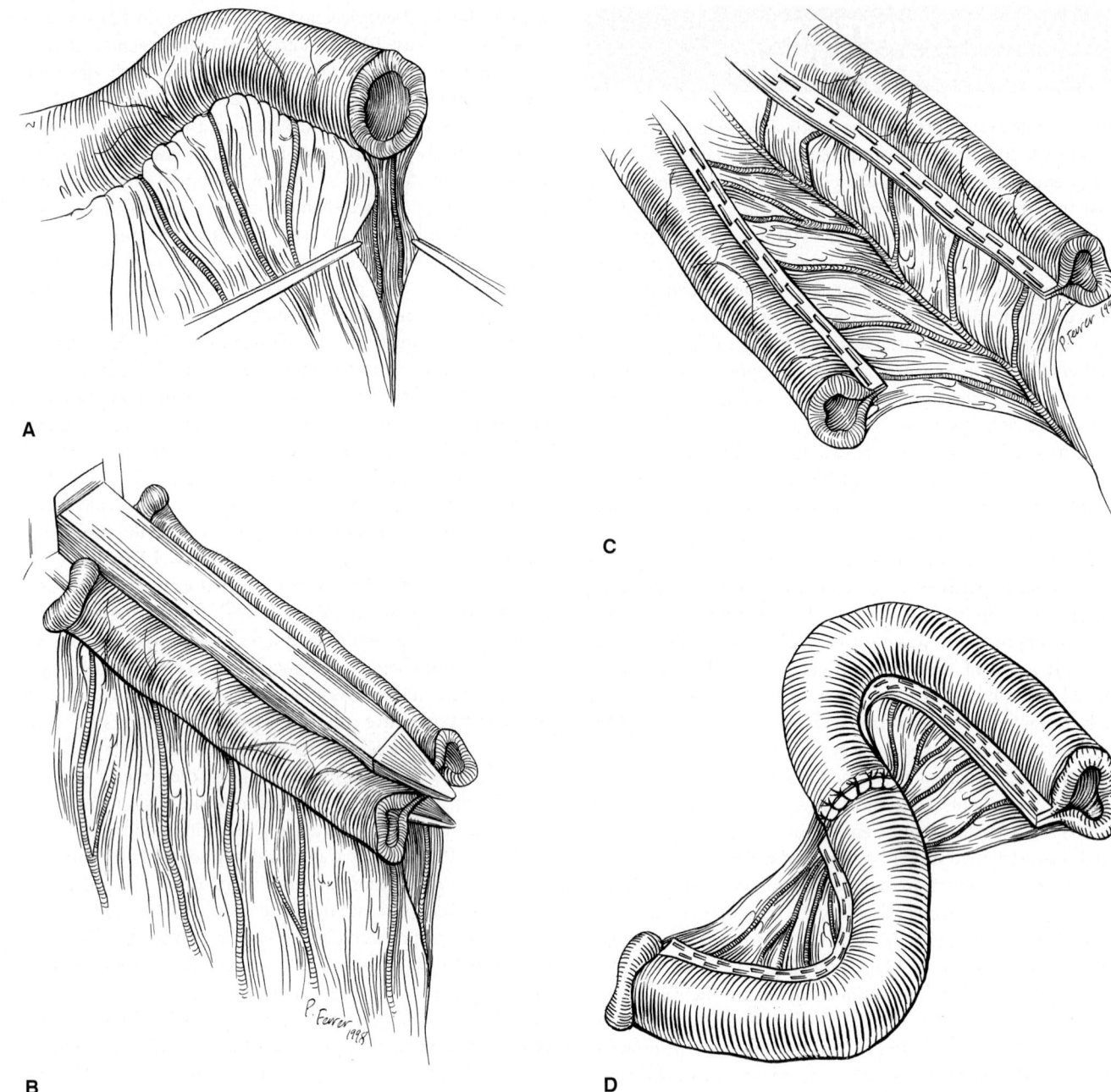

**A**

**B**

**C**

**D**

**FIGURE 50-2** Components of a LILT procedure include division of the mesentery into 2 separate leaflets (**A**), longitudinal division of the bowel (**B**), separation of the 2 leaflets (**C**), and anastomosis of the bowel segments (**D**).

| TABLE 50-1 | Published LILT Results | | | | | |
|---|---|---|---|---|---|---|
| Year | Author | Patients | Mean Follow-up (Years) | Survival (%) | Weaning from PN (%)[a] | Notes |
| 1999 | Waag | 25 | 6 | 72 | 94 (10 mos) | |
| 2000 | Thompson | 16 | 5 | 93.7 | 53 (1 year) | |
| 2003 | Bianchi | 31 | * | 64.5 | 75 | |
| 2006 | Hosie | 49 | * | 82 | 39 | 16 pts lost to follow-up |
| 2008 | Reinshagen | 53 | 6.6 | 77 | 79 | |

*Data not available.
[a]Among survivors.

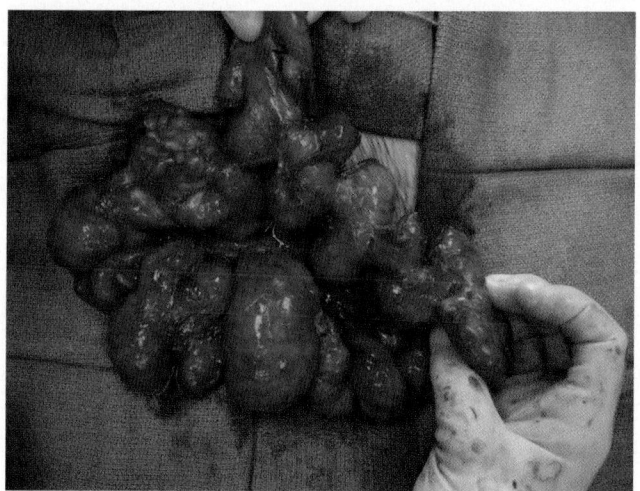

**FIGURE 50-3** Intraoperative photograph of a redo-STEP operation.

patients and as noted by the authors, the small sample size may mask subtle differences between the 2 procedures. Predictive factors for mortality were discussed and include failure to wean from PN, age less than 1 year at the time of surgery, extensive hepatic cirrhosis or bridging fibrosis, and prolonged INR at the time of surgery.

Whatever method of autologous reconstruction is chosen, several important conclusions can be drawn from the careful analysis of the existing data. The goal of surgical intervention should not be to lengthen the intestine per se, but rather to improve the functionality and efficiency of the remaining adapted intestine without further loss of length. This highlights the importance of allowing innate adaptation and growth to take place prior to any discussion of autologous reconstruction. Furthermore, for both LILT and STEP, a dilated bowel is necessary in order to allow for a successful technical operation. Although data on the exact appropriate age are lacking, in the absence of a compelling reason to operate sooner, surgery should be delayed until at least 12 months of age and after dedicated attempts to maximize enteral feeds have reached their full potential. Patient selection needs to include a careful assessment of hepatic function, as severe liver disease is a universal predictor of a poor outcome. Intestinal transplantation can be offered when other methods have failed, such as repeated life-threatening complications associated with PN. Intestinal transplantation has been performed with improved results over the past decade with 75% graft and 80% patient survival at 1 year in 2005. Among patients without pretransplant liver failure, 3-year survival rates as high as 90% have been reported. With improvement in multidisciplinary management of SBS at dedicated centers, hopefully the surgical options available to these patients will continue to improve.

## SUMMARY

The care of patients with SBS is complex and benefits from a multidisciplinary approach. With careful attention to management of growth and nutrition and the prevention of complications, the medical management of these patients has improved over the past decade. In addition, the surgical reconstructive procedures to maximize the function of the remaining bowel have provided another avenue for decreasing PN requirements and improving the quality of life. Scientific advances continue to improve our knowledge of the mechanisms behind intestinal growth and adaptation. The significant growth potential of the remnant bowel after resection often leads to clinical improvement beyond what seems initially possible when faced with a critically ill patient after a major intestinal resection. Further advances in the care of these difficult patients will hopefully lead to improved long-term outcomes in the future.

## SELECTED READINGS

Aguayo P, Fraser JD, Sharp S, St Peter SD, Ostlie DJ. Stomal complications in the newborn with necrotizing enterocolitis. *J Surg Res* 2009;157(2):275–278.

Al-Hudhaif J, Phillips S, Gholum S, Puligandla PP, Flageole H. The timing of enterostomy reversal after necrotizing enterocolitis. *J Pediatr Surg* 2009;44(5):924–927.

Andorsky DJ, Lund DP, Lillehei CW, et al. Nutritional and other postoperative management of neonates with short bowel syndrome correlates with clinical outcomes. *J Pediatr* 2001;139(1):27–33.

Bianchi A. Intestinal loop lengthening—a technique for increasing small intestinal length. *J Pediatr Surg* 1980;15(2):145–151.

Buchman A. Total parenteral nutrition-associated liver disease. *J Parenter Enteral Nutr* 2002;26(5 Suppl):S43–S48.

Buchman AL. Etiology and initial management of short bowel syndrome. *Gastroenterology* 2006;130(2 Suppl 1):S5–S15.

Byrne TA, Morrissey TB, Nattakom TV, Ziegler TR, Wilmore DW. Growth hormone, glutamine, and a modified diet enhance nutrient absorption in patients with severe short bowel syndrome. *J Parenter Enteral Nutr.* 1995;19(4):296–302.

Cober MP, Kovacevich DS, Teitelbaum DH. Ethanol-lock therapy for the prevention of central venous access device infections in pediatric patients with intestinal failure. *J Parenter Enteral Nutr* 2011;35(1):67–73.

Cole CR, Hansen NI, Higgins RD, Ziegler TR, Stoll BJ. Very low birth weight preterm infants with surgical short bowel syndrome: incidence, morbidity and mortality, and growth outcomes at 18 to 22 months. *Pediatrics* 2008;122(3):e573–e582.

Diamond IR, Sterescu A, Pencharz PB, Wales PW. The rationale for the use of parenteral omega-3 lipids in children with short bowel syndrome and liver disease. *Pediatr Surg Int* 2008;24(7):773–778.

Fishbein TM, Matsumoto CS. Intestinal replacement therapy: timing and indications for referral of patients to an intestinal rehabilitation and transplant program. *Gastroenterology* 2006;130(2 Suppl 1):S147–S151.

Fishbein TM. Intestinal transplantation. *N Engl J Med* 2009;361(10):998–1008.

Georgeson K, Halpin D, Figueroa R, Vincente Y, Hardin W Jr. Sequential intestinal lengthening procedures for refractory short bowel syndrome. *J Pediatr Surg* 1994;29(2):316–320; discussion 320–311.

Goday PS. Short bowel syndrome: how short is too short? *Clin Perinatol* 2009;36(1):101–110.

Hoffer EK, Cosgrove JM, Levin DQ, Herskowitz MM, Sclafani SJ. Radiologic gastrojejunostomy and percutaneous endoscopic gastrostomy: a prospective, randomized comparison. *J Vasc Interv Radiol* 1999;10(4):413–420.

Hosie S, Loff S, Wirth H, Rapp HJ, von Buch C, Waag KL. Experience of 49 longitudinal intestinal lengthening procedures for short bowel syndrome. *Eur J Pediatr Surg* 2006;16(3):171–175.

Javid PJ, Malone FR, Reyes J, Healey PJ, Horslen SP. The experience of a regional pediatric intestinal failure program: successful outcomes from intestinal rehabilitation. *Am J Surg* 2010;199(5):676–679.

Kim HB, Fauza D, Garza J, Oh JT, Nurko S, Jaksic T. Serial transverse enteroplasty (STEP): a novel bowel lengthening procedure. *J Pediatr Surg* 2003;38(3):425–429.

Kurkchubasche AG, Smith SD, Rowe MI. Catheter sepsis in short-bowel syndrome. *Arch Surg* 1992;127(1):21–24; discussion 24–25.

Mermel LA, Allon M, Bouza E, et al. Clinical practice guidelines for the diagnosis and management of intravascular catheter-related infection: 2009 Update by the Infectious Diseases Society of America. *Clin Infect Dis* 2009;49(1):1–45.

Miyasaka EA, Brown PI, Kadoura S, Harris MB, Teitelbaum DH. The adolescent child with short bowel syndrome: new onset of failure to thrive and need for increased nutritional supplementation. *J Pediatr Surg* 2010;45(6):1280–1286.

Modi BP, Javid PJ, Jaksic T, et al. First report of the international serial transverse enteroplasty data registry: indications, efficacy, and complications. *J Am Coll Surg* 2007;204(3):365–371.

Modi BP, Langer M, Ching YA, et al. Improved survival in a multidisciplinary short bowel syndrome program. *J Pediatr Surg* 2008;43(1):20–24.

Mouw E, Chessman K, Lesher A, Tagge E. Use of an ethanol lock to prevent catheter-related infections in children with short bowel syndrome. *J Pediatr Surg* 2008;43(6):1025–1029.

Nah SA, Narayanaswamy B, Eaton S, et al. Gastrostomy insertion in children: percutaneous endoscopic or percutaneous image-guided? *J Pediatr Surg* 2010;45(6):1153–1158.

Olieman JF, Penning C, Ijsselstijn H, et al. Enteral nutrition in children with short-bowel syndrome: current evidence and recommendations for the clinician. *J Am Diet Assoc* 2010;110(3):420–426.

Puppala BL, Mangurten HH, Kraut JR, et al. Distal ileostomy drip feedings in neonates with short bowel syndrome. *J Pediatr Gastroenterol Nutr* 1985;4(3):489–494.

Reinshagen K, Kabs C, Wirth H, et al. Long-term outcome in patients with short bowel syndrome after longitudinal intestinal lengthening and tailoring. *J Pediatr Gastroenterol Nutr* 2008;47(5):573–578.

Richardson L, Banerjee S, Rabe H. What is the evidence on the practice of mucous fistula refeeding in neonates with short bowel syndrome? *J Pediatr Gastroenterol Nutr* 2006;43(2):267–270.

Spencer AU, Neaga A, West B, et al. Pediatric short bowel syndrome: redefining predictors of success. *Ann Surg* 2005;242(3):403–409; discussion 409–412.

Struijs MC, Diamond IR, de Silva N, Wales PW. Establishing norms for intestinal length in children. *J Pediatr Surg* 2009;44(5):933–938.

Sudan D, Thompson J, Botha J, et al. Comparison of intestinal lengthening procedures for patients with short bowel syndrome. *Ann Surg* 2007;246(4):593–601; discussion 601–594.

Weber TR, Keller MS. Adverse effects of liver dysfunction and portal hypertension on intestinal adaptation in short bowel syndrome in children. *Am J Surg* 2002;184(6):582–586; discussion 586.

Wu GH, Wu ZH, Wu ZG. Effects of bowel rehabilitation and combined trophic therapy on intestinal adaptation in short bowel patients. *World J Gastroenterol* 2003;9(11):2601–2604.

# CHAPTER 51

## Gastrointestinal Duplications

*Mark F. Brown*

### KEY POINTS

1. Gastrointestinal duplications may occur anywhere from the mouth to the anus.

2. Symptoms may be related to compression of normal structures, such as respiratory distress from compression of the airway or compression of the bowel by a cystic duplication causing obstruction. Symptoms may be related to mass effect with pain or obstruction of the pancreatic duct or common bile duct with either pancreatitis or jaundice.

3. Symptoms may be caused by a mass lesion with subsequent torsion of the intestine.

4. Ectopic gastric mucosa may cause symptoms by acid production in areas where the mucosa is not structured to handle the acid load; this results in bleeding or perforation.

5. Symptoms may be related to a connection from a thoracoabdominal duplication to the spine with meningitis.

6. Duplications may be tubular or cystic.

7. Infection may cause a duplication to rapidly enlarge. This is most significant if the lesion is near the airway.

8. Treatment of duplications is complete resection if possible. In cases where complete resection is not possible the principles of treatment include drainage of the lesion into the gastrointestinal tract and removal or destruction of any ectopic gastric muscoa.

9. If the duplication has a spinal connection, this must be dealt with at the time of resection.

---

Duplications are located throughout the gastrointestinal tract from the mouth to the anus. They vary widely in size and are either spherical or tubular. They possess a well-developed layer of the smooth muscle and a mucous membrane lining derived from some part of the gastrointestinal tract. Most, but not all, lesions are attached to the gastrointestinal tract. Thoracic duplications may share a muscular wall with the esophagus or may lie in a distant position, whereas duplications in the abdomen usually share a muscular wall and lie in the mesentery of the gastrointestinal tract. Table 51-1 summarizes the location of duplications in a number of recently published series.

### EMBRYOLOGY

Multiple theories exist as to the embryologic cause of duplications. None of these theories can completely explain all types and their associated anomalies. It is possible that some combination of these theories is correct or that these lesions occur through some undefined mechanism. Bremer postulated that duplications were caused by aberrant recanalization of the "solid stage" of intestinal development. Lewis and Thyng suggested the diverticular theory, and Bentley developed the split-notochord theory to explain the 15% duplications associated with spinal anomalies and the neuroenteric connections that may exist. Mellish and Koop proposed that environmental factors may be associated with multiple duplications.

### ORAL AND LINGUAL DUPLICATIONS

Oral and lingual duplications present as an asymptomatic mass in the oral region. The diagnosis is usually made by the pathologist after the excision is completed. These lesions may contain ectopic gastric mucosa. The presence of an oral cyst or mass lesion in the mouth or pharynx is an indication for excision. Treatment involves excision with closure of the remaining mucosa.

### ESOPHAGEAL DUPLICATIONS

#### Essentials of Diagnosis

1. Esophageal duplications may present with dysphagia or respiratory symptoms.

2. Esophageal duplications usually present as a cystic lesion of the mediastinum.

3. Esophageal duplications have a 43% incidence of ectopic gastric mucosa.

651

**TABLE 51-1    Distribution of Intestinal Duplications by Anatomic Site in Several Recent Large Series**

| Author | Cervical | Esophageal | Thoracoabdominal | Gastric | Duodenal | Small Intestinal | Colonic | Rectal | Total |
|---|---|---|---|---|---|---|---|---|---|
| Bower | 0 | 15 | 1 | 8 | 4 | 34 | 12 | 2 | 76 |
| Gross | 1 | 13 | 3 | 2 | 4 | 32 | 9 | 4 | 68 |
| Grosfeld | 0 | 4 | 2 | 1 | 0 | 9 | 4 | 0 | 20 |
| Holcomb | 1 | 20 | 3 | 8 | 2 | 47 | 20 | 0 | 101 |
| Ilstad | 0 | 6 | 0 | 1 | 0 | 13 | 0 | 0 | 20 |
| Mellish and Koop | 1 | 6 | 2 | 1 | 0 | 18 | 6 | 4 | 38 |
| Stringer | 0 | 12 | 6 | 7 | 3 | 17 | 3 | 6 | 54 |
| Percent of Total | 1% | 20% | 5% | 7% | 3% | 45% | 14% | 4% | |

## Presenting Signs and Symptoms

Esophageal duplications are relatively uncommon (Table 51-1). In a review of 495 alimentary tract duplications, the esophagus was the site of 19% of the lesions. An additional 4% of the lesions were thoracoabdominal. Most esophageal duplications are cystic in shape and do not have a shared muscular wall with the esophagus although, rarely, they do connect to the esophageal lumen (Fig. 51-1). The mucosal lining of esophageal duplications contains gastric mucosa in 43% of cases, but may contain pseudostratified columnar, small intestinal, or large intestinal mucosa. This gastric mucosa may lead to ulceration, pain, and hemorrhage.

The esophagus can be divided into 3 parts: the cervical third, the middle third, and the lower third. Duplications occur in all segments of the esophagus; however, the presentation may vary. Cervical duplications account for 23% of esophageal duplications. They may present as an asymptomatic neck mass or with symptoms of upper-airway obstruction. These can be confused with cystic hygroma, thyroglossal duct cyst, branchial cleft cyst, or solid tumors such as teratomas. Duplications of the middle portion comprise 17% of esophageal duplications. These usually present with compression of the trachea at a young age. The main differential diagnosis is bronchogenic cysts. Distal esophageal duplications are the most common and are often asymptomatic.

## Complications

The most common complication of esophageal duplications is respiratory distress. In the Holcomb series, 9 of 21 patients presented with respiratory distress. These lesions also present early in childhood, as 18 of 21 patients in this series presented before 2 years of age. Older children presented with dysphagia.

## Diagnosis

The diagnosis is usually suspected based on a chest x-ray revealing a posterior mediastinal mass. Often this x-ray is obtained because of respiratory distress, although it may be part of an evaluation for fever or other respiratory symptoms not related to the duplication. Another study that can be helpful is an esophagogram, which usually reveals an indentation on the esophagus by the lesion. An esophagogram rarely shows a connection between the esophagus and duplication. A computed tomography (CT) scan is the most helpful study because it can provide much better anatomic detail of the relationship of the lesion to other thoracic and mediastinal structures. A CT scan can also reveal other anatomic details, such as a lesion that extends below the diaphragm.

## Associated Conditions

Vertebral lesions including the hemivertebrae, spinal fusion defects, and spina bifida are associated with esophageal duplications in approximately 25% of patients. These vertebral lesions are rarely associated with neuroenteric connections that can lead to meningitis. Abdominal duplications have been reported in up to 25% of patients with esophageal duplications.

## Treatment

The presence of an esophageal duplication or cystic mediastinal mass is an indication for operation. Even if the lesion is an incidental finding and is asymptomatic, it should be removed for diagnostic purposes and to prevent complications such as bleeding, perforation, and airway compromise. Lesions in patients exhibiting respiratory distress or dysphagia should be removed to correct these symptoms.

Resection is the treatment of choice. The majority of esophageal duplications noted in large series were treated with simple resection via thoracotomy and no other techniques were needed. Although neuroenteric connections are unusual, careful observation for these is wise. Thoracoscopic resection of these lesions is an excellent technique that is much more common over the past 10 years. Thoracoscopic resection is technically demanding but these technical skills are much more common than in the past. Other cystic mediastinal

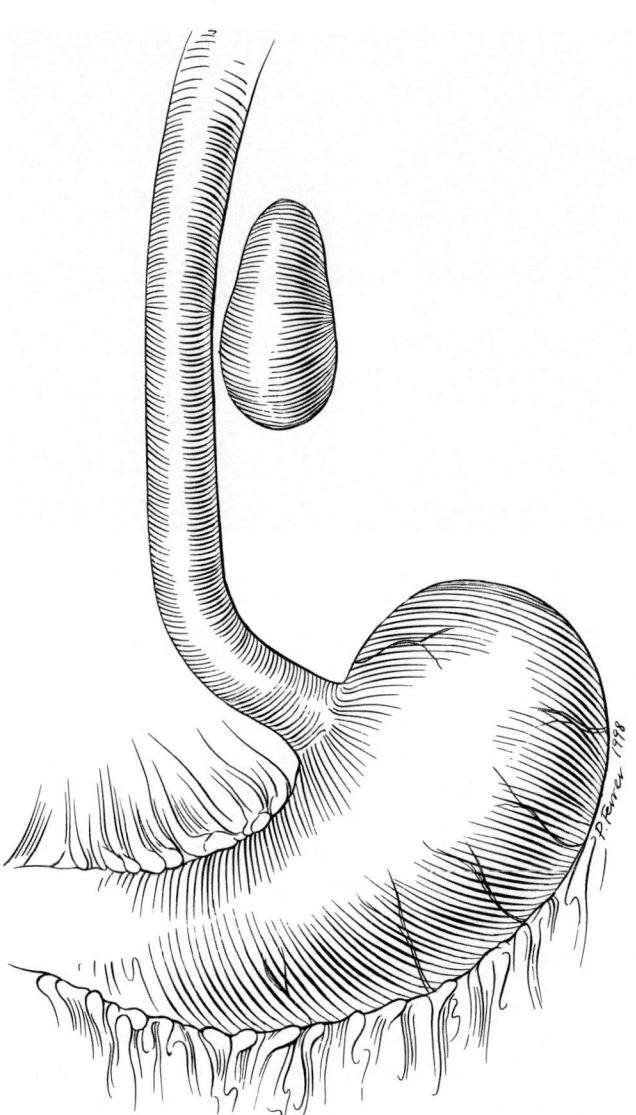

**FIGURE 51-1** Diagram of a midesophageal duplication cyst without a connection to the esophagus. When lined by squamous epithelium, such a bronchopulmonary foregut malformation, presenting as a mediastinal mass, is termed an esophageal duplication; however, when lined by ciliated columnar epithelium, it is a bronchogenic cyst.

lesions, such as bronchogenic cysts, have been removed using thoracoscopic technique. Other options described include resection of the lesion with a segment of esophagus. This should only be needed in unusual circumstances since the surgeon is usually able to separate the duplication from the esophagus. Rarely, when the duplication connects to the esophageal lumen, resection of the duplication with closure of the esophagotomy and buttressing the closure with a pleural or intercostal muscle flap is indicated. Other treatments, such as marsupialization of the cyst to the chest wall and destruction of the mucosa with packing and curettage, are of historical interest only.

The long-term outcome for these patients is excellent if the lesion is resected without complications. Complications of resection include anastomotic strictures if a segment of the esophagus is resected. Phrenic nerve and thoracic duct injuries have also been reported. Deaths from resection are unusual but are reported.

## THORACOABDOMINAL DUPLICATIONS

### Essentials of Diagnosis

1. Thoracoabdominal duplications commonly present with respiratory distress or vomiting.
2. Thoracoabdominal duplications usually present with a tubular lesion that traverses the diaphragm from the chest to the abdomen.
3. Thoracoabdominal duplications may be associated with vertebral abnormalities.
4. Thoracoabdominal duplications have a 29% incidence of ectopic gastric mucosa.

### Presenting Signs and Symptoms

Thoracoabdominal duplications are rare. In a review of several large series on duplications, 364 patients with duplications were identified. Eighty-four had thoracic duplications; 15 of these 84 were thoracoabdominal. Presenting symptoms include respiratory distress, vomiting, gastrointestinal bleeding, and meningitis. The thoracic portion of these lesions occur most commonly on the right side.

### Complications

Serious complications of thoracoabdominal resections have been reported, including incomplete resection with recurrent cysts in the chest, missed tracts from the chest to the abdomen, meningitis, hemothorax, jejunal fistula, incomplete excision of the jejunal tubular component, and ileal necrosis after mucosal excision of an ileal tubular duplication

### Associated Conditions

Thoracoabdominal lesions have a high association of vertebral anomalies and neuroenteric connections. In the chest, the lesions are retropleural and may extend to the neck. The abdominal components may connect to the stomach, pylorus, duodenum, pancreas, jejunum, or ileum (Fig. 51-2).

### Treatment

Resection of thoracoabdominal duplications is more complex than resection of duplications confined to one body cavity. A variety of approaches have been described, including resection of the chest and abdominal portions at separate procedures several weeks apart. Some children require laminectomy in association with the resection. The current trend appears to be a combination of thoracotomy and laparotomy with complete resection of the lesion in 1 stage. Minimally invasive techniques can be used to resect these lesions. The spinal component, if present, must always be considered when planning the operation.

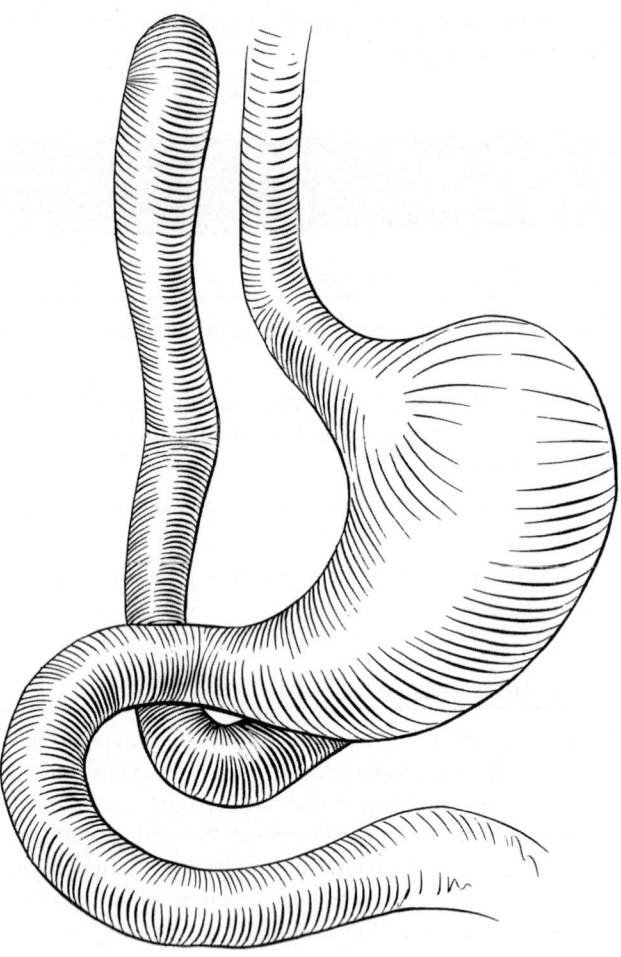

**FIGURE 51-2** Diagram of a thoracoabdominal duplication with an abdominal connection to the gastric antrum.

## GASTRIC DUPLICATIONS

### Essentials of Diagnosis

1. Gastric duplications are twice as common in females as in males.

2. Gastric duplications present with vomiting and GI bleeding.

3. Gastric duplications are usually associated with an upper abdominal cystic lesion.

### Presenting Signs and Symptoms

Gastric duplications usually present before the age of 1 year. They occur twice as often in girls as in boys. The most common symptom at presentation is nonbilious vomiting. Gastrointestinal hemorrhage is frequently seen, either as melena or as hematemesis. Other presenting symptoms include abdominal mass, failure to thrive, and abdominal pain. In a review of 88 gastric duplications, 58 occurred on the greater curve, 7 on the lesser curve, 5 on the anterior wall, 9 on the posterior wall, and 2 in the pylorus.

### Complications

The most common complication of gastric duplications is gastrointestinal bleeding, which occurred in 27 of 55 cases in

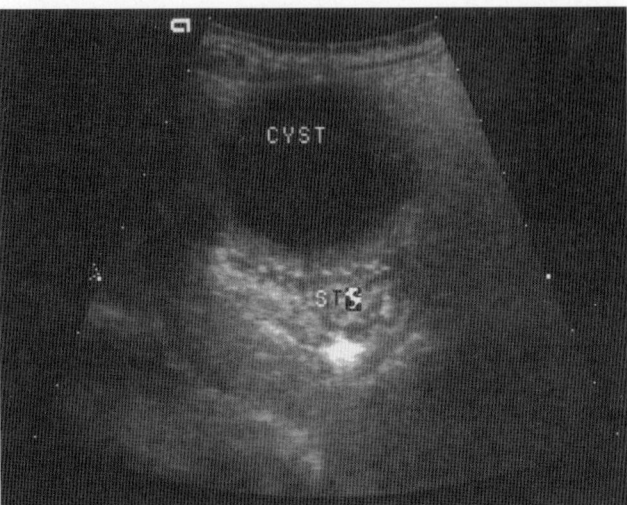

**FIGURE 51-3** Abdominal ultrasound exam demonstrating a gastric duplication. An in utero ultrasound of the fetus had demonstrated an upper abdominal cystic structure.

1 review. Other complications include perforation with peritonitis, recurrence of the cyst after incomplete resection, perforation with fistulous connection to the spleen and left lower lobe of the lung, and fistulous connection to the right lower lobe of the lung. Untreated gastric duplications are associated with malignant degeneration.

### Diagnosis

The suspected diagnosis of gastric duplication has historically been confirmed by upper GI series or by ultrasound (Fig. 51-3). CT scan is an excellent way to delineate the dimensions and anatomic boundaries of the lesion; it has the added advantage of contrast in the GI tract, which will help to determine whether a connection to the stomach is present (Fig. 51-4). Because pancreatic pseudocysts are the most common cysts in the lesser sac, the most common error in diagnosis is mistaking a gastric duplication for a pancreatic pseudocyst.

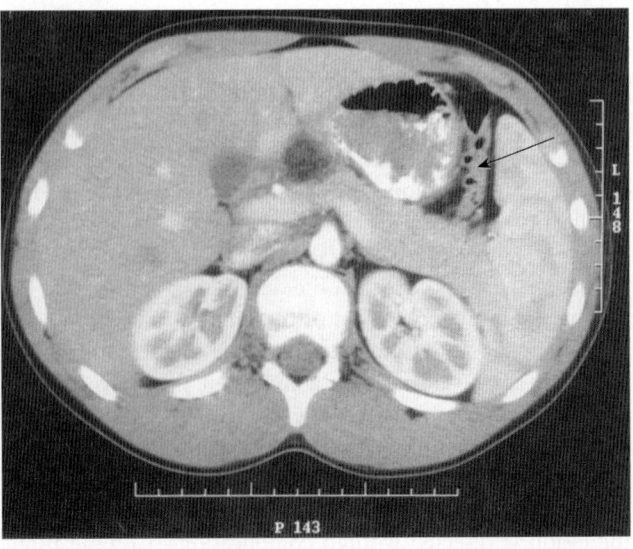

**FIGURE 51-4** Abdominal CT image showing a greater curvature gastric duplication cyst (arrow).

## Associated Conditions

Few specific anomalies are commonly associated with gastric duplications. Case reports of an imperforate anus and vertebral anomalies do appear in the literature. Pancreatitis has been reported in association with gastric or duodenal duplications and will be discussed subsequently.

## Treatment

Because gastric duplications have a high rate of complications, most commonly bleeding, the presence of the lesion is an indication for resection. Most lesions occur on the greater curve of the stomach and share blood supply with the stomach via the gastroepiploic vessels. Excision of the cyst, including its mucosa, and part of the common wall, with closure of the serosal defect, is the simplest treatment (Fig. 51-5). An alternate but similar method is the technique of White. The cyst is first aspirated under direct vision to prevent spillage and to make the excision easier. The cyst is then opened along its entire length. This produces 2 "flaps" of the cyst, with the base of the flaps on the common wall. Each of these flaps is resected back to the common wall, being careful to protect the gastroepiploic vessels. Next, the small mucosal strip at the base is stripped off the stomach. In the original description of this technique, the transverse colon was sutured to the "bed" of the cyst. Lembert sutures may be used to invert the raw area if it is not too large. One other option for resection is to remove the entire common wall and reconstruct the stomach. This option is best for those lesions that connect to the stomach and in which there is difficulty in separating the cyst from the stomach.

If the cyst connects to the lumen of the stomach, the connection must be sutured after the duplication is resected. Care should be taken after any such resection to check the integrity of the stomach by filling it with air through the nasogastric tube and checking for leaks.

## Pyloric Duplications

Pyloric duplications are a rare form of gastric duplication. Figure 51-6 shows a large pyloric duplication attached on

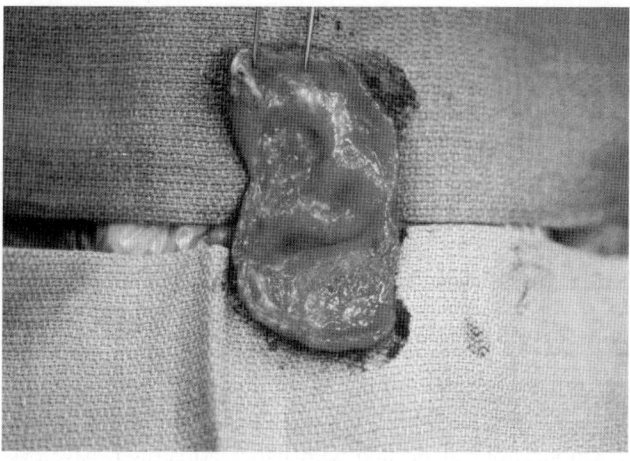

**FIGURE 51-5** Postresection specimen of a greater curvature gastric duplication cyst.

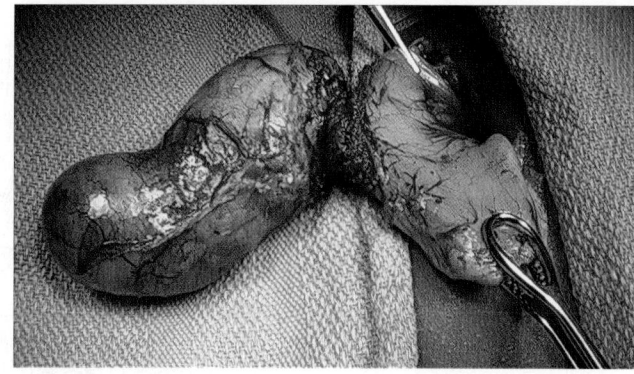

**FIGURE 51-6** A large pyloric duplication attached to the greater curve of the stomach at the pylorus. The ring forceps are on the greater curve of the stomach, and the DeBakey forceps point to the duodenum. The resection is partially complete circumferentially and you can see the separation of the duplication from the pylorus. The duplication was completely removed without opening the gastric mucosa.

the greater curvature of the stomach at the pylorus. A recent review found only 13 reported cases. The average age at presentation was 27 days, with the oldest being 5 months. Unlike gastric duplications that have a significant female preponderance, 7 of 13 patients were male. The size of the cysts ranged from 1 to 8 cm and none of the cysts communicated with the lumen. Most infants were initially felt to have pyloric stenosis. Ten of the 13 patients in the review presented with vomiting, and 7 had a palpable abdominal mass. Upper GI series and ultrasound were the most common diagnostic modalities. The surgical treatment of choice is complete extramucosal excision of the duplication. Other procedures have been done, including gastrojejunostomy and mucosal stripping; however, these more complicated procedures are rarely indicated.

## Duodenal Duplications

### Essentials of Diagnosis

1. Duodenal duplication's male incidence is equal to that in females.
2. Duodenal duplications often present with vomiting and GI bleeding.
3. Duodenal duplications may present with jaundice.
4. Duodenal duplications present with a cystic mass in the pancreatic and duodenal area.

Duodenal duplications are an unusual form of gastrointestinal duplications. In a review of 281 GI duplications, 5% were duodenal duplications. They occur in the first and second portions of the duodenum, are commonly cystic, and usually do not connect to the duodenal lumen. The most common location is on the mesenteric side of the anterior wall (Fig. 51-7). Most duodenal duplications are single, although they have been reported to occur in association with the Meckel diverticulum and other duodenal, gastric, thoracic, and ileal duplications.

### Presenting Signs and Symptoms

Duodenal duplications usually present before the age of 10 years, and at least half present in the first few months of

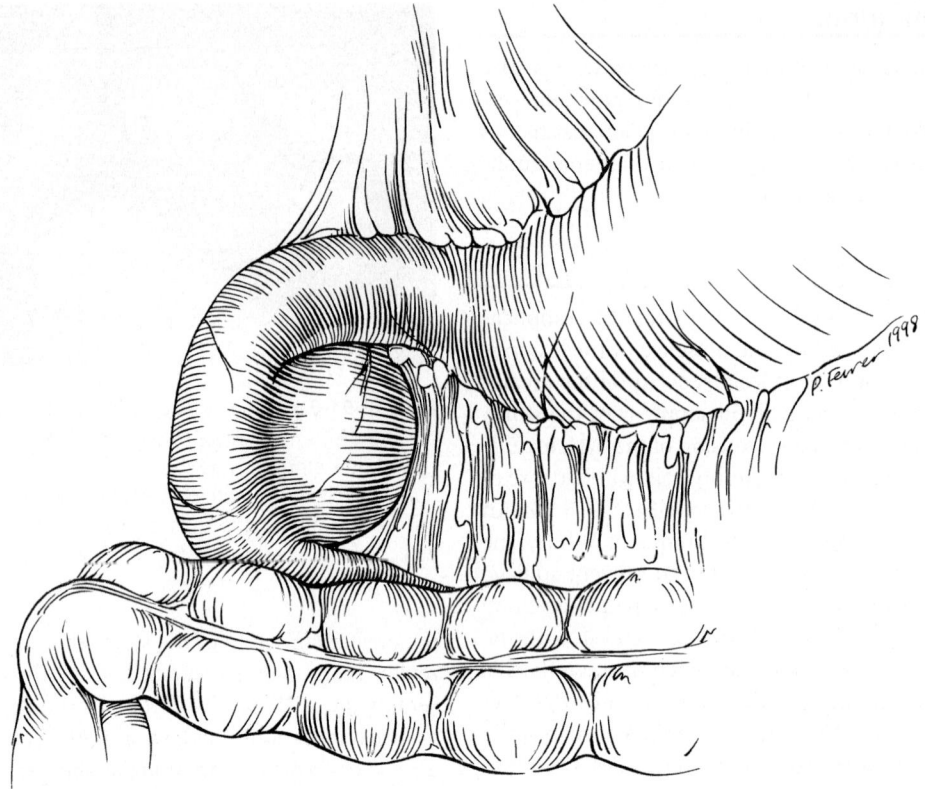

**FIGURE 51-7** Duodenal duplication located within the "C-loop" of the duodenum. The duplication and the duodenum share a common muscular wall.

life. Males and females are equally affected. In a large review of the literature, vomiting and gastrointestinal bleeding were the most common presenting symptoms. A palpable mass was noted in 22 of 55 cases and 1 patient presented with obstructive jaundice. Both biliary colic and pancreatitis have been described in association with duodenal duplications.

## Complications

Complications include duodenal obstruction, biliary obstruction, pancreatitis, necrosis of the duplication, and perforation of the duplication.

## Diagnosis

The diagnosis can be made on upper GI series, although ultrasound and CT scan are excellent, and are better imaging studies for this lesion. The presence of a cyst with motility in its wall as seen on ultrasound is highly suggestive of a duplication. Other helpful studies may include endoscopic retrograde cholangiopancreatography (ERCP) in that some lesions connect to the pancreatic duct, and (2, 6 diisoprepyl acelanilid) technetium-99m iminodiacetic acid scan or magnetic resonance cholangiopancreatography (MRCP) to rule out choledochal cyst.

## Treatment

Several treatment options are available, including resection of the cyst either alone or with the duodenum. Usually, the lesions contain duodenal mucosa; however, they contain gastric mucosa in 21% of cases. The presence of gastric mucosa is an important factor because total resection of those cysts, if possible, may lead to fewer peptic complications in the postoperative period. The original operation described to treat duodenal duplications is the transduodenal opening of a connection or window between the cyst and the duodenum. Care must be taken to protect the bile duct when using this procedure. This same concept has been expanded to include endoscopic creation of a window between the cyst and duodenum. Another option is drainage of the cyst with a Roux-en-Y cystojejunostomy. The advantage of this procedure is its simplicity and a lesser dissection. This option is good if resection of the lesion is likely to compromise the vascularity to the duodenum or disrupt the biliary system. It seems prudent to use this option if the cyst does not contain gastric mucosa on frozen section.

## DUPLICATIONS ASSOCIATED WITH PANCREATITIS

### Essentials of Diagnosis

1. In these duplications recurrent abdominal pain and pancreatitis are common.

2. Duplications associated with pancreatitis often have cystic lesion in the area of the pancreas that may be confused with a pancreatic pseudocysts.

## Presenting Signs and Symptoms

Duplications that are associated with pancreatitis may be gastric, duodenal, or pancreatic in origin. Not all are connected to the gastrointestinal tract, but nearly 100% have a connection either to the normal pancreatic duct of Wirsung or to an aberrant pancreatic lobe. Sixty-two percent of the lesions occur in the head of the pancreas (Fig. 51-8). The pathophysiology of this type of pancreatitis is poorly defined. In 1 review, most of the patients had symptoms of nausea, vomiting, weight loss, and abdominal pain. Often, this pain was associated with food intake. Twenty percent of the patients reviewed had at least 1 of these symptoms and 81% had at least 2 of these symptoms. Most patients had multiple bouts of pancreatitis, although these bouts often went undiagnosed. Fifteen percent of the patients had multiple hospitalizations for undiagnosed abdominal pain, 25% of the patients underwent previous psychiatric evaluations, and 11 of the patients had a previous laparotomy for the pain. Physical exam showed abdominal tenderness and 3% of the patients had a palpable abdominal mass.

## Complications

Complications other than pancreatitis included ascites, stone formation in the duplication, perforation with abscess, erosion into the transverse colon, perforation with pneumoperitoneum, and gastrointestinal bleeding.

## Diagnosis

The diagnosis of this lesion is difficult. Only 50% of the patients in 1 review had an elevated amylase when evaluated. An upper GI study is only helpful if the duplication is large enough and close to the duodenum or stomach so that an indentation is present. CT scan or ultrasound may show the lesion, although these may be confused with the much more common pancreatic pseudocyst. ERCP may be helpful in these lesions. ERCP is helpful in any case of recurrent pancreatitis without a clear cause and in the several cases noted in the literature, ERCP has been useful in delineating the anatomy of the duplication and its connection to the pancreas.

## Treatment

Operative intervention is the only curative treatment for these lesions. No one specific operation can be recommended for their treatment. Procedures used previously in the literature and noted to be curative include simple cystectomy; simple cystectomy with resection of an aberrant pancreatic lobe; partial cystectomy with resection of the mucosa and closure of any pancreatic ductal connection; cystotomy or partial cystectomy and drainage into the stomach, duodenum, or Roux-en-Y jejunal limb; partial pancreatectomy to include the cyst; and a Whipple procedure.

The best procedure for any one lesion is dependent upon the anatomy of the cyst and its connection to the pancreatic duct.

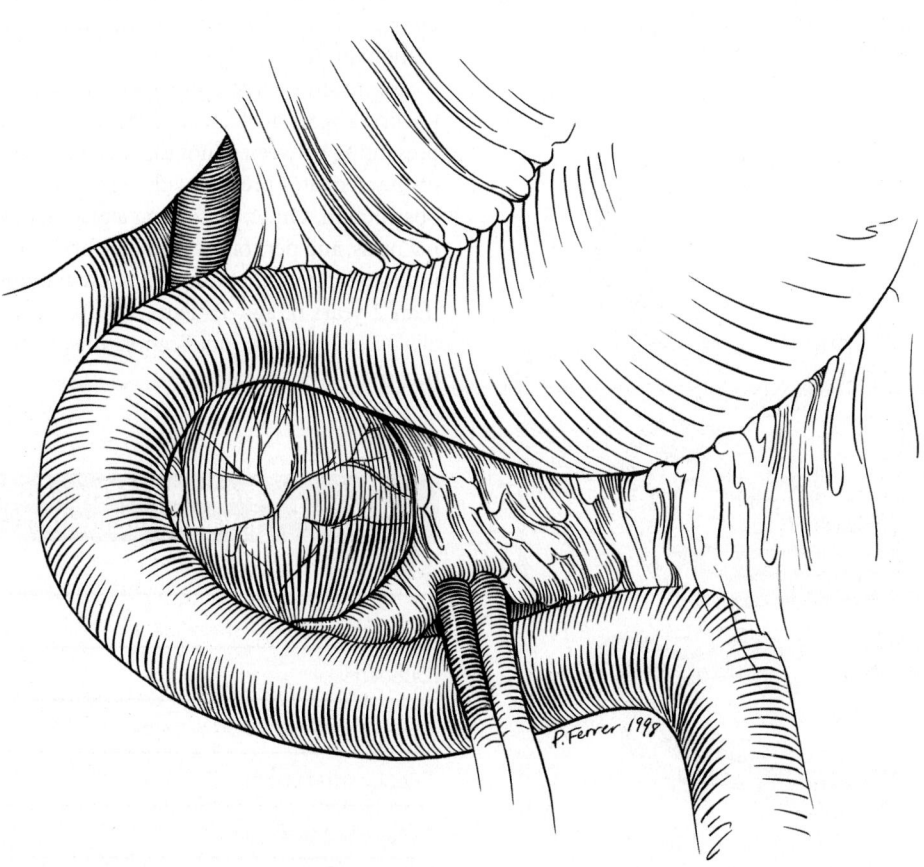

**FIGURE 51-8** Diagram of a duodenal duplication with communication to the pancreatic duct. This may contribute to a recurrent pancreatitis. The optimal treatment is complete excision of the cyst. An alternative therapy is internal drainage of the cyst if ectopic gastric mucosa is not present.

GASTROINTESTINAL DUPLICATIONS

657

Operations for this problem must be individualized; however, several principles are important. Ninety percent of these lesions contain gastric mucosa, so if resection is possible, it is preferable. If resection is not possible, removal of the mucosa to prevent peptic complications is important. Drainage of any dilated and obstructed ducts caused by chronic pancreatitis by using a Puestow procedure or Roux-en-Y limb is indicated, and the surgeon should be guided by the preoperative ERCP.

## SMALL-BOWEL DUPLICATIONS

### Essentials of Diagnosis

1. Small-bowel duplications usually present in the first 2 years of life.

2. In small-bowel duplications an abdominal mass is present most commonly in the ileocecal area.

3. Small-bowel duplications commonly presents with a small-bowel obstruction.

### Presenting Signs and Symptoms

Small-bowel duplications present in 2 forms: tubular and cystic. Tubular duplications follow the intestine for all or part of its length. Tubular duplications may be separate from the bowel, adherent with a separate but attached wall, or may share a common wall. They usually occur on the mesenteric side and share a blood supply with the intestine, although they occasionally have a separate blood supply (Fig. 51-9).

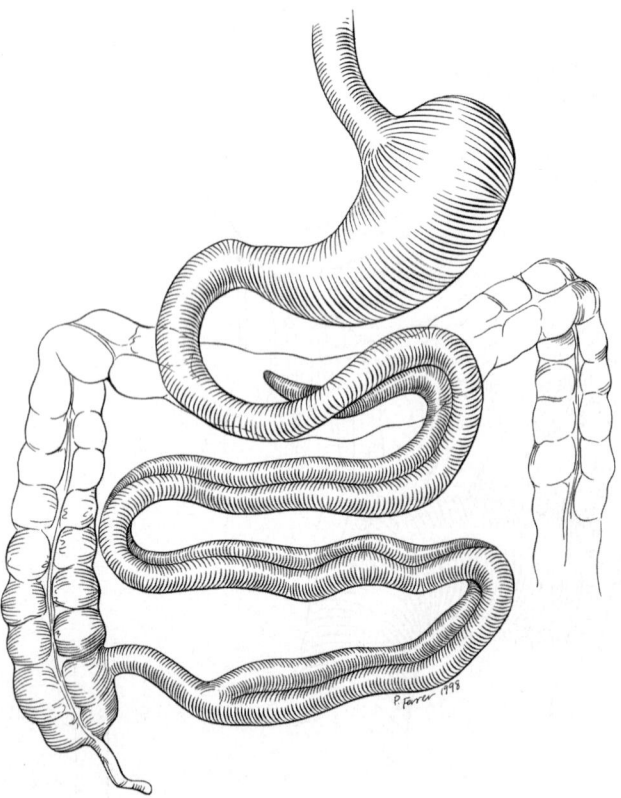

**FIGURE 51-9** Tubular duplication of the small bowel with a shared common wall and a distal communication.

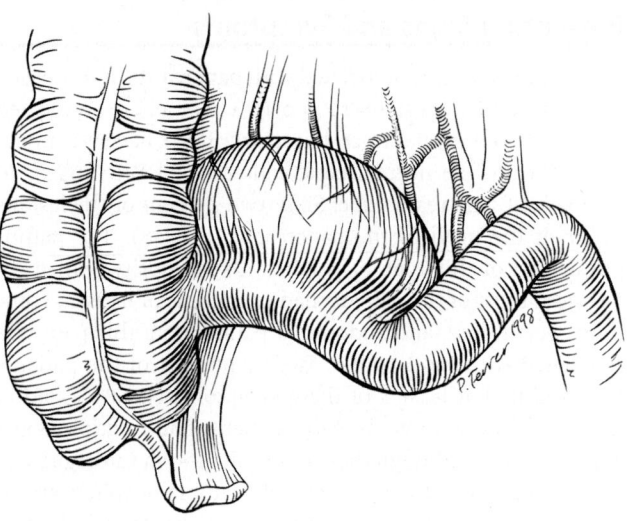

**FIGURE 51-10** Cystic ileal duplication along the mesenteric border of the bowel.

Cystic duplications most commonly occur at the ileocecal junction and share a common blood supply and wall with the ileum (Fig. 51-10). The most common ectopic mucosa is gastric and occurs in 33% of ileal and 50% of jejunal duplications. Ectopic gastric mucosa is more likely to occur in tubular duplications (80%) than in cystic duplications (20%) (Table 51-2). This is a particularly relevant point because tubular duplications are much more difficult to resect and if the ectopic mucosa is left in place, complications are likely. Untreated small-bowel duplications are associated with malignant degeneration.

Seventy-five percent of small-bowel duplications present in the first 2 years of life, with half presenting in neonates and half presenting between 1 month and 2 years of age. Eighty percent of the neonates present with signs and symptoms of a bowel obstruction. Other presenting signs include melena, abdominal mass, and peritonitis from perforation. Rectal bleeding and intussusception are common presentations in children older than 2 years of age. Patients who present with bleeding usually have a tubular duplication that contains ectopic gastric mucosa.

| **TABLE 51-2** | **Frequency of Ectopic Gastric Mucosa in Various Duplications** |
|---|---|
| Esophagus | 43% |
| Thoracoabdominal | 29% |
| Duodenal | 20% |
| Duplications associated with pancreatitis | 90% |
| Tubular small bowel | 80% |
| Cystic small bowel | 20% |
| Colon | 2% |
| Rectum | 10% |

## Complications

Complications of duplications include bleeding or perforation from ectopic gastric mucosa, obstruction, intussusception, and volvulus.

## Diagnosis

Preoperative diagnosis is much more common than in the past. The diagnosis is occasionally made at laparotomy for intestinal obstruction. Ultrasound or CT scan can be helpful in cystic duplications. Occasionally, ectopic mucosa in a duplication is seen on a Meckel scan performed for bleeding. Duplications can be associated with intestinal atresia and are seen as an incidental finding in these cases. Prenatal diagnosis is also possible. Duplications seen on prenatal ultrasound have the double-wall configuration seen in duplications and in the Meckel diverticula. The "Y" configuration of the vasculature entering the duplication is characteristic for a small-bowel duplications.

## Treatment

Operative resection of these lesions can take many forms. The simplest treatment is enucleation of the duplication. Enucleation of some duplications is possible because the blood supply to the small bowel divides and half goes to one side and half to the other side. Because of this, a few of the vessels on one side may be ligated and the bowel remains viable. This can allow resection of the duplication while leaving the normal bowel in situ. Despite this fact, enucleation is rarely possible because the duplications often have a shared blood supply with the intestine and they often share a common wall. For this reason, cystic duplications and short tubular duplications are most easily treated with resection of the duplication and juxtaposed small intestine. The intestine is then reconstructed with an end-to-end anastomosis (Fig. 51-11). In 1 study, 46 of 47 patients with jejunal and ileal duplications were able to be treated with this type of resection.

Long tubular duplications can be a therapeutic dilemma. If resection of the intestine is not an option because of the length of normal bowel that would have to be sacrificed, other options are available. Tubular duplications rarely have an autonomous blood supply, but if present, these can be resected separately from the normal bowel. Because tubular duplications have an 80% incidence of gastric mucosa, simple drainage of the distal end of the duplication into the intestine can cause peptic ulceration of the normal small intestine with bleeding or perforation and should be discouraged. The Wrenn method appears to be very useful in the difficult case of a long small-intestinal tubular duplication. This method includes an incision through the serosa and muscular layers at the distal end of the duplication. The mucosa is separated from the muscular cuff (much like the rectal dissection in a Soave procedure), and this dissection is carried as far proximal as is possible (usually about 15 cm). Multiple incisions may be necessary to strip the mucosa all the way to its proximal end (Fig. 51-12). Any defects made in the mucosa of the native bowel are repaired. Ischemia

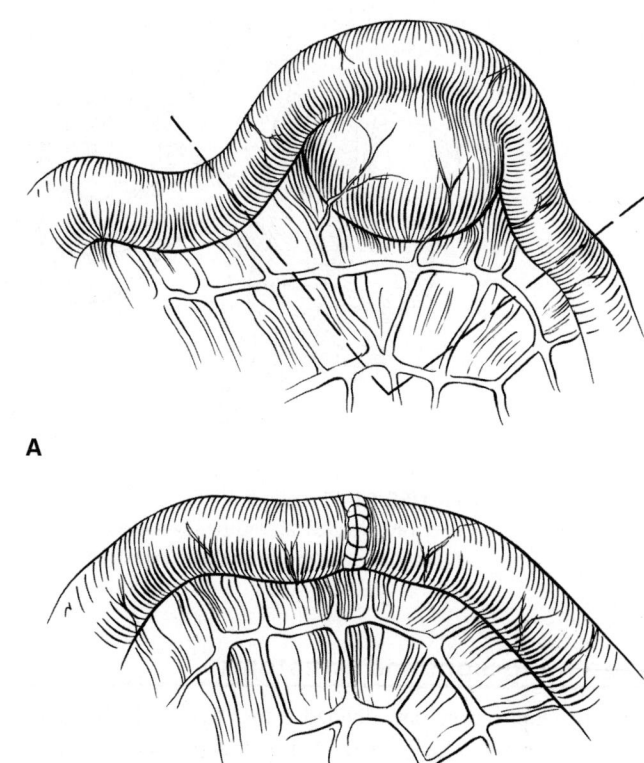

**FIGURE 51-11** Cystic ileal duplication. **A.** Margins of resection outlined taking care to preserve the proximal and distal bowel mesentery. **B.** End-to-end bowel anastomosis completed.

of the adjacent small intestine has been reported following this operation. Gastroduplication is a unique method of treatment of a long tubular duplication. This method was described in a patient in which the distal end of the lumen of the duplication was connected to the ileal lumen. The treatment included resection of the connection between the ileum and duplication with reconstruction of the normal ileum by end-to-end anastomosis (Fig. 51-13A). The distal end of the long duplication was then anastomosed to the stomach. This leaves the long duplication draining into the stomach (Fig. 51-13B). The acid production from any ectopic gastric mucosa is generally well tolerated by the stomach. This procedure has been done successfully and has withstood a 25-year follow-up without complications despite the fact that the duplication has ectopic gastric mucosa seen on the $^{99}$Tc Na-pertechnetate scan.

## COLONIC DUPLICATIONS

### Essentials of Diagnosis

1. Three types of colonic duplications are appendiceal, tubular, and cystic duplications.

2. In colonic duplications abdominal pain is common

3. Colonic duplications may present with either perforation or obstruction.

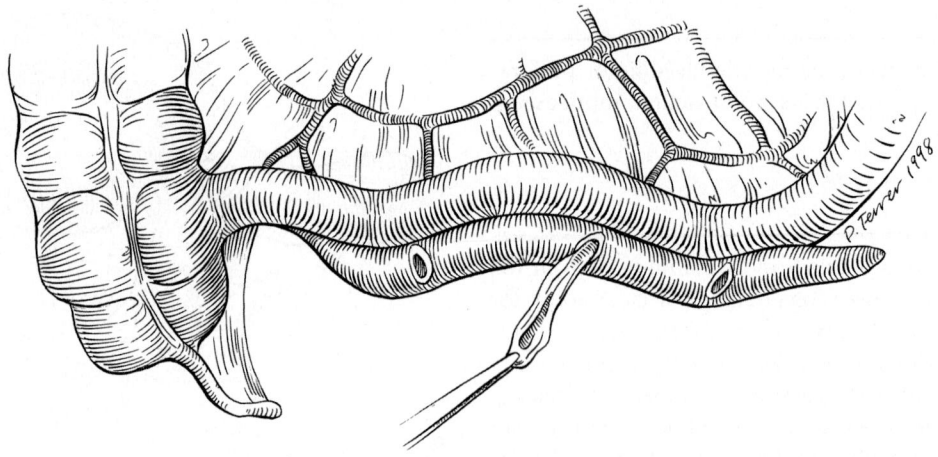

**FIGURE 51-12** Long tubular ileal duplication. Because a complete resection would sacrifice an extensive length of ileum, several enterotomies are made on the duplicated segment and the mucosa is "stripped" from the duplication.

## Presenting Signs and Symptoms

Colonic duplications are divided into 3 types: duplications of the appendix, which are treated with appendectomy; cystic duplications of the colon; and tubular duplications. Rectal duplications will be considered separately. Cystic duplications may present with vomiting, volvulus, abdominal mass, urinary retention, abdominal pain, or perforation presenting as an acute abdomen. Tubular colonic duplications present in various ways. Many are noted at birth in association with duplications of the genitals or bladder. Others present with acute or chronic lower intestinal obstruction, rectovaginal fistula, rectal prolapse, and urinary tract infections. The duplicated colon may be on the mesenteric or antimesenteric side of the colon. Those on the antimesenteric side may terminate as a fistula or

end blindly in the pelvis (Fig. 51-14A), those on the mesenteric side usually terminate as a fistula (Fig. 51-14B). The mucosal lining of these lesions is usually normal colonic mucosa.

Tubular colonic duplications have been divided into 5 groups:

1. *Group 1: Two perineal ani.* This anomaly is diagnostic for long-segment colon duplication. Most of these patients have normal anal sphincters and are asymptomatic. They have the highest rate of genitourinary duplications, malrotation, omphalocele, and the Meckel diverticulum.

2. *Group 2: Duplication in females with fistula(e).* This anomaly is seen if the patient has a rectovaginal or rectoperineal fistula in addition to a perineal anus. Other forms include the patient with 2 fistulae or if a fistula is noted in a patient

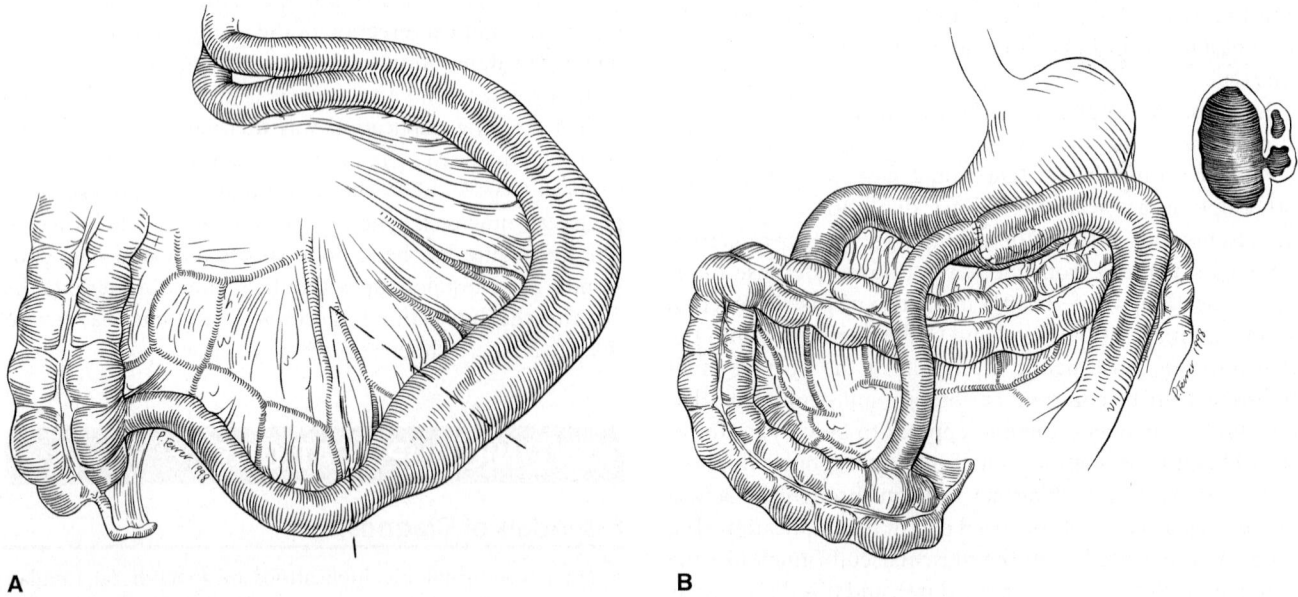

A           B

**FIGURE 51-13** The gastroduplication method of treatment of an obstructed extensive ileal tubular duplication. **A.** The distal end of the duplication is resected and an end-to-end anastomosis is done between the proximal and distal normal ileum. **B.** The distal end of the duplication is then anastomosed in a side-to-side fashion to the stomach to allow duplication content to drain into the stomach. No adverse effect of gastric acid on the small-bowel mucosa was noted after 10 years of patient follow-up.

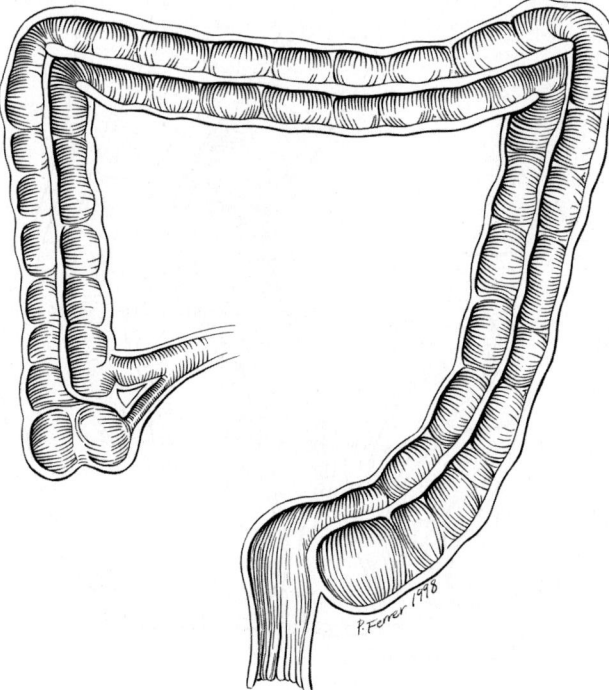

**A**

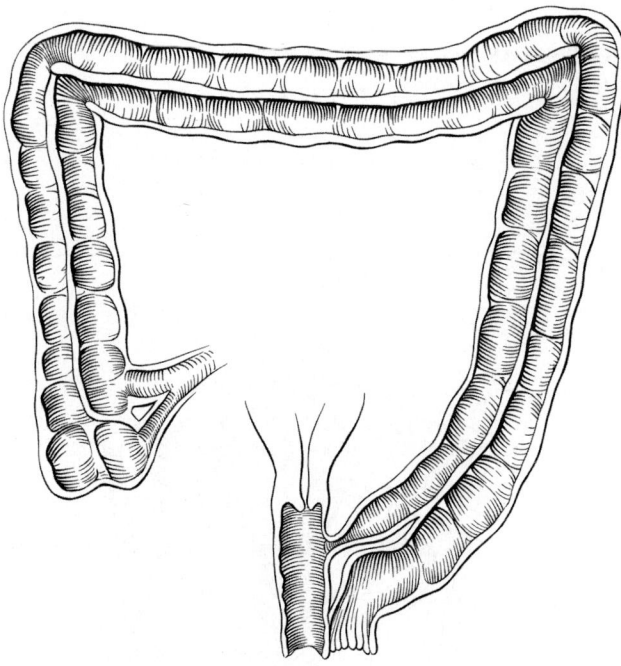

**B**

**FIGURE 51-14 A.** Drawing of a colonic duplication that ends blindly alongside the distal rectum. **B.** Drawing of a tubular duplication of the colon located along the mesenteric side of the bowel with a distal vaginal fistula.

with duplication of the genital organs or bladder. These patients may have constipation because of complete or partial obstruction of the duplicated colon filling with feces and compressing the normal colon.

3. *Group 3: Duplication in males with fistula(e).* Presence of 1 functioning perineal anus and a rectourinary fistula is the hallmark of this group of patients. They may have bifid scrotum or a double penis.

4. *Group 4: Duplication without fistula with imperforate anus.* These patients have the highest incidence of skeletal and urinary anomalies. Almost all have intestinal obstruction. These patients have either an imperforate anus with 2 anal dimples or 1 functioning anus and a second anal dimple. In the latter group, the patent rectum may be obstructed and pushed laterally by a large mass of feces in the obstructed rectum.

5. *Group 5: Single perineal anus with communicating duplication.* Patients with this form may be asymptomatic. The diagnosis may be suspected if the patient has urethral or bladder duplication.

## Complications

Complications of cystic duplications include volvulus, bowel obstruction, or perforation with rupture. Carcinoma has been reported in both cystic and tubular colonic duplications.

## Diagnosis

The diagnosis of cystic colonic duplication is often made at laparotomy. Ultrasound, CT scan, and barium enema may be helpful in evaluating these lesions. The diagnosis is usually made by a combination of perineal inspection, evaluation of the urinary tract, and contrast studies of the 2 colons. Cecal duplications with peristaltic movements have been identified on prenatal ultrasound.

## Associated Conditions

Associated anomalies are common. In 1 review of 57 colonic tubular duplications, only 11 patients had no other anomalies. Fourteen and 16 patients, respectively, had 2 and 3 systems with anomalies. Sixteen patients had anomalies in 4 or 5 systems. Urologic and spinal anomalies were the most common. Twenty-three patients had abnormalities of the bladder, which were usually a double bladder and urethra. Bladder exstrophy and septated bladder were occasionally seen. Thirteen patients had some anomaly of the kidneys themselves, including four with a solitary kidney. Twenty-five patients had genital anomalies, including double vagina, didelphic uterus, and double vulva. Double penis and bifid scrotum were seen in males. Gastrointestinal anomalies were seen in 28 patients and included double appendix, double ileum, omphalocele, the Meckel diverticulum, and malrotation. Eighteen patients had spinal abnormalities.

## Treatment

Surgical treatment of cystic duplications of the colon is much like that of cystic small-bowel duplications. Resection of the adjacent colon is the simplest treatment. The colon is reconstructed with an anastomosis.

Treatment of tubular colonic duplications is operative. Each case must be individualized. The main cause of symptoms is the distal obstructed pouch of the duplication that usually connects to the normal colon proximally and fills with feces, causing compression of the normal colon in the pelvis. This can be treated in either of 2 ways. The distal part of the duplicated colon may be connected to the normal colon with a linear stapler. If this option is chosen, the connection must be distal enough to ensure that the duplication will no longer collect feces and produce an obstructing mass. Alternatively, the distal part of the duplication may be resected. This is an especially good option if the normal rectum and the duplication are separated. If the duplicated colon connects to the urinary tract or vagina, the duplication can be divided and an endorectal mucosectomy of the distal duplication done. The muscular cuff is then closed and an end-to-side anastomosis connects the remaining distal end of the duplication to the normal colon. Because colonic duplications rarely have ectopic gastric mucosa, resection of the duplicated segment is rarely necessary; however, malignancy has been reported in untreated cases of colonic duplication, but no such reports are found in cases treated with distal diversion.

## RECTAL DUPLICATIONS

### Essentials of Diagnosis

1. Rectal duplications are most common in females.

2. Rectal duplications commonly present with constipation.

3. Rectal duplications may present as a posterior rectal mass that must be differentiated from both an anterior meningomyelocele and sacrococcygeal teratoma.

4. Rectal duplications often have a separate anal opening.

### Presenting Signs and Symptoms

Rectal duplications present at a median age of 17 months and are more common in females. Most rectal duplications occur posterior to the rectum, although rarely they may occur anteriorly. Presenting signs and symptoms include an asymptomatic mass, constipation caused by rectal compression, rectal bleeding, rectal prolapse, and tenesmus. Some children have been misdiagnosed as having a perirectal abscess. Others present as fistula in ano. Twenty percent to 40% of these lesions have a fistula to the rectum or the skin. Most of these fistulae occur in the posterior midline as a cone-shaped dimple just above or below the anal verge (Fig. 51-15). Gastric mucosa may occur in these duplications, although they only occur in about 10% of the lesions. Connections to the urinary tract have not been reported, although bladder and ureteral compression have been seen as a result of mass effect. Presentation of these lesions is related to 5 factors: (a) size and mass effect; (b) the presence of a fistula; (c) infection; (d) the presence of ectopic gastric mucosa; and (e) malignant degeneration, which has mainly been reported in adults with untreated duplications.

### Diagnosis

Diagnostic studies include CT or MRI to rule out anterior meningomyelocele.

### Treatment

Treatment includes resection of the entire lesion or its mucosa. The approach to this resection may be transanal or posterior sagittal (Figs. 51-16 and 51-17). Both approaches

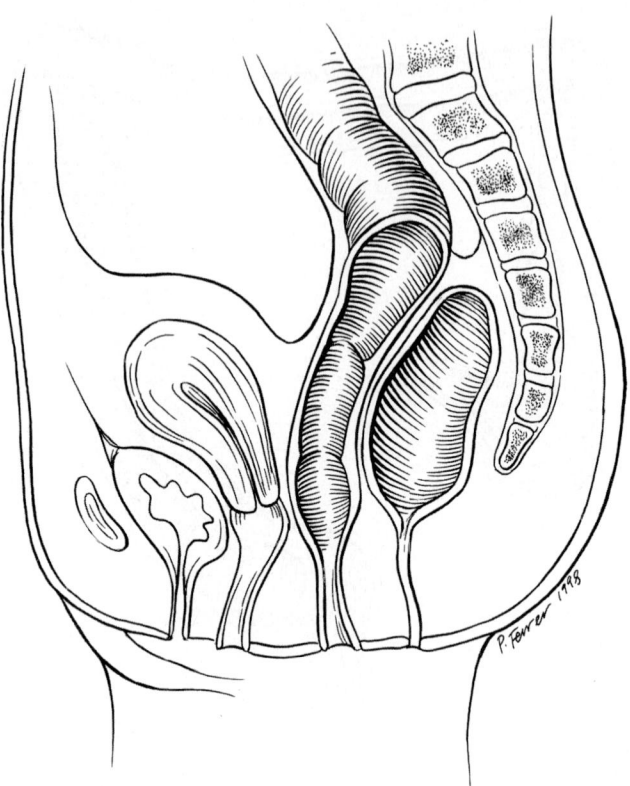

**FIGURE 51-15** Sagittal view of a posterior rectal duplication cyst with a perineal fistula.

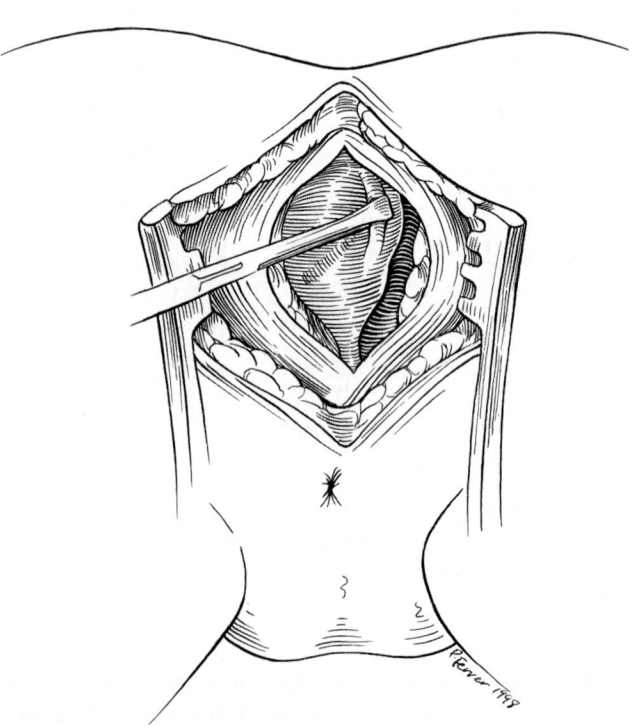

**FIGURE 51-16** Midline posterior sagittal approach to a retrorectal cystic duplication. The duplication is grasped, put on tension, and dissected from the wall of the anteriorly displaced rectum. If the duplication and rectum share a common wall, then this dissection must be carefully done. An alternative is to remove only the mucosal lining of the duplication cyst.

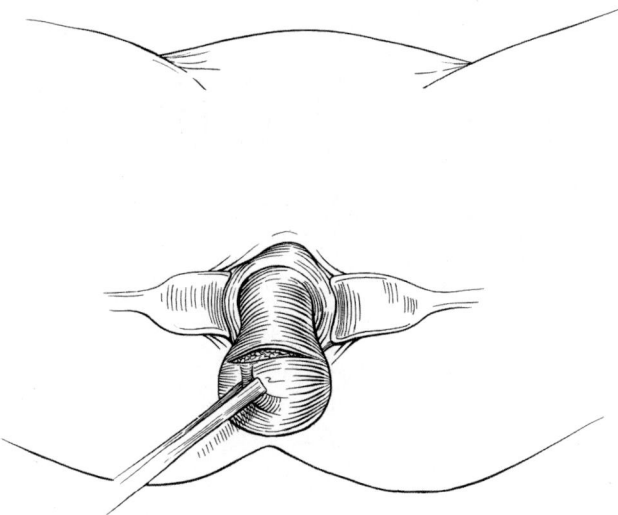

**FIGURE 51-17** An alternate approach to a rectal duplication is a transanal resection. Here the wall of the rectum is incised to allow a submucosal dissection of the mucosal lining of the duplication cyst, removing it completely.

have good results. If the lesions are large, they may require a combination of abdominal and posterior sagittal approaches. Marsupialization of the duplication into the rectum with a stapler has been described. Because adenocarcinoma in rectal duplications has been reported, and its incidence is unknown, mucosal resection should be done if possible. Lesions with ectopic gastric mucosa may cause perineal skin excoriation if the mucosa is not resected. Laparoscopic resection has been reported.

## SELECTED READINGS

Bianchi A. Intestinal loop lengthening—a technique for increasing small intestinal length. *J Pediatr Surg* 1981;16:996–997.

Black PR, Welch KJ, Eraklis EJ. Juxtapancreatic intestinal duplication with pancreatic duct communication: A cause of pancreatitis and recurrent abdominal pain in childhood. *J Pediatr Surg* 1986;21:257–261.

Bower RJ, Sieber WK, Kiesewetter WB. Alimentary tract duplications in children. *Ann Surg* 1978;188:669–674.

Bratu I, Laberge JM, Flageole H, et al. Foregut duplications: is there an advantage to thoracoscopic resection? *J Pediatr Surg* 2005;40:138–141.

Cooksey G, Wagget J. Tubular duplication of the rectum treated by mucosal resection. *J Pediar Surg* 1984;19:318–319.

Drott C, Jansson R. Duplication cyst of the jejunum. *Acta Chir Scand* 1981;147:731–733.

Haratz-Rubinstein N, Sherer DM. Prenatal sonographic findings of congenital duplication of the cecum. *Obstet Gynecol* 2003;101(5 pt 2):1085–1087.

Hartin CW, Stanley TL, Escobar MA, et al. Laparoscopic excision of a newborn rectal duplication cyst. *J Pediatr Surg* 2008;43:1572–1574.

Hoffman M, Sugarman HJ, Heuman D, Turner MA, Kisloff B. Gastric duplication cyst communicating with aberrant pancreatic duct: a rare cause of recurrent acute pancreatitis. *Surgery* 1987;101:369–372.

Holcomb GW III, Gheissari A, O'Neill JA Jr. Surgical management of alimentary tract duplications. *Ann Surg* 1989;209:167–174.

Ildstad ST, Tollerud DJ, Weiss RG, et al. Duplications of the alimentary tract. *Ann Surg* 1988;208:184–189.

Jewett TC, Walker AB, Cooney DR. A long-term follow-up on a duplication of the entire small intestine treated by gastroduplication. *J Pediatr Surg* 1983;18:185–188.

Lang T, Berquist W, Rich E, et al. Treatment of recurrent pancreatitis by endoscopic drainage of a duodenal duplication. *J Pediatr Gastroenterol Nutr* 1994;18:494–496.

LaQuaglia MP, Feins N, Eraklis A, Hendren WH. Rectal duplications. *J Pediatr Surg* 1990;25:980–984.

Lavine JE, Harrison M, Heyman M. Gastrointestinal duplications causing relapsing pancreatitis in children. *Gastroenterology* 1989;97:1556–1558.

Matsumoto S, Hiroyoshi M, Okushima K. Gallstone-containing duodenal duplication communicating with the pancreatic duct. *Hepatogastroenterology* 1995;42:123–125.

McPherson AG, Trapnell JE, Airth GR. Duplication of the colon. *Br J Surg* 1969;56:138–142.

Moss RL, Ryan JA, Kozarek RA, Hatch EL. Pancreatitis caused by a gastric duplication communicating with an aberrant pancreatic lobe. *J Pediatr Surg* 1996;31:733–736.

Murty TVM, Ghargave RK, Rakas FS. Gastroduodenal duplication. *J Pediatr Surg* 1992;27:551–517.

Narasemharao KL, Patel RV, Malik AK, Mitra SK. Chronic perianal fistula: beware of rectal duplication. *Postgrad Med J.* 1987;63:213–214.

Norris RW, Brereton RJ, Wright VM, Cudmore RE. A new surgical approach to duplications of the intestine. *J Pediatr Surg* 1986;21:167–170.

Orr MM, Edwards AJ. Neoplastic change in duplications of the alimentary tract. *Br J Surg* 1975;62:269–274.

Parkash S, Veliath AJ, Chandrasekaran V. Ectopic gastric mucosa in duplication of the rectum presenting as a perianal fistula. *Dis Col Rectum* 1982;25:225–226.

Ravitch M. Hind gut duplication—doubling of colon and genital urinary tracts. *Ann Surg* 1953;137:588–601.

Schwartz DL, So HB, Becker JM, Schneider KM. An ectopic gastric duplication arising from the pancreas and presenting with a pneumoperitoneum. *J Pediatr Surg* 1979;14:187–188.

Schwartz SL, Becker JM, Schneider KM, So HB. Tubular duplication with autonomous blood supply: Resection with preservation of adjacent bowel. *J Pediatr Surg* 1980;15:341–342.

Stringer MD, Spitz L, Abel R, et al. Management of alimentary tract duplication in children. *Br J Surg* 1995;82:74–78.

Williams WH, Hendren WH. Intrapancreatic duodenal duplication causing pancreatitis in a child. *Surgery* 1971;69:708–715.

Wold M, Callery M, White J. Ectopic gastric-like duplications of the pancreas. *J Pediatr Surg* 1988;23:1051–1052.

Wrenn EL Jr. Tubular duplication of the small intestine. *Surgery* 1962;52:494–498.

Young JK, Young KK, Yeon JJ, et al. Ileal duplication cyst: Y-configuration on in vivo sonography. *J Pediatr Surg* 2009;44:1462–1464.

Yousefzadeh DK, Bickers GH, Jackson JH Jr, Benton C. Tubular colonic duplication—review of 1876–1981 literature. *Pediatr Radiol* 1983;13:65–71.

# Cystic Abdominal Disease: Mesenteric, Omental, Solid Organ

# CHAPTER 52

*Harry Applebaum and Roman Sydorak*

## KEY POINTS

1. Most abdominal cysts are asymptomatic and are discovered by prenatal imaging.

2. Diagnosis is made by a combination of ultrasound, CT scans, and MRI.

3. Large size (>5 cm), pain, and signs of intestinal obstruction are the most common indications for intervention.

4. Treatment is aimed at complete excision of the cyst. When not possible, percutaneous drainage with sclerosis or marsupialization is a reasonable alternative.

5. Overall prognosis is excellent except in the rare case of malignant lesions.

Pediatric surgeons are often consulted to evaluate infants and children with cystic lesions of the abdomen. With nearly all pregnant women receiving prenatal ultrasound, requests for evaluation of fetal cystic lesions have also become more commonplace. A variety of cystic lesions have been described in the newborn infant, with most of them now diagnosed with great accuracy in the fetus (Table 52-1). A rather different set of cystic masses is found in the older infant and child, although a large overlap occurs (Table 52-2). While the true nature of a cystic mass can often only be determined at operation, the age of the patient, and the size, location, and mobility of the lesion are important findings that can aid in determining its nature and risk. Imaging studies can further refine the diagnosis, and can sometimes assist in providing temporary, or even definitive, therapy.

The finding of an abdominal cystic lesion in the newborn is rarely an indication for emergency surgery. The exception is the occasional very large mass that causes respiratory embarrassment. Even in this circumstance, temporary ventilation, sometimes accompanied by needle aspiration or percutaneous drainage, will allow time for an adequate preoperative evaluation. Intestinal obstruction is also an occasional presenting symptom that requires more rapid therapy. Palpation of the abdomen, paying particular attention to the mobility of the cyst, may provide a clue to a cyst's etiology. Cysts of the omentum, mesentery, some duplication cysts, and all but the largest ovarian cysts (the attached fallopian tube stretches to allow movement) are often easily manually movable around the abdomen. Rectal exam and pelvic exam in the older child are helpful in determining a pelvic origin of the lesion.

Imaging studies often, although not always, give clues as to the organ or region of origin of a cyst (Fig. 52-1). Ultrasound, computerized tomography (CT), and MRI are used interchangeably to evaluate these lesions. The information obtained such as density, unilocularity or multilocularity, the number of layers in the cyst wall, location, and the presence of calcifications helps narrow the differential diagnosis. For instance, teratomas most often contain characteristic chunky calcifications, whereas meconium cysts in the newborn contain more stippled dystrophic lateral calcifications. Lymphatic malformations of the retroperitoneum present as multiloculated lesions, while those of the mesentery are more frequently unilocular (Fig. 52-2). Duplication cysts present with walls containing multiple layers.

When resection or drainage is indicated, percutaneous intervention and laparoscopy have increasingly replaced traditional open methods. Mobile lesions can often be removed and then aspirated and extracted through a protected "endobag" or removed via a small Pfannenstiel incision with a small skin and subcutaneous tissue flap. Preremoval

| TABLE 52-1 | Diagnosis by Location of Cysts in the Fetus and Infant | |
| --- | --- | --- |
| **Upper Abdomen** | **Mid Abdomen** | **Pelvic** |
| **Intra-abdominal** | **Intra-abdominal** | **Abdominal wall** |
| Choledochal | Mesenteric | Urachal |
| Duplication | Duplication | Hydrocolpos |
| | Meconium cyst | |
| **Retroperitoneal** | **Retroperitoneal** | **Mid pelvis** |
| Adrenal | Teratoma | Ovarian (simple or complex) |
| | Lymphatic malformation | Ovarian teratoma |
| | Renal | |
| | | **Retroperitoneal** |
| | | Sacrococcygeal teratoma |

| TABLE 52-2 | Diagnosis by Location of Cysts in the Older Child | |
| --- | --- | --- |
| **Upper Abdomen** | **Mid Abdomen** | **Pelvic** |
| **Intra-abdominal** | **Intra-abdominal** | **Abdominal wall** |
| Choledochal | Mesenteric | Urachal |
| Duplication | Duplication | |
| | Hydrometrocolpos | **Mid pelvis** |
| | Omental | Ovarian (simple or complex) |
| | Teratoma | |
| | Lymphatic malformation | Ovarian teratoma |
| | Renal | |
| | Pancreatic | |
| | Hepatic | |
| | Splenic | |

aspiration of large lesions often allows for reduced incision size. Intervention is rarely indicated in the fetus as cysts are of insufficient size and can be managed adequately following delivery. Fetal therapy, usually limited to transuterine aspiration, has occasionally been applied where hydrops has developed, where the size of the lesion interferes with the development of other organs, most often the lungs, or where there is thought to be a risk of dystocia during delivery. It has also been used in the therapy of large ovarian cysts, usually >5 cm, where there is a significant risk of antenatal loss of the ovary because of torsion. Antenatal reduction of the size of these lesions is thought to reduce this risk.

## SPECIFIC CYSTIC LESIONS

### Mesenteric Cysts

These cysts (see Fig. 52-3) present as soft lesions of varying size in the midabdominal area and often present with pain

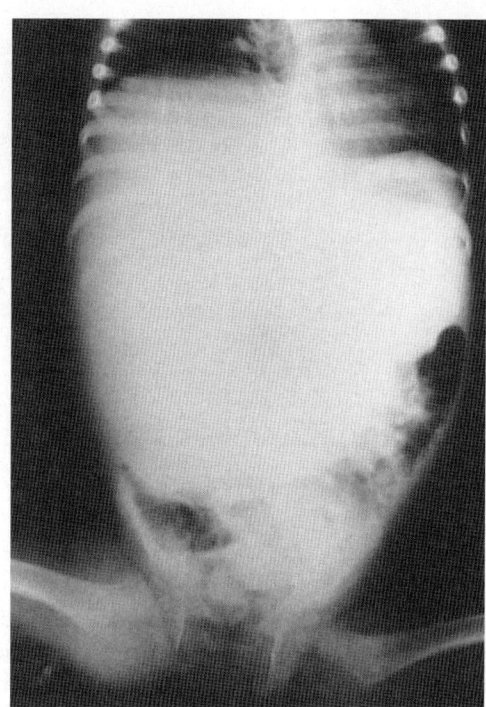

**FIGURE 52-1** Plain abdominal radiograph of an infant who had a distended abdomen at birth. The radiograph revealed a large right-upper-quadrant mass that was displacing intestine inferiorly and to the left, as well as elevating the right hemidiaphragm. This was subsequently found to be a large lymphatic malformation.

and vomiting. They are thought to originate from structural abnormalities of the mesenteric lymphatics that fail to communicate with the remainder of the lymphatic system. The contents are usually straw-colored and proteinaceous in character, with some appearing milky, particularly following fat ingestion. About 60% involve the small bowel mesentery, 25% the large bowel mesentery, and the remainder extend into the retroperitoneum. Those limited to a short segment of the mesentery can be simply excised laparoscopically without bowel resection provided the blood supply to the bowel is not

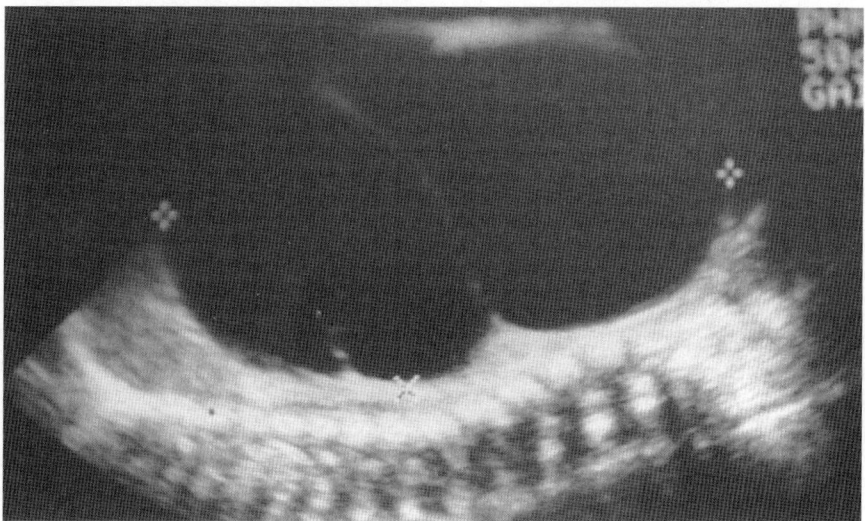

**FIGURE 52-2** Ultrasound of an infant with a large palpable abdominal mass. The ultrasound revealed a multiloculated cystic mass, which was subsequently found to be a large omental cyst.

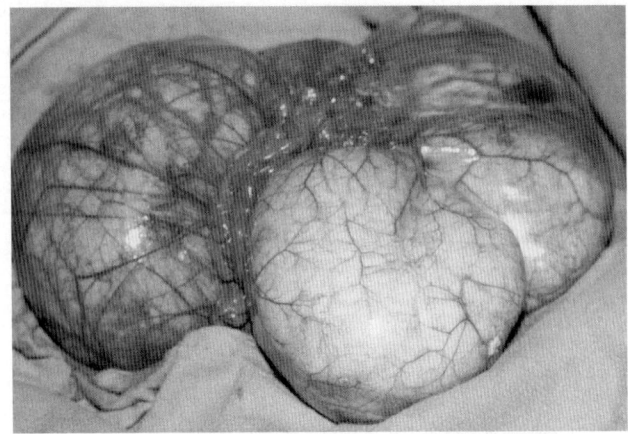

**FIGURE 52-3** Large mesenteric cyst of abdomen.

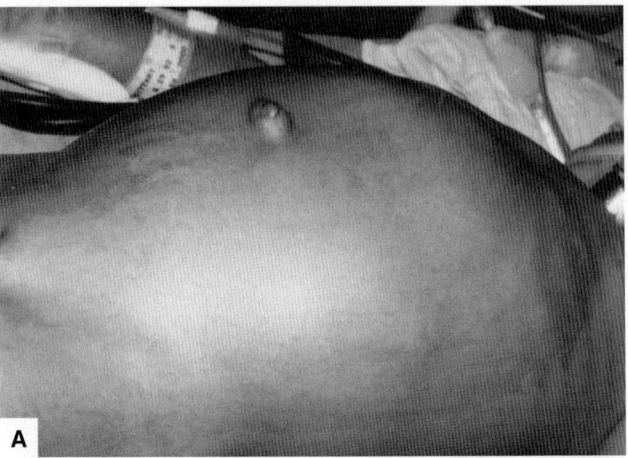

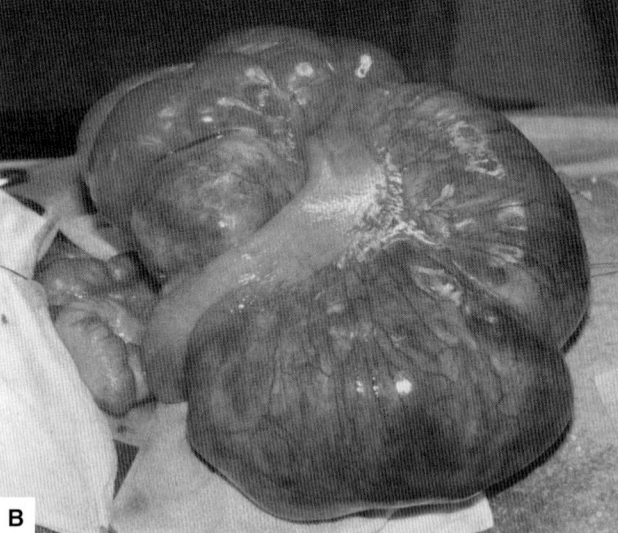

**FIGURE 52-4** **A.** External impression of bulging flanks suggesting an intra-abdominal mass. **B.** Large mesenteric lymphatic malformation.

compromised. More often (50%-60% of the time), resection of a wedge of the mesentery along with the attached small or large intestine, with primary end-to-end anastomosis, is the most practical technique for removal. Simple unroofing of these cysts often results in recurrence. Retroperitoneal extension often proves more challenging and necessitates an open approach to provide exposure and to achieve a complete resection. When resection is not feasible, the only other option is partial excision and marsupialization, which, by definition, has a higher rate of recurrence.

## Lymphatic Malformations

Occasionally, the same type of histologic lesion that is responsible for simple mesenteric cysts is present in a complex multilocular form, and involves a substantial portion of the mesentery and/or retroperitoneum (see Fig. 52-4A and B). These lymphatic malformations are prone to hemorrhage into the cysts either spontaneously or via minor trauma, whereby they become increasingly symptomatic. At times, the cystic structure may take the form of a lymphaticovenous malformation, in which case some or all of the cysts may contain bloody fluid rather than the usual straw-colored variety from the start. Chylous ascites, hypoproteinemia, and malabsorption may be present. Extension of the vascularized portion into the bowel wall has been implicated as a cause of gastrointestinal bleeding. Whenever practical, resection of a limited portion of the intestine and its mesentery remain the procedure of choice. Where involvement is extensive and resection would result in inadequate removal of a large mass or short-gut syndrome, unroofing of the larger lesions has sometimes been beneficial, although ascites may result. Injection of a variety of sclerosing agents into the larger cysts, or use of immunotherapy (OK-432) has sometimes been beneficial. Argon beam coagulation of the base of the malformation may prevent the postoperative development of fluid collections. Extensive lesions have often been problematic over a period of years.

## Omental Cysts

These are lymph-filled cysts similar to mesenteric cysts in presentation and origin. Torsion may occur if the cyst attains a large size because of stretching and twisting of the relatively

insubstantial omentum, in which case the patient presents with severe, acute abdominal pain. Resection of the omentum is curative. Laparoscopic resection is used for smaller mesenteric and omental cysts, and for larger cysts after aspiration. Marsupialization alone has a substantial risk of recurrence and is not recommended.

## Ventriculoperitoneal Shunt Pseudocysts

A shunt-associated pseudocyst is the likely diagnosis in the child with a poorly functioning ventriculoperitoneal shunt and abdominal pain, tenderness, and an abdominal mass. Imaging studies, usually CT scans, will show the abdominal end of the shunt within the cystic structure. The majority are associated with repeated episodes of clinical shunt infection. In this situation, a low-grade localized chronic peritonitis probably causes formation of a pseudocyst around the abdominal end or the shunt, with resultant poor absorption of cerebrospinal fluid. These cysts may grow to a very large size and mimic ascites. Simple drainage of these cysts either percutaneously or intra-abdominally results in a high incidence of recurrence, as well as symptomatic shunt infection. Appropriate treatment usually requires temporary externalization of the shunt. Subsequently, repositioning of the abdominal end of the shunt, with replacement of the entire shunt, is advised. Lysis of adhesions and excision of the some of the pseudocyst may be required to prevent reformation of the pseudocyst and provide for adequate function of the newly placed shunt. The pelvic or suprahepatic, subdiaphragmatic areas are often relatively uninvolved with adhesions. Drainage into the gallbladder, atrium, or pleural cavity can be used when the abdomen is extensively involved with adhesions and multiple repositionings have been unsuccessful.

## Hepatic Cysts

Hepatic cysts may be solitary or multiple, and may be lined with either squamous or biliary epithelium. Depending on the histology, they may contain clear or bilious fluid. Most are idiopathic, although trauma may be the initiating factor in their development. Cysts near the porta hepatis may be confused with choledochal cysts, and are best differentiated from the latter by imaging studies that define a lack of communication or an intrahepatic communication. Upper abdominal pain and compression of the gastrointestinal tract due to the large size of the cyst are the most frequent indications for surgical intervention. Needle aspiration and drainage of the larger cysts are easily accomplished under computed tomography (CT) or ultrasound guidance, although a high incidence of recurrence is the rule. Following aspiration, instillation of a sclerosing agent into demonstrably noncommunicating cysts has been reported to decrease this risk. Operative drainage has resulted in a higher incidence of permanent cure. Marsupialization by open or laparoscopic technique to allow drainage into the peritoneal cavity is most often done, although this also retains a small risk of recurrence. Omental flaps to provide coverage are not necessary. Drainage into a Roux-en-Y limb offers a small chance of recurrence, and is particularly indicated in those that communicate with the biliary tree. Communication is indicated by bilious contents, or by imaging studies including technetium-99m iminodiacetic acid scan, percutaneous injection, transhepatic cholangiogram, or endoscopic retrograde cholongiopancreatography (ERCP) in older children. The risk of future cholangitis must be weighed when contemplating intestinal drainage.

## Pancreatic Cysts

Pancreatic cysts of a congenital nature in infants are rare. They may be either true cysts or pseudocysts, and are most often associated with anomalies of the pancreaticobiliary ductal systems. Correction of the ductal anomalies causing obstruction is required for cure. In older children, traumatic pseudocysts are most common. Approximately two-thirds of these lesions will resolve spontaneously when followed by imaging studies. The remainder will require either external drainage, usually by CT guidance, or internal drainage. This can be accomplished endoscopically, or by surgical cyst-gastrostomy or cyst Roux-en-Y anastamosis. Initial CT scan or ERCP pancreaticogram is useful to rule out ductal transection.

## Splenic Cysts

Splenic cysts (see Fig. 52-5) may be primary or secondary. Primary cysts arise from epithelial rests, while secondary cysts result from nonabsorption of liquified hematomas following

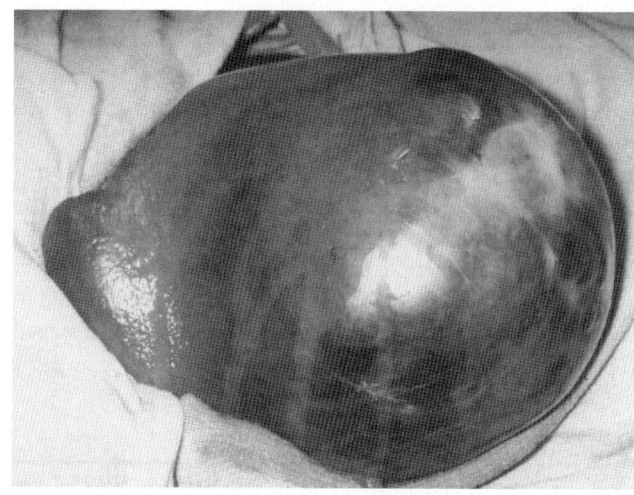

**FIGURE 52-5** Large splenic cyst.

nonoperative management of splenic trauma. Both are of little consequence unless they attain a size substantial enough to cause discomfort. About half of patients present with abdominal pain. The remainder are either asymptomatic, incidentally discovered, or present with rupture, abscess, or compression of adjacent structures. Small simple asymptomatic cysts less than 5 cm can be observed. Larger cysts necessitate open or laparoscopic intervention. Laparoscopic partial splenectomy or cystectomy has appeared adequate, although it may have a slightly higher rate of recurrence, especially if the cyst is only marsupialized. However, benefits of laparoscopy include a shorter length of stay and improved cosmesis. Technically, the Harmonic scalpel (Ethicon Endo-Surgery, Cincinnati, Ohio) or the Ligasure (Covidien, Boulder, Colorado) facilitates division of the splenic parenchyma. Ligation of the main splenic artery and vein may be required with preservation of some of the short gastric vessels to provide perfusion to the normal spleen. Percutaneous drainage with CT guidance for cysts directly beneath the abdominal wall has been described. Splenectomy should rarely be required.

## Adrenal Cysts

Cystic lesions of the retroperitoneum in the newborn are most often the result of neonatal adrenal hemorrhage. This bleeding is thought to be of the Waterhouse–Friedericksen type, resulting from perinatal stress. The lesion may be identified from flank discoloration and/or abdominal mass, with an imaging picture of a complex cystic lesion with indistinct borders that infiltrates the surrounding retroperitoneal tissues. The course is that of spontaneous regression, often with accompanying jaundice from absorption of the blood that it contains. As absorption progresses, a thin pseudo-capsule may appear on imaging studies. Occasionally, this has been confused with the uncommon cystic neuroblastoma. Treatment is expectant, and decreasing size of the lesion rules out a neoplasm. The diagnosis may be confirmed by needle aspiration of the old blood. Exploration is indicated only for lesions that fail to regress. Multiple cystic lesions of the neonatal adrenal glands may occasionally be seen in association with the Beckwith–Wiedemann syndrome.

ABDOMINAL DISEASE

## Meconium Cysts

These cysts appear in the newborn who has had antenatal bowel perforation. A pseudocyst forms around the spilled sterile bowel contents. Characteristic stippled calcifications are present, along with a small-bowel obstruction. Air is present in the cyst if it remains in communication with the proximal end of the atretic bowel. Removal of as much of the cyst as is practical is accomplished at the time of the usually staged correction of the atresia. Removal of the cyst wall can lead to bleeding that can necessitate temporary drainage and staged repair of the atresia.

## Urachal Cysts

Urachal cysts may present as midline swellings of the lower abdomen anywhere along the course of the fetal urachus, from the dome of the bladder to the umbilicus. They sometimes present as a draining umbilicus (urachal sinus), but are more frequently identified when infection (urachal abscess) is present. In this situation, they appear as an erythematous, indurated midline swelling of the mid-lower abdomen. Diagnosis of infected or noninfected cysts is most often made by ultrasound. Primary excision of the cyst or primary drainage and secondary excision of the infected one is required for cure. The entire lesion must be excised, including any attachment to the umbilicus. The lower end must be excised flush with the dome of the bladder. Occasionally, a small piece of attached bladder is removed to insure complete resection. In this situation, the procedure is completed with a double-layer closure of the vesicostomy. A substantial incidence of associated urinary anomalies has been reported in some series. Imaging studies of the kidneys and bladder are therefore indicated.

## Hydrocolpos

Hydrocolpos is a large midline lower abdominal mass in the female neonate that may extend high up into the abdomen and that usually represents a gynecologic lesion. Inspection of the perineum helps in the differential diagnosis. A bulging hymenal membrane indicates hydrocolpos. Cure is achieved by a cruciate hymenal incision, with cauterization of any bleeding edges. Indication of a more complex malformation involving the genitourinary and intestinal systems should be further evaluated and treated on an individual basis. A cystic lesion without perineal abnormalities is usually indicative of a cyst of ovarian origin. For a more extensive discussion of this topic, see the chapter on female genital abnormalities.

## SELECTED READINGS

Charlesworth P, Ade-Ajayi N, Davenport M. Natural history and long-term follow-up of antenatally detected liver cysts. *J Pediatr Surg* 2003;38:1810–1813.

Dequanter D, Lefebvre JC, Belva P, et al. Mesenteric cysts: a case treated by laparoscopy and review of the literature. *Surg Endosc* 2002;16:1493.

Egozi EI, Ricketts RR. Mesenteric and omental cysts in children. *Am Surg* 1997;63:287–290.

Foley P, Ford W, McEwing R, et al. Is conservative management of prenatal and neonatal ovarian cysts justifiable? *Fetal Diagn Ther* 2005;20:454–458.

Kariyattil R, Steinbok P, Singhal A, et al. Ascites and abdominal pseudocysts following ventriculoperitoneal shunt surgery: variations of the same theme. *J Neurosurg* 2007;106:350–353.

Keckler SJ, Peter SD, Tsao K, et al. Laparoscopic excision of splenic cysts: a comparison to the open approach. *Eur J Pediatr Surg* 2010;20:287–289.

Kurrer MO, Ternberg JL, Langer JC. Congenital pancreatic pseudocyst: report of two cases. *J Pediatr Surg* 1996;31:1581–1583.

McCauley RG, Beckwith JB, Elias ER, et al. Benign hemorrhagic adreno-cortical macrocysts in Beckwith Wiedemann syndrome. *AJR Am J Roentgenol* 1991;157:549–552.

Mobley LW 3rd, Doran SE, Hellbusch LC. Abdominal pseudocyst: predisposing factors and treatment algorithm. *Pediatr Neurosurg* 2005;41:77–83.

Ogita S, Tsuto T, Tokiwa K, et al. Intracystic injection of OK-432: a new sclerosing therapy for cystic hygroma in children. *Br J Surg* 1987;74:690–691.

Rich RH, Hardy BE, Filler RM. Surgery for anomalies of the urachus. *J Pediatr Surg* 1983;18:370–372.

Rodgers BM, Vries JK, Talbert JL. Laparoscopy in the diagnosis and treatment of malfunctioning ventriculo-peritoneal shunts in children. *J Pediatr Surg* 1978;13:247–253.

Steyaert H, Guitard J, Moscovici J, et al. Abdominal cystic lymphangioma in children: benign lesions that can have a proliferative course. *J Pediatr Surg* 1996;31:677–680.

Yoder SM, Rothenberg S, Tsao K, et al. Laparoscopic treatment of pancreatic pseudocysts in children. *J Laparoendosc Adv Surg Tech A* 2009;19:37–40.

# CHAPTER 53

# Anorectal Malformations

*Marc A. Levitt and Alberto Peña*

## KEY POINTS

1. The posterior sagittal approach for anorectal malformations, first performed in 1980, led to significant implications in terms of terminology and classification, reduction of complications, and has since been expanded for many other surgical challenges in the pelvis.

2. Correct anatomic terminology, rather than arbitrary descriptions of "low," "intermediate," and "high," are useful in therapeutic and prognostic terms.

3. The key technical points to repairing males with an ARM and a rectourethral fistula are that the lower the rectum, the longer the common wall between the anterior rectum and the posterior urethra, and that the bladderneck fistula is the only defect in which the distal rectum is at or above the peritoneal reflection. The rectum in the rectoprostatic, the rectobulbar, and the no fistula defects lie below the peritoneal reflection and are best approached posterior sagittally rather than transabdominally.

4. An accurate preoperative distal colostogram is vital to ensure proper surgical planning, otherwise the surgeon will be looking for the distal rectum blindly, and can easily injure adjacent structures such as the vas deferens, urethra, seminal vesicles, and the bladder neck.

5. Rectal atresia is a rare anorectal malformation with the unique feature of having a normal-appearing anal canal and dentate line, and being specifically associated with a presacral mass.

6. Rectovestibular fistula is the most common malformation in females. The key technical concern is creating 2 walls out of 1 between the intimately attached rectum and vagina.

7. Cloacal malformations form their own broad spectrum, with a 3-cm common channel being a dividing line between a straightforward repair able to be accomplished with a total urogenital mobilization posterior sagittally, and a complex repair requiring a laparotomy as well as special maneuvers to perform

vaginoplasty, vaginal replacement, sometimes separation of the urinary tract from the gynecologic system, or preservation of the common channel as neourethra.

8. A patient with a good prognosis defect (rectoperineal fistula, rectobulbar urethral fistula, rectovestibular fistula) with a good sacrum and spine should be expected to achieve normal bowel control.

9. When a baby is born with an anorectal malformation, in addition to investigating for associated defects, the surgeon must decide whether to perform a colostomy or if a primary repair can be done. It takes 20 to 24 hours for enough pressure to build in the distal colon to delineate a fistula, and the decision as to what operation to pursue should wait this amount of time.

10. The most trouble-free colostomy for anorectal malformations is a proximal sigmoid diversion, with separated stomas.

11. For patients who cannot achieve voluntary bowel control, a bowel-management program consisting of a tailored daily enema allows the patient to remain completely clean and in normal underwear.

## HISTORICAL REVIEW

Anorectal malformations have been well known for many centuries, and described by, surgeons, sorcerers, and early medical practitioners who attempted to create an orifice in the perineum in children born with these defects. Those patients who were lucky to be born with a rectum located close to the perineum survived those procedures; the others died.

During the first half of the 1900s, patients suffering from the so-called "high" imperforate anus received a colostomy during the newborn period, followed later in life by an abdominoperineal pull-through as a definitive procedure. During this transabdominal pull-through operation, the key maneuver involved pulling the bowel as close to the sacrum as possible to avoid trauma to the genitourinary tract.

Douglas Stephens from Australia made a significant contribution to this field by proposing a sacral approach to create a

669

tunnel behind the urethra and within the puborectalis sling, which he considered a key factor in maintaining fecal continence. Many malformations could be treated with the sacral approach only, but when the rectum was located higher, the patient required an abdominal procedure. All procedures designed till 1980 were based on a few anatomic studies in cadavers, which were not representative of the entire spectrum of anorectal malformations.

One of the few areas of pediatric surgery in which the knowledge of the patient's anatomy was still very limited, even in the 1980s, was that of anorectal malformations. After observing the Stephens technique in his training from 1969 to 1972, brought to the Boston Children's Hospital by Stephen's fellow, Dr. Justin Kelly, the senior author became frustrated with the approach because it involved blind maneuvers in the perineum. From 1972 to 1980 he progressively made the perineal incision longer and longer until for the first time on August 10th, 1980, he opened the buttocks like a book, performing a posterior sagittal approach to find and pull down the distal rectum in a child born with an imperforate anus. The splitting of the "circular" sphincter was radical, but was based on the concept that the sphincter instead was like a funnel, and by staying precisely in the midline, then finding the rectum, separating it from surrounding structures, and then reconstructing the sphincters left them intact and functional. Since 1980, the approach to these defects has been through a posterior sagittal incision, using an electric stimulator, which allowed a better understanding of the basic anatomy of these defects and for the establishment of important correlations among the external anatomy, the internal anatomy, surgical techniques, and clinical results. In the past, the rectum was pulled down through a path that was assumed to be the right one, now the path is more clearly visible and surrounding structures are better preserved. The posterior sagittal approach also led to significant implications in terms of terminology and classification, reduction of complications, and was expanded to be used for a whole host of other applications in the pelvis.

## TYPES OF MALFORMATIONS

Anorectal malformations occur in approximately 1 in 5000 newborns. The most frequent defect in males is an imperforate anus with rectourethral fistula (at the bulbar or prostatic urethral level), followed in frequency by rectoperineal fistulas (traditionally known as low defects). The rectobladderneck fistula defect occurs in 10% of male patients and represents the highest type. The most frequent defect in female patients is rectovestibular fistula, followed by rectoperineal fistula. Persistent cloaca is the third most common defect seen in females, which used to be considered a very unusual defect. A high incidence of "rectovaginal fistulas" were reported in the literature in the past, but in retrospect, it seems that cloaca is a much more common defect in females, as most of the rectovaginal fistulas were actually misdiagnosed cloacae. Rectovestibular fistulas were also frequently erroneously called rectovaginal fistula, which itself is an almost nonexistent defect. Imperforate anus without a fistula occurs in 5% of

| TABLE 53-1 | Classification of Anorectal Malformations |
|---|---|
| **Classification** | |
| Males | |
| Rectoperineal fistula | |
| Rectourethral fistula | |
| Bulbar | |
| Prostatic | |
| Rectobladderneck fistula | |
| Imperforate anus without fistula | |
| Rectal atresia/stenosis | |
| Females | |
| Rectoperineal fistula | |
| Rectovestibular fistula | |
| Persistent cloaca | |
| Imperforate anus without fistula | |
| Rectal atresia/stenosis | |

all anorectal malformations, both in males and in females, which is the only truly "imperforate" type. It is a unique defect in which the rectum is reliably located about 2 cm above the perineum, and in a male, is found at the level of the bulbar urethra.

Anorectal malformations represent a wide spectrum of defects. The terms "low," "intermediate," and "high" are arbitrary and are not useful in therapeutic and prognostic terms. The classification of anorectal malformations now more uniformly used and discussed here is based on therapeutic and prognostic implications (Table 53-1).

## Male Defects

### Rectoperineal Fistula

This is the lowest and simplest defect. The lowest part of the rectum opens anterior to the center of the sphincter (Fig. 53-1). The perineal appearance of this defect may include a subepithelial midline tract with black meconium or white mucous visible, opening somewhere along the midline perineal raphe, scrotum, or even at the base of the penis. Also, the observer may see a prominent midline skin tag called a "bucket handle". All of these are different external manifestations of the same defect and the rectum can reliably be found right below the skin. The sphincter and the sacrum are usually very good and associated defects are rare.

### Rectourethral Fistula

In this defect, the rectum opens into the posterior urethra, most commonly in its lowest part (rectourethral bulbar fistula) (Fig. 53-2). The sacrum and sphincters in these patients are usually good. Associated defects are present more frequently than in rectoperineal fistulas but are still uncommon.

The rectum may open into the upper portion of the posterior urethra: a rectourethral prostatic fistula (Fig. 53-3). The sphincter in these patients is less developed, and the sacrum more frequently abnormal. The chances of having associated defects are higher and the prognosis in terms of bowel and

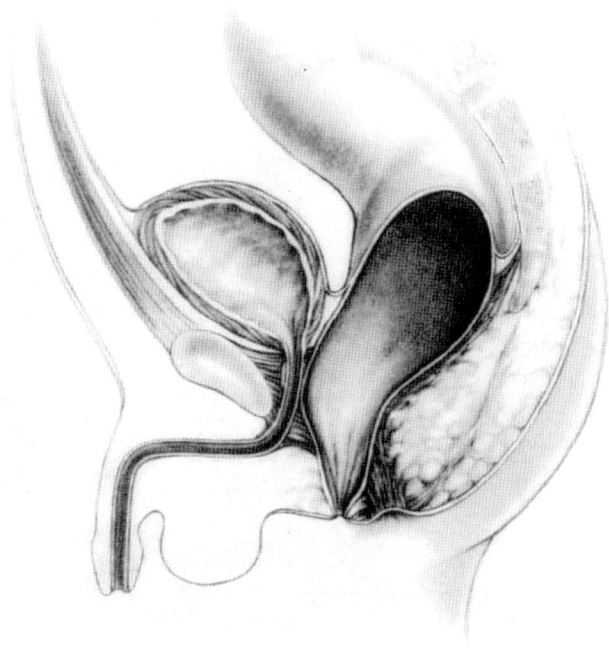

FIGURE 53-1 Rectoperineal fistula (male). (Reprinted with permission from Peña A. *Atlas of Surgical Management of Anorectal Malformations.* New York: Springer-Verlag; 1990.)

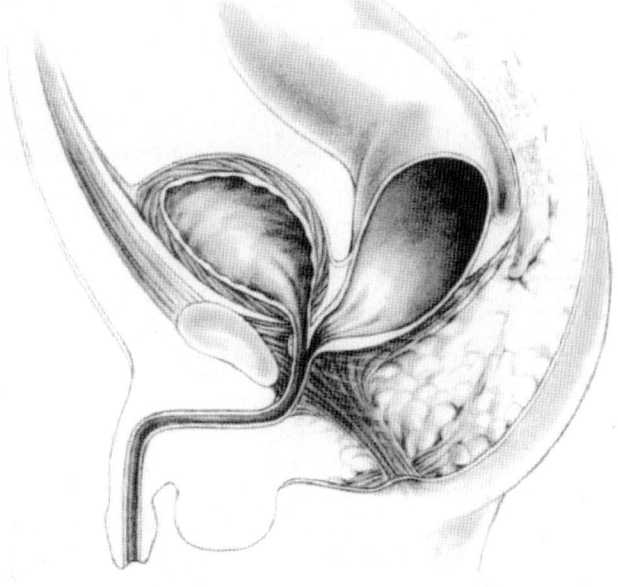

FIGURE 53-3 Rectourethral prostatic fistula. (Reprinted with permission from Peña A. *Atlas of Surgical Management of Anorectal Malformations.* New York: Springer-Verlag; 1990.)

urinary function is not as good as in previously mentioned defects. As can be seen in Figs. 53-2 and 53-3, immediately above the fistula, the rectum and urethra share a common wall. This common wall is shorter in higher defects. Surgeons must keep this important anatomic detail in mind during the repair. The rectum is surrounded laterally and posteriorly by the levator muscle. In both cases, the rectum lies below the peritoneal reflection and passes through the levators. Distal to the end of the rectum (fistula site), a portion of striated voluntary muscle, which is called the muscle complex, is present. At the level of the skin, a group of voluntary muscle fibers, called parasagittal fibers, are located on both sides of the midline. The lower the fistula site, the more prominent is the midline groove between both buttocks and the more prominent is the anal dimple. Higher defects are more frequently associated with poor quality of muscles, and there is a tendency for the patients to have a flat perineum and an almost absent anal dimple.

## Rectobladderneck Fistula

The rectum opens into the bladderneck, well above the sphincter mechanism (at or above the peritoneal reflection). The sphincter mechanism is frequently poorly developed. The sacrum also usually shows signs of severe hypoplasia and/or dysmorphism. The perineum is often flat and the entire pelvis seems to be underdeveloped (Fig. 53-4). The incidence of associated defects is extremely high.

## Imperforate Anus Without Fistula

In this type of defect the rectum ends completely blind at a rather constant location, approximately 2 cm above the perineal skin, which corresponds to the level of the bulbar urethra in male patients. The rectum and the urethra share a common wall, which must be kept in mind during the repair of this defect. More than 90% of patients with Down syndrome and imperforate anus suffer from this specific type of malformation, and about half of the patients with an imperforate anus and no fistula suffer from Down syndrome. Interestingly, the other half of patients who have no Down syndrome suffer from other well-known syndromes demonstrating a genetic

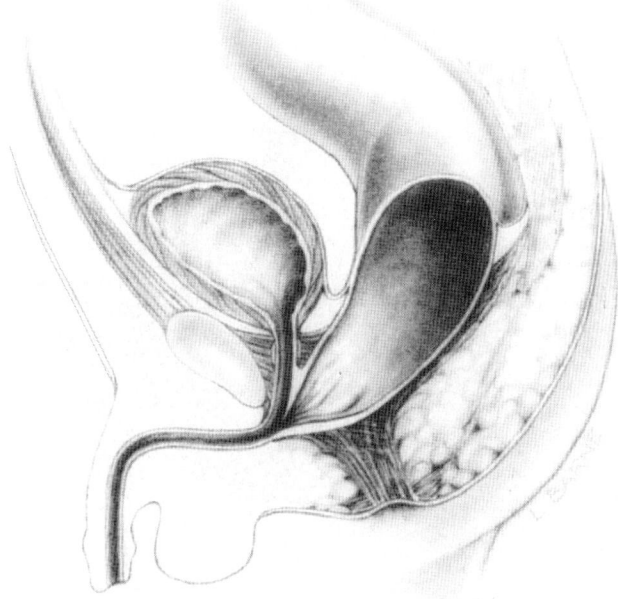

FIGURE 53-2 Rectourethral bulbar fistula. (Reprinted with permission from Peña A. *Atlas of Surgical Management of Anorectal Malformations.* New York: Springer-Verlag; 1990.)

671

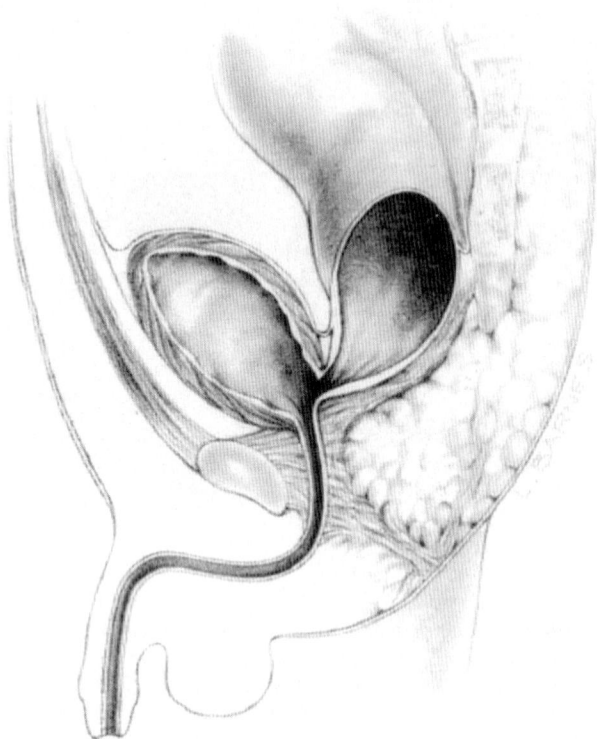

**FIGURE 53-4** Rectobladderneck fistula. (Reprinted with permission from Peña A. *Atlas of Surgical Management of Anorectal Malformations.* New York: Springer-Verlag; 1990.)

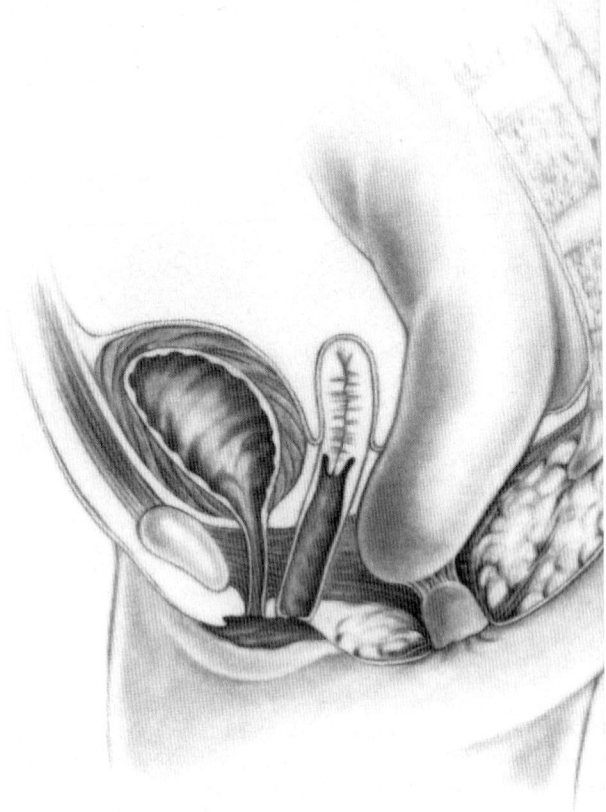

**FIGURE 53-5** Rectal atresia/stenosis. (Reprinted with permission from Peña A. *Atlas of Surgical Management of Anorectal Malformations.* New York: Springer-Verlag; 1990.)

link to this type of anomaly. These patients have good sphincters, good sacrums, and, therefore, good clinical prognosis even if they have Down syndrome.

## Rectal Atresia/Stenosis

Patients who suffer from this unusual, unique defect, represent the only ones who are born with a normal anal canal. Therefore, the perineum in these children looks normal. The anus may appear skin lined (funnel anus) but is correctly located within the pink ellipse, which represents the sphincter. This defect is usually recognized during an attempt to pass a thermometer in the rectum. At the junction of the anal canal and the rectum (about 1 cm above the perineum), there is a total atresia or a severe stenosis (Fig. 53-5). Both the rectum and the anal canal may be separated by a thin membrane or by a dense portion of fibrous tissue. This defect occurs in approximately 1% of all malformations. Because the anal opening and sphincter mechanism is normal, the prognosis is excellent. All such patients must be screened for a presacral mass which in commonly present.

## Female Defects

### Rectoperineal Fistula

In these patients, the rectum opens externally through an abnormal, usually narrow fistulous tract located somewhere between the female genitalia and the center of the sphincter (Fig. 53-6). Prognosis and frequency of associated defects are the same as in the male version.

## Rectovestibular Fistula

The rectum opens within the female genitalia in an area called the vestibule, located immediately outside the hymen. The fistula is usually narrow with a length that varies from a

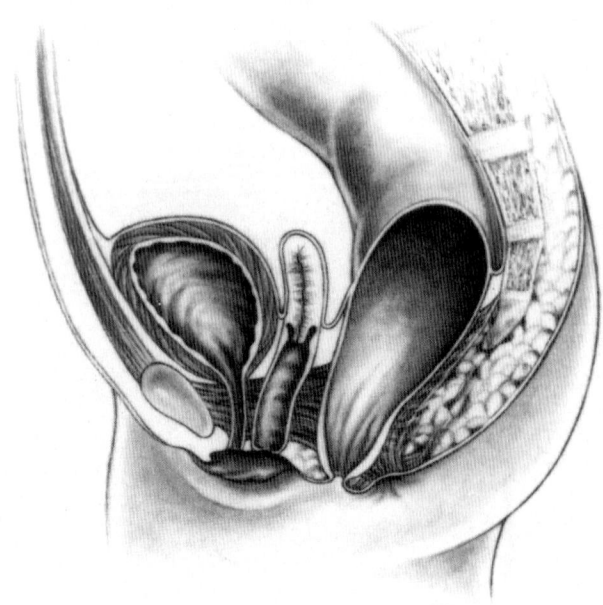

**FIGURE 53-6** Rectoperineal fistula (female). (Reprinted with permission from Peña A. *Atlas of Surgical Management of Anorectal Malformations.* New York: Springer-Verlag, 1990.)

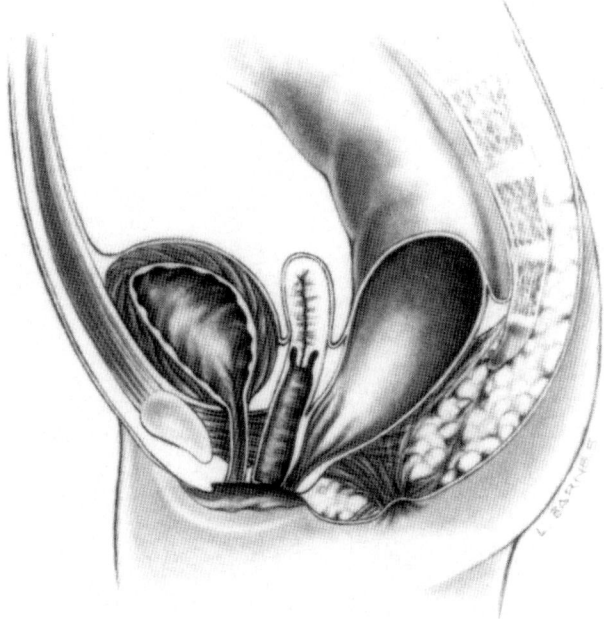

**FIGURE 53-7** Rectovestibular fistula. (Reprinted with permission from Peña A. *Atlas of Surgical Management of Anorectal Malformations.* New York: Springer-Verlag; 1990.)

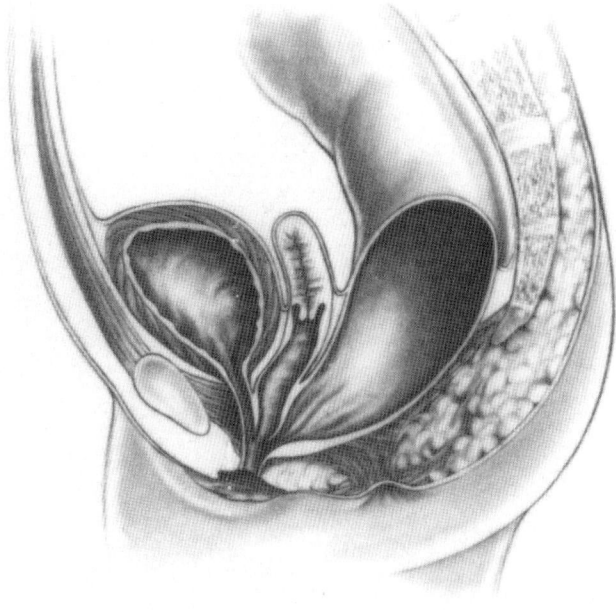

**FIGURE 53-8** Cloaca. (Reprinted with permission from Peña A. *Atlas of Surgical Management of Anorectal Malformations.* New York: Springer-Verlag; 1990.)

few millimeters to 2 to 3 cm. The most important anatomic feature is that the rectum and vagina share a common wall (Fig. 53-7). The sacrum, as well as the sphincters, are usually good. The prognosis for bowel function is excellent. Sadly, this is the group that not uncommonly suffers from a failed attempted repair that negatively impacts the prognosis. The precise diagnosis is a clinical one and requires a meticulous inspection of the newborn genitalia. Many of these patients are still erroneously labeled as having a "rectovaginal fistula." The problem is not only semantic; some of these incorrectly diagnosed patients are subjected to an abdominoperineal procedure, which leads to fecal incontinence.

## Imperforate Anus Without Fistula

The characteristics of this defect in female patients are similar to those for the male counterpart, with the obvious difference that the distal rectum lies contiguous to the posterior wall of the vagina.

## Persistent Cloaca

Cloacal malformations comprise their own wide spectrum of defects. They also represent the most complex types in female patients. A cloaca is defined as a defect in which the rectum, the vagina, and the urinary tract meet and fuse into a single common channel (Fig. 53-8). Externally, one sees a single perineal orifice located where the urethra normally opens. Obviously, there is no anus and the external genitalia look rather small. The length of the common channel varies from 1 to 7 cm (Fig. 53-9). The length of the common channel correlates with the complexity of the malformation and, therefore, with the final functional prognosis. Short common channels represent a defect with a straightforward repair and these patients also have a good functional prognosis. Long common channels represent very high defects, a difficult technical

challenge, and less-than-optimal functional results. The turning point seems to be around 3.0 cm in length.

There are many anatomic variants in this complex type of malformation. Sometimes the rectum opens very high into the dome of the vagina (Fig. 53-10). Very often the vagina is enormously distended and full of mucous fluid; this is called hydrocolpos (Fig. 53-11). The dilated vagina sometimes compresses the trigone of the bladder and interferes with the drainage of the ureters, provoking bilateral megaureters.

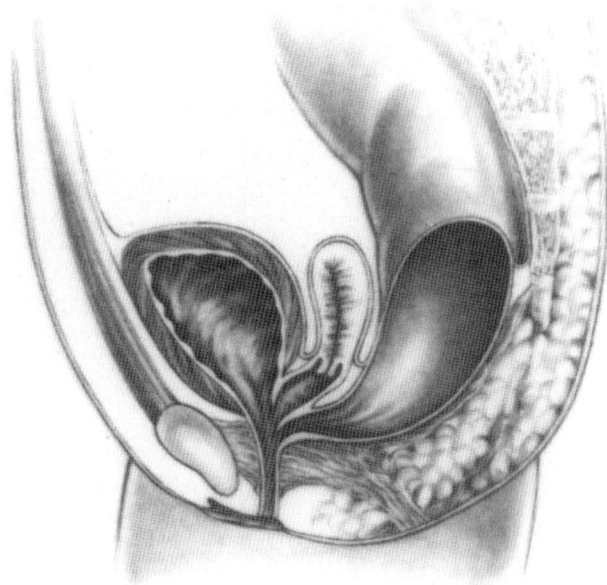

**FIGURE 53-9** Cloaca with a long common channel. (Reprinted with permission from Peña A. *Atlas of Surgical Management of Anorectal Malformations.* New York: Springer-Verlag; 1990.)

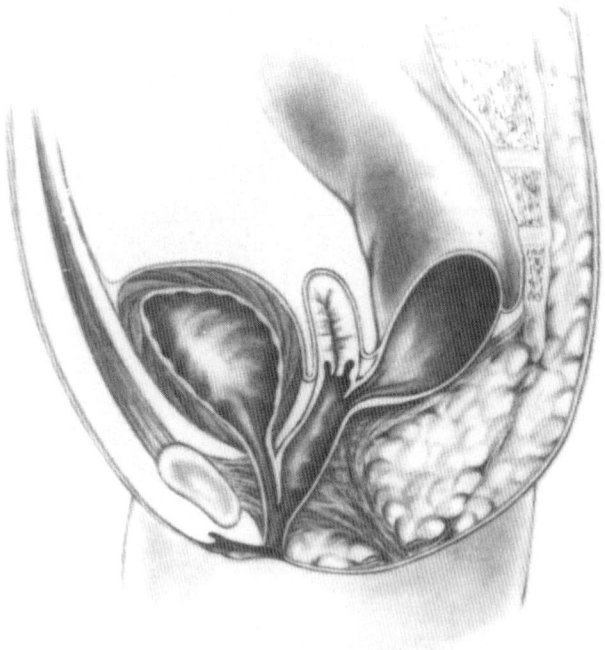

**FIGURE 53-10** Cloaca with a very high rectum. (Reprinted with permission from Peña A. *Atlas of Surgical Management of Anorectal Malformations.* New York: Springer-Verlag; 1990.)

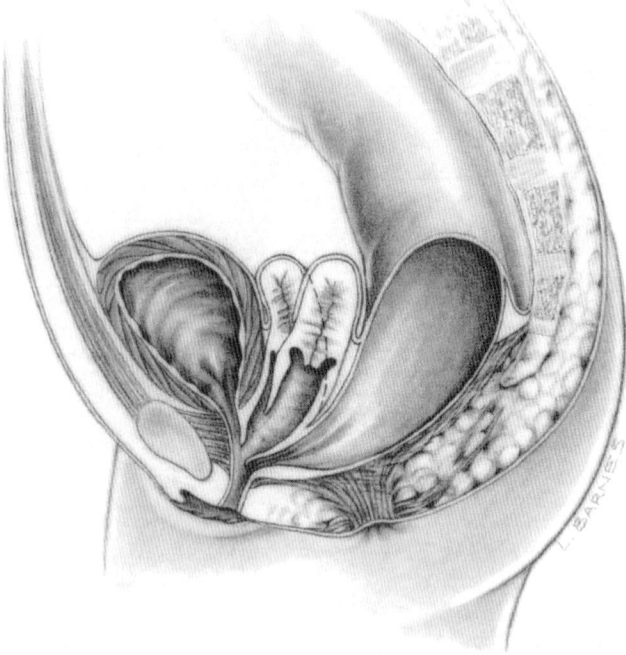

**FIGURE 53-12** Cloaca with 2 hemivaginas. (Reprinted with permission from Peña A. *Atlas of Surgical Management of Anorectal Malformations.* New York: Springer-Verlag; 1990.)

A significant number of patients also suffer from duplex Mullerian systems, with different degrees of septation of the vagina and uterus (Fig. 53-12). In such cases, the rectum usually opens in the lowest part of the septum that separates both hemivaginas. Patients with cloaca may suffer from atresia of the cervix or of the fallopian tubes. Cloaca patients with a short common channel most frequently have a good sphincter mechanism, a normal sacrum, and a relatively low frequency of associated defects, and, therefore, a good functional prognosis. At the other end of the spectrum, one can see patients with cloaca with a long common channel, flat perineum, poor sphincter development, very hypoplastic sacrum, high incidence of associated defects (mainly urologic), and a poor prognosis for bowel and urinary control.

The rectum and the vagina share a common wall as in other types of defects. Also, the vagina and the urinary tract share a very thin common wall, which can be left intact in most cases with a total urogenital mobilization used for reconstruction.

## Complex Malformations

These represent very bizarre, extremely unusual anatomic arrangements of the pelvic structures that are sometimes encountered and are usually associated with a very hypoplastic sacrum, myelomeningocele, tethered cord, and presacral masses. No general guidelines can be drawn for the management of these patients. Each represents a formidable challenge and requires good preoperative imaging and a great deal of expertise to be treated.

## Associated Defects

**Urologic.** Roughly, 50% of patients with anorectal malformations have an additional urogenital defect. The frequency varies depending on the height and complexity of the anorectal malformation. Thus, patients with a cloaca with a long common channel have about a 90% chance of having an associated urologic defect, while for children with perineal fistulas

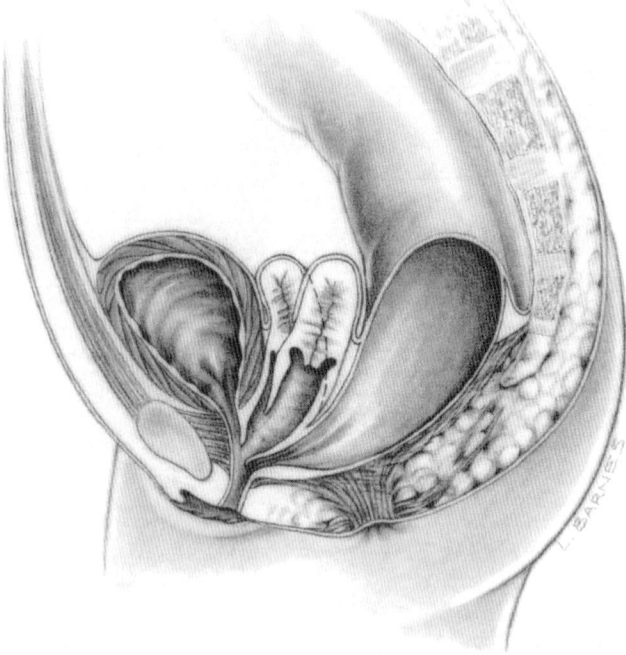

**FIGURE 53-11** Cloaca with hydrocolpos. (Reprinted with permission from Peña A. *Atlas of Surgical Management of Anorectal Malformations.* New York: Springer-Verlag; 1990.)

it is 10%. The risks for other types of defects are about 30% for rectovestibular fistulas, 30% for rectourethral bulbar fistulas, 60% for rectoprostatic fistulas, 90% for rectobladderneck fistulas, 20% for an imperforate anus with no fistula, and less than 10% for rectal atresia. These associated anomalies include a single kidney, vesicoureteral reflux, and hydronephrosis. The risk of poor bladder emptying is significant and must be carefully watched because, in the long term, this can negatively impact kidney function. All patients, therefore, must have some sort of screening test at birth to rule out an associated urologic defect. In very high anorectal malformations and complex defects the main source of morbidity is the urologic condition.

**Gynecologic.** 50% of patients with cloaca have a duplicate Mullerian system, with implications on menses, intercourse, and obstetric potential. Vestibular fistulas have an associated vaginal septum in 5% of cases. The clinician must also be wary of an associated absent vagina, detectable with a careful perineal inspection.

**Spinal and Sacral Defects.** The sacrum is the most frequent bony structure affected in these defects. Sometimes one or several vertebrae are absent. More often, however, even when the number of vertebrae is normal, the sacrum still looks abnormal, smaller, and dysmorphic. Therefore, to objectively evaluate the sacrum its size is compared with bony parameters of the pelvis, creating a ratio that correlates with the final functional prognosis. The sacral ratio of a normal pelvis in a lateral x-ray film is shown in Fig. 53-13. A horizontal line is traced touching the upper portion of the iliac crest. A second line parallel to the upper one is traced, passing through the lowest point of the sacroiliac joint (posterior iliac spine), and a third line is traced parallel to the other 2 touching the lowest radiologic visible point of the sacrum. A ratio is obtained

by dividing the distance between the 2 lower lines by the distance between the 2 upper lines. Among normal children the average ratio is 0.77. Children with anorectal malformations show a spectrum of values; lower ratios represent different degrees of sacral hypodevelopment and correlate with poor sphincters and anal canal sensation, and are associated with defects that have poor functional prognosis. We have never seen a patient who has bowel control with a ratio of less than 0.4.

A hemisacrum associated with an anorectal malformation may mean that there is a presacral mass (usually a teratoma, or an anterior meningocele). The presence of a presacral mass in patients with anorectal malformations usually translates into poor functional prognosis.

Sometimes the sacral vertebrae are abnormal (hemivertebrae). This usually negatively affects the functional prognosis. Hemivertebrae may also affect the lumbar and thoracic spine (scoliosis may result) and are more common in higher defects.

**Other Associated Defects.** Gastrointestinal abnormalities may be present in patients with anorectal malformations. The most frequently seen are esophageal atresia and duodenal atresia. These make newborn management challenging as the child may need multiple procedures and there is no abdominal distention to help demonstrate a rectal fistula.

## DIAGNOSIS AND INITIAL MANAGEMENT IN THE NEWBORN

Fetal diagnoses of anorectal malformations is becoming more common, particularly for cloacas. Polyhydramnios and combinations of renal and sacral/spinal anomalies should make the perinatologist suspicious of a fetus with an anorectal malformation (Fig. 53-14).

### Male Newborn

Once born, 2 important questions must be answered during the first 24 to 48 hours of life in a baby with an anorectal malformation. The first is whether the patient has an associated defect that represents a risk to his or her life. The second decision is related to the modality of treatment that is best for the patient's anorectal malformation: whether the patient can undergo a primary repair or needs a colostomy and a delayed operation for the reconstruction. As previously mentioned, the chances for a baby to have an associated defect are higher the more complex the malformation.

A careful, inspection of the newborn's perineum can, in most cases, determine the type of defect that the patient has. At birth, a baby with an imperforate anus must be kept with nothing by mouth, intravenous fluids administered, and a nasogastric tube inserted to avoid the risk of vomiting and aspiration. An ultrasound of the abdomen is the best screen for obstructive uropathy, and in a female, hydrocolpos. An echocardiogram will rule out an associated cardiac defect. Patency of the esophagus is confirmed when a nasogastric tube is passed.

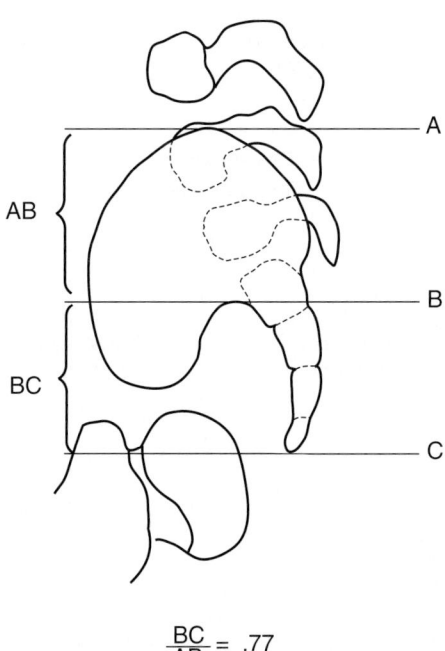

$$\frac{BC}{AB} = .77$$

**FIGURE 53-13** Sacral ratio in a normal individual. (Reprinted from Pena A. Anorectal malformations. *Semin Pediatr Surg* 1995;4(1) with permission from Elsevier.)

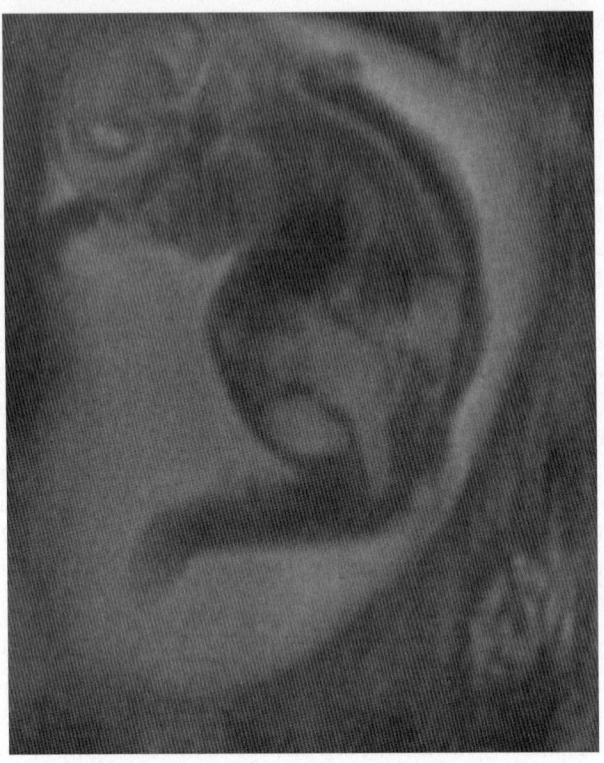

**FIGURE 53-14** MRI image of a 16-week fetus with a cloaca and hydrocolpos.

Figure 53-15 shows the decision-making algorithm for the management of a male newborn with an anorectal malformation. The clinician should wait 24 hours before deciding to open a colostomy or perform repair in a newborn. It is extremely unlikely that a baby will have any problems related to an undiverted, distended bowel during the first 24 hours of life. On the other hand, making this determination too early frequently ends in serious mistakes. At birth, the baby with an imperforate anus usually does not have a distended abdomen. It takes a number of hours for the bowel to become distended. Fistulas to the perineum or to the genitourinary tract are frequently very narrow and abdominal pressure is required to force meconium through them. The presence of meconium in the urine (in males) or through the genitalia (in females) represents information in the diagnosis, and it may take significant time for these to appear. In addition, the lowest part of the rectum passes through the sphincter mechanism in most cases. The sphincter muscle has tone, and that keeps the distal part of the rectum compressed and empty. For the meconium to pass through the fistula, it is necessary to overcome the muscle tone of the sphincter. In more than 90% of males, perineal inspection provides enough clinical evidence to reach a decision about whether to perform a diverting colostomy. The presence of meconium in the perineum, a midline raphe subepithelial black or white ribbon-like tract, a bucket handle

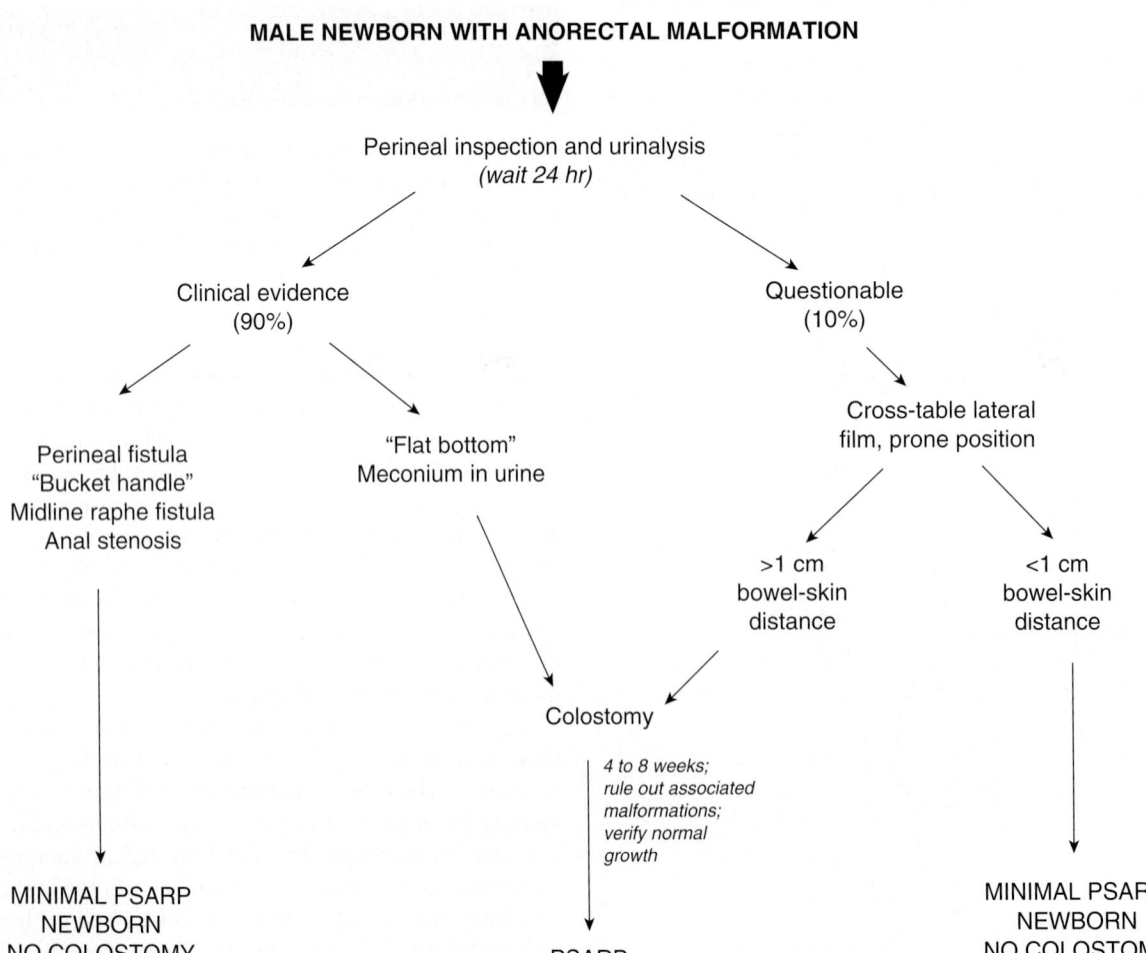

**FIGURE 53-15** Decision-making algorithm for male newborns with an anorectal malformation.

malformation, or an anal membrane are all different manifestations of a perineal fistula. Finding one of these abnormalities establishes the diagnosis. In such cases, the patient can be treated with a newborn anoplasty without a protective colostomy, and no other diagnostic methodology is needed. On the other hand, the presence of a flat bottom (very poor midline groove and absent anal dimple) and/or meconium in urine represents an indication for a diverting colostomy.

The colostomy decompresses the bowel and provides protection during the healing process after the subsequent reconstruction. After the patient recovers from the colostomy, he is discharged from the hospital. If he is growing well and has no other important associated defects such as a cardiac defect that must be repaired, the main repair can be done after he is 1 month of age. This has important advantages for the patient including a shorter time with a colostomy, less size discrepancy between proximal and distal bowel at the time of colostomy closure, and easier to perform anal dilatations.

In less than 10% of patients, the surgeon is unable to determine the location of the distal rectum. Under those circumstances, a radiologic evaluation is indicated. A cross-table lateral film with the baby in the prone position and the pelvis elevated is taken. This study should not be done before 16 to 24 hours of life for the reasons already explained. The presence of air in the blind rectal pouch located more than 1 to

2 cm away from the perineal skin represents an indication for a colostomy. A rectum located closer than 1 to 2 cm from the perineum means that the baby most likely has a perineal fistula, not yet visible, and this patient can undergo a newborn anoplasty.

## Female Newborn

The decision-making process in female newborns is depicted in Fig. 53-16. Ninety-five percent of the time one can make a correct therapeutic-decision based solely on the physical examination. The diagnoses of a rectoperineal fistula, vestibular fistula, and cloaca are simple clinical diagnoses and require only meticulous inspection of the perineum. Only 5% of all patients are born without a fistula and are actually "imperforate." The presence of a perineal fistula means that the patient can be treated with a newborn anoplasty. This operation does not necessarily have to be performed in the first days of life. Frequently, the fistula is competent enough to allow bowel decompression. If this is not the case, fistula dilatations may help the baby pass meconium. Then the repair of the perineal fistula can be done on an elective basis but should not be delayed longer than 2 to 4 months. We prefer if possible to perform the anoplasty during the time that the baby is still passing meconium, as the possibility of infection

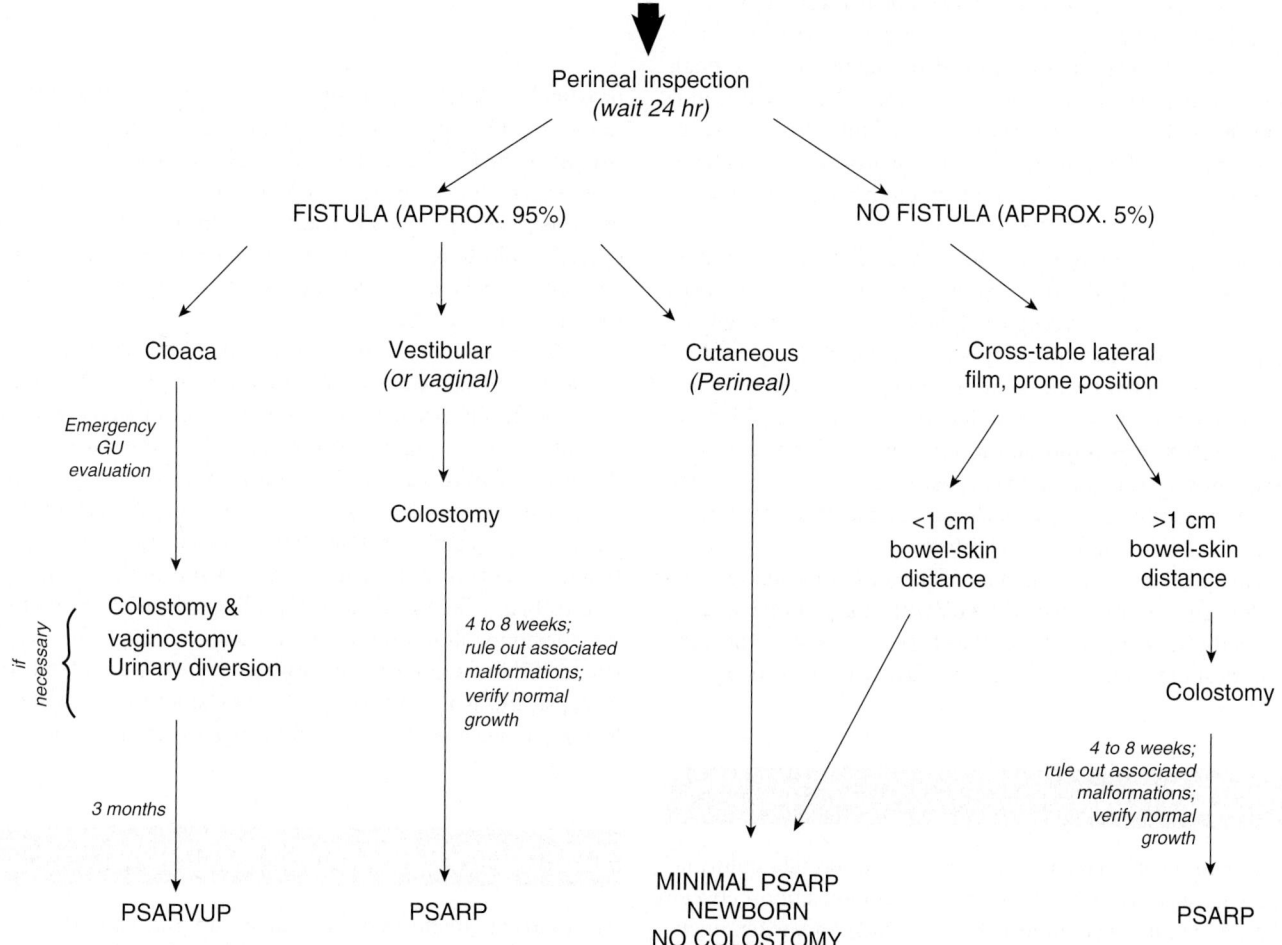

**FIGURE 53-16** Decision-making algorithm for female newborns with an anorectal malformation.

is decreased. If a patient is very sick or if one is dealing with a premature infant, the surgeon should dilate the fistula to allow bowel decompression and postpone the main treatment. Some surgeons prefer not to operate at all on babies with a rectoperineal fistula based on the concept that these patients left untouched can have bowel control. Some others prefer to do a simple cutback procedure to widen the external opening of the fistula in an effort to prevent constipation. We do not recommend these approaches. To maximize bowel control potential (by placing the distal rectum within the sphincter mechanism) and minimize (but never completely eliminate) constipation, (by making the anus an appropriate size) the surgeon will achieve the best results. In a female, the additional indication is to create an adequate perineal body which will allow for a future vaginal delivery, and create a normal-appearing perineum.

For vestibular fistulas, these patients can be operated on early in life without a colostomy and with good results. However, dehiscence and/or stricture after this operation jeopardize the functional prognosis and the clinical results of a reoperation are inferior to those of a good primary procedure. Every effort should be made to avoid complications and a colostomy does help with this. This could be performed before the main repair or simultaneously.

The presence of a single perineal orifice establishes the diagnosis of cloaca. The urologic status is determined before the opening of a colostomy. The presence of a single perineal orifice associated with a palpable lower abdominal midline mass is likely a hydrocolpos that can be delineated by ultrasound. At the time of colostomy opening, the surgeon must be prepared to drain the distended vagina (hydrocolpos). This is done by suturing the vagina to the abdominal wall if large enough, or draining it with a curled tube brought out in the right or left lower quadrant. If the hydrocolpos is bilateral, a portion of the vaginal septum should be removed so both sides are drained.

The main source of morbidity in patients with cloaca during the neonatal period is urosepsis and metabolic acidosis, usually from an unrecognized obstructive uropathy. The importance of decompressing a very distended vagina cannot be overemphasized. Before reaching a decision to create a vesicostomy or ureterostomies in a patient with bilateral megaureters, it is important to decompress the vagina, and frequently, by doing that, the ureters drain well into the bladder. Very rarely patients with cloaca suffer from a very narrow urethra and do require a vesicostomy.

The final repair of a cloaca is called a posterior sagittal anorectovaginourethroplasty (PSARVUP) and is done usually when the patient is 3 to 6 months of age. It represents the most significant technical challenge in pediatric pelvic surgery.

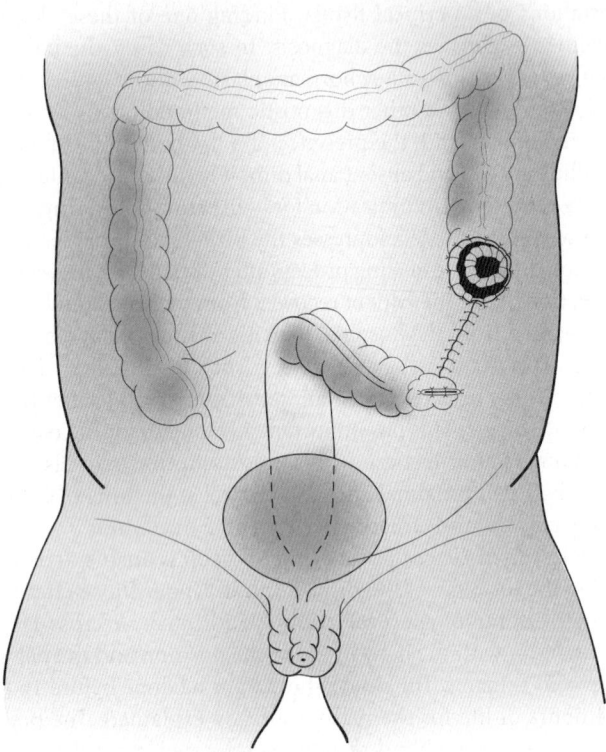

**FIGURE 53-17** Ideal colostomy; proximal end in very proximal sigmoid, distal end, mucous fistula, made tiny and flat, and separated from the functional stoma.

proximal to distal, which could provoke urinary tract infections. A colostomy in the proximal sigmoid with separated stomas created in the left lower quadrant is ideal (Fig. 53-17). The surgeon must be sure to leave enough distal sigmoid colon beyond the mucous fistula. A common mistake is to open the colostomy too distal, which anchors the colon to the abdominal wall and interferes with the subsequent rectal pull through.

At the time of colostomy opening, the distal bowel must be irrigated with saline solution so that the rectal pouch is completely decompressed. A descending colostomy has definite advantages over a right or transverse colostomy. Cleaning of the distal colon is much easier to perform through a descending colostomy than a transverse one. It is not unusual for the patient to pass urine back into the colon through the fistula. In a transverse colostomy the urine remains in the colon and is absorbed, which leads to metabolic acidosis. A more distal colostomy allows the urine to escape through the distal stoma without significant absorption. A loop stoma tends to prolapse and is not diverting, allowing stool to pass distally leading to megarectosigmoid and urinary tract infections.

## COLOSTOMY

Eighty to ninety percent of patients with anorectal malformations have some form of abnormal communication between the colon and the genitourinary tract. Therefore, when opening a colostomy both stomas (proximal and distal) must be completely separated to avoid the passing of stool from

## DEFINITIVE RECONSTRUCTION

All anorectal malformations can be approached posterior sagittally using a posterior anorectoplasty (PSARP). Approximately 40% of patients with cloaca may additionally need a laparotomy to complete the repair. Only 10% of male patients may require entering of the abdomen (via laparoscopy or laparotomy) to mobilize a very high rectum.

The basis of the posterior sagittal approach is the creation of an incision in the midline between both buttocks, the length of the incision varies depending on the type and height of the malformation. The patient is placed in prone position with the pelvis elevated. The sphincter mechanism is divided in the midline. Excellent exposure is obtained, and nerves and muscles are not damaged. The anatomic characteristics of the malformations are recognized, the rectum is separated from the genitourinary tract, the limits of the sphincter mechanism are electrically determined, and the rectum is mobilized sufficiently to reach the perineum and the sphincter mechanism is reconstructed around it. Via a posterior sagittal approach, all these maneuvers are performed under direct vision, which helps to preserve important anatomic structures.

A posterior sagittal approach should not be attempted without a technically adequate distal colostogram, the best study to determine the exact position of the rectum and the fistula. Exploring a patient posterior sagittally without this basic information risks damaging nerves and other important structures. (In perineal and vestibular fistula cases the rectal position is known, so no contrast study is needed). If the rectum is high, at the bladderneck, and the surgeon does not know this, other midline structures (bladderneck, vas deferens, seminal vesicles, prostate, ectopic ureters) can be injured.

## Males with Anorectal Malformations

### Minimal PSARP for Rectoperineal Fistula

In these malformations, the repair serves a dual purpose: first, to move the rectal opening back to be placed within the limits of the sphincter mechanism and, second, to create an adequately sized anus. The fistula is consistently located 1 to 2 cm anterior to the center of the sphincter; thus, the degree of rectal dissection necessary is rather minimal. The most common and feared operative complication is urethral damage. To prevent this, a Foley catheter must be inserted and meticulous technique must be used during the dissection of the anterior rectal wall, as the rectum is intimately attached to the urethra. The patient is placed in the prone position; a 2-cm incision is made dividing the posterior superficial portion of the sphincter. Multiple 6-0 silk sutures are placed at the mucocutaneous junction of the fistula in order to exert uniform traction, which facilitates the dissection. Sometimes the fistula is so small that it requires a lacrimal probe to be demonstrated.

With the lacrimal probe in place, the fistula can be unroofed until a reasonable caliber rectal opening is found, and the multiple silk stitches are placed there. While applying traction to these stitches, a circumferential dissection is performed, trying to stay as close to the rectal wall but still preserving its full thickness. The dissection is performed along the lateral walls first, then continues to the anterior aspect until enough length is gained to move the rectum back to be placed within the limits of the sphincter without tension. A characteristic areolar tissue is reached once the anterior rectal wall is adequately separated from the urethra. The perineal body

## Size Dilators According to Age

| | HEGAR |
|---|---|
| 1 to 4 Months | 12 |
| 4 to 8 Months | 13 |
| 8 to 12 Months | 14 |
| 1 to 3 Years | 15 |
| 3 to 12 Years | 16 |
| More than 12 years | 17 |

FIGURE 53-18 Size dilators according to age. (Reprinted from Levitt MA, Peña A. Imperforate anus and cloacal malformations. In: *Ashcraft's Pediatric Surgery*. 5th ed. 2010, with permission from Elsevier.)

anterior to the center of the sphincter is reconstructed with long-term absorbable sutures up to the anterior limit. This is the space where the fistula had been. The rectum is anchored on its posterior aspect to the posterior edge of the muscle complex and an anoplasty is performed with 16 circumferential stitches. Even when the operation is rather minor, it requires meticulous technique. The operation is performed on an elective basis, but we prefer to do it before the baby is discharged home after birth. If a delayed repair is planned, it should be done within the first several months.

Two weeks after surgery, anal dilatations are started. These dilatations should be done at home following a strict protocol done twice per day. The size of the dilator must be increased every week by 1 mm of the diameter, until the size that is considered normal for the patient's age is reached. Figure 53-18 shows the size of the dilators to be used according to age. Once the correct size is reached, parents must continue doing dilatations twice per day until they feel that the dilator goes in very easily. At that point the frequency of these dilatations can be tapered according to a specific protocol (Fig. 53-19).

Normal bowel control is expected for these patients. Constipation is very common and usually starts after breast feeding has been discontinued. This problem of constipation must be treated aggressively whereby the parents make sure that the baby empties his rectum every day.

### PSARP for Rectourethral Fistula

A foley catheter is inserted through the urethra and the patient is then placed in a prone position with the pelvis elevated. After the skin is prepped, a midsagittal incision is made, from the lower portion of the sacrum to the area of the anal dimple. The skin is divided, as are the subcutaneous tissue, the parasagittal fibers, and the muscle complex (Fig. 53-20). The parasagittal fibers are split in the midline. The muscle complex runs perpendicular to the parasagittal fibers and extends from the skin up to the levator mechanism. The muscle complex joins the levator mechanism forming a nearly 90° angle. Together these muscles form the funnel-like

| ✓ Twice per day, increasing by one unit each week until the desired size is reached, then |
| --- |
| ✓ Once a day for a month |
| ✓ Every other day for 1 month |
| ✓ Every third day for 1 month |
| ✓ Twice a week for 1 month |
| ✓ Once a week for 1 month |
| ✓ Once a month for 3 months |

**FIGURE 53-19** Protocol for dilations.

muscle structure that surrounds the rectum. Deeper to the parasagittal fibers, one finds fat tissue that represents the ischiorectal fossa. Deep to this, one can identify the levator mechanism. The levator muscle is then divided in the midline. The distal colostogram predicts where the rectum will be during this approach (Fig. 53-21). If the patient has a rectobladderneck fistula, the distal rectum is high, at the peritoneal reflection and not visible from this approach. If the patient has a rectoprostatic fistula, the surgeon expects to find the rectum very high (1 cm below the coccyx), and if the distal colostogram shows that the patient has a rectourethral bulbar fistula, the surgeon will find the rectum very low in the incision (Fig. 53-22). Not having this vital information, the surgeon may explore deeper, looking for the rectum. If the patient has a rectobladderneck fistula, the surgeon will not find it, but may instead find the posterior urethra, bladderneck, seminal vesicles, vas deferens, an ectopic ureter, and/or the prostate. The surgeon will also risk damaging important nerves, which can lead to a neurogenic bladder.

Two silk sutures are placed in the posterior rectal wall, and the bowel is opened between both sutures. As the incision in the posterior rectal wall is extended distally and more silk sutures are placed anteriorly taking the bowel edge. The fistula is found at the most distal part. Once the fistula is visualized, a last 5-0 silk suture is placed at the edge of the rectal incision, taking part of the fistula orifice. Immediately above the fistula the anterior rectal wall is intimately attached to the posterior wall of the urethra. The separation of the rectum

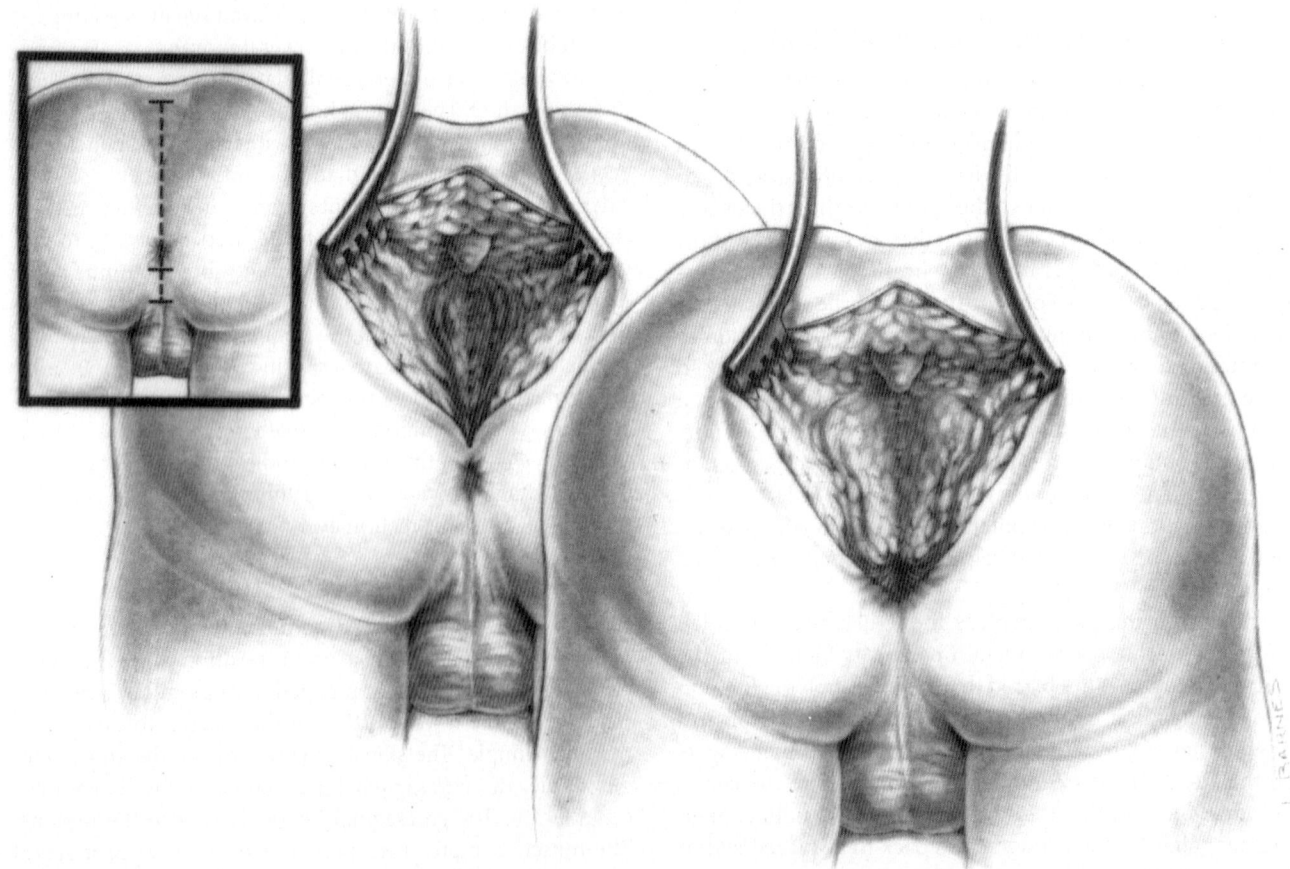

**FIGURE 53-20** Posterior sagittal incision. Division of parasagittal fibers and muscle complex. (Reprinted with permission from Peña A. *Atlas of Surgical Management of Anorectal Malformations.* New York: Springer-Verlag; 1990.)

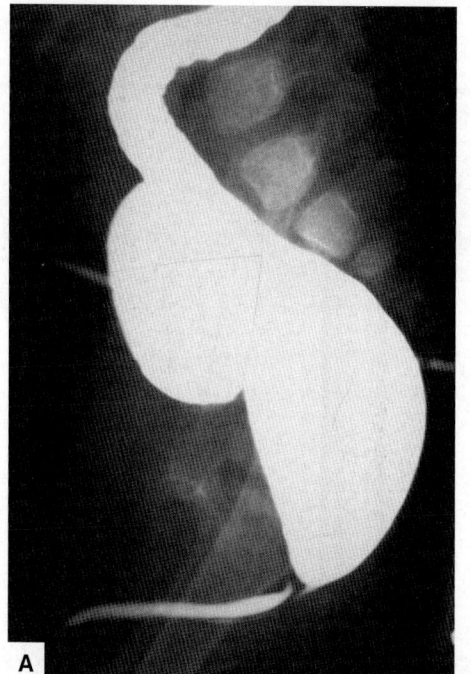

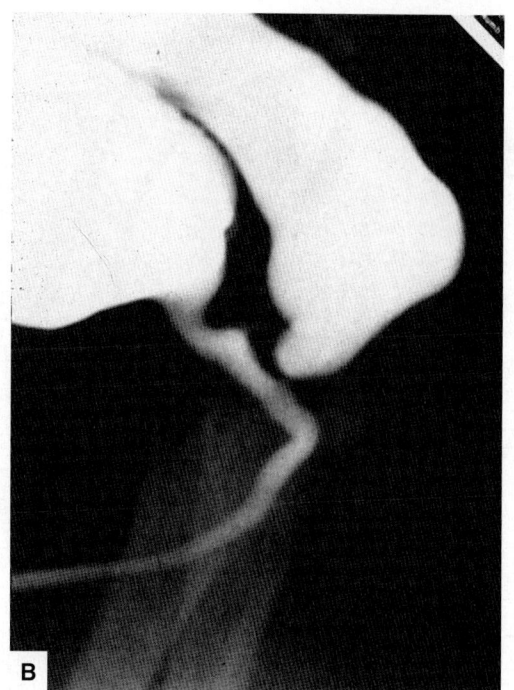

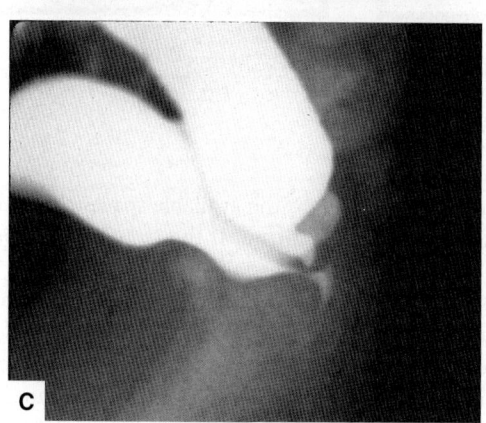

**FIGURE 53-21** Distal colostograms: **A.** Rectobulbar fistula. **B.** Rectoprostatic fistula. (Reprinted from Peña A. Imperforate anus. *Surgery* 1994;115(2), with permission from Elsevier.) **C.** Rectobladderneck fistula.

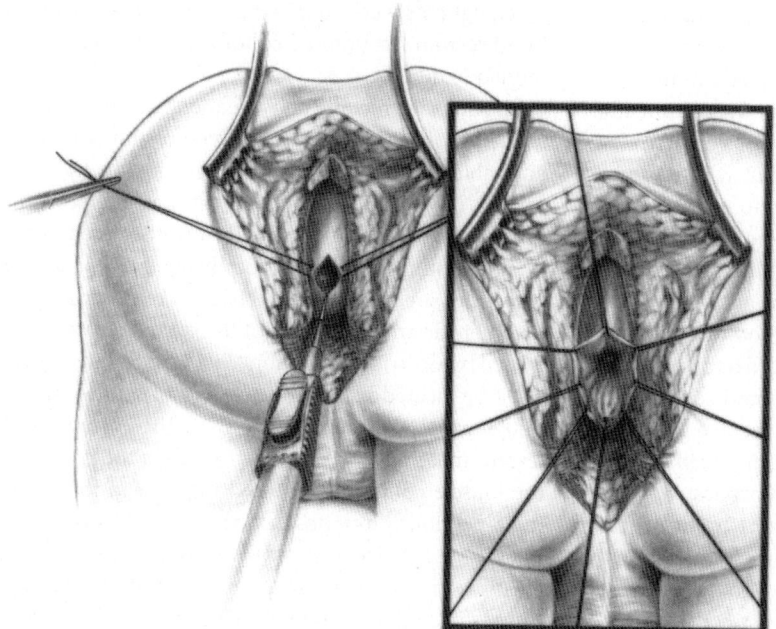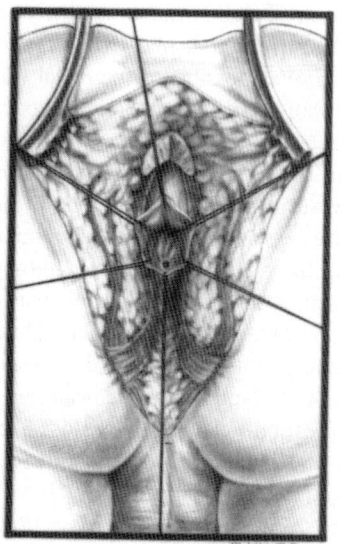

**FIGURE 53-22** Exposure of the rectum. (Reprinted with permission from Peña A. *Atlas of Surgical Management of Anorectal Malformations*. New York: Springer-Verlag; 1990.)

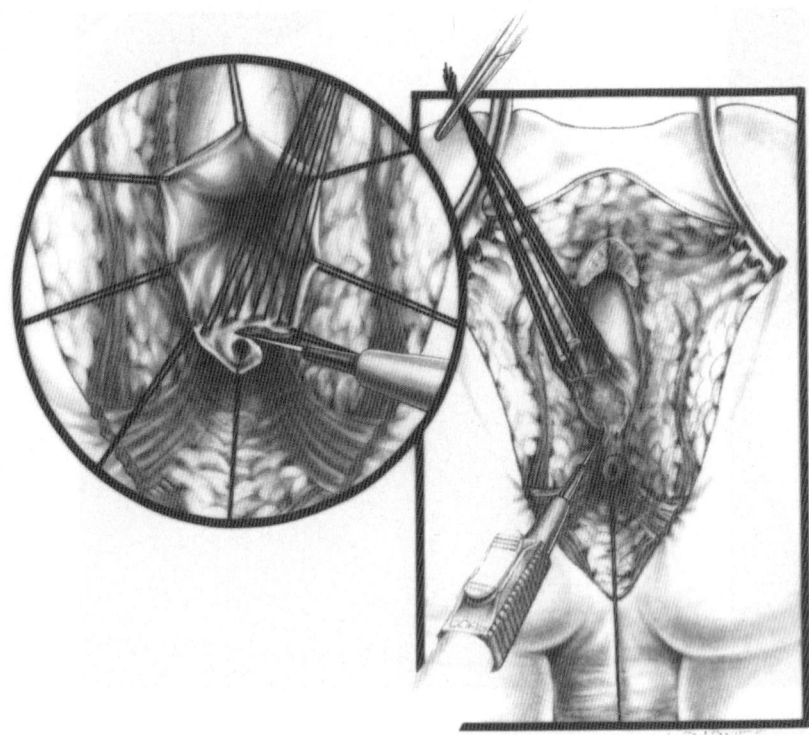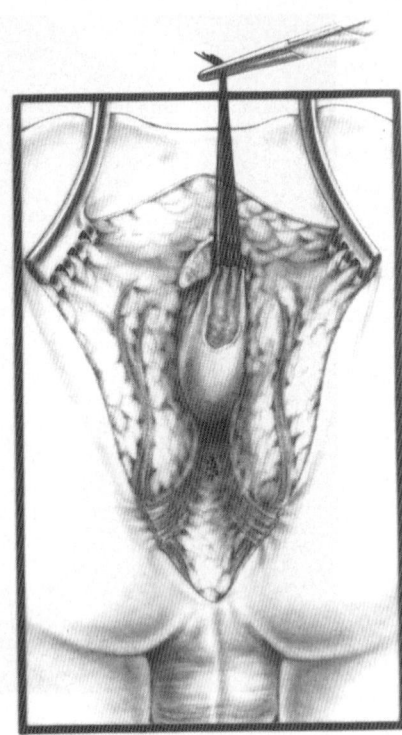

**FIGURE 53-23** Separation of the rectum from the urinary tract. (Reprinted with permission from Peña A. *Atlas of Surgical Management of Anorectal Malformations.* New York: Springer-Verlag; 1990.)

from the urinary tract represents the most delicate part of this procedure. For this, multiple 6-0 silk sutures are placed taking the rectal mucosa immediately above the fistula in a hemicircumferential fashion. These multiple sutures are used to exert uniform traction and to facilitate the separation of the rectum from the urinary tract. The initial part of the dissection is a submucosal one, and about 5 to 10 mm after that, it should become full thickness, separating the rectum completely from the urethra (Fig. 53-23). If this anterior rectal wall dissection is too deep, injury to other structures can easily occur. The rectum is surrounded posteriorly and laterally by a whitish fascia that must be divided before any attempt is made to mobilize the rectum. The circumferential dissection of the rectum after separation from the urinary tract should be performed, staying as close as possible to the rectal wall, but without injuring the wall itself. To do that, it is necessary to recognize that whitish fascia which has vessels that must be cauterized and divided. The rectum has an excellent intramural blood supply, and it is surprising how much length can be gained by dividing these vessels, while still preserving a good blood supply. Injuring the rectal wall, however, provokes damage to those important intramural vessels and may jeopardize the distal rectum. The stitches that were placed in the rectal edge during the opening of its posterior wall, as well as those silk stitches placed in the anterior rectal wall, are incorporated into a single mosquito clamp and are used to exert uniform traction to perform a circumferential dissection of the rectum to gain enough length to bring the rectum down to the perineum (Figs. 53-23 and 53-24). The dissection must continue until the rectum reaches the perineum without tension.

At this point, the need for tapering of the rectum is evaluated (Fig. 53-24). The decision is based on the size of the rectum, as compared to the available space within the limits of the sphincter mechanism. If the rectum is too bulky and does not allow adequate sphincter reconstruction, tailoring of its posterior wall is indicated. In such cases, about 50% of the posterior portion of the rectum is resected and the posterior wall is reconstructed with interrupted long-term absorbable sutures. The amount and length of tapering must be individualized depending on the anatomy of the specific patient. This maneuver is rarely needed. It was more common when patients were operated on at later ages, with a diverted, blind rectum left untouched for a long period of time, which tended to dilate.

The anterior rectal wall is frequently thinned out as a consequence of the separation between rectum and urethra. It is advisable to reinforce this wall, bringing together the smooth muscle layer with interrupted 6-0 absorbable sutures. The urethral fistula is sutured with absorbable suture material. That silk suture placed at the fistula site helps to find and repair this area. The perineal body is reconstructed, bringing together the anterior limits of the sphincter previously determined by electric stimulation (Fig. 53-24). Finally, the rectum must be located in front of the levator and within the limits of the muscle complex (Fig. 53-25). The posterior edge of the levator muscle is sutured together. Then the posterior edge of the muscle complex is sutured together in the midline, taking a portion of the posterior rectal wall in order to anchor it (Fig. 53-26). The rest of the wound is closed and the anoplasty is created with 16 interrupted long-term absorbable sutures in a circumferential manner (Fig. 53-27). Since there is a colostomy, feeds are advanced rapidly and the patient can be discharged in 2 days. The Foley catheter is left in place for 7 days and is removed in an outpatient setting.

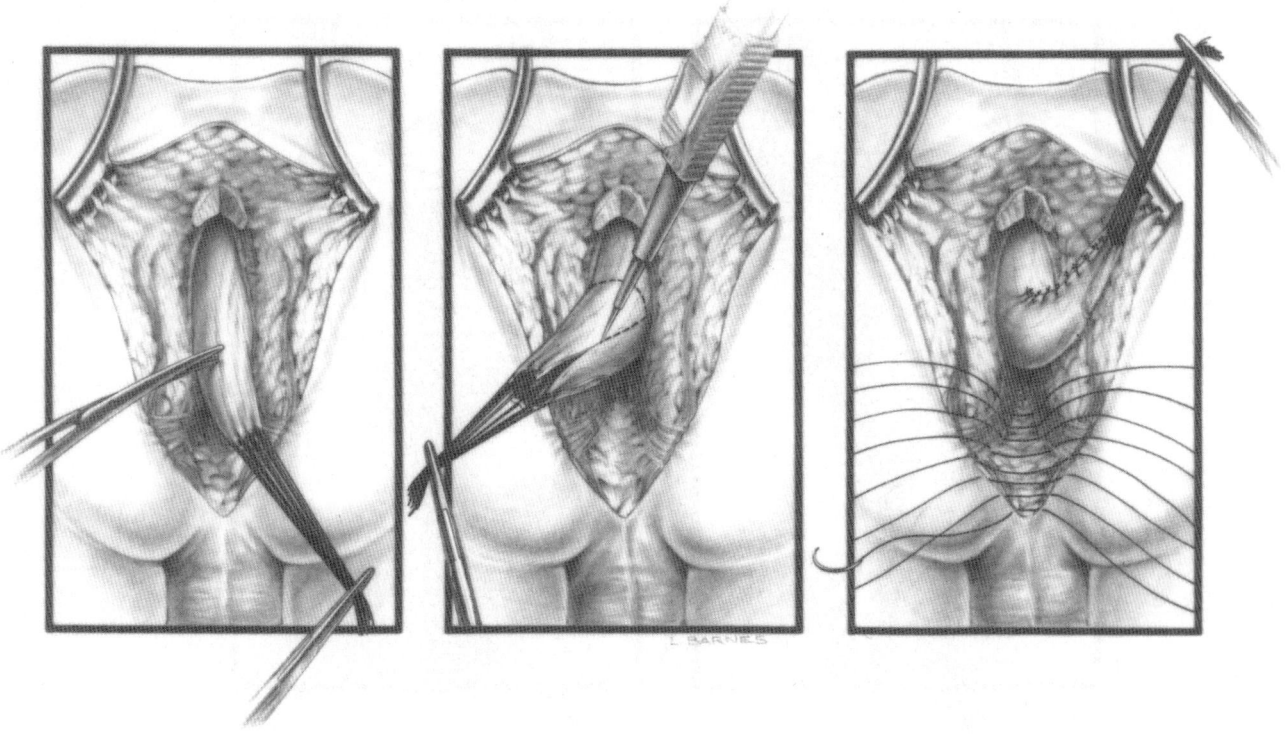

**FIGURE 53-24** Gaining rectal length and tapering the rectum when necessary. (Reprinted with permission from Peña A. *Atlas of Surgical Management of Anorectal Malformations*. New York: Springer-Verlag; 1990.)

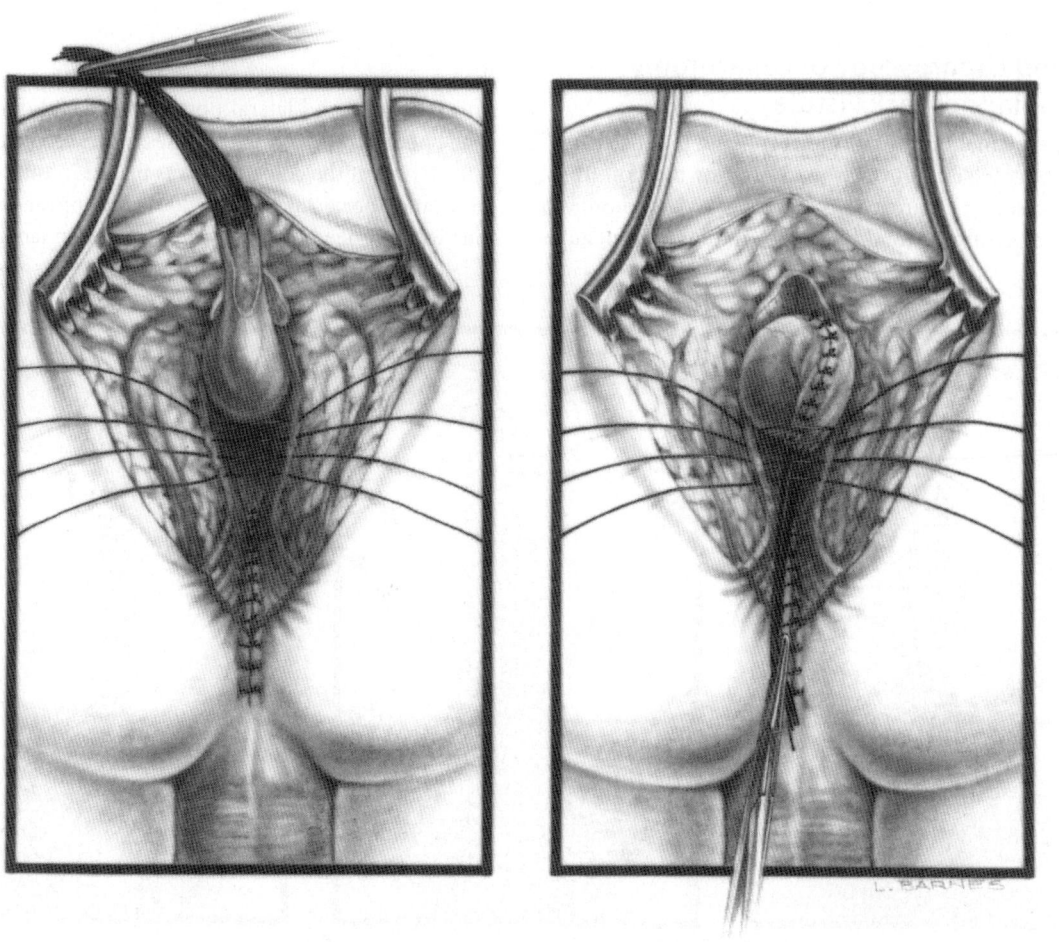

**FIGURE 53-25** Placing the rectum with the limits of the sphincter. (Reprinted with permission from Peña A. *Atlas of Surgical Management of Anorectal Malformations*. New York: Springer-Verlag; 1990.)

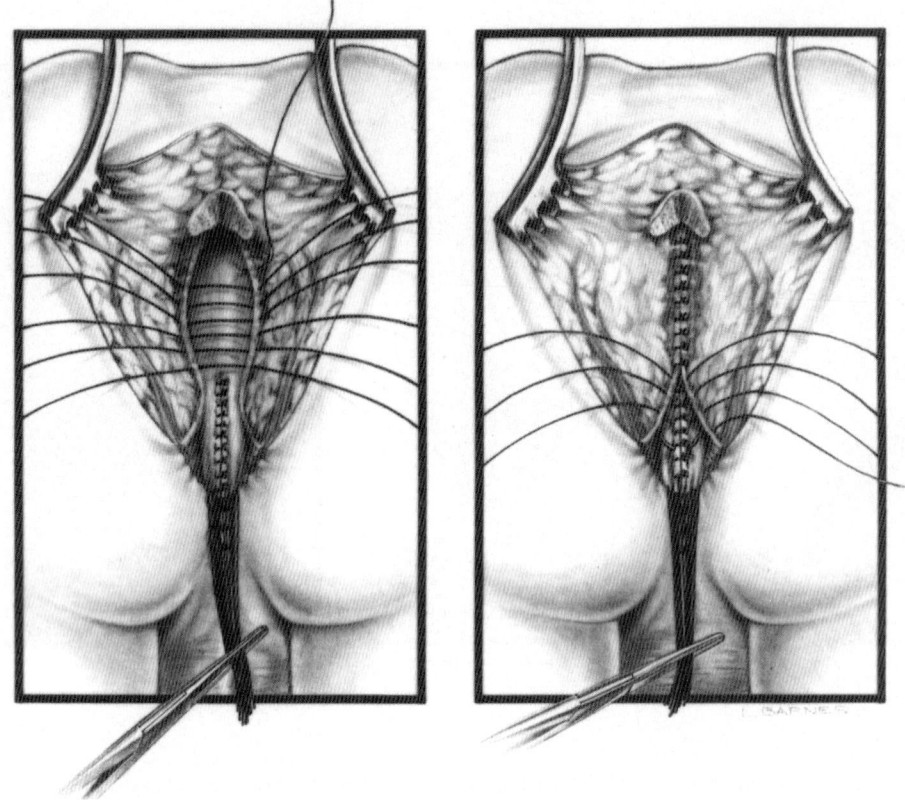

**FIGURE 53-26** Levator and muscle complex sutures. (Reprinted with permission from Peña A. *Atlas of Surgical Management of Anorectal Malformations.* New York: Springer-Verlag; 1990.)

## PSARP and Laparoscopy or Laparotomy for Rectobladderneck Fistula

In this type of malformation, the rectum is found so high that it is not reachable through the posterior incision; thus, the patient needs a laparoscopic approach or laparotomy to mobilize the rectum. A total-body preparation that includes the entire lower part of the patient's body, including anterior, posterior, and lateral portions of the abdomen, as well as the pelvis and lower extremities in the sterile field, is done (Fig. 53-28). If the colostomy was placed in the proximal sigmoid and the distal rectum does not appear bulbous (and thus will not need tapering), we begin with laparoscopy. The

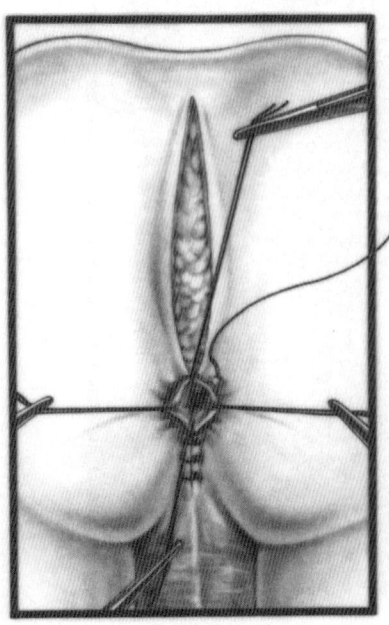
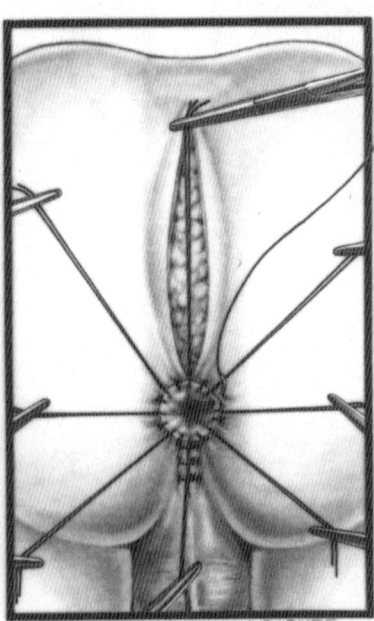
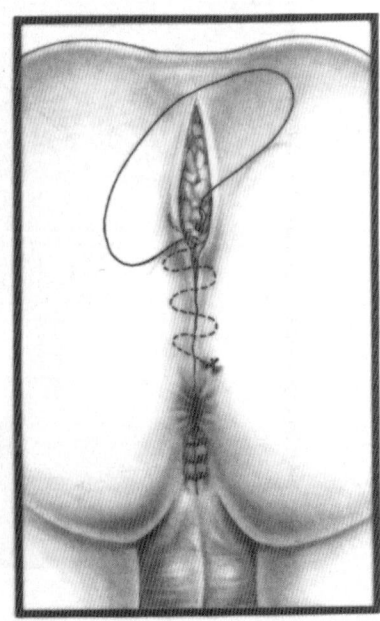

**FIGURE 53-27** Closure of incision and anoplasty. (Reprinted with permission from Peña A. *Atlas of Surgical Management of Anorectal Malformations.* New York: Springer-Verlag; 1990.)

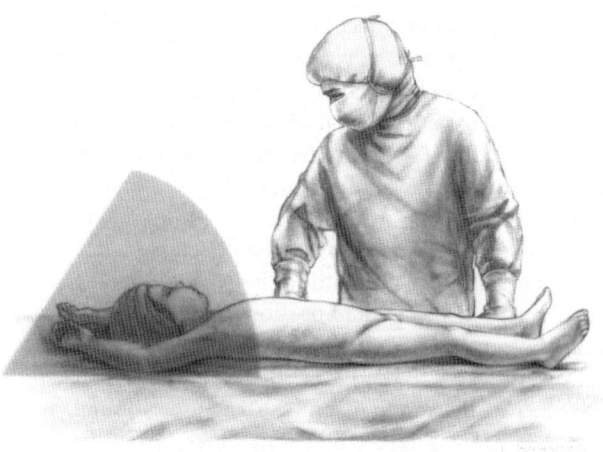

**FIGURE 53-28** Total body preparation. (Reprinted with permission from Peña A. *Atlas of Surgical Management of Anorectal Malformations.* New York: Springer-Verlag; 1990.)

distal rectum is dissected and the fistula ligated. In these very high defects, the rectobladderneck fistula is usually located 1 to 2 cm below the peritoneal reflection, and therefore, the pelvic dissection necessary to mobilize it is minimal. The ureters and vas deferens run very close to the rectum near the trigone of the bladder, and therefore the dissection of the rectosigmoid must be performed very close to the bowel wall. The rectum opens into the bladderneck in a T fashion. This means that there is no common wall above the fistula as seen in lower malformations. Once again the fistula is ligated; gaining adequate length of such a high rectum is very challenging and sometimes not possible laparoscopically. The legs are lifted up and a small perineal incision is made and the rectum is pulled down (Figs. 53-29 and 53-30). The rectum

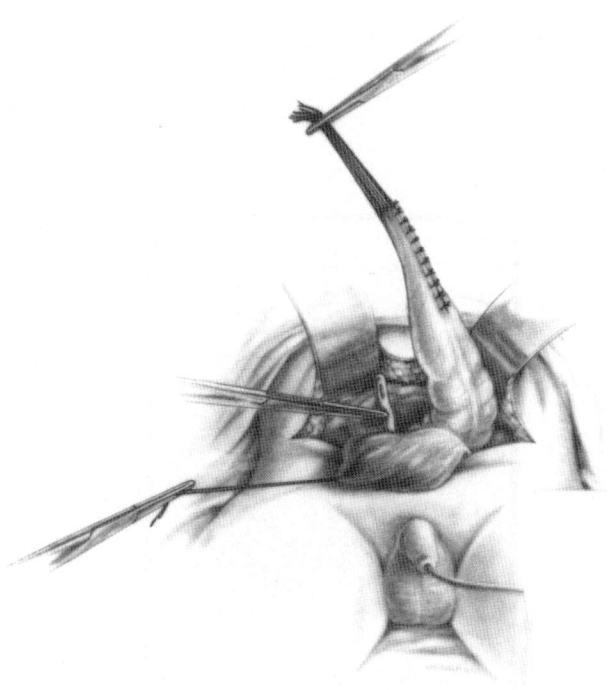

**FIGURE 53-29** Rectal pull-through (Reprinted with permission from Peña A. *Atlas of Surgical Management of Anorectal Malformations.* New York: Springer-Verlag; 1990.)

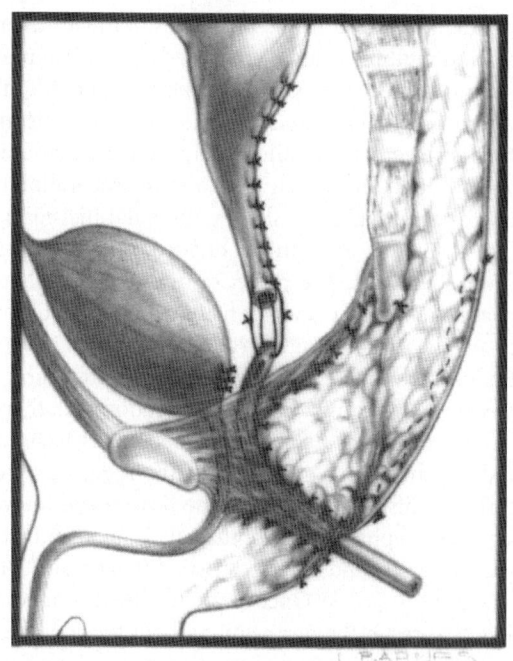

**FIGURE 53-30** Rectal pull-through. (Reprinted with permission from Peña A. *Atlas of Surgical Management of Anorectal Malformations.* New York: Springer-Verlag; 1990.)

is tacked to the posterior edge of the muscle complex and the anoplasty is performed as previously described.

## Imperforate Anus Without Fistula

The technique used to repair an imperforate anus without fistula is very similar to the one described for rectourethral fistula cases. Even when there is no communication between the rectum and urethra, they still share a common wall. Therefore, a plane between both structures has to be established very carefully as previously described.

## Rectal Atresia

Patients who have rectal atresia can also be repaired through this approach. The distal rectum is exposed sagittally posteriorly. The anal canal is opened posteriorly making a circle into a hemicircle. The upper rectum is anastomosed to the anal skin preserving the anterior dentate line and the sphincter mechanism is reconstructed meticulously around the new anorectum.

## Females

### Rectoperineal Fistula

The technique used for the repair of this defect is the same as the one described for the male counterpart. It is somewhat easier because the rectum is not intimately attached to the urethra. Care must be taken to separate the rectum from the posterior wall of the vagina.

### Rectovestibular Fistula

Patients with this malformation have an excellent functional prognosis; thus, every effort should be made to avoid complications that may jeopardize the clinical result.

The patient is placed in the prone position with the pelvis elevated and multiple stitches are placed at the circumference of the fistula orifice (Fig. 53-31). In the case of a deep fistula the posterior sagittal incision is opened first so the fistula site is better visualized. These stitches allow for uniform traction in a caudad direction, which facilitates the separation of the rectum from the vagina. A short midsagittal incision is created, the sphincter mechanism divided, and the posterior rectal wall identified. The posterior and lateral walls of the rectum are identified first, which helps define the anterior wall dissection. The most delicate part of the operation is the separation of the rectum from the vagina. The two structures share a common wall without a plane of separation and, therefore, a significant degree of delicate and meticulous technique is required to achieve that separation without damaging either structure. The dissection between the rectum and the vagina must continue cephalad until both walls (vagina and rectum) are of full thickness and a characteristic areolar plane between them is seen (Fig. 53-32). Once the rectum has been mobilized sufficiently to reach the perineum without tension, the perineal body is repaired, bringing together the anterior limits of the sphincter mechanism previously determined electrically (Fig. 53-33). The levator mechanism is usually not exposed. The posterior edges of the muscle complex are then sutured together in the midline, taking part of the rectal wall as previously described. The wound is closed and the anoplasty is performed with 16 circumferential long-term absorbable sutures.

## Persistent Cloaca

Because of this spectrum of defects, one can expect to find patients who are relatively straightforward to repair with excellent functional prognosis and others who represent an extraordinary technical challenge and may take many hours

of delicate, meticulous technique, and sometimes the functional results may not be very good. This last group of malformations should be repaired by surgeons who have special expertise and experience in dealing with these complex malformations (Table 53-2). A separate endoscopy to define the anatomy outside the newborn period before embarking on the reconstruction is very helpful. A contrast cloacagram, which can be done in 3-D, is also very useful.

The operation starts with a long midsagittal incision extending from the middle portion of the sacrum through the anal dimple and continues down to reach the single perineal opening (Fig. 53-33). The entire sphincter mechanism is divided in the midline until a structure is found, which most of the time is the rectum. Sometimes, however, the anatomic arrangement is sufficiently complex, and the vagina is found posterior to the rectum. The anatomy should have been anticipated by a preoperative cloacagram. The posterior rectal wall is opened, and as the incision continues caudally, 5-0 silk sutures are placed, taking the edges of the open rectum to facilitate the exposure. The entire malformation is exposed. At this point, the length of the common channel is clearly seen. A Foley catheter is introduced into the urethra. The rectum is then separated from the vagina. For this, multiple 5-0 sutures are placed in the anterior rectal wall and the rectum is separated from the vagina, while the surgeon follows the same principles as described for the repair of rectovestibular fistula.

The total urogenital mobilization is then utilized. This consists in the mobilization of both vagina and urethra together as a unit without separating them (Fig. 53-34). For this, multiple silk sutures are placed taking the edge of the vagina and the common channel, in order to apply uniform traction on the urogenital sinus. The urogenital sinus is transected approximately 5 mm from the clitoris and a plane of dissection is created between the pubis and the anterior wall of the

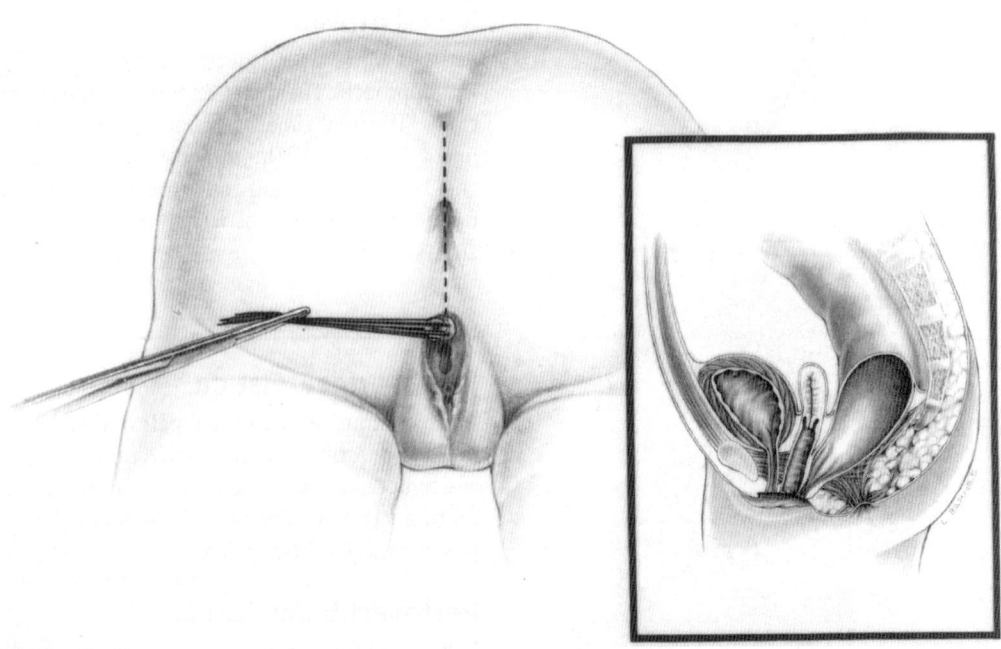

**FIGURE 53-31** Sutures placed at the fistula site. (Reprinted with permission from Peña A. *Atlas of Surgical Management of Anorectal Malformations.* New York: Springer-Verlag; 1990.)

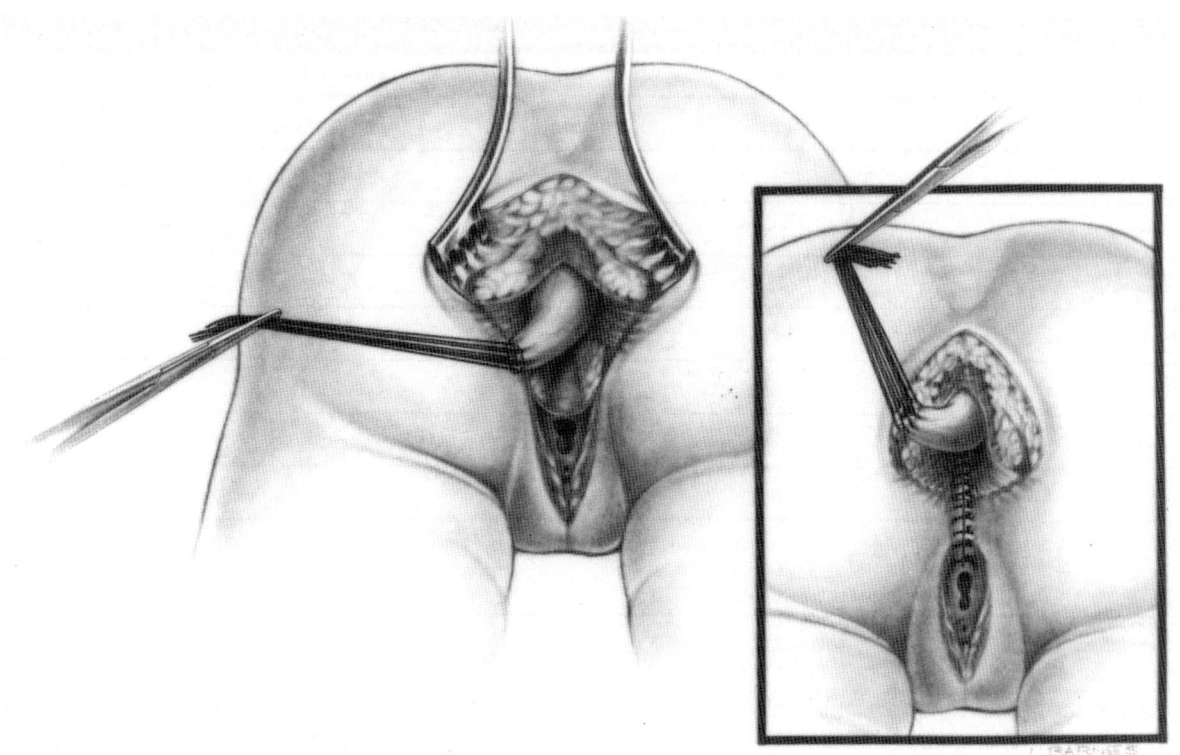

**FIGURE 53-32** Separation of rectum from vagina. (Reprinted with permission from Peña A. *Atlas of Surgical Management of Anorectal Malformations*. New York: Springer-Verlag; 1990.)

urogenital sinus. While applying superiorly directed traction to the multiple sutures, the suspensory ligaments of the urethra and bladderneck (which are avascular) are divided, which provides an immediate significant mobilization of the urogenital sinus (usually 2-3 cm). All cloacae with a common channel length of 2 to 3 cm can be repaired using this maneuver and without opening the abdomen. The advantages of this

mobilization include preservation of an excellent blood supply to the vagina and urethra, an excellent cosmetic appearance, avoidance of urethrovaginal fistula, as well as vaginal strictures.

For those patients who have longer common channels, the total urogenital mobilization through this approach may not be enough to reconstruct the malformation satisfactorily.

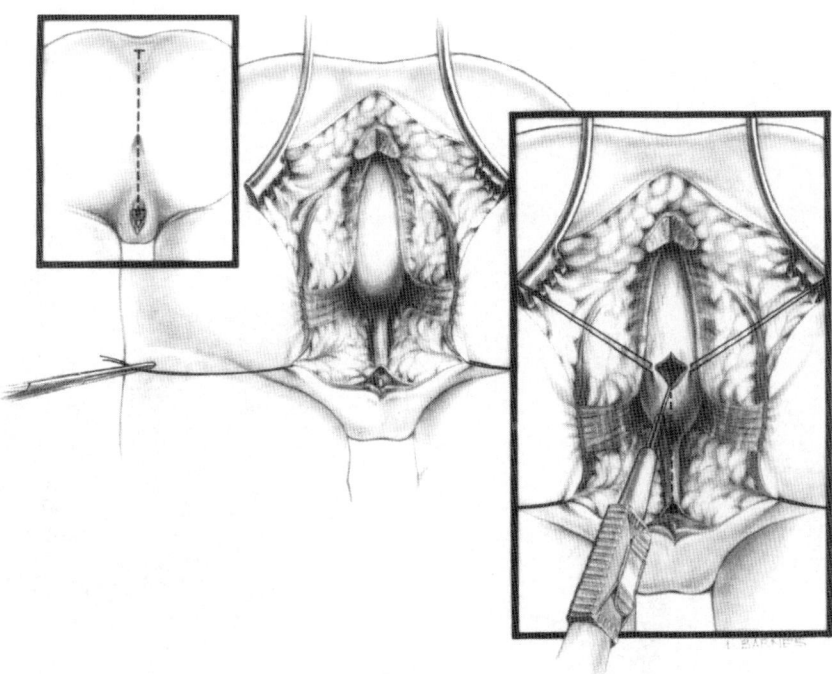

**FIGURE 53-33** Cloaca repair. Incision. (Reprinted with permission from Peña A. *Atlas of Surgical Management of Anorectal Malformations*. New York: Springer-Verlag; 1990.)

**TABLE 53-2    Two Types of Cloacas; our Primary Cloaca Experience, Excluding Redos**

|  | Group A | Group B |
|---|---|---|
| Common channel | Short, <3 cm | Long, >3 cm |
| Type of operation | Only posterior sagittal | Posterior sagittal and laparotomy |
| Length of procedure | 3 hours | 6–12 hours |
| Postoperative hospitalization | 48 hours | Several days |
| Incidence in our series | 193 | 133 |
| Voluntary bowel movements | 66% (n = 93) | 34% (n = 59) |
| Voluntary urinary control | 73%[b] (n = 96) | 26% (n = 70) |
| Intraoperative decision making | Relatively reproducible operation | Complex and technically demanding[a] |

[a]Bladder/vagina separation, ureteral catheterization, vesicostomy, bladderneck reconstruction or closure, vaginal switch, vaginal replacement (with rectum, colon, or small bowel).
[b]The remaining patients are dry on intermittent catheterization.

The mobilized urogenital complex can be delivered up into the abdomen after a laparotomy. Sometimes dissection of its attachments this way allows for it to now reach the perineum. If this is not enough, then through the abdomen, separation of the vagina and urinary tract is performed, which is a tedious and meticulous part of the procedure. To do this, the bladder is first opened and the ureters catheterized, so that the surgeon can palpate them during the dissection of the common wall between vagina(s) and the bladderneck. After the vagina has been completely separated, the surgeon may find (a) that the vagina(s) reaches the perineum, which is rather unusual; or (b) that the patient has 2 hemivaginas located too high to reach the perineum. The transverse length of both hemivaginas together is longer than the vertical one.

In that case, the surgeon can perform a maneuver called a vaginal switch. One of the hemiuteri, as well as the ipsilateral fallopian tube, is resected, preserving the ovary and its blood supply. The blood supply of the hemivagina of that side is sacrificed. The blood supply of the contralateral hemivagina is preserved and provides perfusion for both hemivaginas. The vaginal septum is resected and both hemivaginas are tubularized, creating a long single vagina. What used to be the dome of the hemivagina where the hemiuterus was resected is switched down to the perineum. This is an excellent maneuver but can be performed only when these anatomic characteristics are present (Fig. 53-35).

Sometimes one finds a very high vagina(s) that is also very small; in those cases, one has to use a piece of bowel

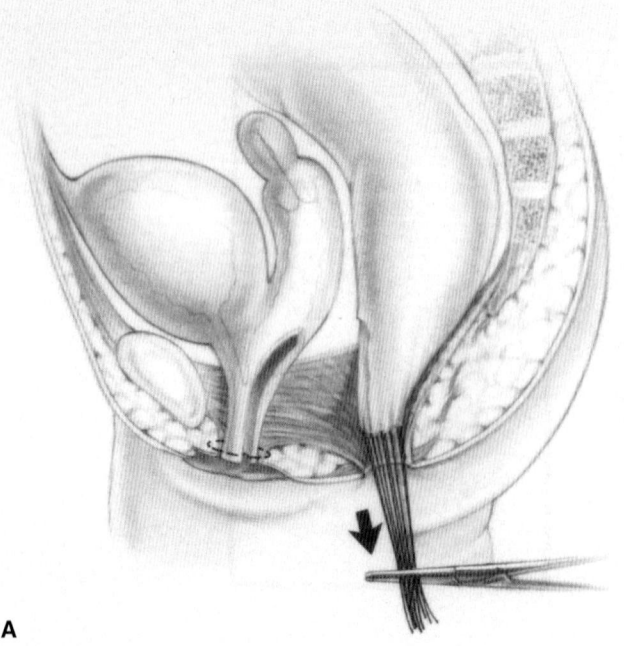

**A**

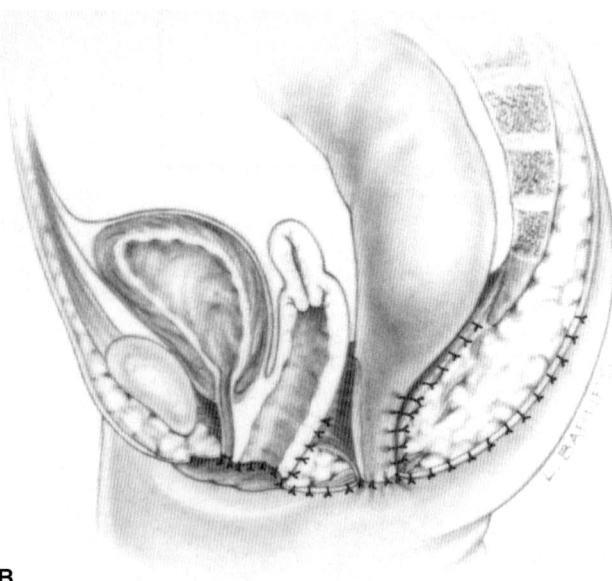

**B**

**FIGURE 53-34** Total urogenital mobilization. **A.** The rectum has been mobilized posteriorly. **B.** After mobilizing the urogenital sinus, the vagina, and urethra are separated. (Reprinted from Peña A. Total urogenital mobilization. *J Pediatr Surg* 1997;32(2), with permission from Elsevier.)

## PERSISTENT CLOACA WITH HYDROCOLPOS, HEMIVAGINAS, & HEMIUTERUS

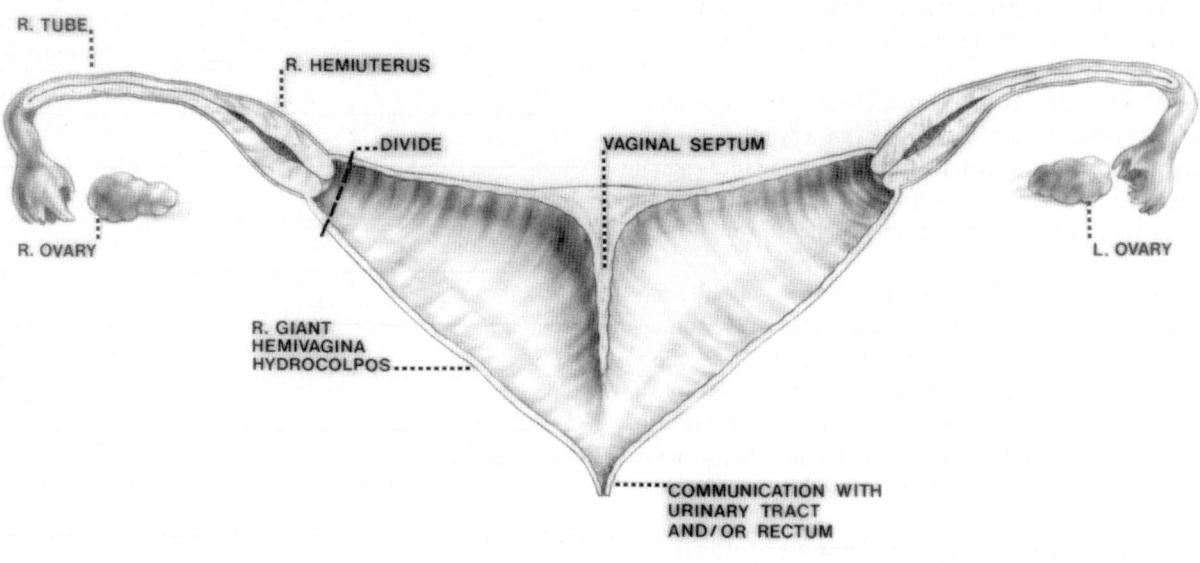

R. TUBE

R. HEMIUTERUS

DIVIDE

VAGINAL SEPTUM

R. OVARY

L. OVARY

R. GIANT
HEMIVAGINA
HYDROCOLPOS

COMMUNICATION WITH
URINARY TRACT
AND/OR RECTUM

PERINEUM

**A**

## VAGINAL RECONSTRUCTION AND SWITCH MANEUVER

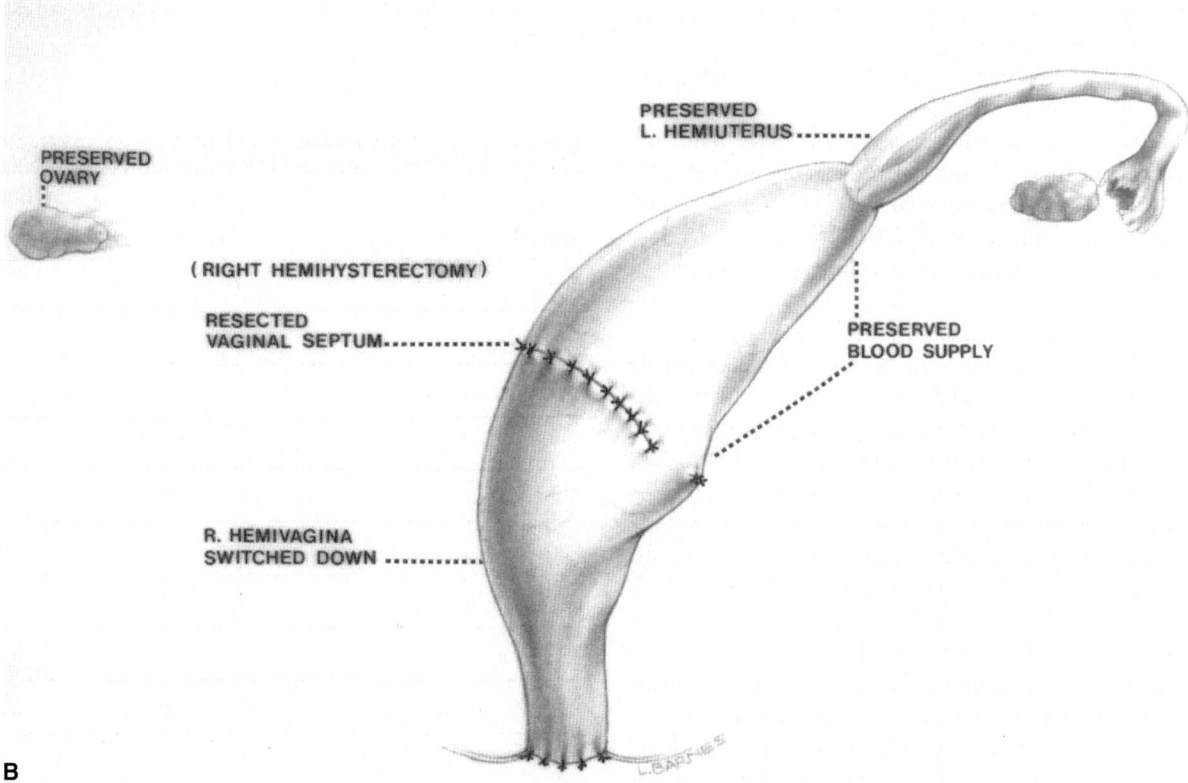

PRESERVED
L. HEMIUTERUS

PRESERVED
OVARY

(RIGHT HEMIHYSTERECTOMY)

RESECTED
VAGINAL SEPTUM

PRESERVED
BLOOD SUPPLY

R. HEMIVAGINA
SWITCHED DOWN

L. BARNES

**B**

**FIGURE 53-35** Vaginal switch. **A.** The right Fallopian tube is removed, preserving the ovary. The right hemi-vagina is mobilized. **B.** The right hemivagina is "switched down" to reach the perineum. (Reprinted from Peña A, et al. Surgical management of cloacal malformations. *J Pediatr Surg* 2004;39(3), with permission from Elsevier.)

to augment or replace the vagina. One can use the colon or the small bowel. Given a choice, the colon sigmoid or the left colon has better characteristics to replace the vagina. The separated urethra is now tubularized and pulled through to the perineum.

A final variant is a long common channel (5 cm or more) and high vagina. In such a case one can leave the common channel untouched to become the neourethra, and separate the vagina(s) from the back of it through the abdomen. The vagina or vaginal replacement is then pulled through to the perineum.

The Foley catheter, after the repair of a cloaca, usually stays for approximately 14 to 21 days, and sometimes even longer in a reconstructed urethra. Vesicostomy may be needed particularly in long common channel cases, and the use of the urethra for intermittent catheterization is delayed until the child is older. Two weeks after the operation, the program of anal dilatations is started. The vagina is not subjected to dilatations.

The colostomy can be closed after the protocol of anal dilatations has been completed. At this setting the cloacal repair is endoscoped, and the assessment for the need and ease of intermittent catheterization is made.

**Functional Results.** Voluntary bowel movements are defined as the act of feeling the urge to use the toilet to have a bowel movement, the capacity to verbalize it, and hold the bowel movement until the patient reaches the bathroom. Soiling is defined as the involuntary leaking of small amounts of stool, which provokes smearing of the underwear. Constipation is defined as the incapacity to empty the rectum spontaneously (every day), which is sometimes manageable with changes in diet, and more often with laxatives. Fecal control is evaluated after the patient is 3 years of age.

Clinical results are different in each type of malformation described. A recent analysis of the authors' series showed that voluntary bowel movements were found in the following percentages: rectal atresia and perineal fistula (100%), vestibular fistula (93.8%), rectobulbar urethral fistula (87.5%), imperforate anus without fistula (85%), cloaca (83.3%), rectourethral prostatic fistula (76.5%), and rectobladderneck fistula (28.6%) (Table 53-3). Table 53-4 shows the percentage of patients who suffer from soiling for each defect. Soiling in patients who have voluntary bowel movements usually represents a manifestation of fecal impaction, and when the constipation is treated properly, the soiling will disappear. Patients who have voluntary bowel movements and never soil are considered "totally continent" (Table 53-5). This includes 100% of perineal fistula cases and 83.3% atresia or stenosis cases, 71.1% of vestibular fistulas, 70.6% of imperforate anus with no fistula, 32.1% of rectourethral bulbar fistulas, 27.3% of cloacae, 28.2% of rectoprostatic fistulas, and no patient in our series with rectobladderneck fistula.

Constipation is a common sequelae seen after the repair of an anorectal malformation. Table 53-6 shows the percentage of patients who suffer from this. Interestingly, patients with lower defects and, therefore, with better prognosis for bowel control, have a higher incidence of constipation and vice versa. Constipation seems to correlate directly with the degree of rectosigmoid dilatation at the time of colostomy

| TABLE 53-3 | Voluntary Bowel Movement and Type of Defect | | |
|---|---|---|---|
| **Defect** | **No. of Cases** | **Voluntary Bowel Movement** | |
| | | **No.** | **%** |
| Atresia or stenosis | 8 | 8 | 100 |
| Rectoperineal fistula | 52 | 50 | 96 |
| Rectovestibular fistula | 113 | 104 | 92 |
| Imperforate anus without fistula | 38 | 31 | 82 |
| Rectobulbar fistula | 97 | 77 | 79 |
| Cloaca, common channel <3 cm | 92 | 61 | 66 |
| Rectovaginal fistula | 5 | 3 | 60 |
| Rectoprostatic fistula | 94 | 61 | 34 |
| Cloaca, common channel >3 cm | 59 | 20 | 34 |
| Rectobladderneck fistula | 44 | 10 | 23 |
| Totals | 602 | 425 | 71 |

602 primary anorectal malformation patients evaluated.

closure. Therefore, every effort should be made to try to keep the rectosigmoid empty and decompressed from day one in these patients. This is accomplished by proactive monitoring and laxative therapy starting right after the colostomy is closed, or soon after the repair if no colostomy is present.

| TABLE 53-4 | Soiling and Type of Defect | | |
|---|---|---|---|
| **Defect** | **No. of Cases** | **Soiling** | |
| | | **No.** | **%** |
| Rectoperineal fistula | 50 | 5 | 10 |
| Rectal atresia or stenosis | 7 | 1 | 14 |
| Recotvestibular fistula | 105 | 35 | 33 |
| Imperforate anus without fistula | 37 | 18 | 49 |
| Rectobulbar fistula | 91 | 46 | 51 |
| Cloaca, common channel <3 cm | 86 | 53 | 62 |
| Rectoprostatic fistula | 95 | 72 | 76 |
| Rectovaginal fistula | 5 | 4 | 80 |
| Cloaca, common channel >3 cm | 44 | 39 | 89 |
| Rectobladderneck fistula | 44 | 39 | 89 |
| Totals | 566 | 312 | 55 |

566 primary anorectal malformation patients evaluated.

ABDOMINAL DISEASE

| TABLE 53-5 | Totally Continent Patients and Type of Defect | | |
|---|---|---|---|
| Defect | No. of Cases | Totally Continent | |
| | | No. | % |
| Rectoperineal fistula | 45 | 40 | 89 |
| Rectal atresia or stenosis | 7 | 6 | 86 |
| Rectovestibular fistula | 105 | 70 | 67 |
| Imperforate anus without fistula | 35 | 18 | 51 |
| Rectobulbar fistula | 87 | 39 | 45 |
| Cloaca, common channel <3 cm | 86 | 31 | 36 |
| Rectoprostatic fistula | 90 | 18 | 20 |
| Rectovaginal fistula | 5 | 1 | 20 |
| Cloaca, common channel >3 cm | 43 | 4 | 9 |
| Rectobladderneck fistula | 42 | 3 | 7 |
| Totals | 547 | 230 | 42 |

547 primary anorectal malformation patients evaluated.

Urinary control can be expected in the overwhelming majority of male patients after repair of the imperforate anus provided a good surgical technique was performed and there is no associated sacral or spinal anomaly. In cloacas where the common channel is shorter than 3 cm, approximately 20% of patients require intermittent catheterization to empty the bladder. The remaining 80% have voluntary urinary control.

| TABLE 53-6 | Constipation and Type of Defect | | |
|---|---|---|---|
| Defect | No. of Cases | Constipation | |
| | | No. | % |
| Rectobladderneck fistula | 46 | 7 | 15 |
| Rectovaginal fistula | 5 | 1 | 20 |
| Cloaca, common channel >3 cm | 49 | 16 | 33 |
| Cloaca, common channel <3 cm | 91 | 36 | 40 |
| Rectoprostatic fistula | 96 | 44 | 46 |
| Imperforate anus without fistula | 39 | 20 | 51 |
| Rectovestibular fistula | 108 | 61 | 56 |
| Rectal atresia or stenosis | 7 | 4 | 57 |
| Rectoperineal fistula | 63 | 36 | 57 |
| Rectobulbar fistula | 96 | 59 | 61 |
| Totals | 600 | 284 | 47 |

600 primary anorectal malformation patients evaluated.

When the common channel is longer than 3 cm, approximately 80% of the patients require intermittent catheterization to empty the bladder. Fortunately, after the repair of a cloaca, patients almost always have a good bladder neck and they are capable of holding urine. The main functional disorder they suffer from is an incapacity to efficiently empty the bladder. Thus, when the bladder becomes completely full, the patients start having overflow urinary incontinence. Intermittent catheterization keeps these patients completely dry, and protects their kidneys from high bladder pressures.

## Functional Sequelae and Their Management

### Constipation

The great majority of patients born with an imperforate anus who undergo a type of repair that includes the preservation of the original rectum (the vast majority these days) will suffer constipation. It seems to be the clinical manifestation of a hypomotility disorder of the rectosigmoid. Patients who at birth underwent transverse colostomies have a greater chance of having dilatation of the rectosigmoid and subsequently suffer from more constipation than patients with more distal colostomies. Patients with loop colostomies, particularly those who allow the passing of stool from the proximal to the distal bowel, will suffer from fecal impaction in the distal rectum, worse megarectosigmoid, and therefore, worse constipation. After the colostomy is closed, proper treatment of the constipation is imperative. Constipation is a self-perpetuating and self-aggravating condition; it produces megarectosigmoid, which, in turn, produces more constipation, creating a vicious cycle, ultimately leading to soiling (overflow pseudoincontinence). It is the surgeon's obligation to make the parents aware of these potential sequelae. The patients should receive a laxative type of diet and/or enough bowel-stimulating laxatives to produce emptying of the rectum every day. Even when the constipation is not curable, it is manageable.

Some patients with severe constipation come late, having never received treatment for constipation early in their lives, and they have a very severe megasigmoid and overflow pseudoincontinence. The laxative requirements in some of these patients is so high that it becomes impossible to administer the medication without producing vomiting. For this group of patients, and provided they have bowel control, an operation is indicated to resect the most dilated part of the colon (sigmoid resection) and create an anastomosis between the normal-size descending colon and the rectum (Fig. 53-36). By doing this, the amount of laxatives that these patients require may decrease, and sometimes, the need for them is eliminated. If a patient suffers from nonmanageable severe constipation and, in addition, belongs to the poor prognosis type of defect (fecal incontinence), then the treatment should consist of the administration of an enema every day; the sigmoid resection is contraindicated, unless the daily enema required to empty the colon is enormous. Usually the right daily enema keeps them clean. Sometimes a Malone appendicostomy and sigmoid resection (when the sigmoid is very dilated) can be done with antegrade enemas given thereafter.

Because of the high incidence of constipation in patients after an imperforate anus repair, some surgeons have thought

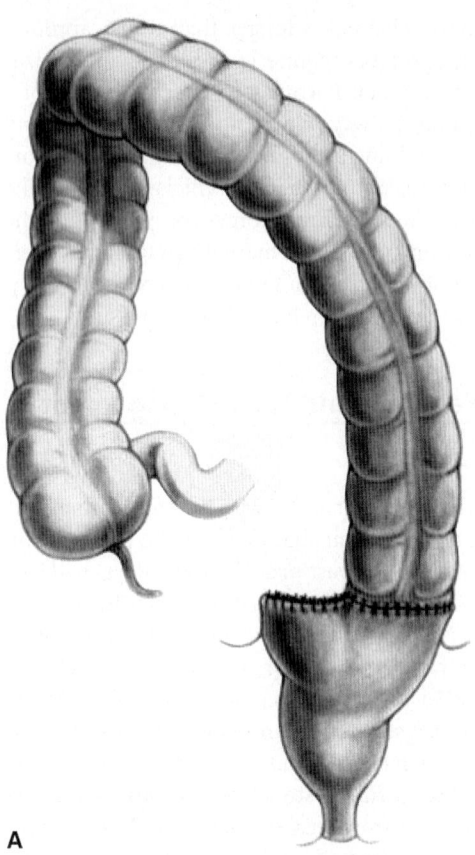

A

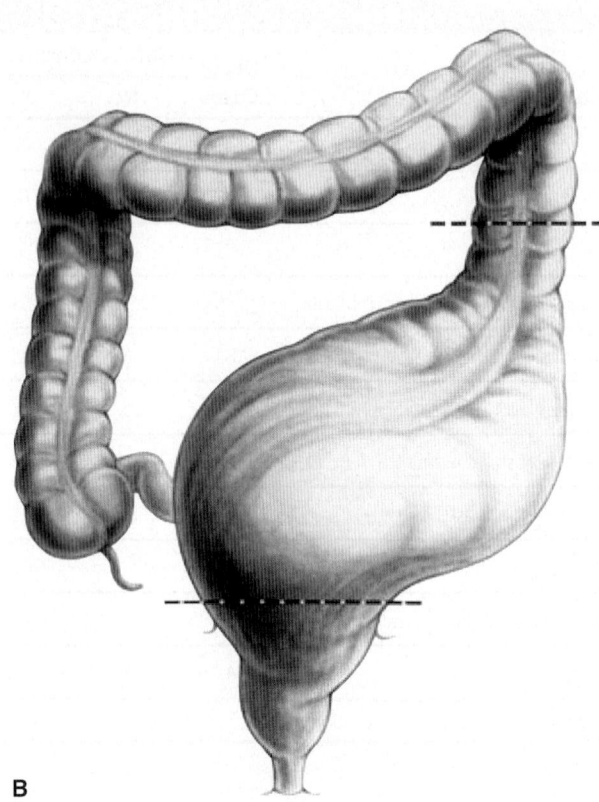

B

**FIGURE 53-36** Sigmoid resection. (Reprinted from Peña A. El-Behery M. Megasigmoid—a source of pseudoincontinence in children with repaired anorectal malformations. *J Pediatr Surg* 1993;28(2), with permission from Elsevier.)

to take rectal biopsies to rule out the presence of concurrent Hirschsprung disease. In our series, Hirschsprung is no more common in patients with anorectal malformation than in the general population. Constipation alone, even severe, without distention, enterocolitis, and failure to thrive is not Hirschsprung. Sadly some of these patients are subjected to a Hirschsprung-like pull-through. An abdomino-perineal pullthrough after an imperforate anus repair does fix the constipation, but they become totally incontinent, even when born with a benign defect because the induced hypermotility is too much for their suboptimal sphincters and anal canal to handle. Therefore, one must be careful to not overdiagnose this disease. A rectal biopsy occasionally may show absent ganglion cells after an imperforate anus repair but the biopsy was likely taken too low, in the transitional epithelium. Without confirmatory hypertrophic nerves, such a biopsy needs to be considered inadequate.

## Fecal Incontinence

It is very important to establish an accurate diagnosis of the specific type of anorectal defect and the quality of the sacrum and spine early in life in order to try to predict the final functional prognosis in terms of bowel control. The parent's expectations can then be adjusted to the reality.

When patients are born with a good prognosis type of defect (rectal atresia, rectoperineal fistula, rectovestibular fistula, rectourethralbulbar fistula with a normal sacrum, imperforate anus without fistula with a normal sacrum), the patient can be expected to develop voluntary bowel movements by the age of 3 years. Soiling is usually avoided by adequately treating constipation. A small percentage of these patients, however, do not develop bowel control, and at around 3 years of age, they should have a bowel-management program to keep them artificially clean with a daily enema.

On the other hand, in patients who were born with a bad prognosis type of defect (rectobladderneck fistula, rectoprostatic fistula with an abnormal sacrum, cloaca with a common channel greater than 3 cm, and an abnormal sacrum), it is anticipated that they will not develop bowel control, and the family can be saved a lot of frustration, time, and expense trying to toilet train the child by directly starting a bowel-management program when the family decides that the child should go into normal underwear (usually at around 3-4 years of age).

With an accurate diagnosis and with knowledge of the status of the sacrum and the spine, it is possible to predict the final result. For those patients who have some chance of having bowel control, there are other prognostic signs that are valuable. For instance, the bowel-movement pattern in an infant frequently indicates the potential for bowel control. When a patient passes stool constantly without any evidence of feeling or pushing, it usually means that the patient is fecally incontinent, whereas a patient who has 1 to 3 bowel movements per day, even when involuntary, but remains completely clean between bowel movements and during the episodes of defecation shows some signs of feelings such as "pushing," is frequently trainable. If a patient has a good bowel movement pattern such as this, the patient deserves a trial of toilet training, whereas a patient with a poor bowel-movement pattern benefits from the bowel-management program with a daily enema.

## Bowel-Management Program

All patients born with an imperforate anus should at the age of potty training be completely clean of stool in the underwear either because they have bowel control (which happens in about 75% of all patients) or because they are subjected to a bowel-management program, a mechanical emptying of the colon.

Bowel management consists in teaching the parents how to clean the colon every day with the use of enemas. By keeping the patient's colon quiet for 24 hours, between enemas, they do not pass stool and thus avoid soiling. To achieve success with the bowel-management program, it is important to first learn which type of colonic motility the patient has; this can be inferred from a contrast enema study done with a hydro-soluble material.

Most patients who underwent a surgical repair that included the preservation of their original rectum will suffer from different degrees of megasigmoid. That means that they also suffer from constipation. Those patients will require large enemas, frequently a mixture of saline solution with added glycerin and/or soap, to be able to clean a large floppy colon. To keep the colon quiet in that group of patients is not a problem; one takes advantage of the fact that they are naturally constipated and, therefore, the patient stays clean 24 hours per day, between enemas.

A small group of patients undergo resection of their original rectum and/or sigmoid. These patients suffer from hypermotility of the colon and have a tendency to have diarrhea. In these patients, it is relatively easy to clean their colon (usually a saline only enema) because it is not dilated. The main problem, however, is trying to keep the colon quiet between enemas, and for that we use a constipating diet and/or medications, such as loperamide and pectin, and fiber additives to slow down the colonic motility.

The bowel-management program is implemented by trial and error. Every patient needs a different type of enema. It usually takes approximately 1 week to implement a working system. To assess whether the enema successfully cleans the colon, we use a daily x-ray film of the abdomen.

## Urinary Incontinence

As previously mentioned, urinary incontinence occurs as an overflow phenomenon in 80% of patients who were born with a cloaca with a common channel longer than 3 cm and in 20% of patients with a shorter common channel. Because the bladderneck is usually competent, intermittent catheterization usually keeps these patients dry.

Urinary incontinence in male patients after an imperforate anus repair may occur because of a poor surgical technique and some sort of nerve damage, or occurs in a patient with an associated sacral or spinal problem.

## SELECTED READINGS

Bischoff A, Levitt MA, Bauer C, Jackson L, Holder M, Peña A. Treatment of fecal incontinence with a comprehensive bowel management program. *J Pediatr Surg* 2009;44(6):1278–1284.

Breech L. Gynecological concerns in patients with anorectal malformations. *Semin Pediatr Surg* 2010;19(2):139–145.

Levitt MA, Kant A, Peña A. The morbidity of constipation in patients with anorectal Malformations. *J Pediatr Surg* 2010;45(6):1228–1233.

Levitt MA, Peña A. Cloacal malformations: lessons learned from 490 cases. *Semin Pediatr Surg* 2010;19(2):128–138.

Levitt MA, Peña A. Pediatric fecal incontinence: a surgeon's perspective. *Pediatr Rev* 2010;31(3):91–101.

Peña A, deVries PA. Posterior sagittal anorectoplasty. Important technical considerations and new applications. *J Pediatr Surg* 1982;17(6):796–811.

Stephens FD. Imperforate rectum: a new surgical technique. *Med J Aust* 1953;1(6):202–206.

# Common Acquired Anorectal Problems of Childhood

# CHAPTER 54

*Robert M. Arensman and Daniel J. Stephens*

## KEY POINTS

1. Hemorrhoidal disease is unusual in childhood and rarely requires operation.

2. Anal fissures are common and related to constipation. Treating the constipation usually cures the fissure.

3. Fistula-in-ano presents frequently as recurrent infection, and should be treated operatively with excision.

4. Rectal prolapse rarely requires operative treatment.

## INTRODUCTION

There are few problems in adult surgical care that create more pain and complaint than perianal problems. By extension, it would seem that children are likely to be as easily disturbed and pained by those conditions that often bear a similar name but may in fact be a little different and require slightly different care. Pain, bleeding, and infection are the common cause of morbidity in these patients, but with prompt evaluation and proper management, prognosis is typically good, except in the rarer cases when these seemingly *minor* ailments represent a harbinger of more serious disease.

## MINOR PERIANAL DISEASE

### Hemorrhoidal Disease

#### Incidence

Hemorrhoids in childhood are fairly rare, and so it is hard to find literature that supports any incidence figures. It suffices to say that true hemorrhoids are not commonly encountered in pediatric surgical practice. So-called sentinel piles associated with fissure are considerably more common and often are misdiagnosed as residual hemorrhoidal disease (this is covered below).

#### Demographics

True hemorrhoids are probably a bit more common in boys, since this group is more likely to have problems with chronic constipation in early life.

#### Presentation

Generally these children present with a history of constipation that is complicated by bleeding, bloody toilet water, or streaks of blood in the stool. Physical examination confirms the presence of bluish varicosities on anal examination or gentle internal anoscopy, or possibly thrombosis with a bluish mass.

#### Diagnostic Evaluation

Little more is needed than a good medical history and physical examination unless there is concern that the hemorrhoid is a manifestation of a considerably more serious problem such as portal hypertension.

#### Treatment

Initial treatment in children should be gentle and directed to the underlying constipation if present. This includes stool softeners, a high fiber diet, good hygiene, Sitz baths, and possibly topical steroids. This proves successful in majority of the cases, so it is generally rare to resort to band ligation, sclerotherapy, cryotherapy, or photocoagulation. On very rare occasions, anesthesia and drainage of a painful thrombosed hemorrhoid are needed, just as is required for adults similarly afflicted.

#### Outcome

Conservative medical management solves hemorrhoidal problems for most children. Rarely will a more aggressive surgical procedure be required for good results, although children need to be observed for the same postoperative complications: abscess, cellulitis, bleeding, and the very rare, but gravely serious necrotizing pelvic sepsis, suggested by the triad of severe pain, fever, and urinary retention.

### Anal Fissure

#### Incidence

Again, it is very difficult to establish an exact incidence for this problem, but this is a more common problem than hemorrhoid disease and one that most pediatric surgeons will encounter several times each year.

## Demographics

The commonest age for appearance if 6 to 24 months which helps define this lesion. This problem is also a little more common in boys than girls, again for the reason that chronic constipation is frequently the inciting cause. However, the possibility of a fissure heralding other diseases is much greater and those should be considered in association with the sex, age, and past medical history of the patient.

## Presentation

Pain and bright red bleeding are the usual presentation. History frequently reveals a history of constipation though not invariably and those cases are hard to explain. Physical examination alone helps in making this diagnosis, but the location of the break in the skin is very important. Ninety percent of fissures in ano occur on the posterior midline. A lateral fissure may more correctly be termed anal abrasion and suggests trauma, abuse, or many forms of anal inflammation with dermal breakdown such as inflammatory bowel disease, tuberculosis, AIDS, Chlamydia, gonorrhea, syphilis, and problems with immunocompentency.

## Diagnostic Procedures

Little is necessary for the posterior midline fissure in ano other than a good medical history and a physical examination. If further studies are needed, they are generally directed toward making an additional diagnosis to explain an unusual fissure. Studies in adults have shown that this problem in adult life is often associated with high resting sphincter pressures. Whether this is the cause or the result of fissure is not clear, but manometric studies are abnormal. Obviously, they are seldom actually done in children.

The presence of a "sentinel pile" is often a clue to problems in the past. The healing of the posterior midline fissure may result in a skin protrusion or raphe, which superficially resembles an external hemorrhoid. If fully epithelialized and without complaints, this is nothing more than a cosmetic inconvenience, but bleeding from a "sentinel pile" is occasionally sufficiently troublesome to warrant excision.

## Treatment

Therapy is conservative and directed toward constipation in most of these children. One begins with stool softeners, a high-fiber diet, Sitz baths, and gentle dilations in the office. In the best-outcome cases, full healing may occur within 10 to 14 days, but the more recalcitrant cases may require up to 6 to 8 weeks. If progress is noted, treatment is continued. If healing fails to occur within 1 to 2 months, one may need to consider alternatives.

The alternatives are not so well studied in children, probably because of the much less common occurrence of this problem in childhood. However, several alternatives are well studied and discussed in the adult surgical literature, and most have been applied to children with safe results to date.

The objective of medical treatment is to achieve a medical sphincterotomy utilizing nitroglycerin, diltiazem, or botulinum toxin. The object is to reduce high sphincteric pressure, improve blood flow to the anal region, and promote healing. All have some degree of success, but recurrence is possible and safety in children has not been fully determined, but risks seem to be low.

Chronic problems may require lateral sphincterotomy, either open or closed. Both are well described, and there actually seems to be little difference in the results, although the open procedure has the benefit of visual control.

## Outcome

Simple medical therapy results in healing for most of these children. Since parents are justifiably concerned about the risks of anesthesia and surgery, medical treatment to achieve a temporary sphincteric relaxation seems well justified. For the recalcitrant cases, the lateral sphincterotomy is indicated and can easily be achieved in the outpatient surgery setting.

## Fistula-in-Ano/Perianal Abscesses

This whole topic is clouded in some uncertainty. Abscesses that occur well over the gluteus maximus muscle and are associated with diaper rash, injuries, bites, or eczema are clearly gluteal abscesses. They are handled easily with antibiotics and drainage procedures if large and fluctuant. However, similar infections that are near the anal canal become a bit more confusing and may actually represent a couple of diseases that present in similar manner.

A true fistula-in-ano should be a congenital lesion that is a fistulous tract from the anal canal to a region of the perianal skin. There should be 2 openings for such a lesion and the intervening tract should be lined with an epithelial lining such as a squamous epithelium similar to the skin of the buttocks (Fig. 54-1). In reality such lesions are quite rare.

Considerably more common is a perianal abscess that falls radially aligned to the anus generally right or left and between the 2 to 5 o'clock location and 7 to 11 o'clock position. When these lesions demand surgical intervention, a probe inserted

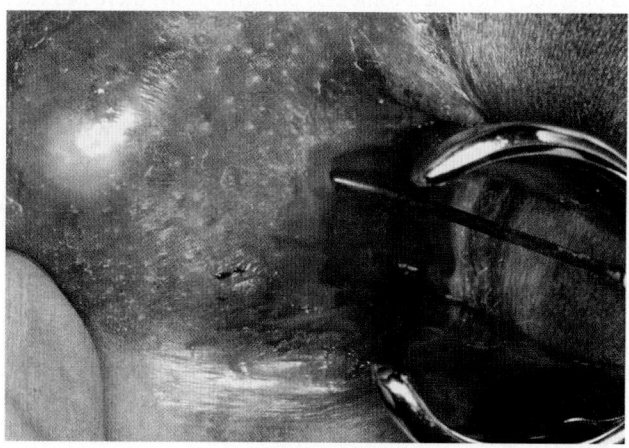

**FIGURE 54-1** True fistula-in-ano with the probe entering and exiting the double orifices, which is characteristic of a complete fistula.

into the abscess often directs toward a crypt of Morgagni in the lower anal canal, but only rarely falls through an opening into the anal canal. When opened, these tracts appear to be filled with granulation tissue and pus. This suggests these lesions arise from a cyptitis or perianal infection that extends from the anal canal. The superficial nature of these lesions—almost none go above the sphincters or into the supralevator space—also suggests a local inflammatory process.

## Incidence and Demographics

Well over 90% of these lesions occur in infants, much more commonly in boys than in girls. They are common problems in any busy pediatric surgical practice but an exact incidence against number of births is not truly known.

## Presentation

First redness and tenderness as in any cellulitis or developing abscess is seen, usually within 2 to 4 cm of the anus. Lesions that occur much further from the anal opening are probably more properly called labial or gluteal abscesses. If allowed to progress, most of the lesions coalesce to form an abscess with fluctulence followed by the development of a "white head" that will eventually spontaneously open and drain.

## Diagnostic Procedures

These lesions generally require nothing other than physical examination. The appearance is characteristic and helps in making the diagnosis. The one diagnostic procedure is culture at the time of drainage. On rare occasions, these abscesses or fistulae are the result of a very unusual infectious organism and might require more than standard antibiotic treatment and drainage. Tuberculosis is probably the more common of these unusual organisms. In addition, these lesions rarely herald an inflammatory bowel disease. Bacterial cultures will not necessarily indicate any unusual organisms but a failure to respond to a combination of antibiotics and drainage should suggest the need for a more extensive search for etiology.

## Treatment

If these lesions are seen, diagnosed, and treated in the very earliest phase, antibiotic therapy alone may be sufficient. This is possible when the problem is phlegmonous, there is a rich blood supply, and drugs are able to penetrate to the core of the problem. More advanced cases require surgical drainage. This can take the form of a simple incision and drainage, but recurrence has proven to be high in many cases so treated. Consequently, many pediatric surgeons use a short period of intravenous sedation or general anesthesia to pass a probe through the abscess toward the nearest crypt of Morgagni and then open a trench along the probe to expose the abscess, to curette the chronic granulation tissue so often encountered at the base, to cauterize the base of the trench, and to leave the wound open so that it heals from the base and obliterates the area of infection completely.

## Outcome

Results are good depending on the stage of the lesion when seen and the aggressiveness of the treatment determined by the stage of advancement. However, even with the more extensive surgical treatment for the larger and more developed abscess, recurrence has been reported, both at the site of the original lesion or contralaterally across the anus. Although bothersome and painful, similar treatment for a recurrent fistula or abscess generally results in good resolution and only a small chance of a third lesion.

# MAJOR PERIANAL DISEASE

## Rectal Prolapse

Rectal prolapse is a compilation of 3 processes seen in childhood and advanced age. Two, procidentia and prolapse, are truly rectal problems. The third is intestinal prolapse associated with intussusceptions. This problem is dealt with in another section of this book and will not be mentioned further in this chapter.

Of the 2 forms of prolapse commonly encountered in children, 1 involves mucosal prolapse through the anal sphincter; the other is a full-thickness rectal wall prolapse. They are obviously different in extent or degree of tissue that has passed through the sphincter. Mucosal prolapse often resembles a small floret of tissue with radial folds, while the more extensive full-thickness prolapse demonstrates the radial folds of colonic mucosa.

Both forms of prolapse are much less frequently seen in the United States today. Good childhood nutrition and hygiene may be partially responsible. The disappearance of parasitic diseases, especially in the warmer, once poorer southern states of the Union and finally the universal testing for cystic fibrosis with prompt initiation of treatment in the infantile period have all reduced what were once considered major causes of prolapse. Although we continue to look for these diseases when unexplained prolapse is encountered, the reality is that only chronic constipation and anal rectal malformation/Hirschsprung disease remain as common inciting reasons for this problem at present.

It is unclear if the anatomical findings in adult prolapse are contributory factors in children: weak sphincter muscle, levator diastasis, a deep space of Douglas, poor posterior fixation, a long rectal mesentery, and redundant rectosigmoid. Only the latter is something that is regularly seen in childhood, confirmed by contrast enemas in very young children that often show a very marked sigmoid loop. In fact, it is unclear whether these findings contribute to prolapse or simply result from the prolapse.

## Incidence and Demographics

The incidence of this problem is not truly known but does appear to be disappearing in the United States. It seems to have a bimodal pattern in children, appearing in infants and then again in children between 2 and 4 years of age. Boys seem to be affected more often than females.

## Presentation

Parents most commonly report the appearance of prolapse because they are assisting a child with stooling or toilet training. They notice the protrusion of a pink to red, mucosal

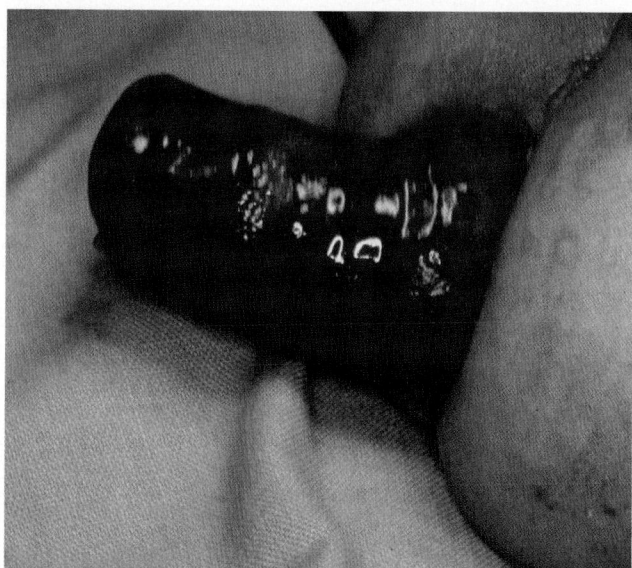

**FIGURE 54-2** True rectal prolapse with eversion of the mucoepidermoid junction.

mass. Parents are less commonly alerted to the problem by a child who complains of rectal bleeding or proctodynia. Parents can often describe the different patterns of mucosal folds that may help in differentiating procidentia from full-thickness rectal prolapse.

Pediatric surgeons know that the lack of a space between the squamomucosal junction differentiates the forms of prolapse from intussusceptions (Fig. 54-2).

## Diagnostic Procedures

Laboratory testing is of little use in these cases unless one believes a parasitic infection may be present in which case stools should be tested for ova and parasites. In addition, if there is any reason to suspect that the afflicted child may be a missed case of cystic fibrosis appropriate testing should be done.

On rare occasions, contrast enemas or video defecography may be indicated to delineate anatomical anomalies, but the latter is particularly difficult to accomplish successfully in children.

## Treatment

Initial treatment in all children is prompt reduction of the prolapse, usually with gentle but constant pressure.

Treatment for children is almost always directed to medical intervention after the first appearance of the prolapse. This is quite reasonable since the majority of children has only one appearance of the prolapse and is quite successfully treated with bulk diet, stool softeners, suppositories, or cleansing enemas. Only a few will have a second prolapse and even fewer will progress to a chronic or recurring problem.

For those children, just as for adults afflicted with this problem, the variety of surgical correction is large. In fact, the abundance of surgical intervention strongly suggests that we do not fully understand the problem and are grappling with the solution. Historically, the infants have often been

subjected to sclerotherapy by injecting into the muscular wall or submucosally. Hypertonic saline, up to 15%, has been the most commonly used agent but a host of others are available, and each has literature supporting its use. Injections are given, especially in the infants, with strapping of the anus for a period after therapy to allow edema and then sclerosis in the rectal wall to solve the problem.

In somewhat older children who have had several recurrences despite medical management, an adaptation of the Thiersch wire technique is probably the most frequently used technique. Adapted from the work of Karl Thiersch who first described the use of a silver thread to prevent prolapse and incontinence, a Thiersch cerclage is now usually done with a nonabsorbable suture placed subcutaneously and tightened over a finger or dilator to produce some degree of anal stenosis (Fig. 54-3). The procedure effectively prevents further prolapse in most cases, but care must be exercised by the family postoperatively to prevent constipation in a child who now has a narrowed anus. The cerclage can usually be cut and removed 3 to 6 months later without the return of prolapse since the cycle of laxity and prolapse has been interrupted.

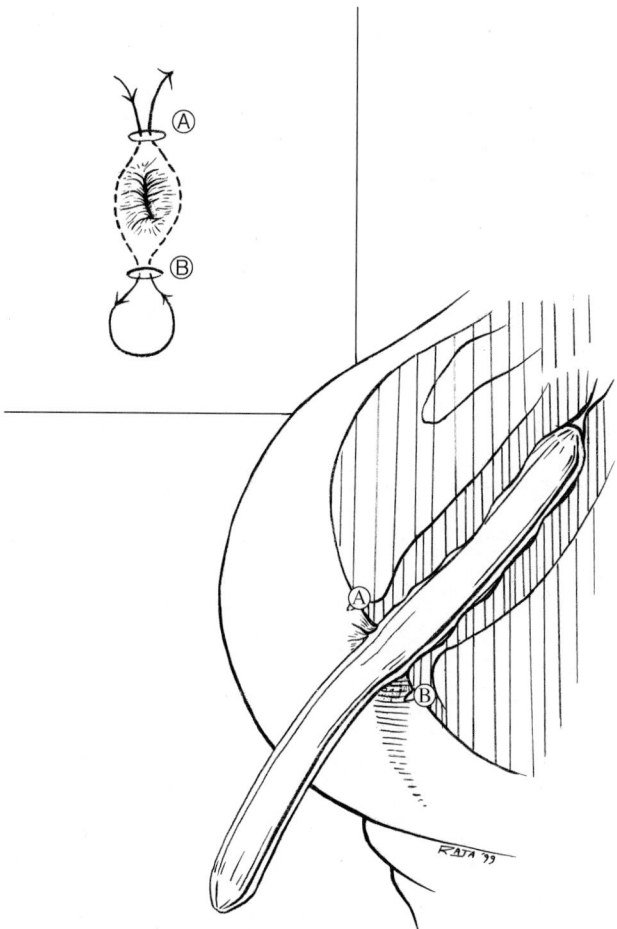

**FIGURE 54-3** The technique of perianal cerclage showing anterior and posterior incisions. A heavy nylon suture is passed circumferentially and tied over an appropriate-sized Hegar dilator inserted into the anal canal.

Only seldom are other perineal (Delorme mucosal sleeve resection or Altemeier perineal rectosigmoidectomy) operations offered to children. The much larger and invasive abdominal procedures are also seldom used in childhood except for the most persistent cases. These include bowel resections to shorten the colon, the presacral suspension procedures such as the Ripstein operation, or a combination of resection and suspension, such as the Frykman–Goldberg operation. Another combination operation, as described by Ashcraft, is suspension coupled with the posterior approximation of the levator complex, essentially treating the prolapse as a hernia of the pelvic sling musculature. All have extensive literature detailing the procedures and reporting the results, usually with reasonably good results but all with some degree of recurrence. However, most are not needed in childhood and seldom have to be offered.

## SELECTED READINGS

Ashcraft KW, Amoury RA, Holder TM. Levator repair and posterior suspension for rectal prolapse. *J Pediatr Surg* 1977;12(2):241–245. PubMed PMID:845769.

Chwals WJ, Brennan LP, Weitzman JJ, Woolley MM. Transanal mucosal sleeve resection for the treatment of rectal prolapse in children. *J Pediatr Surg* 1990;25(7):715–718. PubMed PMID:2199658.

Lewis TH, Corman ML, Prager ED, Robertson WG. Long-term results of open and closed sphincterotomy for anal fissure. *Dis Colon Rectum* 1988;31(5):368–371. PubMed PMID:3366036.

Poenaru D, Yazbeck S. Anal fistula in infants: etiology, features, management. *J Pediatr Surg* 1993;28(9):1194–1195. PubMed PMID:8308691.

Shalaby R, Ismail M, Abdelaziz M, et al. Laparoscopic mesh rectopexy for complete rectal prolapse in children: a new simplified technique. *Pediatr Surg Int* 2010;26(8):807–813. PubMed PMID:20532893.

Tsugawa C, Matsumoto Y, Nishijima E, Muraji T, Higashimoto Y. Posterior plication of the rectum for rectal prolapse in children. *J Pediatr Surg* 1995;30(5):692–693. PubMed PMID:7623230.

# CHAPTER 55

# Gallbladder Disease

*David Juang and George W. Holcomb III*

## KEY POINTS

1. Gallbladder disease in children can arise from a number of underlying conditions, but the disease is due to cholelithiasis in most cases. Cholelithiasis is usually classified as being either hemolytic or nonhemolytic in etiology.

2. Gallbladder contractility can be assessed with radionuclide scanning during CCK injection. Most surgeons utilize a gallbladder ejection fraction of less than 35% as an indicator for cholecystectomy in a symptomatic patient. The normal ejection fraction approximates 75%.

3. Real-time US has an accuracy of approximately 96% for gallbladder disease and is effective in determining hepatic and common bile duct involvement, the presence of thickening of the gallbladder wall, and any abnormalities in the liver or head of the pancreas.

4. We recommend that patients with symptomatic gallbladder disease who are older than 3 years should undergo laparoscopic cholecystectomy. Younger patients, particularly infants, should be individualized.

5. The laparoscopic approach has become the standard method for cholecystectomy in children for the past 20 years.

6. For the majority of pediatric surgeons, the best option may be to perform a preoperative ERCP with sphincterotomy and stone extraction if stones are found preoperatively. If successful, the surgeon can then proceed with laparoscopic cholecystectomy.

7. SSULS is being utilized more frequently, but when compared with traditional 3 and 4-port/incision laparoscopic surgery, the only advantage of SSULS appears to be cosmesis.

Gallbladder disease is being increasingly diagnosed in children, although not nearly as often as in adults. Whether the incidence is actually escalating or the diagnostic accuracy is improving because of the increasing use of ultrasonography (US) and cholescintigraphy remains unclear. The disease processes contributing to gallbladder pathology are different in children compared with adults. Hemolytic disease, which is more common in children, is no longer the only prerequisite for the development of gallstones. Moreover, acute and chronic cholecystitis with severe inflammation and/or scarring of the gallbladder and surrounding tissues are less common in children. Fortunately, lessons gained from the vast published experience in adults can be useful in managing children with gallbladder disease.

## ETIOLOGY

Gallbladder disease in children can arise from a number of underlying conditions, but the disease is due to cholelithiasis in most cases. Cholelithiasis is usually classified as being either hemolytic or nonhemolytic in etiology. Hemolytic disease results in consumption of red blood cells leading to increased hepatic metabolism of bilirubin, which precipitates as stone formation. Nonhemolytic disease includes a variety of causes for stone development or symptomatic gallbladder disease without stones.

### Gallstone Formation

The major chemical components of bile that contribute to its lithogenic potential are bile salts, phospholipids, cholesterol, bilirubin, and electrolyte–water balance. The phospholipid component is mostly lethicin, which, along with bile salts, serve as detergents in the bile. With polar and nonpolar portions to these molecules, they form lecithin–bile acid–cholesterol micelles that keep the cholesterol soluble within the hydrophobic center of the micelle. An imbalance in the concentration of these substances is almost always due to an increase in cholesterol secretion, which results in cholesterol crystal precipitation. These crystals serve as the nidus for further precipitation, resulting in macroscopically detectable gallstones. The addition of physiologic components such as poor gallbladder emptying, inflammation, and bacterial colonization can further precipitate stone formation. This pathway accounts for the majority of adult gallstones, but is less common in children. In addition, cholesterol gallstones are extremely rare in prepubertal children. As in adults, obesity is a common risk factor for cholesterol stone formation in children. Obese children have been found to have an overall 2% incidence of gallstones. Finally, the composition of gallstones in children may be different than that found in adults. Whereas stones in adults are primarily cholesterol in composition, calcium carbonate and black pigment stones are often found in pediatric patients, especially those younger than 10 years of age.

## Hemolytic Disease

Red blood cells are composed of a plasma membrane, the hemoglobin moiety, and a few cytoplasmic enzymes. These 3 basic components provide a functional outline for the major hereditary hemolytic diseases (Table 55-1). Their constant turnover by the reticuloendothelial system leads to the breakdown of hemoglobin to bilirubin. A nearly insoluble molecule, bilirubin requires conjugation by glucuronyl transferase to produce bilirubin diglucuronide, the molecule measured as "direct" bilirubin, which is more soluble. Because the enzymatic process of conjugation is saturable, the hemolytic states may cause an abnormal level of unconjugated (indirect) bilirubin in the bile. This results in the formation of calcium bilirubinate, which polymerizes with bilirubin to form black gallstones. Currently, research suggests that excessive unconjugated hyperbilirubinemia alone is not sufficient to produce pigment gallstones, but it is hypothesized that stasis as a result of incomplete emptying leads to sludge and later to gallstone formation. Because gallbladder sludge is frequently documented in patients with sickle-cell anemia, elective cholecystectomy has been recommended when evidence suggests the presence of sludge, with or without stones. In one study of 35 patients with sickle-cell disease (SCD) and biliary sludge, 23 (65.7%) went on to develop gallstones.

## Hereditary Hemolytic Diseases

Hemolytic cholelithiasis secondary to SCD remains the most common cause of gallstones in children at many institutions. Fifty percent of patients with sickle-cell anemia develop gallstones by 20 years of age. These patients also represent the largest group of patients who develop postoperative complications after cholecystectomy. The total postoperative complication rate reported in the national SCD study group was 39% with sickle events representing 19% of complications; intraoperative or recovery room problems, 11%; transfusion

complications, 10%; postoperative surgical events, 4%; and death, 1%. The open operation was performed in 58% of the patients and the laparoscopic route was used in 42%. The complication rates were similar between the 2 groups. The same study also reported that the incidence of sickle cell events may be higher in patients who were not preoperatively transfused. Meticulous attention and close coordinated efforts with hematologists regarding the perioperative management, transfusion guidelines, and pulmonary care may reduce the incidence of sickle-cell-related complications. Currently, it is now recommended that the laparoscopic approach be utilized for this patient population. Of note, the acute chest syndrome can be seen in up to 20% of sickle-cell patients undergoing abdominal surgery. One study has suggested that the laparoscopic approach does not decrease the incidence of this complication.

Two other hemolytic conditions associated with gallstones are hereditary spherocytosis and thalassemia. The incidence of cholelithiasis in patients with hereditary spherocytosis ranges from 43% to 63% and is slightly more common in girls than in boys. US is recommended before elective splenectomy to determine whether concomitant cholecystectomy should be performed at the time of the splenectomy. The incidence of cholelithiasis in thalassemia has markedly decreased due to more aggressive transfusion management, which prevents the production and release of native red cells containing defective hemoglobin.

## Nonhemolytic Cholelithiasis

In patients without hereditary hemolytic disease, changes to the enterohepatic circulation, whether directly or indirectly, are believed to contribute to stone formation. The most common cause of nonhemolytic cholelithiasis in neonates and infants is the use of total parenteral nutrition (TPN). While many patients requiring long-term TPN have gastrointestinal disease, the complete picture of TPN-associated cholestasis, liver disease, and gallstone formation is not completely understood. Decreased bile flow and gallbladder emptying from a lack of enteral stimulation has been postulated to be an important contribution to TPN-associated gallstones. However, in one study, the use of cholecystikinin (CCK) to prevent stone development in TPN-dependent children had no effect, implying that the role of CCK-mediated bile flow may be less important than previously thought in gallstone formation in these patients. Others postulate that the amino acid infusion from TPN alters bile composition. The administration of fat is believed to ameliorate the deleterious effects of the amino acids in the TPN. TPN has a primary lithogenic effect on bile causing increased bilirubin and calcium concentration. These effects have been shown to be prevented with glutamine supplementation, suggesting there are intermediary steps that still need to be clarified.

A large population of infants and neonates require TPN, but it has been noted that only 43% of children receiving long-term TPN will eventually develop cholelithiasis. This suggests that there are other factors necessary for the development of cholelithiasis in this patient population. Septicemia, dehydration, chronic furosemide therapy, cystic fibrosis, short-bowel syndrome, and ileal resection for necrotizing enterocolitis also are known contributing factors. Cystic fibrosis, the

| TABLE 55-1 | The Major Hereditary Hemolytic Diseases | |
| --- | --- | --- |
| Membrane Defects | Hemoglobin Defects | Enzyme Defects |
| Spherocytosis | Sickle-cell disease | Glucose-6-phosphate deficiency |
| Eliptocytosis | α Thallasemia | Pyruvate kinase deficiency |
| Pyropoikilocytosis | β Thallasemia | |
| Hydrocytosis | | |
| Xerocytosis | | |

phenotype for defective epithelial chloride channels, results in decreased transport of water and chloride, which increases the viscosity of the bile and contributes to stone formation. Cystic fibrosis can also lead to obstruction of the biliary ductules resulting in liver failure. Similarly, patients with bowel dysmotility or dysfunction may have altered bacterial flora, which also affects the enterohepatic circulation. Neonates and premature infants are susceptible to the cholestatic effects of TPN because of the immaturity of their enterohepatic circulation of bile salts.

Possible causes of gallstones in older children include the use of oral contraceptives, cystic fibrosis, pregnancy, obesity, and ileal resection. Cholelithiasis has also been reported in children undergoing cardiac transplantation who are receiving cyclosporine and in patients who have previously required extracorporeal membrane oxygenation as a newborn.

## Acalculous Conditions

The gallbladder can be a source of symptoms in patients without gallstones. Hydrops of the gallbladder, acalculous cholecystitis, biliary dyskinesia, and gallbladder polyps are being seen more frequently.

Acute inflammatory attacks of the gallbladder, called acute acalculous cholecystitis, occur more commonly in association with severe illness such as sepsis, burns, or trauma. This is much less common in children than in adults, but can be seen in critically ill children. In this setting, TPN is often used and, if prolonged, may result in decreased gallbladder contractility with progressive distention, stasis, and possible infection. In a small report of 12 patients, daily US criteria was used to assess the need for cholecystectomy. In the 3 patients who eventually underwent cholecystectomy, progressively increasing gallbladder wall thickness and distention along with pericholecystic fluid were found. In the other patients, the daily US examinations showed progressive improvement. These patients all recovered uneventfully.

## Hydrops

Hydrops is characterized by massive distention of the gallbladder in the absence of stones, infection, or congenital anomalies. It has been most frequently reported in association with the Kawasaki disease and is usually due to a transient obstruction of the cystic duct or to increased mucus secretion by the gallbladder resulting in poor emptying. With additional gallbladder distention, further angulation of the cystic duct may increase the obstruction. Conservative treatment consisting of appropriate antibiotics and early initiation of enteral feedings to stimulate gallbladder emptying often leads to resolution of this condition. If serial US examinations show progressive gallbladder distention with increasing pain, or if the gallbladder appears gangrenous, cholecystectomy is recommended.

## Biliary Dyskinesia

Biliary dyskinesia is becoming a common diagnosis in children. In some centers, it has become the most common reason for cholecystectomy. While the etiology of the symptoms is felt to be gallbladder distension secondary to poor emptying,

bile stasis can also promote sludge, microscopic bile crystallization, and subsequent mucosal irritation. Chronic cholecystitis is often documented on histologic examination of the gallbladder specimen.

Gallbladder contractility and emptying can be assessed with radionuclide scanning during CCK injection. Most surgeons utilize a gallbladder ejection fraction of less than 35% as an indicator for cholecystectomy in a symptomatic patient. Laparoscopic cholecystectomy has been shown to be an effective treatment for this disorder, with expected resolution of symptoms in over 80%. One study examining predictors of successful outcomes after cholecystectomy for biliary dyskinesia found gallbladder ejection fractions of less than 15% most reliably predicted which children would have postoperative symptom relief following cholecystectomy. In that study, children with an ejection fraction greater than 15% did not have predictable resolution of symptoms. Biologic credibility for cholecystectomy in patients with stone disease and dyskinesia has been supported by a recent report from our institution, which found that children with biliary dyskinesia have a marked increased number of mucosal mast cells in the gallbladder mucosa. In a follow-up study, a moderate to high degree of mast cell activation was also found in children with both biliary dyskinesia and gallstones.

## Gallbladder Polyps

Gallbladder polyps are also being seen more frequently in children. Due to the inability to assure life-long follow-up combined with the extremely poor prognosis when gallbladder cancer develops, laparoscopic cholecystectomy is a reasonable option for symptomatic children with gallbladder polyps or for patients with a polyp ≥1 cm.

## RADIOGRAPHIC EVALUATION

Real-time US has an accuracy of approximately 96% for gallbladder disease and is effective in determining hepatic and common bile duct involvement, the presence of thickening of the gallbladder wall, and any abnormalities in the liver or head of the pancreas. Inflammatory changes, as evidenced by gallbladder wall thickening, pericholecystic fluid, or tenderness elicited by probe placement directly over the gallbladder (the sonographic Murphy sign), are indicative of acute cholecystitis. Stones without inflammatory changes must be associated with symptoms to make a diagnosis of symptomatic cholelithiasis.

Although a plain abdominal radiograph is often the initial imaging study used to evaluate abdominal pain in children, it is rarely helpful with gallbladder disease unless the gallstones are calcified (Fig. 55-1). The incidence of radiopaque stones has been reported to be as high as 50% in patients with hemolytic disorders compared with approximately 15% in adolescents with cholesterol stones.

## Hepatobiliary Iminodiacetic Acid Scan (HIDA Scan)

In children who have symptoms suggestive of biliary disease but no findings of stones, hepatobiliary cholescintigraphy

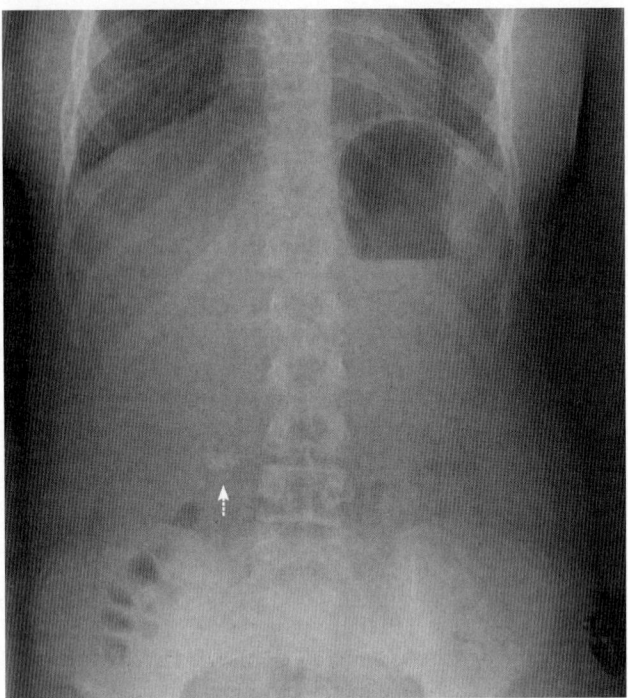

**FIGURE 55-1** A plain abdominal radiograph with radio-opaque gallstones (arrow). The incidence of radiopaque stones has been reported to be as high as 50% in patients with hemolytic disorders compared with approximately 15% in adolescents with cholesterol stones. (From Holcomb III GW, Andrews WS. Gallbladder disease & hepatic infections. In: Grosfeld JL, O'Neill JA, Fonkalsrud EW, et al, eds. *Pediatric Surgery*. 7th ed. Philadelphia, PA: Elsevier, Inc 2011.)

that uses technetium-99m-labeled iminodiacetic acid (IDA) analogues should be obtained (HIDA). With this study, the gallbladder is not visualized in patients with acute cholecystitis. False-positive results can be obtained, especially in critically ill patients, in infants who are fasting or have severe associated illnesses, or are receiving TPN. Intravenous morphine may be useful in this setting because it causes spasm at the sphincter of Oddi, resulting in increased bile duct pressure that enhances visualization of the gallbladder and helps reduce the rate of false-positive studies.

Cholecystokinin-assisted or Lipomul-challenged cholescintigraphy is an accurate predictor of biliary dyskinesia and also suggests the likelihood of symptomatic relief with cholecystectomy. The normal ejection fraction approximates 75%. As mentioned previously, patients with an ejection fraction under 35% are considered to have biliary dyskinesia.

## MANAGEMENT

Historically, gallstones have been treated with nonoperative therapies including oral dissolution agents, direct instillation of these agents, and extracorporeal shockwave lithotripsy, but these measures have been abandoned due to failure, recurrence, and high cost. We recommend that patients with symptomatic gallbladder disease who are older than 3 years should undergo laparoscopic cholecystectomy. Younger

patients, particularly infants, should be individualized. Infant gallstones secondary to prolonged TPN have been reported to dissolve spontaneously. Therefore, in the absence of complications, these patients should be observed for 6 to 12 months following cessation of the TPN and the initiation of enteral alimentation.

The laparoscopic approach has become the standard method for cholecystectomy in children for the past 20 years. The major advantages of this approach include decreased discomfort resulting in a reduced length of hospitalization, an improved cosmetic result, and a faster return to routine activities such as work, school, play, or participation in athletic activities. In most reports, children with noncomplicated disease undergoing laparoscopic cholecystectomy are usually ready for discharge on either the first or the second postoperative day. There have been recent reports of this operation being performed in children as an outpatient procedure.

Patients presenting with an acute episode of cholecystitis and signs of inflammation on laboratory or radiologic studies can be managed with either semiurgent laparoscopic cholecystectomy or antibiotics followed by interval cholecystectomy. In adults, a recent prospective study found no difference in operative complications between early and delayed cholecystectomy, but found that delayed cholecystectomy was associated with more complications from the disease (relapse, choledocholithiasis, pancreatitis). Early intervention has also been shown to be much more cost-effective than interval cholecystectomy. Patients with SCD require special preoperative care to prevent postoperative complications with several reports emphasizing the need for preoperative transfusion. The laparoscopic approach does not appear to be more hazardous for these patients and may be preferred.

Management of cholelithiasis in patients being evaluated and treated for other hematologic diseases such as hereditary spherocytosis also deserves special mention. In these patients, a gallbladder US is recommended before the splenectomy. If gallstones are present, then cholecystectomy should be performed at the time of the splenectomy. However, in a study of 17 patients undergoing splenectomy alone in which cholelithiasis was not seen at the time of the splenectomy, none of the patients subsequently developed symptoms of cholelithiasis with a mean follow-up of 15 years. Thus, prophylactic cholecystectomy at the time of splenectomy is probably not indicated in patients with hereditary spherocytosis who do not have gallstones.

Several unusual conditions merit attention. First, partial external biliary diversion interposing a jejunal loop between the gallbladder and abdominal wall has been described to treat the intractable pruritis in patients with progressive familial intrahepatic cholestasis. We have used this technique as well with resolution of the pruritis. Thus, in these children, cholecystectomy should be avoided. Second, ventriculogallbladder shunts have been performed in patients with a scarred peritoneal cavity from multiple previous operations or severe peritonitis.

### Choledocholithiasis

A number of management strategies for patients with choledocholithiasis are available including: preoperative endoscopic retrograde cholangiopancreatography (ERCP) with sphincterotomy and stone extraction followed by an uncomplicated laparoscopic cholecystectomy; laparoscopic or open common duct exploration at the time of laparoscopic cholecystectomy; or cholecystectomy followed by postoperative endoscopic sphincterotomy with stone extraction. The decision analysis is primarily influenced by the surgeon's experience with laparoscopic choledochal exploration, and also by the availability of an endoscopist experienced in ERCP in children. For the majority of pediatric surgeons, the best option may be to perform a preoperative ERCP with sphincterotomy and stone extraction if stones are located. If successful, the surgeon can then proceed with laparoscopic cholecystectomy. However, if stones are found and cannot be extracted at ERCP and sphincterotomy, then the surgeon will know whether or not laparoscopic or open choledochal exploration is indicated at the time of the cholecystectomy (Fig. 55-2).

## Cholangiography

In patients with cholelithiasis, differing opinions exist in regards to the routine use of cholangiography. In the early to mid-1990s, when there was not much experience with laparoscopic cholecystectomy in children, it was suggested that most, if not all, children undergo a cholangiogram for training purposes as well as to ensure that the correct anatomy has been visualized and to evaluate for the presence of common duct stones, although this is often suspected preoperatively either from symptoms, US, or laboratory studies. As pediatric surgeons have gained more familiarity with the technique of laparoscopic cholecystectomy, routine intraoperative cholangiography for surgeon-training purposes does not appear necessary once the surgeon has become familiar with the

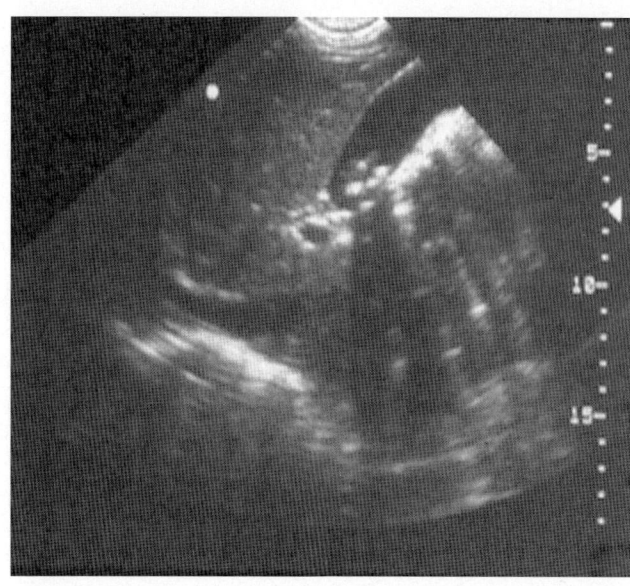

FIGURE 55-3 The abdominal sonogram showing the presence of hyperechoic gallstones. We often obtain an US evaluation a few days before the laparoscopic cholecystectomy to confirm the presence of gallstones and to evaluate for common duct obstruction.

technique. Thus, intraoperative cholangiography is useful primarily to ensure that the correct anatomy is visualized and to evaluate for choledocholithiasis. To decrease operative time and cost at our institution, we will often obtain an US evaluation a few days before the laparoscopic cholecystectomy to confirm the presence of gallstones and to evaluate for common duct obstruction (Fig. 55-3). If cholangiography is needed, we still prefer the Kumar clamp technique, although a number of other techniques in which a catheter is introduced into the cystic duct through a transcystic incision are certainly appropriate. Fluoroscopy is also useful because it is more time efficient than static radiography and allows dynamic assessment of the biliary tree (Fig. 55-4).

## LAPAROSCOPIC CHOLECYSTECTOMY

A modification in the authors' technique over the past several years merits mention before describing a laparoscopic cholecystectomy. For many laparoscopic operations including cholecystectomy, we have adopted a "stab incision" technique for instruments that are not continually exteriorized and reinserted into the abdominal cavity during the operation. In a study of 511 patients undergoing a variety of laparoscopic procedures in which only 1 or 2 Step (Covidien, Norwalk, CT) cannulas were utilized, a reduction of $187,180 was noted in the patient charges. If the Ethicon (Ethicon Endosurgery, Cincinnati, OH) disposable cannulas were used, patient savings of about $123,000 would have been realized. For cholecystectomy, the instruments placed through the 2 right-sided incisions are not routinely changed. Thus, these 2 sites are optimal for the stab-incision technique (Fig. 55-5). The telescope is introduced through the umbilical cannula and the main working port is in the upper abdomen so 2 cannulas are still used in these sites.

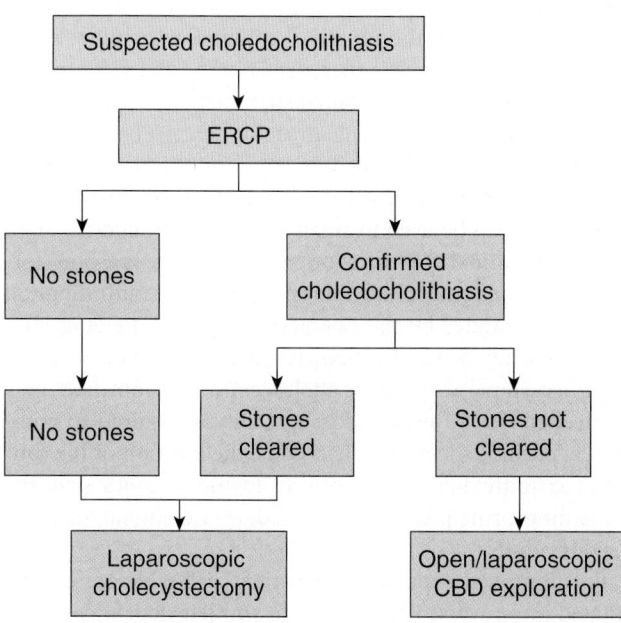

FIGURE 55-2 The algorithm used when choledocholithiasis is suspected pre-operatively at our institution. The decision analysis is primarily influenced by the surgeon's experience with laparoscopic choledochal exploration, and also by the availability of an endoscopist experienced in ERCP in children.

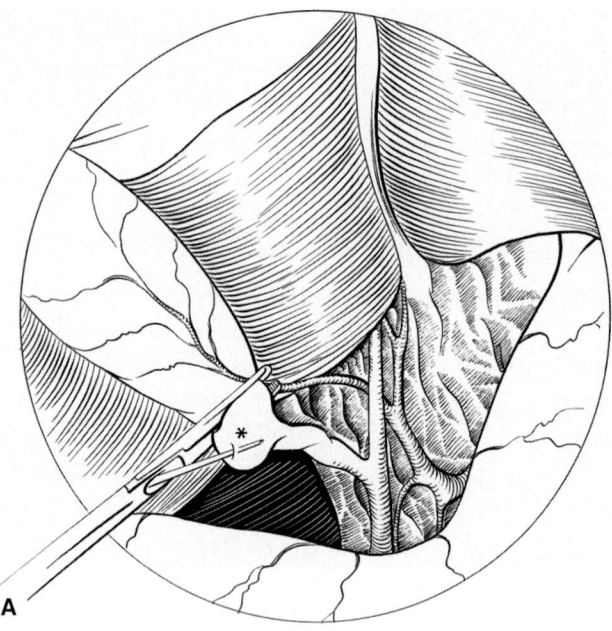
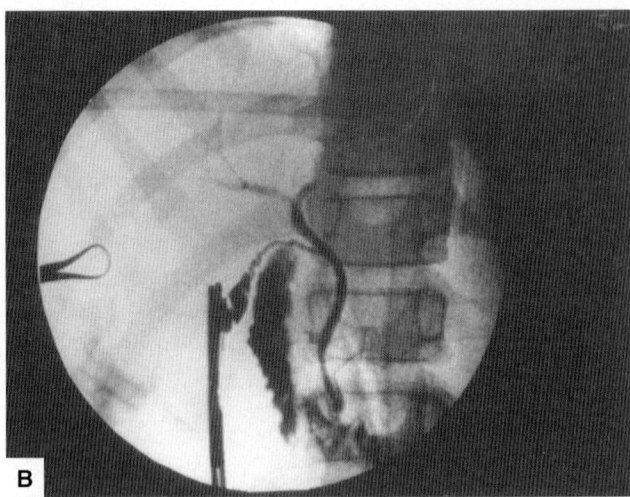

**FIGURE 55-4** The Kumar clamp technique used in conjunction with fluoroscopy. Fluoroscopy is useful because it is more time efficient than static radiography and allows dynamic assessment of the biliary tree. Through a side port of the clamp, a small sclerotherapy needle (asterisk) is inserted directly into the gallbladder and a contrast study is obtained (A). With this method, a lateral incision in the cystic duct, which can be quite difficult for small children, is not necessary. The static image of an operative fluoroscopic cholangiogram depicts a small, long cystic duct entering the common duct with free flow into the duodenum (B). No abnormalities are noted on this study.

## Four-Port Technique

The patient is placed supine on the operating table with 1 or 2 video monitors situated at the head of the table. After induction of anesthesia, an orogastric tube is inserted for gastric decompression and the urinary bladder is evacuated using a Credé maneuver. A 2-cannula and 2 "stab incision" technique is used, but the location of the incisions and the cannulas depends on the patient's age and size (Fig. 55-6). For infants

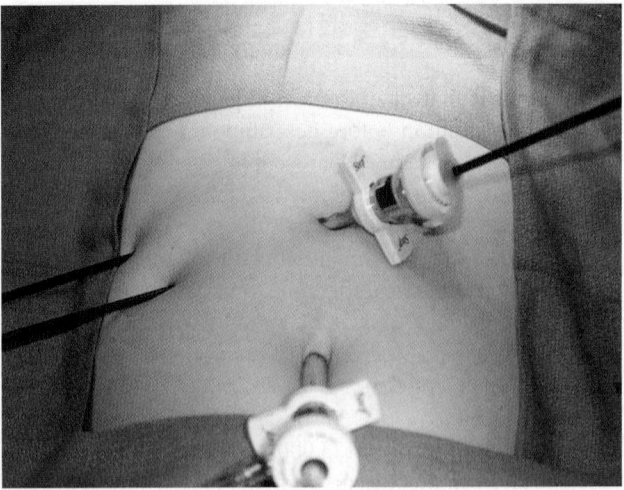

**FIGURE 55-5** The instruments placed through the 2 right-sided incisions are not routinely changed. Thus, these 2 sites are optimal for the stab-incision technique. The telescope is introduced through the umbilical cannula and the main working port is in the upper abdomen so 2 cannulas are still used at these sites.

and small children, the right lower abdominal incision can be positioned in the inguinal crease region and the epigastric cannula should be situated more on the patient's left to allow adequate working space between the instruments.

A 10-mm incision is made in the umbilicus, through which a 10-mm cannula is inserted into the abdominal cavity, and abdominal insufflation is initiated. After creation of an adequate pneumoperitoneum, a 5 or 10 mm 45° telescope is inserted through the umbilical cannula and connected to the camera. The image is then displayed on the video monitors. The right lower abdominal stab incision is created with a No. 11 blade and a locking, grasping forceps is introduced for retraction of the gallbladder superiorly over the liver by the assistant. Usually this is a 5-mm instrument, but a 3-mm instrument can be used in small children. Through the right upper abdominal stab incision, a nonlocking, grasping forceps is also inserted for lateral retraction of the infundibulum of the gallbladder by the operating surgeon. The epigastric port is usually 5 mm in diameter and is the main working site. Occasionally, in larger adolescents, a 10-mm port may be needed if a 10-mm endoscopic clip is required to completely occlude the cystic duct. Once the location of the cannulas is individualized according to the patient's size, the remaining principles of the procedure are similar to those used in adults.

For improved exposure, the patient and table are usually rotated into reverse Trendelenberg and left-dependent positions, which helps the adjacent viscera fall away from the surgical area. In addition, lateral retraction of the infundibulum is important because the cystic duct is then positioned at more of a 90° orientation to the common duct rather than an oblique or even parallel orientation, which occurs without

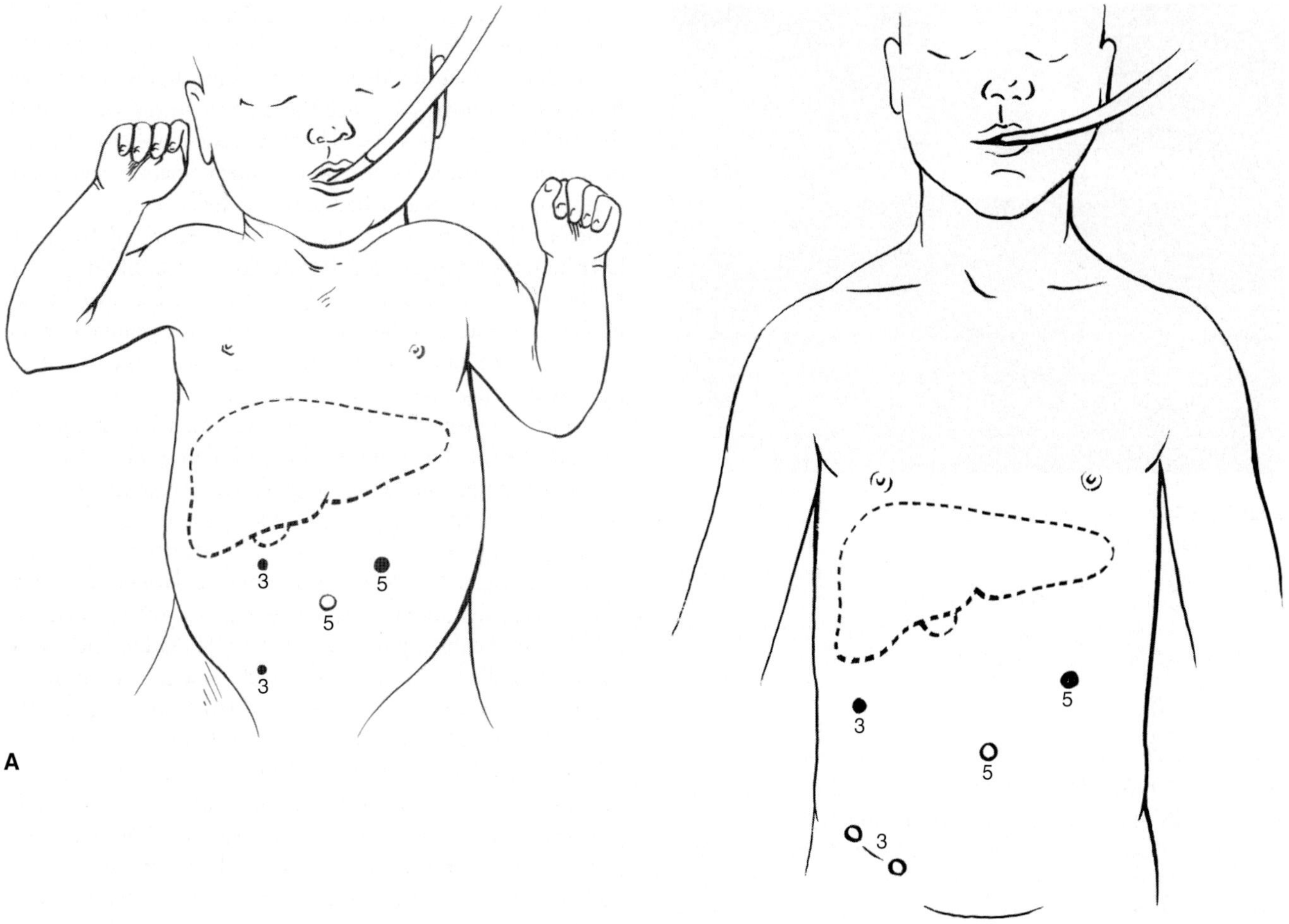

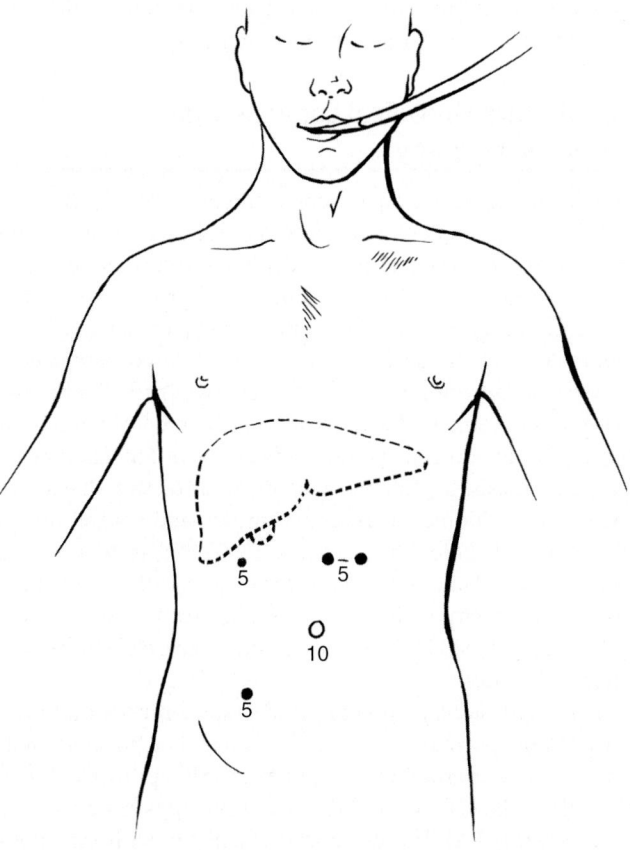

**A**

**B**

**C**

**FIGURE 55-6** Port site locations for the baby, the youth, and the adolescent. The location of the incisions and the cannulas depends on the patient's age and size. For infants and small children, the right lower abdominal incision can be positioned in the inguinal crease region and the epigastric cannula should be situated more on the patient's left to allow adequate working space between the instruments (**A**). In patients between 3 and 12 years of age, the cannulas can be positioned as diagrammed (**B**). Depending on the size of the patient and degree of inflammation of the gall bladder, the umbilical port should be either 5 or 10 mm in diameter. The remaining ports can be 5 and 3 mm. In the teenager, port placement mirrors those used for adults (**C**). At least 1 10-mm port is usually required to withdraw the gallbladder and it can be positioned in the umbilicus for cosmetic purposes.

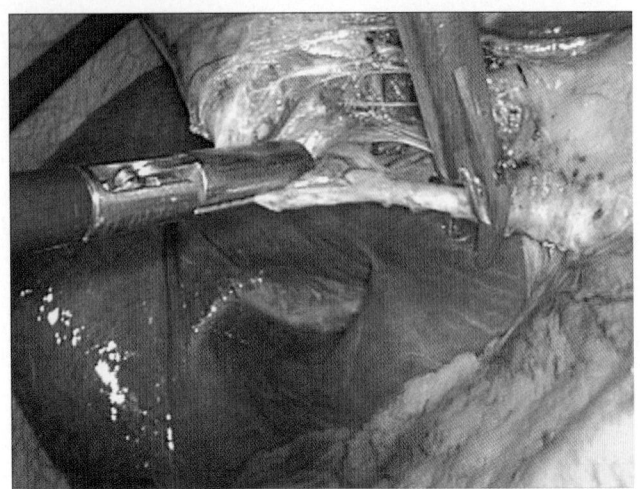

**FIGURE 55-7** Lateral retraction of the infundibulum allows for a 90° orientation of the cystic duct to the common duct. This allows for proper identification of the critical structures. Parallel orientation of these 2 ductal systems can lead to misidentification of the cystic and common bile ducts resulting in injury to the common duct. An endoscopic clip is being placed on the cystic duct.

such lateral retraction (Fig. 55-7). This parallel orientation may lead to misidentification of the cystic and common bile ducts resulting in injury to the common duct.

The initial surgical maneuver is to expose the cystic duct and identify the cystic artery. Adhesions between the duodenum and stomach often require lysis for access to the infundibulum and triangle of Calot. Once the cystic duct is identified, 2 options are available. One is to proceed with cholangiography as previously discussed. If the anatomy is clear and there is no evidence of choledochal obstruction on a preoperative US, we proceed with ligation and division of the cystic duct. Usually 5-mm clips are adequate, although a 10-mm clip may be required in larger patients. Two clips are placed on the cystic duct approximately 5 mm from its insertion into the common bile duct (Fig. 55-8). Another

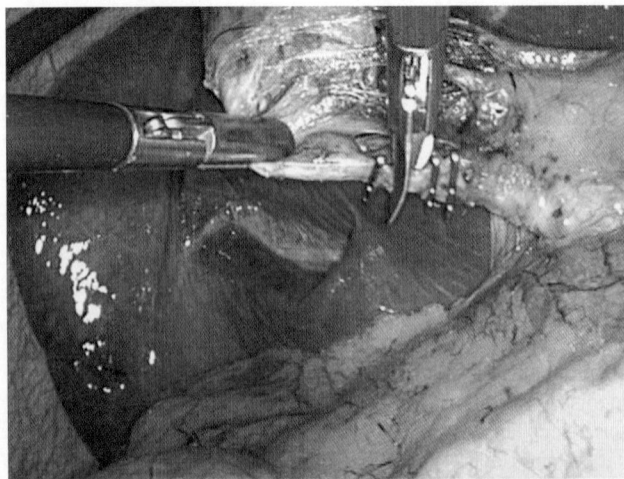

**FIGURE 55-8** Two clips are placed 5 mm from the confluence of the cystic duct and common duct and 1 (or 2) clips are placed distal to these before transaction of the cystic duct. The cystic artery is ligated and divided in a similar fashion.

1 or 2 clips are placed on the cystic duct near the infundibulum to prevent spillage of stones from the gallbladder. The cystic duct is then divided, and the cystic artery is similarly ligated and transected. Once these 2 structures are divided, the gallbladder is detached in a retrograde manner using one of several instruments: the hook cautery, spatula cautery, or endoscopic scissors attached to the cautery.

Before the gallbladder is completely separated from the liver bed, the triangle of Calot should be carefully inspected to ensure that all clips are secure and that there is no evidence of bleeding. After complete detachment of the gallbladder, the telescope is rotated from the umbilical port to the epigastric port. If the epigastric port is 5 mm, then a 5-mm telescope is utilized to visualize the gallbladder and a locking, grasping instrument is introduced through the umbilical cannula to secure the gallbladder. The gallbladder is then extracted through the umbilical port. In older patients, the gallbladder may be too large for removal without further incising the umbilical fascia. This opening should be enlarged in patients with large gallbladders to prevent rupture with spillage of stones and bile during removal of the gallbladder. These gallstones, if spilled, should be removed because complications from retained stones have been reported in adults. After the gallbladder is extracted, the area of dissection is again carefully inspected to ensure adequate hemostasis. All irrigant is evacuated, and bupivacaine is injected into the incisions for postoperative analgesia. In smaller patients, the fascia surrounding the 5-mm cannula sites should be closed. In larger patients, fascial closure for the 5-mm ports or stab incisions is usually unnecessary, but the fascia surrounding the 10-mm cannula sites should be approximated carefully to prevent herniation. For the stab incisions, skin closure is usually all that is needed. The patients are usually hospitalized after the procedure and discharged the next morning.

## Single-Site Umbilical Laparoscopic Cholecystectomy

Single-site umbilical laparoscopic surgery (SSULS) is being utilized more frequently for common surgical procedures and a recent adult consortium was identified to further advances in single-incision surgery. Examples of procedures seeing increased utilization of SSULS include cholecystectomy and appendectomy. It has also been used in children for splenectomy, pyloromyotomy, and ileocecectomy for the Crohn disease. When compared with traditional 3- and 4-port/incision laparoscopic surgery, the only advantage of SSULS appears to be cosmesis. SSULS has become an attractive alternative between traditional laparoscopic surgery and natural orifice transluminal endoscopic surgery (NOTES) as there are a number of real and potential complications with access to the abdominal cavity with NOTES. Similar to SSULS, the only advantage of NOTES over traditional laparoscopic procedures is cosmesis.

For single-site laparoscopic cholecystectomy, an umbilical incision of approximately 2 cm is needed. For this particular indication, our group utilizes either the SILS port (Covidien, Inc, Norwalk, CT) or the TRIPORT (Olympus America Inc., Center Valley PA). The SILS port is a foam port with 3 channels through which the telescope and instruments are introduced.

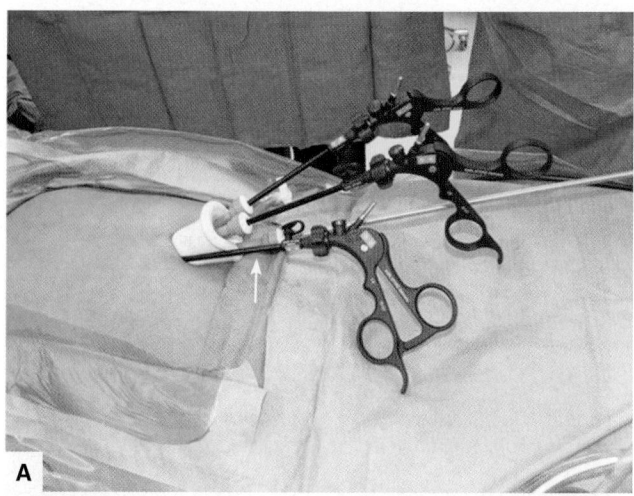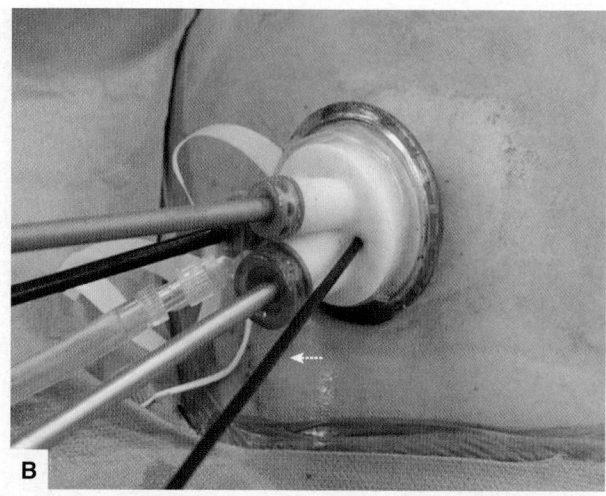

**FIGURE 55-9** For single-site laparoscopic cholecystectomy, an umbilical incision of approximately 2 cm is needed. Our group utilizes both the Covidien SILS port (**A**) and the Olympus Tri-Port (**B**). The SILS port is a foam port with 3 channels through which the telescope and instruments are inserted. A fourth instrument (arrow) is then introduced along the side of the SILS port for retraction of the gallbladder over the liver. The Tri-Port is designed for single-site umbilical surgery as well. We insert a fourth 3-mm instrument through one of the insufflation ports (dotted arrow). (From Holcomb III GW, Andrews WS. Gallbladder disease & hepatic infections. In: Grosfeld JL, O'Neill JA, Fonkalsrud EW, et al. *Pediatric Surgery*. 7th ed. Philadelphia, PA: Elsevier, Inc; 2011.)

A fourth instrument is then introduced along the side of the foam port for retraction of the gallbladder (Fig. 55-9A). There is also a channel for insufflation. The TRIPORT is designed for 3 instruments, but a fourth 3-mm instrument can be introduced through 1 of the insufflation portals (Fig. 55-9B). As with other SSULS procedures, it is helpful to have a long telescope so that the telescope/camera holder can stand away from the operating surgeon. Once the telescope and instruments are introduced, the operation proceeds exactly like a traditional 4-port laparoscopic cholecystectomy. The instrument used to grasp the dome of the gallbladder is introduced at approximately 9 o'clock in the TRIPORT and another instrument is used to retract the infundibulum. With the SILS port, this instrument is introduced along the side of the port in the umbilical incision. The telescope should be angled at 30 to 45°. As with traditional laparoscopic cholecystectomy, it is important to retract the infundibulum of the gallbladder laterally to create a right-angle orientation of the cystic and common bile ducts. Following identification and dissection of the cystic duct and cystic artery, the duct is ligated with endoscopic clips (Fig. 55-10A and B). In a similar fashion, the cystic artery is divided as well. After division of the cystic duct and cystic artery, the gallbladder is dissected free from its liver attachment using electrocautery. A number of instruments can be utilized for this purpose including the hook cautery, spatula cautery, or a Maryland dissector attached to cautery. After complete mobilization of the gallbladder, it is then grasped with an instrument placed through one of the channels in the umbilical port and exteriorized through the umbilical incision along with the port. Prior to extracting the gallbladder, it is helpful to assess for bleeding and to irrigate/suction as it would be necessary to re-introduce the umbilical port to re-create the pneumoperitoneum in order to perform these functions after removing the gallbladder.

The umbilical fascia is then closed with interrupted 0 absorbable sutures. We prefer to close the skin with interrupted 5-0 plain sutures, which is our usual practice for umbilical skin closure for traditional laparoscopic surgery. A nice cosmetic result is achieved using this SSULS approach for cholecystectomy (Fig. 55-11).

## COMPLICATIONS

The most common complications following cholecystectomy occur in children with hemolytic disease as previously described, and are related to the manifestations of the underlying disease. The most significant complication from laparoscopic cholecystectomy is injury to the common bile duct. The rate of ductal injury after laparoscopic cholecystectomy is decreasing, but the number of adult patients who will require a ductal reconstructive operation remains about 1 per 1000 undergoing a laparoscopic cholecystectomy. There are no published reports of ductal complications in children. It would be reasonable to expect that complications in children will remain less than those in adults given the high percentage of adult patients who require an operation due to severe inflammation obliterating the planes of dissection. A relatively few pediatric patients present in this fashion. Regardless, any surgeon performing the operation should be aware of the complications that can occur and how to prevent and manage them.

When ductal injury is recognized at the time of the operation, conversion with open repair should be performed with a low threshold for performing a hepaticojejunostomy. Obstructive ductal injuries and delayed strictures detected after the operation can be temporized with percutaneous transhepatic drainage of the ductal system after which the patient should be referred to a center with a large experience reconstructing these injuries.

Bile leaks after laparoscopic cholecystectomy are usually from the cystic duct stump or from the gallbladder fossa

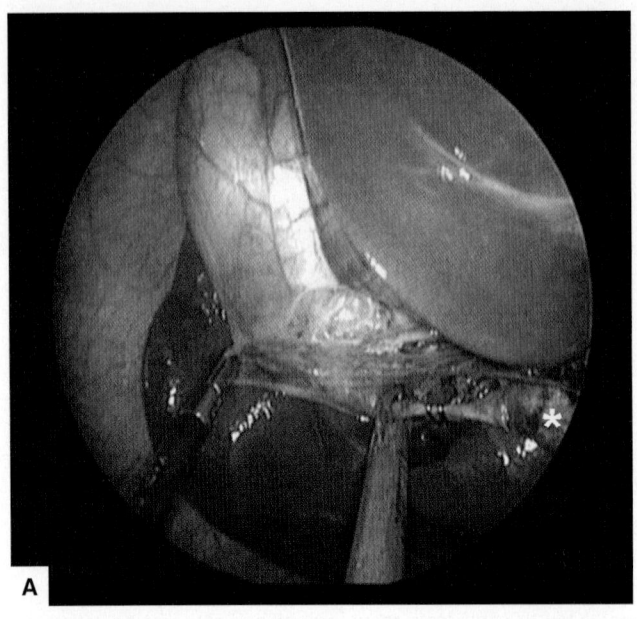
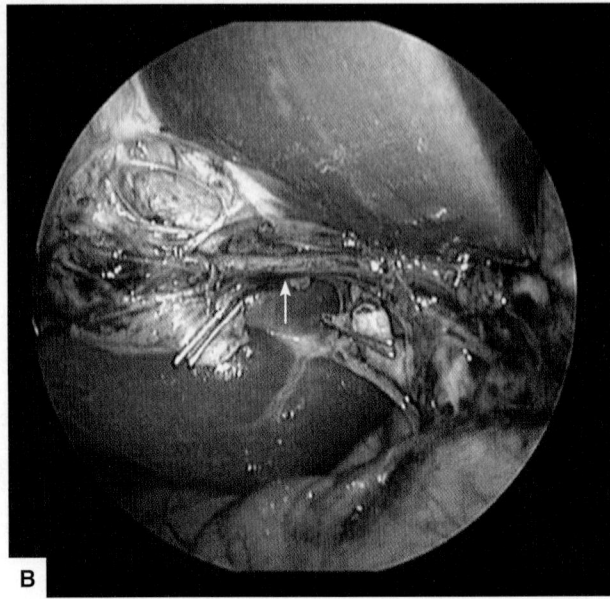

**FIGURE 55-10** Once the telescope and instruments are introduced, the operation proceeds like the traditional 4-port laparoscopic cholecystectomy. It is important to retract the infundibulum of the gallbladder laterally to create a right-angle orientation of the cystic and common bile ducts. In the photograph on the left (**A**), the endoscopic clips are being applied to the cystic duct. Note the right-angle orientation of the cystic and common bile ducts (asterisk). Following ligation and division of the cystic duct (**B**), the cystic artery (arrow) is well visualized and will be similarly ligated and divided. (From Holcomb III GW, Andrews WS. Gallbladder disease & hepatic infections. In: Grosfeld JL, O'Neill JA, Fonkalsrud EW, et al. *Pediatric Surgery*. 7th ed. Philadelphia, PA: Elsevier, Inc; 2011.)

(ducts of Lushka). The sphincter of Oddi maintains a pressure gradient of about 10 mm Hg in the biliary system. Thus, almost all postoperative leaks resolve promptly with sphincterotomy and/or stent placement, which should be performed at the time of the ERCP that is useful for delineating the location of the leak.

Infectious complications are uncommon unless gallstones are spilled. Spilled stones should be removed to reduce these complications.

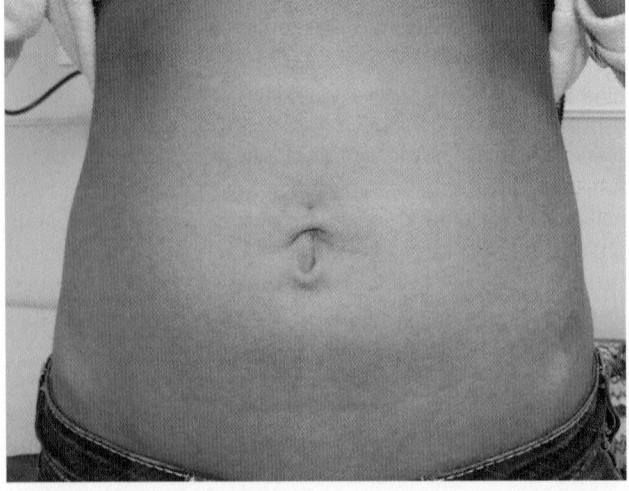

**FIGURE 55-11** After removal of her belly-button ring it is evident that this teenager has achieved a nice cosmetic appearance at 1 month postoperatively from a single-site umbilical laparoscopic cholecystectomy. (From Holcomb III GW, Andrews WS. Gallbladder disease & hepatic infections. In: Grosfeld JL, O'Neill JA, Fonkalsrud EW, et al. *Pediatric Surgery*. 7th ed. Philadelphia, PA: Elsevier, Inc; 2011.)

## CHILDREN'S MERCY HOSPITAL EXPERIENCE

Over the past 10 years, laparoscopic cholecystectomy has become the accepted standard for removal of the gallbladder in children and adolescents. Reported complications have been very few and we can find no reports of choledochal injury in children, although some have undoubtedly occurred. Despite the widespread use of laparoscopic cholecystectomy in children, there are surprisingly few reports in the literature describing a series as large as 100 patients.

Our group recently reported a recent 6-year experience with traditional 4-port laparoscopic cholecystectomy at Children's Mercy Hospital (Table 55-2). Between fall 2000 and June 2006, 224 patients underwent laparoscopic cholecystectomy. The mean age was 12.9 years (range 0-21 years) with a mean weight of 58.3 kg (range 3-121 kg). One hundred and sixty-six children had symptomatic gallstones, 35 children had biliary dyskinesia, 7 patients presented with gallstone pancreatitis, 6 patients were undergoing splenectomy and found to have gallstones, 5 patients had calculous cholecystitis, and 1 patient each had choledocholithiasis, gallbladder polyp, acalculous cholecystitis, and congenital cystic duct obstruction. In this series, there were only 29 patients with hemolytic disease. Eighteen patients had SCD and 11 had hereditary spherocytosis. The mean operative time (excluding patients undergoing a concomitant operation) was 77 minutes (range 30-285 minutes).

Due to preoperative concerns about choledocholithiasis, a preoperative ERCP was performed in 17 patients in this series. Stones were retrieved endoscopically in eight of these patients. Additionally, an operative cholangiogram was

| TABLE 55-2 | Patients Undergoing Laparoscopic Cholecystectomy at Children's Mercy Hospital (September 2000 to June 2006) | | | |
|---|---|---|---|---|
| Symptomatic gallstones (hemolytic disease) | 166 (29) | Mean age (Years) | 12.9 (0-21) |
| Biliary dyskinesia | 35 | Mean weight (kg) | 58.3 (3-121) |
| Gallstone pancreatitis | 7 | Mean operating time (Min) | 77 (30-285) |
| Concomitant splenectomy | 6 | Major complications | 1 |
| Calculous cholecystitis | 5 | | |
| Miscellaneous | 5 | | |
| Total | 224 | | |

*Note:* Reprinted with permission from St Peter SD, Keckler SJ, Nair A, et al. Laparoscopic cholecystectomy in the pediatric population. *J Laparoendosc Adv Surg Tech* A 2008;18:127.

performed in 38 patients and common duct stones (CBD) were identified in 9 patients. CBD stones were cleared intraoperatively in 5 patients while the other 4 patients required postoperative endoscopy and sphincterotomy to retrieve the stones. Due to a postoperative rise in direct bilirubin, 2 patients underwent a postoperative ERCP who did not have an intraoperative cholangiogram. The ERCP was normal in both cases.

There were no conversions, ductal injuries, bile leaks, or mortality. However, 1 sickle-cell patient developed a postoperative hemorrhage, which required laparotomy for control. Interestingly, biliary dyskinesia was diagnosed in only 10% of the first 30 patients in this series, but was diagnosed in 40% of the last 30 patients studied. The mean ejection fraction in these patients was 21%. All of these patients had improvement in their symptoms following the laparoscopic cholecystectomy.

Since the first reported SSULS for cholecystectomy in 1997, the number of reports is increasing in the adult literature. The pediatric literature remains sparse. The most recent and largest retrospective study from Children's Hospital of Alabama describes 25 children who underwent a SSULS cholecystectomy. The most frequent indications were symptomatic cholelithiasis in 17 patients (68%) and biliary dyskinesia in 5 (20%). Five patients had sickle-cell disease. The mean operative time was 73 minutes (range, 30–122). Median hospital stay was 1 day. In 17 patients (68%), a percutaneous 2-mm grasper was needed to retract the gallbladder over the liver. No complications were noted, and no conversion to an open procedure was required. In 5 patients, additional cannulas were added. On follow-up, no complications were noted. No patients were readmitted, and there were no wound infections.

SSULS is also being utilized for gallbladder removal at our institution. A prospective, randomized trial is underway at our hospital comparing single-site umbilical laparoscopic cholecystectomy to traditional 4-port laparoscopic cholecystectomy. Operative time is the primary outcome variable. Using an alpha of 0.05 and a power of 0.80, a total of 60 patients will be enrolled. To date, 50 patients have participated in this trial and results are forthcoming.

## SELECTED READINGS

Aldana PR, James HE, Postlethwait RA. Ventriculogallbladder shunts in pediatric patients. *J Neurosurg Pediatr* 2008;1:284.

Birkett DH. Spilled cells, spilled clips, spilled stones. New problems or old challenges. *Surg Endosc* 1995;9:269.

Carney DE, Kokoska ER, Grosfeld JL, et al. Predictors of successful outcome after cholecystectomy for biliary dyskinesia. *J Pediatr Surg* 2004.;39:813.

Chamberlain RS, Sakpal SV. A comprehensive review of single-incision laparoscopic surgery (SILS) and natural orifice transluminal endoscopic surgery (NOTES) techniques for cholecystectomy. *J Gastrointest Surg* 2009;13:1733.

Ekinci S, Karnak I, Gurakan F, et al. Partial external biliary diversion for the treatment of intractable pruritus in children with progressive familial intrahepatic cholestasis: report of two cases. *Surg Today* 2008;38:726.

Gill IS, Advincula AP, Aron M, et al. Consensus statement of the consortium for laparoendoscopic single-site surgery. *Surg Endosc* 2010;24:762.

Gurusamy K, Samraj K, Gluud C, et al. Meta-analysis of randomized controlled trials on the safety and effectiveness of early versus delayed laparoscopic cholecystectomy for acute cholecystitis. *Br J Surg* 2010;97:141.

Haberkern CM, Neumayr LD, Orringer EP, et al. Cholecystectomy in sickle cell anemia patients: perioperative outcome of 364 cases from the National Preoperative Transfusion Study. Preoperative Transfusion in Sickle Cell Disease Study Group. *Blood* 1997;89:1533.

Holcomb GW 3rd, Morgan WM 3rd, Neblett WW 3rd, et al. Laparoscopic cholecystectomy in children: lessons learned from the first 100 patients. *J Pediatr Surg* 1999;34:1236.

Holzman MD, Sharp K, Holcomb GW, et al. An alternative technique for laparoscopic cholangiography. *Surg Endosc* 1994;8:927.

Mah D, Wales P, Njere I, et al. Management of suspected common bile duct stones in children: role of selective intraoperative cholangiogram and endoscopic retrograde cholangiopancreatography. *J Pediatr Surg* 2004;39:808.

Mendez K, Sabater R, Chinea E, et al. Is there a safe advantage in performing outpatient laparoscopic cholecystectomy in children? *J Pediatr Surg* 2007;42:1333.

Newman KD, Powell DM, Holcomb GW 3rd. The management of choledocholithiasis in children in the era of laparoscopic cholecystectomy. *J Pediatr Surg* 1997;32:1116.

Nougues CP, Harmon CM, Hansen EN, et al. Cholecystectomy using single-incision pediatric endosurgery: technique and initial experience in the first 25 cases. *J Laparoendosc Adv Surg Tech A* 2010 Jun:20(5):493–496.

Ostlie DJ, Holcomb GW 3rd. The use of stab incisions for instrument access in laparoscopic operations. *J Pediatr Surg* 2003;38:1837.

Rau B, Friesen CA, Daniel JF, et al. Gallbladder wall inflammatory cells in pediatric patients with biliary dyskinesia and cholelithiasis: a pilot study. *J Pediatr Surg* 2006;41:1545.

Rothenberg SS, Shipman K, Yoder S. Experience with modified single-port laparoscopic procedures in children. *J Laparoendosc Adv Surg Tech A* 2009;19:695.

Sandler A, Winkel G, Kimura K, et al. The role of prophylactic cholecystectomy during splenectomy in children with hereditary spherocytosis. *J Pediatr Surg* 1999;34:1077.

Sicklick JK, Camp MS, Lillemoe KD, et al. Surgical management of bile duct injuries sustained during laparoscopic cholecystectomy: perioperative results in 200 patients. *Ann Surg* 2005;241:786.

St Peter SD, Keckler SJ, Nair A, et al. Laparoscopic cholecystectomy in the pediatric population. *J Laparoendosc Adv Surg Tech A* 2008;18:127.

Stringer MD, Ceylan H, Ward K, et al. Gallbladder polyps in children—classification and management. *J Pediatr Surg* 2003;38:1680.

Vegunta RK, Raso M, Pollock J, et al. Biliary dyskinesia: the most common indication for cholecystectomy in children. *Surgery* 2005;138:726.

Wales PW, Carver E, Crawford MW, et al. Acute chest syndrome after abdominal surgery in children with sickle cell disease: is a laparoscopic approach better? *J Pediatr Surg* 2001;36:718.

# Biliary Atresia and Choledochal Cyst

CHAPTER 56

*Stephanie A. Jones and Frederick M. Karrer*

## Biliary Atresia

### KEY POINTS

1. Biliary atresia is the most common surgical cause of cholestatic jaundice in the newborn. It is suspected based on laboratory testing demonstrating direct hyperbilirubinemia, elevated alkaline phosphatase, and gamma-glutamyl transferase.

2. Biliary atresia is progressive inflammatory, fibrosing cholangiopathy. Ultrasonography cannot distinguish the obliterated extrahepatic biliary ducts, but can suggest the diagnosis if there is an absent or diminuitive gallbladder or a triangular cord sign.

3. Ultimately, cholangiography is the gold standard for confirming the diagnosis of biliary atresia.

### INTRODUCTION

Biliary atresia is a progressive sclerosis of the extrahepatic biliary tree that, if untreated, leads to cirrhosis, liver failure, and eventually death. It is the most common indication for liver transplant in children. In 1959, Kasai and Suzuki reported a new operation, hepatic portoenterostomy, which achieved biliary drainage even in infants with "noncorrectable" biliary atresia. The Kasai procedure was championed in North America by Lilly and Altman, and now the procedure is accepted worldwide as the initial surgical modality in biliary atresia.

### PATHOPHYSIOLOGY

Embryologically, the extrahepatic biliary tree develops from a hepatic diverticulum (liver bud) of the embryonic foregut. The distal portions of the right and left hepatic ducts develop from the extrahepatic ducts and are clearly defined tubular structures by 12 weeks of gestation. The proximal portions of the main hilar ducts derive from the intrahepatic ductal

plates. These develop from fetal hepatocytes, bipotential progenitor cells, surrounding the branches of the portal vein. These primitive bile duct cells form a ring, the ductal plate, which remodels into mature bile duct structures. The process of intrahepatic bile duct development is dynamic throughout embryogenesis and continues until sometime after birth.

Biliary atresia is classified according to the level of the biliary obstruction into 3 types: Type I—obstruction restricted to the common bile duct (CBD). Type II—obstruction of the common hepatic duct with distal patency. Type III—obstruction of the common hepatic duct and CBD (Fig. 56-1). Associated anomalies include, in about 20% of cases, cardiac lesions, polysplenia, situs inversus, absent vena cava, and a preduodenal portal vein.

The pathogenesis of biliary atresia remains obscure despite numerous etiologic theories and investigations. It has been suggested that the disease is caused by (a) a failure of recanalization, (b) genetic factors, (c) defective morphogenesis, (d) ischemia/vascular lesions, (e) viruses, or (f) toxins. Currently, the most intriguing theory is that biliary atresia is the end result of 1 or more of these insults that then cause the biliary epithelium to become "upregulated" to express the antigen on the cell surface. Recognition by circulating T cells then initiates a cell-mediated immune response, resulting in the fibrosclerotic injury seen in biliary atresia. There seem to be 2 distinct groups of patients with biliary atresia: an early embryonic form associated with the presence of multiple other anomalies and a later fetal/perinatal form that is usually seen in isolation. The etiology of each may be different.

The pathologic findings in biliary atresia are characterized by inflammatory sclerotic obliteration of all or part of the extrahepatic biliary tree as well as of the intrahepatic biliary system. Unlike other atresias of the gastrointestinal tract that have a clearly defined point of obstruction with proximal dilation, in the most common variant of biliary atresia, the bile duct is represented by a fibrous cord without any dilation proximally. Others have residual patency—distally, of the gallbladder, cystic duct, and common duct, or proximally, with hilum cysts. The gallbladder is typically small but may still have a shrunken lumen containing clear fluid ("white bile"). Microscopically, the biliary remnant is represented by dense fibrous tissue, distally. Proximally, minute duct-like structures collecting ducts and biliary glands are surrounded by concentric fibrosis and inflammatory infiltrates. This

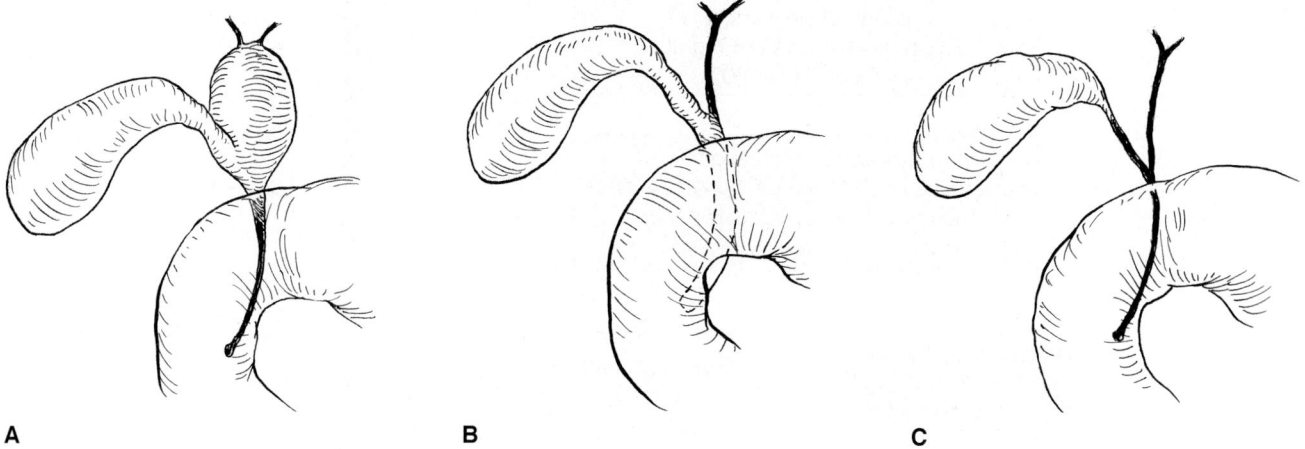

**FIGURE 56-1** The common variants of biliary atresia: Type I (**A**) Distal obliteration with hilar bile cysts (formerly, "correctable" type). Type II (**B**) Patency of the distal biliary tree with proximal obliteration. Type III (**C**) Complete obliteration of the extrahepatic ducts.

sclerosing occlusion of the bile ducts becomes more extensive with increasing age. Kasai and coworkers showed that the intrahepatic ducts communicate with the porta hepatis through minute channels, at least in early infancy. The surgical reconstruction is based on this precept.

## DIAGNOSIS

Jaundice in infants that persists longer than 2 weeks should *not* be considered physiologic, especially if the predominant fraction is conjugated bilirubin. The importance of early diagnosis in achieving success of the Kasai portoenterostomy has been repeatedly emphasized. Because of the myriad causes of cholestasis in infancy, an exhaustive evaluation to exclude *every* possibility can take weeks and should not be undertaken. The goal is to rule out obstructive mechanical causes of jaundice, and rapid work-up is essential. Infants with biliary atresia typically appear normal at birth, becoming clinically jaundiced at 3 to 6 weeks of age. Stool color may be normal or yellow initially, but changes to a light yellow or clay color over time.

Biochemical tests in biliary atresia show hyperbilirubinemia, usually 6 to 12 mg/dL, with 50% as conjugated bilirubin. Transaminases and alkaline phosphates are elevated 2 to 3 times normal. γ-Glutamyl transferase is typically markedly high. Usually, hepatic synthetic function is nearly normal with normal serum albumin levels. Mild elevations of prothrombin time (PT) typically respond to parenteral vitamin K administration. Serologic tests should be performed to exclude infectious etiologies (hepatitis A, B, C, and TORCH titer (toxoplasmosis, rubella, cytomegalovirus, and herpes virus)). α₁-Antitrypsin (AAT) deficiency can mimic biliary atresia and is excluded by determining the AAT level and phenotype. Standard complete blood count with examination of the peripheral smear largely excludes hematologic causes of cholestasis. The diagnostic algorithm for the work-up of a jaundiced infant is shown in Fig. 56-2.

Ultrasound is the imaging diagnostic test of choice. Ultrasonography is a rapid, safe, noninvasive means of evaluating the jaundiced infant. In biliary atresia, ultrasonography may show a small, nondistended gallbladder or a fluid-filled gallbladder that is indistinguishable from normal. The liver may have increased echogenicity. This modality is not sensitive enough to document the presence or absence of the extrahepatic bile ducts. If the bile ducts are grossly dilated, then other diagnoses are suspected (eg, choledochal cyst). The triangular cord sign is an abnormal hyperechogenic triangular area seen in the porta hepatitis that corresponds to the fibrous remnant of the bile duct seen in biliary atresia. This sign has 80% sensitivity and 98% specificity for biliary atresia. Additionally, the presence of polysplenia anomalies (multiple spleens, preduodenal portal vein, situs inversus, and absence of the infrahepatic vena cava) suggest the diagnosis.

Magnetic resonance (MR) cholangiography is less accurate than ultrasound for the diagnosis of biliary atresia. One study reported 90% sensitivity and 77% specificity. It is most useful to further define that anatomy for choledochal cysts or sclerosing cholangitis. Endoscopic retrograde cholangiography has been used to document patency of the extrahepatic biliary tree, but the technique requires considerable technical expertise and a miniature sized side-viewing endoscope that is not widely available.

Hepatobiliary imaging using technetium-99m iminodiacetic acid (IDA) has been used in the past for separating obstructive from parenchymal jaundice. In biliary atresia, particularly early, the uptake of the nucleotide is rapid, but excretion into the gut is absent, even on delayed images. In hepatocellular jaundice, the uptake of the isotope is delayed by parenchymal disease and excretion into the gut may be delayed or not seen. However, visualization of isotope in the bowel excludes biliary atresia, failure to demonstrate gut excretion has only a 50% to 75% specificity for biliary atresia. This modality is not utilized as frequently as in the past because it is time consuming and not very discriminating.

A percutaneous liver biopsy prior to laparotomy has a diagnostic accuracy for biliary atresia between 90% and 95% if interpreted by an experienced pathologist. The histological changes of the liver show preservation of the basic hepatic architecture with bile ductular proliferation, bile plugs, and varying amounts of periportal fibrosis in infants with biliary

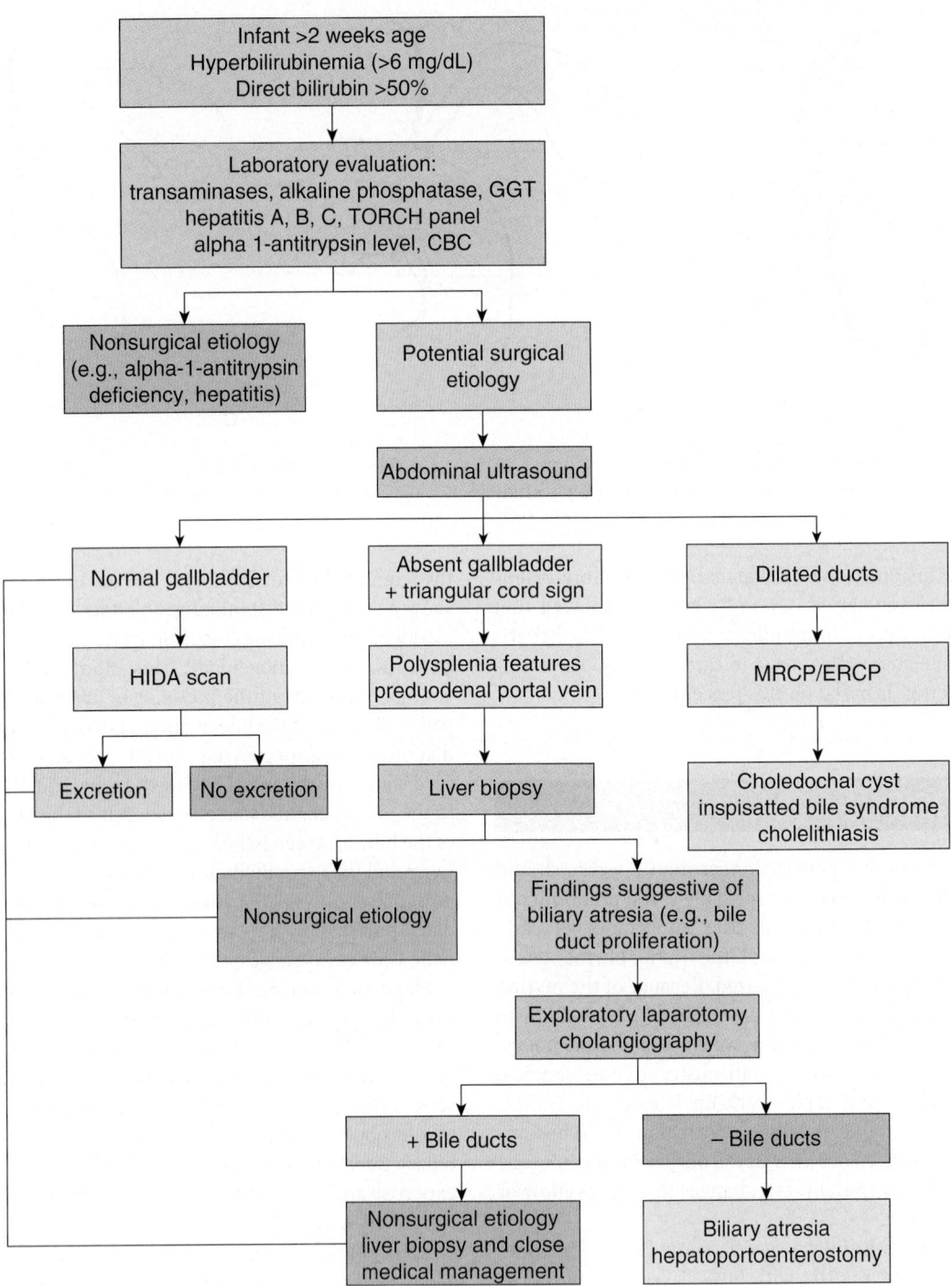

**FIGURE 56-2** Diagnostic algorithm.

atresia. Some will have portal inflammatory infiltrates and giant-cell transformation that makes distinction from the pathologic findings of neonatal hepatitis difficult.

Cholangiography is the final diagnostic maneuver, usually performed as a preliminary step, prior to proceeding to portoenterostomy. Through a small right-upper-quadrant incision, the contracted gallbladder is exposed. It usually has no lumen at all, or only a tiny one that contains a few drops of clear fluid. When a lumen is present, a cholangiogram is obtained by injection of a contrast material (Fig. 56-3). Demonstration of contrast in the duodenum and continuity with the intrahepatic bile ducts excludes biliary atresia (Fig. 56-4). In these circumstances, a generous wedge biopsy (and needle)

of the liver should be performed prior to closing the incision. If cholangiography is impossible (in absent or obstructed gallbladder lumen), then the incision is enlarged to a subcostal laparotomy in preparation for a Kasai portoenterostomy.

## TREATMENT

The only therapies that offer hope of cure for biliary atresia are surgical. Historically, a variety of operations have been devised, including partial hepatic resection with drainage of the cut surface, impalement of the liver with hollow tubes,

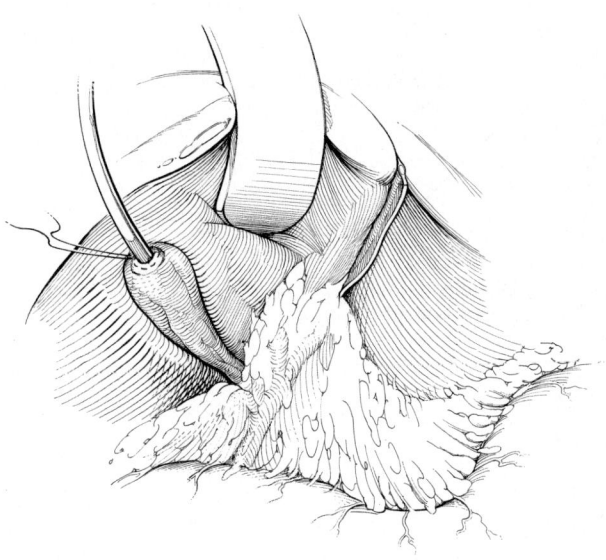

**FIGURE 56-3** Cholangiography is attempted by insertion of a small catheter into the gallbladder lumen (if present).

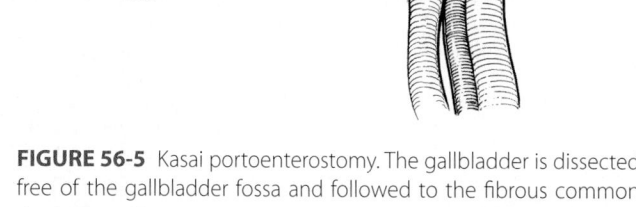

**FIGURE 56-5** Kasai portoenterostomy. The gallbladder is dissected free of the gallbladder fossa and followed to the fibrous common duct remnant.

and diversion of the thoracic duct lymph into the oral cavity. The only procedures to provide long-term success are the portoenterostomy and liver transplantation.

## HEPATIC PORTOENTEROSTOMY

The portoenterostomy procedure begins with mobilization of the gallbladder from the liver bed and dissection of the cystic duct to the fibrous CBD (Fig. 56-5). The superficial peritoneum over the hepatoduodenal ligament is opened to expose the hepatic arteries and biliary remnant. The fibrous common duct is carefully dissected distally and divided at the upper border of the duodenum. The gallbladder and distal ductal remnant are used for traction as the dissection proceeds proximally. The cystic artery is ligated, taking care to

avoid compromise of the right hepatic artery. Proximally, the fibrous biliary duct widens into a cone-shaped mass and enters the liver between the bifurcation of the portal vein (Fig. 56-6). Small bridging veins from the portal vein are meticulously divided. The fibrous cone is amputated flush with the liver substance (Fig. 56-7). No cautery should be used on the amputated hilum. Packing with oxidized cellulose polymer and gauze while the Roux-en-Y is constructed will allow sufficient hemostasis.

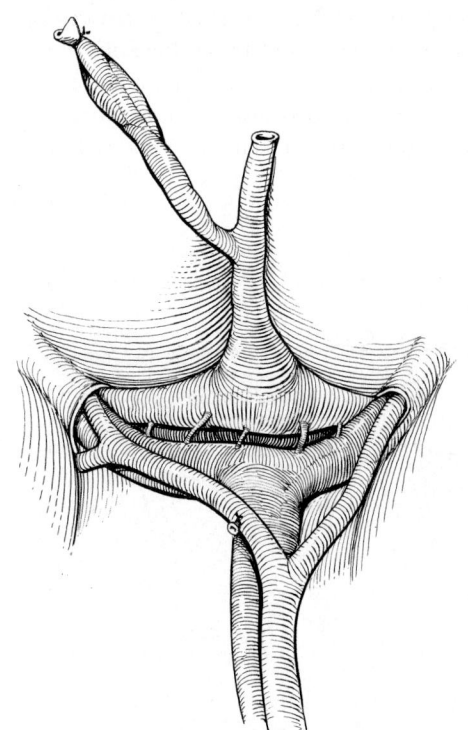

**FIGURE 56-6** After transection of the common bile duct distally, the biliary remnant and gallbladder are used for traction to free them from the underlying structures. The small bridging branches from the portal vein are divided so that the dissection reaches behind the portal vein.

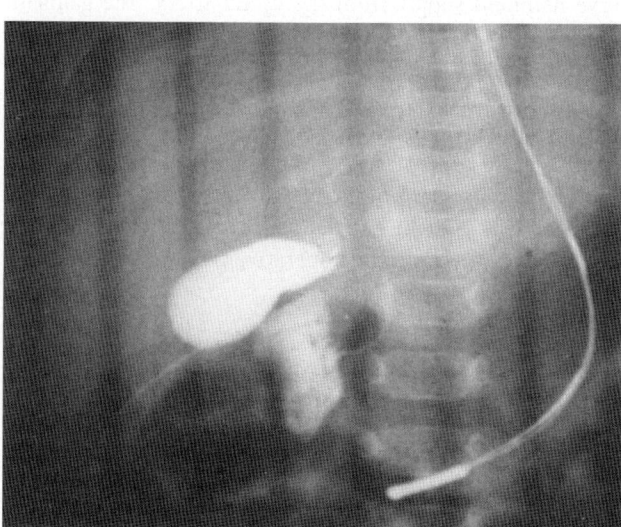

**FIGURE 56-4** Operative cholangiogram showing miniscule but patent intrahepatic and extrahepatic bile ducts with contrast in the duodenum. This patient had Alagille syndrome.

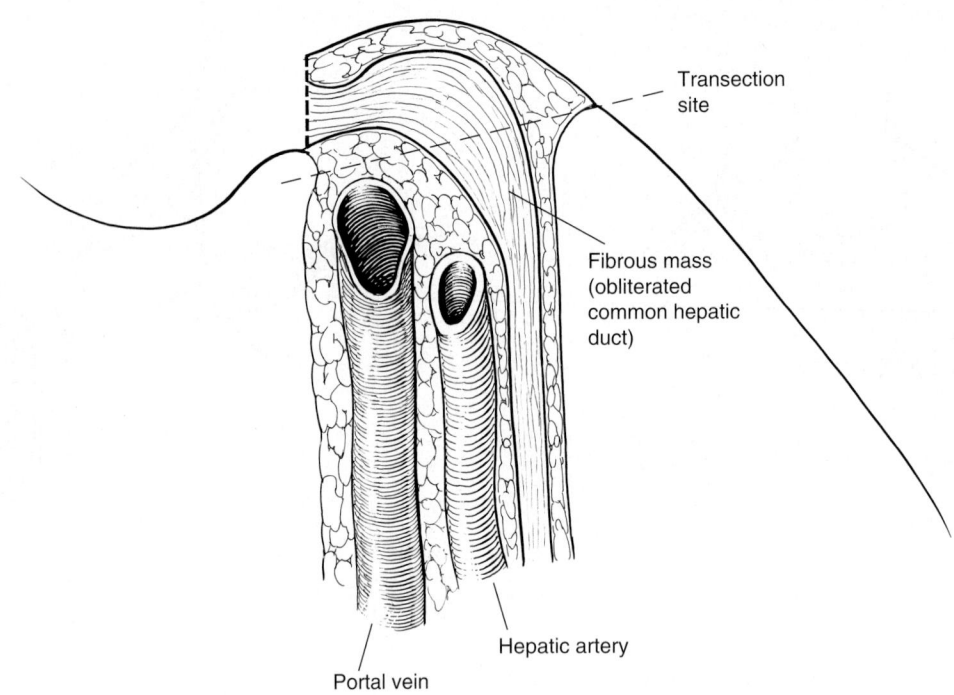

Transection site

Fibrous mass (obliterated common hepatic duct)

Hepatic artery

Portal vein

**FIGURE 56-7** The ductal remnants are transected at the level of the posterior portal vein, flush with the liver surface.

Although a variety of intestinal reconstructions have been described, the traditional Roux-en-Y is now preferred. Most of the other options stem from attempts to reduce the frequency of cholangitis. In general, none of the exteriorization or valve techniques significantly impact the incidence of cholangitis or the long-term outcome.

A 40-cm Roux-en-Y is constructed by transecting the jejunum distal to the ligament of Trietz. The Roux limb is passed retrocolic and a single-layer end-on anastomosis to the transected porta hepatis is made using running absorbable suture (Fig. 56-8). Care must be taken not to place sutures through

the transected tissue in which minute bile ducts are present, especially laterally and posteriorly. A small drain is placed posterior to the porta hepatis in the subhepatic space prior to closure of the incision. This is removed after the patient resumes enteral feeds and there is no sign of a bile leak.

## PORTOCHOLECYSTOSTOMY

In about 20% of patients, patency of the gallbladder, cystic duct, and distal CBD permits its use for reconstruction. The proximal amputation is at the identical level, flush with the liver. The gallbladder must be carefully mobilized to preserve its blood supply from the cystic artery. The gallbladder is opened longitudinally and directly anastomosed to the transected porta (Fig. 56-9). The hypoplastic cystic duct and CBD may be incapable of accepting the full volume of biliary drainage initially. Therefore, temporary tube decompression with a silastic tube placed through the fundus of the gallbladder permits anastomotic healing and gradual dilation of the distal ducts. If the gallbladder is successfully employed for drainage, the risk of postoperative cholangitis is virtually eliminated.

## LIVER TRANSPLANTATION

Improvements in technique and immunosuppression in the 1980s added hepatic transplantation to the available options for treating children with biliary atresia. Although it has been suggested that liver transplantation should replace porto-enterostomy as primary therapy, several arguments to the contrary can be made. A significant percentage of patients

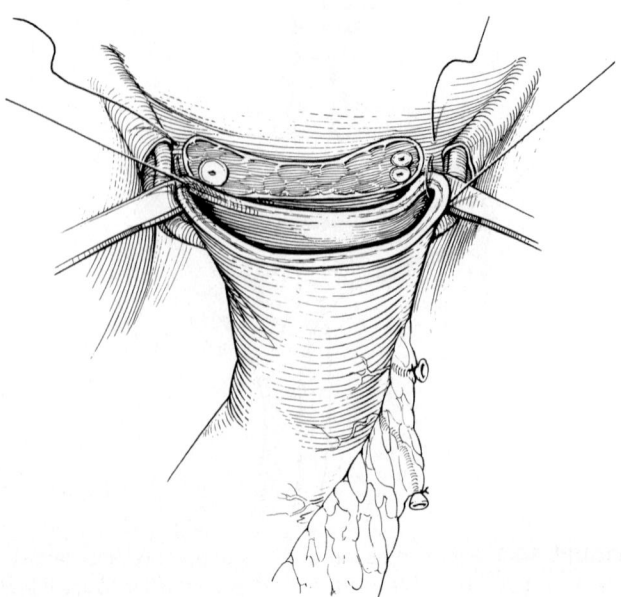

**FIGURE 56-8** After creation of a Roux-en-Y limb of jejunum, an end-to-end anastomosis is created with running absorbable suture.

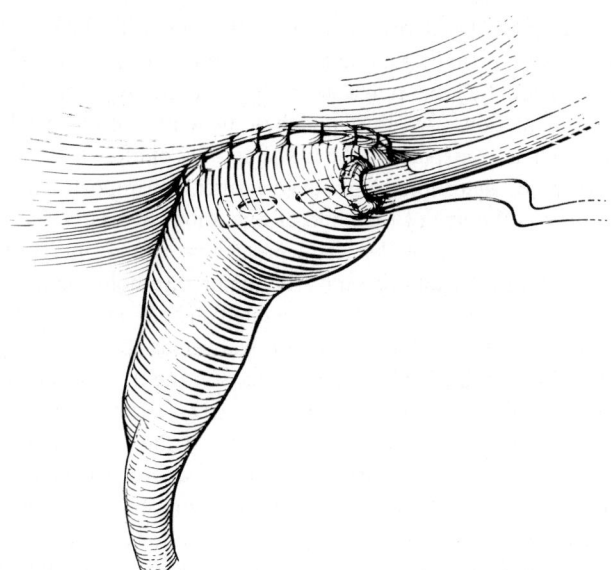

**FIGURE 56-9** When there is residual patency of the distal biliary tree, the gallbladder can be mobilized with its blood supply and anastomosed to the porta. Because of the diminutive size of the unused distal CBD, temporary catheter decompression is recommended.

achieve long-term survival with portoenterostomy alone (50% survival at 5 years and 25% survival into adolescence). Immunosuppression in infancy exposes the child to greater infectious and malignancy risks. The costs of the operation, immunosuppression, monitoring, and follow-up are far greater for transplant recipients. Finally, some have claimed that the Kasai operation adversely affects the outcome of the transplant procedure; however, comparative studies have been unable to show such an effect. Therefore, we believe that transplant should not replace the Kasai operation, but rather should serve as a safety net for early failures or later deterioration of synthetic function or portal hypertensive complications.

## LAPAROSCOPIC TECHNIQUES

With the advent of laparoscopy in pediatric surgery, more surgeons are utilizing this technique for diagnosis and treatment of biliary atresia. Laparoscopic cholecystocholangiography has been evaluated for feasibility in the diagnosis of jaundice in infants. Since its first description several groups have reported variations on this technique. Results have demonstrated the safety and feasibility of laparoscopic cholangiography in this patient population.

There is still controversy regarding laparoscopic portoenterostomy. Technically feasible but often described as challenging, early reported outcomes in small series of patients undergoing laparoscopic portoenterostomy have been equivalent to the open approach. Purported advantages of the laparoscopic approach include less postoperative pain, faster recovery, better cosmesis, and probably most importantly, lower incidence of adhesions. This is an important consideration as one third of these patients go on to require liver transplantation. Several small series have suggested that laparoscopic

portoenterostomy is equivalent to an open portoenterostomy in the hands of an experienced minimally invasive surgeon.

The most disturbing evidence for not performing a laparoscopic portoenterostomy comes from a prospective trial from the European Biliary Atresia Registry in 2011. A consecutive series of patients underwent laparoscopic Kasai procedure from 2006 to 2007. Infants having laparoscopic portoenterostomy were compared to conventionally operated control patients. Forty-two percent of the patients who underwent a laparoscopic portoenterostomy survived 6 months with their native liver, compared to 82% of the control group. Additionally, 82% of patients in the laparoscopic group were transplanted by 24 months, compared with 64% of the conventional group. These results should be interpreted with caution as it was a small series of nonrandomized patients. The authors pointed out that the learning curve for this technically demanding procedure may have adversely influenced the results. Given the significantly unfavorable outcome in the laparoscopic group, any surgeon undertaking the laparoscopic portoenterostomy should be an expert in minimally invasive surgery and proceed with caution.

## RESULTS

The early postoperative course of infants after biliary reconstruction is typical for a major laparotomy. When bowel activity returns, nasogastric decompression can be discontinued and diet reintroduced with formula containing medium-chain triglycerides as the fat source. With timely referral for surgical reconstruction (age <10 weeks), successful bile drainage can be achieved in more than 80% of infants with biliary atresia. Because bile flow is often sluggish in the first few weeks, significant improvement in liver function tests may not occur for 3 to 4 weeks after surgery. The main complications occurring after the Kasai operation are cholangitis, fat malabsorption, and portal hypertension.

## CHOLANGITIS

The development of unexplained pyrexia, accompanied by leukocytosis and bilirubinemia suggests bacterial cholangitis, a common complication after portoenterostomy. Especially common in the first 2 years, the liability of cholangitis wanes thereafter. The combination of bile stasis and bacterial flora present in the intestinal conduit constitutes the prerequisites for the development of cholangitis. Cholangitis is not seen in infants who never drain bile, and is rare after portocholecystostomy. Prompt treatment with broad-spectrum antibiotics (a carbepenem or other agent to control bowel flora) will treat most episodes. Patients with refractory cholangitis and threatened bile shutdown can be successfully managed with intravenous corticosteroids. We have given a short burst of methylprednisone (10 mg/kg) that tapered over 3 to 5 days. Some centers recommend the use of prophylactic antibiotics, low-dose steroids, or choleretics such as ursodeoxycholic acid (UDCA), to reduce or prevent cholangitis episodes. None have been proven to be of statistical benefit, but our preference is UCDA for long-term use (10-20 mg/kg/d). UCDA is a bile acid that modifies the composition of the endogenous bile acid pool, and increases bile flow by stimulating bicarbonate excretion. It also has inherent hepatocytoprotective effects. In our experience, it reduces incidence of cholangitis and bile shutdown.

## FAT MALABSORPTION AND FAT-SOLUBLE VITAMIN DEFICIENCY

Intraluminal bile salts are necessary for micelle formation, permitting normal absorption of fats. Until normal bile drainage is achieved, formulas containing fats as medium-chain triglycerides are preferred (eg, Pregestimil®). Medium-chain triglycerides are absorbed directly through the intestinal mucosa without the need for emulsification, micelle formation, and hydrolysis. Similarly, fat-soluble vitamin deficiencies are common in cholestatic infants. Rickets (vitamin D deficiency), ataxic neuropathy (vitamin E deficiency), keratopathy (vitamin A deficiency), and coagulopathy (vitamin K deficiency) have all been reported in children with biliary atresia. Appropriate supplementation and monitoring of serum vitamin levels can correct or prevent these deficiencies.

## PORTAL HYPERTENSION

Portal hypertensive complications are not uncommon after portoenterostomy, even in the jaundice-free patient. Increased portal pressures can be documented in most infants, even at the time of the initial operation. As a result of ongoing intrahepatic disease or partial biliary obstruction, hepatic fibrosis is often progressive. Portal hypertension manifests clinically as esophageal variceal hemorrhage, hypersplenism, and ascites. Esophageal variceal hemorrhage can be successfully treated by endosclerosis or endoscopic variceal banding. Children with significant hypersplenism can be treated by partial splenic embolization. Ascites is controlled with dietary restrictions and diuretics. In most instances, the development of portal hypertensive complications is a harbinger of hepatic decompensation and should initiate referral for liver transplantation. However, spontaneous reduction of portal pressure can occur, perhaps as a result of spontaneous portosystemic shunts or improvement in liver histology with ongoing bile drainage. This finding justifies the continued management of portal hypertensive complications without transplant, as long as hepatic synthetic function is preserved.

## PROGNOSIS

There is no doubt that the Kasai operation has positively influenced the prognosis of infants with biliary atresia. Without the portoenterostomy, the average life span of patients with biliary atresia is approximately 12 months. Still, the procedure is imperfect. In several studies in the United States, Europe, and Japan, after successful portoenterostomy, a

greater than 50% 5-year survival is attainable with the native liver. Even so, many patients with only transient or partial bile flow benefit by growth to a size sufficient to permit successful transplantation. Two thirds of these patients will ultimately need a liver transplant in the first 2 decades of life.

A major determinant of survival after hepatoportoenterostomy is the age of the child at operation. In nearly every review of success of the Kasai procedure, age at operation strongly influenced outcome. The major threshold seems to be around 60 days old. Infants operated on before that benchmark have about 70% 10-year survival versus approximately 30% if the infant is older than 60 days at the time of operation in the Ohi long-term series. Clearly, the prevention of secondary postoperative complications, namely cholangitis, directly influences outcome. Cholangitis can lead to obstruction of established bile flow and progression of hepatic fibrosis, and has been cited as a risk factor for poor outcome, but not decreased survival. Total serum bilirubin measured 3 months after surgery can help predict those infants who will need to go on to need a liver transplantation.

As important as any single factor, are the experience and operative technique of the surgeon, and the experience of the center in which the procedure is performed. Improved survival has been shown in centers that care for 5 or more patients with biliary atresia a year.

# Choledochal Cyst

## KEY POINTS

1. Choledochal cysts are congenital malformations of the biliary tract commonly associated with anomalous arrangement of the pancreaticobiliary duct. Diagnosis requires recognition of the varied presentation, for example, infants typically present with jaundice, older children present with abdominal pain or pancreatitis.

2. Ultrasound evaluation is the primary step in diagnosis, followed by MRCP or ERCP cholangiography for more accurate definition of the anatomy.

3. Left untreated, choledochal cysts can undergo malignant transformation and promote progressive hepatic fibrosis. Therefore, treatment includes surgical resection, reconstruction of biliary drainage and close surveillance.

## INTRODUCTION

In 1723, Vater first described fusiform dilation of the CBD in his dissertation of normal and abnormal biliary anatomy. Douglas, in 1852, provided the first clinical description of CBD dilation, which he believed to be of congenital origin. In 1959, CBD anomalies were revisited by Alonzo-Lej, who reported 2 clinical cases and reviewed 94 others to form the seminal clinical series describing cystic abnormalities of the biliary ducts. In this series, he formulated a classification of these cystic lesions, outlined their forms, and suggested therapies for each anomaly. Type I malformations, seen in approximately 80% to 90% of patients, represent cystic dilation of the CBD alone. Type II deformities (2%) represent diverticular malformations of the CBD. Type III lesions (1.4%-5%), termed *choledochoceles*, are distal CBD cysts within the substance of the pancreas that generally involve the ampulla. Subsequent to the development of modern imaging modalities and endoscopic retrograde cholangiopancreatography (ERCP), 2 additional cystic malformations have been incorporated into the original classification schema of Alonzo-Lej. This modification, as forwarded by Todani in 1977, includes the Type IVa deformity, a multicystic disease that involves the extrahepatic ducts and extends into the intrahepatic biliary ducts, sometimes affecting 1 lobe of the liver, sometimes both lobes. In most series, type IVa anomalies represent the second most common type. Type IVb lesions include multicystic disease of the extrahepatic ducts only. Type V anomalies, originally described by Caroli in 1958, are characterized by intrahepatic cystic dilation without extension into the extrahepatic biliary ducts. In addition, a forme fruste malformation of generalized, noncystic dilation of the bile ducts and pancreatico-biliary malunion has been described. The Todani modification of the Alonzo-Lej categories of cystic malformations of the biliary ductal system (Fig. 56-10) constitutes the currently accepted classification system for these lesions.

## PATHOPHYSIOLOGY

The etiology of choledochal cystic disease remains ill-defined; however, these malformations are considered congenital because they occur in fetuses and in newborns. Although many theories exist, perhaps the 2 most cited in the literature involve either the anomolous arrangement of the pancreaticobiliary ductal system leading to epithelial damage and subsequent cystic degeneration, or dilation of the biliary ductal system secondary to distal obstruction. Babbitt in 1969, followed by Todani in 1984, identified the common occurrence of anomalous drainage of the pancreaticobiliary ductal system, identified in 65% to 80% of patients with choledochal cysts. In these patients, the pancreatic duct enters the CBD at an abnormal angle and proximal to the circular muscle of the ampulla of Vater. This anomolous arrangement results in a long common channel with no effective sphincter of Oddi about the union of the CBD and the pancreatic duct as normally described. Reflux may then ensue, leading to epithelial damage of the biliary epithelium by pancreatic enzymes and subsequent ductal dilation. A second explanation for the development of choledochal cysts involves the presence of distal ductal obstruction, as proposed by Spitz in 1977. Using a neonatal lamb model, ligation of the distal CBD invoked cystic dilation of the biliary system. In contrast, using the same technique in adult sheep, only dilation of the gallbladder was

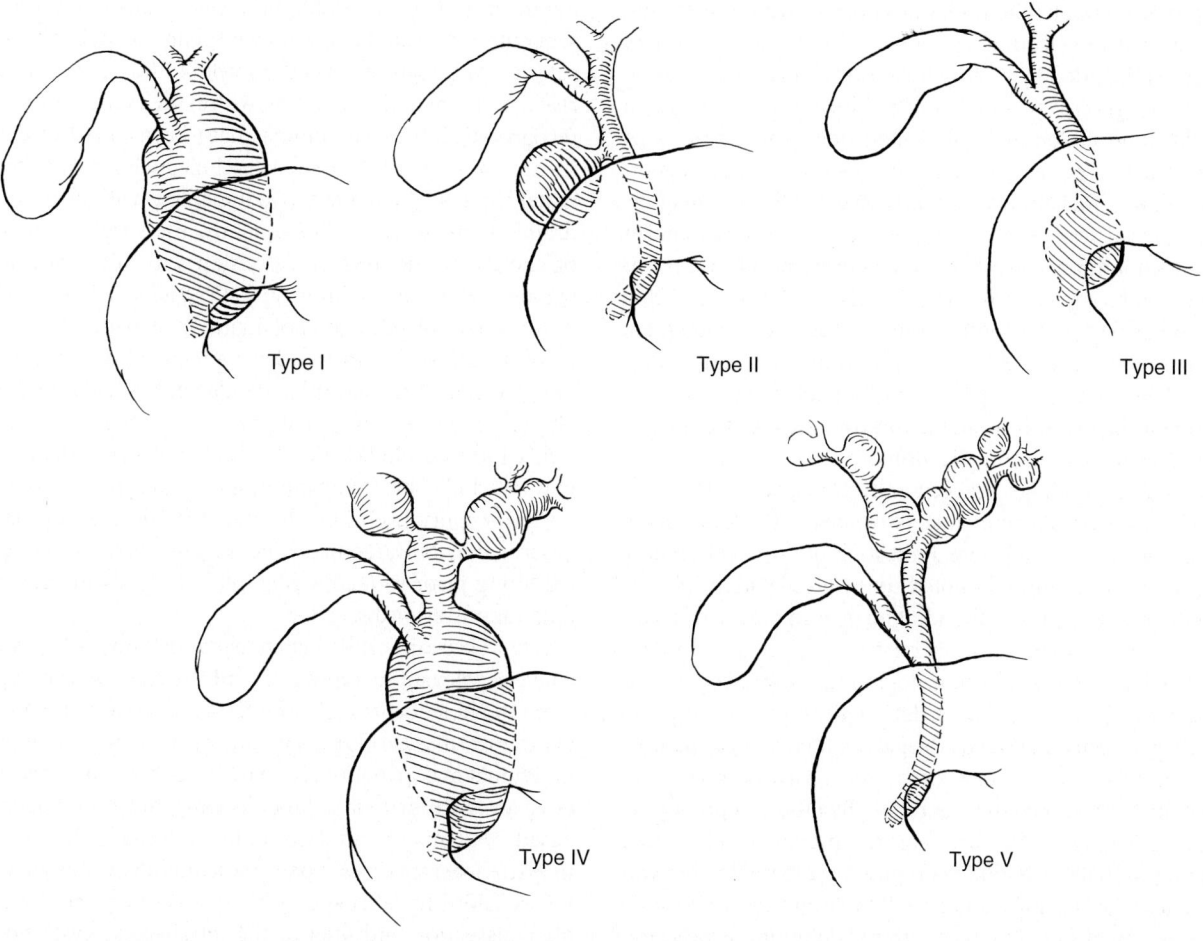

**FIGURE 56-10** The Todani modification of the Alonzo-Lej classification of cystic malformations of the biliary ductal system.

reproducible. It was concluded that immaturity of the ductal epithelium in the neonatal model resulted in cystic dilation secondary to increased intraluminal pressure proximal to the obstructive lesion, albeit from anomolous ductal insertion, congenital stenosis of the distal CBD, ampullary valvar stenosis, or sphincteric dysfunction. In general, the above theories may largely explain the development of Type I and Type IV malformations; however, they fail to explain the pathogenesis of intrahepatic cystic disease or choledochoceles.

## DIAGNOSIS

Choledochal cyst may be diagnosed in all age groups, including in utero with prenatal screening; however, the majority of patients become symptomatic within the first decade of life. The estimated incidence in Western countries varies between 1 in 100,000 and 1 in 150,000. Two-thirds of patients are reported from Japan, with two-thirds of patients being female in the predominant form of disease. No known genetic, metabolic, or environmental basis exists for the development of biliary cystic disease. The classic triad of pain, jaundice, and a palpable mass is noted in less than one-third of afflicted patients. Two distinct populations of patients exist in regard to clinical presentation. An "infantile" group of patients includes those individuals diagnosed prenatally or within the postnatal period of 12 months. In general, unrelenting jaundice from biliary obstruction forms the initial presenting symptom, although infants may be entirely asymptomatic and without screening laboratory abnormality. An "adult" form of disease is heralded by a more insidious clinical presentation and more severe symptomatology, including intermittent jaundice and abdominal pain, often due to pancreatitis. A forme fruste type may present with abdominal pain, hyperamylasemia, and jaundice without a dilated CBD on imaging. Undiagnosed lesions may progress to cholelithiasis and/or choledocholithiasis invoking cholecystitis, portal hypertension secondary to cirrhosis, cholangitis or abscess formation from biliary stasis, peritonitis from cyst rupture, or malignant degeneration. Any child presenting with pancreatitis warrants evaluation for the presence of a choledochal cyst. An expedient diagnosis is desirable to avoid the onset of potentially life-threatening complications.

Laboratory findings are generally nonspecific; however, conjugated hyperbilirubinemia associated with elevations of serum alkaline phosphatase indicative of "surgical" biliary obstruction is commonly noted upon presentation. Hyperamylasemia, generally in the adult form or in the forme fruste anomaly, may also be clinically relevant. The most useful initial screening study is ultrasonography. Regardless of age, ultrasonography is capable of defining the intrahepatic and extrahepatic biliary systems, the gallbladder, and the pancreaticobiliary system. In newborns with obstructive jaundice and a dilated extrahepatic biliary tree by ultrasonography, no further imaging studies are required preoperatively. Other imaging modalities include computed tomography, but this modality provides little additionally relevant information in the majority of individuals. Anatomic definition is best provided by ERCP, generally useful in the evaluation of "adult"

disease where hyperamylasemia and/or clinical pancreatitis is initially encountered. Use in infants is limited by the size of the scope and the need for general anesthesia. Magnetic resonance pancreaticocholangiography (MRCP) is fast becoming the preoperative roadmap of choice. The type of cyst and the anatomy of the pancreaticobiliary junction can be visualized, thereby providing insight for surgical planning.

## TREATMENT

The mainstay of treatment of choledochal cysts remains surgical. Medical therapy alone has an estimated mortality of 97%. The surgical treatment of choledochal cystic disease has evolved and been refined over the past century. Although aspiration and marsupialization were the earliest forms of surgical therapy, the development of external biliary fistulae often led to insurmountable fluid and electrolyte imbalances. Definitive therapy by complete cyst excision and internal drainage by hepaticoduodenostomy was initially described by McWhorter in 1924; however, unacceptable mortality rates were encountered, largely because of the relative extent of this procedure for that era. Given the unacceptably high risk of cyst excision at that time, Gross advocated internal drainage by choledochocystduodenostomy in 1933. This was confirmed as safe in an updated series in 1953. Subsequent patient evaluation, however, revealed morbidity rates approaching 50%, primarily a result of cholangitis from duodenal reflux. The Roux-en-Y cyst jejunostomy was subsequently advocated to circumvent reflux-associated complications. Although the overall morbidity was diminished, the risk of malignant degeneration within the cystic remnant was recognized. Biliary carcinomas have been noted to develop in 2.5% to 4.7% of patients with choledochal cysts, approximately half of which developed in patients with prior internal drainage procedures. Consequently, the surgical procedure of choice is now total cyst excision with internal drainage through a hepaticojejunostomy. Persistent, albeit markedly diminished episodes of cholangitis in hepaticojejunostomy reconstructions led to the development of a valved jejunal interposition. No studies have independently confirmed the efficacy of valved intestinal conduits in the prevention of reflux-induced cholangitis. Finally, pericystic inflammation may preclude safe complete-cyst excision, particularly with posterior (portal vein) involvement. An internal approach, as described by Lilly, requires mucosectomy of the inner epithelial lining prior to reconstruction, but avoids the perils of a difficult posterior dissection.

Cyst excision with hepaticoenterostomy, as described above, is relevant to Types I, II, and IVb lesions. The management of choledochocele (Type III) and variations of intrahepatic cystic disease (Types IVa and V) are dependent upon the individual malformation. In Type III lesions, duodenal-based cysts are unroofed via a duodenotomy; however, pancreatic-based cysts may be excised and/or internally drained, only in extremely rare cases is pancreaticoduodenectomy required for excision. Intrahepatic cystic disease may require lateral hilar dissection and fillet of the intrahepatic cyst and large ostial anastomosis for adequate drainage. Caroli disease, involving a single hepatic lobe, may be amenable to hepatic resection, but generally is curable only with liver transplant.

Differences in management of the forme fruste choledochal cyst exist, mainly on whether or not this anomaly is diagnosed in an adult or a child. Typically, children present with pancreatitis, abdominal pain, and elevated serum amylase. Work-up will show a mildly dilated CBD with pancreatico-biliary malunion. Most groups resected the CBD and reconstructed it with a hepaticojejunostomy or hepaticoduodenostomy in children. There is a preference for hepaticojejunostomy reconstruction as a case report of a patient who underwent a hepaticoduodenostomy developed cholangiocarcinoma 19 years after initial surgery. If a forme fruste choledochal cyst is diagnosed in an *adult* patient, 1 option would be to perform a cholecystectomy with close follow-up, given the high incidence of gallbladder carcinoma in this population (up to 39% in 1 series).

## OPERATIVE TECHNIQUE

### Cyst Excision

Antibiotics, usually a second-generation cephalosporin as a single agent, are administered preoperatively. The patient is positioned supine with a roll placed transversely beneath the upper abdomen. A right-upper-quadrant subcostal or transverse abdominal incision is favored. A self-retaining, abdominal wall retractor is then positioned for exposure. The cyst is readily evident, with further exposure gained by the medial and inferior reflection of the hepatic flexure of the colon (Fig. 56-11). A Kocher maneuver and lateral division of the gastrohepatic ligament accentuate cyst exposure. The cyst frequently extends behind the proximal duodenum. The gallbladder is mobilized from the liver bed (Fig. 56-12). The cystic artery is identified and ligated with silk suture. The degree

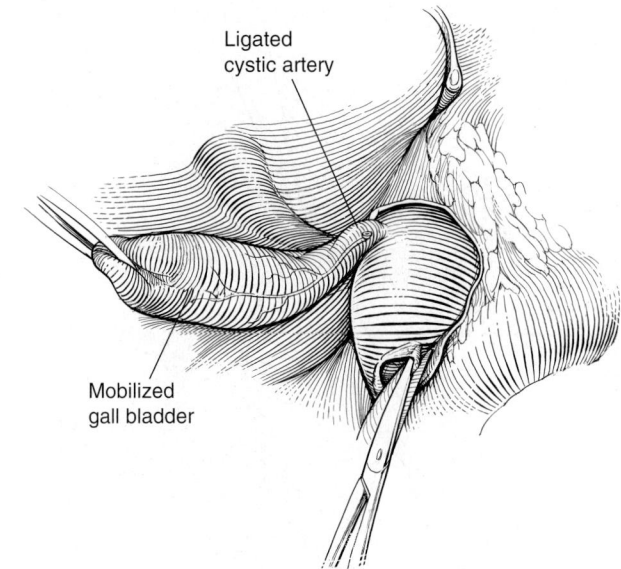

**FIGURE 56-12** The gallbladder is mobilized from the liver bed with ligation of the cystic artery. The duct is left intact for leverage in cyst dissection.

of pericystic inflammation will then dictate circumferential dissection of the porta hepatis structures versus partial excision with posterior mucosectomy (see below). In the usual case, medial reflection of the gallbladder will demonstrate the posterior plane between the cyst and portal vein. Once encircled, the dissection is carried inferiorly to the head of the pancreas. Further dissection can result in pancreatic ductal injury. Therefore, stay sutures are placed at the distal neck of the cyst. The distal duct is then transected and oversewn with a nonabsorbable, monofilament suture (Fig. 56-13). Once transected, the cyst may be reflected cephalad, and the portal vein

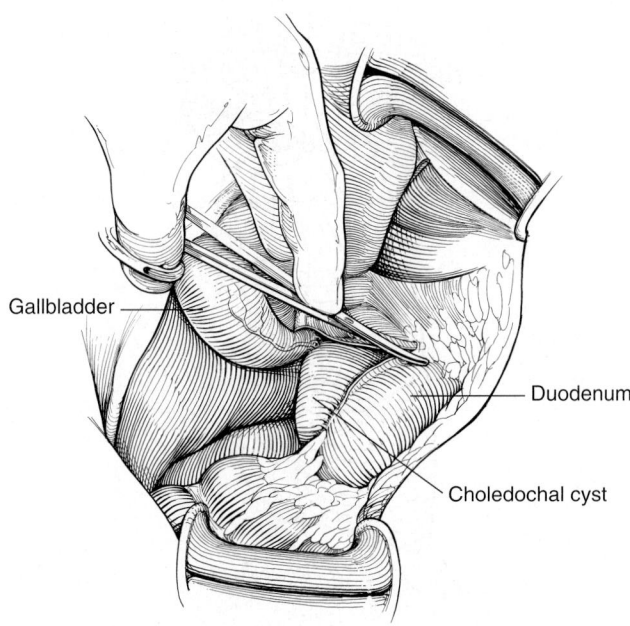

**FIGURE 56-11** Operative therapy of choledochal cyst. Following a right subcostal incision, the hepatic flexure of the colon is mobilized. A Kocher maneuver with lateral dissection of the gastrohepatic ligament will expose the distal choledochal cyst.

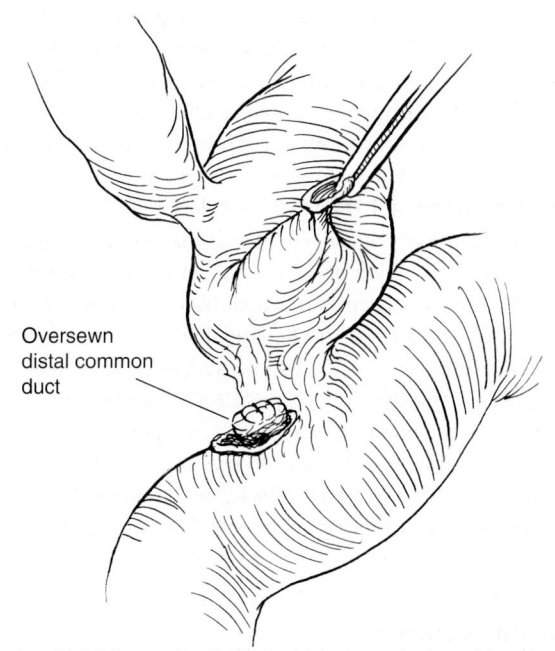

**FIGURE 56-13** The distal choledochal cyst and CBD is identified. The duct is transected as it enters the pancreas with the end oversewn.

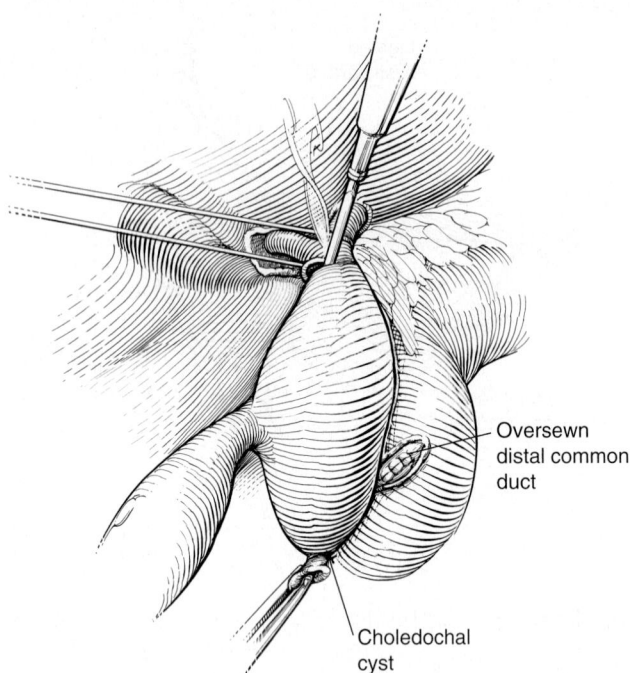

**FIGURE 56-14** The common hepatic duct is transected at the bifurcation.

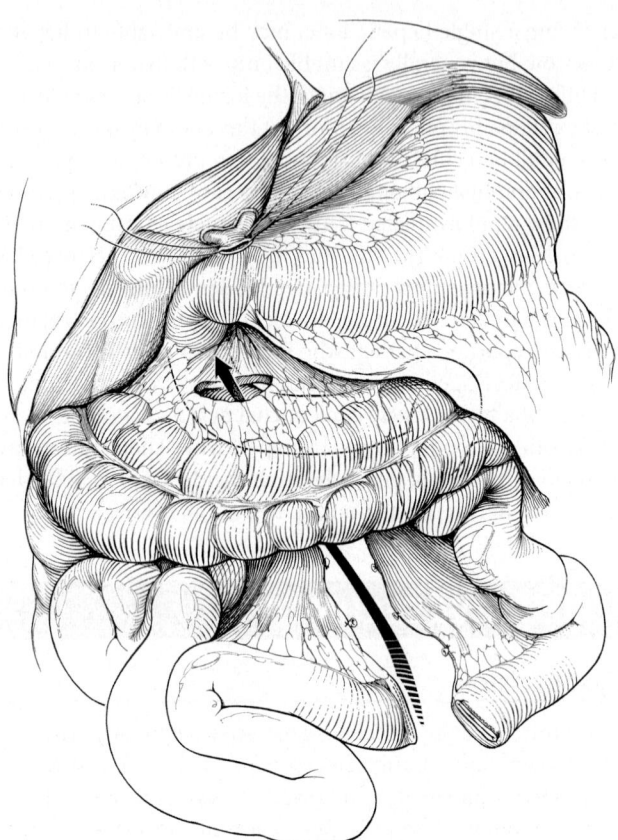

**FIGURE 56-15** A retrocolic Roux-en-Y jejunal limb is used as a conduit for biliary drainage.

and hepatic artery may be dissected free from the back side of the cyst. Dissection is carried to the bifurcation of the hepatic ducts. In the usual case, normal ductal caliber is noted at, or proximal to, the ductal bifurcation. The common hepatic duct is then transected circumferentially, immediately distal to the bifurcation (Fig. 56-14). The choledochal cyst and attached gallbladder may then be removed from the operative field and submitted for pathological examination. Stay sutures are placed laterally to aid in ductal manipulation, avoiding instrument trauma. Reconstruction is then performed with a Roux-en-Y conduit of jejunum. A 40-cm length of jejunum is selected. A jejunojejunostomy is performed in an end-to-side fashion in 2 layers to reestablish bowel continuity. The conduit is brought through a retrocolic window (Fig. 56-15). It should lie easily and without tension in the subhepatic space. The hepaticojejunostomy is then performed in an end-to-end fashion by using full thickness, single-layer, monofilament absorbable sutures (Fig. 56-16). A valve is not used and stents are not placed. Fixation of the jejunal serosa to the transverse mesocolon in 4 quadrants, as it traverses the mesenteric window, avoids tension on the hepaticojejunostomy and internal herniation (Fig. 56-17). Following assurance of adequate hemostasis, a suction drain is positioned in proximity to the anastomosis and externalized through a separate stab wound. The abdominal wound is closed in layers. Antibiotics are only administered perioperatively. The drain is removed in several days following resumption of an oral diet without concomitant bilious drainage.

## Internal Approach

If pericystic inflammation is encountered, precluding the safe dissection of porta hepatis structures, intramural dissection may be performed as described by Lilly. Following

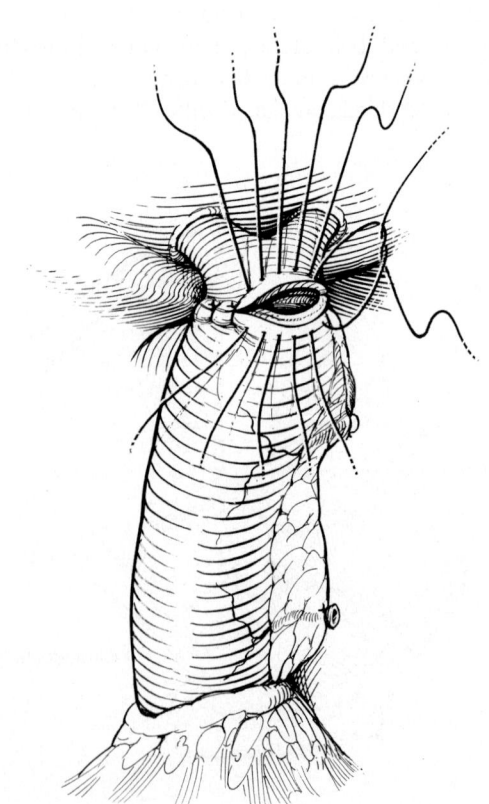

**FIGURE 56-16** The hepaticojejunostomy is constructed in an end-to-end or end-to-side fashion by using full-thickness, absorbable suture.

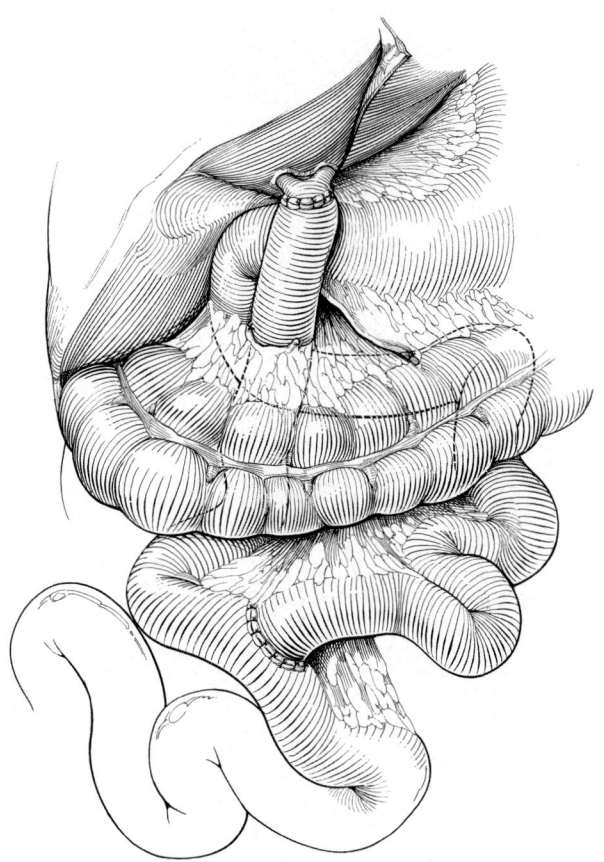

**FIGURE 56-17** The completed reconstruction is shown. Fixation sutures from the jejunal serosa to the transverse mesocolon may be used to secure the retrocolic jejunal limb.

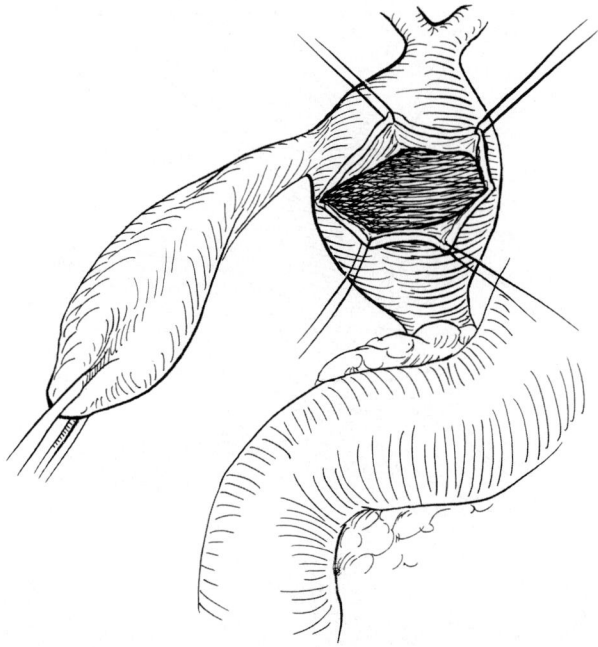

**FIGURE 56-18** If pericystic inflammation precludes circumferential dissection, an internal approach may be used. The anterior cyst wall is first dissected and incised in its midportion.

the portal vein Care is made not to put undo caudal tension on the cyst to avoid division of the hepatic duct too close to the bifurcation. Opening the duct and visualizing the bifurcation from the inside prior to division may help prevent this complication.

Reported benefits of the laparoscopic approach include a magnified view of critical structures, less postoperative pain,

cyst exposure anteriorly, the midportion of the cyst is incised transversely and contents evacuated (Fig. 56-18). Stay sutures are placed in quadrants for traction. A submucosal plane is identified laterally, with dissection then carried posteriorly (Fig. 56-19). The portal vein dissection is avoided by using this technique. A bridging incision is then made within the posterior cyst wall, from which the dissection may be carried cephalad and caudad until normal architecture is encountered (Fig. 56-20). The inflammatory reaction is usually less proximally and distally, whereby transection may be safely performed. The Roux-en-Y reconstruction continues as described (Fig. 56-21).

## Laparoscopic Approach

With new technology, laparoscopic excision of choledochal cysts and Roux-en-Y hepaticojejunosotomy is now feasible. First described by Farello et al in 1995, laparoscopic approach is reported to be increasingly used for pediatric choledochal cyst excision. Most of these series describe a hepaticoduodenostomy or hepaticojejunostomy. The hepaticojejunostomy technique is similar to that of the open approach. Usually 4 or 5 ports are employed: a 10-mm trochar at the umbilicus, 3 5-mm trochars in the left upper quadrant, and mid-right and left abdomen. If there is a large amount of inflammation of the cyst, the anterior wall can be opened to provide a safe window internally to the cyst in order to free the duct from

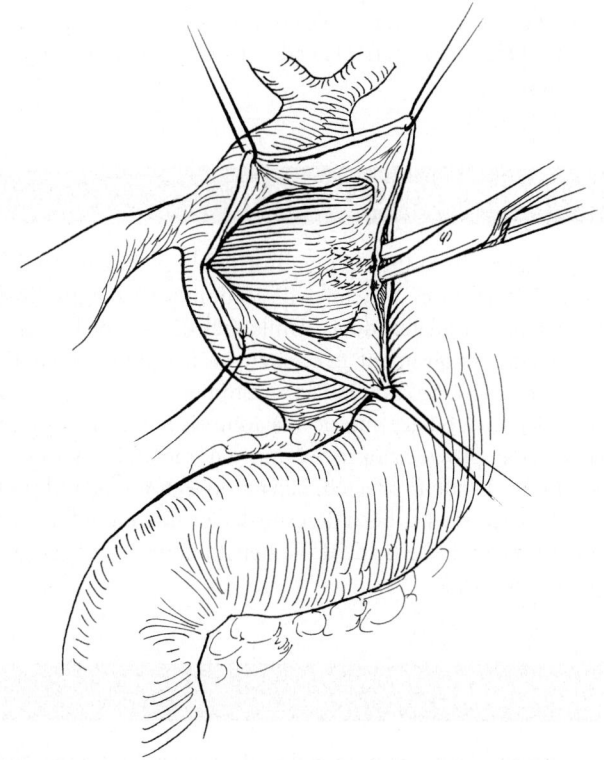

**FIGURE 56-19** A submucosal plane is developed laterally and carried posteriorly, thus avoiding injury to the portal structures.

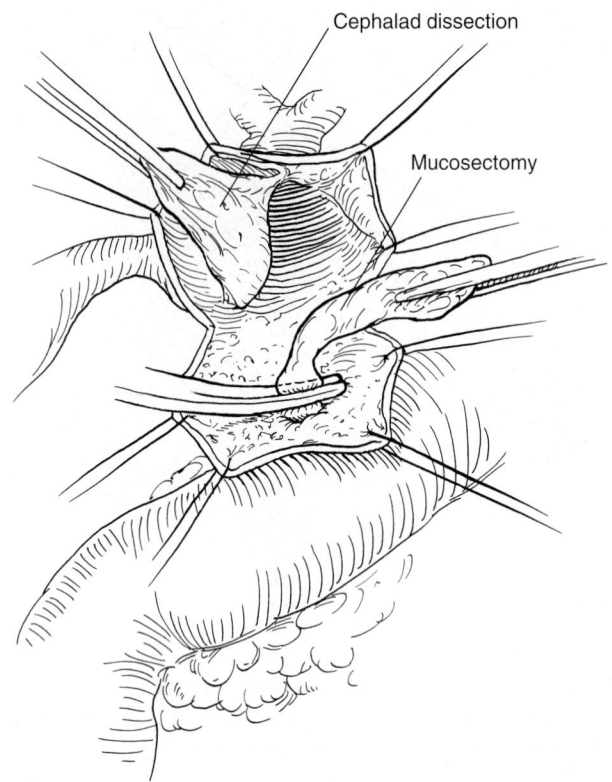

**FIGURE 56-20** Mucosectomy is carried out to the proximal and distal ostia of the cyst.

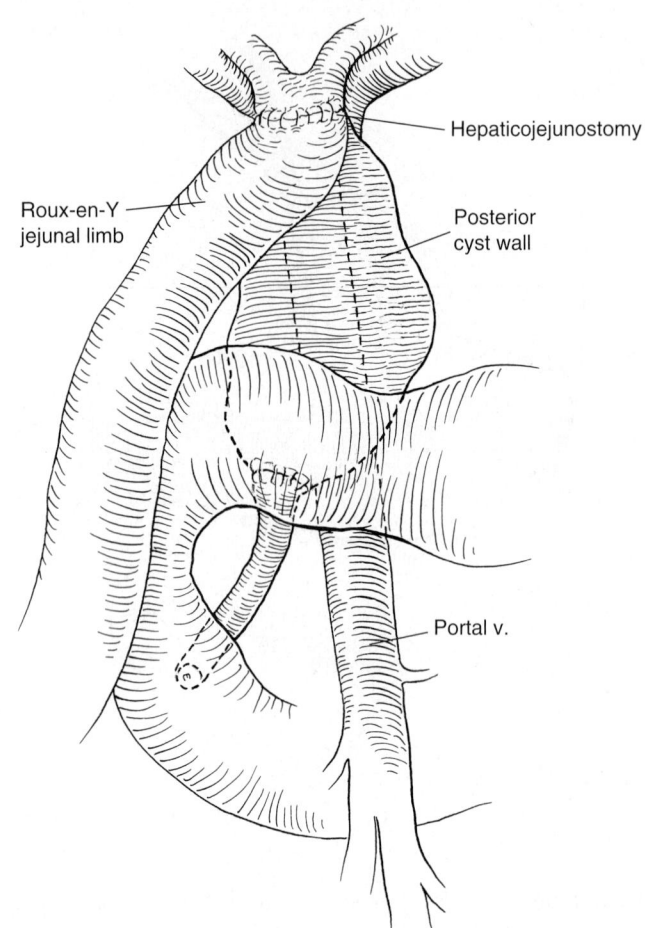

**FIGURE 56-21** Completed Roux-en-Y reconstruction is shown with the posterior submucosal cyst wall left in situ. The distal ostium is oversewn.

shortened hospital stay, and smaller incisions. One series reported the complication of cholangitis in 4/133 patients undergoing a hepaticoduodenostomy, none after hepaticojejunostomy. Other complications reported were pancreatic fistula, postoperative fluid collection requiring drainage, and gastritis. Only 2/190 patients had to be converted to an open procedure.

## INTRAHEPATIC DISEASE

Cystic dilation into the right and/or left branches above the bifurcation requires proximal dissection with longitudinal incision of the dilated ducts. Unilateral disease or bilateral intrahepatic involvement necessitates a longitudinal extension and a more proximal hilar anastomosis (Fig. 56-22). In this situation, a biliary enteric anastomosis in an end-to-side fashion may provide improved, more durable biliary drainage. If only 1 lobe is affected, hepatic lobectomy in addition to the cystectomy has been described. Consideration for liver transplant should be made if the hepatic fibrosis has significantly progressed.

## OUTCOME

A considerable number of publications have outlined the late complications of internal drainage procedures without cyst excision, including suppurative cholangitis, anastomotic

stricture, and malignant change within the retained cyst remnant. Several large series have reported long-term outcomes after excision and hepaticojejunostomy reconstruction for choledochal cysts. Most of these show that with standard treatment of excision and drainage, these patients will have no significant sequelae from this treatment. Ohi, in 1990, encountered neither deaths nor occurrences of malignancy in 100 consecutive patients. One early complication of pancreatic leak was identified. Late complications included 1 liver abscess and 4 cases of intrahepatic stone formation, attributed to long-standing intrahepatic bile duct dilation and stasis proximal to a distal stenosis. A single case of an anastomotic stricture related to technique was encountered. Reoperations were performed a mean of 12 years from the initial excision and drainage procedure, 2 of which required lateral segmentectomy to address intrahepatic disease following stone extraction. More recently, Miyano reviewed a 30-year experience in 180 patients harboring choledochal cyst. Conventional hepaticojejunostomy following cyst excision was performed in 174 patients. Six patients underwent cystenterostomy alone. Neither operative mortality nor malignancy was encountered. Four patients (2.3%) developed postoperative intrahepatic bile duct stone formation, 3 (1.8%) of whom demonstrated associated cholangitis attributable to anastomotic stricture. Of the 121 patients aged 5 years or

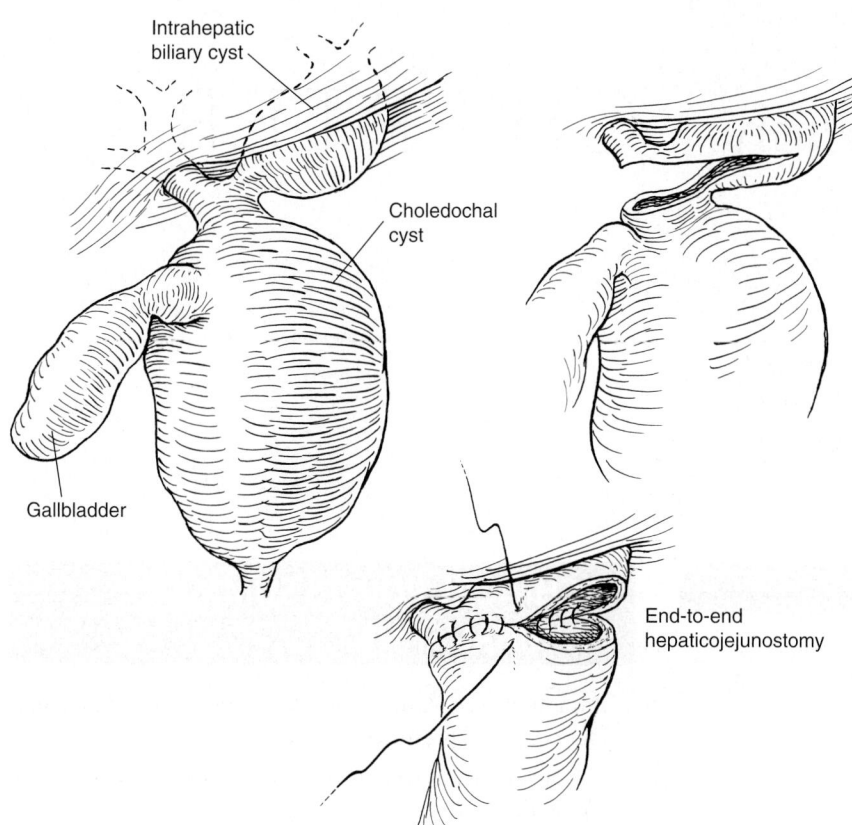

Intrahepatic
biliary cyst

Choledochal
cyst

Gallbladder

End-to-end
hepaticojejunostomy

**FIGURE 56-22** Cystic dilation extending beyond the bifurcation with intrahepatic ductal involvement requires proximal anastomosis, which is performed by longitudinal filleting of the intrahepatic ductal wall. Reconstruction is performed in an end-to-end or end-to-side fashion.

younger, no incidence of stone formation or cholangitis was documented. It would appear that late complications might be significantly age related. In the Ono series from 2010, 2 cases of biliary tract malignancy were noted from 56 children treated and followed for more than 10 years. Overall survival and symptom-free survival rates were 96% (54/56) and 89% (50/56), respectively. In summary, the prognosis of choledochal cyst is excellent if the diagnosis is made expediently prior to the development of irreversible liver disease or malignancy.

## SELECTED READINGS

Chan KWE, Lee KH, Mou J WC, Cheung STG, Tam YHP. The outcome of laparoscopic portoenterostomy for biliary atresia in children. *Pediatr Surg Int* 2011. Published online.

Farello GA, Cerofolini A, Rebonato M, et al. Congenital choledochal cyst: Video-guided laparoscopic treatment. *Surg Laparoscy and Endosc* 1995;5(5):354–358.

Hartley JL, Davenport M, Kelly DA. Biliary atresia. *Lancet.* 2009:374(9702): 1704–1713.

Huang L, Wang W, Liu G, et al. Laparoscopic cholecystocholangiography for diagnosis of prolonged jaundice in infants, experience of 144 cases. *Pediatr Surg Int* 2010;26(7):711–715. Epub May.

Le DM, Woo RK, Sylvester K, Krummel TM, Albanese CT. Laparoscopic resection of type 1 choledochal cysts in pediatric patients. *Surg Endosc* 2006;20:249–251.

Lilly JR. Total excision of choledochal cyst. *Surg Gynecol Obstet* 1978;14(6): 254–256.

Lilly JR, Stellin GP, Karrer FM. Forme fruste choledochal cyst. *J Pediatr. Surg.* 1985;20(4):449–451.

Miyano T, Yamataka A, Kato Y, et al. Hepaticoenterostomy after excision of choledochal cyst in children: a 30-year experience with 180 cases. *J Pediatr Surg* 1996;31(10):1417–1421.

Ohi R, Nio M, Chiba T, et al. Long-term follow-up after surgery for patients with biliary atresia. *J Pediatr Surg* 1990;24(4):442–445.

Ohi R, Yaoita S, Kamiyama T, et al. Surgical treatment of congenital dilatation of the bile duct with special reference to late complications after total excisional operation. *J Pediatr Surg* 1990;25(6):613–617.

Ono S, Fumino S, Shimadera S, Iwai N. Long-term outcomes after hepaticojejunostomy for choledochal cyst: a 10- to 27-year follow-up. *J Pediatr Surg* 2010;45(2):376–378.

Roskams T, Desmet V. Embryology of extra- and intra-hepatic bile ducts, the ductal plate. *Anat Rec(Hoboken)* 2008;291(6):628–635.

Rozel C, Garel L, Rypens F, et al. Imaging of biliary disorders in children. *Pediatr Radiol* 2010;41(2):208–220.

Shimotakahara A, Yamataka A, Kobayashi H, et al. Forme fruste choledochal cyst: long-term follow-up with special reference to surgical technique. *J Pediatr Surg* 2003;38(12):1833–1836.

Sokol RJ, Mack C. Etiopathogenesis of biliary atresia. *Semin Liver Dis.* 2001;21(4):517–524.

Sokol RJ, Mack C, Narkewicz MR, Karrer FM. Pathogenesis and outcome of biliary atresia: current concepts. *J Pediatr Gastroenterol Nutr* 2003;37(1):4–21.

Thanh LN, Hien PD, Dung LA, Son TN. Laparoscopic repair for choledochal cyst: lessons learned from 190 cases. *J Pediatr Surg* 2010;45(3):540–544.

Todani T, Watanabe Y, Narasue M, Tabuchi, K Okajima K. Congenital bile duct cysts: classification, operative procedures, and review of thirty-seven cases including cancer arising from choledochal cyst. *Am J Surg* 1977;134(2):263–269.

Ure BM, Kuebler JF, Schukfeh N, et al. Survival with the native liver after laparoscopic versus conventional Kasai portoenterostomy in infants with biliary atresia: a prospective trial. *Ann Surg* 2011;253(4): 826–830.

# Portal Hypertension

# CHAPTER 57

Jaimie D. Nathan, Kathleen M. Campbell,
Frederick C. Ryckman, Maria H. Alonso,
and Greg M. Tiao

## KEY POINTS

1. Etiology of portal hypertension may be classified as prehepatic, intrahepatic, or posthepatic.

2. Extrahepatic portal vein obstruction (EPVO) is the most common type of prehepatic obstruction.

3. Most cases of acute variceal bleeding can be controlled with fluid resuscitation, correction of coagulopathy, and pharmacologic support.

4. Octreotide is the most commonly used pharmacologic intervention in the management of acute variceal bleeding.

5. Upper endoscopy is an important intervention for both diagnostic and therapeutic purposes in acute variceal bleeding.

6. Endoscopic sclerotherapy or band ligation can be used to control refractory variceal bleeding.

7. Classification of portosystemic shunts: nonselective shunt, selective shunt, direct reconstruction of portal circulation.

8. H-type mesocaval shunt is the most commonly used nonselective shunt.

9. The most common selective shunt is the distal splenorenal shunt.

10. EPVO is optimally managed by the mesentericoportal shunt (Rex shunt).

11. Transjugular intrahepatic portosystemic shunt (TIPS) may be used as a bridge for liver transplantation in patients with intrinsic liver disease who have acute unresponsive variceal bleeding.

12. If significant portal hypertensive complications are accompanied by progressive hepatic synthetic failure, liver transplantation is preferred.

## TECHNICAL POINTS SUMMARY: SURGICAL SHUNTS

1. Intraoperative mesentericoportal venography and measurement of portal pressures.

2. Use of autologous venous conduit (internal jugular vein), if conduit is necessary.

3. Adequate mobilization of inflow and outflow vessels.

4. Fine monofilament suture for anastomoses.

5. Postreconstructive venography is critical.

6. Selective postoperative intravenous anticoagulation in high-risk patients.

7. Antiplatelet therapy for 30 to 90 postoperative days.

## PORTAL HYPERTENSION IN CHILDREN

The management of children with portal hypertension has evolved significantly over the past 2 decades. Improved survival in such patients has resulted secondary to both medical therapies and surgical interventions, including: (a) progress in the pharmacologic control of acute portal hypertensive hemorrhage; (b) improved efficacy and safety of endoscopic methods to treat acute esophageal variceal hemorrhage, which may also reduce the risk of rebleeding; (c) recognition of the role for traditional or innovative surgical therapy (portocaval shunts or reconstruction); and (d) improved outcomes following pediatric liver transplantation as a definitive treatment for children with end-stage liver disease/life-threatening complications of portal hypertension.

### Historical Overview

The principle of the surgical treatment of portal hypertension began with the work of Nikolai Eck in 1877. In dogs, he fashioned a side-to-side portal vein–inferior vena cava anastomosis following which he ligated the hepatic limb of the portal vein, thus creating a functional end-to-side shunt. In 1898, Benti described the portal hypertensive state, a syndrome of splenomegaly and gastrointestinal bleeding. Five years later, Eugene Vidal performed the first successful shunt in humans, an end-to-side shunt that successfully controlled bleeding, but which eventually was complicated by recurrent ascites, encephalopathy, and death. In pediatric surgery, Marion, in 1953, and Clatworthy, in 1955, described a mesocaval shunt in which a divided common iliac vein was turned up and connected to the side of the superior mesenteric vein (SMV). In 1972, Drapanas popularized the use of a prosthetic "H-graft" to bridge the portal-systemic circulation. In 1967, Warren described the distal splenorenal shunt in an effort to separately decompress veins of the esophagus, stomach, spleen, and distal pancreas, leaving flow through the liver via the portal and mesenteric veins. In addition, in an effort to limit encephalopathy, progressively smaller side-to-side shunts were done. Both the splenorenal technique and the application of progressively smaller shunts proved particularly adaptable to the management of portal hypertension in the pediatric patient.

Splenic artery inflow reduction was also recognized as effectively reducing portal pressure. Splenectomy was tried more than 100 years ago as a treatment for ascites secondary to cirrhosis, and it was eventually recognized that as much as two-thirds of portal flow could be reduced by this maneuver. Eventually, however, splenectomy and its hazards, especially for children, was supplanted by both splenic artery ligation and embolization.

A direct attack on varices was begun with coronary vein ligation. Devascularization of the stomach and esophagus was first done in 1950, and a series of modifications followed in an effort to minimize the procedure. The result was a high rebleeding rate. The ingredient then identified to minimize this rebleeding was esophageal or stomach transection and reanastomosis, a technique proposed by Tanner that may have led to the esophagogastrectomy with colon interposition subsequently done in a pediatric series by Koop. A further modification by Sugiura used thoraco-abdominal technique, division, devascularization, splenectomy, vagotomy, and pyloroplasty; it was the most aggressive of the portalazygos system disconnection procedures and was associated with a very low rebleeding rate.

The evolution of liver transplantation followed the initial successful transplant by Starzl in 1967, and the eventual consensus development conference in liver transplantation in 1983. Since that time, advances in liver transplantation have made it the procedure of choice for patients with severe portal hypertension and hepatic decompensation.

## Etiology

Portal hypertension is defined as an elevation of the portal pressure above 10 to 12 mm Hg. In healthy children, portal pressure rarely exceeds 7 mm Hg. Elevation of the portal pressure is most commonly secondary to obstruction of portal venous flow due to prehepatic, intrahepatic, or posthepatic block, although increased splanchnic blood flow may contribute in some cases. Increased pressure within the portal circulation leads to formation of collateral circulatory pathways connecting the high-pressure portal vasculature to the low-pressure systemic venous system. The most common and potentially dangerous communications occur within the

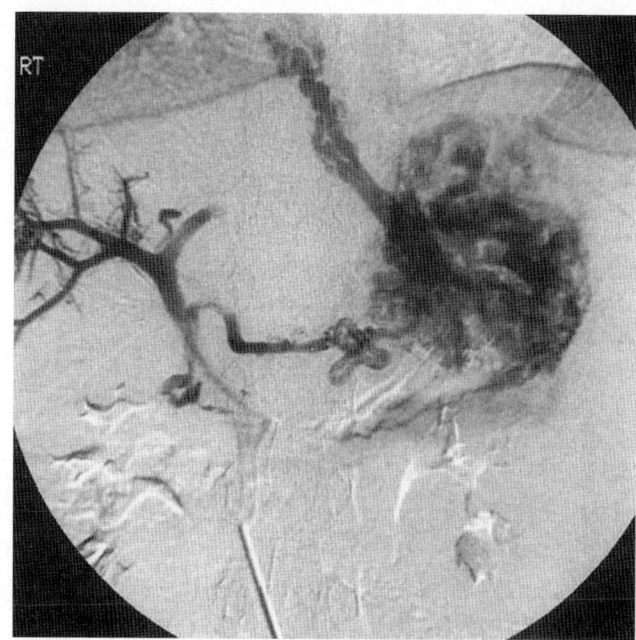

**FIGURE 57-1** Portal venogram demonstrating retrograde flow within the coronary vein to massive gastric and esophageal varicies. Intra-operative exam to confirm vascular anatomy and measure portal pressures prior to shunting.

esophageal wall, connecting the coronary and short gastric veins to the esophageal venous plexus. Esophageal varices developing within this plexus become the site with the highest risk for massive gastrointestinal hemorrhage (Fig. 57-1). Less threatening collateral communications can develop between the recanalized umbilical vein and abdominal wall systemic veins (caput medusa), the inferior rectal veins as hemorrhoids, and in the retroperitoneum. In addition, any surgical union between the portal and systemic venous circulations, such as occurs with intestinal stomas, is a possible, and often problematic, site of variceal development. Favorable collateral vessels developing within the tissues surrounding the pancreas, duodenum and left kidney form "spontaneous" splenorenal shunts. The long-term ability of these collaterals to decompress the hypertensive portal circulation is unproven but suggested.

The progressive development of collateral vessels connecting the portal and systemic circulation has the beneficial effect of decreasing portal pressure. However, this effect is diminished by the concurrent development of a hyperdynamic circulatory state. Portal hypertension has been associated with the presence of autonomic nervous system dysfunction, as well as an excess of circulating cytokines leading to tachycardia, decreased systemic and splanchnic vascular resistance secondary to vasodilatation, plasma volume expansion, increased cardiac output, and, subsequently, increased portal inflow.

The combination of portal venous outflow obstruction, increased portal inflow, and the extensive collateral circulation that develops accounts for many of the complications associated with portal hypertension. Superficial submucosal collateral vessels, especially those in the esophagus and stomach, and to a lesser extent, those in the duodenum, colon, or rectum, are prone to rupture and bleed. In addition,

| TABLE 57-1 | Pediatric Diseases Associated with Portal Hypertension |
|---|---|

**Prehepatic Causes**
Extrahepatic portal vein thrombosis
Cavernous transformation of the portal vein
Splenic vein thrombosis
Congenital portal vein malformation (web or diaphragm)
Extrinsic portal vein compression

**Intrahepatic Causes**
Hepatocellular disease
Autoimmune hepatitis
Hepatitis B, C
Wilson disease
Alpha-1-antitrypsin deficiency
Glycogen storage disease—Type IV
Toxins and drugs
Histiocytosis X
Gaucher disease
Biliary tract disease
Biliary atresia
Cystic fibrosis
Intrahepatic cholestasis syndromes
Sclerosing cholangitis
Congenital hepatic fibrosis
Schistosomiasis
Sinusoidal veno-occlusive disease

**Posthepatic Causes**
The Budd–Chiari syndrome
Inferior vena cava obstructions (web)
Chronic congestive heart failure
Veno-occlusive disease (s/p bone marrow transplantation)
Postoperative hepatic vein stenosis
Prothrombotic disease

**Hyperkinetic Causes (High Flow)**
Arteriovenous fistula (congenital or acquired)

submucosal arteriovenous communications between the muscularis mucosa and dilated precapillaries and veins within the stomach result in vascular ectasia, or congestive hypertensive gastropathy, significantly contributing to the risk of hemorrhage from the stomach.

The elevated portal pressure is a common result of several different mechanisms in children discussed below (Table 57-1).

## Prehepatic Portal Hypertension

The most common type of prehepatic obstruction is extrahepatic portal vein obstruction (EPVO) at any level of the portal vein. Umbilical vein infection in infancy or similar infections in older children, such as perforated appendicitis, primary peritonitis, and inflammatory bowel disease, have historically been identified as predisposing factors, as have primary biliary tract infections and cholangitis. These mechanisms are less commonly seen in children today. Inherited abnormalities predisposing to hypercoagulability, such as factor V Leiden mutation, protein C, protein S, and antithrombin III deficiencies, as well as hyperviscosity/polycythemia in infancy or umbilical vein catheterization, can all lead to secondary thrombosis, especially when accompanied by neonatal dehydration or systemic infection and phlebitis. The common occurrence of these coagulopathies makes their investigation mandatory. Embryological malformations resulting in tortuous, poorly developed portal veins, webs, or diaphragms also can be an uncommon primary cause for EPVO or predispose to an increased risk of thrombosis. The development of periportal collateral vessels, "cavernous transformation of the portal vein," may result from either a disordered embryologic process or longstanding portal vein thrombosis.

Children with EPVO are usually completely healthy prior to an episode of hematemesis or hematochezia. Because their hepatic synthetic function is normal, they are able to recover from their variceal hemorrhage more readily than children with preexisting liver disease. Despite thorough evaluation, over 50% of reported EPVO cases have no identifiable cause.

## Intrahepatic Causes of Portal Hypertension

Portal hypertension in children is commonly related to progressive hepatocellular injury and fibrosis, in the setting of intrinsic liver disease, broadly characterized as hepatocellular disorders and biliary tract disorders. The common final pathway of increased intrahepatic vascular resistance due to hepatic fibrosis and alterations in hepatic microcirculation is the basis for the development of portal hypertension and its associated complications in cirrhosis. The etiologies of chronic liver disease in children are myriad and include recognized disorders such as extrahepatic biliary atresia, metabolic liver diseases such as alpha-1-antitrypsin deficiency, Wilson disease, glycogen storage disease type IV, and cystic fibrosis. When hepatic synthetic failure is not present or only slowly progressive, direct treatment of portal hypertension or its complications is indicated. Because many of these conditions are associated with progressive liver failure, the primary treatment in most cases is liver transplantation. Other rarer intrahepatic causes of portal hypertension include schistosomiasis, in which small intrahepatic portal venules are destroyed, and congenital hepatic fibrosis, a hereditary disorder of interlobar bile duct proliferation and fibrosis.

## Posthepatic Portal Hypertension

Posthepatic portal hypertension is caused by obstruction to the hepatic vein outflow from the liver. Hepatic vein obstruction (the Budd–Chiari syndrome) can occur secondary to obstruction to the hepatic veins at any point from the sinusoids to the entry of the hepatic veins into the right atrium/inferior vena cava. Although a specific etiology is often not found, thrombosis can complicate neoplasms, collagen vascular disease, infection, trauma, or hypercoagulable states. Veno-occlusive disease, microvascular nonthrombotic occlusion of hepatic venules, also has emerged as one of the most

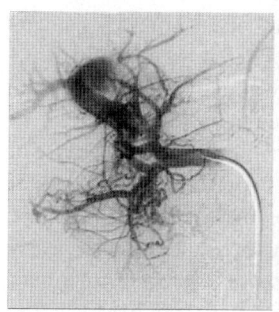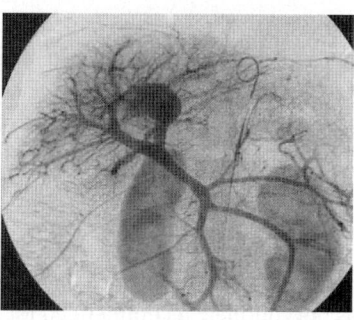

**FIGURE 57-2** Congenital arterial-venous fistula from the left hepatic artery to the left portal vein, with subsequent retrograde filling of the portal venous system. Patient presented with massive diarrhea, protein losing enteropathy and gastrointestinal bleeding. Treated with left hepatic lobe resection.

frequent causes of hepatic vein obstruction in children. Most cases occur after total body irradiation with or without cytotoxic drug therapy associated with bone marrow transplantation. This condition also has occurred after the ingestion of herbal remedies containing the pyrrolizidine alkaloids, which are sometimes taken as medicinal teas.

## Hyperkinetic (High-Flow) Portal Hypertension

Rarely, children present with increased portal inflow resulting in portal hypertension. In our experience, these have been associated with arterial-venous fistulas or malformations between the mesenteric arterial circulation and the portal vein. These children often present with diarrhea, protein losing enteropathy, ascites with significant albumin loss, and bleeding. They are easily recognized on imaging, and primary therapy consists of resection of the malformation and closure of the fistula (Fig. 57-2).

## Diagnosis and Evaluation

Clinical history and physical examination should concentrate on identifying factors that predispose to the development of cirrhosis, including a family history of inherited metabolic disease and possible exposure to viral or toxic pathogens. Clinical examination findings suggesting underlying liver disease (ascites, liver size/contour, nutritional status), hypersplenism (splenomegaly, bruising), or hepatopulmonary syndrome (spider angiomas, clubbing, exercise intolerance, cyanosis) contribute to diagnostic evaluation and therapeutic planning. Hypercoagulability and its complications should be evaluated in both the patient and family members due to the inherited basis for these protein abnormalities.

Imaging tests are essential to confirm the presence of portal hypertension, define the portal venous anatomy, and formulate options for therapy. Initial screening with ultrasonography can suggest the presence of chronic liver disease and should determine portal venous patency. Doppler examination can depict both the direction of portal venous flow and the degree of hepatopetal flow, which correlates with the risk of variceal hemorrhage. Magnetic resonance venography or contrast-enhanced computed tomography has replaced mesenteric angiography to further define portal anatomy, an

essential step when liver transplantation or portosystemic shunt procedures are planned.

Upper gastrointestinal endoscopy is the most accurate and reliable method for detecting both esophageal varices and the source of acute gastrointestinal hemorrhage. This modality is especially valuable in the presence of acute hemorrhage, where up to one-third of patients with known varices may have bleeding from other sources such as portal hypertensive gastropathy or gastric/duodenal ulcerations. In addition, upper endoscopy can identify features associated with an increased risk for hemorrhage, such as large varices, "cherry-red spots" apparent over varices representing fragile telangiectasias within the shallow submucosa, and portal hypertensive gastropathy. Endoscopy is also used to intervene therapeutically when acute bleeding varices are identified and when prophylactic endoscopic treatment of varices is warranted.

Liver biopsy may be helpful in determining the etiology of intrinsic liver disease and in defining further therapy or the need for transplantation. A percutaneous approach may be utilized, unless significant coagulopathy is present, in which case liver biopsy should be performed in the operating room by open or laparoscopic techniques.

## Treatment of Portal Hypertensive Complications

The decision to undertake pharmacologic, endoscopic, or surgical treatment for portal hypertension must be based on the natural history of the disease and the possibility of life-threatening complications. The prognosis is related to the primary etiology of the portal hypertension. In patients with intrinsic liver disease, prognosis is also dependent on the degree of hepatic functional reserve. It has been generally accepted in patients with portal hypertension due to EPVO that the risk of acute variceal bleeding decreases with age, concurrent with the development of spontaneous portosystemic collateral vessels. This postulated natural history has been the primary argument supporting conservative management of hemorrhage in these patients, using endoscopic therapy to obliterate esophageal varices while awaiting the development of favorable retroperitoneal and peripancreatic collateral vessels. However, children who have experienced bleeding complications prior to age 12 and those with grade II or III varices remain at a significantly higher risk for further upper gastrointestinal hemorrhage at a later age. These high-risk populations should be identified and considered for preemptive effective intervention.

In patients with intrinsic liver disease, therapeutic choices are influenced by the probability of progression of their disease and their potential need for liver transplantation in the future. A significant number of these patients require temporizing endoscopic treatment or surgical portosystemic shunt therapy to treat complications or maintain stability prior to undergoing liver replacement.

The most common portal hypertensive complication is gastrointestinal bleeding. Regardless of the site and mechanism of bleeding, initial therapy is directed toward fluid resuscitation and, when necessary, blood replacement. A nasogastric tube should be placed to confirm the upper gastrointestinal tract as the source of bleeding and for evacuation of blood from the stomach. A proton pump inhibitor should be administered to decrease the risk of bleeding from gastric erosions, and antibiotics should be instituted as prophylaxis for bacterial infections or spontaneous bacterial peritonitis. In patients with hepatic synthetic dysfunction and coagulopathy, administration of vitamin K, fresh frozen plasma or cryoprecipitate, and platelets when thrombocytopenia is present also may be necessary. Adequate volume resuscitation is essential; however, volume overload from excessive transfusion or crystalloid administration is counterproductive because this leads to further increase in portal pressure and continued hemorrhage.

## Pharmacologic Treatment

Pharmacologic intervention to decrease portal pressure is essential in patients with continued bleeding, as cessation of hemorrhage is the most critical therapeutic challenge. A variety of pharmacologic options are available when intervention is required.

### Vasopressin

Vasopressin decreases portal venous pressure by increasing the splanchnic vascular tone and by decreasing the splanchnic arterial inflow. Vasopressin infusion has been associated with control of variceal hemorrhage in 53% to 85% of cases in children. However, its clinical utility is limited by its significant side effects.

### Octreotide

Octreotide is an octapeptide synthetic somatostatin analog that reduces splanchnic blood flow by selective mesenteric vascular smooth muscle constriction. Its effects on variceal hemorrhage are similar to those of vasopressin, but it carries a lower risk of adverse systemic side effects. Octreotide can be administered subcutaneously, but is best used as a continuous intravenous infusion (25-50 $\mu g/m^2/h$, or 1.0-3.0 $\mu g/kg/h$). Recent retrospective studies have demonstrated that octreotide is associated with a high rate of bleeding control in children with portal hypertension without significant adverse events.

### Beta Blockers

While beta blockers have no role in the treatment of acute variceal hemorrhage, they have been used in an effort to prevent first variceal hemorrhage in high-risk patients, and as an option for secondary prophylaxis. The goal of therapy is a reduction in heart rate by 25%, thereby decreasing cardiac output, portal inflow, and perhaps blocking $\beta$ receptor-mediated vasodilatation, allowing unopposed $\alpha$ stimulation within the mesenteric arterioles.

Efficacy has been evaluated in 2 groups. In the first, patients with documented varices underwent $\beta$-blocker treatment in an attempt to prevent the first episode of bleeding (primary prophylaxis). In adult patients treated for primary prophylaxis, $\beta$-blockers were associated with significantly lower rates of bleeding and death from bleeding. In the second group, patients were treated following the initial hemorrhage in an attempt to prevent recurrent bleeding (secondary prophylaxis). The results of $\beta$ blockade for secondary prevention of recurrent variceal hemorrhage are more controversial. Low-risk patients appear to enjoy low (3%) rebleeding rates; however, this advantage seems to be lost in Child's class B and C patients, where the risk for recurrent bleeding is reported to be 46% to 72%.

Fewer studies have been performed in children. Because of the presence of extrahepatic portal hypertension in up to half of all children who are candidates for treatment, pediatric results may not correlate directly with adult patients, nearly all of whom have intrinsic liver disease. $\beta$-blocker treatment is not routinely recommended for primary prophylaxis in the pediatric population due to lack of evidence and asthma-like side effects. $\beta$-blockers also inhibit hemodynamic compensation, making them poor choices for pediatric patients.

## Mechanical Tamponade

Mechanical tamponade using balloon catheter tubes (Sengstaken–Blakemore or Minnesota tubes) provides mechanical compression of esophageal and gastric fundal varices. The significant number of complications and high incidence of rebleeding have limited their use to severe uncontrollable hemorrhage as a temporizing measure until a definitive intervention or surgical procedure can be performed. Although balloon tamponade is usually successful in stopping refractory hemorrhage, the effect is often transient, and recurrence following removal is common.

## Endoscopic Intervention for Esophageal Varices

While variceal hemorrhage can usually be controlled using medical therapy, the risk of recurrent hemorrhage and the need for accurate diagnosis of the site of hemorrhage often mandate upper endoscopy during the early posthemorrhage period. When variceal hemorrhage is confirmed or strongly suspected, variceal sclerotherapy or variceal band ligation can be used to eradicate the present or future sites of bleeding.

The use of endoscopic methods to control acute variceal hemorrhage is well established. Endoscopic sclerotherapy (EST) has been widely used as the primary treatment for refractory variceal bleeding due to its high success rate (>90%) and the ability to institute initial treatment at the time of diagnostic endoscopy. Esophageal ulceration at the site of injection is seen in 70% to 80% of patients and serious complications such as esophageal strictures, esophageal perforation, or mediastinitis occur in 10% to 20% of patients. In an attempt to overcome these complications, endoscopic band ligation (EBL) of varices has been developed, using techniques similar to those for banding internal hemorrhoids. Band ligation has the advantage of ligating only the submucosal venous varices, without harming the submucosal lining. Initial variceal obliteration was achieved by EBL in 73% to 100% of children, and rebleeding prior to completion of obliteration occurred less commonly than with EST management.

## Portosystemic Shunts

Numerous surgical procedures have been devised to divert portal blood into the low-pressure systemic venous circulation, thereby decreasing the portal venous pressure. Enthusiasm for the use of portosystemic shunting in children was limited by early reports suggesting that children under 8 years of age, and those with vessels for the shunt anastomosis of less than 8 to 10 mm, would be unsuitable candidates due to the high risk of shunt thrombosis. In addition, Voorhees et al suggested a high incidence of neuropsychiatric disturbances following nonselective shunts in children. More recent experience in centers skilled in pediatric vascular reconstruction has established that a high rate of success can be achieved with minimal complications, even in small pediatric patients. The indications for portosystemic shunting have been altered by the growing success of endoscopic methods to control variceal bleeding and the improvements in pediatric liver transplantation. We now consider the following children to be candidates for portosystemic shunting: (a) children with documented variceal hemorrhage who have progressive or continued esophageal variceal bleeding despite endoscopic intervention and who have preserved hepatic synthetic function; (b) children who fail endoscopic treatment and have intrinsic liver disease, but have adequate liver synthetic function to predict that liver transplantation will not be needed for several years (selective shunt only); (c) severe portal hypertension in patients with cystic fibrosis and variceal hemorrhage whose microbiologic flora compromise liver transplant survival; (d) children with severe portal hypertension who reside a great distance from emergency medical care endangering their survival should significant hemorrhage occur; and (e) children with EPVO and uncontrolled hypersplenism.

In general, portosystemic shunts can be classified into 3 groups: nonselective and selective shunts, and direct reconstructions of the portal circulation using vascular grafts (shunts). We believe that primary reconstruction is the optimum solution when available, followed by selective and lastly nonselective shunts. Nonsurgical shunt options such as TIPS and the Sugiura procedure are used only when other options are not available or as a bridge to transplantation.

Direct reconstruction of the portal circulation in children with EPVO into the left branch of the portal vein represents the ideal solution. This mesentericoportal shunt (Rex shunt) reestablishes normal physiologic portal inflow into the intrahepatic portal vein, either using an interposition jugular venous graft or by transposition of the dilated coronary vein (Fig. 57-3). Candidates for this procedure should fulfill 4 conditions: (a) the liver parenchyma must be normal; (b) they must not have a hypercoagulable state; (c) the umbilical portion of the left portal vein must be accessible and patent; and (d) there must be a suitable vein in the mestentericosplenic venous system to serve as the inflow vessel. The Rex shunt procedure is unique in that it restores hepatopetal portal perfusion and the inflow of hepatotrophic substances to the liver. Patients with diffuse intrahepatic portal vein thrombosis are not candidates for this reconstruction.

Doppler ultrasonography is performed preoperatively to assess the intrahepatic portal veins, and to confirm patency of both internal jugular veins, as the left internal jugular vein is most commonly utilized as a conduit for the Rex shunt. Magnetic resonance angiography is utilized to assess the intrahepatic left portal vein in cases where Doppler ultrasonography

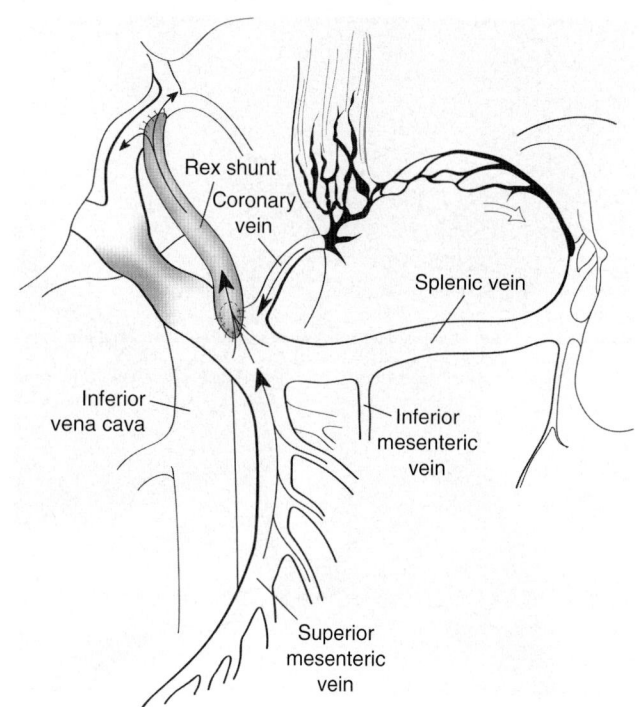

**FIGURE 57-3** Mesentericoportal shunt (Rex shunt)—This shunt returns portal blood flow directly to the hepatic portal circulation via the left branch of the intrahepatic portal vein, and is useful in patients with EPVO and a patent intrahepatic portal venous system. Rex shunt construction usually consists of an interposition internal jugular vein conduit from either the (**a**) SMV, splenic vein, or (**b**) autologous vein (left internal jugular) from the SMV-splenic vein junction to the intrahepatic left portal vein branch (shown in the figure).

is unable to confirm its patency. If the status of the intrahepatic left portal vein still remains unclear, preoperative transjugular retrograde portal venography can be helpful in defining left portal vein patency.

Although experience with Rex shunt construction remains limited, recent studies have documented excellent short-term shunt patency and resolution of episodes of variceal bleeding. In a recent retrospective review of 34 children with EPVO, over 90% of those who underwent exploration had successful construction of a Rex shunt. All Rex conduits remained patent over a follow-up period of up to 7 years, with complete resolution of variceal bleeding and symptoms of hypersplenism. Thus, in appropriately selected patients with EPVO, the Rex shunt represents the optimal solution to provide adequate portal venous decompression, which, in addition, re-establishes hepatopetal portal perfusion (Fig. 57-4).

*Selective shunts* are constructed to divert the "gastrosplenic" portion of the portal venous flow into a systemic vein, most frequently the left renal vein, left adrenal vein, or the immediately adjacent IVC. Communication between the "central" mesentericoportal circulation which perfuses the liver and the gastrosplenic portal circulation is severed by dividing the gastroepiploic veins, the coronary vein, and the retroperitoneal pancreatic collateral vessels. The most common and successful selective shunt is the distal splenorenal shunt (DSRS; Warren Shunt) (Figs. 57-5 and 57-6). We use this shunt as our primary option in children where direct (Rex)

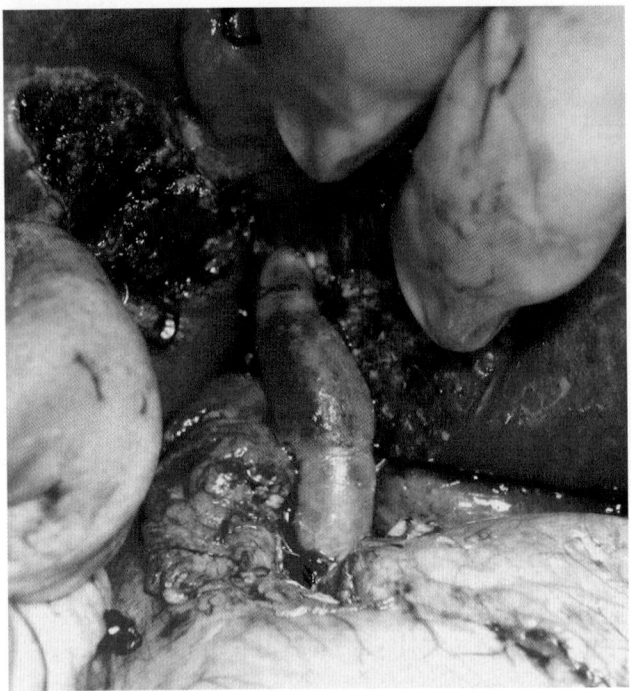

**FIGURE 57-4** Intraoperative photo of Rex reconstruction using an interposition jugular vein graft.

reconstruction of the portal system is not possible. When the left adrenal vein is appropriately located and dilated, it serves as an alternative anastomotic site to access the left renal vein. When performed in centers experienced in complex vascular reconstruction of the portal system, as is necessary in pediatric liver transplantation, shunt patency has ranged from 83% to 100%. Encephalopathy is uncommon in children following

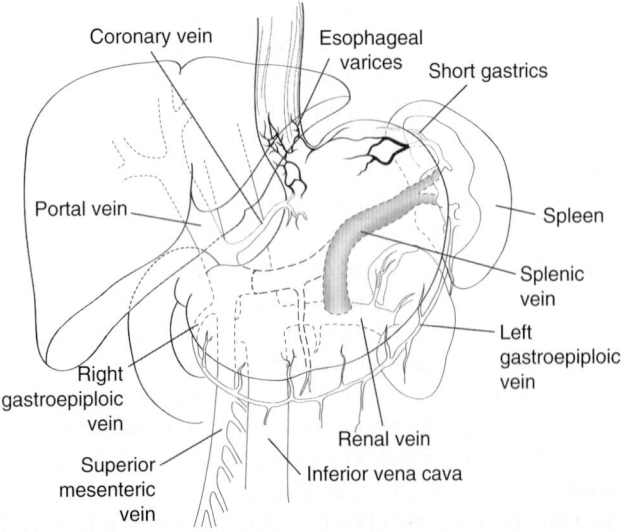

**FIGURE 57-5** Distal splenorenal shunt (DSRS)—A selective shunt allowing communication between the distal splenic vein and the left renal vein. The esophagogastric venous complex communicates via the short gastric veins, decompressing esophageal varices without decreasing perfusion through the mesenteric portal system to the liver.

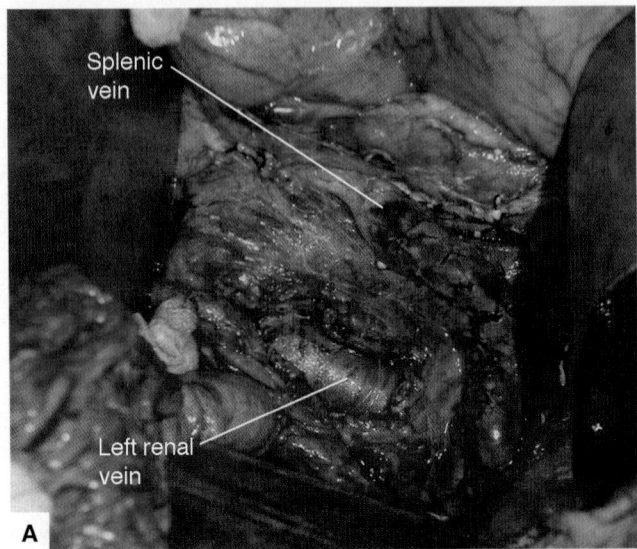

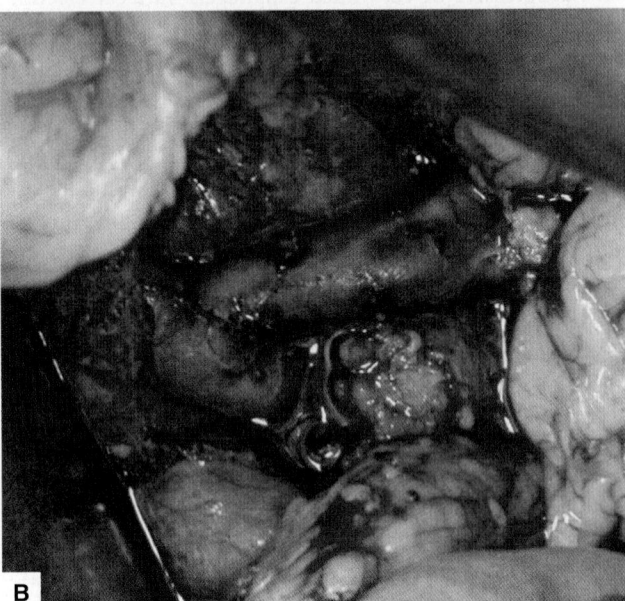

**FIGURE 57-6** Distal splenorenal shunt (DSRS)—**A.** Intraoperative dissection prior to shunt, (**B**) completed end-to-side DSRS. Anterior line on the splenic vein prevents twisting prior to anastomosis.

successful portosystemic shunting, even in patients with intrinsic liver disease.

*Non-selective shunts* are constructed to communicate with the entire portal venous system, and therefore have the potential to divert blood from the normal antegrade perfusion to the liver. Historically, the most commonly used shunt in children was the Clatworthy shunt, a mesocaval shunt in which the distal inferior vena cava (IVC) was ligated and divided, and its proximal portion was then anastomosed to the side of the SMV. This shunt has now been replaced by the H-type mesocaval shunt, which is constructed using a short segment of the internal jugular vein to connect the SMV and the IVC (Fig. 57-7). This shunt retains the advantage of a larger vessel for the anastomosis and avoids ligation of the IVC. The limited intra-abdominal dissection required to construct this shunt contributes to its technical ease, and if liver transplantation is necessary, the shunt can be easily occluded

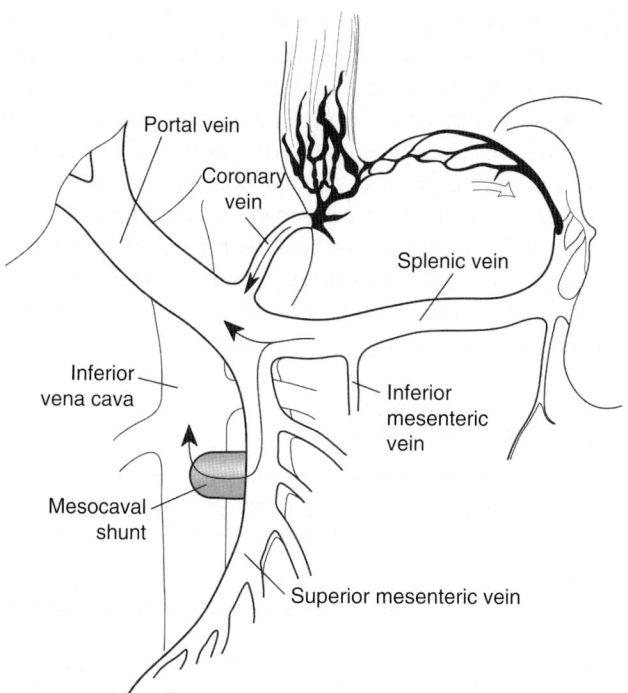

**FIGURE 57-7** Interposition "H"-type mesocaval shunt—A non-selective shunt involving anastomosis of internal jugular vein conduit between the SMV and the infrarenal inferior vena cava. Prosthetic graft can also be used.

| TABLE 57-2 | Portal Hypertension Surgical Options |
| --- | --- |
| **Primary Etiology** | **Preferred Surgical Therapies** |
| Prehepatic Obstruction | Rex shunt construction |
|     Extrahepatic portal vein thrombosis | Direct venous repair |
|     Cavernous transformation of the portal vein | |
|     Congenital portal vein malformation | |
|     Extrinsic portal vein compression | |
| Intrinsic Hepatic Disease | Distal splenorenal shunt |
|     Cirrhosis | H-type mesocaval shunt |
|     Congenital hepatic fibrosis | TIPS |
| Posthepatic Obstruction | H-type mesocaval shunt |
|     The Budd–Chiari syndrome | Cavo-atrial shunt |
|     Veno-occlusive disease | TIPS |
|     Postoperative hepatic vein stenosis | |
| Hyperkinetic Causes (High Flow) | Resection of involved liver |
|     Arteriovenous fistula (congenital or acquired) | |

at that time. Other nonselective shunts have significant disadvantages in children due to the need for splenectomy (proximal splenorenal shunt), or dissection of the main portal vein, which compromises liver transplantation (end-to-side and side-to-side portocaval shunts).

Treatment of the hepatic vein outlet obstruction (the Budd–Chiari Syndrome) can be accomplished through central nonselective shunting, with the addition of caval-atrial shunting if significant retrohepatic IVC obstruction accompanies the extreme liver enlargement often seen in these patients. Any shunt procedure or liver transplantation is complicated by the almost universal hypercoagulability seen in these patients. Because of their small size and significant obstructive symptoms, these children are often better served by liver replacement.

Table 57-2 depicts our preferred surgical options for shunt procedures based on the primary etiology of portal hypertension in children.

## Transjugular Intrahepatic Portosystemic Shunt

The introduction of transjugular intrahepatic portosystemic shunt (TIPS) has added another therapeutic option for the physician confronted with complex portal hypertension. This procedure uses interventional radiologic techniques to place an intrahepatic expandable metallic stent between a portal vein branch and the hepatic vein, forming a central transhepatic nonselective portocaval shunt. Technical difficulties in establishing a safe but large enough tract for sufficient shunt flow limit the utility of this procedure in infants. In children with biliary atresia, the close proximity of the biliary Roux-en-Y limb to the portal vein and the often diminutive size of the portal vein increase the risk of stent occlusion, malposition, or perforation. This procedure provides great benefit in the control of refractory portal hypertensive bleeding unresponsive to pharmacologic intervention and in patients needing temporary portal decompression prior to liver transplantation. The ability to embolize bleeding varices from the coronary vein at the time of TIPS placement assists in achieving primary control of bleeding sites. The 2 principal long-term complications of TIPS are encephalopathy and shunt occlusion. These limitations and risks make TIPS a reasonable and suitable treatment for acute unresponsive variceal hemorrhage in children with established intrinsic liver disease, often while awaiting liver transplantation. It is particularly helpful when used as a bridge to achieve stability by controlling refractory hemorrhage in patients awaiting liver transplantation. Long-term decompression is better achieved through surgical shunts at the present time, and TIPS is not indicated in patients with EPVO.

## Nonshunt Procedures for Portal Hypertension

The use of nonshunt surgical procedures for the management of portal hypertension does not offer the same success as shunt surgery. Historically, these operations have included direct variceal ligation through a transthoracic or abdominal approach, gastroesophageal devascularization procedures (Sugiura Procedure), or, rarely, translocation of the spleen into the thorax (splenopneumopexy). In general, these procedures have been abandoned except in cases where widespread thrombosis of the mesenteric venous vasculature makes shunt therapy or transplantation poor alternatives.

## Liver Transplantation

The progressive improvement in both the operative techniques and the immunosuppression management of children who have undergone liver transplant has led to 1-year survival rates approaching 90% in many centers, with 5-year survival rates of 85%. Regardless of the primary etiology of portal hypertension, liver transplantation successfully resolves the portal flow obstruction and allows the resolution of hypersplenism and hypertensive portal gastropathy. However, the use of primary transplantation as a treatment modality for portal hypertension is limited by the availability of suitable donor organs and the long-term risks of immunosuppression, opportunistic infections, and lymphoproliferative disease. When children have progressive intrinsic hepatic disease, the course of their progression and the amount of hepatic functional reserve should determine the use of primary transplantation compared with temporizing treatments, such as sclerotherapy or surgical shunts. At present, primary transplantation is recommended for children who have significant portal hypertensive complications such as bleeding, hypersplenism, or hepatopulmonary syndrome, and those who have progressive hepatic synthetic failure. Children with intrinsic liver disease but preserved hepatic synthetic function, who may not require transplantation for several years, will achieve excellent palliation with selective DSRS. TIPS is reserved for patients who have unresponsive variceal bleeding as a therapeutic bridge to transplantation, allowing them to achieve suitable stability while awaiting transplant donor organ availability.

## Summary

Therapeutic options for children with portal hypertension now include a broad range of pharmacologic, endoscopic, and surgical procedures. Thoughtful application of all of these options can improve quality of life by decreasing the complications of portal hypertension, and decrease mortality by preventing the consequences of variceal hemorrhage. The development of portal hypertensive gastropathy following palliative procedures such as EST and band ligation may limit their long-term success in children. The excellent results now obtained with selective portosystemic shunts and liver transplantation assure that definitive surgical treatments will continue to be a critical component in the treatment of children with portal hypertensive complications or progressive liver disease. Evolving procedures, such as TIPS, represent excellent short-term life-preserving techniques to stabilize critically ill patients while awaiting liver transplantation. Their role in the future long-term management of children requires continued evaluation.

## SELECTED READINGS

Chaves IJ, Rigsby CK, Schoeneman SE, Kim ST, Superina RA, Ben-Ami T. Pre- and postoperative imaging and interventions for the mes-Rex bypass in children and young adults. *Pediatr Radiol* 2012;42:220–232.

Emre S, Dugan C, Frankenbert T, et al. Surgical portosystemic shunts and the Rex bypass in children: a single-centre experience. *HPB (Oxford)* 2009; 11:252–257.

Garcia-Tsao G, Sanyal AJ, Grace ND, et al. Prevention and management of gastroesophageal varices and variceal hemorrhage in cirrhosis. *Hepatology* 2007;46:922–938.

Laleman W, Van Landeghem L, Wilmer A, et al. Portal hypertension: from pathophysiology to clinical practice. *Liver Int* 2005;25:1079–1090.

Ling SC, Walters T, McKiernan PJ, Schwarz KB, Garcia-Tsoa G, Shneider BL. Primary prophylaxis of variceal hemorrhage in children with portal hypertension: a framework for future research. *J Pediatr Gastroenterol Nutr* 2011;52:254–261.

Ochs A. Transjugular intrahepatic portosystemic shunt. *Dig Dis* 2005;23:56–64.

Scholz S, Sharif K. Surgery for portal hypertension in children. *Curr Gastroenteral Rep* 2011;13:279–285.

Shneider B, Emre S, Groszmann R, et al. Expert pediatric opinion on the report of the Baveno IV Consensus Workshop on Methodology of Diagnosis and Therapy in Portal Hypertension. *Pediatr Transpl* 2006;10:893–907.

Superina R, Shneider B, Emre S, et al. Surgical guidelines for the management of extra-hepatic portal vein obstruction. *Pediatr Transpl* 2006;10:908–913.

Tiao GM, Alonso MH, Ryckman FC. Pediatric liver transplantation. *Semin Pediatr Surg* 2006;15:218–227.

# CHAPTER 58

# Chronic Pancreatitis in the Pediatric Population

*Alex Bondoc and Greg M. Tiao*

## KEY POINTS

1. An unremitting, deranged inflammatory response characterizes chronic pancreatitis (CP) in children and is modulated by environmental and genetic factors.

2. Unlike adults, the etiology of pediatric CP involves congenital or anatomic variants, genetic mutations, or autoimmune disease.

3. The diagnostic work-up of children suspected to have CP should include sweat chloride assessment, genetic assay for *CFTR*, *SPINK1*, and *PRSS* mutations, endoscopic and/or radiographic imaging, and autoimmune testing.

4. Initial therapy for CP includes treatment for symptoms including pain and endocrine and/or exocrine insufficiency. However, more invasive endoscopic or surgical therapy may be necessary and is often predicated on degrees of ductal obstruction and parenchymal disease.

## INTRODUCTION

Chronic pancreatitis (CP) in the pediatric population is uncommon; as a result, its incidence and prevalence are not well established. Studies estimate the disease's prevalence as 3 to 10 cases per 100,000 inhabitants per year. While 70% of adults with CP report a history of alcohol abuse, the etiology in children varies significantly, and the time between onset of symptoms and diagnosis can be months if not years. The clinical consequences include an abdominal pain syndrome, diet intolerance, and the need for repeated hospitalization.

## PATHOGENESIS

Pancreatitis results from significant parenchymal and acinar destruction due to inappropriate activation of digestive enzymes accompanied by varying degrees of inflammation, fibrosis, and loss of function. Duration of symptoms and detectable pathologic gland change determine whether the disease is acute, recurrent, or chronic. In acute pancreatitis (AP), severe, systemic inflammation leads to microvascular ischemia and obstruction of the pancreatic acini, but the process is self-limited. Recurrent pancreatitis is an episode after a period of remission and may represent an inherent problem or susceptibility. In contrast, ongoing pancreatic inflammation and destruction that never fully abates as demonstrated by specific clinical, biochemical, or radiographic abnormalities indicates CP.

The pathogenesis of CP is unknown; however, it has been postulated that repeat episodes of acute pancreatitis led to chronic disease. Recently, Whitcomb and colleagues have proposed that CP arises from an interplay of environmental triggers of pancreatic injury, genetic susceptibilities, and factors leading to a deranged inflammatory response. This process is initiated by a sentinel acute pancreatic event (SAPE). The SAPE activates normally quiescent pancreatic stellate cells into myofibroblast-like cells that express the cytoskeletal protein $\alpha$-smooth muscle actin and produce extracellular matrix. This activation is further potentiated by platelets recruited to the pancreas that release platelet-derived growth factor (PDGF) and transforming growth factor (TGF) $\beta$ as well as damaged ductal and acinar cells release of basic fibroblast growth factor (bFGF). Recent research has demonstrated the increased expression of certain cytokines and activation of the mitogen-activated pathway (MAP) kinase system, both of which are pro-inflammatory, with subsequent down regulation of the anti-inflammatory proliferator-activated receptor pathway (PPAR) $\gamma$ system. Abnormal host genotypes regulating these systems may increase susceptibility to chronic inflammation.

An advanced stage of disease is characterized by pancreatic ductal dilation and/or stricture as well as stone formation. The pain associated with CP correlates with fibrosis of both the main pancreatic ducts and smaller side branches, which may cause increased ductal pressures and inflammatory cell invasion of afferent pancreatic nerves. Progressive destruction of the ductal systems, exocrine acini, and endocrine islets can lead to exocrine insufficiency and diabetes mellitus. Complications of CP include pancreatic pseudocyst or fistula, splenic artery pseudoaneurysm, splenic vein thrombosis, or obstruction of the common bile duct or duodenum. In certain situations, patients may be at higher risk of developing adenocarcinoma.

# ETIOLOGY

As discussed above, a discrete relationship between pediatric AP and CP seems intuitive but limited as the more common causes of AP (Table 58-1) and CP do not directly correlate. Furthermore, up to 30% of pediatric patients suffer from idiopathic CP with no identifiable cause. The TIGAR-O classification (Table 58-2) has been proposed in order to identify possible risk factors, both intrinsic and extrinsic to the patient, of CP. This schema allows for individual patient assessment and identification of potentially interacting etiologies that impact clinical treatment strategies.

## Congenital Anatomic Variants and Anomalies

Pancreaticobiliary anomalies are present in 33% of pediatric patients with CP. These are listed in Table 58-3, classified according to anatomical defect. The majority of patients diagnosed with some of the more common variants never have pancreatitis. In the case of annular pancreas, 70% of patients are asymptomatic. The same is true for pancreas divisum, which is estimated to be present in 10% of all patients, but only 5% of these patients develop pancreatitis. These affected patients seem to have a higher rate of mutation in the gene that encodes serine protease inhibitor Kazal type I (*SPINK1*), which deactivates pancreatic trypsin when prematurely activated.

## Genetic Susceptibility

Hereditary pancreatitis (HP) is associated with a number of known mutations in *PRSS1*, the gene encoding cationic trypsinogen. These mutations are relatively rare, affecting only 1% of the population and cause either gain of function or resistance to inactivation. By studying familial cohorts, this disorder was found to be autosomal dominant with a penetrance of 80% by age 20.

Clinically, these patients suffer from CP with no other explanation and have 2 first- or 3 or more second-degree relatives with CP. A range of 1 to 60 years at time of diagnosis has been reported, but median age of onset for HP is 10 years. Interestingly, this age is younger than that of children with idiopathic CP. Additionally, studies have demonstrated that patients with HP develop more complications of their disease including pseudocyst, steatorrhea, and ascites, and more frequently require surgical intervention. Finally, patients with HP have a 50-fold higher risk of developing pancreatic adenocarcinoma as compared to the general population.

Another gene mutation affecting the regulation of pancreatic trypsin involves *SPINK1*. In contrast to *PRSS1* mutations, *SPINK1* mutations are not believed to directly cause pancreatitis, but rather act as a risk factor and disease modifier lowering the threshold for the development of pancreatitis by exacerbating the subsequent inflammatory response. This theory is based upon genetic studies showing that approximately 2% of the American population carries a *SPINK1* mutation; however, only 1% of carriers develop pancreatitis. Interestingly, 1 study estimated that 25% of patients with idiopathic CP have *SPINK1* mutations and clinically have earlier onset of disease as well as exocrine and endocrine

| TABLE 58-1 | Etiology of Acute Pancreatitis in Children |
|---|---|
| **Acute pancreatitis** | |
| Drugs | Salicylates |
| | Paracetamol |
| | Cytotoxic drugs (ie, L-asparaginase) |
| | Corticosteroids |
| | Immunosuppressives (particularly azathioprine and 6-MP) |
| | Thiazides |
| | Sodium valproate |
| | Tetracycline (particularly if aged) |
| | Erythromycin |
| Periampullary obstruction | Gallstones |
| | Choledochal cyst |
| | Pancreatic duct obstruction |
| | Congenital anomalies of pancreas (especially pancreas divisum) |
| | Enteric duplication cysts |
| Infections | Epstein–Barr virus |
| | Mumps |
| | Measles |
| | Cytomegalovirus |
| | Influenza A |
| | Mycoplasma |
| | Leptospirosis |
| | Malaria |
| | Rubella |
| | Ascariasis |
| | Cryptosporidium |
| Trauma | Blunt injury (handle bar, child abuse, etc) |
| | ERCP |
| Metabolic | α-1 Antitrypsin deficiency |
| | Hyperlipidemias |
| | Hypercalcemia |
| Toxin | Scorpion, Gila monster, tropical marine snakes |
| Miscellaneous | Refeeding pancreatitis |
| Inflammatory/ systemic disease | Hemolytic-uremic syndrome |
| | Reye's syndrome |
| | Kawasaki disease |
| | Inflammatory bowel disease |
| | Henoch–Schonlein purpura |
| | SLE |

ERCP, endoscopic retrograde cholangiopancreatography; G-MP, 6-mercaptopurine; SLE, systemic lupus erythematosus.
Reprinted with permission from Nydegger et al. Childhood pancreatitis. *J Gastroenterol Hepatol* 2006.

failure. Pancreatitis associated with these mutations is more frequently seen in children.

Tropical juvenile pancreatitis bears mention here due to its close association with *SPINK1* mutations. Its etiology is unknown, possibly related to malnutrition, dietary toxins, or

| TABLE 58-2 | Etiological Factors Associated with Chronic Pancreatitis; TIGAR-O Classification System Modified from Etemad et al |
|---|---|
| **Toxic–metabolic** | Isolated autoimmune CP |
| Hypercalcemia | Syndromic autoimmune CP |
| Hyperlipidemia | in association with: Sjogren's |
| Chronic renal failure | syndrome/IBD/PBC |
| Drugs | **Recurrent acute pancreatitis** |
| Toxins (eg, DBTC) | RAP |
| (alcohol and smoking) | Post necrotic |
| **Idiopathic** | Vasculitis |
| Early onset | Post irradiation |
| Late onset | **Obstructive** |
| Tropical | Pancreas divisum |
| **Genetic** | Sphincter of Oddi dysfunction |
| PRSS1 mutations | Duct obstruction (eg, stones, |
| SPINK1 mutations | post inflammatory, |
| ABCC7 (CFTR) mutations | post traumatic) |
| Autoimmune | |

Reprinted with permission from Etemad B. Chronic pancreatitis: diagnosis, classification, and new genetic developments. *Gastroenterology* 2001.

trace element deficiency. This form of CP is more prevalent in developing countries. The pancreas atrophies and calcifies, and exocrine and exocrine failure is common. These patients experience an accelerated clinical course, younger age of onset, and risk of future pancreatic malignancy.

CP was first associated with mutations in cystic fibrosis (CF) transmembrane conductance gene in 1998. *CFTR* encodes an anion channel located at the apical surface of the pancreatic ductal cell and regulates the secretion of bicarbonate-rich fluid that flushes zymogens and calcium from pancreatic ducts. There are over 1500 identified *CFTR* mutations that produce a spectrum of phenotypes; as a result, less than 2% of children with CF develop pancreatitis. CF spans a spectrum of disease that, depending on the type of mutation

| TABLE 58-3 | Anatomic Pancreaticobiliary Anomalies |
|---|---|
| **Pancreatic** | |
| Annular pancreas | |
| **Pancreatic ductal** | |
| Pancreas divisum | |
| anomalous pancreatic junction (or common channel syndrome) | |
| **Biliary ductal** | |
| Choledochal cyst | |
| Choledochocele | |
| **Intestinal** | |
| Duodenal duplication cyst | |
| Ampullary distortion due to malrotation | |

and hetero- and homozygosity, causes variation in pancreatic function from failure to mild dysfunction. Usually pancreatitis occurs in patients with preserved exocrine function, (approximately 10%-15% of patients with CF). One study demonstrated that these patients are diagnosed with CF at a later age and had near normal sweat chloride values. However, 14% of these patients developed CP. Other unique *CFTR* mutations that affect bicarbonate transport and not chloride transport may impact idiopathic CP. Finally, case reports and series have demonstrated instances of pediatric CP in patients with a concurrent *CFTR* mutation and pancreatic anatomic anomalies that are refractory to sphincterotomy which may affect treatment algorithms.

## Autoimmune

Autoimmune CP is characterized by IgG4 hypergammaglobulinemia. Other auto immune disorders such as inflammatory bowel disease and primary sclerosing cholangitis can be present. Auto antibodies such as ANA, anti-SMA, anticarbonic anhydrase, and antilactoferrin can be present. Histologically, the pancreas is edematous, free of calcification, and infiltrated by lymphocytes. A correct diagnosis is critical as autoimmune pancreatitis is steroid responsive.

## Other Risk Factors/Etiologies

Other forms of pancreaticobiliary obstruction can cause CP. Idiopathic fibrosing pancreatitis is characterized by a fibrosed pancreas often with concomitant biliary and pancreatic ductal obstruction. Choledocholithiasis and sphincter of Oddi dysfunction can also cause CP. Metabolic diseases such as hypertriglyceridemia can cause pancreatitis in both pediatric and adult patients. Pediatric-specific conditions such as ornithine transcarbamylase deficiency have also been reported to cause CP. Finally, congenital anomalous pancreatic development related to *Pdx1* gene abnormalities may cause syndromes such as Schwachman–Diamond or Johnson–Blizzard syndromes and may be related to pancreatitis.

## DIAGNOSIS

As with other chronic inflammatory diseases, CP presents a diagnostic challenge to clinicians as timely diagnosis and identification of potentially modifiable disease risk factors may positively impact treatment and improve outcome. In children, several single-institution series indicate that the onset of pain to diagnosis of CP may be delayed by months to even years due to the imperfect diagnostic modalities and the initial inability to differentiate AP from CP.

## Clinical Presentation

Patients with CP most often present with intermittent attacks of epigastric pain. In contrast to adults, constant, unremitting pain is uncommon. The abdominal pain is deep and radiates to the back. On occasion, pain is absent when the pancreas "burns out." Other accompanying symptoms may be nonspecific, including nausea, vomiting, and failure to thrive.

Pancreatic insufficiency, both exocrine and endocrine, may occur, but the incidence of these disease manifestations in children with CP is rare. Case series report small numbers of children complaining of steatorrhea, but insulin-dependent diabetes has not been reported. In comparison, 50% to 80% of adults with CP will develop exocrine insufficiency, heralded by steatorrhea and weight loss due to malabsorption. Forty to 70% of afflicted adults develop diabetes mellitus due to islet cell destruction.

## Laboratory Studies

Laboratory studies may assist in the diagnosis of CP. Elevations of amylase and/or lipase three times greater than normal are suspicious for the diagnosis. Indirect studies of pancreatic function such as measurement of fecal fat elastase may be performed, but the sensitivity of this test is poor. Other direct tests such as small intestine intubation and duodenal sampling have been described but are more invasive and time consuming.

Genetic testing should be considered in certain situations and can be either diagnostic or predictive. Diagnostic testing is utilized in cases when clinical suspicion for CP is high, and genetic testing may provide an etiopathogenesis. Use of predictive testing is less frequently employed due to ethical considerations and the need for genetic counseling. Testing for *PRSS1* mutations in patients with affected first-degree relatives is appropriate in order to provide counseling on environmental risk factor modification and possible future malignancy. Testing for *SPINK1* mutations is not currently recommended.

## Radiologic Studies

A number of modalities can be used to assess parenchymal change, ductal features, and the presence of complications in CP. Each modality has risks and benefits that must be considered. The utility of ultrasound in pediatric diagnosis of pancreatitis is effective as children are smaller, have less intraabdominal fat, and have a prominent left hepatic lobe, which serves as an acoustic window. Ultrasound is able to discern dilated pancreatic ducts, intraductal stones, echotexture irregularity, as well as pseudocysts with reported diagnostic sensitivity and specificity of 50% to 80% and 90%, respectively. There are limitations, as the size and echogenecity are age dependent. Pathologic appearance can be more diverse depending on etiology, clinical disease stage, and presence of complications and the overall result is operator dependent.

Computed tomography (CT) has evolved significantly in the diagnosis of pancreatic pathology with high-resolution techniques and the development of organ-specific protocols, specifically vascular phase in relation to timing of intravenous (IV) contrast injection. CP is characterized by delayed enhancement on arterial phase. Dilation of the main pancreatic duct and/or the common bile duct, the so called "double duct sign," may be present. CT is also helpful for diagnosing complications of pancreatitis. Diagnostic sensitivity and specificity of high-resolution CT approach 90%. Other advantages include relative cost to other diagnostic modalities and less operator dependence. Disadvantages include ionizing radiation and a relative inability in delineating pancreatic ductal anomalies as compared to endoscopic retrograde cholangiopancreatography (ERCP) and now magnetic resonance cholangiopancreatography (MRCP).

Magnetic resonance imaging (MRI) and specifically MRCP protocols have evolved significantly and are now a beneficial modality in the diagnosis of CP. T1, fat-suppressed, gadolinium-enhanced images can demonstrate parenchymal changes due to the loss of normal tissue structure and impaired capillary blood flow. MRCP images obtained from T2, fat-suppressed protocols highlight ductal fluid and do not require IV contrast. Diffusion-weighted images are also able to differentiate between focal areas of fibrosis and tumor due to differential behavior of protons in these histopathologic entities. An IV analogue of secretin, which stimulates pancreatic α and β cell secretion, can be administered as an adjunct to enhance imaging of the pancreaticobiliary junction. Alkaade and colleagues demonstrated retrospectively that in the presence of this adjunct, patients with normal exocrine function had radiographic characteristics of CP by MRI. Furthermore, Testoni et al. demonstrated that secretin administration can increase the detection of small duct disease, typically poorly captured with standard MR, which can be an indicator of early CP. Disadvantages of MRI in pediatric patients include the frequent need for general anesthesia to minimize respiratory motion during a prolonged study as well as the inability to detect parenchymal and intraductal calcification, a hallmark of CP.

## Endoscopic Assessment

ERCP has traditionally been the gold standard in the diagnosis of adult CP; with the improvement in imaging modalities, however, ERCP's diagnostic utility has declined. Specifically, ERCP is able to produce high-resolution images of both the main pancreatic duct as well as smaller side branch ducts. As a result, it can diagnose specific ductal pathology such as the origin of a pseudocyst or the location of malignant stricture. Because of the invasive nature of the procedure, patients undergoing ERCP require sedation. Additional concerns include the overall safety of ERCP in children, although multiple studies demonstrating the safety as well as success of this procedure have been reported. ERCP is associated with morbidity, which ranges from 1% to 11%, with the most common morbidity being post-ERCP pancreatitis. This rate increases to approximately 20% with concomitant therapeutic intervention, which will be discussed in a later section.

The use of endoscopic ultrasound (EUS) has become more common in the diagnosis of pancreatic disease including CP. Several groups have prospectively developed specific parenchymal and ductal criteria indicative of CP (Table 58-4). With 4 or more of these criteria identified, the sensitivity and specificity of EUS approach 91% and 86%, respectively. Furthermore, fine-needle aspiration can be combined with EUS for tissue biopsy. More importantly, Varadarajulu and colleagues were able to demonstrate that EUS was more sensitive than CT in detecting early stage CP in tissue harvested from

**TABLE 58-4  Endoscopic Ultrasound Criteria for the Diagnosis of Chronic Pancreatitis**

| EUS finding | Description | Correlation | Strength |
|---|---|---|---|
| **Parenchymal criteria** | | | |
| Hyperechoic foci with shadowing | Length or width >2 mm | Calcifications | Major A |
| Lobularity with honeycombing (>3 contiguous lobules) | Structures >5 mm with an enhancing rim and echo-poor center | None | Major B |
| Lobularity without honeycombing | As above | None | Minor |
| Hyperechoic foci without shadowing | As above | None | Minor |
| Hyperechoic strand(s) | Lines >3 mm long in at least two different directions with respect to the image plane | None | Minor |
| Intraparenchymal cyst(s) | None | None | Minor |
| **Ductal criteria** | | | |
| Main pancreatic duct calculi with shadowing | None | None | Major A |
| Irregular main pancreatic duct/ectatic contour | None | None | Minor |
| >3 dilated pancreatic duct side branches | None | Side branch ectasias | Minor |
| Main pancreatic ductal dilatation | >4 mm in head, >3.5 mm in body, and >1.5 mm in tail | None | Minor |
| Hyperechoic main pancreatic duct margin | Echogenic, distinct structure covering >50% of entire main pancreatic duct in body and tail | Ductal fibrosis | Minor |
| Stricture(s) | None | None | Minor |

Findings "consistent" with chronic pancreatitis include: 1 major A criterion plus >3 minor criteria; 1 major A plus 1 major B criterion; and 2 major A criteria. Findings "suggestive" of chronic pancreatitis include: 1 major A criterion plus <3 minor features; 1 major B criterion plus >3 minor criteria; and >5 minor criteria. Findings "indeterminate" for chronic pancreatitis include: 3 or 4 minor criteria; and 1 major B criterion alone or with <3 minor criteria. "Normal" findings, not suggestive of disease in the pancreas, include <2 minor criteria.
Data from Catalano MF, et al. EUS-based criteria for the diagnosis of chronic pancreatitis: the Rosemont classification. *Gastrointest Endosc* 2009.

patients already scheduled for pancreatic surgery. In pediatric patients, the disadvantages of EUS are similar to those of ERCP including the need for monitored anesthesia care or even general anesthesia, operator dependence, and the need to use adult instruments in children.

For children suspected to have CP, work-up should include:

1. Sweat chloride test

2. Genetic testing for CFTR, PRSS1, and *SPINK 1* mutation

3. Imaging to rule out structural or anatomic anomalies

4. Assessment for autoimmune causes

## TREATMENT

### Medical Management

The initial treatment of CP is predicated on symptomatic treatment based on the significant inflammation generated by flares that correspond to the usual presenting symptom of abdominal pain. The patient should be made NPO and resuscitated with IV fluids. It is often necessary to administer parenteral narcotics to control pain. Enteric stimulation of the pancreas should be minimized. Traditionally, total parenteral nutrition (TPN) was used to achieve this goal; however, a prospective study in adults with acute pancreatitis demonstrated that enteral nutrition was superior in preventing infectious complications and surgical intervention as compared to those patients receiving TPN. There was no difference in mortality

or other complications. In order to deliver enteral nutrition without stimulating the pancreas, a postpyloric feeding tube should be placed under fluoroscopy. Oral feeds should not be initiated until serum levels of pancreatic enzymes normalize. Special consideration should be given to patients with *CFTR* mutations for, although the patients with CF mutations who also have CP often have preserved pancreatic function, nutritional optimization is important due to the presence of other possible systemic disease and risk of systemic infection. In this case, nutritional status should be optimized with fat-soluble vitamin supplementation.

Other therapies can be initiated that have varying levels of evidence to support their use. Proton pump inhibitors can be administered to alkalinize the gastric and duodenal contents, which, in turn, is thought to decrease pancreatic secretion. A common therapy is the oral administration of replacement pancreatic enzymes, which are thought to play a negative role in the feedback mechanism that regulates cholecystokinin (CCK) release. By preventing CCK release, exocrine pancreatic function is inhibited. A number of randomized controlled trials have been performed demonstrating equivocal pain relief. Of note, pancreatic enzyme replacements come in 2 formulations: nonenteric-coated and enteric-coated microspheres. Studies suggest no benefit of the enteric-coated preparation, which may be absorbed more distally in the small bowel whole the CCK feedback sensitive area is in the more proximal intestine.

The administration of antioxidants has been studied evaluating the benefit in both acute attacks and prevention of flares. Mathew and colleagues have demonstrated that children with

HP have lower serum vitamin E and selenium levels and higher levels of superoxide dismutase activity. Furthermore, it has been shown that higher levels of oxygen free radicals correlate with greater trypsinogen activity. As a result, administration of these micronutrients may benefit patients in a proinflammatory state.

The use of octreotide, a synthetic analogue of the gastrointestinal hormone somatostatin, in acute and CP to control pain has been anecdotal. Conflicting studies exist for its use in adults in prevention of complications related to acute pancreatitis. No study has evaluated its role in children.

## Endoscopic Therapy

Invasive therapy for CP, both endoscopic and surgical, is usually indicated for patients suffering from unremitting pain, especially those children who have known anomalous pancreaticobiliary ductal anatomy. Endoscopic therapy is useful in several fashions with its primary utility being ductal procedures including sphincterotomy, ductal dilation, stent placement, and stone clearance. Celiac plexus blocks can be administered during endoscopy, but this therapy is often ineffective in preventing pain syndrome.

It has been proposed that endoscopic therapy in children with CP may have more long-lasting pain relief as compared to adults due to the fact these younger patients do not engage in harmful lifestyle behaviors such as alcohol and tobacco abuse. Indeed, one of the larger series reporting on ERCP in children with CP demonstrated that only 5 of 42 patients proceeded to surgery due to ongoing pain, while 65% of patients were completely pain free at a mean follow-up period of 5 years. Interestingly, Zhao-Shen and colleagues also suggested that most of the patients in this series were early in their clinical course and hypothesized that endoscopic therapy may be more successful and less invasive in the early-stage disease. Morbidity, specifically post-ERCP pancreatitis, has been reported anywhere from 13% to 25% in therapeutic interventions.

The complications of CP, specifically pseudocyst, have been addressed endoscopically with the creation of cystenterostomies in adults, although the failure and complication rates have been as high as 25%. The literature in pediatric patients is limited to small series, and the results were equivocal.

## Surgical Therapy

As with endoscopic therapy, the primary indication for surgery in children with CP is unremitting pain. Prospective adult data demonstrated that surgery produces more complete and lasting pain relief with fewer procedures as compared to endoscopy. In the pediatric population, given the rarity of CP and surgical therapy for this disease, the data are less robust. Iqbal and colleagues demonstrated retrospectively that children who underwent surgery for CP had fewer episodes of recurrent pancreatitis and fewer hospitalizations as compared to those who underwent ERCP.

As with any operation, preoperative planning is crucial in order to answer 2 important questions: who requires surgery and what is the appropriate procedure for the patient given their specific anatomy. Small series analyzing surgery for CP

in children have demonstrated that earlier pancreatic surgery is much less likely to be successful. As a result, optimization for the individual patient is critical. To date, no algorithm has been identified defining the ideal age, body mass index (BMI), nutritional status, etc, for these patients. Several retrospective studies suggest "earlier surgery" as beneficial, but what this means remains to be defined.

The precise surgical procedure to be performed must address the degree of ductal pathology present (ie, how dilated or strictured is the main pancreatic duct) and the degree of parenchymal disease (ie, should parenchymal resection be performed). Preoperative diagnostic imagining is critical in the determination of the optimal procedure to be performed. The surgeon must also be prepared to modify their approach depending on what is found intraoperatively. As varied as the etiologies and presentations of these patients' disease are, so too are the possible surgical solutions to this complicated problem. From a discussion perspective, the interventions to be performed can be grouped into ductal drainage procedures, parenchymal resections, or a combination of the 2.

## Ductal Drainage Procedures

The longitudinal pancreaticojejunostomy (LPJ) for drainage of the main pancreatic duct was first described by Puestow and Gilbert in 1958. In its original description, the operation also involved splenectomy and amputation of the distal portion of the pancreatic tail. A subsequent Roux limb was anastomosed to the body of the pancreas, and the amputated distal portion was invaginated into the distal Roux limb. In 1960, Partington and Rochelle proposed a modification that spared the spleen and distal pancreatectomy. The pancreatic duct was divided along its length, and the Roux limb was anastomosed to the pancreatic capsule (Fig. 58-1A and B). This procedure provides extensive drainage of a diseased pancreatic duct that may be alternately strictured and dilated relieving pressure along its entire course. A number of retrospective studies have documented the efficacy of this procedure in children with CP improving preoperative IBW and exocrine function as demonstrated by resolved steatorrhea. The modified Puestow procedure may be particularly effective in patients with HP, as these patients often have dilated pancreatic ducts.

## Pancreatic Resections

Resective procedures for pediatric CP are uncommon, although with pancreatic head dominant disease, patients may require a pancreaticoduodenectomy (Whipple procedure). Given the morbidity associated with the procedure and the lack of malignancy, this operation is not the first choice for pediatric patients. A more conservative resection procedure for pancreatic head prominent disease is the Berne modification of the Beger procedure. In this procedure, the head of the pancreas is "cored" out, leaving the dorsal pancreas intact (Fig. 58-2A). A side-to-side pancreaticojejunostomy is then created to restore enteric continuity (Fig. 58-2B). Of note, the common bile duct is often incised and included in the anastomosis. In so doing, the pancreatic parenchymal mass is spared. During the procedure, the main pancreatic

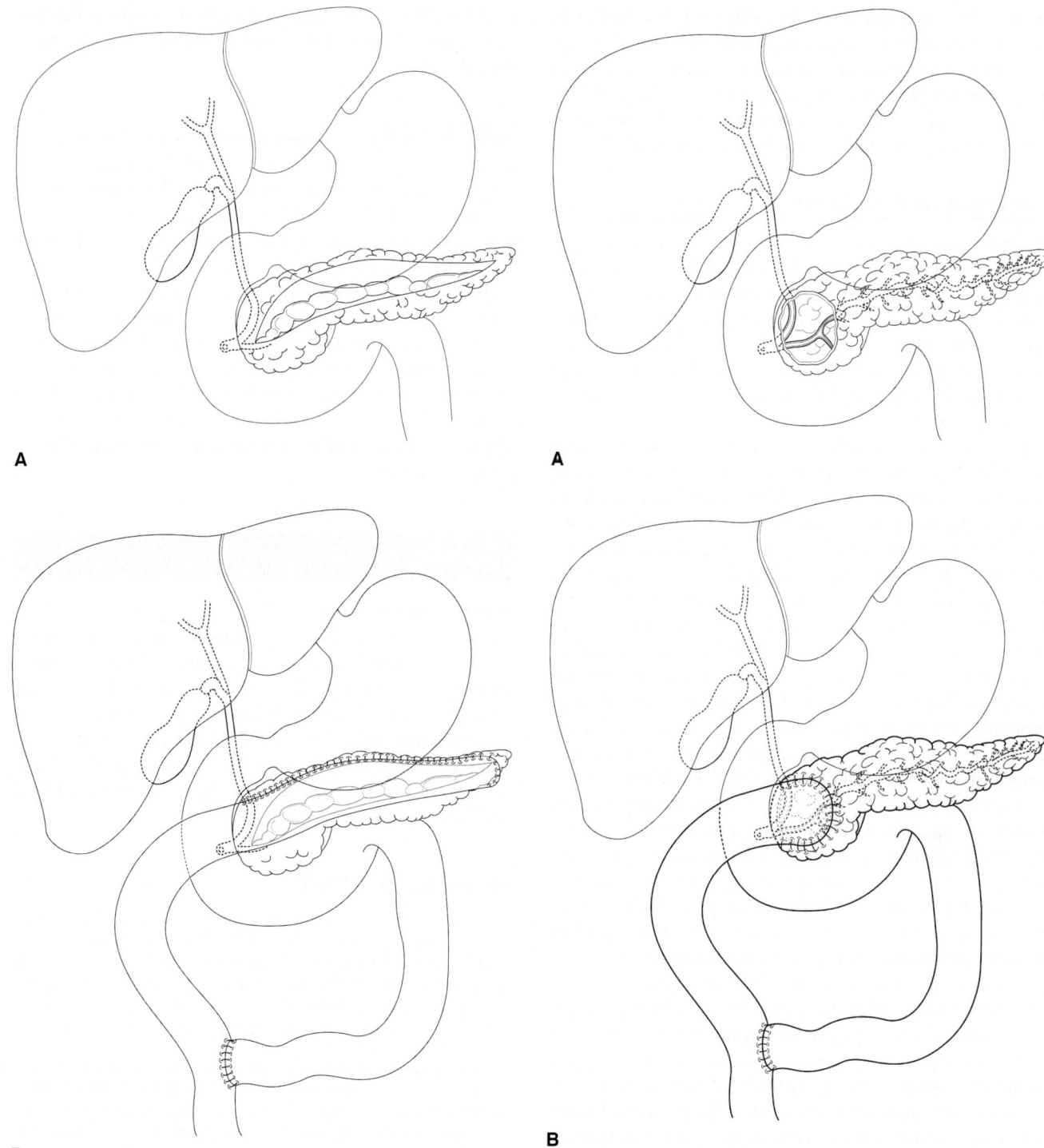

A

B

**FIGURE 58-1** Puestow procedure—Longitudinal pancreaticojejunosotomy.

A

B

**FIGURE 58-2** Berne procedure—Coring of the head of the pancreas with pancreaticojejunostomy.

duct can be explored, and, if stenoses are present, the operation can be modified.

The maximal resective procedure for CP is a total pancreatectomy, which was sometimes used in adults after previous surgical attempts to improve the symptoms related to CP. Total pancreatectomy can be combined with autologous islet cell transplantation to prevent the development of brittle diabetes mellitus. This procedure has been utilized in pediatric patients and the outcomes have been promising. In the largest series published to date, preoperatively, 18 of 24 children used

narcotics chronically, while the remainder used them intermittently. Postoperatively, 60% of the patients were weaned completely from pain medication, while the remaining 40% had significantly lower requirements. Furthermore, unpublished data from this group demonstrated improved quality of life as assessed by the validated Short Form (SF) 36 assessment tool. Fifty-six percent of the patients of were insulin independent after islet infusion with another 26% requiring only 1 daily dose of long-acting insulin. It must be mentioned that in this series, only 1 patient was insulin dependent preoperatively.

Further data were published demonstrating that predictors of success for such a complex surgical procedure include age at surgery <13 years, a shorter duration of symptoms, and a higher islet cell yield. Prior pancreatic surgery, specifically LPJ, distal pancreatectomy, and Frey procedure, which is discussed below, had a significantly negative impact on islet cell yield.

## Combination Procedures

A combination of drainage and resective procedures has utility. The DuVal procedure, first described in 1954, consists of a distal pancreatectomy and splenectomy with subsequent pancreaticojejunostomy. In this case, a single, proximal stricture near the ampulla of Vater can be circumvented with retrograde drainage via the distal pancreas. Weber and Keller used this procedure effectively in 2 patients who also had significant pancreatic tail fibrosis.

Another example of a combination procedure was described by Hans Beger. In this operation, a duodenum-preserving pancreatic head resection is performed, the distal border of which is the junction between the head and body just at the level of the superior mesenteric vein. A small rim of pancreatic head is left in continuity with the duodenum. The exposed end of the pancreatic duct is anastomosed end-to-end to a Roux limb while the remnant pancreas is anastomosed side-to-side to a proximal portion of the Roux limb. The Beger procedure is useful for patients with CP who also have inflammatory disease in the head, common bile duct obstruction, or duodenal stricture. While a technically challenging operation, intestinal continuity is preserved with the requisite milieu of gastrointestinal hormones regulated by the proximal duodenum.

The Frey procedure, a modification of the Beger procedure combines elements of the Puestow procedure with resection. In addition to performing drainage of the pancreatic duct along the length of the gland, the head of the pancreas is cored out. A side-to-side pancreaticojejunostomy is then performed with a Roux limb. Indication for this procedure is a duct of Wirsung dilated >8 mm such that a duct to intestinal mucosal anastomosis can be performed. More recently, Frey advocated use of his procedure for main ducts as narrow as 3.5 mm. The Frey procedure can be helpful in the cases of CP accompanied by complications such as pseudocyst or pancreatic fistula. Rollins and Meyers advocate the Frey procedure as the operation of choice for children who fail medical management of their CP for several reasons: it adequately drains the length of the pancreatic duct and does not carry the morbidity of other operations that entail pancreatic head resection. The Beger as well as the Berne modification bear mention as tailored pancreatic resection procedures insofar as the majority of the pancreatic parenchyma, including both islet and acinar cells, is preserved. Chromik and colleagues postulate that these types of resection can be performed safely, preserve exocrine function, and control pain. By preserving pancreatic mass, these operations may be preferred if a patient will eventually transition to islet cell transplant.

In certain cases, specifically the pancreaticobiliary anomalies, other surgical approaches may be necessary. Neblett and O'Neill describe the utility of transduodenal sphincteroplasty and septoplasty in cases of pancreas divisum with proximal ductal malformations. In several cases, these procedures had to be combined with LPJ in order to identify the dominant duct of Santorini.

## Laparoscopy

Laparoscopic approaches have also been proposed for pancreatic surgery, specifically with regard to complications of pancreatitis. The largest series of published cases has to do with laparoscopic pseudocystgastrostomy. In this multicenter report, pseudocystgastrostomies were created via laparoscopic gastrostomies or via the insertion of gastric trochars. Once the pseudocyst was identified by needle aspiration, it was entered using either the Bovie electrocautery, Harmonic scalpel (Ethicon EndoSurgery), or a combination of both. The cystogastrostomies were then created with either staplers, sutures, or the Harmonic scalpel. In this series, 92% of patients obtained adequate drainage. There were no other major complications.

# CONCLUSION

Pediatric surgical pancreatic diseases are a complex set of disorders, and CP is no different. Changing the clinical outcome for these patients is predicated upon timely diagnosis during the early part of their disease. In order to do so, clinical suspicion must remain high due to the variety of etiologies of this disease process as well as CP's clinical and radiographic heterogeneity. Several studies have demonstrated improved outcomes with multi disciplinary management of these patients and their conditions.

## SELECTED READINGS

Chromik AM. Tailored resective pancreatic surgery for pediatric patients with chronic pancreatitis. *J Pediatr Surg* 2008;43(4):634–643.

Iqbal CW, Moir CR, Ishitani MB. Management of chronic pancreatitis in the pediatric patient: endoscopic retrograde cholangiopancreatography vs operative therapy. *J Pediatr Surg* 2009;44(1):139–143; discussion 143.

Jolley CD. Pancreatic disease in children and adolescents. *Curr Gastroenterol Rep* 2010;12(2):106–113.

Marik PE, Zaloga GP. Meta-analysis of parenteral nutrition versus enteral nutrition in patients with acute pancreatitis. *Br Med J* 2004;328(7453):1407.

Neblett WW 3rd, and O'Neill JA Jr. Surgical management of recurrent pancreatitis in children with pancreas divisum. *Ann Surg* 2000;231(6): 899–908.

Rosendahl J, et al. Hereditary chronic pancreatitis. *Orphanet J Rare Dis* 2007;2:1.

Varadarajulu S, et al. Histopathologic correlates of noncalcific chronic pancreatitis by EUS: a prospective tissue characterization study. *Gastrointest Endosc* 2007;66(3):501–509.

Wang W, et al. Chronic pancreatitis in Chinese children: etiology, clinical presentation and imaging diagnosis. *J Gastroenterol Hepatol* 2009;24(12):1862–1868.

Weber TR, Keller MS. Operative management of chronic pancreatitis in children. *Arch Surg* 2001;136(5):550–554.

Witt H, et al. Chronic pancreatitis: challenges and advances in pathogenesis, genetics, diagnosis, and therapy. *Gastroenterology* 2007;132(4): 1557–1573.

Witt H, et al. Mutations in the gene encoding the serine protease inhibitor, Kazal type 1 are associated with chronic pancreatitis. *Nat Genet* 2000;25(2):213–216.

ABDOMINAL DISEASE

# CHAPTER 59 | The Spleen

*Michael J. Allshouse*

## KEY POINTS

1. Review of basic science, embryology, anatomy, and function.

2. Disorders of the spleen.

3. Treatment options for splenic disease.

4. Splenectomy and partial splenectomy, open and minimal access surgery.

5. Postsplenectomy complications.

## EMBRYOLOGY, ANATOMY, AND FUNCTION OF THE SPLEEN

The spleen arises as a mesenchymal protrusion into the left dorsal mesogastrium that is first seen at the 6 to 8 mm stage of embryogenesis. Incomplete fusion in up to 20% of individuals may result in accessory spleen formation. More unusual events result in asplenia or polysplenia. In human abdominal development, most asymmetric organs began in the midline or were at the outset bilateral, with subsequent suppression of 1 side. The spleen is the exception. It starts on the left and stays there in most cases. As it develops, the spleen lies in the left upper quadrant of the abdomen and has 6 named ligamentous attachments: gastrosplenic, splenorenal, splenophrenic, splenocolic, splenopancreatic, and the presplenic fold. The peritoneum envelops the splenic vessels and the distal pancreas along the concavity of the splenic surface. The splenic artery is a celiac axis branch and travels along the cephalodorsal pancreatic surface. There are usually 2, and sometimes 3 lobular arteries arising from the main splenic artery. These vessels divide further in the parenchyma and are typically end-arteries, although in 10% of specimens there are some cross-connections. The splenic vein accompanies the artery within a number of variant patterns before it joins the superior mesenteric vein to form the portal vein. The "odd number" mnemonic of Harris (1,3,5,7,9,11), as reported in the textbook by Last on anatomy, is a useful tool to recall normal splenic dimension and location: the spleen measures $1 \times 3 \times 5$ inches, weighs 7 ounces and abuts ribs 9 through 11.

The ultrastructure of the spleen is key to its function. The 2 main divisions are termed red and white pulp (Table 59-1). Splenic red pulp filters blood and culls out defective, senescent, or diseased erythrocytes. The red pulp also filters bacteria, parasites, and particulate matter. These functions are supported by the presence of opsonins (fibronectin, properidin, tuftsin) that are produced in the spleen. These agents help activate the complement cascade and induce granulocyte and macrophage phagocytosis. The white pulp contains lymphoid follicles (B cells) and periarteriolar lymphoid sheaths (PALS), which are populated largely by T-lymphocytes. In PALS, antigen presentation by dendritic cells and macrophages to CD4+ T-helper cells activates cell-mediated immune response. Antigen in germinal centers is processed by antigen-presenting cells to B-lymphocytes, resulting in antibody production. The spleen is the largest source of IgM.

Intracellular material is removed from the red blood cells (RBC) as the cells pass through the same tight channels populated along the way by macrophages, which also destroy encapsulated organisms and engulf particulate antigen. The macrophage removes bacteria and transmits the bacteria's identity to the lymphocytes. Without this interaction between macrophages and lymphocytes, the initial protective response of the lymphocytes would be inadequate. The spleen possesses all of the known significant immunoresponsive functions. After splenectomy or, in the spleen's absence, other organs have incomplete compensatory capabilities. The spleen's most important function is its ability to phagocytize unrecognized antigen, especially encapsulated organisms. Congenital asplenia, surgical asplenia, or splenic hypofunction all result in a similar peripheral blood picture (eg, Howell–Jolly bodies) and increase the risk of overwhelming sepsis. Phagocytic function varies directly with the mass of residual perfused and functional splenic tissue.

Within days following splenectomy, abnormal RBCs appear in peripheral blood. The most common finding is the presence of Howell–Jolly bodies. These intracellular inclusions are reliably found in all asplenic patients and serve as indicators of splenic hypofunction or substantial loss of splenic

## TABLE 59-1  Functional Splenic Segments

| Area | Function | Composition |
|------|----------|-------------|
| Red pulp | Mechanical filtration of erythrocytes. Reserve of monocytes | Sinusoids—filled with blood<br>Splenic cords of reticular fibers<br>Marginal zone bordering white pulp |
| White pulp | Active immune response via humoral and cell-mediated pathways | Composed of nodules (malpighian corpuscles) containing lymphoid follicles rich in β-lymphocytes and periarteriolar lymphoid sheaths (pals), rich in T-lymphocytes |

tissue. Significant rises in white blood cell and platelet counts are frequently seen following splenectomy. The leukocytosis improves or returns to normal levels more rapidly than the thrombocytosis. This reversion is proportional to the respective life span of these 2 blood cell lines—white cells exist for hours and platelets 7 to 10 days.

## DISORDERS OF THE SPLEEN

The differential diagnosis of these various disorders is summarized in Table 59-2.

## Anomalies

### Agenesis and Asplenia

Absence of the spleen itself may be clinically insignificant unless life-threatening infection intervenes. It is the association of agenesis of the spleen with a variety of cardiovascular and body isomeric anomalies that most often defines the severity of this condition. Various classifications of splenic agenesis have been suggested but, from a practical viewpoint, there are 2 important groups: simple agenesis and agenesis accompanied by cardiosymmetry aberrations known as the Polhemus–Schafer–Ivemark or "asplenia" syndrome. The congenital cardiac anomalies in this latter group are often severe and life-threatening. Frequently, anomalies of the great vessels as well as abdominal heterotaxy and pulmonary lobar isomerism are seen. Abnormal intestinal rotation with the incumbent risks of obstruction and midgut volvulus are common.

### Accessory Spleen

Accessory spleens are small nodules of splenic tissue that arise in the presence of a normal, dominant spleen. These are the result of an imperfect fusion of splenic elements in the embryonic dorsal mesogastrium. The incidence from autopsy series is about 10%, but they are reported in approximately 20% of patients at the time of splenectomy for hematologic disorders. More than one may be present. Seventy-five percent are found in the region of the splenic hilum, while approximately 20% reside near the pancreatic tail. Rare locations for accessory spleens are the omentum, intestinal mesentery, retroperitoneum, or gonadal region. Splenosis is a term used to describe peritoneal implantation

## TABLE 59-2  Congenital and Acquired Splenic Disorders

| Disorder | Presentation | Diagnosis |
|----------|--------------|-----------|
| Wandering spleen | Palpable, tender, mobile mass in mid-abdomen | Sonogram with color-flow Doppler |
| Accessory spleen | Occult<br>Torsion causing abdominal pain | Discovered at surgery |
| Polysplenia | Seen with preduodenal portal vein in biliary atresia | Ultrasound finding or at exploration for neonatal obstructive jaundice |
| Splenogonadal fusion | Peromelia<br>Asymptomatic<br>GI obstructive symptoms | Preoperative imaging or at surgery |
| Hereditary hemolytic anemia<br>*Membrane Defects*<br>  Hereditary spherocytosis | Jaundice<br>Anemia<br>Palpable spleen | Spherocytes in blood<br>Family history<br>↑ Red cell fragility (rarely necessary) |
|   Hereditary elliptocytosis | Jaundice<br>Anemia | Elliptocytes in blood |

(Continued)

**TABLE 59-2** **Congenital and Acquired Splenic Disorders** *(Continued)*

| Disorder | Presentation | Diagnosis |
|---|---|---|
| *Hemoglobinopathies* | | |
| Thalassemia | Anemia, pallor, retarded growth, maxillary hyperplasia, splenomegaly | Microcytic hypochromic anemia<br>Hemoglobin electrophoresis<br>Family studies |
| Sickle cell disease | Anemia, jaundice<br>Primarily in blacks | Crescent-shaped cells in blood<br>Hemoglobin electrophoresis |
| *Enzyme Defects* | | |
| G-6-PD deficiency | Jaundice<br>Anemia | ↓ G-6-PD activity in RBCs |
| Pyruvate kinase deficiency | Jaundice<br>Anemia | ↓ Pyruvate kinase activity in RBCs |
| *Autoimmune Disorders* | | |
| Idiopathic thrombocytopenic purpura | Bruises, petechiae, bleeding from gums, nose, GI tract, kidneys | Low platelet count<br>Megakaryocytes in bone marrow |
| Autoimmune hemolytic anemia | Anemia<br>Jaundice | Coombs positive<br>Warm antibody—splenic hemolysis<br>Cold antibody—intravascular hemolysis |
| Splenomegaly and hypersplenism | Large spleen with anemia, neutropenia, thrombocytopenia (one or all) | WBC <4000/dL<br>Platelets <50,000 mm$^3$<br>Hgb <9 g/dL |
| Malignancies | Primary: Mass, pain<br>Secondary: Evidence of lymphoma | CT scan or sonogram<br>Staged with MRI or CT scan |
| Benign tumors | Mass<br>Pain<br>Intra-abdominal bleeding | Sonogram<br>CT scan |
| Cysts | Occult if small<br>Left-upper-quadrant pain<br>Palpable mass | Sonogram<br>CT scan |
| Abscess | Fever<br>Left-upper-quadrant pain<br>Predisposing illness | Sonogram<br>CT scan<br>Chest film: effusion |
| Trauma | History of trauma<br>Mechanism of injury appropriate for splenic injury<br>Abdominal pain, distension | Penetrating: wound in proximity of spleen<br>Blunt: sonogram, CT scan |

of splenic fragments following rupture. Accessory spleens rarely confer immune competence but are felt to be a large cause of splenectomy failure in idiopathic thrombocytopenia purpura (ITP). Torsion of an accessory spleen is a rare cause of abdominal pain.

## Polysplenia

As in the asplenia syndrome, polysplenia is often associated with other, more severe anomalies related to cardiovascular development and abdominal heterotaxy. An association exists between polysplenia and extrahepatic biliary atresia. A rare but important anatomic variant is the preduodenal portal vein, which must be suspected and recognized during exploration for portoenterostomy or hepatic transplantation.

## Splenogonadal Fusion

This rare developmental anomaly is seen in 2 basic forms and is frequently linked to aberration in limb embryology known as peromelia. Clinical presentation is typically seen as a left scrotal mass, but this oddity has also presented as intestinal obstruction. Two varieties are seen: 1 with a fibrous band connecting the dominant spleen to the left testis, epididymis, ovary, or mesovarium and 1 that lacks this characteristic band. Splenogonadal fusion is predominantly a male disorder. It has been described in association with ectromelia and micrognathia.

## Wandering Spleen

In this anomaly, the vagabond spleen, untethered by normal ligamentous attachments may migrate to new areas of the peritoneal cavity, often taking the stomach along. Along this peripatetic pathway, torsion, ischemia, infarction, or even gastric volvulus may occur. The itinerant spleen may be palpable on physical exam. It can be seen on ultrasound with Doppler interrogation of splenic vasculature or with CT imaging, where the finding may be glaringly obvious or as subtle as inverse positioning of the splenopancreatic relationship to the stomach. Two-thirds of the cases discovered in children younger than 10 years of age are in boys while in adults, young multiparous women comprise the largest group. Splenomegaly does not appear to be a factor. Approximately two-thirds of children with wandering spleen are asymptomatic before their acute and dramatic presentation with torsion and infarction. For this reason, if wandering spleen is diagnosed, splenopexy, and/or gastropexy are advised.

## HEREDITARY HEMOLYTIC DISORDERS

The hereditary hemolytic disorders of the spleen are autosomally inherited conditions that result in the premature destruction of RBCs. The presence or absence of anemia depends on the ability of the marrow to replace red cell mass. Some of the more severe manifestations of hemolytic anemia vary depending on the release of RBC byproducts. Hereditary hemolytic anemias are classified as defects in the RBC membrane, abnormality of hemoglobin, or enzymatic defects in glucose metabolism.

The increased destruction of erythrocytes can produce anemia and jaundice. Reticulocytosis is common. Increases in indirect bilirubin and elevated serum iron level are noted. The accelerated bilirubin degradation often results in the formation of calcium bilirubinate stones or sludge in the gallbladder and biliary tree. None of these entities are "cured" by splenectomy. The decision to perform surgery must be based on the natural history of the specific disorder, severity, transfusion need, and risk. It is essential to consider factors such as the age of the patient and the impact on global health of the child. Ultimately, the decision must also include consideration of both early and late complications of splenectomy.

## MEMBRANE DEFECTS

### Hereditary Hemolytic Spherocytosis

Hereditary hemolytic spherocytosis (HHS) is a congenital, autosomal-dominant disorder characterized by anemia, intermittent jaundice, and splenomegaly. An intrinsic abnormality of the RBC membrane results in loss of the normal biconcave shape. This spherocytic RBC is presumably the result of a defective membrane sodium pump mechanism. The lack of normal cellular flexibility impedes passage of the

spherocyte through the splenic cords, resulting in premature destruction. The spherocyte's lifespan of about 30 days falls well short of the normal 120-day RBC existence. In many children, the disease is subclinical and is suspected only based on family history. Crises of increased hemolysis may be associated with infection, stress, or fatigue. Newborns may have moderate to severe anemia and hyperbilirubinemia that exceeds physiologic levels. Gallstones may result from saturation of bile with byproducts of hemoglobin pigment metabolism due to accelerated hemolysis.

### Hereditary Hemolytic Elliptocytosis

Hereditary hemolytic elliptocytosis is a Mendelian-dominant trait transmitted by the same chromosome that defines Rh type. The basic pathogenesis is unclear but appears to be due to a defect in RBC membrane similar to HHS. This condition is usually of minor clinical importance. Some patients will experience more severe manifestations and require repeated blood transfusions.

## HEMOGLOBINOPATHIES

### Thalassemia

Thalassemia is caused by a defect in hemoglobin subunit synthesis that results in accumulation of intracellular particles that contribute to accelerated RBC destruction in the spleen. The defective RBCs are small, thin, and misshapen. They have a characteristic resistance to osmotic destruction. This disorder is most common in people of Mediterranean lineage. The thalassemia minor heterozygote is asymptomatic. Thalassemia major is characterized by chronic anemia and jaundice. Associated splenic manifestations include compressive splenomegaly, transfusion dependent anemia, and splenic infarction. Gallstones occur in about one-fourth of these patients, occasionally in children.

### Sickle Cell Disease

In this disorder, which occurs primarily in individuals of African descent, hemoglobin A is replaced by hemoglobin S. Under conditions of reduced oxygen tension, changes in the molecular configuration of the hemoglobin S result in elongation and distortion of the cell morphology. The resultant increase in blood viscosity and intrasplenic stasis leads to small infarcts. Eventually, these multiple sequential infarcts result in autosplenectomy and all of the associated risks of asplenia. Major splenic problems associated with sickle cell disease are sequestration, chronic hypersplenism, and splenic abscess.

## ENZYME DEFECTS

There are 2 enzymatic defects that result in hemolysis: glucose-6-phosphate dehydrogenase (G-6-PD) deficiency and pyruvate kinase deficiency. The first is never, and the second is rarely seen by the surgeon. Both conditions impede the ability of the RBC to metabolize glucose, rendering the cell susceptible to hemolysis. In patients with pyruvate kinase deficiency, the spleen is the primary site of hemolysis.

## AUTOIMMUNE DISORDERS

### ITP

ITP is an acquired disorder that results in platelet destruction by IgG autoantibodies directed against a specific membrane protein on the platelet surface. It is presumed that platelets coated with the IgG are destroyed by macrophages and that this occurs primarily in the spleen. The onset in children tends to be abrupt, severe, and may have been precipitated by a viral illness. The diagnosis is often suspected with onset of purpura. Epistaxis, hematuria, and gastrointestinal bleeding occur less often and 1% to 2% may present with intracranial hemorrhage. A low peripheral platelet count and increased megakaryocyte numbers in bone marrow are characteristic.

### Autoimmune Hemolytic Anemia

Autoimmune hemolytic anemias result from RBC destruction by internal antibodies. Coombs test will usually be positive, with either cold or warm agglutination. In warm antibody anemia, the IgG antibody is directed against the Rh locus and the cell is destroyed by macrophages with receptor sites for the Fc moiety of the IgG molecule. In cold agglutination, an IgM antibody is typically the culprit and the hemolysis is complement mediated, causing intravascular cell destruction.

## TUMORS, CYSTS, AND ABSCESSES

### Malignancies

The Hodgkin lymphoma is the most common malignancy in children that involves the spleen. Splenic involvement is more likely in the presence of systemic symptoms. Primary splenic malignancies are extremely rare, with angiosarcoma and spindle-cell sarcoma in immunocompromised children seen most frequently. Splenic involvement in Juvenile myelomonocytic leukemia is typical and splenectomy continues to be an important aspect of treatment as the child approaches bone marrow or stem cell transplantation.

### Benign Tumors

Benign splenic tumors are quite rare. Cavernous hemangioma and lymphangiomas predominate. Splenic hemangioma may present as splenomegaly, thrombocytopenia, fibrinogen deficiency, and spontaneous rupture. Lymphangioma of the spleen may be part of a more diffuse lymphangiomatosis—a hereditary disorder involving spleen, liver, intestine, kidney, and long bones. Complete resection is not possible. CT and MRI are useful diagnostic adjuncts.

### Splenic Cysts

Splenic cysts are classified as either congenital or acquired. Approximately 75% of cysts are acquired. Worldwide, parasitic cysts caused by *Echinococcus* are the most common variety of acquired, infectious cystic disease. The other major causes are trauma and infarction. Cysts may be simple, unilocular pseudocysts, or epidermal cysts. Patients with large epidermal cysts of the spleen often present with abdominal pain, early satiety, and a palpable mass or fullness. Ultrasound imaging may be sufficient, but CT or MRI may help differentiate these from cystic pancreatic or renal lesions.

### Splenic Abscess

Morbidity from splenic abscess is high. Patients with splenic abscess present with fever and left upper abdominal pain and are often acutely ill, with septic inflammatory response at presentation. Most children have antecedent comorbid condition such as immune deficiency, malignancy, sickle cell disease, intestinal perforation, or typhoid fever. Common organisms are *Staphylococcus*, *Salmonella*, and *Escherichia coli*. Fungal or mycobacterial abscesses may be seen in immunocompromised patients. Ultrasound and CT imaging will help to make the diagnosis and may guide drainage options for treatment.

## TRAUMA

The spleen is one of the most commonly injured intraperitoneal organs in childhood. More than 90% of those injuries are the result of blunt force trauma. The mechanism of injury spans a wide spectrum that includes motor vehicle crashes (pedestrian and passenger), cycling injury, all-terrain vehicle crashes, birth trauma, and nonaccidental trauma. Multisystem injury is common, with head injury as a cause of enormous comorbidity and trauma mortality. The presentation depends on the mechanism, severity of injury, the rate of hemorrhage, and associated injuries. Initial laboratory testing may underestimate severity of injury. Hematuria is an important laboratory finding that generally prompts advanced imaging. Suspicion of splenic injury may be based on focused abdominal ultrasound for trauma (FAST) exam and is best imaged with CT. Hemodynamic stability is a prerequisite for safe CT imaging and nonoperative management.

## TREATMENT OF SPLENIC DISORDERS

### Anomalies

#### Accessory Spleen

Accessory splenic tissue is removed when discovered at the time of splenectomy for immunologic disorders. There is no observed benefit from accessory splenectomy during abdominal surgery for nonsplenic disease (Table 59-3).

#### Wandering Spleen

The wandering spleen is at risk for trauma and torsion. This operation may be done via laparotomy or with a minimally invasive approach. Placement of the spleen in an extra peritoneal pocket, fixation with a polyglycolic acid mesh snood

## TABLE 59-3　Splenic Disorders and Treatments

| | Disorder | Treatment |
|---|---|---|
| Anomalies | Wandering spleen | Splenopexy ± Gastropexy<br>Laparoscopic vs. open |
| | Accessory spleens | Removal at time of splenectomy for hematologic disorder |
| | Splenogonadal fusion | Division of obstructing band<br>Removal of accessory splenic tissue |
| Hereditary anemia | Hereditary spherocytosis | Splenectomy (after age 5) if patient symptomatic<br>Consider laparoscopic or open partial splenectomy |
| Membrane defects | Hereditary elliptocytosis | A. No treatment if asymptomatic<br>B. Splenectomy for rare severe anemia |
| | Thalassemia | A. Transfusion: for Hgb <6 g/dL<br>B. Splenectomy<br>　1. Reduce transfusion requirements<br>　2. Relieve compressive symptoms<br>　3. Relieve abdominal pain caused by splenic infarcts |
| Hemoglobinopathies | Sickle cell disease | A. Transfusion for Hgb <6 g/dL and splenic sequestration<br>B. Splenectomy<br>　1. Splenic abscess<br>　2. Hypersplenism<br>　3. Sequestration more than 2 to 3 episodes per year or 1 life-threatening episode |
| Enzyme defects | G-6-PD deficiency | No treatment |
| | Pyruvate kinase deficiency | Splenectomy for severe anemia |
| Autoimmune disorders | Idiopathic thrombocytopenia purpura (ITP) | A. No treatment if mild<br>B. Steroids or IV immunoglobulin<br>C. Surgery for thrombocytopenia lasting 6 months in patients with low platelet counts interfering with quality of life<br>D. Immunosuppressive agents for surgical failure if no retained accessory spleen is identified |
| | Hemolytic anemia<br>Warm antibody | A. Steroids<br>B. Splenectomy for steroid failure if radioactive RBCs are sequestered in the spleen. |
| | Cold antibody | Immunosuppresion and plasmapheresis |
| Malignancies | Primary | Total splenectomy with chemotherapy |
| | Secondary | Chemotherapy |
| Cysts | Congenital | A. Partial splenectomy or cystectomy<br>B. Total splenectomy if massive<br>C. Aspiration and sclerosis: high recurrence rate<br>D. Observe if small (<4 cm) and asymptomatic |
| | Acquired | Partial or total splenectomy |
| Benign masses | | Partial or total splenectomy |
| Abscess | | A. Antibiotics<br>B. Percutaneous drainage<br>C. Splenectomy |
| Hypersplenism and splenomegaly | | A. Splenectomy for significant clinical illness with WBCs <4000. Platelets <100,000 or Hgb decrease >0.5 g/dL/wk<br>B. Portosystemic shunt for hypersplenism caused by portal hypertension |

(Continued)

**TABLE 59-3  Splenic Disorders and Treatments** *(Continued)*

| | Disorder | Treatment |
|---|---|---|
| Trauma | Penetrating | Laparotomy with splenic salvage if possible |
| | Blunt | A. Supportive care with blood transfusion if necessary |
| | | B. Laparotomy for failure of supportive care |
| | |    1. Suturing of spleen |
| | |    2. Application of hemostatic agent |
| | |    3. Partial splenectomy |
| | |    4. Total splenectomy |
| | |    5. Splenic implant |
| | |    6. Role of laparoscopy evolving: diagnosis and possible clearance of hemoperitoneum to alter inflammatory response. |

or by gastropexy and splenopexy have all been described as successful surgical options.

## Hereditary Hemolytic Disorders

### Hereditary Hemolytic Spherocytosis

Splenectomy has proven to be a safe and effective treatment for HHS. The timing of the surgery depends on multiple factors, including the child's age and the severity of symptoms. Risks of aplastic crisis and cholelithiasis seem to increase with time. Laparoscopic splenectomy is a safe and effective technique. Modifications in the technique continue to evolve, including application of single-site and partial splenectomy options. The presence of gallstones should be investigated prior to operation so that cholecystectomy can be done concomitantly if stones are present. Presence of gallstones, in the absence of other complications of HHS is not a compelling indication for splenectomy.

### Hereditary Hemolytic Elliptocytosis

Hereditary elliptocytosis rarely causes hemolysis and anemia severe enough to warrant splenectomy. Splenectomy is effective treatment, if indicated by severe and persistent symptoms.

### Hemoglobinopathies

Both thalassemia major and sickle cell disease are treated symptomatically, focusing on prevention of infection, provision of appropriate transfusion therapy, and measures to minimize physiologic stress.

Most children with thalassemia major accommodate appropriately to their anemia. Splenectomy may be useful to reduce excessive erythrocyte transfusion requirements. Splenectomy may also be indicated to alleviate compressive symptoms of splenomegaly.

The major indications for splenectomy in sickle cell disease are acute splenic sequestration, hypersplenism, and splenic abscess. In the event of multiple yearly sequestration crises or following one life-threatening splenic sequestration crisis, splenectomy is indicated following transfusion and stabilization. Preemptive vaccination against encapsulated organisms is essential and a surveillance ultrasound exam for cholelithiasis should be obtained. Splenectomy may be performed with either celiotomy or with minimal access approach, depending on the clinical scenario. Splenectomy is effective in treating splenic abscesses in patients with sickle cell disease.

### Enzyme Defects

Most patients with G-6-PD or pyruvate kinase deficiency do not need treatment if they maintain a hemoglobin level above 8 g/dL and are asymptomatic. These entities are rarely severe enough to require splenectomy. G-6-PD deficiency will not respond to splenectomy because the spleen is not the site of hemolysis. Splenectomy may decrease the need for transfusion in patients with pyruvate kinase deficiency.

## Autoimmune Disorders

### ITP

ITP in childhood is often self-limiting. Eighty percent of children with ITP recover spontaneously. Splenectomy is rarely considered in acute ITP unless potentially life-threatening hemorrhage intervenes. In chronic forms of the disease, splenectomy is an option when medical management fails or no longer is effective; or in the child who is symptomatic and whose lifestyle is severely limited by thrombocytopenia. The success rate of splenectomy seems to parallel the clinical response to steroids and intravenous immunoglobulin therapy. Unsuccessful splenectomy should prompt surveillance and elimination of occult or residual splenic tissue, such as accessory spleen, followed by additional immunosuppressive therapy.

### Autoimmune Hemolytic Anemia

Patients with Coombs-positive warm antibody normally respond to steroid therapy. In the event of steroid failure, splenectomy may be considered. Coombs-positive cold antibodies do not benefit from splenectomy, as the site of hemolysis is extrasplenic. The treatment is plasmapheresis and immunosuppression.

## Tumors, Cysts, and Abscesses

### Malignancies

Primary malignant tumors of the spleen are treated with splenectomy and chemotherapy. Splenectomy is no longer part of the staging of Hodgkin lymphoma. Noninvasive imaging studies have supplanted splenectomy in this situation.

## Benign Tumors and Cysts

Benign tumors and acquired cysts are treated with either partial or total splenectomy, depending on the size of the mass. Subtotal or partial splenectomy is optimal if it can be done safely. If there is a suspicion of echinococcal disease, appropriate screening measures and intraoperative precautions should be exercised. Congenital splenic cysts smaller than 4 cm may be observed and are effectively followed with yearly ultrasound examination to document stability of the cyst. Laparoscopic unroofing and subtotal resection of epidermal cysts of the spleen results in an unacceptable rate of recurrence unless the entire cyst wall is excised or complete excision with partial splenectomy is performed. Failure to do so often results in recurrence of a cyst that remarkably resembles the original lesion (Fig. 59-1). Every effort should be made to resect the entire cyst wall. If the epidermal cyst is large, centrally located, or complicated, total splenectomy—either open or via minimal access approach—may be the only option. Guided aspiration and successful sclerosis of a splenic cyst has been documented but is not universally successful and may require multiple treatments.

## Abscesses

In children, splenic abscesses may arise as a manifestation of serious infection in other parts of the body. Multiple, small abscesses may present without specific clinical signs or symptoms. These children are treated with high-dose antibiotics and usually do not need splenectomy unless medical management fails. Image-guided drainage in combination with antibiotics is successful in two-thirds of patients and does not impact the success of subsequent splenectomy.

## Hypersplenism and Splenomegaly

Numerous disorders, both benign and malignant, may cause hypersplenism in children. Hypersplenism due to portal hypertension is best approached by treatment of the underlying cause or with decompression of the portal system. Laparoscopic splenectomy may alleviate symptomatic neutropenia,

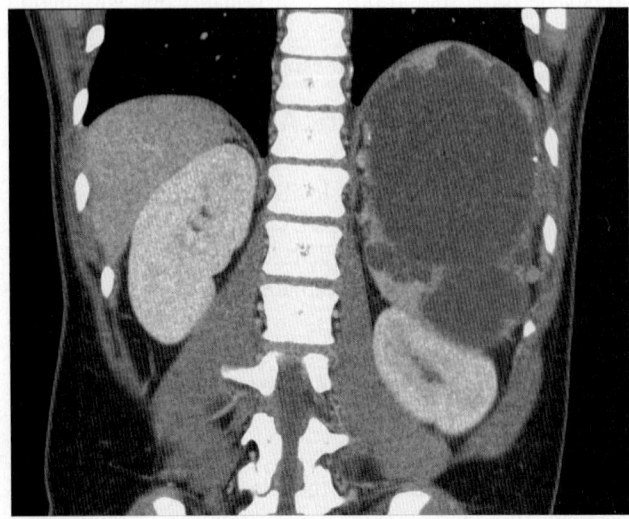

**FIGURE 59-1** Recurrent epidermoid cyst of spleen after laparoscopic unroofing and partial cystectomy.

| TABLE 59-4 | APSA Trauma Committee Guidelines for Isolated Splenic Injury | | | |
|---|---|---|---|---|
| | **CT Grade** | | | |
| | **I** | **II** | **III** | **IV** |
| ICU days | None | None | None | 1 day |
| Hospital days | 2 days | 3 days | 4days | 5 days |
| Predischarge imaging | None | None | None | None |
| Postdischarge imaging | None | None | None | None |
| Activity restriction[a] | 3 weeks | 4 weeks | 5 weeks | 6 weeks |

[a]Return to full-contact sports is at the discretion of the physician. Guidelines for return to unrestricted activity include normal age-appropriate activities.

thrombocytopenia, or anemia in selected cases. Compressive symptoms of splenomegaly can limit the quality of life that may improve with splenectomy. Partial splenectomy in Type I Gaucher disease, unresponsive to enzyme replacement therapy, may improve symptoms even in the face of remnant regrowth.

## Trauma

In the vast majority of children with splenic injury from blunt trauma, hemorrhage is self-limited and non life-threatening. These injuries are nicely imaged with CT scanning. Guidelines for nonoperative management of isolated splenic injury in childhood are published from the American Pediatric Surgical Association (Table 59-4).

The foundation of nonoperative management of splenic injury is hemodynamic stability. All other aspects of care depend on maintenance of adequate tissue perfusion and avoidance of shock. The absolute indication for operation is unrelenting and uncorrectable shock. In children, contrast blush on CT is less significant compared to this finding in adults and is not a harbinger of nonoperative management failure. If there are severe, coexisting injuries that make splenic salvage unsafe or if the child has required transfusion of greater than 40/mL/kg of blood, operative intervention should be considered. Control of hemorrhage and splenic salvage, if possible, are goals.

Routine postinjury imaging of the spleen is unnecessary. The true risk of radiation exposure from CT imaging remains to be defined, but it seems prudent to limit CT exposure unless the information obtained is essential to care. Routine follow-up CT imaging is not part of current evidence-based guidelines. Additional imaging may be important if post injury symptoms of pain, left upper quadrant tenderness or fullness are noted to persist long after the injury.

## POTENTIAL COMPLICATIONS OF SPLENECTOMY

Mortality from splenectomy in childhood has historically been very low. Early morbidity includes perioperative hemorrhage, pancreatitis, gastric injury, abscess, portal vein thrombosis, and other early thromboembolic problems. These are uncommon complications of splenectomy. Two broad but important categories of delayed risk are serious overwhelming infection and vascular disorders.

## Postsplenectomy Infection

Overwhelming postsplenectomy infection (OPSI) was first clearly described in the early 1900s, but the landmark study of King and Schumacher in 1952 was the first to describe fatal meningococcemia in 4 out of 5 children who had splenectomy for hereditary spherocytosis in the first 6 months of life. Subsequent studies clarified the OPSI profile to include age-related risk adjustment and identified that the disease-specific indication for splenectomy was important. Septic death rates 600 times that of the general population have been reported, with half of these deaths reported in children less than 2 years of age. Mortality for this dreaded condition is reported to occur between 50% and 75%. The organisms classically associated with OPSI are *Streptococcus pneumonia, Hemophilus influenza, and Neisseria meningitides. Capnocytophagia* is a common component of canine oral flora and has been curiously associated with bacteremia in asplenic patients. Aggressive wound care and antibiotic treatment should be considered when dog bite injury befalls the asplenic patient. Appropriate vaccination therapy helps reduce the risk to asplenic children. There are published guidelines from the American Academy of Pediatrics for vaccination of the asplenic child. Presplenectomy vaccines are optimally administered three weeks prior to splenectomy

## Chronic Thromboembolic Pulmonary Hypertension and Adverse Vascular Events

There is increasing evidence of an association between splenectomy and prevalence of pulmonary hypertension. The significant increased incidence of thromboembolism and pulmonary hypertension has been documented in thalassemia, hereditary spherocytosis, and several other conditions treated with splenectomy. The term *chronic thromboembolic pulmonary hypertension* is used to describe the most common etiology of the pulmonary hypertension. Other adverse vascular events include increased incidence of myocardial infarction, risk of coronary artery surgery, stroke, and carotid artery surgery in patients following splenectomy for spherocytosis. The role of partial splenectomy and antithrombotic medication to prevent these adverse vascular outcomes has not yet been defined.

## OPERATIVE PROCEDURES

### Open Total Splenectomy

The approach to the spleen via celiotomy may be performed through a number of incisions, based on the size of the spleen, acuity of the costal margin angle, and the necessity of access to other organs such as the gallbladder. Preemptive epidural analgesia or local infiltration blockade prior to incision is recommended if available and coagulation function is satisfactory. A transverse left upper quadrant incision is appropriate in most children (Fig. 59-2). Extension across the upper

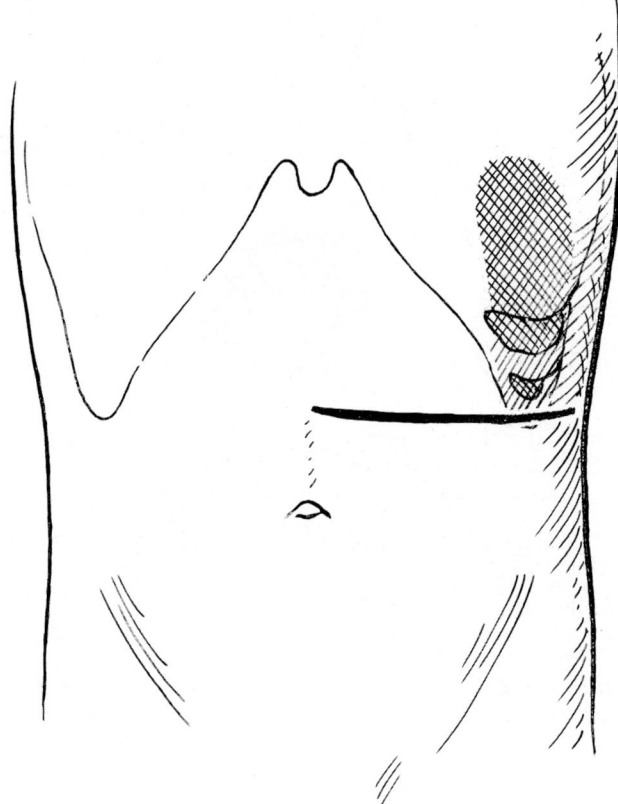

**FIGURE 59-2** In elective splenectomy by open celiotomy, the procedure is started by making a transverse incision in the upper left quadrant beginning at the midline and extending laterally to the midaxillary line.

abdomen may enhance safe exposure in case of massive splenomegaly. Self-retaining retractors are useful adjuncts. Entry into the lesser omental sac allows identification of the main splenic artery, which can be ligated in continuity to minimize risk of blood loss during hilar dissection.

Mobilization of the splenorenal and splenophrenic ligaments allows the spleen and distal pancreas to be medially rotated and delivered into the wound (Fig. 59-3). Splenocolic

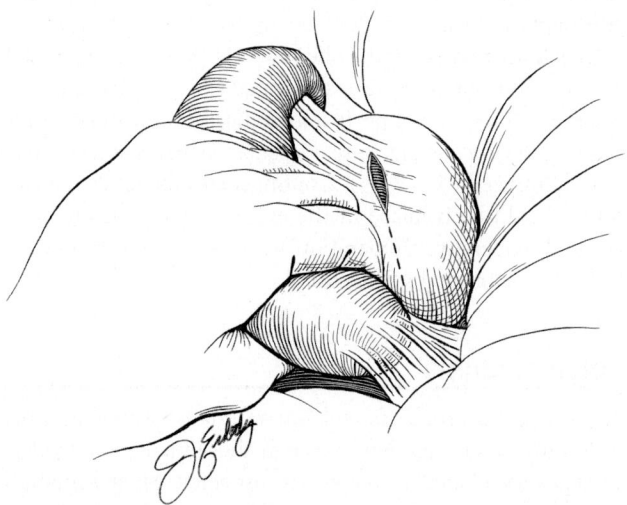

**FIGURE 59-3** To avoid entering the splenic capsule, an incision is made through the splenorenal ligament near the abdominal wall.

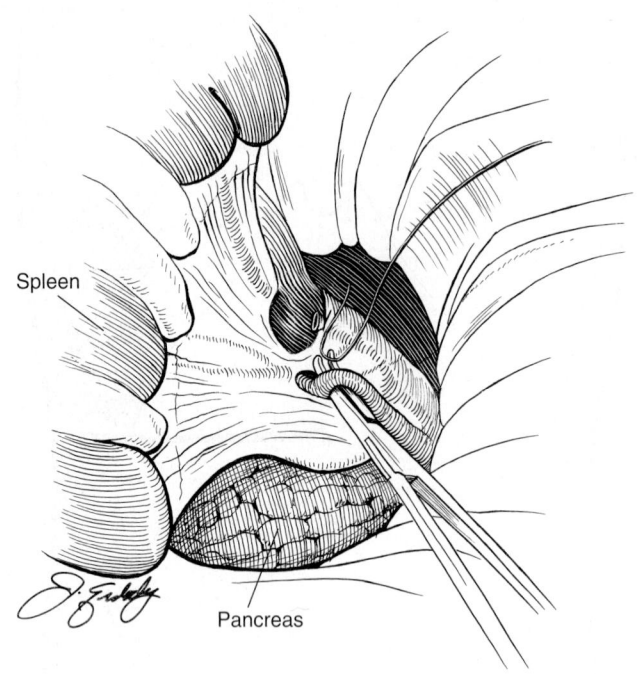

**FIGURE 59-4** The branches of the splenic artery and vein are separates from the pancreas and individually ligated.

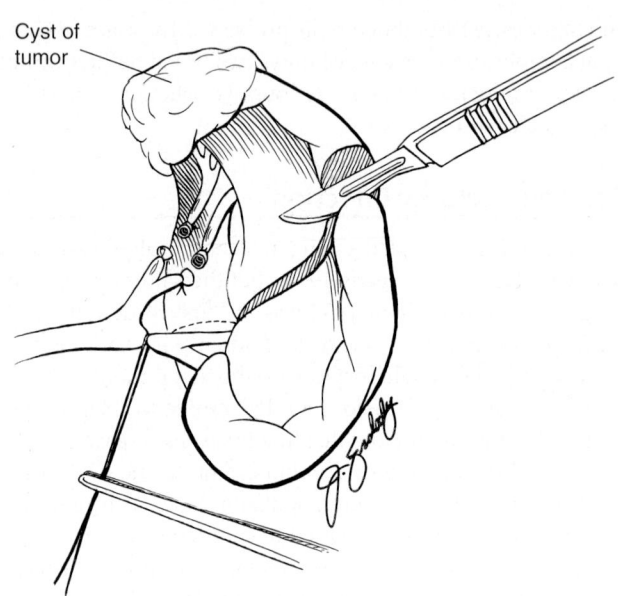

Cyst of tumor

**FIGURE 59-5** For partial splenectomy, a transverse incision is made with a surgical blade and the cautery across the spleen along the line of vascular demarcation. A vessel loop temporarily occludes the inferior pole vessels.

attachments may be divided with cautery, ligatures, or other vessel/tissue sealing tools. The short gastric vessels may be sealed or ligated, based on size and length configuration. The branches of the splenic artery and vein are then individually ligated at the splenic hilum (Fig. 59-4). Careful attention to the distal pancreas prevents parenchymal injury. Drain placement is not necessary and historically has been associated with risk of subphrenic abscess.

## Partial Splenectomy

Exposure for partial splenectomy is similar to that previously described. Temporary vascular control of the main splenic artery is obtained. The segmental vessels to the spleen are carefully examined. The goal of retention of between 10% and 30% of perfused spleen volume seems to be optimal for partial splenectomy in hereditary spherocytosis. After the segmental vessels to the major fraction are ligated (Fig. 59-5), the spleen is cut along the line of perfusion demarcation using cautery, stapling devices, or LigaSure. Capsular mattress sutures may also be utilized (Fig. 59-6). Contingencies for total splenectomy should be in place in the event of dangerous hemorrhage. Preoperative preparation with vaccination should be the same as for total splenectomy.

## Splenic Trauma

The surgical approach for splenic trauma is best via midline celiotomy. After rapid but thorough abdominal and retroperitoneal surveillance, the spleen is inspected. Medial rotation after ligament division—as for splenectomy provides optimum control and visualization. Splenectomy or splenorrhaphy are performed based on severity of the injury, stability

of the child, and major trauma comorbidities. Principles of damage control trauma laparotomy apply. Splenic salvage should only be considered in the hemodynamically stable child without multisystem trauma and who is not coagulopathic, acidotic, and hypothermic.

## Minimal Access Splenic Surgery

Laparoscopic splenic surgery is an established, safe, and effective procedure for the experienced minimal access surgeon.

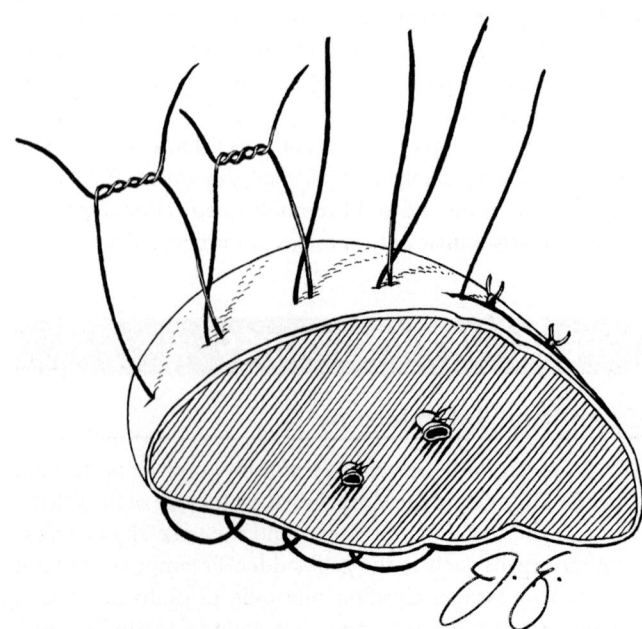

**FIGURE 59-6** Vertical mattress sutures are used to obtain hemostasis from the cut surface of the spleen after partial splenectomy.

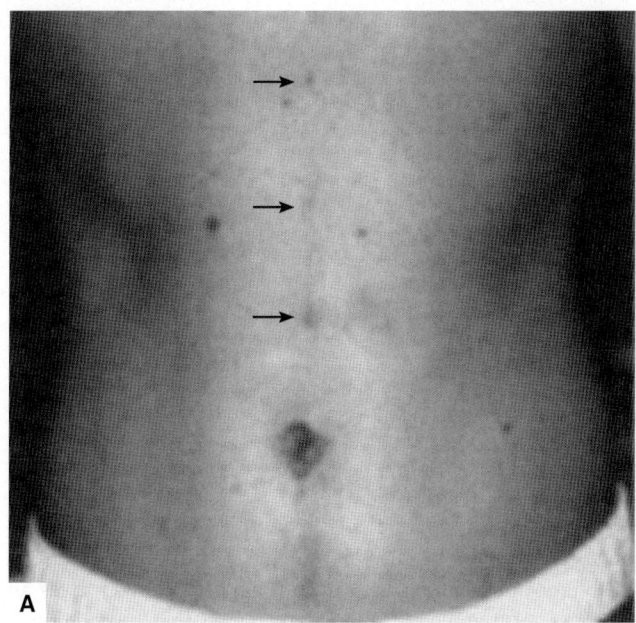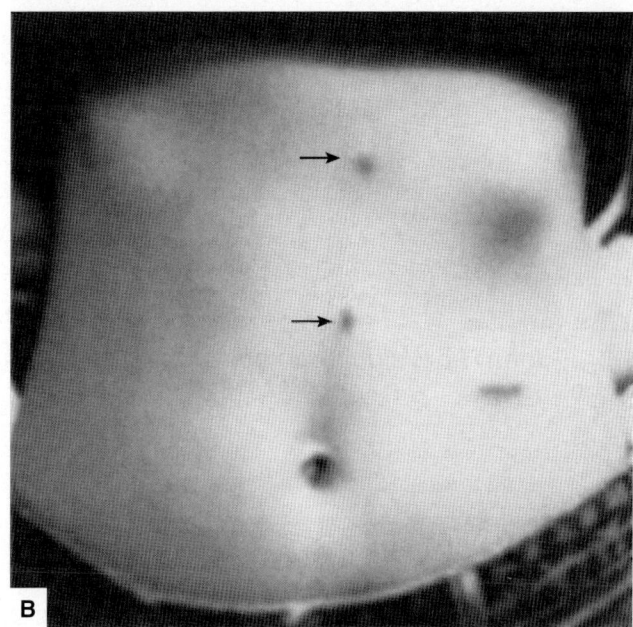

**FIGURE 59-7** Laparoscopic splenectomy port placement options.

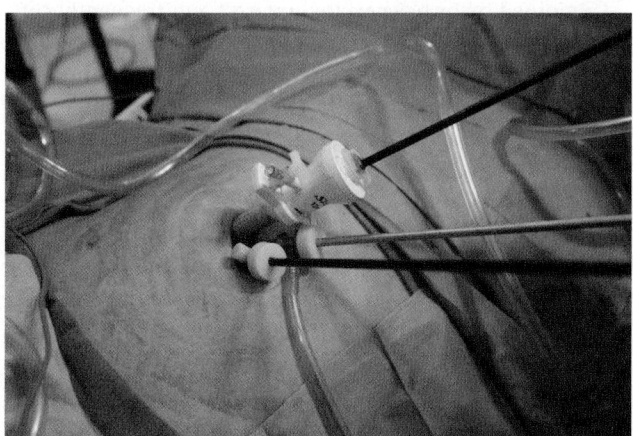

**FIGURE 59-8** Single-site laparoscopic splenectomy.

Port placement may be effective in several array options and depend on the instrumentation and surgeon preference (Fig. 59-7). Initial experience with single-site laparoscopic surgery for splenectomy are encouraging and ideally require specialized, articulating instruments (Fig. 59-8).

## SELECTED READINGS

Abdullah F, Zhang Y, Camp M, et al. Splenectomy in hereditary spherocytosis: review of 1657 patients and application of the pediatric quality indicators. *Pediatr Blood Cancer* 2009;52(7):834–837.

Allen KB, Andrews G. Pediatric wandering spleen: the case for splenopexy—review of 35 reported cases in the literature. *J Pediatr Surg* 1989;24:432–435.

Davies DA, Pearl RH, Ein SH, et al. Management of blunt splenic injury in children: evolution of the nonoperative approach. *J Pediatr Surg* 2009;44:1005–1008.

Fiquet-Francois C, Belouadah M, Ludot H, et al. Wandering spleen in children: multicenter retrospective study. *J Pediatr Surg* 2010;45(7):1519–1524.

Fisher JC, Gurung B, Cowles RA. Recurrence after laparoscopic excision of nonparasitic splenic cysts. *J Pediatr Surg* 2008;43:1644–1648.

Hollingsworth CL, Rice HE. Hereditary spherocytosis and partial splenectomy in children: review of surgical technique and the role of imaging. *Pediatr Radiol* 2010;40:1177–1183.

Jaïs X, Ioos V, Jardim C, et al. Splenectomy and chronic thromboembolic pulmonary hypertension. *Thorax* 2005;60:1031–1034.

Last RJ. Anatomy: regional and applied, 5th Ed. Baltimore: Williams & Wilkins; 1972:470.

Lesher AP, Kalpatthi R, Glenn JB, et al. Outcome of splenectomy in children younger than 4 years with sickle cell disease. *J Pediatr Surg* 2009;44:1134–1138.

Rescorla FJ, West KW, Engum SA, et al. Laparoscopic splenic procedures in children: experience in 231 children. *Ann Surg* 2007;246(4):683–688.

Schilling RF. Risks and benefits of splenectomy versus no splenectomy for hereditary spherocytosis–a personal view. *Br J Haematol* 2009;145:728–732.

Schilling RF, Gangnon RE, Traver MI. Delayed adverse vascular events after splenectomy in hereditary spherocytosis. *J Thromb Haemost* 2008;6(8):1289–1295.

Skandalakis LJ, Gray SW, Ricketts R, et al. The spleen. In: Skandalakis JE, Gray SW, eds. *Embryology for Surgeons*. 2nd Ed. Baltimore: Williams & Wilkins; 1994:334–365.

Slater BJ, Chan FP, Davis K, et al. Institutional experience with laparoscopic partial splenectomy for hereditary spherocytosis. *J Pediatr Surg* 2010;45(8):1682–1686.

Stylianos S, Egorova N, Guice KS, et al. Variation in treatment of pediatric spleen injury at trauma centers versus nontrauma centers: a call for dissemination of APSA benchmarks and guidelines. *J Am Coll Surg* 2006;202:247–251.

Stylianos S, and the APSA Trauma Study Group. Prospective validation of evidence-based guidelines for resource utilization in children with isolated spleen or liver injury. *J Pediatr Surg* 2002;37:453–456.

Watters JM, Sambasivau CN, Zink K, et al. Splenectomy leads to a persistent hypercoagulable state after trauma. *Am J Surg* 2010;199(5):646–651.

THE SPLEEN

751

# Conjoined Twins

# CHAPTER 60

*John H.T. Waldhausen and Mary Hilfiker*

## KEY POINTS

1. There are 8 primary types of conjoined twins. There is a wide variation in anatomy even between these 8 types.

2. Prenatal ultrasound and MRI are useful diagnostic tools. The information gained may help when counseling the family and informing the surgical team in case emergency surgery is needed.

3. Postnatal evaluation depends on the type of twin but should always include an ECHO. Full evaluation allows many (but not necessarily all) of the anatomic issues to be evaluated.

4. Separation is not the only alternative. Not all twins are separable and some parents may not desire separation. All alternatives should be discussed.

5. Surgeons undertaking separation surgeries should be familiar with the literature in order to know how others have dealt with many of the anatomic problems that may be encountered.

6. A team approach to separation is preferable with 1 lead surgeon to coordinate the overall plan of care. Each twin needs his or her own operative team during separation.

7. Planning meetings with all surgeons, nurses, anesthesiologists, and other staff are necessary to help plan and coordinate the separation. Rehearsals may help.

8. Separations may be emergent or elective. In the latter case, separations are most likely to be more successful after 4 months of age.

9. Surgeons should be familiar with the ethical issues surrounding separation and should be prepared to handle attention from the media.

10. Outcome from separation depends on the type of twin but may be excellent. Issues regarding quality of life will vary depending on the type of twin. Surgeons should be able to discuss quality of life concerns with families whether the twins are separated or not.

The topic of conjoined twins is complex. The various types have common characteristics but each set will present unique problems and challenges to overcome. This chapter gives an overview of many of the common themes that surgeons caring for these infants will encounter; however, preparation for the surgery by extensive reading of the literature to examine how others have dealt with these children is essential when caring for these infants.

Conjoined twins have excited interest and frequently conjured an image of the grotesque throughout history because of their uniqueness, compelling appearance, and infrequent occurrence. However, exactly because of this uniqueness, conjoined twins always attract attention. The realization that two individuals are so intimately connected and must share everything they do is both fascinating and somewhat horrifying to most people. The Western desire to provide each twin with a separate existence has spurred medical science to develop methods for accomplishing safe separation. Separations have now become fairly routine, though they involve great care and planning. To date, well over 1000 cases of conjoined twins have been described, as beautifully documented by Rowena Spencer in her 2003 book entitled *Conjoined Twins*. Since 1950, more than 200 surgical separations have been documented with an increasing number of successes. It is also important to note, however, that separation in some cases may not be possible, or that the family may not desire the operation. The manner in which Western societies regard conjoined twins may be different from that of other parts of the world where separation may not be considered important. These children, if not separated, may still need further surgical care to deal with other issues in order to help improve their quality of life. These issues and the techniques and considerations to be considered will be subsequently discussed.

## DISEASE PATHOPHYSIOLOGY

### Incidence

In North America, twins occur in every 80 to 90 pregnancies. Twins may arise either from 2 zygotes resulting in dizygotic twins or from 1 zygote resulting in monozygotic twins. Approximately two-thirds of twins are dizygotic and one-third are monozygotic. Approximately 1 in every 400 monozygotic twin pregnancies have incomplete twinning and result in conjoined twins. The incidence of conjoined twinning varies in different parts of the world. In the United States, the incidence ranges from 1:100,000 to 1:250,000, while in sub-Saharan Africa, it may be as frequent as 1:50,000 with isolated incidences of 1:14,000 in some areas. The higher estimates of incidence are the result of episodes of several births in a circumscribed geographic area over a short period of time. The incidence for live-born conjoined twins is significantly different. Conjoined twins are still-born up to 60% of the time while another 35% die in the first 24 hours of life. This makes the incidence of live-born conjoined twins closer to 1 in 200,000 births. The frequency of monozygotic twins is not affected by racial differences or maternal age. It is reasonable to assume that the frequency of conjoined twins is similarly unaffected. However, autopsy evaluation reveals a predominance of females being affected by conjoined twinning approximately 3 times as frequently as males.

## Embryology

Conjoined twins have been described in many species in both the plant and animal kingdoms. The exact embryology remains theoretical and controversial. There are 2 different theories as to how these twins develop. The first suggests that conjoined twinning results from failure of separation of the embryonic disc late in the blastomere stage at 15 to 17 days gestation, also termed incomplete fission. The second theory suggests that the twins result from partial fusion of 2 embryonic plates at 3 to 4 weeks of gestation. Each theory has strengths and weaknesses and neither has been proved.

Conjoined twins are always monozygotic and monochorionic, though 1 set of diamniotic omphalopagus twins has been reported. Twins are always of the same sex, which would seem to lend more weight to the fission theory as it would seem just as likely that a male and female embryonic plate would fuse; however, this has never been observed. Several cases of pseudohermaphrodites, however, have been documented. Conjoined twins have been reported as part of a set of triplets or quadruplets with the conjoined twins always being isosexual while the other infant or infants may be of the opposite sex. There are also extremely rare sets of conjoined tripling and quadrupling that have been reported as well.

Conjoined twins are always joined in a homologous position, cranially, caudally, ventral to ventral, or dorsal to dorsal. If one accepts fusion as the most likely cause of conjoined twinning, the type of twin that develops depends on where the embryonic discs come into contact. The theory of fusion, which may also be termed the spherical theory, was developed by Dr. Rowena Spencer after analysis of many hundreds of conjoined twins cases. This theory postulates that 2 monovulvar embryonic discs are present floating on either the outer surface (yolk sac) or inner surface (amniotic cavity) of a sphere. These discs may come into contact with each other and fuse either ventrally over a single yolk sac (cephalopagus, thoracopagus, omphalopagus, ischiopagus, and parapagus twins) or dorsally (craniopagus, rachipagus, and pygopagus twins). The orientation of the embryonic disc determines the type of conjoined twinning that develops. The union is not random, however, and may only take place where surface ectoderm is absent or is genetically programmed to break down such as at the oropharyngeal and cloacal membranes or along the neural tube. These unions are always homologous in that the oropharyngeal and cloacal membranes never fuse. Ventral union in general leads to twins sharing 1 abdomen and 1 umbilicus, while dorsal union of the neural tube leads to infants with 2 separate abdomens and 2 umbilical cords.

While the spherical theory of conjoined twin development is appealing in that it can explain almost all types of twinning, additions to the theory must be considered to further explain development. Dr Spencer calls these additions, "adjustments to conjunction," which include aplasia of contiguous lateral anlagen, and division and diversion of midsagittal structures. Division and diversion are best illustrated by cephalopagus twins. With this type of twin, as the oropharyngeal membrane fuses, it splits sagittally, diverts laterally, and fuses with the laterally diverted membrane of the other disc. This results in the Janus type of cephalopagus twin in which there appears to be a face on either side of the body, one half of the face from each twin. Brain imaging demonstrates that in these twins, one half of the frontal lobes derives from each twin as the result of the same process. Aplasia of contiguous lateral anlagen is demonstrated in parapagus twins where the structures in the area of union fail to develop. Using parapagus twins as an example the medial leg for each child is absent because of this process.

There is one other type of twinning that may occur that is not well explained by the above theories: the development of a parasitic or atypical twin. These twins have only a partially formed twin extending from the body of the better developed twin. These parasitic twins cannot survive independently. As many as 20% of conjoined twins have developmental malformations in multiple organ systems. These anomalies are not random, and are typically found in the right-sided twin, and in male sets of twins. The risk of recurrence for conjoined twins in essentially negligible.

## Classification by Types

To classify conjoined twins appropriately requires a common terminology that is all-too-often lacking when these children are described, which thus gives rise to many different terms in the literature. The classification of the type of twin depends on the primary area of union. Since conjoined twins represent a continuum of development in the manner in which the 2 embryologic discs fused or split, it may at times be difficult to classify 1 type of twin based on external appearance only. Picturing a continuum of development is a helpful means of visualizing conjoined twin development. Ventrally united twins may be described by 2 fetuses joined ventrally and then rotated in both the $x$–$y$ axis and the $y$–$z$ axis. By rotating the infants in this manner, one can produce every type of ventrally united conjoined twins. This challenge in classifying twins and the reason there are so many terms in the literature may be due to some overlap between 1 type of twin's external appearance and that of another type.

When referring to a particular infant in a set of conjoined twins it is important to use uniform terminology in describing both the twins and their anatomy. The terms anterior and posterior are not applied to individual twins, but rather refer to the twins as a whole. When the twins are lying in a position such that the abdomen is most fully exposed, right and left are oriented from the twins' perspective and the infants are termed "the twin on the right" and "the twin on the left." Structures within individual twins should be referenced as dorsal and ventral. Using these reference points works well for describing the anatomic relationships of all twins except craniopagus and rachipagus twins.

Conjoined twins are classified into 8 main categories: omphalopagus (umbilicus), thoracopagus (chest), ischiopagus (hip), craniopagus (helmet), and pygopagus (rump), parapagus (side), cephalopagus (head), and rachipagus (spine). Additionally, parasites, teratomas, and fetus-in-fetu may also be

considered part of this process. The Greek term "pagus" means to be fixed or joined, and is preceded by a prefix that describes where the twins are joined. Suffixes are used to describe other aspects of the twins. For example: prosopus refers to the face; brachius to the upper limb; and pus to the lower limb. Other prefixes include di-, tri-, and tetra-, used to describe the number of limbs or heads. The most recent and most logical classification of conjoined twins is based on physical examination with the exception of the important distinction between omphalopagus and thoracopagus twins (Fig. 60-1). Externally, omphalopagus and thoracopagus twins may be

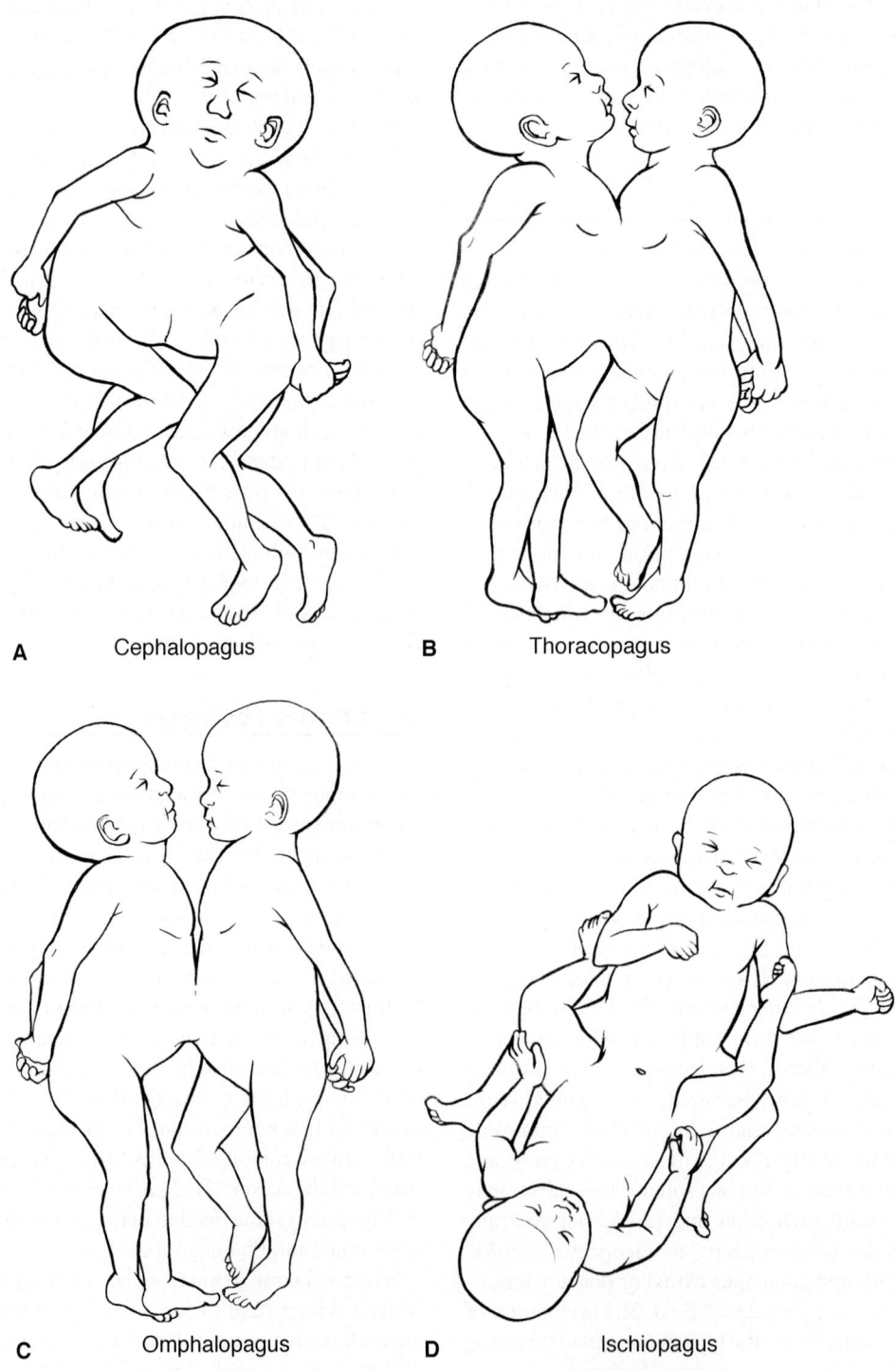

**A** Cephalopagus
**B** Thoracopagus
**C** Omphalopagus
**D** Ischiopagus

**FIGURE 60-1** Classification of conjoined twins based on the anatomy of the shared area. **A.** Cephalopagus. **B.** Thoracopagus. **C.** Omphalopagus. **D.** Ischiopagus.

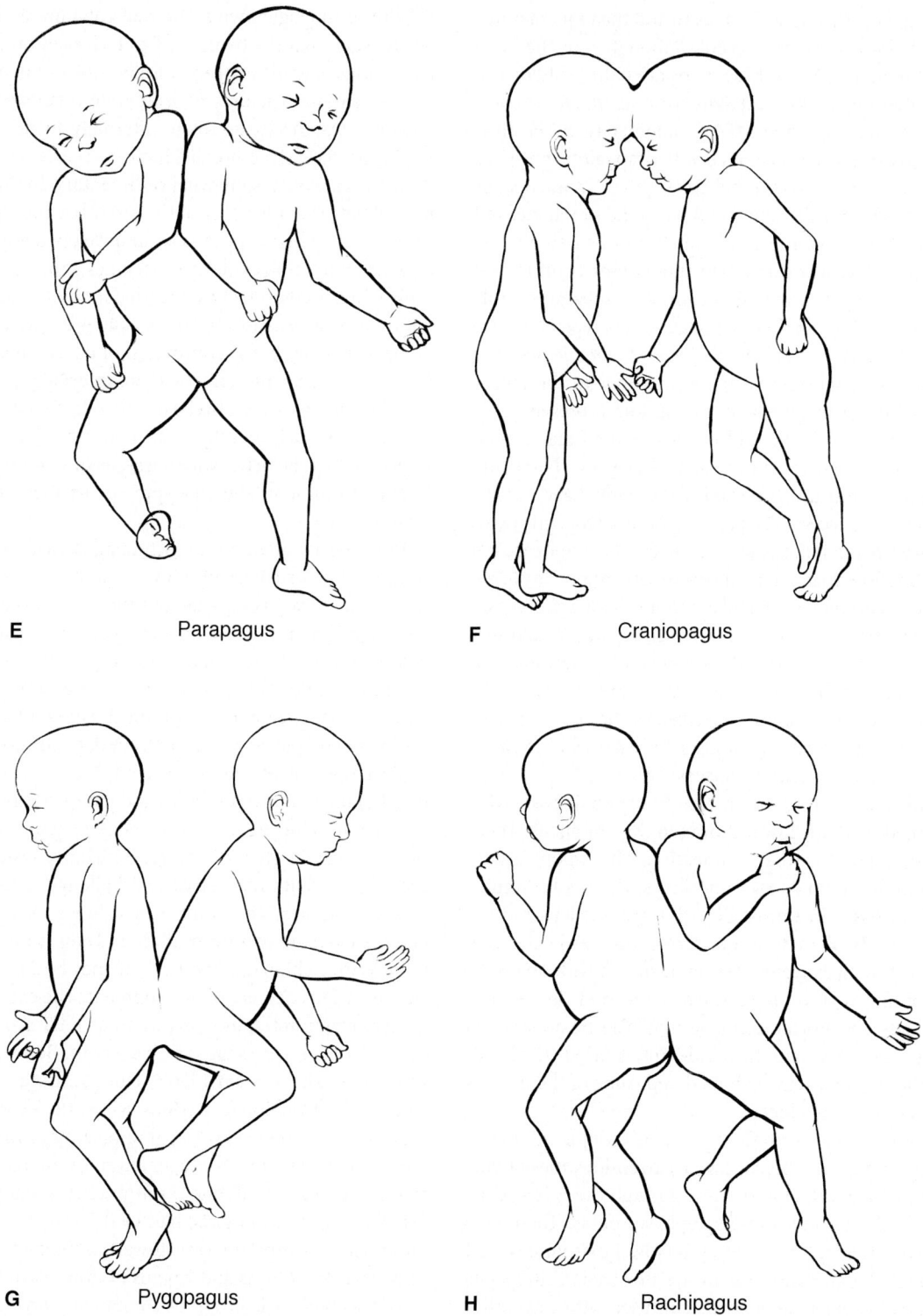

**E** Parapagus  **F** Craniopagus

**G** Pygopagus  **H** Rachipagus

**FIGURE 60-1** (*Continued*) **E.** Parapagus. **F.** Craniopagus. **G.** Pygopagus. **H.** Rachipagus.

indistinguishable. However, thoracopagus twins always have some degree of cardiac union, whereas omphalopagus twins never have a cardiac connection.

The 8 types of twins can be organized into 2 primary groups based on the orientation of the union, either ventral to ventral or dorsal to dorsal. This ventral union includes those twins joined at the rostral and mid-ventral areas, such as cephalopagus infants, to those fused more caudally, such as ischiopagus

and parapagus twins. Infants in this group share some aspect of the gastrointestinal tract and generally have 1 umbilicus. The ventral union of twins often is more typically a ventrolateral orientation as the twins may not directly face each other. Three types of twins in the ventral union group have all 4 extremities present and no pelvic union. These include cephalopagus, thoracopagus, and omphalopagus. The cephalopagus twins are united from the vernix of the head to the umbilicus. These twins share the forebrain, optic chiasm, and the upper aerodigestive tract. Two faces are present, although 1 of the faces may be rudimentary. All of these twins are either stillborn or die shortly after birth. Thoracopagus twins are the most common type of twin comprising 40% of conjoined twins. Historically, they have often been classified with omphalopagus twins because of their common external appearance. Thoracopagus twins are united from the upper thorax to the umbilicus and always have a cardiac connection, even if only by a single vessel. This distinction from omphalopagus twins is important because thoracopagus twins often cannot be separated while omphalopagus twins can. Thoracopagus twins typically share a compound heart of varying degrees of complexity. The upper gastrointestinal tract is shared in 40% and the biliary tree in 22%. The gastrointestinal tract union, if present, usually starts at the level of the mid-duodenum and may extend into the distal small bowel. A portion of the liver is shared and biliary union should be suspected if the twins have a common duodenum. Successful separation of thoracopagus twins with a shared heart is unusual. There are recorded cases of atrial conjunction that have survived separation; however, when there is complex ventricular union, there are no cases described where both twins have survived separation and survival of even 1 twin is rare. All attempts at separation with complex cardiac union, have either attempted to salvage the heart for 1 child with planned sacrifice of the other or have attempted to create 2 cardiac units, 1 for each child. Neither approach has been particularly successful.

Omphalopagus twins account for 35% of conjoined twins and are joined from the lower thorax to the umbilicus. There is never any type of cardiac connection. The union usually extends from the xiphoid to the umbilicus. There is a common bridge of liver tissue in almost all such twins and a part of the diaphragm may be shared. In some cases this may be the only connection. The digestive tract is often shared with one sixth of cases joining in the upper tract at the mid-duodenum. The bile ducts and portal drainage may also be anomalous particularly in cases where the duodenum is fused. The lower aspect of the sternum may be joined and some of these twins will also have an omphalocele.

Ischiopagus twins account for 6% of conjoined twins. Depending on the number of lower extremities these twins may be united from the lower chest through the pelvis. Usually, there are 2 sacrums and 2 symphyses pubis. There may be 2 (dipus), 3 (tripus), or 4 (tetrapus) lower extremities, and external genitalia and anus are always involved. Ischiopagus dipus and parapagus twins may be confused with each other because ischiopagus twins and parapagus twins represent a continuum of rotation along the $x$, $y$, and $z$ axes. Parapagus twins are united laterally and may share parts of the upper gastrointestinal system, while ischiopagus twins will not. In parapagus infants, the developing fetus succumbs to aplasia of contiguous lateral anlagen, such that in the true parapagus twins, the infants are united laterally with no internal rotation along the $z$ axis, and all medial structures from each twin such as the leg or arm, depending on the degree of union, are absent. Parapagus twins may be only united in the lower body and in this case will have 4 arms, while other sets may be more completely united and have only 2 or 3 arms. Parapagus twins always have only 2 legs.

With ischiopagus twins, internal rotation along the $z$ axis occurs such that the twins start to face each other; aplasia of contiguous lateral anlagen lessens and anomalies increase as the various structures of 2 separate infants become more apparent. As the twins rotate internally to face each other, duplicate sets of structures begin to emerge dorsally. The dorsal structures are often somewhat rudimentary. In these cases, the medial buttock or leg of each twin may become apparent. The fused leg may first appear as an undeveloped appendage and, as internal rotation continues, becomes apparent as the tripus limb, comprised of the fused medial limb of each child. Internal rotation also causes the increasing presence of diminutive dorsal genetalia. In the continuum of development, the spine of each twin may not only be more internally rotated toward the opposite twin, but also be oriented farther apart along the $x$ and $y$ axis, such that the twins may face each other but are joined only at the pelvis with 4 legs, as in ischiopagus tetrapus infants. In these infants, the spine is oriented 180º from the other child.

The internal anatomy of ischiopagus twins may be quite complex but usually will allow separation. The upper gastrointestinal tract is separate but the more distal small bowel may be joined at the level of a Meckels diverticulum, leading to a shared distal ileum and colon with a dual mesentery, half from each child. This colon may end as an imperforate anus, cloaca, urogenital sinus, or perineal fistula. One or two anal sphincter complexes may be present depending on the degree of development of the dorsal complex. The liver is usually fused in the ischiopagus tripus and parapagus twins. The biliary tree in ischiopagus twins is separate, while for parapagus twins, it may be shared. The genitourinary system will likely present a difficult reconstructive challenge as the union may be very complex. The number of kidneys varies from 1 to 4, and ureters may cross the midline and empty into the opposite twin. With ischiopagus twins, there may be 2 uteri and 4 ovaries in various degrees of development. The external genitalia in ischiopagus tetrapus twins are rotated 90º from the normal orientation, and are shared by each twin. Between each set of legs there exist a normal labia, clitoris, urethra, and vaginal orifice. With ischiopagus tripus twins, the external genitalia may open on either side of a common anus or may be part of a cloacal malformation or urogenital sinus. In male ischiopagus tetrapus twins, a penis and scrotum are present between each set of legs, but, as in girls, half of the genitalia derives from either twin. As union moves toward ischiopagus tripus, boys may have 2 scrotums and 1 penis or other various anomalies.

The second basic group of conjoined twins includes those united dorsally: twins joined at the neural tube and the cranio-vertebral axis. These infants face away from each other and have 2 umbilical cords, and either separate or nearly separate gastrointestinal tracts. There are 3 types of twins in this group: craniopagus, pygopagus, and rachipagus. All types in this group have 4 arms and 4 legs. The craniopagus twins account for 2% of conjoined twins and may be united at any portion of the skull except the foramen magnum and the face. They are distinctly different from the cephalopagus twins that are ventrally united, with further union in the trunk. Craniopagus union may not be symmetric but may involve the bony skull, meninges, and even the surface of the brain. They can be subclassified in terms of the site of union: frontotemporal/frontoparietal 25%; parietal 45%; and occipital/occipitoparietal 30%. Further categorization of these twins describes either partial or total conjunction. Total conjunction refers to the brains being connected or separated by the arachnoid only. In the partial form, the brain is separated by the bone and dura and each has a separate leptomeninges. The ability to separate these types of twins centers on the degree to which the dural venous sinuses are connected and the subsequent risk of hemorrhage or severe neurologic deficit.

Pygopagus (rump) twins are united at the sacrococcygeal and perineal areas. They account for 20% of conjoined twins. Seven percent of these cases are boys. The twins face away from each other and are joined at the sacrum, buttocks, and perineum. The spinal cord may sometimes be part of the union. Forty percent of these twins will have a common dural tube. Close to 50% of these children have some anomaly of the central nervous system (CNS) and/or vertebral column, which may include hydrocephalus, myelomeningocele and spina bifida, and rachischisis. The pelvis is separate except for osseous fusion in the lateral portion of the sacrum and coccyx. There are usually 2 sets of external genitalia with fusion in the perineum at the area of the posterior forchette in girls. There is only 1 anus, which is posterior to the urogenital fusion. The lower gastrointestinal tracts are separate but the rectum usually unites several centimeters proximal to the anus. Twenty five percent will have renal anomalies including renal agenesis, ectopia, and fusion. Usually these children can be separated, but the perineal reconstruction may be challenging.

Rachipagus (spine) twins are extremely rare and can be categorized as dorsal union from above the sacrum cephalad. The union can include the occiput and segments of the vertebral column. Table 60-1 summarizes the possible unions of conjoined twins.

## Ethical Considerations

The diagnosis of conjoined twins may be emotionally traumatic for the family and an ethical challenge for everyone involved. Many fetuses are likely terminated at the time of diagnosis. For those carried to term and who then survive, decisions must be made regarding their subsequent care. If the diagnosis is known prenatally, it is most helpful to have

| TABLE 60-1 | Possible Unions of Conjoined Twins | | | |
|---|---|---|---|---|
| Group | Type | Cardiac | Liver | Upper Gastrointestinal |
| Ventral | Cephalopagus | + | + | + |
| | Thoracopagus | + | + | + |
| | Omphalopagus | | + | + |
| | Ischiopagus | | + | |
| | Parapagus | + | + | + |
| Dorsal | Craniopagus | | | |
| | Pygopagus | | | |
| | Rachipagus | | | |

| Group | Type | Lower Gastrointestinal | Genitourinary | |
|---|---|---|---|---|
| Ventral | Cephalopagus | | | |
| | Thoracopagus | | | |
| | Omphalopagus | | | |
| | Ischiopagus | + | + | |
| | Parapagus | + | + | |
| Dorsal | Craniopagus | | | |
| | Pygopagus | + | + | |
| | Rachipagus | | | |

| Group | Type | Nervous System | Bony Structures | |
|---|---|---|---|---|
| Ventral | Cephalopagus | + | + | |
| | Thoracopagus | | + | |
| | Omphalopagus | | | |
| | Ischiopagus | | + | |
| | Parapagus | + | + | |
| Dorsal | Craniopagus | + | + | |
| | Pygopagus | + | + | |
| | Rachipagus | + | + | |

discussions with the family before birth so that many of the issues regarding care will have already been decided. In many cases, prenatal evaluation of the children will provide enough information to accurately predict the types of problems the twins are likely to encounter, and the parents may be able to make informed decisions about their children's care. The decision whether to separate the twins or not may be fairly clear if 1 twin has obvious anomalies not compatible with life. If both children can survive, however, the decision to separate the infants is not necessarily straightforward, as some would argue that conjoined twins left together may live long and ful-filling lives. There are numerous historical examples of this. Cultural experience and societal norms all play a role in the decision. How the Western world views conjoined twins may be very different from the viewpoint of other societies, and the parent's background must be taken into consideration. Even if separated, the individual twin's quality of life must be considered as each may have significant medical issues as a result of the separation surgery. In some cases it may well be that if left alone, the children will require little medical care outside of routine health maintenance.

While certain types of conjoined twins are quite likely to survive separation surgery with 2 surviving infants, not all separation surgeries may be so successful. Perhaps the most ethically challenging situation is that in which both twins are born alive but it becomes apparent that both cannot survive in the long term and consideration is given to sacrifice 1 twin to save the other. Numerous ethical studies have addressed this situation. This brings to the forefront ethical arguments regarding what constitutes life, the individual, societal norms, and the law. Christian, Jewish, and Islamic scholars have all written opinions that separation surgeries performed where 1 child is likely to die as a result of the surgery are acceptable if each child has the opportunity to live; in other words, if the surgery is not a planned sacrifice of 1 twin. Arguments for separation in these cases include the doctrine of double effect, 1 twin as an "unjust aggressor," appendage, or surro-gacy and the view that 1 twin has been marked for death by nature. Some ethics scholars have written that separations performed to save 1 twin and cause the demise of the other may be accepted by Western society if the decision was made fairly, for example, by means of anatomy. Each argument has both strengths and weaknesses but none can fully withstand in-depth scrutiny.

Physicians must pay attention to their own moral compass and come to terms with the Hippocratic Oath when dealing with some of these cases. Surgeons need to examine their own motives for offering the surgery and ensure that they are moti-vated to determine and provide what is best for the children and family rather than for any personal gain through notoriety or acclaim. It is crucial in these cases to partner not only with medical colleagues but also with the hospital staff and admin-istration. Not all hospitals may be willing to take on such cases for any of a variety of reasons, including religious beliefs, media exposure, and financial concerns. We have found that for particularly complex cases where ethical concerns may be more prominent, presentation at hospital or university eth-ics boards and hospital forums directed toward and limited to the nurses, physicians, and other health professionals who will be involved with the care of the twins does a great deal to

alleviate concern and allows the development of a common purpose when caring for these children. When the health care team understands up front why certain decisions were made, problems and concerns can be addressed and resolved.

The most important part in the decision-making process is to provide the parents with enough information to allow an informed decision. While entire teams of health care profes-sionals may be involved with these children, the physician–patient relationship with 1 surgeon who is leading the care may allow many of these ethical issues to be resolved. We have often found it useful to have 1 of our neonatologists who is a member of the hospital ethics board involved in these discussions as this allows the parents another perspective and helps ensure that a realistic set of expectations are cre-ated when all of the options are discussed. A practical refer-ence that may be useful to help direct decision-making is the Great Ormand Street Ethical Guidelines for Conjoined Twin Separation. These guidelines state that when separation is fea-sible with a reasonable chance of success with 2 live infants, surgery should be offered and carried out. If surgery is not possible, custodial care should be offered and nature allowed to take its course. If 1 twin is dead or has a lethal anomaly and cannot survive independently from its normal twin, and both would die if not separated, separation to save the healthy twin should be attempted.

## Obstetrical Management

Conjoined twins may be born either by C-Section or transvag-inally. Elective C-Section at 36 to 38 weeks after the lungs are determined to be mature may be preferable, though premature labor is common. At the Red Cross War Memorial Children's Hospital in Cape Town, South Africa, vaginal deliveries are allowed if the combined weight of the infants is predicted to be less than 3.9 kg. Transvaginal deliveries of larger babies may suffer a higher rate of problems with dystocia and stillbirth, while smaller infants including thoracopagus and ischiopagus twins were born transvaginally without injury to the connect-ing bridge with 1 exception of a ruptured omphalocele.

## Postnatal Management and Timing of Surgery

After delivery, the twins need to undergo immediate resus-citation and evaluation for the need for emergent separa-tion. Stable twins are a clear indication for systematic and well-organized evaluation and preparation. In cases requir-ing emergent surgery, infants should undergo echocardiog-raphy and plain skeletal films. Based on these studies and the physical examination much of the expected anatomy may be predicted and specific studies may be obtained as time and circumstances allow. While some have recommended separa-tion in the first 4 to 6 weeks of life, O'Neill notes that emer-gent separation or separation within the first 4 months of life carries a much higher mortality rate, as high as 70% com-pared to elective separation. Emergent surgery is needed if there is injury to the connecting bridge of tissue, the status of 1 infant threatens the life of 1 or both twins, or there is a condition such as a bowel obstruction or a cardiac defect that requires surgical intervention (Fig. 60-2). Procedures needed should be planned with the eventual separation surgery in mind. Infants with imperforate anus, for example, will need

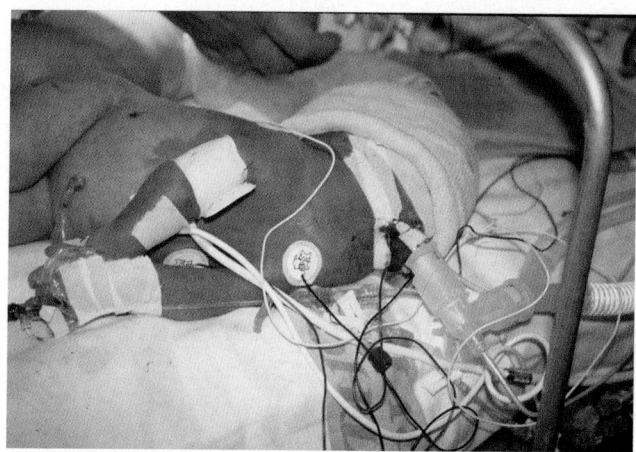

**FIGURE 60-2** Pygopagus twins. The left twin has a life-threatening cardiac anomaly and severe brain anomalies noted on prenatal MRI. This knowledge predelivery allowed the operating team to be ready for emergent separation at birth to save the right twin.

a diverting ostomy and this should be placed with separation planes and eventual tissue flaps and blood supply given due consideration. Placement of an ostomy through the umbilicus or in the midline, for example, may preserve future flap blood supply.

If the twins are stable, a more thorough evaluation is necessary. Elective separation is generally performed 4 to 12 months after birth. In some cases, staged operations may be necessary to achieve the desired results. Delay of the separation surgery allows for growth and for more information on the anatomic union to be obtained. Anesthetic management becomes easier with time and the infants are better able to tolerate blood loss and physiologic derangement. Vascular access becomes easier, though, for some types of twin separations, adequate central venous access will still be needed at the time of separation. It is important to consider the psychologic aspects of the twins as well. There is evidence that twins separated after 1 year of age may have a more difficult time developing a sense of their own individual identity as previously they have identified self as the conjoined state. Not surprisingly, there is frequently a more dominant twin based at least partly on size differences. Sometimes this dominance recedes when the twins are separated.

Attention to nutrition and growth is essential in forming the timeline for surgery. Differential growth rates of the infants are not uncommon despite what would seem to be normal caloric intake for both children. Feeding tubes for either or both infants may at some point be necessary. Differences in portal blood flow and cross-over circulation may account for some of the differences in growth between infants. If there is a distinct difference in growth between the two, separation may be needed in order for the smaller infant to gain weight and grow adequately.

The team described earlier should meet to plan the operation. The operating room nurses and technicians should be chosen and included in the planning sessions. A diagram of the operating room and of the location of necessary equipment should be made. This should include provisions for arranging the operating tables and personnel after the

infants have been separated but also prior to completion of the operation. Sometimes it is also helpful for all the personnel to actually have a dress rehearsal using toy dolls. Surgical skin preparation, draping, placement of electrocautery pads, and monitoring devices may be challenging and should be considered and rehearsed prior to the actual separation surgery.

Conjoined twins often attract media attention. In addition to the considerations and planning involved in designing the actual operation, the team leader must also keep in mind the publicity and security issues. Discussions with the family should be held early to determine what if any media will be involved. If the media is to be involved, it is probably best for the medical team to take charge up front and control the flow of information. The communications department of the hospital can provide help in arranging news conferences and in directing the access of the press to the family and medical staff involved.

Security is related to the decision of how to handle the press and public. If access is limited, which is usually necessary at least for the safety of the infants and personnel, the security staff will need to devise a plan to secure parking access and hospital entrances. In addition, the security staff will need to plan for controlling access to the operating room. Special identification of the medical staff involved should be required. If the media is involved, plans should be made for a postoperative press conference and for periodic conferences as the infants recover. In addition to questions regarding the medical condition of the conjoined twins, the medical staff and hospital representatives should be prepared to answer questions regarding the financial considerations of the care of the infants. The staff may also need to explain difficult considerations regarding the survival of one or both infants.

Plans may also be made for recording the events related to the conjoined twins and the operation to separate them. When the hospital plans to record the operation, the hospital and medical staff can decide what to release to the media. Furthermore, a closed-circuit monitor can be established in a separate but limited-access room for interested medical personnel to view the operation. This limits the number of people in the operating room to only those needed.

## DIAGNOSTIC PRINCIPLES

Most conjoined twins are identified prenatally by ultrasound evaluation. This is frequently a routine prenatal ultrasound or an ultrasound performed to evaluate polyhydramnios, which may occur in conjunction with conjoined twins. Ultrasound diagnosis has been made as early as 12 weeks gestation, though it is more accurate after 20 weeks. Ultrasound findings suggesting conjoined twins include same-sex twins, a single placenta, shared organs, and persistent alignment. Serial ultrasound examinations in the second trimester may further help to define anatomy. Magnetic resonance imaging (MRI) is often used to help define anatomy as it does not involve radiation to the fetus. This may at times add information that ultrasound cannot define because of fetal positioning or the presence of oligo- or polyhydramnios.

**TABLE 60-2** **Diagnostic Evaluation of Conjoined Twins**

| | | |
|---|---|---|
| **Prenatal** | | |
|   Ultrasound | — | Reveals shared areas and other anomalies |
|   Echocardiogram | — | Cardiac anatomy and potential shared structures |
|   MRI | — | As needed to further define anatomy |
| **Postnatal** | | |
|   Physical examination | — | General condition; estimation of shared surface area; vessels of umbilicus; other anomalies |
|   Roentgenograms | — | Overview of possible shared structures |
|   Computerized tomography | — | Details of shared structures; 3D skeletal reconstructions, estimation of shared circulation |
|   Upper gastrointestinal study; barium enema | — | Evaluates extent of shared bowel |
|   Cystogram with retrograde evaluation of ureters | — | Evaluates content of shared renal, bladder, and ureter |
| Liver scan | — | Estimates the extent of shared biliary system and extent of shared liver parenchyma |
| Angiography[a] | — | Anatomy of shared blood vessels and estimation of shared circulation |
| Cardiac catheterization[a] | — | Anatomy of shared hearts and estimation of shared circulation |
| Nuclear medicine flow study | — | Estimates and quantitates shared circulation |
| Magnetic resonance imaging[a] | — | Fine detail of shared bony and soft-tissue structures, including the nervous system |

[a]May require anesthesia.

The ultrasound and MRI should help to define the areas of union. A fetal echocardiogram (ECHO) should also be performed. This will help to identify the degree of cardiac connection in thoracopagus twins and any congenital anomalies present in other conjoined twins. Prenatal evaluation of shared organs and other potential anomalies will aid the surgeon and the neonatologist in consulting with the family regarding possible postnatal outcome and the ability to separate the infants. Some families may opt for termination of the pregnancy especially if the twins have anomalies not compatible with life. These evaluations may also allow the surgical team to identify problems likely to require emergent separation or use of techniques such as the ex utero intrapartum (EXIT) procedure.

Postnatally, the evaluation should be directed by the condition of the twins and by the type of union. The physical examination and condition of the infants is the most important initial information to be gathered. Separate medical records should be kept for each child. For twins who are stable, as much functional and anatomic information as possible should be gathered to help determine separability and functional outcome. Many of the anatomic problems can be predicted from the type of twinning, and some surgeons have proceeded with separation only with the knowledge of prenatal ultrasound and the external anatomy. While in some cases this may be all that is needed, separation surgeries are more likely to be successful if the twins are thoroughly evaluated. Ample literature is available, such that the surgical team should be familiar with the potential anatomic configurations to be expected and the various ways other surgical teams have handled the spectrum of problems. It is important to realize that despite extensive work-up not all anatomic

variations may be identified preoperatively, and the surgical team should be ready to confront unexpected findings. The work-up may be complex, so it is important to have 1 surgeon responsible for the overall care and management of the twins, who can coordinate the evaluation schedule and the various services involved in the care of the infants, pre-, intra-, and postoperatively.

Postnatal evaluation may include routine roentgenograms, computerized tomography, MRI, angiography, gastrointestinal studies, cystograms, and radionucleotide studies to evaluate the biliary system and the degree of blood exchange. Not every set of conjoined twins will need all of these imaging studies performed. Starting with the most basic and then adding studies as needed is the most logical approach (Table 60-2). It may not be possible to define all of the anatomy preoperatively so it is important to expect the unexpected during separation.

## EVALUATION AND TREATMENT OPTIONS

Historically, separation of conjoined twins was often described as the effort of 1 surgeon and 1 team. Successful separation of complex conjoined twins actually takes the efforts of many experts, though all of the activity should be coordinated through 1 lead surgeon. Each twin needs his or her own surgical team, which may include pediatric general, orthopedic, plastic, cardiac, neurologic, and urologic surgeons. In the operating room, 2 separate anesthetic teams and teams of nurses and support staff are needed.

## Anesthesia

Anesthetic management of conjoined twins may be complex, and requires 2 complete anesthetic teams. Cross-circulation may affect how 1 medication or anesthetic affects the infants. Each child should be monitored as if they were a physical individual with pulse oximetry, blood pressure, temperature, electrocardiography, and blood gas monitoring. Adequate venous access for each infant is essential and may require placement of central venous lines. The degree of shared circulation will vary and can be estimated from the preoperative diagnostic studies. General anesthesia is usually induced sequentially while the other infant is monitored for effects of the anesthetic. It may be necessary to synchronize the ventilation in order to ensure adequate ventilation for each infant. Intubation should be performed with the infants lying in as natural a position as possible as cases have been described where if 1 child is suspended above the other to facilitate intubation, vascular collapse may occur in the upper infant due to dependent venous drainage. Adrenal insufficiency is mentioned by several authors for intraoperative consideration. Some authors recommend intraoperative corticosteriods. All of the anesthetic equipment and vascular access needs to be labeled and color-coded to ensure each infant receives the proper medications.

## Cardiovascular System

All sets of conjoined twins should undergo cardiac evaluation. While for some types of twinning, cardiac union will not be present, for others, it is crucial to determine whether 2 separate hearts exist. Echocardiography and electrocardiography are needed in all sets to evaluate any cardiac abnormalities. Twins with 1 QRS complex between them are not separable with 2 survivors, and even the presence of 2 separate QRS complexes does not necessarily mean they can be successfully separated with both twins surviving. Three-dimensional magnetic resonance angiography or CT angiography as well as radionucleide cardioangiography may be used to evaluate cardiac anatomy. In addition, cardiac catheterization may be necessary. Angiography may be necessary to elucidate crossover circulation or to assess blood supply to shared structures such as the tripus leg in ischiopagus tripus twins who may have the dominant blood supply to the leg from 1 infant (Fig. 60-3). Identification of the blood source may be crucial in determining which infant receives a particular structure during separation. Infants with a shared intestine often have a dual blood supply that may allow for allocation of various parts of the intestine to either infant. The degree of the shared circulation is also an important information in terms of the dependence of 1 twin on the other, and with respect to administering medications to each twin. If adequate information is not obtained from the CT, angiograms, and cardiac catherization, a nuclear medicine study can be used to estimate the degree of admixture of the circulatory systems.

The extent of cardiac union is crucial in determining the ability to separate thoracopagus twins. It is often difficult to determine the actual anatomy of many reported cases of conjoined twins as the anatomy is not always clearly described. Spencer and McMahon in 2006 described a series of 1262 conjoined twins with cardiac defects reported in 834 cases (66%).

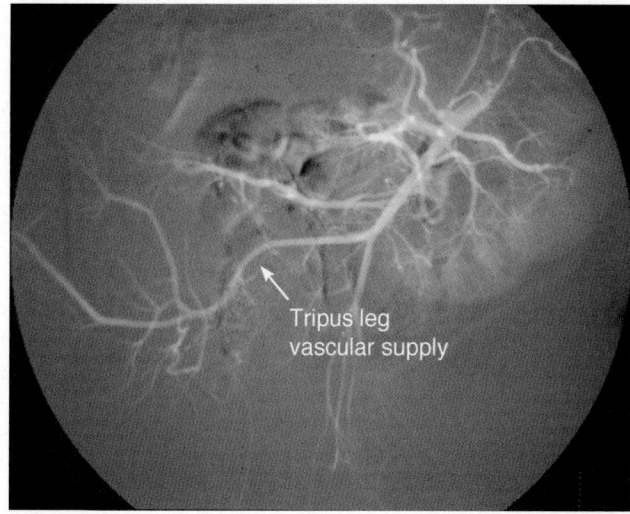

**FIGURE 60-3** Angiogram of ischiopagus tripus twins showing the blood supply to the tripus leg coming from the twin on the left.

Such defects were more common in twins joined ventrally and more frequent with more rostral unions and in the right twin. Transposition of the great vessels and truncus arteriosus predominated defects found in the right twin and laterality defects were more common in the left twin. In cephalopagus twins the posterior heart was noted to often be functionless. Thoracopagus twins share a single compound heart with supernumerary chambers and complex patterns of blood flow. There can be 1 to 4 atria and 1 to 4 ventricles with several variations of great vessel and coronary artery orientation. In the review by Spencer, which reported 14 attempted separation cases with complex atrio-ventricular union, there are no reported cases of 2 surviving twins. Even 1 survivor is extremely unlikely with 2 reported short-term (months) survivors and 1 longer survivor from Cape Town. Infants with only a simple intra-atrial channel have been separated successfully, though mortality remains high. There are 7 reported cases of the twin-reversed arterial perfusion (TRAP) sequence in which 1 twin, the pump fetus, perfused the other twin, the perfused fetus. The latter usually has severe cardiac malformations including acardia.

Omphalopagus and thoracopagus twins have often been lumped into 1 category as externally they may appear similar. Omphalopagus twins, however, never have a shared heart, though they may share a single pericardium but otherwise have separate cardiac structures. There is the rare report of a connecting fibrous band without a lumen in this type of twin. Ischiopagus twins never share the heart but have an increased incidence of cardiac defects (10%) compared to the general population. Parapagus, depending on the subclassification by Spencer (tetrabrachius tripus, tribrachius tripus, tribrachius dipus, dicephalus, dibrachius dipus, and diprosopus), may share a common heart or may be completely separate. Duplication of the heart increases from 60% in dicephalus twins to >80% in tri- and tetrabrachius twins.

## Respiratory System

The lungs are part of foregut development and, with the exception of abnormalities of lobulation, generally develop normally in separable types of conjoined twins including thoracopagus twins. Since most conjoined twins are delivered prematurely, lung function may be an issue for many twins when they are first born. The frequency of cardiac anomalies may also impact lung function of the infants. Omphalopagus, thoracopagus, and parapagus twins may have significant scoliosis or lordosis to the spine or compression of the medial thoracic cages of either or both twins leading to pulmonary hypoplasia or restrictive pulmonary disease. These issues may become important at the time of separation but may also come into play years later with thoracic insufficiency secondary to the spinal and rib deformity.

## Gastrointestinal Tract

### Hepatobiliary

The degree to which the gastrointestinal tract is shared is highly variable between the different types of conjoined twins, and significant variations may exist even within the same category of twins. For twins with shared liver parenchyma, it is necessary to define the biliary system of each infant and the hepatic vasculature. If separation is considered, it is essential that 2 separate hepatic venous systems drain into separate infracardiac vena cavas. The biliary system may be fully separate, but may also be conjoined and require complex reconstruction in order to allow biliary drainage for each infant. CT, MRI, and HIDA scanning may be needed to help establish the nature of the biliary systems, and even with these studies, intraoperative cholangiography may be required. This is particularly true for thoracopagus and omphalopagus twins. Thoracopagus twins have been described with 1 or 2 extrahepatic biliary trees. If there are 2 duodenums, then 2 extrahepatic biliary trees exist, while if there is but 1 duodenum, there are descriptions of either 1 or 2 separate extrahepatic biliary trees. Two extra hepatic systems have been described joining at a common ampulla of Vater. If only 1 pancreas is present, it is best to leave the biliary ducts with that organ and plan reconstruction in the other twin. Up to 17% of thoracopagus twins will have significant biliary anomalies including biliary atresia. Thoracopagus twins with 1 biliary system have been separated using various creative methods for reconstruction. Several of these are nicely outlined in the article by Meyers et al in 2002. Various types of portoenterostomies, suturing bowel to cut surfaces of the liver using a Roux en y reconstruction or the appendix, have been described. Other cases describe other reconstruction methods using hepaticoenterostomies or hepaticoduodenostomies.

Separation of the hepatic parenchyma must be undertaken carefully not only because of concerns for blood loss, but also because hypotension and bradycardia may develop during separation due to distraction and distortion of vessels and blood-flow compromise. Further care must be exercised in separation of the liver in twins with extensive hepatic union, as variations in hepatic arterial supply exist—some of which may preclude separation. Prior to division of the hepatic parenchymal bridge, a complete dissection of the portal structures, including the bile ducts and vascular anatomy, is needed. During hepatic division, careful hemodynamic monitoring is essential as some infants may have significant intrahepatic shunting. Cases have been described in which 1 infant suffered blood loss into the other twin through various intravascular connections when the cross-circulation between the livers was clamped. Blood loss may be minimized by use of circumferential Penrose drains used to compress the parenchyma during division, and large mattress sutures along the cut edge may be placed after division to help ensure hemostasis.

### Intestine

The gastrointestinal tract is shared in all types of conjoined twins except craniopagus and rachipagus twins. Thoracopagus and omphalopagus twins may share a common duodenum, though this would be more likely with thoracopagus twinning. As noted, a shared duodenum should alert one to the likelihood of a common biliary tree. The pancreas is most often separate but may be fused. Ischiopagus and some parapagus twins will have separate upper gastrointestinal systems, and fusion of the bowel at the level of a Meckels diverticulum with a shared colon (Fig. 60-4). Pygopagus twins share a common rectum with separation of the bowel just proximal to that segment. The anus in many of these infants is often oriented more toward one twin and will determine the reconstructive options.

The blood supply to the common sections of the ileum and the colon is from each twin and may likely be separated. Preoperative angiography is important; however, the intestinal blood supply may originate more from one child than the other as the twin's union moves from ischiopagus tripus toward parapagus twinning. While there may be 2 separate GI tracts to the level of the distal small bowel, with each of these types of twins, the blood supply may come primarily from 1 twin or the venous return may be primarily into 1 liver. Either of these anatomic conditions may have significant ramifications for the ability to separate the twins.

Gastrointestinal reconstruction of ischiopagus and some separable parapagus twins should attempt to provide each infant with an intestinal sphincter: the ileocecal valve to one and the anal sphincter to the other, though it is possible that 2 more or less developed anal sphincters may exist. The twin

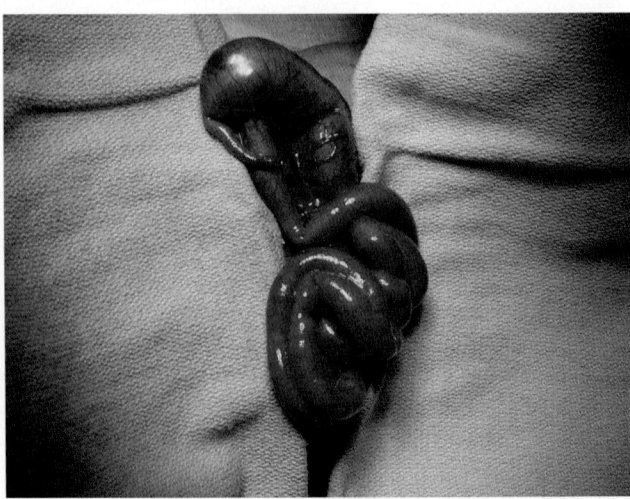

**FIGURE 60-4** Distal small intestine at the area of union into the common terminal ileum and colon in parapagus twins.

with the colon more oriented into their body may be more amenable to receiving the more fully developed anal sphincter. The other twin should receive the ileocecal valve and an attempt made at reconstruction of an anal sphincter. Distribution of the ileocecal valve and the anal sphincter will slow intestinal transit and allow improved nutrition. The colon may be separated longitudinally or divided transversely. We have done the latter with good result. The infant receiving the ileocecal valve then receives the proximal colon, and the distal colon is allocated to the infant with the rectum and anal sphincter. Anoplasties may be performed for each infant at the time of separation. The visualization of the reconstruction is excellent during separation because of the open pelvic rings in some twins, such as ischiopagus. The approach to the levator musculature may be from the anterior approach rather than posteriorly as described in the typical posterior sagittal anorectoplasty. The anal reconstruction has been described both with and without diverting ostomies. Even in children with poorly developed anal musculature, social continence may be achieved through bowel management and the use of further procedures such as an antegrade continence enema (ACE) procedure.

## Genito-Urinary System

The perineum and genitourinary systems of the 2 twins may be quite complex particularly for ischiopagus, parapagus, and pygopagus twins. As the continuum of twinning moves from parapagus dicehpalus, dibrachius to ischiopagus tripus and tetrapus, the perineum also moves through a spectrum of union. In the former type of twin, there is likely a single normal-appearing perineum with associated single set of genitourinary structures. As twins move though the spectrum of parapagus toward the ischiopagus, additional sets of perineal structures will emerge posteriorly, as will the eventual posterior legs of ischiopagus tripus and tetrapus twins (Fig. 60-5). As the structures emerge posteriorly, the anterior structures tend to be more well-developed while the posterior ones may be more rudimentary. As the perineum becomes more complex, so too does the internal associated anatomy. Evaluation with CT, ultrasound, pyelography, cystography, and radionucleid studies may be needed. During separation, cystoscopy is an essential component of the procedure to help define anatomy and place appropriate tubes for identification purposes. Because the cystoscopy may take some time, we have found it advantageous in some cases to tackle this a day prior to the actual separation. Depending on the length of time anticipated for separation, this may be helpful as it may provide additional useful information, though it does require a second anesthetic.

The twins genitourinary system may be quite complex and involve from 1 to 4 kidneys with variations in the number of ureters and cross-over drainage into the opposite twin. Ischiopagus and parapagus twins may have cloacal anomalies, urogenital sinuses, or a mix of the two. Vaginoscopy and vaginography may be helpful in defining this anatomy. The vagina and uterus may carry a dual blood supply with half supplied from each twin. It may be possible to move an entire vagnia/uterus complex into 1 infant or split them and retubularize the structures based on the blood supply. As with the perineum, the posterior genitourinary structures will likely be more rudimentary and may or may not be useful. Male genitalia should be evaluated carefully to determine whether adequate reconstruction may be carried out for a male. The goal of successful urogenital reconstruction is to provide normal renal function and drainage, spontaneous voiding, urinary continence, normal sexual activity, and an acceptable appearance.

## Skeletal System

The skeletal structure of the twins may vary from being almost fully united as in craniopagus twins, to pygopagus twins where the union may only be in the sacrum to a varying degree. Computerized tomographic three-dimensional reconstruction of the skeleton may be very helpful in determining the anatomy (Fig. 60-6). Creation of plastic models to help better visualize the skeletal structures may be needed. For ischiopagus and certain separable types of parapagus twins, 2 separate pelvic rings of varying degrees may exist. Once separated, it may be possible to close the ring in some cases, or it may be necessary to reconstruct the ring with

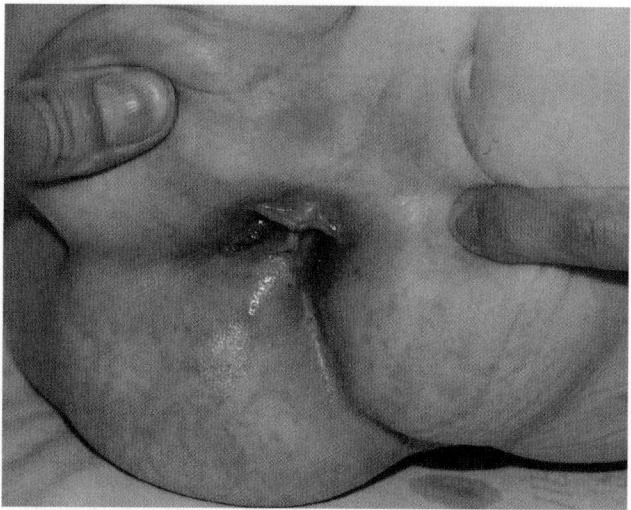

**FIGURE 60-5** Perineum of ischiopagus tripus twins showing 2 separate sets of external urogenital structures and the tripus buttock/leg. The twin on the right had a cloaca while the twin on the left had a urogenital sinus.

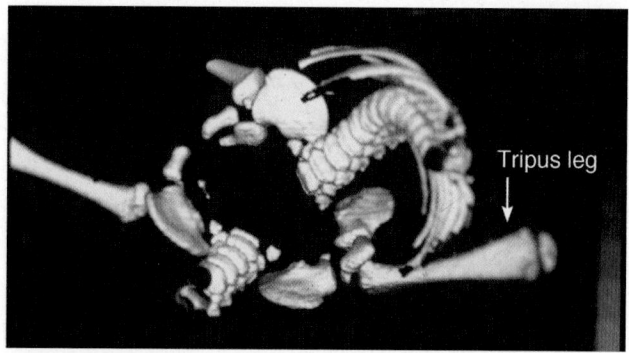

**FIGURE 60-6** CT skeletal reconstruction of ischiopagus tripus twins showing the shared pelvis and shared leg.

native or allograft bone. In some cases, the ring may needed to be left open with closure delayed until later, because of problems with the abdominal domain if the ring is closed at the time of separation. An analogous situation would be the staged closure of cloacal exstrophy in which, after initial closure of the omphalocele and retubularization of the intestinal tract, the abdomen is closed by conversion to bladder exstrophy, and the pelvis is left open until the bladder is closed. Scoliosis may become a significant problem as the children age whether they are separated or not. Initially, the degree of spinal rotation may cause thoracic insufficiency or may compromise the medial lung of each twin. We have eventually done spinal instrumentation for some of these children due to their increasing scoliosis with age.

## Central Nervous System (CNS)

Ischiopagus and pygopagus twins may have no CNS connection or may share a part of the CNS either with fusion of the spinal cord or with sharing of the dural sac. MRI is useful to help delineate this union. Separation of the neural elements should take place prior to any of the intestinal reconstruction to avoid contamination of the neural space. Craniopagus twins are a significant operative challenge with division of the shared blood supply one of the most crucial and life-threatening problems. The operation may be done in either a single stage or multiple stages with gradual rerouting of the blood supply. The latter may be associated with an increased likelihood of success.

## Integument

One of the greatest risks of separation of conjoined twins is the large defect that must be closed at the end. It is important to remember that separation is only half of the operation; reconstruction will dictate the long-term outcome. Measurement of the estimated shared surface area is useful in determining whether adequate skin and soft tissue will be present for closure. If not, consideration may be given to tissue expansion (Fig. 60-7). Both skin and peritoneal expanders have been described. Tissue expansion has been described as performed acutely, but also over a longer 6- to 8-week period of time. Because of the time it may take for adequate tissue expansion, coordination of the timing of surgery and the various procedures that may be needed is crucial. One must also pay

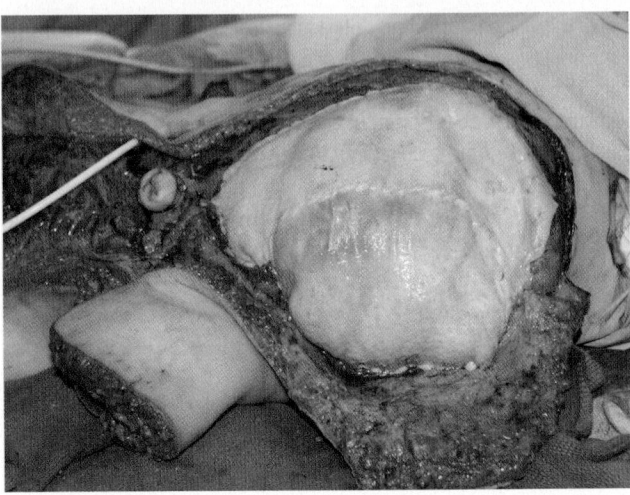

**FIGURE 60-8** Acellular human dermis used to reconstruct the abdominal wall of ischiopagus tripus twins. Ten years after reconstruction there is no evidence of weakening of the abdominal wall or hernia development.

attention to the placement of incisions for other procedures so that tissue planes and blood supply needed for potential flaps and tissue expansion are not disrupted. More rapid tissue expansion may lessen the risk for infection, skin erosion, and loss of a tissue expander. Even with tissue expansion, adequate tissue may not be available for wound closure. Various fascial substitutes including synthetic and processed human and porcine tissue have been used (Fig. 60-8). Additionally, various flaps are described, which can bridge the large tissue gaps that must be filled. For example, the tripus leg in ischiopagus twins may not adequately function as an extremity for either twin. We and others have used the deboned leg successfully as a tissue flap to close the abdomen of one of the twins during separation (Fig. 60-9). We have not found ventral hernias to be a problem with over a 10-year follow-up after use of either the tripus leg or acellular human dermal grafts used for abdominal wall reconstruction.

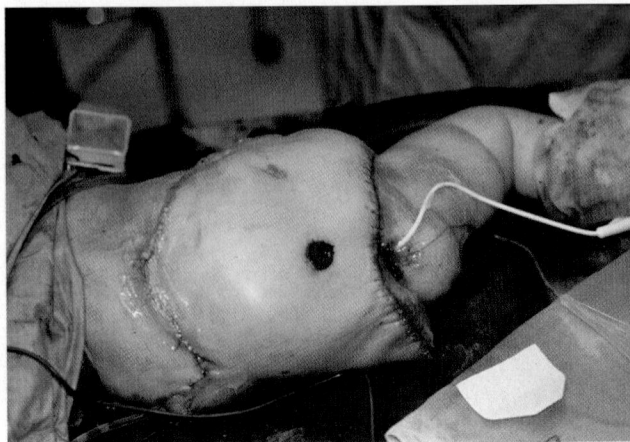

**FIGURE 60-9** Use of the deboned tripus leg to close the abdominal defect of the twin who had the arterial supply to the leg. It was felt the leg would not function well as an extremity and the tissue would be put to better use in this manner.

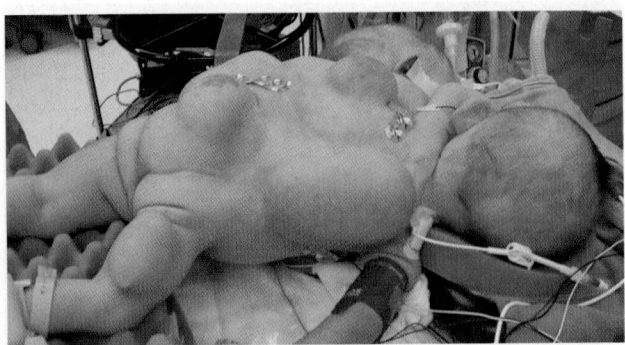

**FIGURE 60-7** Placement of tissue expanders for parapagus conjoined twins.

## TREATMENT OUTCOMES

Initially, medicine had little to offer conjoined twins. Even as recently as the last century, conjoined twins were not considered separable by most physicians and surgeons. As medicine and surgery have advanced, the survivability of conjoined twins has improved. Now complex conjoined twins can be considered for separation and have acceptable long-term outcomes. The outcome is dependent on the type of twinning and the internal anatomy. Separation surgery must pay attention to functional outcome and appearance. Mortality rates are the highest for thoracopagus and craniopagus twins due to the complexity of the vascular anatomy. Ischiopagus and pygopagus twins are likely to survive despite the potential for complex internal anatomy and difficulties with separation. This success is in part the consequence of detailed planning, but even so, the mortality for some types of separation surgeries remains relatively high compared to other pediatric surgical operations.

One area that is not frequently discussed in consideration of conjoined twins is the immediate postoperative care. Depending on the tightness of the abdominal and thoracic closure, the infants may be difficult to ventilate and even have evidence of pulmonary hypertension. Usually this resolves in a matter of days, though some infants will continue to demonstrate problems with restrictive disease. Infection and wound breakdown are the major contributors to morbidity and even mortality in the postoperative period. Nutrition may be an issue, and thus central hyperalimentation or enteral feeding tubes may be needed.

The infants may require future operations either for staged correction of additional congenital anomalies or for problems related to closure and the initial reconstruction. For example, thoracic deformities may exist in both omphalopagus and thoracopagus twins. Scoliosis and torticollis may be present postoperatively and are related to the position of the twins during their conjoined period. These conditions will require physical therapy and possible operative correction. Prostheses and additional extremity operation may be necessary for some types of twins. Further surgery on the urinary or gastrointestinal tract of ischiopagus or pygopagus twins may be needed to help achieve continence or correct other problems. Parents should be made aware of the potential need for further surgeries when they are first considering separation.

The separation of conjoined twins into 2 separate individuals is one of the most unique and challenging situations presented to the pediatric surgeon. Fortunately, with detailed planning and organization and good teamwork, a majority of twins that come to operation may be successfully separated. Long-term follow-up is needed to help ensure a successful outcome.

## SELECTED READINGS

Annas, GJ. Conjoined twins—the limits of law at the limits of life. *N Engl J Med* 2001;344:1104–1108.

Benirschke K, Temple WW, Bloor CM. Conjoined twins: nosology and congenital malformations. *Birth Defects* 1978;14:179–192.

Dreger AD. *One of Us, Conjoined Twins and the Future of Normal.* Cambridge, MA: Harvard University Press; 2004.

Kapur RP, Jack RM, Siebert JR. Dianmiotic placentation associated with omphalopagus conjoined twins: implications for a contemporary model of conjoined twinning. *Am J Med Genet* 1994;52:188–195.

McMahon CJ, Spencer R. Congenital heart defects in conjoined twins: outcome after surgical separation of thoracopagus. *Pediatr Cardiol* 2006;27:1–12.

Meyers RL, Matlak ME. Biliary tract anomalies in thoraco-omphalopagus conjoined twins. *J Pediatr Surg* 2002;37:1716–1719.

O'Neill JA, Holcomb GW, et al. Surgical experience with thirteen conjoined twins. *Ann Surg* 1988;208:299–312.

Rode H, Fieggen AG, Brown RA, et al. Four decades of conjoined twins at Red Cross Children's Hospital—lessons learned. *SAMJ* 2006;96:931–940.

Spencer R. Anatomic description of conjoined twins: a plea for standardized terminology. *J Pediatr Surg* 1996;31:941–944.

Spencer R. *Conjoined Twins, Developmental Malformations and Clinical Implications.* Baltimore MD: The Johns Hopkins University Press; 2003.

Spencer R. Theoretical and analytical embryology of conjoined twins: Part I: Embryogenesis. *Clin Anat* 2000;13:36–53.

Spencer R. Theoretical and analytical embryology of conjoined twins: Part II: Adjustments to union. *Clin Anat* 2000;13:97–120.

Spitz L. The Conjoined Twins. *Med Sci Law* 2002;42:284–287.

Thomas JM, Lopez JT. Conjoined twins—the anesthetic management of 15 sets from 1991–2002. *Pediatr Anesthesia* 2004;14:117–129.

Votteler TP, Lipsky K. Long-term results of 10 conjoined twins separations. *J Pediatr Surg* 2005;40:618–629.

Walker M, Browd SR. Craniopagus twins: embryology, classification, surgical anatomy, and separation. *Childs Nerv Syst* 2004;20:554–566.

PART V

PART V

UROLOGY FOR THE
PEDIATRIC SURGEON

# CHAPTER 61

# The Acute Scrotum

*Heidi A. Stephany and J. Patrick Murphy*

## KEY POINTS

1. The most common causes of pediatric acute scrotal pain and swelling are torsion of the testis and torsion of the testicular or epididymal appendages.

2. Intravaginal testicular torsion, which is associated with abnormal fixation of the testicle within the tunica vaginalis, is most common at puberty. Extravaginal testicular torsion results from twisting of the spermatic cord proximal to the scrotal tunica vaginalis and is thought to occur during descent of the testicle into the scrotum and is seen in the newborn period.

3. There are numerous causes for acute scrotal swelling, but the most important objective is determining and promptly treating any condition that may destroy the testicle. There is approximately a 6-hour window before irreversible ischemic damage occurs.

4. Testicular appendages are mullerian duct remnants on the superior pole of the testis and the epididymal appendages are Wolffian duct remnants. Torsion of the appendages can mimic spermatic cord torsion. Torsion of the appendages is more likely in later childhood. Tenderness of the upper pole of the testicle only, especially with a firm, tender nodule present is characteristic of a torsed appendix testis. The "blue dot" sign is pathognomonic for torsion of an appendage, but is not seen in all cases.

5. A thorough history and physical exam is typically sufficient for determining an operative intervention for the acute scrotum. The absence of a cremasteric reflex is a good indicator of torsion of the cord. In acute epididymitis, the cremasteric reflex is present. Additional studies, including radiography, should be used in cases to confirm the diagnoses of nontorsion.

6. Nonoperative management is aimed at treating the underlying cause. Torsion of the testicular appendages is often nonsurgical and it is treated medically with analgesics, however, if pain persists, surgical exploration is indicated.

7. Suspected testicular torsion requires immediate surgical intervention. While manual detorsion may be attempted, surgical exploration is still indicated. Exploration of the contralateral hemiscrotum should be carried out as it is common to identify a bell-clapper deformity. Fixation of the contralateral testis is recommended to prevent subsequent torsion.

8. A median raphe incision is used with delivery and detorsion of the affected testicle. The contralateral testicle, and if a viable ipsilateral testicle remains, is pexed with nonabsorbable sutures between the tunica albuginea and the scrotal wall. Orchiectomy should be performed if the affected testicle is obviously necrotic.

9. Urgent exploration is not necessary in perinatal torsion when the scrotum is blue and edematous at birth, indicating ischemia has been present for weeks or days. Controversy regarding prompt exploration of the contralateral testis remains. If symptoms have just occurred, exploration is indicated when the infant's anesthetic and overall general condition has been considered.

10. The differential diagnosis of the acute scrotum represents myriad conditions. The astute clinician must determine the need for immediate surgical intervention versus nonoperative treatment in a timely manner to salvage the viable testicular tissue.

## DISEASE PATHOPHYSIOLOGY

Acute scrotal swelling can occur as a result of many conditions. These include testicular (spermatic cord) torsion, torsion of testicular appendages, epididymitis, orchitis, hernia/hydrocele, trauma, tumor, varicocele, and idiopathic scrotal edema. Age is a major factor in the likelihood of any of these diagnoses. Testicular torsion is most common at puberty and in the newborn period. Torsion of the appendages is more likely in later childhood (6-12 years of age) and epididymitis/orchitis in later adolescence.

Testicular or spermatic cord torsion results from twisting of the spermatic cord which compromises the blood supply to the testicle. The number of twists determines the degree of vascular compromise, but in general there is a window of only

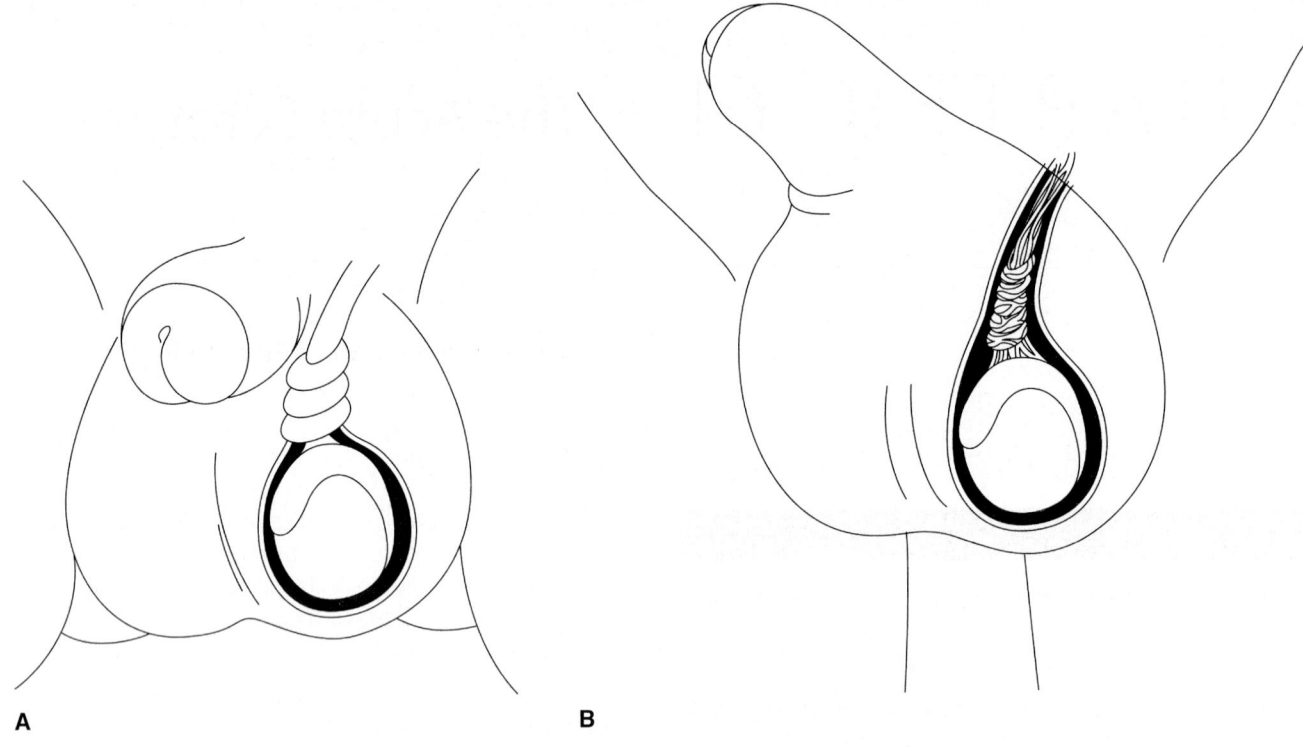

**FIGURE 61-1** Diagram of extravaginal (A) and intravaginal (B) testicular torsion.

about 6 hours before irreversible ischemic damage occurs. The 2 types of testicular torsion are: extravaginal and intravaginal (Fig. 61-1). Extravaginal torsion results from twisting of the spermatic cord proximal to the scrotal tunica vaginalis and is thought to occur during descent of the testicle into the scrotum. As one would expect from this theory, extravaginal torsion occurs in the perinatal period. Intravaginal torsion occurs in the older child and is associated with abnormal fixation of the testicle within the tunica vaginalis. Normally, the tunica will invest the epididymis and posterior surface of the testicle, fixing it to the scrotum and making it unable to twist. When the tunica vaginalis attaches at a more proximal position on the spermatic cord, the testicle and epididymis hang free in the scrotum and can twist within the tunica vaginalis (Fig. 61-2). This abnormal fixation is called the "bell-clapper" anomaly. The incidence in cadavers is 12% and it is often bilateral. The incidence of torsion is significantly less than this; therefore, other factors are important in the etiology of torsion.

Contraction of the cremasteric muscles shortens the spermatic cord and may initiate torsion in males with the "bell-clapper" deformity. Testicular congestion secondary to an inflammatory process or minor trauma may also lead to torsion. The peak incidence at puberty and early adolescence would suggest that the rapid growth and increased vascularity of the testicle associated with the elevated testosterone levels at puberty may also play a role in the initiation of torsion.

The testicular appendages are Mullerian duct remnants on the superior pole of the testis and the epididymal appendages are Wolffian duct remnants. Torsion of these structures is a common cause of acute scrotal pain and swelling, especially in the younger child. Why these structures tend to twist is unknown, but the symptoms often mimic testicular torsion.

Epididymitis and orchitis may be caused by bacterial or viral infection. In the sexually active male, ascending infection by sexually transmitted organisms is the most common etiology. Systemic viral syndromes, especially mumps, can result in orchitis, but is uncommon in young children. Epididymitis in the prepubertal child has a strong association with urinary voiding dysfunction and/or urinary structural anomalies such as ectopic ureters, urethral lesions, or ejaculatory duct anomalies. Pyuria and bacteriuria are often present but not universal. Epididymal inflammation can also be

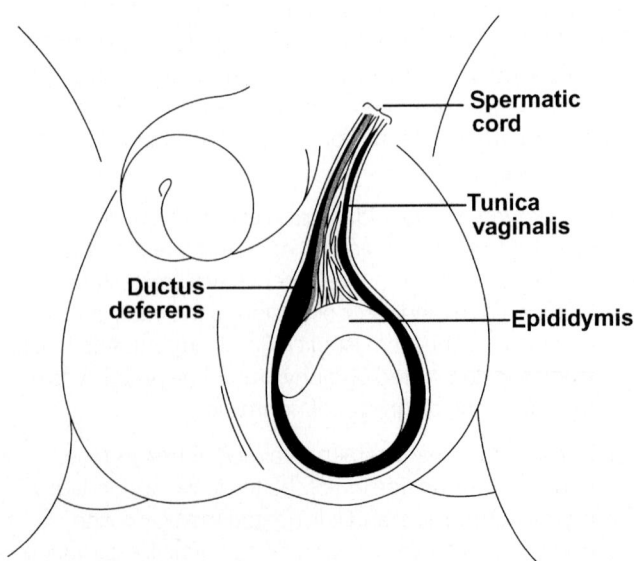

**FIGURE 61-2** Diagram of the "bell-clapper" deformity that predisposes to intravaginal torsion due to failure of the tunica vaginalis to invest the cord and testicle.

secondary to the autoimmune response and vasculitis associated with diseases such as Henoch–Schonlein purpura and polyarteritis nodosum. The scrotal symptoms may precede or be more obvious than the other systemic symptoms. Therefore, a high index of suspicion is necessary to avoid missing the underlying systemic disease.

Hydroceles can be secondary to a patent processus vaginalis or a reactive process in the scrotum. They may occur acutely and may be painful depending on the underlying cause. Incarcerated hernias may cause significant scrotal swelling and may lead to testicular ischemia. Resolution of the scrotal swelling usually follows manual reduction of the hernia. Treating the underlying cause of a hydrocele whether by surgical or medicinal therapy results in its resolution.

Testicular trauma results in scrotal swelling as a result of the direct injury to the scrotal contents or scrotal wall. Surgical treatment is generally not required unless disruption of the tunica albuginea occurs. The traumatic episode may be the first indication of a preexisting condition such as a varicocele or testicular tumor. If the degree of swelling and ecchymosis is significant or seems greater than expected for the level of trauma reported, one should look for an underlying pathologic process such as a tumor or varicocele. It is also important to remember that minor trauma may initiate testicular torsion in some cases. The use of ultrasound with color flow Doppler can help identify such processes.

Another more uncommon cause of acute scrotal swelling is idiopathic scrotal edema. This condition is characterized by edema and erythema of the scrotal wall. It is usually bilateral and it will sometimes involve the penis. The testicle is normal in size and nontender but there may be mild tenderness to the scrotal skin. The etiology is not certain but, it is most likely a reaction to an allergen, bug bite, contact dermatitis, or angioneurotic edema. The condition will resolve spontaneously with symptomatic treatment, but it must be differentiated from a true cellulitis, which would require antibiotic therapy.

## DIAGNOSTIC PRINCIPLES

Acute scrotal swelling can have many causes, and the most important objective is to diagnose and promptly treat any condition that can destroy the testicle. Testicular torsion is the 1 condition that most commonly threatens testicular viability and its diagnosis can most often be made by the history and physical examination. The history of sudden onset of severe unilateral testicular pain, often associated with nausea and vomiting and sometimes abdominal pain, is the classic presentation of testicular torsion. Generally the pain is unrelenting, but there may be a history of previous intermittent attacks of short duration, which would result from torsion–detorsion episodes.

The physical exam should initially address the level of distress the patient exhibits. Torsion of the testicle usually causes the patient to be extremely distressed and he will generally avoid activity. However, some patients can be extremely stoic and the lack of apparent pain does not rule out torsion. The abdomen and inguinal areas should be inspected, looking for other sources of the symptoms such as an incarcerated

inguinal hernia. The scrotum will show various degrees of swelling and erythema depending on the duration of the torsion or an alternate process. Early in the course, landmarks can still be identified in the scrotum but later only a tender phlegmon may be present in the involved hemiscrotum. If the testicle is palpable, examination of the lower pole will generally show marked tenderness on torsion, whereas in epididymitis or torsion of an appendage the lower testicle may not be palpably tender. Tenderness of the upper pole of the testicle only, especially with a firm, tender nodule present is characteristic of a torsed appendix testis. A blue discoloration seen through the scrotal skin overlying the tender nodule is referred to as the "blue dot" sign and is pathognomonic for torsion of an appendage. However, this finding is not identified in all cases of torsed appendix testis. Tenderness of the posterior lying epididymis with a nontender testicle suggests epididymitis; however, an anterior or transverse position of the epididymis suggests torsion. It should always be remembered that testicular torsion can occur subsequent to any of the other conditions that lead to scrotal swelling and this may cloud the presenting history and physical examination.

Diagnostic studies, which may aid in determining the etiology of acute testicular swelling, include urinalysis, radioisotope scanning of the scrotum, and high-resolution ultrasonography with color flow Doppler. Pyuria and bacteriuria are more commonly seen in infectious epididymitis or orchitis, but can be present with torsion. Radioisotope scrotal scanning using a pin hole collimator in experienced hands is a very accurate method of determining testicular ischemia. Its disadvantages include patient exposure to ionizing radiation and the delay involved in obtaining the study. This delay can be significant unless one is at an institution where the study is done frequently. Ultrasonography with color flow Doppler is also an accurate means of detecting testicular ischemia. In general, it is more readily available, can be obtained with minimal delay, and it produces no radiation exposure. Both of these studies have the potential of either a false-positive or -negative result for testicular ischemia. The incidence of error is low, especially in institutions with experienced technicians. However, most clinicians reserve the use of these techniques for those patients who are less likely by history and exam to have testicular torsion, using the flow studies to help confirm the diagnoses of nontorsion. If the clinical history and exam suggest torsion, most surgeons would proceed immediately with scrotal exploration and not delay the procedure to do testicular flow studies.

## TREATMENT OPTIONS

The treatment of the nontorsion causes of scrotal swelling involves management of the underlying condition: antibiotics for infection; reduction and repair of hernias; appropriate detection of and intervention for tumors or trauma diagnosis of any underlying systemic diseases and local care and analgesia for the pain and edema. Torsion of testicular appendages can often be treated nonsurgically, allowing the ischemic structure to become necrotic and then atrophy. The pain is usually short-lived and treatable with oral analgesics. If the

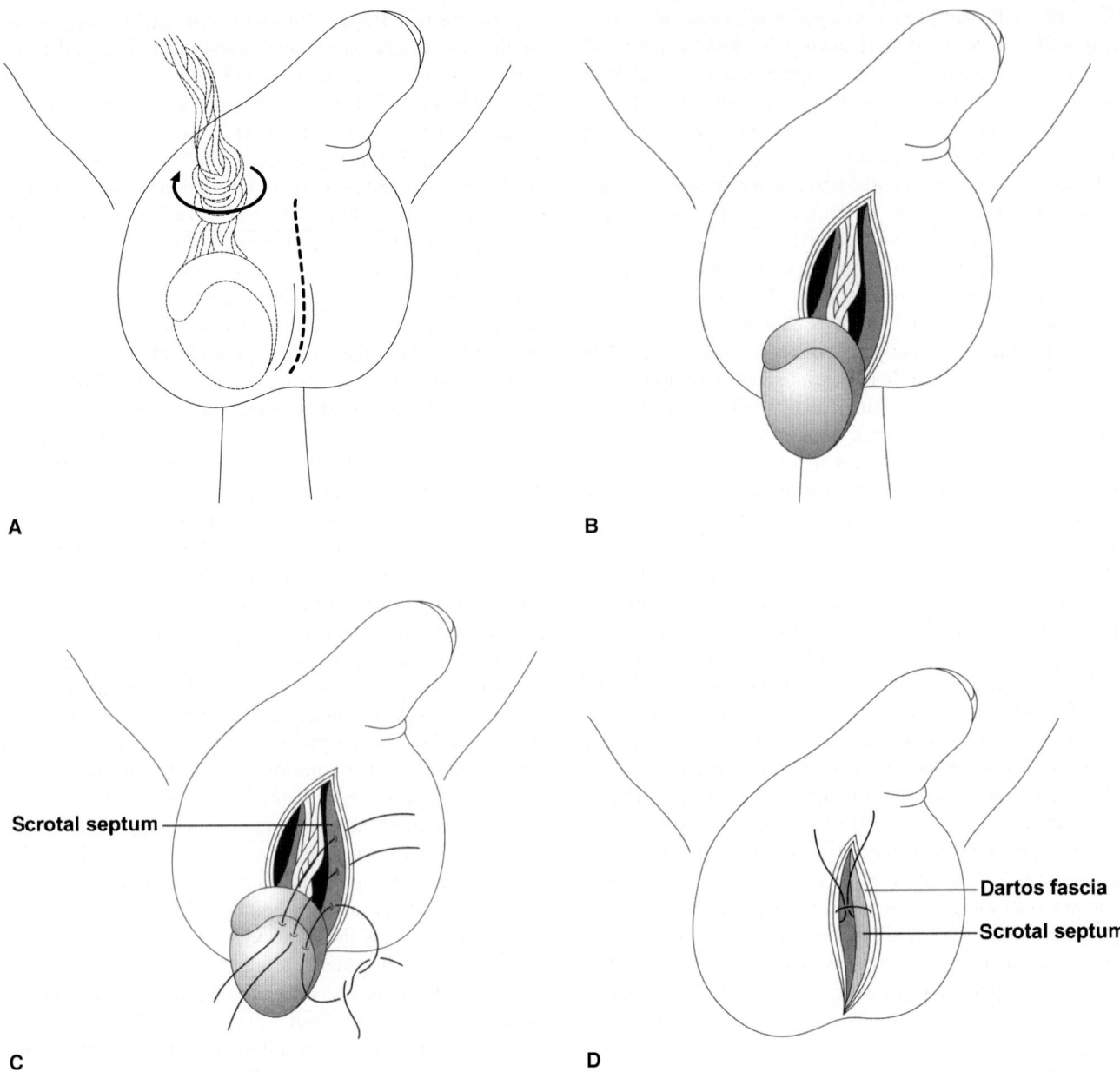

**A**

**B**

**C**

Scrotal septum

**D**

Dartos fascia

Scrotal septum

**FIGURE 61-3** Treatment of testicular torsion. **A.** A midline scrotal incision is made and carried through the fascial layers and through the tunica vaginalis of the involved hemiscrotum. **B.** The testicle is delivered and detorsed. **C.** Fixation is made from the tunica albuginea to the scrotal septum with nonabsorbable sutures in at least 3 different places. It is important to position the epididymis posteriorly and avoid trapping it in the sutures as they are tied. The contralateral testicle is treated in the same fashion. **D.** Closure of the dartos fascia and skin with absorbable sutures.

symptoms persist or increase, surgical treatment is indicated to relieve the symptoms and be sure that a secondary testicular torsion has not occurred.

Suspected testicular torsion warrants immediate surgical intervention. Manual detorsion may be attempted while awaiting the patient's transfer to the operating room. The direction of detorsion should initially be outward (clockwise on the left, counterclockwise on the right), but the direction of torsion can vary. Even if symptoms are relieved after manual manipulation, surgical exploration is still indicated to be certain that complete detorsion is accomplished and retorsion does not occur.

Scrotal exploration is carried out through a median raphe incision, entering the symptomatic scrotal compartment

first and delivering the testicle to allow detorsion (Fig. 61-3). With the torsion relieved, the testicle is placed in warm moist sponges while the opposite scrotal compartment is entered. The contralateral testicle is then fixed with at least 3 nonabsorbable sutures from the tunica albuginea to the scrotal wall. Evaluation of the viability of the involved testis is then made. If it is obviously necrotic, it should be removed. If it appears to be reperfused and bleeding occurs from the cut surface of the testicle, it should be replaced in the scrotum and pexed in the same fashion as the opposite side.

In perinatal torsion, where the scrotum is blue and edematous at birth, usually the testicle has been ischemic for days or weeks and unless symptoms have just occurred in the postnatal period, urgent exploration is not necessary. Most clinicians

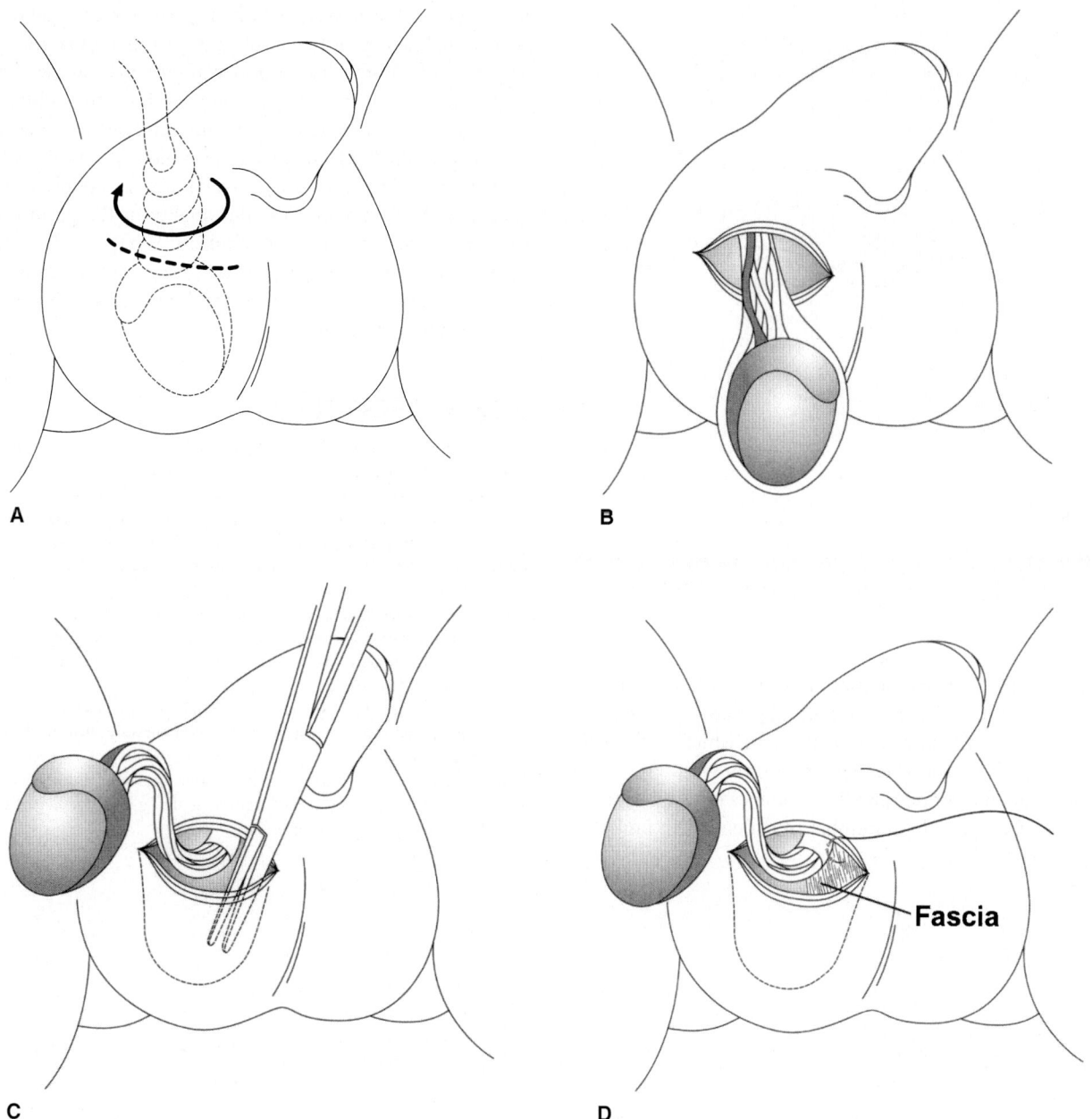

**FIGURE 61-4** Treatment of perinatal testicular torsion. **A.** A transverse incision is made in the upper third of the scrotum. **B.** The tunica vaginalis is opened and the testicle is delivered to the point where the tunica vaginalis invests the cord. **C.** A pouch is created between the dartos and external spermatic fascia large enough to hold the testicle. **D.** The edge of the external oblique fascia is sutured to the tunica vaginalis that overlies the spermatic cord (great care is taken to avoid the spernlatic cord structures).

feel that exploration in the first few days of life is indicated to be certain of the diagnosis. Testicular teratoma or blood and meconium in a hernia sac can mimic perinatal torsion. Also, fixation of the contralateral testis is generally recommended early in life because of reports indicating either synchronous or asynchronous torsion of the opposite side. There is, however, some controversy regarding these recommendations.

This author prefers an inguinal approach to the involved side in perinatal torsion, both because of the possibility of another diagnosis and because it seems easier to deliver and remove the long-term necrotic gonad with extravaginal torsion through this incision (Fig. 61-4). Fixation of the contralateral testes is then done through a transverse scrotal incision

with placement of the gonad in a scrotal pouch between the external spermatic and dartos fascia. This technique is less traumatic to the small, delicate newborn gonad and experimental evidence suggests that anatomic fixation is as good as or better than suture fixation.

## PATIENT OUTCOME

Testicular salvage rates are directly related to the duration and degree of torsion. Testicular atrophy occurs in virtually all testes with duration of symptoms greater than 24 hours.

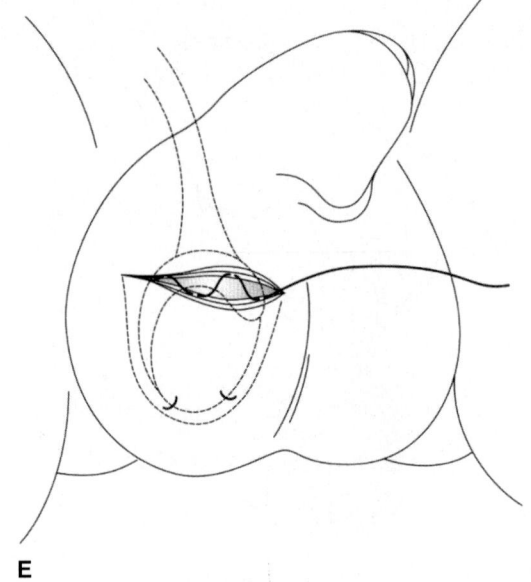

**E**

**FIGURE 61-4** (*Continued*) E. The testicle is placed in the pouch with correct orientation, and the dartos fascia and skin are closed with absorbable sutures.

However, this fact should not dictate a policy of nonexploration in patients with symptoms of greater than 24 hours. Partial or intermittent torsion may occur which could make the testicle salvageable even with long-term symptoms.

Even more important than the incidence of testicular atrophy is the fact that a high number of patients with unilateral testicular torsion have markedly abnormal sperm analyses, indicating bilateral testicular dysfunction in a unilateral disease process. Both clinical and experimental studies have suggested that abnormal spermatogenesis of the contralateral testicle may be related to the infarcted testis remaining *in vivo*, presumably from an autoimmune effect. Other studies have suggested that testes, which are susceptible to torsion, may have an inherent abnormality of the germ cells, similar to that seen in cryptorchidism. Whatever the origin of the abnormality in spermatogenesis, it seems reasonable to remove any testicle that does not show reasonable signs of viability after detorsion.

## SELECTED READINGS

Blyth B. Neonatal testicular torsion. *Dialog Pediatr Urol* 1991;14(5):1–8.

Brandt MT, Sheldon CA, Wacksman J, Matthews P. Prenatal testicular torsion: principles of management. *J Urol* 1992;147:670–672.

Das S, Singer A. Controversies of perinatal torsion of the spermatic cord: a review, survey and recommendations. *J Urol* 1990:143:231–233.

Gatti JM, Murphy JP. Acute testicular disorders. *Pediatr Rev* 2008;29(7): 235–241.

Makela E, Lahdes-Vasama T, Rajakorpi H, et al. A 19-year review of paediatric patients with acute scrotum. *Scand J Surg* 2007;96(1):62–66.

Rabinowitz R, Hulbert WC. Acute scrotal swelling. *Urol Clin N Am* 1995;22(1):101–105.

Soccorso G, Ninan GK, Rajimwale A, et al. Acute scrotum: is scrotal exploration the best management? *Eur J Pediatr Surg* 2010 [Epub ahead of print].

Yagil Y, Naroditsky I, Milhem J, et al. Role of Doppler ultrasonography in the triage of acute scrotum in the emergency department. *J Ultrasound Med* 2010;29(1):111.

# CHAPTER 62

## Cryptorchidism

*Wolfgang Stehr and James M. Betts*

## KEY POINTS

1. Classification of testes falling under the umbrella term "cryptorchidism" includes: intra-abdominal, canalicular, superficial inguinal pouch, ectopic, ascending, vanishing, and absent testis.

2. Orchidopexy is an elective operative procedure best done in the first 6 months of life.

3. Laparoscopic orchidopexy is best reserved for both the diagnosis and treatment of intraabdominal testes, unilateral or bilateral, or for the high canalicular inguinal canal testes. Conventional open orchidopexy is best applied to the palpable superficial inguinal ring area testis or for the testis with a symptomatic inguinal hernia.

4. Testicular descent embryologically is best described by the Hutson 2-phase model. In step one, the abdominal phase (8-15 weeks gestation) is under the influence of MIS; the second inguinoscrotal phase (26-40 weeks gestation) is under androgen stimulation.

## DEFINITIONS

*Cryptorchidism* means hidden or obscure testes and is generally synonymous with undescended testes. *Ectopic testis* defines a condition caused by an abnormally implanted gubernaculum, wherein the testis has descended from the abdominal cavity and settled in the suprapubic area, the thigh, or the perineum instead of the scrotum (a true ectopic testicle is a very rare condition). *Orchidopexy* (synonymous: *orchiopexy*) describes the surgical fixation of the testis in the scrotum and is commonly used to describe the mobilization and fixation of an undescended testis within its respective scrotal compartment.

## EMBRYOLOGY

The primitive gonad begins as coelomic epithelium on the medial aspect of the mesonephros during the fifth week of fetal life. At 7 to 8 weeks of gestation, the primordial germ cells migrate from the embryonic yolk sac to the gonadal cords. Under the influence of SRY (the sex-determining region of the human Y chromosome), which is the testis-determining factor, male differentiation is "switched on." Leydig cells formed from interstitial tissue start secreting testosterone around day 60, and Sertoli cells, under the influence of the follicle stimulating hormone (FSH), start secreting Müllerian inhibiting substance (MIS). MIS enlarges the gubernaculum, induces involution of the ipsilateral Müllerian structures, and increases the number of androgen receptors on the Leydig cell membrane. Testosterone primes the genitofemoral nerve and is responsible for differentiation of the Wolffian duct. The genitofemoral nerve releases the neurotransmitter calcitonin gene related peptide (CGRP) which produces rhythmic gubernacular contractions, and controls migration of the gubernaculum and testes. In the fetus, testosterone shows an initial surge between 12 and 16 weeks of gestation. Later, decreased maternal human chorionic gonadotropin (hCG) and increased maternal estrogen decrease fetal testosterone levels. After birth, decreased maternal estrogens are responsible for the second surge of testosterone, which is seen at around 60 days of life. Hence, most testes which are not descended at birth would descend by 3 months of life.

## DESCENT OF THE TESTES

Several factors have been recognized as important for normal testicular descent: endocrine, mechanical, and neural. In 1985, Hutson proposed a biphasic model for testicular descent. The first phase of testicular descent was described as the transabdominal phase and was thought to be controlled by MIS. During this phase, which takes place at 8 to 15 weeks of gestation, the testis moved from the posterior abdominal wall to the internal inguinal ring. The second phase was described as the inguinoscrotal phase and is assumed to be androgen dependent. During this phase, at 26 to 40 weeks gestation, the testis migrates from the internal inguinal ring to the scrotum. The processus vaginalis bulges into the gubernaculum and elongates to the scrotum. The testis migrates in the processus vaginalis and reaches the scrotum at 35 weeks of gestation. When the testis has descended into the scrotum, the gubernaculum and processus vaginalis involute. An undescended testis may result from a deficiency of various steps in this

**TABLE 62-1** Cryptorchidism in Congenital Malformation Syndromes

**I  Malformation syndromes with endocrine dysfunction**

  1. Syndromes with gonadotropin deficiency
    Kalliman–De Morsier syndrome
    Prader–Willi syndrome
    Laurence Moon and Bardet–Beild syndromes
    LEOPARD syndrome
    Optiz syndrome

  2. Syndromes with primary testicular failure
    Noonans syndrome
    Seckel syndrome
    Enzyme disorders of testosterone synthesis

  3. Persistence of Müllerian duct derivative syndrome

**II  Syndromes with cerebral and/or neuromuscular disorders**

    Pena Schokeir syndrome
    Multiple Pterygium syndrome
    Distal Arthrogryposis syndrome
    Miller–Dicker syndrome

**III  Syndromes with abnormalities of the anterior abdominal wall**

    Prune belly syndrome
    Exomphalos
    Gastroschisis

**IV  Chromosomal Syndromes**

    Syndromes involving chromosomes 4, 8, 9, 10, 13, 15, 18, 21, and 22

testicular descent. An intact hypothalmo-pituitary-testicular axis is considered necessary for normal testicular descent. Androgen insensitivity syndrome results in undescended testes located close to the internal inguinal ring. Various abdominal wall malformations, such as gastroschisis, omphalocele, prune belly syndrome, and bladder exstrophy are associated with undescended testes. Undescended testes may also be encountered in children with neurological defects such as myelomeningocele and microcephaly. Furthermore, cryptorchidism is seen in patients with various endocrine abnormalities and chromosomal aberrations (Table 62-1), as well as in the premature infant.

## INCIDENCE

A prospective study of 7400 male births by the John Radcliffe Hospital Cryptorchidism Study Group found the incidence of cryptorchidism to be 4.9%. Boys with a birth weight of less than 2000 g had a higher incidence (45.4%) compared to those with a birth weight of more than 2500 g (3.8%). At 3 months of age, the overall incidence of cryptorchidism was 1.55%. Another prospective hospital-based cohort study in the United States, consisting of 6935 consecutive male births, reported an incidence of 3.7% cryptorchidism at birth, and

1% at the age of 3 months, and 1% at 1 year of age. In this study, most testes were descended by the age of 3 months.

## CLASSIFICATION AND NOMENCLATURE

Undescended testes can be classified into 3 classes: Those arrested in the line of normal descent, ectopic testes, or absent testes.

## THE INTRA-ABDOMINAL TESTIS

The intra-abdominal testis is one in which inguino-scrotal descent has failed to occur. This testis is located in the abdominal cavity, usually within a few centimeters of the internal inguinal ring. An intra-abdominal testis is always non-palpable. Non-palpable testes comprise 5% to 28% of undescended testis in various series, and are best evaluated laparoscopically (Table 62-2).

## THE CANALICULAR AND/OR EMERGENT TESTIS

A canalicular testis lies within the inguinal canal and may be difficult to palpate. For these patients a laparoscopic inspection/mobilization may be required. However, sometimes it is possible to manipulate this testis distally to the external inguinal ring, in which case it is referred to as an "emergent" testis.

## THE SUPERFICIAL INGUINAL POUCH TESTIS

The superficial inguinal pouch is an areolar space between the external oblique aponeurosis and Scarpa fascia, and is directed obliquely upwards and laterally in front of the pubic

| **TABLE 62-2** | Anatomical Position of 3064 Cryptorchid Testes in 2509 Boys Treated at Our Lady's Hospital for Sick Children, Dublin, Ireland (1969–1995) |
|---|---|
| **Site** | **Number** |
| Superficial inguinal pouch | 2369 (77.3%) |
| Canalicular or abdominal | 547 (17.8%) |
| Vanishing testis | 105 (3.4%) |
| Absent testis | 39 (1.3%) |
| Ectopic | 4 (0.1%) |

tubercle. This is the most common site for an undescended testis (77%) and requires surgical intervention (Table 62-2). A testis situated in this pouch displays great mobility, the range of movement of such a testis being limited only by the areolar margins.

## THE ECTOPIC TESTIS

Ectopic testes are located away from the normal pathway of testicular descent. These testes can be palpated in the perineal, pubopenile, or femoral position. True ectopic testes are very rare (0.1%, Table 62-2).

## THE ASCENDING TESTIS

Testes normally located in the scrotum at birth may later ascend to a higher position and cannot again be manipulated into the scrotum. Ascent of a normally descended testis is an infrequent event and thought to result from cord elongation not keeping up with somatic growth.

## THE VANISHING TESTIS

A vanishing testis is thought to be the result of a vascular or other insult to the developing gonad. The presence of a vas deferens and vessels lying side by side along the normal course of testicular descent, usually in the inguinal canal, strongly suggests that a testis existed at one time and subsequently vanished. Viable testicular remnants have been noted on histological analysis of blind-ending cord structures in 6% to 20% of vanishing testes. It is therefore recommended in order to prevent the risk of future malignancy, that inguinal exploration be carried out in all patients in whom laparoscopy identifies vas and vessels entering the internal ring. It may be prudent to add a contralateral orchidopexy at the time of exploration for the "vanishing testes" if a missed torsion is suspected to have been the likely etiology.

## THE ABSENT TESTIS

For a unilateral or bilateral non-palpable testis, the diagnostic and treatment algorithm is described below (Fig. 62-1).

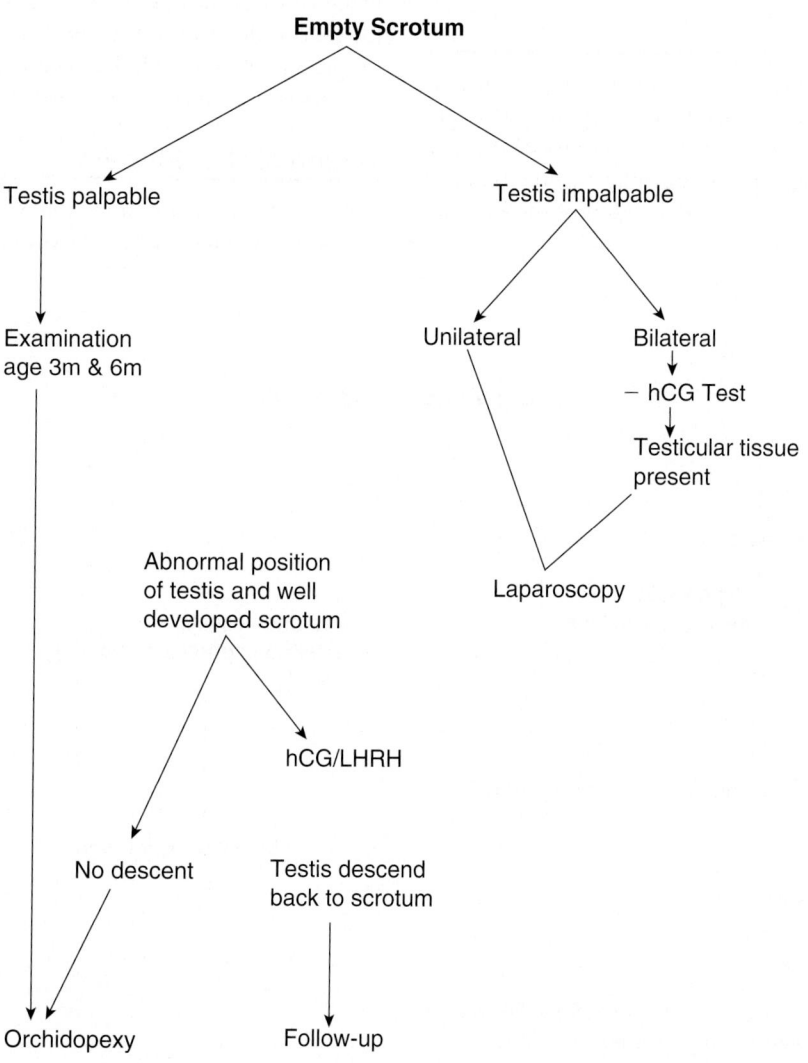

**FIGURE 62-1** Cryptorchidism: diagnostic and treatment algorithm.

# CRYPTORCHIDISM DIAGNOSIS

## Physical Exam

A careful clinical examination is the most important part for the diagnosis of undescended testes. An undescended testis is one that cannot be mobilized to the bottom of the scrotum without overstretching the spermatic cord. A normal testis remains in the scrotum after mobilization even though its initial position was higher. The child should be examined in relaxed and warm surroundings. Boys should be examined at birth, at 3 months of age, and again at 6 months of age, by which time most testes have descended in response to a physiologic postnatal testosterone surge. The position of the testis should be described as either palpable or nonpalpable. If palpable, its location (eg, superficial inguinal pouch testis) should be noted. The appearance of the scrotum should also be assessed and documented (symmetrical/asymmetrical or empty/hypoplastic). A testis that can be brought down to the scrotum (if the scrotum is not hypoplastic) is unlikely to be a true undescended testis. In instances when one cannot determine on physical examination if a testis is retractile or possibly a true undescended testis, a reexamination in 3 months is recommended (Fig. 62-1).

## Imaging

Diagnostic modalities such as ultrasonography, computed tomography (CT), magnetic resonance imaging (MRI) are available; however, the results of these studies rarely influence surgical decision making. Ultrasonography may be useful in locating an extrainguinal testis in the region of the external inguinal ring in obese boys.

## Laparoscopy

Diagnostic laparoscopy was first used for the assessment of a nonpalpable testis in 1976 by Cortesi. It has now become the most widely used and most useful diagnostic modality in the management of the nonpalpable testis. Laparoscopy is by far the most sensitive and specific procedure to localize the nonpalpable testis and to definitively determine, with an accuracy rate of over 95%, whether a gonad is present or absent (Fig. 62-2).

# TREATMENT

## Hormonal Therapy

The use of hormonal treatment for undescended testis has fallen out of favor because of a low success rate in the 20% range, the significant patient/parent discomfort of daily injections, and the possible side effect of androgen hormone administration.

## Indications for Surgical Treatment

The main indications for performing orchidopexy are to: (1) prevent abnormal morphological changes in germ cells that have a potential to reduce fertility and predispose to malignant transformation, (2) repair a concomitant hernia, (3) reduce the risk of torsion, (4) prevent trauma or pain, (5) produce psychological and cosmetic benefit, and (6) provide easier examination for a testicular tumor.

## Timing of Orchidopexy

The optimal time for orchidopexy has been a subject of debate for decades. Despite the conflicting findings as to what

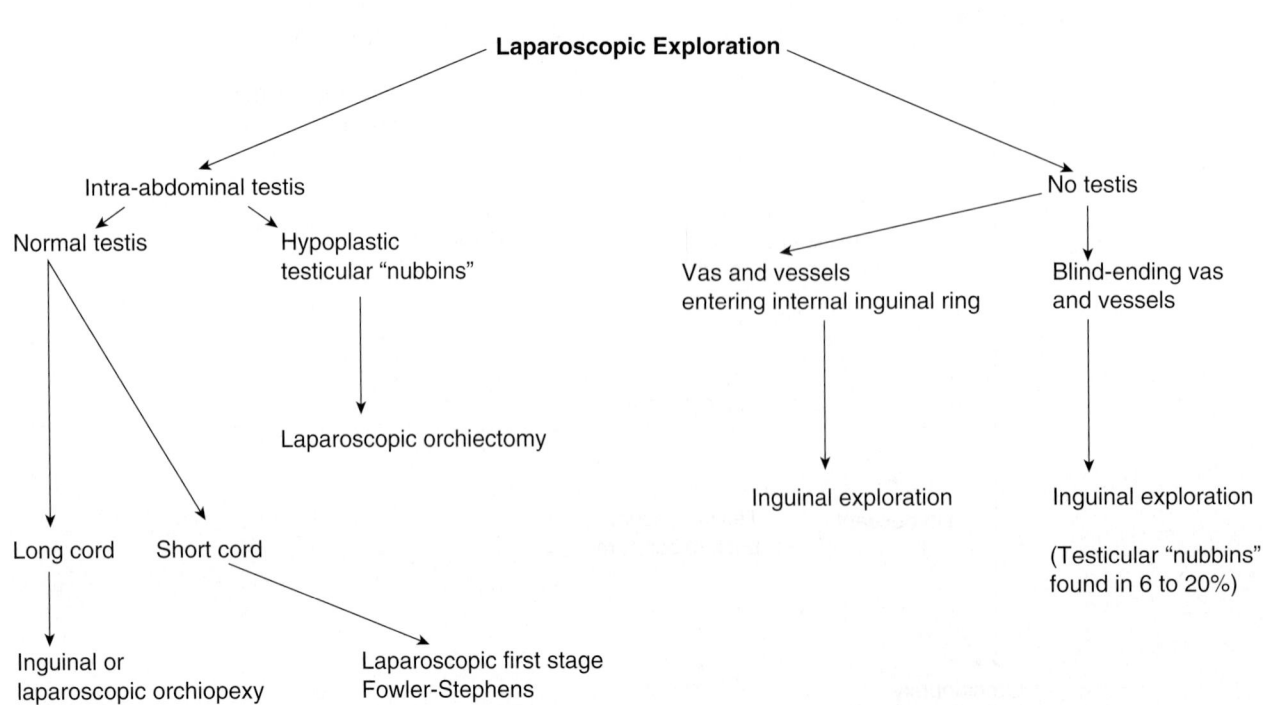

**FIGURE 62-2** Management algorithm based on laparoscopic findings.

degree the operative age influences the fertility potential and what age does the oncologic transformation potential of the cryptorchid testis outweigh the fertility benefit of orchidopexy, it continues to be suggested that there is less trauma from a developmental and psychological point of view when undergoing orchidopexy early during childhood. As spontaneous testicular descent is unlikely to occur after 6 months of age, the current recommendation in many centers is to perform orchidopexy shortly after the child reaches an age of 6 months.

## Anesthesia and Pain Management

Orchidopexy is an outpatient procedure. General anesthesia is supplemented with loco-regional anesthesia (ilioinguinal nerve block or caudal block) to control postoperative pain (See also Chapter 10). In most patients postoperative pain at home can be treated with acetaminophen and/or ibuprofen. Older children occasionally require an acetaminophen–codeine elixir. This is similar to the postoperative pain management for patients after inguinal hernia repair.

## Surgical Technique

The basic steps of an orchidopexy include identification of the testis, mobilization of the cord, isolation of the processus vaginalis, ligation of a hernia sac (if present), and fixation of the testis in the scrotum. There are several techniques to accomplish these goals. We describe an open technique useful for most circumstances, as well as a laparoscopic technique. There continues to be a discussion whether electrocautery is necessary or safe to use during this procedure. We will leave the choice of a hemostatic adjunct up to the individual surgeon, knowing that there is a fine balance between postoperative hematoma and injury to the vas deferens and/or testicular vessels. Administration of prophylactic perioperative antibiotics is not mandated, but can be recommended.

## Open Inguinal Orchidopexy

A transverse incision is made over the lowest skin crease of the abdominoinguinal region lateral to the level of the pubic tubercle (Fig. 62-3A). The incision is carried down through subcutaneous fat and Scarpa fascia. The superficial inferior epigastric vein usually crosses the incision and can be coagulated and divided or avoided. The external oblique aponeurosis is identified as it is exposed, its fibers running parallel to the inguinal canal. A small incision is made in the external oblique aponeurosis over the inguinal canal using the scalpel (Fig. 62-3B). This incision should be placed in line with the fibers running to the external oblique superficial inguinal ring. To avoid injury to the ilioinguinal nerve, which runs parallel to these fibers, a closed pair of scissors is gently introduced through this incision under the fascia, and is bluntly pushed in the direction of the external ring. The aponeurosis fibers can then be sharply opened toward the external ring distally and laterally towards the internal ring. The spermatic cord is identified in the inguinal canal and separated from the external oblique aponeurosis by blunt dissection. The spermatic cord and the testicle are lifted by introducing a forceps or small clamp under these structures. Usually the testicle is attached distally by the gubernaculum testis (Fig. 62-3C). The gubernaculum is divided. At this stage it is very important to avoid a possible aberrant long looping vas deferens, which may make a loop in the gubernaculum distal to the testis. After this mobilization the tunica vaginalis can be opened to examine the testis and epididymis. The size, shape, and consistency of the testes and the relationship of the vas deferens to the vessels of the cord and to the epididymis and testes should be noted. The spermatic cord is then gently put under distal tension. Dissection of the spermatic cord is started by bluntly pushing the cremastric fibers aside. Holding the spermatic cord between the tips of the thumb and the index finger and dissecting with a blunt instrument facilitates this step. The hernia sac is then separated from the vas deferens and vessels by meticulous blunt dissection (Fig. 62-3D). It is

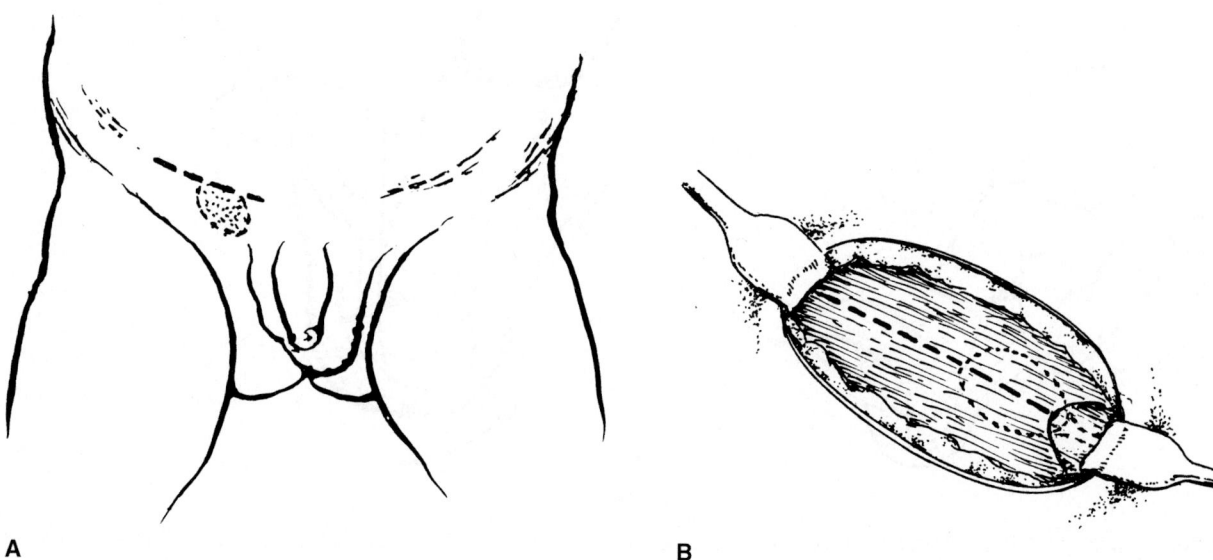

**A**                                      **B**

**FIGURE 62-3** Inguinal orchidopexy. **A.** Skin crease incision. **B.** External oblique aponeurosis is incised exposing the cord structures and the testis.

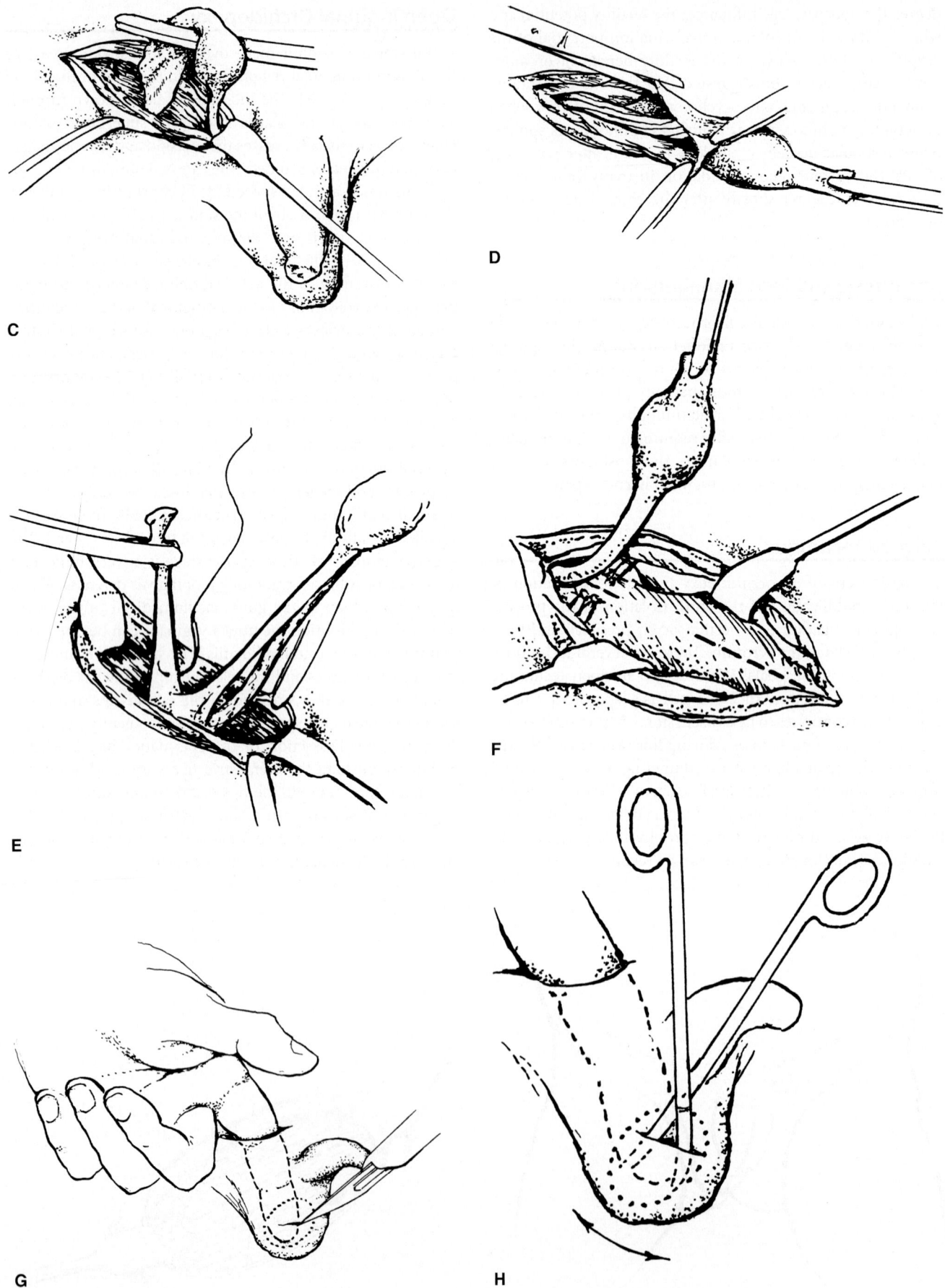

C

D

E

F

G

H

**FIGURE 62-3** (*Continued*) **C.** Testis and spermatic cord are mobilized. The gubernaculum is identified and divided. **D.** The hernia sac is found and dissected free from the vas and vessels. **E.** High ligation of hernia sac by transfixation of a stitch. **F.** At this point further length can be obtained by dividing the transversalis fascia and dividing the inferior epigastric vessels. **G.** A finger is introduced from the wound into the scrotum and a small horizontal incision is made in the scrotal skin. **H.** Subdartos pouch is created using blunt dissection.

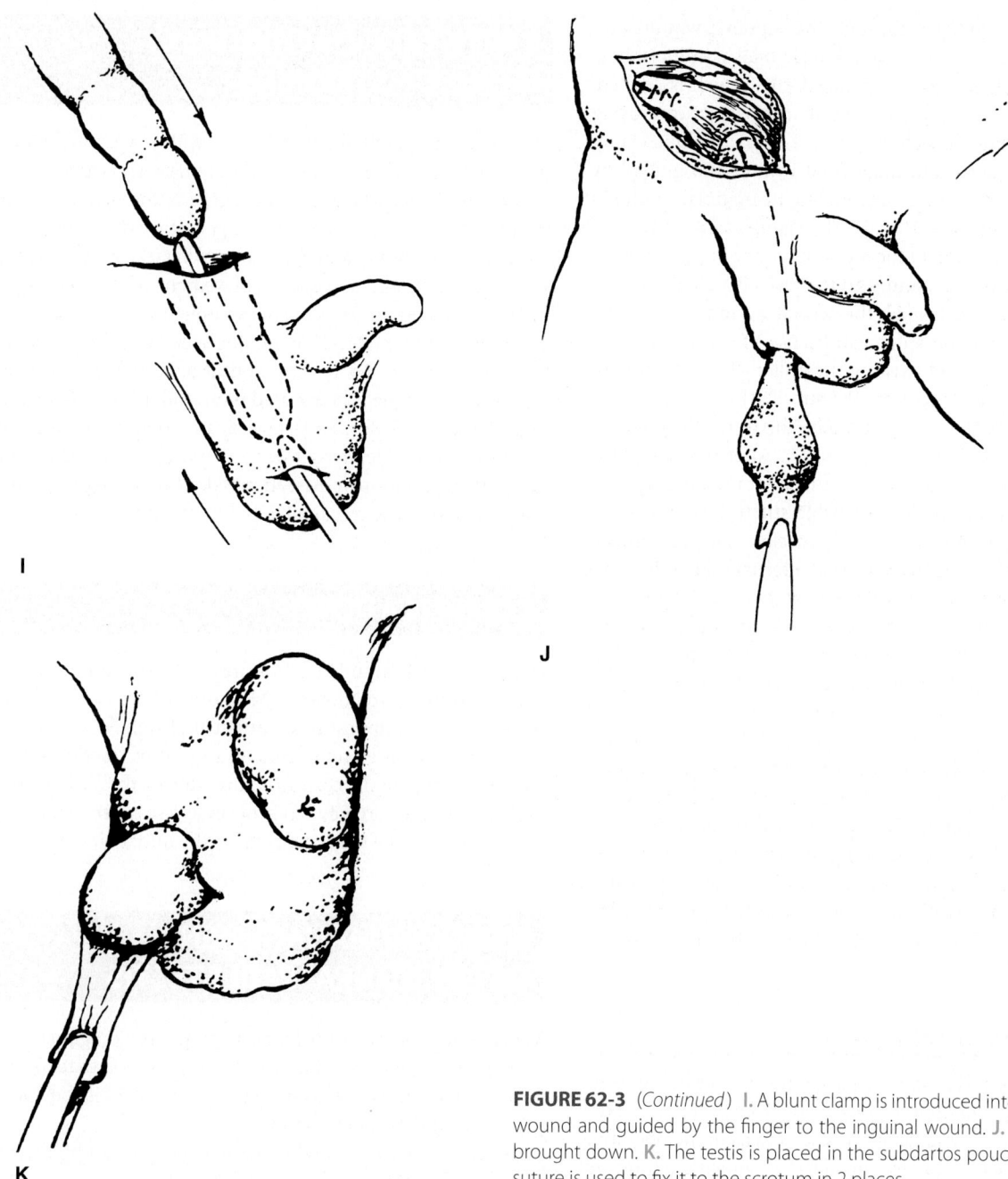

**FIGURE 62-3** (*Continued*) **I.** A blunt clamp is introduced into the scrotal wound and guided by the finger to the inguinal wound. **J.** The testis is brought down. **K.** The testis is placed in the subdartos pouch, and a 5-0 suture is used to fix it to the scrotum in 2 places.

important to avoid disruption of the circumferential integrity of the sac, which is often very fragile. Should a tear in the sac occur, then it should be immediately recognized and repaired with a fine absorbable suture, or incorporated in the "high ligation" of the sac. When the hernia sac has been isolated from the vas deferens and the vessels, it is divided distally and the dissection is continued in a proximal direction. Dissection should be continued to the level where the hernia sac emerges from the peritoneum and the vas deferens turns medially, at or within the deep inguinal ring. It is important to identify the retroperitoneal plane in which the vessels continue in a cranial direction. High ligation of the hernia sac is performed by 3-0 braided suture and the redundant sac tissue can subsequently be excised (Fig. 62-3E). The length of the spermatic cord is now examined, and if the testis does not reach the scrotum, the dissection is continued. Significant care has to be taken to free all cremasteric fibers and fibrous bands from the vas and

vessels. Should this not be sufficient, then the dissection can be continued retroperitoneally. This is facilitated by opening the internal oblique muscle lateral to the internal ring 1.0 to 1.5 cm. A blunt retractor is inserted to expose the retroperitoneal plane. With continuous gentle traction on the spermatic cord it is usually possible to identify additional fibrous bands lateral to the vessels in this retroperitoneal space. These bands are divided under direct vision, carefully avoiding the testicular vessels. (This step is more easily performed laparoscopically, see below). Enough length for the testis to reach the scrotum is usually achieved by this technique, though the rate limiting step is usually related to vascular pedicle length and not the length of the vas. Sometimes it is possible to gain approximately another 1.0 cm by dividing the transversalis fascia and by ligating and dividing the inferior epigastric vessels (Fig. 62-3F). Following this dissection, length should be adequate to reach the bottom of the scrotum. The surgeon's little finger is introduced through the inguinal wound into the scrotum (Fig. 62-3G). A small horizontal skin incision is made over the finger tip, and a sub-dartos pouch is created, big enough to home the testes and its cord structures, using scissors and blunt dissection (Fig. 62-3H). A blunt clamp (Kelly) is introduced into the scrotal wound and guided by the finger through the inguinal canal to the inguinal wound in a retrograde fashion (Fig. 62-3I). The clamp can now be used to grasp a small portion of the tissue surrounding the testis or optimally the gubernaculum, and the testis is pulled down to the scrotum and out through the scrotal wound (Fig. 62-3J). Alternatively a traction stitch can be used for this step. It is very important to avoid twisting the pulled-through remaining spermatic cord structures. The sub-Dartos pouch should be adequate enough to accommodate the testis, the epididymis and remaining tunica (Fig. 62-3K). After passage of the testis through the Dartos window, this tract for a passage can be narrowed with a single absorbable stitch. Fixation of the testis also remains a subject for discussion. We recommend that the testicle be fixed to the medial internal wall of the scrotum in the Dartos pouch with at least 2 stitches near the 2 opposing poles of the testicle with a 5-0 absorbable suture. (There is no reproducible evidence that stitches through the testicular capsule will result in antibodies that will compromise fertility.) The scrotal incision should be closed in 1 or 2 layers, including a subcuticular layer of 5-0 rapidly absorbable suture. In the inguinal wound, after inspection assures that the spermatic cord is not twisted and lies in its anatomic position, the external oblique aponeurosis is closed with 3-0 or 4-0 absorbable sutures avoiding the ileoinguinal nerve and taking care not to narrow the external inguinal ring. Scarpa fascia can be closed with interrupted absorbable sutures. The skin is closed with a rapidly absorbable subcuticular suture (4-0 or 5-0).

### Laparoscopic Orchidopexy

The use of the laparoscope plays a significant role in the treatment of the difficult undescended testis. This is the case in the diagnosis of the nonpalpable testis, as well as in the operative treatment of the high undescended testis requiring significant retroperitoneal mobilization of the vessels.

For most patients a 30° 3- or 5-mm transumbilical laparoscope is ideal, as it allows assessment of the presence of a testis, as well as the vas and vessels at the level of the internal inguinal ring. If a testicle is present, or if a dissection of the vessels is necessary, then 1 or 2 additional instruments should be introduced into the peritoneal cavity for the dissection. Mobilization of the testis and dissection of the previously mentioned fibrous bands can in most cases be performed bluntly after the testicle is carefully grasped and put on tension to tent the peritoneum. The passage into the scrotum can be performed bluntly with one of the laparoscopic instruments, or the procedure can be completed with the open technique (see above). Closure of the internal ring is still a point of controversy; however, available data suggest that the risk for development of a inguinal hernia is not increased after laparoscopic orchidopexy, even if the internal ring is not closed. The scrotal portion of the case is equivalent to the open procedure.

## TWO-STAGE ORCHIDOPEXY (FOWLER–STEPHENS)

Three arterial vessels supply the testis with oxygenated blood: the main testicular, the vasal, and the cremasteric arteries. A key step of the Fowler–Stephens procedure is the ligation of the main testicular artery to allow compensatory development of the arteries of the vas and the collateral vessels. This by design should facilitate the surgeon's achievement of adequate spermatic cord length to reach the dartos pouch in the second stage orchidopexy done typically 6 months later. With the possibility to perform significant retroperitoneal dissection laparoscopically, this technique is being used more and more infrequently. The decision to perform a 1-stage laparoscopic orchidopexy or a 2-stage Fowler–Stephens procedure must be made before any extensive exploration or dissection is done in the inguinal canal that can disrupt the collateral vessels to the testis.

## COMPLICATIONS

Hematoma and wound infection are the 2 most common complications after orchidopexy. Meticulous hemostasis should prevent these complications. Testicular atrophy after inguinal orchidopexy is rare and occurs as a result of traction on the cord or twisting of the cord structures during the orchidopexy. Testicular retraction may rarely occur as a result of inadequate mobilization of the cord and testis at the initial orchidopexy.

## SURGICAL MANAGEMENT OF THE NONPALPABLE TESTIS

Management of the nonpalpable testis poses a diagnostic and therapeutic challenge. The important questions that need to be answered are: Is a testis present or not? What is the appropriate therapeutic approach? (Fig. 62-1).

In patients with bilateral nonpalpable testes, an hCG stimulation test can be performed to determine the presence of testicular tissue. If there is no corresponding rise of testosterone to the stimulation by hCG, and if the basal level of FSH is high, it indicates absence of testicular tissue, and surgical exploration may not be necessary (Fig. 62-1). Alternatively, a diagnostic laparoscopy can be performed immediately.

The various options available are shown in Fig. 62-2. Diagnostic laparoscopy is the preferred first step in the management of a nonpalpable testis. Imaging in the form of ultrasonography, CT, or MRI is possible, but will very rarely influence the decision-making process. The 3 likely findings at laparoscopy are:

1. Blind-ending vas and vessels (vanishing testis): Viable testicular remnants have been noted in 6% to 20% of vanishing testes. It has been suggested that inguinal exploration should be carried out in these patients to remove testicular "nubbins" to prevent future risk of malignancy. Concomitant contralateral fixation orchidopexy is indicated to prevent torsion of the remaining testis.

2. Cord structures entering the internal ring: inguinal exploration is carried out, and if a viable testis is found the testis is relocated to the scrotum. If a remnant "nubbin" is found it is excised in toto to remove the nidus of germ cells to prevent the occurrence of a later malignancy.

3. A viable intra-abdominal testis: the limiting factor to relocate the intra-abdominal testis to the scrotum is the length of the gonadal vessels. Laparoscopic orchidopexy or a 2-Stage Fowler–Stephens procedure should be performed.

## OUTCOMES

### Testicular Size

Most authors have found that testicular volume in adults is lower than normal after childhood orchidopexy. Puri and Sparnon found a significant correlation between the initial position of the cryptorchid testis and subsequent testicular volume in 159 children operated on at a mean age of 9.8 years. Nineteen abdominal testes had an average testicular volume in adult life of 4.9 mL compared to 9.8 mL in canalicular testes and 17 mL in superficial inguinal pouch testes.

### Fertility After Orchidopexy

Successful paternity has been reported in 81% of married men with a past history of unilateral cryptorchidism and in 50% of married men with a past history of bilateral cryptorchidism. Several studies have addressed the outcome for orchidopexy by semen analysis. Puri and O'Donnell performed semen analysis in 142 men who had undergone orchidopexy at ages 7 to 13 years and found that the subsequent quality of semen was dependent upon the original anatomical position of the undescended testes and whether the condition was unilateral or bilateral. Men who had unilateral cryptorchidism produced normal or acceptable semen after orchidopexy. Those with bilateral superficial inguinal pouch testes produced normal or acceptable semen. However, all the men who had bilateral canalicular or bilateral abdominal testes were azospermic.

### Testicular Cancer After Orchidopexy

Cryptorchidism is associated with testicular cancer. About 10% of testicular neoplasms are associated with undescended testes, which implies that the risk of testicular cancer is increased five times compared to the descended testis. The risk of malignancy may also be increased in the contralateral testis. Carcinoma in situ has been reported in about 0.4% of patients undergoing orchidopexy in childhood. The risk of malignancy remains after orchidopexy, although it has been proposed that the risk is lower if orchidopexy is performed at an earlier age. The main role of orchidopexy is, however, to allow easier examination for a putative testicular tumor.

### SELECTED READINGS

Ashley RA, Barthold JS, Kolon TF. Cryptorchidism: pathogenesis, diagnosis, treatment and prognosis. *Urol Clin N Am* 2010;37(2):183–193.

Berkowitz GS, Lapinski RH, Dolgin SE, et al. Prevalence and natural history of cryptorchidism. *Pediatrics* 1993;92:44–49.

Elyas R, Guerra LA, Pike J, et al. Is staging beneficial for Fowler–Stephens orchiopexy? A systematic review. *J Urol* 2010;183(5):2012–2018.

Hutson JM, Balic A, Nation T, Southwell B. Cryptorchidism. *Semin Pediatr Surg* 2010;19(3):215–224.

Hutson JM. Undescended testis. In: Stringer MD, Mouriquand PDE, Oldham KT, Howard ER, eds. *Long-Term Outcomes.* London, Philadelphia; 1998:603–605.

Ismail K, Ashour M, El-Afifi M, et al. Laparoscopy in the management of impalpable testis: series of 64 cases. *World J Surg* 2009;33(7):1514–1519.

John Radcliffe Hospital Cryptorchidism Study Group. Cryptorchidism: a prospective study of 7,500 consecutive male births, 1984–1988. *Arch Dis Child* 1992;67:892–899.

Merry C, Sweeney B, Puri P. The vanishing testis: anatomical and histological findings. *Eur Urol* 1997;31:65–67.

Ritzén EM. Undescended testes: a consensus on management. *Eur J Endocrinol* 2008;159:87–90.

# Circumcision CHAPTER 63

*Marc S. Arkovitz*

## KEY POINTS

1. The preferred 3 techniques for pediatric circumcision are the clamp, the dorsal slit, and the sleeve resection.

2. Clamp techniques are most applicable to the neonatal procedure while dorsal slit and sleeve resections are optimally applied to the older child or young adult.

3. Postoperative bleeding is the most common morbidity of circumcision and is best prevented by meticulous attention to hemostasis.

4. Careful identification of the glans penis and urethral meatus throughout the procedure is the most effective way to avoid inadvertent injury to these structures.

---

. . . And Abraham took Isaac his son, and all that were born in his house, and all that were bought with his money, every male among the men of Abraham's house; and circumcised the flesh of their foreskin in the selfsame day, as God had said unto him. . . .

*Genesis 17:23*

There is probably no other procedure so universally performed by pediatric surgeons as circumcision. Although seemingly mundane, circumcision takes on great personal and religious significance to the pediatric patient and his family. In addition, complications of circumcision can be devastating. Pediatric surgeons must be aware that the majority of neonatal circumcisions performed in the hospital are not performed exclusively by surgeons but that the procedure is performed by a variety of practitioners including obstetricians, pediatricians, urologists, and religious figures.

The debate as to the potential risks and benefits of circumcision is almost as old as the procedure itself. The only universally accepted benefit is an almost absent risk of penile cancer in circumcised males. Other, less widely accepted benefits include a decreased association with sexually transmitted diseases, including HIV, a decreased incidence in urinary tract infections, and a decrease in carcinoma of the cervix in the female sexual partners of circumcised men.

## TECHNIQUE

### Anesthesia

General anesthesia is usually not used for neonatal circumcision unless the procedure is being performed concomitant with other procedures requiring a general anesthetic. Recent evidence supports using a local anesthetic cream to decrease pain; however, many pediatric surgeons will probably not perform the procedure without some form of anesthesia. A general anesthetic is advisable when the boy is more than 6 weeks of age. In adolescents and older boys, the operation is often done with local anesthesia applied as a penile block. This block is produced by infiltration of the dorsal penile nerves at the base of the penis lying between the tunica albuginea and Bucks fascia (Fig. 63-1). Local anesthetics without epinephrine are recommended because epinephrine may cause significant arterial spasm and resultant penile ischemia.

### Operative Techniques

For the purpose of this chapter 3 operative techniques are discussed. It should be noted that prior to the procedure the foreskin must be cleansed thoroughly with a sterilizing solution. Ideally the foreskin should be retracted and the inner layer cleaned as well, however, this is not possible in cases of phimosis or dense preputial adhesions.

### Dorsal Slit

In addition to elective circumcisions, the dorsal slit circumcision (Fig. 63-2) can also be used to release a paraphimosis or when the foreskin cannot be retracted during one of the other procedures. Initial hemostasis in the area where the slit is to be made is achieved by crushing the foreskin for several minutes with a straight hemostat. This is done by placing 1 blade of the hemostat between the glans penis and the preputial skin at the 12 o'clock position and closing the clamp. The foreskin is then incised along the clamped groove using a Metzenbaum scissors. The incision should extend apically to a point 3–5 mm from the coronal sulcus. The foreskin is then retracted, and the inner membrane and glans are cleansed.

The foreskin is then grasped at the 3 o'clock and 9 o'clock positions with either hemostats or stay sutures, and the

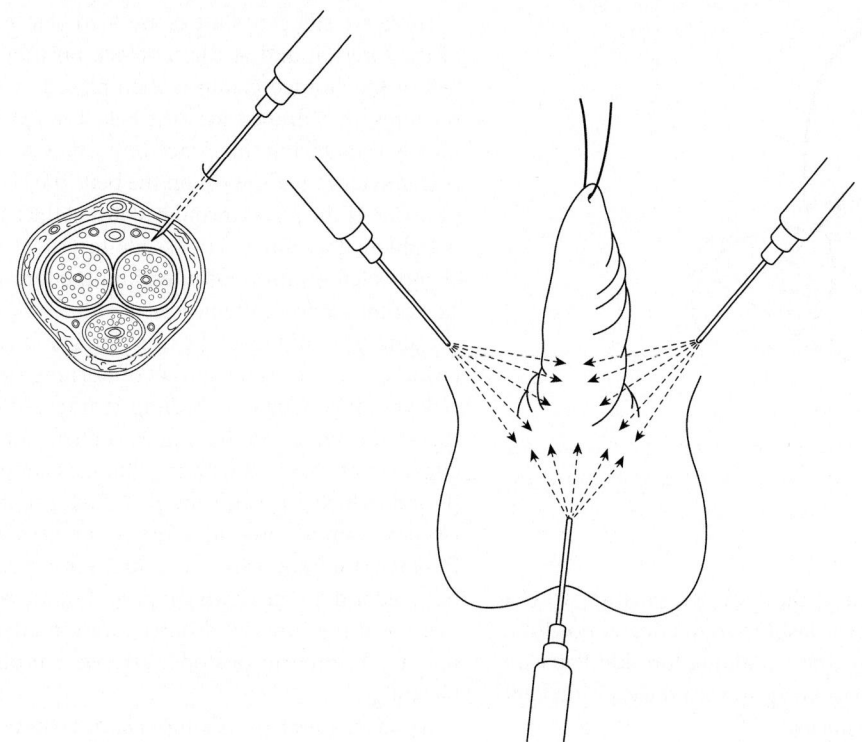

**FIGURE 63-1** The technique for a sensory blockade of the penis. After a dorsal penile injection, a lateral and ventral fanlike distribution of anesthetic agent infiltration is done.

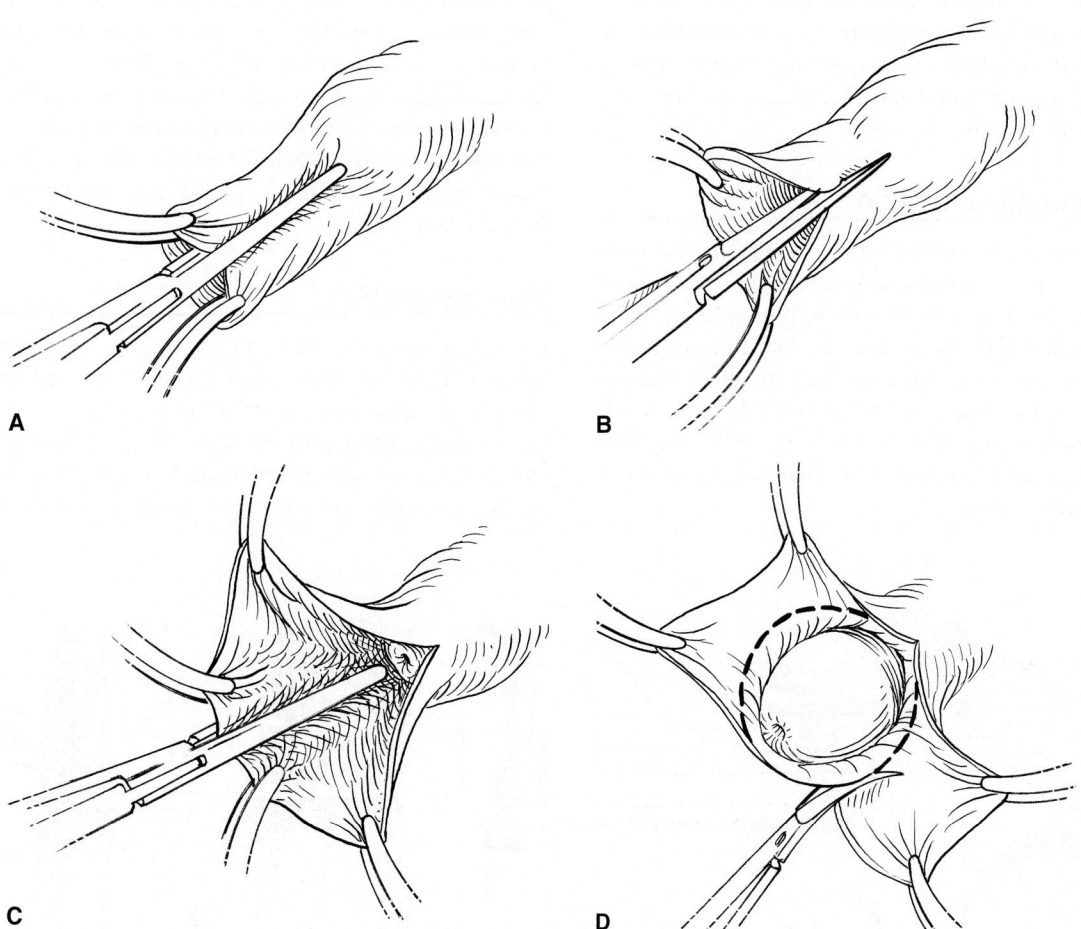

A

B

C

D

**FIGURE 63-2** The dorsal slit circumcision technique. **A.** A straight hemostat is inserted, and the prepuce is crushed in the dorsal midline. Care must be taken to avoid compression and injury of the meatus and glands. **B.** The crushing clamp is removed, and a scissors is used to incise the crush site. **C.** The steps A and B are repeated under direct vision in the ventral midline. The incised prepuce is turned back, allowing inspection and cleansing of the glands. **D.** A circumferential excision of the redundant prepuce is done.

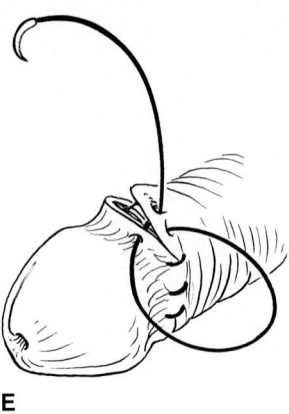

**E**

**FIGURE 63-2** (*Continued*) **E.** The incision line is oversewn with a continuous or interrupted absorbable suture to secure hemostasis.

ventral foreskin is crushed at the 6 o'clock position with a straight hemostat in a similar fashion to the dorsal position. A ventral slit is then made. The remaining foreskin flaps are then excised under direct vision, again with the excision kept 3–5 mm from the coronal sulcus.

The opposing skin edges are then approximated using 4-0 or 5-0 chromic catgut sutures in an interrupted fashion. The first suture is usually placed at the 12 o'clock position, the second at 6 o'clock, and the rest of the sutures are placed in such a fashion as to bisect the remaining paired foreskin flaps with each suture. Similarly, some surgeons prefer a running locking suture approximation of the foreskin in the hope that it will be more hemostatic.

## Gomco Clamp Circumcision

The Gomco clamp procedure (Fig. 63-3) may be the most commonly performed circumcision among all practitioners performing circumcisions. In the newborn population adhesions between the glans penis and the foreskin are gently lysed by spreading in the plane between the glans and the preputial skin with a hemostat. Next a dorsal slit is made following the procedure described above. The foreskin may then be retracted to more thoroughly lyse the adhesions between the foreskin and the glans.

Three 4-0 silk stay sutures are then placed at the cut edges of the foreskin and at the 6 o'clock position. The protective bell of the Gomco clamp is then placed over the glans, and the foreskin is draped over the bell. The stay sutures are used for traction during this procedure, allowing for fairly precise placement of the foreskin on the bell. The clamp is then positioned over the foreskin and bell just at the coronal sulcus and is tightened as much as possible to crush the foreskin. The clamp is left on for 5 minutes, and the foreskin on the distal side of the clamp is then excised with a scalpel.

Cautery should never be used for a Gomco clamp circumcision because of the real risk of burning the entire penis to a degree that repair or healing is impossible. The clamp is then removed, and a dressing is applied. Suturing of the skin edges is not required with the Gomco clamp in the newborn period, which may be why it is such a popular procedure. Gomco clamps come in a variety of sizes and can be used in older children, using the same technique. However, in all boys older than the newborn period, suturing and reapproximating of the inner and outer foreskin are strongly recommended to prevent postoperative wound dehiscence and/or bleeding.

An alternative to the Gomco clamp is the use of a Plastibell®. This disposable device consists of a plastic dome that fits over the glans penis, held by a detachable handle. After a dorsal slit is performed, the bell is placed over the glans, the foreskin is pulled over the bell using traction sutures, and a large suture is tied around the foreskin, in a groove in the bell (Fig. 63-4). Care must be taken to not pull on the foreskin too firmly, as too much skin can be excised in this way. Redundant preputial skin distal to the tie is excised, and the bell is left in place after removal of the detachable handle. The tie and bell will usually spontaneously fall off in 3–7 days, creating a smooth line of separation.

## Sleeve Resection

The advantage of the sleeve resection (Fig. 63-5) is that the entire procedure is done under direct vision, and therefore, injury to the glans penis is almost impossible. Initially, adhesions between the foreskin and glans are gently lysed by either retracting the foreskin and manually lysing them or by gently placing a straight clamp between the glans and the foreskin

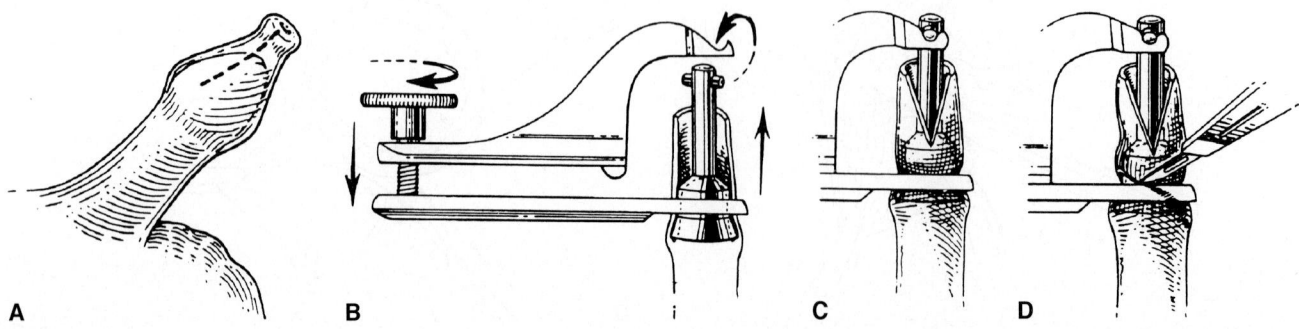

**A**  **B**  **i**  **C**  **D**

**FIGURE 63-3** The Gomco clamp circumcision. **A.** After careful separation of preputial adhesions, a dorsal slit is made following the application of a straight crushing hemostat. **B.** An appropriately sized Gomco bell is placed over the glans of the penis, and the prepuce is drawn over the bell. **C.** The clamp is placed over the bell and prepuce and tightly screwed shut. **D.** The excess prepuce is sharply excised, and the clamp is removed.

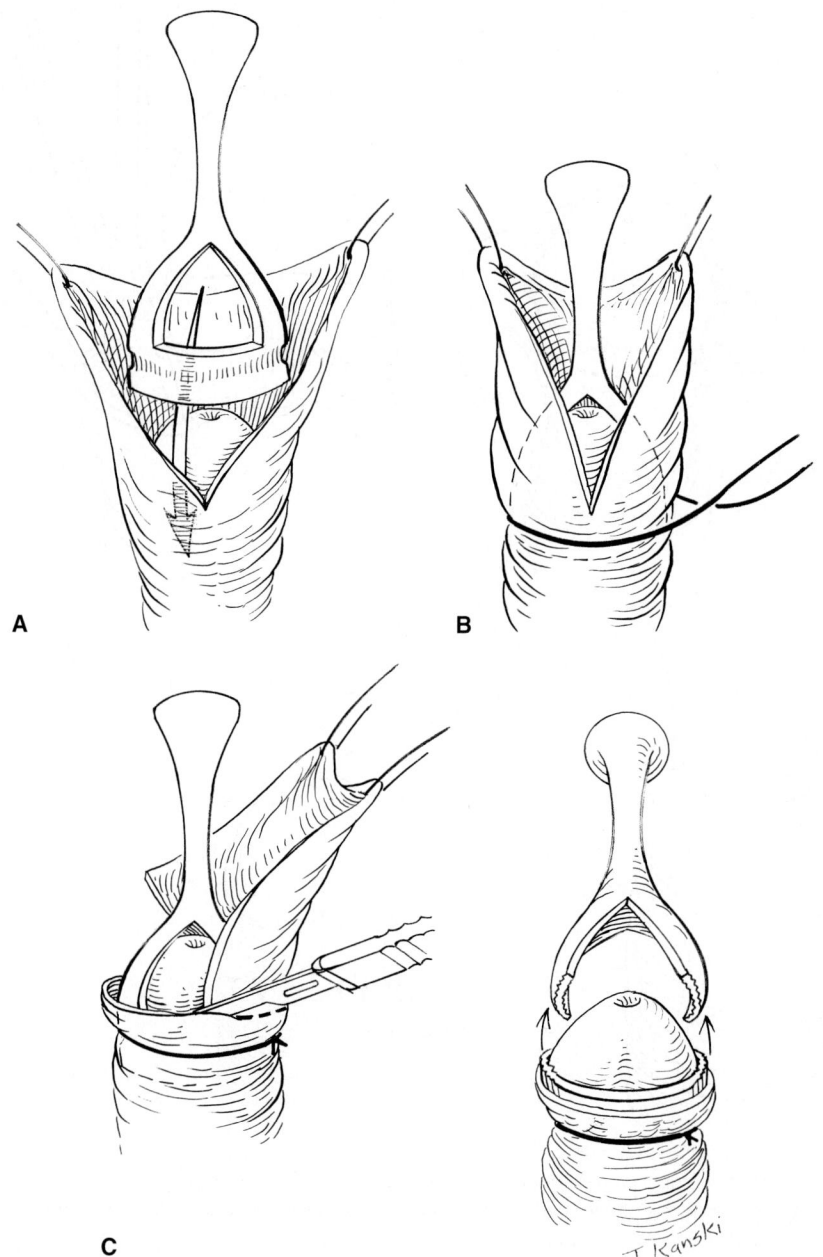

A

B

C

J. Kanski

**FIGURE 63-4** The Plasti-bell technique. **A.** After a dorsal slit is made (Fig. 63-2A), an appropriately sized Plasti-bell is placed over the glans of the penis, and the prepuce is drawn over the plastic ring. **B.** With gentle outward traction on the redundant prepuce, the heavy suture is tied over the prepuce in the groove of the plastic ring. Inspection of the glans assures the proper placement of the suture before the knot is secured. **C.** The breakaway holder is removed, and with the ring in place a portion of the redundant prepuce is excised to expose the underlying glans. This will also assure that the previous suture will not leave the distal prepuce ischemic.

and spreading the jaws of the clamp. The foreskin is then clamped and pulled lengthwise to extend the length of the foreskin. A circumferential incision line is marked with a pen on the outer preputial skin approximately 0.5 cm proximal to the area of the coronal sulcus. The foreskin is then retracted and a line is marked on the inner foreskin also 0.5 cm distal to the coronal sulcus. An incision is then made over both these marked lines with a scalpel, incising the skin and areolar subcutaneous tissues only.

Next, the foreskin is excised using careful sharp cautery, connecting the incisions of the inner and outer foreskin. This ring of foreskin is then resected completely. Hemostasis is

achieved either by individually ligating bleeding points or by precise low-current indirect cautery. The skin edges are reapproximated using either interrupted 4-0 or 5-0 absorbable sutures in the same fashion as described for the dorsal slit.

## POSTOPERATIVE CARE

The circumcision suture line is covered with antibiotic ointment, and a sterile dressing is applied. The initial dressing is usually left on for 24 to 48 hours. The parents are advised to remove the dressing and continue to use antibiotic ointment

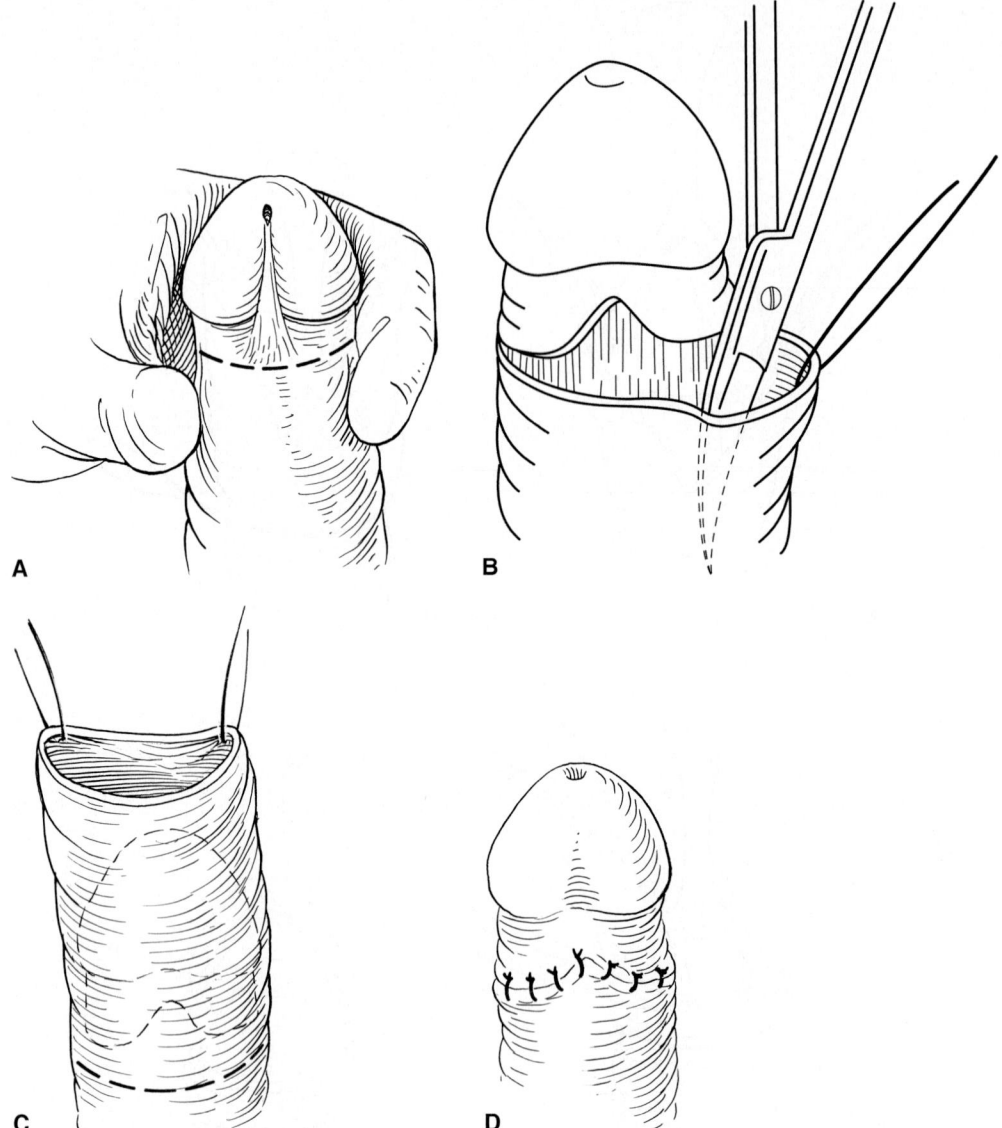

A

B

C

D

**FIGURE 63-5** Free-hand sleeve circumcision. **A.** After separation of preputial adhesions, including at times the ligation of a ventral midline adhesion, a circular incision is made around the penile shaft 1 cm proximal to the corona. **B.** The shaft skin is then bluntly and sharply elevated off of the surface of the corporal bodies around the entire circumference of the penile shaft superficial to Bucks fascia. **C.** The undermined shaft skin and redundant prepuce are then pulled over the glans, and a second circumferential incision is made around the penis, excising the redundant prepuce. Hemostasis must then be secured with forceps and electrocautery, with the bleeding vessels gently raised off of the penile shaft before coagulation. **D.** Interrupted absorbable sutures are then placed in a circumferential fashion between the proximal and the distal shaft skin.

for the first 7 to 10 days to prevent adherence of the sutures to the diapers or underwear.

## COMPLICATIONS

Although rare, there is a real morbidity and even mortality associated with circumcision. Bleeding is the most common postoperative complication of circumcision and can be caused either by a bleeding vessel in subcutaneous areolar tissue that was not ligated or by skin edge bleeding. Often, either of these conditions can be treated by applying direct pressure.

Occasionally the suture line must be opened, and the bleeding point controlled in the operating room.

The next most common complication is an unacceptable cosmetic result secondary to either insufficient or excessive removal of foreskin. This occurs more commonly with clamp techniques of circumcision, when the foreskin is not incised under direct vision. Meticulous attention to detail as well as marking out the coronal sulcus and completely releasing adhesions between the foreskin and the glans penis may help to reduce this complication. Occasionally a circumcision will need to be revised secondary to insufficient foreskin removal or unequal removal whereby the dorsal and ventral parts of the foreskin are uneven and the cosmetic result unacceptable.

Postoperative infection is rare but can occur. This infection is usually minor, with little consequence, but occasionally it can result in generalized sepsis or Fournier gangrene. Diabetic children seem to be particularly prone to postoperative wound infections.

Another complication is damage to the glans or the urethra with resultant fistula formation. This seems to occur more frequently when a clamp method of circumcision is employed as opposed to the open methods of circumcision. Once again, it is important to emphasize the fact that cautery should never be used with a clamp method of circumcision to remove the foreskin. Ignoring this principle has resulted in complete necrosis of the glans and shaft of the penis, requiring gender conversion. Indirect cautery is an equally effective yet safer choice technique that should be used for all shaft bleeding.

Other less common postoperative complications include hypospadius or epispadius, chordee, and meatitis. Again, many of these can be avoided by excising the foreskin under direct vision.

## SELECTED READINGS

Broecker BH. Circumcision. In: Glenn JF, ed. *Urologic Surgery,* 4th ed. New York: JB Lippincott, 1991:841–844.

Brown MR, Cartwright PC, Snow BW. Common office problems in pediatric urology and gynecology. *Pediatr Clin N Am* 1997;44(5):1091–1115.

Cendron M, Elder JS, Duckett JW. Perinatal urology. In: Gillenwater JY, Grayhack JT, Howards SS, Duckett JW, eds. *Adult and Pediatric Urology,* 3rd ed. St Louis: Mosby; 1996:2149–2152.

Cohen MS. Circumcision. In: Fowler JE, ed. *Mastery of Surgery–Urologic Surgery.* Boston: Little, Brown; 1992:422–428.

Docimo SG. Circumcision. In: Marshall FF, ed. *Textbook of Operative Urology.* Philadelphia: WB Saunders; 1996:958–961.

Jordan GH, Schlossberg SM, Devine. Surgery of the penis and urethra. In: Walsh PC, Retik AB, Vaughan ED Jr, Wein AJ, eds. *Campbell's Urology,* 7th ed. Philadelphia: WB Saunders; 1998:3332–3334.

Kaplan GW. Complications of circumcision. *Urol Clin North Am.* 1983;10(3):543–549.

Minninberg DT. Circumcision. In: O'Donnell B, Koff SA, eds. *Pediatric Urology,* 3rd ed. Oxford: Butterworth-Heinemann; 1997:850–853.

Murphy JP. Genitourinary trauma. In: Ashcraft KW, ed. *Pediatric Urology.* Philadelphia: WB Saunders; 1990:444.

Taddio A, Stevens B, Craig K, et al. Efficacy and safety of lidocaine-prilocaine cream for pain during circumcision. *N Engl J Med* 1997;336(17):1197–1201.

# Hypospadias   CHAPTER 64

*Sean Primley and Duncan Wilcox*

## KEY POINTS

1. Higher rates of cryptorchidism and inguinal hernia.

2. Due to the higher incidence of DSD in patients with hypospadias and nonpalpable testicles an evaluation of these patients should be done.

3. Difficulty in passing a catheter at the time of hypospadias repair may be due to the presence of a utricle.

4. Imaging of the upper tracts in hypospadias patients is not routinely done unless there is another indication.

5. The components of hypospadias repair are: correction of chordee, urethroplasty, reconstruction of the glans, and skin coverage.

6. Currently, the repair of most hypospadias is based on the intact urethral plate.

7. The technique used is based on the location of the urethral meatus and the severity of the chordee.

8. Chordee correction should be done prior to urethroplasty.

9. Hypospadias surgeons should be comfortable performing repairs on the full spectrum of hypospadias as findings at the time of operation may reveal a more severe defect.

10. Early complications include bleeding, hematoma, and infection.

11. The rate of late complications is based on the degree of hypospadias and the type of repair used.

12. The overall reoperative rate is 9.8%.

13. Patients with fistulae or urethrocele should be evaluated for distal stenosis.

## INTRODUCTION

Hypospadias represents an arrest in development of the urethral spongiosum that results in hypoplasia of tissues that form the ventral surface of the penis. This manifests as a triangular defect with the apex at the division of the corpus spongiosum, the split corporeal tissue making up the sides, and the glands comprising the base. The result is 3 anatomic anomalies: a proximal location of the urethral meatus, ventral penile curvature, and a dorsal hooded foreskin. The diagnosis is not excluded if one of the above is not present (Fig. 64-1). Uncommonly, a variant of hypospadias is encountered in which the foreskin is completely intact. The diagnosis in these cases is often made at the time of newborn circumcision. This condition is often referred to as the "megameatus" variant of hypospadias.

## Epidemiology

Hypospadias occurs in approximately 1 in 200 to 1 in 300 live births. Registry data show variation in the incidence between countries ranging from 0.2% in Sweden to 0.7% in the Netherlands. Several large registries of birth defects have reported an increase in the incidence of hypospadias over the past several decades. This may be explained by better reporting to registries of minor forms; however, several factors have been cited as causing a true increased incidence. Environmental "estrogen pollutants" which are thought to act as endocrine disruptors that effect fetal virilization have been implicated in this increase as well as an increase in testicular cancer and decreasing semen quality. Maternal estrogens such as diethylstilbestrol (DES) given early have been shown to increase hypospadias rates. Demographic trends such as maternal age >35 and low birth weight have been identified as risk factors for hypospadias. The inability of a single placenta to produce enough human chorionic gonadotropin (hCG) to meet the needs of 2 male fetuses in monozygotic twins may explain the 8.5 fold higher rate of hypospadias when compared to singleton births. Some studies, though not all, have suggested that in vitro fertilization is associated with a higher incidence. There also may be a "larger gene pool" for genetic virilization disorders as a generation of men with hypospadias and cryptorchidism have undergone surgical correction and thus have increased fertility. In most cases, especially in distal forms, hypospadias is a sporadic event. However, hypospadias is seen in 7 to 10% of boys with first-degree male affected relatives, and 10 to 20% in brothers of boys with severe forms.

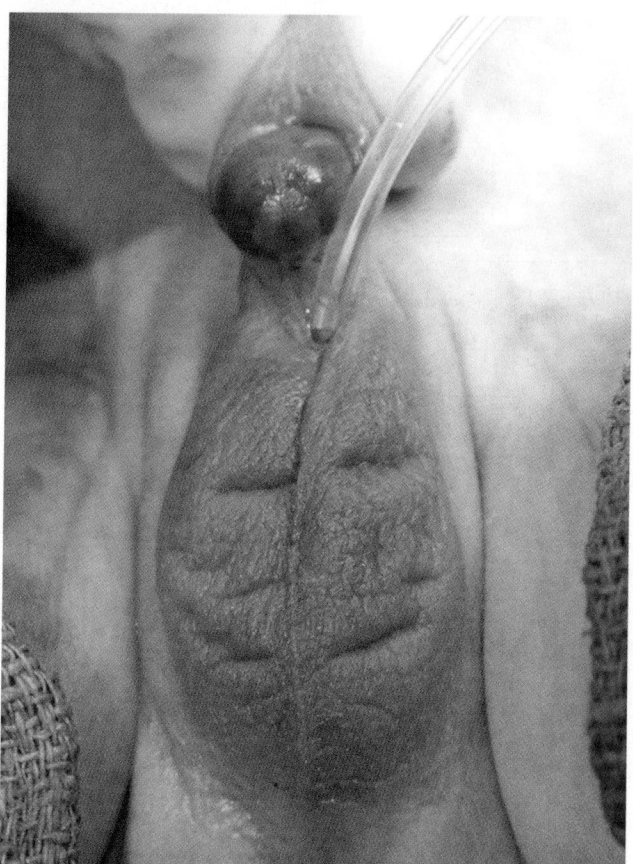

**FIGURE 64-1** A patient with proximal hypospadias showing the typical physical exam finding of a dorsal hooded foreskin, a proximal urethral opening, and ventral chordee.

## Genetic Factors

The etiology of hypospadias remains unknown with less than 5% of cases explainable by androgen metabolism abnormalities, androgen receptor defects, or genetic defects. The masculinization of the urogenital sinus is androgen dependent, and is influenced by testosterone and dihydrotestosterone (DHT). Certain types of congenital adrenal hyperplasia (CAH) can cause genotypic males to show the features of hypospadias.

Such enzymatic defects causing decreased androgen levels include: 3-β-hydroxysteroid dehydrogenase, 17-β-hydroxysteroid dehydrogenase, and 17-α-hydroxylase/17,20-lase. The enzyme responsible for converting testosterone to DHT in the responsive tissue, 5-α *reductase type* II, has also been implicated in certain cases. Some studies have found androgen receptor mutations in patients with hypospadias.

## ASSOCIATED DISORDERS

A higher incidence of cryptorchidism (7-9%) and inguinal hernia (9-16%) is seen in patients with hypospadias (4). While the incidence of inguinal hernia is similar in all degrees of hypospadias, cryptorchid testicles are more common in severe forms. Other than this association, other

abnormalities are rarely seen with hypospadias. The presence of cryptorchidism and any degree of hypospadias should raise the suspicion of a disorder of sexual development (DSD) and should be evaluated fully. In hypospadias patients with unilateral cryptorchidism a nonpalpable testis carries a higher association with DSD conditions than a palpable cryptorchid testis (50% vs 15%). Similarly, in bilateral cryptorchidism those with 1 or 2 nonpalpable testicles are more likely to have a DSD condition than those with palpable testes (47% vs 16%). Furthermore, the incidence of chromosomal abnormalities is higher (22%) in patients with both hypospadias and cryptorchidism than hypospadias (5.6%) or cryptorchidism (4.8%) alone. Up to 20% of severe forms of hypospadias are associated with a persistent prostatic utricle which can make bladder catheterization difficult. Unless symptomatic, routine evaluation with cystoscopy or radiographic studies is not indicated. Abnormalities of the upper urinary tract associated with hypospadias are rare and occur in 2% of patients. This makes *routine* ultrasound evaluation unnecessary.

## Classification

Hypospadias is classified according to the position of the urethral opening from distal to proximal along the ventral surface of the penis. However, care must be taken in this classification as the urethra may be very thin from the meatus to where the corporus spongiosum actually splits revealing a more severe defect. This means that it is important that surgeons be able to repair the full spectrum of hypospadias not just distal forms since the initial diagnosis of distal hypospadias may be false and a more complex repair needed. Prior to performing any hypospadias repair the urethra should be catheterized and the tissue overlaying the urethra evaluated.

## TREATMENT

The goal in surgical repair of hypospadias is the creation of a straight penis with a slit-like meatus which terminates in the ventral aspect of the glans and that allows for normal urination and sexual function. The specific components of the repair are: correction of chordee, urethroplasty, reconstruction of the glans, and skin coverage.

### General Surgical Principles

Timing of initial surgical repair should be between 3 and 6 months of age in the otherwise healthy child, and if possible before 18 months of age. The reason for performing the operation at this age is twofold. First beyond 4 to 5 months, age is not the major risk factor for general anesthesia. Second, treatment in this age group occurs prior to potty training and minimizes the child's separation anxiety. The operation is performed with the patient under general anesthesia to limit patient movement and limit any sensation of pain. Adjuvant analgesia may be given in the form of a caudal block or dorsal penile nerve block. A nationwide review of repeat operations after hypospadias repair did not show that the age at the initial hypospadias repair influenced the need for additional procedures.

A single dose of a broad-spectrum intravenous antibiotic is indicated prior to operation. The authors prefer a first-generation cephalosporin, or gentamicin. Prophylactic antibiotics, given while the urethral catheter is left in after operation have been shown to decrease the incidence of bacteriuria and febrile urinary tract infections after the catheter is removed. An antibiotic with coverage of urogenic pathogens such as a first-generation cephalosporin or trimethoprim–sulfamethoxazole will suffice.

Due to the small and delicate nature of tissues manipulated during hypospadias repair optical magnification is preferred. Most surgeons prefer standard operating loupes which provide 2.5 to 4.3× magnification. Some have advocated for the use of an operating microscope that allows for higher magnification, but it can be cumbersome and may be too powerful for hypospadias repair.

At the start of the operation a monofilament traction suture is placed in the dorsal surface of the glans in the midline. This can later be used to secure the urethral stent. When performing the urethroplasty 7-0 or 6-0 absorbable suture is used. A retrospective review of distal and mid shaft hypospadias patients managed by a single surgeon using either 6-0 polyglactin or 7-0 polydioxanone showed no difference in fistula or stricture rates.

Hemostasis is essential for good hypospadias repair. This can be achieved by placing a tourniquet at the penile scrotal junction after degloving the penis and prior to making any further incision. This provides excellent hemostasis during the operation. Others use epinephrine in a 1:100,000 solution as an injection (1 mL/kg maximum) or on soaked gauze sponges. The theoretical risk is that excessive vasoconstriction would lead to devascularization of skin flaps. Another consideration is electrocautery. Monopolar electrocautery is dispersed to the grounding site along the course of the vessels which may damage the microvasculature. Bipolar electrocautery is preferred for this reason, however, it may be inadequate to stop bleeding from the glans.

The type of dressing used is surgeon dependent and many types of materials are available. The rationale for applying a postoperative dressing is that it decreases swelling, wound infection and disruption, and improves hemostasis. The most common types used are either a compressive wrap or a transparent biomembrane. A randomized prospective trial was undertaken comparing one of the 2 dressing types listed above or no dressing. Both groups applied an antibiotic ointment to the penis postoperatively. There was no significant difference in wound healing, complications, reoperation, or infections postoperatively in the dressing or no-dressing groups.

The indications for urinary diversion depend on the type of repair used. In some minor, distal repairs, the omission of urethral stents did not change overall complications or fistula rates. Repairs may also take place over a 6-8 fr dip stent that is sown in place at the end of the procedure. This is typically left in for a week to 10 days depending on the repair. To aid with bladder spasms the patient is placed on an anticholinergic while the stent is in place.

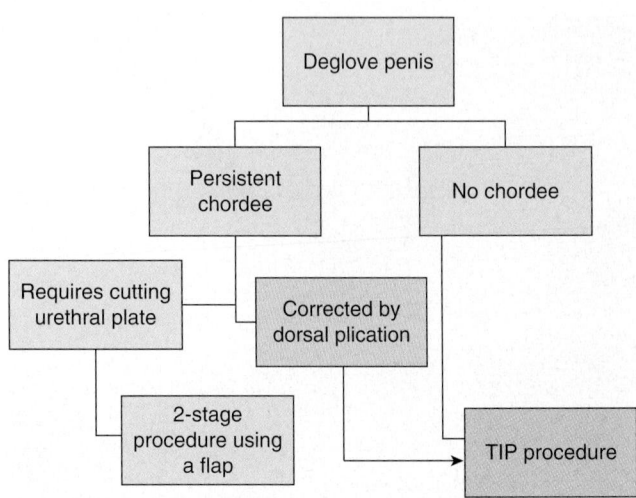

**FIGURE 64-2** Decisional algorithm for primary hypospadias repair.

## Surgical Algorithm

Over 300 different types of surgical repairs are described in the literature. The choice of repair is based on preoperative evaluation and the findings at the time. Currently, most surgeons use the tubularized incised plate (T.I.P.) urethroplasty for distal and mid shaft repairs. This technique is also being applied to some proximal cases. Two-stage repairs are generally reserved for the more complex proximal forms with severe chordee. The algorithm presented here was devised by Snodgrass and is based on 106 primary hypospadias repairs. This algorithm takes into account the principle of preserving the urethral plate whenever possible (Fig. 64-2). Of note, the degree and ability to correct chordee plays a key role in deciding which procedure is performed. Because of the popularity of the T.I.P. procedure, the other techniques described are used less frequently today; however, this is extremely surgeon dependent.

## Correction of Chordee

Penile chordee may result from abnormal tethering of the penile shaft skin to underlying structures, the urethral plate to the corpora cavemosa, or atretic corpora spongiosum tissue extending from the ectopic meatus to the glans. Additionally, chordee can be due to an intrinsic deformity of the corpora spongiosum, or rarely due to a short urethral plate. Addressing this should be done in a stepwise fashion beginning with degloving the shaft skin starting distally and proceeding to the penile scrotal junction. Next, excision of atretic and fibrous corpora spongiosum adjacent to the abnormal meatal position may be done if necessary. Approximately 5% of patients will need an additional straightening procedure after these steps. The urethral plate may then be dissected off the corporeal bodies. Of note, this last step is omitted by some surgeons who proceed directly to dorsal plication. Once complete, the degree of curvature should be assessed using the Gittes artificial erection test using injectable saline. This is accomplished by placing a tourniquet at the penile–scrotal junction and placing a butterfly needle directly into the lateral aspect of the corporeal body directly or distally via the glans.

If chordee persists then surgical straightening is required. Tunica albuginea plication (TAP), described by Baskin and Duckett, corrects chordee by placing a stitch in the dorsal aspect of the penis at the apex of curvature. The dorsal nerve arises from the pudendal nerve and continues distally in 2 bundles superior and slightly lateral to the urethra. As the nerves reach the corporal cavernosal bodies they diverge spreading around the penis. The 12 o'clock position is spared in neuronal structures thus, incising the tunica albuginea in the dorsal midline avoids these nerves and minimizes nerve damage. A 4-0 polydioxanone, or polypropylene stitch is then placed with the knot buried. The incision in the tunica is then closed in a simple interrupted fashion after repeat artificial erection confirms a satisfactory result. The TAP procedure can be applied to mild-to-moderate degrees of chordee. However, if more than 2 rows of plication, or 4 sutures are required then an alternative approach such as complete resection of the urethral plate and corporeal grafting should be considered (see below). In general, if during artificial erection the chordee cannot be corrected with your finger then midline plication is not advised.

While the Nesbit technique is rarely used today it straightens the penis by shortening the convex aspect of the curve. The neurovascular bundles are mobilized off the corporeal bodies prior to making the incision in the posterior lateral portion of the tunica. A transversely orientated ellipse of tunica albuginea from the longer, convex aspect of the penile curvature is removed. The defect is closed in the same orientation. Alternatively, the Heineke–Mikulicz principle can be applied to the ventral surface by making several transverse incisions then closing them in the longitudinal direction. This straightens the penis by lengthening the concave aspect of the curve. The TAP or Nesbit technique can be applied simultaneously with the Heineke–Mikulicz principle on opposing aspects of the penile curvature.

For patients with severe chordee, greater than 40 to 50° where plication would be insufficient to correct the curvature or further shorten the penis, incision of the urethral plate and corporeal grafting is necessary. Curvature this severe is intrinsic to the corpora themselves and transecting the urethral plate rarely, if ever, totally corrects the chordee. Several types of graft materials are used including dermal grafts, tunica vaginalis and single-layer small intestinal submucosa (SIS), all of which have been used with similar success. Once the type of graft material has been selected and harvested a transverse incision is made at the site of maximum curvature on the concave (ventral) aspect of the corpora. The graft is then sutured in place in a running fashion using 6-0 polyglactin suture. The size of the graft harvested should be slightly larger than the defect created to account for any bunching of the graft that occurs during anastomosis.

## URETHROPLASTY

Hypospadias repair can be done either as a 1- or 2-stage operation. Distal, mid-shaft, and proximal hypospadias without significant chordee can be repaired in a single stage and most surgeons choose this approach whenever possible.

Two-stage repairs are reserved for those with perineal hypospadias, severe chordee, and redo operations (the hypospadias cripple). Currently, the most popular single stage operation is the T.I.P. which can be applied to distal, mid-shaft, and proximal defects. This is the modification to the Duplay-type tubularization described by Snodgrass. The incision of the urethral plate allows the urethra to be tubularized around a catheter in a tension free manner, even in those with a shallow urethral groove.

### Tubularized Incised Plate

Once the preputial attachments to the glans are taken down the glans traction stitch is placed. A circumferential subcoronal incision is then marked on the penis starting dorsally and moving around toward the urethral plate. If the current urethral opening is proximal to the circumcising line then a "U" incision is marked thus sparing the plate (Fig. 64-3A). Once the circumcising incision is made, incisions on either side of the urethral plate are made from the current urethral opening and extending distally to the glans where the neo-meatus will be located. The incisions in the glans lateral to the urethral plate should be deep enough to allow for mobilization of the flaps over the neourethra without compromising the vascularity of the urethral plate (Fig. 64-3B). The penis is then degloved and chordee correction can be made as described above.

Next, the urethral plate is incised in the midline from the urethral opening to the glans. This incision should include any urethral web that is present. The depth of the incision is carried down to the corpora cavernosum. In cases of a shallow urethral plate that is inadequate for tubularization a free graft of preputial skin may be placed within the urethral plate incision. The corpus spongiosum lateral to the urethral plate is then dissected off the underlying corpora cavernosa. This can later be used to cover the neourethra as another layer against fistula. The urethral stent is then placed into the bladder. The urethral plate may now be tubularized with the first stitch placed through the epithelium at approximately the level of the mid-glans to create an oval meatus. Tubularization is then carried out from distal to proximal in a running subepithelial closure (Fig. 64-3C). Care should be taken to roll the epithelium into the neourethra. The previously mobilized corpus spongiosum tissue may then be reapproximated over the neourethra in the midline in a running fashion.

A second layer of coverage over the neourethra is recommended to reduce the risk of fistula formation. A vascularized pedicle flap is harvested from the preputial hood and dorsal shaft skin (Fig. 64-3D). The epithelium is removed, and the pedicle buttonholed. The flap is then transferred to the ventral aspect and secured in place with interrupted sutures. Alternatively, the second layer may be harvested from the tunica vaginalis. Glanuloplasty is then done in 2 layers. The skin is then reconfigured using Byars flaps by incising the dorsal hood in the midline down to the level of the mucosal collar of inner preputial skin. This point is sutured; the ventral skin is then trimmed and sutured in the midline, reapproximating the median raphe (Fig. 64-3E). Care should be taken not to remove too much skin to ensure adequate ventral skin coverage. The urethral stent is secured and a dressing is placed.

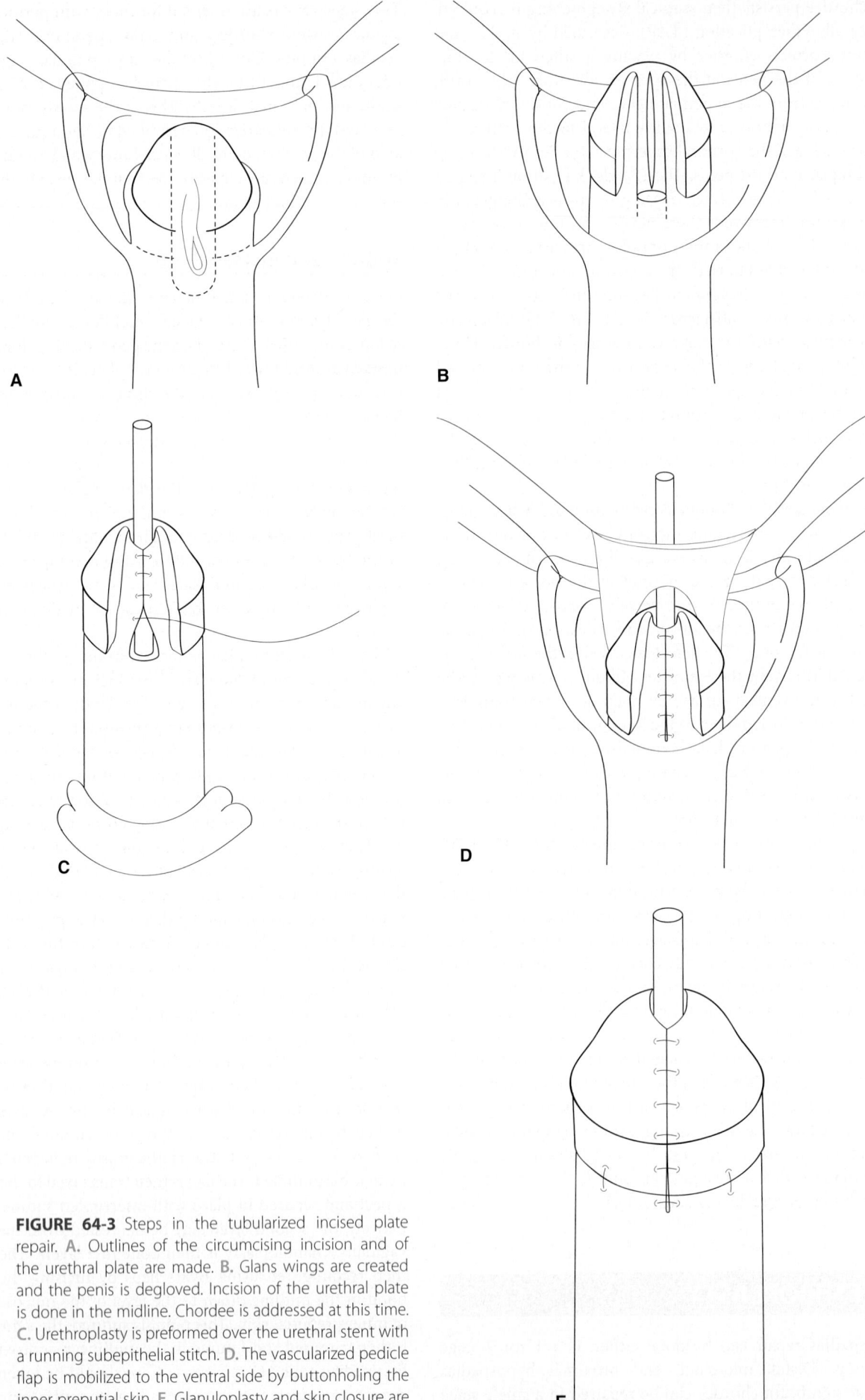

**FIGURE 64-3** Steps in the tubularized incised plate repair. **A.** Outlines of the circumcising incision and of the urethral plate are made. **B.** Glans wings are created and the penis is degloved. Incision of the urethral plate is done in the midline. Chordee is addressed at this time. **C.** Urethroplasty is preformed over the urethral stent with a running subepithelial stitch. **D.** The vascularized pedicle flap is mobilized to the ventral side by buttonholing the inner preputial skin. **E.** Glanuloplasty and skin closure are then preformed.

## URETHRAL REPOSITIONING

The acronym MAGPI that stands for meatal advancement and glanuloplasty was described by Duckett. This is a refashioning of the glans penis with a minor meatal advancement. It is suitable for cases of glandular and subcoronal hypospadias in which the urethra is mobile. A vertical incision is made in the urethral plate with a tenotomy scissors or scalpel to the depth of the corporal bodies. The incision should include any bridge of tissue present in the urethral plate. The incision is then closed in a transverse fashion with 6-0 absorbable suture which advances the meatus to the glans. In effect this repair is based on the Heineke–Mikulicz principle of closing a vertical incision transversely. A circumferential incision is then made below the corona through the inner preputial skin and the shaft skin of the penis is degloved. Glanuloplasty is then performed by retracting the ventral aspect of the meatus distally toward the glans and closing the glans in 2 layers in the midline. The skin is then rearranged using Byars flaps as described above. The use of a catheter for this repair is omitted.

### Meatal-Based Flap

Originally described by Mathieu in 1932 this repair depends on a flap of penile shaft skin proximal to the hypospadiac meatal opening. The length of the defect between the meatal opening and the tip of the glans is measured and an equal length is measured and marked proximally from the meatus. An appropriate width is then marked for the flap.

The circumferential incision of the inner preputial skin is brought around ventrally, the remainder of the shaft skin is degloved and glans wings are developed. The flap is dissected off the underlying corpus spongiosum tissue with a tenotomy scissors and folded over the meatus. The lateral borders are sown to the urethral plate with 7-0 absorbable suture over a stent. A vascularized pedicle flap (see above) is placed over the closure and the glans and ventral skin are reapproximated. While the urethral stent may be left in place for 7 to 10 days some authors suggest that this is not necessary after this repair, showing no difference in overall complications or fistula formation. In general, defects greater than 15 mm cannot be repaired using this technique due to the possibility of incorporating hair-bearing skin of the proximal penis into the repair.

### Onlay Island Flap

This repair is based on a pedicle flap of preputial skin from the dorsal hood. The urethral plate is preserved by marking 2 parallel lines from the urethral opening to the glans. A circumferential incision is also marked on the inner preputial skin below the corona. This is incised, glans flaps are created and the penis is degloved as described above. Chordee, if present, is corrected with a plication stitch. The length of the urethral defect from the glans to the urethral opening is measured. This length is measured transversely along the inner surface of the dorsal hood. The width of the graft is typically 9 to 10 mm. Stay sutures placed in the dorsal hood, outside of the area to be harvested, aid in tissue manipulation. The transverse rectangle of flap is then incised with a scalpel and dissected free from the outer preputial skin and the dorsal shaft skin to the base should be taken to ensure the pedicle is long enough so that the anastomosis can be completed in a tension-free manner. The flap is then brought to the ventral side of the penis and sutured to the urethral plate over a stent using a 6-0 or 7-0 suture in a running fashion. The pedicle is then advanced over the area of anastomosis and secured to the tunica albuginea thus creating a second layer. Glanuloplasty is then preformed and the skin is closed.

In cases where the urethral plate is divided to correct severe chordee, the island flap of preputial skin can be tubularized into a neo-urethra using a Tubularized Preputial Island Flap (TPIF). After the urethral plate has been divided and the penis straightened, creation of the preputial island flap is done as described above. In these cases the width of the graft should be 15 mm as it needs to be rolled around the entirety of the catheter. The graft is then rolled and sutured over the urethral stent in a running fashion. Interrupted sutures at both ends of the anastomosis allow for tailoring of the graft. This is transferred to the ventral side of the penis with the anastomotic line facing the corpora cavernosa. The existing urethral opening is spatulated and sutured to the graft. Dartos tissue is used to cover this anastomosis. The distal aspect of the graft may be tunneled through the glans and sutured in place, or the glans is incised in the midline and glanuloplasty is performed. The skin is then closed.

### Two-Stage Repair

In general, 2-stage repairs are reserved for proximal hypospadias patients with severe chordee, an atretic or "unhealthy" urethral plate, or redo operations. The first stage of the repair involves correction of chordee, preparation of the glans, and harvesting a free flap which will become the neo-urethra. The penis is degloved and the chordee is corrected as above with excision of the urethral plate (Fig. 64-4A). Glans wings are then created by incising the glans deeply in the ventral midline so that the distal ends of the corpora are visible. The material for the free flap is often the preputial skin of the inner dorsal hood (Fig. 64-4B), but bladder mucosa, buccal mucosa from the lower lip or cheek, and postauricular Wolfe skin grafts have also been used. These sites are chosen because they are non-hair-bearing and are easily accessible. Once the graft is harvested the subepithelial tissues and fat are removed. At this stage the graft should have a translucent appearance. The graft is then tacked to the glans and corpora with interrupted absorbable sutures. Quilting sutures are placed in the center of the graft to prevent shearing and to allow for any hematoma to escape (Fig. 64-4C). A Foley catheter is placed in the bladder and a tight dressing is placed over the graft to minimize hematoma formation. A roll of Vaseline gauze is placed over the graft and sutured in place. The catheter and dressing are then removed in 1 week.

The second stage of the operation is preformed 6 months later. At this stage the graft is tubularized into the neo-urethra over a urethral stent (Fig. 64-4D) and covered with a vascular pedicle flap. This is similar to the single-stage tubularized repair described above.

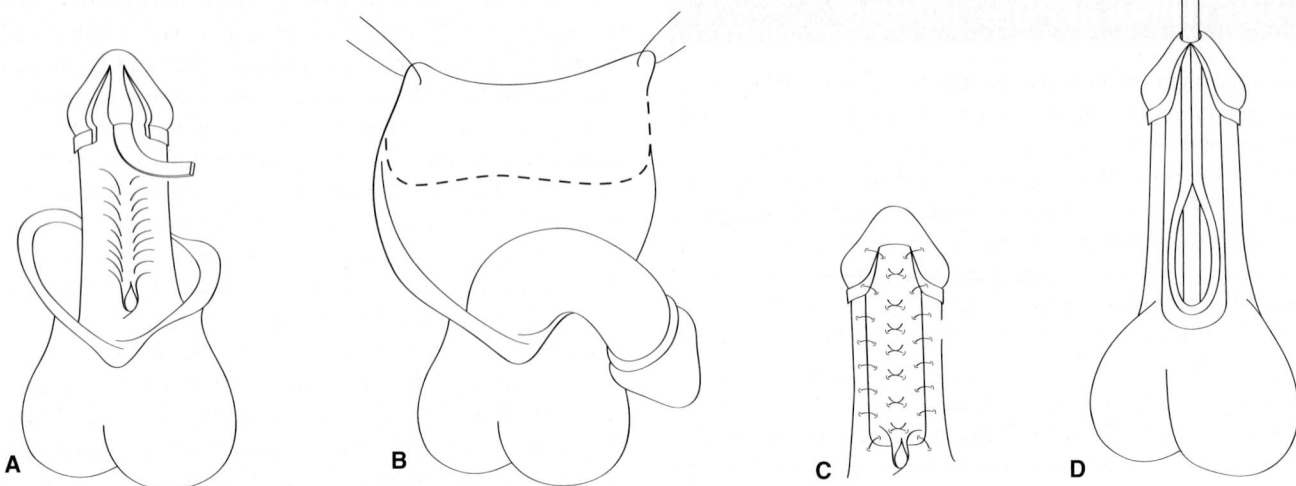

**FIGURE 64-4** The 2-stage repair. **A.** Following degloving of the penis and creation of glans wings the urethral plate is dissected off the corporal bodies. **B.** Free graft is harvested from the dorsal hood. **C.** Free graft is sewn in place. **D.** Tubularization of the urethra at the second stage 6 months later.

## Complications

### Early

Due to the vascularity of the penis, bleeding is a concern. The intraoperative control of bleeding is discussed above, and most surgeons use a compressive dressing to prevent any delayed bleeding. A compressive dressing also serves to limit any postoperative edema. Patients with excessive bleeding postoperatively may require re-exploration to control the source. Hemostasis is also important to prevent hematoma formation which can be a nidus for infection and potentially cause breakdown of the repair. Infection, hematoma, and skin flap ischemia can lead to poor wound healing, fistula formation, or complete wound dehiscence. Good surgical technique such as proper tissue handling, achieving hemostasis, limited use of electrocautery, and maintenance of vascularized pedicle flaps help avoid these complications.

### Late

The incidence of late complications of hypospadias repair depends on the severity of the hypospadias, choice of repair, and surgeon experience. A review of a nationwide database, including 1511 patients, showed the overall reoperation rate following initial hypospadias repair was 9.8%. Of these repeat operations, ~1.3% were repeat hypospadias repairs, 13.9% repair of urethrocutaneous fistula, 12.6% treatment of urethral stricture, 5.3% excision of skin lesion, 3.2% repeat circumcision, and 3.2% release of chordee. This is similar to an analysis of 26 articles including 2035 patients that showed an average reoperation rate of 9%. In general, a period of 6 months should elapse between the initial operation and repair of complications, unless done for bleeding or infection. This will allow for resolution of edema, and complete healing after the first procedure.

### Fistula

Patients can present with an urethrocutaneous fistula at any time following surgical repair. In 1 series 58% of fistulae presented within the first month following operation; however, 23% presented more than 2 years after initial repair. The presence of large or multiple fistulae indicates that the initial urethroplasty will need a complete revision. Prior to repair of fistulae, a distal urethral stricture must be ruled out as this will predispose to recurrence. This may be done with cystoscopy or by passing urethral sounds. While many fistula closures have been described, the underlying principle uses a vascularized pedicle flap between the urethral closure and the skin. In his initial report of this technique Duckett reported a 90% success rate.

### Meatal Stenosis

Meatal stenosis is caused by local ischemia, or fashioning a meatus that is too narrow. It may present as spraying or narrowing of the urinary steam, and difficulty voiding. It can also manifest as recurrent urinary tract infections caused by incomplete bladder emptying. Stenosis can be treated with meatal dilation on an outpatient basis. If this fails, or in cases of severe stenosis a fonnal meatoplasty is done. This involves a cutback of the stenotic urethra and suturing of the skin edges on the glans to the urethra on both sides of the incision. An antibiotic cream can be applied to the meatus after operation.

### Urethral Stenosis

Techniques that involve a circumferential proximal urethral anastomosis such as the TPIF are prone to this complication. Endoscopic procedures such as Direct Vision Internal Urethrotomy (DVIU) have yielded limited success in short segment (<1 cm) strictures following hypospadias surgery. The majority of patients (up to 80%) re-presented with recurrent stricture, and a second attempt at DVIU did not improve outcomes and may lead to longer segmented strictures. Formal repeat urethroplasty is therefore necessary.

### Persistent Chordee

Recurrent chordee is often due to inadequate repair at the time of initial operation. However, it may be caused by fibrosis overlying the site of urethroplasty. In order to exclude the latter the penis is degloved and artificial erection is performed. If persistent chordee is confirmed then a dorsal plication of tunica albuginea may be done to correct it.

## Balanitis Xerotica Obliterans

Balanitis xerotica obliterans (BXO) is a chronic inflammatory process of unknown etiology. It results in scarring and fibrosis of the glans and meatus. The application of topical steroids may help some patients, but formal meatoplasty may be necessary. In severe cases the urethra will need to be removed and replaced with buccal mucosa.

## Intraurethral Hair Growth

Hair within the urethra serves as a nidus for the formation of urinary calculi. This complication is avoided with modem hypospadias repair techniques using non-hairbearing skin in the urethroplasty. For symptomatic patients with a hairy urethra, the only effective option is repeat urethroplasty with a graft of non-hairbearing skin.

## Urethrocele

This condition is a dilated segment of neo-urethra often associated with a distal stricture. Patients can present with a poor urinary stream, post-void dribbling, urinary tract infections, swelling of the penis during urination, or urethral calculi due to stasis. Surgical correction involves excision of the redundant urethra and correction of any distal stenosis that may be present. As in the repair of urethrocutaneous fistula a second layer of closure is advised.

## Outcomes

Outcomes for hypospadias surgery are a function of the degree of hypospadias at initial presentation and the type of repair performed. As expected, the types of repair that are more commonly used in more severe forms of hypospadias are associated with higher rates of complications. Few studies report outcomes in adults after hypospadias surgery. In addition, long-term outcomes are difficult to interpret as newer techniques replace older ones, and ideas about the optimal timing of the first operation and suture material evolve with time. This section will focus on broad outcomes of micturation, cosmetic appearance, and sexual function following different techniques of hypospadias surgery.

## Tubularized Incised Plate

In the initial muticenter report of outcomes in 148 patients following TIP urethroplasty, the overall complication rate was 10%. Five patients had a fistula, 3 had meatal stenosis, and 2 had a partial glans dehiscence. In cases of midshaft (30 patients) and proximal (35 patients) hypospadias repaired using this technique, complications were 13% and 37%, respectively. In a separate series 65 distal and 18 proximal hypospadias repairs were done using the TIP repair. In the patients undergoing a distal repair there were 3 fistulas, 1 glans dehiscence, and 2 skin tags requiring removal. Complications following proximal repair included: 1 fistula, and glans dehiscence in 3 patients.

## MAGPI

Reporting the results of more than 1100 patients following MAGPI repair Duckett found a re-operative rate of 1.2%. Individual complication rates were 0.5%, 0.6% and 0.1% for fistula, meatal retraction, and chordee, respectively. However, the average follow-up for these patients was 2.3 months with a range of 2 weeks to 2 years. Longer term, but smaller series have shown a larger number with partial meatal regression (22%) and complete meatal regression (15%), particularly in those with coronal and subcoronal hypospadias.

## Onlay Island Flap

In a study in which the mean follow-up after onlay island flap was 2.7 years in 374 boys, Baskin reported the reoprative rate was 9% overall. Complications of this repair were: fistula (6%), urethral diverticulum (0.5%), epithelial inclusion cyst (0.5%), and meatal stenosis (1%). In a retrospective review of 189 patients following TPIF, Dewan reviewed patients whose mean follow-up time was 25 months. As this repair is normally reserved for severe cases, complications were common. Fistula occurred in 34%, urethral strictures in 12%, and 18% developed meatal stenosis. The overall reoperation rate was 50%. An additional concern is penile torsion around the flap which was found in 2 of 30 evaluated patients in a separate series.

## Mathieu

Hakim et al reported complications of the Mathieu repair in stented and nonstented patients. The overall complication rate was 3.2% in all 336 patients. There was no difference in overall complications in either group: 3.6% in nonstented patients (8/222), and 2.6% in patients with a stent (3/114). Fistula occurred in 2.7% of the nonstented and 2.6% of the stented group. Additionally, there was 1 meatal stenosis and 1 meatal retraction in the nonstented group.

## Two-Stage Repair

Bracka reviewed 600 of his 2-stage hypospadias repairs. The majority of these had a free flap of preputial skin used in the repair. Revision of the first stage for persistent chordee and/or graft retraction was necessary in 4%. The overall incidence of fistula was 6% and was higher in redo operations, 10% versus 3% for primary repairs. As proof of the importance of a second layer of coverage for any hypospadias repair most of fistulae in this series occurred early prior to the use of a vascularized pedicle flap. Urethral stenosis occurred in 7%. The author concluded that this may be attributed to BXO and suggested that if this were present then a postauricular skin flap or buccal mucosa be used rather than genital skin. In a separate long-term review of free flap patients 27 of an original 44 patients were evaluated after a mean of 12 years following surgery. Ten (44%) had problems with urinary spraying, and 10 needed to "milk" the urethra after urination to prevent post-void dribbling.

## Micturation

The incision of the urethral plate raised concerns over long-term voiding problems. In an intermediate-term study looking at flow rates in toilet-trained boys following TIP repair 33/48 patients had normal peak flow rates and 46/48 had postvoid residuals less than 10% of the expected volume. One of these two patients required meatal dilation. In another study with a mean follow-up of 3.1 years, 18/19 available patients (out of 70) had normal peak flow rates with the remaining patients requiring a meatotomy. These data suggest that TIP repair is not associated with late urethral stenosis and patients may be discharged at 6 months following a normal voiding study or meatal calibration. However, the mean time between initial surgery and reoperation for any cause was 17 months in 1 nationwide review.

## COSMETIC APPEARANCE

Attempts at evaluating the cosmetic appearance of the penis following hypospadias surgery are difficult. Patients and families do not have much to compare to and may cite displeasing factors such as penile size or appearance of the testis/scrotum which cannot be controlled surgically. In studies in which the penis is photographed in a follow-up and reviewed by surgeons who have a vested interest in the repair, observational bias may occur. However, in a study of 27 patients who had undergone a single-stage TIP or Mathieu repair parents rated their sons' penile appearance following surgery on a 0 to 10 scale. Photographs of these patients were also blindly reviewed by 3 surgeons. This study showed concordance between the ranking of the parents and the surgeons with the TIP procedure having superior cosmetic appearance. Similarly, another study had 5 healthcare professionals review photographs of 32 patients. Those that had distal hypospadias underwent either a TIP or Mathieu repair and those with proximal hypospadias underwent a TIP or island onlay. In both cases, the TIP repairs were deemed to have superior cosmetic appearance particularly due to the slit-like appearance of the meatus. Hakim and colleagues reported that 325 of their 336 patients (96.7%) that underwent a Mathieu repair had "excellent cosmetic and function results." In their long-term review of 2-stage repairs after puberty Lam and colleagues found that all patients had "excellent cosmetic results." Of the 27 patients that responded 92% were pleased with their penile appearance and 88% said that they had a normal-appearing penis.

### Sexual Outcome

Following successful hypospadias repair the ability to obtain an erection and sexual function should be normal. Fertility should not be affected unless the patient had associated undescended testicles. Psychosocial function was assessed in 189 boys and men following hypospadias repair using standardized questionnaires. These answers were compared to age-matched controls that underwent inguinal hernia repair.

Psychosocial function did not differ between the 2 groups. In another study of 37 hypospadias repair patients and 39 controls there was no difference in erectile problems or strength of libido. However, there were fewer men in the hypospadias group who were completely satisfied with their sexual life than controls (51.3% and 76.9% respectively). There were also more ejaculatory problems (37%) in the hypospadias group versus none in the control group.

## SUMMARY

Hypospadias is a common problem the rate of which appears to be increasing. Surgical correction is necessary for long-term urinary and sexual function. While surgical planning begins at the time of initial diagnosis, the site of the meatus does not always indicate the complexity of the repair necessary for correction. Therefore, surgeons who perform hypospadias surgery should be prepared to perform more complex repairs if the need arises. Several studies have shown that the reoperation rate following hypospadias repair is about 9%. The types of complications that occur after hypospadias surgery vary depending on the severity of the defect and the technique used to repair it. Further longer-term studies that assess patients' urinary and sexual function are needed to evaluate the durable outcomes of these operative procedures.

### SELECTED READINGS

Baskin LS, Ebbers MB. Hypospadias: anatomy, etiology and technique. *J Pediatr Surg* 2006;41:463–472.

Bubanj T, Perovic S, Milicevic R, et al. Sexual behavior and sexual function of adults after hypospadias surgery: a comparative study. *J Urol* 2004;171(5):1876–1879.

Cimador M, Castagnetti M, Milazzo M, et al. Suture materials: do they affect fistula and stricture rates in flap urethroplasties? *Urol Int* 2004;73:320–324.

Duckett JW. MAG (meatoplasty and glanuloplasty) a procedure for subcoronal hypospadias. *J Urol* 2002;167:2153–2156.

Duckett JW. Transverse Preputial Island Flap Technique for Repair of Severe hypospadias. *J Urol* 2002;167:1179–1182.

Gurdal M, Tekin A, Kirecci S, Sengor F. Intermediate-term functional and cosmetic results of the Snodgrass procedure in distal and midpenile hypospadias. *Ped Surg Int* 2004;20:197–199.

Hammouda H, El-Ghoneime A, Bagli D, McLorie G, Khoury A. Tubularized Incised Plate Repair: functional outcome after intermediate followup. *J Urol* 2003;169:331–333.

Husman DA, Rathbun SR. Long-term follow-up of visual internal urethrotomy for management of short (less than 1 cm) penile urethral strictures following hypospadias repair. *J Urol* 2006;176:1738–1714.

Kolon TF, Goncales ET Jr. The dorsal inlay graft for hypospadias repair. *J Urol* 2000;163(6):1941–1943.

Lam PN, Greenfield SP, Williot P. 2-stage repair in infancy for severe hypospadias with chordee: long-term results after puberty. *J Urol* 2005;174:1567–1572.

Leslie JA, Cain MP, Kaefer M, et al. Corporeal grafting for severe hypospadias: a single institution experience with 3 techniques. *J Urol* 2008;180:1749–1752.

McLorie G, Joyner B, Herz D, et al. A prospective randomized clinical trial to evaluate methods of postoperative care of hypospadias. *J Urol* 2001;165:1669–1672.

Patel RP, Shukla AR, Snyder III HM. The island tube and island onlay hypospadias repairs offer excellent long-term outcomes: a 14 year followup. *J Urol* 2004;172:1717–1719.

Samuel M, Wilcox D. Tubularized incised-plate urethroplasty for distal and proximal hypospadias. *BJU Int* 2003;92(7):783–785.

Scarpa M, Castagnetti M, Musi L, Rigamonti W. Is objective assessment of the cosmetic result after distal hypospadias repair superior to subjective assessment? *J Pediatr Urol* 2009;5:110–113.

Snodgrass WT. Snodgrass technique for hypospadias repair. *BJU Int* 2005;95:683–693.

Snodgrass W, Selcuk Y. Tubularized incised plate for mid shaft and proximal hypospadias repair. *J Urol* 2007;177(2):698–702.

Sozubir S, Snodgrass W. A new algorithm for primary hypospadias repair based on the Tip urethroplasty. *J Pediatr Surg* 2003;38(6):1157–1161.

Thomas DF. Hypospadiology: science and surgery. *BJU Int* 2004;93:470–473.

Utsch B, Albers N, Ludwig M. Genetic and molecular aspects of hypospadias. *Eur J Pediatr Surg* 2004;14(5):297–302.

Ververdis M, Dickson A, Gough D. An objective assessment of the results of hypospadias surgery. *BJU Int* 2005;96:135–139.

Wilcox D, Snodgrass W. Long-term outcome following hypospadias repair. *World J Urol* 2006;24:240–243.

Wilcox DT, Mouriquand PD. Hypospadias. In: Thomas OF, Duffy PG, Rickwood AM, eds. *Essentials of Paediatric Urology.* 2nd ed. London, England: Informica Healthcare; 2008:214–231.

Wood HM, Kay R, Angenneir KW, et al. Timing of the presentation of urethrocutaneous fistulas after hypospadias repair in pediatric patients. *J Urol* 2008;180(4 suppl):1752–1756.

# Urinary Tract Obstruction

# CHAPTER 65

*Michael C. Carr and Howard M. Snyder III*

## KEY POINTS

1. Meatal stenosis is a condition that alters the direction of the urinary stream, but is not worrisome for obstruction of the urinary tract.

2. Posterior urethral valves present as a spectrum, from in utero obstruction which can be lethal due to pulmonary hypoplasia to a boy with persistent bedwetting and daytime incontinence. Long-term follow-up is critical to minimize the complications due to "valve-bladder syndrome."

3. Dilated ureters that are discovered prenatally can be due to ectopic ureters, primary obstructed megaureters, or ureteroceles.

4. The management of megaureters has evolved, with many megaureters showing improvement and complete resolution with expectant management. Long-term follow-up is beneficial through adolescence to look for indolent obstructive changes over time.

5. Antenatal hydronephrosis can represent a ureteropelvic junction (UPJ) obstruction, but the onus is on the clinician to demonstrate the presence of obstruction since the majority of patients detected are asymptomatic.

Urinary tract obstruction in children presents in a variety of fashions, from the child who presents with episodic renal colic secondary to an intermittent ureteropelvic junction (UPJ) obstruction to the prenatal findings of a male fetus with significant bilateral hydroureteronephrosis, a distended bladder, and oligohydramnios that can be the hallmark of posterior urethral valves. This chapter will provide a broad overview of various types of obstruction and their pathophysiology, presentation, and diagnosis along with operative techniques to correct these obstructions.

## MEATAL STENOSIS

### Pathophysiology

Meatal stenosis in boys is an acquired narrowing of the urethral meatus (Table 65-1). It is the result of prior episodes of meatitis in infants which occurs due to chronic irritation and ammoniacal inflammation of the meatus due to contact with urine, stool, or the diaper in infants who have been circumcised. This chronic meatal irritation leads to progressive, indolent scarring of the meatus with subsequent stenosis.

### Presentation and Diagnosis

Most boys with meatal stenosis are not recognized until the time that they attempt to toilet train. Occasionally an astute pediatrician will notice evidence of narrowing of an infant's urethral meatus. Typically, boys with meatal stenosis will have an upwardly deflected urinary stream, and occasionally complain of dysuria. In addition the urinary stream can be very forceful, and smaller and finer in caliber with prolonged voiding. Often times, mothers will question why their sons are having difficulty directing his urinary stream, only to discover that he is pushing his penis downward in order to successfully aim his stream into the toilet.

The diagnosis of meatal stenosis can generally be made with a well-taken history and the findings confirmed at the time of physical examination. Generally, the urethral meatus narrows from the inferior aspect thus leading to the dorsally deflected urinary stream. Once the findings have been confirmed, the family can be offered the option of performing an office meatotomy versus a meatotomy that is performed in the operating room. In over 95% of patients, an office meatotomy can be successfully performed.

### Operative Technique: Meatotomy

With the advent of Emla cream (5% Lidocaine/prilocaine cream, APP Pharmaceuticals), meatotomies can be performed painlessly and very efficiently. A Tegaderm dressing is placed beneath the patients glans, the Emla cream is applied, and the Tegaderm dressing is brought together to maintain contact between the Emla cream and the urethral meatus. After 40 minutes this dressing can be removed and the patient is ready to have the meatotomy performed. Parental involvement is encouraged so that the parent is reading a book to his/her child while the procedure is being performed or the child is allowed to play a video game. A fine straight hemostat is then gently inserted into the urethral meatus to ensure that adequate analgesia is present. The tissue is then crushed

| TABLE 65-1 | Normal Size of the Urethral Meatus in Boys | | | | |
|---|---|---|---|---|---|
| Age | Size | No. (%) | | Size | No. (%) |
| **Group 1** | | | | | |
| 6 wk to 1 yr | Below 8 Fr. | 22/160 (14) | | 10 Fr. | 138/160 (86) |
| 1 yr | Below 8 Fr. | 10/63 (14) | | 10 Fr. | 53/63 (86) |
| 2 yr | Below 8 Fr. | 17/109 (16) | | 10 Fr. | 92/109 (84) |
| 3 yr | Below 8 Fr. | 13/93 (14) | | 10 Fr. | 80/93 (86) |
| **Group 2** | | | | | |
| 4 yr | Tight 8 Fr. | 7/83 (8) | | 12 Fr. | 70/83 (84) |
| 5 yr | Tight 8 Fr. | 10/111 (9) | | 12 Fr. | 92/111 (83) |
| 6 yr | Tight 8 Fr. | 8/87 (9) | | 12 Fr. | 61/87 (82) |
| 7 yr | Tight 8 Fr. | 4/56 (7) | | 12 Fr. | 43/56 (77) |
| 8 yr | Tight 8 Fr. | 4/61 (8) | | 12 Fr. | 41/61 (67) |
| 9 yr | Tight 8 Fr. | 4/69 (7) | | 12 Fr. | 40/60 (67) |
| 10 yr | Tight 8 Fr. | 3/50 (6) | | 12 Fr. | 37/50 (74) |
| **Group 3** | | | | | |
| 11 yr | Below 10 Fr. | 2/45 (4) | | 14 Fr. | 36/45 (80) |
| 12 yr | Below 10 Fr. | 2/40 (5) | | 14 Fr. | 28/40 (69) |

*Note:* From Litvak AA, Morris JD, McRoberts JW. Normal size of the urethral meatus in male children. *J Urol* 1976;115:736. Used by permission.

in the midline allowing the hemostat to remain clamped for 30 seconds. A midline incision is made with straight Iris scissors. This approach will allow for good hemostasis. Puralube, which is ophthalmic Vaseline, is then gently instilled into the urethral meatus and the family is instructed to do this twice daily for 2 weeks. No attempt is made to do any formal dilations as this can be traumatic. The effects of EMLA cream will last for 2 hours, families are instructed to use acetaminophen or ibuprofen as needed and to encourage water drinking for the first 24 hours after the procedure is performed.

A meatotomy that is performed in the operating room involves excising a V-shaped wedge of tissue from the urethral meatus and then fine sutures are placed at 3, 5, 6, 7, and 9 o'clock to oppose the urethral mucosa to the edge of the glans. Once again, families are advised to instill Puralube twice daily for 1 to 2 weeks (Fig. 65-1).

## Surgical Outcome

No restrictions are made on patient's activities. Occasionally, meatal edema following the surgical procedure can cause spraying with voiding, but this almost always resolves spontaneously within a few days. The key is to encourage families to continue to instill Puralube twice daily as the edema resolves. If the parents are compliant with this regimen, recurrent stenosis is extremely rare.

## POSTERIOR URETHRAL VALVES

### Embryology

The embryology of posterior urethral valves is not well understood, and common theories as to the development of valves do not account for the different types of valves clinically seen. Theories include remnants of the urogenital membrane, extreme underdevelopment of normally placed urethral folds, or as a result of anomalous junction of the ejaculatory duct and the prostatic utricle.

Posterior urethral valves were originally classified into 3 different types by H.H. Young (Fig. 65-2). Type I valves are folds that emanate from the distal verumontanum and divide into 2 leaflets and fuse anteriorly. Type II valves arise from the verumontanum and extend proximally as divided membranes. These are extremely rare. Type III valves are a diaphragm in the area of the verumontanum. It is rare to visualize posterior urethral valves prior to any urethral manipulation and therefore passage of a urethral catheter may alter the endoscopic appearance.

### Presentation and Diagnosis

In the past, posterior urethral valves were recognized when newborn males presented with urosepsis or azotemia. Nowadays, with the ubiquitous use of prenatal ultrasonography, the findings of significant hydroureteronephrosis, bladder distension, and dilation of the prostatic urethral (Keyhole sign) alert the perinatologist of the possibility of lower urinary tract obstruction (Fig. 65-3). Ongoing prenatal evaluation following the initial ultrasound focuses on abnormalities within the kidney that suggests underlying renal dysplasia and carefully notes the amniotic fluid index which is a critical parameter. Progressive oligohydramnios that is noted in the second trimester can be a harbinger of pulmonary hypoplasia. This understanding of the relationship between amniotic fluid levels and pulmonary development led to the development of the vesicoamniotic shunt. This device was able to

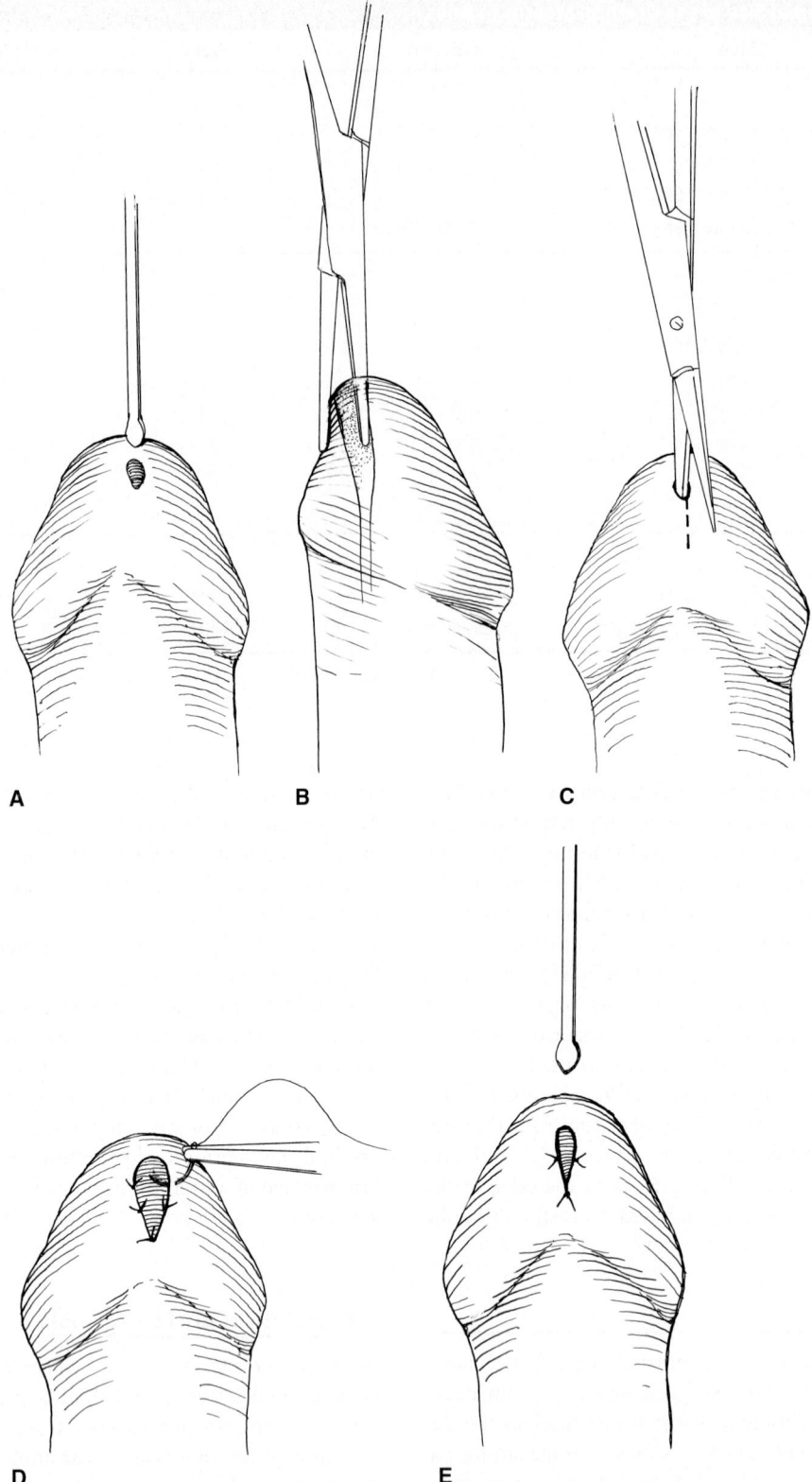

**FIGURE 65-1** Operative repair of meatal stenosis: meatotomy. **A.** The meatus is calibrated serially with a bougie à boule. **B.** The ventral lip of the meatus is crushed in the midline with a fine, straight hemostat for about half a centimeter. **C.** The crushed area is divided with a straight iris scissors. **D.** The urethral mucosa is sewn to the glanular mucosa with interrupted 6-0 chromic sutures. **E.** The meatus is recalibrated serially with a bougie à boule to make sure that the meatotomy has been adequate.

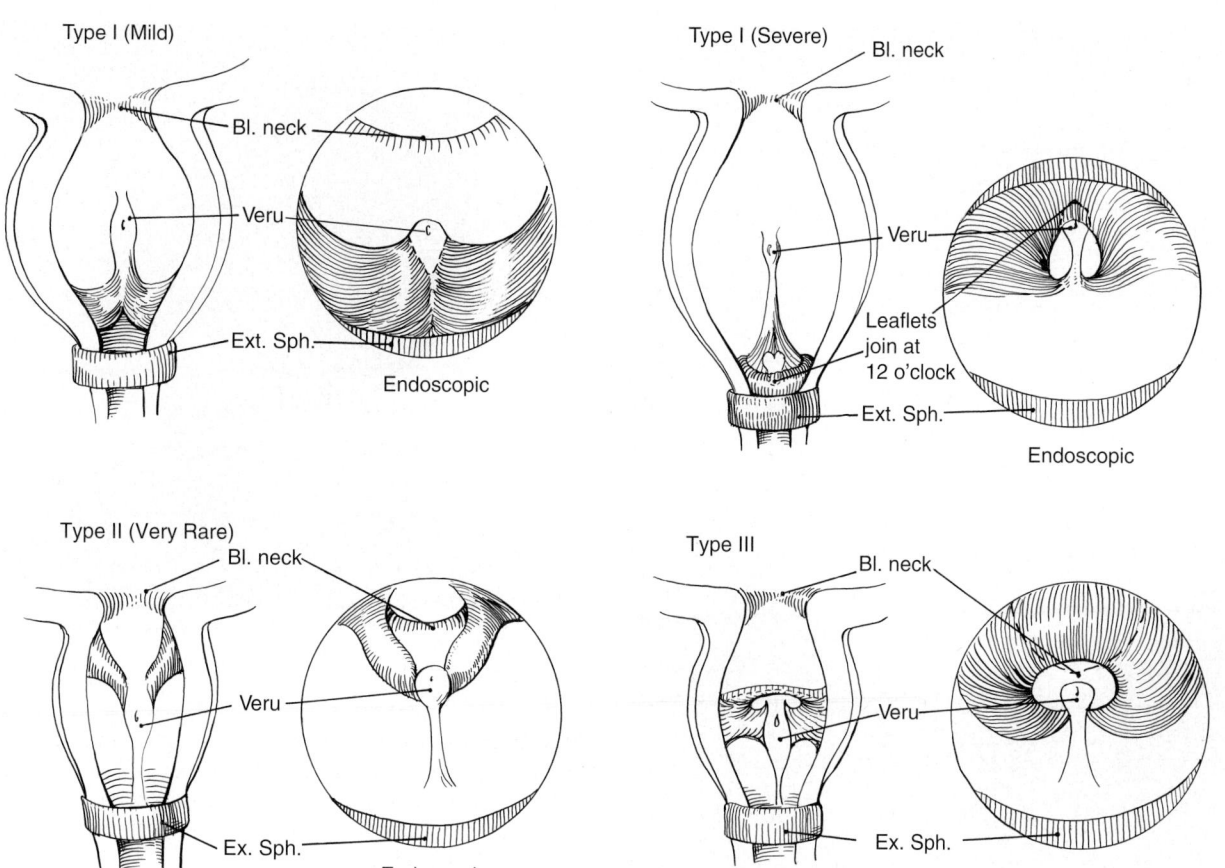

**FIGURE 65-2** Types of posterior urethral valves. (From Hendren WH. Urethral valves. In Ashcraft KW, Holder TM, eds. *Pediatric Surgery*. 2nd ed. Philadelphia: WB Saunders; 1993:665–677. Used by permission.)

successfully bypass the lower urinary tract obstruction and reconstitute the amniotic fluid levels.

The use of fetal bladder aspiration and assessment of electrolytes along with several additional biochemical parameters were used to stratify the renal function of the fetuses. It became apparent that serial bladder aspirations along with

assessment of urine production as well as electrolyte and biochemical analysis provided a better assessment of fetal renal function (Table 65-2).

The placement of vesicoamniotic shunts has become commonplace with the overall complication rate being reported at less than 1%. These shunts, though, can become dislodged and require replacement if oligohydramnios returns. In addition there have been reports of bowel perforation in shunts that were never positioned appropriately within the bladder.

Beyond the newborn period, other symptoms of posterior urethral valves depend on the age of the child and the degree of obstruction. In an extensive review by Hendren, other presenting symptoms included bed wetting, urinary tract

**FIGURE 65-3** Prenatal ultrasound showing markedly distended urinary bladder and dilation of the posterior urethra (arrow), the keyhole sign.

| TABLE 65-2 | Predictive Parameters | |
|---|---|---|
| | **Good** | **Poor** |
| Sodium | <90 mmol/L | >100 mmol/L |
| Chloride | <80 mmol/L | >90 mmol/L |
| Osmolality | <180 mOsm/L | >200 mOsm/L |
| Calcium | <7 mg/dL | >8 mg/dL |
| B2-microglobulin | <6 mg/L | >10 mg/L |
| Total protein | <20 mg/dL | >40 mg/L |

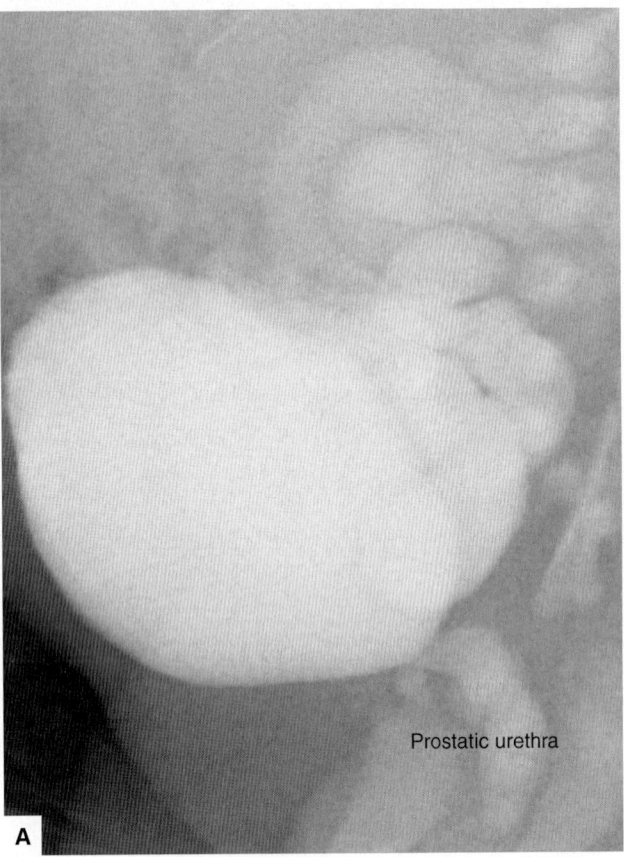

Prostatic urethra

A

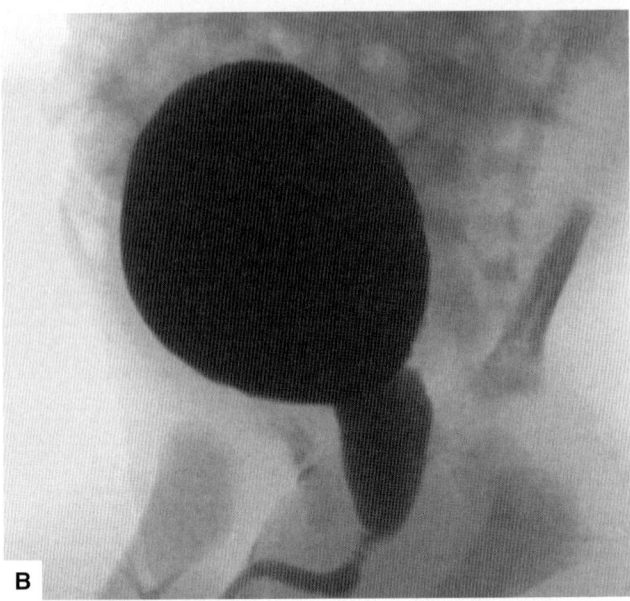

B

**FIGURE 65-4** Two examples of voiding cystourethrograms showing typical features of posterior urethra valves. **A.** Note the presence of a high-volume reflux along with posterior urethral valves. **B.** Classic appearance of posterior urethra, which is dilated, elongated, and associated with bladder-neck hypertrophy.

infection, daytime wetting, poor urinary stream, frequency, dribbling, hematuria, and acute urinary retention. These varied symptoms again underscore that posterior urethral valves present as a spectrum from valves that cause such significant in utero obstruction that end-stage renal disease is to be expected for boys who present with the persistence of daytime wetting despite having successfully toilet trained.

In a newborn with suspected valves, the bladder should be catheterized with a small (4-6 French) feeding tube until the baby is stabilized and further diagnostic studies can be performed. A Coude catheter may be used as well, to decompress the bladder. An initial ultrasound will show the degree of hydronephrosis and the thickness of the bladder wall. Broad-spectrum antibiotics should be started and a basic metabolic panel should be serially monitored to assess renal function as well as electrolyte abnormalities. Initial assessment in the newborn will reflect maternal renal function with subsequent measurements now reflecting the infant's renal function. Once the baby is stable, a voiding cystourethrogram will demonstrate the presence of posterior urethral valves and possibly vesicoureteral reflux (Fig. 65-4). The bladder oftentimes shows trabeculation and the posterior urethra is dilated, elongated with the presence of bladder neck hypertrophy. After the radiographic studies, surgical options depend on the size and the overall stability of the baby. Catheter drainage should be continued until the baby's creatinine has stabilized or until the valves can be endoscopically incised.

In babies who are quite small or who are extremely ill, cutaneous vesicostomy can be considered as well. Upper tract urinary diversion, besides a cutaneous vesicostomy, is not warranted and has been shown to be deleterious to the overall bladder function without improving renal function.

## Operative Technique: Endoscopic Valve Ablation

There are few medical indications for circumcision, but a boy who is born with posterior urethral valves is one situation where circumcision is strongly advised. The baby is placed in a dorsolithotomy position with the use of gel rolls beneath his thighs. Appropriate prepping of the genitalia is performed. The urethral meatus should be calibrated to minimize the risk of injury from an endoscope. A 7.5-French infant cystourethroscope is used to confirm the presence of valves. The bladder should be partially full, and the cystoscopy irrigating bag should be high enough above the patient to distend the urethra for adequate direct visualization of the posterior urethra. Options for endoscopic ablation include the use of a cold knife or hot knife or Holmium laser. The authors preferred method is the use of an 8.5-French resectoscope equipped with a cold knife (Fig. 65-5). The cold knife is initially advanced into the infant's bladder using the 25° lens and the cold knife is visualized while the resectoscope is in the bladder. The sickle blade is used to ablate the valves at the 5 o'clock and 7 o'clock positions under direct visualization. In addition, a triangular blade can be used to further incise the valves at the 12 o'clock position. The idea is to disrupt the annulus so that the valve leaflets no longer cause outlet obstruction. Following successful valve ablation, a Foley catheter or feeding tube can be reinserted which is left in

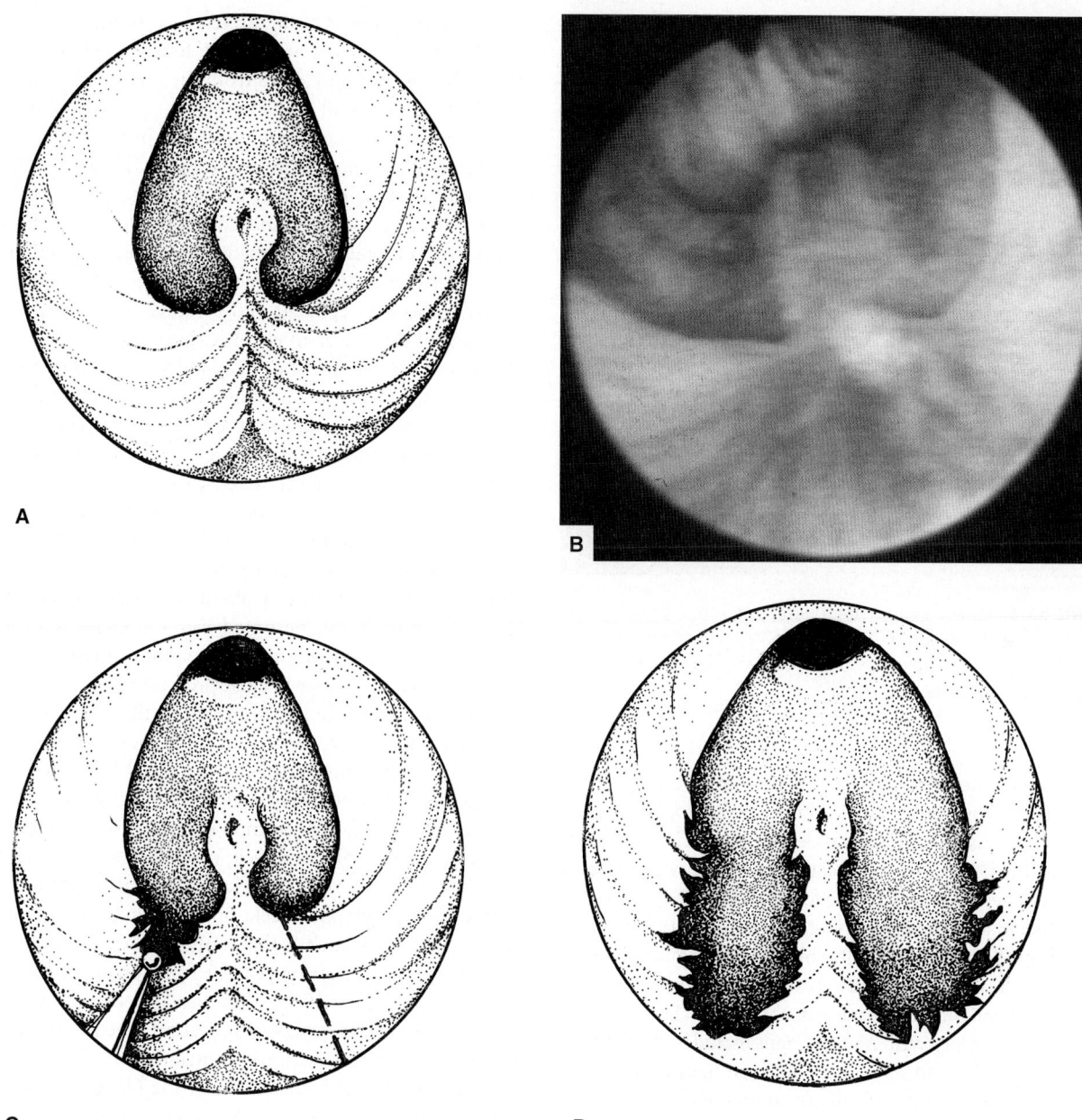

**FIGURE 65-5** Operative repair of posterior urethral valves: endoscopic valve ablation. **A.** With the bladder partly distended, cystourethroscopy demonstrates the sail-like posterior valves emanating from the distal verumontanum. **B.** Artistic rendering of posterior urethral valves. **C.** After passing the cold knife through the cystoscope with the scope in the bladder, the scope is withdrawn to directly visualize the valves. The valve leaflets are cut with the sickle blade (see inset) or a bugbee electrode at the 5 o'clock and 7 o'clock positions on the inferior aspect of the urethra. **D.** The valve leaflets are to be further divided at the 12 o'clock position to further disrupt the annulus and render the valve incompetent. The use of the cold knife avoids any injury due to the use of diathermy.

place overnight. Following removal, the infant's bladder then begins to cycle in a more normal fashion now that the outlet obstruction has been relieved.

## Surgical Outcome

Endoscopic valve ablation is highly successful in eliminating the obstruction in the majority of cases. However, the baby's response to valve ablation needs to be carefully followed. It is not uncommon to see the creatinine continues to rise for a period of time before achieving its nadir as the azotemia resolves. Upper tract imaging with renal and bladder ultrasonography is generally performed 2 months following valve ablation to look for appropriate improvement in the degree of hydroureteronephrosis. A subsequent VCUG study is performed 6 to 12 months following valve ablation to reassess changes to the bladder as well as prostatic urethra and look for improvement or resolution of the vesicoureteral reflux. If upper-tract changes persist and there are still residual abnormalities to the prostatic urethra then a second look endoscopically for residual valves is warranted (Fig. 65-6). With meticulous operative technique, postoperative problems with stricture formation from scarring should not be seen.

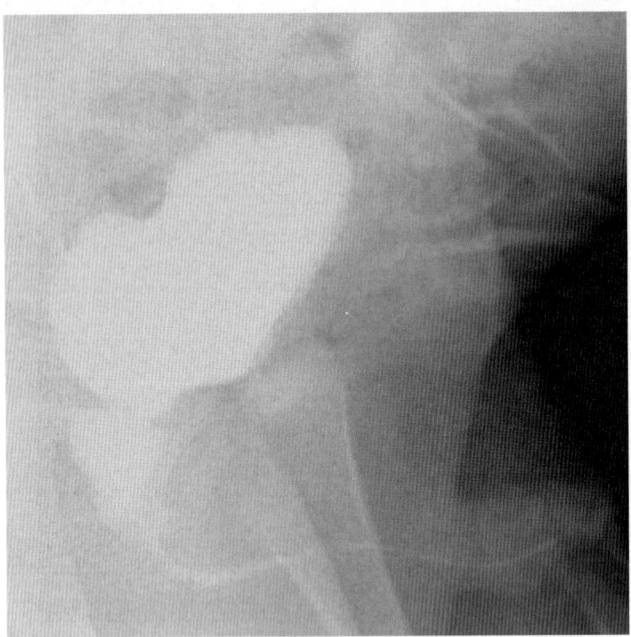

**FIGURE 65-6** Voiding cystourethrogram 12 months following valve incision. Residual dilation and elongation of the posterior urethra warrants a second look to make sure residual leaflets are not contributing to ongoing outlet obstruction.

The initial placement of a feeding tube in an infant who is presumed to have posterior urethral valves should be done by a senior house officer and not left to inexperienced hands as injury to the urethra can occur. An infant who presents with valves deserves appropriate follow-up until adulthood to ensure that bladder function as well as renal function remains appropriate. The so-called "valve bladder syndrome" refers to a boy who has lost the ability to sense appropriate bladder fullness and will oftentimes have an abnormally large bladder that does not empty well. Management includes strict timed voiding schedules and sometimes the need to consider intermittent catheterization to facilitate emptying of the bladder. Some of these boys have underlying renal insufficiency and poor concentrating ability so that they are polyuric. These boys oftentimes will benefit from overnight catheter drainage.

## URETEROVESICAL JUNCTION OBSTRUCTION

Obstruction at the ureterovesical junction is also known as a primary obstructed megaureter. Distal ureteral obstruction can also be seen with renal duplication anomalies, in which the upper pole is either associated with an ectopic ureter or a ureterocele. Each of these entities is different with regard to their pathophysiology, each has characteristic radiographic findings, and each is surgically corrected via different operative approaches.

### Pathophysiology

A basic understanding of the embryology of the ureter is required in order to understand the different types of anomalies that occur at the ureterovescial junction. Ureteral development begins at around the fourth week of gestation, when the ureteral bud arises from the mesonephric or wolffian duct. The ureteral bud lengthens in a cephalad direction, and upon induction of the metanephric blastema the bud will further subdivide into primitive calyces. This area of the ureteral bud eventually forms the collecting system, including the renal pelvis, calyces, and collecting ducts. At about the sixth week of fetal development, the ureteral lumen obliterates, then gradually recanalizes from the midportion of the ureter in both a cephalad and a caudad direction. The last portions of the ureter to eventually reopen are the UPJ and the ureterovesical junction. As bladder development is commencing, the proximal portion of the mesonephric duct, also referred to as the common excretory duct, is absorbed into the developing urogenital sinus as cloacal development continues. By about the eighth week, the ureter and mesonephric duct separates and the portion of the ureter that eventually becomes the ureteral orifice migrates in a cephalad and lateral direction. The ureteral orifices and trigone of the bladder finish their development by about the twelfth week. During this time, muscle can be noted in the ureteral wall. By the fourteenth week, transitional epithelium is present.

If 2 ureteral buds arise in close proximity on the mesonephric duct, a ureteral duplication will result. The distal ureter drains the upper-pole portion of the kidney and the proximal ureter drains the lower pole. If the distal bud develops too far distally, that ureter may have an ectopic insertion. Ectopic ureters are much more common in girls, with the ectopic ureter inserting into bladder neck; urethra; vestibule; vagina; or (rarely) the cervix, uterus, or rectum. In males, ectopic ureters insert into; the bladder neck; prostatic urethra; or (rarely) a wolffian structure such as the seminal vesicles; or the rectum. Ectopic ureteral insertions can be functionally obstructed as the ureter traverses through the pelvic floor musculature or inserts at the bladder neck. The resting tone of bladder neck or pelvic floor musculature contributes to the functional obstruction and with relaxation of the bladder neck, reflux can actually be seen to occur. Most ectopic ureters are associated with renal duplications. The unusual situation of bilateral single-system ectopic ureters is associated with markedly abnormal trigonal and bladder neck development in addition to a bladder that has not cycled normally. With such abnormal development it is virtually impossible to refunctionalize the bladder due to the abnormalities of the bladder neck or intrinsic sphincter complex.

A primary obstructed megaureter is caused by a narrowed, stenotic segment of ureter either in or adjacent to the bladder wall, or by a normal-caliber adynamic, non-peristalsing distal portion of the ureter. This may be the result of failure of recanalization of the distal segment of the ureter, or of abnormal development of the muscle within the ureteral wall.

A ureterocele is caused by an abnormal cystic dilatation of the distal-most portion of the intravesical ureter. The ureterocele usually has a pinpoint obstructing orifice. Ureteroceles are classified into simple (ie, a single ureter) intravesical or ectopic, or duplicated intravesical or ectopic (Fig. 65-7A). Stephens further classified ureteroceles anatomically into stenotic, sphincteric, sphincterostenotic, or cecoureterocele (Fig. 65-7B).

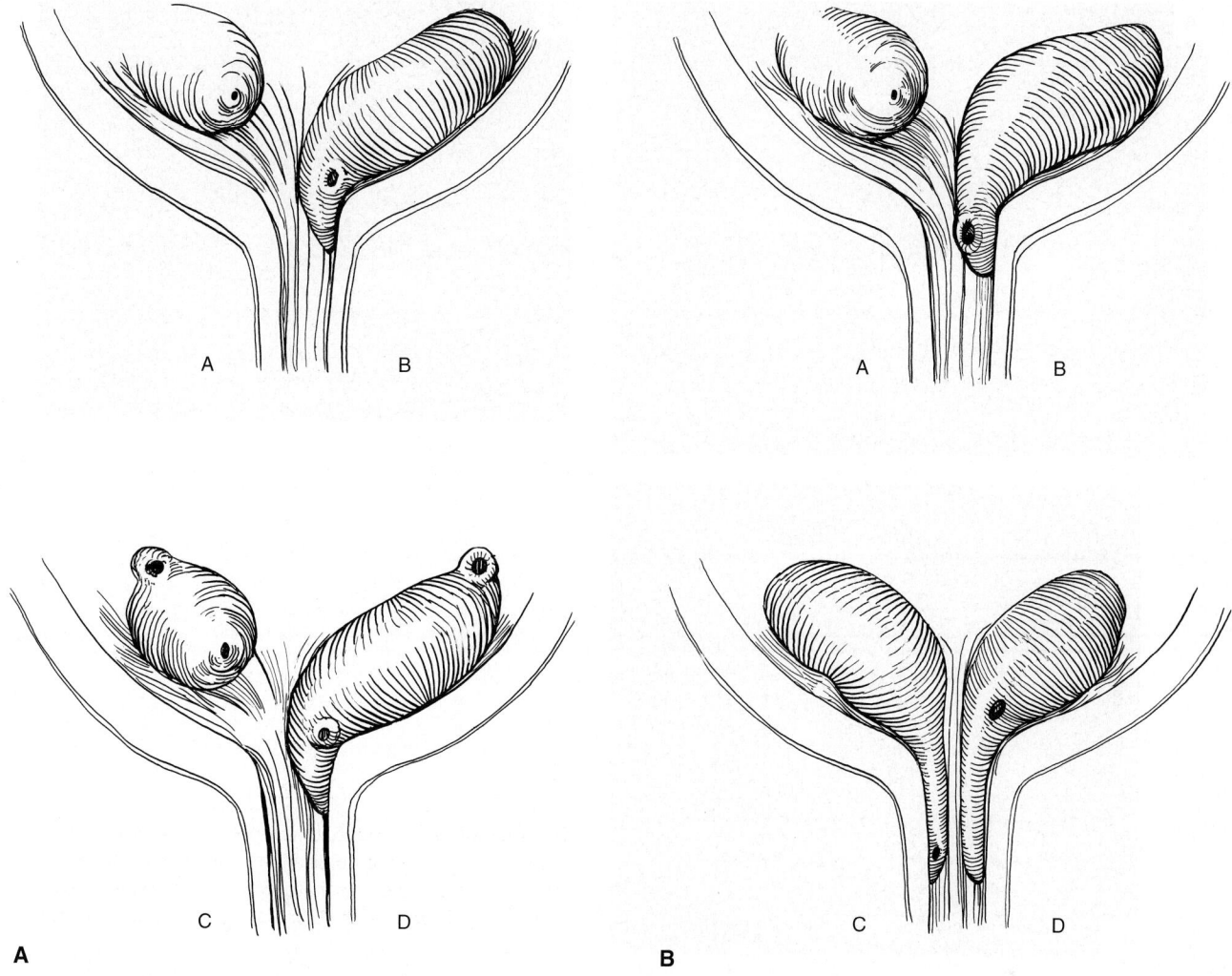

**FIGURE 65-7** **A.** International classification of ureteroceles. *A,* Single, intravesical; *B,* single, ectopic; *C,* duplicated, intravesical; *D,* duplicated, ectopic. **B.** Descriptive anatomic ureterocele classification. *A,* Stenotic; *B,* sphincteric; *C,* sphincterosphincteric; *D,* cecoureterocele. (From Other problems of the upper urinary tract. In Frank JD. Uteral duplication and ureteroceles Rowe MI, O'Neill JA, Grosfeld JL, Fonkalsrud EW, Coran AG, eds. *Essentials of Pediatric Surgery.* St. Louis, MO: Mosby-Year Book; 1995. Used by permission.)

## Presentation and Diagnosis

Prenatal ultrasonography detects the presence of hydroureteronephrosis that can be caused by a primary obstructed megaureter, ectopic ureter, or ureterocele. There still are times when infants will present with a urinary tract infection and are discovered to have hydroureteronephrosis. A ureterocele can prolapse through the urethra and present as a bulging perineal mass. Large ureteroceles may contribute to bladder outlet obstruction, acting as a ball valve at the bladder neck and lead to the development of bilateral hydroureteronephrosis.

The diagnosis of ureterovesical junction obstruction is made radiographically. Various modalities are used in combination to define these anomalies. The majority are noted in an asymptomatic fetus at the time of screening ultrasonography. The clinician is left to prove that there is ongoing obstruction that requires surgical intervention.

An obstructed ectopic upper-pole ureter or obstructing ureterocele in a duplex system can be surmised due to polar hydronephrosis in which the upper-pole moiety demonstrates significant dilation whereas the lower-pole moiety is normal. In this situation, careful assessment of the distal ureter and bladder can differentiate the ectopic ureter from the ureterocele which shows the characteristic cystic filling defect within the bladder (Fig. 65-8). An ultrasound which is carefully performed is oftentimes the only modality that is required to make the diagnosis.

A primary obstructed megaureter in which there is evidence of significant hydroureteronephrosis requires a functional study to prove the existence of obstruction. The use of a Mag III Lasix renogram can provide an assessment of differential renal function, but assessing the washout of the radiotracer is more challenging than in situations of a UPJ obstruction (Fig. 65-9). The use of magnetic resonance urography (MRU) is beginning to gain more widespread acceptance as the protocols for performing the study are increasingly being standardized.

Voiding cystourethrography should always be performed to further delineate the anatomy. In situations where a

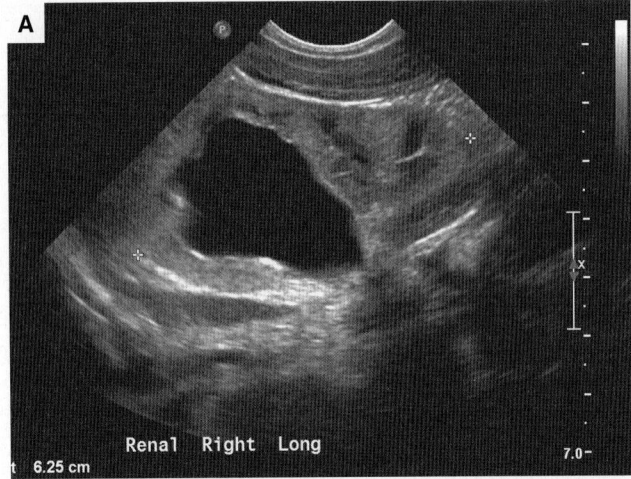

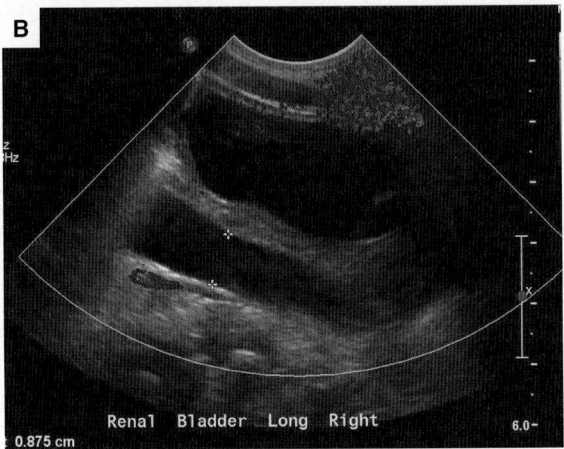

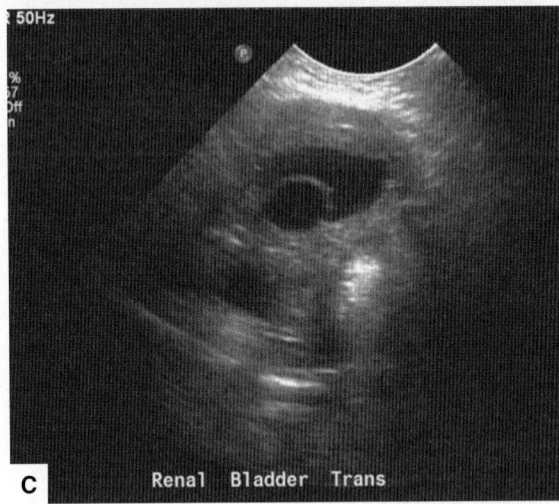

**FIGURE 65-8 A.** Right upper-pole hydronephrosis in association with renal duplication warrants careful evaluation of the distal ureteral anatomy. **B.** A dilated ureter ends with cystic dilatation with (**C**) an intravesical component, the ureterocele.

megaureter is present, the presence of reflux needs to be excluded. A filling defect in the bladder helps to confirm the diagnosis of ureterocele. With an obstructing ureterocele in a duplicated system, reflux is seen 50% of the time into the lower-pole moiety, 25% of the time into the contralateral lower-pole moiety, and 10% into the ipsilateral upper-pole moiety (Fig. 65-10). Rarely are obstructed megaureters both obstructing and refluxing.

A carefully performed physical examination can occasionally reveal the presence of an ectopic ureter or demonstrate that urine is constantly dribbling from a female's perineum. In the past endoscopic inspection was recommended to

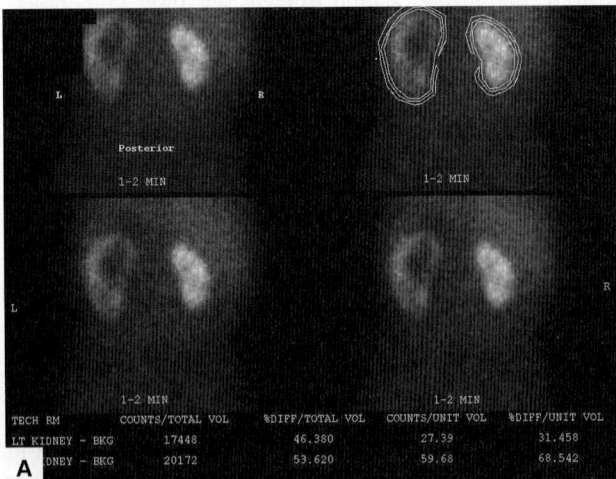

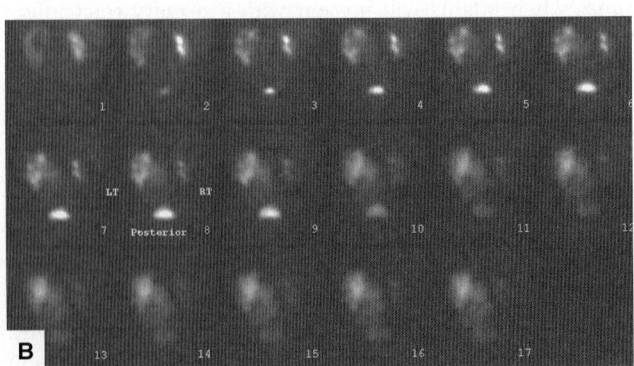

**FIGURE 65-9** MAG_III renal scan. **A.** Differential renal function calculated between 1 and 2 minutes following radiotracer injection is 31.5% in the left kidney based upon unit volume. **B.** Lasix renogram phase demonstrates prompt washout from the right kidney but filling of markedly dilated left ureter.

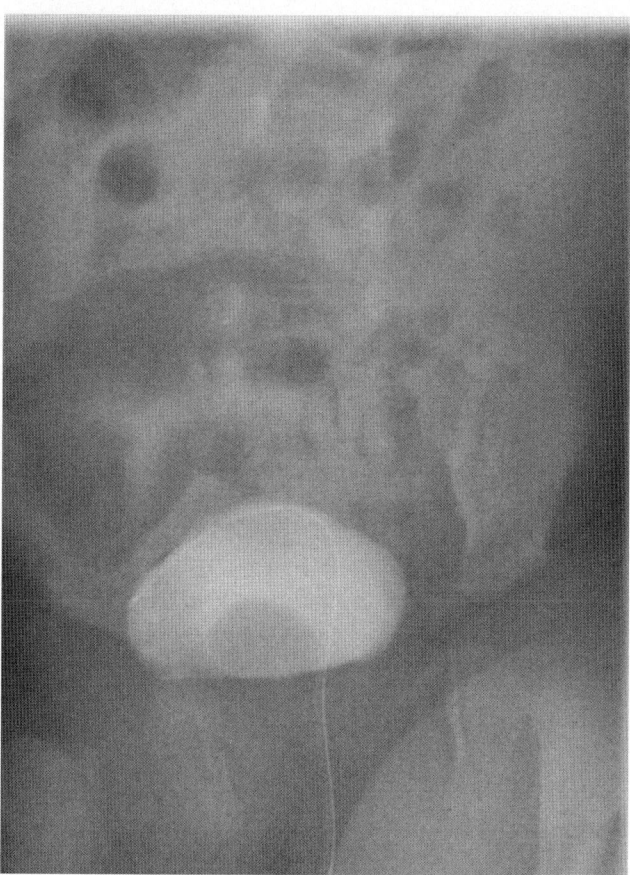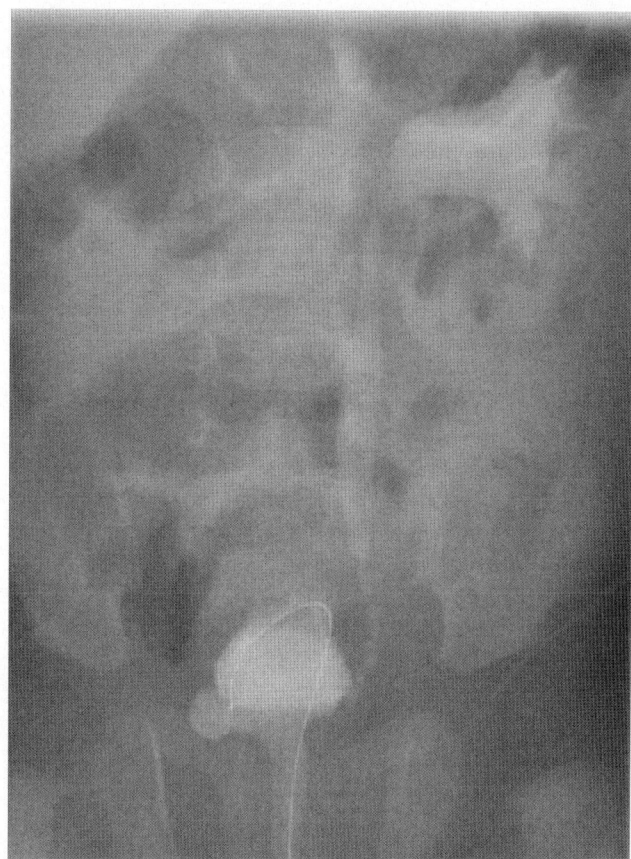

**FIGURE 65-10** Voiding cystourethrogram with the presence of a right ureterocele and reflux into the contralateral lower-pole moiety with voiding.

complete one's diagnostic evaluation. Rarely is this required as a separate procedure anymore. Certainly at the time of definitive surgery one can perform endoscopic evaluation and proceed with definitive repair.

## Surgical Techniques in Ureterovesical Junction Obstruction

### Ectopic Ureter

**Operative Technique.** The surgical approach to an ectopic ureter is partly dependent on one's surgical philosophy. A poorly functioning or dysplastic upper-pole moiety can be dealt with via an upper-pole nephroureterectomy or with a proximal uretero-ureterostomy or uretero-pyelostomy or a distal uretero-ureterostomy. The age of the patient will dictate whether an open surgical approach or a laparoscopic approach can be performed. At our institution, laparoscopic approaches are employed for infants generally over 6 months of age. If the goal is to preserve the upper-pole moiety, a distal ureteroureterostomy can be employed. Initially endoscopy is performed with placement of either an open-ended ureteral catheter into the lower-pole moiety or a guide wire which can then be indentified at the time of the open surgical repair. A Pfannenstiel incision or a modified Gibson incision is used to approach the ureters extravesically. Once the upper-pole ureter is identified, a 5-0 Prolene (Ethicon) suture is placed through the ureter as a traction stitch. The lower-pole ureter is then carefully identified with limited dissection required to separate the 2 ureters. The upper-pole ureter is then carefully transected and mobilized for several centimeters to allow an end-to-side anastomosis to the lower-pole ureter. Traction stitches can be placed through the lower-pole ureter to stabilize this system and facilitate the ureterotomy. A #12-blade (Bard-Parker) can be used for this purpose with care being taken to not back wall the ureter with the scalpel blade. The open-ended ureteral catheter or guide wire is then backed down through the ureter and then brought out the ureterotomy. Anastomosis of the upper-pole ureter to the lower-pole ureter is performed with a running 7-0 Maxon (Covidien) or 7-0 Vicryl (Ethicon) suture. Prior to completion of the anastomosis, an open-ended catheter or a double pigtail stent over the guide wire can be advanced through the anastomosis into the upper-pole moiety. Dilute methylene blue is instilled into the bladder to ensure that the distal stent is positioned appropriately within the bladder. In addition a small Penrose drain is left adjacent to where the uretero-ureterostomy was performed. Overnight drainage of the bladder with a Foley catheter is employed and the stent is left in place for 4 to 6 weeks, to be removed with a brief anesthetic procedure.

If the upper-pole ureter is significantly dilated then a proximal uretero-pyelostomy or uretero-ureterostomy with excision of the distal upper-pole ureter can be performed.

**Operative Technique: Upper-Pole Nephroureterectomy.** If the upper-pole moiety provides little function or shows evidence of dysplastic changes, then an upper-pole nephroureterectomy should be entertained. If the patient is under 6 months

809

of age then the authors preferred approach is an anterior subcostal muscle splitting incision. If the patient is over 6 months of age, a laparoscopic approach can be employed.

Via an anterior approach, the Gerota fascia is opened after the peritoneum is swept medially. Once the kidney is fully exposed, the dilated upper-pole ureter can be identified with the dissection beginning inferior to the renal hilum. The lower-pole ureter should be identified as well and dissected carefully away from the upper-pole ureter. Two traction stitches of 5-0 Prolene can be placed in the upper-pole ureter below the renal hilum and the upper-pole ureter can be transected. By maintaining a handle on the upper-pole ureter dissection can proceed carefully beneath the renal hilum and the lower-pole vessels. Once these are freed up from the ureter, the traction stitch can be passed beneath the lower-pole vessels and any remaining attachments dissected free. One can follow the upper ureter directly to the upper-pole dysplastic cap of renal parenchyma and in so doing, can delineate the margin between the upper and lower-pole moieties. The renal capsule is incised on the upper pole and then reflected off the lower pole using the back of a knife handle to facilitate this dissection. If upper-pole vessels have been encountered they can be divided and ligated. Excision of the upper pole is usually performed with electrocautery, although blunt dissection can be used. The dilated upper-pole pelvis and ureter are carefully separated from the lower-pole hilum and pelvis. The cut surface of the kidney is inspected for communicating calyces from the lower pole and these are oversewn with absorbable suture if noted. If possible, horizontal mattress 3-0 or 4-0 Vicryl sutures are placed to try to close the raw surface of the lower pole, and the renal capsule is reapposed over the cut surface of the lower pole with absorbable suture. The remainder of the upper-pole ureter is then dissected free from the lower-pole ureter with care being taken to dissect on the wall of the upper-pole ureter so as not to disrupt the vascularity of the lower-pole ureter. Dissection continues in a caudad direction on the wall of the upper-pole ureter to a point as low in the pelvis as is possible. The upper-pole ureter is carefully excised and the distal stump of the ureter is left open and drained with a small Penrose drain.

### Obstructed Megaureter

**Operative Technique: Ureteral Tailoring and Reimplantation.** The approach to megaureters has changed considerably with the recognition that the majority of antenatally detected megaureters show gradual improvement over time if patience is employed. This trend has become more and more prevalent over the past 2 decades. There are still situations that require an operative approach which can be dealt with via ureteral tailoring and reimplantation or ureteral imbrication. A massively dilated megaureter may be dealt with via formal ureteral tailoring (Fig. 65-11) whereas imbrication techniques are reserved for less dilated megaureters. Newer descriptions of ureteral stenting of megaureters after gentle dilation of the distal stenotic segment provide an attractive minimally-invasive approach. Long-term results will be eagerly awaited to see if this approach provides durable results.

The bladder is exposed through a Pfannenstiel incision, in which the rectus fascia is incised but the rectus muscle

is preserved. Following a mid-line vertical cystotomy, the obstructed megaureter is catheterized with a small feeding tube and then mobilized both intra- and extravesically, usually up to the level of the iliac vessels. The abnormal distal ureteral segment is excised and cannulated with a larger feeding tube or catheter (usually 8 to 12 French, depending on the size of the patient). With this catheter as a guide, the lateral wall of the ureter is excised for 5 or 6 cm. A running absorbable 5-0 or 6-0 suture is used to tailor the cut edges over the catheter. Interrupted sutures are placed for the last centimeter or so to allow the ureter to be cut to appropriate length before reimplanting it in the bladder. The ureter is brought back into the bladder through a new posterior-cephalad hiatus. The detrusor of the original hiatus is closed with interrupted 4-0 Vicryl sutures. A long submucosal tunnel is developed with tenotomy scissors. Care is taken to not twist the ureter as it comes through the tunnel. The ureter is trimmed to length, if necessary, and reimplanted using interrupted 5-0 chromic sutures. A double pigtail stent is inserted into the ureter for a period of 4 to 6 weeks which is then retrieved during a subsequent brief anesthetic procedure. The bladder is drained with an appropriate-sized Silastic Foley catheter and the bladder closed in layers with absorbable suture.

### Ureterocele

**Operative Technique: Excision of Ureterocele.** A number of factors are considered when dealing with a ureterocele, including the function of the upper-pole moiety, the severity of the associated vesicoureteral reflux, and the presence or absence of bladder outlet obstruction. Over the past 30 years a number of observations have been made and the management of these patients has been streamlined. The fundamental issue is whether the ureterocele is orthotopic or ectopic. In both situations an endoscopic approach can be employed, but those patients who have ectopic ureteroceles will, majority of times, require secondary bladder surgery as well.

Most infants who have ureteral duplication with associated ureterocele are indentified prenatally. These infants are placed on antibiotic prophylaxis at birth and an early ultrasound, 1 to 2 days after birth, can confirm the prenatal findings. Rarely does an infant present with severe urosepsis due to an obstructing ureterocele but fluid resuscitation, institution of broad-spectrum antibiotics, and stabilization of the patient with endoscopic incision of the ureterocele being required. Otherwise a VCUG study can be performed electively at several weeks of age and the infant can be setup for definitive surgical intervention. The premise is to relieve the obstructive uropathy, that is the obstructed upper-pole moiety via incision of the ureterocele.

The infant is positioned in a modified dorsolithotomy position and the genitalia prepped appropriately. A 7.5-French infant cystoscope is used to define the ureterocele and a urine culture is obtained after I.V. antibiotics have been given. The infant cystoscope is then switched for the infant resectoscope that is fitted with a right angled hot knife. The bladder is only partly distended to allow for visualization of the ureterocele and an incision low down on the ureterocele at its medial aspect is performed. An adequate incision will allow the 8.5-French resectoscope beak to be able to be inserted into it. Generally the bladder is then drained overnight via a Foley catheter.

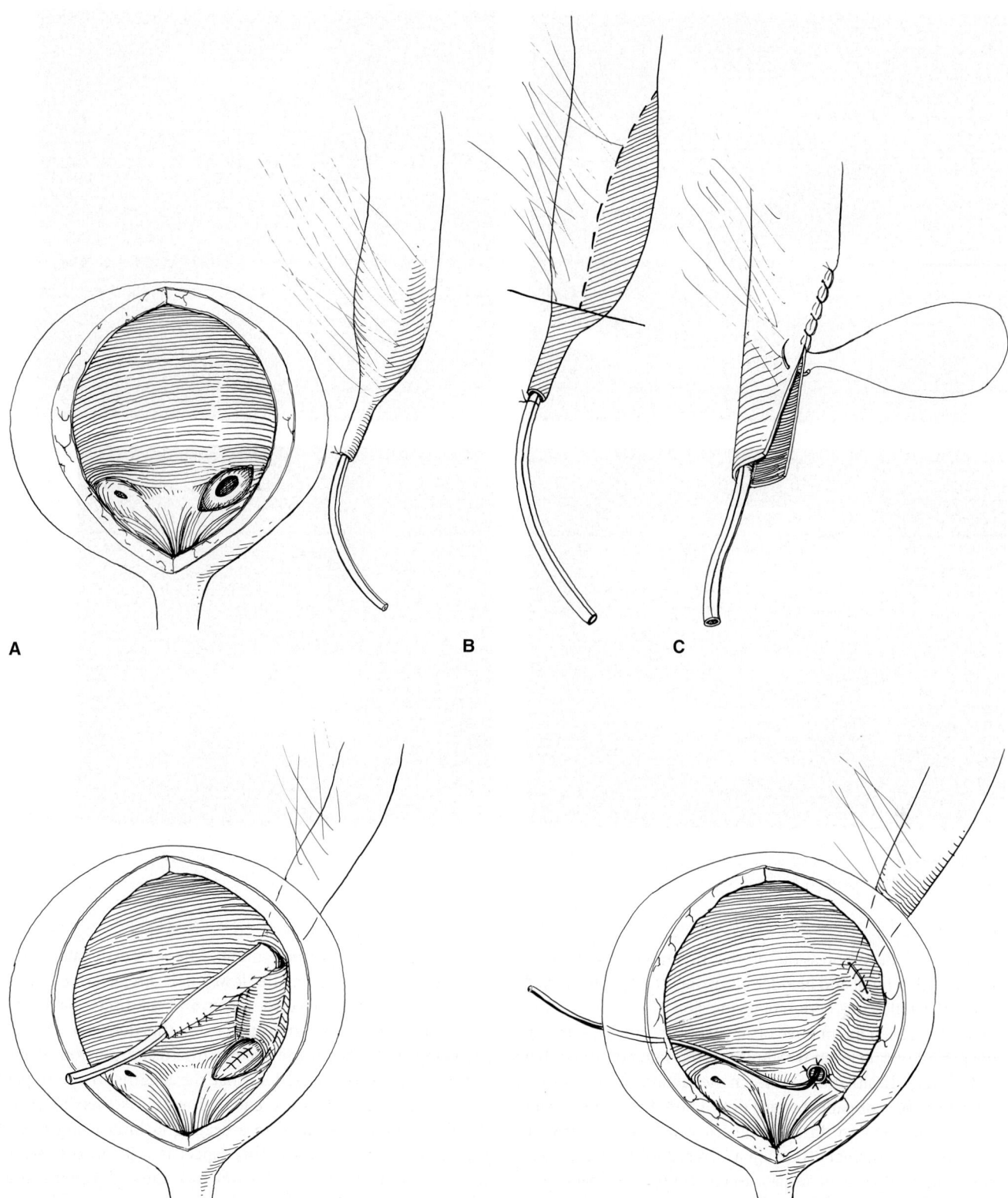

**FIGURE 65-11** Operative repair of obstructing megaureter: ureteral tailoring and reimplantation. **A.** With a small feeding tube in the ureter, the obstructed megaureter is mobilized out of the bladder, usually up to the level of the iliac vessels. **B.** The distal obstructing segment of the ureter is excised. Using a larger catheter as a guide, the lateral wall of the ureter is excised for about 5 or 6 cm. **C.** A running absorbable 5-0 or 6-0 suture is used to tailor the cut edges over the catheter. Interrupted sutures are placed for the last centimeter or so to allow the ureter to be cut to length before reimplantion. **D.** The ureter is brought back into the bladder through a new posterior-cephalad hiatus and a long submucosal tunnel is developed. The original hiatus is closed with interrupted absorbable sutures. **E.** The ureter is trimmed to length and reimplanted with interrupted fine absorbable sutures. A small postoperative stent is placed for 7 to 10 days.

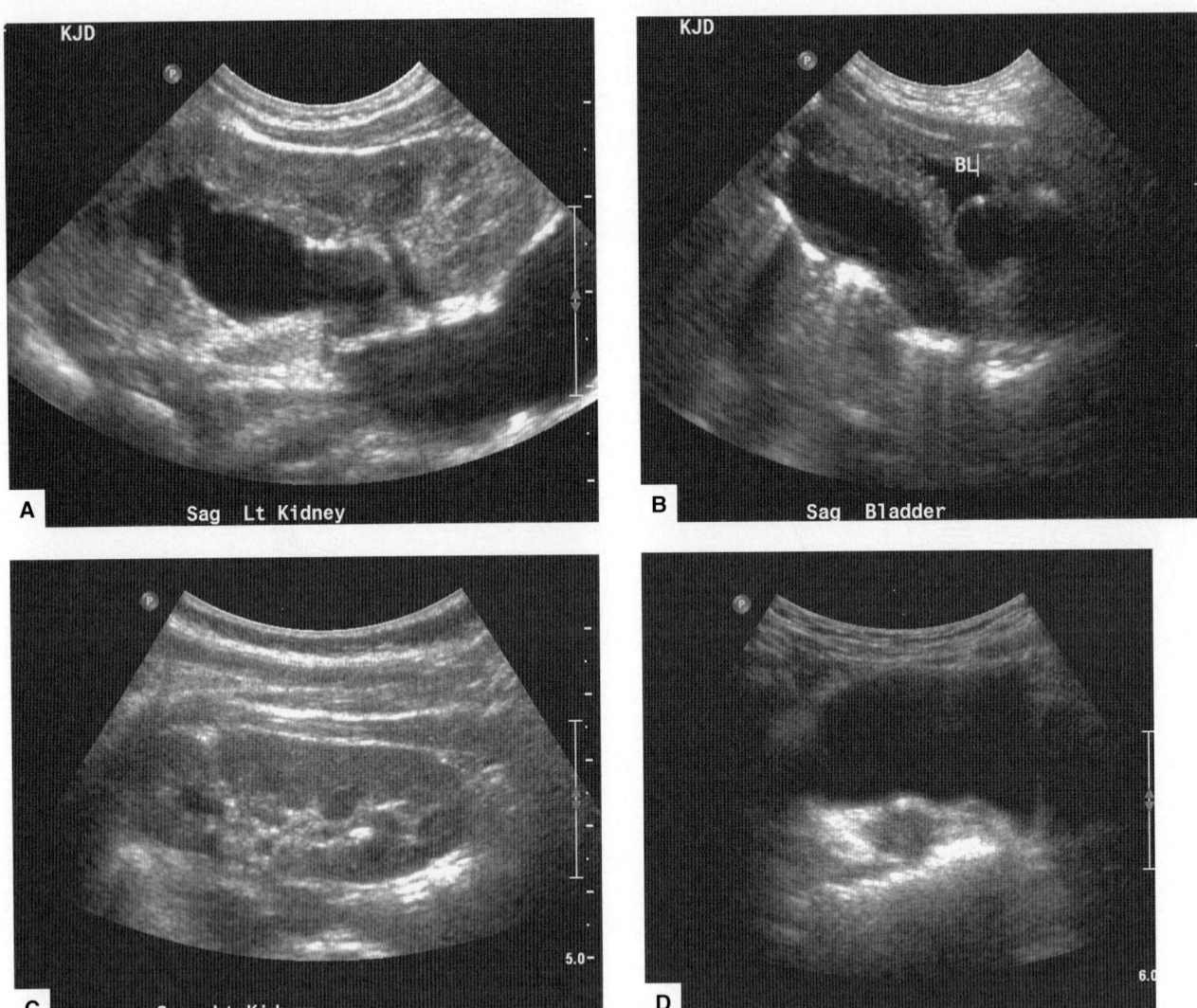

**FIGURE 65-12** Pre-operative appearance (A, B) of the left kidney and bladder and post-operative appearance (C, D) after successful incision of the ureterocele.

Successful decompression of the ureterocele is demonstrated with a renal and bladder ultrasound that is performed 2 months following endoscopic incision (Fig. 65-12). The infants have been maintained on antibiotic prophylaxis during this period of time even if reflux was not noted on the initial VCUG study. In situations in which the ureterocele was orthotopic, over 90% of patients have not required any subsequent surgical intervention. In situations in which the ureterocele is ectopic, the trigonal distortion as a result of the ureterocele will require subsequent surgery to correct the residual defect in the wall of the bladder and the persistence of the vesicoureteral reflux. This assessment is performed between 15 and 18 months of age, when the voiding pressures in the toddler have begun to normalize. If the reflux that was noted previously persists, surgical intervention is recommended to repair the defect in the detrusor as well as reimplant the ureters.

Reconstruction in this situation involves excising the ureterocele remnant, reconstructing the detrusor, and performing a common sheath ureteral reimplantation. The bladder is opened via a midline vertical cystotomy and feeding tubes are placed in the ureteral orifice to the lower-pole moiety and through the defect in the ureterocele that was previously

incised into the upper-pole ureter. The area associated with the ureterocele as well as the lower-pole ureter are circumscribed using needle electrocautery and the ureterocele and lower-pole ureter are dissected from the detrusor muscle following the plane of the ureters. The distal portion of the ureterocele can be excised so that the lengths to the upper and lower-pole ureters are equal. The key is then to close the defect in the detrusor in a keeling fashion using interrupted 4-0 Vicryl sutures. This aspect is critical to provide the appropriate support of the detrusor muscle. The mucosa adjacent to where the ureterocele was is undermined so that the common sheath reimplant of upper and lower-pole ureters can be accomplished. Alternatively if there is not enough length to provide a submucosal tunnel then these ureters can be brought across the trigone in a cross-trigonal fashion and positioned cephalad to the contralateral ureters. The critical aspect is to ensure that the ureterocele has been completely excised and the detrusor defect that has been left is reconstructed appropriately. In situations where the ectopic ureterocele extends well below the bladder neck, consideration can be given to split the pubic symphysis in order to gain adequate exposure. If contralateral reflux was present then a

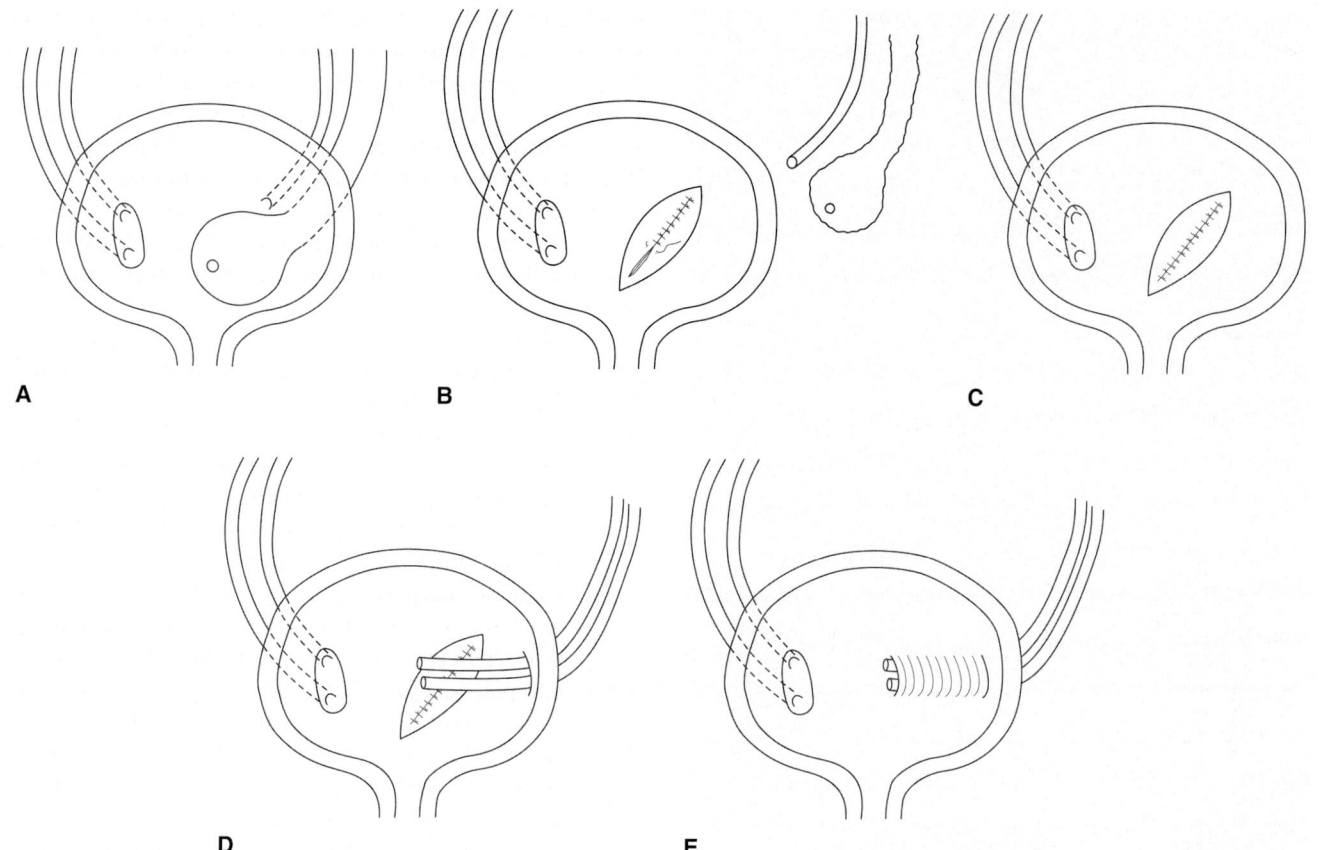

**FIGURE 65-13** Operative repair of the ureterocele. **A.** A Colorado tip cautery is used to circumscribe the area around the ureterocele and lower-pole ureteral orifice. **B.** The ureterocele and the lower-pole ureter are dissected free from the detrusor. The common sheath ureter is then mobilized to completely free them to allow for reimplantation. The large detrusor defect is carefully closed with interrupted absorbable sutures in a keeling fashion to reconstruct the detrusor muscle. **C.** The ureterocele and distal end of both upper-pole and lower-pole ureter are excised and each is cannulated with feeding tubes. Care is taken to not disturb the blood supply to the common-sheath ureters. **D.** The ureters are brought through the posterior bladder and a submucosal tunnel is developed. **E.** The ureters are reimplanted and the mucosal defect is closed. Alternatively, the common-sheath ureters can be reimplanted in a crossed-trigonal fashion. Commonly, the contralateral ureter may also need to be reimplanted because of reflux.

cross-trigonal reimplant of the ureter or ureters is performed as well. A Foley catheter may be left in place for several days in order to facilitate healing, particularly if a large posterior defect was repaired (Fig. 65-13).

## Surgical Outcome of Ureterovesical Junction Obstruction

Postoperative problems with upper-pole nephrectomy for an obstructed ectopic ureter are rare. Urinary leak from communicating lower-pole calyces is unusual with meticulous surgical technique. Infrequently, the distal stump of the ectopic upper-pole ureter acts like a diverticulum causing intermittent recurrent urinary infections. This tends to be the case in situations with gynecologic-ectopy, that is the ectopic ureter inserts into the vagina. In those cases, the stump can be excised or marsupialized into the vagina.

Ureteral tailoring and reimplantation for obstructed megaureter is successful in more than 90% of patients. The main complications are vesicoureteral reflux or obstruction. The incidence of these problems is low.

The success rate of surgery for ureteroceles is variable, depending on the management of the ureterocele. The

success rate of reimplantation is quite high when satisfactory closure of the bladder muscle at the ureterocele defect and an adequate submucosal tunnel are achieved. Recurrent reflux and obstruction are uncommon. Long-term follow-up of the senior author's personal series of patients has not shown any issues with stress urinary incontinence after successful bladder neck surgery with an appropriately-performed keeling reconstruction.

## URETEROPELVIC JUNCTION OBSTRUCTION

### Pathophysiology

UPJ obstruction can be a result of intrinsic or extrinsic etiologies. Much like a primary obstructed megaureter, the most common cause of intrinsic obstruction is focal stenosis as a result of abnormal recanalization of the proximal segment of the ureter, or abnormal development of the muscle within the ureteral wall. Collagen deposition replaces the muscle where there is a congenital absence of the muscular fibers. Less

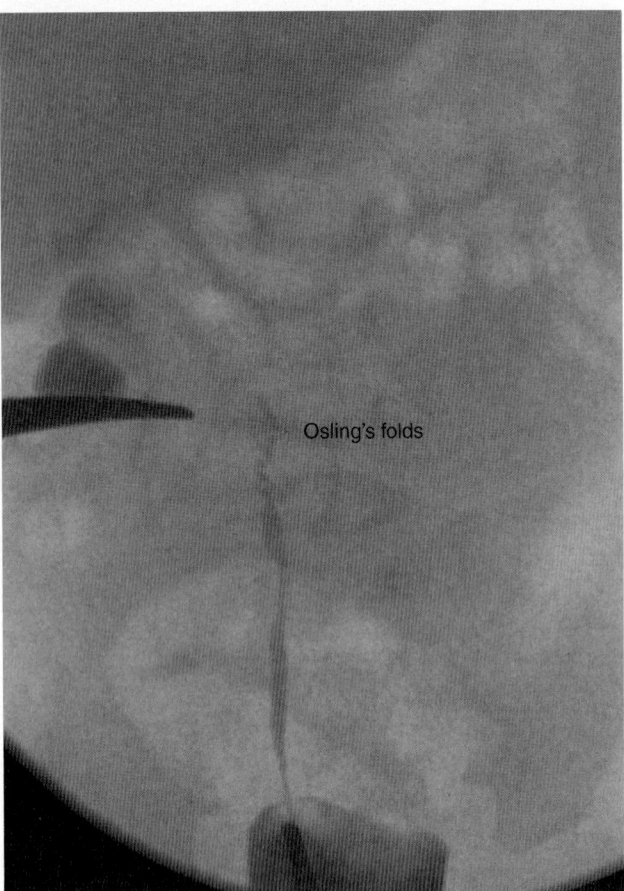

Osling's folds

**FIGURE 65-14** Retrograde pyelogram depicting the Ostling folds that can be seen in association with a ureteropelvic junction (UPJ) obstruction.

commonly, intrinsic narrowing can also be caused by abnormal folds, so-called Östling folds that form valve-like obstructions in addition to obstructing ureteral polyps (Fig. 65-14).

Finally extrinsic obstruction can be due to lower-pole crossing vessels that contribute to intermittent kinking at the UPJ and are found many times in those patients who present with intermittent episodes of renal colic.

## Presentation and Diagnosis

As with other causes of urinary tract obstruction, the most common presentation of UPJ obstruction is hydronephrosis detected via prenatal ultrasonography. This finding leads to postnatal evaluation and ultimately to surgical correction in these kidneys that are deemed to be obstructed. A newborn with an abdominal mass can have an obstructed kidney, although the giant multicystic dysplastic kidney is more commonly noted in newborns. In older infants and children, UPJ obstruction can present with a urinary tract infection, intermittent abdominal pain, hematuria, intermittent episodes of nausea or vomiting, and hypertension. It can also be detected as an incidental finding for radiographic studies such as CT scans, MRI studies, and bone scans. The diagnosis of UPJ obstruction is made radiographically. Renal ultrasonography is the initial diagnostic screening modality that is used to assess the degree of hydronephrosis. Hydronephrosis

detected prenatally, particularly where there is moderate-to-severe hydronephrosis warrants a postnatal evaluation. Many times, minor degrees of hydronephrosis that are detected prenatally do resolve either with subsequent prenatal evaluation or with early postnatal evaluation. Since the infant who is detected with hydronephrosis is generally asymptomatic, it is incumbent to demonstrate that there is evidence of obstruction that warrants surgical intervention. To date, there is not one modality which is considered the gold standard in defining obstruction.

There have been a number of studies assessing different parameters noted with renal ultrasonography that raised the level of concern that obstruction may be present. These include the assessment of the AP diameter of the renal pelvis, ratio of renal parenchymal to collecting system areas, and assessment of the resistive indices of hydronephrotic kidneys. It suffices to say that the degree of caliectasis and evidence of parenchymal thinning are worrisome features that should alert one that obstruction may be present. A functional study is warranted to assess the differential function of the kidneys as well as washout from the kidneys. The Mag III Lasix renogram has supplanted the DTPA Lasix renogram as the study that is utilized most often. It is critical that such a study is done in a reproducible fashion so that the relative degree of hydration is controlled, the Lasix is administered at a time of which peak uptake of radio tracer has occurred and that there is placement of a catheter to ensure appropriate bladder drainage so that an overly distended bladder does not affect the relative washout of the radio tracer from the kidney. The differential renal function is calculated based upon the uptake of the radio tracer into the renal cortex at between 1 and 2 minutes following injection. Generally 15 to 20 minutes following the initial injection, a bolus of Lasix is given and washout of the radio tracer is assessed. Even amongst nuclear medicine experts, there is disagreement with the interpretation of these studies. A kidney in which there is decreased function compared to the contralateral normal kidney and no appreciable washout would be deemed a kidney with relative obstruction. Disagreement occurs as to what the absolute number for relative renal function is and which washout curve truly reflects obstruction.

In the past it was common practice to perform a VCUG study on virtually all infants who presented with antenatal hydronephrosis but recently we have become much more selective in which patient requires a VCUG study to exclude the presence of vesicoureteral reflux. With a well performed renal and bladder ultrasound in which there is no evidence of ureteral dilation and the hydronephrosis is unilateral, a VCUG study is not required.

In the last several years, MRU has made great strides in the assessment of hydronephrosis (Fig. 65-15). This study combines exquisite imaging of the urinary tract as well as providing functional data. The issue has been how to interpret the data that are derived from an MRU, as the analysis requires external postprocessing using relatively complex software. This has proven to be a limiting factor in widespread routine implementation of MRU functional analysis and use of MRU functional parameters similar to nuclear medicine. At our institution, software which was developed in the pediatric radiology department enables comprehensive automated

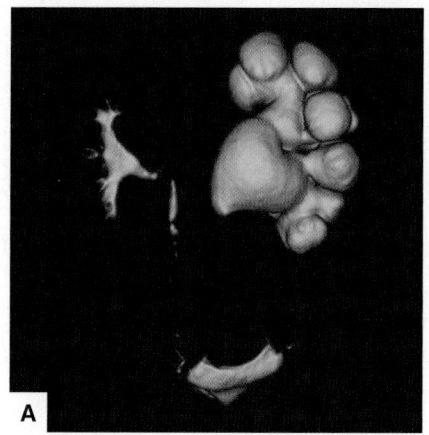

| | Right kidney | Left kidney |
|---|---|---|
| 1. CTT | 1min(s) 30sec(s) | 1 min(s) 50sec(s) |
| 2. RTT | 1min(s) 30sec(s) | X |
| 3. TTP | 2min(s) 50sec(s) | 3min(s) 30sec(s) |
| 4. Whole volume(mL) | 21.02mL | 14.16mL |
| 5. Parenchymal Vol(mL) | 21.02mL | 14.16mL |
| 6a. vDRF | 59.75% | 40.24% |
| 6b. pDRF | 54.68% | 45.31% |
| 6c. vpDRF | 64.17% | 35.82% |
| 7. Difference vDRF pDRF | 5.066% | 5.066% |
| 8. Pallak(mL/min) /mL | 0.30475 | 0.25254 |
| 9. BSA Pallak(mL/min)/mL | 1.74196 | 1.44356 |

**A**  **B**

**FIGURE 65-15** Magnetic resonance urography providing (**A**) exquisite anatomic detail of left UPJ obstruction in addition to (**B**) assessment of the differential glomerulofitration (vpDRF) rate of each kidney, right 64%, left 36%.

functional analysis which is very user-friendly, fast, and easily operated by average radiologists or MR technicians. Such software has the potential to help overcome the obstacles to widespread use of functional MRU in children.

## Operative Technique: Dismembered Pyeloplasty

The timing of surgical intervention is dependent on the concern that ongoing obstruction is present which is or will be detrimental to the overall function of the kidney. In situations with a solitary kidney, the conservative approach may be to consider surgery earlier to prevent the consequences of ongoing obstruction. If the studies are equivocal, then a repeat renal and bladder ultrasound or renal scan done in several months can provide a basis of comparison to look for a change in overall renal function or worsening pelvicaliectasis that would warrant surgical intervention.

The literature is replete with different surgical approaches to the repair of UPJ obstruction. The procedure which has withstood the test of time is the Anderson–Hynes dismembered pyeloplasty (Fig. 65-16) that has been employed for well over 50 years.

The actual repair for the modified Anderson–Hynes dismembered pyeloplasty, as performed through an anterior subcostal incision, is as follows:

1. The anterior subcostal incision is a muscle-splitting incision that is made with the patient supine and a roll placed transversely beneath the patient to elevate the flank (Fig. 65-16).

2. Each muscle layer encountered is split in the direction of the muscle fibers until the Gerota fascia is identified by sweeping the peritoneum medially. The fascia is then incised posteriorly over the lateral aspect of the kidney.

3. The renal pelvis is identified by medial retraction of the peritoneum and lateral traction of the kidney. If the renal pelvis is significantly dilated, an angiocath can be inserted to decompress the pelvis and facilitate identification of the UPJ.

4. Anterior exposure is usually better when a dismembered pyeloplasty is being performed. Once the ureter and UPJ are identified, a traction suture is displaced anteriorly through the proximal ureter to minimize subsequent handling.

5. The area of UPJ is dissected free to allow for a clear area in which to perform the anastomosis. Traction sutures of 5-0 prolene may be placed in the renal pelvis superiorly, medially, laterally, and inferiorly to the UPJ. Once adequate ureteral length is confirmed and the pathology of UPJ identified, the ureter can be transected at the UPJ. If the ureter is short, the kidney is completely mobilized to determine whether it can be brought down sufficiently to allow for a primary tension-free anastomosis.

6. After transection of the UPJ, the renal pelvis may not spontaneously drain until it is incised. This should be done after the site for anastomosis is chosen.

7. The ureter is spatulated on the side opposite to the traction suture using Potts tenotomy scissors. The distance over which the ureter is opened is variable, until healthy ureter is encountered, which springs open when forceps are placed into it.

8. The portion of pelvis is excised, usually a diamond-shaped segment that is present within the traction sutures that were placed in the renal pelvis. It is better to leave too much renal pelvis than too little, especially when resecting along the medial aspect of the renal pelvis. Infundibula can be encountered if one is not careful (Fig. 65-16).

9. The ureter and renal pelvis are aligned to ensure that the anastomosis can be accomplished without tension. If a nephrostomy tube is to be used, it is placed at this time. An inferior calix is chosen, preferably where the overlying parenchyma is not too thick. A Malecot catheter works well and is positioned away from the repair to minimize the chance of the catheter's causing urinary blockage through the reconstructed UPJ.

10. The anastomosis is started by placing the first 7-0 Maxon® (Davis and Geck) suture at the apex of the "V" in the ureter and into the tip of the inferior pelvic flap. As the suture is tied down, the ureter and renal pelvis are brought together to minimize tension on the repair. A small feeding tube

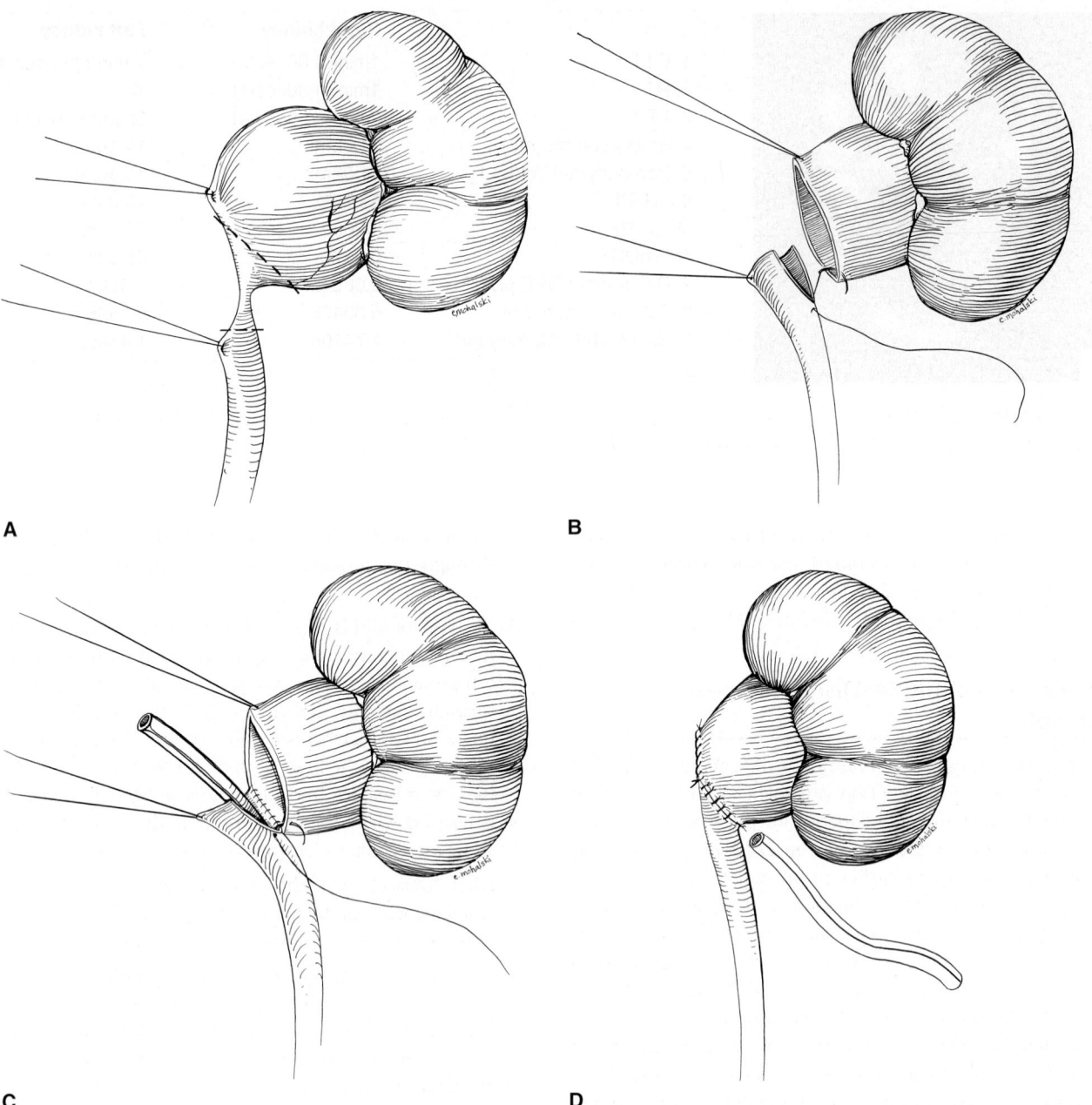

A

B

C

D

**FIGURE 65-16** Operative repair of UPJ obstruction: dismembered pyeloplasty. **A.** The renal pelvis and upper ureter are exposed and their medial aspects are marked with fine Prolene stay sutures above and below the UPJ to maintain proper anatomic orientation. The ureter is transected transversely below the UPJ and spatulated. The renal pelvis is transected obliquely above the UPJ. **B.** Constructing the anastomosis to lie dependently, the lower pelvis is sutured to the "V" at the apex of the spatulated ureter and the back wall of the anastomosis is completed with interrupted fine chromic sutures, placing the knots on the outside of the anastomosis. **C.** A catheter is placed in the ureter and the front wall of the anastomosis is completed with additional chromic sutures. **D.** The upper portion of the pelvis is then sutured with running chromics to shape it in a funnel-like fashion. A penrose drain is placed through a separate stab incision.

is placed into the ureter; it can be used to stabilize the ureter during the anastomosis. A "no-touch" technique is employed with the ureter to minimize trauma and edema to the ureteral tissue. Either interrupted sutures or a running closure may be used, depending on the surgeon's preference. The area of the initial anastomosis is critical to ensuring a watertight closure.

11. Before the repair is completed, the renal pelvis is irrigated to remove any blood clots or debris that could obstruct the UPJ. If an indwelling JJ ureteral stent is employed, it

should be placed now, with care taken to place the stent into the bladder and renal pelvis without kinking it.

12. A Penrose drain is placed adjacent to the repair and brought out through a separate stab wound.

13. The kidney is returned to its native position, and perinephric fat, if available, is placed over the anastomosis.

14. Closure of the three fascial layers is readily accomplished, followed by closure of the Scarpa fascia and subcuticular skin.

15. A Foley catheter, which was placed at the beginning of the procedure, may be left in place for 24 to 48 hours postoperatively. The Penrose drain usually can be removed before discharge or, if left in place, it can easily be removed in the office 7 to 10 days postoperatively.

## Surgical Outcome

Meticulous attention to surgical technique generally results in a pyeloplasty failure rate of well below 5%. With the advent of robotically assisted laparoscopic procedures, the dismembered pyeloplasty is now accomplished in this fashion even in toddlers. The main complications include early postoperative urinary leak and late postoperative stricture formation. There is ongoing debate whether the placement of a JJ stent at the time of an open dismembered pyeloplasty is necessary but it minimizes any concern of postoperative urinary extravasation and is well tolerated in most pediatric patients. It simply requires a brief anesthetic procedure 4 to 6 weeks following surgery to remove the stent. Alternatively with the placement of a Penrose drain, most urinary leaks will tend to resolve over a period of several days following surgery. A postoperative stricture following a pyeloplasty may be approached endoscopically, in which the stricture is either incised carefully with a laser or using a cold knife or cutting wire with appropriate postoperative stenting. A focal stricture that occurs after a well-designed pyeloplasty with a well-constructed funnel is most amenable to this approach. Redo pyeloplasties can also be approached either laparoscopically or in an open fashion and may even require the use of a ureterocalicostomy to correct them. Such procedures are rare if one is careful in their original choice and execution of surgical procedure.

## SELECTED READINGS

### Meatal Stenosis

Noe HN, Dale GA. Evaluation of children with meatal stenosis. *J Urol* 1975;114:455–456.

### Posterior Urethral Valves

Defoor W, Clark C, Jackson E, et al. Risk factors for end-stage renal disease in children with posterior urethral valves. *J Urol* 2008;180:1705–1708.

Smith GH, Canning DA, Shulman et al. The long-term outcome of posterior urethral valves treated with primary valve ablation and observation. *J Urol* 1996;155:1730–1734.

Youssif M, Dawood W, Shabaaan S, et al. Early valve ablation can decrease the incidence of bladder dysfunction in boys with posterior urethral valves. *J Urol* 2009;182:1765–1768.

### Ureterovesical Junction Obstruction.

Ben-Chaim J, Gearhart JP, Peters CA. Collecting system: upper urinary tract. In Oldham KT, Colombani PM, Foglia RP, eds. *Surgery of Infants and Children: Scientific Principles and Practice*. Philadelphia: Lippincott-Raven; 1997:1481–1515.

Kim SH. The ureter. In Ashcraft KW, Holder TM, eds. *Pediatric Surgery*. Philadelphia: WB Saunders; 1993:602–611.

McLellan DL, Retik AB, Bauer SB, et al. Rate and predictors of spontaneous resolution of prenatally diagnosed primary non-refluxing megaureter. *J Urol* 2002;168:2177–2180.

### Ectopic Ureter

Lashley DB, McAleer IM, Caplan GW. Ipsilateral ureteroureterostomy for the treatment of vesicoureteral reflux or obstruction associated with complete ureteral duplication. *J Urol* 2001;165:552–554.

Plaire JC, Pope JC, Kropp BP, et al. Management of ectopic ureters: experience with the upper tract approach. *J Urol* 1997;158:1245–1247.

Smith FL, Ritchie EL, Maizels M, et al. Surgery for duplex kidneys with ectopic ureters: ipsilateral ureteroureterostomy versus polar nephrectomy. *J Urol* 1989;142:532–534.

### Megaureter

Keating MA, Escala J, Snyder H, et al. Changing concepts in management of primary obstructive megaureter. *J Urol* 1989;142:636–640.

Hendren WH. Operative repair of megaureter in children. *J Urol* 1969;101:491–498.

Peters CA, Mandell J, Lebowitz RL, et al. Congenital obstructed megaureters in early infancy: Diagnosis and treatment. *J Urol* 1989;142:641–645.

Shukla AR, Cooper J, Patel RP, et al. Prenatally detected primary megaureter: a role for extended follow up. *J Urol* 2005;173:1353–1356.

Starr A. Ureteral plication. A new concept in ureteral tapering for megaureter. *Invest Urol* 1979;17:153–158.

### Ureterocele

Churchill BM, Sheldon CA, McLorie GA. The ectopic ureterocele: a proposed classification based on renal unit jeopardy. *J Pediatr Surg* 1992;227:497–500.

Cooper CS, Passerini-Glazel G, Hutcheson JC, et al. Long-term follow-up of endoscopic incision of ureteroceles: intravesical versus extravesical. *J Urol* 2000;164:1097–1100.

Hagg MJ, Mourachov PC, Snyder HM, et al. The modern endoscopic approach to ureterocele. *J Urol* 2000;163:940–943.

Shimada K, Matsumoto F, Matsui F. Surgical treatment for ureterocele with special reference to lower urinary tract reconstruction. *Int J Urol* 2007;14:1063–1067.

### Ureteropelvic Junction Obstruction

Braga LH, Lorenzo AJ, Bagli DJ, et al. Risk factors for recurrent ureteropelvic junction obstruction after open pyeloplasty in a large pediatric cohort. *J Urol* 2008;180:1684–1688.

Khrichenko D, Darge K. Functional analysis in MR urography—made simple. *Pediatr Radiol* 2010;40(2):182–199.

Onen A, Jayanthi VR, Koff SA. Long-term follow up of prenatally detected severe bilateral newborn hydronephrosis initially managed nonoperatively. *J Urol* 2002;168:1118–1120.

Rohrmann D, Snyder HM, Duckett JW, et al. The operative management of recurrent ureteropelvic junction obstruction. *J Urol* 1997;158:1257–1259.

Sheldon CA, Duckett JW, Snyder HM. Evolution in the management of infant pyeloplasty. *J Pediatr Surg* 1992;27:501–505.

# Vesicoureteral Reflux

# CHAPTER 66

*Prem Puri and Manuela Hunziker*

## KEY POINTS

1. Primary vesicoureteral reflux (VUR)—the retrograde flow of urine from the bladder into the upper urinary tract—is the most common urological anomaly in children. It occurs in 1% to 2% of the pediatric population and in 30% to 50% of children who present with a urinary tract infection (UTI).

2. The association of VUR, UTI, and renal damage is well known and refluxnephropathy is a major cause of childhood hypertension, growth impairment, and renal insufficiency.

3. It is generally believed that discovering VUR early may prevent exposure to UTI, and this may avoid development or progression of renal parenchymal damage.

4. Sonography should be performed in any infant or child with a suspicion of VUR. VUR is suspected in the presence of a dilated pelvicaliceal system, upper or lower ureter, unequal renal size, or cortical loss and increased echogenicity. Sonography is not sufficiently sensitive or specific for diagnosing VUR.

5. A voiding cystogram remains the gold standard for detecting VUR.

6. Management of VUR is controversial. The various treatment options currently available in the management of VUR are (i) long-term antibiotic prophylaxis, (ii) intermittent antibiotic therapy for UTI, (iii) antibiotic prophylaxis and anticholinergics, (iv) open or laparoscopic reimplantation of ureters, and (v) minimally invasive endoscopic treatment.

7. Continuing antibiotics prophylaxis is reliant on patient's compliance and has the risk of bacterial resistance accompanied by potential breakthrough UTIs. Furthermore, several large, prospective, randomized controlled trials have shown little or no benefit of medical therapy in terms of reducing the incidence of febrile UTI or renal scarring

8. Open surgical treatment of reflux has been the gold standard. However, surgery is not without risks.

9. Minimally invasive endoscopic technique for the correction of VUR has become an established alternative to long-term antibiotic prophylaxis and open surgical treatment. Endoscopic subureteral injection of Deflux® is an excellent first-line treatment in children with 87% success in high-grade VUR after 1 injection. This 15-minute outpatient procedure is safe and simple to perform, and it can be easily repeated in failed cases.

## INTRODUCTION

Primary vesicoureteral reflux (VUR)—the retrograde flow of urine from the bladder into the upper urinary tract—is the most common urological anomaly in children. It occurs in 1% to 2% of the pediatric population and in 30% to 50% of children who present with a urinary tract infection (UTI). The association of VUR, UTI, and renal damage is well known. Refluxnephropathy is a major cause of childhood hypertension, growth impairment, and renal insufficiency. Marra et al reviewed data on children with chronic renal failure who had high-grade VUR in the Italkid project, a database of Italian children with chronic renal failure and found that those with VUR accounted for 26% of all children with chronic renal failure.

The hereditary and familial nature of VUR is now well recognized and several studies have shown that siblings of children with VUR have a much higher incidence of reflux than the general pediatric population. VUR can resolve spontaneously with age, so it is therefore difficult to determine the exact prevalence in family members. Prevalence rates of 27% to 51% in siblings of children with VUR and a 66% rate of VUR in offsprings of parents with previously diagnosed reflux have been reported. It has become evident that familial clustering of VUR must have a genetic basis, but no single major locus or gene for VUR has yet been identified and most researchers now acknowledge that VUR is genetically heterogenous.

## EMBRYOLOGY

Urinary tract development in the embryo begins with the formation of the ureteric bud, which is an outgrowth of the mesonephric duct. Growth of the ureteric bud is stimulated by reciprocal signaling between the bud and the metanephrogenic mesenchyme, and results in the formation of the ureter and branching to form the collecting ducts. Signaling between the bud and the mesenchyme stimulates the metanephrogenic mesenchyme to form the kidney. Apoptosis occurs in the part of the mesonephric duct between the newly developed ureter and the urogenital sinus. The free end of the developing ureter inserts into the bladder wall and forms the vesicoureteric valve.

The ureterovesical junction (UVJ) acts as a valve and closes during micturation or when the bladder contracts. The UVJ is structurally and functionally adapted to allow the intermittent passage of urine and prevent the reflux of urine into the bladder. The main defect in patients with VUR is believed to involve the malformation of the UVJ, in part due to shortening of the submucosal ureteric segment due to congenital lateral ectopia of the ureteric orifice. This leads to retrograde flow of urine into the ureter or kidney. The precise position at which the ureteric bud grows out from the mesonephric duct is critical. Many genes are involved in the ureteric budding and subsequent urinary tract and kidney development. Primary VUR could be due to mutations in 1 or more developmental genes that control these processes.

Secondary VUR is an acquired condition resulting from increased intravesical pressure and is seen in conditions such as neurogenic bladder and bladder outlet obstruction.

## MECHANISM OF RENAL SCARRING

The association between VUR and renal scarring is now widely recognized.

Scarring is directly related to the severity of reflux. Belman and Skoog assessed renal scarring in 804 refluxing units and found renal scars in 5% of those with grade I reflux, 6% of those with grade II reflux, 17% of those with grade III reflux, 25% of those with grade IV reflux, and 50% of those with grade V reflux.

The mechanisms by which reflux produces renal scars is still not clear. Renal parenchymal damage can be congenital or acquired. Congenital reflux nephropathy occurs as a result of abnormal embryological development with subsequent renal dysplasia and is largely seen in male infants with high-grade VUR. Exposure to UTIs in patients with congenital renal dysplasia can lead to progression of renal parenchymal damage. Both experimental and clinical studies have shown that acquired renal scarring associated with VUR is the result of an acute inflammatory reaction caused by bacterial infection of the renal parenchyma. It is well known that the risk of renal scarring after an episode of pyelonephritis is increased in children with high-grade VUR, affecting up to 89% of children with grade IV-V VUR. Parenchymal injury in VUR occurs early, in most patients before the age of 3 years. It is generally believed that discovering VUR early may prevent exposure to UTI and this may avoid development or progression of renal parenchymal damage.

Dimercaptosuccinic acid (DMSA) scans have allowed us to follow sequentially the evolution of a scar from an area of decreased blood flow during the acute inflammatory phase to a parenchymal defect indicative of a mature scar. Yet only half of patients with acute pyelonephritic will have such a scar. What converts an acute inflammatory process into a scar in some patients and not in others is not clearly understood. Factors implicated in the formation of a mature scar include the magnitude of the pressure driving the organisms into the tissues, the intrinsic virulence of the organism itself, and the host-defence mechanisms. Furthermore, some of the worst examples of renal injury associated with VUR are those that are present at birth. As renal damage at that time cannot be the consequence of infection, such injury is assumed to be developmental in origin, but the pathophysiology of this is not entirely clear.

The 3 mechanisms considered potential etiologies for renal scar formation are (1) reflux of infected urine with interstitial inflammation and damage, (2) sterile, usually high-grade reflux, which may damage the kidney through a mechanical or immunological mechanism, and (3) abnormal embryological development with subsequent renal dysplasia. Patients in the latter group may also have UTI in the postnatal period, resulting in extensive parenchymal damage. It is well recognized that in the first 2 groups of renal parenchymal damage, it is essential to discover reflux early before damage can be initiated. In the third group, it is clear that congenital damage currently cannot be prevented. However, in these patients, it is mandatory to discover reflux at the early stages to prevent exposure to UTI and avoid the possible progression of renal parenchymal damage.

## DIAGNOSIS

### Antenatally Diagnosed Reflux

Prenatal ultrasonography has resulted in a dramatic increase in the number of infants detected with significant asymptomatic uropathology, allowing treatment before the potential devastating consequences of UTI occur. An incidental anomaly is detected by antenatal ultrasonography in about 1% of studies and 20% to 30% involving the urinary tract. So far, the commonest abnormal finding is hydronephrosis, comprising over 90% of the urological abnormalities detected. Underlying diagnosis include pelvic–ureteric junction obstruction, vesicoureteric junction obstruction, posterior urethral valves, and VUR.

Although antenatal hydronephrosis is generally considered to represent an obstructive lesion, VUR is not an uncommon cause.

Several studies have investigated outcomes of children diagnosed with antenatal hydronephrosis and VUR has been reported in 10% to 20%. Recently, Skoog et al published guidelines for screening siblings of children with VUR and neonates/infants with prenatal hydronephrosis. They reported a prevalence of VUR of 16.2% in screened populations with prenatal hydronephrosis. Based on review of data and panel consensus, VCUG is recommended for infants with high-grade hydronephrosis, hydroureter, or abnormal bladders on ultrasound, or who develop a UTI on observation.

### Natural History of Prenatally Diagnosed Vesicoureteral Reflux

The vast majority of infants found to have VUR following detection of antenatal hydronephrosis are males. The male preponderance is reported to range from 2:1 to 5:1 in various series. This is in total contrast to the female preponderance that has been consistently reported in later childhood. It is also important to recognize that the calculated ratio between the genders is dependent upon the method of ascertainment. UTIs are more common in females and it is no surprise that when VUR is detected by screening children who presented with symptoms of UTI, more girls than boys are diagnosed with VUR. However, 80% of cases detected by the appearance of antenatal hydronephrosis on prenatal ultrasound are boys and these patients often have high-grade VUR associated renal damage. In approximately two-thirds of the cases, the reflux is bilateral.

It also has been reported that boys are more vulnerable to UTI, especially in the first 6 months of life, where different factors play a significant role. Host factors such as the inner nonkeratinized epithelium of the foreskin create a moist reservoir for uropathogens and contribute to the first contact between the host and the bacteria. Once the prepuce has been colonized, the bacteria can ascend the urinary tract, causing cystitis or pyelonephritis. Rushton and Majd showed a clear predominance of males among infants less than 6 months old with febrile UTI, and a disproportionately high frequency of uncircumcised male infants. Cascio et al showed a pure growth of an uropathogen in 48% of uncircumcised infants with VUR despite the use of prophylactic antibiotics.

A meta-analysis performed by Skoog et al showed that VUR in infants diagnosed by screening after an antenatally detected hydronephrosis was significantly associated with renal damage. Renal abnormalities occurred in a mean of 6.2% versus 47.9% of those with grade I to III versus IV to V reflux.

Yeung et al studied 155 infants with prenatal hydronephrosis and postnatally diagnosed VUR. They observed renal parenchymal damage in 42% of the 135 infants (101 male and 34 female) without a history of UTI. Furthermore, Nguyen et al reported renal parenchymal abnormalities in 65% of predominantly male infants with sterile high-grade reflux. The resolution rate of antenatally diagnosed high-grade VUR (grade IV or V) is approximately 20% by the age of 2 years. However, in approximately 25% of boys followed nonoperatively, UTIs developed by the age of 2 years, despite antimicrobial chemoprophylaxis. Early detection of febrile UTI is critical in infants who are unable to verbally communicate lower urinary tract symptoms. Detection of VUR by screening infants in at-risk population before presentation with febrile UTI is commendable, but its outcomes remain unknown.

## CLINICAL PRESENTATION

It is obviously important to diagnose VUR at the earliest possible age, preferably in infancy. There are a number of clinical presentations, which should raise the suspicion of VUR in an infant and child. As antenatal ultrasound becomes increasingly routine, many cases will be suspected before birth and should be investigated within the first month of life. Infants with a poor urinary stream as in the case of posterior urethral valves or infants with spina bifida have a high incidence

of VUR, while early investigations are indicated in the first-degree relatives of patients with high-grade VUR.

In most cases, VUR is discovered clinically after investigations for UTI. The incidence of VUR in infants with febrile UTI is 30% to 50% with an even higher incidence in male infants. Cascio et al found VUR in 33% of the 57 neonates investigated for first hospitalized UTI with 91% having high-grade VUR.

## RADIOLOGICAL INVESTIGATIONS

### Ultrasound

Sonography should be performed in any infant or child with a suspicion of VUR. The kidneys and upper ureters should be examined both in the B-mode and in real time. The bladder and lower ureters are assessed by real-time examination at each ureterovesical junction for dilatation, configuration, peristalsis, and continuity with the bladder base. Because VUR and UTI may affect renal structure and function, performing renal ultrasound to assess the upper urinary tract is recommended. VUR is suspected in the presence of a dilated pelvicaliceal system, upper or lower ureter, unequal renal size, or cortical loss, and increased echogenicity. Sonography is not sufficiently sensitive or specific for diagnosing VUR. The intermittent and dynamic nature of VUR probably contributes to the insensitivity of routine renal sonography in the detection of even higher grades of reflux.

Phan et al reported a 15% prevalence of VUR in infants diagnosed with antenatal hydronephrosis, many of whom had normal postnatal ultrasound or mild postnatal pelviectasis. They concluded that a VCUG is the only reliable test for detecting postnatal VUR.

### Voiding Cystography

VUR is a dynamic process. Bladder filling and voiding are necessary for its elucidation, which requires catheterization for adequate documentation. A voiding cystogram remains the gold standard for detecting VUR (Fig. 66-1). Despite the unpleasant nature of the procedure, it has a low false-negative rate and provides accurate anatomical detail, allowing grading of the VUR. It is commonly performed as a first-line investigation, together with ultrasound.

Some investigators employ nuclear cystography for diagnosing VUR. This can be either direct or indirect using technetium-labeled diaminotetra-ethyl-pentaacetic acid (DTPA). In direct nuclear cystography, DTPA is instilled into the bladder by urethral catheter or suprapubic injection and the ureters and kidneys are observed on camera during bladder filling and voiding. In indirect nuclear cystography, DTPA is injected intravenously. After the bladder is filled, the patient is instructed to void and the counts taken over the ureters and kidneys are used to assess the presence of VUR. Indirect nuclear cystography requires a cooperative patient and therefore is of no value in infants. The main disadvantage of nuclear cystography is that it does not give anatomical detail and VUR cannot be graded according to international classification.

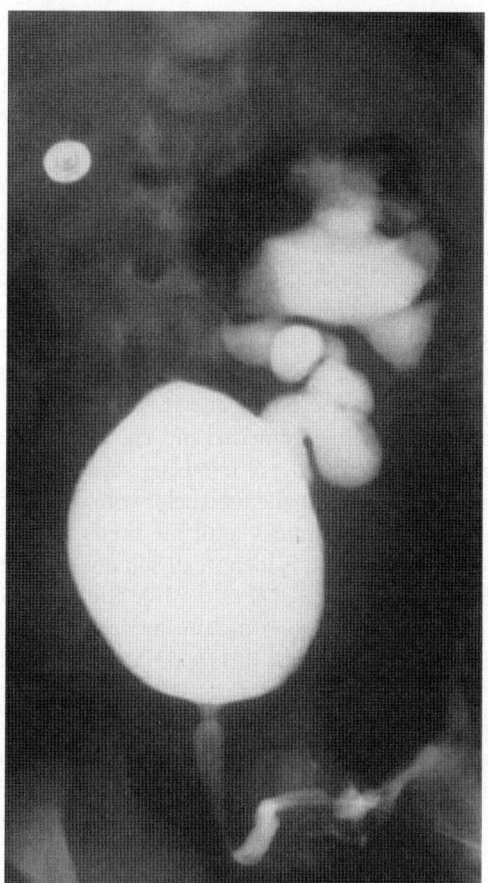

**FIGURE 66-1** Male infant showing grade V left VUR.

According to the international classification of reflux, there are 5 grades of reflux:

1. grade I, ureter only
2. grade II, ureter, pelvis, and calices—no dilatation, normal caliceal fornices
3. grade III, mild dilatation and/or tortuosity of the ureter and mild dilatation of the renal pelvis—minor blunting of the fornices

4. grade IV, moderate dilatation and/or tortuosity of the ureter and moderate dilatation of the renal pelvis and calices—complete obliteration of the sharp angle of fornices but maintenance of the papillary impressions in the majority of calices
5. grade V, gross dilatation of the renal pelvis and calices (Fig. 66-2)

## DMSA Scan

DMSA is the most sensitive technique for detecting renal scarring. When performed in the course of acute UTI, the DMSA scan is currently the most reliable test for the diagnosis of acute pyelonephritis. Several reports have suggested that a normal acute DMSA scan rules out the possibility of high-grade VUR. However, others have reported that acute DMSA scintigraphy has limited overall ability in revealing VUR after first febrile UTI in infants. This has been found to be true even when the findings of the acute DMSA scan were combined with those of renal ultrasonography.

## MANAGEMENT

Management of VUR is controversial. The various treatment options currently available in the management of VUR are (i) long-term antibiotic prophylaxis, (ii) intermittent antibiotic therapy for UTI, (iii) antibiotic prophylaxis and anticholinergics, (iv) open or laparoscopic reimplantation of ureters, and (v) minimally invasive endoscopic treatment.

### Medical Management

This strategy is based on 3 important assumptions: (i) Sterile VUR in most cases is not harmful to the kidneys and has no relevant effect on kidney function. (ii) Children can outgrow VUR, at least the lower grades. (iii) Continuous low-dose antibiotic prophylaxis can prevent infection for many years while VUR is still present.

The patient is required to take low-dose daily antibiotics, and annual ultrasound and VCUG are performed to assess

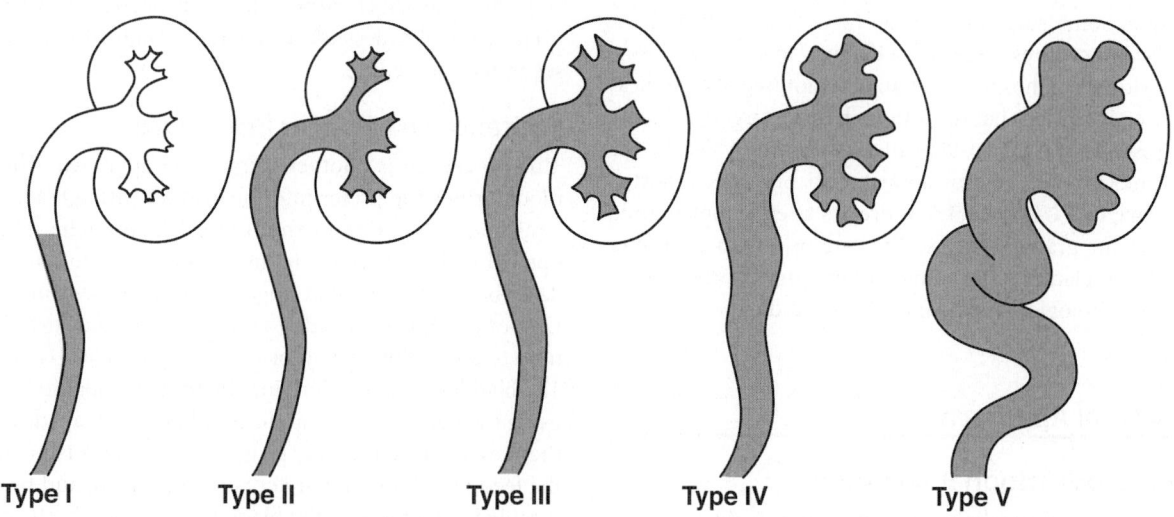

Type I  Type II  Type III  Type IV  Type V

**FIGURE 66-2** International classification of vesicoureteral reflux (grades I-V).

**VESICOURETERAL REFLUX**

821

if the reflux has resolved. Continuing antibiotics prophylaxis is reliant on patient's compliance and has the risk of bacterial resistance accompanied by potential breakthrough UTIs. Compliance of antibiotic therapy has been reported to be poor. Data of 11,000 children under the age of 11 years with a diagnosis of VUR were reviewed with 76% of VUR patients initiated on antibiotic prophylaxis. Only 17% of pediatric VUR patients on prophylactic antibiotics were compliant with therapy. Of patients on prophylactic therapy, 58% had a diagnosis of a UTI within 1 year of treatment. Furthermore, several large, prospective, randomized controlled trials have shown little or no benefit of medical therapy in terms of reducing the incidence of febrile UTI or renal scarring.

Spontaneous resolution is inversely proportional to the initial grade of reflux. Resolution rates for grade I and II VUR have been reported to be between 80% and 68%, respectively. However, the resolution rate for grade III reflux was only 45% and for grade IV/V VUR only 17%.

The European arm of the International Reflux Study Group in children at 10-year follow-up showed that half of the children with grades III and IV reflux randomly allocated to medical treatment still had reflux. In those with bilateral reflux, 61% had persistence of reflux. In a long-term study, Schwab et al reported spontaneous resolution rates of 13% yearly for grade I to III reflux and only 5% for grade IV to V reflux. Median time for resolution under antibiotic prophylaxis was 4.5 years for grade III and 9.5 years for grade IV. Additionally, long-term antibiotic prophylaxis has the risk of bacterial resistance accompanied by potential breakthrough UTIs and antibiotics are usually needed for years.

## SURGICAL TREATMENT

### Open Antireflux Procedures

Open surgical treatment of reflux has been the gold standard. However, surgery is not without risks. The goal of antireflux surgery is to restore the flap-valve mechanism of the UVJ by establishing an adequate submucosal tunnel of intramural ureter. The 2 most commonly used open antireflux procedures are the Cohen technique and the Politano–Leadbetter technique. Some surgeons use the Lich–Gregoir technique. All these procedures, although effective, involve open surgery, prolonged in hospital stay, and are not free of complications, even in the best hands. Although open surgery achieves a success rate of 92% to 98% in grade II to IV VUR, the American Urological Association report on VUR reported persistence of VUR in 19.3% of ureters after reimplantation of ureters for grade V reflux. The rate of obstruction after ureteral reimplantation needing reoperation reported by the American Urological Association in 33 studies was 0.3% to 9.1%.

### Intravesical Approach

### Cohen Cross-Trigonal Technique

A cystoscopy of the lower urinary tract is first recommended. The patient is then positioned supine with a slight break in the table to raise the hips. A transverse suprapubic skin incision (Pfannenstiel) is made. The subcutaneous tissues are incised and the rectus and pyramidalis muscles are split in the middle to expose the anterior bladder wall. A midline cystostomy is performed vertically. In order to flatten and elevate the posterior bladder wall, a Denis Browne ring retractor is positioned. This brings the trigone and the ueretric orifices into the middle of the operative field. Several moistened swabs are placed inside the dome of the bladder in order to stretch the posterior bladder wall and to expose the trigone. A 3 to 5 Fr. soft feeding tube is inserted into the ureteral orifice, as this helps with the dissection. The catheter is passed up to the kidney and fixed with a stay suture. The ureteric orifice is circumcised and the ureter is dissected out circumferentially (Fig. 66-3A) using a needle cautery tip to aid hemostasis. Lifting the tube helps with dissection. The ureteral dissection continues until the ureter is completely free and the peritoneum is identified. Subsequently, the submucosal tunnel is prepared (Fig. 66-3B). The tunnel is positioned just above the trigone, usually horizontal and crossing the midline of the posterior surface of the bladder. After the site of the new ureteric orifice is selected, the bladder mucosa is lifted from underlying bladder muscles using scissors. Through the opening in the mucosa toward the ureteral hiatus, a right-angled or curved mosquito clamp is positioned in order to grasp the tip of the feeding tube. The feeding tube is then gently pulled through the submucosal tunnel, paying attention not to twist or kink the ureter. This brings the ureter into place (Fig. 66-3C). In cases of bilateral reimplantation, the same procedure can be carried out for the opposite ureter and both ureters can be placed in the same submucosal tunnel. It is better to place the ureter with a higher grade of reflux above the ureter with lower reflux grade, as the upper ureter would normally have a slightly longer tunnel. The anastomosis is performed using fine absorbable sutures leaving the feeding tube in position. The feeding tube is then removed and reinserted into the ureter to make sure that the feeding tube passes smoothly through the submucosal tunnel. It is also important to watch for urinary efflux. The feeding tube is exteriorized through the bladder wall, the rectus muscle, and the skin. The cystostomy is closed in 2 layers using running absorbable sutures. The bladder mucosa is closed using running absorbable sutures. It is not necessary to leave the ureter stented unless there is bladder wall oedema or it is a secondary procedure.

### Politano–Leadbetter Procedure

This procedure is another intravesical approach. This technique brings the ureter into the bladder through a new ureteral hiatus superior to the original hiatus. The bladder is opened and the ureters are dissected out in the same way as described above. A right-angle clamp is passed through the UVJ opening from inside to out and the tip of the clamp is used to tent up the posterior wall of the bladder (Fig. 66-4A). The bladder mucosa overlying the tip of the clamp is opened using the needle cautery and a new hiatus is shaped. Through the newly formed hiatus, a right-angle clamp is positioned, the feeding tube in the ureter is then grasped, and the ureter is pulled carefully into the bladder (Fig. 66-4B). The original hiatus is then closed with absorbable sutures and a submucosal

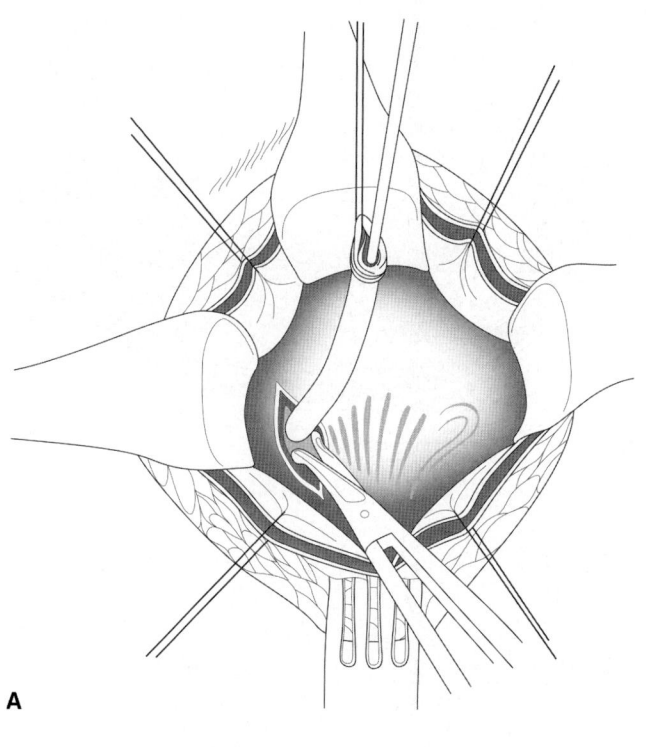

**A**

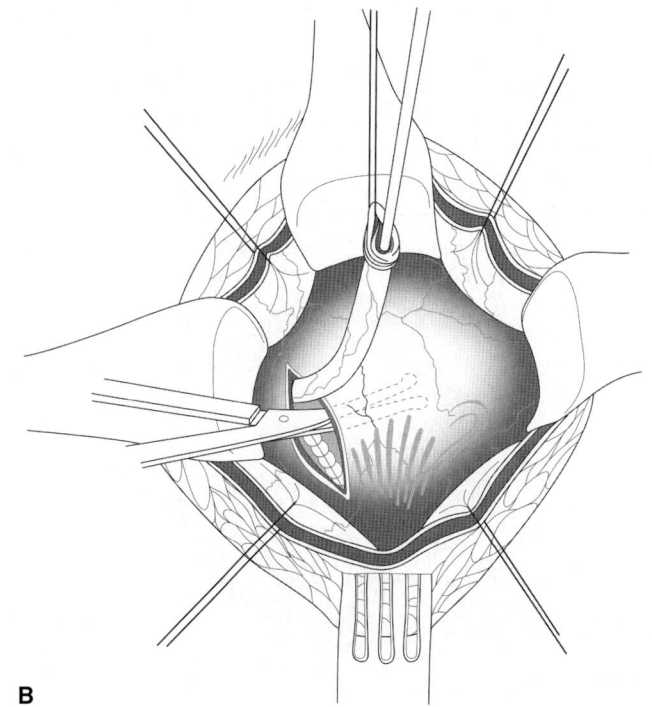

**B**

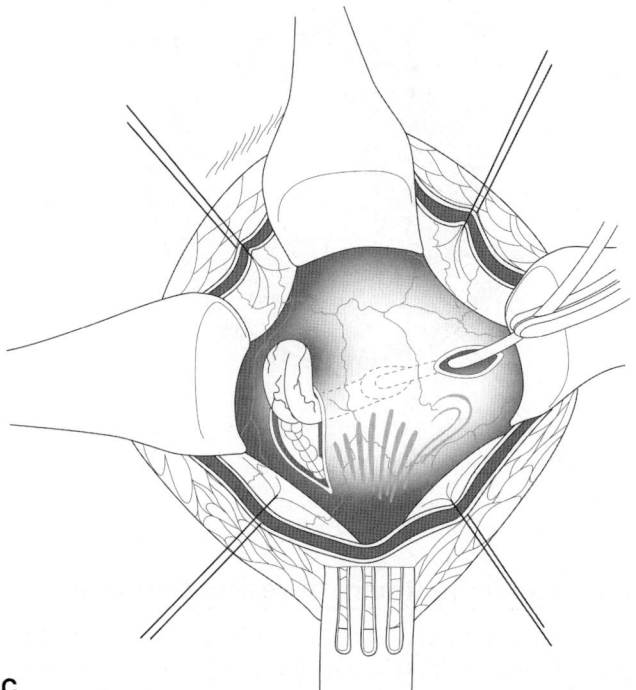

**C**

**FIGURE 66-3** **A.** The ureteric orifice is circumcised and the ureter is dissected out circumferentially. **B.** The submucosal tunnel is prepared. **C.** A right-angled or curved mosquito clamp grasps the tip of the feeding tube and the tip is gently pulled through the submucosal tunnel.

tunnel is made. The ureter is positioned in a submucosal tunnel directed toward the bladder neck and sutured to the bladder mucosa (Fig. 66-4C). The feeding tube is then removed and reinserted into the ureter to make sure that the feeding tube passes easily through the submucosal tunnel. There is no need to leave a feeding tube in the ureter. The cystostomy is closed in 2 layers using running absorbable sutures.

The success rate for Politano–Leadbetter and Cohen Cross-Trigonal Technique are similar. One advantage of the Politano–Leadbetter is the option to create a neo-ostium in an anatomically adequate position and to create a neo-ostium that is easily accessible for future pyelography and ureteral

endoscopy because the ureteral opening of the Cohen procedure is on the opposite side of the bladder. Bowel injury is one of the most feared complications of the Politano–Leadbetter approach, being encountered in approximately 0.5% of cases.

## Extravesical Approach

### Detrusorraphy

This procedure has been developed from the Lich–Gregoir technique. Success rates are similar to intravesical

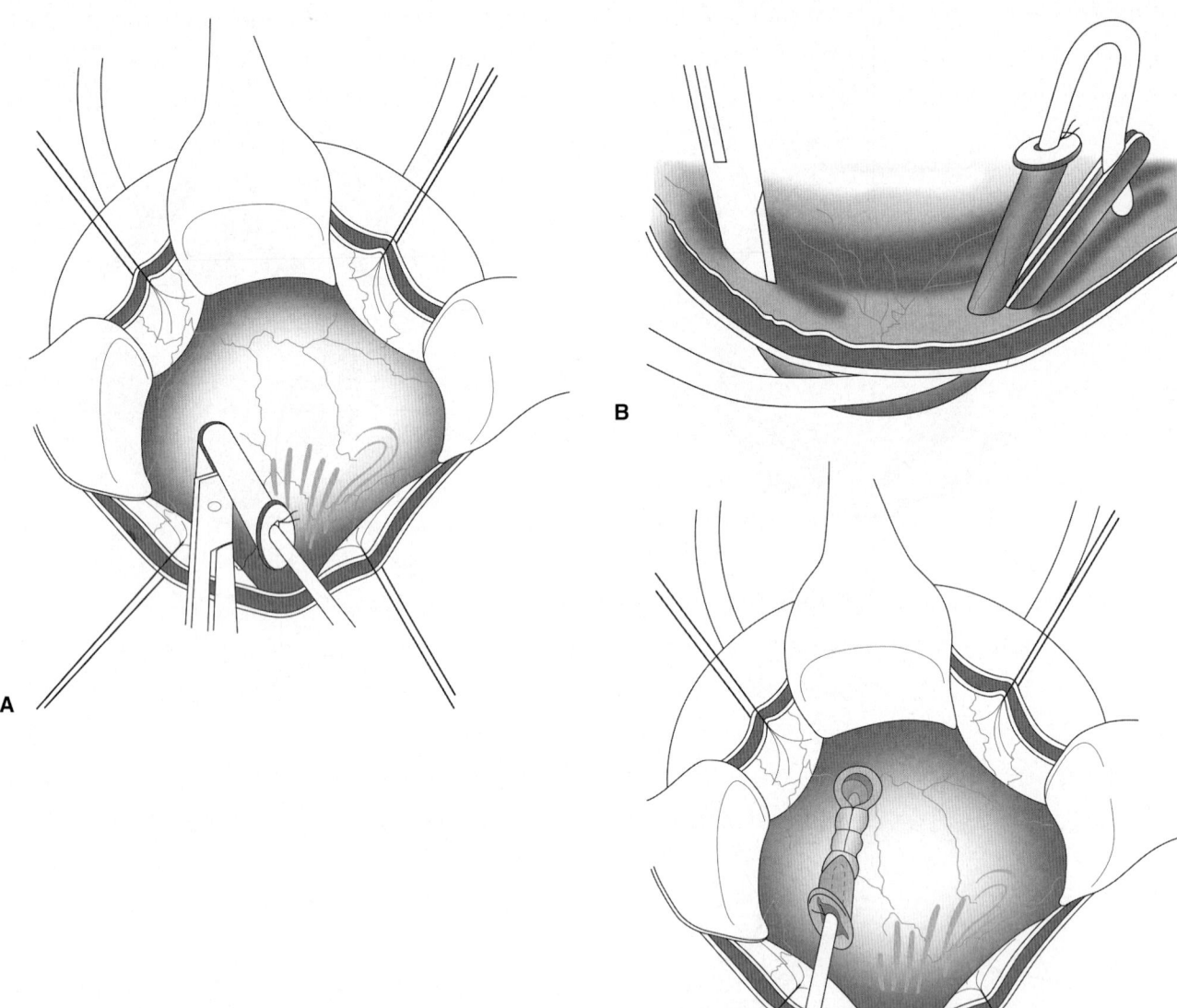

**FIGURE 66-4 A.** A right-angle clamp is passed through the UVJ opening from inside to out and the tip of the clamp is used to tent up the posterior wall of the bladder. **B.** The feeding tube in the ureter is grasped and the ureter is pulled into the bladder. **C.** The ureter is lying in the submucosal tunnel directed toward the bladder neck.

approaches. The most significant complications associated with the extravesical technique of ureteral reimplantation are ureteral obstruction and urinary retention. Ureteral obstruction occurs in about 2% to 4% of the children. Urinary retention is only associated with bilateral reimplantation and is reported to occur in 8% to 15% of the children due to trauma to the pelvic nervous plexus.

## Laparoscopic Ureteral Reimplantation

In recent years, several authors have reported their experience of ureteral reimplantation with laparoscopic extravesical transperitoneal approach as well as pneumovesical approach. This technique results in a shorter hospital stay and less postoperative discomfort compared to open operation. Furthermore, robotic assisted laparoscopic extravesical ureteral reimplantation has shown high success rates similar to open ureteral reimplantation as well as minimal morbidity.

## Endoscopic Treatment of Vesicoureteral Reflux

The concept of endoscopic treatment was introduced by Puri and O'Donnell in 1984 as a minimally invasive treatment for VUR following a successful experimental study in piglets. A minimally invasive endoscopic technique for the correction of VUR has become an established alternative to long-term antibiotic prophylaxis and open surgical treatment. The AUA Guideline recently updated the management of primary VUR in children. They extracted data from 131 articles and data from 17,972 patients were included in their analysis. Success rates are 98.1% for open surgical procedures and 83.0% for endoscopic therapy after 1 injection. With the high success rate of endoscopic treatment, the AUA Guidelines included endoscopic treatment in the management options for VUR.

Endoscopic treatment has several advantages over open surgical treatment or long-term antibiotic prophylaxis. In contrast to long-term antibiotic prophylaxis, it offers immediate cure of reflux with a high success rate, its success does not rely on patient or parent compliance and the procedure is virtually free of adverse side effects. In 2001, Deflux® was approved by the Food and Drug Administration (FDA) as an acceptable tissue-augmenting substance for subureteral injection therapy for VUR. Since then, endoscopic treatment has become increasingly popular worldwide for managing VUR, and Deflux® is the most widely used tissue-augmenting substance.

Recently, the Swedish Reflux Trial in Children recruited children between 1 and 2 years old with grade III to IV VUR for a prospective, open, randomized controlled multicenter study. Children were treated in 3 groups, including low-dose antibiotic prophylaxis, endoscopic therapy, and a surveillance group on antibiotics only for febrile UTI. After 2 years, endoscopic treatment results were significantly better than the spontaneous resolution rate or downgrading in the prophylaxis and surveillance groups.

The technique of endoscopic injection of Deflux® is simple and straightforward. The patients should be placed in a lithotomy position. The cystoscope is passed and the bladder wall, the trigone, bladder neck, and both ureteric orifices are inspected. All cystoscopes available for infants and children can be used for this procedure. The bladder should be almost empty before proceeding with injection, since this helps to keep the ureteric orifice flat rather than away in a lateral field. The disposable Puri flexible catheter (STORZ, Catalogue-No-27201) or a rigid metallic catheter can be used for injection. A 1-mL syringe filled with Deflux® is attached to the injection catheter. Under direct vision through the cystoscope, the needle is introduced under the bladder mucosa 2 to 3 mm below the affected ureteral orifice at the 6 o'clock position (Fig. 66-5). In children with grade IV and V reflux

with wide ureteral orifices, the needle should be inserted not below but directly into the affected ureteral orifice. The needle is advanced about 4 to 5 mm under the mucosa and the injection started slowly. As the Deflux® is injected, a bulge appears in the floor of the submucosal ureter. Most refluxing ureters require 0.4 to 1.0 mL Deflux® to correct reflux. A correctly placed injection creates the appearance of a nipple on the top which is a slit-like or inverted crescent orifice. If the bulge appears in an incorrect place, for example, at the side of the ureter or proximal to it, the needle should not be withdrawn, but should be moved so that the point is in a more favourable position. The noninjected ureteric roof retains its compliance while preventing reflux. Postoperative urethral catheterization is not necessary. Patients are treated as day cases and a voiding cystourethrogram and ultrasound are performed 6 to 12 weeks after discharge. A follow-up renal and bladder ultrasound are obtained 12 months after endoscopic correction.

Figure 66-6A shows a VCUG with right-grade IV VUR and left-grade V VUR in an infant. Complete resolution of VUR after endoscopic treatment in the same infant is shown in Fig. 66-6B.

Procedure-related complications are rare. The only significant complication with this procedure has been failure. There may be initial failure, that is, the reflux is not abolished by the injection, or recurrence, where initial correction is not maintained. About 15% of refluxing ureters require more than 1 endoscopic injection of paste to correct the condition.

Between 2001 and 2010, the authors treated 1551 children with intermediate and high-grade VUR by endoscopic injection of Deflux®. VUR was unilateral in 765 children and bilateral in 786. Renal scarring was detected in 369 (26.7%)

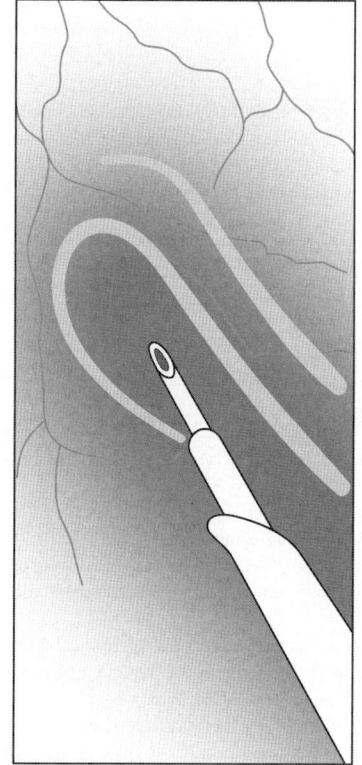 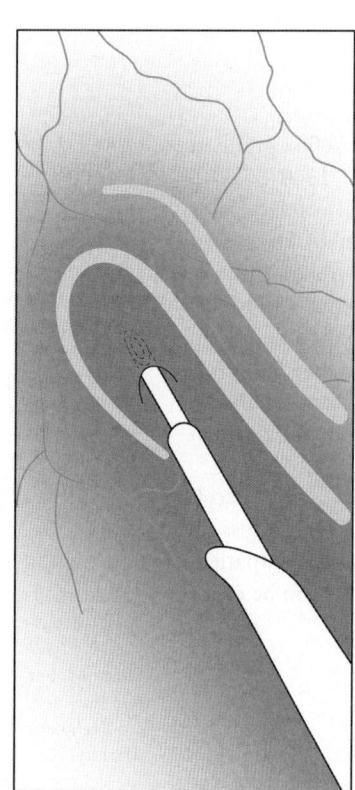 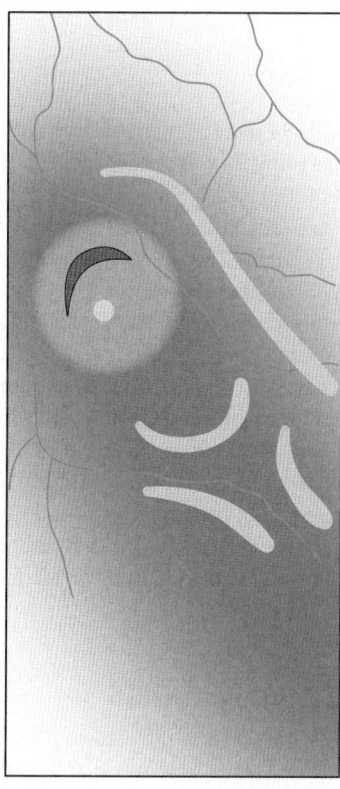

**FIGURE 66-5** Technique of endoscopic subureteric injection: (A) the site of insertion of needle; (B) the needle is advanced 4 to 5 mm before the injection is started; and (C) appearance of the ureteric orifice at completion of injection.

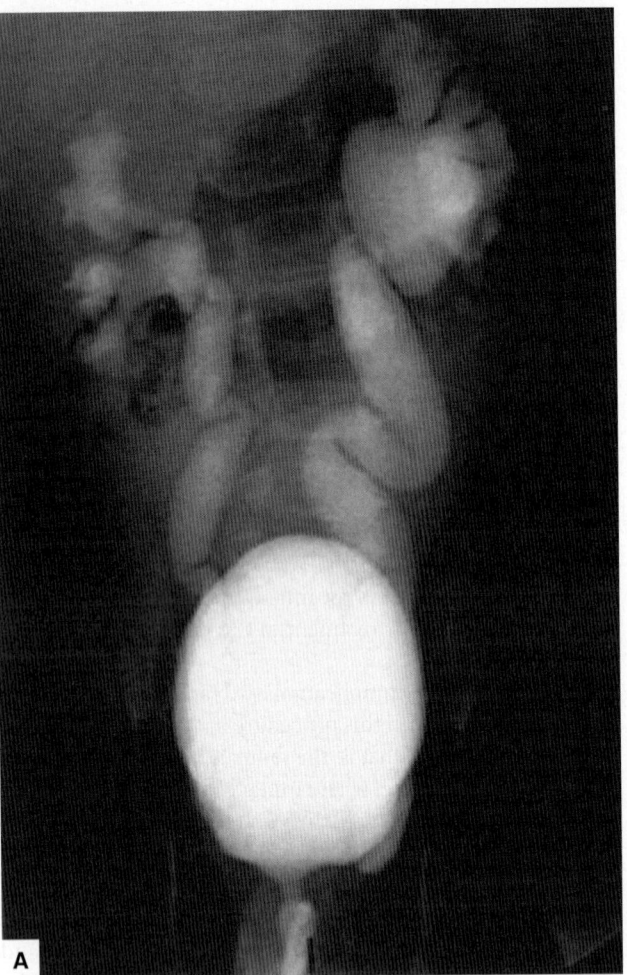
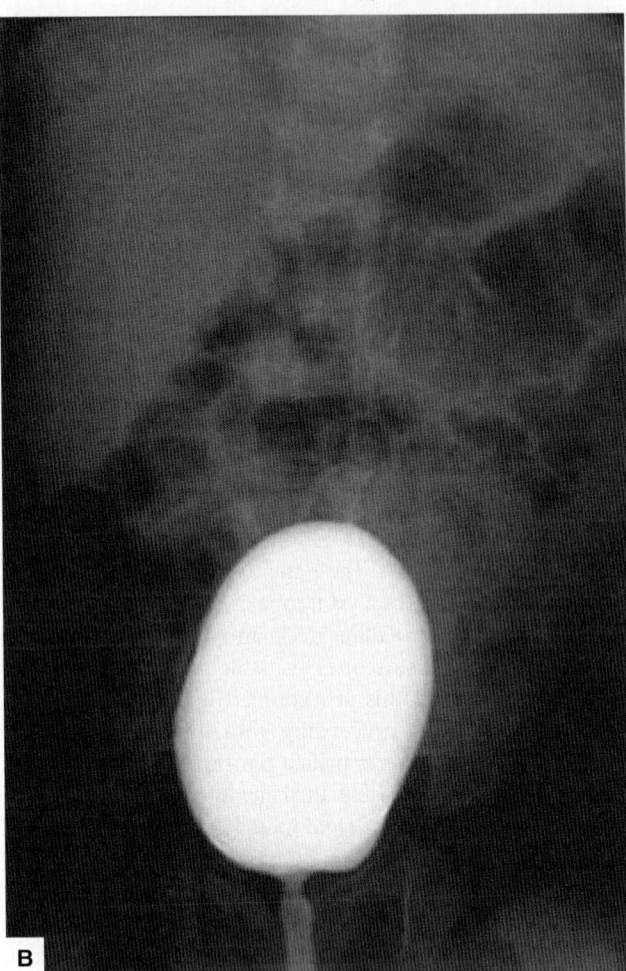

**FIGURE 66-6 A.** VCUG shows right-grade IV VUR and left-grade V VUR in an infant. **B.** VCUG shows complete resolution of VUR after endoscopic treatment in the same infant.

of the 1384 patients who had a DMSA scan. Reflux grade in the 2341 ureters was grade II to V in 98 (4.2%), 1340 (57.3%), 818 (34.9%) and 85 (3.6%), respectively. VUR resolved after first, second, and third endoscopic injection of Dx/HA in 2039 (87.1%), 264 (11.3%), and 38 (1.6%) ureters, respectively. Sixty-nine (4.6%) of the 1512 patients who were followed up developed febrile UTIs during a median follow-up of 5.6 years. None of the patients in the series needed reimplantation of ureters or developed any significant complications, confirming the efficacy and safety in the management of intermediate and high-grade VUR.

Endoscopic subureteral injection of Deflux® is an excellent first-line treatment in children with 87% success in high-grade VUR after 1 injection. This 15-minute outpatient procedure is safe and simple to perform, and it can be easily repeated in failed cases.

## SELECTED READINGS

Cascio S, Colhoun E, Puri P. Bacterial colonization of the prepuce in boys with vesicoureteral reflux who receive antibiotic prophylaxis. *J Pediatr* 2001;139:160.

Cascio S, Chertin B, Yoneda A, et al. Acute renal damage in infants after first urinary tract infection. *Pediatr Nephrol* 2002;17:503.

Chung PH, Tang DY, Wong KK, et al. Comparing open and pneumovesical approach for ureteric reimplantation in pediatric patients—a preliminary review. *J Pediatr Surg* 2008;43:2246.

Cooper CS. Diagnosis and management of vesicoureteral reflux in children. *Nat Rev Urol* 2009;6:481.

Dawrant MJ, Mohanan N, Puri P. Endoscopic treatment for high grade vesicoureteral reflux in infants. *J Urol* 2006;176:1847.

Elder JS. Guidelines for consideration for surgical repair of vesicoureteral reflux. *Curr Opin Urol* 2000;10:579.

Fouzas S, Krikelli E, Vassilakos P, et al. DMSA scan for revealing vesicoureteral reflux in young children with urinary tract infection. *Pediatrics* 2010;126:e513.

Hoberman A, Charron M, Hickey RW, et al. Imaging studies after a first febrile urinary tract infection in young children. *N Engl J Med* 2003;348:195.

Holmdahl G, Brandstrom P, Lackgren G, et al. The Swedish reflux trial in children: II. Vesicoureteral reflux outcome. *J Urol* 2010;184:280.

Knudson MJ, Austin JC, McMillan ZM, et al. Predictive factors of early spontaneous resolution in children with primary vesicoureteral reflux. *J Urol* 2007;178:1684.

Lopez M, Varlet F. Laparoscopic extravesical transperitoneal approach following the Lich–Gregoir technique in the treatment of vesicoureteral reflux in children. *J Pediatr Surg* 2010;45:806.

Marra G, Oppezzo C, Ardissino G, et al. Severe vesicoureteral reflux and chronic renal failure: a condition peculiar to male gender? Data from the ItalKid Project. *J Pediatr* 2004;144:677.

Parekh DJ, Pope JCT, Adams MC, et al. Outcome of sibling vesicoureteral reflux. *J Urol*, 2002;167:283.

Peters C, Rushton HG. Vesicoureteral reflux associated renal damage: congenital reflux nephropathy and acquired renal scarring. *J Urol* 2010;184:265.

Peters CA, Skoog SJ, Arant BS Jr, et al. Summary of the AUA guideline on management of primary vesicoureteral reflux in children. *J Urol* 2010;184:1134.

Phan V, Traubici J, Hershenfield B, et al. Vesicoureteral reflux in infants with isolated antenatal hydronephrosis. *Pediatr Nephrol* 2003;18:1224.

Puri P, Gosemann JH, Darlow J, et al. Genetics of vesicoureteral reflux. *Nat Rev Urol* 2011;8:539.

Puri P, Mohanan N, Menezes M, et al. Endoscopic treatment of moderate and high grade vesicoureteral reflux in infants using dextranomer/hyaluronic acid. *J Urol* 2007;178:1714.

Puri P, O'Donnell B. Correction of experimentally produced vesicoureteric reflux in the piglet by intravesical injection of Teflon. *Br Med J (Clin Res Ed)* 1984;289:5.

Rushton HG, Majd M. Pyelonephritis in male infants: how important is the foreskin? *J Urol* 1992;148:733.

Schwab CW Jr, Wu HY, Selman H, et al. Spontaneous resolution of vesicoureteral reflux: a 15-year perspective. *J Urol* 2002;168:2594.

Skoog SJ, Peters CA, Arant BS Jr, et al. Pediatric vesicoureteral reflux guidelines panel summary report: clinical practice guidelines for screening siblings of children with vesicoureteral reflux and neonates/infants with prenatal hydronephrosis. *J Urol* 2010;184:1145.

Smellie JM, Barratt TM, Chantler C et al. Medical versus surgical treatment in children with severe bilateral vesicoureteric reflux and bilateral nephropathy: a randomised trial. *Lancet* 2001;357:1329.

Smellie JM, Jodal U, Lax H, et al. Outcome at 10 years of severe vesicoureteric reflux managed medically: report of the International Reflux Study in Child *J Pediatr* 2001;139:656.

Sung J, Skoog S. Surgical management of vesicoureteral reflux in children. *Pediatr Nephrol* 2012;27(4):551–561.

Swerkersson S, Jodal U, Sixt R, et al. Relationship among vesicoureteral reflux, urinary tract infection and renal damage in children. *J Urol* 2007;178:647.

Venhola M, Huttunen NP, Renko M, et al. Practice guidelines for imaging studies in children after the first urinary tract infection. *J Urol* 2010;184:325.

# Bladder Exstrophy

# CHAPTER 67

*Douglas A. Canning, Lisa Parrillo,
Kavita Gupta, and Howard M. Snyder III*

## KEY POINTS

1. Bladder exstrophy is rare, occurring about once in 30 to 50,000 live births. Despite a devastating initial appearance, because associated defects are few, many with bladder exstrophy lead near normal successful lives following reconstruction.

2. Goals for repair include providing urinary continence in both sexes and reconstructing the penis in males to provide for standing micturition and vaginal penetration.

3. Two approaches, the staged (Hopkins) repair and the complete repair (Mitchell) are currently in use.

4. If newborn closure is done in early infancy, iliac osteotomy is not always required.

5. A dedicated, experienced, consistent team is required to provide optimal results.

Children with bladder exstrophy are born with the bladder exposed (Fig. 67-1). The defect is obvious. The exposed umbilicus is at the midline. Just inferior to the umbilicus is the exposed bladder, which is surrounded by shiny, transitional para-exstrophy skin. The defect extends from the dome of the bladder to the tip of the urethra in classic bladder exstrophy. In epispadias, the bladder is closed, and only the urethra is exposed. The pubic bones are variably separated, further in bladder exstrophy than in epispadias. The umbilical to anal distance is shortened. If the child is older, the rectum may be prolapsed. In the male, the penis is short. The corporal bodies are separated, drawn apart a variable distance as they pass inferior to the pubic bones. The clitoris in the female is bifid. The vagina may be duplicated and the vaginal introitus may be stenotic.

Despite these dramatic defects, children with bladder exstrophy have surprisingly few other problems. Presuming a successful modern reconstruction is accomplished, most will live rewarding lives and contribute greatly to society.

## SURGICAL HISTORY

### Evolution

The treatment of children with bladder exstrophy has evolved from supportive treatment in primitive times until the early to middle nineteenth century when initial surgical attempts were made to divert the urine to the rectum. The early attempts at ureterosigmoidostomy were fraught with complication, usually infection, and most patients died. A few scattered attempts at bladder closure were made in the middle of the 1800s. One attempt by Richard was made in 1853, and another was performed by Pancoast in 1858 at the Gross Clinic in Philadelphia. These early attempts at bladder closure, coming as they did in the era before antibiotics and suitable upper urinary diversion, failed. Most patients died of overwhelming wound infection or pyelonephritis caused by infection in a poorly emptying upper tract. Because of the severe morbidity of the primitive bladder closures and diversions, most patients were managed expectantly with urinary collection devices that were fashioned to the patient's abdomen (Fig. 67-2). Few patients underwent bladder closure or diversion prior to the beginning of the twentieth century when more modern techniques of ureterosigmoidostomy began to be developed.

The Coffey ureterosigmoidostomy ushered in the "Middle Ages" of exstrophy surgery. His technique implanted the ureter directly through the wall of the sigmoid, advancing the ureter into the lumen of the sigmoid. Despite the preantibiotic period, wound infection rates were low and success was better with this technique. Prior to 1950, nearly all patients with bladder exstrophy underwent primary urinary diversion at about 1 year of age with a ureterosigmoidostomy and cystectomy.

A few surgeons continued to experiment with primary bladder closure. In 1922, Young reported a successful bladder closure in a female patient. The bladder neck was later rolled into a tube, which was designed to increase resistance to drainage at the bladder outlet. According to Young, the patient developed a "3-hour dry interval," which encouraged others to persist in attempts to try for continence without urinary diversion. Modification of the Young continence procedure by Dees 20 years later included incorporation of the bladder neck into the rolled muscular tube. Subsequent

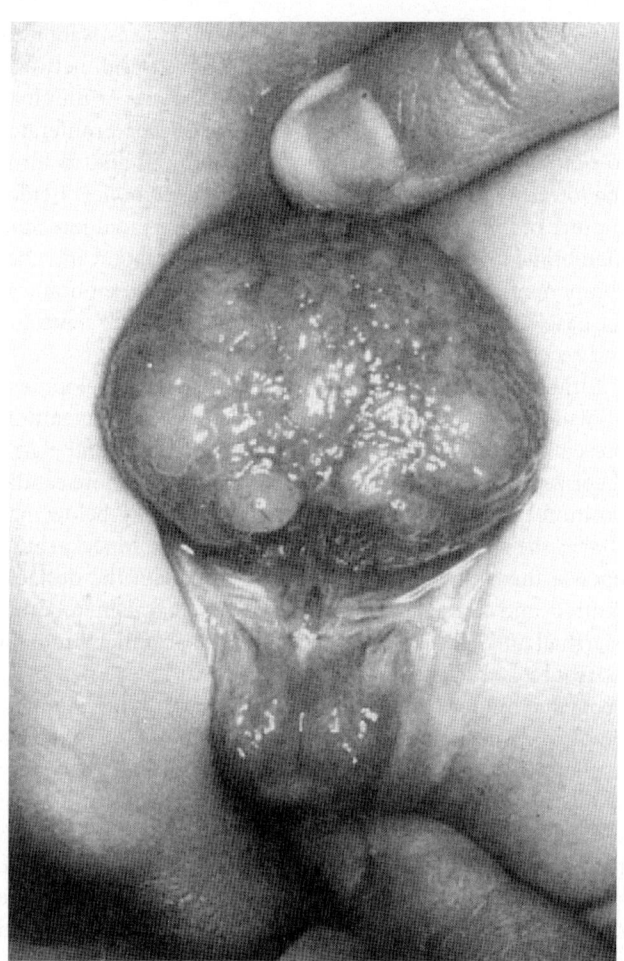

**FIGURE 67-1** Typical appearance of the bladder in classic bladder exstrophy. The bladder has a polypoid appearance with the detrusor prolapsed and the urothelium exposed. The urethral plate is shortened and open. The phallus is small in the male. The umbilical–anal distance is shortened.

modifications by Leadbetter after Dees included ureteral reimplantation superior to the trigone and incorporation of the trigone into the tube combined to result in today's "Young–Dees–Leadbetter bladder-neck plasty." Jeffs modified the Leadbetter technique further with a bladder neck suspension and modification of the incision and closure of the bladder neck. This technique is still widely used to correct urinary incontinence in children with bladder exstrophy. Unfortunately, even today, few patients achieve perfect continence following bladder-neck plasty.

A number of advances over the past 50 years have improved continence following primary bladder closure. Most of the bladder closure operations prior to 1968 were done outside the newborn period. As anesthetic techniques for the newborn improved and experience broadened in bladder-closure techniques, closures in younger infants were attempted. Ansel observed that the more mobile infant pelvis made apposition of the pubic bones easier during primary bladder closure. Bilateral iliac osteotomy, first used in the treatment of bladder exstrophy by Trendelenburg, became more widely used by Jeffs to help approximate the pubic symphysis in hopes of improving continence following the staged bladder repair. Early anatomic bladder closure, which encourages bladder filling and emptying early in life, bilateral iliac osteotomy, which may improve placement of the bladder neck and membranous urethra within the levator complex, and careful postoperative management to treat urinary tract infection and bladder-outlet obstruction early have all contributed to better continence rates and lower incidences of renal deterioration following bladder closure.

Because we now believe that osteotomy is desirable even in the newborn period, we now perform bilateral iliac osteotomy on all children with classic exstrophy at the beginning of the repair. We also acknowledge that the complete anatomical repair, particularly in males is a complicated procedure that

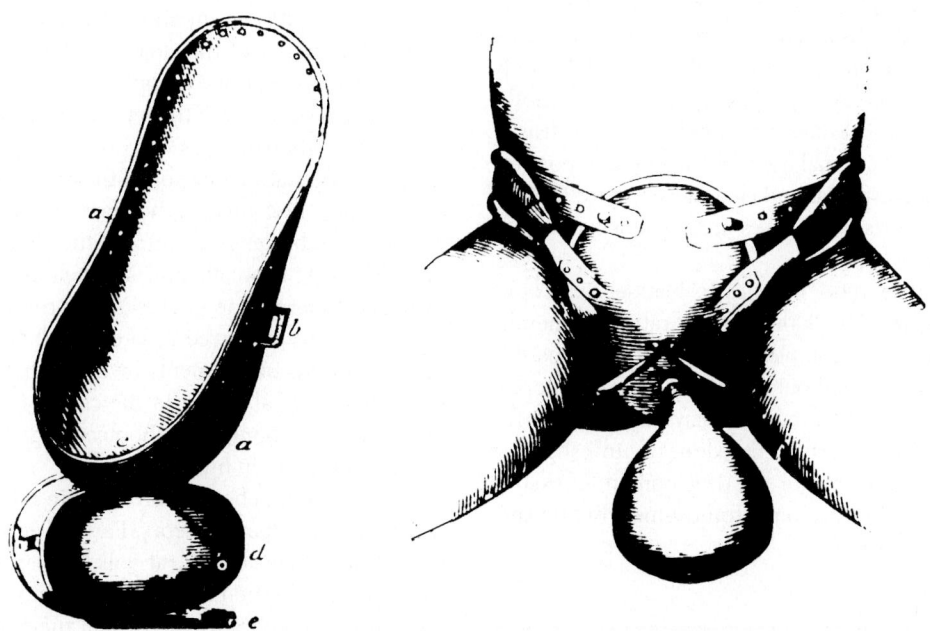

**FIGURE 67-2** Examples of urinary collecting devices used in the eighteenth and nineteenth centuries. (From Murphy, LJT. *The History of Urology*. Springfield, IL: Charles C. Thomas, 1972:333. Used with permission.)

requires great concentration, and meticulous dissection for over 4 to 5 hours. For this reason, at the Children's Hospital of Philadelphia (CHOP), we have a dedicated, consistent team of 2 attending urologists, an anesthesiologist, an orthopedist, and a consistent nursing team performs each closure. Because the osteotomy provides excellent mobility during the pelvic closure, even outside the newborn period, we no longer feel pressure to operate in the first 24 hours, but prefer to convene a rested, consistent team as soon as this can be arranged, rather than emergently on the day of birth.

## Incidence and Inheritance

Bladder exstrophy is rare, occurring once in every 30,000 to 50,000 live births. In a multicenter report from 1968 to 2005 of nearly 26.4 million births, the prevalence at birth of bladder exstrophy was 2.07 per 100,000. The risk of recurrence of bladder exstrophy specifically in a family is 1% and variants can recur in 0.3 to 2.3%. Of 215 children born to parents with exstrophy or epispadias, of a group of 2500 index cases, 3 children inherited bladder exstrophy (1 in 70 or 1.4%). Epispadias is less common, found in 1 in 117 in males and 1 in 484 in females. Although very few patients with classic bladder exstrophy have associated defects, the most common congenital anomaly is a VSD, which occurred in 1.1% of cases. Other defects that have been observed include cleft lip and palate, gastrochisis, omphalocele, hemivertebrae, neural tube defects, maxillary hypoplasia, congenital heart tumor, bilateral pre-auricular fistulas, syndactyly of the toes, and anal defects. In addition, 2 patients with bladder exstrophy have developed Wilms tumor, an exceedingly unlikely event considering the small incidence of the 2 conditions. There is also a report of 3 patients with Down Syndrome.

Despite occasional clustering of individuals with the defect, relatively little is known about the risk factors for bladder exstrophy. In 1 study from 1987, women younger than 20 years of age and high parity (3+) were at increased risk for delivering a child with bladder exstrophy. Another from 2007 found no association with maternal age. Finally, a study from 2011 showed increased prevalence with older mothers. Other risk factors that have been implicated in at least 1 study are high parity, maternal use of estrogens, and possibly antacids in cases of epispadias and cloacal exstrophy. Despite these occasional reports, most cases are not associated with any particular risk factor.

The male-to-female ratio for classic bladder exstrophy lies between 1.5:1 and 2:1. Although the ratio is generally accepted to be higher for complete epispadias, it is possible that complete epispadias without exstrophy is underreported in newborn females, and that the ratio may be closer to 2:1.

There is research currently being done to investigate a genetic mutation responsible for the development of exstrophy. Focus so far has centered on chromosome 9 but no specific locus has been isolated.

## Pathophysiology

Several theories to explain the development of bladder exstrophy revolve around the destabilization of the cloacal membrane at a critical time in development. Before 2 weeks gestation, the cloacal membrane is positioned on the infraumbilical abdominal wall. The membrane is stabilized as mesenchyme migrates from the primitive streak between the 2 endothelial layers of the cloacal membrane. As the cloacal membrane regresses, the mesodermal layer proliferates to reinforce the infraumbilical abdominal wall and to form the lower abdominal wall muscles and pelvic bones. Before rupture of the cloacal membrane, the urorectal fold joins the membrane to separate the cloaca into the urogenital and anal components. Subsequent rupture of the cloacal membrane at the base of the genital tubercle establishes the urethral meatus and rectal orifice.

Although several theories exist to explain the development of bladder exstrophy, no one theory satisfies all the features present in patients born with the defect. Patton and Barry theorized that the genital hillocks developed in a more caudal position than was typical with fusion occurring below, not above, the cloacal membrane. Marshall and Muecke built upon a theory by Patton and Barry to explain the destabilization and subsequent rupture of the cloacal membrane. Marshall and Muecke believed that the cloacal membrane in exstrophy is thickened. They theorized that the normal mesenchymal migration between the leaflets of the cloacal membrane in exstrophy is truncated, owing to increased thickness of the membrane. According to Marshall and Muecke, subsequent rupture of the membrane without reinforcement of the mesodermal layer would result in exstrophy. If the rupture occurs after the descent of the urorectal septum, classic bladder exstrophy would result. If rupture occurred before descent of the urorectal septum, cloacal exstrophy would result with resultant exposure of the hindgut as well as the bladder halves.

Lending support to the Marshall and Muecke theory, in utero ultrasound has documented the late rupture of the cloacal membrane in a fetus subsequently born with cloacal exstrophy. The observation that rupture of the membrane can occur late in gestation in a fetus with cloacal exstrophy suggests that the presence or absence of the urorectal septum, as well as the timing of the cloacal rupture, may be important to the development of exstrophy. The Muecke chick embryo experiments support his theory. Chicks with surgical implantation of plastic triangles onto the cloacal membrane at 48 to 52 hours gestation developed the characteristic appearance of exstrophy. Presumably, the plastic prevented mesodermal migration. Subsequent rupture of the deficient cloacal membrane ensued. Thomalla and Mitchell used a laser to injure the cloacal membrane in chicks. Exstrophy developed when the laser injury occurred as late as 61 hours (before curling of the tailbud). Experiments by both Muecke and Thomalla show that surgical injury to the cloaca results in exstrophy. Little is known about the pathophysiology of abnormal mesodermal migration in humans.

One additional observation made in rat embryos may further refine the Muecke theory. Early in development, marked cranial movement of the rat yolk sac separates the yolk sac from the cloacal membrane. In the region between the yolk sac and the membrane, the genital tubercle proliferates and forces the cloaca into a dorsal caudal position. A thick plate of mesenchymal tissue lies at the base of the genital tubercle. Failure of the cranial progression of the yolk sac in exstrophy would prevent migration of the genital tubercle and posterior displacement of the cloaca. The abdominal wall muscle and genital hillocks (labioscrotal or genital folds) would then fail to meet at the midline. The subsequent superficial cloacal membrane, poorly reinforced with mesoderm, would then be prone to rupture, resulting in exstrophy. This theory, which refines rather than refutes the work in chick embryos, may explain the shortened umbilical–anal distance seen in nearly all patients with exstrophy or epispadias, as well as the clinical appearance of several of the exstrophy variants.

Other theories include that of Sadler and Feldkamp who suggested that one, and perhaps both, of the lateral body wall folds fail to move ventrally enough to fuse appropriately in the midline. Depending whether the failure to close includes the abdomen, either cloacal exstrophy or classic bladder exstrophy will occur. Another hypothesis involves an abnormal insertion of the body stalk and the following lack of mesenchymal tissue in the midline. The cloaca therefore never is positioned posteriorly, is weak, and ruptures inappropriately. A final suggestion from Beaudoin and colleagues suggests that inadequate development of the bony pelvis is the principal cause of the exstrophy: the pelvis does not rotate appropriately preventing the soft tissues adherent to the pelvic ring from fusing at the midline.

## ANATOMY

The defect in bladder exstrophy can be thought of as a hernia, with the herniated tissue including the bladder, the trigone, and the bladder neck, as well as the urethra in males. The defect in the abdominal wall extends from the umbilicus superiorly, laterally along the separated rectus muscles to the level of the laterally displaced pubic bones to the level of the anus. An intersymphyseal band of fascial tissue represents the laterally displaced walls of the divergent urogenital diaphragm.

The umbilicus is displaced inferiorly, perhaps because of incomplete migration of the mesodermal layer during development. The area between the displaced rectus muscles and the exposed bladder is covered with shiny fibrous tissue, the "paraexstrophy skin" that Duckett showed could be used to augment urethral length during the primary bladder closure. The rectus muscle inserts normally at the pubic tubercle; the displaced pubic bones carry the rectus muscles to a lateral position. This displacement of the rectus muscles widens the internal inguinal canal and places the internal inguinal ring just beneath the external inguinal ring. For this reason, indirect inguinal hernia and incarceration are common, particularly in boys.

The bladder size is variable, from a small patch to a larger bladder plate, which, when reduced into the pelvis, will hold 15 to 30 cc. The bladder is almost never normal-sized. The bladder size may reflect the degree of pubic diastasis with the larger bladder plates associated with wider pubic diastasis. When exposed to air, the urothelium develops a polyploid appearance almost immediately. The severity of the polypoid change seems to be related to the amount of trauma the urothelium is exposed to. The longer the bladder is out and exposed to salves, diapers, or clothing, the more severe the change. Microscopic changes in the transitional epithelium

are present at birth or shortly thereafter, and may be present in utero. In patients in whom the bladder is left exposed, these changes may result in squamous or adenomatous metaplasia, which may later progress to squamous carcinoma or adenocarcinoma in patients who live for long periods with the bladder exposed. Trauma to the bladder surface tends to irritate the epithelium and is painful.

Rectal prolapse is occasionally seen before the bladder is closed or if the closure fails. Poor support of the displaced levator muscle complex, along with the Valsalva effect of crying in these unhappy children, results in rectal prolapse in some. Reclosure of the bladder with osteotomy to provide better approximation of the pelvis and levator sling prevents further rectal prolapse.

Few renal anomalies occur in patients with bladder exstrophy or epispadias. Duplication of the ureter may occur (as it can in normal patients) and is of no consequence as long as it is recognized prior to closure. Because of the deepened peritoneal cul-de-sac beneath the bladder, the ureters course deeply within the bony pelvis to emerge through the bladder muscle with almost no submucosal tunnel. The result is vesicoureteral reflux in nearly all patients with classic bladder exstrophy.

The penis in boys with exstrophy is short. The separation of the pubic bones prevent the corpora cavernosa from joining at the mid-line at the usual position at the inferior margin of the pubic symphysis. The corporal bodies are shortened in absolute length as compared with normal children. Marked dorsal chordee with a shortened urethral plate is present. The corporal shortening seems to occur most dramatically in the corporal segment distal to its attachment to the inferior margin of the pubic ramus. These 2 observations suggest that closure of the pelvis may improve the cosmetic appearance of the penis, but that the penis is congenitally short, and will appear so in most cases, despite an excellent reconstructive effort.

The superficial neurovascular bundles are displaced laterally. The pudendal nerves innervating the corpora emerge from the sacral trunk (S2 through S4) and pass posterior to the pelvic floor muscles, medially to the ischial spines, and into the Alcock canal. A duplicate urethra has been reported, which may be incorporated into the epispadias repair. In most cases of epispadias, the urethral meatus is at the penopubic junction. A few children have incomplete degrees of epispadias with the urethral meatus partly or nearly completely out to the tip of the meatus. Some degree of dorsal chordee is almost universally present despite the severity of the epispadias.

A 10-fold higher-than-normal incidence of cryptorchidism has been reported in patients with exstrophy or epispadias. In our experience, many of these testes can be manipulated into the scrotum following the initial bladder closure. Prior to closure, the epididymis, vas deferens, ejaculatory ducts, and seminal vesicles are normal. This suggests that the undescended testis in bladder exstrophy is more anatomic (or mechanical) than endocrinologic in origin.

Females with bladder exstrophy have a hemiclitoris on each side. The vagina may be duplicated. The vaginal orifice is usually narrowed and displaced anteriorly, located just distal to the urethral plate. The uterus may be duplicated, but the fallopian tubes and ovaries are usually normal. Females with epispadias may have a bifid or 2 separate clitoral bodies. The mons pubis in exstrophy or epispadias is flattened.

The pubic diastasis that is present in all patients with the exstrophy–epispadias complex results in outward rotation of the hips. Despite the rotation, children and young adults have few hip or gait problems. The degree of external rotation of the hips is greater in patients with bladder exstrophy than in those with epispadias. In young children with bladder exstrophy, an abnormally externally directed foot progression angle (a "waddling" gait) has been noted, which seems to improve with age. Unlike in cloacal exstrophy, few spinal defects are noted.

## DIAGNOSTIC PRINCIPLES

Occasionally, the diagnosis of bladder exstrophy is made in utero. The sonographic absence of a normal bladder in association with an anterior abdominal mass and low-set umbilicus suggests bladder exstrophy, omphalocele, or gastroschisis. In some cases, the diagnosis can be made as early as 20 weeks gestation. In most cases, despite the potential for antenatal diagnosis, the family is not prepared to deal with what is a considerable surgical undertaking in the newborn period.

## TREATMENT OPTIONS

### Goals of Treatment

Today's bladder exstrophy reconstruction attempts to provide urinary continence while preserving renal function. In males, penile reconstruction must correct the dorsal chordee to allow vaginal penetration, and provide a urethral meatus that is distal enough to provide for micturition while the boy is standing without spraying. In females, the clitoral bodies should be reconstructed without injuring the nerve supply or the erectile tissue. In both sexes, the cosmetic appearance of the genitalia must be good.

The standard for excellence in bladder exstrophy reconstruction has evolved from many excellent centers. The staged approach of Jeff, modified by his successor, Gearhart through his team's experience with more than 1000 patients at Johns Hopkins has provided for micturition with continence for a large number of children without renal compromise. The Hopkins reconstruction stresses the importance of early-bladder closure with subsequent epispadias repair and, finally, bladder-neck reconstruction for continence.

Mitchell has described an approach that combines the bladder closure with the epispadias repair in the newborn. Mitchell believes the improved mobility of the bladder neck when the epispadias is corrected at the time of bladder closure aids in placement of the bladder neck and proximal urethra deep within the pelvis. In the hands of these excellent technicians, both the Hopkins and the Mitchell techniques have yielded good results. Both approaches stress the importance of a vigorous bladder-neck dissection designed to place the bladder, bladder neck, and proximal urethra deep within the levator complex in hopes of achieving urinary continence with voiding.

## PRIMARY BLADDER CLOSURE

Unless an osteotomy is used, the bladder is best closed within the first 24 to 48 hours. If the team plans an osteotomy, the closure, as mentioned above may be delayed as much as 3 months without harm as long as the exposed bladder is carefully managed. The infant should be transferred to a center where the closure is to be performed. The umbilicus should be ligated with a large suture ligature rather than the commonly used plastic clamp to reduce trauma to the bladder. The bladder is covered with a square of clear plastic wrap, or if available, a nonadherent hydrogel sheet dressing (Vigilon®—Bard Medical, Covington, GA). No gauze or salves are placed in contact with the bladder. A renal ultrasound should be performed to identify hydronephrosis or renal duplication.

### Staged Approach

Jeffs noted that the renal preservation and, ultimately, continence depended on achievement of adequate bladder volumes and normal micturition. Continence rates and bladder function with preserved renal function were consistently reported to be better in patients with epispadias when compared with patients with classic bladder exstrophy. The idea of Jeffs was to convert bladder exstrophy to complete epispadias with an initial bladder closure. Bladder-neck reconstruction was postponed until years later. This gave the bladder a chance to "cycle" without creating bladder outlet obstruction. Cendron pursued a similar approach.

### Osteotomy

In 1958, Shultz revisited the Trendelenburg idea of rotation of the innominate bones to reduce the pubic diastasis. He reported the use of a bilateral iliac osteotomy, followed 2 weeks later by bladder closure and approximation of the pubic symphysis in a female. The patients reportedly became continent within a week of removing the bladder catheter and remained so. Schultz believed that closer apposition of the pubic bones would better recreate the normal anatomy of the pelvic musculature. Better function of the urogenital diaphragm appeared to provide urinary continence in this one patient. The initial success of Schultz led to a strong advocacy for osteotomy. Lattimer and Chisholm each reported a large series of patients using osteotomy at the time of bladder closure. The bladder closure at this time was done with bladder-neck repair to provide continence. The long-term results in these series were discouraging, with low continence rates and upper-tract deterioration in many children.

The goal of osteotomy, of course, is to recreate a more normal configuration of the bony pelvis, which theoretically will provide for better levator function and better subsequent volitional control of the external urethral sphincter. As good as the theory is, in practice, 2 problems occur that somewhat reduce the benefit of the osteotomy. First, following osteotomy closure, there is considerable progressive separation of the pelvic bones over time because the bones of the infant do not stabilize well, regardless of the technique used to attach the pubic bones together. Second, in the newborn, the bones of the baby may be malleable enough to provide for good approximation of the pelvis without the need for osteotomy, thereby obviating the need for the additional surgery. Nevertheless, osteotomy is recommended in infants closed outside of 48 hours because the osteotomy seems to provide additional mobility of the pelvis, which helps secure a pubic closure with minimal morbidity, and a pubic symphyseal approximation, which may be more permanent.

Proponents of osteotomy suggest that improved continence rates can be expected following the bladder-neck reconstruction if osteotomy is used in the bladder closure. Patients closed after 48 hours without osteotomy seem to have had a more difficult time achieving continence after completing staged reconstruction. The routine use of osteotomy has contributed to many teams now closing the bladder exstrophy as a more elective procedure rather than in the first 48 hours.

## Bladder Closure

After the initial evaluation, which should have included a renal and bladder ultrasound to rule out hydronephrosis and ureteral duplication, the child is well hydrated with intravenous fluids. At least 6 to 8 hours of intravenous antibiotics, usually ampicillin and gentamycin, are given to assure adequate tissue levels of antibiotic prior to starting the bladder closure. The osteotomy is performed first, followed by the bladder closure. In the older child, the external fixation device is placed at the conclusion of the procedure, followed by the traction, which is used for 10 days to 4 weeks following the repair.

Prior to the osteotomy, the infant is prepared and draped to provide access to the entire infant inferior to the sternum anteriorly and inferior to the second lumbar vertebrae posteriorly. This preparation provides sterile access to the anterior and posterior surfaces, which will provide the opportunity for manipulation of the infant's thighs at the time that the pubic suture is tied.

Several osteotomy techniques have been used: posterior iliac osteotomy; anterior innominate osteotomy; a combination of posterior and inferior; and osteotomy through the superior or superior and inferior pubic rami (Fig. 67-3). Posterior iliac osteotomy was performed more frequently in the past. More recently, the anterior (Salter) approach has been used, which can be done through an anterior incision. After exposure of the sacral notch, the innominate bone is cut. Additional exposure of the anterior surface of the iliac bone may make it possible to incise the anterior table of the iliac bone which may provide additional mobility and a better pelvic closure. In patients older than 1 year of age, pins that will subsequently attach to an external fixator are placed. Attention is then turned to the bladder closure.

There are 2 approaches to the initial surgery for bladder exstrophy currently performed in North America: the traditional staged (Hopkins) approach and a newer combined approach that has been advocated by Mitchell. Both approaches have delivered excellent relative success rates. Both techniques will be described and the similarities and differences outlined.

In the Hopkins approach, following the osteotomy, the ureters are catheterized with small infant feeding tubes that will remain in place for 4 to 6 weeks following the bladder closure.

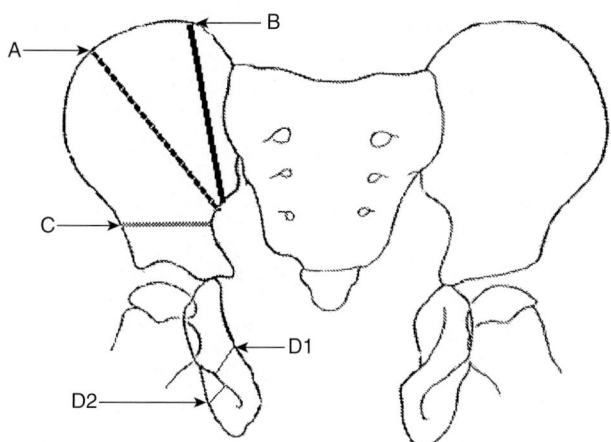

**FIGURE 67-3** Types of osteotomies. (A) Anterior diagonal iliac osteotomy (Wedge). (B) Posterior iliac osteotomy. (C) Anterior transverse (Salter) osteotomy; D1, Anterior pubic ramus osteotomy, superior ramus only (Frey); D1 and D2, Complete anterior pubic ramus osteotomy (Montagnani). (C, B): Combined anterior and posterior osteotomy. (Sponseller). (From McKenna P, et al. Iliac osteotomy: A model to compare the options in bladder and cloacal exstrophy reconstruction. *J Urol* 1994;151:182; and Gearhart JP, et al. A combined vertical and horizontal pelvic osteotomy approach for primary and secondary repair of bladder exstrophy. *J Urol* 1996;155:689.)

These small tubes are sewn in place with fine chromic suture. Effective drainage of the upper tracts may reduce the risk of bladder prolapse or dehiscence. An incision made along the lateral edge of the exposed urothelium extends from superior to the umbilicus to the base of the bladder. This incision removes the umbilicus (Fig. 67-4A). We prefer to remove the umbilicus because we think that the risk of infection if the umbilicus is moved superiorly rather than removed does not warrant the cosmetic benefit of leaving the umbilicus. We fashion a new umbilicus in a more normal position at the level of the anterior superior iliac crest. Creation of the umbilicus is postponed until the conclusion of the bladder closure.

Following the skin incision, the retroperitoneal space is entered superior to the umbilicus, and the bladder is widely mobilized from the rectus fascia. The peritoneum is separated from the posterior wall of the bladder and elevated to allow the bladder to drop deeper into the retroperitoneum. The dissection is carried inferior to the pubis. The fibromuscular attachments of the corporal bodies to the pubis bilaterally are dissected away from the bone in a subperiosteal plane taking care to prevent injury to the neurovascular bundle, which is lateral (Fig. 67-4B,C).

In the past, the next step was to divide the urethral plate distal to the prostate, separate the corporal bodies from the intercrural prostate, and deliver the bladder and prostatic urethra back into the pelvis, untethering it from the distal urethra and penis. To bridge the gap of the separation, paraexstrophy skin flaps were developed from the adjacent shiny skin and brought together on the midline (Fig. 67-4D,E). The distal flaps were sutured to the prostatic urethra and the bladder neck to widen the prostatic urethra. This assured a wide-open bladder neck when the bladder and the proximal urethra were closed. The paraexstrophy flaps were tubularized

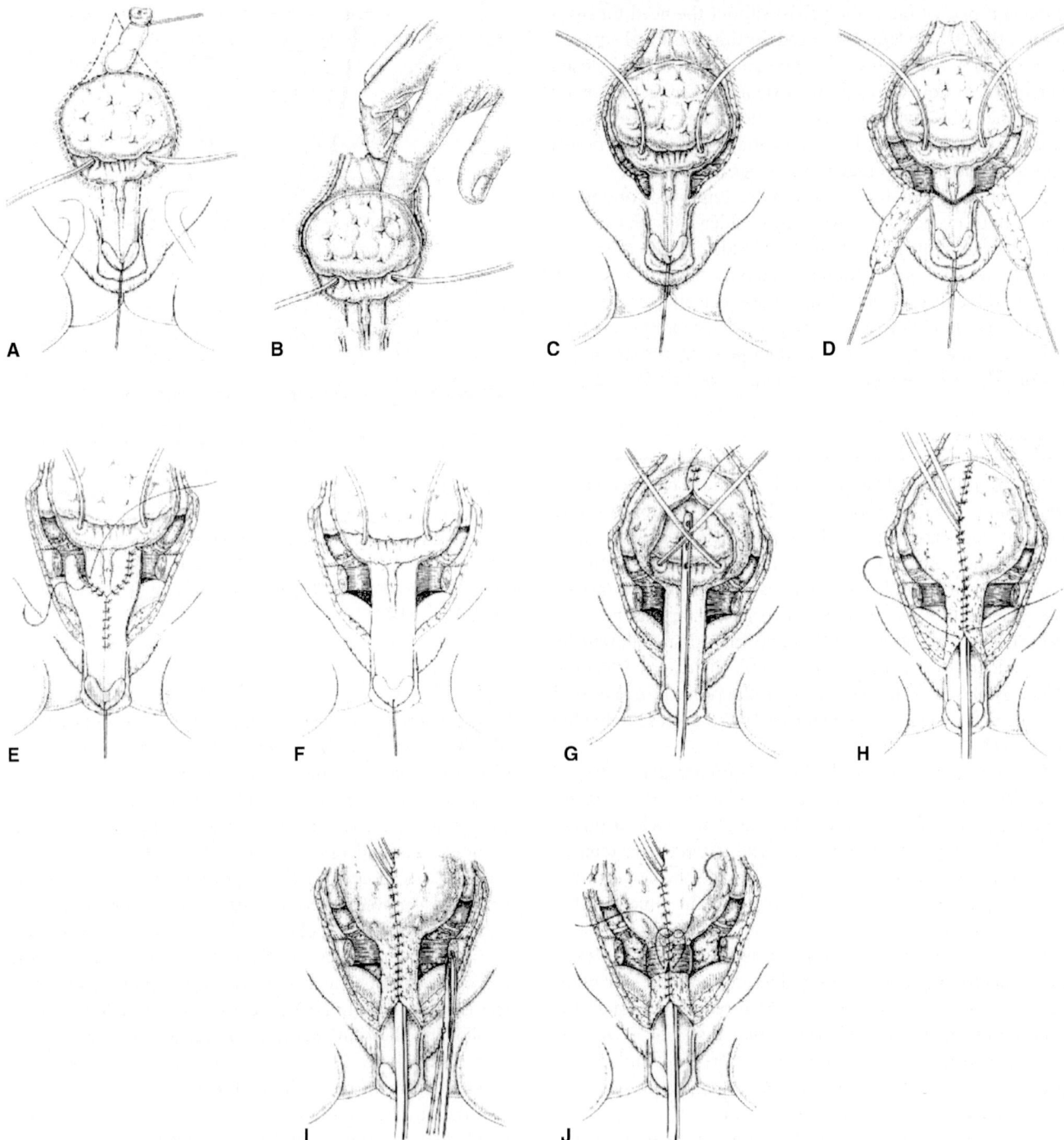

**FIGURE 67-4** Bladder closure. **A.** Incision. After placement of ureteral catheters, the umbilicus is removed and the incision is carried well distal to the verumontanum. Care is taken to prevent incorporation of the squamous tissue lateral to the bladder. **B.** The bladder is mobilized off of the peritoneum superiorly and inferolaterally. **C.** The dissection is carried inferior to the pubis. **D, E.** Paraexstrophy flaps can be used to import additional tissue to assure a wide-open bladder neck when the bladder and proximal urethra are closed. If flaps are used, they should be made no longer than a 3:1 length-to-width ratio. In practice, we rarely use flaps. **F.** The corporal bodies are freed from the urethra and the prostatic urethra is mobilized from the intersymphyseal band to allow the urethral and the bladder neck to recess posteriorly deep within the pelvis. In the Seattle (Mitchell) repair, this step is made much easier by the additional exposure provided by splitting the corpora, which allows an excellent view of the anterior and posterior aspects of the bladder neck and posterior urethra. The dissection of the corpora is designed to provide additional penile length and is taken to the inferior margin of the pubis but not beyond. **G, H.** The bladder is closed with 2 layers of PGA suture. In the Hopkins technique, the urethra is closed to the bladder neck only over a 12 French sound. No stents are placed through the urethra. In the Mitchell repair, the male urethra is closed to the level of the glans penis and the corpora are reapproximated dorsal to the urethra, replacing the urethra to a normal ventral anatomic position. The female urethra in the Mitchell technique is closed without mobilizing it from the surface of the vagina. The urethra and the vagina are then advanced posteriorly as a unit with a "Y" to "V" closure. **I, J.** The tissue inferolateral to the pubic arch is freed further (and the urethral incision extended) to allow more posterior displacement into the pelvis. Closure of the intrasymphyseal tissue over the urethra as depicted in J is not always possible, and probably not necessary as long as the lateral dissection is adequate enough to allow posterior displacement. PGA; polyglycolic acid. (From Ransley PG, Duffy PG. Bladder exstrophy closure and epispadias repair. In: Spitz L, Coran AG, eds. *Rob and Smith's Operative Surgery: Pediatric Surgery.* 5th ed. London: Chapman and Hall; 1995. Used with permission.)

as a urethral extension distally to the abdominal wall closure when the bladder and proximal urethra were closed. Penile lengthening was accomplished by incising the anterior attachments of the corporal bodies to the pubis. The distal epispadias remained for later reconstruction.

Since the advent of the Cantwell Ransley epispadias repair, and the Mitchell single-stage bladder closure, the need for urethral lengthening during the initial bladder closure is less clear. In the event that the urethra does not reach the glans following placement of the bladder neck into the space between the levator muscles in the pelvic diaphragm, the urethra can be brought to the penoscrotal junction for subsequent hypospadias repair.

We have been impressed that the urethra, particularly the anterior urethra in bladder exstrophy or epispadias, is expansible and when completely detached from the corporal bodies, will allow the bladder neck to drop posteriorly *and allow the urethra to reach the glans*. This observation, made independently by both Mitchell and Ransley, has simplified the bladder-neck reconstruction and may result in fewer urethral strictures and better bladder cycling during the initial period following bladder closure. The "bladder cycling," natural cyclic filling and emptying of the bladder that is provided by the additional resistance at the bladder neck may stimulate bladder growth early in the first months. The additional bladder volume may result in improved compliance and continence later.

It has been surmised that the intersymphyseal band of tissue that traverses the bladder neck area has in it the rudimentary urogenital diaphragm (external sphincter) muscle complex. Therefore, lateral dissection frees this band from the pubis; a wraparound of the bladder neck is often depicted in the diagrams (Fig. 67-4I,J). In execution, however, this may neither be so clear-cut nor physiologically sound. Dissection inferolateral to the pubic arch will free the levators for more posterior displacement into the pelvis when the prostatic urethra is released from its intercrural position. This posterior displacement of the bladder neck and posterior urethra that is accomplished with extensive inferolateral dissection is essential to a successful closure. Following mobilization of the urethral plate, the bladder and proximal urethra are closed in 2 layers with absorbable suture. The bladder is closed with a vertical suture line in an attempt to draw the bladder dome superiorly and thereby minimize risk of prolapse through the bladder neck after closure. The bladder neck is closed to a 12 French diameter tube. This size is wide enough to provide good drainage, but is small enough to prevent bladder prolapse.

## Complete Anatomic Closure

The complete newborn anatomic repair by Mitchell treats the bladder, bladder neck, and urethra as a single unit. The concept is to treat the exstrophic defect as a hernia and therefore to close the bladder and the urethra by delivering the entire defect posteriorly. To do this, the Mitchell repair disassembles the penis into its 3 components, allowing access to the intersymphyseal ligament. The urethra is dissected away from the separate corporal bodies, which allows the bladder neck and prostatic urethra to drop posteriorly as the corpora

are rotated superiorly over the closed urethra (Fig. 67-5A–I). In females, the urethra and the vagina are treated as a unit and are often moved further posteriorly with a "Y-V" posterior advancement. The bladder closure and superior dissection are as described above. The ureteral stents are taken through the urethral closure to act as a urethral splint and are removed at 10 to 14 days.

The Seattle group performed this operative correction on 29 patients from the years 1989 to 2002. They achieved continence, which they defined as maintaining a dry interval for longer than 2 hours and being able to void spontaneously without catheterization, in 76% of these patients. Prior to 1989, 27% of patients undergoing exstrophy repairs would require augmentation, but only 3% of the 29 patients repaired with the Mitchell approach need augmentation. It is thought that the Mitchell repair properly positions the bladder neck in the pelvis with the pelvic urethra within the diaphragm, thereby allowing the bladder to cycle earlier.

## Herniorrhaphy

Because the abdominal muscles are displaced laterally in boys and girls with bladder exstrophy, the external inguinal ring tends to lie just anterior to the internal inguinal ring. This anatomic relationship results in an increased incidence of inguinal hernia, with a pronounced risk of incarceration. In 1 study, 56% of boys and 15% of girls developed inguinal hernias over a follow-up period of 10 years. Forty-six percent of the boys presented with incarceration requiring emergent management. Another retrospective review of 70 consecutive patients with bladder exstrophy noted that 42 (86%) boys and 3 (15%) girls developed inguinal hernias, which were bilateral in 78% of the cases. No recurrence following correction occurred in females, whereas 17% of boys developed a recurrence. Although a hernia is rarely noted prior to closure, we recommend closure of the patent processus vaginalis on each side at the time of the initial closure. A preperitoneal approach through the abdominal incision is usually possible, and obviates a second abdominal incision. If the testis appears tethered, orchiopexy can be done as well.

## Umbilicoplasty

Because the umbilicus is usually removed in the initial closure of bladder exstrophy, a cosmetic umbilicus must be constructed. This is usually done at the time of the initial closure. Various types of umbilicoplasties have been described. We prefer creation of a circular flap surrounding the suprapubic tube. The edges of the medial aspect of this flap are sewn to the fascia to provide a dimpled appearance. The suprapubic tube is taken through the new umbilicus. Alternatively, no umbilicus is created at the time of the initial closure deferring the umbilicoplasty to the time of the hypospadias repair if necessary.

## Pelvic Immobilization

After bladder and urethral closure in the newborn, an assistant manually rotates the greater trochanter on each side to approximate the pubic bones. A heavy nylon or PDS/Vicryl

835

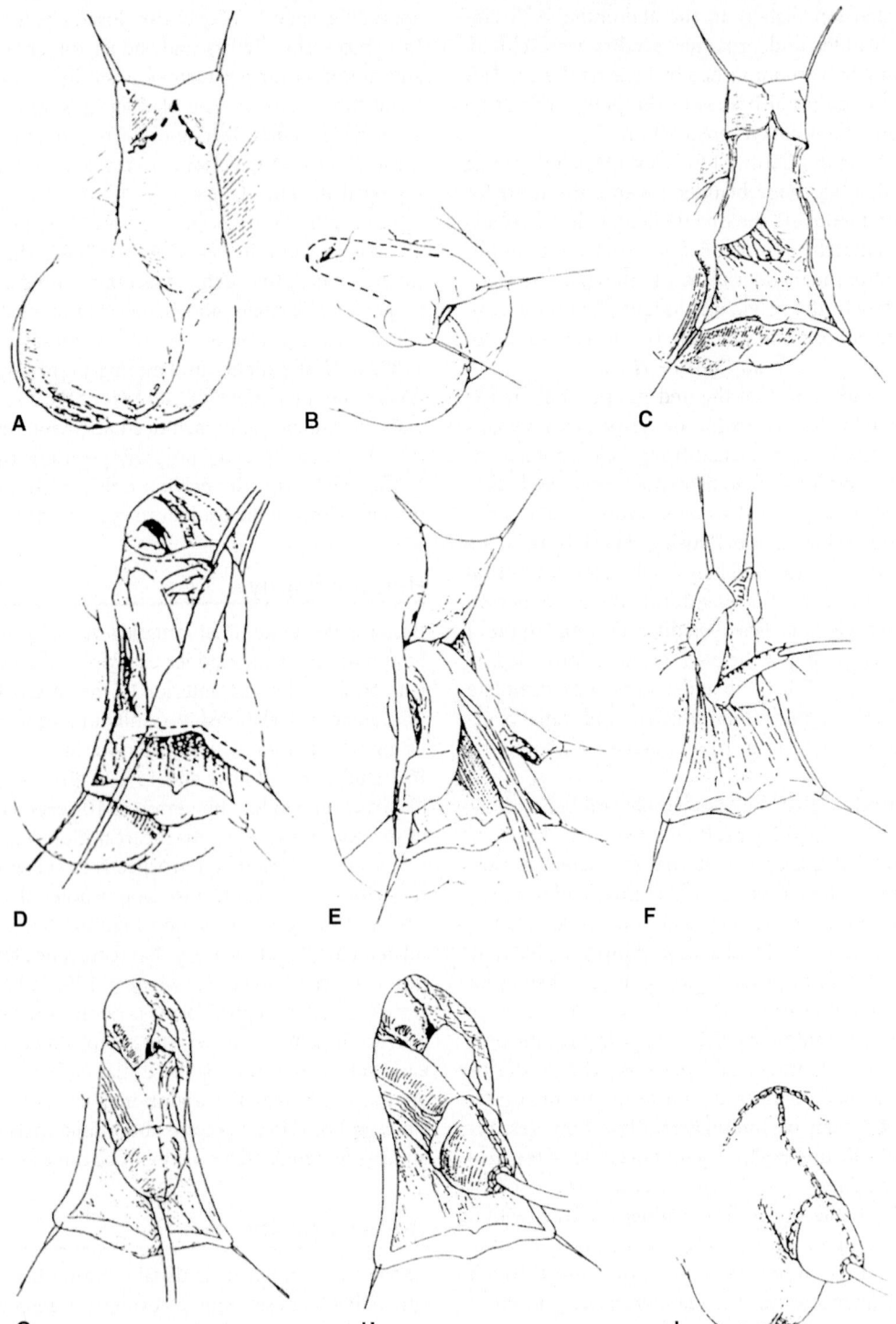

**FIGURE 67-5** The Mitchell epispadias repair. **A.** Traction sutures are placed into each hemiglans, oriented horizontally. These stay sutures will become vertical in orientation following later corporal rotation. **B.** A circumcising incision is made ventrally and the urethral plate is outlined dorsally to allow later tubularization. **C.** The remainder of the penile shaft skin is dissected off the lateral and ventral aspects of the paired corporal bodies. The neurovascular bundles, which are found on the lateral face of each corpora, should be carefully avoided during the degloving of the shaft skin. **D.** The urethra is then dissected off the corporal bodies. **E.** The entire urethra, based on its proximal blood supply, is lifted off of the glans and corporal bodies. The 2 corporal bodies, each with the respective hemiglans attached, are separated completely on the midline. The glans is divided into 2 halves, each supplied by the vessels of the paired lateral neurovascular bundles. **F.** The urethra is closed and positioned ventral to the entire length of the corporal bodies. **G.** The corpora are freely rotated to correct dorsal chordee. **H.** The corpora cavernosa are sutured together with fine absorbable suture on the dorsum. The urethra is positioned in the ventral groove between the corpora cavernosa and sutured to each glans. If the closed urethra is too short, it can be matured to the ventral aspect of the penis to form a hypospadiac urethral meatus, which can be subsequently corrected. **I.** Final appearance after skin closure. (From Mitchell ME, Bagli DJ. Complete penile disassembly for epispadias repair: Mitchell technique. *J Urol* 1996;155:300–304. Used with permission.)

suture is placed, tied with the knot anterior to prevent erosion into the urethra. The rectus muscles are brought together with fascial sutures for a solid abdominal wall closure. The urethral meatus opens at the base of the epispadias in the Hopkins staged approach, along the ventral shaft of the penis, or at the tip of the glans in the Mitchell approach.

In infants, the Hopkins team advocates a modified Bryant traction, which seeks to lift the buttocks just off the bed with minimal applied weight. At Hopkins, this traction is maintained for 4 weeks in infants and up to 6 weeks in older children. In patients older than 1 year, the iliac and innominate bones have matured sufficiently to allow for placement of pins and an external fixation device is used to stabilize the closure. If an external fixator is used, care must be taken to prevent overzealous compression on the device. Usually, light tension is used which is gradually increased over the first 2 weeks postoperatively. Too much medial rotation initially results in tension on the sciatic nerve with resulting transient weakness or reflex-induced vasoconstriction and hypertension.

Mitchell also uses the Bryant traction, but only for 2 to 3 days and then has patients placed in an exstrophy splint, which will maintain adduction of the hips. Spica cast immobilization is also used for 3 weeks.

The suprapubic tube and the ureteral catheters are maintained during the period of traction. If the one-stage (Mitchell) technique is used, the ureteral catheters are taken through the reconstructed urethra and maintained for 7 to 10 days. Prior to removal of the suprapubic tube, patency of the urethra is assessed by measuring residual urine in the bladder. If the bladder fails to drain at low pressure, the outlet may be gently dilated under sedation.

## Incontinent Period

For the 3 to 5 years following bladder closure, the bladder gradually increases capacity awaiting bladder-neck reconstruction. During this period the bladder must not be permitted to develop high pressures. High-pressure bladder emptying results in 3 problems: urinary tract infection, upper tract deterioration, and loss of bladder compliance. Enthusiasts of the 1-stage anatomic closure think that the increased visibility of the bladder neck at the time of the initial closure provides for better reconstruction of the continence mechanism at a time when bladder cycling is essential for detrusor development, which is essential to subsequent continence. Both the Jeffs staged approach and the Mitchell repair rely on the early cycling and "accommodation" of bladder volume over the first few years to allow for a compliant bladder at the time of the continence surgery. Additionally, the size of the bladder template at birth will affect continence rate.

Bladder and renal ultrasound are obtained frequently during the first year following closure. If hydronephrosis or urinary tract infections occur during the incontinent period, the outlet should be dilated or intermittent catheterization should be initiated. Because all patients with exstrophy have vesicoureteral reflux, urinary tract infection, if it occurs after bladder closure, will usually result in renal scarring, particularly if the bladder pressure is high.

In several studies (Perlmutter et al, Mollard et al, McMahon et al, Lottman et al, Purves et al) continence rate is on average 70%. The fewer attempts at closure the better. Novak et al showed that if a patient had 2 repairs there was only a 60% chance the patient would have adequate bladder capacity for a bladder neck repair and only 17 % would be continent.

## Other Epispadias Repairs

Before the bladder-neck plasty is performed in the staged repair, the bladder should have volume in excess of 70 to 90 cc. Epispadias repair may increase the outlet pressure slightly in cases where the bladder volume remains small following bladder closure. Many North American programs have adopted the 1-stage anatomic (Mitchell) repair, which corrects the epispadias at the time of the original closure. Others continue with the *Cantwell–Ransley epispadias repair,* which is described next. This approach spawned the Mitchell repair and remains the gold standard for long-term results.

The epispadias repair should lengthen and straighten the penis to a dependent position and should provide a urethra adequate for normal voiding and for easy catheter passage. Several different techniques have been described to correct epispadias. Because penile lengthening (separation of the corporal attachments to the pubic rami) often is performed during the initial bladder closure, a dorsal tubularization of the urethral plate or a modification of the Young urethroplasty is adequate, in some cases. In most cases, however, the urethra is still ventral after the initial penile lengthening and a modification of the Cantwell–Ransley repair is a better choice. The ability to detach the urethra from the corporal bodies without disruption of the urethral plate to allow the urethra to drop ventrally may result in lower fistula rates in epispadias.

## Cantwell–Ransley Epispadias Repair

After placement of glans-holding sutures, a Heineke–Mikulicz advancement of the urethral plate is performed at the tip of the spade-like glans to advance the new meatus to a more ventral position. The urethral plate is then outlined and incised after a circumcising incision is carried around the shaft of the penis and the penis is degloved of shaft and ventral foreskin. Beginning in the middle of the ventrum of the penis, a plane is developed between the corporal bodies and the urethra. This plane is carried dorsally and ventrally from the middle of the penis proximally to the pyramid of the prostatic bed and distally to the glans tissue. This dissection effectively separates the paired corporal bodies from the urethra from prostate to the glans (Fig. 67-6A,B). Glanular wedges are excised to facilitate approximation of glans wings over the tubularized glanular urethra. The urethra is closed over a soft silastic tube. Fine interrupted PGA sutures are used.

Separate tourniquets are placed on each corpus and separate injections with saline are made to determine the concavity of the location of maximal curvature. The corporal bodies will be rotated medially to a dorsal position that will correct most or all of the curvature. In some cases, transverse incision into each tunica albuginea to the point of maximal bend will be needed to further lengthen the corpora. These incisions are converted to diamond-shaped defects (Fig. 67-6C).

When these 2 diamonds are approximated with dorsomedial rotation, the curvature will be greatly improved and a dependent penis will result. This also places the urethra beneath the corporal and neurovascular bundles at the dorsal midline (Fig. 67-6D). The ventral prepuce may then be used to form an island flap for dorsal skin coverage (Fig. 67-6E).

Baird et al (2005) followed 129 patients that underwent the Cantwell–Ransley Repair. In the immediate postoperative period 16% developed a urethrocutaneous fistula. Nine patients developed urethral stricture. Twelve patients had minor skin separation of the dorsal skin closure and eight patients required penile straightening surgery.

## Continence Surgery: Bladder-Neck Reconstruction

Reconstruction of the open bladder neck is necessary in the staged reconstruction of bladder exstrophy. A few patients may develop continence following the Mitchell repair without additional surgery. The continence surgery endeavors to provide voluntary voiding with day and nighttime continence without jeopardizing renal function. Before undertaking continence surgery, the child must be motivated to be dry and old enough to cooperate with both parents and physicians. Considerable time and effort are required to train the child to recognize the feeling of a full bladder and to faithfully urinate when the bladder feels full. The family must be committed to a period of training, during which frequent telephone calls and occasional office visits to the medical center, monitoring with urinalysis, intermittent catheterization, and periodic cystoscopy may be necessary.

Several factors need to be considered prior to planning the bladder-neck reconstruction: bladder size, presence of chronic infection, renal scarring or hydronephrosis, and severity of pubic diastasis. In some cases, if the bladder volume is small or if the bladder is thick-walled and poorly compliant, augmentation with construction of a Mitrofanoff stoma may be in the child's best interest.

If the bladder size is sufficient, if the kidneys are not hydronephrotic or scarred, and if the pubis is well approximated, bladder-neck reconstruction without augmentation is appropriate. If the pubis is still markedly widened, repeat osteotomy may be helpful to place the urethra within the pelvic ring and to achieve voluntary control of urination. Many believe that urethral support from the striated muscles of the urogenital diaphragm and bladder-neck suspension results in better continence rates. An effective osteotomy is felt to optimize this advantage. Although many procedures to increase outlet resistance have been described, the two described here seem to be the most straightforward and effective in our hands: the Young–Dees Leadbetter–Jeffs procedure and the Mitchell procedure.

## Young–Dees–Leadbetter–Jeffs–Gearhart Procedure

The bladder is opened through a low, transverse incision placed near the bladder neck with a vertical extension. The urethral orifices are identified and stents are placed. In the past, a cross-trigonal reimplantation procedure was used. More recently, the reimplanted ureters have been directed in a cephalad direction with success. The new reimplant allows

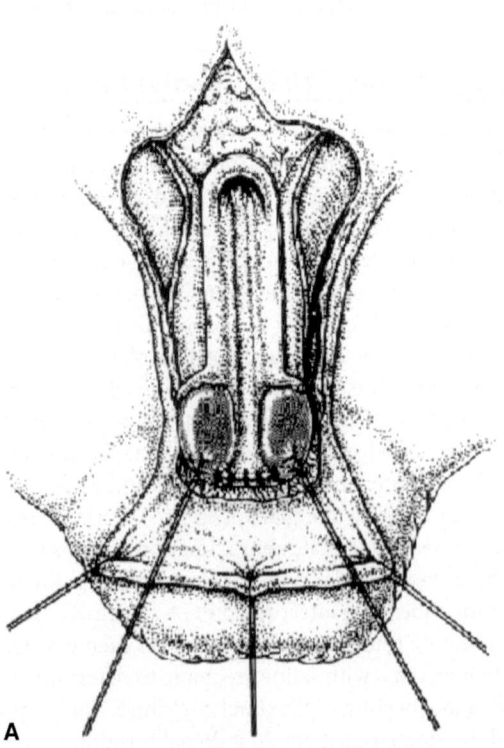
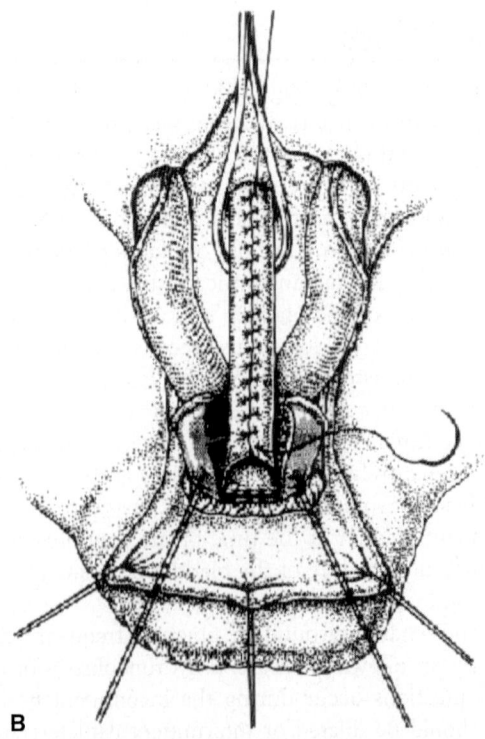

**A**  **B**

**FIGURE 67-6** Cantwell–Ransley epispadias repair. **A.** Glans-holding sutures have been placed and the Heineke–Mikulicz advancement has been performed to move the urethral meatus ventrally. The urethral strip has been mobilized and the penile shaft skin has been separated from the corpora. **B.** Careful dissection separates the urethral plate from the corporal bodies. The dissection extends from prostatic to glanular urethra. Glanular wedges facilitate approximation of glans wings over the tubularized glanular urethra.

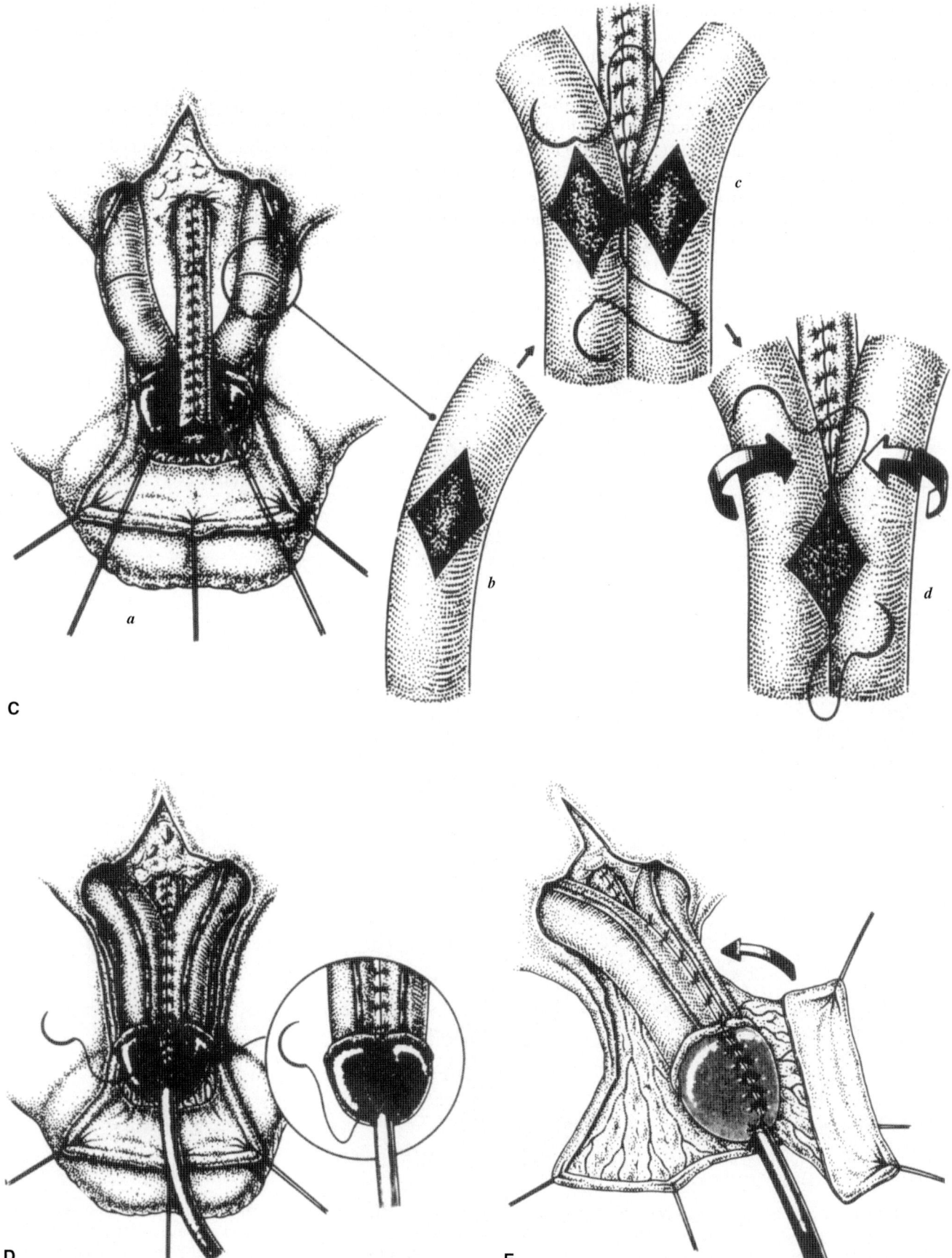

**FIGURE 67-6** *(Continued)* **C.** If necessary to correct corporal curvature, dorsal incision at the point of maximal curvature are made. These are joined as the corpora are rotated. **D.** A series of interrupted sutures approximates the corpora. The glans is brought together in layers. **E.** The inner prepuce is isolated on a vascular pedicle and brought to the dorsum for skin coverage. The ventrum is covered with the outer prepuce. (From Snyder HM III. The surgery of bladder exstrophy and epispadias. In: Frank JD, Johnston JH, eds. *Operative Pediatric Urology*. Edinburgh, Churchill-Livingstone; 1990:214–217. Used with permission.)

a greater proportion of the trigone to be safely incorporated into the bladder neck repair (Fig. 67-7A–C). The Young–Dees portion of the bladder-neck plasty is created after the reimplantation is completed. A 30 × 14-mm wide strip is outlined in the posterior urethra and into the trigone. This strip begins at the penile urethra and extends superior to the trigone. After a solution of epinephrine (1:100,000) is injected beneath the mucosa, the epithelium is removed adjacent to the strip. The detrusor is notched in a series of Z-plasties to lengthen the bladder neck with minimal reduction of bladder volume (Fig. 67-7D–F). The strip is rolled into a tube over an

8-French stent. The deepithelialized detrusor is closed over the tube in a double-breasted fashion to provide 3 functional layers (Fig. 67-7G–M).

## The Mitchell Modified Bladder-Neck Plasty

The team of Mitchell has substantially modified the bladder-neck repair. The distal margin of the dilated prostatic urethra is incised transversely as in the Young–Dees–Leadbetter–Jeffs procedure. Instead of extending the transverse incision vertically, a "V" flap of bladder neck is incised anteriorly leaving a

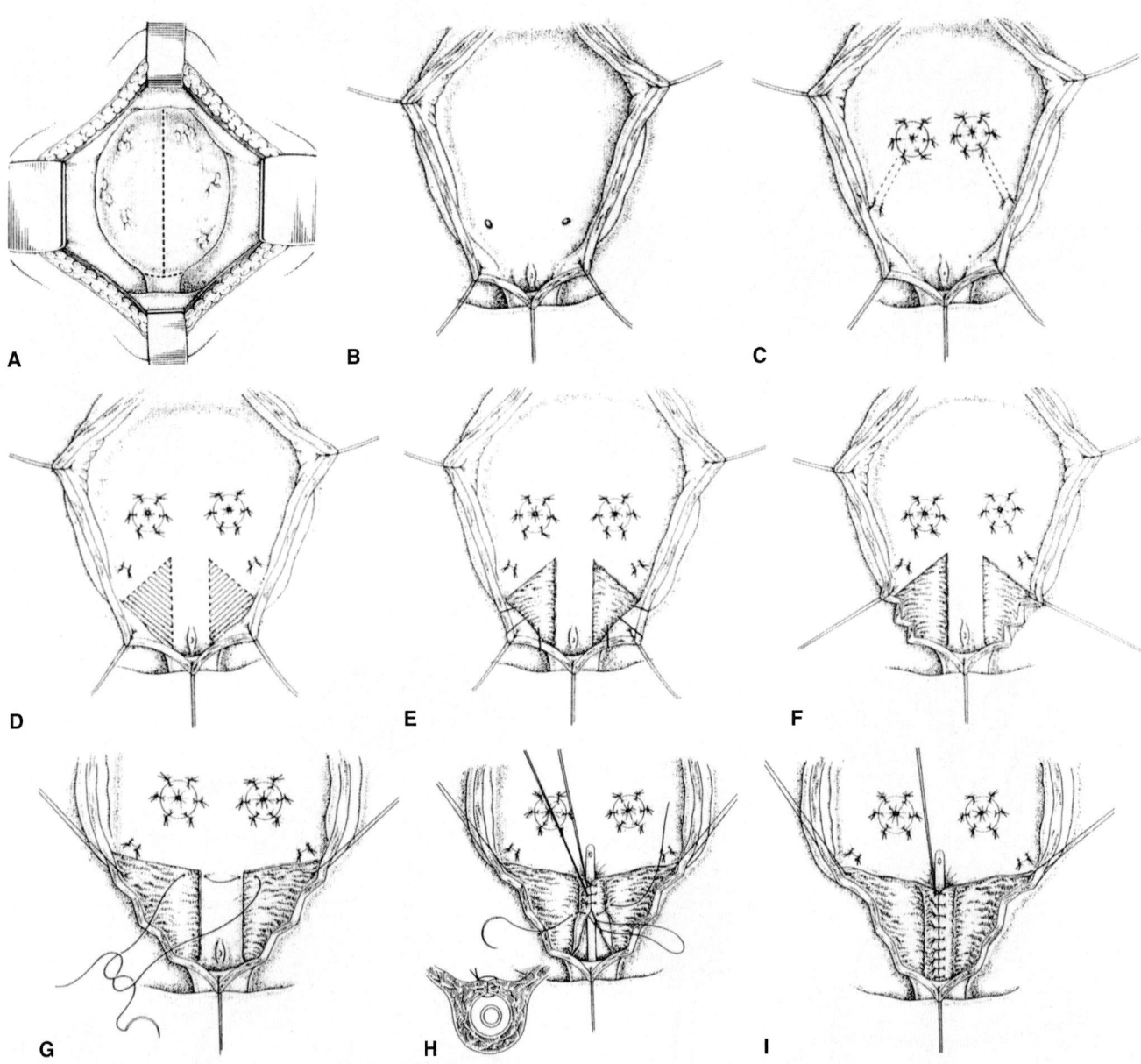

**FIGURE 67-7** The Young–Dees–Leadbetter–Jeffs bladder-neck reconstruction. **A.** After mobilization of the bladder neck and proximal urethra, a low transverse incision is extended vertically exposing the ureteral orifices and the entire trigone and proximal urethra. **B.** The bladder muscle lateral to the mucosal strip is denuded by sharp dissection. **C.** Ureteral reimplantation is performed using either a cross-trigonal technique or a cephalotrigonal technique to provide additional trigonal tissue for the repair. **D.** A strip of mucosa approximately 15 to 20 mm in width by 30 mm in length that extends from the midtrigone to the prostatic urethra is outlined. **E, F.** Multiple small incisions into the bladder muscle in the area of the denuded lateral triangles allow lengthening of the bladder neck area and allow the bladder to retract into a more cephalad position. **G, H.** The bladder neck is closed, beginning with a suture that incorporates detrusor muscle and urothelium. Each suture is placed on traction to draw up more of the strip to allow for easier subsequent placement of the more distal sutures. **I.** The completed mucosal layer of the repair.

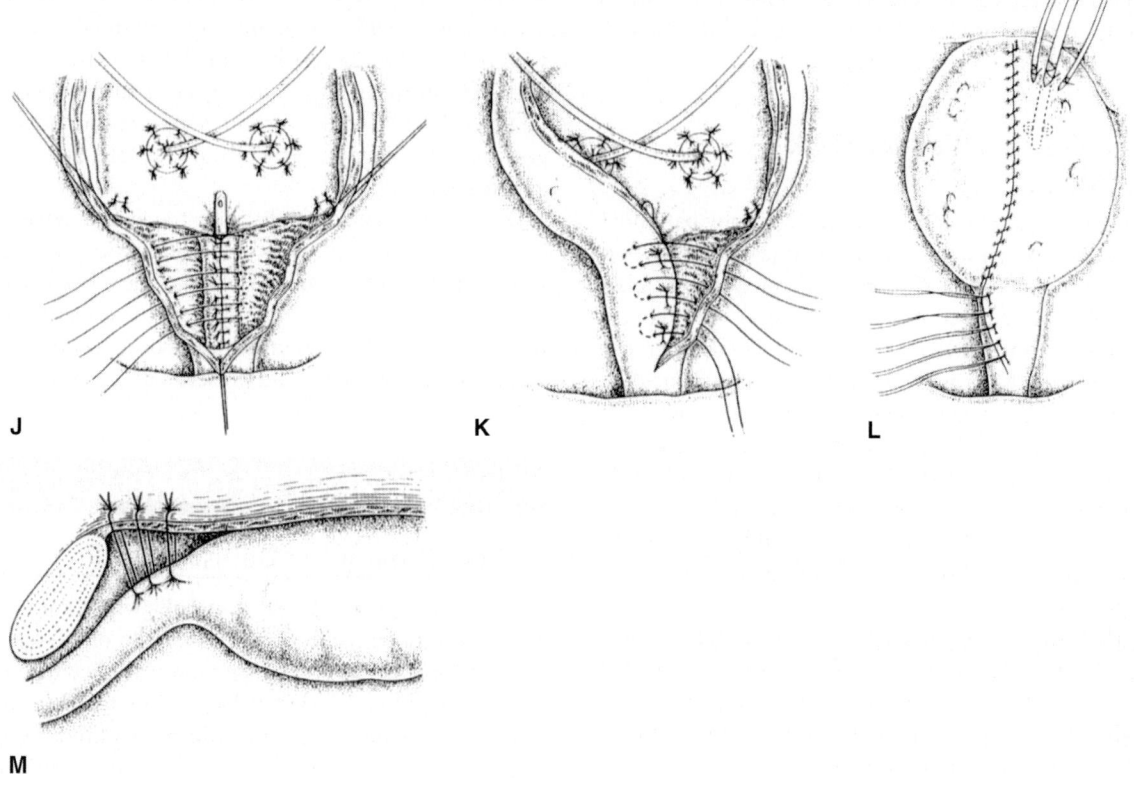

**FIGURE 67-7** *(Continued)* **J.** Ureteral stents, which will be left for 10 to 14 days, are placed and sutured. The first layer of the double-breasted bladder-neck plasty is placed. **K.** The second layer of horizontal mattress sutures is placed. **L.** The bladder is closed after placement of a suprapubic catheter, which will remain in place for 3 weeks. **M.** The outer layer of the vest-over-pants repair is brought anteriorly as a Marshall–Marchetti–Krantz bladder-neck suspension. (From Gearhart JP. Bladder neck reconstruction in the incontinent child. In: Frank J, Johnston JH, eds. *Operative Paediatric Urology.* Edinburgh: Churchill Livingstone; 1990:228–231. Used with permission.)

strip of urethra and bladder neck posteriorly, approximately 15-mm wide. After ureteral reimplantation, the urethra, bladder neck, and trigone are tubularized over an 8 to 10-French stent for a distance of 3 to 4 cm while the anterior bladder is closed vertically. The point of the V ends at the superior extent of the closure. In this way, the bladder neck is narrowed without loss of bladder volume. This repair does not buttress the bladder neck area with extra layers of deepithelialized detrusor. Mitchell does not add the Marshall–Marchetti–Kranz fixation to the abdominal wall.

## Outcomes of Reconstruction Stages

### Results Following Bladder Closure

Although the bladder is closed successfully in most patients, dehiscence, stone formation, and hydronephrosis requiring urethral dilatation or vesicostomy can occur. Of 75 patients completing staged repair, some for the second time at Johns Hopkins Hospital, 52 had a successful closure. Sixteen (21.3%) developed a major complication, such as prolapse, dehiscence, or hydronephrosis, and required a repeat closure. Seven had minor complications such as bladder stone, pubic suture infection, or squamous metaplasia along the suture line at the dome of the closed bladder. At CHOP, of 48 patients closed with the staged repair, there were no complications in 32 (67%). Five patients suffered a dehiscence

and 8 patients had bladder-outlet obstruction. Five patients developed bladder stones, which may have been a result of poor bladder emptying. Unfortunately, few patients who fail the initial bladder closure go on to develop continence. Since adopting osteotomy for all children, we have had no dehiscences at CHOP with the complete repair.

### Results Following the Epispadias Repair

In 1 series from the Mayo Clinic, 2 groups of patients were followed into adulthood following epispadias repair. One group included 44 patients with classic bladder exstrophy. Another group of 42 patients had complete epispadias. Fifty-five percent of the exstrophy patients had a straight penis as compared with 67% of the epispadias patients. In another series of 18 boys with exstrophy who had completed epispadias repair, the flaccid penis was directed horizontally or downward in all but three. Recent results with the Cantwell Ransley repair and with the Mitchell repair are even better.

Despite extensive dissection during epispadias repair, most patients are potent following reconstruction of the penis. Unfortunately, a large number of patients in most series have difficulty with ejaculation and ejaculate very small volumes or not at all. This may be caused by extensive dissection at the level of the bladder neck in the initial closure. Better ejaculatory function was reported in diverted patients in the Mayo Clinic series. In their group of 53 patients, 25 older patients

BLADDER EXSTROPHY

841

who had been diverted to a ureterosigmoidostomy could be evaluated for ejaculatory function; 16 of these had antegrade ejaculation and 9 were anejaculatory.

## Results Following Bladder-Neck Reconstruction

Despite major advances, continence in exstrophy patients is far from perfect. Even in centers with large exstrophy populations, fewer than 50% of all patients operated for bladder exstrophy are truly continent, defined as voiding with day and night continence. In most centers, the percentage is even lower. Most patients require intermittent catheterization or bladder augmentation with bowel to achieve suitable dry intervals. Of 45 patients who had closure and continence procedures at the Children's Hospital of Philadelphia (excluding those patients who had undergone urinary diversion), only 13 (29%) have a suitable (3-hour) dry interval and only 7 (16%) are truly continent with day and night dryness.

The early results of Mitchell are very encouraging following the primary anatomic closure. Of 16 infants with bladder exstrophy closed with the complete primary repair at birth, 10 have dry intervals of greater than 2 hours. Only 1 patient required a subsequent bladder-neck plasty.

Mouriquand and colleagues (2003) followed 80 children with bladder exstrophy who underwent Young–Dees–Leadbetter–Jeffs bladder neck repairs. Forty-five percent of these patients had a dry interval longer than 3 hours. Lottman and colleagues (1998) followed 57 patients for an average follow-up of 12 years. Seventy-one percent of the male patients and 53% of the female patients were continent. As previously noted, the bladder capacity at the time of the reconstruction is directly correlated with achievement of continence.

The difficulty achieving continence is related to the importance of a near-perfect bladder closure as a newborn in order to stimulate bladder growth without compromising compliance. Too much bladder-outlet resistance will result in poor emptying and increased bladder muscle stiffness, as well as urinary tract infection. The combination of urinary infection and high bladder pressures can be devastating to the infant kidney.

Identifying factors that correlate with success from retrospective reviews is difficult. Nevertheless, two observations seem worthy of mention. First, patients who had a successful initial bladder closure more frequently became continent following bladder-neck reconstruction than did patients who required a second bladder closure. Only 7 of 18 (39%) patients who failed initial closure were dry for more than 3 hours after completing reconstruction, as compared with 43 of 57 (75%) patients who had successful initial closure. This suggests that an early, successful closure may begin to stimulate bladder growth so that capacity is maximized and bladder wall fibrosis is minimized, leading to better compliance at the time of the bladder-neck plasty.

Second, even though bilateral iliac osteotomy has not been proven to reduce dehiscence rates at the time of the initial closure, it does seem to contribute to continence in patients closed later than the first 72 hours of life. In the same study,

49 of 67 (73%) who underwent closure before 72 hours of age or closure with osteotomy were continent, as compared with only 2 of 8 (25%) who had closure without osteotomy after 72 hours of age. The study by Husmann from the Hospital for Sick Children in Toronto supports this and even suggests no advantage to early closure, as long as osteotomy is performed.

Despite reasonable results with the staged repair at some centers, in most centers overall continence rates following reconstruction of the native bladder have been depressing. This has resulted in a turn away from the staged approach to one relying mainly on augmentation or diversion as a means of achieving continence and preserving renal function.

## MANAGEMENT OF COMPLICATIONS

### Bladder Prolapse or Dehiscence

Once bladder prolapse begins, usually with a minor appearance of urothelium at the inferior margin of the repair, complete dehiscence is a near certainty. A second attempt at closure should be delayed at least 6 months. A formal osteotomy using external fixation will be required. Even with a successful second closure, continence without augmentation is rare. In 38 patients referred to Johns Hopkins Hospital with a failed bladder closure, no patient developed bladder capacities enabling the patient to void on his or her own.

### Complications of the Epispadias Repair

Even with today's superior suture material and improved approaches to reconstruction, urethral strictures and urethrocutaneous fistulas are still common following epispadias repairs. Most of the small fistulas can be closed with a second procedure with good results. There are still a few patients, however, who will require extensive reconstruction or replacement of the urethra. In the past, urethral replacement with ureter has been used, as well as full-thickness skin grafts and bladder mucosal grafts. Unfortunately, few patients can donate a segment of ureter; and full-thickness skin grafts and bladder mucosal grafts have not been effective in long-term follow-up. Our free graft of choice today is buccal mucosa. Buccal mucosa is easy to harvest and seems to take more readily than bladder mucosa or split-thickness skin flaps.

### Small Capacity Bladder/Failed Bladder-Neck Plasty

Despite successful bladder closure, a group of patients will fail to gain suitable bladder capacity for bladder-neck reconstruction. If epispadias repair has not yet been performed, urethroplasty may add enough passive resistance to the urinary outlet to increase bladder capacity further. In many cases, even with adequate bladder volumes prior to bladder-neck plasty, acceptable postoperative continence does not occur. If these patients undergo another bladder-neck plasty, the success rate is no better than 35% for the restoration of urinary continence.

The decision to proceed with repeat bladder-neck plasty should be individualized. Many exstrophy patients do not seem to initiate a good detrusor contraction after bladder-neck repair. At the Great Ormond Street Hospital in London, Hollowell and coworkers studied the 21 non-augmented patients and found only 6 (28.6%) who could initiate a sustained detrusor contraction for voiding. These data are dissimilar to the Hopkins experience where a significant number of patients (57%) void. The reasons why remain elusive, but they probably relate to a combination of difficulty with primary closure, subsequent accommodation, and problems following the bladder-neck plasty rather than with intrinsic problems with the detrusor or innervation of the exstrophic bladder. As we improve our surgical procedures, continence rates should improve.

Nearly all patients can be made dry by augmentation of the bladder coupled with the initiation of intermittent catheterization. Large series from several centers report more than 90% of the patients dry. Procedures employing the Mitrofanoff principle provide consistent, durable dryness and are the preferred approach. If the appendix is not available, a tapered or reconfigured segment of small or large bowel can be used in its place.

In some cases, there is so little bladder available that a complete urinary pouch from bowel is better than trying to preserve the small bladder. Many combinations of small- and large-bowel configurations have been used in the creation of the pouch. Stomach segments have been used alone or in combination with other bowel segments to help maintain better electrolyte balance and to reduce the risk of chronic urinary tract infection and stone formation. In this case, the small native bladder is left in place for seminal secretions in the male.

Bladder stones occur in all types of reservoirs, especially those infected with *Proteus mirabilis*. Patients with exstrophy have a higher risk of stone formation when intestinal mucosa has been added to the urinary tract. To avoid stones, we have our patients irrigate their bladder/reservoir with 300 cc of tap water each night to clear the mucus. If stones develop in the pouch, they should be removed without fragmentation through a small incision. Fragmentation to facilitate endoscopic removal only results in difficulty in rendering the patient stone free.

Perforation is perhaps the most concerning risk in patients with an augmented bladder or a continent pouch. Chronic infection and chronic distension are the common denominators that lead to perforation. Even though patients with exstrophy have normal sensation and should feel a distended pouch, the rupture rate is still high in this group of patients. Any patient who experiences abdominal discomfort, should be treated as an emergency and be evaluated for possible rupture. Ultrasound and cystography will sometimes show evidence of extravasation on the drainage film. Perforations, however, are often not detectable with radiologic study. Failure to recognize and treat bladder perforation promptly results in significant morbidity and even death.

Ureterosigmoidostomy is the oldest form of urinary diversion to provide continence for patients with exstrophy. The concept is simple: the ureters are tunneled into the tinea of the sigmoid colon and the urine and feces mix. The anus provides the continence mechanism for both urine and feces. When a successful antirefluxing ureterocolonic anastomosis is made, few upper-tract problems occur. This procedure generally has been well tolerated and anal continence is usually achieved. It may be the best alternative for patients in developing countries where the day-to-day management of more complicated composite bladders is difficult to achieve.

Despite the advantages of a relatively efficient means to continence in patients with bladder exstrophy, ureterosigmoidostomy should not be used if the patient has hydronephrosis following a failed bladder-neck plasty. In a review of 103 patients undergoing various types of reconstruction for bladder exstrophy, patients undergoing ureterosigmoidostomy had the highest continence rate as well as the highest rate of renal deterioration, with 10% dying of renal failure and 23% with loss of 1 kidney because of hydronephrosis and urinary tract infection.

A long-term review of 27 patients performed at CHOP focused on the complications that can potentially occur after ureterosigmoidostomy. These patients' upper urinary tracts have been closely monitored and 18% have developed changes such as cortical thinning, scarring, renal calculi, and caliectasis; however, all 27 have maintained normal renal function. Only 3 patients were plagued with metabolic acidosis. Twenty-five patients were continent during the day and 15 achieved nighttime continence. Four of the patients suffering from nighttime incontinence underwent conversion of their ureterosigmoidostomy to a Mainz 2 pouch, which successfully treated this issue. Finally, there is a known risk of colonic tumors. In this series, 4 patients needed to undergo the removal of benign polyps.

The lifelong risk of colonic tumor in these patients is about 10%. Deaths have occurred in some of those who are diagnosed late. Tumors that develop within the colon are dependent on the presence of urine, feces, urothelium, and colonic epithelium in close apposition along a suture line. Tumors in humans tend to occur along the suture line between the ureter and the colon, but have occurred elsewhere in the colon and have even occurred after defunctionalization of the ureterosigmoidostomy.

Because of the reports of tumor, urologists felt compelled to recommend conversion of the ureterosigmoidostomy to a continent catheterizable pouch in hopes of reducing the long-term risk. However, most patients are satisfied with the continence afforded by the ureterosigmoidostomy without the inconvenience of intermittent catheterization and refuse conversion. This state of affairs may make the long-term follow-up for tumor difficult in this group of patients.

## THE EXSTROPHY PATIENT AS AN ADULT

### Sexual Function

As children born with exstrophy mature, issues of sexual performance and fertility assume particular importance. Males with exstrophy and epispadias seem to do well despite what appears to be a severe sexual handicap. At least 70% of males with repaired epispadias followed into adulthood achieved satisfactory erections for sexual intercourse; however, despite adequate sexual function, Woodhouse and coworkers, in a long-term follow-up of 27 reconstructed boys with exstrophy, noted only 6 who successfully fathered children. Lattimer and colleagues reported decreased sperm counts in 7 of 9 reconstructed exstrophy patients. In a more recent review by Stein of 88 patients reconstructed in Mainz, all adults engage in sexual intercourse. Thirty of 32 male adults were satisfied with the cosmetic result of the reconstructed external genitalia. Penile deviation was present in 11, which was distressing in 2 patients. After genital reconstruction, 9 men developed epididymitis, necessitating 2 orchiectomies and 3 vasectomies. No patient with reconstruction of the external genitalia ejaculated normally or has fathered children, whereas the ejaculation was normal in 3 who did not undergo genital reconstruction.

Wittmeyer et al followed 25 patients with bladder exstrophy from 1957 to 1990, 10 with urinary diversion and 15 with bladder reconstruction. Only 1 of the men considered his penis to be of normal size. All of the 12 men were capable of achieving an erection and 11 could ejaculate. Seven men had fathered children, but only 1 spontaneously. For the females, 3 of 6 had successfully given birth to children.

Ebert and colleagues evaluated 17 men with bladder exstrophy–epispadias complex, 5 of whom had a 1-stage reconstruction. At a mean follow-up of 19 years, 15 of the men had a preserved bladder. Sixteen of the men were capable of ejaculating. Sperm analysis was performed: 3 had normospermia, 7 had oligasthenospermia, and 6 had azospermia. Normospermia was significant in patients after only 1 bladder neck procedure. In the literature, there have been semen analyses performed on approximately 80 adult males with a history of extrophy. Half of these patients had azospermia and only 10% had normospermia.

There are 2 main problems that are thought to contribute to decreased fertility: an incompetent bladder neck with retrograde ejaculation, and scarring of the seminal vesicles or ampulla of the vas. In cases of retrograde ejaculation, artificial insemination may be successful by retrieving sperm from the urine or by passing a catheter into the often-dilated retrourethral space. Patients with scarring at the ampulla of the vas, which leads to vasal obstruction are not without hope. Harvesting sperm from the ampulla, the vas, or even the epididymal head might be accomplished in these patients. Females, in general, have few problems with sexual intercourse. Many develop uterine prolapse and some require unique positioning for successful and comfortable coitus. Fertility in reconstructed females is much more common than in males. A survey of 2500 exstrophy patients identified only 38 males who had fathered children; yet, 132 females had given birth to 156 children. In another report of 29 females with exstrophy, 8 had borne 11 children.

In general, females with exstrophy should deliver through a cesarean section. In 1 report, 4 patients, each with an augmented bladder and an orthotopic urethra, carried a healthy child to term. Mild to severe hydronephrosis occurred and persisted throughout the pregnancy but resolved spontaneously in all cases after delivery. A few patients had progressive difficulty with urethral catheterization and ultimately required indwelling catheters. Those who diverted to abdominal stomas, who had delivered vaginally, developed postpartum uterine prolapse 75% of the time.

An observational study by Deans et al evaluated 52 women with bladder exstrophy, 38 of whom had attempted to become pregnant, and 19 who had succeeded. Of a total of 57 pregnancies, there were 34 live births all of which were delivered by C-section. Complications occurred in 4 deliveries and included ureteral transection, fistula formation, and postpartum hemorrhage.

## Bladder Cancer

Adenocarcinoma of the bladder occurs in patients with exstrophy approximately 400 times more frequently than in the normal population and accounts for about 90% of bladder tumors in these patients. Adenocarcinoma is the most commonly reported tumor in untreated cases of bladder exstrophy. It also occasionally occurs in adults who have had bladder closure after infancy, but has not yet been reported in a patient whose bladder was successfully closed at birth. Chronic irritation of the exposed bladder is thought to cause metaplastic transformation of the urothelium to cystitis glandularis, with later malignant degeneration to carcinoma. A more recent description likened the histochemical and immunohistochemical appearance to colorectal carcinoma.

Although adenocarcinoma is most common, squamous carcinoma, rhabdomyosarcoma, and undifferentiated urothelial carcinoma also are reported in patients with bladder exstrophy. Until a large number of patients who have completed modern staged reconstruction are followed into adulthood, it is difficult to quantify the risk of tumors in patients closed in infancy. As a result, long-term monitoring with cytologic evaluation is recommended.

Now that patients who have undergone modern exstrophy treatment techniques have been followed into adulthood, it is gratifying to see the successful lives many of them enjoy. Many of these treated patients have become scholars, business people, athletes, and happily married parents. Progress in continence procedures and in techniques to enlarge and safely catheterize the bladder are largely responsible. Nevertheless, this complex problem remains a challenge, and room exists for greater advances in the future.

## SELECTED READINGS

Baird AD, Gearhart JP, Mathews RI. Applications of the modified Cantwell–Ransley epispadias repair in the exstrophy–epispadias complex. *J Pediatr Urol* 2005;1(5):331.

Canning DA, Gearhart JP, Peppas DS, Jeffs RD. The cephalotrigonal reimplant in bladder neck reconstruction for patients with exstrophy or epispadias. *J Urol* 1993;150(1):156–158.

Cendron J. Bladder exstrophy from an external to an internal diversion. *Birth Defects* 1977;13(5):197–199.

Connor JP, Hensle TW, Lattimer JK, Burbige KA. Long-term follow-up of 207 patients with bladder exstrophy: an evolution in treatment. *J Urol* 1989;142(3):793–795.

Davillas N, Thanos A, Liakatos J, Davillas E. Bladder exstrophy complicated by adenocarcinoma. *Br J Urol* 1991;68(1):107.

de la Hunt MN, O'Donnell B. Current management of bladder exstrophy: a BAPS collective review from eight centres of 81 patients born between 1975 and 1985. *J Pediatr Surg* 1989;24(6):584–585.

Deans R, Banks F, Liao LM, Wood D, Woodhouse C, Creighton SM. Reproductive outcomes in women with classic bladder exstrophy: an observational cross-sectional study. *Am J Obstet Gynecol* 2012;206(6):496.

Duckett J, Snyder H. The Mitrofanoff principle in continent urinary reservoirs. *Semin Urol* 1987;5(1):55–62.

Duckett JW. Use of paraexstrophy skin pedicle grafts for correction of exstrophy and epispadias repair. *Birth Defects* 1977;13(5):175–179.

Ebert AK, Reutter H, Ludwig M, Rösch WH. The exstrophy–epispadias complex. *Orphanet J Rare Dis* 2009;4:23.

Ebert AK, Schott G, Bals-Pratsch M, Seifert B, Rösch WH. Long-term follow-up of male patients after reconstruction of the bladder–exstrophy-epispadias complex: psychosocial status, continence, renal and genital function. *J Pediatr Urol* 2010;6(1):6–10.

Jaureguizar E, Draaken M, Lakshmanan Y, et al. Phenotype severity in the bladder exstrophy-epispadias complex: analysis of genetic and nongenetic contributing factors in 441 families from North America and Europe. *J Pediatr* 2011;159(5):825–831.

Gearhart J, Jeffs R. Exstrophy–epispadias complex and bladder anomalies. In: Walsh P, Retik A, Vaughan E, Wein A, eds. *Campbell's Urology.* Vol 2. Philadelphia: WB Saunders; 1998:1949–1987.

Gearhart JP, Forschner DC, Jeffs RD, Ben-Chain J, Sponseller PD. A combined vertical and horizontal pelvic osteotomy approach for primary and secondary repair of bladder exstrophy. *J Urol* 1996;155(2):689–693.

Gearhart JP, Jeffs RD. Bladder exstrophy: Increase in capacity following epispadias repair. *J Urol* 1989;142(2 Pt 2):525–526.

Gearhart JP, Sciortino C, Ben-Chaim J, Peppas DS, Jeffs RD. The Cantwell–Ransley epispadias repair in exstrophy and epispadias: lessons learned. *Urology* 1995;46(1):92–95.

Gittes RF. Carcinogenesis in ureterosigmoidostomy. *Urol Clin N Am* 1986;13(2):201–205.

Goyanna R, Emmett J, et al. Exstrophy of the bladder complicated by adenocarcinoma. *J Urol* 1951;65:391–400.

Husmann DA, McLorie GA, Churchill BM. Closure of the exstrophic bladder: an evaluation of the factors leading to its success and its importance on urinary continence. *J Urol* 1989;142(2 Pt 2):522–524.

Husmann DA, McLorie GA, Churchill BM, Ein SH. Inguinal pathology and its association with classical bladder exstrophy. *J Pediatr Surg* 1990;25(3):332–334.

Jeffs R, Charrios R, et al. Primary closure of the exstrophied bladder. In: Scott R, ed. *Current Controversies in Urologic Management.* Philadelphia: WB Saunders; 1972:235.

Jeffs RD. Exstrophy, epispadias, and cloacal and urogenital sinus abnormalities. *Pediatr Clin N Am* 1987;34(5):1233–1257.

Koo HP, Avolio L, Duckett JW Jr. Long-term results of ureterosigmoidostomy in children with bladder exstrophy. *J Urol* 1996;156(6):2037–2040.

Kramer S, Mesrobian H, Kelalis PP. Long-term follow-up of cosmetic apperance and genital function in male epispadias. *J Urol* 1986;135: 543–547.

Lottmann H, Melin Y, Lombrail P, Cendron J. Reconstruction of bladder exstrophy: retrospective study of 57 patients with evaluation of criteria in favor of the acquisition of continence. *Ann Urol (Paris)* 1998;32(4):233–239.

Langer JC, Brennan B, Lappalainen RE, et al. Cloacal exstrophy: prenatal diagnosis before rupture of the cloacal membrane. *J Pediatr Surg* 1992;27(10):1352–1355.

Lattimer JK, MacFarlane MT, Puchner PJ. Male exstrophy patients: a preliminary report on the reproductive capability. *Trans Am Assoc Genitourin Surg* 1978;70:42–44.

Lepor H, Jeffs RD. Primary bladder closure and bladder neck reconstruction in classical bladder exstrophy. *J Urol* 1983;130(6):1142–1145.

Mesrobian HG, Kelalis PP, Kramer SA. Long-term follow up of 103 patients with bladder exstrophy. *J Urol* 1988;139(4):719–722.

Mouriquand PD, Bubanj T, Feyaerts A, et al. Long-term results of bladder neck reconstruction for incontinence in children with classical bladder exstrophy or incontinent epispadias. *BJU Int.* 2003;92(9): 997–1001.

Novak TE, Costello JP, Orosco R, Sponseller PD, Mack E, Gearhart JP. Failed exstrophy closure: management and outcome. *J Pediatr Urol* 2010;6(4):381–384.

Reutter H, Boyadjiev SA, Gambhir L, et al. Phenotype severity in the bladder exstrophy-epispadias complex: analysis of genetic and nongenetic contributing factors in 441 families from North America and Europe. *J Pediatr* 2011;159(5):825–831.

Siffel C, Correa A, Amar E, et al. Bladder exstrophy: an epidemiologic study from the International Clearinghouse for Birth Defects Surveillance and Research, and an overview of the literature. *Am J Med Genet Part C Semin Med Genet* 2011;157:321–332.

Silver RI, Yang A, Ben-Chaim J, Jeffs RD, Gearhart JF. Penile length in adulthood after exstrophy reconstruction. *J Urol* 1997;157(3):999–1003.

Wittmeyer V, Aubry E, Liard-Zmuda A, et al. Quality of life in adults with bladder exstrophy–epispadias complex. *J Urol* 2010;184(6): 2389–2394.

# Cloacal Exstrophy

# CHAPTER 68

*Charles G. Howell Jr and Jeffrey Donohoe*

## KEY POINTS

1. Initial total repair versus staged repair has shown no difference in outcome.

2. Preservation of the hindgut is critical to avoiding nutritional and metabolic issues.

3. Gender reassignment is controversial and all phallic structures should be preserved if there is any possibility of raising the 46xy infant as a male.

4. Posterior sagittal anorectoplasty is a viable option in selected patients with help of an ACE procedure for bowel management.

5. Urinary reconstruction is preferable with a plan for a catheterizable stoma in a urinary reservoir.

## INTRODUCTION

More than 50 years have elapsed since the report by Rickham describing the first successful repair of this complex problem. Today, treatment has evolved such that survival approaches 90 to 100%; however, what is now apparent is that a team approach to treatment is essential—pediatric surgeons, urologists, orthopedic surgeons, neurosurgeons, endocrinologists, geneticists, etc.—and the outcome must include a focus on the child's quality of life.

## DISEASE PATHOPHYSIOLOGY

### Anatomy

The anatomy of this complex problem is usually readily visible to the experienced surgeon. The usual case consists of a moderate-sized omphalocele, a prolapsed terminal ileum (elephant-trunk deformity), 2 exposed hemibladders, 1 or 2 appendiceal orifices, and 2 ureteral orifices (Figs. 68-1 and 68-2). The anus is usually imperforate. The hemibladders may join superior or inferior to the prolapsed intestine. The genitalia of the male infant is usually manifested as a bifid penis

that is widely separated, intra-abdominal testes, and either an absent scrotum or widely separated scrotal halves. The genitalia of the female infant are most commonly manifested as a bifid clitoris, but like the penis in males, it may be absent. Duplication of the uterus and vagina is usually present with the ovaries being normal.

Not all cases of cloacal exstrophy fit into 1 classical category. Hurwitz et al developed a classification system, summarized in Table 68-1, which describes the variations of cloacal exstrophy by using the bladder and bowel surface patterns as the basis for this system. The coding system developed by Manzoni et al emphasizes the surface anatomy and is very useful for the comparison of cases between institutions. Table 68-2 illustrates the coding symbols and all of the potential differences that may exist in a particular patient.

### Embryology

Abnormal embryogenesis involving the cloacal membrane has been the hallmark of the etiology of this disorder. Traditional theories of embryogenesis share a common theme: the abnormalities seen in cloacal exstrophy arise from the early rupture of the cloacal membrane (Fig. 68-3). One theory holds that the basic defect is a caudal displacement of the paired primordia of the genital tubercle allowing persistence of a more cephalad cloacal membrane and a simultaneous incomplete internal urorectal septal division. Another explanation holds that the cloacal membrane overdevelops, preventing the appropriate separation of the endodermal and ectodermal tissue, and then ruptures. Regardless, all of these theories have a common theme, namely, early rupture of the cloacal membrane. Hurwitz et al proposed an interesting correlation between the timing of the disruption of the cloacal membrane, hindgut eversion, and the subsequent type of cloacal exstrophy. Table 68-3 summarizes these patterns. When further correlated with genital configuration, the more cranial the bladder plate is noted to be, the wider the separation of the genitalia. The more confluent the bladder plate is below the intestinal plate, the more likely the cloacal exstrophy pattern will have a single genital configuration.

Modern technology that allows us to see the development of the fetus in utero has challenged the traditional theories of embryogenesis. Prenatal ultrasounds have noted the persistence of the cloacal membrane for greater than 22 weeks

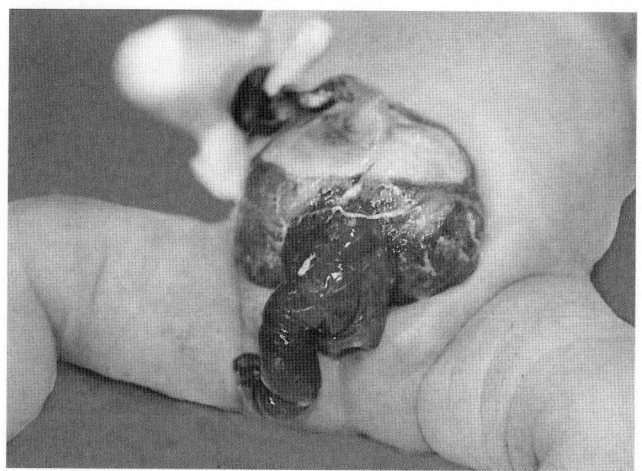

**FIGURE 68-1** An infant with classic cloacal extrophy characterized by a large omphalocele and prolapsing terminal ileum (elephant-trunk deformity).

gestation. Previous theories suggested that the cloacal membrane ruptured at approximately 5 to 8 weeks of gestation. The presence of an intact membrane after 8 weeks gestation is in sharp contrast to these traditional theories. Further investigation into this fascinating area is possible but currently the embryology is unknown. A chick and a mouse model have been developed and may lead to a more sophisticated understanding of the embryology.

## Spectrum of Anomalies

The spectrum of anomalies that is associated with cloacal exstrophy is vast. In our previous series, 21 different anomalies were seen in 11 patients. In a comparable series, 29 of the

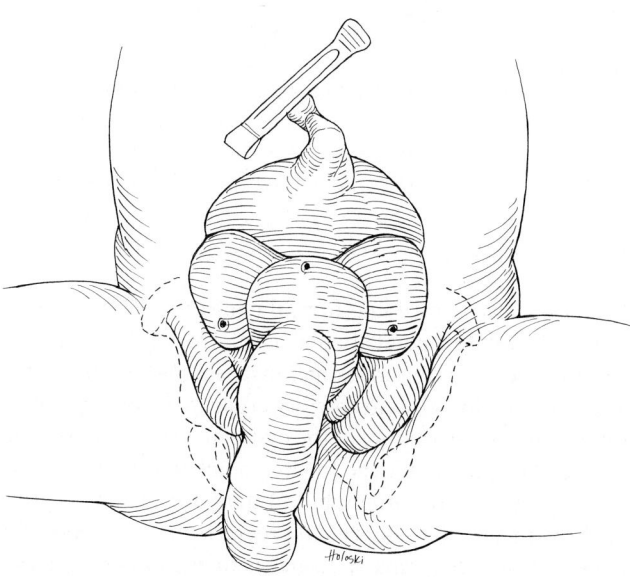

**FIGURE 68-2** Major components of classic cloacal extrophy: omphalocele, exstrophied bilateral hemibladders with ureteric or Müllerian remnant orifices; central exstrophied ileocecal bowel plate with superior orifice of the terminal ileum, inferiorly, the colon, and centrally, the appendix; bifid rudimentary external genitalia; separated pubic rami.

| TABLE 68-1 | Cloacal Exstrophy Classification |
|---|---|
| Type I, | A—Hemibladders confluent cranial to bowel |
| | B—Hemibladders lateral to bowel |
| | C—Hemibladders confluent caudal to bowel |
| Type II, | A—Bladder variation |
| | B—Bowel variation |
| |     1. Distal bowel exstrophy |
| |     2. Fistulous communication without bowel exstrophy |
| | C—Mixed forms (bladder and bowel variation) |

| TABLE 68-2 | Cloacal Exstrophy Coding Symbols | | |
|---|---|---|---|
| | **Coding** | **Exstrophied** | **Covered** |
| **Omphalocoele** | | | |
| Present | 0 | | |
| Absent | — | | |
| **Bladder** | | | |
| Complete | BL | $BL_E$ | $BL_C{}^b$ |
| Hemi | HBL | $HBL_E$ | $HBL_C{}^b$ |
| **Bowel** | | | |
| Primary | | | |
|   Ileocecal | B1 | $B1_E$ | $B1_F{}^a$ |
|   Colonic | B2 | $B2_E$ | $B2_F{}^a$ |
|   Rectosigmoid | B3 | $B3_E$ | $B3_F{}^a$ |
| Duplication | | | |
|   Ileocecal | D1 | $D1_E$ | $D1_C{}^b$ |
|   Colonic | D2 | $D2_E$ | $D2_C{}^b$ |
|   Rectosigmoid | D3 | $D3_E$ | $D3_C{}^b$ |
| Anus | | | |
|   Present | A | | |
|   Absent | — | | |
| **Female Genitalia** | | | |
| Vagina | | | |
|   Present | V | $V_E$ | |
|   Absent | — | | |
| Clitoris | | | |
|   Complete | CL | | |
|   Hemi | HCL | | |
| **Male Genitalia** | | | |
| Phallus | | | |
|   Complete | P($P_E$—epispadiac; $P_N$—normal; $P_H$—hypospadiac) | | |
|   Hemi | HP | | |
| Testes | | | |
|   Descended | T↓ | | |
|   Undescended | T↑ | | |

[a]F-plus fistula
[b]If fistula is associated add (F), for example BLC(F)
*Note:* Reprinted from Manzoni GM, Ronsky PG, Hurwitz RS. Cloacal exstrophy and cloacal exstrophy variants: a proposed system of classification. *J Urol* 1987;138:1065–1068.

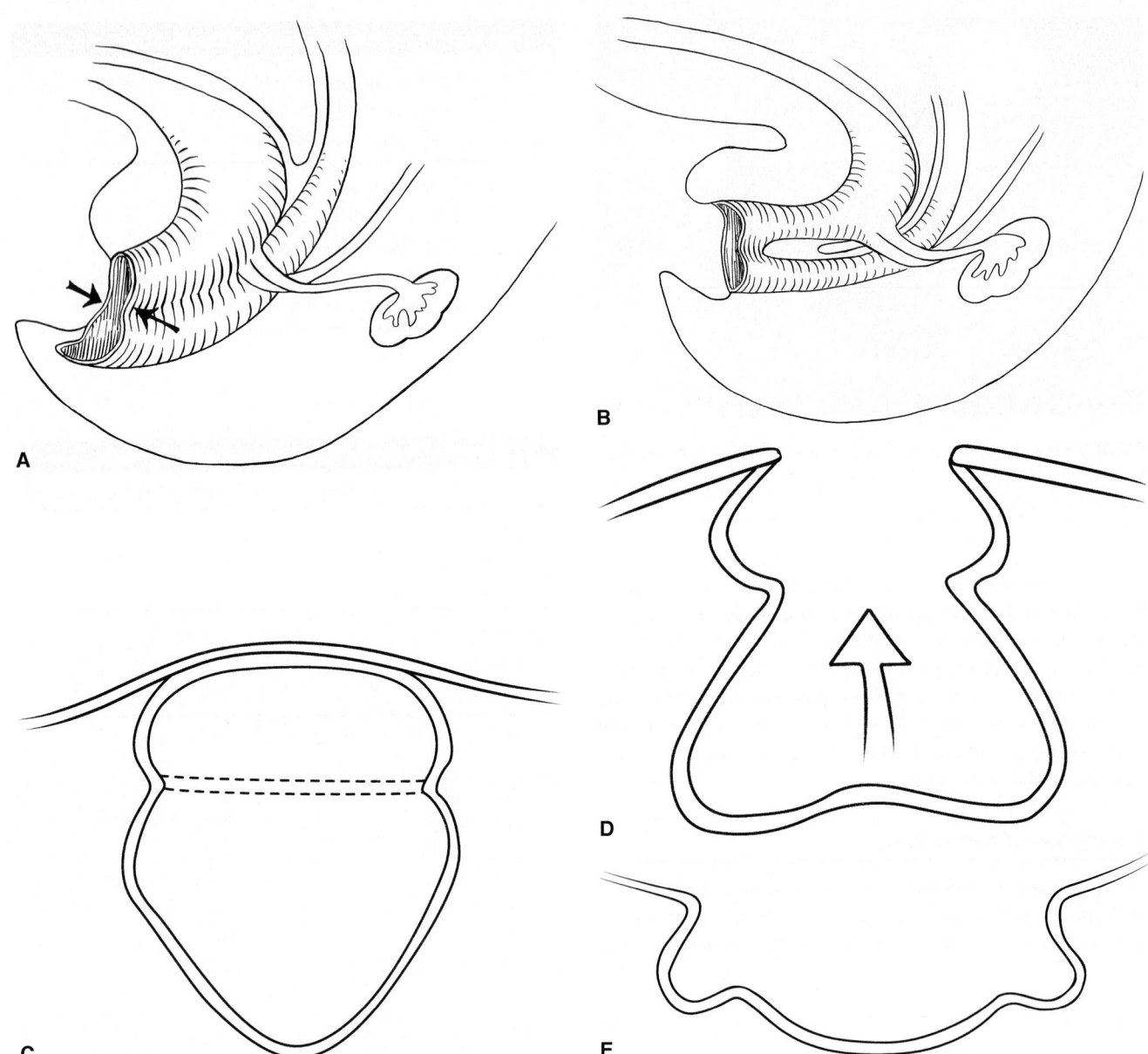

**FIGURE 68-3** Embryologic basis for cloacal extrophy in the 5-week embryo. **A.** If the cloacal membrane ruptures before the urorectal septum descends, extrophy of a central bowel field flanked by exposed mucosa of the hemibladders is the result. **B.** If cloacal separation begins by downward growth of the urorectal septum (6-week embryo) and the cloacal membrane disintegration occurs, the exstrophied gut may lie caudal to a single exstrophied bladder. **C–E.** Rupture of the cloacal membrane as late as the seventh week produces classic bladder exstrophy.

34 patients reviewed had a total of 66 associated anomalies. More recently a series of 77 cases was highlighted with over 200 anomalies. Despite the severity of the associated anomalies, they almost always occur in the abdomen or pelvis, with life-threatening anomalies of the heart and lungs being very rare. Table 68-4 depicts a list of such associated anomalies.

## DIAGNOSTIC PRINCIPLES

### Diagnosis

Increasingly, the perinatologist is able to diagnose the condition prior to birth. Both major and minor criteria have been reported, which assist in the prenatal diagnosis. The presence of a large mass protruding from the lower abdomen associated with widely separated pubic rami, "rocker bottom feet," and the presence of a myelomeningocele (MMC) make the diagnosis of cloacal exstrophy a certainty. Follow-up ultrasounds may show rupture of the cystic mass with no demonstrable bladder, a moderate to large omphalocele, and bowel protruding from the infraumbilical area with a lumbar MMC. Elevated maternal α-fetoprotein provides further support for the diagnosis. The prenatal diagnosis then allows for referral of the parents for prenatal surgical and maternal–fetal consultation and planned delivery in a tertiary referral center, making available the appropriate team of specialists to manage the infant's problems. Very important decisions can then be made with regards to the severity of the particular defect, the potential survival, and management of this severe anomaly

| | Correlation of Embryology of Cloacal Exstrophy with the Surface Pattern of Bladder and Bowel |
|---|---|
| **TABLE 68-3** | |

Type I-A: Cloacal membrane extends below the caudal margin of the bladder primordial area; after eversion of the hindgut, the bladder plate extends above and to the sides of the intestinal plate.

Type I-B: Cloacal membrane overlies both the caudal and cranial areas of the bladder primordium. After eversion of the hindgut, the intestinal plate extends above and below bladder plates with hemibladders on each side.

Type I-C: Cloacal membrane overlies only the cranial margin of the bladder primordium. When hindgut eversion occurs, the bladder plates are confluent caudal to the intestinal plate and may extend upwards on the sides of the intestinal plate.

Type II-A: Small cloacal membrane contained within borders of bladder primordium. Hindgut eversion is limited by the small membrane, which helps to avoid prolapse.

Type II-B: Large caudal-extending cloacal membrane with rupture after more complete descent of the uro-rectal septum.

| **TABLE 68-4** | **Spectrum of Anomalies** |
|---|---|

I. Abdominal Wall
   A. Omphalocele
   B. Abdominal-wall deficiency syndrome

II. Gastrointestinal Anomalies
   A. Ileocecal exstrophy
      1. With superior orifice prolapsed ileum
      2. Single or duplicate inferior orifice with blind-ending hindgut
      3. Duplicate appendiceal stumps with duplication of hindgut
   B. Imperforate anus
   C. Malrotation
   D. Bowel duplication
   E. Duodenal atresia
   F. Meckel's Diverticulum
   G. Short-bowel syndrome

III. Upper Urinary Tract
   A. Agenesis or multicystic kidneys
   B. Megaureter
   C. Hydronephrosis and hydroureter
   D. Fusion anomalies
   E. Ectopia of ureter into vas or vagina, uterus or fallopian tube
   F. Pelvic kidney
   G. Ureteral duplications

IV. Reproductive Tract Anomalies
   A. Bifid external genitalia (penis, clitoris, labia, or scrotum)
   B. Diminutive penis
   C. Cryptorchidism
   D. Duplication of uterus and vagina
   E. Vaginal agenesis

V. Central Nervous System Anomalies
   A. Myelomeningocele
   B. Meningocele
   C. Lipomeningocele

VI. Skeletal System
   A. Split symphysis
   B. Congenital dislocated hips
   C. Talipes equinovarus
   D. Agenesis of the lower extremities
   E. Deformity of the leg or foot
   F. Vertebral anomalies

including very important early discussions regarding gender assignment, especially if the infant is XY. If, however, the infant is born in a hospital that cannot provide the physicians or support personnel for such a complicated undertaking, there is ample time for transfer to an appropriate children's hospital.

## Immediate Management

Once delivered, immediate stabilization, including intubation and resuscitation is provided, if necessary. The omphalocele can then be wrapped with a few warm, moist gauze sponges and the exstrophy and omphalocele can then be covered with plastic wrap to keep the surface moist and the infant normothermic. From shortly after birth, special care should be taken to preserve the bladder mucosa and to avoid drying or maceration. Vaseline gauze or saline-soaked gauze should not be applied to the bladder mucosa.

The infant is then taken to the neonatal intensive care unit for further stabilization, including intravenous access, baseline cultures, and the institution of antibiotics. Examination of the infant at this time will be helpful in determining the sex of the infant (prenatal chromosome analysis is helpful), the magnitude of the defect with regards to size of the omphalocele, exstrophied bowel and the hemibladders, the number and location of appendiceal and ureteral orifices, the presence of spinal dysraphism, and the movement of the lower extremities. Ultrasound examination of the head for cranial anomalies, the spine for tethered cord or less-pronounced types of spinal dysraphism, and the abdomen for the presence of kidneys and ureters is helpful. Rarely does one see cardiac or unusual respiratory anomalies with this disorder. A baseline chest x-ray with a naso-gastric tube in the stomach, an abdominal radiograph of the kidneys, ureters, and bladder (KUB) and an abdominal ultrasound can then be obtained

for evaluation of even more unusual anomalies prior to the usual planned surgical intervention. Preoperative contrast studies and endoscopic evaluations are not necessary in the more common types of cloacal exstrophy. In the vast majority of cases, we do not feed these infants prior to surgical intervention. Prior to any definitive treatment, the team of surgeons, neonatologists, endocrinologists, and psychiatrists will require a planned extensive educational session with the family. The most critical topics in this initial discussion will be gender assignment (most infants in the past were raised as females, but in recent years this has changed with strong consideration for assignment based on genotype), fecal and urinary incontinence (most will have a permanent colostomy and can be kept clean and dry with modern-day urinary tract reconstruction), reproductive capability (no cases of fertility have been reported), and ambulation (most are ambulatory depending on the presence and degree of spinal dysraphism and lower-limb involvement).

## DEFINITIVE TREATMENT OPTIONS

If the infant is small-for-gestational age with a very large omphalocele that will be difficult to close primarily, and if the infant has severe associated anomalies, then consideration for a staged correction becomes the priority. However, if the infant is a vigorous, term infant with a small to moderate-sized omphalocele and large, more normal appearing hemibladders, then total correction is considered. Preoperative stabilization is almost always possible, with appropriate time for the pediatric surgeon, urologist, orthopedist, and neurosurgeon to plan the operative sequences. Other consultants who may have been involved in the prenatal evaluation may also gather to assist the family and the team leader with crucial decisions. Regardless, planned initial intervention is usually recommended in the first 24 to 48 hours prior to bacterial colonization and while the pubis can be primarily approximated, aiding in the bladder and omphalocele closure without requiring an osteotomy. However, there are a number of reasons why this may not be possible or advisable. First, the pubic rami may be so widely separated or the conformation of the pelvis so "shallow" that early pubic closure is not possible. Second, the child may not be sufficiently stable to undergo more than an initial separation of bowel from bladder segments and closure of the omphalocele. Third, closure of the pubis over an insufficient bladder outlet may render future reconstructive procedures more difficult. In a series reported by Smith, 7 of 11 bladders were closed secondarily along with pubic osteotomy at a mean age of 23 months. There appeared to be no difference in long-term outcome.

### Primary Closure

The initial operative procedure begins with a preparation of the entire lower half of the infant in the operative field. The omphalocele membrane is initially excised, being careful to leave any portion that is attached to the liver. The majority of infants will be closed with a primary fascial closure, whereas, larger defects may require placement of a temporary silastic pouch. Once the umbilical vessels are ligated and divided, the abdominal cavity is then explored. Assessment of the length of the intestine is particularly important. Associated uppergut anomalies are managed as they are encountered. More frequently, however, our attention is directed to the pelvis where an assessment is made of the ileocecal plate, a single or duplicate hindgut is evaluated, and the number and location of appendices is noted. The intra-abdominal testicles or

ovaries are noted. All 46xx infants are raised as females. In the past, most 46xy infants were also gender converted to the female phenotype. More recent reports have surfaced supporting raising xy infants as males unless the phallic structure is very rudimentary and not amenable to functional reconstruction. Male imprinting of the brain in early life may lead to extreme psychological issues in adolescence if the xy infant has gender re-assignment to female. Assessment of the size of the hemibladders and their estimated urine volume capacity after primary closure is also important to note.

The management of the bowel is usually then undertaken. Preservation of the entire intestinal length is the obvious goal with careful measurement of the small intestine and hindgut length. Reduction of the exstrophied ileocecal junction and closure by tubularizing the effaced bowel plate is then performed. Once complete, the hindgut, or terminal end of the colon, is carefully mobilized with attention to its blood supply to create a left mid-to upper-quadrant colostomy. During this mobilization of the hindgut, careful attention is afforded to the ureters, and stents are usually placed for ease in dissection. If the hindgut is duplicated, the two may be anastomosed in a pro-grade fashion prior to exteriorization of the most distal end; or one of the duplicated hind gut remnants can be used to create a vagina (now or later), or be used later to augment the bladder, if necessary. The appendix (one or more) is also preserved for later use in reconstruction of the urinary tract should a Mitrofanoff-catheterizable stoma be necessary for future bladder management. Some authors recommend a primary pull-through to construct a functioning anus, depending on the other conditions of the infant. Most often this decision is delayed until a later evaluation and examination under anesthesia can establish a future feasibility of anorectal stool continence.

After resection of the omphalocele and establishment of continuity of the bowel with an end-colostomy in the left upper quadrant, a decision with regard to approximation of the pubis and primary bladder closure is usually made. Factors influencing this decision are the size of the infant, projected difficulty of abdominal wall closure (silo or not), severity of the other anomalies, and the infant's tolerance of the surgical procedures that are nearly complete. If the infant is doing well and adequate hemibladders are present for a good closure, then progression to completion of a total correction seems justified. After completion of a bilateral anterior osteotomy or approximation of the pubis if possible without the osteotomy, the bladder halves are separated from the adjacent tissue, avoiding damage to the nerve supply to the bladder. This facilitates both the closure of the bladder as well as the abdominal wall. Rarely, if sufficient bowel exists and there is a small bladder plate, the vesicoenteric plate may be left intact to facilitate closure of the bladder rather than excising the plate. Alternatively, this may be done at a separate operation at a later date. Bladder closure is most difficult in the area of reconstruction of the urethra. Once bladder closure is completed, temporary drainage of the bladder is usually accomplished with bilateral ureteral stents and a suprapubic catheter. In the female, duplicate vaginas can rarely be joined (1, however, may be larger and can be placed posterior to the urethra). Adjacent tissue is tubularized to create a urethra. In the genotypic male with inadequate phallic tissue (very controversial) for rearing as a phenotypic male, a perineal urethra may be constructed using portions of the phallic remnants. Furthermore, with the decision to raise the infant as a female, bilateral gonadectomy in the genotypic male is indicated at this time. (Very controversial!) Alternatively, in light of the continued controversy about gender assignment, it may be more prudent to defer the gender question to a later decision and instead, do the primary reconstruction, deferring any external genital reconstruction or plan for gonadectomy.

## Staged Closure

Either planned staged repair of the cloacal exstrophy or an aborted primary closure can be necessary for a variety of reasons. As mentioned earlier, the size of the infant, extent of prematurity, size of the omphalocele, degree of anomalies, or stability of the infant can require that the infant has a staged correction. During the first stage of the correction, the omphalocele is either closed primarily or with placement of a silo followed by closure of the fascia over the next 7 to 10 days. Giant omphaloceles may be managed by scarification with topically applied agents (dilute iodine-containing solutions, topical silver sulfadiazine) followed by ventral hernia repair with myocutaneous flap; use of silo with subsequent fascial closure; or use of an artificial tissue construct material covered with skin flaps. The ileocecal plate is separated from the hemibladders and tubularized, the bladder halves are then re-approximated in the posterior midline, and then an end-colostomy as previously described is created (Fig. 68-4). Gender assignment and a decision regarding the status of the gonads are best deferred at this time.

After several months have elapsed and the infant is in a stable condition, the second stage of the procedure is accomplished. After adequate bowel cleansing and preparation, the infant's lower body is again totally prepped and draped in the operative field. Bilateral anterior and sometimes posterior, iliac osteotomies are required. The 2 bladder halves are then re-approximated anteriorly and construction of a urethra is

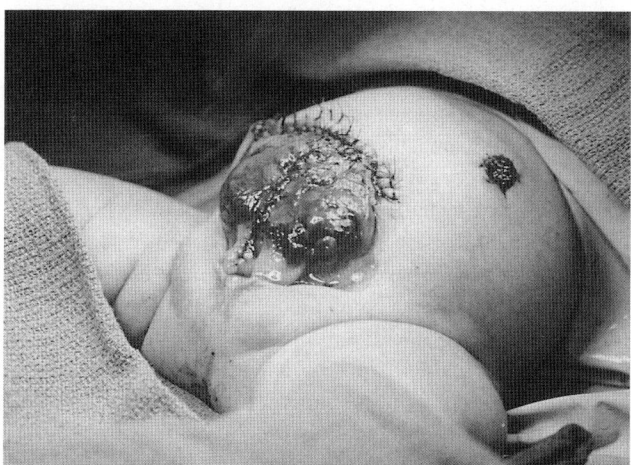

**FIGURE 68-4** An infant with cloacal extrophy after the first stage of closure with resection of the omphalocele, tubularization and closure of the ileocecum, preservation of the appendix, creation of an end colostomy in the left upper quadrant, and the reapproximation of the hemibladders.

dependent on the anatomy available at the time. Reconstruction of the external genital anatomy of the perineum can also be done at this time.

Unfortunately, in male infants, the penis is either bifid, very small as a micro-penis, or absent. Whatever phallic tissue is present is usually very rudimentary and widely separated, making an adequate functional correction difficult. If a decision is made to reassign the gender to female, reconstruction of the external genitalia may use the urethral plate from the corporal bodies to develop a urethral opening, use the glans for the clitoris and the widely separated scrotum for the labial folds, thus enhancing the female appearance.

The decision to repair the perineum in the female infant is usually made at the time of bladder closure, especially if this is the second stage in the correction of the genital anomalies. Because the clitoris is usually bifid, incorporating the 2 halves into one and recessing the end is usually straightforward. Reconstruction of the vagina may be very difficult. The hemivaginas do not always enter the perineum separately from the bladder and definition of the actual anatomic circumstance can be challenging. The 2 hemivaginas may actually enter the posterior wall of the hemibladders, be very small and eventually neglected, and remain part of the bladder without sequelae as long as there is agenesis of the cervix and uterus. Most duplicated vaginas are so far apart that they cannot be combined into one. Therefore, the smaller one is sacrificed and the larger of the 2 is placed posterior to the urethral opening and bladder. Regardless of the management of the hemivaginas, if they are connected to the cervix and uterus with a potentially functioning reproductive system, the decision will be to either bring them to the perineum as 1 organ or to surgically remove them. Repairing what is functionally a "cloacal deformity" in the imperforate anus spectrum, may best be approached by the midline sagittal prone approach that is used for reconstruction of the urogenital organs as well as the anorectal deformity.

## Urinary Reconstruction

Urinary continence and vaginal reconstruction are the most common unresolved issues after the initial stages of reconstruction of the infant with cloacal exstrophy. Urinary continence is not as crucial in the first several years of life and can be managed satisfactorily with diapers. After successful closure of the bladder via a staged or complete primary approach, care is simply taken to provide renal preservation and growth. However, as the child becomes older and can participate in actual self-care, and perhaps in the decision-making processes, the need to be diaper-free and dry becomes more important. The timing of continence procedure for the bladder depends on the readiness of the child and social factors at home. Any continence operation will require a commitment to intermittent catheterization by patient and parents. It is wise to invest in teaching preoperatively to assess readiness for this procedure. Depending on the bladder capacity, presence or absence of a catheterizable urethra, and the willingness of the child or parent, multiple different types of procedures may be considered. Taking such an individualized approach becomes imperative for successfully achieving the aforementioned goals.

The goals of urinary reconstruction in the management of cloacal exstrophy patients are the same as those of classic bladder exstrophy: renal preservation via a compliant bladder with modest capacitance; prevention of recurrent ascending urinary tract infections from vesicoureteral reflux and subsequent pyelonephritis; and urinary continence, the latter being particularly challenging. Voided urinary continence and continence of stool is relatively rare due to the multifactorial nature of the disease process. One must keep in mind that significant spinal defects and spinal cord tethering may contribute to the nonfunctional status of the bladder by providing a neurogenic component which compounds the already existing anatomic and functional limitations of the bladder.

Medical diagnostic and treatment management to optimize bladder growth and capacity includes the following: frequent upper-tract sonography; urodynamic studies, particularly in children with concerns for spinal dysraphism and/or tethered cord; anticholinergic medication; and intermittent catheterization if it is required to ensure bladder emptying and cycling. Bladder growth is evaluated with cystographic examination under anesthesia via gravity-fill. Urinary continence via voiding or intermittent catheterization of the urethra is possible, but unlikely, and most patients require eventual incontinent or continent urinary diversion.

Incontinent diversion is best to preserve the upper tracts in children who are unable to catheterize or be catheterized due to physical or mental limitations. Continent diversions include procedures where the native bladder is preserved and those where the ureters are diverted to a catheterizable pouch made of bowel segments. Preserving the bladder is preferred in that bilateral ureteral anastomosis to bowel segments is not required and the native bladder neck remains as a pop-off mechanism. When preserving the bladder, in addition to the creation of a catheterizable cutaneous channel for intermittent bladder emptying, such diversion will likely require a bladder augmentation to improve the capacitance and compliance and a bladder-neck reconstruction to increase urethral resistance and improve the chances of being continent for timed intervals. Again, the timing of such continence surgery depends on the readiness and willingness of the child and family to incorporate frequent intermittent catheterization protocols into their lives. Individualized approaches are paramount for success.

The use of augmentation to increase bladder capacity and decrease intravesical pressures, along with the presence of either a catheterizable urethra or appendicovesicostomy becomes of significant interest to the young child approaching adolescence. We have been hesitant to use either colon (hindgut) or ileum in the child younger than 1 year of age for anything other than bowel absorption because of the significant problems that we have encountered with short-bowel syndrome. Once the child is past potential problems with short-bowel syndrome, a portion of ileum could be used with less fear of exacerbating malabsorption, fluid losses, and acidosis. The stomach as a gastrocystoplasty has been used in the past but the incidence of complications has almost led to the total abandonment of this organ for this purpose. Despite the attractiveness of the stomach as the substitute of choice for reconstruction, complications are frequent. Ulceration with pain and hematuria, perforation of the reservoir, stricture formation of ureterogastric anastomoses, low reservoir compliance with increasing hydronephrosis, and metabolic aberrations have all complicated the use of the stomach in the reconstruction in these children. Whether primary bladder closure is undertaken initially or as a second operation, additional operative procedures are almost always necessary to achieve urinary continence. Exstrophy bladders rarely have normal compliance or contractility. In a study by Shapiro, the histology of exstrophied bladders was shown to be highly fibrotic and lacking in normal smooth-muscle architecture. Moreover, the pelvic floor and sphincteric musculature is widely separated or missing. Furthermore, most patients have a tethered cord and abnormal neurologic function. In fact, most patients with cloacal exstrophy will not achieve functional continence.

Although ureterosigmoidostomy is not a realistic option for patients with cloacal exstrophy, its use for classic exstrophy was formerly common. From this experience, we learned that 11% of patients with urine diverted into the fecal stream will develop colon cancer, and it is uncertain how many patients with bladders enhanced by bowel augmentation will develop adenocarcinoma.

As with classic bladder exstrophy, the issues involved in achieving urinary continence are final bladder wall compliance, capacity, and method of emptying the bladder. Currently, no suitable synthetic material exists for bladder augmentation. Of the available tissues for augmentation, the most biocompatible is transitional epithelium. The most readily available source is the ureter, although renal pelvis has also been used for augmentation in patients with nonfunctional kidneys. The advantages are less long-term risk for development of adenocarcinoma of the augmented segment, and remarkably good compliance. The disadvantage is that it may simply not be available in many of these patients who may be born with a solitary or a pelvic kidney.

There is less concern in classic exstrophy than in cloacal exstrophy about using small or large bowel for bladder augmentation. The bowel available for augmentation for the cloacal exstrophy patient is almost limited to small intestine only, because all segments of colon should be left in continuity with the ileum if possible to improve enteric absorption. There appears to be less concern with electrolyte abnormalities when the ileum is used to augment the bladder rather than colon. Compliance is equivalent to or better than that achieved with stomach, and the urine is less acidic; however, mucous is a larger problem with ileum than with stomach.

The newest alternative for bladder augmentation is still in the experimental phase, but successes with in vitro tissue-engineered neobladders have been reported, both in canines and in humans. Atala et al performed augmentation cystoplasty on 7 MMC patients with autologous urothelial and smooth muscle cells (obtained from biopsy specimens) which were cultured and seeded onto a biodegradable composite matrix consisting of collagen and polyglycolic acid. They reported improvement in urodynamic parameters and no complications regarding mucous production, urolithiasis, or bowel function. Augmentation using autologous tissue-engineered cells has been reported in dogs that have undergone partial cystectomy in order to simulate bladder exstrophy. This study showed promising results; however, an exstrophic bladder is more than just simply, a smaller capacity bladder. There are no reports of autologous tissue-engineered augments being used on patients or animals with either bladder or cloacal exstrophy. More data are required before this procedure can be widely recommended and used.

The continence mechanism for patients with any but the most favorable exstrophy variants will depend on creation of a catheterizable stoma as described by Mitrofanoff. This can be achieved by using the appendix, ureter, stomach, ileum, or fallopian tube. If the ileum is used, a new modification of the Mitrofanoff principle as described by Monti, and subsequently modified by Gerharz, allows for the formation of a channel of variable length by adding segments of tubularized ileum linearly while using a minimal total length of ileum.

Bladder-neck reconstruction is ideal in that it increases outlet resistance enough to prevent urinary leakage over a specified timed interval, while preserving the native urethral channel as a pop-off mechanism. It is most often used in conjunction with a continent catheterizable channel such as a Mitrofanoff, since spontaneous voided continence is possible but unlikely. The most commonly employed techniques are the Young–Dees–Leadbetter technique which primarily narrows the urethra, but requires ureteral mobilization and reimplantation; and urethral lengthening procedures such as the Kropp and Pippi/Salle repairs. Complete division and closure of the bladder neck are used infrequently as an initial procedure, and more commonly as a follow-up procedure after one or several attempts at reconstructing the bladder neck have proven unfruitful in gaining complete continence. It has been shown that this procedure is not as definitive in gaining continence as previously thought, and it comes with the potential cost of upper-tract deterioration and bladder perforation due to failure of compliance with catheterization schedules. It cannot be overemphasized that without the urethra as a pop-off mechanism, timed catheterization and proper irrigation and drainage is critical to prevent such life-threatening situations.

## Vaginal Reconstruction

Vaginal reconstruction even in the genotypic female with rudimentary, bifid, vaginas is extremely difficult. Occasionally, the opportunity to create a vagina from an unused, duplicate hindgut seems to be the most prudent option at the time of bladder closure and osteotomy. Frequently, however, we care for a genotypic male patient reared as a female who is approaching puberty, and it is now time to create a vagina from intestine, skin, or bladder. The same problem exists for a genotypic female patient who had inadequate vaginal structures from the beginning. Vaginoplasty may be the last great hurdle that these children and their surgeons have to accomplish. This procedure, however, is usually delayed until the child is believed to be mature enough to handle the psychosocial ramifications and the need for repeated and consistent dilatations. Successful vaginal reconstruction is difficult to achieve using the original vaginal tissue in severe variants because the bifid vaginas are widely displaced laterally and they are difficult to mobilize to the midline. It is preferable to select the best vagina in the case of duplication. If 1 vagina

is removed, its corresponding hemiuterus should also be removed to prevent hematocolpos at puberty. In the case of gender conversion or a poor quality native vagina, alternatives include tubularizing the bladder plate into a vagina while creating a neobladder from a bowel segment, or creating a neovagina from bowel at a later time (puberty). Duplicated colonic segments or ileum can be used and are preferable to molded skin grafts. This can be done by a combined anterior/posterior sagittal approach when it is determined whether or not to perform a pull-through operation. Alternatively, bowel can be pulled through at a later date. Multiple studies support the superiority of colon over ileum for vaginal reconstruction.

## Gender Reassignment

At one time, gender reassignment was recommended in all genetic males at birth. Multiple studies confirm that the inadequate and widely displaced hemiphalluses are generally too short and inadequate for male functional reconstruction. However, major psychosocial issues have led us to reconsider this decision.

Cloacal exstrophy is not, by definition, an intersex disorder; however, aphallia and phallic inadequacy are structural anomalies. Using the new term "disorder of sexual differentiation," cloacal exstrophy males would be included due to the improper differentiation and development of their phallic structures; however, the testes of male exstrophy patients are histologically similar to normal males without exstrophy and dissimilar to patients with severe cryptorchidism and disorders of sexual differentiation (DSD). With cloacal exstrophy, there is no evidence of a disorder of gonadal differentiation and the cryptorchidism is more likely due to the mechanical factor of the severe abdominal wall defect. Considering this lack of abnormal gonadal differentiation, it is debatable that cloacal exstrophy males can be considered as having an intersex disorder or DSD.

Besides the nomenclature, evidence from long-term studies of genetic males with cloacal exstrophy who underwent sexual reassignment to female shortly after birth, suggests that exposure of the brain to prenatal testosterone and subsequent "imprinting" prior to puberty contributes to the development of male sexual identity. Reiner et al found that only 5 of 14 such patients had unwavering female sexual identity. In fact, 6 of 14 had unwavering male identity, despite being raised as girls and 8 wished for surgical reconstruction of a penis. They concluded that routine gender assignment of XY males to phenotypical female sex can result in unpredictable sexual identification and that such intervention on these children should be reexamined. Due to this, there has been a growing non-consensus among pediatric urologists as to gender assignment in newborn males with cloacal exstrophy. A 2005 survey of active fellows in the Urology Section of the American Academy of Pediatrics support this lack of consensus. On cursory interpretation of the data, over 2/3 (70%) agreed or strongly agreed that male sexual assignment was most appropriate. However, on closer inspection, clinicians with more than 15 years of experience were twice as likely to select a female assignment compared to those respondents with less than 15 years of experience, as were respondents affiliated with residency/fellow training programs. Furthermore a multivariate analysis considering both of the above demographic factors had an additive effect, resulting in a female assignment nearly four-times more often.

A recent case report further confounds all of the above findings. Mirheydar reported on a sexually reassigned, genetically male cloacal exstrophy patient who was unintentionally exposed to testosterone at puberty. She was assigned a female sex and identified as a female her entire life but at puberty started showing signs of virilization. An exhaustive search revealed a gonad that was not previously removed despite what the parents were told at birth. Despite the presence of a testis, the virilization from puberty until the age of 17, and the expected androgen imprinting of the brain, this patient always identified as female, was uncomfortable with her testosterone surge and subsequent virilization, and elected to have the gonad removed so that she could remain female. She had an unwavering female sexual identity despite still having a gonad for several years postpuberty.

Needless to say, deciding whether or not to remove the gonads and subsequently perform vaginoplasty in genotypically male patients with cloacal exstrophy is a unique and challenging problem for pediatric urologists, from whom there is no general consensus on how to proceed. It cannot be overemphasized that a team approach is required and that the parents need to be appropriately counseled so that they can make an informed decision, or lack of one if they decide to delay gender assignment until puberty. Additionally the parents, and the child, eventually and especially as puberty nears, should seek counseling from specialists who are qualified in the psychosocial and behavioral aspects of this clinical problem.

The options remain: bilateral abdominal orchidopexy with phallic reconstruction, bilateral orchiectomy with phallic reduction, and vaginoplasty and delaying gender assignment until puberty. Perhaps testes should be preserved, at least at the initial operation, so that the family and the gender assignment team can have time to discuss the necessary issues.

## Myelodysplasia

More than 50% of children with cloacal exstrophy will have some form of myelodysplasia—either a frank MMC, lipomyelocystocele, or a lipomeningocele. Lipomyelocystocele is repaired as soon as reasonable after the initial surgery to repair the cloacal exstrophy. If the open MMC is closed, a shunt for hydrocephalus may also be needed. In a review of neurologic implications of cloacal exstrophy, a magnetic resonance image (MRI) of the lumbosacral spine in all infants with cloacal exstrophy is recommended since a combination of vertebral and spinal cord anomalies were present in nearly 100% of their patients. The presence of a tethered cord is a common finding and repair is usually delayed until after the more pressing abdominal operations are completed. Late development of tethering is also possible and yearly neurologic exams, as well as urgent attention to complaints of lower back pain or lower extremity pain, is indicated.

The treatment of the orthopedic anomalies with splinting and prosthetics is an integral part of the rehabilitation of these children. Chronic rehabilitative support is a necessity, and treatment is usually conducted in centers that offer multidisciplinary clinics, psychiatrists, enterostomal therapists, social services, and support groups led by other parents.

## AUTHORS' PREFERRED OPERATIVE PROCEDURE

Our preferred operative procedure for cloacal exstrophy (Fig. 68-5A) is done during the first 48 hours after delivery so as to allow for reapproximation of the pubic rami without the need for a bilateral anterior osteotomy. Initially, the omphalocele sac is resected. The ileocecal plate is separated from the hemibladders and tubularized. The appendix (one or more) and duplicate hindgut, if present, are preserved (Fig. 68-5B). Figure 68-5B illustrates a lateral view with end-colostomy and ureteral stents and a Foley catheter exiting the neourethra and draining the bladder. Figure 68-5C illustrates the end result after the first stage of a staged closure, with the hemibladders reapproximated. Most often the anterior surface of the bladders is not closed, they lie on the anterior abdominal wall, and the mucosa is left exposed. The ileocecal plate has been tubularized, preserving the entire gastrointestinal tract with appendix (one or more) still attached. Figure 68-5D illustrates the colostomy exiting the left upper quadrant, the bladder halves reapproximated with osteotomies having been done, and the bladder in the pelvis with the appendix having been used for an appendicovesicostomy. Figure 68-6 illustrates an infant after a total correction with resection of the omphalocele; tubularization and closure of the ileocecal plate; creation of a left-upper-quadrant colostomy; preservation of the appendix; closure of the bladder; bilateral anterior osteotomies; placement of bilateral ureteral stents; placement of a suprapubic cystostomy; creation of a urethra; placement of a Foley catheter to drain the bladder; salvage of the larger of the hemivaginas; and resection of the tiny hemivagina, atretic cervix, and uterus.

## TREATMENT EFFECTIVENESS/ PATIENT OUTCOME

This group of patients represents the most difficult and challenging of all the abdominal-wall defects. The major goal is no longer survival, but quality of life. The goal of fecal and urinary continence may theoretically be possible in all infants with cloacal exstrophy, but the infants who have had gender reassignment will not be able to reproduce. Furthermore, gender assignment has turned into a very controversial subject. These patients require a commitment from the surgeon for a lifelong relationship in order to manage the many necessary problems and subsequent operations. The effectiveness of establishing normal urinary continence is extremely rare, as only 10% of children are able to void spontaneously. Therefore, our goal for urinary continence in the remaining 90% of patients is to establish a continent urinary diversion with the patient learning to perform intermittent catheterization. Fecal continence in this group of patients is found only in 1 to 2 cases (usually a variant of exstrophy with more developed

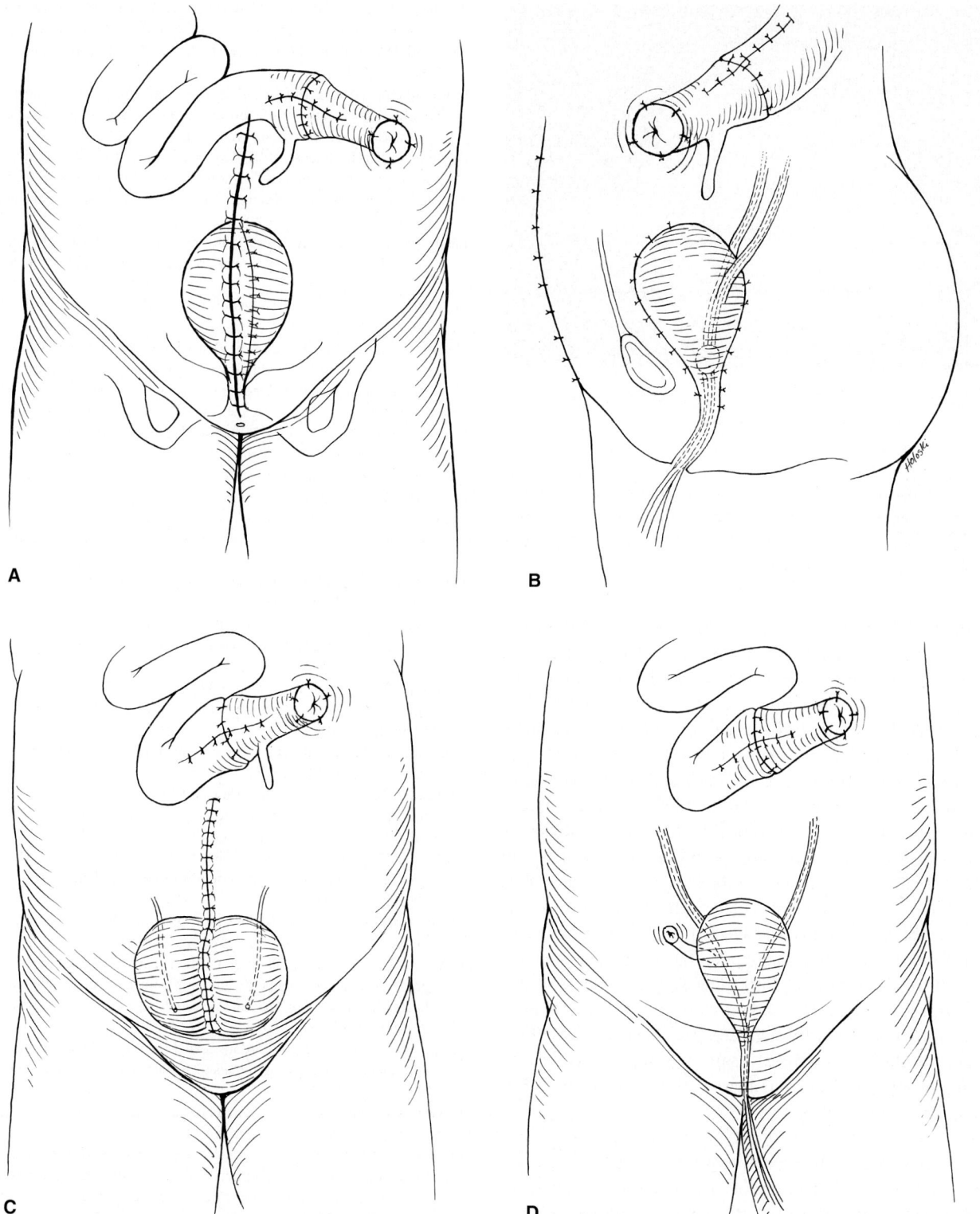

**FIGURE 68-5** Drawings of the preferred operative procedure, single or multiple stages. **A.** The ileocecal plate is closed demonstrating preservation of the appendix, and the pubic rami have been reapproximated. **B.** Lateral illustration of the end-colostomy with appendix, stents in the ureters, and the Foley catheter exiting a reconstructured urethra. The ureteral stents more often would exit the bladder, along with a suprapubic tube, if the anterior surface of the bladder is completely closed. Stents may also exit on the abdominal wall if the anterior surface of the bladder cannot be closed. **C.** The common end result of the first stage of a closure with the hemibladders reapproximated in the posterior midline and the bladder mucosa exposed on the lower abdominal wall. A urethral reconstruction will be deferred, the appendix is still attached to the cecum, and the end colostomy exits the left upper quadrant. **D.** The end colostomy in the left upper quadrant. The appendix has now been used to create an appendicovesicostomy for the intermittent catheterization of the bladder.

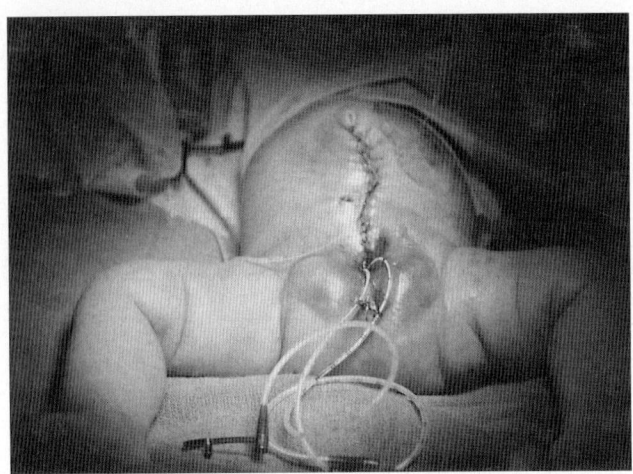

**FIGURE 68-6** Postoperative view of an infant following total correction of cloacal extrophy. The omphalocele is closed and covered; the ileocecal plate has been tubularized and closed, exiting the bowel as a left upper quadrant colostomy; the bladder is closed, bilateral ureteral stents are in place exiting through a suprapubic cystotomy, and the appendix has been preserved for future reconstruction; a vagina has been salvaged; and, with the aid of bilateral anterior osteotomies, the pubis has been closed.

hindgut or anterior perineal fistula). The results of abdominoperineal pull-through in this group of patients report normal fecal continence in approximately 10%. The remaining 90% of the patients in this group are either committed to permanent fecal ostomies or have had a pull-through and now require daily bowel-management programs. Establishment of a functional reproductive system has also been challenging and as of yet has not been accomplished in the majority of patients. Genotypic males converted to females obviously cannot bear children, and large series of patients in whom a functional vagina has been established are not available. Genotypic and phenotypic females who have an adequate vagina at birth and who also have a normal-appearing uterus or hemiuterus have the greatest potential to have a normal sex life and to bear children. Unfortunately, the numbers of this best-case scenario are few, and most are born with inadequate tissue for vaginal pull-through and may have nonfunctional or absent uterine structures. Again, vaginoplasty is delayed until puberty and data from a large series of patients in this category are not available.

In summary, this group of patients needs the most-experienced surgeons possible from the very beginning. These pediatric surgeons, pediatric urologists, pediatric orthopedists, and pediatric neurosurgeons must be committed to long-term care to improve the quality of life for these patients.

## SELECTED READINGS

Atala A. Autologous cell transplantation for urologic reconstruction. *J Urol* 1998;159:2–3.

Atala A, Bauer SB, Soker S, Yoo JJ, Retik AB. Tissue-engineered autologous bladders for patients needing cystoplasty. *Lancet* 2006;367:1241–1246.

Bruch SW, Adzick NS, Goldstein RB, Harrison MR. Challenging the embryogenesis of cloacal exstrophy. *J Pediatr Surg* 1996;31:768–770.

Diamond DA, Jeffs RD. Cloacal exstrophy: a 22-year experience. *J Urol* 1985;133:779–782.

Diamond DA, Burns JP, Mitchell C, et al. Sex assignment for newborns with ambiguous genitalia and exposure to fetal testosterone: attitudes and practices of pediatric urologists. *J Pediatr* 2006;148:445–449.

Docimo SG, Jeffs RD, Gearhart JP. Bladder, cloacal exstrophy, and prune belly syndrome. In: Oldham KT, Colombani PM, Foglia RP, eds. *Surgery of Infants and Children: Scientific Principles and Practice.* Philadelphia: Lippincott-Raven; 1997:1095–1122.

Elbahnasy AM, Shalhav A, Hoenig DM, Figenshau R, Clayman RV. Bladder wall substitution with synthetic and nonintestinal organic materials. *J Urol* 1998;159:628–637.

Frey P. Bilateral anterior pubic osteotomy in bladder exstrophy closure. *J Urol* 1996;156:812–815.

Gearhart JP, Forschner DC, Jeffs RD, Ben-Chaim MJ, Sponseller PD. A combined vertical and horizontal pelvic osteotomy approach for primary and secondary repair of bladder exstrophy. *J Urol* 1996;155:689–693.

Hurwitz RS, Manzoni GM. Cloacal exstrophy. In: O'Donnell B, Koff SA, eds. *Pediatric Urology.* Oxford: Butterworth-Heinemann; 1997:514–525.

Langer JC, Brennan B, Lappalaineu RE, et al. Cloacal exstrophy: prenatal diagnosis before rupture of the cloacal membrane. *J Pediatr Surg* 1992;27:1352–1355.

Levitt MA, Mak GA, Falcone RA, et al. Cloacal Exstrophy-pull-through or permanent stoma? A review of 53 patients. *J Pediatr Surg* 2008;43:164–170.

Lund DP, Hendren WH. Cloacal exstrophy: experience with 20 cases. *J Pediatr Surg* 1993;28:1360–1369.

Manzoni GM, Ransley PG, Hurwitz RS. Cloacal exstrophy and cloacal exstrophy variants: a proposed system of classification. *J Urol* 1987;138:1065–1068.

Matthews RI, Perlman E, Marsh DW, Gearhart JP. Gonadal morphology in cloacal exstrophy: implications in gender assignment. *BJU Int* 1999;84:99–100.

Matthews RI. Achieving urinary incontinence in cloacal exstrophy. *Semin Pediatr Surg* 2011;20(2):126–129.

McKenna PH, Khoury AE, McLorie GA, Churchill BM, Babyn PB, Wedge JH. Iliac osteotomy: a model to compare the options in bladder and cloacal exstrophy reconstruction. *J Urol* 1994;151:182–187.

Mirheydar H, Evason K, Coakley F, Baskin LS, DiSandro M. 46, XY female with cloacal exstrophy and masculinization at puberty. *J Pediatr Urol* 2009;5(5):408–411.

Mitrofanoff P. Cystomie continente trans-appendiculare dans le traitement des vessies aneurologues. *Chir Pediatr* 1980;21:297.

Rangel SJ, Lawal TA, Bischoff A, et al. The appendix as a conduit for antegrade continence enemas in patients with anorectal malformations: lessons learned from 163 cases treated over 18 years. *J Pediatr Surg* 2011;46:1236–1242.

Reiner WG, Gearhart JP. Discordant sexual identity in some genetic males with cloacal exstrophy assigned to female sex at birth. *N Engl J Med* 2004;350:333–341.

Ricketts RR, Woodard JR, Zwiren GT, et al. Modern treatment of cloacal exstrophy. *J Pediatr Surg* 1991;26:444–450.

Rickham PP. Vesico-intestinal fissure. *Arch Dis Child* 1960;35:97–102.

Sawaya D, Goldstein S, Seetharamaiah R. Gastrointestinal ramifications of the cloacal exstrophy complex: a 44 year experience. *J Pediatr Surg* 2010;45:171–176.

Smith EA, Woodard JR, Broecker BH, et al. Current management of cloacal exstrophy: experience with 11 patients. *J Pediatr Surg* 1997;32:256–262.

Welch KJ. Cloacal exstrophy (vesicointestinal fissure). In: Ravitch MM, Welch KJ, Benson CD, et al., eds. *Pediatric Surgery.* Chicago: Year-Book Medical Publishers; 1979:802–808.

Ziegler MM, Duckett JW, Howell CG. Cloacal exstrophy. In: Welch KJ, Randolph JG, Ravitch MM, et al., eds. *Pediatric Surgery.* Chicago: Yearbook Medical Publishers; 1986:764–771.

# CHAPTER 69

# Urinary Tract Reconstruction for Continence and Renal Preservation

*Curtis A. Sheldon and Eugene Minevich*

## CONCEPTUAL APPROACH TO URINARY TRACT RECONSTRUCTION AND PREOPERATIVE EVALUATION

There are 4 components to balanced urinary tract function that must be achieved in order to ensure long-term success with urinary reconstruction. The first component is that of adequate bladder (reservoir) capacity and sufficient compliance to provide low-pressure storage. The maintenance of storage pressures below 35 to 40 cm $H_2O$ will optimize upper-tract preservation. Optimal bladder capacity should allow a 4-hour catheterization or voiding interval during the day, and an 8-hour interval at night without reaching excessive pressure or precipitating incontinence.

The second component is that of adequate bladder outlet resistance to maintain urinary continence. Third, there must be a convenient, reliable mechanism for bladder (reservoir) emptying. Ideally, this should be achieved by spontaneous voiding, otherwise intermittent catheterization is necessary. The native urethra may represent an acceptable conduit for this maneuver, although should its catheterization prove excessively difficult or uncomfortable (preventing patient compliance), an alternative catheterizable conduit may be necessary. Fourth, unobstructed and nonrefluxing sterile upper-tract drainage of urine into the bladder (reservoir) is desirable in order to protect the upper tracts.

When contemplating urinary tract reconstruction, meticulous preoperative evaluation is critical. It is essential to tailor the reconstruction to the individual needs of the patient. Renal function is assessed by measurement of serum creatinine and glomerular filtration rate. Anatomy is assessed by intravenous urography or ultrasound, contrast voiding cystourethrography, and careful preoperative endoscopic evaluation. Evaluation of bladder and sphincteric function is of paramount importance. Here, detailed urodynamic investigation, as well as upright cystography to evaluate the competence of the bladder neck, are performed. A careful history, physical examination, and counseling of the patient and family allow an assessment of the patient's intellect, dexterity, and potential for self-care. After this assessment is completed, an exhaustive trial of nonoperative therapy is undertaken. This trial may include the use of pharmacologic agents (anticholinergics, sympathomimetics, or sympatholytics) in an attempt to achieve safe intravesical pressure from the perspectives of upper-tract preservation and continence. This trial of therapy may also include intermittent catheterization, which may result in sufficient stabilization of the urinary tract, thereby avoiding any surgical reconstruction. Moreover, this important therapeutic modality indicates the need for urinary tract reconstruction where spontaneous voiding would be unlikely.

## COMPENSATING FOR INADEQUATE BLADDER CAPACITY OR COMPLIANCE

### Physiologic Considerations

There are several important reconstructive concepts pertinent to bladder augmentation. The first regards the management of the recipient bladder. If bowel augmentation is performed,

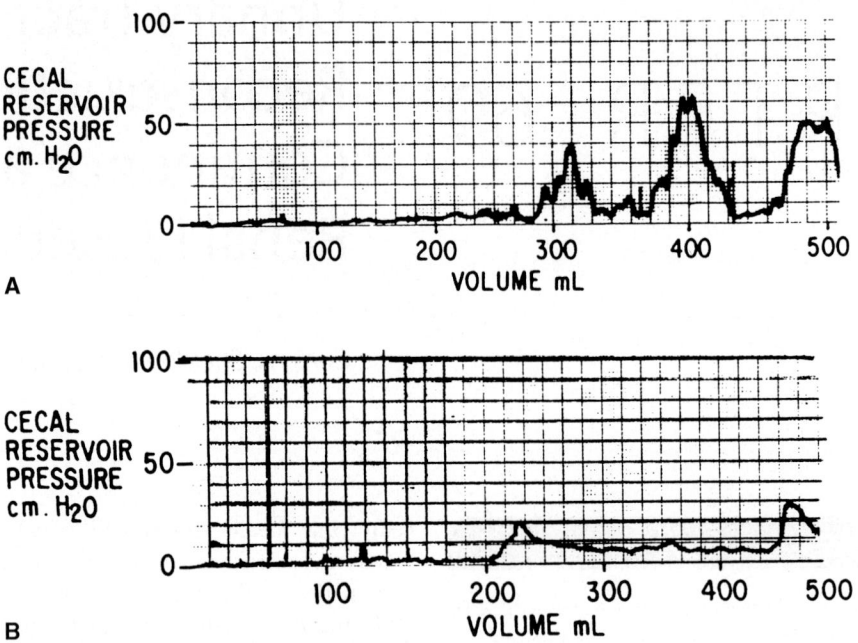

**FIGURE 69-1** Urodynamics of cecal reservoir. **A.** Tubular bowel produces high-pressure peristaltic waves. **B.** Cup patch bowel with peristalsis disrupted stores large volume without pressure rise. (From Goldwasser HR, Webster GD. Augmentation and substitution enterocystoplasty. *J Urol* 1986;135:215. Used with permission.)

leaving the detrusor essentially intact to generate high pressures, the augmented segment will act urodynamically as a capacious diverticulum. This type of diverticular decompression instead of augmentation can occur if bowel is added to either a neurologically intact or impaired bladder. The problem can be avoided by an extended sagittal opening of the bladder ("clam cystoplasty"). Essentially, this is a reconfiguration of the bladder from a sphere into a flat plate, so that the detrusor is no longer capable of generating a contraction that produces a significant pressure elevation.

Just as pressure generated by the bladder detrusor is an important contributor to the pressure generated in an augmented urinary reservoir, so also is the pressure generated by the bowel segment itself. With peristaltic contractions, pressures ranging from 60 to 100 cm $H_2O$ may be encountered. This observation led Kock to develop his concept of turning the intact bowel into a reservoir incapable of effective peristalsis by creating a "pouch." Opening the bowel along its antimesenteric border and closing it with disruption of the circular muscle ("detubularization") inhibits peristalsis. Once unable to undergo peristalsis, the reservoir dilates and stores urine at a low pressure (Fig. 69-1). Additionally, there is a very significant increase in the geometric capacity of the intestinal segment. A third important concept is that of accommodation (Fig. 69-2). It is well known that the reconstructed bladder will gradually enlarge over time. At a constant pressure, a structure with a larger radius will accommodate a greater volume—again, an advantage of detubularized bowel segments.

Bladder augmentation can be performed with various donor tissues such as ileum, colon, ileocecal region, stomach, and ureter. There are a large variety of continent urinary diversions that have greatly increased the number of patients who are candidates for continent reconstruction. Such diversion may be either external, involving a variety of segments of the gastrointesinal tract or internal, such as ureterosigmoidostomy, its multiple variations, and the rectal bladder.

There are several considerations to be entertained when choosing an augmentation donor site. There are anatomic considerations, such as mobility of blood supply, which favor the use of ileum, sigmoid, the ileocecal region, and the greater

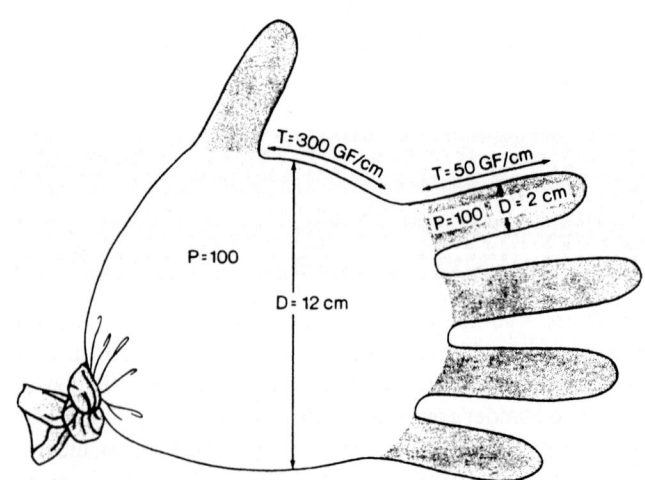

**FIGURE 69-2** Inflated surgeon's glove illustrates the LaPlace relationship. Although pressure (*P*) is equal throughout, tension (*T*) is greater in the portion with greater diameter (*D*). (From Hinman F. Selection of intestinal segments for bladder substitution: physical and physiological characteristics. *J Urol* 1988;139:522. Used with permission.)

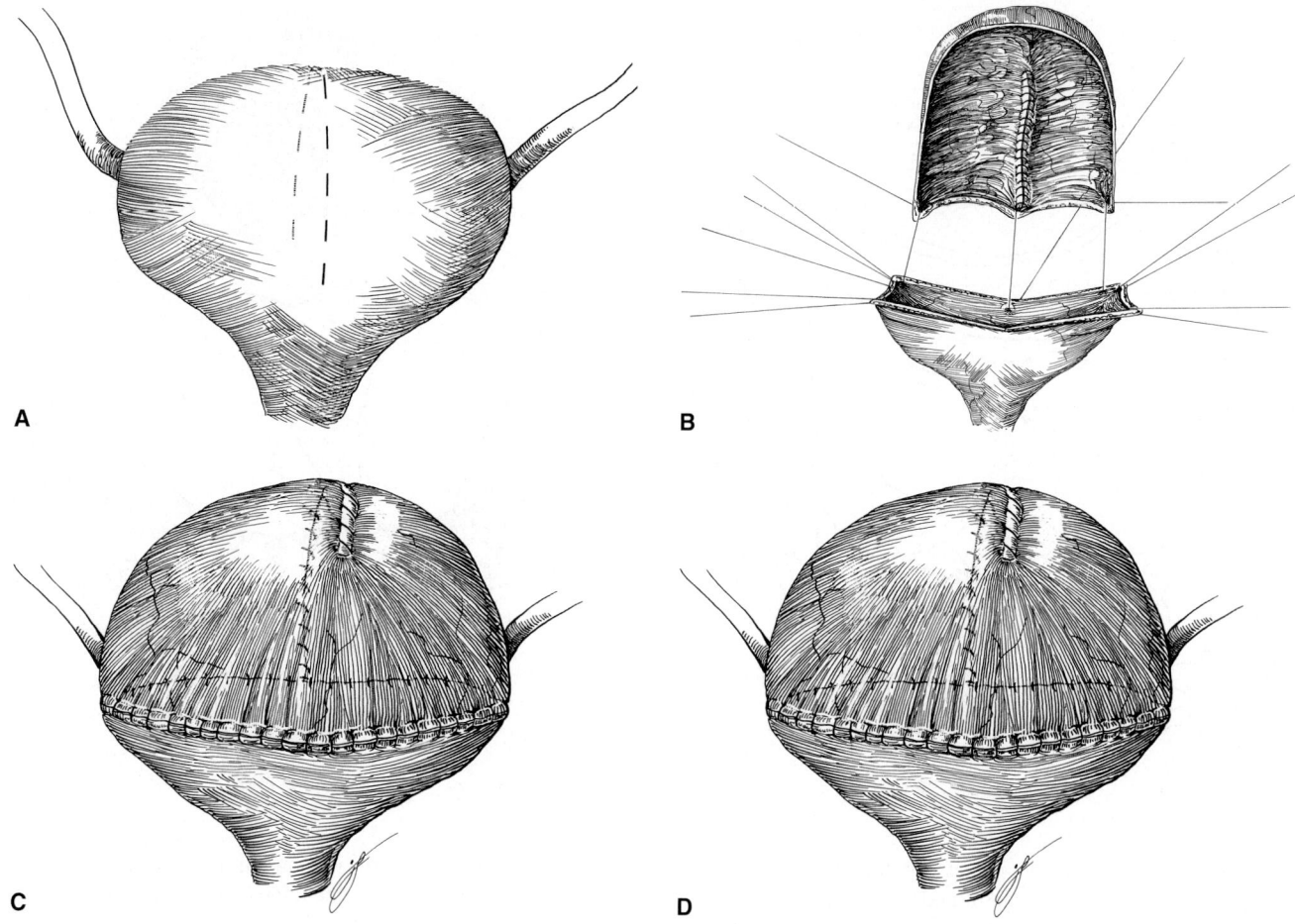

**FIGURE 69-3** Bladder augmentation employing an intestinal segment. **A.** The bladder is opened as a "clam shell." **B.** The intestinal segment is detubularized by longitudinal incision along the antimesenteric border. A cup-patch is fashioned by suturing one edge of the resultant rectangle to itself. **C.** The cup-patch is sutured to the remnant bladder plate. **D.** Final appearance.

curvature of the stomach. The ability to implant a ureter or a Mitrofanoff neourethra may also be a consideration. Additionally, it may be important to avoid the peritoneal cavity so as to preserve peritoneal dialysis or a ventricular peritoneal shunt. Such considerations favor the use of ureteral augmentation or autoaugmentation.

The choice of an augmentation donor site may be limited by the patient's primary disease. Patients with a short gut may not tolerate a loss of the ileocecal region or a significant length of ileum. Patients with borderline fecal continence (such as those with an imperforate anus or myelodysplasia) may not tolerate loss of the ileocecal valve or the water reabsorptive capacity of the right colon. Metabolic consequences may assume an overriding influence: the risk of absorptive acidosis and growth retardation, which may be exacerbated by chronic renal insufficiency, may favor the use of autoaugmentation, ureteral augmentation, or gastrocystoplasty techniques.

Because the reconstruction must be tailored to the individual needs of the patient, the surgeon must be familiar with a wide variety of reconstructive alternatives and prepare the patient accordingly. This includes bowel preparation, even when gastrocystoplasty, autoaugmentation, or ureteral augmentation are anticipated.

## Small-Bowel Procedures

Ileocystoplasty is the most frequently used augmentation technique. A 20- to 40-cm segment of ileum is selected, such that it will easily reach the bladder. After the segment is resected, detubularized, and reconfigured, it is anastomosed to the bladder using a 2-layer closure with running 3-0 Vicryl sutures (inner-layer interlocking) (Fig. 69-3). Voiding in augmented bladders occurs primarily through a pressure rise generated through abdominal straining and incomplete emptying is common. Intermittent self-catheterization may be required for effective emptying.

Other techniques of bladder augmentation or replacement using small bowel include the Camey procedure (Fig. 69-4), Kock pouch (Fig. 69-5), and ileal neobladder. These procedures are less successful in achieving continence and have a significant rate of complications and reoperation.

## Ileocecal Segment Procedures

Urologists favor the ileocecal bowel segment for bladder reconstruction because of the natural configuration of the cecum, which gives it the appearance of an ideal substitute

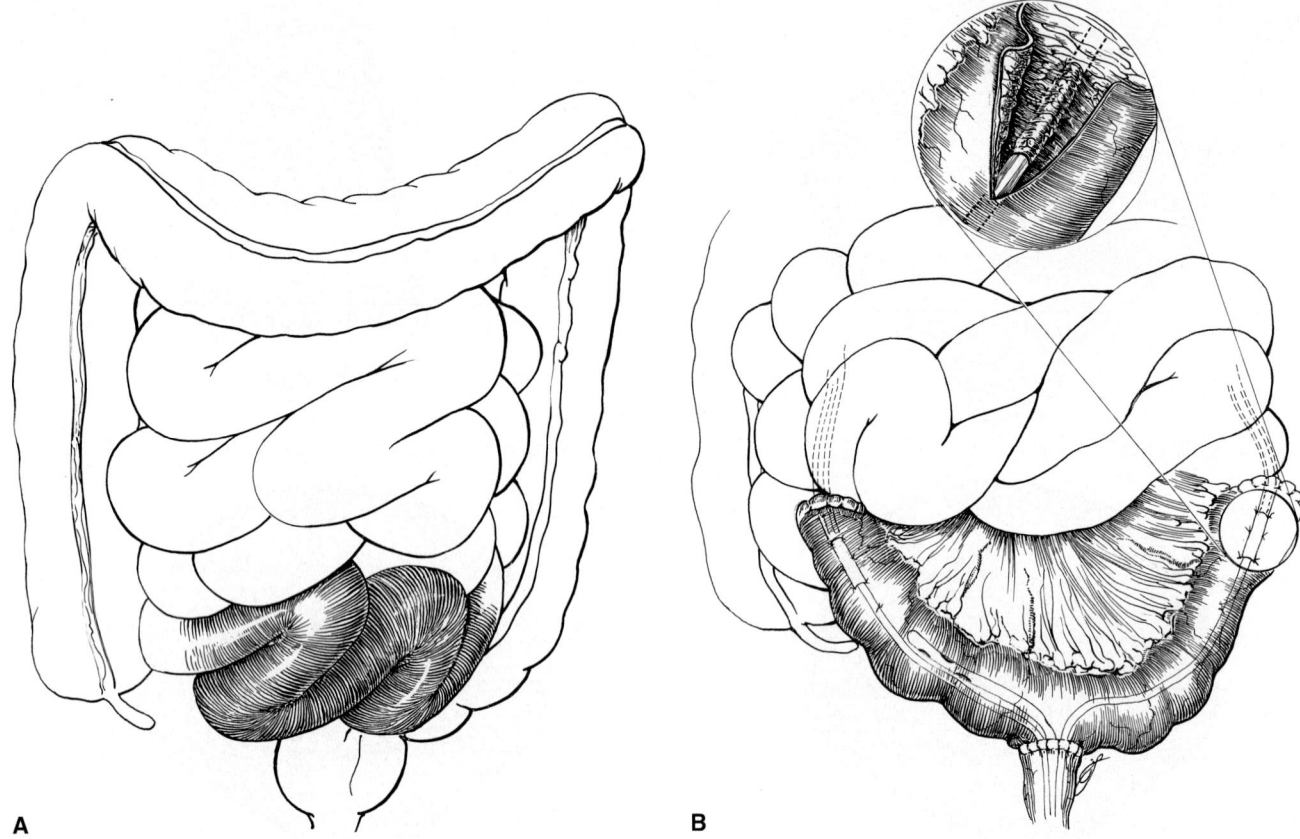

**A**

**B**

**FIGURE 69-4** Camey enterocystoplasty: **A.** A 35- to 40-cm length of intact ileum is anastomosed to the urethral stump to create a continent intestinal reservoir. **B.** Ureters are sutured into a 3- to 4-cm trough in the bowel mucosa in each limb of the reservoir to create effective anti-reflux flap valves.

for the bladder. Experience with the native ileocecal valve as an adequate antireflux mechanism, however, has not been encouraging. Consequently, various surgical modifications of the ileocecal valve have been introduced in an effort to try to lessen the incidence of reflux.

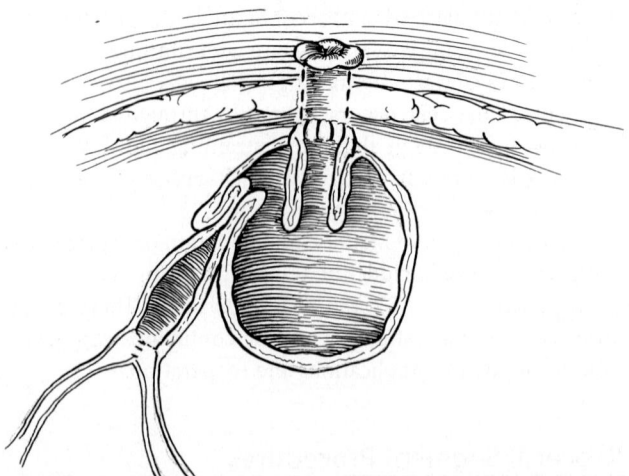

**FIGURE 69-5** Kock pouch. A 70-cm segment of ileum is reformed into a peristaltic pouch with 2 nipple valves. Most recent modification involves fixation of nipple valve to reservoir wall, changing it to a fixed flap valve.

When the cecal or ileocecal segment has been used intact for bladder augmentation, nighttime incontinence has been a significant problem in most series. This problem most likely reflects peristaltic waves in the intact bowel segment, because enuresis is rare when the cup patch technique is used. Other continent diversions employing the ileocecal valve include the Maintz pouch, the Penn pouch, the Indiana pouch, and the Florida pouch. Of these techniques, the Indiana pouch has been applied most frequently in pediatric practice and has met with variable results.

## Large-Bowel Procedure

Mathisen reported sigmoid augmentation of the bladder by the "open loop" technique in 1955, which is, in essence, the cup-patch technique of Goodwin discussed earlier. This technique did not appear to differ from other bowel segments with respect to the ability to empty, infections, electrolyte abnormalities, or other significant variables. Positive experiences with construction of a colonic neobladder have been reported, although nocturnal incontinence remains a problem in up to 33% of patients.

## Gastric Segment Procedures

The work of Mitchell and coinvestigators ushered in the modern era of the use of stomach in urinary reconstruction

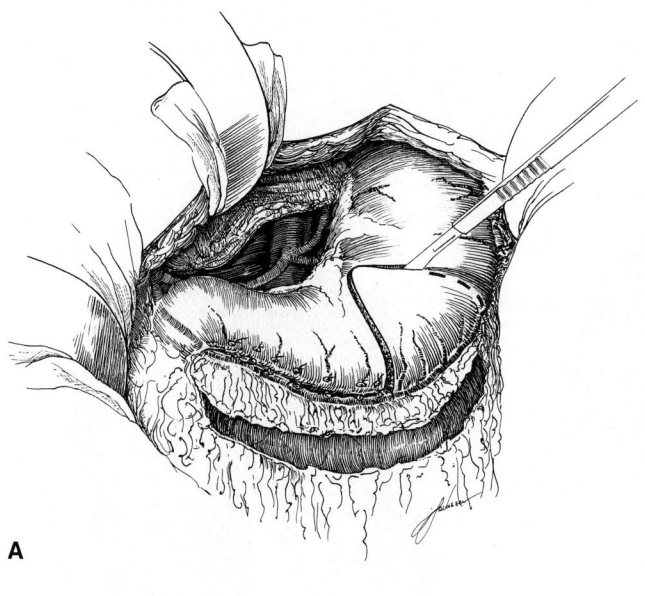

A

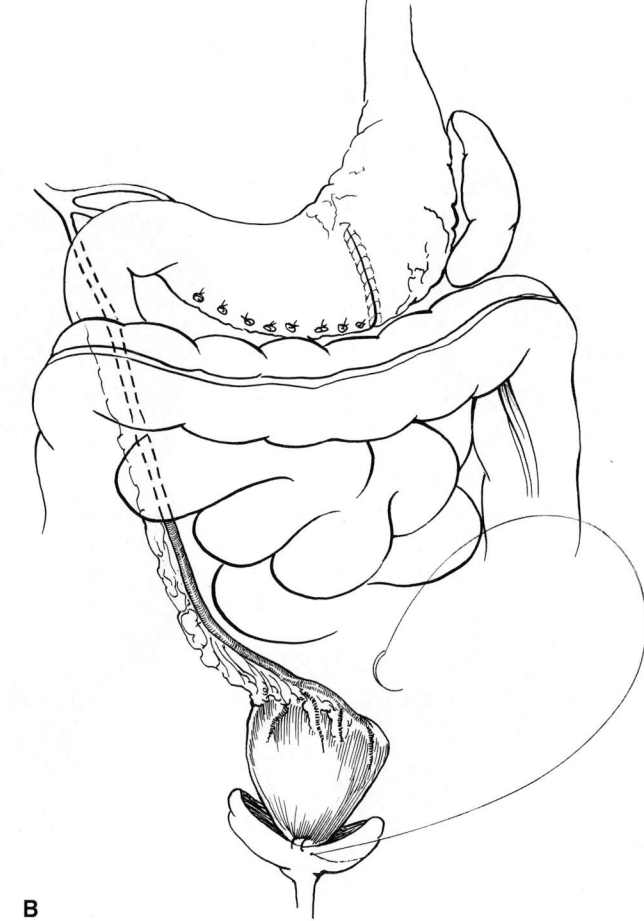

B

**FIGURE 69-6** Gastrocystoplasty. **A.** Development of right gastro-epiploic pedicle and isolation of wedge of gastric fundus. **B.** Mobilization of right gastroepiploic pedicle through retroperitoneal plane into augmentation position. The stomach is closed.

(Fig. 69-6). They demonstrated gastrocystoplasty to be highly successful, versatile, and well tolerated, even in the face of azotemia. Our long-term follow-up with gastrocystoplasty or gastric neobladder reveals a continence rate of 91%, stable renal function in all patients, and upper-tract deterioration in only 1 patient who became noncompliant with intermittent catheterization.

Additionally, gastrocystoplasty has proven to be an excellent alternative for patients with end-stage renal disease facing subsequent transplantation. The gastric neobladder has been successfully employed for reconstruction with the native urethra, the orthotopic ureteral neourethra, and with the orthotopic appendiceal neourethra. Gastric composite continent reconstructions have been reported as employing stomach and colon and as employing stomach and ileum, although long-term follow-up will be necessary to assess their effectiveness.

## Ureteral Augmentation and Autoaugmentation

Ureteral augmentation (Fig. 69-7) and autoaugmentation (Fig. 69-8) hold great promise because of their ability to prevent absorptive metabolic disorders and to be performed by an entirely extraperitoneal approach. However, these procedures are more likely to fail to attain adequate capacity and compliance because of inherent restriction in available surface area.

## INTERNAL DIVERSION: PROCEDURES PROVIDING URINARY CONTINENCE VIA AN INTACT ANORECTAL CONTINENCE MECHANISM

### Ureterosigmoidostomy

Although abandoned by most institutions because of the risks of malignancy, acidosis, and upper-tract deterioration, some centers continue to employ versions of ureterosigmoidostomy as a preferred modality for reconstruction in bladder exstrophy. Reports of series employing modern reconstructive techniques reveal quite acceptable results even with relatively long-term follow-up. In 1 series of 46 patients, long-term follow-up revealed 1 tubular adenoma, which was removed endoscopically. Upper-tract deterioration sufficient to require conversion to a colonic conduit was encountered in 3 additional patients. These authors use as an argument for employment of ureterosigmoidostomy in the exstrophy patient, a high incidence of unsatisfactory outcome in patients reconstructed with conventional means, including bladder-neck reconstruction and augmentation. Also noted is a significant incidence of upper-tract deterioration with primary exstrophy reconstruction on long-term follow-up and what appears to be a significant risk of adenocarcinoma developing in the bladder exstrophy plate itself.

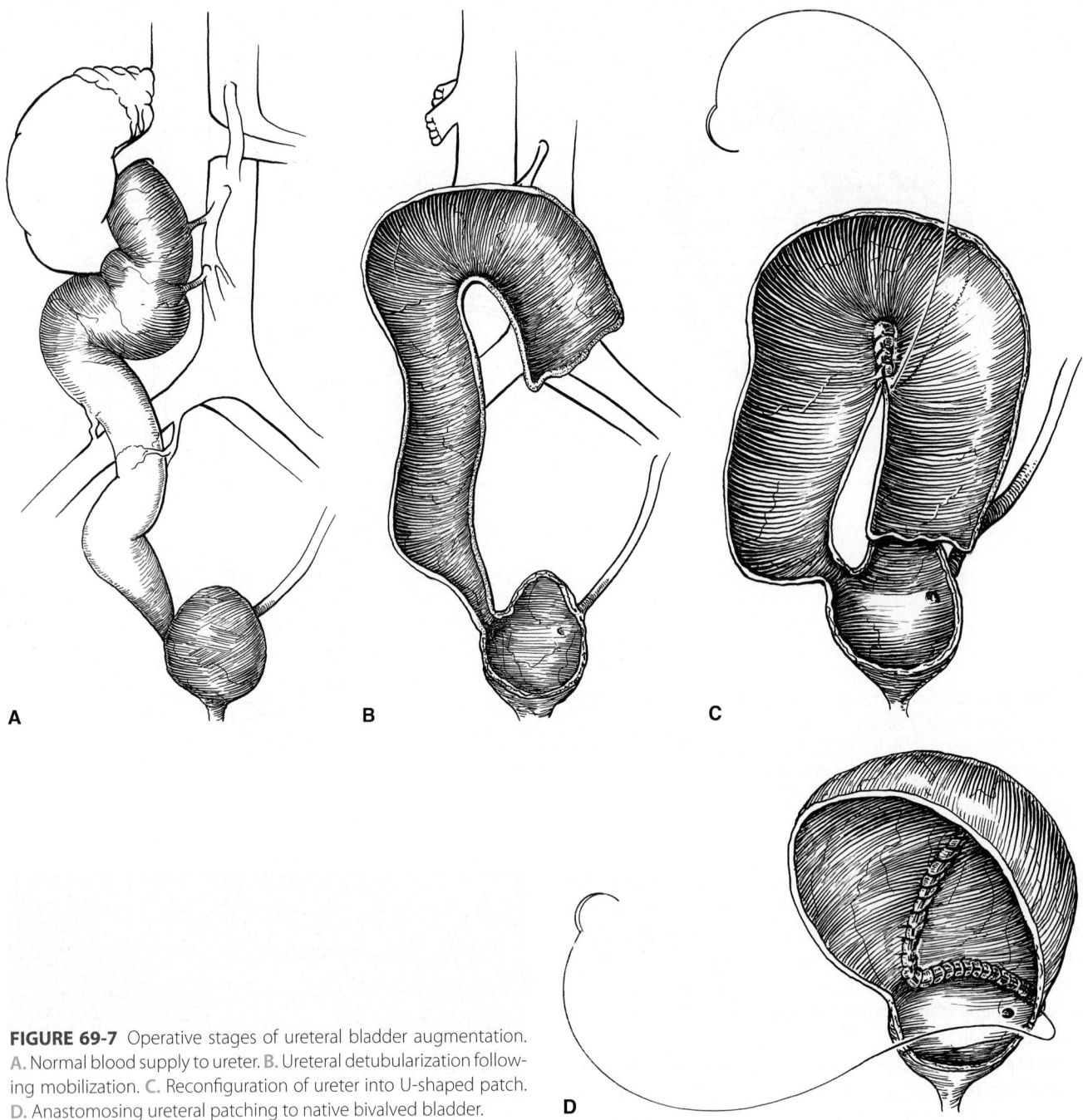

**FIGURE 69-7** Operative stages of ureteral bladder augmentation. **A.** Normal blood supply to ureter. **B.** Ureteral detubularization following mobilization. **C.** Reconfiguration of ureter into U-shaped patch. **D.** Anastomosing ureteral patching to native bivalved bladder.

## Sigma Rectum

The incidence of nocturnal incontinence with ureterosigmoidostomy has been addressed by procedures designed to provide a detubularized segment of sigmoid colon at the level of the ureteral reimplantation. Examples include the Mainz sigma rectum (Fig. 69-9). A similar approach has been taken with the ileorectal Kock pouch, in which a Kock pouch is anastomosed to the side of the sigmoid colon.

It is, of course, imperative that anorectal competence be documented prior to such procedures. Sufficient anorectal competence to allow continence can be assumed if the patient can comfortably maintain continence, holding an enema of volume equal to approximately 8 to 10 hours worth of urine output during normal activities without leakage.

## Rectal Neobladder

Some interest has been generated with respect to various modifications of the rectal bladder. These procedures have a reliance upon the anorectal sphincter for continence in common. Additionally, the urinary reservoir is more compartmentalized. Figure 69-10 depicts the augmented and valved rectum. This procedure was performed in 83 patients with a 100% daytime continence rate and a 99% nighttime continence rate.

## Artificial Bladder

A permanently implanted, nonbiologic substitute for the bladder has been tried with such diverse materials as Vitallium,

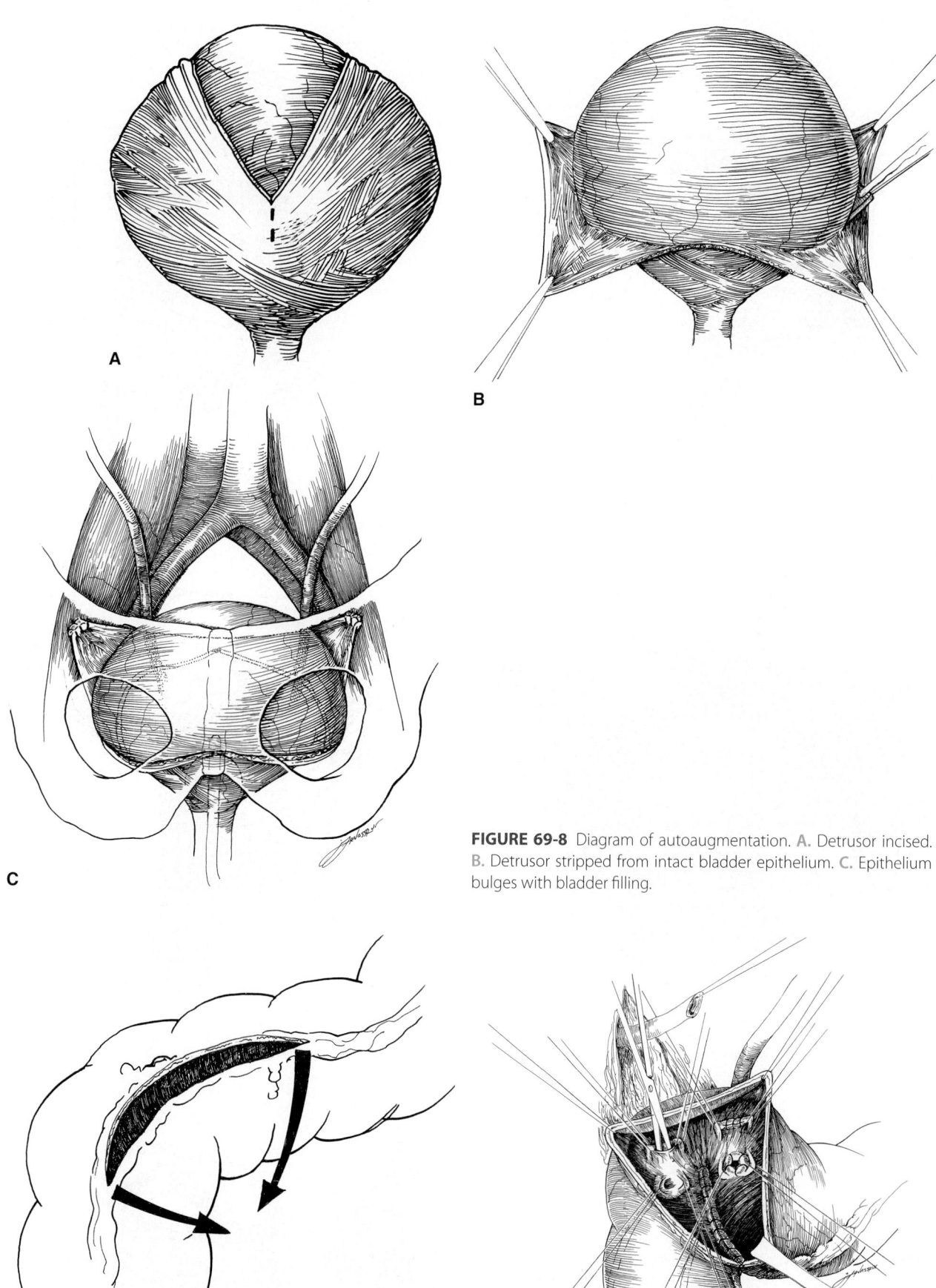

**FIGURE 69-8** Diagram of autoaugmentation. **A.** Detrusor incised. **B.** Detrusor stripped from intact bladder epithelium. **C.** Epithelium bulges with bladder filling.

**FIGURE 69-9** The Mainz pouch II (sigmoid rectum). **A.** A longitudinal incision in the sigmoid colon is followed by a side-to-side anastomosis to create a detubularized segment. **B.** Sacral fixation is achieved and long ureteral reimplantation is performed in the Goodwin fashion.

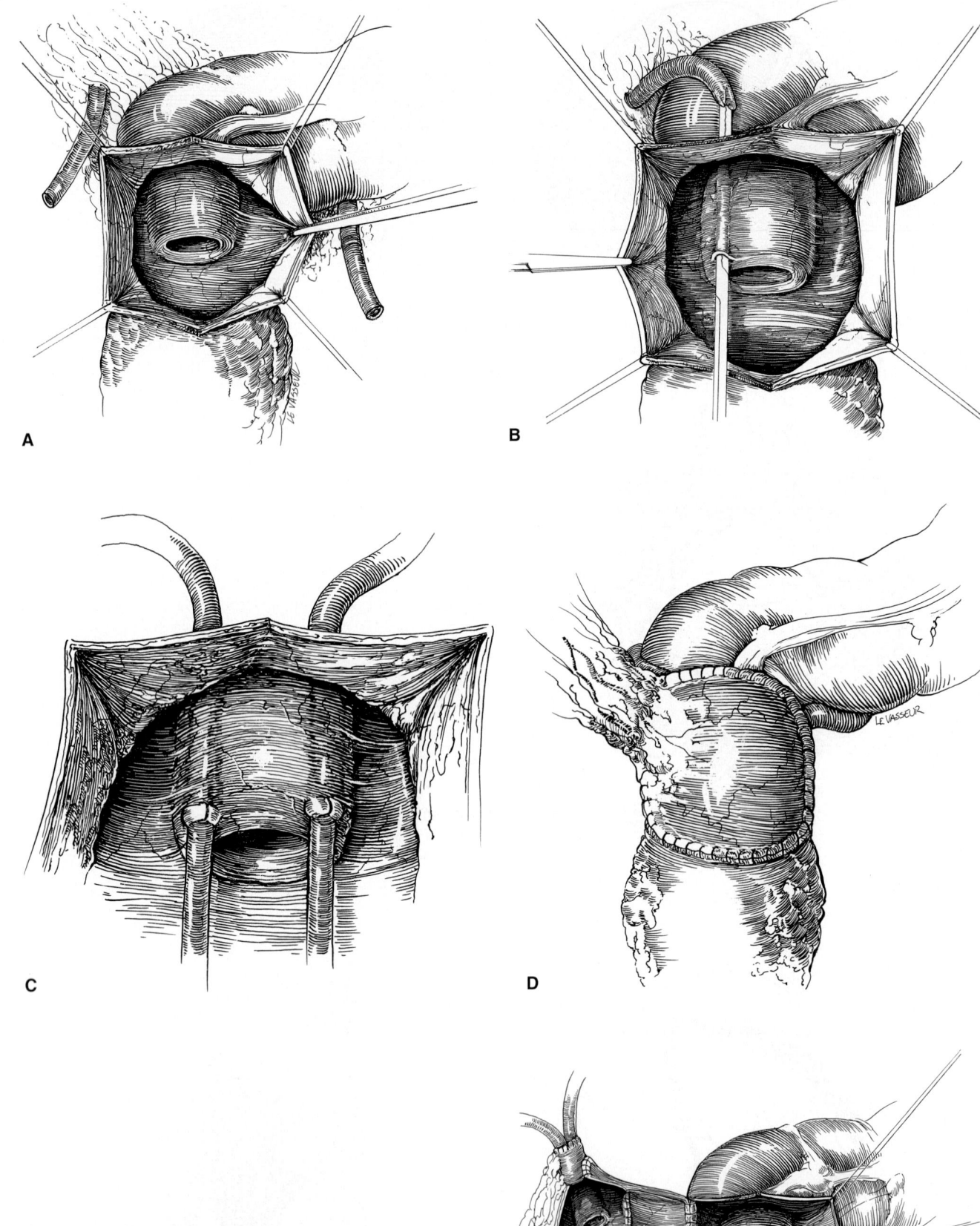

A

B

C

D

E

**FIGURE 69-10** The augmented and valved rectum. **A.** The anterior wall of the rectosigmoid is opened and a colorectal intussusception valve is created. **B.** The ureter is passed between the 2 layers of the intussusceptum. **C.** A stented mucosa-to-mucosa anastomosis is completed on both sides. An alternative (currently the method of choice) is to reimplant the ureters through a submucosal tunnel by using the Goodwin technique. **D.** The opened rectum is closed with an ileal patch. **E.** With dilated ureters, a second intussusception valve from ileum is used for reflux prevention.

polyethylene, Teflon, polyvinyl, silicone rubber, Ivalon, Dacron, silver, Tantalum, and expanded polytetrafluoroethylene (Gor-Tex). All efforts have failed because of the development of an inflammatory reaction with or without active bacterial infection. Autologous tissue bladders remain experimental.

# COMPENSATING FOR INADEQUATE BLADDER OUTLET RESISTANCE

Urinary continence is maintained by a complex relationship between bladder outlet resistance and pressure. To maintain dryness, the bladder outlet resistance must exceed intravesical pressure not only at rest but during changes in posture, coughing, sneezing, and straining. There are several components to this mechanism. Certainly, intrinsic urethral resistance caused by inherent tension in the urethral wall as well as the length and diameter of the urethra play an important role. Other components include smooth and striated muscular activity and the fact that intra-abdominal pressure may be reflected on the proximal urethra. This latter mechanism provides a *mechanism* to compensate for elevated intravesical pressure caused

by applied intra-abdominal pressure by simultaneously applying similar pressure to the proximal urethra.

Based on these components of continence, it is not surprising that most surgical interventions designed for the achievement of incontinence include procedures to lengthen the urethra, suspend the bladder neck, and compress the urethra. It is clear that, in males, pubertal changes can assist in creation of outlet resistance after a detrusor tube repair.

## Urethral Lengthening Procedures

### Young–Dees–Leadbetter Procedure

Efforts to proximally lengthen the existing urethra through tubularization of the posterior detrusor grew out of the early work of Young. In the procedure, which was later modified by Dees and Leadbetter, the urethra is lengthened by tubularization of a long (4-5 cm) segment of the posterior bladder wall. Two triangular sections of urothelium are excised, and the resultant urothelial strip is approximated over a small catheter (8 or 10 French) to fashion the neourethra. The adjacent detrusor is approximated to itself over this mucosal tube to add muscular support (Fig. 69-11).

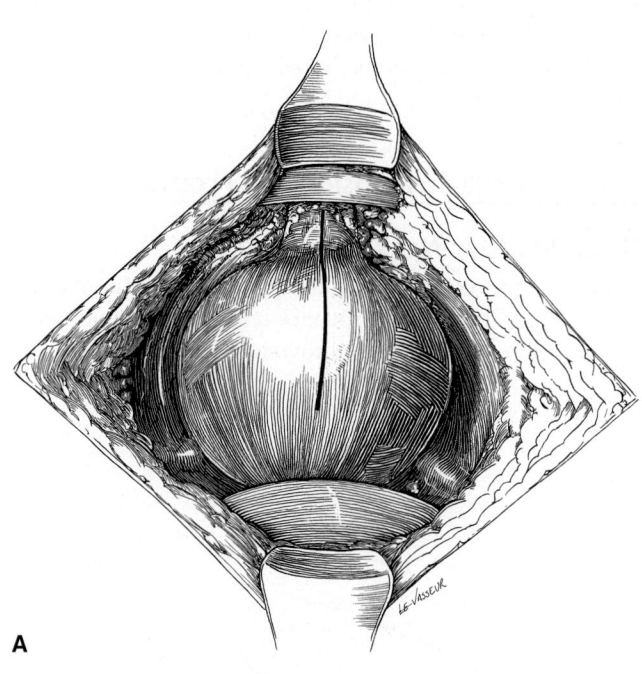

**A**

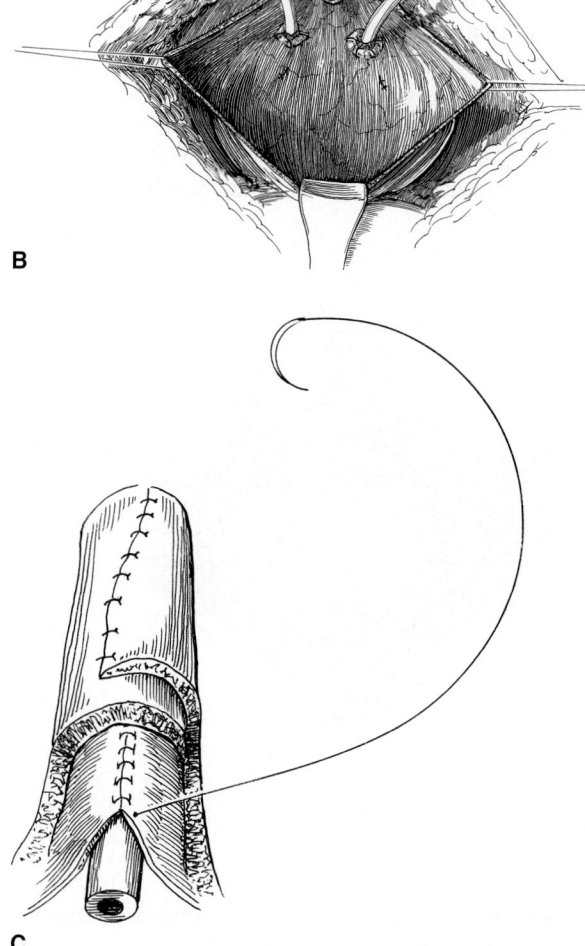

**B**

**C**

**FIGURE 69-11** **A.** Bladder incision. The Leadbetter technique of tubularization of posterior detrusor. **B.** Ureters are reimplanted higher in the bladder to permit creation of a long detrusor tube. **C, D.** The detrusor is overlapped over the mucosal tube.

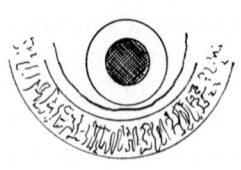 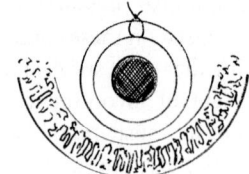 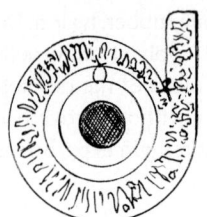 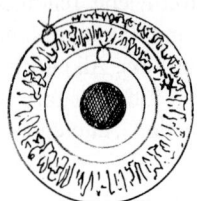

**D**

**FIGURE 69-11** (*Continued*)

Other authors have had better success with the Young–Dees–Leadbetter-type reconstruction by using several modifications. Lepor and Jeffs attributed their success to a urethral suspension (Marshall–Marchetti–Krantz type of procedure) and the use of urodynamic control at the time of surgery to assure adequate urethral resistance (Fig. 69-12).

The placement of an adjuvant Mitrofanoff neourethra in patients undergoing Young–Dees–Leadbetter bladder-neck reconstruction allows a channel for intermittent catheterization, which has been useful for all such reconstructions, especially in the early postoperative period. With time, as the patient learns to void through the reconstructed urethra, the Mitrofanoff neourethra can be removed in a simple outpatient surgical procedure or, if it does not leak, it can be left in situ.

## Kropp Procedure

Kropp described another approach to produce a competent urethra: turning the junction of the urethra with the bladder into an effective flap-valve as is seen at the normal ureterovesical junction (Fig. 69-13). A detrusor tube is formed anteriorly or posteriorly in continuity with the bladder neck and urethra, and reimplanted submucosally in the bladder. Compression of the detrusor tube as the bladder fills creates an effective flap-valve mechanism, producing continence. Although excellent continence is achieved with such a flap-valve mechanism, spontaneous voiding is not possible in this situation, and intermittent catheterization is required for bladder emptying. The main postoperative problem is difficulty with catheterization.

## Pippi Salle Procedure

Problems with catheterization after the Kropp procedure were addressed by Pippe Salle. In his technique, the mucosa of an anterior bladder wall-flap based on the urethra is sutured to posterior wall mucosa in an onlay fashion. A second layer of sutures approximates the muscle of the flap to the posterior detrusor. The remaining mucosal edges are approximated over the lengthened urethra. Initial reports of this procedure are encouraging.

## Bladder-Neck Suspension and Fixation

### Open Bladder-Neck Suspension

These procedures were designed primarily for the correction of stress urinary incontinence related to an abnormally low positioning of the urethrovesical junction. Increased

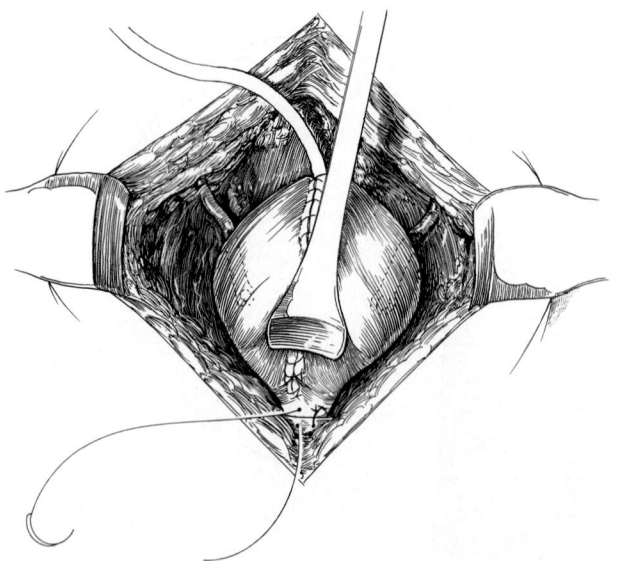

**A**

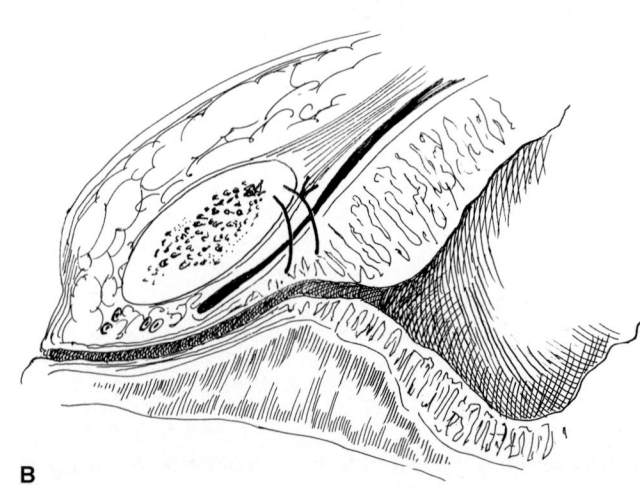

**B**

**FIGURE 69-12** **A.** Posterior detrusor tube suspended from posterior surface of pubic bone and rectus muscle. **B.** Suspension helps preserve both length and position of detrusor tube.

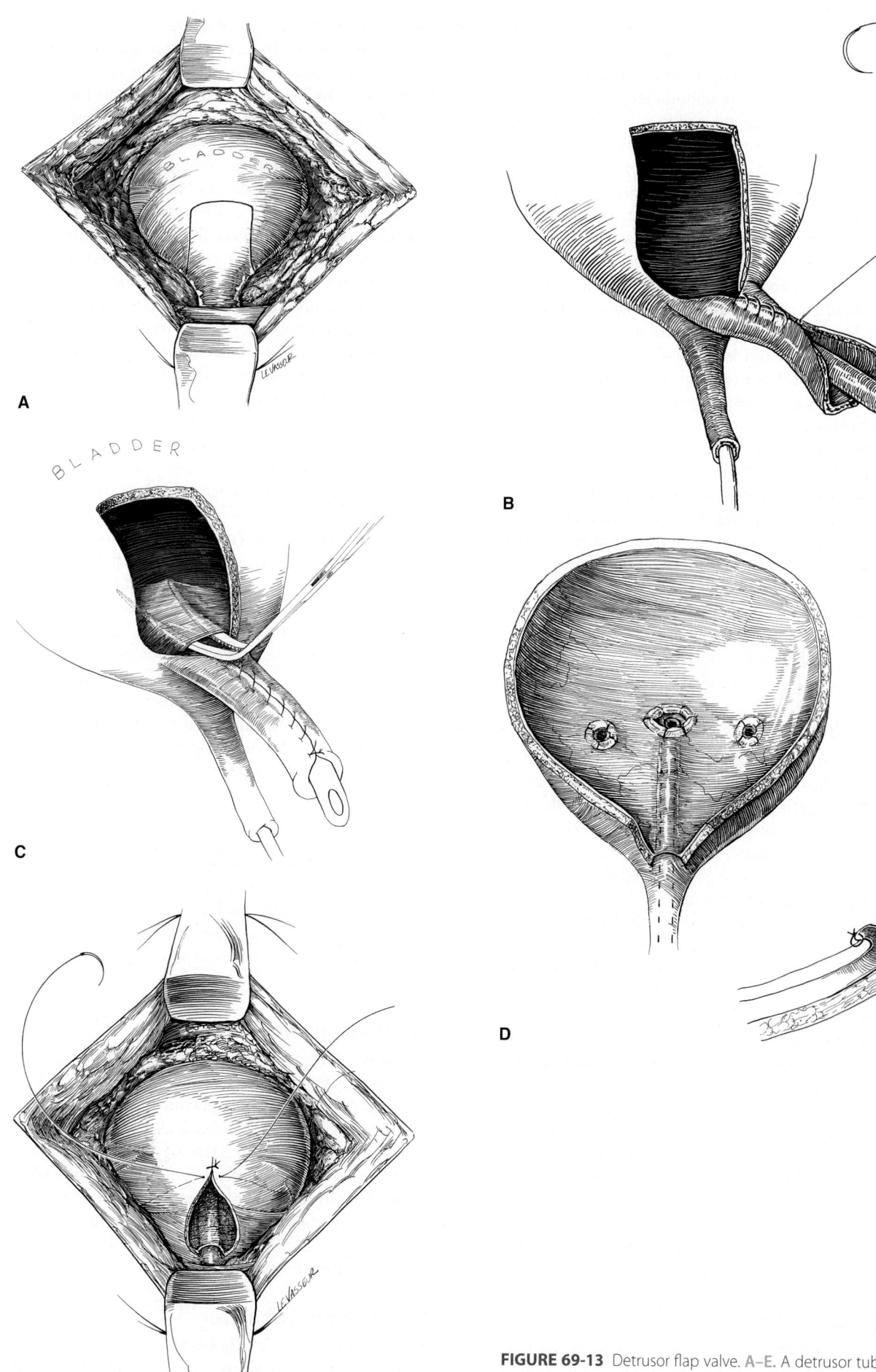

**A**

**B**

**C**

**D**

**E**

**FIGURE 69-13** Detrusor flap valve. **A–E.** A detrusor tube is created (anterior shown, posterior tube also possible) and tunneled submucosally in bladder to create a competent flap valve.

intra-abdominal pressure could not be transmitted to the urethra, with a resultant low-pressure gradient between the bladder and the urethra, leading to stress urinary leakage during periods of increased intra-abdominal pressure. Restoration of normal anatomy should lead to correction of stress incontinence without the production of problems with bladder emptying, provided that detrusor function is normal. The urethral suspension procedures may also produce urethral stretch and thus lengthening, urethral narrowing, and/or urethral compression, which may also increase bladder outlet resistance.

The urethral suspension and fixation procedure that has become the standard against which others have been compared is the Marshall–Marchetti–Krantz operation. In this open operation, the urethra is suspended from the posterior aspect of the pubic bone or rectus fascia with a series of absorbable sutures, which most surgeons today place into the periurethral tissues adjacent to the urethra. In elevating this tissue, the endopelvic fascia is also tightened. This suspension brings the urethrovesical junction to a position where increases in intra-abdominal pressure are directly transmitted to the urethra, thus correcting stress incontinence.

The Burch procedure is a similar operation to elevate the urethrovesical angle; however, in this operation, vaginal fascia near the urethra is sutured to the Cooper ligament (ileopectineal ligament). The possible advantage of this operation is that the ileopectineal ligament may provide a more reliable anchor for sutures than the periosteum of the pubic bone. Additionally, osteitis pubis is avoided.

## Endoscopic Bladder-Neck Suspension

As it became clear that urethral suspension operations had much to offer in the treatment of stress urinary incontinence, the development of semiclosed needle suspensions offered a logical progression. The original Pereyra procedure has been modified in a number of ways.

Endoscopic suspension was first described by Stamey. His innovation was to emphasize the use of the cystoscope to control accurate placement of the suspending sutures exactly at the urethrovesical junction so as to ensure appropriate urethral suspension. In the Raz needle suspension procedure, the Stamey technique is further modified. During vaginal dissection the retropubic space is entered and mobilization of the urethra and bladder neck is performed to be certain that the urethra can be moved sufficiently intra-abdominally to expose it to intra-abdominal pressure. To ensure adequate fixation of the suspension sutures to the periurethral tissues, a serial helical stitch is placed to encompass the endopelvic fascia, as well as the full thickness of the vaginal wall, except for the epithelium. This enables a broadly secured anchoring of the suture to the periurethral tissues. Suprapubically, the suspending sutures are elevated to be certain that closure of the bladder neck is occurring (as confirmed by cystoscopic inspection) and these are then tied to one another.

## Fascial Sling Procedures

There is a significant difference between the suspension-type procedures and those procedures that involve some form of sling suspension of the urethra. This type of approach dates to the Millan suspension. In this operation, the rectus fascia is exposed, and 2 longitudinal strips of rectus fascia are dissected just above the insertion of the rectus into the pubic bone, maintaining their continuity with the rectus fascia laterally on each side. The Retzius space is dissected and the bladder-neck region and urethra are separated from the vaginal wall. The rectus strips are brought into the Retzius space lateral to the rectus muscle, passed beneath the urethra at the bladder neck, brought back suprapubically through the midline incision between the rectus muscles, and then sutured to the anterior rectus fascia with sufficient elevation of the bladder neck to ensure intra-abdominal positioning of the urethra. The biggest drawback of this procedure has been a significant problem with long-term urinary retention. Direct compression of the urethra by the fascial strip would add to bladder outlet resistance and explain the different outcome from simple suspension. Sling procedures, particularly with the use of foreign material, can occasionally result in erosion of the urethra or bladder neck.

Sling urethral suspension procedures have been modified by combining them with needle suspension. In the Raz technique of transvaginal needle suspension of the bladder neck with a fascial sling, a rectus fascial patch is fashioned like a hammock to cover the length and width of the urethra. Four polypropylene (Prolene) sutures are placed at each corner of the graft and are drawn suprapubically with a Stamey-type needle as in an endoscopic suspension. Upward elevation of the suspending sutures lifts the entire urethra and/or bladder neck unit and compresses it through the action of the patch. McGuire modified this technique by using only 2 sutures with bolsters to pull upward a smaller rectus fascial strip with the same technique as a Stamey suspension.

## Direct Urethral Compression by Foreign Body

There has been considerable interest and progress in the production of increased bladder outlet resistance through the use of external compression of the urethral lumen during the last 20 years, as non-reactive polymers of varying types have been developed.

## Periurethral Injection

Direct passive urethral compression through the periurethral injection of Teflon (polytetrafluoroethylene) or Deflux® (dextranomer/hyaluronic acid copolymer) was suggested by some authors. The raising of a submucosal wheal of bulking agent coapts the urethral wall, increasing bladder outlet resistance and preventing the transmission of intra-abdominal pressure to the urethra through a column of urine in an open bladder neck and/or posterior urethra. The Food and Drug Administration has not yet cleared the use of any bulking agent for periurethral injection.

## Artificial Urinary Sphincter

The artificial urinary sphincter has been shown to be effective for compressing the urethra and thus contributes to bladder

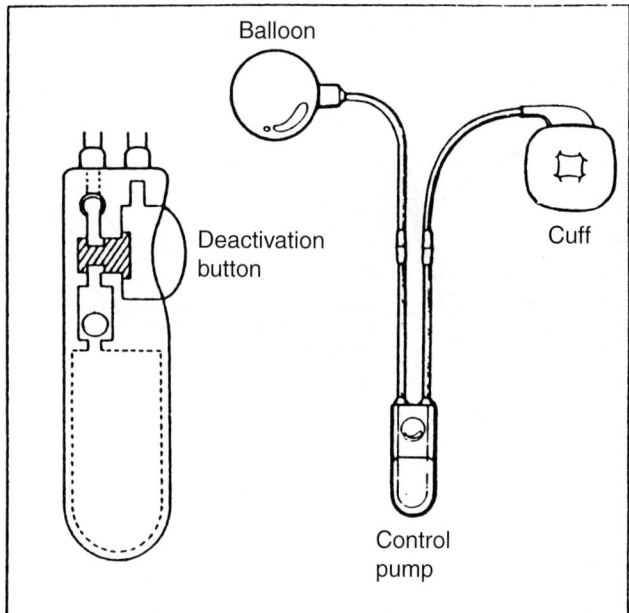

**FIGURE 69-14** The American Medical Systems model 800 artificial urinary sphincter. It is a simplified model with deflation pump, delay-fill resistor, and deactivation button in 1 control unit that can be implanted in the scrotum or labia. (From American Medical Systems, Minnetonka, MN, Publication 30831. Used with permission.)

outlet competence. The most popular model consists of a cuff placed around the bladder neck or bulbar urethra, a reservoir placed intra-abdominally, and an activating pressure bulb located in the scrotum or labia (Fig. 69-14). Controlled pressure is maintained in the cuff until the pump is squeezed, transferring fluid from the cuff into the reservoir balloon and permitting bladder emptying to take place. A delay-fill resistor in the control mechanism provides 1 to 2 minutes of lowered intraurethral pressure before automatic refilling of the cuff takes place from the reservoir balloon. Pressure-regulating balloons of various pressure ranges are available, and a 60 to 70 cm $H_2O$ balloon is generally selected for pediatric reconstruction.

Multiple mechanical problems have occurred in patients with the artificial sphincter in place. The most common problems have been fluid leaks from the cuff or tubing kinks requiring surgical revision. The most serious complications are erosion of the sphincter into the urethra or the development of infection around the cuff. The latter problems generally require removal of the device.

It is critical that patients recognize that compliance with a program of regular bladder emptying is essential to avoid the transmission of high intravesical pressures to the upper tracts. Paradoxically, compliance has been worst in children who were rendered incompletely dry with a sphincter. Patients may become discouraged and simply stop opening the sphincter, resulting in a high-pressure bladder with secondary upper-tract damage. Long-term surveillance is critical in patients with a genitourinary sphincter in place, as late changes in the dynamics of the bladder have been reported and silent damage to the upper tracts can follow.

## PROVIDING FOR ALTERNATE CONTINENT URINE DRAINAGE

### Physiologic Considerations

Procedures directed at urethral functional replacement are based on the creation of a tubular conduit of sufficient length that is exposed to external compressive forces, thereby providing outlet resistance that cannot be overcome by intravesical (intrareservoir) pressure. The success of these procedures in terms of continence relies upon attaining controlled reservoir–neourethral balance. Neourethral resistance to reservoir outflow must be sufficient to exceed both resting and intermittently elevated intravesical pressure associated with gravity (upright posture), as well as episodic additive intra-abdominal pressure spikes (coughing, sneezing, straining, and sudden postural changes). The creation of neourethral resistance must be complemented by low intravesical (intra-reservoir) pressure. This may entail bladder augmentation or replacement by bowel, and should include reconfiguration by detubularization. A large capacity is imperative, as is intermittent catheter drainage before the low compliance portion of the reservoir's pressure–volume curve is entered. Because the reconstruction of outlet resistance to permit spontaneous balanced voiding is most difficult, the construction of a neourethra should not be undertaken if spontaneous voiding is anticipated. The patient should, however, be prepared for a possible permanent need for intermittent catheterization.

A transabdominal tube of bladder, bowel, appendix, or ureter with a sufficient length exposed to intra-abdominal pressure may provide continence through hydraulic principles. However, greater success is achieved by supplementation with a valve mechanism, whereby a portion of the neourethral length is exposed to intravesical hydrostatic pressure. Nipple- and flap-valve mechanisms are used most commonly.

A nipple valve is a lumen within a reservoir created by the inversion of a tubular conduit. This most commonly takes the form of ileocecal or ileal–ileal intussusception. The circumferential application of intrareservoir pressure causes luminal collapse and sufficient resistance to prevent egress of urine. This valve is subject to an inherent instability resulting from the fact that the same forces that achieve luminal collapse cause anatomic distraction at the base of the nipple, resulting in valve shortening and, often, eventual incompetence (Fig. 69-15).

The flap valve is also a lumen within a reservoir, but in this instance, all or a portion of the conduit is supported against the inner surface of the wall of the urinary reservoir. Here, intrareservoir pressure collapses the internal lumen and, if the compressed channel is well-anchored to the reservoir wall, additional intrareservoir forces simply add to compression of the channel and are not disruptive to the flap-valve mechanism. This is the mechanism that underlies the normal competence of the ureterovesical junction.

Probably the most important adjunct to the efficiency and longevity of these valvular mechanisms is their exposure to low reservoir pressures. Thus, the creation of a low-pressure reservoir, as reviewed previously, is an essential

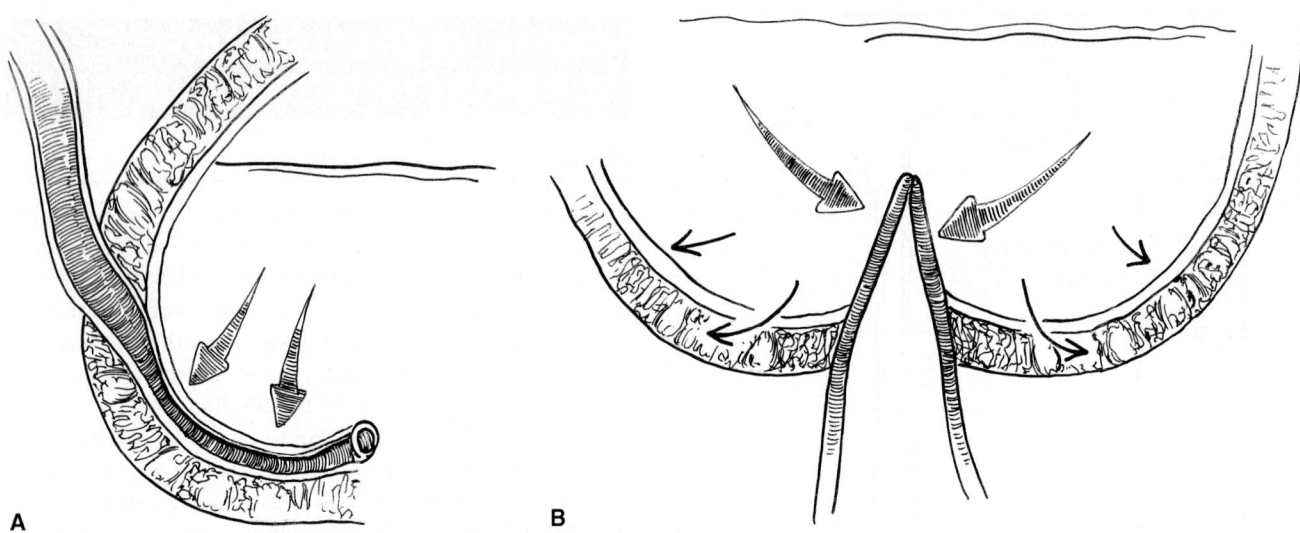

**A** **B**

**FIGURE 69-15** **A.** Flap valves; (**B**) nipple valves. Nipple valves (B) are continent because the nipple is circumferentially compressed by pressure within the reservoir. Unfortunately, the intrareservoir pressure also has a laterally destructive force on the base of the nipple, causing a shortening or total effacement of the valve with loss of the continence mechanism. Flap valves (A) are continent because the submucosal segment is compressed by filling of the reservoir (as for a reimplanted ureter for vesicoureteral reflux). Unlike nipple valves, flap valves are stable because they are fixed to the wall of the reservoir. Thus, reservoir filling does not tend to cause loss of the continence mechanism.

component in the construction of a competent neourethra. Once constructed, these neourethras have the potential for anastomosis to the residual native urethra (if present) or for the creation of a continent anterior abdominal or perineal stoma.

## Mitrofanoff Principle

The Mitrofanoff neourethra is an example of a flap-valve mechanism that is particularly applicable to children. The Mitrofanoff principle can be summarized as consisting of 2 components: (a) a narrow supple conduit is brought to the skin as a catheterizable stoma; and (b) antirefluxing insertion of this conduit into the reservoir provides continence by a flap-valve mechanism (Fig. 69-16). In this procedure, a continent, catheterizable tubular conduit (neourethra) connecting the urinary bladder to the skin is achieved. This provides a 1-way flap-valve mechanism that permits a catheter to be easily passed into the bladder. The flap valve is also a secure mechanism to prevent incontinence.

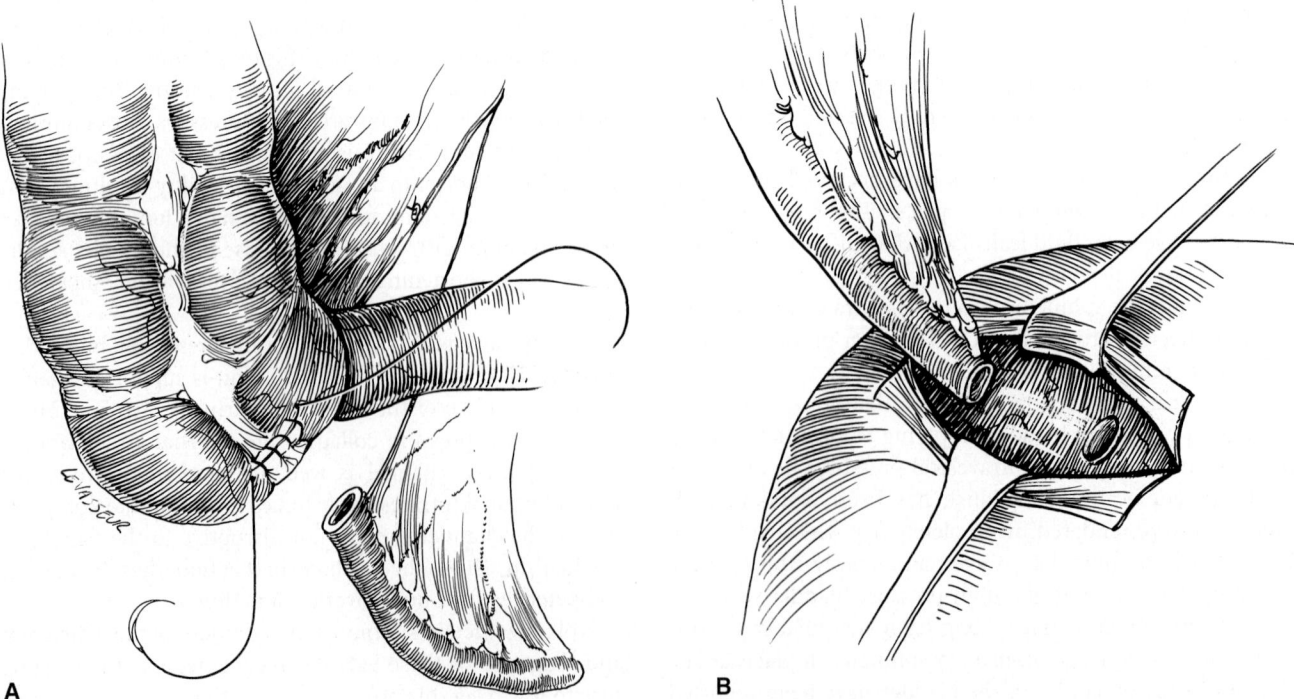

**A** **B**

**FIGURE 69-16** The Mitrofanoff procedure. **A.** Appendix has been mobilized on its mesentery and cecal segment is closed. **B.** Extravesical dissection shows mucosal orifice in which distal end of appendix will be implanted.

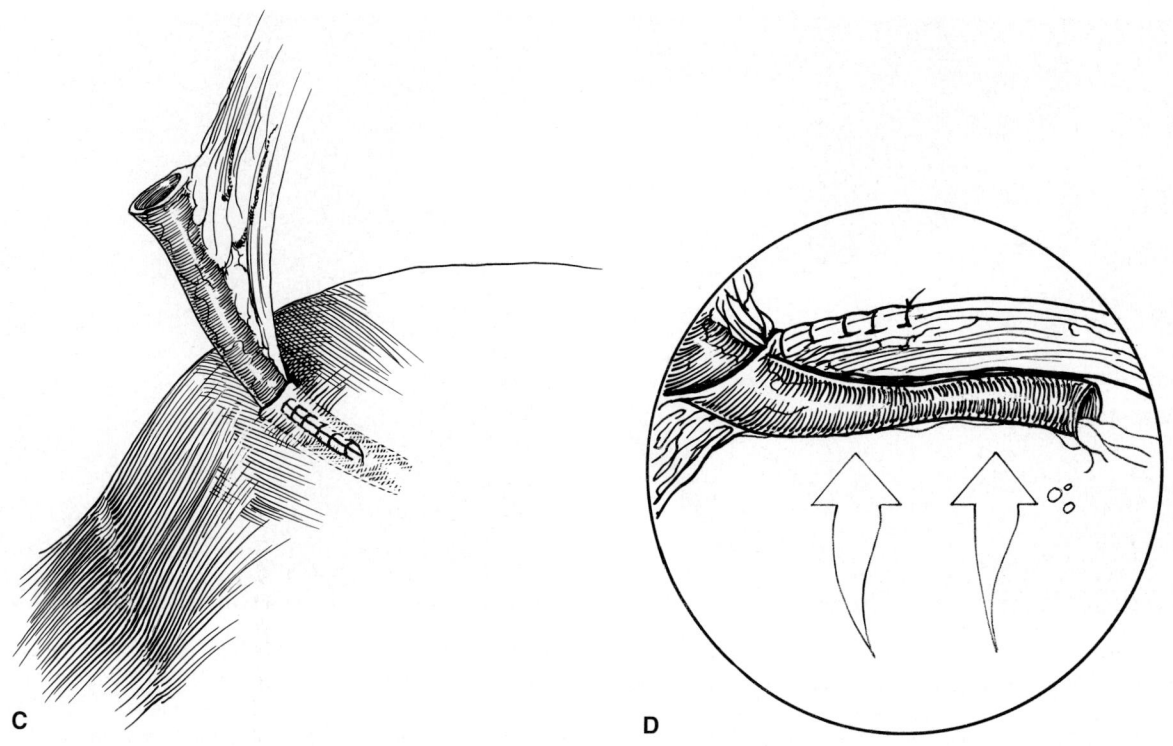

C                                                    D

**FIGURE 69-16** (*Continued*) **C.** Finally, the detrusor is closed over implanted appendix and its proximal end is then brought to skin to serve as catheterizable stoma. **D.** This diagram depicts resulting continent flap-valve mechanism of the Mitrofanoff procedure. Similar to the reimplanted ureter, a rise in intravesical pressure compresses conduit against detrusor, occluding its lumen, and achieving continence.

The appendix, the most common type of Mitrofanoff tube used, is removed from its cecal origin, and the appendiceal mesentery is preserved. A submucosal plane is developed in the bladder by either detrusor incision or cystotomy with creation of a long submucosal tunnel. The cecal end of the Mitrofanoff neourethra is exteriorized to the skin; a U-insertion flap technique is used to help minimize the risk for stomal stenosis. If the appendix is unavailable, a tapered segment of ileum (over a 12- to 14-French catheter) can be used, although, currently, a transverse retubularized segment of ileum is more commonly used. The length of these ileovesicostomies is limited by the circumference of the bowel segment used, which is inadequate in some cases. Casale introduced a technique which allows a doubling in length of the continent conduit. The ureter also provides a source for a Mitrofanoff conduit when available (this conduit can be created if nephrectomy had been or is being done or if a transureteroureterostomy is being performed). Because an ileal conduit is readily constructed, a transureteroureterostomy is not recommended unless otherwise indicated. If the ureteral segment is refluxing, concomitant ureteral reimplantation may be required.

The Mitrofanoff neourethra concept has proven extremely versatile and has been implanted into bladder, colon, and stomach with equal efficiency. The flexibility of this technique is also exemplified by the ability to externalize the Mitrofanoff neourethra at either the anterior abdominal wall (Fig. 69-17), the umbilicus (Fig. 69-18), or the perineum (Fig. 69-19). The versatility of this technique has been enhanced by extending the length of the appendix by using tubularized cecum. The concept of Mitrofanoff and extension of these principles have permitted successful continent reconstruction of the lower urinary tract in a wide variety of situations.

An important potential complication, subsequent to noncompliance with catheterization, is rupture of the urinary reservoir. Patients and families should be strongly cautioned regarding such an eventuality, and this possibility argues for preserving the native urethra as a "pop-off" mechanism, rather than simply dividing the native bladder outlet.

Total urethral replacement in the female and partial urethral replacement in the male is possible by employing cutaneous tubularized pedicle grafts, ureter, and appendix extended with cecum that employs a flap-valve principle.

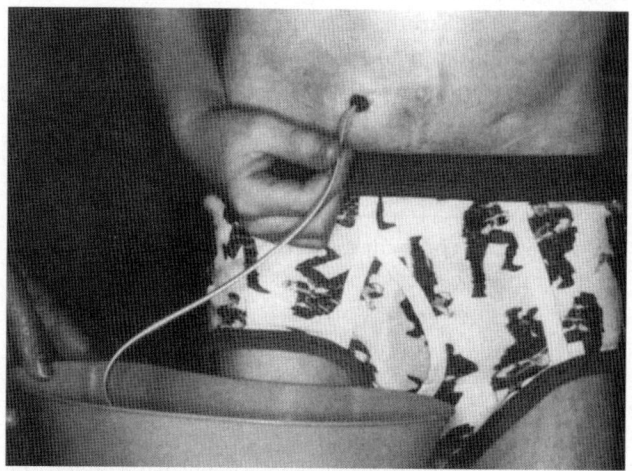

**FIGURE 69-17** Typical Mitrofanoff neourethra with catheter in position. (From Sheldon CA, Gilbert A. Use of the appendix for urethral reconstruction in children with congenital anomalies of the bladder. *Surgery* 1992;112:805–812. Used with permission.)

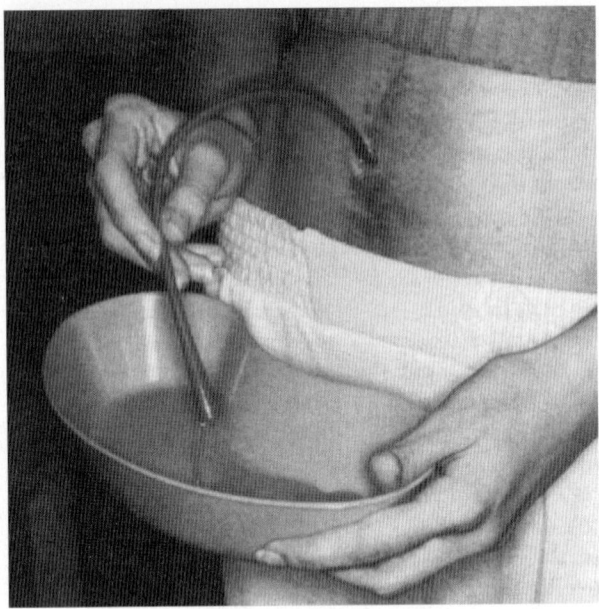

**FIGURE 69-18** Inconspicuous umbilical stoma is easily catheterized by the patient. (From Sheldon CA, Gilbert A. Use of the appendix for urethral reconstruction in children with congenital anomalies of the bladder. *Surgery* 1992;112:805–812. Used with permission.)

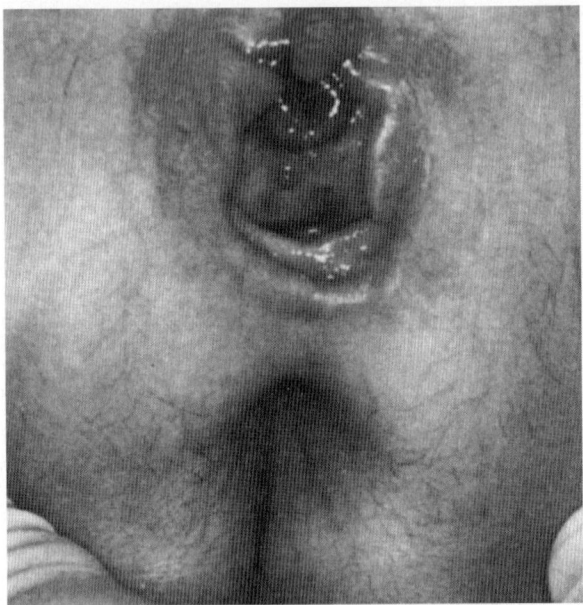

**FIGURE 69-19** Neourethra brought to perineum in the orthotopic position. (From Sheldon CA, Gilbert A. Use of the appendix for urethral reconstruction in children with congenital anomalies of the bladder. *Surgery* 1992;112:805–812. Used with permission.)

Successful replacement of the entire lower urinary tract with substitution of both bladder and urethra is now possible.

## COMPENSATING FOR INADEQUATE URETERAL LENGTH

In reconstructing the urinary tract, the method by which the upper urinary system is connected to the reservoir is of great importance. Owing to the high number of patients who have had continent reconstruction and who require clean intermittent catheterization, the incidence of bacteriuria is high. It seems wise, particularly in children, to protect the upper urinary tract by a nonrefluxing attachment of the ureter or ureteral substitute to the reservoir. When the ureter is short or abnormal, this can pose a considerable challenge; this section reviews a number of techniques that have been used to deal with this problem.

### Nephropexy

Every effort must be made to attach the upper urinary tract to the lower urinary tract without tension. Hendren showed that by wide mobilization of the kidney and ureter as a unit, an additional several centimeters can be obtained in the infant, or up to 2 to 3 inches in an older individual. Meticulous dissection is essential to the success of this technique; all retroperitoneal tissue is swept toward the ureter and kidney, to avoid damaging the segmental blood supply of the ureter. The gonadal vessels may be divided distally and also kept with the ureter, helping to preserve a segmental blood supply. The kidney is mobilized as it would be for a radical nephrectomy and maintains its attachments only through the renal hilus. With this extended mobilization, the kidney can be displaced to some extent in virtually all cases. The lower pole of the kidney is sutured to the psoas muscle with nonabsorbable sutures as low as possible without placing undue tension on the pedicle. As a major increase in length is not achieved with this extensive surgery, it is appropriate to reserve this maneuver for those cases in which some of the techniques to be mentioned below cannot be used and a small amount of further ureteral length is all that is required to ensure a good result.

### Transureteroureterostomy

One of the most useful techniques in urinary tract reconstruction is that of transureteroureterostomy (TUU) (Fig. 69-20). Most reports regarding this technique have been overwhelmingly favorable. In a review of these experiences, several principles essential to the successful execution of a TUU have emerged. Wide exposure is essential and usually should be achieved transabdominally. Wide mobilization of the donor ureter (including the gonadal vessels in some cases) permits a tension-free anastomosis. If the ureter is too short to lie comfortably under the inferior mesenteric artery, then the ureter should be placed above this vessel. The anastomosis should be placed on the medial wall of the recipient ureter and, whenever possible, the latter should be left in situ without mobilization to ensure a better blood supply to the anastomosis area. Spatulation of the donor ureter should ensure a generous anastomosis with the recipient ureter. If the donor ureter is larger than the recipient ureter, it is simply cut straight across. In a TUU, either an internal stent to divert the urine from each kidney or a nephrostomy tube is advisable to avoid extravasation of urine and subsequent fibrosis with wound contracture around the anastomosis. Meticulous attention to technique clearly contributes to the achievement of this goal.

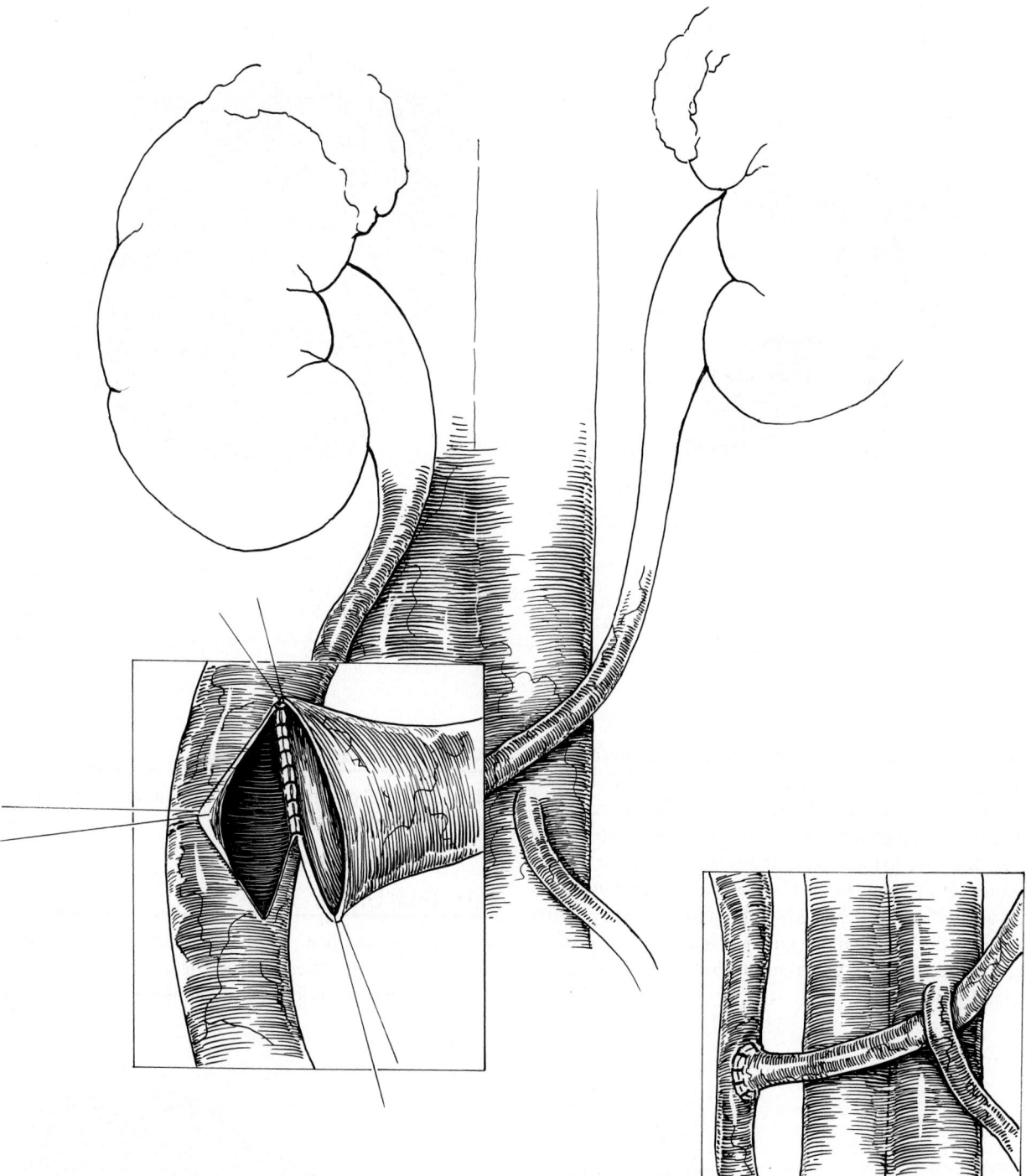

**FIGURE 69-20** Transureteroureterostomy. Meticulous attention to technical detail and avoidance of tension gives a high success rate. Insert demonstrates passage of ureter inferior to the inferior mesenteric artery.

The usefulness of TUU lies primarily in letting one good ureter provide effective drainage for two renal units. One good, long reimplant with a TUU is better than 2 compromised reimplants. In general, the best ureter with the least dilatation should be reimplanted into the bladder.

## Psoas Hitch and Boari Flap

The bladder can often be gently stretched and surgically reshaped to permit ureteral reimplantation. The immobilization of a portion of the bladder by suturing it upward against the psoas fascia above the iliac vessels was popularized to facilitate reimplantation of a shortened ureter and permits replacement of at least the distal third of the ureter without difficulty (Fig. 69-21).

In performing a vesicopsoas hitch, it is useful to open the bladder on the side away from the proposed hitch to permit more bladder to be stretched up toward the psoas muscle. We prefer nonabsorbable sutures placed through a generous bite of the bladder wall but excluding the mucosa. With a little care, injury or entrapment of the genitofemoral nerve can be avoided.

The Boari flap is an extension of the concept of a vesicopsoas hitch. In this procedure, a bladder flap is formed from

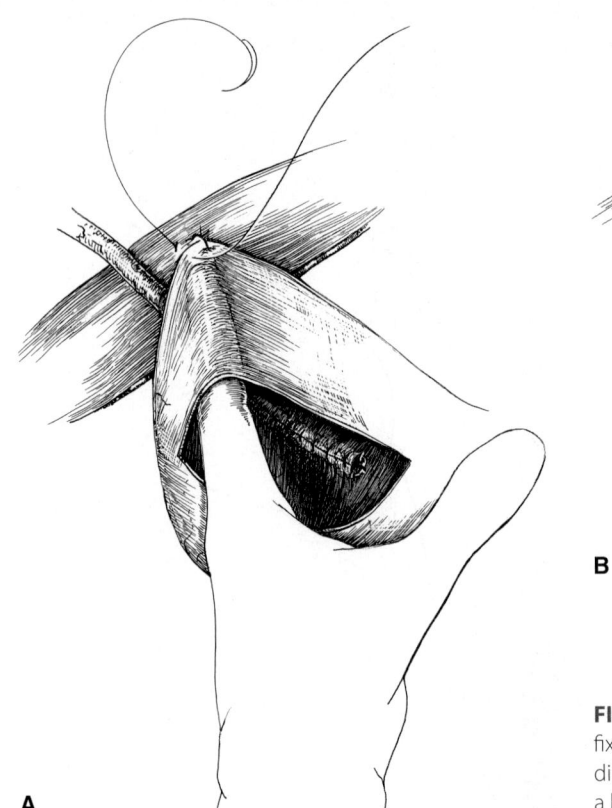

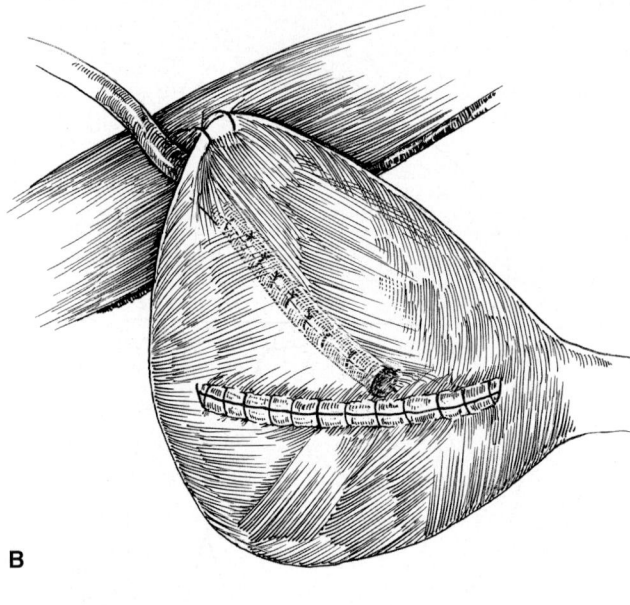

**FIGURE 69-21** Vesicopsoas hitch. **A.** Stretch of the bladder and fixation to psoas muscle permits a good reimplant of a short or dilated ureter. **B.** The Boari flap is an extension of this technique, with a broad flap of detrusor hinged at the bladder dome.

the front wall of the bladder with its hinge at the lateral dome of the bladder, permitting the flap to be rotated upward toward the kidney. By combining this flap with a vesicopsoas hitch, a nearly complete replacement of the ureter can be performed. Essential to the success of this flap is the preservation of a good blood supply to the bladder muscle that constitutes it. It is advisable to fix the length of this muscular flap posteriorly against the muscle of the gutter to maintain its position. After the attachment of the ureter it is tubularized as part of the bladder closure.

## Renal Autotransplantation

Although renal autotransplantation is a relatively rare way of dealing with the short ureter it may be the only approach in certain situations.

## Intestinal Ureter

In recent years, there has been an increased use of small bowel (ileum) for ureteral replacement as part of urinary tract reconstruction in children and young adults (Fig. 69-22). It

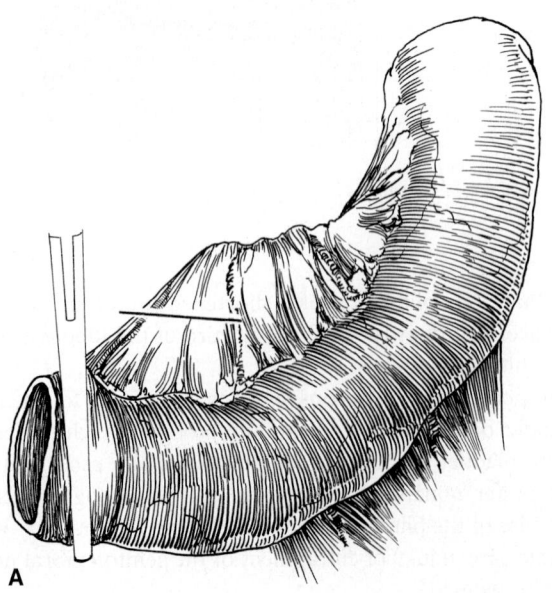

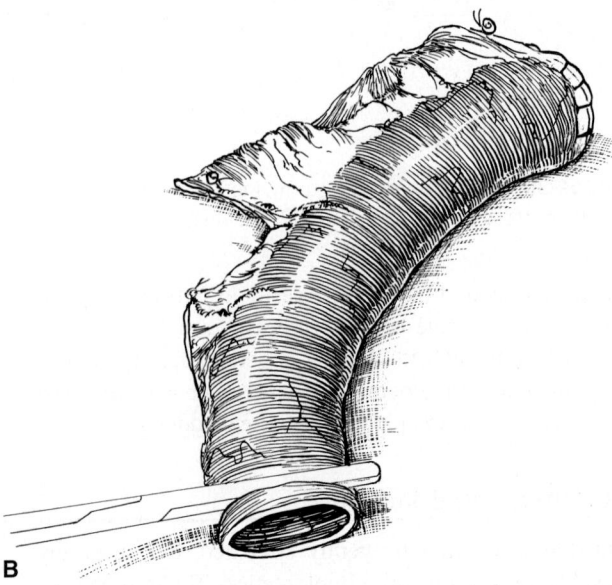

**FIGURE 69-22** Tapered intestinal ureter (A–E): the Hendren technique. Despite meticulous technique, persistent reflux is common and late strictures occur.

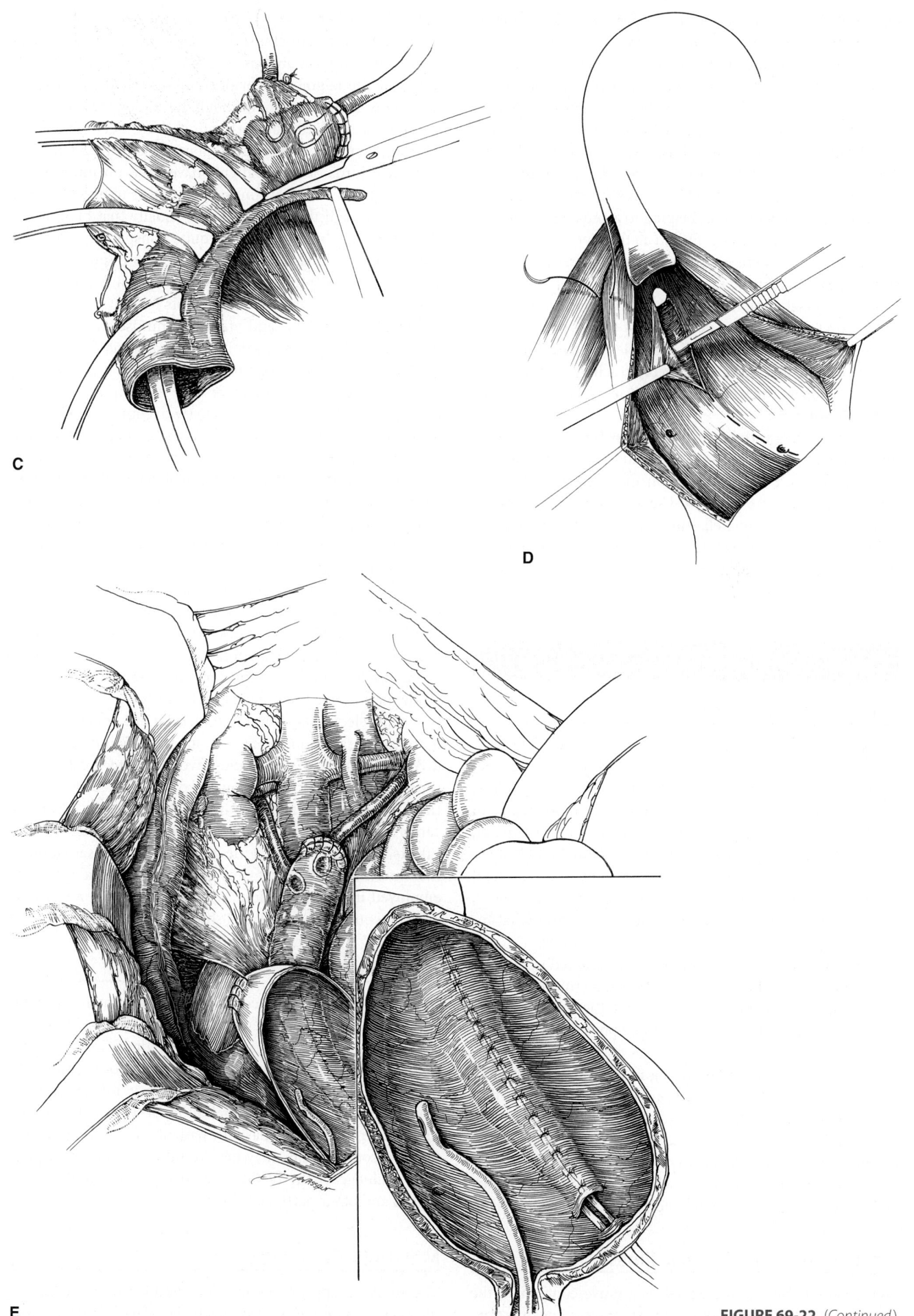

C

D

E

**FIGURE 69-22** (Continued) 875

is critical that the ileal ureter be isoperistaltic. For replacement of the right ureter, the mesentery of the ileum must be rotated 90°. A widely spatulated anastomosis to the renal pelvis or lower-pole infundibulum and a direct anastomosis to the back wall of the bladder near the trigone is usually performed. Distal tapering appears to be important in achieving an antirefluxing anastomosis of the ileal ureter to the bladder. A suitable bladder is, however, critical. The use of the vesicopsoas hitch not only permits a longer submucosal tunnel, but also fixes the new hiatus, helping to avoid angulation and kinking with bladder filling. Even if all these points are meticulously followed, there is a 25% reflux rate after ileal ureter tapering and implanting into the bladder.

An additional complication that is emerging with the use of ileal ureters is the late development of stricture. Perhaps the problem could be avoided if urine sterility could be maintained consistently, but this is difficult to achieve in the reconstructed urinary tract that is emptied by clean intermittent catheterization.

Greater success with bowel ureters may be achieved if they do not require anastomosis to the bladder. Casale et al have had success with the interposition of a bowel segment to bridge a ureteral gap. The bowel segments were not tapered and appeared to drain well. This may be a promising technique when there is a useful distal ureteral segment that cannot be joined to the upper urinary tract by the means covered earlier.

## COMPLICATIONS

### Reconstructive Failure

Reconstructive failure encompasses upper-tract deterioration, failure to store, and/or failure to empty. Upper-tract deterioration may be associated with obstruction, reflux, infection, or inadequate reservoir function. Obstruction of the kidney may be caused by acute angulation of the ureter, ischemic contracture, urolithiasis, or inflammatory changes. The need for resectional ureteral tapering, extensive ureteral mobilization, division of the ureter at more than 1 level, and reconstruction resulting in other than a urothelial-to-urothelial anastomosis appears to enhance this risk.

Ureteral reflux is most commonly encountered because of failure to achieve sufficiently low intravesical (intrareservoir) pressures. Additional risk factors include the employment of nipple valve antireflux techniques as opposed to flap-valve techniques.

Bacteriuria is a common finding in patients who undergo major urinary tract reconstruction. This may supply further evidence for those who argue that, at least in children, an antirefluxing attachment of the upper urinary tract to the reservoir is appropriate. When a symptomatic infection occurs, a careful search for an anatomic obstruction, calculus, reflux, or inadequate reservoir compliance/emptying is appropriate.

### Acute Abdominal Surgical Illness

Acute abdominal surgical illness is a grave concern in the patient who has undergone urinary tract reconstruction,

particularly when associated with bladder augmentation or creation of an intestinal reservoir. The most common causes of an acute surgical abdomen in this setting include perforation of the augmented bladder or intestinal reservoir or small-bowel obstruction. Although the etiology remains conjectural, the majority of perforations have been associated with augmentation of a remnant of neurogenic bladder. More than two-thirds of such patients have been on intermittent catheterization and total continence appears to be a common factor. Although the presentation is usually that of an acute abdomen, the symptoms may be quite nonspecific; therefore, a high index of suspicion is essential. It is important to be aware that the rupture may occur many years after reconstruction. Altered sensation in patients with dysraphic states or spinal cord injury, and steroid administration in renal transplant patients may confound the diagnosis. In establishing the diagnosis, a cystogram is essential, but it is associated with a significant false-negative rate. A computerized axial tomographic study of the abdomen (with contrast in the bladder or reservoir) may be the most accurate method of making the diagnosis. However, any patient with an augmented bladder on intermittent catheterization who has abdominal pain, fever, or vomiting should be presumed to have a bladder perforation unless the symptoms can be conclusively attributed to another etiology. Exploratory laparotomy may be required to make the diagnosis.

Less common, but important, diagnoses in the differential diagnosis include small-bowel obstruction, pseudomembranous enterocolitis, toxic shock syndrome, and ventricular-peritoneal shunt complications.

The performance of a postoperative repeat laparotomy following urinary tract reconstruction is of critical concern. Certainly, elective laparotomy should be preceded by formal bowel preparation in the face of augmentation or continent diversion. The surgeon should have access to a catheter in the bladder to allow insufflation and desufflation for leak identification purposes, and a catheter should be placed in any catheterization conduit, such as a Mitrofanoff neourethra. Efforts must be directed at identification and preservation of mesenteric blood supply to any gastric or intestinal segments employed in reconstruction. Whenever possible, an experienced reconstructive urologist should be present.

### Urolithiasis

In patients with augmented bladders or continent intestinal reservoirs, the development of reservoir or bladder stones (often a number of years after the procedure) is fairly common. The most successful therapies have been found to be extracorporeal shock wave lithotripsy for upper-tract stones and open surgical extraction for reservoir stones. The increased risk of urolithiasis in patients undergoing Mitrofanoff reconstructions may be a result of the loss of dependent drainage of the bladder, resulting in accumulation of mucus and other particulate debris.

### Metabolic Complications

The multiple and potentially devastating metabolic consequences of employing gastrointestinal segments in the urinary tract were recently reviewed. These metabolic derangements are caused by solute flux (both active and passive) between the urine and blood across the gastrointestinal segment wall. The character and severity of such derangements are dependent upon the nature of the segment employed, the absorptive surface area, the dwell time, and the metabolic reserve of the individual patient. Compensatory mechanisms for metabolic changes are provided by the kidneys, liver, and lungs. Significant compromise of function of any of these organ systems may exacerbate an underlying metabolic defect. Syndromes include alterations in the acid–base status, disorders of serum electrolyte composition, hyperammonemia, and bone demineralization.

Systemic acidosis may result from the incorporation of jejunal, ileal, or colonic segments into the urinary tract. Jejunal conduits are associated with hypochloremia, hyponatremia, hyperkalemia, and acidosis in 20% to 40% of instances. In the jejunum, passive diffusion of solutes occurs along their concentration gradients. The passage of hypertonic urine into a jejunal segment will result in a loss of sodium, chloride and water, resulting in hyponatremia, hypochloremia, and volume contraction, with subsequent contraction acidosis. Additionally, diminished renal blood flow results in secondary hyperaldosteronism, resulting in a more hypertonic urine and hyperkalemia. The latter is further aggravated by the potassium shift as a result of acidosis.

The metabolic consequences of interposing ileal and colonic segments within the urinary tract relate to the active secretion of sodium (in exchange for hydrogen) and bicarbonate (in exchange for chloride), as well as the reabsorption of ammonium, hydrogen, and chloride. Ammonium absorption appears to be quantitatively the most important, explaining many of the abnormalities encountered when ileal or colonic segments have an interface with urine. Hydrogen ion, generated from ammonium, is buffered by serum bicarbonate producing water and $CO_2$. The latter is readily eliminated by the lungs, resulting in a chronic compensatory respiratory alkalosis. Additional buffering is provided by bone, resulting in a variable degree of demineralization and secondary hyperparathyroidism. This is manifested by hypercalciuria, hyperphosphaturia, hyperoxaluria, hypocitraturia, hypocalcemia, and hypomagnesemia. Osmotic diuresis and acidosis combine to result in total-body potassium depletion. Of great concern is the recent observation that the conventional measurement of serum electrolytes alone fails to detect many cases of absorptive acidosis.

Ureterosigmoidostomy places the patient at risk for the development of hyperchloremic metabolic acidosis. This is particularly problematic because of the massive surface area and the tendency for prolonged periods between evacuation.

Metabolic alkalosis is a unique complication of gastrocystoplasty. Although uncommon, hypokalemic–hypochloremic metabolic alkalosis has been reported. Excessive bicarbonate absorption is postulated to occur secondary to the combination of mineralocorticoid excess and potassium/chloride depletion.

Hypokalemia, hypocalcemia, and hypomagnesemia are significant potential sequelae of incorporating intestinal segments within the urinary tract. Sufficiently severe hypokalemia that results in muscular paralysis has been reported. While hypocalcemia is rarely severe enough to be symptomatic, it

may present with irritability, tremors, tetany, or coma, and may even prove fatal. Hypomagnesemia is also rarely severe enough to be symptomatic but it may present with altered sensorium, personality changes, delirium, psychosis, weakness, tremors, tetany, or seizures, and may also be fatal.

Hyperammonemia complicating urinary tract reconstruction with intestine may cause altered sensoria and coma. As previously noted, ammonium ions are actively absorbed from intestinal segments and may be present in large amounts in urine because of its generation by renal tubules and production from urea by urea-splitting organisms.

The overriding concern of incorporating intestinal segments is the effect on childhood growth and development. Several studies provide data strongly suggestive of defective linear growth in such cases. This concern is particularly worrisome in those patients with diminished renal function. Here, the metabolic insult is both more likely and more severe because growth and development are often already significantly impaired. Strong evidence exists for a primary effect of incorporating intestinal segments into the urinary tract on bone mineralization. Metabolic acidosis results in defects in bone mineralization, bone disease, and linear growth failure through decreased renal tubular calcium reabsorption, depressed intestinal absorption of calcium and phosphorous, and vitamin D metabolism. Treatment with alkalinating agents has been partially successful in preventing or reversing demineralization disease both experimentally and in patients with urinary intestinal diversion.

## Malignancy

A majority of our understanding of urointestinal malignancy following reconstruction comes from the experience with ureterosigmoidostomy. Although the risk of neoplasia in this population is clearly much greater than in the general population, the exact risk has been somewhat difficult to quantitate. There is a substantial interval between the performance of ureterosigmoidostomy and the presentation of malignancy (Fig. 69-23). The mean interval is 24 years, with malignancy being detected in 69% of patients 15 to 30 years following reconstruction. This latency interval has several important implications; a carcinogenic effect is clearly implied. Moreover, there is a potential for early surveillance diagnosis. Clearly, long-term follow-up is mandatory. Importantly, these data raise a concern as to the risk of malignancy with newer modalities of reconstruction for which follow-up is much shorter.

The incidence of malignancy developing in conduits and continent diversion has been comparably small. Of interest, is the observation that exclusion of urine or feces from the urointestinal anastomosis has a protective influence. Additionally, the placement of an interposed segment of intestine between the urointestinal anastomosis and the fecal stream is protective.

## Hematuria–Dysuria Syndrome

An important complication of bladder reconstruction using stomach is the hematuria–dysuria syndrome. This is a syndrome of severe pain and urinary bleeding caused by

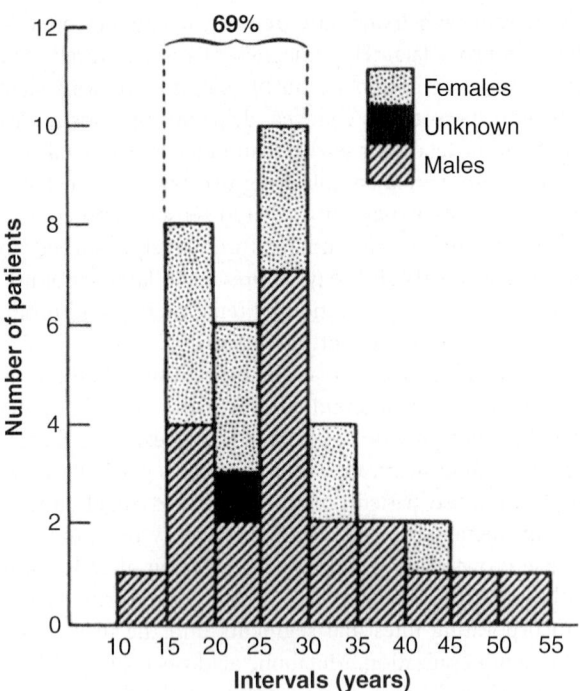

**FIGURE 69-23** Interval between ureterosigmoidostomy and diagnosis of malignancy. (From Sheldon CA, McKinley RD, Hartig PR, Gonzalez R. Carcinoma at the site of ureterosigmoidostomy. *Dis Colon Rectum* 1983;26:58. Used with permission.)

urothelial erosion from acid secreted in the urine following gastrocystoplasty. Endoscopic evaluation of children with the hematuria–dysuria syndrome suggests greater involvement of the urethra than the bladder itself.

Three major factors appear to be of importance in the genesis of this complication: acid hypersecretion, profound oliguria, and bladder-neck incompetency. True acid hypersecretion appears to be quite rare and, presumably, the predominant mechanism for this is hypergastrinemia, which has been reported in some instances.

## Altered Gastrointestinal Function

Finally, the incorporation of intestinal segments into the urinary tract may result in significant alterations in gastrointestinal tract function. Alterations in gastric function have been reported following gastrocystoplasty. Functional alterations reported include weight loss, feeding intolerance, dumping syndrome, delayed gastric emptying, and esophagitis. Our own review of gastrocystoplasty with emphasis on long-term follow-up (minimum follow-up of 5 years) failed to demonstrate any significant incidence of altered gastric function or altered acid base status in 44 consecutive patients. Technical emphasis must be placed on avoiding the vagus nerves, avoiding significant dissection in the region of the gastric pylorus, and avoiding traction-distortion of the angle of His (eg, by a gastrostomy tube) that may predispose to gastroesophageal junction incompetence and reflux. Another theoretical concern is the potential for removing sufficient parietal cell mass to interfere with vitamin $B_{12}$ absorption secondary to decreased intrinsic factor production. Long-term follow-up is necessary to make this determination.

Several potentially important sequalae of intestinal malabsorption may accompany intestinal resection. These include diarrhea, vitamin deficiency, and fecal incontinence. Diarrhea is most frequently caused by alterations in bacterial colonization and impairment of bile acid reabsorption (with or without accompanying steatorrhea).

Malabsorption from ileal resection is directly related to the length of resection. Resections of greater than 100 cm of ileum (adult equivalent) diminish bile acid reabsorption to a degree that cannot be compensated by increased hepatic synthesis. As a result, the bile salt pool is diminished and steatorrhea develops. Another important sequelae of the diminished bile salt pool in this population is cholelithiasis, which, like urolithiasis, is clinically seen at a significantly increased incidence following ileal resection. Diarrhea induced by altered bile acid reabsorption (with or without accompanying steatorrhea) is further enhanced by the rapid emptying of ileal contents into the colon, causing a tendency for osmotic diarrhea.

The ileum is also the sole site of vitamin $B_{12}$ absorption and ileal resection is associated with vitamin $B_{12}$ deficiency. This deficiency is manifested by macrocytic anemia and spinocerebellar degenerative disease, but it may take many years to become manifest because of the body stores of vitamin $B_{12}$.

Although most of the data involve adult patients, it is estimated that 10% of children undergoing resection of ileocecal valve segments will experience chronic diarrhea. This may be resolved after restoring intestinal continuity by returning the ileocecal segment to its normal position within the gastrointestinal tract.

Despite these data, the use of intestinal and gastric segments appears to be extremely well tolerated in most children. It would, however, appear prudent to avoid removal of large segments of ileum or removal of the ileocecal valve for purposes of urinary reconstruction, particularly in those patients already compromised. Such patients would include those with preexisting malabsorption or short-gut syndromes and patients with marginal fecal continence where fecal soilage may become incapacitating by loss of stool consistency. Such patients include those with myelomeningocele and imperforate anus who commonly require urinary tract reconstruction.

## SELECTED READINGS

Adams RC, Vachha B, Samuelson ML, et al. Incidence of new onset metabolic acidosis following enteroplasty for myelomeningocele. *J Urol* 183(1):302–305.

Bauer SB. Long-term efficacy of artificial urinary sphincters in children. *J Urol* 2008;180(2):441.

Cain MP, Dussinger AM, Gitlin J, et al. Updated experience with the Monti catheterizable channel. *Urology* 2008;72(4):782–785.

Dave S, Salle JL. Current status of bladder neck reconstruction. *Curr Opin Urol* 2008;18(4):419–424.

DeFoor W, Minevich E, Reddy P, et al. Bladder calculi after augmentation cystoplasty: risk factors and prevention strategies. *J Urol* 2004; 172(5 Pt 1):1964–1966.

DeFoor W, Minevich E, Reeves D, et al. Gastrocystoplasty: long-term followup. *J Urol* 2003;170(4 Pt 2):1647–1649; discussion 49–50.

DeFoor W, Tackett L, Minevich E, et al. Risk factors for spontaneous bladder perforation after augmentation cystoplasty. *Urology* 2003;62(4): 737–741.

DeFoor WR, Heshmat S, Minevich E, et al. Long-term outcomes of the neobladder in pediatric continent urinary reconstruction. *J Urol* 2009; 181(6):2689–2693; discussion 93–94.

Djakovic N, Wagener N, Adams J, et al. Intestinal reconstruction of the lower urinary tract as a prerequisite for renal transplantation. *BJU Int* 2009;103(11):1555–1560.

Farrugia MK, Malone PS. Educational article: the Mitrofanoff procedure. *J Pediatr Urol* 6(4):330–337.

Hafez AT, McLorie G, Gilday D, et al. Long-term evaluation of metabolic profile and bone mineral density after ileocystoplasty in children. *J Urol* 2003;170(4 Pt 2):1639–1641; discussion 41–42.

Husmann DA, Rathbun SR. Long-term follow-up of enteric bladder augmentations: the risk for malignancy. *J Pediatr Urol* 2008;4(5):381–385; discussion 86.

Johal NS, Hamid R, Aslam Z, et al. Ureterocystoplasty: long-term functional results. *J Urol* 2008;179(6):2373–2375; discussion 76.

Lopez Pereira P, Moreno Valle JA, Espinosa L, et al. Enterocystoplasty in children with neuropathic bladders: long-term follow-up. *J Pediatr Urol* 2008;4(1):27–31.

MacNeily AE, Afshar K, Coleman GU, et al. Autoaugmentation by detrusor myotomy: its lack of effectiveness in the management of congenital neuropathic bladder. *J Urol* 2003;170(4 Pt 2):1643–1646; discussion 46.

Vemulakonda VM, Lendvay TS, Shnorhavorian M, et al. Metastatic adenocarcinoma after augmentation gastrocystoplasty. *J Urol* 2008;179(3):1094–1096; discussion 97.

# Pediatric and Adolescent Gynecology

# CHAPTER 70

*Lesley Breech and Akilah Weber*

## KEY POINTS

1. It is important for pediatric surgeons to collaborate as a team with adolescent gynecologists, pediatric urologists, and endocrinologists for the diagnosis and management of complex gynecologic problems from infancy to late adolescence.

2. Introital masses in infants with urinary symptoms are diagnosed by introital inspection done in either the frogleg or the knee/chest position, the differential diagnosis including aurethral prolapse or a prolapsed ureterocele.

3. Hymenectomy is typically not necessary for mucocolpos in infancy because accumulated fluid will typically spontaneously resorb; however, in menarchal girls with breast development who present with pelvic and abdominal pain with failure to menstruate, hymenectomy is necessary to relieve the hematocolpos behind the obstructing hymen.

4. Labial adhesions/agglutination that also obstruct the free flow of urine are best treated by topical estrogen or corticosteroids for a 4 to 6 week course to induce labial separation.

5. Both simple and complex ovarian cysts diagnosed in utero or in the early neonatal period by ultrasound exam are best observed for 4 to 6 months if they are 5 cm or less in diameter and if they are asymptomatic, with the expected outcome being a complete spontaneous resolution.

6. Ovarian preservation operative technique is the key directive when planning and carrying out excision of ovarian cysts or benign neoplasms, whether by open or laparoscopic technique.

## INTRODUCTION

Only a few decades ago, pediatric and adolescent gynecology was not recognized as a separate and distinct field in medicine; it was often considered a small focus of general gynecology. Since then, however, it has evolved into a growing subspecialty encompassing both medical and surgical management of gynecologic conditions. This development stems from an awareness that pediatric and adolescent females are not "little women" and conditions affecting this population are unique in both presentation and management. Additionally, attention to the reproductive tract is critical to preserve options for future fertility in young females. Although in many cases it was necessary for surgical gynecologic needs to be managed by the pediatric surgeon alone, now such concerns are often managed by a multidisciplinary team that can involve pediatric and adolescent gynecologists, pediatric surgeons, gynecologic oncologists, and urologists. This chapter will discuss the most common conditions that may affect the pediatric and adolescent age group and may present to a practitioner who surgically manages pediatric and adolescent females. We describe the presentation, evaluation, and surgical techniques with an emphasis on fertility sparing treatment options for this population.

## EXTERNAL ANATOMY

As in other areas of medicine, it is important to take a thorough age-appropriate history. Depending on the age of the patient and the nature of the complaint, it may be pertinent to also take a sexual history and inquire about possible abuse. Given that some questions or topics may be uncomfortable for you and the patient, it is important to establish a good rapport initially with the patient and parent to help ease the interaction. While taking the history, it might also be necessary to ask the parent(s)/guardian(s)/accompanying individual(s) to step out of the room so that you may speak to the patient alone. If the patient is menarchal then it is important to always ask the date of her last menstrual period. Additionally it is important to know what type, if any, of birth control she is taking.

The chief complaint will determine the appropriate exam required. If inspection of the vulva is required, it is important to reassure the patient and parent that no instruments will be placed into the vagina (if the patient is not sexually active). It is also important to reassure parents and family members that most vulvar complaints can be evaluated in the office and do not require evaluation under anesthesia. Knowledge

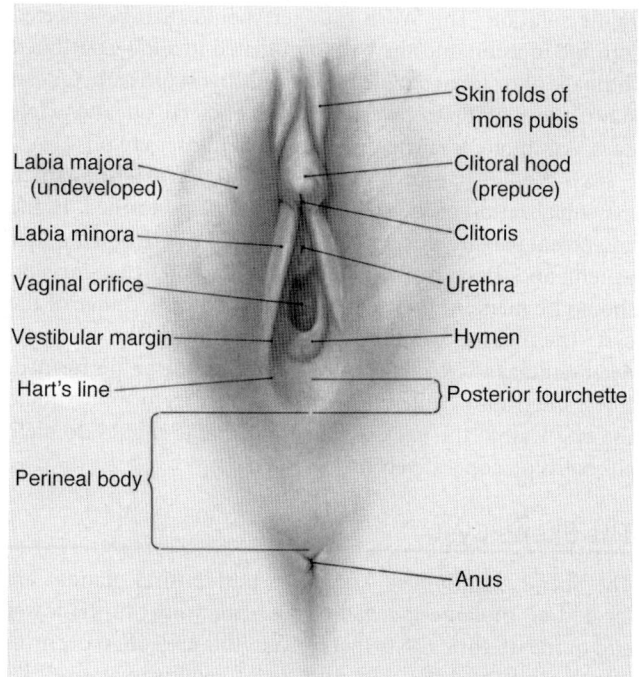

**FIGURE 70-1** Anatomic details of the external genitalia will render a diagnosis in the majority of pediatric gynecologic disorders.

Labels in figure:
- Skin folds of mons pubis
- Clitoral hood (prepuce)
- Clitoris
- Urethra
- Hymen
- Posterior fourchette
- Anus
- Labia majora (undeveloped)
- Labia minora
- Vaginal orifice
- Vestibular margin
- Hart's line
- Perineal body

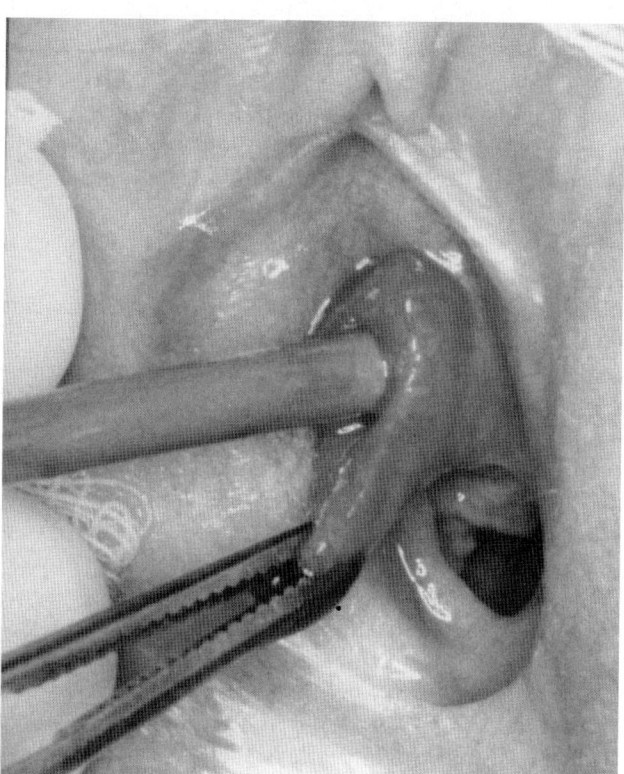

**FIGURE 70-2** Urethral prolapse. Identification of the base of the prolapsed tissue is important. It must be excised entirely or else necrotic tissue will be left in the incision line.

of the female vulva and the distribution of certain conditions can assist in your assessment and diagnosis (Fig. 70-1). The pediatric patient can be placed in the frog leg position for examination of the external genitalia. Gentle downward traction of the labia majora is often all that is required to visualize the hymen and lower vagina. Asking the patient to cough, or making her laugh, will often cause the hymen to gently move and open to confirm patency, if not obvious with labial traction alone. An alternative position is placing the pediatric patient in the knee-chest position. Taking deep breaths in this position also allows visualization of the lower vaginal canal. Adolescent patients can be placed in stirrups to visualize the external anatomy; however, techniques used in pediatric patients can sometimes be useful at this age as well.

## INTROITAL MASSES

The vaginal introitus, that is, the vaginal opening, is the site for the development of various masses in the neonate, child, and adolescent female. Knowledge of the normal female external genitalia is essential for accurate diagnosis and management.

### Urethral Prolapse

Urethral prolapse can occur from evagination of the urethral mucosa in a partial or circumferential fashion. In the former situation it presents as an exophytic periurethral lesion while in the latter situation it resembles a donut or a "small prolapsing cervix" around the urethral meatus. It is distinct from the vagina; however, in some circumstances the vagina cannot be seen. Urethral prolapse occurs more commonly in

Black females, especially if there is history of constipation or forceful coughing. It can present with painless bloody spotting on the underwear or difficulty urinating. Conservative therapy with sitz baths and topical estrogen cream twice a day is usually effective in treating urethral prolapse. The prolapse, particularly if large, may take 4 to 6 weeks to resolve. If the prolapse is recurrent, urethral necrosis develops or urinary retention occurs, then the prolapse should be excised.

When a urethral prolapse is excised, a Foley catheter is placed in the urethra, and the base of the prolapsed tissue is identified and excised by sharp circumferential dissection (Fig. 70-2). It is important to remove all of the necrotic tissue. Using interrupted 4-0 or 5-0 Vicryl to approximate the urethral mucosa to the periurethral mucosa is recommended. This area is quite vascular and hemostasis is important. The foley catheter can be removed and the patient can go home that same day with instructions to do sitz baths and topical estrogen cream for the next 1 to 2 weeks. Activity should be restricted for at least the next 36 hours, with an emphasis on prevention of straddle trauma (such as riding a tricycle on the day of surgery) at the incision site.

### Prolapsed Ureterocele

Prolapsed ureteroceles appear as a purplish congested mass that can often make it difficult to visualize the urethra. Gentle labial traction allows visualization of a normal hymen. The prolapse can cause bladder outlet obstruction or urosepsis, therefore urgent urologic consultation is warranted once the diagnosis is made to allow for prompt surgical intervention.

## The Bartholin Gland Cyst

The Bartholin glands are located in the labia minora at the 4- and 8-o'clock positions. They secrete mucus to provide lubrication for the vagina and when obstruction occurs, a cyst forms. Bartholin gland cysts will usually resolve using conservative management with sitz baths. However, if symptomatic, making a small incision to allow drainage is appropriate.

Usually after puberty, a Bartholin gland cyst can become infected and develop an abscess. The patient will begin to complain of pain and swelling at the site and it may become erythematous. These do not resolve spontaneously and will need to be drained. The area should be cleaned and anesthetized with 1% lidocaine. A stab incision should be made at the site that is most tense. Cultures should be taken of the drainage for *Chlamydia trachomatis* and *Neisseria gonorrhoeae*, since most abscesses develop with the onset of vaginal intercourse. A hemostat clamp, small forceps, or sterile Q-tip should be inserted into the incision to break any septations and adequately drain any loculated area. The incision can be extended slightly but should not exceed the size of a Word catheter. The Word catheter is small and made out of rubber. At its tip is an inflatable balloon, which holds about 3 mL of sterile water. Its purpose is to keep the incision from prematurely closing prior to complete drainage. After complete drainage, the cavity should be irrigated with sterile saline solution. The Word catheter should then be inserted into the incision and the balloon inflated to allow continued drainage of residual purulent material. The Word catheter can stay in place for up to 2 weeks, but will often fall out after a few days. Antibiotic treatment is needed if cultures are positive.

If a Bartholin gland cyst or abscess continues to reoccur, then marsupialization of the cyst wall should be performed. In the adolescent patient, this procedure should be performed under general anesthesia in the operating room. A vertical incision should be made in the vaginal mucosa over the center of the cyst. The incision should be extended through the cyst wall. After drainage is complete, irrigation should be performed. Interrupted absorbable sutures should be used to approximate the cyst wall to the vaginal mucosa. Patients should do daily sitz baths postoperatively for several days.

## The Skene Cyst

The Skene glands (also known as periurethral glands) are located on the anterior wall of the vagina next to the lower end of the urethra. Cysts that form in this area often occur in infancy and appear as a smooth clear to whitish paraurethral mass (Fig. 70-3). Most will resolve within a few months; however, if it is symptomatic or persistent, then surgical intervention with needle drainage or a simple incision is necessary. If the cyst reoccurs after surgical intervention, then marsupialization of the cyst wall should be performed.

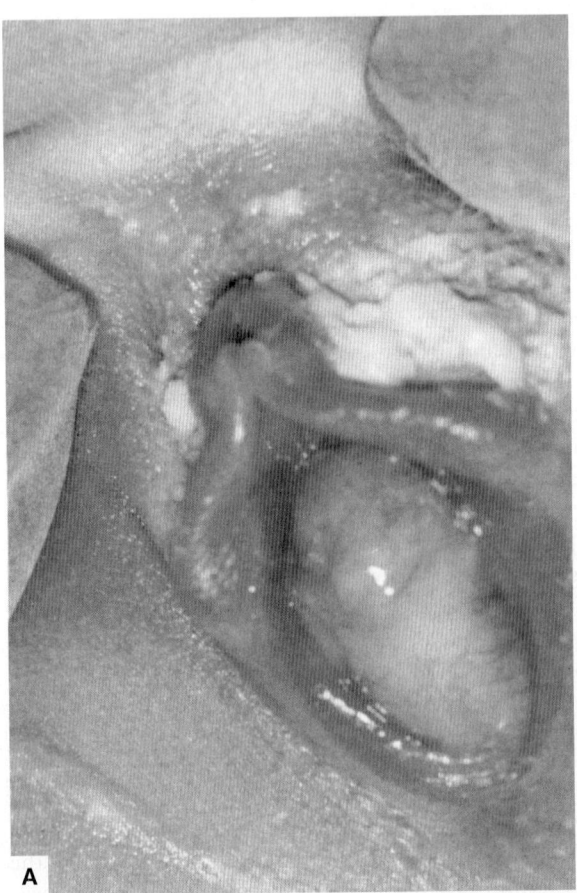
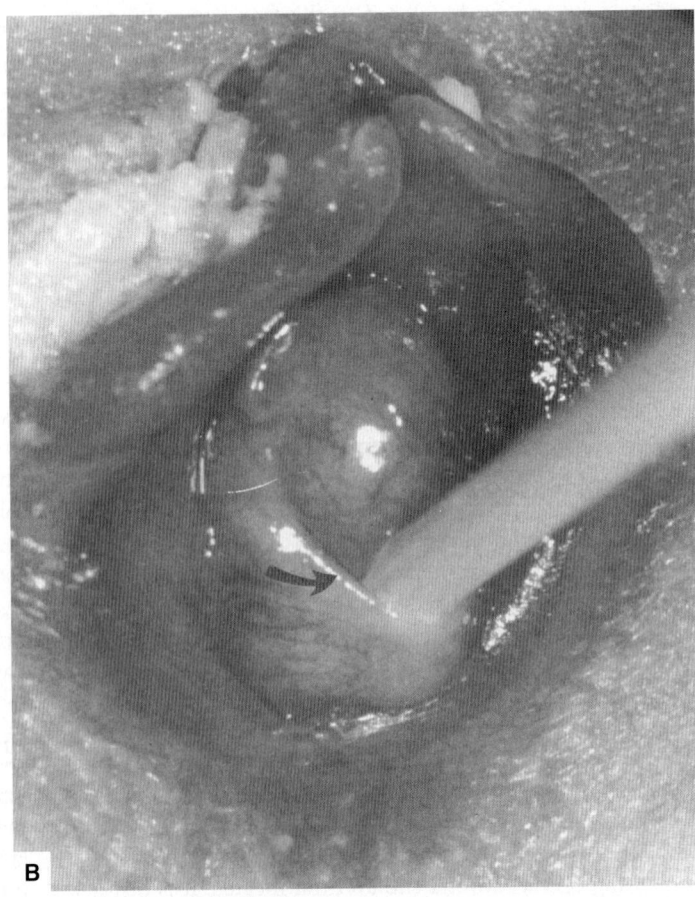

**FIGURE 70-3** **A.** A suburethral cyst in a newborn can be confused with an imperforate hymen. **B.** A small catheter can usually demonstrate the patent hymen stretched thin over the suburethral cyst.

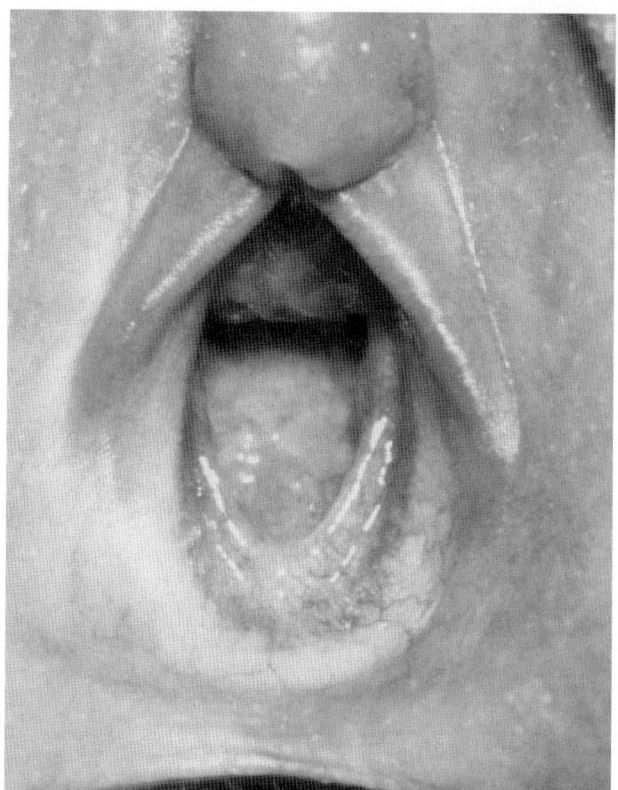

**FIGURE 70-4** Capillaries can be seen on this thin unestrogenized hymen and vestibule. The hymen in this child is of a low posterior rim configuration.

## Other Introital Cysts

Other introital cysts include hymenal and vaginal cysts. These are usually inclusion cysts and will resolve spontaneously over time. If the cyst is symptomatic then it should be marsupialized.

## HYMENAL ABNORMALITIES

The mucosa of the hymen appears as thin, erythematous, capillary-covered mucosa in the young child due to the hypoestrogenic state (Figs. 70-4 and 70-5). During puberty the hymen thickens, the color is pink, and the tissue becomes elastic (Fig. 70-6). It is important for physicians to understand the normal appearance of the hymen based on the presence or absence of estrogen.

The hymen is composed of endoderm from the urogenital sinus epithelium. It separates the vaginal lumen from the urogenital sinus. During embryological development, canalization of the junction between the sinovaginal bulbs and the urogenital sinus establishes a patent hymen. Failed or incomplete canalization results in hymenal abnormalities.

A microperforate hymen occurs when the tissue almost completely covers the vaginal opening. There is usually a very small opening at 12 o'clock below the periurethral tissue (Fig. 70-7). The hymenal tissue in the cribiform hymen covers the entire vaginal opening but has microperforations throughout. In the septate hymen, a band of tissue divides the vaginal opening (Fig. 70-8).

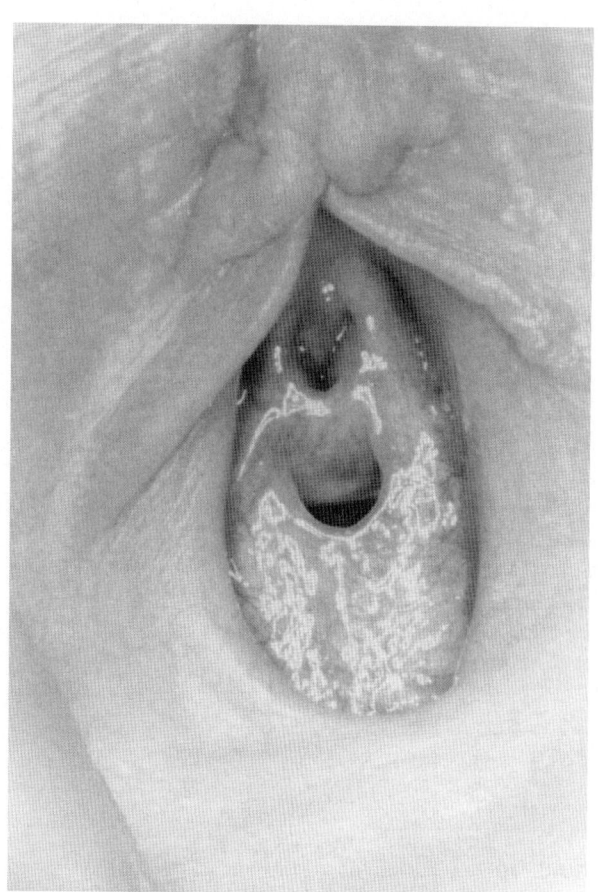

**FIGURE 70-5** A prepubertal child's vulva with a high collar of hymenal tissue. The vaginal orifice is placed anteriorly in the suburethral area.

In all of the above cases, there is no obstruction to menstrual flow; however, tampon use or sexual intercourse may be painful or impossible. If that is the case, surgical intervention is recommended to achieve an adequate hymenal opening. The hymen is exquisitely sensitive; thus significant resection should be performed under general anesthesia.

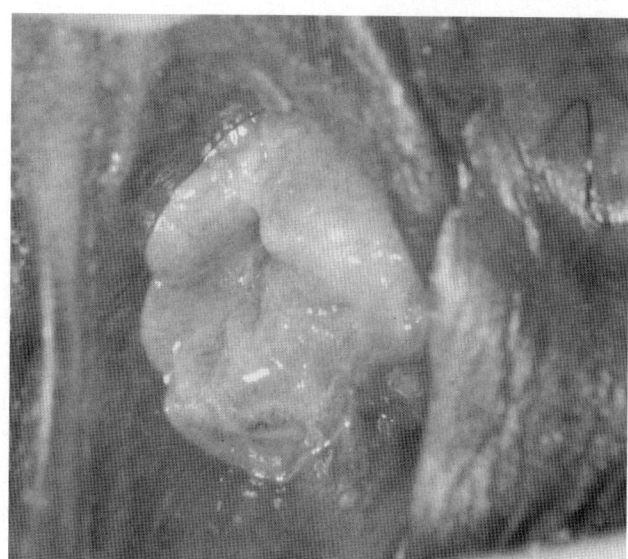

**FIGURE 70-6** This 9 ½-year-old child's hymen is pink covered in white mucous, thickened, and redundant. These are all signs of estrogen stimulation.

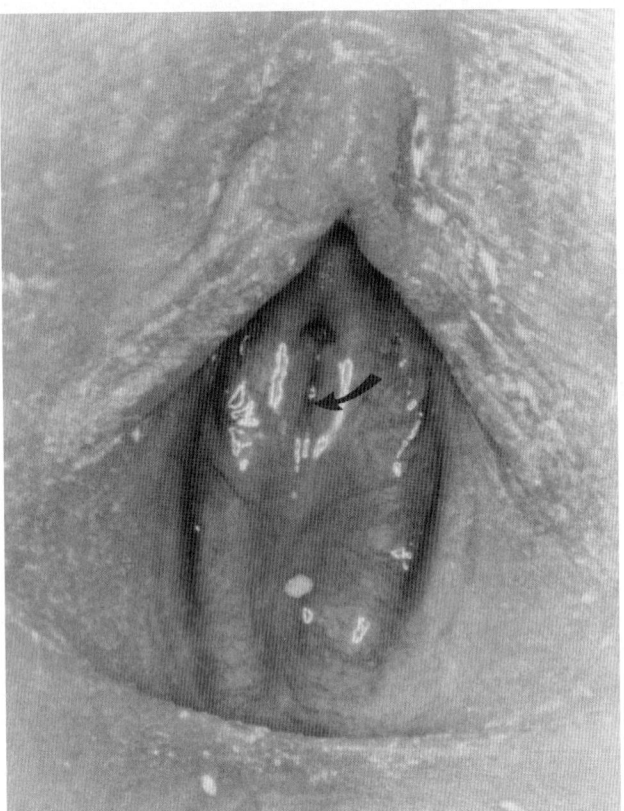

FIGURE 70-7 A microperforate hymen in which the anteriorly placed suburethral orifice precludes direct visualization into the vagina. This is frequently confused with an imperforate hymen in the prepubertal child.

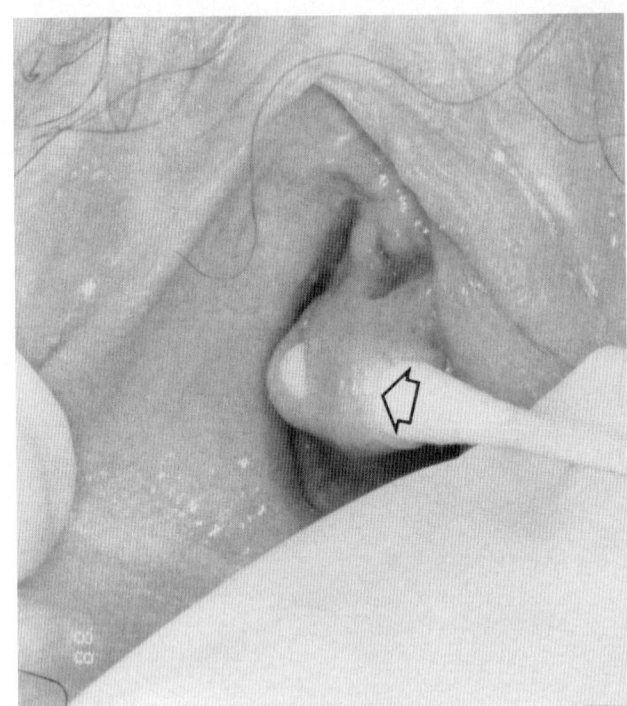

FIGURE 70-8 The septated hymen.

Needle point electrocautery is recommended to resect the redundant tissue. Interrupted absorbable suture should be used to approximate the vaginal mucosa to the hymenal ring. Postoperative care should include use of nonsteroidal anti-inflammatory drugs (NSAIDs) and topical lidocaine gel for the first 24 hours.

An imperforate hymen occurs when canalization of the distal portion of the vaginal plate does not occur, thus leaving a thin membrane that completely covers the entire vaginal opening. This prevents the drainage of mucus and blood. There are 2 time periods when this condition can have important clinical ramifications: shortly after birth and at menarche. Shortly after birth, the hymenal tissue may be visualized bulging from the introitus. Mucus secretion is stimulated by maternal estradiol production and accumulates within the obstructed vagina and creates a mucocolpos. If small, it will resorb over time and the patient can undergo a hymenectomy once she becomes pubertal and begins breast development. However, if this is not recognized prior to onset of menarche, this will again become an issue. Concealed menstrual blood accumulates behind the hymen, causing distension of the vagina along with abdominal and pelvic pain. On exam, one can often see a bluish-colored hymen bulging from the introitus (Fig. 70-9). A pelvic ultrasound will often confirm the presence of hematocolpos. Usually, visualization of a bulging hymen and ultrasound findings of hematocolpos are sufficient to diagnose an imperforate hymen and rule out other causes for hematocolpos (see "Vaginal Abnormalities").

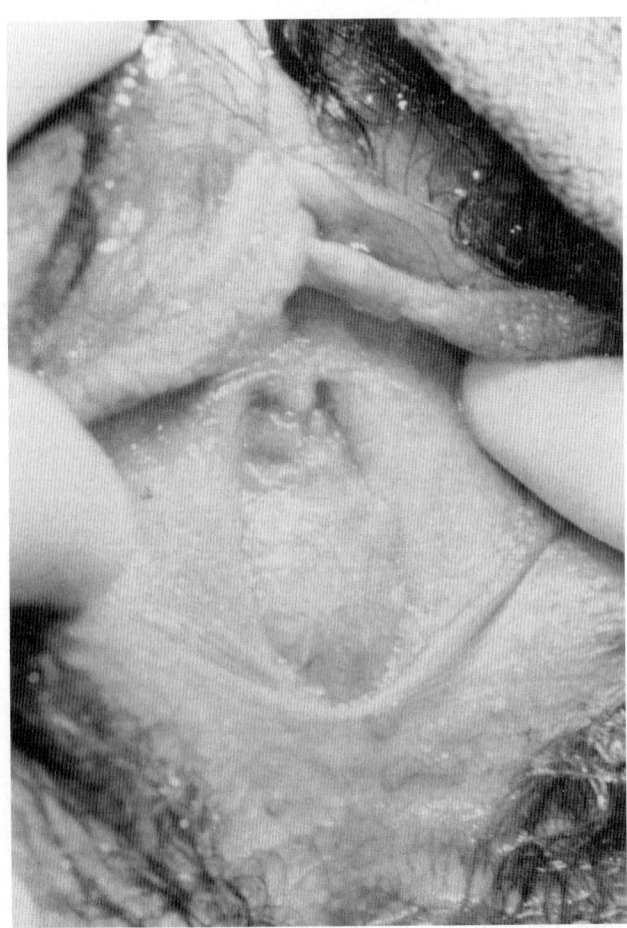

FIGURE 70-9 Imperforate hymen with bulging caused by the associated hematocolpos.

In a menarchal girl, once the diagnosis is made, she should be taken to the OR as soon as possible for evacuation and hymenectomy. In the OR a foley catheter should be placed to avoid injury to the urethra. Needlepoint cautery may be used to make a cruciate incision into the hymenal tissue. The hematocolpos may then be drained, followed by copious irrigation of the vagina. The excess hymenal tissue is then excised, and care is taken not to excise too close to the vaginal mucosa. The vaginal mucosa is then approximated to the hymenal ring using interrupted 4-0 vicryl sutures. The patient can generally be discharged to home the day of surgery with the same postoperative instructions as with other hymenal resection procedures. Continued antibiotics are not mandated; however, they are an option to decrease the risk of an ascending infection into the dilated reproductive tract.

## VULVAR LESIONS

### Lipoma

Lipomas are slow growing, benign tumors of fat cells. In the vulva they are usually less than 3 cm in diameter and rarely transform into a malignant lesion. It is often easy to clinically diagnose a lipoma based on its asymptomatic presentation and its soft consistency. It is rare to find a vulvar lipoma in the newborn. If this occurs, the clinician should look for a possible anorectal malformation (ARM) due to the reported association of perineal lipomas and ARM in newborn females.

If the lipoma is symptomatic, large, or causing emotional distress for the patient and/or family, then it should be excised. Recurrence is not common.

### Vascular Anomalies

Vascular anomalies may occur at any age and are rarely found on the external genitalia. They are generally classified as vascular tumors or vascular malformations. Vascular tumors occur when there is an error in endothelial proliferation. Infantile hemangiomas are the most frequently occurring vascular tumor. Although most infantile hemangiomas regress over time, there is a higher risk of ulceration for those located in the genital area. Additionally, infantile hemangiomas located in the vulvar area have been associated with the SACRAL syndrome (spinal dysraphism, anogenital anomalies, cutaneous anomalies, and renal and urologic anomalies associated with angioma of lumbosacral location) and the PELVIS syndrome (perineal hemangioma, external genitalia malformations, lipomyelomeningocele, vesicorenal abnormalities, imperforate anus, and skin tag). Treatment of vascular tumors should be performed by a specialist.

Vascular malformations are congenital lesions of vascular dysmorphogenesis. These include capillary-lymphaticovenous malformation (ie, the Klippel–Trenaunay syndrome), venous malformation, and lymphatic malformation. These will often grow over time and may cause pain, bleeding and local obstruction. Treatment options include sclerotherapy and resection. Recurrence is common.

### Genital Condyloma

Genital condylomas, also called genital warts, are caused by the human papilloma virus (HPV). Although over 200 types of HPV have been identified, only about 30 types cause anogenital infections. HPV types 6 and 11 are the causative agents for more than 90% of cases of genital condyloma. Although HPV is a sexually transmitted infection, the presence of genital condyloma in children (especially those under the age of 3) in most likely due to vertical transmission during childbirth and not a result of sexual abuse. In adolescent females, the presence of genital condyloma is most likely the result of sexual contact and a thorough evaluation of the vulva, vagina, cervix, and perirectal area should be performed to evaluate for the presence of other condyloma. This is especially important in patients who are immunocompromised (Fig. 70-10).

The majority of patients with genital condyloma from maternal transmission will have regression of their lesions within 5 years. For adolescent females or persistent condyloma in the child, options for removal often depend on the size of the lesion and the age of the patient. In smaller lesions, topical imiquimod cream is FDA approved for use in patients 12 years and older. Although some clinicians may use topical imiquimod is patients younger than 12 years, its safety and efficacy in that age group has yet to be established. Another nonsurgical option is the use of trichloracetic acid, but the caustic nature is too painful for children. For larger lesions and for children, electrocauterization and laser vaporation are the techniques of choice. The goal is to remove only the epidermal layer. If electrocautery is used, the base of the condyloma should be charred, and the char rubbed away with gauze. The resulting wound should not bleed. If bleeding occurs, the destruction of the epidermis is too deep. The key is to remove the major wart load without structural damage; it is advisable to leave some lesions behind if there is danger of scarring. For example, if total excision of lesions at the urethral meatus might result in a deep wound and ultimately stenosis, it would be preferable

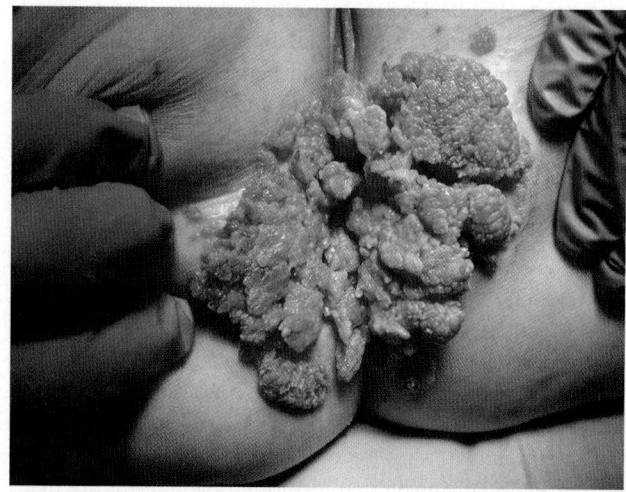

**FIGURE 70-10** An 8-year-old liver transplant patient with diffuse perineal and perianal condylomata. She underwent intraoperative laser treatment and aggressive postoperative wound care.

to leave some residual condylomata. Usually the extensive inflammation caused by removal of lesions in adjacent sites will result in regression of the residual lesion and if not, topical therapy can be used.

## Trauma

Trauma to the vulva is often caused by a straddle-type injury. This occurs when a child straddles an object as she falls, causing injury to the urogenital structures. This injury is usually superficial and rarely involves the hymen. In fact, hymenal and intravaginal trauma should raise suspicion regarding the possibility of abuse. Most do not require surgical intervention, only compression to stop bleeding followed by ice packs and NSAIDs. However, deeper lacerations should be repaired with interrupted absorbable sutures. The extent of the laceration and the age of the child will determine if this should be repaired in the emergency room (with sedation) or in the operating room. A child with an injury around or involving the urethra should be monitored longer to ensure her ability to urinate.

Blunt trauma to any portion of the vulva may cause a hematoma instead of a laceration. The size of a vulvar (or intravaginal) hematoma varies; however, it can become quite large, due to the extensive blood supply of the perineal structures. Such lesions can potentially continue to expand for several hours after the injury, thus continued observation is indicated. If rapid expansion is noted an arterial laceration is probable and therefore surgical exploration is warranted. Otherwise adequate observation, ice packs, and sitz baths are the treatment for nonexpanding vulvar hematomas. If the trauma is to the clitoral area, it is also important to ensure that the patient can void prior to discharge.

## LABIAL LESIONS

### Labial Adhesions

Labial adhesions, or labial agglutination, often initially appear between the ages of 3 months to 6 years and can recur or persist, despite treatment, until puberty. It is normally asymptomatic and an incidental finding. On examination, a thin, membranous line is seen between the labia minora starting at the posterior forchette and extending anteriorly. If the adhesion does not cover the urethra and the patient does not have recurrent urinary tract infections or post void dribbling, then treatment is optional. Reassurance should be provided to the family regarding the high resolution rate with puberty.

However, if the adhesion does extend to the urethra, or the patient is symptomatic, the use of topical estrogen or steroid cream, most commonly betamethasone cream, for 4 to 6 weeks usually results in separation of the adhesions (Fig. 70-11). It is very traumatic to the child to have the agglutinated tissues forcefully separated in an outpatient setting, especially given that resulting raw margins are likely to reagglutinate. Due to similar recurrence rates, even sharp adhesiolysis in the operating room is inferior to medical management.

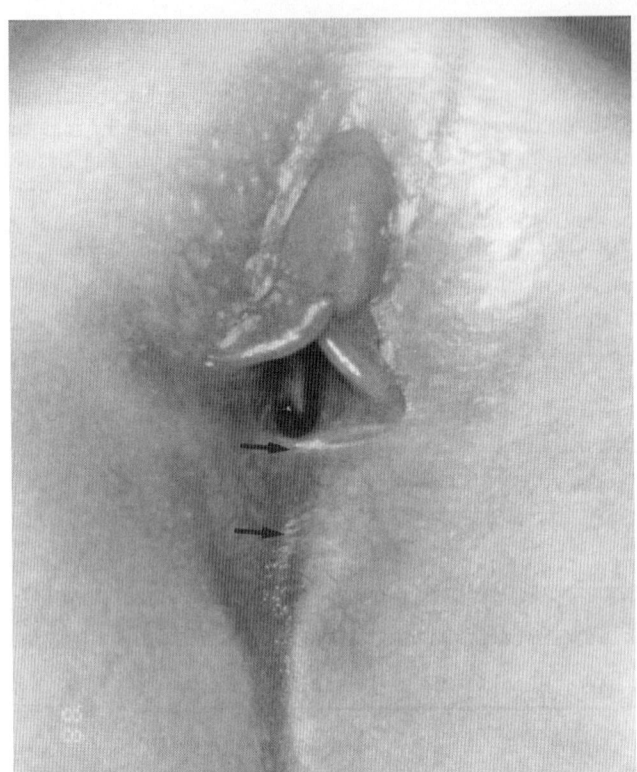

**FIGURE 70-11** Agglutination of the vulva.

### Labial Hypertrophy

Labial enlargement, of one or both of the labia minora, is an increasingly common complaint among adolescent females. The management in the adolescent female is controversial for 2 main reasons. The first is that the physician must distinguish between labial enlargement and labial hypertrophy. Labial enlargement is considered a normal variant in female anatomy and usually does not require surgical intervention. Instead the patient needs reassurance and a discussion on the variations of normal female genitalia; reserving surgical intervention to those who are symptomatic (labial/vulvar pain, swelling, or discomfort). Labial hypertrophy is defined, depending on the source, as labia that both or individually measure 4 to 5 cm in length. Not all patients with true labial hypertrophy will need or want surgical intervention. The second issue is determination of the best time for surgical intervention. Since the labia could continue to grow through the adolescent period of development, any benefit from surgical intervention may be negated, especially if performed early in puberty. In patients who suffer from objective labial hypertrophy with pain, surgical debulking should be delayed until the completion of the majority of pubertal development.

For those labia that are obviously hypertrophic, or those >4 cm in length and symptomatic in a patient who desires surgical intervention, there are 2 main techniques for performing a labioplasty. The first technique is to resect the excess, redundant labial tissue at the distal pigmented border and create symmetric appearing labia. The second technique aims to preserve blood supply and minimize denervation using a W- or V-shaped wedge resection at the base of the hypertrophic labia(s) and re-approximate the remaining tissue, thus retaining the pigmented border. Postoperatively, the edema and pain may be decreased by the use of ice packs for 24 to 36 hours. Patients should wear loose fitting clothing to protect the incision site and labia from friction. Additionally, the area should be kept clean and dry. Finally, prior to any surgical intervention it is imperative that a full discussion regarding risks and benefits be held with the adolescent patient and her family. Both should be fully informed of the potential for recurrence after surgery and future impairment in perineal sensation, especially if there is any concern regarding the elective nature of the procedure.

## INTERNAL ANATOMY

### Vagina

#### Foreign Body

Curiously, history is not as helpful in cases of intravaginal foreign objects as one would think. It is uncommon for a young girl to spontaneously disclose placing an object in her vagina; however, directed questioning, especially regarding a history of foreign body placement in other parts of the body, can be beneficial. Therefore, one should consider a foreign body when a prepubertal girl comes in with the complaint of vaginal spotting and/or persistent vaginal discharge despite treatment. If the foreign body cannot be confirmed by visualization with the application of gentle labial traction, then a generous lavage of the vagina should be the next step. This can be done in the ER or in the office without the need for sedation. If nothing is found after the lavage and the symptoms persist or the initial history is very suspicious for a foreign body, the next step is to perform a vaginoscopy under sedation or general anesthesia (Table 70-1).

In the operating room, the patient should be placed in the lithotomy position with either stirrups or an assistant holding the patient's legs. The cystoscope (usually #7 or 10 French) should be placed into the vagina. The labia majora may be compressed together to prevent evacuation of the fluid administered to distend the vagina. A thorough inspection of the entire vagina is then performed. Vaginal foreign objects should be removed cautiously because the hypoestrogenic environment may increase the likelihood that the object will become embedded into the adjacent vaginal wall(s), causing inflammation and possible formation of granulation tissue. Such inflammatory processes will resolve after removal of the foreign object. Some advocate using a short 2-week course

| TABLE 70-1 | Vaginoscopy |
|---|---|
| 1. Topical or general anesthetic |
| 2. Place endoscope into vagina |
| 3. Allow irrigating fluid to lavage the vagina |
| 4. Apply gentle but firm pressure on the vulva to impede the egress of fluid |
| 5. Identify the cervix at the vaginal apex |
| 6. Slowly remove the endoscope examining the entire vaginal canal |

of estrogen cream topically to help decrease the inflammation; however, intravaginal application is never indicated in a prepubertal girl.

### Trauma

Accidental wounds are usually lateral to the midline and only rarely transect the hymen. When the wound is midline and/or transects the hymen, sexual abuse should be suspected and the child advocacy team should be activated. Injuries that enter the vagina are dangerous because the apex of the vagina can be avulsed and the peritoneal cavity entered, and/or deep pelvic blood vessels can be injured with subsequent intra-abdominal hemorrhage. Patients with vaginal trauma should be evaluated under general anesthesia in the operating room to isolate the site and extent of injury. The laceration should be copiously irrigated prior to repair. A laparoscopy may be required to rule out perforation into the abdominal cavity. If the injury is extensive, vital signs and hematocrit should be monitored postoperatively until both are stable.

### Vaginal Septa

The fallopian tubes, uterus, and upper vagina develop from the Müllerian ducts which fuse and migrate caudally to reach the urogenital sinus. The fusion of the Müllerian ducts with the urogential sinus form the uterovaginal canal. The vaginal plate forms and then elongates. Canalization of the vaginal plate begins caudally and continues in the cephalad direction and creates the lower vagina. Canalization is complete by the 22nd week of gestation. Failure of fusion and/or canalization of the Müllerian ducts and urogenital sinus results in the creation of a vaginal septum.

**Longitudinal Vaginal Septum.** This is perhaps the easiest of the vaginal septa to correct, but may be the most difficult to detect because it usually does not cause obstruction. It is caused by a failure of fusion of the 2 Müllerian ducts into a single vagina and therefore it is commonly associated with duplication of the cervices and uteri. Less commonly, a longitudinal vaginal septum may be present in association with a complete uterine septum through a single uterus. Females with a longitudinal vaginal septum may complain of persistent vaginal bleeding despite tampon use, due to bleeding from the other side. Additionally, they may have difficulty with sexual intercourse. The length of the septum can vary from extending the complete length of the vagina to partial separation at the apex of the vagina. In some cases, 1 side of the septum will be obstructive resulting in hematocolpos and pain after menarche. When this occurs, it is often associated with ipsilateral renal agensis and is referred to as OHVIRA (obstructed hemi-vagina and ipsilateral renal agenesis).

In pubertal females, diagnosis can be made in the office by performing a pelvic exam and visualizing the septum with the speculum or by feeling the septum on the bimanual exam. A pelvic and renal ultrasound should be ordered to evaluate for uterine duplication and renal abnormalities. If there is no obstruction of either hemivagina, then septum resection is elective and should only be performed if it interferes with sexual intercourse, causes difficulty with tampon use, or if removal is desired by the patient. Surgical intervention should be done in the operating room under general anesthesia. Traditionally, the patient is placed in lithotomy position utilizing stirrups to elevate the legs. However, we recommend consideration of placing patient in the prone position with the pelvis elevated for excellent visualization and less restriction for the surgeon. A foley catheter should be placed into the urethra at the beginning of the case. The septum is removed by using electrocautery or harmonic technology to wedge out the septum. At the apex of the vagina, care should be taken to avoid injury to either cervix. When in doubt, it is better to leave a small amount of vaginal septum behind rather than to cause injury to the cervix. Once the septum is removed the vaginal mucosa should be reapproximated using interrupted absorbable sutures.

If one hemivagina is obstructed then timely surgical resection is required. This procedure should be performed shortly after diagnosis and in the operating room under general anesthesia. The patient is placed in lithotomy position and a foley catheter is placed. A large bore angiocath is placed through the center of the vaginal bulge to correctly identify the obstructed hemivagina. Once correct placement is confirmed by aspirating the hematocolpos, the needle point cautery or scalpel is used to make an incision at the site of the angiocath. The edges of the incision should be stabilized with traction sutures while evacuating the hematocolpos. The excess septum should be excised, carefully avoiding extension outside the wall of the vagina. The vaginal mucosa should be reapproximated using interrupted absorbable sutures. Postoperatively, nothing should be placed into the vagina for the next 4 to 6 weeks. Postoperative antibiotic treatment is not required, yet may be beneficial to decrease the risk of an ascending infection and possible endometritis.

**Transverse Vaginal Septum.** A transverse vaginal septum is caused by failure of a portion of the vagina to canalize during development. The presence of a transverse vaginal septum is often discovered after menarche due to the development of hematocolpos. Not uncommonly, the septum may have microperforation(s) which allow for minimal release of menstrual flow. If a transverse vaginal septum is suspected, it is important to request a pelvic MRI to evaluate the thickness and location of the septum and to rule out the diagnosis of vaginal agenesis or segmental vaginal atresia (see "Vaginal Agenesis").

Transverse vaginal septa are classified as low, mid, or upper vaginal in location. Low transverse vaginal septa account for approximately 14% of all transverse septa. On physical exam it may be confused with an imperforate hymen due to the presence of a bulge protruding from the vagina. However, unlike the imperforate hymen, this protrusion does not move with Valsalva maneuvers. Low transverse vaginal septa are the easiest type to correct surgically. The patient should be placed in the lithotomy position under general anesthesia. A large bore angiocath is placed into the center of the septum. Once correct placement is confirmed by aspirating the hematocolpos, the needle point cautery is used to make an incision at the site of the angiocath. The edges of the incision should be grasped with traction sutures while evacuating the hematocolops. The excess septum should be removed, carefully avoiding entry into the lateral wall of the vagina. The upper and lower vaginal mucosa should then be anastomosed using interrupted absorbable sutures.

The incidence of a mid vaginal transverse septum is 40% and on examination a shortened vagina is noted with a bulge felt (but not protruding from the vagina) if hematocolpos is present. Mid vaginal transverse septa are often the most challenging surgically because they can be too high to easily access from the perineum, via a vaginal approach, and too low to easily access abdominally. The traditional positioning for this procedure is to place the patient in the lithotomy position with a foley in place. Once again, a large bore angiocath is placed into the center of the septum. Aspiration of menstrual blood confirms correct placement and confirms the direction of the axis of the vagina. After safely entering and draining the upper vagina, needle point cautery is used to excise the entire septum. The upper and lower vaginal mucosa should then be mobilized and approximated with interrupted delayed absorbable sutures. If the septum is thin and/or the vaginal mucosa is well approximated, without tension, then postoperative vaginal molds are not necessary.

Another option for positioning when surgically managing a mid-vaginal transverse septum is the prone position with the pelvis elevated. A midline incision is made through the perineal body and the dissection is continued until the vagina is reached. An incision is made into the posterior vaginal wall and continued well above the level of the transverse septum. The septum is excised and the upper and lower vaginal mucosa are mobilized and approximated. Careful attention should be paid to the path of the urethra; the use of an indwelling Foley catheter can be quite helpful. The posterior vaginal wall is then closed using interrupted sutures. The perineal body is closed in layers using interrupted absorbable sutures.

A transverse septum in the upper vagina is estimated to occur 46% of the time. It is important to evaluate these patients with an MRI to help differentiate between a high tranvsverse vaginal septum versus cervical atresia (see "Uterine Anomalies"). These anomalies are often too high to safely approach in the lithotomy or prone position. Thus they are often repaired via laparotomy. A Pfannesteal incision should be made approximately 2 cm above the pubic symphysis. Once the fascia and peritoneum are entered, abdominal retractors should be placed to allow good visualization of the pelvis. The bladder is then gently dissected off the uterus and vagina. Placing a Hegar dilator into the vagina will help determine the location of the transverse septum. Needle point cautery is then used to make a longitudinal incision that extends above and below the location of the septum. Once the vagina is entered and the septum is identified it is completely resected. The proximal portion of the lower vagina should also be mobilized to approximate its mucosa edges to the upper vagina. Once again, if the septum was thin and/or the vaginal mucosa is well approximated, without tension, then postoperative vaginal molds are not necessary.

## Vaginal Agenesis

**Distal Vaginal Agenesis.** Distal vaginal agenesis occurs when the lower portion of the vagina does not form from the urogenital sinus. The Müllerian structures (the upper vagina, cervix, and uterus) develop normally. Young women usually present after puberty and complain of cyclical abdominal pain due to accumulating hematocolpos. A pelvic ultrasound is a good first-line imaging technique to determine upper-tract anatomy. A transperineal ultrasound can also be helpful to demonstrate the distance from the perineal skin to the obstructed upper vagina. An MRI may also be considered to rule out cervical dysgenesis, especially if the obstruction is located fairly high in the vagina, and may help determine the thickness of the segment of vaginal agenesis. If the patient presents during the newborn period with a hydrocolpos, consideration of a persistent urogenital sinus is important. A combination of both urine and mucus constitutes the hydrocolpos, which requires persistent drainage until the definitive repair.

In newborns, repair can be delayed until 6 to 12 months of age if there is good continued drainage of the hydrocolpos with the avoidance of hydroureter and hydronephrosis. In young women with an inflamed, painful hematocolpos, many believe the patient should undergo surgical repair as soon as possible. However, it is often advantageous to treat the patient with hormonal suppression to allow a decrease in inflammation, and improve pliability of the native vagina during surgical mobilization. During surgical repair, the patient is placed in the lithotomy position with a foley through the urethra, in the bladder. Careful dissection should be performed in the space between the urethra/bladder and rectum until the upper vagina is reached. The hematocolpos is drained and the vagina is mobilized distally and approximated with interrupted sutures to the introitus. An interposition graft to connect the introitus to the upper vagina may be required if the distance is too far or if the vagina will not reach the introitus.

**Complete Vaginal Agenesis.** Complete vaginal agenesis is also referred to as the Mayer–Rokitansky–Kuster–Hauser syndrome (MRKH) when patients have congenital absence of the organs formed by the Müllerian system (vagina, uterus, cervix). A small percentage of patients, approximately 7% to 10%, will have a normal uterus or a rudimentary uterine horn with a functional endometrium. Unlike patients with androgen insensitivity syndrome, these patients have a normal 46 XX karyotype and have normal ovaries. Therefore, at puberty they will have normal progression of secondary sexual characteristics. Most patients present with primary amenorrhea; however, those with a functional endometrium will develop pain at varying rates depending on the amount of endometrium within the uterine remnant. A renal ultrasound or abdominopelvic MRI should be obtained to evaluate for associated renal anomalies.

If a diagnosis is made in childhood, the most important goal for the pediatric surgeon is to support the creation of a psychological milieu in which a successful neo-vagina can be created after the girl has reached sexual maturity. In spite of the pressure from parents who may want to proceed with correction before the girl reaches her teenage years, they need to understand that both the operative and the nonoperative approaches require that the patient be a full participant and that the rudimentary vaginal dimple will respond most favorably when under the influence of estrogen.

When the patient is ready for creation of a neo-vagina, the American Congress of Obstetricians and Gynecologists (ACOG) recommends vaginal dilation as the first-line therapy for adolescents and young women with vaginal agenesis. The use of vaginal dilators has a success rate that is greater

| TABLE 70-2 | Frank Procedure for Neovagina |
|---|---|
| Best suited for the patient with a vaginal dimple |
| Not appropriate for cloacal anomalies |
| First educate the patient about her own anatomy |
| Use hand-held mirrors and digital exploration |
| Dilators are 3-13 cm long and 2-5 cm wide |
| Start with the shortest and smallest dilator |
| Place steady pressure at a 30° angle posteriorly |
| Pressure should be for 20 minutes, 3 times a day |
| Close supervision and constant encouragement are necessary, especially in the first few weeks |
| A modified bicycle seat has been recommended to facilitate the procedure |
| Sexual intercourse may be attempted at any stage during the therapy if the patient has an understanding sexual partner |

than 90% and avoids any morbidity associated with surgical care (Table 70-2). For patients who fail dilation, there are several surgical techniques for creation of a neo-vagina.

Historically, the method most commonly performed by gynecologists in the United States for creation of a neo-vagina is the modified Abbe–McIndoe procedure. In this procedure a split thickness skin graft is harvested and sutured over a vaginal mold. Usually the graft is taken from the buttock, but other sites have also been used. The patient is placed in the lithotomy position and a space is created between the bladder and the rectum which is continued upward to the peritoneum. The mold, with the graft, is sutured into this space and kept in place by temporarily sewing the labia minora together (Fig. 70-12). The patient is kept in the hospital and on bed rest for 7 days after which the mold is removed and a stent is worn for 3 to 6 months. To prevent stenosis, the patient should continue to wear the vaginal mold, use dilators, or engage in vaginal intercourse.

Buccal mucosa is another option for graft material used to create a neo-vagina. As in the Abbe–McIndoe procedure, the patient is placed in the lithotomy position and a space is created between the bladder and the rectum. The buccal mucosa is then cleaned and the openings to the Stensen duct and parotid gland duct are identified. The graft is then harvested, meshed, and lengthened. It is then sutured into the newly created vaginal space. A rigid vaginal mold is placed for 7 days followed by a larger mold which is kept in place for 3 months. To prevent stenosis, the patient should wear the mold at night or engage in vaginal intercourse.

The Vecchietti procedure uses active traction instead of passive dilation to stretch the native vaginal dimple and create a functional vaginal space within 6 to 9 days. Laparoscopic modifications have increased interest in the use of the technique. A mold, referred to as an "olive," is placed at the vaginal dimple. Sutures attached to the olive are brought through the vesico-rectal space into the peritoneal cavity with needle guidance. Specialized laparoscopic instrumentation is utilized to guide the sutures retroperitoneally until they are pulled out though the abdominal wall at the level of the umbilicus. The sutures are then attached to a traction device

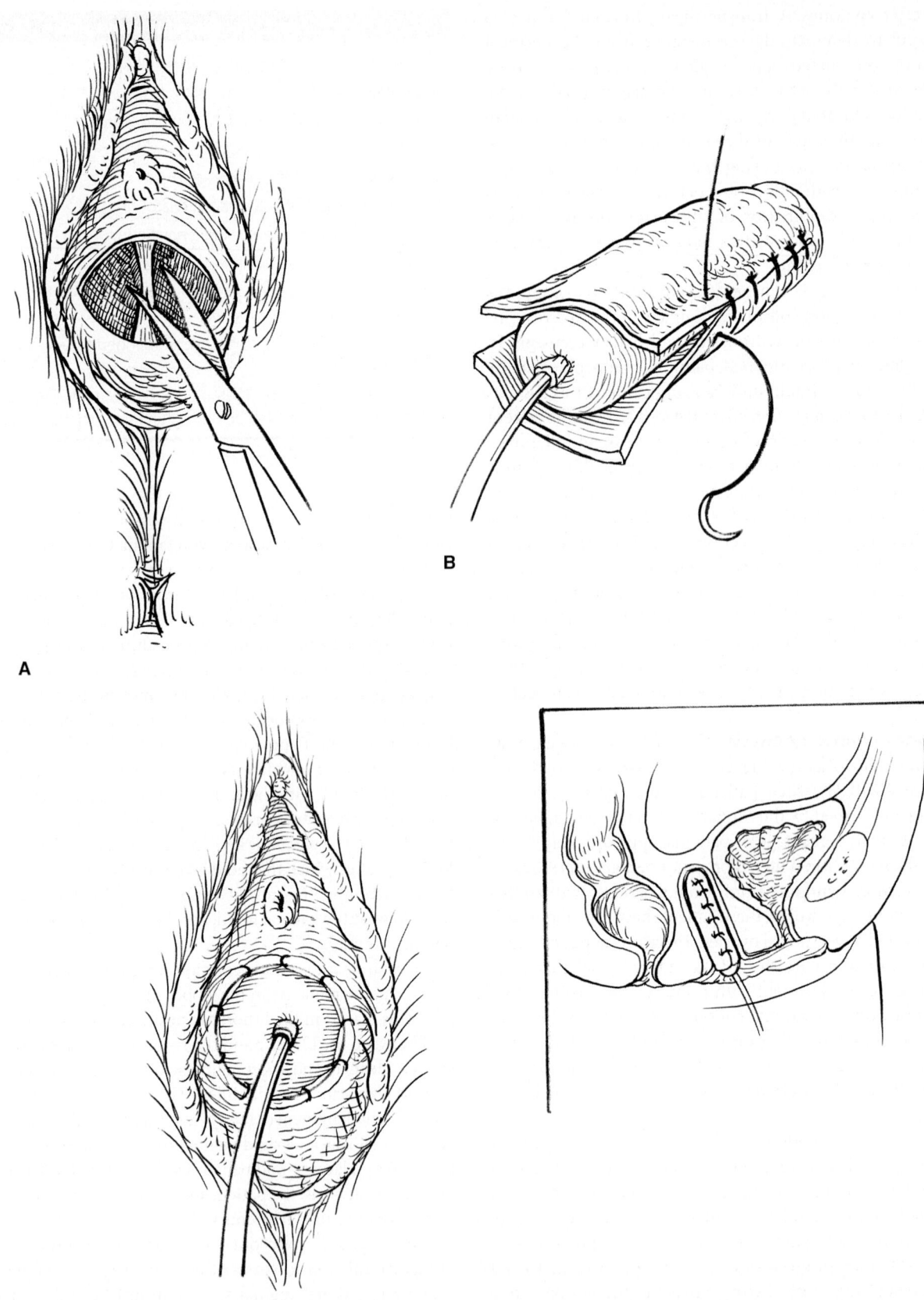

**FIGURE 70-12** Congenital absence of the vagina. **A.** In the McIndoe procedure the midline septum that marks the site of the projected vagina is incised, and a space is bluntly developed between the anterior bladder and the posterior rectum. **B.** An autologous split-thickness skin graft is harvested and sutured over an inflatable silicone rubber stent. **C.** The stent and graft are then inserted into the vesicle-rectal space and secured by suture technique at the introitus.

on the patients' abdomen which is tightened 1.0 to 1.5 cm a day. This traction device applies constant upward traction on the olive which creates the vaginal space. The patient is kept in the hospital for 6 to 9 days after which daily use of the vaginal mold is essential until she is sexually active.

Bowel vaginoplasty is often used for patients with a history of an ARM or a more complex anomaly, but this technique has also been used for patients with MRKH. Sigmoid colon is the most commonly utilized portion of the bowel for vaginoplasty. At least 10 cm of bowel should be mobilized with its vascular pedicle down to the perineum. A space is created between the rectum and the bladder and the bowel neovagina is sutured to the introitus. Most patients do not require vaginal dilation; however, occasionally dilation may be indicated especially in patients who undergo repair many years prior to use of the neovagina for sexual intercourse.

If a patient has a rudimentary Müllerian remnant, it should be removed either laparoscopically or during the laparotomy, if indicated during vaginal reconstruction. If the Müllerian structure appears normal with the potential for function to carry a future pregnancy, then it should be anastomosed to the neovagina to allow for menstrual outflow.

## Malignancy

Clear-cell adenocarcinoma of the vagina has been associated with in utero exposure to DES (diethylstilbestrol). For women exposed in utero to DES, their overall risk for developing clear cell carcinoma of the vagina is 1 out of 1000; giving them a relative risk of 40.7 when compared to the general population. Most cases are diagnosed in the teenage years to mid 20s. However, there are reports of women diagnosed in their 30s and 40s. Initial treatments were quite radical for these very malignant tumors, but more recently, in order to preserve reproductive function, the combination of a wide local incision with retroperitoneal pelvic lymphadenectomy to rule out lymph node metastasis, followed by local radiation, has been reported with good success for small vaginal tumors.

Vaginal rhabdomyosarcoma, also known as Sarcoma Botryoides, is rarely diagnosed after the age of 8. The classic presentation is a young girl who presents with vaginal bleeding and on exam, a grape like lesion is visualized coming from the introitus. Previous treatment for this tumor was a radical surgical procedure, such as pelvic exenteration. Recently, however, either multiagent chemotherapy alone or less radical surgery with adjuvant multiagent chemotherapy±radiation therapy has been just as effective. Follow-up to ensure vaginal patency is essential to ensure adequate menstrual egress in the future.

## Uterus

There are rare indications for surgery of the uterus in the pediatric or adolescent patient. In the younger girl, the uterus is hormonally inert and protected from complications of bleeding seen in menarchal females. Neoplasm and infection are rare as well. Uterine anomalies are often found either incidentally or during evaluation for infertility as young women. Typically uterine anomalies with otherwise normal menstrual function do not require surgical intervention. It is only after documented pregnancy wastage has occurred that most uterine anomalies should be considered for surgical correction. Two anomalous conditions that require surgical correction in adolescents are the rudimentary uterine horn and cervical agenesis.

### Rudimentary Uterine Horn

A rudimentary uterine horn occurs embryologically due to the failure of fusion of the Müllerian ducts in the midline or the failure of 1 side to fully develop. In patients with a fully developed single Müllerian duct located in the midline (unicornuate uterus), the opposite rudimentary horn may be communicating or noncommunicating. Patients with a communicating rudimentary horn are at risk for pregnancy implantation in that horn resulting in pregnancy loss or ectopic pregnancy. Therefore, to decrease such risks, communicating atretic uterine structures should be removed. Additionally, even noncommunicating rudimentary structures that are found to have a functional endometrium will develop hematometra once the patient becomes menarchal. A pelvic ultrasound or an MRI may be helpful in demonstrating the presence of a functional endometrium. If hematometra develops, the rudimentary uterine horn should be removed.

In patients with complex anomalies, such as a cloaca, it is not uncommon to find the Müllerian remnants located on opposite sides of the pelvis. During surgical reconstruction, we recommend antegrade saline perturbation of the fallopian tubes and uterus to assess patency of the Müllerian system. If saline is unable to flow from the fallopian tube through the uterus and out of the cervix, there is a suspicion that the structure is not patent and could develop hematometra once the patient becomes pubertal. At that time, the options are to either remove that Müllerian structure, or to ensure an adequate outflow tract by anastomosing it to the vagina. With retention of Müllerian structures, it is essential to closely monitor the patient with serial pelvic ultrasound after pubertal development. Our recommended guideline is to begin ultrasound surveillance about 6 to 9 months after breast development, signifying ovarian estrogen production, and continuation with at least one after the onset of menarche.

### Cervical Agenesis and Dysgenesis

Cervical anomalies are rare; however, differentiating the diagnosis from others is crucial to provide proper management. A pelvic MRI is essential to help rule out the presence of a high vaginal septum or complete vaginal agenesis. Patients often present with amenorrhea, abdominal pain, and imaging demonstrating hematometra. In patients with cervical agenesis, cervical development is variable with the lower uterine segment terminating abruptly in a peritoneal sleeve. It is often also accompanied by the absence of the upper portion of the vagina. Patients will have variable amounts of cervical development, often requiring intraoperative assessment to determine if reconstruction can safely be performed or if hysterectomy is the safest alternative. Any assessment should be deferred until after puberty when the full extent of growth and development after hormonal stimulation can be determined. Most importantly, surgeons should be prepared for either reconstruction or the possibility of a more definitive intervention, like hysterectomy.

There have been reported cases of sepsis and death in patients with cervical agenesis who underwent connection of the uterine structure to the more developed portion of the native vagina. This is presumed to be due to the increased risk of ascending infections and recurrent obstruction in the absence of a well-developed cervix. It is unknown if this risk is additionally increased by the presence of a neovagina created from a piece of bowel, skin, or another type of tissue. As a result, the traditional surgical treatment has been to perform a hysterectomy. There have, however, been reported cases of successfully using skin and mucosa grafts to create an endocervical tract. Even in our practice, we have anastomosed native vagina and bowel neovagina to a dysgenetic cervix with anecdotal success. We have not experienced any infections; however, most of our patients are not yet menarchal. Due to the controversy in management of these patients, a thorough discussion should be held with the patient and her family about the various options, including the risks and benefits of each, if cervical agenesis/dysgenesis is suspected.

## Ovary

### Ovarian Cyst

Pelvic ultrasound is the best imaging modality to evaluate the female adnexa (ovary and fallopian tube). CT scan is generally reserved for lesions that are highly suspicious for malignancy, with the additional benefit of evaluation of possible nodal and/or metastatic disease.

**Fetus.** Fetal reproductive abnormalities may be detected by ultrasound during routine obstetric exams. Cystic structures are the most common lesions found in this group. Fetal gonadotropins (FSH, LH produced at the pituitary gland) stimulate the development of fetal ovarian cysts before 28 weeks of gestation. Around that time, a negative hypothalamic–pituitary feedback loop develops as a result of a combination of both fetal and maternal hormones and thus, produces decreased levels of fetal gonadotropins during the third trimester of pregnancy. After delivery, there is a high rate of resolution of these cysts during the neonatal period. In addition, since there is such a low risk of antenatal complications, the current recommendation is to observe with serial imaging and avoid aspiration or removal antenatally.

**Neonate and Infant.** After birth and the withdrawal of maternal hormones, an elevation in gonadotropins is seen which persists for the first year or two of life; however, circulating levels of estradiol remain low, and the neonatal response is minimal. Consequently, with time there is a steady decrease of gonadotropins as the hypothalamic–pituitary axis becomes accustomed to the low circulating levels of estradiol.

Cysts during this period are usually unilateral and may be characterized as either simple or complex based on ultrasound characteristics. Both simple and complex cysts have been demonstrated to regress within the first 4 months of life. Therefore, if the patient is asymptomatic and the cyst is less than 5 cm, observation with repeat imaging every 1 to 2 months over a 4 to 6 month period is recommended. If the cyst enlarges or changes in consistency on imaging, the infant becomes symptomatic (poor feeding, failure to thrive, or appears to be in pain), or the cyst persists after the 4 to 6 month observation period, then surgical intervention is warranted. An ovarian-sparing procedure is recommended, attempting to only remove the lesion and retain any possible ovarian tissue for future fertility. The procedure can be performed via laparotomy or laparoscopy, depending on the experience of the surgeon. In all cases, minimizing any spill is essential, since a final diagnosis will not be available intraoperatively. Although most cysts in this age group are benign, performing a fine needle aspiration alone is not favored as it has a high recurrence rate.

**Childhood.** The childhood hormonal milieu is similar to that of the postmenopausal period. This developmental phase is characterized by a low-estrogen state. The ovaries are virtually inactive, and the pituitary secretes less gonadotropin than at any other point in life. As a result, the incidence of cysts is low during this time. They tend to be mostly benign and resolve without surgical intervention. Neoplastic cysts do occur, though less frequently, and of these, mature cystic teratomas are the most common.

Simple cysts are thought to be follicular in nature and tend to be small, unilocular, and thin-walled. They are hormonally inactive and benign. Large cysts (>4 cm) or those that persist or are symptomatic should be surgically removed. The infundibulopelvic ligament is longer in the child, making the risk of torsion more of a concern with larger cysts. The surgical goal is ovarian cystectomy only, with removal of the entire cyst wall and leaving the remaining ovarian tissue intact.

It is necessary to consider alternative diagnoses when an ovarian mass is associated with other symptoms. Signs and symptoms associated with precocious puberty such as rapid growth spurt, early breast development, early pubic or axillary hair growth requires evaluation. The patient should be referred to a pediatric gynecologist or pediatric endocrinologist for hormonal evaluation.

**Pubertal.** Ovarian cysts are very common in this age group due to hormonal stimulation of ovarian follicles. Most are benign and are either follicular cysts, corpus luteal cysts, or hemorrhagic functional cysts. Management of these cysts includes observation of clinical status and repeat imaging in at least 4 to 6 weeks, to allow cyclic changes to occur with some improvement in the ovary. Since these cysts develop from physiologic changes, they usually resolve with time and surgical intervention is only needed if torsion is suspected, the symptoms persist (worsen) or the mass persists. Again, the aim of surgical intervention is removal of the cyst only with preservation of ovarian tissue.

If the patient has a history of an obstructive reproductive anomaly, the presence of an adnexal mass should raise the suspicion of an endometrioma. Otherwise, endometriomas are rare in the adolescent population. An endometrioma should be managed with surgical excision of the entire cyst wall to prevent recurrence. The adolescent should be referred to a gynecologist for hormonal treatment to treat any microscopic disease and suppress the possibility of a recurrent lesion.

If a patient has been sexually active and the adnexal lesion appears complex, one should consider a tubo-ovarian abscess (TOA). These are usually a complication of pelvic inflammatory disease (PID) and can have devastating long-term reproductive consequences if not recognized and treated early. On ultrasound imaging, septations within the lesion are often visualized along with a hyperemic blood flow pattern to the periphery of the mass on Doppler studies. On CT imaging, a multi-loculated, fluid filled cystic area is seen with thickening of the walls. Treatment consists of admission to the hospital with broad-spectrum IV antibiotic therapy. The CDC recommends that IV antibiotic therapy should be continued for 24 hours after improvement if clinical symptoms occur. She can then be discharged to home with oral antibiotics that should continue for a total of 14 days of therapy. If, after 48 to 72 hours, the patient's symptoms or clinical status (persistent high fever, high level of leukocytosis, or the size of the abscess increases) does not improve, surgical intervention may be warranted. Recent literature supports the role of percutaneous drainage as a less invasive approach. In many cases, interventional radiology may be helpful for US or CT guided percutaneous drainage. If unsuccessful or unavailable, then the TOA should be incised and drained with copious irrigation of the abdomen with saline, using a laparoscopic approach, if possible. Surgical care should be performed with hesitation as unilateral salpingo-oophorectomy may be unavoidable depending on the extent of the inflammation and adhesions.

If the radiographic evidence demonstrates multiple loculations with papillations, increased blood flow or a significant solid component, a thorough evaluation for malignancy should be performed (see "Ovarian Malignancy").

## Ovarian Torsion

Torsion of the adnexa (ovary and/or fallopian tube) is a true surgical emergency due to the significant risk to the viability of the ovary. Torsion appears to be more common in the pediatric population because the mesovarian and fallopian tubes are significantly more mobile before descent into the pelvis with puberty. The pain is often acute in nature and can be described as colicky. Venous occlusion occurs initially with persistent arterial perfusion of the tissues leading to edema, distension, and hemorrhage. Eventually the pressure within the ovarian capsule prohibits arterial flow, with resultant hypoxemia. If ovarian torsion is not recognized, the potential for development of necrosis is significant.

In a prepubertal child an enlarged ovarian volume, with accompanying abdominal pain and vomiting is highly suspicious for ovarian torsion. When evaluating a menarchal female, discrepant ovarian volume, abdominopelvic pain, and vomiting are also findings concerning for torsion. In a study of 107 girls with suspected torsion evaluated in the emergency department at our facility, 46 girls were found to have surgically confirmed torsion. None of the menarchal females with an ovarian volume less than 20 mL were torsed. However, the decision to surgically evaluate for torsion should be based both on ultrasound findings of an enlarged ovary and the clinical presentation. Consistent with previous literature, in our review, the most common symptom in both premenarchal and menarchal girls was vomiting. Although many centers have the capability to perform duplex Doppler and color-flow imaging, the presence or absence of flow cannot definitively identify torsion. Any surgical intervention taken should be conservative. Most cysts that incite adnexal torsion

are benign and therefore treatment should be detorsion alone. A follow-up ultrasound is recommended a few months later to ensure resolution of the inciting cyst. If persistent, complex in consistency, or large size, surgical intervention is indicated for treatment. Cystectomy at the time of detorsion is not routinely recommended due to the substantial risk of trauma to the ovarian stroma, if performed in the presence of both hemorrhage and edema.

In patients with recurrent ovarian torsion, a prophylactic oophoropexy should be considered. This is particularly important for patients who have torsion of an otherwise normal ovary, which is reported to occur in 25% of cases in the pediatric population. This can be accomplished laparoscopically by shortening the utero-ovarian ligament or by suturing the ovary to the uterosacral ligament.

## Ovarian Autoamputation

The autoamputated ovary is frequently an incidental finding. A small mobile calcified mass is discovered in a child with an abdominal or pelvic imaging study for some other indication. Such a mass is associated with the absence of an ovary. If identified before the age of 2 years, the mass is more likely to retain some of the cystic nature. In the older child, the cystic fluid is completely absorbed, and the mass is firm and likely calcified. These differing findings in different age groups suggest the most likely mechanism for development is either prenatal or neonatal torsion with subsequent infarction in utero or during the neonatal period. These masses can easily be removed laparoscopically when discovered.

## Ovarian Neoplasms

Ovarian neoplasms are rare in the pediatric population, and account for approximately 1% of all neoplasms in premenarchal girls. They arise from 1 of 3 cell lines: the germinal epithelium covering the urogenital ridge, the stromal components of the urogenital ridge, and the germ cells from the yolk sac. These cell lines produce several types of ovarian neoplasms and the frequency of each is age dependent. Germ cell tumors are the most common ovarian neoplasm in the pediatric and adolescent population, and benign mature teratomas occur most frequently. Patients with an ovarian neoplasm can present with abdominal pain, increasing abdominal girth, nausea, and vomiting (suspect torsion of the neoplasm), or have an asymptomatic abdominopelvic mass incidentally found on routine examination.

Ultrasound is an excellent initial imaging modality. Ultrasound distinguishes among cystic, solid and more complex lesions. Important findings include a thickened wall, internal debris, visible fluid levels, and mural nodules. Malignant tumors may contain cystic areas; however, more commonly they have solid components with evidence of necrosis on pathologic analysis. Coarse calcification, teeth, bone, or calcified cartilage are seen in malignant or benign teratomas, whereas stippled calcifications have been associated with dysgerminomas. For malignant metastatic disease, CT or MRI is superior in demonstrating the extent of the tumor.

Some ovarian neoplasms produce markers that can be measured and evaluated from serum samples. These markers are helpful in determining the risk of malignancy; thereby influencing surgical planning, including the approach and the

| TABLE 70-3 | Laboratory "Markers" for Ovarian Neoplasms |
|---|---|
| **Tumor Marker** | **Ovarian Neoplasm** |
| CA-125 | Epithelial |
| Alpha feto-protein | Endodermal sinus tumor |
| | Mixed germ cell |
| | Immature teratoma |
| HCG | Dysgerminoma |
| | Choriocarcinoma |
| | Placental site tumor |
| | Embryonal carcinoma |
| Inhibin | Granulosa theca-cell |
| Mullerian-inhibiting substance (MIS) | Granulosa theca-cell |
| LDH | Dysgerminoma |
| | Mixed germ cell |
| Estradiol | Granulosa cell |
| Testosterone | Sertoli–Leydig tumor |
| Carcinoembryonic antigen (CEA) | Epithelial |
| | Germ cell |

surgical team present. CA-125 is a marker for epithelial ovarian cancer, however, it is relatively nonspecific with an elevation with other intraperitoneal processes such as the Crohn's disease, endometriosis, and PID. Alpha-fetoprotein (AFP) is produced by endodermal sinus tumors (ESTs), mixed germ cell tumors, and immature teratomas. Human chorionic gonadotropin (HCG) can be elevated in patients with a dysgerminoma, but is more often elevated in patients with choriocarcinoma, placental site tumors, and embryonal carcinomas. Inhibin and Müllerian inhibiting substance (MIS) are elevated in association with granulosa-theca cell tumors. Lactate dehydrogenase (LDH) is elevated in patients with a dysgerminoma or a mixed germ cell tumor. Estradiol levels are high in patients with granulosa cell tumors and testosterone is elevated in Sertoli–Leydig tumors. Carcinoembryonic antigen (CEA) is produced by both epithelial and germ cell tumors (Table 70-3).

Staging of ovarian cancer is based on the Federation of International Gynecologic Oncologists (FIGO) and is based on surgical findings (Table 70-4). If preoperative suspicion of a malignancy is high, the surgeon should strongly consider collaborating with a surgical oncologist or at least assure that the surgical procedure performed is in accordance with recommended guidelines from the Children's Oncology Group. For potential ovarian malignancies, a vertical abdominal incision should be made in the event that metastatic disease is present and para-aortic lymph node sampling is required. Prior to any significant surgical intervention, peritoneal washings should be obtained from the pelvis and right and left paracolic gutters for cytologic analysis. The remainder of the surgical procedure is dictated by

| TABLE 70-4 | FIGO Staging Classification for Ovarian Cancer | |
|---|---|---|
| **FIGO Stages** | | **TNM Categories** |
| | Primary tumor cannot be assessed | TX |
| | No evidence of primary tumor | T0 |
| I | Tumor limited to the ovaries | T1 |
| IA | Tumor limited to one ovary; capsule intact, no tumor on ovarian surface; no malignant cells in ascites or peritoneal washings | T1a |
| IB | Tumor limited to both ovaries; capsule intact, no tumor on ovarian surface; no malignant cells in ascites or peritoneal washings | T1b |
| IC | Tumor limited to one or both ovaries with any of the following: capsule ruptured, tumor on ovarian surface, malignant cells in ascites or peritoneal washings | T1c |
| II | Tumor involves one or both ovaries with pelvic extension | T2 |
| IIA | Extension and/or implants on uterus and/or tube(s); no malignant cells in ascites or peritoneal washings | T2a |
| IIB | Extension to other pelvic tissues; no malignant cells in ascites or peritoneal washings | T2b |
| IIC | Pelvic extension (IIA or IIB) with malignant cells in ascites or peritoneal washings | T2c |
| III | Tumor involves one or both ovaries with microscopically confirmed peritoneal metastasis outside the pelvis and/or regional lymph node metastasis | T3 and/or N1 |
| IIIA | Microscopic peritoneal metastasis beyond pelvis | T3a |
| IIIB | Macroscopic peritoneal metastasis beyond pelvis 2 cm or less in greatest dimension | T3b |
| IIIC | Peritoneal metastasis beyond pelvis more than 2 cm in greatest dimension and/or regional lymph node metastasis | T3c and/or N1 |
| IV | Distant metastasis (excludes peritoneal metastasis) | M1 |

*Note:* Liver capsule metastasis is T3/Stage III, liver parenchymal metastasis M1/Stage IV. Pleural effusion must have positive cytology for M1/Stage IV.

| TABLE 70-5 | World Health Organization Classification of Neoplastic Ovarian Tumors |
|---|---|

I. Common "epithelial" tumors
  A. Serous[a]
  B. Mucinous[a]
  C. Endometrioid[a]
  D. Clear cell[a]
  E. Brenner[a]
  F. Mixed epithelial
  G. Undifferentiated
  H. Mixed mesodermal tumors
  I. Unclassified

II. Sex cord stromal tumors
  A. Granulosa stromal cell
    1. Granulosa cell
    2. Thecoma-fibroma
  B. Androblastomas; Sertoli–Leydig cell tumors
    1. Well-differentiated (Pick adenoma, Sertoli cell tumor)
    2. Intermediate differentiation
    3. Poorly differentiated
    4. With heterologous elements
  C. Lipid cell tumors
  D. Gynandroblastoma
  E. Unclassified

III. Germ cell tumors
  A. Dysgerminoma
  B. Endodermal sinus tumor
  C. Embryonal carcinoma
  D. Polyembryoma
  E. Choriocarcinoma
  F. Teratomas
    1. Immature
    2. Mature (dermoid cyst)
    3. Monodermal (struma ovarii, carcinoid)
  G. Mixed forms
  H. Gonadoblastoma

IV. Soft tissue tumors not specific to the ovary

V. Unclassified tumors

VI. Secondary (metastatic) tumors

VII. Tumor-like conditions (eg, pregnancy luteoma)

[a]Benign, borderline, or malignant.

the type of ovarian neoplasm present and the extent of the disease process.

**Types of Tumors.** This section will discuss the most common ovarian neoplasm in each of the 3 main types of ovarian neoplasms seen in the pediatric and adolescent population. For a complete list of the types of ovarian neoplasms, please see Table 70-5.

**Germ Cell Tumor.** As previously described, germ cell tumors are the most common ovarian neoplasm in childhood and adolescence. The vast majority are benign, however, germ cell tumors account for approximately two-thirds of malignant tumors in children and about 60% of ovarian neoplasms in girls under the age of 20.

**Teratoma.** Teratomas are neoplasms that contain tissue that is foreign to the anatomic site or organ that is affected. These tumors are composed of ectodermal, mesodermal, and endodermal elements and arise from totipotential primordial germ cells. There are various levels of maturation and as a result, teratomas are divided into 2 groups.

*Mature Teratoma.* Mature teratomas, also known as benign cystic teratoma or simply a dermoid cyst, is the most common type of germ cell tumor. In children, they can be bilateral in up to 10% of cases. Presentation may include acute symptoms (from torsion, hemorrhage, or rupture) or chronic complaints. Not uncommonly, the patient is asymptomatic and the dermoid is an incidental finding identified on imaging for another indication, that is, renal, bladder ultrasound for reflux or spine films for scoliosis. An ultrasound may show the "tip of the iceberg" sign, which consists of cystic and solid echoes with areas of acoustic shadowing that obscure the back of the cyst wall. Plain abdominal films may demonstrate calcifications.

Dermoid cysts will not resolve spontaneously and therefore surgical intervention is necessary. Treatment includes removal of the entire lesion while preserving as much ovarian tissue as possible. Careful enucleation of the cyst is recommended. Aspiration of the cyst should be avoided due to the uncertainty of malignancy and the risk of peritoneal irritation with spillage of even benign cyst fluid. In cases of a presumed mature teratoma, the choice of surgical approach, laparoscopically versus laparotomy, remains unclear. Historically, a small laparotomy approach has been recommended to decrease the risk of spillage of the cyst fluid which can cause a chemical peritonitis, adhesion formation, and subsequent infertility. However, more recent literature regarding the safety of laparoscopy for this indication supports consideration of this technique, especially in cases with a small, more simple appearing mass with normal tumor markers. Regardless of the technique, if spillage occurs, copious irrigation of the abdomen and pelvis should be performed as soon as the mass has been removed from the abdominal cavity. When deciding on an approach, consideration should be given to surgeon experience with laparoscopic ovarian cystectomy (in lieu of aspiration), as this has been associated with less spillage, shorter operating room time, and a more complete resection.

*Immature Teratoma.* Immature teratomas are more common in younger patients. They can be highly malignant and AFP may serve as a marker. The AFP levels may also be elevated in patients with mixed germ cell tumors, which contain components of both an immature teratoma and other germ cell tumors. The surgical staging for an immature teratoma should include unilateral pelvic and para-aortic lymph node sampling and a distal omentectomy. Immature teratomas are graded based on a histologic grading system and the most important component for grading is the neural component.

Although in the past these patients were often given chemotherapy postoperatively, current recommendation from the Children's Oncology Group supports using chemotherapy only in those patients who have relapsed. Additionally, second-look surgery is rarely required.

**Dysgerminoma.** Dysgerminomas are malignant neoplasms arising from primordial, sexually undifferentiated germ cells. They are the most common ovarian malignancy in the female adolescent and account for 50% of all ovarian germ cell malignancies. It is less common prior to menarche. Presentation may include abdominal/pelvic pain, or symptoms of pelvic pressure as these are large, bulky tumors. Torsion, hemorrhage, and rupture may also occur secondary to the size of the tumor. Most patients have Stage I disease and therefore only require surgical therapy without the need for adjuvant chemotherapy. For patients with Stage IA disease, a unilateral salpingo-oophorectomy is the treatment of choice. The opposite ovary should be closely inspected and if it appears normal, it should be left alone. However, any suspicious areas should be biopsied. Dysgerminomas are bilateral in 10% to 20% of cases and therefore if disease is present in the opposite ovary, it should be removed along with the fallopian tube. The uterus should be left in place for future childbearing with assisted reproductive technology. Dysgerminomas spread through the lymphatic system, therefore ipsilateral pelvic and paraaortic lymph nodes should be sampled. For patients with greater than Stage I disease, chemotherapy in addition to operation will be necessary. Though these tumors are radiosensitive, this method of treatment compromises fertility and is generally not utilized. Recurrence rates for dysgerminomas are as high as 17%. Survival is dictated by stage.

**Endodermal Sinus Tumor.** EST, also known as yolk sac tumor, arises from undifferentiated and multipotential embryonal cells and is the second most common malignant germ cell tumor in girls. This rapidly growing and highly aggressive tumor affects the ovary in primarily postmenarchal girls. AFP is the serum marker for this tumor. As with most malignancies, treatment depends on stage. For Stage I and IA disease, unilateral salpingo-oophorectomy is adequate. For higher stages, multiagent chemotherapy is recommended as an adjuvant to surgery. These tumors are not radiosensitive and have a tendency to metastasize. EST has a notably poor survival rate.

**Sex Cord Stromal Tumor.** Sex cord stromal tumors arise from uncommitted mesenchymal stem cells that exist below the surface epithelium of the urogenital ridge. These stem cells are able to differentiate into several different lines, hence the variable malignant cells that arise from this progenitor. Sex cord stromal tumors are functional neoplasms associated with hormonal activity. They comprise 10 to 20% of childhood and adolescent ovarian tumors, and their incidence is correlated with age.

**Granulosa Cell Tumor.** The proportion of granulosa cells present determines the malignant potential; pure granulosa cells are quite malignant, a mixture of granulosa and theca cells are less malignant and pure theca cells are benign.

Granulosa cell tumors are divided into adult and juvenile subtypes. The juvenile form has a higher mitotic index and produces a larger size tumor than the adult subtype, but they are usually unilateral and thus have a more favorable prognosis. Juvenile granulosa cell tumors produce estrogen and therefore the presenting symptoms may mimic precocious puberty with vaginal bleeding and even premature thelarche or menarche. Although the gonadotropin levels remain low, increases in estrogen are evident in the serum and urine, distinguishing this process from true precocious puberty. Post menarchal females may present with complaints of irregular menstrual cycles, amenorrhea, abdominal pain or discomfort, increased abdominal girth or an abdominopelvic mass. Presentation usually occurs at Stage I and treatment is limited to unilateral salpingo-oophorectomy. Recurrence is rare and chemotherapy is usually only used at that time.

**Sertoli–Leydig Tumor.** Sertoli–Leydig cell tumors were previously known as arrhenoblastomas or androblastomas. They are androgen producing tumors and account for less than 0.5% of all malignant ovarian neoplasms in children. They are usually unilateral and present most commonly as early stage disease (Stage IA). Histology and staging of this tumor are integral to prognosis. Histology is based on the presence and differentiation of heterologous, endodermal, and mesenchymal components.

The androgen effects occur in 2 stages: first a defeminization process occurs with amenorrhea, followed thereafter by virilization. Prepubertal girls may experience accelerated somatic growth, and post pubertal girls experience irregular menstrual cycles, body masculinization, and hirsutism. Gonadotropin levels are low and testosterone is a useful marker. AFP may be produced by Sertoli–Leydig tumors, and, thus, has also been used as a neoplastic marker.

Treatment consists of unilateral salpingo-oophorectomy. Bilateral tumors, poorly differentiated tumors or metastatic disease all require more aggressive therapy. Multiagent chemotherapy has shown some benefit in this population.

**Epithelial Cell Tumor.** Epithelial tumors arise from the surface epithelium of the ovary. Although they are the most common type of ovarian malignancy in adult females, they are rarely malignant in the pediatric and adolescent population. They are classified as benign, borderline, or malignant. Malignant epithelial tumors in childhood are better differentiated and earlier stage, with a better prognosis, than in older patients.

Benign epithelial cell tumors are generally classified as a serous cystadenoma or a mucinous cystadenoma. Treatment of epithelial tumors is based on classification. Benign tumors are usually confined to the ovary and managed conservatively. Unilateral cystectomy is preferable only if it can be performed completely and safely without compromise to the tumor capsule, otherwise, oophorectomy or salpingo-oophorectomy may be necessary. Follow-up imaging is essential because the risk of recurrence persists, especially with mucinous cystadenomas.

Even malignant epithelial tumors in the pediatric and adolescent population can be managed conservatively if it appears that the tumor is confined to one ovary. However, a thorough surgical staging is mandatory to evaluate for microscopic disease elsewhere (including pelvic and para-aortic lymph node sampling, omentectomy, and peritoneal biopsies). In these situations, collaboration with a gynecologic oncologist may be beneficial; literature in the adult population supports such collaboration as outcomes are demonstrably better with such involvement. Our group recently reported the management of a 13-year-old with a mucinous cystadenocarcinoma who was managed conservatively. She underwent a unilateral salpingo-oophorectomy with full surgical staging in collaboration with a gynecologic oncologist. She was found to have Stage IC ovarian cancer. Postoperatively, she received chemotherapy and has done well since.

## Fallopian Tubes

During embryogenesis, the upper portion of the Müllerian ducts develops to form the fimbria and fallopian tubes. The purpose of the fallopian tubes is to transport the egg, once released from the ovary, to the endometrial cavity. Additionally, fertilization occurs within the fallopian tubes. Therefore, any pathology affecting the fallopian tubes can have significant long-term reproductive consequences if not addressed early and appropriately.

### Paratubal Cyst

Paratubal cysts are often incidental findings identified either during a surgical procedure for another abnormality or on abdominal/pelvic imaging for another indication. They appear thin walled, contain clear fluid, and can be found at any location along the fallopian tube. When the cysts are pedunculated at the fimbrial end of the fallopian tube, they are referred to as hydatid cysts of Morgagni. Paratubal cysts are usually asymptomatic and do not cause significant abdominal/pelvic pain. However, the size can vary from 0.5 cm to greater than 20 cm in diameter. Those that are >4 cm diameter in size may significantly increase the risk of adnexal torsion; thus, elective removal should be considered to decrease the risk of torsion. If a paratubal cyst is the working diagnosis, laparoscopy is the recommended approach. If the paratubal cyst is <4 cm, stable in size, and asymptomatic, then no intervention is required.

### Broad Ligament Cyst

The broad ligament is the fold of peritoneum located on each side of the uterus that attaches it to the walls and the floor of the pelvis. It covers the fallopian tubes and connects to the anterior aspect of the ovaries. It has been described as a blanket over the reproductive structures in the pelvis. As a variation of the paratubal or Wolffian duct cyst, this type can form in the broad ligament and its size can vary. Since these lesions are benign fluid filled embryologic remnants, laparoscopy and cystectomy, with or without drainage, is an acceptable technique. The cyst can be easily dissected from within the leaves of the broad ligament; however, attention to the course of the fallopian tube is imperative. The fallopian tube is often stretched around larger cysts, and thus, may be at risk of trauma during resection.

## Hydrosalpinx/Hematosalpinx/Pyosalpinx

The hormonal stimulation which accompanies the onset of puberty triggers the production of small amounts of fluid within the fallopian tube. Occlusion of the fimbriated end or a segment of the fallopian tube prevents the normal outflow of tubal secretions. Adhesions may develop at the fimbriae from previous surgical treatment or subsequent to peritoneal inflammation involving the fimbriae, thus prohibiting the usual egress of fluid. In cases of hydrosalpinx, the fallopian tube becomes distended with the collection of sterile fluid. In cases of fallopian tube damage subsequent to Müllerian outflow obstruction, retrograde menstruation from an obstructed uterus or vagina may produce unilateral or bilateral hematosalpinx. A pyosalpinx occurs when the obstructed fluid becomes infected.

Management of pure hydrosalpinx in adolescents is more controversial than in adults. The long-term sequelae to the fallopian tube is unknown; therefore, conservative management is initially recommended. Hydrosalpinges, if asymptomatic, can be observed; and if over time it does not continue to increase in size, it should not be treated surgically. Hematosalpinges generally resolve once the uterovaginal obstruction is relieved. Pyosalpinges are most commonly a result of PID/TOA and the management is the same as the previously discussed CDC recommendations for treatment of TOA (see above).

If the hydrosalpinx or hematosalpinx continues to enlarge or becomes symptomatic after initial observation, then intervention is indicated. Drainage of the obstructed fluid will relieve symptoms of pain. An attempt should be made to create persistent patency for continued outflow from the fallopian tube with techniques such as fimbrioplasty or neosalpingostomy. If this is not possible due to the amount of anatomic distortion, or the fluid recurs after an initial attempt, a salpingectomy may be warranted. If symptomatic pyosalpinx is resistant to medical therapy with antibiotics, drainage of the purulent material is beneficial. Less invasive techniques may be attempted with the assistance of image-guided drainage. Rarely, when surgical management of a TOA becomes necessary, then a salpingectomy should be considered. Bilateral salpingectomy should be avoided whenever possible.

## Torsion

Isolated fallopian tube torsion is rare. There are both intrinsic and extrinsic causes of tubal torsion. Intrinsic causes include excessively long fallopian tubes and the presence of a hydrosalpinx or hematosalpinx. Extrinsic causes include ovarian and peritubal masses or other congenital abnormalities (long pelvic ligaments allowing excess mobility of the adnexa).

Signs of tubal torsion mimic that of ovarian torsion. Often, there is an acute onset of abdominal pain with accompanying nausea and vomiting. It can be difficult to distinguish tubal torsion from ovarian torsion on preoperative imaging, but if the patient has a history of tubal pathology it should be highly suspected. In patients with a known large broad ligament or peritubal cyst, fallopian tube torsion should be strongly suspected with the development of acute abdominopelvic pain and vomiting, even with a normal appearing ovary on ultrasound. Surgical management should be laparoscopic detorsion of the fallopian tube with treatment of the underlying cause.

## SELECTED READINGS

Brotherton J, Yazdany T. Resection of vulvar arteriovenous malformation in a premenarchal patient. *Obstet Gynecol* 2010;115(2 Pt 2):426–429.

CareM. ACoAH. ACOG Committee Opinion No 355: Vaginal agenesis: diagnosis, management and routine care. *Obstet Gynecol* 2006;108:1605–1609.

Doyle JO, Laufer MR. Mayer–Rokitansky–Kuster–Hauser (MRKH) syndrome with a single septate uterus: a novel anomaly and description of treatment options. *Fertil Steril* 2009;92(1):391.e17–391.e19.

Emans JS, Laufer MR, Goldstein DP. *Pediatric and Adolescent Gynecology*. 5th ed. Philadelphia. Lippincott Williams and Wilkins; 2005.

Guthrie BD, Adler MD, Powell EC. Incidence and trends of pediatric ovarian torsion hospitalizations in the United States, 2000–2006. *Pediatrics* 2010;125(3):532–538.

Hatch EE, Pamler JR, Titus-Ernstoff L, et al. Cancer risk in women exposed to diethylstilbestrol in utero. *JAMA* 1998;280(7):630–634.

Karpelowsky JS, Hei ER, Matthews K. Laparoscopic resection of benign ovarian tumours in children with gonadal preservation. *Pediatr Surg Int* 2009;25(3):251–254.

Linam L, Darolia R, Naffaa L, et al. US findings of adnexal torsion in children and adolescents: size really does matter. *Pediatr Rad* 2007;37(10):1013–1019.

Melnick S, Cole P, Anderson D, et al. Rates and risks of diethylstilbestrol-related clear cell adenocarcinoma of the vagina and cervix. *Am J Epidemiol* 1986;124(3):518–519.

Michelotti B, Segura BJ, Sau I, Perez-Bertolez S, et al. Surgical management of ovarian disease in infants, children, and adolescents: a 15-year review. *J Laparoendosc Adv Surg Tech* 2010;20(3):261–264.

Oh JT, Choi SH, Ahn SG, et al. Vulvar lipomas in children: an analysis of 7 cases. *J Pediatr Surg* 2009;44(10):1920-1923.

Perlman S, Nakajima S, Hertweck SP. *Clinical Protocols in Pediatric and Adolescent Gynecology*. New York: Parthenon Publishing Group; 2004.

Reddy J, Laufer MR. Hypertrophic labia minora. *J Pediatr Adolesc Gynecol* 2010;23(1):3–6.

Schnee DM. Pelvic inflammatory disease. *J Pediatr Adolesc Gynecol* 2009;22(6):387–389.

Sexually Transmitted Disease Treatment Guidelines 2006. http://www.cdc.gov

Shaul DB, Monforte HL, Levitt MA, et al. Surgical management of perineal masses in patient with anorectal malformations. *J Pediatr Surg* 2005;40(1):188–191.

Shimada T, Miura K, Gotoh H, et al. Management of prenatal ovarian cysts. *Early Hum Dev* 2008;84(6):417–420.

Sinal SH, Woods CR. Human papillomavirus infections of the genital and respiratory tracts in young children. *Semin Pediatr Infect Dis* 2005;16(4):306–316.

Smith NA, Laufer MR. Obstructed hemivagina and ipsilateral renal anomaly (OHIVRA) syndrome: management and follow-up. *Fertil Steril* 2007;87(4):918–922.

Wang S, Lang JH, Xhou HM. Venous malformations of the female lower genital tract. *Eur J Obstet Gynecol Reprod Biol* 2009;145(2):205–208.

Wester T, Rintala RJ. Perineal lipomas associated with anorectal malformations. *Pediatr Surg Int* 2006;22(12):979–981.

# CHAPTER 71

## Disorders of Sexual Differentiation

*Mary E. Fallat and Jeannie Chun*

## KEY POINTS

1. The infant born with the greatest discordance between genetic sex and phenotypic appearance is at most risk for psychological consequences as a result of confusion of gender identity.

2. Congenital adrenal hyperplasia (CAH) or the adrenogenital syndrome due to excessive endogenous androgen production in genetic females is the main cause of masculinization of the external genitalia in 46XX individuals.

3. Mutations of variable type and severity in the AR gene result in a spectrum of forms of the androgen insensitivity syndrome (AIS), the most common cause of a male DSD.

4. An abnormality of the sex chromosomes usually results in failed, incomplete, or asymmetric gonadal differentiation.

5. Female and male DSD disorders (DSDs) have symmetric gonads, and ovotesticular DSDs or children with mixed gonadal dysgenesis have asymmetric gonads.

6. Female children with DSD and most children with ovotesticular DSD are chromatin positive and lack a fluorescent Y. A fluorescent Y chromosome is found in children with male DSD and mixed gonadal dysgenesis.

As defined by the Intersex Society of North American, "intersex" is a general term used for a variety of conditions in which a person is born with a reproductive or sexual anatomy that does not seem to fit the typical definitions of female or male. Caring for a child with a Disorder of Sexual Differentiation (DSD) requires skill and compassion. These disorders are statistically uncommon and are caused by a variety of conditions. The estimated incidence of true intersex is 0.018%. When conditions such as the Klinefelter syndrome and the Turner syndrome are included in the definition of intersex, the incidence may be as high as 1.7%. Although an atypical appearance of the genitalia is most often seen at birth, this is not always the case and the diagnosis may be made at a remote time from birth, including at puberty and into adulthood.

The overall management of an infant or child with an intersex disorder is complex and necessitates the involvement of a team, which may include a neonatologist, geneticist, pediatric endocrinologist, pediatric surgeon, pediatric urologist, pediatrician, gynecologist, and/or psychiatrist. The infant born with the greatest discordance between genetic sex and phenotypic appearance is at most risk for psychological consequences as a result of confusion of gender identity. Gender assignment in these children or the process by which the sex of rearing is decided is something that ideally should be done expeditiously but in the future best interests of the child and family. This assignment depends on many factors including the etiology of the disorder, the magnitude of anatomic abnormalities, the potential for future sexual and reproductive function, and the capabilities and/or limitations of surgical reconstruction. The issue of gender assignment in some circumstances has been refined based on increasing knowledge of the natural history of certain disorders and the ultimate prediction of gender identity, which is the person's conscious and unconscious feelings of belonging to one sex or the other. In the 1920s, Bernice L. Hausman described intersexuality as a "continuum of physiological and anatomical sex differences," contesting the notion of a "true sex" concealed in the tissues of the body. The historic term "hermaphrodite" is burdened by the implications of the anomaly, and "intersexuality" is a neologism that tries to "naturalize various sexes, which themselves are naturally occurring." The nomenclature of DSD has changed to be more respectful of these individuals for whom sexual identity may continue to be challenged by environment and appropriate resources and support groups. For purposes of this chapter, gender role is what a person does or says to communicate his or her status to others. Gender dysphoria is the feeling that one's gender identity may be incorrect.

## PERSPECTIVES ON DISORDERS OF SEXUAL DIFFERENTIATION

The origins and contemporary perceptions and realities of DSD are important to understand in the context of current treatment options and the implications of management strategies. The discrimination and biases historically shown toward persons with DSD inevitably shaped their medical care, even as it contributed to a better understanding of the emotional, psychological, anatomic, and functional consequences of these disorders. The earliest impressions of DSD were cast in a favorable light. Herodotus (484-425 BC) is credited with the first description of women-like men, describing them as soothsayers who foretold the future. Half a century later, Plato (427-347 BC) described an ambisexual tribe with no mystical power, forming a third sex that was a union of man and woman and the original perfect human form. Hermaphroditus was created as the son of Hermes, the god of invention, athletics, secrets, and occult philosophy and Aphrodite, the goddess of love. The emergence of this bisexual god as a patron saint of the attributes of sex was felt to be a divine representation of all of humanity. However soon thereafter, the connotation of hermaphrodite changed, the origin of a hermaphrodite was ascribed to a "freak of nature that mixed genders," and the Romans saw sexual ambiguity as a threatening omen deserving of punishment. Most ancient people eliminated children with doubtful gender. Although the fate of bisexual beings became less cruel with time, the status for such persons was on the borderline of society. Generally speaking, human beings with 2 sexes were not able to find their place in any of the early societies, since they represented a threatening gap with regard to the norm, implying a clear biological differentiation between men and women, and thus a differentiation in roles. In periods of crisis, hermaphrodites became scapegoats for fear and uncertainty.

In 1937, the urologist Hugh H. Young of Johns Hopkins University published "*Genital Abnormalities, Hermaphrodites and Related Adrenal Diseases.*" The book records the clear and unbiased description of several case histories that illustrate the unique reproductive health of intersex individuals. Young neither passed judgment on the people he studied nor attempted to coerce into treatment those who rejected this option. He referred to people who had sexual experiences as both men and women as "practicing hermaphrodites," and described cases where this arrangement was socially optimal as long as discretion was employed. His enlightenment of intersexuality unfortunately also marked the beginning of its suppression, as the book detailed the surgical and hormonal methods of changing intersex individuals into either males or females. Young may have differed from his successors in being less judgmental and controlling of the patients and their families, but he laid a foundation on which intervention practices were built.

Intersex has permeated and influenced our culture and behavior in many ways, both subtle and overt. These traditions and beliefs may shape the way that individuals with DSD feel about themselves and how others treat them.

## Intersex in Religion

Beings that are simultaneously male and female have stirred the human imagination since ancient times. According to Christian theologians and Jewish rabbis, Adam was the first hermaphrodite, a self-sufficient being, like his creator. After the original sin, Adam was divided into 2 imperfect sexes, each incapable of reproducing on their own. The cult of the dual being is also found in the mystical religions and philosophy of Hindu peoples, exemplifying the belief that the sacred ultimate power of the universe is both feminine and masculine. Hermaphroditism was considered to be the embodiment of sexual excess for some, while for philosophers, it represented the 2-fold nature of the human being, considered as the original being. However, both the Talmud and the Tosefta, the Jewish books of law, list extensive regulations for people of mixed sex.

## Intersex in Literature

The idea of transformation goes very far back in Greek literature. It was already present in the Iliad and in the Odyssey, and was perpetuated in the poetry of the 5th and 4th centuries BC. The poet Homer was one of the first persons to be captivated with the nature (sexual identity is inherited) versus nurture (sexual identity can be modified by environmental influences) debate. In *Banquet*, by Plato, Aristophanes states that the human race was originally of 3 genders: male, female, and androgyn. The androgyns had both male and female sexual organs, male and female bodies, and 2 converse faces on the same head. The androgyns were aware of their physical perfection, their total independence since they were able to reproduce alone, and their invulnerability.

The contemporary *Middlesex* is a Pulitzer Prize-winning novel by Jeffrey Eugenides published in 2002. The narrator and protagonist is an intersexed man of Greek descent with 5-alpha-reductase deficiency, which causes him to have certain feminine traits. Initially reared as female, the book describes an ultimate coming to terms with a modified gender identity. The novel portrays the journey of a mutated gene through 3 generations of a Greek family, causing momentous changes in the protagonist's life in the context of the nature versus nurture theme of intersex ideology.

## Intersex in Pop Culture and the Media

There are protean examples of intersex individuals in pop culture. Jabba the Hutt and the entire fictional race of Hutts in *Star Wars* are hermaphrodites. The mother of Cartman in *South Park* is rumored to be a hermaphrodite. The Hermats in *Star Trek: New Frontier* are a species of hermaphrodites. Lieutenant Commander Burgoyne 172 is a Hermat and displays characteristics of both genders. All of the creatures created in the Electronic Arts video game *Spore* are hermaphrodites.

## Intersex in Other Societies

Third genders, intersexuality, and transgender are groups that have been part of societies since the beginning of time. Many communities accept the third sex, including Thailand, Samoa, the American Indians, and the Philippines. Examples include the *hijra* people of the Indian subcontinent, and the *katoey* or *kathoey* people of Thailand, which are mixed groups of many sex, gender, and sexual orientation variations. Katoey and hijra originally referred to intersex people, but the terms have expanded in recent years to include transvestites, transgenders, transsexual women, and gay males. Individuals who are born and raised in other cultures may have entirely different views of DSD and acceptance of both their anatomic and functional differences.

## Intersex in the Military

Societies that have accepted intersex individuals culturally may still have issues with whether or not to accept them in the military. The outsized transgender population of Thailand presents a dilemma for the military, which considers kathoeys eligible for conscription at 21 years old like every other male citizen. Officially, Israel Defense Forces policy does not prohibit intersex patients' draft. In a case from Israel, a combat Israeli Defense Forces female soldier, whose complete androgen insensitivity syndrome (CAIS) diagnosis was not reported to the military health authorities before her recruitment, was allowed to fulfill 2 years of duty service. Medical and other professional issues were discreetly handled. Ironically, the recommendation was to allow intersex patients military service, but not in combat units.

The Department of Defense in the US formalized World War II-era policies banning homosexuals from military service in 1982, in what would come to be called the "Don't Ask Don't Tell" military ban. Transgenders, intersex individuals, gays, and lesbians were effectively banned from serving in the US military. They were allowed to serve only in the Coast Guard Auxiliary or the US Air force Civil Air patrol. The lack of willingness to accept an intersex-identified individual was predicated mainly on the basis of a medical disqualification. A popular assertion was that intersex people would be a burden to both the military and the military health care system, although there is a lack of identification of any regulatory, legal, or policy basis for this claim. The legislation was repealed in 2011, although as of this writing, there is no designated process to help those who were "thrown out" of the military to regain their status.

## Intersex in Sports

Sex determination in individuals with sexual ambiguity has created difficulties in the arena of international sports for years. The Olympic Games in Berlin in 1936 conducted by Hitler generated much controversy around the issue of racial and religious discrimination, but it also brought the complexities of gender verification to the forefront of competitive sport for the first time. The lead up to the Berlin Olympics was blighted by attempts of Hitler to disadvantage Jewish competitors, preventing them from training and issuing threats to discourage their entry to the competition. Controversy continued during the games, most notably in the women's 100-metre sprint. Two women had competed fiercely in prior competitions. Physically, both women appeared virilized, with muscle patterns and facial features more characteristic of the male sex. Rumors circulated that both were men, competing with the wrong sex to gain unfair advantage. Since no formal gender verification program existed at this time, the Olympic committee felt compelled to perform a sex check, but only on the Polish-born athlete. This sex test was a crude physical examination involving the gross inspection of the external genitalia. Although it confirmed a normal external appearance, years later a post-mortem examination showed that this athlete had both ambiguous genitalia and abnormal sex chromosomes, although the exact DSD was not established.

In the following 30 years, the sporting media speculated that several other female athletes had DSDs because they possessed physical attributes that would generally be associated with the male sex. As media hype escalated, compulsory gender verification in the form of a gynecological examination was introduced prior to the 1966 European athletics championship. In these so-called "nude parades," athletes were forced to stand naked in front of a committee and were subjected to an inspection of their external genitalia. For the 1968 Olympics, Barr body detection was introduced and was widely proclaimed to be the solution to gender misrepresentation in sport. The Barr Body is only found in cells with XX sex chromosomes and represents a chromatin clump occurring as a consequence of deactivation of 1 of the paired sex chromosomes. However, the introduction of Barr body analysis created more problems than it solved, as confirming or refuting sex purely via a chromosomal test fails to take account of the complexities of sex determination. Women with CAIS would have been barred from competing due to the presence of XY sex chromosomes despite an entirely female phenotype. Men with the Klinefelter syndrome (XXY) would be eligible to compete as females due to the presence of the Barr body on cytological analysis and would potentially gain clear sporting advantage because of their physique. In 1991, Barr body analysis was replaced with PCR analysis for the SRY locus using DNA extracted from a buccal smear. The SRY gene was previously considered essential for differentiation of the indifferent fetal gonad into the male testis. It is now accepted that other genes are prerequisites for the normal development of the testes and male internal and external genitalia. Indeed, certain 46XX individuals have testes but do not possess the SRY gene, implying that male differentiation of the indifferent fetal gonad can be induced by alternative sex determining genes alone.

All women were screened in Olympic competition beginning in 1992, with over 2000 tests performed at the 1992 Barcelona games. Fifteen tests were reported positive, and 8 more were positive out of over 3000 tests at the Atlanta games in 1996. Of the eight athletes found to have the SRY locus in Atlanta, 7 had AIS and the final athlete had 5-alpha-reductase deficiency. All athletes were allowed to compete in their respective competition. The morphological status of those who tested positive in Barcelona is strictly confidential and it is not known whether these athletes were allowed to compete. In short, testing has created controversy and embarrassment for a significant number of female athletes competing, often unknowingly, with some form of intersex disorder. Indeed, there is no evidence that female athletes with DSDs have displayed any sports-relevant physical attributes that have not been seen in biologically normal female athletes.

## Ethical Considerations

The nature versus nurture debate has fueled intersex ethics since the time of the poet Homer, who was captivated with this debate. The 1876 system devised by Edwin Klebs used gonad tissue to determine sex (nature). In the 1920s, Bernice L. Hausman described intersexuality as a "continuum of physiological and anatomical sex differences", contesting the notion of a "true sex" concealed in the tissues of the body. John Money perpetuated the nurture part of the debate with his classic and somewhat notorious work that predicted gender identity would be based on nurture. The truth is that an individual's traits are due neither solely to nature nor solely to nurture and gender often cannot be defined solely as male or female, but it is both and may change over the lifetime of an individual with a DSD.

In March 1993, publications by Anne Fausto-Sterling in the *New York Times* and a parallel, more technical article on "The Five Sexes: Why Male and Female Are Not Enough" in *The Sciences* (New York Academy of Sciences) made headlines and the topic of intersex was moved to the forefront of ethical discussions. Cheryl Chase emerged as an intersex champion and leader when she responded with news of the creation of the Intersex Society of North America (ISNA), an intersex support group on the World Wide Web, and Hermaphrodites with Attitude, ISNA's newsletter. In early 1997, the American Academy of Pediatrics (AAP) refused to let Cheryl Chase present the viewpoint of intersex patients and she turned to the Lawson Wilkins Pediatric Endocrine Society. Her talk challenged the near-universal practice of doing "corrective" surgery on infants with ambiguous genitals in preference for doing procedures or interventions only that were medically necessary or for life-threatening conditions: hernia repair, gonadectomy for pre-malignant conditions, medical therapy for salt imbalance.

The psychological consequences of taking the alternative road, that is raising children as intersexuals, is not without challenges for both children and parents. These include the inevitable questions encountered at day care, at school, showering in gym class, and pubertal development that may be decidedly different from the individual's chosen peer group. It has been increasingly recognized that individuals with a DSD should have the opportunity to be evaluated and managed by a multidisciplinary team.

## NORMAL PROCESS OF SEXUAL DETERMINATION

Sexual determination is a 3-part process occurring sequentially with an end product of genital differentiation. *Chromosomal* sex is determined by the union of maternal and paternal haploid gametes at fertilization. Chromosomal sex dictates *gonadal* sex, which directs the formation of testes or ovaries. In normal individuals, *phenotypic* sex is concordant with genetic sex, and is the result of the presence or absence of testicular hormones acting on the undifferentiated genitalia. Each part of the genital tract may differentiate more or less independently from the other parts, depending on the local physiologic or paracrine conditions during development. This makes it possible for the phenotypic sex to develop in the opposite direction to the genetic sex. Any discordance between the 3 parts of sexual determination can result in an individual with a form of intersex.

### Molecular Biology

The molecular biology in intersex has enhanced our understanding of the process of sexual differentiation and confirmed its complexity. An expanding number of genes on both sex chromosomes and autosomes are implicated in the control of sex determination and differentiation (Table 71-1). Many recent discoveries have resulted from the study of

| TABLE 71-1 | Genes Involved in Sexual Differentiation | | | |
|---|---|---|---|---|
| Gene | Name | Chromosome | Function | Deletion or Duplication Results |
| SRY | *Sex* determining *Region* of the *Y* chromosome | Y | Causes bipotential gonad to develop into a testis | Gonad develops into an ovary |
| SF-1 | *Steroidogenic Factor* 1 | 9 | Hypothesized to control biosynthesis of all steroid hormones in both adrenal glands and gonads | Deletion lethal: complete absence of both adrenals and gonads |
| WT-1 | Wilms tumor suppressor gene | 11 | Necessary for gonadal development prior to sexual dimorphism | Deletion lethal: bilateral renal and gonadal agenesis |
| SOX 9 | SRY-box 9 | 17 | Expressed on chondrogenic, early gonadal and testicular tissue | Haploinsufficiency results in campomelic dysplasia and testicular dysgenesis |
| DSS | Dosage sensitive sex reversal locus | X (XP21) | Putative "ovarian determining gene" | Duplication in 46,XY individuals leads to testicular dysgenesis and sex reversal |
| DAX1 | Deleted in adrenal hypoplasia on the X chromosome | X (with DSS locus) | | Mutations cause adrenal hypoplasia but do not affect testicular development |
| MIS | Mullerian inhibiting substance | 19 | Causes regression of Mullerian duct in male embryos | Deletion results in full or partial retention of Mullerian duct derivatives |
| MIS receptor | Mullerian Inhibiting Substance receptor | 12 | Necessary for function of MIS | Deletion results in full or partial retention of Mullerian duct derivatives |

(Continued)

| Gene | Name | Chromosome | Function | Deletion or Duplication Results |
|------|------|-----------|----------|--------------------------------|
| CYP21 | P450c21 (21-hydroxylase) | 6 | Converts progesterone to DOC | Enzymatic defect can result in congenital adrenal hyperplasia |
| CYP11A | P450 scc (cholesterol side chain cleavage enzyme) | 15 | Convert cholesterol to pregnenolone | Defects result in male DSD |
| CYP17 | P450c17 (17 $\alpha$-hydroxylase, 17, 20-lyase) | 10 | Converts pregnenolone to 17-OH pregnenolone to dehydroepiandrosterone (DHEA) and progesterone to 17-OH progesterone to androstenedione | Defects result in male DSD |
| CYP11B1 | P450c11 (11-hydroxylase) | 1 | Converts DOC to corticosterone and 11 deoxycortisol to cortisol | Enzymatic defect can result in congenital adrenal hyperplasia |
| CYP11B2 | P450c11 (18-hydroxylase) | | Converts corticosterone to aldosterone | |
| HSD17B3 | 17-ketosteroid reductase (17-KS OH) (17$\beta$- hydroxysteroid dehydrogenase) | 9 | Converts androstenedione to testosterone | Defect results in male DSD |
| CYP19 | P450 aromatase | 15 | Can metabolize 3 substrates into estrogen species | Mutations result in female DSD |
| SRD5A1 SRD5A2 | 5-$\alpha$-reductase-1 5-$\alpha$-reductase 2 | 5 2 | Converts testosterone to DHT | Gene abnormalities result in male DSD |
| HSD3B2 | 3$\beta$-hydroxysteroid dehydrogenase | 8 | Converts pregnenolone to progesterone and 17-OH, pregnenolone to 17-OH progesterone and DHEA to androstenedione | Enzymatic defect can result in congenital adrenal hyperplasia or male DSD |
| AR | Androgen receptor | X | Binds with androgen and alters transcription of target gene | Defect results in a syndrome of androgen insensitivity (male DSD) |
| CFTR | Cystic fibrosis transmembrane conductance regulator | 7 | Encodes transmembrane protein of chlorine channels | Abnormalities of epididymis and ducti deferentes |
| StAR | Steroidogenic acute regulatory protein | 8 | Cholesterol transfer from outer to inner mitochondrial membrane | Lipoid congenital adrenal hyperplasia |
| POR | p450 oxidoreductase | 7 | Electron transfer protein for microsomal p450s | Antley–Bixler syndrome |

**TABLE 71-1   Genes Involved in Sexual Differentiation** (Continued)

sex-reversed individuals. Development of the mammalian male phenotype is dependent on the testes. In 1959, the Y chromosome was proven to be male-determining. The H-Y male specific histocompatibility chromosome antigen became the leading candidate for the putative testis determining factor (TDF) until it was discovered that some male mice lacked this antigen. The next candidate was zink finger Y (ZFY), a DNA binding transcriptional regulator whose gene is on the short arm of Y. This hypothesis was also refuted when another subset of males lacking ZFY but containing a segment of the Y chromosome was discovered. In 1990, Sinclair and Gubbay described genes in humans and mice with TDF properties named SRY, which is the current best candidate for directing

testicular determination. The SRY gene encodes a DNA binding protein whose expression is specific to the Y chromosome of all mammals, with appropriate specificity in the gonadal ridge just prior to testis differentiation.

Male sex differentiation is also dependent upon a number of autosomal genes. The WT1 (*Wilms tumor suppressor*) and SF-1 (*steroidogenic factor one*) genes both play a critical role in the development of the bipotential gonad. Mutations in the WT1 gene cause Denys–Drash syndrome, a form of dysgenetic male DSD. SF-1 is critical to the synthesis of steroid and anti-Mullerian hormone. Translocations on the long arm of the autosomal chromosome 17q in the SRA1 locus are closely related to SRY, belong to the SOX gene family, and haploinsufficiency causes campomelic dysplasia with sex reversal. Additional genes on 9p and 10q also affect testicular determination.

Female differentiation appears to be constitutive, although one presumptive "ovarian determining gene" or the DSS locus (dosage sensitive sex reversal) has been localized to Xp21. Duplication of this locus is required for female differentiation. Several 46, XY females with partial duplication of the short arm of the X chromosome and intact SRY have been described who have testicular dysgenesis and lack of male differentiation. Mutations of another gene within the DSS locus, DAX1 (deleted in adrenal hypoplasia on the X chromosome) cause adrenal hypoplasia without affecting testicular development.

## Internal and External Sexual Differentiation

Male and female human embryos have an initial ambisexual stage, possessing bipotential gonadal tissue, the mesodermally derived Wolffian and Mullerian ducts within the gonadal ridge, and undifferentiated external genitalia. Differentiation of the testes begins at around 6 weeks gestation and is directed by SRY. The fetal testis produces 2 products necessary for male differentiation, androgens and Mullerian inhibiting substance (MIS).

The events stimulating male sex differentiation require the presence of androgens and a functional androgen receptor (AR). Androgens stimulate the Wolffian ducts (WD) to develop into epididymis, vas deferens, and seminal vesicle (SV). Testosterone is the major androgen secreted by the testis, but it is metabolized to a more active metabolite, 5α-dihydrotestosterone (DHT) by the enzyme $\Delta^4$-3-ketosteroid-5α-reductase (5α-reductase) in various androgen target tissues. Testosterone is metabolized from cholesterol via 4 enzymatic conversions. Cholesterol is converted to pregnenolone by P450scc; P450c17 converts pregnenolone to 17-OH pregnenolone and then to dihydroepiandrosterone (DHEA); 3β-hydroxysteroid dehydrogenase converts DHEA to androstenedione, and this is converted to testosterone by 17-ketosteroid reductase. Mutations of any of these genes can result in deficient masculinization of a 46, XY individual.

Testosterone secretion by fetal Leydig cells begins at around 8 weeks under control of unknown factors, and peaks between 11 and 18 weeks gestation, under control of maternal chorionic gonadotropin. Development of Wolffian duct structures occurs between 9 and 13 weeks gestation and is induced by testosterone. The enzyme DHT is expressed at about 13 weeks gestation, and is the active androgen involved in masculinization of the embryonic urogenital sinus into prostate and prostatic urethra; and genital tubercle, urethral folds and labioscrotal swellings into penis, penile urethra, and scrotum. The latter events also require the expression of 5-α reductase 2. The hormone DHT has a ten-fold greater affinity for ARs than testosterone. Androgen action in target organs is mediated by ARs that are mainly located in the mesenchyme during fetal life, and at least partially seems paracrine in nature.

MIS is a glycoprotein hormone produced by the Sertoli cells that causes the regression of the anlagen of the fallopian tubes, uterus, and upper vagina. Production of MIS is felt to be regulated in vivo by the SRY gene. The MIS gene has been localized to chromosome 19 and the MIS receptor to chromosome 12. Abnormalities of either gene can result in the retained Mullerian duct syndrome.

The uterus, fallopian tubes, and upper third of the vagina autonomously develop from the Mullerian ducts in the absence of the testis, and the external genital primordia develop into clitoris, labia minora, and labia majora. The role of estrogens in sexual differentiation is unclear, and ovaries are unnecessary for female sexual differentiation.

# PATHOPHYSIOLOGY OF SEXUAL DETERMINATION

Developmental abnormalities causing intersex conditions are conventionally categorized into three main groups: genetic females with phenotypic masculinization (Female DSD), genetic males with phenotypic feminization (Male DSD), and gonadal ambiguities or absence resulting from chromosomal abnormalities.

## Female DSD

Congenital adrenal hyperplasia (CAH) or the adrenogenital syndrome due to excessive endogenous androgen production in genetic females is the main cause of masculinization of the external genitalia in 46, XX individuals. The etiology in the majority (90%) of cases is a deficiency of the P450c21 oxidase enzyme on chromosome 6. A small number of cases occur because of deficiencies of the p450c11 or 3β-hydroxysteroid dehydrogenase enzymes. Formation of the ovaries, uterus, and fallopian tubes is normal, but the vagina is foreshortened and joins the urethra. In the severely masculinized forms of CAH (high vaginal atresia), the vagina ends in a fistula at approximately the location of the external urethral sphincter. In less severe forms, the vagina ends more distally in a common urogenital sinus. The external genitalia are characterized by clitoral enlargement ranging from minimal to an almost normal-appearing phallus and labial masculinization ranges from labioscrotal folds to complete scrotal fusion (Fig. 71-1). Gonadal descent never occurs because the ovaries are normal. Infants with bilateral undescended testes should be evaluated with a karyotype to confirm the presence of a Y chromosome.

The defect in the adrenogenital syndrome resides in the adrenal glands and all of the enzymatic deficiencies result in deficient cortisol biosynthesis. Release of feedback inhibition results in increased corticotropin production and stimulation of the adrenal gland, resulting in adrenal hyperplasia and overproduction of products proximal to the enzymatic defect. Preferential overproduction of androgenic steroids results in the variable degrees of masculinization.

## Male DSD

Mediation of the effects of both testosterone and DHT requires a functional AR to induce expression of androgen-dependent genes. Mutations of variable type and severity in

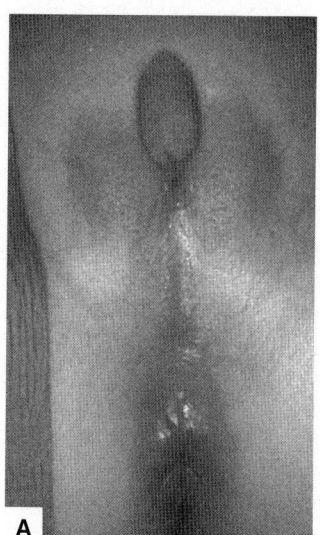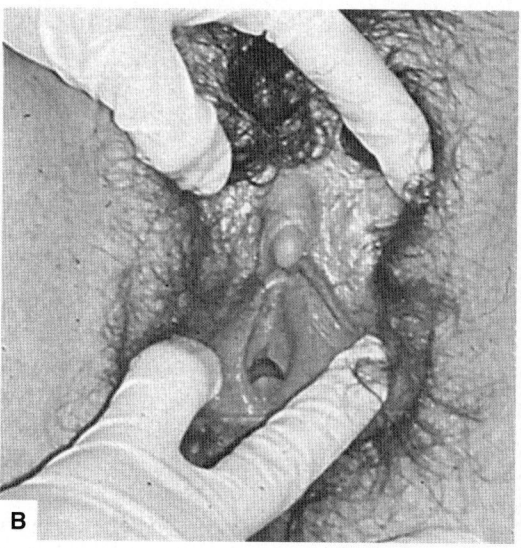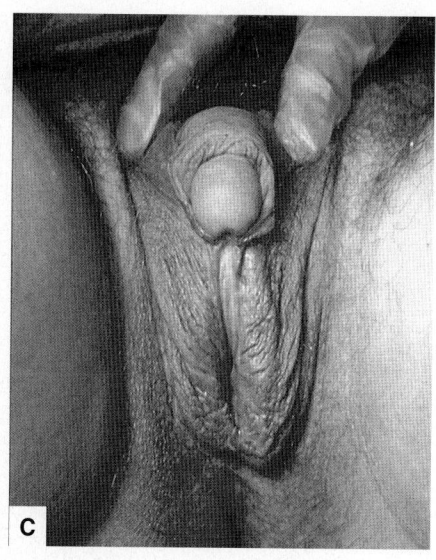

**FIGURE 71-1** **A.** A 46, XX child with congenital adrenal hyperplasia (CAH), clitoral hypertrophy, and a urogenital sinus. **B.** An adolescent girl with CAH who was no-compliant with her medical regimen and has clitoromegaly and an unrepaired urogenital sinus. **C.** An adolescent girl with CAH who was noncompliant with her medical regimen and has severe masculinization including an uncorrected urogenital sinus, labioscrotal fusion, and clitoromegaly.

the AR gene result in a spectrum of forms of the AIS, the most common cause of a male DSD. Affected individuals have a 46, XY karyotype and normal symmetric testes that may be intraabdominal or descended, with the external genital phenotype varying from normal male (partial or PAIS) to normal female (complete or CAIS). Approximately 250 mutations in the AR gene have been identified and characterized in individuals with AIS. The 2 primary types of AR defect associated with AIS are attributed to either abnormalities of androgen binding or abnormalities of DNA binding. Although some individuals with AIS will have defects of androgen binding detected in cultured genital skin fibroblasts, this is not uniform and there is no reliably consistent correlation between the quantity and quality of androgen binding and the external genital phenotype of affected individuals.

Prepubertal children with AIS generally have normal serum concentrations of testosterone and LH. Limited studies indicate that these values may be increased in newborns and infants with PAIS but not CAIS. Estrogen production increases to about twice normal in individuals with AIS, mainly by the testes due to increased LH stimulation of Leydig cells, but also due to aromatization of androstenedione and testosterone in peripheral tissues. MIS may be normal or elevated and Mullerian structures are normally regressed. In spite of advances in molecular analysis of AR defects, clinical factors remain of primary importance in assigning the sex-of-rearing for an infant with AIS. This is straightforward for those with the mildest or most severe degrees of feminization, but remains the subject of greatest concern for individuals whose phallic size is considered "inadequate," as some individuals with PAIS have successfully responded to high-dose testosterone treatment.

Other causes of insufficient masculinization of a 46-XY genetic male include insufficient testosterone production or an inability to convert testosterone to dihydrotestosterone. Deficiency of androgen production may occur because of genetic

defects in the enzymes responsible for the ultimate conversion of cholesterol to testosterone. The 4 P450 enzymes involved in adrenal steroidogenesis include P450scc or cholesterol side chain cleavage enzyme; P450c11, which mediates both 11-hydroxylase and 18-hydroxylase; P450c17, which mediates the 17 α-hydroxylase and 17,20-lyase activities; and P450c21, which mediates the 21-hydroxylase of both the glucocorticoid and mineralocorticoid pathways. These children produce little or no serum testosterone but MIS levels are normal for age. The testes may be undescended, small, or both, and Mullerian structures are absent. The penis may be small and hypospadic.

Other enzymes that may be responsible for deficient androgenization include 3 β-hydroxy-steroid dehydrogenase and 17-ketosteroid reductase. The former enzyme controls essential steps in the production of both glucocorticoids and mineralocorticoids, as well as converting DHEA to androstenedione in the testis. The latter converts androstenedione to testosterone. Type II male DSD due to 5 α-reductase deficiency causes failure of conversion of testosterone to dihydrotestosterone in peripheral target tissues. This is an autosomal recessive disorder that includes severe hypospadias, undescended testes, a prepenile scrotum, and enlarged prostatic utricle. The Type 2 isoform located on chromosome 19 is the one that is predominantly expressed in the external genitalia.

The persistent Mullerian duct syndrome (PMDS) due to deficient MIS or its receptor occurs when usually phenotypic males, often with undescended testes, have persistent Mullerian structures (Fig. 71-2). The gonads in this condition are normal, although the undescended gonads pose a risk for future testicular cancer. The descended testis may pull the Fallopian tube and uterus into the track through which it has descended (hernia uteri inguinalis) or the undescended testis from the other side of the body may be pulled into the same track (transverse testicular ectopia). The vas deferens may enter the retained Mullerian duct structures accounting for future infertility.

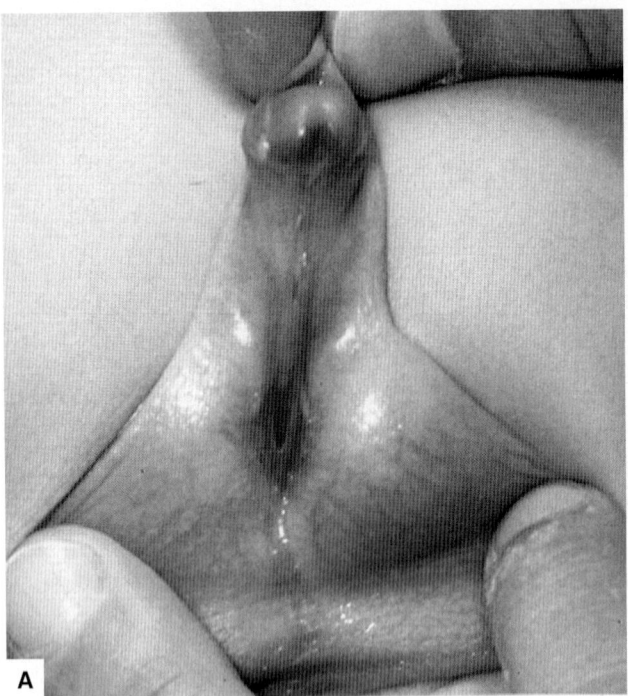

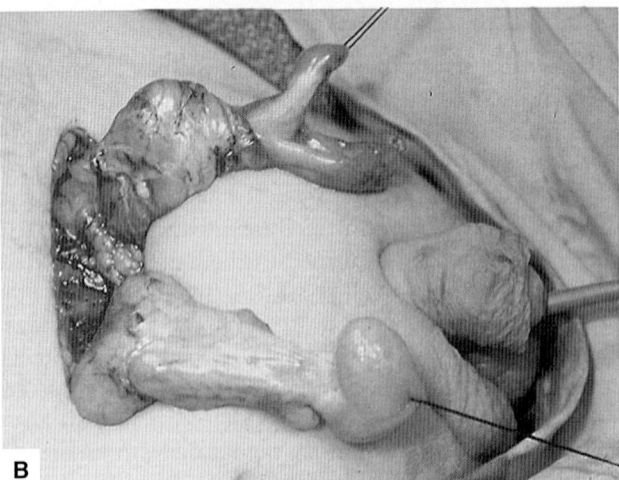

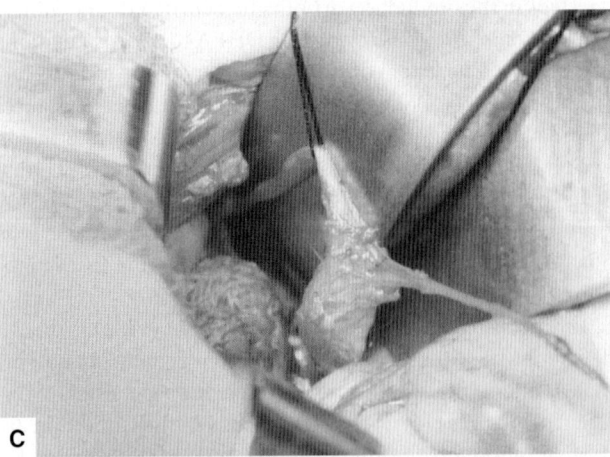

**FIGURE 71-2** **A.** A 46, XY child with symmetric descended gonads and penoscrotal hypospadias who has retained Müllerian duct structures. **B.** Inguinal exploration in the same child revealed a normal-sized right testis, a small left testis, and a uterus. **C.** The vas deferens on each side entered the uterus.

## Gonadal Ambiguities Resulting from Chromosomal Abnormalities

An abnormality of the sex chromosomes usually results in failed, incomplete, or asymmetric gonadal differentiation. The most common of these abnormalities is mixed gonadal dysgenesis associated with a 45X/46XY karyotype. In this condition, there is usually a small dysgenetic testis on one side and a streak gonad on the other. In spite of its size, the small testis produces sufficient testosterone to cause masculinization and clitoral hypertrophy. There is a urogenital sinus defect. In individuals with a 46XY karyotype or pure gonadal dysgenesis, a defective Y chromosome may result in bilateral streak gonads. Both testosterone and MISs are low or absent resulting in a phenotypic female and preservation of Mullerian duct structures. Gonads containing testicular tissue in this condition have a propensity to neoplastic transformation as early as the neonatal period.

Ovotesticular DSDs are rare and usually characterized by asymmetric gonads. They may have nondysgenetic ovarian and testicular differentiation that is separated on both sides or combined in one or both gonads as an ovotestis. In a combined gonad, the testis is always centrally located, and is not prone to neoplastic transformation. The Mullerian structures are regressed on the side of testicular tissue. The vagina enters the urethra as a urogenital sinus defect.

## DIAGNOSTIC EVALUATION

The syndromes that present at birth with sexual ambiguity are female DSD, male DSD, ovotesticular DSD, and mixed gonadal dysgenesis. Two screening criteria can be used to expeditiously diagnose which of the 4 disorders is responsible for the phenotypic differentiation. The first criterion is the presence of gonadal symmetry or asymmetry. Symmetry is determined by the position of 1 gonad relative to the other with the external inguinal ring as a reference point. If a diffuse biochemical etiology underlies the abnormality, the gonads should both lie above or below the ring. Female and male DSD disorders have symmetric gonads, and ovotesticular DSD or children with mixed gonadal dysgenesis have asymmetric gonads.

The second criterion is the presence of sex chromosome markers that now include staining of the Barr body that denotes an inactivated second X chromosome, or fluorescence to detect the distal end of the long arm of the Y chromosome, Yq. A buccal smear was historically used to look for an inactivated X chromosome, although fluorescence to detect the distal arm of the Y chromosome has replaced chromatin analysis in most centers. Female children with DSD and most children with ovotesticular DSD are chromatin positive and lack a fluorescent Y. A fluorescent Y chromosome is found in children with male DSD and mixed gonadal dysgenesis. The accuracy of sex assignment using these 2 criteria approaches 80 to 90%. Table 71-2 lists the additional information that may permit completion of the diagnosis and gender assignment. Table 71-3 is a summary table of specific conditions, diagnosis, and management schemes.

| TABLE 71-2 | Newborn Evaluation of the Intersex Infant |
|---|---|
| History | Familial syndromes or developmental anomalies of prenatal drug ingestion |
| Physical Exam | External genitalia—Phallus or clitoral size |
| | Urethral orifice |
| | Vaginal introitus |
| | Scrotal abnormalities |
| | Gonadal symmetry or asymmetry |
| | Rectal exam to palpate uterus |
| Laboratory | Electrolytes |
| | Buccal smear, Y fluorescence |
| | Serum and urinary steroids |
| | High-resolution chromosomes (karyotype) |
| | MIS assay |
| | hCG stimulation test |
| Radiography | Urethrogram/genitogram |
| | Ultrasound of the pelvis and urinary tract |
| | MRI of the pelvis |

Radiographic assessment is an instrumental part of diagnosis and management. Options include ultrasound, which poses no radiation risk and is a screening test that allows evaluation of both the genital and urinary tracts looking for abnormal dilation of normal or abnormal structures and presence of intra-abdominal gonads. MRI scan allows for more definitive evaluation of individual structures and the pelvic floor, although it requires sedation (Fig. 71-3). Contrast genitogram and urinary tract evaluation in both the AP and lateral views with catheters in place allows delineation of the reproductive and urinary tracts in relation to each other (Fig. 71-4). Ultimately, a careful cystoscopy and vaginoscopy done under anesthesia before an operation is planned is integral to defining any surgical procedure and counseling parents.

## PERIOPERATIVE POSITIONING

The patient's position during surgery should provide both exposure for the procedure and access to IV lines, tubes, and monitoring devices. Attention should be given to the patient's safety and comfort, as well as to the circulatory, respiratory, neurological, and musculoskeletal systems. Injury potential occurs due to the alteration of normal defense mechanisms and forced prolonged immobility during the procedure. The surgeon, anesthesiologist, and nursing staff should work as a team to do the preoperative assessment to determine the patient's tolerance to the planned position, including age, skin condition, height and weight, nutritional status, preexisting conditions, and physical/mobility limits. Intraoperative factors include type of anesthesia, length of operation, and position(s) required.

Properly functioning equipment and devices contribute to patient safety and provide adequate surgical site exposure.

Use of gel pads decreases pressure at bony prominences by redistributing overall pressure across a larger surface area. Pillows, blankets, and molded foam devices may produce only a minimum of pressure reduction. Special precautions must be taken when the patient is positioned in lithotomy. Extreme thigh flexion may increase intra-abdominal pressure and impair respiratory function by decreasing tidal volume. With the legs in stirrups, venous return from the lower extremities is enhanced and blood pools in the splancnic bed. Blood loss during the procedure may not immediately manifest until the legs are repositioned at the end of the case. The legs should be repositioned slowly at the same time by 2 persons to allow for physiologic adjustment to extra volume circulating through the lower extremities again. Arms are best extended on arm boards or folded across the torso rather than positioned at the sides, where hands will be at risk of getting caught in the lower table as it is raised at the end of the case.

There are 3 described lithotomy positions. These are: high, medium, and low. The high lithotomy position is often used in the adult for vaginal hysterectomy or for patients with frozen joints. The low lithotomy position is used for surgical procedures that require excellent exposure to both abdomen and perineum. Stirrups are secured in holders on each side of the operating table at the level of the patient's upper thighs. They are adjusted at equal height so that symmetry will be achieved when the legs are raised. Each of 2 persons raises 1 leg by grasping the sole of a foot in 1 hand and supporting the calf at the knee with the other. The knees are flexed and the legs placed inside the stirrup posts. If loop (candy cane) stirrups are used, the feet are placed in the canvas slings at a 90° angle to the abdomen. One loop encircles the sole and the other goes around the ankle. If the legs are properly positioned, both undue abduction and external rotation are avoided, and the lower leg or ankle does not contact the metal part of the stirrup. After the patient is positioned, the lower section of mattress is removed and the bed lowered. The buttocks must not extend beyond the end of the operating bed. For lengthy procedures, antiembolic stockings or sequential compression devices are used in adolescents or obese children to minimize the risk of venous stasis and deep vein thrombosis. Other potential risks include pressure sores, and nerve damage or compartment syndrome from prolonged immobilization. When using universal stirrups with a boot, the toe, knee, and opposite shoulder should be in a relatively straight line and knee abduction avoided.

## TREATMENT OPTIONS

### Clitoral Recession and Reduction

This procedure is usually contemporaneously reserved for the age-appropriate patient who can understand and give assent, although each case should be considered individually. There is still some controversy about the severely masculinized female patient with CAH. These patients generally choose a female gender identity and repair, including the high vaginal atresia requiring flaps, that may be optimally done during a complete

**TABLE 71-3  DSD Conditions: Diagnostic and Management Strategy**

| Condition | Karyotype | Enzyme or Gene Defect | Diagnostic Criteria | Physical Findings | Assign Gender | Medical Therapy | Surgical Therapy |
|---|---|---|---|---|---|---|---|
| **FEMALE DSD** | | | | | | | |
| Congenital adrenal hyperplasia (CAH, adrenogenital syndrome) | 46XX | P450c21 P450c11 3b-OH steroid dehydrogenase POR | ↑K, ↓Na ↑ androgen ↑ 17-OH progesterone MIS absent | Gonadal symmetry Clitoral hypertrophy Urogenital sinus Labioscrotal fusion and enlargement | F | Hydrocortisone or cortisone acetate and Florinef | Clitoral reduction and recession Vaginoplasty Labioscrotal reduction |
| **MALE DSD** | | | | | | | |
| Testosterone deficiency | 46XY | 17-KS OH 3B-OH steroid dehydrogenase P450c17 | ↓ testosterone | Small undescended testes (symmetric) Severe hypospadias No Mullerian structures | If M | Presurgical testosterone stimulation Testosterone at adolescence | Staged hypospadias repair Prepenile scrotal repair Orchiopexy |
| | | | | Female phenotype | If F | Estrogen/Progesterone at puberty | Gonadectomy |
| Androgen receptor deficiency Complete androgen insensitivity (CAIS) Testicular feminization syndrome | 46XY | Androgen receptor gene | ↑ testosterone ↑ MIS | Female phenotype without mullerian structures. | F | Estrogen/Progesterone at puberty | Gonadectomy in infancy Vaginal replacement in adolescence |
| Androgen receptor deficiency Reifenstein syndrome Partial androgen insensitivity (PAIS) | 46XY | Androgen receptor gene | Normal testosterone Slight ↑of MIS | Feminization No Mullerian structures | If F | Estrogen/Progesterone at puberty | Gonadectomy, clitoral reduction/recession, labioscrotal reduction in infancy |
| | | | | Gonadal symmetry, small undescended testes Hypospadias No Mullerian structures | If M | Presurgical testosterone stimulation Testosterone at adolescence | Hypospadias repair Prepenile scrotal repair Orchiopexy |
| 5α reductase deficiency | 46XY | Dihydrotestosterone gene (DHT) | ↑ testosterone ↑ MIS ↓ DHT | Gonadal symmetry, undescended normal testes Severe penoscrotal hypospadias Prepenile scrotum | M | Presurgical testosterone replacement DHT replacement | Hypospadias and prepenile scrotal repair |

## CHROMOSOMAL ABNORMALITIES

| Condition | Karyotype | Genes | Hormones | Phenotype | Sex | Hormone therapy | Surgery |
|---|---|---|---|---|---|---|---|
| Ovotesticular DSD | 46XX | SRY<br>SOX 9<br>DSS | ↓ or normal testosterone<br>↓ or normal MIS | Gonadal asymmetry: testis, ovary, or ovotestis<br>Urogenital sinus<br>Clitoral hypertrophy | If F | Estrogen/progesterone at puberty | Clitoral recession<br>Vaginoplasty<br>Labioscrotal reduction<br>Preserve ovarian tissue |
| | | | | | If M | Presurgical testosterone stimulation<br>Testosterone at adolescence | Staged hypospadias repair<br>Prepenile scrotal repair<br>Remove mullerian structures preserve vas and normal testis<br>? orchiopexy |
| Pure gonadal dysgenesis | 46XY | SRY<br>SF-1<br>SOX 9<br>DSS | Testosterone absent<br>MIS absent | Phenotype female<br>Vagina present<br>Gonads absent<br>Symmetric appearance | F | Estrogen/progesterone at adolescence | Gonadectomy of residual tissue |
| Mixed gonadal dysgenesis | 45X/46XY or 46XY | SRY<br>SF-1<br>SOX 9<br>DSS | ↓ testosterone<br>↓ MIS | Gonadal asymmetry: testis and streak gonad<br>Urogenital sinus<br>Clitoral hypertrophy | If F | Estrogen/progesterone at adolescence | Clitoral recession<br>Vaginoplasty<br>Labioscrotal reduction<br>Gonadectomy |
| | | | | | If M | Presurgical testosterone stimulation<br>Testosterone at adolescence | Staged hypospadias repair<br>Prepenile scrotal repair and remove Mullerian structures<br>Preserve vas and normal testis<br>? orchiopexy |

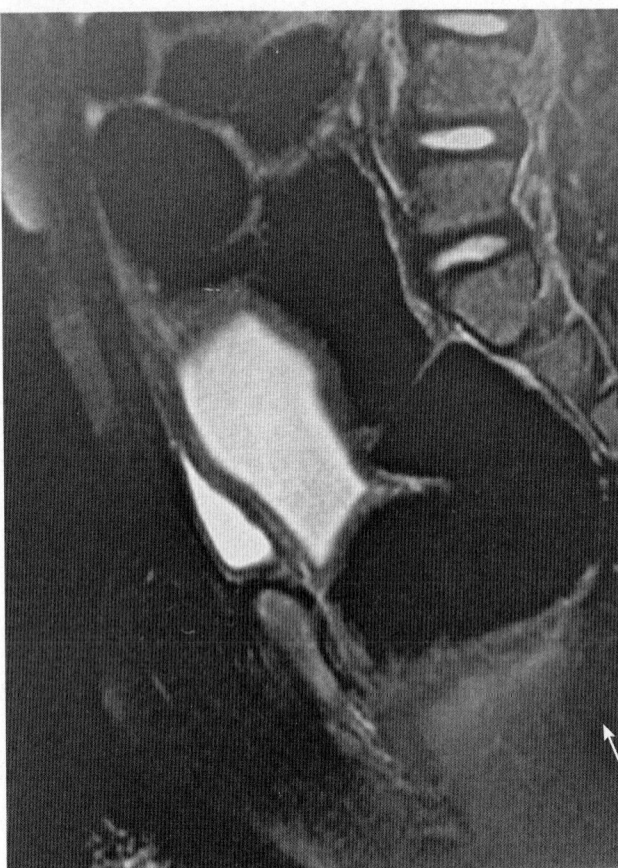

**FIGURE 71-3** The T2-weighted contrast MRI image of the pelvis showing a decompressed bladder and large vagina anterior to the rectum. The child had a vaginal atresia with a fistula entering a long urogenital sinus at the bladder neck. At birth, she required a vaginostomy tube for decompression. An abdominal perineal approach for reconstruction and perineal pull-through was done at age 3 years.

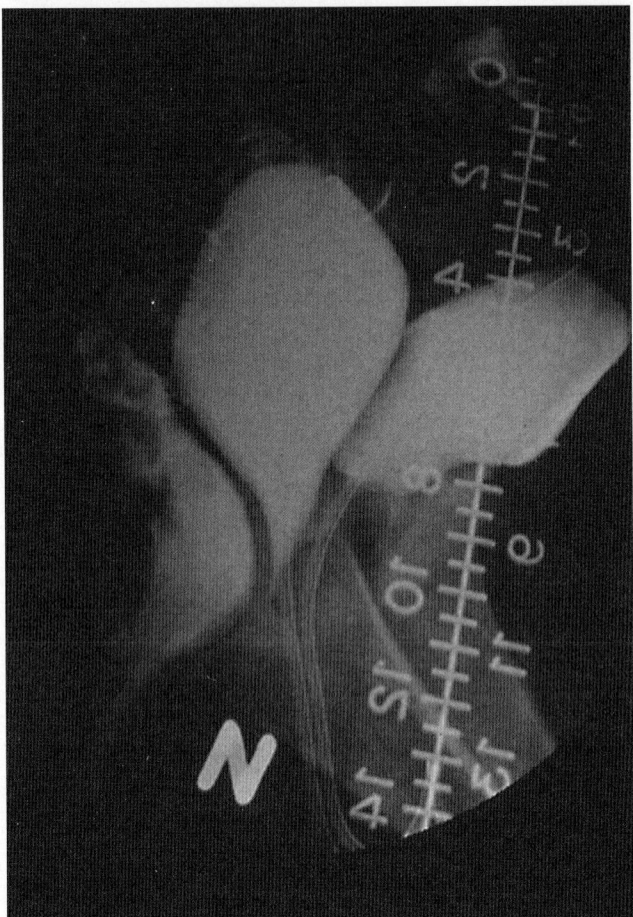

**FIGURE 71-4** A contrast genitogram with catheters in place showing the rectum, vagina, and bladder from left to right. The N marker is on the child's perineum. The ruler aids in estimating the distance between the lower vagina to the skin. In this case, there is a distance of nearly 3 cm between the lower vagina and the skin.

rather than staged reconstruction of the genitalia. The patient is positioned in lithotomy. A Foley catheter is inserted as part of the procedure after prepping unless cystoscopy and vaginoscopy is done first as part of a planned total reconstruction. If clitoral recession only is to be carried out, a dorsal incision may be adequate (Fig. 71-5A–H and Fig. 71-6A–E). The incision begins at the prominence of the mons veneris in the midline approximately 2.0 cm above the base of the clitoris. This incision is deepened to the periosteum of the pubis and the intersymphyseal ligament. A separate connecting incision is made near the subcoronal sulcus, carried 180° around and just behind the dorsal aspect of the glans, leaving a few millimeters of mucus membrane. Dissection proceeds at the level of the Buck fascia, exposing the shaft of the clitoris dorsally and laterally. The ventral elements of the clitoris do not require dissection. The suspensory ligament of the clitoris is isolated and divided, freeing the structure from the pubis. The corporal division is located, and each extension followed beneath the right and left pubic rami. Recession is accomplished by placing 3 sutures of 3-0 Vicryl in the fascial covering of the mid-shaft of the clitoris and the periosteum beneath the pubis. The mons veneris and hood of the clitoris are reconstructed to allow only minimal exposure of the glans. The glans can also be separately reduced in a coronal configuration if it is large and this is the desire of the patient (Fig. 71-7).

If reduction clitoroplasty is also desired, a circumferential incision is made around the glans, and dorsally created Byar flaps divided for future creation of labia minora (Fig. 71-8A–D). This procedure requires precise anatomic definition of the dorsal neurovascular bundles, which are depicted in Fig. 71-8B–D. After dissecting the plane of the Buck fascia described as above, an incision is made into the fascia over the neurovascular bundles, which are isolated and retracted. The corpora are then divided and excised from a point just proximal to the entry of the neurovascular bundles into the glans, up to approximately the bifurcation. An end-to-end interrupted anastomosis joins the remaining clitoral tissue using 5-0 or 6-0 Vicryl. The dorsal clitoris is reconstructed by approximating the circumscribed glans to the skin of the mons pubis. The divided skin flaps are draped around the sides of the clitoris to create labia minora. In many cases, a clitoral reduction will be done in conjunction with a vaginoplasty and reconstruction of the labia minora, coordinated with other skin flaps used to widen the vaginal orifice.

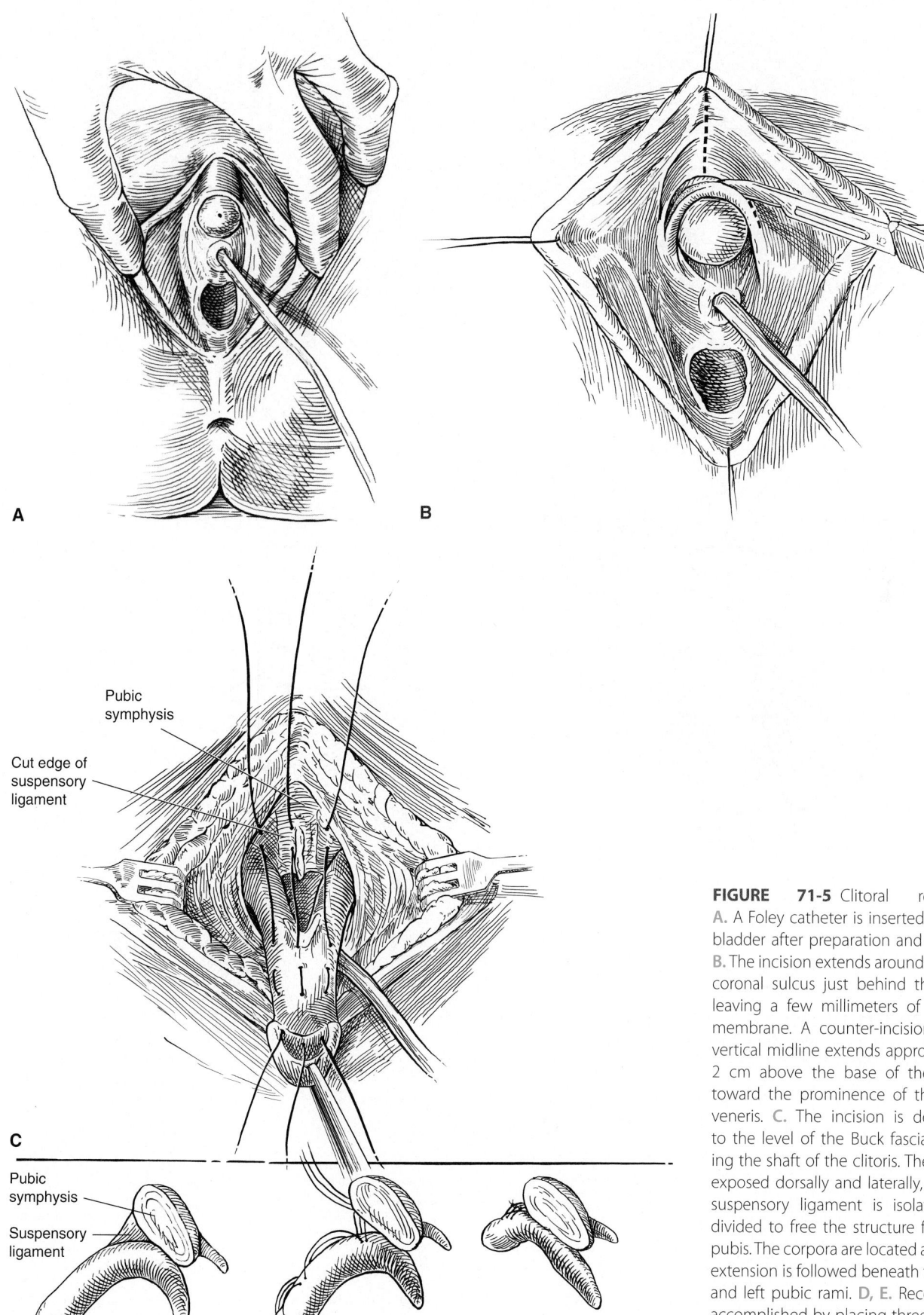

A

B

Pubic
symphysis

Cut edge of
suspensory
ligament

C

Pubic
symphysis

Suspensory
ligament

D

**FIGURE 71-5** Clitoral recession. **A.** A Foley catheter is inserted into the bladder after preparation and draping. **B.** The incision extends around the subcoronal sulcus just behind the glans, leaving a few millimeters of mucous membrane. A counter-incision in the vertical midline extends approximately 2 cm above the base of the clitoris toward the prominence of the mons veneris. **C.** The incision is deepened to the level of the Buck fascia, exposing the shaft of the clitoris. The shaft is exposed dorsally and laterally, and the suspensory ligament is isolated and divided to free the structure from the pubis. The corpora are located and each extension is followed beneath the right and left pubic rami. **D, E.** Recession is accomplished by placing three sutures of 3–0 Vicryl in the fascial covering of the midshaft of the clitoris and the periosteum beneath the pubis.

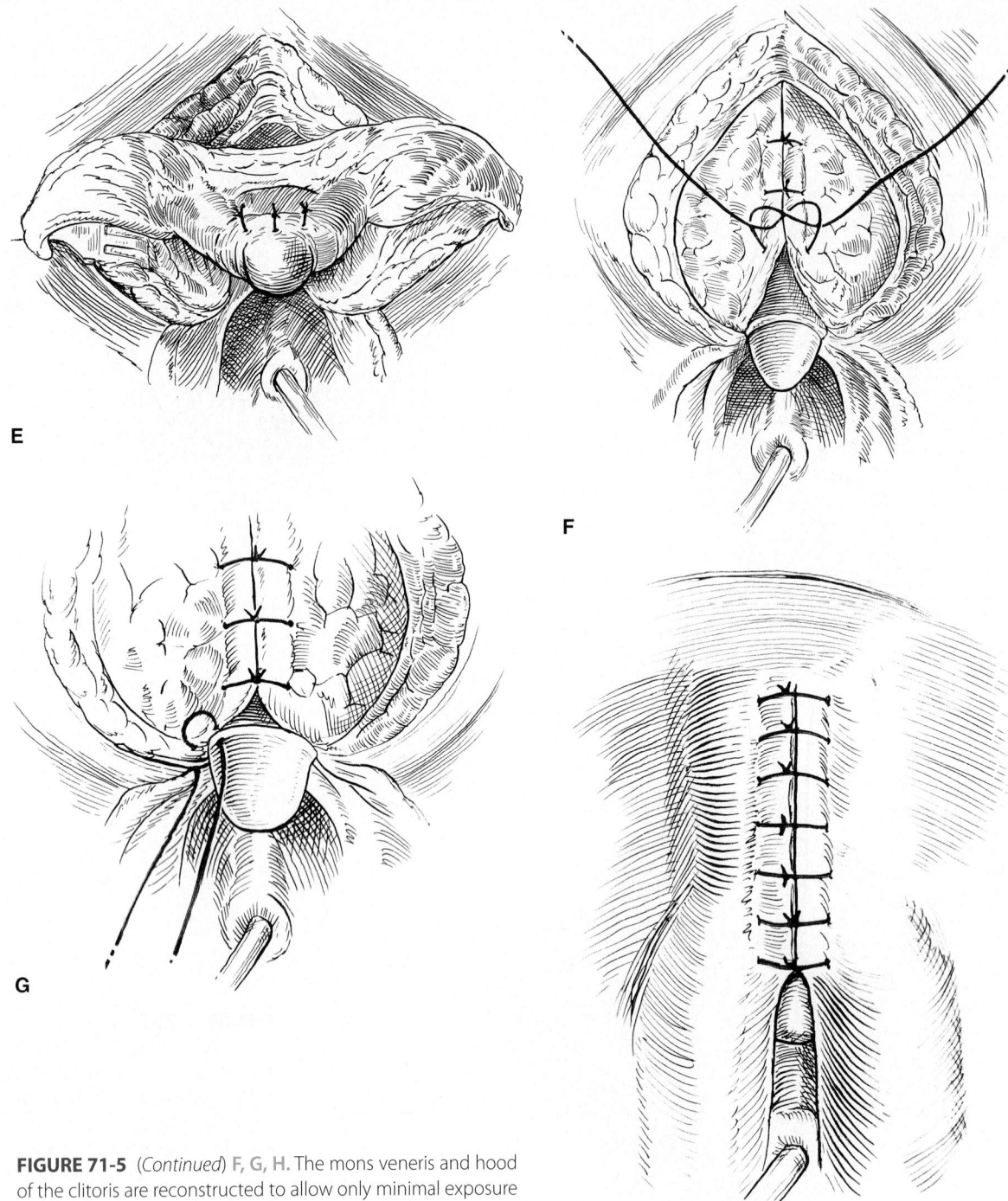

E

F

G

H

**FIGURE 71-5** (*Continued*) **F, G, H.** The mons veneris and hood of the clitoris are reconstructed to allow only minimal exposure of the glans.

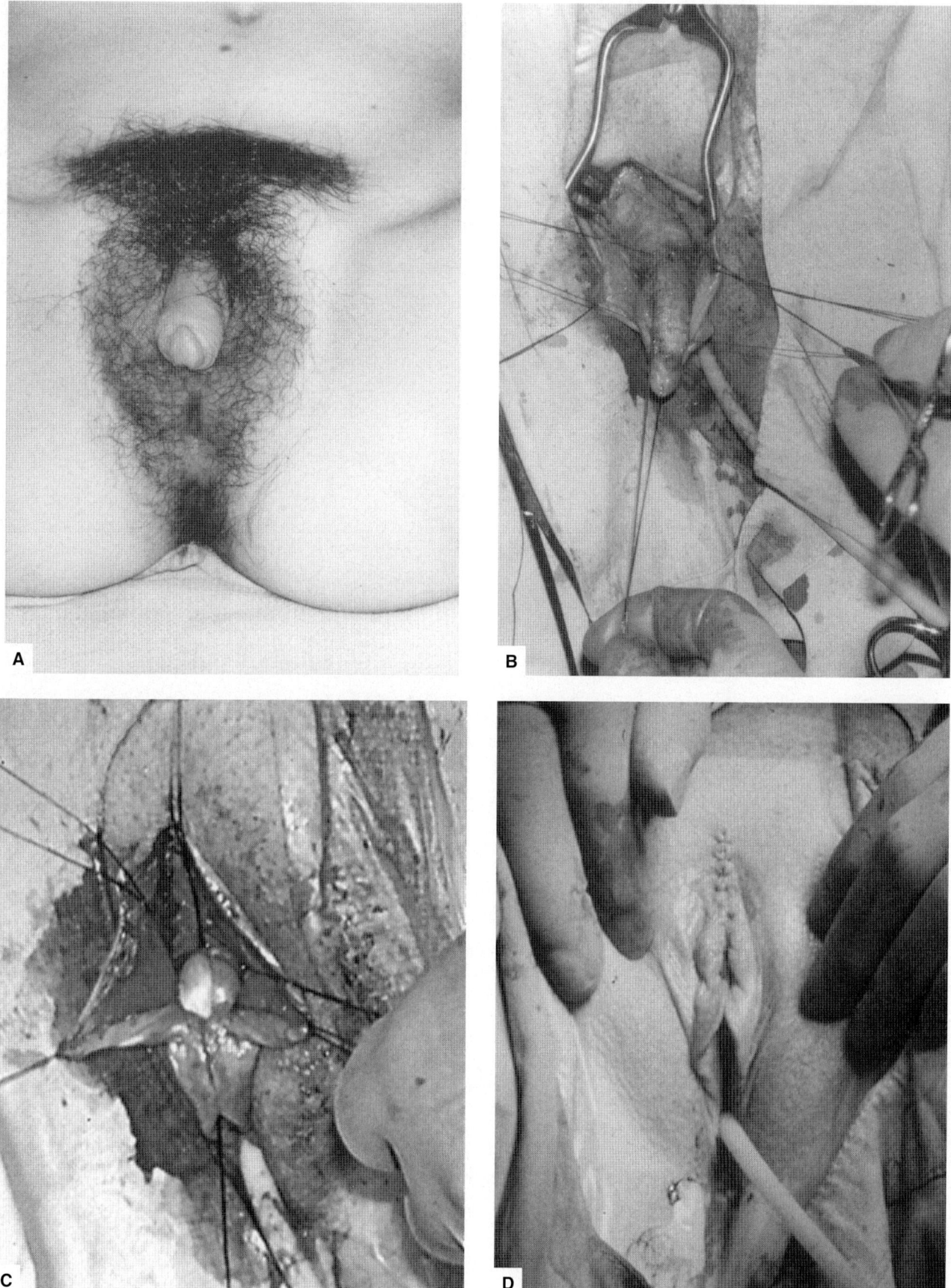

**FIGURE 71-6** **A.** A 46, XX female adolescent with CAH and clitoral hypertrophy. **B.** The operative view of clitoral shaft dissection. **C.** Glanulo-plasty and reconstruction of the clitoral hood. **D.** Postoperative appearance.

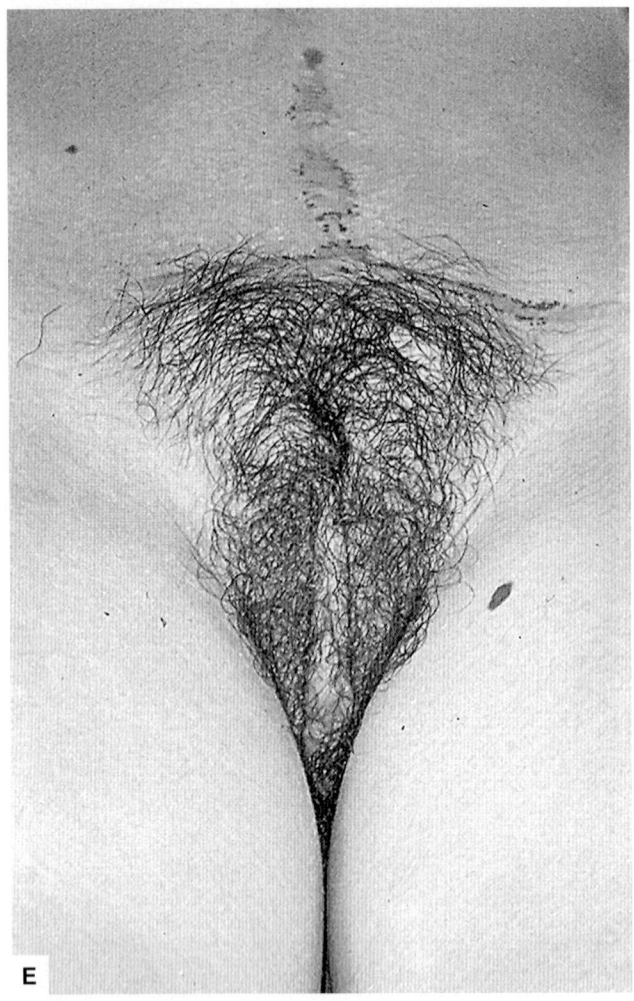

**FIGURE 71-6** (*Continued*) **E.** Late postoperative appearance.

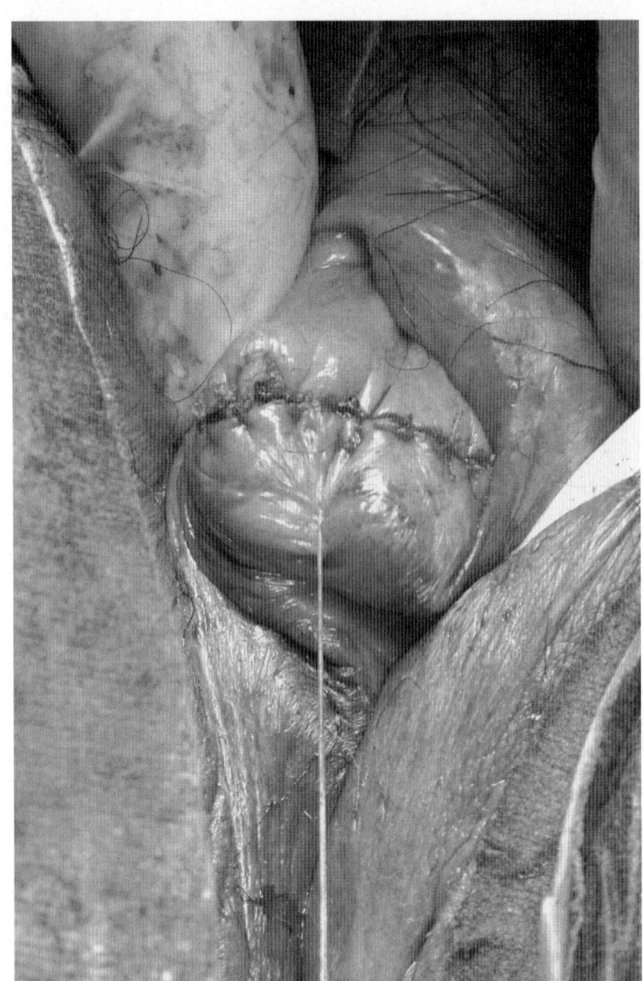

**FIGURE 71-7** Wedge glanuloplasty done to reduce the size of the glans.

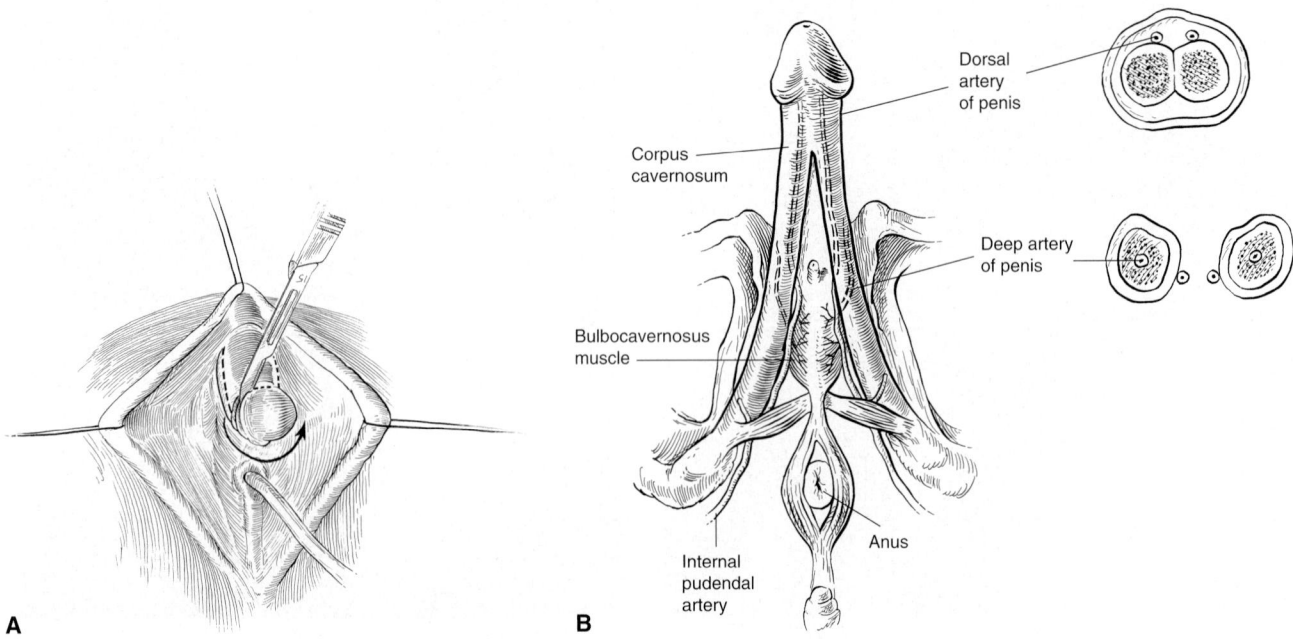

**FIGURE 71-8** Clitoral reduction. **A.** If clitoral reduction is needed, a near circumferential incision leaving only a ventral strip of tissue, *or* a circumferential incision if an island flap is needed, is made around the glans. The incision is carried dorsally onto the mons veneris to create a skin flap that will later be divided in the midline for creation of labia minora. **B.** Clitoral reduction requires anatomic definition of the dorsal neurovascular bundles. After dissecting in the plane of the Buck fascia described previously, an incision is made into the fascia over the neurovascular bundles, which are then isolated and retracted.

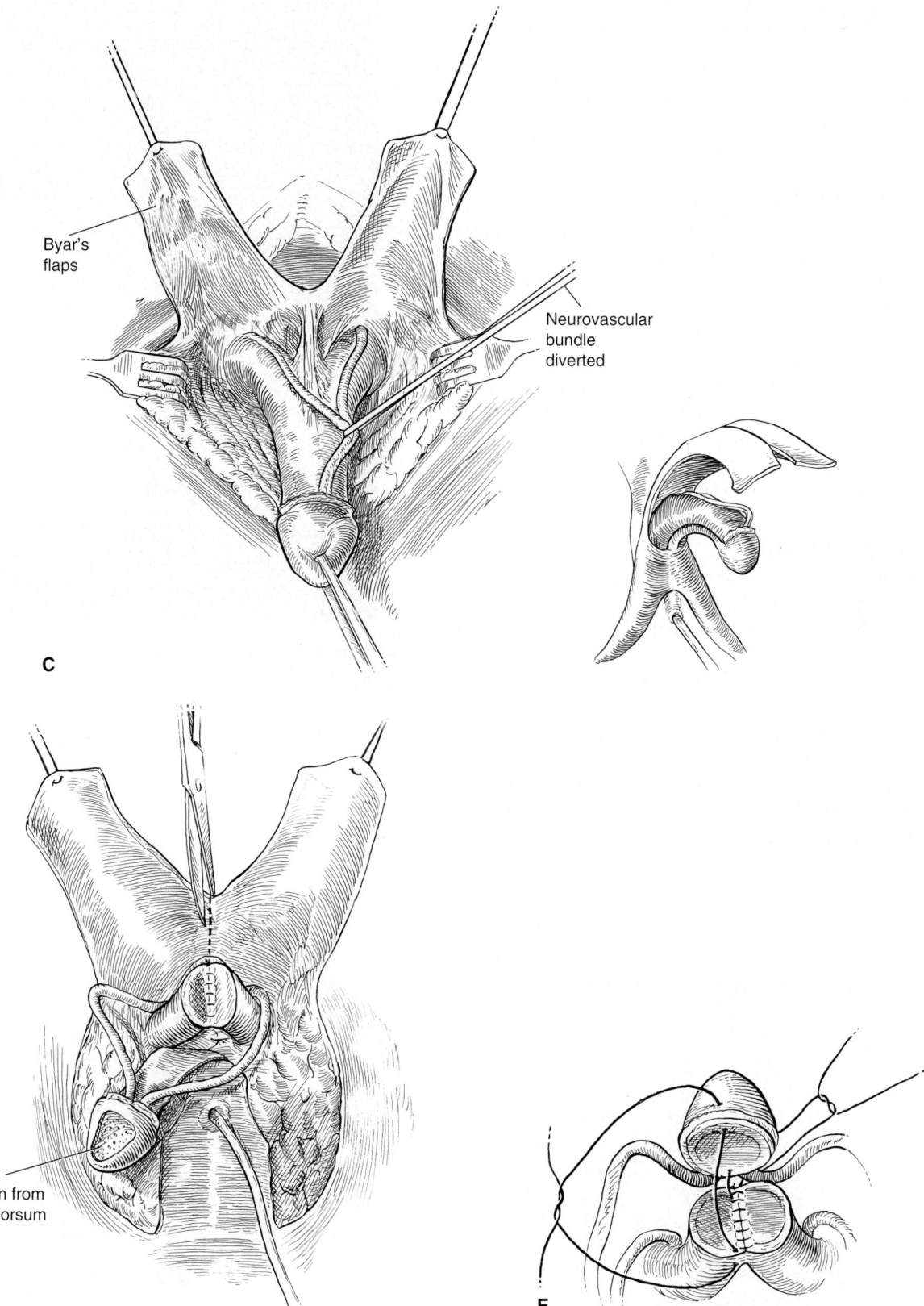

**FIGURE 71-8** (*Continued*) **C.** Ventral and lateral (*inset*) views of the clitoris showing dissection of the neurovascular bundles. Shaft and corpora are exposed and the suspensory ligament will be divided. **D.** The corpora are divided and excised from a point just proximal to the entry of the neurovascular bundles into the glans and up to approximately the bifurcation. **E.** An end-to-end anastomosis joins the remaining clitoral tissue to the shaft using 5-0 or 6-0 Vicryl suture (*inset*). A small wedge excision may be used to reduce the size of the glans and it is closed with a fine absorbable suture. The dorsal clitoris is reconstructed by approximating the remaining mucous membrane distal to the glans to the skin of the mons pubis, and draping the divided skin flaps around the sides of the clitoris to create labia minora (see Fig. 75-10G).

## Vaginoplasty

### Preoperative Preparation

All children who require vaginoplasty, however simple or complicated, undergo a mechanical bowel preparation similar to that used for intestinal surgery.

### Cystoscopy and Vaginoscopy

A careful and thorough cystoscopic and vaginoscopic evaluation precedes reconstruction, usually done after radiographic studies are obtained but prior to planning any reconstruction. Cystoscopy and vaginoscopy are repeated on the day of surgery, both for anatomic definition and to place catheters in the bladder and vagina. The urogenital sinus is entered, and the external urinary sphincter identified with specific reference to the location of the vaginal orifice. The presence or absence of a cervix is noted. A Foley catheter is placed in the bladder and a Fogarty or foley catheter in the vagina, and the catheters are secured together or separately (Fig. 71-9).

### Low Vaginoplasty

This procedure can be done in conjunction with a clitoral recession or reduction. The vagina must enter the urogenital sinus distal to the external urethral sphincter. A series of U-flaps (Fig. 71-10A–D and Fig. 71-11A–D) are outlined in the labioscrotal folds. After raising the labioscrotal flaps, the Byar flaps are rotated around the clitoris and sutured in place. The vagina is opened in the midline posteriorly and the labioscrotal flaps are advanced. Small incisions may also be needed in the lateral walls of the vagina to enhance the vaginal opening. The broad-based U-flap is placed into the posterior vagina.

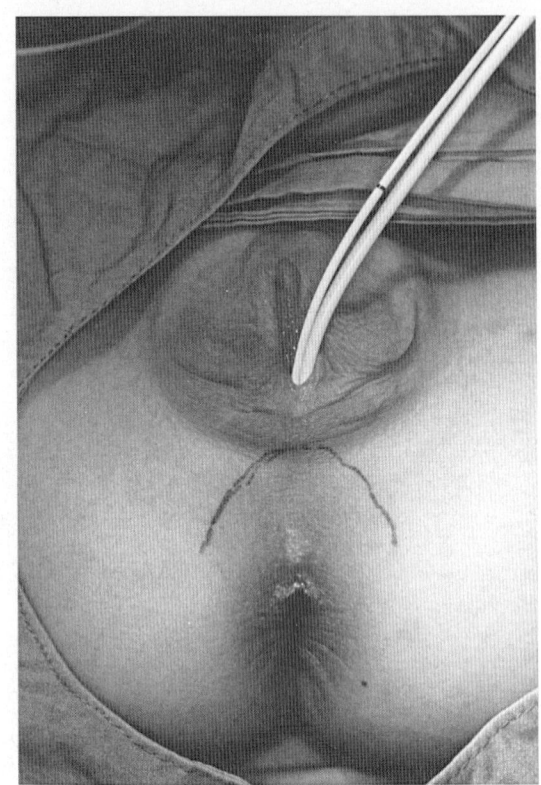

**FIGURE 71-9** In preparation for vaginal reconstruction, a cystoscopy has been performed, a Foley catheter placed in the bladder, and a Fogarty catheter placed in the vagina by cannulating the vaginal fistula in the urogenital sinus.

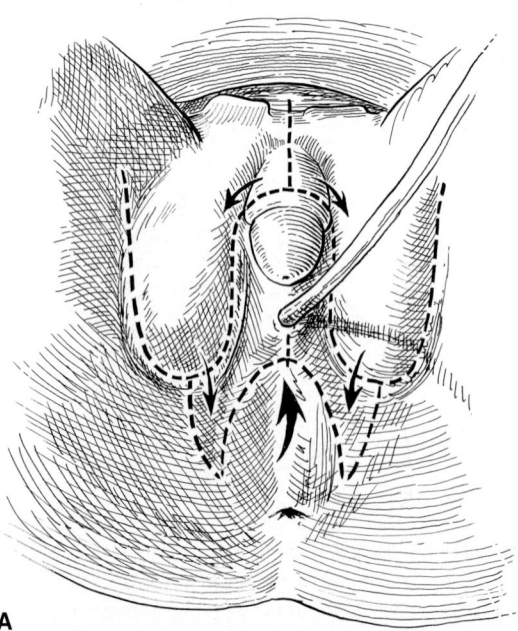

A

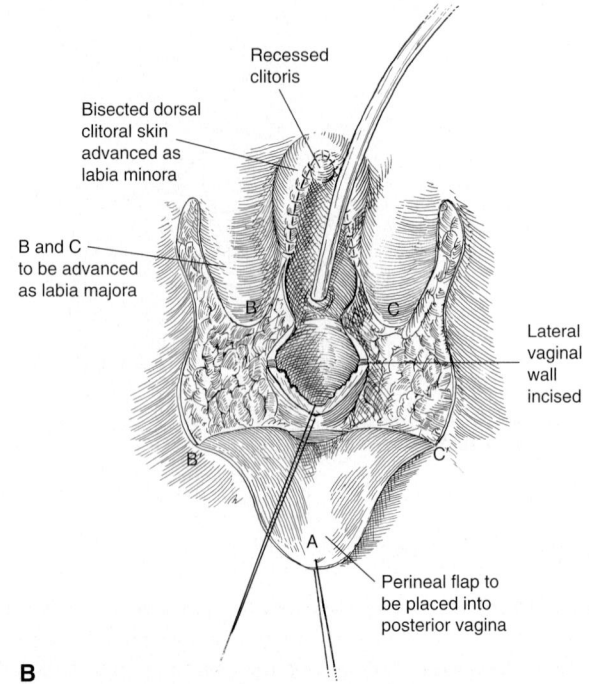

B

**FIGURE 71-10** Low vaginal atresia. **A.** A series of U-flaps are outlined in the labial scrotal folds. A broad-based posterior U-flap is developed and the urogenital sinus delineated. **B.** Clitoral recession or reduction is carried out and the Byar flaps rotated around the recessed clitoris and sutured in place (B to B' and C to C'). The vagina is opened in the midline posteriorly and small incisions may also be made in the lateral walls of the vagina to enhance the vaginal introitus. The broad-based U-flap is placed into the posterior vagina and the labial scrotal flaps are advanced into the lateral recesses of the vagina.

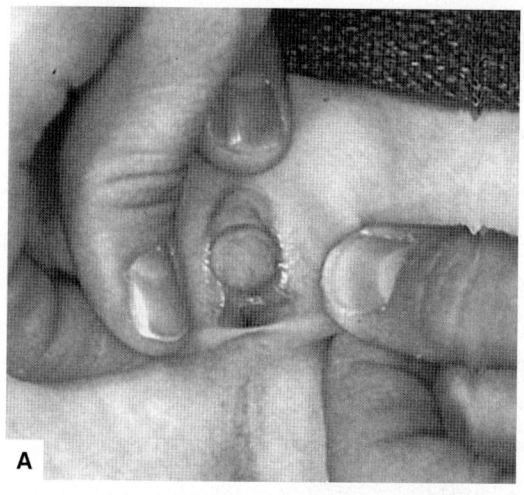

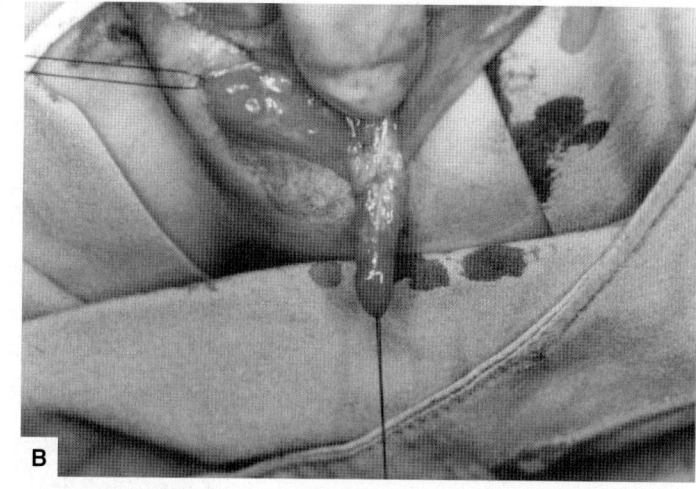

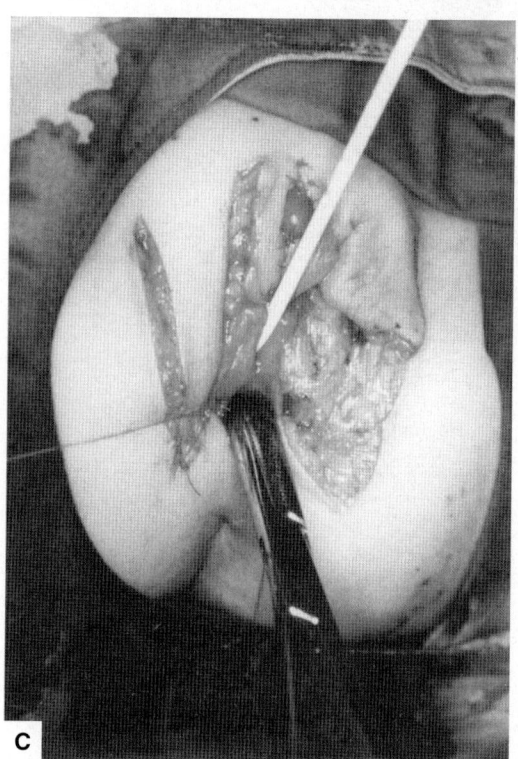

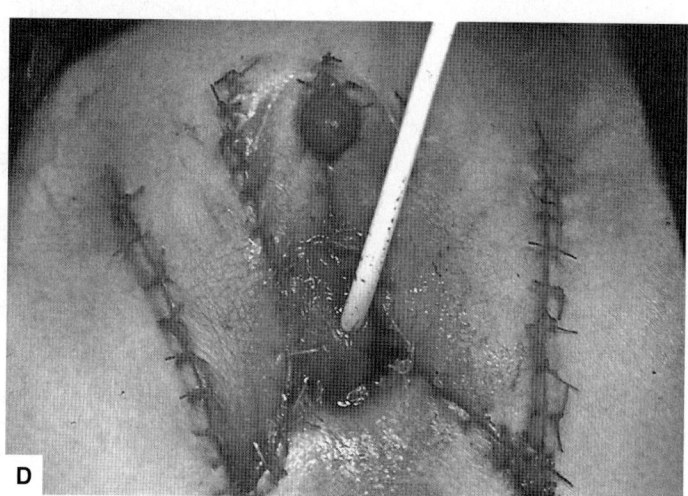

**FIGURE 71-11 A.** A 46, XX female with CAH and low vaginal atresia. **B.** Dissection of the clitoral shaft. **C.** The clitoris and labia minora have been reconstructed and the urogenital sinus opened. The clamp is in the vaginal introitus, and the catheter is in the urethra. **D.** Completed suture lines.

## High Vaginal Atresia Repair

In this situation, the vagina enters the urethra proximal to or at the external sphincter. In the technique advocated by Donahoe, an anterior island flap is used to augment the anterior wall of the mobilized vagina (Fig. 71-12A–G). A clitoroplasty may be done in conjunction with the vaginoplasty. After making all incisions, a finger is placed in the rectum to allow safer mobilization of the posterior vagina from the rectum. The Fogarty catheter previously placed in the vagina allows localization of the vaginal fistula. A nerve stimulator is used to locate the external urinary sphincter prior to opening the vaginal fistula over the Fogarty balloon. The fistula is circumscribed after deflating the balloon and the cuff closed with fine interrupted sutures. Next, the anterior vagina must be mobilized off the bladder. A ventral skin incision made below the clitoris during reduction clitoroplasty releases an island flap, which can be moved inferiorly into the anterior

vagina (Fig. 71-13). The Byar and labioscrotal flaps are then moved into position to create labia minora and majora. An abdominal approach may also be needed to mobilize a high vagina, divide the fistula, and mobilize the vagina toward the perineum (Fig. 71-14).

## Posterior Approach

A posterior approach to the urogenital sinus using techniques described by Pena may aid in the dissection and avoid the urinary sphincter. This total urogenital mobilization technique may also be done with the patient supine. The technique emphasizes placement of multiple fine sutures around the urogenital sinus at the perineum, which allows traction and mobility as the entire unit is dissected and mobilized (see Chapter 53, "Anorectal Malformations"). High insertions of the vagina into the urogenital sinus will still require dissection around the urinary sphincter and may require opening

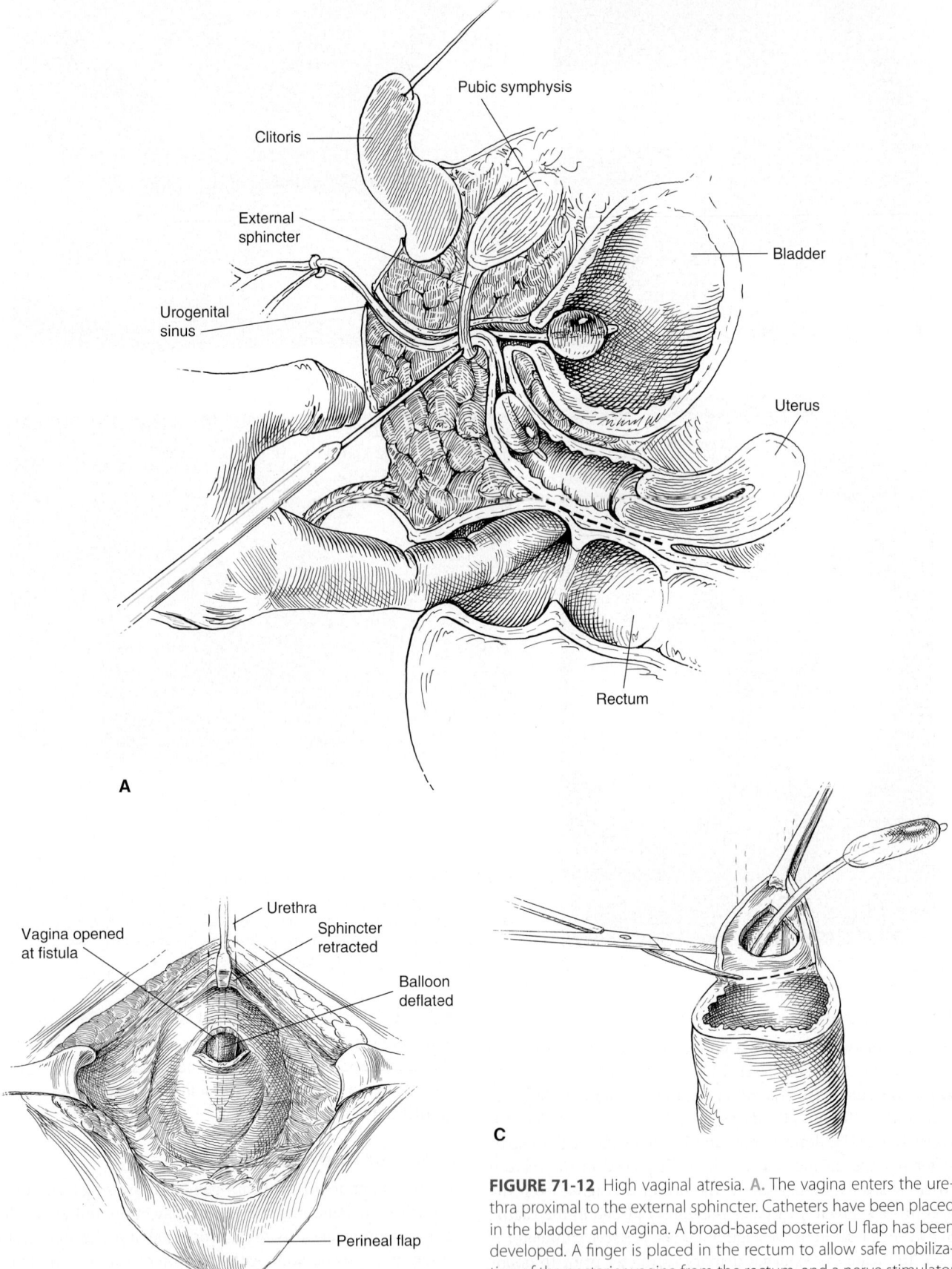

**A**

Pubic symphysis

Clitoris

External
sphincter

Urogenital
sinus

Bladder

Uterus

Rectum

**B**

Vagina opened
at fistula

Urethra

Sphincter
retracted

Balloon
deflated

Perineal flap

**C**

**FIGURE 71-12** High vaginal atresia. **A.** The vagina enters the urethra proximal to the external sphincter. Catheters have been placed
in the bladder and vagina. A broad-based posterior U flap has been
developed. A finger is placed in the rectum to allow safe mobilization of the posterior vagina from the rectum, and a nerve stimulator
is used to locate the external urinary sphincter prior to opening the
vaginal fistula. The fistula can be identified by palpating the Fogerty
balloon in the vagina. **B.** The fistula is opened over the Fogerty balloon. **C, D.** The fistula is circumferentially dissected after deflating the
balloon and the adjacent urogenital sinus opening is closed with
fine interrupted Vicryl.

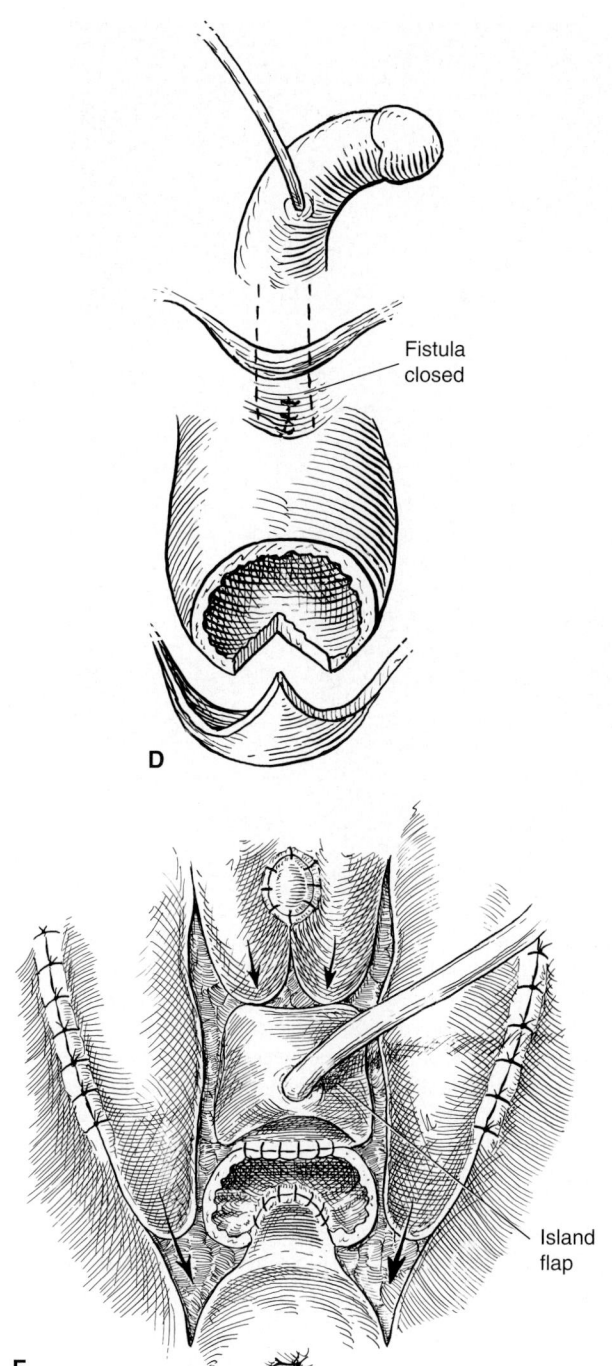

Fistula closed

**D**

Island flap

**F**

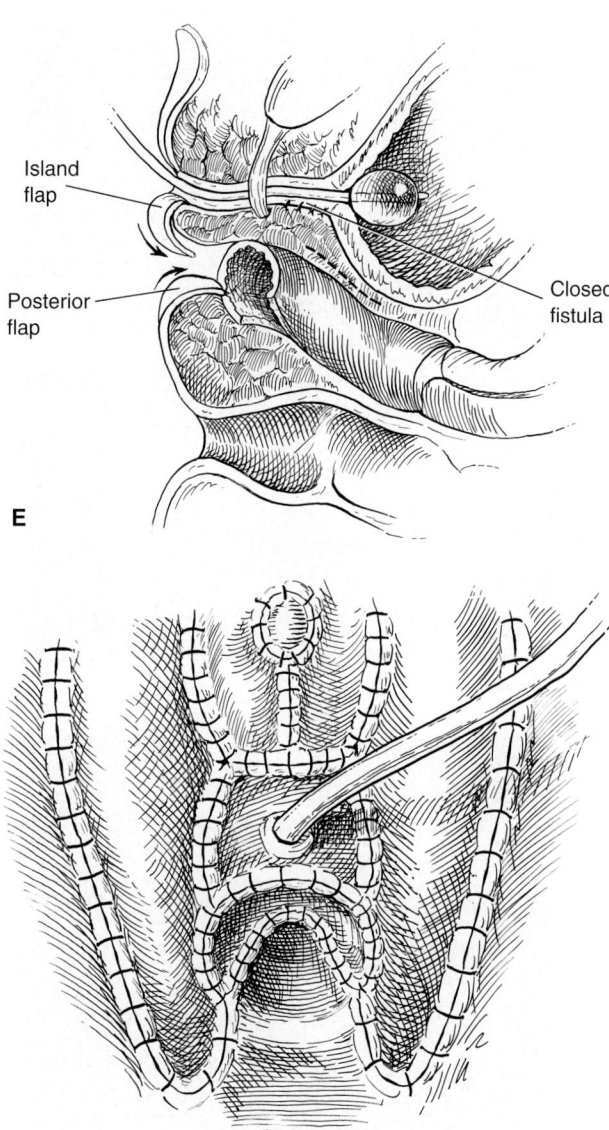

Island flap

Posterior flap

Closed fistula

**E**

**G**

**FIGURE 71-12** (*Continued*) **E.** The anterior vagina is mobilized distally. **F.** A ventral skin incision made below the clitoris during reduction clitoroplasty releases an island flap that can be moved inferiorly into the anterior vagina. **G.** The Byar and labial scrotal flaps are moved into position to create labia minora and majora.

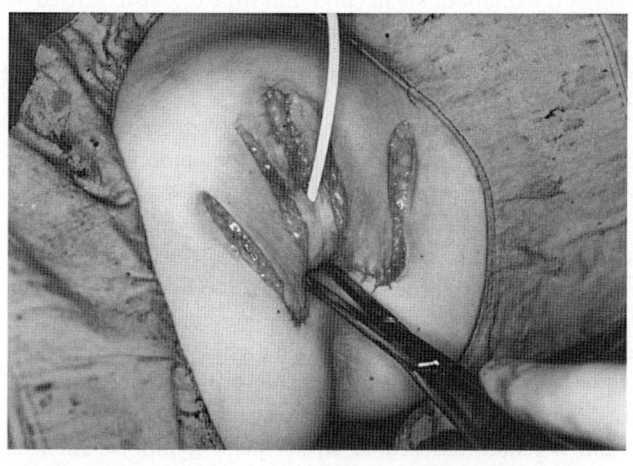

**FIGURE 71-13** A child with high vaginal atresia undergoing reconstruction. An island flap has been released and is used to reconstruct the anterior wall of the vagina.

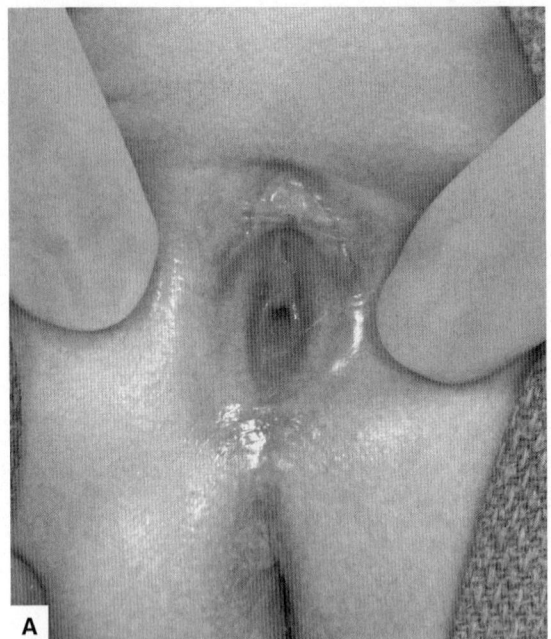

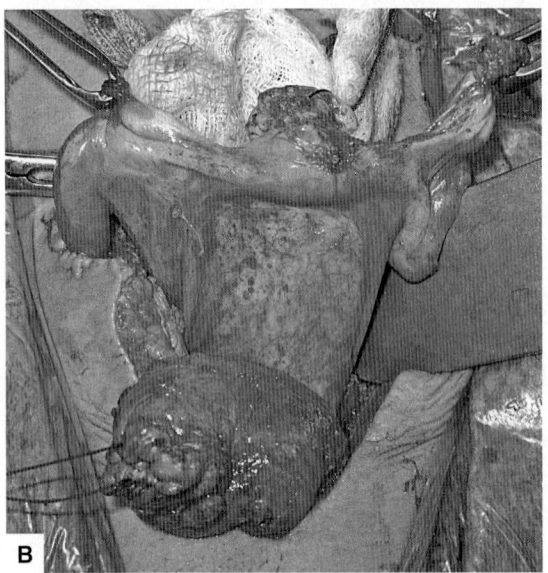

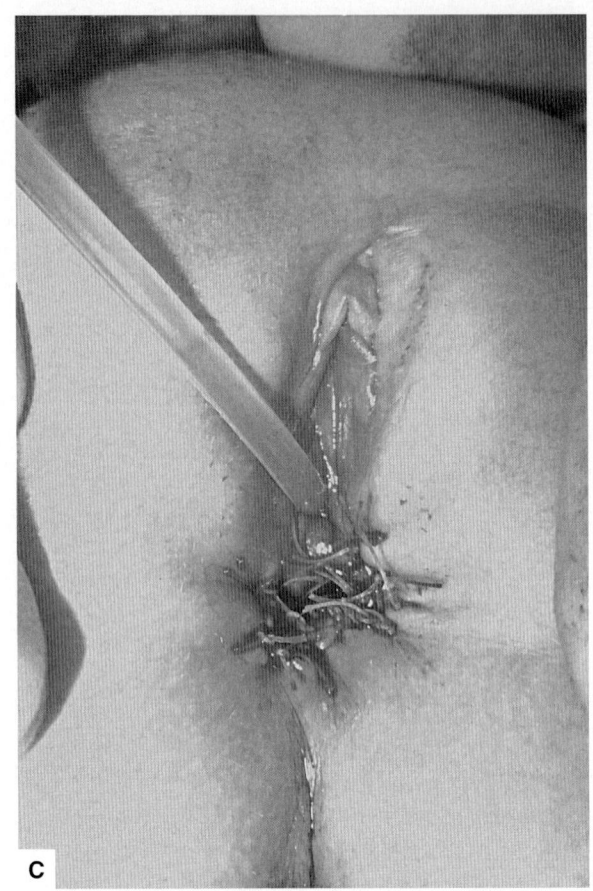

**FIGURE 71-14** A child with vaginal atresia and fistula entering the bladder neck. The vagina had been drained with a vaginostomy tube at birth due to associated hydrocolpos and was also tethered by scar in addition to being high in the pelvis. The child required an abdominal and perineal approach to mobilize the vagina and bring it into the pelvis where it could then be accessed from the perineum. **A.** Appearance of the perineum showing urogenital sinus. The vaginal fistula could not be identified cystoscopically. **B.** Abdominal view of the reproductive tract after separation from the bladder (foreground). The clamps hold the fallopian fimbriae. The child proved to have a large obstructed vagina. **C.** Postoperative appearance of the perineum.

the abdomen to achieve enough length to bring the vagina down to the skin. Alternatively, vaginal augmentation may be needed using one of the techniques described below for the absent vagina (Fig. 71-15).

## Absent Vagina

There are several techniques that may be used to construct, augment, or enhance the caliber of a vagina that is congenitally absent or inadequate. In some patients with only a rudimentary lower vagina or vaginal dimple and absence of Mullerian structures, prolonged external dilatation is successful. The use of myocutaneous flaps or tubularized skin grafts are advocated by some authors, and their use is generally delayed until adulthood in anticipation of intercourse. Particularly with the skin graft technique, a mold must be

used until coitus begins, precluding this type of reconstruction in the infant or small child. Intestine can also be used to bridge the gap between a high vagina, inadequate vagina, or to create a neovagina. This technique may be used at virtually any age.

Sigmoid vaginoplasty (Fig 71-16A–B) is done by first identifying a segment of distal sigmoid with a blood supply that will reach the perineum. The bowel segment is divided only at the distal end initially, and is pulled through to the perineum and sutured. This ensures adequate length with no tension on the mesentery. The upper end of the bowel segment is then divided, avoiding injury to the mesentery. A short segment of bowel above the neovagina may be resected to preclude adjacent suture lines that might predispose to fistula formation. However, all of the mesentery is preserved. The colon is reanastomosed. If an adequate colonic segment is

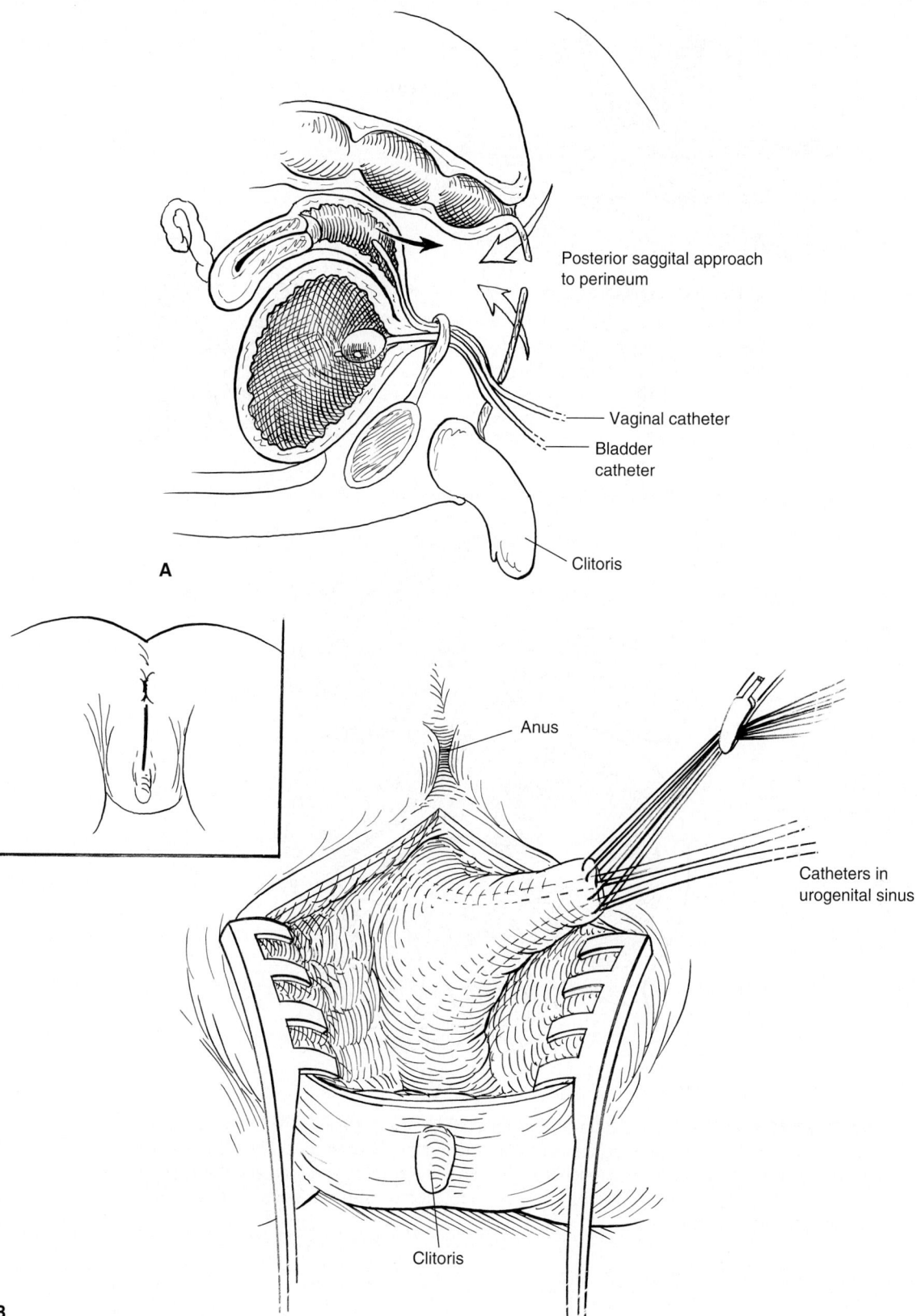

**Posterior saggital approach to perineum**

**Vaginal catheter**

**Bladder catheter**

**Clitoris**

**A**

**Anus**

**Catheters in urogenital sinus**

**Clitoris**

**B**

**FIGURE 71-15** **A.** Posterior total urogenital mobilization approach to high vaginal atresia. Catheters are placed. The child is positioned prone with the legs spread and the pelvis elevated on rolls. **B.** A posterior sagittal midline incision is made from the anterior anus to the urogenital sinus, using the muscle stimulator to define the anatomic midline. The edges of the urogenital sinus are dissected and controlled with multiple fine silk traction sutures. The sutures are held together with a single clamp, to facilitate pulling the vagina in different directions as it is mobilized circumferentially. Traction applied on the vagina allows precise identification of the dissecting plane posteriorly and laterally. The urogenital sinus is opened in the posterior midline from meatus to vaginal confluence.

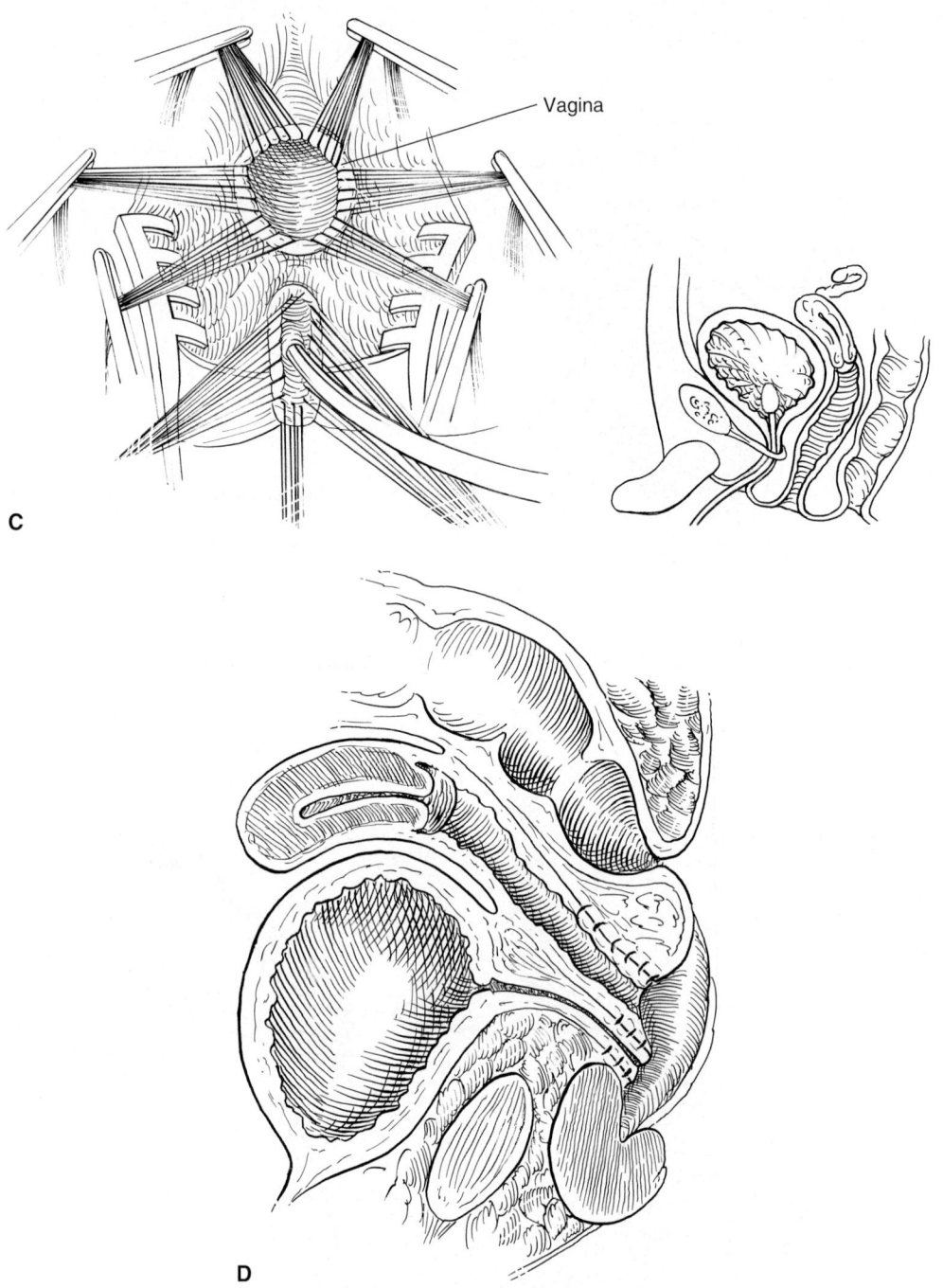

C

Vagina

D

**FIGURE 71-15** (*Continued*) **C.** The distal atretic vagina is opened posteriorly, exposing the confluence of the anterior vaginal wall and proximal urethra and facilitating their separation. **D.** The urethra is tabularized around the foley catheter using the urogenital sinus with a fine absorbable suture, and the vagina and ure-thra are sutured to the perineum. The muscles are anatomically reconstructed, using electrical stimulation to verify appropriate reapproximation.

not available, small bowel may be used for the vaginoplasty (Fig. 71-16C–D). After isolating an appropriate segment, the intestine is folded on the antimesenteric border and a stapling device used to make a more appropriately sized tube to bring down to the pelvis. Another modification is the use of cecum to create a vagina (Fig. 71-16E). After removing the appendix, this obviates the need for separate closure of the proximal end, as the cecum can be inverted and the open colon sutured to the perineum.

## TREATMENT EFFECTIVENESS AND PATIENT OUTCOMES

### Psychologic Implications for Child and Family

*Gender identity* is defined as the consistency and persistence of one's self-awareness as an individual man, woman, or ambivalent. *Gender role* is the behavior, both verbal and

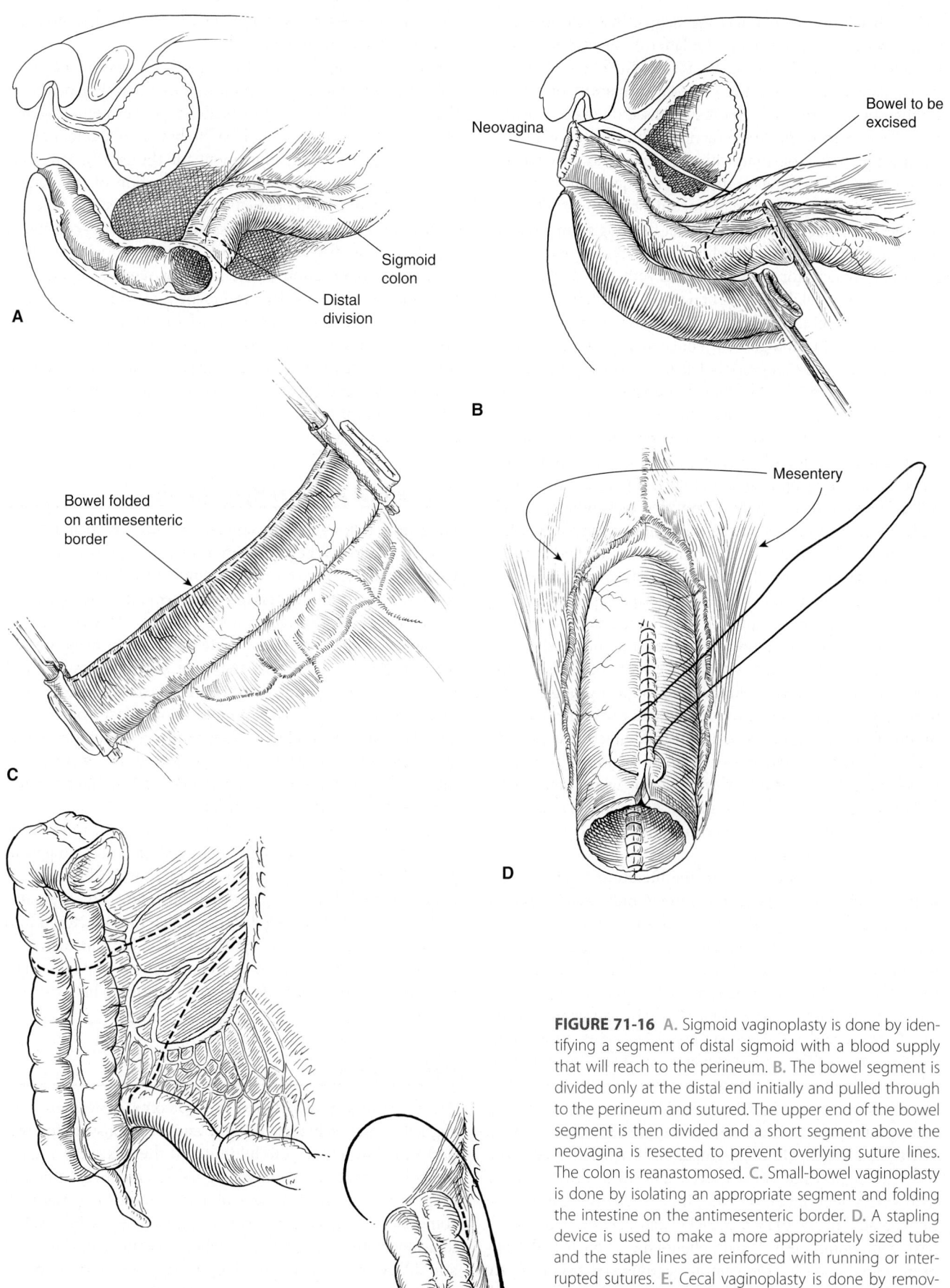

**A**

Sigmoid colon

Distal division

Neovagina

Bowel to be excised

**B**

Bowel folded on antimesenteric border

**C**

Mesentery

**D**

**E**

**FIGURE 71-16 A.** Sigmoid vaginoplasty is done by identifying a segment of distal sigmoid with a blood supply that will reach to the perineum. **B.** The bowel segment is divided only at the distal end initially and pulled through to the perineum and sutured. The upper end of the bowel segment is then divided and a short segment above the neovagina is resected to prevent overlying suture lines. The colon is reanastomosed. **C.** Small-bowel vaginoplasty is done by isolating an appropriate segment and folding the intestine on the antimesenteric border. **D.** A stapling device is used to make a more appropriately sized tube and the staple lines are reinforced with running or interrupted sutures. **E.** Cecal vaginoplasty is done by removing the appendix and mobilizing the cecum towards the perineum (*inset*). The appendix is removed and the terminal leal side of the cecum is sutured closed. The open colon is sutured to the perineum. An ileo-ascending colostomy is performed.

active, that indicates publicly the degree that one is either man, woman, or ambivalent. The latter is capable of changing and is responsive to social forces. In follow-up studies available, it is apparent that the large majority of gender ambiguous patients are heterosexual based on sex of rearing. Nevertheless, an intricate interaction of hormonal forces and rearing practices, together with medication as dictated by pathogenesis of the intersex disorder, is required to maintain the feelings and appearance of unequivocal gender. There is no objective evidence to indicate that the long-term psychosexual outcome of a woman who has undergone major genital surgery is superior to that of a man with a small penis.

There are several developmental stages in childhood, and it is best to counsel the parents and educate the child in a way that parallels chronologic and conceptual growth. Historically, children were commonly left uninformed until someone judged them old and mature enough to comprehend how they were different. These attempts to protect children from knowledge may leave them vulnerable to a personal crisis at exactly the age when sexual identity and identity with a peer group are important. A child less than 2 years old is self-centered and incapable of thinking in another person's terms. At 2 to 6 years, he or she will continue to be somewhat egocentric, and minimize differences between individuals. Over the age of 6, deductive reasoning improves, and with it the ability to discern differences in external appearance. Traditional ages of noncompliance with medication begin at 6 to 8 years old, when children might resist taking medication since "no one else needs to do it." The early to mid-adolescent years are another time when the need for peer group conformity may take precedence over compliance with medication. By this time, it is essential that the child grasp that therapy is essential for maintenance of personal health. With this in mind, the defined periods of family crisis where counseling and education become important are at the time of diagnosis, at the time of any surgical procedure, and at the beginning of major developmental stages.

There is some controversy in the literature regarding the ultimate expression of gender identity in individuals exposed to prenatal androgen. Money et al most consistently established the effects of prenatal androgens on genetic females, including an increase in physical energy, more active play, less interest in dolls and maternal goals, choosing of opposite sex peer choices in play, and more ambivalent gender identity. The exposure of the brain to normal levels of testosterone in utero, neonatally and at puberty are major contributors to formation of gender identity in males. Money found that there was an increase in bisexual and homosexual tendencies among females with CAH who were exposed in utero to high levels of androgen. Other investigators have failed to confirm this. The highest rates of sex reversal occur in genetic males with single gene mutations that impair testosterone formation or action (17-βHSD, 5-αRD) and genetic males who have a predominantly female phenotype at birth and have been reared as girls. The central nervous system androgen effect and exposure to sex-determining genes is pervasive and overrides sex assignment/rearing in these cases. The least rate of sex reversal is seen in genetic males with mutations that impair the function of the AR including CAIS. Individuals

with partial AIS seem to adapt fairly well to the assigned sex, whether it be male or female.

Several decades ago after the Hugh Young case studies were published, there was an evolution toward operation, believing that this was the best way to establish gender identity. Early operation purportedly would lead to better adjustment of the child as well as easier adjustment for the family. Surgeons learned techniques that allowed preservation of the neurovascular bundle during reduction and/or recession of the clitoris. Long-term failures of recession resulted from continued secretion of androgens and poor compliance with medical regimens. Appreciation of the need for regular appraisal of the endocrine, metabolic, and biochemical elements in each patient was recognized as essential for procedural success. Follow-up studies indicate that women who had removal of the clitoris often fail to achieve orgasm, whereas those who have a clitoral preserving operation generally achieve orgasm without painful or unusual sensations in the clitoris if they are sexually active.

## Congenital Adrenal Hyperplasia

Long-term follow-up of patients with CAH has been detailed in a few reports. When compared with control women, individuals with CAH are more often single and childless. At least some of the women experience impairments with regard to body image and attitudes toward sexuality. However, many follow up studies do not indicate an increase in homosexual preference among even the most severely masculinized women. At least 1 study documented a self-admission compliance rate of only 50% with medication. Most women have a final height that is below average for the mean of the control group. Many of the women are felt to be well adjusted, having developed excellent social networks and coping strategies commensurate with their disorder.

In a study where the salt-losing and non-salt-losing forms of CAH were compared, individuals with the salt-losing form generally had decreased pregnancy rates and a higher incidence of hirsutism and poor medical follow-up. They also had more menstrual irregularities, which likely factored into a decrease in overall fertility. There was a high incidence of stenosis of the introitus in women who had previous vaginal reconstruction, contributing to a decrease in heterosexual activity.

## Vaginal Atresia

A few reports have detailed the outcome of women with vaginal atresia. Whether or not a vaginal reconstruction was performed in infancy or childhood, if there is some vaginal stenosis present or a de novo vaginal dimple, the method of dilation with increasing sizes of acrylic molds has met with some success. This method requires the patient to be psychologically mature and motivated when it is initiated. Daily care and dilatation is also required for any type of surgical neovagina to achieve and maintain function. Results following the McIndoe with dilatation or the Frank dilatation method of a vaginal dimple can be excellent, as the neovagina responds to cyclic stimulation by the ovary or exogenous hormones.

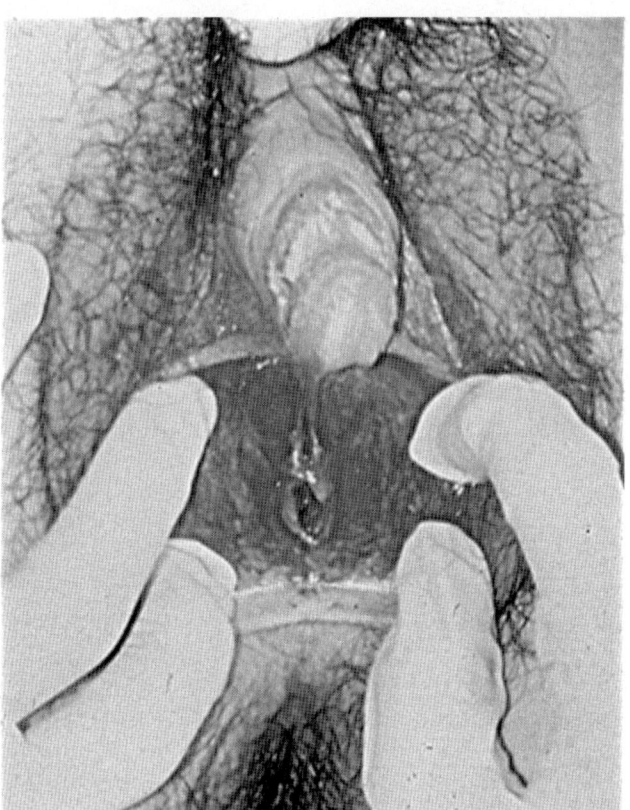

**FIGURE 71-17** A 46, XY individual reared as a female who developed clitoral hypertrophy at puberty. At exploration, she had a fallopian tube and absent gonad on one side, a hypoplastic uterus and an undescended testis on the opposite side, with histology compatible with dysgerminoma.

Distention and lubrication may be less than normal, but does not seem to detract from sexual satisfaction. The major inconvenience of a bowel vagina is the production of mucus. Daily vaginal irrigations are usually required due to the odor and concretions that tend to accumulate.

## Neoplasia Arising in Dysgenetic Gonads

Many long-term studies have detailed the incidence of neoplasia arising in abnormal gonads. Occurrence of neoplasia and dysgenetic gonads is primarily associated with the Y chromosome containing karyotypes, and is less common in patients with 45, XO gonadal dysgenesis (Fig. 71-17). If the Mullerian system is developed and a Y chromosome or fragment is present, there is approximately a 25% incidence of neoplasia. Early exploration and gonadectomy should be performed in these children. Adult patients presenting with primary or secondary amenorrhea and abnormal sexual development, such as infantile external or internal genitalia and atrophic vaginal mucosa, should be thoroughly evaluated for an intersex disorder and gonadectomy if indicated. In individuals with mixed gonadal dysgenesis who lack 2 gonads at laparotomy, a yearly pelvic or abdominal ultrasound evaluation is indicated. Of interest, scrotal testes are not likely to become neoplastic in such patients. An association of the Wilm tumor and genital ambiguity has also been reported.

## SELECTED READINGS

Bhangoo A, Buyuk E, Oktay K, et al. Phenotypic features of 46,XX females with StAR protein mutations. *PER* 2007;5:633.

Belgorosky A, Guercio G, Pepe C, et al. Genetic and clinical spectrum of aromatase deficiency in infancy, childhood and adolescence. *Horm Res* 2009;72:321–330.

Brain CE, Creighton SM, Mushtaq I, et al. Holistic management of DSD. *Best Practice Res Clin Endocrinol Metab* 2010;24:335–354.

Chavhan GB, Parra DA, Oudjhane K, et al. Imaging of ambiguous genitalia: classification and diagnostic approach. *Radiographics* 2008;28:1891–1904.

Crouch NS, Creighton SM. Long-term functional outcomes of female genital reconstruction in childhood. *Paediatr Urol* 2007;100:403–406.

Dacou-Voutetakis C. A multidisciplinary approach to the management of children with complex genital anomalies. *Nat Clin Practice* 2007;3(10):668–669.

deVries AL, Steensma TD, Doreleijers TA, et al. Puberty suppression in adolescents with gender identity disorder: a prospective follow-up study. *J Sex Med* 2011;8:2276–2283.

deVries AL, Doreleijers TA, Cohen-Kettenis PT. Disorders of sex development and gender identity outcome in adolescence and adulthood: understanding gender identity development and its clinical implications. *Pediatr Endocrinol Rev* 2007;4(4):343–351.

Eugenides J. *Middlesex.* New York, NY: Farrar, Straus & Giroux; 2002.

Fallat ME, Donahoe PK. Intersex genetic anomalies with malignant potential. *Curr Opin Pediatr* 2006;18:305–311.

Fausto-Sterling A. The five sexes: why male and female are not enough. *The Sciences.* New York Academy of Sciences; 1993:20–24.

Garel L. Abnormal sex differentiation: who, how and when to image. *Pediatr Radiol* 2008;38(Suppl 3):S508–S511.

Hughes IA. Disorders of sex development: a new definition and classification. *Best Practice Res Clin Endocrinol Metab* 2008;22(1):119–134.

Hughes IA, Nihoul-Fékété C, Thomas B, et al. Consequences of the ESPE/LWPES guidelines for diagnosis and treatment of disorders of sex development. *Best Practice Res Clin Endocrinol Metab* 2007;21(3):351–365.

Intersex Society of North America (ISNA), www.isna.org.

Johnsdotter S, Essén B. Genitals and ethnicity: the politics of genital modifications. *Reprod Health Matters* 2010;18(35):29–37.

Jones HW, Scott WW. *Hermaphroditism, Genital Anomalies and Related Endocrine Disorders.* Baltimore, MD: Williams and Wilkins Company; 1958.

Kuhnle U, Krahl W. The impact of culture on sex assignment and gender development in intersex patients. *Perspect Biol Med* 2002;45(1):85–103.

Lee PA, Houk CP. Disorders of sexual differentiation in the adolescent. *Ann NY Acad Sci* 2008;1135:67–75.

MacLellan DL, Diamond DA. Recent advances in external genitalia. *Pediatr Clin N Am* 2006;53:449–464.

Maharaj NR, Dhai A, Wiersma R, et al. Intersex conditions in children and adolescents: surgical, ethical and legal considerations. *J Pediatr Adolesc Gynecol* 2005;18:399–402.

Mazur T. Gender dysphoria and gender changes in androgen insensitivity or micropenis. *Arch Sexual Behav* 2005;34(4):411–421.

Mendonca BB, Costa EMF, Belgorosky A, et al. 46,XY, DSD due to impaired androgen production. *Best Practice Res Clin Endocrinol Metab* 2010;24:243–262.

Mieszczak J, Houk CP, Lee PA. Assignment of the sex of rearing in the neonate with a disorder of sex development. *Curr Opin Pediatr* 2009;21:541–547.

Miller WL, Auchus RJ. The molecular biology, biochemistry, and physiology of steroidogenesis and its disorders. *Endocrin Rev* First published ahead of print November 4, 2010 as doi.10.1210/er.2010-0013.

Nabhan ZM, Lee PA. Disorders of sex development. *Curr Opin Obstet Gynecol* 2007;19:440–445.

Nihoul-Fékété C. How to deal with congenital disorders of sex development in 2008 (DSD). *Eur J Pediatr Surg* 2008;18:364–367.

Thyen U, Richter-Appelt H, Wiesemann C, et al. Deciding on gender in children with intersex conditions. *Treat Endocrinol* 2005;4(1):1–8.

Wisniewski AB, Migeon CJ, Meyer-Bahlburg HF, et al. Complete androgen insensitivity syndrome: long-term medical, surgical, and psychosexual outcome. *J Clin Endocrinol Metabolism* 2000;85(8):2664–2669.

Yang JH, Baskin LS, DiSandro M. Gender identity in disorders of sex development: review article. *Urology* 2010;75:153–160.

Young HH. *Genital Abnormalities, Hermaphroditism and Related Adrenal Disorders.* London, England: Bailliere, Tindall and Cox; 1937.

# PART VI

## VASCULAR SYSTEM ANOMALIES

# CHAPTER 72

## The Surgical Treatment of Patent Ductus Arteriosus and Aortic Coarctation

*Andrew C. Fiore, Michael Hines, and D. Glenn Pennington*

## Patent Ductus Arteriosus

### KEY POINTS

1. Full-term neonates, infants, and older children should have patent ductus arteriosus (PDA) closed even in the absence of symptoms, provided the pulmonary vascular resistance is less than 8 to 10 wood units/m$^2$.

2. Ligation is reserved for preterm infants and small newborns.

3. In full-term newborns and older children, the ductus arteriosus is divided whenever possible to avoid the rare complications of ductal recanalization or aneurysm formation following ligation.

4. Closure using the midline sternotomy approach is most commonly employed for patients requiring cardiopulmonary bypass to correct a coexisting cardiac lesion.

5. On rare occasions when the PDA cannot be encircled, it can be closed from inside the main pulmonary artery.

6. The double-umbrella and vascular occluder are currently used for percutaneous catheter closure of PDA and Gianturco coils are becoming increasing popular.

7. Endoscopic ductal closure can be applied to patients less than 3 to 5 kg, an important distinction from transcatheter closure, where femoral vessel size may be prohibitive.

8. Complications of PDA closure include bleeding and aneurysm of the ductus arteriosus after ligation or division.

9. The high complication rate following ductus ligation in preterm infants is related more to prematurity than to the surgery. About 5% to 10% of these premature patients develop sequellae, including retrolental fibroplasia, blindness, and cerebral palsy.

### INTRODUCTION

The ductus arteriosus is a vessel 5 to 10 mm in length that connects the main pulmonary trunk with the descending aorta just distal to the origin of the left subclavian artery. An embryologic remnant of the distal portion of the sixth left branchial arch, the ductus arteriosus is usually on the left side, but in cases of right aortic arch, it can be on either side. It is rarely completely absent or bilateral.

### EMBRYOLOGY AND PATHOLOGIC ANATOMY

The media of the ductus at birth is composed of circularly arranged smooth muscle cells that contract in response to increasing oxygen tension. The first stage of postnatal closure occurs at 10 to 15 hours after birth and the final stage is complete at 2 to 3 weeks in 88% of full-term infants. Although final closure may occur at any age, it is distinctly uncommon beyond 6 months of life. Beyond 1 year of age, about 1% of all ducti remain open and very few close after that.

In the premature newborn with a birth weight of 1000 g or less, the incidence of patent ductus arteriosus (PDA) is 80% to 90%. This high incidence is related to decreased smooth muscle in the ductal wall, diminished response of the muscle to oxygen, and increasing levels of E series prostaglandins, which vasodilate the ductal muscle and prevent closure.

### NATURAL HISTORY, MORTALITY, AND MORBIDITY

The incidence of isolated PDA in a full-term infant is 1/2000 live births and represents 5% to 10% of all types of congenital heart disease. Etiologic factors include maternal rubella and living in high altitudes, prematurity, neonatal hypoxia, and respiratory distress of the newborn. The prevalence is higher in girls by a ratio of 2:1.

PDA causes a high mortality in infants and it has been estimated that 30% of patients with isolated untreated PDA die in the first year of life. Congestive heart failure is the mode of death in infants with a large PDA. Beyond infancy, death from a large PDA is secondary to right heart failure from severe pulmonary vascular disease or intractable left ventricular failure secondary to chronic volume overload. A large PDA can cause elevated pulmonary vascular resistance by age 5 or older.

Premature infants can have a higher mortality with PDA because the left to right shunt can aggravate problems of prematurity such as bronchopulmonary dysplasia, necrotizing enterocolitis, and intraventricular hemorrhage.

The use of antibiotics has reduced the incidence of bacterial endocarditis, a complication formerly associated with a small PDA.

## CLINICAL FEATURES

The clinical features of PDA depend on the size of the ductus and the degree of pulmonary vascular occlusive disease.

## TERM INFANTS AND OLDER CHILDREN

Symptoms of congestive heart failure, including tachypnea, tachycardia, poor feeding, slow weight gain, and recurrent pulmonary infections, are seen within the first 6 months of life. If the shunt is moderate to large, the classic continuous murmur is present in systole and diastole. The liver is enlarged and the jugular venous pressure is elevated. The peripheral pulses may be bounding. The chest radiograph demonstrates cardiomegaly with an enlarged main pulmonary artery and lung plethora. The electrocardiogram is consistent with left atrial and ventricular enlargement.

The echocardiogram with Doppler color flow imaging will confirm the diagnosis and establish any coexisting cardiac lesions. This technique has replaced cardiac catheterization except in special circumstances of elevated pulmonary vascular resistance or associated cardiac anomalies.

If the ductus is small, left ventricular failure and symptoms of congestive heart failure do not occur until later in life. Although a continuous murmur is rarely heard in neonates, typically a murmur (short, systolic, or possibly continuous) is detected by 2 or 3 months of age and subsequent Doppler echocardiography confirms the diagnosis.

## PREMATURE INFANTS

The incidence of PDA is higher in premature infants because hypoxia secondary to coexisting respiratory distress syndrome inhibits ductal closure. The premature infant has limited ability to increase cardiac output and excessive pulmonary blood flow through the patent ductus leads to hypoperfusion of the vascular tree. This may lead to sepsis, renal failure, necrotizing enterocolitis, metabolic acidosis, and death. The murmur is usually systolic and may be associated with bounding peripheral pulses. The Doppler echocardiogram is diagnostic.

## INDICATIONS FOR CLOSURE

Full-term neonates, infants, and older children should have the PDA closed even in the absence of symptoms, provided the pulmonary vascular resistance is less than 8 to 10 wood units/$m^2$. Congestive heart failure is an indication for closure in infancy. Otherwise closure should be performed in the first year of life. The authors believe that the PDA should be closed to avoid the risk of pulmonary arteriolar occlusive disease and the small but definite risk of bacterial endocarditis. In adulthood, a persistent ductus can become aneurysmal with associated luminal calcification, thus increasing the operative risk for closure.

In premature infants, a more conservative approach is recommended. Aspirin or indomethacin, shown to be effective in ductal closure by inhibiting prostaglandin synthesis, is used first. If medical closure is contraindicated (as in the premature infant with renal insufficiency or large intraventricular hemorrhage) or if the ductus remains patent after 2 courses of indomethacin, then surgical closure is performed. A recent randomized trial demonstrated that necrotizing enterocolitis in preterm infants is strongly associated with a large PDA and that ductal closure is beneficial.

## SURGICAL CLOSURE

For surgical closure of PDA, the patient is positioned for a left posterior lateral thoracotomy. Intra-arterial monitoring by catheter is unnecessary. A curvilinear incision is made 1 fingerbreadth below the tip of the left scapula. The serratus anterior muscle is preserved and the left hemithorax is opened through the fourth intercostal space. The lung is retracted inferiorly using damp gauze and 2 ribbon retractors. The posterior mediastinal pleura is opened along the descending aorta and the incision carried cephalad until the origin of the transverse aortic arch and the left subclavian arteries are identified (Fig. 72-1). The hemiazygos vein is ligated and divided. The anterior edge of pleura is held on slight traction with stay sutures (Fig. 72-2). This improves ductal exposure, keeps the vagus and recurrent laryngeal nerves medially, and permits removal of 1 ribbon retractor. The tissue plane close to the aortic wall above and below the ductus is opened parallel with the PDA. With the aortic end of the PDA held on traction superiorly, a blunt tip right-angled clamp is placed under the ductus. The ductal tissue is fragile and therefore an attempt to come around the ductus with the curved clamp is made only when dissection is deep enough above and below.

The clamp should be applied from below upward. Frequently, a small band of tissue needs sharp dissection as the metal tip of the instrument is seen emerging from the cephalad end of the ductus (Fig. 72-3). The clamp is then gently spread parallel to the ductus to improve exposure. The left recurrent laryngeal nerve is identified and gently dissected off

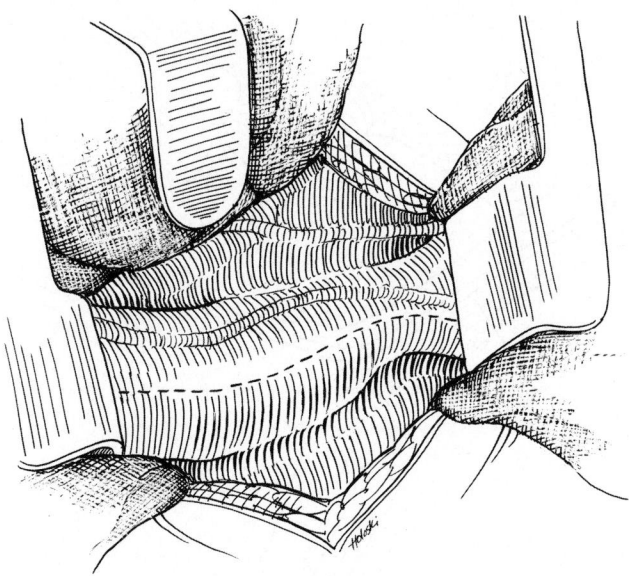

**FIGURE 72-1** Left thoracotomy through the fourth intercostal space. The lung is retracted inferiorly and the posterior mediastinal pleura incised (dotted line). The phrenic and vagus nerves can be seen.

the posterior plane of the ductus to avoid entrapment by the ligaclip, suture, or the vascular clamp.

At this point, a test occlusion of the PDA for 30 to 60 seconds is made with vascular forceps. The thrill should disappear. The systemic pressure may rise. Bradycardia with

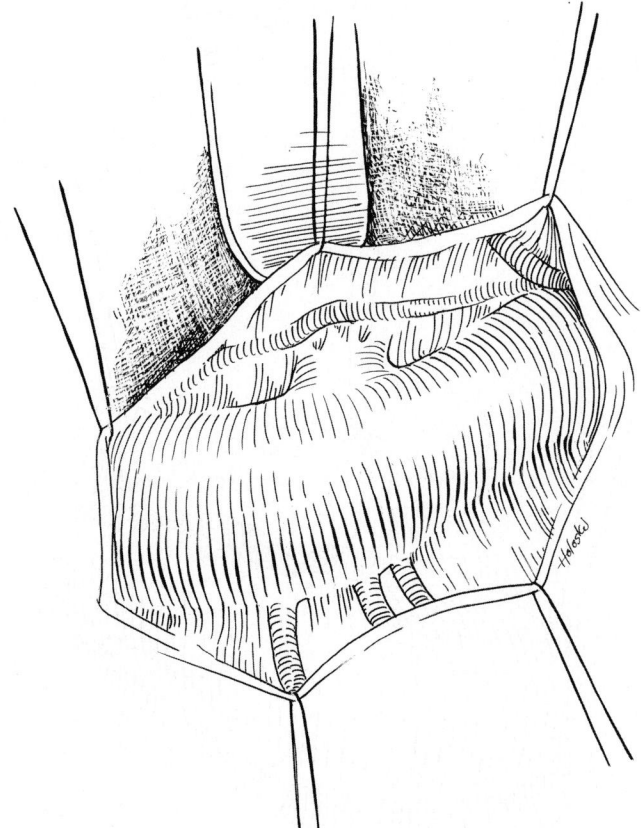

**FIGURE 72-2** Stay sutures are placed on the anterior edge of the pleura and the ductus is encircled in a plane close to the aortic wall. The recurrent laryngeal nerve is on the pleura flap which is retracted medially.

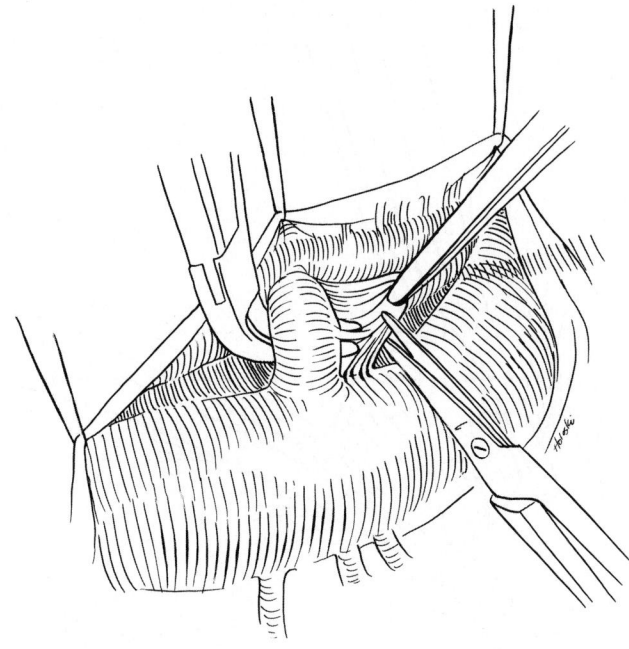

**FIGURE 72-3** The right angle clamp is placed around the ductus. Adhesive bands are cut sharply.

desaturation should not be seen unless the ductus is the sole source of pulmonary blood flow.

## DIVISION

Division avoids the rare but reported complications of ductal recanalization or aneurysm formation following ligation. Therefore the authors prefer to divide the ductus in full-term newborns and all older children whenever possible.

The aortic end of the patent ductus is occluded first with a vascular clamp applied as close to the aortic wall as possible. With this clamp used as traction towards the surgeon, the pulmonary artery side of the ductus is occluded with a second vascular clamp, applied carefully to avoid injury to the recurrent laryngeal nerve, which is now free posteriorly. If more ductal length is desired, a partial occlusion clamp may be used at the aortic end (Fig. 72-4). The ductus is divided and the aortic end is oversewn first using a continuous horizontal mattress followed by an over-and-over polypropylene suture. The aortic clamp is removed and the suture is held on traction. Gentle downward traction on the aorta as the aortic clamp is released allows the clamp to be fully reapplied if bleeding is noted. The pulmonary end is closed analogously and both sutures cut after hemostasis is established (Fig. 72-4).

## LIGATION

Ligation is reserved for preterm infants and small newborns. Thick ligatures of braided silk are moistened and carefully passed around the ductus. The pulmonary site is ligated first, placing both index fingers deep in the chest parallel to the aorta (Fig. 72-5). Usually 2 or 3 ligatures are used (Fig. 72-6).

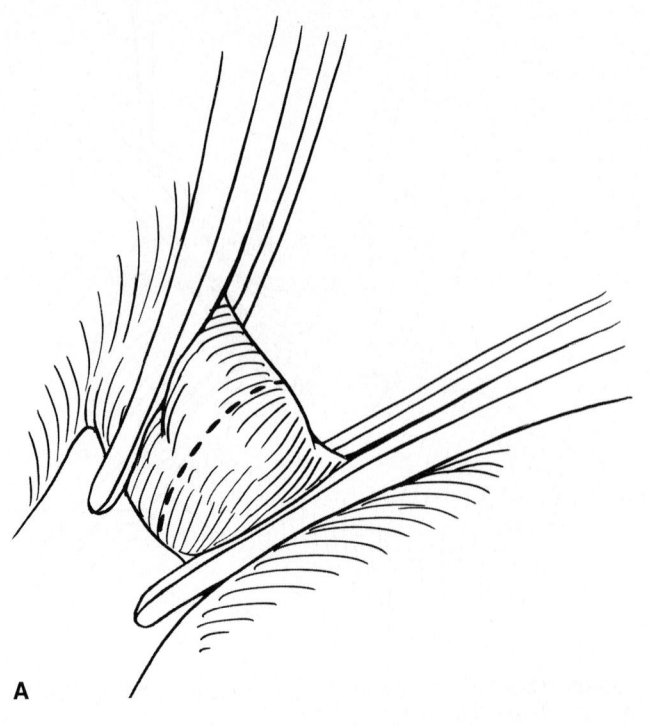

A

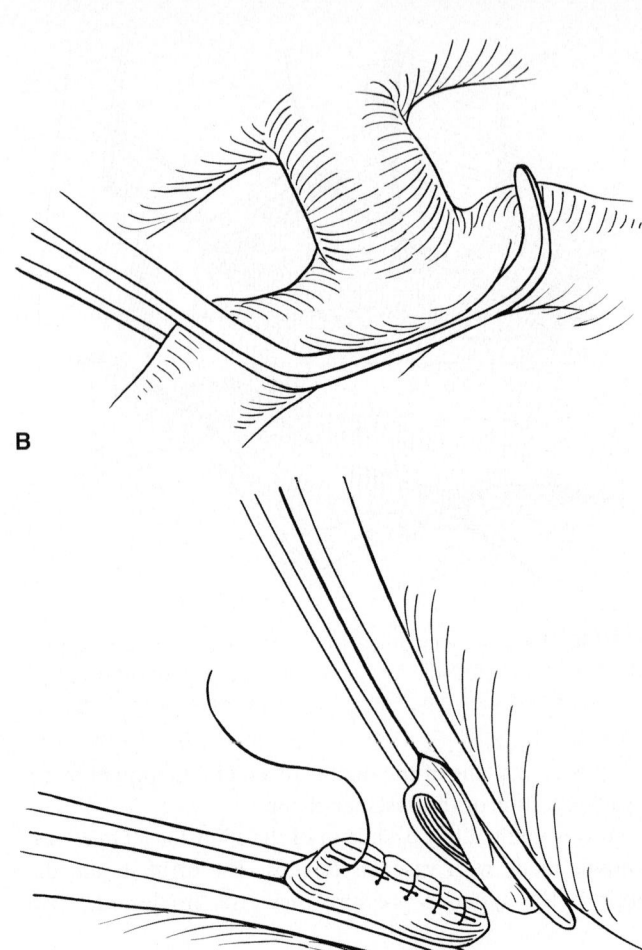

B

C

**FIGURE 72-4** **A.** Straight vascular clamps are applied and the ductus is divided. **B.** Alternatively, a partial occlusion clamp may be used at the aortic end to obtain more length for division. **C.** Both ends are oversewn with a running mattress suture in 1 layer and then a continuous over-and-over stitch in the second layer.

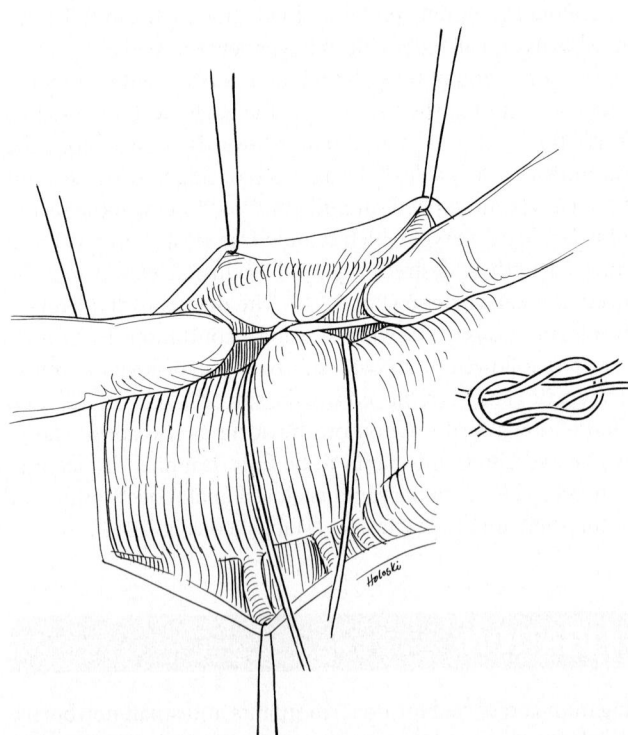

**FIGURE 72-5** The ligature close to the pulmonary artery is tied first. Both index fingers should be deep in the chest in the plane of the PDA.

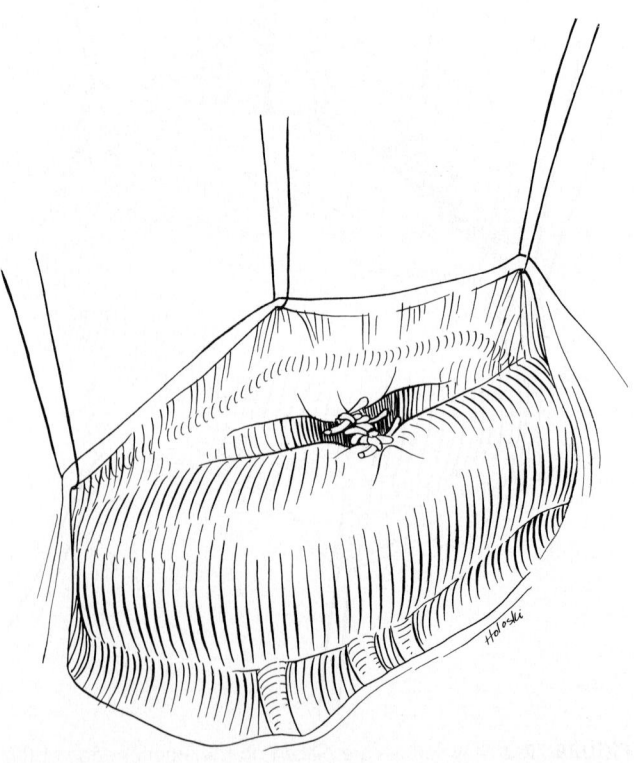

**FIGURE 72-6** The lumen of the PDA is completely abolished with 2 or 3 ligatures.

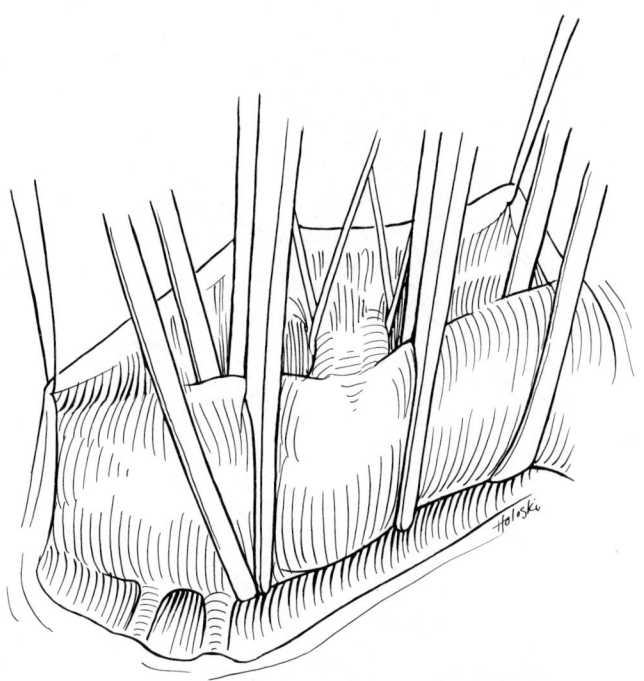

**FIGURE 72-7** For patients with pulmonary hypertension, the aorta is cross-clamped above and below the PDA before the first knot is tied.

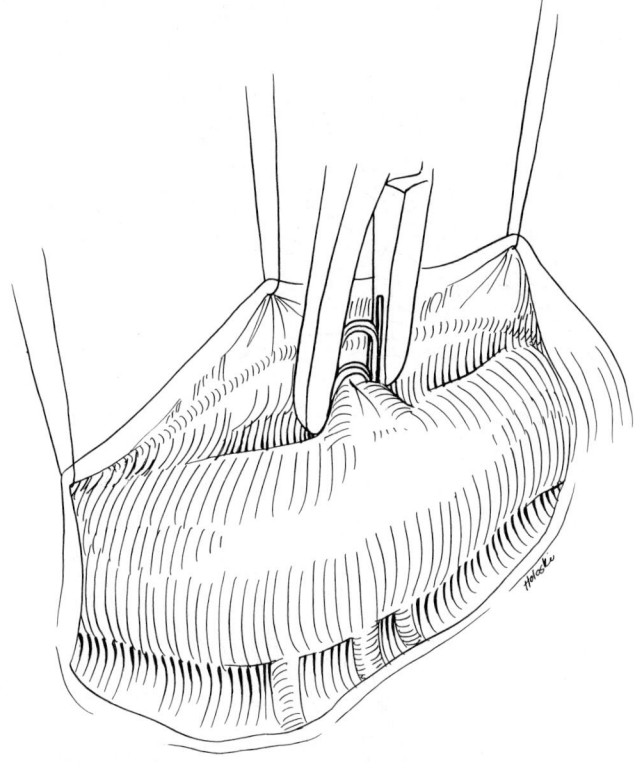

**FIGURE 72-8** In premature neonates, the PDA is occluded with 2 small or medium hemoclips. The recurrent laryngeal nerve is retracted medially.

If the patient has pulmonary hypertension, the aorta is temporarily clamped above and below the ductus, as shown in Fig. 72-7. After the clamps are applied, the PDA is ligated and the clamps immediately removed.

An alternative technique of ductal ligation in the premature infant is ligaclip occlusion. The exposure of the PDA is the same, except that the dissection is made only above and below the ductus, working perpendicular to the aorta. The friable duct is not encircled, but the recurrent laryngeal nerve is dissected free posteriorly. A safe and fast occlusion is achieved with the application of 2 ligaclips, taking care to avoid entrapment of the recurrent laryngeal nerve (Fig. 72-8).

In older children, the PDA can be short and wide, making clamp application for ductal division difficult and dangerous. An acceptable alternative is suture ligation as described by Blalock. Using double-armed 5-0 polypropylene suture, adventitial stitches are taken into the superior, inferior, and anterior aspects of both ends of the ductus. Pledgets can be incorporated into this purse string if necessary. The aortic end is snugly tied first, followed by the pulmonary side. A transfixion suture ligature at the middle of the PDA completes the repair (Fig. 72-9). An alternative technique for the short, wide ductus is to place a side-biting clamp across the aortic end of the ductus (Fig. 72-4) and a straight vascular clamp across the pulmonary artery end. The ductus is easily divided and both ends oversewn, followed by clamp removal.

Following division or ligation, the posterior mediastinal pleura may be approximated using interrupted or continuous suture. The chest is closed in the standard manner with 1 intercostal chest tube in place.

## CLOSURE FROM MIDLINE STERNOTOMY

This approach is most commonly employed when the patient requires cardiopulmonary bypass to correct a coexisting cardiac lesion. The midline sternotomy can also be used to operate on patients with a recanalized or calcified aneurysmal ductus, who may require cardiopulmonary bypass for closure.

The pericardium is opened longitudinally with the edges held on traction sutures. The aorta and pulmonary artery are separated using the cautery. The origin of the right and left pulmonary branches are clearly defined. A clamp is placed on the adventitia of the ascending aorta and gentle traction is applied to the right and toward the inferior vena cava. The assistant may place a small ribbon retractor inside the pericardium over the left pulmonary artery branch if needed to adequately visualize the location of the ductus. With ventilation temporarily discontinued, the surgeon places a blunt tip right-angled clamp around the PDA from the patient's right side, keeping the origins of both right and left pulmonary branches under direct vision (Figs. 72-10 and 72-11). The ductus can be ligated or divided just before or after instituting cardiopulmonary bypass.

If the ductus is short or if adhesions from attempted ligation through a previous thoracotomy make encirclement difficult, the patient is placed on cardiopulmonary bypass. A straight vascular clamp occludes the aortic end. The ductus is divided and bleeding from the pulmonary end is controlled

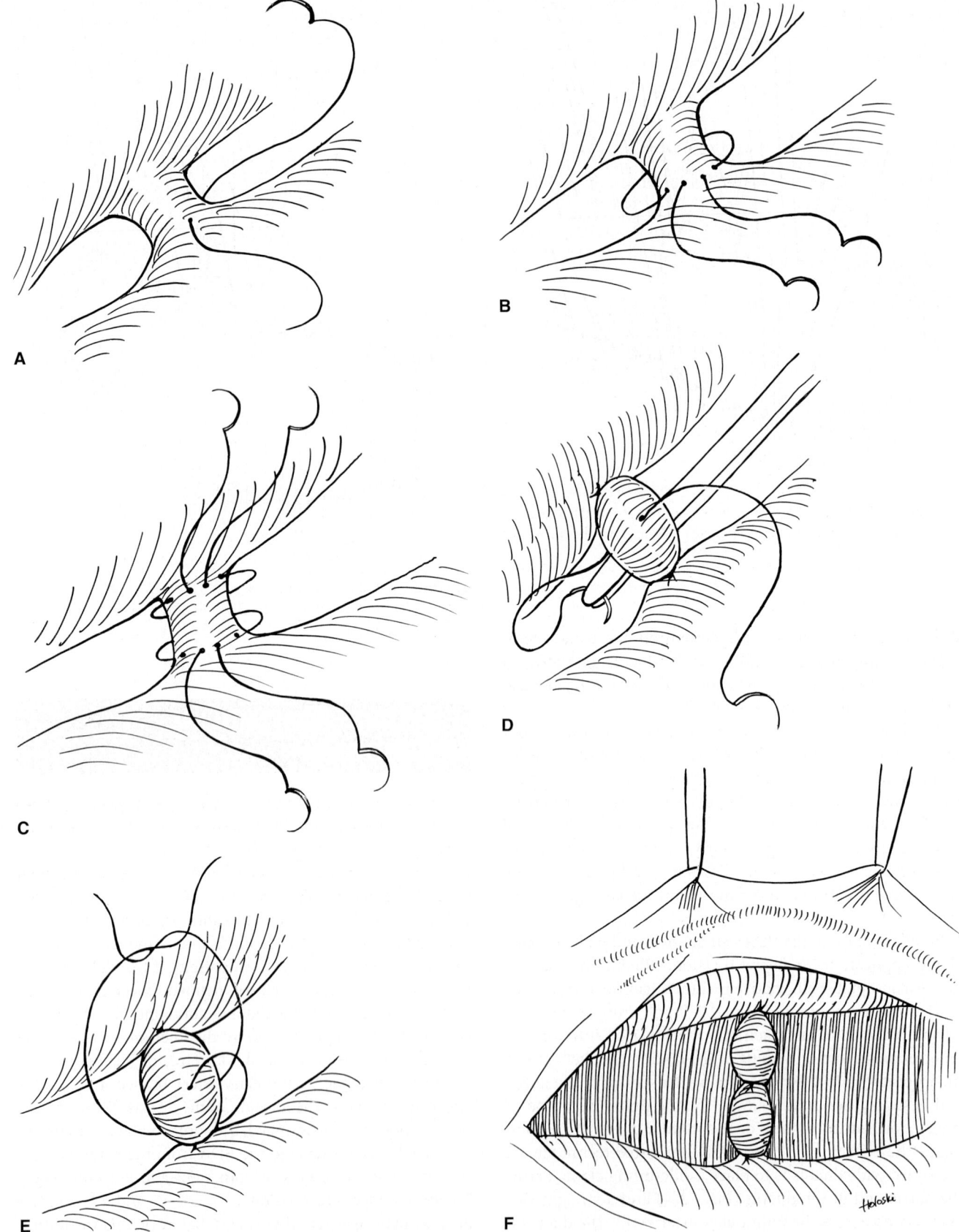

**FIGURE 72-9** The patent ductus may be obliterated using suture ligation technique. Usually 3 suture ligatures are placed, as shown in **A–F**.

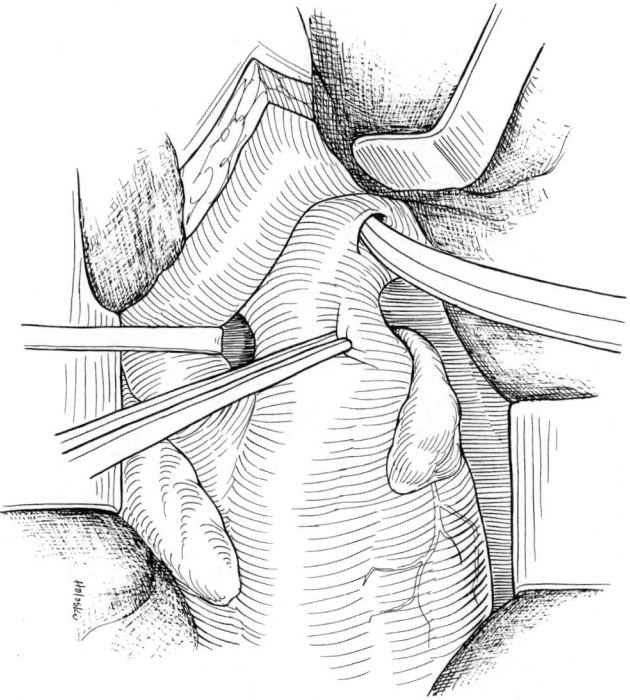

**FIGURE 72-10** The PDA is closed from a midline sternotomy. The left and right pulmonary arteries are carefully identified. The aorta is retracted to the right and inferiorly.

with pump suction and reduction of perfusion flow as the patient is cooled. The aortic end is oversewn first and the clamp removed. The pulmonary side is inspected and either closed primarily or augmented with a small patch of autologous pericardium to avoid stenosis at the origin of the left pulmonary artery.

## CLOSURE FROM INSIDE THE PULMONARY ARTERY

On rare occasions, the PDA cannot be encircled due to dense intrapericardial adhesions, previous surgery on the ductus, or in patients with a ductal aneurysm. In these cases, the PDA can be closed from inside the main pulmonary artery. Cardiopulmonary bypass is begun using 2 venous cannula. The pulmonary artery branches are snared to prevent lung flooding through the PDA. A small vent is placed through the right superior pulmonary vein into the left atrium and the air vent needle inserted into the ascending aorta is kept on continuous suction. The patient is cooled to 25°C. After the heart fibrillates, the caval snares are secured and the patient is placed head down. The main pulmonary artery is opened and the ductus is inspected. If the opening is small, it may be closed using interrupted pledgeted mattress sutures and intermittent low-flow bypass to improve visibility. A balloon-tipped catheter can be inflated and employed to reduce flow through the ductus as sutures are placed (Fig. 72-12).

Alternatively, the patient can be cooled to 18°C. The head is packed in ice and 3 arch vessels are snared. The pump is turned off following 20 to 25 minutes of cooling and the ductus closed under direct vision with a patch of Dacron or Gore-Tex, using continuous or interrupted pledgeted sutures (Fig. 72-13). Aortic cross-clamping with cardioplegia may be employed at the surgeon's discretion.

Prior to tying of the last suture, the patient is placed in a head-down position and the lungs inflated to expel any air from the duct. The heart, great vessels, and aorta are deaired as perfusion is commenced. The main pulmonary artery is closed, with the heart beating as the patient is warmed.

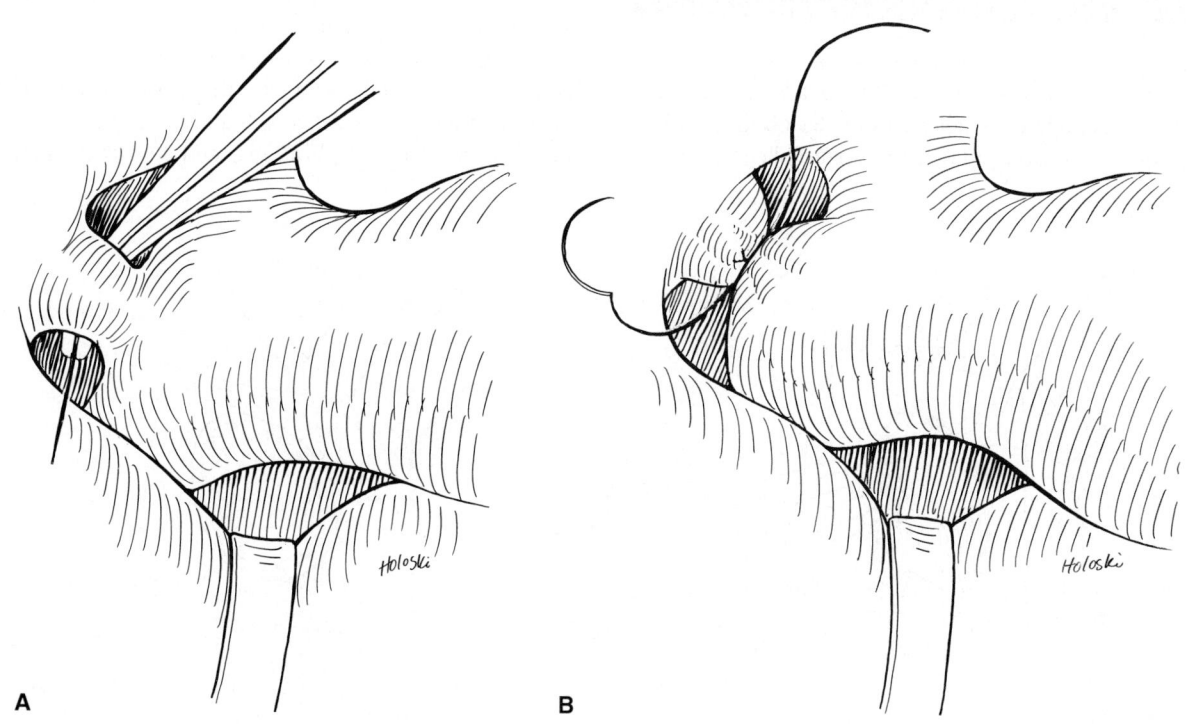

**A**          **B**

**FIGURE 72-11** The PDA is encircled with 1 or 2 ligatures of silk (**A**) and ligated just before the institution of cardiopulmonary bypass (**B**).

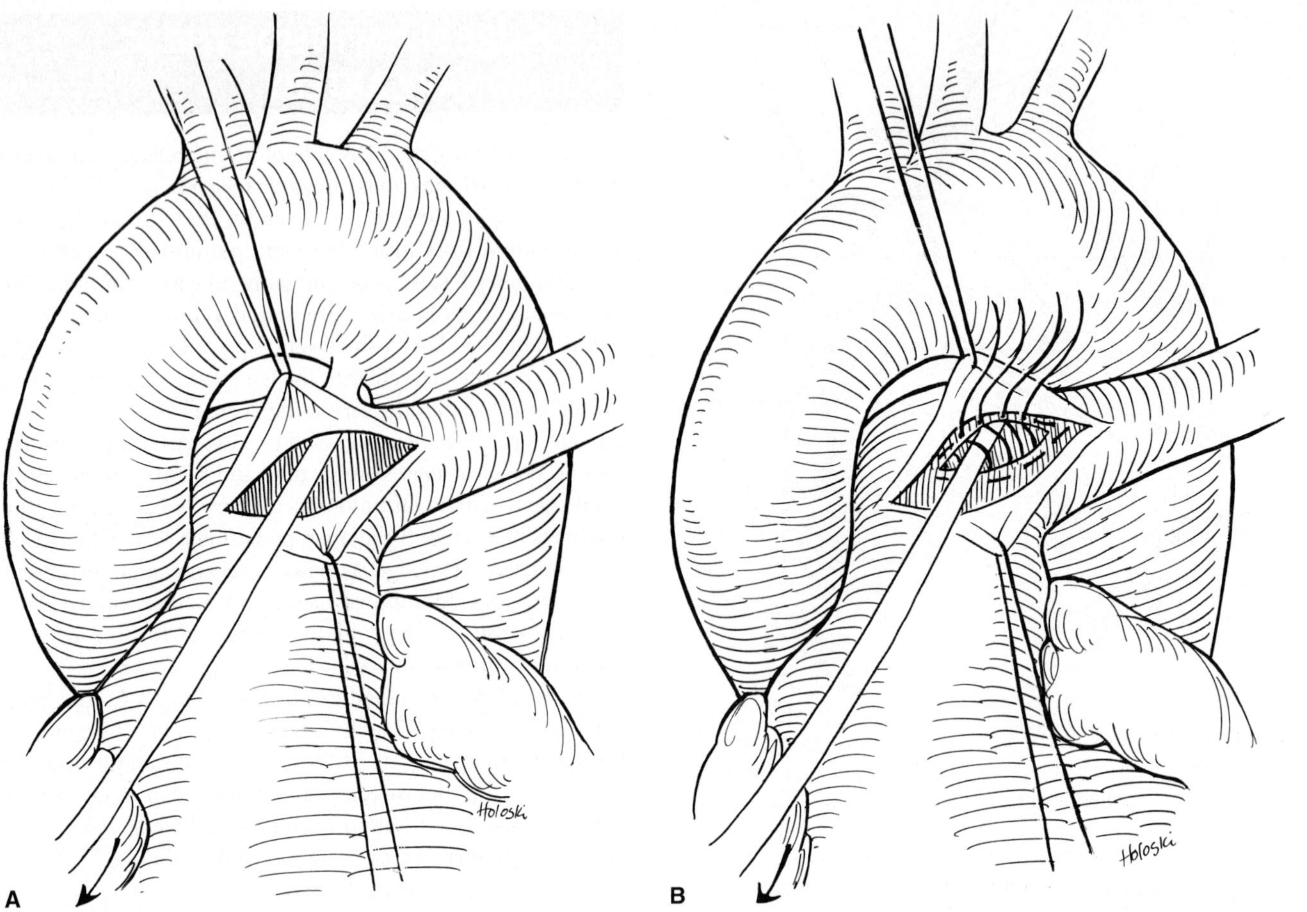

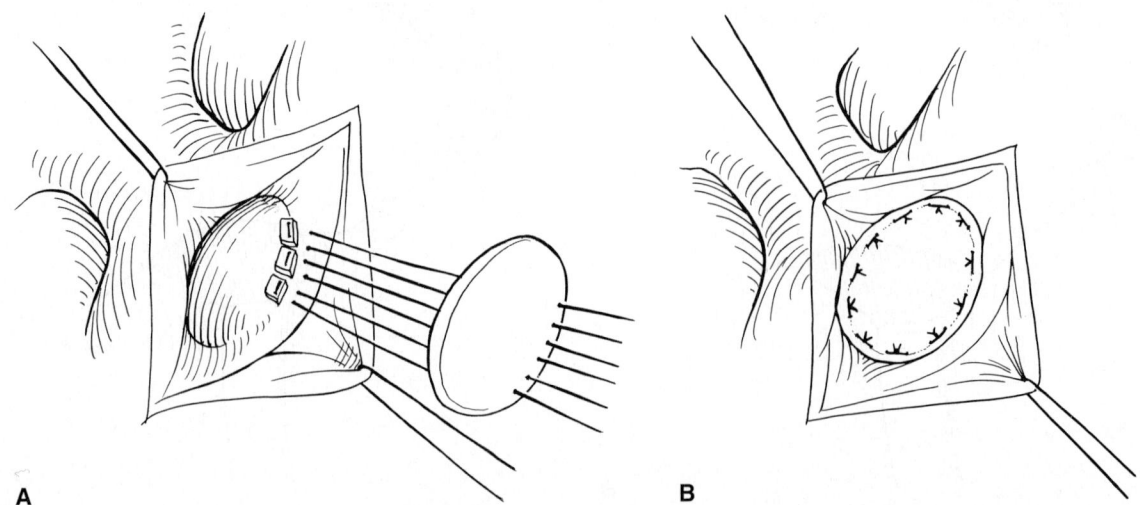

**FIGURE 72-12** The PDA is closed from inside the pulmonary artery. **A.** A balloon catheter occludes the PDA while (**B**) interrupted sutures are precisely placed on the pulmonary artery side of the ductus.

## PERCUTANEOUS CATHETER CLOSURE OF PDA

Transcatheter closure of the PDA for patients beyond the neonatal period was first reported by Porstmann and Rashkind. They developed the double-umbrella occluder, which consists of 2 foam disks attached to a steel skeleton, and is implanted by an antegrade approach through the femoral vein (Fig. 72-14). Complete and secure closure has been obtained in about 95% of patients. Currently, both this device and the vascular occluder are used.

Closing a patent ductus with Gianturco coils has become increasingly popular owing to the small sheath requirements, relative ease of delivery, high rate of successful occlusion, low rate of complications, and low cost. Successful

**A**                    **B**

**FIGURE 72-13** The PDA is closed from within the main pulmonary artery using interrupted pledgeted mattress sutures and a Dacron or Gore-Tex patch.

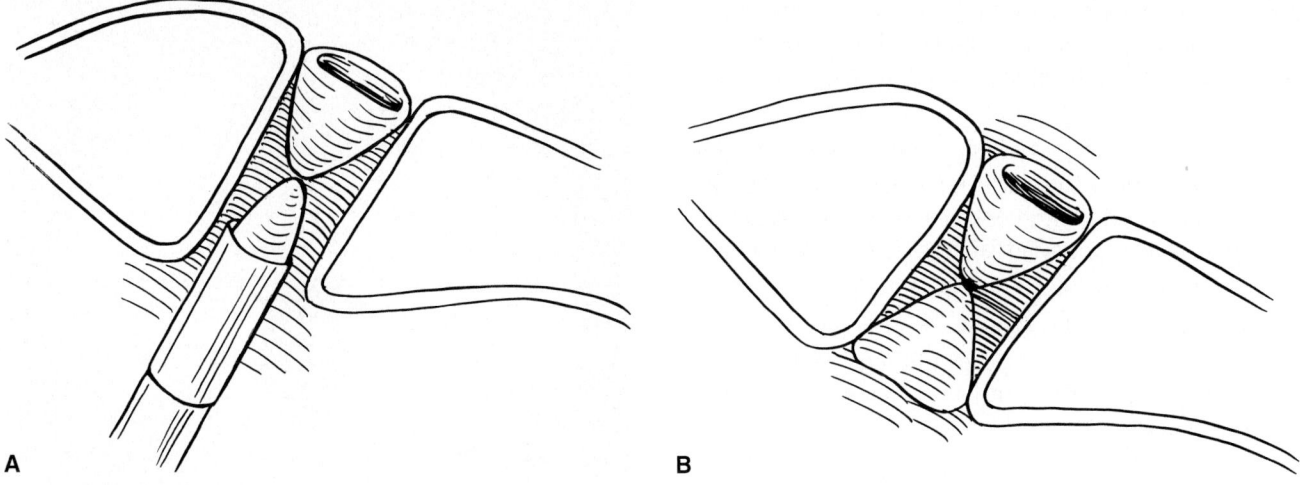

**FIGURE 72-14** The PDA is closed using a double umbrella device introduced percutaneously through the common femoral vein.

closure has been limited to PDAs up to 3.5 mm in diameter. The success rate is 90% to 95%, as judged by color doppler echocardiography.

## THORACOSCOPIC CLOSURE OF PDA

Laborde and his associates pioneered PDA closure without thoracotomy. Using thoracoscopic techniques in 332 patients, Laborde and associates achieved complete closure in all but 6 patients, with no deaths and hospital stays of 2 to 3 days. Endoscopic ductal closure can be applied to patients less than 3 to 5 kg, an important distinction from transcatheter closure, where femoral vessel size may be prohibitive. Contraindications to the endoscopic approach include calcified ductus, which should not be clipped, ductus diameter beyond 1 cm, and dense pleural adhesions from previous infection or prior surgery. The current technique is elegantly described by Burke and associates.

## ROBOTIC DUCTAL LIGATION

Robotic surgical systems represent a further refinement in the evolution of endoscopic instrumentation. This computer-augmented technology offers 3-dimensional visualization that mimics depth perception and significantly improves instrumentation with motion scaling, which enhances intra-corporeal dexterity. The lack of tactile feedback remains a dis-advantage. The indications for the robotic approach to PDA surgery are evolving. The current technique is described in detail by Bacha and associates.

## COMPLICATIONS OF PDA CLOSURE

Bleeding associated with the repair of patent ductus may occur due to a tear in the aorta, pulmonary artery, or ductus. Should the aortic end bleed, clamps can be temporary applied above and below the ductus. Bleeding from the lower

pressure pulmonary side is controlled with digital pressure while the proximal segment of the duct is clamped inside the pericardium. Rarely, ligation of the left pulmonary artery or aorta has been reported. Careful attention to anatomical landmarks will decrease the risk of mistaking the pulmonary artery or aorta for the ductus.

Damage to the phrenic, vagus, and recurrent laryngeal nerves is avoided by gentle technique and proper exposure of the ductus.

Postoperative chylothorax can be avoided by limiting the cephalad dissection and ligating all lymphatic tissue, especially in the area of the thoracic duct.

Aneurysm of the ductus arteriosus has been observed after ligation or division. Sequelae include rupture, embolization, infection, and thrombosis of the pulmonary artery. Excision of the aneurysm, removal of thrombus, and primary closure of aorta and pulmonary artery are essentials of treatment.

Preterm infants have particularly high morbidity, ranging between 50% and 80%, following ductus ligation. Approximately 30% of patients have bronchopulmonary dysplasia and at least 5% to 10% develop sequelae related primarily to their prematurity and to a lesser degree to long-term ventilation and oxygen toxicity. These include retrolental fibroplasia, blindness, and cerebral palsy.

# Aortic Coarctation

## KEY POINTS

1. Coarctation of the aorta is a relatively common congenital cardiac defect caused by constriction of abnormally located ductal tissue within the wall of the aorta, just beyond the aortic arch. It may be an isolated lesion or associated with the most severe forms of congenital heart disease.

2. Early recognition in the neonate can allow safe effective surgical intervention with low morbidity and mortality. Surgery in the older child is also very successful.

3. Percutaneous techniques in primary coarctation remain experimental and should be approached cautiously because of the high morbidity and mortality associated with rupture.

4. Early surgical repair remains the gold standard for treating aortic coarctation. Surgical techniques include resection with end-to-end anastomosis, with or without partial arch augmentation, subclavian flap repair, patch aortoplasty, and resection with graft insertion.

5. Recurrent coarctation occurs most commonly after neonatal repair and approaches 10% regardless of the technique used, with the majority of recurrences in the first year of life.

6. Percutaneous techniques have allowed many children with recurrences to avoid a second surgical procedure.

7. The incidence of postoperative paralysis after coarctation repair reported is approximately 0.4% and is directly related to ischemic time.

8. Other effects of surgical repair include hypertension and postcoarctation abdominal pain.

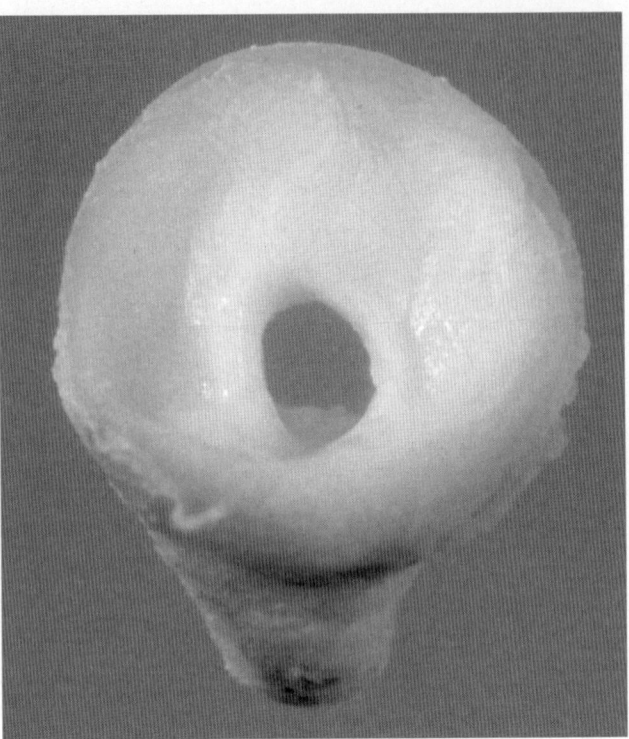

**FIGURE 72-15** Resected coarctation segment demonstrating the focal obstruction created by the ductal shelf.

# DEFINITION AND ETIOLOGY

Coarctation is a discrete narrowing of the thoracic aorta that occurs in the region of the ductus arteriosus, just beyond the takeoff of the left subclavian artery. Other rarer forms of coarctation of the aorta can occur in the midthoracic aorta, abdominal aorta, or midaortic arch. These are extremely uncommon and are not discussed in this section.

There has been a great deal in the literature over the years about the distinction of preductal, juxtaductal, and postductal coarctation, but from the standpoint of etiology and treatment, common forms of coarctation can be considered juxtaductal. The constriction of the aorta adjacent to the ductus is believed to be secondary to an abnormal infiltration of ductal cells into the wall of the aorta. The fetal ductus arteriosus provides a path for right-side blood, already oxygenated within the placenta, to bypass the pulmonary circulation and go directly into the aorta. At birth, expansion of the lungs, increased pulmonary blood flow, a drop in pulmonary vascular resistance, and reversal of the direction of the shunt through the ductus all stimulate contractile elements within the ductal tissue and lead to physiological and anatomic closure of this fetal communication. Under normal circumstances, the aorta is unaffected. However, in some neonates there is excessive migration into the adjacent aortic wall of these specialized ductal cells, which contract at the same time that the ductus closes, creating a shelf within the lumen of the aorta and leading to varying degrees of obstruction to flow (Fig. 72-15). Perhaps the best evidence for this theory is the phenomenon seen with the administration of prostaglandin to infants with early coarctation. As evaluated with echocardiography, not only does the ductus reopen, but frequently the coarctation relaxes, at times to the extent that it is difficult to see the shelf or measure a gradient.

In infants with a great deal of aortic narrowing, the decrease in distal aortic perfusion pressure can be severe, acute, and life-threatening. In others, the amount of narrowing may be minimal, and there may not be any significant pressure gradient across the shelf for many years. However, with continued growth of the normal aorta and poor growth in the area of the shelf, the obstruction worsens, the gradient increases, and symptoms may appear. The timing of the occurrence of symptoms leads some to categorize patients with coarctation into 2 types referred to as the infantile type and the adult type. However, these are clearly categories that describe clinical events rather than anatomic subsets.

Coarctation of the aorta constitutes about 5% to 6% of all congenital heart defects. Several other cardiac anomalies are associated with coarctation, including PDA, bicuspid aortic valve, ventricular septal defect, and mitral valve abnormalities such as parachute mitral valve. These associated defects are most often seen in patients presenting with symptoms during infancy but may be found in patients with later presentation of their coarctation.

Coarctation of the aorta was first discovered on autopsy in the 1700s and described by several authors. The first repair was not performed until 1945, independently by both Crafoord and Gross. Significant advancements in the surgical treatment of coarctation were subsequently reported. Gross described the use of aortic homografts in 1951. The use of prosthetic grafts was reported by Vossschulte and the subclavian flap technique was described by Waldhausen and Nahrwold in 1966. More recent work has centered on development of percutaneous angioplasty techniques for recurrent coarctation.

## PRESENTATION AND DIAGNOSIS

Patients who present in infancy with isolated coarctation frequently do so at several days of age, after closure of the ductus arteriosus and severe narrowing of the aorta. Perfusion of the viscera and extremities below the coarctation becomes uniformly poor, with acidosis, oliguria to anuria, absent distal pulses, and often frank cardiovascular collapse and shock. Reopening the ductus arteriosus with prostaglandin infusion restores perfusion to the viscera and legs. With reperfusion, diuretics, treatment of the acidosis, and inotropic drugs, most infants can recover, be stabilized, and undergo surgical repair.

Other findings in infants with severe coarctation may include the presence of a systolic murmur (especially over the left chest and posteriorly), a gallop rhythm, electrocardiographic evidence of right ventricular hypertrophy with or without left ventricular hypertrophy, and cardiomegaly with pulmonary edema as observed by chest x-ray. The definitive diagnosis is made with echocardiographic demonstration of the shelf and estimation of the gradient. In complicated cases, especially in the presence of other congenital heart disease, a cardiac catheterization may be required.

Older children who develop significant coarctation as they grow may present with symptoms of upper extremity hypertension. More often, these children are asymptomatic and have the diagnosis made when upper extremity hypertension is detected by routine examination, such as during school physical examinations. Hypertension is thought to be related to stimulation of the renin-angiotensin system by low perfusion pressures distal to the obstruction. Femoral pulses may be noticeably weak, depending on the degree of collateralization. Gradients in blood pressures between the right arm and either leg may be significant; however, there may be a minimal gradient if collateralization has been extensive.

Frequently the gradient can be detected only during exercise. The electrocardiogram usually demonstrates left ventricular hypertrophy, depending on the degree of hypertension. Rib notching on chest x-ray from expansion of developing intercostal collateral arteries has classically been described in coarctation, but is seen only after long-standing upper extremity hypertension and rarely before the age of 8 years. With current healthcare practices and diagnostic techniques, it is unusual for a child with coarctation to go undiscovered for several years.

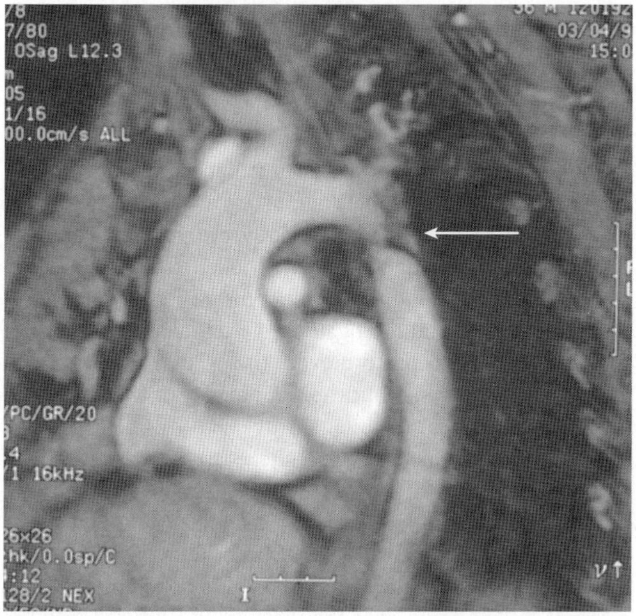

Cardiac catheterization is frequently indicated in the older child to measure the degree of obstruction, define the site of coarctation, and delineate the collateral arterial development. In more recent years magnetic resonance imaging (MRI) has been used to define the anatomy of the coarctation, collaterals, and even to estimate the gradient (Fig. 72-16). At some centers this has become the study of choice for evaluation of coarctation in the older child, thereby avoiding the more invasive catheterization.

## TREATMENT

Once the infantile type is diagnosed, prostaglandin infusion and other supportive measures usually achieve complete resuscitation, with restoration of normal distal perfusion, resolution of the metabolic acidosis, and complete recovery of cardiac, renal, and neurologic function. Prostaglandin infusion should be maintained until the defect has been repaired. Older children require control of hypertension and, after evaluation of collaterals, should undergo repair. Although there is no medical treatment that will correct the defect, there has been recent interest in primary percutaneous transcatheter balloon dilatation of coarctation. Issues include the risk of rupture, the recurrence rate, and failure to deal with the ductus arteriosus. Unlike dilatation of a recurrent obstruction surrounded by adhesions and scar from the previous intervention, dilatation of a primary coarctation may involve an unacceptably high rate of aneurysm formation or uncontained rupture and death. Currently this should be considered experimental, and the gold standard for primary coarctation remains surgical relief of the obstruction.

Surgical techniques of repair include resection with end-to-end anastomosis, with or without partial arch augmentation, subclavian flap repair, patch aortoplasty, and resection with graft insertion (Fig. 72-17). Each technique differs in its approach and has advantages and disadvantages.

## RESECTION WITH END-TO-END ANASTOMOSIS

In this operation the aorta is mobilized from the arch to the descending aorta, including the ductus arteriosus or ligamentum arteriosum. The dissection is extended to include 4 or 5 sets of intercostals, but collaterals are left intact. Those within the 2 clamps may be temporarily occluded. Once clamped proximally and distally, the segment of aorta containing the coarctate segment is excised, including the ductus, which is separately ligated and divided. It is crucial that all ductal tissue be removed to minimize recurrence. If the

**FIGURE 72-16** MRI demonstration of a typical juxtaductal aortic coarctation.

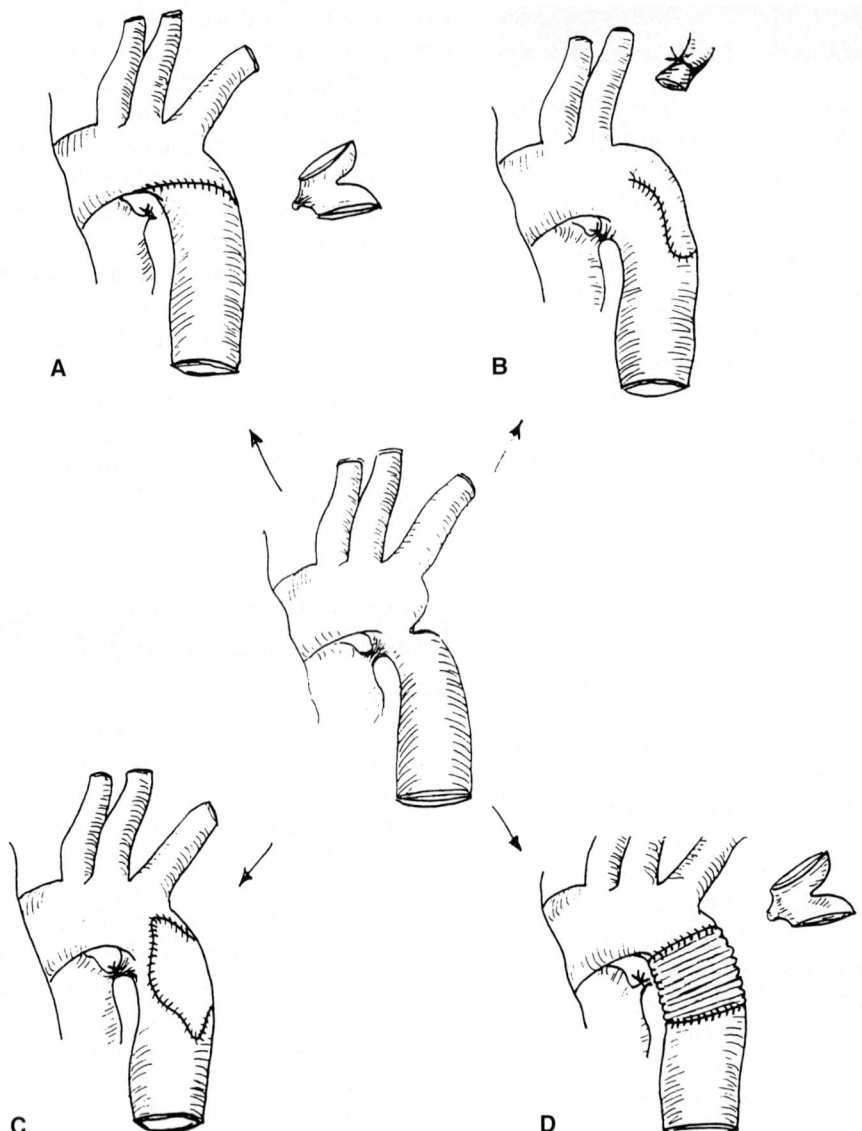

**FIGURE 72-17** Illustration of the 4 classic repair techniques for coarctation. **A.** Resection with end-to-end anastomosis. **B.** Subclavian flap aortoplasty. **C.** Patch aortoplasty. **D.** Resection with graft insertion.

isthmus of the aorta is small, this technique allows augmentation of the arch by extending the arteriotomy proximally along the underside of the arch, cutting the distal end at a slight bevel, and bringing it up under the arch for a wide anastomosis. Frequently, the aorta distal to the coarctate segment is somewhat enlarged secondary to poststenotic dilatation, facilitating the arch augmentation. Although this can easily be done with a running technique with good results, some surgeons prefer a semiinterrupted technique or use interrupted sutures for the anterior part of the anastomosis.

Resection of the coarctate segment with primary reanastomosis has several advantages over other techniques. During initial experiences, there was concern about the potential for growth with a continuous suture line, but experience with the arterial switch operation proved that the aorta grows sufficiently, and the fine polypropylene suture usually breaks under the tension of arterial pressure and growth. In addition, the resection technique allows complete excision of the coarctate segment and all ductal tissue from the aorta.

## SUBCLAVIAN FLAP REPAIR

In this repair, the aorta is similarly mobilized, but the dissection includes the left subclavian artery up to the takeoff of the vertebral artery. Once the clamps are in place, the ductus is ligated and usually divided. The left subclavian artery is ligated at the level of the vertebral branch. Many surgeons feel that it is important to ligate the vertebral artery as part of the subclavian division to prevent the occurrence of subclavian steal phenomena, but the significance of this and need for vertebral ligation remain controversial.

Once divided distally, the subclavian artery is opened along its outer wall down across the coarctate segment and onto the descending aorta. The incision is continued down the lateral wall of the aorta for a distance approximately equal to the length of the subclavian artery. The opened subclavian artery is folded down over the incision and sutured into the aorta, creating a flap repair. If a longer aortic occlusion time is expected during coarctation repair, or if the infant has multiple defects, a Silastic® intraluminal shunt can be placed that allows for distal aortic perfusion to prevent paraplegia and unloads the ventricle to avoid heart failure.

## PATCH AORTOPLASTY

After left thoracotomy and aortic mobilization as described above, the clamps are applied, and the aorta is opened with a longitudinal incision across the coarctation. With a variety of materials including pericardium, homograft, polytetrafluoroethylene (PTFE) or Dacron, the aorta is augmented at the level of the coarctation, relieving the obstruction. Although clearly none of these materials undergoes growth, sewing to healthy aortic tissue and proving adequate relief of the obstruction may allow sufficient expansion to prevent recurrence. However, this technique probably presents a higher risk of pseudoaneurysm formation than the techniques not employing prosthetic material.

## RESECTION WITH GRAFT INSERTION

Through a left thoracotomy, the aorta is mobilized, providing proximal and distal control. The aorta is clamped, the coarctate segment is completely excised, and an appropriate size tube graft is inserted, bridging the gap between the proximal and distal aorta. Graft materials may include various forms of Dacron and PTFE. Because the graft material will not grow, the use of a graft is usually limited to older children and young adults, though it may be used in larger patients with recurrent coarctation, especially with significant periaortic scarring. In rare circumstances with complex long-segment coarctations, surgeons have reported the use of a tube graft to bypass the obstruction rather than resect it.

## COMBINED REPAIR

When aortic coarctation exists in conjunction with another cardiac defect, approach and timing of the repair depend on the type and significance of the associated defects. Patent ductus is easily repaired as part of the coarctation repair. Treatment of coexisting large ventricular septal defects (VSD) is more controversial. Many centers choose to correct the coarctation first and in some cases place a band on the pulmonary artery to protect the pulmonary vascular bed from the large left-to-right shunt. The VSD is addressed at a later date with debanding of the pulmonary artery if necessary and patching or reconstruction as required.

Considerable experience with palliation for hypoplastic left heart syndrome has demonstrated that correction of coarctation and aortic arch reconstruction are readily performed from a sternotomy incision. Some centers currently approach patients with coarctation associated with significant VSD with sternotomy, cardiopulmonary bypass, a short period of deep hypothermic circulatory arrest for the coarctation repair, followed by VSD patching after reinstitution of cardiopulmonary bypass. This allows immediate correction of the VSD, with removal of the high-pressure load on the right ventricle,

and avoids the need for pulmonary artery reconstruction and the potential complications of pulmonary artery banding. This approach does, however, require a short period of circulatory arrest not required with a staged approach. Both strategies have been shown to work satisfactorily, and current management depends on the surgeon and institutional preference and experience.

Patients with coexisting aortic and mitral valve abnormalities are significantly more complicated. Those with severe aortic and mitral hypoplasia are treated as are those with hypoplastic left heart syndrome, with repair of the coarctation as part of the hypoplastic ascending aorta and arch reconstruction. However, many patients have varying degrees of multilevel left-sided obstruction, including coarctation, as seen in the Shone complex. Because repair of aortic stenosis in the face of persistent obstruction at the arch level will do little to improve distal perfusion, the coarctation usually is repaired first to improve distal perfusion. More important, perhaps, is the difficulty in accessing true aortic and mitral valve gradients in the presence of distal aortic obstruction and an open ductus arteriosus. With closure of the ductus, relief of the coarctation obstruction, and the subsequent improvement in cardiac output and forward flow, aortic valve gradients may be much higher than previously measured.

## RISKS AND OUTCOMES

### Recurrence and Pseudoaneurysm

Recurrent coarctation occurs most commonly after neonatal repair and approaches 10% regardless of the technique used. The majority of recurrences present in the first year of life, although they may not require intervention for several years. In the past, many surgeons avoided end-to-end repairs in newborns for fear of high recurrence rates from restriction of growth by a continuous circumferential suture line. This led to increased use of the subclavian flap technique. Subsequent review, however, demonstrated that the rate of recurrence was essentially equal with the 2 techniques when used in the neonate. Selection of the technique between subclavian flap and resection and reanastomosis remains the surgeon's preference in the neonate, although most surgeons avoid dividing the subclavian artery in children over 1 year of age.

Early reports of pseudoaneurysm formation after patch angioplasty led to a reduction in the use of this technique. Although many debated the proper choice of patch material in preventing this complication, most of the pseudoaneurysms formed on the inner side of the aorta opposite the patch and were most likely caused by overresection of the ductal shelf with weakening of the aortic wall and subsequent aneurysm formation. Currently this technique has fallen out of favor except in some complicated repairs in conjunction with another technique or in the larger child with a recurrent coarctation.

Treatment of recurrent coarctation has been improved significantly with the introduction of percutaneous balloon angioplasty techniques. Because the recurrence site is surrounded by adhesions and scar from the previous repair, the occurrence of postdilatation aneurysm has remained very low. In the patients who fail balloon dilatation of a recurrent coarctation, surgery is feasible and can usually be accomplished with minimal morbidity using a resection, patch angioplasty, or graft technique.

Mortality with coarctation repair is highest in the neonatal group and may approach 10% to 15%. Death most often occurs in infants with associated left-sided lesions, such as the Shone complex or variants of hypoplastic left heart syndrome, or in children who suffer cardiac arrest or a period of shock with multisystem dysfunction. Mortality in the non-neonate with a routine coarctation and no associated cardiac anomalies is generally less than 1%.

# PARAPLEGIA

Any temporary interruption of flow through the descending aorta is associated with some risk of postprocedure paraplegia. Large variability in sources of spinal cord blood flow patterns may be responsible, primarily the artery of Adamkiewicz, which has been shown to arise from the aorta anywhere between T-5 and L-1 and therefore makes preservation of collaterals during coarctation repair essential in preventing paralysis. The incidence of postoperative paralysis after coarctation repair reported in the literature is around 0.4% and is directly related to ischemic time. There has been no reported occurrence with clamp times less than 15 minutes, but the incidence is essentially 100% if the clamp time exceeds 1 hour, unless some form of circulatory support is used.

Numerous techniques to maintain perfusion to the spinal cord during the repair to eliminate the risk of paraplegia include various shunts and cardiopulmonary bypass. However, as long as the aortic clamp time is less than 30 minutes, these perfusion techniques do not reduce the incidence of cord injury. For more complex repairs that will clearly require more than 30 minutes of interruption of flow, perfusion techniques are clearly warranted, and the intraluminal Silastic shunt works well when used in conjunction with the subclavian flap repair.

Several simpler techniques to improve cord perfusion and reduce the risk of injury during the repair include mild passive hypothermia, systemic steroids, local hypothermia, and intrathecal papaverine. Early reports of paraplegia associated with intraoperative hyperthermia give credence to the use of passive hypothermia. Probably most important in coarctation repair is the maintenance of existing collaterals and the avoidance of overtreating proximal hypertension during an expedient repair.

# HYPERTENSION

The persistence of hypertension after surgery to repair coarctation is seen with increasing frequency as the age at time of repair increases. Long-term hypertension is rare in patients repaired as neonates, unless they develop a recurrent coarctation. Rebound hypertension in the immediate postoperative period is much more common and may occur in 30% of patients. It is most likely an effect of reperfusion and splanchnic vasospasm and responds well to systemic vasodilators, usually subsiding within 24 to 48 hours. Children over 5 years of age at the time of repair who have required medical treatment for hypertension preoperatively are more likely to require medication postoperatively and have a significantly increased risk for permanent hypertension.

# POSTCOARCTATION ABDOMINAL PAIN

In addition to temporary postoperative hypertension, another effect of the reperfusion phenomena is seen primarily in older children. The return of high-pressure pulsatile perfusion can stimulate mesenteric vasospasm and temporary intestinal ischemia, leading to a recognized syndrome of postcoarctation abdominal pain. It may be predisposed by inappropriate treatment of postoperative hypertension. Excessive vasodilation may decrease perfusion pressure in an already tight and vasospastic mesenteric vascular bed, and inadequate control of hypertension may exacerbate the problem. This is rarely observed in patients under 2 years of age and usually subsides gradually over the first day or 2. Treatment usually involves restricting oral intake and the appropriate use of vasodilators along with adequate volume loading to improve intestinal perfusion.

## SELECTED READING

### Patent Ductus Arteriosus

Bacha EA, Bolotin G, Consilio K, Raman J, Ruschhaupt DG. Robotically assisted repair of sinus venous defect. *J Thorac Cardiovasc Surg* 2005;129:442–443.

Bacha EA. Introduction to "recent advances in congenital heart surgery" for surgical review "pediatric cardiology." *Pediatr Cardiol* 2007;28:77–78.

Burke RP. Video-assisted thoracoscopic surgery for patent ductus arteriosus. *Pediatrics* 1994;93:823–825.

Burke RP, Jacobs JP, Cheng W, et al. Video assisted thoracoscopic surgery for patent ductus arteriosus in low birth weight neonates and infants. *Pediatrics* 1999;104:227–230.

Laborde F, Folliguet TA, Etienne PY, Carbognani D, Batisse A, Petrie J. Videothoracoscopic surgical interruption of patent ductus arteriosus. Routine experience in 332 pediatric cases. *Eur J Cardiothorac Surg* 1997;11:1052–1055.

Porstmann W, Wierny L, Warnke H, Gerstberger G, Romaniuk PA. Catheter closure of patent ductus arteriosus. 62 cases treated without thoracotomy. *Radiol Clin North Am* 1971;9:203–218.

Rashkind WJ, Mullins CE, Hellenbrand WE, Tait MA. Nonsurgical closure of patent ductus arteriosus: clinical application of the Rashkind PDA Occluder System. *Circulation* 1987;75:583–592.

### Aortic Coarctation

Craaford C, Nylan G. Congenital coarctation of the aorta and its surgical treatment. *J Thorac Surg* 1950;37:46.

Crawford FH, Sade RM. Spinal cord injury associated with hyperthermia during aortic coarctation repair. *J Thorac Cardiovasc Surg* 1984;87:616.

Gross RE. Surgical correction for coarctation of the aorta. *Surgery* 1945;18:673.

Pennington DG, Liberthson RR, Jacobs M, et al. Critical review of experience with surgical repair of coarctation of the aorta. *J Thorac Cardiovasc Surg* 1979;77:217.

Pennington DG, Dennis HM, Swartz MT, et al. Repair of coarctation of the aorta in infants: experience with an intraluminal shunt. *Ann Thorac Surg* 1985;40:35.

Shinebourne EA, Tam ASY, Elseed AM, et al. Coarctation of the aorta in infancy and childhood. *Br Heart J* 1976;38:375.

Waldhausen JA, Nahrwold DL. Repair of coarctation of the aorta with a subclavian flap. *J Thorac Cardiovasc Surg* 1966;51:532.

# CHAPTER 73

## Vascular Compression Syndromes

*Peter B. Manning*

## KEY POINTS

1. Vascular compression syndromes are often collectively referred to as vascular rings and slings, but this characterization does not represent the true diversity of the group of conditions.

2. Compromise of the trachea and/or esophagus in the upper mediastinum by adjacent vascular structures is a common feature of vascular compression syndromes.

3. Because of this shared feature, vascular compression syndromes often present with similar clinical pictures of stridor and/or dysphagia and their diagnostic evaluation relies on similar strategies.

4. The developmental embryology of vascular compression syndromes is quite different, however, and this may influence the presence or absence of associated anomalies and cause treatment strategies to differ dramatically.

## INTRODUCTION

Vascular compression syndromes are most easily segregated into 3 main groups:

1. Anomalies of aortic arch branching (which include the true vascular rings in addition to anomalous origin of the right subclavian artery)

2. Left pulmonary artery sling

3. Innominate artery compression syndrome

Vascular rings include a number of anatomic variations of anomalous development of the aortic arch complex, resulting in vascular structures completely encircling both the trachea and the esophagus. Pulmonary artery sling refers to the anomalous origin of the left pulmonary artery (LPA) from the right pulmonary artery that courses between the trachea and esophagus to the left hilum. This is often associated with significant tracheal stenosis or hypoplasia. The innominate compression syndrome refers to tracheal compression by the adjacent, developmentally normal innominate artery. The

primary pathology is more likely to be tracheomalacia than malformation or malposition of an artery.

## VASCULAR RINGS

True vascular rings exist when the trachea and esophagus are completely encircled by vascular structures associated with altered development of the aortic arch and its branches. These surrounding vascular structures may include the aorta and its branches as well as the ductus/ligamentum arteriosus, and the pulmonary artery.

### Embryology and Anatomy

The thoracic aorta originally develops from the bilaterally symmetrical fourth aortic arches. By the end of the second month of gestation, components of the arch complex have regressed leaving the "typical" anatomy of a left aortic arch with 3 arch branches (innominate, left common carotid, and left subclavian) and a left-sided ductus arteriosus from the proximal LPA to the aorta in the general vicinity of the left subclavian artery origin (Fig. 73-1). Virtually all vascular rings can be explained by anomalous regression or persistence of different components of the bilateral aortic arch complex.

The two most common variants of true vascular rings are persistent double aortic arch and right aortic arch with left ligamentum. These occur with near equal frequency. In most cases of vascular ring, the right arch is dominant. In cases of persistent double arch, the left component may be completely atretic distally, is most often hypoplastic compared to the right component, occasionally is similar in size to the right component, and is dominant in a small percentage of cases (Figs. 73-2 and 73-3). There is typically a ligamentum arteriosus in a normal location between the proximal LPA and the left arch near the origin of the left subclavian artery. This ligamentum contributes to the ring, and as explained later, should also be divided in the management of the ring.

In cases of right aortic arch and left ligamentum, the left subclavian artery typically arises anomalously as the last branch off the arch, coursing in a retroesophageal position to reach the left arm. Its origin is characteristically bulbous and known as a Kommerell diverticulum, which represents

943

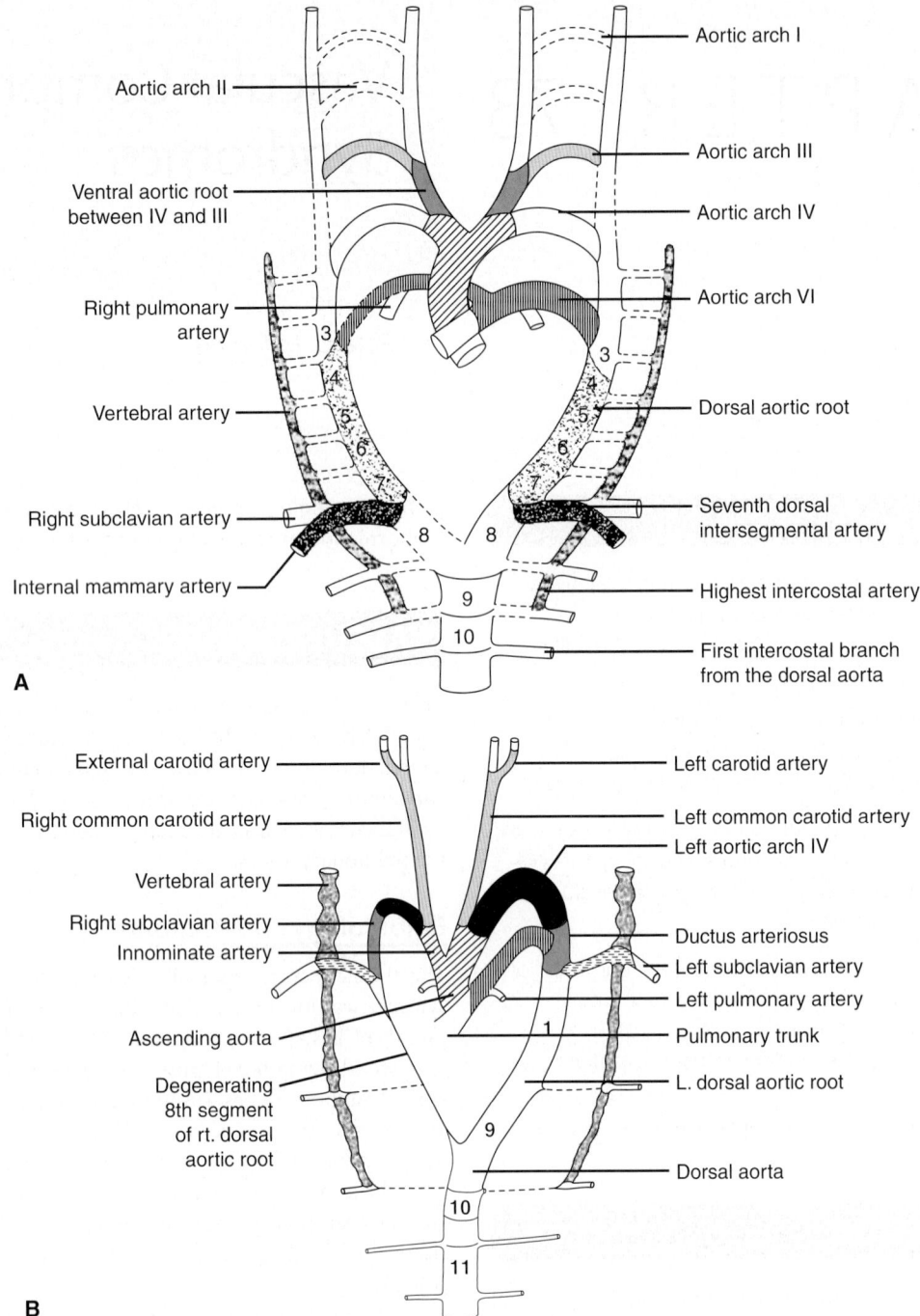

**FIGURE 73-1** Depiction of the developmental embryology of the aortic arch in (**A**) an early stage of development and (**B**) a later stage after involution of the right aortic arch.

the remnant of the distal left fourth arch (Fig. 73-4). The left side of the ring is completed by the pulmonary artery and the ligamentum, which courses from the LPA to join the left arch remnant at the junction of the Kommerell diverticulum and the origin of the left subclavian artery. In some cases, the left subclavian artery arises anteriorly with the left carotid in a "mirror image" pattern compared to the normal left arch branching, but the ligamentum may still course to the left of the trachea and esophagus to join an isolated Kommerell diverticulum from the proximal descending aorta.

## Presentation and Evaluation

The age at which patients are diagnosed with vascular ring may be quite variable. The most common symptoms are those related to airway compression and are reported in most patients. Stridor, a persistent cough, or frequent respiratory infections are most commonly reported. A third of patients will have dysphagia. Sometimes the respiratory symptoms will be noted most prominently during feeding, or may first become evident when an infant is transitioned from formula to a more solid diet.

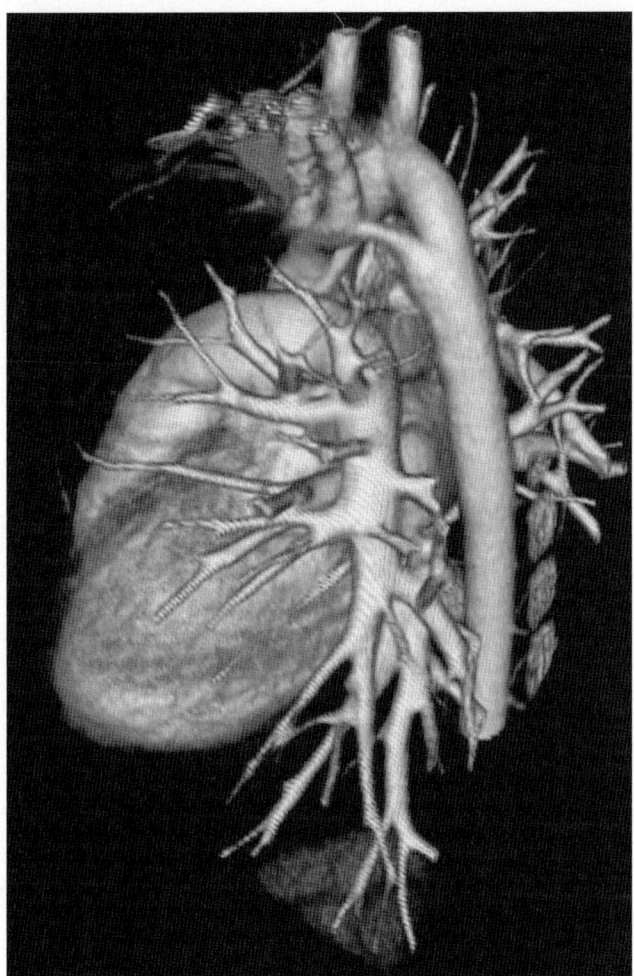

FIGURE 73-2 Three-dimensional reconstruction of contrast computed tomography (CT) demonstrating double aortic arch with hypoplastic left arch.

The majority of vascular rings are symptomatic early in life, with double aortic arch variants typically symptomatic at a younger age, even in the neonatal period. Because of the variety of presentations that may be seen with vascular rings and the similarity of these symptoms to more common problems, such as laryngomalacia or gastroesophageal reflux, a high index of suspicion must be maintained to consider vascular rings in the evaluation of these complaints.

Physical examination may be helpful in raising the index of suspicion for a vascular ring. Correlating the phase of the ventilation cycle and "noisy breathing" may help localize the level of obstruction. More proximal airway obstruction causes inspiratory stridor, while more distal airflow problems lead to expiratory stridor. In patients with vascular rings, the obstruction is mid to distal tracheal, which typically results in inspiratory and expiratory stridor. If there is a discordance of the peripheral pulses and 4 extremity blood pressures, this may suggest anomalies of aortic arch branching, although such differences are uncommon.

Chest x-rays, often obtained to evaluate for pulmonary parenchymal disease, are frequently part of the initial evaluation. A chest x-ray suggesting a dominant right aortic arch or a right-sided descending aorta should direct further evaluation for vascular ring. The absence of an obvious right

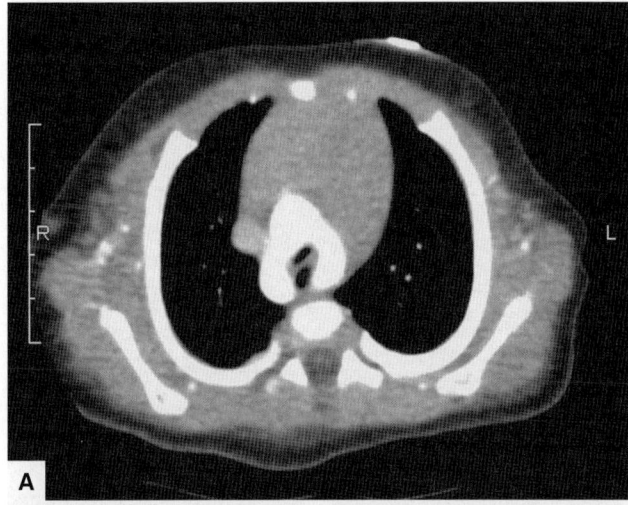

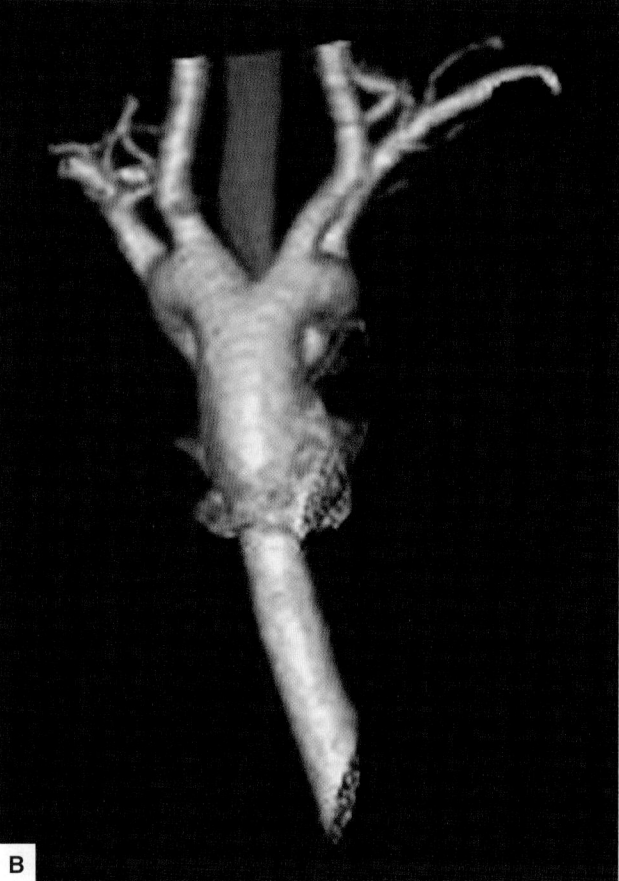

FIGURE 73-3 A. Axial and (B) 3-D reconstruction of contrast CT demonstrating double aortic arch with near equal right and left arch segments.

dominant arch does not rule out a vascular ring. The side of the arch is often quite difficult to identify in infants due to the large thymic shadow in the upper mediastinum. Barium swallow, demonstrating characteristic lateral and posterior indentation of the barium column, has often been advocated as a confirmatory study for vascular rings.

While some patients may undergo these studies as part of an evaluation of gastrointestinal symptoms, other imaging modalities are far superior for demonstrating these anomalies.

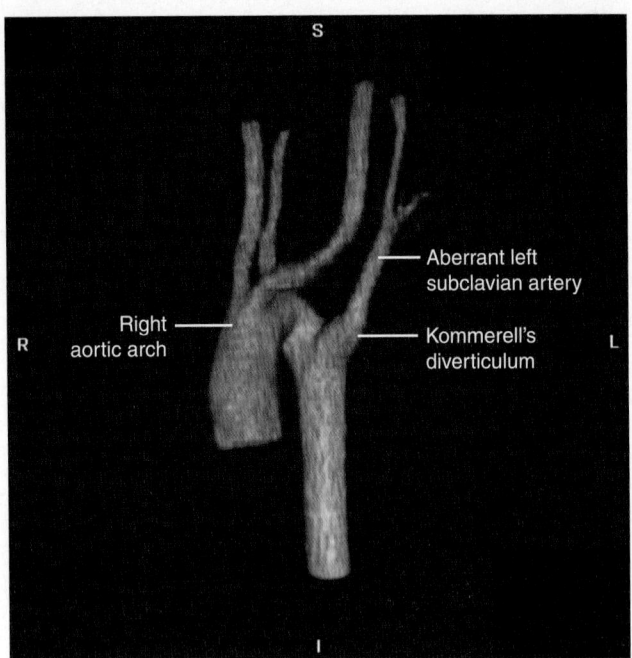

**FIGURE 73-4** The three-dimensional reconstruction of contrast CT demonstrating right aortic arch with aberrant left subclavian artery originating from a Kommerell diverticulum.

Contrast computed tomography (CT) angiography or magnetic resonance imaging (MRI) scans have become the preferred method for demonstrating vascular ring anatomy. These scans are able to display excellent details of the vascular anatomy, simultaneous imaging of airway, esophagus, and vascular structures in a single study, and allow 3-dimensional reconstructions of images. Since both CT and MRI only visualize vessels with blood flow, neither will demonstrate the entire anatomy if the ring is completed by a ligamentum arteriosus or an atretic arch segment. CT scans can be obtained with very short acquisition times, resulting in very little need for sedation, though the patient is exposed to radiation. MRI avoids radiation exposure, but typically requires sedation or general anesthesia, which may be more risky in a child with a compromised airway.

## Surgical Management and Outcomes

Surgical intervention is indicated in all symptomatic patients. Vascular rings are occasionally detected as "incidental findings" in patients without classic symptoms. Given the low risk of the operations, correction is generally recommended in any patient, particularly in younger children, with even vague symptoms that may be related to the vascular compression.

The primary goal of surgery is to open the vascular ring in at least 1 site to allow expansion of the trachea and esophagus. This conceptually changes an "O" to a "C." Consideration must be given, however, to avoiding situations where the persistent anomalous course of a blood vessel might continue to cause compressive symptoms. Since most patients have a dominant right arch, recreating a "normal" aortic arch anatomy is never a goal. A goal of creating a right arch with mirror-image branching will be more than satisfactory.

In planning a site for division of the ring, it is important to be cognizant of the potential impact on distal circulation supplied by the arch branches as well as the descending aorta. Intraoperative monitoring of pulse oximetry and blood pressures in both arms and a leg allow for objective decision-making before permanently dividing a blood vessel. This is particularly important in cases of a double aortic arch where both arches are nearly equal in size. Test occlusion at a proposed site of division and measurement of arm and leg oximetry and blood pressure allow assessment of the ultimate impact on distal perfusion. In cases where there is confusion about the identity of specific branches of the arch, test occlusion and observation of the impact on pulse oximetry will assist in elucidating the exact anatomy. This was often very useful when a chest x-ray and barium swallow constituted the entire preoperative evaluation. Careful dissection and definition of the anatomic detail was imperative in such cases, but with the uniform use of CT and MRI imaging, anatomic detail is typically well understood before entering the operating suite.

In cases of double aortic arch, the nondominant arch should ideally be divided distally, between the take-off of the subclavian artery and the connection of the distal arch to the descending aorta. In the majority of cases, this is the left arch, and it is often most hypoplastic at this level. The ligamentum arteriosus is also typically divided as it joins at this segment of the left arch and its division allows the vessels to be mobilized farther off the trachea and the esophagus (Fig. 73-5). In cases where both arches are similar in size, it is usually best to preserve the arch that is on the same side as the descending aorta to prevent the persistence of a retroesophageal aortic course.

In right arch/left ligamentum cases, the classic repair involves a simple division of the ligamentum. Some surgeons would advocate mobilization and posterior pexy of the Kommerell diverticulum to avoid esophageal compression. Recent experience has demonstrated that in patients with persistent symptoms following division of a ligamentum only, reoperation with excision of Kommerell's diverticulum and reimplantation of the anomalous left subclavian artery onto the left common carotid artery has resulted in relief of symptoms. Many surgeons now advocate resection of the diverticulum with subclavian reimplantation as a routine component of the primary procedure for such patients.

Posterolateral thoracotomy through the fourth interspace on the side opposite the dominant arch (usually a left thoracotomy) gives excellent exposure for these cases. The author has found that if subclavian reimplantation to the carotid artery is to be performed, a higher approach via the third interspace facilitates this portion of the procedure. Thoracoscopic division of vascular rings has been advocated by some, particularly in cases in which the segment to be divided is atretic or a ligamentum. Since the dominant arch and descending aorta are on the opposite side of the chest, the ipsilateral subclavian artery is often the only arterial structure immediately identifiable on inspection of the mediastinum. The pleura is opened beginning over the subclavian artery and extended inferiorly enough to allow dissection of the distal arch or the connection to the descending aorta of the Kommerell diverticulum, which is found behind the esophagus. Care must be taken to avoid injury to the vagus nerve anteriorly during this initial

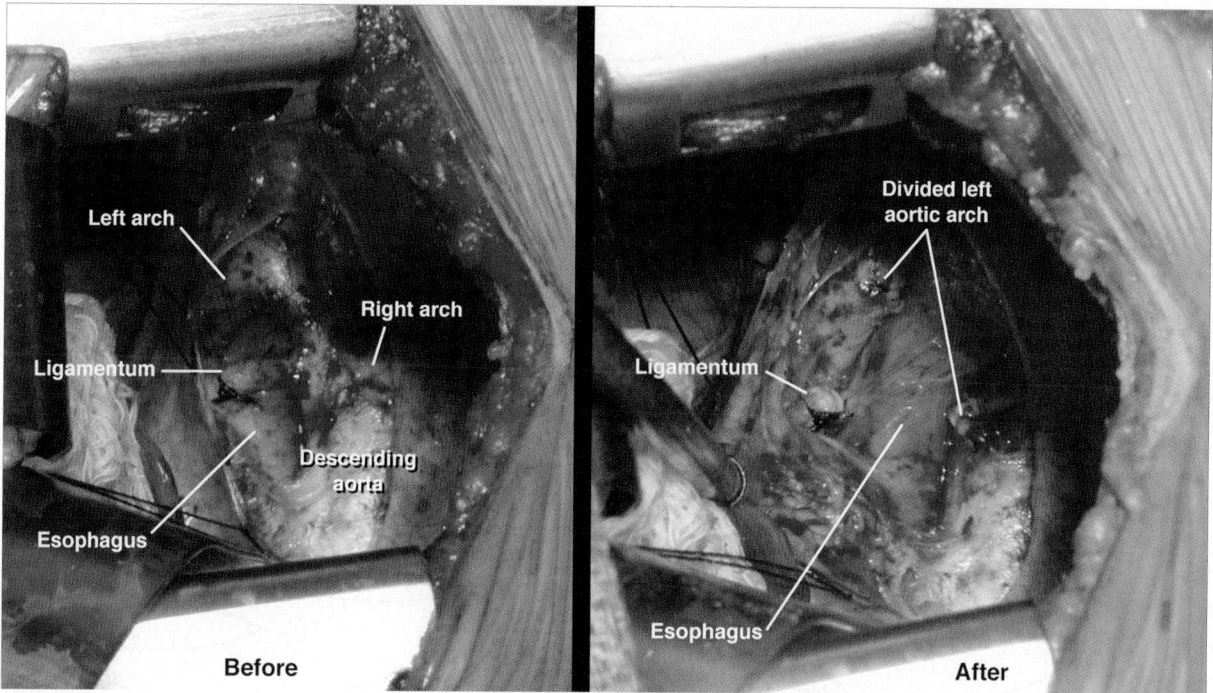

**FIGURE 73-5** Surgical images of double aortic arch before and after division of distal left arch and ligamentum (same patient as in Fig. 73-2).

dissection and to its recurrent laryngeal branch when dissection proceeds to the ligamentum arteriosus. Judicious use of cautery during dissection will control lymphatic leak and lessen the potential for a postoperative chylothorax.

When reimplantation of the subclavian artery onto the carotid artery is to be performed, the carotid artery is found via the same pleural opening in the superior portion of the chest. Avoiding excessive cautery in mobilizing the carotid will help decrease the risk of creating a Horner syndrome, which is associated with injury to the ansa cervicalis nerve branches that accompany the carotid artery.

The majority of patients experience significant improvement in symptoms immediately following operation although persistence of some stridor, particularly in infants, is common due to some degree of associated tracheomalacia. Further gradual improvement in symptoms should be expected, but there are few long-term follow-up studies of patients with vascular rings that document this. One study showed abnormalities in flow-volume loops during objective pulmonary function studies in nearly half of clinically asymptomatic patients an average of 6 years after surgery.

## ABERRANT RIGHT SUBCLAVIAN ARTERY

Anomalous origin of the right subclavian artery from the distal left aortic arch is a relatively frequently seen abnormality of arch branching, but does not represent a vascular ring, since the esophagus and trachea are not completely encircled by vascular structures. The aberrant subclavian artery in this anomaly does not originate from a Kommerell diverticulum.

In the majority of cases, this anomaly is completely asymptomatic. When it does create problems, they more commonly involve swallowing (classically referred to as "dysphagia lusoria"). Airway symptoms have been described, although rarely. When all other potential etiologies for the symptoms have been ruled out, reimplantation of the anomalous subclavian onto the right carotid artery via right thoracotomy is recommended.

## PULMONARY ARTERY SLING

While included in most discussions of vascular compression syndromes, LPA sling does not represent a complete vascular ring. It is, however, associated with the highest morbidity and mortality of all compression anomalies due to the frequency of its association with tracheal stenosis.

### Embryology and Anatomy

In patients with a pulmonary artery sling, the LPA arises anomalously from the posterior aspect of the right pulmonary artery, courses between the trachea and esophagus just above the carina, and enters the left pulmonary hilum in a nearly normal position (Fig. 73-6). Cases of hypoplasia of the artery are described, but in most cases, it is of normal caliber. The anomalous pulmonary artery has no hemodynamic impact on cardiac function. The morbidity associated with this anomaly is completely related to its impact on the adjacent airway.

Although older studies suggest an incidence of tracheal stenosis with LPA sling to be 50%, more current experience suggests that this association is much higher, likely in the 80% to

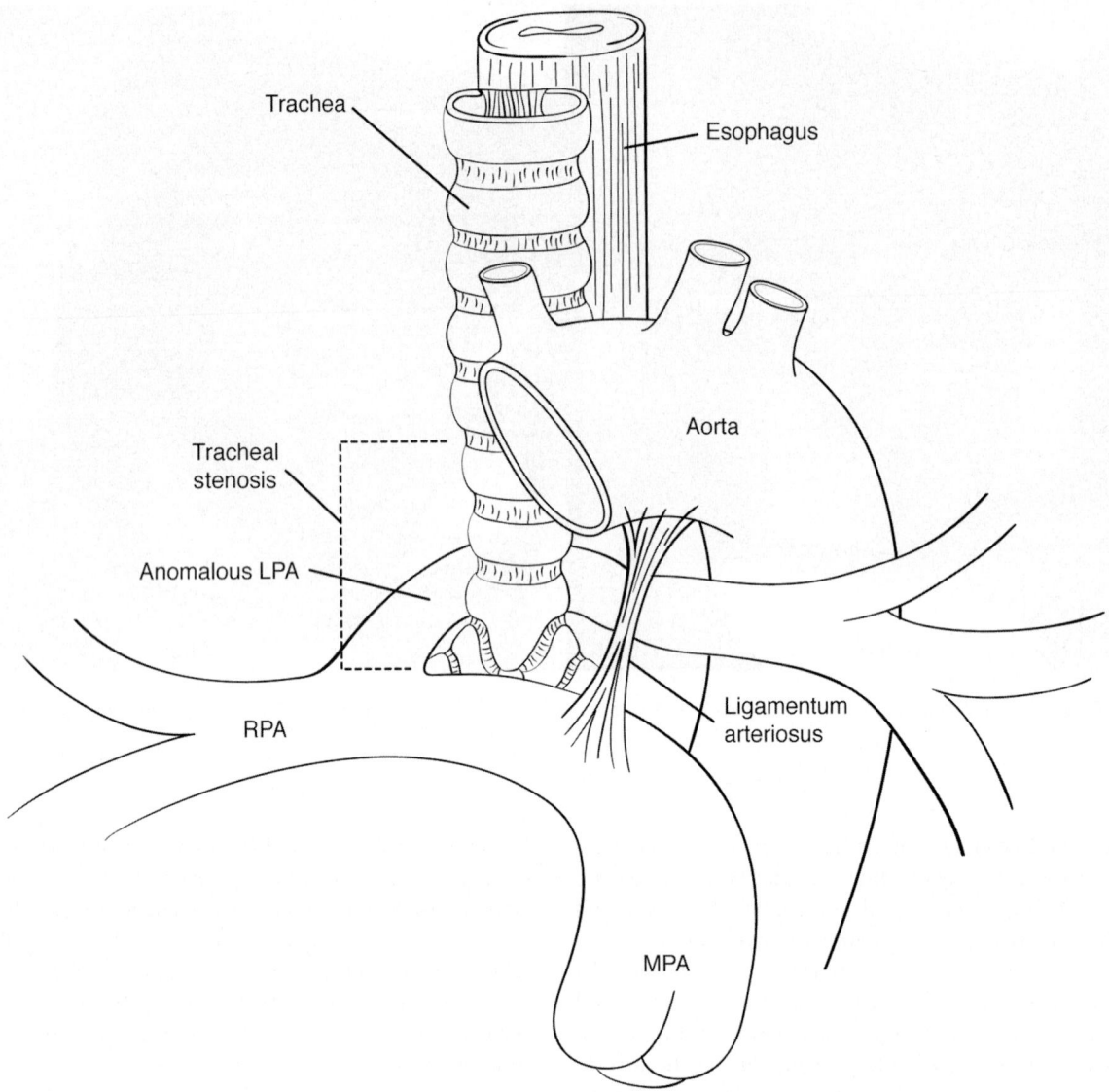

**FIGURE 73-6** Illustration of left pulmonary artery (LPA) sling and its relationship to the trachea.

90% range. Anatomic tracheal stenosis characterized by complete tracheal rings is likely a developmental consequence of the vascular malformation. Surprisingly, the tracheal stenosis seen in these patients is not typically isolated to the segment encircled by the pulmonary artery, but usually extends for a significant distance proximally, even to the extent of involving the entire tracheal length. Also commonly seen are anomalies of tracheal arborization, such as the presence of a right bronchus suis.

## Presentation and Evaluation

Infants with LPA sling typically are noted to have stridor in the first weeks of life, though significant symptoms that prompt further evaluation often arise after a few months. A common clinical scenario is the child who develops an unusually severe degree of respiratory distress with stridor as a consequence of what would otherwise appear to be a mild upper respiratory infection. The time of onset and severity of symptoms are entirely determined by the degree of tracheal pathology. Feeding difficulties are not typically seen with this anomaly aside from challenges imposed by stridor or the increased work of breathing.

Chest x-rays are typically normal. Echocardiography will demonstrate the pulmonary artery anomaly and is an important study to rule out the presence of other intracardiac anomalies that have been seen in up to one third of children with this problem. Contrast CT angiogram or MRI demonstrate the vascular anatomy very well and can also delineate branching anomalies of the airway, when present (Fig. 73-7). These studies often demonstrate the significant reduction of tracheal caliber in these patients, but cannot adequately differentiate between anatomic stenosis and extrinsic compression by vascular structures.

Careful bronchoscopic examination is essential in all patients with pulmonary artery sling to investigate for the presence of complete tracheal rings. This study may be particularly hazardous in the presence of significant airway

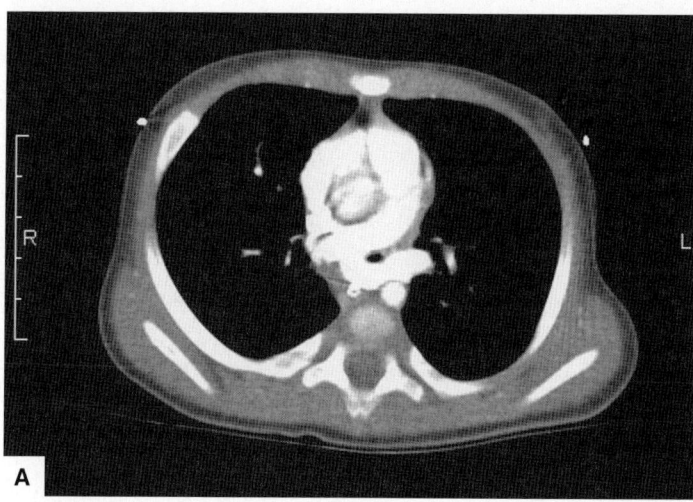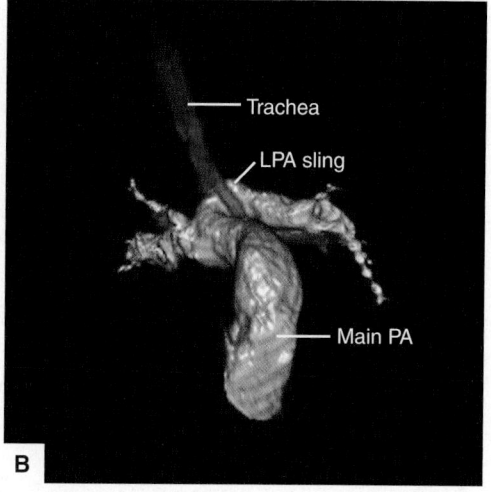

**FIGURE 73-7** The axial view (A) and the 3-D reconstruction (B) of contrast CT demonstrating LPA sling and tracheal hypoplasia.

hypoplasia and should be limited to investigating only as far as the proximal extent of the stenosis. Barium swallow is not usually obtained in these patients, although visualizing an anterior indentation of the barium column between esophagus and trachea is virtually pathognomonic of pulmonary artery sling.

## Surgical Management and Outcomes

Reimplantation of the anomalous LPA has been performed via left thoracotomy, but current practice is to correct this anomaly via sternotomy, utilizing cardiopulmonary bypass support. Simultaneous repair of the tracheal stenosis using the slide tracheoplasty technique should be performed in virtually all cases where complete rings are present. Associated intracardiac defects can be repaired as well. Direct reimplantation of the LPA onto the main pulmonary artery adjacent to the divided stump of the normal left ligamentum has resulted in excellent long-term patency rates of this structure. Some authors have advocated anterior translocation of the anomalous pulmonary artery performed when the trachea is divided for repair, but this may result in acute angulation of the LPA or anterior compression of the reconstructed airway (Fig. 73-8).

Restenosis or late hypoplasia of the reimplanted pulmonary artery has been reported rarely in recent series and may be detected by echocardiography or nuclear medicine pulmonary perfusion scan. Virtually all morbidity and mortality associated with pulmonary artery slings are due to the related tracheal pathology. Current experience with simultaneous reimplantation and slide tracheoplasty has yielded survivals of 90% or better in centers dedicated to the management of this complex population.

## INNOMINATE ARTERY COMPRESSION SYNDROME

Like pulmonary artery sling, the innominate compression syndrome is included in most discussions of vascular rings even though it does not represent a complete vascular ring.

Innominate compression syndrome involves only anterior compression of the trachea and typically causes only airway symptoms.

## Embryology and Anatomy

Use of the term "innominate artery compression syndrome" is, in most cases, a misnomer that contributes to the lack of understanding of the multifactorial etiology of this entity. The name implies an anomaly of the innominate artery, which is almost never the case. Anatomic studies using CT or MRI have clearly demonstrated that the normal course of the innominate artery begins at its aortic origin to the left of midline, crosses anterior to the trachea, and ultimately bifurcates into the right common carotid and right subclavian arteries on the right.

Tracheomalacia is most likely the most significant factor contributing to innominate artery compression syndrome. Multiple structures share a relatively limited space in the midline of the upper mediastinum, bounded by the vertebral bodies posteriorly and the sternum anteriorly. The thymus typically occupies the greatest amount of this space in the infants in whom this syndrome is noted. The innominate artery crosses the mid to distal trachea just behind the thymus, and with some degree of tracheomalacia, the airway is most likely to be deprived of its domain. In most infants this syndrome is self-limited, analogous to what is often seen with gastroesophageal reflux in infancy. The thymus will gradually regress in size, and the increased caliber of the airway and stiffness of its cartilages will result in resolution of symptoms, often by 1 year of age.

## Presentation and Evaluation

The innominate artery compression syndrome typically presents in the first months of life with stridor that is similar to that seen with true vascular rings and the more commonly seen laryngomalacia. The stridor is characteristically inspiratory and expiratory, suggesting a tracheal level of obstruction to airflow. Apnea or similar near life-threatening events often prompt further evaluation.

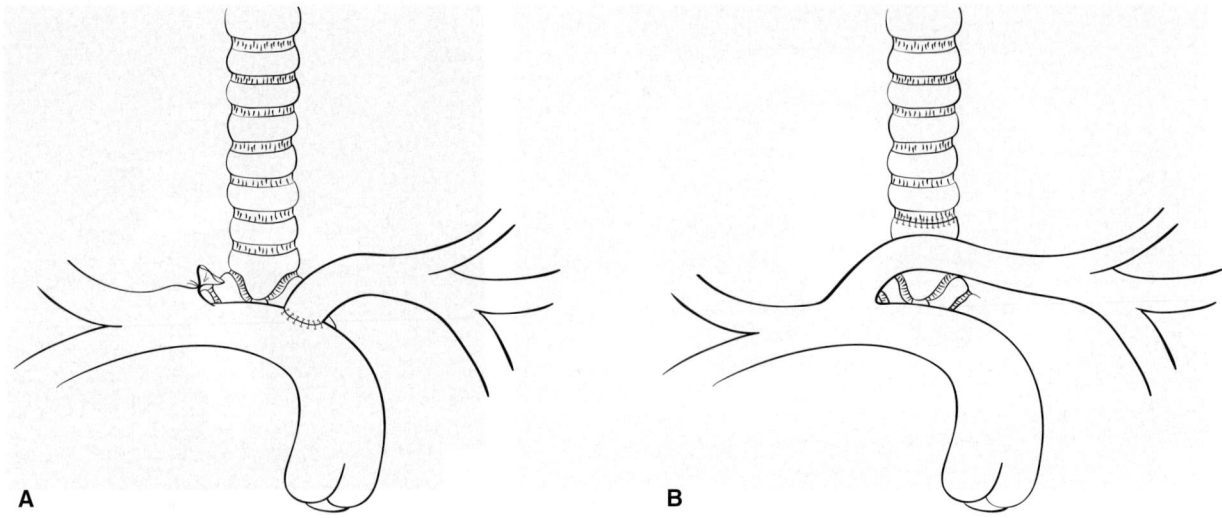

**FIGURE 73-8** Reimplantation (A) and anterior translocation (B) techniques of LPA sling management.

Bronchoscopy is the principal method of diagnosis and may demonstrate pulsatile anterior compression of the mid to distal trachea, which may compromise the lumen by as much as 80% to 90%. Swallowing symptoms are absent as the esophagus is not compromised by any vascular structure, although the airway symptoms may be accentuating during feeding when a swallowed bolus adds to the loss of domain of the floppy trachea.

When symptoms are not severe, observation is warranted, as many infants will improve spontaneously over time. When apnea or near life-threatening events are noted, or if the airway lumen is compromised by more than 50%, operative intervention should be considered.

Bronchoscopy is important in characterizing the location and severity of tracheal collapse, as well as to rule out other causes of stridor such as anatomic tracheal stenosis, foreign body aspiration, or laryngomalacia. Contrast CT or MRI will aid in ruling out anomalies of the great vessels, and will often demonstrate the level of tracheal compromise in relationship to the innominate artery origin from the aorta. These imaging modalities will also demonstrate the size of the thymus and aid in assessing the degree to which the spatial relationships might be changed with an aortopexy procedure.

## Surgical Management and Outcomes

When surgical intervention is considered, aortopexy with complete or partial thymectomy is most commonly recommended. Aortopexy may be performed via right or left thoracotomy and open and endoscopic techniques have been described. An anterior approach via the bed of the resected second costal cartilage may also be considered.

The thymus is removed carefully to avoiding injury to the phrenic nerves. Then the aortic-innominate artery junction is sutured to the posterior aspect of the sternum. Creating a small flap of pericardium, which is based on the natural pericardial reflection at the aortic-innominate junction, avoids suturing the blood vessel itself, reducing the risk of its injury. It also allows adjustment of the degree of anterior translocation

in the unusual case where mobilizing the innominate artery all the way to the sternum would cause distortion of the vessel. Dissection of the plane between vasculature and the airway must be avoided to allow the anterior translocation of the vessels to not only create space for the floppy trachea, but also suspend it open.

Pulse oxymetry or blood pressure monitoring in the right arm should be performed during the procedure to ensure that there is no compromise of the caliber of the innominate artery. Bronchoscopy during or immediately after suspension may be helpful in assessing the adequacy of the relief of tracheal compression. Reimplantation of the innominate artery onto a more proximal and rightward location on the ascending aorta via sternotomy may be considered in unusual cases where aortopexy is not likely to create a significant improvement in room for the airway. This situation is more often considered in older children where the thymus has already involuted to some degree and the distance between innominate artery and sternum is small, as shown on CT or MRI studies.

Persistent stridor, particularly during agitation or associated with upper airway infections, is commonly seen in the months following surgery, as nothing specifically is done to address the tracheomalacia itself, which is likely the most important component in the pathophysiology of this syndrome. The stridor typically improves with growth of the airway, as it does in patients who can be safely managed nonoperatively,

## SELECTED READINGS

Alsenaidi K, Gurofsky R, Karamlou T, Williams WG, McCrindle BW. Management and outcomes of double aortic arch in 81 patients. *Pediatrics* 2006;118:e1336–e1341. Epub 2006 Sep 25.

Applebaum H, Woolley MM. Pericardial flap aortopexy for tracheomalacia. *J Pediatric Surg* 1990;25:30–31; discussion 31–32.

Backer CL, Hillman N, Mavroudis C, Holinger LD. Resection of Kommerell's diverticulum and left subclavian artery transfer for recurrent symptoms after vascular ring division. *Eur J Cardiothorac Surg* 2002;22:64–69.

Backer CL, Mavroudis C, Rigsby CK, Holinger LD. Trends in vascular ring surgery. *J Thorac Cardiovasc Surg* 2005;129:1339–1347.

Chen SJ, Lee WJ, Lin MT, et al. Left pulmonary artery sling complex: computed tomography and hypothesis of embryogenesis. *Ann Thorac Surg* 2007;84:1645–1650.

Fawcett SL, Gomez AC, Hughes JA, Set P. Anatomical variation in the position of the brachiocephalic trunk (innominate artery) with respect to the trachea: a computed tomography-based study and literature review of Innominate Artery Compression Syndrome. *Clin Anat* 2010;23:61–69.

Gardella C, Girosi D, Rossi GA, et al. Tracheal compression by aberrant innominate artery: clinical presentations in infants and children, indications for surgical correction by aortopexy, and short- and long-term outcome. *J Pediatr Surg* 2010;45:564–573.

Hernanz-Schulman M. Vascular rings: a practical approach to imaging diagnosis. *Pediatr Radiol* 2005;35:961–979. Epub 2005 July 29.

Kogon BE, Forbess JM, Wulkan ML, Kirshbom PM, Kanter KR. Video-assisted thoracoscopic surgery: is it a superior technique for the division of vascular rings in children? *Congenit Heart Dis* 2007;2: 130–133.

Manning PB, Rutter MJ, Lisec A, Gupta R, Marino BS. One slide fits all: the versatility of slide tracheoplasty utilizing cardiopulmonary bypass support for airway reconstruction in children. *J Thorac Cardiovasc Surg* 2011;141:155–161. Epub 2010 Nov 5.

Marmon LM, Bye MR, Haas JM, Balsara RK, Dunn JM. Vascular rings and slings: long-term follow-up of pulmonary function. *J Pediatr Surg* 1984;19:683–692.

Ruzmetov M, Vijay P, Rodefeld MD, Turrentine MW, Brown JW. Follow-up of surgical correction of aortic arch anomalies causing tracheoesophageal compression: a 38-year single institution experience. *J Pediatr Surg* 2009;44:1328–1332.

Strife JL, Baumel AS, Dunbar JS. Tracheal compression by the innominate artery in infancy and childhood. *Radiology* 1981;139:73–75.

# Abdominal Aortic Pathology

## CHAPTER 74

*Jaimie D. Nathan*

## KEY POINTS

1. Aortic thrombosis in neonates is usually a complication of umbilical artery catheterization, and its diagnosis can be confirmed by ultrasonography. Management options include anticoagulation, thrombolysis, and surgical thrombectomy, and choice of therapy should be individualized.

2. Abdominal aortic aneurysms in children are most commonly caused by infection, often in association with a history of umbilical artery catheterization.

3. The radiologic modalities used to define anatomic details of abdominal aortic aneurysms and guide surgical planning include magnetic resonance angiography, computed tomography angiography, and conventional aortography.

4. The decision to proceed with surgical repair of an abdominal aortic aneurysm is based on the likelihood of rupture or other complications.

5. Takayasu arteritis causes an inflammatory aortitis, characterized by an early acute phase and a late occlusive phase. Conventional arteriography has been the gold standard for diagnosis, but magnetic resonance arteriography is becoming the preferred technique in many centers.

6. Corticosteroids are used to treat the inflammation associated with Takayasu arteritis in its early phase and prevent the late occlusive complications. Surgical revascularization may be required and include aortoaortic bypass grafting or patch aortoplasty, with renal artery or visceral artery reconstruction.

7. Hypertension is the cardinal presenting feature of congenital abdominal aortic coarctation. Conventional aortography remains the gold standard for evaluating the location and extent of disease, with selective arteriography to determine involvement of the renal or visceral arteries.

8. The surgical approaches for repair of abdominal aortic coarctation are varied and individualized based on the location and length of the stenotic segment and involvement of renal arteries. Resolution of hypertension following surgical repair is reported in 95% of children.

9. Conventional abdominal aortogram with selective renal arteriography is the gold standard for diagnosing renovascular hypertension, which is surgically correctable in children.

10. Percutaneous transluminal renal angioplasty (PTRA) is usually the first revascularization option considered, particularly for short nonostial lesions of the main renal artery. Surgical revascularization, individualized based on extent and location of the renal artery disease, is appropriate for complex lesions or lesions in which PTRA has failed.

## AORTIC THROMBOSIS

Although very rare, aortic thrombosis carries a high risk of morbidity and mortality. In the pediatric population, aortic thrombosis most commonly affects neonates, usually as a complication of umbilical artery catheterization. Studies have reported that a high percentage of neonates with an umbilical artery catheter develop some degree of arterial thrombosis, but only about 25% of these patients have resultant clinical symptoms. While the use of an umbilical artery catheter is the main predisposing condition in neonates with aortic thrombosis, 46% of affected neonates have multiple risk factors, including polycythemia, arrhythmias, a thrombophilic disorder, congenital heart disease, sepsis, dehydration, and maternal diabetes. In older children, spontaneous aortic thrombosis may occur in association with coarctation or other aortic pathology.

In patients with spontaneous aortic thrombosis, particularly in the absence of identifiable risk factors, it is imperative to perform a complete evaluation for possible coagulation disorders, such as antithrombin III, protein C, or protein S deficiencies. The presence of lupus anticoagulant, usually maternal in origin, may also lead to spontaneous thrombosis. Earlier reports of cases of aortic thrombosis in the pediatric population have likely underestimated the true incidence of thrombophilic disorders, as numerous new thrombophilic disorders have been identified recently.

## Symptoms of Aortic Thrombosis

The most common symptoms and signs of aortic thrombosis in the neonate are discoloration and decreased perfusion of the lower extremities, decreased or absent femoral pulses, and decreased temperature of the lower limbs or feet. Other common clinical features include hypertension, acute renal failure, and congestive heart failure.

## Diagnosis of Aortic Thrombosis

The clinical triad of a history of umbilical artery catheter, hypertension, and reduced lower-extremity perfusion is highly suggestive of aortic thrombosis. The diagnosis of aortic thrombosis is usually confirmed by ultrasonography, although magnetic resonance angiography (MRA) may also be utilized.

Conventional angiography is rarely feasible in neonates due to size considerations and the degree of critical illness in such patients. In 86% of patients, thrombus is identified in the infrarenal aorta, with extension into the iliac arteries in 72%. Over 50% of neonates with aortic thrombosis have involvement of one or both renal arteries.

## Treatment of Aortic Thrombosis

Due to the high risk of morbidity and mortality, treatment is indicated in all neonates with acute aortic thrombosis. Therapeutic options include anticoagulation, thrombolysis, and surgical thrombectomy. The choice of therapy should be individualized, and guided by the patient's underlying comorbidities and the risks of treatments, the extent of thrombosis, the degree of ischemic compromise, and the underlying etiology of thrombosis.

In neonates without severe vascular compromise, many authors recommend removal of the umbilical artery catheter and anticoagulation as initial management. Unfortunately, anticoagulation in the neonate, particularly in the premature newborn, is difficult and has many associated risks, including intracranial hemorrhage. Low-molecular-weight heparin has numerous advantages over unfractionated heparin and recently has gained acceptance in children. Klinger et al have described the successful management of severe aortic thrombosis in 2 neonates with the use of low-molecular-weight heparin therapy. If the degree of extremity ischemia is severe or if there is progression of symptoms with the use of anticoagulation alone, either catheter-directed or systemic thrombolytic therapy with recombinant tissue plasminogen activator or urokinase must be considered.

If contraindications to medical therapy exist or attempts at thrombolysis have failed, surgical thrombectomy is indicated. Several surgical approaches to neonatal aortic thrombectomy have been described, including transperitoneal, retroperitoneal, and left thoracotomy.

## Outcomes and Complications

Regardless of the treatment modality utilized, the mortality of acute neonatal aortic thrombosis remains high, and complications, such as renal dysfunction, necrotizing enterocolitis, limb amputation, and hemorrhage, are common.

Long-term morbidity in survivors includes hypertension, renal atrophy, unequal limb length, and neurologic sequelae.

# ABDOMINAL AORTIC ANEURYSM

Abdominal aortic aneurysms in children are exceedingly rare, with fewer than 200 cases reported in the literature. The most frequent cause of aortic aneurysms in the pediatric population is infection, particularly in association with umbilical artery catheterization. These mycotic aneurysms are most commonly caused by *Staphylococcus aureus,* although a variety of bacterial and fungal organisms have been reported. Other underlying etiologies for abdominal aortic aneurysms in children include connective tissue disorders (eg, Ehlers–Danlos syndrome and Marfan syndrome), neurocutaneous syndromes (eg, tuberous sclerosis and neurofibromatosis), inflammatory arteritides (eg, Takayasu arteritis, Kawasaki disease, polyarteritis nodosa, and giant cell arteritis), and trauma (either as a complication of umbilical artery or cardiac catheterization or accidental).

Fewer than 10 true idiopathic congenital abdominal aortic aneurysms have been reported in the literature. These are usually seen in children younger than 5 years of age and have been reported to occur in the newborn period. Congenital aortic aneurysms have been diagnosed antenatally, and in 1 case, fetal demise was attributed to prenatal rupture of a congenital abdominal aortic aneurysm. Histologically, congenital aneurysms exhibit fibromuscular dysplasia (FMD) of the aortic wall, with no other clues to the cause of this rare disorder.

## Symptoms of Abdominal Aortic Aneurysms

Abdominal aortic aneurysms in the pediatric population may present with nonspecific abdominal symptoms and hypertension or as an asymptomatic pulsatile abdominal mass. Aneurysm rupture in children is uncommon, although several cases have been reported, and patients with mycotic aneurysms are at greatest risk. The thrombotic and embolic complications that are often seen with atherosclerotic abdominal aortic aneurysms in adults rarely occur in children. The exceptions are children with aneurysm formation due to Takayasu arteritis or Kawasaki disease, who are at increased risk for complications related to thrombosis and distal embolization.

## Diagnosis of Abdominal Aortic Aneurysms

Abdominal ultrasonography is typically performed as the initial radiologic study in the evaluation of a palpable pulsatile abdominal mass. MRA, computed tomography angiography (CTA), or conventional aortography can be performed to define the specific anatomic details of the aneurysm and to plan subsequent surgical repair. These studies are critical for evaluating the abdominal aortic visceral branches, as abdominal aortic aneurysms may present with associated aneurysms or stenosis of the celiac, superior mesenteric, or renal arteries (Fig. 74-1).

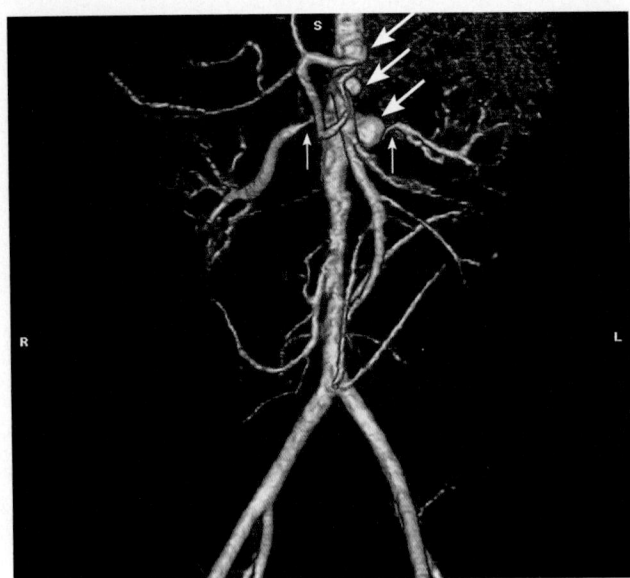

**FIGURE 74-1** Magnetic resonance angiogram (3-dimensional reconstruction) demonstrating aneurysms (*thick arrows*) of the abdominal aorta and the origins of the celiac axis and superior mesenteric artery, with associated bilateral renal artery stenosis (*thin arrows*).

## Repair of Abdominal Aortic Aneurysms

The decision to repair an abdominal aortic aneurysm in a child is similar to that in an adult and is based on the likelihood of rupture or other complications. Although there are no definitive indications for surgery, most authors would consider as a candidate for surgical repair any patient with a symptomatic aneurysm, a rapidly enlarging aneurysm, or a mycotic aneurysm.

Surgical options for repair include replacement with a prosthetic vascular graft, resection and end-to-end anastomosis, and lateral resection with primary patch repair. The surgical approach must be individualized in each patient, based on the anatomy of the aneurysm and any associated aneurysm or stenosis of visceral branches. Due to the rarity of abdominal aortic aneurysms in the pediatric population, long-term outcomes are very difficult to determine.

## TAKAYASU ARTERITIS

Inflammatory disorders of the aorta constitute a highly uncommon cause of abdominal aortic pathology in children. Recognized as the only form of large-vessel vasculitis in childhood, Takayasu arteritis is characterized by granulomatous inflammation of the aorta and its major branches. Although Takayasu arteritis most commonly affects females in their second and third decades of life, it can occur at any age and has even been reported in children as young as 6 months.

Histologically, Takayasu arteritis is a pan-arteritis, with involvement of all layers of the arterial wall. In its acute phase, the inflammatory infiltrate of lymphocytes and giant cells involves the media and the adventitia, including the vasa vasorum, with progressive loss of elastic fibers and smooth muscle cells in the media. In the late phase, intimal fibroproliferation

and fibrosis of the media result in segmental stenosis of the involved arteries, as well as poststenotic dilations and other localized aneurysms. The pathophysiology of the arterial injury in Takayasu arteritis is not well elucidated, but evidence suggests that an autoimmune mechanism via humoral or cell-mediated pathways likely plays a central role.

## Symptoms of Takayasu Arteritis

Approximately 70% of children with Takayasu arteritis present with an early acute phase, consisting of nonspecific constitutional signs and symptoms, including low-grade fever, malaise, fatigue, night sweats, and weight loss. Mild anemia and a marked elevation in the erythrocyte sedimentation rate may be found. These clinical features lack specificity and may remit spontaneously within 2 to 3 months, often delaying definitive diagnosis.

In the late occlusive phase of the disease, the most common presenting features of Takayasu arteritis in children are hypertension (with abdominal aorta and/or renal artery involvement), congestive heart failure, or a neurologic event (with aortic arch and/or carotid artery involvement). It is uncommon for an otherwise asymptomatic child to present with diminished or absent pulses, vascular bruits, or claudication. Importantly, the clinical presentation of Takayasu arteritis is highly variable, due to recurrence and potential coexistence of disease phases, unpredictable intervals between acute and occlusive phases, and geographical variation in the patterns of vascular involvement.

## Diagnosis of Takayasu Arteritis

Isolated midaortic involvement of Takayasu arteritis may mimic congenital abdominal aortic stenosis. An accurate diagnosis is critical, however, since Takayasu arteritis is initially treated medically with corticosteroids to relieve inflammation, and congenital abdominal aortic stenosis is managed by surgical revascularization. Although the concentrations of acute-phase reactants, such as C-reactive protein and erythrocyte sedimentation rate, correlate poorly with disease activity in Takayasu arteritis, they are usually elevated during the active phase of disease.

Historically, the gold standard for the diagnosis of Takayasu arteritis has been conventional arteriography, with the delineation of luminal irregularity, stenotic segments, occlusion, and dilation or aneurysms in the aorta or its major branches. However, MRA is becoming the preferred technique for diagnosis and monitoring during the course of therapy because of ability of MRA to detect mural thickening and aortic wall edema, acute inflammatory phase lesions not often identifiable by conventional aortogram. MRA noninvasively delineates the extent of vascular involvement. This is critical to surgical planning in the late occlusive phase, since the renal arteries are involved in more than 80% of children with Takayasu arteritis and the mesenteric vessels are involved in more than 60% of these children.

## Treatment of Takayasu Arteritis

The goal of therapy in Takayasu arteritis is to relieve inflammation and thereby prevent its late occlusive complications.

Corticosteroids serve as the principle medical therapy, although methotrexate, cyclophosphamide, mycophenolate mofetil, and infliximab have been utilized in refractory cases or to reduce the dose intensity of steroids that need to be administered. In the setting of occlusive disease, the indications for surgical revascularization of midaortic Takayasu arteritis include hypertension due to aortic stenosis or associated renovascular disease, severe lower-extremity claudication, and mesenteric ischemia.

It is critical that systemic hypertension be well controlled prior to surgery. The predominant revascularization techniques include either aortoaortic bypass grafting or patch aortoplasty, with renal artery or visceral artery reconstruction as necessary.

## Outcomes and Complications

The best outcomes of surgical revascularization for Takayasu arteritis are achieved if surgery is performed when the acute inflammatory disease is quiescent. It is also important that anastomosis not be performed at a diseased area of the artery, as recurrence of active disease at anastomotic sites can lead to restenosis and aneurysmal dilation. Other postoperative complications following surgical vascularization include graft occlusion, recurrent hypertension, and relapsing disease with progressive end-organ ischemia, such as renal failure. Although surgical results demonstrate improved hypertension in 90% of patients postoperatively, life-long follow-up is mandatory.

# CONGENITAL ABDOMINAL AORTIC COARCTATION

Congenital abdominal aortic coarctation, also referred to as midaortic syndrome, is an uncommon condition that is characterized by significant luminal narrowing of the abdominal aorta and frequently involves ostial stenosis of its major branches. Renal artery stenosis occurs in approximately 80% of patients with abdominal aortic coarctation, and the celiac axis and superior mesenteric artery are stenotic in up to 25% of cases. Abdominal aortic coarctation is an important cause of renovascular hypertension in the pediatric population, and males and females are equally affected.

Accounting for less than 2% of all coarctations, the midaortic syndrome may affect a short segment of abdominal aorta or a long diffuse segment, and is often termed aortic hypoplasia. The pathogenesis of congenital abdominal aortic coarctation is poorly understood. Most authors favor a developmental defect, and several developmental mechanisms have been proposed. One of the earliest proposed mechanisms described is that incomplete fusion of the paired primitive dorsal aortas during embryological development results in kinking and permanent constriction. Another proposed hypothesis is that overfusion of the paired dorsal aortas results in coarctation. This mechanism is supported by studies demonstrating decreased aortic diameters in patients with single origins of the lowest pair of lumbar arteries, an anomaly considered a result of overfusion. Others have proposed that the

very high incidence of multiple renal arteries suggests that abdominal aortic coarctation is due to abnormal migration of the kidneys. The development of obstructing luminal fibrous clefts and ridges secondary to anomalous mesenchymal cell maturation has also been hypothesized as a developmental etiology of congenital abdominal aortic stenosis. Congenital viral infections have been proposed as a pathogenetic mechanism, as prenatal exposure to rubella has been shown to disturb the growth of a developmentally normal aorta. Finally, the association of genetic disorders (eg, neurofibromatosis and Williams syndrome) with abdominal aortic coarctation suggests a possible genetic component to its etiology.

## Symptoms of Congenital Abdominal Aortic Coarctation

Most patients with congenital abdominal aortic coarctation present within the first 2 decades of life, and there are even reports of newborns with symptomatic abdominal aortic coarctation. Hypertension is the cardinal presenting feature, and it is often asymptomatic and found incidentally. In cases of symptomatic hypertension, patients may present with headaches, dizziness, sleep disturbance, palpitations, and fatigue. Blurred vision, epistaxis, and cardiac and cerebrovascular events may also occur, and longstanding severe hypertension can precipitate renal failure and left ventricular hypertrophy and congestive heart failure. Physical signs in patients with abdominal aortic coarctation may include cardiac murmurs, abdominal bruits, reduced or absent femoral pulses, and differential blood pressures between the upper and lower extremities.

The pathophysiology of hypertension in abdominal aortic coarctation is based on renal hypoperfusion, with consequent activation of the renin–angiotensin–aldosterone system. Stenosis of the renal arteries is most often responsible for the clinical presentation with hypertension; however, in cases in which the renal arteries are normal, hypertension will also develop if the abdominal aortic stenosis or hypoplasia is suprarenal in location. As would be expected, patients with infrarenal coarctation and normal renal arteries typically do not have hypertension. A classification system for abdominal aortic coarctation has been developed by Hallett et al based on the relationship of the coarctation to the renal arteries and on the presence or absence of renal artery stenosis (Table 74-1). Lower-extremity claudication and symptomatic mesenteric ischemia have been reported in abdominal aortic coarctation, but are rare, due to the formation of effective collateral circulation.

| TABLE 74-1 | The Hallett Anatomic Classification of Abdominal Aortic Coarctation |
|---|---|
| Type I | Suprarenal coarctation with renal artery stenosis |
| Type II | Infrarenal coarctation with renal artery stenosis |
| Type III | Suprarenal coarctation with normal renal arteries |
| Type IV | Infrarenal coarctation with normal renal arteries |

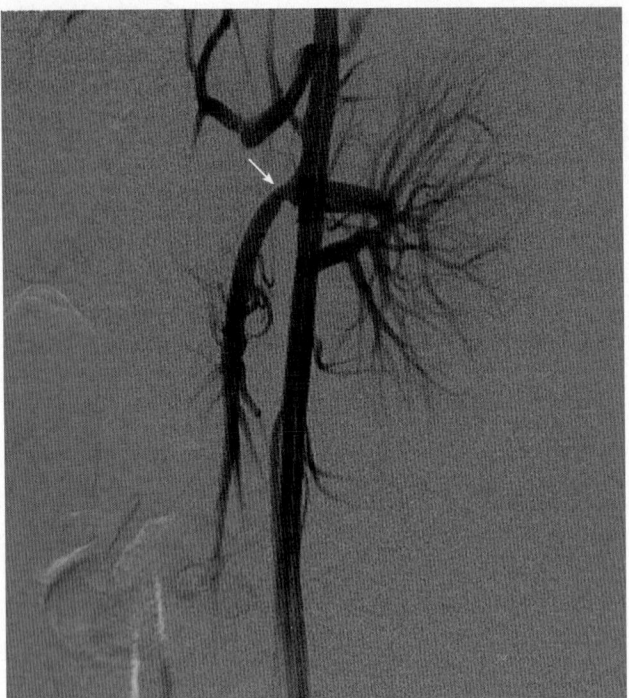

**FIGURE 74-2** Conventional aortogram (lateral view) demonstrating findings of midaortic syndrome in an 8-year-old boy. The abdominal aorta is narrowed to approximately 60% of its expected diameter. An approximately 50% stenosis of the superior mesenteric artery is identified just anterior to its origin from the aorta (*arrow*). A moderate stenosis of the celiac axis was also identified in this patient (*not demonstrated on this image*).

## Diagnosis of Congenital Abdominal Aortic Coarctation

Doppler ultrasonography to evaluate the abdominal aorta, renal arteries, and renal parenchyma is often the initial radiologic modality performed in children with hypertension. It provides information about renal artery stenosis, estimates resistive indices in the renal hilum, and may also provide evidence of visceral artery stenosis. The gold standard for evaluating the location and the extent of abdominal aortic coarctation has been conventional aortogram, with selective views to determine involvement of the renal and visceral arteries (Fig. 74-2). Hemodynamic significance of stenotic lesions can be assessed by direct measurement of pressure gradients. Recently, MRA and CTA have been used with increasing frequency, as they are able to delineate the vascular anatomy of the aorta and its branches with a high level of accuracy and can provide additional information regarding the presence of associated inflammatory changes, which may be suggestive of Takayasu arteritis or other inflammatory process. Inflammatory changes are often not discernible on conventional aortography.

## Management of Congenital Abdominal Aortic Coarctation

Initial therapy for the child with congenital abdominal aortic coarctation is medical control of hypertension, but the definitive management is surgical correction. The principle

indication for operative intervention is persistent severe hypertension uncontrolled by medications, and the goals of surgical management are control of hypertension and preservation of renal function. In some patients, surgical intervention may be delayed by achieving an effective antihypertensive regimen, allowing the child to reach full growth potential prior to operation.

## Surgical Treatment

Numerous surgical techniques may be utilized in the repair of abdominal aortic coarctation. In patients with short segment aortic lesions, resection of the involved segment may be performed with either end-to-end anastomosis or placement of an interposition graft. Alternatively, patch aortoplasty using a polytetrafluoroethylene patch is a good option for short-segment disease, when technically feasible (Fig. 74-3). This approach has been shown to result in normal growth of the aorta with no pressure gradient.

In patients with diffuse and lengthy aortic lesions, aortoaortic bypass from above the stenosis to below it offers the best technical approach. If the coarctation reaches the level of the diaphragm, thoracoabdominal aortic bypass is indicated. Renal artery revascularization is performed as necessary, and autogenous saphenous vein or internal iliac artery grafts are utilized if feasible. In patients with abdominal aortic coarctation involving the visceral arteries, revascularization of the celiac axis and superior mesenteric artery may also be necessary.

The operative approach to congenital abdominal aortic coarctation is individualized and is determined principally by the location and length of the lesion and whether one or both of the renal arteries are involved (Fig. 74-4). Most patients with a Type I lesion will require a thoracoabdominal aortoaortic bypass (or patch aortoplasty) and simultaneous renal artery revascularization. In patients with Type II lesions, the aortic coarctation can be left alone if it is not hemodynamically significant, and the renal artery stenosis can be bypassed or reconstructed by a number of different autogenous approaches. An additional approach for Type II lesions involves infrarenal aortic reconstruction

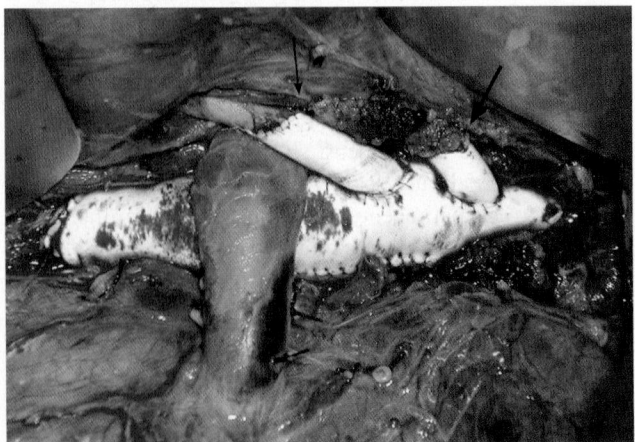

**FIGURE 74-3** Patch aortoplasty repair of abdominal aortic coarctation, using a polytetrafluoroethylene graft, with concomitant revascularization of the celiac axis (*thick arrow*) and superior mesenteric artery (*thin arrow*).

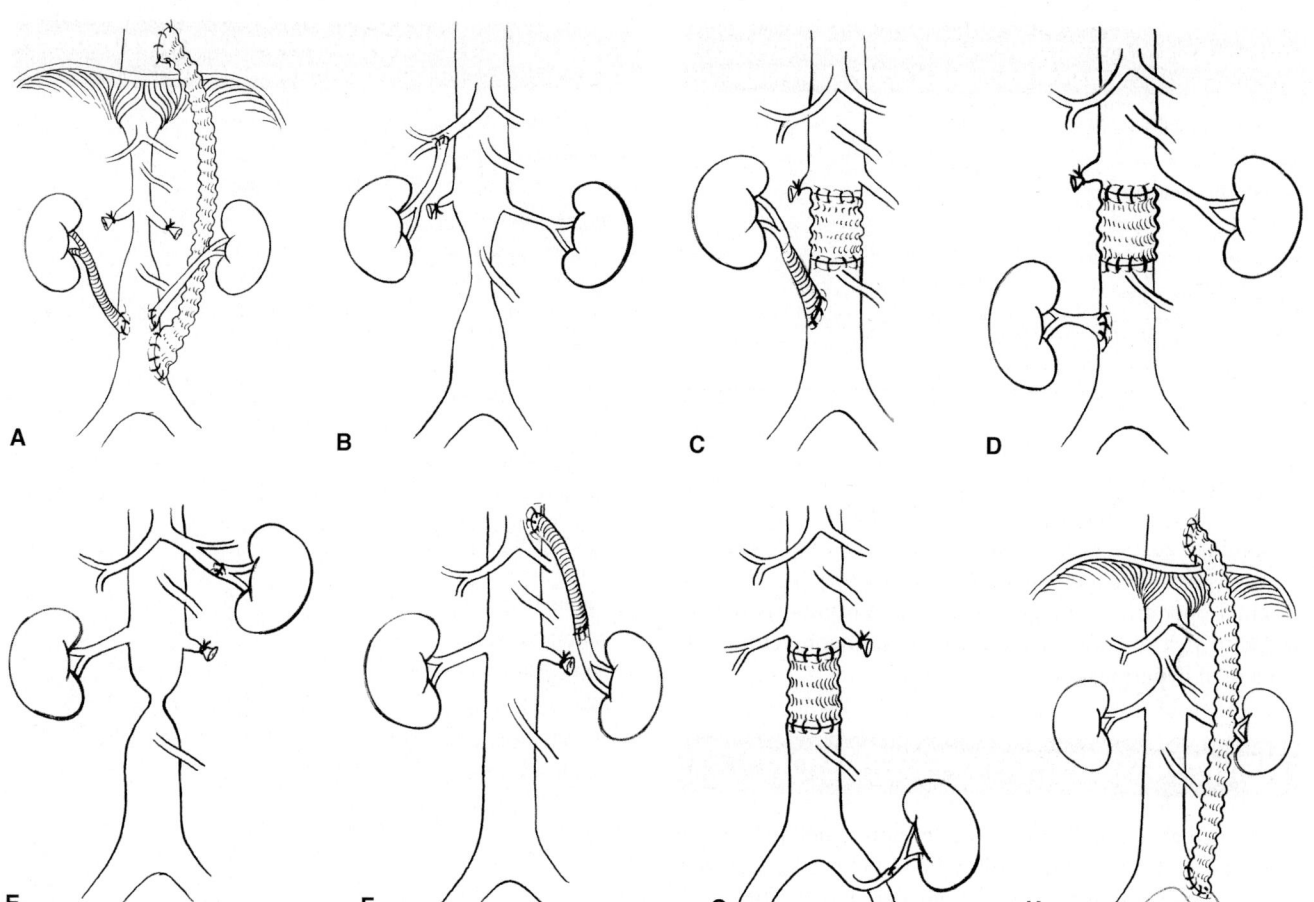

**FIGURE 74-4** Operative strategies for abdominal aortic coarctation with or without concomitant renal artery stenosis. **A.** Type I lesion repair with thoracoabdominal aortoaortic bypass and simultaneous renal artery revascularization by autogenous vein graft bypass (right kidney) and by direct aortorenal reimplantation (left kidney). **B.** Type II lesion with reconstruction only of right renal artery stenosis by hepatorenal bypass technique using autogenous vein graft. **C.** Type II lesion repair by infrarenal aortic interposition graft and right renal artery aortorenal bypass. **D.** Type II lesion repair by infrarenal aortic interposition graft and right renal autotransplantation. **E.** Type II lesion with reconstruction only of left renal artery stenosis by end-to-end splenorenal arterial anastomosis. **F.** Type II lesion with reconstruction only of left renal artery stenosis by suprarenal aortorenal bypass using autogenous vein graft. **G.** Type II lesion repair by infrarenal aortic interposition graft and left renal autotransplantation with revascularization via the internal iliac artery. **H.** For a severe type III lesion, a thoracoabdominal aortoaortic bypass will provide retrograde flow up the aorta into normal renal arteries.

with autotransplantation of either kidney. For patients with Type III lesions, a thoracoabdominal aortoaortic bypass will provide retrograde flow up the aorta into normal renal arteries. Alternatively, patch aortoplasty may be performed in the setting of a short segment Type III lesion. In Type IV lesions (not depicted in Fig. 74-4), aortic reconstruction is indicated only for severe claudication or lower-extremity ischemia and is often amenable to patch aortoplasty.

The underlying principle of surgical treatment of congenital abdominal aortic coarctation is to control hypertension while preserving renal function by revascularization of the affected kidney(s). This usually requires repair or bypass of the stenotic aorta along with the renal artery reconstruction. Most authors favor a single procedure to correct the aortic coarctation and renal artery stenosis. In particularly small children, an initial operation to bypass the renal artery, followed in a staged fashion by the aortic reconstruction, may be a preferable strategy. In patients in whom renal artery reconstruction is not feasible, nephrectomy may be considered as a last resort to control persistent, severe hypertension.

## Complications Following Surgical Repair of Congenital Abdominal Aortic Coarctation

Complications following surgery for congenital abdominal aortic coarctation occur in fewer than 10% of patients, but can result in significant morbidity (Table 74-2). Surgical mortality in most series is less than 5%, but mortality up to 8% has been reported. A small number of children develop marked abdominal pain and a form of necrotizing enterocolitis following repair of a coarctation, presumably as a result of a reperfusion injury. Although more common following repair of a thoracic coarctation, this syndrome can develop following repair of a suprarenal abdominal aortic coarctation as well. Patients who develop this syndrome have been shown to have paradoxical hypertension, particularly diastolic hypertension and elevated plasma catecholamines.

Resolution of hypertension following surgical repair of congenital abdominal aortic coarctation is reported in up to 95% of patients. This response is durable, as approximately 70% to 85% of patients remain normotensive over

| TABLE 74-2 | Postoperative Complications Following Repair of Abdominal Aortic Coarctation |
|---|---|

Necrotizing enterocolitis

Leak

Anastomotic aneurysm

Aortic rupture

Thrombosis

Recurrent stenosis

Acute paradoxical hypertension

Persistent sustained hypertension

long-term follow-up. Lifelong follow-up is critical in children who have undergone surgical repair of congenital abdominal aortic coarctation because recurrent stenosis and anastomotic aneurysms can occur many years after the original operation. Late graft failure or thrombosis occurs in 5% to 10% of patients and may require nephrectomy for control of hypertension.

# RENOVASCULAR HYPERTENSION

In the pediatric population, hypertension is defined as systolic blood pressure and/or diastolic blood pressure greater than the 95th percentile for age, gender, and height, on at least 3 occasions. Renovascular hypertension is defined as hypertension occurring as a direct physiologic result of impaired blood flow to a part or all of one or both kidneys. Approximately 1% to 5% of all children and adolescents have hypertension and 10% of those children and adolescents have renovascular hypertension.

The pathophysiology of renovascular hypertension involves activation of the renin–angiotensin–aldosterone axis by hypoperfusion of the affected kidney. Etiologies of renovascular hypertension in children and adolescents are numerous (Table 74-3), and diagnosis is critical, since renovascular hypertension is a potentially surgically correctable cause of hypertension and renal failure. Children who are younger than 10 years of age are most likely to have a surgically correctable cause of hypertension and among children younger than 5 years of age, up to 80% will have a surgically correctable cause of hypertension.

The most common etiology of pediatric renovascular hypertension is FMD, a noninflammatory and nonatherosclerotic disorder of medium-sized arteries. FMD characteristically involves the mid or distal portion of the renal artery, and can affect the intima, media, and adventitia, although its cause is unknown. A significant number of children, approximately 30% in reported series, have renal artery stenosis in association with congenital abdominal aortic coarctation. Although uncommon in North America and Europe, Takayasu disease is an important cause of renovascular hypertension in children and adolescents in Asia and Africa.

Several syndromes are associated with renovascular hypertension in children, including neurofibromatosis and tuberous sclerosis, and renal artery lesions in patients with such disorders are usually multiple and complex, with long-segment

| TABLE 74-3 | Etiologies of Renovascular Hypertension in Children and Adolescents |
|---|---|

Congenital

   Fibromuscular dysplasia

   Congenital abdominal aortic coarctation

   Renal artery aneurysm

   Renal hypoplasia/dysplasia

Vasculitis

   Takayasu arteritis

   Kawasaki disease

   Moyamoya disease

Syndromic

   Neurofibromatosis

   Tuberous sclerosis

   Williams syndrome

Extrinsic compression

   Neuroblastoma

   Wilms' tumor

   Other tumors

Other

   Traumatic renal artery thrombosis/stenosis/aneurysm

   Umbilical artery catheterization

   Unilateral atrophic pyelonephritis

   Radiation

   Congenital rubella syndrome

stenosis and involvement of second-order and third-order branches. Renal artery stenosis has also been reported in association with Williams syndrome. Various tumors, including neuroblastoma and Wilms tumor, can extrinsically compress the renal artery, thereby activating renin release and causing hypertension. Hypertension may occur in up to 5% of children with renal trauma. Posttraumatic renovascular hypertension, which may occur years after the initial injury, can be caused by direct vascular injury with subsequent segmental renal infarction or by stenosis resulting from renal artery disruption.

## Symptoms of Renovascular Hypertension

The diagnosis of renovascular hypertension is often delayed because most children with hypertension are asymptomatic and it is not common for children to have routine blood pressure measurements. In up to 70% of children with renovascular disease, hypertension is an incidental finding in an asymptomatic child. The blood pressure at the time of presentation of a child with renovascular hypertension is usually extremely high, and management with antihypertensive medications is very difficult.

Some children will present with relatively nonspecific symptoms, such as lethargy and headaches in adolescents and failure to thrive and irritability in younger children. Others may present with complications arising from long-standing severe hypertension, including congestive heart failure, stroke, and seizures. On rare occasions, children

| TABLE 74-4 | Clinical Factors Highly Suggestive of Renovascular Hypertension |
|---|---|

Extremely high blood pressure

Refractory hypertension (requiring ≥2 medications)

Secondary signs and symptoms of hypertension (cardiac; neurologic)

Diagnosis of a syndrome with high risk of associated vascular disease

Signs or symptoms of arteritis

History of vascular injury (prior trauma; umbilical artery catheterization)

Bruit heard over renal artery

Elevated peripheral plasma renin, moderate hypokalemia, metabolic alkalosis

with renovascular hypertension may present with metabolic abnormalities due to renal dysfunction.

Once a child is identified as hypertensive, a meticulous history and physical examination must be performed to determine the likelihood that a renovascular etiology is the cause. A history of abdominal trauma should suggest the possibility of posttraumatic renovascular hypertension. A history of umbilical artery catheterization in the neonatal period may also be consistent with a renovascular etiology. Symptoms of claudication, or the finding of decreased femoral pulses, should suggest an abdominal aortic coarctation. Constitutional symptoms, such as fevers, fatigue, and weight loss, may point to Takayasu disease as a potential etiology. The presence of an abdominal bruit, which is present in only 30% of children with renal artery stenosis, should also suggest renovascular disease. Evidence of an abdominal mass should suggest one of the tumor types that can cause hypertension. The presence of specific clinical factors predicts a high probability of renovascular disease (Table 74-4).

## Diagnosis of Renovascular Hypertension

The evaluation of the hypertensive child begins with a urinalysis and serum BUN and creatinine because the most frequent medical cause of hypertension is renal insufficiency. Peripheral plasma renin levels are usually not helpful because renin is elevated in a variety of causes of hypertension. In the setting of severe hypertension, evaluation for end-organ injury should also be performed, including echocardiography and fundoscopic examination. Approximately 60% of children with renovascular hypertension will have evidence of left ventricular hypertrophy, and 60% will have hypertensive retinopathy.

Doppler ultrasound of the abdominal aorta, renal arteries, and renal parenchyma is usually the initial diagnostic imaging study ordered to evaluate for renovascular disease. Several Doppler parameters may be used to assess for evidence of renal artery stenosis, including peak systolic velocity, acceleration time, and resistive index. Doppler ultrasound is not sensitive or specific enough, however, to accurately diagnose most cases of renal artery stenosis in children, since false-positive and false-negative results are not uncommon. A major limitation is the inability of Doppler to detect stenosis in small renal artery branches and accessory renal arteries. Nevertheless, Doppler ultrasound is an important study to evaluate for nonvascular causes of hypertension (eg, tumors and intrinsic renal abnormalities).

Captopril-augmented renal scintigraphy with 99m-technetium-dimercaptosuccinic acid (DMSA) or with 99m-technetium-mercaptoacetyltriglycine (MAG3) is a functional study that can potentially be used to localize renal artery stenosis in children. In practice, however, the accuracy of such functional studies is limited in the presence of significant renal insufficiency or bilateral disease. The sensitivity of renal scintigraphy in detecting renovascular disease in children ranges from 59% to 73%, and its specificity is reported to be 68% to 88%. For optimal accuracy, such studies require the discontinuation of antihypertensive medications that affect the renin–angiotensin–aldosterone axis prior to the procedure. For these reasons, functional studies have fallen out of favor among many clinicians in the evaluation of renovascular hypertension in children.

The gold standard for the diagnosis of suspected renovascular hypertension in children is the conventional abdominal aortogram with selective renal arteriography. The aortogram provides the best assessment of the ostia of the renal arteries, but selective angiography of each renal artery, including accessory arteries, is required to fully evaluate for stenosis of the distal renal arteries and the smaller branch vessels. Lateral views of the aortogram are also performed to assess for concomitant stenosis of the celiac axis or the superior mesenteric artery. Three-dimensional images can be generated by rotational angiography, a recent technical advance being utilized by interventional radiologists. In appropriate cases of renal artery stenosis, therapeutic angioplasty can be performed under the same anesthetic as the arteriogram. Renal arteriography can also identify the rare case of a renal artery aneurysm, which can be treated by selective transcatheter embolization.

Renal vein renin sampling, another diagnostic technique in the evaluation of renovascular hypertension, may be performed via femoral vein approach at the same time as the diagnostic arteriogram. This technique can lateralize the renin-producing focus, and more precise localization can be achieved by selective sampling from segmental venous tributaries. Renal vein renin sampling in children is most useful in 2 settings: (1) to confirm an otherwise equivocal diagnosis in patients who do not have the typical appearance of a hemodynamically significant renal artery stenosis on arteriography; and (2) to identify which side to address first in a staged procedure in bilateral disease, which occurs in approximately 40% to 50% of patients.

Because conventional renal arteriography is invasive and carries a risk of vascular and renal complications, recent attention has been given to CTA and MRA as noninvasive imaging modalities for evaluating renovascular hypertension. Both CTA and MRA provide good accuracy for the diagnosis of renal artery stenosis in adults, but have significant limitations in evaluating renovascular causes of hypertension in children due the small size of their vessels, particularly in the detection of lesions distal to the main renal artery. Selective renal arteriography provides the best spatial and temporal resolution in children and maintains

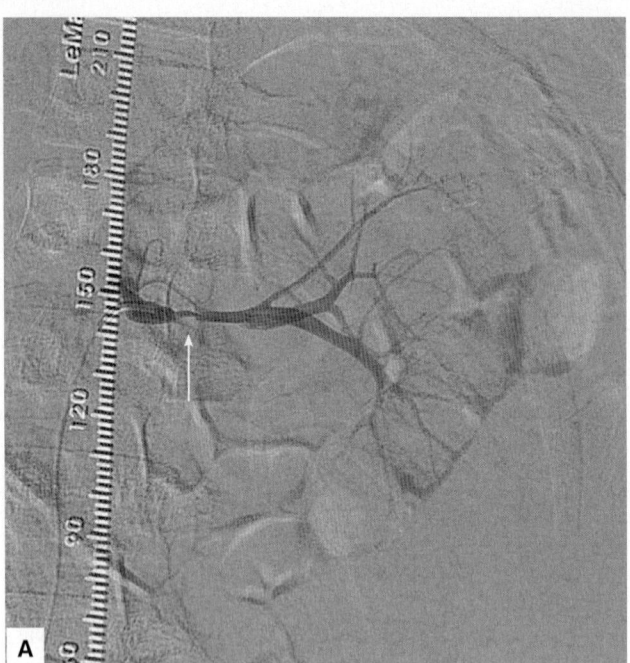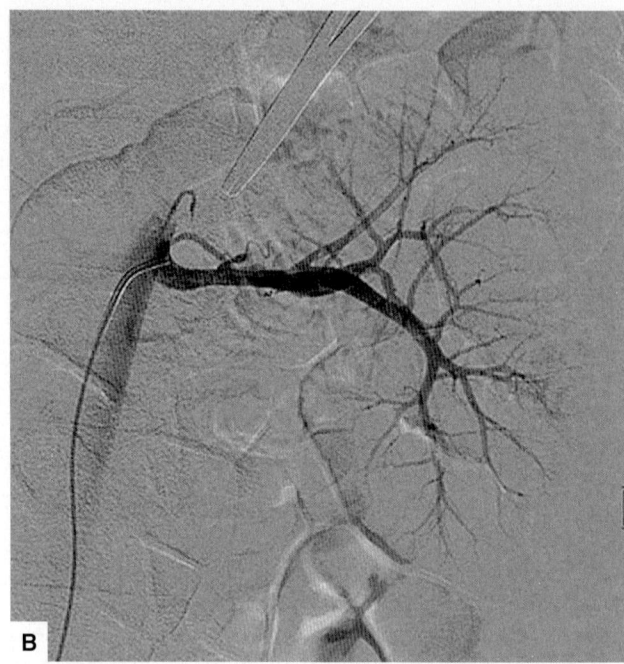

**FIGURE 74-5** **A.** Selective renal arteriogram demonstrating a high-grade focal stenosis (*arrow*) of the midportion of the left main renal artery. **B.** Following percutaneous transluminal renal angioplasty, there is no residual stenosis of the left renal artery.

superior sensitivity for the detection of stenosis in the renal artery branch vessels or in an accessory renal artery. If the clinical suspicion for renovascular hypertension is high and noninvasive studies are inconclusive, conventional renal arteriography must be pursued.

## Treatment of Renovascular Hypertension

The overall goals of treatment of renovascular disease in children are adequate blood pressure control to avoid symptoms and complications of hypertension, the preservation of renal function, and the avoidance of adverse effects of treatment. These patients characteristically present with very high blood pressure, and it is important to assure a gradual reduction in blood pressure as antihypertensive medications are initiated. The antihypertensive regimen typically includes a calcium channel blocker or a beta-blocker, although a combination of multiple medications is often necessary. Medications that affect the renin–angiotensin axis, such as angiotensin-converting-enzyme inhibitors and angiotensin-receptor blockers, should be avoided because of the risk of renal insufficiency and renal failure, related to severe reductions in the glomerular filtration rate.

Renovascular hypertension often responds poorly to medical management, and long-term use of antihypertensive medications leads to complications and renal parenchymal damage. Endovascular or surgical interventions should be considered when 2 or more medications are required to maintain adequate blood pressure control or when medications have unacceptable adverse effects.

## Percutaneous Transluminal Renal Angioplasty

Percutaneous transluminal renal angioplasty (PTRA) is usually the first revascularization option considered in children

with renal artery stenosis. The location, length, and underlying etiology of the stenotic lesion are important factors for the success of this interventional approach. Discrete short nonostial lesions of the main renal artery secondary to FMD are the most likely lesions to be successfully dilated using PTRA (Fig. 74-5). Stenotic areas involving the ostium or adjacent to an aneurysm should not be dilated because of the increased risk of arterial rupture. Approximately 10% of pediatric patients will have an associated renal artery aneurysm. In addition, renal artery lesions secondary to systemic arteritis (eg, Takayasu disease), associated with neurofibromatosis, or in the setting of concomitant mid-aortic syndrome, are unlikely to have successful outcomes with PTRA.

Although single focal nonostial stenotic lesions of the main renal artery have traditionally been identified as the most amenable to successful PTRA, recent studies in adults have demonstrated success with PTRA for renal branch artery lesions. At this time, however, the outcomes of PTRA for branch vessel lesions in children have not yet been evaluated. Most authors agree that focal stenosis of unilateral or bilateral main renal arteries constitutes an appropriate indication for PTRA in children. When the appropriate lesions are treated with PTRA, the success rate in achieving cure or improvement in renovascular hypertension in children is greater than 90%. Even when PTRA does not result in normalization of blood pressure, this intervention may allow reduction of antihypertensive medications and preservation of renal parenchyma, thereby delaying surgical revascularization until a young child has grown, making definitive operation easier.

## Complications of Percutaneous Transluminal Renal Angioplasty

Arterial spasm is a common complication of PTRA, and can be treated with intra-arterial nitroglycerine. Major

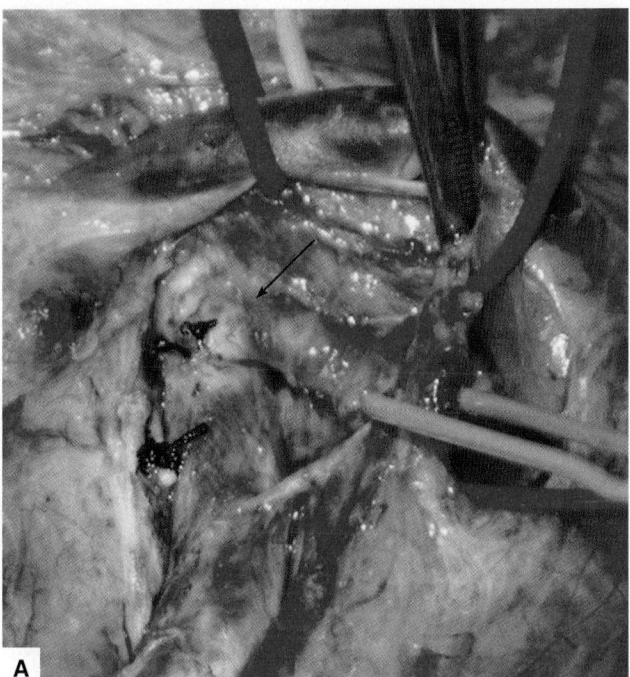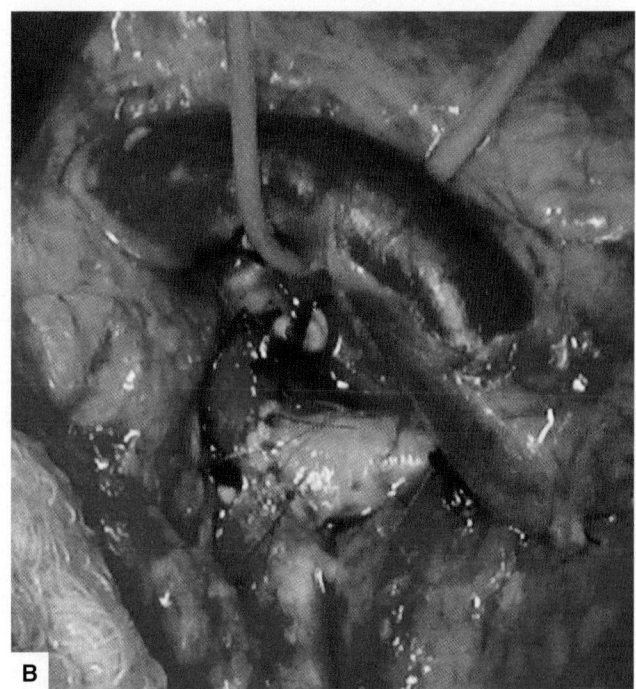

**FIGURE 74-6** **A.** Stenosis of the ostium (*arrow*) of the left renal artery. **B.** Direct aortic reimplantation of the left renal artery was performed using interrupted monofilament sutures after resecting the stenotic ostial segment of the artery.

complications of PTRA are uncommon, and include thrombosis, arterial dissection, arterial rupture, and intrarenal arteriovenous fistula. Restenosis of renal artery lesions has been reported to occur in less than 25% of children who have undergone PTRA. Restenosis most frequently occurs within 1 year of PTRA and can be treated by repeat angioplasty.

## Surgical Revascularization

Surgical revascularization is appropriate in children with renal artery lesions that are too complex for PTRA or if PTRA fails to achieve long-term control of hypertension. The revascularization approach is individualized based on the extent and location of the renal artery disease of each child. Surgical options for revascularization include direct aortic reimplantation, resection of the stenotic segment with primary reanastomosis, aortorenal bypass with autogenous (or rarely, prosthetic) grafts, and autotransplantation.

For ostial renal artery lesions, resection of the stenosis with direct aortic reimplantation is usually possible (Fig. 74-6). It is important to ensure that the reimplantation of the renal artery beyond the stenosis is performed under no tension. In order to accomplish this, the Gerota fascia is incised laterally to allow the kidney to be mobilized medially. Midrenal artery stenosis can be managed by resection of the stenosis with primary reanastomosis or more commonly, by aortorenal bypass, using autogenous graft, either the saphenous vein or the internal iliac artery.

In children, saphenous vein grafts have been shown to become aneurysmal with time. Although most saphenous veins will dilate with time, approximately 25% will become truly aneurysmal. This usually occurs within the first 2 years after surgery. Therefore, for most surgeons, the first choice of autogenous graft, particularly for patients with unilateral

disease, is the internal iliac artery. In patients with complex lesions or midaortic syndrome, the internal iliac arteries may be insufficient in length or may be involved by the disease process. In addition, only 1 internal iliac artery can be used, as the sacrifice of both arteries may lead to impotence. When the internal iliac artery is not appropriate, or if bilateral renal artery stenosis is present, saphenous vein grafts may be used.

The use of a Dacron graft to wrap the saphenous vein may decrease the risk of aneurysm formation. Prosthetic grafts are usually avoided for renal artery revascularization in children because such conduits cannot change in size with normal vessel growth, thereby compromising long-term patency of small-caliber prosthetic grafts. Although direct revascularization via the splenic artery or other major branches of the celiac axis has been used in the past, this is a risky approach due to the possibility of future development of celiac axis ostial stenosis, and therefore recurrent hypertension. In select cases, the kidney can be autotransplanted into a new position after resection of the stenotic renal artery segment.

Approximately 90% to 97% of children who undergo surgical revascularization for renovascular hypertension have cure or significant improvement of their hypertension after surgery.

## Complications of Surgical Revascularization

Surgical complications may include graft thrombosis, anastomotic stenosis, aneurysms, persistent hypertension, and renal failure. In the youngest patients, many surgeons utilize an interrupted monofilament suture technique for the anastomosis, in order to reduce the risk of thrombosis or stenosis. Internal iliac artery bypass grafts have only rarely been reported to develop late stenosis. Graft stenosis occurs in fewer than 5% of autogenous saphenous vein grafts, although aneurysmal dilation of the venous graft can also complicate long-term outcomes. Stenosis is most likely to occur in small patients because the vascular anastomosis can become insufficient as the patients grow. In cases of anastomotic stenosis, PTRA may be attempted, but often surgical revision is required. Due to the technical challenges in reconstructing renal arteries that are less than 2 mm in diameter, it may be reasonable to defer revascularization, if feasible, in the youngest of patients, as the best outcomes after renal artery revascularization are reported in children older than 3 years.

## Primary Nephrectomy

Primary nephrectomy may be necessary to control severe hypertension in children with renal artery disease that is irreparable by PTRA or surgical revascularization. Cases deemed irreparable are usually those with multiple intrarenal stenoses or aneurysms, as well as cases in which a diminutive, poorly functioning kidney is driving the hypertension. Nephrectomy is a last resort alternative in patients who have failed attempts at renal artery revascularization. Nephrectomy may be necessary to achieve a surgical cure in children with hypertension caused by unilateral chronic atrophic pyelonephritis or unilateral renal hypoplasia or dysplasia. For post-traumatic causes of renal artery stenosis, if a segmental intraparenchymal artery was injured, a partial nephrectomy may result in cure of the patient's hypertension.

## Surveillance and Outcomes

Life-long surveillance of children with renovascular hypertension who have undergone PTRA or surgical revascularization focuses on blood pressure control, renal function, and assessment for other vascular involvement. Postoperative monitoring should include routine measurements of blood pressure and serum creatinine levels, as well as interval renal Doppler ultrasounds at 3, 6, 12 months, and yearly thereafter. Patency of the revascularized renal artery, as well as the contralateral side, must be assessed, as a contralateral renal artery stenosis may develop at a later time. Optimal outcomes in children with renovascular hypertension are achieved in centers with a multidisciplinary care team that includes pediatric nephrology, surgery, and interventional radiology.

## SELECTED READINGS

Delis KT, Gloviczki P. Middle aortic syndrome: from presentation to contemporary open surgical and endovascular treatment. *Pers Vasc Surg Endovasc Ther* 2005;17:187–206.

Gulati A, Bagga A. Large vessel vasculitis. *Pediatr Nephrol* 2010;25:1037–1048.

Hallett JW, Brewster DC, Darling RC, O'Hara PJ. Coarctation of the abdominal aorta: current options in surgical management. *Ann Surg* 1980;191:430–437.

Hendren WH, Kim SH, Herrin JT, Crawford JD. Surgically correctable hypertension of renal origin in childhood. *Am J Surg* 1982;143:432–442.

Huang Y, Duncan AA, McKusick MA, et al. Renal artery intervention in pediatric and adolescent patients: a 20-year experience. *Vasc Endovasc Surg* 2008;41:490–499.

Johnston SL, Lock RJ, Gompels MM. Takayasu arteritis: a review. *J Clin Pathol* 2002;55:481–486.

Kaye AJ, Slemp AE, Chang B, et al. Complex vascular reconstruction of abdominal aorta and its branches in the pediatric population. *J Pediatr Surg* 2008;43:1082–1088.

Kimura H, Sato O, Deguchi JO, Miyata T. Surgical treatment and long-term outcome of renovascular hypertension in children and adolescents. *Eur J Vasc Endovasc Surg* 2010;39:731–737.

Klinger G, Hellmann J, Daneman A. Severe aortic thrombosis in the neonate—successful treatment with low-molecular-weight heparin: two case reports and review of the literature. *Am J Perinatol* 2000; 17:151–158.

Lin Y, Hwang B, Lee P, Yang L, Meng CCL. Mid-aortic syndrome: a case report and review of the literature. *Int J Cardiol* 2008;123:348–352.

Malikov S, Delarue A, Fais PO, Keshelava G. Anatomical repair of a congenital aneurysm of the distal abdominal aorta in a newborn. *J Vasc Surg* 2009;50:1181–1184.

Martin JE, Moran JF, Cook LS, Goertz KK, Mattioli L. Neonatal aortic thrombosis complicating umbilical artery catheterization: successful treatment with retroperitoneal aortic thrombectomy. *Surgery* 1989; 105:793–796.

McLaren CA, Roebuck DJ. Interventional radiology for renovascular hypertension in children. *Tech Vasc Interv Radiol* 2003;6:150–157.

Mehall JR, Saltzman DA, Chandler JC, et al. Congenital abdominal aortic aneurysm in the infant: case report and review of the literature. *J Pediatr Surg* 2001;36:657–658.

Mendeloff J, Stallion A, Hutton M, Goldstone J. Aortic aneurysm resulting from umbilical artery catheterization: case report, literature review, and management algorithm. *J Vasc Surg* 2001;33:419–424.

Morales JP, Sabharwal T, Tibby SM, Burnand KG. Successful thrombolysis of a symptomatic neonatal aortic thrombosis associated with hypernatremic dehydration—case report and literature review. *Int J Clin Prac* 2008;62:502–505.

Nagel K, Tuckuviene R, Paes B, Chan AK. Neonatal aortic thrombosis: a comprehensive review. *Klin Padiatr* 2010;222:134–139.

Reddy E, Robbs JV. Surgical management of Takayasu's arteritis in children and adolescents. *Cardiovasc J Afr* 2007;18:393–396.

Sethna CB, Kaplan BS, Cahill AM, Velazquez OC, Meyers KEC. Idiopathic mid-aortic syndrome in children. *Pediatr Nephrol* 2008;23: 1135–1142.

Sparks SR, Chock A, Seslar S, Bergan JJ, Owens EL. Surgical treatment of Takayasu's arteritis: case report and literature review. *Ann Vasc Surg* 2000;14:125–129.

Stadermann MB, Montini G, Hamilton G, et al. Results of surgical treatment for renovascular hypertension in children: 30-year single-centre experience. *Nephrol Dial Transplant* 2009;25:807–813.

Stanley JC, Criado E, Upchurch GR, et al. Pediatric renovascular hypertension: 132 primary and 30 secondary operations in 97 children. *J Vasc Surg* 2006;44:1219–1229.

Terramani TT, Salim A, Hood DB, Rowe VL, Weaver FA. Hypoplasia of the descending thoracic and abdominal aorta: a report of two cases and review of the literature. *J Vasc Surg* 2002;36:844–848.

Tullus K, Brennan E, Hamilton G, et al. Renovascular hypertension in children. *Lancet* 2008;371:1453–1463.

Tullus K, Roebuck DJ, McLaren CA, Marks SD. Imaging in the evaluation of renovascular disease. *Pediatr Nephrol* 2010;25:1049–1056.

Vo NJ, Hammelman BD, Racadio JM, et al. Anatomic distribution of renal artery stenosis in children: implications for imaging. *Pediatr Radiol* 2006;36:1032–1036.

# CHAPTER 75 — Vascular Anomalies

Richard G. Azizkhan, Aliza P. Cohen,
Roshni Dasgupta, and Denise Adams

## Part I: Vascular Tumors

### KEY POINTS

1. Vascular anomalies comprise 2 distinct disease entities—vascular tumors and vascular malformations. These entities differ in their biology, presentation, and natural history.

2. Hemangiomas are the most common vascular tumors of childhood. These lesions are subdivided into 2 broad classifications—hemangiomas of infancy and congenital hemangiomas.

3. Many patients with hemangiomas of infancy do not require treatment; however, those with life- or function-threatening lesions require pharmacologic and/or surgical interventions.

4. Hemangiomas of infancy sometimes arise in specific patterns (eg, cervicofacial and lumbosacral) that may be associated with airway or spinal cord involvement respectively.

5. Multiple cutaneous hemangiomas of infancy may be associated with visceral hemangiomas, particularly liver hemangiomas. Patients with this presentation should therefore undergo diagnostic screening.

6. Propranolol and corticosteroids are the mainstays of pharmacotherapy. Lasers are used primarily for the treatment of ulcerated hemangiomas and telangiectasias following involution.

7. Surgical excision is most commonly performed when hemangiomas present a threat to function or are associated with complications and do not respond to pharmacotherapy or other less-invasive alternatives, and when they cause periorbital or significant airway symptomatology and are unlikely to respond quickly to medical management.

## INTRODUCTION

The field of vascular anomalies comprises a broad spectrum of lesions with dissimilar pathobiology and clinical behavior. Some of these lesions are easily recognizable and can be managed in a relatively straightforward fashion; however, many others are complex and often require the combined expertise of numerous specialists. Prior to the 1980s, progress in this field was stymied by the use of imprecise and inconsistent nomenclature, which led to confusion among professionals and poor communication between physicians and the research community. A seminal article by Mulliken and Glowaki (1982) marked a clear turning point. These authors proposed a nosologic system that designated vascular anomalies as either tumors or malformations, based on their clinical appearance, histopathologic features, and biologic behavior. Vascular tumors were defined as lesions arising by endothelial proliferation, whereas vascular malformations were thought to be developmental abnormalities that exhibit normal endothelial turnover. This system provided a basic framework that precipitated discussion among specialists and set the stage for demystifying the field. In 1996, the International Society for the Study of Vascular Anomalies reached a consensus on nosology, making only minor modifications to the classification system proposed more than a decade earlier. This revised system (Table 75-1) has been adopted by vascular anomaly experts worldwide and has had a crucial impact on progress in research and patient care.

Given the scope of pathology within the field of vascular anomalies and the need to limit our chapter, our discussion of vascular tumors will focus primarily on hemangiomas—the most frequently encountered lesion. We will provide a brief overview of information relevant to proper diagnosis and management, highlighting patterns of presentation and anatomic sites that are complex and difficult to manage. Additionally, we will describe the most common vascular malformations diagnosed and managed by pediatric surgeons.

## HEMANGIOMAS

Hemangiomas comprise 2 broad tumor types: hemangiomas of infancy and congenital hemangiomas. Hemangiomas of infancy (also referred to as infantile hemangiomas or simply hemangiomas) are far more common, affecting approximately 10% of white children in North America and having a predilection for females (3:1). These benign lesions generally arise cutaneously in the cervicofacial region (60%), and

963

| TABLE 75-1 | Classification of Vascular Anomalies |
| --- | --- |

**Vascular Tumors**

Hemangiomas

   Infantile

   Congenital

   Spindle cell

   Epitheliod

Hemangioendothelioma

   Kaposiform hemangioendothelioma

   Epitheliod hemangioendothelioma

   Tufted angioma

Angiosarcoma

Other tumors

**Vascular Malformations**

*Simple*

Low flow

   Capillary

   Lymphatic

   Venous

Fast flow

   Arterial

*Combined*

   Arterio-venous (AVM)

   Capillary arterio-venous (CAVM)

   Capillary venous (CVM)

   Capillary venous lymphatic (CVLM)

   Capillary arterio-venous lymphatic (CAVLM)

   Venous lymphatic (VLM)

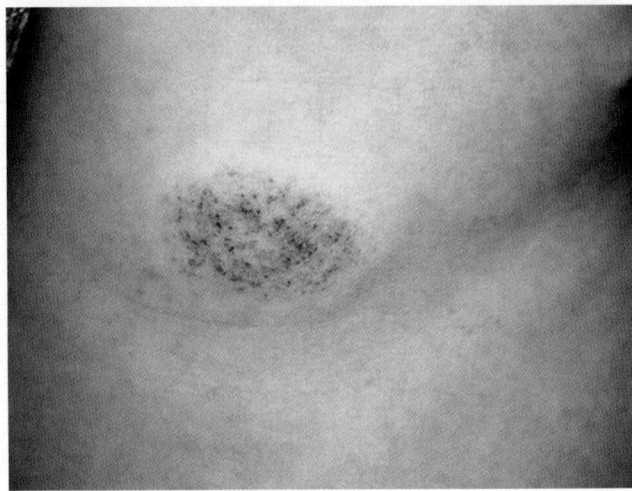

**FIGURE 75-1** RICH with a pale halo surrounding a violaceous cutaneous and subcutaneous mass.

may appear as focal, segmental, solitary, or multiple lesions. They can also involve any anatomic site and may affect the extremities, thoracoabdominal walls and cavities, solid organs, hollow viscera, and brain. Hemangiomas of infancy typically undergo a phase of active growth and later tumor regression over the first decade of life. Research indicates that GLUT-1, a marker for glucose transport, is unique to infantile hemangiomas in all stages of their lifecycle.

Congenital hemangiomas are an uncommon subset of vascular tumors. Unlike hemangiomas of infancy, these lesions present as fully grown at birth and do not undergo additional postnatal growth. Two subtypes of congenital hemangioma have been described: rapidly involuting congenital hemangiomas (RICHs) and noninvoluting congenital hemangiomas (NICHs). RICHs generally spontaneously regress by 12 to 14 months of age, leaving a residual patch of thin skin with prominent veins and little, if any, subcutaneous fat. NICHs do not undergo involution. These 2 tumor subtypes have similar morphology and usually appear as solitary lesions arising on the head, trunk, or limbs. Both RICHs and NICHs are generally violaceous in color with either fine or coarse telangiectasias. A pale halo frequently encircles the lesion, and in some cases, a central ulceration, a linear scar, or central nodularity is seen (Fig. 75-1). It is often difficult to determine at presentation if the hemangioma is a RICH or NICH, and close

follow-up is needed to monitor the progression of the lesion as the child grows. Unlike hemangiomas of infancy, neither congenital tumor subtype stains positive for GLUT-1.

## Incidence, Risk Factors, and Associations

Hemangiomas of infancy are estimated to occur in 1% to 3% of white neonates and upwards of 10% of children by age 1. These lesions are more frequently encountered in premature infants with a birth weight less than 1000 g (23%). A lower incidence is reported in darker-skinned and Japanese infants. Prenatal associations include older maternal age, placenta previa, and pre-eclampsia. Hemangiomas are also 3 times more common in infants born to mothers who have undergone chorionic villus sampling, thus raising the question of whether placental cellular elements are the possible progenitors of these lesions. Although most hemangiomas arise sporadically, a family history is reported in approximately 10% of patients. Familial transmission in an autosomal dominant inheritance pattern has been reported for both hemangiomas and vascular malformations.

## Presentation and Appearance

Most hemangiomas appear within the first few weeks of life; however, at least one third of tumors are observed at birth with premonitory signs such as a red macule, a blanched spot, bruising, or localized telangiectasia. Hemangiomas are clinically categorized as superficial (50% to 60%), deep (15%), or combined (25% to 35%), based on their anatomic depth (Fig. 75-2A–C). Superficial hemangiomas generally occur cutaneously and vary from compressible bright red to purple nodules or plaques that are present at birth or appear shortly after. Superficial hemangiomas can also be macular or telangiectatic, mimicking a capillary malformation, or can exhibit arteriovenous shunting, masquerading as an arteriovenous malformation. Lesions that originate in the deeper tissues often present later than superficial lesions, generally at 1 to 3 months of age. They typically appear as firm, rubbery,

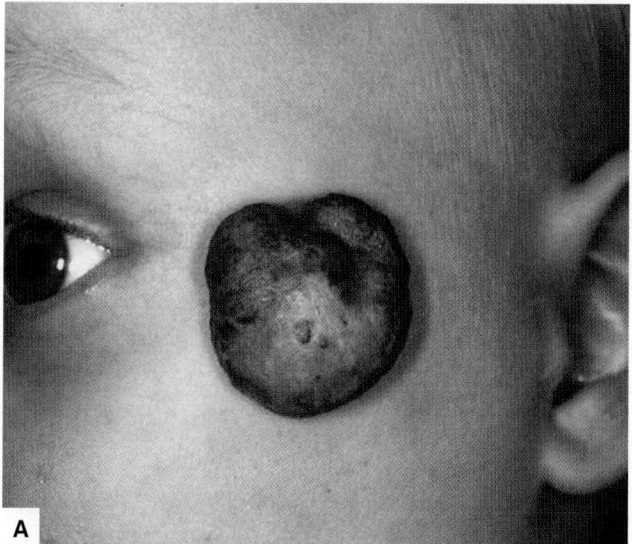

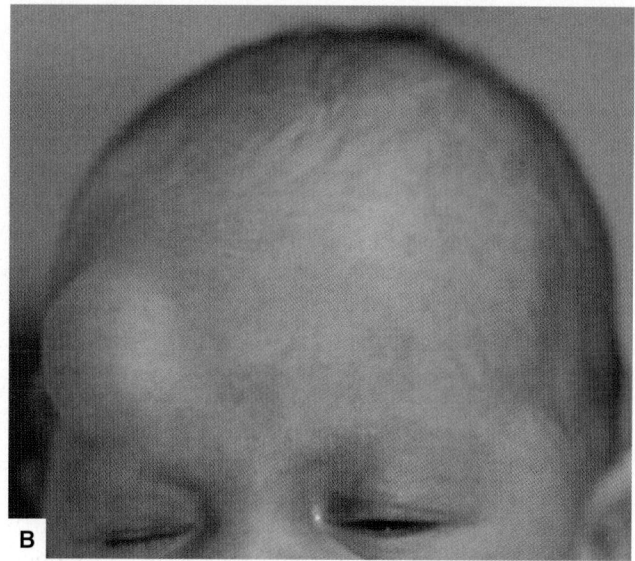

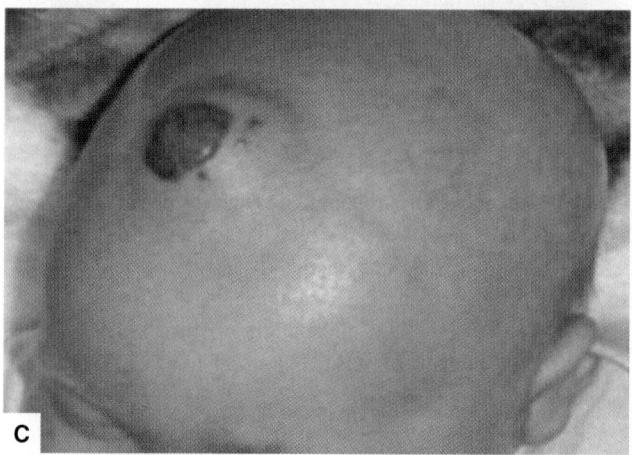

**FIGURE 75-2** Spectrum of localized infantile hemangiomas. **A.** Superficial; (**B**) deep; (**C**) combined.

subcutaneous masses with a blue-purple hue and no overlying superficial component. In patients with deep lesions, the overlying skin is often normal, except for superficial draining veins. As such, these lesions may be difficult to distinguish from venous or lymphatic vascular malformations or other rare tumors. As with superficial hemangiomas, deep hemangiomas are warm to the touch. Combined hemangiomas appear as obvious red dermal tumors with a deeper subcutaneous mass.

## Clinical Course

Hemangiomas of infancy generally follow a predetermined course of proliferation and involution, but exhibit wide variation in the rate, duration, and degree of growth and spontaneous tumor regression. The proliferative phase is characterized by increased endothelial cell hyperplasia. This phase begins the first few weeks after birth and typically continues for 6 to 9 months. Rapid growth of lesions during this time can cause a wide variety of complications, including ulceration, infection, hemorrhage, necrosis, airway obstruction, loss of vision, and cardiac failure. The likelihood that a specific complication will occur is frequently associated with the location of the lesion. For example, hemangiomas in perioral and perineal locations are particularly at risk of ulceration, which can be caused by recurrent friction with feeds and diaper changes

as well as moisture and the presence of bacterial flora. Also, periorbital lesions may cause loss of vision.

Following proliferation, the growth rate of lesions generally stabilizes and the gradual involutive process begins. Most hemangiomas undergo some degree of involution. In 50% of patients, this occurs by age 5, and in 70%, it occurs by age 7. Other lesions may continue to regress until ages 9 to 10. The rate of involution is not related to the anatomic site of the lesion or to the size or appearance of the lesion. Approximately 50% of patients have normal skin once regression is complete. The skin can, however, exhibit varying degrees of skin atrophy, a fibrofatty residuum, wrinkling, telangiectasias, yellowish inelastic patches, or scars where previous ulceration occurred during proliferation.

## Pathogenesis

Although the molecular events associated with the clinical course of infantile hemangiomas are yet to be elucidated, a number of mechanisms of pathogenesis have been proposed. Some authors purport that these lesions are the result of the clonal proliferation of endothelial cells. The origin of these endothelial cells is, however, still unclear. One theory suggests that primitive angioblasts may give rise to the clonal expansion of endothelial cells. There is also evidence to support the premise that endothelial cells may be derived from distant

**965**

sources (eg, the placenta or bone marrow) that travel into the local tissue environment. The placental theory is especially appealing, as it explains the transcriptional and immunophenotypical similarities between placental and infantile hemangioma tissues and vasculatures. A number of predisposing factors directly implicate the placenta in the pathogenesis of infantile hemangiomas. These factors include the increased incidence of infantile hemangiomas following placental complications or placental trauma, such as placenta previa, preeclampsia, and chorionic villi sampling. Also, several markers of hemangiomas (ie, GLUT-1, Lewis Y antigen, Fcγ-RIIb, and type 3 iodothyronine deiodinase) are uniquely coexpressed in placental tissue. Nonetheless, although this theory may provide the source for the cells that give rise to hemangiomas, it does not account for why infantile hemangiomas occur in some, but not all cases, since placental shedding occurs in all pregnancies.

While the mechanisms of proliferation and involution remain unclear, it is likely that the proliferative period is secondary to an imbalance of angiogenic vascular growth factors, and the involution process is secondary to increased apoptotic factors. Hemangiomas undergo distinct histopathologic changes during each phase of their lifecycle. During proliferation, there is extensive angiogenesis and endothelial cell proliferation. Also, within the hemangioma, there are increased levels of the basic fibroblast growth factor, vascular endothelial growth factors (VEGFs), type IV collagenase, and proliferating cell nuclear antigen. During the involutive phase, the stigmata of rapid growth give way to cellular apoptosis and the replacement of hemangioma tissue with fatty tissue. Additionally, there are increased levels of the angiogenesis inhibitor metalloproteinase.

## Diagnosis

Owing to the widespread use of prenatal screening, congenital hemangiomas have been detected as early as the 12th week of gestation. These tumors initially exhibit a fast-flow pattern by ultrasound (US) and magnetic resonance imaging (MRI).

The diagnosis of infantile hemangiomas is generally based on clinical presentation, history, and physical examination. When the diagnosis is unclear, a variety of noninvasive imaging modalities are essential. US with color flow Doppler can be extremely useful in differentiating hemangiomas from similarly appearing vascular malformations that have diminished to absent flow characteristics, such as lymphatic or venous malformations. On US, an infantile hemangioma appears hypoechoic, well-defined, and heterogeneous in texture, with small cystic and sinusoidal spaces. In most proliferating hemangiomas, a characteristic fast-flow pattern is seen on Doppler US.

Computed tomography (CT) defines the extent and involvement of the hemangioma and is also useful in distinguishing hemangiomas from lymphatic anomalies; however, it indicates only qualitative differences in blood flow. In the proliferative phase, a hemangioma appears as a well-circumscribed tumor with homogeneous parenchymatous density and intense enhancement (Fig. 75-3). In the involutive phase, it appears heterogeneous, with distinct lobular architecture and large draining veins in the center and the periphery.

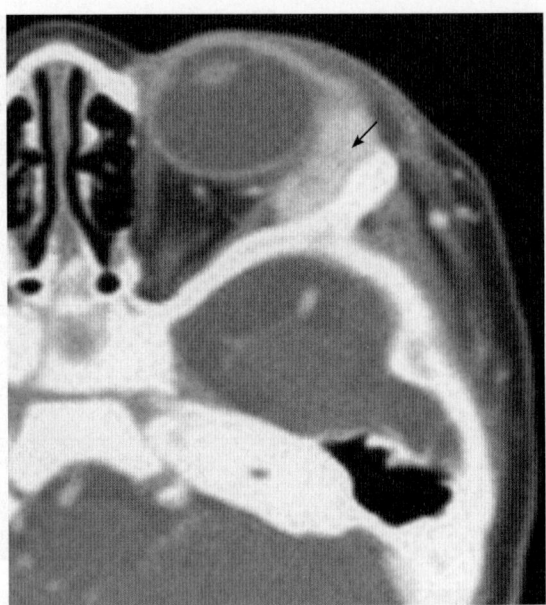

**FIGURE 75-3** CT image of a proliferating infantile hemangioma lateral to the globe within the right orbital cone. The hemangioma has a homogeneous density with enhancement.

MRI and magnetic resonance angiography (MRA) are especially useful for craniofacial, visceral, and extremity lesions, as they reveal both the extent of involvement with tissue planes and rheological characteristics (Fig. 75-4). As with CT, MRA can also be helpful in distinguishing hemangiomas and other vascular tumors from vascular malformations.

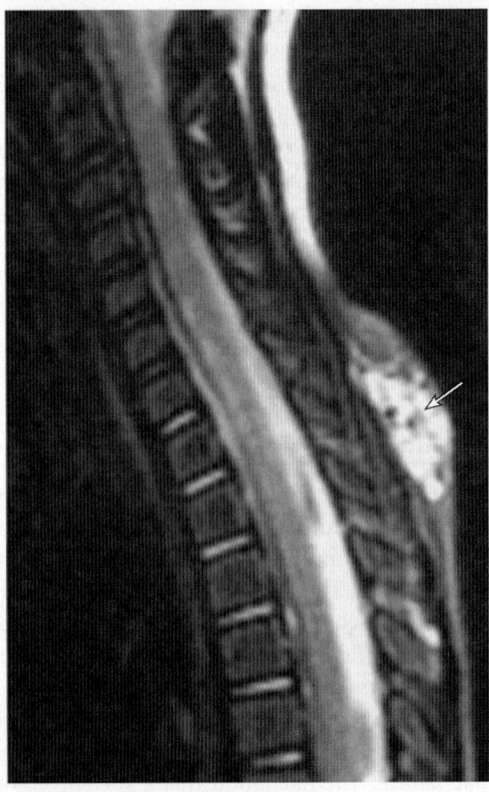

**FIGURE 75-4** MRI of hemangioma of the lower lumbar region documenting extent of involvement of the skin and subcutaneous tissues. Note the degree of vascular enhancement. The spinal cord and attachments were normal in this infant.

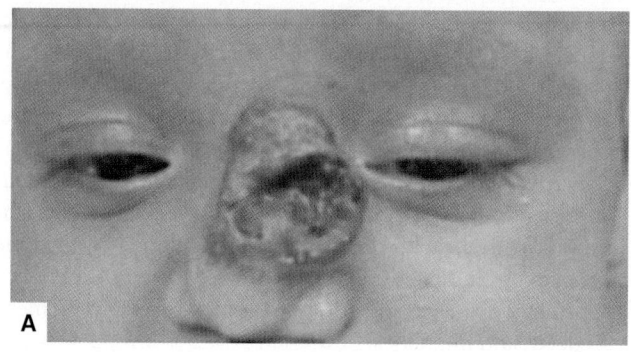
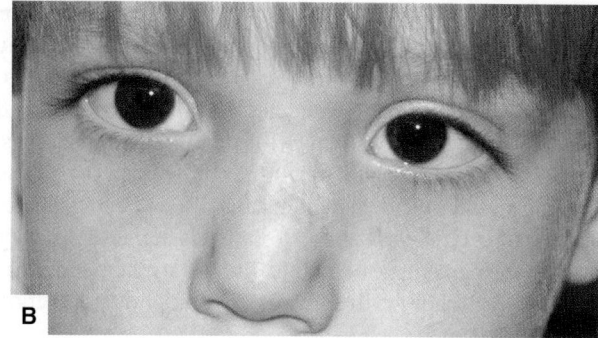

**FIGURE 75-5** **A.** Ulcerated infantile hemangioma treated with oral prednisolone and topical care. **B.** Long-term outcome following therapy. A residual scar is present but is esthetically acceptable.

## Differential Diagnosis

Differential diagnosis includes malignant tumors such as infantile fibrosarcoma, rhabdomyosarcoma, neuroblastoma, and angiosarcoma, as well as other benign vascular tumors (eg, KHE, tufted angioma, and hemangiopericytoma). Biopsy is indicated only when the diagnosis is uncertain or the clinical history is incompatible with the known life cycle of a hemangioma.

Although Glut-1 staining can occur focally in several conditions, it is diffusely positive only in infantile hemangiomas and other tumors of mesenchymal origin (eg, perineuromas) that are not part of the clinical or histologic differential diagnosis of this lesion. As such, it is an extremely useful marker, allowing for precise histopathologic diagnosis, particularly in cases in which clinical or radiologic findings are equivocal.

## Ulceration

Ulcerations are the most common complication of hemangiomas, occurring in 10% to 15% of superficial lesions (Fig. 75-5). Most ulcers develop during a phase of rapid growth, and all leave behind some degree of scarring. They are commonly quite painful and can become infected. As mentioned earlier in the chapter, lesions in perioral and perineal locations are particularly at risk of this complication. Similarly, lesions in intertriginous areas such as neck folds, thighs, and the posterior auricular area are more prone to ulceration.

## PROBLEMATIC PATTERNS OF PRESENTATION

### Multiple Hemangiomas

Although most affected infants have only one hemangioma, up to 30% have more than 1. A recent (2011) relatively large (*n* = 151) prospective multicenter study supports the long-held notion that the presence of multiple cutaneous lesions is a marker for liver hemangiomas. The authors report that infants younger than 6 months of age with 5 or more cutaneous hemangiomas are at risk for hepatic hemangiomas and that this risk is significantly higher than in infants with fewer than 5 cutaneous lesions (Fig. 75-6A,B). These findings underscore the need for screening with abdominal US when 5 or more cutaneous hemangiomas are present. While the reason for this association is unknown, the authors hypothesize that a greater number of circulating endothelial progenitor cells would result in the development of hemangiomas in the skin and the liver.

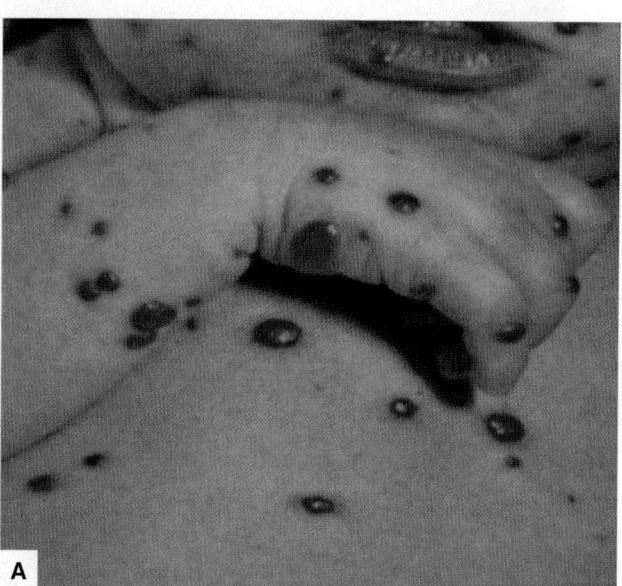

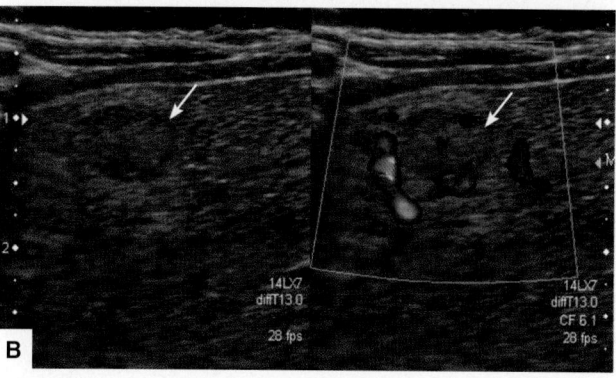

**FIGURE 75-6** **A.** Infant with multiple cutaneous hemangiomas and multifocal hepatic hemangiomas. **B.** Hepatic ultrasound documenting multiple hepatic lesions—arrow points out a specific hepatic lesion with Doppler flow characteristics of a fast flow vascular anomaly.

The additional reported findings that infants with 5 or more cutaneous infantile hemangiomas had a significantly lower gestational age and birth weight than those with 1 to 4 cutaneous lesions further validates the previously discussed risk factors for the development of infantile hemangiomas. Prematurity and low-birth-weight not only increase the risk of having an infantile hemangioma, but also of having greater numbers of cutaneous lesions. Despite this higher frequency, however, the percentage of infants with hepatic hemangiomas requiring treatment for liver disease in this study population was low (8%).

## Segmental Lesions and PHACE Syndrome

Hemangiomas that present in developmental segments are referred to as *segmental* lesions. These lesions are far less common than localized hemangiomas and are associated with a higher risk of being life or function threatening and of having associated structural abnormalities. Segmental hemangiomas in locations other than the face can be associated with visceral hemangiomas. Large cervicofacial segmental hemangiomas, particularly those on the forehead, temple, upper cheek, and around the periorbital area can be accompanied by one or more of a constellation of anomalies known as PHACE syndrome, which is uncommon though not rare. These anomalies include: *p*osterior fossa brain malformations, *h*emangiomas, *a*rterial abnormalities, *c*ardiac and aortic arch defects, and *e*ye abnormalities. Sternal clefts or supraumbilical raphes have also been documented in some patients. Additionally, more than 50% of patients experience neurologic sequelae, including seizures, stroke, developmental delay, and migraines.

Segmental hemangiomas are plaque-like in contour. They generally undergo a prolonged proliferative phase (18 months) and do not completely involute. Also, they are at a higher risk of ulceration and residual scarring. Close monitoring of these lesions is essential. When there is an index of suspicion for PHACE syndrome, referral should be made for ophthalmologic and neurologic examination, screening echocardiogram, and MRI of the head, neck, and chest (Fig. 75-7A–C). The frequency of repeated imaging studies generally depends on symptom presentation and disease progression.

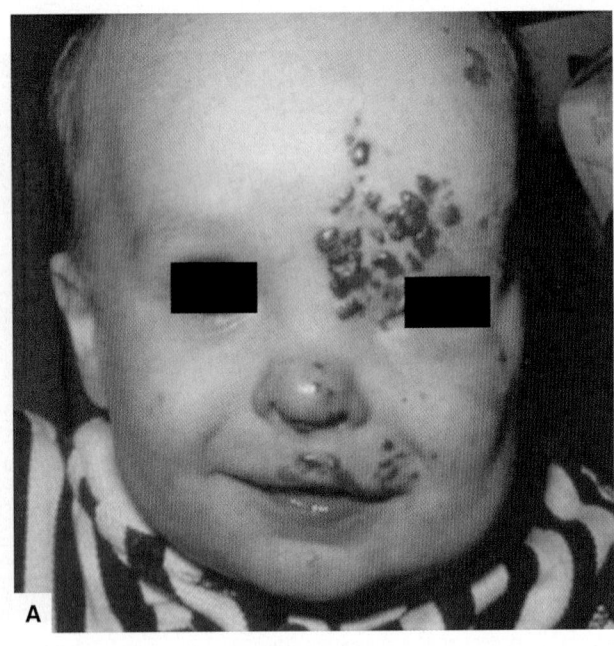

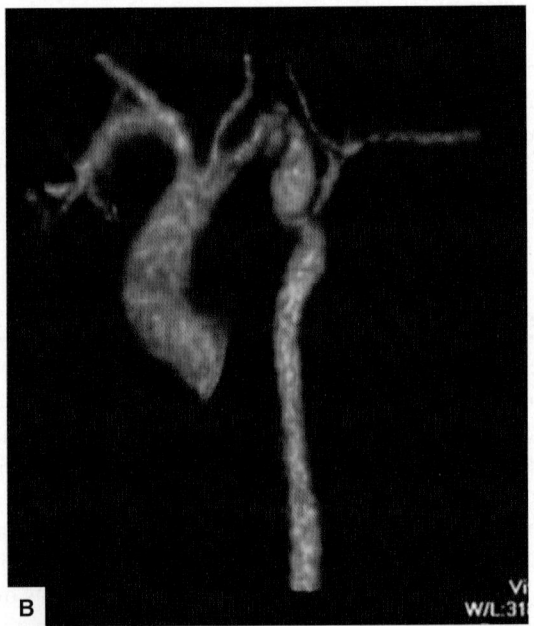

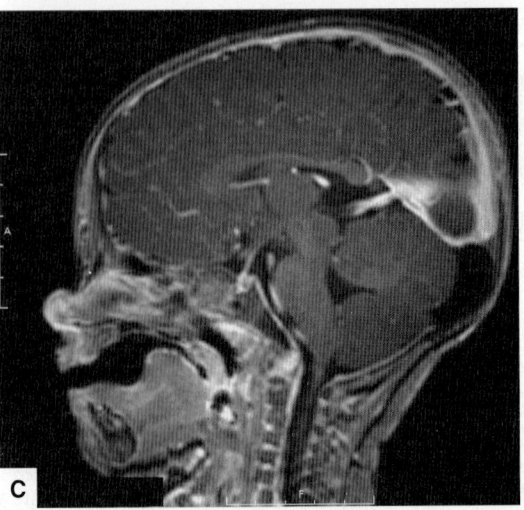

**FIGURE 75-7** PHACE Syndrome: (**A**) facial hemangioma with microophthalmia; (**B**) MRA of aortic arch demonstrating and interrupted arch anomaly. **C.** MRI of brain showing abnormality of the cerebellum.

## Lumbosacral Hemangiomas

Lumbosacral hemangiomas can be associated with underlying spinal cord abnormalities such as tethered spinal cord and lipomeningocele. In males, these hemangiomas are often associated with genitourinary malformations such as bifid scrotum. Children younger than 5 months of age should undergo a screening spinal US to rule out associated anomalies. Older children, who are unable to undergo US, should receive an MRI of the spine.

The parents of infants with perineal hemangiomas should be advised regarding diaper care. A barrier cream and metronidazole cream is generally recommended to help prevent ulcerations.

## PROBLEMATIC ANATOMIC SITES

### Hepatic Hemangiomas

The liver is the most common visceral site of hemangiomas, and hepatic hemangiomas are the most common benign liver tumors of infancy. These lesions follow a natural history similar to that of cutaneous lesions and are generally GLUT-1 positive on histologic examination. Most infants present within the first 2 months of life. The spectrum of severity associated with hepatic hemangiomas is variable, ranging from asymptomatic to life threatening. Clinical presentations may include hepatomegaly, high-output congestive heart failure, anemia, thrombocytopenia, respiratory distress, and jaundice.

Hepatic hemangiomas arise in 3 main patterns of presentation: focal, multifocal, and diffuse (Fig. 75-8A–C). Focal hepatic hemangiomas are solitary, spherical lesions that exhibit hypoechoic density on US. US, CT, MRI all demonstrate evidence of high flow. Multifocal hepatic hemangiomas are individual spherical lesions. On imaging, they may have indications of arteriovenous shunting. Diffuse hepatic hemangiomas differ from multifocal lesions in that they have extensive replacement of the hepatic parenchyma with innumerable centripetal enhancing lesions. Diffuse lesions have the potential to cause the most morbidity and mortality. Baseline determination of extent of lesion, cardiac function, thyroid function, and coagulation factors should be obtained. The growth of a hepatic hemangioma can be rapid, and the managing clinician must be aware of numerous medical issues associated with this tumor. These patients can rapidly develop life-threatening complications. Evidence of severe shunting,

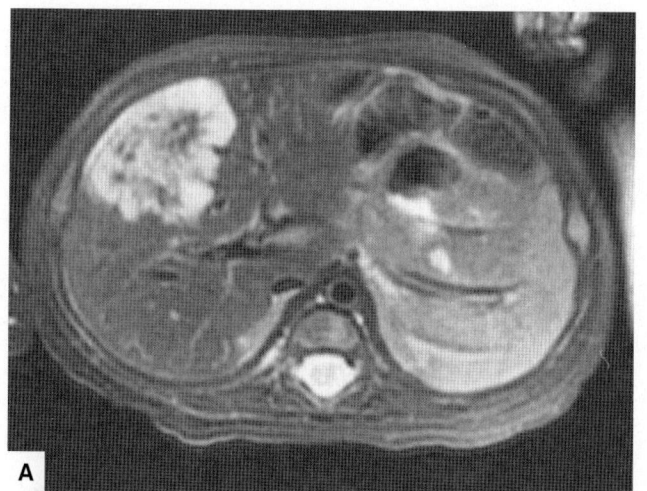

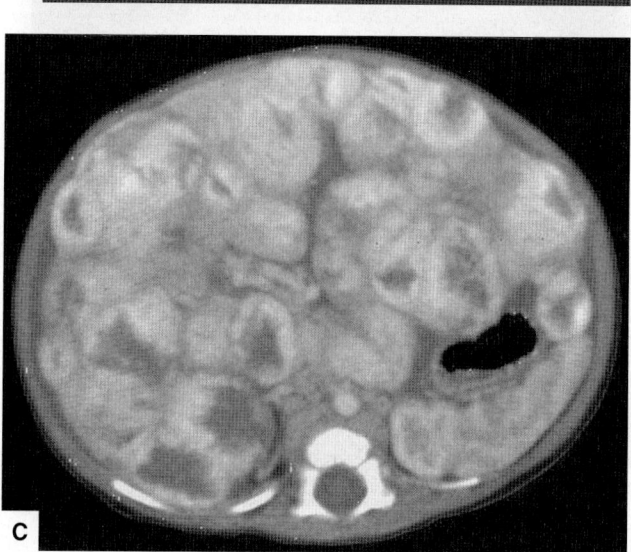

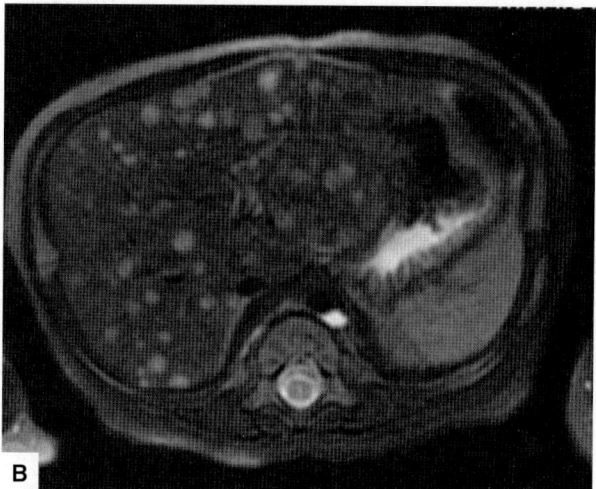

**FIGURE 75-8** Hepatic hemangioma main patterns as seen on MRI imaging. **A.** Focal; (**B**) multifocal; (**C**) diffuse, note the centripetal vascular staining of the lesions.

abdominal compartment syndrome, congestive heart failure, or hypothyroidism warrants early multimodal intervention.

Hypothyroidism in this setting is thought to be a consumptive disorder caused by the increased activity of type 3 iodothyronine deiodinase within the hemangioma. The rapid rate of inactivation of the thyroid hormone by the deiodinase enzyme produced by the hemangioma surpasses the synthetic capacity of the neonatal thyroid; this is more likely to occur in patients with diffuse hepatic lesions. Nevertheless, based on our clinical experience, we screen all patients with either multiple or diffuse hepatic hemangiomas. These patients undergo T3, T4, and TSH testing. Patients who require treatment are started on thyroxine and Cytomel therapy, often at doses much higher than required in patients with congenital hypothyroidism. These infants should be followed carefully by a pediatric endocrinologist.

As mentioned above, patients with hepatic hemangiomas may also present with anemia and coagulopathies. Anemia is thought to be secondary to the shunting and loss and the coagulopathy is secondary to the lesion and also lack of functional liver tissue to produce adequate tissue factors. The true Kasabach–Merritt phenomenon of an intravascular coagulopathy secondary to platelet trapping is not associated with hepatic hemangiomas, but rather with tufted angiomas and kaposiform hemangioendotheliomas (KHEs). High-output cardiac failure is a well-recognized sequela in patients with hepatic hemangiomas secondary to the extensive arteriovenous shunting of the lesions. An initial CT or MRI scan is helpful in these symptomatic patients, as it provides a more comprehensive image of the lesions and also helps in evaluating the degree of shunting. An echocardiogram should be performed on all patients with diffuse and multifocal lesions as well as in patients with focal lesions who show evidence of shunting. Patients should be followed closely by cardiologists throughout the course of treatment of the hemangioma.

Some focal liver hemangiomas are extremely large and are associated with high-output cardiac failure (Fig. 75-8A). These lesions may be diagnosed both pre- and postnatally and are thought to be congenital hemangiomas. This has been confirmed by Glut-1 negative staining of biopsies as well as by a clinical course of rapid involution, which is a key characteristic of the congenital tumor subtype RICH. Additionally, a recent report documents a new subgroup of infants with small and extensive (>30) involuting cutaneous hemangiomas and liver hemangiomas in which the cutaneous lesions are Glut-1 negative.

## Diagnosis of Hepatic Hemangiomas

Occasionally, hepatic hemangiomas are diagnosed on a screening antenatal US or found incidentally during an US performed for other indications. Also, there is an increased risk for visceral hemangiomas in patients with large solitary segmental hemangiomas, and a screening US in these patients usually detects liver hemangiomas early in their proliferative phase. Most hepatic hemangiomas, however, are identified by US screening of patients with 5 or more cutaneous lesions. This is followed by CT or MRI imaging. The CT scan typically reveals areas of diminished parenchymal density in the absence of administered contrast. Following infusion of contrast in both CT and MRI, lesions exhibit centripetal enhancement from their periphery towards their center (Fig. 75-8C).

The treatment strategy for a child with the diagnosis of hepatic hemangioma can range from simple observation to a series of complicated interventions requiring input from an interdisciplinary team of medical, radiological, and surgical subspecialists.

## Hemangiomas in a Beard Distribution

More than 60% of patients with cervicofacial hemangiomas that occur in a beard distribution (ie, the, chin, jawline, and preauricular areas) have associated airway hemangiomas (Fig. 75-9A,B). The larynx, specifically the subglottis, is the most common site of presentation. These patients should undergo a screening endoscopy to determine if there is airway involvement, as subglottic hemangiomas may cause significant airway compromise during the proliferative period. Imaging modalities, particularly MRI, are useful

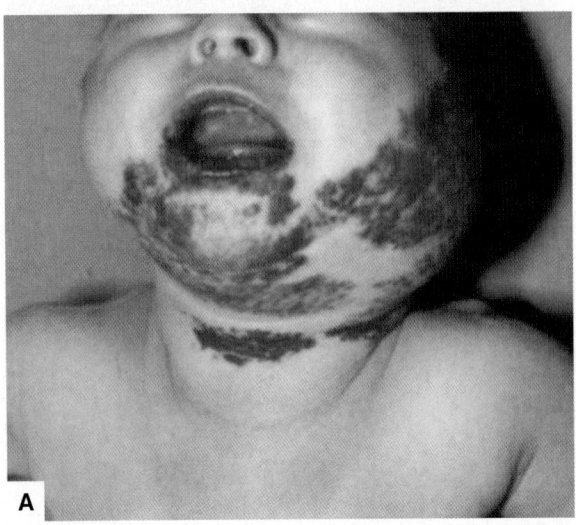

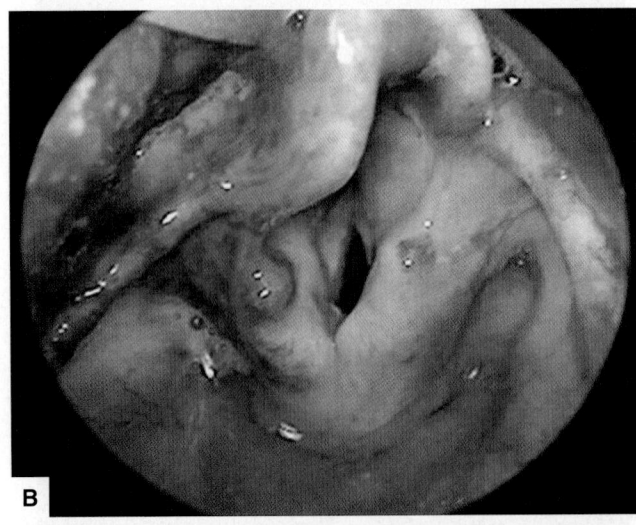

**970**   **FIGURE 75-9** **A.** Beard distribution of segmental facial hemangioma in an infant. **B.** Airway involvement observed on endoscopy.

in confirming the diagnosis and the extent of involvement. MRI with T2-weighted contrast (gadolinium) images reveal an isointense or hypointense soft tissue mass, whereas T1-weighted contrast images reveal uniformly intense enhancement of the lesions. If the diagnosis is uncertain, a biopsy should be done to confirm the histology and Glut-1 positivity. Patients must be closely followed and treatment should be initiated in the presence of airway involvement. (See section on management.) Tracheotomy placement is used only in refractory cases or in cases in which the airway is significantly compromised.

Airway hemangiomas can also occur in the absence of cutaneous involvement or in association with lesions of the chest. Presentation generally occurs within the first 6 months of life, and the earlier the presentation, the greater the risk of airway compromise and the need for intervention. Symptoms include progressive stridor and retractions. The diagnosis is made by laryngotracheobronchoscopy, and although an MRI scan is indicated, it rarely demonstrates extension of the lesion beyond the subglottis. Children with mild-to-moderate symptoms can be effectively treated with open surgical resection of the subglottic hemangioma; however, many of these patients are currently managed effectively with propranolol. (See section on management.) In patients with extensive airway involvement, tracheotomy placement may be required to prevent airway compromise during the proliferative period.

## Problematic Facial Hemangiomas

Periorbital lesions, particularly those that involve the upper and lower lid and/or the retrobulbar space, may cause proptosis with corneal exposure, strabismus and amblyopia, optic atrophy, and bony malformation (Fig. 75-10A,B). Periodic ophthalmologic evaluation is therefore required both during the proliferative and involutive phases. Early ophthalmologic evaluation and treatment is indicated for periocular

hemangiomas to avoid deprivation amblyopia, which can occur with only 1 to 2 weeks of deprivation during key developmental periods. If lesions occlude the visual fields, the long-term development of visual pathways may be compromised.

Hemangiomas involving the nose occur in close to 16% of facial hemangiomas. Proliferation of lesions on the tip of the nose can cause permanent distortion of normal anatomy and splaying of the nasal cartilage. Lesions located on the pinna of the ear can also deform normal structures and result in ulceration with focal destruction of the auricle. Lesions obstructing the auditory canal can cause temporary conductive hearing loss. Lip hemangiomas frequently involute slowly, often resulting in residual skin changes. Also, lip ulcerations can cause feeding difficulties, secondary infection, and significant scarring.

# MANAGEMENT STRATEGIES

## Overview

Decisions regarding intervention are based on the size and location of the tumor, the presence of complications, the age of the patient, and the rate of tumor growth. The management of complex lesions must be individualized and planned by clinicians with special expertise in treating vascular anomalies. Closely monitoring tumor growth, particularly during the proliferative phase, is essential. Because many hemangiomas of infancy leave little or no functional disability and have only a minimal cosmetic impact, premature intervention in stable, regressing, or noncomplicated lesions may be unwarranted; furthermore, intervention may result in scarring that is worse than would occur if the lesion was left untreated. Given the aesthetic concerns of parents, ongoing emotional support and education about the natural history of the lesion are crucial.

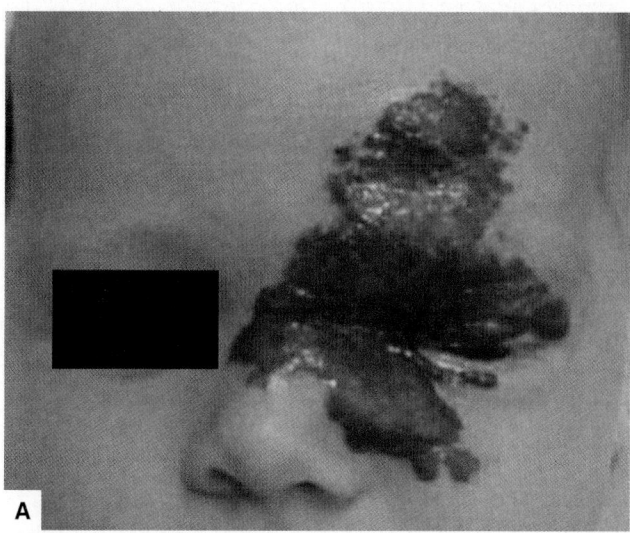

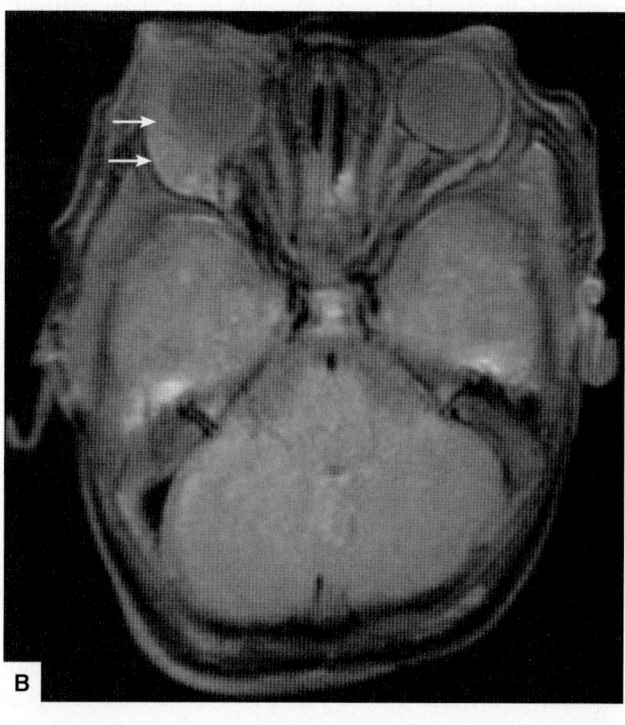

**FIGURE 75-10** **A.** Infantile hemangioma with periorbital involvement impacting visual acuity; (**B**) MRI documenting extent of the hemangioma within the orbit.

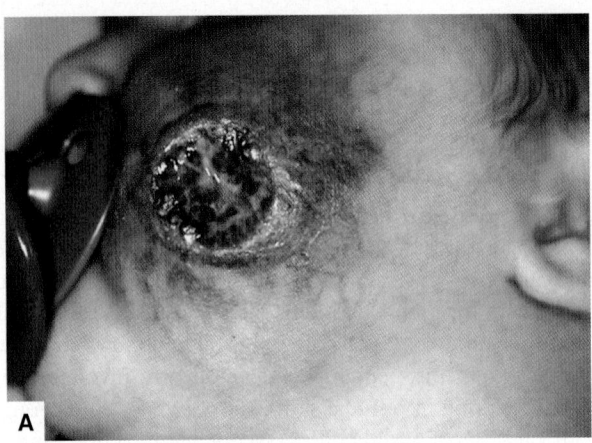
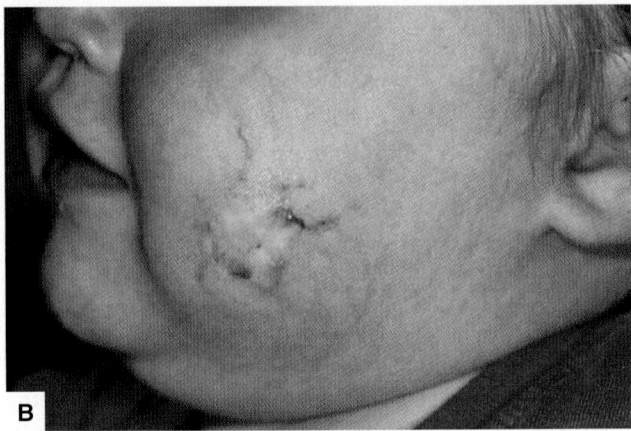

**FIGURE 75-11** Ulcerated hemangioma (**A**) before and (**B**) after PDL treatment and topical care.

Additionally, clinicians should convey expected short- and long-term outcomes to parents and ensure that they have an appropriate understanding and realistic expectations.

Immediate treatment is imperative when lesions affect vital structures, cause congestive heart failure, or are ulcerated. A number of treatment options are currently used and multimodal therapy is often essential. These treatment modalities are described below.

## Treatment of Ulcerations

Once ulcerations develop, treatment should focus on decreasing pain, preventing secondary infections, and promoting reepithelialization. Superficial ulcerations generally respond to supportive wound care. Topical antibiotic and barrier creams are used. In addition, oral medications such as acetaminophen or acetaminophen with codeine are sometimes necessary to alleviate pain. If cellulitis occurs, oral systemic antibiotics should be administered. Ulcerations on localized cervicofacial lesions and lesions on the trunk and extremities are generally resectable and can result in excellent cosmetic outcomes. When resection is not feasible or desirable, the pulsed-dye laser (PDL) is used to decrease pain and promote reepithelialization (Fig. 75-11A,B). This approach is particularly helpful in anatomic areas that are not amenable to resection, such as extensive facial or perineal lesions.

## Pharmacotherapy

### Propranolol

Propranolol, a nonselective beta-blocker used to treat infants with cardiovascular conditions, has become the first line of treatment for function-threatening and potentially disfiguring hemangiomas. Although the mechanism of action of propranolol is still speculative, it is thought to involve the downregulation of VEGF and bFGF (beta fibroblast growth factor) gene expression and to trigger apoptosis of capillary endothelial cells.

The dramatic effect of propranolol on hemangiomas was first described in 2008 by Léauté-Labrèze and colleagues, who serendipitously discovered that it induced early involution during the proliferative phase. Their reported findings in a small series of infants sparked the enthusiasm of clinicians eager to replicate their outcomes and identify appropriate uses and dosages of the drug. Although subsequent reports and case series have demonstrated that propranolol therapy is generally safe and effective for both cutaneous and airway lesions, many questions remain unanswered and multicenter trials to determine long-term results and appropriate dosing regimens are underway. In our experience, a response rate of greater than 90% can be achieved, and this often occurs within several days of propranolol administration. Treatment is typically maintained for several months, and patients are then weaned off the propranolol (Fig. 75-12A,B). As premature cessation of this therapy may result in hemangioma regrowth, careful monitoring during the weaning process is essential.

Because propranolol is a nonselective beta-blocker, it antagonizes both B1 and B2 receptors. It therefore can have adverse effects, including hypotension, hypoglycemia, and bradycardia. Seizures have also been reported and are likely secondary to hypoglycemia. In view of these potential effects, our institutional protocol for the initiation of propranolol therapy requires an inpatient setting for 48 hours. The patient must receive a pretreatment echocardiogram and electrocardiogram. Initial doses range from 1 to 3 mg/kg/day, which is far lower than the doses administered to cardiac patients. Caregivers are keenly aware of clinical warning signs, including lethargy, labored breathing, and diaphoresis. To prevent hypoglycemia, they must ensure that infants are frequently fed and go no longer than 4 to 6 hours between feeds.

Recently, topical propranolol has been shown to be effective in stabilizing localized lesions. The agent has no significant adverse effects and is particularly favored in patients with small lesions that do not warrant the risks of systemic therapy.

### Corticosteroids

Prior to the introduction of propranolol, corticosteroids had been the mainstay of medical therapy for life-threatening or function-threatening hemangiomas, as well as for hemangiomas likely to result in disfigurement. When used during the proliferative phase, they induce regression of the hemangioma. These agents may be administered orally, intralesionally,

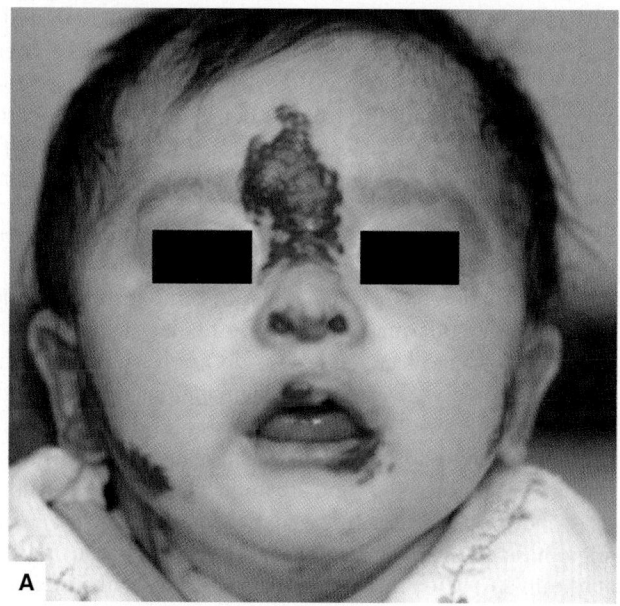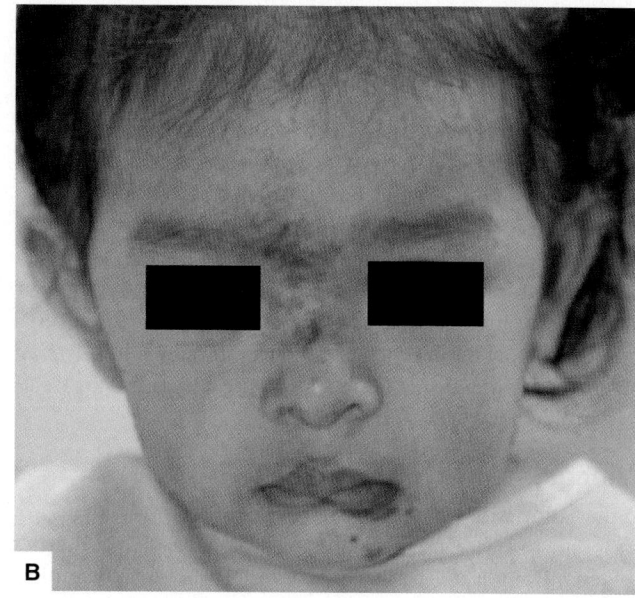

**FIGURE 75-12** Rapidly proliferating infantile hemangioma in a 7-week-old infant: **A.** Pre-propranolol treatment. **B.** After 5 months on propranolol.

or topically. Although the mechanism of action of corticosteroids is uncertain, it is thought that they have an antiangiogenic effect that decreases endothelial cell proliferation and causes apoptosis of these cells.

**Systemic Corticosteroids.** When used for life- of function-threatening hemangiomas, the authors' experience is that systemic corticosteroids result in an overall response rate of approximately 70%. In particularly complicated cases, a combined regimen of corticosteroids and propranolol is sometimes used because of a perceived synergistic effect. Given that prospective randomized controlled studies of dosing have not yet been conducted, current dosing regimens are based on retrospective studies. The standard dosing regimen for prednisolone begins with 2 to 3 mg/kg/day. This dose is continued for 1 month. If the response is positive, the patient is continued on this dose for another 2 to 4 weeks. The daily dose is then gradually lowered to 1 mg/kg and is generally maintained for up to 4 months, and occasionally, up to 6 months. A positive response to therapy is indicated by softening of the lesion, lightening and graying of its color, and slowing of growth within 2 months of initiating therapy. If no response is seen, an attempt is made to titrate the dose to effect a response. If this fails, the dose is tapered and the child is taken off the medication. As with propranolol, rebound growth can occur if the steroids are discontinued before the end of the proliferative phase. In this situation, hemangiomas usually respond to a dose slightly higher than that used immediately before steroid discontinuation.

Although systemic steroids are considered a safe and effective treatment when used over several months, potential transient side effects commonly include the development of cushingoid facies, insomnia, irritability, restlessness, and immunosuppression. Live vaccines should not be given during systemic corticosteroid therapy or for 3 to 4 months after cessation of therapy. In the setting of longer term steroid use, it is prudent to prescribe trimethoprim/sulfamethoxazole

to prevent *Pneumocystis jiroveci* (formerly called *P. carinii*) pneumonia.

Other less frequently encountered side effects include adrenal suppression, hypertension, hyperglycemia, and myositis. Children who receive systemic corticosteroids for more than 12 months are at high risk for growth retardation and osteoporosis. A growth delay is noted in most patients; however, by age 2, nearly all children are back on their normal growth curve.

Corticosteroids have been used to treat congenital hemangiomas antenatally when there is evidence of impending fetal hydrops. The benefits of treatment must, however, be balanced with the potential adverse effects, which may include premature closure of the ductus arteriosus and diminished glomerular filtration with salt retention. Long-term effects remain unknown.

**Intralesional Corticosteroids.** Intralesional steroids are best used for small localized problematic hemangiomas rather than larger segmental lesions. This therapeutic approach is especially effective in managing lesions in the periorbital region, nasal tip, and subglottic region. One to three injections are given at 4- to 6-week intervals. A long-acting steroid (eg, triamcinolone acetonide) and a short-acting steroid (eg, betamethasone acetate) can be combined in a total volume that does not exceed 2.5 mL. The dose and volume are individualized according to the size of the lesion. Injections with a 26- to 30-gauge needle are made directly into the hemangioma in different directions through the same needle site. Direct pressure is then applied for 2 to 10 minutes to prevent bleeding. For subglottic lesions, direct injection into the cricoid plate should be avoided, as cartilage resorption may occur.

Although success rates associated with intralesional injections are similar to those associated with systemic corticosteroid therapy, injections have fewer side effects. They are, however, known to cause fat necrosis and depigmentation. Also, injections in periorbital lesions carry the risk of retinal artery embolization and thrombosis, with resulting blindness. To minimize this risk, fundoscopic retinal examinations should be performed as the lesion is slowly injected so to observe early signs of retinal arterial flow interruption.

**Topical Corticosteroids.** The short-term application of ultrapotent topical steroids (eg, clobetasol propionate) is useful in treating smaller localized craniofacial lesions, and typically accelerates involution. Good or partial response to treatment has been reported in close to 75% of cases. Although topical ointments have some degree of systemic absorption, they are not associated with significant adrenal pituitary axis inhibition, as are systemically administered agents. They therefore offer an appealing alternative for treating problematic localized lesions.

## Vincristine

Vincristine is an option reserved only for patients who do not respond to other medical therapies or have medical issues that contraindicate the use of propranolol or corticosteroids. This mitotic inhibitor acts by preventing tubulin polymerization and spindle formation and inducing apoptosis in tumor cells. In that endothelial cells are known to have a high tubulin content, hemangiomas are thought to be especially susceptible to vincristine. Patients are started on doses of 0.5 to 1 mg/m$^2$ of body surface area/kg/week.

Although vincristine is known to be associated with acute neurotoxicity in adults, its neurotoxic effects in children are reportedly mild. Even with prolonged use (ie, 2 or more years) in treatment regimens for children with malignancies, there are no apparent long-term risks. Optimally, a pediatric oncologist should participate in the care of patients receiving chemotherapy.

## Interferon

Interferon-alpha is an antiangiogenic agent that decreases endothelial cell proliferation by downregulating bFGF. It is considered a tertiary therapy for patients with life-threatening hemangiomas that are unresponsive to other medical therapies. However, given that its neurotoxicity can produce spastic diplegia and other motor development disturbances in children, and that some patients experience permanent spastic diplegia, interferon has generally fallen out of favor and is rarely used.

## Surgical Management

**Laser Therapy.** Although the PDL has been used by some clinicians for more than 2 decades, its routine use has long been controversial. Given the limited depth of vascular injury achieved with this laser, when it is used early in the proliferative phase, it does not prevent the growth of a deep subcutaneous component and nor is it beneficial for treating lesions with a deep component. There are, however, a number of specific indications for PDL treatment. We advocate its use for the treatment of ulcerated hemangiomas that are refractory to medical treatment, as it decreases pain and promotes more rapid reepithelialization. In a very small number of patients, particularly those with segmental lesions, ulceration may, however, worsen with laser treatment. The PDL is also effective for treating residual telangiectasias

left after tumor involution. The $CO_2$ laser and the ND:YAG (neodymium:yttrium–aluminum–garnet) lasers have been used to ablate airway hemangiomas, though, when used too aggressively, they can induce scar deposition and subglottic stenosis. Both the $CO_2$ laser and the Er:YAG (erbium) laser can be used for resurfacing scarred skin following involution.

**Surgical Excision.** Surgical excision is indicated in the following clinical settings: (1) when hemangiomas present a threat to function or are associated with complications and do not respond to pharmacotherapy or other less-invasive alternatives; (2) when ulcerated lesions do not respond to medical management; (3) when large hemangiomas have a high probability of leaving significant fibrofatty residuum or excess skin; (4) when periorbital or airway hemangiomas cause significant symptomatology and are unlikely to respond quickly, or do not respond to medical management; (5) when hemangiomas persist beyond a reasonable period of time or grow atypically; (6) when there is a perceived emotional burden on the child or family and the lesion can easily be removed, leaving no significant cosmetic deformity.

Because the outcome of spontaneous involution is difficult to predict, the timing of surgery is controversial. If surgical excision is required in order to avoid the psychosocial consequences of a visible hemangioma, the operation should be performed during the preschool period, prior to the development of body awareness.

The surgical approach depends on the size and location of the hemangioma. Although lenticular excision enclosure is a well-established approach for localized lesions, the length of scarring can be a disadvantage. A particularly useful technique for localized lesions in many anatomic sites is circular excision and purse-string closure (Fig. 75-13A–D). This technique can be used at any phase in the clinical course of a lesion. It reduces both the longitudinal and transverse dimensions and converts a large circular lesion into a small ellipsoid scar. No other excision and closure technique result in a smaller scar. Because normal skin and subcutaneous tissue are relatively lax, this technique is unlikely to result in significant distortion of surrounding structures. In the presence of a residual puckered scar, revision using an elliptical incision can result in a more linear scar. In patients who have complicated hemangiomas, multiple specialized procedures are required to restore normal facial contours, especially in the lips, nose, and ears.

**Hepatic Hemangiomas.** Surgical treatment for hepatic hemangiomas may include hepatic vascular embolization, resection, or transplantation. These approaches all require the close collaboration of an interdisciplinary team comprising an interventional radiologist, a pediatric surgeon with hepatobiliary expertise, and an oncologist.

Patients are often stable and require only monitoring and observation. In patients with high-output congenital heart failure, embolization is used to decrease arteriovenous shunting and porto-hepatic venous shunting. This procedure may be effective for focal lesions and can be an important temporizing measure until systemic pharmacotherapy can take effect. Embolization may, however, result in hepatic infarction, sepsis, and cirrhosis. Regardless, patients with profound

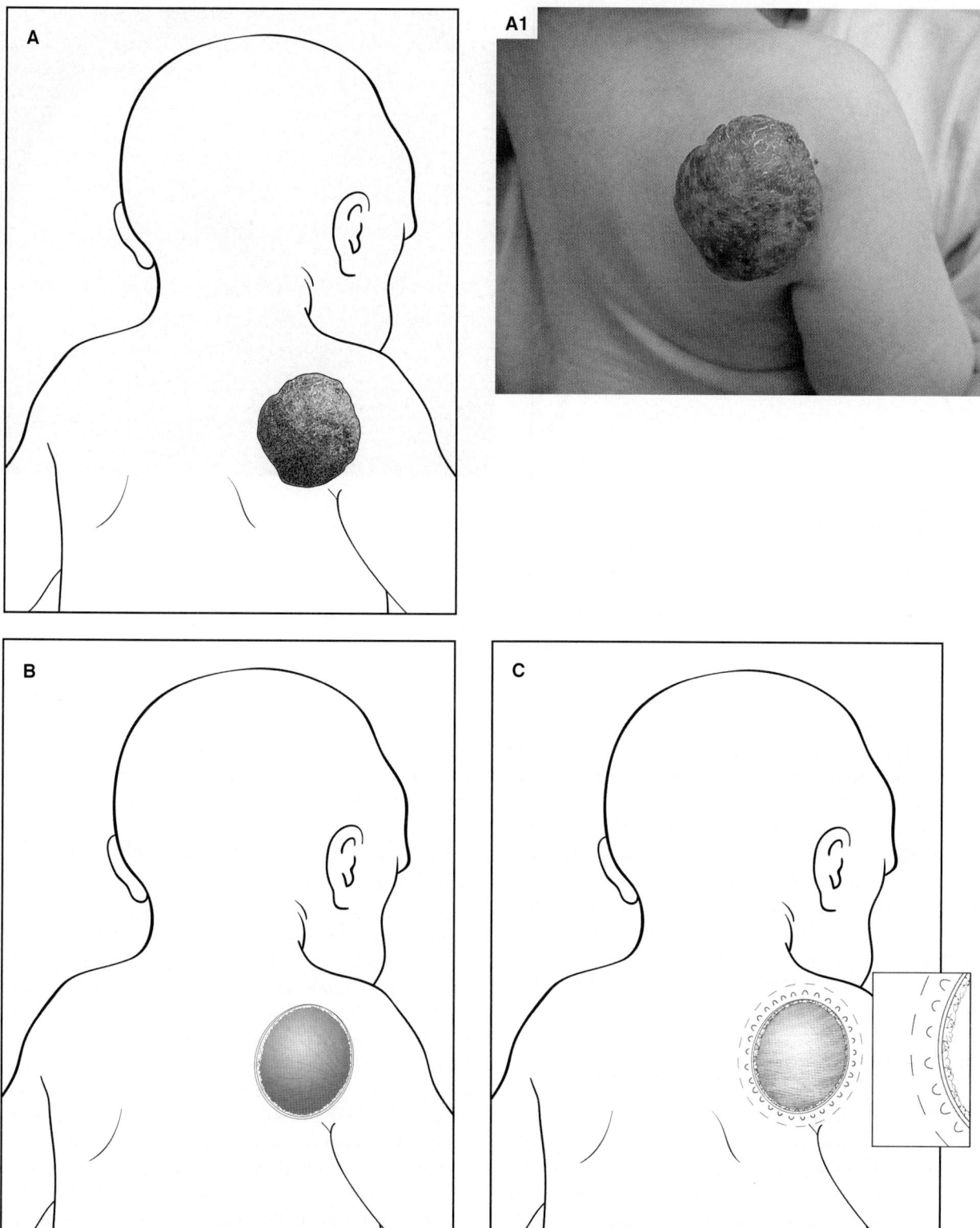

**FIGURE 75-13** Localized convex surface hemangioma amenable to circular excision and purse string closure: (**A**) lesion over the scapular region; (**A1**) actual patient; (**B**) after circular excision of lesion, the edges of the wound are sequentially undermined to create skin mobility for wound closure; (**C**) a double purse string suture is placed circumferentially; (**D**) the purse string sutures are approximated creating wound closure; (**D1**) patient 2 weeks after surgery.

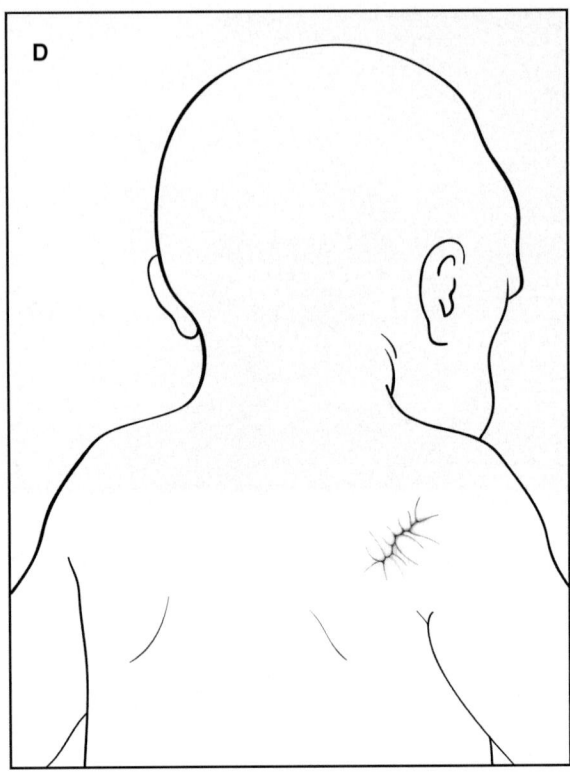

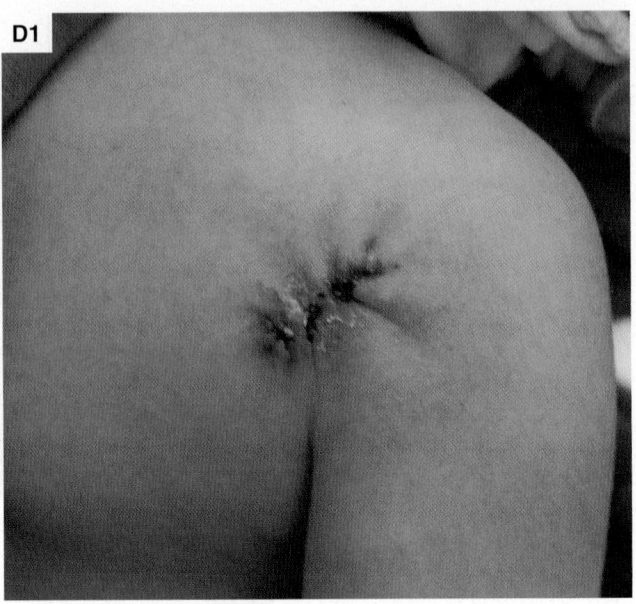

**FIGURE 75-13** (*Continued*)

hypothyroidism related to their hepatic hemangiomas require large doses of thyroid hormone replacement to achieve a stabilizing euthyroid status.

Surgical management depends on the type of hepatic lesion (focal, multiple, or diffuse), the overall physiologic status of the patient, and the success of other therapies. Resection is rarely appropriate but is performed when lesions are focal and not amenable to other approaches. Liver transplantation is an option that we have used successfully in two patients with diffuse lesions that were unresponsive to embolization and pharmacotherapy.

## Other Vascular Tumors

### Pyogenic Granuloma

Pyogenic granulomas are acquired inflammatory proliferative lesions that sometimes resemble superficial hemangiomas. Although the term implies an infective origin, the etiology of these lesions is unknown. They can occur early in infancy as rapidly growing masses, and typically begin as solitary red papules that assume a pedunculated appearance. Lesions present primarily on the head and neck but can occur at any skin site. They are also commonly seen in association with capillary malformations. Unlike hemangiomas, pyogenic granulomas have a higher incidence in males. They also differ histologically, showing a lobular arrangement of capillaries and no increase in mast cells. As with hemangiomas, however, these lesions have a proliferating endothelium. Whereas bleeding is rare in patients with hemangiomas, it is a common presenting symptom in patients with pyogenic granulomas. Chemocautery with silver nitrate is a first-line

office procedure, but it often fails. Electrocautery or laser fulguration is often successful. However, in rare cases in which lesions are persistent, resection is required.

## Kaposiform Hemangioendothelioma and Tufted Angioma

KHE is an aggressive vascular tumor that presents at birth in approximately 50% of cases and appears within the first year of life in most other cases. The tumor is usually solitary, and multifocal lesions rarely occur. Unlike hemangiomas of infancy, KHE has no female preponderance and usually occurs in the proximal arms and legs and the trunk, including the retroperitoneum. KHE typically manifests as a plaque-like mass with a deep red-purple hue. It is associated with surrounding subcutaneous edema and induration (Fig. 75-14A–E), the degree of which depends on the amount of trapped blood elements and the extent of intralesional bleeding in tissue. In contrast to hemangiomas of infancy, KHE is often highly infiltrative and diffuse, involving the skin and subcutaneous tissues and adjacent muscle and bone. Although it is locally aggressive, reports of metastasis are rare. The mortality rate of this tumor is high (20% to 37%), and bleeding is the primary cause of death. Retroperitoneal involvement is associated with a particularly poor outcome.

Tufted angioma usually presents as an erythematous, slightly tender, indurated macule, or plaque in a child younger than age 5. As with KHE, tufted angioma is typically located along the midline axis of the neck, upper trunk, and extremities. Unlike KHE, tufted angioma is characterized by rounded nodules or tufts of densely packed capillaries and pericytes in the mid-dermis, which bulge into and compress large,

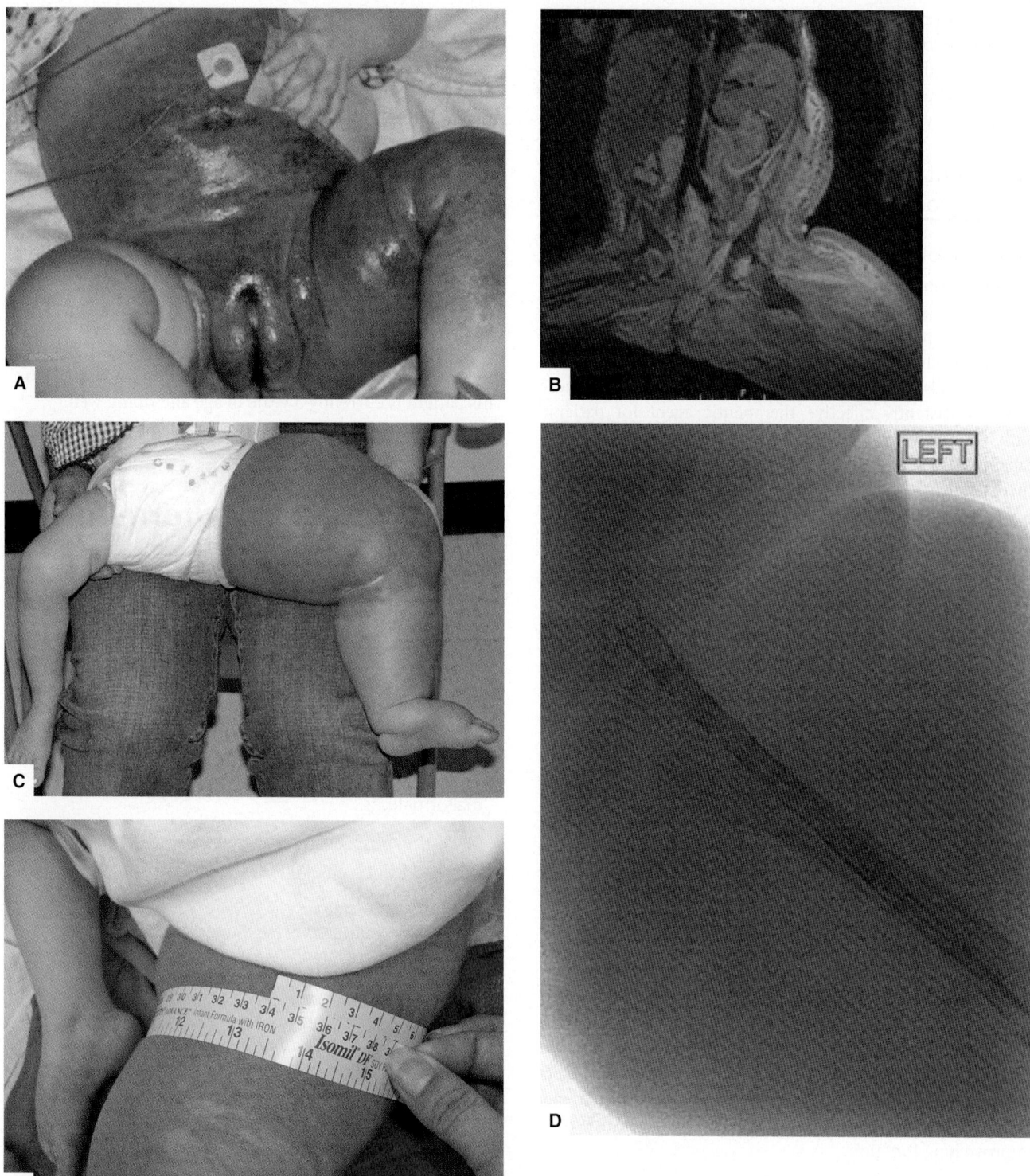

**FIGURE 75-14** KHE in an infant: **A.** Extensive involvement of the extremity. **B.** MRI demonstrating extensive involvement of all tissue planes. **C.** The patient had high-output cardiac failure with a massive extremity. **D.** Endoluminal iliac artery covered stents were placed in the left iliac and femoral arteries to decrease collateral arteriovenous flow and shunting. **E.** Postembolization and rapamycin treatment with shrinkage of left leg to a more normal size. The child remains well and fully functional 4 years later.

thin-walled vessels at the periphery of the nodules. Tumors exhibiting gradations between KHE and tufted angioma have been described. Because both can be associated with the Kasabach–Merritt phenomenon (KMP), they may represent variations of the same tumor.

KHE, and to a lesser extent, tufted angioma, can cause a coagulopathy called the KMP. KMP involves platelet trapping that results in profound thrombocytopenia, an enlarging lesion, and a consumptive coagulopathy with significant hypofibrinogenemia. Although KHE and tufted angioma do not always result in KMP, KMP is thought to be primarily responsible for the significant morbidity and mortality associated with these disorders. A number of treatments have been used; however, none have been uniformly effective and are yet to be validated in prospective clinical trials.

## Treatment of Kaposiform Hemangioendothelioma and Tufted Angioma

### Pharmacotherapy

Although most patients initially receive high-dose steroids, this therapy is associated with only a 30% response rate; furthermore, a positive response may not be long lasting. Vincristine, cyclophosphamide, and other chemotherapeutic agents are also used with limited success. At present, there is no consistently effective therapeutic agent for patients with KHE or tufted angioma; however, sirolimus (also called rapamycin) is a promising novel therapy that has been used successfully with several patients in our institution.

An ongoing clinical trial examining the effectiveness of sirolimus for the treatment of KHE has yielded favorable preliminary results, demonstrating control of lesion growth and control of KMP. This agent works through regulating the mTor (mammalian target of sirolimus) pathway, which controls several cellular processes, including catabolism, anabolism, cellular motility, angiogenesis, and growth. In mammals, mTOR is a serine/threonine kinase regulated by phosphoinositol 3 kinase (PI3K).

Our current understanding is that the VEGFR-3 receptor on the surface of lymphatic endothelium results in the activation of the mTOR pathway during lymphangiogenesis. Sirolimus is a lymphangiogenesis inhibitor. It blocks the mTOR pathway, thereby preventing downstream protein synthesis and subsequent endothelial cell proliferation. It has been postulated that mTOR inhibitors such as sirolimus may be beneficial in the treatment of a variety of complicated vascular anomalies in which lymphangiogenesis is a prominent feature of the malformation. Sirolimus is currently the only FDA-approved mTOR inhibitor indicated for prevention of kidney allograft rejection in adults and children 13 years or older; however, it is commonly used to manage organ rejection in younger children, and is generally well tolerated. Also, in a recent clinical trial in patients with lymphangioleiomyomatosis, sirolimus was shown to improve lung function.

**Vincristine.** Vincristine is widely recognized for its use in treating childhood malignancies such as leukemia and retinoblastoma and hematologic conditions such as thrombocytopenic purpura. In patients with KMP, it is often added to steroids, creating a synergistic effect. Vincristine is best delivered through central venous access, with an initial weekly dose of 0.5 to 1 mg/m$^2$ administered by intravenous injection; this dose is then tapered, increasing the interval between injections depending on the clinical response. Treatment is generally administered for 4 to 6 months.

### Embolization and Endovascular Management

Arterial embolization has been used for high-flow tumors (including KHE) in patients who have high-output cardiac failure that has not responded to aggressive pharmacologic management. Occlusion of the blood vessels can be temporary or permanent, depending on the material injected. If a lesion is resectable, embolization can be performed prior to resection to minimize intraoperative blood loss. At our institution, we have also successfully placed covered stents to redirect blood flow in a KHE patient with KMP who had pelvic and lower extremity involvement and fulminant high-output cardiac failure (Fig. 75-14D).

### Surgical Management

If a patient is in high-output heart failure and the lesion is resectable, resection may be a life-saving procedure. We recently used this approach in a neonate with a KHE lesion of the arm who had medically resistant fulminant heart failure. This patient is currently 3 years of age and doing well.

# Part II: Vascular Malformations

## KEY POINTS

1. Vascular malformations are relatively common lesions that are present at birth and often expand or grow in response to trauma, infection, or hormonal changes.

2. Depending on the predominant channel type involved, vascular malformations are designated as capillary, venous, lymphatic, arterial, and combined malformations.

3. MRI is the most useful diagnostic tool for determining the location, extent, and complexity of vascular malformation involvement.

4. Capillary malformations are the most commonly occurring vascular lesion; they may be associated with other vascular anomalies or congenital malformations.

5. Venous malformations are slow-flow lesions that generally appear bluish, with discrete veins often visible through the skin.

6. Lymphatic malformations comprise a broad range of slow-flow lesions, including common cystic lymphatic lesions, lymphangiomatoses, lymphangiectasias, and lymphedema.

7. Arteriovenous malformations are fast-flow communications between arteries and veins; these lesions are among the most dangerous vascular connecting channels.

8. Complex combined vascular malformations should be classified by the anatomic description of the abnormal vascular channels within the lesion.

9. For all vascular malformations, multimodal therapeutic approaches must be tailored to the individual needs of each patient.

## OVERVIEW

Vascular malformations are the second major category of vascular anomalies. Although the specific molecular mechanisms that underlie the formation of these lesions have not yet been elucidated, they are known to result from abnormal morphological development of the vascular system. Vascular malformations are relatively common; unlike vascular tumors, however, they have no gender predilection and are immunonegative on Glut-1 staining. Vascular malformations are present at birth and lesions often expand or grow in response to trauma, infection, or hormonal changes. Although most lesions occur sporadically, some families exhibit inherited lesions. Genetic studies of these families have begun to identify causative gene mutations.

Depending on the predominant channel type involved, vascular malformations are designated as capillary, venous, lymphatic, arterial, and combined malformations. The severity of lesions varies significantly both within and among these clinical subgroups. Lesions with an arterial component are rheologically fast flow, and can be associated with cardiac failure secondary to high-output cardiac states, and disproportionate growth of involved organs and extremities. Capillary, lymphatic, venous, and combined venolymphatic malformations are slow-flow lesions. Venous malformations and combined lesions with a venous component predispose to venous stasis and localized intravascular coagulopathy. The risk of these complications is increased in large, diffuse, or multifocal lesions, which have a higher likelihood of significant consumptive coagulopathy. Malformations containing a lymphatic component also can lead to significant disfigurement from soft tissue hypertrophy and skeletal overgrowth, bony abnormalities, and/or infection. A wide range of treatment options is available, and decision making must consider the anatomic location, presenting symptoms, effect on function, aesthetics, and prognosis.

## CAPILLARY MALFORMATIONS

Capillary lesions are the most common type of vascular malformation. These lesions often present at birth as a macular capillary stain (colloquially referred to as stork bite, angel kiss, or salmon patch) and are commonly found on the forehead, eyelids, nose, and nuchal region. Because these stains often fade quite quickly or disappear during childhood, they are generally of little long-term concern. Other capillary malformations referred to as port-wine stains persist throughout life (Fig. 75-15). At birth, these lesions are usually flat and bright pink. As the infant's hemoglobin falls over the first few weeks of life, the color of lesions may fade slightly. With age, these stains can become thickened or nodular and often darken.

Depending on location of the capillary malformation, it may be associated with other vascular anomalies or congenital malformations. Capillary malformations that overlie the eyelid may indicate a unilateral arteriovenous malformation of the retina and intracranial optic pathway associated with the Wyburn–Mason syndrome. A high

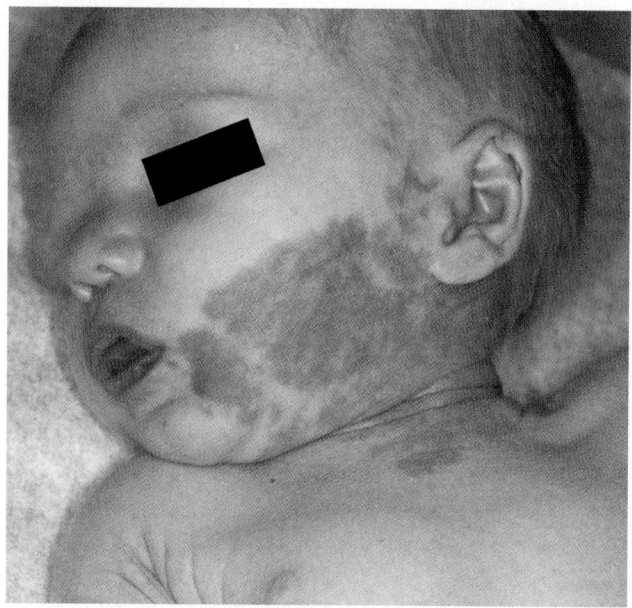

**FIGURE 75-15** Neonatal capillary malformation (port-wine stain) that will persist and may hypertrophy as the child ages.

index of suspicion warrants examination by an ophthalmologist, as this pattern of presentation is associated with a 10% risk of glaucoma. Capillary malformations may also overlie a deep arteriovenous malformation anywhere on the body. Lesions on the trunk or extremities may coexist with venous and lymphatic malformations (the Klippel–Trenaunay syndrome). Lesions located over the lower lumbar midline may indicate the presence of underlying spinal dysraphism, lipomeningocele, tethered spinal cord, and diastematomyelia. If there is craniofacial or lumbar involvement, an MRI or CT scan is required to rule out central nervous system abnormalities.

### Sturge Weber Syndrome

Sturge Weber syndrome (SWS) is a rare neurocutaneous disorder associated with a characteristic facial port-wine stain in the ophthalmic distribution of the trigeminal nerve, glaucoma (10%) and vascular eye abnormalities, and an ipsilateral intracranial vascular malformation (Fig. 75-16A). Children with SWS often develop progressive neurologic problems, including seizures, migraines, stroke-like episodes, learning difficulties or significant developmental delay, visual field impairment, and hemiparesis.

The specific genetic and environmental factors that result in SWS are unknown, but the localized abnormalities of blood vessel development and function affecting the facial skin, eye, and brain suggest that a disruption occurs during the first trimester of pregnancy. A number of associated genetic abnormalities have been documented in patients SWS, and a mutation in the *RASA1* gene, which encodes a GTPase activating protein, has been reported. This gene has been implicated in the normal proliferation, migration, and survival of vascular endothelial cells.

The spectrum of symptoms is highly variable, as is the constellation of organs involved and the severity of involvement. Some patients present with facial port-wine stains and seizures

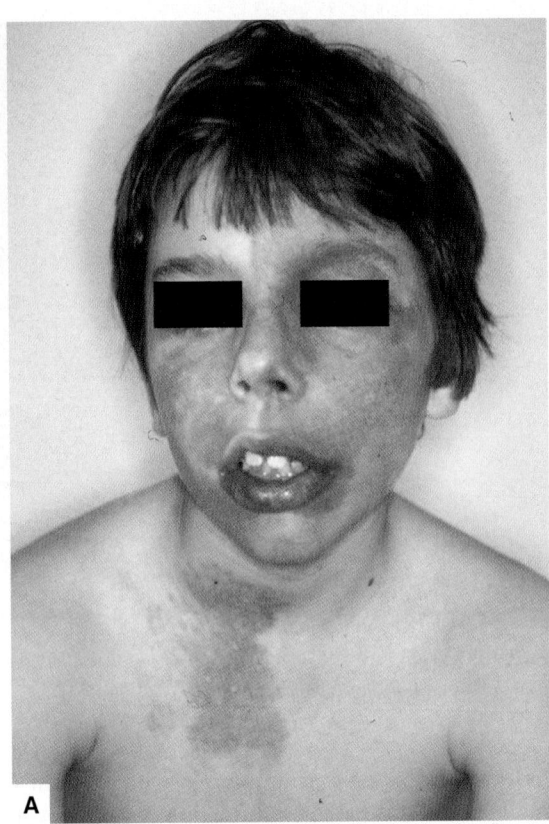

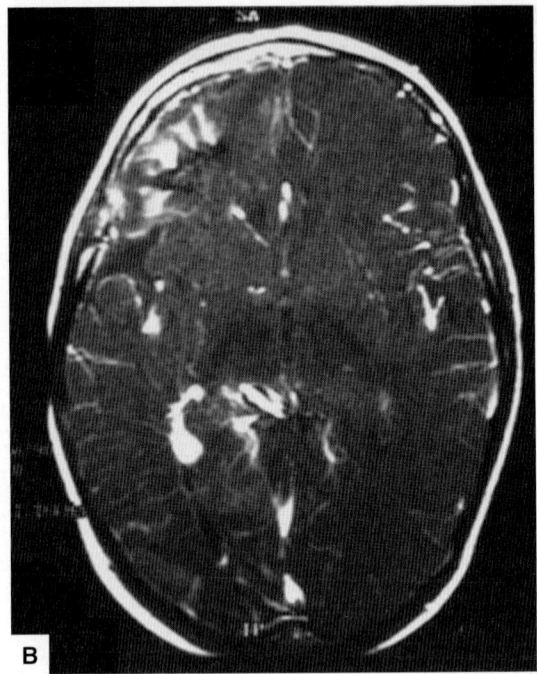

**FIGURE 75-16 A.** Patient with SWS. Note the left facial asymmetry from overgrowth; (**B**) cranial MRI documenting intracranial vascular malformations.

as the only manifestation of an intracranial vascular malformation, whereas others also have severe cognitive and neurologic deficits, intractable seizures, increased intracranial pressure, and intractable glaucoma with visual loss, and dental problems.

Patients should be followed closely for evidence of developmental delay. If delay is noted, it is prudent to refer patients for a neurologic evaluation and an MRI of the brain. SWS can be associated with progressive neurologic deterioration secondary to leptomeningeal involvement of the brain. A baseline MRI is therefore typically obtained in early childhood. For patients who have significant intracranial disease or progressive neurologic symptoms, an annual MRI is obtained (Fig. 75-16B).

The management of patients with SWS depends on the clinical manifestation and severity of symptoms, with the treatment of seizures and glaucoma being of primary concern. Treatment of the port-wine stains is actually the least problematic aspect of overall management. Long-term neurodevelopmental outcomes are highly variable, and patients must be followed by an experienced neurologic team. Treatment for neurologic complications comprises the control of seizures with anticonvulsants or epilepsy surgery for seizures refractory to pharmacologic management.

## Management of Capillary Malformations

Decisions regarding if, when, and how to treat patients with capillary malformations should consider the size and location of the lesion. Lesions on extra-facial locations that are not an aesthetic concern may not require treatment. The gold standard for the treatment of lesions on visually prominent areas is the PDL at the 595-nm wavelength; however, several other lasers are now also being used. Laser therapy should be initiated before the progression of lesions that occurs after puberty and during adulthood. Treatments can begin at 6 months of age, and require sedation or a general anesthetic.

Laser therapy often prevents the progression of the capillary malformation; however, several treatments and yearly monitoring are essential. Although long-term successful lightening is achieved in approximately 25% of patients, approximately 30% show little or no improvement. The remainder may require periodic treatment throughout their lifetime. Furthermore, pyogenic granulomas and residual scarring have been documented in areas treated with laser. Worthy of note, preliminary data suggest that using topical rapamycin may improve the efficacy of treatment with PDL. In capillary lesions that have thickened and become darker with age, the Nd:YAG laser has been used to decrease the intensity of the stain; however, patients are often left with residual scarring.

Interestingly, there is currently no prospective evidence that early laser treatment reduces complications such as overgrowth of the underlying bone or soft tissue or darkening/thickening of the lesion with time. Nonetheless, given the stigma associated with facial lesions in particular, there is a definite psychosocial benefit to early intervention. Families must be counseled as to all of these issues and the spectrum of possible short- and long-term outcomes associated with laser therapy.

A treatment option that is currently used for hypertrophied lip and eyelid tissue is surgical debulking. Skin grafting in facial aesthetic units has been used to achieve satisfactory cosmesis. Surgical resection may be necessary in patients with lesions that are resistant to laser therapy.

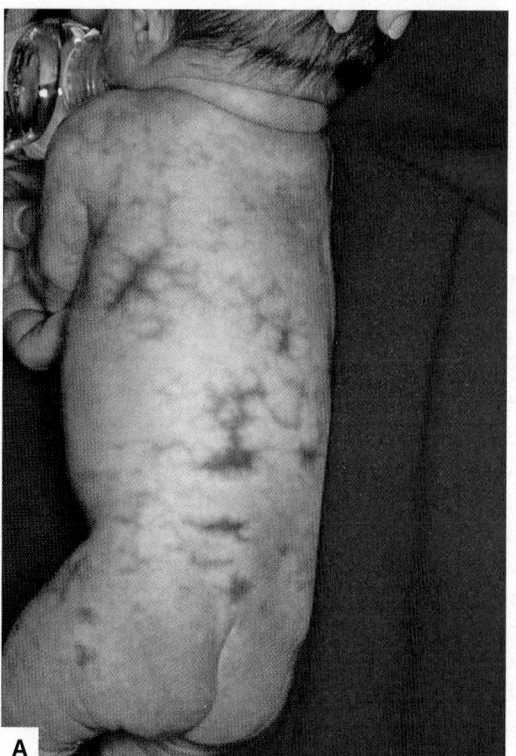
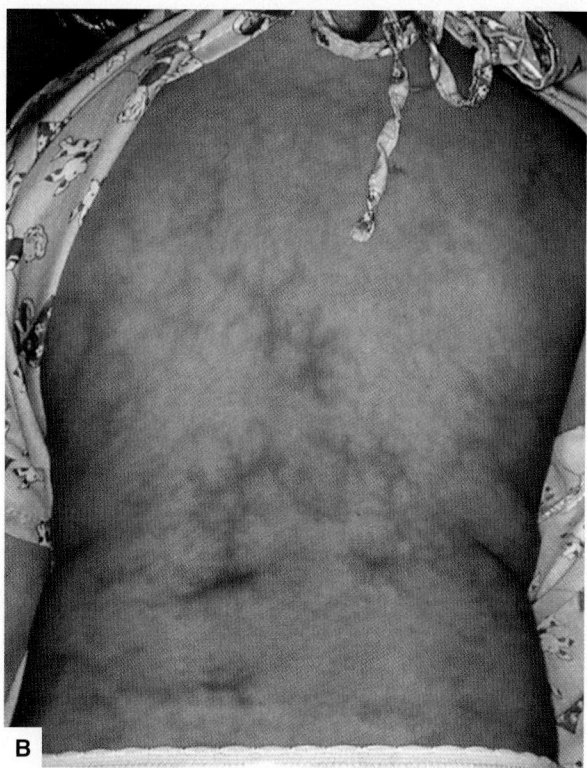

**FIGURE 75-17** **A.** Cutis marmorata telangiectatica congenita in a newborn child. Note the reticulated pattern of the capillary malformation in the skin. **B.** The same child at 4 year of age. These lesion is still present but less prominent.

## Cutis Marmorata Telangiectatica Congenita

Cutis marmorata telangiectatica congenita (CMTC) is an uncommon vascular anomaly characterized by persistent violaceous skin marbling, phlebectasia, telangiectasia, and superficial ulceration. Occasionally, superficial ulceration and cutaneous atrophy are also seen. The skin marbling occurs in a characteristic reticulated pattern and is generally evident at birth. It may become more pronounced in response to cold temperatures, physical activity, or crying; however, it does not disappear. CMTC may be limited to certain anatomic regions (localized) or may be distributed over large areas of the body (generalized) (Fig. 75-17A,B). It frequently occurs on the extremities and the trunk but may involve the face.

The precise genetic cause of CMTC is unknown and both sporadic inheritance and familial inheritance have been reported. CMTC often occurs in association with a variety of other congenital anomalies, including but not limited to hypertrophy or hypotrophy of an involved extremity. Patients who present with "true" limb hemihypertrophy are at increased risk of hepatic and renal malignancies and should therefore undergo screening US every 3 months up to approximately age 8. Other reported abnormalities include syndactyly, club foot, scoliosis, cleft palate, dystrophic teeth, glaucoma, hypothyroidism, and hypospadias. In view of limb length differences, patients should be followed closely by an orthopaedist with special expertise.

The skin pigmentation associated with CMTC often lightens with time; if persistent, however, it can be treated with PDL therapy. The outcome with laser therapy is variable.

## Macrocephaly-Capillary Malformation Syndrome

Macrocephaly-capillary malformation syndrome (formerly referred to as macrocephaly-CMTC) is a rare congenital syndrome of unknown etiology. The syndrome is characterized by macrocephaly and vascular lesions, reticulated or confluent port-wine stains, and persistent centrofacial capillary malformations. Diagnosis requires the presence of macrocephaly and capillary formations in addition to at least 2 of the following minor criteria: asymmetry or overgrowth, developmental delay, midline facial capillary malformations, neonatal hypotonia, syndactyly/polydactyly, frontal bossing, joint hypermobility or hyperelastic skin, and hydrocephalus, and Chiari malformations. The extent of the cutaneous malformation does not correlate with the severity of other associated abnormalities. Patients with macrocephaly-capillary malformation syndrome and hemihypertrophy are at increased risk of Wilms tumor and should therefore be closely monitored.

## VENOUS MALFORMATIONS

Venous malformations are slow-flow lesions composed of localized or diffuse ectatic veins with abnormal collections of irregular venous channels having flat, mitotically inactive endothelia and scant mural smooth muscle. These malformations are generally present at birth but may not be observed until later in childhood or in adolescence, when lesions expand and become visible or symptomatic. Venous malformations usually occur sporadically; however, a number of families with these lesions have been identified. Some kindreds that express a phenotype with multiple lesions in different anatomic regions have a mutation in the gene encoding the endothelial-specific receptor tyrosine kinase TIE2.

Lesions usually appear bluish, with discrete veins that are often visible through the skin. Many lesions are confined to the subcutaneous tissues, whereas others are more infiltrative and often involve deeper muscles. Superficial lesions can be symptomatic due to periodic thromboses, painful phleboliths, or pain from venous congestion and swelling. Deeper lesions with muscle infiltration are often painful with activity. Patients who require treatment should undergo more extensive investigation, including Doppler US, MRI, and direct-puncture angiography; these tests will confirm the diagnosis and assess the extent of the lesion.

Phleboliths are often seen on plain radiographs. Patients with diffuse and multiple venous malformations have a higher risk of coagulation disorders, including localized or disseminated intravascular coagulation. If these disorders are unrecognized or inadequately managed, they may lead to serious thromboembolic events such as pulmonary emboli. These clotting abnormalities are presumably caused by venous stasis, vascular tortuosity, and/or structural abnormality of the veins. Patients should therefore be screened with a basic coagulation profile including a complete blood count (CBC), platelet count, prothrombin time (PT), partial thromboplastin time (PTT), D-dimer, and fibrinogen. Additionally, they should be screened for genetic polymorphisms associated with an increased risk of aberrant clotting (ie, factor V Leiden, plasminogen activator inhibitors, and methylenetetrahydrofolate reductase). Because they are particularly at risk for increased bleeding and a pulmonary embolus following surgery, we recommend prophylactic antithromboembolic treatment in anticipation of prolonged bed rest. We are currently using a protocol of low-molecular-weight heparin administered 2 weeks prior to surgery or interventional procedures and continued for 2 weeks postoperatively.

Rarely, pulmonary hypertension may be a manifestation of chronic pulmonary emboli. A recent study has shown that patients with Klippel–Trenaunay syndrome or extensive venous malformations of greater than 15% of body surface area have pulmonary hypertension. A correlation between levels of D-dimer and degree of pulmonary hypertension was also noted. These patients should therefore undergo a screening echocardiogram to investigate possible pulmonary hypertension.

## Treatment of Venous Malformations

### Overview

Treatment varies considerably depending on the severity of symptoms and the location and extent of the lesions. Many children do not require treatment at the time of diagnosis, and nonproblematic lesions can initially be managed with observation alone. However, because a venous malformation gradually expands, patients may become symptomatic and seek intervention in childhood or adolescence. Less commonly, a lesion involving an anatomically sensitive area or causing gross deformity necessitates management as early as infancy. If possible, however, intervention should be delayed until the risks associated with anesthesia decrease (6 to 12 months of age). To lessen the psychological impact of a noticeable deformity, operative intervention is optimally performed before 3.5 years, when long-term memory and self-esteem begin to develop. If the deformity is minor, parents often prefer to postpone therapy until the child is able to independently make the decision to proceed with operative intervention.

Patients with extremity lesions generally benefit from tailored compression garments. Although this is supportive therapy, it is useful for controlling swelling and pain and may also help in managing disease progression. To improve compliance, garments should be initiated at an early age. Growing children require refitting for garments at least twice each year to ensure adequate fit and therapeutic benefit. Patients who develop painful superficial phlebitis and areas with clot formation within the malformations should be treated with a course of anti-inflammatory medication.

Extensive venous malformations that are not amenable to resection or only partially resectable can be managed with sclerotherapy (Fig. 75-18A–C). To preserve function when vital structures are involved, a series of sclerotherapy procedures with sodium tetradecyl sulfate is often performed with US and fluoroscopic guidance. Alternatively, other sclerosants such as polidocanol (Aetoxisclerol), alcoholic solution of zein (Ethibloc), bleomycin, sodium morrhuate, or ethanolamine oleate are sometimes used. Although ethanol was formerly a first-line sclerosant, it has fallen out of favor due to severe adverse effects, including neurotoxicity and skin breakdown. The sclerosing agent is injected through a percutaneously placed injection needle into the venous malformation to obliterate its channel lumen by damaging the endothelium with subsequent inflammation and fibrosis. Approximately 75% of patients benefit from this treatment modality; however, 50% of patients experience recanalization of the vascular malformation within 6 months of a single treatment. Patients with complicated lesions generally require a series of treatments at 6- to 8-week intervals.

When a lesion is localized and accessible and does not involve vital structures, surgical excision yields excellent outcomes. More extensive lesions are generally only partially resectable. In this setting, other modalities such as preoperative sclerotherapy are useful to facilitate resection and improve surgical outcomes. For lesions that involve a joint, we recommend resection of the intraarticular component of the lesion using an open approach. This operation can help to prevent hemarthroses and further degeneration of the articular cartilage. Although the long-term results of this practice are unknown, it is thought that it may prevent progressive joint damage and pain. Superficial lesions or the superficial component of deep lesions can be treated with the Nd:YAG laser.

## Glomuvenous Malformation

Glomuvenous malformation is the most common known inherited venous malformation. It is an autosomal dominant condition that is caused by a loss-of-function mutation in the

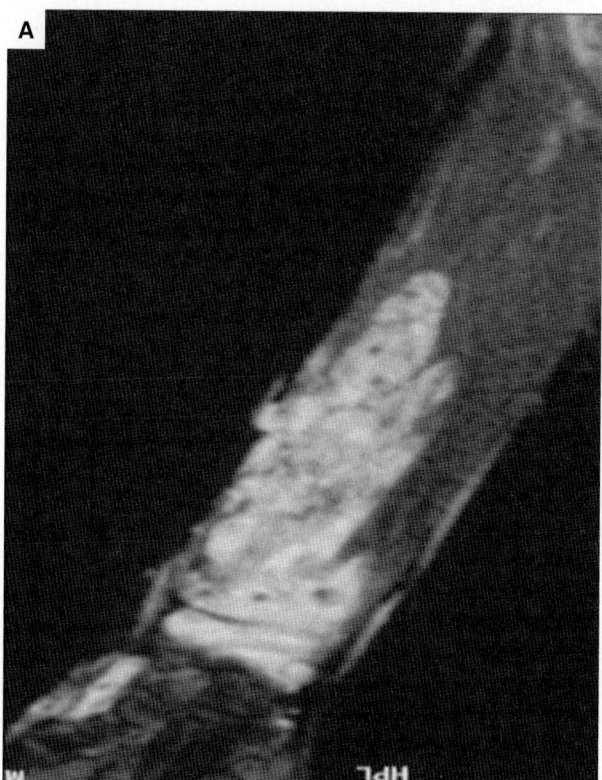

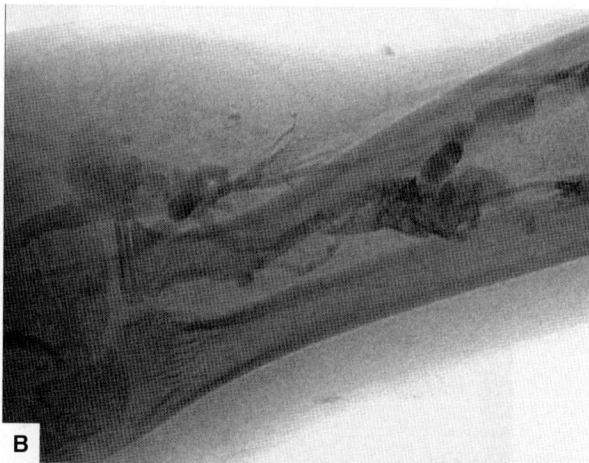

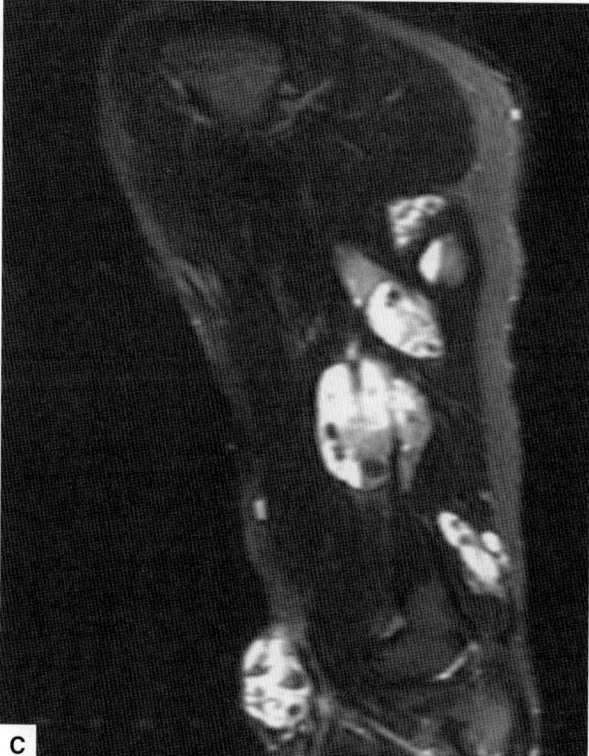

**FIGURE 75-18 A.** MRI image of large venous malformation involving radial extensor and flexor muscles of the right wrist and forearm. **B.** Sclerotherapy of the venous malformation combined with intravenous contrast to outline the vascular anatomy during the injection. **C.** MRI demonstrating multiple enhancing venous malformations involving the musculature of the thigh.

glomulin gene. Lesions are frequently multiple (70%), small, and located in the skin and subcutaneous tissue (Fig. 75-19). They involve the extremities (75%), trunk (14%), or head/neck (10%) and present as raised bluish-purple nodules with a cobblestone appearance. Glomuvenous malformations can be clinically differentiated from the more commonly seen venous malformations in that they are painful on palpation. If possible, symptomatic lesions are best managed by complete surgical excision.

## Blue Rubber Bleb Nevus Syndrome

Blue rubber bleb nevus syndrome is a rare disorder characterized by discrete venous malformations of varying size and appearance that most frequently involve the skin, soft tissue, and gastrointestinal tract. Lesions typically present on the

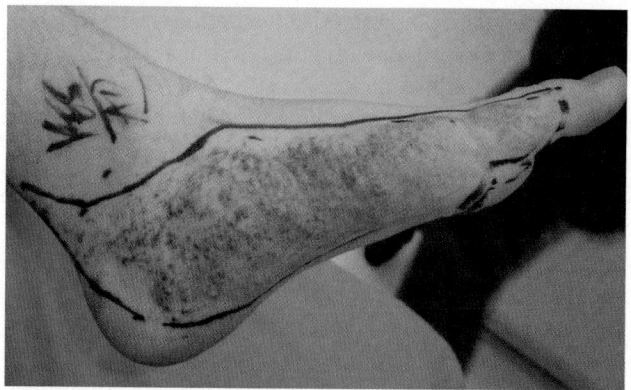

**FIGURE 75-19** Painful glomuvenous malformation of the foot. This was resected and grafted with a split thickness skin graft. The patient is now 8 years post resection with no further impairment or symptoms.

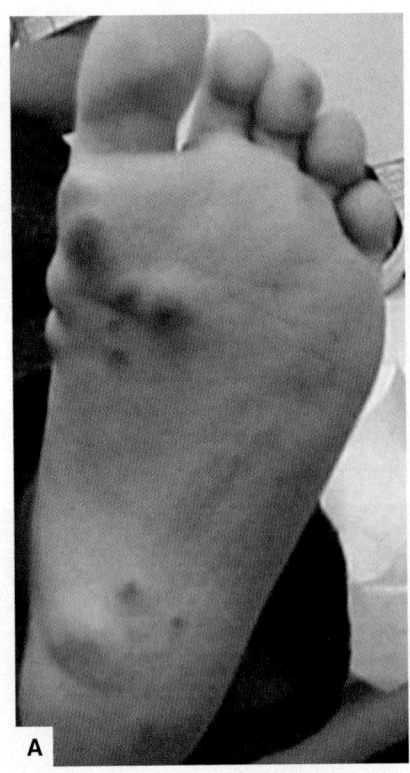

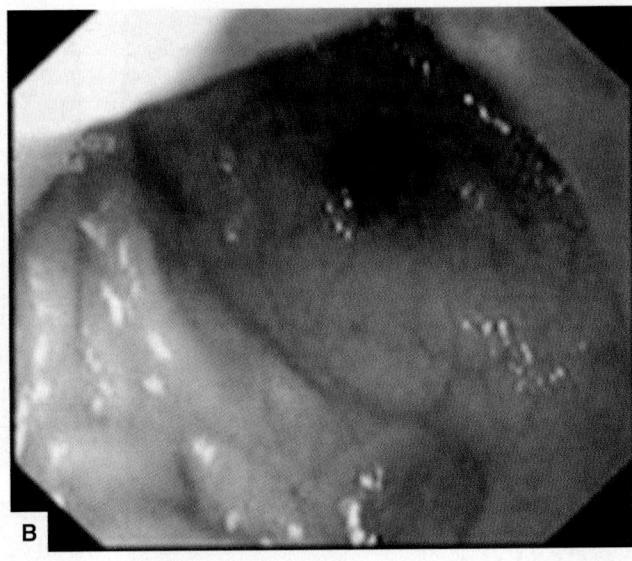

**FIGURE 75-20** Blue rubber bleb nevus syndrome. **A.** Blue venous nodules involving many areas of the body including the feet. **B.** Involvement of the small intestine is common as seen on this endoscopic picture.

plantar and palmar surfaces, but can also occur anywhere on the body (Fig. 75-20A). The morbidity and mortality associated with this syndrome depend on the extent of visceral organ involvement. Lesions within the gastrointestinal tract may be associated with significant bleeding (Fig. 75-20A). In this setting, patients do not have large volume spontaneous bleeds but tend to develop an indolent chronic anemia. In patients who require multiple transfusions, surgical resection is indicated. This is usually accomplished using a push enteroscopy technique, with a gastroenterologist performing an endoscopy in the open abdomen. To ensure complete visualization of the lumen, the surgeon sequentially advances the bowel over the endoscope. The lesions are marked as they are encountered and subsequently resected. Resection is accomplished either by wedge resections, intussusception of the bowel, or full thickness small bowel resections and anastomoses, aiming to minimize the amount of intestine lost. Given that our experience indicates that new lesions may form during puberty, we recommend these resections should be performed following this period. Most patients have a normal life span, though they require long-term monitoring.

### Maffucci Syndrome

Maffucci syndrome is a rare disorder that presents in childhood and is characterized by venous malformations, vascular anomalies, multiple enchondromas, and dyschondroplasia of the limbs. The venous malformations are superficial or deep and are often seen throughout the body, including the brain and the oral and abdominal cavities. Enchondromas are benign cartilaginous tumors that can develop at any site but usually involve the long bones, with the hands and feet being the most commonly involved. Reports estimate that as many as 20% to 40% of enchondromas transform

into chondrosarcomas. Enchondromas should therefore be watched carefully for changes that may indicate transformation. If the venous malformations are symptomatic, they can be treated with sclerotherapy or surgical resection. Limb length discrepancies and pathologic fractures have also been documented. Bone union is slow and unsatisfactory, and curved and uneven bones bring about secondary deformities that increase throughout the developmental period. In severe cases, the hands and feet become almost unrecognizable and are transformed into huge tumor masses. Patient management is complex and patients are best managed in a multidisciplinary setting.

## LYMPHATIC MALFORMATIONS

Lymphatic malformations are benign vascular lesions thought to arise from embryologic disturbances in the lymphatic system. They comprise a broad range of slow-flow lesions, including common cystic lymphatic lesions, lymphangiomatoses, lymphangiectasias, and lymphedema. These lesions can be isolated or can occur as part of a constellation of vascular lesions in patients with complex vascular anomalies. Additionally, they can be associated with syndromes. Our discussion will be limited to the most frequently seen lesions that pediatric surgeons are called upon to evaluate.

### Lymphatic Development

Lymphatic malformations are thought to be the result of abnormal development of the embryonic lymphatics or lymphatic jugular sacs, with failure of these structures to connect or drain into the venous system. Two mechanisms are believed to play a role in lymphatic development. The centrifugal theory postulates that primitive lymph sacs bud from venous endothelia early in embryogenesis. Endothelial sprouting of these sacs to the periphery, which may occur through the expression of factors such as VEGFR-3 and Prox-1, form the large deep lymphatics. The second mechanism, referred to as the centripetal theory, postulates that the lymphatic system derives from mesenchymal progenitor cells or lymphangioblasts that develop independent of the venous system. It is likely that fusion of the peripheral and deep lymphatics occurs. More recent molecular studies of lymphangiogenesis support both theories and maintain that superficial lymphatics develop from mesenchymal lymphoblasts, whereas deep lymphatics develop from veins. The homeobox *gene Prox 1* has been identified as the first lymphatic-specific marker central to lymphatic budding, sprouting, and migration, and it is seen in all lymphatic malformations.

## Common Cystic Lymphatic Malformations

Cystic lymphatic malformations are the most common lymphatic malformations that occur in children. Three morphologic patterns are seen within this classification: microcystic, macrocystic, and combined. Microcystic lesions arise as clear, small (<2 mm to 1 cm) vesicles that infiltrate the subcutaneous tissue and muscles. These vesicles are often firm and may give the impression of a brawny edema. Macrocystic lymphatic malformations are often large (≥2 cm), compressible or noncompressible masses under normal or bluish skin. Most of these lesions are multilobular, multilocular masses that consist of numerous cysts that vary in size. Unlike fast-flow lesions such as hemangiomas and arteriovenous malformations (AVMs), these lesions are not warm to the touch. Combined cystic lymphatic malformations have both microcystic and macrocystic components; these lesions are the most frequently encountered common cystic malformation.

It is important to note that the often seen term *cystic hygroma* refers to a large cervical or axillary lesion identified in the perinatal period. However, because the term does not encompass the morphology and anatomic distribution of most cystic lymphatic malformations, its use is inaccurate and best avoided in describing lymphatic malformations.

Although cystic lymphatic malformations can arise in any anatomic region, they more commonly appear in rich lymphatic areas, such as the head and neck, axilla, mediastinum, groin, and retroperitoneum. They have no known racial or sex predilection.

## Diagnosis

**Prenatal.** Large cystic lymphatic lesions can be diagnosed in utero as early as the beginning of the second trimester, and prenatal diagnosis has significant implications. Large anterior cervical and lingual lesions may be associated with airway obstruction, and prenatal diagnosis can influence the mode, timing, and place of delivery (Fig. 21A,B). It can also signal the need to prepare for possible interventions to control a precarious airway in the delivery room. These patients often require the presence of a skilled surgical team capable of performing an EXIT (ex utero intrapartum treatment)

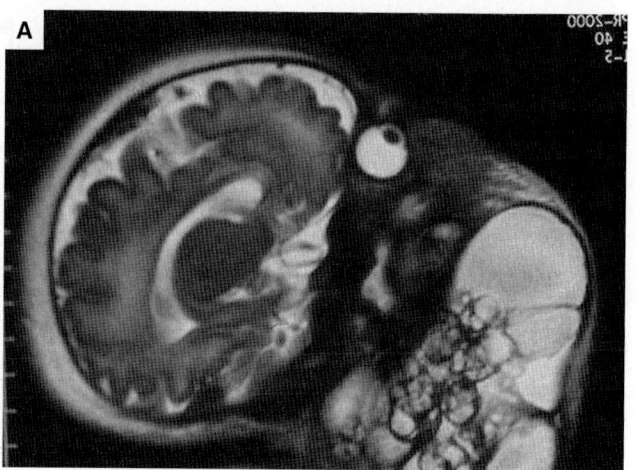

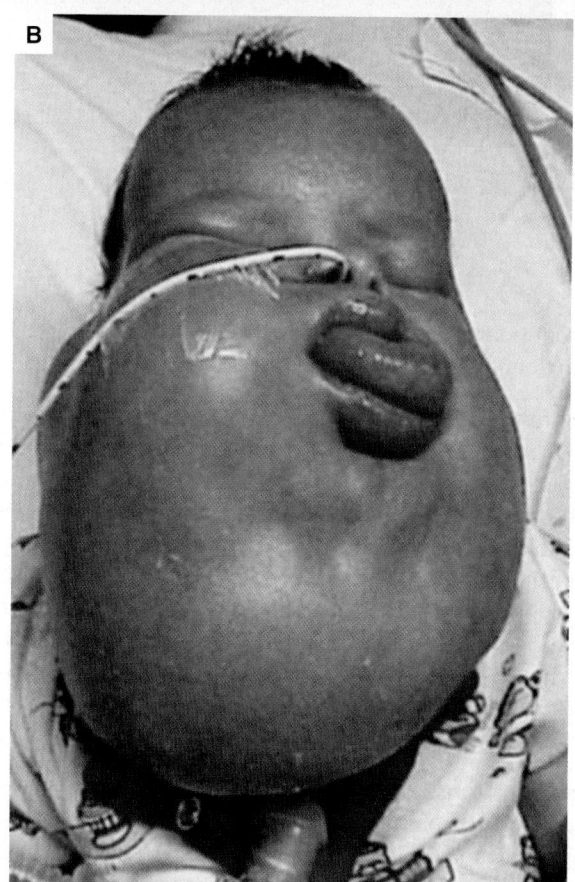

**FIGURE 75-21** **A.** Prenatal MRI of a fetus with a macrocystic lymphatic lesion involving the anterior cervical region of the fetus. **B.** The airway was temporarily secured with fiberoptic endoscopic intubation during the EXIT delivery. The child required a tracheostomy to maintain a safe airway.

procedure. A recent study at our institution suggests that the postnatal outcome of these prenatally diagnosed patients is poor. Infants who survive are often left with permanent nerve palsies, somatic growth abnormalities of the jaws, and abnormal dentition. Additionally, lesion regrowth and re-expansion may occur.

Large posterior cervical lesions have been associated with Turner or Noonan syndrome, as well as other congenital anomalies. They carry a high prenatal mortality rate, particularly with hydrops and diffuse lymphedema. Fetal

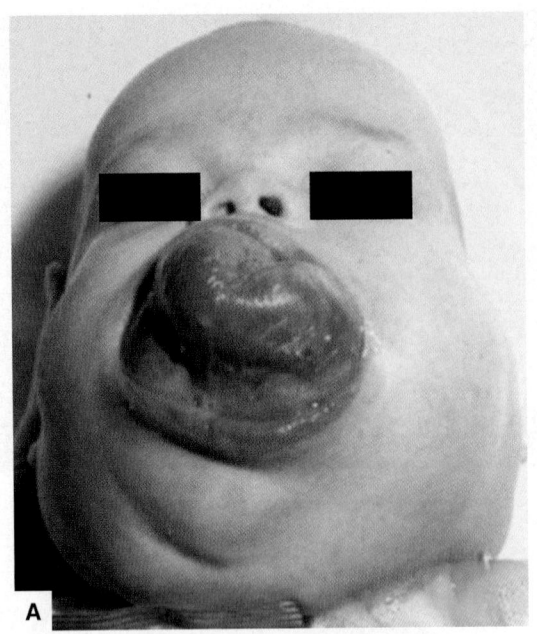
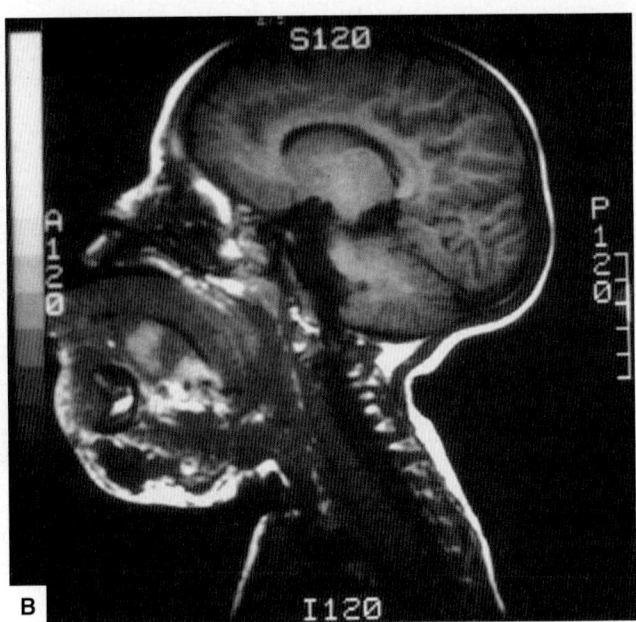

**FIGURE 75-22** **A.** Large cervicofacial lymphatic malformation (LM) with macro and microcystic components. **B.** MRI documenting the complexity and severity of the LM as it involves the anterior cervical region, tongue, and floor of mouth.

chromosomal analysis should therefore be performed and genetic and family counseling should be provided.

**Postnatal.** Although some cystic lesions are noted at birth, most become evident by age 2 and are readily diagnosed by physical examination. However, all patients with cervical cystic lesions should receive a chest radiograph to exclude possible mediastinal involvement. Although US is helpful in confirming the diagnosis of superficial lesions, it is less beneficial for revealing extension into deep structures of the neck, thoracic cavity, and retroperitoneum. MRI is the modality of choice for determining the extent of cystic lesions and their relationship to soft tissues, nerves, muscle, and vascular structures (Fig. 75-22A,B).

**Complications.** Patients can experience numerous complications. Cutaneous involvement can be associated with spontaneous lymphatic leakage from pathologic vesicles. Bacteria can readily enter through these vesicles and spread through affected tissue. Patients with extremity malformations are thus instructed on proper foot hygiene and are often given a prophylactic prescription for a broad-spectrum antibiotic. They are advised to initiate therapy as soon as the first symptoms of infection appear and seek medical attention immediately. In the worst clinical scenario, leakage can be associated with acute cellulitis and life-threatening sepsis. Recurrent and generally painful cellulitis can also occur, causing loss of function and aesthetic disfigurement. Given that such infections can be life threatening, aggressive antimicrobial therapy is essential.

Large cystic lesions of the head and neck are also associated with respiratory obstruction of the larynx and trachea. In early childhood, some affected patients have difficulty swallowing and are at high risk for aspiration. These patients may require gastrostomies to maintain adequate enteral nutrition. Proper management is extremely difficult and requires staged

operative procedures, speech therapy, physical therapy, and long-term follow-up, preferably by a multidisciplinary team.

Other complications include localized hemorrhage into cysts and nerve compressions that can cause paresthesias and pain. Although rare, dysphagia, chylothorax, and chylopericardium have been reported in patients with mediastinal involvement.

## Treatment

The treatment of patients with lymphatic malformations depends on the clinical presentation, the size of the lesion, the location of the lesion, and the presenting complications. For complicated or extensive lesions, multimodal therapy is commonplace.

Patients with malformations of the trunk and extremities benefit from tailored compression garments, which are useful for controlling swelling and pain and may also help in managing disease progression. Garments should be tailored for the patient by an experienced practitioner, with close attention paid to areas of the malformation that are symptomatic.

In a small percentage of patients with localized lymphatic malformations, lesions appear to resolve spontaneously. This is likely due to a sclerosant effect on the lymphatic malformation related to trauma or infection. Therefore, only lesions that are persistently symptomatic, functionally limiting, or aesthetically disfiguring require intervention.

Sclerotherapy is currently the primary treatment for most localized symptomatic macrocystic lymphatic malformations. Although it is not curative, many (approximately 80%) patients benefit significantly from this approach. A number of sclerosing agents have been used, including doxycycline, ethanol, bleomycin, and OK-432 (also known as Picibanil). Doxycycline, an antimicrobial agent that inhibits protein synthesis, is used to treat most lymphatic malformations in our practice. Lymphatic cysts are aspirated and sclerosed under image guidance (Fig. 75-23A–C). The doxycycline concentration used is 10 mg/mL; a maximum dose of 150 mg (less in infants) is administered. Both US and fluoroscopic imaging are useful to ensure against venous embolization of the sclerosant. When lesions are large, a closed suction drain is placed for 24 hours in order to aspirate ongoing fluid drainage. Treatments are often scheduled 4 to 6 weeks apart, depending on the results. A recent (2008) study of 41 patients reported an 83% overall reduction in lesion size; however, most patients with complicated or extensive lesions required multiple treatments. Because doxycycline is a tetracycline antibiotic, it can be associated with staining of the teeth. Complication rates range from 2% to 10% and are more common in microcystic and combined lesions and with the administration of higher doxycycline doses.

OK-432 is a common sclerotherapy agent used outside of the United States, but not yet approved for use in the United States. It is derived from a lyophilized mixture of group A *Streptococcus pyogenes* incubated with benzylpenicillin. In a recent (2009) prospective randomized study, it was shown to have a 94% response rate with macrocystic lesions in the head and neck. Bleomycin, a chemotherapeutic agent that inhibits DNA synthesis, is another sclerosant widely used outside the United States, primarily in Europe and the Middle East. Although it is most successful with macrocystic lesions, it reportedly improves 40% of microcystic lesions. The administration of bleomycin is associated with dose-related and idiopathic forms of pulmonary fibrosis. Two recent studies suggest that genetic polymorphisms increase the risk of idiopathic pulmonary fibrosis. However, pulmonary fibrosis is extremely rare in patients with lymphatic malformations treated with bleomycin.

In certain anatomic regions, swelling of the malformation is a dangerous side effect of sclerotherapy. It can cause airway compromise, especially when the lesion is located in the cervical area and mediastinum. The procedure is usually performed in the hospital with the patient under general anesthesia, and patients are observed for at least 24 hours. Common adverse effects include fever for 2 to 4 days and a localized inflammatory reaction with tenderness, erythema, or swelling of the lesions, lasting 1 to 3 weeks. If the initial response to any sclerosant is unsatisfactory, treatment is often repeated at 6-week to 3-month intervals. When treatment is unsuccessful or yields only a partial response, surgery may be required.

Although complete surgical excision is optimal for large lesions that extend through multiple anatomic regions, this is generally impossible to achieve. However, smaller and superficial malformations unresponsive to sclerotherapy are amenable to complete excision with excellent results body. Larger lesions that involve deep structures of the neck, tongue, and mediastinum entail the risk of multiple complications, including fistula formation, infection, damage to nerves and vascular structures, and aesthetic disfigurement (Fig. 75-24A–C). In some patients with extensive microcystic disease, lymphatic vesicles may become apparent in or around the scar years after excision.

Persistent disease manifests in close to one third of patients who have undergone what was thought to be gross total resection. If asymptomatic, these patients may not require

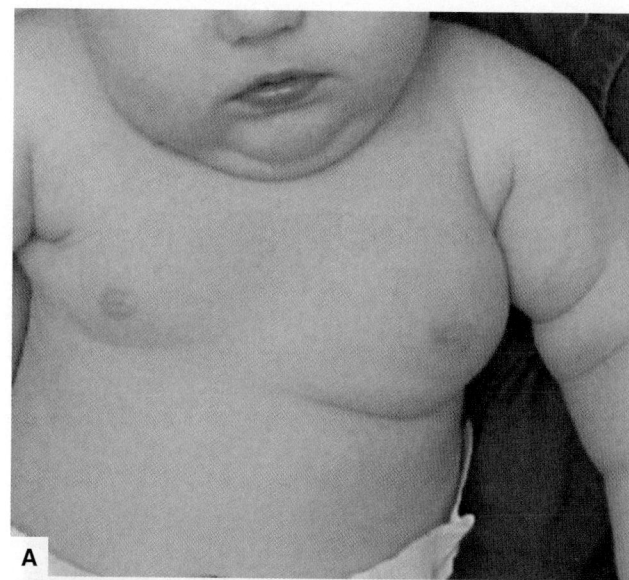

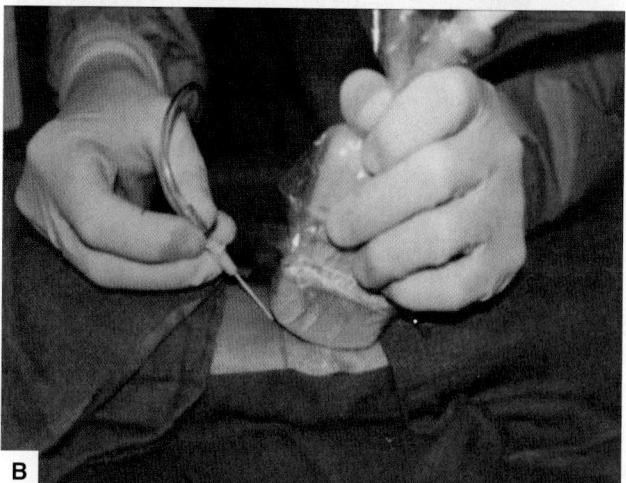

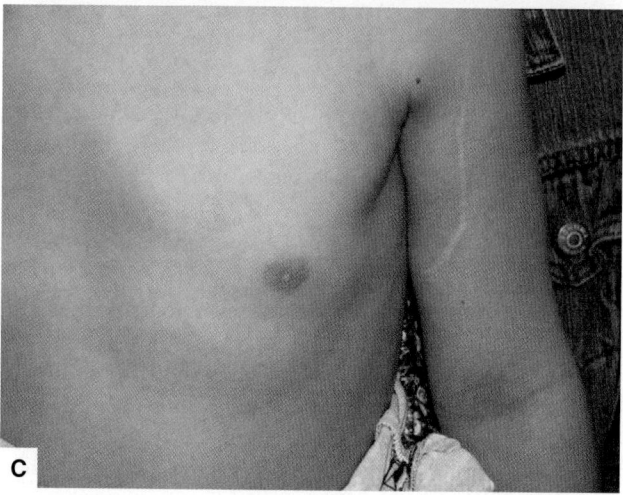

**FIGURE 75-23** Macrocystic lymphatic malformation in the left anterior chest wall and axilla in a 2-month-old infant. **A.** Presclerotherapy photograph; (**B**) ultrasound guided sclerotherapy. This child had 5 procedures to control all the macrocystic components. **C.** At 6 years of age, the child has a normal chest wall appearance. The child had also an excision of a microcystic LM involving the upper arm—note the longitudinal scar on the left upper arm.

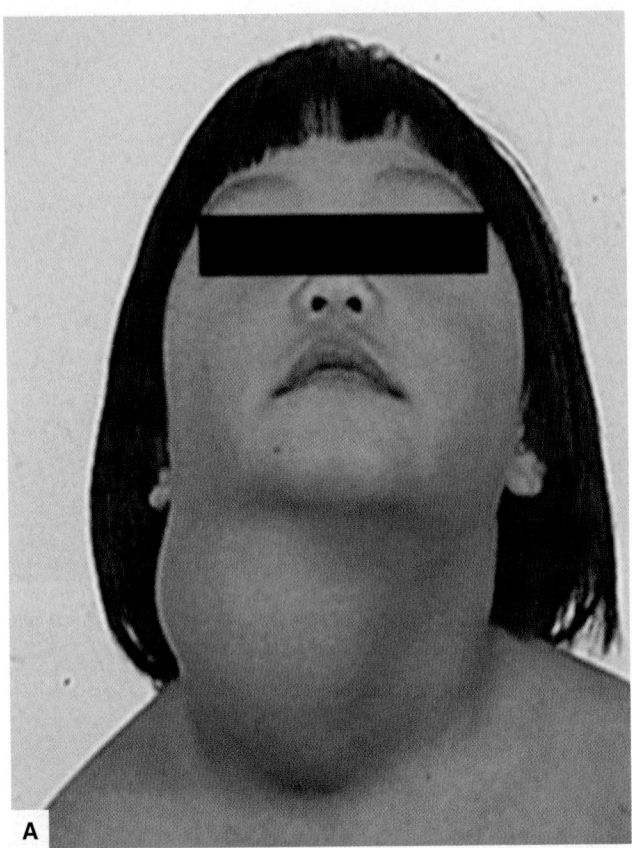

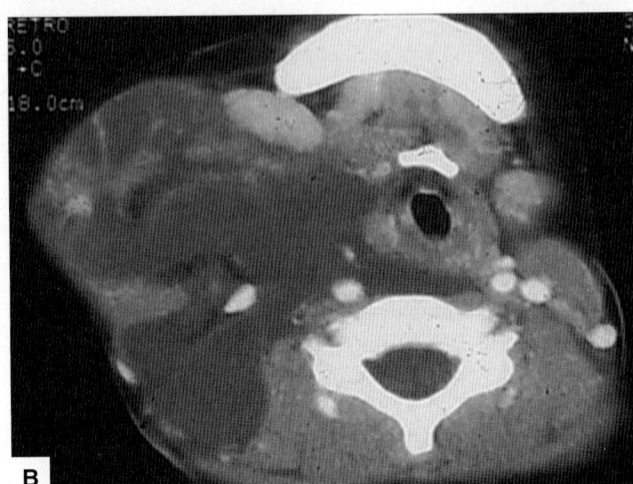

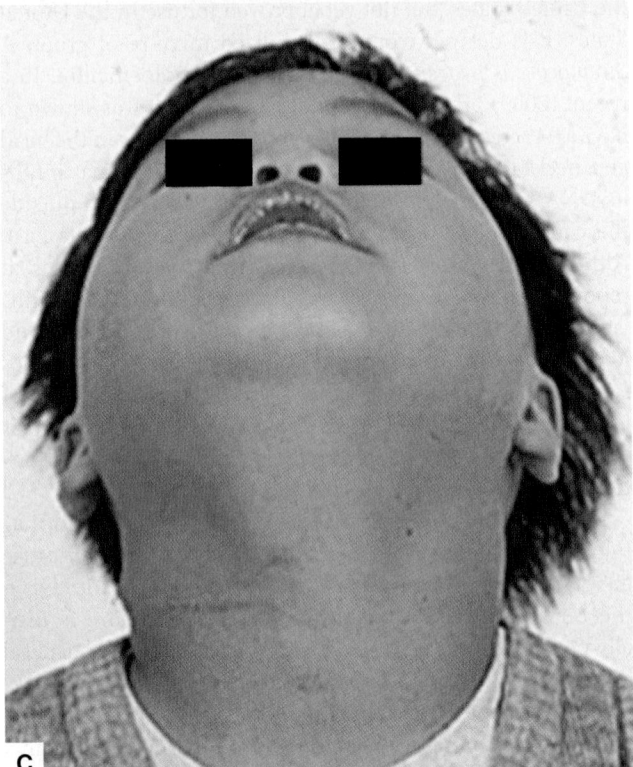

**FIGURE 75-24** Macrocystic cervical lymphatic malformation. **A.** Preoperative photo; (**B**) CT image demonstrating extensive macrocystic lesions in the anterior cervical region; (**C**) 12 months postsurgery, the scar is acceptable and there is no evidence of recurrence.

additional treatment. Those who are symptomatic, however, may require additional procedures.

Debulking in patients with overgrowth is important to facilitate function and improve mobility. This often involves staged procedures. Closed suction drains may be required in the setting of prolonged lymphatic leakage that occurs following surgical debulking.

Laser therapy is often helpful in treating the cutaneous lymphatic blebs that overlie lymphatic malformations and are often within resection scars. These blebs often leak lymphatic fluid. Laser ablation helps prevent leakage and may prevent cellulitis, as the blebs can be a bacterial portal of entry. Lymphatic vesicles often recur and annual retreatment is often necessary.

Sirolimus (rapamycin), a pharmacologic agent described previously in this chapter has been used at our institution for the management of patients with pleural and visceral lesions and lesions with bone involvement, and an ongoing prospective clinical trial is underway. To date, our experience indicates that when sirolimus is used as an adjunct to surgery, it improves overall outcome and helps resolve chylothoraces. Moreover, soft-tissue lesions improve dramatically. Because sirolimus is known to impair wound healing, it must be used with caution in patients undergoing extensive surgery.

## LYMPHANGIOMATOSES

In an effort to establish a classification schema and uniform nomenclature for the spectrum of diseases historically referred to as *lymphangiomatoses*, a consensus group comprising both clinicians and vascular biologists was formed in 2011. Although the group has yet to complete its work, there is general agreement that lymphangiomatoses are extremely rare, are characterized by a profuse proliferation of lymphatic vessels, and can affect internal organs, bones, soft tissue, and/or skin. Additionally, they are most common in children and young adults. Other names for lymphangiomatoses or similar conditions that appear in the literature include generalized lymphangioma, systemic cystic angiomatosis, multiple lymphangiectasis, generalized lymphatic malformation, generalized lymphatic anomaly, and diffuse lymphatic malformation. Being mindful of the widespread confusion that exists, we will present an overview of 3 related clinical entities thought to fall within the broad spectrum of lymphangiomatoses (Fig. 75-25A–E).

## The Gorham Disease

Initially described in 1955, the Gorham disease (also referred to in the literature as the Gorham–Stout disease, vanishing

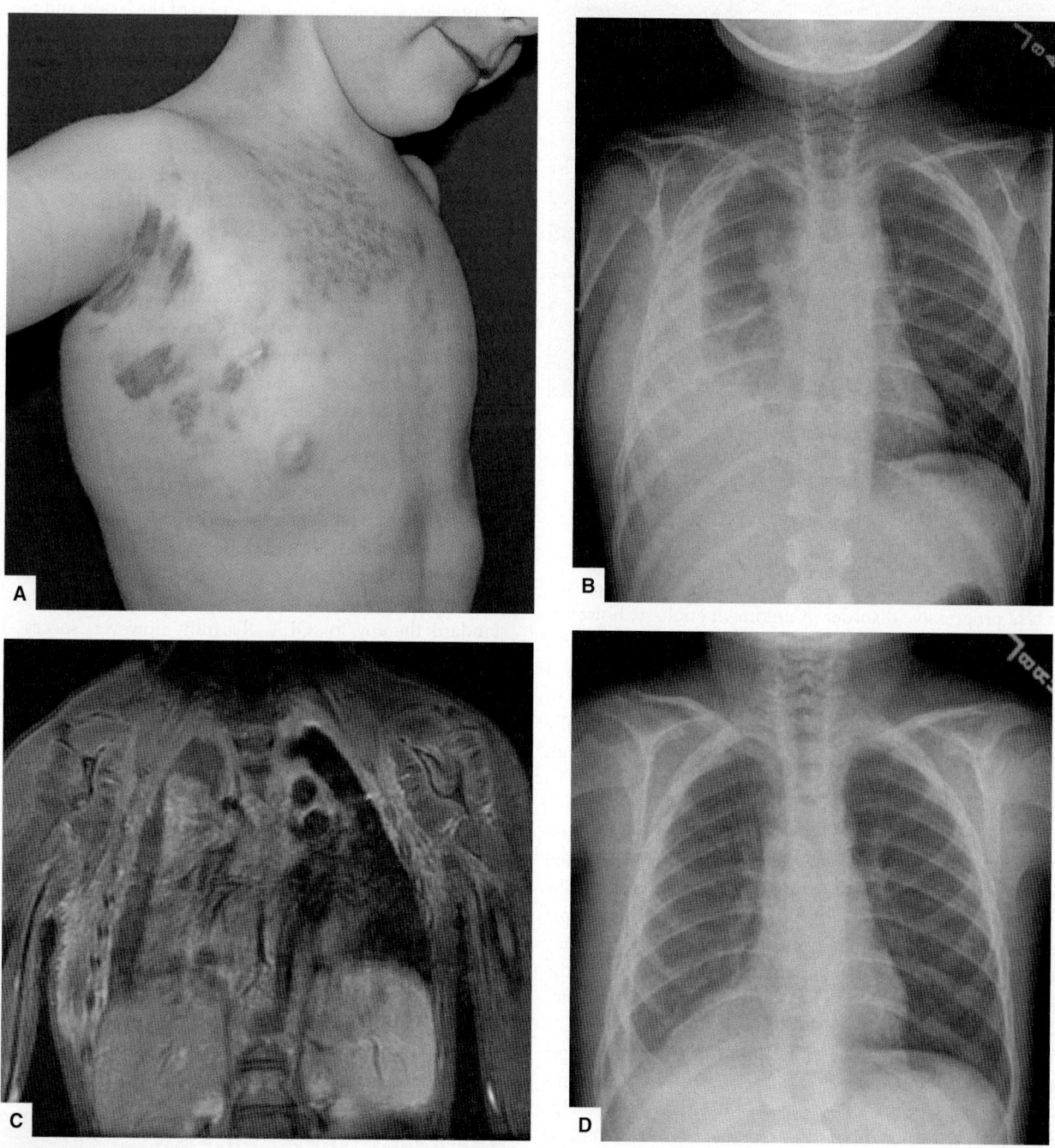

**FIGURE 75-25** Diffuse lymphangiomatosis. **A.** A 7-year-old boy with rapidly progressive microcystic lymphatic malformation involving chest wall and mediastinum. **B.** A chest radiograph clearly demonstrating chylous effusions on the right. **C.** MRI confirming the wide extent through the entire anterior and posterior chest wall and mediastinum. The pleural effusions recurred after thoracoscopic debridement, mechanical, and chemical pleural abrasion, and prolonged chest drainage; (**D**) following rapamycin treatment, the effusions resolved within 3 weeks and the malformation regressed over several months. The patient is now 6 years following therapy and requires maintenance rapamycin to prevent recurrence.

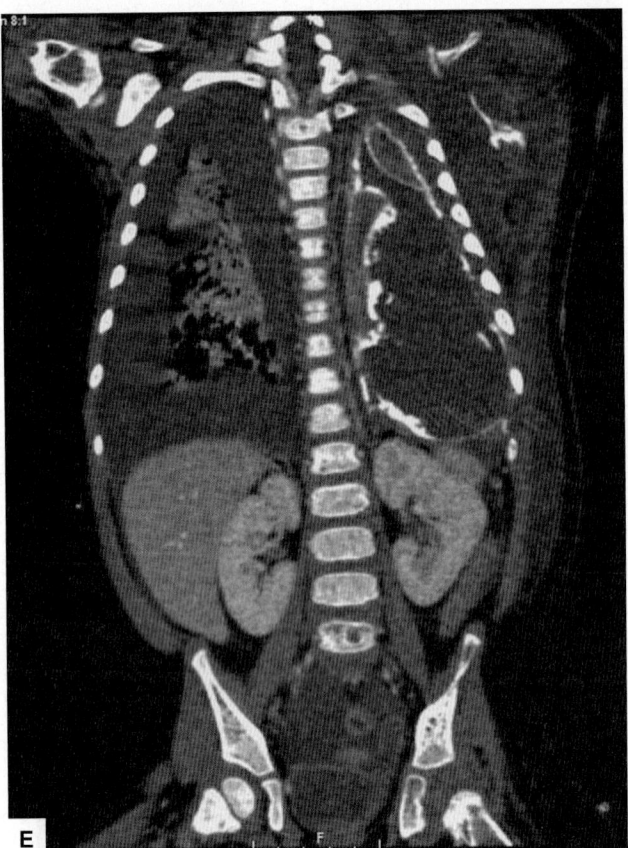

**FIGURE 75-25** (*Continued*) E. MRI documenting lumbar vertebral and left scapula lytic bone involvement in another child the Gorham disease associated with extensive pleural and mediastinal LM.

bone disease, phantom bone, idiopathic or progressive massive osteolysis, hemangiomatosis, and lymphangiomatosis) is a rare progressive disorder of unknown etiology; however, in some patients, the onset of the disorder is associated with a minor traumatic event. The disease is characterized by a proliferation of thin-walled lymphatic channels, resulting in destruction and resorption of the osseous matrix. It usually occurs in children and adults younger than age 40, although most patients are diagnosed around the onset of puberty. To date, no genetic or familial link has been described.

The clinical presentation of the Gorham disease varies, depending on the site of involvement. It may develop at any site, but commonly involves the shoulder, spine, pelvic girdle, and skull. Patients can present with pain, swelling, pathologic fractures, or skeletal deformity. Additionally, the disease may involve chylous pericardial and pleural effusions due to the mediastinal extension of the lesions within the ribs or vertebrae (Fig. 75-25E).

The diagnosis is based on clinical examination, radiologic imaging studies, and histopathologic examination. Plain films may reveal osteolytic lesions, whereas MRI is extremely helpful in assessing the extent of soft tissue and bony involvement as well as possible visceral involvement. If possible, biopsy of the lesion is the most definitive means of establishing the diagnosis. Thoracentesis confirms the presence of chylothorax in patients with pleural effusions.

Because there is no standard therapy for the disease, multimodal treatment is required. Until recently, interferon alfa-2b therapy along with the administration of anti-osteoclastic medications such as bisphosphonates, were used to stabilize patients and prevent disease progression. Unfortunately, however, outcomes with this combined regimen are inconsistent. Patients may also respond to sirolimus and are being included in the prospective clinical trial that is currently underway; a complete analysis of study results is not yet available. Radiation therapy with moderate doses (30 to 45 Gy) may arrest endothelial cell proliferation, thereby limiting the spread of the disease. Also, it may aid in the management of resistant chylothoraces. Nevertheless, the long-term outcome of radiation treatment is unknown. The surgical management of bony lesions can include resection of the lesion and reconstruction using bone grafts or prosthetics. The surgical management of chylothorax can be quite challenging and is often unsuccessful. Pleurodesis, ligation of the thoracic duct, and pleurectomy have all been successful in the management of effusions, though recurrence of pleural effusion is common. Although disease progression is unpredictable, spontaneous regression has been reported. Many lesions stabilize; however, reossification of the affected bone is rare.

## Generalized Lymphatic Anomaly

A number of comparisons between generalized lymphatic anomaly (GLA) and the Gorham disease have been proposed. Whereas GLA is thought by some to be a multifocal, multisystem disorder that may have diffuse bony involvement, the Gorham disease is characterized by progressive regional osteolysis. Unlike the Gorham disease, GLA is not always progressive. The onset of GLA is thought to be more insidious than the onset of the Gorham disease. Additionally, GLA is associated with more visceral involvement as well as a greater number of macrocystic lymphatic malformations, particularly splenic. As with the Gorham disease, there is no standard therapy for GLA. Recently, however, success has reportedly been achieved in several patients with the use of sirolimus.

## Kaposiform Lymphangiomatosis

Of the 3 disease entities included in our discussion of lymphangiomatoses, kaposiform lymphangiomatosis (KLA) is the least well characterized. KLA is a diffuse lymphatic anomaly, usually arising with skeleton and lung involvement; however, it may also involve large anatomic areas. Histopathologic examination reveals spindled lymphatic endothelial proliferation. These spindled cells resemble other kaposiform vascular tumors such as KHE. Patients may have mild thrombocytopenia and hemorrhage in the lungs, which may be fatal. A wide variety of chemotherapeutic agents, including vincristine, have been used.

## LYMPHANGIECTASIAS

### Diffuse Lymphangiectasia

Children with extensive lymphatic malformations of more than 1 extremity sometimes have diffuse lymphangiectasia, which may involve the lungs, liver, and gastrointestinal tract.

In this setting, malabsorption and protein-losing enteropathy become a life-threatening problem. Treatment is primarily supportive and the outcome is poor.

## Primary Intestinal Lymphangiectasia

Primary intestinal lymphangiectasia (also called the Waldmann disease) is a rare disorder of unknown etiology that is characterized by the presence of dilated intestinal lacteals and lymphatic channels throughout all intestinal layers and the mesentery. The disorder can be congenital or secondary to other disorders. Symptoms may include abdominal pain, nausea, vomiting, diarrhea, steatorrhea, failure to thrive, growth retardation, and hypocalcemic seizures. The disorder can be associated with lymphedema of the extremities and chylous effusions in the peritoneum and pleura, in addition to other abnormalities such as lymphoma, lymphopenia, impaired neutrophil function with impaired cell-mediated immunity, and splenic atrophy. Also, syndromes are known to be associated with intestinal lymphangiectasia. These include von Recklinghausen, Turner or Noonan, Klippel–Trenaunay, and Hennekam syndromes.

Radiologic studies are useful in establishing the differential diagnosis; however, the diagnosis is confirmed by endoscopic intestinal biopsy. The diagnosis is generally established by age 3.

The primary treatment of intestinal lymphangiectasia is supportive, consisting of the correction of fluid and electrolyte imbalance and dietary manipulation. A low-fat, high-protein diet supplemented with medium-chain triglycerides is recommended. The absence of fat prevents engorgement of intestinal lymphatic vessels and helps prevent rupture of the lacteals. Other treatments that have been used include steroids, octreotide, and anti-plasmin. Surgical resection of localized disease can be helpful in controlling symptoms. Small bowel transplantation holds promise for patients in whom medical management fails.

## Congenital Pulmonary Lymphangiectasia

Congenital pulmonary lymphangiectasia is a rare disorder thought to be caused by a diffuse dysplasia of the lymphatic network. It is characterized by dilation of the pulmonary lymphatics that drain from the subpleural and interstitial spaces of the lung. Autopsy results suggest that 0.5% to 1% of infants who die in the neonatal period have pulmonary lymphangiectasia. Cases are thought to be sporadic, although associations with Noonan syndrome, Down syndrome, and Ulrich Turner syndrome have been described. Patients can present in utero with hydrops fetalis and pleural effusions. Many newborns present with intractable respiratory distress, which is often associated with significant chylous pleural effusions. The disease may also present as an isolated pulmonary lesion, as part of generalized lymphangiectasias, or as secondary to severe pulmonary venous hypertension or venous obstruction.

The diagnosis is made through the correlation of clinical presentation with radiologic and pathologic studies. Increased interstitial markings, hyperexpansion, and pleural effusions may be evident on a chest radiograph. Chest CT scans show ground-glass infiltrates, interstitial densities, and pleural effusions. Lung biopsy is the most definitive means of establishing a definitive diagnosis; biopsy reveals dilated lymphatics within the interstitium of the lung.

Treatment of this disease is primarily supportive and includes gentle ventilation strategies, extracorporeal membrane oxygenation (ECMO), and nutritional support. Localized lesions are sometimes amenable to surgery. For patients who present during the neonatal period, the prognosis is especially poor despite advances in neonatal intensive care.

# LYMPHEDEMA

Lymphedema is a general term that refers to specific pathologic conditions characterized by regional accumulation of excessive amounts of interstitial protein-rich fluid. It can be either a primary (ie, idiopathic) condition or a secondary condition caused by trauma, neoplasia, infection, filariasis, radiotherapy, or excision of lymph nodes. Lymphedema generally involves abnormalities in the lymphatic drainage of the extremities, although visceral lymphatic abnormalities can also occur.

Primary lymphedemas are frequently classified according to the age at which the edema becomes apparent. Two types of primary lymphedemas are seen in the pediatric population—congenital lymphedema and lymphedema praecox. Both types are rare and generally affect patients younger than age 20. Congenital lymphedema (Milroy disease) infrequently presents in the antenatal period with pleural effusions or hydrops fetalis. It is usually evident at birth or becomes apparent within the first 2 years of life (Fig. 75-26). Lymphedema praecox is most commonly noticed during puberty, though it may appear as late as the third decade of life. It is the most common form of primary lymphedema, accounting for up to 94% of cases in large reported series. The estimated female preponderance (10:1) suggests the involvement of estrogenic hormones.

In patients with congenital lymphedema, the swelling can involve only a single lower extremity; however, edema of multiple limbs, the genitals, and even the face is sometimes seen. Bilateral leg swelling and involvement of the entire lower extremity is reportedly more common in patients with congenital lymphedema than in those with other forms of primary lymphedema. When presentation occurs early in the postnatal period, painless, soft, nonpitting swelling is observed. An autosomal dominant pattern of transmission is frequently described for cases that cluster in families. Mutations in the VEGFR3, FOXC2, SOX18, and CCBE1 genes have been identified as possible molecular causes in some of these kindreds.

Primary lymphedema is associated with other congenital anomalies as well as several genetic syndromes. Associated anomalies include intestinal and thoracic lymphangiectasias, chylous ascites, chylothorax, lymphangiomatosis, congenital heart disease, and Fabry disease. Genetic syndromes include Noonan and Turner syndrome, yellow-nail syndrome, cerebrovascular malformations, and distichiasis (duplication of eyelashes).

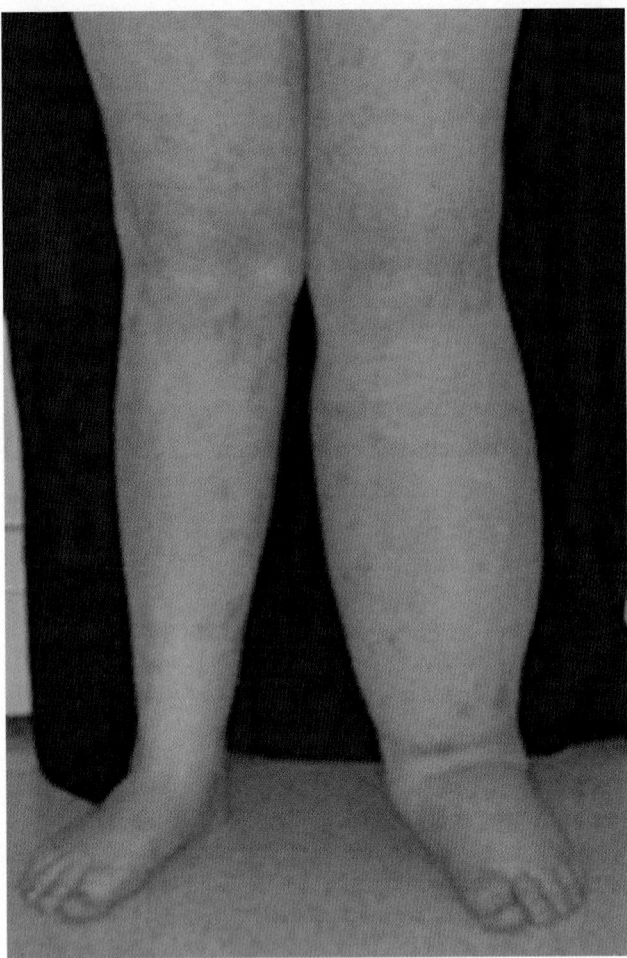

**FIGURE 75-26** Congenital lymphedema.

The clinical course of primary lymphedema is unpredictable, with some cases remaining stable and others progressing to a huge deforming extremity with functional impairment. Anatomic, postural, and lifestyle factors (eg, physical activity level) may act in a congenitally deficient lymphatic system, causing stasis of lymphatic fluid and exacerbating lymphedema. Complications include lymphangitis, cellulitis, functional disabilities, and cosmetic and psychological problems.

The diagnosis of primary lymphedema is established by a thorough clinical history and physical examination. Additionally, a Doppler venous study and a complete assessment of the vascular system should be performed to exclude the possible presence of associated venous and arterial abnormalities. Lymphoscintigraphy can be used to confirm the diagnosis. In older children and adolescents, it is important to rule out extraabdominal and iliofemoral compression by a pelvic mass as a secondary etiology of the lymphedema. CT venography and biopsy of the mass may be helpful in making the distinction.

Most patients with lymphedema respond to nonsurgical treatment. Supportive stockings and elastic garments worn throughout the day, combined with intermittent pneumatic compression used overnight, are also effective in controlling disease. Skin care is extremely important, and infection must be promptly treated with antibiotics. If infection is not managed aggressively, it can lead to progressive and irreversible swelling over time.

Surgical debulking may be necessary to improve function and allow for mobility in most debilitated patients. This is done by creating vascularized cutaneous flaps and resecting excess skin and subcutaneous tissue but preserving underlying fascia and muscle; the redundant skin is then trimmed, leaving the patient with an improved, functional extremity contour. Medial and lateral reductions are accomplished with a staged approach, leaving a 6- to 9-month interval between procedures. When preserving the involved skin is unfeasible, skin and subcutaneous tissue are excised and split thickness skin grafts are used to cover underlying muscle and fascia. Complications are common and include poor wound healing, lymphatic leakage, and postoperative infection. Families should be made aware of these potential problems before surgical debulking procedures are undertaken.

## ARTERIAL MALFORMATIONS

Arterial malformations are almost always asymptomatic until late in life, when their presence may be revealed by coexistent acquired arterial disease. True generalized dilatation occurring primarily without evidence of arteriovenous fistulae or of atherosclerosis is extremely rare.

## ARTERIOVENOUS MALFORMATIONS

AVMs are congenital vascular lesions associated with a variable degree of arteriovenous shunting. Some of these lesions are thought to originate from arteriovenous connections that have failed to regress during development. No clear genetic etiology has been described; however, a mutation in the *PTEN* gene (a tumor suppressor gene) has been described in some patients with extracranial AVMs.

These fast-flow communications between arteries and veins are among the most dangerous vascular connecting channels. They vary in diameter from several millimeters to the size of the normal precapillary anastomosis. The length of the channels between the arteries and the veins can vary from millimeters to centimeters, and convoluted or cavernous abnormal vascular structures may be intercalated between the arterial and venous ends of the malformation. The fast-flow character of AVMs usually becomes evident in childhood or during puberty (Fig. 75-27). Rapid expansion has been reported following pregnancy, trauma, or inadequate surgical intervention. AVMs most commonly occur in the head and neck, but trunk and extremity involvement is also seen. Diffuse AVMs are encountered particularly in the limbs and more frequent in lower than in upper limbs. Localized malformations are composed of a mass of abnormal intercalated tissues and can occur in any organ.

Owing to variations in position, size, length, and number, there is a wide pattern of clinical appearance. Nevertheless, these malformations are recognizable by warmth, a palpable thrill, and an audible bruit. MRA demonstrates the location and extent of the anomalous anatomy and is useful for developing a treatment plan. In some patients, angiograms clearly delineate the nidus and multiple connections between the arterial and venous systems.

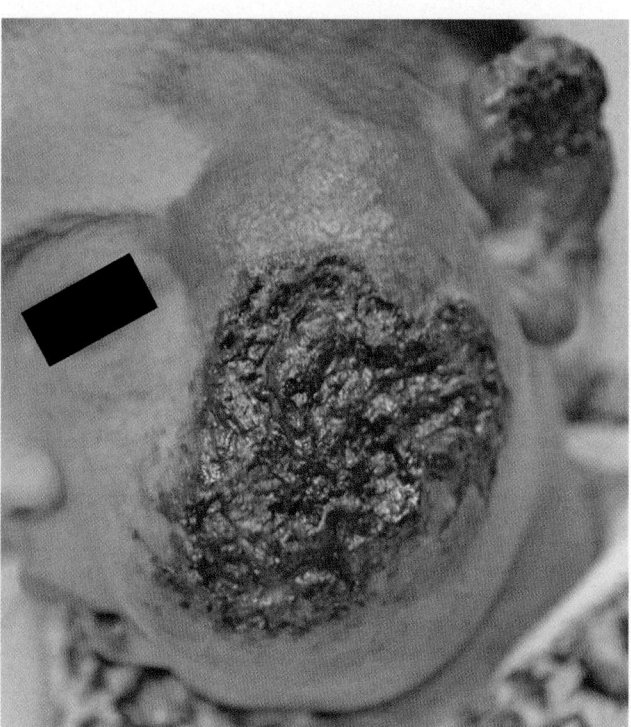

**FIGURE 75-27** Massive arteriovenous malformation involving the entire left face and neck. Patient shows ulceration and breakdown of the malformation with congestive heart failure (Schöbinger Stage IV).

Once the diagnosis has been established, patients should be closely monitored and a baseline echocardiogram should be performed. When a lesion is small and asymptomatic, a period of observation is often the most prudent initial strategy. Often, pain, expansion of the lesion, ulceration, bleeding, or cardiac decompensation may occur after a quiescent period. If patients are symptomatic, active treatment is indicated. Intraarterial embolization of the nidus combined with surgical excision offers the best chance for cure; however, complete excision may be impossible because of location and extent of the malformation. Complex lesions require creative operations, tailored to individual pathology and anatomy. When lesions cannot be excised, palliative embolization may be appropriate to control symptoms. Embolization techniques include the use of metal coils, particles, and glues such as Onyx® (ethylene vinyl alcohol copolymer) (Fig. 75-27). Close follow-up is important, as lesions often recur. For extremity lesions, amputation may eventually be required. Long-term complications include cardiac hypertrophy, cardiac failure, and cardiac instability, as well as hemorrhage and stroke.

## OTHER COMPLEX COMBINED VASCULAR MALFORMATIONS

### Capillary-Lymphatico-Venous Malformations

Capillary-lymphatico-venous malformations (CLVMs) are the most common complex combined vascular anomaly. This constellation of findings was first reported by French physicians, Maurice Klippel and Paul Trénaunay, in 1900, and for more than a century, the eponym, *Klippel–Trénaunay syndrome*, has been used to describe patients with CLVM. In contemporary literature, CLVM is also sometimes incorrectly referred to as *Klippel–Trénaunay–Weber* syndrome—a designation that implies an association with Parkes Weber syndrome. As discussed later in this chapter, however, Parkes Weber syndrome is a fast-flow lesion composed of a capillary-arteriovenous malformation (CAVM) or a capillary-arteriovenous-lymphatic malformation (CAVLM) in association with limb hypertrophy.

CLVM is a slow-flow anomaly that occurs sporadically and with equal gender distribution. To date, no linkage with a causative gene has been identified; however, the angiogenic growth factor gene *AGGF1* has been identified as a putative gene. The classic presentation is an infant with an enlarged lower extremity with lateral capillary malformations, lymphatic vesicles, and visible varicosities. Nonetheless, morphologic variability is quite common. More specifically, a large ($n = 252$) study of CLVM patients conducted at the Mayo Clinic found lower extremity involvement, upper extremity involvement, and trunk involvement in 88%, 29%, and 23% of patients, respectively. The disfigurement can range from light capillary staining with mild soft tissue overgrowth to gross deformity of the anatomic area of involvement. Soft tissue and skeletal hypertrophy of the extremity predominate; however, in 10% of patients, this extremity may be short or hypotrophic. Although severe cases are sometimes detected on antenatal imaging, CLVM is usually diagnosed at birth. Congenital lymphedema, CAVM, CLOVES (described later in this chapter), and Proteus syndromes are included in the differential diagnosis.

Lymphatic malformations may arise in the buttock/perineum and in the pelvis, presenting as lymphedema or lymphatic cysts. As the child ages, lymphatic blebs frequently appear, most commonly arising in areas of the capillary malformation.

Venous malformations are heterogeneous. They can arise as focal lesions, varicosities, phlebectasias, hypoplastic or aplastic vessels, or veins with absent or incompetent valves. These malformations can extend into the perineum, pelvis, and retroperitoneum. Most patients in our practice have persistent embryonic veins, most common of which are the vein of Servelle (the lateral marginal vein) and the sciatic vein.

A wide spectrum of severity is seen in the degree of soft tissue and bony hypertrophy. Some patients exhibit severe bony hypertrophy combined with significant soft tissue overgrowth of fatty tissues, whereas others have only mild overgrowth of subcutaneous tissue. The presence of macrodactyly, syndactyly, clinodactyly, polydactyly, or ectrodactyly has also been documented (Fig. 75-28A–C).

Given that high-quality imaging studies in infants and young children require general anesthesia, unless there is an urgent indication for imaging, it is generally delayed until the child is 6 years of age. Such an indication may include hematochezia, bladder outlet obstruction, and a required surgical intervention. Radiographs are useful in evaluating bony deformities and delineating limb length discrepancies. Duplex US provides morphologic information regarding the size of veins, perforators, and venous valve competence. MRI

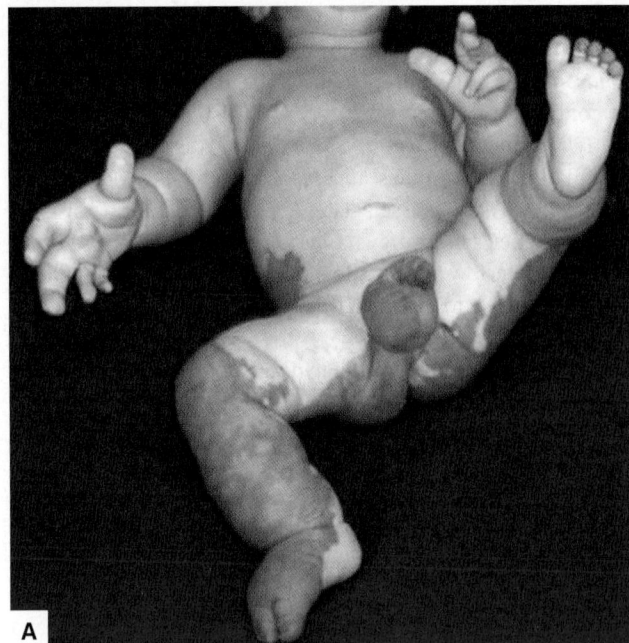

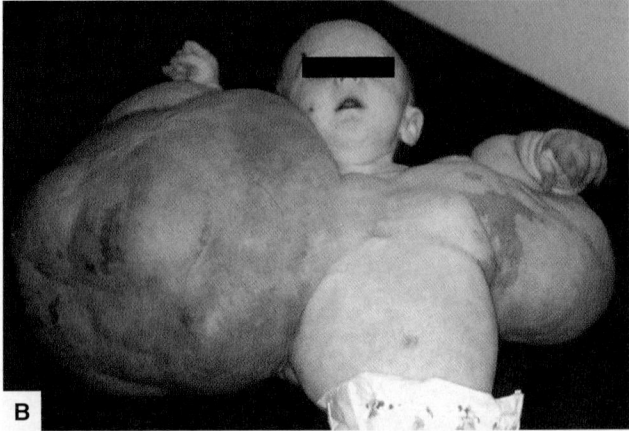

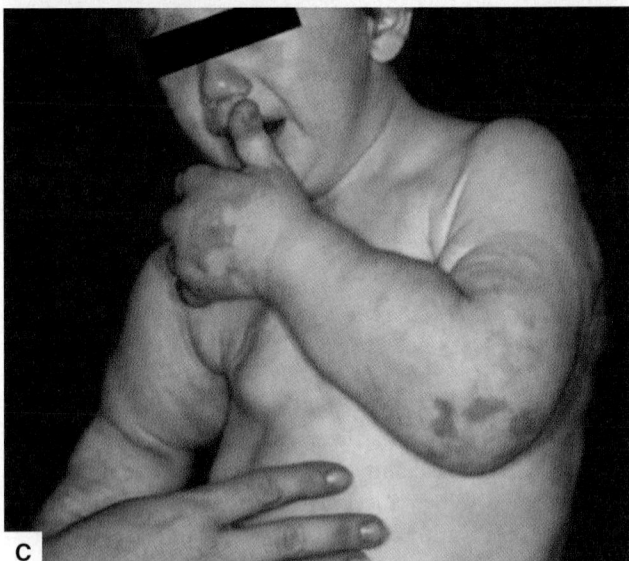

**FIGURE 75-28** Two infants with extensive CVLMs. **A.** Extensive involvement of the torso and both lower extremities. This child has overgrowth and macrodactyly of his fingers in addition to his CVLM; (**B**) this second infant has bilateral torso, axillary, and upper extremity involvement. **C.** The child required multiple sequential resections but has highly functional extremities and an excellent quality of life.

and MR venography (MRV) are the best imaging modalities for assessing the type, location, and extent of the vascular malformation. Soft tissue and bony overgrowth can also be characterized. MRV delineates the extremity veins and demonstrates the anomalous venous channels. Conventional venography can be particularly helpful in confirming the continuity of any deep venous system before undertaking endovascular or surgical intervention.

## Management

Patients with CLVM often have low-grade coagulopathies with elevated D-dimer levels and low fibrinogen levels. Complications such as deep venous thrombosis and pulmonary embolism are not uncommon. Patients with these complications are routinely screened for genetic polymorphisms associated with prothrombotic tendencies. Those who undergo elective surgical procedures and who have identified coagulation abnormalities require both mechanical and pharmacological antiembolism prophylaxis with low-molecular-weight heparin. Lovenox® is thus commonly administered daily for 2 weeks preoperatively and 2 weeks postoperatively, or until the patient regains full mobility. High-risk patients with previously documented pulmonary emboli may require the

placement of retrievable inferior vena cava filters prior to complex surgical procedures.

Chronic lymphedema, poor skin integrity, venous stasis, and open lymphatic vesicles predispose CLVM patients to cellulitis. To minimize this risk, patients are counseled on proper skin hygiene. Patients with recurrent cellulitis may require antibiotic prophylaxis.

Management of these complex patients requires the close collaboration of an interdisciplinary team. Wearing tailored compression garments that provide 30 to 40 mm Hg compression is the mainstay of nonoperative treatment, as this minimizes swelling from lymphedema, chronic venous insufficiency, and lymphatic vesicles. Early initiation of compression therapy generally fosters better adherence during adolescence and adulthood. Pneumatic lymphatic pumps are also useful when there is a significant lymphedema component.

## Procedural Management

Surgical resection of anomalous superficial veins that are often symptomatic can be undertaken using cardiovascular radiofrequency ablation or open surgical techniques. Prior to resecting or ablating symptomatic embryonic veins, care must be taken to ensure there is a patent deep venous system.

Depending on symptoms and the location, extent, and type of malformation, sclerotherapy can be an important adjunctive therapy.

In view of the psychological benefit of minimizing the child's disfigurement as well as the advantage of minimizing soft tissue infections, surgical debulking is also undertaken when appropriate. The primary criterion for deciding whether debulking of an extremity is a viable approach is the location of the overgrowth. Debulking of intrafascial overgrowth is imprudent due to morbidity associated with muscle resection and possible injury to neurovascular structures. Because of morphologic variations in the presentation of CLVM, debulking procedures must be individually tailored, with the aim of removing as much excess weight and bulk as possible (Fig. 75-28B,C). Nonetheless, for some anatomic sites (eg, genitalia), adopting a "less is more" approach to debulking may achieve the best long-term functional outcomes. Sclerotherapy can also be used preoperatively to facilitate debulking.

Most patients with CLVM require an orthopedic consultation to assess (1) the need for and timing of procedures to correct leg length discrepancies, (2) the need for extremity amputation, and (3) the need for management of intra-articular disease. Limb length discrepancies are known to occur in close to 70% of patients, and these patients have an average limb length discrepancy of 1.75 cm. In that prediction of limb length discrepancies is extremely difficult, annual orthopaedic assessments should begin in infancy. Patients with upper extremity discrepancies and leg discrepancies of <1.0 cm require no therapeutic interventions. Those with leg discrepancies ranging from 1.0 to 2.5 cm are typically managed with heel lifts. Those with leg discrepancies >2.5 cm are frequently managed with epiphysiodesis at the distal femoral and/or proximal tibial growth plates at 11 to 12 years of age.

Amputation is indicated for patients in whom lower-extremity deformities prevent ambulation. The level of the amputation is determined by the extent of the deformity. For example, marked foot enlargement and the inability to wear shoes may require digit or transmetatarsal amputations to facilitate ambulation. Venous malformations are sometimes associated with an intra-articular extension, most commonly in the knee joint. This can limit range of motion and cause pain, and can also be associated with hemarthroses, arthropathy, and significant arthritis. Sclerotherapy to adjacent aberrant vessels, together with the removal of the intra-articular malformation, has become the mainstay of managing these difficult problems.

## Capillary-Arteriovenous Malformation and Capillary Arteriovenous Fistulae

Formerly referred to as *Parkes Weber syndrome*, CAVM and capillary-arteriovenous fistulae (CAVF) are combined malformations characterized by the presence of a confluent capillary malformation with underlying multiple micro-arteriovenous fistulae in association with soft tissue and skeletal hypertrophy of the affected limb (Fig. 75-29A,B).

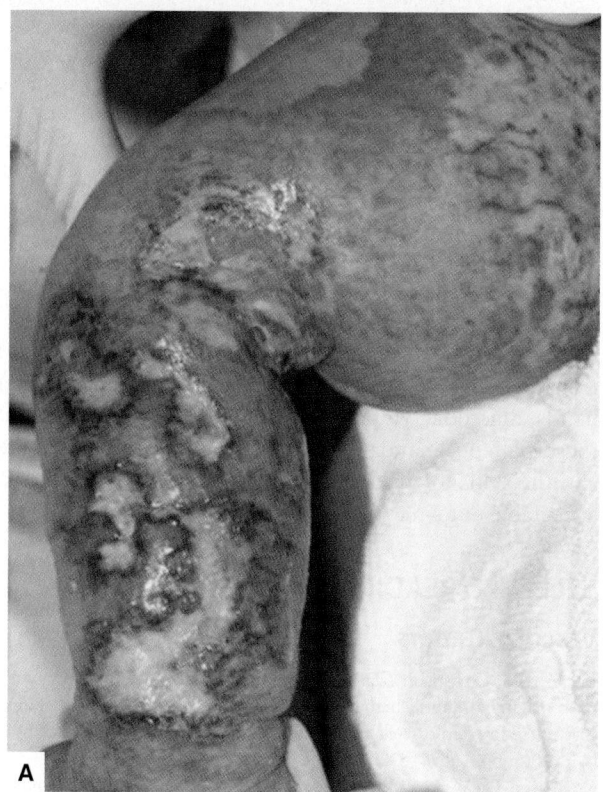
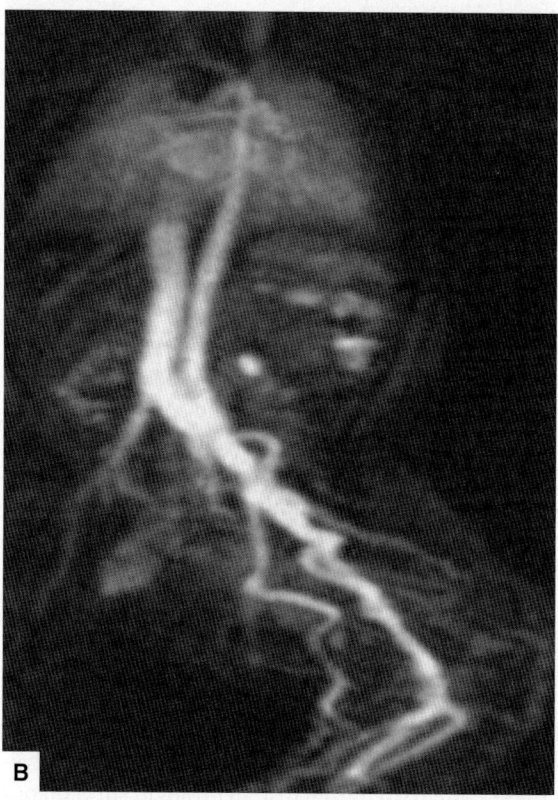

**FIGURE 75-29** The Parkes Weber syndrome: CAVM. A. Extensive ulcerations in the involve extremity from arteriovenous shunting and a steal phenomenon causing skin ischemia and necrosis. B. MRA documenting rapid shunting from the left iliac and femoral arterial tree into the iliac veins and inferior vena cava.

Commonly, there is also an associated lymphatic component (CAVLM). Mutations in the *RASA-1* gene, either de novo or inherited, have been identified in patients with CAVM who have multifocal capillary malformations. According to a recent report of 44 families with *RASA-1* mutations, all patients had capillary malformations and one third had fast-flow malformations.

At birth, the affected infant is noted to exhibit diffuse enlargement of the involved limb, which is most commonly a lower extremity. The stained areas are usually warm, with a palpable thrill. Doppler US demonstrates fast flow and low-resistance runoff in the areas of capillary staining. Radiographs can document limb length discrepancies and lytic lesions within the bone. Contrast-enhanced T2-weighted MRI sequences reveal arteriovenous shunting flow voids and the extensive diffuse nature of the malformation. Angiography more precisely reveals discrete arteriovenous shunts. This is particularly useful when endovascular treatment is being considered.

CAVM and CAVLM patients are optimally managed in an interdisciplinary setting. Management is based on presenting symptoms and functional issues and is tailored according to individual needs; however, cardiac function, extremity overgrowth, and pain and ulceration related to ischemia are always closely monitored. Patients have a risk of developing cardiac overload over their lifetime. Although this is generally well tolerated, hypertrophic cardiomyopathy can develop secondary to massive arteriovenous fistulae. If this occurs, patients may require repetitive superselective embolization, and occasionally, surgical debulking or amputation.

## CLOVES SYNDROME

CLOVES syndrome is a newly recognized constellation of anomalies that consists of *c*ongenital *l*ipomatous *o*vergrowth, *v*ascular malformations, *e*pidermal nevi, and *s*keletal anomalies. Truncal lipomatous masses, vascular malformations, and acral/musculoskeletal anomalies typically predominate, although the diagnosis can be established without the presence of all of these characteristic clinical features (Fig. 75-30A,B).

Lipomatous masses in patients with CLOVES are hypervascular and can exhibit rapid recurrence following surgical resection. These masses are infiltrative and commonly extend from the trunk into adjacent areas such as the retroperitoneum, mediastinum, and thoracic cavity. In many patients, involvement of the spinal column and extension into the epidural space is associated with nerve root and spinal cord compression.

Capillary malformations, lymphatic malformations, and lymphatic vesicles are often seen over and abutting truncal lipomatous masses. Ectatic veins may cause deep vein thrombosis or pulmonary emboli during postoperative convalescence. Close to one third of patients are known to have perispinal AVMs in the region of truncal involvement. These patients require close neurologic surveillance and may need interventional and/or surgical procedures to mitigate neurologic morbidity. Embolization is an essential adjunct in managing these patients. Scoliosis has been

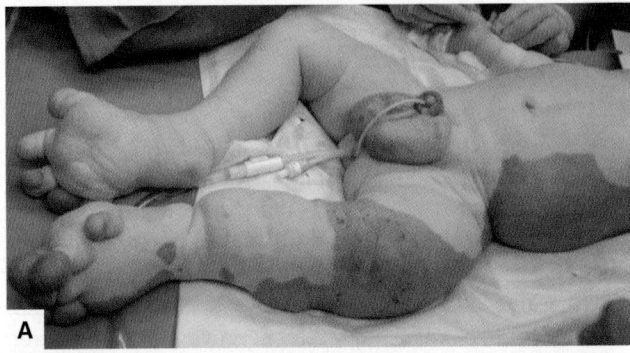

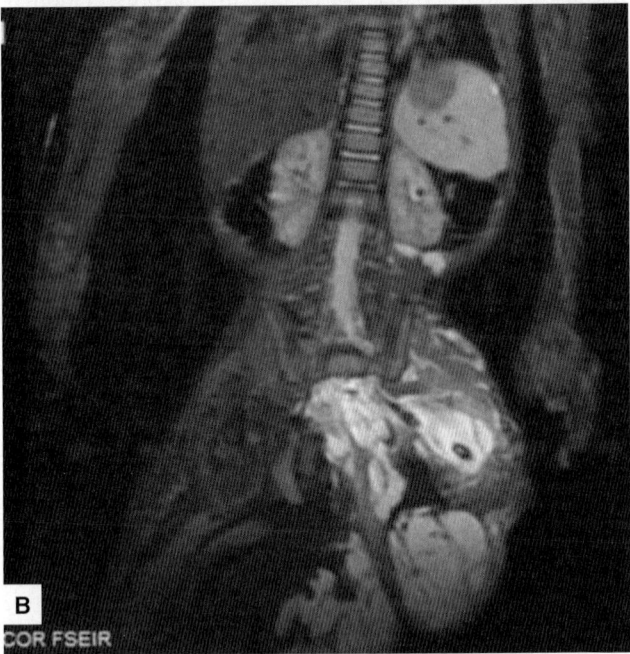

**FIGURE 75-30** An infant with CLOVES syndrome. **A.** The patient has features of dramatic somatic overgrowth. Some of the malformation is composed hamartomatous and excessive adipose tissue in addition to the macrodactyly and complex CVLM. **B.** MRI demonstrates extensive infiltration of the venous lymphatic malformation throughout the involved extremities and torso.

observed in close to 50% of patients with CLOVES, and many require spine stabilization.

Musculoskeletal abnormalities most commonly involve the feet and hands. Acral deformities include large, wide feet and hands, macrodactyly, and a wide sandal gap. Management of these patients mandates special expertise, good judgment, and the skills to ensure that the patient has a functional and acceptable outcome.

## SELECTED READINGS

### Vascular Tumors

Barnés CM, Christison-Lagay EA, Folkman J. The placenta theory and the origin of infantile hemangioma. *Lymphat Res Biol* 2007;5:245–255.

Bischoff J. Progenitor cells in infantile hemangioma. *J Craniofac Surg* 2009; 20(Suppl 1):696–697.

Christison-Lagay ER, Burrows PE, Alomari A, et al. Hepatic hemangiomas: subtype classification and development of a clinical practice algorithm and registry. *J Pediatr Surg* 2007;42:62–68.

Dickie B, Dasgupta R, Nair R, et al. Spectrum of hepatic hemangiomas: management and outcome. *J Pediatr Surg* 2009;44:125–133.

Drolet BA, Chamlin SL, Garzon MC, et al. Prospective study of spinal anomalies in children with infantile hemangiomas of the lumbosacral skin. *J Pediatr* 2010;157:789–794.

Frieden IJ, Rogers M, Garzon MC. Conditions masquerading as infantile haemangioma: part 1. *Australas J Dermatol* 2009;50:77–99.

Frieden IJ, Rogers M, Garzon MC. Conditions masquerading as infantile haemangioma: part 2. *Australas J Dermatol* 2009;50:153–170.

Gruman A, Liang MG, Mulliken JB, et al. Kaposiform hemangioendothelioma without Kasabach–Merritt phenomenon. *J Am Acad Dermatol* 2005;52:616–622.

Lyons LL, North PE, Mac-Moune Lai F, et al. Kaposiform hemangioendothelioma: a study of 33 cases emphasizing its pathologic, immunophenotypic, and biologic uniqueness from juvenile hemangioma. *Am J Surg Pathol* 2004;28:559–568.

Metry DW, Haggstrom AN, Drolet BA, et al. A prospective study of PHACE syndrome in infantile hemangiomas: demographic features, clinical findings, and complications. *Am J Med Genet A* 2006;140:975–986.

Mulliken JB, Enjolras O. Congenital hemangiomas and infantile hemangioma: missing links. *J Am Acad Dermatol* 2004;50:875–882.

North PE, Waner M, James CA, et al. Congenital nonprogressive hemangioma: a distinct clinicopathologic entity unlike infantile hemangioma. *Arch Dermatol* 2001;137:1607–1620.

Sarkar M, Mulliken JB, Kozakewich HP, Robertson RL, Burrows PE. Thrombocytopenic coagulopathy (Kasabach–Merritt phenomenon) is associated with Kaposiform hemangioendothelioma and not with common infantile hemangioma. *Plast Reconstr Surg* 1997;100:1377–1386.

The Hemangioma Investigator Group: Haggstrom AN, Drolet BA, Baselga E, et al. *J Pediatr* 2007;150:291–294.

## Vascular Malformations

Azizkhan RG. Vascular anomalies of childhood. In: Fischer JE, Bland KI, editors. *Master of Surgery*, 5th ed., vol 1. Philadelphia: Lippincott Williams & Wilkins; 2007:343–357.

Blei F. Congenital lymphatic malformations. *Ann NY Acad Sci* 2008;1131:185–194.

Bruder E, Perez-Atayde AR, Jundt G, et al. Vascular lesions of bone in children, adolescents, and young adults. A clinicopathologic reappraisal and application of the ISSVA classification. *Virchows Arch* 2009;454:161–179.

Donaldson JS. Pediatric vascular anomalies: the role of imaging and interventional radiology. *Pediatr Ann* 2008;37:414–424.

Elluru R, Azizkhan RG. Cervicofacial vascular anomalies. II. Vascular malformations. *Sem Pediatr Surg* 2006;15:133–139.

Greene AK, Alomari AI. Management of venous malformations. *Clin Plastic Surg* 2011;38:83–93.

Hammill AM, Wentzel M, Gupta A, et al. Sirolimus for the treatment of complicated vascular anomalies in children. *Pediatr Blood Cancer* 2011;57:1018–1024.

Jacob AG, Driscoll DJ, Shaughnessy WJ, et al. Klippel–Trénaunay syndrome: spectrum and management. *Mayo Clin Proc* 1998;73:28–36.

Kulungowski AM, Fishman SJ. Management of combined vascular malformations. *Clin Plastic Surg* 2011;38:107–120.

Maguiness SM, Liang MG. Management of capillary malformations. *Clin Plastic Surg* 2011;38:65–73.

Poldervaart MT, Breugem CC, Speleman L, Pasmans S. Treatment of lymphatic malformations with OK-432 (Picibanil): review of the literature. *J Craniofac Surg* 2009;20:1159–1162.

Rockson SG. Lymphedema. Review. *Am J Med* 2001;110:288–295.

Ruggiere P, Montalti M, Angelini A. Gorham–Stout disease: the experience of the Rizzoli Institute and review of the literature. *Skeletal Radiol* 2011;40:1391–1397.

# PART VII

## NEUROSURGERY FOR THE PEDIATRIC SURGEON

# CHAPTER 76

## Neurosurgery for the Pediatric Surgeon

*Daniel von Allmen*

This chapter focuses on clinical topics in which there is overlap between pediatric neurosurgeons and pediatric general surgeons. Included are discussions on hydrocephalus, congenital spine and brain malformations, and dumbbell spinal tumors.

## HYDROCEPHALUS

Hydrocephalus is defined as a pathologic condition in which ventricular enlargement is associated with elevated intracranial pressure (ICP) that occurs when the amount of cerebrospinal fluid (CSF) produced exceeds the amount absorbed. It is among the most common conditions that pediatric neurosurgeons treat. About 40% of the neurosurgical procedures performed at our institution are directed toward the treatment of hydrocephalus.

### Etiology of Hydrocephalus

CSF is produced at a rate of 0.3 cc/min, regardless of age. The CSF flows from the lateral ventricles to the third ventricle via the foramen of Monro, from the third ventricle to the fourth ventricle through the aqueduct of Sylvius, and out of the fourth ventricle either through the laterally placed foramina of Luschka or through the midline foramen of Magendie. Once out of the ventricular system, the CSF flows into the spinal and cerebral subarachnoid spaces and, ultimately, becomes absorbed into the venous system. The chief site for CSF absorption into the venous system is along the superior sagittal sinus via the arachnoid granulations.

Under ordinary circumstances, CSF production and absorption are matched. Hydrocephalus represents an imbalance between the rate of production and the rate of resorption. Overproduction of CSF (usually by choroid plexus tumors) is very rare. Much more frequently, it is CSF absorption that is impaired. Impairment of CSF absorption can result from a mechanical obstruction within the ventricular system (ie, blockage of flow from 1 ventricle to another) or obstruction within the subarachnoid space at the arachnoid granulations where CSF is absorbed into the bloodstream. The former is known as noncommunicating hydrocephalus, and the latter is referred to as communicating hydrocephalus.

Noncommunicating hydrocephalus can result from obstruction anywhere within the ventricular system but usually occurs at the foramen of Monro, the aqueduct of Sylvius, or the fourth ventricle and its outlet channels. Causes of noncommunicating hydrocephalus include tumors, cysts, inflammatory scarring, intraventricular hemorrhage, and rarely, genetic disorders. Ventricular obstruction at the foramen of Monro can be caused by colloid cysts, subependymal giant cell astrocytomas (in tuberous sclerosis), choroid plexus papillomas and carcinomas, central neurocytomas, and infrequently, intraventricular meningiomas. Obstruction at the aqueduct of Sylvius by a mass lesion can result from gliomas of the midbrain or tectum, pineal region masses, and posterior third ventricular tumors. The fourth ventricle can be obstructed by tumors including medulloblastomas, ependymomas, cerebellar astrocytomas, and brainstem gliomas. Intraventricular or arachnoid cysts located around the third ventricle (ie, suprasellar) or the fourth ventricle can sometimes block CSF flow. Inflammatory responses that lead to scarring can be induced by intraventricular hemorrhage or infection. These stimuli initiate an ependymal reaction leading to obstruction of the CSF pathway. Finally, an X-linked disorder associated with aqueductal stenosis has been identified. This syndrome includes mental deficiency and spasticity and can be associated with other central nervous system anomalies, including agenesis of the corpus callosum, fusion of the thalami, and atrophy of the pons and corticospinal tracts.

Causes of communicating hydrocephalus include meningitis, trauma, and intraventricular hemorrhage. Each of these processes is thought to cause an inflammatory reaction that impedes the flow of CSF from the subarachnoid space to the venous system. In some cases of communicating hydrocephalus, there is no identifiable predisposing factor.

## Signs and Symptoms

The signs and symptoms of hydrocephalus depend greatly on the age of the child. The clinical course for children less than 2 years is relatively benign because infants can expand the size of their cranial vault, thereby minimizing the elevation in ICP. Head growth is abnormally fast, and the head circumference crosses percentiles. The anterior fontanelle is full, the sutures are split, and the scalp veins may be prominent. Poor feeding or vomiting may occur. Development may be delayed, or there may even be loss of developmental milestones. Increased tone and/or hyperreflexia may be apparent, particularly in the legs. Late signs include lethargy, sixth nerve palsy, and limitation of the up gaze with a chronic downward deviation of the eyes, or "sunsetting."

In the older child, the cranium is less able to expand to offset the mounting volume of CSF; thus, the signs and symptoms are more typical of an adult with raised ICP. Headaches, especially those that awaken children while sleeping, are a classic symptom of raised ICP. Nausea, vomiting, lethargy, difficulty with school performance, loss of developmental milestones, and behavioral changes can all be a part of the symptom complex. On examination, papilledema, sixth nerve palsy, or sunsetting of the eyes are particularly telling signs.

## Diagnostic Studies

Hydrocephalus can be confirmed radiographically by cranial ultrasound (if the anterior fontanelle is still open), computed tomographic (CT) scans, or magnetic resonance imaging (MRI) (Fig. 76-1). The latter 2 options, especially MRI, provide the best visualization of the brain and may identify an underlying structural cause for the hydrocephalus. A special technique, cardiac-gated cine-flow MRI, can dynamically measure the flow of CSF through the cerebral aqueduct during the cardiac cycle and is helpful in diagnosing aqueductal stenosis.

## Treatment

Medical treatment options for hydrocephalus are extremely limited. Agents that reduce CSF production, such as acetazolamide or furosemide, can be used but are associated with electrolyte and pH imbalances and rarely provide a long-term solution. Available surgical options are dictated by the type of hydrocephalus (noncommunicating vs communicating) and the child's age. Ventricular shunting has been the mainstay of surgical treatment since the 1950s and is the only available option for children with communicating hydrocephalus and for infants with noncommunicating hydrocephalus. For older children with noncommunicating hydrocephalus, neuroendoscopy offers an alternative treatment option (see below).

If placement of a ventricular shunt is deemed to be the best treatment option, the proximal end of the system is inserted into a CSF reservoir, most commonly the lateral ventricle,

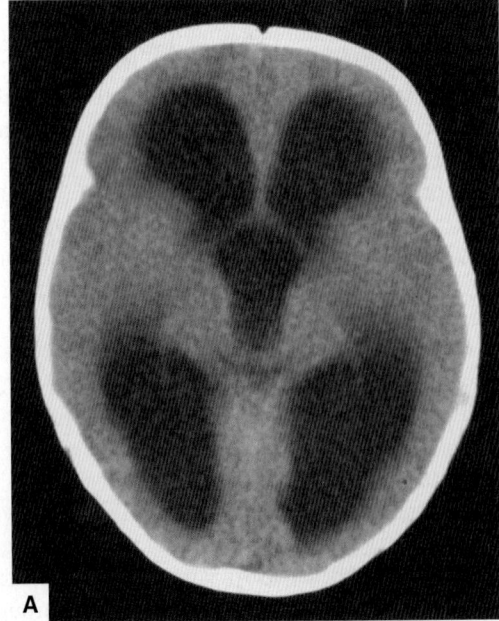
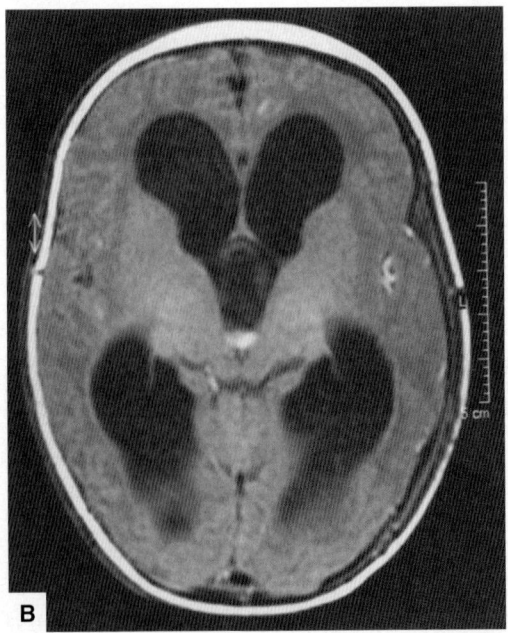

**FIGURE 76-1** **A.** CT scan in an infant with communicating hydrocephalus. **B.** MRI scan in the same child demonstrating greater anatomic detail.

which can be approached through either a frontal, occipital, or posterior temporal trephine. Another possible site in patients with communicating hydrocephalus is the lumbar subarachnoid space. The proximal catheter is usually connected to a valve that serves to regulate flow through the shunt system. A wide variety of valves are available, and further discussion about the mechanics of each type of valve is beyond the scope of this chapter. (The interested reader is referred to an excellent monograph by Drake for more detailed information.) The valve, in turn, is connected to a distal catheter, which is inserted into a cavity that will serve as a receptacle for the CSF and ultimately allows it to be absorbed into the bloodstream. Possible sites for placement of the distal catheter are the peritoneum, pleural cavity, central venous system, and gallbladder.

Among pediatric neurosurgeons, the favored location for the distal catheter is the peritoneum. The peritoneal cavity readily absorbs the CSF, and placement is technically simple and carries minimal risk. The peritoneal cavity can be accessed via an open technique or by utilizing a trocar. The standard length of the distal catheter is about 90.0 cm, and all of this catheter can be inserted into the peritoneal cavity, regardless of the patient's size or age, to compensate for the eventual growth of the patient.

The central venous system is another possible site for the distal catheter and is the second most preferred location. Veins that can be cannulated to gain access to the central venous system include the external jugular, internal jugular, facial, and subclavian. This can be accomplished by either an open or percutaneous procedure; some neurosurgeons will seek the assistance of a pediatric surgeon to insert the distal catheter. Open techniques usually require a cervical incision to expose the common facial or internal or external jugular vein. The jugular and subclavian veins can be approached percutaneously via any of the standard approaches. With the Seldinger technique and a peel-away sheath, the distal catheter can be advanced into the central venous system. Intraoperative fluoroscopy is invaluable for optimizing proper placement of the catheter tip (ideally at or near the junction of the right atrium and the superior vena cava). When a shunt is placed into the venous system, it is imperative to use a 1-way valve that permits flow only distally (almost all commercially available valves are constructed this way), to prevent retrograde flow of blood into the cerebral ventricular system.

The third possible location for distal shunt catheters is the pleural cavity. Typically, the catheter is inserted into the pleural cavity using a trocar, through a small skin incision along the anterior axillary line over one of the middle ribs (T-5–T-8). Age is a limitation of this technique, since children less than 5 years often do not adequately absorb the CSF from the pleural space, producing a symptomatic pleural effusion.

The gallbladder is a surprising but effective site for the distal catheter, provided that a preoperative ultrasound reveals no stones or sludge within it (Fig. 76-2A). Through a right subcostal incision, the gallbladder is isolated, opened, and about 4.0 cm of catheter is inserted. A purse-string suture is passed around the opening to secure the catheter in place (Fig. 76-2B). Additionally, the catheter can be secured to fibrous tissue in and around the gallbladder, which helps to minimize the risk of migration out of the gallbladder. Ample tubing is left in the peritoneal space to accommodate for growth of the child.

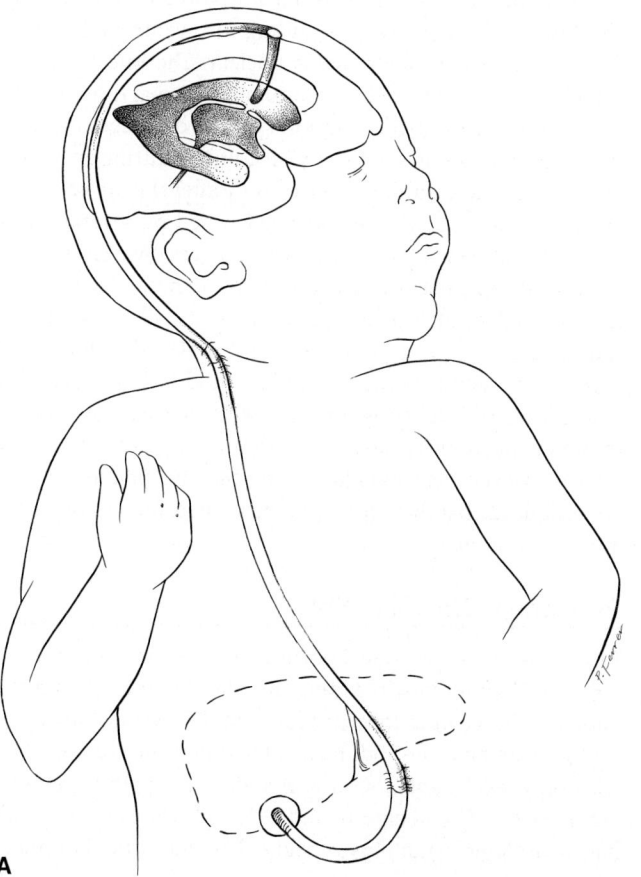

**A**

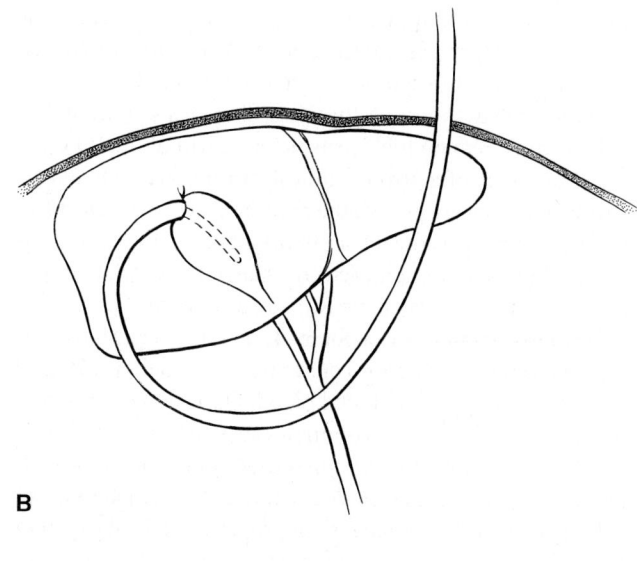

**B**

**FIGURE 76-2** **A.** Diagram demonstrating ventriculogallbladder shunt in an infant. **B.** Enlargement of the abdominal portion demonstrating the redundant peritoneal portion of the shunt catheter and placement of the distal catheter in the gallbladder.

## Complications of Ventricular Shunts

### Shunt Malfunction

Shunts can treat but cannot cure hydrocephalus and are associated with a number of complications, which commonly include, shunt malfunction. The incidence of shunt malfunction in several large series is 30% to 40% within 1 year and 50% within 5–6 years following insertion. The signs and symptoms of shunt malfunction are similar to those of untreated hydrocephalus and can mimic a flulike illness with headache, nausea, and vomiting. It is critical to listen carefully to the parents, as they often can tell from experience when the shunt has malfunctioned. Although a child can deteriorate rapidly (over minutes to hours) to lethargy, coma, and impending cerebral herniation, this is rare. Symptoms more commonly develop over several days, weeks, or even months. Symptoms may be steadily progressive or may occur intermittently. Examination may disclose papilledema *even in the absence of any clinical signs or symptoms*. Pumping the shunt gives little useful information and may actually suck debris or choroid plexus into the shunt; we therefore do not recommend routinely pumping the shunt to make a diagnosis.

Ancillary diagnostic studies may be helpful in confirming the diagnosis. A CT scan usually (but not always) shows ventricular enlargement. Changes in ventricular size may be subtle, and a comparison should always be made with prior baseline scans if available. Unfortunately, some patients have no discernible change in ventricular size even with clear-cut shunt malfunction. Radionuclide shunt flow studies are often abnormal in cases with obvious shunt malfunction, but unfortunately are of little benefit in questionable cases. A shunt tap can be performed by inserting a small-gauge needle into the shunt reservoir and may show poor proximal flow from the ventricular catheter, an elevated opening pressure, or consistent improvement in symptoms after removal of CSF.

Unfortunately, none of these ancillary tests is infallible, and one must remain highly suspicious of shunt malfunction in the presence of a strong clinical history. When pediatric neurosurgeons were polled, the clinical history was most frequently identified as the most important determinant in diagnosing shunt failure, followed by change in ventricular size on CT scans and elevated pressure on a shunt tap.

The most common reason for malfunction is occlusion of the proximal catheter by debris consisting of choroid plexus, glial or ependymal tissue, or clotted blood. Occlusion of the distal catheter is the next most common cause for shunt malfunction. Valves appear to be an infrequent source of shunt malfunction. Other causes include fracture of the catheter system with or without disconnection, improper placement of either the proximal or distal end, and migration of the distal end out of the appropriate location. In some cases, the exact source of shunt malfunction cannot be determined. Shunt function can be restored by replacing the part of the shunt system that has failed or by replacing the whole system.

Proper function of the distal portion of the shunt is dependent on placing the tip in an area of the peritoneal cavity with sufficient surface area of peritoneum to effectively absorb the CSF. The presence of extensive adhesions from previous operations or infections can make this a significant problem that might prompt one to consider one of the other options for distal catheter placement. However, in some cases, the use of laparoscopy can help to identify and direct the catheter to an acceptable site within the peritoneal cavity.

### Shunt Infection

The most exasperating complication of shunts is infection. Reported incidences of shunt infection range from 3% to 29%, with an average of 5% to 15% per shunt operation. The source of infection is usually intraoperative contamination. Thus, 70% of infections occur within 2 months of surgery, and 80% to 90% within 6 months. The age of the patient plays an important role in determining the risk for infection because children less than 6 months face a 15% risk, whereas the risk for children older than 6 months is only 5%. At least half of the patients with shunt infection present with shunt malfunction. Other symptoms can include fever, meningismus, erythema or swelling along the shunt tract, cellulitis at the site of incisions, and abdominal pain or tenderness. The specifics of possible abdominal symptoms are discussed later. The diagnosis of shunt infection can be established by aspirating CSF from the shunt system for culture, Gram stain, cell count, glucose, and protein. A shunt infection typically causes a CSF leukocytosis with a predominance of neutrophils and bands, low CSF glucose, and elevated CSF protein. Lumbar puncture is not an effective method of evaluating for shunt infection because the lumbar CSF is positive for infection in only 50% of documented shunt infections.

Shunt infections are most frequently caused by *Staphylococcus epidermis*, followed by *Staphylococcus aureus*, gram-negative rods (especially in neonates), and *Propionibacterium acnes*. Shunt infections are treated with intravenous antibiotics. Although some advocate adding intraventricular antibiotics, the utility of this remains unclear. The infected shunt usually must be removed. A temporary external drain is usually inserted to provide temporary CSF drainage and also serves as an ongoing source of CSF cultures during antibiotic treatment. A new shunt is inserted only after the infection has been adequately eradicated, as determined by several negative CSF cultures. This regimen was universally successful in treating shunt infections in a study by James. Alternatively, the infected shunt can be treated in situ and subsequently removed at the end of treatment and replaced immediately with a new shunt. However, this method is less successful, eradicating the infection in only 90% of cases. Antibiotic treatment without replacing the shunt is successful in only 30%. However, *Haemophilus influenzae* and pneumococcus are unique in that they may often be treated successfully with antibiotics alone.

### Peritoneal Complications

Infections of the peritoneal portion of the shunt can produce abdominal symptoms, including an acute abdomen. Among 19 patients with ventriculoperitoneal shunt (VPS) infections presenting with an acute abdomen, all had peritoneal signs (59% with only local signs). Fever and abdominal pain were present in 74%, 47% had emesis, and 26% had anorexia. Only half had neurologic symptoms or signs. Patients with abdominal symptoms and shunts should be evaluated with abdominal ultrasound or CT, looking for a pseudocyst or an abscess.

Pseudocysts are loculated pockets filled predominantly with unabsorbed CSF, and in most cases there is a concomitant low-grade shunt infection with *S. epidermidis* or *Proprionobacter acnes*. The cyst wall is a peritoneal serous membrane thickened by chronic inflammatory tissue rather than formed mesothelial tissue, thus the term pseudocyst. In addition to infection, multiple previous abdominal operations and chronically elevated CSF protein have been identified as risk factors for the development of pseudocysts. They can occur in a delayed fashion, even years following the last shunt operation. Patients may present with abdominal pain, distension, vomiting, fever, or anorexia. It is important to note that 80% to 100% of patients have no symptoms of shunt malfunction. The diagnosis is established with abdominal ultrasound. Typical findings include a loculated fluid collection with small amounts of debris within it, located immediately adjacent to the distal end of the shunt catheter. Infection has been identified as the causative factor in 30% to 100% of pseudocysts, with most series reporting a rate over 60%; thus, CSF should be aspirated from the shunt system and cultured before the start of antibiotics. Treatment of the pseudocyst involves removing the peritoneal catheter. During the procedure, fluid from the pseudocyst can be aspirated retrogradely through the catheter and sent for culture. Whether or not the whole shunt is removed initially depends on the index of suspicion for a shunt infection. If it is low, some authors recommend converting the peritoneal shunt to an atrial or pleural shunt immediately. Others assume that the shunt is infected and remove the entire shunt initially and begin antibiotic therapy. The pseudo-cyst typically subsides once the peritoneal catheter is removed, and aspiration is rarely necessary. There are no contraindications to reinserting the shunt into the peritoneal cavity after adequate treatment has been completed.

If an abscess is identified, the shunt is removed, and the abscess is treated. Occasionally, a drain may need to be inserted, either through an open procedure or percutaneously, to evacuate the residual purulent material. Once the infection has been adequately cleared, the shunt may be reinserted; however, if there is any concern for residual peritoneal infection, it may be wise to select a different site for the distal catheter.

Perforation of viscera can occur either at the time of shunt insertion or later, from erosion of the tubing through the visceral wall. If the injury occurs at the time of insertion, and there is spillage of visceral contents, the laceration should be repaired, and the shunt removed from the peritoneal cavity. If the shunt was in contact with visceral contents, it is best to externalize the shunt to a closed drainage system, drain the ventricles for a few days while sampling CSF for infection, and revise the shunt only when it is clear that CSF infection is not a concern. If, however, the shunt tubing was well isolated and uncontaminated, one could consider inserting it into another cavity, such as the venous system or pleural space. Delayed erosion of the shunt catheter through the visceral wall is a well-documented phenomenon. It is thought to be more common with catheters that are spring reinforced. Perforations of the stomach, small or large intestine, bladder, and uterus have been reported. In addition to the typical symptoms of pain, fever, nausea, vomiting, and anorexia, a unique symptom is a long history of watery stools. The diagnosis can be confirmed with an abdominal CT or by injecting a contrast agent down the shunt tubing. If the latter is done, the proximal end of the shunt should be occluded to avoid contrast material refluxing into the ventricles. Treatment may depend on the mode of presentation. Snow recommends that if there is evidence of peritonitis at the time of presentation, the patient is best served by abdominal exploration and repair of the visceral injury. Alternatively, if the abdominal exam is benign, the catheter may simply be removed. The hope is that the fibrous tract that typically forms around the catheter may seal off the opening in the visceral wall.

Less common peritoneal complications include extrusion of the catheter into the scrotum through a hernia, volvulus, and ascites. If the catheter enters a hernia sac, the catheter may be carefully pushed back into the peritoneal cavity during the herniorrhaphy.

## Central Venous Complications

Complications from inserting the distal shunt catheter into the venous system include thrombosis, bacteremia, and other sequelae of shunt infection. Ventriculoatrial catheters are typically very soft and have a small outer diameter and present a minimal risk of vessel injury or thrombosis. The greatest concern is the potentially serious consequences of an infected venous shunt. In addition to causing bacteremia, venous shunt infections can induce endocarditis, cor pulmonale, cardiac arrhythmia, and shunt nephritis. The latter is acute renal failure that occurs as a result of deposition of immune complexes into the kidneys, which results in a diffuse glomerulonephritis.

## Pleural Complications

Complications unique to pleural shunts include empyema, noninfectious pleural effusions, and pneumothorax. An empyema can develop in response to a shunt infection and usually responds to antibiotics and removal of the shunt. If the pleural lining is not able to absorb the CSF, an effusion will form and may affect respiratory function. These can be treated by exposing the shunt catheter in the subcutaneous space and aspirating fluid through the distal portion of the catheter. Obviously, another site for the distal catheter must be selected. Finally, there is a risk of a pneumothorax during the insertion of the pleural catheter. This risk can be minimized by having the anesthesiologist hold respiration in the expiratory phase as the trocar is introduced into the pleural cavity. Once the stylette is removed, the assistant can flood the wound with irrigant as the catheter is being passed through the trocar. Another Valsalva maneuver is performed as the trocar is removed.

## Intra-abdominal Surgery in the Presence of a Ventriculoperitoneal Shunt

The major concern for performing an intra-abdominal operation in a patient with a VPS is infection. There are a number of studies in pediatric patients examining the risk of intra-abdominal surgery and the safety of laparoscopic procedures surgery in patients with shunts in place, Fraser et al, reported on 99 intra-abdominal procedures (51 laparoscopic and 48 open) in patients with VPSs. The most common operation performed was a fundoplication and gastrostomy tube. After 6 months of follow-up, they identified 1 shunt infection in the laparoscopic group, 3 infections in the open group, and no cases of air embolism into the central nervous system. The authors concluded that open and laparoscopic intra-abdominal operations are safe and carry a small but acceptable risk of infection and no neurologic risk when using laparoscopy. However, there is some evidence to suggest that laparoscopy is not completely benign. Uzzo studied this problem in 2 patients who had a VPS and underwent a laparoscopic bladder augmentation. The shunts were thoroughly evaluated before the procedure with a head CT and a shunt tap. In both cases, the shunt was deemed to be functional by the neurosurgeons. ICP was monitored throughout the case by inserting a 23-gauge needle into the shunt and attaching it to a transducer. Immediately after insufflating the peritoneum, ICP began to rise, taking about 30 minutes to reach 25 mm Hg, at least 10 mm Hg greater than the baseline recordings. There was a corresponding decrease in cerebral perfusion pressure to about 60 to 65 mm Hg. In each of these cases, aspirating CSF during the procedure effectively reduced the ICP back to baseline. The possible mechanism for these findings includes diminished intracranial venous outflow and reduced CSF flow through the shunt, both as a result of increased intra-abdominal pressure. He concluded that strong consideration should be given to intraoperative ICP monitoring for any patient with a VPS undergoing a laparoscopic procedure.

For an emergent case with a high probability of contamination such as perforated appendicitis, the distal catheter can be externalized at the time of the abdominal procedure. This provides access to the CSF for daily cultures to rule out an infection while the intraperitoneal process is being treated. The shunt can then be reinternalized once the inraperitoneal process resolves.

## Endoscopic Third Ventriculostomy

A relatively new and exciting surgical technique that can be offered as an alternative to patients with obstructive hydrocephalus is endoscopic third ventriculostomy (ETV). This procedure is performed with the aid of an endoscope, which is passed through a small burr-hole into the lateral ventricle, through the foramen of Monro, and into the third ventricle. Under direct vision, a fenestration can be made in the floor of the third ventricle between the infundibular recess anteriorly and the mammillary bodies posteriorly, communicating with the ventricular and subarachnoid spaces and bypassing the ventricular obstruction. ETV is effective in 60% to 80% of patients. Patient selection is crucial and only patients with noncommunicating hydrocephalus are reasonable candidates for the procedure. In addition, most series report a lower success rate (60% to 70%) in children under 2 years of age, although this limitation is not universally recognized. Younger children may respond less readily to ETV because they have relatively underdeveloped arachnoid granulations

with less efficient CSF absorption; third ventriculostomy in these patients may therefore simply convert a noncommunicating to a communicating hydrocephalus. For children less than 2 years who require treatment for obstructive hydrocephalus, we prefer to place a VPS initially and reserve ETV for later, perhaps at the time of shunt failure.

Potential complications of ETV include a vascular injury to the basilar artery with devastating consequences, as the basilar tip and its perforating vessels are very close to the area of the fenestration. Other potential complications include transient or permanent pituitary insufficiency (most commonly diabetes insipidus) as a result of injuring the hypothalamus or pituitary stalk and short-term memory loss from damage to the mammillary bodies. Fortunately, complications are rare. The long-term failure rate for third ventriculostomy is very low.

# CONGENITAL CRANIOSPINAL MALFORMATIONS

Developmental malformations present the most frequent reasons for collaboration between pediatric surgeons and neurosurgeons, for at least 4 reasons. First, the juxtaposition of neuroectoderm and endoderm during early embryonic development produces a number of malformations involving both neural and gastrointestinal tissues (such as combined spina bifida) in ways that require a collaborative effort to repair. Second, certain malformations of the gastrointestinal system (such as imperforate anus or certain gastrointestinal duplications) or chest (such as neurenteric cysts of the posterior mediastinum) may serve as markers for additional developmental malformations involving the nervous system. Third, certain central nervous system abnormalities (such as myelocystocele or spinal lipomas) may be mistaken for malformations involving other organ systems (such as sacrococcygeal teratoma). Finally, seemingly innocuous malformations involving the face (such as nasal dermal sinuses) or back (such as midline skin tags, hemangiomata, or hairy patches) that may be referred to a pediatric surgeon for removal may have occult intracranial extension or serve as sentinel markers of important underlying central nervous system malformations that, if not properly addressed, may lead to complications involving the central nervous system. Although these relationships cannot always be predicted in advance, knowing the developmental anatomy of the nervous system and understanding the ways in which the neuroectoderm and endoderm can interact will eliminate a number of unpleasant surprises.

## Normal Development of the Nervous System

It is very helpful to have a basic understanding of early neural development. The human embryo at 2 weeks of gestation is a bilaminar structure containing an epiblast and hypoblast (Fig. 76-3A). During the third week, cells in the epiblast migrate toward the mid-line primitive streak and ingress through the primitive groove to form the endoderm (these cells displace the hypoblast cells laterally) and the intervening

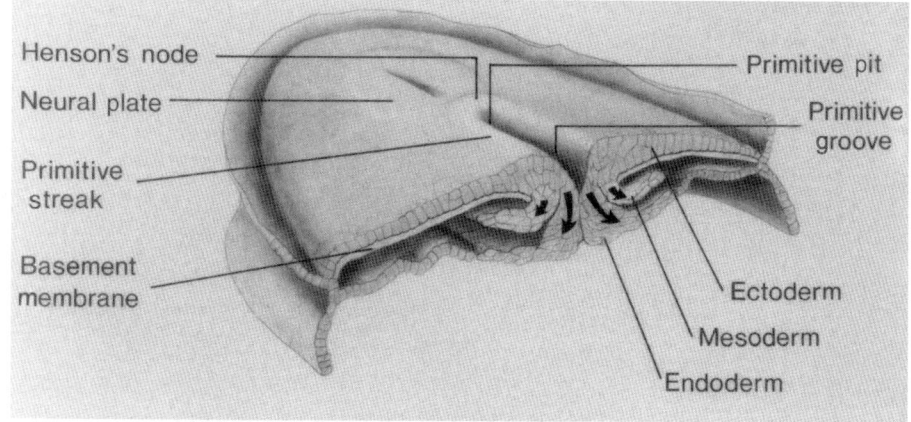

**A**

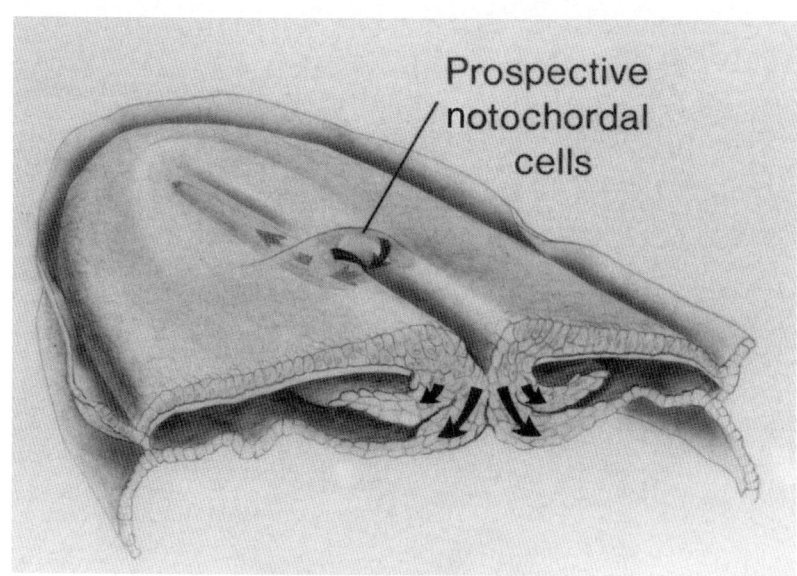

**B**

**FIGURE 76-3** Normal human gastrulation. **A.** Prospective endodermal and mesodermal cells of the epiblast migrate through the primitive groove; remaining epiblast cells will become the neuroectoderm and cutaneous ectoderm. **B.** Prospective notochordal cells located in Hensen node ingress through the primitive pit (the rostral end of the primitive streak) to become the notochordal process. (From Dias MS, Walker ML. The embryogenesis of complex dysraphic malformations: a disorder of gastrulation? *Pediatr Neurosurg* 1992;18:229–253.)

mesoderm; the remaining epiblast cells form the ectoderm (Fig. 76-3A). These cell movements, termed *gastrulation*, convert the embryo from a bilaminar to a trilaminar structure containing ectoderm, mesoderm, and endoderm.

Cells at the rostral end of the primitive streak in the Hensen node ingress through the primitive pit (the cranial end of the primitive groove) and become the notochordal process (Fig. 76-3B). The notochordal process initially is hollow, consisting of a ring of cells radially arranged about a central lumen (the notochordal canal), which, in turn, is in communication with the primitive pit (Fig. 76-4A). During the third week of embryogenesis, the notochordal process fuses (intercalates) with the underlying endoderm for a period of about 3 days; during this period, the notochordal canal is contiguous with both the amnion and the yolk sac and creates a "through and through" hole in the embryo termed the primitive neurenteric canal (Fig. 76-4B). At the end of this period, the notochordal canal separates (excalates) from the endoderm, and the primitive neurenteric canal is obliterated (Fig. 76-4C).

The ectoderm is subdivided into neuroectoderm (the forerunner of the central nervous system), which occupies the medial ectoderm, and cutaneous ectoderm (the future integument), to which the neuroectoderm is bound along its lateral and rostral borders. During the fourth week of embryogenesis, the neuroectoderm undergoes a complex series of morphologic changes that convert the flattened neuroectoderm (or neural plate) to a closed tubular structure (the neural tube) through a process called *primary neurulation* (Fig. 76-5A, B, and C). The flattened neural plate undergoes midline bending to form the neural groove; elevation and convergence of the lateral portions of the neural plate (the neural folds) and their fusion in the midline produce the closed neural tube. As the neural folds fuse, the cutaneous ectoderm separates and becomes the overlying skin. Abnormalities of neural tube closure often produce additional cutaneous abnormalities such as midline hemangiomata, hairy patches, dimples, or appendages that serve as markers for the underlying abnormality of the neural tube. Neurulation begins in the hindbrain or upper spinal cord and proceeds both cranially and caudally; the last areas to close are the anterior and posterior neuropores, which are located at the lamina terminalis (just anterior to the optic chiasm) and the second sacral spinal cord segment, respectively.

The more caudal portions of the neural tube (the spinal cord caudal to the second sacral segment and the filum terminale) are formed from the caudal cell mass (the caudal

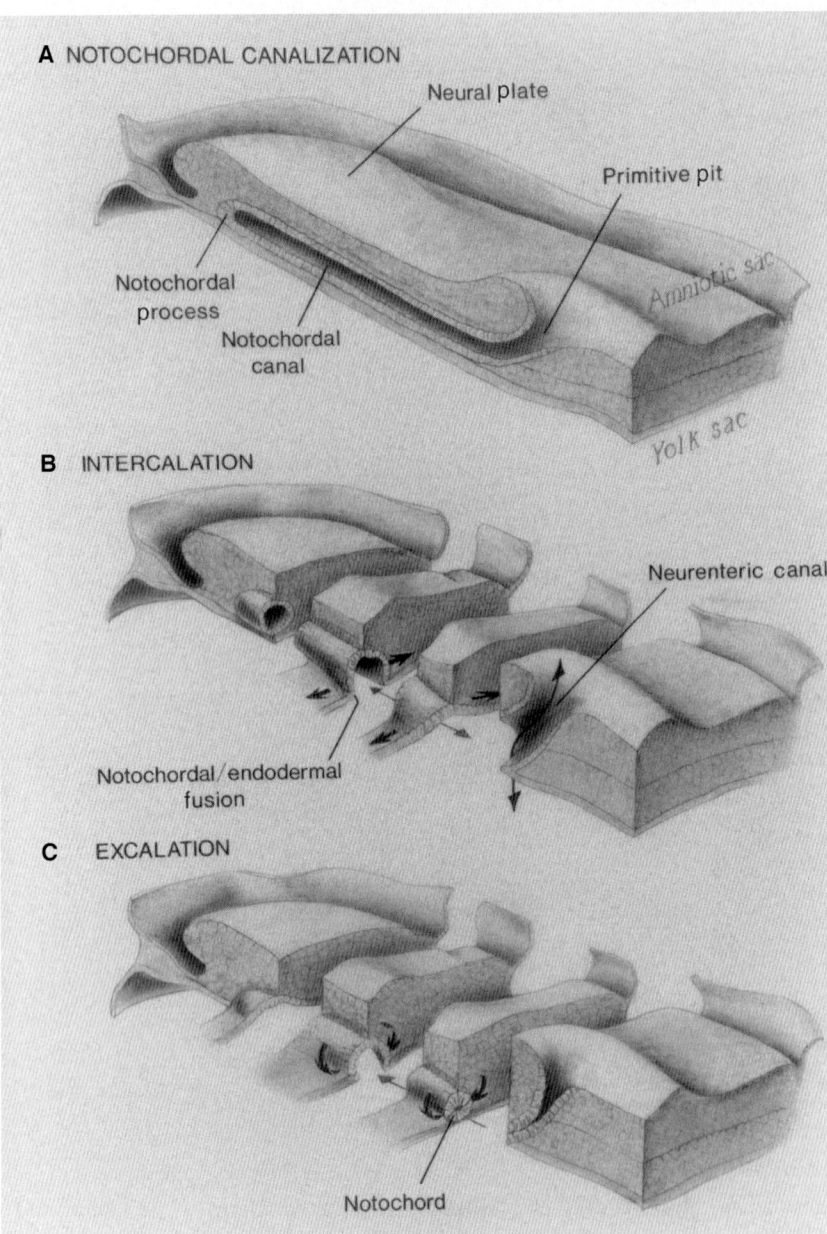

**A** NOTOCHORDAL CANALIZATION

Neural plate

Primitive pit

Notochordal process

Notochordal canal

Amniotic sac

Yolk sac

**B** INTERCALATION

Neurenteric canal

Notochordal/endodermal fusion

**C** EXCALATION

Notochord

**FIGURE 76-4** Notochordal development. **A.** The notochordal process contains a central lumen (the notochordal canal), which is continuous with the amnionic cavity through the primitive pit. **B.** During intercalation, the notochordal process fuses with the underlying endoderm; the communication of the amnion with the yolk sac is called the neurenteric canal. **C.** During excalation, the notochord rolls up and separates from the endoderm; the neurenteric canal is obliterated. (From Dias MS, Walker ML. The embryogenesis of complex dysraphic malformations: a disorder of gastrulation? *Pediatr Neurosurg* 1992;18:229–253.)

embryonic remnant of the primitive streak and Hensen node) through a different process termed *secondary neurulation* (Fig. 76-6). Multipotent cells in the caudal cell mass that are destined to form the caudal nervous system, the mesenchyme of the lower sacrum and coccyx, and the caudal embryonic pole are in juxtaposition with both the posterior notochordal and hindgut endodermal cells (the portion of endoderm that is destined to form anorectal structures). During secondary neurulation, cells of the caudal cell mass become radially arranged into multiple "tubules"; these structures later coalesce to form the secondary neural tube and eventually fuse with the neural tube formed from primary neurulation. The juxtaposition of the caudal cell mass and the underlying hindgut endoderm produces a variety of congenital abnormalities that may involve both anorectal structures and the caudal neuraxis.

Beginning at about the sixth gestational week and continuing into postnatal life, the neural tube undergoes several morphogenetic changes, which ultimately result in an "ascent of the conus medullaris"; this is accomplished through 2 distinct mechanisms. Before embryonic day 54, the caudal end of the neural tube undergoes a number of histoanatomic changes collectively referred to as retrogressive differentiation, becoming more slender and fibrous and eventually being transformed into the filum terminale. Beyond embryonic day 54, differential growth of the vertebral column relative to the neural tube results in a progressive length discrepancy so that the conus medullaris ascends during development (Fig. 76-7). The conus in the majority of neonates (particularly those beyond 3 months of age) lies opposite or cranial to the disc space between the first and second lumbar vertebrae (the L1-2 disc space). A spinal cord that ends more caudally, with the conus at or below the L1-2 disc space, is generally considered to be radiographically tethered.

Although brief, this overview of early embryology will provide a background for a more complete understanding of

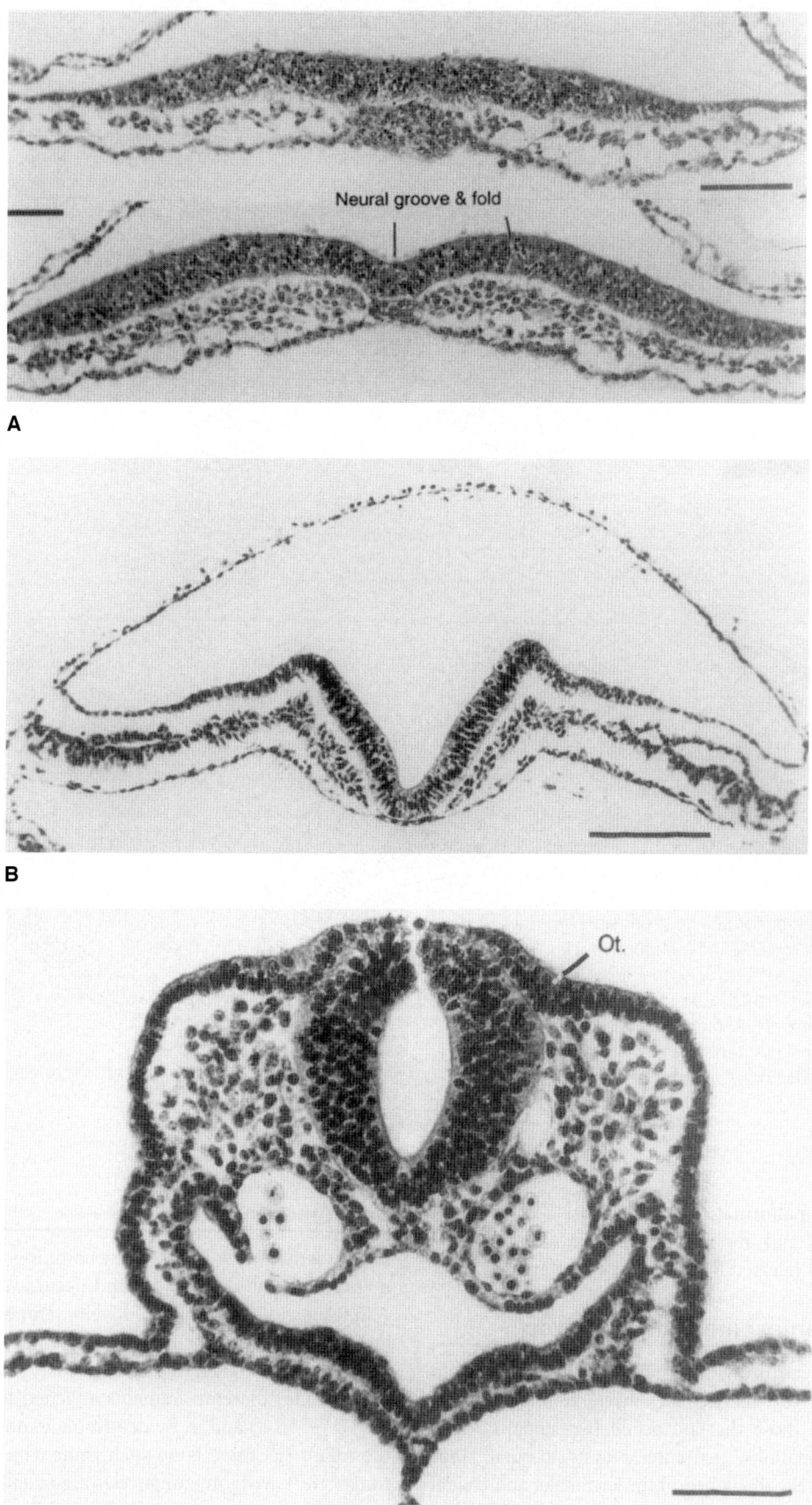

**FIGURE 76-5** Photomicrographs of human neuroepithelium during neurulation. **A.** The neuroepithelium is a pseudostratified columnar epithelium. The neural groove is well seen in the midline overlying the notochord, and the neural folds are slightly elevated. **B.** Later stage shows further elevation of the neural folds about the midline neural groove. **C.** Still later stage shows a nearly closed neural tube; the cutaneous ectoderm (the future integument) is still attached to the neural folds. Ot, otic placode. (From O'Rahilly R, Müller F. *The Embryonic Human Brain. An Atlas of Developmental Stages.* New York: Wiley-Liss; 1994.)

## Secondary Neurulation

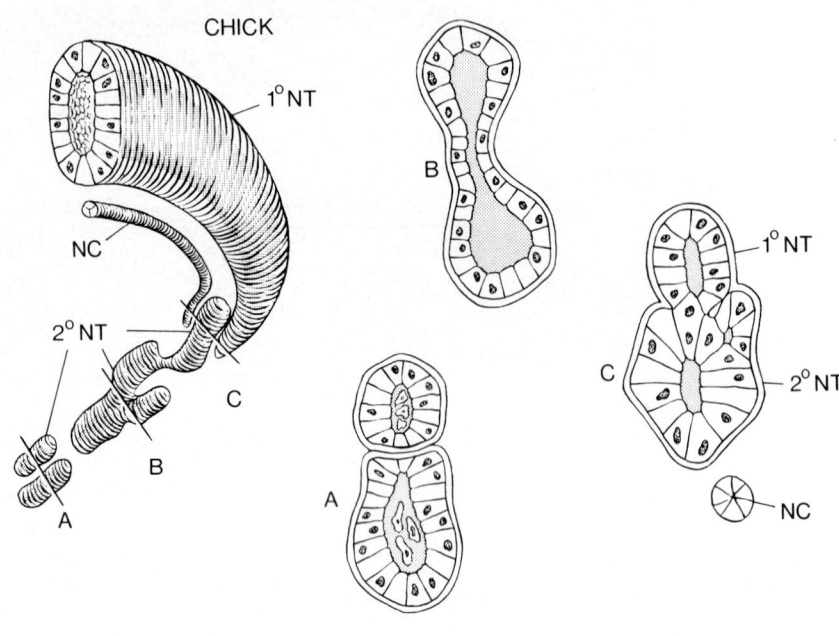

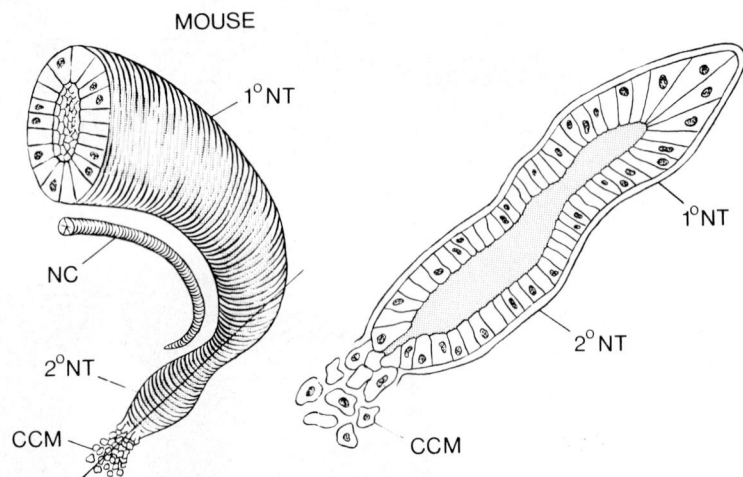

**FIGURE 76-6** Secondary neurulation in chick embryos. **A.** Cells of the caudal cell mass (ccm), located at the neural tube formed from primary neurulation (1° NT) form multiple independent vesicles. **B.** These vesicles fuse to form a secondary neural tube. **C.** The secondary neural tube then fuses with the primary neural tube (NC, notochord). (From Dias MS, McLone DG. Spinal dysraphism. In: Weinstein SL, ed. *The Pediatric Spine: Principles and Practice.* New York: Raven Press; 1994.)

congenital neural malformations. For a more complete discussion of normal and abnormal neural development, the interested reader is referred to several recent references.

### Congenital Craniospinal Malformations

Most contemporary texts divide dysraphic malformations into those that are open (eg, anencephaly, myelomeningocele, and meningocele), and those that are occult (eg, spinal lipoma, split cord malformations, neurenteric cysts, dermal sinus tracts, myelocystocele, thickened filum terminale, and caudal agenesis). Although superficially attractive, this classification scheme is confusing in that many of the "occult" malformations have clinically apparent midline skin markers (hemangiomas, sinuses, appendages, or tufts of hair) that, for the astute clinician, serve as markers for the underlying spinal cord anomaly. We have instead recently begun to emphasize a classification based on reputed embryogenetic mechanisms (Table 76-1).

### Myelomeningocele

Myelomeningocele is the most common dysraphic malformation compatible with life and occurs with a frequency of 1 in 1200–1400 live births. Myelomeningocele represents a localized failure of primary neurulation—a portion of the neural tube has failed to properly close, and the neural tissue (or placode) therefore remains attached to the surrounding skin (Fig. 76-8) and is, by definition, exposed on the back of the infant (ie, there is no such thing as a "closed myelomeningocele"). Myelomeningoceles are usually cystic appearing because of the accumulation of spinal fluid beneath the placode. Although some reserve the term myeloschisis for a large or flat lesion, myelomeningoceles and myeloschisis both represent the same embryonic problem, failure of primary neurulation. The use of 2 terms to describe essentially the same disorder is confusing, and it has been suggested that the term myeloschisis be discarded.

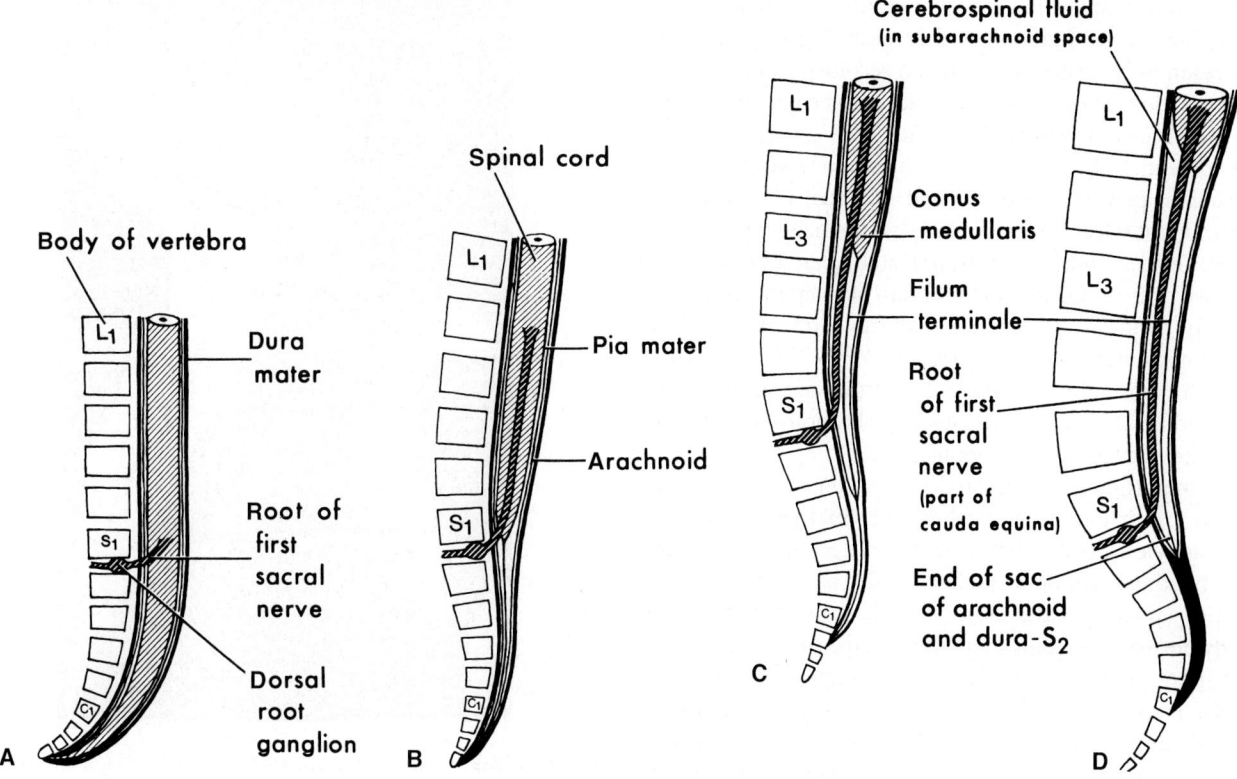

**FIGURE 76-7** Ascent of the conus medullaris. **A–C.** Throughout prenatal development, the caudal spinal cord comes to lie at progressively more cranial levels as a result of retrogressive differentiation before embryonic day 54, and differential growth of the spinal cord and vertebral column. At birth (**D**), the cord normally lies opposite or craniad to the disc space between the first and second lumbar vertebrae. A conus, which is more caudally located, is considered to be tethered.

Although the pediatric surgeon is not usually involved initially, many children with myelomeningocele eventually develop problems for which the pediatric surgeon may be called on to assist with management. Many patients with myelomeningocele require shunt placement and complications of shunt operations (see Fig. 76-8) are the most common reasons for consultation. Assistance with vascular access for placement of ventriculoatrial shunts, access to the pleural space for ventriculopleural shunts, or surgical exposure to the gallbladder for ventriculogallbladder shunts may be requested. Children with multiple abdominal adhesions or distorted anatomy from multiple previous operations or infections may require lysis of adhesions during shunt placement. Some children with myelomeningocele and chronic constipation may benefit from creation of a cecostomy or appendicostomy for bowel lavage. Placement of gastrostomy

| TABLE 76-1 | Embryogenetic Classification of Spinal Developmental Malformations |
|---|---|
| **Malformation** | **Reputed Embryogenetic Mechanism** |
| Myelomeningocele | Segmental failure of primary neurulation |
| Lipomyelomeningocele | Premature dysjunction (separation of the neuro-and-cutaneous ectoderm) |
| Dermal sinus | Incomplete dysjunction |
| Split spinal cord malformations | Failure of midline axial integration during gastrulation |
| Thickened filum terminate | Disordered development of caudal cell mass |
| Sacral agenesis | Failure of caudal cell mass development |

*Note:* Adapted from Dias MS, Li V. *Pediatric Clinics of North America* 1998;45:1539–1578.

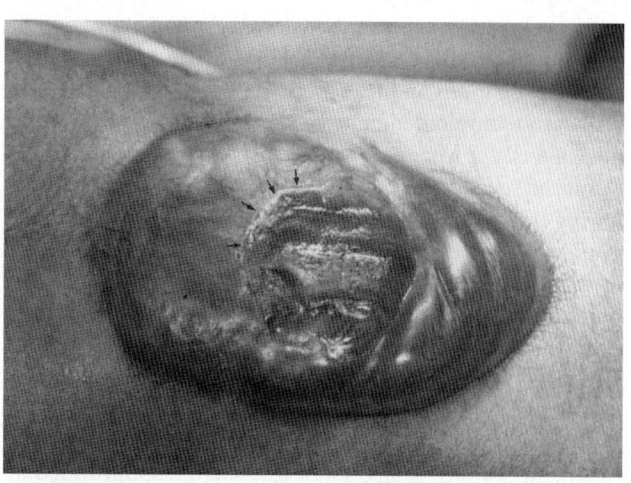

**FIGURE 76-8** Photo of a child with a myelomeningocele. The placode is located in the central portion of the malformation and is circumferentially connected along its lateral borders (*arrows*) with dystrophic skin.

tubes and fundoplication may be required for complications of swallowing dysfunction and/or gastroesophageal reflux as a result of brainstem dysfunction secondary to the Chiari malformation. These procedures may also be complicated by the presence of the ventricular shunt.

A potential therapeutic intervention offered by highly specialized pediatric surgeons and maternal fetal medicine physicians at select centers involves the prenatal repair of the defect. In a randomized study, prenatal repair was shown to improve hydrocephalus and hindbrain herniation, reduce the need for ventriculoperitoneal shunting, and improve distal neurologic function in some patients. While there was some maternal morbidity reported, the results are encouraging for avoiding some of the serious complications faced by the myelomeningocele patient population.

It is important to understand and to convey accurate and reliable information when dealing with children with myelomeningoceles. Most children with isolated myelomeningoceles (ie, those without associated major anomalies of other organs) survive to adulthood, and their life expectancy is nearly normal (although a few children die each year, usually from unrecognized shunt failure or complications of treatment). Eighty percent have normal intelligence; although 60% of these have some learning disability (verbal scores are better than performance scores, and math and problem solving are particularly difficult). Hydrocephalus requiring a ventricular shunt is present in 85% of children but bears little relationship to intelligence. Sixty percent of preadolescents are capable of ambulating, either with or without assistance (although this number drops during adolescence), and about 80% are "socially continent" (meaning they are dry, although many perform clean intermittent catheterization).

Myelomeningocele is a static disease, and any deterioration in a child with myelomeningocele should prompt a search for an underlying cause. Unfortunately, most children with myelomeningocele experience 1 or more episodes of clinical deterioration sometime during their lives. By far, the most common cause of deterioration is a shunt malfunction, which can present in a bewildering number of ways. Nowhere else in pediatric neurosurgery is clinical judgment so important (and misjudgment so treacherous) as in the evaluation of a child with myelomeningocele and suspected shunt malfunction. In addition to the usual triad of headache, nausea, and vomiting, these children may present with neck or back pain (especially at the myelomeningocele closure site), seizures (either new in onset or a change in a preexisting pattern of seizures), significant changes in behavior or school performance, swallowing or other evidence of hindbrain dysfunction, changes in upper or lower extremity strength, coordination, balance, or tone, changes in urinary or bowel habits, and scoliosis or other orthopedic deformities. Finally, as discussed above, the child with shunt malfunction may have papilledema without any symptoms. In short, shunt malfunction in this population can be the root cause for *any deterioration*, and the clinician should always check the shunt before entertaining any other treatment options. If any doubt exists about shunt function, the shunt should be explored operatively before any other procedures are undertaken.

Other causes of deterioration in children with myelomeningoceles include hindbrain and spinal cord dysfunction from

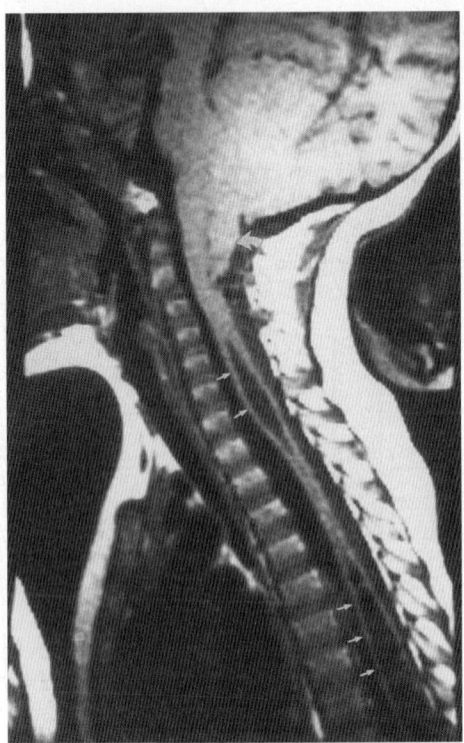

**FIGURE 76-9** Sagittal $T_1$-weighted MRI showing a Chiari malformation and syringomyelia in a child with myelomeningocele. The midline vermis (*curved arrow*) and medulla are located within the spinal canal below the level of the foramen magnum. Two syringomyelic cavities (*small arrows*) occupy the cervical and thoracic spinal cord.

the Chiari malformation and/or syringomyelia (occurring in 15% to 20% of children) and spinal cord tethering (occurring in about one-third of children). The Chiari malformation (Fig. 76-9) refers to a constellation of brain malformations, part of which involves a descent of the cerebellar vermis, caudal brainstem, and the fourth ventricle through the foramen magnum at the skull base and into the rostral spinal canal, which may produce symptoms by compressing the brainstem and rostral spinal cord. Although it is radiographically present in nearly every child with a myelomeningocele, only about 15% to 33% of children develop significant symptoms from the Chiari malformation. Symptoms and signs most commonly (up to 90% of symptomatic children) develop during the first year of life and generally consist of lower cranial nerve dysfunction (swallowing abnormalities, regurgitation, recurrent aspiration pneumonia, hoarseness or vocal cord palsy, obstructive or central apnea); upper-extremity weakness; ataxia, dyscoordination, or gait disturbance; or scoliosis.

Those children with symptomatic Chiari malformations should undergo a cervicomedullary decompression of the brainstem and upper spinal cord with a dural patch graft to create additional space for the spinal cord and descended cerebellar and brainstem tissue. The laminae at all vertebral levels overlying the descended cerebellar tonsils are removed, the dura is opened widely, and a graft of pericranium, cadaver dura, bovine pericardium, or other material is sutured circumferentially to the dural opening. Although a small portion of the occipital bone at the foramen magnum is often removed, a wide bony removal is not necessary because children with Chiari II malformations already have a large foramen magnum. Similarly, opening the fourth ventricular outlets, plugging the obex (the opening from the fourth ventricle to the central canal of the spinal cord), and other maneuvers are probably of little additional value in most cases and significantly increase the operative risk.

Postoperatively, pain, sensorimotor deficits, and cerebellar function improve in the majority, but swallowing dysfunction and/or vocal cord palsies, particularly if severe, may not improve significantly, and fundoplication, gastrostomy feeding tubes, and tracheostomies may be necessary to prevent pulmonary aspiration.

Syringomyelia (Fig. 76-9) refers to a cystic collection of spinal fluid within the substance of the spinal cord and is present in 20% to 40% of children with myelomeningocele. Treatment is generally reserved for those whose collections are either very large or causing symptoms. Syringomyelia produces symptoms by stretching and compressing the adjacent spinal cord tissue. Symptoms may include progressive weakness in upper and/or lower extremities, loss of sensation, back or radicular pain, or scoliosis. Changes in bowel or bladder function are rare.

Syringomyelia is generally treated with a laminectomy over the largest portion of the syrinx, opening the syrinx either in the midline raphe or, alternatively, dorsolaterally at the dorsal root entry zone (taking care to avoid the cervical enlargement if possible), and placing a shunt tube from the syrinx cavity to either the peritoneal (syringoperitoneal) or pleural (syringopleural) space. Cervicomedullary decompression of the Chiari malformation is less frequently successful in treating syringomyelia in children with Chiari II malformations.

Spinal cord tethering is identified radiographically by an abnormally low-lying position of the spinal cord terminus, below the L1-2 disc space. Again, spinal cord tethering is radiographically evident in virtually every child with myelomeningocele but produces symptoms in only about a third. The pathophysiology of tethering has been studied both in humans and in animal models by Yamada and colleagues; the stretching of the spinal cord produces changes in spinal cord blood flow, which, in turn, lead to ischemia and changes in mitochondrial oxidative metabolism in the caudal spinal cord.

Symptoms and signs of spinal cord tethering may include back and/or leg pain, weakness or loss of leg function, deteriorating gait, deterioration in bowel or bladder function, and increasing scoliosis or other lower-extremity orthopedic deformities such as pes cavus and equinovarus deformities. Symptoms are thought to arise because the repaired myelomeningocele placode is scarred at the site of the previous closure and cannot ascend with the child's growth and movements; unrecognized associated malformations such as split cord malformations or thickened filum terminale (see below) may provide additional sources of tethering. Surgery is reserved for those children with symptomatic tethering and involves exploration and untethering of the placode and any associated tethering elements from the dura and surrounding structures such that the spinal cord lies free within the thecal sac. The dura is closed primarily or with a dural patch graft. A number of synthetic grafts have been tried to prevent retethering, but none has met with significant long-term success.

Although the radiologic abnormalities of the tethered cord, Chiari malformation, and syringomyelia are present radiographically in many children with myelomeningocele, the mere presence of any of these malformations does *not*, by itself, suggest the need for treatment. Rather, treatment is reserved for children having evidence of clinical deterioration.

## Spinal Lipomas (Lipomyelomeningocele)

Spinal lipomas are the most frequent of the closed congenital spinal cord malformations, accounting for 35% of skin-covered lumbosacral masses. An associated subcutaneous fatty mass (Fig. 76-10A, B, and C) is present in 70% of patients. Rarely, the mass is mistaken for a sacrococcygeal teratoma, although spinal lipomas are almost always more rostrally located in the mid- or upper sacrum. Infrequently, they may involve the thoracic or cervical spine. Other cutaneous markers may include midline lumbosacral hemangiomas, dimples, skin tags, or appendages. The subcutaneous component of the lipoma virtually always extends through a dorsal defect in the spine (often, but not always, between dysplastic laminae) and ends within the intramedullary portion of the spinal cord (Fig. 76-10C). Rarely, the lipoma may be purely intradural, having no subcutaneous component, but still tethers the spinal cord to the dura. Spinal lipomas are thought to arise through premature separation (dysfunction) of the neural tube from the cutaneous ectoderm (skin); this allows mesenchymal cells access to the inside of the neural tube, where they are induced to form fat. Lipomas that originate caudal to the second sacral spinal cord segment (from neural tube derived from secondary neurulation) are thought to arise through a different, as yet undefined, mechanism involving the caudal cell mass, sometimes in association with disorders of cloacal derivatives (urogenital system and hindgut, see below).

Spinal lipomas, as with all of the congenital spinal cord malformations, produce signs and symptoms of spinal cord dysfunction because of spinal cord tethering at the level of the malformation. Signs and symptoms of tethering include back and/or leg pain; progressive sensorimotor deficits; urologic changes (incontinence, difficulties initiating a urinary stream, frequent bladder infections, or changes on urodynamic studies suggestive of a neurogenic bladder) or defecatory difficulties; orthopedic abnormalities of the feet such as pes cavus, equinovarus deformities, hammer toes, or asymmetric feet; and scoliosis. Current thinking is that most children with spinal lipomas will eventually deteriorate because of tethering, and operation is recommended as soon as the malformation is identified, preferably *before* the child becomes symptomatic.

Lipomas are readily visible as hyperintense lesions on $T_1$-weighted images (Fig. 76-10B). The spinal cord is low lying, consistent with tethering. The preoperative evaluation includes a formal assessment of lower extremity muscle function (preferably a manual muscle test), a urologic evaluation including urodynamic studies, and an orthopedic assessment of lower-extremity and spinal deformities. Surgery involves excising the lipoma, isolating its underlying attachment with the dorsal spinal cord, and untethering the spinal cord. Most pediatric neurosurgeons also excise some part of the lipoma within the spinal cord substance. It should be emphasized that *simply excising the subcutaneous*

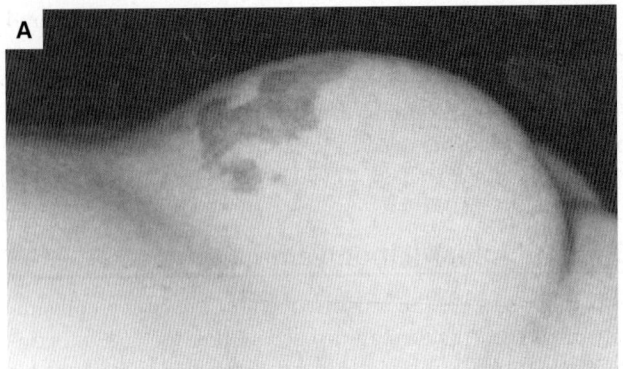

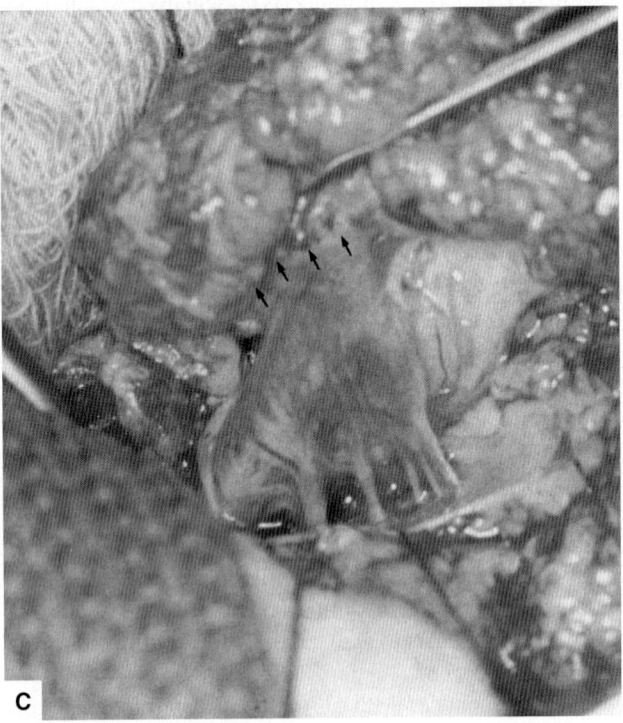

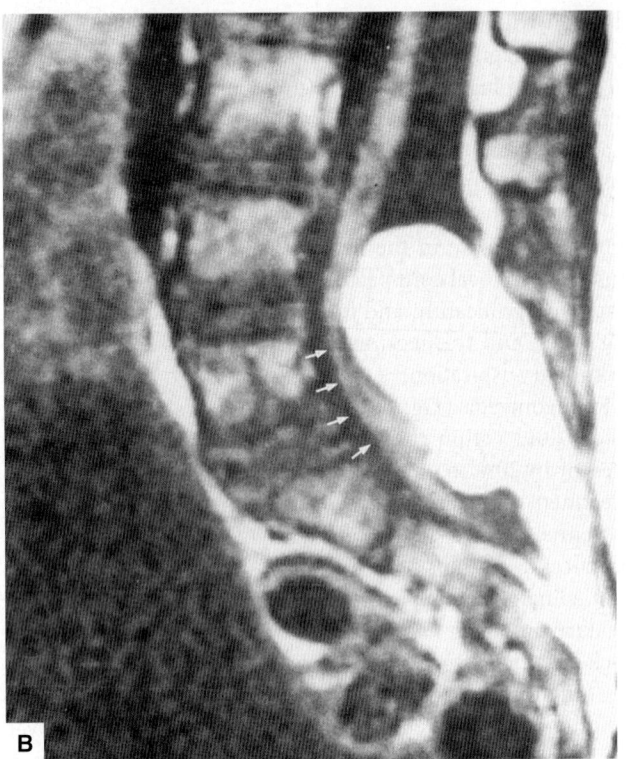

**FIGURE 76-10** Spinal lipoma. **A.** Photograph of a child with a spinal lipoma. A subcutaneous fatty mass is located on the sacrum above the gluteal cleft. A small hemangioma is evident. **B.** Sagittal T₁-weighted MRI scan shows the fatty mass extending to the spinal canal. The spinal cord (*arrows*) is low lying. **C.** Intraoperative photograph shows the fatty mass extending down to, and contiguous with, the spinal cord (*arrows*). Several spinal nerve roots are evident ventrolateral to the lipoma.

*lipoma without addressing its relationship to the underlying spinal cord is not adequate treatment.*

The outcome is generally excellent when the lesion is dealt with prophylactically; in a series of 71 asymptomatic patients by McLone and colleagues, none were made worse by surgery, and 66 (93%) remained clinically stable at long-term follow-up. In contrast, among 87 children operated on at the time of clinical deterioration, 2 suffered operative complications, 26% improved (only 11.5% returned to normal), and 51% were stable at long-term follow-up; at long-term follow-up, 41% deteriorated in a delayed fashion and required further untethering operations.

## Dermal Sinus Tracts

Dermal sinus tracts are thought to represent incomplete dysjunction of the neural tube from the cutaneous ectoderm during neurulation. As a result, a tract of cutaneous tissue remains attached to the nervous system. The lumbosacral dermal sinus tract often extends deep to the ostium, through or between the lamina(e) immediately beneath (Fig. 76-11), penetrates the dura, and ascends within the

thecal sac to end on the dorsal aspect of the spinal cord at the level of the posterior neuropore (the second sacral spinal cord level), just above the tip of the conus medullaris. In addition to tethering the spinal cord, dermal sinus tracts can cause symptoms and signs through at least 3 other mechanisms. First, they can serve as a portal of entry for bacteria, leading to recurrent infections (bacterial meningitis or spinal abscess). Second, desquamation of epithelial cells and debris from the dermoid tumor can produce an intense inflammatory response, resulting in aseptic meningitis. Third, dermoid tumors can develop within the spinal cord or canal and compress the spinal cord.

Dermal sinus tracts almost always have some associated cutaneous marker, usually the tract itself, which produces a lumbosacral dimple. Dermal sinus tracts are usually easy to differentiate from the benign coccygeal dimple, which is present in about 4% of normal infants. As its name implies, the benign coccygeal dimple is located at or just above the tip of the coccyx within the gluteal cleft. The tip of the coccyx is readily palpated deep to the dimple. In contrast, the dermal sinus tract is located higher, in the "flat" of the lumbosacral area, well rostral to the coccyx and almost always cranial to

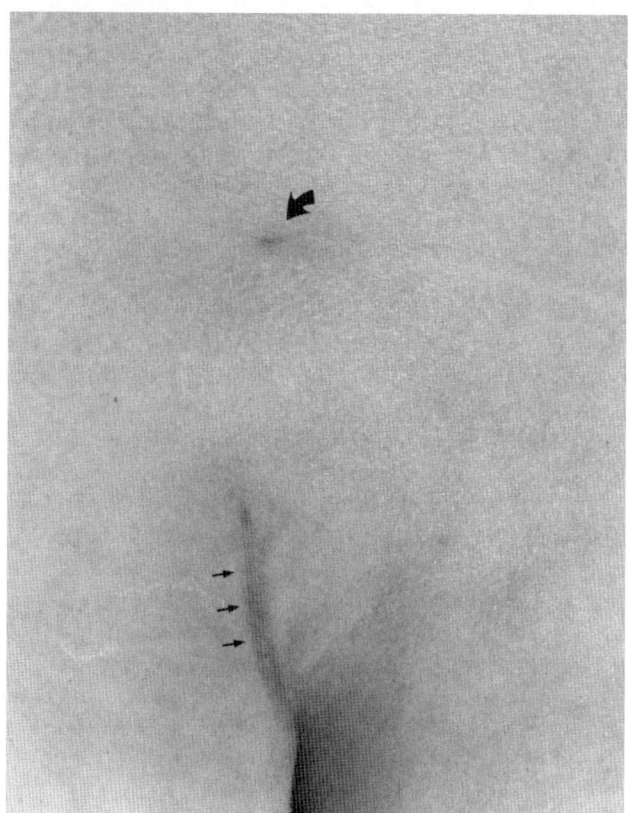

**FIGURE 76-11** Photograph of a dermal sinus tract (*curved arrow*) in the sacral region. The gluteal cleft (*small arrows*) is abnormally deviated toward the left.

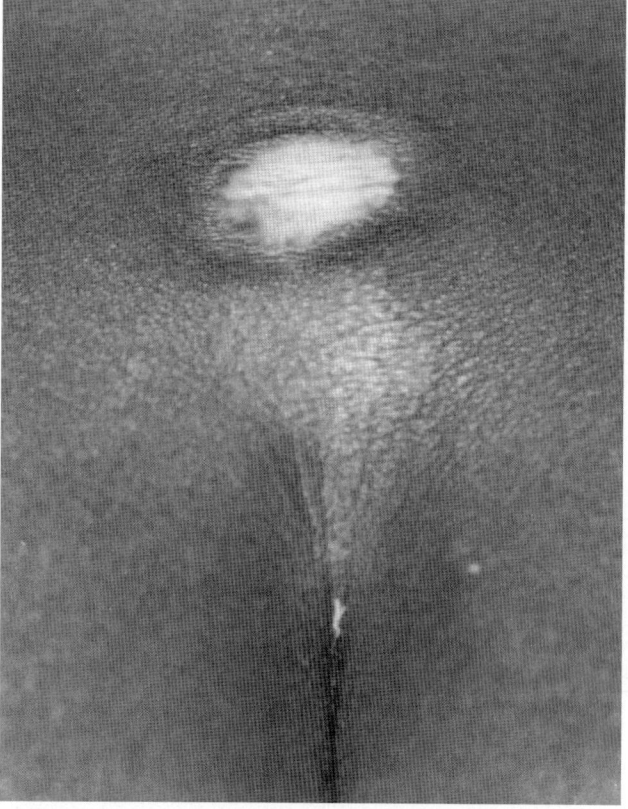

**FIGURE 76-12** Myelomeningocele manqué. Photograph shows a scarified area of skin. At surgery, nerve roots extended from the skin lesion to the spinal cord.

the end of the gluteal cleft (Fig. 76-11). Dermal sinus tracts may be irregular, surrounded by heaped-up areas of skin or small dermal masses, or associated with cutaneous hemangiomas, skin tags, or tufts of hair within the ostium. Abnormal or asymmetric forking of the gluteal cleft is common; the dermal sinus tract may be located at the end of one fork. Finally, dermal sinus tracts may be associated with focal neurologic deficits, a neurogenic bladder, or orthopedic deformities. Benign coccygeal dimples are never associated with any of these findings.

An MRI of the lumbar spine will show the spinal cord to be tethered. Dermoid tumors, if present, may be seen within the thecal sac or spinal cord parenchyma but may be isointense to spinal fluid or spinal cord and therefore difficult to visualize. Unfortunately, dermal sinus tracts are not always visible on MRI, and the absence of a visible tract does not exclude a connection. If the lesion appears clinically suspicious, especially if the conus is abnormally low, the malformation should be explored regardless of whether a tract is visible on MRI. The tract is followed down to the underlying spine, a laminectomy is performed, and the tract is followed to its terminus at the conus medullaris; any associated dermoid tumors are also removed.

Rarely, the "tug of war" between cutaneous and neuroectoderm may instead be won by the cutaneous ectoderm, pulling the neuroectoderm toward the skin and producing a myelomeningocele manqué. The involved neuroectoderm usually is in the form of dorsal roots that leave the underlying spinal cord, penetrate the dura, and end either in the subcutaneous

tissues or even within the skin. The skin overlying the malformation is usually somewhat thinned and scarified and has been referred to as a "cigarette burn" (Fig. 76-12); it is sometimes painful and tender. The skin malformation again serves as a marker for the underlying spinal cord malformation; rather than simple excision of the skin lesion, the entire malformation should be dealt with to treat spinal cord tethering. Again, for both dermal sinus tracts and myelomeningoceles and manqué acute, *simply removing the cutaneous component without addressing the underlying spinal cord malformation is not sufficient.*

Dermal sinus tracts may also be visible at the cranial end of the neural tube, most commonly either frontally (frontonasal sinus tracts) or in the occiput (occipital sinus tracts); they rarely occur in a midline parietal location. Dermal sinus tracts between the nasion and the midparietal region may penetrate the bone of the skull and end perilously close to the sagittal sinus but should never have an intradural extension. The reason for this is embryologic—the explosive growth of the cerebral hemispheres after neural tube closure should sweep any malformation involving neural tube closure posterior to the area just behind the vertex.

Frontonasal dermal sinus tracts typically begin along the dorsum of the nose anywhere between the tip and the nasion (Fig. 76-13) and travel between the skin and nasal cartilage to end at or near the anterior skull base (Fig. 76-14). Although they often appear innocuous and may end harmlessly in the extracranial space, some sinuses extend intracranially through a tiny defect in the anterior skull base near the foramen cecum

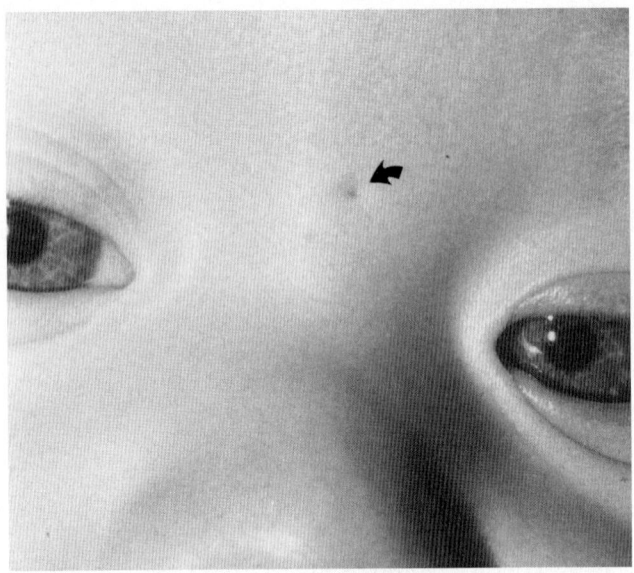

**FIGURE 76-13** Frontonasal dermal sinus tract in an infant. The ostium of the tract is located at the glabella (*curved arrow*).

and serve as a portal of entry for intracranial infection (meningitis or brain abscess), or as a source of intracranial dermoid tumors. The occipital dermal sinus tract similarly can have intracranial extension into the supratentorial compartment, the posterior fossa, or both, with intracranial complications.

The radiographic workup of cranial dermal sinus tracts should include both enhanced cranial MRI and CT scans with bone windows and coronal views through the anterior skull base. The frontonasal dermal sinus tract and/or associated dermoid tumors are best visualized on MRI scans with gadolinium-enhanced sagittal and coronal views, but a small bony defect may be visible only on coronal CT scans with bone windows, even though an intracranial abnormality on MRI cannot be found. Unfortunately, some intracranial connections may not be visible even with high-resolution imaging studies. As with the lumbosacral dermal sinus tracts, all suspicious lesions should be explored even if radiographic studies are negative. These lesions are best approached in a combined fashion with a pediatric surgeon, otolaryngologist or plastic surgeon, and a pediatric neurosurgeon. If there is a known intracranial extension, the entire tract is explored and removed, either in a combined extra- and intracranial procedure or in 2 separate procedures (with the intracranial portion

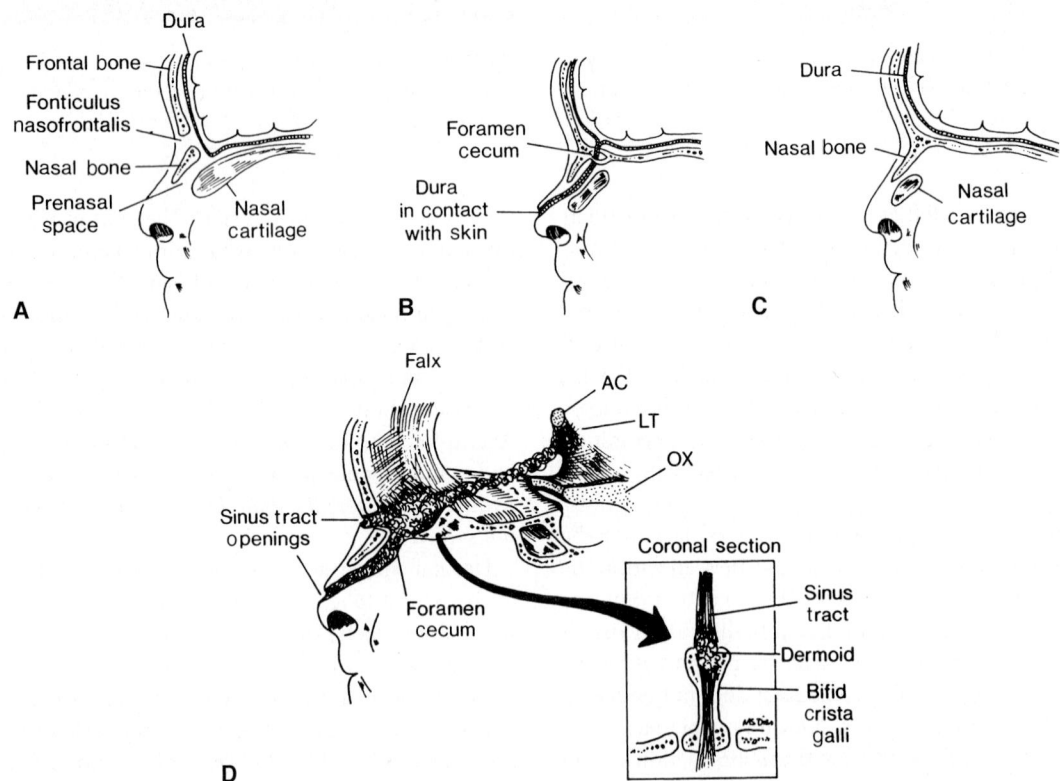

**FIGURE 76-14** Normal frontonasal development (A–C) and the embryology of frontonasal dermal sinus tracts (D). **A.** During normal embryogenesis, the fonticulus nasofrontalis forms between the frontal and nasal bones; the prenasal space forms between the nasal bone and nasal cartilage. **B.** A tongue of dura extends through the foramen cecum toward the midline nasal skin. **C.** Later, this tongue of dura is obliterated, and the anterior cranial base is formed; the foramen cecum remains as a vestige of this embryonic tract. **D.** Abnormal dysjunction during closure of the anterior neuropore leaves a tract of cutaneous ectoderm between the commissural plate and the midline nasal skin. Formation of the anterior frontobasal structures results in a tract whose cutaneous opening may be located at the fonticulus nasofrontalis or anywhere along the dorsum of the nose, and that extends through the foramen cecum, between the two halves of a bifid crista galli, and along the anterior cranial base; in rare instances, the tract extends all the way to the commissural plate. (Adapted from Sessions RB. Nasal dermal sinuses: new concepts and explanations. *Laryngoscope* 1982;92(Suppl 29):1–28.)

usually being performed first). If there is no visible intracranial extension, the extracranial tract may be excised locally, and the tract followed toward the skull base, with the pediatric neurosurgeon on stand-by; an intracranial exploration may be necessary if intracranial extension is found at the time of surgery.

## Split Cord Malformations, Neurenteric Cysts, the Split-Notochord Syndrome (Combined Spina Bifida), and other Complex Dysraphic Malformations

A number of spinal cord malformations involve concomitant anomalies of the gastrointestinal system, posterior mediastinum, and/or retroperitoneum as neurenteric cysts or certain enteric or bronchial duplications, diverticula, or fistulaes. The key to understanding these malformations lies in properly appreciating the embryonic relationship between the developing neural tube and the endoderm during early development.

Most of these malformations involve a split-cord malformation (SCM) in which the spinal cord is split or clefted over a portion of its length. The terms diastematomyelia and diplomyelia were used in the past but have generated a great deal of confusion; these terms have therefore been largely supplanted by the common term SCM. Two types of SCMs are recognized. Type I lesions are double dural sac malformations in which both the spinal cord and dural sac are split, and there is an extradural bony or fibrocartilaginous spur interposed between the 2 thecal sacs (Fig. 76-15A). Type II malformations are single dural sac malformations in which the spinal cord, but not the thecal sac, is clefted, and both hemicords are therefore contained within a common dural sac (Fig. 76-15B).

Although the earlier literature suggested that the type II malformations did not contain any tethering elements, at surgery, fibrous bands of tissue (analogous to the bony or cartilaginous spurs of the type I malformations) are usually found between the 2 hemicords. In addition, both types contain aberrant nerve roots that exit from the medial aspects of one or both hemicords and end blindly on the midline mesenchymal elements, which can additionally tether the spinal cord. Both types of malformations therefore contain tethering elements, which can produce neurologic deterioration. Associated congenital spinal cord malformations such as lipomas, dermal sinus tracts, and thickened filum terminale may be present and present additional tethering elements.

An associated enteric malformation may also be present and may be the feature that prompts medical attention. The most common malformation is a posterior mediastinal (foregut) or retroperitoneal "dorsal enteric cyst" often (in about 50% of cases) associated with an adjacent clefted vertebral body ("butterfly" vertebra) or other vertebral anomaly. The enteric cyst may contain either enteric tissues (gastric, small intestinal, or colonic) or bronchial tissues (in the mediastinal cases), suggesting that these malformations arise before the normal separation of the gut from the tracheobronchial tree. Posterior mediastinal cysts are usually associated with the middle or lower thirds of the esophagus. Duplications of the small intestine may also be present.

A tract may extend between the enteric malformation and the adjacent vertebrae, and the enteric malformation often is adherent to the vertebral column. The tract may extend between the two halves of a cleft vertebra and even into the spinal canal; associated intraspinal neurenteric cysts may be present. In rare cases, the spinal cord and vertebral columns are split widely apart, forming 2 "neuraxial columns" between

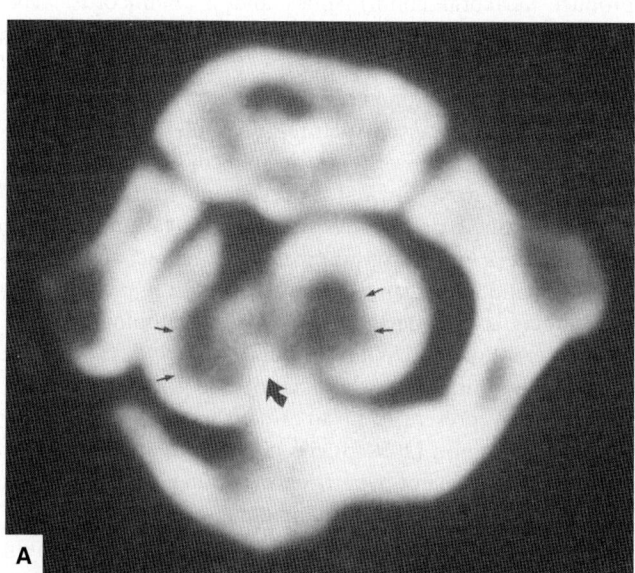

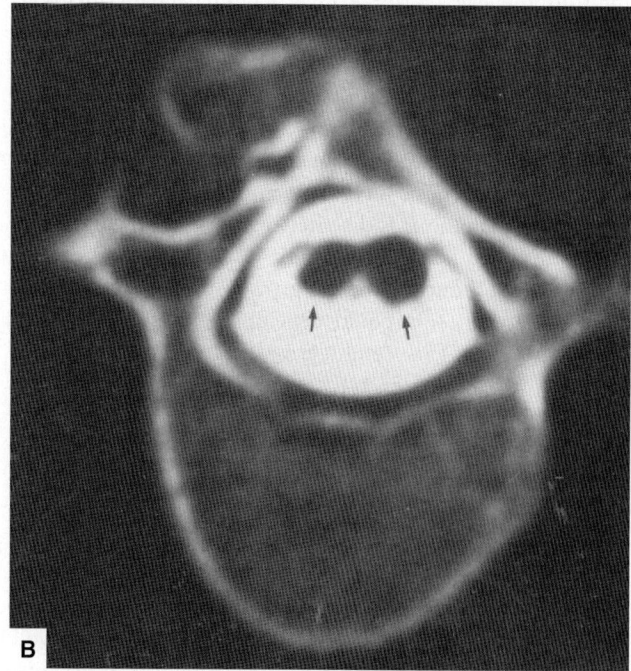

**FIGURE 76-15** Split-cord malformations (SCM). **A.** Axial metrizamide myelogram of a type I SCM shows 2 hemicords (*small arrows*), each ensheathed in its own dural sac, and separated by a midline bony spike (*curved arrow*). **B.** Axial T$_1$-weighted MRI scan of a type II SCM shows 2 hemicords (*black arrows*) within a single dural sac. A midline tethering band is not visible in the MRI but was found at surgery.

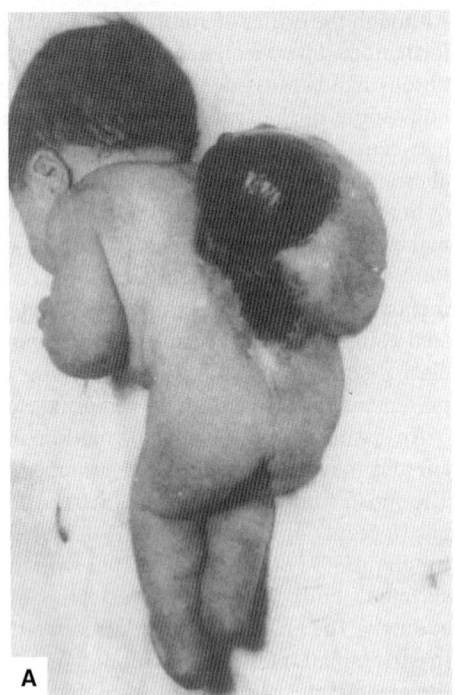
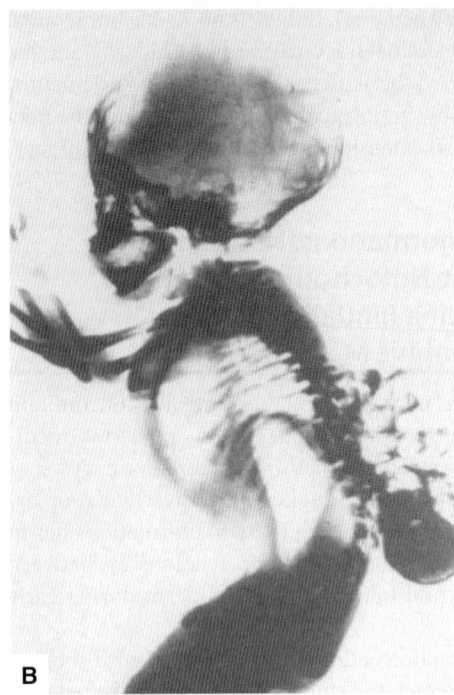

**FIGURE 76-16** Combined spina bifida (split notochord syndrome). **A.** Photograph of infant shows a huge, covered dorsal mass. **B.** Lateral x-ray shows multiple loops of bowel within the sec. (From Saunders RL. Combined anterior and posterior spina bifida in a living neonatal human female. *Anat Rec* 1976;87:255–278.)

which lies a central cleft containing a variable amount of enteric tissue ranging from an enteric cyst to entire loops of bowel that pass through the midline cleft and lie posteriorly on the back of the child; this malformation is referred to as the "split notochord syndrome" or combined (anterior and posterior) spina bifida (Fig. 76-16). Associated intra-abdominal enteric duplications may also be present; in the extreme, complete hindgut duplication occurs with twinned colons extending from the level of Meckel diverticulum caudally, including double anuses. Girls additionally may have 2 vaginas, bilateral unicornuate uteri, and 2 bladders, each having a single ureter and urethra, which ends in its own urethral opening. Some girls have a bifid clitoris, and boys have a bifid penis. The spinal column also is doubled, with an associated split spinal cord.

The embryogenesis of SCMs and other complex dysraphic malformations is disputed, and several theories have been advanced. Beardmore and Wigglesworth proposed that before or during the outgrowth of the notochordal process, an adhesion could develop between the epiblast and hypoblast. This "endodermal–ectodermal adhesion" would provide a barrier to the elongating notochord, which would then become split around the adhesion; independent development of paired neuroepithelial anlagen would then form 2 "hemicords." Associated remnants of the adhesion could give rise to endodermal remnants located anywhere between the gut and cutaneous ectoderm.

Noting the similarities between the central cleft in the split notochord syndrome and the neurenteric canal of normal embryos, both of which connect the amnion with the yolk sac, Bremer, proposed that these malformations must arise through the formation of an "accessory neurenteric canal" caused by a dorsal herniation of endoderm that splits the notochord and neuroepithelium. McLetchie and Saunders

suggested that the initial malformation involves duplication of the notochord, which secondarily allows a endodermal–ectodermal interaction between the duplicated notochords.

Dias and Walker proposed that these and related complex dysraphic malformations arise during a time when prospective anlagen from all three germ layers are in intimate association, while they are being laid down during *gastrulation*. According to this theory, the notochordal and spinal cord precursors during gastrulation remain separate rather than integrating to form a single midline neuraxis and develop independently over a variable portion of their length to produce vertebral abnormalities and 2 "hemicords." The intervening space between the paired "hemicords," being comprised of pluripotent primitive streak cells, could form tissues derived from one or more of the three primary germ layers, including enteric structures (neurenteric cysts, intestinal duplications or diverticula, or loops of bowel within the central cleft), mesenchymal tissues (bony spurs or fibrous midline bands, blood vessels, muscle, and fat encountered between the 2 hemicords; anomalous vertebrae; and immature renal and Müllerian tissues), ectodermal tissues (dermal sinus tracts and/or dermoids), and even pathologic tissues such as teratomas and Wilms tumors.

Clinically, cutaneous stigmata of the underlying malformation are present in up to 80% of patients with SCMs. The most common (20% to 55% of patients) and specific of these is a focal area of hypertrichosis. Other cutaneous stigmata include cutaneous hemangiomata, dimples, lipomas, and bony abnormalities. Symptoms of spinal cord tethering occur because the 2 hemicords are transfixed by the intervening bony, cartilaginous, or fibrous tissues between the two hemicords. Sensorimotor deficits, changes in bowel or bladder habits, and orthopaedic deformities result. A "suspended" sensorimotor deficit (in which neurologic deficits are referable only to the involved spinal cord segments without more distal deficits) may arise presumably from local traction at the level of the malformation.

Radiographic evaluation of SCMs includes an MRI and/or a spinal CT scan with intrathecal contrast (a CT myelogram). Although the sensitivity of spinal MRI is improving, CT myelography is better to evaluate the fine details of these malformations for surgical planning. High-resolution CT myelography is particularly good at identifying thin intradural fibrous tethering bands in the type II malformations that may not be visible on MRI. About 15% of SCMs involve tandem lesions, so the entire spinal cord should be studied.

Prophylactic repair of the malformation and untethering are recommended by most before the child develops signs and symptoms because neurologic deficits, once they develop, are usually stabilized but may not improve with surgery. At surgery, the tethering bony spurs (type I) or fibrous bands (type II) are resected, and, in the type I malformations, the dural cuff between the two hemicords is excised and a single dural sac is reconstituted (described as "converting pants to a dress"). Any associated tethering elements should be dealt with as well. In particular, the filum terminale is almost always short and thickened and should be sectioned. Any associated enteric tracts should also be dealt with by the pediatric surgeon, usually following or concurrent with the neurosurgical repair.

## Thickened Filum Terminale

The filum terminale is a nonfunctional strand of tissue that projects from the end of the conus to the bottom of the thecal sac and is formed from secondary neurulation. A thickened filum terminale is defined as one that is greater than 2-mm thick on MRI scans or CT myelography. The embryogenesis is unknown but likely involves a disturbance of the caudal cell mass during early embryogenesis. Up to 90% of malformations have fat within the filum terminale (the so-called "fatty filum"), and 86% are associated with a low-lying conus medullaris. Although as many as 6% of normal individuals have some fat within the filum, the association of a thickened, fat-infiltrated filum and a low-lying conus suggests a tethering lesion. As many as 50% of patients have cutaneous manifestations of the anomaly but in many, the initial presentation is with sensorimotor findings or a neurogenic bladder.

Plain x-rays sometimes demonstrate a defect in one or more vertebral laminae (spina bifida occulta). Spinal MRI demonstrates the low-lying spinal cord and a filum terminale that is thickened and infiltrated with fat (producing a hyperintense strand of tissue connecting the conus and the distal thecal sac on $T_1$-weighted images). Surgical treatment involves a limited incision, sacral laminectomy, and simple section of the filum terminale near the end of the thecal sac.

## Terminal Myelocystocele

A myelocystocele is a rare caudal spinal cord malformation in which there is dilation (terminal syringomyelia) of the caudal end of the spinal cord, with a corresponding dilatation of the caudal thecal sac, giving a "double bubble" appearance (Fig. 76-17) to the distal neuraxis on MRI. There

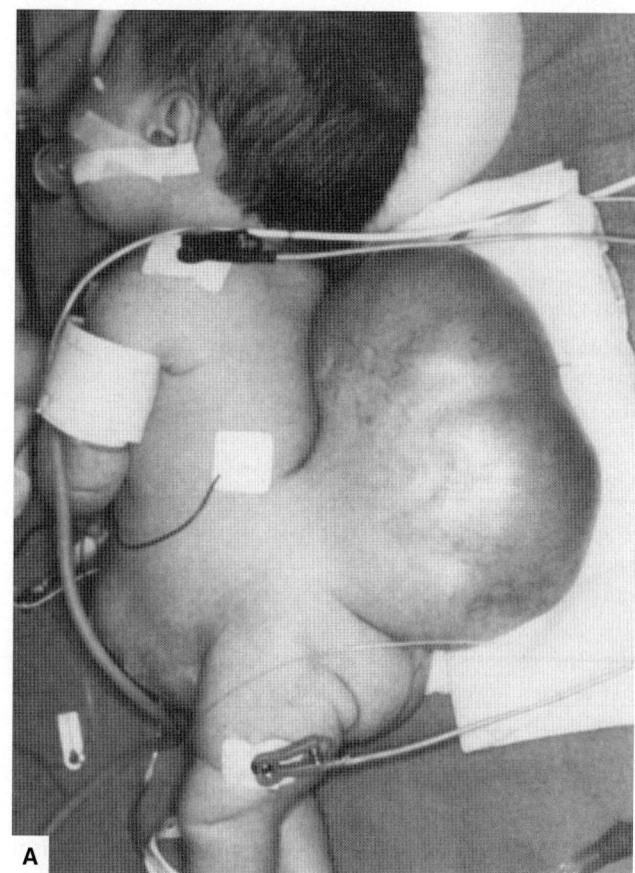

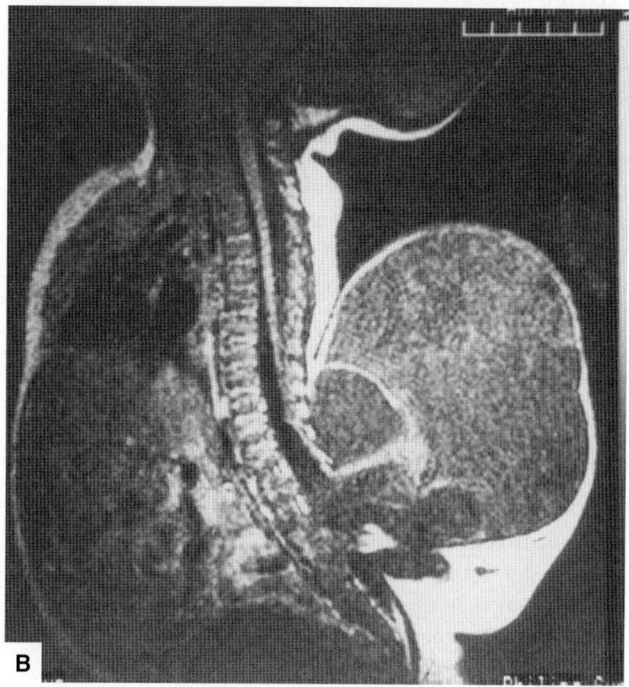

**FIGURE 76-17** Myelocystocele. **A.** Photograph of an infant with cloacal exstrophy (repaired) and a huge skin-covered dorsal mass. **B.** Sagittal $T_1$-weighted MRI shows a double compartment sac containing a dilated terminal spinal cord contained within a larger spinal fluid containing dural sac. (Photograph courtesy of Keith Aronyk, MD.)

is also usually an associated terminal spinal lipoma. The size of the malformation is variable, but some can reach a monstrous size (Fig. 76-17). The embryogenesis is unknown but again probably involves a disorder of caudal cell mass development. Clinically, the lesions appear as closed, skin-covered lumbosacral masses that resemble a spinal lipoma or sacrococcygeal teratoma. Many of these have erroneously been termed "closed myelomeningoceles" (a misnomer because, as previously discussed, a myelomeningocele cannot, be closed). Surgical treatment involves excising the redundant and nonfunctional dilated neural tissue, imbricating the remaining spinal cord, untethering the cord from the lipoma, and closing the thecal sac.

## Caudal Agenesis

The syndrome of caudal agenesis is usually included in the spectrum of dysraphic malformations, although tethering or other neurosurgical lesions are less frequent in these patients. The coccyx and part or all of the sacrum are usually missing. The agenesis rarely extends rostrally to involve the lumbar or even lower thoracic segments. The syndrome is more common in the offsprings of diabetic mothers (1% of the offsprings born to diabetic mothers will have sacral agenesis, and 16% of children with sacral agenesis are offsprings of diabetic mothers); both hyperglycemia and ketones have been implicated in the embryopathy. The embryonic mechanism is unknown, but a disorder of a caudal "embryonic field" has been implicated.

Clinically, the child with sacral agenesis has varying degrees of paralysis and atrophy of the distal leg musculature, producing an "inverted champagne bottle" appearance. The buttocks are flattened and atrophic as well. A neurogenic bladder is almost universal. Sensory function is curiously preserved. Lumbosacral spine x-rays reveal absence of a variable portion of the caudal spinal column, most commonly including part or all of the sacrum; hemivertebrae or fused vertebrae may also be seen. All children with sacral agenesis should undergo a baseline lumbosacral MRI to exclude important associated spinal cord malformations. The spinal cord ends bluntly within the thecal sac (Fig. 76-18), confirming the failure of caudal spinal cord development. Although sacral agenesis is a static malformation that need not be treated, associated tethering lesions (myelomeningoceles, SCMs, lipomas, dermoid tumors, fibrous bands, and thickened filum terminale) can all cause neurologic deterioration in these patients and should be treated if found. In addition, bony or dural stenosis of the spinal canal may cause progressive deterioration and may also require treatment.

## The Association of Imperforate Anus, Cloacal Exstrophy, OEIS, VACTERL, and Currarino Triad With Congenital Spinal Cord Malformations

The juxtaposition of the caudal neural tube (the conus medullaris below the second sacral spinal cord segment and the filum terminale) and the caudal spinal mesenchyme from the caudal cell mass, along with the hindgut endoderm and caudal urogenital system from the prospective cloaca during early development, results in the association between

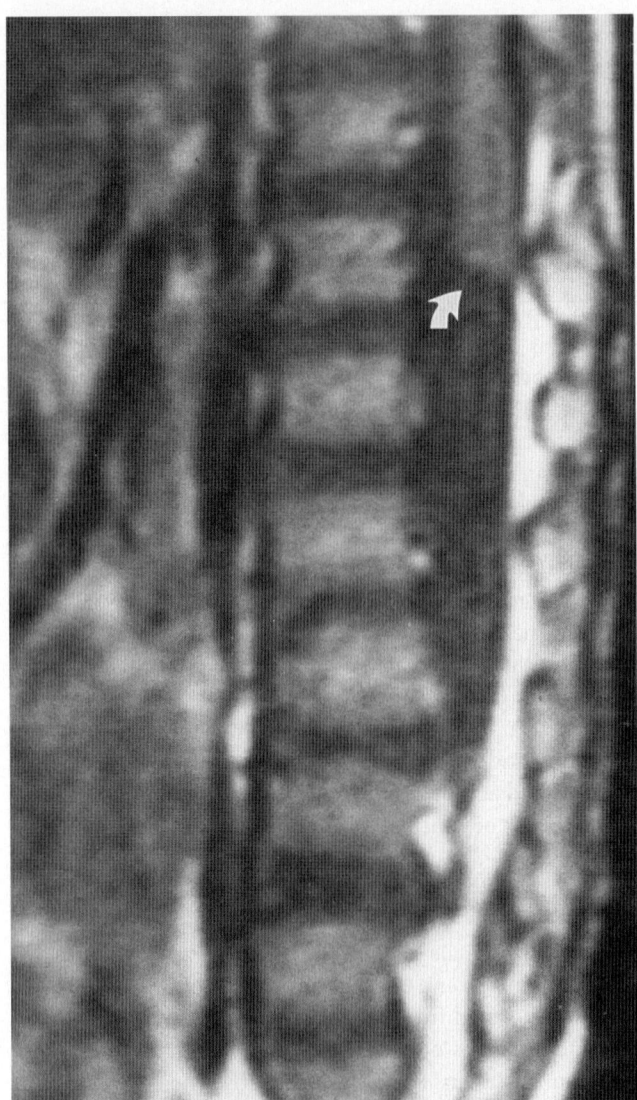

**FIGURE 76-18** Sagittal T$_1$-weighted weighted MRI in a child with sacral agenesis shows absence of the bony sacrum and a blunted caudal spinal cord (*curved arrow*).

congenital anomalies involving cloacal derivatives and spinal cord malformations. Bony malformations of the sacrum (including agenesis, dysplasia, and/or asymmetry) are present in 30% to 38% of children with imperforate anus, including 48% of those with high imperforate anus; and 15% of those with low imperforate anus; genitourinary malformations are present in 20%. Associated congenital spinal cord anomalies are present in 10% to 14% of children with imperforate anus. Although more frequent in children with high imperforate anus, congenital spinal cord malformations also occur in children with low imperforate anus. Thickened filum terminale, spinal lipoma, and myelocystocele most commonly occur in association with anorectal malformations; less common anomalies include anterior meningoceles, syringomyelia, and dural stenosis. Caudal spinal cord anomalies also occur in association with the VACTERL (vertebral anomalies, imperforate anus, cardiac defects, tracheoesophageal fistula, renal anomalies, and limb reduction anomalies).

Caudal spinal cord malformations occur with even greater frequency in patients with cloacal exstrophy, where the spinal cord anomalies tend to be more complex than in those with isolated imperforate anus. Spinal cord malformations can also be seen as part of the OEIS (omphalocele, exstrophy, imperforate anus, and spinal defects) sequence, with 4 of 6 cases described by Carey as having skin-covered "meningoceles." Among 13 patients with cloacal exstrophy and caudal spinal cord malformations described by Warf, 5 had myelocystoceles, 4 had spinal lipomas, and 3 had a thickened filum terminale.

The diagnostic evaluation for every patient with imperforate anus, anorectal stenosis, or cloacal exstrophy, regardless of the type, should include a spinal imaging study such as an MRI. Unfortunately, the associated problems with genitourinary and defecatory functions in this group of patients makes a proper clinical evaluation difficult; serial urodynamic studies are valuable for detecting occult urologic changes. In addition, particular attention should be given to the presence of associated neurologic deficits. Children with congenital tethering lesions should be offered neurosurgical repair and prophylactic untethering before symptoms and signs intervene.

Currarino triad is a distinct malformation sequence consisting of anorectal stenosis, a presacral mass, and an anterior sacral bony defect. The most common enteric malformations include anal or anorectal stenosis, although anorectal agenesis, anorectal stenosis with rectovaginal fistula, and rectal ectopia have also been described. An associated hemisacral or "scimitar" sacral defect (Fig. 76-19) is present; segmentation anomalies are less frequent. The presacral mass is most frequently a presacral teratoma or anterior meningocele;

neurenteric cysts, or dermoid tumors are unusual. At least 50% of cases are familial, and both X-linked and autosomal dominant inheritance patterns have been described.

This constellation of anomalies has been thought to arise through an abnormal adhesion or fistula between the neuroectoderm and endoderm in a manner analogous to the split-notochord syndrome, SCMs, and other complex dysraphic malformations described above. However, these embryonic mechanisms do not adequately fit our current understanding of caudal axial development because, unlike split-cord variants that involve more rostral regions of the neuroectoderm formed from primary neurulation, the Currarino triad involves neuroectoderm and caudal endodermal structures that are normally formed from the caudal cell mass. We encountered a child with the Currarino triad and a type II caudal SCM in which one hemicord was contiguous, through the sacral defect, with a presacral teratoma and an enteric duplication. This association of a caudal SCM with Currarino triad recently led us to propose that the Currarino triad arises through an incomplete dorsoventral separation of the caudal cell mass from the hindgut endoderm during late gastrulation.

Children with the Currarino triad most often present with constipation of varying degrees. Perirectal abscesses and fistula and meningitis are less common. Neurologic evaluation should include plain lumbosacral spine x-rays, which will demonstrate the scimitar sacrum to good advantage, and a lumbosacral MRI to evaluate the spinal cord and caudal

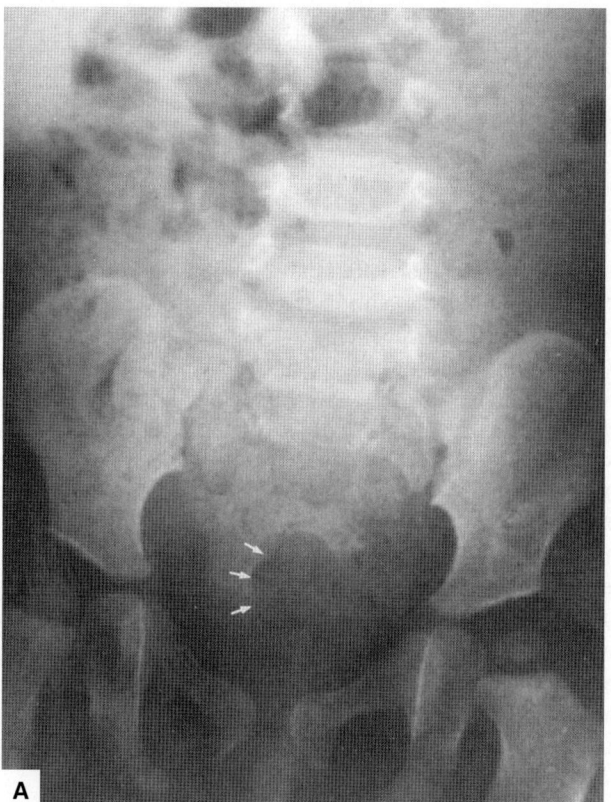
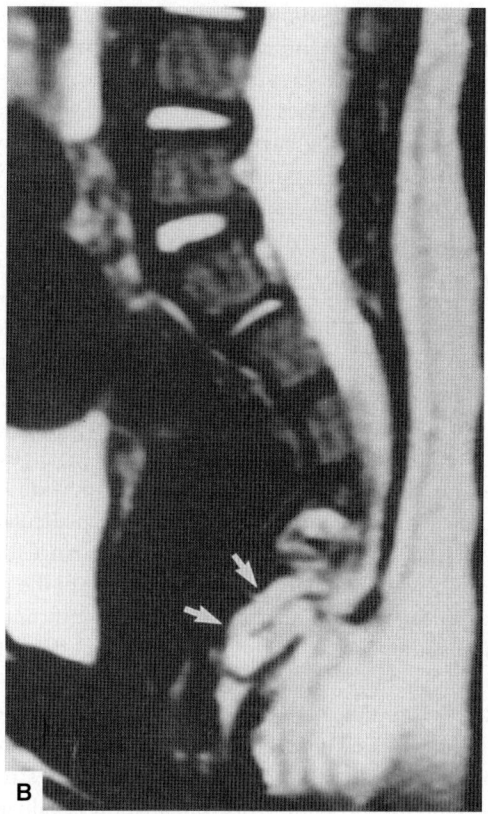

**FIGURE 76-19** Unusual case of the Currarino triad. **A.** Anterior–posterior lumbosacral x-ray shows a scimitar defect in the bony sacrum. **B.** T₂-weighted MRI shows a presacral teratoma (*white arrows*) and a low-lying spinal cord. At surgery, the spinal cord was split caudally, with one of the hemicords extending through the sacral defect to become contiguous with the presacral teratoma. (From Dias MS, Azizkhan RG. A novel embryogenetic mechanism for Currarino's triad: inadequate dorsoventral separation of the caudal eminence from hindgut endoderm. *Pediatr Neurosurg* 1998;28:223–229.)

neuraxial structures. A meningocele is most easily repaired via a posterior approach, ligating the opening of the thecal sac into the meningocele to seal it from the abdominal contents. Any tethering spinal cord elements should be dealt with before neurologic deficits intervene. Presacral teratomas should be treated as any sacrococcygeal teratoma.

In summary, congenital malformations of the central nervous system present a number of opportunities for interaction between the pediatric neurosurgeon and pediatric surgeon. We have emphasized the developmental anatomy of congenital malformations in this chapter because a thorough understanding of this anatomy helps one to best understand the intimate associations, as well as the borderland, between the central nervous system and other organ systems.

## "DUMBBELL" TUMORS

"Dumbbell" tumors have both intraspinal and extraspinal components that are connected by an isthmus of tissue that traverses the neural foramina. Although the soft tissue mass can be quite large, there is usually minimal or no bone destruction except for widening of the neural foramina, and the stability of the spine is therefore commonly preserved. The thoracic region is most commonly involved, followed by the lumbosacral and cervical spine. Tumors that can grow in this fashion include ganglioneuroma, ganglioneuroblastoma, neuroblastoma, sarcoma, schwannoma, neurofibroma, lymphoma, and primitive neuroectodermal tumors. Most of the literature on "dumbbell" tumors is devoted to ganglioneuromas, ganglioblastomas, and neuroblastomas; between 10% and 15% of these tumors have extension into the spinal canal. In the larger reported series, of those with growth into the spinal canal, at least 64% have neurologic signs and symptoms at the time of presentation. The most common symptom is pain, and the most common sign is weakness.

### Diagnosis

The diagnosis of a "dumbbell" lesion can be established through a variety of radiographic studies; however, there are strengths and limitations to each modality. Because these tumors do not cause bone destruction, plain spine radiographs are capable of showing only indirect changes that occur as a result of growth of the intraspinal portion of the lesion. Typical findings include a widened interpedicular distance, widening of the neural foramina, and changes in the contour of the vertebral body, that is, scalloping of the posterior or lateral surfaces of the body. The most significant limitation of this study is that it fails to image the soft tissue mass. The major advantage is that the stability of the spine can be assessed by examining the alignment of the spine and the severity of osseous change. Furthermore, dynamic flexion–extension films can measure the effects of physical stressors on the stability of the spine. This information is valuable in deciding whether or not a spinal fusion is necessary.

CT scanning is the best means of demonstrating osseous changes in the spine. Axial images are obtained, and images in the sagittal and coronal planes can be reconstructed. Though the extraspinal soft tissue is often well visualized,

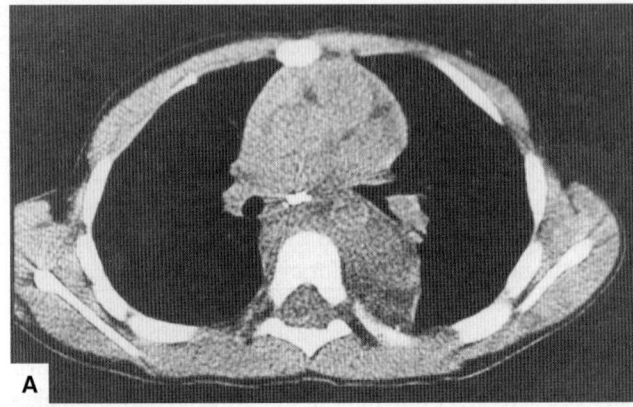

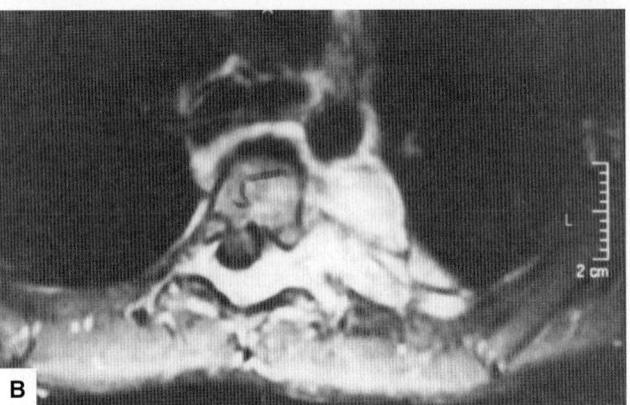

**FIGURE 76-20** Dumbbell tumor. **A.** An axial CT of the T-5 vertebral body showing no destruction of the body. The extraspinal soft tissue mass is well delineated; however, the intraspinal extension is not well visualized. **B.** An axial MRI after intravenous contrast through the same level. The full extraspinal and intraspinal growth is much more clearly defined than on CT. Note that the tumor is growing through the foramina, lying dorsolateral to the spinal cord, and pushing it ventrally and to the opposite side.

the intraspinal soft tissue component is very poorly outlined, even after the administration of intravenous contrast, making MRI the most effective modality for imaging "dumbbell" lesions that traverse the neural foramina. This study not only demonstrates the extraspinal soft tissue mass, it is far and away the best means of visualizing the intraspinal component (Fig. 76-20). The use of intravenous contrast and multiple imaging sequences will almost always provide excellent distinction between tumor and neural elements and can provide information as to whether the tumor is purely extradural or whether there is intradural extension. The major limitation of MRI is that osseous structures are not as well visualized as on CT scan; however, one can always supplement the MRI with plain spine radiographs if necessary. Regardless of the imaging technique utilized, it is imperative to identify the full extent of intraspinal growth to optimize the planning of an appropriate operative strategy.

### Treatment

Since the most appropriate treatments for all the various types of "dumbbell" lesions are beyond the scope of this chapter, we focus only on operative management. Potential

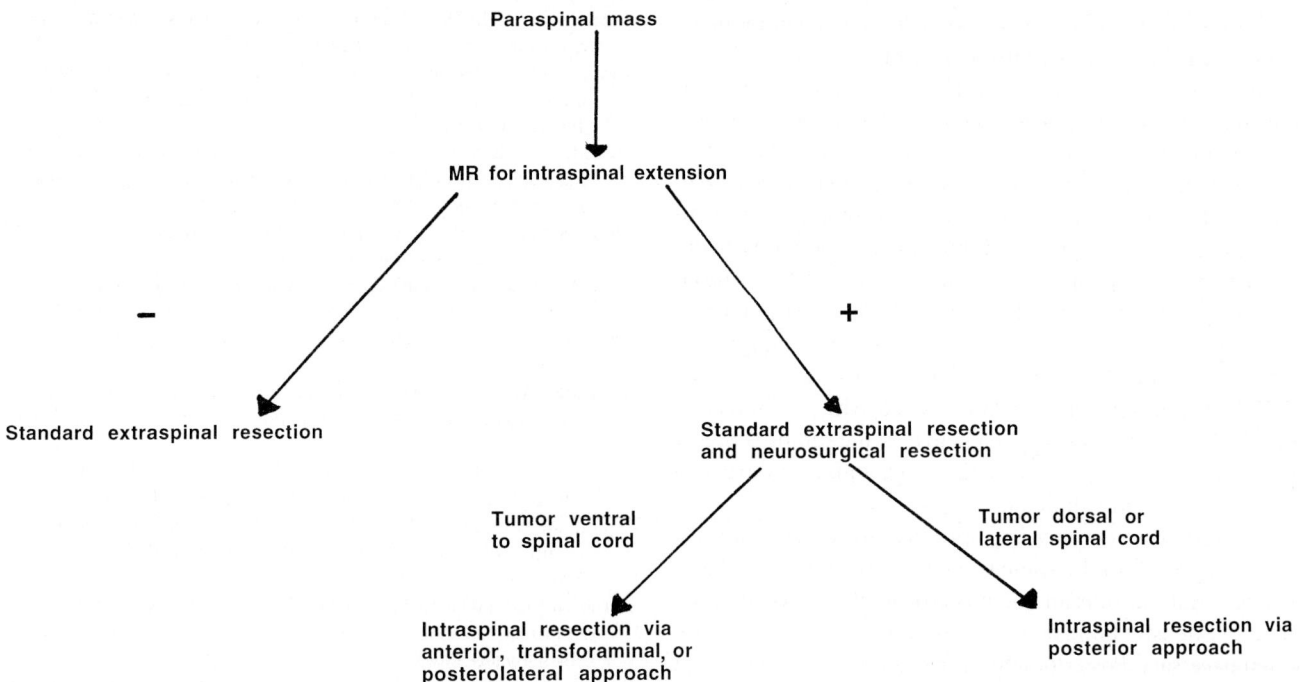

**FIGURE 76-21** One algorithm for the surgical management of patients with dumbbell spine tumors, with an emphasis on the role of the pediatric neurosurgeon in these cases.

indications for removal of the intraspinal component of the tumor include rapid neurologic deterioration, progressive neurologic deterioration despite adjuvant therapy, tumor that occupies more than 50% of the spinal canal, tumors in which the chance for cure is maximized by surgical resection, and the lack of a diagnosis despite biopsy of the extraspinal component. There are several approaches to the spine, and the selection of the most appropriate approach depends heavily on the findings from the preoperative imaging studies. The most important variables are the underlying diagnosis, the extent of growth into the intraspinal space and the position of the tumor relative to the spinal cord. If there is only minimal encroachment of the tumor through the foramen and the tumor is ganglioneuroma or neurblastoma, removal of the foraminal extension is unnecessary. The tumor is divided at the paravertebral margin leaving the tumor in the foramin to regress spontaneously. If removal is indicated based on tumor histology, it may be possible to remove the intraforaminal piece through a standard exposure used to excise the extraspinal component. However, one must remember that, invariably, these tumors are adherent to or arise from a component of the spinal nerve. Any manipulation of the extraspinal portion, thus, has the potential of placing undesired traction on the spinal cord. If there is significant intraspinal extension, that is, to the dural sac, it is prudent to resect the intraspinal portion via a standard neurosurgical approach to the spine. The type of approach utilized depends on the position of the tumor relative to the spinal sac. If the tumor is ventral, the two possible approaches are an anterior approach in which the access to the spinal canal is accomplished by resecting the vertebral body or a posterolateral approach in which the pedicle is removed. Either of these approaches can usually be performed via the same exposure used to remove

the extraspinal component. If the tumor is lateral or dorsal to the spinal sac, a posterior approach through a separate midline incision, followed by a laminectomy or laminoplasty, is the most logical choice. Most "dumbbell" tumors lie dorsal or lateral to the spinal sac. The posterior approach is therefore, usually most effective (Fig. 76-21). With any of the aforementioned approaches, it is possible to open the dura and examine the intradural space if the preoperative studies suggest there is extension into the dural sac.

Whether the neurosurgical procedure to remove the intraspinal tumor is performed in conjunction with the procedure to excise the extraspinal portion depends on the preferences of the surgeons involved. Certainly, if the tumor lies ventral to the spinal sac, the only reasonable alternative is a 1-stage operation utilizing the same exposure. However, if a posterior approach to the spine is selected, one has the option of excising the tumor in 1 or 2 stages. We have found that a combined approach is the most effective in achieving a total resection of the intraspinal portion because we can often look from one side of the foramen to the other to insure that the entire tumor is removed.

If a posterior spinal approach is selected, 2 questions should be asked preoperatively: First, what is the ideal position of the patient for the approach to the spine? Second, should the intraspinal or extraspinal portion be resected first? The posterior approach to the spine can be performed with the patient in either the lateral or prone position. If the intraspinal extension is extensive, the prone position affords the neurosurgeon the maximal amount of working room and visualization but will likely require that the intraspinal and extraspinal portions be removed with different operative setups (the exception being if the extraspinal portion can be removed with only a minimal exposure of the paraspinal space). If the intraspinal portion is small, the lateral position allows both components to be reached in the same operative setup.

The issue of which component to resect first is a difficult one. If the extraspinal portion is removed first, there is potential for spinal cord injury, and manipulation and traction of the foraminal component of the tumor should be minimized. One strategy to minimize the risk of neurologic injury is to disconnect the extraspinal and intraspinal portions early on, so that the extraspinal portion can be manipulated without restriction. The major benefit to resecting the intraspinal portion first is that the tumor can be removed as far out of the foramen as possible, and the involved nerve or nerves can be detached from the spinal cord if needed. The risk of resecting the intraspinal portion first is that, if the tumor is highly vascular, controlling the bleeding as it extends into the extraspinal space is more difficult.

In addition to neurologic compromise, the other major risk of any approach to the spine is the potential for delayed spinal deformities. Anterior and posterolateral approaches often require extensive bone removal: An immediate fusion is thus, often necessary. Posterior approaches, however, are more apt to preserve stability and negate the need for a fusion providing certain precautions are taken. First, although it is often necessary to remove some or most of the facet on the side ipsilateral to the tumor, it is rarely necessary to do the same on the opposite side. Care must be taken to preserve the facet capsules and limit the facet removal on the contralateral side to less than the medial one-third of the facet. Second, some believe a laminoplasty (where the lamina are replaced at the end of the resection) offers better long-term stability than multilevel laminectomies.

In summary, the operative management of "dumbbell" tumors often requires a team approach, including pediatric surgeons, neurosurgeons, and sometimes orthopaedic surgeons. An essential component of the team approach is complete identification of intraspinal extension with appropriate preoperative imaging studies. This will optimize the team's ability to formulate an operative strategy that will maximize the potential for a successful outcome (Fig. 76-21).

## SELECTED READINGS

Akwari OE, Payne WS, Onofrio BM, Dines DE, Muhm JR. Dumbbell neurogenic tumors of the mediastinum. *Mayo Clin Proc* 1978;53:353–358.

Barson AJ. The vertebral level of termination of the spinal cord during normal and abnormal development. *J Anat* 1970;106:489–497.

Beardmore HE, Wigglesworth FW. Vertebral anomalies and alimentary duplications. *Pediatr Clin North Am* 1958;5:457–474.

Bickers DS, Adams RD. Hereditary stenosis of the aqueduct of Sylvius as a cause of congenital hydrocephalus. *Brain* 1949;72:246.

Blount JP, Campbell JA, Haines SJ. Complications in ventricular cerebrospinal fluid shunting. *Neurosurg Clin North Am* 1993;4:633–655.

Burchianti M, Cantini R. Peritoneal cerebrospinal fluid pseudocysts: a complication of ventriculoperitoneal shunts. *Child's Nerv Syst* 1988;4:286–290.

Carey JC, Greenbaum B, Hall BD. The OEIS complex (omphalocele, extrophy, imperforate anus, spinal defects). *Birth Defects* 1978;14(6B): 253–263.

Chapman PH, Borges LF. Shunt infections: prevention and treatment. *Clin Neurosurg* 1984;23:652.

Chestnut R, James HE, Jones KL. The Vater association and spinal dysraphia. *Pediatr Neurosurg* 1992;18:144–148.

Currarino G, Coln D, Votteler T. Triad of anorectal, sacral, and presacral anomalies. *Am J Roentgenol* 1981;137:395–398.

Davidoff AM, Thompson CV, Grimm JK, Shorter NA, Filston HC, Oakes WJ. Occult spinal dysraphism in patients with anal agenesis. *J Pediatr Surg* 1991;26:1001–1005.

Dias MS, Azizkhan RG. A novel embryonic mechanism for Currarino's triad: inadequate separation of the caudal eminence from hindgut endoderm. *Pediatr Neurosurg* 1998;28:223–229.

Dias MS, McLone DG. Hydrocephalus in the child with myelomeningocele. *Neurosurg Clin North Am* 1994;4:715–726.

Dias MS, McLone DG. Spinal dysraphism. In: Weinstein SL, ed. *The Pediatric Spine: Principles and Practice.* New York: Raven Press; 1994:96–125.

Dias MS, Pang D. Split cord malformations. *Neurosurg Clin North Am* 1995;6:339–358.

Dias MS, Walker ML. The embryogenesis of complex dysraphic malformations: a disorder of gastrulation? *Pediatr Neurosurg* 1992;18: 229–253.

Drake JM, Sainte-Rose C. Shunt complications. In: Drake JM, Sainte-Rose C, eds. *The Shunt Book.* Cambridge, MA: Blackwell; 1995:121–192.

Fallon M, Gordon ARG, Lendrum AC. Mediastinal cysts of fore-gut origin associated with vertebral abnormalities. *Br J Surg* 1954;41: 520–533.

Fernbach SK, Naidich TP, McLone DG, Leestma JE. Computed tomography of primary intrathecal Wilms tumor with diastematomyelia. *J Comput Assist Tomogr* 1984;8:523–528.

Fox RJ, Walji AH, Mielke B, Petruk KC, Aronyk KE. Anatomic details of intradural channels in the parasagittal dura: a possible pathway for flow of cerebrospinal fluid. *Neurosurgery* 1996;39:84–91.

Gaskill SJ, Marlin AE. Pseudocysts of the abdomen associated with ventriculoperitoneal shunts: a report of twelve cases and a review of the literature. *Pediatr Neurosci* 1989;15:23–27.

Gaskill SJ, Marlin AE. The Currarino triad: its importance in pediatric neurosurgery. *Pediatr Neurosurg* 1997;25:143–146.

Graham SM, Flowers JL, Scott TR, Lin F, Rigamonti D. Safety of percutaneous endoscopic gastrostomy in patients with a ventriculoperitoneal shunt. *Neurosurgery* 1993;32:932–934.

Gutierrez FA, Oi S, McLone DG. Intraspinal tumors in children. Clinical review, surgical results and follow-up in 51 cases. *Concepts Pediatr Neurosurg* 1983;4:291–305.

Harlow CL, Partington MD, Thieme GA. Lumbosacral agenesis: clinical characteristics, imaging, and embryogenesis. *Pediatr Neurosurg* 1995;23:140–147.

James HE, Walsh JW, Wilson HD, Connor JD, Bean JR, Tibbs PA. Prospective randomized study of therapy in cerebrospinal fluid shunt infection. *Neurosurgery* 1980;7:459–463.

Karrer FM, Flannery AM, Nelson MD, McLone DG, Raffensperger JG. Anorectal malformations: evaluation of associated spinal dysraphic syndromes. *J Pediatr Surg* 1988;23:45–48.

Kelly PJ. Stereotactic third ventriculostomy in patients with nontumoral adolescent/adult onset aqueductal stenosis and symptomatic hydrocephalus. *J Neurosurg* 1991;75:865–873.

King D, Goodman J, Hawk T, Boles ET, Sayers MP. Dumbbell neuroblastomas in children. *Arch Surg* 1975;110:888–891.

Kolye MA, Kaji DM, Duque M, Wild J, Galansky SH. The Malone antegrade continence enema for neurogenic and structural fecal incontinence and constipation. *J Urol* 1995;154:759–776.

La Marca F, Grant JA, Tomita T, McLone DG. Spinal lipomas in children: outcome of 270 procedures. *Pediatr Neurosurg* 1997;26:8–16.

Marlin AE, Gaskill SJ. Cerebrospinal fluid shunts: complications and results. In: Cheek WR, ed. *Pediatric Neurosurgery: Surgery of the Developing Nervous System.* Philadelphia: WB Saunders; 1994:221–233.

McComb JG. Congenital dermal sinus. In: Pang D, ed. *Disorders of the Pediatric Spine.* New York: Raven Press; 1995:349–360.

McLendon R, Oakes W, Heinz E, Yeates AE, Burger PC. Adipose tissue in the filum terminale: a computed tomographic finding that may indicate tethering of the spinal cord. *Neurosurgery* 1988;22:873–876.

McLetchie NGB, Purves JK, Saunders RL. The genesis of gastric and certain intestinal diverticula and enterogenous cysts. *Surg Gynecol Obstet* 1954;99:135–141.

McLone DG. Myelomeningocele. In: Y JR, ed. *Neurological Surgery.* Vol 2. 4th ed. Philadelphia: WB Saunders; 1996:843–860.

McLone DG, Dias L, Kaplan WE, Sommers MW. Concepts in the management of spina bifida. In: Humphreys RP, ed. *Concepts in Pediatric Neurosurgery.* Vol 5. Basel: S Karger; 1985:14–28.

McLone DG, Naidich TP. The tethered spinal cord. In: McLaurin RL, Venes JL, Schut L, Epstein F, eds. *Pediatric Neurosurgery.* Philadelphia: WB Saunders; 1989:71–96.

McQuown SA, Smith JD, Gallo AE. Intracranial extension of nasal dermoids. *Neurosurgery* 1983;12:531–535.

Novelli PM, Reigel DH. A closer look at the ventriculo-gallbladder shunt for the treatment of hydrocephalus. *Pediatr Neurosurg* 1997;26:197–199.

Oakes WJ, Worley G, Spock A, et al. Surgical intervention in twenty-nine patients with symptomatic type II Chiari malformations: clinical presentation and outcome. *Concepts in Pediatric Neurosurgery.* Vol 8. Basel: S Karger; 1988:76–85.

Oshio T, Matsumura C, Kirino A, et al. Recurrent perforations of viscus due to ventriculoperitoneal shunt in a hydrocephalic child. *J Pediatr Surg* 1991;26:1404–1405.

Pang D. Split cord malformation: part II: the clinical syndrome. *Neurosurgery* 1992;31:481–500.

Pang D. Sacral agenesis and caudal spinal cord malformations. *Neurosurgery* 1993;32:755–779.

Pang D, Dias MS, Ahab-Barmada M. Split cord malformation: part I: a unified theory of embryogenesis for double spinal cord malformations. *Neurosurgery* 1992;31:451–480.

Pedersen H. Mediastinal enterogenous cyst with spinal malformations: case report. *Acta Paediatr Scand* 1965;54:392–396.

Petrak RM, Pottage JC Jr, Harris AA, Levin S. *Haemophilus influenzae* meningitis in the presence of a cerebrospinal fluid shunt. *Neurosurgery* 1986;18:79–81.

Plantaz D, Hartmann O, Passagia JG, et al. The treatment of neuroblastoma with intraspinal extension with chemotherapy followed by surgical removal of residual disease. A prospective study of 42 patients—results of the NBL 90 study of the French Society of Pediatric Oncology. *Cancer* 1996;78:311–319.

Pollack IF, Pang D, Albright AL, Krieger D. Outcome following hindbrain decompression of symptomatic Chiari malformations in children previously treated with myelomeningocele closure and shunts. *J Neurosurg* 1992;77:881–888.

Raffel C, Neave VCD, Lavine S, McComb JG. Treatment of spinal cord compression by epidural malignancy in childhood. *Neurosurgery* 1991;28:349–352.

Rush DS, Walsh JW. Abdominal complications of CSF-peritoneal shunts. *Monogr Neural Sci* 1982;8:52–54.

Sakoda TH, Maxwell JA, Brackett CE Jr. Intestinal volvulus secondary to ventriculoperitoneal shunt. *J Neurosurg* 1971;39:95–96.

Saunders RL. Combined anterior and posterior spina bifida in a living neonatal human female. *Anat Rec* 1943;87:255–278.

Uzzo RG, Bilsky M, Mininberg DT, Poppas DP. Laparoscopic surgery in children with ventriculoperitoneal shunts: effect of pneumoperitoneum on intracranial pressure—preliminary experience. *Urology* 1997;49;753–757.

Warf BC, Scott RM, Barnes PD, Hendren WH. Tethered spinal cord in patients with anorectal and urogenital malformations. *Pediatr Neurosurg* 1993;19:25–30.

Wen DY, Bottini AG, Hall WA, Haines SJ. The intraventricular use of antibiotics. *Neurosurg Clin N Am* 1992;3:343.

Wolfe S, Schneble F, Tröger J. The conus medullaris: time of ascendence to normal level. *Pediatr Radiol* 1992;22:590–592.

# PART VIII

## TRAUMA

# CHAPTER 77

# Trauma Epidemiology, Scoring and Triage Systems, and Injury Prevention

*Thane A. Blinman and Michael Nance*

## KEY POINTS

1. Children follow different patterns of injury than adults.

2. Commonly used scoring systems have decreased predictive power in injured children because, among other problems, few systems take into account size-based differences in pediatric physiology.

3. Despite these problems, scoring systems decrease subjective evaluation of trauma, and therefore play a critical role in pediatric trauma research and quality improvement (QI).

4. Injury prevention is a key component of any trauma system and trauma center. The priorities for prevention initiatives are best decided at the community level based on measured needs.

## INTRODUCTION

In the United States, more children will die from trauma than any other cause—more than from cancer, more than from AIDS, more than from congenital anomalies, more than from all other causes combined. Injury-related death is responsible for nearly 30% of all years of potential life lost. Mortality is but the tip of the injury iceberg. For every injury-related death in the pediatric population, there are 12 children hospitalized for injury, and more than 60 treated for an injury in an emergency department (Table 77-1). Development of trauma systems, optimization of trauma care, and institution of injury prevention measures have not been successful at eliminating this problem. However, such efforts have not been without benefit.

In the IOM report on pediatric emergency care (including trauma), deficiencies in current practices were highlighted. In addition, the IOM stated that the ideal system would "...ensure that each patient receives the most appropriate care, at the optimal location, with the minimum delay." That same IOM report recognized the system of hospitals (trauma centers) established to care for injured Americans as a "model of care." However, while the evidence is clear that trauma systems improve the care of the adult trauma patient, it is less clear that such is the case for the pediatric trauma patient. In this chapter, we describe pediatric trauma systems, epidemiology, injury scoring, and prevention, with special attention on how pediatric injury differs from adult injury.

## TRAUMA SYSTEMS

Organized trauma systems were developed largely through federal legislation, especially the National Highway Safety Act of 1966 and the Emergency Medical Services Act of 1973. Later, several state trauma systems were established (eg, Maryland, Illinois), and these served as models for other states interested in creating an organized trauma system. The American College of Surgeons, through their Committee on Trauma, published "Optimal Care for the Injured Patient," a document designed to outline the standards for the organization of trauma centers. Absent from this document was specific language describing the needs of centers caring for injured children. Official recommendations regarding the optimal resources for trauma centers caring for children were not incorporated into the document for another decade.

Despite progress toward creation of an organized trauma system, there is no national agency or entity (eg, American College of Surgeons) singly responsible for the regulation and verification of trauma centers. Instead, this responsibility is left to the individual states, as is the decision to establish any organized trauma system. This deficiency was noted by the IOM in their characterization of the current national trauma system.

Modern organized care of the injured child took shape with the federal Emergency Medical Services for Children Program in 1984. The goal of this program was to ensure optimal prehospital care for ill and injured children and adolescents, and to integrate pediatric services into the general EMS system. However, despite efforts to improve readiness of emergency departments for the care of critically ill and injured children, deficiencies remain common and systems are less organized than those available for adult care. The fragmentation and variation in the delivery of pediatric emergency care was noted and again, The Institute of Medicine strongly

| TABLE 77-1 | Annual Pediatric Trauma Volume in the United States |
|---|---|
| **Type of Injury** | **Number of Children Injured** |
| Fatal injury | 14,537 |
| Hospitalized injuries | 185,935 |
| Emergency department treated injuries | 8,797,338 |

recommended coordination, regionalization and accountability for pediatric emergency and trauma care. However, the cost of establishing a pediatric trauma system is substantial both in terms of human resources and capital. For this reason, it is imperative that the value of a pediatric trauma center be clarified.

Trauma centers are categorized based on level of resources available for the treatment of the trauma patient. The highest category (eg, Level 1) typically have the immediate availability of both personnel and hospital resources for management of the most acutely ill trauma patients. These highest level trauma centers are commonly affiliated with academic medical centers with training programs, maintain a high volume of patients and have research and outreach responsibilities. The next tier of trauma centers (eg, Level 2) are also designed to provide immediate care to the severely injured patient but often are established in non teaching centers and have lower patient volume that level 1 trauma centers. In some states or systems, separate verification and designation exists for pediatric trauma centers. These pediatric centers typically are associated with a children's hospital and provide access to pediatric-focused specialists. Not all trauma centers are equipped to care for injured children.

## BENEFIT OF PEDIATRIC TRAUMA CENTERS

Remarkably, it has been difficult to clearly demonstrate a survival benefit of a trauma center over a non trauma center. The best evidence of a survival advantage is provided by the National Study on the Costs and Outcomes of Trauma (NSCOT) project. This adult-only study compared the mortality for a cohort of more than 18,000 patients treated at either a designated trauma center or a non trauma center in 14 states across the US. A significant reduction in in hospital (RR 0.80) and 1-year (RR 0.75) mortality was noted for patients treated at a designated trauma center. A similar study in the pediatric population, comparing care provided at a pediatric trauma center to that at a non trauma center, has not been performed. However, there are many studies, often limited in scope by geography, injury type or center type, that demonstrate outcome benefits for children treated at pediatric-focused trauma centers. For example, studies limited to outcomes for pediatric patients treated for splenic injuries demonstrated benefit to treatment at a pediatric

trauma center (or free-standing pediatric hospital) as compared to non trauma center or adult-focused trauma center. In analysis of a statewide trauma system, management of the head-injured patient has been shown to be superior at designated pediatric trauma centers as compared to either adult trauma centers or adult trauma centers with added qualifications for pediatric trauma. In addition, for children treated in designated pediatric trauma centers, a significant reduction in overall mortality (above that for treatment at a designated trauma center vs non trauma center) was noted. When comparing all injury outcome rather than organ-specific analyses, the youngest pediatric trauma patients (aged 0 to 10 years) and those with more severe injuries (injury severity score [ISS] of greater than 15) were noted to have a lower in hospital mortality, and a shorter length of stay, when pediatric hospitals were compared to adult hospitals. The reason for this improved outcome is not known. The availability of specialized resources, whether that be human or equipment, or hospital units (eg, pediatric intensive care or pediatric emergency department) are possible explanations.

## ACCESS TO CARE

If pediatric trauma centers are of benefit, then in an ideal system, access to that care would be equal across the land. Such is not the case, however. In fact, the minority of pediatric trauma care is rendered in pediatric trauma centers. For all injured children, nearly two thirds are treated at non pediatric centers. More importantly, even one third of the youngest (age 0 to 10 years) and/or sickest (injury severity score >15) were treated outside of pediatric-focused institutions. This may be due in part to access to specialized trauma care. In the adult population, nearly 47 million Americans were not within 60 minutes of a designated trauma center by air or ground transportation. Similar deficiencies were noted in a pediatric-focused analysis, which demonstrated a lack of access to pediatric trauma centers within an hour by air or ground for nearly 14 million children (Fig. 77-1). However, a direct correlation between timely access to this specialized care and improved outcomes has not been demonstrated.

## PEDIATRIC TRAUMA EPIDEMIOLOGY

Annual trauma mortality has declined over the decades in the pediatric population. However, more than 15,000 children still die each year as a result of injury, leaving room for improvement (Fig. 77-2). Injury mechanisms vary by patient age, but falls and motor vehicle-related injuries predominate (Fig. 77-3). The case fatality rate by injury mechanism varies greatly. By far, firearm injuries are the most lethal with a case fatality rate of nearly 12% (Fig. 77-4). Body region of injury varies with age and injury mechanism. Overall, in children hospitalized in trauma centers, head injuries are most common and the most likely to be lethal (Fig. 77-5).

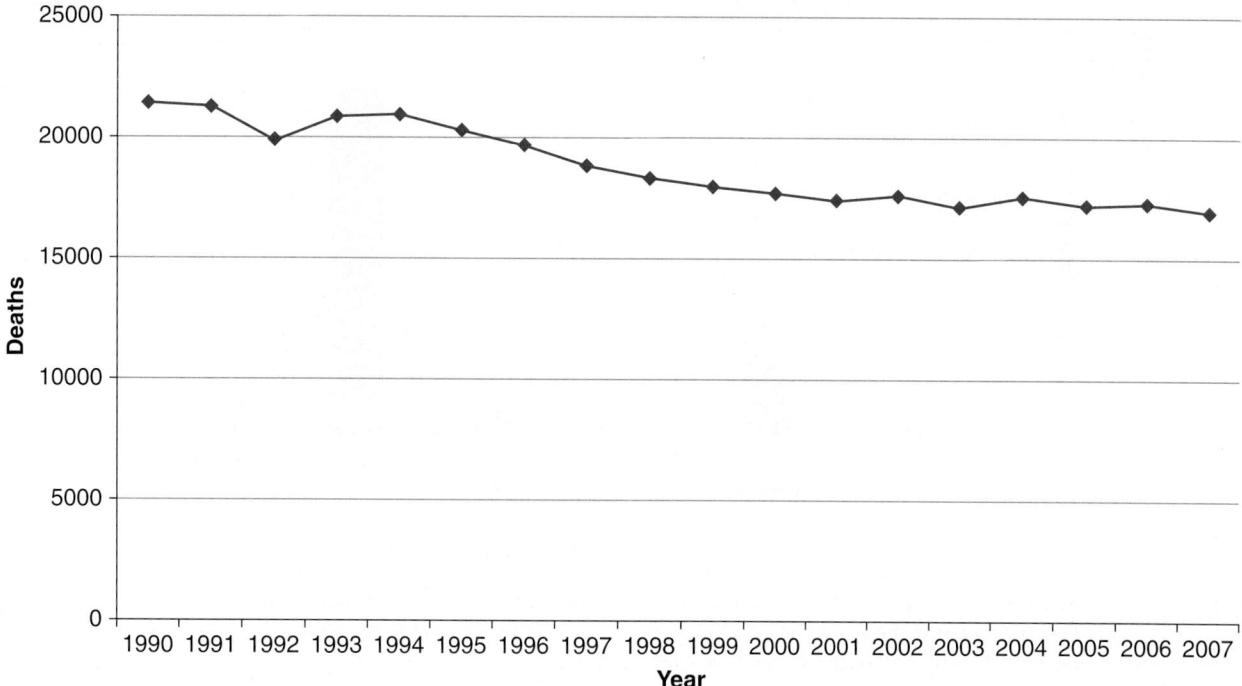

**Annual injury mortality (age, 0–19)**

**FIGURE 77-1** Annual injury-related mortality for the pediatric population (age 0 to19 years) for the period 1990 to 2007. (Data from Centers for Disease Control and Prevention, National Center for Injury Prevention and Control. Web-based Injury Statistics Query and Reporting System (WISQARS). Department of Health and Human Services Web site: http://www.cdc.gov/ncipc/wisqars. Accessed March 16, 2011.)

## PEDIATRIC INJURY SCORING

Injury severity scales and scores attempt to provide an objective means of describing or classifying individual injuries and overall degree of "injured-ness." By linking these measures to outcomes, scales and score promise a probabilistic estimate of survival or other outcome. Such measurements, if valid, would allow the following:

▶ **Decision Support**: Ideally, injury measurements support bedside decisions. For example, some injury scores (eg, the Revised Trauma Score [RTS]) have been imagined as triage tools that would allow rescuers to

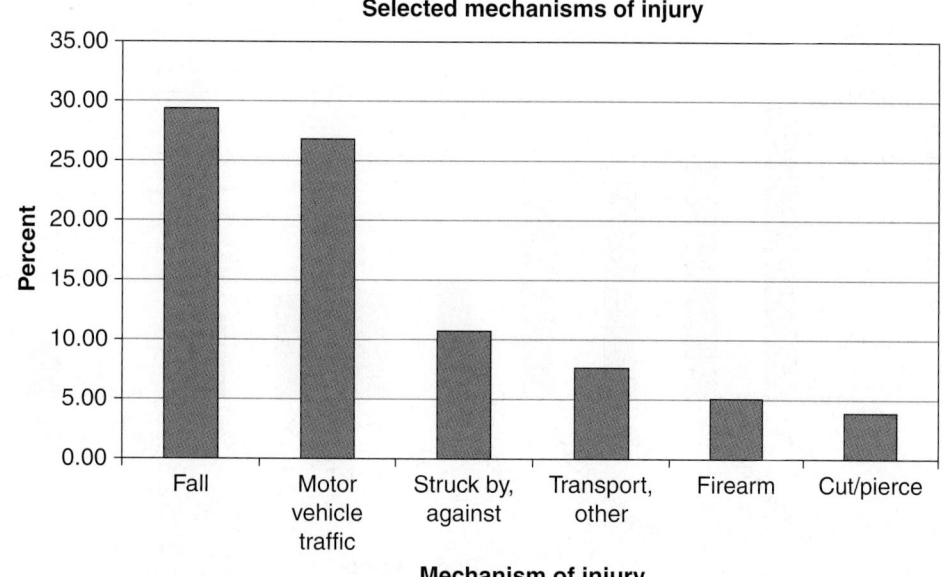

**Selected mechanisms of injury**

**FIGURE 77-2** Most common injury mechanisms for children admitted to selected trauma centers in the United States (2010). (Data from from National Trauma Data Bank Annual Pediatric Report, 2010. American College of Surgeons, 2010.)

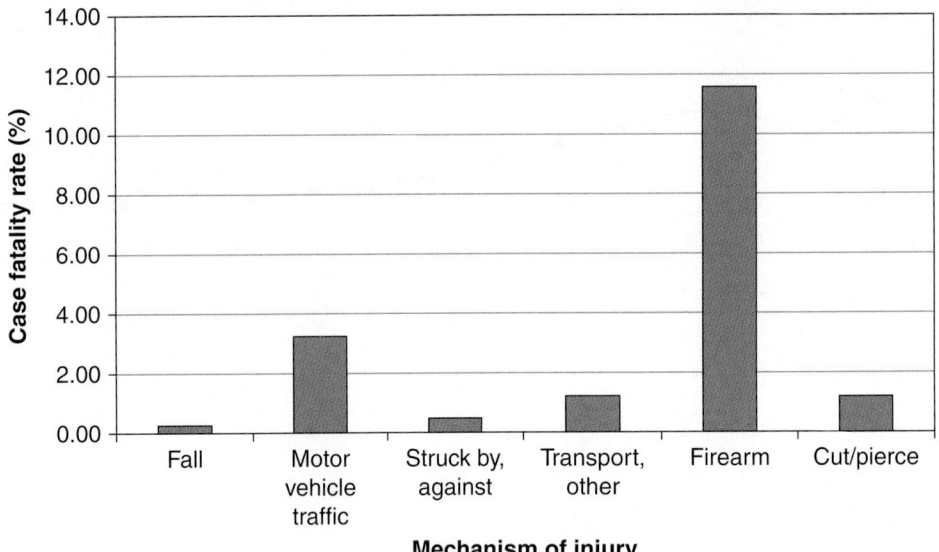

**FIGURE 77-3** Case-fatality rate for selected injury mechanisms for children admitted to selected trauma centers in the United States (2010). (Data from National Trauma Data Bank Annual Pediatric Report, 2010. American College of Surgeons, 2010.)

decide quickly if a given patient should be transported to a Level 1 trauma center. Similarly, injury scales can drive decision nodes of clinical algorithms. For example, if the Glasgow Coma Scale (GCS) is ≤8, then intubate the patient. Or, if the Organ Injury Scale (OIS) for a spleen laceration is grade 3 or worse, then follow the solid organ injury pathway. However, while some scoring tools give the probability of survival, decisions

regarding withdrawing care cannot be made with these tools.

▶ **Hospital QI**: Objective measures of injury allow evaluation of clinician and hospital performance compared to other hospitals with similar populations of injured patients. In particular, QI projects increasingly use measures of observed/expected (O/E) outcomes, especially mortality.

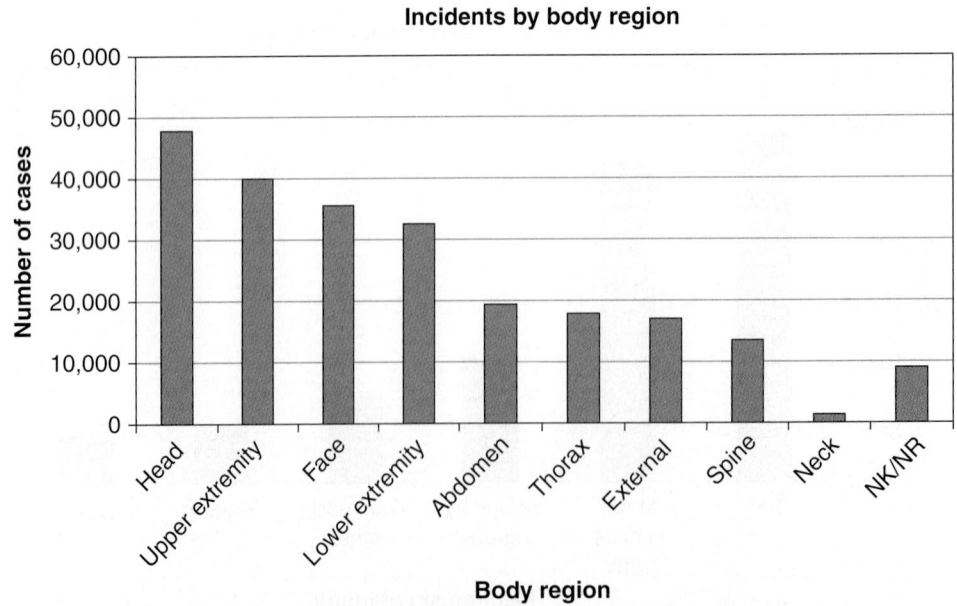

**FIGURE 77-4** Body region of injury for children admitted to selected trauma centers in the United States (2010). (Data from National Trauma Data Bank Annual Pediatric Report, 2010. American College of Surgeons, 2010.)

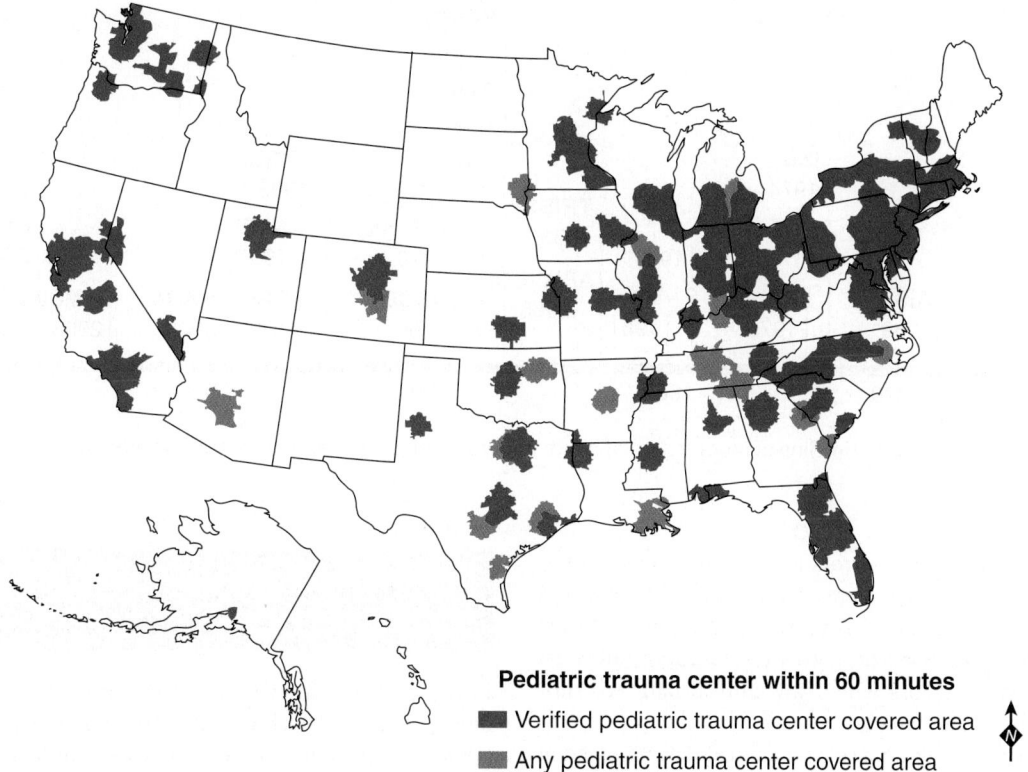

**FIGURE 77-5** Pediatric population with 60-minutes access (by air or ground) including verified pediatric trauma centers (red) and/or pediatric capable, self-designated pediatric trauma centers (blue). (Reprinted with permission from Nance ML, Carr BG, Branas CC. Access to pediatric trauma care in the United States. *Arch Pediatr Adolesc Med* 2009;163:512–518.)

▶ **Utilization**: Prediction about patient length of stay, consumption of hospital resources (beds, nurses, etc), and costs follows from historical data relating these scores to cost data.

▶ **Epidemiology**: How are injury patterns (anatomy and severity) changing across populations in time and space?

Injury measurement in pediatric patients has followed the development of tools intended for adults. Because children exhibit different responses to injury, tend to present with different patterns of injury, and are mostly free from the comorbidities (especially vascular disease) of injured adults, the tools designed for adults hold less validity and predictive power for children. Several attempts to incorporate these differences have been introduced, with varying success.

In this section, we will describe several important injury scales and scores, their use in pediatric trauma, and some criticism of the methods upon which they rely.

## SCORES AND SCALES

While "scale" and "score" are used interchangeably in casual use, they are not the same.

A measurement *scale* maps a number onto a physical object. In the most general terms, scales come in 4 types:

▶ **Nominal**: numbers (sometimes letters or even words) are used only for labels (eg, ICD-9)

▶ **Ordinal**: numbers denote a rank order, but do not imply equal differences between rank, or even any kind of 0 (eg, Abbreviated Injury Scale [AIS], OIS)

▶ **Interval**: a scale with a constant interval between ticks on the scale, but with a 0 point that is arbitrary (eg, temperature)

▶ **Ratio**: equal intervals and an absolute 0 (eg, agee, systolic blood pressure, respiratory rate, cardiac output, etc)

*In general, injury scales are ordinal scales.* For example, there is no reason to expect a grade III splenic laceration to be worse, to the same degree, than a grade II as a grade IV is to a grade III. In fact, it is generally recognized that there is a *qualitative* difference between grade II and III and a big increase in severity (as measured by probability of the need for intervention such as transfusion, operation, or embolization) that is not seen between III and IV.

Injury severity *scores* (not to be confused with the score named the "Injury Severity Score") are composites of several injury scales, and sometimes other scores or even components of other scores. These are combined according to a scheme that is intended to predict outcome (particularly mortality). Virtually all are the product of mulitivariate linear or logistic regression, techniques that became easy to use (and abuse) with the widespread availability of fast computers in the 1970 (Fig. 77-6). Because injury scales are generally ordinal-type scales, few statistical measures are properly used with these. For example, it is not strictly correct to report a mean or standard deviation with these, and it is certainly not correct to report *p*-values from

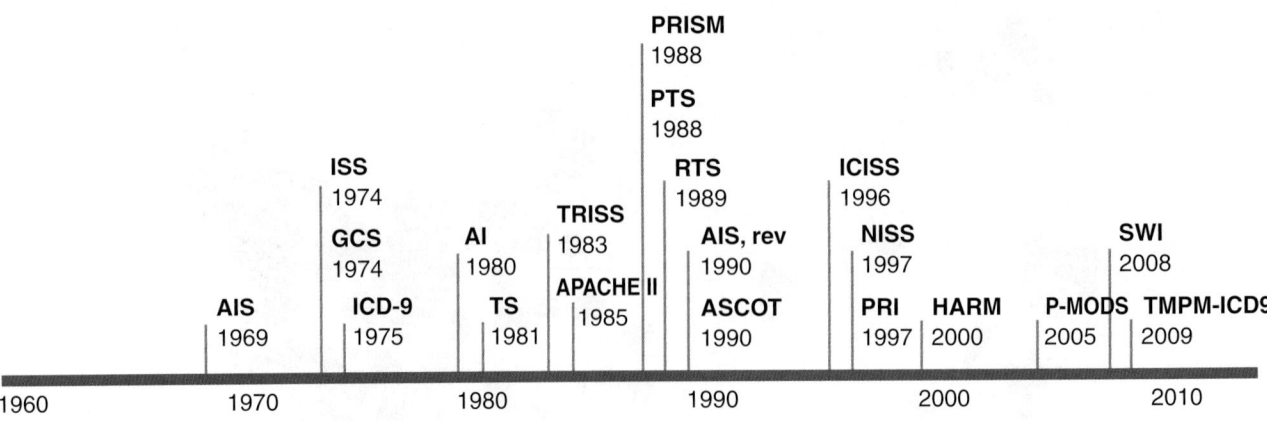

**FIGURE 77-6** Timeline of introduction of major injury scoring tools. See text for abbreviation names.

*t*-tests. Nevertheless, these errors are common, and propagate through to the injury *scores*, which derive their values from the injury *scales*. For this reason, and because almost all injury scoring is based on regression methods, all must produce information loss when raw clinical data are subsumed by indexes and weights.

Scales and scores rely on available clinical data assessed at the bedside on admission, throughout the hospital course, and sometimes, at autopsy. This *post hoc* nature of data acquisition shows why nearly all of these complex scores are useless for bedside management (with the notable exceptions of the GCS, and, less successfully, the RTS). Not only are data required to calculate these scores usually not available until the *end* of treatment, but the algorithms that produce most scores require computations that are infeasible to the bedside clinician. Driven by hospital benchmarking and retrospective outcomes research, the emphasis of these scores is mostly on accuracy rather than on triage. Even if all the data and the calculations were available prognostic scores could not morally be used for end-of-life decisions: these crude probabilistic tools imperfectly predict mortality, as the large annual number of pediatric "unexpected survivors" demonstrates. One of the oldest criticisms of the statistical methodology is that methods that follow the law of large numbers cannot account for individual variation and stochastic events, so cannot be validly applied to the individual.

Data for scores and scale come from anatomic observations, physiologic measurements, or both. Implicit in the methodology of these tools is the premise that recovery after injury depends upon some function of "physiological reserve," physiologic injury, and severity of the injuries (Fig. 77-7).

As will be seen, injury scoring methods almost never account for measures of physiological reserve, a somewhat nebulous concept rendered even less clear by children's well-known ability to compensate, obscuring impending physiological collapse. Moreover, there is really no accounting for synergistic action between 2 or more severe injuries; mathematically, injury scoring systems treat injuries as if they were independent. Finally, for children, physiological scaling effects (eg, a normal heart rate for a 70-kg patient is dangerous bradycardia in an infant) are neglected. The wary pediatric trauma surgeon should view these tools with extra skepticism.

## IMPORTANT INJURY SEVERITY SCORING TOOLS

In this section, we will look at the more important tools in detail. Figure 77-8 shows how the major scales and scores relate to each other. Scores and scales can be classified several ways (eg, triage vs outcome scores, etc), but here these tools will be grouped according to whether they measure anatomic data, physiological data, or both in a combined score (Table 77-2).

## ANATOMIC

### Abbreviated Injury Scale

The Abbreviated Injury Scale (AIS) is an anatomic scale devised and owned by the Association for the Advancement of Automotive Medicine (AAAM). The scale, first introduced in 1971 and periodically revised, groups injuries by body

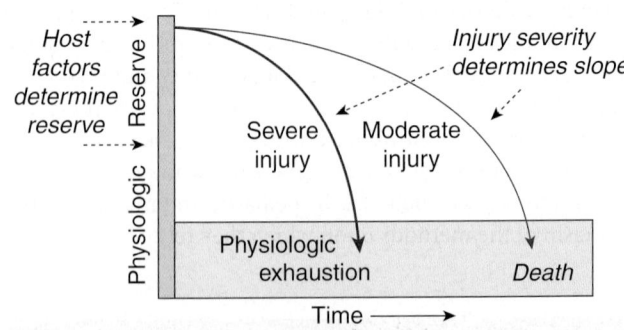

**FIGURE 77-7** Outcome after injury is a function of the severity of injury and the victim's response, or the nebulous concept of "physiologic reserve." Children often have more reserve than adults with chronic debilitating illness, but they also exhibit a more precipitous decline once they have exhausted their ability to compensate. This tendency to "fall off the cliff" or suddenly decompensate from apparently "stable" vitals can fool practitioners unaccustomed to pediatric physiology, making accurate prehospital scoring even more valuable.

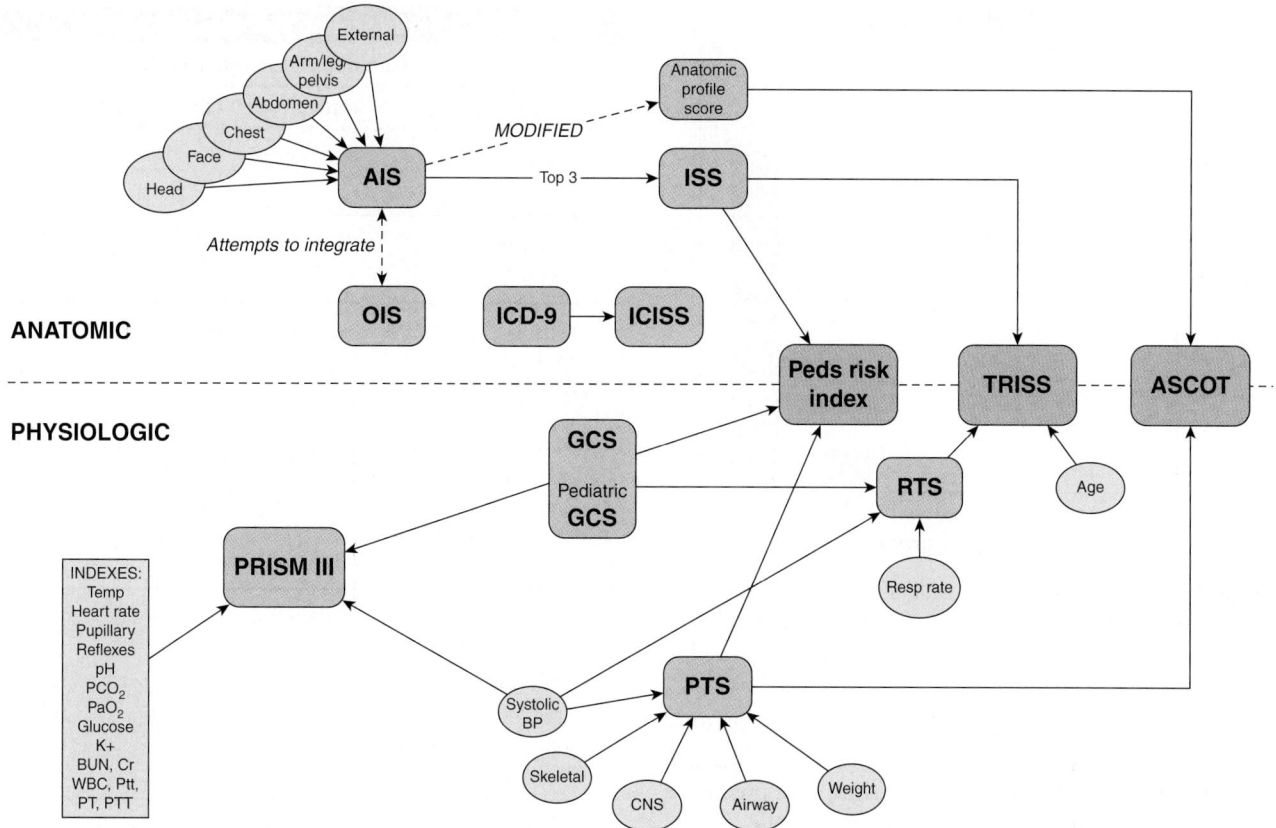

**FIGURE 77-8** Relationships between clinical data and common scores and scales. See text for abbreviations.

region (eg, head, thorax, extremity, etc) and rates specific injuries according to a 6-point score: 1 = minor, 2 = moderate, 3 = serious, 4 = severe, 5 = critical, 6 = fatal or untreatable. The AIS forms the basis of the Injury Severity Score (see below). Organized into 9 "chapters" or body regions (head, face, neck, thorax, abdomen/pelvis, spine, upper extremities, lower extremities, burns/other trauma), the "AIS dictionary" gives structured injury descriptions for each region. Importantly, the AIS does not include complications (eg, pneumonia) or other outcomes

(eg, death, hearing loss, etc) as injuries. Not until 1990 was any account for age or size included in the AIS descriptors when "Age <15" was added as a descriptor to some injuries.

## Organ Injury Scale

The AIS is a proprietary injury measurement tool, and while it forms the basis of the ISS, trauma surgeons are taught and use the OIS clinically. The OIS was developed when in 1987, the AAST appointed a committee of trauma surgeons tasked to develop a comprehensive scale of specific organ injuries. These organ-specific scales grade injuries, as with the AIS, as 1 = minimal, 2 = mild, 3 = moderate, 4 = severe, 5 = massive, and 6 = lethal. The main difference between the OIS and the AIS was an attempt to describe a magnitude of anatomic disruption, excluding any estimate of blood loss or effect of intervention. In children, the OIS is most useful as a guide to protocol-driven, non operative management of solid organ injuries, particularly spleen, liver, and kidney. While the OIS does predict some outcome, these ordinal scales are non monotonic: As the renal OIS demonstrates, there is a much larger difference in risk of nephrectomy between grades 3 and 4 than between grades 2 and 3 (Fig. 77-9).

## Anatomic Profile

The Anatomic Profile (AP) was introduced in 1990 in response to perceived weaknesses in the AIS and, more particularly, in the ISS (described below), but is still derived from the AIS. In general, the AP uses a 4-component model

| TABLE 77-2 | Injury Severity Scoring Systems |
|---|---|
| Anatomic | |
| AIS | |
| OIS | |
| Anatomic Profile | |
| ICD-9 (Single Worst Injury, ICISS, TMPM-ICD9) | |
| ISS and NISS | |
| Physiologic | |
| GCS | |
| RTS and TS | |
| Pediatric Trauma Score | |
| Severity of Illness Scores: PRISM | |
| Composite Scores | |
| Trauma and Injury Severity Scores | |
| A Severity Characterization of Trauma | |
| Pediatric Risk Indicator | |

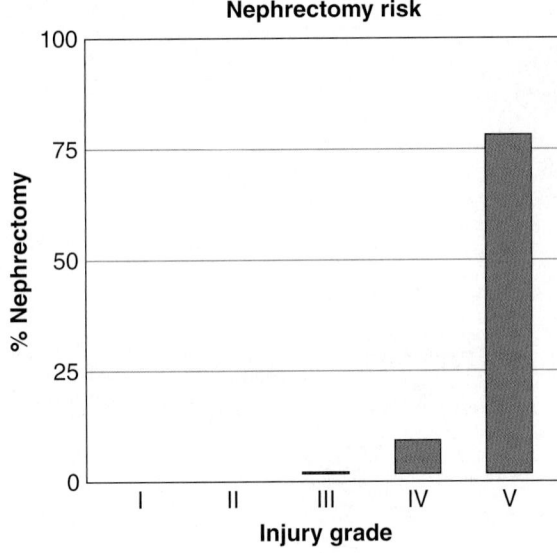

**FIGURE 77-9** The OIS is only an ordinal scale, not an interval scale. The risk of nephrectomy increases sharply above grade 3.

emphasizing the brain/spinal cord, thorax/neck, and all other remaining injuries (with the fourth component a summary of minor injuries, typically neglected as having little predictive power). The AP is the square root of the sum of the squares of these components, similar to (but not exactly the same as) the square root of the ISS, and was posited as being analogous to the resultant or norm of several vectors. The AP is a score, and carries predictive information that forecasts mortality when mapped to a logistic regression model of survival probability. It is rarely used in pediatric trauma, but does form an essential component of another composite score, A Severity Characterization of Trauma (ASCOT) (see below).

## ICD-9 Codes and ICD-9 Derived Scores

The International Classification of Diseases, version 9, is essentially a nominal scale, with codes that roughly map to OIS and AIS grades (see Table 77-3). The American College of Surgeons now requires International Classification of diseases ninth Edition (ICD-9-CM) codes for injury coding in the National Trauma Databank, offering a chance to develop new injury scoring methods from large computerized database. The ICD-9 Injury Severity Score (ICISS) was developed by first calculating survival risk ratios (SRR) for every injury type described in the ICD-9. Each individual SRR is calculated by dividing the number of survivors by the total number of patients with a particular ICD-9-CM. The ICISS for any individual patient is then calculated as the product of all survival risk ratios for an individual patient's traumatic ICD-9 codes ($SRR_1 \times SRR_2 \times SRR_3 \times \cdots \times SRR_{last\ injury}$). This score is reported to yield better survival prediction than the ISS, while avoiding the numerical curiosities of the ISS.

The ICISS appears to give good results in children (and functions well as a hospital benchmarking tool), but a simpler method (Single Worst Injury, SWI) predicts outcome by taking the survival risk ratio of the individual child's single worst (ICD-9 described) injury. Since release of the

| TABLE 77-3 | Injury Scaling Methods Comparison |||||
|---|---|---|---|---|---|
| **Comparison of Spleen Injury Scales** ||||||
| **Injury Description** | **Injury Type** | **OIS** | **AIS-90** | **ICD-9** ||
| Subcapsular, <10% of surface area | Hematoma | I | 2 | 865.01 865.11 ||
| Capsular tear, <1 cm of parenchymal depth | Laceration | I | 2 | 856.02 865.12 ||
| Subcapsular, 10% to 50% of surface area Intraparenchymal, <5 cm in diameter | Hematoma | II | 2 | 865.01 865.11 ||
| Capsular tear, 1 to 3 cm parenchymal depth that does not involve a trabecular vessel | Laceration | II | 2 | 865.02 865.12 ||
| Subcapsular, >50% of surface area; Ruptured supcapsular or parenchymal Intraparenchymal ≥5 cm or expanding | Hematoma | III | 3 | ||
| >3 cm parenchymal depth, or involving trabecular vessels | Laceration | III | 3 | 865.03 865.13 ||
| Laceration involving segmental or hilar vessels producing major devascularization (>25% of spleen) | Laceration | IV | 4 | ||
| Completely shattered spleen | Laceration | V | 5 | 865.04 ||
| Hilar vascular injury which devascularizes spleen | Vascular | V | 5 | 865.14 ||

ICISS, the Osler group reported their updated method, the Trauma Mortality Prediction Model (TMPM-ICD9), based on a repeated probit regression algorithm to yield a probability of death. In particular, the TMPM-ICD9 maps the 5 worst injuries (or really, the severity measures of the ICD-9 codes of the 5 worst injuries) onto a standard cumulative distribution function. It has not yet been validated in pediatric patients, but promises accurate mortality prediction in a way that leverages billing data already being collected nationwide. Another interesting approach based on ICD-9 criteria is the Bayesian Logistic Injury Severity Score (BLISS). In general, it is expected that ICD-9 based systems will gain in importance, not only because they give monotonic predictions of mortality (unlike older methods like ISS; see below), but because the American College of Surgeons has adopted the ICD-9 coding as the National Trauma Data Standard (Table 77-3).

## Injury Severity Score

The ISS is one of the most commonly used measures of injury severity, despite its oddities. Originally conceived to describe blunt trauma (automatically giving it a theoretical advantage for use in children where blunt trauma is predominant), revisions to the AIS dictionary improved the performance of the ISS in penetrating trauma. The ISS is calculated as

$$ISS = A^2 + B^2 + C^2$$

where $A$, $B$, and $C$ are the 3 highest AIS values from *different* body regions. In general, an ISS > 15 is considered "severe," that is, associated with a high mortality risk. An AIS code of 6 for any body region automatically raises the ISS to the maximum value of 75. The ISS does not allow measurement of multiple injuries to any single region, and for this reason, the New Injury Severity Score (NISS) was introduced. The NISS is defined as the sum of the squares of the Abbreviated Injury Scale scores of each of a patient's 3 most severe AIS injuries even if they are in the same body region. However, the NISS does not appear to predict mortality much better than the ISS, and if anything violates assumptions of monotonicity even more than the ISS (see below).

Several authors have pointed out other flaws in the ISS. Chief among these is the nonmonotonic relationship of ISS scores to actual mortality. In part, this is because of the odd sum-of-squared-scores method that excludes a number of values (yielding not 75, but only 44 discrete values). Worse, the values are not evenly distributed across the scale (clustering most reachable values below 50, with just 6 above 50). Meanwhile, because the ISS allows some values to be reached in several ways, there is both information loss, and an implication that there is equal mortality for these combinations, something that has not been shown. For these reasons, the ISS is plainly not an interval measure, and really follows something less than an ordinal scale. Moreover, the ISS frequently overestimates the mortality risk in children. For example, a child with a pulmonary contusion (AIS 4) automatically has an ISS of at least 16 and a high implied mortality, yet this injury is often revealed on now-common CT scans, and children typically recover.

## PHYSIOLOGIC

### Glasgow Coma Scale

The GCS was the product of international studies funded by several US government agencies. First released in 1974, it was revised in 1976 to include a sixth point in the motor scale ("withdrawal from painful stimuli"). The main advantages of the GCS are its simplicity and powerful triage and prognostic power. The GCS is still misunderstood, and misunderstanding of the elements of its components can degrade its usefulness.

The GCS returns a value from 3 (worst) to 15 (best) based on simple addition of measures of 3 scales (Table 77-4).

This composite of ordinal scale data makes the GCS not a scale but in fact a kind of score, subject to the same information loss as all scores (there are 120 possible combinations, but

| TABLE 77-4 | Glasgow Coma Scale | |
|---|---|---|
| **Eye Opening** | **Best Verbal Response** | **Best Motor Response** |
| | | 6: obeys commands |
| 4: spontaneous | 5: oriented | 5: localizes |
| 3: to speech | 4: confused | 4: withdraws |
| 2: to pain | 3: inappropriate words | 3: abnormal flexion |
| 1: none | 2: incomprehensible sounds | 2: extension |
| | 1: none | 1: none |

only 12 possible discrete scores, creating the same information loss problem seen with the ISS, and no 0). Of the 3 scales, the motor response gives the most information regarding severity, both for adults and children. Obviously, the verbal scale presents a problem for young, preverbal children and infants. In this circumstance, a pediatric GCS was introduced that modifies the elements of the scales (Table 77-5).

As with the adult scale, a GCS of 13 to 15 = "minor"; 9 to 12 = "moderate"; 5 to 8 = "severe," and 3 to 4 = "very severe." Comparison of the 2 sets of scales reveals the dependence of the pediatric score on painful stimuli, and herein lays the main source of error in its use. Not only are the responses more subjective (and therefore more prone to misinterpretation), but poor clinical technique can give bad answers. For example, painful stimulation applied to the leg or nail-bed can elicit simple reflex flexion (yielding an erroneous 3 for motor response), while classic methods used in adults like the "sternal rub" can actually *cause* injury. For these reasons, the best method for eliciting motor and verbal responses in babies is to pinch the pectoralis or trapezius muscles. Regardless of method, the clinician has to remember to record the *best* value for each index.

Despite its pitfalls, the GCS gives reliable bedside guidance. For example, it has been demonstrated that a patient exhibiting a GCS ≤8 (or motor ≤4) cannot protect his or her airway and should be intubated. The GCS gives a less subjective measure of level of consciousness (LOC) and coma; allows tracking of changes in LOC; allows faster response to changes in LOC (eg, suggesting exacerbation of intracranial hemorrhage). The pediatric GCS has been validated in children under age 2, predicting the need for operative intervention and the probability of complications (including death, with a GCS below 8 tracking strongly with mortality).

| TABLE 77-5 | Modified Pediatric Glasgow Coma Scale | |
|---|---|---|
| **Eye Opening** | **Best Verbal Response** | **Best Motor Response** |
| | | 6: obeys commands |
| 4: spontaneous | 5: coos or babbles | 5: withdraws to touch |
| 3: to speech | 4: irritable, cries | 4: withdraws to pain |
| 2: to pain | 3: cries to pain | 3: flexion to pain |
| 1: none | 2: moans to pain | 2: extension to pain |
| | 1: none | 1: none |

| TABLE 77-6 | Code Values for the Revised Trauma Score | | |
|---|---|---|---|
| **Revised Trauma Score: Code Values** | | | |
| Glasgow Coma Scale | Systolic Blood Pressure | Respiratory Rate | Coded Value |
| 13 to 15 | >89 | 10 to 29 | 4 |
| 9 to 12 | 76 to 89 | >29 | 3 |
| 6 to 8 | 50 to 75 | 6 to 9 | 2 |
| 4 to 5 | 1 to 49 | 1 to 5 | 1 |
| 3 | 0 | 0 | 0 |

## Revised Trauma Score

The RTS is a modification of the original Trauma Score (TS) described in 1981. Intended to provide an objective triage tool that could aid medical command centers in directing injured patients to trauma centers, the RTS is calculated as:

$$A = 0.9368 \text{ (GCS code value)} + 0.7326 \text{ (SBP code value)} + 0.2908 \text{ (RR code value)}.$$

Notice that the raw values for GCS, SBP, and RR are not used, but instead each of these is given a scale value (Table 77-6) that is then weighted (with weights derived from linear regression). This returns a raw score that can be used to predict survival when fed into a logistic regression function:

$$P(s) = -\left( \frac{1}{1 + e^{-A}} \right).$$

The RTS does not yield pediatric-specific values. For example, a 3-kg infant with a normal systolic blood pressure and respiratory rate would appear more seriously injured, despite having no injury at all. While the RTS and TS were conceived as ambulance transport triage tools, their use as such depends on the premise that diversion to a trauma center is demonstrably better for any given injury; as noted above, this has not been shown.

## Pediatric Trauma Score

Introduced in 1987, the Pediatric Trauma Score (PTS) borrows the methods of the RTS, but changes the weights in an effort to improve the predictive and triage power of the RTS for children. Later, an age-specific PTS (AS-PTS) was described, again using the logistic regression equation, but now altering the calculation of A as

$$A = W_0 + W_{1GCS} + W_{2SBPc} + W_{3PULSE} + W_{4RR},$$

where the $W_i$s are the regression weights corresponding to indexes (not raw vital sign readings) of each variable (GCS, SBP, PULSE, and RR) and $W_o$ is added to create a 0-intercept for the logistic curve. While not in widespread use, this AS-PTS is an early attempt to incorporate some notion of scaling into the physiological data that feed the equation (with age as a stand-in for body mass). Like other trauma scores, the AS-PTS was intended as a triage tool

(ie, a PTS ≤8 is recommended as an indicator for diversion to a trauma center). However, it cannot be demonstrated that use of the PTS (or the RTS) is superior to clinical judgment for this decision.

## Other Pediatric Physiologic Scores in Critical Care

These injury scores are not the only methods used for critically injured children. Many nonspecific physiologic injury prediction models have been described including PRISM, P-MODS, PIM, PELOD, and others. The Pediatric Risk of Mortality (PRISM, now in its third revision, PRISM-III) is the prototype for these scores, and is the most commonly used PICU score in the United States. Intended more for medical patients in the pediatric intensive care unit than the trauma bay, it uses physiological data to control for severity of illness rather than injury. Like other scores, PRISM is the product of mulitvariate regression, including indexed laboratory and vital sign data from either the first 12 or 24 hours into a weighted logistic regression model. Further description of these (and other) models is beyond the scope of this chapter, but most are reviewed.

# COMPOSITE SCORES

## Trauma and Injury Severity Scores

Of all the composite trauma prediction scores, none is as widely used or as frequently modified, as the Trauma and Injury Severity Scores (TRISS). TRISS gives a probability of survival ($P_s$) using a logit model, the same logistical equation used for RTS, PRISM, etc:

$$P(s) = -\left( \frac{1}{1 + e^{-A}} \right).$$

However, here

$$A = A_0 + A_1 \text{ (RTS)} + A_2 \text{ (ISS)} + B_3 \text{ (age index)},$$

where the $A_i$s are weights. In other words, TRISS is a composite score, taking into account anatomic data (ISS) and physiological data (RTS, or more particularly, the indexes of GCS, SBP, and RR) plus a ranking of age (limited to greater than or less than 54 years old). Moreover, there are different weights for blunt and penetrating trauma, and another set of weights for pediatric patients. Weights are periodically revised in order to try to fit data mortality data better. Because the TRISS is derived from ISS, RTS, and GCS, plus some vital sign data not adjusted for body size, all of the errors in these methods carry forward into the TRISS calculation for pediatric patients, making TRISS relatively unreliable overall for pediatric injury. Furthermore, like most measures of injury severity, TRISS does not incorporate any measure of "patient reserve" or preexisting disease that could alter a child's ability to recover from an injury. Despite these weaknesses, TRISS remains the most commonly used score for both adults and children.

| TABLE 77-7 | ASCOT Age Indexes |
|---|---|
| Age | Index |
| 0 to 54 | 0 |
| 55 to 64 | 1 |
| 65 to 74 | 2 |
| 75 to 84 | 3 |
| >85 | 4 |

## A Severity Characterization of Trauma

ASCOT was introduced by Champion et al in 1990 as a means to overcome the weaknesses inherent in TRISS. Like TRISS, ASCOT uses both anatomic and physiological data as well as some consideration for age. For anatomic data, ASCOT substitutes AP scores, eliminating reliance on AIS and ISS. Physiological data mirror data used for the RTS (GCS, SBP, RR). Age is included, but still only really discriminates among those older than 54 years old (Table 77-7).

As with other systems, ASCOT relies upon a logistic function of weighted data to calculate a probability of survival:

$$P(s) = -\left(\frac{1}{1 + e^{-k}}\right),$$

where

$$k = k_1 + k_2 \text{BCS} + k_3 \text{SBP} + k_4 \text{RR} + k_5 A + k_6 B + k_7 C + k_8 \text{Age}.$$

The indexes (not raw values) of GCS, SBP, RR, A, B, C, and Age are individually weighted by a specific $k_i$. ASCOT is quite similar to TRISS structurally, including components of the physiological components of RTS and the GCS, but for anatomic data ASCOT substitutes the A, B, and C components from the AP in place of the ISS. Additionally, like TRISS, blunt and penetrating mechanisms are weighted differently (Table 77-8).

Despite this added complexity, ASCOT is not a superior scoring tool. Not only is ASCOT more difficult to calculate, but it does not carry better predictive power than TRISS. Moreover, ASCOT offers no large advantage in pediatric patients, even with a slightly lower propensity to underestimate probability of survival. Like TRISS, ASCOT cannot be used for triage or for end-of-life decisions. Perhaps for all these reasons, ASCOT has not gained widespread use in pediatric trauma.

## Pediatric Risk Indicator

One of the few pediatric specific scores, the Pediatric Risk Indicator (PRI) was introduced in 1997 as an attempt to provide a better pediatric-specific injury measurement tool. Although it borrows heavily from other methodologies, it is essentially a simple composite of several other scores:

$$PRI = \frac{ISS}{(GCS + |PTS|)}.$$

In this way, the PRI returns a simple ratio in which PRI >1 suggests severe injury. Incorporation of the PTS gives the PRI age-based validity for children, and inclusion of the GCS correctly emphasizes the outsize effect of head injury in pediatric trauma mortality. Still, like other composite scores, the PTS shares the flaws of the ISS, but unlike TRISS or ASCOT, it does not return a survival probability. It is rarely used.

# FUTURE DIRECTIONS FOR INJURY DESCRIPTION

Examination of the various scoring systems reveals interesting errors and flaws that degrade the ability of these tools to predict trauma outcomes. First, as shown with many scores, risk often does not rise monotomically with score values (Fig. 77-10), meaning that a worse score may not really correlate with more risk or the same increase in risk. These effects are amplified in children. Meanwhile, reliance on logistic regression and "weight jiggling" in order to fit predictions to data leaves the major scores vulnerable to overfitting of the models to large data sets. Worse, the nested layers of indexes of raw physiologic data ineluctably produces information loss. Forcing physiological measures (interval or ratio data) into indexes (ordinal scores) essentially amounts viewing the data through low-bit encoders. Worse, these highly pixelated "pictures" of anatomic or physiological injury are then combined according to computer-generated weights that are medically meaningless (eg, the $W_0$ weight in RTS, included solely to achieve a 0-intercept).

When used in children, their predictive power appears to be even more suspect. It is well recognized that compared to adults, children follow different patterns of injury (eg, seat-belt injuries, nonaccidental trauma, distribution of cervical spine injury, etc) and exhibit very different physiological responses (eg, trivial increase in energy expenditure in response to injury, but a far higher baseline energy expenditure, etc). Because size-specific alterations in baseline physiology across the normal range of human body mass is

| TABLE 77-8 | ASCOT Blunt and Penetrating Weights | | |
|---|---|---|---|
| k | Variable | Blunt | Penetrating |
| $k_1$ | Constant | −1.1570 | −1.1350 |
| $k_2$ | GCS | 0.7705 | 1.0626 |
| $k_3$ | SBP | 0.6583 | 0.3638 |
| $k_4$ | RR | 0.2810 | 0.3332 |
| $k_5$ | A | −0.3002 | −0.3702 |
| $k_6$ | B | −0.1961 | −0.2053 |
| $k_7$ | C | −0.2086 | −0.3188 |
| $k_8$ | Age | −0.6355 | −0.8365 |

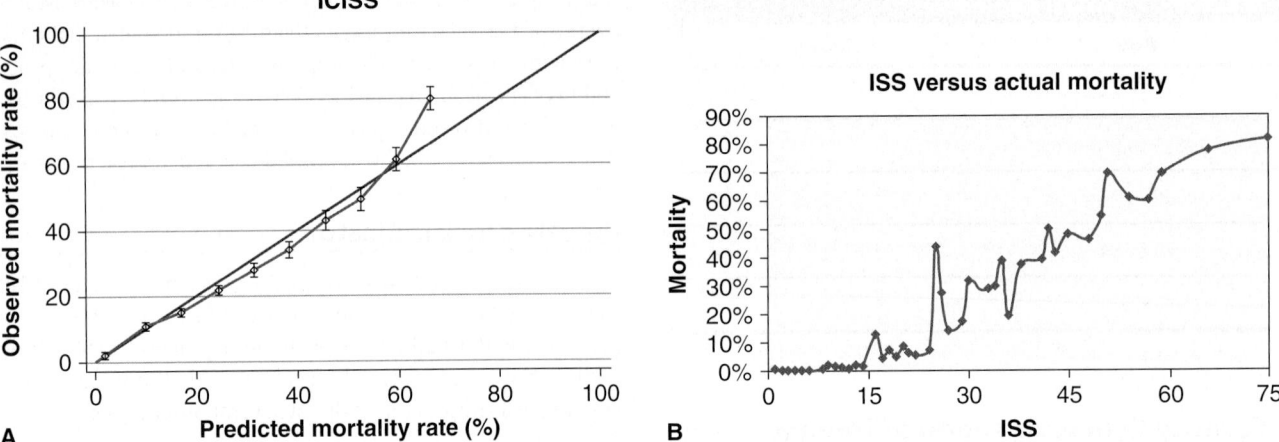

**FIGURE 77-10** Comparison of mortality risk for different injury scoring systems reveals the difference between a nearly monotonic score such as ICISS (A) and a non monotonic score such as the ISS (B) where actual mortality risk does not rise smoothly with increasing score values.

poorly understood, it is not surprising that scoring systems fail to explicitly incorporate allometric scaling into their derivations. Nevertheless, because of the extensive use of weighted variables, some of this size-dependent information must contribute to the probability computations, however, indirectly. Consequently, comparisons of prediction models in children that focus on physiologic measures (eg, the best motor response of the GCS) appear to perform best in children. Despite these weaknesses, scores like TRISS and ISS appear to perform fairly well (with caveats) for benchmarking purposes for pediatric patients. For now, these remain the *de facto* standards. However, ICD-9-based methods will likely supplant TRISS and ISS.

Still, some researchers are beginning to look beyond simple black-box regression methods in order to objectively rank injury and measure "injured-ness." For example, improved resolution of now universally available CT scans allows improved interrater reliability of OIS-, AIS-, and ICD-9-based scores, and even holds out the possibility of volumetric approaches that would allow an actual measurement of the degree of disruption of an organ. Advanced imaging promises to add critical data to pediatric trauma measures, particularly in brain and cervical spine injury where simple CT scans lack sensitivity.

Meanwhile, computerized medical records, especially of automatic recording of vital-sign data, is increasingly used experimentally to create new predictors of outcome. For example, it was long ago noticed that beat-to-beat spacing variability in cardiac rate follows a power-law distribution stemming from fractal-like spacing in the time domain (similar effects have been shown in ventilatory regulation). What was once regarded as noise, was later recognized as the summed effect of multiple regulatory feedbacks on the cardiac rhythm. Interestingly, when regulatory mechanisms begin to fail, the heart rate becomes *more* regular. In this way, it has been shown that measures of this increasing regularity give clinicians a possible means to quantify "physiological reserve," measures that can be tied to increasing intracranial pressure in closed head injury, or to overall mortality. Recently, one group has used this methodology in

combination with the now-familiar logistical regression to calculate a severity of illness score for sick newborns and to give unprecedented predictive power for outcomes. Because pediatric physiology is so varied over the range of size from infant to teens, these and other mathematically sophisticated techniques (such as classification trees, Bayesian methods, and even clustering methods from bioinformatics) promise to improve injury scoring in children.

## INJURY PREVENTION

Prevention is the most logical solution to injury-associated morbidity and mortality. Unfortunately, prevention measures alone are unlikely to eradicate this epidemic. The classic approach to injury prevention was first outlined by William Haddon in the 1970s. Haddon believed, contrary to popular principles, that injury was the natural result of predictable circumstances. Haddon postulated that injuries could be considered in 3 phases (Haddon matrix), preevent, event and postevent, each presenting opportunities for modulation. Each phase had modifiable aspects including host factors, agents, physical environment, and social environment (Table 77-9).

This approach is still applicable to almost any injury circumstance. Modification of the preevent circumstances (primary prevention) typically involves education, and/or safety design measures that prevent the injury from occurring at all. For example, gating areas around a swimming pool to prevent inappropriate access and subsequent drowning would constitute primary prevention. Measures designed to mitigate the injury despite occurrence of the event (secondary prevention) would include airbag deployments in frontal collisions. Finally, postevent or tertiary injury prevention involves optimizing the outcome of the injured patient despite the event. This is the approach practiced by all health care providers involved in management of the trauma patient. The most successful prevention measures incorporate steps to address all 3 event phases.

| | **Host Factors** | **Agent** | **Physical Environment** | **Sociocultural Environment** |
|---|---|---|---|---|
| TABLE 77-9 | The Haddon Conceptual Framework of Factors Determining Risk of Head Injury Caused by a Motor Vehicle–Bicycle Collision | | | |
| Preevent phase | Age<br>Lights, reflective clothing | Driving while intoxicated | Bicycling lanes<br>Nontraffic bicycling facility | Parental education<br>Family income<br>Helmet law |
| Event phase | Helmet use<br>Riding skill<br>Riding speed | Driving skill<br>Motor vehicle speed | Speed limits<br>Weather<br>Lighting | |
| Postevent phase | Comorbidity | | Weather 911 | Trauma System |

Prevention initiatives variably implement the 3 "E's" of prevention: education, enforcement, and/or engineering. An example of a successful injury prevention initiative is that directed against motor vehicle-related mortality. Motor vehicles are the most common cause of injury morbidity and mortality in the pediatric population (6703 deaths and >150,000 injuries in children aged 0 to 19, for year 2007). Prevention efforts have resulted in a 36% reduction in motor vehicle-related injury mortality from the first half of the 1980s (crude death rate, 14.64/100,000) to the first half of the 2000s (crude death rate, 9.39/100,000). The success is due to educational efforts to inform the public about the proven efficacy of child-restraint systems and their proper use, engineering modifications to provide child appropriate restraints (eg, booster seats, tethering for car seats), and enforcement through seatbelt and child-restraint laws.

Though generally well-meaning, not all prevention initiatives are beneficial. Given the limited pool of resources available for prevention efforts, measuring the success of an injury prevention program or prevention initiative is imperative. Ideally, success is measured through comparisons of outcome (eg, proper utilization of car seats) conducted before, during, and after the intervention. Efforts demonstrated to be effective may then be exported to other communities for implementation. However, proven success in one population may not necessarily be successful (or appropriate) in another. For example, violence prevention efforts in a community with high rates of interpersonal violence may not be useful in a community with low rates of crime. Similarly, helmet laws may decrease head injury, but may also decrease bike riding.

## SELECTED READINGS

ACS-COT. *Resources for Optimal Care of the Injured Patient: 2006.* Chicago, IL: American College of Surgeons; 1986.

ACS-COT. *Resources for Optimal Care of the Injured Patient: 2006.* Chicago, IL: American College of Surgeons; 2006.

Buckley JC, McAninch JW. Revision of current American Association for the Surgery of Trauma Renal Injury grading system. *J Trauma* 70(1): 35–37.

Centers for Disease Control and Prevention, National Center for Injury Prevention and Control. Web-based Injury Statistics Query and Reporting System (WISQARS). Department of Health and Human Services Web site: http://www.cdc.gov/ncipc/wisqars. Accessed March 16, 2011.

Champion HR, Copes WS, Sacco WJ, et al. A new characterization of injury severity. *J Trauma* 1990;30(5):539–545; discussion 545–546.

Champion HR, Sacco WJ, Copes WS, et al. A revision of the Trauma Score. *J Trauma* 1989;29(5):623–629.

Committee on Trauma, American College of Surgeons. Optimal hospital resources for care of the seriously injured. *Bull Am Coll Surg* 1976;61(9): 15–22.

Davis DH, Localio AR, Stafford PW, Helfaer MA, Durbin DR. Trends in operative management of pediatric splenic injury in a regional trauma system. *Pediatrics* 2005;115:89–94.

Densmore JC, Lim HJ, Oldham KT, Guice KS. Outcomes and delivery of care in pediatric injury. *J Pediatr Surg* 2006;41:92–98.

Gausche-Hill M, Wiebe RA. Guidelines for preparedness of emergency departments that care for children: a call to action. *Ann Emerg Med* 2001;37:389–391.

IOM. *Hospital Based Emergency Care: At the Breaking Point.* Washington, DC: National Academies Press; 2006.

IOM report Emergency Care for Children: Growing Pains. Washington, DC: National Academies Press; 2006.

Kilgo PD, Meredith JW, Hensberry R, Osler TM. A note on the disjointed nature of the injury severity score. *J Trauma* 2004;57(3):479–485; discussion 486–487.

Lacroix J, Cotting J. Severity of illness and organ dysfunction scoring in children. *Pediatr Crit Care Med* 2005;6(3 Suppl):S126–S134.

MacKenzie EJ, Rivara FP, Jurkovich GJ, et al. A national evaluation of the effect of trauma-center care on mortality. *N Engl J Med* 2006;354: 366–378.

Mackenzie EJ, Rivara FP, Jurkovich GJ, et al. The national study on costs and outcomes of trauma. *J Trauma* 2007;63:S54–S67.

Mooney DP, Rothstein DH, Forbes PW. Variation in the management of pediatric splenic injuries in the United States. *J Trauma* 2006;61: 330–333.

Morris JA Jr, Norris PR, Ozdas A, et al. Reduced heart rate variability: an indicator of cardiac uncoupling and diminished physiologic reserve in 1,425 trauma patients. *J Trauma* 2006;60(6):1165–1173; discussion 1173–1174.

Nance ML, Carr BG, Branas CC. Access to pediatric trauma care in the US. *Arch Pediatr Adol Med* 2009;163(6):512–518.

Osler T, Rutledge R, Deis J, Bedrick E. ICISS: an international classification of disease-9 based injury severity score. *J Trauma* 1996;41(3):380–386; discussion 386–388.

Potoka DA, Schall LC, Ford HR. Development of a novel age-specific pediatric trauma score. *J Pediatr Surg* 2001;36(1):106–112.

Saria S, Rajani AK, Gould J, Koller D, Penn AA. Integration of early physiological responses predicts later illness severity in preterm infants. *Sci Transl Med* 2(48):48ra65.

Schluter PJ, Nathens A, Neal ML, et al. Trauma and Injury Severity Score (TRISS) coefficients 2009 revision. *J Trauma* 68(4):761–770.

Tepas JJ 3rd, Leaphart CL, Celso BG, et al. Risk stratification simplified: the worst injury predicts mortality for the injured children. *J Trauma* 2008;65(6):1258–1261; discussion 1261–1263.

Voss A, Schulz S, Schroeder R, Baumert M, Caminal P. Methods derived from nonlinear dynamics for analysing heart rate variability. *Philos Transact A Math Phys Eng Sci* 2009;367(1887):277–296.

# Child Abuse   CHAPTER 78

*Arthur Cooper, Leslie Ann Taylor,*
*and David Merten*

## KEY POINTS

1. Physicians and other health, education, social service, and public safety providers are mandated by law to report suspected child abuse to local child protective authorities.

2. Child battering remains the most common cause of homicide in infants and toddlers.

3. The term "shaken baby syndrome" has been superseded by the term "abusive head trauma", recognizing the importance of factors such as detailed mechanistic history and developmental age and stage in addition to classic physical findings, radiographic imaging, and laboratory data.

4. Unique "patterns" of body system injury often represent findings suspicious for child abuse.

5. Any unexplained alteration in mental status may indicate child abuse due to inflicted closed head injury.

6. Pediatric surgeons have a personal, professional, and public responsibility to provide testimony in court when called upon to do so, as either an expert, or a witness to the facts.

## INTRODUCTION

The inauguration of pediatric subspecialty certification in Child Abuse Pediatrics in 2010 was an historic development in the maturation of the field of child maltreatment. As a result, pediatric surgeons will less often find themselves called upon to testify in court on behalf of battered children. Yet, as the recognized experts in the mechanisms, patterns, responses, and outcomes of physical injury in children, pediatric surgeons can still be expected to be subpoenaed as fact witnesses to the injuries sustained by children under their care, as well as their likely long-term consequences. Hence, a working knowledge of the common manifestations of abusive injuries in childhood must be a key component of the cognitive armamentarium of every pediatric surgeon, for purposes both of early recognition and reporting, and of timely diagnosis and treatment.

## HISTORY

Children have certainly been victims of inflicted injury from the dawn of humankind. Instances of what today would be recognized as child abuse are recorded even in *The Bible*, while nursery rhymes are replete with additional examples. The earliest medical acknowledgment of child abuse appeared in 1860, when the French forensic physician Auguste Ambroise Tardieu reported 32 cases in his "Medico-legal Study of Cruelty and Brutal Treatment Inflicted on Children," followed in 1868 by his fulsomely illustrated "Medico-legal Study of Infanticide." Both were virtually forgotten until 1946, when the pediatric radiologist John Caffey first called the widespread attention of the English-speaking medical world to a then-unrecognized association of injuries—multiple long-bone fractures in infants with chronic subdural hematomas—and alerted physicians to the then-unbelievable notion that these injuries may have been inflicted by their caretakers.

His former fellow, Frederic Silverman, soon expanded upon this body of work, followed thereafter by the pediatric surgeon Morton Woolley. It only remained for Henry Kempe, in 1962, to publish the landmark article that coined the term *battered child syndrome*. Since that time, pediatricians, pediatric radiologists, and pediatric surgeons have all become increasingly involved in the identification and management of child abuse, and in all North American states, provinces, and territories, as in most nations of the developed world, physicians and other health, education, social service, and public safety providers are mandated by law to report suspected child abuse to local child protective authorities.

## EPIDEMIOLOGY

Despite increased efforts to prevent child abuse, inflicted injuries still exact a staggering toll from youth worldwide. Maltreated children still comprise about 10% of all injured patients younger than 6 years of age presenting to the emergency department, while about 2.5% are victims of frank physical abuse. A 1995 Gallup poll suggests that potentially abusive physical discipline is widespread, with more than

3 million American children being disciplined by being struck with an object somewhere other than the buttocks, or being punched, kicked, thrown, shaken, knocked down, or beaten up. Child battering remains the most common cause of homicide in infants and toddlers. According to the United States Department of Health and Human Services Administration for Children and Families Children's Bureau, some 750,000 total child abuse cases were "indicated" and 1500 total child abuse deaths were reported in the United States in 2010, although the total number of cases is likely much higher, since the majority of registered cases of suspected abuse are later determined to be "unfounded," many for lack of evidence.

DiScala et al reported the results of the largest trauma registry based study of physically abusive injuries to date in 2000. They found that 1997 of 18,828 (10.6%) cases in children <5 years were caused by abuse. When compared to unintentionally injured children, they were half as old (mean age 12.8 mo vs 25.5 mo), 4 times more likely to have had significant prior medical histories (53% vs 14.1%), 4 times more likely to have sustained severe (ISS ≥20) injuries (22.6% vs 6.3%), and 5 times more likely to have died as a result of their injuries (12.7% vs 2.6%). Battering (53%) and shaking (10.3%) were the most common injury mechanisms, as opposed to the falls (58.4%) and motor vehicle crashes (37.1%) that most often harmed unintentionally injured children, with the result that twice as many abused children sustained intra-abdominal injuries (11.4% vs 6.8%), while thrice as many sustained intrathoracic (12.5% vs 4.5%) and intracranial (42.2% vs 14.1%) injuries. As such, it is hardly surprising that abused children consumed more hospital resources than unintentionally injured children (use of ICU 42.5% vs 26.9%, LOS 9.3 da vs. 3.8 da), had more than 3 times the functional limitations at hospital discharge (8.7% vs 2.7%), and were discharged home less than half as often (43.4% vs 96.1%). Of note retinal hemorrhages were observed in 27.8% of physically abused children, but in only 0.1% of unintentionally injured children, making the presence of this finding all but diagnostic of intentional injury in children.

# PATHOPHYSIOLOGY

Most inflicted injuries result from "discipline" gone awry, following a triggering crisis that pits an exaggerated response by a highly stressed, typically immature, caretaker, against a child young and small enough to be unable to effectively resist. Boys are more commonly abused than girls by a ratio of 2:1, premature infants than term infants by a ratio of 3:1, and stepchildren than other children by a ratio of 4:1. A related caretaker is the abuser in approximately 85% of cases, the mother's paramour in 10%, a babysitter in 4%, and a sibling in 1%. Underlying the triggering crisis may be any number of factors, most often psychological and social. The result is a battered child—bruised in some 70%, or broken, burned, or beaten in another 10% each—not to mention his shattered family.

Relatively few inflicted injuries in children are life-threatening and require emergent operation. In addition, early recognition and reporting of child abuse can prevent the predictable progression to more serious injury and death. Pediatric surgeons play a vital role in the detection of child abuse, as they typically examine the child totally unclothed in the course of the primary survey applied to all victims of significant injury, including child abuse. Typical abusive injuries encompass bruises, lacerations, bites, dental and ocular trauma, fractures, poisonings, and drownings. Common patterns of abusive injury are described below, in the order most often encountered in pediatric surgical practice.

## Soft Tissue Injury

Most bruises and lacerations sustained by children occur over bony prominences during the course of play. Bruises and lacerations usually involving better protected body parts, such as the cheeks, buttocks, and genitalia, are suspicious for abuse. Multicolored bruises imply repetitive contusions sustained at several different points in time, owing to the generally predictable rates of progression in breakdown and metabolism of hemoglobin pigments. Unfortunately, despite this fact, the precise "age" of a bruise cannot be determined with accuracy as was previously held, due to slight differences in the rates of disappearance. The radius and configuration of "bite" marks afford important clues to the identity of the perpetrator. "Whip" and "strangulation" marks are usually self-evident. So, respectively, are "slap" and "grip" marks, the former most often found in the shape of hand print on the face or the buttocks, the latter most often observed bilaterally, both anteriorly and posteriorly on the lower lateral chest wall of young infants, in association with violent shaking. The presence of a "cauliflower" ear suggests repetitive pulling or twisting. An abnormal coagulogram will certainly increase the likelihood of bruising following trivial injury, but does not automatically exclude the possibility of abuse in the absence a consistent account. Nor does a past history of "easy bruisability" exclude the possibility of abuse.

## Skeletal Injury

Inflicted fractures, most often produced by a sudden, forceful torqueing motion applied to a limb, will typically present as spiral, greenstick, or torus fractures, which usually can be managed by an orthopaedic surgeon without the need for operative reduction or fixation. Occult bony injuries regarded as highly suggestive of skeletal abuse include "bucket-handle" fractures, metaphyseal "chip" fractures, and subperiosteal hematomas. Fractures of the acromion process of the scapula or the proximal humerus in a child are additionally suspect. Spiral extremity fractures in children younger than 9 months of age and femur fractures in children younger than 2 years of age are particularly suspicious for abuse. However, such fractures, while still seen as suggestive of abuse, are no longer considered pathognomonic if there exists a credible history of unintentional torsion, as may occur during a fall associated with entrapment and twisting of the affected limb. Paraspinal fractures of the lower ribs in infants suggest the possibility of violent shaking, as forceful bilateral compression of the lower chest wall will be necessary for the perpetrator to maintain a grip.

Callus formation may provide the only evidence of skeletal abuse, but it does not typically begin to appear on plain radiographs for some 7 to 10 days following injury. A careful history must always be obtained to exclude occult traumatic, metabolic, and infectious causes for the observed skeletal injury. Conditions such as obstetrical trauma, rickets, scurvy, hypervitaminosis A, osteogenesis imperfecta, infantile cortical hyperostoses, and syphilis can all mimic child abuse, but can generally be excluded on radiographic evaluation by an experienced pediatric radiologist. Again, however, a history consistent with unintentional injury is paramount, since inflicted injury can occur in spite—or because—of the above diagnoses.

## Burn Injury

Inflicted burns, ranging from small superficial brandings, such as cigarette burns, through moderate-sized scald burns, to large life-threatening immersion burns, most often require surgical management by a burn specialist. Any scald burn in an unusual location, such as the back, or with a sharp border, especially of the hands, feet, or buttocks—particularly those which present with a "glove," "stocking," or "doughnut" pattern of distribution, in which the perineum itself is burned while a circular "sparing" of tissues surrounding the perineum is evident. Such a pattern indicates that the victim's buttocks were "pressed" onto the bottom of the tub or basin and held there for several moments while being exposed to scalding water—hence must be regarded as highly suspicious for abuse. Patterned burns, such as iron burns and radiator burns, may occur unintentionally if the history clearly so suggests, but the larger and more regular the area of exposure to the pattern, the greater the likelihood of abuse.

## Head Injury

Among the more serious inflicted injuries are those that may require the expertise of a neurosurgeon. They include blunt head trauma, skull fractures, and subdural hematomas from "abusive head trauma," the term now preferred over "shaken baby syndrome." Such head injuries in young infants may be associated with mechanisms other than, or in addition to, violent shaking. Controversy continues to exist regarding the role of violent shaking in the pathophysiology of abusive head trauma. Many experts, perhaps even a majority, believe that shaking alone is sufficient to produce the classic findings—of bilateral subdural hematomas and multiple retinal hemorrhages. Originally described by Caffey in association with long bone fractures, far more frequent are variable degrees of alteration in mental status that putatively results from diffuse axonal shearing. However, some experts continue to maintain that at least some level of impact—for example, violent shaking against bedding, or a perpetrator's thigh—is necessary to produce a profound enough increase in acceleration–deceleration forces to shear both the fragile "bridging" veins that traverse the infant's meninges and the delicate, developing axons within the white matter of the infantile internal capsule. That said, care must be taken to differentiate the intracranial effects of violent shaking from a recently described condition known as "benign enlargement of the subarachnoid space" (BESS) which, although most commonly unilateral, can also occur bilaterally, and may predispose the thinned, extended "bridging" veins to tear upon minor injury. Skull fractures are rarely, if ever, associated with violent shaking as a sole mechanism. Moreover, those attributed to falls of less than 4 feet are unlikely to have been inflicted, even if associated with a small, linear fracture, unless they are associated with a history of unconsciousness, which is rarely, if ever, observed in association with such low falls—for example, those from bed or sofa height. However, depressed skull fractures, or those that exhibit a "shattered eggshell" pattern, are more suspicious for abuse, and they suggest the added possibility that the child may also have been a victim of a direct blow to the head. Here, as always, history is paramount. Finally, traumatic brain injury due to abusive head trauma is a late manifestation in the progression of child abuse. Unfortunately, these head injuries, occurring predominantly in infants, are the leading cause of fatal child abuse.

## Abdominal Injury

Although abdominal abuse is rare as compared to other forms of child abuse, it can be life-threatening or lethal. Inflicted abdominal injuries are the second leading cause of fatal child abuse. McCort et al reported 4 of 10 children with abdominal abuse dying of their injuries. Touloukian found a 50% fatality rate. O'Neill et al reported on 110 children with inflicted injuries. Nine had abdominal injuries and all were life-threatening. One child died from abdominal abuse. In 1988, Cooper et al found that of some 10,000 injured children, 360 (2.8%) had suffered inflicted trauma. Twenty-two children (6% of the abused children) suffered significant abdominal abuse, and 10 children died due to abdominal trauma, of whom 4 were dead on arrival. Remarkably, the 4 observed patterns of injury—duodenal and pancreatic hematomata, duodenal and jejunal rupture, minor solid visceral injuries, major solid visceral injuries—could have been predicted based on admitting vital signs.

Children are particularly susceptible to severe internal injury from inadvertent or inflicted abdominal trauma because of several anatomic factors. They have a thin abdominal wall with poorly developed musculature. Widely splayed lower ribs provide little coverage for lower riding upper abdominal viscera, while the more exposed liver extends across the upper abdomen. Similarly, the shallower pelvis provides scant protection to the higher riding urinary bladder. In addition, the anteroposterior diameter of the abdomen is short as compared to adults, increasing the exposure of the duodenum and pancreas to serious injury when a sharp blow to the upper abdomen crushes them against the spinal column.

Blows or kicks to the abdomen cause predictable injuries to the solid and hollow viscera. Blunt abdominal injuries, which should always be considered suspicious for child abuse, include gastric rupture, duodenal hematoma, or duodenal perforation (Figs. 78-1 and 78-2). Intestinal shearing injuries leading to bowel wall or mesenteric

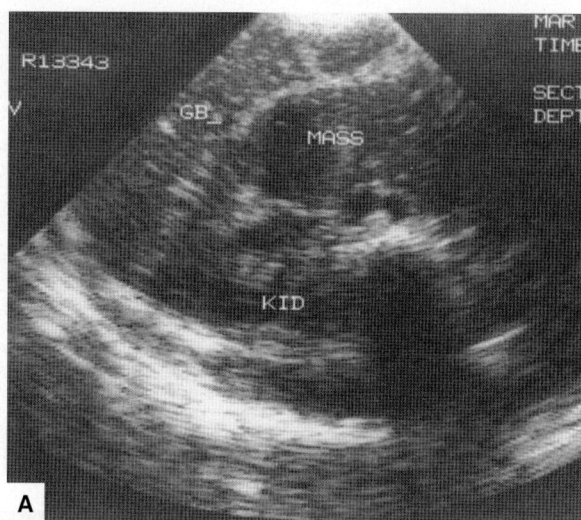
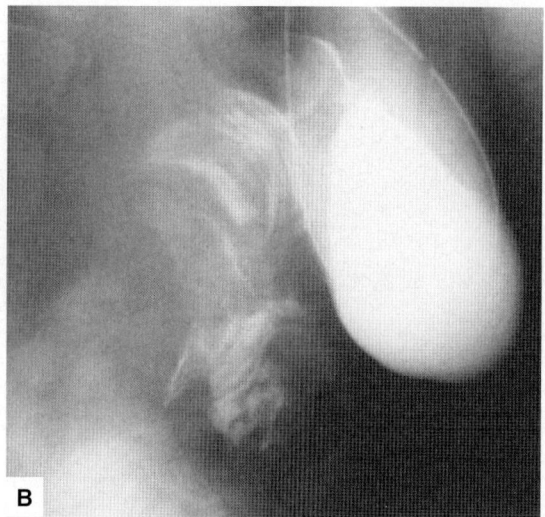

**FIGURE 78-1** Ten-year-old boy presenting with vomiting. There was a recent history of being "punched in the stomach" by his stepmother. **A.** Transverse sonography of the epigastrium in projection shows a predominantly sonolucent hematoma (MASS) of the descending duodenum lying medial to the gallbladder (GB) and anterior to the kidney (KID). **B.** An upper gastrointestinal series shows partial duodenal obstruction and distortion producing the typical "coiled spring" appearance of intramural duodenal hematoma.

hematoma or bowel perforation are nearly always indicative of abdominal abuse, which, in recent years, has eclipsed epigastric bicycle handlebar injury as the predominant mechanism of injury. As stated, the most common site for intestinal shearing injuries is at the duodenojejunal junction, with isolated duodenal injuries being next most common (Fig. 78-3). Chylous ascites may also arise from mesenteric injury. Pancreatic contusion or transection from a blow to the epigastrium should also arouse suspicion (Figs. 78-4 and 78-5). Pancreatic pseudocysts have been reported as a late presentation of child abdominal

abuse. Colonic rupture and avulsion of the common bile duct have also been reported from abdominal abuse as have complete avulsion of the superior mesenteric artery and aortic pseudoaneurysm.

The mechanism of injury is usually a direct blow from a fist or knee, or kneeling on or kicking the child's abdomen (Fig. 78-6). The characteristic midline injuries occur when viscera are crushed against the spine by the adult fist, knee, or foot. The surgeon should suspect child abuse when a hollow viscus injury is found in a child and, conversely, suspect hollow viscus injury in a child presenting with abdominal

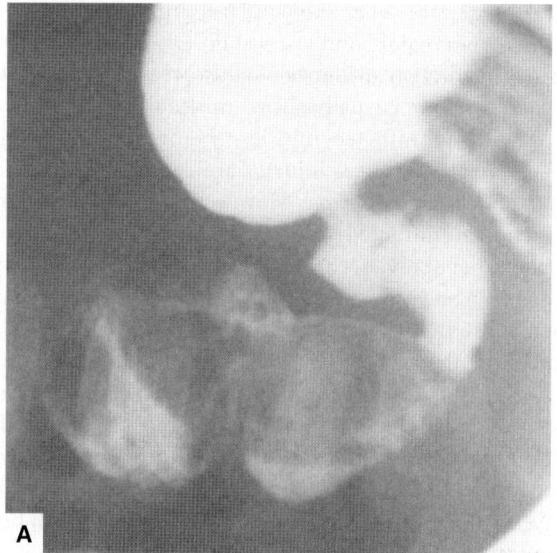
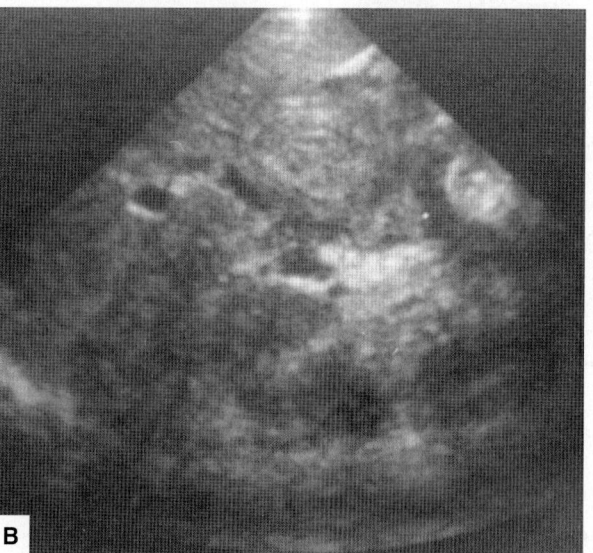

**FIGURE 78-2** A 19-month-old male with bilious vomiting and no history of trauma. **A.** An upper gastrointestinal series with the child in a prone position shows a typical "coiled spring" appearance of an intramural duodenal hematoma with relative obstruction of the proximal duodenum. **B.** Longitudinal sonography of the epigastrium reveals the hematoma as a mass of mixed echogenicity.

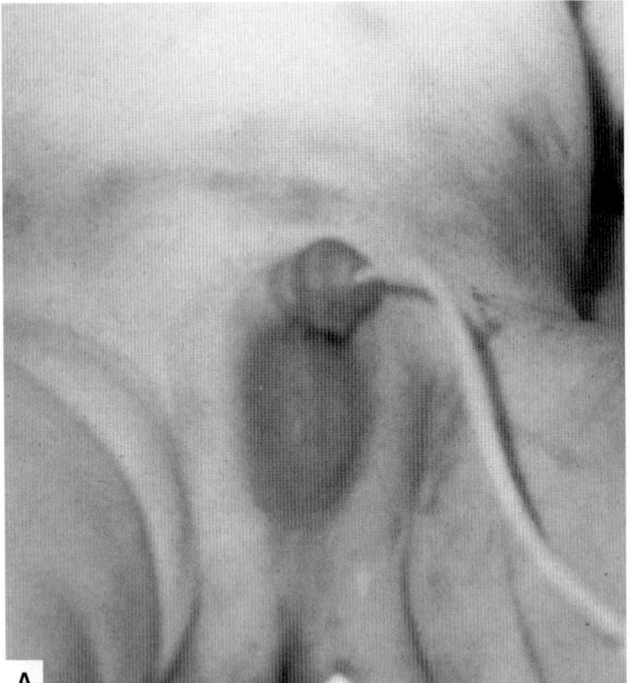

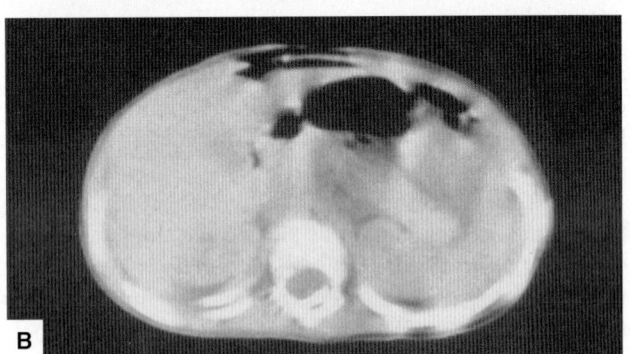

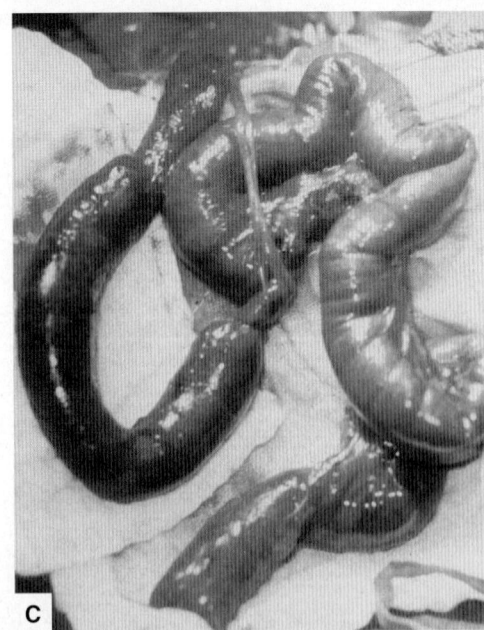

**FIGURE 78-3** A 15-month-old boy presented with scalp lacera-tion and vomiting. There was abdominal distension and bruising and blood per rectum. His abdomen had been kneeled on by his mother's boyfriend. **A.** Abdominal bruising. **B.** CT scan shows free air. **C.** At operation, 42 cm of duodenum and jejunum had been stripped of mesentery.

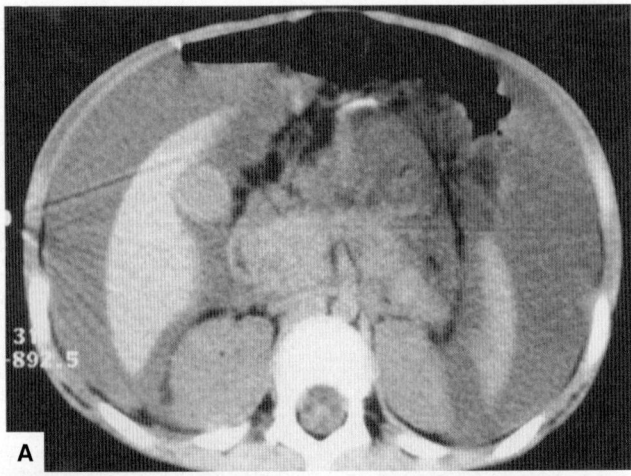

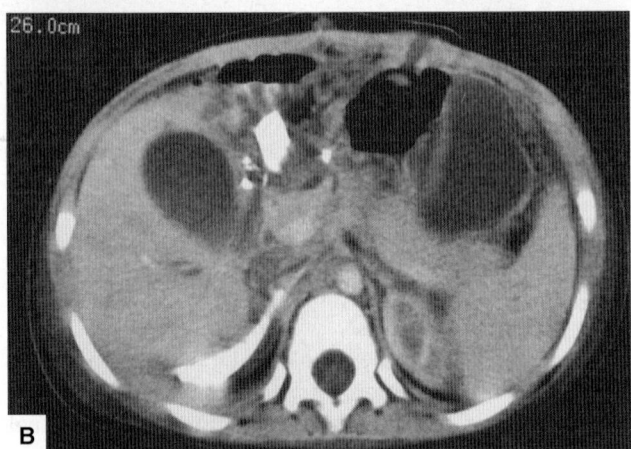

**FIGURE 78-4** A 2-year-old female with multiple bruises and abdominal distension. **A.** Abdominal CT shows a pneumoperito-neum with air beneath the anterior abdominal wall and extensive hemoperitoneum. No pancreatic injury could be identified. **B.** A follow-up CT scan 8 days later because of continued abdominal distress shows a large retrogastric pancreatic pseudocyst anterior to the pancreas. (Courtesy of George S. Bissett III, MD, Duke University Medical Center, Durham, NC.)

findings and other evidence of abuse, recalling that histories in such cases are virtually always misleading.

As with noninflicted injuries, the overwhelming major-ity of inflicted truncal injuries are caused by blunt rather than penetrating trauma. However, inflicted injuries dif-fer from noninflicted injuries in almost every other way. Ledbetter et al reviewed 156 children younger than 13 years of age who had blunt abdominal trauma. Eleven percent had been abused. Boys were twice as likely to be abused as girls, similar to the gender incidence in unintentional trauma. However, the abused children were younger, with a mean age of 2.5 years, making toddlers the most likely victims of abdominal abuse. Children suffering unintentional trauma had a mean age of 7.6 years, consistent with the school-age child as the frequent victim of a motor vehicle crash both as a pedestrian or as a passenger.

While late presentation is hardly unknown in cases of unintentional abdominal trauma, children with abdominal abuse are often delayed in presentation to the medical facil-ity, either because the abuser fails to realize the severity of

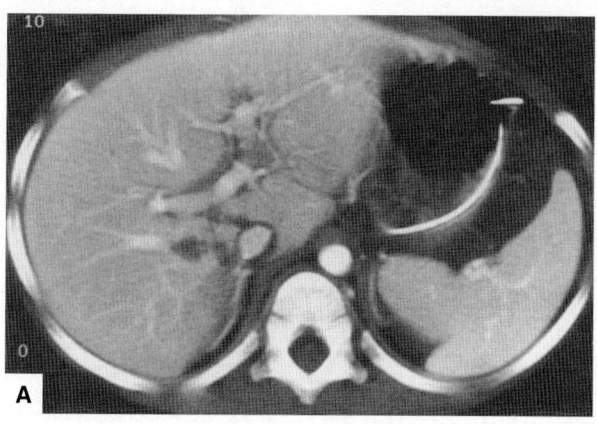
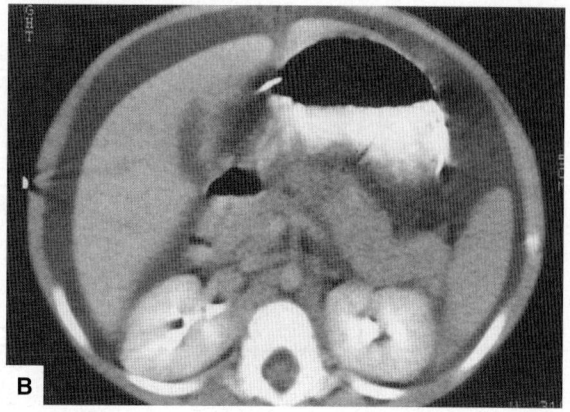

**FIGURE 78-5** A 3-year-old boy presented with vomiting and left-upper-quadrant bruising and fracture of the first metatarsal. Serum amylase and lipase were elevated. He had been punched in the midepigastrium by his mother's boyfriend. Eleven days after the injury, he required exploration for pancreatic ascites from pancreatic transection. **A.** CT scan shows periportal edema from liver trauma. **B.** CT scan shows pancreatic ascites and pancreatic transection.

the injury inflicted or has tried to conceal the injury until the child is in extremis. Delay in presentation may also be caused by late rupture of crushed and ischemic intestine. Abdominal abuse is also characterized mostly by male perpetrators, typically either the child's father or the mother's paramour.

With rare exceptions, a misleading history inconsistent with the injury observed will be offered. Common explanations for abusive injuries are that no injury occurred, that the child fell from a bed or sofa, was dropped by a sibling, inadvertently self-inflicted the injury, or fell onto furniture. Because the most common victims of abdominal abuse are in

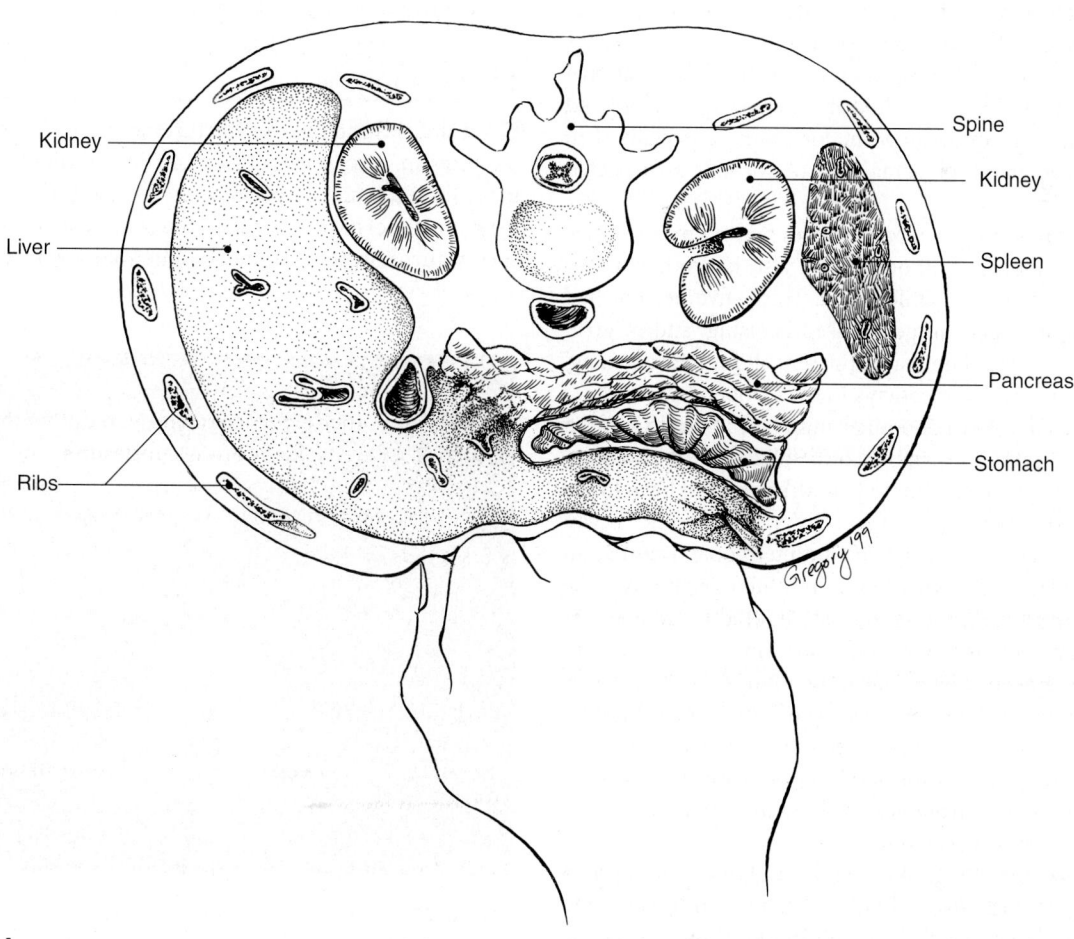

Kidney

Liver

Ribs

Spine

Kidney

Spleen

Pancreas

Stomach

**A**

**FIGURE 78-6** **A.** Mechanism of blunt injury to the liver, pancreas, and duodenum.

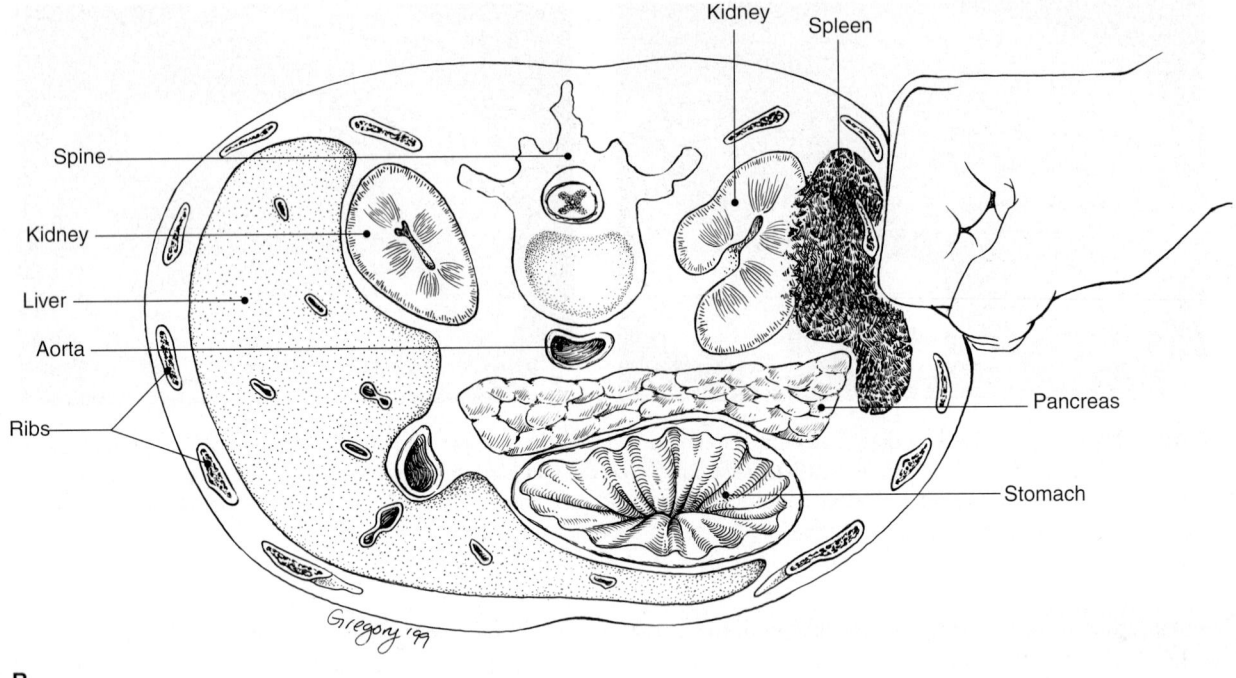

Spine

Kidney

Liver

Aorta

Ribs

Kidney    Spleen

Pancreas

Stomach

Gregory '99

**B**

**FIGURE 78-6** (*Continued*) **B.** Mechanism of injury to the spleen.

the toddler age group or younger, it is rare that the patient can contribute to the history. This misleading history may create confusion about the diagnosis before and after the child has reached the medical facility, compounding the delay in appropriate treatment. Therefore, child abuse should be considered in any child with unexplained major injury, especially if in shock, cardiac arrest, or coma with or without a suspected head injury.

Most children in the Ledbetter series had no major injury outside the abdomen, although most also had other minor injuries consistent with child abuse. Thirty-five percent had no other injuries and no generalized bruising, and of great significance, most did not have apparent abdominal bruising. This was also true of the patients in the Cooper series.

The most common abdominal injury in abused children is an upper midline disruption of a solid or hollow viscus, whereas unintentionally injured children tend to have lower abdominal injuries or an injury to a single solid organ (Figs. 78-4A and 78-7). Unlike unintentional trauma, in which the spleen is the most common solid organ injured, the liver is the most common solid organ injured in child abuse, and children may die from exsanguination (Figs. 78-5A and 78-8A). The spleen is less likely to be injured in child abuse, as blows tend to be midline, but a splenic injury in a child too young to walk should be considered to be inflicted (Figs. 78-9 and 78-10). Renal contusion and laceration are less-common solid-organ injuries from inflicted trauma, but can occur. Bladder rupture is also possible.

The cause of death in children with abdominal abuse is hemorrhagic shock from solid organ disruption or septic shock from visceral perforation and peritonitis. The abused children in the study by Ledbetter et al had a fatality rate twice as high as the unintentional group—53% of the abused children died and only 21% of those inadvertently injured

died. Some abused children had an associated head injury that contributed to their ultimate demise.

## Thoracic Injury

Chest injuries include rib fractures and lung contusion. Rib fractures in infancy should be considered highly suspicious for inflicted injury, especially if posterior. The mechanism may be a direct blow or striking the child against a solid object such as furniture, but also can be anteroposterior compression

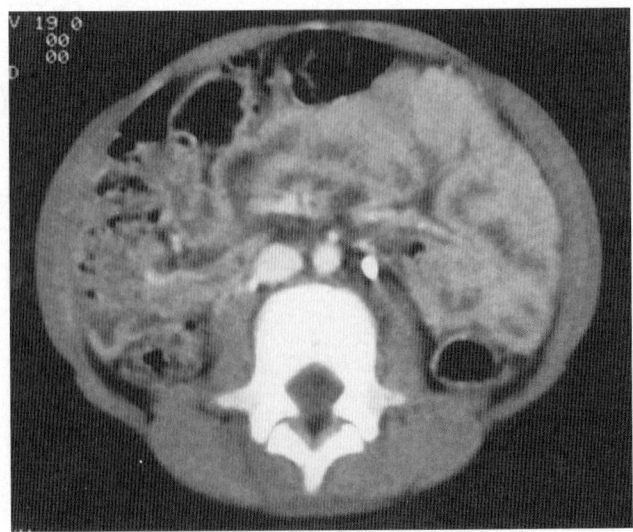

**FIGURE 78-7** A 2-year-old abused female with abdominal pain and distension. Abdominal CT with intravenous contrast reveals enhancing thick-walled bowel with free peritoneal fluid. At laparotomy, a jejunal perforation was found. (Courtesy of George S. Bissett III, MD, Duke University Medical Center, Durham, NC.)

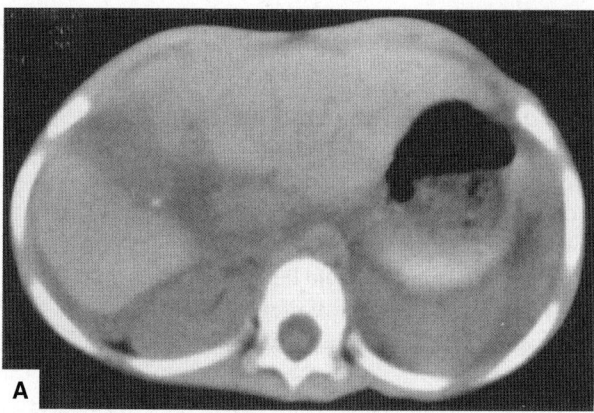 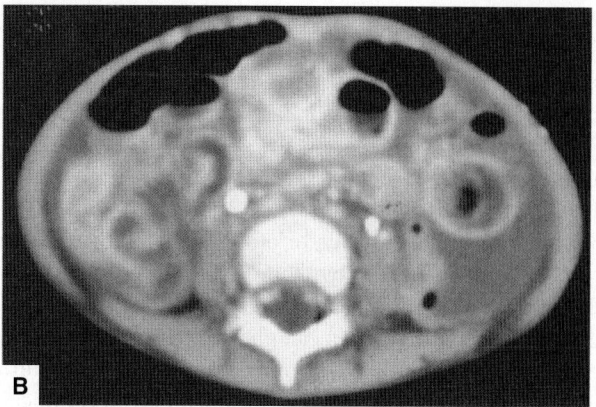

FIGURE 78-8 A 3-year-old girl with multiple bruises and sudden abdominal distension following a "fall" against the coffee table. A. Abdominal CT shows a hemoperitoneum and a large laceration through the right lobe of the liver. B. Following intravenous contrast, there is prolonged small-bowel wall enhancement caused by hypovolemia and shock.

of the chest, as may occur during a severe shaking or an abusive "bear hug." There may be associated trunk encirclement bruising, which is a pattern of bilateral thumbprints on one side of the torso and multiple bilateral fingerprints on the opposite side. Pneumothorax and hemothorax are much less commonly reported inflicted injuries. Both traumatic chylothorax and cardiac laceration and rupture have been reported as resulting from abuse. A child presenting with unexplained subcutaneous emphysema should prompt immediate evaluation of the pharynx and chest for injuries.

## Rectal Injury and Sexual Abuse

Child abuse and deviant sexual activity account for most anorectal and intravaginal injury in children. Although child sexual assault rarely requires the intervention of a surgeon, all children presenting with vaginal tears, straddle injuries, and rectal trauma or condylomata-acuminata or -lata should be evaluated carefully for the possibility of abuse—which, in

the case of young children, may require examination under anesthesia—although straddle injuries clearly associated with unintentional injury mechanisms do occur. Noninflicted wounds tend to be asymmetric without transection of the hymen, while abusive injuries are more likely to be midline. Symmetric wounds that transect the hymen and may also penetrate the peritoneal cavity. Rectal abuse can be unrelated to sexual activity. For example, sharp or blunt objects deliberately inserted into the rectum can cause rectal or sigmoid laceration and perforation.

## Caregiver Fabricated Illness

Caregiver fabricated illness, formerly called Munchausen syndrome by proxy, is a special category of child abuse that may present to the pediatric surgeon. Serious disease entities or symptoms are produced or fabricated in the child by the caregiver, almost always the mother, so as to gain the attention of medical professionals. Induced vomiting may lead to the involvement of the surgeon for surgical management of gastroesophageal reflux. Reflux symptoms persist despite

FIGURE 78-9 A 3-year-old boy who was struck in the left flank by his mother's boyfriend. Abdominal CT with intravenous contrast including the lower thorax shows a shattered spleen with hemoperitoneum. There is also a left pleural effusion with left-lower-lobe contusion. (Courtesy of George S. Bissett III, M.D., Duke University Medical Center, Durham, NC.)

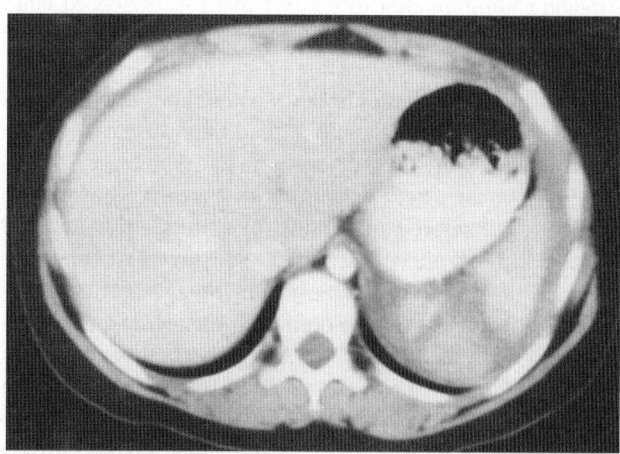

FIGURE 78-10 A 9-year-old girl with abdominal distension and pain following a kick in the abdomen by her father. Abdominal CT with oral and intravenous contrast reveals hemoperitoneum associated with a fractured spleen.

marginally positive pH probe results and seemingly adequate medical management. Reoperation for persistent reflux which has been fabricated has also been described in this population.

Caregiver fabricated illness patients may also present with requests for central line placement. Feldman et al emphasize that once in place, the central line can become the portal for life-threatening manipulation by the perpetrator with injection of infectious material, air, or other debris. Catheters can be used to induce anemia by blood withdrawal. Intentional catheter clotting or dislodgement may lead to multiple catheter placements. The surgeon can play a vital role in preventing this type of abuse by questioning the indications for line placement and replacement in children with atypical indications for central lines.

## DIAGNOSTIC PRINCIPLES

The medical diagnosis of child abuse is based upon the totality of the historical, physical, and clinical findings. Since physical signs alone are seldom, if ever, truly pathognomonic for child abuse, the astute clinician must additionally rely on narrative and interactive cues, ascertained during an interview with the child's caretakers, to determine whether or not a threshold is reached that arouses reasonable suspicion for child abuse. If so, it obliges both additional medical workup and a report to local child protective authorities. While such reports are legally required to be made in most jurisdictions, the mandated reporter is protected from liability if the report is made in good faith, even if abuse is disproven. On the other hand, a report intentionally withheld exposes the physician to legal sanction.

Pediatric surgeons play a vital role in identifying possible abuse, since early recognition is aided by their familiarity with unintentional trauma. Forensic concerns are also crucial during medical evaluation of the child for suspected abuse because inappropriate return of an abused child to an unsafe environment may subject the child to ongoing, possibly lethal, injury, while medical substantiation of inflicted injury is essential to successful prosecution in child abuse cases. However, the primary concern of the pediatric surgeon must always remain the safety, health, and welfare of the abused child. As such, the surgeon should be alert to the fact that inexperienced child protective agents may ask for diagnostic evaluation that is not medically indicated. Such requests should be politely but firmly declined, as these may also expose both the physician and the hospital to legal action, in addition to the avoidable inconvenience or risk, however slight, to the child.

Injuries inconsistent with the stated mechanism or time frame are considered suspicious for child abuse and a full evaluation is therefore warranted. A history that is evasive for the injury or implausible given the age and developmental stage of the child, conflicting histories from different caregivers, histories that change with time, histories in which the caretakers protect each other or blame the child, a sibling, or a third party for the injury, or a history of hospital or doctor "shopping" should be also be considered suspicious, and fully and carefully documented in the medical record. In such cases, the child should be admitted to the hospital for protection and observation during the subsequent workup.

Meticulous documentation of all physical findings, as well as immediate photographs of the injuries, is imperative in all child abuse cases. Bruises should be measured and their color described. Fresh bruises will generally have a bluish-red appearance, while bruises 3 to 4 days old will generally have brown, yellow, or green color. Bruising can take up to 14 days to fade. As such, accurate "dating" of bruises is impossible. Even so, a child who presents with a single explanation for multicolored bruises should be suspected of being abused.

Any unexplained alteration in mental status may indicate child abuse due to inflicted closed head injury, which must be considered as part of the differential diagnosis. Other causes of altered mental status, while far more common, are also more obvious. In all cases involving an unexplained alteration in mental status, history is likely to be vague, since there may be no identifiable onset or precipitating event. As such, inflicted injury should continue to be considered, until such time as a definitive diagnosis is established.

Child abuse is a frequently unrecognized cause of thoracic trauma. The young child's soft ribs tend to bend rather than break, while lung contusions are seldom identified on routine chest examination owing to the nonspecificity of auscultatory signs of pulmonary consolidation. That said, a great number of rib fractures encountered in young children will be abusive in nature. Suggestive findings include multiple adjacent bruises over adjoining ribs, and in severe cases, flail chest. However, many such injuries manifest no external signs. Bony rib calluses in different stages of healing are indicative of abuse when identified, often as an incidental finding on a chest film obtained for an unrelated indication.

Symptoms and signs of abdominal trauma include fever, vomiting, abdominal pain, abdominal distension, abdominal discoloration, and abdominal tenderness. The history in abusive abdominal injury, as always, is vague, and typically suggestive of either trivial injury—which is a distinctly unusual cause of significant intra-abdominal injury—or nonspecific gastrointestinal illness that ultimately leads to bilious vomiting. Although external bruising may be present, serious internal injuries can occur with no external evidence thereof, and are more likely if found in association with traumatic brain injury or malnutrition. Acute scrotal swelling with bluish discoloration from intra-abdominal bleeding has been described as a presenting sign of abdominal abuse. Hematuria should raise the question of renal contusion or avulsion. Myoglobinuria from rhabdomyolysis, which may precipitate acute renal failure, can result from a severe beating. Elevated liver transaminases or amylase should prompt investigation for hepatic or pancreatic injury.

Children with major blunt abdominal trauma due to child abuse may present in traumatic cardiac arrest when major visceral injury, such as a shattered liver, hepatic vein avulsion, or cavomesenteric disruption, has occurred, and can be preceded by a generalized seizure. The likelihood that cardiopulmonary resuscitation itself causes such injuries is very low. When preceding seizure activity is present, definitive diagnosis may be seriously delayed. Children may also be in septic or hypovolemic shock if there is delayed presentation of an intestinal perforation. Peritonitis usually develops within 6 to 12 hours of an intestinal perforation. A crush injury of the jejunum may not present for 3 to 4 days, during which time bowel wall necrosis progresses, leading to perforation and peritonitis. Distal bowel perforations may not present with pneumoperitoneum, which is more typical of proximal bowel perforations. An occult distal small-bowel perforation may be difficult to discover with radiologic techniques. If suspected, peritoneal lavage can be diagnostic by showing bacteria, bile, intestinal debris, or elevated amylase. Duodenal and pancreatic injuries can remain occult for days and may be difficult to diagnose even with computed tomography.

A patulous anus and blood in the rectal vault are suggestive of abusive rectal injury, but in chronic cases, can occasionally be difficult to distinguish from inflammatory bowel disease if lacerations mimicking rectal fissures are observed. If a rectal perforation extending above the peritoneal reflection has occurred, pelvic or lower abdominal pain may be the presenting symptom. Sedation and analgesia may be needed to obtain an adequate examination. Examination under anesthesia will likely also be needed if sigmoidoscopy, cystoscopy, or vaginoscopy are contemplated. Photographs of the perineum are essential. Colposcopic examination and documentation are ideal in cases of possible vaginal injury.

Inflicted extremity trauma is a common presentation of child abuse. Most such injuries occur in infants too young to walk. Typical findings include swelling, deformity, and point tenderness, usually without visible bruising, as well as limitation of motion in the affected extremity. In the upper extremity, abusive injury can be difficult to differentiate from nursemaid's elbow. Diagnosis is frequently delayed by hours or days, even weeks. In one recent investigation by Farrell et al, delayed presentation occurred in 21% children with unintentional fractures, 15% showed no external signs of injury, and 12% used the injured extremity normally, delay being more common among the latter. However, while 83% of these children remained irritable >30 months after their fractures, and 91% of them cried immediately thereafter, all of them manifested at least 1 symptom or sign of injury.

## LABORATORY TESTS

Hematocrit, urinalysis, and coagulogram constitute the basic "child abuse series" of laboratory tests that should routinely be obtained in cases of suspected child abuse. A low or falling hematocrit—the trend is no less important than the absolute value—may herald occult or ongoing hemorrhage. Gross or microscopic hematuria indicates potential renal trauma, suggesting the possibility of blows to the flanks. An abnormal coagulogram may suggest an underlying hematologic cause for observed bruising, but cannot definitively exclude the possibility of abuse, if all other diagnostic parameters suggest its presence.

Hepatic transaminases, amylase, and lipase should be obtained if there is a significant likelihood of abdominal injury. Enzyme leaks suggest subclinical injury to these organs even in the absence of confirmatory imaging. Biochemical tests to rule out metabolic bone diseases may be particularly helpful if pathologic fractures are being considered. However, most such diseases can be ruled in or out based on radiographic examination.

## IMAGING STUDIES

After the detailed history, careful and thorough examination of the unclothed child, and appropriate laboratory tests, diagnostic imaging is performed, and is the foundation of definitive diagnosis in cases of suspected physical child abuse. Additional consent must always be obtained from the child's caretakers for all invasive studies, most particularly radiographic studies, whether or not the child's caretakers may be the perpetrators.

In some jurisdictions, obtaining invasive radiologic studies solely for forensic purposes is illegal. The pediatric surgeon must be familiar with local laws pertaining to child abuse evaluation. Most invasive radiologic studies can easily be justified for medical reasons, if only to identify occult injuries known to be associated with physical child abuse. Early treatment can then be initiated when needed. Child protective authorities are responsible for obtaining judicial consent for forensic evaluations if not medically indicated or justifiable.

Photographs are the most fundamental, and most essential, of all imaging studies. They allow documentation not only of initial manifestations and subsequent changes, so later examiners can follow the progression of key clinical findings. All such photographs should be labeled and signed by the maker, with the date and time they were taken duly noted, either on the margin or on the reverse. Photographs in color are greatly preferred. In the absence of photographic documentation, simple but carefully and accurately drawn diagrams of relevant clinical findings should be entered into the medical record in a timely fashion, duly noting size, shape, location, coloration, as well as other distinguishing features.

Most children with suspected abusive injuries will be clinically stable, so diagnostic imaging can proceed in a routine manner. However, for those who are clinically unstable, diagnostic imaging should proceed in accordance with *Advanced Trauma Life Support® (ATLS®)* guidelines, which call for an initial "trauma series" consisting of supine anterior radiographs of chest and pelvis, and a lateral radiograph of the cervical spine as indicated.

Radiographic survey for fractures is a standard evaluation for child abuse, although the entire survey should not be completed emergently if the child is unstable. The complete survey should consist of plain films of the skull, cervical spine, thoracolumbar spine, chest, pelvis, and extremities. Radiographs of both extremities must be obtained to permit bilateral comparison, and should include shoulders, elbows, wrists, hands, knees, ankles, and feet. Fractures in different stages of healing or symmetric fractures are suspicious, as are fractures of ribs, clavicle, sternum, or spine in a very young child. Radionuclide bone scanning may also be employed in equivocal cases.

Noncontrast computed tomography (CT) of the head should be obtained if there is any question of a clinically important traumatic brain injury. All children with any history or findings of alteration in mental status who also meet the Field Trauma Triage Guidelines for trauma center transfer established by the United States Centers for Disease Control Prevention (CDC) and the American College of Surgeons (ACS) should be assigned to this category.

Noncontrast CT can safely be omitted in children younger than 2 years with less severe injury if they exhibit normal mental status, no scalp hematoma except frontal, no loss of consciousness or loss of consciousness for less than 5 seconds, nonsevere injury mechanism, no palpable skull fracture, and who act normally according to their parents. The noncontrast CT can safely be omitted in children 2 years and older with less severe injury if they exhibit normal mental status, no loss of consciousness, no vomiting, nonsevere injury mechanism, no signs of basilar skull fracture, and no severe headache.

The course of diagnostic imaging in children with suspected truncal injury is determined by the clinical presentation. Imaging studies should be selected based on careful clinical radiologic consultation, and should only be performed if the child is clinically stable. A hemodynamically unstable child may require immediate surgical exploration without preoperative radiologic evaluation. In no case, however, should a child who is less than clinically stable undergo CT unless accompanied by providers skilled in resuscitation.

Postero-anterior and lateral chest radiographs reveal the great majority of significant intrathoracic injuries. Rib fractures, pleural effusion, and pulmonary contusion rarely require surgical intervention. Conventional supine and erect or left lateral decubitus abdominal radiographs usually serve as a convenient starting point for abdominal imaging and may, in certain cases, provide definitive evidence of intra-abdominal injury. Examples include pneumoperitoneum, hemoperitoneum, or gastric or intestinal obstruction. Gastric perforation typically presents with massive pneumoperitoneum. However, partial or complete duodenal or proximal jejunal transections will sometimes require air injected via a gastric tube as a contrast medium in order to demonstrate pneumoperitoneum.

"Double contrast" CT, utilizing both intravenous and oral contrast, is generally the most useful imaging examination in evaluating children with suspected abdominal trauma. CT is both sensitive and specific in delineating the presence and extent of solid viscus injury. Injuries to the liver, spleen, and kidneys are readily detected by CT. Pancreatic injury may be more difficult to identify acutely by CT, and delayed sequelae, such as pancreatitis and pseudocyst formation, may be the first indication of significant pancreatic trauma. The diagnosis of hollow viscus injury usually depends upon the identification of free intraperitoneal air and/or leak of oral contrast material. CT is especially useful in distinguishing uncomplicated duodenal hematoma from duodenal perforation. Unsuspected injuries to the liver and spleen are occasionally identified in patients with only minor or nonspecific abdominal signs and symptoms, or none at all. As always, however, the advantage of precise diagnosis must be weighed against the small but significant risk of late malignancy following exposure to CT. Children who present with no history of abdominal pain, vomiting, or altered mental status, and no evidence of chest or abdominal wall bruising or tenderness, or decreased breath sounds, are highly unlikely to require an acute therapeutic intervention, and should not be referred for CT.

The role of sonography in evaluation of blunt abdominal trauma remains controversial. Focused Assessment by Sonography in Trauma (FAST) is an integral part of the primary survey of seriously injured children, and should routinely be performed to exclude the presence of intraperitoneal fluid in patients meeting the CDC-ACS Field Trauma Triage Guidelines for trauma center transfer. For patients not meeting these criteria, routine sonography in lieu of CT is sensitive for identification of duodenal hematoma as well as solid organ injuries. As such, advocates of this diagnostic approach point out that the injuries missed by this technique are usually clinically unimportant. Even so, most experts believe that the high diagnostic sensitivity and specificity of CT provide the greatest diagnostic yield for intra-abdominal injury. In summary, in cases of suspected abuse, where CT is available, ultrasonography should not be considered an adequate screening alternative. Even so, given the concern for the development of late malignancy in children undergoing CT, the *Image Gently®* protocols promulgated by the Alliance for Radiation Safety in Pediatric Imaging, sponsored by the Society for Pediatric Radiology and several other professional organizations, should routinely be employed whenever CT is utilized.

Other imaging techniques have limited and specific diagnostic application. Excretory urography (EUG)—previously known as intravenous pyelography or urography (IVP or IVU)—as well as voiding cystourethrogram (VCUG) may be useful in children with suspected urinary tract trauma, although EUG is less sensitive than CT for detection of renal injuries. Gastrointestinal contrast examination—esophagogram (barium swallow), upper gastrointestinal (UGI) series with or without small-bowel follow-through (SBFT)—and barium enema (BE) may be helpful in demonstrating possible sites of hollow organ injury, as well as the degree of obstruction, if present. When there is clinical suspicion of perforation, nonionic water-soluble contrast agents should be substituted for barium. In children with symptoms suggesting possible resolving duodenal hematoma, UGI series or sonographic examination should be performed to identify the traumatic nature of the problem and potentially prevent further abuse.

Liver–spleen scintigraphy, while sensitive for detection of hepatic and splenic trauma, provides limited information as to the extent of intra-abdominal injury. It is rarely used, except in follow-up of solid organ injuries owing to its lower radiation dose versus CT. Angiography should be reserved for cases of specific vascular injury or active bleeding that may require embolization or surgical intervention. Magnetic resonance imaging (MRI) is rarely applicable in the acute evaluation of injured children due to constraints of time, logistics, and availability, but this technique can be extremely useful in definitive evaluation of neurotrauma.

## TREATMENT OPTIONS

Severely abused children should be managed by a pediatric or general trauma surgeon in accordance with current *ATLS®* guidelines, in consultation with a neurosurgeon or orthopedic surgeon or other appropriate subspecialist, as for any case of serious trauma. That said, the majority of abusive injuries can be successfully managed medically by the pediatrician.

A child abuse pediatrician, if available, should additionally be consulted for assistance with the medicolegal and psychosocial aspects of diagnosis and treatment. Children's Advocacy Centers (CACs) recognized by the National Children's Alliance (NCA) are an excellent resource in identifying such physicians. Even so, the treating physician is ultimately responsible to assure that the report of suspected child abuse is made to local child protective authorities. Social services must also be involved in the ongoing evaluation and management of potentially abused children. In addition to interaction with child-protective services and support for the families of these youngsters, social services share the primary responsibility to assure that they return to a safe environment.

Major traumatic brain injury should be managed in accordance with protocols established by the Brain Trauma Foundation (BTF). Minor traumatic brain injury should be managed in accordance with protocols established by the American Academy of Pediatrics (AAP) and the American Academy of Family Physicians (AAFP). Subtle cognitive dysfunction is increasingly recognized as a significant issue following minor head trauma, especially when it results in concussion. If so, a pediatric neurologist or developmental behavioral pediatrician should likely become involved in long-term follow-up as early as possible.

Lung contusion and rib fracture, the most commonly encountered abusive intrathoracic injuries, are treated conservatively with analgesia, and rarely require intubation and ventilation. Pneumothorax, hemothorax, and chylothorax should be treated with chest tube drainage. Thoracotomy is rarely needed in the acute phase, and is seldom needed in the convalescent phase, except in exceptional cases when persistent air leak, trapped lung, or persistent chylothorax has failed to respond to conservative management.

Most abusive abdominal injuries result from blunt trauma that afflicts the epigastrium. Duodenal hematoma is managed with bowel rest and total parenteral nutrition (TPN). Late small intestinal stricture, thought to be caused by bowel ischemia from mesenteric vascular injury, has been reported following abusive injury, and may require operative management. Pancreatic contusion should also be treated nonoperatively. The majority of pancreatic pseudocysts resolve with nonoperative management, including bowel rest and TPN, although major pancreatic duct transection may require resection of the body or tail of the pancreas. Intestinal shearing injury may require sleeve bowel resection if the mesentery is usually too damaged to be salvaged. Primary anastomosis can be performed if exploration has been carried out early and the patient is stable. If severe peritonitis and shock are present, however, creation of enterostomies is safer management. Mesenteric biopsy can be performed for staging of the age of the injury. Blunt hepatic, splenic, and renal trauma can usually be successfully managed nonoperatively, as in unintentional trauma, if isolated injury is confirmed and the child remains hemodynamically stable.

Penetrating abdominal trauma should be managed by standard techniques of exploratory laparotomy for suspected perforated viscus. Rectal perforations below the peritoneal reflection can on selective occasions be treated with bowel rest and antibiotics alone, while those extending above the peritoneal reflection usually require closure of the laceration and diverting colostomy. Abusive perineal injuries may contain sperm as well as organisms known to cause sexually transmitted infections. The wound and the vagina should be irrigated and the irrigation fluid sent for sperm analysis and culture. Debridement and loose primary closure of deep perineal wounds under general anesthesia may be required.

Treatment of child abuse has always required more of the physician and surgeon than optimal medical and surgical management. Complying with mandatory reporting and remaining available for testimony in child abuse cases, although time-consuming and potentially disruptive for surgeons, is critical for the proper management of child abuse.

## EXPERT TESTIMONY

Aside from missed diagnosis due to simple ignorance, obstacles to physician involvement in child abuse cases may include fear of angry parents, fear of potential liability, fear of damage to one's medical practice, and even simple reluctance to "get involved." Weighed against the potential harm, or even death, that may befall the abused child, such concerns are trivial. Physicians caring for children owe it to their young patients to permit nothing to stand in the way of accurate diagnosis and expert treatment. Such physicians must also realize they are not police officers, prosecuting attorneys, judges, or juries. Rather, they are the protectors of the child, and advisors to their parents, even if they are the abusers. Nevertheless, they have a personal, professional, and public responsibility to provide testimony in court when called upon to do so, as either an expert, or a witness to the facts.

Pretrial preparation is critical. The most senior responsible physician should testify. He or she must personally review all medical records and imaging studies, and become familiar with the most recent and relevant scientific literature regarding the case being considered. Pretrial conference with legal staff to review testimony is mandatory. The physician must also be prepared to undergo *voir dire*, the process through which his or her qualifications to testify are established. During trial, the physician should answer questions directly, simply, and factually, without volunteering unrequested information or interpretations. The role of the medical expert is to provide medical interpretation and opinion; the role of the fact witness is to offer the details of the case history and findings; and the role of the court is to obtain permissible evidence and determine legal intentionality. The task of the physician is therefore to assist the court in learning the truth, regardless of who issues the subpoena, for it is the judge or jury who will decide the case. Answers to questions from attorneys litigating in court should therefore be directed *at* the questioner, but *to* the judge or jury.

## SUMMARY

For most cases of child abuse, psychosocial implications, rather than medical or surgical considerations, will predominate. That said, detection of the stigmata of child abuse in their early stages will prevent children from being returned to homes where they may be severely or lethally injured. For those sustaining serious or life-threatening abusive injury, optimal outcome depends on maintaining a high level of suspicion for child abuse, such that rapid identification and timely management can follow in the most effective manner.

## SELECTED READINGS

Alliance for Radiation Safety in Pediatric Imaging. *Image Gently®*. Accessed November 20, 2012 at http://www.pedrad.org/associations/5364/ig.

American Academy of Pediatrics Committee on Quality Improvement and American Academy of Family Physicians Commission on Clinical Policies and Research. The management of minor closed head injury in children. *Pediatrics* 1999;104:1407–1415.

American College of Surgeons Committee on Trauma. *Advanced Trauma Life Support® (ATLS®) Student Course Manual*. Chicago: American College of Surgeons; 2012.

Barnes PM, Norton CM, Dunstan FD, Kemp AM, Yates DW, Sibert JR. Abdominal injury due to child abuse. *Lancet* 2005;366:234–235.

Black CT, Pokorny WJ, McGill CW, Harberg FJ. Anorectal trauma in children. *J Pediatr Surg* 1982;17:501–504.

Bratu M, Dower JC, Siegel B, Hosney SH. Jejunal hematoma, child abuse, and Felson's sign. *Conn Med* 1970;34:261–264.

Buchino J. Recognition and management of child abuse by the surgical pathologist. *Arch Pathol Lab Med* 1983;107:204–205.

Caffey J. Multiple fractures in the long bones of infants suffering from chronic subdural hematoma. *Am J Roentgenol* 1946;56:163–173.

Cameron CM, Lazoritz S, Calhoun AD. Blunt abdominal injury: simultaneously occurring liver and pancreatic injury in child abuse. *Pediatr Emerg Care* 1997;13:334–336.

Caniano DA, Beaver BL, Boles ET. Child abuse: An update on surgical management in 256 cases. *Ann Surg* 1986;203:219–224.

Children's Advocacy Centers. *National Children's Alliance*. Accessed November 20, 2012 at http://www.nationalchildrensalliance.org/index.php?s=24.

Coant PN, Kornberg AE, Brody AS, Edwards-Holmes K. Markers for occult liver injury in cases of physical abuse in children. *Pediatrics* 1992;89:274–278.

Cooper A, Floyd T, Barlow B, et al. Major blunt abdominal trauma due to child abuse. *J Trauma* 1988;28:1483–1487.

DiScala C, Sege R, Li G, Reece RM. Child abuse and unintentional injuries: a 10-year retrospective. *Arch Pediatr Adolesc Med* 2000;154:16–22.

Duhaime AC, Genarelli TA, Thibault LE, Bruce DA, Margulies SS, Wiser R. The shaken baby syndrome. A clinical, pathological, and biomechanical study. *J Neurosurg* 1987;66:409–415.

Duhaime AC, Alario AJ, Lewander WJ, et al. Head injury in very young children: mechanisms, injury types, and ophthalmological findings in 100 hospitalized patients younger than 2 years of age. *Pediatrics* 1992;90:179–185.

Einstein EM, Delta BG, Clifford JH. Jejunal hematoma: an unusual manifestation of the battered child syndrome. *Clin Pediatr* 1965;4:436–440.

Farrell C, Rubin DM, Downes K, Dorman J, Christian CW. Symptoms and times to medical care in children with accidental extremity fractures. *Pediatrics* 2012;129:e128–e133.

Feldman KW, Brewer DK. Child abuse, cardiopulmonary resuscitation, and rib fractures. *Pediatrics* 1984;73:339–342.

Feldman KW, Hickman RO. The central venous catheter as a source of medical chaos in Munchausen syndrome by proxy. *J Pediatr Surg* 1998;33:623–627.

Gaines BA, Shultz BS, Morrison K, Ford HR. Duodenal injuries in children: beware of child abuse. *J Pediatr Surg* 2004;39:600–602.

Gornall P, Ahmed S, Jolleys A, Cohen SJ. Intra-abdominal injuries in the battered baby syndrome. *Arch Dis Child* 1972;47:211–214.

Grosfield JI, Ballantine TV. Surgical aspects of child abuse (trauma-X). *Pediatr Ann* 1976;658–665.

Guleserian K, Gilchrist B, Luks F, Wesselhoeft C, DeLuca FG. Child abuse as a cause of traumatic chylothorax. *J Pediatr Surg* 1996;31:1696–1697.

Helfer RE, Slovis TL, Black M. Injuries resulting when small children fall out of bed. *Pediatrics* 1977;60:533–535.

Hobbs CJ. Abdominal injury due to child abuse. *Lancet* 2005;366;187–188.

Holmes JF, Lillis K, Monroe D, el. al, for the Pediatric Emergency Care Applied Research Network (PECARN). Identifying children at very low risk of clinically important blunt abdominal injuries. *Ann Emerg Med* 2013;62(2):107–116.

Kempe CH, Silverman FN, Steele BF, Droegemueller W, Silver HK. The battered-child syndrome. *JAMA* 1962;181:17–24.

Kirks DR. Radiologic evaluation of visceral injuries in the battered child syndrome. *Pediatr Ann* 1983;12:888–893.

Kochanek PM, Carney N, Adelson PD, et al. Guidelines for acute medical management of severe traumatic brain injury in infants, children, and adolescents-second edition. *Pediatr Crit Care Med* 2011;13(Suppl):S1–S82.

Kuppermann N, Holmes JF, Dayan PS, et al, for the Pediatric Emergency Care Applied Research Network (PECARN). Identification of children at very low risk of clinically-important brain injuries after head trauma: a prospective cohort study. *Lancet* 2009;374:1160–1170.

Lacey SR, Cooper C, Runyan DK, Azizkhan RG. Munchausen syndrome by proxy: patterns of presentation to pediatric surgeons. *J Pediatr Surg* 1993;286:827–832.

Ledbetter DJ, Hatch EI, Feldman KW, Fligner CL, Tapper D. Diagnostic and surgical implications of child abuse. *Arch Surg* 1988;123:1101–1105.

McCort J, Vaudagna J. Visceral injuries in battered children. *Radiology* 1964;82: 424–428.

McCoy CR, Applebaum H, Besser AS. Condyloma acuminata: An unusual presentation of child abuse. *J Pediatr Surg* 1982;17:505–507.

McNeely PD, Atkinson JD, Saigal G, O'Gorman AM, Farmer JP. Subdural hematomas in infants with benign enlargement of the subarachnoid spaces are not pathognomonic for child abuse. *AJNR Am J Neuroradiol* 2006;27:1725–1728.

O'Neill JA, Meacham WF, Griffin PP, Sawyers JL. Patterns of injury in the battered child syndrome. *J Trauma* 1973;13:332–339.

Pena SDJ, Medovy H. Child abuse and traumatic pseudocyst of the pancreas. *J Pediatr* 1973;83:1026–1028.

Price EA, Rush LR, Perper JA, Bell MD. Cardiopulmonary resuscitation-related injuries and homicidal blunt abdominal trauma in children. *Am J Forens Med Path* 2000;21:307–310.

Rivara FP, Kamitsuka MD, Quan L. Injuries to children younger than 1 year of age. *Pediatrics* 1988;81:93–97.

Sasser SM, Hunt RC, Faul M, et al, for the Centers for Disease Control and Prevention. Guidelines for field triage of injured patients: recommendations of the National Expert Panel on Field Triage, 2011. *Morbidity Mortality Weekly Rep* 2012;61(RR-1):1–21.

Schechner SA, Ehrlich FE. Gastric perforation and child abuse. *J Trauma* 1974;14:723–725.

Shah P, Applegate K, Buonomo C. Stricture of the duodenum and jejunum in an abused child. *Pediatr Radiol* 1997;27:281–283.

Sivit CJ, Taylor GA, Eichelberger MR. Visceral injury in battered children: a changing perspective. *Radiology* 1989;173:659–661.

Tardieu A. Etude medico-legale sur les sevices et mauvais traitements exerces sur des enfants. *Ann D Hyg Publ et Med-Leg* 1860;13:361–398.

Tardieu A. *Etude medico-legale sur l'infanticide*. Paris: J.-B. Bailliere et Fils; 1868.

Touloukian R. Abdominal visceral injuries in battered children. *Pediatrics* 1968;42:642–646.

Trokel M, DiScala C, Terrin NC, Sege RD. Blunt abdominal injury in the young pediatric patient: child abuse and patient outcomes. *Child Maltreatment* 2004;9:111–117.

Trokel M, DiScala C, Terrin NC, Sege RD. Patient and injury characteristics in abusive abdominal injuries. *Pediatr Emerg Care* 2006;22:700–704.

United States Department of Health and Human Services Administration for Children and Families Children's Bureau. *Child Abuse 2010*. Accessed November 20, 2012 at http://www.acf.hhs.gov/programs/cb/resource/child-maltreatment-2010.

Wood J, Rubin DM, Nance ML, Christian CW. Distinguishing inflicted versus accidental abdominal injuries in young children. *J Trauma* 2005;59:1203–1208.

# CHAPTER 79

# Head Injury

*Charles B. Stevenson and Kerry R. Crone*

## KEY POINTS

1. The predominant mechanism of head injury in children varies with age. The leading cause of severe head injury in infants is nonaccidental, or inflicted, trauma.

2. The physiologic processes resulting from acute head injury are divided into primary brain injury and secondary brain injury.

3. Children with extensive cerebral shear injury on admission often have protracted hospitalizations with permanent neurologic deficits and poor functional outcomes.

4. Avoidance of systemic hypotension, hypercarbia, hypoxemia, hyperglycemia, intracranial hypertension, and seizure activity can significantly minimize secondary injury following moderate or severe traumatic brain injury, thereby substantially reducing morbidity/mortality and improving functional outcomes.

5. Children with a post-resuscitation GCS of ≤8 should generally undergo continuous ICP monitoring as part of their management.

6. The classic triad of findings in children with inflicted injury includes subdural hematomas, retinal hemorrhages, and evidence of skeletal injury.

Three out of four children hospitalized for trauma have sustained a head injury. While most pediatric head injuries are minor, requiring only brief hospital stays for observation, injuries to the central nervous system still represent the most common cause of mortality in pediatric trauma patients. Management of the child with severe head injury requires special consideration be given to fundamental differences in pediatric and adult neurophysiology. In addition, certain mechanisms of traumatic brain injury (TBI), such as the "shaken baby syndrome," are unique to infants and young children and can be quite devastating to the developing brain. Similarly, recovery patterns and potential following brain injury differ significantly between children and adults,

affecting long-term rehabilitation strategies in the pediatric population. This chapter characterizes the major types of pediatric head injury and their treatment, highlighting similarities and differences between pediatric and adult management strategies where appropriate.

## EPIDEMIOLOGY

TBI results in an estimated 3000 deaths, 29,000 hospitalizations, and 400,000 emergency department (ED) visits annually among children aged 0 to 14 years, a figure that is progressively increasing. Perhaps not surprisingly, of all types of traumatic injuries in children, TBI is the most likely to result in death or permanent disability. This is particularly the case in infants and younger children, in whom severe head injury is commonly nonaccidental, or inflicted, in nature.

The predominant mechanism of pediatric head injury varies with age. Sadly, the leading cause of severe head injury in infants continues to be child abuse, or non-accidental trauma (NAT), with at least 25% of children under the age of 2 years admitted to the hospital for head injury having sustained NAT. Falls and drops from caregivers' arms or infant carriers placed on countertops are also quite common, but typically result in minor injuries such as nondepressed skull fractures or small, nonoperative extra-axial hematomas. Toddlers (1-3 years old) are particularly prone to falls from heights around the home, such as staircases, furniture, and out of nonsecured windows, given their ability to ambulate and climb independently. Intracranial injuries sustained from such freefalls, particularly from significant heights, can be quite serious.

Children 3 to 12 years of age frequently sustain TBI in transportation-related incidents: bicycle accidents, in which an unhelmeted child crashes or is hit by a car, are commonplace. Similarly, children in this age group are commonly unsuspecting pedestrians struck by cars. Motorbike and all-terrain vehicle (ATV) accidents are alarmingly frequent in children and teenagers alike and are a cause of significant facial and intracranial injury. Finally, as in the adult population, motor vehicle collisions are the most common cause of injury deaths in teenagers, killing more teens than all other causes combined.

1055

# TREATMENT OF SPECIFIC INJURY TYPES

## Cephalohematomas and Subgaleal Hematomas

Cephalohematomas and subgaleal hematomas both result from bleeding underneath the scalp secondary to local trauma and occur almost exclusively in infants and young children. Despite the apparent similarities, they represent clinically distinct injuries with differing sequelae and management strategies.

### Cephalohematomas

Cephalohematomas accumulate between the skull and overlying periosteum. These subperiosteal hematomas are commonly encountered in newborns as a result of birth trauma related to forceps- or vacuum-assisted delivery, or from use of a neonatal scalp monitor. Their extension is limited by the insertion of the periosteum at suture lines, a distinguishing feature of these lesions.

Cephalohematomas rarely require operative treatment: the majority reabsorb spontaneously within 3 to 6 weeks. Occasionally, they may calcify over time, leading to local cosmetic deformity. In certain cases, local surgical removal may be reasonable to remove the mass effect and normalize the appearance of the child. However, even in cases of calcified cephalohematomas, the calcified tissue is generally absorbed and remodeled by the maturing calvarium over several months, with return of the normal bony contour.

### Subgaleal Hematomas

In contrast to their subperiosteal counterparts, subgaleal hematomas collect in the loose connective tissue layer deep to the galea aponeurotica but superficial to the periosteum. Thus, their size is not limited by periosteal insertions, and they freely cross suture lines. As these lesions are most often seen in infants, quickly enlarging subgaleal hematomas may result in enough blood loss to cause hemodynamic instability, even after relatively minor trauma. Such patients should therefore be followed with serial hemoglobin and hematocrit checks until stabilization of the hematoma, as transfusion may be necessary for larger collections in very young children.

Like cephalohematomas, subgaleal hematomas rarely require operative management. Percutaneous aspiration of these collections in order to relieve mass effect is generally not recommended, as removal of the blood can result in unexpected anemia, particularly in newborns.

## Skull Fractures

Perhaps the most common head injury encountered in the pediatric ED is a solitary fracture of the calvarium or skull base detected on a routine skull X-ray or CT scan of the head. While the vast majority of skull fractures in children require no specific therapy, a few exceptions warrant discussion.

### Linear, Nondepressed Skull Fractures

As many as 90% of skull fractures in pediatric patients are non-depressed and involve the calvarium, particularly the frontal and parietal bones. They commonly occur in isolation, although CT may demonstrate an underlying cortical contusion, extra-axial hematoma, or small amount of subarachnoid hemorrhage in association with the injury. These fractures heal quickly in children and do not require operative management. Even when a small amount of depression is present at the fracture site, surgical elevation is generally not required, as infants and children have a remarkable capacity for naturally remodeling the contour of their calvarium due to the plasticity inherent in the bone. In children old enough to ambulate and school-age children, strong consideration should be given to activity restrictions (eg, no jumping on trampoline; no contact sports) for a set time period (eg, 3 months) to allow for proper healing of the bony injury.

## Depressed Skull Fractures

Depression of a fracture fragment greater than the thickness (or 1.5× the thickness in infants and young children) of the skull generally requires operative elevation. This is especially true when the fracture involves the frontal bone in front of the hairline, as a visible depression on the patient's forehead is unacceptable from a cosmetic standpoint. Depressed skull fractures are typically accompanied by overlying abrasion, laceration, and swelling of the scalp. If present, a scalp laceration may be incorporated into the operative incision. For fractures of the forehead, the incision is placed just behind the hairline.

At surgery, the scalp is incised and retracted to expose the fracture. Depending on the degree of depression of the bone fragment, the underlying dura may be lacerated with associated cortical injury. As such, exploration is recommended at the time of elevation. A high-speed drill is used to fashion an appropriately-sized bone flap incorporating the fracture fragment. The flap is removed and the dura carefully inspected for any puncture or laceration—if present, the underlying brain is checked for any clot or active hemorrhage and the dura closed primarily with nonabsorbable suture. Epidural bleeding is carefully controlled to avoid development of a postoperative epidural hematoma. The bone flap is then secured into place, taking care to ensure the bone edges are flushed with the contour of the skull. The choice of fixation system for the bone flap varies with the age of the patient. In children over the age of 6 years, permanent titanium fixation plates are generally utilized. Younger children, however, may experience limitation of skull growth, with subsequent local deformation, with use of permanent plates. Commercially available absorbable craniofacial fixation plates, or simple sutures such as 0 or 2-0 silk, are therefore preferred for securing bone flaps in infants and toddlers.

In the presence of an overlying full-thickness scalp laceration, a depressed skull fracture is said to be open, or compound (Fig. 79-1). Compound fractures are more often associated with underlying dural and brain injury, and as such, portend a worse overall prognosis. In addition, they pose significant infectious risk to the patient, as epidural/subdural abscesses and/or meningitis may result if not managed properly. Expiditious surgical exploration and debridement, preferably within 6 hours of the injury, is essential to minimize infectious complications. Prophylactic antibiotics are typically administered in the ED and continued through the postoperative period.

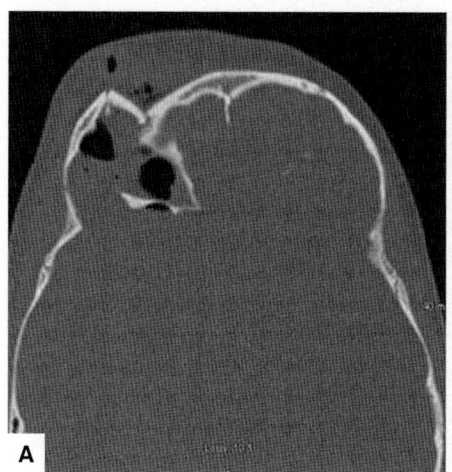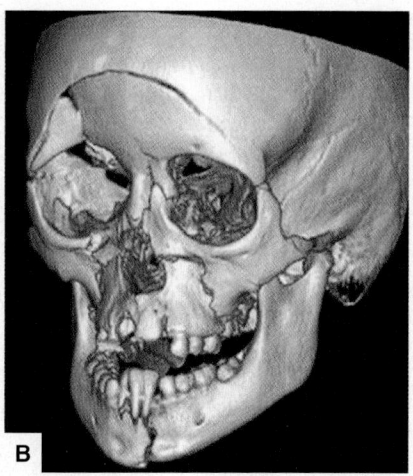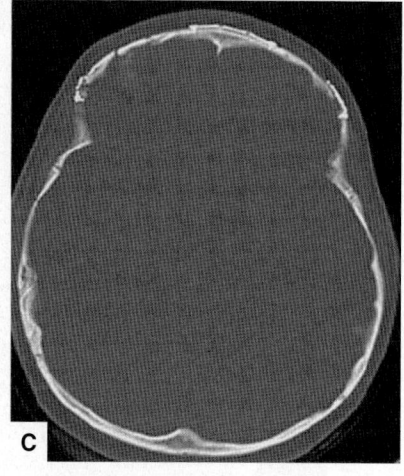

**FIGURE 79-1** Axial (**A**) and 3D-reconstruction (**B**) CT images demonstrating extensive craniofacial injuries in a 6-year-old child involved in an unhelmeted ATV accident in which she was thrown face-first into a tree. A bicoronal craniotomy was performed to elevate and fixate the bifrontal bone fractures, including the comminuted and depressed right orbital fracture, which demonstrated significant underlying dural lacerations. **C.** Axial CT image obtained after craniofacial repair.

## Primary Brain Injury

The deleterious effects seen with acute TBI can be classified as either primary injuries or secondary injuries according to the pathophysiologic processes involved. Primary brain injury refers to the direct mechanical insult, or impact damage, to the brain that occurs at the moment of injury. It can be focal or diffuse in nature, resulting in irreversible injury to neuronal and vascular structures with typically permanent loss of tissue in severe cases. Cerebral contusions, epidural hematomas (EDH), and subdural hematomas are common examples of focal primary injuries. Diffuse primary injury results from rapid angular acceleration–deceleration movement of the head and ranges in severity from simple concussions to extensive axonal disruption in the form of diffuse axonal injury.

## Cerebral Contusions

The most common focal brain injury is a cerebral contusion, in which the surface of the brain impacts against the skull during a forceful acceleration–deceleration motion. They may occur directly at the point of impact (coup), or at a point directly opposite to the vector of impact (contracoup), and are typically located in areas of the brain residing over bony prominences of the skull: the inferior frontal lobes overlying the orbits, the inferior temporal lobes resting upon the petrous ridge, and the frontal and temporal poles. Contusions represent small areas of brain in which there has been disruption of cortex and underlying white matter, with subsequent petechial hemorrhage and surrounding edema. In the setting of penetrating trauma, such as an overlying open, depressed skull fracture, these lesions warrant operative exploration, primarily for debridement and proper closure of the open defect. Otherwise, the vast majority of contusions do not require surgical intervention.

Rarely, individual petechiae within a contusion(s) can progress and coalesce, or "blossom," to form intracerebral hematomas. If large, and associated with adjacent cerebral edema, these intraparenchymal hematomas may exhibit significant mass effect, become symptomatic, and require local craniotomy for surgical evacuation. More commonly, contusions blossom to a lesser extent and develop progressive edema in the immediate postinjury period. Because of this risk, management of mild to moderate-sized contusions includes admission for close neurologic observation and follow-up CT examination. Occasionally, hyperosmolar medical therapy may be required to manage elevated intracranial pressure (ICP) due to large contusions.

## Epidural Hematomas

EDH are present in approximately 2.5% of neonates and infants sustaining head trauma, and roughly 5% of older children and adolescents with TBI. The relatively lower incidence of EDH in neonates and infants is believed to be due, in part, to the tight dural attachments adhering to the overlying periosteum, thereby helping to prevent formation of collections in the epidural space, as well as their relatively soft, pliable calvarial bones that serve to effectively dissipate energy from trauma. As children grow older, the cortical bone of their skull matures and becomes less pliant, with deepening of the middle meningeal artery groove and eventual encasement of the artery, making the vessel more susceptible to tearing during fractures of the squamous temporal bone—the classic mechanism for EDH formation.

Acute EDH have a characteristic lenticular, biconvex hyperdense appearance on CT, and they are most commonly located in the temporoparietal region with an associated skull fracture (Fig. 79-2). Most children with acute, expansile EDH present with a progressively declining level of consciousness secondary to the compression and resulting deformity of brain tissue caused by the mass effect of the clot itself. Depending on the severity of the injury mechanism, patients may already be obtunded with an ipsilateral blown pupil upon arrival to the ED, and therefore not display the so-called "lucid interval." Small EDH in awake, asymptomatic children may be watched carefully in an ICU setting with serial CT scans and close neurological observation.

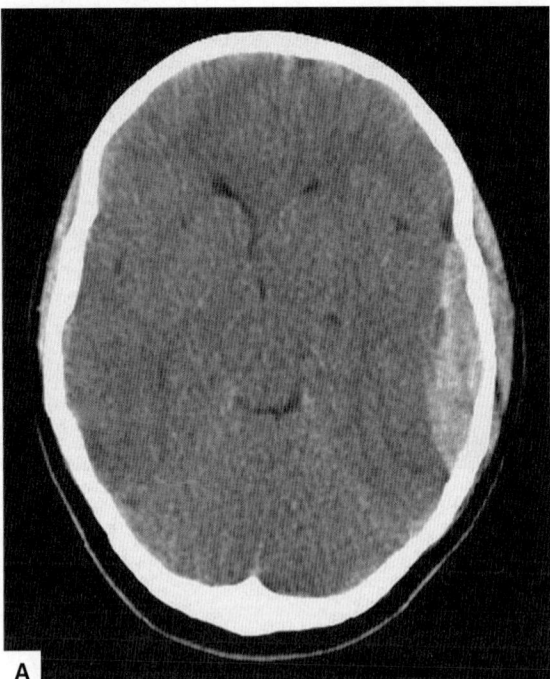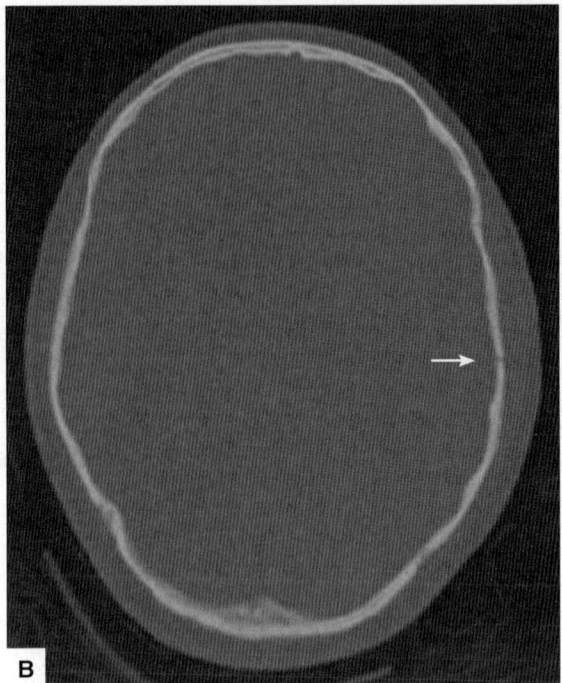

**FIGURE 79-2** (A) Axial CT image revealing a left-sided acute epidural hematoma with local mass effect and shift of the underlying brain in an 18-month-old child witnessed to fall from a countertop. Bone window imaging (B) demonstrated a linear, nondepressed skull fracture *(arrow)* extending through the left squamous temporal and parietal bones. The child was taken for emergent craniotomy and evacuation of the hematoma, at which time laceration of a branch of the middle meningeal artery was discovered beneath the fracture site.

However, most EDH are large upon initial evaluation; consequently, they represent a true neurosurgical emergency, and the majority of patients presenting with acute EDH are taken for urgent craniotomy and evacuation of the hematoma.

At surgery, a linear, curvilinear, or "question mark" incision is centered over the hematoma, typically in the frontotemporal or temporoparietal region. The temporalis muscle is incised with monopolar cautery and reflected in subperiosteal fashion. At this point, any associated skull fracture will likely be apparent. A generous craniotomy flap is fashioned with a high-speed drill. Once the bone flap is removed, the clot is able to be evacuated with gentle suction and irrigation. Following complete evacuation, it is critical to identify the original source of the epidural hemorrhage. As noted above, the source of bleeding is most often a lacerated middle meningeal artery associated with a fracture of the overlying squamous temporal bone. The vessel is typically completely coagulated with bipolar cautery and sectioned. In neonates and infants, the source of the hemorrhage may in fact be venous rather than arterial—collections of small epidural veins should be coagulated or hemostasis established with topical thrombin and an applied hemostatic matrix such as gel foam. Meticulous hemostasis is required to prevent postoperative accumulation of the EDH, and, if necessary, a small temporary epidural drain may be placed.

Patients undergoing operative evacuation of isolated EDH generally do quite well postoperatively. A postoperative CT, obtained the morning after surgery, is generally prudent to verify clot evacuation, resolution of mass effect, and absence of any associated cerebral edema. These patients are allowed to resume a regular diet and ambulate the day after surgery and are generally discharged home within 2 to 3 days. Long-term cognitive or developmental sequelae are not typically encountered.

## Subdural Hematomas

In general, acute subdural hematomas (SDH) are associated with more complex and severe underlying primary brain injury than EDH and, as such, these lesions typically portend a much worse prognosis. Like EDH, acute SDH account for only a minor portion of intracranial pathology in childhood trauma; however, SDH are seen more commonly than EDH, with an incidence ranging from 3.5 to 10.8% in the pediatric population. Two common sources of subdural hemorrhage include tearing of cortical or bridging veins during rapid, violent acceleration–deceleration movements of the head, as well as accumulation of subdural blood around significant cortical hemorrhagic contusions and/or lacerations. The latter mechanism belies severe primary injury, and the resulting SDH is often accompanied by profound cerebral edema and midline shift. The pathophysiology of these injuries involves compression of the underlying brain with stretch and shearing of axons, cellular membrane disruption, and extensive injury to the cerebral microvasculature.

The characteristic CT appearance of an acute SDH is a hyperdense-appearing crescentic mass overlying the cerebral convexity, adjacent to the inner table of the skull. Depending upon the specific mechanism of injury, children with an acute SDH wider than 5 mm in diameter often have significant cerebral edema on initial CT, with loss of gray matter–white matter differentiation and extensive midline shift measuring more than the width of the SDH itself (Fig. 79-3). These

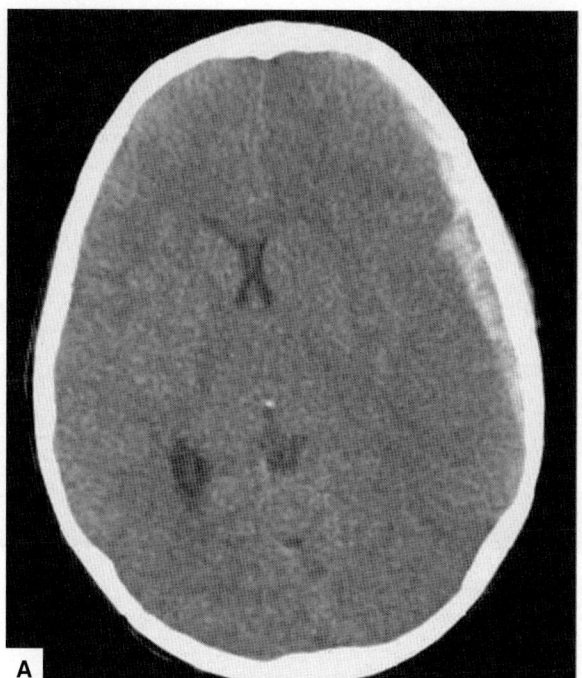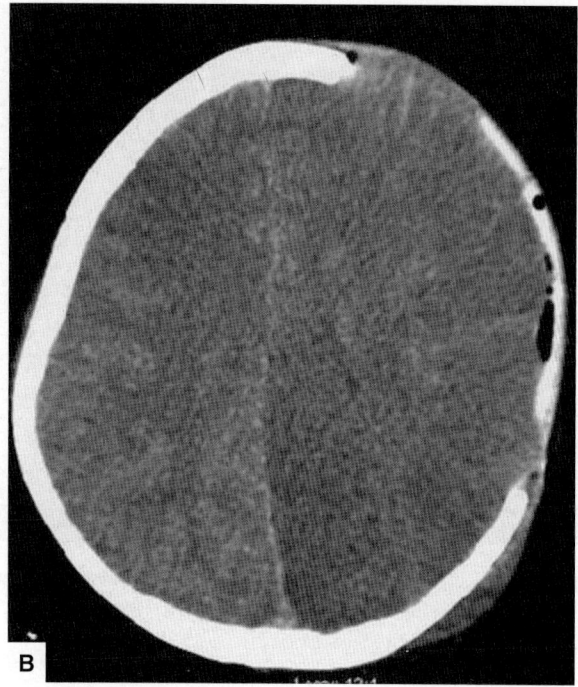

**FIGURE 79-3 A.** Axial CT image demonstrating a left-sided hemispheric acute subdural hematoma in a 7-year-old boy struck by a car while riding his bicycle. While there is only minimal mass effect and midline shift underlying the SDH, there is already evidence of edema and loss of gray–white matter differentiation in the left cerebral hemisphere to suggest extensive brain injury. **B.** CT image obtained following decompressive craniectomy and evacuation of the SDH revealing evolution of the primary brain injury, with extensive hypoxic–ischemic changes throughout the left cerebral hemisphere and herniation of infarcted brain out of the craniectomy site.

children present with a severely depressed level of consciousness and require emergent open craniotomy. Patients harboring smaller SDH, or SDH layering in the interhemispheric fissure or along the tentorium cerebelli, are generally asymptomatic and rarely require operative intervention. Children with such injuries may simply be admitted for close neurologic observation with repeat scans as necessary to insure spontaneous resolution of the hemorrhage.

For those children presenting with an acute SDH (regardless of size) over the convexity, extensive brain swelling on the side of the SDH, and decreased level of consciousness, rapid surgical decompression of the brain and evacuation of the hematoma are usually indicated. At surgery, many of these hematomas will actually be found to be larger than indicated on CT. As such, a generous craniotomy incorporating as much of the frontal, parietal, and temporal bones is performed. The dura is opened widely, typically in a cruciate fashion, and any clot encountered is removed. Careful exploration for bleeding veins is undertaken and meticulous hemostasis obtained. In most cases, edematous brain will begin to expand and herniate through the craniectomy defect. In these instances, the bone flap is left out, thereby providing additional intracranial volume for the injured brain to swell, and a parenchymal ICP monitor placed prior to closure of the scalp flap. For these cases of severe injury, an ICP monitor can be useful in guiding postoperative management of elevated ICP.

Postoperatively, these patients generally undergo extended stays in the ICU. Malignant cerebral edema may be difficult to control, resulting in prolonged periods of intracranial hypertension with resulting coma and ventilator dependence.

Patients with significant underlying brain injury are at increased risk for post-traumatic seizures and are therefore routinely administered prophylactic antiepileptic drugs in the immediate postinjury period. The mortality rate in this patient population approaches 30% in some series, with many survivors remaining physically disabled with moderate to severe neurocognitive deficits. Many of these children will also develop post-traumatic hydrocephalus requiring eventual placement of a permanent cerebrospinal fluid shunt. Optimal treatment strategies, including appropriate nutrition, ICP management, neuroprotective measures, and long-term cognitive rehabilitation, remain an area of continuous research as investigators look to reduce morbidity and improve the functional outcome of patients sustaining severe head injury.

## Diffuse Axonal Injury

Diffuse axonal injury (DAI) represents the most severe form of diffuse primary brain injury and is generally seen in children sustaining high-velocity injuries, such as passengers in high-speed motor vehicle collisions and pedestrians hit by cars. The proposed pathophysiologic mechanism is extensive shearing forces applied to bundles of axons within the deep white matter of the cerebral hemispheres or to the interface of gray and white matter just below the cortical surface. Patients with DAI present with very poor neurologic exams, often unresponsive or posturing. Extensive shear injury of neurons in the midbrain or pons may also result in focal cranial nerve deficits, such as a fixed pupil or absent corneal reflex. Depending upon the status of the child's airway and

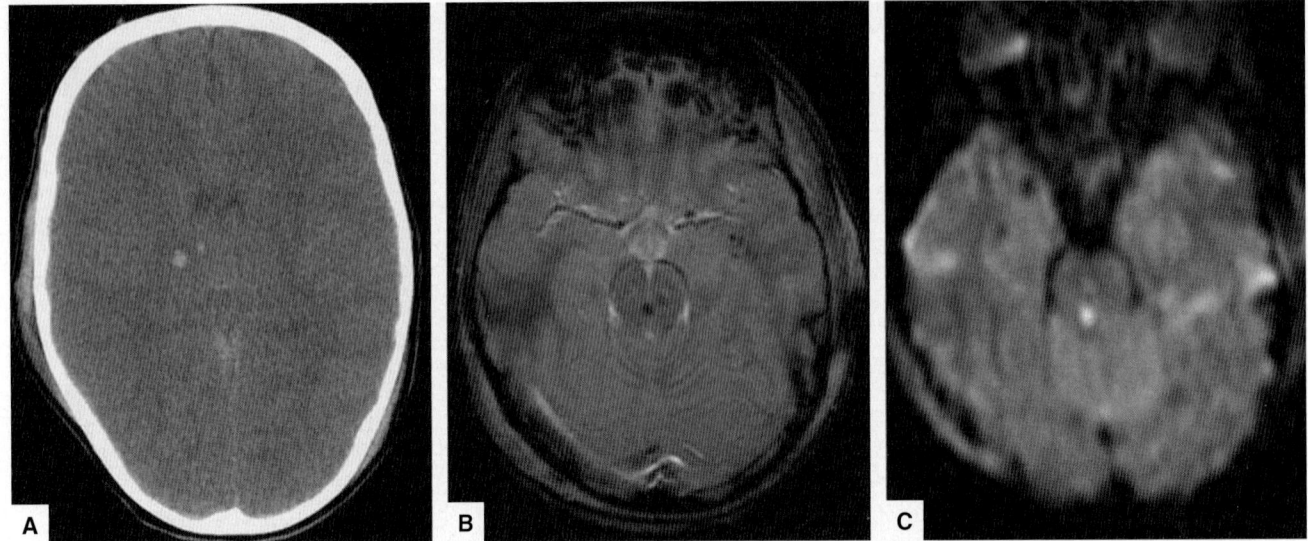

**FIGURE 79-4** (A) Axial CT image demonstrating small, hyperdense shear hemorrhages deep within the right hemisphere. MRI revealing areas of hemorrhagic shear injury within the brainstem as dark, punctuate lesions on gradient echo images (B) and as bright areas of restricted diffusion on diffusion-weighted imaging (C).

breathing, and ready availability of emergency medical services, cerebral anoxic insult may accompany DAI.

Findings of DAI on initial CT scan are often subtle, such as small, punctate shear hemorrhages or discrete hypodense regions of edema in or around the gray–white junction, corpus callosum, or brainstem. A small amount of traumatic subarachnoid hemorrhage may be present along the cortical surface or in the basal cisterns. If indicated, MRI is a far more sensitive modality to detect the changes of DAI, as areas of shearing are easily appreciated on T2 and FLAIR imaging sequences (Fig. 79-4). In patients with prolonged episodes of unresponsiveness, MRI is often utilized to assess the extent of these changes in order to help determine prognosis.

Clinical management of patients with DAI can be quite frustrating, as there are few interventions available to speed recovery. As with any type of significant head injury, treatment of DAI centers around control of ICP and prevention of secondary injury to the brain. In unresponsive patients, this generally includes placement of an ICP monitor or external ventricular drain (EVD); however, ICP in patients with DAI is usually not significantly elevated unless accompanied by cerebral edema. In patients with more mild-to-moderate DAI, recovery may take several days. The injury may or may not be associated with long-term neurocognitive deficits, and formal neuropsychological follow-up is typically arranged. In contrast, recovery from severe DAI is exceedingly slow, with lengthy hospitalizations, protracted courses of inpatient and outpatient rehabilitation, and permanent disability.

## Secondary Brain Injury

Secondary brain injury refers to a multitude of physiologic alterations that occur in response to, or as a result of, the primary injury. Common examples of such factors include intracranial processes, such as cerebral edema and intracranial hypertension, as well as systemic processes, including hypoxemia, hypercarbia, and hypotension, any of which may serve to exacerbate the primary injury and significantly worsen

prognosis and clinical outcome. As such, the importance of secondary brain injury cannot be overemphasized. In contrast to the primary injury, the deleterious effects of secondary brain injury can be minimized or even avoided altogether by understanding and anticipating the pathophysiologic processes responsible, vigilant monitoring of intracranial and systemic events, and appropriate clinical interventions.

## Intracranial Processes: Cerebral Edema and Intracranial Hypertension

Intracranial hypertension is a common secondary brain injury, most commonly resulting from cerebral cytotoxic and vasogenic edema. Cerebral edema may occur in the setting of almost any head injury and is a result of multiple pathophysiologic processes at the cellular level. Vasogenic edema is a result of disruption of the blood–brain barrier (BBB), with resulting rapid influx of intravascular proteins and fluid from plasma into the extracellular space of the cerebral parenchyma. Conversely, cytotoxic edema is due to derangement of cellular metabolism of neurons and glial cells, with resultant retention of intracellular sodium and water and swelling of affected cells in the setting of an intact BBB. Together, these 2 mechanisms of cerebral edema can combine to worsen local primary brain injury and lead to increased ICP. Excessive, uncontrolled cerebral edema (malignant cerebral edema) may result in uncal or tonsillar herniation and ultimately brain death. On CT examination, cerebral edema is easily identified as relative hypodensity surrounding areas of contusion or hemorrhagic shearing. If complicated by anoxic injury, as is frequently the case with severe TBI, larger regions of hypodensity, the so-called finding of "black brain," with concomitant loss of the gray-white junction may be present and portend irreversible injury with extremely poor prognosis (Fig. 79-5).

The Monro–Kellie doctrine states that the volume of the intracranial contents (brain tissue, CSF, and blood) within the skull must remain constant for the ICP to remain constant. Therefore, the presence of cerebral edema, hydrocephalus,

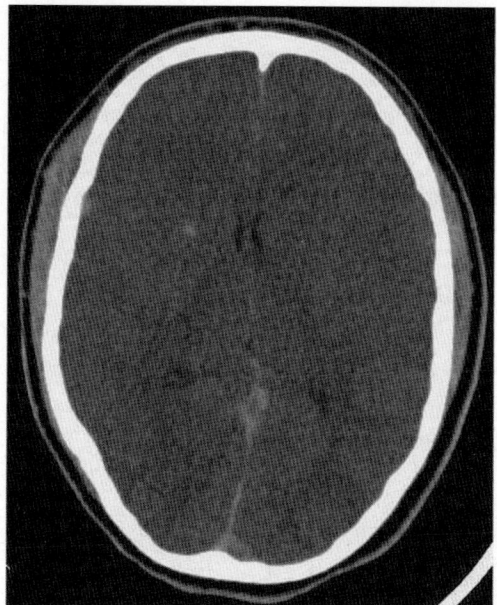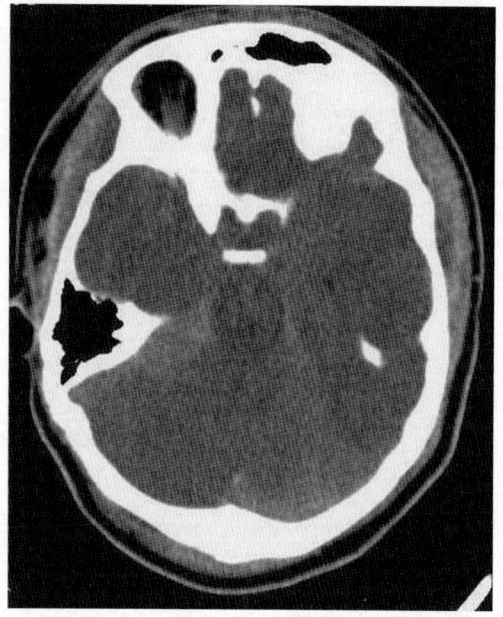

**FIGURE 79-5** Axial CT images demonstrating homogeneous hypodensity of the brain with loss of the gray–white junction and diffuse cerebral edema (so-called "black brain"), indicative of severe hypoxic–ischemic brain injury. There is diffuse effacement of cerebral sulci and the basal cisterns, with scattered areas of traumatic subarachnoid hemorrhage. This patient was involved in an unhelmeted motorbike accident and was found to have a clinical examination consistent with brain death upon arrival to the emergency department.

hyperemia, or hematoma resulting from trauma requires the volume of 1 of the intracranial components to decrease in order to maintain normal ICP. Assuming the amount of brain tissue is a constant, one can infer that when the increase in intracranial volume seen in acute TBI cannot be compensated for by a decrease in blood or CSF, the ICP rises, resulting in intracranial hypertension (Fig. 79-6).

Uncontrolled and prolonged intracranial hypertension is frequently associated with serious morbidity or death in head-injured patients, making aggressive ICP control of paramount importance to the management of these patients. Normal ICP in infants and small children typically averages less than 6 to 8 mm Hg, whereas in older children and teenagers, ICP is generally less than 10 to 15 mm Hg in the noninjured state. Most studies of head injury in adults have used 20 to 25 mm Hg as a threshold for instituting therapy for intracranial hypertension, as this level has been shown to be a predictor of long-term outcome. Studies of severe TBI in children have used the benchmark of 20 mm Hg to define intracranial hypertension, although some authors advocate using 10 to 15 mm Hg as a threshold to institute appropriate therapy in younger children and infants.

## Systemic Processes

Systemic factors such as hypotension, hypercarbia, hypoxemia, and hyperglycemia can significantly affect outcome following TBI. Early hypotension (from the time of impact through resuscitation) doubles the mortality following severe TBI, while late hypotension in the ICU carries a fourfold risk of death or survival in persistent vegetative coma as compared with adult patients who remain normotensive. Similarly, hypoxemia is associated with increased morbidity and mortality in patients with severe TBI, an effect which is

compounded when associated with concomitant hypotension. Hyperglycemia has also been found to have adverse effects on the injured brain, with even 1 isolated episode of hyperglycemia (defined as blood glucose >200 mg/dL) being shown to more than triple mortality rates in patients with severe TBI. Although definitive algorithms for optimal ICU management of children with TBI remain to be elucidated, a reasonable strategy for reducing secondary brain injury due to systemic factors is vigilant maintenance of intravascular volume and cardiac output (normotension), normal pulmonary gas exchange, and tight glucose control. In addition, adequate nutrition plays an essential role in promoting healing of the critically injured child with TBI.

## Clinical Evaluation of Children Sustaining Trauma to the Head

Evaluation and management of the head-injured child begins at the time of initial resuscitation in the field. The mechanism and timing of injury, attempted resuscitative efforts at the scene of the injury, and the response of the child to those efforts can all affect the severity of head injury and overall prognosis. A careful history, including exact mechanism of injury (eg, height of fall, helmeted vs unhelmeted bicycle crash), presence or absence of a loss of consciousness or seizures, and progression of the neurologic exam immediately following the injury are all important parameters that should be obtained by first responders from available witnesses.

Concurrent with primary assessment for concomitant life-threatening injuries, initial examination in the ED should include particular attention to the evaluation of head trauma. External signs of head injury (eg, bruising, lacerations, scalp swelling) should be actively sought. A bulging fontanelle in

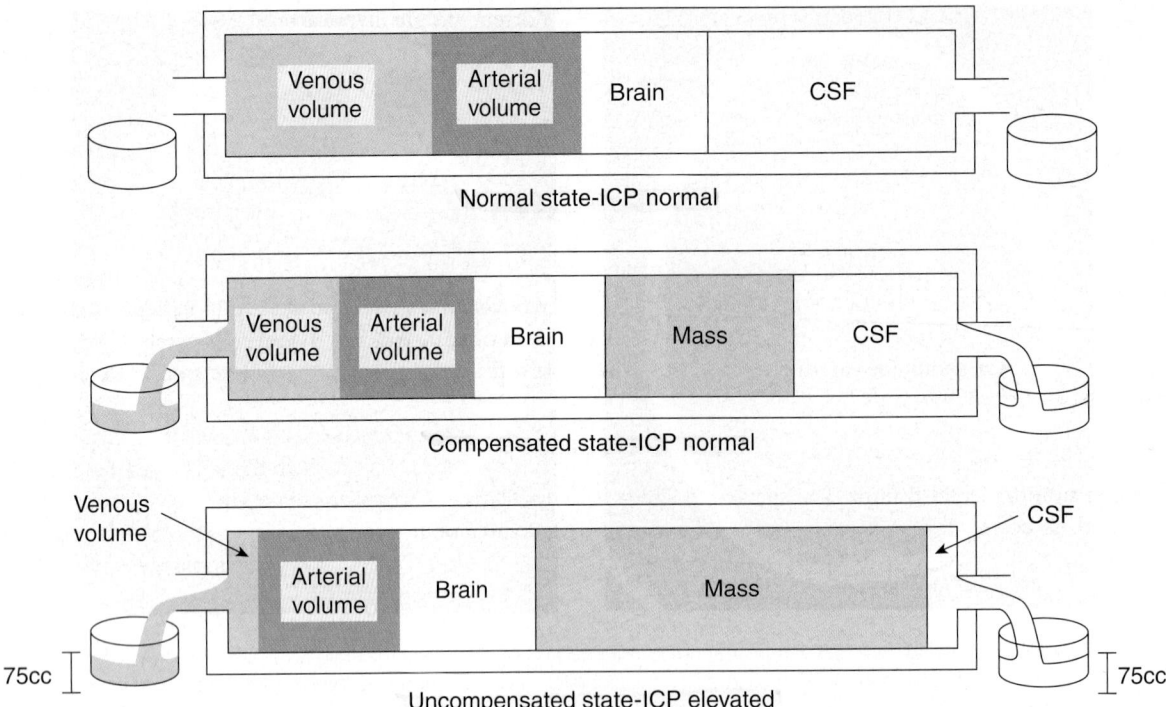

**FIGURE 79-6** Compensating for an expanding intracranial mass lesion. (From Kanter MJ, Narayan RK. Intracranial pressure monitoring. *Neurosurg Clin North Am* 1991;2:257–265. Used with permission.)

an infant suggests increased ICP and may be indicative of an underlying TBI. The evaluation of the child's neurologic status should be rapid but descriptive, and may be tailored depending on the age as well as level of consciousness of the patient. In universal terms, the postresuscitation Glasgow coma score (GCS) has demonstrated utility and general applicability as a prognostic indicator and should be calculated (Table 79-1). A GCS of 8 or less is considered severe TBI, while patients with a GCS of 13 to 15 have only minor injury with an expectation for full recovery.

In addition to reporting GCS, confounding factors to the overall neurological assessment, such as pharmacologic sedation or administration of paralytics, should be noted by the examiner. In an unresponsive/comatose patient, examination of brainstem reflexes is of critical importance to ascertain the anatomic level and extent of neurologic injury. Pupillary response (optic and oculomotor nerves) is easy to assess and indicates functioning at the level of the midbrain. Pupil size results from a balance of sympathetic and parasympathetic stimuli: loss of input from 1 source causes unopposed activity of the other stimuli. Unilateral mydriasis ("blown pupil") can result from transtentorial or uncal herniation as the pupillary constrictor fibers of the oculomotor nerve are compressed. Direct trauma to the orbit, with injury to the eye itself or cranial nerves, can also cause mydriasis. The corneal reflex (trigeminal and facial nerves) tests pontine function. The cough and gag reflexes test the glossopharyngeal and vagus nerves and assess the integrity of the medulla.

Additional focal neurologic deficits suggest localized brain injuries and should be noted if present. For instance, unilateral facial palsy may indicate peripheral facial nerve injury and can occur in the setting of a basilar skull fracture.

Corneal –
Pontine

Cough
+ Gag –

Medulla

**TABLE 79-1    Glasgow Coma Score and Pediatric GCS**

| | Infant <1 yr | Child 1-4 yrs | Age 4-Adult |
|---|---|---|---|
| **Eyes** | | | |
| 4 | Open | Open | Open |
| 3 | To voice | To voice | To voice |
| 2 | To pain | To pain | To pain |
| 1 | No response | No response | No response |
| **Verbal** | | | |
| 5 | Coos; babbles | Oriented; speaks; interacts | Oriented and alert |
| 4 | Irritable cry; consolable | Confused speech; disoriented; consolable | Disoriented |
| 3 | Cries persistently to pain | Inappropriate words; inconsolable | Nonsensical speech |
| 2 | Moans to pain | Incomprehensible; agitated | Moans; unintelligible |
| 1 | No response | No response | No response |
| **Motor** | | | |
| 6 | Normal, spontaneous movement | Normal, spontaneous movement | Follows commands |
| 5 | Withdraws to touch | Localizes pain | Localizes pain |
| 4 | Withdraws to pain | Withdraws to pain | Withdraws to pain |
| 3 | Decorticate flexion | Decorticate flexion | Decorticate flexion |
| 2 | Decerebrate extension | Decerebrate extension | Decerebrate extension |
| 1 | No response | No response | No response |

Deep-tendon reflexes may be frequently exaggerated after head injury because of loss of cortical inhibition, and are absent in spinal cord injury. Asymmetric reflexes may suggest a local intracranial or spinal lesion. Although a Babinski response is normal in an infant younger than 6 months of age, it is abnormal in older children and suggests CNS injury.

Radiographic evaluation of a patient after head injury includes a CT scan of the head and generally includes plain films of the neck to assess for potential accompanying cervical spine injury. In addition to noting areas of acute hemorrhage, edema, or infarction on the standard brain tissue images, the bone windows of the CT should be carefully analyzed for any calvarial or basilar skull fractures. Occasionally, additional studies, including MRI, MR angiogram, or CT angiogram, are necessary to further evaluate potential cerebrovascular injury. When nonincidental trauma is suspected, a skeletal survey should be performed to examine skull, long bones, spine, and ribs for evidence of healing or acute fractures.

## Treatment of Children with Severe Traumatic Brain Injury

Aggressive, age-appropriate neurocritical care of children with severe head injury can decrease mortality and improve functional outcome in survivors. Such care typically involves a multidisciplinary team of trauma providers, including pediatric surgeons, neurosurgeons, intensivists, as well as critical care nurses, nurse practitioners, respiratory therapists, and social workers. Together this team must understand the pathophysiology of head injury, and be able to monitor critically injured patients as well as respond appropriately to rapidly changing clinical situations.

## Basic Neurophysiologic Principles of Resuscitation

Children who suffer significant head trauma are often apneic. If this apnea is prolonged, hypoxemia and hypercarbia will occur with a subsequent rise in ICP and exacerbation of cerebral ischemic injury. The airway must be cleared of obstruction, and the adequacy of ventilation and oxygenation assessed. It is our practice to intubate by rapid sequence induction those children with severe TBI (GCS ≤8), those who lack airway protective reflexes, and those who are at risk for ineffective respirations from their injuries. While the ultimate goal for rapid sequence intubation is CNS protection, ICP can rise from 15 mm Hg to 100 mm Hg with laryngoscopy and intubation. Administration of CNS-protective sedatives and anesthetics can facilitate the intubation and make it safer by decreasing $CMRO_2$, CBF, and ICP.

After the airway is secured, adequate oxygenation and ventilation must be assured. We attempt to maintain pulse oximetry saturation at >95% and $Pa_{O_2}$ >80 torr while maintaining relative normocarbia with a $Pa_{CO_2}$ of 35 ± 2 torr. Hypercarbia should be avoided as it increases cerebral blood volume and ICP. Conversely, extreme or prolonged periods of hyperventilation should be avoided as it is well known to paradoxically induce localized or global cerebral ischemia. Hyperventilation causes constriction of cerebral blood vessels, lowers cerebral blood volume, and temporarily lowers ICP. However, after prolonged periods of hyperventilation, CBF returns to normal despite hypocarbia. At this point, CSF buffering capacity is lost and small increases in $Pa_{CO_2}$ cause rebound intracranial hypertension. This premise was confirmed in a randomized controlled study of severe head injury, in which patients who were prophylactically hyperventilated to a $Pa_{CO_2}$ of 25 torr had worse outcomes due to increased incidence of cerebral ischemia than did patients who received normal ventilation.

As articulated earlier in this chapter, hypotension and hypovolemia should be avoided in patients sustaining severe head trauma. Autopsy evidence of cerebral ischemia is found in a majority of patients who die from TBI. Early measurements of CBF after injury demonstrate that 33% of patients will have ischemia (CBF ≤18 mL/100 g/min) in the first 6 hours following injury. In the uninjured state, central autoregulatory mechanisms maintain CBF at a constant level over a mean blood pressure range of 50 to 150 mm Hg (Fig. 79-7). This autoregulation is a myogenic response of the blood vessels to changes in pressure. However, CNS injury diminishes the capacity of the body to maintain CBF over moderate swings in blood pressure, compounding the risk of cerebral ischemia in the setting of increased ICP. Thus, circulating blood volume should be restored quickly with judicious volumes of isotonic intravenous fluids to maintain adequate CBF. Hypotonic fluids should always be avoided as they may increase cerebral edema. If a patient remains hemodynamically unstable after adequate fluid resuscitation, vasopressors and/or inotropic agents may be necessary. Critically injured children require vigilant hemodynamic monitoring during acute head injury, including continuous arterial and often central venous pressure monitoring.

Fever should be aggressively controlled in these patients, as it generally results in increased metabolic rate and CBF. Patients with fever are treated with acetaminophen and cooling blankets, typically with administration of paralytics to prevent shivering. Prolonged induction of hypothermia in children with severe TBI is controversial due to its questionable efficacy and known systemic morbidity, and is currently the subject of a multicenter randomized clinical trial (Cool Kids). Children with significant head injury will also often have seizures. Seizures can cause abrupt increases in ICP and significantly exacerbate the primary injury. We opt to treat all patients with a GCS ≤8, or those with documented seizure activity, with phenytoin (15-20 mg/kg bolus, then 5 mg/kg/d, titrated to maintain therapeutic serum levels) for the first week following injury or until intracranial hypertension resolves.

## Intracranial Pressure Monitoring and Treatment

Most patients with severe TBI receive some type of ICP monitoring. In general, children with a post-resuscitation GCS of ≤8 should undergo placement of either an EVD or fiberoptic ICP monitor. EVDs allow for both continuous monitoring of ICP as well as continuous drainage of CSF for ICP reduction and management. This therapeutic capability of EVDs gives them a clinical advantage over fiberoptic parenchymal ICP monitors, which simply transduce pressure and do not allow for removal of CSF. However, EVDs must be placed through brain parenchyma into the lateral ventricle, which can be difficult if the ventricles are small or collapsed. Furthermore, ventriculostomy catheters may become obstructed with brain matter, blood, or debris in the CSF, or from collapse of the ventricle itself, rendering them ineffective.

Several agents are available for medical management of elevated ICP. Mannitol is commonly employed for its diuretic and rheologic properties. In patients with intact pressure autoregulation, the viscosity changes induced by mannitol cause increased CBF with subsequent constriction of cerebral blood vessels, which reduces cerebral blood volume and ICP. In patients without intact pressure autoregulation, mannitol is still effective in decreasing ICP through its osmotic and diuretic effects. Similarly, hypertonic saline, most commonly 3% saline, has potent osmotic and diuretic properties resulting in reduction of cerebral edema and ICP, and its use has gained in popularity over the last several years.

Barbiturates can lower ICP by lowering $CMRO_2$ and CBF via inhibition of free radicals. Because of the systemic side effects of barbiturates (hypotension, anergy, infections/sepsis), these agents are reserved until failure of other therapies. Clinical trials investigating use of barbiturates for TBI have demonstrated widely disparate results, and in general, these agents have failed to clearly demonstrate clinical efficacy. We use barbiturate coma as salvage therapy when other methods to manage ICP fail. Pentobarbital is typically titrated to desired ICP or to burst suppression on bedside EEG.

There is currently no indication for routine use of steroids in head-injured patients, as available data suggest no therapeutic benefit and demonstrate worse outcomes with corticosteroid administration. Possible exceptions would include appropriate stress dosing of steroids to patients with preexisting hypopituitarism or baseline steroid dependence for concomitant illness (eg, arthritis or asthma).

## Nonaccidental Head Injury

Unfortunately, inflicted injury continues to be the most common cause of traumatic mortality in infants. While a complete discussion of this challenging and often controversial topic is beyond the scope of this chapter, the following provides a brief overview on the scope of the problem. The exact incidence of inflicted neurotrauma is difficult to ascertain, yet certain risk factors and trends can be extracted from available data. It is a syndrome of young children, with mean age younger than 1 year. Cases are generally more common in urban areas and during the colder months in autumn and winter. In addition, a history of young parents, low socioeconomic status, and socially unstable households is common. Perpetrators are most frequently fathers, boyfriends, and female babysitters. The classic triad of findings in children with inflicted injury includes subdural hemorrhages, retinal hemorrhages, and skeletal injury.

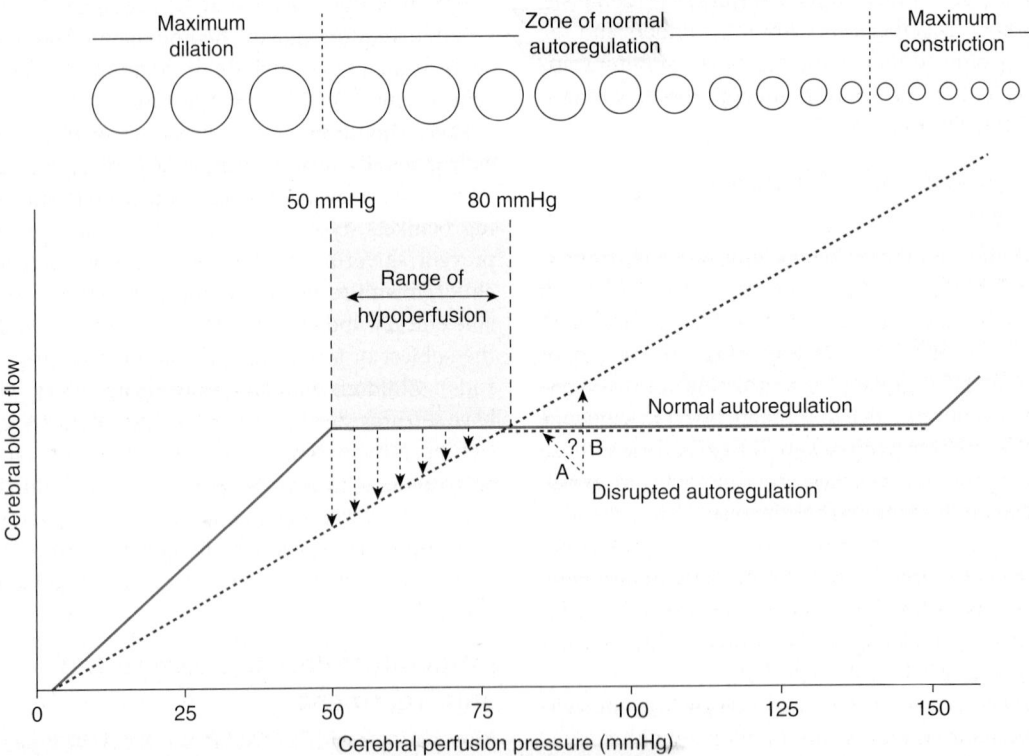

**FIGURE 79-7** Normal pressure autoregulation and two possible degrees of disruption because of severe head injury. The solid curve represents normal pressure autoregulation, with lower and upper breakpoints of 50 and 150 mm Hg, respectively. Disrupted pressure autoregulation is represented by the dashed line. The pressure-passive nature of complete disruption is illustrated by the straight curve where CBF is directly proportional to CPP (*Line A*). In the situation of partial disruption, the system is pressure-passive up to the reset breakpoint of 80 mm Hg after which pressure auto-regulation occurs between 80 and 150 mm Hg (*Line B*). In either case, there is a range of hypoperfusion between 50 and 80 mm Hg where ischemia may occur despite normal CPP. (From Lang EW, Chesnut RM. Intracranial pressure: Monitoring and management. *Neurosurg Clin North Am* 1994;5:573–605, 1994. Used with permission).

In cases of inflicted injury, the most common histories provided by caretakers include a history of trivial blunt trauma, such as short fall from a bed, or no history of trauma. Low-height falls in infants and young children are generally very well tolerated and result in only minor injury; therefore, a child with serious injuries from this purported mechanism should raise suspicion. In those children brought to medical attention without a history of specific trauma, vomiting, lethargy, irritability, seizures, apnea, and unresponsiveness are the most common presenting symptoms reported. Infants in particular may present with varying levels of consciousness, ranging from normal to comatose. Initial physical examination may reveal scalp contusions, tense or bulging fontanelle, splayed cranial sutures, or patterned bruising over the chest and abdomen. Retinal hemorrhages are present in the vast majority of children with inflicted head injury, and should be documented by a pediatric ophthalmologist on dilated exam.

Fractures of the ribs and long bones are characteristic findings of abusive injury, and are best characterized on a dedicated full skeletal survey. The most common intracranial injury reported is of course acute or subacute subdural hematomas extending over the surface of 1 or both cerebral hemispheres. In severe cases, parenchymal hypodensities indicative of tissue injury and infarction may be present and portend poor prognosis (Fig. 79-8). MRI may be helpful in identifying lesser degrees of injury, such as small areas of subdural bleeding or

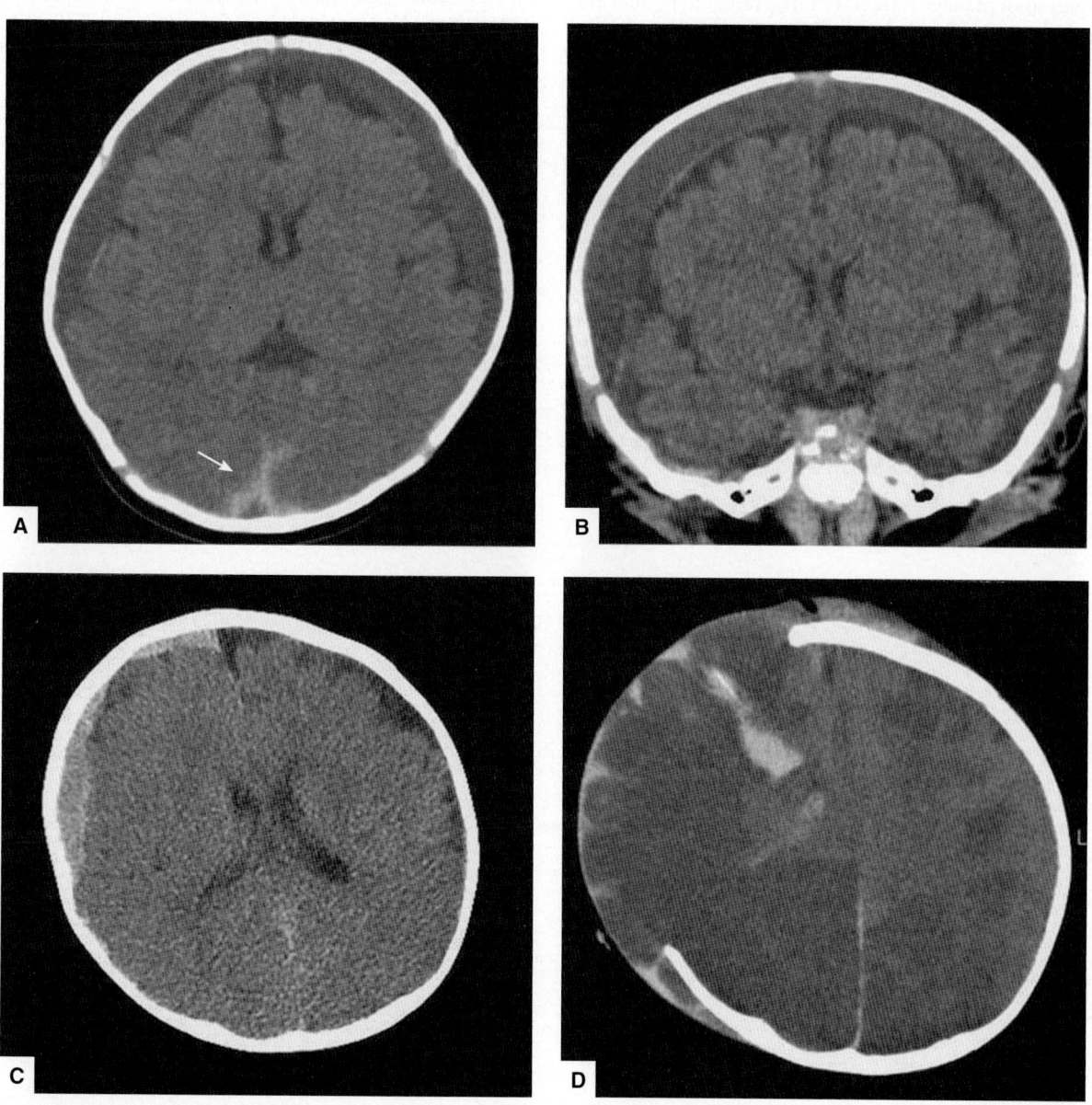

**FIGURE 79-8** Axial (A) and coronal (B) CT images from an infant confirmed to have sustained nonaccidental trauma demonstrating large, bilateral subacute subdural hematomas with mass effect on the underlying brain and splaying of the overlying cranial sutures. Note the area of acute subdural hemorrhage within the interhemispheric fissure posteriorly (*Arrow in A*). Axial preoperative CT image (C) from an abused infant revealing a seemingly small, right-sided acute SDH with mild-moderate mass effect on the underlying brain. Postoperative CT imaging (D) obtained following emergent decompressive craniectomy and SDH evacuation reveals the full extent of the primary injury, with large areas of hypodense, infarcted brain evident bilaterally. There is acute hemorrhage deep within the frontal lobe and herniation of brain outside of the cranial vault on the right.

parenchymal contusions, not easily identified on CT. In addition, MR easily distinguishes chronic subdural hematomas from extraaxial CSF collections, thereby verifying a traumatic etiology when there is clinical concern for inflicted injury.

Medical and surgical treatment of acute brain injury secondary to inflicted injury does not differ from that associated with other mechanisms. General principles of neurocritical care are applied, with ICP monitoring and management as appropriate. Seizures, whether generalized or subclinical, are common in this patient population and strong consideration should be given to prophylactic use of anticonvulsants. In the event of subdural hematomas with significant mass effect, operative evacuation is generally indicated. For those children with large areas of bilateral hypodense brain and significant cerebral edema, decompressive craniectomy may be employed to manage refractory intracranial hypertension, although debate still surrounds the utility of this strategy given the uniformly poor outcomes in these children despite aggressive intervention.

## SELECTED READINGS

Alberico AM, Ward JD, Choi SC, et al. Outcome after severe head injury: relationship to mass lesions, diffuse injury, and ICP course in pediatric and adult patients. *J Neurosurg* 1987;67:648–656.

Berger MS, Pitts LH, Lovely M, et al. Outcome from severe head injury in children and adolescents. *J Neurosurg* 1985;62:194–199.

Chesnut RM, Marshall SB, Piek J, et al. Early and late systemic hypotension as a frequent and fundamental source of cerebral ischemia following severe brain injury in the Traumatic Coma Data Bank. *Acta Neurochir Suppl* 1993;59:121.

Dias MS, Borchers J, Hernan L, et al. Evaluation and management of pediatric head trauma. In: Fuhrman BP, Zimmerman JJ, eds. *Pediatric Critical Care*. 2nd ed. St. Louis, MO: Mosby; 1998:1221.

Duhaime AC, Christian CW, Rorke LB, et al. Nonaccidental head injury in infants—the "shaken baby syndrome." *N Engl J Med* 1998;338: 1822–1829.

Ersahin Y, Mutluer S, Mirzai H, Palali I. Pediatric depressed skull fractures: analysis of 530 cases. *Childs Nerv Syst* 1996;12:323–331.

Griesdale DEG, Tremblay MH, McEwen J, et al. Glucose control and mortality in patients with severe traumatic brain injury. *Neurocrit Care* 2009;11(3):311–316.

Langlois JA, Rutland-Brown W, Thomas KE. *Traumatic Brain Injury in the United States: Emergency Department Visits, Hospitalizations, and Deaths*. Atlanta, GA: Centers for Disease Control and Prevention, National Center for Injury Prevention and Control; 2004.

Levin HS, Aldrich EF, Saydjari C, et al. Severe head injury in children: Experience of the Traumatic Coma Data Bank. *Neurosurgery* 1992;31(3): 435–443.

Marmarou A. Increased intracranial pressure in head injury and the influence of blood volume. *J Neurotrauma* 1992;9(Suppl 1):S327–S332.

Muizelaar JP, Lutz HA, Becker DP. Effect of mannitol on ICP and CBF and correlation with pressure autoregulation in severely head-injured patients. *J Neurosurg* 1984;61:700–706.

Muizelaar JP, Marmarou A, Ward JD, et al. Adverse effects of prolonged hyperventilation in patients with severe head injury: A randomized clinical trial. *J Neurosurg* 1991;75:731–739.

Muizelaar JP, Ward JD, Marmarou A, et al. Cerebral blood flow and metabolism in severely head-injured children Part 2: Autoregulation. *J Neurosurg* 1989;71:72–76.

Rosomoff HL, Kochanek PM, Clark R, et al. Resuscitation from severe brain trauma. *Crit Care Med* 1996;24(2 Suppl):S48–S56.

Sharples P, Stuart A, Matthews D, et al. Cerebral blood flow and metabolism in children with severe head injury. Part 1: Relation to age, Glasgow coma score, outcome, intracranial pressure, and time after injury. *J Neurol Neurosurg Psychiatry* 1995;58:145–152.

Skippen P, Seear M, Poskitt K, et al. Effect of hyperventilation on regional blood flow in head-injured children. *Crit Care Med* 1997;25(8): 1402–1409.

Taylor G, Myers S, Kurth CD, et al. Hypertonic saline improves brain resuscitation in a pediatric model of head injury and hemorrhagic shock. *J Pediatr Surg* 1996;31(1):65–70.

# CHAPTER 80

# Thoracic Injuries

*Marianne Beaudin and Richard A. Falcone Jr*

## KEY POINTS

1. The initial approach to thoracic trauma is no different from that employed for any child who is seriously injured. Priorities includes securing the airway, maximizing breathing, and ensuring that circulation is adequate.

2. Mortality from blunt trauma is usually related to associated injuries.

3. Emergency department (ED) thoracotomy should be performed solely for patients having suffered a penetrating injury with signs of life either at the scene or on arrival.

4. The most important principle in managing children with rib fractures is adequate control of pain.

5. The majority of injuries to the lung and pleura are successfully managed with tube thoracostomy and rarely require thoracotomy.

## EPIDEMIOLOGY

Thoracic injuries occur in 4.4% of children with serious injuries, making them relatively uncommon among children admitted to a major trauma center. The most common injuries are pulmonary contusions, pneumo- and hemothorax, and rib fractures, representing 48%, 39%, and 32% of chest injuries, respectively.

Blunt trauma is by far the most common mechanism of injury; motor vehicle crashes and intentional injuries are the most common etiologies. Penetrating chest injuries, mostly caused by firearms, had increased through the early 90s, although more recent data suggest that this trend may be reversing.

Reported mortality rates associated with thoracic injuries vary from 7% to 26%. In blunt trauma, isolated thoracic injuries are only associated with a 5% mortality. However, mortality increases to 25% when head or abdominal injuries are also present, and increases to as much as 40% when both head and abdominal injuries are present. In our experience, approximately 20% of children with a thoracic injury will require a tube thorocostomy. Life-threatening isolated chest injuries are rare, and immediate thoracotomy is necessary in only 3% to 6% of patients.

## DIAGNOSIS

Although the physical examination may reveal important markers of injury, alone it is inexact in definitively establishing the presence or absence of thoracic injuries. Concerning physical findings, examination should prompt further diagnostic studies. The initial assessment including physical examination and chest x-ray should be performed in a timely manner in order to promptly identify patients with life-threatening injuries such as tension pneumothorax, tracheobronchial injuries, massive hemothorax, and aortic injuries.

Physical examination should start with visual inspection for symmetric chest wall rising and evidence of abrasions, hematoma, or open wounds. The neck should also be inspected for signs of tracheal deviation and venous jugular distension. The chest wall is then palpated to identify bony abnormalities, hematomas, subcutaneous epmphysema, and areas of tenderness. Finally, the chest is auscultated keeping in mind that breath sounds in a small child can be easily transmitted across the mediastinum resulting in the delayed recognition of hemo- or pneumothorax.

In patients sustaining penetrating injuries, the chest should be carefully examined to identify all wounds. A cardiac injury is suggested by parasternal wounds and an associated intra-abdominal injury is suggested by penetrating wounds below the fourth and fifth intercostal space anteriorly, or the tip of the scapula posteriorly.

An anterior–posterior chest x-ray should be obtained in the emergency department shortly after arrival of the patient. The chest x-ray may be delayed only in the patient in extremis who needs urgent placement of an endotracheal tube or chest tube. In an intubated patient, performing the chest x-ray after quickly placing an oro- or nasogastric tube can help in diagnosing an aortic injury. For penetrating wounds, the entrance and exit sites should be marked with radiopaque markers prior to the chest x-ray.

Most clinically significant injuries will be apparent on chest x-ray within 6 hours after injury. The child with a penetrating

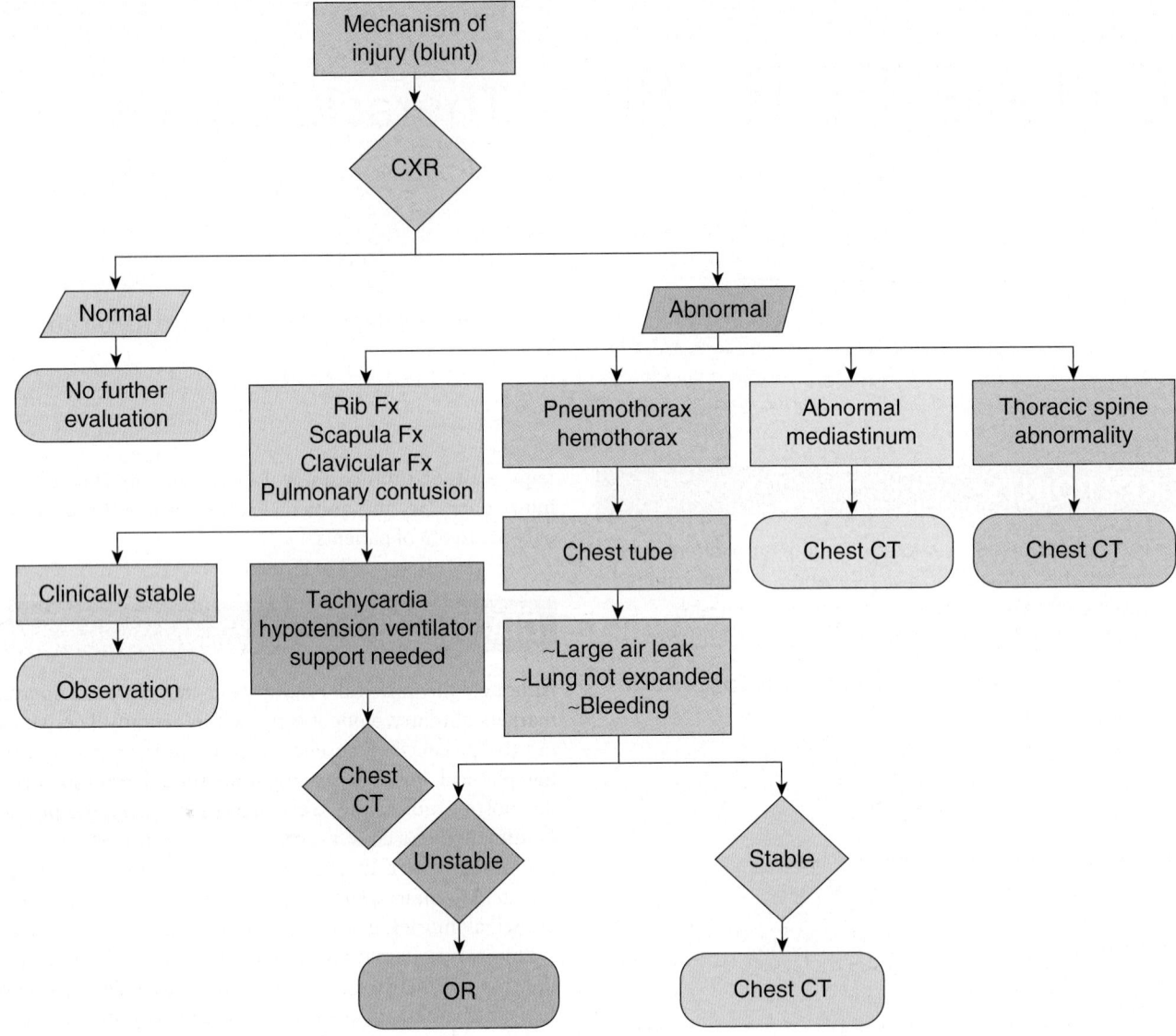

**FIGURE 80-1** Algorithm for imaging of pediatric chest trauma with CT.

injury and an initially normal chest x-ray should have a repeat chest x-ray about 6 hours after initial evaluation.

The presence of hemo- or pneumothorax or concern for mediastinal injury on chest x-ray should prompt consideration of a chest CT to identify underlying injury. The utility of routine chest CT in the setting of high-impact trauma in the pediatric population is controversial. Studies in adults suggest that injuries initially missed on chest x-ray are often found on chest CT altering subsequent management. This has not been confirmed in children as the findings on CT scan did not alter clinical management in three recent studies. Moreover, most abnormal findings on chest CT that led to a change in management were in the lower chest and would have been seen on a CT of the abdomen.

A "funny looking" mediastinum and loss of the aortic knob on chest x-ray are suspicious for an injury to the thoracic aorta. A helical CT angiography of the thorax is a useful screening tool in stable patients. A helical CT angiography of the chest that fails to demonstrate any mediastinal hemorrhage rules out an aortic injury. Rarely, in patients in whom the diagnosis remains uncertain, an arch aortography needs to be performed.

In summary, the decision to perform a chest CT in the pediatric trauma population should be based on several considerations: mechanism of injury (high-impact blunt trauma and penetrating trauma), clinical status, and findings on chest x-ray suspicious of tracheobronchial, esophageal, or major vascular injuries (Fig. 80-1). The role of ultrasound is evolving in the evaluation of chest trauma. The most important application is in the evaluation of possible pericardial effusion in the trauma bay as a component of the focused assessment with sonography for trauma (FAST) examination. The use of FAST for detection of hemothorax has been reviewed retrospectively and found to be more rapidly performed and have a sensitivity and specificity similar to portable chest x-ray. However, it is currently not recommended as a substitute for a portable chest x-ray. Similarly, FAST examination has been described for detection of pneumothorax with a good sensitivity and specificity when performed by surgeons in the trauma bay, although the presence of massive subcutaneous emphysema limits visualization. Ultrasound may also play a role in the evaluation of cardiac injuries as we will see later in this chapter.

# MANAGEMENT OF IMMEDIATELY LIFE-THREATENING THORACIC INJURIES

The priorities for treatment are, in order, the airway, breathing, and circulation. Whether the child is agonal, unstable, or stable determines how one meets these priorities.

The most reliable way to secure the airway is endotracheal intubation employing a rapid sequence intubation technique. Emergent intubation may be required in the trauma bay for several reasons. First, a decreased level of consciousness, typically a Glasgow Coma Scale (GCS) score of less than 8; second, impaired ventilation and oxygenation related to a chest injury such as a massive hemothorax, flail chest, or severe pulmonary contusions; and finally, patient agitation that interferes with diagnostic studies and treatment.

Pulse oximetry to continuously monitor oxygenation and inline capnography to monitor $CO_2$ levels are important adjuncts in the management of the airway in the trauma bay. Inline capnography to detect excessive or inadequate ventilation is especially useful for the child with an associated head injury in whom improper ventilation can further reduce already compromised cerebral perfusion.

## Emergency Thoracotomy

Emergency department (ED) thoracotomy should be performed solely for patients having suffered a penetrating injury with signs of life either at the scene or on arrival. A meta-analysis of 2399 patients in 22 different series found a 35% survival rate following ED thoracotomy in victims of penetrating trauma with signs of life on arrival, and a 14% survival rate for those with signs of life at the scene that were lost prior to arrival at the ED. Victims of penetrating trauma with no signs of life at the scene and all victims of blunt trauma had a poor outcome after ED thoracotomy, with a collected survival rate of less than 1% (Table 80-1).

As the airway and breathing are secured, the left chest is incised from the midclavicular line to the posterior axillary line through the inframammary crease. The incision is carried sharply through the fifth interspace and the pleura is incised with scissors. A rib spreader is placed, the inferior pulmonary ligament is divided, and the left lung is retracted superiorly (Fig. 80-2). Once inside the pleural cavity, the

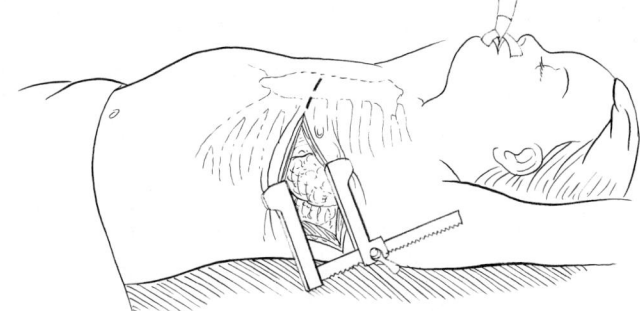

**FIGURE 80-2** Location of incision for left resuscitative thoracotomy.

pericardium is inspected for bulging and/or discoloration, which may indicate pericardial tamponade. The pericardium is incised vertically with scissors anterior to, and with care taken to protect, the phrenic nerve. This incision must be large enough to allow manual internal cardiac compression (Fig. 80-3). Extension of the left anterolateral thoracotomy through the sternum and into the right chest will allow full exposure of the heart for penetrating cardiac injuries, or should significant right-sided hemothorax be noted after the left chest has been opened. Depending upon the bony maturation of the child, heavy scissors or a saw may be used to traverse the sternum (Fig. 80-4). To diminish ongoing hemorrhage during resuscitation, the thoracic aorta may be clamped just above the diaphragm. The parietal pleura overlying the aorta just above the diaphragm should be incised vertically and the nearby mesenchymal tissue dissected bluntly to separate the esophagus. The aorta is then clamped with a large vascular clamp. Care should be taken, if possible, to locate and avoid the anterior spinal artery to decrease the chance of paraplegia (Fig. 80-5).

## Pericardial Tamponade

If the child has a parasternal penetrating wound and is hemodynamically stable, echocardiography should be performed to detect pericardial fluid. Transthoracic and transesophageal approaches are the ones most commonly employed in the trauma setting. If bandages, chest tubes, or massive subcutaneous emphysema preclude the more expeditious transthoracic approach, the transesophageal echocardiography should be considered to detect the presence of pericardial fluid and to identify aortic injury. Parenthetically, pericardial fluid may also be identified in the course of a FAST examination of the injured child. Children and adolescents have extraordinary compensatory means and can harbor cardiac tamponade and appear well for some time, only to decompensate rapidly and die unless appropriate interventions take place. Clinical signs consisting of hypotension, muffled heart sounds, and distended neck veins are insensitive and are infrequently seen in children with pericardial tamponade.

The stable patient with evidence of pericardial fluid should undergo an expeditious subxiphoid pericardotomy in the controlled setting of the operating room. This approach is preferred over pericardiocentesis in the trauma bay. However, pericardiocentesis can be easily performed in the trauma bay

| TABLE 80-1 | Meta-Analysis of Collected Series of Patients Undergoing ED Thoracotomy | | |
|---|---|---|---|
| Injury Type | No Signs of Life at the Scene | Signs of Life at the Scene, not on Arrival | Signs of Life on Arrival to ED |
| Penetrating | 0/635 | 111/770 (35%) | 126/365 (14%) |
| Blunt | 0/154 | 1/187 (<1%) | 1/228 (<1%) |

*Note:* Adapted from Rhee PM, Acosta J, Bridgeman A, et al. Survival after emergency department thoracotomy: review of published data from the past 25 years. *J Am Coll Surg* 2000;190(3):288–298.

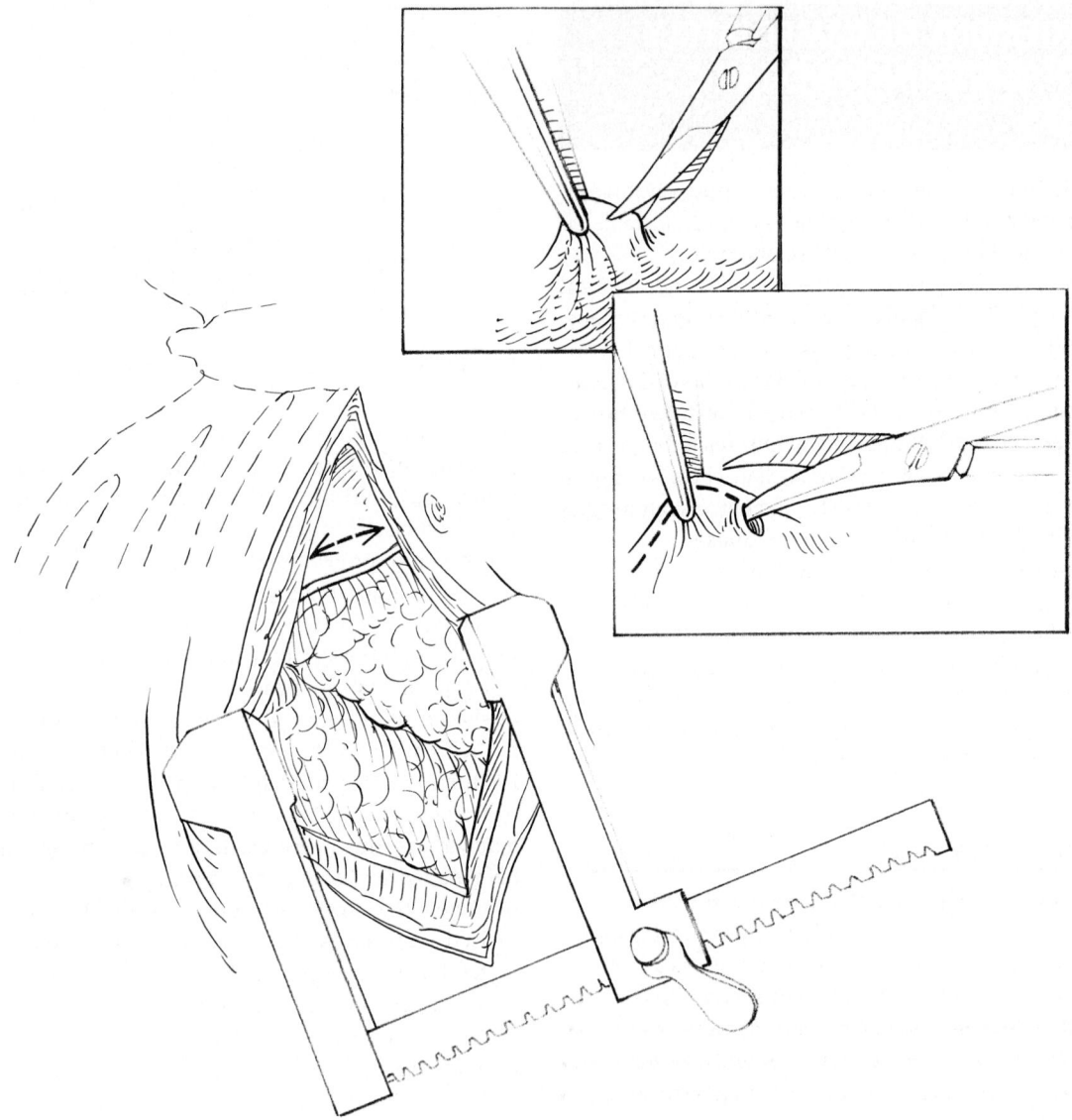

**FIGURE 80-3** Evacuation of pericardial tamponade.

and can serve as a bridge therapy while preparing to do the subxiphoid window in the operating room.

Operating instruments should be available for potential sternotomy, as should blood products, in case significant hemorrhage is encountered. A vertical midline upper-abdominal incision is made and is carried down through the midline fascia and to the left of the xiphoid, which is either retracted to the right or resected. The lowest anterior aspect of the pericardium is grasped and a small, controlled, pericardiotomy is made (Fig. 80-6). If extensive hemorrhage is encountered, the pericardiotomy is held closed while the incision is carried up through the sternum. If controlled hemorrhage is encountered, then the pericardial fluid is evacuated and a drain is placed.

## RIB FRACTURES

In contrast to the adult experience, where rib fractures are noted in 33% of adult injured patients, rib fractures were noted in only 1.6% of injured children.

Motor vehicle-related injuries account for nearly 70% of all rib fractures; intentional injuries account for 21% of rib fractures. The fourth through ninth ribs are the most commonly fractured ribs. Fractures of the ninth through 12th ribs should raise concerns about associated liver and/or spleen injury. For children younger than 3 years of age, intentional injury accounts for nearly two-thirds of rib fractures and of all the cases of child abuse documented in the United States, 5% to 27% of the children between the age of 0 and 3 sustained rib injuries. These children most often present with posterior arch rib fractures and rib fractures in this age group should raise the concern for nonaccidental trauma prompting further evaluation including a skeletal survey.

Fractures of the first and second ribs no longer are regarded as sensitive markers of injuries to the mediastinal vessels as recent data demonstrate no increased risk for aortic injuries in these patients. Great vessel disruptions are no greater with the first and second rib fractures than with any other rib fractures. However, first and second rib fractures should still be regarded as indicating a high-impact mechanism of injury and consideration should be given to performing a chest CT

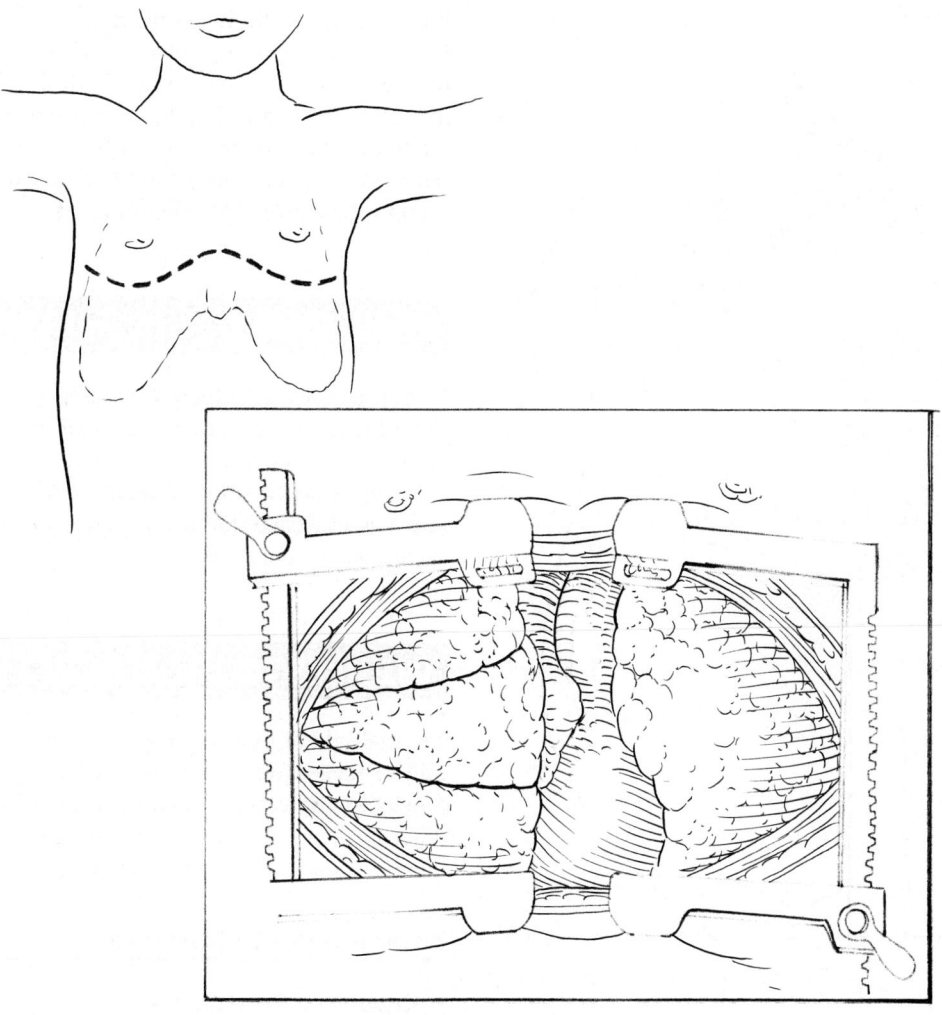

**FIGURE 80-4** Extension of the left anterolateral thoracotomy to the right, the "clam shell" thoracotomy.

in search of other injuries. The most important principle in managing children with rib fractures is adequate control of pain. Judicious use of nonsteroidal anti-inflammatory agents, narcotics, intercostal nerve block, and epidural analgesia has a clear role in this regard.

## STERNUM

Sternal fractures in children are uncommon. The vast majority of sternal fractures are isolated and nondisplaced fractures of the upper midportion of the sternum. The shoulder harness of the seat belt restraint system and direct impact are the most common mechanisms of injury. Associated injuries are seen in 50% to 60% of patients with sternal fractures. These include rib fractures in 40%, long-bone fractures in 25%, and head injuries in 18% of patients. Fortunately, most sternal fractures are not associated with cardiac injuries. Sternal fractures are best diagnosed by lateral chest x-ray, although they may at times be seen with an AP view.

Patients with sternal fracture should have an electrocardiogram upon evaluation in the emergency room. If the EKG is normal, the patient does not require admission and can be discharged with adequate analgesics. However, if the EKG is

abnormal, then admission is appropriate and cardiac monitoring for at least 24 hours is provided along with adequate analgesics. If there is gross displacement of the sternal fracture or disabling pain, the sternal fracture should be stabilized operatively.

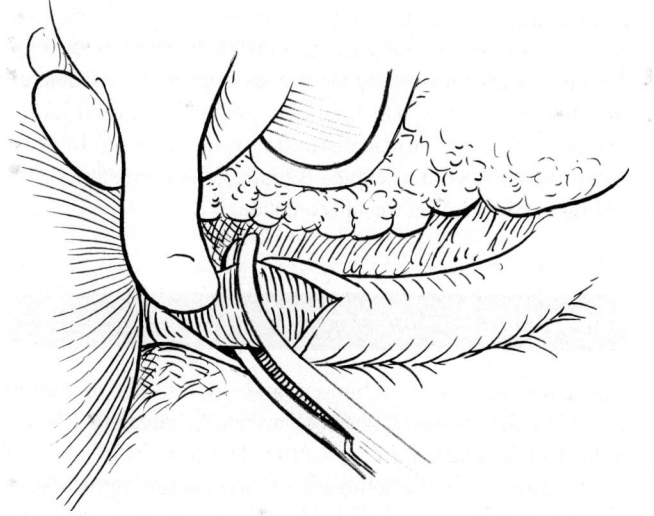

**FIGURE 80-5** Clamping of the aorta.

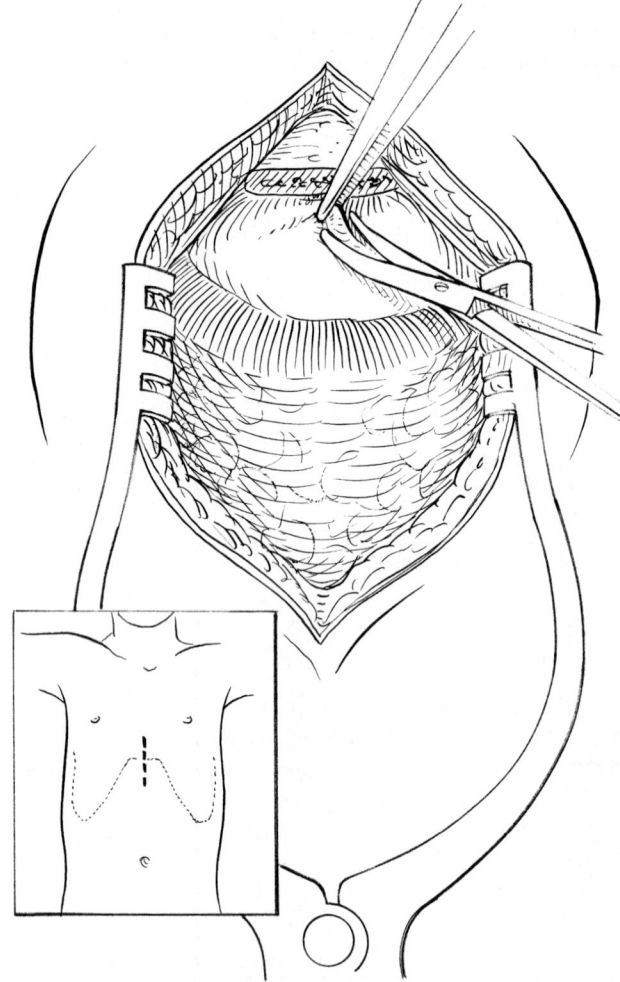

Marker
for force
+ Assoc.
Injury

**FIGURE 80-6** Subxiphoid approach for pericardial fluid or for placement of a pericardial window.

## SCAPULA

Fractures of the scapula are uncommon because of the scapula's posterior location and the significant force required to cause an injury. The body and neck of the scapula are the most common sites of fracture and associated injuries are seen in 80% to 90% of patients with scapula fractures. Pulmonary contusions are by far the most common associated injuries, followed by rib fractures, brachial plexus injuries, and arterial injury. Aortic disruption is uncommon. In most cases, the child with a scapula fracture can be managed with a sling for the arm on the affected side.

## CLAVICLE

Clavicular fracture in children and adolescents are often caused by direct impact or fall on an outstretched arm. Treatment will depend on the age of the child and the location of the fracture. Medial fractures are treated with only immobilization in a sling for 7 to 14 days. These types of fractures in newborns and infants can be treated without a sling and

require only careful handling of the child. A midclavicular fracture, typically seen in older children, can be treated either nonoperatively or operatively. Typically, patients required immobilization in a sling for 1 to 4 weeks, although recent reports in the pediatric trauma literature suggest that open reduction and internal fixation results in shorter time to union with a low rate of complications.

## FLAIL CHEST

Flail chests are uncommon in children, principally because of the compliant nature of the chest wall, and diagnosis is based on the clinical observation of paradoxical motion of the chest wall. Intubation is only necessary if oxygenation cannot be maintained despite the use of narcotics, anti-inflammatory agents, and epidurals to provide analgesia.

## INJURIES TO THE LUNG

The majority of injuries to the lung and pleura are successfully managed with tube thoracostomy and rarely require thoracotomy. Because penetrating and blunt injuries to lungs differ in their pathophysiology and treatment, the management of these injuries is addressed separately.

### Blunt Injuries to the Lung

#### Pulmonary Contusion

Pulmonary contusion is the most common consequence of blunt trauma to the lung and is seen in 48% of patients with blunt thoracic trauma. Pulmonary contusions may not be apparent on the initial chest x-ray and may not appear for 48 to 72 hours after injury. External signs are often absent, so a high index of suspicion is necessary given that 40% of patients with pulmonary contusion have a delayed presentation.

Injuries to other organ systems are common in children who present with lung injury and a thorough patient evaluation is warranted to avoid missing associated trauma. Most clinical reports suggest that children with pulmonary contusion have an excellent outcome and rarely require ventilatory support. However, because of the likelihood of associated intrathoracic injury, it is useful to repeat a chest x-ray in 6 to 48 hours to identify other intrathoracic injuries in children with pulmonary contusion.

Although a chest x-ray is the best radiologic modality to evaluate the child with chest trauma, its limitations are well recognized. Lung contusions can be confused with aspiration pneumonia, which most commonly occurs in the right lower lobe. CT scans are more sensitive and frequently will show evidence of pulmonary contusion and pneumohemothorax that are not evident on chest x-ray. However, a chest CT for the sole purpose of evaluating lung contusions seen on chest x-ray should be done only in patients with serious respiratory compromise.

The management of pulmonary contusion consists of careful fluid administration and adequate pulmonary toilet.

Although as many as 20% of the children with lung contusions will eventually develop pneumonia, there has been no demonstrated benefit to antibiotic prophylaxis. In children who have severe lung contusions, mechanical ventilation with an oscillator using lateral decubitus with the least-affected side up can be useful. Another technique is to use differential lung ventilation employing a double-lumen endobronchial tube connected to two ventilators. For the best results, this technique, employing synchronized independent lung ventilation, should be an early consideration.

## PNEUMOTHORAX

Pneumothorax and hemothorax account for 39% to 50% of intrathoracic injuries in children, respectively. Blunt trauma-related pneumothoraces may result from (a) rib fractures penetrating the lung itself leading to air leak; (b) deceleration injuries that tear the lung; (c) crush injury with disruption of alveoli; and (d) increase in intrathoracic pressure resulting in ruptured alveoli as seen in traumatic asphyxia. Generally, pneumothoraces following blunt trauma resolve more quickly than do those following penetrating injury.

The size of a pneumothorax is traditionally expressed as a function of the distance the lung is collapsed from the chest wall as compared with the total lung diameter. For example, if the hemithorax measures 10 cm and the lung is collapsed by a pneumothorax to 6 cm, the percent of pneumothorax is expressed as 40. However, an alternative method, which some consider to be more accurate, considers the lung as a cylinder and uses the formula $\pi R^2$ to calculate the volume loss.

The standard treatment for traumatic pneumothorax is tube thoracostomy in order to remove the trapped air and to allow for complete reexpansion of the lung. In a hemodynamically unstable patient with a probable tension pneumothorax, a chest x-ray should not delay insertion of the chest tube. Most importantly, in the face of a tension pneumothorax, needle decompression of the chest should not be delayed. In the stable patient, obtaining a chest x-ray is valuable because it confirms the diagnosis; demonstrates additional injuries such as diaphragmatic rupture; and demonstrates other findings that would change the site of the chest tube, such as a large hemothorax.

In blunt trauma, the pneumothorax usually has little or no associated hemothorax and a small chest tube is usually sufficient. However, if there is an associated hemothorax, a larger chest tube should be placed to ensure complete evacuation of the accumulated blood. In cases of an extremely large hemothorax, 2 chest tubes may be necessary, 1 placed anteriorly and superiorly for removal of air and 1 placed inferiorly and posteriorly for removal of the fluid. The chest tube is connected to a water-seal device that is put on suction. A chest x-ray obtained following placement of the chest tube determines whether both air and fluid are completely evacuated and the lung is fully expanded.

Children who have isolated small pneumothoraces involving only the apex of the lung and who are essentially asymptomatic may be managed without a chest tube. A similar course of management may be appropriate for patients whose pneumothorax is not evident on the chest x-ray but is seen as an incidental finding on the CT scan obtained for evaluation of associated abdominal injuries. However, if air can be seen around the entire lung, then tube thoracostomy is preferred. If observation alone is used as management of a small pneumothorax, then a follow-up chest x-ray should be done at 6 and 24 hours after diagnosis to ensure stability and/or resolution of the pneumothorax. Children with small pneumothoraces who are undergoing general anesthesia with positive ventilation should have a chest tube placed prior to induction of anesthesia.

Removal of a chest tube should be based on clinical criteria. The cessation of air leak is reliable evidence that the torn-lung parenchyma has sealed against the parietal pleura. The chest tube should be placed to underwater seal without suction for a minimum of 4 hours. That period of observation without an air leak suggests that the lung is adequately sealed against the parietal pleura and will likely stay expanded without suction. A chest x-ray at that time confirms that the lung is fully expanded.

Imaging following chest tube removal is controversial in the literature. The adult trauma literature suggests that omitting routine chest x-ray after chest tube removal is safe in selected trauma patients who are able to communicate respiratory symptoms and are not mechanically ventilated. The same findings were corroborated in a pediatric study of postoperative cardiac surgery patients. Prospective studies are needed to establish clear guidelines on chest tubes removal in children in the trauma setting. In the meantime, a safe approach is to put the chest tube on water seal only and monitor for an air leak. Large and persistent air leaks suggest the disruption of a major airway, which requires additional intervention. In the absence of a leak, a chest x-ray can then be performed to confirm that the lung is still inflated. If there is no respiratory distress and the lung remains fully expanded on chest x-ray, the tube can be removed and a follow-up film is obtained in 6 hours with the patient upright and with forced expiration.

## TRACHEOBRONCHIAL INJURIES

Intrathoracic tracheobronchial injuries are rare in children, accounting for less than 1% of all thoracic trauma. In a review of the National Pediatric Trauma Registry, all of the reported bronchial injuries were secondary to blunt trauma. Tracheal injuries resulting from penetrating trauma most often occur in the neck and are extremely rare in children. Bronchial injuries may present without external signs other than a pneumothorax on chest x-ray. A large and persistent air leak on placement of the chest tube suggests the disruption of a major airway. If ventilation and oxygenation are compromised because of the size of the air leak, a double-lumen tube and single-lung ventilation may acutely reduce the size of the air leak and permit adequate ventilation and oxygenation.

Subcutaneous emphysema, dyspnea, substernal tenderness, and hemoptysis are the most common presenting signs of tracheobronchial disruption. Subcutaneous emphysema, pneumomediastinum, pneumothorax, and air surrounding

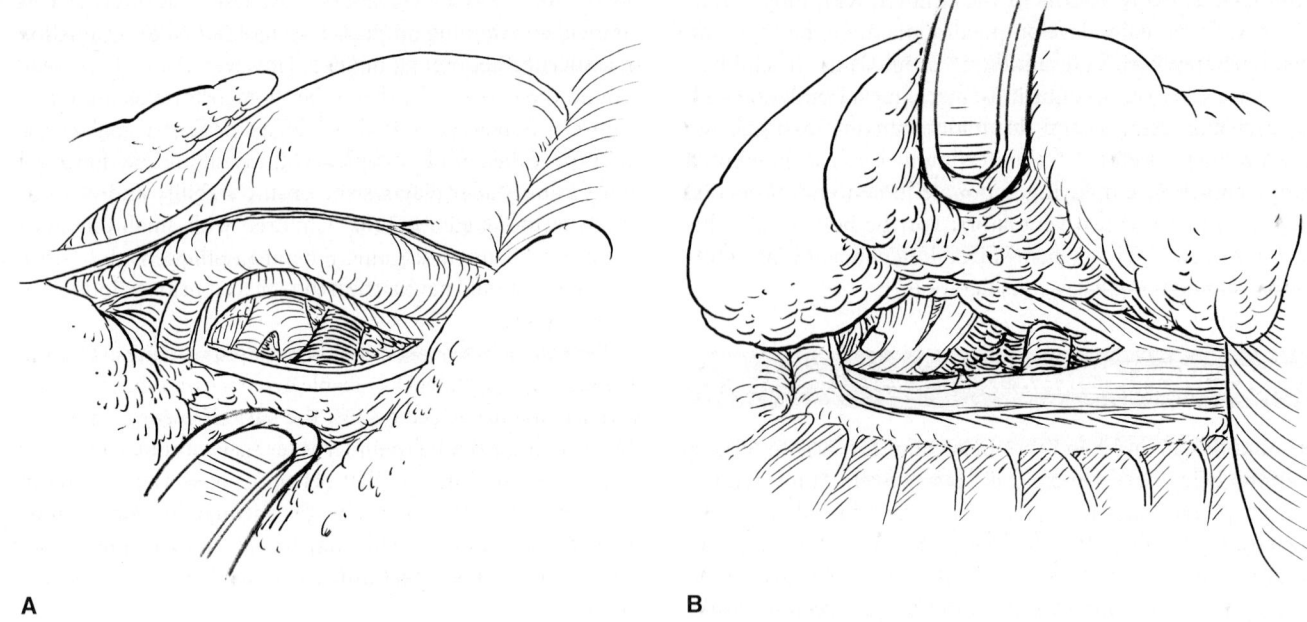

**A**

**B**

**FIGURE 80-7** Right thoracic approach to tracheal and right bronchial injuries. **A.** Anterior hilar exposure. **B.** Posterior hilar exposure.

the bronchus on chest x-ray are the most common associated radiographic findings. Collapse of the lung toward the chest wall and away from the hilum is an uncommon but highly suggestive finding of bronchial disruption. Although pneumomediastinum may be seen without damage to the mediastinal organs, its identification on x-ray warrants consideration of injury to the tracheobronchial tree or to the esophagus.

Early diagnosis of tracheobronchial injuries is essential. If possible, flexible or rigid bronchoscopy should be performed to confirm both the location and the extent of airway disruption. If the size of the endotracheal tube permits, the bronchoscope should be passed through the endotracheal tube and the bronchus and trachea examined.

Primary repair and reconstruction of the disrupted tracheobronchial tree should be performed as early as possible. Delayed surgery is a recognized risk factor for stenosis, often necessitating repeated operations. However, some injuries can be managed nonoperatively such as small lacerations in the membranous trachea and some partial bronchial tears that involves approximately one third of the circumference.

A standard posterior lateral thoracotomy is done and the lung is retracted anteriorly. The hilum of the lung may be clamped if the air leak is too large to allow ventilation. Otherwise, the injured trachea or bronchus should be repaired with interrupted simple sutures (preferably monofilament absorbable) after the edges have been debrided (Figs. 80-7 and 80-8).

## HEMOTHORAX

Most children with trauma-related hemothorax require only tube thoracostomy. In contrast to instances of pneumothorax in which a small chest tube suffices to expand the lung, the child with a hemothorax usually requires a chest tube

large enough to evacuate blood to avoid the development of a hemofibrothorax and subsequent entrapment of the lung (Table 80-2). In general, urgent chest tubes for trauma should be placed with the assumption that there will be some degree of hemothorax.

The chest tube should be inserted caudally and posteriorly. However, placement of the tube more posterior than the midaxillary line predisposes to obstruction of the tube when the child is in a supine position. If possible, a finger should be inserted to ensure intrathoracic placement and to identify the possibility of a diaphragmatic tear.

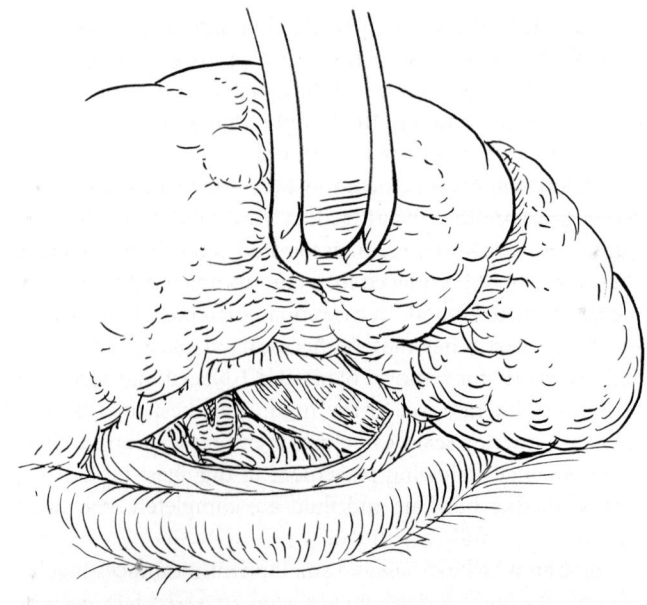

**FIGURE 80-8** Left thoracic approach to left bronchial injuries. (Posterior hilum.)

| TABLE 80-2 | Thoracostomy Tube Size by Weight |
| --- | --- |
| Weight (in kg) | Chest Tube Size (in Fr) |
| 3 to 5 | 10 to 12 |
| 6 to 9 | 12 to 16 |
| 10 to 11 | 16 to 20 |
| 12 to 14 | 20 to 22 |
| 15 to 18 | 22 to 24 |
| 19 to 22 | 24 to 28 |
| 23 to 30 | 24 to 32 |
| >32 | 32 to 40 |

Upon placement of the tube, attention should then be given to the color and quantity of the blood evacuated. Massive bleeding from lung parenchyma following blunt trauma is uncommon and thoracotomy is rarely needed. Pulmonary or pleural bleeding requiring surgery is usually the result of rib fractures that lacerate intercostal vessels or puncture and lacerate the lung. Fortunately, because of the low arterial pressure in the pulmonary circulation, bleeding from the lung parenchyma usually stops after the lung is fully reexpanded.

The need for thoracotomy is suggested by chest tube output more than 2 to 3 mL/kg/hour or an initial chest tube output exceeding 20% to 30% of the child's blood volume (approximately 15 to 20 mL/kg). In the older child or adolescent, comparable volumes suggesting the need for surgery are 200 to 300 mL/hour or 1500 mL in the initial chest tube output.

## PENETRATING INJURIES TO THE LUNG

Penetrating injuries to the lung are usually a result of stab wounds and gunshot wounds. Stab wounds are low-velocity injuries and have a better outcome as compared with gunshot wounds. Gunshot wounds may be low or high velocity. High-velocity gunshot wounds (projectiles traveling greater than 1500 to 2000 ft/sec) often result in substantial tissue destruction from cavitation or blast effect or from secondary missiles such as fragments of rib.

Children with penetrating thoracic injuries are more likely to require operative intervention than those with blunt chest injuries. The clinician is challenged by having to distinguish between "simple" penetrating chest and a "nonsimple" penetrating chest injury based on clinical findings and the chest x-ray.

Examples of a simple chest injury include stab wounds with minor chest wall injury, stab wounds with a simple pneumothorax or minor lung laceration, or a gunshot wound that produces minimal lung parenchymal damage or disruption of a distal bronchus.

Examples of a "nonsimple" chest injury are stab wounds with injuries to the heart; a major injury to the lung or major vessel; a stab wound with open or tension pneumothorax; a

stab wound with a hemothorax of greater than 1500 mL in an adolescent or 30% of blood volume in a child; a gunshot wound with injury to the heart, proximal bronchus, great vessels, or esophagus; or a transmediastinal gunshot wound with any of the above injuries.

A large percentage of stab wounds to the chest do not penetrate a muscular chest wall. Eighty percent of asymptomatic stab wounds of the chest can be successfully managed as outpatients. A chest x-ray should be obtained initially and 6 hours after presentation to the ED. If normal, the patient may be discharged. Twelve percent of patients with no pneumothorax on the initial chest x-ray subsequently develop a hemopneumothorax, underscoring the importance of the 6-hour observation period and the follow-up chest x-ray.

In the instance of gunshot injuries to the chest, pneumo- and hemothorax should be assessed with a chest x-ray and a chest tube inserted if needed. The heart and mediastinum should be evaluated with a quick surface echocardiogram (FAST) to rule out a pericardial effusion. If air leak and the bleeding from the chest tube are minimal and the echocardiogram is negative, the patient can be admitted and observed in a monitored setting.

Patients with penetrating injuries to the tracheobronchial tree present with respiratory distress in 59% to 73%, subcutaneous emphysema in 17% to 41%, pneumothorax in 16% to 60%, and hemoptysis in 14% to 25%. Air leak is usually massive. These injuries are frequently diagnosed at the time of operation for other reasons, usually massive bleeding. However, if the patient's condition is stable, bronchoscopy should be performed. Repair of tracheobronchial injuries is best approached via a lateral thoracotomy with debridement and repair using interrupted monofilament absorbable sutures.

Massive bleeding from the lung and/or pulmonary vessels, as well as air leakage from the bronchial tree, requires rapid control of the hilum. During an ED thoracotomy, a maneuver that can be applied quickly to control massive bleeding from the lung consists in twisting the lung around its hilum. In a more controlled OR setting, application of Satinsky or Debakey clamps at the hilum allows for intrapleural dissection of the pulmonary vessels. If the injury is proximal, then dissection of the pulmonary vessels within the pericardium is an option. Another maneuver that can be used for deeper parenchymal or vascular injury associated with penetrating trauma is dividing the parenchyma above the tract of the injury using a stapling device to gain access to the source of bleeding.

## BLUNT CARDIAC INJURIES

Most cardiac injuries in children result from blunt trauma, with motor vehicle crashes being the most common mechanism. Abnormal ventricular wall motion, decreased ejection fraction, or elevated cardiac enzymes and isoenzymes have been identified in 43% of children with lung contusion or rib fractures following blunt chest injury. However, the incidence of clinically significant blunt cardiac injury (BCI) is rare; it is observed in less than 5% of patients. Myocardial contusion is by far the most common cardiac injury.

## Cardiac Contusion

In its extreme, it may mimic myocardial infarction with depressed myocardial function as well as supraventricular and ventricular arrhythmias. The right ventricle is more commonly involved because of his location. The compression and acceleration force that are applied to the heart after blunt trauma can also, more rarely, cause injury and rupture of the cardiac free wall, the ventricular septum, and the cardiac valves.

The application of significant force to the thoracic cage is the greatest risk factor for BCI. In the case of motor vehicle crashes, relevant information includes the direction of impact, speed of the vehicle, steering wheel deformation, air bag deployment, and passenger restraint system used. However, BCI has been reported with motor vehicle speeds of less than 20 miles/hour.

Anterior chest wall tenderness, pain, contusion, or anterior rib fractures are consistent but not specific for BCI. Although imperfect, the electrocardiogram (EKG) is the simplest and fastest way to diagnose BCI. An EKG should be performed on any patient with a significant impact on the chest from blunt trauma to rule out BCI. Concerns about the sensitivity of the EKG to diagnose BCI center around 2 points. First, the EKG principally reflects abnormalities of the left ventricle and BCI is generally regarded as a right-ventricular phenomenon. Second, comparisons of EKG with an echocardiography suggest that the EKG may not detect significant abnormalities detectable by echocardiography. Nonetheless, cardiac irritability, evidenced by arrhythmias and conduction delays (Table 80-3), is the pathognomonic consequence of BCI.

An admission EKG and a 6-hour period of observation identify most of the patients who require treatment of BCI. Low-risk patients who are identified as minimally injured, who have a normal EKG, and who are hemodynamically stable may be discharged from the ED. A normal EKG in an otherwise stable patient with no other reason for a monitored bed requires no further evaluation for BCI.

CPK/MB levels and cardiac troponin T&I assays have not proved useful in the diagnosis of clinically relevant BCI. Similarly, echocardiography may be useful in the hemodynamically unstable patient, but adds little in the evaluation of the hemodynamically stable patient suspected of having a BCI. *Echo IF unstable*

Complications of BCI are rare and occur early in the patient's clinical course. The hemodynamically stable patient with an abnormal EKG may be observed in the ICU or in a telemetry-monitored bed for 24 to 48 hours. Patients with BCI and persistent hypotension not accounted for by associated injuries should undergo additional studies (echocardiography or transesophageal echocardiography) to delineate cardiac abnormalities (Fig 80-9). *Commotio cordis* is a pattern of injury that was initially described in the pediatric population. It involves sudden impact on the anterior chest that subsequently causes severe malignant arrhythmia, more commonly ventricular fibrillation. It is thought to be more prevalent in children due to the compliance of the chest wall that allows transmission of the high-energy impact to the heart. It is associated with sports such as baseball and football. Survival is quoted to be as low as 15% but has now increased in the recent years after automatic external defibrillators were made more readily available in schools and athletic facilities.

# PENETRATING INJURIES TO THE HEART

Penetrating injuries to the heart are most often related to stab wounds and bullets and the right ventricle is the chamber most often injured. Clinical manifestations of penetrating injuries to the heart are dependent upon the relative roles of pericardial tamponade and massive hemorrhage. The severity of pericardial tamponade is a function of the size of the pericardial tear, the rate of bleeding from the cardiac wound, and the chamber involved. Eighty to 90% of patients with stab wounds to the heart present with tamponade. With small knife wounds, the pericardial laceration seals quickly and blood accumulates to contribute to the development of life-threatening tamponade.

In contrast to stab wounds, gunshot wounds result in comparatively large openings in the pericardium and in the cardiac chambers. Hemorrhage in these instances is usually massive and rapid and pericardial tamponade is often absent. Gunshot wounds to the heart are frequently lethal unless intervention is prompt and effective.

Any child with a parasternal entrance wound, in the area defined as the "cardiac box," should be suspected of having a cardiac injury (Fig. 80-10). A FAST examination can be performed quickly in the trauma bay and can be quite effective at excluding a hemopericardium. In a recent study in adults who sustained penetrating trauma to the chest, sensitivity and specificity for a FAST examination to detect a hemopericardium was 100%. In the child who is stable, a transthoracic echocardiography can also be useful to diagnose penetrating cardiac injuries in tamponade.

The definitive treatment for a penetrating cardiac injury is cardiorrhaphy through a thoracotomy or sternotomy. The left anterior or anterolateral thoracotomy is the most frequently chosen incision site. Further exposure can be obtained by transsternal extension into the right chest. The pericardium is opened, taking care not to injure the phrenic nerve, and the tamponade is relieved. Bleeding from the heart is controlled

| TABLE 80-3 | Pathognomonic Consequences of Blunt Cardiac Injury | |
|---|---|---|
| **Supraventricular** | **Ventricular** | **Conduction Abnormalities** |
| Sinus tachycardia | Premature ventricular contractions | Right bundle branch block (RBB) |
| Atrial flutter | Ventricular tachycardia | First-degree heart block |
| Atrial fibrillation | Ventricular fibrillation | RBB with conduction delay |
| | | Third-degree heart block |

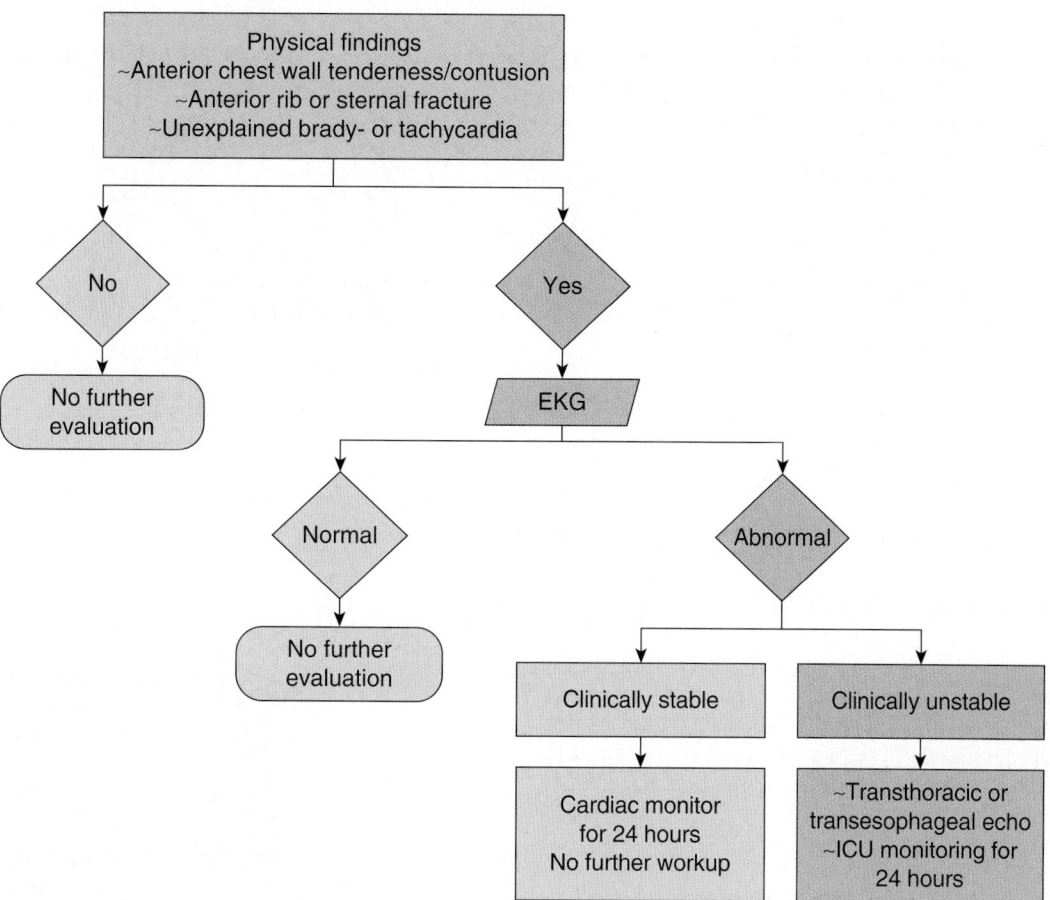

**FIGURE 80-9** Algorithm for blunt cardiac trauma investigation.

by digital occlusion and the laceration is closed with nonabsorbable mattress sutures over Teflon pledgets (Fig. 80-11). In the absence of Teflon pledgets, strips of pericardium may be used to buttress the sutures. For larger wounds, a Foley catheter with a balloon inflated with saline may be inserted into the opening as a temporizing measure to control hemorrhage (Fig. 80-12). With wounds near the coronary arteries, care must be taken not to obstruct the coronary flow. Wounds of the atria, cava, or aorta may be controlled with partial occluding clamps. If a subxiphoid window was a preliminary approach, then that incision may be extended into a median sternotomy offering superb exposure to the heart, great vessels, and pulmonary hilum.

## AORTIC AND GREAT VESSEL INJURIES

Aortic injuries are uncommon in children and are seen in approximately 1% to 3% of children who have made it to a major trauma center. The mortality rate observed in children with aortic and great vessel injuries is 75%. The most common great vessel injury is aortic disruption, usually seen in the older adolescent patient as an occupant in motor vehicle crashes. Fifty percent of patients with aortic disruption who survive the prehospital phase of care will die from hemorrhage within 24 hours of hospitalization.

The mechanisms of aortic disruption include (a) sheer forces caused by the relative mobility of a portion of the vessel; (b) compression of the aorta and great vessels over the vertebral column; and (c) intraluminal hyperextension.

Fifty percent of patients with thoracic vascular injury from blunt trauma present without external physical signs of injury. The most common clinical signs include palpable fracture of the sternum, expanding hematoma at the thoracic outlet, infrascapular murmur, upper-extremity hypertension, diminished or absent peripheral pulses, palpable fracture of the thoracic spine, hypotension, and elevated central venous pressure.

Radiographic signs suggestive of great vessel injury include massive hemothorax, a widened superior mediastinum, depression of the left mainstem bronchus more than 140°, obliteration of the aortic knob, deviation of the nasogastric tube, and endotracheal tube or trachea to the right and left apical hematoma. The most reliable radiographic marker is a "funny looking mediastinum" and the loss of the aortic knob contour.

Because of the high likelihood of associated injuries, priorities in management are an important concern. Hemodynamically unstable patients who have intra-abdominal hemorrhage should undergo laparotomy before any other procedure. Patients that are stable enough to undergo imaging should undergo chest CT angiography, which has become the diagnostic study of choice over aortography.

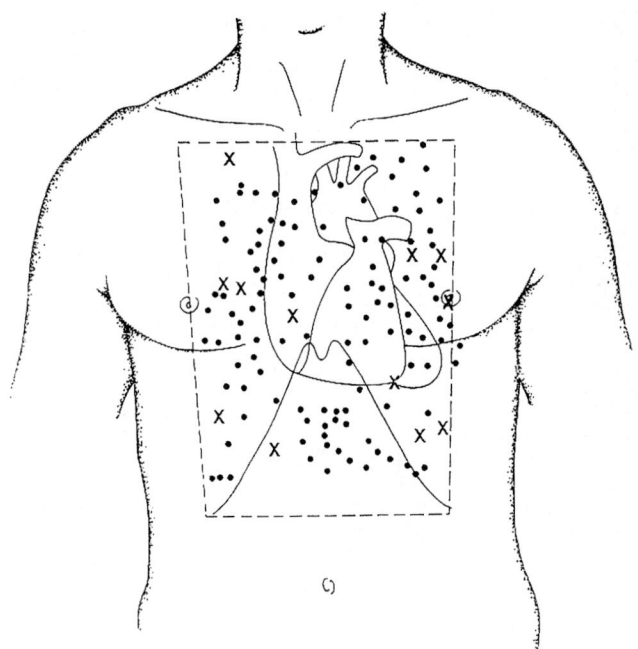

**FIGURE 80-10** The "cardiac box". Definition of proximity to the heart for penetrating injuries. X = wounds that produced cardiac injuries. (Reprinted with permission from Nagy KK, Lohmann, C, Kim DO, et al. Role of echocardiography in the diagnosis of occult penetrating cardiac injury. *J Trauma Injury Infect Crit Care* 1995;38(6):859–862.)

Control HTN c̄ β-blockade

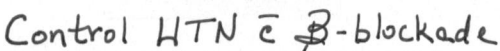

During diagnostic testing and once an injury is confirmed, hypertension needs to be controlled with β-blockade, but care must be taken not to underperfuse these patients, as many also suffer from traumatic brain injuries. Until recently, most thoracic aortic injuries in children were repaired surgically using primary repair or grafting. These surgeries necessitate the use of a shunt, a bypass, or a clamp-and-sew technique. The main associated risk is paraplegia due to spinal cord ischemia during the procedure. In the last 10 years, new techniques of endovascular stenting have been used based on the adult experience. Successful treatment of blunt aortic injuries has been reported in the pediatric trauma literature. More studies are needed to evaluate the long-term outcome of this procedure.

In contrast to aortic injuries associated with blunt trauma, aortic and subclavian vessel injuries secondary to penetrating trauma most often require operative intervention. Several approaches can be used depending on the location of the entry wound or trajectory of the bullet (Fig. 80-13). A resuscitative thoracotomy should always be via a left anterolateral approach. It can then be extended to gain access to the other side with the so-called "clam-shell" incision. In the more controlled OR setting, a median sternotomy provides good exposure to the anterior mediastinum and great vessels. It can then be extended on either side as the "trap-door" incision. The upper component of the "trap-door" incision can help in gaining control of the subclavian and carotids vessels. The median sternotomy can also be extended in the neck along the sternocleidomastoid muscle. Access to pulmonary hilum, azygos system, and esophagus is made easier with a posterolateral thoracotomy.

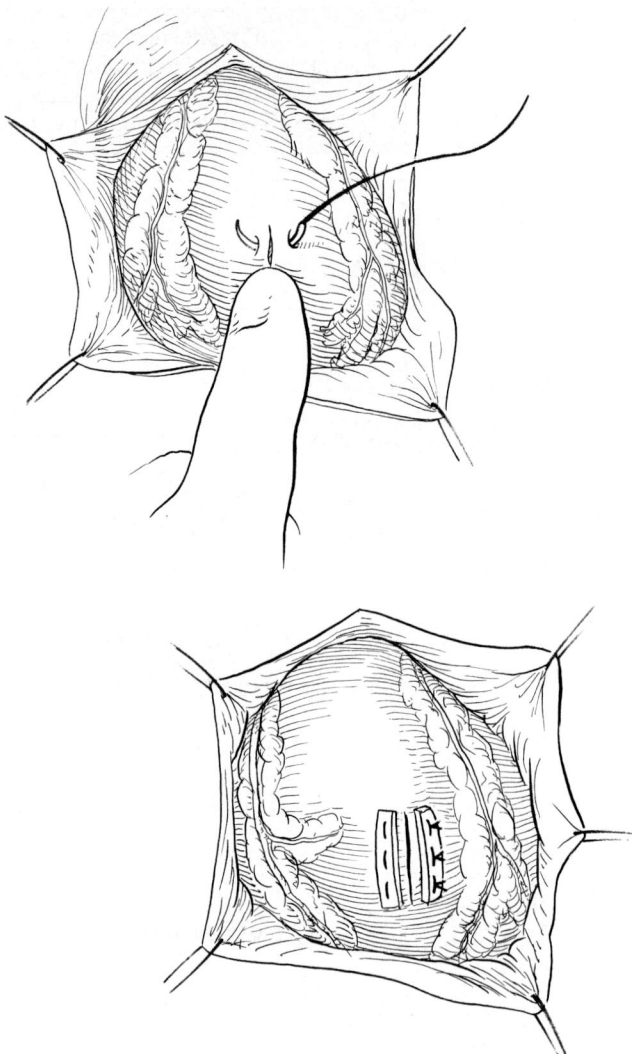

**FIGURE 80-11** The penetrating wound of the heart is controlled by digital compression after pericardiotomy while pledgeted sutures are prepared for direct cardiac repair.

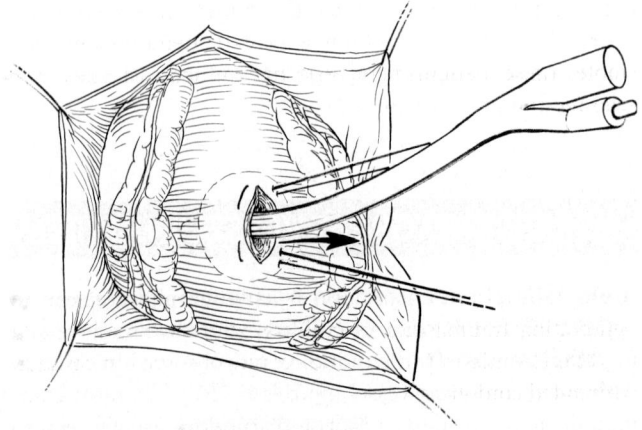

**FIGURE 80-12** For larger penetrating cardiac injuries, a Foley catheter under direct vision is inserted into the heart. After balloon inflation, traction on the Foley temporarily controls the bleeding while suture repair is prepared.

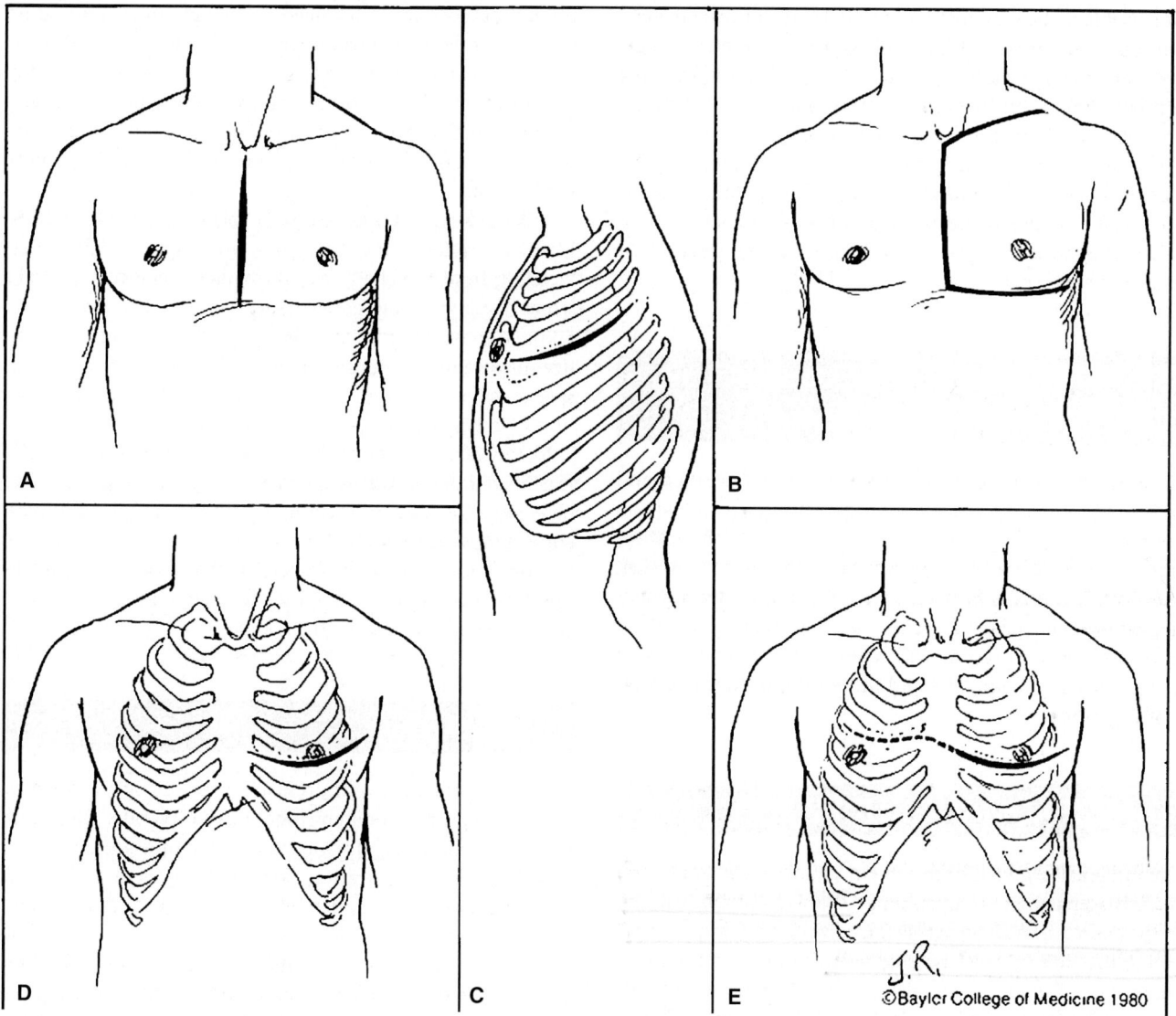

**FIGURE 80-13** Different approaches for thoracic trauma depending on location of injury: **A.** median sternotomy, **B.** book thoracotomy, **C.** posterolateral thoracotomy, **D.** anterolateral thoracotomy, and **E.** extension of an anterolateral thoracotomy across the sternum. (Reprinted with permission from Wall, Jr. MJ, Huh J, Mattox KL. Chapter 25. Indications for and techniques of thoracotomy. In: Moore EE, Feliciano DV, Mattox KL, eds. *Trauma.* 6th ed. New York: McGraw-Hill; 2008.)

It can be very useful to perform a chest x-ray with the entry and exit wounds with a radio-opaque marker prior to planning the type of thoracotomy. If hemodynamically stable, these patients can also benefit from a chest CT angiography.

## ESOPHAGEAL INJURIES

Intrathoracic esophageal injury is seen in less than 1% of pediatric trauma patients and is most likely secondary to penetrating trauma due to gunshot injuries. The diagnosis can often be missed initially and delayed recognition can lead to dreaded complications.

In hemodynamically stable patients following penetrating trauma, pneumomediastinum can be seen on the initial chest x-ray. A chest CT can also show air in the pleura or mediastinum. The CT is also useful to evaluate the trajectory of the penetrating object. This can be useful to determine the likelihood of esophageal injury and thus deciding on the need for esophagram or esophagoscopy. If esophageal injury is suspected, evaluation is continued with a contrast study, usually first with waster-soluble contrast followed by barium, which is more sensitive. In cases where the esophogram is normal but there is high suspicion based on trajectory, rigid esophagoscopy should be performed to reach a combined sensitivity of 100%.

Although rare, esophageal trauma should be considered in the blunt trauma patient with odynophagia or pneumomediastinum. If pneumomediastinum is the only finding, a CT scan showing no other signs of esophageal injury is an adequate evaluation for esophageal injury. If there is both pneumomediastinum and clinical symptoms/signs related to a potential esophageal injury, CT as well as esophogram and esophagoscopy should be considered.

Treatment of esophageal injuries will depend on timing of presentation and diagnosis. If diagnosed early (typically less than 24 hours), primary repair can usually be achieved.

Non-viable tissue is debrided as needed and end-to-end anastomosis is performed. If diagnosis is delayed or local conditions are not favorable, drainage with T-tube or proximal esophagostomy can be done. A chest tube is also left in the pleural cavity. Repair is then done in a delayed fashion.

If a patient undergoes immediate thoracic exploration for a penetrating chest trauma without prior radiologic studies, care must be taken to ensure the esophagus is intact.

Late diagnosis can present with fever, tachycardia, chest pain, and empyema.

## SPONTANEOUS PNEUMOMEDIASTINUM

Spontaneous pneumomediastinum is a well-described and rare medical entity that can be sports-related. It can be seen with several sports and is not related to blunt chest trauma secondary to the activity, but rather to the physical exertion. It can also be seen after a respiratory tract infection or bronchospasm. Patients who seek medical attention most commonly present with chest pain. A simple chest x-ray is usually diagnostic and there is no need for further investigations.

## DIAPHRAGMATIC INJURIES

Diaphragmatic injuries are rare in children and more frequently seen in penetrating trauma. With a penetrating injury to the chest beneath the nipple line, diaphragmatic and intra-abdominal injury must be suspected. Blunt diaphragmatic rupture has a reported prevalence of 0.1%. Injuries are more commonly seen on the left side due to the protective effect of the liver on the right side. There is also a strong association with intra-abdominal injuries.

A chest x-ray should be performed initially. Signs associated with diaphragmatic injuries include an elevated hemidiaphragm, an abnormal diaphragmatic contour, and herniated contents in the chest. If a diaphragmatic injury is strongly suspected, a normal chest CT alone is not sensitive enough to exclude the diagnosis. The next step is to proceed to a diagnostic laparoscopy or thoracoscopy to evaluate the diaphragm. Depending on the clinical context, if other intrathoracic or intra-abdominal injuries are also present, thoracotomy and laparotomy are other acceptable approaches. Repair of the diaphragmatic defect can often be accomplished primarily with nonresorbable monofilament sutures. Rarely, a prosthetic patch is required.

## THORACOSCOPY IN TRAUMA

Experience with video-assisted thoracoscopy has popularized the use of this minimally invasive technique to evaluate and manage patients with thoracic injuries. The experience with children is limited but still promising. Many regard thoracoscopy as being no more invasive than tube thoracostomy. The need for single-lung ventilation may be a relative contraindication in some patients. Most consider single-lung ventilation necessary for optimal visualization of the thoracic cavity, the mediastinum, and diaphragm; however, in children, low levels of insufflation may allow for adequate visualization without single-lung ventilation.

Video-assisted thoracoscopy is most commonly used to identify injuries to the diaphragm, to diagnose and manage bleeding from the chest wall, to manage persistent air leaks from damaged lung parenchyma, and to evacuate blood retained in the chest cavity. The use of thoracoscopy to identify diaphragmatic injuries is nearly 100% successful. It has special value in patients suspected of diaphragmatic penetration following thoracoabdominal wounds.

In the case of chest-wall bleeding, even if control is not feasible via the thoracoscope, the identification of the site of bleeding allows for more limited thoracotomy to definitively control the bleeding. Finally, evacuation of the posttraumatic hemothoraces is successful in 60% of the cases. The likelihood of success is enhanced if the intervention takes place earlier rather than later in the course.

## SUMMARY

Thoracic injuries in children are rare but are associated with a disproportionately high mortality rate. This high mortality rate is usually a consequence of associated injuries. Blunt and penetrating thoracic injuries differ in their associated mortality and require thorough evaluation and management.

The initial approach is no different from that employed for any child who is seriously injured and includes securing the airway, maximizing breathing, and ensuring that circulation is adequate.

## SELECTED READINGS

Avarello JT, Cantor RM. Pediatric major trauma: an approach to evaluation and management. *Emerg Med Clin N Am* 2007;25(3):803–836.

Bliss D, Silen M. Pediatric thoracic trauma. *Crit Care Med* 2002; 30(11 Suppl): S409–S415.

Carson S, Woolridge DP, Colletti J, Kilgore K. Pediatric upper extremity injuries. *Pediatr Clin North Am* 2006;53(1):41–67.

Cooper A, Barlow B, DiScala C, String D. Mortality and truncal injury: the pediatric perspective. *J Pediatr Surg* 1994;29(1):33–38.

Dissanaike S, Shalhub S, Jurkovich GJ. The evaluation of pneumomediastinum in blunt trauma patients. *J Trauma* 2008;65(6):1340–1345.

Eber GB, Annest JL, Mercy JA, Ryan GW. Nonfatal and fatal firearm-related injuries among children aged 14 years and younger: United States, 1993–2000. *Pediatrics* 2004;113(6):1687–1692.

Feliciano DV, Rozycki GS. Advances in the diagnosis and treatment of thoracic trauma. *Surg Clin North Am* 1999;79(6):1417–1429.

Grant WJ, Meyers RL, Jaffe RL, Johnson DG. Tracheobronchial injuries after blunt chest trauma in children—hidden pathology. *J Pediatr Surg* 1998;33(11):1707–1711.

Inci I, Ozcelik C, Nizam O, Eren N, Ozgen G. Penetrating chest injuries in children: a review of 94 cases. *J Pediatr Surg* 1996;31(5):673–676.

Karmy-Jones R, Hoffer E, Meissner M, Bloch RD. Management of traumatic rupture of the thoracic aorta in pediatric patients. *Ann Thorac Surg* 2003;75(5):1513–1517.

Moore MA, Wallace EC, Westra SJ. The imaging of paediatric thoracic trauma. *Pediatr Radiol* 2009;39(5):485–496.

Naggy KK, Lohmann C, Kim DO, Barrett J. Role of echocardiography in the diagnosis of occult penetrating cardiac injury. *J Trauma* 1995;38(6):859–862.

Nance ML, Sing RF, Reilly PM, Templeton JM Jr, Schwab CW. Thoracic gunshot wounds in children under 17 years of age. *J Pediatr Surg* 1996;31(7):931–935.

Neal MD, Sippey M, Gaines BA, Hackam DJ. Presence of pneumomediastinum after blunt trauma in children: what does it really mean? *J Pediatr Surg* 2009;44(7):1322–1327.

Pabon-Ramos WM, Williams DM, Strouse PJ. Radiologic evaluation of blunt thoracic aortic injury in pediatric patients. *AJR* 2010;194(5):1197–1203.

Patel RP, Hernanz-Schulman M, Hilmes MA, Yu C, Ray J, Kan JH. Pediatric chest CT after trauma: impact on surgical and clinical management. *Pediatr Radiol* 2010;40(7):1246–1253.

Rhee PM, Acosta J, Bridgeman A, Wang D, Jordan M, Rich N. Survival after emergency department thoracotomy: Review of published data from the past 25 years. *J Am Coll Surg* 2000;190(3):288–298.

Ruddy RM. Trauma and the paediatric lung. *Paediatr Respir Rev* 2005;6(1):61–7.

Sayers RD, Underwood MJ, Bewes PC, Porter KM. Surgical management of major thoracic injuries. *Injury* 1994;25(2):75–79.

Sheikh AA, Culbertson CB. Emergency department thoracotomy in children: Rationale for selective application. *J Trauma* 1993;34(3):323–328.

Sisley AC, Rozycki GS, Ballard RB, Namias N, Salomone JP, Feliciano DV. Rapid detection of traumatic effusion using surgeon-performed ultrasonography. *J Trauma* 1998;44(2):291–296.

# Abdominal Trauma

# CHAPTER 81

*Alex Stoffan and David P. Mooney*

## KEY POINTS

1. Most solid organ injuries can and should be managed nonoperatively.

2. Laparotomy is still indicated for hemodynamic instability or peritonitis.

3. Diaphragmatic injuries, once diagnosed, are often associated with thoracic and abdominal injuries, and should be explored and repaired from the abdomen.

4. Splenorrhaphy remains the surgery of choice for unstable patients with splenic injury.

5. Angioembolization may supplant operation for hemodynamically stable patients with persistent hemorrhage.

6. Exploration for liver injury is rarely necessary, though some patients may require later interventional procedures for complications.

7. Gastric injury is uncommon, though it may occur more often in children than in adults, and usually occurs along the greater curvature.

8. The management of pancreatic ductal injury remains controversial: nonoperative, resection, or drainage.

9. The duodenum is more exposed and more prone to injury in pediatric patients.

10. Intestinal injuries are best diagnosed on physical examination, and therapeutic delay of less than 24 hours only mildly increases morbidity.

Although trauma remains the leading cause of mortality among children, emergency abdominal operations are infrequently required. The typical surgeon caring for injured children can expect to perform 1 or fewer emergency abdominal operations per year. This infrequency may diminish the experience of most surgeons and increases the utility of a chapter such as this.

## HISTORY OF OPERATIVE MANAGEMENT

With the publication of the United States War Manual in 1918, operative management of abdominal injuries became the treatment of choice and resulted in a marked decrease in mortality rate. With the report from Toronto of a series of children with the signs and symptoms of splenic injury who did not require operation, the era of nonoperative management began more than 30 years ago. The widespread use of computerized tomography (CT) has increased the number of abdominal injuries diagnosed. Many severe solid-organ injuries, previously thought to require laparotomy, have also been found to resolve nonoperatively. Despite this, every surgeon who cares for children should be facile with the skills needed for prompt laparotomy in the management of injured children. Completion of training courses, such as the Advanced Trauma Operative Management (ATOM) course® (TM ACS) may help surgeons acquire and retain operative trauma skills.

## INDICATIONS FOR OPERATIVE MANAGEMENT

The primary indications for laparotomy in injured children include hemodynamic instability despite adequate volume resuscitation, peritoneal findings, pneumoperitoneum, and evisceration. While the presence of an abdominal gunshot or stab wound penetrating the peritoneum has traditionally been managed with laparotomy, this has recently been called into question in adults. In a stable child, select stab and gunshot wounds to the abdomen may be managed expectantly in a center experienced in this strategy. In a hemodynamically stable patient, it may be difficult to differentiate an intestinal injury that requires repair from one that will heal without intervention, leading to exploration.

The large majority of solid-organ injuries in children do not require operation and many pediatric centers have reported operative rates of 1% or less. The majority of children with a hollow viscus injury requiring operation may be diagnosed by physical examination. CT of the abdomen and pelvis with intravenous, but without enteral contrast, is the diagnostic study of choice to evaluate the abdomen in injured children, although concerns over radiation exposure in children have led to attempts to limit this modality. Diagnostic peritoneal lavage is rarely indicated in children and its ability to locate peritoneal blood has been supplanted by the focused abdominal sonography for trauma (FAST) examination. While the FAST examination appears to be inadequately sensitive in detecting solid-organ injury, it may be helpful to determine the presence or absence of peritoneal and/or pericardial fluid.

## PREPARATIONS FOR LAPAROTOMY

If the patient is hemodynamically unstable, preoperative preparations will need to be expedited, but not so much as to jeopardize patient safety. The use of a preoperative checklist has been shown to improve patient mortality and decrease complications. The rapid completion of a checklist may help ensure that the patient has adequate large-caliber vascular access, has blood available, and has received any indicated antibiotics, that necessary equipment is available, and that the correct patient is having the correct procedure. The expenditure of 60 to 90 seconds to complete this process may give long-term dividends. If time allows, an arterial line as well as a Foley catheter and nasogastric tube should be inserted, though these may be placed once control of hemorrhage has been achieved and resuscitation is underway. Central venous lines are rarely helpful in this situation and should be reserved for the occasion when no other access, including by the cut-down or intraossesous route, can be achieved. The use of a warming blanket and warmed resuscitation fluids will help to prevent hypothermia. Tetanus prophylaxis should be considered.

Laparoscopy may be indicated as an initial maneuver under certain conditions: a hemodynamically stable patient with physical examination findings concerning for hollow viscus injury. A thorough laparoscopic exploration may avoid laparotomy, especially when it is possible to demonstrate that the peritoneum has not been violated in penetrating trauma.

The child is placed supine on the operating table and the skin is prepped from the suprasternal notch to the middle thigh level. A vertical midline incision provides excellent exposure to all quadrants of the abdomen. In children younger than 5 years of age, a transverse supraumbilical incision is an alternative, but the midline approach is the best option where speed is a critical factor. In dire circumstances, the skin may be prepped and the surgical field draped as the patient is being induced for the procedure. The surgeon should be prepared to incise the skin immediately should the patient become hypotensive if peripheral vascular resistance is diminished by the anesthetic agents used.

Upon opening the peritoneum, the surgeon may be greeted with massive intraperitoneal bleeding. This may be decreased by compression of the infradiaphragmatic aorta at the hiatus with a small Richardson retractor, a sponge stick, or manual compression, while the 4 quadrants of the abdomen are packed. After they are packed, the vascular compression may then be released. Once the patient has been resuscitated, systematic exploration of each quadrant, with the presumed bleeding quadrant carefully unpacked last, allows the demonstration of the injury while maintaining hemodynamic stability. A retroperitoneal hematoma should be left undisturbed unless it is found to be expanding or overlies the duodenum and pancreas. If the bleeding is controlled with packing and the patient is hypothermic, coagulopathic, or acidotic, the abdominal wall should be expeditiously covered. This may be done using a variety of techniques including the zipper, the Bogota bag, or towels covered with adhesive plastic wraps. The patient should then receive additional resuscitation and stabilization prior to reexploration and completion of injury repair in 12 to 36 hours.

## DIAPHRAGM INJURY

Diaphragmatic tears from a blunt mechanism may be difficult to diagnose, and their diagnosis and management are often delayed. Injuries of the left hemidiaphragm are more often diagnosed, possibly secondary to the protective effect of the liver. Diagnosis is suggested by distortion of the diaphragm on chest radiograph and may be confirmed by ultrasonography. Tears that result from a penetrating injury are more evident on exploration, and the diaphragm should be carefully inspected in any patient undergoing exploration for a penetrating upper abdominal or thoracic injury. During repair of diaphragmatic injury, an inspection should be performed for any associated abdominal or thoracic injuries (Fig. 81-1). Repair of diaphragmatic tears should be done by a transabdominal approach to inspect for any associated intra-abdominal injuries. Either a transverse upper abdominal or subcostal incision is preferred. The diaphragm is exposed and inspected by pulling the stomach and spleen downward on the left and the liver downward on the right. The edges of the diaphragmatic tear are débrided and the tear closed with an interrupted nonabsorbable suture. Pledgets or U-stitches may be used to

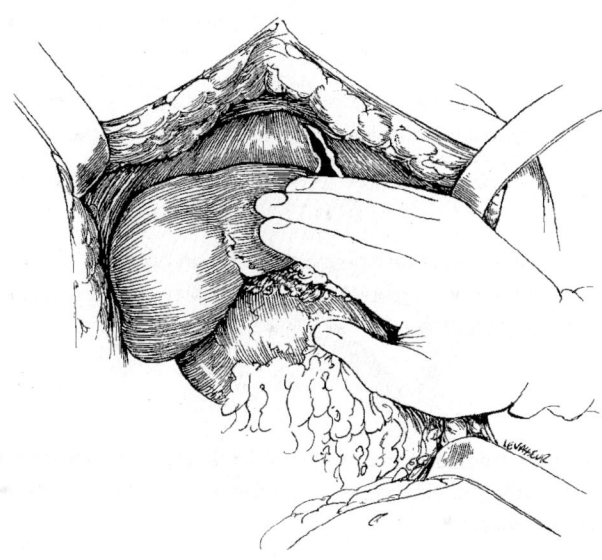

**FIGURE 81-1** The upper quadrant and the diaphragmatic surfaces are inspected by pulling the liver down on the right and the stomach and spleen down on the left.

which may be removed during sustained positive-pressure peak inspiration as the final closure suture is secured (Fig. 81-3). Associated pulmonary injuries when hemostatic may be treated by tube thoracostomy, placed prior to diaphragmatic repair.

## SPLEEN INJURY

The large majority of splenic injuries resolve with nonoperative management. Splenic injuries that cause hemodynamic instability despite resuscitation and lead to laparotomy are likely to be massive with hilar vascular disruption. Ongoing hemorrhage in hemodynamically stable patients is more likely to be from trabecular arterial injuries.

In general, splenic bleeding is best controlled initially by packing all 4 abdominal quadrants, followed by careful exploration of each to rule out associated significant injury, finishing with the left upper quadrant. Access to the vascular pedicle of the spleen is best obtained by division of the greater omentum at its attachment to the colon and retraction of the stomach and omentum superiorly (Fig. 81-4). This maneuver allows the splenic artery and vein to be controlled where they separate from the superior–posterior aspect of the pancreas, prior to mobilizing the spleen. The spleen is then mobilized by division of its 3 avascular attachments: the splenocolic, splenorenal, and lateral ligaments (Fig. 81-5).

The majority of splenic injuries requiring laparotomy may be addressed by splenorrhaphy. Splenic immune function may be preserved if one-third or more of the splenic tissue remains viable. A variety of techniques are available to achieve this end, and the proper technique will depend upon the specific

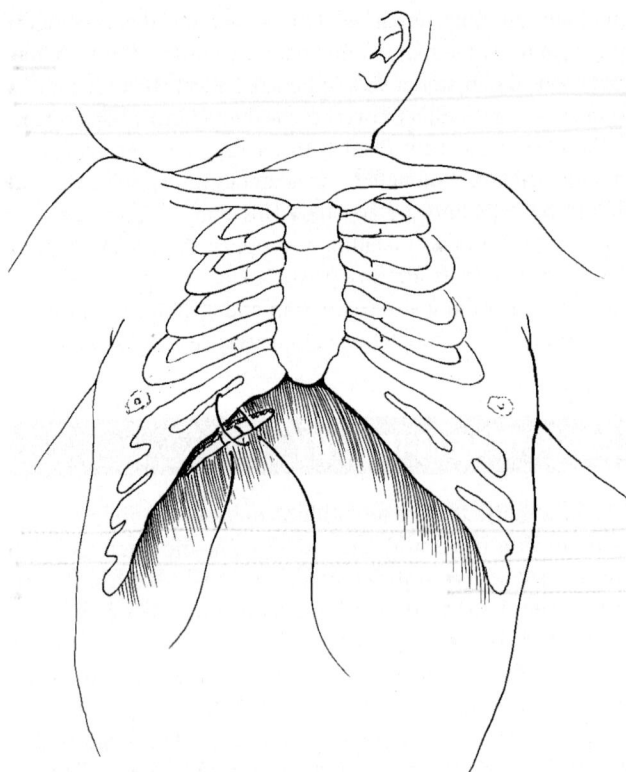

**FIGURE 81-2** A laceration in the diaphragm is débrided and then closed with permanent suture. A simple, mattress, or pericostal suturing technique is used.

reinforce the diaphragmatic edges as necessary (Fig. 81-2). Buttressing the repair with a layer of absorbable patch material may help decrease the recurrence rate. Including the nearby costal cartilage in the closure may reinforce lateral diaphragmatic tears. In the absence of any associated pulmonary injury, a pneumothorax may be evacuated by the placement of a soft, rubber catheter through the defect,

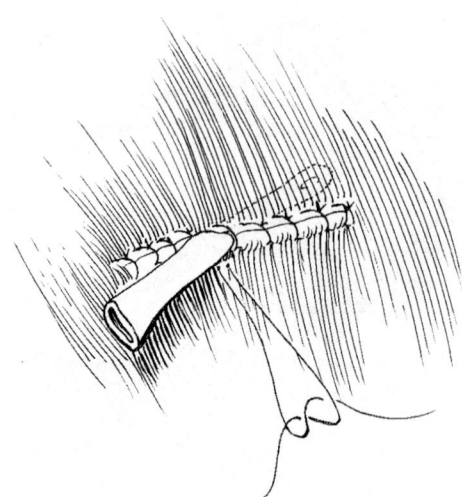

**FIGURE 81-3** To reestablish a vacuum in the pleural cavity, the diaphragm laceration is closed around a rubber catheter. A positive inspiration is combined with catheter aspiration followed by catheter removal as the last suture is tied securing an airtight closure.

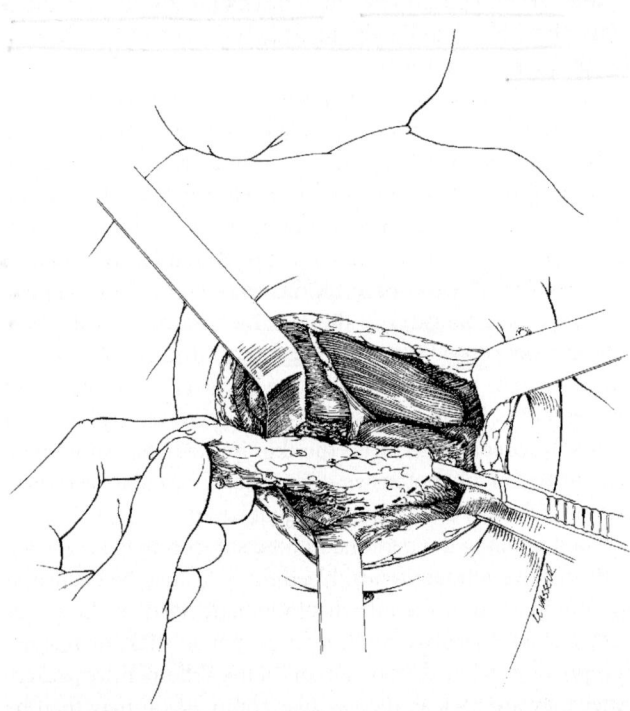

**FIGURE 81-4** Entering the lesser sac to gain control of the splenic artery and vein is done by incising the gastrocolic omentum adjacent to its attachment to the transverse colon.

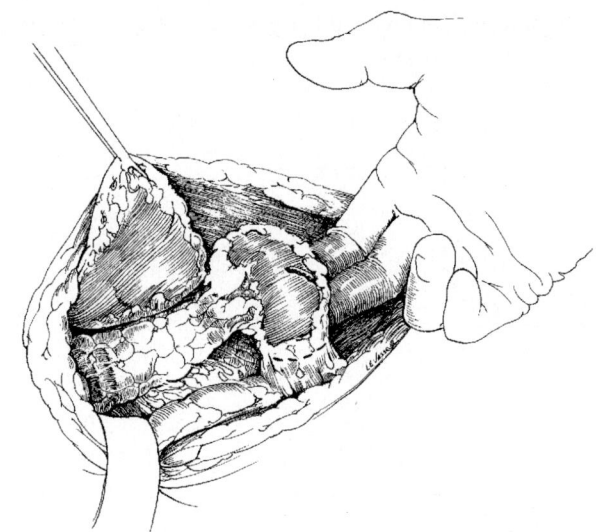

**FIGURE 81-5** By dividing the splenocolic, splenorenal, and the lateral ligaments, the spleen is mobilized out of the left upper quadrant.

injury encountered. For a simple, peripherally based laceration, horizontal mattress sutures of a large absorbable material on an atraumatic needle may be placed across the defect. Teflon pledgets may be used to prevent tearing of the splenic capsule (Fig. 81-6A, B, and C). Alternatively, a simple laceration may be approximated with deep figure-of-eight sutures to close the parenchymal deep space with capsular simple sutures in between. <u>Omentum may be incorporated into the simple sutures to improve hemostasis</u> (Fig. 81-6D, E, and F). An injury of the lower splenic pole may be repaired using horizontal "through-and-through" mattress sutures of large absorbable material on an atraumatic needle. Incorporation of the omentum or the use of Teflon pledgets may help to support the splenic capsule (Fig. 81-6G, H, and I). Historically, a technique is described that uses a spinal needle to introduce long longitudinal sutures through the splenic parenchyma. The sutures are placed in a horizontal mattress fashion, approximating the splenic parenchyma (Fig. 81-6J, K, and L). A chromic "ladder" may be constructed and wrapped around

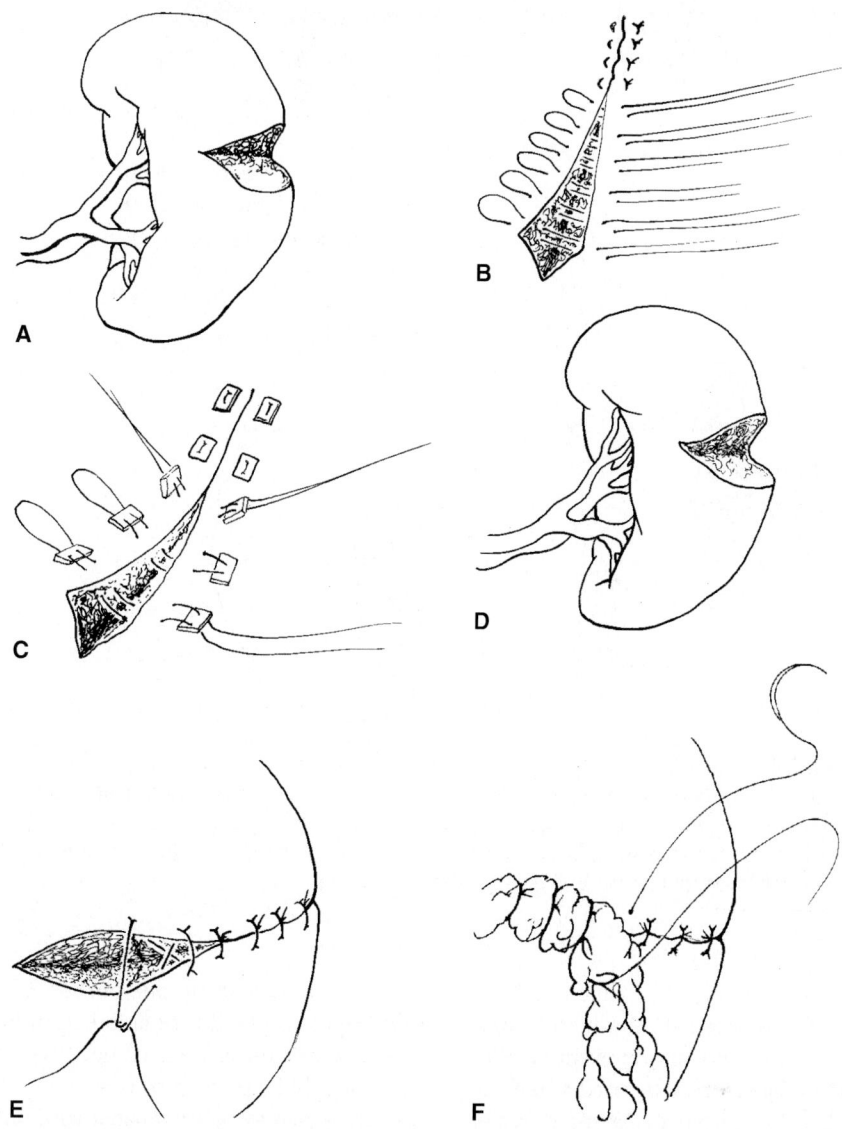

**FIGURE 81-6** **A, B, C.** For a simple peripheral splenic laceration, splenorrhaphy is done with horizontal mattress sutures with or without using pledgets. **D, E, F.** Figure-of-eight sutures placed deeply into the splenic parenchyma will effectively approximate the sides of a peripheral splenic laceration. A portion of greater omentum can be incorporated into the ties.

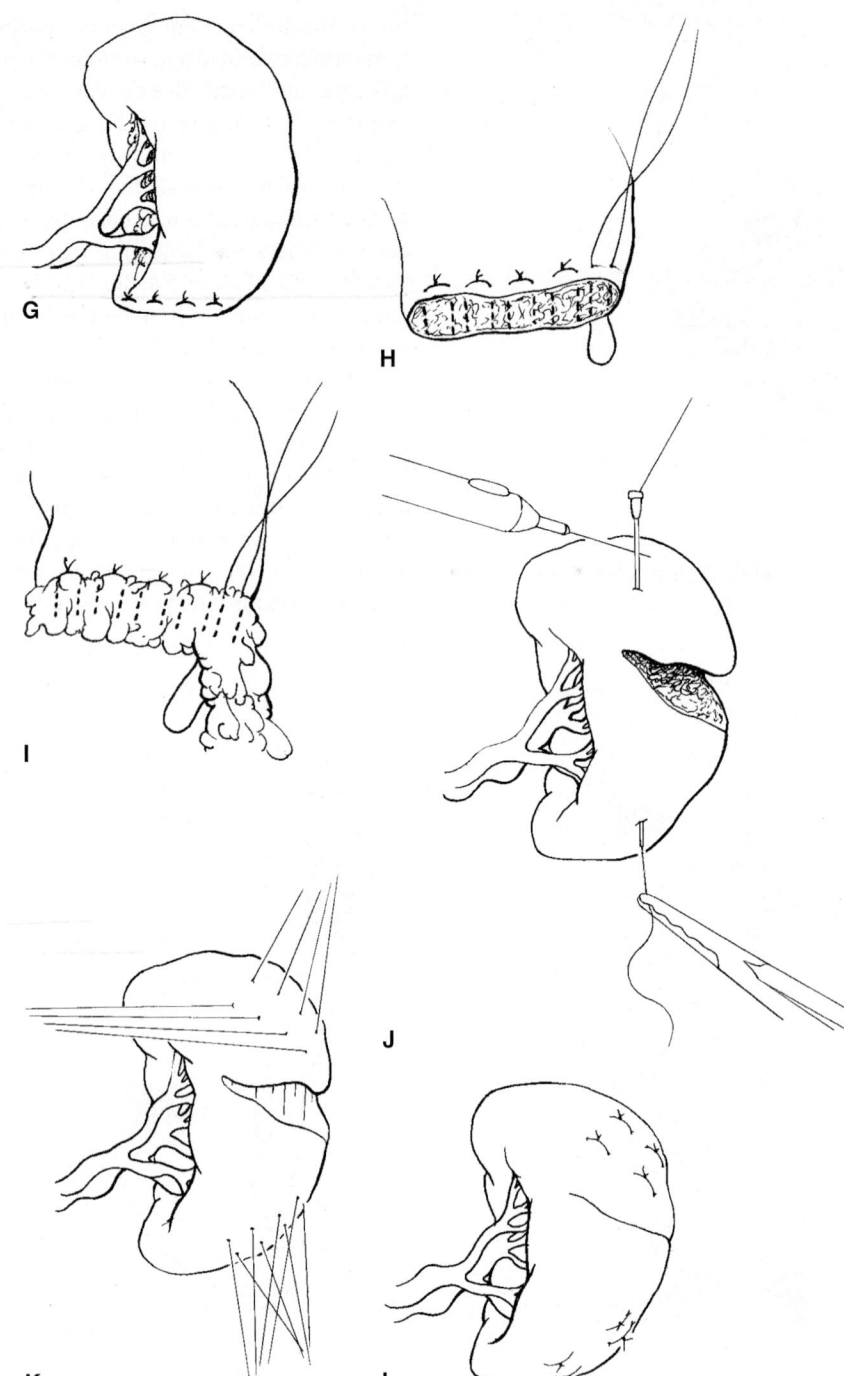

**FIGURE 81-6** (*Continued*) **G, H, I.** A lower-pole splenic laceration can be controlled with through-and-through horizontal mattress sutures, which may include omentum as a seal over the raw surface. **J, K, L.** A spinal needle is introduced across a splenic laceration. Cauterization aids hemostasis, and the needle serves as a suture passage guide for mattress sutures, which when tied, will approximate the wound edge.

the greater curvature of the spleen (Fig. 81-6M and N). Tying the chromic ladder ends together across the hilum compresses the splenic parenchyma and may prevent further bleeding. Topical hemostatic agents may be used when the capsule of the spleen has been torn from an extensive area of the surface. The spleen may then be wrapped in an absorbable mesh, compressing bleeding parenchyma (Fig. 81-6O and P). The mesh may be used to help compress other parenchymal defects with or without hemostatic agents.

Significant damage to one portion of the spleen may preclude repair. Under this situation, ligation of the involved segmental vessels and excision of the damaged, and now ischemic, tissue should be performed (Fig. 81-7). The resultant splenic edge may then be approximated with horizontal sutures and covered with omentum as demonstrated previously.

In unstable children, especially with multiple other significant injuries, who may not tolerate the time necessary to perform splenorrhaphy, splenectomy remains the procedure

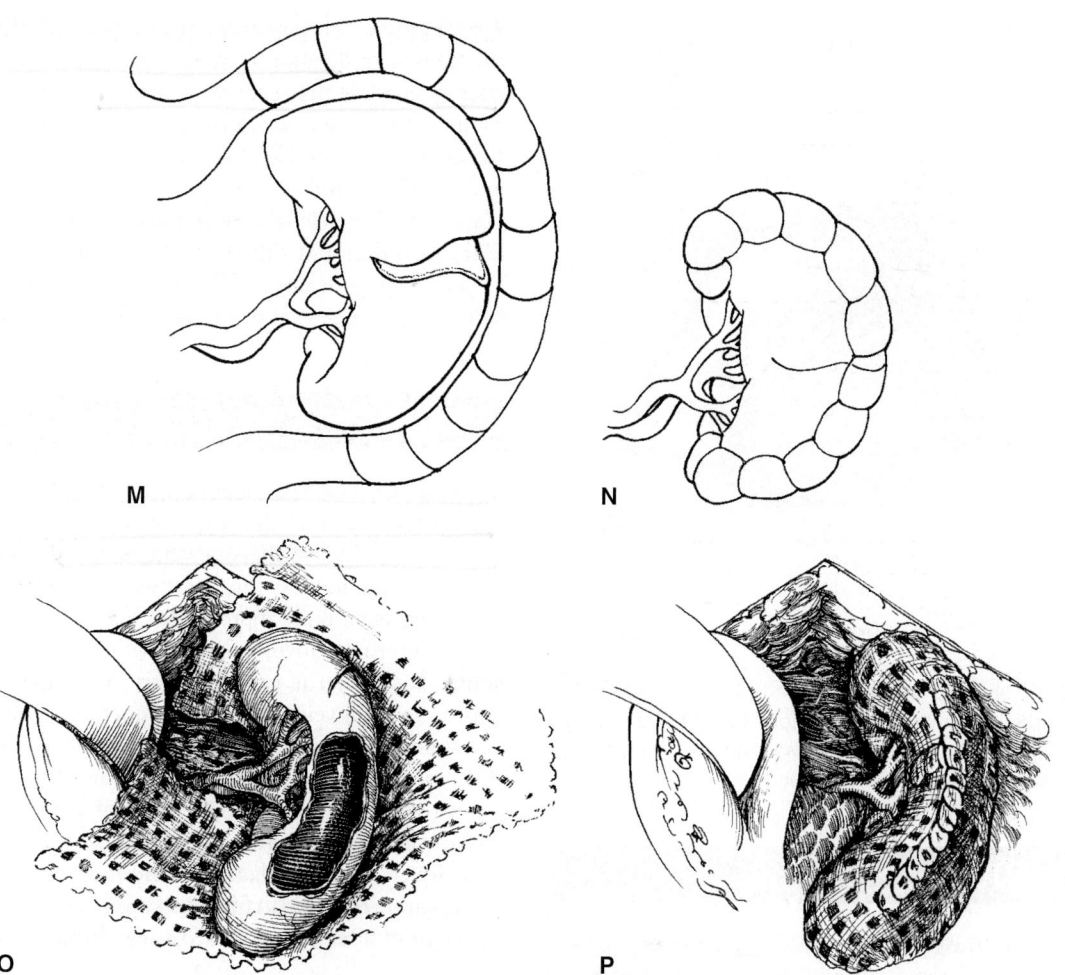

**FIGURE 81-6** *(Continued)* **M, N.** A chromic "ladder" may be constructed and wrapped around the curvature of the spleen and tied in front of or behind the splenic hilum, thus compressing the splenic parenchyma. **O, P.** The spleen is enwrapped in an absorbable mesh to compress or "tamponade" the bleeding parenchyma.

of choice. The spleen is mobilized by the above techniques and the splenic vessels are exposed through the lesser sac. The splenic artery and vein are ligated separately with large non-absorbable sutures. The short gastric vessels must be ligated carefully or divided using tissue-sealing devices to prevent postoperative bleeding.

## LIVER INJURY

Liver injury is less common than splenic injury and its anatomy is far more complex. An understanding of the varying hepatic vascular anatomy is necessary to manage these injuries properly. The arterial supply of the liver is from 2 sources: systemic and portal. The venous drainage is via 3 main hepatic veins and some short veins draining the posterior surface of the liver directly into the vena cava. The right hepatic vein is most frequently injured in blunt trauma. Liver injury results from blunt or penetrating trauma to the right upper quadrant or lower right chest. An intravenous contrast-enhanced CT scan confirms the diagnosis. Abdominal distension and hypovolemia are cardinal signs that laparotomy is imminent. However, both may be missing in children with significant hepatic injury.

Emergent laparotomy for liver injuries in children is increasingly uncommon, and is reserved for patients who remain hemodynamically unstable despite aggressive resuscitation. Later percutaneous or endoscopic interventional procedures for complications of liver injury, such as biliary leak, are more common.

In children requiring urgent laparotomy for a liver injury, preparations should be made for possible sternotomy or inguinal incision to allow the passage of an intracaval shunt. As large hemorrhage must be presumed, adequate vascular access and immediately available blood products are necessary. A generous midline incision provides excellent exposure and allows a sternal extension as necessary. Blood loss may be decreased by a variety of maneuvers, including packing. Once significant hemorrhage has been controlled, a more careful exploration for the source of bleeding and any associated injuries may be conducted. In unstable patients, complex injuries are best approached by hemorrhage control and closure, resuscitation to correct hypothermia and coagulopathy, and then, once stable, arteriography and embolization. Intricate biliary repairs and biliary-enteric bypasses are performed much less often than previously and are best reserved for when the patient is stable. Clearly nonviable tissue should be resected, but marginal tissue may prove viable on re-exploration.

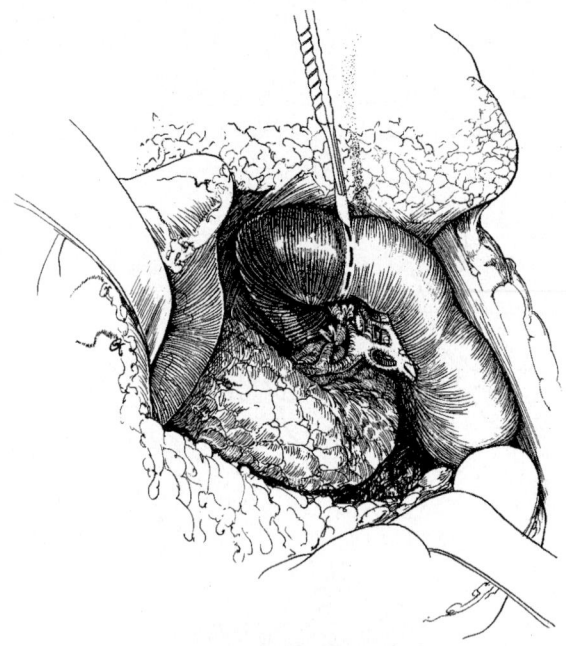

**FIGURE 81-7** Damaged portion of the spleen not repairable. Segmented resection can be safely done following the selective ligation of splenic artery and vein branches, and the cut splenic surface is managed as depicted in Fig. 81-6G, H, and I.

## TRACT INJURIES

Tract injuries are the result of penetrating injuries. Hemorrhage from these lesions typically stops spontaneously, or may be aided by manual compression of nearby liver parenchyma. This may be assisted by the use of hemostatic agents applied into the tract prior to compression. If compression does not lead to hemostasis, the wound should be opened and bleeding points isolated and ligated (Fig. 81-8). Closure of the ends of the tract may lead to hepatic rupture if there is ongoing bleeding within the tract.

## LACERATIONS

Hemorrhage from hepatic lacerations typically stops spontaneously. The surface of actively bleeding lacerations should be gently held with compression with the addition of hemostatic agents as needed. If not successful, then the laceration may be explored by using the finger-fracture technique to identify specific bleeding points and severed biliary radicals that are ligated. Deep suture ligation of the laceration without exploration is not recommended because of the risk of injury to biliary structures. Autotransfusion is useful if bowel injury is absent. If hemorrhage continues, the use of the Pringle maneuver may be useful to enable improved visualization of the laceration, and it may aid in determining the source of the hemorrhage (Fig. 81-9). If the liver hemorrhage slows in response to the Pringle maneuver, then the hemorrhage is more likely from a portal vein or hepatic artery source. If it does not decrease, then it is more likely from the hepatic veins or the retrohepatic vena cava. The maneuver may be maintained for several minutes to aid in dissection.

If a dramatic decrease in hemorrhage is obtained through the maneuver, ligation of the hepatic artery as close to the liver as possible may achieve hemostasis. An alternate technique for the control of bleeding from a liver laceration is through the use of packing placed between the diaphragm and against the inferior surface of the liver (Fig. 81-10). After hemostasis has been achieved, the laceration should be filled with omentum and sutured to the capsule with absorbable material. Large drains should be placed above and below the laceration in the event of a biliary leak (Fig. 81-11).

## PERIHEPATIC VENOUS INJURY

Voluminous dark venous bleeding that persists despite the Pringle maneuver, or that worsens with manipulation, raises the suspicion of a perihepatic venous injury. The correct surgical approach to these injuries remains controversial and the mortality rate for any approach is high.

One approach involves the placement of an atrial caval shunt. Dissection is carried around the inferior vena cava above the renal veins and a tourniquet is loosely placed. The abdominal incision is carried up through the sternum and dissection is carried out through the lowest posterior-medial aspect of the pericardium. The inferior vena cava is isolated within the lowest portion of the pericardium and a second tourniquet is loosely placed around it at that level. A purse-string suture is placed in the right-atrial appendage and a multiply fenestrated shunt is passed down through the atrium and

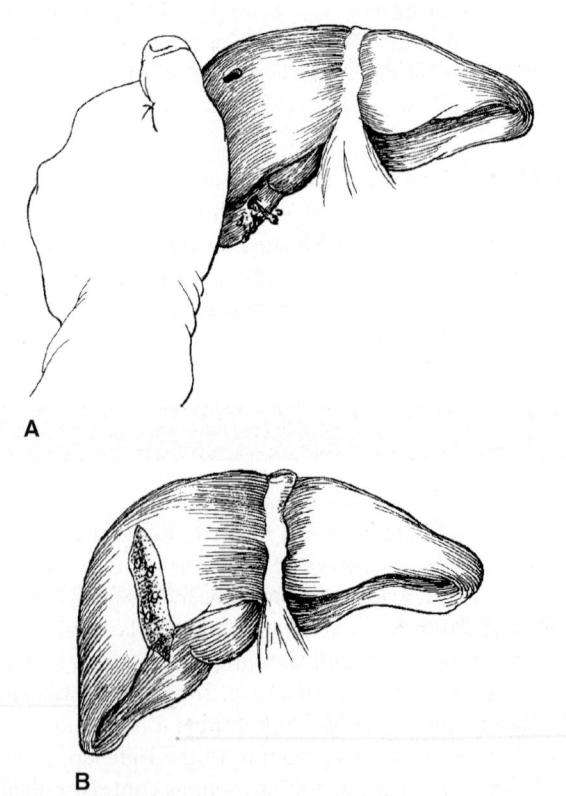

**FIGURE 81-8** A liver puncture tract injury. **A.** Compression of the parenchyma overlying the tract is often effective in achieving hemostasis. **B.** The tract has been opened, the bleeding points have been directly visualized, and suture ligatures control bleeding.

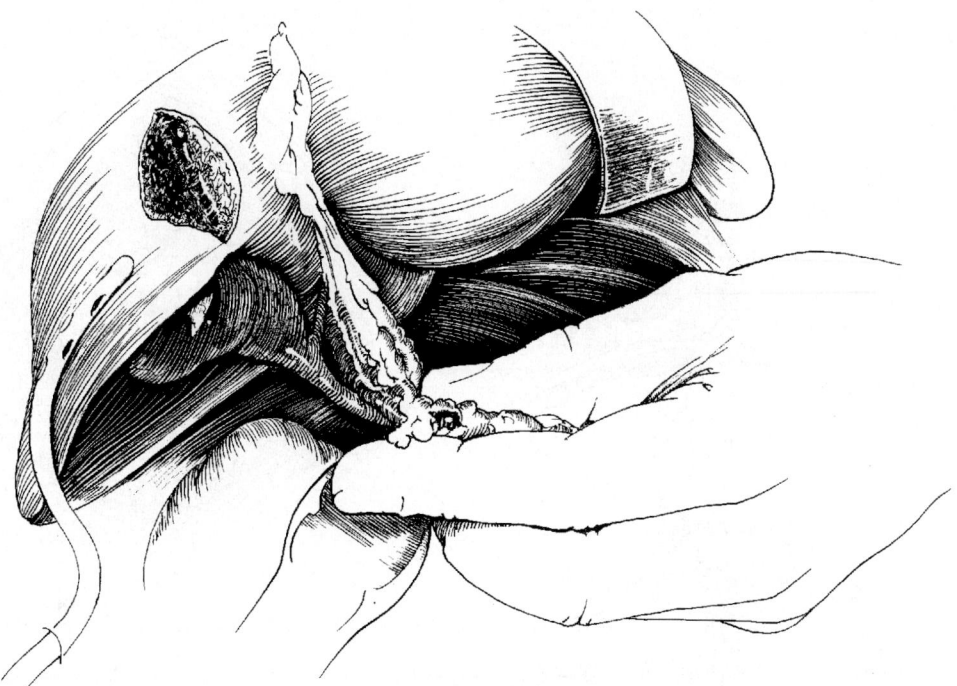

**FIGURE 81-9** Pringle maneuver by which the hepatic portal structures are compressed between the surgeon's thumb and index finger to temporarily occlude the hepatic artery and portal vein. Placement of an atraumatic vascular clamp can be used to replace the compressing fingers.

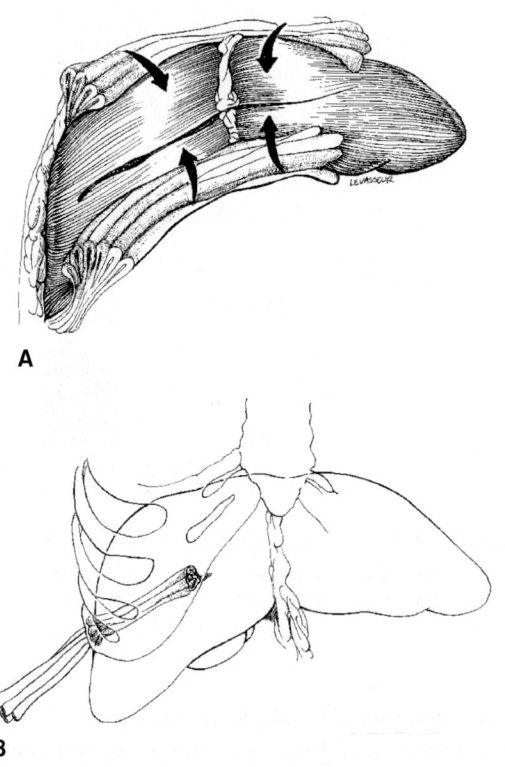

A

B

**FIGURE 81-10** An alternate technique to control liver laceration bleeding is to place packs behind the liver between the liver and diaphragm and against the inferior surface of the liver. **A.** The packs are in place and compress the laceration. **B.** Penrose drains are placed into the laceration and they are exited laterally, providing an ongoing assessment of the amount of bleeding.

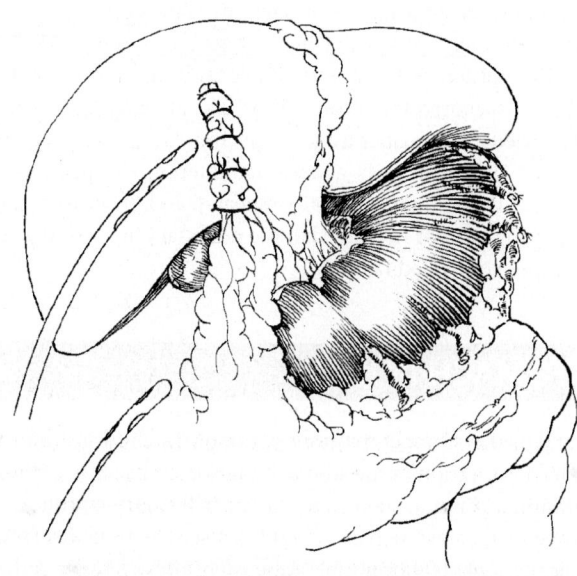

**FIGURE 81-11** The omentum stuffed into a laceration is an effective hemostatic agent. Regional drains will help quantify ongoing blood loss.

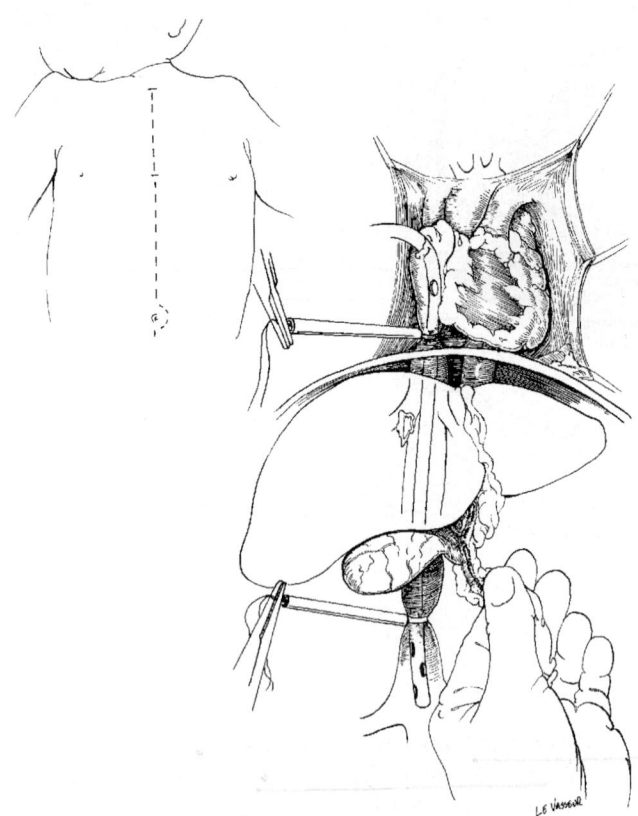

**FIGURE 81-12** Placement of an atriocaval shunt. A firm multifenestrated, large-bore plastic tube is inserted through a right-atrial appendage purse-string suture and tourniquets are secured around the vena cava just above the diaphragm and above the renal veins.

inferior vena cava and the tourniquets secured (Fig. 81-12). A modified chest tube may be used for this purpose as may an endotracheal tube, depending upon the patient's size. The top of the tube may be used as a route for large volume infusion. In combination with the Pringle maneuver, this will decrease, but not eliminate hemorrhage. The liver is then rotated medially and direct vascular repair is performed.

An alternate approach is to pack the right upper quadrant of the abdomen until visible hemostasis is obtained and closing. The patient is then resuscitated and any coagulopathy and acidosis corrected. From 24 to 72 hours later, the patient is returned to the operating room and the packs carefully removed. If bleeding is again encountered, the packing is replaced. This sequence may be repeated and, if suture repair of the vena cava or hepatic vein are necessary, it is conducted in a more controlled fashion.

## STOMACH INJURY

Injury to the stomach is more common in children than in adults. Perforation of the stomach may occur because of blunt abdominal trauma, such as in the lap belt injury complex, or iatrogenic factors, such as forceful nasogastric tube insertion. Typically, a plain abdominal radiograph shows free air and an abnormal position of the nasogastric tube.

Rupture of the stomach occurs along the greater curvature in the region of the fundus. If this injury is discovered,

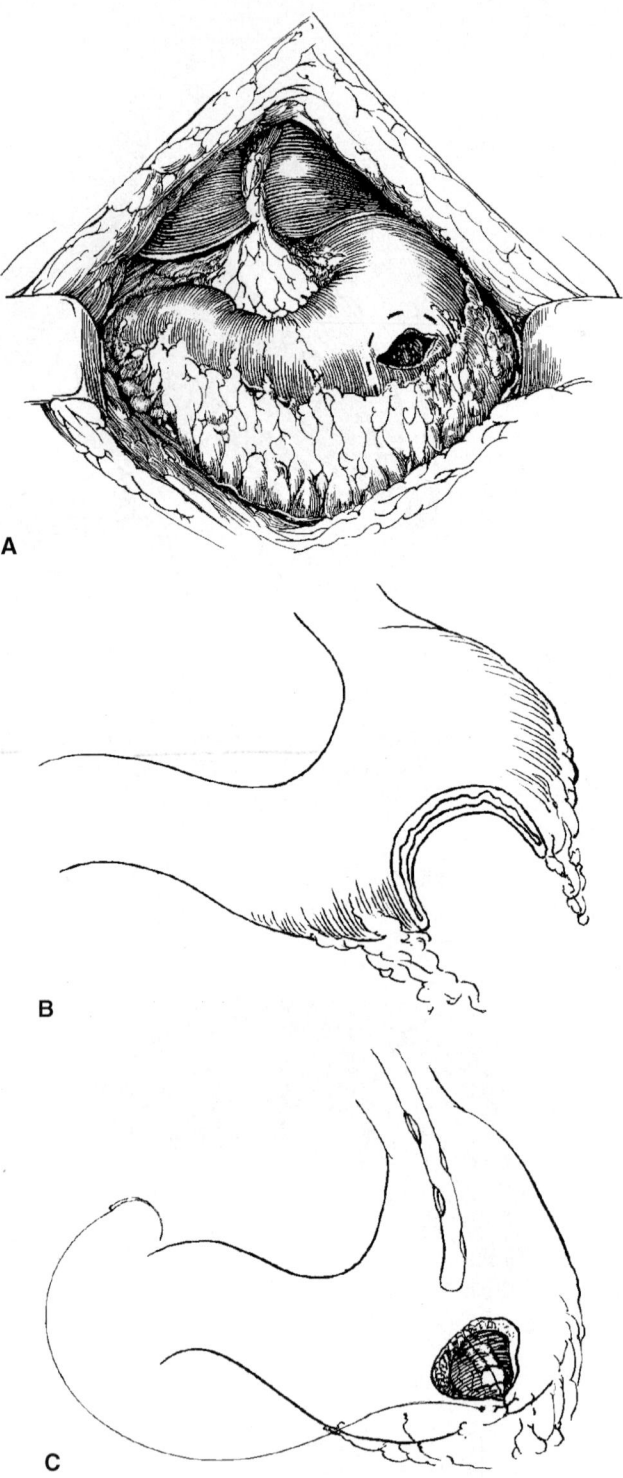

**FIGURE 81-13** A gastric injury. **A.** Typical anterior wall greater curvature blow out injury. **B.** A 2-layer closure is preferred after débridement of devitalized tissue. **C.** Postoperatively, a nasogastric tube is left in place.

a careful exploration should be performed to exclude other injuries. Elevation of the left lobe of the liver with a retractor allows exposure of the stomach from the esophagus to the duodenum. The gastrocolic ligament is divided and the lesser sac is entered to inspect the posterior surface of the stomach and pancreas. The edges of a gastric perforation are debrided to viable tissue and approximated in 2 layers. A nasogastric tube should be placed (Fig. 81-13).

## PANCREATIC INJURY

The pancreas may be injured through a variety of means, but blunt trauma from a handle bar, a punch, or compression by the lap belt during a motor vehicle crash are the usual mechanisms of injury. Signs of pancreatic injury may be subtle. Plain radiographs of the abdomen are likely to be normal. Patients often present with increasing epigastric discomfort hours after a seemingly minor event or occult intentional injury. Serum amylase may be normal initially, only to rise significantly over the following hours. Abdominal CT scan with intravenous contrast is typically diagnostic, but initial CT scan findings, prior to significant retroperitoneal inflammation, may be subtle.

The management of pancreatic injuries remains controversial, as many resolve without operation. Nonoperative management has been practiced successfully even for children with proven ductal injury. Prompt endoscopic retrograde cholangiopancreatography with laparotomy and distal pancreatectomy has been shown to shorten the length of stay in children with suspected ductal injury in a small number of patients. However, patients with distal ductal injuries have been also managed successfully with external or delayed internal drainage of resultant pancreatic pseudocysts, sparing many children laparotomy. One report describes the successful management of pancreatic ductal injuries through the use of an endoscopically placed pancreatic ductal stent. On occasion, the diagnosis of ductal injury is delayed for several days, and surrounding inflammation may make resection more difficult. The presence of bile staining, gastrointestinal contents, or air in the retroperitoneum indicate associated intestinal injury.

The entire abdomen should be prepped and draped. A broad transverse upper abdominal incision should be used in younger children and a vertical midline incision in older children. Mobilization and inspection of the upper abdominal contents should be performed to rule out associated injuries. This should include a wide Kocher maneuver and inspection of the entire gland (Fig. 81-14). The lateral attachments of the second portion of the duodenum are divided and the duodenum is retracted medially, exposing the vena cava and the head of the pancreas, which is palpated. The gastrocolic omentum is divided and the anterior surface of the pancreas is inspected after the stomach is retracted superiorly.

## DISTAL PANCREATIC DUCTAL INJURY

Pancreatic ductal lacerations distal to the superior mesenteric artery and vein may be treated by distal pancreatectomy with splenic preservation. The gastrocolic and splenocolic ligaments are divided. The stomach is retracted upward and the colon downward. The inferior border of the pancreas is separated from the retroperitoneal tissues by blunt dissection from the superior mesenteric vein to the splenic hilum (Fig. 81-15).

Distal pancreatic tributaries of the splenic artery and vein are then carefully identified, ligated, and divided. In certain patients, the time required for this meticulous dissection may

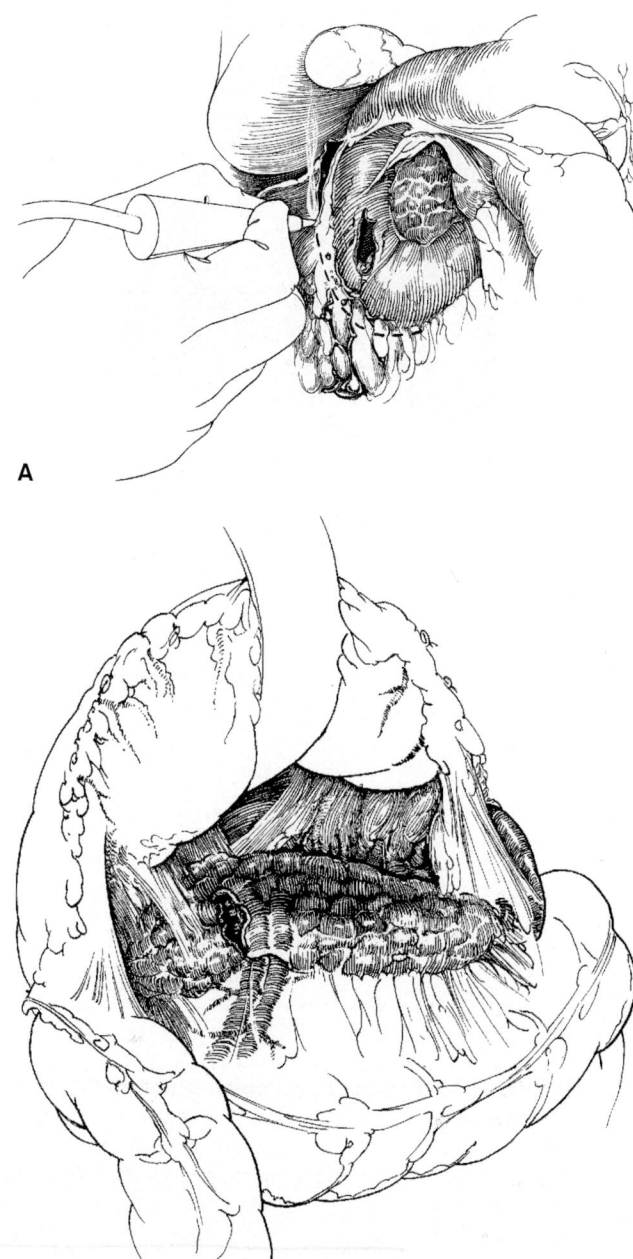

**A**

**B**

**FIGURE 81-14** Exposure to assess the injured pancreas. **A.** A Kocher maneuver is done, incising the peritoneum along the lateral duodenal wall. Medial retraction will expose the pancreatic head as well as the retroduodenal vena cava. **B.** After division of the gastrocolic ligament and superior retraction of the stomach and inferior traction on the colon, the anterior surface of the pancreas is exposed.

not be available, or the splenic artery and vein may be injured. In these situations, the splenic artery and vein may be ligated and divided as they depart the posterior–superior surface of the pancreas.

The pancreas is divided proximal to the injury and the main pancreatic duct is ligated with nonabsorbable suture. The parenchyma is closed with mattress sutures and external drains are placed. The spleen should then be inspected at the completion of the pancreatic resection to ensure its viability based upon the short gastric vessels. If not, a splenectomy is performed.

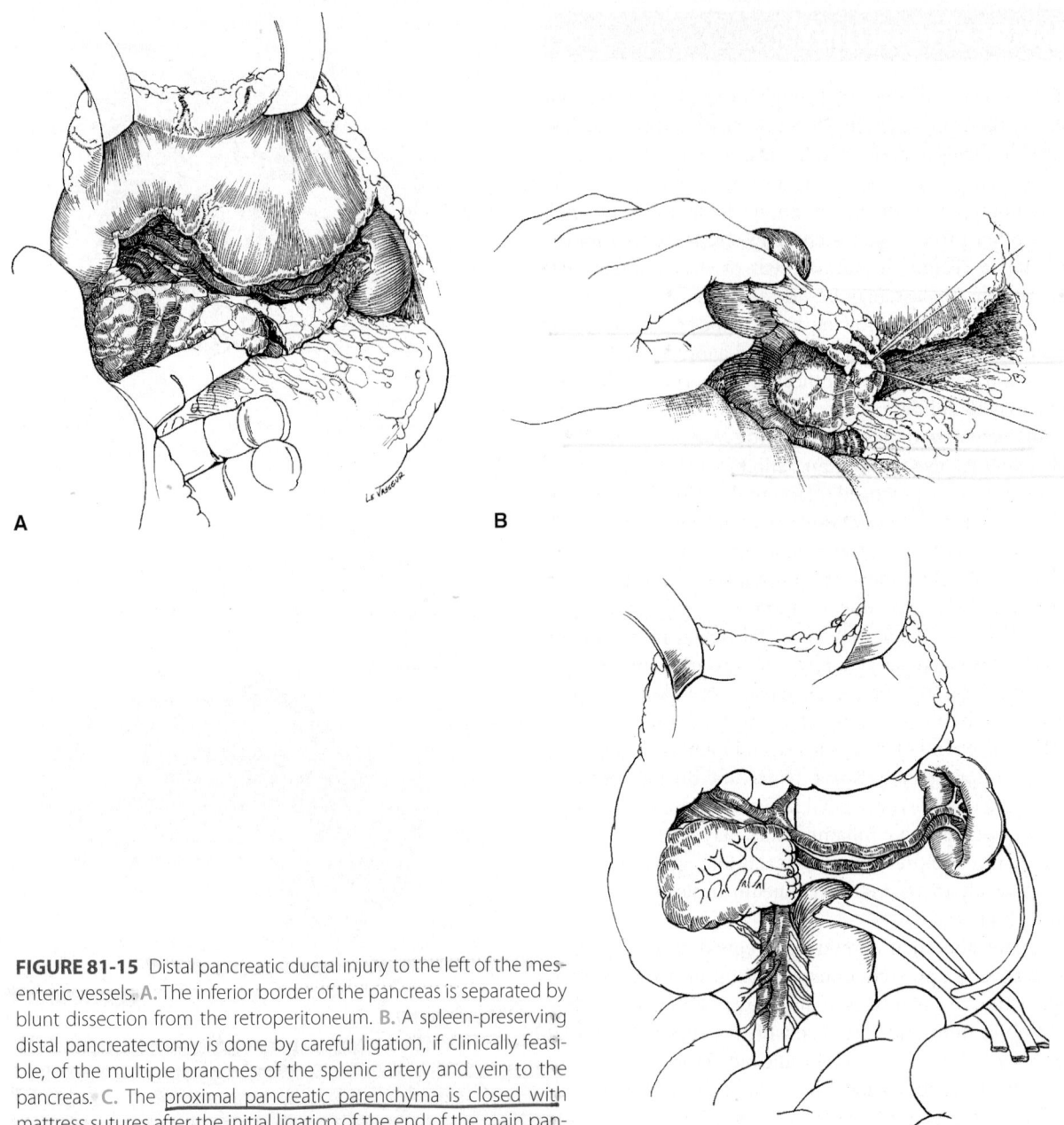

**FIGURE 81-15** Distal pancreatic ductal injury to the left of the mesenteric vessels. **A.** The inferior border of the pancreas is separated by blunt dissection from the retroperitoneum. **B.** A spleen-preserving distal pancreatectomy is done by careful ligation, if clinically feasible, of the multiple branches of the splenic artery and vein to the pancreas. **C.** The proximal pancreatic parenchyma is closed with mattress sutures after the initial ligation of the end of the main pancreatic duct with a nonabsorbable suture. Drains are placed in the pancreatic bed.

# PROXIMAL PANCREATIC DUCTAL INJURY

An injury to the pancreatic duct proximal to the superior mesenteric artery and vein is a difficult problem, and its repair is fraught with complications, including anastomotic stenosis, pancreatic fistulae and possible pancreatic insufficiency after extensive resection. Operation should be reserved for those patients in whom other measures are deemed insufficient, and resection should be avoided at initial operation, whereas extensive simple drainage is a viable alternative.

If operation is necessary, an attempt should be made to preserve the distal pancreatic segment with a Roux-en-Y pancreaticojejunostomy. The proximal severed end of the pancreatic duct is carefully identified, and then ligated with nonabsorbable suture. The proximal parenchyma is oversewn with mattress sutures. A Roux loop of jejunum is then fashioned (Fig. 81-16). The open end of the distal jejunal limb is closed and an end-to-side pancreaticojejunostomy is performed with a posterior row of 3-0 silk sutures to approximate the pancreatic capsule to the jejunal serosa. The posterior wall of the duct is then anastomosed to the jejunal mucosa with interrupted 5-0 prolene sutures and the anastomosis is stented using a shortened 5-French

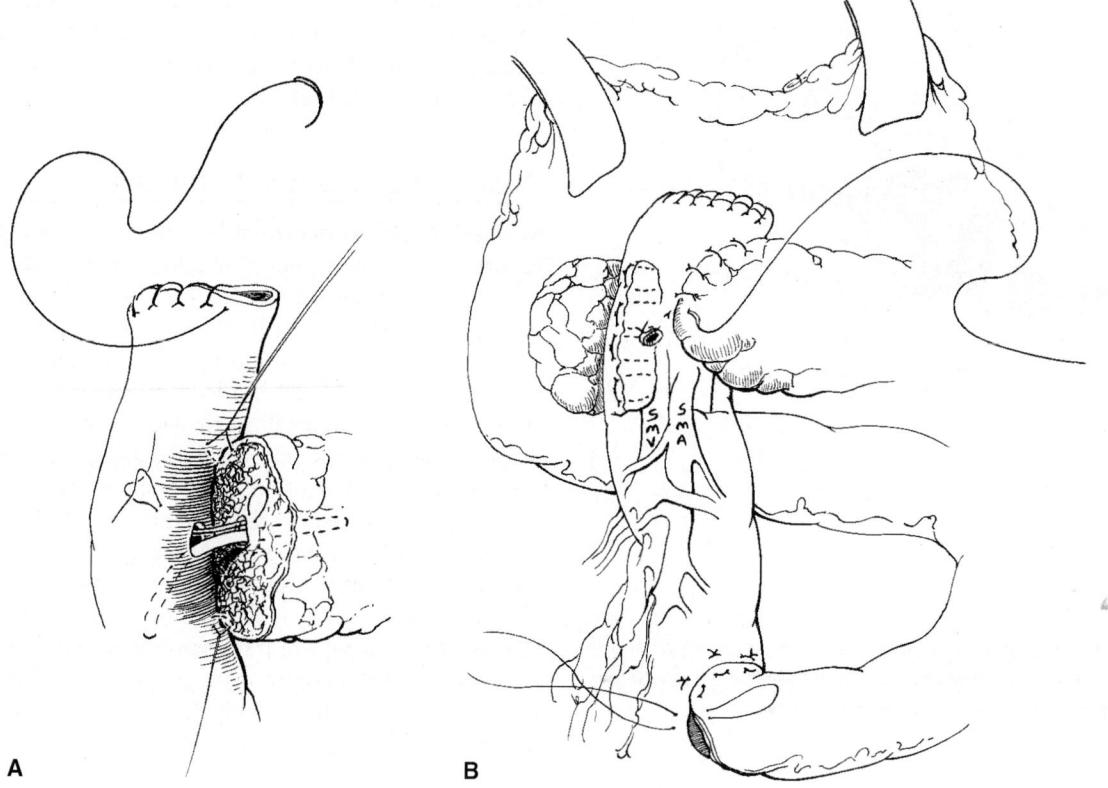

**FIGURE 81-16** Repair of a proximal pancreatic ductal injury. **A.** A Roux-en-Y pancreaticojejunostomy is done using an intraductal stent. **B.** A second row of Lembert sutures buries the pancreas into the side of the jejunum and the Roux-en-Y connection is completed.

feeding tube, which is tacked to the jejunal mucosa by using an absorbable suture. The ductal anastomosis is then completed. An anterior row of Lembert sutures is used to bury the pancreas into the jejunum and the creation of the Roux loop is completed. The area is covered with omentum and drained well.

## COMBINED DUODENAL, COMMON BILE DUCT, AND MAJOR PANCREATIC DUCT INJURY

This is a devastating injury that can be fatal if treated with drainage alone; it requires aggressive management. The repair performed will depend on the specific injuries encountered, as well as on the stability of the patient. In the rare situation that a patient suffers extensive duodenal and pancreatic injuries yet is able to tolerate a protracted operation, and the surgical team is experienced in the procedure, a pancreatic–duodenal resection with immediate reconstruction can be considered. An alternative to extensive resection includes exclusion of the pylorus with a pursestring of large nonabsorbable suture material, primary duodenal repair, and loop gastrojejunostomy with extensive external regional drainage.

In either instance, a generous Kocher maneuver is performed and careful inspection of the duodenum and pancreas is performed to adequately assess the anterior and posterior surfaces of each structure. The gastrocolic ligament is then divided and the pancreas is exposed through the lesser sac to inspect the front of the gland. If resection is chosen, the common bile duct is identified. A plane is developed between the neck of the pancreas and the anterior aspect of the portal and superior mesenteric vessels by finger dissection. The inferior border of the pancreas is dissected free and the pancreas is rotated cephalad. Tributaries from the splenic artery and vein to the pancreas are ligated and divided. Two noncrushing intestinal clamps are then placed, and the pancreas is divided between them. The first part of the duodenum is preserved if possible, and the distal duodenum is divided. A noncrushing bulldog clamp is placed on the common bile duct and it is divided distal to the clamp. Finally, a cholecystectomy is performed. The third and fourth portions of the duodenum are mobilized and the jejunum is divided distal to the ligament of Treitz. The arterial and venous branches to the uncinate process are divided and the specimen is then removed. The completed reconstruction is with an end-to-side pancreaticojejunostomy, end-to-side choledochojejunostomy, and an antecolic duodenojejunostomy (Fig. 81-17). The biliary and pancreatic anastomoses are performed as stated previously with interrupted 5-0 prolene interrupted sutures to the jejunal mucosa, stented to minimize anastomotic stenosis.

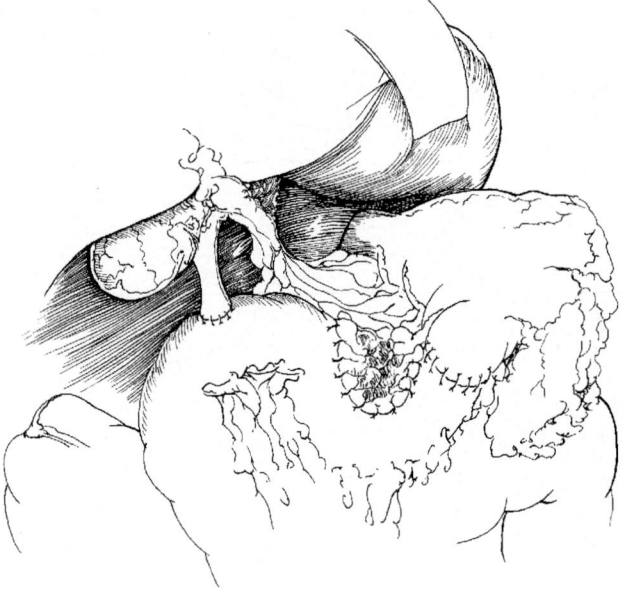

**FIGURE 81-17** Management of a combined duodenal, common bile duct, and major pancreatic duct injury. Reconstruction is completed with a pancreaticojejunostomy, end-to-side choledochojejunostomy, and an antecolic duodenojejunostomy.

## DUODENUM INJURY

### Duodenal Hematoma

Children have weaker abdominal muscles, a wider costal arch, and a narrow anteroposterior diameter. Consequently, the duodenum lies in a more exposed position and is prone to injury in abdominal trauma. Intramural duodenal hematoma can result from a direct blow to the epigastrium, such as a bicycle handlebar, which compresses the duodenum against the spine. Symptoms are those of proximal intestinal obstruction. The diagnosis may be suspected on physical examination and, although CT scan is helpful, the diagnosis is best confirmed by upper gastrointestinal series or ultrasonography. The management is nonoperative as the hematoma resolves over 2 to 3 weeks. If a large duodenal hematoma is encountered during laparotomy, it should be evacuated (Fig. 81-18). The serosa is incised and the clot

gently removed. The submucosa is usually intact and any obvious bleeding points on it are carefully cauterized. The serosa with attached muscularis is then reapproximated with interrupted 4-0 sutures.

### Duodenal Laceration/Perforation

Most full-thickness duodenal lacerations can be closed primarily. A Kocher maneuver should be performed to carefully inspect for any associated injuries. Extensive injuries may require exclusion of the pylorus to protect the duodenal repair, or may be addressed using a "patch" of jejunum using either a Roux-en-Y limb or a loop of jejunum (Fig. 81-19). Breakdown of a duodenal repair with uncontrolled leakage of duodenal contents may be devastating, and any repair with an increased risk of breakdown should be drained both internally and extensively. Longitudinal or oblique tears are closed in the direction of the injury to prevent narrowing of the duodenal lumen. Mucosal approximation is imperative and is accomplished by a vertical mattress suture in 1 layer (Fig. 81-19). A complete transection is repaired with a primary end-to-end anastomosis using a 2-layer closure, with care taken to ensure that the bile and pancreatic ducts are not involved.

## JEJUNOILEAL INJURIES

Injury to the small intestine can result from penetrating injuries, or may follow even mild blunt trauma. Children involved in motor vehicle collisions who are restrained solely by a lap seat belt may suffer the lap belt complex of injuries, which includes abdominal-wall ecchymosis, lumbar spine injury, and intra-abdominal injury. While the majority of patients with intestinal injury have signs of peritoneal irritation on presentation, the diagnosis may prove difficult, especially in children with a brain injury. Free air is commonly not seen on initial plain radiographs and is present only 25% of the time on initial abdominal CT scan, which may reveal free peritoneal fluid without solid-organ injury. Demonstration of intestinal injury mandates prompt laparotomy, as mortality increases with a delay in operative management of more than 24 hours.

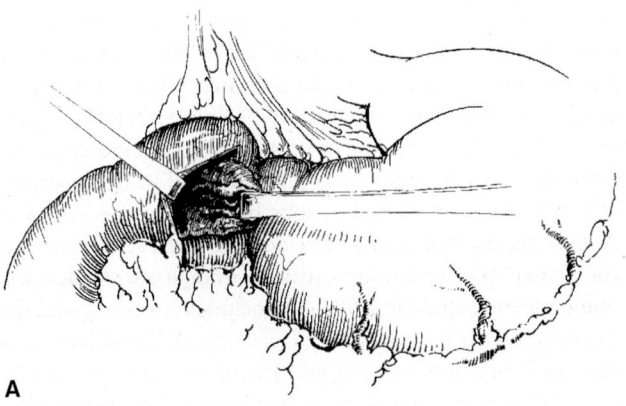
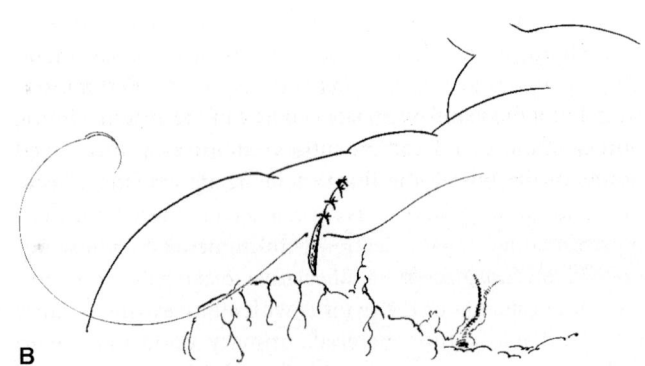

**A**    **B**

**FIGURE 81-18** Evacuation of a duodenal hematoma found at laparotomy. **A.** A serosal incision is made and the clot is pulled or sucked out of its intramural location. **B.** The seromuscular area is then reapproximated.

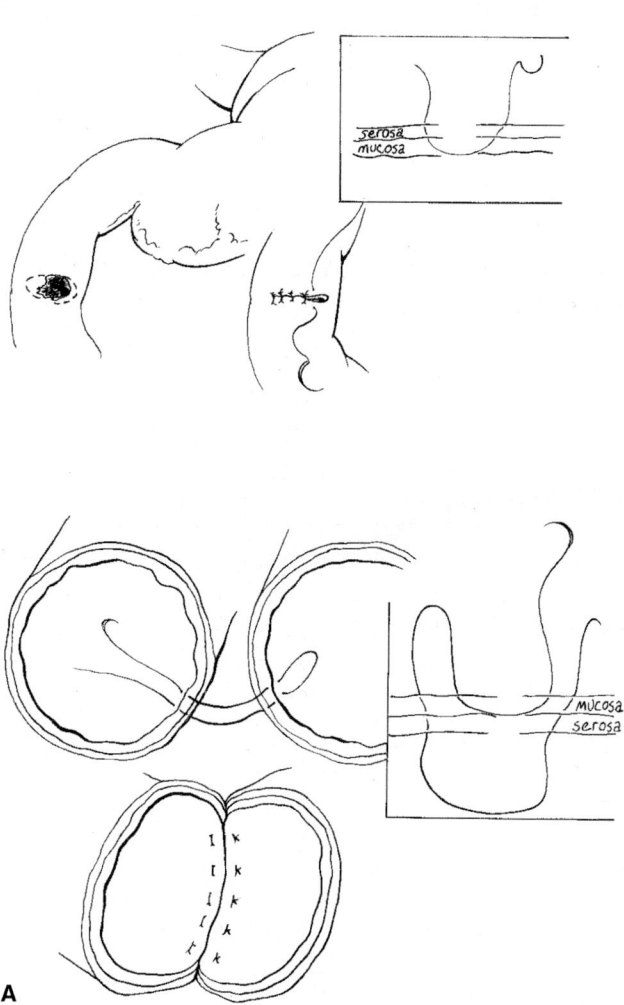

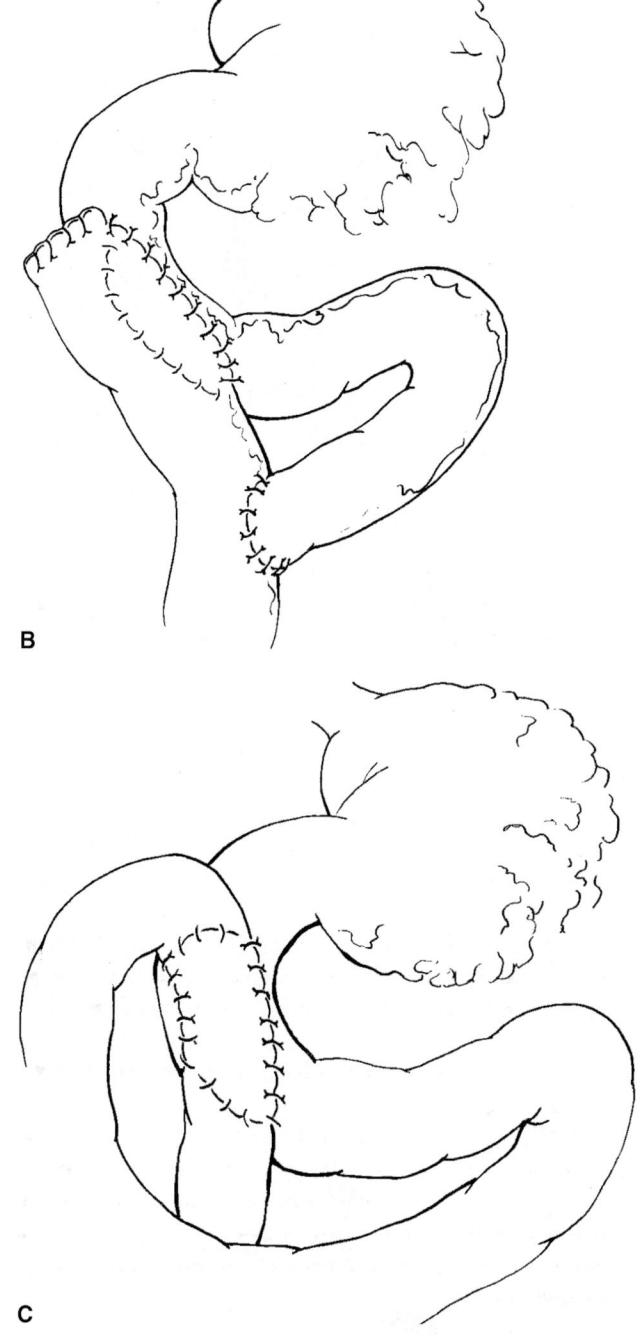

**FIGURE 81-19** Repair of a duodenal laceration. **A.** Mucosal approximation is critical, and the use of a 1-layer vertical mattress suture is an effective technique. **B.** A Roux-en-Y loop of jejunum is used to form a duodenojejunostomy and to restore gastrointestinal continuity. **C.** A loop of jejunum can also be used as a patch duodenojejunostomy either for luminal continuity or for reinforcing coverage.

Laparotomy is performed as described earlier. Perforations from blunt mechanisms typically occur in the antimesenteric border of the bowel and are most common near the 2 fixed points of the bowel: the ligament of Treitz and the cecum. Serosal injuries should be repaired or, when extensive, the injured segment of intestine resected. The majority of injuries may be repaired primarily, or resected and a primary anastomosis performed without the creation of an intestinal stoma (Figs. 81-20 and 81-21). In patients with multiple intestinal perforations amid otherwise viable bowel, such as from a shotgun blast, the perforations may be rapidly approximated using a skin-stapling device.

## MESENTERIC INJURY: MESENTERIC HEMATOMA

A mesenteric hematoma is a common finding in blunt abdominal trauma. A hematoma should not be opened unless it is expanding, which may indicate significant vascular injury. If a hematoma is opened, bleeding vessels should be ligated and the adjacent bowel inspected to assess viability (Fig. 81-22). If the bowel viability is questionable, a resection and primary anastomosis is performed (Fig. 81-23).

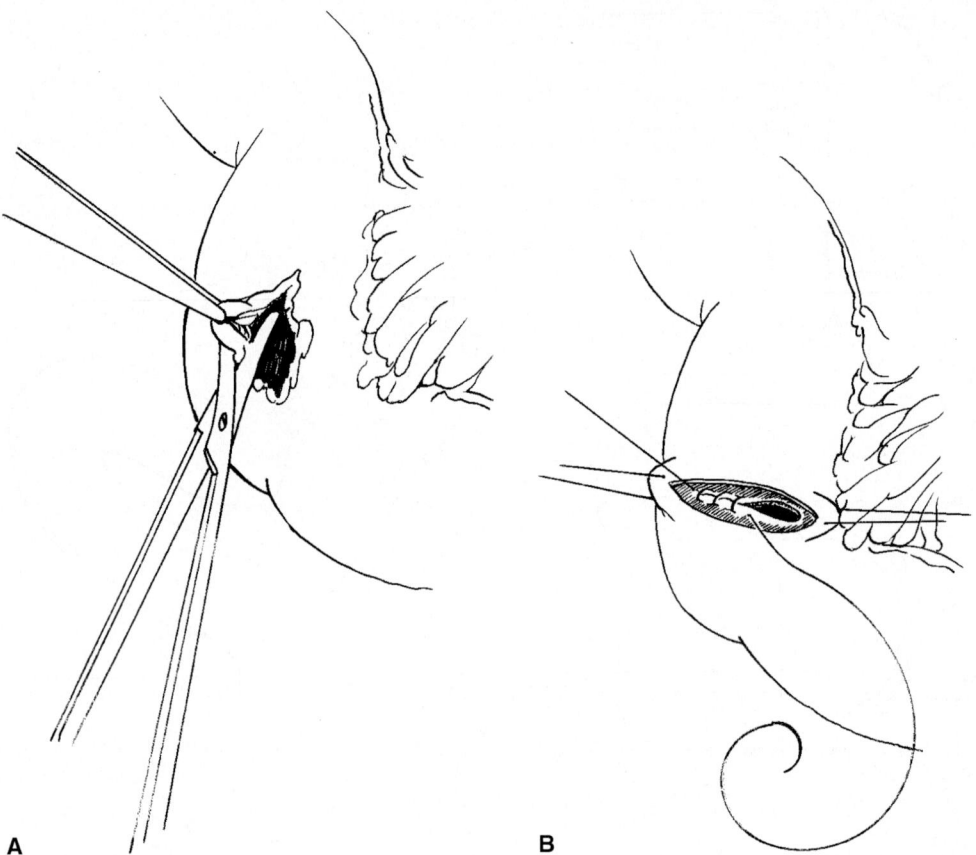

A                              B

**FIGURE 81-20** Penetrating intestinal injuries or blunt blowout injuries are débrided (A) and primarily closed transversely, typically in 2 layers. **B.** With a loss of mesentery, resection and anastomosis is more typically done.

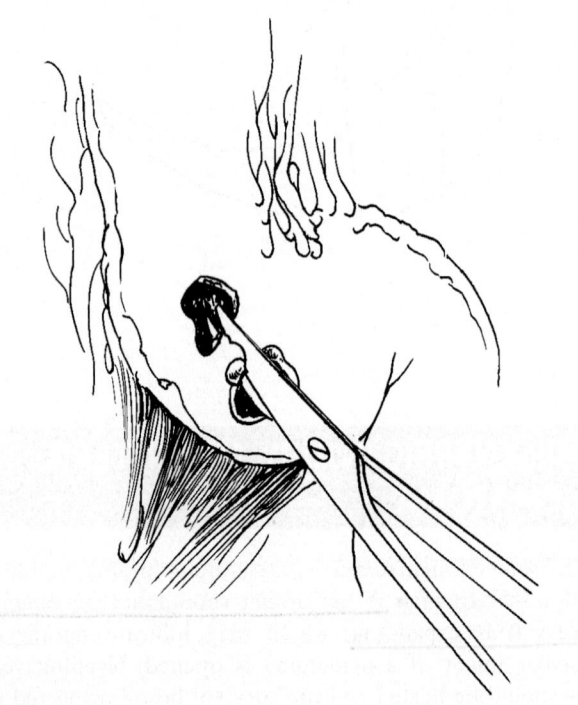

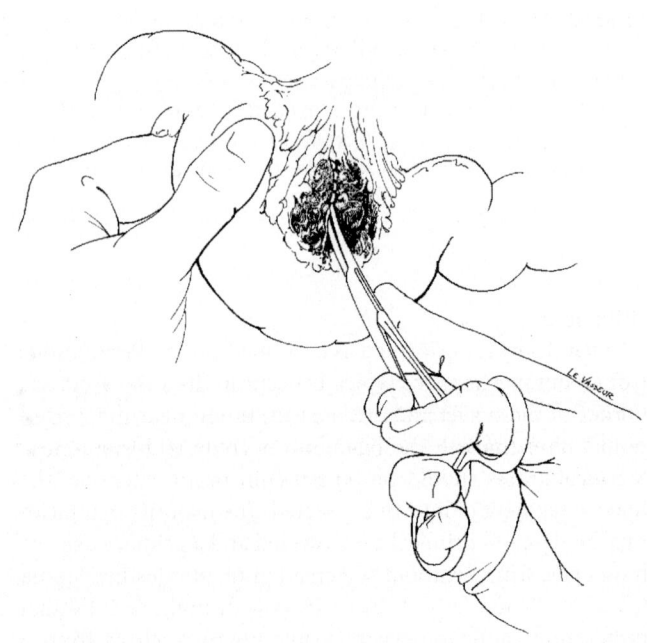

**FIGURE 81-21** Following multiple intestinal perforations, intervening short bridges of intestinal wall are best excised and débrided, and wall reconstruction is incorporated into a single repair.

**FIGURE 81-22** If a mesenteric hematoma is expanding, it should be opened, evacuated, and the bleeding vessels ligated or coagulated.

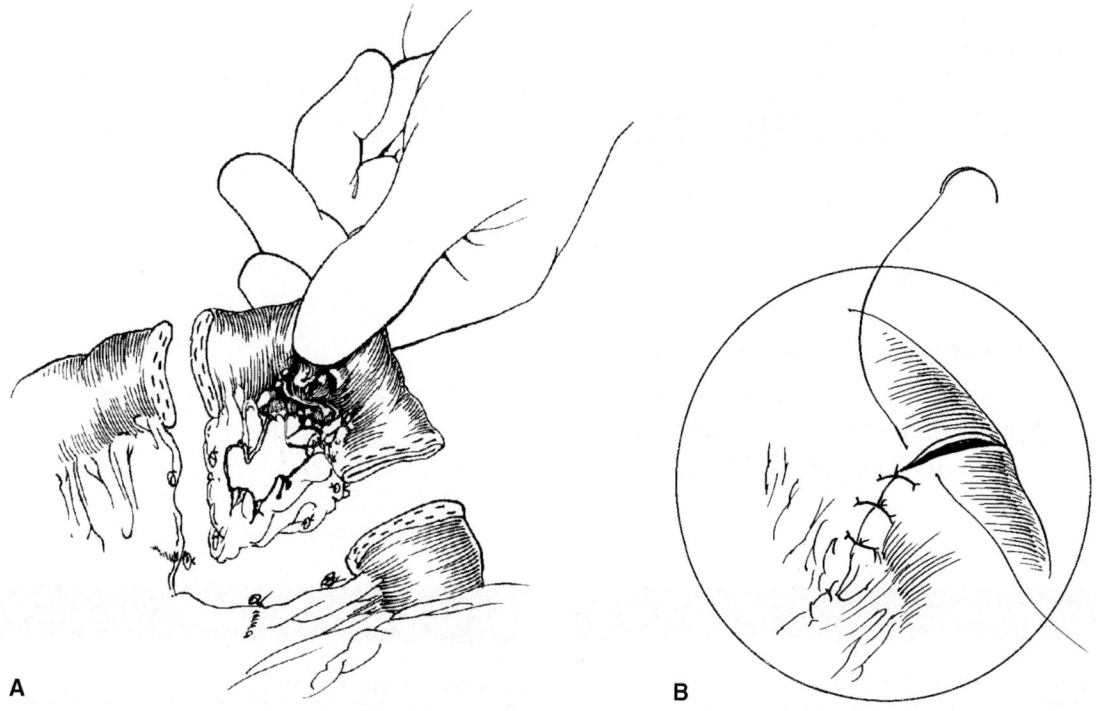

**FIGURE 81-23** If following a mesenteric injury, there is compromise of the circulation to the bowel, a segmental resection (**A**) should be done followed by primary end-to-end anastomosis (**B**).

## COLON

Colonic injuries are uncommon in children and are usually the result of penetrating trauma. Primary repair is appropriate for most colonic injuries, even with peritoneal contamination, and diverting colostomy is rarely necessary. Small puncture wounds are closed with interrupted Lembert sutures. For larger wounds, the edges are débrided and the perforation is closed in 2 layers in a transverse direction. For more extensive injuries with a devitalized segment of bowel, a colon resection and primary anastomosis is done.

## RECTUM

Penetrating rectal trauma most commonly results from child abuse, but may occur from falling on posts or other sharp objects. The diagnosis may be suspected on physical examination, but may require examination under anesthesia and proctoscopy to adequately determine the depth of injury. Full-thickness rectal injuries require diversion of the fecal stream with a proximal colostomy, although this has been questioned. A layered closure of the rectal wall is done and the retrorectal space anterior to the coccyx is drained. Associated vaginal tears are repaired primarily in layers. Significant rectal injuries commonly involve the anal sphincter mechanism, and a careful evaluation and repair of the sphincter mechanism is performed at the initial operation.

## ACKNOWLEDGMENTS

The authors thank Dr. Martin Eichelberger for his extensive contributions to previous editions of this chapter.

## SELECTED READINGS

Bonnard A, Zamakhshary M, Wales PW. Outcomes and management of rectal injuries in children. *Pediatr Surg Int* 2007;23(11):1071–1076.

Canty TG Sr, Weinman D. Treatment of pancreatic disruption in children by an endoscopically placed stent. The Fifth International Conference on Pediatric Trauma. Beaver Creek, CO, June, 2000.

Christiano JG, Tummers M, Kennedy A. Clinical significance of isolated intraperitoneal fluid on computerized tomography in pediatric blunt abdominal trauma. *J Pediatr Surg* 2009;44(6):1242–1248.

Civit CJ. Imaging children with abdominal trauma. *Am J Roentgenol* 2009;192(5):1179–1189.

Gaines BA. Intra-abdominal solid organ injury in children: diagnosis and treatment. *J Trauma* 2009;67(2 Suppl):S135–S139.

Gaines BA, Rutkoski JD. The role of laparoscopy in pediatric trauma. *Semin Pediatr Surg* 2010;19(4):300–303.

Kiankhooy A, Sartorelli KH, Vane DW, et al. Angiographic embolization is safe and effective therapy for blunt abdominal solid organ injury in children. *J Trauma* 2010;68(3):526–531.

Letton RW, Worrell V, Tuggle DW, et al. Delay in diagnosis and treatment of blunt intestinal perforation does not adversely affect prognosis in the pediatric trauma patient. *J Trauma* 2010;68(4):790–795.

Lynn KN, Werder GM, Callaghan RM, et al. Pediatric blunt splenic trauma: a comprehensive review. *Pediatr Radiol* 2009;39(9):904–916.

Malek MM, Shah SR, Kane TD. Video. Laparoscopic splenic-preserving distal pancreatectomy for trauma in a child. *Surg Endosc* 2010;24(10):2623.

Paris C, Brindamour M, Ouimet A, et al. Predictive indicators for bowel injury in pediatric patients who present with a positive seat belt sign after motor vehicle collision. *J Pediatr Surg* 2010;45(5):921–924.

Stylianos S. Liver injuries and damage control. *Semin Pediatr Surg* 2001; 10(1):23–25.

Walker ML. The damage control laparotomy. *J Natl Med Assoc* 1995;87:119.

*Roger Cornwall, James C. Gilbert,*
*Peter F. Sturm, Robert S. Hatch,*
*Richard M. Schwend, William W. Robertson Jr,*
*and Douglas G. Armstrong*

## KEY POINTS

1. Accurate diagnosis of injuries to the growth plate in extremity injuries is critical to avoiding growth arrest in pediatric extremity injuries.

2. Vascular injuries are associated with knee and elbow injuries. Patients with stable orthopaedic injuries should undergo repair of the vascular injury first. With unstable injuries, temporary arterial bypass can provide time for stabilization of the bony injury followed by definitive vascular repair.

3. In children, compartment syndrome is characterized by analgesia, agitation, and anxiety. Normal pulses and capillary refill do not rule out compartment syndrome.

## INTRODUCTION

This chapter discusses a broad array of injuries to the extremities, covering general principles, specific injuries, and complications, and highlighting in particular the areas in which the fields of pediatric surgery and pediatric orthopaedic surgery intersect. The content is divided into 7 sections: (a) general principles (b) vascular injuries; (c) compartment syndrome; (d) fractures and dislocations of the upper extremity; (e) fractures and dislocations of the lower extremity; (f) the mangled extremity and amputation; and (g) nonaccidental trauma (NAT). This chapter will provide a framework for approaching the child with an extremity injury as well as specific strategies for treating common injuries and their complications. Familiarity with an overall approach to the identification, classification, and management of various injuries, as well as with certain unique aspects of growing bone in children, is essential to an understanding of the content presented. Thus, we briefly discussed this information below.

## GENERAL PRINCIPLES

### Patient Evaluation

Initial evaluation requires that all injured extremities be completely exposed. The presence of wounds, the shape, size, and deformity of the extremity, as well as its color and any spontaneous movement should be noted. If present, shortening of the lower extremities with external rotation should also be noted. Areas of localized pain, crepitus, or instability often herald an underlying fracture. The vascular evaluation includes assessment of the temperature, color, and capillary refill. While the motor examination may be significantly limited in certain types of injuries secondary to pain, spontaneous movement should be noted and attempts must be made to assess nerve-specific motor function in the awake patient. Similarly, sensory function should be examined in the conscious patient, although it is often difficult to assess reliably in the young child. The patient should be asked to move through the range of motion at each joint, proceeding from the proximal to the distal aspect of the extremity. Radiographic assessment should include anterior/posterior and lateral views. Additionally, it is sometimes necessary to obtain bilateral extremity views to avoid confusion between injury and the normal growth pattern.

### Multiple Injuries

Although individual extremity fractures may not be threatening to life or limb, multiple fractures in an extremity increase the risk of complications synergistically, and the coexistence of concomitant skeletal and visceral injuries increases overall morbidity and mortality. The probability of death in a child with multiple rib fractures and a head injury is 71%. Lower extremity and spine injuries account for about 33% of the long-term disability seen in the multiply injured child.

Early surgical stabilization (performed before 72 hours after injury) of long-bone fractures in the multiply injured child is known to decrease ICU and hospital stays, to decrease time on mechanical ventilation, and to decrease the number of complications. Therefore, the detection of skeletal extremity injuries is important early in the evaluation of the multiply injured child. The initial evaluation of injured extremities occurs during the secondary survey, at which time perfusion, soft tissue coverage, neurological function, deformity, and tenderness are assessed. However, due to distracting injuries, less obvious extremity injuries may escape the secondary survey. If deformity, swelling, crepitus, or tenderness is noted during the subsequent hospital stay, radiographs of that site should be obtained.

## Physeal Fractures

Perhaps the most obvious distinction between skeletal trauma in the child and that in an adult is the presence of growth plates, or physes, in the skeletally immature patient. While the growing skeleton can remodel substantial deformity, the physes present diagnostic and therapeutic challenges when injured.

Diagnosis of a physeal fracture may be difficult. The physis, composed of cartilage, is radiolucent and can vary in appearance between locations and patients. Those unaccustomed to examining pediatric skeletal radiographs may mistake a normal physis for a fracture line. Isolated fractures of the physis present with normal radiographs when the fracture is nondisplaced, as the fracture line cannot be seen through the radiolucent cartilage. Tenderness, swelling, and a history of a mechanism of injury capable of causing a physeal fracture should warrant treatment of an occult fracture of the pertinent physis. Clinical suspicion must be high to detect occult physeal fractures, as the morbidity of a missed injury in this area of the bone is significant, with partial or complete growth arrest and articular damage. Partial growth arrest can result in an angular deformity as the remainder of the physis continues to grow. Complete arrest can cause limb-length deficiency in a young child.

Fractures involving the physes often extend through the metaphysis and/or epiphysis on either side, as classified by Salter and Harris (Fig. 82-1). Salter–Harris Type I and II fractures are the most common types in most locations and have the lowest rate of growth arrest. Salter–Harris Type IV fractures are notorious for partial growth arrest, and Salter–Harris Type V fractures, although rare, can cause sufficient compressive damage and complete arrest. The fracture extends into the articular surface with Type III and Type IV fractures, which often require operative reduction and stabilization to avoid intra-articular malunion and resulting posttraumatic arthrosis. The treatment of physeal fractures must be prompt, as repeated or late attempts to reduce a displaced

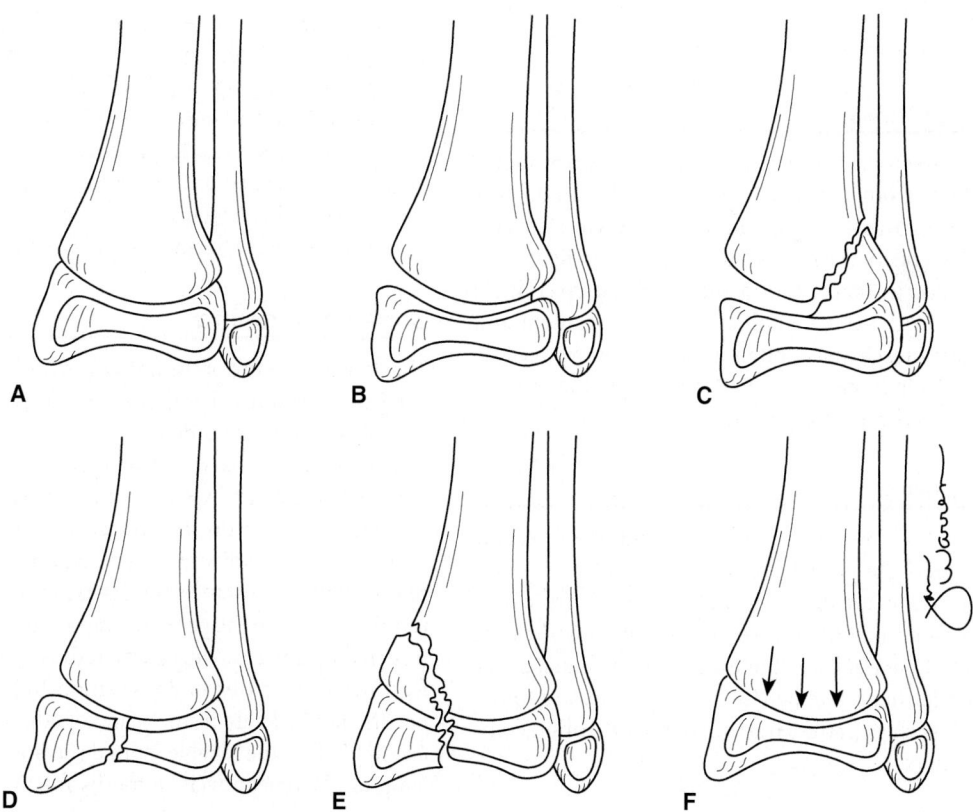

**FIGURE 82-1** Salter–Harris classification of epiphyseal injuries. **A.** Normal physeal anatomy and configuration. **B.** *Type I:* This is a transverse fracture through the hypertrophic zone of the growth plate. The growing zone of the physis is usually not injured and growth disturbance is uncommon. **C.** *Type II:* This fracture is essentially similar to Type I, but toward the edge it deviates away from the physis and splits off a triangular fragment of metaphyseal bone. **D.** *Type III:* The fracture splits the epiphysis and then passes through the hypertrophic layer of the physis; it inevitably damages the reproductive layer of the physis and may lead to growth disturbance. **E.** *Type IV:* This fracture resembles Type III, but it extends into the metaphysis. **F.** *Type V:* There is a longitudinal compression of the physis. Although there may be no visible fracture, the growth plate is crushed; this may result in growth arrest.

physeal fracture (beyond 7-10 days postinjury) can substantially increase the risk of growth arrest.

The most common physeal fractures are in the upper extremity, including the proximal phalanx of the finger, distal radius, and lateral condyle of the humerus. Physeal fractures are seen twice as often in boys at or just before the peak growth spurt. Lower-extremity physeal injuries are most frequently at the ankle.

## Intra-articular Fractures

As mentioned above, fractures that involve the articular surface of a bone require anatomic healing in order to restore joint function. Incongruity of the joint surfaces due to malunion of an intra-articular fracture restricts joint motion and increases the mechanical stress at the cartilage surfaces, leading to arthritic degeneration. Healing of an intra-articular fracture with as little of 2 mm of step-off at the articular surface has been associated with the development of permanent post-traumatic arthritis. Intra-articular fractures typically present with hemarthrosis. Radiographs generally should include anteroposterior, lateral, and internal and external rotation oblique views to discover possible osteochondral fragments that may be quite small. Other causes of an acute hemarthrosis at the knee in a child that must be considered include cruciate ligament injury, patella dislocation, meniscal injury, or an unrecognized bleeding disorder.

## Avulsion Fractures

Avulsion fractures occur when attached soft tissues pull a fragment of bone from its normal location. In the child, most avulsion fractures involve the apophyses, or growth plates for bony prominences that serve as attachments for ligaments and muscles. For instance, the medial humeral epicondyle can be avulsed by the attached ulnar collateral ligament and flexor–pronator muscle mass, often during an elbow dislocation. Some avulsion fractures require anatomic reduction and union in order to restore proper function.

## Stress Fractures

Stress fractures are common in growing children, especially in those who actively participate in sports. The most commonly affected bones are the tibia, fibula, and femur. The tibia is affected in about half of all cases and usually involves the proximal shaft. Other affected bones include the metatarsals, distal radius, calcaneus, and pelvis. Unusual bones are sometimes affected, such as a stress fracture of the first rib in competitive swimmers.

## Open Fractures and Dislocations

Open fractures are often caused by high-energy trauma, and up to 50% of children with an open fracture have an associated injury. These fractures are classified into 3 types, according to the Gustilo classification system (Table 82-1). The grading is based on the degree of soft-tissue injury accompanying the fracture. Prognosis worsens as the grade increases. General treatment priorities for these fractures include control of external hemorrhage, splinting and traction, application of a sterile

| TABLE 82-1 | Gustilo Classification of Open Fractures |
|---|---|

**Type 1:** The wound is generally a small, clean puncture through which a bone spike has protruded. There is little soft tissue damage and the fracture is not comminuted.

**Type 2:** The wound is more than 1 to 2 cm long, but there is no skin flap. There is not much soft tissue damage, and there is no more than moderate crushing and comminution at the fracture.

**Type 3:** There is extensive damage to the skin, soft tissue, and neurovascular structures, and considerable contamination of the wound. There are 3 subdivisions of this fracture:

Type 3a: Soft tissue is available for wound coverage.

Type 3b: Because of extensive soft tissue injury, the fractured bone cannot be covered by soft tissue; there is also evidence of periosteal stripping.

Type 3c: There is evidence of vascular disruption that requires surgical repair.

dressing, and evaluation of other associated injuries. Prior to operative intervention, antibiotics are given and the tetanus status is verified. Multiple-wound débridements, stabilization of fracture fragments, wound care, and flap coverage are the immediate operative goals. The traumatic wound should be extended, dead tissue removed (including completely devascularized bone fragments), and questionable tissue cleaned and irrigated with up to 10 L of fluid. Gustilo recommends a repeat débridement within 24 to 72 hours for all Type 2 and Type 3 open fractures. In general, open fractures should be operatively irrigated and debrided urgently, although recent studies have challenged the strict requirement of six hours from time of injury for lower-grade open fractures.

## Bone Remodeling

The dynamic nature of the growing skeleton can allow remodeling of substantial deformity. Several principles govern the remodeling of fracture deformities. First, the closer a fracture is to an active physis, the greater the capacity for remodeling. For instance, metaphyseal fractures have a higher remodeling potential than do diaphyseal fractures. Second, the rate of growth of the adjacent physis determines the capacity for remodeling. For instance, the distal radius physis grows significantly faster than the proximal radius, whereas the opposite is true in the humerus. Thus, distal radius and proximal humerus fractures display tremendous remodeling. Third, remodeling occurs most reliably in the plane of adjacent joint motion, as exemplified by the reliable sagittal (flexion–extension) remodeling of a supracondylar humerus fracture in the absence of coronal plane (varus–valgus) remodeling. Finally, the amount of growth remaining impacts the degree of possible remodeling, and remodeling can rarely be reliably used to correct deformities in children approaching skeletal maturity. Conversely, growth stimulation from fractures in the skeletally immature can actually lead to deformity, such as angular deformity from asymmetric proximal tibia overgrowth or leg-length discrepancy from femoral shaft overgrowth. For these reasons, treatment of fractures in the child must take into account the complex dynamics of the growing skeleton.

# VASCULAR INJURIES

## Background

Eighteen percent of arterial injuries in children are associated with fractures, and the injury is usually a crush injury or segmental fracture. Although significant limb ischemia is an uncommon complication of fractures of the long bones in children, it is significant in that its consequences can be devastating. Unrecognized and untreated cases may result in ischemic contracture or limb loss.

Relationships of bony anatomy, soft-tissue anatomy, and circulatory pathophysiology affect the genesis, severity, and final outcome of vascular injury. For instance, the proximity of the brachial artery and its branches to the distal humerus accounts for the ischemia that can accompany severely displaced supracondylar humerus fractures. Similarly, the tethered nature of the popliteal artery predisposes it to injury with a displaced proximal tibia physeal fracture. Knowledge of these relationships allows early detection of altered perfusion in the setting of an extremity injury. Such early detection is critical, as ultimately, the extent and duration of altered perfusion determine the viability of an injured extremity.

The degree of fracture displacement on examination may not accurately reflect displacement occurring in the field. Thus, understanding and identifying the mechanism of injury are critical. Fracture patterns at higher risk for vascular compromise, such as displaced supracondylar humerus fractures and displaced fractures/dislocations about the knee, should heighten suspicion for vascular injury.

## Diagnostic Considerations

Mechanism of injury, anatomic site, and fracture pattern should be elucidated in order to determine the ischemic potential of the injury. The time of injury should be determined as precisely as possible. In some cases, the onset of ischemia does not correspond to the time of the injury, as ischemia can develop with movement of fracture fragments during splinting and transport, or following postinjury swelling. Nonetheless, both animal studies and clinical reviews indicate a direct correlation between time of ischemia and outcome, with 6 hours being a threshold time for good prognosis. Therefore, early recognition of vascular compromise is a key determinant of outcome.

A thorough physical examination should include observations of the degree of local and distal swelling, skin color, temperature, and integrity, and spontaneous movements of the distal extremity. Gentle palpation may demonstrate tense, swollen areas. Vascular examination should reliably identify classic signs of limb ischemia such as absent distal pulse, pallor, decreased skin temperature, decreased capillary refill, and decreased venous filling. Because many patients may have a concomitant injury of a peripheral nerve that is in close proximity to the traumatized vessel, a complete neurologic exam of the extremity should be performed. Conversely, identification of a nerve injury should heighten the suspicion for the development of ischemia. For instance, in the setting of a displaced supracondylar humerus fracture, the presence of a median nerve injury increases the likelihood for concomitant vascular complications.

The Doppler arterial pressure index has been successfully used to clinically evaluate the risk of vascular injury. The Doppler arterial pressure in the injured limb is divided by the arterial pressure in the opposite limb. A value of less than 0.90 is highly significant for a vascular injury that is affecting flow to the extremity. Intimal tears may not, however, be detected by this test. Angiography is suggested in patients with a pulse deficit, a moderate hematoma, unexplained transient shock, or adjacent nerve injury. When the neurovascular examination is normal, the use of angiography for evaluating proximate injuries is controversial. In addition, in the setting of a displaced supracondylar humerus fracture with distal ischemia, angiography is unnecessary and will only delay fracture reduction, which restores perfusion in most cases. Even if perfusion is not restored following fracture reduction and fixation, the predictable level of arterial injury obviates the need for time-consuming and invasive angiography. Immediate exploration is recommended instead.

## Diagnostic Pitfalls

The early recognition of vascular injury generally avoids otherwise late complications. Each of the following errors, however, may delay the diagnosis:

- Failing to determine time of injury
- Failing to suspect vascular injury in head trauma or unresponsive patients
- Assuming that normal pulse or capillary refill indicates adequate perfusion throughout the limb
- Failing to repeat the examination in a timely fashion, if warranted
- Misinterpreting nerve injury (ie, neuropraxia vs ischemia)
- Focusing solely on the bony injury, without evaluating soft-tissue injury

## Penetrating Extremity Trauma

There is currently an increase in penetrating injuries in children, particularly in adolescents. Extremity gunshot wounds may compromise perfusion, nerve function, or soft-tissue coverage. Penetrating injuries to the lower extremity are more likely to cause perfusion deficits than are penetrating injuries to the arm. All wounds must be thoroughly débrided and vital structures covered with soft tissues. The course of the penetrating wound should be determined visually and radiographically. Prior to obtaining the radiograph, penetrating injuries should be marked with radiopaque markers. Foreign bodies should be identified on film. The upper limb is rarely threatened if only the radial or ulnar artery is involved. If both the radial and ulnar arteries are occluded, then arterial reconstruction is mandatory.

## Patient Management

When there is a combined orthopedic and vascular injury, the vascular repair should be carried out first if the fracture is stable. Perfusion is often restored by placement of a temporary shunt to allow fracture stabilization before completing

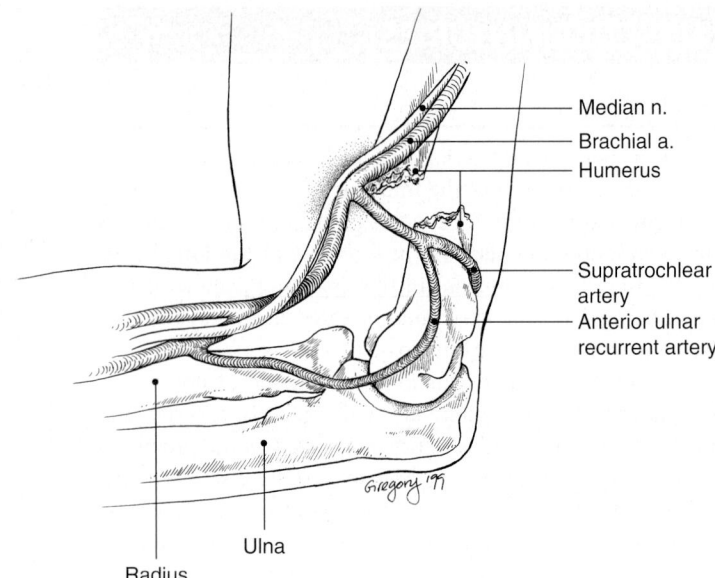

**FIGURE 82-2** The intimate relationship between the brachial artery and its branches and the distal humerus predisposes to vascular insufficiency following severely displaced supracondylar humerus fractures.

the arterial repair. If the orthopedic injury is an unstable fracture, fracture stabilization should be employed prior to the vascular repair. Such fixation may be definitive, such as the percutaneous pinning of a reduced supracondylar humerus fracture, or temporizing, such as a spanning external fixator across an unstable knee dislocation.

The nature of the vascular repair depends on the nature and location of the injury. In the case of a supracondylar humerus fracture, often the brachial artery is tethered and kinked by entrapment of its supratrochlear branch at the fracture site (Fig. 82-2). In such a case, ligation and transection of this branch will release the brachial artery from its tether and restore flow once associated vasospasm has subsided. If an isolated thrombus is identified within an injured artery, a thrombectomy and primary arterial repair can restore flow. In the setting of an arterial transection, the vascular repair may be accomplished by primary anastomosis or interposition

grafts of autogenous saphenous vein or polytetrafluoroethylene (PTFE). If reconstruction of a venous injury is not possible, the injured vein is ligated. Arterial injuries below the popliteal trifurcation are repaired so that at least 1 vessel is complete distally with adequate flow. When indicated, completion angiograms and prophylactic fasciotomies are performed after vascular repairs.

Follow-up of vascular injuries is important, as subacute complications may develop. For instance, a penetrating injury that causes bleeding controlled by local pressure alone can result in the formation of a pseudoaneurysm (Fig. 82-3). A pseudoaneurysm presents as an expanding pulsatile mass and can rupture and hemorrhage or cause ischemia distally through arterial emboli. Angiography (invasive or magnetic resonance) can be used for preoperative evaluation. Upon surgical exploration, the damaged portion of the artery can be repaired or resected and grafted.

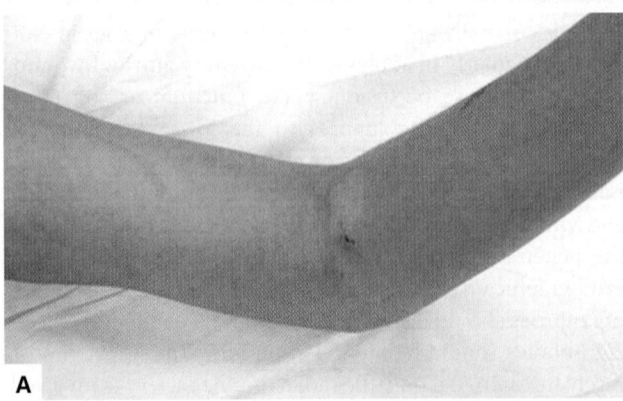

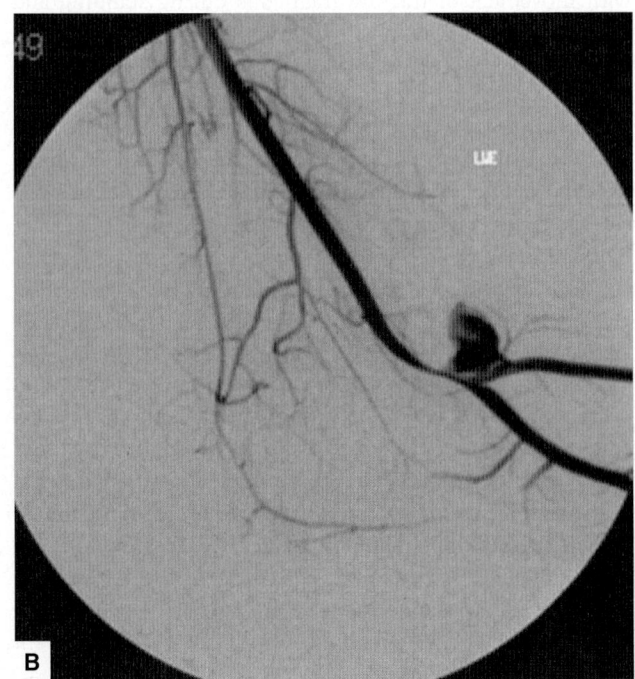

**FIGURE 82-3** Brachial artery pseudoaneurysm resulting from a small puncture wound with a pocketknife in the antecubital fossa. A 9-year-old boy presented with pulsatile bleeding that was stopped with local pressure. He returned 5 days later with a painful, pulsatile mass, and underwent pseudoaneurysm resection and primary arterial repair.

# COMPARTMENT SYNDROME

Both endogenous and exogenous factors can cause the increased hydrostatic tissue pressure within a compartment. The following conditions put patients at high risk:

▶ Limb ischemia for more than 4 hours

▶ A high-energy fracture

▶ Multiple fractures in the same limb (eg, ipsilateral distal humerus and distal radius)

▶ An open fracture

▶ Crush injuries

▶ Multisystem injury and shock

▶ Altered mental status or prolonged anesthesia (sustained extremity position)

▶ Bleeding disorders, electrical burns, or snake bites

## Pathophysiology

Increased hydrostatic pressure within a closed anatomic area results in decreased tissue perfusion and subsequent loss of function. Fascial binding of muscle groups creates the potential site for the development of compartment syndrome. The 4 muscle groups of the lower leg (anterior, lateral, superficial posterior, and deep posterior) and the 3 muscles groups of the forearm (volar, dorsal, mobile wad) are particularly subject to compartment compromise, but this is also seen in many other areas, including the thigh, the buttocks, and the intrinsic muscles of the hand and foot.

Compartmental tamponade results in a decrease in arteriolar pressure. The resulting loss of tissue perfusion leads to tissue necrosis, if the pressure is not decreased within 6 hours. Tissue necrosis leads to further capillary permeability and to interstitial fluid leakage. An irreversible cycle of damage and necrosis is begun (Fig. 82-4).

## Clinical Symptoms and Diagnosis

The most important point of management is recognizing the child who is at risk and instituting prevention. All too often, the "seven Ps" of limb ischemia are used erroneously to assess the presence of a compartment syndrome. Instead, the 3 As: analgesics, agitation, and anxiety should be used in children. Clinically, increasing pain or analgesic requirements are the first and most common symptom in the conscious patient. However, children may not complain of pain but will appear anxious and have tachycardia. As the compartment becomes fully involved, the nerves travelling through the compartment become ischemic. The patient may complain of paresthesia or weakness in the distribution of the nerve.

Because the compartment pressure remains below the systolic blood pressure, a palpable pulse remains present distal to the involved compartment. Thus, it is critical to understand that *normal pulses and capillary refill distal to the involved compartment does not rule out a compartment syndrome.* If, however, the pulse is absent, evaluation for a concomitant vascular injury should be done, especially if the history supports this possibility.

An elevated interstitial fluid pressure within the compartment is the earliest sign of compromise. Direct measurement of elevated compartment pressures is thus an important element in the diagnosis; this is done with the use of needles inserted into the muscle group that is at risk. Concurrent arterial pressures determine the perfusion gradient of the compartment. Differences of less than 30 mm Hg between

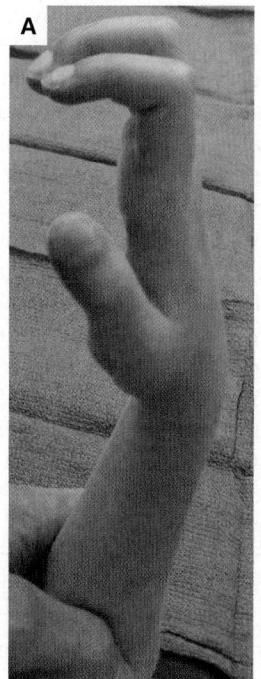
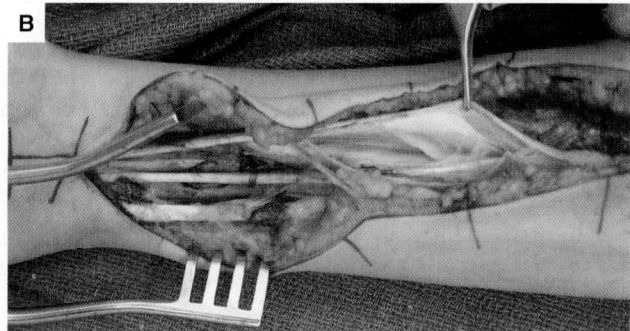
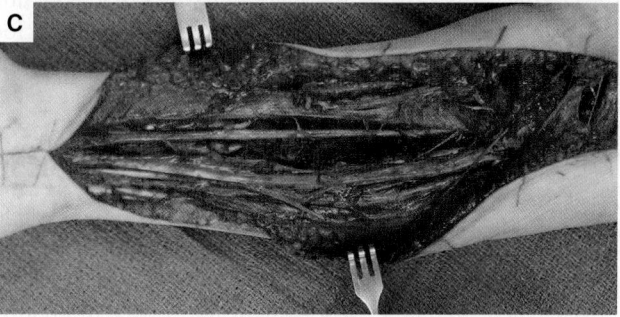

**FIGURE 82-4** The Volkmann ischemic contracture of the forearm from an untreated compartment syndrome following a displaced supracondylar humerus fracture. Note the flexion deformities of the digits (**A**), the severe myonecrosis (**B**). Radical debridement and neurolysis (**C**) was followed by free functioning gracilis transfer to restore finger flexion.

the diastolic arterial pressure and the intracompartmental pressure indicate the need for decompressive fasciotomy. In young children, compartment pressures can be obtained in the operating room before and after the decompressive fasciotomy. For the child with a head injury or for the older child in whom the clinical findings are inconsistent, compartment pressure measurements can be performed at the bedside. One limitation of the use of pressure measurements in the assessment of compartment syndrome in children is the typically low arterial pressures in infants and young children. Conventional pressure criteria for fasciotomies cannot be reliably used, for instance, when the normal diastolic pressure is only 40 mm Hg. In such cases, compartment syndrome should be diagnosed and treated on clinical grounds.

## Patient Management

The outcome of treatment depends on the duration of symptoms prior to release of the abnormal compartment pressure. The first step in treatment of the compression is the relief of constricting bandages or casts. If the symptoms of the compartment compromise are not improved with the removal of external causes, then relief of the internal cause is indicated.

If the elapsed ischemic time from vascular injury or occlusion is less than 4 hours, a limb should be evaluated, and repeated examinations and pressure measurements should be carried out. If the duration of ischemia is greater than 4 hours, prophylactic fasciotomy of the involved compartments is indicated. At the time of prophylactic fasciotomy, release of all compartments distal to the injury should be performed, including the intrinsic compartments of the hands and feet.

## Decompression of the Lower Leg

The double-incision technique of Mubarak and Hargens is preferred to the alternate transfibular/4-compartment fasciotomy. Although the Mubarak technique requires both lateral and medial incisions, it avoids the potential instability created by removal of the fibula. The medial dissection is started approximately 2 cm posterior to the medial tibial edge. The medial dissection is started approximately 2 cm posterior to the medial tibial edge. The saphenous nerve and vein are kept anterior to the fasciotomy. A transverse fascial incision will show the division between the superficial and deep compartments. The fascia of the superficial compartment is released proximally along the medial edge of the gastrocnemius belly and distally along the Achilles tendon. The flexor digitorum longus lies in the deep compartment. Its tendon is the guide to the release of the deep structures. Again, any dead muscle should be removed. Skin and subcutaneous tissues are left open in order to inspect the wounds and to reduce circumferential pressure.

## Wound Aftercare

External or internal fixation of fractures may facilitate aftercare. Continuing management requires débridement of necrotic muscle, coverage of bone segments with muscle or skin flaps, delayed skin closure, and possible skin grafting. Ultimate function can be facilitated with the use of splints and physical or occupational therapy.

## Outcomes

The treatment of a compartment syndrome leaves no residual functional deficit. There may, however, be scarring from the delayed closure of the surgical wounds or skin grafting. However, the outcome of an unrecognized or incompletely treated compartment syndrome is an ischemic contracture. Dead muscle contracts, healing into fibrous scar tissue. The physical contractures of the soft tissues, as well as any residual nerve dysfunction, limits function. In mild cases, a more functional extremity may result after surgical release of contractures and neurolysis of the involved nerves. In more severe cases, free functioning muscle transfers may be required to restore even rudimentary function to the extremity. Loss of the involved limb is the greatest complication of a compartment syndrome. Although untreated compartment syndrome in the absence of concomitant arterial injury does not itself threaten the viability of the entire limb, secondary infection or permanent neural damage may render the extremity useless and amputation may be indicated.

# FRACTURES AND DISLOCATIONS OF THE UPPER EXTREMITY

## Proximal Humerus Fractures

Fractures of the proximal humerus in children aged 5 to 12 are generally through the metaphysis. In adolescents these fractures are usually Salter–Harris Type II physeal injuries. The mechanism of injury is commonly a fall onto the outstretched hand, but a direct blow is sometimes responsible. Patients may present holding the elbow to their side, appearing to have a shoulder dislocation. The diagnosis is made with plain radiographs, with advanced imaging rarely required. Treatment depends on the displacement and the age of the patient. Most fractures in this region are nondisplaced or minimally displaced, and can be treated with simple immobilization consisting of a sling and swathe or other such devices. A great deal of deformity can be tolerated in this location, given the fast growth of the proximal humerus to correct the deformity and the abundant motion in all planes at the glenohumeral joint to compensate for residual deformity. However, in adolescents with severely displaced fractures, reduction is necessary, often requiring open reduction and percutaneous or internal fixation. Other indications for surgery include ipsilateral limb injury, concomitant brachial plexus injury, multiple trauma, rare intra-articular fractures, and open fractures.

## Humeral Shaft Fractures

Humeral shaft fractures occur more frequently in multiply injured children, and causes tend to vary with age. In the neonate, these fractures can occur from a difficult delivery. In children under 3 years of age, they may be a result of child abuse. In the older child or teenager, they can occur with pathologic fracture through a bone cyst. Children often present holding the affected arm by their side. A careful neurologic examination, paying particular attention to radial nerve function, is essential, as the radial nerve may be injured during fracture displacement. The patient's skin must also be carefully examined for wounds because small punctures may be indicative of an open fracture.

Radial nerve injury is typically a neuropraxia, and spontaneous resolution occurs in 80% of cases. However, if the radial nerve is intact prior to closed reduction and a deficit is later noted, then exploration is indicated as entrapment of the nerve within the fracture could have occurred.

## Supracondylar Humerus Fractures

Supracondylar humerus fractures account for 60% of all elbow fractures in children, occurring most frequently between 5 and 8 years of age. The mechanism of injury is usually a fall onto the outstretched hand. Supracondylar humerus fractures are of particular importance to the general surgeon in that they are the fracture in children that is most commonly associated with neurovascular complications. A comprehensive management regimen includes bony stabilization and treatment of the soft-tissue injury. With every fracture, some component of soft-tissue injury exists.

Nondisplaced fractures heal reliably with 3-4 weeks of cast immobilization. Type II fractures generally require reduction except in the youngest patients with minimal angulation. Type III extension fractures and all displaced flexion type fractures require percutaneous pinning following reduction, given their inherent instability. Open reduction is more often required for these fractures as well. Several controversies still exist regarding timing of surgery, pin configuration, and post-operative regimens, but these discussions are beyond the scope of this text.

Type III extension-type supracondylar fractures are associated with neurovascular deficits in up to 13% of cases. The neurovascular bundle anteriorly is subjected to traction injury and, less likely, to puncture from a sharp bony prominence (Fig. 82-5). Open supracondylar fractures (flexion and extension) and extension-type supracondylar fractures in which the distal fragment lies anterior to the proximal fragment, should elicit increased suspicion for vascular injury.

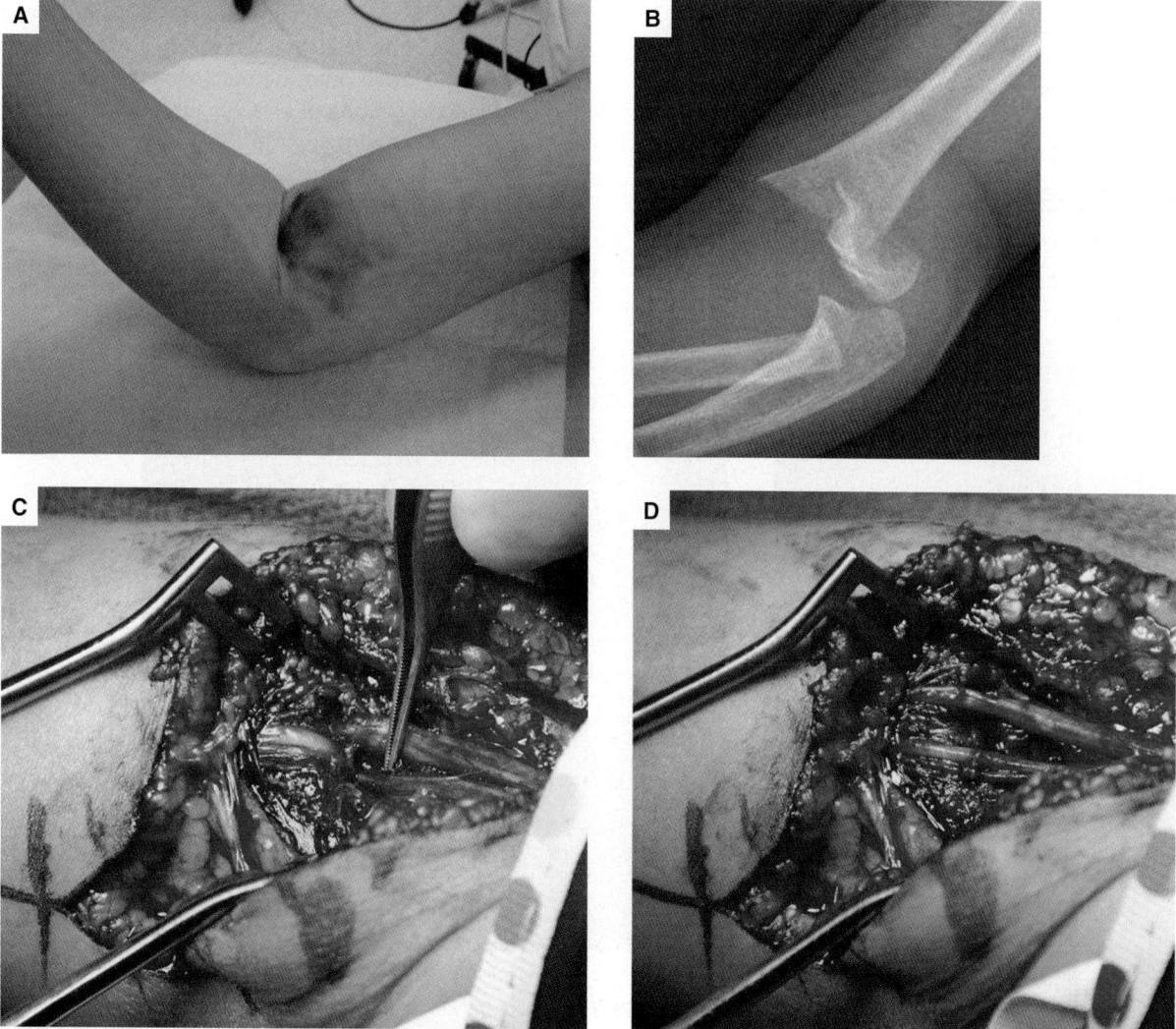

**FIGURE 82-5** A 2-year-old boy presenting with a type III supracondylar humerus fracture (B) has ecchymosis and dimpling in the antecubital fossa (A) suggesting tenting of the neurovascular structures. After fracture reduction and pinning, the vascularity of the limb did not improve, warranting open exploration. The brachial artery was found kinked by tethering of the supratrochlear artery in the fracture site (C). Ligation and sectioning of this branch allowed reconstitution of brachial artery flow (D).

Similarly, given the proximity of the median nerve and brachial artery, preoperative median nerve deficit can be a harbinger of brachial artery injury and should raise suspicion for impending vascular complications.

In patients who present with a supracondylar humerus fracture and impaired vascularity to the limb, emergent fracture reduction is indicated. While splinting the elbow in slight flexion may temporarily restore circulation, definitive fracture reduction and stabilization is emergently needed. In some cases, trauma to the brachial artery requires thrombectomy, direct repair, or excision and grafting using standard vascular surgical techniques. It is important to note appropriate tension on a vein graft if one is used. Excessive length of the vein graft placed with the elbow extended can lead to kinking once the elbow is flexed post-operatively. Concomitant injury to the median nerve can be noted at the time of vascular repair, although rarely does such an injury require repair. Prophylactic fasciotomies can be performed following vascular repair at the discretion of the surgeon, based on degree of swelling, length of ischemia, and compartment pressure measurements.

Postoperative care of the supracondylar humerus fractures should include a period of observation to monitor for the development of compartment syndrome, even if ischemia or severe swelling did not exist at presentation or surgery. Reduction and stabilization of the fracture provide remarkable pain relief, so any severe pain postoperatively should be evaluated as a possible sign of compartment syndrome.

## Lateral Condyle Fractures

Although common, lateral condyle fractures of the humerus can be difficult to diagnose. The mechanism of injury is commonly a fall onto the outstretched hand. As with supracondylar fractures, these occur most frequently in children 5 to 8 years of age. These fractures cross the physis of the distal humerus and enter the joint, making them prone to several complications, including nonunion, valgus deformity, late ulnar nerve palsy, avascular necrosis of the capitellum, lateral condyle overgrowth, cubitus varus, and loss of elbow motion. Most, but not all, of these problems are avoidable by early diagnosis and proper treatment. The child presents with a painful, swollen elbow. The elbow should be examined carefully because marked swelling and lateral bruising may be the only signs of an unstable injury.

Nondisplaced fractures may be treated in a cast, although with careful weekly monitoring to detect late displacement. Fractures that are displaced at the lateral metaphyseal aspect of the fracture more than 2 mm vertically or 1 mm horizontally require fixation (Fig. 82-6). Whether treated nonsurgically or surgically, the time to healing is substantially longer for lateral condyle fractures than for supracondylar humerus fractures.

## Medial Epicondyle Fractures

Medial epicondyle fractures commonly occur in adolescence, and more frequently in boys. The mechanism of injury is most commonly a fall onto the outstretched hand with the elbow extended, resulting in a valgus force across the elbow. The flexor/pronator muscle origin and ulnar collateral ligament, originating at the medial epicondyle, cause the avulsion. Continuation of such forces with this mechanism may result in additional fractures of the olecranon and radial neck as well as elbow dislocation. As many as 50% of medial

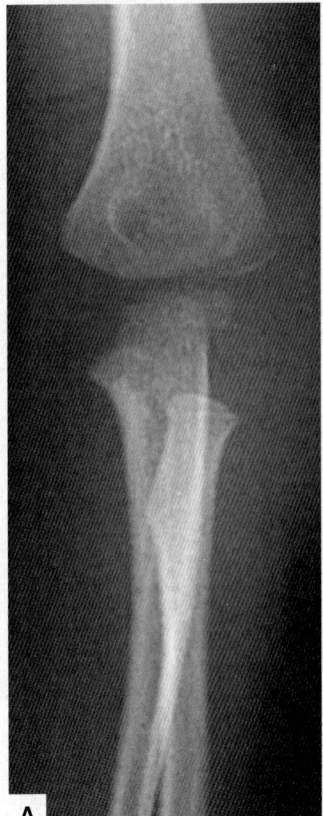
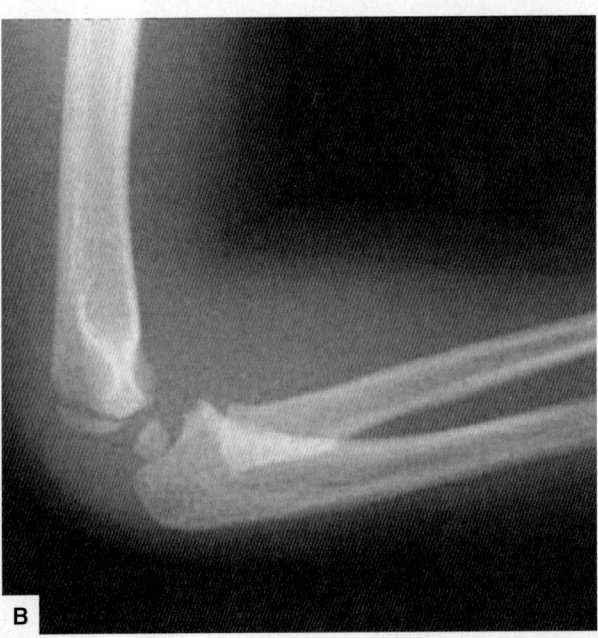

**FIGURE 82-6** Lateral condyle fracture in a 2-year-old child. **A.** The AP view shows a fracture gap of 2 to 3 mm, which can be followed from lateral to the center of the elbow where it disappears running vertically through the epiphysis into the joint. **B.** The significant posterior gap is an ominous sign. The child required open reduction and internal fixation.

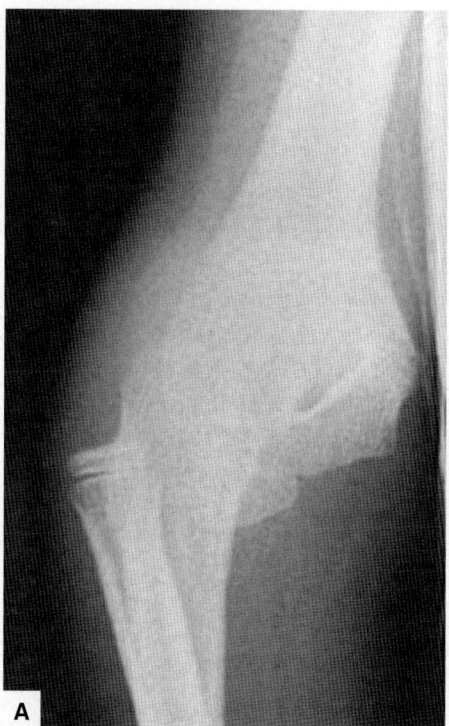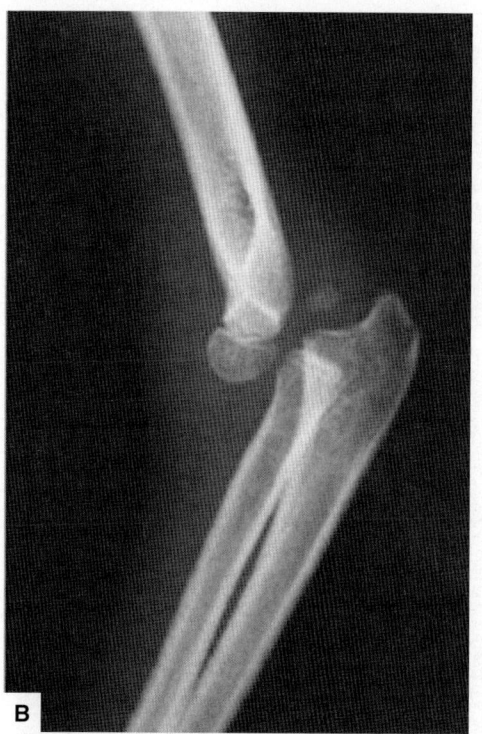

**FIGURE 82-7** **A.** Anterior posterior view of the elbow to a 10-year-old child who had fallen. Note the absence of the medial epicondyle. **B.** Lateral view showing posterior dislocation of the elbow and the medial epicondyle entrapped in the joint. Open reduction and internal fixation of the epicondyle is required for this type of injury. Early motion is necessary.

epicondyle fractures occur with an elbow dislocation, including those dislocations that spontaneously reduce prior to arrival in the emergency department (Fig. 82-7).

## Monteggia Fracture-Dislocation

The classic Monteggia lesion is a fracture of the proximal third of the ulna associated with a dislocation of the radial head from its radiocapitellar and proximal radioulnar articulations. The radial head can dislocate anteriorly, posteriorly, or laterally, with the ulna fracture angulating in a parallel manner. Of importance in children is the fact that the ulna can fail in plastic deformation, where the ulna is bent rather than broken. Similarly, the ulna fracture can be a fairly subtle and minimally angulated greenstick fracture. In both of these circumstances, the radial head dislocation can be missed if not suspected. It is therefore imperative to properly radiographically assess the radiocapitellar joint in all children with forearm injuries. A line drawn along the radius should intersect the capitellum. The posterior interosseous branch of the radial nerve can be stretched by either anterior or lateral dislocation of the radial head. Therefore, function of the finger extensors and thumb abductors must be documented prior to treatment.

Most Monteggia fracture dislocations in children can be treated successfully by closed reduction and casting, provided the ulna and radial head dislocation can be reduced anatomically and the diagnosis is made early enough. However, it is not uncommon for the diagnosis to be missed until after the fracture of the ulna has healed in a malunited position with the radial head still dislocated. In such a situation, osteotomy of the ulna and open reduction of the radial head is required (Fig. 82-8). However, if the radial head is left dislocated too long in a growing child, it will lose its normal concavity, precluding later realignment with the capitellum. The age or time-from-injury cut-off has not been fully defined, although reconstructions of this nature have been successful more than 2 years following the injury.

## Radius and Ulna Fractures

Fractures of the radius and ulna, especially at their distal ends, are the most common fractures seen in children. The outcome is typically determined by the location and type of fracture as well as the age of the child. Associated neurovascular injuries are uncommon, although compartment syndrome can follow severely displaced forearm fractures and acute carpal tunnel syndrome can complicate severely displaced distal radius fractures. It is important to note, however, that an ipsilateral distal radius and distal humerus fractures (the so-called "pediatric floating elbow") can lead commonly to compartment syndrome despite each fracture not being severely displaced. It is therefore important to examine the entire extremity when a wrist injury is evident.

Most radius and ulna shaft fractures can be treated with closed reduction and casting, although there has been a recent rise in the rate of surgical treatment of these fractures. First, the more distal the fracture, the better. Second, younger children have substantially more remodeling potential than older children and can thus tolerate more deformity at fracture healing. Third, forearm shaft fractures take longer to heal

**1107**

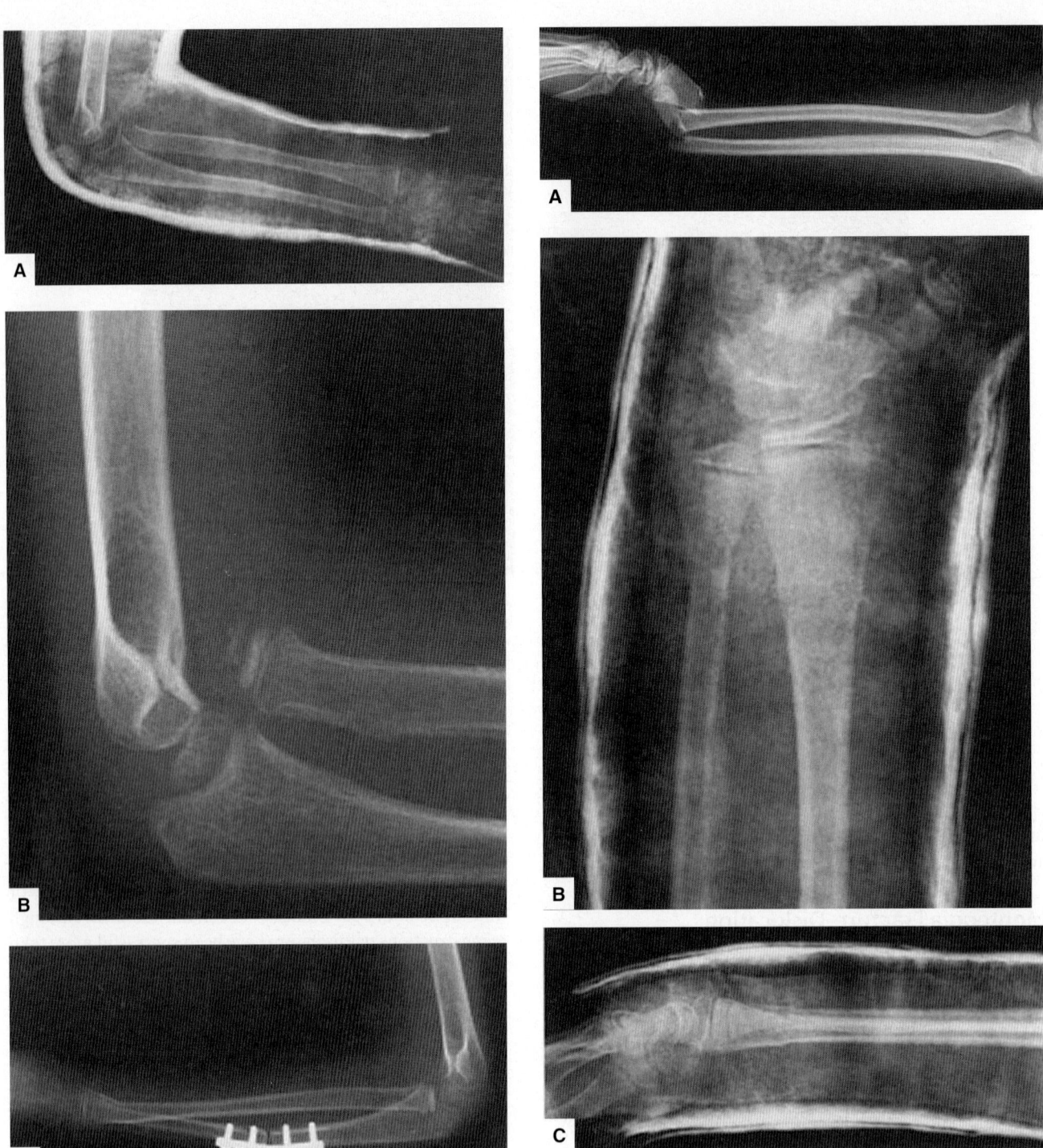

FIGURE 82-8 Monteggia fracture. A. AP view of the forearm of a 6-year-old treated with an above elbow cast for an apparent greenstick fracture of the ulna. Note that the radial head does not line up with the capitellum of the elbow. B. Lateral view of the elbow out of the cast showing anterior dislocation of the radial head. C. Osteotomy of the ulna and open reduction of the radial head were required.

FIGURE 82-9 A. Lateral view of the forearm of an 11-year-old boy who had fallen from a basketball hoop. Note the complete displacement dorsally of the lower radius, resulting in a "dinner fork" deformity. The patient had pain and numbness along the median distribution. The ulna appears to be almost penetrating the skin. B. AP view after closed reduction and casting. C. Lateral view after closed reduction and casting.

than metaphyseal fractures of the radius and ulna, and can thus displace over several weeks during cast immobilization. Finally, refracture is not uncommon after fracture healing.

Distal radius fractures, with or without a concomitant distal ulna fracture, are very common. The fracture may involve the metaphysis or the physis, but it rarely involves the articular surface. Most distal radius fractures are dorsally displaced

and result from a fall onto the outstretched hand with the wrist in an extended position at impact. Buckle fractures of the metaphysis, where the cortex fails in compression on the concave side, can be treated symptomatically with a brace or cast with reliable healing and no need for follow-up radiographs. Conversely, displaced fractures may require reduction and casting or pinning (Fig. 82-9), although young children can remodel substantial deformity over time. Fractures that involve the distal radius physis have an approximately 5% risk of affecting the growth of the distal radius. Fortunately, most growth disturbances occur in adolescents nearing the end of normal growth, although it is often advisable to surgically stop ipsilateral ulnar growth to prevent ulnar overgrowth and painful impaction into the carpus.

## Hand Fractures and Dislocations

Fractures are extremely common in the child's hand. While most fractures are minimally displaced and heal well with minimal treatment, several fractures can cause significant complications if not treated more aggressively.

The most common carpal fracture in children, as with adults, is that of the scaphoid. The peak age is 13-15 years. Occult fractures should be suspected if a patient presents with snuffbox tenderness after a fall on an outstretched hand. Magnetic resonance imaging can confirm the diagnosis acutely. Nondisplaced fractures of the distal pole or waist can be treated with casting, although displaced waist fractures and any fracture of the proximal pole require surgical reduction and fixation. As many as two thirds of these fractures present as established nonunions, which require open reduction, internal fixation, and bone grafting.

Metacarpal fractures are common and generally easily treated. Thumb metacarpal fractures can remodel well, given the motion at the thumb carpometacarpal joint, although intra-articular fractures at this joint are unstable and require surgical fixation. Finger metacarpal base fractures in young children often result from crush injuries and compartment syndrome should be excluded. Small finger metacarpal neck fractures (boxer's fractures) can remodel well given their proximity to the distally located physis. Closed reduction and casting is typically sufficient to achieve an excellent functional outcome.

Proximal phalanx base fractures are the most common finger fractures and are generally easily reduced and casted. A particularly troublesome fracture in the child's finger is the so-called Seymour fracture (Fig. 82-10). This injury includes a displaced physeal fracture of the distal phalanx and a nailbed laceration with avulsion of the proximal end of the nail plate. This open fracture is at risk for infection, growth arrest, and nail deformity if the diagnosis is missed. The nail must be removed to allow irrigation of the fracture, removal of the interposed torn nailbed, and reduction of the fracture with or without pinning and/or nailbed repair.

Finger amputations commonly involve the distal tip of the distal phalanx. Nonvascular reattachment of the amputated tip as a composite graft can at the least provide a biological dressing to allow healing by secondary intention. Such healing can reliably cover even exposed bone in a young child. Replantation should be considered for any injury at or proximal to the distal interphalangeal joint. Survival rates in pediatric finger replantation are lower than that for adults, given the typical crush/avulsion mechanisms and the small size of the vessels. Similarly, leeches are often required for venous congestion post-operatively given the often distal level of the amputation and the crushing of the dorsal veins. However, functional results can be excellent following replantation in a child, and skeletal growth can approach normal.

# FRACTURES AND DISLOCATIONS OF THE LOWER EXTREMITY

## Fractures and Dislocations of the Hip

Young children with ligamentous laxity and a largely cartilaginous acetabulum can sustain a hip dislocation with relatively

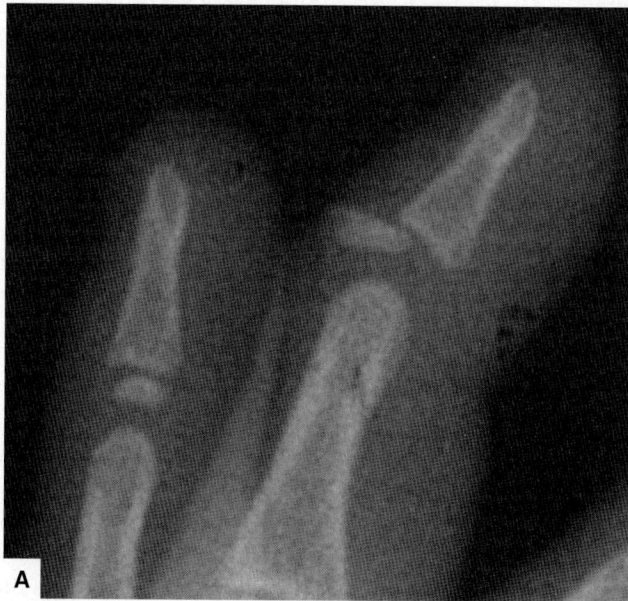
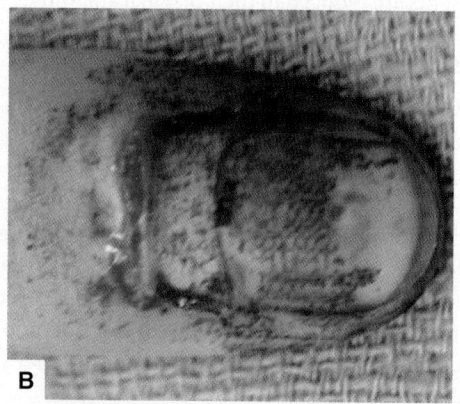
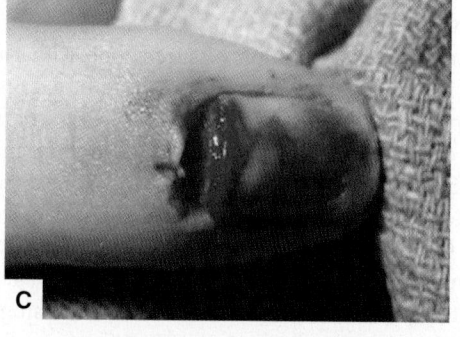

**FIGURE 82-10** (A) Lateral radiograph and (B) clinical appearance of a Seymour fracture. After nail plate removal (C), the open physeal fracture is evident.

little force. However, in adolescents, hip dislocations typically result from higher-energy trauma. The vast majority of traumatic hip dislocations are posterior, with the hip presenting in a flexed, adducted, internally rotated position and the thigh appearing shortened. Because compromise of the tenuous blood supply to the femoral head continues while the hip remains dislocated, this is considered a true orthopedic emergency. Closed reduction under conscious sedation is typically successful, although the reduction must be confirmed carefully as nonconcentric reductions may indicate entrapped osteochondral fragments or soft tissue. Computed tomography or MRI should be used in the case of any imperfect congruity on post-reduction radiographs. Neurovascular evaluation of the limb before and after reduction is crucial, as a sciatic nerve injury may accompany the dislocation. Small children may have postreduction instability, and a spica cast for several weeks can prevent loss of the reduction. Surgery is required if an incongruent reduction is caused by interposed tissue, or if an associated acetabular rim fracture is sufficiently large or displaced. In the long term, the hip in the younger child is at risk for Perthes-like changes and growth arrest. In the child older than 12 years of age, osteonecrosis resembling the adult pattern may develop.

## Fractures and Dislocations of the Femur

### Femoral Neck Fractures

Femoral neck fractures are high-energy injuries and are usually displaced. The transcervical vessels that travel up the femoral neck to the femoral head may be injured, leading to avascular necrosis rates between 30 and 60%. The vascular damage is considered to be from the initial trauma, so immediate open reduction may have little beneficial effect. Nevertheless, these fractures are treated emergently with open reduction and internal fixation. Vascularity is best restored if the fragments are reduced to their original anatomic position.

### Intertrochanteric and Subtrochanteric Fractures

Intertrochanteric and subtrochanteric fractures are below the circumflex vessels and are at less risk of osteonecrosis. Unless markedly displaced and unstable, they are typically treated by skeletal traction, usually in a 90-degree hip and knee position. Spica casting should follow several weeks later. For severely displaced or irreducible fractures, open reduction and internal fixation may be required. For the adolescent, ORIF is considered the treatment of choice in order to allow early mobility.

### Femoral Shaft Fractures

The femoral shaft is a commonly injured bone, with a bimodal age distribution peaking at 2 and 17 years of age. Its treatment depends on the age of the child and the type of fracture. Because associated injuries can occur in the hip and knee, these joints must be adequately evaluated. Physeal fractures, ligamentous injuries, and effusions can all occur in the knee, and the hip can have an associated fracture or dislocation. In the infant who is younger than 4 months of age, Pavlik harness treatment is successful and easier than using a spica

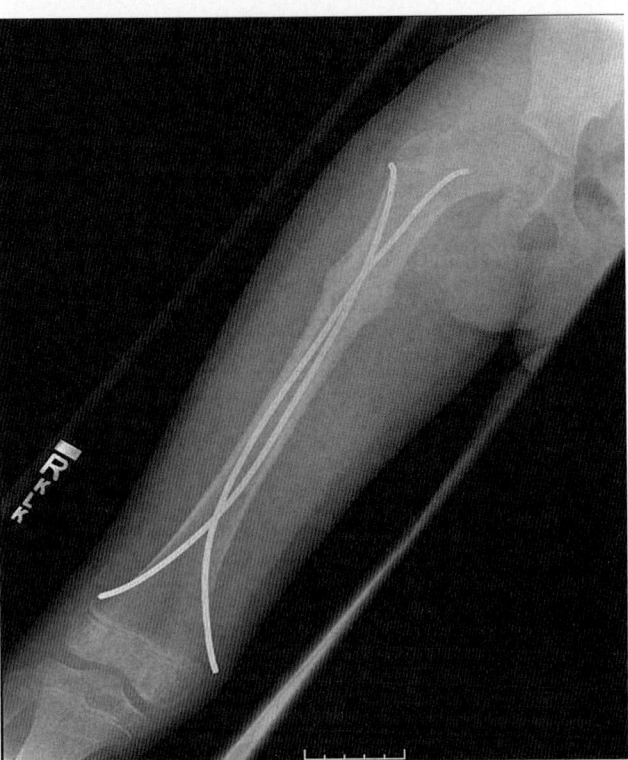

**FIGURE 82-11** Anteroposterior radiograph following flexible intramedullary nailing of a femoral shaft fracture.

cast. In children who are younger than 5 years of age, early spica cast treatment for 6 weeks is adequate. In school-age children, the historically used skeletal traction followed by spica casting has been largely abandoned, due to the socioeconomic disadvantages of the required prolonged hospital stay as well as the development of minimally invasive internal fixation techniques. Flexible intramedullary nailing has now become the treatment of choice for the majority of femoral shaft fractures in children aged 6-10 years, although certain unstable fracture patterns require other fixation techniques, such as submuscular plating or external fixation (Fig. 82-11). The adolescent is typically treated with rigid intramedullary nailing, although with modification of the implant design and entry site from the adult type fixation in order to accommodate the particular vascular anatomy of the developing proximal femur. Femoral shaft fractures in children heal reliably with few complications, although overgrowth may occur and cause a limb-length discrepancy.

### Distal Femur

The distal femur contributes about 70% of the growth of the femur and about 40% of the total growth of the lower extremity. Fractures through the distal femoral physis are resisted by the undulating nature of the physis and by the strong fibrous tissue of the zone of Ranvier surrounding it. Typically, the child is hit from the side and the deformity is in the coronal plane (Fig. 82-12). The limb is often acutely angulated and can be quite difficult to reduce, even under general anesthesia. Because the risk for displacement is high after reduction, internal fixation or percutaneous pin fixation is advised, depending on the age of the child and fracture pattern.

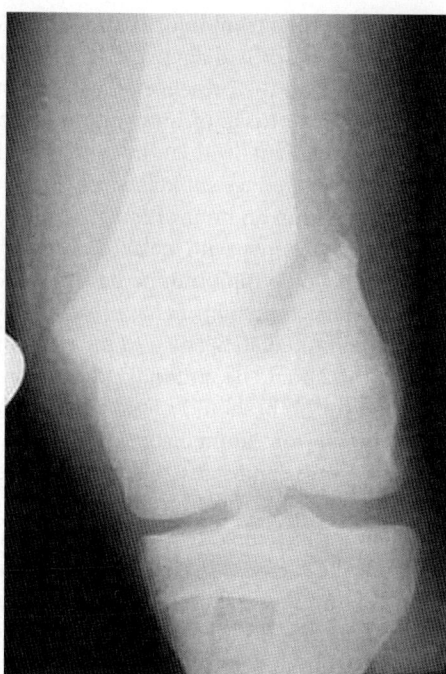

**FIGURE 82-12** AP radiograph of a displaced Salter II fracture of the distal femur.

Growth disturbance has been reported in up to 50% of these fractures, and can lead to limb length discrepancy if complete or angular deformity if partial. Therefore, close follow-up is advised in order to detect the physeal dysfunction early.

## Vascular Injuries in Pediatric Knee Trauma

Knee dislocations and displaced fractures of the distal femur and the proximal tibia jeopardize the vascular integrity of the pediatric knee. In the immature skeleton, knee dislocations occur less commonly than in adults because of the relative weakness of the physes. Assessment of vascular integrity begins with a complete patient evaluation, relating to the

fracture/dislocation pattern and to the vascular anatomy peculiar to the knee.

The vulnerable anatomy of the popliteal artery accounts for its predisposition to injury (Fig. 82-13). The artery is anchored at the femur by the adductor hiatus and anchored below the knee by the fibrous arch of the soleus. Five genicular arteries are given off in the popliteal space. These include the medial and lateral superior and inferior genicular arteries and the middle genicular artery. Artery branches anastomose with the anterior tibial recurrent artery, but do not provide adequate circulation in cases of popliteal occlusion. In its course, the popliteal artery remains intimately associated with the posterior distal femur and proximal tibia.

The popliteal artery and vein lie against the posterior aspect of the distal femur at the level of the epiphyseal plate. Anterior distal fragment displacement from a hyperextension injury is the most likely cause of vascular injury, but threat of altered perfusion is present with any displaced knee injury. In cases of vascular compromise, external fixation crossing the knee provides bony stability prior to vascular repair.

Fractures of the proximal tibial epiphysis are rare (Fig. 82-14). Popliteal artery occlusion in these injuries is also very rare. Nonetheless, the peripheral neurovascular status of each patient should be assessed as previously described. As with fractures of the distal femur, proximal tibial physeal injuries that are associated with vascular injury require stabilization of the knee, usually with external fixation crossing the knee.

Treatment algorithms for vascular injuries about the knee have been developed primarily from experience with knee dislocations. Direction of the displaced tibia describes the knee dislocation. Posterior and anterior dislocations are most common. Clinical examination demonstrates gross instability with the anterior and posterior drawer test, Lachman examination, and collateral ligaments stressed with the knee in 20 to 30 degrees of flexion. Anterior dislocations are more likely to cause traction injury to the popliteal artery, whereas posterior dislocations are more likely to cause a ruptured

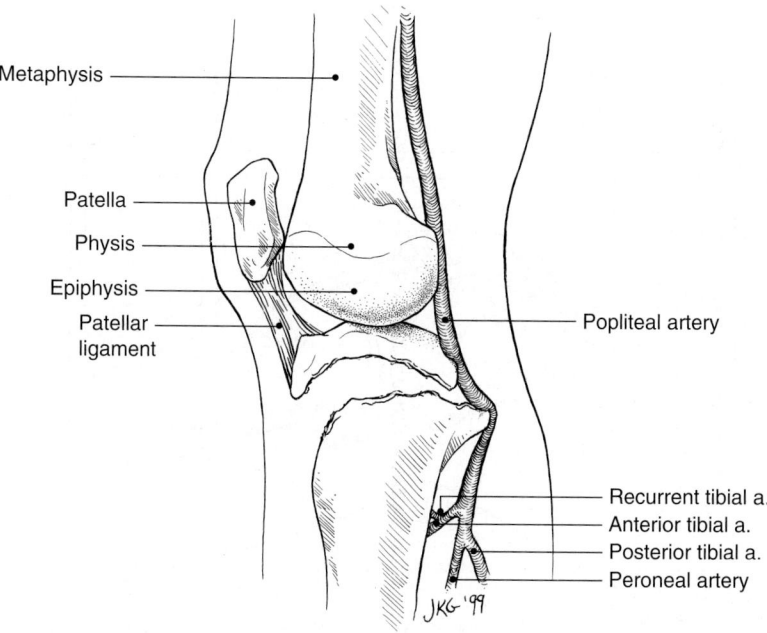

Metaphysis

Patella

Physis

Epiphysis

Patellar ligament

Popliteal artery

Recurrent tibial a.
Anterior tibial a.
Posterior tibial a.
Peroneal artery

JKG '99

**FIGURE 82-13** Drawing demonstrating the relationship of the distal femur and the proximal tibia to the popliteal artery and its branches.

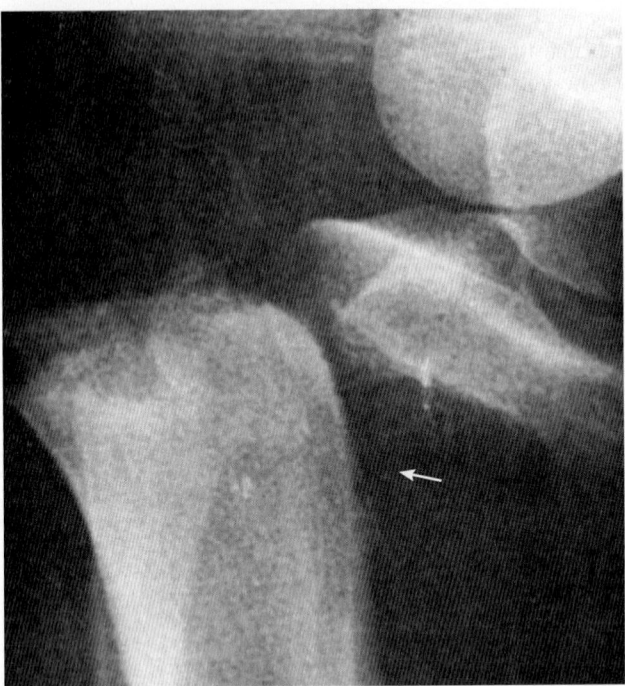

**FIGURE 82-14** Lateral radiograph of a markedly displaced fracture of the proximal tibial epiphysis.

artery. Vascular injury is equally likely with all directions of dislocation.

A study of 245 knee dislocations conducted by Green and colleagues found that approximately 40% of anterior and 40% of posterior dislocations were associated with a vascular lesion. The rationale for emergent treatment is supported by the findings of Green that vascular injuries treated within 8 hours from time of injury had an 87% salvage rate and a 13% amputation rate. In sharp contrast, vascular injuries untreated within 8 hours from time of onset resulted in an 85% amputation rate. A frequent clinical pitfall was erroneously correlating a warm but pulseless foot with good perfusion. In these cases, despite the fact that cutaneous circulation seemed brisk, significant muscular ischemia persisted.

The importance of time from injury cannot be overstated. Once a severe knee injury is diagnosed, observation of the limb is a luxury, even in the presence of a strong pulse and negative ischemic signs. Risks of observation outweigh the risks of exploration. Patients with an uncomplicated clinical picture whose fractures reduce spontaneously or are reduced with manipulation within an hour of injury, can be followed clinically. However, patients with delayed recognition of a serious injury, such as the multitrauma patient with spontaneous reduction whose limb injuries have received secondary priority, should be immediately taken to the operating room for exploration. This should be undertaken by a team capable of revascularizing the limb, should a lesion be found.

Other indications for immediate exploration include absence of a strong pulse and signs of ischemia. Patients with diminished pulse should be taken to the operating room by the vascular team for intraoperative arteriogram. Those with signs of ischemia should be explored through a posteromedial approach for direct evaluation of the popliteal artery. Immediate exploration is justified because of the overwhelming likelihood that the injury causing ischemia occurred in the popliteal region.

Bony stabilization with expeditious external fixation precedes definitive vascular repair (Fig. 82-15). Exploration then may proceed through a posteromedial incision. Ligamentous repair or reconstruction can be performed simultaneously in ideal circumstances. Either end-to-end anastomosis or a reverse saphenous vein graft repairs excised damaged portions of the artery. An arteriogram will locate suspected distal thrombus for removal by a Fogarty balloon catheter. Most, if not all, patients with a revascularization procedure should receive fasciotomies of all compartments in the lower leg. A two-incision approach for the fasciotomies is the preferred technique.

## Fractures of the Tibia and Fibula

### Tibia Intercondylar Eminence Fractures
The tibia intercondylar eminence is the insertion site of the anterior cruciate ligament, and avulsion fracture of this

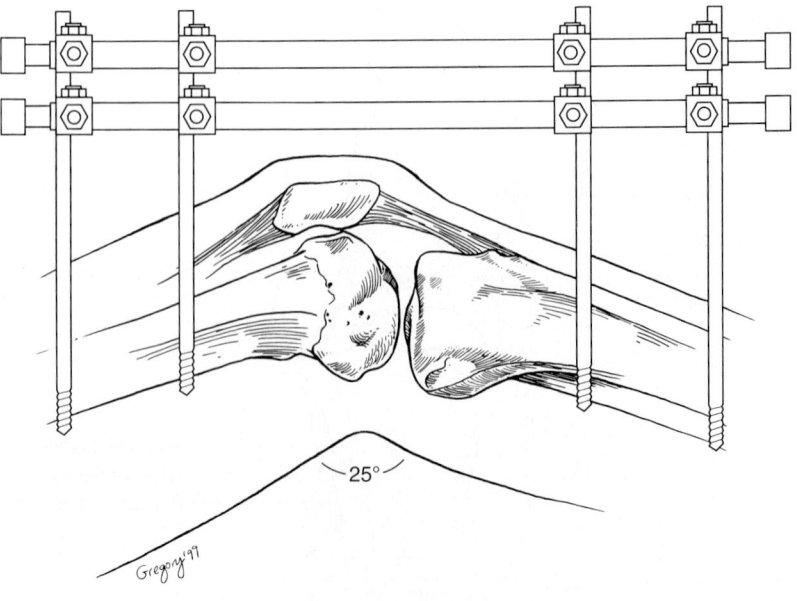

**FIGURE 82-15** Drawing of an external fixator spanning the knee joint.

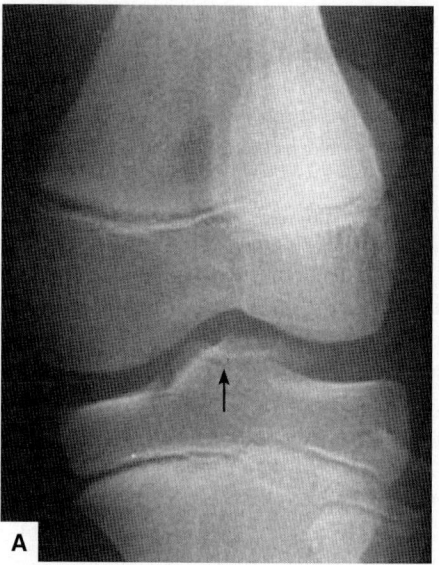 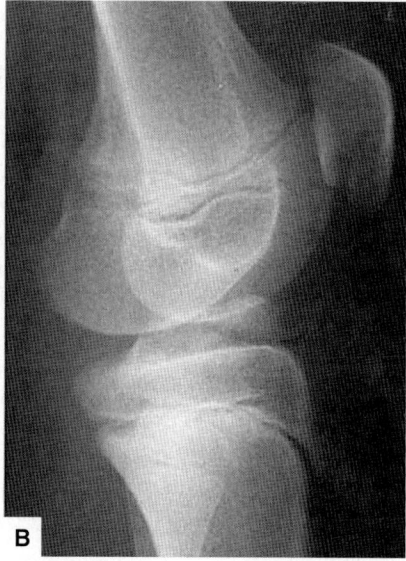 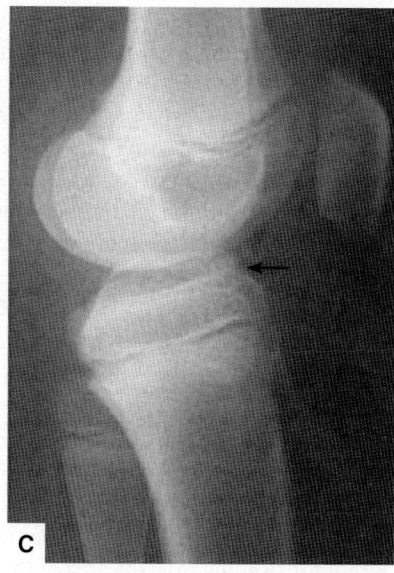

**FIGURE 82-16** **A.** An 11-year-old boy was riding his bicycle and fell off onto his left foot. The knee was swollen and had a hemarthrosis. The AP radiograph shows a displaced intercondylar eminance fracture at the attachment of the anterior cruciate ligament (arrow). **B.** Lateral radiograph shows the displaced fragment impinging into the joint. **C.** Reduction required arthroscopy to free the medial meniscus from under the fragment, suture repair of the fragment, and knee extension to help to hold the fragment reduced. The patient had mild anterior cruciate ligament laxity after the fracture was healed, but no clinical symptoms.

eminence is analogous in injury mechanism and presentation to an anterior cruciate ligament tear (Fig. 82-16). Nondisplaced fractures can be treated in a cast in slight knee flexion, whereas minimally displaced fractures require reduction and casting with the knee in full extension. More than minimal displacement requires surgical treatment, with either open or arthroscopic reduction and fixation.

## Proximal Tibia Physeal Fractures

Salter–Harris Type I and Type II proximal tibial physeal fractures are typically seen in teenagers as a result of a twisting injury during sports. While nondisplaced fractures may be successfully treated with nonoperative means, displaced fractures require more aggressive treatment. Displacement of the proximal tibial epiphysis presents a risk to the popliteal artery in the same manner as does a knee dislocation, and careful vascular evaluation should be performed as above. Intraarticular fractures require anatomic reduction and fixation. Occult fractures may occur, and MRI or stress radiographs can be helpful in confirming the clinical diagnosis.

The tibial tubercle may be avulsed by the patellar tendon during eccentric contraction of the quadriceps muscle in knee flexion, such as occurs during a landing from a jump. This fracture constitutes an injury to the proximal tibial physis and epiphysis. Nondisplaced fractures may be treated nonoperatively, but displaced fractures, especially those entering the knee joint, require surgical stabilization. Although rare, anterior compartment syndrome of the leg may occur following this fracture.

## Proximal Tibia Metaphysis Fractures

Fractures of the proximal tibia metaphysis are typically stable fractures with minimal displacement. The fibula is intact in approximately 50% of cases. During the healing and remodeling stages there is a generalized overgrowth of both the distal and the proximal physes. There is also asymmetric overgrowth of the medial side of the proximal tibia physis that can cause a progressive valgus deformity of the tibia. Although the mechanism is unknown, it is unlikely to result from a direct injury to the tibial physis, as an identical deformity can follow any cortical penetration of the proximal tibial metaphysis.

## Tibial Shaft Fractures

The tibia is the third most fractured long bone in children, after the forearm bones and the femur. The most common type of tibia fracture is the isolated tibia shaft fracture with the fibula intact. This is caused by indirect rotational forces. In the toddler, this fracture is often difficult to detect. Physical examination can be unremarkable, as can be the radiograph, unless oblique views are obtained. The fracture usually has a spiral or oblique pattern in the distal tibia, and because of the thick periosteal sleeve, significant instability or displacement is unusual. Generally, healing is uneventful with nonoperative treatment.

Most displaced fractures are amenable to closed treatment as well, although the tolerances of acceptable deformity are narrow. Closed reduction is often successful, although the fractures may displace, especially into varus, during cast treatment and close follow-up is required. While the specific indications for surgical intervention are beyond the scope of this text, fractures that cannot be successfully treated by closed means can be treated with external fixation or flexible intramedullary nailing.

Because of the thin soft tissue envelope of the tibia and the direct trauma mechanism of many tibia fractures, open tibia fractures are not uncommon. Principles of open fracture treatment are followed as described previously. External

**1113**

fixation is typically used for fracture stabilization in order to allow access to the wound for repeated debridements or coverage as needed.

Ipsilatreal femoral shaft fractures occur in 6% of tibial shaft fractures, usually occurring as a result of high-energy trauma. Complications are more common than for isolated fractures of either bone. Surgical stabilization of both fractures allows early mobilization of the multiply injured patient.

## Distal Tibia and Fibula Physeal Fractures

Ankle injuries in children can be very different from those in adults. Although ankle sprains involving the lateral ligaments do occur, children with open physes are more likely to sustain a fracture through the physis of the distal fibula during an inversion injury to the ankle. An ankle sprain can be differentiated from a distal fibula physeal fracture by the point of maximal tenderness. In either case, radiographs are normal except for swelling over the area of the lateral malleolus.

The most common distal tibia physeal fracture is a Salter–Harris Type II injury that does not involve the articular surface. This fracture can often be significantly displaced and can put pressure on the adjacent medial skin. If the skin is compromised, urgent reduction is required. The fracture is occasionally quite difficult to reduce, even in the operating room, because of entrapment of the tibialis posterior tendon. The physis is at risk for complete or partial growth arrest, particularly in the young child, and parents must be cautioned about this complication.

There are several physeal ankle fractures in children that also affect the articular surface. The Tillaux fracture is a Salter–Harris Type III pattern. It occurs when the lateral tibia physis is still open and the medial physis has closed. The mechanism is a rotational injury to the planted foot, with the anterior tibiofibular ligament avulsing the anterolateral aspect of the tibia epiphysis. The child presents with a swollen ankle and a hemarthrosis on clinical examination. If the fracture is displaced more than 2 mm, operative treatment is recommended.

## Foot Injuries

Metatarsal fractures are the most common pediatric foot fractures. The first metatarsal is most often injured in young children, and the fifth metatarsal is most often injured in adolescents. Nondisplaced fractures generally heal well with cast immobilization, with the exception of the Jones fracture in the proximal diaphysis of the fifth metatarsal, which is prone to delayed union. The secondary apophysis of the fifth metatarsal can be confused with a fracture, although avulsion fractures at the peroneus brevis insertion can occur. Lisfranc injury of the midfoot is a disruption of the ligaments at the metatarsal cuneiform joints. On first glance, the radiograph is often incorrectly believed to be normal, although the ligamentous injury may be accompanied by seemingly innocuous metatarsal base fractures. Nondisplaced injuries may be casted, whereas displaced injuries require reduction and pin or screw fixation. Metatarsal fractures resulting from crush injuries to the foot typically present with severe pain and swelling and should be evaluated for possible compartment syndrome.

Hindfoot fractures are rare in children. Fractures of the talus generally involve the talar neck and can threaten the vascularity of the talar dome, leading to osteonecrosis and collapse. Surgical treatment is required for all displaced fractures, and healing time may be slow. A child can sustain a nondisplaced calcaneal fracture, such as a low-energy compression fracture, from a minor fall. The child may limp for no obvious reason. Although the calcaneus may be tender, the radiograph initially may be normal. Healing is not apparent until several weeks after the injury. Treatment is with cast immobilization.

Toe phalanx fractures are not uncommon, and most are amenable to buddy taping for symptomatic relief. However, several fractures, such as intra-articular fractures, Seymour fractures (as described earlier in the hand), and malrotated fractures, warrant more aggressive treatment.

# THE MANGLED EXTREMITY AND AMPUTATION

The mangled extremity is a severe injury characterized by extensive bone and soft-tissue loss with major vascular injury and loss of innervation. This type of injury occurs from mechanisms such as crush injuries, motor vehicle crashes, motorcycle crashes, or train/pedestrian accidents. Because the rate of infection in severely mangled extremities is quite high, adequate débridement is essential to decrease the risk of infection. Also, fasciotomy should be performed to decrease the risk of compartment syndrome, although, in some cases, the injury may have already caused disruption and decompression of the fascial compartments.

Although the extent of soft-tissue loss often correlates with the need for amputation, this potential need is best predicted by the loss of innervation and failure to restore an adequate blood supply. However, the degree of soft-tissue injury does not necessarily correlate with the degree of bony injury. Thus, severely fractured extremities with intact soft tissue may be salvaged, whereas extensive destruction of soft tissue with minimal loss of bone often results in amputation.

## Lawn Mower Injuries

It is estimated that about 16,000 children younger than age 16 years are injured by a lawn mower each year, and 85% of these injuries occur in children younger than 14 years of age. Although the injured child is typically a bystander, injuries also occur to children operating a mower and to children who are passengers that fall from a mower. Injuries generally involve posterior and plantar aspects of the foot and carry a traumatic amputation rate of 20% to 50%. Such amputations are also more common in younger children.

Lawn mower injuries are considered high-energy injuries. The kinetic energy at 3000 rpm is 2000 ft-lbs, which is equal to 3 times the power of a 0.357 magnum gun. Such explosive wounds can propel highly infectious contaminants deep into the soft tissues. Wounds should be extended proximally and distally until normal tissue is encountered and contaminants lodged in various areas should undergo débridement.

Copious irrigation should then be delivered. For young children, a small external fixator across the area of injury provides excellent stabilization without constricting splints. It allows fracture fragments to be left in a reduced position, while still leaving the wounds exposed enough for repeat débridements. Several procedures spaced 1 or 2 days apart may be needed to attain a stable wound. Marginal tissue can be cleaned and reinspected after the initial surgery. After the wound is stable, definitive fixation of the fracture fragments can be performed if closure, skin grafting, or flap coverage is feasible. In many cases, revision amputation planning obviates the need for fracture fixation.

## Amputation

The length of time and emotional trauma associated with limb salvage often make early amputation and rapid rehabilitation a more workable solution for the child with massive extremity injury. Several injury scores have been useful indicators of successful limb salvage in the face of negative prognostic factors such as crush injury, massive soft-tissue damage, vascular compromise, irreversible neurologic loss, complex fractures, sepsis, and burns. Although these scales are not universally accepted, their use serves as a guideline to amputation in the severely injured patient. In some cases, however, reimplantation of certain amputated extremities can be successfully performed through the collaborative efforts of orthopaedic, plastic, and vascular surgeons. One of the most useful predictive scales is the Johansen Mangled Extremity Severity Score, which is presented in Table 82-2. If the combination of points in the 4 categories of this scale exceeds 7, this indicates that the extremity in question is nonsalvageable.

| TABLE 82-2 | Mangled Extremity Severity Score Variables | |
| --- | --- | --- |
| | | Points |
| Skeletal/soft tissue injury | | |
| Low energy (stab, simple fracture, civilian gunshot wound) | | 1 |
| Medium energy (open or multiple fractures, dislocation) | | 2 |
| High energy (close range shotgun or military gunshot wound) | | 3 |
| Very high energy (above + gross contamination, soft-tissue avulsion) | | 4 |
| Limb ischemia | | |
| Pulse reduced or absent but perfusion normal | | 1[a] |
| Pulseless, paresthesia, diminished capillary refill | | 2[a] |
| Cool, paralyzed, insensate, numb | | 3[a] |
| Shock | | |
| Systolic pressure >90 mm Hg | | 0 |
| Transient hypotension | | 1 |
| Persistent hypotension | | 2 |

Modified for children; that is, no age variable.
[a]Double points for ischemia >6 hours.

The category carrying the greatest weight, and therefore the worst prognosis, is limb ischemia, with points doubling after 6 hours.

## Amputation Techniques

Because preservation of extremity length is a primary goal in children, and because of the risk of terminal overgrowth of trans-diaphyseal amputations, the recommended levels of amputation differs from that in adults. Self-image, energy efficiency, and improved proprioception are important in the child amputee. New reconstructive techniques, such as tissue expansion and bone lengthening (Ilizarov) technology, can be employed to enhance a short amputation stump.

Flaps to cover the amputation do not have to be the traditional anterior and posterior based flaps if the available skin has good vascularity. Neuromuscular pedicle flaps (such as the latissimus dorsi flap in the upper extremity or the lateral proximal gastrocnemius flap in the lower extremity) can be used to improve distal skin coverage. Rotation of sensate flaps to the weight-bearing surface from nonweight-bearing portions of the stump is a good strategy. In the nonweight-bearing surfaces, large open wounds can be covered with split thickness grafts. The uncertain sensory return in free neurovascular pedicle grafts makes them less desirable for weight-bearing surfaces.

If possible, joint disarticulations are recommended in the growing child, preserving an intact epiphyseal/physeal unit at the end of an amputated limb in order to preserve the growth of the bone and prevent overgrowth of the transected bone. This overgrowth phenomenon causes the development of terminal spurs, which grow through the stump of 12% to 20% of children who have had trans-diaphyseal amputations. This is a frequent problem with amputations at the level of the humerus, but can occur in any long bone, including the femur and the tibia. Treatment of the overgrowth phenomenon is challenging and no technique is universally successful. It is therefore highly recommended to avoid trans-diaphyseal amputations in growing children.

A Syme amputation through the ankle joint, leaving the distal tibia epiphysis, is well tolerated. If a below-knee amputation is required, it can be useful to save one of the bones of the foot, such as the head of the talus, and attach it to the proximal tibia. This provides an osteocartilaginous distal amputation site that may prevent overgrowth. Through-the-knee amputations also prevent overgrowth and give some added length to the limb, rather than having an amputation through the level of the femoral diaphysis. However, a knee disarticulation level amputation makes it awkward to place a hinged prosthesis because the hinge is positioned too low to the ground. Acute shortening of the femur, leaving the articular surface of the knee intact, adjusts the height of the knee and can allow improved soft-tissue coverage. If the limb is expected to be too long, a distal femur epiphysiodesis can be performed.

## Prosthetics

Early rehabilitation in the young amputee is of paramount importance. If a lower extremity wound is not contaminated at the time of débridement, primary wound closure and fitting of an "instant prosthesis" is possible. At the time of surgery, a plaster socket is molded to the stump. A pylon is attached to this temporary socket. A prosthetic foot allows weight bearing within 24 hours. A permanent prosthesis is constructed once the amputation stump has healed and edema has subsided. If weight bearing is not possible, then physical therapy mobilization on crutches should begin as soon as the patient's condition permits.

Children accept and adapt to lower-extremity prostheses rapidly. However, because the volume of the stump increases, growth is a problem in the lower-extremity amputee. As the normal leg outgrows the prosthesis in length, the prosthesis can be lengthened. Advances in technology have resulted in prostheses that weigh less, that allow better motion, and that provide energy "storage" in the prosthetic mechanism.

Upper extremity prosthesis acceptance is low in children. The functionality of a prosthetic terminal device may be helpful in specific circumstances, such as sports activities. However, a sensate stump tends to be much more functional for activities of daily living than an insensate prosthesis. Despite advances in the control of the motor functions of the prosthesis, upper extremity prostheses are rarely worn.

## Nonaccidental Trauma

The greatest suspicion for NAT must be in younger children, particularly those younger than 1 year of age. A radiologic skeletal survey is especially useful in this age group because fractures in various stages of healing may not be recognized and because associated unsuspected fractures are commonly found. The tibia has been reported to be the most frequent long-bone fracture in these children, and in a series of postmortem fractures in infants, the distal tibia metaphysis was reported to be the most common fracture. Fractures of the rib, femur, humerus, and skull are also commonly seen in infants who have sustained nonaccidental injury. Because rib fractures are not easily seen on radiographs, they may be underreported.

Fractures are typically seen in the shaft of the long bones, either transverse or spiral/oblique. The classic NAT fracture pattern has been described as a corner fracture through the metaphysis adjacent to the physis, but extending through the diaphysis. The age at which a fracture occurs can be estimated by the amount of callus present in a diaphyseal fracture or by the amount of focal radiolucent extension of the physis into the metaphysis in a metaphyseal fracture.

Although 51% of fractures detected in a postmortem study involved the rib, only 36% of these were apparent on a skeletal survey. Rib fractures are commonly caused by thoracic compression and typically involve the posterior aspect of the rib or the costochondral junction. Early after injury, these fractures, especially those of the costochondral junction, are often not visible on radiographs. As fracture callus forms and new bone formation occurs, injuries gradually become more apparent.

Fractures of the femur in children under the age of 1 year or not yet walking should raise suspicion for NAT. For children older than 1 year of age who are walking, the likelihood of a femur fracture occurring from NAT is low, reported in only

1 of 42 fractures. Children older than 1 year of age are quite active and can generate enough force to fracture the femur during a fall. Falls of less than 3 to 4 feet, however, do not generally cause a serious injury. In children younger than 3 years of age, even falls from a height of less than 10 feet rarely result in severe or life-threatening injuries.

In young patients, humeral shaft fractures have historically been felt to be strongly associated with child abuse, whereas supracondylar humerus fractures have been considered accidental. However, recent studies have found that the majority of these fractures in young children are not caused by abuse.

## SELECTED READINGS

### General Principles

Armstrong PF. Initial management of the multiply injured child: the ABC's. *Instr Course Lect* 1992;41:347–350.

Cheng JC, Shen WY. Limb fracture pattern in different pediatric age groups: a study of 3,350 children. *J Orthop Trauma* 1993;7:15–22.

Gustilo RB, Merkow RL, Templeman D. Current concepts review. The management of open fractures. *J Bone Joint Surg Am* 1990;72:299–304.

Loder RT. Pediatric polytrauma: orthopaedic care and hospital course. *J Orthop Trauma* 1987;1:48–54.

Murray DW, Wilson-MacDonald J, Morscher E, Rahn BA, Käslin M. Bone growth and remodeling after fracture. *J Bone Joint Surg Br* 1996;78:42–50.

Pape HC, Tornetta P III, Tarkin I, Tzioupis C, Sabeson V, Olson SA. Timing of fracture fixation in multitrauma patients: the role of early total care and damage control surgery. *J Am Acad Orthop Surg* 2009;17:541–549.

Peterson HA. Partial growth plate arrest and its treatment. *J Pediatr Orthop* 1984;4:246–258.

Wilkins KE. Principles of fracture remodeling in children. *Injury* 2005;36: A3–A11.

### Vascular Injuries

Blakey CM, Biant LC, Birch R. Ischaemia and the pink, pulseless hand complicating supracondylar fractures of the humerus in childhood: long-term follow-up. *J Bone Joint Surg Br* 2009;91:1487–1492.

Halvorson JJ, Anz A, Langfitt M, et al. Vascular injury associated with extremity trauma: initial diagnosis and management. *J Am Acad Orthop Surg* 2011;19:495–504.

Kauvar DS, Sarfati MR, Kraiss LW. National trauma databank analysis of mortality and limb loss in isolated lower extremity vascular trauma. *J Vasc Surg* 2011;53:1598–1603.

Klinkner DB, Arca MJ, Lewis BD, Oldham KT, Sato TT. Pediatric vascular injuries: patterns of injury, morbidity, and mortality. *J Pediatr Surg* 2007;42:178–183.

Mangat KS, Martin AG, Bache CE. The 'pulseless pink' hand after supracondylar fracture of the humerus in children: the predictive value of nerve palsy. *J Bone Joint Surg Br* 2009;91:1521–1525.

Patterson BM, Agel J, Swiontkowski MF, Mackenzie EJ, Bosse MJ, LEAP Study Group. Knee dislocations with vascular injury: outcomes in the Lower Extremity Assessment Project (LEAP) Study. *J Trauma* 2007;63: 855–858.

Shah SR, Wearden PD, Gaines BA. Pediatric peripheral vascular injuries: a review of our experience. *J Surg Res* 2009;153:162–166.

White L, Mehlman CT, Crawford AH. Perfused, pulseless, and puzzling: a systematic review of vascular injuries in pediatric supracondylar humerus fractures and results of a POSNA questionnaire. *J Pediatr Orthop* 2010;30:328–335.

### Compartment Syndrome

Bae DS, Kadiyala RK, Waters PM. Acute compartment syndrome in children: contemporary diagnosis, treatment, and outcome. *J Pediatr Orthop* 2001;21:680–688.

Flynn JM, Bashyal RK, Yeger-McKeever M, Garner MR, Launay F, Sponseller PD. Acute traumatic compartment syndrome of the leg in children: diagnosis and outcome. *J Bone Joint Surg Am* 2011;93:937–941.

Hovius SE, Ultee J. Volkmann's ischemic contracture. Prevention and treatment. *Hand Clin* 2000;16:647–657.

Matsen FA 3rd. Compartment syndrome. An unified concept. *Clin Orthop Relat Res* 1975;(113):8–14.

Prasarn ML, Ouellette EA. Acute compartment syndrome of the upper extremity. *J Am Acad Orthop Surg* 2011;19:49–58.

Stevanovic M, Sharpe F. Management of established Volkmann's contracture of the forearm in children. *Hand Clin* 2006;22:99–111.

## Fractures and Dislocations of the Upper Extremity

Bahrs C, Zipplies S, Ochs BG, et al. Proximal humeral fractures in children and adolescents. *J Pediatr Orthop* 2009;29:238–242.

Blakemore LC, Cooperman DR, Thompson GH, Wathey C, Ballock RT. Compartment syndrome in ipsilateral humerus and forearm fractures in children. *Clin Orthop* 2000;376:33–38.

Brauer CA, Lee BM, Bae DS, Waters PM, Kocher MS. A systematic review of medial and lateral entry pinning versus lateral entry pinning for supracondylar fractures of the humerus. *J Pediatr Orthop* 2007;27:181–186.

Cornwall R, Ricchetti ET. Pediatric phalanx fractures: unique challenges and pitfalls. *Clin Orthop Relat Res* 2006;445:146–156.

Davidson JS, Brown DJ, Barnes SN, Bruce CE. Simple treatment for torus fractures of the distal radius. *J Bone Joint Surg Br* 2001;83:1173–1175.

Kamath AF, Baldwin K, Horneff J, Hosalkar HS. Operative versus non-operative management of pediatric medial epicondyle fractures: a systematic review. *J Child Orthop* 2009;3:345–357.

Nakamura K, Hirachi K, Uchiyama S, et al. Long-term clinical and radiographic outcomes after open reduction for missed Monteggia fracture-dislocations in children. *J Bone Joint Surg Am* 2009;91:1394–1404.

Ring D, Jupiter JB, Waters PM. Monteggia fractures in children and adults. *J Am Acad Orthop Surg* 1998;6:215–224.

Song KS, Kang CH, Min BW, Bae KC, Cho CH. Internal oblique radiographs for diagnosis of nondisplaced or minimally displaced lateral condylar fractures of the humerus in children. *J Bone Joint Surg Am* 2007;89:58–63.

Van der Resi WL, Otsuka NY, Moroz P, Mah J. Intramedullary nailing versus plate fixation for unstable forearm fractures in children. *J Pediatr Orthop* 1998;18:9–13.

## Fractures and Dislocations of the Lower Extremity

Arslan H, Kapukaya A, Kesemenli C, Subaşi M, Kayikçi C. Floating knee in children. *J Pediatr Orthop* 2003;23:458–463.

Butcher CC, Hoffman EB. Supracondylar fractures of the femur in children: closed reduction and percutaneous pinning of displaced fractures. *J Pediatr Orthop* 2005;25:145–148.

Cassinelli EH, Young B, Vogt M, Pierce MC, Deeney VF. Spica cast application in the emergency room for select pediatric femur fractures. *J Orthop Trauma* 2005;19:709–716.

Herrera-Soto JA, Price CT. Traumatic hip dislocations in children and adolescents: pitfalls and complications. *J Am Acad Orthop Surg* 2009;17:15–21.

Ho CA, Skaggs DL, Tang CW, Kay RM. Use of flexible intramedullary nails in pediatric femur fractures. *J Pediatr Orthop* 2006;26:497–504.

Kay RM, Matthys GA. Pediatric ankle fractures: evaluation and treatment. *J Am Acad Orthop Surg* 2001;9:268–278.

Kensinger DR, Guille JT, Horn BD, Herman MJ. The stubbed great toe: importance of early recognition and treatment of open fractures of the distal phalanx. *J Pediatr Orthop* 2001;21:31–34.

Kocher MS, Sink EL, Blasier RD, et al. Treatment of pediatric diaphyseal femur fractures. *J Am Acad Orthop Surg* 2009;17:718–725.

Lynch JM, Gardner MG, Gains B. Hemodynamic significance of pediatric femur fractures. *J Pediatr Surg* 1996;31:1358–1361.

Moon ES, Mehlman CT. Risk factors for avascular necrosis after femoral neck fractures in children: 25 Cincinnati cases and meta-analysis of 360 cases. *J Orthop Trauma* 2006;20:323–329.

Myers SH, Spiegel D, Flynn JM. External fixation of high-energy tibia fractures. *J Pediatr Orthop* 2007;27:537–539.

Pape JM, Goulet JA, Hensinger RN. Compartment syndrome complicating tibial tubercle avulsion. *Clin Orthop Relat Res* 1993;295:201–204.

Ribbans WJ, Natarajan R, Alavala S. Pediatric foot fractures. *Clin Orthop Relat Res* 2005;432:107–115.

Song KM, Sangeorzan B, Benirschke S, Browne R. Open fractures of the tibia in children. *J Pediatr Orthop* 1996;16:635–639.

Yang JP, Letts RM. Isolated fractures of the tibia with intact fibula in children: a review of 95 patients. *J Pediatr Orthop* 1997;17:347–351.

## Mangled Extremities and Amputation

Davids JR, Meyer LC, Blackhurst DW. Operative treatment of bone overgrowth in children who have acquired or congenital amputation. *J Bone Joint Surg* Am 1995;77:1490–1497.

Gregory RT, Gould RJ, Peclet M, et al. The mangled extremity syndrome (MES): a severity grading system for multisystem injury of the extremity. *J Trauma* 1985;25:1147–1150.

Hervé C, Gaillard M, Andrivet P, Roujas F, Kauer C, Huguenard P. Treatment of serious lower limb injuries: Amputation versus preservation. *Injury* 1987;18:21–23.

Johansen K, Daines M, Howey T, Helfet D, Hansen ST. Objective criteria accurately predict amputation following lower extremity trauma. *J Trauma* 1990;30:568–573.

Lawn mowing injuries common in children and teens. *Science Daily.* June 3, 2008. http://www.sciencedaily.com/releases/2008/06/080603091342.htm.

Poole GV, Agnew SG, Griswold JA, Rhodes RS. The mangled lower extremity: Can salvage be predicted? *Am Surg* 1994;60:50–55.

Vollman D, Smith GA. Epidemiology of lawn-mower-related injuries to children in the United States, 1990-2004. *Pediatrics* 2006;118:e273–e278.

## Non-Accidental Trauma

Blakemore LC, Loder RT, Hensinger RN. Role of intentional abuse in children 1 to 5 years old with isolated femoral shaft fractures. *J Pediatr Orthop* 1996;16:585–588.

Dalton JH, Slovis T, Helfer RE, Comstock J, Scheurer S, Riolo S. Undiagnosed abuse in children younger than 3 years with femoral fracture. *Am J Dis Child* 1990;144:875–878.

Garcia VF, Gotshall CS, Eichelberger MR, Bowman LM. Rib fractures in children: A marker of severe trauma. *J Trauma* 1990;30:695–700.

Kleinman PK, Marks SC, Spevak MR, Belanger PL, Richmond JM. Extension of growth plate cartilage into the metaphysis: A sign of healing fracture in abused infants. *Am J Roentgenol* 1991;156:775–779.

Loder RT, Bookout C. Fracture patterns in battered children. *J Orthop Trauma* 1991;5:33–42.

Novacheck TF. The role of the orthopaedic surgeon in diagnosing child abuse. In: Morrissy RT, Weinstein SL, eds. *Lovell and Winter's Pediatric Orthopaedics.* 6th ed. Philadelphia: Lippincott Williams & Wilkins; 2006.

Williams RA. Injuries in infants and small children resulting from witnessed and corroborated free falls. *J Trauma* 1991;31:1350–1352.

# Burn Injury

# CHAPTER 83

*John P. Crow*

## KEY POINTS

1. Most children survive a burn injury regardless of the size of cutaneous injury.

2. Sepsis, respiratory failure, and anoxic brain injury are the leading causes of death in pediatric burn victims.

3. The Parkland formula with modifications for size and presence of inhalational injury is the resuscitation formula of choice.

4. Colloid is often used to prevent crystalloid over-resuscitation despite a lack of evidence regarding outcome.

5. *Early burn wound excision* with skin coverage is the most important therapeutic maneuver with full-thickness injury to the skin.

6. Silver-impregnated products provide excellent wound coverage for exposed dermis present in donor sites and partial-thickness wounds and limited full-thickness burn wounds.

7. Dermal replacement products are valuable in extensive burn injury for wound coverage and neodermal development.

8. *Optimal nutrition* is essential in the management of moderate and large surface area burn injury.

9. Pharmacological therapy is helpful in optimizing nutrition and blunting the hypermetabolic response.

## BURN CARE IN THE TWENTY-FIRST CENTURY

There have been many advances in the care of the burn victim since the middle part of the twentieth century. Current survival rates indicate how successful burn care has become. A 50% mortality rate for a 20% body surface area burn in the late 1940s can be compared to at least a 65% survival rate currently reported in 85% body surface area burn. Survival is nearly assured in a child with any size burn who arrives to a burn unit alive with published mortality rates of less than 3%. In a 20-year autopsy study of 145 children dying of burn injury, 47% died of sepsis, 29% from respiratory failure, and most of the remainder from anoxic brain injury.

## RESUSCITATION

The first task, when presented with a newly burned child, is to follow the ABCs of trauma. Assessment of the airway is paramount in a patient with burn injury of the face and neck or with exposure to smoke in an enclosure. Intubation may be necessary because of neurologic changes from carbon monoxide poisoning, airway obstruction, or for airway protection (Table 83-1). The edema of the burned airway will peak at 12 hours post injury, converting a routine intubation at time of arrival into a difficult one. The burned child with impending upper airway obstruction will only become symptomatic moments before disaster. *"When in doubt, intubate!"* Figure 83-1 is an algorithm for airway management.

There are 2 considerations when dealing with flame burns to the airway. First is the consideration of flame injury to the airway itself. The inhaled flame will only burn as deeply as the vocal cords. Injury proximal to the vocal cords must be considered when there are deep burns of the face and neck, soot in the mouth, singed nasal hairs, and, most importantly, glottic swelling. The second consideration is the development of respiratory failure from the hundreds of components found in the smoke that is inhaled. This is a chemical injury to the proximal airways of the tracheobronchial tree from water-soluble compounds formed from the smoke. Lipid-soluble compounds are harmful to the lung at the alveolar level. The lung injury itself may be delayed in presentation up to 3 days post exposure. The treatment follows standard respiratory protocols with special attention to the unplugging of the smaller airways.

Carbon monoxide is a leading cause of death in a fire. Any patient that is exposed to smoke in an enclosed environment is at risk. The keystone of treatment is 100% oxygen from the prehospital phase through the immediate burn period until the carboxyhemoglobin level is in an acceptable range. An arterial blood sample is the only reliable way to monitor progress because bedside pulse oximetry is erroneously normal in carbon monoxide toxicity. There is no evidence-based

1118

| TABLE 83-1 | Absolute and Relative Indications for Endotracheal Intubation of the Burned Child | |
|---|---|---|
| **Absolute Indications for Intubation** | **Relative Indications** | |
| Full-thickness burns to face, lips, mouth, and neck | Soot in oropharynx | |
| Smoke inhalation seen by endoscopy | Singed nasal hairs | |
| Airway obstruction | Exposure in closed space | |
| Carbon monoxide toxicity with neurologic change | Partial-thickness burns to face | |
| Massive body burns with circumferential chest-wall injury | | |

wall excursion (Fig. 83-2). This procedure is done with the electrocautery at the bedside in the massively burned child, usually with intravenous anesthesia. Otherwise, general anesthesia may be needed if the patient has more limited burn injury and is awake.

Next is the assessment of the burn wound. The volume of resuscitation fluid needed depends on the amount of body surface area injured (partial- and full-thickness burn only) and the association with inhalation injury. The amount of body surface area injured can be estimated easily by simple proportions. The "rules of nine" provide a crude estimate of burn size injury in the adolescent. Smaller children and infants have a higher proportion of skin in the head relative to their legs (Fig. 83-3). Accurate documentation of the burn injury is essential for immediate and late therapy. Computer diagrams are now available and extremely valuable in estimating fluid needs. First-degree burns are not counted and are of no acute clinical significance.

Resuscitative fluids are based on the amount of burned skin. Resuscitation is needed when more that 10% of body surface area in a child is injured and 15% in the teenager. The most commonly used formula is the Parkland formula that estimates the fluid needs at 4 mL/kg/% burn for the first 24 hours using lactated ringers (LR), a balanced salt solution. Half of the fluid is given during the first 8 hours when there is a massive outpouring of fluid into the burn wound and surrounding tissues and the other half is given over the remaining 16 hours. A total of 6 mL/kg/% burn is used with concomitant inhalation injury. This formula will underestimate total fluid needs in the infant and small child because there is a proportionally larger maintenance fluid need.

literature supporting the use of hyperbaric oxygen with carbon monoxide toxicity from burn injury.

Following airway assessment is the preservation of the circulation. Warmed fluids and a hot environment are vital to the resuscitation process. There is a high risk of hypothermia in the triage area. The patient with a burn has often been exposed to the environment for long periods of time prior to arrival in the burn center. Stress on the patient, as well as inadequate perfusion of the burned tissues, may lead to further loss of viable dermis in the zone of ischemia, bordering the burn injury. Escharotomies may be necessary to preserve distal limb perfusion and permit adequate chest

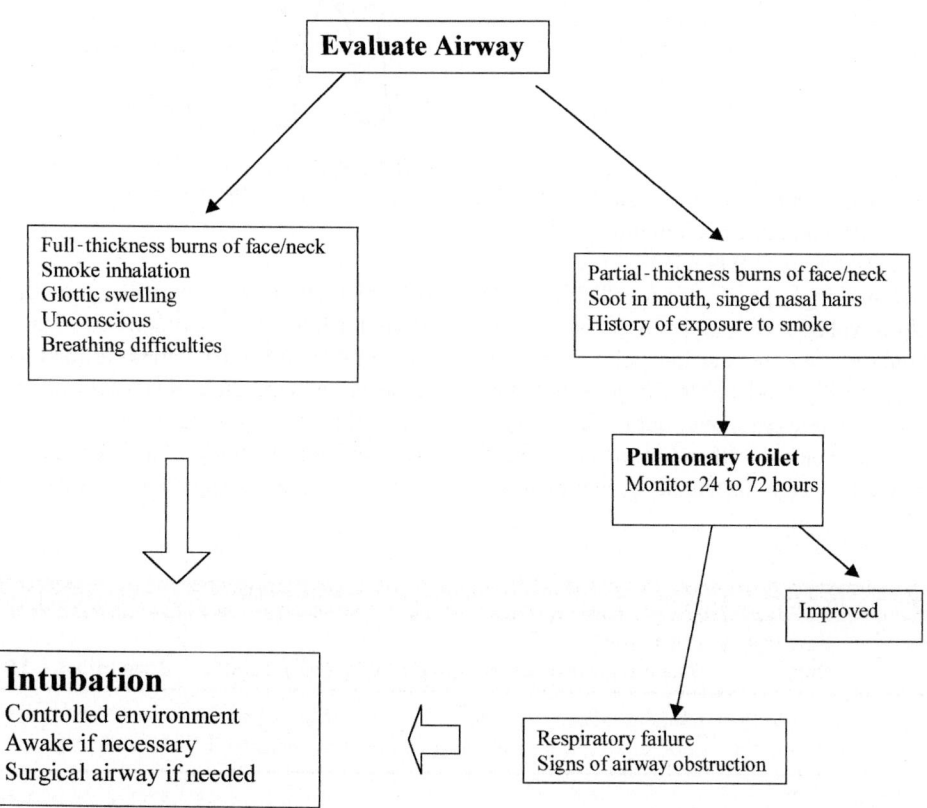

**FIGURE 83-1** Algorithm for airway management of the burned child.

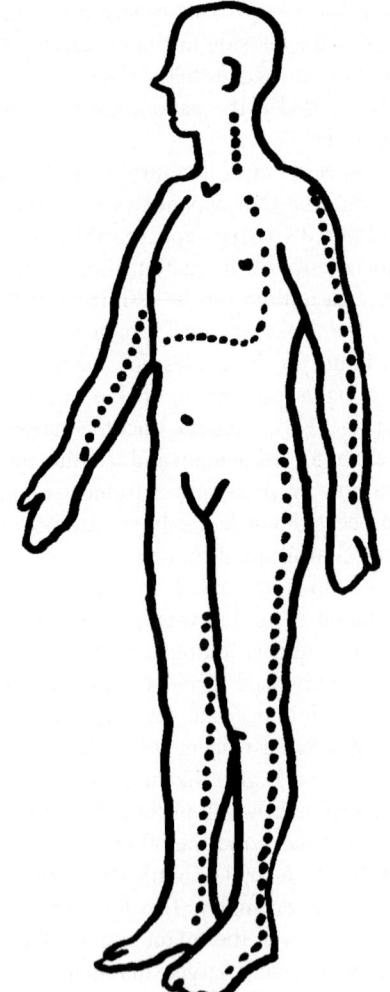

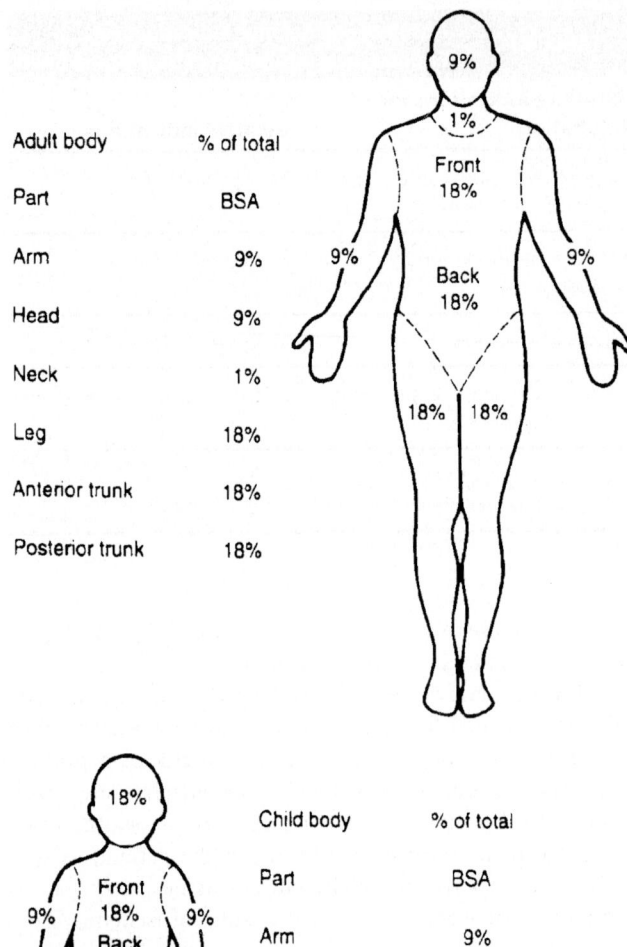

| Adult body | % of total |
|---|---|
| Part | BSA |
| Arm | 9% |
| Head | 9% |
| Neck | 1% |
| Leg | 18% |
| Anterior trunk | 18% |
| Posterior trunk | 18% |

**FIGURE 83-2** A diagram of the sites used for escharotomy. Depending on the area of burn involved, medial and lateral incisions can be made down each extremity as well as down the lateral trunk, across the lower chest, and down the neck.

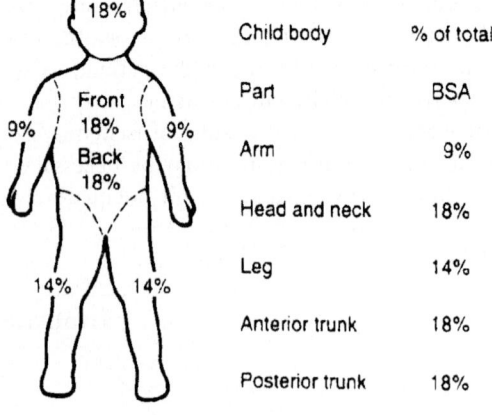

| Child body | % of total |
|---|---|
| Part | BSA |
| Arm | 9% |
| Head and neck | 18% |
| Leg | 14% |
| Anterior trunk | 18% |
| Posterior trunk | 18% |

**FIGURE 83-3** A diagram of the "rules of nine" to estimate burn size in the adult and how it differs on the child.

Maintenance fluids must be added to the total in kids less than 30 kg (<5 years old) while dextrose should be added to infants less than 15 kg (<2 years old) (Table 83-2).

There is currently no single parameter to reliably guide the appropriate fluid volume in the resuscitative phase. The Parkland formula defines the starting point and is an estimate of the likely hourly fluid needs. Urine output has been the most commonly used parameter but is often a poor indicator of intravascular volume. Other parameters include central venous pressure, serum lactate level, hemoglobin level, mental status, tachycardia, and others. There is no substitute for frequent assessment by a clinician in the care of a moderate or large burn patient in the first 24 hours where all of the parameters can be reviewed with appropriate modification of the burn resuscitation rate.

Colloid administration has been extensively studied in the burn patient, but considerable controversy still exists regarding

| TABLE 83-2 | Parkland Formula for Burn Injury with Modifications for Weight and Presence of Inhalational Injury | | | |
|---|---|---|---|---|
| | Burn Injury Only | Burn Injury plus Inhalation | Burn Injury < 30 kg (<5 yrs Old) | Burn Injury < 15 kg (< 2 yrs Old) |
| Lactated Ringers (LR) | 4 mL/kg/% burn | 6 mL/kg/% burn | 4 mL/kg/% burn plus maintenance IVF (6 mL/kg/% burn with inhalation) | |
| $D_5$ LR or LR and $D_5$ 0.45 NS in split amounts | | | | 4 mL/kg/% burn plus maintenance IVF (6 mL/kg/% burn with inhalation) |

## Anatomy of Normal Skin

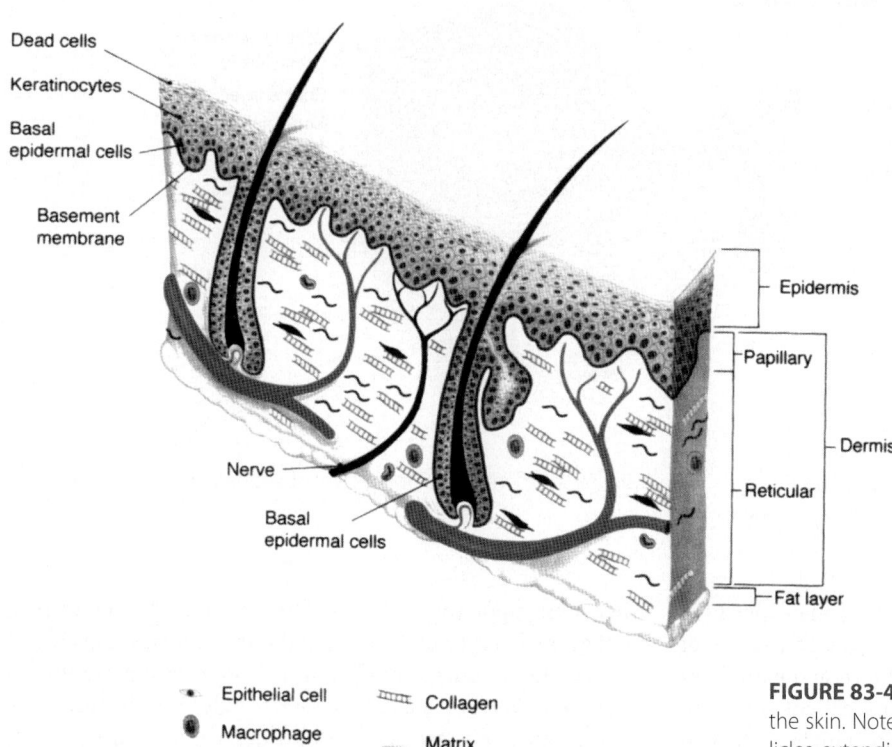

Dead cells
Keratinocytes
Basal epidermal cells
Basement membrane

Epidermis
Papillary
Dermis
Reticular
Fat layer

Nerve
Basal epidermal cells

- Epithelial cell
- Macrophage
- Fibroblast
- Neutrophil
- Collagen
- Matrix (glycosaminoglycans)
- Matrix protein (fibronectin)

**FIGURE 83-4** This is a diagram of the normal anatomy of the skin. Note the epidermis and how it lines the hair follicles extending deep into the dermis, the proportion of dermis to epidermis (4:1 or more), the nerves and blood vessels in the dermis, and outer lining of dead cells in the epidermis, which provides the barrier to the outside.

its use, particularly in the immediate postburn period. The addition of exogenous albumin is discouraged in the first 8 to 12 hours after burn injury because of capillary leak of all noncellular fluids. Albumin is helpful in replenishing the plasma proteins in the burned child after the cellular junctions have tightened at the 12th hour. This will restore vascular oncotic pressure, reducing the amount of peripheral edema, and may preserve gut motility. There is a strong argument for the use of colloid in the prevention of "fluid creep" where a large volume of crystalloid resuscitation alone leads to complications of edema. Massive edema can cause poor perfusion, worsening respiratory compliance, and the development of intraabdominal compartment syndrome. In a recent survey of 101 burn center staff, (49% directors, 19% staff physicians, and 23% nurses), 70% used the Parkland formula for burn resuscitation while 50% used colloid in the first 24 hours. Evidence providing the effectiveness of albumin in overall outcome is lacking.

## BURN WOUND

The assessment of the burn wound in a child requires patience and vigilance. The wound is in the early stages of evolution when first seen in the triage area. It is prudent to decide about skin grafting on the second or third day and not in the triage room unless the skin appears thick white, brown, or black. A thick white appearance is typical of a full-thickness injury. Brown or black eschar is worrisome for a fourth-degree

component with necrosis of the fat and deeper tissues. With a full-thickness circumferential injury particularly from flame injury, escharotomy is needed. This is best done at the time of initial evaluation. A hot water burn is notorious for appearing deep in the first week, yet healing without surgery. By the 10th post burn day, most partial-thickness hot water burns will be closed while open wounds will benefit from prompt graft closure. Immersion burns are usually deeper than accidental burns due to the prolonged exposure to hot water.

An understanding of the anatomy of the skin is essential in the treatment of burn injury (Fig. 83-4). The epidermis is the thin layer of skin that is destroyed in all partial- and full-thickness injuries. This thin layer provides the most important immediate functions of the skin. When it is gone, the barrier to the outside world is lost. Therefore, tissue fluids evaporate continuously through the wound and bacteria can enter the host. The dermis is the thick supporting structure for this important outer layer. The dermis is thickest at the palms and soles of the feet and thinnest in the eyelids. A burn injury heals because of the keratinocytes lining the adnexal structures of the dermis. These epithelial cells that ultimately produce keratin resurface the exposed dermis over time. If all of the dermis is destroyed, healing must occur from the lateral edges at an incredibly slow rate. Therefore:

1. If the dermis is destroyed (a third-degree burn), then the wound must be replaced with a skin graft or heal by secondary intention from the lateral edge (around 4 weeks for a wound the size of a silver dollar).

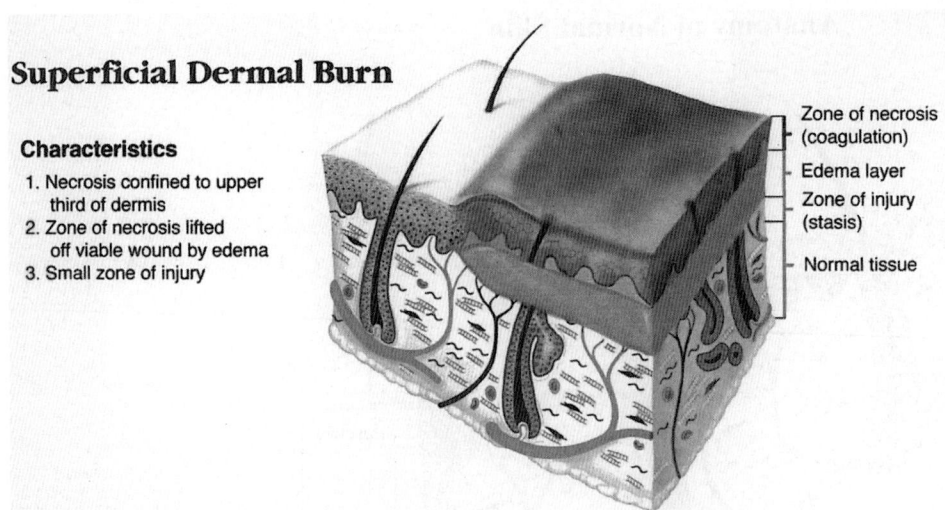

## Superficial Dermal Burn

### Characteristics

1. Necrosis confined to upper third of dermis
2. Zone of necrosis lifted off viable wound by edema
3. Small zone of injury

- Zone of necrosis (coagulation)
- Edema layer
- Zone of injury (stasis)
- Normal tissue

**FIGURE 83-5** A superficial partial-thickness injury with involvement of the upper layer of dermis and blister formation. Note the different zones of injury.

2. A burn wound in an area of thick dermis may appear to be full thickness but will heal once the deepest layers of the dermis are exposed (back, soles of feet, and palms). In contrast, in areas of thin dermis or in a patient with thin skin (infants), grafting is needed at a much higher rate with granulation present by 14 days postburn.

3. It is important to protect the exposed dermis until it heals with an antimicrobial cream in a moist environment. The always present bacteria, if allowed to proliferate, will deepen a partial-thickness burn into a full-thickness injury.

4. The appearance of the adnexal structures in the burn wound, particularly hair follicles with surrounding skin islands, indicates partial-thickness injury.

The telltale sign of a full-thickness injury is the presence of a white eschar, indicating the coagulation of the dermal proteins. Careful and repeated examination of the wound is more reliable in assessing the need for skin grafting. Sensation can vary depending upon the thickness of the skin, how it is performed, and over what area of the body and is therefore less reliable.

First-degree burns are obvious to everyone and require no treatment. With only a red but intact epidermis, the functions of the skin are preserved. Second-degree burns are a spectrum that can be arbitrarily divided into superficial and deep.

In a superficial second-degree injury, the texture of the skin is preserved so that the skin lines are visible in the dermal bed. Often, there is blister formation that disrupts on its own (Fig. 83-5). With deeper but still superficial partial-thickness injury, the outer skin is gone but the contour of the skin is preserved. When providing the proper environment in this type of burn wound, healing should occur with little or no scar formation in 10 days or less. These wounds manifest severe pain as a result of exposure of the nerve endings in the wound, particularly during dressing changes.

Deep second-degree burns have a more homogenous, but still red, appearance in the dermal bed (Fig. 83-6). The area

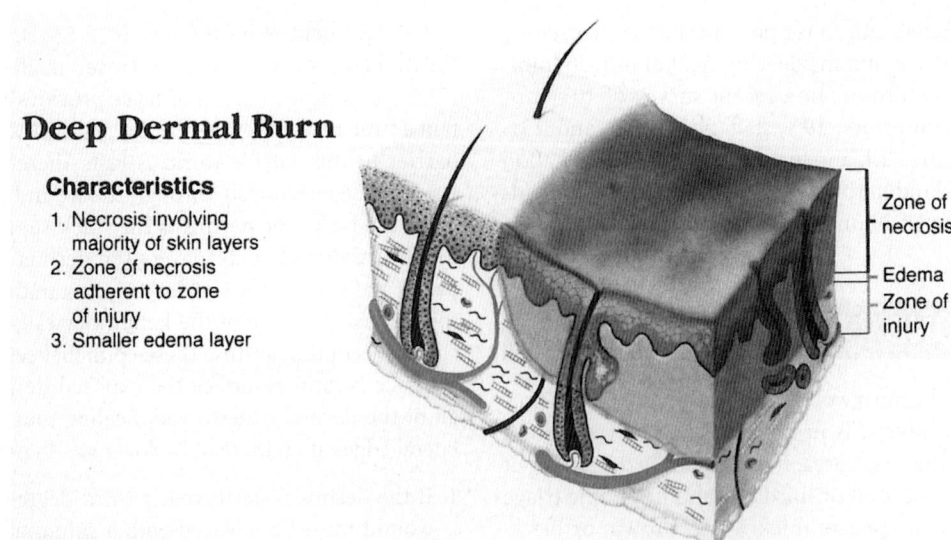

## Deep Dermal Burn

### Characteristics

1. Necrosis involving majority of skin layers
2. Zone of necrosis adherent to zone of injury
3. Smaller edema layer

- Zone of necrosis
- Edema
- Zone of injury

**FIGURE 83-6** A deeper but still partial-thickness injury. Dermal elements are still present.

## Full-Thickness Burn

**Characteristic**

No remaining
viable dermis

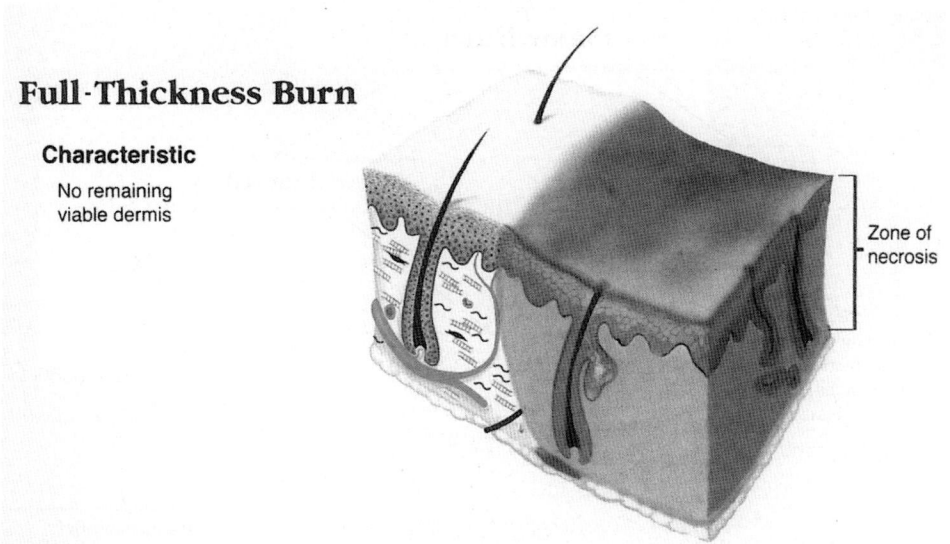

Zone of
necrosis

**FIGURE 83-7** A full-thickness injury of the dermis. There are no epidermal cells left to resurface the wound.

may even be covered with a white eschar for the first 10 days that eventually thins and disappears. The healing process takes from 10 to 21 days for epithelial coverage and may leave a significant scar. The use of enzyme therapy, collagenase in this type of burn will dissolve the white eschar in a shorter period of time with better evaluation of the injury by the surgeon and possible earlier spontaneous wound closure. Critical areas of the body with deep partial-thickness burns, particularly the hands and feet, are better treated with an early skin graft rather than to risk the scar formation from a burn that heals in a 10- to 21-day period.

Third-degree burns have thick, white eschar and tend to have less pain compared to second-degree burn injury (Fig. 83-7). Brown or black eschar is always third degree with extension of the thermal injury into the fat and deeper tissues. Once it is clear that a burn is third or fourth degree, grafting should be planned and performed as expeditiously as possible.

## EARLY HOSPITAL CARE

After the initial resuscitative phase is complete, careful attention to fluids, nutrition, and the burn wound is paramount in the successful care of the burn victim. Respiratory toilet is also vital in any patient exposed to smoke or flame injury to the face.

Evaporative losses continue until the burn wound is covered. Free water loss is expected and appropriately treated by adding free water to the enteral formula. After the initial phase of resuscitation, urine output is a poor indicator of fluid status. Higher-than-normal urinary output is required to return the patient to a euvolumic state. Body weight and serum electrolytes are the best guide for fluid replacement. Careful monitoring and replacement of phosphorus and zinc is needed as well as vitamin supplementation.

Virtually all children can be sustained with enteral feedings. It is the standard of care in a large burn (>30% body surface area) to start enteral feedings in the first 24 hours after the burn injury. It is harmful and counterproductive to wait until there is evidence of bowel function. Even one day of bowel rest causes villous blunting and an ileus. A nasojejunal tube is usually needed, particularly in the massively burned victim. There is recent evidence demonstrating an improved immune response, a less severe hypermetabolic response, and a decrease in the need for central venous access when enteral nutrition is started early and sustained throughout the burn stay. Even a moderately sized partial-thickness burn that does not require skin coverage may need enteral supplementation because of a decrease in appetite and increased caloric needs.

The burn wound must be examined daily. Flame burns that may initially appear to be of partial thickness will often progress over the first 3 days. Hot water burns are even more difficult to predict on first examination. Figures 83-8 and 83-9 outline algorithms for the management of flame and hot water burn wounds.

Daily hydrotherapy is a time-tested and often overlooked treatment of the burn wound, especially in the care of the child in a nonburn unit setting. The dead tissue, as well as the wound byproducts, must be cleaned off daily as much as the patient will tolerate. Procedural sedation is essential with short-acting anxiolytic and analgesic therapy. Proper protocols need to be developed and followed to protect the child during hydrotherapy when procedural sedation is used.

Topical antimicrobial cream is the primary treatment in the prevention of burn wound sepsis (Table 83-3). Silver sulfadiazine is an ideal agent in a deep partial- and full-thickness burn. It has a broad antimicrobial and antifungal spectrum, moderate eschar penetration, and can be applied daily without pain. It can cause profound neutropenia but is of uncertain clinical significance. Silver sulfadiazine will often arrest the late phases of healing if used in a partial-thickness injury. Mefanide is a much more potent agent with a broad spectrum of antimicrobial activity and excellent eschar penetration but is used primarily to prevent chondritis of the ear due to its systemic complications. Bacitracin is ideal for the superficial partial-thickness wound and for the deep partial-thickness wound in the last phases of healing. Collagenase is an enzyme that can be added to bacitracin to accelerate eschar removal, especially with thin, white eschar.

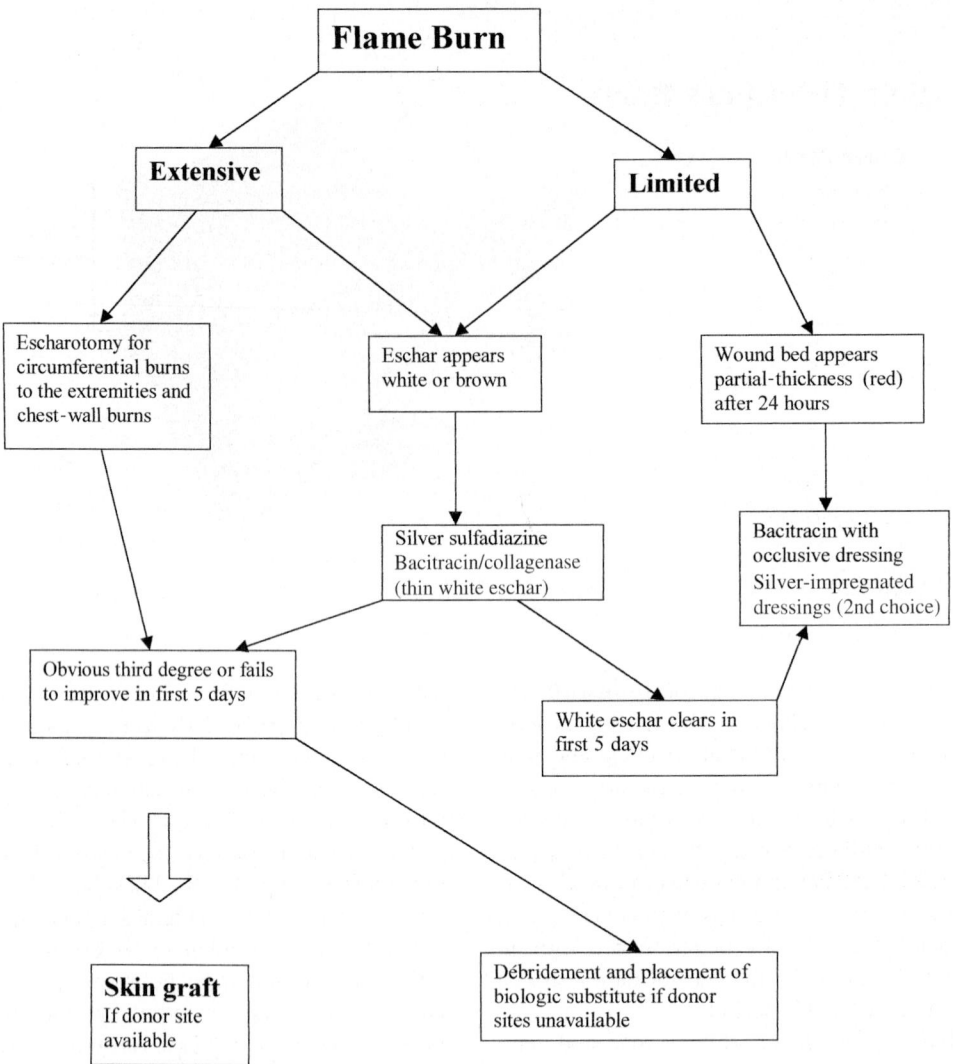

**FIGURE 83-8** Algorithm for the evaluation and early management of the flame burn.

## SKIN GRAFTS

Once it is obvious that the burn wound is third degree or a deep second degree in a critical body site, skin grafting is indicated. Early grafting is done in the first week after the burn injury even within 48 hours in some burn units. The burn wound itself becomes inflamed in the second week of the postburn course causing more intraoperative blood loss and later scar formation.

The ideal coverage of the burn wound is a full-thickness graft but its use is limited to late reconstruction, particularly in the areas of the palm and the face. Partial-thickness sheet grafts obtained with a mechanically powered dermatome are used to obtain autologous skin tissue for transplantation over large surface areas (Fig. 83-10). Potential donor sites in the child include the thigh, buttock, back, and scalp (Fig. 83-11). The scalp or anterior chest is recommended when coverage of the face is needed. This will provide skin with a reddish blush instead of a yellowish hue from grafts obtained elsewhere.

There is a tradeoff with any partial-thickness graft. A thicker skin graft with a greater proportion of transplanted dermis gives a better result in the burn wound but requires more time for the

donor site to heal. Re-cropping of the donor site is more delayed and the likelihood of donor scar formation increases. A good rule of thumb is to use grafts of 0.010–0.012 inches for infants and 0.012–0.014 inches for a child. A sheet graft obtained at 0.014–0.016 inches in the teenage patients is acceptable when a thick graft is desirable. Donor sites at these depths require a minimum of 3 weeks to heal before a new graft can be harvested.

A split-thickness graft shrinks 30% at the time of harvest. An unmeshed graft is the most functional and cosmetic of the partial-thickness graft but requires careful and frequent examination in the immediate postoperative period. A meshed graft can be wrapped in a bulky dressing and left alone until the 3rd to 5th postoperative day. A wet dressing, intermittently bathed with an antimicrobial solution, will help to protect the tissue in the interstices of the meshed graft from desiccation and infection. Mefanide solution (5%) is now available for post grafting wound irrigation. It has an excellent antimicrobial spectrum without the systemic side effects seen when mefanide cream is used on an open wound.

To get more skin coverage, a skin graft can be meshed at different ratios: 1:1, 1.5:1, 2:1, 3:1, and even 6:1. A 1.5:1 meshed graft will expand the skin graft to its original size. The tradeoff with any meshed graft is that the mesh pattern is

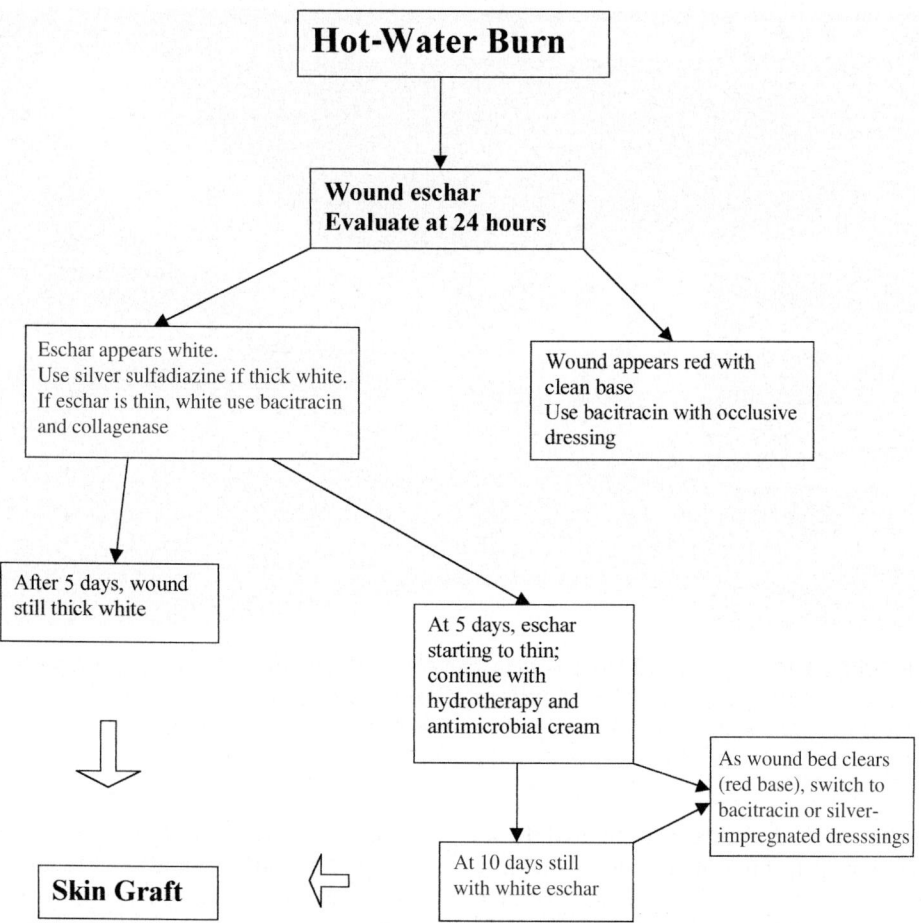

**FIGURE 83-9** Algorithm for the evaluation and early management of the hot-water (scald) burn.

visible lifelong. This pattern is least noticeable with a 1:1 graft. As the mesh size increases, more scar formation is required for wound closure with a higher incidence of late contracture. A mesh pattern greater than 2:1 is used only for wound coverage in the large burn injury. Other options exist for wound coverage in this population.

Preparation of the wound bed is paramount to successful skin grafting. Tangential excision of the nonviable skin is performed until healthy tissue is exposed (Fig. 83-12). The 2 hallmark signs of viable tissue are punctate bleeding and the healthy appearance of the deeper tissues. In most cases, this is down to the level of healthy fat. Always look for thrombosis of dermal and subcutaneous vessels to indicate the deeper levels of thermal injury and need for deeper débridement. Punctate bleeding is less reliable than the appearance of the tissues. A tourniquet placed on an extremity at the time of the initial débridement will help to lower intraoperative blood loss but is safe only in experienced hands. Mechanical devices exist to assist in débridement. They are particularly helpful over irregular surfaces.

Fixation of the graft to the wound bed is done expeditiously with staples around the periphery of the graft and in the seams. Fibrin sealants can be used for hemostasis of the burn wound and fixation of the graft. Repositioning of the graft with fibrin glue however becomes more difficult with

| TABLE 83-3 | Table of Antimicrobial Creams | | | | | | |
|---|---|---|---|---|---|---|---|
| | Spectrum | Application | Eschar penetration | Complications | Other | Uses |
| Silver sulfadiazine | Gram (+) gram (−) fungus | Daily Painless Closed technique | Moderate to poor | Transient neutropenia Allergy | Pseudo eschar Arrests late-stage healing | Deep 2nd and 3rd-degree burns |
| Mefanide cream | Gram (+) gram (−) | Twice daily Painful | Excellent and immediate | Systemic Metabolic acidosis | Minimal fungal activity | Invasive burn sepsis (short term) Ear coverage |
| Bacitracin | Gram (+) | Daily Open or closed | Poor or none | Allergic rxn commonly seen | Can be combined with collagenase | Minimal or no eschar |

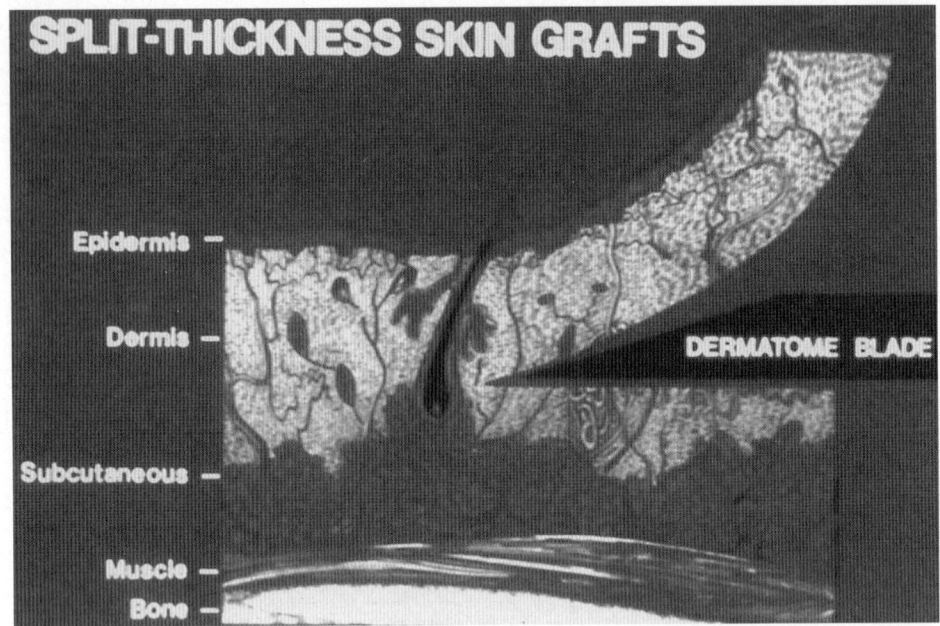

**FIGURE 83-10** This demonstrates the dermatome blade cutting through the dermis to obtain a partial-thickness graft. The graft is then made up of epidermis and portion of the dermis, but most of the graft is dermis. The ideal thickness is 0.010 to 0.014 inches.

time. Grafts to the fingers, toes, and face are sutured. Bulky dressings with splints help to prevent shifting of the graft in the immediate postoperative period. Neovascularization and adherence is nearly complete by the fifth postoperative day when the staples or sutures can be safely removed. Graft loss due to infection or motion is much less likely once the graft has turned red and is adherent to the wound bed. Negative pressure wound therapy (NPWT) is very helpful with skin grafting. Its uses are expanding but it is most helpful in traumatic wounds and deep wounds, both burned and non-burned, where excessive wound exudate and graft adherence are common causes of graft loss.

Proper physical and occupational therapy is important to start just after admission to the burn unit. It is usually stopped over joint areas after grafting but must resume once the autologous tissue has engrafted. Post discharge compression therapy with a custom-fit garment is needed over areas of skin grafting, burn wounds that require more than 2 weeks to heal, and in any individual prone to hypertrophic reaction. Compression garments must be worn continuously for 1 year or until scar maturation is seen. Silicone pads, facial masks, steroid injection, laser therapy, and skin creams are all used to help with hypertrophic skin reaction. No single therapy is completely efficacious, particularly in children where hypertrophic reaction is more common, and can be devastating.

## ALTERNATIVE WOUND COVERAGE

The ultimate goal of the burn surgeon is wound closure. There are products for temporary wound closure used in areas of partial-thickness injury, donor sites, and over limited areas of

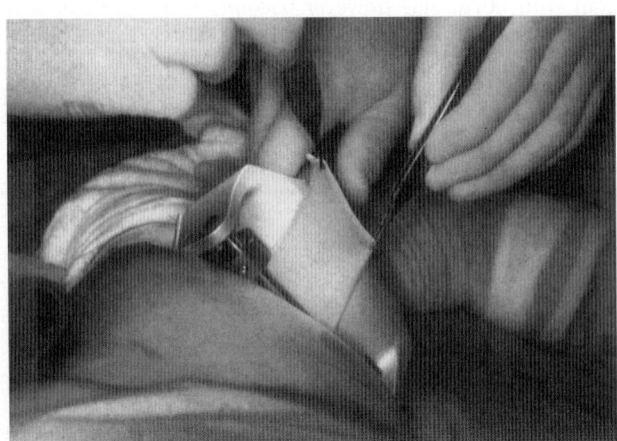

**FIGURE 83-11** A photo of a graft being taken from the thigh of a child.

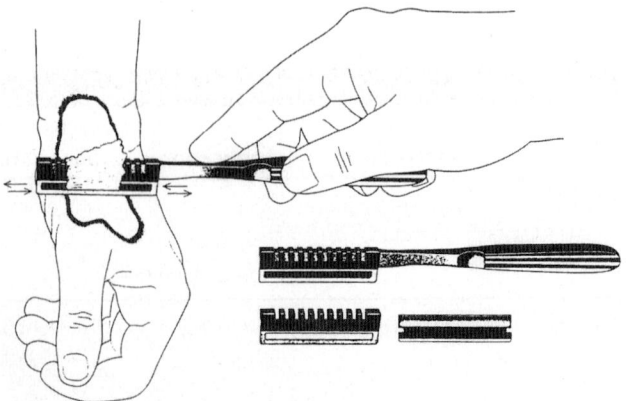

**FIGURE 83-12** The sequential removal of the burned tissue with a Goulian dermatone in the process of tangential excision of the burn wound.

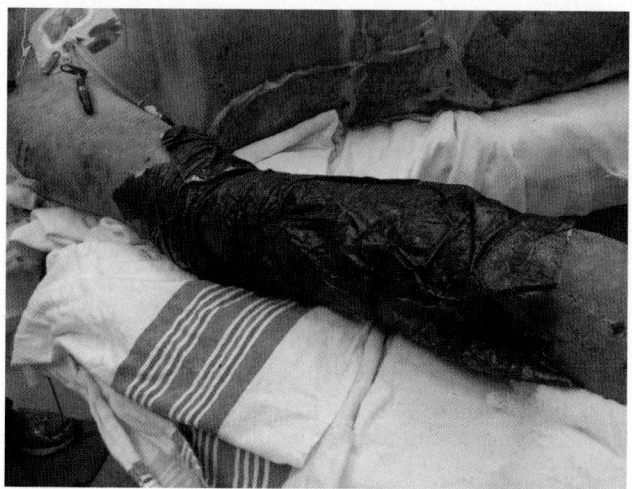

**FIGURE 83-13** Photo of patient with Acticoat on arm. It is used as an inner layer and changed every 2–3 days.

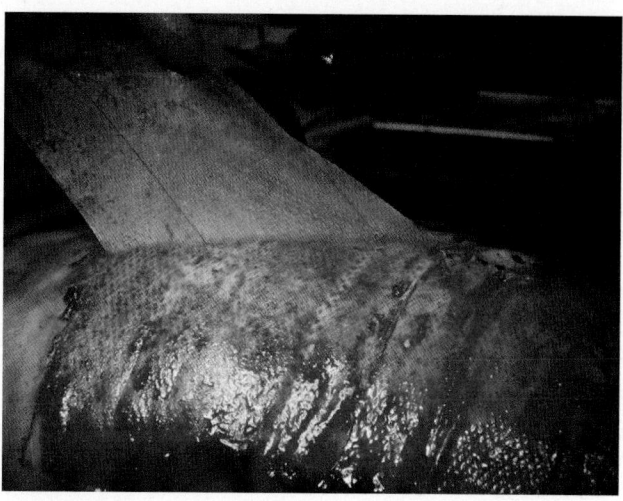

**FIGURE 83-14** Operative photo of the second stage of wound closure using Integra where outer layer is peeled off, exposing the healthy neodermis. Thin autograft is then applied to neodermis.

full-thickness injury. In addition, there are more permanent products for full-thickness burn injury.

Temporary products are useful in the partial-thickness wound, either from a burn injury or from a donor site. When a product such as this adheres to the wound, it replaces the functions of the skin until such time that the wound has healed. Post injury pain is diminished, as is the loss of fluid through the wound. The patient can then be discharged and followed in the outpatient setting. It is essential to evaluate adherence 24 hours after placement of the product and to remove it or replace it if loose. Biobrane (Dow-Hickman, Sugarland, TX) can be used early in the course of a superficial partial-thickness wound with excellent wound adherence as described above. Many newer products exist for dermal wound coverage, whether it is a partial-thickness burn, donor site, or open areas around previous grafting. The 2 common factors in these products are that they are impregnated with the silver ion that has broad antimicrobial spectrum and they do not adhere to the wound. Acticoat (Smith & Nephew, London, England) is a silver-impregnated polyethylene net changed every 2 to 3 days and works best in the inpatient arena (Fig. 83-13). Mepilex Ag (Molnlycke Health Care, Goteborg, Sweden) and Aquacel Ag (Convatec, Skillmam, NJ)

have a sponge type of backing, excellent for fluid absorption. Either product can be left in place for a week or longer and is useful for exposed dermis, particular donor sites, and superficial partial-thickness burn wounds (Table 83-4).

More permanent alternatives to wound coverage replace the dermis. These dermal replacement products are used in the massively burned patient. They provide the supporting structure of skin that is difficult to obtain when forced to reuse donor sites.

The first product was developed and used clinically in a controlled, prospective fashion in the late 1970s. Integra (Integra LifeSciences Corp., Plainsboro, NJ) was reintroduced and approved by the Food and Drug Administration in the 1990s. Extensive experience is now available for this product. Integra promotes the ingrowth of fibroblasts creating a new dermis that is then covered by ultrathin skin grafts in a second stage. It provides early wound closure with the luxury of elective graft coverage when donor sites are available (Fig. 83-14). In addition, the skin grafts used for the second stage are ultrathin (0.005-0.008 in) and can be widely meshed (Fig. 83-15). The donor area will heal quickly and can be reused within 7 to 10 days. Finally, there is at least comparable if not improved results in scar

| TABLE 83-4 | Table of Types of Silver Impregnated Dressings | | | | |
|---|---|---|---|---|---|
| | **Product** | **Uses** | **Frequency** | **Advantages** | **Limitations** |
| Acticoat (Smith/ Nephew) | 2 layers of silver-coated polyethylene mesh | Inner layer on open wounds | Change every 2–3 days | Can use to cover large areas of wound Can cover fresh skin grafts | Limited outpatient use Requires bulky outer dressings |
| Mepilex Ag (Molnlycke Health Care) | Soft silicone sponge with silver and safetec adhesive | Donor sites Partial-thickness burns | Change every 7 days or when saturated | Patient comfort Outpatient coverage Absorbs fluid | Must have wide edge of normal skin |
| Aquacel Ag (Convetec) | Hydrofiber with ionic silver | Donor sites Partial-thickness burns | Hardens and can remain for 14 days | Patient comfort Works well with wound exudate | Once hardens, cannot lift for inspection |

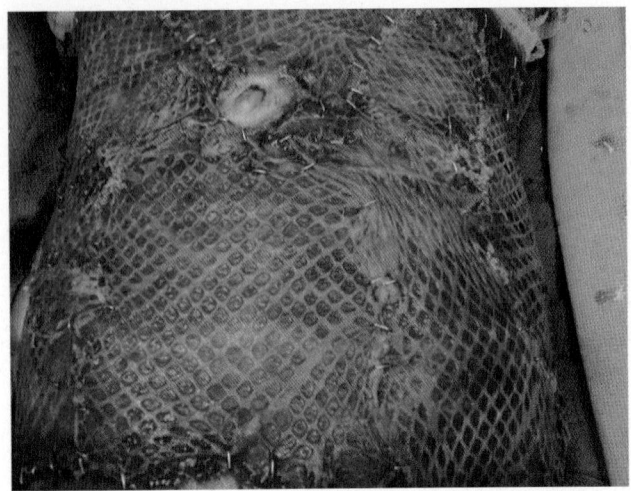

**FIGURE 83-15** Operative photo of the second stage of wound closure by Integra. Thin, widely meshed autograft is placed over neodermis.

formation. Additional uses of Integra include reconstruction for scar contracture, exposed bone and tendon coverage when used in conjunction with a NPWT and for nonburn reconstruction.

Homograft is another excellent product used for early wound closure. It, however, must be changed biweekly, provides no additional dermal replacement, and must be eventually replaced by standard-thickness skin grafts. Alloderm (LifeCell Corporation, Branchburg, NJ) is a dermal replacement product that can be used in conjunction with thin grafts. Another product available for the massively burned patient is cultured epithelial autograft. As the name implies, this is grown *in vitro*, is a few cell layers thick, and is placed over a dermal bed. Its use is limited by a low take rate and high cost.

## NUTRITION AND THE HYPERMETABOLIC RESPONSE

Nutrition is second only to wound closure in importance in the burn injured child. Early initiation of enteral nutrition is essential in the care of all moderate and large burn patients. Proper hyperglycemic control is standard in any critically ill patient.

The burn injury takes a toll on the patient's lean body mass unlike any other injury. Pharmacologic agents have been studied to blunt the hypermetabolic response and subsequent loss of lean body mass. Oxandrolone, an anabolic steroid, improves nutrition, weight gain, and serum protein levels and may decrease donor site healing time. Additionally, there is improved muscle strength when combined with exercise in the rehabilitation phase. Treatment can be continued for 1 year.

Propranolol has been shown to be effective in blocking the hypermetabolic response. It reduces the upregulated metabolic rate and increases net protein balance. In addition, it decreases hepatic cell fatty infiltration and increases lean body mass with a corresponding decrease in muscle wasting.

Both of these pharmacologic agents have been studied in a controlled fashion in children with favorable results.

## SUMMARY

Burn injury is a devastating event that changes the lives of its victims. Now that survival is almost assured, careful, yet aggressive evaluation and therapy is needed by the pediatric surgeon caring for these burn survivors in order to improve their overall outcomes.

## SELECTED READINGS

Greenhalgh, DG. Burn resuscitation. *J Burn Care Res* 2007;28(4):555–565.

Greenhalgh DG. Burn resuscitation: the results of the ISBI/ABA survey. *Burns* 2010;36(2):176–182.

Jeng JC, Fidler PE, et al. Seven years' experience with Integra as a reconstructive tool. *J Burn Care Res* 2007;28(1):120–126.

Jenschke MG, Finnerty CC, et al. The effects of oxandrolone on the endocrinologic, inflammatory, and hypermetabolic responses during the acute phase postburn. *Ann Surg* 2007;246:351–362.

Lawrence A, Faraklas I, et al. Colloid administration normalized resuscitation ratio and ameliorates "fluid creep". *J Burn Care Res* 2010;31(1):40–47.

Miller JT, Btaiche IF. Oxandrolone in pediatric patients with severe thermal burn injury. *Ann Pharmacother* 2008;42(9):1310–1315.

Saffle, JR. The phenomenon of "fluid creep" in acute burn resuscitation. *J Burn Care Res* 2007;28(3):382–395.

UpToDate. Emergency care of moderate and severe thermal burns in children. Author: Joffe MD. Available at www.uptodate.com. Last updated May 11, 2010. Assessed Nov 11, 2010.

Williams FN, Herndon DN, et al. The leading cause of death after burn injury in a single pediatric burn center. *Crit Care* 2009;13(6):183.

Wolf, SE. Nutrition and metabolism in burns: state of science, 2007. *J Burn Care Res* 2007;28(4):572–576.

# CHAPTER 84

## Animal Assaults: Bites and Stings

*Marcene R. McVay and Charles Wagner*

## KEY POINTS

1. Identification of the offending organism is of paramount importance in determining the most appropriate course of treatment.

2. The administration of antibiotic prophylaxis should be based on the degree of wound contamination or documented microbiology, but is mandated for bites from cats and humans.

3. Verbal reports of spider bites are often erroneous, and surgeons should have a high index of suspicion for other causes.

4. The only antivenins readily available in the United States are for indigenous snakes and black widow spiders. Arizona has an antivenin for scorpions.

5. Be alert for secondary injuries in the patient who has sustained an animal bite, as it is not uncommon and can be life-threatening.

6. Human bite wounds may raise suspicion of child abuse, and HIV/hepatitis infection must be considered.

7. The efficacy of negative pressure wound therapy has been shown, and it is an appropriate addition to the wound care armamentarium.

8. The symptoms of envenomation progress more rapidly in young children due to their low body weight, and the importance of timely treatment cannot be overstated.

## GENERAL PRINCIPLES

Despite the wide variability in offending organisms and specific considerations related to each, adoption of a systematic approach to the evaluation and treatment of all bite injuries is possible. Three basic concepts should be addressed, and the use of common sense cannot be overemphasized.

(1) *Type of bite.* This includes identification of the offender, when possible, and determination of whether or not envenomation took place. Geography often dictates the incidence and exposure to a specific animal, and knowledge of the regional population is extremely helpful in determining the type of agent injected. Proof of envenomation includes both a visible injection site (fang marks, stingers, and bites) and local tissue reaction (swelling, local hemorrhage, pustules, erythema). The exceptions are direct venous injection or coral snake envenomation which cause little, if any, local reaction.

(2) *Degree of injury.* An assessment should be made of the extent of both local and systemic damage. The mechanism of the injury may influence the intensity of treatment. An uncomplicated dog bite injury to the hand can be treated with cleansing and closure, while a bite from a large mammal such as a horse can be both cutting and crushing, and contaminated with bacterial flora of soil and plant origin. In cases involving a large attacker, the possibility of secondary traumatic injuries must also be considered.

Signs and symptoms of systemic illness due to envenomation include coagulopathy, neurologic involvement, respiratory compromise or failure, or even cardiovascular collapse. Awareness of these signs will give the clinician a high index of suspicion in appropriate situations and guide timely intervention. When envenomation is documented by local wound criteria, admission for observation and further treatment is appropriate.

(3) *Treatment.* Treatment is also focused on both local and systemic effects of the injury. Although the choice of antibiotics plays a critical role in treatment, the basic principle of cleansing and débridement of the wound is paramount. Topical anesthetic agents and conscious sedation techniques are indeed valuable tools for the care of both the wound and the child's discomfort and fear. The clinician must assess the need for and type of mechanical intervention (primary or staged repair, need for débridement) as well as consider the options for closure (suture or cyanoacrylate glue, conventional wound dressings, or negative pressure wound therapy). Location of the injury will often dictate the aggressiveness or method of surgical treatment. Wounds of the face have a better outcome with primary closure, but conservative wound care with delayed reconstruction may be most appropriate when faced with significant tissue loss from a large animal bite to an extremity. Long-term form and function must be considered when making these decisions.

Systemic treatment concerns include the determination of whether or not antibiotic or tetanus prophylaxis or the administration of antivenin is indicated. All bite wounds are considered contaminated and antibiotic therapy was once the standard-of-care for every bitten patient. Although familiarity with several uncommon but predictable bacteria that colonize the mouths of specific animal attackers is important, current practice would challenge the notion that all bite wounds must be treated with systemic antibiotic therapy. Rabies and tetanus, however, must always be considered. Therefore, an assessment of the patient's immunization status and the potential need for tetanus prophylaxis is indicated. And although there are specific antivenins available, evidence-based protocols exist for the purpose of ensuring that they are administered in a judicious manner.

## SNAKEBITES

### Epidemiology

No other animal injury conjures up more fear, misunderstanding, and untested treatments than snakebites. The actual incidence of snakebite injuries is difficult to determine because there is no mandatory reporting. However, the 2009 annual report from the American Association of Poison Control Centers' National Poison Data System (AAPCC NPDS) revealed 6629 total reported snakebites, 54% of which involved documented envenomation. Only 3 deaths were reported, all from rattlesnake bites, which

comprised 35% of the total venomous snakebite injuries. Copperheads were the most common venomous snake offenders (37%) followed by rattlesnakes, cottonmouths, coral snakes, and least commonly, poisonous exotic snakes (1%). Of those bitten, 30% were under the age of 19 years. Not surprisingly, the majority of bites occur on the extremities as the snake attempts to defend itself against a perceived attempt to handle or harm it.

Although a range of exotic snakes exist in the United States, bites from these are readily identified because they are mostly captive creatures. Of the 120 indigenous snake species in the United States, only 20 are venomous and all are included in the families Viperidae (or Crotalinae, pit vipers including rattlesnakes, cottonmouths/water moccasins, and copperheads) and Elapidae (coral snakes). Maine, Hawaii, and Alaska are the only states without native, venomous snakes, and the vast majority of bites occur in the southwestern region of the country during the summer months.

### Evaluation

Positive identification of the snake is required for appropriate diagnosis and treatment, and understanding the regional distribution of various species of snakes will help determine the most likely offender (Fig. 84-1). In the 25% of cases when an offender cannot be established, a clinical evaluation for signs and symptoms of envenomation becomes the focus of diagnosis and treatment. Symptoms related to an autonomic

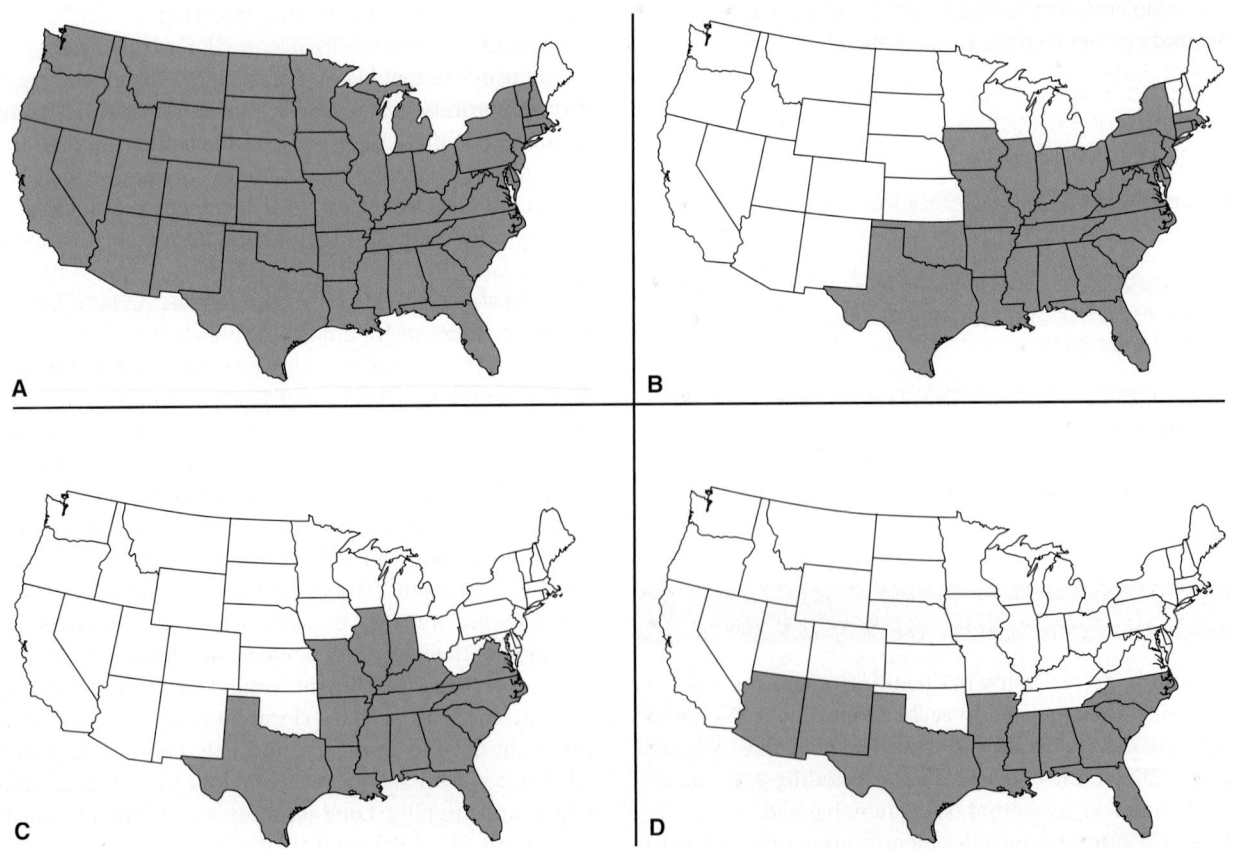

**FIGURE 84-1** U.S. map of regional snakes. **A.** Rattlesnake, (**B**) Copperhead, (**C**) Cottonmouth, (**D**) Coral snake. (Alaska, Hawaii, and Maine have no indigenous snakes.)

response to anxiety or fear (sweating, cool/clammy skin, tachycardia, nausea, vomiting, diarrhea, or even syncope) must be differentiated from those of systemic illness.

The venom of a pit viper contains a mixture of peptides and enzymes that increase capillary membrane permeability resulting in a range of effects from local soft tissue reaction to shock and disseminated intravascular coagulation (DIC). The hallmark of envenomation is fang marks, pain, and rapid onset of swelling. Drops of nonclotting blood are often seen at the strike site. Localized pain is felt immediately in practically all envenomated bites, and edema, erythema, and ecchymosis emerge at 30 minutes and can progress for hours. Since these snakes inject a consistent concentration of venom with each strike, toxic effects will be greater in small children because their dosage is higher.

## Management

A number of outdated and harmful treatments are reviewed in Table 84-1. Appropriate field treatment includes immobilization of the affected area below the level of the heart, removing constricting jewelry or clothing, placing the victim at rest, and transporting to the nearest medical facility. The use of tourniquets is discouraged. In the emergency department, a standard assessment of airway, breathing, and circulation should be undertaken, and an AMPLE history obtained (Allergies, Medications, Past medical history, Last meal and Events surrounding the incident) according to the ATLS protocol (Advanced Trauma Life Support®). A complete examination including cardiovascular, pulmonary, and neurologic systems should be followed by a detailed assessment of the wound. If no envenomation has occurred, gentle cleansing of the wound and appropriate tetanus prophylaxis are the only treatments indicated. Though once advocated, antibiotic coverage (with ampicillin–sulbactam or ampicillin–clavulanate) should only be used for wounds with documented infection or heavy contamination.

If envenomation has occurred, the patient is admitted and observed. Laboratory studies include CBC, electrolyte and renal function panels, CPK, coagulation studies (PT/PTT,

| TABLE 84-1 | Outdated and Unproven Treatments for Snakebites |
|---|---|

Tourniquets
Incision and oral suction
Mechanical suction devices
Immersion in warm water or sour milk
Application of potassium permagnatate
Cryotherapy
Electric shock therapy

fibrinogen, and split products), and urinalysis. A tube of blood for type and crossmatch is obtained and saved for possible later use. Polyvalent Crotalinae ovine immune Fab (FabAV, Crofab©) is the mainstay of treatment in the United States for significant Crotalinae envenomation. A patient with moderate to severe toxicity or with a significant possibility for airway obstruction from local swelling of bites to the head and neck should receive FabAV therapy (Table 84-2). Consultation with a medical toxicologist via a regional poison control center is strongly recommended prior to antivenin administration (national hotline: 800-222-1222). For optimum effectiveness, antivenin should be given within 6 hours of injury and repeated every 6 hours for 3 doses as necessitated by subsequent clinical and laboratory investigations. These patients should be admitted to a monitored setting in the hospital. Patients meeting only minor criteria for envenomation should be observed in the emergency department for 8 to 12 hours with repeat laboratory investigations prior to discharge home. No antivenin therapy is indicated in such cases (Fig. 84-2).

The clinician should be prepared to manage other side effects of envenomation including coagulopathy and rhabdomyolysis with resultant renal failure. The coagulopathy associated with envenomation is pathophysiologically different than in conventional DIC, and clotting factors and platelets are an ineffective therapy because they are inactivated on entering the bloodstream. The treatment is antivenin.

| TABLE 84-2 | Clinical Classification of U.S. Crotalinae Envenomation to Guide FabAV Administration | | |
|---|---|---|---|
| Category | Tissue Effect | Systemic Signs | Coagulopathy and Bleeding |
| Minimal | Swelling, pain, and ecchymosis adjacent to the bite site | None | Normal coagulation parameters; no bleeding |
| Moderate | Swelling, pain, and ecchymosis less than full extremity or less than 50 cm if bite on head, neck, or trunk | Present but not life-threatening (eg, nausea, vomiting, diarrhea, oral parasthesia, unusual tastes, tachycardia, tachypnea, mild hypotension [systolic BP >90 mm Hg in an adult]) | Abnormal coagulation parameters; no bleeding or minor hematuria, gum bleeding and/or epistaxis |
| Severe | Swelling, pain, ecchymosis involving more than the entire extremity; greater than 50 cm if bite on head, neck, or trunk; threatens the airway; OR signs of compartment syndrome | Present and life-threatening (eg, respiratory insufficiency, marked tachycardia for age with severe hypotension, obtundation, seizures) | Markedly abnormal coagulation parameters with serious bleeding |

Note: BP, blood pressure.

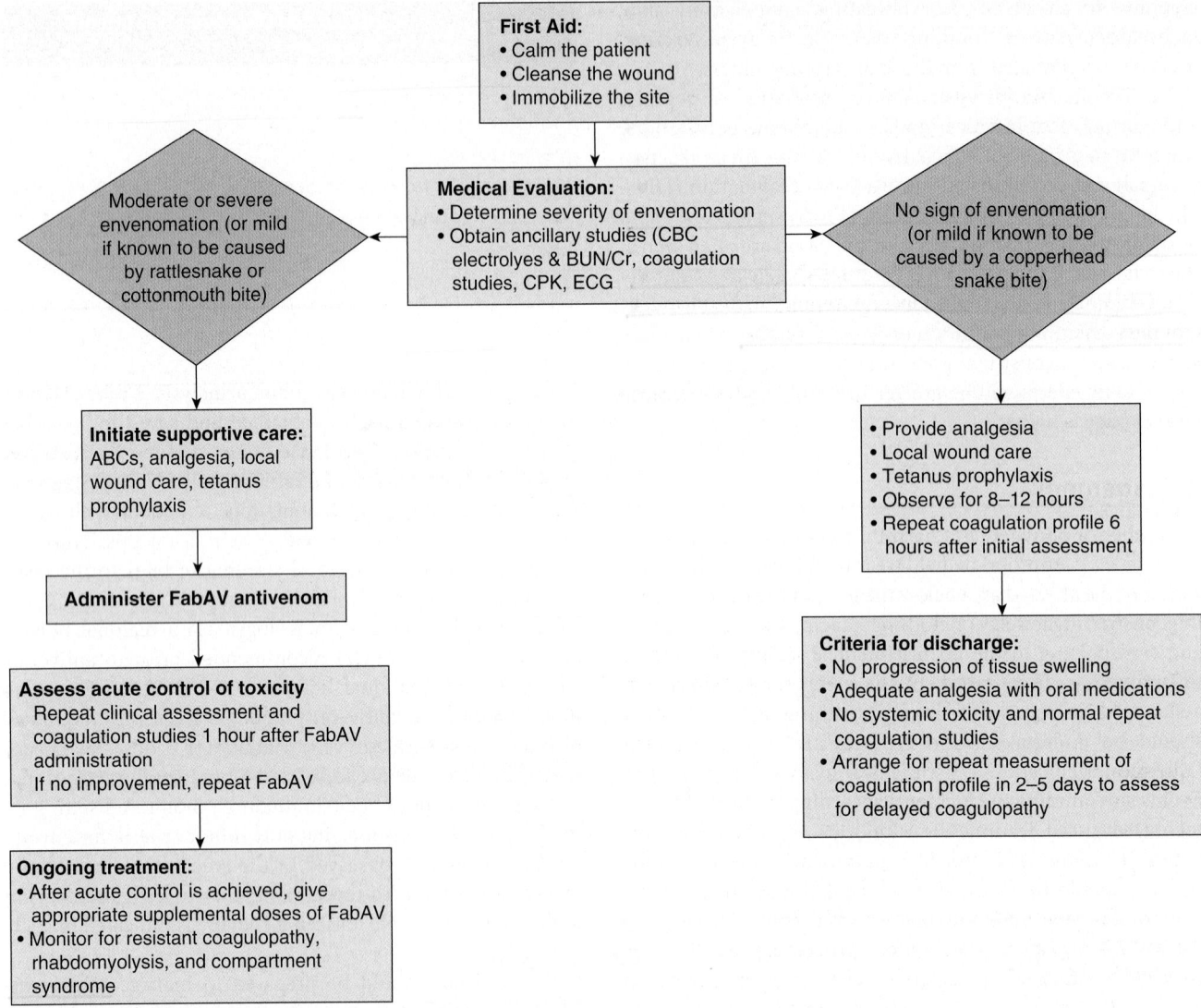

**First Aid:**
• Calm the patient
• Cleanse the wound
• Immobilize the site

**Medical Evaluation:**
• Determine severity of envenomation
• Obtain ancillary studies (CBC electrolyes & BUN/Cr, coagulation studies, CPK, ECG

**Moderate or severe envenomation (or mild if known to be caused by rattlesnake or cottonmouth bite)**

**No sign of envenomation (or mild if known to be caused by a copperhead snake bite)**

**Initiate supportive care:**
ABCs, analgesia, local wound care, tetanus prophylaxis

**Administer FabAV antivenom**

**Assess acute control of toxicity**
Repeat clinical assessment and coagulation studies 1 hour after FabAV administration
If no improvement, repeat FabAV

**Ongoing treatment:**
• After acute control is achieved, give appropriate supplemental doses of FabAV
• Monitor for resistant coagulopathy, rhabdomyolysis, and compartment syndrome

• Provide analgesia
• Local wound care
• Tetanus prophylaxis
• Observe for 8–12 hours
• Repeat coagulation profile 6 hours after initial assessment

**Criteria for discharge:**
• No progression of tissue swelling
• Adequate analgesia with oral medications
• No systemic toxicity and normal repeat coagulation studies
• Arrange for repeat measurement of coagulation profile in 2–5 days to assess for delayed coagulopathy

**FIGURE 84-2** Algorithm for the management of Crotalinae snakebites. (Reprinted with permission from uptodate.com. http://www.uptodate.com/contents/management-of-crotalinae-rattlesnake-water-moccasin-cottonmouth-or-copperhead-bites-in-the-united-states.)

Clotting abnormalities that should prompt re-dosing of antivenin are outlined in Table 84-3.

Acute hypersensitivity reactions can occur with use of antivenin (up to 15%), and epinephrine, diphenhydramine and albuterol should be available during administration. The incidence of serum sickness, once as high as 80% to 90% with the antivenin introduced in the 1950s, is less than 15% with FabAV. It presents 1 to 3 weeks after completion of treatment and is manifested by fever, rash, joint pain, and

lymphadenopathy. A standard taper of oral steroids is an appropriate treatment with a reliable response rate.

Wound care is primarily supportive, and early aggressive débridement or excisional therapy is not advocated. The wound should be cleansed and covered with a loose, dry dressing. The periphery of the affected area should be outlined with a marker, and circumference measurements of the extremity documented every 15 to 30 minutes until local progression has halted. Elevation of the affected extremity aids in reduction of edema, pain, and parasthesias, but should be avoided until after the administration of antivenin. Though rarely required, the decision to perform a dermotomy or fasciotomy should be based on documented compartment pressures and not strictly clinical findings. In the case of vascular compromise to the digits, digital dermotomy can be performed by making an incision through the subcutaneous tissue of the finger beginning at the webspace. Secondary closure may or may not be required.

The majority of patients admitted with pit viper bite victims can be discharged within 24 to 72 hours. Range-of-motion exercises are started. Elevation of the involved extremity

| TABLE 84-3 | Clotting Factor Abnormalities to Guide FabAV Redosing |
|---|---|

Fibrinogen <50 mcg/Ml

Platelet count <25,000/mL

INR >3.0

aPTT >50 sec

Multiple defects in coagulation

Comorbid conditions that predispose to hemorrhage

should continue for several more days, and patients/families should be warned that swelling may persist in some form up to 6 months after the bite. There have been reports of anaphylactic reactions to a second envenomation and antivenin administration, so counseling regarding prevention is indeed the key in this situation.

Several pertinent exceptions to the above presentation and treatment of Crotalinae bites must be noted when dealing with the Mojave rattlesnake. Significant local tissue reaction including ecchymosis is unlikely to develop at the inoculation site. Unlike other pit viper envenomations, neuromuscular weakness and respiratory depression are more common and may be delayed. Therefore, neuromuscular checks should be performed for a minimum of 12 hours after injury. Administration of FabAV is based on the same indications as for other Crotalinae bites.

## Coral and Exotic Snakes

Coral snake bites differ from pit viper bites in several ways. The marks appear as a row of teeth, not fangs, and the local reaction is minimal to absent. Identification of the snake by its distinctive ring marking ("red on yellow, kill a fellow") is most helpful. Coral snake venom has a potent neurotoxin component, and envenomation can present acutely 8 or so hours after the injury with CNS changes and respiratory depression. The only coral snake antivenin approved by the FDA (Wyeth, lot 4030026) expired in October 2011, and it is only approved for Texas and Eastern coral snakes. The University of Arizona Viper Institute is working on development of a new antivenin, but it will not be available soon. Neostigmine has shown some promise in reversing neuromuscular compromise in Mexico, but no therapies are approved here in the United States. Mechanical ventilation for up to 1 week may be required as a supportive measure. Patients with possible or documented coral snake bites need to be observed for 24 to 48 hours for maximum safety.

Management of non-native venomous snakebites can present a particular challenge. Consultation with a local zoo and the poison-control hotline listed above are the 2 best resources to guide care or referral.

# SPIDER BITES

## Epidemiology

Of 11,000 spider bites reported by the 2009 NPDS, the majority (65%) were from non- or minimally venomous spiders, such as the jumping spider, which is the most common biting spider in the United States. Black widow and brown recluse spiders, the most common source of spider bites requiring medical intervention in the United States, caused roughly 20% and 12% of envenomations, respectively, with exotic spiders such as tarantulas causing less than 1%. There were no deaths reported, but an equivalent number of major outcome events occurred due to the black widow and brown recluse. Though the overwhelming majority of bites affect adults over 20 years of age, there is an increased incidence in children under the age of 5 years in comparison to other age groups.

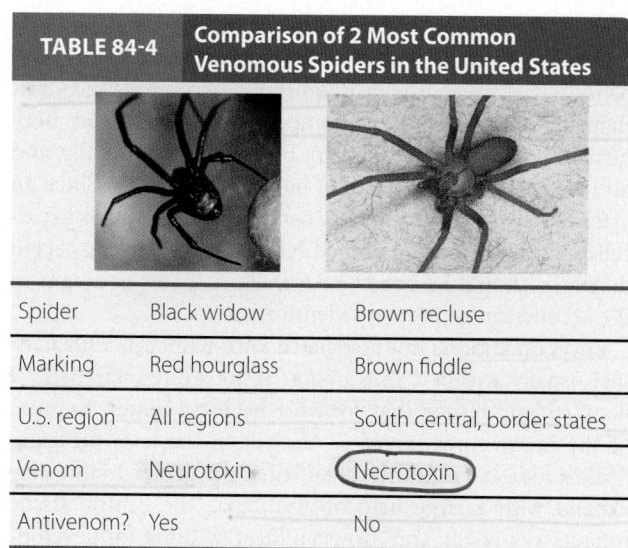

| TABLE 84-4 | Comparison of 2 Most Common Venomous Spiders in the United States | |
|---|---|---|
| Spider | Black widow | Brown recluse |
| Marking | Red hourglass | Brown fiddle |
| U.S. region | All regions | South central, border states |
| Venom | Neurotoxin | Necrotoxin |
| Antivenom? | Yes | No |

## Evaluation

Determination of spider envenomation is much more difficult than with snakes, since the attacker is often missed and never located. Assuming that a reported injury was caused by a spider bite is not advised, since skin and soft tissue infections from methicillin-resistant *Staphylococcus aureus* (MRSA) have been widely reported to mimic the appearance of brown recluse bites. Misdiagnosis in this regard could have severe consequences.

The most common offending spiders in the United States have distinctive appearances and the human body's response to their venom differs slightly (Table 84-4).

## Brown Recluse     NECROtoxin

The necrotoxic bites of the brown recluse spider (*Loxosceles*) were not recognized until reports appeared in the 1950s. It is indigenous to the central and southern United States (except Florida) and in states bordering Mexico (Fig. 84-3). The accuracy of reported bites outside of these areas should be questioned and another diagnosis sought. As the name

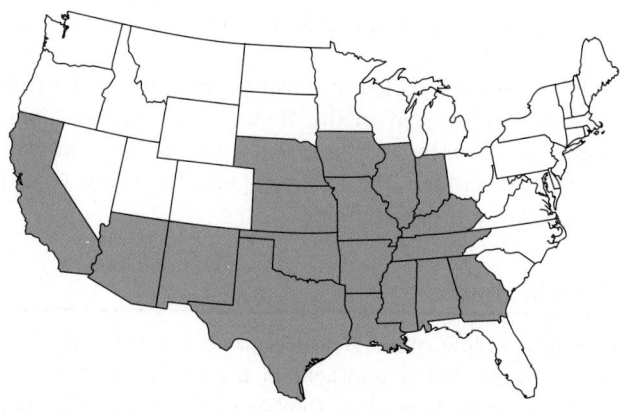

**FIGURE 84-3** Regional distribution of *Loxosceles* spider (brown recluse).

implies, the spider sequesters itself in secluded areas such as cellars and woodpiles, indoors and outdoors, and behind and beneath dark areas. The distinguishing marking is the violin-shaped band over the cephalothorax. Because they are nocturnal hunters, the bite may not be appreciated initially, and up to 90% of verbal reports of bites are unreliable. Since an extensive list of dermatologic conditions can mimic loxoscelism and actual documented bites are rare, any suspected diagnosis should be questioned unless a spider is caught in the act and can be properly identified.

Envenomation is not associated with pain, but with itching, usually within 2 to 8 hours. Serious bites start with a hemorrhagic blister that forms a necrotic center. Because of the many components of the venom such as protease, hyaluronidase, and other cytotoxins, the center lesion may expand with a large halo of erythema. The central tissue infarcts as a result, and forms an ideal medium for development of a secondary infection. The wound may take up to several days to form an eschar. Systemic symptoms such as fever, DIC, and hemoglobinuria, are rare. Because of the slow progression of the signs of envenomation, delayed presentation is the norm.

Basic first-aid treatment including elevation of the affected extremity, application of ice, tetanus prophylaxis, and gentle wound cleansing are generally all that is required for treatment, as this injury is usually self-limited and frequently heals without surgical intervention. Certain specific treatments have been touted, including dapsone, hyperbaric oxygen, antihistimines, intralesional or systemic steroids, excision, among others. No human prospective trials have been performed to determine the efficacy of these therapies, and the side effects of each should be weighed against the possible benefit before undertaking any intervention. There is no approved antivenin in the United States. As with snakebites, antibiotic prophylaxis is not required. However, if MRSA infection is more strongly suspected than a spider bite and the patient has systemic symptoms such as a fever, a culture of the wound should be obtained and empiric treatment with clindamycin or trimethoprim/sulfamethoxazole initiated, with treatment tailored to microbiology results. Early excision and grafting of lesions on functional areas like the hand may be indicated, and negative pressure wound therapy with a vacuum-assisted closure (VAC) device can be considered in both acute and chronic wounds to truncate healing time. Otherwise, delayed excision of the resulting contracted scar can be performed on an elective basis for improved cosmesis.

Other spiders reported to cause necrotic skin ulcers that could be encountered in the United States include hobo spiders (northwestern region), yellow sac spiders, and wolf spiders (worldwide). The treatment outlined above is also appropriate for these arachnids.

## Black Widow

The black widow spider (*Latrodectus*) is found in all states except Alaska, but is prevalent in the South, Ohio Valley, and West Coast. Legends of the bite of the black widow are grounded in that the mortality from severe bites was once as high as 5%. Since a lyophilized equine antivenin has been made available, the mortality rate has significantly declined, with no deaths being reported by the NPDS in over 10 years. The distinguishing mark of the spider is the red hourglass on the underbelly. Only the female is toxic.

Envenomation is recognized by intense pain with a small wheal and erythema at the site. After a few hours, this smudge mark becomes a dime-sized target lesion with a tiny central fang mark. It is surrounded by blanched skin and an outer pink, nonraised circle. The injected volume of venom is small, but the neurotoxin is very potent and stimulates a massive release of acetylcholinesterase. Systemic symptoms are rare, but progress rapidly with the onset of muscle rigidity, altered mental status, and seizures.

Most spider bites are harmless, and require minimal supportive treatment only. The wound is cleansed, and cold compresses and anti-inflammatory drugs are used to control the pain. Antibiotics are not recommended unless a secondary bacterial infection is present. Muscle spasms and rigidity are treated with diazepam. Narcotics will complicate the effects of the venom and should not be used. When symptoms are not controlled or progress to life-threatening events, antivenin is administered. One must observe the usual precautions for this therapeutic agent. Surgical intervention is rarely, if ever, required. Once the symptoms are controlled, the long-term outcome is good.

# INSECT STINGS

Insects inflict a greater number of venomous bites than any other species but are reported less often. Most stings occur during the summer months, and severe reactions are noted more often in children.

## Bees and Wasps

The stings of bees and wasps produce a local tissue reaction with a wheal and flare. The more serious constitutional symptoms develop within 20 minutes after the sting and include urticaria, syncope, and respiratory distress. The most serious and well-known effect is anaphylaxis, which may occur with an initial insult or because of hypersensitivity from prior exposure. Direct toxicity is not fatal.

Treatment involves both local care and systemic support. Prompt removal of the stinging mechanism by any method limits the amount of venom injected. This is most effective within the first 20 minutes of injury. Yellow jackets, wasps, and hornets have colonized stingers, while honey bees do not. Antibiotic treatment should be initiated based on evaluation of the wound. Cold compresses to the site will aid in pain management, and the use of baking soda baths may help alleviate the itching. A number of home and medical remedies to reduce the swelling and neutralize the venom have been attempted, including applications of aspirin paste, tobacco paste, papain, onion, meat tenderizer, toothpaste, and a copper coin. No topical therapy has been proven effective.

The systemic support of a child with initial or delayed hypersensitivity includes airway control, IM epinephrine,

| TABLE 84-5 | Treatment of Acute Anaphylaxis |
|---|---|

*Clinical Diagnosis:*

▶ Most common signs and symptoms: urticaria, angioedema, flushing, pruritis, vomiting

▶ Critical signs: rapid progression of symptoms, respiratory distress (wheezing, stridor, increased work of breathing), arrhythmias, syncope

*Acute Management:*

▶ Airway

▶ *Epinephrine*ᵃ (0.01 mg/mL IM, max dose 0.5 mg)

▶ Place in recumbent position with legs elevated

▶ Oxygen

▶ Crystalloid bolus (rapid 20 mL/kg), monitor urine output

▶ Albuterol (for bronchospasm)

▶ Antihistimine (1–2 mg/kg diphenhydramine IM or IV, max 50 mg)

▶ Steroids (consider 2 mg/kg methylprednisolone IV, max 125 mg)

*Treatment of Refractory Symptoms:*

▶ Epinephrine infusion

▶ Large volume IV fluid resuscitation with vasopressors

ᵃEpinephrine is the mainstay of treatment for anaphylactic reactions.

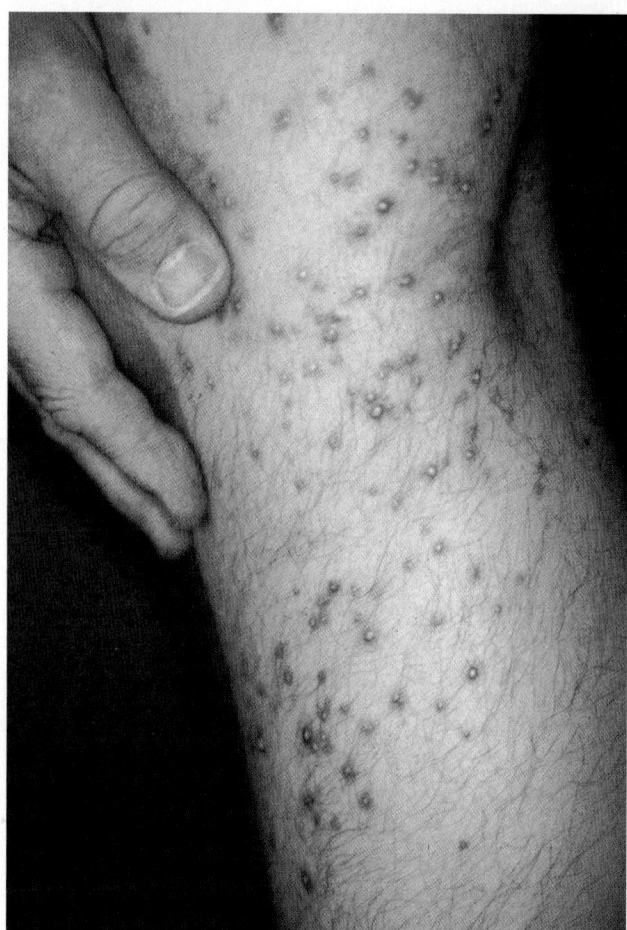

**FIGURE 84-4** Fire ant bites, 2 days after injury.

volume expansion, and albuterol updrafts for bronchospasms (Table 84-5). Consideration should be given to intravenous glucocorticoids in severe cases. The major problem is that these systemic symptoms will sometimes present early, before medical attention can be obtained. Patients with demonstrated hypersensitivity may benefit from a desensitization regimen. Metered injection "pens" loaded with epinephrine allow for rapid treatment of anaphylaxis in the field. Medical alert bracelets are also recommended.

## Fire Ants

Fire ants can be extremely aggressive if disturbed in their ant hills. They will continue to attack once they are disturbed. Envenomation causes edema, pruritis, erythema, pain, and burning from an alkaloid toxin. The initial flare becomes a wheal that develops into a clear vesicle within a few hours and over 1 to 2 days forms a sterile pustule (Fig. 84-4). Cool compresses, topical steroids, and oral antihistimines are generally the only treatments required. Death in children from fire ant envenomation is related to both hypersensitivity and anaphylaxis, which should be treated in the same manner as bee stings.

## Scorpions

Of 30 species of scorpions found in the United States only 1, *Centruroides*, is dangerous to humans. It is found primarily in Arizona and portions of surrounding states. Less than 1% of adults die from its sting, but that percentage increases with decreasing age to 20% mortality in infants. The venom of this "bark scorpion" is primarily a neurotoxin, and it manifests with neuromuscular, neuroautonomic, and local tissue effects. The progression to systemic symptoms ranges from

5 minutes to 4 hours after the sting, and death can occur within 24 hours. Local effects include an initial sharp burning pain at the site followed by pruritis, erythema, swelling, and ultimately ascending hyperesthesias. Classic systemic signs include mydriasis, nystagmus, hypersalivation, dysphagia, and restlessness, but any organ system can be affected. Treatment is supportive, with ice, immobilization of the site below the heart, topical or local anesthetic agents instead of narcotics, a topical antibiotic, tetanus prophylaxis, and benzodiazepines for muscle spasms. Atropine can be used to treat parasympathetic effects, and other medications supplied as needed to treat other systemic symptoms. There is an antivenin, and consultation with the Arizona Poison and Drug Information Center (800-362-0101) is encouraged to help guide its use.

# ANIMAL BITES

## Dog Bites

It is estimated that 1.5% of the U.S. population sustains dog bites every year (4.7 million). In children under the age of 15 years, dog bites are the reason for approximately 20% of injury-related doctor visits. Persons living in a household with dogs are more than twice as likely to be bitten as those

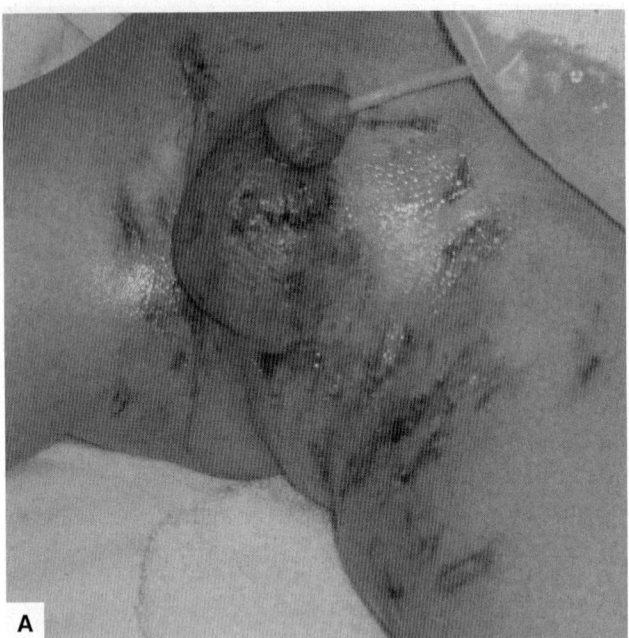
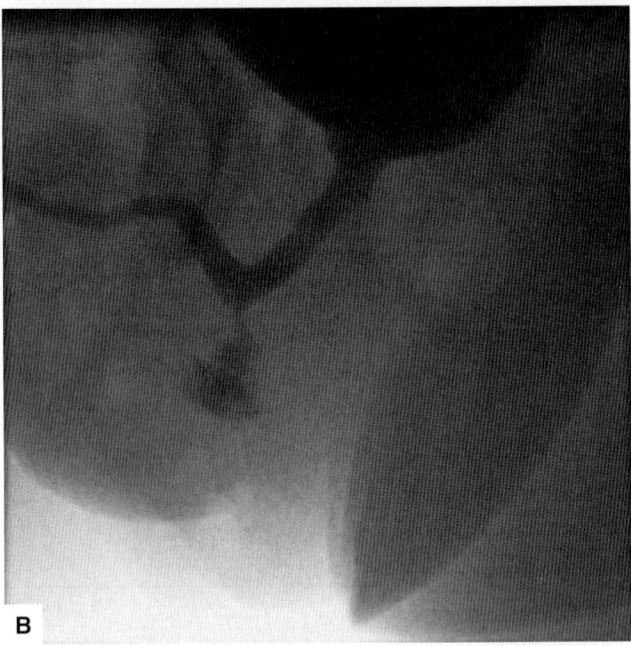

**FIGURE 84-5** **A.** Dog bite injury to the perineum in a 4.5-year-old boy by an Akita. There was also a rectal injury. **B.** VCUG showing occult urethral injury from same attack.

without. It is promising among prevention groups that the overall incidence of dog bites in children has decreased by nearly half since the mid-1990s, but hospitalizations as a result of an attack have increased. The most common breeds implicated are pit bulls (over 50%) and Rottweilers (9%), though other breeds have been consistently implicated including chows, German shepherds, akitas, and mixed breeds involving all of the above.

Injuries in school-aged children are usually on the extremities, whereas facial wounds are more common in infants and toddlers. Death is uncommon, but is directly related to hemorrhage. Wounds can range from small, punctate wounds to large, slashing, devitalized soft tissue injuries (Fig. 84-5).

In cases of isolated extremity injury, treatment is first related to the wound. Small wounds, punctate in nature, are cleansed with soap and water. The vicinity of the wound to the neurovascular structures is evaluated and requires the surgeon to rule out injuries involving these structures. Closure of facial wounds is always performed, and delayed closure of all wounds is avoided if possible. Any patient whose wound has been closed as an outpatient should be re-evaluated in 48 to 72 hours. Large wounds require operative débridement, and management with a VAC device is encouraged for wounds that cannot be primarily closed. When injury is not isolated to a specific area of the body, a complete evaluation of the patient should be undertaken to rule out more serious secondary trauma. Bony and solid organ injuries resulting in significant internal injury can occur if the dog-to-victim ratio is large enough. We have seen major artery lacerations, pneumothoraces, splenic lacerations, and urethral injuries that were overlooked until a secondary assessment was made.

Like humans, canine saliva harbors a variety of both aerobic and anaerobic bacteria. The most common bacterial isolate from dog bite wounds is *Pasturella canis*, but other species include *Staphylococcus*, *Streptococcus*, *Moraxella*, *Klebsiella*, and numerous others. Although the trend is toward minimizing antibiotic usage, only uncomplicated superficial wounds do not require prophylaxis. Amoxicillin/sulbactam (Unasyn) is the IV antibiotic of choice, and after a single dose in the emergency department, a 3 to 5 day course of oral amoxicillin/clavulanate (Augmentin) is an appropriate treatment. Tetanus immunization status should be updated. An additional infectious consideration is rabies. Working with the proper governmental agencies, the status of the dog's vaccination history should be determined. If up to date, observation for a prescribed amount of time (dictated by local law) provides the information needed for treatment of the patient. If the dog develops signs of rabies, is known to be rabid, or if there is a high suspicion for rabies, treatment using rabies immunoglobulin and human diploid-cell vaccine is instituted based on recommendations from local and state health department officials.

## Cat Bites

Wounds inflicted by cats are either punctate injuries from sharp incisor teeth and/or scratches from the animal's claws, which may be very superficial or deep through the dermis. Sequelae from these injuries are almost solely infectious in nature, as these bites are considered heavily contaminated. The wound is examined and rarely requires more than just cleansing. Antibiotic, tetanus, and rabies prophylaxis are administered as outlined for dog bites. The most common bacteria causing infection in a cat bite is *Pasturella* multilocida. It causes erythema, edema, tenderness, and a seropurulent discharge. Regional adenopathy, chills, and fever can ensue. More complex problems include septic arthritis, osteomyelitis, and tenosynovitis. Cat-scratch disease (caused by *Bartonella henslae*) is not uncommon, and manifests by regional lymphadenopathy, fever, chills, arthrosis, and oculoglandular syndrome. This may progress to a suppurative adenitis requiring drainage.

# HUMAN BITES

The etiology of a human bite injury varies from an accidental biting of the tongue to intended violent assault. Pediatric bite wounds are usually caused by aggressive play with another child, and are rarely of any consequence because they generally do not break the skin. Any bite with an intercanine distance of greater than 3 cm, however, should raise concern that the bite was inflicted by an adult. The "fight injury" presents with lacerations over the third and fourth metacarpophalangeal and proximal interphalangeal joints of the dominant hand, and arise when an assailant's clenched fist meets the teeth of another person. The effect can be a crush-type injury, as well as a laceration with penetration of the joint or injury to the tendon. The wound needs to be extensively cleansed and consultation with a hand surgeon is advised, as these wounds are highly prone to infection from organisms invading the deep compartment and planes of the hand. All human bite wounds with the exception of those on the face should be cleansed and left open. *Eikenella corrodens* is a common contaminant, and Augmentin is again the antibiotic of choice for prophylaxis. Follow-up within 48 hours is recommended.

A special consideration regarding human bites is the risk of infection by HIV or hepatitis. The risk is related to the size of the inoculums. Serologic testing for HIV and hepatitis B and C should be performed on the assailant, if known. If the biting human is not identified, consultation with a specialist in infectious disease is recommended follow-up serologic testing for HIV can be arranged. Hepatitis B immune globulin and vaccination should be considered.

Lastly, the events or circumstances of the human bite must be elicited. The differentiation between adult and child bites is important because this may be an unrecognized form of child abuse. If necessary, recognizable dental abnormalities outlining the skin may be an aid in identifying the abuser. Knowledge and proper documentation of this (including photographs) and reporting to the appropriate government agencies is necessary for the long-term care of the patient.

## SELECTED READINGS

Boyer LV, Theodorou AA, Berg RA, et al. Antivenom for critically ill children with neurotoxicity from scorpion stings. *N Engl J Med* 2009;360:2090–2098.

Bronstein AC, Spyker DA, Cantilena LR, et al. 2009 Annual Report of the American Association of Poison Control Centers' National Poison Data System (NPDS): 27th Annual Report. *Clin Toxicol* 2010;48:979–1178.

Diaz JH. The global epidemiology, syndromic classification, management and prevention of spider bites. *Am J Trop Med Hygeine* 2004;71(2):239–250.

Gilchrist J, Sacks JJ, White D, Kresnow M-J. Dog bites: still a problem? *Inj Prev* 2008;14:296–301.

Glaser, D. Are bee stings acid and wasp stings alkali? Does neutralizing their pH give sting relief? www.insectstings.co.uk.

Gold BS, Dart RC, Barish RA. Bites of venomous snakes. *N Engl J Med* 2002;347(5):347–356.

Kaye AE, Belz JM, Kirschner RE. Pediatric dog bite injuries: a 5-year review of the experience at The Children's Hospital of Philadelphia. *Plast Reconst Surg* 2009;124:551–558.

Likes K, Banner W, Chavez M. *Centruroides exilicauda* envenomation in Arizona. *West J Med* 1984;141:634–637.

Swanson DL, Vetter RS. Bites of brown recluse spiders and suspected necrotic arachnidism. *N Engl J Med* 2005;352(7):700–707.

Warrell DA. Commissioned article: management of exotic snakebites. *Q J Med* 2009;102:593–601.

Wong SL, Schneider AM, Argenta LC, Morykwas MJ. Loxoscelism and negative pressure wound therapy (vacuum-assisted closure): an experimental study. *Int Wound J* 2010;7(6):488–492.

# PART IX

## SURGICAL ENDOCRINOLOGY

# CHAPTER 85

# Neonatal Hypoglycemia

*Daniel von Allmen*

## KEY POINTS

1. Hyperinsulinemic hypoglycemia is the common cause of persistent hypoglycemia in the newborn.

2. Mutations in the ABCC8 and KCNJ1 genes are most common and impact the function of the ATP – Potassium Channel in the Beta cell of the islet.

3. Medical therapy includes treatment with continuous feedings, diazoxide and somatostatin analogs.

4. The 2 primary manifestations of the disease are focal and diffuse.

5. Patients with diffuse disease failing medical therapy are treated with 95% pancreatectomy.

6. Patients with focal disease failing medical therapy are treated with complete enucleation of the lesion.

7. Minimally invasive approaches to surgery have been described.

## HYPERINSULINEMIC HYPOGLYCEMIA OF INFANCY

Hypoglycemia is a common finding in neonates, infants, and children and is most commonly a secondary response to other systemic conditions such as sepsis, central nervous system pathology, congenital heart disease, drug effects, and asphyxia or anoxia. Most of these episodes are transient and very few patients require evaluation for persistent or intermittent hypoglycemia. In approximately 1% to 2% of all newborns with hypoglycemia, low serum glucose levels persist despite high rates of infusion of intravenous glucose. Within this very small subgroup, one must consider several possible etiologies including metabolic disease due to inborn errors of metabolism, hormonal deficiencies related to pituitary aplasia or hypoplasia, and persistent hyperinsulinemic hypoglycemia of infancy (HHI).

Despite its rarity, HHI is the most common cause of persistent hypoglycemia in the newborn. The incidence is reported to be 1:50,000 in the general population although it can be significantly more common in some in-bred populations. Gray and Feemster first described the condition in 1924 and in 1938 Laidlaw coined the term nesidioblastosis to describe the histologic findings of an overabundance of islets in the pancreas. Since then a number of different histologic manifestations of beta-cell abnormalities have been described and over the past 2 decades we have gained a more complete understanding of the underlying genetic and molecular processes that characterize the various subtypes of the disease. This chapter will outline our current understanding of the disease variants and the medical and surgical approaches to treatment.

## PATHOPHYSIOLOGY

Dysregulation of beta-cell production and release of insulin is the primary abnormality resulting in persistent hypoglycemia. The current understanding of the basis for the dysregulation began with the cloning of the sulfonylurea receptor gene, *SUR1*, in 1995. SUR1 is closely linked functionally to a potassium channel (Kir6.2) and the genes for both SUR1 and Kir6.2 are in close proximity on chromosome 11. Mutations in the ATP-regulated potassium channel alter the calcium dependent release of insulin from storage granules in the beta-cell resulting in various forms of the disease.

Beta-cell dysfunction can be diffused throughout the pancreas or can be present as a focal lesion related to clonal expansion of a single beta-cell defect. In large series, diffuse disease is far more common and accounts for about 80% of cases. Focal disease is far less common but important to identify given the significant impact on the surgical therapy to be discussed later in the chapter.

Specific genetic mutations can be identified in 45% to 55% of cases of HHI and 7 different molecular mechanisms have been described. Knowledge of the underlying genetic mutation can be helpful in determining the morphologic manifestations of the disease which in turn impacts the potential response to medical therapy and magnitude of the procedure for those that require an operation. The 7 genes currently identified that can harbor mutations resulting in clinical disease are *ABCC8, KCNJ11, GLUD1, GCK, HADH, HNF4A,* and *SLC16A1*. Recessive mutations are most common and are characterized by diffuse disease with a more treatment-resistant clinical course. Dominant mutations are described

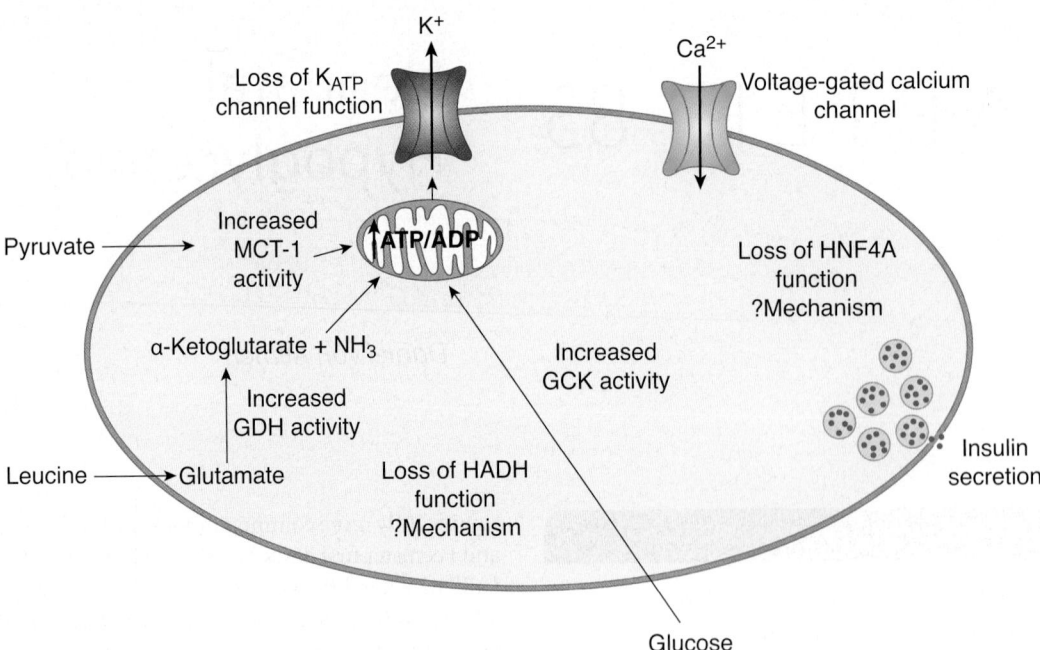

**FIGURE 85-1** Schematic representation of the known causes of HHI in the pancreatic Beta-cell. Loss of function mutations in the genes encoding the Kir6.2 (dark gray) and the SUR1 (light gray) subunits of the KATP channel are the commonest cause of HH. Gain-of-function mutations in the *GCK* and *GLUD1* (encoding GDH) genes have been described in patients with HH and *SLC16A1* gene mutations, which cause an increase in MCT-1 activity result in exercise-induced hyperinsulinism. The molecular mechanisms that lead to HH in patients with *HADH* and *HNF4A* mutations are not known. (From Flanagan SE, Kapoor RR, Hussain K. Genetics of congenital hyperinsulinemic hypoglycemia. *Seminars in Pediatr Surg* 2011;20:13–17.)

for a number of the genes and are typically more responsive to medical therapy. Mutations in the ABCC8 and KCNJ11 genes account for the majority of the known defects (45%) while all of the other known mutations represent only 5% to 10% of cases. In 45% to 55% of cases the etiology remains unknown (Fig. 85-1).

The *ABCC8* and *KCNJ11* genes encode the SUR1 and Kir6.2 subunits of the pancreatic-cell adenosine triphosphate (ATP)-sensitive potassium (KATP) channel previously mentioned. Loss of function at these genes is the most common known cause of congenital HHI. The KATP regulates insulin secretion by precipitating membrane depolarization and subsequent insulin secretion. The mutations in ABCC8 and KCNJ11 seen in HHI result in continuous depolarization of the cell and inappropriate insulin secretion. Most of the patients with mutations in these genes have 2 recessively acting mutations that result in diffuse disease that is difficult to control with medical therapy and ultimately requires an aggressive operation. The minority of patients have a single paternally inherited KATP channel mutation identified which can result in a focal lesion amenable to local resection. Mutations in the *GCK*, *HADH*, *GLUD1*, *HNF4A*, and *SLC16A1* genes are much rarer and generally cause diazoxide responsive disease.

## DIAGNOSIS

There are a number of clinical findings that should prompt one to look for hypoglycemia in the newborn. Patients are often macrosomic from high insulin levels in-utero.

Jitteriness, pallor, sweating, apathy, irritability, poor feeding, seizures, or coma should all prompt an investigation of serum glucose levels along with other tests. The importance of early diagnosis and treatment cannot be overemphasized given the devastating neurologic impact of delayed intervention. The diagnosis of HHI is based primarily on the demonstration of inappropriate plasma insulin levels in the face of hypoglycemia. Normal insulin levels should be low to immeasurable during periods of systemic hypoglycemia and even fasting levels of insulin are distinctly abnormal when serum glucose levels are abnormally low. These findings clearly indicate a defect in insulin control. Serum insulin levels of 10 microunits per mL in the face of plasma glucose levels less than 40 mg/dL are distinctly abnormal. The glucose infusion rate (mg/kg/min) required to maintain an adequate serum glucose level is more helpful information. A normal newborn requires a minimum glucose infusion of 6 to 8 mg/kg/min to maintain normal serum glucose levels. Those with defective insulin control frequently require glucose infusions up to 25 mg/kg/min to keep the serum glucose concentration higher than 40 mg/dL.

Hypoglycemia normally results in the release of the counter regulatory hormones, glucagon, somatostatin, growth hormone, cortisol, and catecholamines, which promote the mobilization of fat and the generation of ketone bodies. However, insulin is a strong inhibitor of lipolysis and the high level of insulin present in HHI prevents mobilization of fats effectively blocking ketone body formation. Thus the absence of ketone bodies during periods of hypoglycemia also strongly suggests the diagnosis of hyperinsulinemic hypoglycemia.

In HHI the high insulin level results in deposition of abnormally large amounts of glycogen in the liver and inhibition of glucagon release. Administration of glucagon to patients with islet cell dysplasia results in a breakdown of the abnormal glycogen stores and a greater increase in the serum glucose level than would be expected if normal glycogen stores were depleted. An increase of more than 30 mg/dL in serum glucose concentration following administration of glucagon is abnormal.

Determining whether a patient has diffuse or focal disease as accurately as possible is important from a prognostic and therapeutic standpoint. Prior to elucidation of the genetic factors outlined above, only invasive venous sampling studies available at a few institutions could provide information on the histologic variant of disease. However, with the advent of more sophisticated genetic analysis and advanced imaging capabilities, invasive studies may be avoided. Recently, [18F]FDOPA PET-CT has been identified as a valuable tool to assist in the differentiation of diffuse and focal disease. The affected pancreatic islet tissue metabolizes L-DOPA to dopamine by decarboxylase action, the increased islet cell activity can be identified with (18F)fluoro-L-DOPA ([18F]FDOPA) providing imaging evidence of diffuse involvement or help with localizing a specific focal lesion. Studies using this technique have proven effective when combined with the information gained through genetic analysis in guiding surgical interventions.

## TREATMENT OPTIONS

Many patients with persistent hypoglycemia respond to medical therapy and never require operative intervention. The mainstays of medical therapy for HHI are frequent or continuous feedings, diazoxide and somatostatin analogs. Diazoxide therapy can be used on a chronic basis if the initial response is adequate to keep the patient asymptomatic. It also has some benefit in the management of patients with recurrent hypoglycemia following partial pancreatectomy. Unfortunately, long-term therapy with diazoxide is not without risk. Cases of cardiac failure and ataxia have been described with long-term use of even submaximal doses of diazoxide. These cases are rare, however, and many patients have received long-term therapy without sequelae.

The somatostatin analogue octreotide has also been used successfully for the treatment of HHI. The mechanism of action involves direct inhibition of beta cells by interfering with calcium-mediated insulin release. The use of somatostatin analogs is made somewhat more difficult because of difficulty in administration and short duration of action. In addition, octreotide is known to reduce splachnic blood flow and cases of necrotizing enterocolitis have been reported associated with its use.

## SURGICAL MANAGEMENT

Given the devastating neurologic sequalae of severe hypoglycemia, surgical intervention is clearly indicated in those patients who fail to respond adequately to medical therapy.

However, extensive pancreatectomy is not without short- and long-term risk leading to a long-standing struggle to determine the appropriate operation for the disease. Patients in whom focal disease is suggested by preoperative workup and confirmed at the time of operation benefit from limited resection of the diseased pancreas alone. Those with diffuse disease require a more extensive resection. The dilemma that surgeons face when treating diffuse disease with subtotal pancreatectomy is the nagging issue of how much of a pancreatic resection is enough. In early surgical series, most patients were treated with a 60% to 80% pancreatectomy. Unfortunately, 30% to 50% of patients have recurrent hypoglycemia that is not controlled with medical therapy requiring re-exploration with resection of additional pancreatic tissue. In several experienced centers, the operation of choice has evolved into a sub-total 95% to 98% pancreatectomy while others advocate a lesser resection followed by a near total pancreatectomy in those that recur. To further complicate the issue, there are a number of case reports and small series that describe the successful use of minimally invasive techniques to perform the resection.

## SURGICAL TECHNIQUE

### Preoperative Preparation

Reliable intravenous access for the administration of glucose solutions during the operation is the most important step in preparing an infant for surgery for islet cell dysplasia. A central line can be placed at the beginning of the procedure to provide intravenous access if necessary. Blood for transfusion should be available but significant blood loss is unusual. During the procedure serum glucose levels should be followed closely.

### Open Procedure

The patient is positioned supine on the operating room table and the abdomen is entered through a transverse supraumbilical incision. Infants with hyperinsulin induced hypoglycemia are typically large and a moderate-sized incision extending to the left mid-abdomen is required to provide adequate exposure. After an initial exploration of the abdomen, the pancreas should be exposed through the gastrocolic ligament. A careful examination of the pancreas is then performed. In cases where the preoperative workup suggests a focal lesion, the area is carefully inspected using loupe magnification for evidence of visible disease. For lesions of the tail of the pancreas, a spleen sparing distal pancreatectomy can be performed using bipolar cauterization to divide branches to the pancreas from the splenic vein and either a stapler or other energy source to divide the pancreas. The specimen must be sent to pathology for frozen section confirmation of the diagnosis. Lesions of the head or body can be enucleated where possible with frozen sections done to confirm complete excision of the abnormal tissue. More extensive lesions in the head of the pancreas may require pancreaticojejunostomy for drainage of the tail of the pancreas following resection. Confirmation that the lesion has been removed based upon intraoperative examination by pathology is necessary prior to closure.

# SUBTOTAL (95%) PANCREATECTOMY

Wide exposure to the pancreas, duodenum, and spleen are required. Exposure is obtained by mobilizing the hepatic flexure of the colon and taking down the gastrocolic ligament to give wide exposure to the lesser sac (Fig. 85-2). The colon is retracted inferiorly and a wide Kocher maneuver is done to mobilize the duodenum and head of the pancreas. The common bile duct is identified in the hepatoduodenal ligament along with the portal vein. A replaced right hepatic artery coming from the superior mesenteric artery may also be found. The tail of the pancreas is mobilized off the splenic vein by dividing the short pancreatic branches with bipolar cautery (Fig. 85-3). There can be a number of small arterial branches from the splenic artery to the body of the pancreas that must also be divided. The pancreas is carefully elevated off the superior mesenteric artery as it enters the celiac trunk. The confluence of the superior mesenteric vein and splenic vein to form the portal vein is exposed as the junction of the body and tail of the pancreas is elevated off the vessels (Fig. 85-4). Dissection of the medial portion of the pancreas begins with mobilization of the uncinate process from its attachments to the third portion of the duodenum. The goal of the 95% pancreatectomy is to resect all pancreatic tissue except the small amount of tissue between the common bile duct and the duodenum. This is accomplished by identifying the common bile duct as it enters the pancreas posteriorly and dividing the pancreatic parenchyma just lateral to the common duct using a right angle clamp and ties. The parenchyma is divided using care to preserve the common bile duct and

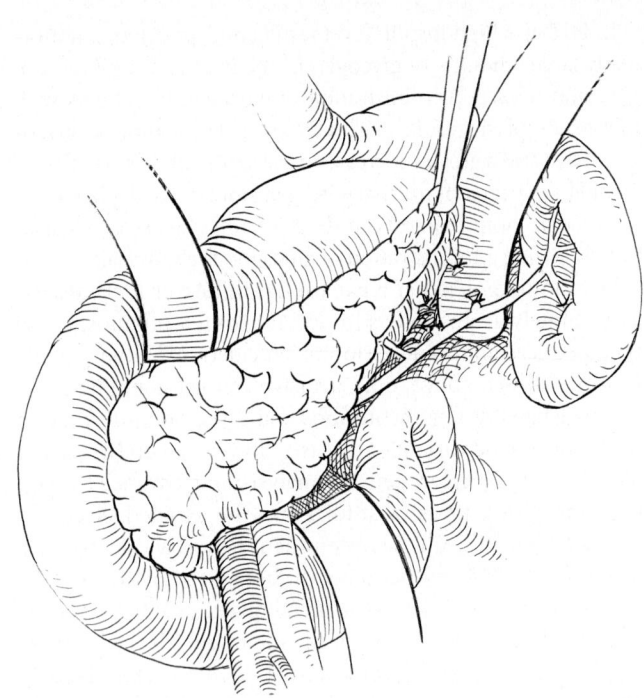

**FIGURE 85-3** The dissection is carried out beginning at the distal pancreas where the tail of the gland is mobilized off of the splenic vein, dividing the short venous branches from the pancreas with silk ties or the bipolar electrocautery.

the pancreaticoduodenal artery. If the bile duct is difficult to visualize, it can be opacified with methylene blue dye through a needle cholangiogram. Avoiding injury to the common bile duct, preserving duodenal blood flow, and resecting as much pancreas as possible are accomplished by following the course of the common bile duct along the posterior pancreas

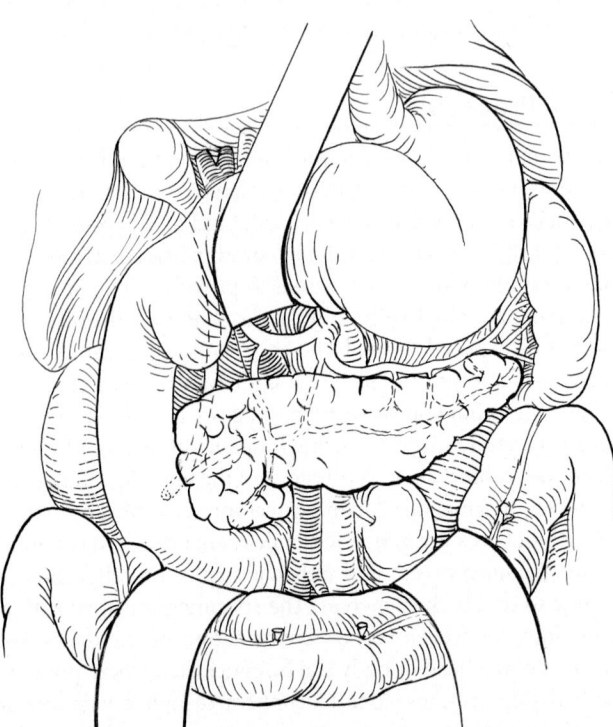

**FIGURE 85-2** Wide exposure of the pancreas and its relation to the splenic artery and vein, the spleen, mesenteric vessels, and duodenum, and the portal triad is done by mobilizing the colon flexures, dividing the gastrocolic ligament, and entering the lesser sac.

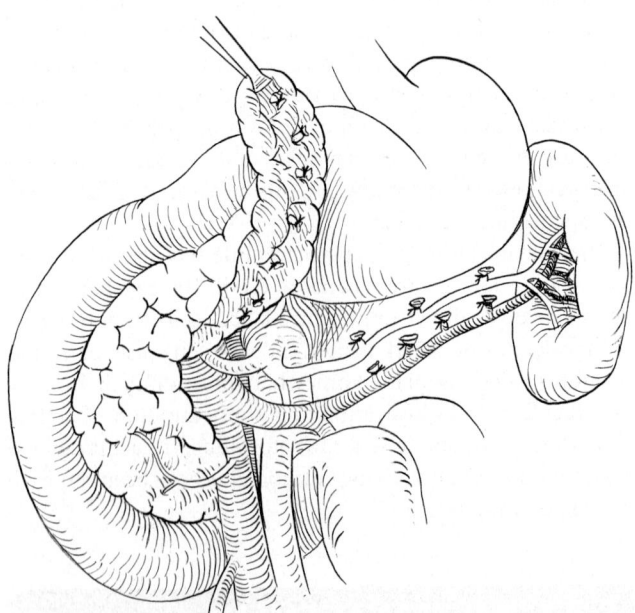

**FIGURE 85-4** The tail and body of the pancreas are mobilized lateral to the spine. Separation of the splenic vessels from the pancreas exposes the confluence of the splenic vein and superior mesenteric vein where the portal vein is formed.

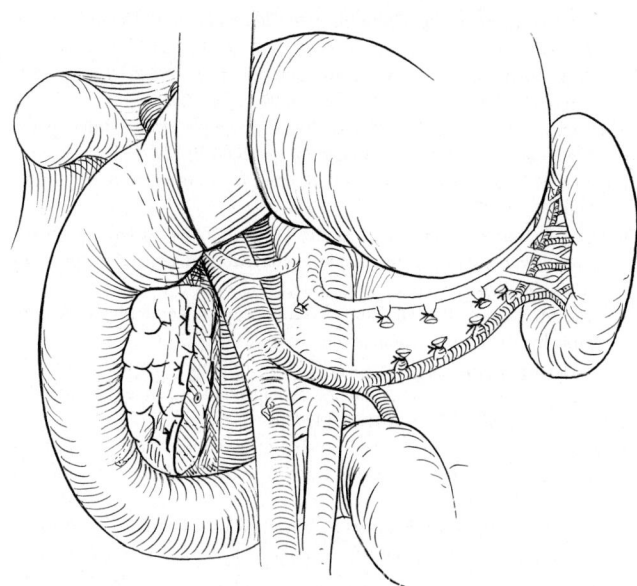

**FIGURE 85-5** A 95% pancreatectomy is completed by extending the dissection beyond the mesenteric vessels to just lateral to the common bile duct.

toward the ampulla of Vater. A small rim of pancreatic tissue is left along the duodenum between the duodenum and the common bile duct (Fig. 85-5).

In patients with persistent hypoglycemia following a 95% pancreatectomy, the tissue between the common bile duct and pancreas is resected leaving only small bits of pancreatic tissue along the blood supply to the duodenum and the common bile duct. Total pancreatectomy carries not only the risks of devascularizing the duodenum and injuring the common bile duct, but also the obvious risks of lifelong diabetes and exocrine pancreatic dysfunction.

Any ectopic pancreatic tissue identified during the initial exploration should be excised prior to closing the abdomen. A close suction drain is brought out through a separate stab wound and the abdomen is closed in layers.

## LAPAROSCOPIC APPROACH

The laparoscopic approach has been described by several authors who report acceptable results. It is particularly applicable in cases of focal disease in the distal pancreas. The technique has been described by various authors and the method proposed by Klaas Bax follows. The patient is positioned supine on the table with the legs in a frog-leg orientation. The surgeon stands at the end of the table which is placed in reverse Trendelenberg. The camera port is introduced at the umbilicus and two additional ports are introduced in the right and left mid-abdomen. Following insufflation with $CO_2$, the greater curve of the stomach is suspended to the anterior abdominal wall with 2 transabdominal stay sutures. The pancreas is exposed in the lesser sac by division of the gastrocolic ligament. The pancreas is easily seen and inspected. Focal lesions can be identified and enucleated. If the lesion cannot be identified, the pancreas is mobilized for a more detailed

inspection. In patients with diffuse disease or persistent hypoglycemia after initial operation, a 95% pancreatectomy can be achieved with "surprising ease" laparosocopically.

## POSTOPERATIVE CARE

In the early postoperative period serum glucose levels must be followed very closely and an adequate infusion of glucose maintained to avoid hypoglycemia. Feedings can be initiated early in the postoperative course and as feedings increase the glucose infusion can be slowly decreased and discontinued. If necessary, diazoxide or octreotide therapy may be required to maintain adequate glucose levels. If the patient cannot be weaned from a continuous glucose infusion, resection of additional pancreatic tissue is necessary.

Initially feedings are started as a continuous drip and are later switched to bolus feedings as the patient demonstrates the ability to maintain adequate serum glucose levels.

## RESULTS

Patients with focal disease and a clearly identified and resected mass at the time of operation do very well. In a single large series from the Children's Hospital of Philadelphia, 82% of patients with focal disease had a complete response, defined as not requiring any medical therapy with normal glucoses. In contrast, a complete response was achieved in only 33% of patients with diffuse disease (50% in those undergoing >95% pancreatectomy). In the immediate post-op period, approximately 10% to 30% of patients in most series developed transient hypoglycemia. Frequently these patients require short-term treatment with diazoxide and the hypoglycemia eventually resolves. The number of patients with diffuse disease who have persistent severe hypoglycemia requiring aggressive medical therapy varies with the amount of pancreas resected at surgery. While the overall impression is that patients tolerate subtotal (95%) pancreatectomy remarkably well, some long-term follow-up studies suggest significant morbidity from the onset of diabetes during adolescence. About 50% of patients with a resection limited to the pancreas to the left of the mesenteric vessels have sufficient persistence of symptoms to require additional surgery. However, those who do not develop recurrent hypoglycemia have little long-term risk of diabetes. Conversely, 30% to 70% of patients treated with a subtotal (95%) pancreatectomy develop diabetes by early adolescence. Patients undergoing a near total pancreatectomy (>95%) develop diabetes earlier. In light of the data regarding the risk of recurrent symptoms and diabetes, some centers have moved to an algorithm in which patients initially undergo an 85% pancreatectomy (resection of all pancreatic tissue to the left of the mesenteric vessels) to reduce the incidence of diabetes. In the patients with persistent hypoglycemia after the initial procedure, the remaining pancreas is resected to complete a near total pancreatectomy.

From a technical standpoint, preservation of the spleen during resection of the tail of the pancreas has reduced some of the long-term morbidity related to infection. In the early experience prior to splenic preservation, a significant number of the patients treated with pancreatectomy plus splenectomy subsequently dies of sepsis.

From an exocrine standpoint, patients do remarkably well following this procedure. In most recent studies none of the patients experience steatorrhea or require pancreatic enzyme replacements. Dunger et al examined exocrine and endocrine function in 7 patients who were 1 to 2 years status post 95% pancreatectomy and found that although the activities of pancreatic enzymes and bicarbonate concentrations were reduced in approximately half the children, they were clinically well with no evidence of malabsorption. If hyperinsulinemic hypoglycemia is diagnosed early and treated aggressively, growth and neurologic development will also be normal.

## SUMMARY

In summary, HHI is a rare developmental abnormality of the pancreas, which presents as persistent nonketotic hyperinsulinemic hypoglycemia in the newborn. Work over the past 2 decades has helped to significantly improve our understanding of the genetic and molecular basis for the disease. Once the diagnosis is made, the initial treatment options include diazoxide, glucocorticoids, glucagon, and octreotide. Eventually many patients will require surgery and the procedure of choice is tumor enucleation for focal disease and 95% pancreatectomy for those with diffuse disease and/or persistent hypoglycemia. Following the procedure, many patients will have some degree of endocrine dysfunction of the pancreas and there is a high incidence of later diabetes.

## SELECTED READINGS

Al-Shanafey S. Laparoscopic vs open pancreatectomy for persistent hyperinsulinemic hypoglycemia of infancy. *J Pediatr Surg* 2009;44:957–961.

Barthlen W, Blankenstein O, Mau H, et al. Evaluation of [18F] Fluoro-L-DOPA positron emission tomography-computed tomography for surgery in focal congenital hyperinsulinism. *J Clin Endocrinol Metab* 2008;93:869–875.

Bax KMA, van der Zee DC. The laparoscopic approach toward hyperinsulinism in children. *Semin Pediatr Surg* 2007;16:245–251.

Dekelbab BH, Sperling MA. Hyperinsulinemic hypoglycemia of infancy: the challenge continues. *Diab/Metab Res Rev* 2004;20:189–195.

de Lonlay P. Hyperinsulinemic hypoglycemia in children. *Ann Endocrinol* 2004;65:96–98.

Dunger DB, Burns C, Ghale GK, Muller DP, Spitz L, Grant DB. Pancreatic exocrine and endocrine function after subtotal pancreatectomy for nesidioblastosis. *J Pediatr Surg* 1988;23:112–115.

Flanagan SE, Kapoor RR, Hussain K. Genetics of congenital hyperinsulinemic hypoglycemia. *Semin Pediatr Surg* 2011;20:13–17.

Laje P, Halaby L, Adzick NS, Stanley CA. Necrotizing enterocolitis in neonates receiving octreotide for the management of congenital hyperinsulinism. *Pediatr Diab* 2010;11:142–147.

Lovvorn HN III, Nance ML, Ferry RJ Jr, et al. Congenital hyperinsulinism and the surgeon: lessons learned over 35 years. *J Pediatr Surg* 1999;34:782–793.

Marquard J, Palladino AA, Stanley CA, Mayatepek E, Meissner T. Rare forms of congenital hyperinsulinism. *Semin Pediatr Surg* 2011;20:38–44.

Martin LW, Ryckman FC, Sheldon CA. Experience with 95% pancreatectomy and splenic salvage for neonatal nesidioblastosis. *Ann Surg* 1984;200:355–362.

Pierro A, Nah SA. Surgical management of congenital hyperinsulinism of infancy. *Semin Pediatr Surg* 2011;20:50–53.

Rahier J, Guiot Y, Sempoux C. Morphologic analysis of focal and diffuse forms of congenital hyperinsulism. *Semin Pediatr Surg* 2011;20:3–12.

Schonau E, Deeg KH, Huemmer HP, Akcetin YZ, Bohles HJ. Pancreatic growth and function following surgical treatment of nesidioblastosis in infancy. *Eur J Pediatr* 1991;150:550–553.

Shilyansky J, Fisher S, Cutz E, Perlman K, Filler RM. Is 95% pancreatectomy the procedure of choice for treatment of persistent hyperinsulinemic hypoglycemia of the neonate? *J Pediatr Surg* 1997;32:342–346.

Stanley CA. Hyperinsulinism in infants and children. [Review] [34 refs]. *Pediatr Clin N Am* 1997;44:363–374.

Stringer MD, Davison SM, McClean P, et al. Multidisciplinary management of surgical disorders of the pancreas in childhood. *J Pediatr Gastroenterol Nutr* 2005;40:363–367.

Thomas PM, Cote GJ, Wohllk N, et al. Mutations in the sulfonylurea receptor gene in familial persistent hyperinsulinemic hypoglycemia of infancy [see comments]. *Science* 1995;268:426–429.

Warden MJ, German JC, Buckingham BA. The surgical management of hyperinsulinism in infancy due to nesidioblastosis. *J Pediatr Surg* 1988;23:462–465.

# CHAPTER 86

## Disorders of the Thyroid, Parathyroid, and Adrenal Glands

*Corey W. Iqbal and David C. Wahoff*

## KEY POINTS

1. Total thyroidectomy should be performed for all primary thyroid malignancies with the exception of anaplastic thyroid cancer.

2. Protection of the recurrent laryngeal nerves is critical in thyroid and parathyroid procedures. Understanding of the anatomy and its potential variations can help prevent iatrogenic injuries.

3. Ectopic and supernumerary parathyroid glands can pose a significant challenge to the surgeon. The surgeon should be prepared with sufficient preoperative imaging and knowledge of where to search for missing parathyroid glands.

4. Minimally invasive adrenalectomy is less painful and associated with a quicker recovery in appropriately selected patients.

5. Pheochromocytoma needs to be ruled out prior to resection of an adrenal mass. Patients with a pheochromocytoma require specific preoperative management with alpha-blockade.

## INTRODUCTION

Functional endocrine neoplasms in the pediatric patient are rare; however, these lesions are the most frequent indication for surgical resection of endocrine glands. Oftentimes, the surgeon may need to perform a resection not only to alleviate symptoms due to hormone hypersecretion but to distinguish between benign and malignant neoplastic processes as well, particularly in this age where advanced radiographic imaging is bringing more incidental lesions to the clinician's attention. Other disorders of the endocrine glands may come to the surgeon's attention due to pathologic hyperfunction, enlargement, or for risk reduction. The surgeon should feel comfortable in the technical aspects of the surgical management of endocrine neoplasms and other endocrinopathies. In this chapter we focus on operative techniques for the management of thyroid, parathyroid, and adrenal neoplasms and endocrinopathies.

## THYROID GLAND

### Essentials of Diagnosis

1. While thyroid nodules are less common in childhood compared to adults, the incidence of malignancy is higher.

2. Medullary thyroid carcinoma may be indicative of multiple endocrine neoplasia syndrome IIA or IIB and pheochromocytoma should be ruled out in these patients.

3. Ultrasound-guided fine needle aspiration is useful to evaluate a thyroid nodule in the adolescent but sampling error makes it a less useful diagnostic test in the pre-adolescent.

4. The MACIS score is a prognostic tool for papillary and follicular variant thyroid cancers that is well established in adults. Its utility in the pediatric patient is not well studied.

### Embryology

During the third fetal week, the thyroid gland originates as an outpouching from the foramen cecum at the base of the tongue. This outpouching solidifies into a bilobed structure as it descends below the cricoid cartilage, anterior to the trachea. Fibrous connective tissue, known as the ligament of Berry, anchors the thyroid gland to the trachea. The fourth branchial pouch gives rise to the para-follicular C-cells which will produce calcitonin. These cells are found laterally at the junction of the upper two-thirds of the thyroid gland, and for this reason, medullary thyroid carcinomas (which arise from the para-follicular C-cells) tend to be localized to this region.

### Anatomy

The thyroid gland is a bilobed structure with superior and inferior poles bilaterally. It receives its blood supply from the superior and inferior thyroid arteries bilaterally. The superior thyroid artery arises as the first branch of the external carotid artery. It has a significant anatomic relationship to the superior laryngeal nerve. Infrequently, the superior thyroid artery may branch from the common carotid artery just proximal to the carotid artery bifurcation. The inferior thyroid artery arises from the thyrocervical trunk which is a branch of the subclavian artery. Understanding the relationship of the inferior thyroid artery to the recurrent laryngeal nerve (RLN) is critical in preventing iatrogenic injury during thyroid procedures.

Venous drainage is via the superior, middle, and inferior thyroid veins bilaterally. The superior and middle thyroid veins drain directly into the internal jugular vein. Drainage of the inferior thyroid veins can be variable. The right inferior thyroid vein can drain into either the right subclavian vein or the left brachiocephalic vein. The left inferior thyroid vein drains directly into the left brachiocephalic vein.

As mentioned previously, the anatomic relationship of the RLN to the inferior thyroid artery and thyroid gland is critical in safely conducting thyroid surgery. The RLN innervates all of the muscles of the larynx (with the exception of the cricothyroid muscle). Unilateral injury results in hoarseness from vocal cord adduction while bilateral injury can result in airway compromise necessitating a tracheostomy. The RLN arises as a branch of the vagus nerve. The right RLN descends and courses around the right subclavian artery; the left RLN courses around the aortic arch. In most patients both nerves then ascend through the mediastinum along the tracheo-esophageal groove, posterior to the inferior thyroid artery, and to the larynx. However, the relationship of the RLN to the inferior thyroid artery can vary and care should always be taken to identify and protect the nerve prior to ligating the inferior thyroid artery. In most cases the RLN is posterior to the inferior thyroid artery; however, the nerve can be anterior or even course between the small branches of the inferior thyroid artery (see later in *Operative Techniques* section). A non-RLN can be present in as many as 1% of the population. In this variation, the laryngeal nerve (typically on the right) does not descend into the mediastinum but takes a direct course from the cervical portion of the vagus nerve to the larynx.

The superior laryngeal nerve innervates the cricothyroid muscle of the larynx which regulates vocal cord tension. Injury to this nerve results in voice fatigue and impaired pitch. In general, the superior laryngeal nerve follows the superior thyroid artery and care should be taken to protect this nerve when ligating the superior thyroid artery during thyroidectomy. The course of the superior laryngeal nerve can also be variable, and in 20% of patients the nerve will be lateral to the superior thyroid artery.

## Physiology

Within the thyroid gland, the follicular cells synthesize triiodothyronine (T3) and thyroxine (T4) from tyrosine residues of thyroglobulin and iodine. These hormones are important in neurological development and in the regulation of the body's metabolic state. T3 is a deiodinated form of T4 and although T4 is secreted in greater abundance, nearly 80% is converted peripherally to T3, which is a much more active form. Most circulating thyroid hormone is in the bound state either to thyroxine-binding globulin, transthyretin, or albumin. In fact, less than 1% of either T3 or T4 is circulating in an unbound (or active) state.

Regulation of T3 and T4 production and secretion from the thyroid gland is via a negative feedback loop that involves the hypothalamus and anterior pituitary gland. Neuronal cells in the paraventricular nucleus of the hypothalamus release thyrotropin-releasing hormone which passes to the anterior pituitary gland through the superior hypophyseal artery and stimulates the release of thyroid stimulating hormone (TSH). TSH acts directly on the thyroid follicular cells increasing T3 and T4 production. T3 and T4 feedback in a negative feedback fashion to inhibit TSH production whereas low levels of T3 and T4 stimulate TSH production.

The para-follicular C-cells secrete calcitonin which is a hormone involved in calcium regulation. Secretion is stimulated by hypercalcemia, gastrin, and pentagastrin. Calcitonin works in opposition to parathyroid hormone to lower calcium by decreasing gut absorption of calcium, inhibiting osteoclast activity, and inhibiting renal phosphate and calcium absorption.

## Indications for Thyroidectomy

### Work-Up of Thyroid Nodule

Thyroid nodules occur in children with an incidence of 1% to 2% and are the most common indication for thyroid resections. These nodules are malignant in as many as 27% of cases but can represent a spectrum of various benign and malignant conditions (see Table 86-1). While there is poor correlation between a hyperfunctioning nodule and the presence of malignancy versus a "cold," non-functioning nodule, these lesions oftentimes come to surgical resection regardless. A history of radiation exposure or a family history of thyroid malignancies, parathyroid disease, pheochromocytoma, or other traits consistent with multiple endocrine neoplasia (MEN) should raise the suspicion for potential malignancy—specifically medullary thyroid carcinoma. Other important variables in the history include change in size over time and signs or symptoms of hypo- or hyperthyroidism.

Physical examination should focus on palpation of the mass, the presence of any other thyroid masses, and careful palpation for lymphadenopathy. Thyroid function tests can confirm the presence or absence of hyperthyroidism; however, as previously stated, the correlation between a hyperfunctioning nodule and malignancy is poor. Ultrasonography is an important diagnostic modality in the evaluation of a thyroid nodule. It can distinguish between solid and cystic masses and although it cannot differentiate between benign and malignant lesions, ultrasound-guided fine needle aspiration (FNA)

| TABLE 86-1 | The Differential Diagnosis of Thyroid Nodules Categorized as Benign or Malignant | |
| --- | --- | --- |
| **Malignant** | | **Benign** |
| Papillary | | Follicular adenoma |
| Follicular | | Thyroiditis |
| Mixed type | | Thyroglossal cyst |
| Anaplastic | | Colloid nodule |
| Medullary | | Branchial cyst |
| Lymphoma | | |

| TABLE 86-2 | Characteristics of Primary Thyroid Malignancies | | | |
|---|---|---|---|---|
| | **Papillary** | **Follicular** | **Medullary** | **Anaplastic** |
| Presentation | Thyroid nodule | Thyroid nodule | Thyroid nodule | Rapidly enlarging neck mass |
| FNA | Positive or suspicious | Suspicious | Positive | Positive |
| Preoperative Studies | Ultrasound<br>Thyroglobulin | Ultrasound | Ultrasound<br>Serum calcitonin<br>*RET* protooncogene<br>Urinary metanephrines &<br>catecholamines | — |
| Treatment | Total thyroidectomy<br>Central compartment<br>lymph node dissection | Total thyroidectomy*a* | Total thyroidectomy<br>Central compartment lymph<br>node dissection | Palliative radiation |
| Mode of Spread | Lymphatic | Hematogenous | Lymphatic<br>Hematogenous | Locally invasive<br>Lymphatic<br>Hematogenous |

*a*Central compartment lymph node dissection not routinely recommended due to low incidence of nodal involvement.

is important for cytologic analysis particularly in adolescents. Malignancy on cytologic evaluation warrants a total thyroidectomy with central lymph node dissection. Indeterminate findings are managed with a thyroid lobectomy proceeding to a total thyroidectomy if histologic examination confirms the presence of a malignancy (see Table 86-2). A benign nodule by FNA can be observed unless it is hyperfunctioning. FNA in preadolescents is far less reliable due to increased sampling error and proceeding to a resection in this population is advisable. All patients with a suspected malignancy should have a chest radiograph.

## Thyroid Malignancies

Papillary thyroid cancer is the most common thyroid malignancy and is characterized by the presence of psammoma bodies on histology (see Table 86-2). This form of primary thyroid cancer carries a very favorable prognosis even in the setting of metastases with a survival of 86% to 100% at 30 years despite a lifelong recurrence rate of 30%. The MACIS score may be useful to determine the prognosis and is based upon: Metastases, Age, Completeness of resection, Invasion, and Size. The mechanism of metastasis is via the lymphatics to regional lymph nodes. Metastases to the lung and bone are uncommon.

Follicular adenocarcinoma is a more aggressive form of thyroid malignancy with a potential for vascular invasion with subsequent metastases to the lung, liver, and bone. In the United States, lymphatic spread is uncommon; however, in European studies as many as 25% of patients have nodal involvement. The inability to differentiate a follicular adenoma from an adenocarcinoma on a fine needle aspirate is oftentimes an indication for resection. Using the MACIS score to determine prognosis for follicular adenocarcinoma may be of use in the pediatric patient but has not been well studied.

Medullary thyroid cancer (MTC) arises from the parafollicular C-cells and is associated with familial MTC or as a manifestation of MEN IIA or IIB (see Table 86-3). There are also sporadic forms of the disease but this is less common and patients with MTC should undergo *RET* protooncogene analysis. Serum calcitonin levels are usually elevated; however, this is a poor screening tool for patients with known familial MTC or MEN II. MTC is far more aggressive than papillary or follicular thyroid carcinoma with 5- and 10-year survival rates of 86% and 68%, respectively, and therefore in kindreds with known *RET* protooncogene mutations early, prophylactic thyroidectomy should be offered. Recurrence rates are reported to be as high as 25%.

Anaplastic thyroid cancers are rare and carry a grim prognosis with a survival of less than 12 months. This malignancy presents as a rapidly growing mass that is locally invasive. Resection, even palliative, is not recommended.

As eluded to previously, when the presence of malignancy is unknown preoperatively, lobectomy can be undertaken with a completion thyroidectomy reserved if malignancy is confirmed on pathologic examination. However, if multifocal or bilobar disease is known preoperatively then proceeding initially with a total thyroidectomy is appropriate. It is important, in the setting of a malignancy, to perform a total thyroidectomy to prevent local recurrence, to facilitate surveillance using iodine uptake scans and thyroglobulin, and to make radioablation of residual disease postoperatively more effective.

## Other Thyroid Disorders

Other less common indications for total or sub-total thyroidectomy include diffuse goiter, toxic diffuse goiter, and thyroiditis. The most common etiology for goiter currently is Hashimoto thyroiditis (also known as chronic lymphocytic thyroiditis) which is characterized by autoantibodies to thyroid peroxidase, thyroglobulin, and TSH receptors. The most common indication for resection in the presence of a goiter is to rule out a malignancy but other indications include impending airway compromise or failure to respond to medical therapy.

| TABLE 86-3 | Characteristics of the Multiple Endocrine Neoplasia Syndromes | | | |
|---|---|---|---|---|
| | **MEN 1** | **MEN 2A** | **MEN 2B** | **FMTC**[a] |
| Eponym | Werner syndrome | Sipple syndrome | Williams–Pollock syndrome | — |
| Gene | MEN1 | RET | RET | RET NTRK1 |
| Parathyroid hyperplasia | Yes | Yes | No | No |
| Pancreatic neoplasms | Yes | No | No | No |
| Pituitary neoplasms | Yes | No | No | No |
| Medullary thyroid carcinoma | No | Yes | Yes | Yes |
| Pheochromocytoma | No | Yes | Yes | No |
| Mucosal neuromata | No | No | Yes | No |

[a]Familial medullary thyroid carcinoma.

Thyroiditis encompasses a spectrum of disease (see Table 86-4). Hashimoto thyroiditis is an autoimmune disorder that results from chronic lymphocytic infiltration involving antibodies to thyroid peroxidase. The gland becomes firm and enlarged. Subacute thyroiditis (also known as the DeQuervain thyroiditis) is the painful enlargement of the thyroid gland associated with hyperthyroidism. The etiology is unclear but it is felt to be viral in origin. This disease is usually self-limiting. Suppurative or bacterial thyroiditis is usually caused by oral flora that seed the left thyroid lobe via a persistent piriform sinus from the pharynx. Management with antibiotics that cover oral flora is usually adequate; however, if the infection progresses to abscess formation then incision and drainage are necessary.

## Preoperative Considerations

If the patient has had a prior cervical exploration, a preoperative vocal cord check should be performed to document whether or not both RLNs have been preserved. Furthermore, if malignancy has been confirmed or is suspected an ultrasound assessing for suspicious lymph nodes should be performed to prepare for the possibility of needing to perform an extended lymph node dissection. This assessment can typically be performed with the initial ultrasound-guided FNA. Patients with papillary thyroid cancer should have a preoperative thyroglobulin obtained while patients with MTC should have a serum calcitonin obtained in addition to screening for a pheochromocytoma if a MEN syndrome is suspected.

## Operative Technique

### Positioning

The patient is placed supine on the operating room table and general endotracheal anesthesia is used. Depending on the patient's size, the arms may or may not need to be tucked. The critical component to positioning is adequate neck extension to provide adequate exposure—this may be difficult in large or obese adolescents (see Fig. 86-1). A soft roll can be placed underneath the shoulders to help obtain adequate

| TABLE 86-4 | Characteristics of Thyroiditis in Children | | |
|---|---|---|---|
| | **Acute** | **Subacute** | **Lymphocytic** |
| Types | Bacterial thyroiditis | The DeQuervain or granulomatous thyroiditis Subacute lymphocytic thyroiditis | The Hashimoto thyroiditis Chronic lymphocytic thyroiditis |
| Etiology | Bacterial | Viral (coxsackie, adenovirus) | Autoimmune |
| Presentation | Tender neck mass | Tender neck mass if it is the DeQuervain thyroiditis Non-tender neck mass for SLT | Signs of hyper- or hypothyroidism |
| Thyroid Status | Euthyroid | Hyperthyroid (early) Hypothyroid (late) | Hypothyroid with bouts of hyperthyroidism |
| Treatment | Antibiotics I&D if abscess present | Symptomatic if hyperthyroid NSAIDs | Thyroid replacement |

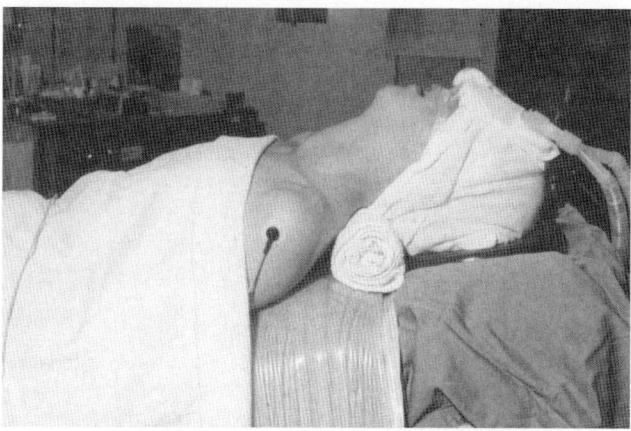

**FIGURE 86-1** Positioning for cervical exploration with appropriate neck extension.

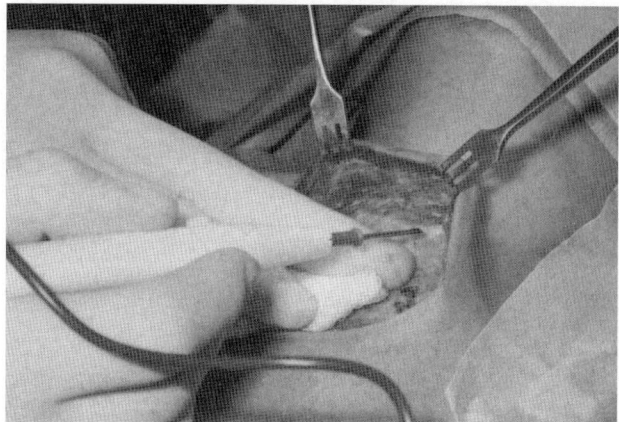

**FIGURE 86-3** Skin retractors facilitate raising the subplatysmal flaps.

neck extension. The prep should extend from the ears and chin cephalad, to the nipples caudally, and to both shoulders laterally.

## Operative Technique

A Kocher incision is used to perform an adequate cervical exploration and expose the thyroid gland. The landmarks are 2 to 3 cm above the sternal notch extending laterally to include the medial borders of the sternocleidomastoid muscles approximately 1 cm above the clavicles. A silk suture can be used to mark out the incision (see Fig. 86-2). A skin incision is made sharply and electrocautery is used to divide the platysma muscle which lies superficially. Flaps are then created just below the platysma superiorly to the level of the thyroid cartilage and inferiorly to the manubrium. Skin retractors can be used to facilitate dissection in this plane (see Fig. 86-3). After elevation of these flaps a self-retaining retractor is placed (see Fig. 86-4). The anterior jugular veins are encountered in this dissection and can usually be preserved; if they are injured they can be ligated. The strap muscles (a collection of the sternohyoid, omohyoid, and sternothyroid muscles) are then identified and opened in the midline in a longitudinal fashion to allow retraction laterally along with the sternocleidomastoid muscles. This will expose the deep

cervical fascia which is opened to expose the thyroid gland (see Fig. 86-5).

The thyroid gland should then be mobilized by carrying the dissection laterally towards the carotid sheath (see Fig. 86-6). This plane between the strap muscles and the thyroid gland can be opened with a combination of gentle, blunt dissection and electrocautery. Opening this space will allow the surgeon to begin mobilizing the lateral-most aspect of the thyroid gland and start to retract it medially. Being able to pull the lateral borders of the thyroid gland medially will facilitate exposure of the thyroid vasculature.

If the planned operation is a thyroid lobectomy, then a right-angle clamp can be used to bluntly dissect the thyroid isthmus away from the trachea and allow division. The thyroid gland is a highly vascularized organ and therefore we prefer to suture ligate both ends of the isthmus with polyglactin suture. If a pyramidal lobe is present, this should be included in the resection.

Downward traction is placed on the thyroid gland and the superior thyroid artery and vein can then be identified and ligated (see Fig. 86-6). Care must be taken to avoid injury to the superior laryngeal nerve, which supplies the cricothyroid muscle and runs in close proximity to the superior thyroid artery. Injury can be avoided by ligating the vasculature close

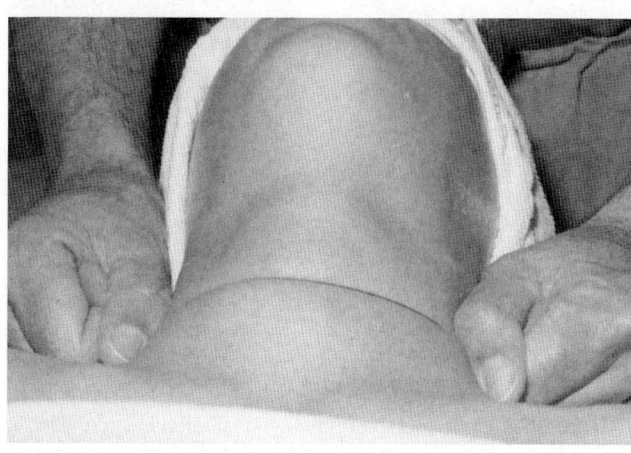

**FIGURE 86-2** A silk suture is used to mark the incision.

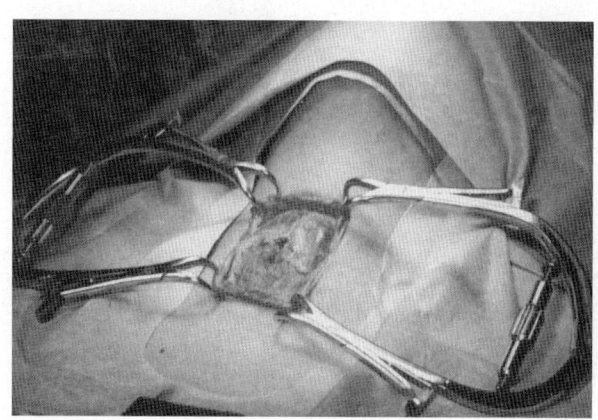

**FIGURE 86-4** A self-retaining retractor can be used to facilitate exposure.

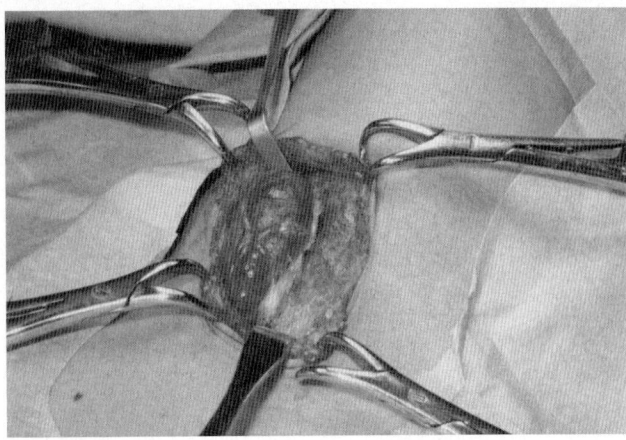

**FIGURE 86-5** Opening the deep cervical fascia exposes the thyroid gland.

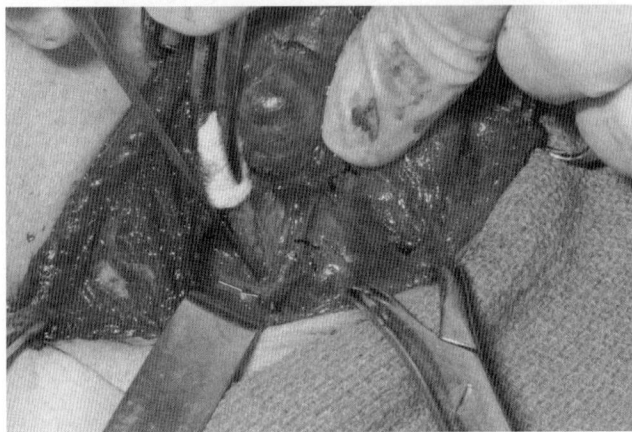

**FIGURE 86-7** The inferior thyroid artery (arrow) and vein are identified. The inferior thyroid artery shares an important relationship to the RLN.

to the thyroid gland. Ligation of the vessels close to the gland can also help prevent devascularizing the parathyroid glands. Whether the surgeon starts the dissection at the superior pole or at the inferior pole is based on preference.

Once the superior lobe has been mobilized, the dissection should be carefully continued inferiorly towards the lower pole to identify the inferior thyroid artery (see Fig. 86-7). The middle thyroid vein can often be identified and ligated during this dissection which allows further rotation of the thyroid gland medially. This mobilization allows the parathyroid glands and the RLN, both of which are posterior, to be visualized. Dissection of the inferior thyroid artery is then required but must be undertaken with extreme caution because of the risk of injury to the RLN but it can typically be identified at the inferolateral aspect of the thyroid (see Fig. 86-8).

Both RLNs run in close proximity to the inferior thyroid artery and this relationship must be understood to avoid inadvertent injury. The left RLN branches off of the vagus nerve and wraps around the aorta from where it ascends along the trachea. It may lie in the tracheo-esophageal (TE) groove or lateral to the TE groove. In most cases the left RLN will lie posterior to the artery in the TE groove; in 20% of cases the nerve is anterior to the vessel; and in the remaining 30% of

cases the nerve courses between the branches of the inferior thyroid artery. The right RLN arises from the right vagus, courses around the right subclavian artery, runs obliquely towards the trachea, and then ascends along the trachea. It is usually more lateral to the TE groove than the left nerve

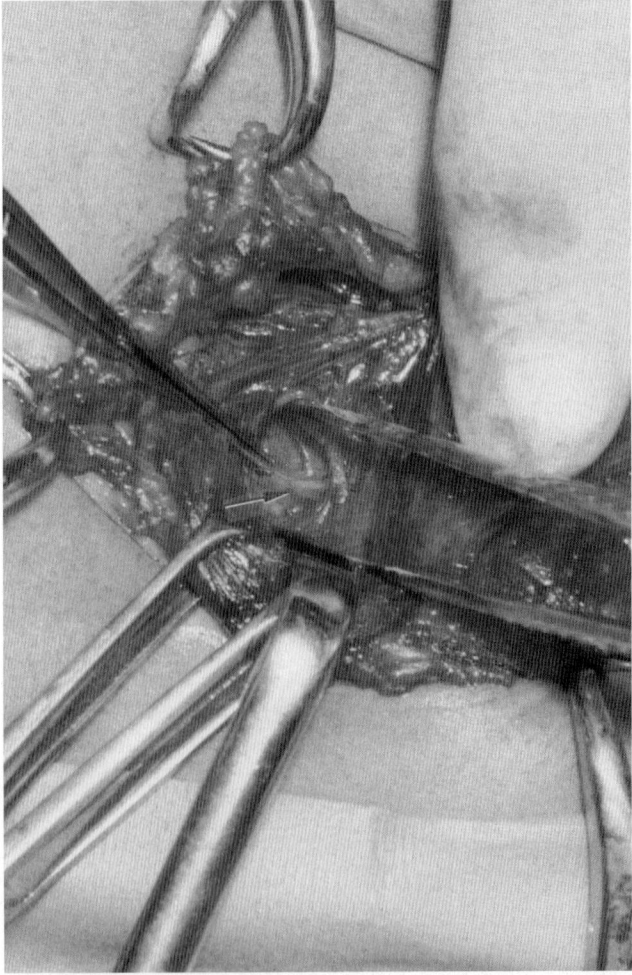

**FIGURE 86-8** Once the recurrent laryngeal (arrow) is identified it should be carefully dissected away from the gland minimizing handling of the nerve to prevent injury.

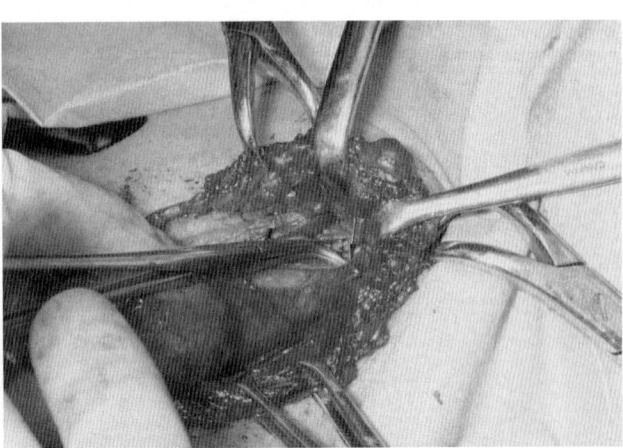

**FIGURE 86-6** Lateral dissection exposes the remainder of the thyroid and allows identification of the superior thyroid artery and vein.

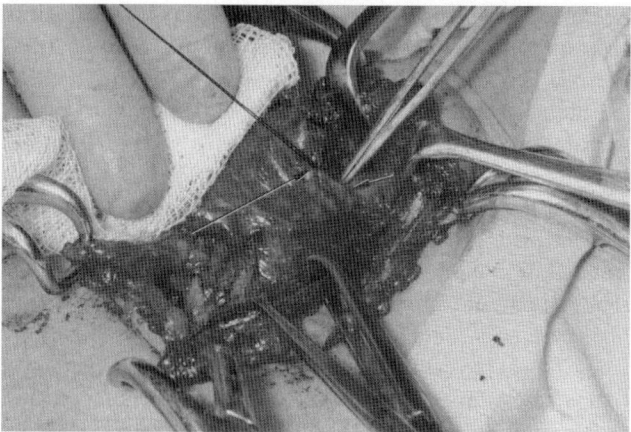

**FIGURE 86-9** The thyroid vessels should be ligated close to the gland to preserve the vascular supply to the parathyroid glands.

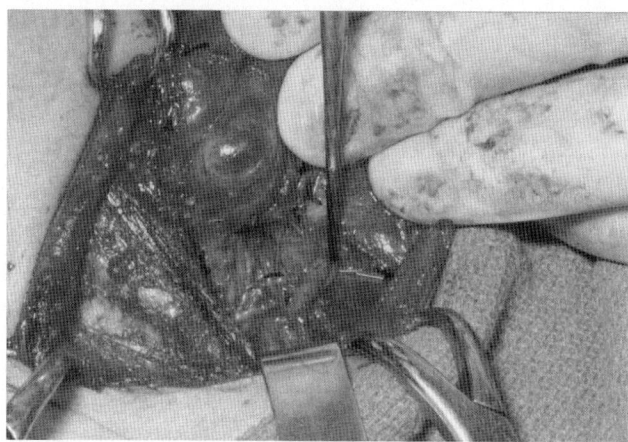

**FIGURE 86-10** The left inferior parathyroid gland (arrow) is visualized and its end-arterial supply from the inferior thyroid artery.

and its anatomic relationship to the inferior thyroid artery is also different in that it is anterior to the artery only 30% of the time, deep to the artery 20% of the time, and in 50% of cases courses between the inferior thyroid artery branches. The surgeon must also be wary of a non-RLN on the right side in which case the nerve arises from the cervical portion of the vagus and courses directly to the larynx.

Once the RLN has been identified the surgeon should take care to avoid excessive handling of or unnecessary dissection around it. Excessive traction can result in a neuropraxia with temporary nerve dysfunction and should also be avoided. With the nerve protected, the inferior thyroid artery can be ligated. Similar to the superior thyroid artery, the inferior thyroid artery should also be ligated close to the gland (see Fig. 86-9). This avoids injury to the RLN but also preserves the end-artery blood supply to the parathyroid glands which is predominately through the inferior thyroid artery.

Care in preserving the parathyroid glands, as well as their vascular supply is critical to avoid postoperative hypoparathyroidism and subsequent hypocalcemia, particularly when total thyroidectomy is being performed. Two parathyroids (inferior and superior) are present on both the left and right thyroid lobes. The parathyroid glands are readily identified by their tan coloration that distinguishes them from the remainder of the thyroid gland—although they are easily confused with adjacent adipose tissue. Most commonly the parathyroids measure 4 to 5 mm and are found on the posterior surface of the thyroid gland with the inferior parathyroid gland residing toward the lower pole and the superior parathyroid gland residing in the middle to upper pole of the thyroid. However, the parathyroid glands are prone to significant variability in their location which will not be addressed in this section as it is discussed elsewhere in this chapter. Their vascular supply is most commonly from end-arterial branches from the inferior thyroid artery (see Fig. 86-10). However, end arteries can also arise from the superior thyroid artery therefore both arteries should be ligated close to the thyroid gland to prevent devascularization of the parathyroids.

If the parathyroid cannot be safely dissected free of the thyroid gland and preserved or if the gland is inadvertently devascularized, autotransplantation of the gland should be undertaken. The devascularized gland is minced and autotransplanted into a pocket made in the sternocleidomastoid muscle. We then close this pocket with a polypropylene suture with the tails cut long to facilitate access to this tissue should re-exploration be necessary. Other authors have reported autotransplanting the parathyroid tissue into the chest wall or the forearm. If we do not suspect that the parathyroid tissue is abnormal, we autotransplant the parathyroid tissue into the sternocleidomastoid to avoid an additional incision. When autotransplanting diseased parathyroid tissue (such as MEN patients) we prefer the chest wall or forearm for easier access in the future (see Parathyroid section). In performing a total thyroidectomy for malignancy a small portion of thyroid tissue can be left on the parathyroid gland to prevent devascularization if postoperative radioactive iodine is anticipated.

Removal of the thyroid gland is then completed by taking down the posterior thyroid attachments to the trachea known as the ligament of Berry (see Fig. 86-11). Due to the anatomic location of the RLN in the TE groove, it can be inadvertently pulled up and injured during division of this ligament. Therefore, care should still be exercised to protect the RLN.

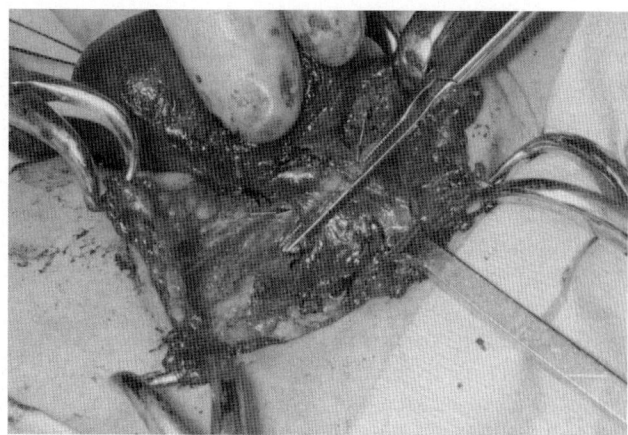

**FIGURE 86-11** The ligament of Berry (arrows) anchors the thyroid gland to the trachea and must be taken down with care as the RLN can easily be pulled up during this dissection.

If only a lobectomy is being performed, the specimen should be marked and sent fresh to pathology. For a total thyroidectomy the steps are repeated on the contralateral side.

If a malignancy is suspected, a central lymph node dissection should be carried out by excising the lymph nodes in the lower aspect of cervical lymph node level VI: from the cricoid cartilage to the level of the manubrium and between both carotid sheaths. If preoperative ultrasound identified suspicious lymph nodes outside of the central compartment then those lymph nodes should be removed as well. This may require extension of the cervical incision cephalad to access lymph nodes along the carotid sheath and sternocleidomastoid muscle.

After excision of the specimen, hemostasis should be ensured as a cervical hematoma can lead to life-threatening airway compromise. We have a low threshold to use topical hemostatic agents and inspect the operative field for bleeding with the patient in Valsalva. Drains are placed at the surgeon's discretion based on the extent of the dissection (lobe versus total thyroidectomy) and the size of the thyroid gland (ie, goiter). Once hemostasis has been ensured, the strap muscles are reapproximated in the midline with interrupted absorbable sutures. The platysma is closed with a running absorbable suture, and the skin is closed with a running, absorbable monofilament suture. Taking the patient's head out of flexion may facilitate reapproximation of the platysma and skin during closure.

Minimally invasive techniques including video-assisted and robot-assisted thyroidectomy have been described and are being applied in less than 15% of all thyroidectomies. While these techniques are associated with smaller, less visible scars, application is not universal. Thyroid gland and nodule size are important considerations as well as the need for lymph node excision; patients with thyroiditis, cervical radiation, or prior cervical operation are also poor candidates. Furthermore, these techniques have not been well studied in the pediatric population.

## Postoperative Considerations

Postoperatively, the patient's voice is assessed to ensure there is no evidence of RLN injury by having the patient pronounce a long "E." Hoarseness does not always indicate an irreversible nerve injury, as neurapraxia can result from traction injuries. In this setting, re-evaluation in 4 to 6 weeks is appropriate as most patients will show improvement over time. Bilateral nerve injury oftentimes necessitates emergent tracheostomy. A cervical hematoma is a life-threatening complication and should be managed with emergent airway protection, cervical decompression, and operative re-exploration to identify a bleeding source.

A serum calcium should be checked on the first postoperative day in all patients having a total or subtotal thyroidectomy to ensure that the parathyroid glands are functioning. These patients, even with autotransplantation of the parathyroid glands, can experience a transient state of hypoparathyroidism and may require supplemental calcium. Mild symptoms such as circum-oral or limb parasthesia can be managed with oral calcium supplementation but routine supplementation in asymptomatic patients is not necessary. If the hypocalcemia is profound and the patient is severely symptomatic, central access should be obtained and intra-venous calcium administered to prevent cardiac dysrhythmias.

Patients are hospitalized overnight and allowed to restart per oral intake. Pain is usually controlled with oral analgesics and patients may be dismissed home on postoperative day one. If a drain was placed, it is removed on postoperative day one prior to dismissal. Additionally, patients undergoing subtotal or total thyroidectomy will require thyroid hormone replacement and indefinite follow-up with TSH assays but replacement is not started for 4 to 6 weeks postoperatively when repeat thyroid studies are obtained and, if indicated, radioactive iodine is given. Replacement can begin after this. If a thyroid lobectomy has been performed, the residual thyroid tissue should be adequate, however, we routinely obtain a TSH level 6 weeks post-operatively.

# PARATHYROID GLANDS

## Essentials to Diagnosis

1. Primary hyperparathyroidism is most commonly associated with a solitary adenoma (up to 85%).

2. Imaging with a sestamibi nuclear scan with subtraction and ultrasound are critical to localize the lesion preoperatively.

3. Secondary hyperparathyroidism due to hyperplastic parathyroid glands is seen in end-stage renal disease. Failure of the hyperparathyroidism to resolve after transplant is indicative of tertiary hyperparathyroidism which may require operative therapy.

## Embryology

The parathyroid glands arise during the fifth week of gestation from neural crest mesenchyme and the endoderm of the third and fourth branchial pouches. The third branchial pouch descends and gives rise to the 2 inferior parathyroid glands. The fourth branchial pouch gives rise to the 2 superior parathyroid glands. The glands are comprised of 2 cell types: chief cells which produce parathyroid hormone and oxyphil cells.

## Anatomy

Typically, there are a total of 4 parathyroid glands: 2 superior and 2 inferior parathyroid glands. These glands are tan in color, are 4 to 5 mm in size, and are found on the posterior surface of the thyroid gland with the inferior parathyroid gland residing in the lower pole and the superior parathyroid gland residing in the middle to upper pole of the thyroid. The primary vascular supply is from the inferior thyroid artery, but they may also be supplied by the superior thyroid artery and/or thyroidea ima artery.

The parathyroid glands can be variable in their location and number. An ectopic gland may be present in 20% to 32% of cases and usually involves the inferior glands. Possible locations for an ectopic inferior parathyroid gland can include: near the hyoid bone, within the carotid sheath, intrathyroidal, intrathymic, and mediastinal. Common locations for ectopic superior glands include: tracheoesophageal groove, retro-esophageal space, within the carotid sheath, or the posterior mediastinum. Furthermore, up to 15% of patients may have a fifth gland, usually present in the thymus.

## Physiology

The primary function of the parathyroid glands is to maintain calcium homeostasis. PTH is released in response to low serum calcium. PTH functions by stimulating osteoclast activity (to release calcium from bone), increasing intestinal calcium absorption through vitamin D, and increasing renal calcium absorption. Its secretion is inhibited by high serum calcium levels.

## Indications for Parathyroidectomy

Surgical resection of parathyroid glands is exclusively limited to states of hyperparathyroidism. Hyperparathyroidism is classified as either primary, secondary, or tertiary hyperparathyroidism. All are associated with high or inadequately suppressed serum PTH levels. The signs and symptoms of hypercalcemia can be non-specific (see Table 86-5) and there can be other causes of hypercalcemia during childhood (see Table 86-6).

### Primary Hyperparathyroidism

Primary hyperparathyroidism is the most frequently encountered disorder of the parathyroid gland and is due to a hyperfunctioning adenoma in 70% to 85% of cases. The remaining patients have either multiple adenomas or 4-gland hyperplasia. Hyperplasia is usually seen in the setting of MEN I or IIA but can be sporadic. Parathyroid adenomas are rare in the pediatric population with an incidence of less than 1%. Parathyroid cancer in children is recognized and is associated with hypersecretion of PTH as well, but this entity is exceedingly rare in children and the literature is limited to few case reports. Rarely ectopic PTH secretion from a malignancy may be the source of hypercalcemia.

The diagnosis of primary hyperparathyroidism is made by an elevated total serum calcium level with an inadequately

| TABLE 86-6 | Causes of Hypercalcemia |
|---|---|
| Hyperparathyroidism | |
|   Primary hyperparathyroidism | |
|   Secondary hyperparathyroidism | |
|   Tertiary hyperparathyroidism | |
|   Ectopic parathyroidism | |
| Hypervitaminosis A | |
| Sarcoidosis | |
| Familial hypocalciuric hypercalcemia | |
| Williams syndrome | |
| Subcutaneous fat necrosis | |
| Thyrotoxicosis | |
| Hypophosphatemia | |
| Prolonged immobilization | |
| Thiazide diuretics | |

suppressed PTH level. In other words, if the PTH is elevated or not adequately suppressed by elevated total serum calcium level (ie, a high normal PTH level) then the diagnosis of primary hyperthyroidism is made. Adequate imaging using ultrasonography and a sestamibi nuclear subtraction scan is critical to localize the adenoma in preparation for resection and possibly performing a minimal access parathyroidectomy. These imaging modalities will not be helpful in the setting of hyperplasia. The possibility of an MEN syndrome should always be entertained especially with a strong family history and appropriate work-up undertaken.

If the patient has persistent or recurrent primary hyperparathyroidism after a previous parathyroidectomy, the operative notes should be reviewed carefully to ascertain which gland or glands may have been removed. In evaluating a patient with hypercalcemia and hyperparathyroidism, the clinician should be sure to exclude familial hypocalciuric hypercalcemia (FHH). In FHH the urine calcium will be low in contrast to primary hyperparathyroidism where urine calcium levels are elevated.

### Secondary and Tertiary Hyperparathyroidism

Secondary hyperparathyroidism arises in the setting of end-stage renal disease (ESRD) where hypocalcemia results from decreased levels of vitamin D and elevated phosphate levels. This chronic state of hypocalcemia causes persistent stimulation of the parathyroid glands with resultant hyperplasia. Elevated PTH stimulates ongoing osteoclast activity which can lead to renal osteodystrophy.

Patients with chronic renal disease should be treated with supplemental vitamin D, restriction of dietary phosphate, and oral phosphate binders. Cinacalcet is a calcium analogue that is approved for use in patients with ESRD requiring dialysis and can be used as well. Ultimately, most patients with

| TABLE 86-5 | Symptoms of Hypercalcemia and Associated End-Organ Damage | |
|---|---|
| **Symptoms** | **End-Organ Damage** |
| Fatigue | Renal insufficiency |
| Weakness | Cardiac bradyarrhythmias |
| Confusion/memory loss | Bone demineralization |
| Restlessness | |
| Nausea and/or emesis | |
| Loss of appetite | |
| Polyuria/polydypsia | |
| Abdominal pain | |

secondary hyperparathyroidism will experience resolution with kidney transplantation.

Tertiary hyperparathyroidism is seen in those patients with ESRD who do not have resolution of their hyperparathyroid state despite successful kidney transplantation. In this condition the parathyroid glands continue to autonomously secrete hormone despite normal circulating calcium levels. If kidney function has been optimized and medical therapy is failing, three and a half gland excision is required.

## Operative Technique

### Positioning

Positioning for a parathyroidectomy is similar to thyroidectomy—the patient is supine with the neck in extension and general endotracheal anesthesia is used (see Fig. 86-1). The prep should be extended inferiorly if a median sternotomy for ectopic mediastinal glands is possible. The major caveat depends on whether or not intraoperative parathyroid hormone assay is planned and whether or not a full cervical exploration will be undertaken or minimal access. For intra-operative parathyroid hormone assay to be conducted vascular access is needed for blood draws. However, when a full cervical incision is used, the internal jugular vein can be easily accessed by the surgeon for subsequent blood draws. If minimal access parathyroidectomy is planned an arterial line may be necessary.

### Cervical Exploration

To conduct a full cervical exploration, the thyroid gland is exposed as previously described. The thyroid is mobilized being sure to protect the RLN and inferior and superior thyroid arteries and veins—the middle thyroid vein must often be ligated to help mobilize the thyroid gland. Large parathyroid adenomas are readily identified while modest-sized adenomas or hyperplastic glands may not be as apparent.

The parathyroid glands can be variable in their anatomic location. The inferior glands arise from the third branchial pouch and are usually found on the posterior aspect of the lower pole of the thyroid. However, during embryogenesis the inferior glands can fail to separate from the thymus (approximately 1%) placing them either intrathymic or elsewhere in the mediastinum, and therefore the surgeon should be prepared to mobilize the thymus or even perform a transcervical thymectomy if the inferior glands cannot be identified. If there is failure of the inferior parathyroid glands to migrate, then they may be found high in the neck above the thyroid gland even as high as the hyoid bone. Ectopic inferior parathyroid glands can also be intrathyroidal (which requires lobectomy for excision) or within the carotid sheath.

The superior parathyroid glands arise from the fourth branchial pouch. The fourth branchial pouch also gives rise to the thyroid. When the superior parathyroid glands cannot be found they may be intra-thyroidal and require a thyroid lobectomy for excision. Ectopic superior parathyroid glands can also be found in the TE groove, in the retroesophageal space, in the carotid sheath, and in the posterosuperior mediastinum. The variability in parathyroid gland location

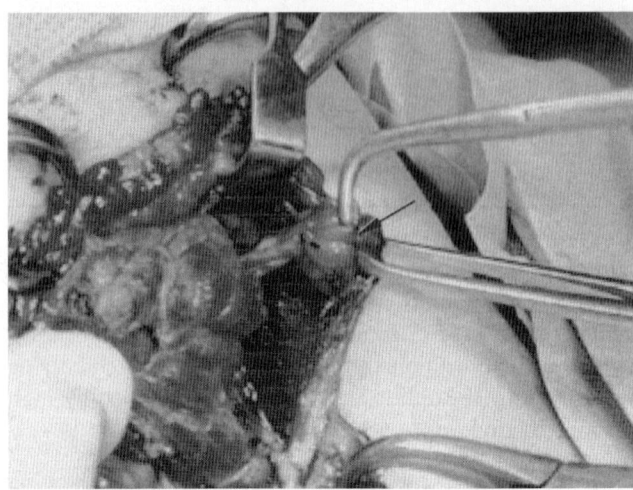

**FIGURE 86-12** A hyperplastic parathyroid gland on its vascular pedicle.

re-emphasizes why satisfactory imaging is paramount prior to proceeding to the operating room. The surgeon should be prepared to chase ectopic parathyroid glands including the possibility of a median sternotomy and so the patient and family should be appropriately counseled pre-operatively.

Once the parathyroid glands are identified frozen section should be used to confirm whether normal, adenomatous, or hyperplastic parathyroid tissue is present. If the surgeon is unsure on visual inspection of the gland, a biopsy should be taken and sent for frozen section prior to excision. The parathyroid gland is easily mobilized from the surrounding thyroid tissue and its vascular pedicle ligated (see Fig. 86-12).

We routinely use intraoperative parathyroid hormone assay. If a full cervical exploration is being conducted then we access the internal jugular vein for each draw. If a minimal access approach is being used, and the internal jugular vein is not readily accessible then anesthesia may need to obtain serial blood samples for analysis—although this is unusual. A baseline value is obtained once the carotid sheath is exposed to avoid a falsely elevated value due to manipulation of the adenoma. The half-life for parathyroid hormone is 3 to 4 minutes, therefore samples are then collected at 5 and 10 minutes post excision. At 10 minutes, a drop in the parathyroid hormone level of more than 50% from baseline value is considered curative.

When the clinician is confident in the diagnosis of primary hyperparathyroidism due to a solitary parathyroid adenoma based on biochemical and radiographic studies, minimal access parathyroidectomy in conjunction with intraoperative parathyroid hormone assay should be considered. This approach avoids a full cervical exploration and therefore requires a smaller incision compared to a standard cervical incision. Intraoperative parathyroid hormone assay is always used in conjunction with minimal access parathyroidectomy. This approach is associated with less pain, preservation of the structures on the contralateral side, and can be performed on an outpatient basis. However, if the PTH does not normalize then full cervical exploration is indicated. Minimally invasive video- and robot-assisted techniques similar to those used for thyroidectomy have been described for parathyroidectomy.

However, these techniques have not been well studied in the pediatric population.

When multiple adenomas or hyperplastic glands are felt to be the source of hyperparathyroidism then full cervical exploration should be undertaken with excision of any abnormal glands. If all 4 glands are abnormal then either 3.5 glands should be resected or all 4 glands should be resected with autotransplantation of one-half gland into either the chest wall or the brachioradialis muscle of the forearm. When autotransplanting benign parathyroid tissue during a 4-gland excision we use the sternocleidomastoid to avoid an additional incision. However, when transplanting diseased parathyroid tissue, a site that is readily accessible should be utilized to facilitate easy and safe access in the future should the patient have recurrent disease. We prefer autotransplantation into the subcutaneous tissue just below the clavicle. It is readily accessible without having to prep the forearm, and we have found it easier to re-access the parathyroid tissue here compared to the forearm. If 3.5 gland excision is performed with a remnant portion of a parathyroid gland intact, this area should be marked with a stitch to facilitate future explorations should there be recurrent parathyroid disease.

When all 4 glands cannot be identified and only normal parathyroid tissue is present in the identified glands the surgeon must consider ectopic glands. A thyroid lobectomy should be performed on the side of the missing gland to diagnose and possibly treat an abnormal intrathyroidal gland. Furthermore, transcervical thymectomy should be considered as well. Some surgeons advocate routine removal of the thymus in the setting of hyperplastic glands due to a 15% incidence of an intrathymic fifth gland, although this has not been our practice.

## Postoperative Considerations

As with thyroidectomy, injury to the RLNs and post-operative hematoma are serious potential complications. All patients should have serum calcium checked on post-operative day one to ensure that hypocalcemia is not present prior to discharge from the hospital. The risk for this is greatest in those patients undergoing 3.5 or 4 gland excision as the remnant parathyroid or autotransplanted tissue may be slow to produce parathyroid hormone. Patients with a solitary adenoma are also at risk as the remaining glands have been suppressed during the hypercalcemic state and may not produce parathyroid hormone immediately. Cure rates are reported to be as high as 95%. Failure in patients with histologically proven adenomas is usually due to the presence of an unrecognized parathyroid adenoma. Patients with hyperplastic parathyroid glands due to MEN, secondary hyperparathyroidism, and tertiary hyperparathyroidism are at higher risk for recurrence.

## ADRENAL GLANDS

### Essentials to Diagnosis

1. Most adrenal masses in children will be functional and evaluation should include evaluation for hypersecretion of cortisol, sex hormones, aldosterone, and catecholamines.

2. Differentiating between a benign or malignant adrenal cortical tumor preoperatively is difficult.

3. MRI or CT is useful to localize adrenal lesions. For cortical lesions a radiolabelled iodo-cholesterol (NP-59 scan may be required; for medullary lesions a MIBG scan may be necessary). If these imaging techniques fail to localize the lesion, adrenal venous sampling should be considered.

4. Patients with pheochromocytoma require premedication with phenoxybenzamine preoperatively.

### Embryology

The adrenal gland arises from the mesoderm and neural crest cells. During the fifth gestational week mesodermal cells migrate into the mesenchyme forming thick buds of fetal cortical cells. This is followed by a second migration of mesoderm that envelops the fetal cortical cells and will become adult cortical cells. Shortly after birth the fetal cortical cells degenerate and the adult cortical cells proliferate. The cortex then forms 3 layers (listed from deep to superficial): zona reticularis, zona fasciculate, and zona glomerulosa. The adrenal medulla arises from neural crest cells migrating to the initial fetal cortical mass. There is a close relationship between primordial adrenal cells and the genital ridge which can lead to ectopic adrenal tissue (cortical or medullary) along the course of gonadal descent.

### Anatomy

Both adrenal glands are situated in the retroperitoneum within the Gerota fascia superior to the kidneys reflecting the early nomenclature for these glands as suprarenal glands (see Fig. 86-13A). The arterial supply to both glands is primarily through multiple small branches from the posterior inferior phrenic arteries. Branches of the sympathetic chain and the celiac plexus course along the adrenal vessels to innervate the medulla. Despite similar arterial blood supply, venous drainage and the anatomic relationships to adjacent organs is very different between the right and left adrenal glands. These differences must be understood by the surgeon undertaking adrenalectomy.

The right adrenal gland sits atop the right kidney, behind the right lobe of the liver, and is in contact with the posterior diaphragm (see Fig. 86-13B). The venous drainage is directly into the inferior vena cava (IVC) via the right adrenal vein (see Fig. 86-14A). The left adrenal gland is situated superior to the left kidney, posterior to the pancreas and the splenic vessels (see Fig. 86-15). It is also in contact with the posterior diaphragm. Venous drainage of the left adrenal gland is via the left adrenal vein which drains directly into the left renal vein (see Fig. 86-14B).

### Physiology

The adrenal cortex synthesizes and secretes the corticosteroids which are inclusive of mineralocorticoids, glucocorticoids, and sex hormones all of which are derived from cholesterol (see Fig. 86-16). The outermost layer of the cortex is the zona glomerulosa which produces the mineralocorticoid, aldosterone. Secretion of aldosterone is tightly regulated by

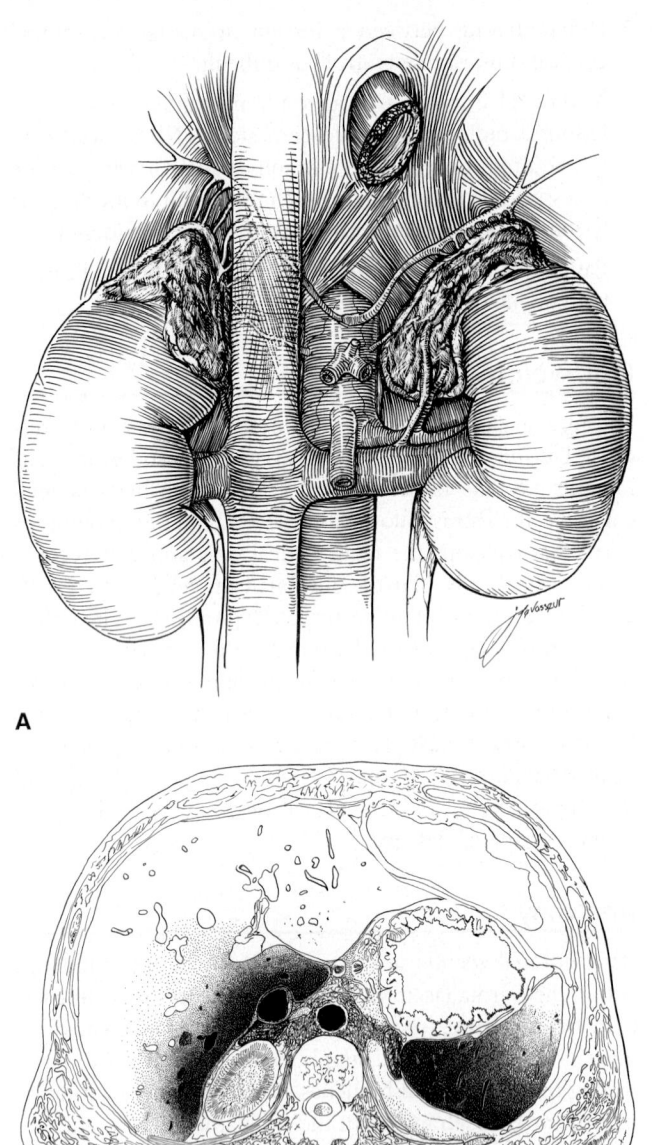

**A**

**B**

**FIGURE 86-13** Anatomy of the adrenal glands: **A.** The adrenal glands are superior to the kidneys bilaterally and derive their arterial supply from branches of the inferior phrenic artery. **B.** AXIAL view of the right adrenal gland and its anatomic relationships to the liver, IVC, and diaphragm.

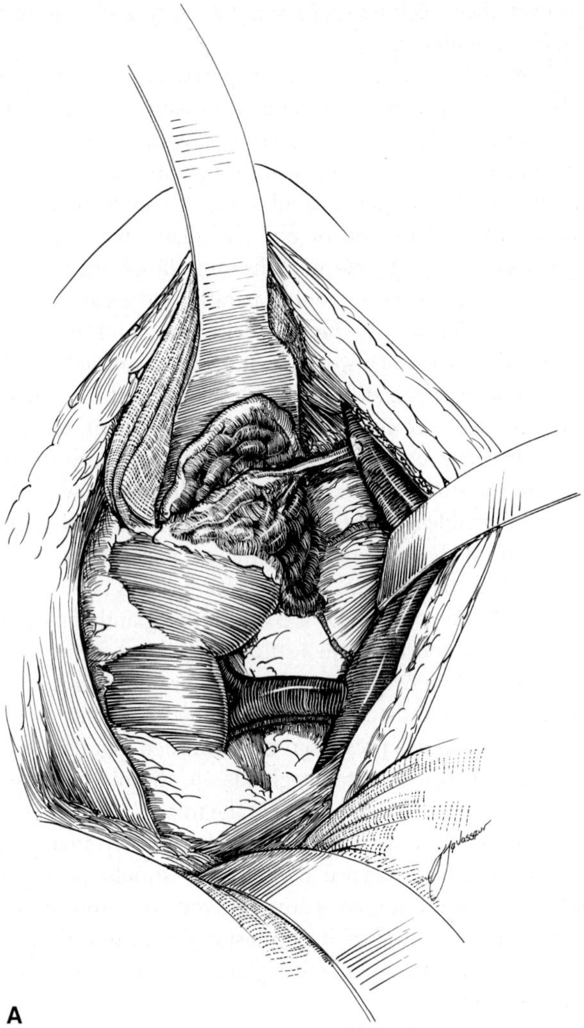

**A**

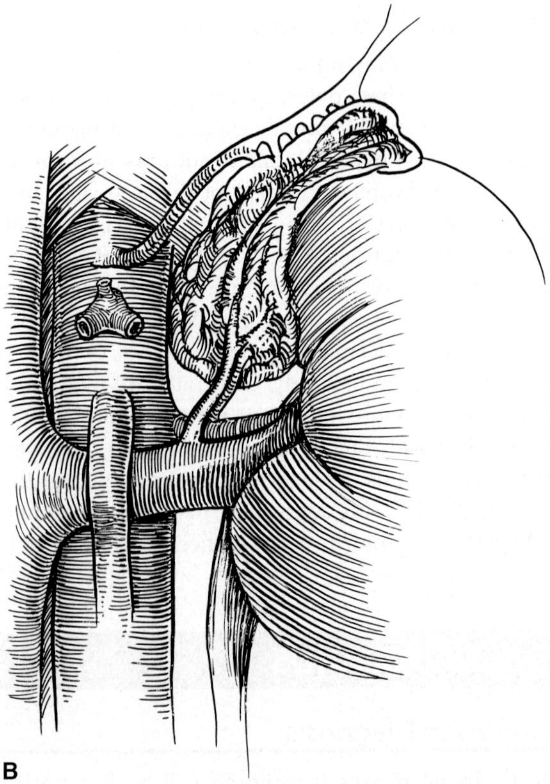

**B**

**FIGURE 86-14** **A.** The right adrenal vein drains into the inferior vena cava. **B.** The left adrenal vein drains into the left renal vein.

extracellular potassium levels and angiotensin II through the rennin–angiotensin system which is activated by decreased renal blood flow. Aldosterone maintains fluid and electrolyte balances via increased renal resorption of sodium, increased renal resorption of water, and increased renal excretion of potassium.

The middle layer of the adrenal cortex is the zona fasciculate which primarily produces the glucocorticoids, primarily cortisol, in response to stimulation from adrenocorticotropic hormone (ACTH) which is released from the anterior pituitary gland. ACTH release is in turn controlled by corticotrophin-releasing hormone (CRH) from the hypothalamus which is either enhanced or suppressed by blood cortisol levels as part of a negative feedback loop.

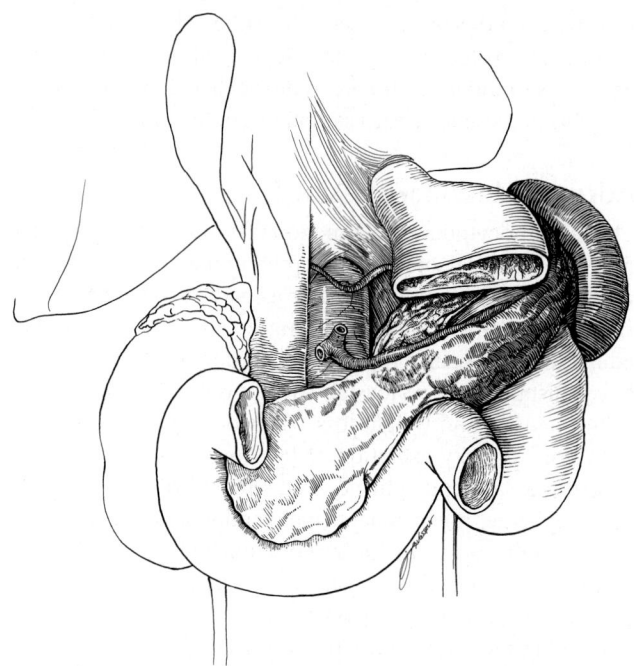

**FIGURE 86-15** The left adrenal gland and its anatomic relationship to the pancreas and spleen.

The innermost layer of the adrenal cortex is the zona reticularis which produces the sex hormones, primarily the androgens dihydroepiandrosterone (DHEA) androstenedione. These prescursors are converted to testosterone and estrogen in the testes and ovaries.

The adrenal medulla synthesizes and secretes epinephrine and norepinephrine (see Fig. 86-17). In humans, epinephrine

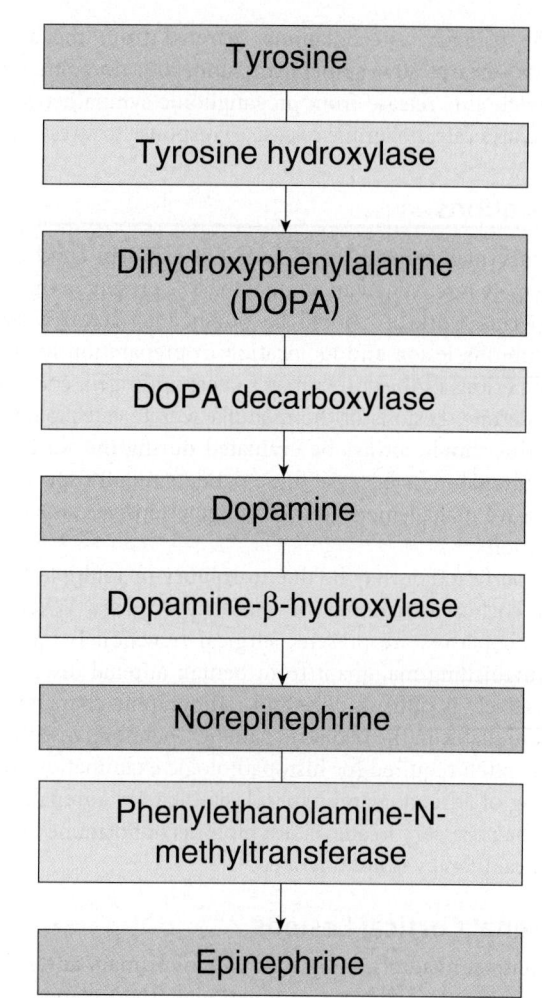

**FIGURE 86-17** Catecholamine synthesis in the adrenal medulla.

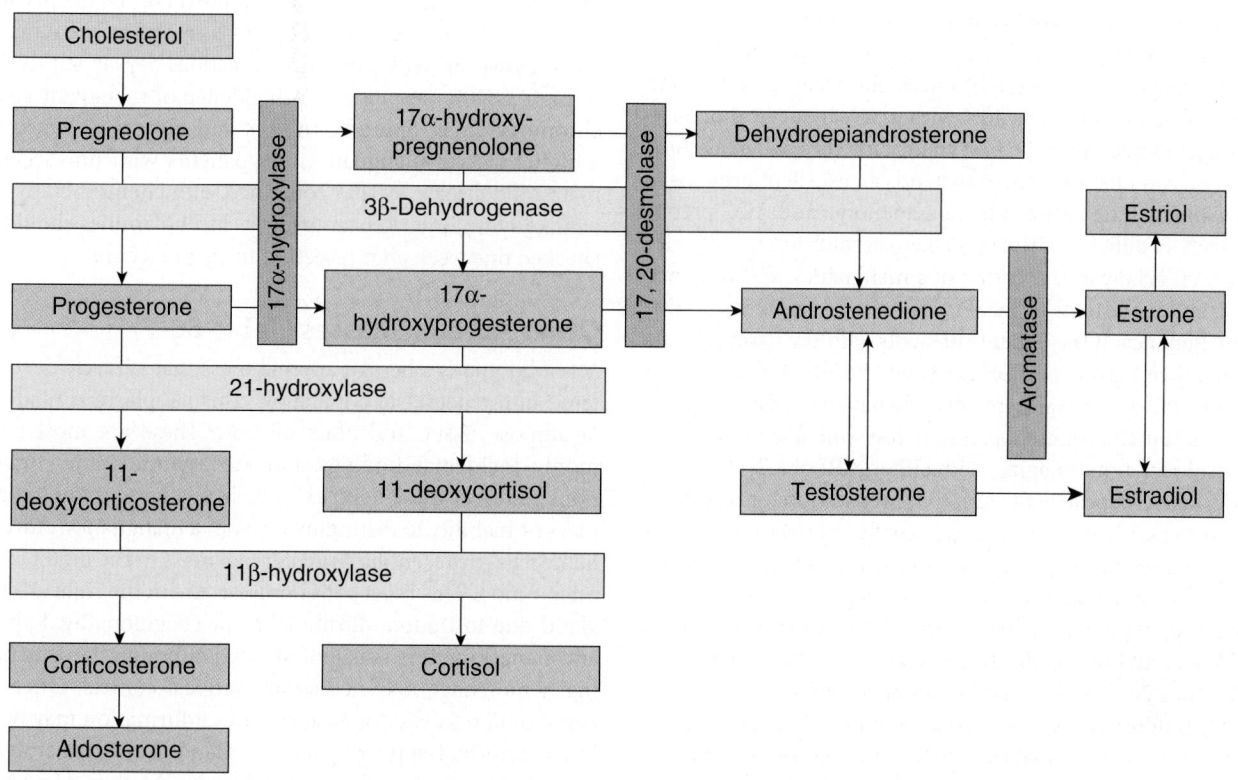

**FIGURE 86-16** Hormone synthesis from cholesterol in the adrenal cortex.

is the primary catecholamine secreted from the adrenal glands—nearly 80% epinephrine and 20% norepinephrine. Acetylcholine release from preganglionic sympathetic fibers stimulates catecholamine release in response to stress.

## Indications

Primary malignancies of the adrenal gland in children are extremely rare. When an adrenal mass is present, a thorough endocrine work-up should be pursued to detect a hyperfunctioning lesion and its location in preparation for resection. Lesions of the cortex may secrete androgen, cortisol, or aldosterone. Lesions of the medulla secrete catecholamines, and this should always be evaluated during the work-up of any adrenal mass because these patients require special preoperative management to avoid a hypertensive crisis during resection.

Hyperfunction may be due to solitary or multiple adenomas, cortical carcinoma, or gland hyperplasia. When solitary neoplasms are present, surgical resection is indicated. Distinguishing malignant from benign adrenal disease preoperatively is difficult. Size and radiographic characteristics are unreliable in the pediatric patient. Therefore, resected tissue is often required for histopathologic examination. In the setting of adrenal gland hyperplasia bilateral adrenalectomy may be necessary to alleviate symptoms of hormone excess if medical therapy is not tolerated.

## Adrenal Cortical Lesions

In contrast to adults, more than 95% of primary adrenal cortical lesions in children are functional. These patients typically present with signs and symptoms of virilization due to overproduction of androgens but can also present with cushingoid features due to cortisol excess. Hypersecretion can be due to an adrenal adenoma (or adenomas) or adrenal cortical carcinoma (ACC). ACC tend to be advanced at the time of diagnosis and even with resection recurrence rates are reported to be as high as 40% with a 5-year survival of 34%. Complete resection is the best chance for cure, whereas complete excision for adenomas portends an excellent prognosis.

Distinguishing between benign adenoma and ACC preoperatively is difficult. Urinary 17-ketosteroids are usually elevated, especially in the setting of a malignancy. The presence of distant metastases or local invasion is certainly suggestive of malignancy. If the patients presents with the Cushing syndrome then plasma cortisol levels will be elevated as well. In the setting of adrenal-dependent hypercortisolism, a high-dose dexamethasone suppression test will fail to suppress cortisol secretion. Imaging, with either MRI or CT, should be undertaken to localize the lesion in preparation for resection. In rare cases, hypercortisolism can be due ectopic ACTH secretion. In this instance of hypercortisolism, plasma cortisol levels are not suppressed during a high-dose dexamethasone suppression test. Treatment of the source of ectopic ACTH should be sought. Bilateral adrenalectomy, may need to be considered if a source cannot be found.

Hyperaldosteronism, or Conn Syndrome, is rare in the pediatric patient. In children, this is most commonly associated with hyperplasia as opposed to an adenoma. However, in the setting of an adenoma or, very rarely, a carcinoma, resection is indicated. Imaging with either MRI or CT should be pursued to localize a lesion. If one cannot be identified with these modalities then a radiolabelled iodo-cholesterol (NP-59) or adrenal venous sampling can be utilized.

## Adrenal Medullary Lesions

Pheochromocytomas are functional tumors of the adrenal medulla. These neoplasms are predominately sporadic but may arise in familial kindreds or as part of the MEN IIA or IIB syndromes. The mean age of onset is 11 years and, unlike adults who have paroxysmal hypertension, pediatric patients have sustained hypertension with vision changes, headaches, nausea, and weight loss. The work-up should include a 24-hour urinary excretion of fractionated catecholamines (dopamine, norepinephrine, and epinephrine) as well as metanephrine, normetanephrine, vanillymandelic acid, and homovanillic acid. Including fractionated catecholamines helps the clinician distinguish pheochromocytoma and paraganglioma from neuroblastoma.

Imaging should include either CT or MRI. A $^{131}$I metaiodobenzylguanidine (MIBG) scan can also be useful to localize small (<1 cm) or extra-adrenal lesions. Up to 10% of pheochromocytomas will be familial or associated with MEN IIA or IIB and in this circumstance there is a 25% incidence of bilateral lesions. Once localized, resection should be undertaken as complete excision is the most effective treatment.

Prior to resection, patients with a pheochromocytoma should be premedicated with phenoxybenzamine to achieve adequate alpha-blockade for 7 to 10 days preoperatively. If rebound tachycardia develops then a beta-blocker should be added. The night prior to resection patients should be preadmitted for intravenous volume repletion as their long-standing vasoconstriction has led to volume depletion and places them at risk for hypotension after removal of the neoplasm.

Up to 47% of pheochromocytomas in children are malignant. However, with complete resection, 5-year survival is as high as 90% despite a 47% incidence of malignant pheochromocytomas. Sporadic tumors and tumors >6 cm carry a higher risk of malignancy. For patients with unresectable metastatic disease, MIBG combined with chemotherapy can palliate symptoms. Repeat urinary catecholamines should be checked one week after resection to ensure a cure.

## Other Adrenal Masses (Table 86-7)

Myelolipoma is a benign adrenal mass that is rarely encountered in the pediatric population. This neoplasm is made up of adipose tissue and bone marrow. These are most commonly incidental findings and are asymptomatic. Indications to resect these neoplasms include a large, symptomatic mass or inability to distinguish it from a malignancy. Adrenal hemorrhage presenting as an adrenal mass in the infant is not uncommon. This most commonly occurs in the right adrenal gland due to trauma during labor or coagulopathy. Expectant management is usually indicated although life-threatening hemorrhage may necessitate surgical control. Once the hematoma resolves calcification or cyst formation may result in an abnormal-appearing adrenal gland. If the hematoma is seeded hematogenously an abscess may develop. Metastatic lesions to the adrenal gland can also occur.

| TABLE 86-7 | Differential Diagnosis for an Adrenal Mass Categorized as Functional and Nonfunctional | |
| --- | --- | --- |
| **Functional** | **Nonfunctional** | |
| Adrenal adenoma | Neuroblastoma | |
| Adrenal cortical carcinoma | Adrenal cyst | |
| Pheochromocytoma | Hemangioma | |
| Metastatic disease | Leiomyoma/leiomyosarcoma | |
| | Lymphoma | |
| | Melanoma | |
| | Metastatic disease | |
| | Myelolipoma | |

## Operative Techniques

The approaches to adrenalectomy are highly variable and include open approaches that consist of: anterior, posterior, trans-peritoneal, retroperitoneal, and even thoracoabdominal exposures. Since the original description by Gagner in 1992, laparoscopic adrenalectomy is being utilized more frequently and provides a less invasive approach that hastens recovery. Most adrenalectomies can be performed laparoscopically, however, local extension or invasion, concern for malignancy particularly with lymph node involvement, large neoplasms, major vascular invasion, or extensive adhesions from prior abdominal procedures are relative contraindications to a minimally invasive approach. Furthermore, the anatomy of the right versus the left adrenal gland is different and can change the degree of difficulty of adrenalectomy. The surgeon should tailor his or her approach based on the patient, the tumor characteristics, and the tumor location.

## Laparoscopic Right Adrenalectomy

Laparoscopic adrenalectomy is performed under general endotracheal anesthesia with the patient in a lateral decubitus position. For a right adrenalectomy the left lateral decubitus position is used, a bean bag helps maintain the positioning and flexion is used on the operating room table to open the space between the iliac crest and the costal margin. All pressure points should be carefully padded and straps should be used to secure the patient. An orogastric tube should be placed to decompress the stomach and an indwelling urinary catheter is placed to monitor urine output.

The surgeon is positioned behind the patient and the assistant is situated in front of the patient. The monitors are placed at the patient's head. The first trocar is a 5-mm camera port made half-way between the anterior iliac spine and the umbilicus. We favor an open cut-down although some surgeons prefer use of the Veress needle. A 5-mm 45° angled scope is used to explore the abdomen. Additional ports are then placed including a 10-mm working port just lateral to the initial port (which will be used for specimen retrieval); cephalad to the camera port in the mid-axillary line an additional 5-mm trocar is placed for liver retraction; the final port site is a 5-mm working port placed in the posterior axillary

line (see Fig. 86-18). It is important to keep the port sites close to the costal margin so that the iliac crest does not prohibit manipulation of the laparoscopic instruments.

Initially the right colon may need to be mobilized to facilitate placement of the lateral most trocar. The right colon is then reflected medially and the triangular ligament of the right hepatic lobe is divided with the Harmonic scalpel. Once the right lobe of the liver has been mobilized the liver retractor is used to reflect it medially exposing the right adrenal gland. The Harmonic scalpel is then used to dissect the adrenal gland. Oftentimes it is easier to mobilize the adrenal gland's lateral, superior, and inferior attachments to allow lateral retraction. In doing this the arterial supply is usually taken and the lateral retraction exposes the right adrenal vein which drains directly into the inferior vena cava (IVC). Care must be taken to gently retract the gland to avoid avulsing the adrenal vein from the IVC which leads to brisk bleeding and requires conversion to an open procedure. A 5-mm clip applier is used to ligate the adrenal vein. After division

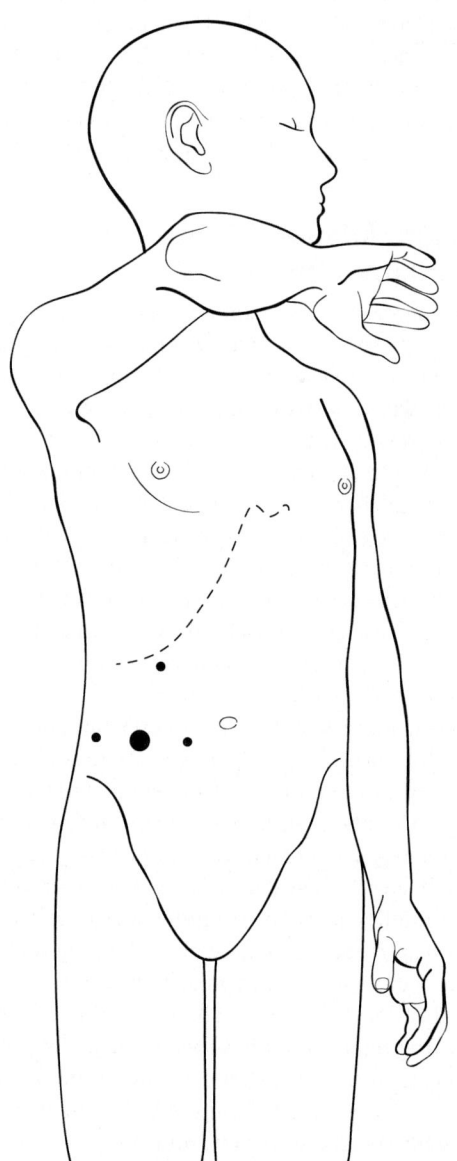

**FIGURE 86-18** Port placement for laparoscopic right adrenalectomy with the patient in the lateral decubitus position.

of the adrenal vein, care should still be taken in retracting the gland laterally as there may be accessory veins from the IVC that require ligation. The remainder of the dissection is then completed with the Harmonic scalpel and the specimen is removed in an EndoCatch bag through the 10-mm port site. The surgical site is then re-explored to ensure hemostasis. The skin of all 5-mm trocar sites is then closed with absorbable suture; the 10-mm trocar site fascia is closed with absorbable suture prior to skin closure.

Laparoscopic adrenalectomy can be performed with the patient supine; however, retraction of the abdominal viscera medially can make this approach more cumbersome. We find that the supine approach is more suitable for bilateral disease to avoid repositioning of the patient (see below). An endoscopic retroperitoneal or posterior approach has also been described. With the patient in the prone jackknife position a balloon dissector is placed through a 10-mm trocar placed into the retroperitoneal space just lateral to the 12th rib and is insufflated to create a working space. Three additional 5-mm ports are then placed: the first one just lateral to the 11th rib, another more lateral between the 9th and 10th ribs, and the third just below the 12th rib. This approach may be useful for bilateral disease as it avoids repositioning of the patient as well as avoiding complications related to trans-peritoneal access, yet the working space is tight and can make the operation more difficult especially for larger masses.

## Open Right Adrenalectomy—Anterior Approach

An open approach to the right adrenal gland is occasionally required to perform an adrenalectomy and can include an anterior trans-peritoneal approach, a retroperitoneal approach, flank approach, a posterior approach, or even a thoracoabdominal approach. When using an open technique, we prefer a transabdominal approach. This allows a thorough abdominal exploration and, because an en bloc resection may be required when performing an open adrenalectomy, the anterior, trans-peritoneal approach makes en bloc resection technically much easier than a retroperitoneal or posterior approach. We reserve a thoracoabdominal approach for very large tumors with major vascular involvement where access to the suprahepatic inferior vena cava may be necessary.

Under general endotracheal anesthesia the patient is placed supine with a roll under the right flank. An indwelling urinary catheter is placed to monitor urine output and an orogastric or nasogastric tube is used decompress the gastrointestinal tract. An anterior approach to the right adrenal gland can include a bilateral subcostal incision, a right subcostal incision, or a midline incision. We prefer a right subcostal incision. Upon entry into the abdomen, exploration is conducted. Similar to the laparoscopic approach, the triangular ligament of the right liver is divided to allow the liver to be retracted medially. The right colon is also reflect medially (which may require taking down the hepatic flexure in the case of larger tumors) to expose the duodenum which is then Kocherized to expose the right adrenal gland and IVC.

If the mass is large or there is a high suspicion for malignancy, the dissection is typically started on the medial portion to ensure that there is a plane between the neoplasm and the IVC. If a plane cannot be created, the surgeon must determine if the extent of invasion precludes resection. If an IVC resection is required and distal control of the IVC cannot be achieved below the liver then extension of the incision to the chest may be necessary to allow access to the suprahepatic IVC. If a free plane is present between the adrenal gland and the IVC, the right adrenal vein and any accessory branches can readily be identified and ligated. The remainder of the dissection is then carried medial to lateral to complete the adrenalectomy. Hemostasis is then ensured and the subcostal incision is closed in layers with absorbable suture including the posterior fascia, the anterior fascia, and skin.

## Open Right Adrenalectomy—Posterior Approach

For patients who have had extensive abdominal procedures who are not laparoscopic candidates and in whom an anterior approach would be difficult due to adhesions, a posterior approach is an option. However, a posterior approach should not be utilized for large tumors with local invasion. The posterior approach requires prone positioning of the patient under general endotracheal anesthesia. A Hugh–Young paraspinous incision is made to the right side of the midline from the 12th rib in a hockey-stick fashion carrying the curve towards the iliac crest (see Fig. 86-19). This approach requires removal of a portion of the 12th rib (and sometimes excision of the 11th rib) as well as division of the latissimus dorsi muscle to facilitate exposure. The pleura is then encountered and must be dissected away from the diaphragm. Care should be taken to not violate the pleura during this mobilization. After opening the diaphragm, the Gerota fascia is then divided to expose the right kidney and adrenal gland. The adrenal gland is then dissected free ligating the adrenal vein and arteries as described above. If the pleura had been violated, at the conclusion of the case the incision should be closed over a red rubber catheter placed into the pleural space and hooked to suction which is then removed quickly with the patient in Valsalva. The incision is closed in layers and a post-operative chest radiograph should routinely be obtained.

## Laparoscopic Left Adrenalectomy

For a laparoscopic left adrenalectomy the patient is placed in the right lateral decubitus position under general endotracheal anesthesia. As previously mentioned, an orogastric tube is placed along with an indwelling urinary catheter. The

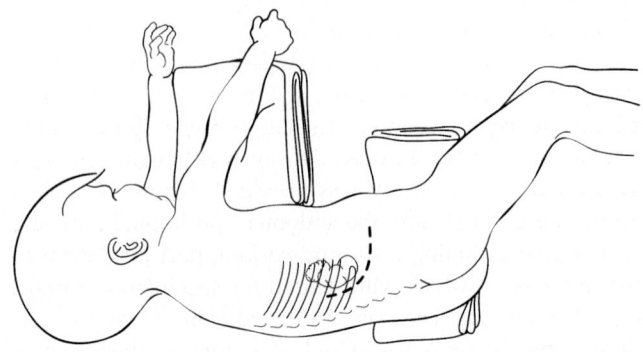

**FIGURE 86-19** Incision for posterior approach to right adrenalectomy.

surgeon operates form the patient's back, the assistant is at the patient's front, and the monitors are positioned towards the patient's head. With appropriate padding, straps, and flexion of the bed an initial 5-mm camera port is placed halfway between the anterior iliac spine and the umbilicus. We prefer an open technique versus the Veress needle for this initial trocar. The port sites are similar as for a laparoscopic right adrenalectomy; however, the medial most 5-mm port may not be necessary unless the spleen and pancreas need to be retracted medially for exposure. Rotating the patient face down will allow gravity to pull the spleen and pancreas medially—therefore it is critical to ensure the patient is adequately strapped to the table. A 10-mm working port is placed just lateral to the camera port, and a 5-mm working port is placed lateral to this in the posterior axillary line (see Fig. 86-20). Again, placement of the fourth trocar for retraction is at the surgeon's discretion.

The abdomen is initially explored and then a Harmonic scalpel is used to mobilize the left colon medially. This maneuver

may be necessary to create room for the lateral most trocar. Contrary to the right side, on the left side the left adrenal vein can be identified early on at the inferior-medial aspect of the adrenal gland which is ideal in the setting of a pheochromocytoma. Once the adrenal vein has been ligated, the remainder of the gland can be mobilized using the Harmonic scalpel including ligation of the arterial supply. The specimen is then removed via an EndoCatch bag and the incisions are closed as previously described. During dissection of the adrenal gland care must be taken to avoid injury to the pancreas. If a pancreatic injury occurs, a surgical drain should be left.

## Open Left Adrenalectomy— Anterior Approach

As mentioned previously, an open approach may be necessary for large tumors with local invasion, vascular involvement, suspicious lymph nodes, or adhesive disease where laparoscopy may not be feasible. Open approaches include an anterior trans-peritoneal approach, a retroperitoneal approach (through an anterior or flank incision), or a posterior approach. As for right adrenalectomies, when using an open technique for a left adrenalectomy, we prefer a transabdominal approach for the same reasons.

The patient is placed supine and under general endotracheal anesthesia a roll is positioned under the left side. An indwelling urinary catheter is placed and the gastrointestinal tract is decompressed with either an orogastric or nasogastric tube. Multiple incisions can be used including a bilateral subcostal, a left subcostal, or midline incision. We prefer a left subcostal incision. Upon entry to the abdomen manual exploration is undertaken. The splenic flexure is taken down and along with the spleen and tail of the pancreas is reflected medially. If an en bloc resection involving the spleen and/or pancreas is required, the gastrocolic ligament will need to be divided to allow access into the lesser sac for mobilization of these organs.

Reflection of the splenic flexure, pancreatic tail, and spleen will expose the Gerota fascia and the left kidney and adrenal gland (see Fig. 86-15). The retroperitoneal fat may make it difficult to readily identify the adrenal gland. The lateral and medial attachments should then be taken down with particular care at the inferomedial border of the adrenal gland where the left adrenal vein drains into the left renal vein (see Fig. 86-14B). Once identified this should be ligated. The left inferior phrenic vein drains into the left adrenal vein and may need to be divided as well. For hyperfunctioning neoplasms, particularly pheochromocytomas, the adrenal vein should be ligated first to avoid ongoing catecholamine release. While mobilizing the medial and lateral portions of the left adrenal gland the surgeon will encounter the arterial branches which should be ligated as well. At this point the posterior and superior attachments can be divided completing the adrenalectomy. After hemostasis has been ensured closure of the subcostal incision with absorbable suture should include 3 layers: the posterior fascia, the anterior fascia, and the skin.

## Open Left Adrenalectomy— Posterior Approach

For patients who have had extensive abdominal procedures who are not laparoscopic candidates and in whom an anterior

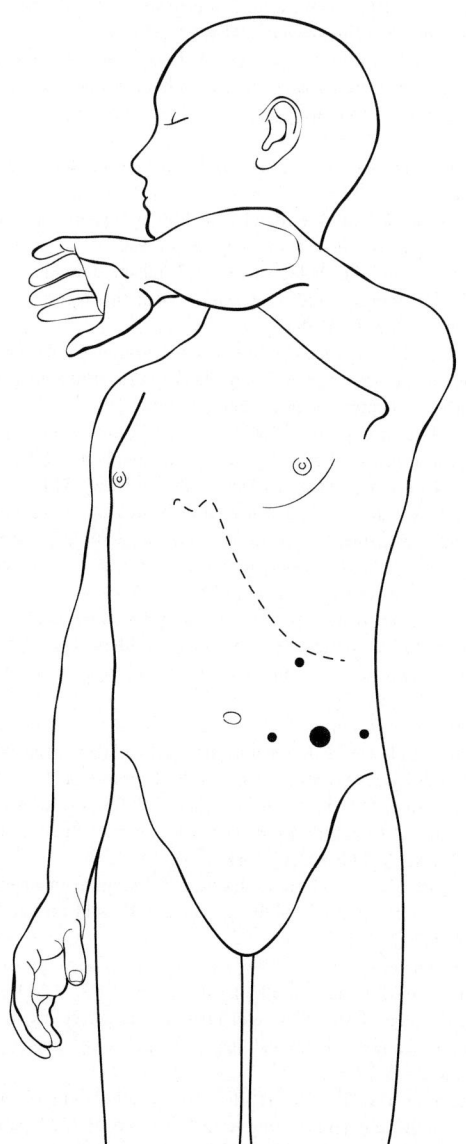

**FIGURE 86-20** Port placement for laparoscopic left adrenalectomy with the patient in the lateral decubitus position.

SURGICAL ENDOCRINOLOGY

approach would be difficult due to adhesions, a posterior approach is an option (exclusive of large tumors and/or local invasion). For a left adrenalectomy the posterior approach is performed in similar fashion as described above for the right adrenalectomy except that the incision will be to the left side of the midline. As for right adrenalectomies, a retroperitoneal approach either anterior or through a flank incision is rarely needed. We feel that the exposure is better through a trans-peritoneal approach for larger tumors with local invasion. Lesions that would be easily excised through a retroperitoneal approach are best approached laparoscopically.

## Bilateral Adrenalectomy

Patients with bilateral disease (most commonly bilateral adrenal hyperplasia) may require a bilateral adrenalectomy. We still favor a minimally invasive approach in this subset of patients. A lateral approach can be used, however, this requires that the patient be repositioned. As mentioned above, the posterior minimally invasive approach allows for a bilateral adrenalectomy to be performed without repositioning the patient, however, most surgeons are not familiar with this approach.

One alternative is to use a laparoscopic anterior approach with the patient in the supine position. A 10-mm camera port is placed in an open fashion at the umbilicus. A 5-mm port for retraction is placed sub xiphoid and 2 additional 5-mm working ports are placed subcostally (one at the anterior axillary line and the other at the mid-clavicular line) on the right and left hand side. The procedure is performed in a similar fashion to the lateral approach; however, further mobilization and retraction of the colon, liver, spleen, and pancreas are required to obtain adequate visualization of the operative field. It is helpful to have the patient securely strapped to the operating table to allow for right and left "air planing" of the bed to facilitate exposure. An additional 5-mm working port in the upper midline can also be useful to help retract the viscera medially.

If a minimally invasive approach cannot be offered, then an open approach should be utilized. Bilateral adrenalectomy can be performed through an anterior approach using either a bilateral subcostal incision or a midline celiotomy. A posterior approach for bilateral disease has also been advocated to avoid the potential complications from a trans-peritoneal approach although this requires 2 separate incisions.

## Postoperative Considerations

Hemorrhage is the most worrisome complication of adrenalectomy, particularly for right adrenalectomies where the dissection occurs along the IVC. The anterior approaches (either laparoscopic or open) lend themselves to the pitfalls of accessing the peritoneal cavity including adhesion formation, iatrogenic injuries to the viscera, and post-operative ileus. Most patients undergoing laparoscopic adrenalectomy have minimal pain and can be dismissed the following day. Patients having an open procedure require a longer hospitalization of 3 to 5 days for recovery. Patients having bilateral adrenalectomies must have appropriate hormone replacement to avoid an adrenal crisis.

## SELECTED READINGS

Caty MG, Coran AG, Gaegen M, et al. Current diagnosis and treatment of pheochromocytoma in children. Experience with 22 consecutive tumors in 14 patients. *Arch Surg* 1990;125:978–981.

Corrias S, Einaudi E, Chiorboli G, et al. Accuracy of fine needle aspiration biopsy of thyroid nodules in detecting malignancy in childhood: comparison with conventional clinical, laboratory, and imaging approaches. *J Clin Endocrinol Metab* 2001;86:4644–4648.

Cupisti K, Wolf A, Raffel A, et al. Long-term clinical and biochemical follow-up in medullary thyroid carcinoma: a single institution's experience over 20 years. *Ann Surg* 2007;246:815–821.

Grigsby PW, Gal-or A, Michalski JM, et al. Childhood and adolescent thyroid carcinoma. *Cancer* 2002;95:724–729.

Hanna AM, Pham TH, Askegard-Giesman JR, et al. Outcome of adrenocortical tumors in children. *J Pediatr Surg* 2008;43:843–849.

Harman CR, van Heerden J, Farley DR, et al. Sporadic primary hyperparathyroidism in young patients. *Arch Surg* 1999;134:651–656.

Harness JK, Thompson NW, McLeod MK, et al. Differentiated thyroid carcinoma in children and adolescents. *World J Surg* 1992;16:547–554.

Haveman JW, van Tol KM, Rouwe CW, et al. Surgical experience with differentiated thyroid carcinoma. *Ann Surg Onc* 2003;10:15–20.

Holcomb III GW. Laparoscopic adrenalectomy. In: Holcomb III GW, Georgeson KE, Rothenberg SS. *Atlas of Pediatric Laparoscopy and Thoracoscopy.* 1st ed. Philadelphia, PA: Elsevier Saunders; 2008:135–141.

Iqbal CW, Wahoff DC. Diagnosis and management of pediatric endocrine neoplasms. *Curr Opin Pediatr* 2009;21(3):379–385.

Jacobson SR, van Heerden J, Farley DR, et al. Focused cervical exploration for primary hyperparathyroidism without intraoperative parathyroid hormone monitoring or use of the gamma probe. *World J Surg* 2004;28:1127–1131.

Josefson J, Zimmerman D. Thyroid nodules in children. *Pediatr Endocrinol Rev.* 2008;6:14–23.

Kollars J, Zarroug AE, van Heerden J, et al. Primary hyperparathyroidism in pediatric patients. *Pediatrics* 2005;115:974–980.

Palmer BA, Zarroug AE, Poley RN, et al. Papillary thyroid carcinoma in children: risk factors and complications of disease recurrence. *J Pediatr Surg* 2005; 40:1284–1288.

Pham TH, Moir CR, Thompson GB, et al. Pheochromocytoma and paraganglioma in children: a review of medical and surgical management at a tertiary care center. *Pediatrics* 2006;118:1109–1117.

Powers PA, Dinauer CA, Tuttle RM, Francis GL. The MACIS score predicts the clinical course of papillary thyroid carcinoma in children and adolescents. *J Pediatr Endocrinol Metab* 2004;17(3):339–343.

Puligandla P. The Canadian Pediatric Thyroid Nodule Study: an evaluation of current management practices. *J Pediatr Surg* 2008;43:826–830.

Roman S, Mehta P, Sosa JA. Medullary thyroid cancer: early detection and novel treatments. *Curr Opin Oncol* 2008;21:5–10.

Saint-Vil D, Emran MA, Lambert R, et al. Cumulative doses of adjunct 131I treatment depend on location of residual thyroid tissue after total thyroidectomy in differentiated thyroid cancer. *J Pediatr Surg* 2007;42:853–856.

Seehofer D, Rayes N, Ulrich F, et al. Intraoperative measurement of intact parathyroid hormone in renal hyperparathyroidism by an inexpensive routine assay. *Langenbeck's Arch Surg* 2001;386:440–443.

Skinner MA, Safford SD. Endocrine disorders and tumors. In: Ashcraft KW, Holcomb III GW, Murphy JP. *Pediatric Surgery.* 4th ed. Philadelphia, PA: Elsevier Saunders: 2005;1088–1104.

Thompson GB, Hay ID. Current strategies for surgical management and adjuvant treatment of childhood papillary thyroid carcinoma. *World J Surg* 2004;28:1187–1198.

Turner MC, Lieberman E, DeQuattro V. The perioperative management of pheochromocytoma in children. *Clin Pediatr.* 1993; 31:583–589.

Van Wyk JJ, Ritzen EM. The role of bilateral adrenalectomy in the treatment of congenital adrenal hyperplasia. *J Clin Endocrinol Metab* 2003;88:2993–2998.

Zimmerman D, Hay ID, Gough IR, et al. Papillary thyroid carcinoma in children and adults: long-term follow-up of 1039 patients conservatively treated at one institution during three decades. *Surgery* 1988;104:1157–1166.

# PART X

# CHAPTER 87

*Rebecca J. McClaine and Daniel von Allmen*

## INTRODUCTION

Survival of pediatric malignancies has improved dramatically over the past half-century due to advances in the safety and efficacy of chemotherapeutic agents and radiation therapy. Additionally, although strategies to limit toxicity have likewise been developed, cancer therapy during childhood can be associated with lifelong morbidity. Chemotherapy and radiation serve as adjuncts to surgery in the treatment of neuroblastoma, the Wilms tumor, rhabdomyosarcoma, and hepatoblastoma; optimization of these regimens is the subject of ongoing clinical trials. A basic understanding of these topics is essential for all providers who care for the child with cancer.

## EPIDEMIOLOGY AND SURVIVAL STATISTICS FOR PEDIATRIC CANCERS

The incidence of cancer in children is relatively low, 133 cases per million children under age 15 years, compared with that of adults, 4620 cases per million, in the United States. The incidence bimodal, with an incidence rate of 200 cases per million in children age 2 years or younger, and a second peak during adolescence. Before age 2 years, central nervous system (CNS) malignancies, neuroblastoma, acute myeloid leukemia (AML), the Wilms tumor, and retinoblastoma account for the majority of diagnoses, while Hodgkin lymphoma, osteosarcoma, and the Ewing sarcoma become more prevalent during adolescence. Overall, the most common cancers in children under 15 years are acute lymphoblastic leukemia (ALL, 24.5% of cases), CNS tumors (20.2%), neuroblastoma (7.5%), and the Wilms tumor (6.1%) (Table 87-1). In contrast to adult tumors, less than 10% of pediatric cancers are epithelial in origin.

Despite the low incidence of cancer in children, cancer remains the leading cause of nonaccidental death among children less than 15 years, overall accounting for 10% of pediatric deaths. The cancer mortality rate among children decreased by about 40% between 1975 and 1995 largely due to improved survival from ALL (Table 87-2). The current 1-year and 5-year relative survival rates for all pediatric cancers are 90% and 71%, respectively (Fig. 87-1).

## CHEMOTHERAPY

The first successful treatment of a pediatric malignancy with chemotherapy was documented in 1948 by Sidney Farber, who utilized the folic acid antagonist aminopterin in children with ALL, leading to brief periods of remission. Since then, the development of additional therapeutic agents, the use of such agents in combination, the ongoing refinement of

| TABLE 87-1 | Distribution of Cancer Types in Children Less Than age 15 Years |
|---|---|
| **Type of Cancer** | **% of Total Cases** |
| Acute lymphoblastic leukemia | 24.5 |
| Central nervous system tumors | 20.2 |
| Neuroblastoma | 7.5 |
| The Wilms tumor | 6.1 |
| Hodgkin lymphoma | 4.4 |
| Non-Hodgkin lymphoma | 4.0 |
| Rhabdomyosarcoma | 3.4 |
| Acute myeloid leukemia | 3.2 |
| Retinoblastoma | 3.1 |
| Osteosarcoma | 2.4 |
| The Ewing sarcoma | 1.7 |
| Gonadal germ cell tumors | 1.7 |
| Fibrosarcoma | 1.7 |
| Thyroid cancer | 1.2 |
| Hepatoblastoma | 1.0 |

*Note:* Modified from Ries LAG, Percy CL, Bunin GR. Introduction. In: Ries LAG, Smith MA, Gurney JG, et al., eds. *Cancer Incidence and Survival among Children and Adolescents: United States SEER Program 1975-1995. NIH Pub. No. 99-4649.* Bethesda, MD: National Cancer Institute, SEER Program; 1999:2–3.

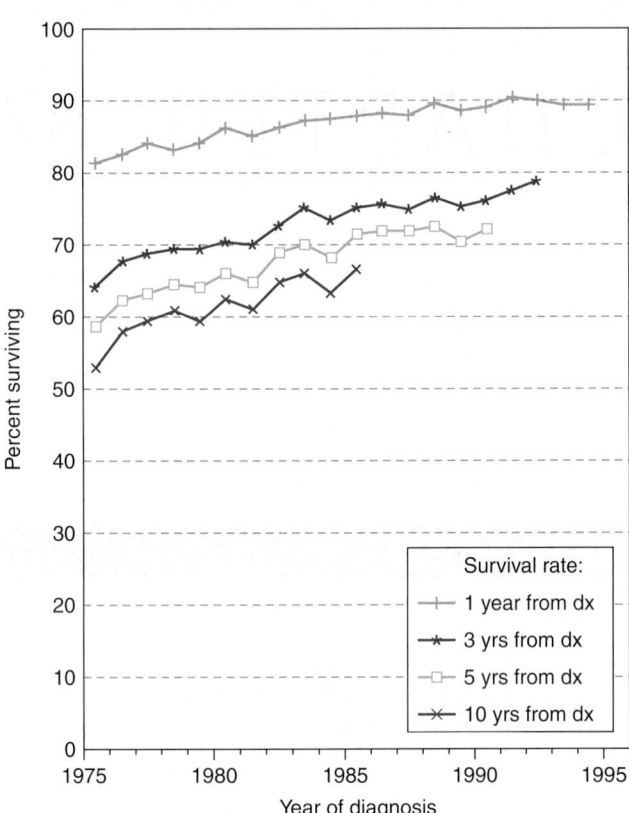

**FIGURE 87-1** Trends in relative survival rates for all pediatric cancers in children less than age 20 years, 1974 to 1995. Substantial increases in survival have been noted since the 1970s in all pediatric cancers. (Reproduced with permission from Ries LAG, Percy CL, Bunin GR. Introduction. In: Ries LAG, Smith MA, Gurney JG, et al., eds. *Cancer Incidence and Survival among Children and Adolescents: United States SEER Program 1975-1995. NIH Pub. No. 99-4649.* Bethesda, MD: National Cancer Institute, SEER Program; 1999:9.)

| TABLE 87-2 | Trends in Relative 5-Year Survival Rates for Cancer in Children Less than Age 15 Years | | | |
|---|---|---|---|---|
| | **Year of Diagnosis** | | | |
| **Type of Cancer** | 1960-1963 | 1970-1973 | 1980-1982 | 1986-1992 |
| All sites | 28 | 45 | 65 | 71 |
| Acute lymphoblastic leukemia | 4 | 34 | 70 | 79 |
| Central nervous system | 35 | 45 | 55 | 61 |
| Neuroblastoma | 25 | 40 | 53 | 63 |
| The Wilms tumor | 33 | 70 | 86 | 93 |
| Hodgkin lymphoma | 52 | 90 | 91 | 92 |
| Non-Hodgkin lymphoma | 18 | 26 | 62 | 71 |
| Soft tissue | 38 | 60 | 65 | 72 |
| Acute myeloid leukemia | 3 | 5 | 21 | 33 |
| Bone or joint | 20 | 30 | 54 | 65 |

*Note:* Modified from Parker SL, Tong T, Bolden S, et al. Cancer statistics, 1997. *CA Cancer J Clin* 1997;47:25.

treatment protocols, and the introduction of toxicity-limiting agents have been largely responsible for the increased pediatric cancer survival seen over the past 3 to 4 decades. Continued improvement in these areas, along with the expanded development and use of biologic chemotherapeutic agents, will likely result in future gains in pediatric cancer survival.

## Administration, Dosing, and Response

Children often tolerate chemotherapy better than adults, due to a more robust and rapid recovery from the toxic effects of treatment. In general, chemotherapy administration schedules are less frequently altered in children due to dose-limiting toxicities, compared to adults. These findings may explain the recent recognition that adolescents and young adults with pediatric cancers do better when treated in pediatric centers where they receive more aggressive pediatric dosing regimens than when treated at adult centers. Still, doses may be delayed or reduced due to hematologic toxicity (neutropenia with absolute neutrophil count <750 or 1000/mm³, or thrombocytopenia with platelet counts <75,000 to 100,000/μL), nephrotoxicity or hepatotoxicity based upon laboratory evaluation, or side effects such as mucositis or diarrhea.

Recent protocols in the treatment of pediatric cancers have focused on increasing chemotherapy dose intensity by increasing dose, frequency of administration, or both. The goal is to administer the highest dose that falls within the linear phase of the dose–response curve, in the shortest possible interval, while maintaining tolerable toxicity. Even small shortcomings in the delivery of maximal dose can have substantial clinical implications. In osteosarcoma, patients receiving less than 80% of the proposed chemotherapy had a threefold increased risk of relapse. Supportive therapy measures, such as granulocyte colony-stimulating factor (G-CSF) to counteract neutropenia or dexrazoxane to minimize cardiac toxicity, can facilitate achieving successful increases in dose intensity.

Response to chemotherapy is typically defined as a complete response (CR) when there is disappearance of all clinical, radiographic, and biochemical evidence of cancer, for 4 weeks. Partial response (PR) implies a >50% reduction in the sum of the areas of all lesions visible on cross-sectional imaging, lasting 4 weeks; stable disease represents <50% reduction or <25% growth of lesions measured in the same manner, for 8 weeks. Finally, progression is defined as >25% growth of the area of any 1 lesion. Typically, chemotherapy courses are prescribed for a set number of cycles, but radiographic evaluation of the disease may be scheduled after 2 to 3 cycles to evaluate response. If a PR has occurred, therapy is continued for the prescribed number of cycles, or for 2 cycles beyond a radiographic CR. Stable disease or progression necessitates re-evaluation and possible change of the prescribed therapy.

## Adjuvant versus Neoadjuvant Chemotherapy

Adjuvant therapy refers to the administration of chemotherapy following local treatment of a tumor with surgery or radiation, for the treatment of subclinical micrometastases. The use of adjuvant chemotherapy following tumor resection has been shown to improve survival in several adult and pediatric tumors, including osteosarcoma and advanced the Wilms tumor. The survival benefit of chemotherapy after surgical resection of nonmetastatic osteosarcoma was demonstrated in a randomized cooperative group trial; patients who received adjuvant chemotherapy had a 66% disease-free survival, as compared with a 17% disease-free survival in patients who received surgical intervention alone. The decision to employ such therapy after local control is based upon both tumor characteristics that predict the risk of metastasis. Most current regimens recommend that chemotherapy commence within 2 weeks of surgical resection.

In contrast to adjuvant chemotherapy administered after surgical resection, neoadjuvant therapy is given prior to the operation. This strategy may result in shrinkage of an initially unresectable tumor making a more complete resection possible. Reducing the size of the tumor may also result in a less morbid definitive operation.

Neoadjuvant administration also allows for assessment of tumor response to the chemotherapeutic agent. Further individualized therapy can then be guided by this information; osteosarcoma is often treated neoadjuvantly for this reason. Disadvantages to neoadjuvant chemotherapy include: (1) ineffective chemotherapy could allow the tumor to grow and become unresectable, and (2) response to the therapy could lead to tumor shrinkage or conversion of lymph nodes to negative, effectively downstaging the tumor and leading to eventual undertreatment.

## Chemotherapeutic Agents

Chemotherapy agents are divided into classes based upon their mechanism of action. Each class of agents targets malignant cells at different points within the cell cycle (Fig. 87-2). The most common agents, along with their mechanism of action, affected tumors, and side effects, are listed in Table 87-3.

### Alkylating Agents

Alkylating agents were the first modern chemotherapeutic agents used. These drugs are cytotoxic as a result of covalent bonding of an alkyl group (alkylation) to cellular DNA macromolecules, preventing DNA repair. During the cell cycle, this occurs predominantly in the G1–S transition; however, these agents are able to kill cells in any phase. Cyclophosphamide is a classic nitrogen-mustard derivative utilized in protocols for a number of pediatric cancers. The major dose-limiting toxicity of alkylating agents is myelosuppression; cyclophosphamide and ifosfamide are also associated with hemorrhagic cystitis, which can be prevented by treatment with mesna, a compound that binds toxic urinary metabolities.

### Platinum Agents

Cisplatin and carboplatin are heavy-metal compounds that bind DNA in a similar fashion to alkylation. Cisplatin, utilized routinely in the treatment of hepatoblastoma and many other tumors, can produce significant nephrotoxicity, ototoxicity, and neurotoxicity that can be cumulative and may not resolve with discontinuation. Carboplatin is associated with more profound myelosuppression, especially thrombocytopenia, and less neuro- and nephrotoxicity.

### Antimetabolites

Antimetabolites function as chemotherapeutic agents by becoming incorporated into DNA macromolecules, thus rendering the molecule defective. The maximal cytotoxic effect of the antimetabolites occurs in cells that are synthesizing DNA (S phase). Fluorouracil, a pyrimidine, has limited application in the pediatric population but is used in treatment of hepatoblastoma.

### Antibiotics

Antibiotics with antineoplastic activity have been isolated from a variety of microbial organisms. Anthracyclines, such as doxorubicin, inhibit topoisomerase II, thereby interfering with the winding and unwinding of the DNA molecule. In addition to inhibiting topoisomerase II, anthracyclines also intercalate between base pairs of DNA and create free radicals that damage DNA, and can work throughout the cell cycle in this manner. The most common and severe toxicity associated with these agents is cardiomyopathy, both acute and chronic.

Bleomycin, which is used commonly in the treatment of germ cell tumors, is associated with development of an interstitial pneumonitis that can lead to pulmonary fibrosis. Dactinomycin (actinomycin D) has a broad range of

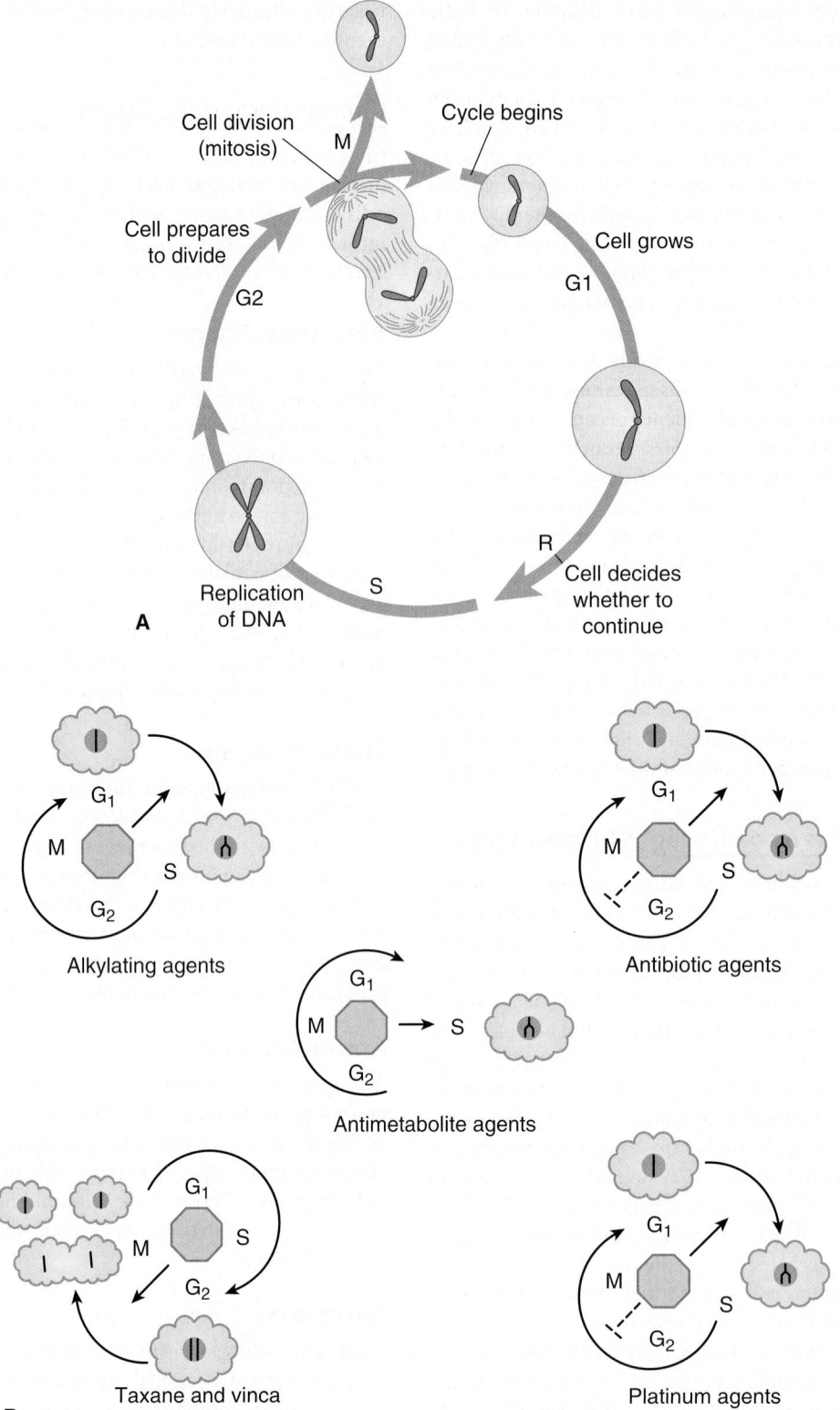

**FIGURE 87-2** **A.** Cell cycle. In G1, the cell grows and repairs DNA damage. If the cell is healthy and DNA has been repaired, the cell progresses through this checkpoint to synthetic (S) phase. In the S phase, the cell replicates its DNA. The cell prepares to divide in G2 phase, then divides during mitosis (M) phase. **B.** Activity of chemotherapy agents at points in the cell cycle. Alkylating agents facilitate transfer of alkyl groups to DNA, disrupting the G1/S transition. Antibiotic agents deregulate normal DNA and RNA processing, slowing progression through G1/S and G2/M transitions. Antimetabolites result in faulty base insertion into replicated DNA or specifically inhibit rate-limiting enzymes that are needed to produce deoxyribonucleotides for DNA replication during the S phase. Taxane and vinca alkaloid agents alter the mitotic spindle during mitosis, preventing cell division. Platinum agents work throughout the cycle, forming DNA structural adducts limiting progression at various cell-cycle checkpoints. (A: Reproduced with permission from The internet encyclopedia of science: Cell cycle. Available at: http://www. daviddarling.info/encyclopedia/C/cell_cycle.html. Accessed October 30, 2010; B: Reproduced with permission from Kunos C, Waggoner SE. Chapter 26—Principles of radiation therapy and chemotherapy in gynecologic cancer: basic principles, uses, and complications. In: Katz VL, Lobo RA, Lentz G, et al., eds. *Comprehensive Gynecology*. 5th ed. Philadelphia: Mosby Elsevier; 2007:723.)

| TABLE 87-3 | Chemotherapeutic Agents | | |
|---|---|---|---|
| **Class of Agent** | **Mechanism of Action** | **Therapeutic Uses** | **Acute Toxicities** |
| **Alkylating Agents** | | | |
| *Classic* | | | |
| Cyclophosphamide | DNA alkylation, crosslinking | ALL, CNS, Ewing, Hodg, NB, NHL, osteo, rhabdo, Wilms; HSCT | Alo, cystitis, myelo, n/v, infertility |
| Ifosfamide | DNA alkylation, crosslinking | Ewing, NB (rec), rhabdo (rec), Wilms (rec) | Alo, CNS, cystitis, hepatic, myelo, n/v, renal |
| Melphalan | DNA alkylation, crosslinking | Rhabdo; HSCT | Alo, diarrhea, mucositis, myelo, n/v |
| *Nitrosureas* | | | |
| Lomustine | DNA alkylation, crosslinking | CNS | Myelo, n/v, pulmonary fibrosis |
| *Other* | | | |
| Procarbazine | DNA methylation, free radical formation | CNS, Hodg | Infertility, myelo, n/v, rash, seizures |
| **Platinum Agents** | | | |
| Carboplatin | DNA/platinum adduct formation, DNA crosslinking | CNS, NB, rhabdo, Wilms | Myelo, n/v, ototoxicity, renal |
| Cisplatin | DNA/platinum adduct formation, DNA crosslinking | CNS, HB, NB, osteo | Alo, diarrhea, hepatic, mucositis, myelo, n/v, ototoxicity, peripheral neuropathy, renal |
| **Antimetabolites** | | | |
| Cytarabine | Pyrimidine analog | ALL, CNS | Diarrhea, hepatic, mucositis, myelo, n/v, renal |
| 5-Fluorouracil | Inhibitor of thymidine synthesis | HB | Dermatitis, diarrhea, mucositis, myelo |
| Mercaptopurine | Inhibitor of purine synthesis | ALL, CNS | Diarrhea, hepatic, mucositis, myelo, n/v, renal |
| Methotrexate | Inhibitor of dihydrofolate reductase | ALL, NHL, osteo | Diarrhea, hepatic, mucositis, myelo, n/v |
| **Antibiotics** | | | |
| *Anthracyclines* | | | |
| Daunorubicin | DNA intercalation, free radical formation, topoisomerase II inhibitor | AML | Alo, cardiac, diarrhea, hepatic, mucositis, myelo, n/v, vesicant |
| Doxorubicin | DNA intercalation, free radical formation, topoisomerase II inhibitor | Ewing, HB, Hodg, NB, NHL, osteo, Wilms | Alo, cardiac, diarrhea, hyperpigmentation, mucositis, myelo, n/v, vesicant |
| *Camptothecin derivatives* | | | |
| Irinotecan | Topoisomerase I inhibitor | Rhabdo (rec) | Alo, diarrhea, hepatic, mucositis, myelo, rash |
| Topotecan | Topoisomerase I inhibitor | NB, rhabdo (rec) | Alo, diarrhea, hepatic, mucositis, myelo |
| *Others* | | | |
| Bleomycin | DNA intercalation, free radical formation | Hodg | Fever, rash, mucositis, myelo, n/v, pulmonary fibrosis |
| Dactinomycin | DNA intercalation, free radical formation, topoisomerase II inhibitor | Rhabdo, Wilms | Alo, diarrhea, hepatic, hyperpigmentation, mucositis, myelo, n/v, vesicant |
| **Plant Alkaloids** | | | |
| *Vinca alkaloids* | | | |
| Vinblastine | Inhibitor of microtubule formation | Hodg | Myelo, vesicant |
| Vincristine | Inhibitor of microtubule formation | ALL, CNS, Ewing, HB, Hodg, NB, NHL, osteo, rhabdo, Wilms | Myelo, peripheral neuropathy, vesicant |
| *Epipodophyllotoxin* | | | |
| Etoposide | Topoisomerase II inhibitor | CNS, Ewing, NB, rhabdo (rec), Wilms; HSCT | Alo, diarrhea, hepatic, mucositis, myelo, n/v, peripheral neuropathy |

*Note:* ALL, acute lymphoblastic lymphoma; AML, acute myeloid leukemia; alo, alopecia; CNS, central nervous system tumors; HSCT, hematopoietic stem cell transplantation; HB, hepatoblastoma; Hodg, Hodgkin lymphoma; myelo, myelosuppression; n/v, nausea and vomiting; NB, neuroblastoma; NHL, Non-Hodgkin lymphoma; osteo, osteosarcoma; rec, recurrent; rhabdo, rhabdomyosarcoma.

clinical applications and was one of the first agents to demonstrate antitumor activity. It remains a cornerstone of adjuvant chemotherapy for both the Wilms tumor and rhabdomyosarcoma.

## Plant Alkyloids

Vincristine and vinblastine are similar alkaloids with a wide range of clinical activity in pediatric cancers. These vinca alkaloids disrupt microtubule formation, interfering mostly during the mitotic and G2 phases of the cell cycle. Neurotoxicity, specifically peripheral and autonomic neuropathy, is the dose-limiting toxicity of vincristine; while this usually resolves when therapy is ended, it can be permanent. The vinca alkaloids are among the more caustic agents when extravasation occurs.

Etoposide is a plant-derived agent that inhibits topoisomerase II activity; it functions similarly to the anthracycline antibiotics, in disrupting DNA unwinding, especially during the G2-S transition. This agent is included in regimens for many pediatric cancers, including neuroblastoma, the Wilms tumor, and recurrent rhabdomyosarcoma.

## Biologic Agents

Over the past 2 decades, basic science research has led to an explosion of information regarding genetic carcinogenesis, tumor development and sustainment, and the interaction of the immune system with malignant entities. As a result, a number of biologic chemotherapeutic agents have been developed to more specifically target cancer via these biologic mechanisms. These agents tend to fall into 1 of several broad categories. Inhibition of cellular signalling pathways interferes with normal cell function; Gefitinib and Avastin, which inhibit EGFR and VEGF, respectively, are examples. Intracellular signaling pathways, such as ras, p53, and Bcl-2, have also been targeted with specific inhibitors. Biologic response modifiers, such as tumor vaccines, bacterial component preparations, and cytokines, are utilized to enhance the patient's innate immune response to the tumor. Finally, monoclonal antibodies have been designed to target tumor-specific cell surface proteins; these antibodies can be derived from mice (murine), or designed as chimeric, containing both murine and human elements. Antibodies targeted to human T-cell cytokines, such as rituximab (chimeric anti-CD20) have been shown to improve survival in adult lymphoma patients.

Multiple biologic agents are currently undergoing phase I or II testing for pediatric cancers. To date, 2 such agents have demonstrated a survival advantage when added to traditional chemotherapeutic regimens.

The biologic response modifier muramyl tripeptide phosphatidylethanolamine (MTP-PE), a preparation of bacterial cell walls, has been associated with improved overall survival in children with nonmetastatic osteosarcoma. When combined with standard chemotherapy agents, MTP-PE has shown an increase in 6-year overall survival from 70 to 78%.

A recent trial published by Yu and the Children's Oncology Group has demonstrated increased disease-free and overall survival for children with high-risk neuroblastoma treated with a monoclonal antibody to the tumor-associated protein disialoganglioside GD2. The antibody was utilized in the maintenance phase of therapy, along with granulocyte-macrophage colony-stimulating factor (GM-CSF), interleukin (IL)-2, and isotretinoin, and compared to a control group treated with isotretinoin alone.

# RADIATION THERAPY

The use of radiation to treat cancer was first described by Roentgen more than 100 years ago. As in adult malignancies, the goal of radiation therapy in pediatric cancers is local tumor control, with minimal toxicity to surrounding normal tissues.

## Principles, Dosing, and Administration

Radiation therapy is the use of ionizing radiation to control malignant cells. Radiation kills cells by causing double-strand breaks in cellular DNA, both directly, by ionizing the atoms within cellular DNA, and, more importantly, by causing the production of reactive free radicals from cellular atoms that indirectly damage genetic material. After this damage has occurred, cell death occurs when intrinsic cellular DNA repair mechanisms fail, and the cell undergoes apoptosis, cell cycle arrest, or aberrant mitosis. Malignant cells are more sensitive to the effects of radation than normal tissue due to impaired DNA repair mechanisms in the tumor cells. Ionizing radiation initially results in sublethal damage to cells, with subsequent cell death occurring both acutely and in delayed fashion. Early-responding tissues are those with increased cell turnover; this includes malignant cells, but also includes skin, mucosa, and bone marrow. In contrast, late-responding tissues such as muscle and kidney are susceptible to damage from radiation, but this tends to occur in a more delayed fashion.

The dosing of radiation therapy is designed to maximize killing of malignant cells while preserving normal tissue. Fractionation of radiation doses refers to the technique of administering divided doses that are separated by periods of time. Fractionation allows time for both normal cells and tumor cells to repair cellular damage, limiting toxicity in normal tissues, but also allowing tumor cells to recover; fractionation strategies obviously must balance these factors. Typical schemes divide the total intended dose into weekday treatments, for a total time course of 6 weeks. Hyperfractionation schemes may employ twice-daily smaller fractions to further limit tumor cell recovery.

The total dose of radiation that can be administered to a tumor is limited by the toxicity imparted to surrounding normal tissues. Typically, toxic doses are those that have historically imparted late radiation effects (occurring 3 months or more after the conclusion of therapy) that progressed to permanent end-organ damage. For normal tissue, this dose depends upon the total dose of radiation and the volume of healthy tissue exposed; this volume is minimized with the use of techniques that more precisely deliver radiation to the tumor. The Gray (Gy) is the unit of absorbed dose; 1 Gy represents 1 joule/kg of water, and 1 Gy is equivalent to 100 centigray (cGy).

Several aspects of radiation therapy in pediatric patients deserve special consideration. Often children must be immobilized or sedated to safely deliver ionizing doses precisely to the desired treatment area. Also, because the tissues of pediatric patients are developing, subtherapeutic doses may be used, which may result in higher recurrence rates, but also ensure lower toxicity.

# HEMATOPOIETIC STEM CELL TRANSPLANTATION

Hematopoietic stem cell transplantation (HSCT), or bone marrow transplantation, is the process by which hematopoietic stem or progenitor cells are infused intravenously to restore hematopoiesis. For malignancy, this therapy is utilized following the administration of myeloablative therapy, consisting of chemotherapy, typically etoposide or cyclophosphamide, and/or total body irradiation, in doses of 8 to 14 Gy. The source of the cells can be the patient himself (autologous), or a human leukocyte antigen (HLA)-matched donor (allogenic).

Among pediatric malignancies, HSCT has demonstrated a survival benefit only in the treatment of high-risk neuroblastoma. In a randomized trial, children undergoing autologous HSCT following consolidation chemotherapy, compared with those receiving continued chemotherapy alone, demonstrated improved event-free survival.

# COMMON SHORT-TERM TOXICITIES AND SUPPORTIVE CARE

Most acute toxicities associated with childhood cancer therapy are reversible. Toxicity is greatest in normal cells with the highest rate of turnover, such as those found in bone marrow, skin, gastrointestinal tract mucosa, and hair follicles. Side effects can range from mild, such as alopecia, nausea, or oral mucositis, to life-threatening effects associated with specific regimens, like cardiotoxicity with anthracyclines or hemorrhagic cystitis with alkylating agents. Myelosuppressive effects, specifically neutropenia, often may be dose-limiting.

Alopecia is a side effect associated with many agents used in protocols for pediatric malignancies. Chemotherapeutic agents associated with alopecia include doxorubicin, daunorubicin, cyclophosphamide, etoposide, and ifosfamide. Alopecia typically occurs 2 to 3 weeks after the first treatment, occurs over 3 to 4 weeks, and lasts 3 to 5 months.

Nausea and vomiting are common side effects. The most highly-emetogenic agents include cisplatin, cyclophosphamide, cytarabine, and doxorubicin, with more effects seen with higher doses. 5-HT3 receptor antagonists, such as ondansetron, have been shown to both prevent and treat chemotherapy-associated nausea and vomiting; this effect is augmented by the concurrent use of steroids, such as dexamethasone. Oral mucositis, characterized by painful ulcerations of the oral mucosa, is another common side effect of both radiation and chemotherapy, specifically methotrexate, 5-FU, doxorubicin, cisplatin, cytarabine, etoposide, and irinotecan.

The use of anthracyclines is associated with both acute and long-term cardiac toxicity in the pediatric population. The anthracycline drug complexes with iron, leading to the formation of reactive oxygen species that target myocytes. Children treated at a young age and females are at higher risk for long-term complications. Children treated with anthracyclines should undergo echocardiography to assess cardiac function, both routinely and prior to administration of general anesthesia.

Myelosuppression is an expected side effect of almost every pediatric chemotherapeutic and radiotherapy regimen. Leukocyte and platelet nadirs typically occur at 7 to 10 days following therapy administration, and recover by 10 to 14 days. Chronic anemia is more common than acute and transfusions of packed red blood cells and platelets are common.

Neutropenia, along with the accompanying risk of severe bacterial or fungal infections, continues to represent a serious risk to life during cancer therapy. In dose-intensive regimens, more than 75% of chemotherapy courses result in hospitalization for fever, with a 10% to 20% incidence of bacteremia per course. Routine use of recombinated G-CSF (filgrastim) during the expected leukocyte nadir has been associated with more rapid granulocyte recovery and fewer hospitalizations for febrile neutropenia. Pegfilgrastim, a modified G-CSF, provides similar benefits with the advantage of one-time dosing. Febrile neutropenia is defined as absolute neutrophil count <500/mm$^3$ or <1000/mm$^3$ with anticipated 50% decrease, and fever >38.5 or >38.0 on 2 occasions.

# LONG-TERM SEQUELAE OF PEDIATRIC CANCER THERAPY

Because of the advances in cancer therapy over the past decades, the number of long-term survivors has increased exponentially. In the Childhood Cancer Survivor Study, pediatric cancer survivors and their siblings have been followed in retrospective cohort fashion and the adjusted relative risk of severe or life-threatening condition 20 to 36 years after diagnosis, compared to sibling controls, was 8.2 for survivors; the overall rate of severe condition or death at 30 years following diagnosis was 42%.

A number of CNS side effects have been reported following the use of cranial irradiation including global neurocognitive deficit and specific functional impairments or seizures secondary to leukoencephalopathy. More than 50% of childhood brain tumor patients treated with 30 Gy or more will have severe growth retardation. Radiation doses exceeding 12 Gy for whole-lung irradiation and 40 Gy for focal lung therapy have been associated with both acute pneumonitis and decreases in lung volumes. These affects are intensified with concomitant use of anthracyclines.

Although the incidence of severe or debilitating renal failure for survivors of childhood cancers is relatively low (0.5%), this represents a relative risk of 9 compared to sibling controls, 25 years after treatment. Both acute and chronic renal insufficiency is associated with cisplatin therapy, at doses >200 mg/m$^2$. Ifosfamide likewise is associated with proximal and distal tubular dysfunction in the acute setting, especially when utilized in combination with cisplatin, and in children under 5 years old.

Diminished fertility in both male and female pediatric cancer survivors is known to be associated with specific therapy protocols. In males, treatment with cyclophosphamide is associated with infertility. In girls, cyclophosphamide, procarbazine, and the alkylating agent busulfan are likewise associated with infertility and early menopause later in life.

The incidence of secondary neoplasm among survivors has been evaluated in a number of studies, and reported to be 2 to 10%, or 3 to 20 times relative risk, compared to age-matched controls. Friedman et al have reported data from the largest cohort study of pediatric cancer survivors, who are now a mean of 23 years out from cancer diagnosis. Increased risk of secondary cancer was seen with all primary cancer diagnoses, but was most marked for Hodgkin lymphoma (SIR 8.7) and the Ewing sarcoma (8.5).

## ADJUVANT THERAPY FOR SPECIFIC PEDIATRIC CANCERS

While surgical resection remains the mainstay in the treatment of most pediatric solid tumors, adjuvant therapy protocols have accounted for substantial improvements in survival. Staging and risk assessment models for these malignancies have also helped to limit toxicity for low-risk patients. The specifics of therapeutic regimens for various tumors are discussed in more detail in subsequent chapters but brief summaries are presented here.

## Neuroblastoma

Patients with low-risk neuroblastoma have a cure rate of 90% (Table 87-4). Almost all of these children can be treated with observation or surgical resection alone; even patients with incompletely resected tumors in this group demonstrate a survival rate of 95% without chemotherapy. However, children with intermediate-risk neuroblastoma typically undergo surgical resection and therapy with carboplatin, cyclophosphamide, doxorubicin, and etoposide. The duration of treatment is 12 and 24 weeks, respectively, for tumors with favorable and unfavorable biology.

High-risk neuroblastoma is treated aggressively with surgery, chemotherapy and radiation; however, only 30% to 40% of patients historically have survived long-term. The addition of HSCT and treatment with isotretinoin and anti GD-2 therapy in the setting of minimal residual disease has been associated with increases in survival.

## The Wilms Tumor

The Wilms tumor, or nephroblastoma, was the first reported solid pediatric tumor to respond to chemotherapy, and one of the first pediatric solid tumors treated with radiotherapy (Table 87-5). In the current treatment of the Wilms tumor, risk stratification based upon pathology and staging continue to guide treatment protocols with patients receiving surgery alone, surgery and chemotherapy, or surgery, chemotherapy, and radiation based on stage. In the United States, patients undergo biopsy or nephrectomy followed by adjuvant therapy, while in Europe surgery typically follows neoadjuvant therapy.

| TABLE 87-4 | Children's Oncology Group (COG) Neuroblastoma Risk-Assessment Schema | | | | |
|---|---|---|---|---|---|
| INSS Stage | Age | *MYCN* Status | INPC Classification | DNA Ploidy | Risk Group |
| 1 | 0-21 y | Any | Any | Any | Low |
| 2A/2B | <1 y | Any | Any | Any | Low |
| | 1-21 y | Nonamplified | Any | — | Low |
| | | Amplified | Favorable | — | Low |
| | | | Unfavorable | — | High |
| 3 | <1y | Nonamplified | Any | Any | Intermediate |
| | | Amplified | Any | Any | High |
| | 1-21 y | Nonamplified | Favorable | — | Intermediate |
| | | | Unfavorable | — | High |
| | | Amplified | Any | — | High |
| 4 | <18 m | Nonamplified | Any | Any | Intermediate |
| | <1 y | Amplified | Any | Any | High |
| | 18 m-21 y | Any | Any | — | High |
| 4S | <1 y | Nonamplified | Favorable | >1 | Low |
| | | | Unfavorable | Any | Intermediate |
| | | | Any | =1 | Intermediate |
| | | Amplified | Any | Any | High |

*Note:* Modified from Stage information—neuroblastoma treatment. National Cancer Institute, U.S. National Institutes of Health. Available at: http://www.cancer.gov/cancertopics/pdq/treatment/neuroblastoma/HealthProfessional/page3. Accessed October 30, 2010.

| TABLE 87-5 | Current Adjuvant Treatment Guidelines for the Wilms Tumor | | |
|---|---|---|---|
| Stage | Histology | Overall Survival | Treatment |
| Stage I | FH | 98% | OR, VinDac18 |
| | FA or DA | 83% | OR, VinDac 18, XRT |
| Stage II | FH | 96% | OR, VinDac18 |
| | FA | 80% | OR, abd XRT, VinDacDox24 |
| | DA | 82% | OR, abd XRT, VDCE24 |
| Stage III | FH | 95% | OR, abd XRT, VinDacDox24 |
| | FA | 71-100% | OR, abd XRT, VinDacDox24 **OR** |
| | | | VinDacDox24, OR, abd XRT |
| | DA | 53-67% | OR, abd XRT, VDCE24 **OR** |
| | | | VDCE24, OR, abd XRT |
| Stage IV | FH | 90% | OR, abd XRT[a], pulm XRT[b], VinDacDox24 |
| | FA | 72% | OR, abd XRT[a], pulm XRT[b], VinDacDox24 |
| | DA | 33-44% | OR, abd XRT[a], whole lung XRT, VDCE24 **OR** |
| | | | VDCE24, OR, abd XRT[a], whole lung XRT |
| Stage V | FH | 78% | B renal bx, VinDac18 **OR** |
| | | | VinDacDox24, 2nd look surgery, possible continued chemo/XRT |
| | AH | 55% | B renal bx, VDCE24, 2nd look surgery, possible continued chemo/XRT |

*Note:* AH, anaplastic histology; DA, diffuse anaplastic; FA, focal anaplastic; FH, favorable histology; OR, nephrectomy with lymph node sampling; VDCE24, vincristine/doxorubicin/cyclophosphamide/etoposide × 24 weeks; VinDac18, vincristine/dactinomycin × 18 weeks; VinDacDox24, vincristine/dactinomycin/doxorubicin × 24 weeks; XRT, radiation therapy.
[a]Possible, depending upon local stage of tumor.
[b]If CXR evidence of metastases.
Modified from Standard treatment options for Wilms tumor. National Cancer Institute, U.S. National Institutes of Health. Available at: http://www.cancer.gov/cancertopics/pdq/treatment/wilms/HealthProfessional/page5. Accessed October 30, 2010.

## Rhabdomyosarcoma

The prognosis of rhabdomyosarcoma diagnosed in childhood is substantially better than for adults, with 5-year overall survival rates of 61% versus 27%. The most common sites are the head, genitourinary tract, and extremities. Factors associated with good prognosis include younger age, favorable site, smaller tumor, complete resection, and embryonal histology. These factors are used to guide adjuvant therapy.

Current adjuvant treatment protocols for childhood rhabdomyosarcoma continue to focus on the use of chemotherapy in all patients for treatment of micro- or gross metastatic disease, and surgery and radiation for local control.

The lowest-risk patients achieve 90% survival with vincristine and dactinomycin alone. Cyclophosphamide is added to the drug regimen in low-risk patients, such as those in a favorable location with gross residual disease following resection, or resected tumors in an unfavorable location with lymph node spread or >5 cm in size. Radiation therapy at 41 Gy is administered to any patient with microscopically residual tumor.

The survival for intermediate-risk patients is 55% to 70%. The current recommended chemotherapy regimen consists of vincristine, dactinomycin, and high-dose cyclophosphamide. All children with alveolar histology, regardless of completeness of resection, undergo radiation therapy, with total treatment dose of 41 Gy. Because children with grossly positive margins following resection are most likely to recur locally, aggressive radiation is utilized (50 Gy).

High-risk patients are those with distant metastases at diagnosis; 5-year survival rate is around 50%. Current treatment regimens are identical to those for intermediate-risk patients.

Recurrent rhabdomyosarcoma in children carries a relatively poor prognosis. High-dose chemotherapy with HCST has been attempted in this population, with no reported survival benefit.

## Hepatoblastoma

Hepatoblastoma represents the majority of liver tumors in children, and 90% of those diagnosed in children aged 4 years or younger. Cure is possible only with complete surgical excision of the primary tumor. Patients with very low-risk hepatoblastoma, those with stage I disease with pure fetal histology, may be treated by surgical resection alone, or with doxorubicin following surgery. All other stage I or II cancers are currently treated with 4 total courses of cisplatin/doxorubicin or cisplatin/vincristine/fluorouracil. Stage III tumors universally undergo neoadjuvant chemotherapy with the above agents, followed by resection (for responsive tumors) or evaluation for liver transplantation (for tumors that have not responded favorably). Children with stage IV tumors are treated neoadjuvantly with one of the same chemotherapeutic regimens, and response of the primary and metastatic lesions assessed.

## Other Pediatric Malignancies

The survival of children with osteosarcoma has been shown to be improved substantially with the use of neoadjuvant or adjuvant chemotherapy with resection, compared to resection alone. Typical adjuvant chemotherapy regimens consist of high-dose methotrexate, cisplatin, and doxorubicin, or cisplatin, doxorubicin, cyclophosphamide, and vincristine. At diagnosis, 20% of tumors have already metastasized to the lung, and the lung is the most common site of recurrence. Because resection of all disease remains the only option for cure of osteosarcoma, lung metastases should be resected when possible.

In patients with the Ewing sarcoma, the incidence of occult micrometastatic disease is high. Therapy regimens typically begin with neoadjuvant chemotherapy, consisting of vincristine, doxorubicin, and cyclophosphamide alternating with ifosfamide and etoposide. Local control is then achieved with either surgery or radiation, with doses of approximately 56 Gy; surgical resection has never been shown to be superior to radiation in improving recurrence-free survival. Radiotherapy may also be utilized in treating metastatic or recurrent lesions. Pulmonary lesions or metastases are typically treated with whole-lung irradiation followed by resection of residual tumor.

## CONCLUSION

Although survival of pediatric malignancies has improved substantially over the past 40 years, several aspects of pediatric oncology continue to present challenges. Future research will undoubtedly continue to evaluate the role of reducing therapy in low-risk patients to prevent long-term morbidity, develop biologic agents as adjuncts to current standard chemotherapy regimens for high-risk and recurrent tumors, and expand upon methods of radiation delivery to minimize damage to healthy tissue. While surgery will always play a vital role in the treatment of pediatric cancer, these and other advances in adjuvant therapies will dramatically improve outcomes in the decades to come.

## SELECTED READINGS

Ammann RA, Bodmer N, Hirt A, et al. Predicting adverse events in children with fever and chemotherapy-induced neutropenia: the prospective multicenter SPOG 2003 FN study. *J Clin Oncol* 2010;28:2008–2014.

Barrett D, Fish JD, Grupp SA. Autologous and allogeneic cellular therapies for high-risk pediatric solid tumors. *Pediatr Clin N Am* 2010;57:47–66.

Bhatia M, Davenport V, Cairo MS. The role of interleukin-11 to prevent chemotherapy-induced thrombocytopenia in patients with solid tumors, lymphoma, acute myeloid leukemia and bone marrow failure syndromes. *Leukemia Lymphoma* 2007;48:9–15.

Cetingul N, Midyat L, Kantar M, et al. Cytoprotective effects of amifostine in the treatment of childhood malignancies. *Pediatr Blood Cancer* 2009;52:829–833.

Fox E, Widemann BC, Hawkins DS, et al. Randomized trial and pharmacokinetic study of pegfilgrastim versus filgrastim after dose-intensive chemotherapy in young adults and children with sarcomas. *Clin Cancer Res* 2009;15:7361–7367.

Friedman DL, Whitton J, Leisenring W, et al. Subsequent neoplasms in 5-year survivors of childhood cancer: the childhood cancer survivor study. *J Natl Cancer Inst* 2010;102:1083–1095.

Haas-Kogan DA, Fisch BM, Wara WM, et al. Intraoperative radiation therapy for high-risk pediatric neuroblastoma. *Int J Radiat Oncol Biol Phys* 2000;47:985–992.

Kayton ML, Delgado R, Busam K, et al. Experience with 31 sentinel lymph node biopsies for sarcomas and carcinomas in pediatric patients. *Cancer* 2008;112:2052–2059.

Kuhn A, Porto FA, Miraglia P, Brunetto AL. Low-level infrared laser therapy in chemotherapy-induced oral mucositis: a randomized placebo-controlled trial in children. *J Pediatr Hematol Oncol* 2009;31:33–37.

Link MP, Goorin AM, Miser AW, et al. The effect of adjuvant chemotherapy on relapse-free survival in patients with osteosarcoma of the extremity. *N Engl J Med* 1986;314:1600–1606.

Lipshultz SE, Scully RE, Lipsitz SR, et al. Assessment of dexrazoxane as a cardioprotectant in doxorubicin-treated children with high-risk acute lymphoblastic leukemia: long-term follow-up of a prospective, randomized, multicentre trial. *Lancet Oncol* 2010;11:950–961.

Malogolowkin MH, Stanley P, Steele DA, Ortega JA. Feasibility and toxicity of chemoembolization for children with liver tumors. *J Clin Oncol* 2000;18:1279–1284.

Matthay KK, Reynolds CP, Seeger RC, et al. Long-term results for children with high-risk neuroblastoma treated on a randomized trial of myeloablative therapy followed by 13-*cis*-reinoic acid: a children's oncology group study. *J Clin Oncol* 2009;27:1007–1013.

Meyers PA, Schwartz CL, Krailo MD, et al. Osteosarcoma: the addition of muramyl tripeptide to chemotherapy improves overall survival—a report from the Children's Oncology Group. *J Clin Oncol* 2008; 26:633–638.

Nag S, Martinez-Monge R, Ruyman F, et al. Innovation in the management of soft tissue sarcomas in infants and young children: high dose brachytherapy. *J Clin Oncol* 1997;15:3075–3084.

Nakamura L, Ritchey M. Current management of Wilms' tumor. *Curr Urol Rep.* 2010;11:58–65.

Oeffinger KC, Mertens AC, Sklar CA, et al. Chronic health conditions in adult survivors of childhood cancer. *N Engl J Med* 2006;355:1572–1582.

Park JR, Eggert A, Caron H. Neuroblastoma: biology, prognosis, and treatment. *Hematol Oncol Clin N Am.* 2010; 24:65–86.

Parker SL, Tong T, Bolden S, et al. Cancer statistics, 1997. *CA Cancer J Clin* 1997;47:5–27.

Perilongo G, Maibach R, Shafford E, et al. Cisplatin versus cisplatin plus doxorubicin for standard-risk hepatoblastoma. *N Engl J Med* 2009; 361:1662–1670.

Ries LAG, Percy CL, Bunin GR. Introduction. In: Ries LAG, Smith MA, Gurney JG, et al., eds. *Cancer Incidence and Survival among Children and Adolescents: United States SEER Program 1975-1995. NIH Pub. No. 99-4649.* Bethesda, MD: National Cancer Institute, SEER Program; 1999:1–16.

Sredni ST, Gadd S, Huang CC, et al. Subsets of very low risk Wilms tumor show distinctive gene expression, histologic, and clinical features. *Clin Cancer Res* 2009;15:6800–6809.

Wharam MD, Meza J, Anderson J, et al. Failure pattern and factors predictive of local failure in rhabdomyosarcoma: a report of Group III patients on the Third Intergroup Rhabdomyosarcoma Study. *J Clin Oncol* 2004;22:1902–1908.

Yu AL, Gilman AL, Ozkaynak F, et al. Anti-GD2 antibody with GM-CSF, interleukin-2, and isotretinoin for neuroblastoma. *N Engl J Med* 2010;363:1324–1334.

# CHAPTER 88

# Nephroblastoma (Wilms Tumor)

*Andrew M. Davidoff*

## KEY POINTS

1. Wilms tumor is the second most common abdominal tumor in children and accounts for 95% of the renal tumors in children.

2. The overall survival for all patients with Wilms tumor is >90%.

3. For unilateral tumors, upfront resection with lymph node biopsy is the current recommendation from the Children's Oncology Group.

4. Children with bilateral renal masses require no biopsy; they are begun on 3-drug chemotherapy for 6 to 12 weeks prior to local control with nephron-sparing surgery.

5. Patients are treated on risk-based protocols with molecular risk factors being integrated into the assessment that includes stage and histology.

## PATHOPHYSIOLOGY

### Epidemiology

Wilms tumor is the second most common intra-abdominal cancer of childhood and the fifth most common pediatric malignancy overall. It represents approximately 6% of all pediatric cancers and accounts for more than 95% of all tumors of the kidney in the pediatric age group. In the United States, there is an annual incidence of 8 cases per million children younger than 15 years of age, with the total incidence estimated at about 500 cases per year. Approximately 75% of the cases occur in children younger than 5 years of age, with a peak incidence at 2 to 3 years of age. Because of the rarity of this tumor, clinical investigation conducted in an organized manner was begun in 1969 through the establishment of the National Wilms Tumor Study Group (NWTSG). This represented a cooperative effort among several groups to treat patients in a clearly defined manner so that statistically relevant comparisons of treatment variations could be made. Due, in large part to this effort, survival for patients with Wilms tumor, when considered as a whole, once less than 30%, is currently greater than 90%. In 2001, the NWTSG was incorporated into the larger Children's Oncology Group (COG).

### Pathology

Classic Wilms tumor has a triphasic appearance, with the 3 cell types being stromal, epithelial, and blastemal. All 3 elements are not required, however, to have a diagnosis of Wilms tumor. The neoplastic cells can often be seen to be forming primitive tubules and glomeruli. One of the major contributions of the NWTS was a report by Beckwith and Palmer that separated Wilms tumors into distinct histopathologic categories based on prognosis. An analysis of 427 specimens found that 11% of the total patients in this study contributed to 52% of the mortality. Since that study, Wilms tumors have been classified into favorable and unfavorable histologic groups. The unfavorable histologic group includes Wilms tumors with anaplasia and 2 distinct renal tumors: clear-cell sarcoma of the kidney (CCSK) and malignant rhabdoid tumor of the kidney. Anaplasia can be focal or diffuse in nature, with the focal subtype being somewhat more favorable, and is characterized by cells with large, polyploid nuclei and multipolar mitotic figures. Anaplasia was present in 4.5% of cases entered on NWTS-III and is more common in older children, reaching a peak at approximately 5 years of age. This histopathologic variant is also more frequent in African American patients than in white patients.

CCSK and rhabdoid tumors of the kidney are now considered separate entities rather than variants of Wilms tumor, but these 2 histologies continue to be registered on therapeutic COG protocols. The CCSK (bone-metastasizing renal tumor of childhood) is associated with a very high rate of skeletal metastases, but its site of origin and age distribution are identical to favorable histology Wilms tumor. These tumors are associated with a very high rate of tumor relapse, which suggests that micrometastases occur in the early stages of tumor growth. Rhabdoid tumor of the kidney was seen in 2% of NWTS-III patients and presents earlier with a median patient age of 13 months at diagnosis. In addition to its early age of presentation, many cases are also associated with an apparently separate primary neuroectodermal tumor of the brain. These tumors are very aggressive and are associated with a mortality of approximately 90%, even in patients with early stage tumors.

| TABLE 88-1 | Syndromes Related to the WT1 and WT2 Loci | | |
|---|---|---|---|
| **Syndrome** | **Locus** | **Genetic Lesion** | **Phenotype** |
| WAGR | 11p13 | Deletion *WT1* gene | Aniridia, genitourinary anomalies, delayed-onset renal failure |
| Denys–Drash | 11p13 | Point mutation in zinc-finger regions of *WT1* gene | Ambiguous genitalia, diffuse mesangial sclerosis |
| Beckwith–Wiedemann | 11p15 | Precise genetic lesion unclear; loss of imprinting of several genes including IGF2, H19, and $p57^{kip2}$ implicated | Organomegaly, large birth weight, macroglossia, omphalocele, hemihypertrophy, ear pits and creases, neonatal hypoglycemia |

## Molecular Biology

Childhood tumors, including Wilms tumor, have long been favorite models for study to investigate the molecular events of carcinogenesis because the early age of onset suggests that only a few events are required to establish a neoplastic phenotype. As with many cancer genes, the first clue to the location of a Wilms tumor gene came from the cytogenetic analysis of DNA from patients with Wilms tumor in whom there were commonly associated, genetically determined anomalies (Table 88-1). Because of the association of seemingly unrelated phenotypic abnormalities, a large chromosomal disruption would be predicted. This strategy revealed a constitutional deletion of band 13 of the short arm of chromosome 11 in patients with the rare congenital WAGR syndrome. Patients with this syndrome have aniridia, genitourinary malformations, and mental retardation as well as Wilms tumor. The fact that loss of expression of this gene appeared to lead to the activation of its oncogenic potential suggested that this Wilms tumor gene was a "tumor-suppressor" gene. Candidate genes were sought from the minimum deletion region of chromosome 11 p13 and, ultimately, the *WT1* gene was isolated and cloned. Sequence analysis suggests that *WT1* is a transcriptional regulator whose protein product binds to specific DNA motifs. Although the exact function of the WT1 protein has not been clearly defined, the pattern of WT1 expression suggests that it has a role in metanephric stem cell differentiation. This may explain the finding of associated genitourinary abnormalities. In patients with isolated Wilms tumor, however, evidence for WT1 mutation exists in only about 5% to 10% of the cases.

Another syndrome associated with constitutional abnormalities of the WT1 gene is the Denys–Drash syndrome. In this syndrome, patients have severe genitourinary abnormalities (eg, male pseudohermaphroditism) and renal failure secondary to progressive, diffuse glomerular nephropathy. Fifty percent to 90% of these patients will develop Wilms tumor. The alteration of the *WT1* gene in patients with this syndrome appears to be a missense mutation within the DNA-binding region of this transcription factor.

The Beckwith–Weidmann syndrome (BWS) is another syndrome of which Wilms tumor is a common component. This syndrome consists of a number of abnormalities, including macroglossia, macrosomia, hypoglycemia, visceromegally, and omphalocele, in addition to a predisposition to a number of tumors, most commonly Wilms tumor. The locus for BWS seems also to be located on the short-arm of chromosome 11 but at a site distinct from WT1, that being 11p15, as

identified by large karyotypic abnormalities and linkage analysis of BWS families. In sporadic Wilms tumor, there appears to be a small percentage of patients with loss of 1 copy of genetic material in the 11p15 region. Nearly always, there has been a loss of the maternal allele, suggesting that genetic imprinting occurs at this locus. In rare patients, uniparental paternal disomy has occurred whereby there is inheritance of 2 paternal copies of this region. Several genes have been identified within the 11p15 region, which demonstrates genomic imprinting; alterations of one of these may be responsible for the development of BWS.

Familial Wilms tumor occurs at an incidence of approximately 5%. Linkage analysis shows however, that the locus for this predisposition is not WT1 or WT2, suggesting that there are other loci involved in the genesis or predisposition for Wilms tumor. An additional Wilms tumor locus at 16q was suggested by loss of heterozygosity (LOH) (loss of 1 of 2 copies of a chromosomal region) for chromosome 16q markers in about 20% of Wilms tumors. LOH at a locus mapping to the distal chromosome 1p has also been found in a small group of patients with Wilms tumor (~12%) and at 11p in 33% of Wilms tumor patients. Patients with LOH for chromosome 16q have relapse rates 3.3 times higher and a mortality rate 12 times higher than patients without LOH for chromosome 16q, suggesting that a gene within this site may be involved in disease progression to a more malignant phenotype.

Another gene that seems to have some prognostic importance when activated in Wilms tumors is p53. The *p53* gene encodes a protein which, among many functions, appears to play a role in cell-cycle arrest in cases in which DNA damage has occurred. When the damage cannot be corrected, p53 induces the cell to apoptose. Although p53 alterations are the most common genetic abnormality detected in adult tumors, they are rare in pediatric malignancies, including Wilms tumor. However, there is a high incidence of *p53* gene mutation in the anaplastic histologic subtype of Wilms tumor. This may explain why these tumors do not respond well to chemotherapy, as their p53-dependent apoptotic pathway may have become inactivated.

Determining additional prognostic factors will be important so that refinements in Wilms tumor therapy can continue. Further genetic studies may identify those patients at high risk for relapse so that intensification of therapy can be instituted in this select group of patients. Similarly, genetic characterization of patients with Wilms tumor will likely lead to the identification of subgroups of patients with a more favorable prognosis who can be managed according to a minimal therapeutic regimen.

## DIAGNOSIS

### Presentation

Children with Wilms tumor typically present with an asymptomatic abdominal mass. It is not uncommon for the tumor to be discovered by a parent while bathing the child, or by a relative who notices a protuberant abdomen. Associated signs and symptoms such as malaise, pain, and either microscopic or gross hematuria are found in approximately 20% to 30% of the children. Hypertension, presumably because of increased renin activity, is present in approximately 25% of children with Wilms tumor. Occasionally, a child will present with a rapidly enlarging abdominal mass, anemia, hypertension, pain, and fever. These children usually have a subcapsular hemorrhage within the tumor that leads to these symptoms.

The main differential diagnosis is often between a Wilms tumor and neuroblastoma. Usually this distinction is relatively easy because a Wilms tumor is intrarenal with a characteristic intrinsic abnormality of the urinary collecting system. Neuroblastomas arise within the adrenal gland or the paravertebral sympathetic ganglia and these masses displace rather than distort the kidney. Benign conditions such as multicystic kidneys and obstructive uropathy should be considered in the differential diagnosis of an abdominal mass in a child. Wilms tumor presenting as an abdominal mass on the left side must be distinguished from an enlarged spleen. Tumors that cross the midline are more likely to be neuroblastoma, although very large Wilms tumors can present as midline abdominal masses. The physical examination should include inspection for hemihypertrophy, aniridia, or findings associated with Beckwith–Wiedemann syndrome. The presence of bone pain suggests a neuroblastoma, but bony metastases are seen in children with CCSK tumors. Neurologic changes suggesting brain metastases are rare in children with Wilms tumor but can be seen in infants with rhabdoid tumors or CCSK.

### Evaluation

The work-up of a child with an intraabdominal mass suspected of being a Wilms tumor should proceed in a systematic fashion. Real-time ultrasonography is usually the initial study and can determine whether or not the mass is intrarenal or extrarenal, and also whether the lesion is cystic or solid. Computed tomography (CT) of the abdomen and pelvis is generally the imaging study of choice for those patients suspected of having a renal tumor. This will confirm the presence of a solid renal mass and will also afford the opportunity to visualize the contralateral kidney to confirm its presence (and function), and to exclude synchronous bilateral disease with a high degree of sensitivity.

Intravascular tumor extension into the inferior vena cava occurs in about 6% of Wilms tumor cases. Therefore, this should be specifically investigated in the preoperative evaluation of all children with a renal mass, as it may alter the conduct of surgery. This can generally be done most easily and accurately with Doppler ultrasonography. Magnetic resonance imaging (MRI) can also be used to assess intravascular tumor extension but usually requires sedation in young children, and so is not routinely used. However, it may be helpful

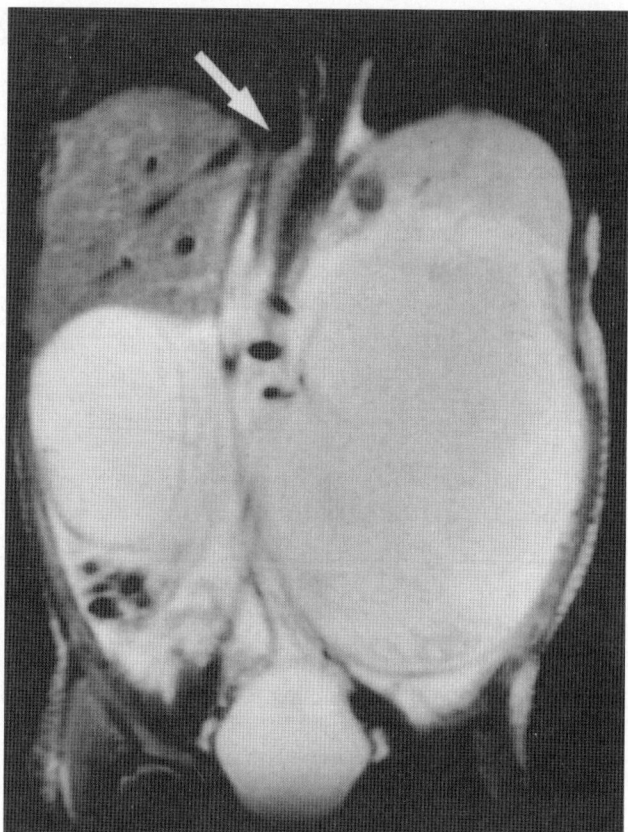

**FIGURE 88-1** An MRI scan demonstrating intra-atrial extension of tumor thrombus.

in defining an extensive tumor thrombus that extends up to the level of the hepatic veins or even into the right atrium (Fig. 88-1). In addition, MRI may be useful in distinguishing Wilms tumor from nephrogenic rests (see below). Finally, echocardiography may be useful in rare circumstances to demonstrate (or exclude) intracardiac tumor extension.

The most common site of metastatic spread of Wilms tumor is the lungs; chest CT is the preferred imaging modality for evaluating this site. Other rare sites of metastases, such as the liver, are usually well evaluated with the initial abdominopelvic CT scan.

Once the histology of the tumor has been determined following resection or, rarely biopsy, a postoperative MRI of the brain should be performed in children with rhabdoid tumor and CCSK and a skeletal survey or bone scan should be carried out in patients with CCSK. In the absence of specific symptoms, these studies should not be performed preoperatively because of the rarity of these histologies.

### Staging

Accurate staging of patients with Wilms tumor is imperative and the staging system developed by the NWTS and currently in use in the COG is a surgicopathologic staging system (Table 88-2). Because appropriate therapy, as well as prognosis, is based on tumor stage, accurate staging of patients with Wilms tumor at the time of diagnosis is imperative. At the time of surgery, a thorough abdominal exploration should be carried out because the presence of disease beyond the

| TABLE 88-2 | Wilms Tumor Staging System |
|---|---|

I   Tumor limited to kidney and completely excised. The surface of the renal capsule is intact. Tumor was not ruptured before or during removal. There is no residual tumor apparent beyond the margins of excision

II   Tumor extends beyond the kidney, but is completely excised. There is regional extension of the tumor; ie, penetration through the outer surface of the renal capsule into perirenal soft tissues. Vessels outside the kidney substance are infiltrated or contain tumor thrombus. There is no residual tumor apparent at or beyond the margins of excision

III   Residual nonhematogenous tumor confined to abdomen. Any one or more of the following occur:

    1. Lymph nodes on biopsy are found to be involved in the hilus, the periaortic chains, or beyond

    2. There has been peritoneal contamination by tumor such as by biopsy or rupture of the tumor before or during surgery, or by tumor growth that has penetrated through the peritoneal surface

    3. Implants are found on the peritoneal surfaces

    4. The tumor extends beyond the surgical margins either microscopically or grossly

    5. The tumor is not completely resectable because of local infiltration into vital structures

IV   Hematogenous metastases. Deposits beyond Stage III; ie, lung, liver, bone, and brain

V   Bilateral renal involvement at diagnosis. An attempt should be made to stage each side according to the above criteria on the basis of extent of disease prior to biopsy

kidney will significantly affect therapy and prognosis. Careful regional lymph node sampling is important because the presence of nodal involvement is associated with an increased incidence of tumor relapse and a poorer prognosis.

## TREATMENT

### Surgery

The role played by the surgeon in the therapy of Wilms tumor is paramount because a meticulous and well-performed procedure will accurately determine the stage of the tumor and the patient's future therapy. A poorly performed procedure can lead to inadequate therapy if patients are not appropriately staged, or to unnecessarily intensive therapy if operative spill of the tumor occurs or if incomplete resection of the primary tumor is carried out. The main responsibility of the surgeon is to remove the primary tumor completely, without spillage, and to accurately assess the extent to which the tumor has spread.

### Preoperative Planning

Approximately 25% of children with Wilms tumor will present with hypertension. Therefore, a preoperative assessment of blood pressure should be performed in all patients, with hypertension being medically controlled prior to surgery. In many patients, but not all, the hypertension will resolve after radical nephrectomy, although it may take some time. Patients with Wilms tumor rarely present with renal insufficiency and so formal preoperative assessment of renal function is usually not required. Although patients with a Wilms tumor-predisposition syndrome may have intrinsic renal disease, it is usually not of clinical significance until a few years later. Appropriate genetic testing may be done, as indicated. Children with Wilms tumor will occasionally present with pulmonary insufficiency due to extensive metastatic disease in the lungs. The clinical assessment of a patient is generally sufficient to determine whether they can tolerate general anesthesia; formal pulmonary function studies are not required. As Wilms tumor is generally very chemosensitive, the tumor burden in the lungs and the functional pulmonary status should improve fairly promptly once chemotherapy has been initiated.

Preoperative, as well as intraoperative, biopsies are generally contraindicated and should only be performed when a tumor is deemed inoperable, or the patient is unable to tolerate a laparotomy. Therefore, if a solid renal mass is unilateral, it should simply be resected (along with the kidney). Wilms tumor can often grow to a very large size prior to detection. However, even large tumors rarely invade surrounding structures, they simply push them away (and may efface them). Because of this, most Wilms tumors are resectable at presentation. A tumor that is completely resected may be a stage I or II tumor and therefore the patient will not require doxorubicin and flank irradiation, thereby avoiding their associated toxicities. Those patients that receive neoadjuvant therapy are assigned a local stage of III and so will receive doxorubicin in addition to vincristine and dactinomycin, and ionizing irradiation, regardless. Similarly, patients who undergo a preoperative or intraoperative biopsy are assigned a local stage of III. Therefore an attempt at primary resection should usually be made, even if the tumor is large.

Indications for delayed resection of the primary tumor include: bilateral disease, disease in a solitary kidney, unilateral disease in a patient with a Wilms tumor predisposition syndrome (such as WAGR, Beckwith–Weidmann and Denys–Drash), pulmonary insufficiency from a heavy metastatic burden in the lungs, extensive intravascular thrombus above the level of the hepatic veins, clear evidence of preoperative rupture (a circumstance unreliably determined by preoperative imaging), unresectable, in the surgeon's judgment, without resection of adjacent organs (an assessment generally made at laparotomy).

### Timing of Surgery

One of the main controversies in the treatment of children with Wilms tumor is whether or not to administer preoperative chemotherapy, as suggested by the International Society of Pediatric Oncology (SIOP). The surgeon considering the use of preoperative chemotherapy should realize that there can be significant adverse effects on staging and histological evaluation in children who receive preoperative chemotherapy which could lead to either overtreatment or undertreatment. Proponents of preoperative therapy suggest that the tumor is easier to resect with a decreased incidence of tumor spill and a lower mortality and morbidity.

Despite the arguments against the use of preoperative therapy, as previously described, specific patient groups can be identified who would seem to benefit from preoperative chemotherapy. These are patients with bilateral tumors, those patients with IVC and intra-atrial involvement and patients with massive tumors considered by the operating surgeon to be unresectable without undue risk to the patient.

## Surgical Approach

As nearly all children with Wilms tumor will receive adjuvant chemotherapy, a central venous access device is generally placed at the time of nephrectomy, usually just before the start of the operation, to ensure secure intravenous access for the procedure. Patients are placed at a supine position with a bump under the appropriate flank. A radical nephrectomy should be carried out through a generous transverse, transperitoneal incision that allows for adequate exposure and complete exploration of the abdomen (Fig. 88-2). Some surgeons prefer a midline incision. A thoracic extension may be necessary but has been associated with a higher complication rate. Whichever incision is used, however, it should be large enough so that the integrity of the specimen is not compromised upon its removal from the abdominal cavity, as tumor rupture and spill have significant consequences.

Upon entering the peritoneal cavity, the presence of preoperative rupture should be documented, with bloody peritoneal fluid being considered a sign of rupture, whether or not gross or microscopic tumor is identified in the fluid. Isolation of the hilar vessels *prior* to mobilization of the primary tumor is no longer recommended since major vascular injury to the mesenteric arteries, celiac vessels, and aorta has been reported.

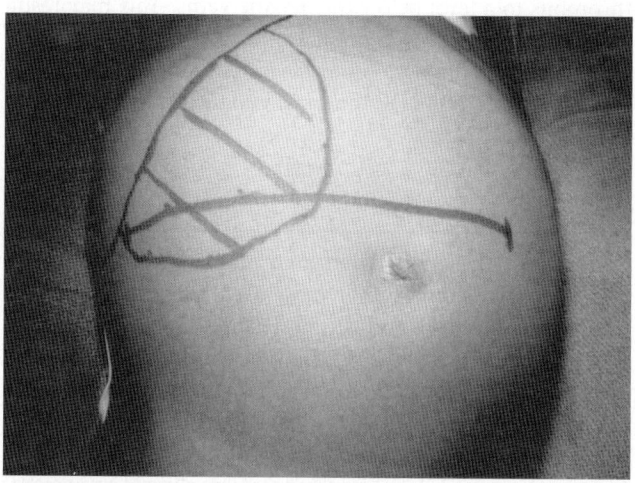

**FIGURE 88-2** Typical transabdominal incision.

Dissection generally begins at the lateral margin after the colon and its mesentery have been mobilized medially to more completely expose the kidney and tumor. The posterior surface of the tumor/kidney is also usually an avascular, safe plane of dissection. Exposure of the superior extent of right-sided tumors may benefit from mobilization of the right hepatic lobe while exposure of the superior extent of left-sided tumors may benefit from medial mobilization of the pancreas and spleen. Generally, the normal adrenal gland can be separated from the tumor and preserved; however, the ability to remove the tumor mass without rupture should not be compromised in an attempt to preserve the adrenal gland. The inferior tumor dissection should include removal of the ureter in continuity with the kidney. The ureter should be followed from the renal hilum to as low as conveniently possible, where it should be ligated and divided after palpating for the possible presence of intraureteral tumor. Once the kidney and tumor have been mobilized laterally, posteriorly, superiorly and inferiorly, the only remaining attachments are medial; these attachments contain the renal artery(s) and vein(s) (Fig. 88-3). Palpation of the renal vein prior to dividing it is recommended to exclude the possibility of a tumor thrombus, as occurs in about 10% of cases. Once the artery and vein have been tied and divided, the kidney and tumor should be free and can be passed off the field. Biopsy of the primary tumor should *not* be carried out prior to removal and a meticulous dissection to avoid rupture of the tumor capsule with spillage of tumor cells is imperative, as tumor spill is strongly associated with recurrence. Spillage refers to transgression of the tumor capsule during operative removal, whether accidental, unavoidable or by design. Spill can be "local," confined to the renal fossa, or "diffuse," occurring beyond those limits. The degree of spill will change the field of adjuvant radiation therapy, and so should be reported in the operative note.

Intraoperative inspection of the liver and the contralateral kidney is no longer required, unless lesions had been identified on preoperative imaging studies, because of the high accuracy of current imaging modalities. However, lymph node sampling is *critically* important, despite the absence of abnormal nodes on preoperative imaging, or upon gross inspection during operative exploration, since a review of lymph node sampling by the NWTS demonstrated a false negative rate of 31% and a false positive rate of 18% based on preoperative and intraoperative assessment. Unfortunately, there is currently a fairly high incidence of inadequate intraoperative staging, primarily due to failure to sample lymph nodes. Lymph nodes in the pericaval (right-sided tumors) and periaortic region (left-sided tumors) should be removed and submitted for histologic evaluation; visual assessment alone of the lymph nodes poorly predicts their pathologic involvement.

Wilms tumors rarely invade surrounding structures but frequently adhere to adjacent organs. If the tumor cannot be cleanly separated from adjacent structures then excision of the tumor with surrounding structures can be carried out in continuity if the operating surgeon feels that all tumor tissue can be completely removed. Since patients with small residual disease respond well to present chemotherapy and ionizing radiation, and since an increased incidence of complications

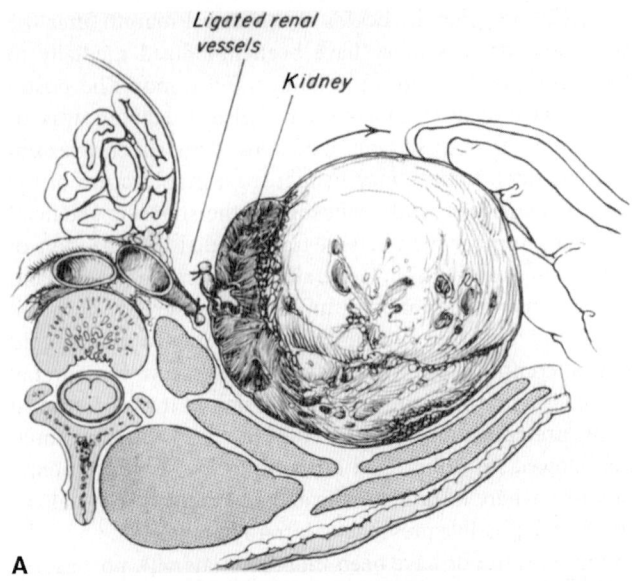

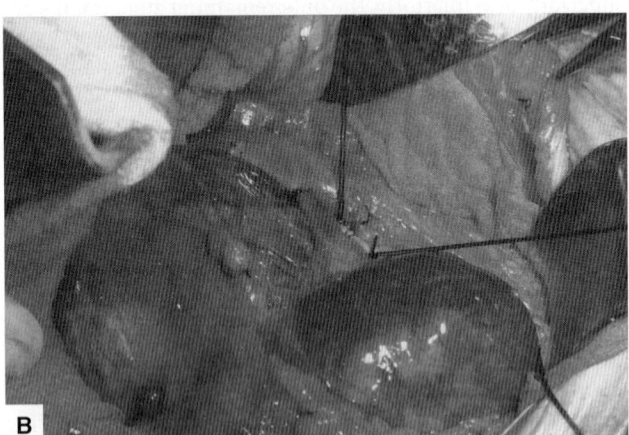

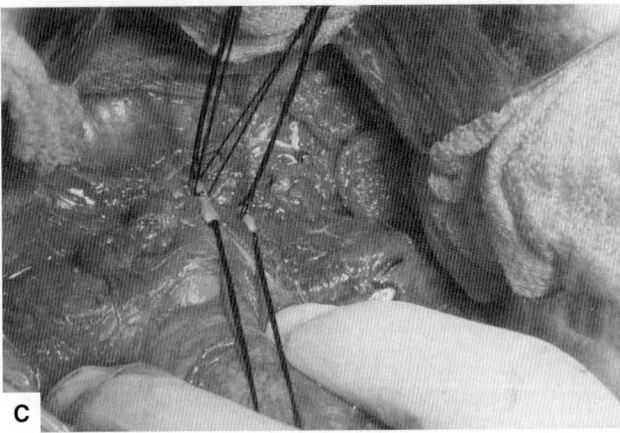

**FIGURE 88-3** A–C. Identification of the hilar vessels.

has been associated with tumor resections that include adjacent structures, radical resection is only indicated if all tumor can be removed. In the case of hepatic invasion a resection of part of the liver along with the primary tumor can usually be carried out. However, a formal hepatectomy is rarely indicated. The use of titanium clips is strongly recommended to identify gross residual tumor and the margins of the resected primary tumor.

There are reports of surgeons performing unilateral partial nephrectomy and laparoscopic nephrectomy (radical or partial) for Wilms tumor, particularly in Europe where children routinely receive preoperative chemotherapy. However, the appropriateness and adequacy of these approaches has not been confirmed and they are not currently endorsed by COG.

A complication rate of approximately 20% is seen following primary nephrectomy for Wilms tumor. The most frequent complication is small-bowel obstruction followed by major intraoperative hemorrhage, wound infection, vascular injury, and injury to other organs. In the majority of cases, the etiology of the small-bowel obstruction is adhesions, followed by intussusception and internal hernia. Most of the cases occur within the first 3 months following nephrectomy; nearly all cases of intussusception occur within the first 3 weeks after surgery. The incidence of small-bowel obstruction does not appear to be increased in children who receive postoperative radiation therapy.

## Tumor Thrombus

Vascular extension into the renal vein, cava and atrium presents special surgical challenges. Intravascular tumor extension can occur in Wilms tumor cases; renal vein involvement has been noted in 11% of cases (most often detected at operation) and caval and atrial involvement in about 6% of Wilms tumor cases. It should be sought by preoperative imaging and its presence or absence confirmed intraoperatively. Tumor extension into the renal vein and proximal inferior vena cava can in most cases be removed en-bloc with the kidney. Thrombus that extends into the vena cava can often be withdrawn from the IVC by opening the IVC (after gaining proximal and distal control). If the thrombus is not adherent to the wall of the IVC and is removed intact, the tumor may still be stage II if none of the other criteria for assigning a higher stage are met. Proximal and distal control of the IVC can generally be achieved if the superior extent of the thrombus is below the level of the hepatic veins. However, primary resection of tumors with extension into the inferior vena cava above the level of the hepatic vein or into the atrium is associated with higher operative morbidity. Thrombus that extends above the hepatic veins may require cardiopulmonary bypass to safely remove the full extent of disease. Alternatively, neoadjuvant chemotherapy may be given in an attempt to shrink the thrombus to a level below the hepatic veins. This may result in tumor adherence to the wall of the IVC, however, thereby precluding its complete removal. In this circumstance, ionizing radiation to the IVC and residual tumor thrombus may be indicated.

## Adjuvant Therapy

Historically, the most important prognostic variables for patients with Wilms tumor have been the histopathologic tumor classification and surgical stage. Survival statistics based on these factors, which have largely guided treatment, are shown in Table 88-3. However, more recently, it has been recognized that a Wilms tumor risk stratification system based on histology and stage alone does not accurately identify all patients at risk for recurrence. New clinical and genetic risk factors for recurrence have been validated and have now

| TABLE 88-3 | Ten-Year Outcomes for Patients with Wilms Tumor Treated on NWTS-4 | | |
|---|---|---|---|
| **Histology** | **Stage** | **10 yr Relapse Free Survival (RFS)%** | **10 yr Overall Survival (OS)%** |
| Favorable | I | 91 | 96 |
| | II | 85 | 93 |
| | III | 84 | 89 |
| | IV | 75 | 81 |
| | V | 65 | 78 |
| Anaplastic | I | 69 | 82 |
| | II–III | 43 | 49 |
| | IV | 18 | 18 |

been incorporated into the assigning of therapy in the current COG clinical trials for patients with Wilms tumor. These factors include patient age at the time of diagnosis, tumor weight, histologic response to therapy, and the allelic status of chromosomes 1p and 16q in resected tumors. Since 2006, several new clinical trials have opened within COG for the treatment of patients with Wilms tumor. Together these protocols cover the entire spectrum of Wilms tumor. Central to the approach to therapy for these patients is a risk classification scheme, which is defined in Table 88-4. To facilitate accurate and timely risk assessment, enrollment in an overarching tumor collection and biology classification protocol, "AREN03B2: Renal Tumors Classification, Biology, and Banking Study," is a prerequisite. Patients are then enrolled on one of the therapeutic protocols.

Surgery alone is proscribed as definitive treatment for children less than 2 years of age with Stage I, favorable histology disease where the tumor weight is less than 550 g, as these patients are at "very low risk" for recurrence. Children with Stage I (or II) disease who do not qualify for surgery alone are still considered "low risk" for recurrence, but, in addition to surgery, are treated with 22 weeks (7 cycles) of 2-drug chemotherapy (vincristine and dactinomycin) on regimen EE-4A. However, if the tumor from these patients is subsequently found to have LOH of both 1p and 16q, these patients are switched to "standard" risk therapy consisting of 28 weeks (9 cycles) of 3-drug chemotherapy, in which doxorubicin is added to vincristine and dactinomycin, on regimen DD-4A. Stage III patients whose tumors do not have 1p and 16q are also treated with "standard risk" DD-4A, plus radiation therapy. However, if their tumor is subsequently found to have both 1p and 16q LOH, these patients with Stage III disease are considered "higher risk" and are treated as described below.

Patients with favorable histology Wilms tumor that is either Stage III disease with 1p and 16q LOH, or Stage IV (metastatic) disease are at "higher-risk" of recurrence. Those with Stage III disease and 1p and 16q LOH are treated for 33 weeks (11 cycles) with vincristine, dactinomycin, and doxorubicin plus cyclophosphamide and etoposide on regimen M, as well as abdominal irradiation. Patients with Stage IV disease without 1p and 16q whose pulmonary lesions respond "rapidly and completely" (see later discussion) are treated with regimen DD-4A chemotherapy and no pulmonary irradiation. All other patients with metastatic disease (those with 1p and 16q LOH, those with "slow, incomplete" response of their pulmonary disease (see later discussion), or those whose

| TABLE 88-4 | Risk Stratification and Treatment Study Assignment for Patients with Favorable Histology Wilms Tumor | | | | | |
|---|---|---|---|---|---|---|
| **Patient Age** | **Tumor Weight** | **Stage** | **LOH** | **Rapid Response** | **Final Risk Group** | **COG Treatment Study** |
| <2 yrs | <550 g | I | Any | N/A | Very Low | AREN0532 |
| Any | >550 g | I | None | N/A | Low | None |
| >2 yrs | Any | I | None | N/A | Low | None |
| Any | Any | II | None | N/A | Low | None |
| >2 yrs | Any | I | LOH | N/A | Standard | AREN0532 |
| Any | >550 g | I | LOH | N/A | Standard | AREN0532 |
| Any | Any | II | LOH | N/A | Standard | AREN0532 |
| Any | Any | III | None | N/A | Standard | AREN0532 |
| Any | Any | III | LOH | N/A | Higher | AREN0533 |
| Any | Any | IV | LOH | Any | Higher | AREN0533 |
| Any | Any | IV | None | Yes | Standard | AREN0533 |
| Any | Any | IV | None | No | Higher | AREN0533 |
| Any | Any | V | Any | Any | Bilateral | AREN0534 |

metastases are extra-pulmonary are treated with regimen M and radiation to the site(s) of metastatic disease.

All patients with anaplastic Wilms tumor are at "high risk" for tumor recurrence. For risk assessment and treatment purposes, a distinction is made between focal (anaplasia confined to one or a few discrete foci within the primary tumor, with no anaplasia or marked nuclear atypia elsewhere) and diffuse anaplasia. Patients whose tumors have focal anaplasia, Stages I–III, or diffuse anaplasia, Stage I, are treated with regimen DD-4A. Patients with Stage IV focal anaplasia, Stages II–III, diffuse anaplasia, and Stage IV diffuse anaplasia without measurable disease are treated for 30 weeks with cyclophosphamide/carboplatin/etoposide and vincristine/doxorubicin/cyclophosphamide plus radiation therapy (regimen UH-1). Patients with Stage IV diffuse anaplasia with measurable disease are treated with 1 to 2 cycles of irinotecan/vincristine as window therapy to evaluate tumor response and determine whether this combination should be added to the backbone treatment with UH-1.

## OUTCOME

The survival statistics for NWTS-IV are shown in Table 88-3. Survival for patients with stages II to IV focal anaplasia was 100% but represented a small fraction of the total group of patients with anaplasia. Stages II to IV diffuse anaplastic tumors had a 4-year survival rate of 27% with 3-drug chemotherapy versus a 52% survival rate in children treated with actinomycin-D, vincristine, Adriamycin, and cyclophosphamide. Unfortunately, the 4-year survival for malignant rhabdoid tumors was 25%.

Although the overall survival for patients with Wilms tumor is favorable, adverse side effects are associated with therapy. Second malignant neoplasms have been reported with a cumulative risk at 10 years of 1%. Most of the second malignancies have occurred in irradiated areas. Although no significant cardiovascular problems have been reported in NWTS patients with Adriamycin, this drug is a cardiotoxic agent and there are reports of cardiac abnormalities in long-term survivors associated with Adriamycin. While refinements in radiation therapy have significantly decreased the musculoskeletal abnormalities, scoliosis and musculoskeletal abnormalities in early-stage patients not receiving postoperative radiation therapy is approximately 7 times less frequent than in patients who previously received postoperative radiation therapy.

## BILATERAL WILMS TUMOR

Due to an increased risk of renal failure in patients with bilateral Wilms tumor, these patients receive neoadjuvant therapy with 3-drug chemotherapy (regimen DD-4A) in an effort to shrink the tumors prior to surgery and facilitate the preservation of renal parenchyma, thereby preserving renal function. Also treated in this manner are patients with Wilms tumor arising in a solitary kidney or those patients with a unilateral Wilms tumor who are at an increased risk for developing a metachronous tumor. Patients with a number of genetic syndromes, particularly those associated with abnormalities of the Wilms tumor 1 (WT1) and Wilms tumor 2 (WT 2) genes on the short arm of chromosome 11, carry this risk. Patients with unilateral Wilms tumor and a Wilms tumor predisposition syndrome are treated with regimen EE-4A if their disease is stage I-II but DD-4A if the disease is stage III–IV.

A biopsy is not required in a child with bilateral, solid renal masses, as bilateral Wilms tumor is the certain diagnosis. Although the histologic subtype will not be known, studies have shown that biopsies of bilateral renal masses rarely detect anaplasia, even when present. However, a biopsy, if performed, does not mandate subsequent radiation therapy, as it does in patients with unilateral Wilms tumor. Neoadjuvant therapy consisting of vincristin, actinomycin-D, and doxorubicin should be initiated. Bilateral nephron-sparing surgery should be considered in all patients with bilateral Wilms tumor, even if preoperative imaging suggests the lesions are unresectable. This approach, when combined with adjuvant therapy, provides the opportunity to preserve renal function while maintaining a high probability of cure. Often, large lesions compress adjacent normal kidney parenchyma such that at the time of exploration more uninvolved renal parenchyma exists than might have been anticipated by the preoperative imaging. Operative intervention for local control should be done early, by 6, or at latest 12, weeks after initiation of chemotherapy, since little significant further change in tumor size is likely and it is important to determine the exact tumor histology (favorable vs anaplastic). When possible, a small rim of normal kidney (0.5–1 cm) is included around the resected lesion. At times, however, resection proceeds in the generally well-defined plane between the tumor and kidney. Despite this approach, tumor rarely extends to the surgical margins because there is often a fibrous rim or capsule that surrounds Wilms tumors. In cases where there are numerous small lesions in the kidneys that appear by imaging to be nephrogenic rests or cysts, representative biopsies can be obtained. During the conduct of the operation, it is important to determine whether the collecting system has been entered, which occurs commonly. When such a breach is identified, the cut edges of the violated calyx are closed with absorbable suture, often after placing a "double-J" ureteral stent. The decision to place a ureteral stent is based on the degree of disruption of the collecting system and the complexity of its closure. A flank penrose drain is also commonly placed. The penrose drains are generally removed prior to patient discharge; internal stents are removed cystoscopically 4 to 6 months later. If the tumor histology is anaplastic, consideration of performing a completion nephrectomy should be entertained, especially if the surgical margins were positive.

## NEPHROBLASTOMATOSIS

*Nephrogenic rests* are foci of embryonic tissue retained in the kidney after embryonic development has been completed. These rests can be intralobar or perilobar depending upon their location within the kidney. Perilobar nephrogenic rests do not appear to be precursor lesions of Wilms tumor, but intralobar nephrogenic rests are rarely seen except in association with Wilms tumor. Nearly half of unilateral Wilms tumor are associated with nephrogenic rests, while almost all cases of bilateral Wilms tumor are associated with nephrogenic rests. A more important finding is that nephrogenic rests have been found in nearly all of the kidneys resected in unilateral cases that go on to eventually develop metachronous contralateral Wilms tumor. For this reason, any child with nephrogenic rests within the resected specimen after removal of unilateral Wilms tumor should be monitored particularly carefully with imaging studies for the development of subsequent tumor in the contralateral kidney.

The term *nephroblastomatosis* is used for cases in which there is a diffuse or multifocal presence of nephrogenic rests. The treatment of children with nephroblastomatosis is not clearly established. Children with a diagnosis of nephroblastomatosis should be followed carefully with imaging studies (ultrasound, CT scan) to determine the status of the lesions within the kidneys, looking for changes.

## METASTATIC WILMS TUMOR

The primary distant site for Wilms tumor metastases is the lungs; hepatic metastases are much less common. Approximately 12% of Wilms tumor patients will have evidence of hematogenous metastases at diagnosis, with 80% having pulmonary metastases. Patients with Stage IV favorable histology tumors at diagnosis have a very good prognosis while unfavorable histology patients and patients who relapse with metastatic disease have a grave prognosis. Approximately 20% of favorable histology patients will relapse following therapy with a majority of relapses being in the lungs. Patients with pulmonary metastases usually can be managed by combined chemotherapy and radiation therapy; pulmonary resection is rarely indicated because chemotherapy is extremely effective. Although histologic confirmation of pulmonary relapse may be indicated, complete removal of pulmonary metastases at relapse does not increase survival.

A new response-based approach is being taken for patients with stage IV disease in the COG. Those patients, treated with regimen DD-4A, who have complete radiographic disappearance of their lung metastases (or who have tissue confirmation that residual nodules do not contain viable tumor) at the week 6 reevaluation will be considered "rapid responders," will continue on DD-4A and will not receive pulmonary irradiation. Patients who do not have complete resolution of pulmonary nodules will be considered "slow, incomplete responders," will be switched to regimen M and will receive whole-lung irradiation. Those patients who, at the time of diagnosis have pulmonary metastases confirmed histologically and have the lesions completely resected (and therefore have no residual disease available for response monitoring) will be treated with DD-4A but will be required to receive whole lung irradiation. Therefore, consideration must be given to the implications of resecting pulmonary lesions at the time of diagnosis. If the lesions are found to be benign, the patient will have been spared doxorubicin (if local stage I–II) and pulmonary irradiation. However, if the lesions

are metastatic Wilms tumor and are removed completely, the patient will have lost the opportunity to be considered a rapid responder and avoid whole lung irradiation.

## CONCLUSION

Significant improvement has been made in the treatment of children with Wilms tumor. New protocols in place are designed to maintain a high rate of cure for these patients while minimizing toxicity, based on the refinement of the risk stratification system. This risk stratification is certain to undergo further refinements in the coming years as advances in technology lead to increased understanding of the molecular biology of Wilms tumor. In addition, as new critical factors and pathways in Wilms tumor oncogenesis are identified, new druggable targets will be found, leading to targeted, potentially patient-specific therapies that will improve the probability of cure while minimizing toxic side effects. Surgeons will continue to play a critical role in the management of children with Wilms tumor, however, and it is imperative that they understand the directives of these new protocols and how the conduct of an operation can influence therapy and outcome for these patients.

## SELECTED READINGS

Beckwith JB, Kiviat NB, Bonadio JF. Nephrogenic rests of nephroblastomatosis and the pathogenesis of Wilms' tumor. *Pediatr Pathol* 1990;10:1–36.

Beckwith JB, Palmer NF. Histopathology and prognosis of Wilms' tumor. *Cancer* 1978;41:1927–1948.

Breslow NE, Beckwith JB. Epidemiological features of Wilms' tumor: results of the National Wilms' Tumor Study. *J Natl Cancer Inst* 1982;68:429–436.

Breslow NE, Sharples K, Beckwith JB, et al. Prognostic factors in non-metastatic, favorable histology Wilms' tumor. *Cancer* 1991;68:2345–2353.

Coppes MJ, Haber DA, Grundy PE. Genetic events in the development of Wilms' tumor. *N Engl J Med* 1994;331:586–590.

D'Angio GJ, Breslow N, Beckwith JB, et al. Treatment of Wilms' tumor: results of the Third National Wilms' Tumor Study. *Cancer* 1989;64:349–360.

Davidoff AM, Giel DW, Jones DP, et al. The feasibility and outcome of nephron-sparing surgery for children with bilateral Wilms tumor: the St. Jude Children's Research Hospital experience: 1999–2006. *Cancer* 2008;112:2060–2070.

Davidoff AM. Wilms tumor. *Curr Opin Pediatr* 2009;21:357–364.

de Kraker J, Lemerle J, Voute PA, Zucker JM, Taunade MF, Carli M. Wilms' tumor with pulmonary metastases at diagnosis: the significance of primary chemotherapy. *J Clin Oncol* 1990;8:1187–1190.

Dome JS, Cotton CA, Perlman EJ, et al. Treatment of anaplastic histology Wilms' tumor: results from the fifth National Wilms' Tumor Study. *J Clin Oncol* 2006;24(15):2352–2358.

Evans AE, Norkool P, Evans MS, Breslow N, D'Angio GJ. Late effects of treatment of Wilms' tumor. A report from the National Wilms' Tumor Study. *Cancer* 1991;67:331–336.

Green DM, Breslow N, Ii Y, et al. The role of the surgical excision in the management of Wilms' tumor patients with pulmonary metastases: a report from the National Wilms' Tumor Study. *J Pediatr Surg* 1991;26:728–733.

Green DM, Breslow NE, Beckwith JB, et al. Comparison between single dose and divided dose administration of dactinomycin and doxorubicin. A report from the National Wilms' Tumor Study Group. *J Clin Oncol* 1998;16(1):237–245.

Green DM. Controversies in the management of Wilms tumour—immediate nephrectomy or delayed nephrectomy? *Eur J Cancer* 2007;43(17):2453–2456.

Grundy PE, Telzerow PE, Breslow N, Moksness J, Huff V, Patterson MC. Loss of heterozygosity for chromosomes 16q and 1p in Wilms' tumors predicts an adverse outcome. *Cancer Res* 1994;54:2331–2333.

Hamilton TE, Green DM, Perlman EJ, et al. Bilateral Wilms' tumor with anaplasia: lessons from the National Wilms' Tumor Study. *J Pediatr Surg* 2006;41(10):1641–1644.

Larsen E, Perez-Atayde AR, Green DM, et al. Surgery only for the treatment of patients with stage I (Cassady) Wilms' tumor. *Cancer* 1990;66:264–266.

Othersen HB Jr, deLorimer A, Hrabousky E, Kelalis P, Breslow N, D'Angio GJ. Surgical evaluation of lymph node metastases in Wilms' tumor. *J Pediatr Surg* 1990;25:330–331.

Ritchey ML, Shamberger RC, Haase G, et al. Surgical complications after primary nephrectomy for Wilms' tumor: report from the National Wilms' Tumor Study Group. *J Am Coll Surg* 2001;192(1):63–68.

Shamberger RC, Guthrie KA, Ritchey ML, et al. Surgery-related factors and local recurrence of Wilms tumor in National Wilms Tumor Study 4. *Ann Surg* 1999;229(2):292–297.

Shamberger RC, Ritchey ML, Haase GM, et al. Intravascular extension of Wilms tumor. *Ann Surg* 2001;234(1):116–121.

Weeks DA, Beckwith JB. Relapse-associated variables in stage I favorable histology Wilms' tumor. *Cancer* 1987;60:1204–1212.

ONCOLOGY

# CHAPTER 89

# Neuroblastoma

*Eric Long and Dai H. Chung*

## KEY POINTS

1. As the second most frequent solid cancer of childhood, neuroblastoma remains an enigmatic tumor with a dismal outcome for advanced stage disease.

2. Patient age and tumor stage at the time of diagnosis are the 2 most important variables contributing to neuroblastoma progression and relapse.

3. Neuroblastoma stage is not only dependent on tumor location but also the presence of nodal and/or metastatic disease along with patient risk factors.

4. The operative goal in neuroblastoma treatment is complete tumor removal of both the primary tumor and its adjacent involved lymph nodes (for stage I and II disease). There may also be considerable value in the cytoreductive removal of the maximum tumor burden that is both safe and feasible in more advanced stage disease.

5. Surgical resection is not recommended in stage IV-S disease where the neuroblastoma is prone to spontaneous regression.

6. Multimodal therapy-operation, chemotherapy and irradiation is key for neuroblastoma treatment depending on patient age, disease stage, response to therapy, and tumor relapse. The treatment goal remains both local control, metastatic control, and the prevention of relapse.

## INTRODUCTION

Neuroblastomas exist as a spectrum of solid tumors that arise from primitive cells of fetal neural crest origin. These progenitor cells or neuroblasts localize along the sympathetic chain during embryological development and are destined to differentiate into nerve tissue cells as well as the tissue comprising the adrenal medulla. Neuroblastic tumors, therefore, can originate anywhere along the developmental pathway of the neural crest cell-derived sympathetic nervous system, including the adrenal medulla. Neuroblastoma accounts for 97% of all neuroblastic tumors. There is a wide spectrum of tumor phenotype, ranging from the benign differentiated form of ganglioneuroma to intermixed type of ganglioneuroblastomas to undifferentiated neuroblastoma. Clinically, they exhibit a broad range of tumor behavior that can span from a localized mass (which can undergo spontaneous regression), to an aggressive phenotype with disseminated disease involving distant organ metastases; and to disease relapse in the face of comprehensive multimodal treatment protocols. Accounting for 15% of all pediatric cancer-related deaths, neuroblastoma remains as one of the most difficult cancers to treat effectively for cure as reflected by the minimal gains made in overall survival after the treatment of high-risk disease. With research advances intensifying over the past decade, much has been discovered regarding the pathophysiology and molecular mechanisms underlying the tumorigenicity of neuroblastoma, and many novel therapies are currently in clinical trials. Yet in spite of this, neuroblastoma remains as an enigmatic cancer with an unpredictable clinical course and dismal overall outcome for advanced-stage disease.

## EPIDEMIOLOGY

With between 600 and 700 new cases diagnosed in the United States each year, neuroblastoma is the third most common childhood cancer, trailing only leukemia and brain tumors. Responsible for approximately 10% of all childhood tumors, it is the most common extra-cranial solid tumor in the pediatric population. The clinical incidence in North America is roughly 1 in 10,000 live births, with 90% of new cases occurring in children under the age of 5. With nearly 30% of new cases occurring in infants less than 1 year, neuroblastoma is the most frequently diagnosed malignancy in the first year of life, almost twice that of leukemia (58 vs 37 per one million infants). The median age at diagnosis is between 17 and 22 months. Almost exclusively a disease of infants and children, neuroblastoma rarely presents in adolescence and adulthood where outcomes are progressively worse with increasing age at diagnosis. Race predilection of neuroblastoma is marginally greater among Caucasian than African-American infants, but this ethnic difference tends to disappear with increasing age of patients. Neuroblastoma is slightly more common among boys than girls. Approximately 1% of neuroblastoma patients present as a familial type. Study of the inheritance patterns of these families supports an autosomal dominant mode of transmission with incomplete penetrance. Patients with familial neuroblastoma tend to present at an earlier age when compared with the sporadic form (9 vs 18 months), and they are more likely to have multiple primary tumors. The degree of disease expression is variable, frequently with both benign and malignant tumors arising within the same family.

Patients with a low or intermediate risk group of neuroblastoma have survival rates surpassing 90%, yet outcomes remain dismal for the high-risk group despite maximal medical therapy. In patients with high-risk disease, approximately 15% to 20% of patients demonstrate refractory or chemoresistant disease, and roughly 50% experience relapse following treatment. The 5-year overall survival rate in these patients is very poor at ~20%. The National Cancer Institute Surveillance Epidemiology and End Results group estimated 5-year survival rates for all neuroblastoma patients at 74% during a period from 1999 to 2005. While this represents a significant improvement from prior decades when 5-year survival estimates were 52%, this improved survival is likely attributable to strides in overall survival of patients in the low-risk group of neuroblastomas. Specifically, the overall survival rate for the high-risk group of neuroblastoma patients has only been modest at best with recent reports estimating event-free survival (EFS) approaching 40% to 50% in those children completing multiagent chemotherapy with autologous stem cell rescue.

## CLINICAL PRESENTATION

As a result of their neural crest lineage, neuroblastomas may occur anywhere along the sympathetic chain, most commonly in the adrenal medulla. The clinical manifestations of neuroblastoma are multifactorial and closely related to the site of the primary tumor as well as to the extent of metastatic disease, when present. Neuroblastoma is most frequently found in the retroperitoneal cavity, with 50% in the adrenal medulla and 25% originating from the paraspinal ganglia. In roughly 20% of cases, the primary tumor is in the posterior mediastinum followed by the pelvis, head, and neck regions in the other 5%. Age at diagnosis has significant implications due to the fact that in children less than 1 year of age, over half of the tumors will present as intra-abdominal masses while approximately one-third will have thoracic lesions at diagnosis. In comparison, older children (1-5 years) are more likely to have a primary abdominal tumor roughly 75% of the time with the thoracic location accounting for only 10% to 15% of primary tumors.

Initial symptoms typically are due to the mass effect from the tumor and are likely to be nonspecific; and therefore, it can easily be overlooked by the clinician. Moreover, the inability of patients from such a young age group to effectively communicate their symptoms is additionally confounding. Intra-abdominal neuroblastomas may reach significant size and tend to present as asymptomatic masses that are incidentally discovered by parents and/or physicians during routine clinic visits. Commonly reported symptoms of abdominal neuroblastomas are vague in nature such as

general malaise, abdominal pain, distention, weight loss, failure to thrive, irritability, unexplained fever, and anemia. Some (approximately 25%) may demonstrate hypertension as a result of excess catecholamine production. On physical exam, neuroblastomas presenting in advanced-stage disease may be detectable as a firm, nodular, and occasionally painful mass. Severe, acute symptoms are less common and usually relate to metastatic disease or compression from a profoundly enlarged tumor. Spontaneous rupture of tumor leading to acute abdominal pain, anemia, and hypotension has also been reported. Though less common, pelvic neuroblastomas can enlarge to the point of bladder and colon compression resulting in urinary retention and constipation. These tumors are usually palpable on digital rectal exam and must be differentiated from a presacral teratoma as well as other potential spine pathologies that are common in this age group. Thoracic neuroblastomas often present as an incidental mass on chest radiograph performed for unrelated or mild respiratory symptoms. The lesion may involve the stellate ganglion leading to Horner syndrome, characterized by miosis, anhydrosis, ptosis, and occasionally ophthalmic heterochromia on the affected side. Patients with enlarging mediastinal neuroblastomas can present with respiratory insufficiency, distress, or even dysphagia due to a mass effect on the lung parenchyma and esophagus.

Paraspinal neuroblastomas are of particular concern due to the risk of tumor extension into the spinal canal through the intervertebral foramina that can potentially lead to extradural compression of the spinal cord. These dumbbell- or hour glass-shaped tumors can manifest clinically as new onset paraplegia, which underscores the importance of performing a thorough neurological exam in any patients with suspected neuroblastoma. Evidence of spinal cord compression, including weakness, pain, and sensory loss, is seen in 5% of all neuroblastoma cases and must be treated emergently. Cauda equina syndrome may be observed, as manifested by bowel and bladder dysfunction, loss of anal tone, saddle anesthesia, or absent extremity reflexes. Though some controversy exists over the most appropriate treatment for these patients with devastating neurological symptoms, currently emergent chemotherapy is recommended as opposed to laminectomy because of the risk of serious complications associated with the emergent surgical decompression approach.

Metastatic dissemination of neuroblastoma can occur via direct invasion of adjacent structures or by hematogenous or lymphatic spread. Frequently, metastases with complete bone marrow infiltration can occur involving all of these processes of disease spread. At the time of diagnosis, 50% of patients will have metastatic lesion with regional lymph node involvement occurring in nearly 35%. Neuroblastoma most commonly metastasizes to the bony skeleton, particularly the long bones, spine, skull, pelvis, and ribs. Periorbital ecchymosis or "raccoon eyes" and proptosis are classic signs of metastatic disease and are related to the propensity of neuroblastoma to metastasize to the bony orbit. These signs can often be mistaken for a basal skull fracture resulting from trauma; therefore, one must be diligent with obtaining a detailed history and exam. Localized pain, limping, irritability, or a change in physical activity suggests potential bony involvement. Metastasis to the bone marrow can present with anemia, leukopenia, and thrombocytopenia with or without frequent infections depending on the degree of bone marrow failure. Invasion into major renal vasculature can present with hypertension secondary to vascular compression and subsequent renin secretion. The propensity to grow locally to surround vasculature emanating from the aorta–celiac axis or superior mesenteric artery is a therapeutic challenge. The local growth potential of para-spinal neuroblastoma to grow via vertebral foramina into the spinal canal has been detailed above.

## Paraneoplastic Conditions

Opsoclonus-myoclonus syndrome (OMS), also known as "dancing eye syndrome" or "dancing eyes, dancing feet syndrome" is a paraneoplastic, immune-mediated encephalopathy which is characterized by rapid, chaotic, conjugate eye movements in all directions along with involuntary muscle contractions. Occurring in 2% to 4% of all neuroblastoma patients, OMS may be the initial symptom triggering the diagnosis of an occult neuroblastoma. While the etiology of this syndrome remains unknown, recent studies suggest an immune-mediated response by antibody-antigen complexes of IgG3 and IgG4 against neural crest-like cells in the tumor that cross-react with neuronal cells in the cerebellum. Unfortunately, 70% to 80% of patients will have long-term neurological deficits in the form of cognitive, motor, and developmental or behavioral delay, which underscores the importance of prompt recognition and treatment. Once diagnosed, OMS should be treated aggressively. There are no randomized clinical trials to guide specific therapy and controversy exists over the combination therapy of glucocorticoids, adrenocorticotropic hormones, intravenous immunoglobulin, chemotherapy, and immunosuppression. Despite intense treatment protocols, many children will relapse once corticosteroid therapy is terminated. The Children's Oncology Group (COG) is evaluating a number of combination therapies to determine the standardized treatment regimen that will optimize neurological outcome. Although morbidity is high, children presenting with OMS have uniformly favorable tumor outcomes in regards to disease-free survival and eventual cure, with some studies estimating survival upwards of 90%.

As an endocrine tumor, neuroblastoma is capable of secreting biologically active substances, including vasoactive intestinal peptide (VIP) among many others. Hypersecretion of VIP is characterized by intractable watery diarrhea along with dehydration and hypokalemia. The severity of diarrhea is related to the level of VIP secretion, which is known to correlate with more differentiated tumors. Representing approximately 4% of all neuroblastomas, these patients may present with an infectious or malnutrition condition with weight loss, electrolyte imbalances, and failure to thrive. Symptoms are often refractory to medical treatment, but resolve following tumor resection. A recent retrospective analysis of a single country experience with VIP-secreting neuroblastomas revealed less than 80 cases over a 30-year period. The majority of cases were low-risk, differentiated tumors; however, approximately 10% of these patients continued to exhibit symptoms of clinically aggressive tumor behavior following initiation of chemotherapy and were subsequently found to

have poorly differentiated tumors. Surgical excision of the primary tumor led to symptom improvement in the vast majority of cases.

## 4S Disease

A particular subset of neuroblastoma, known as 4S disease (stage IV-S), is characterized by stage I disease with metastatic lesions localized to skin, liver, and/or bone marrow. The diagnosis of 4S disease is limited to infants less than 1 year of age with a localized primary tumor and skin, liver, and/or bone marrow involvement (<10% malignant nucleated cells in marrow). It is present in 5% of all neuroblastoma cases. The 4S disease is considered to be of low-risk group category and typically carries an excellent prognosis due to its propensity to regress spontaneously. Several retrospective and prospective studies have shown overall survival surpassing 92%. Patients present with a distinctive pathologic and clinical picture distinguished by a small primary tumor with numerous metastases to the liver, skin, and bone marrow. Liver metastases may be substantial and expand rapidly, resulting in significant hepatomegaly and possibly respiratory compromise. The characteristic nontender subcutaneous nodules have a bluish hue, and have been described on exam as "blueberry muffin" spots due to their similarity in color to rubella in newborns. Of note, these nodules may be discerned from infectious etiology by their characteristic blanch response in which they leave a surrounding rim of erythema following palpation.

Infants with 4S disease should undergo a diagnostic tissue biopsy to assess for tumor biology. Since resection of the primary tumor has not been shown to influence overall outcome, simple removal of a subcutaneous nodule for tissue evaluation should be performed. Respiratory compromise in these patients signifies aggressive tumor growth and chemotherapy with or without radiation can be used to mitigate tumor expansion. Patients with 4S disease can exhibit unfavorable biologic features such as *MYCN* amplification, diploidy, and their management should follow the guidelines for intermediate-risk (diploidy) or high-risk (*MYCN* amplification) category treatment algorithms.

# DIAGNOSIS

## Tissue Evaluation

The evaluation of any mass or lesion that is suspicious for neuroblastoma requires tissue sampling. A definitive diagnosis of neuroblastoma can only be made by histopathological assessment of tissue, which includes immunohistochemical analyses. Obtaining an adequate volume of tissue for thorough histopathological evaluation is paramount and is best accomplished through open and/or laparoscopic biopsy. However, CT- and/or ultrasound (US)-guided percutaneous core needle biopsy is being employed with increasing frequency; however, such a technique is done with some reservation due to limited tissue sampling. A recent retrospective review compared US-guided core needle biopsy to traditional open biopsy for the diagnosis of intermediate- and high-risk groups of neuroblastomas and demonstrated comparable efficacy with no significant difference in adequacy of tissue biopsy or the need for repeat biopsy. Of note, the group that underwent core needle biopsy had a significantly lower rate of major complications compared to the open biopsy group. When direct access to tumor tissue is not feasible, or if the diagnosis is unclear as in cases of smaller lesions, a concordantly positive bone marrow biopsy with aspiration showing immunocytologically positive aggregates of neuroblastic cells, along with elevated urinary catecholamine metabolites, can establish the diagnosis. However, tissue diagnosis is still preferred since it affords a more accurate molecular evaluation. Regardless of the initial diagnostic approach, the bone marrow compartment should be assessed for involvement once the diagnosis of neuroblastoma has been confirmed. Bilateral bone marrow aspirates with trephine biopsies (usually posterior iliac crest) are recommended to exclude metastatic disease before initiation of a treatment protocol. Sufficient sampling of the marrow is necessary to allow for immuno-histochemical and molecular immunocytologic evaluation. However, in general, infants younger than 6 months of age do not require bone marrow biopsy.

## Laboratory Testing

As noradrenergic derivatives of neural crest cell lineage, neuroblastomas are capable of secreting catecholamine metabolites and are known to produce a number of biologically active products including homovanillic acid (HVA), vanillylmandelic acid (VMA), adrenaline, noradrenaline, dopamine, metanephrine, and vanillylglycolic acid. The most useful of these products are HVA and VMA, as studies have shown that they have the highest sensitivity and specificity for neuroblastoma detection from urine (or serum) samples. HVA and VMA, which are elevated in more than 90% of patients with neuroblastoma, have implications not only at the time of diagnosis, but also during the course of treatment, including the detection of disease relapse. Higher levels of HVA at initial diagnosis tend to be associated with more immature, undifferentiated tumors, while increased levels of VMA are secreted by more mature tumors. Other serum biomarkers that have been proposed as prognostic indicators or which have the ability to estimate treatment response include lactate dehydrogenase (LDH), neuron-specific enolase (NSE), and ferritin. Though nonspecific, LDH can indicate a large tumor burden or increased tumor cell proliferation. NSE is a cytoplasmic marker of neuronal differentiation and increased levels are known to correlate with advanced stage and tumor burden. A rapid increase in serum ferritin level can signify tumor proliferation and suggest disease progression.

## Radiographic Studies

Many patients will have undergone a myriad of imaging studies leading up to identification of a neuroblastic tumor. Often, plain radiographs of the chest and abdomen are obtained and may show a widened mediastinum due to a posterior mediastinal mass, frequently with calcifications, which is particularly characteristic of neuroblastoma. Paraspinal widening above the diaphragm can be due to a thoracic tumor or extension from an abdominal tumor. Ultrasonography is

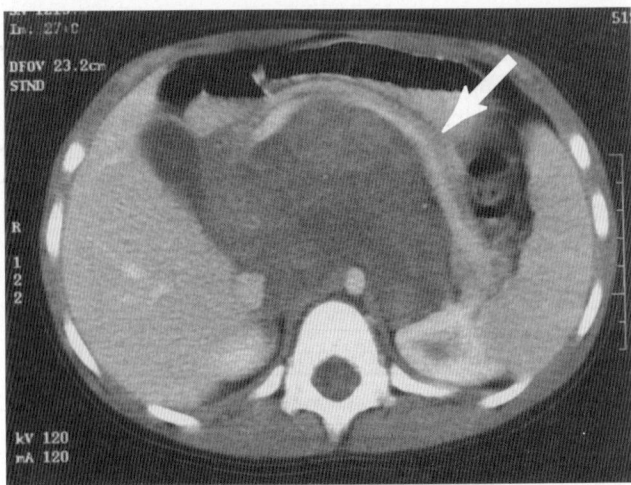

**FIGURE 89-1** A computed axial tomogram of a patient with a large central neuroblastoma. The splenic vessels and pancreas are draped over the anterior border of the tumor.

frequently used as an initial study to delineate a cystic from a solid abdominal mass.

Computed tomography (CT) is considered the gold standard for the initial evaluation of a primary tumor in patients with neuroblastoma (Fig. 89-1). CT is capable of tumor localization while also allowing for determining adjacent tissue involvement and disease burden. The use of intravenous contrast enhancement is essential in order to distinguish tissue planes between visceral organs, local vasculature, as well as to identify possible metastatic lesions in distant organs. A characteristic CT image feature for neuroblastoma is a retroperitoneal mass with calcifications (paraspinal or adrenal) that displaces the ipsilateral kidney downward. This finding is not to be confused with the "claw-like" projections of a Wilms tumor that may be seen emanating from the kidney as an intrarenal mass, yet lacking the downward displacement as seen in neuroblastoma.

Magnetic resonance imaging (MRI) is a useful adjunct to CT scan, especially for delineating major vessel involvement as well as for assessing extension into the spinal canal. Intra- and paraspinal tumors are best evaluated with MRI given its superiority over other modalities for evaluating intraforaminal "dumbbell" tumor extension with potential spinal cord compression. One prospective study of newly diagnosed neuroblastoma patients found MRI to be more accurate than CT for the detection and characterization of stage IV disease, showing that MRI is 83% sensitive compared to 43% by CT scan, while its specificity is 97% compared to 88% with CT scan alone. Three-dimensional reconstruction images based on CT or MRI should be considered when available in order to enhance measurements of tumor size and extension. It is recommended that sites of metastatic disease undergo CT or MRI imaging so that future treatment responses and/or relapses can be more accurately documented. Tumors arising in the head or neck region are also better assessed with either CT or MRI.

Scintigraphy using radiolabeled [123]iodine-metaiodobenzyl-guanidine (MIBG) has an important role in the initial evaluation of neuroblastoma since it permits a whole-body disease

1190

assessment. As a norepinephrine analog, MIBG preferentially localizes to catecholamine-secreting tissues and is selectively concentrated in over 90% of all neuroblastomas. Some centers routinely perform [123]I-MIBG scintigraphy in every patient prior to initiation of treatment, including a surgical procedure, though this practice varies among institutions. Scintigraphy is also considered the imaging study of choice for initial staging given its sensitivity for the detection of soft tissue and bone marrow disease. Any distant site harboring an unequivocally positive lesion on MIBG scintigraphy is considered metastatic disease. Lymph node metastases are also detectable by [123]I-MIBG, making it the standard recommendation in some institutions for the surveillance of recurrence and for reassessing treatment response in the high-risk category of patients. The longer-acting radioisotope, [131]iodine-MIBG, has also been targeted for high-dose, tumor-specific delivery in advanced-stage and refractory disease; but, no formal treatment protocols have been implemented.

## CLASSIFICATION AND STAGING

### Classification AGE + STAGE @ DX

Of patients with neuroblastoma, the two most important variables that contribute to the risk of disease progression and relapse are age and stage at diagnosis. It is easier to define risk for the extremes of age and disease stage. As would be expected, older children with stage IV disease carry the highest risk of death and relapse, while localized tumors in infants less than 1 year of age are nearly all cured, many times without the need for chemotherapy. It is the children in the middle of this spectrum that are the most difficult to treat by consensus.

The fundamental basis of neuroblastoma classification is tumor pathology. As a peripheral neuroblastic tumor, neuroblastomas exist along a spectrum that includes intermixed ganglioneuroblastomas, ganglioneuromas, and nodular ganglioneuroblastomas. The degree to which these tumors are classified as benign or malignant is mainly related to the extent of blastic differentiation (undifferentiated, poorly differentiated, and differentiating). Histopathologically, the microscopic evaluation of neuroblastoma depends not only upon differentiation, but also on the presence and extent of Schwannian cells, stroma, and the morphologic feature of the nucleus, described as the mitosis-karyorrhexis index (MKI). The MKI is a quantitative measure of tumor cell nuclear atypia that accounts for the number of cells in mitosis with pyknotic nuclei, and necrotic tumor cells. MKI values are measured microscopically (per 5000 cells) and are expressed as percentages of a viewing field. Criteria for increased values are age-dependent (<18 months, 18-60 months, >60 months).

Historically, the histopathologic characteristics of neuroblastoma tumors were used to classify patients into prognostic groups. Reported in 1984, the Shimada classification system considers the patient age, the presence of Schwannian stroma, the degree of cellular differentiation, and the MKI to distinguish "favorable" and "unfavorable" prognostic groups. Under the Shimada system, a "favorable" classification consists of younger patients with well-differentiated tumor containing abundant Schwannian stroma, while "unfavorable"

characteristics include older patients (>5 years of age) and poorly differentiated neuroblasts with a high MKI amongst a paucity of stroma. While the Shimada classification offers a standardized system for staging and prognosis, the advent of high-resolution imaging modalities with advances in molecular techniques have allowed for improved pathologic disease classification and staging.

In 1999, the International Neuroblastoma Pathology Classification (INPC) was released from the Children's Cancer Group to aid in the prognostic evaluation of patients with neuroblastoma. Using the Shimada classification as a framework, this INPC system incorporates patient age, degree of Schwannian development, level of differentiation, MKI, and the microscopic/macroscopic morphologic features of maturing tumors to classify neuroblastic tumors into three categories (ganglioneuroma, ganglioneuroblastoma, and neuroblastoma) with either favorable or unfavorable histology (UH) (Fig. 89-2). The INPC has been prognostically validated by a large, retrospective study in 2001 by Shimada et al. In this classification scheme, the neuroblastoma subgroup with favorable histology (FH) consisted of poorly differentiated and differentiating tumors with low or intermediate MKIs in patients less than 18 months of age as well as differentiating tumors with low MKIs in patients with ages between 18 months to 5 years. The FH group had 5-year EFS of 90.4%. In contrast, the UH subgroup consisted of undifferentiated tumors with or without high MKIs in patients of any age, poorly differentiated tumors with or without intermediate MKIs in patients with ages between 18 months to 5 years, or tumors with any level of differentiation and/or MKI in patients older than 5 years. The 5-year EFS in this group was 26.9%. The INPC has allowed for improved concordance among pathologists worldwide by creating a standardized, histology-based prognostic system.

### Staging INSS

Staging of neuroblastoma is not only based on tumor location and the presence of nodal and/or metastatic disease, but also on the patient's risk group stratification, which is used to predict response to therapy. Although various staging classifications have been developed over past decades, the International Neuroblastoma Staging System (INSS) is currently the standard and most widely accepted system for classifying newly diagnosed neuroblastomas (Table 89-1). Developed in 1986, the INSS has established consistency in the staging of neuroblastoma patients across the world. Based on the classic tumor, node, and metastasis (TNM) system, the INSS considers the location and extension of the primary tumor, the status of local/regional lymph nodes, and the presence/location of distant metastases. Stage I and II tumors are localized, do not cross the midline, and are generally amenable to primary resection. Complete gross excision of tumors in these stages may not always be possible and there may be positive ipsilateral lymph nodes in IIB tumors. Stage III tumors may be unilateral and unresectable, they may infiltrate across the midline, even without regional lymph node involvement, or they may have positive contralateral regional lymph nodes, except in the case of an unresectable midline tumor with bilateral extension by infiltration. Stage IV tumors are classified

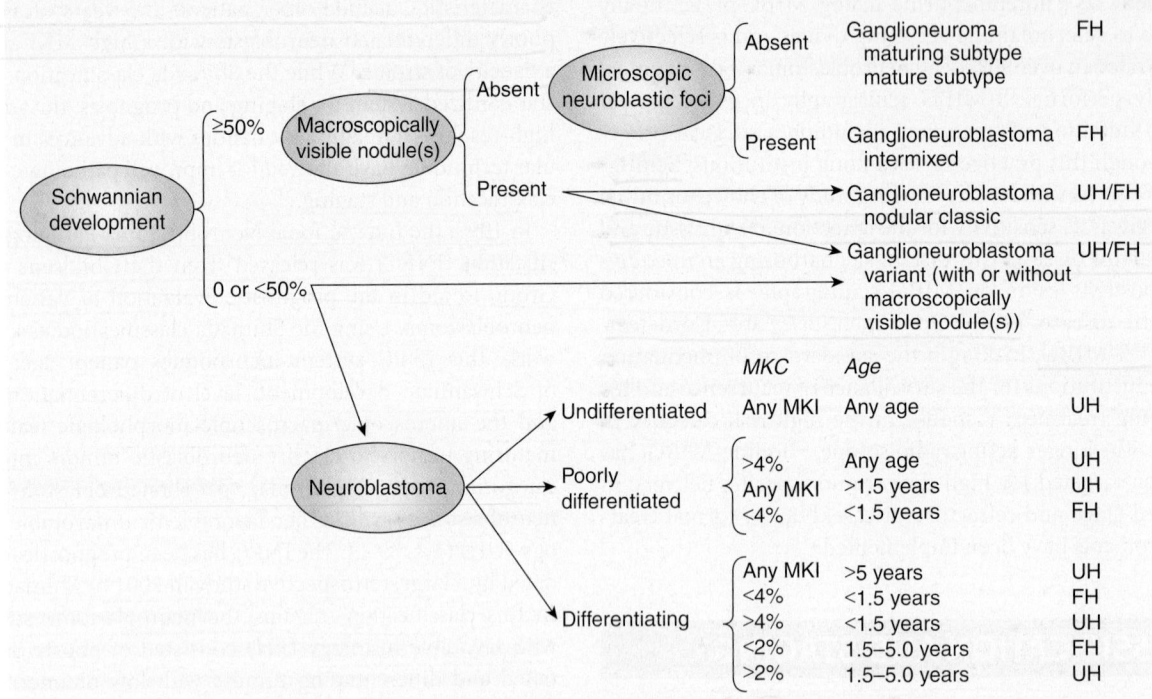

**FIGURE 89-2** International neuroblastoma pathology classification. MKC, mitotic and karyorrhectic cells; MKI, mitotic-karyorrhectic index, 2% = 100 of 5000 tumor cells, <4% = >100 to 200 of 5000 tumor cells, >4% = >200 of 5000 tumors cells; FH, favorable histology; UN, unfavorable histology (Reprinted with permission from Husain AN, Stocker JT, eds. *Color Atlas of Pediatric Pathology*. New York: Demos Medical Publishing; 2011).

| TABLE 89-1 | The International Neuroblastoma Staging System |
|---|---|

**Stage I**

Localized tumor with complete gross excision with or without microscopic residual disease; ipsilateral and contralateral lymph nodes (LN) negative for tumor microscopically

**Stage IIA**

Unilateral tumor with incomplete gross resection; ipsilateral and contralateral LN negative for tumor microscopically

**Stage IIB**

Unilateral tumor with or without complete gross excision with ipsilateral LN positive for tumor; contralateral LN negative microscopically

**Stage III**

Tumor infiltrating across the midline with or without regional LN involvement, localized unilateral tumor with contralateral regional LN involvement, or midline tumor with bilateral extension by infiltration (unresectable) or by LN involvement

**Stage IV**

Any primary tumor with dissemination to distant LN, bone, bone marrow, liver, skin, or other organs (except as defined for stage 4S)

**Stage IV-S**

Localized primary tumor (as defined for stage I or II) with dissemination limited to skin, liver, or bone marrow (limited to infants younger than 1 year)

as any primary tumor with evidence of distant lymph node, bone marrow, or organ/skin dissemination. The exception to Stage IV classification, known as Stage IV-S, is when an infant less than 1 year of age with a stage I or II tumor presents with disseminated disease that is limited to the skin, liver, or bone marrow (<10% replacement). In general, patients with Stage IV-S disease, despite having metastases, have high rates of spontaneous disease regression usually leading to an excellent overall prognosis. The Children's Oncology Group risk stratification uses INSS stage, age, *MYCN* status, tumor histopathology, and DNA index to classify patients into low-, intermediate-, or high-risk categories. Estimates of probable disease-free survival from this group are greater than 95% for low-risk disease, greater than 90% for intermediate-risk disease, and less than 30% for high-risk disease.

The INSS is fundamentally based on the degree and extent of surgical resection of the primary tumor and is therefore subject to the surgeon's varying ability to achieve margins and lymph node excision. To illustrate the variability in the staging system, a patient with a primary tumor extending across the midline and no obvious nodal involvement on imaging would be classified as stage III; however, if at the time of operation the surgeon is able to achieve complete resection of the tumor with negative contralateral lymph nodes, then this patient would be considered stage I and unlikely to require any further treatment.

To answer the need for a consistent pretreatment risk stratification scheme, a new clinical staging system known as the International Neuroblastoma Risk Group Classification System (INRGCS) was developed (Fig. 89-3). Based on

| INRG Stage | Age (months) | Histologic Category | Grade of Tumor Differentiation | MYCN | 11q Aberration | Ploidy | Pretreatment Risk Group |
|---|---|---|---|---|---|---|---|
| L1/L2 | | GN maturing; GNB intermixed | | | | | A very low |
| L1 | | Any, except GN maturing or GNB intermixed | | NA | | | B very low |
| | | | | Amp | | | K high |
| L2 | <18 | Any, except GN maturing or GNB intermixed | | NA | No | | D low |
| | | | | NA | Yes | | G intermediate |
| | ≥18 | GNB nodular; neuroblastoma | Differentiating | NA | No | | E low |
| | | | | NA | Yes | | H intermediate |
| | | | Poorly differentiated or undifferentiated | NA | | | H intermediate |
| | | | | Amp | | | N high |
| M | <18 | | | NA | | Hyperdiploid | F low |
| | <12 | | | NA | | Diploid | I intermediate |
| | 12 to <18 | | | NA | | Diploid | J intermediate |
| | <18 | | | Amp | | | O high |
| | ≥18 | | | | | | P high |
| MS | <18 | | | NA | No | | C very low |
| | | | | NA | Yes | | Q high |
| | | | | NA | | | R high |

FIGURE 89-3 International neuroblastoma risk group classification. EFS, event-free survival; L1, localized tumor confined to 1-body compartment and with absence of image-defined risk factors (IDRFs); L2, locoregional tumor with presence of one or more IDRFs; M, distant metastatic disease (except stage MS); MS, metastatic disease confined to skin, liver, or bone marrow in children younger than 18 months; NA, not applicable (Reprinted with permission from Cohn SL, Pearson AD, London WB, et al. The International Neuroblastoma Risk Group [INRG] Classification System: An INRG Task Force Report. *J Clin Oncol* 2009;27(2):295, Fig. 2).

analysis of data from over 8800 neuroblastoma patients, the INRGCS classification system incorporates 7 clinical and biological variables into a risk-based pretreatment classification scheme. The statistically significant variables that are factored into the classification are patient age, INRG stage, histologic category, grade of tumor differentiation, *MYCN* amplification status, chromosome 11q aberration, and DNA ploidy. The INRG stage used in this classification system is termed the International Neuroblastoma Risk Group Staging System (INRGSS), which is based on a set of preoperative, diagnostic imaging criteria termed image-defined risk factors (IDRFs), rather than operative findings. In comparison to the INSS, the INRGSS stratifies local–regional disease into 2 stages instead

of three. Under the INRGSS, patients can be divided into 1 of 4 categories: L1 (localized disease that does not involve vital structures and is confined to 1-body compartment); L2 (localized disease with IDRFs); M (distant metastatic disease); and MS (metastatic disease confined to the skin, liver, and/or bone marrow in children < 18 months of age). Using the INRGCS, patients can be categorized into pretreatment very low-, low-, intermediate-, and high-risk groups based on 5-year EFS rates of >85%, >75 to ≤85%, ≥50 to ≤75%, and <50%, respectively (Fig. 89-4). International implementation of this system has facilitated the comparison of risk-based clinical trials and has led to improved treatment protocols, especially for high-risk patients. It should be noted that the INRGSS is not intended to replace the INSS, but rather to be used in conjunction with the INSS for risk group stratification.

## MULTIMODALITY TREATMENT

Because of the heterogeneity of disease presentation and tumor stage, no single treatment regimen can be used to effectively treat all neuroblastomas. Patient management should be individualized and protocol based using risk-group stratifications and the biologic characteristics of the tumor as predictors of outcome. An even greater challenge for clinicians is the fact that more than 50% of children will have locally advanced or metastatic disease at the time of diagnosis. Therefore, a comprehensive therapeutic protocol is directed towards complete reduction of primary tumor

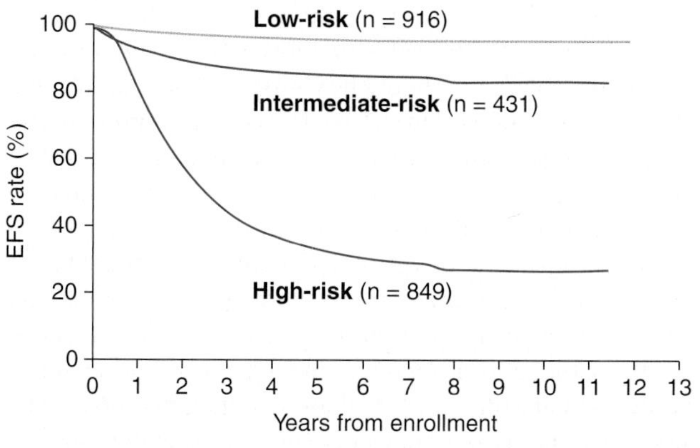

FIGURE 89-4 Event-free survival based on risk-group categorization.

burden and elimination of metastatic disease using a combination of surgery, chemotherapy, radiation therapy, and bone marrow/stem cell transplantation.

## Surgery

The role of surgery in the treatment of neuroblastoma is based on INSS staging as well as the associated risk-group stratification. A surgical procedure may be used not only as primary therapy, but also for diagnostic and staging purposes. Although the timing of operation has been debated in "intermediate-" and "high-risk" groups of patients with neuroblastoma, it is generally accepted that surgical resection alone is the treatment of choice for a "low-risk" category of disease. For early-stage cancers (I, IIA, and IIB), complete surgical excision of the primary tumor is recommended as the initial treatment, and often it may be the only therapy that is required. A complete curative resection based on fundamental surgical oncology principles should always be the goal. In "low-risk" patients, survival correlates with the ability to maintain local control. The ability to obtain a complete gross resection, which is defined by the macroscopic removal of all visible tumor and clinically abnormal regional lymph nodes, distinguishes stage I from stage IIA. The presence of residual microscopic tumor does not preclude a complete gross excision. A near-complete excision is defined as excision of the tumor with minimal residual macroscopic disease, which corresponds to stage IIA. Stage IIB is defined by complete gross or near-complete excision of the primary tumor with the presence of infiltrated regional ipsilateral lymph nodes. For localized disease that is limited to stages I and IIB, treatment with resection alone has yielded promising results. Multiple studies have shown that a "surgery-only" approach is safe for low-risk tumors. In further evaluating "surgery-only" for INSS stage I disease, other studies have found a 2-year survival rate of nearly 90%, even when microscopic residual disease is present. Another study comparing complete vs. subtotal resection of localized, non-metastatic tumors determined 2-year disease-free survival to be 93% in the complete resection group vs. 54% in the subtotal resection group. Interestingly, studies have also shown that local recurrence following resection of stage I neuroblastoma can be safely treated with re-excision and rarely requires additional therapy.

The timing of operation and the degree of resection vary with stage III and IV tumors. These lesions often involve multiple contiguous structures along with a component of metastatic disease. For intermediate-risk patients, surgical management consists of complete tumor resection if possible, including all regional lymph nodes, while preserving major vascular structure and vital organ function. In stage III tumors, it has been shown that significant improvement in overall survival can be observed when gross surgical resection corresponds to microscopic completeness. Performing a complete or near-complete gross resection may be technically difficult, and thus, an incomplete excision corresponds to a situation in which gross macroscopic disease remains, or when contralateral lymph nodes are positive despite a complete gross excision. Incomplete resections can be further classified into subtotal resection (STR; removal of >50% but <95% of the visible tumor) or less than STR (removal

of <50% of the visible tumor). In 1 study, stage III patients with no *MYCN* amplification were successfully treated with operation without the need for radiotherapy or chemotherapy, as reflected by a 10-year EFS and overall survival (OS) of 74.9 ± 16.9% and 92.6 ± 5.5%, respectively. For those with *MYCN* amplification, a multimodal treatment consisting of chemotherapy, surgery, and radiotherapy was associated with improved complete response (CR) or very good partial response (VGPR) of 81% as well as 10-year EFS and OS (75 ± 10.8%). Since most intermediate-risk patients receive neoadjuvant chemotherapy, identifying tumors with favorable biologic features pre-operatively allows for a higher rate of gross total resection in this group.

Although chemotherapy is the mainstay of treatment for advanced, high-risk neuroblastoma, operative therapy still has a definitive role. Early surgical intervention for advanced disseminated disease should focus on obtaining an adequate volume of tissue for cytogenetic and pathologic analysis, while documenting the degree of metastases if present. Studies have shown that tumor volume reduction is greatest between the second and fourth cycle of chemotherapy, and therefore, operative intervention for primary tumor resection is usually timed after the fourth or fifth cycle of induction chemotherapy. While it is generally agreed that "operation post-chemotherapy" approach to advanced disease offers the greatest chance for local control and possibly improved survival, the extent of surgical resection has been debated. However, most agree that complete gross resection of all macroscopic disease is appropriate in the vast majority of cases, citing that resection correlates with a reduced risk of local recurrence, especially in combination with induction chemotherapy and local radiotherapy. It has been suggested that there may be some survival benefit for attempting complete gross resection at the initial operation in stage IV neuroblastomas, though the numbers have not been significant and this approach carries an increased risk of patient morbidity. An exception to the management paradigm of stage IV disease is in infants with stage IVS neuroblastoma. Surgical resection is not recommended given the propensity for these tumors to spontaneously differentiate and regress.

## Operative Considerations

Thorough preoperative planning is crucial prior to any operation for neuroblastoma. Multidisciplinary collaboration should be obtained to formulate a comprehensive treatment plan. Tumor features such as size, extent of adherence and/or extension into adjacent structures, and the likelihood of "operation-only" cure should be considered carefully. As with all cancer operations, dependable IV access is important since neuroblastomas can be highly vascular making the risk for blood loss substantial. Reliable, size-appropriate modalities for hemodynamic monitoring should be used given the potential for significant alterations in hemodynamics as a result of intra-operative catecholamine extravasation during tumor manipulation. Because neuroblastomas can arise in multiple anatomic locations, the surgical approach and technique will vary based on the primary tumor. More than half of all neuroblastomas arise from the retroperitoneal portion of the abdominal cavity. Given that visceral and/or vascular tumor involvement is likely, the need for wide exposure is usually necessary and facilitated by patient size. Standard midline or transverse abdominal incisions are frequently used with some surgeons preferring bilateral subcostal (chevron) incisions for access to the upper retroperitoneum. For tumors involving major midline vessels, particularly on or near the celiac axis and diaphragm, a thoracoabdominal approach maybe best suited. For example, large right-sided tumors adherent to the diaphragm will require a wide exposure that can be optimally obtained through a thoracoabdominal approach. This affords the surgeon the ability to visualize and obtain control of major blood vessels, including the aorta, inferior vena cava, and renal vessels, which is of particular importance with encasing tumors (Fig. 89-5). Exploration of the abdominal cavity should be performed to assess the primary tumor, lymph nodes, and other involved structures. Dissection is often tedious and should be approached with meticulous caution to prevent hemorrhage, since it is generally acceptable to leave residual tumor if it avoids bleeding complications. As part of the dissection, the renal vein and artery should be mobilized and controlled. A dissection plane should be established between the tumor and the IVC, and proper exposure and ligation of the right adrenal venous drainage to the IVC and left adrenal venous drainage to the left renal vein is imperative. A nephrectomy should be avoided unless substantial tumor burden will be left behind. En bloc resection of adjacent organs is rarely needed unless significant tumor involvement is encountered.

Laparoscopic adrenalectomy in adults and children with benign disease has become the standard of care, yet the role of the laparoscopic approach in children with malignant tumors remains controversial. The use of laparoscopic approach for smaller periadrenal neuroblastomas is growing in certain centers along with the employment of minimally invasive techniques for the initial management and diagnosis of primary tumors. Laparoscopic biopsy of infiltrating abdominal lesions is becoming more common as well. A retrospective review from a single institution analyzing 7 consecutive laparoscopic adrenalectomies for small neuroblastic tumors over a 1-year period was recently reported. All tumors were well-circumscribed and noninfiltrating with an average tumor size of 2.8 cm. Three of the patients were INSS stage I while the other 4 were INSS stage IV (all 4 patients received preoperative chemotherapy). There were no deaths or late complications and the average hospital stay was 3 days. Other groups have reported similar results related to the feasibility of the laparoscopic approach for small, well circumscribed, noninvasive adrenal neuroblastomas.

## Chemotherapy

Multiagent chemotherapy is the basis of all treatment regimens for advanced stage and high-risk neuroblastomas. In spite of advances in combination therapy, a well-defined, proven chemotherapeutic regimen capable of achieving complete remission in these patients has not been found. Initial tumor response to induction chemotherapy demonstrates a 50% to 80% CR or VGPR to dose-intensive, multiagent regimens. The most commonly used agents are cyclophosphamide,

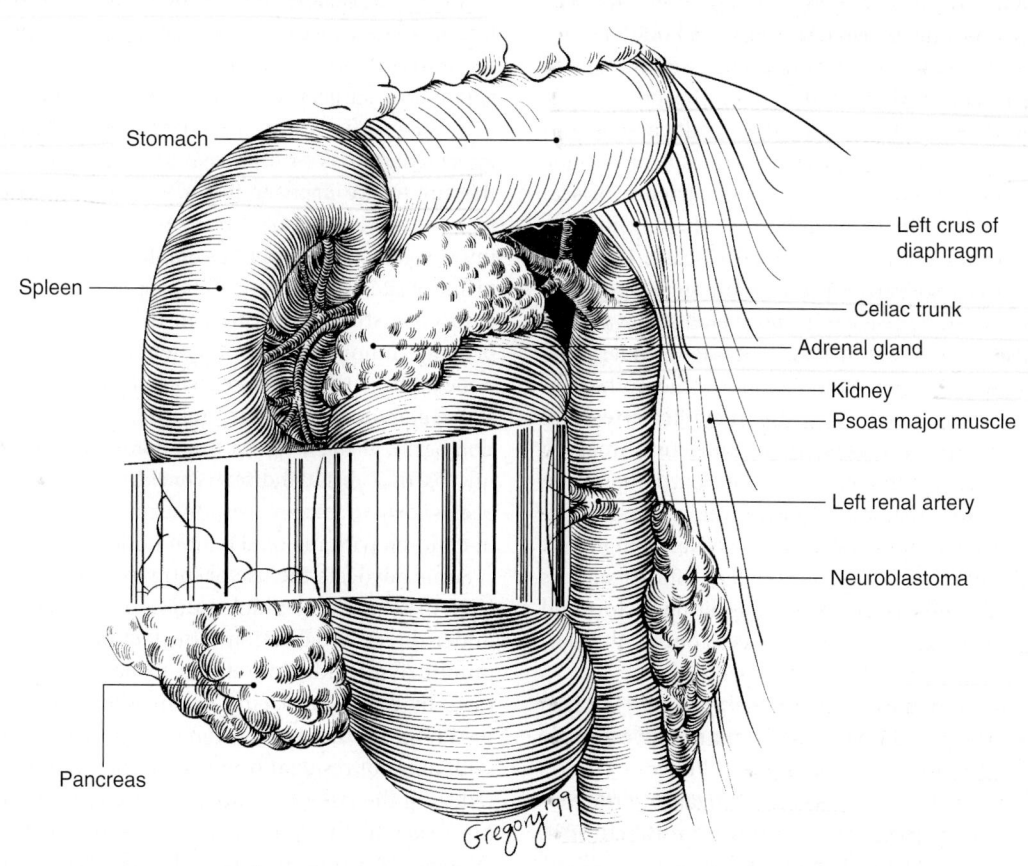

**FIGURE 89-5** Thoracoabdominal exposure with mobilization of the kidney out of the renal fossa to expose tumor along the lateral border of the aorta. The spleen and pancreas were previously mobilized.

Labels in figure: Stomach, Spleen, Pancreas, Left crus of diaphragm, Celiac trunk, Adrenal gland, Kidney, Psoas major muscle, Left renal artery, Neuroblastoma

doxorubicin, cisplatin, melphalan, carboplatin, etoposide, topotecan, ifosfamide, and vincristine. The most important therapeutic goal is local disease control. Unfortunately, tumor resistance to chemotherapeutic agents is common with disseminated disease, as exhibited by aggressive neuroblastoma phenotypes with high rates of relapse. To decrease the risk of developing tumor resistance to chemotherapy, it is recommended that surgical resection of any primary or local–regional disease is performed as soon as there is radiographic evidence of resectability, even if the patient has not completed their full course of induction therapy. The rationale for this approach is based on the hypothesis that chemotherapeutic agents with different mechanisms of action are most effective when given together against the most-minimal volume of tumor burden possible.

Recent estimates are that 50% to 60% of children with high-risk neuroblastoma will develop a recurrence. The management scheme in these patients has traditionally been induction chemotherapy followed by myeloablative consolidation therapy with stem cell rescue. A multicourse regimen of 13-*cis*-retinoic acid (RA) then follows for eradication of residual disease. Any persistent disease, or recurrence, is treated with multiagent chemotherapy, though these are likely to be clonally selected aggressive phenotypes, and the long-term survival in this population is poor. Stem cell harvesting is performed during induction chemotherapy, usually after the 2nd cycle, while surgical resection of the primary tumor and any metastatic disease is done after the 5th cycle of chemotherapy or when there is radiographic evidence of resectability.

After induction, treatment is consolidated with 1 or more courses of high-dose chemotherapy to eradicate minimal residual disease, but this unavoidably induces bone marrow ablation, which necessitates autologous stem cell transplant (ASCT). Rescue is not without risk since the presence of tumor contamination of the bone marrow graft can contribute to relapse. Complications of such a transplant include growth failure, endocrinopathy, and the occurrence of secondary malignancies. Finally, maintenance therapy may be incorporated to target minimal residual disease. Unfortunately, relapse and poor survival are common in high-risk patients, as evidenced by event-free and overall survival rates of 26% and 37%, respectively, in stage IV patients undergoing chemotherapy/ASCT. Upon completion of chemotherapy, patients may receive six courses of RA to eradicate residual disease that may still be present despite meeting imaging criteria for complete remission. This treatment is based on reports that high-dose therapy with RA given after chemoirradiation significantly improved overall survival in high-risk neuroblastoma (59% vs 37% at 5 years). Side effects, such as skin dryness and cheilitis, are the dose-limiting factor; and consequently, RA therapy consists of 2-week courses alternating with 2 weeks for mucocutaneous recovery.

Trials involving myeloablative chemotherapy and [131]I-MIBG have been underway in an effort to minimize adverse side effects by making therapies more targeted. Previous studies have shown that [131]I-MIBG exhibits activity against refractory neuroblastoma with response rates ranging from 10% to 50%. In a phase I trial of [131]I-MIBG therapy for relapsed neuroblastoma, myelosuppression was the most significant toxicity at doses >15 mCi/kg, with nearly half of the patients requiring hematopoietic cell transfusion. Despite this, the response rate (36%), event-free survival (18% at 1 year), and overall survival (49% at 1 year; 29% at 2 years) were found to be significantly higher in patients older than 12 years and those who had fewer than three prior treatment regimens. Subsequently, a phase I dose escalation study of [131]I-MIBG with myeloablative chemotherapy and stem cell rescue reported a significant response rate of 25% in patients with primary refractory disease. Given these findings, [131]I-MIBG may prove to be useful in conjunction with other treatment modalities.

Despite using independent prognostic variables to tailor treatment, many high-risk neuroblastomas have developed resistance to chemotherapeutic agents, making the likelihood of relapse quite high. The total length of therapy averages nearly 1 year and most treatment failures are due to minimal residual disease that was not eradicated following high-dose chemotherapy. While the aim of further treatment is remission, prolonged disease stabilization is usually the reality, and most patients who relapse eventually die from disease progression. Even patients who achieve a cure with initial therapy remain at risk for developing long-term complications related to treatment, including hearing loss, infertility, and second malignancies.

## Radiotherapy

External-beam radiotherapy (EBRT) is an important part of the treatment paradigm in both intermediate and high-risk neuroblastomas. As a radiosensitive malignancy, neuroblastoma cells can be targeted at sites of residual primary tumor, regional lymph node involvement, and metastatic beds. For intermediate-risk disease, radiotherapy is typically reserved for unresectable or residual disease following chemotherapy and/or surgery, or in the case of tumors with unfavorable prognostic features/histology. Nearly all patients with intermediate-risk or high-risk disease receive focused radiotherapy to the primary tumor site for increased local control. Several institutional retrospective studies have reported improved local control rates employing 21 Gy or more to the primary site. Though not statistically significant, a small retrospective study found that in the absence of EBRT to the primary tumor site, 44% of patients recurred locally, whereas none of the patients who received 20 Gy to the primary tumor site experienced a primary relapse. This suggests that radiation of the primary tumor in patients with gross residual and microscopic residual disease may be of value. EBRT has also been shown to improve response rates and event-free survival in children with regional lymph node metastases.

Some advocate the use of intraoperative radiation therapy (IORT), which allows higher doses of irradiation to be applied under direct visualization. This technique has the benefit of minimizing irradiation effects to nearby, uninvolved structures by either displacing or shielding them at the time of resection. Furthermore, it can deliver high-radiation doses to both areas of residual tumor and microscopic disease, while reducing the risk of irradiation toxicity to uninvolved structures such as the spinal cord. In 1 retrospective study, stage IV neuroblastoma patients who underwent chemotherapy, resection, and IORT had similar recurrence rates to their stage I, II, or III counterparts while their survival remained quite poor. With stage III or less, the overall survival rate was 78% at 2 and 5 years, but with stage IV, the overall survival rate was 71% and 21% at 2 and 5 years, respectively. The local recurrence rate with stage III or less was 31% at 5 years, while it was 33% at 2, 5, and 10 years with stage IV. Thus, IORT appears to promote local control in advanced neuroblastoma.

## SELECTED READINGS

Carpenter EL, Mosse YP. Targeting ALK in neuroblastoma-preclinical and clinical advancements. *Nat Rev Clin Oncol* 2012;9:391–399.

Cohn SL, Pearson AD, London WB, et al. The International Neuroblastoma Risk Group (INRG) Classification System: An INRG Task Force Report. *J Clin Oncol* 2009;27(2):289–297

Hara J. Development of treatment strategies for advanced neuroblastoma. *Int J Clin Oncol* 2012;17:196–203.

Matthay KK, George RE, Yu AL. Promising therapeutic targets in neuroblastoma. *Clin Cancer Res* 2012;18:2740–2753.

Nuchtern JG, London WB, Barnewolt CE, et al. A prospective study of expectant observation as primary therapy for neuroblastoma in young infants: a Children's Oncology Group Study. *Ann Surg* 2012;256(4):573–580.

Yu AL, Gilman AL, Ozkaynak MF, et al. Children's Oncology Group. Anti-GD2 antibody with GM-CSF, interleukin-2, and isotretinoin for neuroblastoma. *N Engl J Med* 2010;363(14):1324–1334.

NEUROBLASTOMA

# Teratoma CHAPTER 90

*Frederick J. Rescorla*

## KEY POINTS

1. Fifty percent of pediatric germ cell tumors are extragonadal.

2. Teratomas (mature and immature) are the most common germ cell tumor and are benign lesions requiring only complete surgical resection.

3. Yolk sac (endodermal sins) is the predominant prepubertal malignant histology and alpha fetoprotein (AFP) is a marker of disease.

4. Accurate staging is essential as Stage I gonadal tumors are treated without chemotherapy.

5. The survival for malignant germ cell tumors treated with surgery and selective use of chemotherapy is excellent.

6. Current chemotherapy is extremely effective, thus resection of adjacent involved organs or structures is not indicated.

7. Initially unresectable extragonadal tumors treated with neoadjuvant chemotherapy and delayed resection have equivalent survival compared to initial resection.

Pediatric germ cell tumors are rare tumors with malignant germ cell tumors accounting for 1% to 3% of all malignant tumors in childhood. Several unique features distinguish these tumors: the nongonadal sites are more common than gonadal sites in children compared to adults where only 10% are extragonadal; yolk sac tumor is the most common malignant histology and alpha fetoprotein (AFP) serves as a marker to follow response to therapy and monitor recurrence; and, the introduction of modern chemotherapy with cisplatin, etoposide, and bleomycin has markedly improved survival and allowed the successful use of neoadjuvant therapy with preservation of vital organs.

Primordial germ cells arise near the allantois during the fourth fetal week and then migrate to the genital ridge where they develop into the gonads. Arrested migration is thought to result in the deposition of cells in extragonadal locations such as the retroperitoneum whereas aberrant migration results in the deposition at sites such as the pineal gland, mediastinum, and sacrococcygeal region.

## CLASSIFICATION

The totipotential nature of germ cells results in a wide variety of histologic patterns (Fig. 90-1). Seminoma or dysgerminoma, a primitive germ cell tumor is unusual in childhood occurring primarily in the adolescent years. Embryonal carcinoma is capable of further differentiation into embryonic and extraembryonic tumors. Teratomas are the most common germ cell tumors and are classified as mature or immature teratomas. Teratomas contain elements from 1 or more of the embryonic layers: ectoderm, endoderm, and mesoderm.

Mature teratomas contain well-differentiated tissues whereas immature teratomas contain neuroepithelium and are graded between 1 and 3 based on the number of low-power fields of primitive tissue. Although both mature and immature teratomas are considered benign lesions, accurate histologic evaluation is imperative as up to 25% of some malignancies are mixed tumors with more than one type of tissue. In addition, grade 3 immature teratomas are associated with microscopic foci of yolk sac tumor. Yolk sac tumor, a highly malignant tumor also known as endodermal sinus tumor is the most common malignant histology and occurs commonly in the prepubertal extragonadal sites such as the sacrococcygeal, retroperitoneal, genital, and mediastinal regions as well as the prepubertal testes. Choriocarcinoma is relatively rare in childhood.

The survival for malignant germ cell tumors was poor prior to the introduction of cisplatin in 1977. The early pediatric trials combined cisplatin and bleomycin with other less effective chemotherapeutic agents thus likely limiting the survival. The Intergroup germ cell tumor studies conducted by the Pediatric Oncology Group (POG) and Children's Cancer Group (CCG) between 1990 and 1996 utilized cisplatin, etoposide and bleomycin (PEB) with overall excellent survival. The treatment schema was risk-based (Fig. 90-2) and survival by stage was excellent (Fig. 90-3).

Based on the results of this study the current study from the Children's Oncology Group was opened in 2003 (Fig. 90-4). There is no current open protocol for Stage IV ovarian tumors

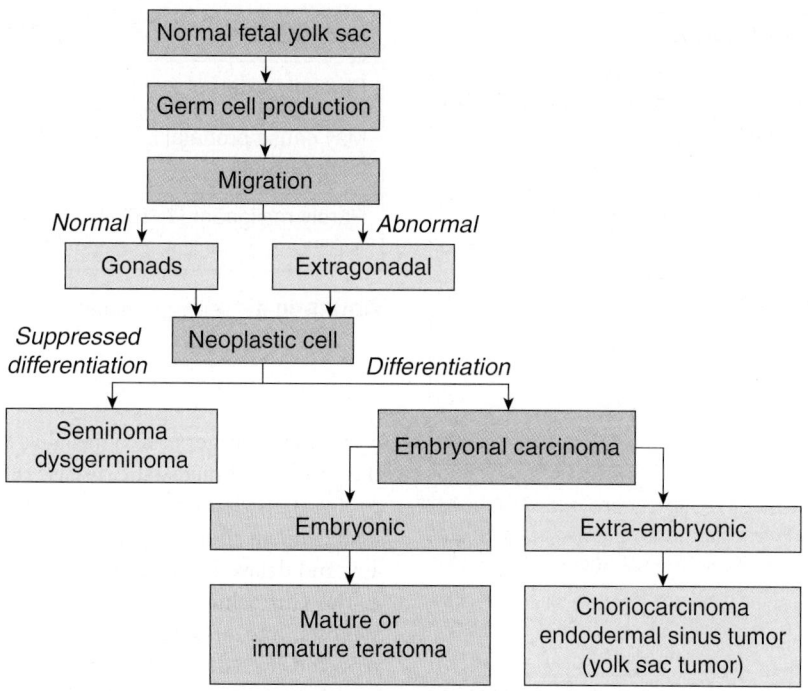

**FIGURE 90-1** The developmental schema for germ cell tumors.

or Stage III and IV extragonadal tumors and standard PEB would be administered.

## Sacrococcygeal Tumors

Germ cell tumors at this site are the most common extragonadal tumor in neonates. They can also present later in infancy and the clinical presentation is quite different based on age (Fig. 90-5). Altman et al reported the commonly utilized classification system for tumors at this location (Fig. 90-6) and noted the higher malignancy rate in the less apparent lesions (Type III and IV). In neonates, preoperative evaluation should seek to determine the degree of pelvic or abdominal extension and may also be useful to determine the vascular supply. In some cases, abdominal exploration may be required initially to resect or mobilize the pelvic portion with division of middle sacral artery prior to resection of the external portion. In addition, in cases with very high flow, it may be useful to have abdominal vascular control as shown in Fig. 90-7.

The basic steps of surgical excision for primarily external lesions are shown in Fig. 90-8. Removal of the coccyx is still considered an essential step and a drain is often placed. Fishman et al described a buttock contouring closure as shown in Fig. 90-9. As noted above, most of the neonatal lesions are benign (mature or immature teratomas) and require no further therapy. Follow-up should consist of serial AFP levels every 3 months to ensure that they are normal by 9 months of age along with rectal examinations until 3 years of age. Follow-up is essential as recurrence after resection of an initial benign lesion occurs in 10% to 20% of children, and of these, 50% are malignant. Long-term follow-up studies of newborns and older children have identified bladder and bowel abnormalities including neuropathic bladder and constipation and soiling in some children.

| Low risk | Stage I testes Immature teratomas (any site) | Surgery only |
|---|---|---|
| **Intermediate risk** | Stage II testes Stage I–II ovary | PEB × 4 (5 days) |
| **High risk** | Stage III–IV testes + ovary Stage I–IV extragonadal | High dose vs standard dose platinum × 4 + Etoposide Bleomycin |

**FIGURE 90-2** Risk-based treatment schema for the POG/CCG Intergroup Study, 1990-1996. P, cisplatin; E, etoposide; B, bleomycin; HDP, high-dose cisplatin.

| 1990–96 | CCG8891/POG9048 CCG8882/POG9049 | 515 pts |
|---|---|---|
| Stage | EFS | Survival |
| I | 87.7% | 96.9% |
| II | 93.8% | 96.9% |
| III | 86.5% | 90.8% |
| IV | 82.4% | 85.9% |

**FIGURE 90-3** Event-free survival (EFS) and survival by stage in the POG/CCG Intergroup Study, 1990-1996.

**Low risk – COG AGCT 0132 (5/03)**

| Stage I | | Surgery | |
|---|---|---|---|
| Testes | Ovary | alone | Closed 1/10 |
| All immature | Teratomas | | |

**Intermediate risk – COG AGCT 0132 (5/03)**

| Stage II–III | Ovary | Platinum (3d) |
|---|---|---|
| | + | Etoposide × 3 |
| **Stage II–IV** | Testes | Bleomycin |
| Stage I–II | Extragonadal | |

**High risk**

| Stage III–IV | Extragonadal | |
|---|---|---|
| | | PEB |
| Stage IV | Ovary | |

**FIGURE 90-4** Children's Oncology Group, current study AGCT 0132 (opened 2003). Low and intermediate risk treatment of pediatric germ cell tumors. High-risk tumors, no open protocol.

| Neonatal | Older child |
|---|---|
| Primarily external | Primarily internal |
| May cause prenatal hydrops compression | Present with symptoms of rectal/bladder |
| Rarely malignant (7–10%) | High malignancy rate (>70%) |

**FIGURE 90-5** Clinical presentation of SCTs.

Older infants and children often present with extensive unresectable lesions (Fig. 90-10). These are usually yolk sac tumors and are chemosensitive allowing initial biopsy, neoadjuvant chemotherapy, organ preservation, and post chemotherapy tumor resection. In the CCG/POG study of 74 infants, 59% had metastatic disease at presentation and most had initial biopsy only. Post chemotherapy resection was sacral only in 63% (Fig. 90-10C) and combined abdominal-sacral in 35%. Four year survival (Fig. 90-11) was not affected by timing of surgery (90% initial vs 83% delayed, $p = 0.50$) or the presence of metastatic disease (88% mets vs 80% no mets, $p = 0.48$). In view of this, if an extensive lesion is noted, initial management should be biopsy only, neoadjuvant chemotherapy, and delayed resection.

The Currarino triad consists of presacral teratoma, anal stenosis, and a sacral defect. This association was initially reported by Ashcraft and Holder who recognized the autosomal dominant nature of this condition. These defects are often difficult and neurosurgical assistance with resection or repair of neural defect with simultaneous anoplasty after initial colostomy is often required.

## Mediastinal Germ Cell Tumors

These tumors are usually located in the anterior mediastinum and most have a benign histology. Some however are

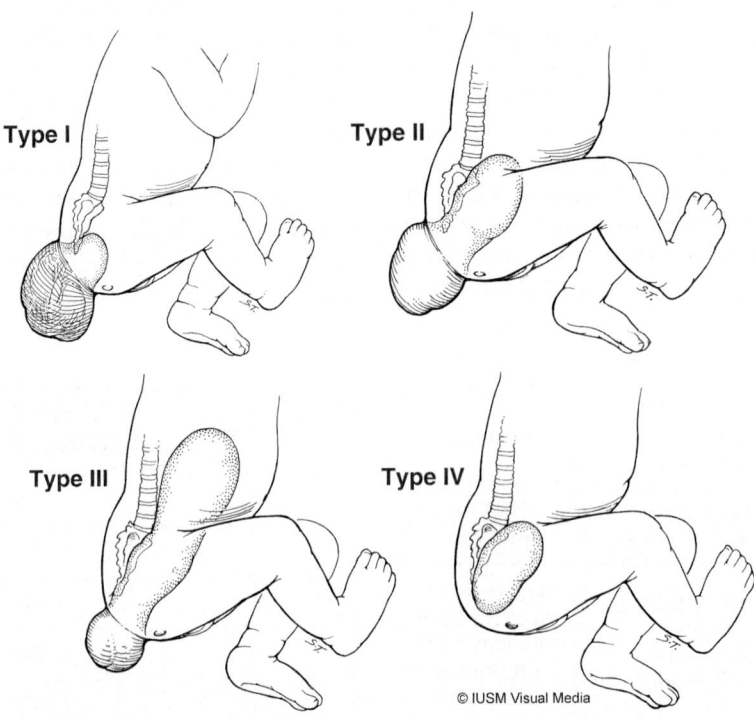

© IUSM Visual Media

**FIGURE 90-6** Classification of sacrococcygeal teratomas based on Altman's American Academy. **A.** Type I (46.7%) predominantly external. **B.** Type II (34.7%) external with intrapelvic extension. **C.** Type III (8.8%) visible externally but predominantly pelvic and abdominal. **D.** Type IV (9.8%) entirely presacral.

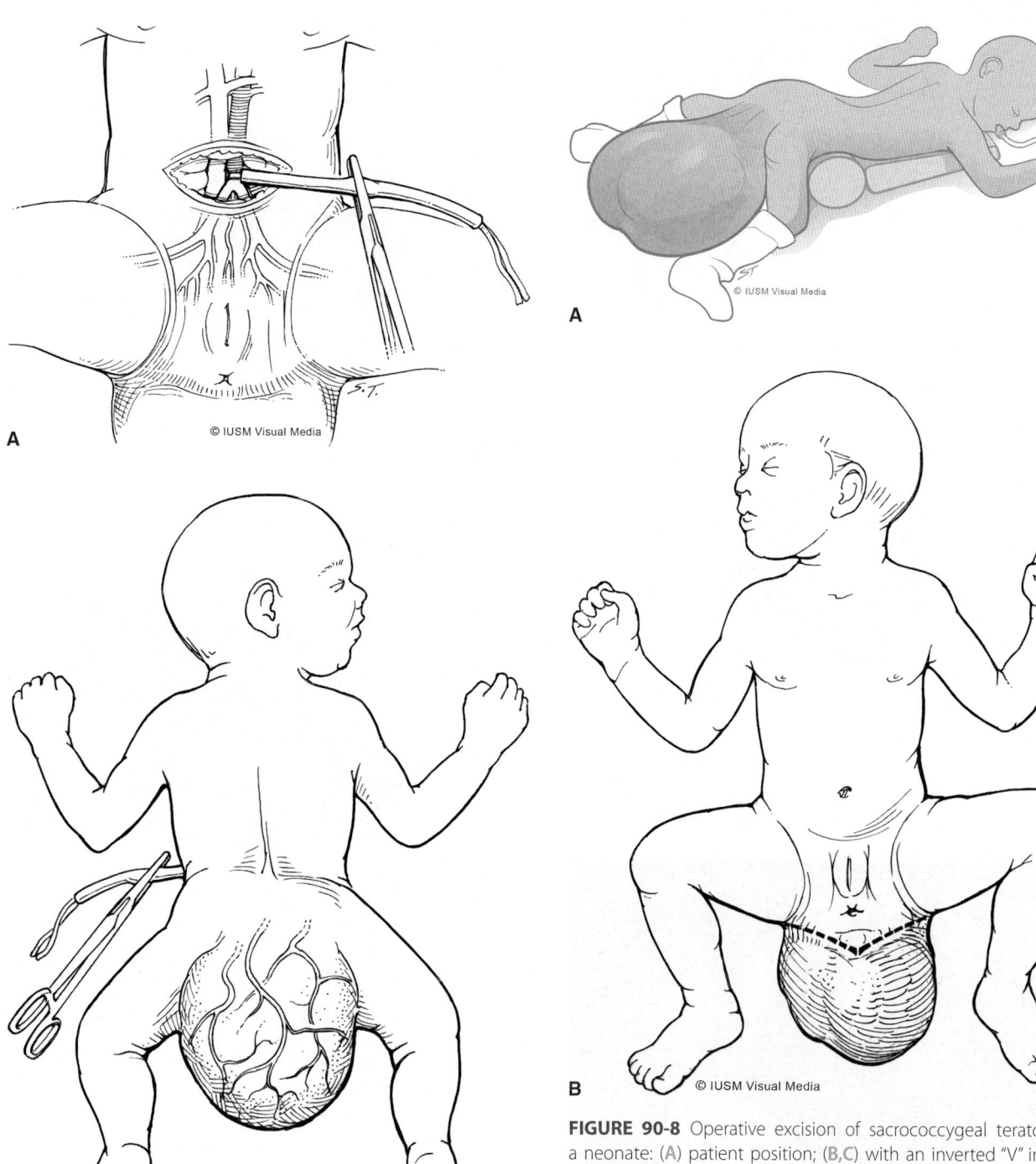

A

B

**FIGURE 90-7** **A,B.** A method of controlling the aorta to allow temporary vascular occlusion in high-flow tumors.

A

B

**FIGURE 90-8** Operative excision of sacrococcygeal teratoma in a neonate: (**A**) patient position; (**B,C**) with an inverted "V" incision; (**D**) the tumor along with the coccyx is excised; (**E**) use of a Hegar dilator to avoid injury to the rectum; (**F**) placement of sutures between the anal sphincter and presacral fascia.

malignant and can enlarge to cause respiratory symptoms and chest pain as well as symptoms of superior vena caval obstruction. Large tumors can cause airway obstruction and are associated with significant risk if a general anesthetic is utilized due to loss of spontaneous ventilation. If the tracheal area and peak expiratory flow rate are both greater than 50%, a general anesthetic is usually well tolerated. However, if this is not the case, alternative diagnostic procedures include aspiration of

pleural fluid, needle biopsy, or open biopsy utilizing an anterior thoracotomy (Chamberlin procedure) with excision of costal cartilage providing access to the mass (Fig. 90-12).

Many larger tumors can be treated with neoadjuvant chemotherapy with significant resolution in size allowing subsequent resection (Fig. 90-13). Median sternotomy or thoracotomy can be utilized for resection. In the COG/POG intergroup Study of 38 patients, 22 underwent biopsy followed by subsequent resection. Of a total of 31 resections, 20 were median sternotomy and 11 with thoracotomy. This is often a difficult procedure due to adherence to major vessel as well as

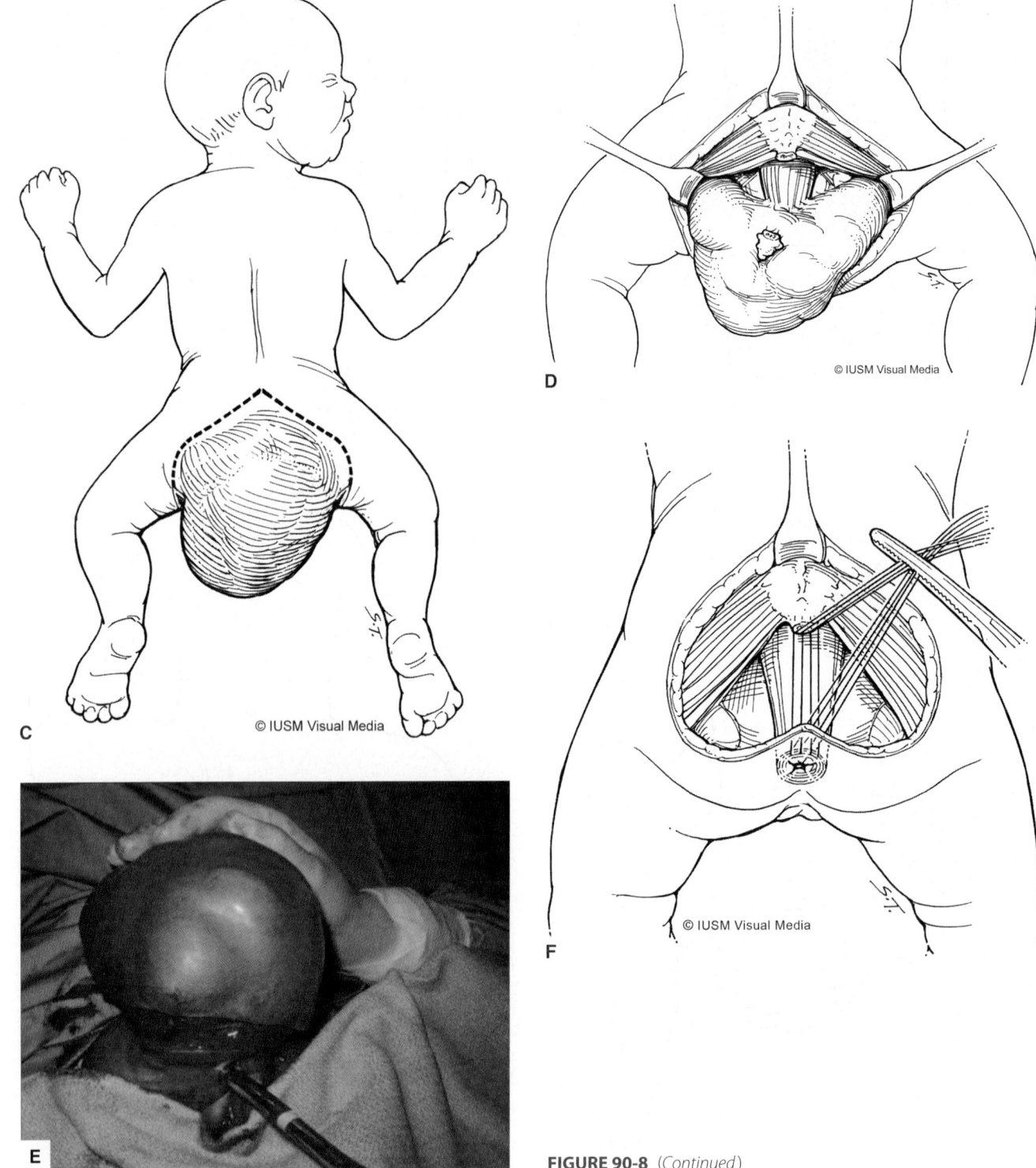

C

D

© IUSM Visual Media

E

F

© IUSM Visual Media

© IUSM Visual Media

**FIGURE 90-8** (*Continued*)

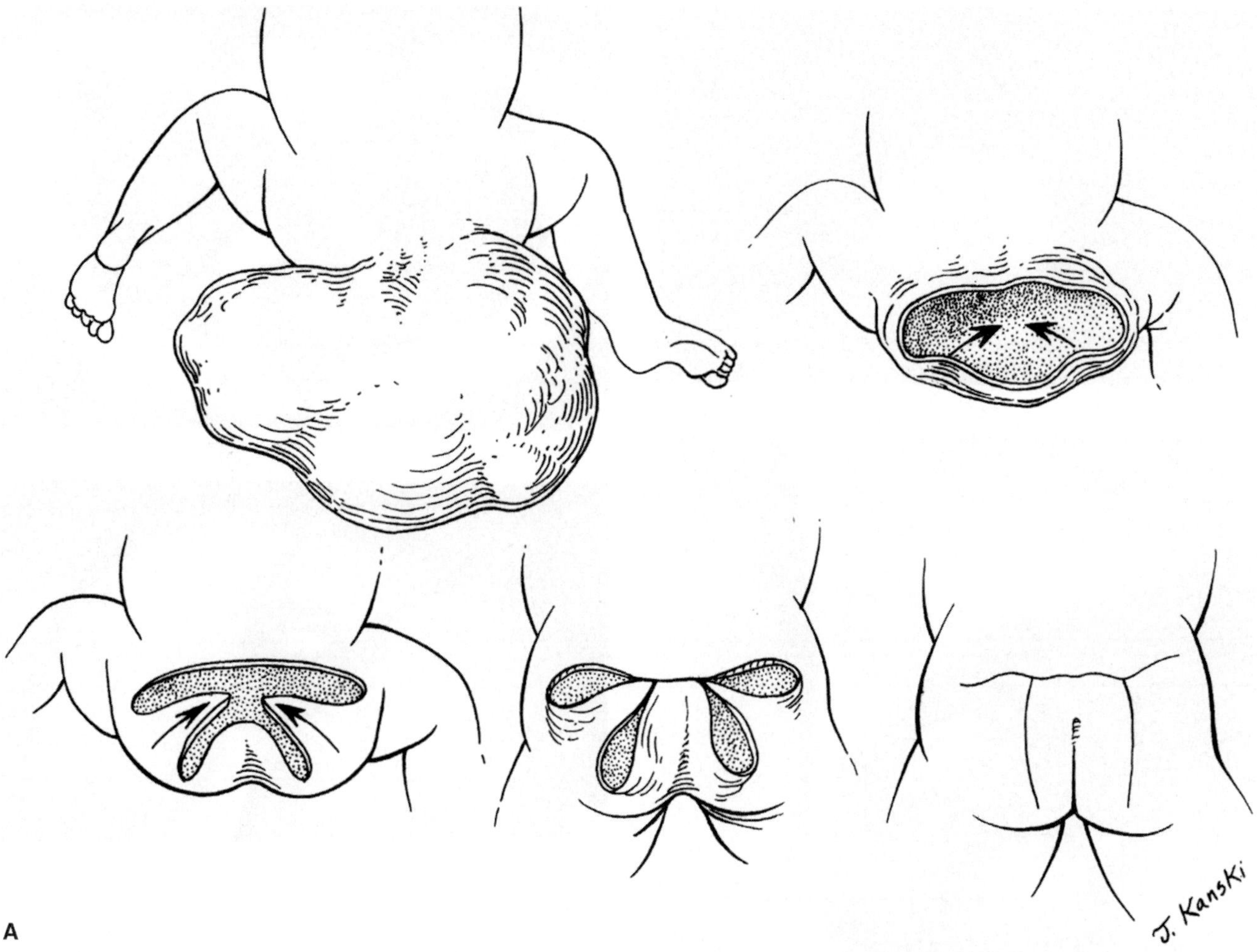

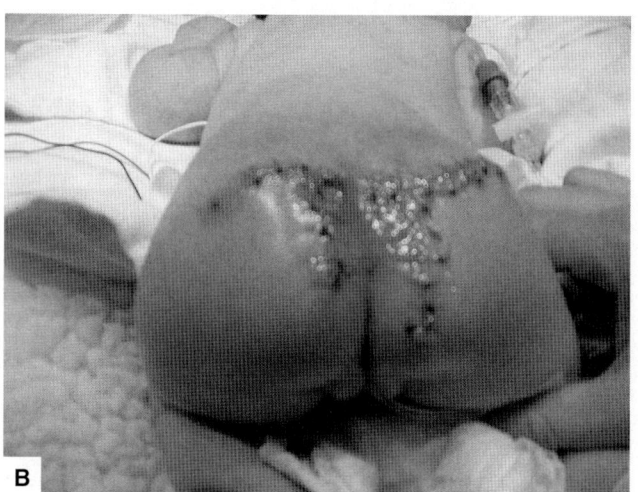

**A**

**B**

J. Kanski

**FIGURE 90-9 A.** Buttocks contouring closure as described by Fishman et al. **B.** Child treated with this technique. (A) (Reprinted with permission from Fishman SJ, Jennings RW, Johnson SM, et al. Contouring buttock reconstruction after sacrococcygeal teratoma resection. *J Pediatr Surg* 2004;39:439–441.)

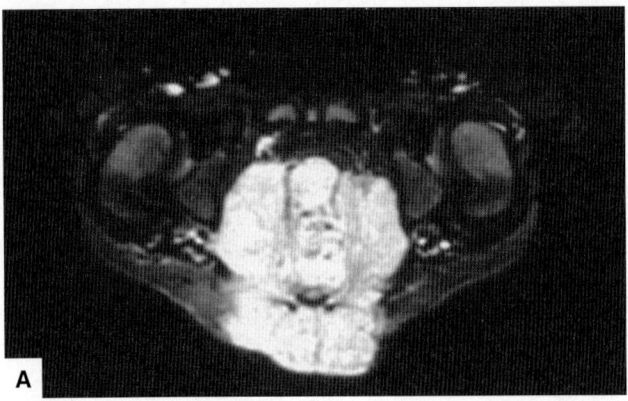

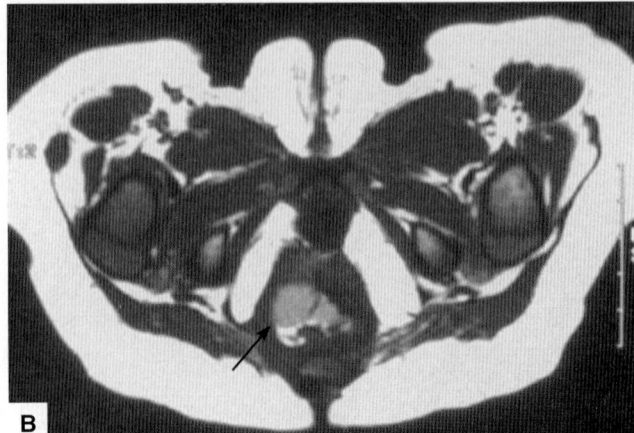

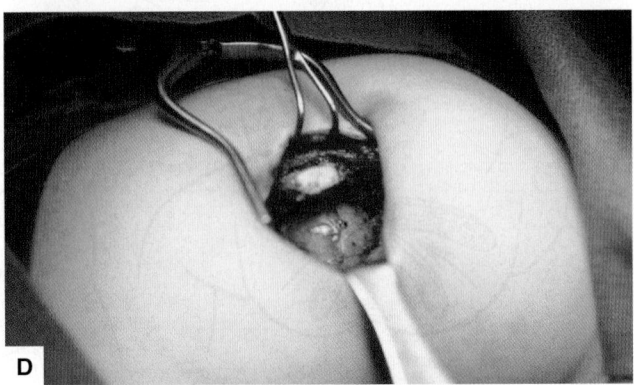

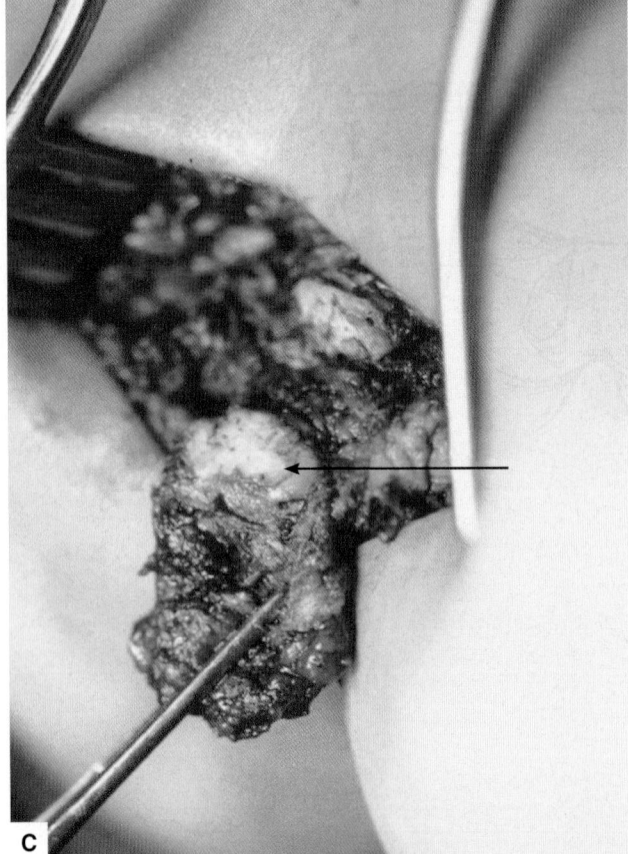

**FIGURE 90-10 A.** Large unresectable malignant SCT yolk sac histology, AFP 272,000 ng/mL in a 15-month-old girl. **B.** Post PEB chemotherapy CT of same tumor (arrow) AFP 22 ng/mL. **C.** Photograph of limited posterior resection with resection of residual tumor and coccyx (arrow). **D.** View of rectum in the base of wound.

the phrenic and vagus nerves. The survival in the Intergroup Study was 71% which is higher than historical series but lower than tumors at the other extragonadal sites (Fig. 90-11).

## Abdominal and Retroperitoneal

Most germ cell tumors at these sites present in infancy with an abdominal or pelvic mass and pain, the most common presenting symptoms. Most tumors at this location are mature and immature teratomas with rates of malignancy ranging from 0% to 24%. A rare type within this group is the infantile choriocarcinoma which is thought to be a placental tumor with metastases to the fetal liver.

The histologic pattern of the malignant tumors at this site is usually the yolk sac but can also include choriocarcinoma and mixed tumors. In the POG/CCG Study, 19 of 24 had elevated

AFP levels and of these 15 were pure yolk sac tumors, 4 mixed histology tumors and 5 other histology. Primary resection should be performed if the tumor can be removed without injuring or removing other uninvolved organs. Several studies have demonstrated the hazardous nature of these procedures with major vascular, intestinal, and bile duct injuries. In the Intergroup Study, only 5 underwent complete initial resection and the remaining had postchemo resections. Of interest, 4 had no residual post-chemo tumor. The survival with chemotherapy and surgery has risen from 20% to the current survival of 87% (Fig. 90-11).

## Genital (Vaginal)

This rare site has served as an example of the ability of neoadjuvant chemotherapy to not only eliminate a large volume of

| | N | Treatment | 6 yr. EFS (%) | 6 yr. Survival (%) |
|---|---|---|---|---|
| Retroperitoneal/ Abd | 26 | HDP/EB vs PEB | 82.8 | 87.6 |
| Sacrococcygeal | 74 | HDP/EB vs PEB | 4yr. EFS (%) 84 | 4yr. survival (%) 90 |
| Mediastinal | 38 | HDP/EB vs PEB | 69 | 71 |
| Genital | 13 | HDP/EB vs PEB | 76.2 | 91.7 |

**FIGURE 90-11** Event-free survival (EFS) for malignant extragonadal tumors by site.

disease but to change the residual to a benign histology, usually mature teratoma. These girls are less than 3 years of age and present with a mass or vaginal bleeding (Fig. 90-14). The girl in Fig. 90-14 had an AFP of 85,000 ng/mL. She underwent biopsy of the protruding vaginal mass demonstrating yolk sac tumor and after chemotherapy had minimal vaginal residual which was removed by a partial vaginectomy. Pathology at resection revealed mature teratoma. On the recent Intergroup Study, vaginal preservation was possible in 10 of 12 girls. There is no role for initial total vaginectomy or hysterectomy.

## Cervicofacial

This rare site generally consists of mature or immature teratomas presenting in the neonatal period. Approximately

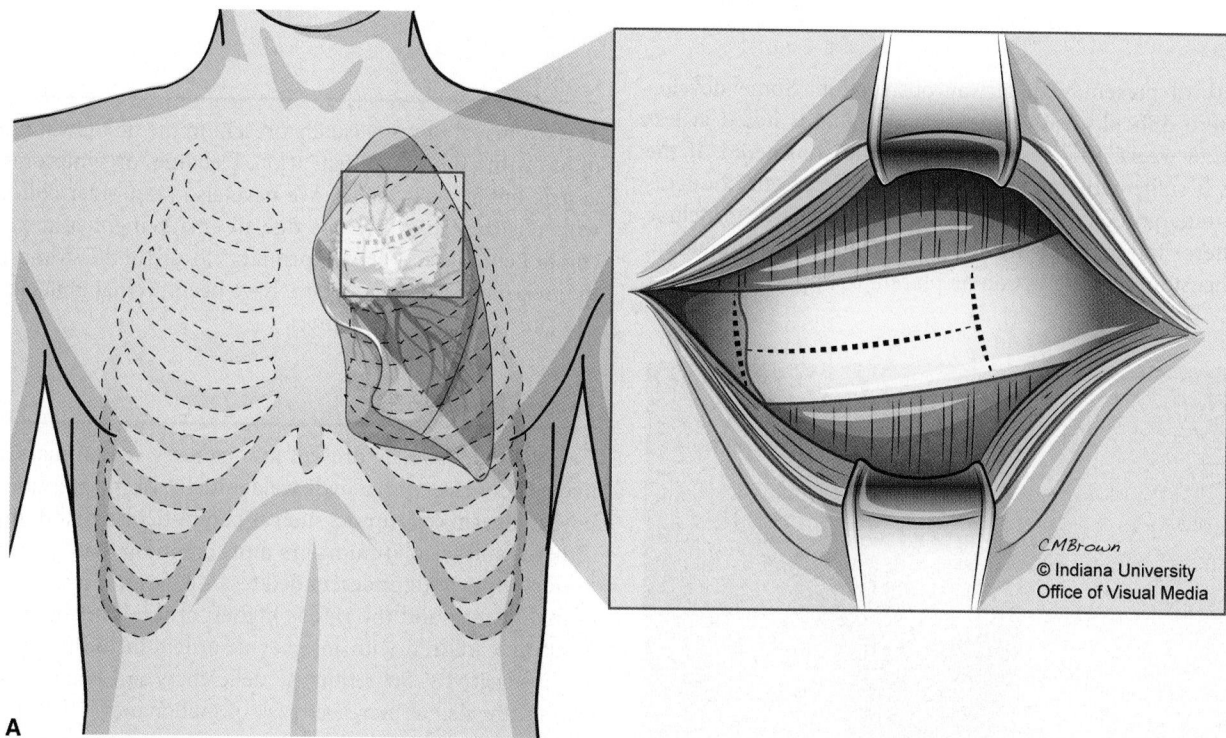

A

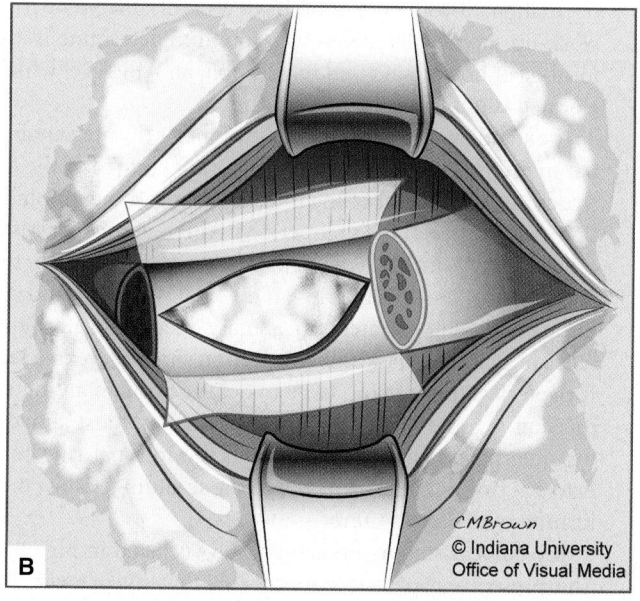

B

**FIGURE 90-12** A,B. Chamberlin procedure for biopsy of an anterior mediastinal tumor.

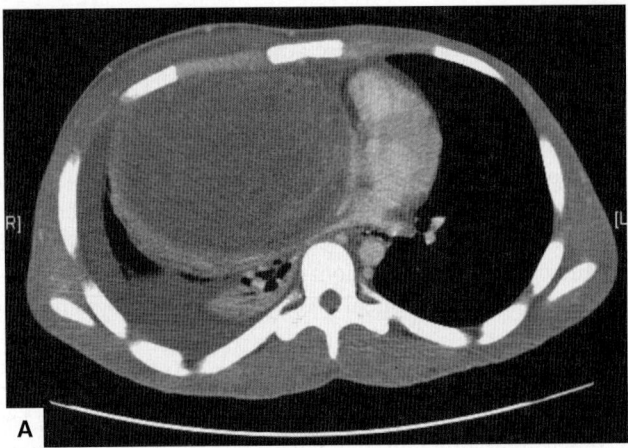
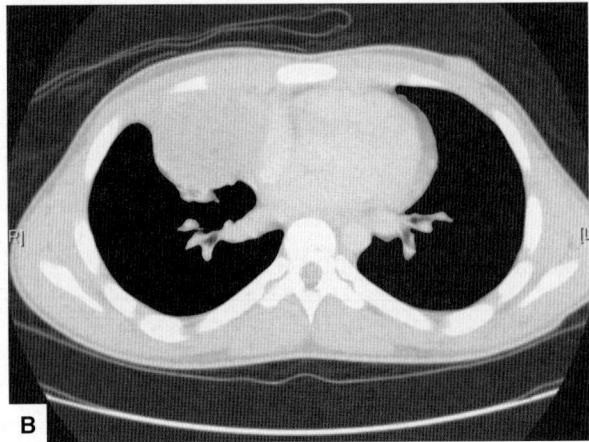

**FIGURE 90-13** **A.** Mediastinal malignant germ cell tumor at diagnosis with pleural effusion; diagnosed with needle biopsy demonstrating germ cell tumor. **B.** post neoadjuvant chemotherapy with significant size reduction, resected through a thoracotomy.

one-third present with airway obstruction. Some develop in-utero difficulty with hydrops and if this is noted at less than 28 weeks fetal resection should be considered. If the fetus is sufficiently mature and hydrops is present, the fetus can undergo delivery. Options to assist at delivery include ex-utero intrapartum treatment (EXIT) with intubation, tracheostomy, and resection on placental support.

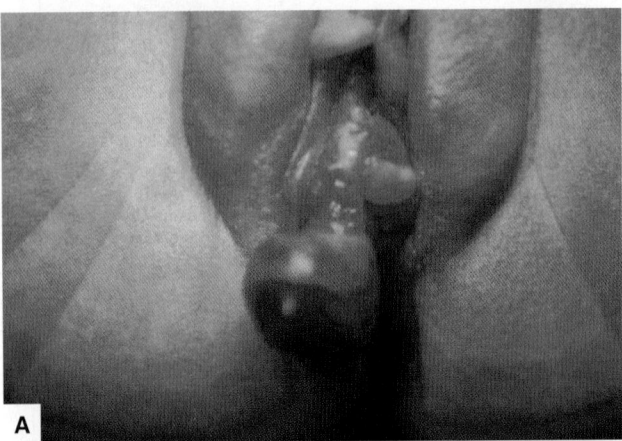

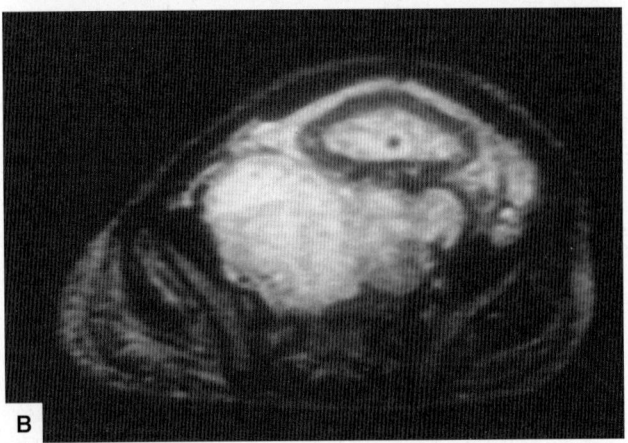

**FIGURE 90-14** **A.** A 16-month-old girl with vaginal bleeding and a mass. **B.** CT scan demonstrates a large pelvic tumor that encases the upper vaginal and uterus.

## Gastric

These unusual tumors usually present in the first few months of life with abdominal distention, bleeding, or symptoms of gastric outlet obstruction. We have also seen older children with obstructive symptoms due to enlargement of a cystic component. Resection with primary closure of the stomach is the treatment of choice. There have been no malignancies at this site as most are teratomas.

## Testes Tumors

Testes tumors usually present as a painless scrotal mass and maybe confused with a hydrocele initially. In the prepubertal boys nongerm cell tumors such as paratesticular rhabdomyo-sarcoma and sertoli tumors are more common than germ cell tumors. Boys with undescended testes have an increased risk of malignancy and the risk is highest at the intraabdominal location. Children with intersex disorders including andro-gen insensitivity, 5α reductase deficiency, and gonadal dys-genesis are also at increased risk of malignancy. Of all germ cell tumors, teratoma (a benign lesion) is more common than the malignant yolk sac tumor. In view of this, the preoperative work-up should include an ultrasound to determine if it is a focal or uniform mass and in addition, an AFP level which if elevated is indicative of yolk sac tumor.

The standard approach to testes tumors is through an inguinal incision (Fig. 90-15) with temporary control of the cord structures at the level of the internal ring and then mobilization of the testes. If the preoperative AFP is elevated, a radical orchiectomy is undertaken with ligation of all cord structures at the level of the internal ring. If the AFP is normal, and if the ultrasound demonstrates a focal mass, there is greater probability of a benign mass and enucleation should be considered. If the testes tumor is too large to deliver through an inguinal incision, a more oblique incision parallel and just above the inguinal ligament can extend from the internal ring to the external ring and then down onto the scrotum to allow mobilization of the testes tumor.

The current staging system of COG is listed in Fig. 90-16. The presence of retroperitoneal adenopathy of over 4 cm

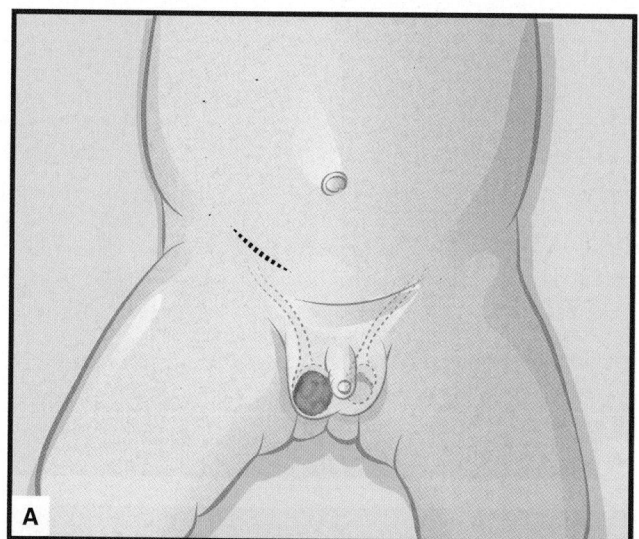

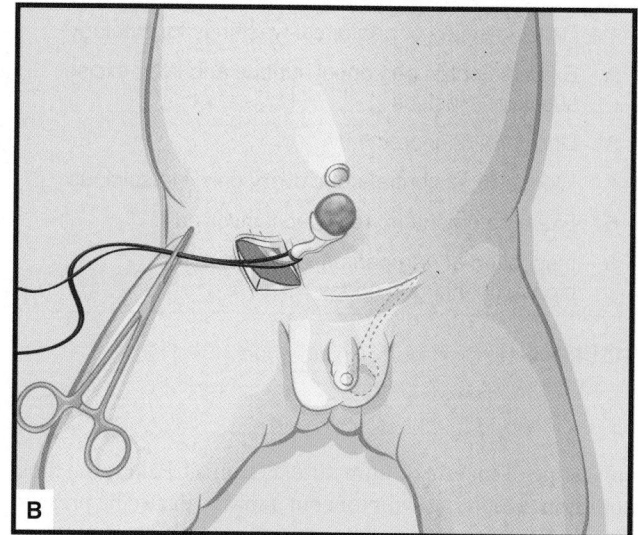

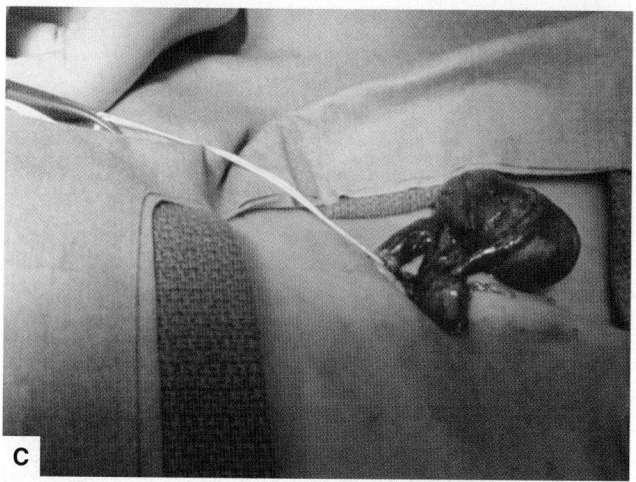

**FIGURE 90-15** A,B. Surgical approach to a testes tumor with control of vessels at the internal ring. C. Operative photo.

in size is assumed to be malignant whereas nodal disease between 2 and 4 cm requires biopsy. There is no role for RPLND in prepubertal boys. The surgical treatment and survival from the recent study are listed in Fig. 90-17. As noted all Stage I patients with relapse were successfully salvaged with chemotherapy. The current treatment algorithm for

testes tumors is shown in Fig. 90-4. Compared with the Intergroup Study (1990-1996), this protocol decreases the number of treatment days by 55% and total dose of chemotherapy by 25% in those with a complete response.

## Ovary

The ovary is the most common site for germ cell tumors in children and adolescents and 80% to 90% of these are benign

| | |
|---|---|
| **I** | • Limited to testis<br>• Completely resected by high inguinal orchiectomy<br>• No clinical, radiographic, or histologic evidence of disease beyond the testes<br>• Markers normal after appropriate half life decline.<br>• Transscrotal orchiectomy |
| **II** | • Microscopic disease in scrotum or high in spermatic cord (≤5 cm from proximal end)<br>• Increased tumor markers after appropriate half life decline. |
| **III** | • Retroperitoneal lymph node involvement (>4 cm by CT, or 2–4 cm with biopsy proof).<br>• No visceral or extra-abdominal involvement |
| **IV** | • Metastatic |

**FIGURE 90-16** COG testes staging system.

| | | Testes | | |
|---|---|---|---|---|
| | **N** | **Treatment** | **6 yr. EFS (%)** | **6 yr. Survival (%)** |
| Stage I | 63 | Surgery alone | 78.5 | 100 |
| Stage II | 17 | PEB x4 | 100 | 100 |
| Stage III | 17 | HDP/EB vs. PEB | 94.1 | 100 |
| Stage IV | 43 | | 88.3 | 90.6 |

**FIGURE 90-17** Treatment schema and results for malignant testes tumor, on Intergroup Study 1990-1996, P, cisplatin; E, etoposide; B, bleomycin; HDP, high-dose cisplatin.

1. Collect ascites or peritoneal washings for cytology

2. Examine entire peritoneal surface and liver; excise suspicious lesions

3. Unilateral oophorectomy

4. Wedge Bx of contralateral ovary only if suspicious

5. Examine omentum, removed if involved

6. Inspection of retroperitoneal lymph nodes, biopsy of enlarged nodes

**FIGURE 90-18** Ovarian staging procedure.

consisting of mature or immature teratomas. Pain is the most common presenting symptom but a mass can also be present. Ten percent present with torsion. Preoperative assessment usually includes an ultrasound and/or abdominal and pelvic CT scan and tumor markers should be determined prior to surgical exploration.

The ability to differentiate benign from malignant lesions preoperatively is difficult. Although benign lesions are primarily cystic and a 2% risk of malignancy is frequently quoted in the adult literature for these lesions, the Intergroup Study of 131 girls noted that 57% of malignant tumors had cystic components. In addition, elevated markers are only noted in around 57% of malignant tumors. One recent study noted that the best predictor of malignancy is a solid mass greater than 8 cm. The recommendation of the COG surgeons is to approach all lesions with any solid component as a potential malignant lesion and plan a proper staging procedure as listed in Fig. 90-18. The COG staging system is noted in Fig. 90-19. In view of the chemosensitive nature of these tumors, the current recommendation for tumors which invade surrounding structures is to avoid resection of such structures as the uterus and simply to perform a biopsy. The recommendation for bilateral lesions is to attempt ovarian preservation on the least affected side. Initial biopsy and neo-adjuvant chemotherapy followed by delayed resection with an attempt of ovarian preservation is the preferred approach.

**Stage I:** Limited to ovary (ovaries) peritoneal washings negative; tumor markers normal after appropriate half-life decline, (AFP 5 days, HCG 16 hours); *omentum (-) by inspection.*

**Stage II:** Microscopic residual, negative lymph nodes, peritoneal washings negative for malignant cells, tumor markers positive or negative.

**Stage III:** Lymph node involvement; gross residual or biopsy only; contiguous visceral involvement (omentum, intestine, bladder); peritoneal washings positive for malignant cells; tumor markers positive or negative.

**Stage IV:** Distant metastases, including liver.

**FIGURE 90-19** COG ovarian staging system.

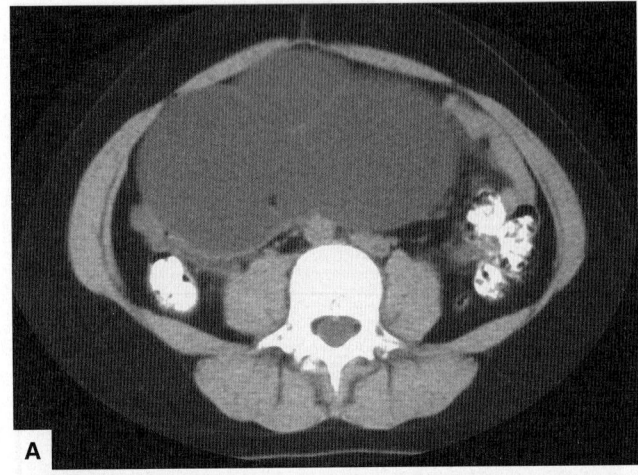

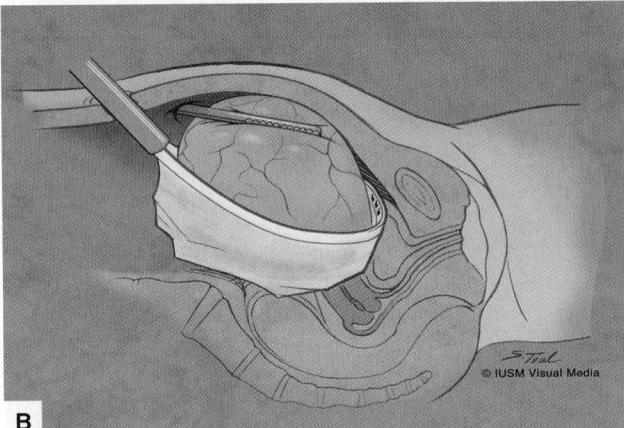

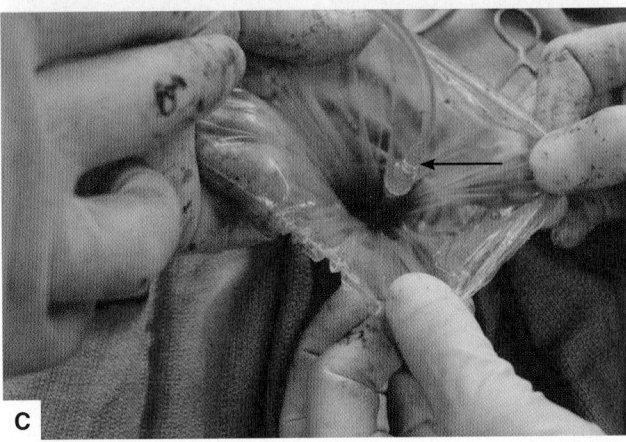

**FIGURE 90-20** **A.** Large multicystic ovarian tumor. **B.** Laparoscopic removal of ovarian tumor. **C.** Decompression of the cystic component inside of a retrieval bag.

It is reasonable to approach completely cystic lesions with a laparoscopic approach. The primary concern is to avoid spill of a malignant tumor leading to upstaging of the tumor. There are several techniques to avoid spill. One option is to place the lesion in a retrieval bag with delivery of the neck of the bag through the umbilicus and then decompression of the cyst allowing removal of the bag and contained empty cyst (Fig. 90-20). Another option for larger cysts is to utilize an adhesive (cyanoacrylate) to glue a bag to the cyst through a small (5 cm) incision thus allowing delivery of the mass

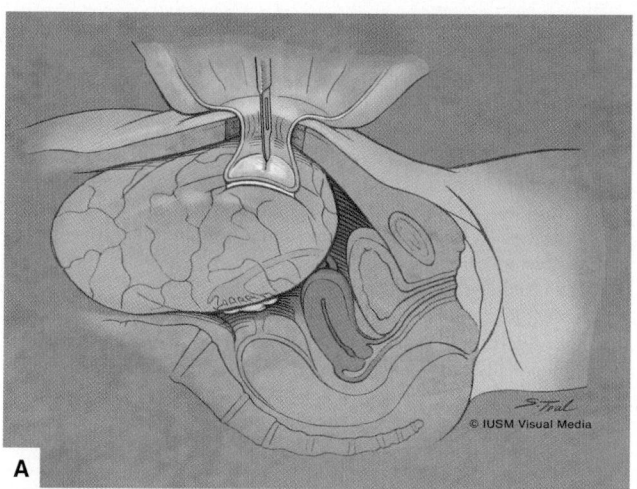

A

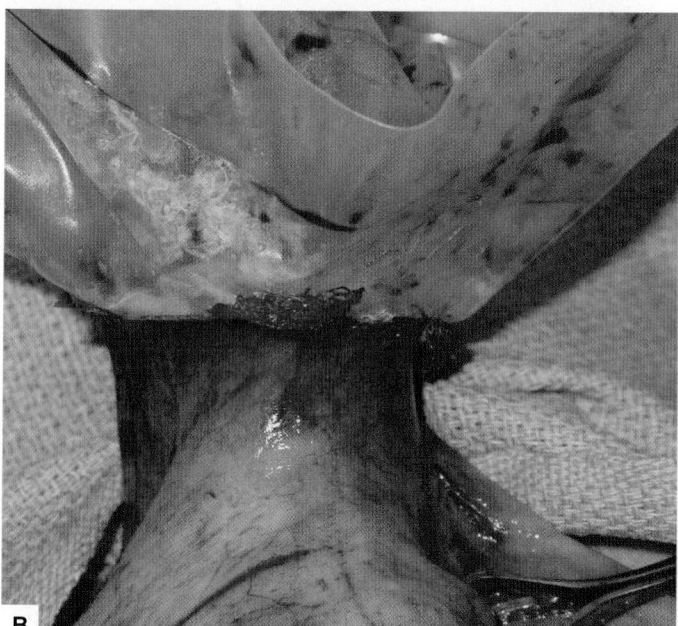

B

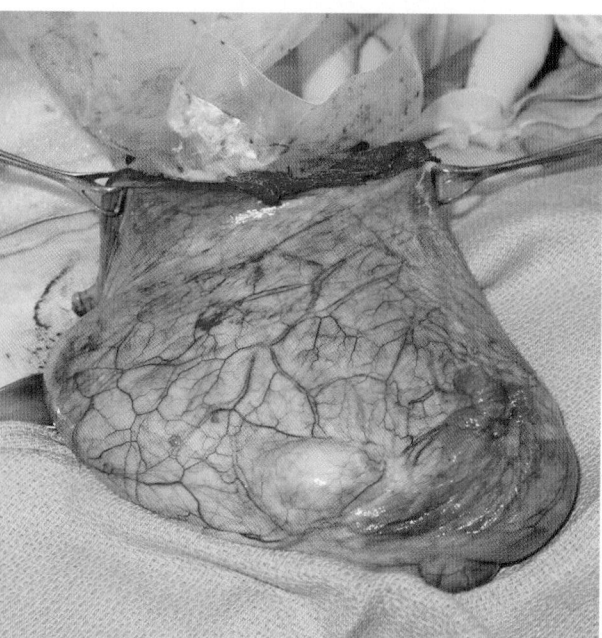

**FIGURE 90-21** **A.** Technique of gluing a bag to the cyst allowing decompression of the cyst. **B.** Operative photograph of the technique with delivery of a large cystic lesion through a small incision.

TERATOMA

(Fig. 90-21). This can also allow delivery of the ovary into the incision and consideration of an ovary preserving procedure.

The Intergroup Study results are listed in Fig. 90-22. Based on the excellent results of the Stage I patients, as well as 2 European studies utilizing surgery alone for Stage I tumors with very good salvage rates with chemotherapy for relapse,

the current protocol (Fig. 90-4) was established in 2003 to treat Stage I ovarian tumors with surgery alone. Unfortunately, the low-risk stratum has been closed due to higher than anticipated recurrence rate in these girls.

## SELECTED READINGS

Altman RP, Randolph JG, Lilly JR. Sacrococcygeal teratoma: American Academy of Pediatric Surgical Section Survey—1973. *J Pediatr Surg* 1974;9:389–398.

Ashcraft KW, Holder TM. Hereditary presacral teratoma. *J Pediatr Surg* 1974;9:691–697.

Billmire D, Vinocur C, Rescorla F, et al. Malignant mediastinal germ cell tumors: an intergroup study. *J Pediatr Surg* 2001;36:18–24.

Billmire D, Vinocur C, Rescorla F, et al. Malignant retroperitoneal and abdominal germ cell tumors: an intergroup study. *J Pediatr Surg* 2003;38:315–318.

Billmire D, Vinocur C, Rescorla F, et al. Outcome and staging evaluation in malignant germ cell tumors of the ovary in children and adolescents: an intergroup study. *J Pediatr Surg* 2004;39:424–429.

Cushing B, Giller R, Cullen JW, et al. Randomized comparison of combination chemotherapy with etoposide, bleomycin, and either high-dose or standard-dose cisplatin in children and adolescents with high-risk

| | N | Treatment | 6 yr. EFS (%) | 6 yr. Survival (%) |
|---|---|---|---|---|
| Stage I | 41 | PEB x4 | 95 | 95.1 |
| Stage II | 16 | | 87.5 | 93.8 |
| Stage III | 58 | HDP/EB vs PEB | 96.6 | 97.3 |
| Stage IV | 16 | | 86.7 | 93.3 |

**FIGURE 90-22** Treatment schema and EFS and survival of ovarian tumors from the Intergroup Study (1990-1996). P, cisplatin; E, etoposide; B, bleomycin; HPD, high-dose cisplatin.

malignant germ cell tumors: a Pediatric Intergroup Study-Pediatric Oncology Group 9049 and Children's Cancer Group 8882. *J Clin Oncol* 2004;22:2691–2700.

Einhorn LH, Donohue J. *Cis*-diamminedichloroplatinum, vinblastine, and bleomycin combination chemotherapy in disseminated testicular cancer. *Ann Intern Med* 1977;87:293–298.

Fishman SJ, Jennings RW, Johnson SM, et al. Contouring buttock reconstruction after sacrococcygeal teratoma resection. *J Pediatr Surg* 2004;39:439–441.

Gothard JWW. Anesthetic considerations for patients with anterior mediastinal masses. *Anesthesiology Clin* 2008;26:305–314.

Hirose S, Sydorak RM, Tsao K, et al. Spectrum of intrapartum management strategies for giant fetal cervical teratoma. *J Pediatr Surg* 2003;38:446–450.

Rescorla F, Billmire D, Stolar C, et al. The effect of cisplatin dose and surgical resection in children with malignant germ cell tumors at the sacrococcygeal region: a pediatric intergroup trial (POG 9049/CCG8882). *J Pediatr Surg* 2001;36:12–17.

Rescorla F, Billmire D, Vinocur C, et al. The effect of neoadjuvant chemotherapy and surgery in children with malignant germ cell tumors of the genital region: a pediatric intergroup trial. *J Pediatr Surg* 2003;38:910–912.

Rogers PC, Olson TA, Cullen JW, et al. Treatment of children and adolescents with stage II testicular and stages I and II ovarian malignant germ cell tumors: a Pediatric Intergroup Study-Pediatric Oncology Group 9048 and Children's Cancer Group 8891. *J Clin Oncol* 2004;22:3563–3569.

Schlatter M, Rescorla F, Giller R, et al. Excellent outcome in patients with stage I germ cell tumors of the testes: a study of the Children's Cancer Group/Pediatric Oncology Group. *J Pediatr Surg* 2003;38:319–324.

# CHAPTER 91

# Diagnosis and Treatment of Rhabdomyosarcoma

*Felicia N. Williams and David A. Rodeberg*

## KEY POINTS

1. Overall 5-year survival for rhabdomyosarcoma has increased from 25% to 70% over the past 50 years.

2. Embryonal rhabdomyosarcoma (ERMS) occurs in younger children and has a more favorable survival rate of 60%.

3. In patients with alveolar tumors (ARMS), the presence of regional nodes disease indicates a significantly worse prognosis, similar to metastatic disease, whereas in ERMS tumors the outcomes for patients with regional node disease is not any different than localized disease.

4. All patients with RMS receive some form of chemotherapy. Standard therapeutic regimens consist of a combination of vincristine, actinomycin-D, and cyclophosphamide (VAC).

5. Radiotherapy (RT) is an important adjunct to therapy for many children diagnosed with RMS, offering improved local control and outcomes.

6. A more aggressive surgical approach may be warranted for recurrent RMS and debulking is indicated in retroperitoneal tumors.

## INTRODUCTION

Prior to 1960, the pillar of therapy for rhabdomyosarcoma (RMS) was aggressive surgical resection, often including removal of a significant amount of normal tissue. Operations were often disfiguring and outcomes disappointing, with survival rates from 7% to 70% depending on tumor location. The addition of chemotherapy to the RMS treatment algorithm in 1961 improved these outcomes. The addition of radiotherapy (RT) in 1965 to select patients further improved outcomes and decreased the need for aggressive radical operations. Recognition of the crucial contribution of multimodal therapy to the treatment of RMS led to the establishment of the Intergroup Rhabdomyosarcoma Study Group (IRSG) in 1972. Subsequently, IRSG merged with other pediatric cooperative oncology groups in North American to form the Children's Oncology Group (COG). RMS studies were continued by the Soft Tissue Sarcoma Committee (STS) of the COG. With all of these efforts, the overall 5-year survival rate of RMS has increased from 25% to 70% (Fig. 91-1). However, these improvements in outcome have plateaued and now appear limited by the poor outcomes experienced in patients with metastatic or relapsed RMS.

## RMS PATIENT DEMOGRAPHICS

In the first 2 decades of life, RMS is the most common form of soft-tissue sarcoma accounting for 4.5% of all cases of childhood cancer. It is the third most common extracranial solid tumor of childhood after Wilms tumor and neuroblastoma. Age at presentation follows a bimodal distribution with peak incidences between 2 and 6 years and again between 10 and 18 years of age. This distribution reflects the occurrence of the 2 major histologic subtypes of RMS: embryonal (ERMS) and alveolar (ARMS). The incidence of ERMS is highest at birth and extends through childhood but declines in adolescence. In contrast, the frequency of ARMS is low in infants and peaks during childhood and adolescence. Approximately 65% of all cases of RMS occur in children younger than 6 years of age. Slightly more males (58.4%) are affected than females (41.6%) and Caucasians have a higher incidence than African Americans (rate ratio 1.2).

## RMS TUMOR BIOLOGY

RMS is a malignant tumor of mesenchymal origin. It is included in the group of small blue, round cell tumors of childhood along with neuroblastoma, lymphoma, and primitive neuroectodermal tumors (PNET). The 2 major histologic subtypes of RMS are embryonal and alveolar. ERMS is the most common histology affecting two-thirds of all patients. ERMS can be further divided into spindle-cell and botryoid subtypes. Spindle-cell histology is common in paratesticular lesions whereas botryoid lesions are generally polypoid masses filling the lumen of a hollow viscus such as the vagina, bladder, and extrahepatic bile ducts. Histologically ERMS is typically comprised of spindle shaped cells with a rich stroma. ERMS tumors occur more frequently in the head

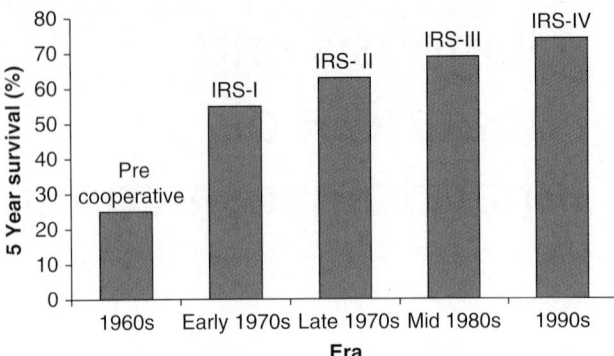

**FIGURE 91-1** Improvement in survival for RMS over the past 40 years.

and neck region as compared to the extremities. In addition to occurring in younger patients, ERMS has a more favorable survival rate of 60%.

ARMS tumors occur in older children and tumors are most commonly located on the trunk or extremities. Histologically these lesions are comprised of small round densely packed cells arranged around spaces resembling pulmonary alveoli. However, this histologic classification of RMS may in the near future be supplanted by gene array analysis. Prognosis is worse in ARMS with a 5-year survival rate of 54%.

The pathogenesis of RMS remains unclear, however, many hypotheses exist. It is largely thought that RMS arises as a consequence of regulatory disruption of skeletal muscle progenitor cell growth and differentiation. Pathogenic roles have been suggested for the MET proto-oncogene, involved in migration of myogenic precursor cells, and the p53 proto-oncogene responsible for tumor suppression.

Translocations of the FKHR transcription factor gene (chromosome 13) with either PAX3 (chromosome 2) or PAX 7 (chromosome 1) transcription factor genes occur in approximately 75% of ARMS tumors. In these PAX/FKHR fusions, the DNA binding domain of PAX is combined with the regulatory domain of FKHR. This results in increased PAX activity leading to the undifferentiation and proliferation of myogenic cells. Understanding the role of these fusion proteins in tumor development may provide insight into treatment strategies and potential biomarkers for the diagnosis of RMS. Approximately 25% of ARMS tumors are translocation negative. By gene array analysis these fusion negative ARMS tumors more closely resemble ERMS and have a prognosis similar to ERMS. Therefore, it has been proposed that tumors should be divided into PAX/FKHR fusion positive and negative tumors rather than by the more ambiguous alveolar and embryonal histologies.

Although most cases of RMS occur sporadically, the disease is associated with familial syndromes, including Li Fraumeni and Neurofibromatosis I. Li Fraumeni is an autosomal-dominant disorder usually associated with a germline mutation of p53. Patients with this syndrome present with RMS at an early age and have a family history of other carcinomas, especially premenopausal breast carcinoma. Neurofibromatosis is an autosomal dominant genetic disorder characterized by optic gliomas, café-au-lait spots, and neurofibromas. The association of RMS with Li Fraumeni and Neurofibromatosis appears to involve malignant transformation

through the inactivation of the p53 tumor suppressor gene, and hyperactivation of the RAS oncogene. While no specific carcinogens have been identified, benzenediazonium sulfate has been shown to induce RMS in mice. Maternal marijuana or cocaine use in pregnancy may be an environmental factor that contributes to the development of RMS. There are ongoing trials looking at the correlation between birth weight and the risk of RMS.

## PRESENTATION AND EVALUATION OF RMS

### Presentation of RMS

RMS typically presents as an asymptomatic mass found by the patient or the parents of younger children. Specific symptoms vary based on the site of occurrence and extent of disease and are generally related to mass effect or complications of the tumor. The most common sites of primary disease are the head and neck region, the genitourinary tract, and the extremities.

### Preoperative Evaluation

Patients with suspected RMS require a complete workup prior to surgical intervention. Standard lab work, including complete blood counts (CBC), electrolytes, renal function tests, liver function tests (LFTs), and urinalysis (UA) should be performed. In addition, imaging studies of the primary tumor should be performed with computed tomography (CT) or magnetic resonance imaging (MRI). CT is advantageous for the evaluation of bone erosion and abdominal adenopathy, whereas MRI frequently provides better definition of the primary tumor and surrounding structures. MRI may be preferable for limb, pelvic, and paraspinal lesions. Evaluation for metastatic disease includes a bone marrow aspirate and bone scan, CT of the brain, lungs, and liver, and lumbar puncture for cerebrospinal fluid collection.

Imaging of the primary tumor defines the proximity of the tumor to vital structures and determines size. Proximity to vital structures is important for the determination of whether or not the tumor can be primarily resected or if neo-adjuvant therapy is required to potentially decrease the morbidity of resection and improve the chances for complete resection. It has been demonstrated that the size of the primary tumor, with a cut point of tumor diameter at 5 cm as determined by pretreatment imaging, carries prognostic significance.

Evaluation of regional and distant lymph nodes, by clinical and radiographic means should be performed since this is an important component of pretreatment staging. Determination of lymph node involvement is important since positive regional nodes are irradiated and distant nodes are considered metastatic disease. Recent evidence suggests that in-transit nodes for extremity tumors may need to be more aggressively evaluated since the incidence of positivity is higher than anticipated and failure to include these nodal basins in the radiation field increases the chances for local/regional tumor failure. In addition, for patients with ARMS tumors, the presence of regional nodes disease indicates a significantly worse prognosis, similar to metastatic disease, whereas in ERMS

| TABLE 91-1 | TNM Pretreatment Staging Classification | | | | | |
|---|---|---|---|---|---|---|
| Stage | Sites | T | | Size | N | M |
| 1 | Orbit Head and neck (excluding parameningeal) GU nonbladder/nonprostate | $T_1$ or $T_2$ | | a or b | $N_0$ or $N_1$ or $N_x$ | $M_0$ |
| 2 | Bladder/prostate, extremity, cranial parameningeal, other (includes trunk, retroperitoneum, etc.) | $T_1$ or $T_2$ | | a | $N_0$ or $N_x$ | $M_0$ |
| 3 | Bladder/prostate, extremity, cranial parameningeal, other (includes trunk, retroperitoneum, etc.) | $T_1$ or $T_2$ | | a b | $N_1$ $N_0$ or $N_1$ or $N_x$ | $M_0$ $M_0$ |
| 4 | All | $T_1$ or $T_2$ | | a or b | $N_0$ or $N_1$ | $M_1$ |

**Definitions:**

| | | |
|---|---|---|
| Tumor T (site)$_1$ - | | confirmed to anatomic site of origin (a) <5 cm in diameter (b) >5 cm in diameter |
| T (site)$_2$ | | extension and/or fixed to surrounding tissue (a) <5 cm in diameter (b) >5 cm in diameter |
| Regional Nodes | | |
| $N_0$ | | regional nodes not clinically involved |
| $N_1$ | | regional nodes clinically involved by neoplasm |
| $N_x$ | | clinical status of regional nodes unknown (especially sites that preclude lymph node evaluation) |
| Metastasis - | | |
| $M_0$ | | no distant metastasis |
| $M_1$ | | metastasis present |

*Note:* Staging before treatment requires thorough clinical, laboratory, and imaging examinations. Biopsy is required to establish histologic diagnosis. Pretreatment tumor size is determined by external measurement or MRI or CT, depending on anatomic location. For less accessible primary sites, CT also will be used for lymph node assessment. Metastatic sites will require some form of imaging confirmation (but not histologic confirmation, except for bone marrow examination).

tumors the outcomes for patients with regional node disease is not any different than localized disease.

Metabolic imaging using $^{18}$F-fluorodeoxyglucose positron emission tomography (FDG PET) has become widely used in the adult population to determine the extent of disease in the setting of many cancers, however, there is limited experience in the pediatric population. Recent studies have suggested that FDG PET would be both a sensitive and specific tool in the clinical determination of the extent of disease in childhood sarcomas. Further, when combined with CT, it may be more accurate than conventional imaging modalities in staging patients or restaging patients at the time of recurrence.

## Pretreatment Clinical Staging

Staging of RMS is determined by the site of the primary tumor, primary tumor size, degree of tumor invasion, nodal status, and the presence or absence of metastases and is based solely on the preoperative workup of imaging and physical exam. This is expressed in a TNM classification system, modified for the site of tumor origin (Table 91-1). Adequate pretreatment clinical staging requires a thorough physical examination and preoperative imaging. The TNM staging system has been validated as a reliable predictor of patient outcome.

## Clinical Group   Post-Resection

The extent of residual disease after resection is one of the most important prognostic factors in RMS. Currently, patients are assigned to a Clinical Group based on the completeness of

tumor excision and the evidence of tumor metastasis to the lymph nodes or distant organs after pathologic examination of surgical specimens (Table 91-2). This system differs from TNM staging in that determination of each patient's Clinical Group is based on the extent of the surgical resection instead of tumor size and site. Data from IRS-III and IRS-IV demonstrate that 5-year failure-free survival rates vary according to clinical grouping and by histologic type (Fig. 91-2). One

| TABLE 91-2 | Clinical Grouping for RMS Patients |
|---|---|
| Group | Criteria |
| I | Localized disease, completely resected a. Confined to organ or muscle of origin b. Infiltrating outside organ or muscle of origin; regional nodes not involved |
| II | Compromised or regional resection including: a. Grossly resected tumors with microscopic residual tumor b. Regional disease, completely resected, with nodes involved and/or tumor extension into an adjacent organ c. Regional disease, with involved nodes, grossly resected, but with evidence of microscopic residual tumor |
| III | Incomplete resection or biopsy with gross residual disease remaining |
| IV | Distant metastases present at outset |

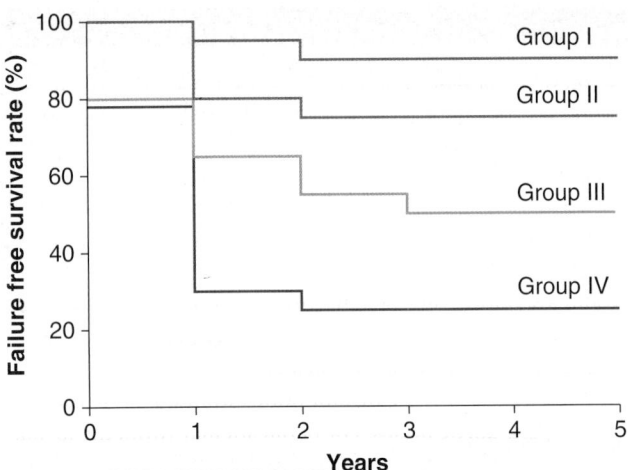

**FIGURE 91-2** Rhabdomyosarcoma survival based on completeness of surgical resection (Clinical Group). Clinical group is determined by extent of surgical excision and presence of metastatic disease. Data from the IRS IV study are shown. Patients with Group I (completely excised tumors) and Group II (microscopic residual disease) have the most favorable outcome. Over half of all patients have gross residual disease (Group III tumors) and have an intermediate outcome. Patients with established metastases (Group IV) are at highest risk for treatment failure.

criticism of Clinical Grouping is that variations of surgical techniques make comparisons of Clinical Grouping between different institutions problematic. Nonetheless, this system offers a tremendous companion to preoperative staging in determining patient risk assessment and prognosis (Table 91-3).

## Risk Stratification

In an effort to tailor the intensity of therapy to patient outcomes, the STS has developed a risk-stratification system that incorporates pretreatment staging (based on anatomic site and TNM status) and extent of disease after surgical resection

(clinical group). This stratification system is constantly changing as new information becomes available. Categorization of patients into low, intermediate and high risk provides a good predictor of patient outcome and should allow better correlation between intensity of therapy and outcome (Table 91-3).

## RMS TREATMENT

### Biopsy

Open biopsy of a mass suspected to be RMS should be performed in order to confirm the diagnosis. Care should be taken to obtain adequate specimens for pathologic, biological, and treatment protocol studies. For small lesions in areas that will be treated with only chemotherapy and radiation or for metastatic disease, core needle biopsy may be appropriate for diagnosis. While less invasive than open biopsy, core needle biopsy obtains a smaller tissue sample which increases sampling error and the number of inconclusive findings. In addition, this smaller volume of tissue may prevent the performance of adequate molecular biology studies. Image guidance with ultrasound may increase the accuracy of sampling while helping to avoid inadvertent puncture of surrounding structures. Clinical and radiographic positive lymph nodes should be confirmed pathologically. Open biopsy is recommended, however, fine-needle aspiration or core needle biopsy of lymph nodes may be performed at the discretion of the surgeon's judgment and pathologist's recommendations. Sentinel lymph node biopsy may offer a safe and less invasive means of lymph node evaluation for extremity and truncal lesions, although its role in RMS has yet to be determined.

### Resection of the Mass

In cases where the operative procedure was only a biopsy of a resectable primary tumor, or a nononcologic operation for tumor removal, or the status of the surgical margins are

| TABLE 91-3 | Categorization of Patients into Risk Group Allow Better Correlation between Intensity of Therapy and Outcome | | | |
|---|---|---|---|---|
| **Risk Group** | **Pretreatment Stage[a]** | **Clinical Group[b]** | **Site[b]** | **Histology** |
| Low 1 | 1 or 2 | I or II | Favorable or unfavorable | EMB |
| | 1 | III | Orbit only | EMB |
| Low 2 | 1 | III | Favorable | EMB |
| | 3 | I or II | Unfavorable | EMB |
| Intermediate | 2 or 3 | III | Unfavorable | EMB |
| | 1-3 | I-III | Favorable or unfavorable | ALV |
| High | 4 | IV | Favorable or unfavorable | EMB |
| | 4 | IV | Favorable or unfavorable | ALV |

*Note:* Patients at lowest risk are those with favorable histology tumors in favorable sites and lower group/stage, about 35% of the patient population. About 50% have intermediate risk tumors. This group includes nonmetastatic alveolar tumors and more advanced stage embryonal tumors. Patients with metastatic disease (excluding the ERMS patients less than 10 years of age) have a poor outcome—representing about 15% of the population.
[a]Pre-treatment stage dependent on site of disease.
[b]Favorable Sites: Orbit, Genitourinary tract, biliary tract, nonparameningeal head, and neck.

unclear, pretreatment re-excision (PRE) is advisable. PRE is a wide re-excision of the previous operative site with adequate margins of normal tissue prior to the initiation of adjuvant therapy. PRE is most commonly performed on extremity and trunk lesions, but should be considered the treatment of choice whenever technically feasible. Outcomes for patients who undergo PRE and are rendered Group I (complete excision) have the same outcomes as other Group I patients.

The primary goal of surgical intervention for RMS is wide and complete resection of the primary tumor with a surrounding rim of normal tissue. A circumferential margin of 0.5 cm is considered adequate, however, there is minimal data to support this recommendation. Such a margin may be unobtainable especially with head and neck tumors. Because of these limitations, adequate margins of uninvolved tissue are required *unless* excision would compromise adjacent organs, results in loss of function, poor cosmesis, or is not technically feasible. All margins should be marked and oriented at the operative field to enable precise evaluation of margins. If a narrow margin occurs, several separate biopsies of "normal" tissue around the resection margin should be obtained. These specimens should be marked and submitted separately for pathologic review. Communication between the pathologist and surgeon is critical to assure that all margins are accurately examined. The surgeon should not bisect or cut the excised tumor into specimens prior to sending it to the pathologist. Any areas of unresectable residual microscopic or gross tumor should be marked with small titanium clips in the tumor bed to aid RT simulation and subsequent re-excision. Published analyses have shown that outcomes resulting from a clear margin and no residual disease (Group I) are superior to residual microscopic margins (Group II) or gross residual disease (Group III). Tumors that are removed piecemeal are considered Group II even if all gross tumor is removed.

## Lymph Node Sampling/Dissection

Lymph node status is an important part of pretreatment staging and therefore directly impacts risk-based treatment strategies in RMS. Regional lymph node disease (N-1) is present in 23% of all RMS patients, predominantly in primary tumor sites such as perineum, retroperitoneum, extremity, bladder/prostate, parameningeal, and paratesticular. Data from IRS-IV would suggest that N-1 disease in patients with ARMS is associated with tumor characteristics that carry a poor prognosis but independently is a prognostic factor for both failure free survival (FFS) and overall survival (OS). In addition, it has been shown previously that in patients with otherwise localized disease, such as an extremity, N-1 disease may be associated with an inferior outcome. Clinical and radiographic positive nodes should therefore be biopsied to confirm tumor involvement thus ensuring correct assessment of disease risk and assignment of optimal therapy. Lymph node removal has no therapeutic benefit, therefore, lymph node resection, as opposed to biopsy, plays no role in therapy. Clinical and/or radiographic negative nodes do not require pathologic evaluation except in extremity tumors and for children older than 10 years of age with paratesticular tumors. In both of these sites the high incidence of nodal disease and false negative

*Extremity + Paratesticular > 10 y o*

imaging necessitates pathologic evaluation of regional nodal basins.

The use of sentinel node mapping to determine regional node status has proven to be beneficial in adult breast cancer and melanoma. For childhood RMS, sentinel node mapping is not yet the standard of care but appears to be very effective. If regional nodes are positive, then distant nodes should be harvested for pathologic evaluation. Tumor identified in these nodes would be considered metastatic disease and would therefore alter therapy using the current risk-based protocols. For upper extremity lesions, the distant nodes would be the ipsilateral supraclavicular (scalene) nodes. In the lower extremity, the distant nodes would include the iliac and/or para-aortic nodes. For paratesticular RMS, the ipsilateral para-aortic lymph nodes above the renal vein are considered distant nodes.

## Second-Look Operations and Resection for Recurrence

During, or after completing, adjuvant therapies, patients with RMS are reimaged with CT or MRI. If residual tumor remains, or if the outcome of therapy remains in doubt, a second-look operation (SLO) may be considered. SLO can be performed to confirm clinical response, to evaluate pathologic response, and to remove residual tumor in order to improve local control. As with the initial operation, the goal of SLO is complete resection of disease without causing loss of function or cosmesis. Data from IRS III suggested that SLO results in the reclassification of 75% of partial responders to complete responders after excision of residual tumors. These operations were most effective in extremity and truncal lesions. More recently, data from IRS-IV showed that patients with no visible tumor at the time of SLO had a 7% incidence of viable tumor compared to 53% for patients with a mass visible on imaging. Outcomes were better for patients with no viable tumor and patients who had negative margins after SLO.

A more aggressive surgical approach may be warranted for recurrent RMS. Data would suggest that resection of recurrent RMS confers a 5-year survival of 37% compared to 8% survival in a group of patients without aggressive resection.

However, aggressive resection of a residual mass after completion of adjuvant therapy may not be warranted. Associated morbidity of resection and the inability to achieve complete resection in some cases must be considered. Further, it is not uncommon to find an absence of viable tumor tissue in resected samples. This brings into question the utility of aggressive reresection and suggests that better means of detecting viable tumor is crucial. As discussed, PET/CT may provide the crucial information required to make these decisions.

## Chemotherapy  *VAₒC*

Today, all patients with RMS receive some form of chemotherapy. Standard therapeutic regimens consist of a combination of vincristine, actinomycin-D, and cyclophosphamide (VAC). Although tremendous advances have been made in improving the outcomes of patients with isolated local and regional disease, little progress has been made in improving survival outcomes for children with advanced RMS. The limiting factor has been an inability to improve significantly upon standard chemotherapeutic regimens. Dose intensification of vincristine and actinomycin-D is not possible due to their neurotoxic and hepatotoxic side effects. Studies evaluating dose intensification of cyclophosphamide found that although patients tolerate higher doses, outcomes of intermediate-risk tumors are not improved. These findings have stimulated the evaluation of new drug combinations and the development of risk-based treatment protocols.

## Radiation Therapy

RT is an important adjunct to therapy for many children diagnosed with RMS, offering improved local control and outcomes. Candidates for RT primarily include those with Group II (microscopic residual) or Group III (gross residual) disease. The impact of therapy is influenced by the location of the primary tumor and the amount of local disease at the time RT is initiated. Among patients with Group II disease, low-dose radiation (40 Gy at 1.5-1.8 Gy per fraction) is associated with local tumor control rates of at least 90%. For patients with Group III disease, radiation doses are more commonly 50 Gy.

Radiation therapy in very young children with RMS poses a unique therapeutic challenge. Efforts to improve RT compliance, to prevent reduced or omitted radiation dose or volume that occur in an attempt to avoid late effects, may significantly improve outcomes. Million et al found that over half of the operative bed recurrences were associated with noncompliance and that omission of radiation therapy was the most common protocol deviation. Three fourths of children die when local-regional disease is not controlled, emphasizing the importance of radiation therapy in RMS.

## Assessment of Response to Treatment

European RMS trials have demonstrated that tumor response to induction therapy was a significant predictor of survival, however, these findings have not been duplicated in the United States. The significance of persistent radiographic masses in patients treated for RMS is unknown. Conventional imaging modalities offer no information about the biology of these masses and are unable to differentiate between active tumors and scar. It is possible that FDG-PET may offer useful clinical information in patients treated or partially treated for RMS. While PET/CT has a limited role in early diagnosis (lesions smaller than 5 mm, well-differentiated tumors or those with a low metabolic rate) it may play a pivotal role in the initial staging, treatment response evaluation, and detection of metastatic disease.

# SPECIFIC ANATOMIC SITES

RMS is unique among most solid tumors in that it may occur in many different areas of the body. Tumors at different sites may behave differently than those in other areas. In addition, some areas of the body offer unique obstacles to surgical resection. As such, some specific anatomic sites of tumor occurrence will be discussed separately.

## Head and Neck (Superficial Nonparameningeal)

Approximately 35% of all RMS arises in the head and neck region. Of these tumors, 75% occur in the orbit. Other sites include the buccal, oropharyngeal, laryngeal, or parotid areas. RMS histology correlates to some extent with the location of the orbital tumor. ERMS more commonly arise in the superior nasal quadrants, whereas ARMS generally originate within the inferior orbit. For all head and neck RMS, biopsy is required for diagnostic confirmation. Resection may be limited by the inability to obtain an adequate margin; therefore, the success of resection is heavily dependent on location with superficial parotid being most amenable to resection. Lymph nodes that are clinically or radiographically involved must be biopsied. Given this information it is not surprising that most tumors are treated mainly with RT and chemotherapy. Outcomes correlate strongly with tumor location. Orbital RMS carries the best prognosis and is least likely to extend to the meninges. These tumors generally present earlier in the course of disease. Tumors arising in nonorbital parameningeal locations have a high likelihood of meningeal extension. If this occurs after chemotherapy and radiation therapy, the outcome is often fatal.

## Parameningeal

Parameningeal RMS includes tumors arising in the middle ear/mastoid, nasal cavity, parapharyngeal space, paranasal sinuses, or the pterygopalatine/infratemporal fossa region. These tumors are considered high-risk because of their propensity to cause cranial nerve palsy, bony erosion of the cranial base, and intracranial extension. Wide local excision is recommended, but is often not feasible due to the location of the tumors. Craniofacial resection for tumors of the nasal areas, paranasal sinuses, temporal fossa, and other deep sites are appropriate for resection by experienced surgical teams. For patients with unresected tumors and/or lymph node-positive disease, the use of 3-drug chemotherapy regimens (including an alkylating agent) plus local or regional radiation may be beneficial. The optimal dosing and timing of radiation have not been determined. The recognition of poor outcomes associated with meningeal extension has led to a propensity for early radiation therapy of primary tumors and adjuvant chemotherapy. The accurate prediction of the small subset of patients who achieve local control without radiation is not possible and in 1 study only 12% of patients were cured without radiation therapy.

## Trunk, Abdominal Wall, Chest Wall

Accounting for only 4% to 7% of tumors, RMS of the trunk is associated with a poor prognosis. Symptoms for RMS of the trunk often occur late in the progression of disease resulting in extensive involvement at diagnoses. Complete surgical resection is difficult, particularly when the pleura and peritoneum are involved. In addition, resections are frequently morbid and associated with poor cosmetic outcomes. Resection may require major chest wall or abdominal wall reconstruction with prosthetic materials or with flaps. Indicators of poor prognosis include advanced stage at presentation, alveolar histology, recurrent disease, tumor size greater than 5 cm, lymph node involvement, and the inability to undergo gross total resection.

Abdominal wall RMS generally presents as a painless, firm mass. Many abdominal wall primaries can be removed completely at presentation or following neoadjuvant chemotherapy. However, tumors arising from the deep layers of the abdominal wall may not be noticed until significant tumor progression has occurred, thus rendering resection much more challenging. Tumor excision should include full thickness resection of the abdominal wall including the skin and peritoneum with a margin of normal tissue. Reconstruction of the abdominal wall may require mesh or myocutaneous muscle flaps to optimize function and cosmesis. Data suggest that localized tumors of the abdominal wall can be resected with favorable outcomes. If the size or location prevents adequate excision, neoadjuvant chemotherapy should be initiated to reduce tumor size and facilitate subsequent resection.

The differential diagnosis for malignant chest wall masses includes the Ewing sarcoma, PNET, and RMS. Diagnostic biopsies are performed in the long axis of the tumor, parallel to the ribs. Wide local excision of chest wall lesions with a 0.5 cm margin including the previous biopsy site, involved chest wall muscles and involved ribs, as well as wedge excision of any involved underlying lung is recommended. Thoracoscopy performed at the time of resection may be helpful in determining the extent of pleural involvement and tumor extension to the underlying lung. Chest wall reconstruction can be performed using a number of techniques employing prosthetic mesh, myocutaneous flaps, and titanium ribs. Chest wall lesions have a worse prognosis than other trunk lesions with a 1.8 year survival rate of only 42%. Although RT may be beneficial for local control of tumor, this option is associated with significant morbidity and is not associated with improved survival.

## Biliary Tract

Classically, patients with biliary RMS present at a young age (average age 3.5 years) with jaundice and abdominal pain, often associated with abdominal distension, vomiting, and fever. Work-up reveals a significant direct hyperbilirubinemia and a mild elevation of hepatic transaminases. Gross total resection of biliary tract RMS is rarely possible and is often unnecessary due to favorable outcomes with treatment by chemotherapy and radiation alone. Currently, biopsy is the only role of surgery in the treatment of biliary RMS. The histology of biliary RMS is often the botryoid variant of embryonal RMS which carries a good overall prognosis. Biliary obstruction can be relieved by stenting; external biliary drains should be avoided due to infectious complications. Overall, outcomes are good unless distant metastases are present at the time of diagnosis.

## Paraspinal

Paraspinal RMS is rare (3.3% of all cases of RMS) and carries a poor prognosis due to its frequent spread along anatomic structures such as neurovascular bundles and fascial sheaths. It occasionally produces spinal cord compression. Complete excision of paraspinal lesions is often difficult to achieve due to large tumor size at presentation and involvement of the vertebral column and spinal canal. Recurrence rates for paraspinal RMS are high (55%) with the majority

of these occurring at distant locations. The lung is the most common site of distant metastasis followed by the central nervous system.

## Retroperitoneum/Pelvis

Like paraspinal tumors, retroperitoneal/pelvic lesions are often discovered at an advanced stage and thus generally carry a poor prognosis. RMS at this site can envelop vital structures, making complete surgical resection challenging. Neoadjuvant chemotherapy may play a role in tumors that cannot be safely resected at the time of diagnosis. With the exception of Group IV metastatic disease, aggressive resection is recommended and has been shown to enhance survival. Group IV patients with embryonal histology and those who present at less than 10 years of age may also undergo surgical debulking. It has been demonstrated that excising greater than half of the tumor prior to chemotherapy resulted in improved rates of FFS when compared to patients who did not undergo debulking. This is the only setting in which surgical debulking of RMS has shown any benefit. *NOTE Debulking*

## Perineum/Perianal

Perineal tumors are rare and usually present at an advanced stage. Characteristics associated with improved survival include a primary tumor size less than 5 cm, less advanced clinical group and stage, negative lymph node status, and age less than 10 years. Interestingly, histology does not affect overall outcome at this site. Resection can be challenging due to proximity to the urethra and anorectum. At resection, particular care should be taken to preserve continence. If anorectal obstruction exists, a temporary colostomy may be necessary. Patients presenting in Clinical Group I had 100% OS at 5 years compared to 25% for Group IV patients.

## Extremity *20% New Dx*

RMS of the extremity accounts for 20% of all new diagnoses. The majority have alveolar histology and thus a poor prognosis. The cure rate for children with extremity RMS has, however, improved steadily from 47% in IRS I to 74% in IRS III. As with many sites of RMS, complete gross resection at initial surgical intervention is the most important predictor of FFS. The primary goal of local tumor control in extremity tumors is limb-sparing complete resection. Amputation is rarely necessary for tumor excision. Positive regional lymph nodes are found in 20% to 40% of patients and are associated with decreased OS (46% survival rate for node-positive patients compared to 80% survival for node-negative patients). Seventeen percent of IRS-IV patients with clinically negative nodes were found to have microscopic nodal disease on biopsy. In light of this, surgical evaluation of lymph nodes is necessary to accurately stage children with extremity RMS, even in the absence of clinically positive nodes. Currently, axillary sampling is recommended for upper extremity lesions and femoral triangle sampling is recommended for lower extremity lesions. Sentinel lymph node mapping may be a useful adjunct in the setting of extremity RMS. If regional nodes are involved, XRT fields are adjusted to incorporate the regional lymph node basins. This approach is associated with

*Impact of ⊕ Nodes*

*NOTE*

decreasing rates of local and regional recurrence. In-transit nodal involvement at the time of diagnosis, present in 4% of IRS IV patients, has also been identified as a factor contributing to regional treatment failure. This may be evaluated by MRI or possibly FDG-PET at the time of diagnosis. XRT should be used at regional lymph node sites in these patients.

## Genitourinary: Bladder/Prostate

RMS of the bladder or prostate typically presents with urinary obstructive symptoms. These lesions are typically of embryonal histology (73%). The major goal of surgery is complete tumor resection with bladder salvage. This can be achieved in 50% to 60% of patients. Partial cystectomy has resulted in similar survival rates and improved bladder function compared to more aggressive resections. Tumors in the dome of the bladder frequently can be completely resected, whereas more distal bladder lesions frequently require ureteral reimplantation or bladder augmentation. Prostatic tumors require prostatectomy, often combined with an attempt at bladder salvage with or without ureteral reconstruction. Continent urinary diversion may be necessary if tumors are unresectable or have a poor response to medical therapy. Lymph nodes are involved in up to 20% of cases. Therefore, during biopsy or resection, iliac and para-aortic nodes should be sampled, as well as any other clinically involved nodes. An analysis of patients with bladder or prostate RMS in IRS IV revealed that 70% arose from the bladder with an overall 6-year survival of 82%. Bladder function was preserved in 55% (36/66) of event-free survivors. Of all patients entered on study, 40% (36/88) survive event-free with apparently normal functioning bladders.

## Genitourinary: Vulva/Vagina/Uterus

Traditionally, females with primary tumors of the genital tract underwent aggressive resection followed by chemotherapy with or without radiation. Current treatment approaches rely more heavily on neoadjuvant chemotherapy to reduce tumor size and minimize the extent of resection in an attempt to preserve organ function. These tumors respond well to chemotherapy with impressive tumor regression that often precludes the need for radical operations like pelvic exenteration. Vaginectomy and hysterectomy are performed only for persistent or recurrent disease. Primary uterine tumors require resection with preservation of the distal vagina and ovaries if they do not respond to chemotherapy. Oophorectomy is indicated only in the setting of direct tumor involvement. For those patients presenting with nonembryonal RMS of the female genital tract, more intensive chemotherapeutic regimens are recommended to reduce the risk of recurrence. Prognosis for this site with only loco-regional disease is excellent with an estimated 5-year survival of 87%.

## Paratesticular

Paratesticular RMS generally presents as a painless scrotal mass. Histology is generally favorable with most tumors showing the spindle cell subvariant of embryonal histology. Survival rates are >90% for patients presenting with Group I or II disease. Radical orchiectomy via an inguinal approach with resection of the spermatic cord to the level of the internal ring is the standard of care. Open biopsy should be avoided because the flow of lymphatics in this region facilitates spread of the disease. If a trans-scrotal biopsy/resection has been performed, subsequent resection of the hemiscrotum is required. If unprotected spillage of tumor cells occurs during tumor resection, patients are considered Clinical Group IIa regardless of the completeness of resection. The incidence of nodal metastatic disease for paratesticular RMS is 26% to 43%. Unfortunately, studies have demonstrated that CT is a poor means of evaluating lymph node involvement in the retroperitoneum. Patients older than 10 years of age or those with enlarged nodes have a much higher incidence of node involvement. Those patients should, therefore, undergo an ipsilateral retroperitoneal lymph node resection. Advances in surgical techniques have demonstrated promising results with laparoscopic retroperitoneal lymph node dissection for high-risk pediatric patients with paratesticular RMS, allowing for expedited convalescence and rapid initiation of adjuvant chemotherapy. Suprarenal nodes should be evaluated since positive nodes in this area place a patient in Group IV with disseminated metastatic disease.

## Metastatic Disease

Blood
Lymph

RMS metastasizes both through hematogenous and lymphatic routes. Children with metastatic RMS have very poor rates of survival. For the IRS studies I to III, children with metastatic disease had a 5-year disease-free survival of 20, 27, and 32%, respectively in each of the successive studies.

## Prognosis

The prognosis of patients with RMS is dependent on many factors. Favorable prognostic factors include embryonal/botryoid histology, primary tumor sites in the orbit and non-parameningeal head/neck region and genitourinary excluding the bladder/prostate regions, a lack of distant metastases at diagnosis, complete gross removal of tumor at the time of diagnosis, tumor size less than or equal to 5 cm, age less than 10 years at the time of diagnosis, and time to relapse. For all histologic types of RMS, outcome is heavily dependent on age at diagnosis, the primary anatomic site, extent of disease (tumor size, invasion, nodal status, metastatic disease), and the completeness of surgical excision. The STS Committee is investigating the outcomes of patients by disease characteristics and tumor biology to refine risk-adapted therapy for the treatment of RMS.

For Group I patients, local recurrence was the most common site of first failure in nonirradiated patients. Patients with Stage 1-2 ARMS had slightly but statistically insignificantly improved local control, event-free survival, and OS rates when local radiation therapy was given. The need for local radiation therapy in Stage 1-2 patients deserves evaluation in a randomized study.

For Group II patients those patients at highest risk for treatment failure had alveolar/undifferentiated histology, unfavorable primary sites, regional disease with residual tumor after gross resection and node involvement, or were treated with early therapeutic regimens (IRS-I or II). Current therapy for patients with group II tumors results in 85% survival long-term, indicating that risk-based therapeutic strategies have assisted with achieving failure-free survival.

Data from the COG patients suggest that patients with intermediate-risk RMS that have early treatment failure occurring fewer than 120 days from study entry had local failure. The group suggests that earlier RT could potentially improve outcome by preventing early local progression. Their goal was to determine the frequency and clinical features of early treatment failure during induction chemotherapy before protocol radiation therapy for children with intermediate-risk RMS. A small proportion of patients with intermediate-risk RMS suffer an early failure as a result of early progression (2.2%) or treatment-related mortality (0.3%).

Patients with Group III disease have incomplete resection or biopsy only prior to chemotherapy and irradiation. Wharam et al determined that predictors of failure-free survival in Group III include tumor size <5 cm, primary sites of orbit and bladder/prostate, and TNM staging equivalent to T1/N0Nx tumors in stage I or stage II. RT is important for local control of Group III disease. A report from the COG focused on the prognostic significance of tumor response at the end of therapy in clinical group III patients. They found that despite standard of care, some patients achieve less than a complete response, but this was not associated with poorer outcomes or decrease in survival. Thus, aggressive alternative therapy may not be warranted for patients with clinical group III RMS.

Approximately 15% of patients with RMS present with metastases (Group IV) at the time of diagnosis. Patients in Group IV have poor outcomes despite aggressive multimodality treatments with only 25% expected to be free of disease 3 years after diagnosis. A review of prognostic factors and outcomes for children and adolescents with metastatic RMS in IRS-IV found that three-year OS and failure-free survival was improved if there were two or fewer metastatic sites and the histology of the tumor was embryonal. Compared to patients without metastatic disease, Group IV patients in the IRS-IV study were more likely to be older (median age 7 years vs 5 years), had a higher incidence of alveolar histology (46% vs 22%), had tumors that were more invasive (T2: 91% vs 49%) and larger (>5 cm: 82% vs 51%), a higher incidence of lymph node involvement (N1: 57% vs 16%), and had a greater proportion of extremity and truncal/retroperitoneal primary sites (48% vs 25%). This study concluded that not all children with metastatic RMS have uniformly poor prognoses suggesting that therapy should be tailored according to these factors.

Future clinical trials focusing on the molecular biology driving RMS tumor behavior may assist with customized clinical therapies that will improve outcome and FFS in patients diagnosed with RMS.

## SELECTED READINGS

Blakely ML, Andrassy RJ, Raney RB, et al. Prognostic factors and surgical treatment guidelines for children with rhabdomyosarcoma of the perineum or anus: a report of Intergroup Rhabdomyosarcoma Studies I through IV, 1972 through 1997. *J Pediatr Surg* 2003;38:347–353.

Blakely ML, Lobe TE, Anderson JR, et al. Does debulking improve survival rate in advanced-stage retroperitoneal embryonal rhabdomyosarcoma? *J Pediatr Surg* 1999;34:736–741; discussion 41–42.

Breneman JC, Lyden E, Pappo AS, et al. Prognostic factors and clinical outcomes in children and adolescents with metastatic rhabdomyosarcoma—a report from the Intergroup Rhabdomyosarcoma Study IV. *J Clin Oncol* 2003;21:78–84.

Chui CH, Billups CA, Pappo AS, Rao BN, Spunt SL. Predictors of outcome in children and adolescents with rhabdomyosarcoma of the trunk—the St Jude Children's Research Hospital experience. *J Pediatr Surg* 2005;40:1691–1695.

Ferrari A, Bisogno G, Casanova M, et al. Is alveolar histotype a prognostic factor in paratesticular rhabdomyosarcoma? The experience of Italian and German Soft Tissue Sarcoma Cooperative Group. *Pediatr Blood Cancer* 2004;42:134–138.

Ferrari A, Bisogno G, Macaluso A, et al. Soft-tissue sarcomas in children and adolescents with neurofibromatosis type 1. *Cancer* 2007;109:1406–1412.

Gow KW, Rapkin LB, Olson TA, Durham MM, Wyly B, Shehata BM. Sentinel lymph node biopsy in the pediatric population. *J Pediatr Surg* 2008;43:2193–2198.

Grufferman S, Wang HH, DeLong ER, Kimm SY, Delzell ES, Falletta JM. Environmental factors in the etiology of rhabdomyosarcoma in childhood. *J Natl Cancer Inst* 1982;68:107–113.

Hayes-Jordan A, Doherty DK, West SD, et al. Outcome after surgical resection of recurrent rhabdomyosarcoma. *J Pediatr Surg* 2006;41:633–638; discussion 633–638.

Hays DM, Lawrence W Jr, Wharam M, et al. Primary reexcision for patients with 'microscopic residual' tumor following initial excision of sarcomas of trunk and extremity sites. *J Pediatr Surg* 1989;24:5–10.

Huh WW, Skapek SX. Childhood rhabdomyosarcoma: new insight on biology and treatment. *Curr Oncol Rep* 2010;12:402–410.

Kleis M, Daldrup-Link H, Matthay K, et al. Diagnostic value of PET/CT for the staging and restaging of pediatric tumors. *Eur J Nucl Med Mol Imaging* 2009;36:23–36.

La TH, Wolden SL, Rodeberg DA, et al. Regional nodal involvement and patterns of spread along in-transit pathways in children with rhabdomyosarcoma of the extremity: a report from the Children's Oncology Group. *Int J Radiat Oncol Biol Phys* 2011;80(4):1151–1157.

Leaphart C, Rodeberg D. Pediatric surgical oncology: management of rhabdomyosarcoma. *Surg Oncol* 2007;16:173–185.

Mandell L, Ghavimi F, LaQuaglia M, Exelby P. Prognostic significance of regional lymph node involvement in childhood extremity rhabdomyosarcoma. *Med Pediatr Oncol* 1990;18:466–471.

Million L, Anderson J, Breneman J, et al. Influence of noncompliance with radiation therapy protocol guidelines and operative bed recurrences for children with rhabdomyosarcoma and microscopic residual disease: a report from the Children's Oncology Group. *Int J Radiat Oncol Biol Phys* 2011;80(2):333–338.

Minn AY, Lyden ER, Anderson JR, et al. Early treatment failure in intermediate-risk rhabdomyosarcoma: results from IRS-IV and D9803—a report from the Children's Oncology Group. *J Clin Oncol* 2010;28:4228–4232.

Pappo AS, Shapiro DN. Rhabdomyosarcoma: biology and therapy. *Cancer Treat Res* 1997;92:309–339.

Parham DM, Qualman SJ, Teot L, et al. Correlation between histology and PAX/FKHR fusion status in alveolar rhabdomyosarcoma: a report from the Children's Oncology Group. *Am J Surg Pathol* 2007;31:895–901.

Puri DR, Wexler LH, Meyers PA, La Quaglia MP, Healey JH, Wolden SL. The challenging role of radiation therapy for very young children with rhabdomyosarcoma. *Int J Radiat Oncol Biol Phys* 2006;65:1177–1184.

Raney RB, Anderson JR, Barr FG, et al. Rhabdomyosarcoma and undifferentiated sarcoma in the first two decades of life: a selective review of intergroup rhabdomyosarcoma study group experience and rationale for Intergroup Rhabdomyosarcoma Study V. *J Pediatr Hematol Oncol* 2001;23:215–220.

Raney RB, Anderson JR, Brown KL, et al. Treatment results for patients with localized, completely resected (Group I) alveolar rhabdomyosarcoma on Intergroup Rhabdomyosarcoma Study Group (IRSG) protocols III and IV, 1984-1997: a report from the Children's Oncology Group. *Pediatr Blood Cancer* 2010;55:612–616.

Raney RB, Jr., Gehan EA, Hays DM, et al. Primary chemotherapy with or without radiation therapy and/or surgery for children with localized sarcoma of the bladder, prostate, vagina, uterus, and cervix. A comparison of the results in Intergroup Rhabdomyosarcoma Studies I and II. *Cancer* 1990;66:2072–2081.

Rodeberg D, Paidas C. Childhood rhabdomyosarcoma. *Semin Pediatr Surg* 2006;15:57–62.

Rodeberg DA, Anderson JR, Arndt CA, et al. Comparison of outcomes based on treatment algorithms for rhabdomyosarcoma of the bladder/prostate: combined results from the Children's Oncology Group, German Cooperative Soft Tissue Sarcoma Study, Italian Cooperative Group, and International Society of Pediatric Oncology Malignant Mesenchymal Tumors Committee. *Int J Cancer* 2010;128:1232–1239.

Rodeberg DA, Garcia-Henriquez N, Lyden ER, et al. Prognostic significance and tumor biology of regional lymph node disease in patients with rhabdomyosarcoma: a report from The Children's Oncology Group. *J Clin Oncol* 2011;29(10):1304–1311.

Rodeberg DA, Stoner JA, Hayes-Jordan A, et al. Prognostic significance of tumor response at the end of therapy in group III rhabdomyosarcoma: a report from the children's oncology group. *J Clin Oncol* 2009;27:3705–3711.

Soyer T, Karnak I, Ciftci AO, Senocak ME, Tanyel FC, Buyukpamukcu N. The results of surgical treatment of chest wall tumors in childhood. *Pediatr Surg Int* 2006;22:135–139.

Spunt SL, Lobe TE, Pappo AS, et al. Aggressive surgery is unwarranted for biliary tract rhabdomyosarcoma. *J Pediatr Surg* 2000;35:309–316.

Tefft M, Lindberg RD, Gehan EA. Radiation therapy combined with systemic chemotherapy of rhabdomyosarcoma in children: local control in patients enrolled in the Intergroup Rhabdomyosarcoma Study. *Natl Cancer Inst Monogr* 1981;56:75–81.

Wharam MD, Meza J, Anderson J, et al. Failure pattern and factors predictive of local failure in rhabdomyosarcoma: a report of group III patients on the third Intergroup Rhabdomyosarcoma Study. *J Clin Oncol* 2004;22:1902–1908.

Williamson D, Missiaglia E, de Reynies A, et al. Fusion gene-negative alveolar rhabdomyosarcoma is clinically and molecularly indistinguishable from embryonal rhabdomyosarcoma. *J Clin Oncol* 2010;28:2151–2158.

# CHAPTER 92

# Nonrhabdomyosarcoma Soft Tissue Sarcomas

*Andrea Hayes-Jordan*

## KEY POINTS

1. Nonrhadomyosarcomas are a heterogeneous group of soft tissue tumors that comprise 4% of all childhood malignancies.

2. Degree of surgical resection and age are important prognostic variables.

3. NRSTSs are relatively chemo-insensitive.

4. Synovial sarcoma and malignant peripheral nerve sheath tumors are the most common pediatric NRSTS.

5. Surgical resection is the mainstay of successful treatment of malignant peripheral nerve sheath tumors.

6. Radiotherapy may be indicated in the setting of positive surgical margins.

## BACKGROUND AND OVERVIEW

Approximately 8% of childhood malignancies are soft tissue sarcomas. Half of these are nonrhabdomyosarcoma soft tissue sarcomas NRSTS. There are over 50 histologic types and genetic patterns are poorly understood. When surgical resection is feasible, about 60% of patients are expected to achieve long-term survival with or without radiation therapy. Patient outcome is largely based on age, the presence of metastasis at diagnosis, and size and depth of the lesion. Here we focus on the most common primary histologies and differences in presentation and surgical treatment of childhood NRSTS and other common pediatric soft tissue tumors.

The treatment for children and adolescents with NRSTS has not previously been standardized, nor have there been any pediatric cooperative group trials as in rhabdomyosarcoma (RMS). Because there are many histological subtypes of NRSTS, standardization of treatment is difficult. The first risk-based prospective trial of NRSTS in children and adolescents is completing soon. In this trial patients with NRSTS are treated as low-, intermediate-, or high-risk based on criteria previously ascertained in a thorough review of 121 patients by Spunt. In patients with surgically resected NRSTS, univariate analysis revealed clear risk factors. Positive surgical margins ($p = 0.004$), tumor size greater than or equal to 5 cm ($p < 0.001$), invasiveness ($p = 0.002$), high-grade ($p = 0.028$), and intra-abdominal primary site ($p = 0.055$) had a negative impact on event free survival EFS. Multivariate analysis verified all of these risk factors except for invasiveness. Local recurrence was predicted by intra-abdominal primary site ($p = 0.028$), positive surgical margins ($p = 0.003$), and the omission of radiation therapy (0.043). As expected, the biology of the tumor, that is tumor size $\geq 5$ cm, invasiveness, and high grade, predicted distant recurrences. Children and adolescents with initially unresectable NRSTS are a subgroup of pediatric NRSTS that are particularly high risk. These are large tumors, greater than 5 cm, which involve critical neurovascular structures of the extremity, trunk, abdomen, or pelvis. In these patients, the 5-year estimated overall survival and EFS were 56% and 33%, respectively and post relapse survival was poor, 19% despite multimodality therapy.

In addition to unresectability, age is a prognostic indicator in pediatric NRSTS. Patients less than 1 year of age have an excellent prognosis whereas, the adolescents and young adults have the worse prognosis compared to younger patients or older adults. A 34-year review of patients treated at St Jude Children's Research Hospital, (SJCRH) revealed the overall 5-year survival estimate for children less than one year of age was 92%, compared to 36% in those 15 to 21 years of age. Patients between 1 and 15 years had an intermediate survival of approximately 60%. Survival after relapse was poor in all age groups less than 18 years except those less than 1 year of age. The 5-year estimate of post relapse survival in patients 0 to 1 year of age was 80% compared to the 15 to 25 years in which survival was 21%. Although the type of chemotherapy in these patients was variable, surgical excision was completed for lesions less than or equal to 5 cm and for most patients, incisional biopsy of lesions greater than 5 cm.

## INFANTILE FIBROSARCOMA

Patients in the study above that were less than 1 year of age had infantile fibrosarcoma (IF). This is a very rare form of NRSTS that occurs mostly during the first year of life but can be present up to year 4. IF presents as a rapidly occurring mass in the trunk or extremities; it can erode bone and usually reaches a large size.

Most cases of IF have a specific translocation t(12;15) (p13;q25) leading to fusion of *ETV6 (TEL)*, a member of the ets family of transcription factors, on chromosome 12p13, and *NTRK3 (TRKC)*, which encodes a receptor tyrosine kinase for neurotropin- on chromosome 15q25. Other complex cytogenetic abnormalities include trisomy 11, random gains of chromosomes 8, 11, 17, and 20, deletion of the long arm of 17 and a t(12;13) translocation. The helix–loop–helix dimerization domain of *ETV6* fuses to the protein tyrosine kinase domain of *NTRK3*. The fusion protein results in ligand-independent chimeric protein tyrosine kinase activity with autophosphorylation. This leads to constitutive activation of Ras-MAPK and P13K-AKT pathways via insulin receptor substrate-1, which is tyrosine-phosphorylated, and through the activation of *c-Src*. The fusion protein also associates with TGF-betaII receptor, which can be oncogenic by leading to inhibition of TGF-beta receptor signals that mediate tumor suppression.

Identical genetic findings have been reported in the cellular variant of congenital mesoblastic nephroma, a microscopically similar tumor of the kidney, and in secretory carcinoma of breast and acute myeloid leukemia, implying oncogenesis by lineage-independent activation of kinase-related signaling pathways.

## SYNOVIAL SARCOMA

Synovial sarcoma (SS) and malignant peripheral nerve sheath tumor (MPNST) are the most common pediatric NRSTS. SS is the most common NRSTS of childhood. It is characterized by a very specific fusion gene and X and 18[t(X;18) (p11.2;g11.2)]. Its etiology is unknown. In evaluating the 3 largest reviews of pediatric SS, common principles are evident. For children 0 to 16 years and tumors less than 5 cm in size, overall 5 year survival (OS) is 71% to 88%. In this group, the addition of chemotherapy did not correlate with survival. In patients 17 to 30 years the addition of chemotherapy does correlate with metastasis free survival. In patients with SS tumors greater than 5 cm, that are deep and invasive, without metastasis, OS is 50% to 75% and chemotherapy responsiveness is 50% to 60%. It is clear that for SS survival does not depend on surgical margins but depends on size (>5 cm) and local invasiveness. Brecht et al found, event-free survival was 92% and 56%, respectively, when SS tumors are less than or equal to 5 cm or greater than 5 cm. Radiotherapy does have a role in this disease and is recommended after marginal resection, or before anticipated marginal resection.

## MALIGNANT PERIPHERAL NERVE SHEATH TUMOR

Malignant peripheral nerve sheath tumor (MPNST), also called schwannoma or neurofibrosarcoma, usually arises in proximity to nerve sheaths. MPNST may develop in a pre-existing neurofibroma in approximately 40% of patients, particularly those with neurofibromatosis type 1. In a review of

171 patients 5 yr OS and progression free survival was 51% and 37%, respectively. Multivariate analysis revealed absence of NF-1, and tumor invasiveness to be poor prognostic variables. The overall response of the patients who received neoadjuvant chemotherapy was 45%. Some partial responses were seen in patients with initial unresectable disease because of neurovascular involvement. Neoadjuvant radiotherapy failed to maintain or achieve local control in 45% of patients (26 of 58). Neither chemotherapy nor radiotherapy showed any statistically significant difference in outcome. This article concludes by stating "…complete surgical resection is the mainstay of successful treatment." In another much smaller series, the same patterns in outcome were seen.

## Clinical Characteristics

Unlike RMS, NRSTSs are relatively chemo-insensitive. In the above pediatric studies and in adult multi-institutional studies the impact of chemotherapy on outcome is minimal. In large American Joint Commission on Cancer (AJCC) stage 3 tumors, overall survival was no different between patients who received surgery and neoadjuvant or adjuvant radiation therapy, or if chemotherapy was added. Complete surgical excision provides the best outcome. Patients usually present with a painless mass, sometimes identified after a recent episode of trauma. Pediatric patients who have an extremity or trunk mass that is greater than 5 cm, should have an MRI examination followed by core needle or open biopsy (Fig. 92-1). If NRSTS is identified and nonmutilating limb sparing surgical excision is feasible, resection should be completed. If margins are microscopically positive, postoperative radiotherapy should be given in high-grade tumors and tumors larger than 5 cm. Low-grade tumors that are less than 5 cm can be re-excised or just watched closely. If surgical excision is not feasible without amputation or severe morbidity, whether less than or greater than 5 cm, preoperative chemotherapy and radiotherapy should be administered. If surgical excision is feasible but R1 resection is anticipated, the type of radiotherapy whether pre- or postoperative brachytherapy, proton beam therapy, or external beam should be discussed with the radiation oncologist with the goal in pediatric extremity tumors to avoid the growth plate in younger patients who are still growing. In tumors less than 5 cm, complete surgical excision with negative microscopic margins is the goal. In the case of unexpected malignant pathology, primary re-excision is recommended. For all NRSTS, negative microscopic margins should be achieved; however, there is no consistent reliable evidence to indicate the width of acceptable margins.

NRSTS are graded histologically to help predict outcome. Grade 1 is any NRSTS with low malignant potential, such as IF, with mitotic activity less than 5 per high powered filed. NRSTS with tumor necrosis less than 15% and mitotic activity of 5 to 10 per HPF were graded 2, and specific histologic subtypes with known aggressive behavior and/or any sarcoma with tumor necrosis of more than 15% or mitotic activity of more than 10 per HPF were graded 3.

Cytotoxic chemotherapy (Adriamycin, Ifosfamide, Vincristine, Dactinomycin etc), at best will be effective in 45% to 50% of patients. (This does not include targeted therapy as

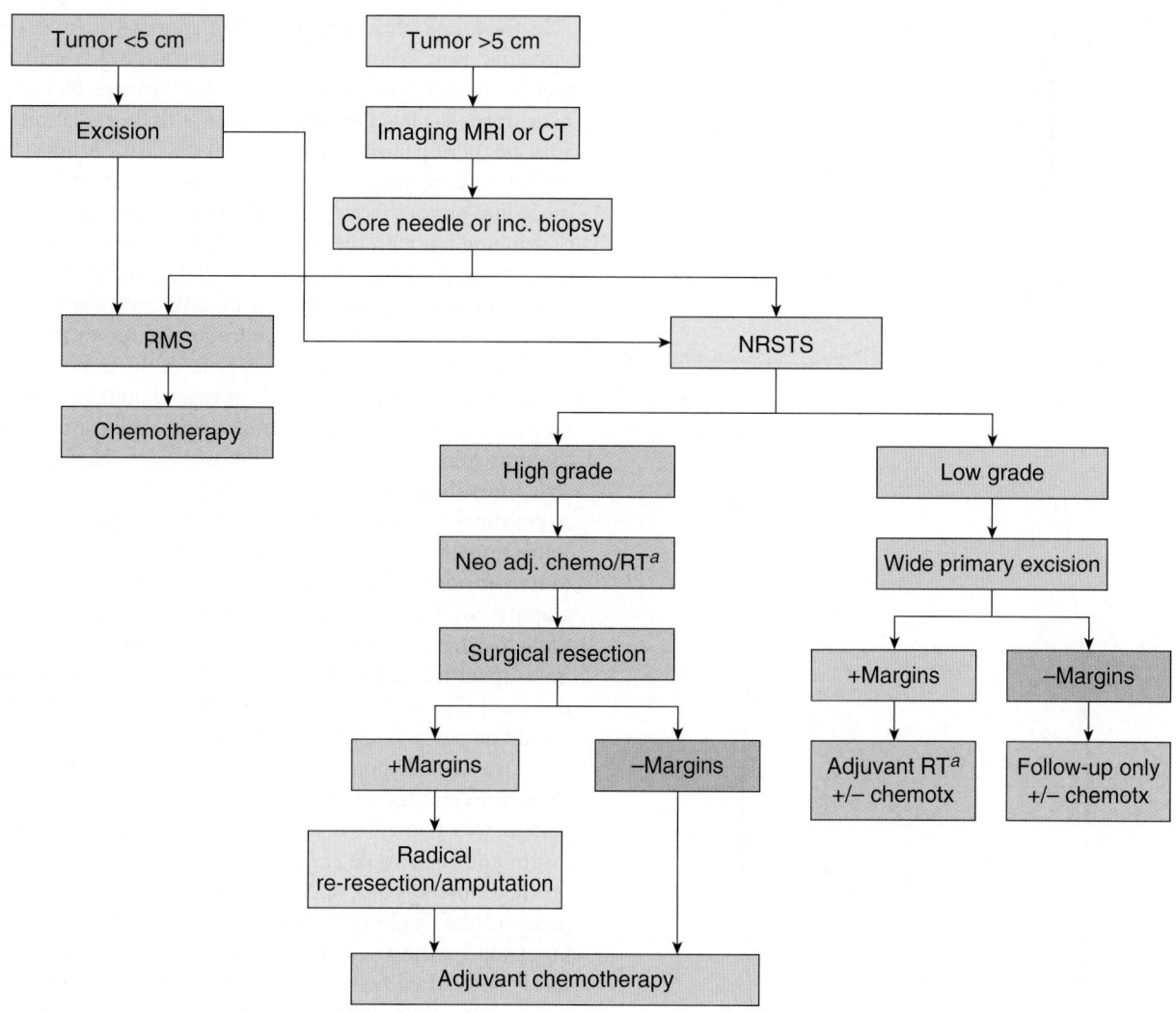

**FIGURE 92-1** Flow chart for management of nonrhabdomyosarcoma soft tissue sarcomas. [a]RT, radiation therapy—avoid radiation at growth plates in young pediatric patients.

there are not yet sufficient data to analyze the efficacy of this mode of treatment at this time.) Very close observation by imaging is warranted if neoadjuvant chemotherapy is chosen, since an increase in tumor size may preclude limb sparing, nonmutilating surgery or in the case of abdominal or pelvic tumors, may become unresectable.

## Metastatic Disease

Sentinel lymph node biopsy, although recommended for RMS to evaluate normal appearing lymph nodes, is only recommended in histologic subtypes of NRSTS which have high risk of lymph node metastasis. These include epitheliod sarcoma and clear cell sarcoma which have an approximate incidence of lymph node metastasis of up to 30%. SS metastasizes to the lymph nodes about 15% of the time.

Computed tomography (CT) scan of the chest is a necessary part of the work-up to excluded lung metastasis. Lung metastases occur in approximately 30% of patients with NRSTS. Since NRSTS are relatively chemo-insensitive, surgical resection of lung metastases is recommended. Thoracotomy is the recommended approach in order to palpate the lung for any tumors that may have been missed on imaging.

## Operative Resection of Extremity Soft Tissue Tumors

The goal of tumor resection in pediatric nonrhabdomyosarcoma soft tissue sarcoma is an R0 (negative microscopic margins) resection with at least 1 cm margins circumferentially. Unfortunately, there are no prospective randomized trials to provide the recommended width of the margins but 1 cm is adequate. Surgical resection of the entire muscle where the tumor resides from origin to insertion is not necessary.

Surgical approach to these tumors should be age and size dependent. After a soft tissue sarcoma type has been verified by incisional or core biopsy, surgical resection should be completed. In all cases, an axial incision should be made as seen in Fig. 92-2. The direction of the incision for biopsy and resection is critical. If a transverse incision is made instead of an axial incision, and after final pathologic evaluation positive microscopic margins are found, closure after re-excision of a transverse incision would be very difficult and likely require the help of a plastic reconstructive surgeon. Pediatric patients with extremity NRSTS, who have not completed their growth, especially those less than 5 years of age, require an approach that aims to omit radiation therapy. External

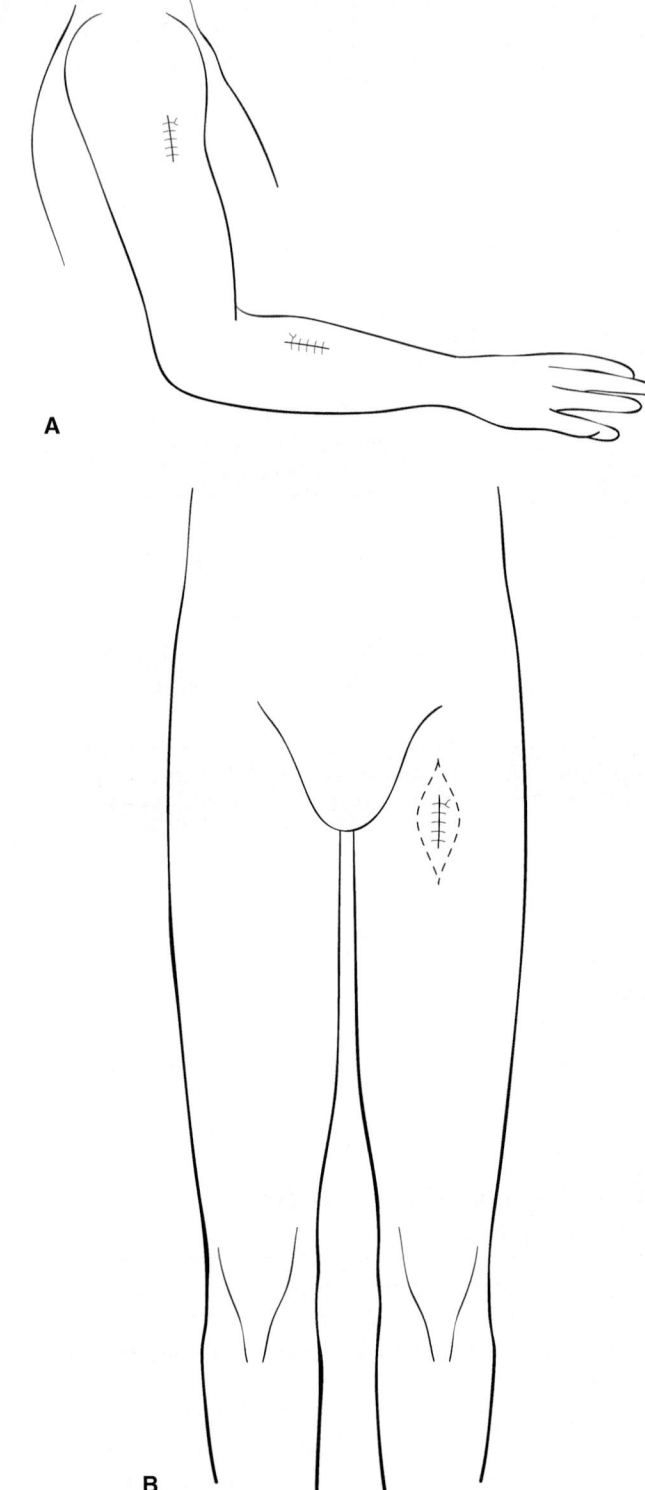

**FIGURE 92-2** Orientation of incisions in extremity soft tissue sarcoma operative resection. (**A**) Upper extremity, (**B**) Lower extremity.

In the trunk and extremities, the approach to soft tissue sarcomas is as follows. (Preoperative planning is critical in that if a positive margin is anticipated because of a critical neurovascular structure, consultation with the radiation therapist for perioperative planning is necessary.) A linear incision is made to match the length of the tumor beneath. The incisional or core biopsy site should be excised as an ellipse of skin and left with the specimen if the tumor is superficial, or sent separately if the tumor is deep. Medial and lateral subcutaneous flaps should then be fashioned deep into the scarpas layer. Throughout the procedure extreme care should be taken not to actually see the capsule of the tumor. Normal subcutaneous adipose tissue or muscle should be used as a margin. When dividing muscle, anticipate the contraction of the muscle and take at least a 2 cm margin. Neurovascular structures should be identified an isolated with a vessel loop. A proximal tourniquet is not necessary but is preferred by some surgeons. Vascular reconstruction may be necessary if tumor invades the artery or vein and is preferred in lieu of amputation. Neurolysis may be possible in some cases as a limb-sparing technique. Decisions regarding pre-, post-, or intra-operative radiation therapy for anticipated R1 resections are crucial. Suction drains are usually necessary and should be put in line with the incision.

Figure 92-3 demonstrates the surgical excision of a neurofibrosarcoma of the upper extremity in a teenager. The patient was treated with initial biopsy, followed by Adriamycin and Ifosfamide chemotherapy. The tumor progressed on chemotherapy and operative excision was necessary. Skin incision was made including excision of the biopsy site as indicated by the arrow in Fig. 92-3B. Neurovascular structures were identified and isolated with vessel loops. The tumor was primarily in the biceps muscle. Care to preserve the neurovascular structures while removing the tumor with at least a 1 cm margin required unipolar cautery as well as bipolar cautery. Gross total resection was achieved, however, proximally, at the level of the brachial plexus, positive microscopic margins necessitated postoperative radiation therapy in this region.

## Sentinel Lymph Node Biopsy

The sentinel lymph node biopsy technique is similar to the one used for melanoma and extremity RMS. Lymphatic mapping is required prior to intraoperative sentinel lymph node biopsy. Lymphatic mapping is begun by the nuclear medicine physician who injects radioactive colloid at the biopsy or tumor site. This determines the location of the sentinel node and nodal basin. The sentinel node is the first node that drains the tumor area. If the tumor metastasized, this would be the node it would metastasize to initially. This is especially important for trunk lesions since their drainage can be unpredictable. Flank lesions can drain to either the axilla or groin. Once the nodal basin has been identified the patient should proceed to the operating room where lymphazurin blue (LZB) dye will then be injected. We prefer to inject the colloid in the nuclear medicine department under a general anesthetic and then transfer the patient to the operating room still anesthetized for injection of the LZB. Ideally, less than 12 hours should elapse between injection and operative time.

beam radiation to the growth plates will result in a limb that is 1/3 shorter than the other and thus a severe limb-length discrepancy. Complete surgical excision with negative margins is preferred in these patients. If complete surgical excision is not possible, a detailed discussion with the radiation therapist is required. Brachytherapy at the time of operative excision, when positive margins are anticipated is an option. Pre- or postoperative proton beam or other precise growth plate sparing approaches may be required.

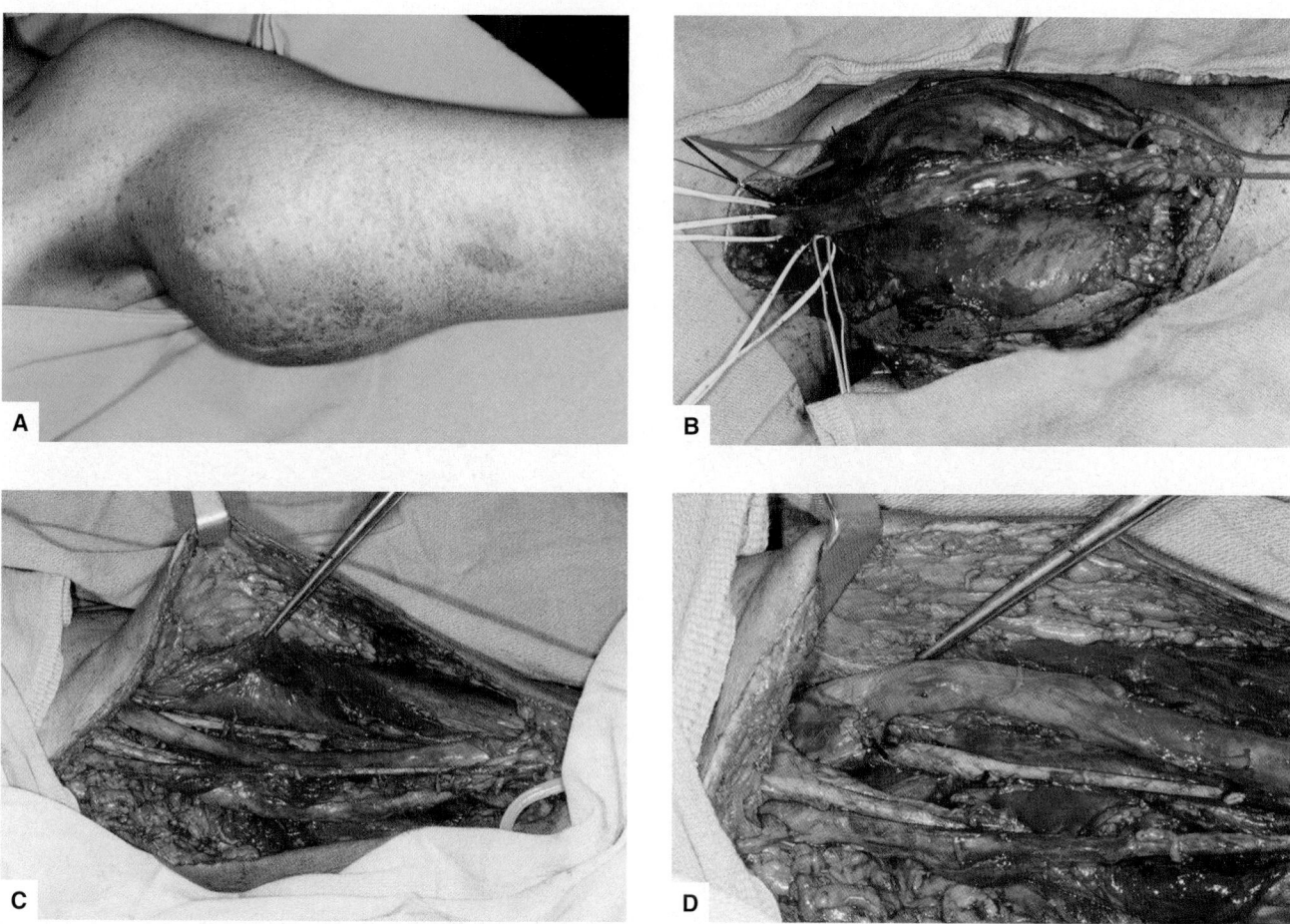

**FIGURE 92-3** **A.** Neurofibrosarcoma in the upper extremity/axilla after failed chemotherapy (a) a 14-cm mass. Note café-au-lait lesions. **B.** Vessel loops encircle arteries, veins, and nerves. **C.** After completed resection, preservation of major brachial artery and vein. **D.** Magnified view of brachial artery, axillary vein, and hypertrophied radial nerve and sheath.

In the operating room a hand-held probe reading the radioactive counts is placed on the skin at the suspected nodal basin to verify where to make the incision for the sentinel lymph node excision (Fig. 92-4D). Then 2 to 3 mL (milliliters) of LZB is injected subdermally with multiple small injections circumferentially around the tumor or biopsy site (Fig. 92-4A and C). There is a small risk of allergic reaction and patients are premedicated with steroids and diphenhydramine before the LZB is injected. The patient is prepped and draped and the probe prepped into the field. At least 10 minutes should elapse between LZB injection and incision at the nodal basin. An axial incision is made in the appropriate nodal basin and careful gentle blunt dissection is used to identify the afferent blue lymphatic and blue lymph node while continually using the probe to guide the surgeon to the lymph node that is both blue and has high radioactive counts (Fig. 92-4B and E). Radioactive counts should be 10% or less of the counts at the primary injection site. Once the node has been identified that has both high counts and is blue, a "figure-of-8" suture is placed through the node to elevate it into the operative field (Fig. 92-4B and E). This allows preservation of architecture of the lymph node. Grasping the lymph node with a forceps or other instrument may destroy the architecture of the lymph node and impair the pathologist's ability to identify subcapsular metastatic disease. The lymph node is then excised using standard electrocautery.

## Desmoid Tumors

Desmoid tumors are very different than desmoplastic small round cell tumors (DSRCT). They are intermediate grade sarcoma-type tumors which are locally very aggressive and can be fatal, but usually do not metastasize. Desmoid fibromatosis is a mesenchymal neoplasm. It is encountered in 2 settings, within the context of familial adenomatous polyposis (FAP) and sporadically. Here we focus on the sporadic group. Desmoid tumors can arise in any body site and are much more common in women. Surgery has been the therapeutic mainstay, but radiotherapy plays an important role in treatment as do systemic therapies such as tamoxifen and suilindac combination and non-steroidal anti-inflammatory drugs (NSAID). Desmoids have a very unique course in that they can recur locally and be more aggressive or regress spontaneously. However, they have no capacity for metastasis. Resecting recurrent tumors can become potentially mutilating. Some large retrospective studies demonstrated that microscopically positive (or grossly positive) margins were predictive of increased local recurrence on retrospective multivariate analysis, although radiation improved outcome in one. Other studies have failed to demonstrate an effect of microscopic margin on recurrence. Some of these differences may result from the mixture of disease sites, pattern of adjuvant radiotherapy application, and selection of patients

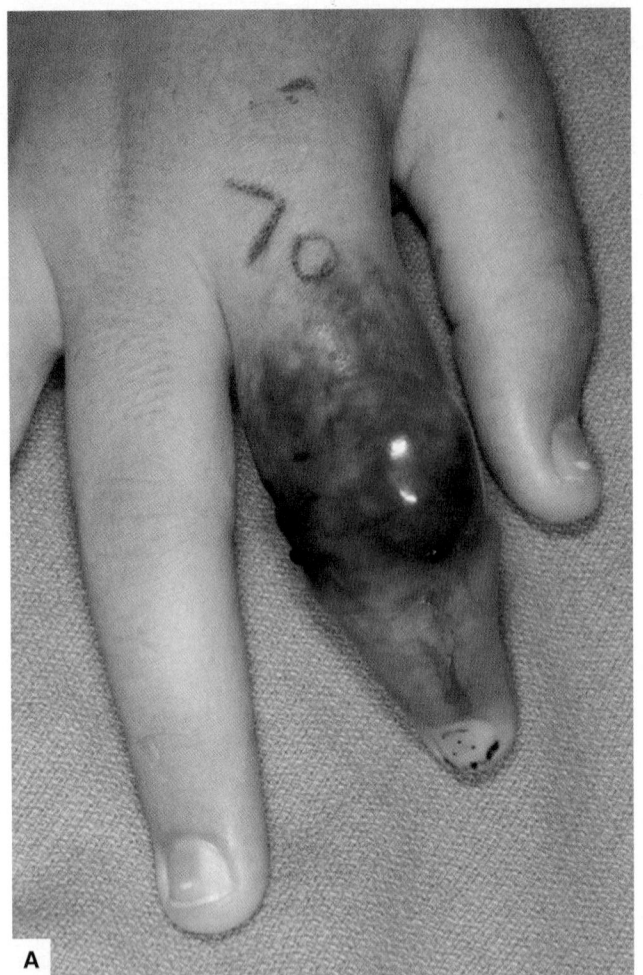

A

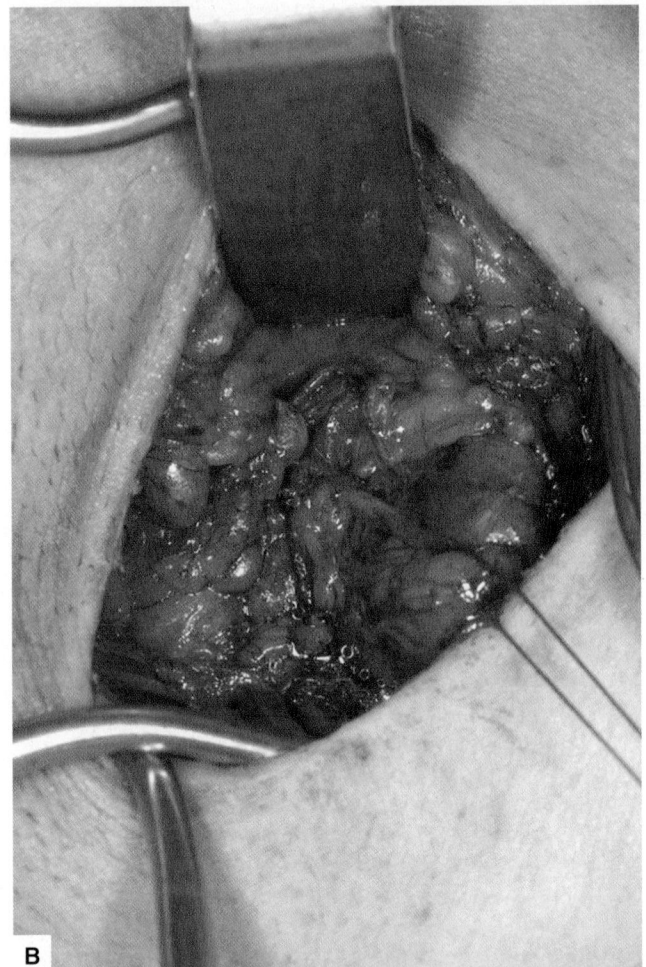

B

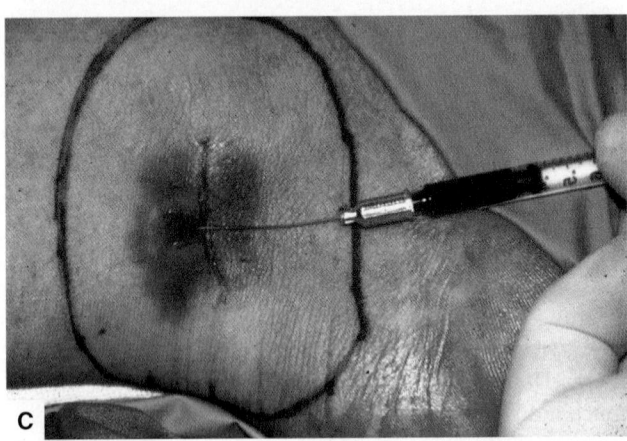

C

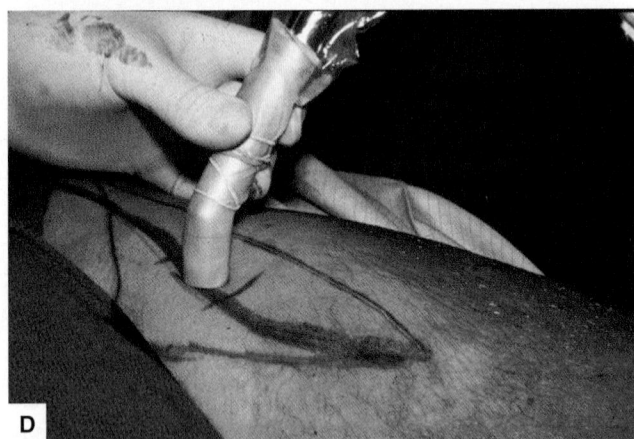

D

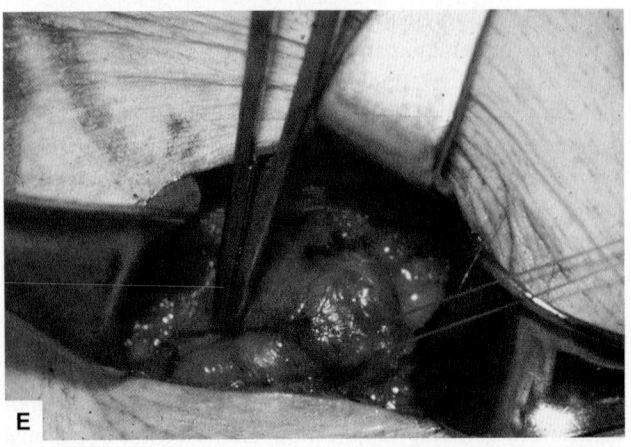

E

**FIGURE 92-4** Operative technique of sentinel lymph node biopsy—axillary and inguinal approach. **A.** Intradermal Lymphazurin blue (LZB) injection of SS of the index finger in a 12-year-old. Two to three milliliters are used. **B.** Blue enhanced afferent lymphatic leading to lymph node. "Figure-of-8" vicryl suture used to elevate lymph node into the operative field. Lymph node is then excised using electrocautery. **C.** Method of injection when previous biopsy or excision scar is present. Intradermal injection of LZB around incision. **D.** Radioactive colloid injected prior to LZB, allows detection by the gamma probe. **E.** Incision is then made at the site of maximal radioactive counts where afferent blue lymphatic and lymph node are identified. Gamma probe is used to verify radioactive counts in blue lymph node. The use of both the LZB dye and radioactivity, provide 98% accuracy of lymphatic mapping and sentinel lymph node biopsy.

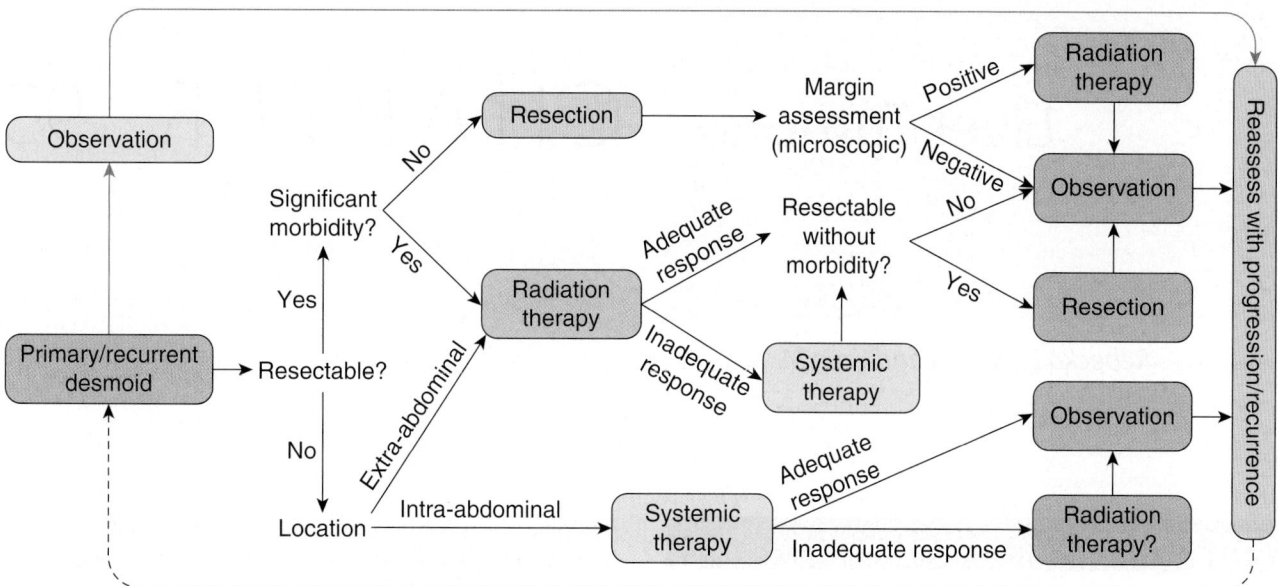

**FIGURE 92-5** General treatment protocol for desmoid tumors at the University of Texas M.D. Anderson Cancer Center. The route of initial observation for certain cases to avoid overtreatment advocated by some is depicted above in gray. Given the propensity for progression on treatment and local recurrence, all treatment pathways ultimately end in observation. Radiation therapy can be preceded, and even precluded, by systemic therapy in certain cases of initially unresectable extra-abdominal desmoid tumors.

treated by the surgical approach. In the end, surgical therapy must be tailored to what is achievable in terms of margins with preserving functional status for the individual patient. Incomplete resection or positive microscopic margins in desmoid tumors should be treated with adjuvant radiotherapy. Figure 92-5 provides a helpful algorithm to follow.

## Operative Resection of Desmoid Tumors

Operative excision of desmoid tumors optimally achieves a negative microscopic margin. In the operating room, tissue adjacent to the tumor may appear grossly normal but can harbor microscopic diseases. As noted above, negative microscopic margins are the most important factors in determining local recurrence. However, it is not uncommon for desmoid tumors to abut or encroach upon critical neurovascular structures, especially in the abdomen or head and neck. In these cases, marginal resection should be completed followed by intra-operative radiation therapy or external beam radiation therapy.

## Summary

Nonrhabdomyosarcoma soft tissue sarcomas are a heterogeneous group of neoplasms that account for approximately 4% of all childhood tumors. Surgical resection is the mainstay of treatment and long term survival can be expected in 60% of patients.

## SELECTED READINGS

Ballo MT, Zagars GK, Pollack A, Pisters PW, Pollack RA. Desmoid tumor: prognostic factors and outcome after surgery, radiation therapy, or combined surgery and radiation therapy. *J Clin Oncol* 1999;17(1):158–167.

Carli M, Ferrari A, Mattke A, et al. Pediatric malignant peripheral nerve sheath tumor: the Italian and German soft tissue sarcoma cooperative group. *J Clin Oncol* 2005;23(33):8422–8430.

Coindre JM. Grading of soft tissue sarcomas: review and update. *Arch Pathol Lab Med* 2006;130(10):1448–1453.

Cormier JN, Huang X, Xing Y, et al. Cohort analysis of patients with localized, high-risk, extremity soft tissue sarcoma treated at two cancer centers: chemotherapy-associated outcomes. *J Clin Oncol* 2004;22(22):4567–4574.

Ferrari A, Casanova M. New concepts for the treatment of pediatric nonrhabdomyosarcoma soft tissue sarcomas. *Expert Rev Anticancer Ther* 2005;5(2):307–318.

Friedrich RE, Hartmann M, Mautner VF. Malignant peripheral nerve sheath tumors (MPNST) in NF1-affected children. *Anticancer Res* 2007;27(4A):1957–1960.

Hayes-Jordan AA, Spunt SL, et al. Nonrhabdomyosarcoma soft tissue sarcomas in children: is age at diagnosis an important variable? *J Pediatr Surg.* 2000;35(6):948–953; discussion 953–944.

Lev D, Kotilingam D, Wei C, et al. Optimizing treatment of desmoid tumors. *J Clin Oncol* 2007;25(13):1785–1791.

Spunt SL, Poquette CA, Hurt YS, et al. Prognostic factors for children and adolescents with surgically resected nonrhabdomyosarcoma soft tissue sarcoma: an analysis of 121 patients treated at St Jude Children's Research Hospital. *J Clin Oncol* 1999;17(12):3697–3705.

Stoeckle E, Coindre JM, Longy M, et al. A critical analysis of treatment strategies in desmoid tumours: a review of a series of 106 cases. *Eur J Surg Oncol* 2009;35(2):129–134.

*Rebecka L. Meyers and Greg M. Tiao*

## HISTORICAL CONTEXT

Liver tumors in children encompass a wide spectrum of entities ranging from the congenital and acquired non-neoplastic masses to benign growths to the frankly malignant lesion. Complete surgical excision remains a therapeutic cornerstone in the management of most childhood liver tumors. From a historical standpoint, it is enlightening to realize how far techniques in liver resection have evolved. An early report on liver resection in children by Howat from the 1960s described 14 resections for malignant "hepatoma" of childhood with only 3 survivors and an operative mortality due to hemorrhage of 31%. The main risks of liver surgery, even though segmental vascular and biliary anatomy had been described by Couinaud in 1954 were bleeding and biliary fistula. In 1974, in a landmark survey of the American Academy of Pediatrics (AAP) Surgical Section examining outcomes following liver resection, Exelby reported over a 10% mortality rate following surgical intervention. Two-thirds of the children underwent incomplete tumor excision and none survived. Over the subsequent decade, various technical procedures were established to minimize bleeding including the Pringle maneuver (clamping of the afferent vascular pedicle), total vascular occlusion (clamping of the aorta and balloon occlusion of the inferior vena cava), hypothermia, preresection ligation of the hepatic inflow and outflow vasculature, and hypotensive anesthesia. The result was improved perioperative survival such that in 1982, Price reported a series of 11 pediatric tumor resections with no operative deaths.

With the continued evolution of techniques, development of new technology and a better understanding of the disease process, perioperative mortality following surgical resection of liver tumors have been substantially reduced. Treatment strategies have evolved such that multidisciplinary input should be employed in the management of virtually all children diagnosed with a liver tumor. In that context, outcomes for children afflicted with liver lesions continue to improve.

## DIFFERENTIAL DIAGNOSIS

The differential diagnosis of a liver mass in a child includes malignant tumors, benign tumors, and both congenital and acquired non-neoplastic masses (Table 93-1). Liver tumors are rare in children accounting for about 1.5% of all childhood malignancies. Primary pediatric malignant tumors include HB, HCC, rhabdoid tumors, and sarcomas. More rarely one may encounter metastatic lesions or contiguous invasion from primary pediatric solid tumors such as neuroblastoma, Wilms tumor, or pancreatoblastoma. Hepatic involvement in hematologic malignancies such as hemophagocytic lymphohistiocytosis (HLH), Langerhans cell histiocytosis (LCH), megakaryoblastic leukemia may occasionally mimic a primary hepatic malignancy. Benign tumors

## TABLE 93-1 Differential Diagnosis of Pediatric Liver Masses

| Malignant Tumors | Benign Tumors | Other Masses |
|---|---|---|
| ▶ Hepatoblastoma (HB) | ▶ Mesenchymal Hamartoma | ▶ Vascular Malformations |
| ▶ Hepatocellular Carcinoma (HCC) | ▶ Biliary Cystadenoma | ▪ AV malformation |
| ▶ Sarcoma | ▶ Focal Nodular Hyperplasia (FNH) | ▪ Blue Rubber Nevus Syndrome |
| ▪ Biliary Rhabdomyosarcoma | ▶ Infantile Hemangioma | ▶ Congenital/Acquired Cysts |
| ▪ Angiosarcoma | ▶ Hepatic Adenoma | ▪ Simple |
| ▪ Rhabdoid | ▶ Nodular Regenerative Hyperplasia (NRH) | ▪ Ciliated Foregut Cyst |
| ▪ Undifferentiated | ▶ Teratoma | ▪ Polycystic liver disease |
| ▶ Metastatic/Other | ▶ Inflammatory Myofibroblastic Tumor | ▪ Choledochal Cyst |
| ▪ Wilms Tumor | | ▪ Inspissated Bile Lake/Biliary Atresia |
| ▪ Neuroblastoma | | ▪ Parasitic Cysts |
| ▪ Colorectal | | • Hydatid |
| ▪ Carcinoid tumor | | • Amoebic |
| ▪ Pancreatoblastoma | | ▶ Abscess |
| ▶ Hematologic | | ▪ Bacterial |
| ▪ Hemophagocytic Lympho-Histiocytosis (HLH) | | ▪ Fungal |
| ▪ Langerhans Cell Histiocytosis (LCH) | | ▪ Chronic Granulomatous Disease (CGD) |
| ▪ Megakaryoblastic Leukemia | | ▪ Hematoma |
| ▪ Lymphoma | | ▪ Fatty liver |

include vascular tumors which are most common and others such as mesenchymal hamartoma, biliary cystadenoma, hepatic adenoma, focal nodular hyperplasia (FNH), nodular regenerative hyperplasia (NRH), teratoma, and inflammatory myofibroblastic tumors. Non-neoplastic masses include vascular malformations, congenital and acquired cysts, abscess, hematoma, and fatty infiltration of the liver.

For many of the non-neoplastic masses the key to diagnosis lies in the underlying medical condition. For example, one might expect to find a bacterial hepatic abscess in a child with chronic granulomatous disease, a fatty deposit in the liver of a child with hyperlipidemia or obesity, or an inspissated bile lake in a child with biliary atresia (Fig. 93-1). Hepatic hematoma or infarction should be suspected in any child with a history of hepatic trauma or in newborns with sepsis and coagulopathy; especially if there is a history of perinatal birth trauma.

Age at presentation and level of alpha fetoprotein (AFP) are often the keys to differential diagnosis (Table 93-2). The most common tumor in infants is infantile hepatic hemangioma. Rare malignant tumors in neonates are teratoma, rhabdoid tumor, and biliary rhabdomyosarcoma. Most cases of HB occur in children under the age of 3. Mesenchymal hamartoma is seen in toddlers and school-aged children. In adolescents, malignant liver tumors include HCC and undifferentiated sarcoma. HCC in this age group is comprised of a heterogeneous group of tumors including transitional cell tumors with features of both HB and HCC, *de novo* HCC tumors, HCC developing in a setting of underlying metabolic or cirrhotic liver disease, and fibrolamellar carcinomas.

Although elevation of AFP argues in favor of malignancy, elevation in AFP is not specific. Several conditions may be associated with an elevated AFP level and without biopsy, may lead to errors in diagnosis. At birth the AFP level is high and decreases rapidly in the first 6 months of life. AFP is often secreted at very high levels in the regenerating liver and/or after ischemic liver injury. A spontaneous decline in the AFP level without treatment favors a physiologic origin. An elevated AFP may be associated with other tumor types including germ cell tumors, mesenchymal hamartoma, or infantile hepatic hemangioma. Other conditions such as viral hepatitis or tyrosinemia may be associated with a high AFP level.

# BENIGN TUMORS

## Hepatic Hemangioma

Infantile hepatic hemangioma is the most common benign tumor of the liver in infancy. Figure 93-2 illustrates the striking variability of focal, multifocal, and diffuse subtypes. Many focal lesions are discovered incidentally, and if localized, may be small enough to be of little clinical significance. Symptoms seen with larger lesions include abdominal distention, vomiting, hepatomegaly, congestive heart failure, anemia, thrombocytopenia and consumptive coagulopathy, jaundice secondary to biliary obstruction, and associated cutaneous or visceral hemangiomas. The diagnosis of infantile hepatic hemangioma is usually straightforward and based on the combination of clinical symptoms and radiographic appearance on ultrasound and CT scan. Contrast enhanced CT scan shows an area of diminished density, and after injection of intravenous contrast, enhancement from the periphery toward the center of the lesion, which after a short delay, results in progressive isodense filling of the lesion. MRA has been used in complex cases to identify atypical radiographic features that may portend a poor prognosis. Unfavorable

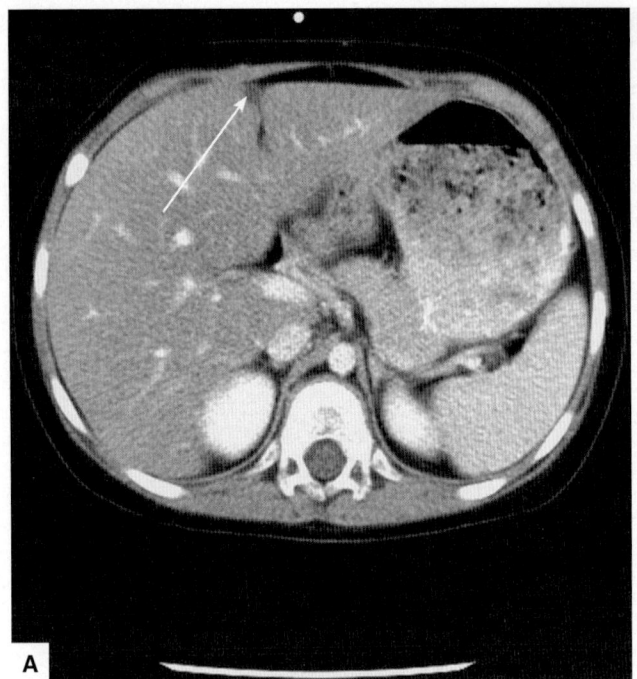

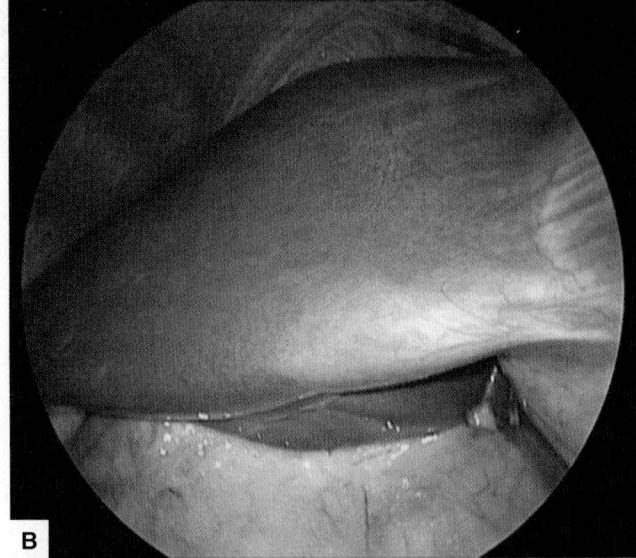

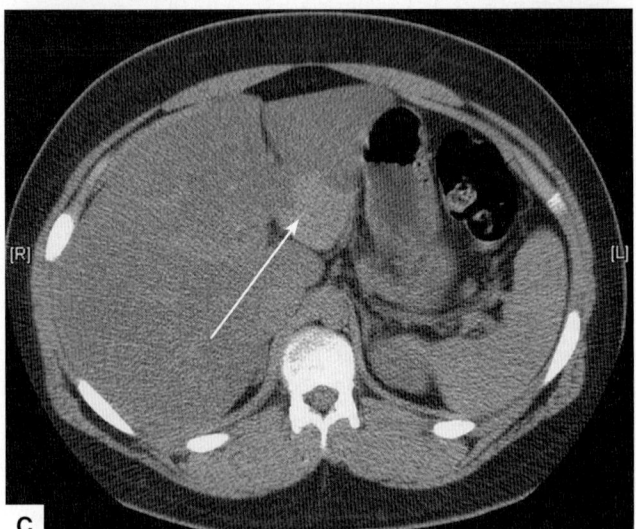

**FIGURE 93-1** Fatty infiltration of liver. **A.** Fatty deposit adjacent to falciform in patient with hyperlipidemia. **B.** Laparoscopic appearance of fatty deposit adjacent to falciform. **C.** Rapid weight gain in obese adolescent, geographic deposition of fat with island of normal liver not infiltrated by fat.

radiographic features include: central varix with arteriovenous shunt, central necrosis or thrombosis, and diffuse hemangiomatous involvement of the liver with abdominal vascular compression. Angiography may be used in infants with refractory symptoms in whom either hepatic artery

| TABLE 93-2 | Age at Presentation, Primary Liver Tumors of Childhood | |
|---|---|---|
| **Age Group** | **Malignant** | **Benign** |
| Infant/Toddler | Hepatoblastoma 43%<br>Rhabdoid tumor 1%<br>Malignant germ<br>cell 1% | Hemangioma/vascular 14%<br>Mesenchymal<br>hamartoma 6%<br>Teratoma 1% |
| School Age/<br>Adolescent | Hepatocellular (and<br>transitional cell<br>tumors) 23%<br>Sarcomas 7% | Focal nodular<br>hyperplasia 3%<br>Hepatic Adenoma 1% |

*Note:* Data from Von Schweinitz D. Management of liver tumors in childhood. *Semin Pediatr Surg* 2006;15:17–24.

ligation or embolization is considered. If a definitive diagnosis of simple infantile hepatic hemangioma can be made, patients are observed because spontaneous regression occurs frequently. With large symptomatic tumors, the terminology is confusing, with lesions described as hepatic hemangioma, infantile hepatic hemangioma, infantile hepatic hemangioendothelioma (IHEE), and kaposiform hemangioendothelioma interchangeably. A European pathologic classification recognizes 2 types in IHEE. Type I is more common and is composed of a single layer of plump but bland endothelial cells with rare mitotic figures. Type 2 has more pleomorphic endothelial cells and is considered by some to be a low-grade angiosarcoma. The Boston Vascular Tumor Study Group prefers to refer to all tumors confined to the liver as infantile hepatic hemangioma.

A treatment algorithm has been proposed and can be reached at www.liverhemangioma.org (Fig. 93-3). About 65% of tumors are solitary or unifocal with a survival of 86% and death caused by a co-morbidity. Thirty-five percent of tumors are multifocal or diffuse with a survival somewhere between 60% and 100% with death due to cardiorespiratory compromise from tumors refractory to medical and interventional

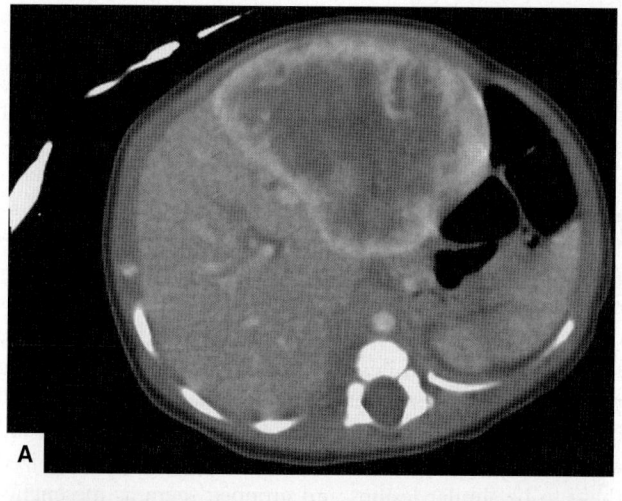

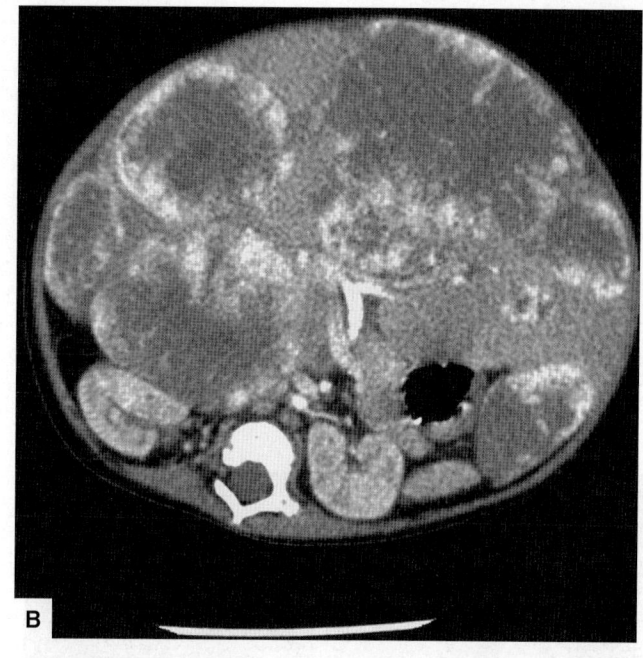

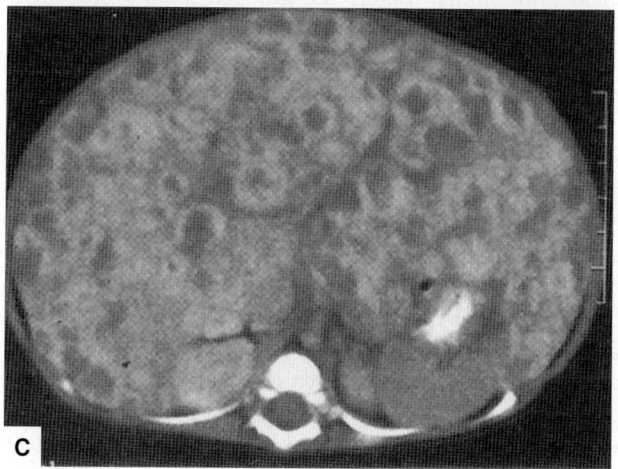

**FIGURE 93-2** Three sub-types of infantile hepatic hemangioma. A. Focal. B. Multifocal. C. Diffuse.

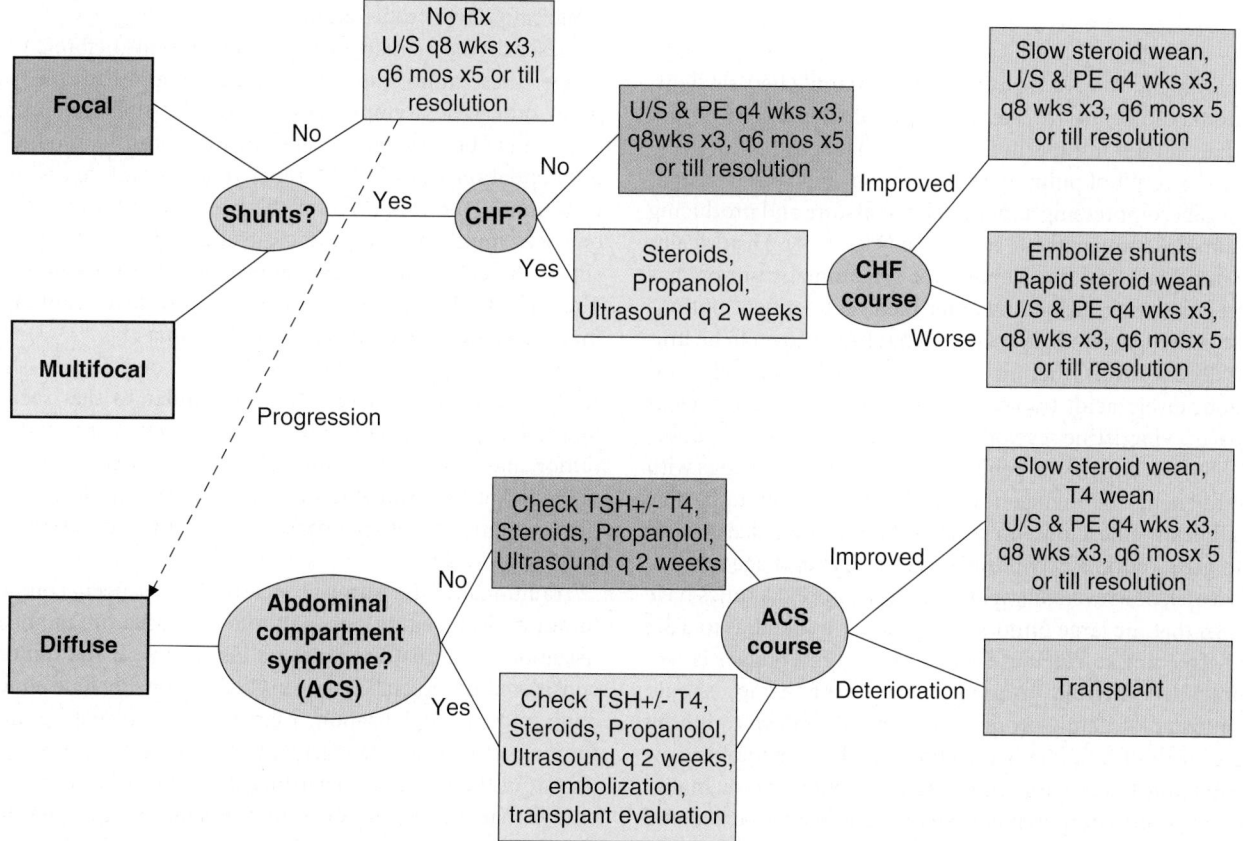

**FIGURE 93-3** Treatment algorithm: infantile hepatic hemangioma. (Adapted from Fishman S et al. www.liverhemangioma.com.)

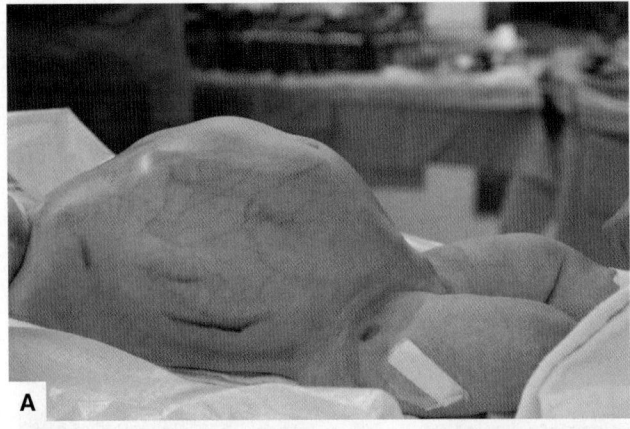

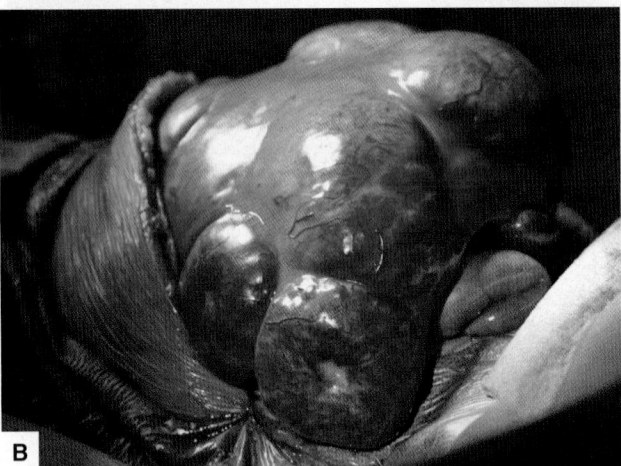

**FIGURE 93-4 A,B.** Large infantile hemangioma with abdominal compartment syndrome.

management. A large rapidly growing infantile hepatic hemangioma can be life-threatening with intractable high-output cardiac failure, intraperitoneal hemorrhage, respiratory distress as a result of pulmonary congestion, and massive hepatomegaly compressing abdominal vasculature and producing abdominal compartment syndrome (Fig. 93-4). Historically, the initial medical intervention for symptomatic tumors has been corticosteroids. Many other medical treatment options exist, although no single treatment has been shown to be universally effective. Other medications utilized include epsilon-aminocaproic acid, tranexamic acid, low-molecular-weight heparin, vincristine, cyclophosphamide, interferon 2-alpha, AGM-1470, and newer-generation antiangiogenic drugs with some benefit. The angiogenesis inhibitor interferon-alpha may be clinically efficacious; however, it should be avoided or used with great caution in children less than 1 year of age because of the risk of irreversible spastic diplegia. Recent studies have shown that the large tumors may produce antibodies to TSH and screening to rule out secondary hypothyroidism is recommended. Thyroid hormone replacement therapy should be initiated. Recently propranolol has been shown to inhibit the growth of infantile hemangioma and propanolol is now the first line treatment in most centers. Although rare, malignant transformation to angiosarcoma has been reported and close follow-up is recommended. In infants who fail medical management, symptomatic solitary tumors may be treated by excision, hepatic arterial ligation, or selective angiographic embolization. Although potentially hazardous, hepatic arterial embolization is beneficial in tumors causing high-output cardiac failure. Liver transplantation may be life-saving for cases with diffuse angiomatous change.

## Mesenchymal Hamartoma

Although mesenchymal hamartoma of the liver is the second most common benign liver tumor in children, its biology and pathogenesis are poorly understood. Mesenchymal hamartoma has been described by various names including pseudocystic mesenchymal tumor, hepatic and giant cell lymphangioma, cystic hamartoma, bile cell fibroadenoma, and cavernous lymphangiomatoid tumor. Edmondson recognized these to be similar lesions and grouped them as mesenchymal hamartomas. The pathogenesis of mesenchymal hamartoma is unclear. The 3 leading theories postulate (1) abnormal embryologic development of the mesenchyme producing obstruction of the developing biliary tree that results in cystic, anaplastic, and proliferating bile ducts with most of the proliferative growth just before or after birth, because no mesenchymal mitotic activity is seen histologically; (2) abnormal development of blood supply with ischemic necrosis and reactive cystic changes; (3) abnormal proliferation of embryologic hepatic mesenchyme with increased expression of fibroblast growth factor-2 (FGF-2). Microscopically, the tissue consists of a mixture of bile ducts, liver cell cysts, and mesenchyme. The cysts may simply be dilated bile ducts, dilated lymphatics, or amorphous fluid surrounded by mesenchyme. Elongated or tortuous bile ducts surrounded by connective tissue are unevenly distributed with the bile ducts at the periphery often exhibiting active proliferation.

Mesenchymal hamartoma typically presents before 2 years of age. These tumors are usually detected as a palpable mass in an otherwise asymptomatic child. The alpha-fetoprotein (AFP) may be variably elevated in this tumor confounding differentiation from HB. Mesenchymal hamartoma is more common in the right lobe of the liver. On ultrasonography one sees multiple echogenic cysts although, if the cysts are small, the entire tumor may appear as an echogenic mass. The typical CT scan shows a well-circumscribed, multicystic mass separated by solid septae and stroma (Fig. 93-5). The stroma and septae may be vascular and occasionally show contrast enhancement on CT scan similar to that seen in infantile hepatic hemangioma. When the cysts are small the tumor may appear solid and biopsy is required to rule out malignancy. Occasionally, a highly vascular tumor in a neonate may present with hydrops, high output heart failure, and respiratory distress.

Traditionally, the surgical treatment has been complete tumor excision, either nonanatomically with a rim of normal tissue or as an anatomic hepatic lobectomy. If the tumor is considered unresectable, the surgical options include enucleation and marsupialization. Marsupialization may result in tumor recurrence. Management continues to evolve, with debate in the literature regarding the advisability of nonoperative management in the asymptomatic patient. Caution is warranted if expectant management is chosen due to reports of association with undifferentiated (embryonal) sarcoma.

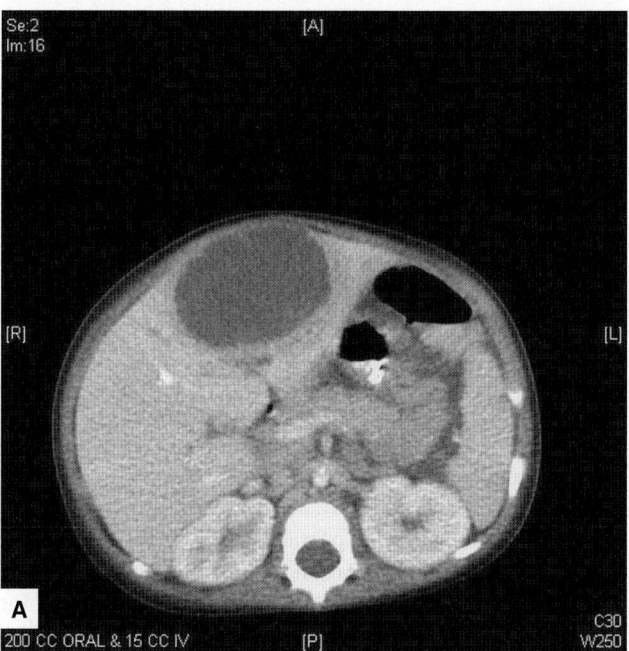

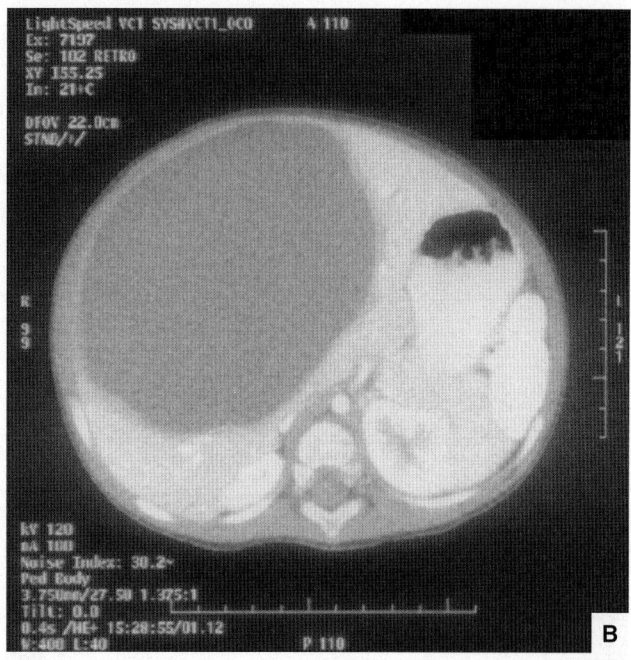

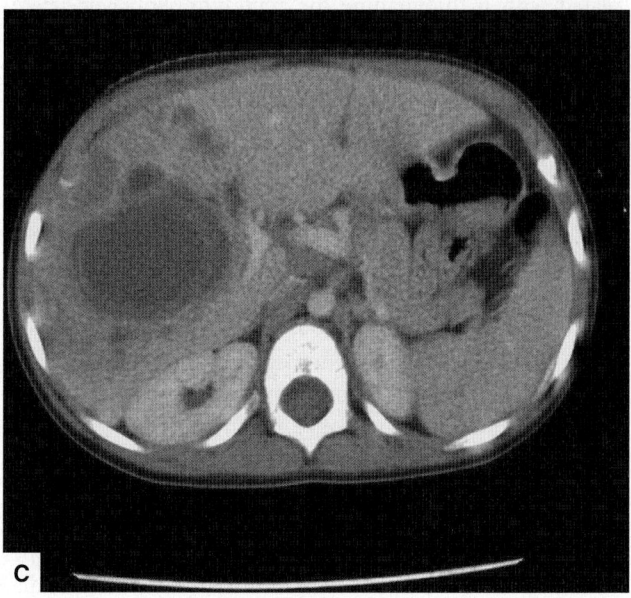

**FIGURE 93-5** Congenital and acquired cystic masses and tumors. **A.** A 4-year-old from Central America with acquired cyst, amoebic abscess. **B.** A 1-month-old with a Congenital Simple Hepatic cyst so large that it causes symptoms (pain, compression of stomach and duodenum, and upward pressure on diaphragms). **C.** A 2-year-old with Mesenchymal Hamartoma: complex multicystic mass with cysts separated by thick solid septae.

## Benign Epithelial Tumors

Benign epithelial tumors that are common in adults may occur in childhood. These include FNH, NRH, and hepatic adenoma.

## Focal Nodular Hyperplasia

FNH may be diagnosed at any age, from newborns to the elderly. In children, it usually is diagnosed between 2 and 5 years of age. It is a benign epithelial tumor that has been referred to by various names including benign hepatoma, solitary hyperplastic nodule, focal cirrhosis, cholangiohepatoma, and mixed adenoma. FNH has been seen in association with a variety of different conditions including previous trauma to the liver, other liver tumors, hemochromatosis, the Klinefelter syndrome, itraconazole, smoking, oral contraceptives, congenital absence of the portal vein (Abernathy

syndrome), and a history of pediatric treatment with chemotherapy for a Wilms tumor or neuroblastoma. Grossly, FNH tumors are well-circumscribed and lobulated with the architecture of bile ducts and a central stellate scar containing blood vessels that supply the hyperplastic process. Usually, there is no real capsule, but exuberant fibrous tissue may surround the lesions. Lesions are often multiple, and vary in size from a few millimeters to more than 20 cm in diameter.

Small FNH lesions are asymptomatic incidental findings. Larger lesions typically present with abdominal pain. The diagnosis of FNH is suggested by ultrasound showing a well-demarcated, hyperechoic, and homogenous lesion; the tumor may be better seen on CTA or MRA after intravenous contrast enhancement. Although approximately 50% of FNH will have normal accumulation of the [9m]Tc sulfur colloid on liver scintigraphy, this finding is not universally specific and there have been many reports of scintigraphic findings suggestive

**1233**

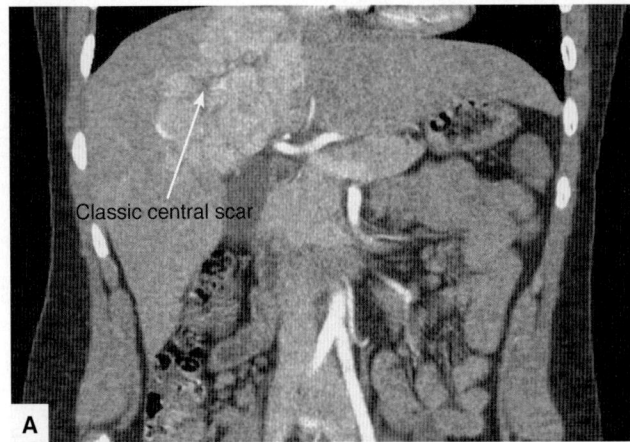

Classic central scar

**A**

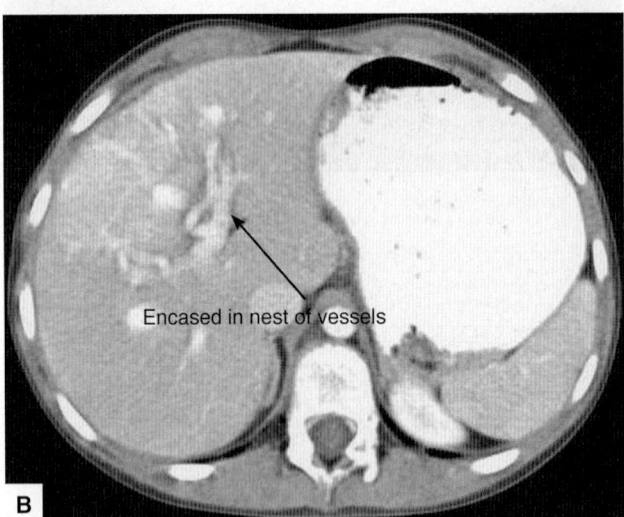

Encased in nest of vessels

**B**

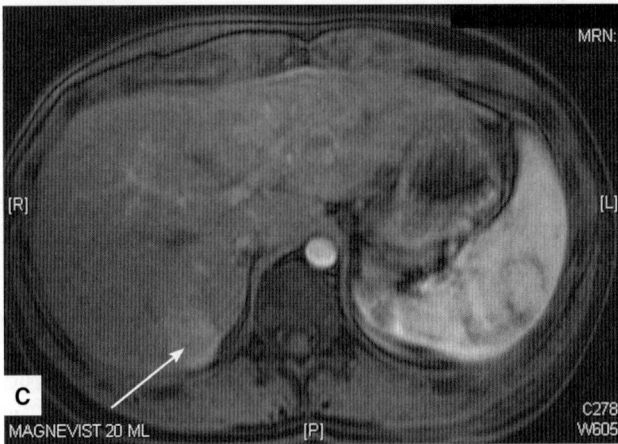

MRN:

[R]                    [L]

**C**

MAGNEVIST 20 ML      [P]      C278 W605

**FIGURE 93-6** Focal Nodular Hyperplasia (FNH) with variable radiographic appearance. **A.** FNH with classic findings (well demarcated with a central stellate scar). **B.** Hypervascular with an unusual nest of dilated vessels encasing the tumor. **C.** Tumor was isodense with liver on MRI T1, and T2 (seen here only after gadolinium contrast enhancement).

of FNH in children who turned out to have HB or HC. FNH can be a radiographic chameleon and although a radiographic "central stellate scar" is considered a "classic" finding, the radiographic appearance can be quite variable (Fig. 93-6). If biopsy does not definitively confirm the diagnosis, excision may be necessary.

Complete surgical resection of biopsy-proven FNH is not mandatory in asymptomatic patients. Spontaneous regression is rare although it may be seen after cessation of oral contraceptives. Symptomatic patients in whom the diagnosis of malignancy has not been definitively ruled out will require surgical excision. Symptomatic patients in whom the benign diagnosis has been confirmed may be candidates for ablative therapy with transcatheter arterial embolization or percutaneous ablative techniques.

## Nodular Regenerative Hyperplasia (NRH)

NRH of the liver is a multiacinar regenerative nodular lesion in a noncirrhotic liver. It is a rare entity of unknown etiology but has been associated in children with a variety of other diseases and drugs. In about half of the children there is some component of associated portal hypertension. NRH has been reported in children with portal hypertension and hepatopulmonary syndrome, celiac disease, mimicking metastatic nodules in children with prior treatment of Wilms tumor or neuroblastoma, azathioprine treatment of inflammatory bowel disease, intrahepatic occlusive venopathy in children treated with 6 thioguanine for acute lymphoblastic leukemia, Budd–Chiari Syndrome, pulmonary arterial hypertension and connective tissue disorders, chronic granulomatous disease, and a spectrum of other disorders many of which involve some sort of perturbation of the hepatic vasculature. Radiologically its nodular appearance may look like neoplasia and open wedge biopsy is often required to definitively rule out malignancy. Prognosis in the absence of portal hypertension is good and complications are rare.

## Hepatic (Hepatocellular) Adenoma

Rare in children, hepatic adenoma, sometimes called hepatocellular adenoma, is most common in young women in their twenties, especially in response to birth control hormonal therapy. The differential diagnosis from FNH can be difficult but with newly developed cross-sectional imaging techniques such as MR with Eovist, this difficulty has been reduced. Adenomas are associated with glycogen-storage disease types 1 and 3, galactosemia, hyperthyroidism, polycythemia, diabetes, Fanconi anemia, polycystic ovary syndrome, and anabolic steroids. When associated with oral contraceptives or anabolic steroids the tumor may regress with cessation of the hormonal therapy. Recent studies have shown that adenomas with mutations in HNF1 or the beta catenin pathway have increased risk of malignant degeneration. Biopsy of adenoma with assessment of these markers is increasingly recognized as a necessary intervention. If these mutations are present, ablation or resection may be considered. Persistent or progressive adenomas are at risk of rupture and bleeding, and surgical excision is often recommended. Percutaneous ablation may also be considered but patients will require close follow-up.

## Other Benign Tumors

### Hepatobiliary Cystadenoma

Cystadenomas of the liver are benign tumors most commonly found in middle-aged women. Rare case reports include a

4-year-old boy who had a large mucin-hypersecreting hepatobiliary cystadenoma that caused a hepato-colo-cutaneous fistula, resulting in significant external fluid loss. Total excision and repair of the fistula was possible after shrinkage of the tumor via selective embolization of the feeding artery.

## Hepatic Teratoma

True hepatic teratoma is extremely rare. Twenty-four cases have been reported in the literature; 18 of which were in children less than 3 years old. About half of these tumors have been malignant. The characteristic histological finding is a predominance of hepatic tissue. Inflammatory myofibroblastic tumor is a rare entity formerly known as inflammatory pseudotumor. These tumors occur throughout the body. This tumor has been associated with underlying chronic infections from mycobacterium avium intracellulare, immunodeficiency, biliary obstruction, and autoimmune sclerosing cholangitis. Treatment of symptomatic lesions is excision.

# MALIGNANT TUMORS

Contemporary research efforts focus primarily on the 2 most common malignant liver tumors in children, HB and HCC. In the late 1970s and early 1980s, the introduction and use of chemotherapy in patients diagnosed with HB induced the most dramatic improvement in outcome. Improvements recently have been more modest, and are mainly due to increasingly sophisticated surgical techniques based on more accurate anatomic knowledge and an increasing breadth of experience in complex liver resection.

## Hepatoblastoma (HB)

### Epidemiology, Biology, Genetics

HB accounts for about 80% of the malignant tumors in children. The incidence has increased from 0.6 to 0.8 per million to 1.2 to 1.5 per million over the past 2 decades. The increased incidence may be due to the growing prevalence of premature birth and very low birth weight babies, known risk factors for HB. Unproven, but postulated environmental risk factors include parental exposure to smoking, welding fumes, petroleum products, and paint. Increased risk of HB is found in children afflicted with Trisomy 18, Beckwith Weideman syndrome (BWS), and familial adenomatous polyposis (FAP). The association with BWS is so strong that it is recommend that affected children be screened with ultrasound and AFP regularly until the age of 7. Familial case reports of HB with FAP suggest a role in the pathogenesis of HB for chromosomes 5 and 11.

During the last 2 decades several signal transduction cascades that govern proliferation, differentiation, and maturation have been implicated in HB pathogenesis including the Wnt, Hedgehog, Insulin like growth factor axis, and hepatocyte growth factor (HGF)/c-Met pathways. One of the most provocative genetic findings has been the association between HB and mutations of the beta-catenin and activation of the Wnt/beta-catenin signaling pathway. Microarray analysis has defined 2 distinct tumor subclasses with regard to Wnt signaling and corresponding to distinct phases in liver development. Histologic subtypes of HB such as small cell undifferentiated (SCU) appear genetically distinct. Hedgehog signaling is known to contribute to tumor growth in adult HCC and recent studies have shown a similar association in HB.

## Pathology

The gross and histologic work-up of HB is well-described. A detailed gross description should include information about which Couinaud segments are involved, number and size of tumor nodules, and macroscopic vascular involvement. For the evaluation of surgical resection margins and the assessment of microscopic residual disease, it is recommended that surgeons and pathologists work closely together using colored sutures and/or inking to identify critical margin areas. Currently, there is not an internationally agreed upon pathologic classification system. The criteria for the various modern classification schemes were recently reviewed. About 55% of HB are epithelial (30% fetal, 20% fetal embryonal, 3% macrotrabecular, 2% small cell undifferentiated (SCU)), and 45% are mixed epithelial and mesenchymal (Table 93-3). Subtypes are rarely homogeneous and about 85% of all HB contain at least some fetal and embryonal components. In pure fetal histology (PFH) there is very little mitotic activity and these tumors appear to carry very favorable prognosis. A subset of fetal HB shows increased mitotic activity and is sometimes called mitotically active fetal, or crowded fetal HB. Originally termed "anaplastic," Haas et al proposed the term SCU subtype. Sometimes found in only a few small foci within the tumor, this subtype portends a poor prognosis. A subset of SCU HB displays rhabdoid features and shares lack of INI1 expression with malignant rhabdoid tumors.

## Imaging, Staging, PRETEXT, Risk Group Stratification

Ultrasound is the best screening technique for the evaluation of an abdominal mass. In most liver tumors, the hepatic origin of the mass will be confirmed. Subsequent imaging with computed tomography (CT) and/or magnetic

| TABLE 93-3 | Pathologic Classification of Hepatoblastoma by Histologic Subtype |
|---|---|
| Epithelial Hepatoblastoma | |
|   Fetal | |
|   Embryonal/mixed fetal and embryonal | |
|   Macrotrabecular (MT) | |
|   Small cell undifferentiated (SCU) | |
|     -formerly anaplastic | |
|     -shares features of Rhabdoid Tumor of Liver | |
| Mixed Epithelial and Mesenchymal Hepatoblastoma | |
|   Without teratoid features | |
|   With teratoid features | |

*Note:* This is the classification used by the SIOPEL liver tumor study group, goal of international pathologic classification system subject of International Pathology Symposium Hepatoblastoma, Los Angeles, March 2011.

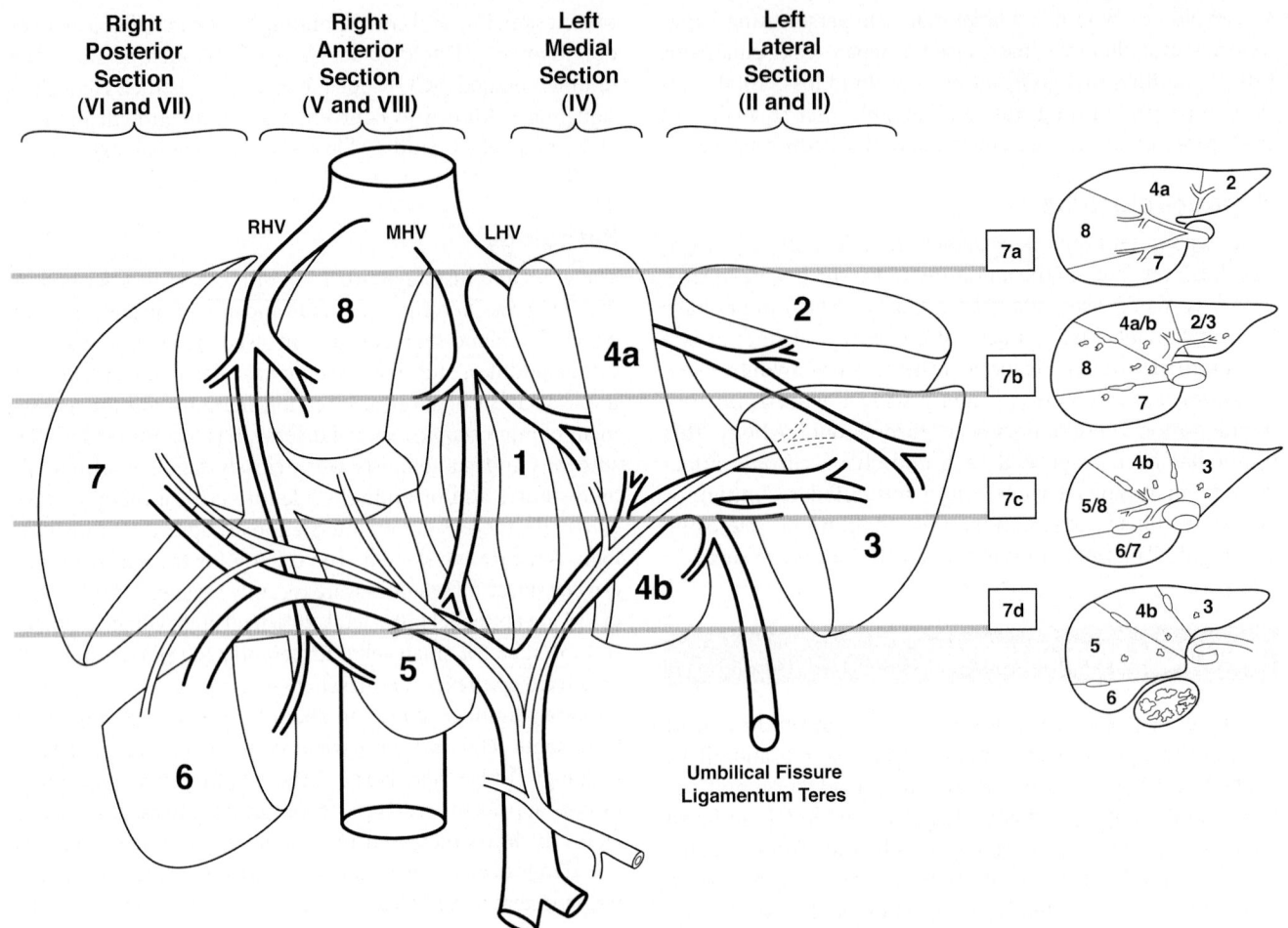

Right Posterior Section (VI and VII)  Right Anterior Section (V and VIII)  Left Medial Section (IV)  Left Lateral Section (II and II)

RHV    MHV    LHV

Umbilical Fissure
Ligamentum Teres

**FIGURE 93-7** PRETEXT defines tumor involvement of 4 Liver "Sections."

resonance imaging (MRI) is best performed by radiologists with experience in pediatric oncology. The importance of high-quality imaging in children with liver tumors is paramount because staging and treatment are dependent on the findings. Chest CT is essential to rule out metastatic lesions. CT of the abdomen should be done in 3 phases: noncontrast, arterial, and venous. The arterial phase shows the hepatic arterial supply and may be useful for the detection of small hypervascular lesions (ie, small HCC or metastasis). Images in the venous phase maximize the margins of primary tumors and are best for assessment of portal and hepatic venous involvement. Most pediatric oncology centers will have an MRI protocol for liver tumor imaging. Conventional MRI contrast agents (gadolinium chelates) are used routinely.

Pre-treatment extent of disease (PRETEXT) is based on cross-sectional imaging assessment of the extent of tumor involvement of the 4 main sections of the liver: right posterior section (Couinaud 6, 7); right anterior section (Couinaud 5, 8); left medial section (Couinaud 4a, 4b); left lateral section (Couinaud 2,3) (Fig. 93-7). Cross-sectional anatomy of these segments can be challenging, and is shown in (Fig. 93-7A ). PRETEXT (Fig. 93-8) was devised by the Liver Tumor Strategy Group (SIOPEL) of the International Society of Pediatric Oncology (SIOP) for their first trial, SIOPEL 1 and revised for SIOPEL 3 in 2007. Assignment to one of 4 PRETEXT groups

(PRETEXT I, II, III, or IV) is determined by the number of contiguous uninvolved sections of the liver. PRETEXT is further annotated with a V, P, E, M, or C depending upon extension of tumor beyond the hepatic parenchyma of the major sections. Caudate involvement is annotated as "C." Tumor extension outside the liver to a contiguous intraabdominal organ (eg, stomach, diaphragm) is annotated as "E." Distant metastatic disease (usually lungs) is annotated as "M." Major vascular involvement is annotated as a "V" (all 3 hepatic veins or the vena cava) or "P" (portal bifurcation or the main portal vein).

Since the 1990s all SIOPEL trials have used PRETEXT as a tool to stratify treatment, define risk categories, and report outcomes in HB. Although the risk stratification schema differ between groups, all of the major multicenter pediatric liver tumor study groups, Childrens Oncology Group (COG), SIOPEL, German Pediatric Oncology Hematology (GPOH), and Japanese Pediatric Liver Tumor study group (JPLT), have adopted PRETEXT into their risk stratification (Tables 93-4 and 93-5). PRETEXT can over-stage but will show good interobserver agreement (reproducibility) (Aronson et al, 2005). When applied serially it provides an opportunity to monitor the effect of preoperative chemotherapy to assess tumor response to adjuvant chemotherapy (Fig. 93-9). In the current COG trial, AHEP0731, surgical resection guidelines use PRETEXT to define treatment algorithm. PRETEXT is assigned at diagnosis, POST-TEXT after neoadjuvant chemotherapy.

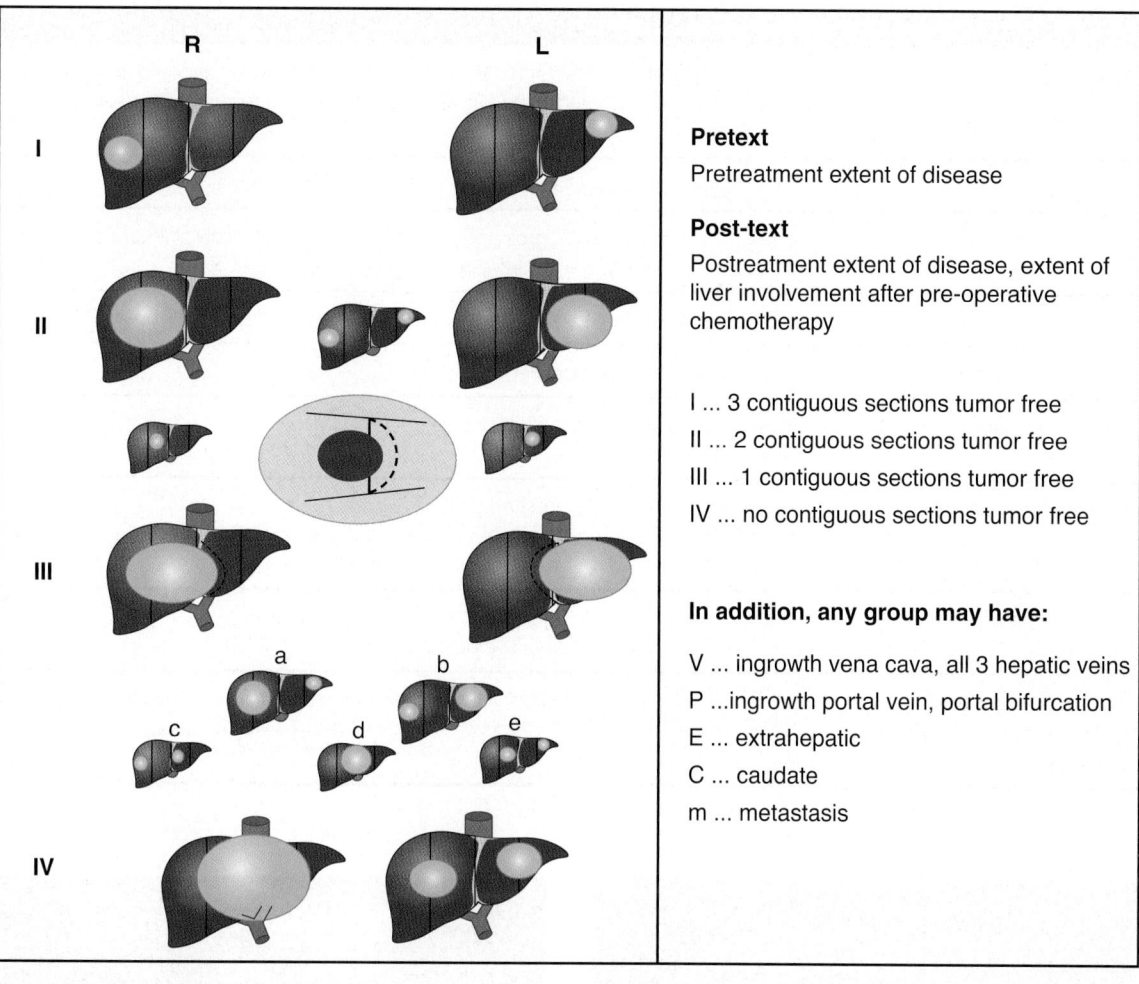

**Pretext**

Pretreatment extent of disease

**Post-text**

Postreatment extent of disease, extent of liver involvement after pre-operative chemotherapy

I ... 3 contiguous sections tumor free

II ... 2 contiguous sections tumor free

III ... 1 contiguous sections tumor free

IV ... no contiguous sections tumor free

**In addition, any group may have:**

V ... ingrowth vena cava, all 3 hepatic veins

P ...ingrowth portal vein, portal bifurcation

E ... extrahepatic

C ... caudate

m ... metastasis

**FIGURE 93-8** PRETEXT. *Pre*treatment *Ext*ent of Disease. POST-TEXT. *Post*reatment *Ext*ent of Disease, extent of liver involvement after pre-operative chemotherapy.

| TABLE 93-4 | Hepatoblastoma Staging and Risk Stratification | | | | |
|---|---|---|---|---|---|
| **CHIC International Risk Stratification System** | **COG** | **SIOPEL** | **JPLT Japanese** | **GPOH German** | |
| Low Risk = PRETEXT I, II, III, with no V, P, E, Rupture, or Mulifocal | Very Low-Risk: Pure fetal histology resected at diagnosis, PRETEXT I or II | | Very Low Risk: PRETEXT I Primary Resection | | |
| Intermediate risk = Same as low risk plus age >6 years old, AFP100–1000 | Low-risk: any histology resected at diagnosis, PRETEXT I or II | Standard risk: PRETEXT I, II, III | Low-risk: PRETEXT II Limited preop chemo | Standard risk: PRETEXT I, II, III | |
| High Risk = PRETEXT IV, or any PRETEXT with V, P, E, Rupture, Multifocal | Intermediate Risk: PRETEXT III and IV Extrahepatic tumors (+VPE); SCU | | Intermediate Risk: PRETEXT III and IV Extrahepatic tumor (+VPE) | | |
| Very High Risk = metastatic, AFP <100, or SCU histology | High-Risk: Metastatic disease at diagnosis, AFP <100 at diagnosis | High-Risk: PRETEXT +VPEM, IV, metastasis at diagnosis, SCU histology, AFP <100 at diagnosis | High-Risk: Metastatic disease Stem Cell Transplant | High-Risk: PRETEXT +VPEM, IV, metastasis at diagnosis, SCU histology, AFP <100 at diagnosis | |

**TABLE 93-5    COG Staging and Risk Stratification, AHEP 0731**

| | |
|---|---|
| Stage I | Tumor completely resected at diagnosis by segmentectomy or standard anatomic lobectomy, recommended for PRETEXT I and PRETEXT II tumors with clear vascular margins on preoperative imaging |
| Stage II | Complete gross resection at diagnosis with microscopic residual |
| Stage III | Biopsy only at diagnosis, or, gross total resection with nodal involvement or tumor spill or incomplete resection with gross intra-hepatic disease |
| Stage IV | Distant metastatic disease at diagnosis, irrespective of local extent of tumor |
| Very-low-risk hepatoblastoma | Stage I Pure Fetal Histology (PFH) |
| Low-risk hepatoblastoma | Stage I Any histology except PFH or SCU<br>Stage II non-SCU |
| Intermediate-risk hepatoblastoma | Stage I Small Cell Undifferentiated (SCU)<br>Stage II SCU<br>Stage III |
| High-risk hepatoblastoma | Stage IV<br>AFP <100 at diagnosis, irrespective of Stage |
| Refer for possible liver transplant (at diagnosis or after 2nd cycle of chemotherapy) | POST-TEXTIII +V, +P (after first 2 cycles of chemotherapy)<br>PRETEXT III extensive multifocal<br>Any PRETEXT IV |

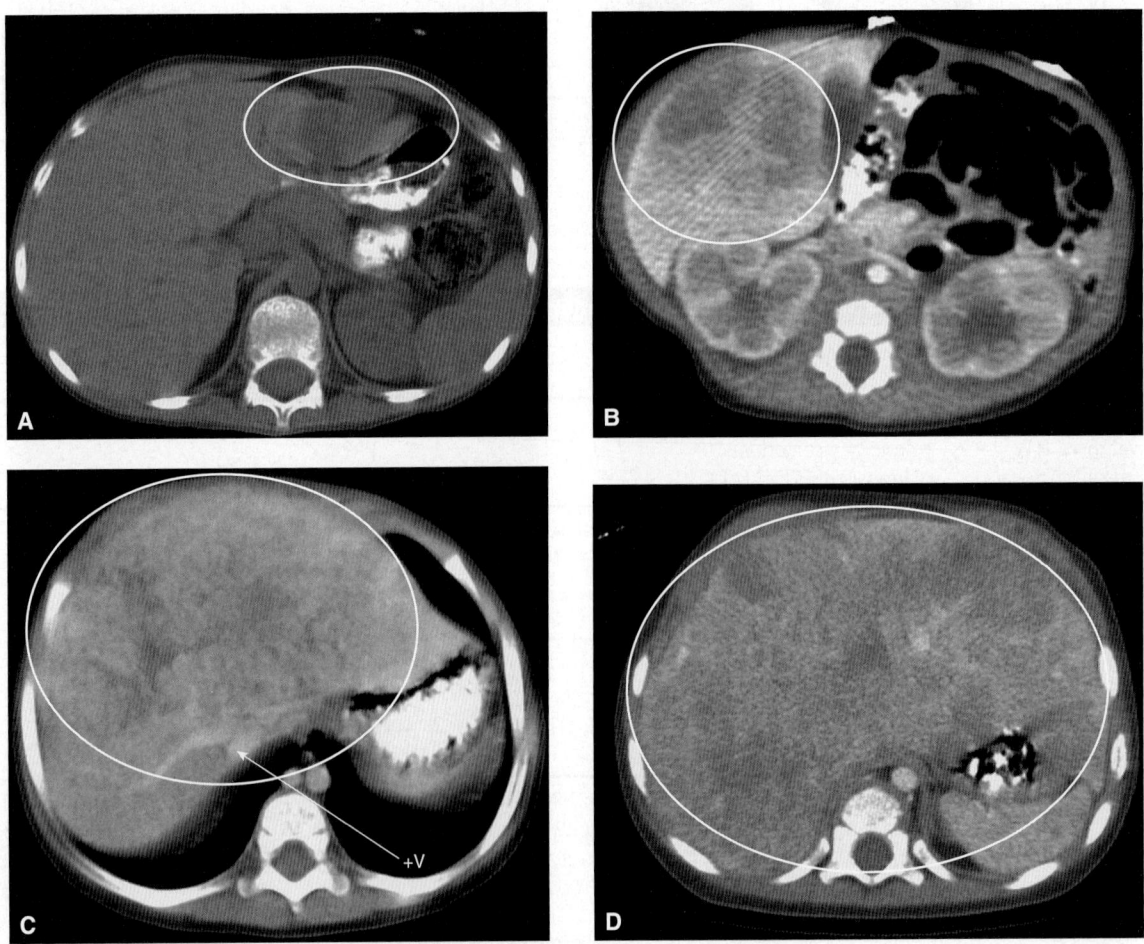

**FIGURE 93-9** Examples of PRETEXT for hepatoblastoma risk stratification. **A.** PRETEXT I: left lateral section. **B.** PRETEXT II: right anterior and posterior sections. **C.** PRETEXT III, +V: left lateral section, left medial section, and right anterior section with invasion all three hepatic veins (+V). **D.** PRETEXT IV, +V, +P: Tumor involves all 4 sections and invades vena cava and portal bifurcation.

| TABLE 93-6 | Summary Results Recent Hepatoblastoma Cooperative Trials | | |
|---|---|---|---|
| **Study** | **Chemotherapy** | **Number of Patients** | **Outcomes** |
| INT0098 (CCSG, POG) Ortega 2000 | C5V vs CDDP/DOXO | Stage I/II: 50; Stage III: 83; Stage IV: 40 | 4-year EFS/OS: I/II = 88%/100% vs 96%/96% III = 60%/68% vs 68%/71% IV = 14%/33% vs 37%/42% |
| P9645 (COG) Malogolowkin 2006 | C5V vs CDDP/CARBO | Stage I/II: *pending publication* Stage III: 38; Stage IV = 50 | 1-year EFS[a]: Stage III/IV: C5V 51%; CDDP/Carbo 37% [a]Study closed early due to inferior results CDDP/CARBO arm |
| HB 94 (GPOH) Fuchs 2002 | I/II: IFOS/CDDP/DOXO III/IV: IFOS/CDDP/DOXO + VP/CARBO | Stage I: 27; II: 3; III: 25; IV: 14 | 4-year EFS/OS: I = 89%/96%; II = 100%/100%; III = 68%/76%; IV = 21%/36% |
| HB 99 (GPOH) VonSch 2007 | SR: IPA HR: CARBO/VP16 | SR: 58 HR: 42 | 3-year EFS/OS: SR: 90%/88% HR: 52%/55% |
| SIOPEL 2 Perilongo 2004 | SR: PLADO HR: CDDP/CARBO/DOXO | PRETEXT: I = 6; II = 36; III = 25; IV = 21; Mets: 25 | 3-year EFS/OS: SR: 73%/91% HR: IV = 48%/61% HR Mets: 36%/44% |
| SIOPEL 3 Perilongo 2010, Zsiros 2011 | SR: CDDP vs PLADO HR: SUPERPLADO | SR: PRETEXT I = 18; II = 133; III = 104 HR: PRETEXT IV = 74; +VPE = 70; mets = 70; AFP <100 = 12 | 3-year EFS/OS: SR: CDDP 83%/95%; PLADO 85%/93% HR: overall 65%/69%; mets 57%/63% |
| JPLT1 Sasaki 2002 | I/II: CDDP(30)/THPA-DOXO III/IV: CDDP(60)/THPA-DOXO | Stage: I: 9; II: 32; IIIa: 48; IIIb 25; IV: 20 | 5-year EFS/OS: I = ?/100%; II = ?/76%; IIa = ?/50%; IIIb = ?/64%; IV = ?/7% |

C5V, cisplatin, fluorouracil and vincristine; CDDP, cisplatin; DOXO, doxorubicin; IFOS, ifosfamide; VP, etoposide; CARBO, carboplatin; IPA, Ifosfamide, cisplatin, adriamycin; SR, standard risk; HR, high risk; PRETEX, Pretreatment extent of disease staging system; +VPE Mets, metastatic disease; SUPERPLADO, CDDP/CARBO/DOXO; EFS, event-free survival; OS, overall survival.

## Chemotherapy

Although complete surgical resection is the cornerstone of any cure, chemotherapy plays a critical role facilitating surgical resection and reducing tumor relapse. The role of chemotherapy can be traced to the early 1970s when members of the Children's Cancer Study Group (CCSG, legacy group of today's COG) launched the very first cooperative group studies for the treatment of children with malignant liver tumors. These trials produced the first evidence that chemotherapy might reduce tumor volume allowing resection.

The role of chemotherapy changed dramatically with the introduction of cisplatin in the 1980s. Response rates of HB to cisplatin-based chemotherapy soared and the resection rate increased. Corresponding 3-year overall survival increased and now approaches 80%. The chemotherapy regimens used by each of the major multicenter trials, as well as the outcomes of these trials, are listed in (Table 93-6). Cisplatin-based chemotherapy has become the gold-standard for the treatment of HB in all multicenter trials, but the drug combinations have evolved. PLADO (a combination of cisplatin and doxorubicin) was once the mainstay of therapy for the SIOPEL studies, but has now been supplanted with cisplatin monotherapy. SIOPEL 4 recently showed improved survival for high risk tumors with dose dense weekly cisplatin, and every 3 week doxorubicin (Zsiros et al 2013). This is similar to the results of the INT-0098 study from America a decade ago which showed equivalent results between Cisplatin/5FU/Vincristine (C5V) and Cisplatin/Doxorubicin for low-risk tumors. For higher risk tumors Doxorubicin and Carboplatin continue to play a role. Other agents that have been tested include Ifosfamide, VP-16, and Etoposide. The chemotherapy strategy employed in the current COG AHEP-0731 study is shown in (Fig. 93-10). Considerable effort has been made by most recent studies to reduce cisplatin-induced ototoxicity. The risk of cisplatin-induced bilateral moderate-to-severe high-frequency hearing loss is significantly increased in the young developing ear. SIOPEL 6 is investigating the potential otoprotective effect of sodium thiosulfate, which competitively binds at the cisplatin receptor site.

In patients with unresectable recurrent disease, chemotherapy is the only option to achieve clearance and render the relapse resectable. Salvage regiments using various

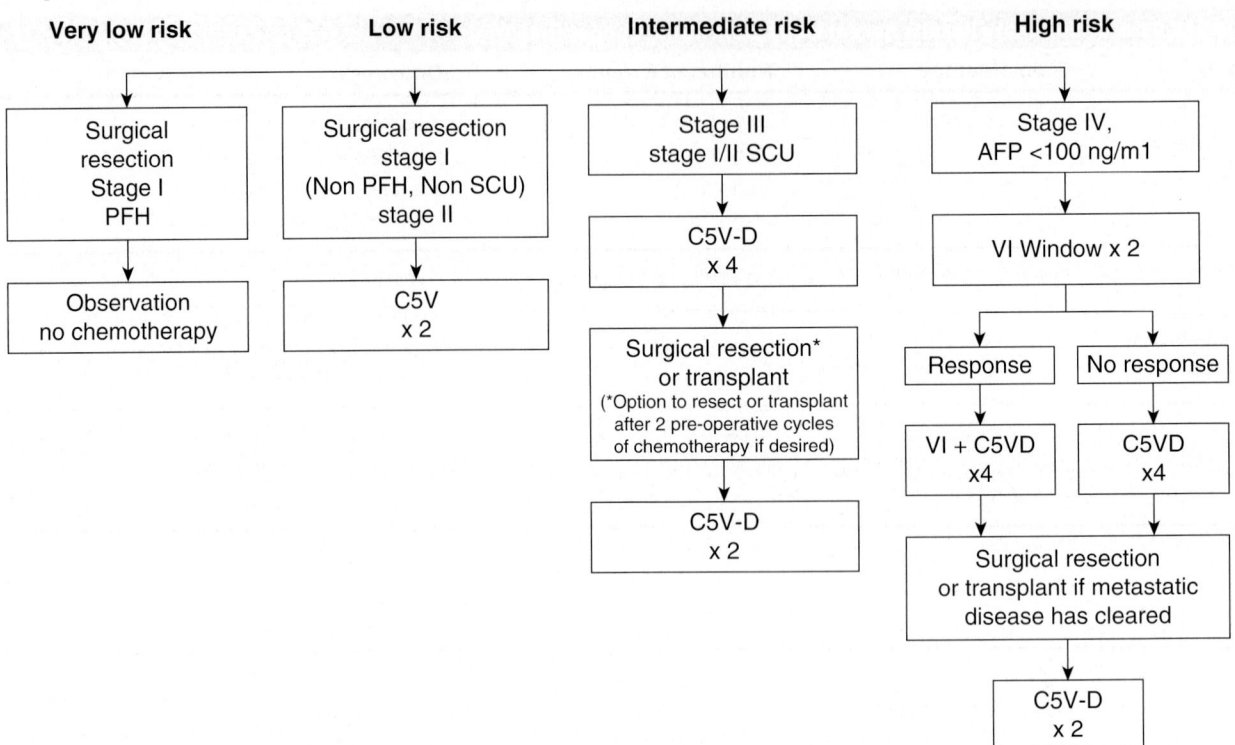

**FIGURE 93-10** Current COG hepatoblastoma protocol (AHEP-0731) treatment scheme. PFH, pure fetal histology; C5V, cisplatin; 5FU, vincristine; C5V-D, cisplatin; 5FU, vincristine + doxorubicin; SCU, small cell undifferentiated; AFP, alpha-feto protein, VI, vincristine irinotecan.

combinations include carboplatin/doxorubicin, carboplatin/etoposide, and irinotecan/vincristine. Malogolowkin showed increased ability to achieve salvage with doxorubicin combinations in patients not initially treated with doxorubicin. Irinotecan as a single agent was used in a SIOPEL phase II study with significant anti-tumor activity.

## Surgery

Contrary to earlier trials where decisions about surgical resection were made by individual surgeons, the surgical guidelines of the current COG trial AHEP-0731 use PRETEXT to define the timing and extent of surgical resection. Surgical resection is recommended (1) by lobectomy or segmentectomy at diagnosis for PRETEXT I and II, (2) by lobectomy or trisegmentectomy after neoadjuvant chemotherapy for PRETEXT III (or POSTTEXT I, II, or III and no major venous involvement –V and –P), and (3) by liver transplant or extreme resection for POSTTEXT III+V+P, and for any PRETEXT IV. Resection at diagnosis is recommended only when a segmentectomy or nonextended lobectomy will predictably yield a complete resection—that is, PRETEXT I or II tumors with at least a 1 cm margin and no concern for macrovascular involvement. Alternatively, in the European SIOPEL and GPOH study groups, neoadjuvant chemotherapy is given to ALL patients with a rare patient going directly to transplant depending upon the recommendation of the transplant center.

**Tumor Biopsy or Resection at Diagnosis.** In the past COG recommended for all patients, exploratory laparotomy at diagnosis to either resect or perform open biopsy. Laparotomy and resection are now recommended in patients with

PRETEXT I and PRETEXT II tumors as long as a safe, margin free resection by either segmentectomy or standard anatomic lobectomy is felt to be feasible. If not, percutaneous or laparoscopic biopsy can be considered but, sufficient tissue for pathologic subtyping is of paramount importance as even a single focus of SCU histology in a histologically heterogenous tumor, will upstage the patient to high risk.

**Resectability and Technical Aspects of Resection.** A thorough understanding of liver anatomy is essential in planning any liver resection (Fig. 93-7). Division between the upper and lower Couinaud segments is marked by the bifurcation of the portal vein. Vertical margins between right posterior, right anterior, left medial and left lateral sections are marked by hepatic veins and umbilical fissure. PRETEXT can be used to predict tumor resectability. Lovorn has recently shown that the majority of chemotherapy response occurs in response to the first 2 cycles of chemotherapy. The first POST-TEXT assessment should therefore be obtained about 10 days after the second cycle of chemotherapy. There are limitations of the PRETEXT system; distinction between real invasion beyond the anatomic border of a given hepatic section and its compression and displacement by the tumor can sometimes be very difficult, especially at diagnosis. Tumor resectability depends upon surgical expertise and the resection/transplant of most PRETEXT III and IV tumors, is probably best done at a center with technical expertise and experience in liver resection. Specialized equipment which can be helpful includes ultrasonic CUSA-type dissector, Ligasure (Covidien), water knife (Hydro-jet, ERBE), argon beam coagulator, and intraoperative ultrasonography. Intraoperative ultrasonography may be helpful in extensive tumors, making sure resection margins are 1 cm if possible and evaluating for any satellite lesions.

The procedure begins with mobilization of the liver and anatomic definition of the extent of the tumor, satellite lesions, and of suspicious areas of vascular involvement. Portal vein and hepatic artery inflow and suprahepatic cava outflow are fully defined prior to any parenchymal dissection. Complete safety and protection of the inflow and outflow to the remaining liver must be maintained. Sampling of lymph nodes from the hepatoduodenal ligament should be performed. Division of the portal, arterial, and hepatic venous branches to the tumor usually precedes parenchymal dissection, but *this is done only after the surgeon is certain that the remaining inflow and outflow vessel branches are protected.* If possible, parenchymal dissection is performed along the line of ischemia minimizing blood loss with meticulous technique. Blood loss can be minimized by maintenance of a central venous pressure below 5. Intermittent vascular inflow occlusion with Pringle maneuver, outflow occlusion with hepatic venous clamping, or both can safely be applied for short periods. Warm ischemia in short 10- to 15-minute intervals with intervening 5- to 10-minute periods of perfusion and recovery is much better tolerated than longer periods of occlusion. During and after dissection of the parenchyma various techniques of local hemostasis can be utilized including LigaSure, harmonic scalpel, vascular clips, bipolar coagulation, argon beam, infrared coagulation, and topical thrombostatic agents such as thrombin soaked Gelfoam, Surgicel, Tisseel.

Incomplete tumor resection and macroscopic residual have been associated with worse outcome. Whenever there is any doubt, and particularly when one suspects macroscopic residual, the surgeon should biopsy and re-resect the margin of liver. It should be stressed that while microscopic positive foci at the resection margin may, in select cases, still be compatible with survival, the goal is a complete tumor resection with negative margins. If the ability to obtain a resection free margin cannot be anticipated with a high degree of confidence, referral for liver transplantation is preferred.

Atypical, nonanatomic, or wedge resections are *not recommended.* In 2 consecutive German multicenter trials, HB89 and HB94, 38% of the patients with an atypical resection were found to have post resection residual tumor and this was associated with a worse outcome. Possible explanations are the dissemination of tumor cells in the liver after atypical resection, the presence of unappreciated microscopic vascular invasion, and the known role of HGF stimulating post resection liver regeneration and residual tumor cell proliferation. Atypical liver resections are justified in very select cases mainly of multifocal tumors, when liver transplantation is not an option due to uncontrolled metastatic disease.

**Liver Transplant for HB.** After the pioneering work of Reyes, Superina, and AlQabandi in the late 1990s, transplant for HB entered a new era. Long-term survival ranging from 55% to 100% has been reported over the past decade in over a dozen single center series. Cases of "unresectable" HB due to involvement of the entire liver, extensive multifocality, or major hepatic venous or portal venous involvement comprises 10% to 20% of all HB treated in multicenter trials. The best results for high risk HB reported to date were

in SIOPEL 3 and the improvement in outcome seen in this study appears to be at least partly due to an increase in the use of liver transplant. In accordance with the most recent SIOPEL 3 protocol—*"The commonest reasons for a tumor being deemed unresectable (except via total hepatectomy) are: (a) tumor clearly involving all four sections of the liver as judged by MRI or CT angiography; (b) location so close to the main vessels at the hilum of the liver and/or the hepatic veins that it is unlikely that a tumor-free excision plane will be achieved. These patients should be identified at diagnosis and their clinical course and imaging followed closely throughout their initial chemotherapy, in conjunction with a liver transplant surgeon."*

It is important that consultation with a transplant center with special expertise in pediatric liver surgery be considered early in the treatment in order to prevent delays and unwanted extended courses of chemotherapy while awaiting resection and transplantation. Extended and prolonged pretransplant exposure to chemotherapy risk the induction of chemotherapy resistance genes, a well-described phenomenon in HB. An occasional patient with an extensive PRETEXT IV tumor might be treated with primary transplant, but most patients receive preoperative chemotherapy. Multifocal PRETEXT IV HB in the absence of any metastatic disease after chemotherapy (POSTEXT III or IV, multifocal, M) is a clear indication for liver transplantation. Apparent clearance of tumor from one section of liver after preoperative chemotherapy should not distract from transplant because of the high probability of persistent microscopic viable neoplastic cells despite radiographic "clearance." Clinicians should resist the temptation to intensify chemotherapy in a vain effort to avoid transplant because of the high likelihood of inducing tumor resistance to chemotherapy. In a subgroup of PRETEXT III tumors there will be major vascular invasion that does not clear with neoadjuvant chemotherapy. A POST-TEXT III tumor with persistent +V and/or +P may preclude safe and prudent performance of a trisegmentectomy. Resection in the face of major venous invasion runs the risk of leaving viable neoplastic tissue behind if the surgeon must peel viable tumor directly off from the involved vein. Some have argued in favor of venous resection and reconstruction ("extreme" or "complex" resection) as opposed to transplant in these cases. There are no trials comparing the results of partial resection with extensive venous dissection versus complete resection with transplantation. Complex resection carries an increased risk of surgical complication, including bleeding and/or venous outflow obstruction and positive tumor margin. Multiple series have shown superior outcome with primary transplant (about 80% overall survival) compared to rescue transplant (about 30-40% overall). The basis for this is undoubtedly multifactorial but 2 important concerns are the likelihood of chemotherapy resistance in relapse tumors, and the debilitated state of the patients when transplanted in the face of end-stage disease.

An absolute contraindication to liver transplant is persistent pulmonary metastases unresponsive to adjuvant chemotherapy. The tumor should show at least partial response to chemotherapy (decrease in tumor size, decrease in serum AFP, and decrease in size or disappearance of pulmonary nodules). Lung metastasis that do respond to chemotherapy, but do not entirely clear, should be surgically resected.

SIOPEL, together with support from COG, GPOH, Study of Pediatric Liver Transplantation (SPLIT), and individual pediatric liver transplant centers all over the world, has established a worldwide electronic registry for liver transplant for childhood tumors (HB, HC, infantile hemangioma, and others) the *Pediatric Liver Unresectable Tumor Obervatory (PLUTO)* (Otte 2010). The link to this registry is: http://pluto .cineca.org.

### Trans Arterial Chemoembolization (TACE).
Trans Arterial Chemoembolization (TACE) is a technique that has fallen out of favor in recent year due to the successes with liver transplantation, but does continue to be quite popular in China. Recent experience reported from China shows mean tumor shrinkage of 59%, mean decrease in AFP of 60%, and mean tumor necrosis in the surgical specimens of 87% (Li et al, 2008). Widespread use has been somewhat limited by toxicity. Chemotherapeutic cocktails have included pirarubicin, doxorubicin eluting beads, mitomycin, lipiodol, and followed by occlusive agents such as Gelfoam particles or stainless steel coils. It is most often used as palliation for large unresectable tumors in the presence of uncontrolled metastatic disease.

### Preoperative Portal Venous Embolization.
Preresection portal venous embolization has been used in adults with HCC to induce hypertrophy of the remaining liver remnant and case reports of this technique have been reported in children. This technique may be useful in children with large tumors. The portal venous branch on the side of the tumor is cannulated percutaneously and polyvinyl alcohol and coils are inserted to induce occlusion of the portal vein branch feeding the tumor under fluoroscopic control. This has a dual effect of alcohol thrombosis of the embolized tumor and compensatory hypertrophy of the unharmed opposite liver lobe increasing the potential hepatic functional reserve in patients with cirrhosis and underlying liver dysfunction in preparation for hepatic resection of the tumor.

### Surgery for Pulmonary Metastases.
Aggressive surgery seems to have an important role in the resection of pulmonary HB metastases, either persisting or relapse lesions. The optimal approach and the timing of surgery are debatable. Optimal approach for a unilateral lesion might be unilateral thoracotomy with wedge resection. If there are multiple lesions in the same area of lung, some have advocated extended wedge or lobectomy in the hope of defining presence or absence of adjacent micrometastases. Some have advocated sternotomy with bilateral lung palpation, especially prior to liver transplantation. Fuchs et al reported that preoperative imaging detected about 76% of the total number of metastases when compared to intraoperative findings. The timing of lung resection, before or after resection of the primary tumor has also been debated. Lung resection may be preferable before liver resection in order to avoid the effects of metastases growth stimulation and tumor cell proliferation triggered by hepatic growth factors secreted after major liver surgery. Alternatively, waiting until after this growth stimulation has occurred may aid in the detection of previously undetectable micrometastasis. Thoracotomy and resection for pulmonary metastatic relapse are not futile; as 30% may achieve a durable cure.

### Surgery for Tumor Relapse in the Liver.
In SIOPEL 1, 5 locally relapsed patients underwent a redo liver resection, 2 of 5 became long-term survivors. In JPLT 1, 4 locally relapsed patients underwent a redo liver resection with short-term survival (17 months) in all 4, long-term follow-up not reported. In the liver transplant experience overall survival for "rescue" transplant, transplant for a local relapse, was 30%, compared to 82% for patients transplanted at the first operation.

### Preoperative Tumor Rupture.
Bleeding from a preoperative tumor rupture occurs in about 2% to 3% of HB resulting in an intracapsular hematoma and may stop spontaneously. Occasionally a preoperative tumor rupture may present with free rupture into the peritoneal cavity with hypovolemic shock. Correction of clotting factors should be followed either by an attempt at percutaneous embolization or operative control of the hemorrhage with delayed resection. Inadvertent injury to vital structures can be minimized if heroic, uncontrolled procedures are avoided. It is particularly important to avoid, if possible, massive blood loss, as massive blood transfusion during liver tumor resection has been correlated with an increased risk of tumor recurrence.

### Surgical Complications.
Surgical complications which may require operative intervention encompass a wide spectrum including bleeding, impairment of blood flow in or out of the liver, blockage or leaking of bile flow, liver failure, infection, and others (Table 93-7).

*Bleeding and Major Vessel Injury.* Bleeding from liver tissue at the site of a needle biopsy can almost always be stopped with appropriate correction of clotting factors and with direct pressure. In contrast, massive bleeding during or after a complex tumor resection may be life-threatening. Uncontrolled bleeding at the time of tumor resection is most often caused by inadvertent injury to one of the major vessels. Inappropriate

| TABLE 93-7 | Potential Surgical Complications of Major Liver Resection |
|---|---|
| Bleeding | Intraoperative hemorrhage; postoperative hemorrhage; intrahepatic hematoma; hemobilia; gastrointestinal bleeding; side effects of massive transfusion |
| Blood flow | Obstructed venous outflow; hepatic artery injury or thrombosis; portal venous injury or thrombosis; hepatic necrosis |
| Liver failure | Too small-for-size liver remnant (<25% of normal liver, <50–60% cirrhotic liver), coagulopathy; hypoglycemia; encephalopathy; ascites |
| Bile drainage | Bile leak; biliary fistula; biloma; bile peritonitis; biliary stricture; cholangitis |
| Infection | Sepsis; cholangitis; wound infection; hepatic or perihepatic abscess; pneumonia; peritonitis |
| Other | Adhesive bowel obstruction; diaphragm injury; pleural effusion; would dehiscence; recurrent or persistent tumor |

aggressive attempts at tumor resection in proximity to major vessels risks bleeding and residual tumor. In the event of a failed initial resection reoperative resection may be associated with increased perihepatic blood loss because of adhesions to the diaphragm, retroperitoneum, and right adrenal gland. Unrecognized anatomic origin of a replaced right or left hepatic artery may lead to bleeding and inappropriate ligation. A normal liver can occasionally survive permanent interruption of arterial inflow or portal venous inflow, but not both. In the rare instance that both portal and arterial inflow of the remaining liver tissue has been disrupted, survival requires immediate revascularization or transplant. Hepatic failure will progress rapidly with total devascularization. Even in the absence of obvious ligation, if these vital vessels are not handled gently, postoperative thrombosis can occur. Loss of adequate venous drainage from the residual liver remnant will cause congestion and loss of parenchymal viability. Protection of venous drainage includes judicious planning of anticipated surgical resection margins.

*Cardiac Arrest.* Intraoperative cardiac arrest occurs in 1% to 2% of major liver resection procedures. The most common cause is uncontrolled massive blood loss. Cardiac arrest may also occur from tumor emboli or, more commonly, an air embolus. Risk of an air embolism can be minimized by meticulous dissection of the suprahepatic veins and retrohepatic vena cava, avoidance of inappropriately aggressive or uncontrolled attempts at resection, suction on the central venous catheter if an embolus has occurred, and prevention to some degree by the use of higher PEEP (Positive End-Expiratory Pressure) setting during the suprahepatic vein and IVC dissection portion of the procedure. It is also very important to preoperatively screen all patients who have been treated with doxorubicin as their baseline cardiac function may be compromised.

*Liver Failure.* Potential causes of postoperative liver failure include small liver remnant, liver devascularization, interruption of venous drainage, excessive liver warm ischemia due to prolonged vascular occlusion or massive bleeding, major bile duct obstruction, halogenated anesthetic agents, viral infections, and drug reactions. Unless definitive signs of improvement are seen in the first few days, liver transplantation should be considered. Small-for-size residual liver remnant is a relatively rare cause in children because of the low incidence of underlying cirrhosis in most children with liver tumors. Long-term survival and appropriate liver regeneration can be anticipated with a remnant volume of 25% to 30% of normal liver, or 60% to 75% of cirrhotic liver. If vascular occlusion is used intraoperatively "ischemic preconditioning" techniques can expand its safety. Although warm ischemia can theoretically be "tolerated" for up to 60 minutes, most experienced liver surgeons will limit inflow occlusion to periods of 15- to 20-minutes interspersed with 5- to 10-minute periods of reperfusion.

*Bile Leak.* Persistent bile leak is one of the most frequent complications in liver surgery occurring in 2% to 12% of cases and its frequency has not decreased over the years. The bile ducts, particularly at the level of the hilum as they enter the hepatic parenchyma, are more easily disrupted than the vessels. If a minor injury is recognized it can usually be directly repaired. Major injury with loss of ductal wall, complete division, or loss of length mandates debridement back to healthy, well-perfused ducts and drainage with a roux-en-y jejunal limb. Bile leak from the cut surface can be minimized by meticulous dissection, avoidance of nonanatomic resections, and closure of all sites of bile drainage on the raw surface of the liver. Although placing drains at the time of operation does not lessen the rate of bile leakage, it facilitates postoperative management. Bile leaks that do not respond to appropriate drainage are almost always associated with distal obstruction, such as a retained section of viable liver excluded from the biliary drainage system, iatrogenic occlusion (clip, ligature, thermal injury), hematoma, stone, residual obstructing tumor, or ischemic stricture.

## Outcome

So far, no controlled comparison has been done between the therapeutic strategies of SIOPEL and COG, primary chemotherapy for-all versus primary surgery for some. In terms of overall survival rates, the results of the different study groups have been similar (Table 93-6). The improved results seen in the high-risk arm of SIOPEL 3 highlight some important lessons learned over the past 2 decades: (1) With standard treatment only about 25% of children who present with metastatic disease are ultimately cured. Alternative chemotherapy and surgical resection of pulmonary metastatic disease should be considered in children who do not show an early clearance of the pulmonary metastasis with chemotherapy. (2) The presence of a positive microscopic margin may not portend a poor prognosis in patients who had had an excellent response to chemotherapy; and (3) liver transplant or extreme resection (eg, mesohepatectomy or resection with major venous resection and reconstruction) should be considered in every child with unresectable HB (about 15% of cases).

## Hepatocellular Carcinoma

### Epidemiology

Although described previously, it was not until 1967 that childhood HCC was identified by Ishak and Glunz as an entity to be distinguished from HB. In 1974 Exelby et al analyzed the clinical course of childhood HCC and found an overall dismal outcome. Due to the rarity of HCC in the pediatric age group and its relative chemotherapy resistance, the history of clinical research for this tumor is much less rich than for HB.

More than two-thirds of pediatric HCC occur in children older than 10 years of age, but only 0.5% to 1% of all HCC manifest before 20 years of age. Very few HCCs are diagnosed in children less than 5 years old, and in this young age group, transitional-type tumors are seen. About 20% to 35% of children with HCC have underlying chronic liver disease. Compared to adults, de novo tumors without underlying cirrhosis are more common in children. Conditions associated with HCC in children including ataxia/telangiectasia and Fanconi anemia may predispose to *de novo* tumors in an otherwise healthy liver; however, the majority of conditions that predispose to HCC involve chronic hepatic inflammation such as alpha 1 antitrypsin deficiency, total anomalous venous return, Alagille's syndrome, biliary atresia, congenital hepatic fibrosis, FAP, FNH, hemochromatosis, hepatic adenoma, hepatitis B and C, glycogen storage disease, neurofibromatosis, oral contraceptives, parenteral nutrition associated cholestatic liver failure, progressive familial intrahepatic cholestasis (PFIC), Bloom syndrome, and tyrosinemia. In East Asia and Africa, HCC is more common than HB due to the widespread prevalence of hepatitis B and C. In Taiwan, where HCC is most often seen in carriers of the hepatitis B virus, vaccination programs targeted against hepatitis have led to a significant decrease in the incidence of HCC. In contrast to hepatitis B, the cirrhosis and the subsequent development of HCC in the hepatitis C population usually takes several decades to develop.

## Pathology

It is disputed whether HCC in children versus HCC in the adult are the same disease. Zimmermann and others have suggested that HCC forms a tumor family, consisting of adult-type HCC and its variants, fibrolamellar HCC, and a novel entity occurring in young children and adolescents, transitional liver cell tumor (TLCT). The gross presentation is in the form of solitary or multifocal lesions with four main growth patterns, expanding mass lesions, pedunculated/hanging lesions, invading tumors with poor delineation, and multifocal tumors resembling metastatic disease. These growth patterns exert a considerable influence on the surgical resectability of the tumors.

**Fibrolamellar Hepatocellular Carcinoma (FL-HCC).** This tumor usually arises in noncirrhotic livers of adolescents or young adult patients and is encountered more frequently in Western countries. Overall, FL-HCC accounts for less than 10% of all HCCs. Recent data show that FL-HCC has a biology similar to that of adult-type HCC. FL-HCC shows vascular invasion in up to 35% of cases, frequently metastasizes into locoregional lymph nodes (about 50% of cases), and tends to show unusual spreading patterns, including intraperitoneal spread. FL-HCC is typically a solitary lesion which has a predilection for the left liver lobe (two thirds; unusual for hepatic primary tumors). It reveals well-defined margins and a central scar in 70%. The cut surface often shows a firm and tan to brown tissue with radiating septa. Histologically the cells form strands embedded in fibrosclerotic stroma which may form a central stellate scar.

**Transitional Liver Cell Tumor (TLCT).** TLCT is a recently identified liver neoplasm that occurs in younger children. The term, transitional, had been proposed to denote a putative intermediate position of the tumor cells between hepatoblasts and more mature hepatocyte-like cells. TLCT are highly aggressive lesions that have a treatment response pattern different from HB. The usual presentation is that of a large or very large solitary hepatic tumor (mostly in the right liver lobe), commonly associated with very high serum AFP levels. Grossly, the tumors display an expanding growth pattern and sometimes exhibit central necrosis. Histologically, the tumor cells vary between HCC-type cell and the cells found in HB, sometimes with formation of multinuclear giant cells. Beta-catenin is typically expressed in a mixed nuclear and cytoplasmic pattern.

## PRETEXT and Staging

No staging or grading system has been found which accurately predicts prognosis in pediatric HCC. In the pediatric multicenter trials, HCC has been the ugly stepsister of HB, usually treated on the same protocols, but analyzed separately. PRETEXT has been used because of its utility in HB and the crossover between these 2 tumors in the intermediate age group. In adults, the Edmondson and Steiner histologic grading system seems to add prognostic value to the TNM grading system, which is now in its 6th edition. COG has no current open trials for HCC, prior trials have used the traditional Evan staging system (I, II, III, IV).

## Chemotherapy

HCC is relatively chemoresistant and therefore carries a poor prognosis with a dismal cure rate. Complete surgical resection or transplantation is often the only hope. Unfortunately, HCC is most often advanced at diagnosis. Even with aggressive attempts at surgical resection, tumor relapse is common and tumor-free survival rates of not more than 25% to 30% can be achieved. The first multicenter clinical trials on pediatric liver tumors were conducted in the USA by the CCSG and POG, and usually included both HCC and HB. These early trials showed the poor response of HCC to chemotherapy and radiation and had dismal cure rates in the majority of patients.

The more recent North American cooperative study (INT-0098) included 46 children and adolescents with HCC. There were no differences regarding response or survival rates between the two chemotherapy regimens. Seven of the eight stage I patients (88%) with complete tumor excision at time of diagnosis followed by adjuvant cisplatin-based chemotherapy, survived. This result suggests that adjuvant chemotherapy may be of benefit for patients with completely resected HCC. However, since one-third of these initially resected patients have responded well without any additional chemotherapy, the question of the necessity for adjuvant chemotherapy will only be answered in a randomized trial. In contrast, outcome was uniformly poor for patients with advanced-stage disease. The 5-year event-free survival for stage III and IV patients was 23% and 10%, respectively (Table 93-8).

HCC patients have been treated in 3 consecutive studies of the GPOH (Table 93-8). In the first study, HB89, ifosfamide, cisplatin, and doxorubicin (IPA), did not show benefit. Four of 12 patients survived, all had completely resected tumors. In the second study, HB94, patients with nonresectable HCC received conventionally dosed carboplatin and etoposide in addition to IPA, which seemed to produce at least short-term partial benefit. Of the registered 25 patients, nine had locally unresectable and 11 metastatic HCC. Three of the nine and one of the 11 patients survived free of disease in addition to 4 of 5 patients with resectable tumor (total 8 of 25 = 32%).

HCC was treated along with HB in SIOPEL 1, 2, and 3, and results are shown in Table 93-8. Only 2 of the 39 HCC patients entered into the SIOPEL-1 study underwent complete resection of the tumor at diagnosis. The remainder received preoperative chemotherapy and tumor response to chemotherapy was actually seen in 49% (18 of 37), which is very high for HCC. Despite this, complete tumor resection was achieved in only 36% (14 of 39) with a 5-year survival

| TABLE 93-8 | Summary Results Hepatocellular Carcinoma (HCC) Cooperative Trials | | | |
|---|---|---|---|---|
| Study | Chemotherapy | Number of Patients | | Outcomes |
| INT0098 (CCSG, POG)<br>Katzenstein 2002 | CDDP/DOXO | Stage I: 8;<br>Stage II: 0<br>Stage III: 25<br>Stage IV: 13 | | 5-year EFS/OS:<br>I/II = 88%/88%<br>III = 8%/23%<br>IV = 19%/34% |
| HB89 (GPOH)<br>VonScwein 2004 | CDDP/DOXO | Stage I/II/IIIa: *6*<br>Stage IIIb, IV: 6 | | 5-year DFS:<br>Stage I/II/IIIa = 50%<br>Stage IIIb, IV = 17% |
| HB 94 (GPOH)<br>VonSc 2004 | CDDP/DOXO | Stage I/II/IIIa: *5*<br>Stage IIIb, IV: 20 | | 5-year DFS:<br>Stage I/II/IIIa = 60%<br>Stage IIIb, IV = 25% |
| HB 99 (GPOH)<br>VSchw 2004 | CDDP/DOXO | Stage I/II/IIIa: 14<br>Stage IIIb,IV: 27 | | 5-year DFS:<br>Stage I/II/IIIa = 71%<br>Stage IIIb, IV = 15% |
| SIOPEL 1<br>Czauderna 2002 | CDDP/DOXO | PRETEXT: I = 1; II = 14; III = 11; IV = 13; +VPEM = 8 | | 5-year EFS/OS: 17%/28% |
| SIOPEL 2<br>Czauderna 2002 | CDDP/DOXO | PRETEXT: I = 1; II = 3; III = 1; IV = 7; +VPEM = 5 | | 5-year EFS/OS: 23%/23% |
| SIOPEL 3<br>Zsiros 2009 | CDDP/DOXO | PRETEXT: I = 4; II = 22; III = 14; IV = 21; +VPEM = ? | | 3-year EFS/OS: 10%/16% |

CDDP, cisplatin; DOXO, doxorubicin; IFOS, ifosfamide; VP, etoposide; CARBO, carboplatin; IPA, Ifosfamide, cisplatin, adriamycin; PRETEXT, Pre-treatment extent of disease staging system; +VPEM, Vena Cava, Portal vein, Extrahepatic, Metastatic disease; EFS, event-free survival; OS, overall survival; DFS, disease-free survival.

of 17%. In SIOPEL 2, 13 of the 16 treated patients received preoperative chemotherapy with cisplatin, carboplatin, and doxorubicin. Response to preoperative chemotherapy was observed in 6 of 13 cases (46%). Gross total tumor resection was achieved in half the patients (47%) but overall long-term survival was only 22%.

## Surgery

Given the poor response of HCC to chemotherapy and radiation, the mainstay of treatment is surgery. This means that in contrast to HB, a primary radical tumor resection should be considered and all available techniques should be used to achieve this goal. Of particular relevance are TACE and preoperative portal vein embolization. Patients with the clinical constellation of advanced HCC should always be treated in consultation with a specialized center with experience in liver surgery.

**Liver Transplantation for HCC in Children.** The role of liver transplantation in pediatric HCC is in greater evolution than in pediatric HB. Liver transplantation is contraindicated in the presence of any extrahepatic tumor, even in the occasional patient where it clears with chemotherapy. Some argue that an exception might be made in the intermediate case of children with transitional cell liver tumors (TCLT). Outcome for transplant in adult HCC has improved over the years due to our recognition that strict selection criteria are important in preventing post-transplant tumor relapse. The

Milan criteria introduced by Mazzaferro in 1996 work well *in adults with advanced cirrhotic liver disease.* The Milan criteria restrict transplant for HCC in adults: (1) single tumor <5 cm; (2) not more than 3 nodules; (3) no angioinvasion; (4) no extrahepatic involvement. The problem with applying the Milan criteria to children is that 50% to 70% of children present with large *de novo* tumors in an otherwise noncirrhotic liver. Two recent series of pediatric liver transplantation questioned the relevance of Milan criteria to pediatric HCC. In a series from Stanford, 10 children were transplanted for HCC and neither the number of tumors, nor the size of tumor, nor the presence of gross vascular invasion was correlated with the risk of post-transplant tumor relapse (Beaunoyer et al 2007). Of the 4 Milan criteria evaluated in children in a transplant series from Poland: 3 children did not fulfill 4 criteria; 3 children did not fulfill 2 criteria; and 2 children did not fulfill 1 criteria. The only child in their series who fulfilled all 4 Milan criteria was a child with tyrosinemia with a small incidental tumor found on surveillance screening. In view of this, some centers will offer transplantation to children with large de novo tumors, regardless of size, as long as there is no evidence of extrahepatic spread.

## New Agents and Treatment Modalities

**Sorafenib.** New treatment modalities including metronomic chemotherapy and adjuvant antiangiogenic therapy are the target of investigation based upon some early promising results. Most promising is Sorafenib, an antiangiogenic tyrosine kinase inhibitor, where a survival advantage has clearly been shown in prospective trials in the treatment of HCC in adults with unresectable tumors. This also may be the case in some in childhood HCC.

**TACE and Theraspheres.** TACE using the drugs doxorubicin (including newly available doxorubicin eluting beads) mitomycin and cisplatin is employed in the treatment algorithm of HCC. Intra-arterial injection of cytotoxic agents results in higher local concentration of drugs with reduced systemic side effects, while the intra-arterial embolization causes ischemic necrosis of the tumor. This therapeutic strategy has been used in a small number of children and adolescents with HCC as adjuvant therapy in an attempt to facilitate tumor resection, or as palliative therapy in children with metastatic or extrahepatic disease. There are no large trials in children, however, in a study of adult HCC patients without liver failure or cirrhosis, TACE successfully reduced tumor growth. A related approach that combines radiation therapy with angiographic embolization has been the intraarterial injection of 90Yttrium radioactive microspheres, called Theraspheres.

**Percutaneous Ablative Therapies.** Ablative percutaneous methods are more relevant to pediatric HCC than HB, as HCC is more often advanced at diagnosis, and therapy often more directed toward palliation than cure. Techniques include percutaneous radiofrequency ablation (RFA), percutaneous ethanol injection (PEI), and cryotherapy. Cryotherapy although once popular in adults has now fallen out of favor due to superior results achieved with RFA and PEI. RFA and PEI are suitable for smaller size tumors only, generally below 3 to 4 cm in maximum diameter. RFA provides slightly better tumor kill than PEI (90% vs 80% complete tumor necrosis) with less sessions (mean of 1.2 vs 4.8). RFA is also associated with fewer side effects; thus in many centers, RFA is now preferred. Caution is needed in nodules located adjacent to the major bile ducts or to bowel loops. Complications of these ablative techniques occur in about 8% to 9% of cases, mainly in the form of pain, fever, bleeding, tumor seeding, thermal injury, and gastrointestinal perforation.

# OTHER LIVER TUMORS

## Rhabdoid Tumor

The definition of a rhabdoid tumor classically relies on a characteristic morphology and loss of hSNF5/INI1 tumor suppressor gene expression. In cases lacking the typical histological features, the loss of expression of the *INI1* gene product is the essential diagnostic tool. Although pediatric rhabdoid tumors are most common in the kidney and brain, they do occur in the liver. A rhabdoid liver tumor is difficult to distinguish from the SCU variant of HB. Given the aggressive biologic behavior and poor prognosis seen with the SCU variant of HB, it has been suggested that tumors previously classified as SCU-HB were actually rhabdoid tumors.

The differentiation of an SCU-HB from a rhabdoid tumor is challenging and is important in terms of research, but possibly clinically irrelevant as both are biologically aggressive with poor response to chemotherapy. This tumor is rare and aggressive which may present with spontaneous rupture. These rare tumors are often chemoresistant although a recent case report achieved a potential cure with multimodal therapy including ifosfamide, vincristine, and actinomycin D. As with all locally aggressive liver tumors that respond poorly to chemotherapy, the most important treatment goal is complete surgical excision.

## Hepatic Sarcomas

Primary hepatic sarcomas are rare, and their outcome depends primarily on tumor histology, sensitivity to chemotherapy and/or radiotherapy, and the ability to achieve complete tumor resection.

## Biliary Rhabdomyosarcoma

The classic presentation of biliary rhabdomyosarcoma is in young children with jaundice and abdominal pain, and is often associated with abdominal distension, vomiting, and fever. Histology is either embryonal or botryoid, subtypes of rhabdomyosarcoma that have a favorable prognosis. Because the tumor most often involves the central biliary tree and porta hepatis, the ability to achieve gross total resection is rare. Fortunately, the tumor is sensitive to both chemotherapy and radiation and long-term survival is seen in 60% to 70% of patients. Surgical intervention has 2 goals: to establish an accurate diagnosis and to determine the local–regional extent of disease. Although chemotherapy is generally effective at relief of the associated biliary obstruction, patients remain at risk for biliary sepsis until the obstruction abates as the tumor shrinks with chemotherapy.

## Undifferentiated Embryonal Sarcomas

Undifferentiated (embryonal) sarcoma of the liver is a rare tumor in children. Historically, it was an aggressive neoplasm with an unfavorable prognosis. These tumors may arise in a solitary liver cyst. Survival has improved with recent multimodal approaches designed for patients with soft tissue sarcomas at other sites, including conservative surgery at diagnosis, multiagent chemotherapy, and second-look operation in cases of residual disease. Using these techniques several series have reported survival in up to 70% of children.

## Angiosarcoma

Although rare, several case reports in the literature support the potential for malignant transformation of an infantile hepatic hemangioma to angiosarcoma. Histologic verification of malignancy can be difficult and angiosarcoma should be suspected if the biologic behavior of an infantile hepatic hemangioma shows unusual progression or recurrence after a period of relative quiescence. Relatively chemoresistant, prognosis is generally poor unless diagnosed early. There are case reports of successful transplantation.

## Metastatic Liver Tumors

Unlike the large body of literature addressing liver resection for metastatic colorectal tumors in adults, there are little published data on the treatment of metastatic tumors in the liver from abdominal solid tumors in childhood. A recent series from a Children's Hospital Los Angeles reported only 15 such patients over a 17-year period including: neuroblastoma (7); Wilms tumor (3); osteogenic sarcoma (2); gastric epithelial (1); and desmoplastic small round cell tumor (2). Eleven of the 15 patients died of progressive disease; 4 had a local recurrence. The overall prognosis in these children was poor and the decision to perform hepatic metastasectomy should be made with caution. A tumor not reported in the series from Los Angeles is metastatic pancreatoblastoma. We recently treated a child who presented with multiple, large bilobar hepatic metastases from pancreatoblastoma who is alive at last follow-up (1 year post transplant) following chemotherapy, subtotal pancreatectomy, and liver transplant. Not all liver lesions in children with abdominal solid tumors turn out to be metastatic disease. Both NRH and FNH have been reported to mimic hepatic metastasis in children. Definitive diagnosis requires biopsy and/or resection.

## Hepatic Involvement in Hematologic Malignancies

### Hemophagocytic Lymphohistiocytosis

HLH may occasionally present as an abnormal liver mass in a newborn with coagulopathy. Predisposing factors include familial, herpes simplex virus, and severe combined immunodeficiency. Diagnostic criteria include fever, splenomegaly, bicytopenia, hypotriglyceridemia, hypofibrinogenemia, hemophagocytosis, low NK cell activity, hyperferritinemia, and high IL-2 receptor levels. Treatment is with combination chemo-immunotherapy, including etoposide, dexamethasone, cyclosporine A.

### Megakaryoblastic Leukemia

Rarely congenital acute megakaryoblastic leukemia (AMKL) may present isolated to the liver with ascites caused by massive infiltration of hepatic sinusoids by leukemic cells. The bone marrow by microscopy and flow cytometry and the peripheral blood smear may not initially show the presence of blasts. Because the marrow fibrosis may not manifest until after the massive hepatic infiltration it may initially be difficult to diagnosis as leukemia. In most children with liver involvement the spleen, lymph nodes, and marrow will also be involved at diagnosis. But even in these cases the diagnosis may be difficult both clinically and pathologically and the hepatic and lymph node involvement is not uncommonly misinterpreted as solid tumor.

## SELECTED READINGS

Aronson DC, Schnater JM, Staalman CR, et al. Predictive value of the pretreatment extent of disease system in hepatoblastoma: results from the international society of pediatric oncology liver tumor study group SIOPEL-1 study. *J Clin Oncol* 2005;23:1245–1252.

Avila LF, Encinas JL, Leal N, et al. Liver transplantation for malignant tumors in children. *Cir Pediatr* 2007;20:189–193.

Barnhart D, Hirschl R, Garver K, et al. Conservative management of mesenchymal hamartoma of the liver. *J Pediatr Surg* 1997;32:1495–1498.

Beaunoyer M, Vanetta JM, Ogihara M, et al. Outcomes of transplantation in children with primary hepatic malignancy. *Pediatr Transplant* 2007;12:1–3.

Czauderna P, Otte JB, Aronson DC, et al. Guidelines for surgical treatment of hepatoblastoma in the modern era: Recommendations from the childhood Liver Tumour Strategy Group of the International Society of Paediatric Oncology (SIOPEL). *Eur J Cancer* 2005;41:1031–1036.

Dickie B, Dasgupta R, Rair R, et al. Spectrum of hepatic hemangiomas: management and outcome. *J Pediatr Surg* 2009;44:125–133.

Faraj W, Dar F, Marangoni G, et al. Liver transplantation for hepatoblastoma. *Liver Transpl* 2008;14:1614–1619.

Fuchs J, Rydzynski J, vonSchweinitz D, et al. Pretreatment prognostic factors and treatment results in children with hepatoblastoma: A report from the German Cooperative Pediatric Liver Tumor Study HB94. *Cancer* 2002;95:172–182.

Gupta AA, Gerstle JT, Ng V, et al. Critical review on the management of advanced pediatric liver tumors. *Pediatr Blood Cancer* 2010, Wileyonlinelibrary.

Hery G, Franchi-Abella S, Habes D, et al. Initial liver transplantation for unresectable hepatoblastoma after chemotherapy. *Pediatr Blood Cancer* 2011;57:1270–1275.

Horton JD, Lee S, et al. Survival trends in children with hepatoblastoma. *Pediatr Surg Int* 2009;25:407–412.

Howat JM. Major hepatic resections in infancy and childhood. *Gut* 1971; 12:212–217.

Huang SA, Tu HM, Harney JW, et al. Severe hypothyroidism caused by type 3 iodothyronine diodinase in infantile hemantioma. *N Engl J Med* 2000;343:185–189.

Isaacs H Jr. Fetal and neonatal hepatic tumors *J Pediatr Surg* 2007;42: 1797–1803.

Katzenstein HM, Krailo MD, Malogolowkin MH, et al. Hepatocellular carcinoma in children and adolescents: results from the Pediatric Oncology Group and the Children's Cancer Group Study. *J Clin Oncol* 2002;29:2890–2897.

Katzenstein HM, Malowgolowkin MH, Meyers RL, et al. Biology and treatment of children with all stages of hepatoblastoma: COG protocol AHEP-0731. Approved by CTEP and NCI 2008, open for enrollment September 2009, www.childrensoncologygroup.org

Katzensten HM, Rigsby C, Shaw PH, et al. Novel therapeutic approaches in the treatment of children with hepatoblastoma. *J Pediatr Hematol Oncol* 2002;24:751–755.

Lewis Ms, Kaicker S, Strauchen JA, Morotti RA. Hepatic involvement in congenital acute megakaryoblastic leukemia: a case report with emphasis on the liver pathology findings. *Pediatr Dev Pathol* 2008;11:55–58.

Li JP, Chu JP, Yand JY, et al. Preoperative transcatheter selective arterial chemoembolization in treatment of unresectable hepatoblastoma in infants and children. *Cardiovasc Intervent Radiol* 2008;31:1117–1123.

Lopez-Terrada D, Alaggio R, DeDavila MT, et al. Towards an international pediatric liver tumor consensus classification: proceedings of the Los Angeles COG International Pathology Pediatric Liver Tumors Symposium. *Modern Pathology* 2013, epub ahead of print.

Lopez-Terrada D, Zimmermann, A. Current issues and controversies in the classification of pediatric hepatocellular tumors. *Pediatr Blood Cancer* 2012;59:780–784. PMID 22648938.

Malogolowkin MH, Katzenstein HM, Meyers RL, et al. Complete surgical resection is curative for children with hepatoblastoma with pure fetal histology: a report from the Children's Oncology Group. *J Clin Oncol* 2011;29(24):3301–3306.

Malogolowkin MH, Katzenstein HM, Meyers RL, et al. Complete surgical resection is curative for children with hepatoblastoma with pure fetal histology: a report from the Children's Oncology Group. *J Clin Oncol* 2011;29:3301–3306.

Meyers RL, Czauderna P, Otte JB. Surgical treatment of hepatoblastoma. *Pediatr Blood Cancer* 2012;59:800–808.

Meyers RL, Katzenstein HM, Krailo M, et al. Surgical resection of pulmonary metastatic lesions in hepatoblastoma. *J Pediatr Surg* 2007;42: 2050–2056.

Meyers RL, Katzenstein HM, Malogolowkin MH. Predictive value of staging systems in hepatoblastoma. *J Clin Oncol* 2007;25:737–738.

Meyers RL, Otte JB. Liver transplant for unresectable liver tumors in children. In *Pediatric Liver Tumors*, Zimmermann A, Perilongo G, eds. Berlin, Heidelberg: Springer Verlag; 2010:133–153.

Meyers RL, Rowland JH, Krailo M, et al. Pretreatment prognostic factors in hepatoblastoma: A Report of the Children's Oncology Group. *Pediatr Blood Cancer* 2009;53:1016–1022.

Meyers RL. Tumors of the liver in children. *Surg Oncol* 2007;16:195–203.

Otte JB. Progress in the surgical treatment of malignant liver tumors in children. *Cancer Treat Rev* 2010;36:360–371.

Otte JB, deVille de Goyet J. The contribution of transplantation to the treatment of liver tumors in children. *Semin Pediatr Surg* 2005;14:233–238.

Otte JB, Meyers RL. Liver transplantation *J Pediatr Surg* 2006;41:607–608.

Otte JB, Pritchard J, Aronson DC, et al. Liver transplantation for hepatoblastoma: Results from the International Society of Pediatric Oncology (SIOP) Study SIOPEL-1 and Review of the World Experience. *Pediatr Blood Cancer* 2004;42:74–83.

Perilongo G, Maibach R, Shafford E, et al. Cisplatin versus cisplatin plus doxorubicin for standard risk hepatoblastoma. *N Engl J Med* 2009;361:1662–1670.

Perilongo G, Malogoloowkin M, Feusner J. Hepatoblastoma clinical research: lessons learned and future challenges. *Pediatr Blood Cancer* 2012;59:818.

Roebuck DJ, Aronson D, Clapuyt P, et al. 2005 PRETEXT: a revised staging system for primary malignant liver tumours of childhood developed by the SIOPEL group. *Pediatr Radiol* 2007;37:123–132; 1096–1100.

Schnelldorfer T, Chavin KD, Lin A, et al. Inflammatory myofibroblastic tumor of the liver. *J Hepatobil Pancreat Surg* 2007;14:421–423.

Semeraro M, Branchereau S, Maibach R, et al. Relapses in hepatoblastoma patients: clinical characteristics and outcome—experience of the International childhood lliver tumor strategy group SIOPEL. *Eur J Cancer* 2013;49:915–922. PMID 23146961.

Tannuri AC, Tannuri U, Gibelli NE, et al. Surgical treatment of hepatic tumors in children: lessons learned from liver transplantation. *J Pediatr Surg* 2009;44:2083–2087.

Tiao GM, Bobey N, Allen S, et al. The current management of hepatoblastoma: a combination of chemotherapy, conventional resection, and liver transplant. *J Pediatr* 2005;146:204–211.

Towu E, Kiely E, Pierro A, Spitz L. Outcome and complications after resection of hepatoblastoma. *J Pediatr Surg* 2004;39:199–202.

Von Schweinitz D. Hepatoblastoma recent developments in research and treatment. *Semin Pediatr Surg* 2012;21:21–30.

Von Schweinitz D, Byrd DJ, Hecker H, et al. Effciency and toxicity of ifosfamide, cisplatin, and doxorubicin in the treatment of childhood hepatoblastoma. Study committee of the Cooperative Paediatric Liver Tumour Study HB89 of the German Society of Paediatric Oncology and Haematology. *Eur J Cancer* 1997;33:1243–1249.

Von Schweinitz D, Hecker H, Harms D, et al. Complete resection before development of drug resistance is essential for survival from advanced hepatoblastoma—a report from the German cooperative pediatric liver tumor study HB-89. *J Pediatr Surg* 1995;30:845–852.

Zsiros J, Brugieres L, Brock P, et al. Dose-dense cisplatin-based chemotherapy and surgery for children with high risk hepatoblastoma (SIOPEL 4): A prospective, single-arm, feasibility study. *Lancet Oncol* 2013;14:834–842.

Zsiros J, Maibach R, Shafford E, et al. Successful treatment of childhood high-risk hepatoblatoma with dose-intensive multiagent chemotherapy and surgery: final results of the SIOPEL-3HR study. *J Clin Oncol* 2010;28:2584–2590.

ONCOLOGY

# CHAPTER 94

# Gastrointestinal Polyps/Intestinal Cancer

*Artur Chernoguz and Jason S. Frischer*

## KEY POINTS

1. Presence of colorectal adenomas in children mandates evaluation for familial polyposis syndromes.

2. The first presenting symptoms of polyposis syndromes are often secondary to extraintestinal manifestations and unrelated to gastrointestinal polyps.

3. Polyposis syndrome treatment involves a number of surgical options which allow patients to maintain satisfactory lifestyles.

4. Despite a number of surgical options, including total colectomy, cancer risks remain, and lifetime surveillance is mandatory.

5. With improved survival, surveillance for extraintestinal manifestations is critical.

6. Small intestinal malignancies are rare, but diagnosis in the pediatric population is often delayed secondary to low suspicion.

7. Colorectal cancer in the pediatric population is extremely rare, but children with polyposis syndromes are at an extremely high risk of eventually developing colorectal cancer.

## JUVENILE POLYPS

The most common polypoid intestinal lesion in the pediatric population is a colorectal polyp, an intraluminal protrusion of the intestinal epithelium and submucosa. The entity of a juvenile polyp refers to the type of polyp, rather than the age at the onset of the disease, and is synonymously termed a hamartomatous, inflammatory, or retention polyp. The incidence of juvenile polyps is estimated at 1% in children, and a vast majority is not associated with familial syndromes. While solitary juvenile polyps have traditionally not been considered premalignant, evidence of adenomatous changes suggests otherwise. Careful investigation is required to differentiate sporadic polyps from those linked to familial syndromes in order to guide the treatment and cancer prevention strategy.

## Isolated Juvenile Polyps

### Presentation

Juvenile polyps typically present in the first decade of life, but are rarely identified prior to 2 years of age. The most frequent presenting symptom is lower intestinal bleeding, followed by intermittent abdominal pain. Occasionally, polyps can move by intestinal peristalsis to produce an intussusception of the bowel. Up to one third of patients with juvenile polyps present with anemia secondary to chronic blood loss, even in cases of a solitary polyp.

### Diagnosis

The diagnostic methods of intestinal polyps largely depend on their suspected location. Distal colonic polyps that manifest with hematochezia prompt a rectal examination and lower endoscopic investigation, which can be both diagnostic and therapeutic. Although a complete colonoscopy may be viewed as a particularly invasive procedure in children, the need to examine the proximal colon necessitates such a thorough investigation. Recent studies advocated the use of colonoscopy, as 8% to 40% of patients were found to harbor proximal colon polyps. The location and number of polyps discovered on endoscopy may indicate risk of familial polyposis syndromes and the need for a more extensive evaluation. Juvenile polyps are not always isolated (typically 1-3 polyps), ranging from 0.5 to 5 cm. Finding more than 3 to 5 lesions may suggest the diagnosis of juvenile polyposis syndrome (JPS) and requires further work-up, including upper endoscopy. Microscopically, juvenile polyps are hamartomas, but often contain inflammatory and cystic features secondary to retained mucus.

### Treatment

Conservative treatment with observation may be reserved for those patients who have a solitary bleeding event without evidence of anemia due to chronic blood loss. Often, these occurrences are self-limited and symptoms resolve when the polyp outgrows its blood supply or self-amputates secondary to torsion around its pedicle. If the symptoms persist, or are accompanied by pain, endoscopic polypectomy can be therapeutic. Polyps located in the distal portion of the rectum may be readily visualized in an anesthetized patient. We prefer the prone position using the Lone Star Retractor

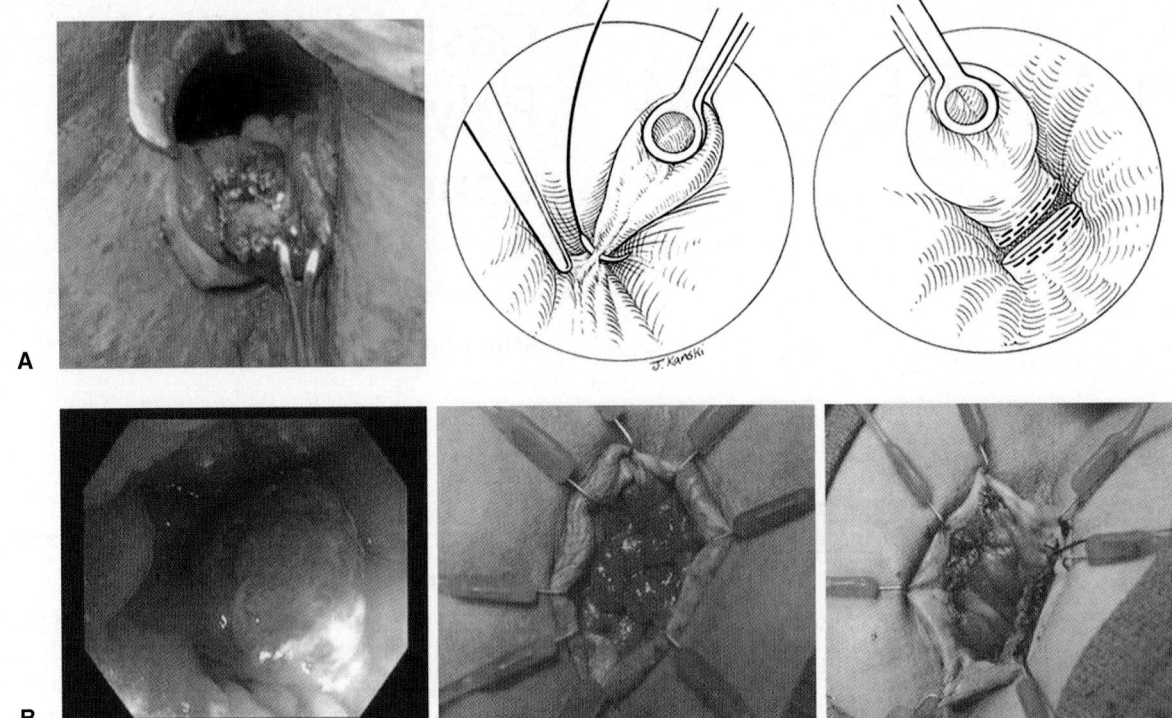

**FIGURE 94-1** **A.** Exposure using the Hill–Ferguson rectal retractor. Transrectal excision of a distal rectal polyp can be accomplished using suture ligature or endoscopic stapling techniques. **B.** Rectal polyp identified on endoscopic examination. Exposure was provided using the Lone Star Retractor System™, allowing the removal of the polyp using suture ligature. Courtesy of Dr. Randolph M. Steinhagen, Mount Sinai School of Medicine, New York, NY.

System™ (CooperSurgical, Inc.) to optimize visualization, though the lithotomy position or use of the Hill–Ferguson Rectal Retractor is also feasible. Polypectomy by suture ligation or using a surgical stapler can be undertaken without the need for performing endoscopy (Fig. 94-1). Polyps located in the proximal rectum or colon need to be addressed with the help of a skilled endoscopist. After visualization of the lesion during colonoscopy, polypectomy can be performed using a cauterizing wire-snare. Following the polypectomy, the specimen is directed for histologic examination to evaluate for adenomatous changes, features suggestive of a familial disorder, dysplasia, or malignant transformation. Positive findings mandate investigation for polyposis syndromes.

## Surveillance

No evidence-based formal surveillance guidelines exist. However, based on the observations of recurrence and dysplasia in patients with even a single polyp, some authors suggest repeat colonoscopy within 1 to 3 years, depending on the polyp burden, the presence of adenomatous changes, or with recurrent bleeding. It should be recognized, that while the risk of malignancy is low, cases of cancer arising from a single polyp have been described. Genetic testing may raise suspicion of a familial disorder and guide the need for follow-up.

## Juvenile Polyposis Syndrome

JPS is an autosomal dominant process with an incidence of approximately 1:16,000-100,000 (Table 94-1). This disorder typically affects the large bowel, but associated small bowel and gastric lesions have been described. Polyps associated with this disorder carry a significant risk of early malignancies including colorectal, gastric, duodenal, and pancreatic cancer. The overall risk of cancer approaches 70% by 60 years of age and many patients present in their teens. Thus, suspected cases require vigilant and active follow-up.

## Presentation

There are 3 general sub-types of JPS. The *infantile* form typically manifests as rectal prolapse, anemia, persistent GI bleeding, intussusception, hypoproteinemia, and electrolyte imbalance, leading to failure to thrive. Patients afflicted with the *infantile* form of JPS usually succumb to the disease at an early age (<2 years), despite aggressive nutritional support and bowel resections. The *diffuse* form of JPS affects children 6 months to 5 years of age and usually presents with similar, but often milder symptoms, as compared to the *infantile* subtype. The polyps are distributed throughout the gastrointestinal tract, but are most commonly found in the stomach, distal colon, and rectum. *Juvenile polyposis coli*, the sub-type affecting 5 to 15 year-olds, presents with anemia, as a result of rectal bleeding. Severe malnutrition is uncommon. Despite its name, Juvenile Polyposis patients can present as adults. Nevertheless, most patients are diagnosed before the second decade of life with a mean age at diagnosis of 6 years. A number of associated anomalies have been described, including intestinal malrotation, polydactyly, as well as cranial and cardiac defects.

| TABLE 94-1 | Hereditary Gastrointestinal Polyposis Syndromes | | | | | | | |
|---|---|---|---|---|---|---|---|---|
| Syndrome | Incidence | Gene | Gene Location | Mutation Identified (%) | Number of Polyps | Histology | Associated Tumors | Risk (%) |
| Juvenile Polyposis Syndrome | 1:16,000-1,100,000 | SMAD4 BMPR1A MPSH | 18q21 10q23 9q34 | 60 | >5-100s | Juvenile Polyps | Colon Stomach Small Intestine Pancreas | 20-70 21 Low Low |
| Familial Adenomatous Polyposis (FAP) | 1:8,000-10,000 | APC | 5q21 | 70-90 | 100-1000s | Adenomatous | Colon Duodenum Desmoid Liver (Hepatoblastoma) Pancreas Thyroid Stomach CNS | 100 4-12 3.5-32 1-2 1-2 1-2 <1 <1 |
| Attenuated FAP | <1:10,000 | APC | 5q21 | 20-30 | 10-100 | Adenomatous | Colon Duodenum Thyroid | 70-100 4-12 1-2 |
| Gardner's Syndrome | 1:1,000,000 | APC | 5q21 | >90 | >1000 | Adenomatous | Colon Desmoid Duodenum Thyroid Brain Pancreas Hepatoblastoma Stomach | 100 3.5-32 5-12 2 2 <2 <2 <1 |
| Peutz-Jeghers Syndrome | 1:8,300-1:280,000 | LKB1/STK 11 | 19p13 | 50-90 | <20 | Peutz-Jeghers Polyps | Breast Colon Pancreas Stomach Ovary Lung Small Intestine Uterine/Cervix Testicle | 45-54 40 11-36 29 18-21 15-17 13 9-10 9 |
| Cowden Syndrome | 1:200,000-250,000 | PTEN | 10q23 | >80 | Multiple | Hamartomatous | Breast Thyroid Endometrial | 25-50 3-10 5-10 |

## Diagnosis

Diagnostic features of JPS have undergone several modifications, but currently require: (a) ≥3 to 5 colorectal polyps (usually 50-200), (b) multiple polyps throughout the GI tract, or (c) any number of polyps with a family history of JPS (Fig. 94-2). Microscopically, the polyps appear similar to benign sporadic lesions, but some may be multilobated, papillary, or villous, and without lamina propia expansion. Reports have commented that up to 30% of lesions contain dysplastic changes or frank isolated adenomas. While the genetic basis of Juvenile Polyposis has been linked to the SMAD4 gene on chromosome 18q21 or the BMPR1A

gene on chromosome 10q23, but approximately half of the patients have no identifiable mutations. Deletions in BMPR1A and PTEN have been linked to the severe form of JPS of infancy. Since no identifiable mutations exist in approximately half of the patients, genetic testing is not routinely employed to diagnose JPS. Upper and lower endoscopic evaluation examining the stomach, proximal duodenum, and the entire colon is critical for the diagnosis and follow-up in cases of suspected juvenile polyposis. Recently, capsule endoscopy has gained favor in identification of small bowel polyps, but may be limited by the patient's inability to cooperate with the study.

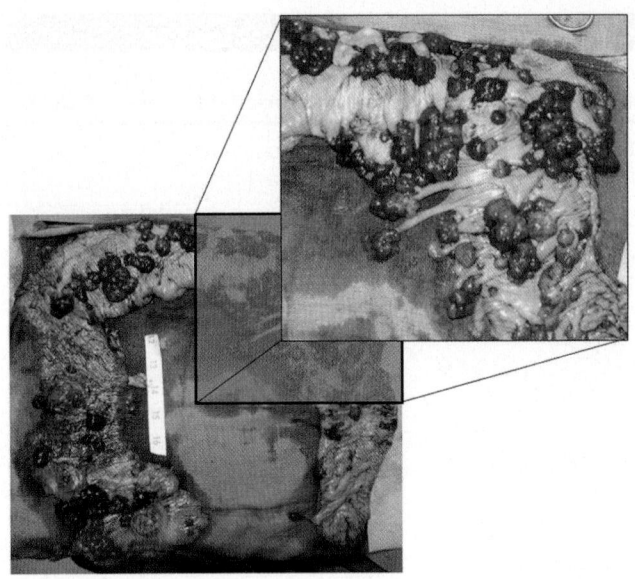

**FIGURE 94-2** Surgically excised colon specimen from a patient diagnosed with Juvenile Polyposis Syndrome. Polyps are distributed throughout the colon.

## Treatment

Nutritional deficiencies caused by chronic blood loss occasionally require parenteral nutritional support, as well as blood transfusions in preparation for surgical treatment. Interventions must be individualized to the patient, based on the location and extent of the disease and overall health status. Endoscopic polypectomies can achieve symptomatic relief. However, cases involving prohibitively large polyps and significant potential for bleeding necessitate surgical intervention. Often, treatment requires laparotomy or laparoscopy in order to perform multiple enterotomies/polypectomies, and, in selected cases proctocolectomy with ileorectal or ileoanal anastomosis. Some have advocated aggressive approaches towards the disease distributed throughout the colon and rectum by performing a total abdominal procto-colectomy and ileal pouch-anal anastomosis. However, the potential surgical morbidity, may predispose the patient to a change in bowel habits, including increased frequency and compromise in continence, with associated psychosocial consequences. One must also take into account the risk of recurrence in the remaining rectal mucosa as well as the small bowel pouches, which often needs to be addressed with additional resections and reconstruction. Unfortunately, no clear prognostic factors have been identified to reliably determine which patients may benefit from rectum-sparing surgery and which should undergo a more aggressive initial resection. This precludes the development of clear surgical guidelines, but provides a number of operative options which can be tailored to the individual patient. It should be stressed that the success of such an approach heavily relies on close follow-up and willingness to undergo additional diagnostic and operative procedures. Gastric polyps commonly found in JPS patients require upper endoscopic exploration. Exploration may reveal significant involvement of gastric mucosa, which is not amenable to polypectomy, necessitating total or subtotal gastrectomy.

## Surveillance

Due to a clinically significant risk of malignancy, recommended follow-up with upper and lower endoscopy is done every 1 to 3 years beginning at age 10 to 15 (Table 94-2). However, a recent 10-year review of children diagnosed with JPS revealed adenomatous changes in <1% of polyps, and no malignant changes were detected. The authors propose that the interval between follow-up colonoscopies be extended. The need for upper endoscopy is less clear, but is currently recommended. First-degree relatives of the patient should be offered genetic testing.

# FAMILIAL POLYPOSIS SYNDROMES

Identification of patients with familial polyposis syndromes is crucial for their treatment, surveillance, and genetic counseling of family members. A detailed family history may reveal a higher than usual incidence of colorectal cancers, or frequent polyps. Positive findings should prompt further investigation, including, in many cases, genetic testing. Work-up requires upper and lower endoscopic investigation in almost all cases. Adequate small bowel surveillance remains a challenge, but may improve with increased use of capsule endoscopy. Due to a great degree of overlap in diagnostic features, clinical and pertinent historical findings may prove invaluable in assisting to accurately making a histologic diagnosis.

## Familial Adenomatous Polyposis

Familial Adenomatous Polyposis (FAP) is an autosomal dominant disorder which occurs in approximately 1 in 8000 to 10,000 live births. While this condition accounts for <1% of colorectal cancers, 100% of untreated individuals afflicted with this syndrome develop a colorectal malignancy. Median age of cancer development is thought to be in the third to fourth decade, but earlier onset may occur in severe phenotypes. In 70% to 90% of patients, a mutation in the *APC* (Adenomatous Polyposis Coli) gene located on chromosome 5q, coding for a multifunctional protein involved in tumor suppression, can be identified (Table 94-1).

## Presentation

Typical presenting symptoms of rectal bleeding, abdominal pain, anemia, and diarrhea vary in severity and are uncommon until the adenomas significantly increase in size and number. Patients typically develop symptoms in their teens, while malignant transformation occurs approximately 10 years following the appearance of adenomas. However, with increasing counseling, a number of patients are identified as a result of genetic testing, which is often prompted by the diagnosis of FAP in a family member. Colonoscopy usually reveals multiple (hundreds to thousands) adenomatous polyps. FAP presents along a spectrum of severity, ranging from milder phenotypes to severe disease with extra-intestinal manifestations, including desmoid tumors, hepatoblastomas, gliomas, congenital hypertrophy of retinal pigmentation (CHRPE), and absence of or supernumerary teeth. Close to 90% of patients with FAP will develop fundic gastric polyps,

| TABLE 94-2 | Surveillance Recommendations in Patients with Gastrointestinal Polyposis Syndromes | |
| --- | --- | --- |
| | Age (Years) | Interval (Years) |
| **Juvenile Polyposis Syndrome** | | |
| Colonoscopy | 10-15 | 1-3 |
| Upper endoscopy | 10-15 | 1-3 |
| Capsule endoscopy | a | a |
| Abdominal ultrasound | a | a |
| Thyroid ultrasound | a | a |
| **Familial Adenomatous Polyposis (FAP)** | | |
| Colonoscopy | 10-12 | 1-2 |
| Colonoscopy post-IRA colectomy | | 0.5-1 |
| Colonoscopy post-IPAA | | 0.5-3 |
| Upper endoscopy | 20-30 | 1-3 |
| Capsule endoscopy | a | a |
| Abdominal ultrasound[a] | 10-12 | 1 |
| Thyroid ultrasound[a] | 10-12 | 1 |
| Abdominal-Pelvic CT/MRI | b | b |
| **Attenuated FAP** | | |
| Colonoscopy | 16-20 | 1-2 |
| Upper endoscopy | 25-30 | 3 |
| Capsule endoscopy | a | a |
| Abdominal ultrasound | 10-12 | 1 |
| Thyroid ultrasound | 18-20 | 1 |
| **Peutz-Jeghers Syndrome** | | |
| Colonoscopy | 8 | 3 Years until 50[c] |
| | 50 | 1-2 |
| Video capsule endoscopy/MRE | 8 | 3 |
| Upper endoscopy | 8 | 3 Years until 50[c] |
| Clinical breast exam | 25 | 0.5 |
| Mammogram/Breast MRI | 25 | 1 |
| Testicular exam | Birth-12 | 1 |
| Cervical smear | 18-20 | 1 |
| Transvaginal ultrasound | 18 | 1 |
| MRCP/Endoscopic ultrasound | 30 | 1-2 |

IPAA, Ileal pouch, anal anastomosis; IRA, ileorectal anastomosis; CT, computed tomography; MRI, magnetic resonance imaging; MRE, magnetic resonance enterography; MRCP, magnetic resonance cholangiopancreatography.

[a]These studies may be considered, but data supporting this recommendation are lacking.
[b]1-3 years post colectomy, then 5-10 years and immediate, if symptoms suggest (desmoid surveillance).
[c]If initial screening is (–), follow-up endoscopy at age 18.

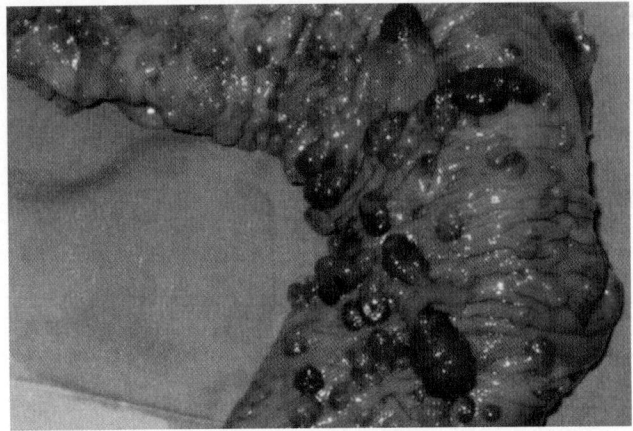

**FIGURE 94-3** Colon specimen of a patient with familial adenomatous polyposis demonstrating multiple polyps of variable sizes and at different stages of development. Courtesy of Dr. Randolph M. Steinhagen, Mount Sinai School of Medicine, New York, NY.

which have a limited risk for malignant transformation, but dysplasia can occur. Frequently, duodenal polyps are noted on endoscopic imaging. They are commonly found in the periampullary region and represent a significantly higher threat of malignancy later in life.

## Diagnosis

Diagnosis of FAP is made upon identification and pathologic confirmation of >100 colonic polyps (Fig. 94-3). These adenomas vary in size and stages of development and can be identified in patients as early as in their teens. While a majority of the patients with FAP have an identifiable truncating mutation in the *APC* gene, the severity of the disease and presence of extraintestinal symptoms heavily depend on the location of the mutation. Over 700 *APC* mutations have been identified, yet nearly a third of the patients present with *de novo* mutations.

## Treatment

Individuals affected by FAP are at risk for early development of a colorectal malignancy. If left untreated, 100% of patients will develop cancer by the time they are in their thirties. However, several reports suggest that aggressive cases can lead to the development of cancer in children and teenagers with FAP. Nonoperative treatments have not yet reliably been proven to prevent malignant transformation. A recent trial with a selective cyclooxygenase inhibitor demonstrated safety and potential benefit as an adjunct to current therapy in reducing the number of colorectal polyps in the pediatric population. It is not yet known if this approach can address the malignant potential of the disease process. While medical treatment regimens are being explored, surgery remains the mainstay of therapy. Timing and type of surgery is determined for individual patients based on the genetic and phenotypic severity, as well as patient's wishes. It is usually recommended that patients undergo a colectomy in the teenage years or in early adulthood. Patients with advanced histology, >20 adenomas, or adenomas exceeding 1 cm in size, should be considered for colectomy at an earlier age, since premature malignancy is almost assured in this population. Conversely, the presence of desmoid tumors may delay surgery.

Several effective surgical options exist for patients with FAP. The traditional approach of total abdominal proctocolectomy with end-ileostomy is rarely used today because of the psychosocial impact of having an ileostomy and the availability of surgical techniques capable of achieving satisfactory results. Total abdominal colectomy with ileorectal anastomosis decreases surgical morbidity associated with a pelvic dissection (sexual dysfunction, reduced fertility) and allows for improved bowel function. These advantages are provided at the expense of a higher risk of malignancy, necessitating continued regular endoscopic surveillance. Over the past 3 decades, total proctocolectomy with ileal pouch endorectal pull-through has become a more popular option. This procedure may require the creation of a temporary diverting ileostomy at the time of abdominal colectomy, and ileoanal anastomosis, although recent data reports excellent results without fecal diversion. If created, the ileostomy can usually be closed after several weeks. This procedure can be approached with or without transrectal mucosal proctectomy.

Recent advances in surgical equipment have produced an option of performing a double-stapled anastomosis, which typically involves leaving a rectal cuff. The potential improvement of functional outcomes using this technique must be weighed against the increased risk of development or recurrence of malignancy in the remaining rectal mucosa. It is important to remember that if mucosal proctectomy is not performed at initial operation, it may be necessary at a later time if the disease progresses.

Despite diversion, the immediate postoperative period can be complicated by bowel obstruction and anastomotic breakdown, leading to pelvic abscess formation, and potentially life-threatening pelvic sepsis. Extended follow-up is necessary to assess for the development of anastomotic strictures and pouchitis. Pouchitis, or inflammation of the ileal pouch, can manifest with abdominal pain, change in bowel habits and continence, as well as fever. The rates of this complication are considered to be lower in FAP patients undergoing ileoanal anastomosis, compared to those with ulcerative colitis. However, recent evidence highlights the great variability in defining pouchitis, and suggests similar rates, reaching 20%. Despite these discrepancies, patients affected with pouchitis tend to respond to treatment with antibiotics or probiotics and rarely require re-operation. It is believed that the size of the pouch is directly related to the risk of developing pouchitis. Multiple pouch options are available, but the size of the pouch may be limited by the narrow pelvises of pediatric patients.

Younger patients may be candidates for straight pull-through ileoanal anastomosis. Over time, the distal ileum can expand and, together with well-preserved anal sphincter function, can provide a substantial degree of continence without the associated risk of pouchitis. Furthermore, some authors found that after a 2-year follow-up, continence was significantly better following the creation of a J-pouch, while pouchitis rates were decreased with straight pull-through. The straight pull-through technique can be especially beneficial in select complex cases when the J-pouch configuration would produce significant tension on the anastomosis, or compromise vascular supply. Nevertheless, the clinically significant differences can be considered minimal and decisions should be made on a case-by-case basis.

As mentioned previously, recent studies have also challenged the traditional requirement for diversion as a part of restorative proctocolectomy procedures. It has been shown that omitting a diverting ileostomy from the procedure does not increase the complication rates related to the pouch and avoids the potential issues related to the ileostomy, such as prolapse, skin breakdown, bowel obstruction, and the need for second operative procedure.

Finally, recent technological advances have enabled the completion of a proctocolectomy and reconstruction with ileal pouch using laparoscopy, as well as a single incision approach, potentially further minimizing the morbidity of the operation and improving cosmesis.

## Surveillance

Despite the complete or near-complete resection of colonic tissue, malignant transformation can occur in the neoreservoir or retained rectal tissue following mucosectomy or the double-stapled anastomosis. Recent reports have shown consistently high rates of adenoma development in the retained rectal cuff, as well as the ileal pouch. The rate of cancer development has been quoted as high as 4% in long-term follow-up studies. We believe that the cancer rates will increase as more double-stapled pouches are created and long-term data becomes available. Therefore, vigilant life-long endoscopic surveillance of the pouch and anastomosis is imperative.

Upper endoscopy follow-up is an essential part of surveillance in FAP. It is recommended that upper endoscopic investigation begin at the time of identification of colonic lesions, or by 20 to 30 years of age and should continue every 1 to 3 years. This recommendation stems from the observations that upper gastrointestinal malignancies do not typically occur in the pediatric population of FAP patients. Yet, evidence of dysplastic and adenomatous changes in the ampullary and gastric polyps has led some to advocate earlier endoscopy. Biopsies of the upper gastrointestinal tract should be taken to evaluate for dysplastic changes. FAP patients are at a significantly increased risk of developing hepatoblastoma, adrenocortical, pancreatic, and thyroid malignancies (Table 94-1). A number of laboratory and imaging options are proposed for these devastating extra-intestinal manifestations of FAP. Some authors recommend thyroid and abdominal ultrasounds to be performed yearly starting at 10 to 12 years of age (Table 94-2).

## Attenuated FAP

Attenuated FAP (AFAP) is a poorly understood variant of FAP, typically characterized by fewer adenomas (~30), primarily located in the proximal colon, with a later onset of extra-intestinal manifestation, as well as a more delayed malignant transformation within the polyps.

## Diagnosis

Diagnosis of AFAP is made based on the reduced number of colonic polyps (<100) and older age at presentation. Genetic analysis is more challenging in this population, since the *APC* mutation is identified in only 20% to 30% of the patients (Table 94-1).

## Treatment

Once the polyps are identified, endoscopic polypectomy should suffice in most cases, unless the lesions grow larger than 1 cm, >20 in number, or demonstrate features of advanced histology. In such cases, colectomy, including proctectomy with ileal pouch anal anastomosis has been advocated.

## Surveillance

Due to milder symptomatology of AFAP, recommended endoscopic screening starts later than in typical FAP patients (16-20 years old), but should continue at 1 to 2 year intervals thereafter. Importantly, the screening emphasis should lie on the exploration of the ascending colon, the common location of AFAP lesions. Upper endoscopic exploration is recommended to begin at the age of 25 to 30 years old and to continue every 3 years (Table 94-2).

## The Gardner Syndrome

The Gardner Syndrome is considered a variant of FAP. Symptoms commonly develop in patients <20 years of age, but may be evident as early as 2 months of age. Extraintestinal symptoms such as bone and skin abnormalities typically precede gastrointestinal symptoms by approximately 10 years.

The Gardner Syndrome is associated with extra-colonic osteomas, most commonly affecting the skull and facial bones, as well as fibromas, lipomas, and epidermoid cysts. Malignant tumors of the ampulla of Vater, adrenal gland, and thyroid gland are associated with this syndrome (Table 94-1).

One of the characteristic features of the Gardner phenotype is the desmoid tumor. A desmoid tumor is a proliferation of unencapsulated fibromatous tissue, characterized by a unique infiltrative growth without metastases. Despite their benign characterization, desmoids can pose to be of significant morbidity due to compression and infiltration of surrounding tissues. They are notoriously difficult to treat primarily due to their significant infiltrative nature and recurrence potential.

Up to 32% of FAP patients develop desmoid tumors and may be seen as early as adolescence. These commonly occur in the abdominal cavity, most often affecting the mesentery. Desmoid tumors are most often seen in FAP patients who have previously undergone colonic resection. These patients have a substantially higher recurrence rate, often making subsequent resections more difficult. Since desmoids do not metastasize, these neoplasms are not considered malignant; however, they envelop and compress normal viscera, causing obstructive symptoms and making surgical resection quite treacherous. When feasible, local resection may be successful in the pediatric population, but is typically plagued by high rates of recurrence. The primary goal of surgery, in the management of desmoid tumors, is to achieve resection with negative margins. However, when such a procedure endangers nearby vital structures, a more localized resection is accepted in order to preserve function. In advanced cases non-surgical treatment with radiation therapy, as well as corticosteroids, anti-inflammatory, and anti-estrogen agents is occasionally met with success.

Gastrointestinal adenomatous polyps are typically located in the colon, small bowel, and stomach and usually go undiagnosed until the patient is in his 30s. Of utmost importance is the fact that malignant transformation is virtually universal and occurs by the 4th decade of life. Prophylactic colon resection with reconstruction has been recommended in the 2nd decade, but may be beneficial earlier, depending on the severity of phenotype. Life-long surveillance for gastrointestinal and extraintestinal malignancies is mandatory.

## The Turcot Syndrome

This FAP-related syndrome is characterized by the appearance of intestinal polyps and neoplasms in the central nervous system, such as glioblastoma, medulloblastoma, and ependymoma. Thyroid malignancy has also been described in association with the Turcot Syndrome.

## The Peutz–Jeghers Syndrome

The Peutz–Jeghers Syndrome (PJS) is a rare (1 in 8300-280,000) autosomal dominant syndrome characterized by gastrointestinal polyps, mucocutaneous pigmented lesions, and increased risk of malignancy. Approximately one third of patients will experience symptoms in the first decade of life and 50% before the age of 20 years. PJS patients are at an increased risk of developing tumors of the intestinal tract, as well as breast, uterus, and ovaries (Table 94-1).

### Presentation

Gastrointestinal polyps begin to cause symptoms in one third of the affected patients <10 years old and in one half of those under 20 years of age. The most common presenting symptom is abdominal pain. Other symptoms include GI bleeding, anemia, intussusception, and small bowel obstruction. A vast majority of patients (95%) also present with the characteristic mucocutaneous pigmented lesions, which can be noted in infancy. Polyps can be present throughout the GI tract, but the majority (60-90%) of the polyps are found in the small intestine, followed by the colon. The respiratory and urinary tracts, as well as the gall bladder have occasionally been shown to harbor polyps.

### Diagnosis

The diagnosis of PJS is made when ≥2 of the following are discovered: (a) ≥2 Peutz–Jeghers polyps of the small bowel, (b) mucocutaneous hyperpigmentation of the mouth, lips, nose, eyes, fingers, genitalia, or (c) a family history of PJS. Gastrointestinal polyps are traditionally classified as hamartomas, but they display characteristic features, such as arborization and pseudoinvasion, placing them into a unique category. A mutation in the tumor suppressor *LKB-1* gene can be identified in over 50% of the patients. The role of genetic testing is controversial at this time. Since approximately 25% of the PJS patients do not have an identifiable mutation, diagnosis is made based on clinical features even in the setting of negative genetic testing (Table 94-1).

### Treatment

Medical therapy has not been an active part of PJS treatment. Recent trials exploring the role of cyclooxygenase inhibitors and metformin demonstrate a potential benefit, but strong evidence and definitive protocols are lacking. The role of endoscopic polypectomy has been advocated and is thought to reduce the risk of polyp-related symptoms. Patients presenting with intussusception or obstruction frequently require operative intervention. The severity of bowel compromise dictates the need for resection, but intraoperative enteroscopy is recommended in order to remove the polyps and reduce the risk of reoperation.

### Surveillance

PJS is associated with the greatest risk of malignancy among the hamartomatous polyp syndromes. Cancer primarily arises in the gastrointestinal tract, but can also be identified in the breasts and lungs. Benign tumors can affect the testes and ovaries. While rare in the pediatric population, cases of gastrointestinal malignancy occurring in childhood and teenage years have been reported. The exact pathway of malignant transformation has not been fully elucidated and appears to differ from the classic sequence seen in FAP. Screening aims to identify not only those at risk for cancer, but also to prevent the development of symptoms associated with large polyps. A recent review recommends that patients undergo upper and lower endoscopic evaluation at the age of 8 years and every 3 years thereafter, this is provided that polyps are identified. Otherwise, the follow-up should be deferred until 18 years of age, or sooner if symptoms develop (Table 94-2). Capsule endoscopy is recommended at the same intervals to assess the small bowel. This recommendation is aimed to prevent the need for emergent laparotomy secondary to obstructive symptoms. The role of Magnetic Resonance Enterography (MRE) in monitoring is not clear at this time, but may become a reasonable diagnostic or surveillance option for small bowel polyps in PJS. Debate continues over the preferred age of initial screening, with some advocating deferring the upper and lower endoscopy to 20-30 years of age. Polypectomy may successfully resolve the symptoms, while reducing the risk of cancer. Potential at-risk relatives of PJS patients should undergo examination for typical features of the disease, as well as the necessary cancer screening, even while the risk status is not confirmed.

## Cowden Syndrome

Cowden Syndrome is a rare autosomal dominant disorder (1:200,000-250,000), linked to the mutation in the *PTEN* gene on chromosome 10q23 (Table 94-1). The role of PTEN is not completely understood, but it is thought to act as a tumor suppressor.

### Presentation

This pathology usually manifests with cutaneous lesions, including trichelemmomas and acral keratosis, as well as hamartomatous gastrointestinal lesions (>50%) and vascular malformations. Mental impairment and microcephaly are not uncommon. Cowden syndrome is associated with an increased risk for a number of malignancies, including breast and thyroid cancer. While these typically do not manifest until the third or fourth decade of life, thyroid malignancy has been reported in children.

## Diagnosis

Detailed diagnostic criteria, based on the presence of certain combinations of mucocutaneous, gastrointestinal, and soft tissue lesions have been outlined and continue to undergo revisions according to the latest genetic and diagnostic developments.

## Treatment and Follow-Up

Management of Cowden Syndrome is primarily aimed at the prevention of the development of malignant features. Gastrointestinal polyps do not represent a significant risk of malignancy; however, the polyps may serve as markers of potential internal malignancy. Increased rates of extra-intestinal malignancies require close follow-up with surgical interventions later in life. It is generally recommended that these patients undergo thyroid cancer screening starting from 18 years of age and breast cancer screening starting at 25 years.

## The Bannayan–Riley–Ruvalcaba Syndrome

The Bannayan–Riley–Ruvalcaba Syndrome is a hamartomatous polyp disorder phenotypically similar to the Cowden Syndrome and is characterized by macrocephaly, intestinal polyps, lipomas, and penile pigmentation. These lesions can be evident and symptomatic in childhood. Sixty percent of the patients have a mutation in the PTEN gene, linking this disorder to the Cowden Syndrome. Hamartomatous polyps are primarily identified in the colon or rectum, but are not considered a risk for malignancy.

## COLORECTAL CANCER

While traditionally considered a disease of adulthood, colorectal malignancy can present in childhood and even, in some cases, infants. As many as 0.5% of new cases of colorectal cancer are diagnosed in patients <20 years of age. Colorectal carcinoma is the most common pediatric tumor of the colon, followed by the Burkitt lymphoma. Pediatric colorectal cancer tends to present in more advanced stages and is associated with dismal outcomes (<15% survival at 5 years). The incidence in patients <20 years old is approximately 1/1,000,000. Due to its rarity, treatment and outcome data in the pediatric population is scarce.

The development of colorectal cancer in the pediatric population is poorly understood at this time. The stepwise progression model culminating in malignant transformation of a polyp to carcinoma appears to apply in patients afflicted with familial syndromes such as FAP. These patients demonstrate an accelerated pattern of progression. However, most pediatric patients with colorectal malignancy present with sporadic disease. Predisposing conditions, such as FAP and JPS, can be identified in approximately 10% of patients. Hamartomatous polyps are typically not considered pre-cancerous, whereas adenomatous polyps are associated with a higher risk of malignant transformation. Nevertheless, the Peutz–Jeghers Syndrome and JPS, both hamartomatous polyp diseases, have been linked to the development of malignancy. Environmental factors, such as individual history of abdominal irradiation, usually for treatment of another malignancy, are associated with an increased risk of colorectal carcinoma in children.

## Presentation

Similar to adults, pediatric patients with colorectal cancer tend to present with abdominal pain, bloody stools, anemia, change in bowel habits, and weight loss. Low index of suspicion of colorectal malignancy in children often delays treatment, leading to advanced stage of the disease at the time of the diagnosis. However, it is unclear if the natural course of the disease is accelerated in the pediatric population, making a timely diagnosis in this group even more challenging.

## Diagnosis

Abdominal X-ray, barium enemas, Computed Tomography (CT), and Magnetic Resonance Imaging (MRI) are all used in cases of suspected intra-abdominal malignancy, eventually leading to colonoscopic evaluation. Depending on the size of the lesion, colonoscopy with polypectomy, or biopsy, which serves to guide further work-up and treatment, is usually undertaken. After thorough exploration of the entire colon in patients suspected of harboring a colorectal malignancy, a metastatic work-up, consists of CT of the chest, abdomen, and pelvis, as well as a bone scan.

## Treatment

While no definitive pediatric guidelines for treatment are currently agreed upon, surgical resection is an essential component of treatment in pediatric colorectal cancer. Due to increased risk of recurrence, a total proctocolectomy is required for patients with ulcerative colitis or a polypoid syndrome. While the appropriate number of sampled lymph nodes needed for staging in the pediatric population is not known, there is evidence that an aggressive approach may be beneficial. Adult literature recommendations state that a minimum of 12 sampled lymph nodes are needed for adequate staging and this has often been extrapolated to the pediatric population. Chemotherapeutic regimen including oxiplatin, irinotecan, fluorouracil, as well as antiangiogenic agents, may be used; however, with limited success. Radiation therapy is usually reserved for rectal malignancy, as well as for palliation.

## SMALL INTESTINAL TUMORS

Primary pediatric GI neoplasms are exceptionally uncommon, combining to make up less than 5% of pediatric tumors. The majority of these patients are identified in their teens. A recent review at a major children's hospital has identified 58 cases of gastrointestinal tumors in 33 years, with 67% of those representing malignancies. The exact distribution of types of malignancies in the small bowel is not known, in part owing to the recent diagnostic technology developments, allowing a more accurate re-classification of histological entities. Diagnosis of small bowel malignancies in the pediatric population is even more challenging since the index of suspicion for this pathology is traditionally low. Surgical resection is commonly utilized in the treatment of these tumors, but the role of lymph node resection or follow-up is less clear. Definitive data on the associated symptoms is lacking, but some evidence that Inflammatory Bowel Disease may predispose to the development of small bowel cancer has emerged recently.

## Presentation

Small bowel malignancies present with relatively nonspecific symptoms and often consist of abdominal pain, vomiting, weight loss, change in bowel habits, and intussusception.

## Diagnosis

Despite the presence of symptoms, the diagnosis is often made as a result of surgical exploration. Imaging studies, such as CT, MRI, ultrasound, double balloon enteroscopy, and upper GI series with small bowel follow-through may be useful, but do not reliably identify a primary tumor. Nevertheless, imaging and biopsy should be attempted.

## Lymphoma

The Non-Hodgkin Lymphoma remains the most common primary bowel tumor in children. It is typically found in the distal small bowel, but may occur in all portions of the GI tract. The most common tumor of the small intestine, in the pediatric population, is the Burkitt lymphoma which is a subtype of the non-Hodgkin lymphoma. This is in contrast to adult small intestinal lymphomas where Diffuse Large B-Cell Lymphoma is the most common sub-type.

## Presentation

Lymphoma can present with abdominal pain, which is sometimes accompanied by a palpable mass, symptoms of intestinal perforation, or obstruction. On occasion, the tumor may cause intestinal intussusception.

## Diagnosis

Tissue biopsy is required for definitive diagnosis and may be obtained intra-operatively. Lymph node analysis helps determine the course of treatment.

## Treatment

Surgical resection may be urgent and, with regional lymphadenectomy, provides favorable survival rates in cases of localized GI lymphoma. Chemotherapy and radiotherapy, combined with surgery may be required in disseminated cases, though results are mixed. The survival is heavily dependent on the ability to perform a sufficient resection. Patients treated for localized tumors can achieve a 2-year survival of 80%, while widespread disease confers a more dismal prognosis (33% 2-year survival).

## Gastrointestinal Stromal Tumor (GIST)

These tumors are uncommon in the pediatric population. Similar to adults, they tend to occur in the stomach, followed by small bowel. In adults they have been linked to overexpression of *c-kit* or Platelet-Derived Growth Factor Receptor Alpha and arise from the precursors of the cells of Cajal located primarily in the myenteric plexus of the intestine. This appears to be true for the rare intestinal pediatric GISTs as well. They may also be associated with systemic diseases such as Neurofibromatosis I.

## Presentation

GISTs can present with symptoms of intestinal obstruction, gastrointestinal bleeding, or an incidentally identified abdominal mass.

## Diagnosis

Definitive diagnosis is accomplished by histologic analysis using the surgical specimen.

## Treatment

The curative strategy includes en bloc resection of tumor and involved structures, as well as assessment of the regional lymph nodes and liver for metastatic spread. Follow-up imaging is necessary, as recurrence of tumor has been described, but formal guidelines are not available due to the rarity of the tumor. Adult protocol of adjuvant imatinib mesylate (Gleevac, Novartis Pharmaceuticals) has been used in the pediatric population, but is still in the trial phase. The success of this therapy may be influenced by the presence of the *c-kit* mutation within the tumor.

## Carcinoid Tumor

Pediatric carcinoid tumor is an exceptionally rare entity, comprising approximately 0.1% of pediatric malignancies. These tumors have been described along the GI tract from stomach to rectum, but most commonly involve the appendix, followed by the small intestine. In rare cases, carcinoid tumors may invade surrounding structures and metastasize to distal organs (liver, lung, bone), but the majority are benign.

## Presentation

Carcinoid may present with abdominal pain, signs of obstruction, rectal bleeding, as well as anemia from chronic blood loss. Symptoms of carcinoid syndrome (diarrhea, respiratory distress, cutaneous flushing) are exceedingly rare and are present in the literature as occasional reports. Most carcinoid tumors in children are discovered at the time of appendectomy, with a rate of <0.1%.

## Diagnosis

Since the elevated serum levels of 5-hydroxyindoleacetic acid (5-HIAA) may be absent even in metastatic disease, the diagnosis is typically made incidentally from the surgical specimen. Octreotide scintigraphy and 24-hour urinary 5-HIAA may be useful in diagnosis of a suspected carcinoid tumor.

## Treatment

Surgical resection with negative margins is adequate treatment in localized disease <2.0 cm. Tumors that are noted to penetrate the serosa should undergo full metastatic survey and require resection of the involved bowel and mesentery. Tumors measuring >2.0 cm in size, which are exceptionally rare, also prompt metastatic survey with CT, MRI, and $^{99}$Tc bone scan. The role of an extended colon resection for tumors >2.0 cm is not clear and may not be indicated in localized disease. Metastatic disease is treated with adjuvant chemotherapy, though the efficacy is limited.

## SELECTED READINGS

Adolph VR, Bernabe K. Polyps in children. *Clin Colon Rectal Surg* 2008;21(4):280–285.

Aretz S. The differential diagnosis and surveillance of hereditary gastrointestinal polyposis syndromes. *Dtsch Arztebl Int* 2010;107(10):163–173.

Barnard J. Screening and surveillance recommendations for pediatric gastrointestinal polyposis syndromes. *J Pediatr Gastroenterol Nutr* 2009;48(Suppl 2):S75–S78.

Beggs AD, Latchford AR, Vasen HF, et al. Peutz–Jeghers syndrome: a systematic review and recommendations for management. *Gut* 2010;59(7):975–986.

Beliard A, Prudhomme M. Ileal reservoir with ileo-anal anastomosis: long-term complications. *J Visc Surg* 2010;147(3):e137–e144.

Calva D, Howe J. Juvenile polyposis. *Cancer Syndromes* [Internet edition] Bethesda, MD: National Center for Biotechnology Information (US); 2009.

Durno C, Monga N, Bapat B, Berk T, Cohen Z, Gallinger S. Does early colectomy increase desmoid risk in familial adenomatous polyposis? *Clin Gastroenterol Hepatol* 2007;5(10):1190–1194.

Fairley TL, Cardinez CJ, Martin J, et al. Colorectal cancer in U.S. adults younger than 50 years of age, 1998–2001. *Cancer* 2006;107(5 Suppl):1153–1161.

Friederich P, de Jong AE, Mathus-Vliegen LM, et al. Risk of developing adenomas and carcinomas in the ileal pouch in patients with familial adenomatous polyposis. *Clin Gastroenterol Hepatol* 2008;6(11):1237–1242.

Groen EJ, Roos A, Muntinghe FL, et al. Extra-intestinal manifestations of familial adenomatous polyposis. *Ann Surg Oncol* 2008;15(9):2439–2450.

Half E, Bercovich D, Rozen P. Familial adenomatous polyposis. *Orphanet J Rare Dis* 2009;4:22.

Huang SC, Erdman SH. Pediatric juvenile polyposis syndromes: an update. *Curr Gastroenterol Rep* 2009;11(3):211–219.

Jasperson KW, Tuohy TM, Neklason DW, Burt RW. Hereditary and familial colon cancer. *Gastroenterology* 2010;138(6):2044–2058.

Jass JR. Colorectal polyposes: from phenotype to diagnosis. *Pathol Res Pract* 2008;204(7):431–447.

Kartheuser A, Stangherlin P, Brandt D, Remue C, Sempoux C. Restorative proctocolectomy and ileal pouch-anal anastomosis for familial adenomatous polyposis revisited. *Fam Cancer* 2006;5(3):241–260; discussion 261–242.

Ladd AP, Grosfeld JL. Gastrointestinal tumors in children and adolescents. *Semin Pediatr Surg* 2006;15(1):37–47.

Lowichik A, Jackson WD, Coffin CM. Gastrointestinal polyposis in childhood: clinicopathologic and genetic features. *Pediatr Dev Pathol* 2003;6(5):371–391.

National Comprehensive Cancer Network Available at: http://www.nccn.org Accessed May 19, 2011.

Pilarski R. Cowden syndrome: a critical review of the clinical literature. *J Genet Couns* 2009;18(1):13–27.

Ryan DP, Doody DP. Restorative proctocolectomy with and without protective ileostomy in a pediatric population. *J Pediatr Surg* 2011;46(1):200–203.

# The Lymphomas

## CHAPTER 95

*Peter Ehrlich*

## KEY POINTS

1. Staging laparotomy is no longer necessary for work-up of lymphomas.

2. Hodgkins Disease accounts for 6% of pediatric malignancies and is the most commonly diagnosed cancer among adolescents aged 15 to 19.

3. The initial step to diagnosis of the Hodgkin lymphoma is lymph node biopsy. If a surgeon decides to approach a mediastinal mass thorascopically, they must ensure that adequate specimens are obtained as up to 50% of mediastinal cases required a second diagnostic biopsy when a thoracoscopic biopsy was performed.

4. Non-Hodgkin Lymphomas (NHL) are a varied group of tumors with almost 60 unique subtypes, accounting for 7% of tumors and are typically high grade.

5. For the Burkitt lymphoma, the prognosis is dependent on the extent of disease rather than on completeness of surgical resection.

The treatment for a child with Lymphoma requires a multidisciplinary team of healthcare professionals. Outcomes have improved and current multimodality therapy is focused on reducing the toxicity of treatment. The main role of surgery is for diagnosis. However, there are several key issues that a surgeon must be cognizant of when treating a child with a presumptive lymphoma. For example, extreme caution must be used in a child with respiratory compromise due to a large mediastinal mass suspected to be a lymphoma, alternatively, emergency surgery may be necessary in a child with a gastrointestinal lymphoma.

## THE HODGKIN LYMPHOMA

The Hodgkin lymphoma is named after Thomas Hodgkin a British pathologist who in 1832 described the disease in a paper titled, "On Some Morbid Appearances of the Absorbent Glands and Spleen." It was not until years later that Sternberg (1898) and Reed (1902) described the distinctive multinucleated giant cell with prominent nucleoli that are characteristic of HD (Fig. 95-1). Reed–Sternberg cells are derived from germinal center B cells and are the pathognomonic cells of HL. Cure rates for pediatric HL are excellent approaching 90% to 95% (Fig. 95-2).

## INCIDENCE AND EPIDEMIOLOGY

HL accounts for 6% of all pediatric malignancies, with an incidence of about 6 cases per 1 million. HL has a bimodal distribution with peaks in adolescence (15-19 yrs) and after age 55 years. Epidemiologic studies identify 3 forms of HL; Childhood HL, Adolescent Young Adults (AYA) and Older Adult HL. Childhood HL is found in children less than 14 years and accounts for 10-12% of cases. It is more common in males and the histological subtype is more likely to be mixed cellularity or nodular lymphocyte predominant. Risk factors for childhood HL include increasing family size, lower socioeconomic status and exposure to the Epstein-Barr virus (EBV).

AYA is defined as HL in those aged 15 to 35 and accounts for over 50% of the cases. It is the most commonly diagnosed cancer among adolescents aged 15 to 19. AYA HL has no gender preference and the most common form is nodular sclerosis. Risk factors include higher socioeconomic status, early birth order, and smaller family size, and EBV. Older Adults HL occurs in those older than 55 and comprises 35% of the cases.

## HISTOLOGY

The current World Health Organization (WHO) classification system separates HL into 2 broad categories: classical and lymphocyte predominant Hodgkin Lymphoma. Classical HL has 4 subtypes: lymphocyte depleted, nodular sclerosing, mixed cellularity and classical lymphocyte rich and accounts for 90% of all cases. Nodular sclerosis is the most common subtype (65% of cases). Immunomarkers are very helpful in diagnosing HL. Classical Hodgkin is characterized by CD15 and CD30 positive Reed–Sternberg cells. CD30 is a marker of activated B- and T-lymphoid cells, and is present in almost

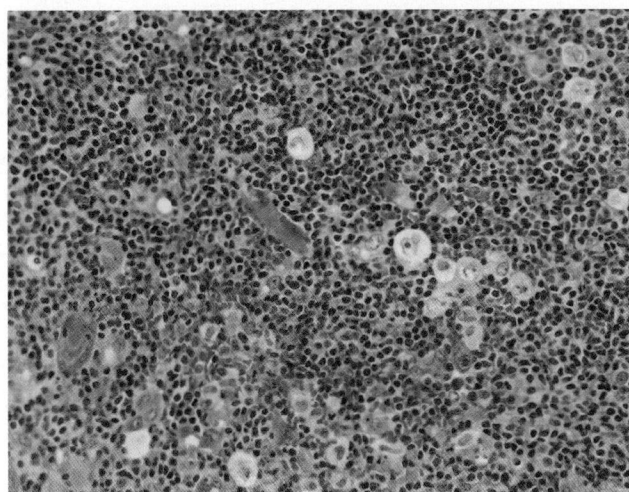

**FIGURE 95-1** High-power hematoxylin and eosin stained slide of a patient with Hodgkin Lymphoma and typical Reed Sternberg cells.

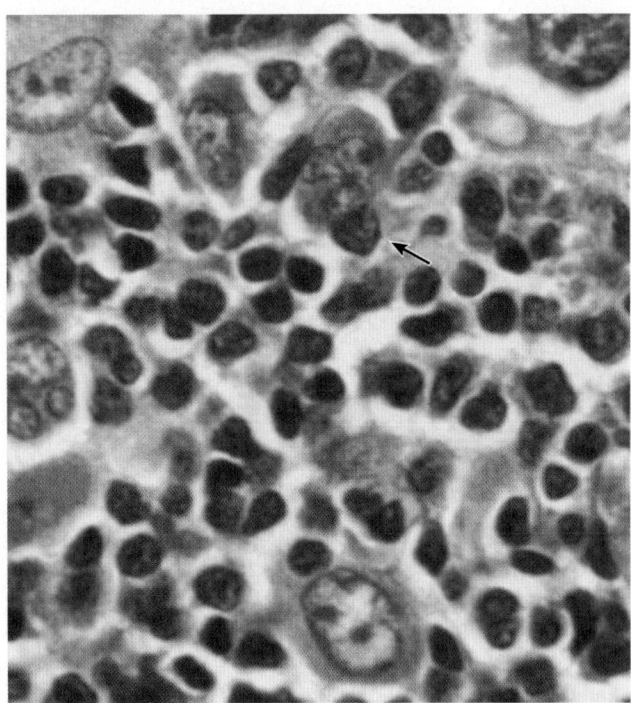

**FIGURE 95-3** High-power hematoxylin and eosin stained slide of a patient with lymphocyte predominate Hodgkin Lymphoma. Arrow points to classical "popcorn cell."

all cases. About 87% of classical Hodgkin lymphomas express CD15, the carbohydrate X hapten. Classical Hodgkin lymphoma rarely expresses CD45, also known as common leukocyte antigen, which is expressed by nearly all non-Hodgkin lymphomas. CD45 serve as a useful differential marker between HL and non-Hodgkin lymphoma.

The lymphocyte predominant (LPHD) subtype accounts for 10% of all cases and is characterized by lymphocytic and histiocytic (L&H) cells which express markers not typically seen in the "classical" subtype (Fig. 95-3). These cells are also known as "popcorn cells" and are CD20 positive. Other B cell immunomarkers found in LPHD include CD79a, CD75, epithelial membrane antigen, and CD45. The lymphocyte-predominance subtype historically carries the best prognosis.

Lymphomas are a malignant clonal expansion of cells. In HL, the origin of the malignant Reed–Sternberg cells and their mononuclear variants is likely to be the interdigitating reticulum cell. This antigen-presenting cell is located in the paracortex of the lymph node. Epstein–Barr virus exposure is associated with HL (and NHL). In the childhood form the EBV viral infection appears to precede tumor cell expansion, and EBV may act alone or in conjunction with other carcinogens. In the AYA form it is thought that EBV exposure is delayed suggesting that delayed exposure to EBV, or some other unidentified common infectious agent, may be a risk factor for AYA HL. Immunodeficiency is also strongly associated with HL. Since the development of highly effective multiagent and multidisciplinary treatment regimens, all histologic subtypes have become responsive to therapy.

## CLINICAL PRESENTATION

Lymphoma must be considered in any child with lymphadenopathy. Patients most frequently present primarily with cervical and/or supraclavicular lymphadenopathy (80%).

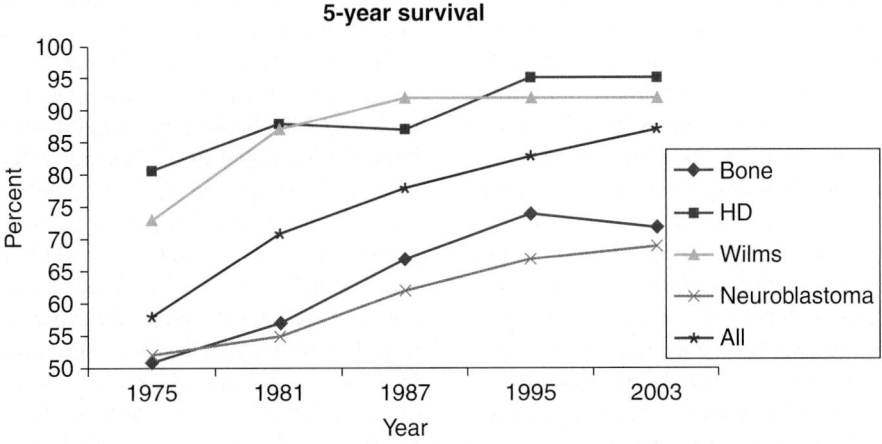

**FIGURE 95-2** Graph shows survival statistics of different pediatric cancers from 1975 to 2003.

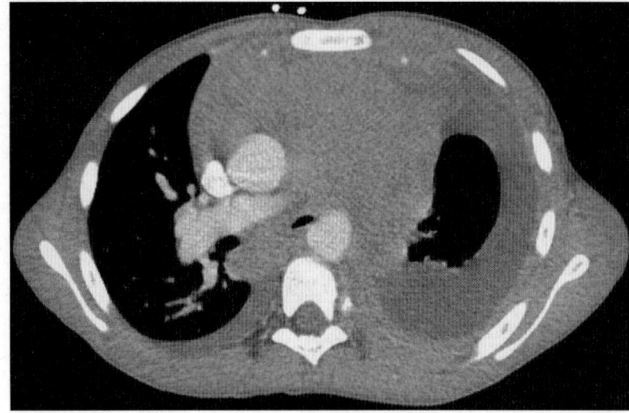

**FIGURE 95-4** A computed tomography scan of a large anterior mediastinal mass with pleural effusion.

| TABLE 95-1 | HL Staging Ann Arbor Classification with Cotswolds Modification |
|---|---|
| Stage I | Involvement of a single lymph-node region or lymphoid structure (eg, spleen, thymus, the Waldeyer ring), or involvement of a single extralymphatic site |
| Stage II | Stage II Involvement of 2 or more lymph-node regions on the same side of the diaphragm |
| Stage III III1 III2 | Indicates that the cancer has spread to both sides of the diaphragm, including 1 organ or area near the lymph nodes or the spleen. With or without involvement of splenic, hilar, celiac, or portal nodes With involvement of para-aortic, iliac, and mesenteric nodes |
| Stage IV | Indicates that the cancer has spread to both sides of the diaphragm, including 1 organ or area near the lymph nodes or the spleen. |

*Note:* Modifiers
- *A or B:* the absence of constitutional (B-type) symptoms is denoted by adding an "A" to the stage; the presence is denoted by adding a "B" to the stage.
- *E:* is used if the disease is "extranodal" (not in the lymph nodes) or has spread from lymph nodes to adjacent tissue.
- *X:* is used if the largest deposit is >10 cm ("bulky disease"), or whether the mediastinum is wider than 1/3 of the chest on a chest X-ray.
- *S:* is used if the disease has spread to the spleen.

The nature of the staging is (occasionally) expressed with:
- CS, clinical stage as obtained by doctor's examinations and tests.
- PS, pathological stage as obtained by exploratory laparotomy (surgery performed through an abdominal incision) with splenectomy (surgical removal of the spleen). *Note:* exploratory laparotomy has fallen out of favor for lymphoma staging.

Enlarged axillary nodes (25% of all cases) or inguinal nodes (5%) are less common. A key factor for the surgeon to assess in any child with lymphadenopathy is the presence of mediastinal disease. Respiratory symptoms, dyspnea on exertion, or orthopnea, may result from large mediastinal masses. Mediastinal disease is found in up to 75% of adolescents and 33% of children. A simple chest radiograph is mandated because mediastinal involvement may be extensive and produce major complications upon the induction of anesthesia (Fig. 95-4).

Patients may also have "B symptoms" in up to 33% of cases. B symptoms include a fever greater than 38°C, soaking night sweats, and weight loss of 10% or more. These symptoms are not specific to HL and can occur in non-Hodgkin lymphoma. B symptoms have prognostic significance reflected in the staging of HL (Table 95-1).

## DIAGNOSIS

A full history and physical examination focusing on nodal areas and the abdomen should be performed. Prior to surgery, a chest radiograph must be obtained to assess the presence of mediastinal disease. If a mediastinal mass is detected, a CT scan of the chest is mandated to assess the tracheal area and pulmonary function tests further define the extent of respiratory impairment (Fig. 95-4). An excisional biopsy of a suspicious lymph node should be the initial step to diagnosis of Hodgkin lymphoma. In some cases, the procedure may need to be performed under local anesthesia due to the size of the mediastinal mass and the resultant respiratory compromise (Fig. 95-5). Minimally invasive techniques have been used to biopsy mediastinal masses if no suspicious extrathoracic lymph nodes are available for biopsy. However, if a surgeon decides to approach the mass thorascopically or laparoscopically, they must ensure that adequate specimens are obtained. A report from the Children Oncology Group (COG) Hodgkin Lymphoma committee demonstrated that up to 50% of mediastinal cases required a second diagnostic biopsy when a thoracoscopic biopsy was performed. An anterior mediastinotomy (the Chamberlain procedure) is a useful approach when the diagnosis of lymphoma cannot be made using less invasive techniques (Fig. 95-6).

## STAGING

The Ann Arbor staging system and its Cotswolds modification remain the standard for adult and pediatric HL (Table 95-1). The original Ann Arbor staging system developed in 1974 was based principally upon the use of staging laparotomy and lymphangiogram, both of which have been abandoned.

Complete staging has both clinical and pathology components. Basic tests should include a complete blood cell count with differential, lactate dehydrogenase (LDH), alkaline phosphatase, erythrocyte sedimentation rate, or C-reactive protein (CRP), hepatic and renal function tests, and electrolytes. Radiographic studies include a chest radiograph and a computed tomography (CT) of the neck, chest, abdomen, and pelvis. If mediastinal disease is found on chest radiograph, the ratio of its maximal diameter to that of the thoracic cavity on a posteroanterior view is measured. A mass with a ratio greater than 1:3 places the patient in the subcategory of bulky mediastinal disease associated with a worse prognosis. Bone marrow (BM) biopsy is reserved for those patients with B symptoms or stage III–IV disease. [18F]-2 fluoro-D-2-deoxyglucose positron emission tomography (PET) is replacing gallium scans and recent studies have assessed the ability of PET scans

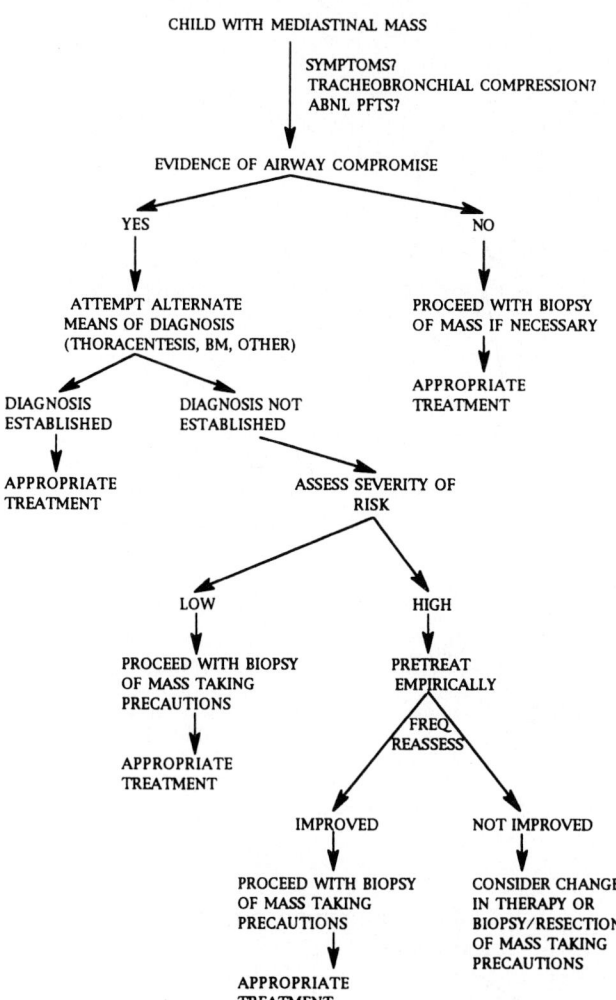

CHILD WITH MEDIASTINAL MASS

SYMPTOMS?
TRACHEOBRONCHIAL COMPRESSION?
ABNL PFTS?

EVIDENCE OF AIRWAY COMPROMISE

YES — ATTEMPT ALTERNATE MEANS OF DIAGNOSIS (THORACENTESIS, BM, OTHER)

NO — PROCEED WITH BIOPSY OF MASS IF NECESSARY → APPROPRIATE TREATMENT

DIAGNOSIS ESTABLISHED → APPROPRIATE TREATMENT

DIAGNOSIS NOT ESTABLISHED → ASSESS SEVERITY OF RISK

LOW → PROCEED WITH BIOPSY OF MASS TAKING PRECAUTIONS → APPROPRIATE TREATMENT

HIGH → PRETREAT EMPIRICALLY → FREQ REASSESS

IMPROVED → PROCEED WITH BIOPSY OF MASS TAKING PRECAUTIONS → APPROPRIATE TREATMENT

NOT IMPROVED → CONSIDER CHANGE IN THERAPY OR BIOPSY/RESECTION OF MASS TAKING PRECAUTIONS

**FIGURE 95-5** Simplified algorithmic approach to the treatment of a child with a mediastinal mass. Biopsy refers to an incisional or excisional biopsy of the mediastinal mass performed with a general anesthetic. Alternate means of diagnosis may include a lymph node biopsy performed with a local anesthetic only. At great risk are patients with orthopnea, >50% tracheobronchial narrowing, and truncation of the expiratory flow loop. Precautions taken when performing a biopsy include proper positioning and airway management, availability of a rigid bronchoscope in the room, and the presence of surgeons when anesthesia is induced.

to replace CT scans and as possible prognostic indicators for response to therapy. Magnetic resonance imaging (MRI) provides a more accurate evaluation of disease in the abdomen compared with CT, with better visualization of fat-encased retroperitoneal nodes but whether or not this provides clinically significant information has yet to be established.

## SURGERY

Historically, a staging lapaprotmy played a primary role in the diagnosis of HL. With the wide application of chemotherapy in all stages of HL, surgical staging has become irrelevant because the additional information it provides does not alter treatment. The surgeon's primary role is to obtain tissue for diagnosis. Biopsies should be taken from the most easily accessible site and adequate tissue must be obtained and sent fresh to pathology for immunohistochemistry, immunophenotyping, cytogenetics, and flow cytometry. Fine needle aspiration is generally discouraged as it is often not accurate nor is sufficient tissue obtained to properly stage and classify the patient. A thoracoscopic biopsy or a Chamberlain procedure (Fig. 95-6) can be used to obtain tissue for diagnosis in patients with only mediastinal involvement. Retroperitoneal lymphadenopathy is often accessible through laparoscopic biopsy. A second role for surgery is to provide central venous access for chemotherapy. Bilateral oophoropexies are also performed in girls who will receive abdominal radiotherapy.

## TREATMENT

### Risk Classification

Treatment is based on risk classification. Children and adolescents with HL are divided into 3 risk categories (low, intermediate, and high-risk disease) based on clinical and pathologic staging data. These include; histological subtype, stage at presentation, presence or absence of B symptoms, number of involved sites, and/or presence of bulky of disease (>10 cm). Although in various clinical trials the definitions may slightly change, in general, *low-risk* disease is defined as "classical" Hodgkin lymphoma patients, with clinical stage I or II disease, no B symptoms or bulky nodal involvement, and disease in fewer than 3 nodal regions. *Intermediate-risk* disease includes stage I, II, and sometimes IIIA disease with criteria and some trials have included: B symptoms, bulky disease, a large number of involved nodal regions, and extranodal involvement of disease. *High-risk* patients are those with stage IIIB, IVA/B disease. LPHD is considered a low-risk disease but is often separated from the classical HL studies.

### Chemotherapy and Radiation Therapy

Although the outcomes for children with HL have improved dramatically, the short- and long-term toxicity of therapy has been substantial. Current therapeutic protocols for HL have focused on maintaining excellent outcomes, but reducing toxicity. Ideal chemotherapy regimens use drugs that are individually effective with different mechanisms of action and toxicities to allow for a maximal dose. Radiotherapy was the first reported "curative" treatment for HL in the 1930s. Radiation therapy was based on the concept of contiguous lymph node basin involvement and treatment was focused on the whole nodal region plus adjacent regions which may be uninvolved. This treatment is called extended field radiotherapy (EFRT) and resulted in significant toxicity and late effects. EFRT has been supplanted by involved field radiation therapy (IFRT) which has reduced the exposure of uninvolved areas for example the heart. A further reduction of RT volume to cover just the nodal tissue involved by disease, without any attempt to include whole nodal region(s), is termed involved node radiation therapy (INRT). Using FDG PET analysis of residual disease and advances in radiation planning, it is possible now to confine the radiation to the initially involved nodal tissues rather than the whole nodal chain. Preliminary

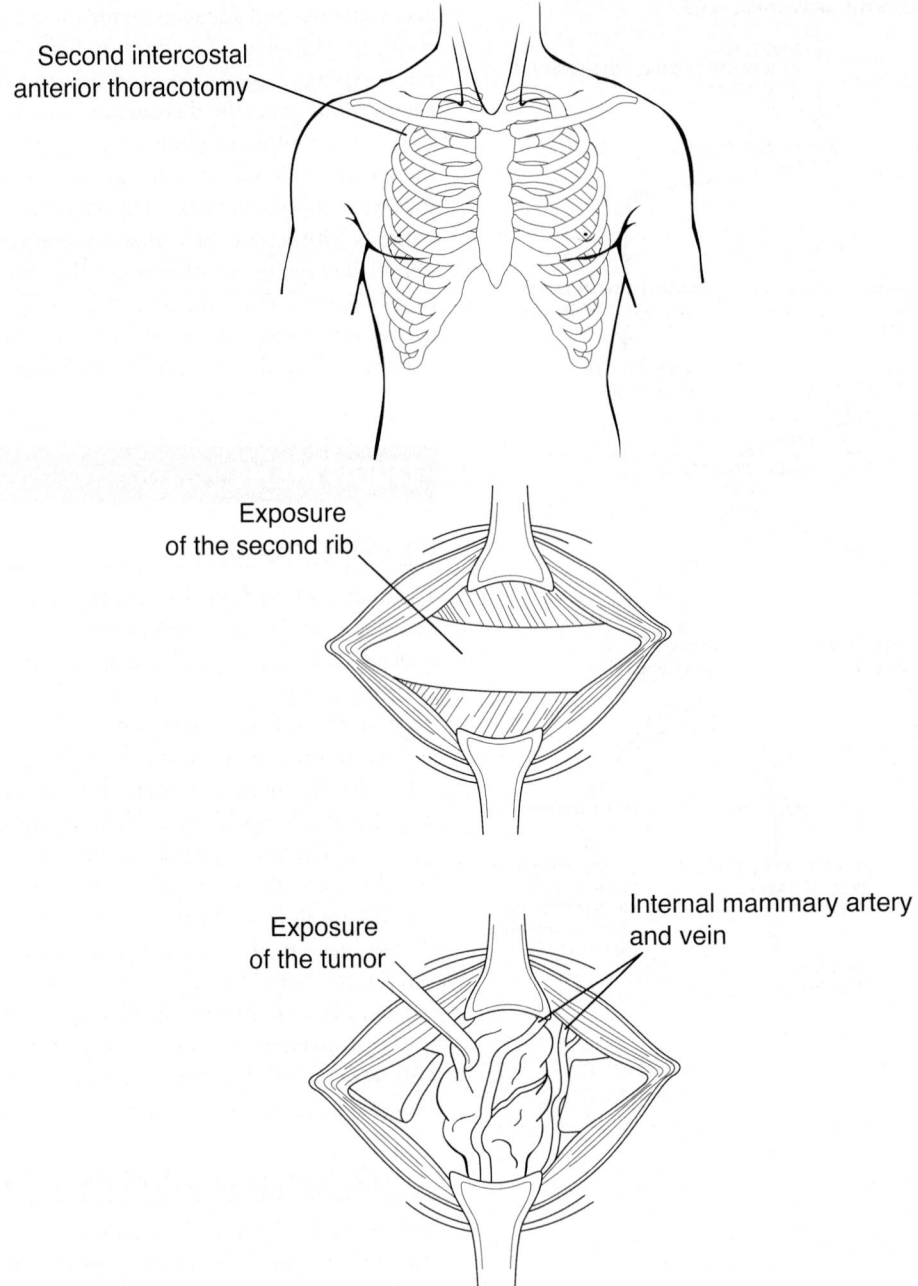

**FIGURE 95-6** The technique of the Chamberlain procedure; anterior thoracotomy at second rib and exposure of the tumor.

data reported from British Columbia in Canada indicated no increase in relapses with INRT compared with IFRT or EFRT using a current multiagent chemotherapy regimen.

## Therapy for Low-Risk Disease

Several multiinstitutional trials demonstrate that children and adolescents with low-risk HL can be effectively treated with 2 to 4 cycles of chemotherapy followed by 15 to 25 Gy IFRT, with series reporting 90% or better event-free survival (EFS), with overall survival (OS) greater than 95%.

## Therapy for Intermediate-Risk Disease

Intermediate-risk trials for HL have documented the need for adjuvant radiotherapy in most patients. In the CCG 5942

trial, intermediate-risk children with complete response were randomized to receive either IFRT or no further treatment. Three-year EFS was 82% with OS 93%, but the patients who received IFRT had 3 year EFS of 88%. Both these studies support the need for IFRT with most intermediate HL patients. The current intermediate-risk COG trial is a randomized trial to see if early complete responders can have a dose reduction of both chemotherapy and radiation therapy without a decrease in their EFS. Induction chemotherapy consists of ABVE-PC (Adriamycin;doxorubin, bleomycin, vincristine, etopside, prednisone, and cyclophosphamide) for 2 cycles. It is a double randomized response based protocol with both IFRT and chemotherapy intensifications following induction. This study closed in the fall of 2010.

## Therapy for High-Risk Disease

Patients with high-risk tumors require both intensification of chemotherapy and radiation therapy. The most recent studies suggest that outcome of patients with high-risk factors can be improved with intensification of chemotherapy and lowering RT based on response. Pediatric Oncology Group (POG) 9425 study reported 2 year EFS for intermediate and high-risk disease in response-based paradigm. In this study, 63% of patients received 9 weeks of chemotherapy and 21 Gy of IFRT because of good response whereas the others received more intensive therapy. The most current COG high-risk study recently opened. This is a nonrandomized response based protocol. Induction therapy is with ABVE-PC and patients will be divided into rapid early responders, and slow early responders. Response will be determined by PET scan and further chemotherapy and radiotherapy targets are based on the PET scan.

## Therapy for Lymphocyte-Predominant Hodgkin Disease

Lymphocyte-Predominant Hodgkin disease (LPHD) is recognized as a distinct clinical-pathological entity, with a favorable outcome, but also associated with a higher risk of late relapse and subsequent development of NHL. Interestingly, treatment by surgical resection alone has been reported in adult and pediatric patients. The outcomes suggest that patients with low-stage disease may be effectively treated with surgery alone, particularly considering the toxicity of treatment. In 2007, the Europeans reported 100% survival in 58 LP patients treated initially with surgery alone; 50 had a CR and received no adjuvant therapy. A recently completed COG protocol treated patients with stage I single node disease with surgery only. Results have not been published.

## Treatment Toxicities

RT (35-44 Gy) produces bone and soft-tissue hypoplasia in prepubertal children. In the chest this results as spinal and clavicular shortening and under development of the soft tissues in the neck. Long-term survivors of HL treated with full-dose RT have an increased risk of atherosclerotic heart disease, valvular dysfunction, and pericardial disease. Heart disease and valvular disease tend to occur late 8 to 10 years after therapy. Bleomycin results in both short- and long-term lung toxicity with impaired diffusion capacity and restrictive lung disease. RT can also produce breast hypoplasia and contribute to the pulmonary fibrosis. Hypothyroidism, hyperthyroidism, as well as benign and malignant thyroid nodules have been recognized as problems occurring in long-term survivors of HL. Sterility/infertility is a significant risk of alkylating agents, most commonly cyclophosphamide and/or procarbazine. The risk of second malignancies is significantly increased in the long-term survivors of HL treated with full-dose RT. The Late Effects Study Group estimated the 30-year cumulative incidence of SC to be 26.3% among survivors diagnosed before age 16. The 2 most frequent cancers are breast cancer (20% risk at 45 years of age) followed by thyroid carcinoma (36-fold increased rate). It is thought that modern IFRT should lead to lower second malignancy rates.

## NON-HODGKIN LYMPHOMA

NHL is a varied group of tumors with almost 60 unique subtypes based on morphologic, immunophenotypic, and genetic differences as well as clinical behavior (Table 95-2). A detailed review of all the different types of NHL is beyond

| TABLE 95-2 | World Health Organisation (WHO) and Clinical Classification of Selected Subtypes of Non-Hodgkin Lymphoma | | |
|---|---|---|---|
| | **Clinical Behavior** | | |
| **WHO Pathologic Category** | **Indolent** | **Aggressive** | **Highly Aggressive** |
| Mature B-cell neoplasms | Follicular lymphoma | Diffuse large B-cell lymphoma, NOS | The Burkitt lymphoma |
| | Chronic lymphocytic leukemia/small lymphocytic lymphoma | Primary mediastinal large B-cell lymphoma | |
| | Hairy cell leukemia | Mantle cell lymphoma | |
| | Extranodal marginal zone lymphoma | | |
| | Lymphoplasmacytic lymphoma/ Waldenstrom macroglobulinemia | | |
| | Splenic B-cell marginal zone lymphoma | | |
| Mature T-cell and NK-cell neoplasms | Mycosis fungoides | Hepatosplenic T-cell lymphoma | |
| | Szary syndrome | Peripheral T-cell lymphoma, NOS | |
| | | Angioimmunoblastic T-cell lymphoma | |
| | | Anaplastic large cell lymphoma, ALK+ type | |
| | | Anaplastic large cell lymphoma, ALK-type | |

ALK, anaplastic lymphoma kinase; NK, natural killer; NOS, not otherwise specified; WHO, World Health Organisation.

*Note:* Adapted from Jaffe E, Harris NL, Stein H, et al. Introduction and overview of the classification of lymphoid neoplasms. In: Swerdlow SH, Campo E, Harris NL, et al. eds. *WHO Classification of Tumours of Haematopoietic and Lymphoid Tissues.* Lyon: IARC; 2008:158–166.

the scope of this chapter. The most common subtypes of NHL accounting for 90% of cases found in children are presented.

NHL can be roughly divided based on the cell of origin (B-cell or T-cell) or on clinical behavior (indolent, aggressive, or highly aggressive). The most common NHL in children and adolescents are precursor B- and T-lymphoblastic lymphoma, anaplastic large cell lymphoma, and Burkitt lymphoma. Indolent lymphomas are slowly progressive but incurable diseases, with a median survival time of 8 to 10 years. Aggressive lymphomas, such as the Burkitt and Burkitt-like lymphomas, are rapidly progressive at presentation, but curable in 70% to 90% of patients.

## Incidence Epidemiology and Classification

NHL accounts for 7% of cancer in children and adolescents with an incidence of 10 per 1 million populations annually in the United States. NHL is rare in children less than 5 but increases dramatically after age 20. NHL is more common in males (1.1–1.4 to 1) with a higher frequency in whites than blacks or Asians. Certain NHL types cluster according to race, for example the natural killer (NK) T-cell lymphomas are most frequently encountered in Asian populations. A family history of a hematologic malignancy produces an increased risk, but it is not NHL-disease specific.

DNA and RNA viruses are thought to be critical triggers in the pathogenesis of NHL. The Epstein–Barr virus (EBV) is the most well-known trigger. EBV was first detected in cultured African Burkitt lymphoma (BL) cells and is known to be present in over 90% of such cases. EBV is important as an initiator for lymphoproliferations/lymphomas occurring in congenital immunodeficiencies, immunosuppressed organ transplant recipients, patients receiving maintenance chemotherapy, and patients receiving combined immunosuppressive therapy for collagen disorders. Other viruses involved in the pathogenesis of NHL include the retrovirus human lymphotropic virus type 1 (HTLV-1) and human herpes virus 8 (HHV-8). Bacterial overgrowth can also promote the occurrence of a lymphoma. In gastric lymphoma of mucosa-associated lymphoid tissue (MALT) type, *Helicobacter pylori* infection has been shown to be necessary for the development and early proliferation of the lymphoma.

NHLs in children are typically high grade. Ninety percent are from 3 main groups. These are: (1) mature B cell NHL which includes BL, Burkitt-like lymphoma (BLL) or diffuse large B-cell lymphoma (DLBCL); (2) lymphoblastic lymphoma (LL) or (3) anaplastic large T-cell lymphoma (ALCL). The other 10% are similar to types seen in adults such as MALT and mature T-cell natural killer (NK) cell lymphoma (Table 95-2). NHL subtypes have different cell lineages and cell cycle kinetics with different propensity to invade the BM and central nervous system (CNS).

## Clinical Presentation and Staging and Surgery

NHL must be considered in any child with lymphadenopathy. Most children with B cell lymphoma present with either abdominal symptoms such as a mass, pain, intussusception, bleeding, ascites, or a bowel perforation or may present with respiratory symptoms from a mediastinal tumor. As with HL the presence of mediastinal disease must be assessed

(Fig. 95-5). Superior vena cava syndrome, respiratory distress, and pleural effusions are more common in patients with NHL. In these cases immediate treatment with corticosteroids with or without cyclophosphamide or radiation may be required. The fear in these cases is that the treatment will make it difficult to establish the pathologic diagnosis. Alternatively, there is some thought that treatment for up to 48 hours is beneficial and unlikely to obscure subsequent pathologic diagnosis. Children with NHL tend to present with advanced stage disease including BM involvement and malignant pleural or pericardial effusions. Pleural fluid and pericardial fluid often require drainage and cytologic examination of the fluid can be diagnostic. Patients may also present with B symptoms (see Hodgkin section).

## Staging

Although no staging system is entirely satisfactory, the most widely used staging system for NHL is the St Jude Murphy system (Table 95-3). The Children's Oncology Group divides NHL into 2 categories: limited and extensive. Limited disease corresponds to stages I and II in the St. Jude system, and extensive correlates with stages III and IV.

## Surgery

Staging laparotomy is also not needed anymore for NHL because all patients receive systemic chemotherapy. There are 2 main reasons a surgeon will encounter a patient with NHL. The first is an incisional or excisional biopsy for diagnosis. Tissue is required to identify the biological subgroups. Specimens must be sent fresh for routine histology, cytology, immunopathology, cytogenetics using fluorescence *in situ* hybridization (FISH—looking for chromosomal translocation), polymerase chain reaction (PCR), and growth patterns. Small, easily resectable lesions can be excised in total and in a rare situation will not require further therapy but resection

| TABLE 95-3 | The St. Jude Murphy Staging System for Non Hodgkin Lymphoma |
|---|---|
| Stage | Description |
| I | A single extranodal tumor or single anatomic nodal area with exclusion of mediastinum and abdomen. |
| II | A single extranodal tumor with regional nodal involvement ≥2 involved nodal regions or localized involvement of extranodal disease on the same side of diaphragm.<br>A primary gastrointestinal tract tumor that is completely resected. |
| III | ≥2 nodal or extranodal tumors on opposite sides of the diaphragm.<br>Any primary intrathoracic tumor.<br>Unresectable primary intra-abdominal disease.<br>Any paraspinal or epidural disease. |
| IV | Involvement of central nervous system and/or bone marrow. |

of big retroperitoneal or mediastinal masses contraindicated. For example, in Burkitt lymphoma, the prognosis is dependent on the extent of disease rather than on completeness of surgical resection. Alternatively, the surgical committee of the Children's Cancer Group (CCG) evaluated the role of surgical therapy in 68 patients with non-Hodgkin lymphoma in the CCG-551 study. Tumor burden was the most important prognostic factor. However, in disease that can be completely resected it may improve EFS and prevent complications such as bowel perforation. In the setting of localized disease data do support a role for complete resection. The second reason a surgeon may encounter is a child with NHL results from abdominal complications such as intussusception or bleeding, perforation or obstruction.

## B Cell Tumors

The subtypes of NHL are determined by the stage of differentiation at which malignant transformation occurs. B cells originate in the BM and through many intermediate cell types to eventually become antibody-producing plasma cells. Malignant transformation can occur at any point along the path of differentiation.

## THE BURKITT LYMPHOMA, BURKITT-LIKE LYMPHOMA (BL, BLL)

BL and BLL account for about 40% of childhood NHL. It was first described in Uganda in 1958. There are 3 variants of BL; endemic, sporadic and immunodeficiency related. In the United States, BL most frequently occurs in the abdomen. BL can also be found in the CNS and BM. BL is characterized by a distinct c-myc gene rearrangement. In 80% of the translocations this involves the locus at 14q32, in 15% of cases it is 2p11, and in 5% it is 22q11. BL is the most rapidly growing tumor in children, with a doubling time of approximately 24 hours. The apoptosis rate is also substantial which contributes to a characteristic low power microscopic "starry sky" appearance thought to be secondary to dead cells being taken up by pale histiocytes (Fig. 95-7). BL cells are mature B-cells

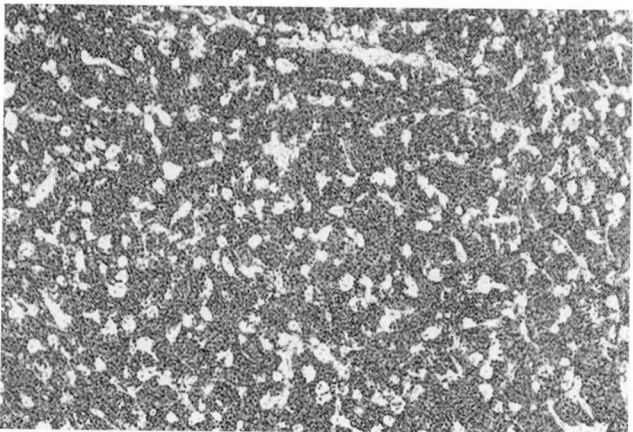

**FIGURE 95-7** Hematoxylin and eosin stained slide of a patient with Burkitt Lymphoma demonstrating the "starry sky" appearance.

that are positive for CD19, CD20, CD22, and CD79a, and have a monotypic surface IgM. BLL is an aggressive highly proliferative variant with features that overlap classical BL and DLBCL. BLL is treated on BL regimens. The distinction between BL and BLL is often difficult and controversial.

## DIFFUSE LARGE B-CELL LYMPHOMA (DLBCL)

DLBCL accounts for 10% of pediatric lymphomas. It is more frequent in adolescents. DLBCL is derived from transformed mature B cells of the peripheral lymphoid organs. DLBCL tumors are characterized by larges cells often 4 to 5 times bigger than small lymphocytes. About 20% of pediatric DLBCL present as a mediastinal mass, but the tumors can occur anywhere. Symptoms are based on tumor location and the presence of an enlarging mass. Increased LDH, pleura effusions, and ascites are less frequently observed than in other NHL. The BM and the CNS are rarely involved. The tumors do express c-myc like BL as well as genes from the NF kappa-beta pathway, but there is no specific marker of DLBCL or a specific genetic signature in children. The tumors express CD19, CD20, CD22, and CD79a. Gene expression profiling has identified 2 subtypes Germinal Center B-cell like (GC) and Activated B-cell (ABC). The most common subtype, GC, has a more favorable outcome.

## T CELL TUMORS

### Lymphoblastic Lymphoma (LL)

LL makes up approximately 30% of childhood NHL. In pediatric patients with LL, 75% will have T-cell immunophenotype. The remaining LL patients have a precursor B-cell phenotype more commonly presenting as disease localized in skin and bone. Whether the LL is a T cell or B cell does not affect prognosis. LL tumors have a precursor lymphoblast phenotype (TdT [terminal deoxynucleotidyl] positive) and express T-cell markers, including CD7 or CD5. T cell rearrangements are common as well as several cytogenetic and molecular changes. Because T development begins in the thymus, it is not surprising that 50% to 70% of patients with T cell LL present with an intrathoracic tumor. Pleural effusions are common, superior vena cava syndrome and airway compression can occur. Abdominal involvement is uncommon and, when observed, usually includes hepatosplenomegaly and BM infiltration. This makes LL difficult to distinguish it from acute lymphoblastic leukemia (ALL). There is some thought that LL is ALL in an extra medullary site. In these cases, survival may be better after treatment with a lymphoblastic leukemia-type regimen.

### Anaplastic Large T Cell Lymphoma (ALCL)

ALCL is a mature T cell cancer and accounts for 10% of NHL in children. Clinically, ALCL has a broad range of presentations, including involvement of lymph nodes and a variety of extranodal sites, particularly skin and bone. ALCL is often associated with "B" symptoms and a nonspecific set of symptoms that come and go and a broad range of presentations including skin and bone. This often complicates and often delays diagnosis.

ALCL are characterized by large cells with a big cytoplasm and horseshoe or kidney shaped nuclei called hallmark cells. Ninety percent of ALCL cases are CD30-positive (Ki- antigen) and have the translocation t(2;5) (p23;q35). This results in production of a fusion protein NPM/ALK. ALCL is classified into systemic (ALK + and ALK −) and Cutaneous lymphomas. ALK + prognosis is good with an 80% OS survival. ALK− is predominantly found in adults with a poorer prognosis OS 45%. The cutaneous form is extremely rare in children and only accounts for 1.7% of ALCL. Its OS is 90%.

## POSTTRANSPLANT LYMPHOPROLIFERATIVE DISORDERS (PTLD)

The risk of PTLD in following solid organ transplantation (SOT) corresponds to the intensity and exposure to immunosuppression. The lowest frequency is reported in renal transplant recipients (1%) and the highest in heart–lung or liver–bowel allografts (5%). EBV seronegativity at time of transplant and young age are the 2 greatest risk factors for subsequent PTLD. In children, PTLD may occur early because of their risk for a primary EBV infection. PTLD can be an EBV-induced monoclonal or, more rarely, polyclonal B-cell or T-cell proliferation as a consequence of immune suppression. The diagnosis can be difficult and patients tend to present with nonspecific findings such as episodic and unexplained fever, weight loss, fatigue. The tumors can occur both within and outside the allograph, including, lymphoid tissue, GI tract, lung, and liver. Involvement of the GI tract may present with vomiting, diarrhea, bleeding, intussusception, or obstruction. Perforation may occur at presentation or immediately following initiation of therapy secondary to transmural necrosis.

## TREATMENT AND OUTCOMES

### Chemotherapy for NHL

Chemotherapy is the primary treatment modality. Each regimen is divided into phases of induction, consolidation, re-intensification, and maintenance. There are 3 core treatment regimens for NHL in children. These are; LSA2-L$_2$ (cyclophosphamide, vincristine, methotrexate, daunorubicin, prednisone, cytarabine, thioguanine, asparaginase, carmustine, hydroxyurea) regimen, and the COMP (cyclophosphamide, Oncovin [vincristine], methotrexate, prednisone) regimen. The third is the Berlin–Frankfurt–Münster (BFM). This is a similar regimen to LSA$_2$-L$_2$. The main difference is the earlier application of L-Asp and high-dose methotrexate (MTX) in the BFM regimen. Despite the different disease processes, stages, and stratification, most treatment regimens are based on one of the 3 regimens above with adjustment made for stage, histology, and phases of therapy. For example, LBL protocols are a continual exposure to cytostatic agents over a long period of time; BL/BLL and DLBCL are treated with rapid repeated short, dose-intense chemotherapy courses. ALCL has a completely different strategy. Although these regimens are effective, they are toxic even with use of granulocyte colony-stimulating factor (G-CSF) as up to 3% can die from treatment complications. One particular threat is acute tumor cell lysis syndrome (ATLS). Depending on the size of the tumor, the acute lysis of many tumor cells places a tremendous metabolic load on the kidneys, composed of phosphates, potassium, purines, and protein. Patients may present with elevated serum uric acid, lactate, and potassium levels. This syndrome may be further aggravated during the initial massive cell lysis caused by chemotherapy. ATLS can result in hyperuricemic nephropathy and renal shutdown.

### Radiation Therapy

Radiation therapy has been shown to add toxicity with limited therapeutic benefit in NHL in stage I disease. Radiation is used for CNS disease with limited effects and is controversial.

### BL and BLL and DLBCL

Most BL and BLL regimens are derived from the LSA$_2$-L$_2$ or BFM regimens with the use of methotrexate (MTX) for CNS disease. Patients with localized resected tumors have nearly 100% EFS with 2 5-day therapy courses. Recent trials report OS rates of 98%, 90%, and 86% in stage I/II, III, and IV disease, respectively. DCLC also has excellent outcomes when treated on BL and BLL protocols with EFS reaching 97%.

### Lymphoblastic Lymphoma (LL)

EFS for children with LL ranges from 60% to 90% with lower stages reaching 90%. Most current treatments are based on the LSA$_2$-L$_2$ protocol or the BFM group strategy. The main differences between the protocols are earlier application of L-Asp and high-dose MTX in the BFM regimen. Treatment intensity is stratified according to stages I and II versus stages III and IV. Children with stage I/II are rare and achieve EFS rates higher than 90% with reduced-intensity (omission of re-intensification in the BFM protocol) and full-length maintenance therapy. Most relapses occur early. A current COG study is looking at the benefit of high-dose MTX with added cyclophosphamide and anthracycline during induction with the regimen from the BFM-95. The study is still open and accruing patients.

### Anaplastic Large Cell Lymphoma

ALCL uses different treatment for local and systemic disease. Patients with localized disease show the best results with pulsed multiagent chemotherapy similar to the regimen used in mature B-cell NHL reporting OS of 93%. Children and adolescents with disseminated ALCL have a poorer survival of 60% to 75%. It is unclear which strategy is best for the treatment of disseminated ALCL. COG is testing the replacement of vincristine with vinblastine in the maintenance phase of the APO regimen (doxorubicin, vincristine, and prednisone).

## TOXICITES

The long-term toxicity profile for patients with NHL is very similar to HL. Acutely, the NHL regimens, due to their intensity tend to be more toxic.

## SELECTED READINGS

Bhatia S, Yasui Y, Robison LL, et al. High risk of subsequent neoplasms continues with extended follow-up of childhood Hodgkin's disease: Report from the Late Effects Study Group. *J Clin Oncol* 2003;21:4386–4394.

Burkitt D. A sarcoma involving the jaws in African children. *Br J Surg* 1958; 46:218–223.

Cader FZ, Kearns P, Young L, Murray P, Vockerodt M. The contribution of the Epstein-Barr virus to the pathogenesis of childhood lymphomas. *Cancer Treatment Rev* 2010;36:348–353.

Donaldson SS, Link MP. Combined modality treatment with low-dose radiation and MOPP chemotherapy for children with Hodgkin's disease. *J Clin Oncol* 1987;5:742–749.

Ehrlich PF, Friedman DL, Schwartz CL. Monitoring diagnostic accuracy and complications. A report from the Children's Oncology Group Hodgkin lymphoma study. *J Pediatr Surg* 2007;42:788–791.

Fredd J, Kelly K. Current approach to the management of Pediatric Hodgkin Lymphoma. *Pediatr Drug* 2010;12:85–98.

Harris NL, Jaffe ES, Diebold J, et al. World Health Organization classification of neoplastic diseases of the hematopoietic and lymphoid tissues: report of the Clinical Advisory Committee meeting—Airlie House, Virginia, November 1997. *J Clin Oncol* 1999;17:3835–3849.

La Quaglia MP, Stolar CJ, Krailo MD, et al. The role of surgery in abdominal non-Hodgkin's lymphoma: Experience from the Children's Cancer Study Group. *J Pediatr Surg* 1992;27:230–235.

Lister TA, Crowther D, Sutucliffe SB, et al. Report of a committee convened to discuss the evaluation and staging of patients with Hodgkin's disease: Cotswolds meeting. *J Clin Oncol* 1989;7:1630–1636.

Meyers Pa, Potter VP, Wollner N, Exelby P. Bowel perforation during initial treatment for childhood non-Hodgkin's lymphoma. *Cancer* 1985; 56:259–261.

Nachman J, Sposto R, Herzog G, et al. Randomized comparison of low-dose involved field radiation after complete remission in Hodgkins disease who achieve a complete response to chemotherapy. *J Clin Oncol* 2002; 20:1500–1507.

Punnett A, Tsang RW, Hodgson DC. Hodgkin lymphoma across the age spectrum: epidemiology, therapy, and late effects. *Sem Rad Oncol* 2010; 20:30–44.

Reddy KS, Perkins SL. Advances in the diagnostic approach to childhood lymphoblastic malignant neoplasms. *Am J Clin Pathol* 2004;122:S3–S18.

Reiter A. Diagnosis and treatment of childhood non-Hodgkin lymphoma. *Hematology* 2007;1:285–296.

Schellong G, Potter R, Bramswig J, et al. High cure rates and reduced long-term toxicity in pediatric Hodgkin's disease: the German Reiter Austrian multicenter trial DAL-HD-90. The German-AustrianPediatric Hodgkin's Disease Study Group. *J Clin Oncol* 2010;17:3736–3744.

Schwartz CL, Constaine LS, Villaluna D, et al. A risk adapted, response based approach using APVE-PC for children and adolescents with intermediate and high risk Hodgkin's lymphoma: the results of P9425. *Blood* 2009;114:2051–2059.

Shamberger RC, Weinstein HJ. The role of surgery in abdominal Burkitt's lymphoma. *J Pediatr Surg* 1992;2:236–240.

Swerdlow SH, Webber SA, Chadburn A, et al. Post-transplant lymphoproliferative disorders. In Swerdlow SH, Campo E, Harris NL, eds. *WHO Classification of Tumours of Haematopoietic and Lymphoid Tissues.* Lyon: IARC; 2008:343–351.

Travis LB, Hill D, Dores GM, et al. Cumulative absolute breast cancer risk for young women treated for Hodgkin lymphoma. *J Natl Cancer Inst* 2005;97:1428–1437.

# Pigmented Lesions and Melanoma

# CHAPTER 96

*Brian S. Pan and David A. Billmire*

## KEY POINTS

1. Ninety-eight percent of Caucasian children have at least 1 nevus by early childhood. In contrast, melanoma accounts for only 2% of all pediatric malignancies.

2. Physical features that may raise suspicion for malignant transformation include **a**symmetry, irregularity of the **b**orders, variability in the **c**olor, and **d**iameter greater than 5 mm (ABCD criteria).

3. A Spitz nevus in its typical form is a benign melanocytic lesion that is a diagnostic and management challenge for both pathologists and clinicians secondary to the histologic features it can potentially share with melanoma.

4. The nevus sebaceous of Jadassohn is a benign epidermal nevus most commonly encountered on the scalp and face with a reported incidence of basal cell carcinoma of 0.8%.

5. Giant congenital nevi carry a lifetime malignancy risk ranging from 2.8 to 8.5% and 60% of these malignancies occurred within the first decade of life.

6. Melanomas less than 1-mm thick should be excised with a 1-cm margin while for those greater than 1 mm in thickness, a 2-cm margin is acceptable.

7. Surgical treatment options for large pigmented lesions include serial excision, skin grafting, and tissue expansion.

## INTRODUCTION

The frequency of pigmented lesions in childhood as well as the rising incidence of melanoma in adults has raised awareness of screening for cutaneous malignancy. These concerns, however, are not completely justified in the pediatric population. Melanocytic nevi are highly prevalent amongst Caucasian children, with over 98% possessing at least 1 nevus by early childhood. In contrast, melanoma accounts for only 2% of all pediatric malignancies. Further, cutaneous melanoma prior to puberty is extremely rare with only a 0.3% to 0.4% incidence in the United States. Due to these factors and the cumulative risk of malignant transformation in adulthood, a working knowledge of the clinical spectrum of the most common pediatric pigmented lesions, their natural history, risk of malignant transformation, and treatment options is important to possess.

## PATHOPHYSIOLOGY

A nevus is a benign skin lesion defined by its sharply circumscribed borders. The differential diagnosis of these pigmented lesions is based on the lesion's gross morphologic characteristics, the patient history, and microscopic examination. In general, a nevus' characteristics are derived from its cell line of origin and include melanocytic nevi (derived from melanocytes), epidermal nevi (derived from keratinocytes), connective tissue nevi (derived from fibroblasts and other connective tissue cellular elements), and vascular nevi (derived from vascular elements). With the exception of the nevus sebaceous of Jadassohn, an epidermal nevus, the focus of this chapter will be directed towards melanocytic nevi. Melanocytic nevi are composed of melanocytes whose embryologic origins are from the neural crest. The tan to black coloring of melanocytic nevi is the product of enzymatic reactions within the endoplasmic reticulum that convert tyrosine to melanin. This pigment is then packaged into melanosomes and in normal melanocytes, released from their dendritic processes to evenly color the skin.

Melanocytic nevi arise when melanocytes lose their dendritic processes (with the exception of blue nevi) and aggregate into nests of cells at the dermal–epidermal junction. Melanocytic nevi can be further stratified based upon their histological location in the skin. Junctional nevi are believed to represent an early developmental stage in the natural history of a nevus, positioned along the dermal–epidermal junction where native melanocytes are typically found. As the name implies, the nevus cells of intradermal nevi are confined within the dermis, deep to the epidermis. The transitional entity between the junctional and intradermal nevus is the compound nevus subsiding within both the epidermis and dermis. Clinically, as the melanocytes composing the nevus migrate deeper into the dermis, the lesion will become more papular (elevated) and less pigmented. Unfortunately,

| TABLE 96-1 | Characteristics of Acquired Nevi, Atypical Nevi, Melanoma | | |
|---|---|---|---|
| Characteristics | Acquired Melanocytic Nevus | Atypical Melanocytic Nevus | Melanoma |
| A—Asymmetry | Symmetrical | Mildly asymmetrical | Asymmetrical |
| B—Border | Regular, well demarcated | Mildly irregular | Irregular, ill-defined |
| C—Color | Regular, homogenous | Variegated | Variegated |
| D—Diameter | <1 cm (generally <5 mm) | <1 cm (generally 5-10 mm) | <1 cm (generally >6 mm) |
| E—Evolution | Stable | Stable | Unstable, changes with time |

the sequence of molecular events that cause melanocytes to undergo malignant transformation to malignant melanoma remains poorly understood.

## ACQUIRED MELANOCYTIC NEVUS

Acquired melanocytic nevi or acquired moles are extremely common during childhood, appearing after 6 months of life and increasing in number throughout childhood and adolescence. They arise as tan to dark brown, flattened macules that can become more elevated, assuming the form of a papule. Typically with a diameter less than a centimeter, acquired nevi are benign, characteristically round, symmetrical, and sharply demarcated with an evenly pigmented surface (Table 96-1). The environment and a genetic preponderance both contribute to the development of these lesions. Intense, intermittent sun exposure from an outdoor lifestyle increases the incidence of nevi in exposed, unprotected areas. In addition, individuals with lightly pigmented complexions tend to develop more acquired nevi than more heavily pigmented individuals. Although acquired melanocytic nevi are benign, clinical signs suggestive of malignant transformation to melanoma should be monitored for and if encountered, prompt a biopsy.

## ATYPICAL MELANOCYTIC NEVUS

Atypical melanocytic nevi are essentially benign, acquired melanocytic nevi that possess physical features that may raise suspicion for malignant transformation. Asymmetry, irregularity of the borders, variability in the color and a diameter greater than 5 mm (ABCD criteria) are clinical features consistent with melanoma that atypical nevi can possess without the histologic changes diagnostic of melanoma (Table 96-1). These lesions initially arise during puberty and continue to develop throughout life, especially in sun-exposed areas. With both environmental and genetic factors contributing to their development, these lesions have a prevalence ranging from 2% to 10% in Caucasians. The environmental factors contributing to the development of acquired nevi are similar to those responsible for atypical nevi with the number of atypical nevi rising in proportion to the total number of acquired nevi. Germline mutations in CDK2NA, CDK4, CMM1, and other genetic factors have also been shown to play a role in the development of atypical nevi and melanoma.

FAMM syndrome (Familial atypical mole and melanoma) is associated with these germline mutations and as the name indicates, an increased risk for the development of melanoma. The criteria for FAMM syndrome include the occurrence of malignant melanoma in 1 or more first- or second-degree relative, the presence of multiple melanocytic nevi (including atypical nevi), and melanocytic nevi demonstrating histologic atypia. Given the clinical similarities between atypical nevi and melanoma, routine surveillance is critical in patients with multiple atypical nevi. An excisional biopsy of atypical nevi should also be performed as an initial diagnostic measure in patients with new lesions.

## SPITZ NEVUS

A Spitz nevus in its typical form is a benign melanocytic lesion that is a diagnostic and management challenge for both pathologists and clinicians secondary to the histologic features it can potentially share with melanoma. For this reason, it has also been referred to as juvenile melanoma, benign melanoma, and an epithelioid or spindle cell nevus. These nevocellular lesions most commonly occur in the head and neck region of children and young adults, with two-thirds presenting in fair-skinned individuals less than 20 years of age. In its typical form, Spitz nevi appear as small (less than 1 cm in diameter), symmetric, dome-shaped, pink papules due to their relative lack of melanin; however, variants occur with darker hues ranging from tan to black (Fig. 96-1). These variations in presentation and

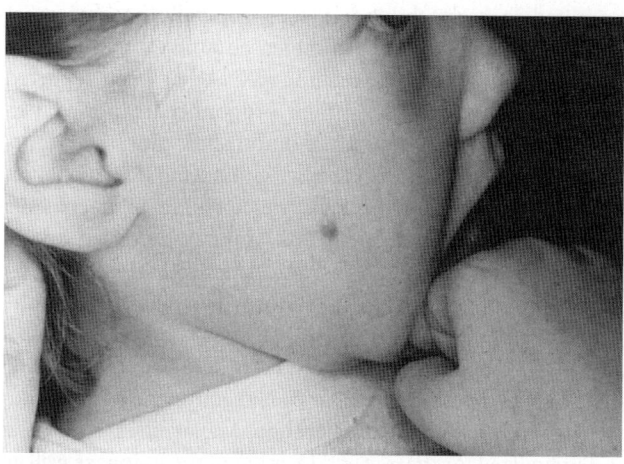

**FIGURE 96-1** Two-year-old child with a typical Spitz nevus.

1271

clinical history often lead to misdiagnosis where the lesion is initially believed to be a pyogenic granuloma, hemangioma, dermatofibroma, or verruca vulgaris.

The histologic hallmark of a Spitz nevus is the presence of compound, uniformly organized, large or spindle-shaped melanocytes arranged in nests. Although distinguishing between a Spitz nevus and melanoma is straightforward in its classic presentation, an accurate diagnosis can become problematic when the lesion in question becomes less characteristic. For these reasons, the majority of clinicians recommend a full-thickness excisional biopsy with 1 to 2 mm margins.

Owing to documented cases of metastasis and death, atypical Spitz nevi are treated with the same oncologic excisional principles as melanoma to avoid under-treatment. The use of sentinel lymph node biopsy for atypical lesions remains controversial given a high incidence of positive biopsies, the questionable significance of a positive result, and the overall excellent prognosis in these patients.

## HALO NEVUS

Halo nevi are benign melanocytic lesions that develop a circumferential inflammatory infiltrate peripherally, resulting in a zone of depigmentation. Commonly referred to as Sutton nevi or leukoderma acquisita centrifugum, these lesions tend to arise during adolescence and can spontaneously involute. While not all halo nevi undergo involution, this feature is attributed to a poorly understood autoimmune mechanism involving elements of both the humoral and cell-mediated immune system. This process is not unique to halo nevi, having also been observed with congenital melanocytic nevi (CMN), giant CMN, and Spitz nevi. Observational management is appropriate unless the central pigmented area demonstrates signs of atypia, prompting a biopsy of the lesion.

## BECKER NEVUS

Becker melanosis or a Becker nevus is identified by the presence of its characteristic hair growth within an irregularly bordered hyperpigmented macule. While Becker nevi can be noted in early childhood, they generally become most apparent during puberty. An increased number of androgen receptors and androgen receptor mRNA has been reported in these lesions, explaining their pronounced expression in males. Multiple developmental anomalies can be concurrently expressed with Becker nevi, prompting its description as a syndrome. The musculoskeletal (spina bifida, pectus excavatum, sciolosis), cutaneous (supernumerary nipples, accessory scrotum), and breast anomalies (breast hypoplasia) that can occur, tend to be regionally associated with the location of the nevus.

While Becker nevi are generally considered benign melanocytic lesions, routine surveillance is recommended given the potential for malignant degeneration. Management should be individualized for the size and location of the lesion, as well as for any associated deformity.

## BLUE NEVUS

The common blue nevus presents as an acquired, papular, bluish-black solitary lesion less than 1 cm in diameter. It is most often encountered on the dorsum of either the hands or feet. The cellular blue nevus, another subtype of blue nevi, tends to be slightly larger in diameter and presents commonly in the scalp or near the sacrum as an elevated plaque. Cellular blue nevi can be either congenital or acquired unlike the common blue nevus. Histologically, blue nevi are benign nests of melanocytes that have retained their dendritic processes unlike other melanocytic nevi. The bluish hue of these nevi is attributed to the Tyndall effect in which melanin preferentially absorbs longer wavelengths of light, scattering the shorter wavelengths (representing the blue portion of the spectrum). The coloration of the nevus of Ota and Mongolian spots can also be attributed to the Tyndall effect. Although generally confined to the dermis, these lesions can extend deeper into the subcutaneous tissue and even into bone. As previously stated, blue nevi are benign lesions; however, changes in the cutaneous behavior of these lesions or evidence of aggressive local extension should prompt surgical intervention.

## NEVUS OF OTA AND ITO

The nevus of Ota is a benign dermal melanocytic hamartoma with an increased incidence in patients of Asian descent ranging from 0.014% to 0.034%. Interestingly, a bimodal distribution in the presentation of this lesion seems to exist, with 48% developing in the perinatal period and 36% developing during adolescence. With a predilection for the female sex, the nevus of Ota generally presents as a unilateral, bluish-gray macule within the distribution of the first and second branches of the trigeminal nerve. Concomitant involvement of the tympanic membrane, oral and nasal mucosa is common, however, ophthalmologic complications have been reported with the highest frequency. In one study, glaucoma was reported with a frequency of 10.3%.

The nevus of Ito is also a benign dermal melanocytic hamartoma, similar to the nevus of Ota except for its area of distribution. This lesion typically presents in the posterior supraclavicular and lateral cutaneous brachial nerve distributions, involving the neck, scapular, and shoulder regions. The incidence of the nevus of Ito is unknown, however, it too occurs more commonly in people of Asian descent.

Although the nevus of Ota and Ito are generally considered a benign lesions, dermatologic surveillance is warranted given the risk for malignant degeneration to melanoma.

## NEVUS SPILUS (SPECKLED LENTIGINOUS NEVUS)

Nevus spilus, also commonly referred to as speckled lentiginous nevus, is a compound nevus clinically recognized by its characteristic light brown background staining with darker macules and papules superimposed within the lesion. The background staining is usually recognized around the time of birth, suggesting that the lesion is perhaps related to CMN. Macules and papules that arise within this background can vary within the spectrum of pigmented melanocytic lesions, ranging from lentigines, nevi, Spitz nevi, and blue nevi. Similar to CMN, these lesions present with a frequency between 2% and 3% and warrant observation given the risk of malignant transformation to melanoma. If an area within the nevus appears suspicious, an excisional biopsy should be performed down to the level of the fascia given the potential extension of nevus cells into deeper subcutaneous planes.

## NEVUS SEBACEOUS OF JADASSOHN

The nevus sebaceous of Jadassohn is a benign epidermal nevus most commonly encountered on the scalp and face. This lesion is usually recognized soon after birth, presenting as a verrucous, riveted plaque of varying shapes with a yellowish hue (Fig. 96-2). It is theorized that postzygotic mutations lead to mosaicism in pluripotent stem cells, resulting in the formation of these hamartomas with epidermal, follicular, sebaceous, and apocrine elements. The natural history of nevus sebaceous of Jadassohn involves several stages of development ultimately leading to secondary benign and malignant neoplastic changes (Table 96-2). However, a review of the literature suggests that malignant transformation of these lesions is much less than previously thought, with a reported incidence of basal cell carcinoma of 0.8%. Multiple large case series have demonstrated an absence of malignant degeneration in children under the age of 16, with reported cases of basal cell and sebaceous carcinoma in older adults. The data suggest that observation is an acceptable alternative to early excision with the caveat that the risk of malignant transformation increases with age and surveillance can be complicated as the lesion evolves.

## CONGENITAL MELANOCYTIC NEVUS

CMN are classically defined as benign nevomelanocytic proliferations that are present at birth. Nevi arising between 1 month and 2 years of age are termed tardive nevi and are

| TABLE 96-2 | Tumors Associated with Nevus Sebaceous of Jadassohn |
|---|---|
| **Tumors** | |
| Syringocystadenoma papilliferum | |
| Trichoblastoma | |
| Trichilemmoma | |
| Sebaceoma | |
| Nevocellular nevus | |
| Keratoacanthoma | |
| Seborrheic keratosis | |
| Viral Warts | |
| Basal cell carcinoma | |

clinically and histologically indistinguishable from CMN. These lesions have an estimated frequency between 1 and 6% according to several large clinical series, with an increased incidence in individuals with darker pigmentation.

Presenting as round, well-demarcated lesions with tan to black coloring, CMN can theoretically be differentiated from common acquired nevi histologically and by their clinical history (Fig. 96-3). Histologically, CMN demonstrate nevocellular elements infiltrating the deeper layers of the dermis, subcutaneous tissues, and skin appendages which is not universally true in smaller lesions. Growing in near direct proportion to its regional location, these lesions can become variegated and change in pigmentation as the child grows. Several classification schemes exist for categorizing these nevi and although arbitrary, the most commonly employed method is according to size. Small nevi (less than 1.5 cm in diameter) and intermediate-sized nevi (1.5-19.9 cm in diameter) are generally grouped together while giant CMN (greater than 20 cm in diameter) are considered separately secondary to their association with melanoma, neurocutaneous melanosis, and the complexity of their treatment.

While the association between giant congenital nevi and melanoma is well established, the precise risk of malignant transformation in smaller nevi is controversial. The report by Rhodes et al is frequently cited in the literature, estimating a 2.6% to 4.9% cumulative risk for malignant transformation

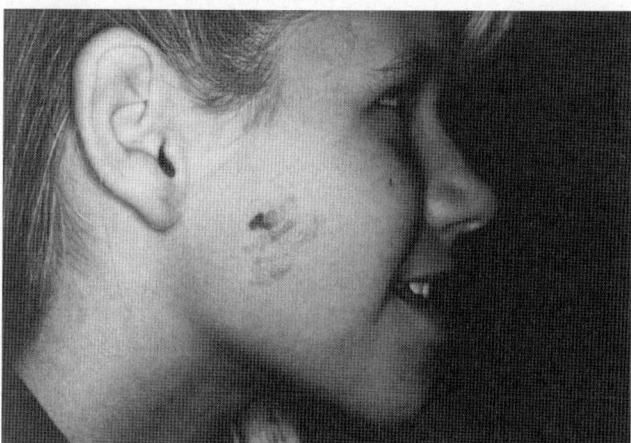

**FIGURE 96-2** Nevus Sebaceous of Jadassohn.

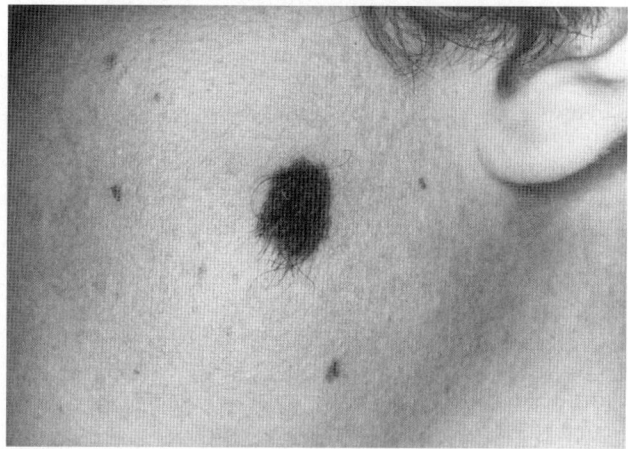

**FIGURE 96-3** Congenital melanocytic nevus.

to melanoma in patients by the age of 60. When malignant transformation does occur, it tends to present around the onset of puberty in contrast to the earlier presentation of melanoma in giant CMN. Thus routine surveillance and patient/parent examination is advised unless the lesion exhibits signs and symptoms of malignant transformation, prompting an excisional biopsy.

## GIANT CONGENITAL MELANOCYTIC NEVUS

Giant CMN are rare disfiguring melanocytic lesions with a reported incidence of 1 in 20,000 births. Giant congenital nevi possess histologic characteristics nearly identical to CMN that differentiate them from acquired nevi. However, it is the extent of their subcutaneous and cutaneous involvement that

distinguishes them from congenital nevi. Unlike congenital nevi, giant congenital nevi can extend beyond the subcutaneous tissues, with nevus cells infiltrating into fascia, muscle, as well as extracutaneous regions such as the gastrointestinal tract, the retroperitoneum, and the leptomeninges. The involvement of these extracutaneous structures is secondary to the path of migration of melanoblasts from their embryologic origins at the neural crest.

While multiple criteria have been proposed, a congenital nevus is defined as "giant" if it measures greater than 20 cm in diameter or is predicted to be greater than 20 cm in diameter by adulthood. For example, a 6-cm lesion on the body of an infant corresponds to a 20-cm lesion in an adult. Giant congenital nevi most commonly present in the distribution of the trunk (Fig. 96-4) followed by the extremities, head, and neck. Visible at the time of birth, the entire extent of the lesion may not be readily apparent as the pigmentation and character of the nevus change with time. Over the course of the lesion's

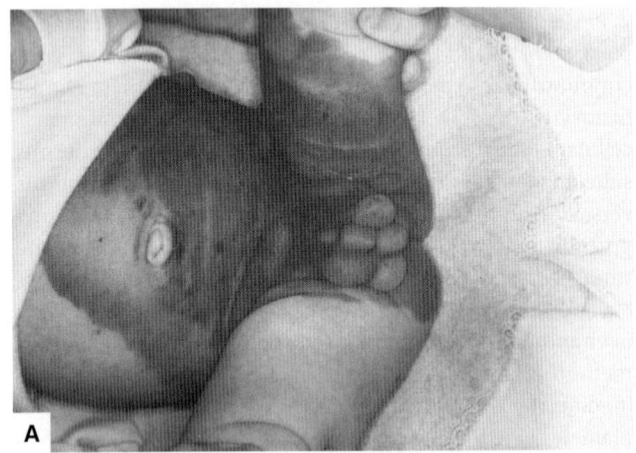
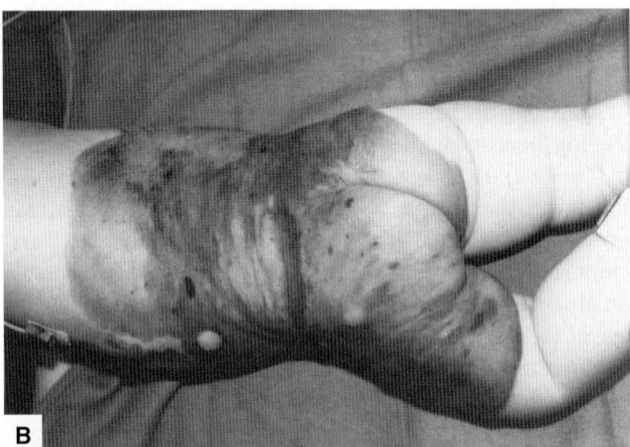
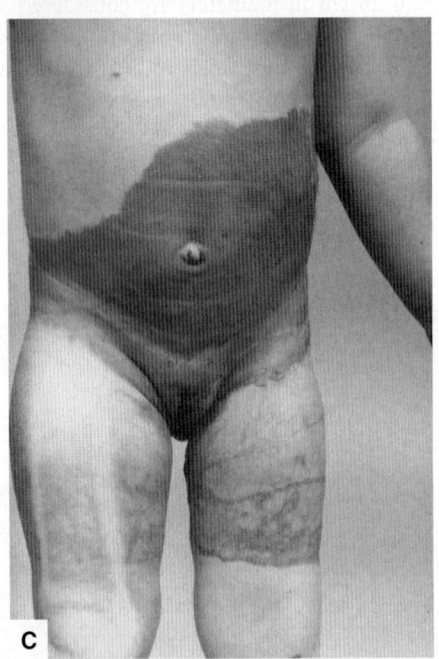
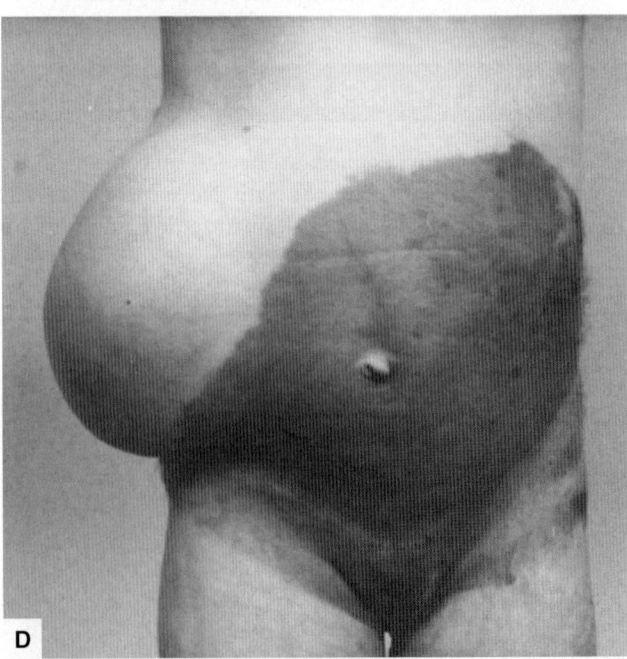

**FIGURE 96-4** Female infant with a bathing trunk distribution giant congenital melanocytic nevus. **A.** Perineal view of the nevus demonstrating a neural component of the nevus in the labia. **B.** Dorsal thorax and gluteal distribution of the nevi with neural components. **C.** Postoperative view after excision of anterior abdominal wall and labial neural nevi and left thigh resurfacing with a split thickness skin graft. **D,E.** Expansion of the flank and trunk. **F-H.** Postoperative view after tissue expander removal, nevus excision, and flap advancement.

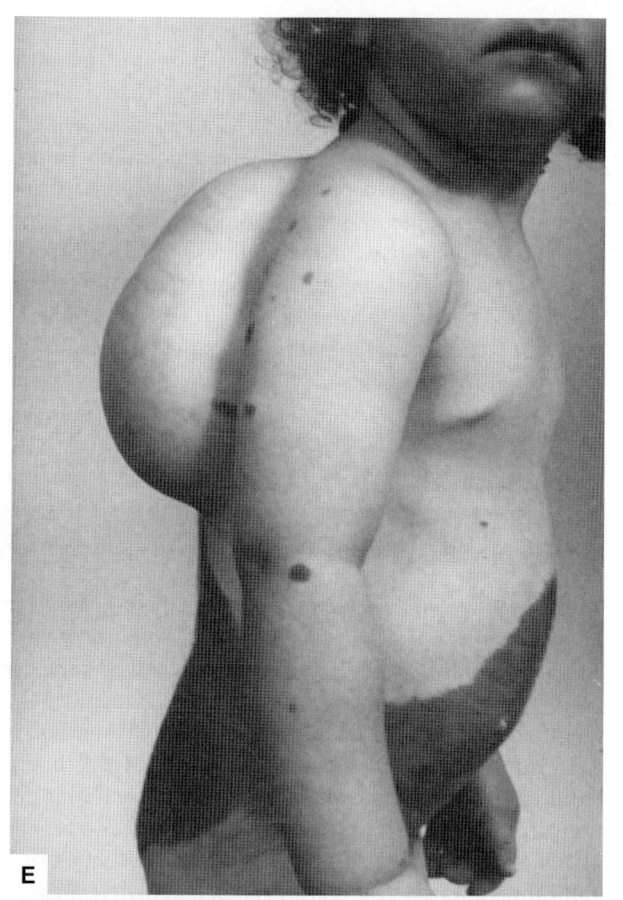

E

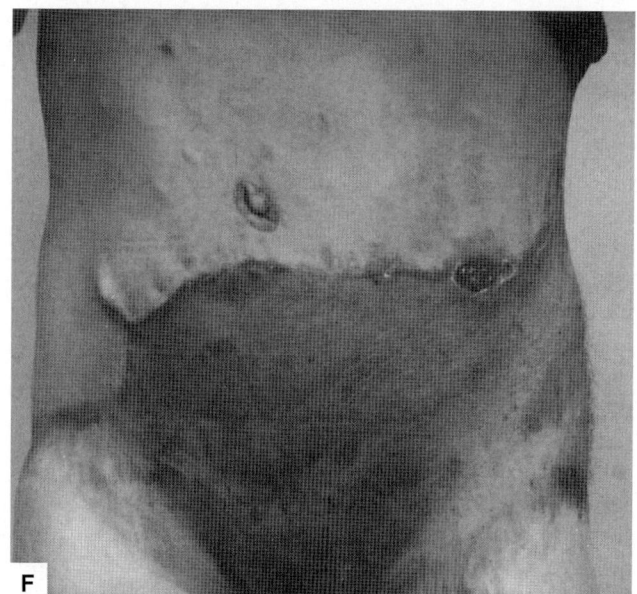

F

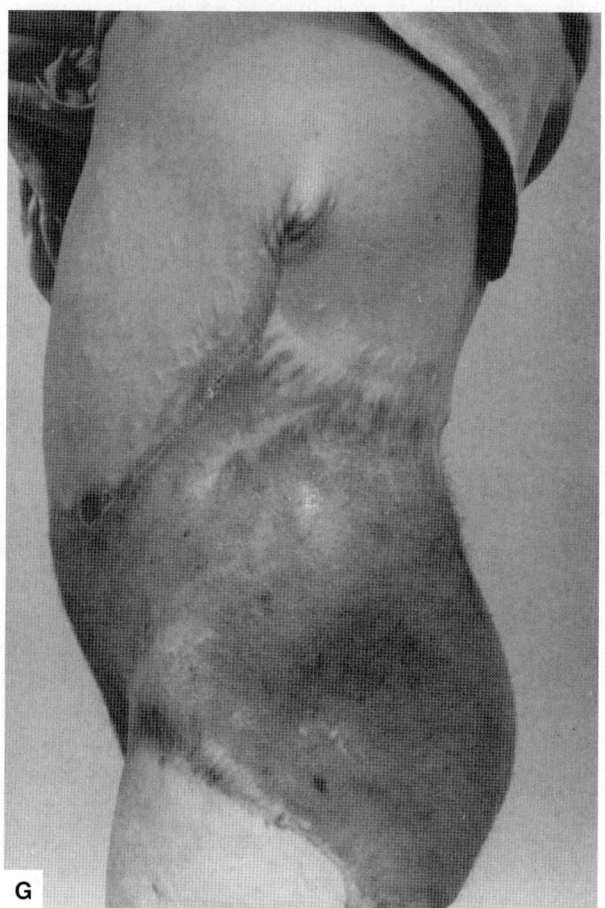

G

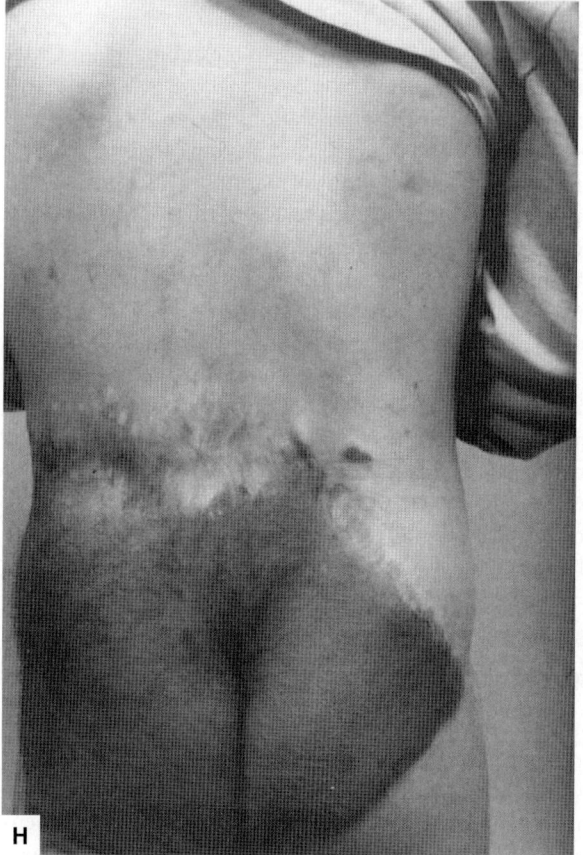

H

**FIGURE 96-4** *(Continued)*

natural history, it may become hyperpigmented, develop hypertrichosis and satellite lesions can become more apparent. Giant congenital nevi will also expand in direct proportion to their regional location.

Observation is imperative to monitor for signs and symptoms of either malignant transformation to melanoma or neurocutaneous melanosis in patients with giant congenital nevi. Ulceration, tenderness, itching, pain, or bleeding should prompt a biopsy of the area to rule out malignant transformation. Unfortunately, monitoring for extracutaneous malignancies is challenging given the potential for involvement of the gastrointestinal tract, the retroperitoneum, and leptomeningeal structures.

The exact risk of malignant transformation to melanoma is difficult to define because of the variable definitions for a "giant" congenital nevus in the literature, the low incidence of these nevi, and the effects of reporting bias. Recent reports have suggested a lifetime risk ranging from 2.8% to 8.5%. Supporting the rationale for early surgical intervention, a study by Kaplan found that 60% of these malignancies occurred within the first decade of life.

In addition to the increased risk of melanoma, giant CMN are associated with neurocutaneous melanosis. These extracutaneous melanocytic proliferations reside in the central nervous system and may remain asymptomatic, manifest secondary to malignant transformation, or as a neurologic complication. A more detailed review of this topic will be discussed in the next section.

The management of giant CMN is a controversial subject given the uncertain malignant potential of the lesion, the possibility of extracutaneous malignancies despite cutaneous extirpation, and the inability to completely excise the infiltrating subcutaneous elements of the nevus. However, early surgical intervention is generally recommended as a means of prophylaxis against local malignant transformation as well as for the favorable surgical properties of an infant's skin. Unfortunately, despite significant reconstructive efforts, the aesthetic outcome can be as unfavorable as the lesion itself.

## NEUROCUTANEOUS MELANOSIS

Neurocutaneous melanosis is a rare syndrome defined by the presence of melanocytic proliferations in the central nervous system in association with giant CMN, multiple satellite lesions, or 3 or more smaller congenital nevi. These leptomeningeal deposits of melanocytes result from the same neuroectodermal embryologic migration errors responsible for CMN. The physical presence of these proliferations is benign and asymptomatic unless malignant transformation occurs or if their presence leads to malfunction of the normal leptomeningeal architecture. The mass effect of these lesions can cause hydrocephalus and its sequelae, cranial nerve palsies, developmental delay, and seizures. The presentation of this syndrome has a bimodal distribution, first around 2 years of age and then later between the second and third decade of life.

Symptomatic neurocutaneous melanosis is fortunately rare, with an estimated incidence of 4% in patients with nevi that are of high-risk for the development of this syndrome; however, when symptoms do occur, the prognosis is poor with death occurring within 2 to 3 years. Screening is advocated in patients with high-risk nevi, defined as those with giant CMN with satellite lesions, patients with greater than 3 medium-sized CMN, and especially when these lesions are midline over the posterior axis. If possible, a gadolinium-enhanced MRI of the brain and spine should be obtained prior to 6 months of age before myelination of the brain masks the presence of melanosis. If detected, asymptomatic patients with neurocutaneous melanosis should be serially examined and imaged not only to monitor for the development of melanoma but to prevent potential neurologic morbidity from undetected hydrocephalus. Symptomatic patients should be referred for management of their underlying symptoms and the sequelae of these lesions.

## MELANOMA

While the incidence of melanoma in adults has significantly increased in the last 30 years with a lifetime occurrence in 1 of 58 individuals, childhood cases are relatively rare. Melanoma accounts for only 2% of all pediatric malignancies and the incidence prior to puberty is between 0.3% and 0.4% in the United States. Secondary to its low incidence in childhood, and prior diagnostic difficulties differentiating melanoma from Spitz nevi, the true natural history and prognosis of this malignancy is still being clarified. Recent European clinical reviews suggest that in general, pediatric melanoma behaves similarly to melanoma in adults, with comparable 5-year survival rates (79% vs 77%), histologic features (the most common type is superficial spreading), and overall mortality (10%).

Malignant melanoma is classified histologically into 4 major subtypes: superficial spreading, nodular, lentigo maligna, and acral lentiginous melanoma (listed from the most common subtype to the least common). In the pediatric population, it is further subdivided into conditions unique to this age group. These 6 categories include: transplacental melanoma, malignant degeneration from giant CMN, melanoma arising secondary to predisposing conditions (xeroderma pigmentosa, FAMM syndrome, albinism, immunosupression), malignant transformation from normal skin, and finally from preexisting lesions.

Commentary on several of these categories is warranted. Transplacental melanoma is exceedingly rare and is the result of malignant seeding of the fetus from the mother. The prognosis unfortunately is invariably poor given the extent of dissemination of the disease at the time of discovery. As previously mentioned, the estimated lifetime risk of melanoma arising from a giant congenital nevi ranges from 2.8% to 8.5%. Screening for melanoma in these patients is complicated and the disease is often advanced at the time of diagnosis. Melanoma arising deep within the subcutaneous extent of giant nevi complicates clinical detection as well as the irregular, variegated surface of the lesion itself. These factors coupled with high incidence of melanoma prior to 3 years of age support the rationale for early surgical intervention.

Irrespective of the patient's age or preexisting conditions, any report of a pigmented lesion undergoing rapid physical change should invoke suspicion for malignant transformation. The classic clinical signs that should raise suspicion include the ABCDE checklist: asymmetry, borders that are ill-defined, color variegation, diameter >0.6 cm, and evolution of lesion's characteristics (Table 96-1). In addition to these clinical signs, bleeding or ulceration should prompt an excisional biopsy. The lymph node basin draining the confines of the lesions should also be examined for evidence of adenopathy.

## TREATMENT

Multiple factors must be considered when counseling the patient and/or parent about the treatment options for pigmented lesions. The variables to be considered include the age of the patient at their initial presentation, the risk of malignant degeneration of the lesion, the physical and psychological stress of the lesion for the patient and the corrective surgery. Many aspects regarding the treatment options remain controversial including the timing of intervention and the appropriateness of the technique for the particular lesion.

Regardless of the diagnosis, a general principle of evaluation for pigmented lesions is the acquisition of a full thickness biopsy. Excisional biopsies should be performed by obtaining a 1 to 2 mm margin of nonaffected skin with a depth at the level of the subcutaneous tissue surrounding the lesion. Minimally invasive techniques such as shave biopsies, curettage, dermabrasion, chemical peels, and laser ablation are not recommended for diagnostic purposes, as they do not allow for full histologic evaluation. Further, if these techniques are employed, they are no-extirpative, potentially leaving behind residual cells which in certain lesions can undergo malignant degeneration.

## SMALL NEVI

Small-pigmented lesions that are amenable to primary closure are most appropriately excised in an elliptical fashion parallel to the Langer lines. Alternatively, lesions can be excised in a circular fashion and converted to a straight-line closure by excising the remaining dog-ears. This technique can be useful in aesthetically sensitive areas such as the face to decrease the length of the scar that is often overestimated with elliptical designs. In situations where the long axis of the nevus is not parallel to the Langer lines, the axis of the nevus should be used to design the orientation of the excision. Excess soft tissues are otherwise needlessly sacrificed if this consideration is not incorporated into the design. In addition to design, closure of the skin edges under minimal tension after undermining the subcutaneous plane adjacent to the incisions can aid in decreasing the morbidity of the resulting scar.

In general, small lesions without evidence of malignant transformation can be observed until the child's cooperation can be elicited to undergo the procedure under local anesthesia. Clearly, if the lesion appears suspicious or develops worrisome features prior to this ideal time, an excisional biopsy should be obtained under general anesthesia.

## MODERATE, LARGE, AND GIANT NEVI

Early surgical consultation is imperative for pigmented lesions that cannot be closed in a primary fashion. In ideal circumstances, the family is educated about the surgical risks, potential benefits, and the available procedures for their child soon after birth. The complexity of the surgical options, potential morbidity, and possible need for multiple procedures can make these discussions difficult for the family, and their expectations whenever they opt for an intervention must be managed appropriately.

As previously stated, early consultation and operative intervention is ideal when managing larger lesions for several reasons. First, the risk of malignant transformation to melanoma for giant CMN is greatest during the first decade of life with over 50% occurring before 3 years of age. Secondly, the elasticity of the skin in younger children, especially infants can allow for fewer procedures and more aggressive single-stage excisions (Fig. 96-5). Finally, the psychological benefits of operating prior to entering school, coupled with the ability to tolerate multiple operations or tissue expansion, further strengthen the argument for early intervention. The current armamentarium in the treatment of large pigmented lesions includes serial excisions, skin grafting, and tissue expansion. Autologous free tissue transfer and other flap reconstruction techniques are also available in select cases yet their description is outside the scope of this chapter.

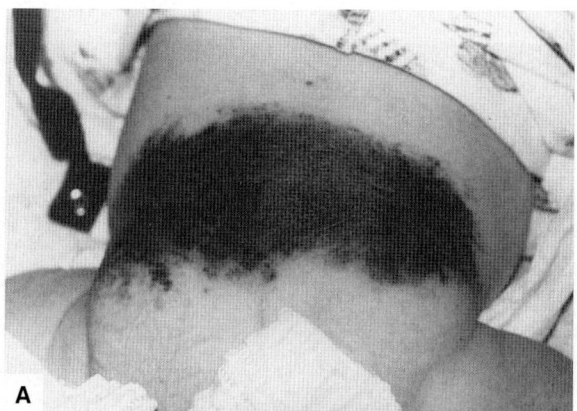

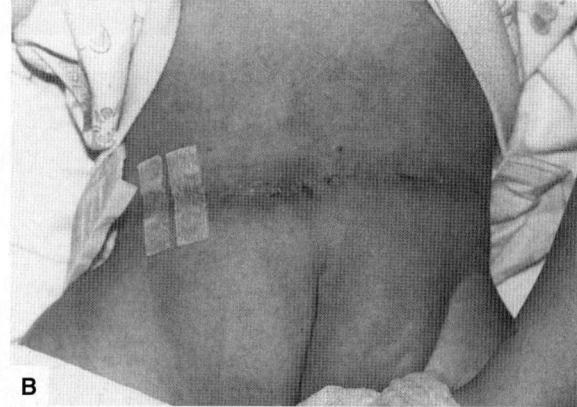

**FIGURE 96-5** **A.** Large congenital melanocytic nevus involving the dorsal thorax in a 6-week-old infant. **B.** Postoperative view after a single stage excision in an outpatient setting.

Serial excision is a relatively straightforward, reliable technique that is best reserved for lesions that can be addressed 2 stages or less. The recommended interval between stages is generally between 3 and 12 months to allow for adequate healing and relaxation of the adjacent tissues to permit another operation. The simplicity of this technique is its primary advantage and it is particularly useful for patients and families who cannot tolerate the psychosocial stress of undergoing tissue expansion. The potential for scar spread and hypertrophy is certainly a risk given that incisions are closed under some tension; however, it does obviate the need for multiple visits and the potential complications associated with tissue expansion.

The utilization of skin grafts is another reliable technique for reconstructing the deficit left after the excision of large lesions. The primary advantage of skin grafting is the ability to resurface large areas in a single stage. The aesthetic results are further enhanced with the use of nonmeshed split-thickness grafts and full-thickness grafts taken from strategic donor sites to obtain an acceptable color match. Unfortunately, the morbidity associated with skin graft based reconstructions limits its utility. With the exception of full thickness grafts, the donor site can be extensive, leaving another wound not exempt from potential healing and scarring problems. In addition, skin grafts applied to fascial excisions are significantly disfiguring unless the lesion is merely resurfaced. As previously mentioned, resurfacing techniques leave behind residual nevus cells with the potential for malignant degeneration. For these reasons and the availability of other techniques, the widespread use of skin grafts is limited.

Tissue expansion provides versatility that techniques based upon serial excision or skin grafting fail to offer. Its application should be advocated if 3 or more stages are anticipated to complete a reconstruction. The primary advantage of this technique is its ability to increase the availability of soft tissue with properties that are identical to the normal adjacent tissue. Thus, the skin color, texture, and in the scalp, hair can be incorporated into the reconstruction. For these reasons, tissue expansion is an ideal technique for large pigmented lesions in the scalp (Fig. 96-6) and trunk (Fig. 96-4). For particularly large lesions, multiple expansions can be performed including the previously expanded flap. In most circumstances, the expansion process is undertaken in an outpatient setting over the course of 3 months with weekly office visits. It is our practice to overinflate the expander beyond the manufacturer's guidelines and to proceed with expansion until the time of removal. Despite these advantages, tissue expansion is not without its drawbacks and potential complications. The complication rates reported in the literature range from 13% to 20% that include reports of pain with expansion, seroma formation, hematoma, infection, and flap loss.

The most critical practical consideration is the ability of the family and the patient to cooperate throughout the expansion process. This includes multiple office visits and the psychosocial stress for the patient and the family associated with having an implanted expander. Additionally, tissue expansion has not been universally successful in all anatomic locations. Corcoran, Kryger, and Bauer have reported the successful use of tissue expansion of the extremities in association with

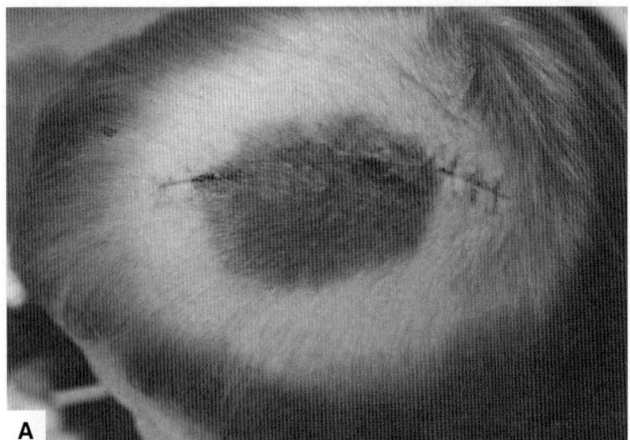

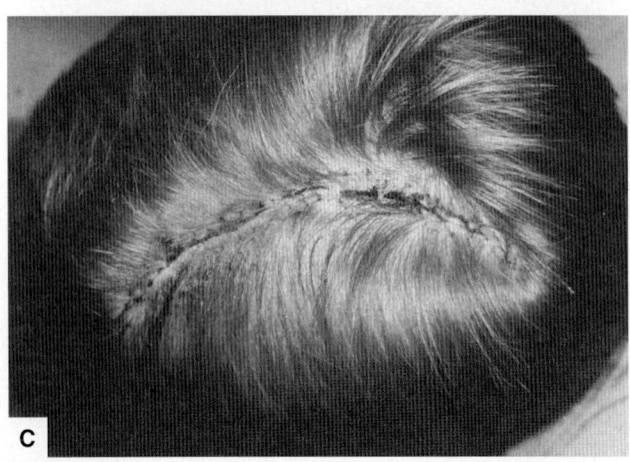

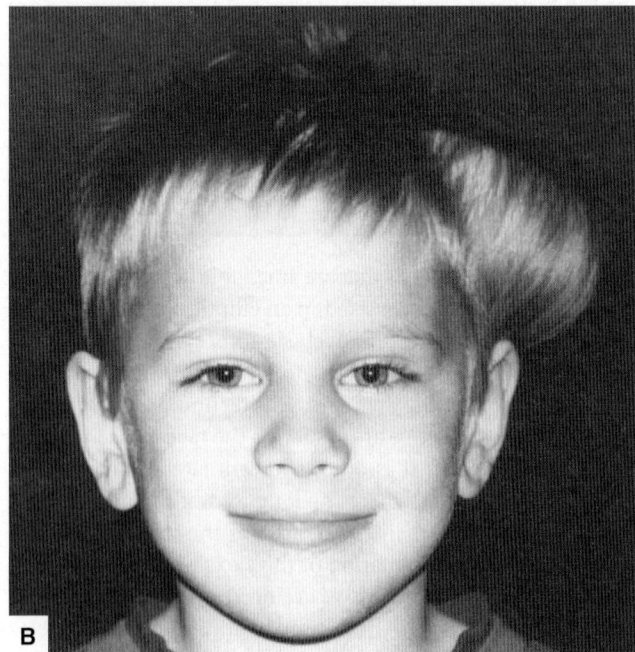

**FIGURE 96-6 A.** Initial result after a planned staged excision of a moderately sized congenital melanocytic nevus. **B.** Postoperative view after placement and subsequent expansion of a scalp expander. **C.** Following removal of scalp expander, excision of nevus and flap advancement.

transposition flaps, free flaps and full thickness skin grafts. It has been our experience that the use of tissue expanders in the extremities is limited. The ability to recruit adjacent tissue, the potential for compartment syndrome and high complication rates has changed our approach in the extremity to subcutaneous excision and skin grafting (Fig. 96-4B,C).

The scalp is another anatomic site that warrants special consideration before undergoing expansion. Approximately 50% of the scalp can be reconstructed with tissue expansion without significantly thinning the hair. This technique should be used with caution; however, in younger children given the thinning of the calvarium that can occur with expansion. In a clinical series by Bauer, and in our experience, there has been no evidence of permanent calvarial deformity, nor any detrimental effects to open cranial sutures after expansion. Remodeling of thinned calvarium and areas of deformation at the site of the inflated expander generally occurs within 3 to 4 months.

## MELANOMA

In the initial evaluation of suspected melanoma, a full-thickness excisional biopsy of the lesion including a narrow margin of normal skin excised at the level of the subcutaneous tissue should be obtained. We recommend that the specimen be reviewed by an experienced pediatric dermatopathologist to avoid confusion with Spitz nevi and its atypical variants. Upon confirmation of the diagnosis, 3 therapeutic issues require consideration: re-excision of the primary site, management of regional lymph nodes, and the use of systemic therapy.

## MANAGEMENT OF THE PRIMARY SITE

Following the initial excisional biopsy, the primary site requires re-excision with wider circumferential margins based on the depth of invasion. Multiple trials analyzing the local recurrence rates in patients randomized to narrow versus wider margins suggest that narrower margins are sufficient. Extrapolated from this data, the following margins are recommended: 0.5 to 1 cm margin for melanoma in situ is sufficient. Melanomas less than 1 mm thick should be excised with a 1-cm margin. For lesions greater than 1 mm in thickness, margins ranging from 1.5 to 3 cm have traditionally been recommended; however, a 2-cm margin is acceptable.

## MANAGEMENT OF REGIONAL LYMPH NODES

The development and refinement of lymphoscintigraphy and sentinel lymph node biopsy for staging melanoma and determining management of regional lymph nodes have been critical in the treatment of this disease, especially in adult patients. Its application for the pediatric population has also gained acceptance. Current indications for performing sentinel lymph node biopsy include melanomas greater than 1 mm in thickness or thinner melanomas displaying more aggressive behavior. In large adult series, sentinel node status has proven to be the most important prognostic factor predicting both locoregional recurrence and survival. In the Gershenwald multicenter series, negative sentinel lymph node status was associated with a 60% increase in 3-year disease free survival for stage I and II cutaneous melanoma. Although sentinel lymph node biopsy has become a useful tool in determining these factors as well aiding in the decision whether to perform regional lymphadenectomy, its effect on overall survival has yet to be determined.

## ADJUVANT THERAPY

Systemic adjuvant therapy for patients with biopsy-proven spread to regional lymph nodes is still under investigation. Multiple chemotherapeutic regimens, radiation therapy, non-specific immunotherapy, and biologic therapy used in adult trials have been applied to pediatric melanoma without demonstrating any survival benefit. Evidence from several large clinical trials investigating interferon alfa-2b, the only FDA approved adjuvant therapy, demonstrate improved relapse-free survival yet only a moderate improvement in overall survival. Smaller pediatric trials have also been conducted; however, the significance of the data is limited by small patient populations. Despite this supporting evidence, the benefits of interferon therapy must be weighed against the systemic side effects and potential toxicity which include myelosuppresion and hepatotoxicity. At this time, aggressive screening, early detection, and surgical excision prior to regional or systemic spread remain the most successful management tools.

## SELECTED READINGS

Arneja JS, Gosain AK. Giant congenital melanocytic nevi. *Plast Reconstr Surg* 2009;124(1 Suppl):1e–13e.

Bittencourt FV, Marghoob AA, Kopf AW, et al. Large congenital melanocytic nevi and the risk for development of malignant melanoma and neurocutaneous melanocytosis. *Pediatrics* 2000;106(4):736–741.

Corcoran J, Bauer BS. Management of large melanocytic nevi in the extremities. *J Craniofac Surg* 2005;16(5):877–885.

Cribier B, Scrivener Y, Grosshans E. Tumors arising in nevus sebaceous: a study of 596 cases. *J Am Acad Dermatol* 2000;42(1):263–268.

Downard CD, Rapkin LB, Gow KW. Melanoma in children and adolescents. *Surg Onc* 2007;16(3):215–220.

Huynh PM, Grant-Kels JM, Grin CM. Childhood melanoma: update and treatment. *Int J Dermatol* 2005;44(9):715–723.

Lyon VB. The spitz nevus: review and update. *Clin Plast Surg* 2010;37(1):21–33.

Schaffer JV. Pigmented lesions in children: when to worry. *Curr Opin Pediatr* 2007;19(4):430–440.

Watt AJ, Kotsis SV, Chung KC. Risk of melanoma arising in large congenital melanocytic nevi: A systematic review. *Plast Reconstr Surg* 2004;113(7):1968–1974.

# PART XI

# CHAPTER 97

# Immunology and Transplantation

*Sara K. Rasmussen and Paul M. Colombani*

## KEY POINTS

1. Though nonspecific host defenses are somewhat deficient in the infant and pediatric patient, the effector arm of the specific immunologic response to alloantigens of clinical organ transplants is intact at the time of birth.

2. Effective organ allograft immunosuppression requires a balance of prevention of rejection of the graft while avoiding the toxicity of excessive immunosuppressing agents.

3. Immunosuppressive agents can be categorized into those used for induction (rabbit anti-thymocyte globulin, corticosteroids), those for maintenance (mycophenolate mofetil, tacrolimus), and those used to treat acute rejection (corticosteroids).

## INTRODUCTION

Infections are a leading cause of pediatric morbidity and mortality, particularly in the neonatal period. Explanations for this phenomenon include a lack of previous antigenic experience on the part of pediatric patients; an intrinsic immaturity of lymphocyte functions in this age group; and, for neonates, an active cellular suppression mechanism. In addition, several specific inherited defects of the immune system may manifest themselves in early infancy and continue to plague these patients through childhood and on into adulthood. Acquired defects in the immune defenses occur in transplantation and oncology patients. This chapter will review the specific and nonspecific components of the immune system with particular reference to the pediatric patient's ability to fight infection (see also Chapter 13—"Surgical Infection: Classification, Diagnosis, Treatment and Prevention"). Emphasis will be placed on the differences in these responses in neonates and children compared to the responses in adult subjects. The ability of children to mount an immune response against alloantigens in the transplantation setting will be discussed. In addition, this chapter will review current methods of clinical immunosuppression for the pediatric age group.

## COMPONENTS OF THE IMMUNE SYSTEM

Immune responses are generally divided into specific and nonspecific components. Each of these components is further subdivided into humoral and cellular compartments (Table 97-1).

### Nonspecific (Nonimmune) Host Defenses

#### Humoral Components

The humoral components of nonspecific host defense systems include the classic complement pathway and the alternate, or properdin, pathway. The complement cascade is made up of 9 serum proteins which are activated during the inflammatory response. The proteins react with immunoglobulins (Ig)—IgM or IgG—and antigen. Activated complement (C′) liberates mediators of the inflammatory response, and the levels of the C3/C5 component correlate with susceptibility to infection. The C3 level determines the rate of phagocytosis or lysis of invading organisms. In the presence of immunoglobulins, the C142 component (the membrane attack complex) activates C3, the binding of immunoglobulins, and eventual opsonization of the organism by the phagocytic system. Complement is detectable at 1% of adult levels at 5 weeks of gestation. By 26 to 28 weeks of gestation there is a rapid increase in complement levels in the serum of the fetus. By term, complement levels are 30% to 50% of adult levels. Complement levels in term infants are subnormal in approximately 50% of neonates, but the mean level of activation may approach 70% to 90% of adult activity following activation.

The properdin or alternate pathway also appears early in gestation during the first trimester. By term, this activity is 30% to 60% of adult levels and is therefore more suppressed in neonates than the levels of proteins in the complement cascade. Quantitatively, preterm infants have a lower level of properdin. Opsonizing activity by the properdin pathway is determined by factor B levels, and because these levels are lower in term and preterm infants overall, opsonizing activity is limited.

| TABLE 97-1 | Summary of Immune System Components |
|---|---|

Nonspecific immunity
    Humoral components
        Complement pathway
        Properdin pathway
    Cellular components
        Polymorphonucleocytes
        Monocytes/macrophages
        Reticuloendothelial system

Specific immunity
    Humoral components
        Immunoglobulins: IgM, IgG, IgA, IgE, IgD
    Cellular components
        B cells
        T cells
            T helper
            T cytotoxic
            T suppressor
            Natural killer

## Cellular Components of the Nonspecific System

The cellular components of nonspecific host defense include polymorphonucleocytes (PMN), monocytes, macrophages, and the modified macrophages of the reticular endothelial system (RES). In response to chemotactic factors, PMN migrate to areas of infection. There is a clear deficiency in chemotaxis because of the decreased elasticity of neonatal PMN, which are also responsible for killing bacteria after phagocytosis. The phagocytic ability of these cells is probably normal at birth, but in vitro assays of phagocytosis are diminished in the cells of term and preterm infants compared to adult cells. The addition of adult serum to these neonatal cells normalizes their activity, which suggests that neonates are simply more deficient in opsonizing factors as alluded to above. The result, however, is that the phagocytic ability of these cells is diminished, particularly in stressed infants and children.

Following engulfment and phagocytosis of organisms, PMNs kill these organisms primarily by peroxidation by oxygen-free radicals produced by the cells. Neonatal PMN clearly have a decreased ability to generate oxygen-free radicals for intracellular killing. Also, under stress conditions, even though phagocytosis may be relatively intact, there is decreased intracellular killing.

Migratory macrophages and monocytes are similarly deficient in chemotactic ability and phagocytosis in the neonatal period. Beyond that, macrophage function appears to be normal.

The RES is a system of fixed macrophages or monocytes in a variety of sites including the liver, spleen, and bone marrow. These cells serve to remove particulates from the bloodstream, including viral, bacterial, and fungal organisms. The RES system is intact in both term and preterm infants. This system is able to respond at maximum levels at term, but serum opsonizing factors are required for optimal function.

Important adjunct components of the nonspecific immune system in neonates are the mononuclear phagocytes in maternal milk ingested during breast feeding. These mononuclear cells comprise 80% of the cells found in colostrum and breast milk. On the first day of breast milk production, there are approximately 2 million cells/mL of breast milk. This number of phagocytes declines to approximately 1.3 million cells/mL by approximately 3 months following birth. These activated cells secrete components of complement and possess immunoglobulin Fc receptors and complement receptors. They also contain and may secrete intracellular IgA. They may also be responsible for the phagocytosis and intracellular killing of swallowed organisms with which neonates have had no previous immune experience. In addition, these cells may elaborate and secrete a number of lymphokines which may be important for the development of optimal function of the gut-associated immune responses in infants.

In summary, there are a number of nonspecific, nonimmune components for host defenses that are all qualitatively present in preterm and term infants as well as in children. In general, the humoral components are deficient in quantity which may lead to a decreased level of serum opsonization factor in neonatal and infant blood. Cellular components of this system are highly dependent on these opsonic factors for optimal function. As a result, overall nonspecific host defenses are somewhat deficient in the pediatric age group, particularly in neonates as compared to adults. This deficiency is primarily due to limiting opsonic activity when infants are under stress, as well as other potential deficiencies in chemotaxis and intracellular killing.

## Specific Immune Defenses

Most important in developing specific immunity against infections and mounting an immune response to alloantigens in the transplantation setting are the humoral and cellular components of the immune system.

### Humoral Components

The humoral components of the immune system are primarily the immunoglobulins elaborated by B lymphocytes. In addition to specific immunoglobulin production in response to antigenic stimulus, which is termed active immunity, there is also passive maternally-derived IgG, conferring some immune protection in the first few months of life.

### Passive Humoral Immunity

The principal immunoglobulin conferring passive immunity in the neonatal period is maternally derived IgG. In neonates, the levels of IgG in the serum correlate well with maternal IgG levels. Immunoglobulin G freely crosses the placental barrier and this transfer of immunoglobulin increases with gestational age. The absolute half-life, on a gram percent basis, of maternally derived IgG is approximately 3 to 4 weeks, but specific protective titers of antibody may last up to 12 months. This duration of protective effect depends on the initial levels at birth. The more premature the infant at birth, the shorter the time duration for maternal transfer of IgG and the result is lower levels of maternally derived IgG in the circulation. The advantage of this maternally transferred IgG is that it provides a transfer of specific immunoglobulin protection against tetanus, diphtheria, pertussis, measles, rubella, and varicella, as well as a wide variety of organisms including streptococci, staphylococci, toxoplasmae, and salmonellae (H-type). These protective immunities reflect the circulating immunoglobulins most adults have in their plasma vascular compartment. Unfortunately there is little transfer of protective antibodies for influenza, poliovirus, and shigella, salmonella (O-type), and *Escherichia coli* organisms.

## Active Humoral Immunity

Besides IgG there are 3 principal antibodies in host defenses: IgM, IgA, and IgE. All 4 immunoglobulins are active in newborn and preterm infants and are synthesized in response to a specific antigenic challenge.

Immunoglobulin M is the first component elaborated in response to a specific antigen or infection. It comprises approximately 15% of the immunoglobulin in adults and is the major immunoglobulin elaborated against gram-negative organisms and viruses. There is no placental transfer of IgM, and therefore any IgM present requires *de novo* synthesis by the fetus or infant. Immunoglobulin M is first present at 10 to 15 weeks of gestation, and any level of IgM >20 mg/mL signifies an in utero infection.

Immunoglobulin G, the most prevalent component of the immunoglobulin system, as stated above, is primarily transferred from the maternal circulation. Fetal production of IgG begins in the third trimester; low levels are observed at term, followed by a steady increase in endogenous IgG by 3 to 4 months postpartum. By 24 months of age, infants have achieved normal adult production levels of IgG.

The third immunoglobulin component, IgA, also comprises approximately 10% to 15% of adult immunoglobulins. It is the primary immunoglobulin found in secretions, particularly in the gut. Fetal production of IgA begins at 12 weeks of gestation, and there are very low levels throughout the first 2 years of life. As with IgM, there is no placental transfer of IgA, and elevated levels of IgA also indicate *de novo* synthesis and an in utero infection. In normal term infants at 1 month of age, there are detectable levels of IgA in the circulation. Most children have normal levels of IgA by age 10.

The last humoral component, IgE, is present in infants. As for IgM and IgA, there is no placental transfer, and IgE levels are elevated in skin-sensitizing activity and allergic phenomena.

A very minor component of the humoral immunity is IgD. It is probably purely a marker of immature B cells because it is usually seen early in B-cell development both intracellularly and on the cell surface. With the development of more mature B cells and isotype switching from IgD to IgM, IgG, IgA, or IgE is produced and IgD is no longer expressed.

## Cellular Immune Defenses

The 2 principal specific active components of the cellular immune system are B and T lymphocytes, including natural killer cells.

## B Lymphocytes

B lymphocytes are derived from the bursal equivalent which in humans is most likely the fetal liver and bone marrow.

The first B cells identified are pre-B cells which contain cytoplasmic IgM only. These cells are present in the fetal liver at 8 weeks of gestation and then are found in the bone marrow at later stages of gestation. The first true B cells that have only surface IgM are found at 10 weeks of gestation, and by 10 to 12 weeks cells containing both IgG and IgM on their cell surface are present, indicating isotype switching from IgM to IgG. Beyond 12 weeks of gestation, both IgA- and IgG-only positive cells are present. By 20 weeks of gestation the fetus can develop specific antibody production in response to infection. Development of the full repertoire of B cells is beyond the scope of this chapter, but it is probably complete by term. This generation of cell lines that react to different antigens (clonal diversity or idiotype generation) is required for the full expression of B-cell immune responses and is present at birth.

Antigen modulation, a peculiarity of fetal B cells, allows a specific antigen to bind to the immunoglobulin on the surface of the B cell. This binding causes capping (internalization) of the antigen-immunoglobulin complex, which produces inactivation of that particular cell. Following this inactivation, there is no reexpression of that specific immunoglobulin on future clonally elaborated B cells, providing a possible explanation for the elimination of forbidden autoreactive clones that react to self cells and also for neonatal tolerance. Antigen modulation is very rare in adults and in children. Its failure in pediatric patients was not appreciated in early organ transplantation and led to severe rejection episodes.

## T Lymphocytes

T lymphocytes, which are derived from the thymus (or processed through the thymus), are the effector arm of the cell-mediated immune response. They also provide help for each other and for B cells in differentiating and proliferating through the elaboration of a myriad of cytokines. There are 3 subsets of T lymphocytes: helper, suppressor, and cytotoxic. In addition there is a subset of cytotoxic T cells called natural killer cells, which are nonspecific killer cells. Basically, helper T lymphocytes are primarily responsible for the elaboration of lymphokines which help to induce differentiation and proliferation of other T-cell subsets and B cells. Suppressor T lymphocytes appear to down-regulate immune responses by direct inhibition. Cytotoxic T lymphocytes are stimulated in response to specific antigen activation and are responsible for direct cell cytotoxicity.

The T-cell repertoire is generated and/or matures in the thymus. The thymus gland is derived from the third branchial pouch and is present as early as 6 weeks of gestation. The thymic epithelium is clearly demarcated by 6 weeks of gestation, with the initial invasion of lymphocytes occurring by 8 to 9 weeks of gestation. These lymphocytes have presumably migrated from the fetal liver and bone marrow. By the ninth week of gestation, specific T cells can be identified in the embryonic thymus. And by the 11th week of gestation, these T cells have generated their cell surface markers: CD4 for helper cells and CD8 for cytotoxic and suppressor cells. By 12 to 14 weeks of gestation, the thymus is histologically identical to that in older children and adults. By 15 to 20 weeks of gestation, there are circulating peripheral T cells with mature markers on their cell surface (CD3). T-cells derived either from the thymus or from the circulation of the 18- to 20-week fetus are fully functional T lymphocytes which respond normally to specific antigens as well as to nonspecific mitogenic stimulatory responses.

As a result of this early maturation of T cells, specific cell-mediated immunity is present in term infants. There is an overall decrease in the numbers of T cells in preterm infants who are both small for gestational age and appropriate in size for gestational age. Infants who are small for gestational age, however, may retain decreased proliferative responses up to 12 months after birth.

Of interest is the presence of suppressor cells in the neonatal circulation. These neonatal suppressor cells are probably CD4 suppressors and can cause nonspecific inhibition of the cell-mediated responses of adult T lymphocytes in coculture. There apparently is no *in vivo* or *in vitro* inhibition of neonatal cells. These suppressor cells secrete a soluble suppressor factor which is active only against adult cells (both T and B cells). This suppression is not related to the major histocompatibility complex (MHC) and does not cause direct cytotoxicity. It is possible that these circulating cells prevent any maternal immunocompetent cells that may cross the placenta from causing an immune reaction (rejection) in the growing fetus.

## TRANSPLANTATION IMMUNOLOGY

As stated above, both the specific and nonspecific immune systems of infants and children are intact at birth. Qualitatively, all components of these systems are present and functioning. The numbers of cells that can be recruited to respond to any given antigen whether it is infectious or an alloantigen are, however, somewhat deficient in the pediatric age group. In the transplantation situation, pediatric patients, even in the first few months of life, are capable of mounting an immune response to alloantigens. The vigorousness of this response based on absolute numbers of specific responding cells is somewhat decreased, and the younger the child, the slower the response that may develop.

It is well known that the MHC, made up of both class I and class II antigens, is present on virtually all mammalian cells. The various numbers of class I and II antigens present on any cell within an organ determine its antigenicity and lead to various degrees of reactivity by the transplant recipient toward the specific organ transplanted. This explains the variability in rejection rates seen when different vascularized solid organs are transplanted. Pediatric patients have all the cellular and humoral components needed to mount a response to foreign MHC antigens. In addition, they can mount immune reactions to ABO blood groups as well as to minor tissue-specific antigens. The MHC is divided into 2 groups: class I, the A, B, and C loci; and class II, the D and DR loci. In response to an alloantigen, pediatric recipients mount both a humoral and a cell-mediated response.

The humoral response may take the form of a preformed antibody in the case of ABO incompatibility or when the recipient has previously been sensitized to specific MHC antigens (a previous transplant or a blood transfusion). A preformed antibody provides the basis for clinical hyperacute

rejection. In addition, first-set reactions occur in an alloantigen situation where B lymphocytes are activated by MHC antigens and produce specific antibodies in response to these antigens.

Cell-mediated responses are also restricted by cell type: CD4 helper cells and CD8 cytotoxic T cells. CD4 cells respond only to class II antigens, and CD8 cells respond to class I antigens. The phenomenon of MHC restriction also applies to these alloantigen responses and basically means that foreign class I and class II antigens must be presented to the responding T cells in relationship to self MHC antigens. For practical purposes monocyte/macrophages process foreign MHC antigens and present these antigens to T or B cells along with self MHC. The result is the activation of CD4 cells in response to class II antigens with the release of cytokines which potentiate cell proliferation, maturation of cells, and recruitment of new T cells into the response. These recruited cells include CD8 cytotoxic T cells and CD8 suppressor T cells which respond to self-class I plus antigen. The theory is that suppressor cells are also elaborated in this immune response and begin to downregulate the overall response and modulate the reaction. In addition to these suppressor cells, there are other varieties of regulatory cells that come into play to downgrade both T- and B-cell responses. These include anti-idiotypic antibodies which are elaborated in response to a large production of a particular IgM or IgG antibody. There are also CD8 T cells with specific T-cell receptors that function as autoregulatory cells to downgrade the overall T-cell responses by direct cytotoxicity.

As stated above, all these components of the effector arm of the specific immune response are present at birth and are involved in the response of pediatric patients to alloantigens of the clinical transplantation situation.

### Immunodeficiency

A large number of congenital immunodeficiencies have been described. These clinical entities are usually secondary to point mutations of genes responsible for enzymes or other proteins required for optimal function of the immune system. All components of the immune system can be involved singly for some enzymes or multiply if the proteins affected are critical for common functions of the immune system.

In addition to these inherited or sporadically acquired point mutations immunodeficiency can be acquired after infection with the human immunodeficiency virus.

A detailed description of congenital and acquired immunodeficiency is beyond the scope of this discussion. A summary of the more commonly seen clinical immunodeficiency states appears in Table 97-2.

### Clinical Immunosuppression

Advances in immunosuppressive therapy have led to the remarkable success of clinical organ transplantation over the past 3 decades. As clinical experience with organ transplantation in children grew, it became apparent that these patients required similar, if not greater, immunosuppression and surveillance for rejection than adult transplant recipients. This requirement for active immunosuppression has also led to a

**TABLE 97-2 Common Immunodeficiencies**

| Disorder | Functional Deficiency | Mechanic/Mutation |
|---|---|---|
| Acquired immunodeficiency syndrome | T cell | Human immunodeficiency virus |
| Primary immunodeficiency states | | |
| Cellular/humoral | | |
|     X-linked agammaglobinemia | Antibody | Tyrosine kinase deficiency |
|     Common variable | Antibody | ? |
|     Selective IgA | IgA | ? |
|     DiGeorge syndrome | T cell | Mutation Xp21.1 |
|     Severe combined immunodeficiency including ADA deficiency | T cell/antibody | Proline-rich protein |
|     CD3 deficiency | T cell | CD3 |
|     CD8 deficiency | T cell | ZAP70 |
|     Ataxia telangiectasia | T cell/antibody | Phospholipus 3-like kinase |
| Humoral | | |
|     Complement properdin pathways (all protein deficiencies described); early: C1g, C1r, C1s, C2, C4, C3; late: C5, C6, C7, C8 | Complement cascade | Multiple |
| Phagocytic cells | | |
|     Congenital neutropenia | PMN | ? |
|     Leukocyte adhesion defects (1 and 2) | PMN | CD18/? |
|     Chronic granulomatous disease | PMN | Multiple inhibition of intracellular killing |

ADA, adenosine deaminase; PMN, polymorphonuclear leucocyte.

greater frequency of opportunistic infections and secondary malignancies in this population of immunologically naive patients.

Over the years, a variety of agents have been used to provide immunosuppression in transplant recipients. The first clinically used agents were primarily antiproliferative agents developed for cancer chemotherapy and were used with high-dosage corticosteroids. Over the past 2 decades, more-specific agents have become available to provide direct suppression of the responding immune cells actually responsible for rejection.

As our understanding of the specific mechanism of action of these agents has grown, there has been a gradual trend away from the use of high dosages of single or double agents and toward the use of multiple drug combinations in lower dosages to affect different compartments of the humoral and/or cellular immune response to alloantigens. Table 97-3 lists the agents currently used for clinical immunosuppression in the pediatric age group as well as their proposed cellular sites of action.

## Corticosteroids (Solumedrol, Medrol)

Corticosteroids, both methylprednisolone and prednisone, have been in clinical use for 4 decades, and they provide potent anti-inflammatory effects by inhibiting transcription of cytokine-encoding genes. At higher dosages there may be a direct cytotoxic effect on lymphocytes. Steroids can be used for both induction therapy and in the treatment of an acute rejection episode. The first dose is given intravenously

**TABLE 97-3 Classification of Immunosuppressive Drugs by Mechanism of Action**

| Agent | Mechanism of Action |
|---|---|
| Nonspecific | |
|   Corticosteroids (Solumedrol, Medrol) | Antiinflammatory, lympholytic, inhibition of gene activation |
|   Azathioprine (Imuran) | Inhibition of purine biosynthesis, (competitive inhibition of phosphoribosylpyrophosphate aminotransferase) |
| Specific | |
|   Mycophenolate mofetil (Cell-Cept) | Inhibition of purine synthesis in purine salvage pathway in lymphocytes only (competitive inhibition of inositol monophosphate dehydrogenase) |
|   Cyclosporine (Sandimmune, Neoral) | Calcineurin inhibitor |
|   Tacrolimus (Prograf) | Calcineurin inhibitor |
|   Anti-CD3 monoclonal antibody (Orthoclone) | Binding a murine monoclonal antibody to CD3 receptors on mature T cells (promoting C'-dependent cell cytotoxicity or receptor capping) |
|   Antithymocyte globulin | Binding of polyclonal antibody to multiple sites on T-cell surface (promoting C'-dependent cytotoxicity or receptor capping) |

(Solumedrol 10 mg/kg) during the transplantation procedure, and the dose is decreased with a relatively rapid taper over time. Eventually maintenance therapy is achieved with steroid doses of between 0.1 and 0.3 mg/kg per day by 3 to 6 months posttransplantation. With the availability of more potent immunosuppressive agents, a number of centers have been successful in either reducing steroid use to every-other-day dosing or completely eliminating them from long-term immunosuppressive protocols. The impetus for this trend to eliminate corticosteroid use is the high morbidity and mortality secondary to opportunistic infections, as well as the potent salt and water retention seen with secondary hypertension. The long-term use of steroids also leads to osteoporosis and affects gastric acid production, resulting in gastritis or ulcer formation, and is significantly associated with the development of post-transplant diabetes mellitus. Recent use of induction agents, like thymoglobulin, have allowed for "steroid free" protocols which really comprise a very rapid 4-day taper and discontinuance of steroids post-transplant.

## Azathiaprine (Imuran)

Azathiaprine is a purine analog which is metabolized to 6-mercaptopurine by the liver. This agent inhibits DNA synthesis in all mammalian cells. Azathiaprine competes with the enzymes necessary for purine biosynthesis, with the end result that there are fewer purines available for DNA synthesis, a decrease in DNA synthesis, and a decrease in cell division. Azathiaprine can be given intravenously or orally, and the usual starting dose is 1 to 2 mg/kg per day in a single dose. The major toxic side effect of azathiaprine is bone marrow suppression affecting all cell lines in the marrow. Neutropenia is the first evidence of azathiaprine toxicity. Therefore, patients should have their white blood cell counts followed and dose adjustments made for white blood cell counts falling below 5000/mm³. Late toxicity of azathiaprine may include red cell aplasia, hepatitis, and pancreatitis. Mycophenolate mofetil has replaced azathioprine as a first-line immunosuppression agent.

## Mycophenolate Mofetil (Cell-Cept)

Mycophenolate mofetil (Cell-Cept) is an antimetabolite similar to azathiaprine. Its potential advantage over azathiaprine is that it competitively inhibits inositol monophosphate dehydrogenase, which is a critical enzyme in the purine salvage pathway. This specific inhibition of the purine salvage pathway is exploited in the clinical transplantation situation because purine biosynthesis through this pathway is the *only* way that lymphocytes can synthesize purines. Other mammalian cells are able to synthesize purines through a *de novo* synthetic pathway and are not affected by mycophenolate mofetil. Mycophenolate is well absorbed orally. In the pediatric population, patients are given 600 mg/M² every 12 hours each day. The principal toxic side effects of mycophenolate mofetil are gastrointestinal upset with anorexia, nausea, vomiting, and diarrhea. As a result, patients may develop crampy abdominal pain secondary to its use. High doses may cause bone marrow suppression with anemia and neutropenia.

MMF has been shown to be effective in the prevention of acute rejection episodes in adult renal transplant patients, as well as improved graft survival in pediatric patients. MMF has an important role in induction as well as maintenance immunosuppression.

## Calcineurin Inhibitors

### Cyclosporine (Sandimmune, Neoral)

Cyclosporine is an intracellular fungal metabolite whose immunosuppressive activity was identified and immediately used in clinical transplantation situations. It appears to impart its immunosuppressive effect by inhibiting calcium-dependent T-lymphocyte activation. This inhibition of early activation results in a failure of helper T cells to elaborate cytokines, particularly interleukin 2, a potent inducer of cytotoxic T-cell activity. Cyclosporine can be administered intravenously or orally. It is poorly absorbed from the gastrointestinal tract and must be dissolved in various lipid carriers to facilitate absorption. After transplantation, patients may initially receive 5 mg/kg per day administered intravenously in 3 divided doses or as a continuous intravenous infusion. The usual oral dose for pediatric organ transplant recipients is 10 mg/kg per day divided into 2 doses. Depending on the preparation of cyclosporine used, trough levels are followed on a daily basis until a steady state is achieved. Trough levels between 150 and 500 ng/mL are commonly acceptable in most clinical situations. A microemulsion preparation of cyclosporine (Neoral) offers improved oral absorption and greater ease of dosing. The area under the curve or 2-hour postdose levels appear to be better indications of immunosuppression than trough levels for this preparation. A number of side effects occur secondary to the use of cyclosporine, including neurologic symptoms (tremors, seizures), hypertension, hirsutism, hypercholesterolemia, gingival hyperplasia, hepatotoxicity, and nephrotoxicity. All these side effects can be alleviated by dosage reduction.

### Tacrolimus (Prograf)

Tacrolimus is a macrolide antibiotic also derived from a fungus. This drug is 100-fold more potent than cyclosporine on a per-milligram basis. Tacrolimus can be administered intravenously or given orally. Because it is rapidly absorbed in the gastrointestinal tract with good pharmacologic activity, there is little indication for intravenous administration. A typical dose for pediatric patients is 0.15 mg/kg divided into every 12 hour administration. The occasional patient who requires intravenous administration can receive the drug by continuous infusion or by intermittent doses of 0.05 mg/kg per day given every 12 hours. As with cyclosporine, trough levels of tacrolimus are followed daily until stable levels are achieved. Individual pediatric patients may have widely disparate levels when given standard dosing, and doses must therefore be altered based on trough levels. Trough levels between 5 and 10 mg/mL are initially obtained with the higher levels used during rejection episodes. The principal toxic side effects of tacrolimus are neurologic symptoms (tremors, nervousness, sleepiness, and nightmares), hypertension, dyslipidemia, gastric problems (nausea, vomiting, and diarrhea), and development of diabetes mellitus, hyperkalemia, and nephrotoxicity. As in the case of cyclosporine, these toxic side effects are dose-related and usually respond to dose adjustment. There has been an increasing interest in minimizing the use of calcineurin inhibitors, mainly because of the long-term nephrotoxicity and risk for diabetes.

## Sirolimus

Sirolimus, or rapamycin, is an inhibitor of the mammalian target of rapamycin (mTOR). It is a macrocyclic lactone that is produced by a strain of *Streptomyces hygroscopicus*. Sirolimus is a potent inhibitor of B- and T-lymphocytes, as well as an inhibitor of smooth muscle proliferation and inhibitor of intimal hyperplasia. Unlike in adults, rapid metabolism of this drug in the pediatric population necessitates drug-level monitoring. Sirolimus does have an adverse effect on wound healing, with a significant incidence of lymphoceles requiring surgical drainage in 1 study. Additionally, use of sirolimus is associated with dyslipidemia. Currently, sirolimus is used as rescue therapy in patients with chronic allograft nephropathy. A major concern regarding usage of sirolimus was a potential increased incidence of PTLD in young, EBV-naïve patients. Currently, sirolimus is mainly used in pediatric liver transplant patients to reduce the nephrotoxicity from calcineurin inhibitor exposure, as well as treatment of rejection episodes.

## Anti-CD3 Monoclonal Antibody (Orthoclone OKT3)

Anti-CD3 monoclonal antibody is a murine antibody raised against the T-cell receptors of mature human lymphocytes. Because all mature T lymphocytes have a CD3 receptor, OKT3 monoclonal antibody is extremely effective in eliminating mature T cells from circulation, including activated T lymphocytes in a transplanted organ. The principal toxicity of this agent is directly related to the intravenous administration of foreign protein. There is a known infusion-related cytokine release syndrome that is problematic for patients, causing fever, myalgias, and capillary leakage. This can lead to pulmonary edema and respiratory distress. Furthermore, studies have failed to demonstrate that it has superior efficacy to other agents. Use of OKT3 has fallen out of favor as an induction agent in pediatric solid organ transplantation. It has instead been replaced by newer IL-2 antibody and polyclonal antilymphocyte preparations. The North American Pediatric Renal Transplant Cooperative Study in 2004 reported that none of the pediatric renal transplants performed in 2003 received OKT3 therapy.

## Antithymocyte Globulin

Antithymocyte globulin is a polyclonal antibody derived from rabbits that is specific for human T lymphocytes. The polyvalent nature of the antibody eliminates all T lymphocytes from the circulation. CD2 and CD11 are receptors found on immature T lymphocytes, and CD2/CD11 levels are followed in the blood. The agent is given intravenously at doses of 15 to 20 mg/kg per day as a single intravenous dose. There has been a resurgence of the use of polyclonal antibodies as part of an induction regimen for post-transplant immunosuppression.

The use of rabbit anti-thymoglobulin has been demonstrated as an effective induction agent for all types of transplants. As with OKT3, there are significant side effects related to foreign protein administration, and patients are pretreated with steroids, diphenhydramine, and acetaminophen to alleviate these effects.

## IL-2 Receptor Antibodies

Anti-IL2 receptor blockers target a single antigen on the T-cell, inhibiting the IL-2 induced clonal expansion of activated T cells. Because their target is so narrow, they may offer a more specific suppression than the polyclonal antibodies. Use of these agents is well tolerated, with avoidance of the cytokine release syndrome. Statistically significant lower incidence of graft thrombosis occurred when induction was performed using an IL-2 antibody induction. The main advantage of IL-2 receptor blockers appears to be a decreased incidence of acute rejection episodes; ultimately it is hopeful that this will translate into prolonged allograft survival. The number and severity of acute rejection episodes significantly impacts the incidence of chronic rejection, and hence, graft loss. Use of these antibodies is contraindicated in hepatitis-related liver transplants.

Finally, there is an anti-CD-52 monoclonal antibody, alemtuzumab (Campath H-1) that has seen increasing use. Its administration leads to a profound depletion of peripheral lymphocytes, NK cells, and monocytes. Currently its use is restricted mostly to high-risk transplant recipients.

## Treatment Strategies

The agents described above are usually prescribed in combination to provide immunosuppression adequate to maintain a graft in a transplant recipient without rejection or significant toxicity. Each of these agents is used to provide effective immunosuppression at 3 different stages in the posttransplantation period. The first stage is the induction stage at the time of implantation of the organ, followed by a maintenance period. The treatment of any rejection episodes that may occur also demands a change in treatment strategy. Common immunosuppression protocols are listed in Table 97-4.

### Induction Therapy

Currently, most kidney, heart, pancreas, intestine, and lung-transplant recipients receive induction therapy. Induction therapy begins at the time of implantation of the graft and continues for the first few weeks after transplantation. The most common induction therapy utilized is rabbit-anti-thymocyte globulin combined with intravenous steroids. In contrast, there is little use of induction antibodies for liver transplantation.

### Maintenance Therapy

Maintenance therapy involves maintaining a steady level of conventional immunosuppression while diminishing the overall dosage to obtain the minimal immunosuppressive dosage necessary to achieve a rejection-free patient. Increasingly, there have been attempts to avoid steroids in the maintenance therapy. With the introduction of cyclosporine- and

**TABLE 97-4** | **Immunosuppression Protocols**

Induction

 *Corticosteroids:* 10 mg/kg intraoperatively and every day for 2 days; then decrease dose to 2 mg/kg per day every 2 days until it is
  1 mg/kg per day

 *Steroid-sparing Induction:* ATG preparation on induction and daily until POD #4

 *Mycophenolate mofetil:* 300 mg/M² every 12 hours orally

 *Tacrolimus[a]:* 0.15 mg/kg every 12 hours orally to obtain trough levels of approximately 10 ng/mL or

 *Cyclosporine[a]:* 2 mg/kg per day every 8 hours intravenously with gradual conversion to 10 mg/kg per day every 12 hours orally;
  target trough levels ~200 ng/mL

 *Anti-thymocyte globulin:* 1.5 mg/kg daily intravenously for 5 days

 *Basilixumab:* Day 0 and Day 4 post transplant

Maintenance

 *Corticosteroids:* Prednisone gradually tapered to 0.2–0.3 mg/kg per day orally by 3–6 months and every-other-day dosing
  by 6–12 months

 *Tacrolimus:* Maintain trough levels at 5–7 ng/mL or

 *Cyclosporine:* Maintain trough levels ~100–150 ng/mL, used primarily in early post-transplant patients when Tacrolimus needs
  to be avoided and wound healing is still an issue

 *Mycophenolate mofetil:* 600 mg/m² per day for 6–12 months; may continue for problem rejection or to decrease dosing of other drugs

Rejection

 *Corticosteroids:* Methylprednisolone 10 mg/kg intravenously every day for 3 days; then taper 2 mg/kg per day every other day
  until 1 mg/kg per day and hold (may convert to oral prednisone during taper)

 *OKT3 monoclonal antibody[b]:* 2.5–5.0 mg/day intravenously for 10–14 days (use 2.5 mg if the patient weighs <20 kg, and 5.0 mg
  if weight is >20 kg

 *Antithymocyte globulin polyclonal antibody[b]:* 15 mg/kg per day intravenously for 10–14 days

 *Basilixumab*

[a]May need to withhold tacrolimus/cyclosporine dosing at induction if significant liver or kidney dysfunction.
[b]Usually given for steroid-resistant rejection.

tacrolimus-based therapies, there has been significant ability to withdraw steroids in transplant recipients. While steroid-minimizing regimens have shown improvement in growth markers, longer term follow-up demonstrates a significant decrease in graft function and an increase in rejection episodes. Newer studies that utilize antibody-based induction regimens have shown more promise. The best results with steroid withdrawal have been based on extended induction with IL-2 antibodies and complete steroid avoidance. Currently, most maintenance regimens target various T-cell activation mechanisms.

Tacrolimus trough levels are maintained at 10 ng/mL for the first 3 months following transplantation with a gradual reduction to approximately 5 to 7 ng/mL after that time. Long-term maintenance levels of tacrolimus are gradually decreased, and many patients receive very low detectable levels, 1 to 3 ng/mL, on a long-term basis.

Mycophenolate mofetil dosing continues for the first-year post-transplantation with dose adjustments made for any gastrointestinal toxicity or bone marrow suppression. The use of a mycophenolate/tacrolimus combination is the most frequently used discharge regimen in kidney and liver recipients. More rarely, mycophenolate/sirolimus, tacrolimus/sirolimus, and mycophenolate/cyclosporine combinations have been used. Tacrolimus has virtually replaced the use of cyclosporine in most centers. Discharge without steroid therapy is more common in liver than kidney recipients; 20% of liver recipients and 27% of intestinal recipients in 2004 were discharged without steroids.

## Antirejection Strategy

Despite induction therapy, a significant number of patients develop rejection episodes during the first few weeks following transplantation. Fortunately, the incidence of rejection has been decreasing overall. Most episodes of acute kidney and liver rejection are treated with corticosteroids, administered at a dose of 10 mg/kg/day. Some centers are using antithymocyte globulin with success.

## Complications of Immunosuppression

The clinical immunosuppressive strategies currently used attempt to strike a balance between rejection prevention and the infectious or toxic complications of immunosuppressive drugs. The individual immune response of pediatric patients to the antigen load with a transplanted organ unfortunately establishes the degree of immunosuppression necessary to achieve freedom from rejection. For a small number of patients who respond vigorously to the transplanted organ, this converts to more severe complications and toxicities from higher doses of immunosuppressive drugs. Table 97-5 summarizes the common complications of immunosuppression. The problem seen most often in pediatric patients undergoing significant chronic immunosuppression involves opportunistic infections, which translates into more frequent problems with bacterial and fungal sepsis often related to indwelling catheters. In addition, children lack specific immunity to a number of parasitic and viral pathogens. Pediatric transplant recipients, therefore, must be aggressively assessed for

| TABLE 97-5 | Complications of Immunosuppression |
|---|---|

**Infection**
  Bacterial, fungal (*Staphylococcus* and *Candida* organisms)
  Protozoans (*Pneumocystis carinii*, toxoplasmosis)
  Viral (cytomegalovirus, Epstein–Barr virus, herpes virus, adenovirus)

**Secondary malignancy**
  Posttransplant lymphoproliferative disorder (PTLD)
  Kaposi sarcoma
  Other lymphoma/leukemia
  Other primary cancers (skin, colon, breast, lung)

**Toxicity**
  Corticosteroids: osteoporosis, femur avascular necrosis, cataracts, gastritis
  Azathioprine: neutropenia, red cell aplasia, pancreatitis, hepatitis
  Cyclosporine: hypertension, nephrotoxicity, hirsutism, hypercholesterolemia, neurotoxicity
  Tacrolimus: hypertension, nephrotoxicity, neurotoxicity, hyperkalemia, insulin-dependent hyperglycemia

opportunistic infection in the post-transplantation period; they commonly require prophylactic agents to prevent these infections. Table 97-6 summarizes the prophylactic regimen used at the Johns Hopkins Hospital for pediatric patients during the first 6 months posttransplantation. In general, prophylaxis for *Pneumocystis carinii* pneumonia, as well as for opportunistic herpes virus infections including cytomegalovirus and Epstein–Barr virus (EBV), is used in patients who are at risk for these infections. This population of pediatric patients includes those who undergo induction or receive OKT3 or antithymocyte globulin therapy, as well as those who receive a cytomegalovirus- or EBV-mismatched organ from a viral positive adult donor. One potential advantage of the IL2-receptor antibodies is a decrease in the incidence of

| TABLE 97-6 | Infection Prophylaxis |
|---|---|

**Immunizations (pretransplantation)**
  Diphtheria–tetanus–pertussis, poliovirus, hepatitis B, measles-mumps-rubella, varicella, influenza

**Immunizations (posttransplantation)**
  Diphtheria–tetanus–pertussis (heat-killed oral polio virus); avoid any live virus vaccines

**Prophylaxis**
  *Pneumocystis carinii* pneumonia: Bactrim (Monday, Wednesday, Friday weekly schedule)
  Herpes viruses
    Cytomegalovirus: immunoglobulin G, acyclovir, or ganciclovir
    Epstein-Barr virus: immunoglobulin G, acyclovir, or ganciclovir
    Herpes simplex virus: acyclovir
    Varicella-zoster virus: varicella-zoster virus immunoglobulin within 72 hours of exposure; acyclovir for active infection

PTLD, as well as overall better tolerance of its infusion compared to OKT3 and ATG.

In addition to developing a primary mononucleosis syndrome secondary to EBV activation or infection, pediatric transplant recipients are at higher risk for EBV associated post-transplantation lymphoproliferative disorder. A primary mononucleosis syndrome characterized by lymphadenopathy, hepatosplenomegaly, pharyngitis, and fever may progress to frank lymphoma or to a leukemic state secondary to unchecked proliferation of transformed B lymphocytes. In an immunologically normal individual, cytotoxic T cells are generated, which presumably eliminates these clones of transformed B cells and downregulates the mononucleosis syndrome. With significant immunosuppression, pediatric transplant recipients are unable to mount an effective T-cell response to these EBV-transformed B lymphocytes and essentially develop Burkitt-type lymphoma or leukemia. These patients must be aggressively treated with withdrawal of immunosuppression. If they have significant bulky lymphomatous disease or leukemia, they may require cytoreduction therapy to eliminate the majority of proliferating B cells. Withdrawal of immunosuppression following adequate cytoreduction presumably allows for recovery of the T-cell arm of the immune system and provides long-term cellular control of the transformed B lymphocytes.

## Effects of Immunosuppression

As increasing numbers of pediatric transplant recipients survive and require long-term treatment with immunosuppressive agents, we will see more evidence of significant long-term toxicity. The primary late effects of corticosteroids include Cushing syndrome, osteoporosis, impaired growth, avascular necrosis of the femoral head, cataracts, glaucoma, cardiovascular disease, and gastritis or peptic ulcer disease. Long-term use of azathioprine can cause hepatitis, pancreatitis, and red cell aplasia. Cyclosporine used on a long-term basis can lead to hypercholesterolemia, arteriosclerosis, hypertension, nephrotoxicity, neurotoxicity, hyperkalemia, and hyperglycemia. The effects of long-term use of tacrolimus include hypertension and nephrotoxicity, diabetes mellitus, and dyslipidemia as described above. Adverse effects of sirolimus include impaired wound healing and dyslipidemia. It is minimization of these adverse effects which drives investigation into immunosuppression minimization.

Secondary malignancies also are a fact of life for long-term immunosuppressed transplant recipients. A small number of patients may develop Kaposi sarcoma, which is presumably related to an EBV-like virus. Posttransplantation lymphoproliferative disorder secondary to EBV infection also can occur in chronically immunosuppressed patients. Patients are also at higher risk for the common malignancies seen in non-immunosuppressed patients, such as Hodgkin disease, non-Hodgkin lymphoma, and skin cancer. Our pediatric transplant recipients at the Johns Hopkins Hospital undergo yearly cancer surveillance including a chest radiograph and a general physical examination to screen for skin lesions and any other problems. Teenaged female recipients should undergo yearly pelvic examinations and Papanicolaou tests when appropriate.

# CONCLUSIONS

Fortunately for pediatric surgeons and their patients, neonates and children have a competent immune system at birth that provides significant responses in the face of infection and surgical stress. All the features of the immune system are qualitatively present in newborns and in older children, but there are significant quantitative differences between children and adults.

A variety of congenital and acquired immunodeficiency states may occur in the pediatric age group that complicates their treatment.

In the transplantation clinical population an intact immune system requires significant immunosuppression to prevent rejection. The overall naivete of the pediatric immune system and the difference in how medications are metabolized in the transplantation clinical situation results in a higher incidence of secondary complications of immunosuppression than in adults, and therefore greater vigilance for complications of immunosuppression must be maintained. There have been great strides in long-term transplant patient and graft survival, which has led to increasing interest in producing immunosuppression regimens that minimize adverse effects on the patients. Ultimately, the goal is to induce a tolerant state for the transplanted organ, but until this is achieved, careful tailoring of the medications to the individual patient must be maintained.

## SELECTED READINGS

Abbas AK, Lichtman AH, Prober JS. *Cellular and Molecular Immunology, Updated Edition*. Philadelphia, PA: WB Saunders Co; 2009.

Agarwal A, et al. Immunosuppression in pediatric solid organ transplantation. *Semin Pediatr Surg* 2006;(15):142–152.

Colombani PM. Clinical immunosuppression. In: Oldham KT, Colombani PM, Foglia RP, eds. *Surgery of Infants and Children: Scientific Principles and Practice*. Philadelphia, PA: Lippincott-Raven; 1997:671–700.

Hannet I, Erkeller-Yuksel F, Lydyard P, Deneys V, DeBruyere M. Developmental and maturational changes in human blood lymphocyte subpopulations. *Immunol Today* 1992;13:215–218.

Meier-Kriesche H-U, et al. Immunosuppression: evolution in practice and trends, 1994–2004. *Am J Transpl* 2006:(6, part 2):1111–1131.

Schonder K, Mazareigos G, Weber R. Adverse effects of immunosuppression in pediatric solid organ transplantation. *Pediatr Drugs* 2010;12(1): 35–49.

Yang I, et al. Immunosuppressive strategies to improve outcomes of kidney transplantation. *Semin Nephrol* 2007;27(4):337–392.

# CHAPTER 98

## Surgery and End-Stage Renal Disease

*Khashayar Vakili and Craig W. Lillehei*

## KEY POINTS

### Essentials of Diagnosis

1. Congenital or inherited disorders are the most common causes of renal failure in children.

2. The etiology of renal failure plays a very important role in the management of patients with ESRD.

### Essentials of Management

1. RRT includes hemodialysis, peritoneal dialysis, and renal transplantation.

2. The decision of the modality to be used is multifactorial and based on the individual patient.

3. For long-term dialysis, an arteriovenous fistula or graft is preferable to a hemodialysis catheter.

4. Peritoneal dialysis catheters are preferred in small children with small caliber vessels.

5. Renal transplantation is ultimately the best treatment for children with ESRD.

## INTRODUCTION

The surgical management of pediatric patients with end-stage renal disease (ESRD) is generally focused on providing means for renal replacement therapy (RRT), namely dialysis or renal transplantation. Many patients with ESRD will alternate between the various modalities of renal replacement therapies throughout their lifetime. Initiation of RRT is usually based on the presence of complications such as fluid overload, acidosis, symptomatic uremia, electrolyte abnormalities, failure to thrive, profound bone disease, or developmental delay. The decision regarding the most suitable RRT modality for each patient is based on a number of factors such as the acuity of renal failure, etiology of renal disease, patient size, anatomy, and family support. Currently, kidney transplantation is the treatment of choice for children with ESRD since it provides several advantages when compared

to long-term dialysis. Such transplant-related benefits include improvements in quality of life, improved growth and development, and avoidance of the morbidity and mortality associated with long-term dialysis.

Pediatric kidney transplantation should be performed at specialized centers with a dedicated multidisciplinary team to achieve optimal long-term graft and patient survival.

The surgeon is intimately involved in the care of pediatric patients with ESRD to address such challenges as creation and maintenance of dialysis access, construction of urinary conduits, native nephrectomy, and transplantation. This chapter focuses on surgical decision making and techniques that are used in the care of the pediatric patient with ESRD.

## PATIENT CHARACTERISTICS AND PATHOPHYSIOLOGY OF CHILDREN WITH ESRD

The most common etiologies of renal failure in children who have undergone kidney transplantation are listed in Table 98-1. Congenital or inherited disorders are the most common causes in younger children. The leading cause of renal failure is related to abnormalities of renal genesis closely followed by conditions resulting in obstructive uropathy. In older children, acquired renal disease becomes more common.

Renal insufficiency in the pediatric patient is usually secondary to chronic kidney disease (CKD) as opposed to acute renal failure (ARF). Stage 1 and 2 CKD are considered mild disease with normal or near normal renal function. Patients with a glomerular filtration rate (GFR) below 60 mL/min/1.73 m² for ≥3 months are considered to have Stage 3 CKD. Patients with Stage 4 CKD (GFR of 15-30 mL/min/1.73 m²) should undergo preparation for RRT since once the GFR is <15 mL/min/1.73 m² (Stage 5 CKD), RRT is indicated.

In ARF, the indications for dialysis are usually hypervolemia, hyperkalemia, or metabolic acidosis. The most common causes of ARF in the pediatric population include congenital heart disease, sepsis, acute tubular necrosis, or nephrotoxic agents. In addition, ARF can be encountered following complex congenital heart surgery with a long duration

| TABLE 98-1 | Diagnoses and Demographics of Pediatric Patients Undergoing Renal Transplantation Based on Data from North American Pediatric Renal Trials and Collaborative Studies (NAPRTCS) | |
|---|---|---|
| **Primary Diagnosis** | | **%** |
| Aplasia/hypoplasia/dysplasia | | 15.9 |
| Obstructive uropathy | | 15.6 |
| Focal segmental glomerulosclerosis | | 11.7 |
| Reflux nephropathy | | 5.2 |
| Chronic glomerulonephritis | | 3.3 |
| Polycystic disease | | 2.9 |
| Medullary cystic disease | | 2.8 |
| Hemolytic uremic syndrome | | 2.6 |
| Prune Belly | | 2.6 |
| Congenital nephrotic syndrome | | 2.6 |
| Familial nephritis | | 2.3 |
| Cystinosis | | 2.0 |
| Pyelo/interstitial nephritis | | 1.8 |
| Membranoproliferative glomerulonephritis-Type I | | 1.7 |
| Idiopathic crescentic glomerulonephritis | | 1.7 |
| SLE nephritis | | 1.5 |
| Renal infarct | | 1.4 |
| The Berger (IgA) nephritis | | 1.3 |
| Henoch–Schonlein nephritis | | 1.1 |
| Membranoproliferative glomerulonephritis-Type II | | 0.8 |
| The Wegener granulomatosis | | 0.6 |
| Wilms tumor | | 0.5 |
| Drash syndrome | | 0.5 |
| Oxalosis | | 0.5 |
| Membranous nephropathy | | 0.4 |
| Other systemic immunologic disease | | 0.3 |
| Sickle cell nephropathy | | 0.2 |
| Diabetic glomerulonephritis | | 0.1 |
| Other | | 9.8 |
| Unknown | | 6.2 |
| *Gender* | | |
| Male | | 59.4 |
| Female | | 40.6 |
| *Race* | | |
| White | | 59.8 |
| Black | | 16.9 |
| Hispanic | | 16.7 |
| Other | | 6.6 |

*Source:* North American Pediatric Renal Trials and Collaborative Studies (NAPRTCS) Annual Report (2008). Available at: *https://web.emmes.com/study/ped/annlrept/annlrept.html* (Accessed 1 March 2010). Reprinted with permission.

of cardiopulmonary bypass. Once it has been determined that a patient with renal insufficiency requires RRT, the most appropriate modality needs to be selected.

## CHOICE OF RRT

Based on the 2009 US Renal Data System Annual Report, the incidence of dialysis initiation in 2007 was about 1245 children with a prevalence of about 7200 children receiving treatment for ESRD through transplantation or dialysis. Greater than 60% of RRT is initiated via a hemodialysis catheter. In older patients with ARF, hemodialysis via a percutaneous catheter is the most common approach for initiation of dialysis. In smaller patients, due to the small size of their vessels, peritoneal dialysis (PD) is favored.

The decision for initiation of dialysis or RRT is usually made in conjunction with the nephrologist. The choice of RRT modality is dependent on several factors which include: (1) cause of renal failure, (2) anticipated recovery of renal function, (3) size of patient, (4) suitability of the peritoneum, (5) suitability of vasculature, (6) patient/family compliance and convenience.

### Hemodialysis

Hemodialysis is usually performed via a central venous catheter, arteriovenous fistula, or arteriovenous graft. The choice of hemodialysis access modality is primarily based on the urgency for dialysis and suitability of vessels. In patients who require urgent or emergent dialysis, the placement of a central venous hemodialysis catheter is the only real option. Since arteriovenous fistulas usually require 6-8 weeks for adequate maturation before use, they do not provide immediate access for dialysis. Nonetheless, if possible, they are the preferred access for long-term dialysis. If a patient is anticipated to require dialysis within the subsequent 3 to 6 months, creation of an arteriovenous fistula is recommended to eliminate the need for a central venous catheter. Despite the increasing focus on the morbidity associated with central venous catheters, greater than 85% of children under the age of 13 and 60% of children between the ages of 13 to 19 are initiated on hemodialysis via a central venous catheter. Based on the North American Pediatric Renal Trials and Collaborative Studies (NAPRTCS), the modality and distribution of hemodialysis access is: central venous catheter (79%), arteriovenous fistula (12%), and arteriovenous graft (9%).

The percentage of children with ESRD on hemodialysis increases with age. Less than 10% of children under 1 year of age are managed via hemodialysis whereas close to 50% of children over 12 years receive hemodialysis. This trend is due to the small size of the vessels in younger patients which makes the creation of a fistula or placement of a hemodialysis catheter technically challenging and, at times, impossible.

### Central Venous Hemodialysis Catheters (See also Chapter 9, Vascular Access Procedures)

Central venous catheters provide the advantage of immediate access for emergent or urgent dialysis. They may also be used as a bridge to eventual renal transplantation, PD, or until maturation of an arteriovenous fistula or graft. Usually, the central venous hemodialysis catheter is placed via the internal jugular or subclavian vein. The preferred position of the tip of the catheter is just into the right atrium. Venous thrombosis or stricture is one of the complications associated with long-term indwelling catheters. Thrombosis or stricture of the subclavian veins can preclude a successful future arteriovenous fistula or graft in the corresponding upper extremity. This concern is especially important in patients with CKD who will require life-long RRT and may be dependent on the availability of suitable access for dialysis. For this reason, use of the internal jugular or occasionally the external jugular vein as a site of catheter insertion is recommended. The right internal jugular vein provides a straight route to the right atrium and has been shown to have lower long-term malfunction rate when compared to catheters placed via the left internal jugular vein. Accessing the internal jugular vein under ultrasound guidance can minimize the risk of carotid artery injury and has therefore become the routine practice at our institution. If the internal jugular veins are not suitable, the next option is via a subclavian approach.

Catheter diameter sizes range from 7-12 French and the selection of the appropriate catheter is dependent on the patients' size. The catheter should be of a caliber which will permit adequate blood flow during dialysis so that effective hemodialysis can be achieved in a reasonable time period. A crucial factor to optimize blood flow through the catheter is placement of the tip within the right atrium but avoiding the tricuspid valve.

Dialysis catheters have 2 lumens designated as "arterial" and "venous." The arterial lumen provides the inflow to the dialysis circuit through multiple side holes along the catheter while the venous lumen is situated at the tip of the catheter to provide outflow. The separation between the outflow and inflow lumens minimizes recirculation.

If the patient is expected to require long-term dialysis as an outpatient, placement of a tunneled catheter is advisable. The majority of tunneled catheters have a cuff which is placed in the subcutaneous tunnel. It provides an anchor for tissue in-growth minimizing the risks for dislodgement and infection. The 1-year secondary patency rates of cuffed tunneled catheters vary widely, ranging from 25% to 90% in different series. Early catheter malfunction is usually mechanical in origin and may be secondary to twisting of the catheter within the tunnel, constriction of the catheter by suture, or poor positioning of the distal tip. Later catheter malfunction is usually secondary to thrombus formation within the catheter, development of a fibrin sheath around the catheter, or dislodgment.

Even though catheters provide numerous advantages such as immediate use for dialysis and avoidance of repeated venipuncture, the potential morbidities of infection, vascular thrombosis and stricture should generally preclude their long-term use. Nonetheless, in the pediatric population, the use of catheters for long-term (>3 months) hemodialysis is generally acceptable in the following cases: (1) the child is too small (<20 kg) for the creation of an arteriovenous fistula, (2) the catheter is used as a bridge to peritoneal dialysis, or (3) kidney transplantation is anticipated in the near future.

A more permanent vascular access is recommended for any pediatric patient who is anticipated to have greater than a 1-year waiting period for kidney transplantation.

## Arteriovenous Fistulae (AVF) or Arteriovenous Grafts (AVG)

AVF is the best long-term option for hemodialysis access. Every patient who is anticipated to require long-term dialysis should be evaluated for the creation of an AVF.

National Kidney Foundation/Kidney Disease Outcomes and Quality Initiative (NKF/KDOQI) guidelines recommend a 50% AVF rate for initiation of dialysis and at least 40% for prevalence in all patients on hemodialysis. These rates are challenging to achieve in the pediatric population, especially given the technical challenges in children weighing less than 10 kg. If suitable vessels are not available for the creation of AVF then AVG placement should be considered. National Kidney Foundation's recommendations regarding the preference for the location of AVF or AVG in descending order are: (1) Radiocephalic fistula (wrist level), (2) Brachiocephalic fistula (elbow level), (3) Transposed brachial-basilic vein fistula, (4) Forearm loop AVG (preferred to straight), (5) Upper arm graft, (6) Chest-wall or lower-extremity AVF or AVG (Figs. 98-1 to 98-4).

Evaluation of a candidate for creation of an AVF or AVG should be directed at identifying suitable arterial inflow and venous outflow. It is also important to rule out any central venous outflow obstruction. The nondominant extremity should be considered first for the creation of the fistula. Careful physical and ultrasound examination of the target vessels should be performed, preferably by the surgeon. Patients with a long-term history of subclavian catheters or those with significant venous collateral formation may need examination of the more central venous system using duplex ultrasound or venography.

A minimum diameter of 2 mm for the inflow artery and a vein diameter of 2.5 mm with a tourniquet in place are usually acceptable vessel calibers. The entire length of the vein should be examined carefully using ultrasound to evaluate any areas of narrowing or sclerosis which would decrease the prospects for successful maturation of the fistula. If there is no suitable autogenous vein for the creation of a direct AVF, the next option is use of an AVG. Several types of graft material are available including Dacron, bovine, polyurethane, cryopreserved vein, and PTFE. The most common prosthetic graft currently used is PTFE. It is generally used in a tapered 7- to 4-mm size with the smaller end used at the arterial anastomosis to limit excessive flow which might result in a steal syndrome. The graft should be tunneled superficially through the subcutaneous tissue so that it can be easily accessed for insertion of the dialysis needles. Most commonly, the grafts are placed in the forearm and in a loop configuration with anastomoses to the brachial artery and the basilic or brachial veins. Grafts placed in the upper arm are usually in a straight configuration between the brachial artery near the elbow and the basilic or axillary vein near the axilla (Fig. 98-4). If creation of an upper extremity AVG is not possible, a lower extremity AVG would be the next reasonable option. Lower extremity AVGs are placed between the femoral artery and

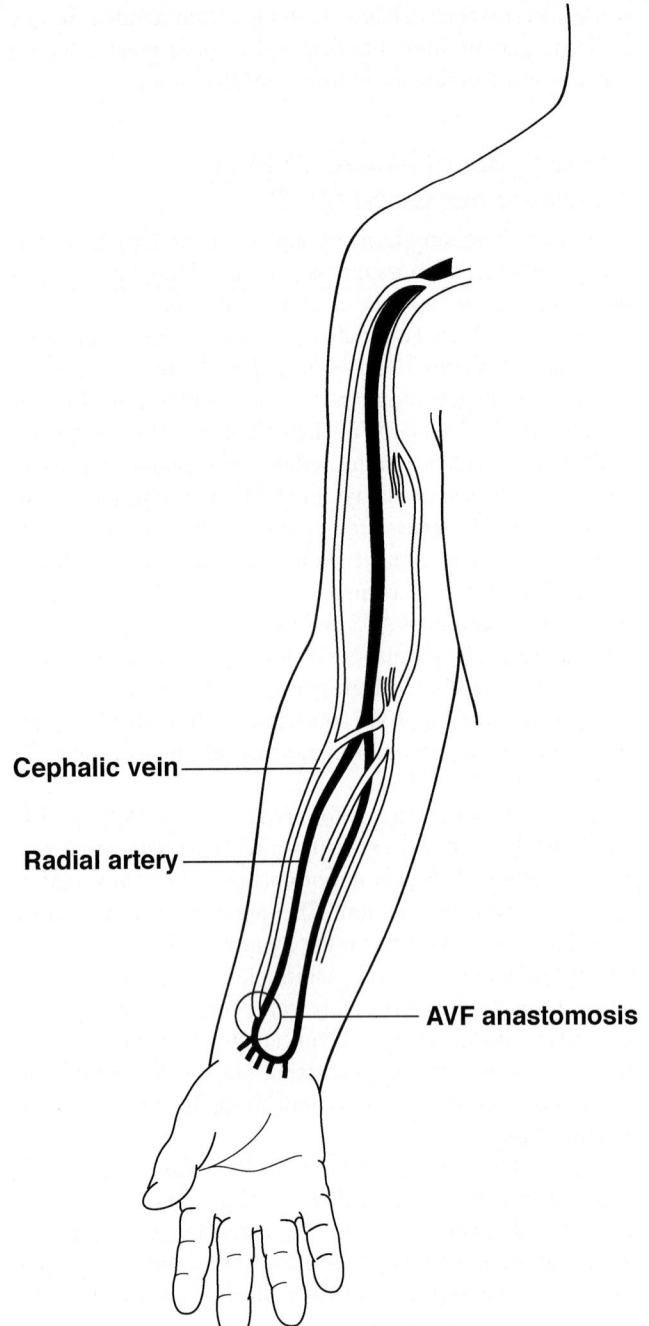

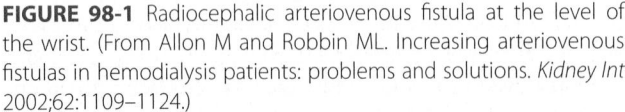

**FIGURE 98-1** Radiocephalic arteriovenous fistula at the level of the wrist. (From Allon M and Robbin ML. Increasing arteriovenous fistulas in hemodialysis patients: problems and solutions. *Kidney Int* 2002;62:1109–1124.)

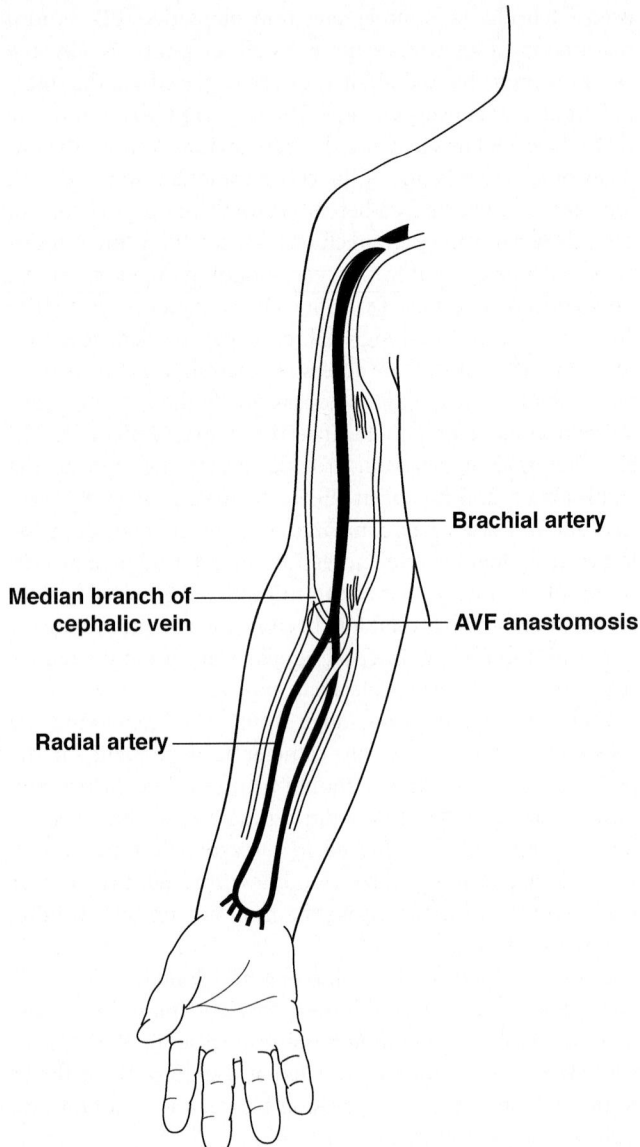

**FIGURE 98-2** Brachiocephalic arteriovenous fistula. (From Allon M and Robbin ML. Increasing arteriovenous fistulas in hemodialysis patients: problems and solutions. *Kidney Int* 2002;62:1109–1124.)

femoral vein. They are tunneled subcutaneously in a loop configuration over the anteromedial thigh. It should be noted that in children a femoral AVG may result in enlargement of the extremity due to increased venous pressure and flow.

## Peritoneal Dialysis (PD)

Based on the NAPRTCS 2008 report, about 60% of pediatric patients with ESRD are initiated on peritoneal dialysis. PD is particularly favored in the 0 to 5 age group because it avoids placement of hemodialysis catheters within small vessels. PD also provides the ability to perform dialysis at home which is considered an advantage by some patients and families.

The majority of PD catheters registered in the NAPRTCS database are either curled (62%) or straight (27%) Tenckhoff catheters. The catheters may have 1 or 2 cuffs. The most common configuration of PD catheter placement is a curled catheter with a single cuff, placed through a straight tunnel with a lateral exit site. The cuff closest to the intraperitoneal tip of the catheter should be placed in an extraperitoneal position, preferably within or beneath the rectus muscle and anchored to the fascia (Fig. 98-5). In infants, a subcutaneous cuff is at risk of erosion through the overlying skin and therefore avoided. Double cuff catheters are used when the child's size permits placement of the second cuff within the subcutaneous tunnel and allows a 1.5 to 2 cm distance from the skin exit site. The methods used for the placement of PD catheters include open, percutaneous Seldinger, and laparoscopic techniques.

purse-string is secured and the cuff is positioned between the peritoneum and the anterior fascia. The overlying muscle and anterior fascia may be closed over the cuff. The catheter is tunneled through the subcutaneous tissue for a distance of at least 5 cm.

Once the catheter is in its final position, 10 mL/kg of saline should be instilled through the catheter into the peritoneum and allowed to drain by gravity. A properly functioning catheter should return greater than 80% of the instilled fluid. The skin incision is then closed with a subcuticular absorbable suture.

The catheter can be used immediately after surgery. However, if possible, we prefer to wait to allow for adequate wound healing to minimize the risk of leakage through the incisions. In addition, we typically start with low dwell volumes of 10 mL/kg for several days before gradually increasing to the final dialysis volumes. This strategy allows for less stress on the incisions while healing in order to minimize patient discomfort and the potential risk for leakage.

Laparoscopic PD catheter placement is thought to have several advantages over the open or percutaneous techniques which include the ability to position the catheter in

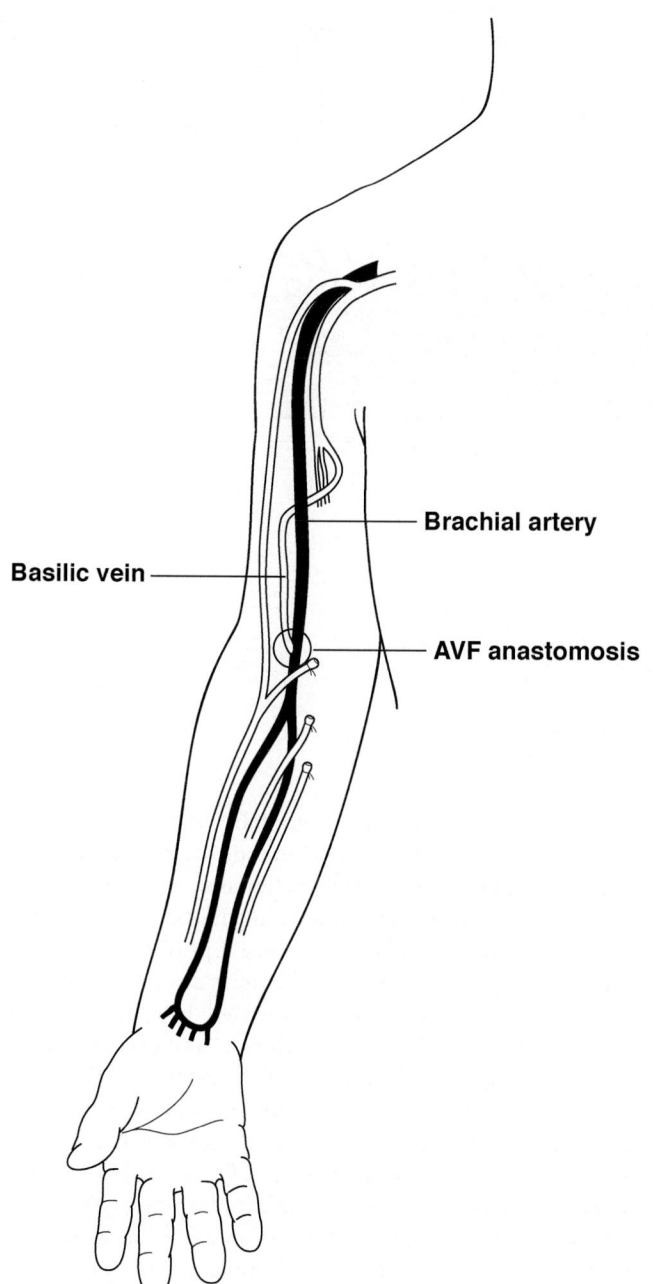

**FIGURE 98-3** Basilic vein transposition with brachial artery–basilic vein anastomosis. This AVF may be performed in one or two stages (arteriovenous anastomosis first followed by basilic vein transposition after maturation of fistula). (From Allon M and Robbin ML. Increasing arteriovenous fistulas in hemodialysis patients: problems and solutions. *Kidney Int* 2002;62:1109–1124.)

The open technique for the placement of a peritoneal dialysis catheter is performed under general anesthesia. A 2 to 4 cm transverse incision is made over the rectus muscle in the lower abdomen. The anterior fascia is incised transversely and the muscle is split along its fibers. The peritoneum is then incised. Partial omentectomy can be performed through this incision to lessen the risk for subsequent occlusion of the catheter. A purse-string suture is placed in the peritoneum/posterior fascia. The catheter is guided towards the pelvis over a wire or stylet with care to avoid injury to any abdominal organs or structures. After the removal of the stylet, the

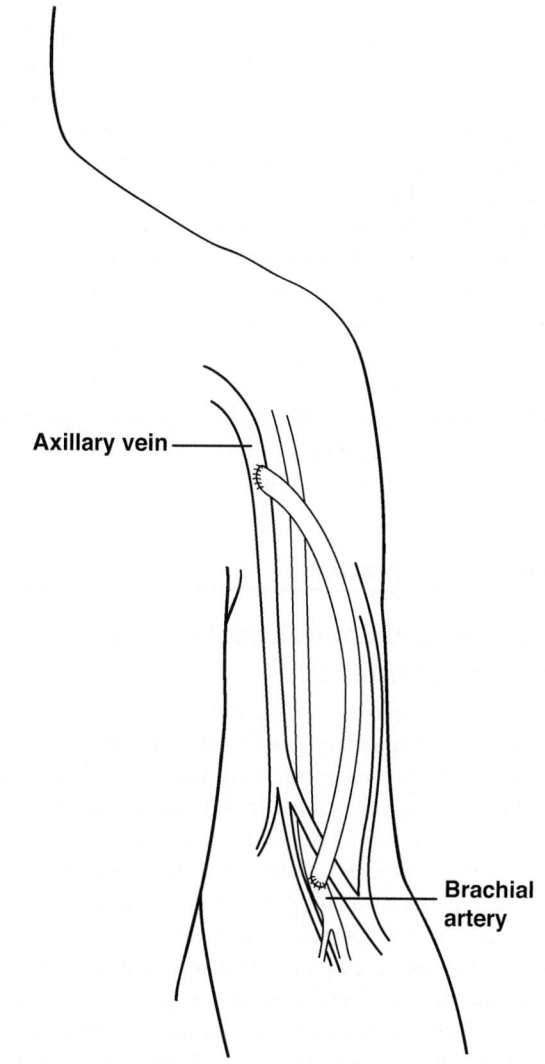

**FIGURE 98-4** Upper arm straight polytetrafluoroethylene graft from the brachial artery to the basilic or axillary vein.

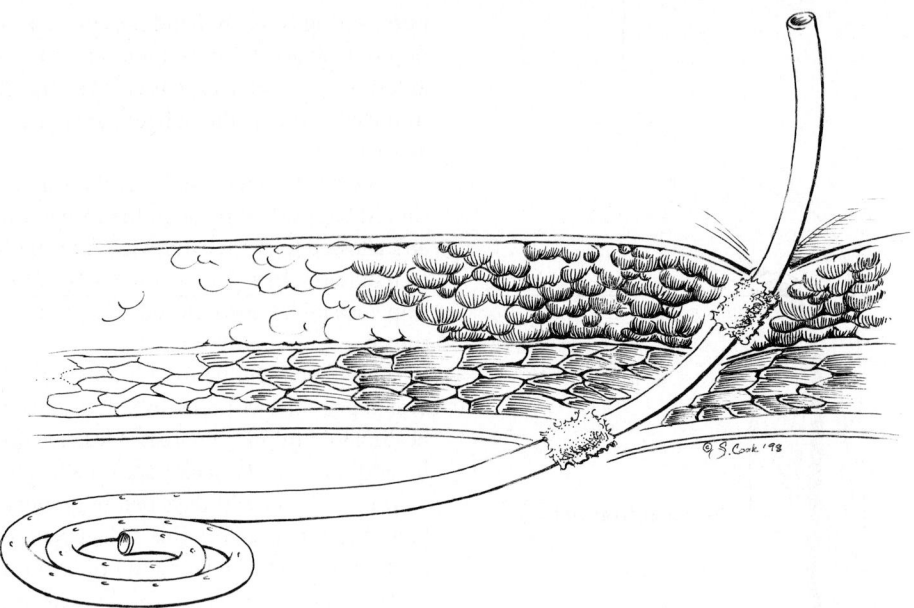

**FIGURE 98-5** Proper location of the cuffs when a 2-cuff peritoneal dialysis catheter is used. One cuff is between the posterior sheath and the anterior sheath and the second cuff is within in the subcutaneous tissue.

the abdomen can be visualized directly, a more complete omentectomy can be done, and assessment can be made for hernias as well as abdominal adhesions secondary to a previous operation. These advantages may become more important in patients with prior abdominal operations. The issue of omentectomy at the time of PD catheter placement remains controversial. Studies report a 15 to 60% reduction in the risk of catheter occlusion following omentectomy. However, this risk reduction needs to be weighed against the operative risks of omentectomy. Overall, about 60% of surgeons perform omentectomy at the time of PD catheter placement.

Based on a Cochrane review, there is no evidence in the literature demonstrating a superiority of catheter type, placement, or insertion technique in decreasing the rate of peritonitis, exit site, or tunnel infections.

## Renal Transplantation

### Indications and Contraindications for Renal Transplantation

The primary diagnoses and demographics for pediatric patients undergoing renal transplantation in 2008 are shown in Table 98-1. The causes of renal failure in children are quite different than in adults. In general, the etiologies of ESRD in children can be divided into obstructive, congenital, or acquired. The exact etiology of ESRD has an important impact on the pretransplant preparation of the patient, operative approach, postoperative management, and long-term outcomes. For example, patients with obstructive uropathy may require bladder reconstruction surgery prior to transplantation. Failure to provide a suitable urinary reservoir and a reliable mode for drainage can place the graft at jeopardy. Some conditions such as focal segmental glomerulosclerosis may require special protocols to decrease the risk of disease recurrence in the transplant allograft. In Type 1 primary hyperoxaluria or atypical hemolytic uremic syndrome, simultaneous liver and kidney transplantation may be necessary.

Every child with ESRD or impending ESRD should be considered for renal transplantation since it provides significant long-term benefits to the child. Therapies directed at the correction of the numerous ESRD-associated disturbances using growth factors, nutritional supplements, and erythropoietin analogs are important; however, they do not achieve the benefits provided by renal transplantation, particularly in children under 2 years of age. Furthermore, renal transplantation in infancy may prevent the detrimental effects of CKD on neurologic development. Therefore, only in the presence of clear-cut contraindications, should transplantation not be offered as an option. Absolute contraindications to transplantation include presence of metastatic malignancy, active infection with hepatitis B, severe multiorgan failure, positive direct immunologic cross-match, or irreversible debilitating brain injury. Relative contraindications include ABO incompatibility, previous positive direct cross-match, active autoimmune disease (lupus erythematosus, anti-glomerular basement membrane disease), HIV infection, psychomotor or psychiatric illness necessitating custodial care, chronic hepatitis C viral infection, and significant history of noncompliance, lack of family support, or inadequate home supervision.

### Evaluation for Renal Transplantation

The evaluation process for transplantation involves a thorough assessment of the patient by a multidisciplinary team which includes a nephrologist, transplant surgeon, urologist, transplant nurse coordinator, social worker, psychologist, dietician, and pharmacist. Psychosocial evaluation and pretransplant education of a patient's family are also necessary. A complete history and physical should be performed with special attention to the identification of associated anomalies in children with congenital renal anomalies. The surgeon needs to assess the potential recipient for the adequacy of inflow and outflow vessels as well as a satisfactory urinary reservoir or conduit. Evaluation of femoral arterial pulses is important to assess the adequacy of the iliac vessels for arterial inflow. Prior history of femoral catheters, pelvic malformations, or any other findings suggestive of vascular abnormality should prompt a radiographic evaluation (US, CT, or MRI) to assess the abdominal arterial and venous systems. Some congenital malformations may result in vascular aberrations such as left-sided vena cava, intraperitoneal aorta, or an absence of the abdominal vena cava. In these cases, careful preoperative vascular mapping using CT or MR angiograms is necessary for operative planning. Such imaging can be quite helpful in delineating the presence of adequate retroperitoneal or paravertebral venous drainage.

In the presence of inferior vena cava (IVC) thrombosis, iliac vessels, or even the distal patent segment of vena cava may be used for venous outflow of the graft. There is a higher risk of renal vein thrombosis following transplantation into a recipient with a thrombosed IVC and therefore many clinicians favor using deceased donor grafts rather than living donor grafts in this circumstance. The presence of vascular anatomic variations certainly provides an additional challenge to the surgeon but should not necessarily preclude transplantation.

Pre-transplant laboratory tests include blood typing, HLA typing, complete blood count, electrolytes, BUN, creatinine, coagulation parameters, liver function tests, urinalysis, urine culture, and panel reactive antibody. Minimum cardiac and pulmonary evaluation should include a chest radiograph and an electrocardiogram. When clinically indicated, pulmonary function testing or echocardiogram should be obtained. Routine serologic tests include CMV, EBV, HIV, toxoplasmosis, hepatitis B, hepatitis C, MMR, VZV, and HSV. Patients should have up-to-date vaccinations (Hep B, tetanus, HIB, IPV, MMR, varicella, pneumococcal vaccine, influenza, and hepatitis A) prior to transplantation if at all possible. Live virus vaccines should be administered at least 4 weeks prior to transplantation. Immunosuppressed individuals following transplantation may have a blunted response to killed-vaccines and should not be exposed to live-virus vaccines. Serum cross-match should be performed between the recipient and the donor prior to transplantation. Nutritional deficits and metabolic derangements should be corrected prior to transplantation in order to minimize post-operative complications. Since the majority of the pediatric patients receive adult-size kidneys, the size of the child should be sufficient to receive the intended organ. Due to these size constraints, we try to avoid transplanting an adult-size kidney into infants weighing less than 6.5 kg or with a length less than 65 cm. Our general approach has been to allow infants to be supported with dialysis until they reach an appropriate size for transplantation.

In the majority of cases, pediatric kidney transplantation is performed once a patient has developed ESRD and is on maintenance dialysis. However, about 25% of children undergo pre-emptive transplantation with the highest rate in the 6 to 12 year old age group. Pre-emptive transplantation is thought to have many potential benefits which are directly related to avoidance of dialysis and the morbidities associated with ESRD including uremia, metabolic acidosis, secondary hyperparathyroidism, malnutrition, anemia, and hormonal imbalance. Pre-emptive transplantation is usually achieved using living donor kidney grafts. Overall, 60% of all kidney grafts are from living donors with the parents constituting the majority (81%) of these donors. The remainder of donors are comprised of deceased donors; either after brain death (DBD) or after cardiac death (DCD). DBD donors generally yield better quality grafts and constitute the majority of pediatric kidney deceased donors.

## Pretransplant Urologic Considerations

Lower urinary tract anomalies are a common cause of renal failure in children and are present in about 25% of pediatric kidney recipients. Common diagnoses include vesicoureteral reflux, posterior urethral valves, neurogenic bladder, Prune belly syndrome, and bladder or cloacal exstrophy. In these cases, a thorough pretransplant urologic evaluation should be conducted. The presence of a suitable reservoir or well functioning urinary conduit is essential to prevent allograft injury secondary to hydronephrosis or ureteral reflux.

Pretransplant urologic work-up may include determination of postvoid residual volume, cystoscopy, urodynamics, or voiding cystourethrogram. Bladder pressures above 40 cm of water have been associated with allograft damage following kidney transplantation. Anticholinergics and intermittent catheterizations can be used to decrease bladder pressures in patients with high post-void residuals.

It may be challenging to maintain a bladder of adequate size and suitable compliance prior to transplantation, particularly in patients without substantial urine production or with prior urinary diversion. Intermittent catheterization and bladder cycling may be used to maintain capacity and compliance. In selected cases, undiversion of the urinary tract prior to transplantation can be used for such bladder cycling if there is sufficient urine output.

If the bladder size or compliance remain unsatisfactory, bladder reconstruction or augmentation may be required prior to transplantation. Bladder augmentation is usually accomplished using small intestine, colon, or stomach. In patients who do not have a bladder available for transplantation, an intestinal urinary conduit may be constructed. In general, intestinal conduits have a higher rate of complications including infections, acidosis, ureteral stricture, and urolithiasis. (See also Chapter 69, "Urinary Tract Reconstruction for Continence and renal Preservation.") Therefore, efforts should be made to rehabilitate the native bladder if possible.

## Indications and Approach to Native Nephrectomy

The indications for native nephrectomy include intractable hypertension, severe nephrotic syndrome, very enlarged kidneys (eg, infantile polycystic kidney disease), recurrent urinary tract infections, or pyelonephritis. Native nephrectomy may also be indicated to decrease the total urine volume following transplantation. If there is excessive urine output from the native kidneys, younger patients may have difficulty drinking enough fluids following transplantation to remain adequately hydrated.

Native nephrectomy can be performed either in advance of transplantation or at the time of the transplant. The timing is dependent on multiple factors and should be made on an individualized basis. For example, severe nephrotic syndrome results in the loss of numerous proteins in the urine including endogenous anticoagulants. As a result, these patients develop a hypercoagulable state and are more prone to vascular thrombosis. Bilateral native nephrectomy prior to transplantation allows time for recovery of normal plasma protein levels. Obviously, dialysis would need to be initiated following bilateral native nephrectomy.

Native nephrectomy prior to transplantation can often be performed via a laparoscopic approach, even in infants. In small patients undergoing intraabdominal placement of the renal allograft, native nephrectomies can be performed at the time of transplantation, just prior to implantation of the graft. In larger patients for whom an extraperitoneal iliac fossa placement of the allograft is planned, an ipsilateral native nephrectomy can be performed by cephalad extension of the incision.

## Surgical Technique and Intraoperative Management

In the pediatric population, the size of the patient as well as the suitability of the inflow and outflow vessels dictates the position of the renal allograft. The majority of grafts used in pediatric patients are adult-sized kidneys. In patients of an adequate size the preferred approach is placement of the renal allograft in the iliac fossa via an extraperitoneal approach with vascular anastomoses to the iliac vessels (Fig. 98-6). However, in children <20 kg, an adult-sized allograft may not comfortably fit within the iliac fossa and therefore intraabdominal graft placement is preferred. In this circumstance,

the distal aorta and vena cava are typically used for inflow and outflow, respectively, since the iliac vessels are small in caliber (Fig. 98-7). In the case of a small pediatric donor (<15 kg), both kidneys may be transplanted in an en-bloc fashion (pexing to prevent postoperative vascular pedicle torsion may be needed). Both kidneys are left connected to the aorta and vena cava after procurement. The suprarenal openings of the aorta and vena cava are oversewn and the inferior ends are used for anastomoses to the recipient vessels.

Intraoperative fluid and blood pressure management are important to optimize outcome following renal transplantation. A central venous line is placed for monitoring of central venous pressures (CVP) as well as providing reliable intravenous access and frequent laboratory monitoring. We generally aim to maintain the CVP in the 5 to 12 mm Hg range. However, this strategy needs to be individualized based on the hemodynamics, graft perfusion, and postoperative function of the graft. Close monitoring of blood pressure is also important. The goal is to maintain a systolic blood pressure over 90 to 100 or a mean arterial pressure over 60 to 65 which is usually achieved by assuring adequate volume status. However, in those patients with suboptimal blood pressures and adequate circulating volume, we use intravenous dopamine drip for the first 24 to 48 hours to achieve satisfactory perfusion pressures. Excessive fluid overload that may result in pulmonary edema and prolonged intubation, especially in patients with slow graft function should be avoided.

A Foley catheter is placed in the bladder with a 3-way system to allow for bladder filling at the time of the ureteral anastomosis. In anuric patients with prior bladder augmentation, the reservoir should be irrigated with antibiotic solution until the effluent fluid is reasonably clear. This detail is particularly important in patients who have not been performing intermittent irrigations at home and who are therefore at risk for purulence within their reservoir.

**Extra-Peritoneal Iliac Fossa Approach.** In the iliac fossa approach, a "hockey-stick" or curved incision is made from the midline, 1 finger-breadth above the pubic bone, extending laterally and cephalad just lateral to the border of the rectus muscle and 1 to 2 finger-breadth medial to the anterior superior iliac spine. Following incision of the subcutaneous tissues, the external oblique fascia lateral to the rectus muscle is carefully divided along with the internal oblique and transversus abdominus muscle until the peritoneum is identified. The inferior epigastric vessels can be ligated and divided if they interfere with the exposure. Injury to the spermatic cord in males should be avoided; however, the round ligament in females can be divided. The peritoneum is carefully mobilized medially off of the ilio-psoas muscle, a useful landmark. The iliac vessels reside medial to the psoas muscle. The iliac vessels are dissected from the surrounding tissues. Large lymphatic channels overlying the vessels should be ligated if divided. The renovascular anastomoses are usually to the iliac artery and vein in an end-to-side fashion using running 5-0 or 6-0 non-absorbable monofilament sutures. If the external iliac vessels are of unsatisfactory caliber, the common iliac vessels should be used. The venous anastomosis is usually performed first in order to minimize arterial clamp time. However, if technically preferable, the arterial anastomosis

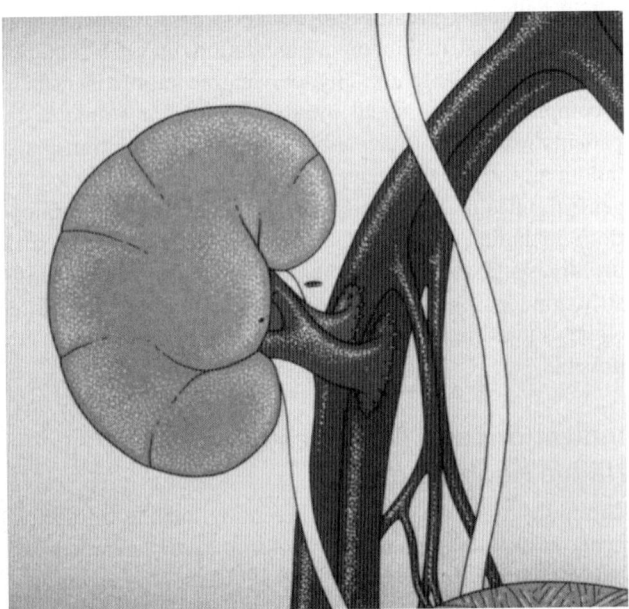

**FIGURE 98-6** End-to-side vascular anastomosis between the renal vessels and the external iliac vessels when the renal graft is placed in the iliac fossa through a retroperitoneal approach.

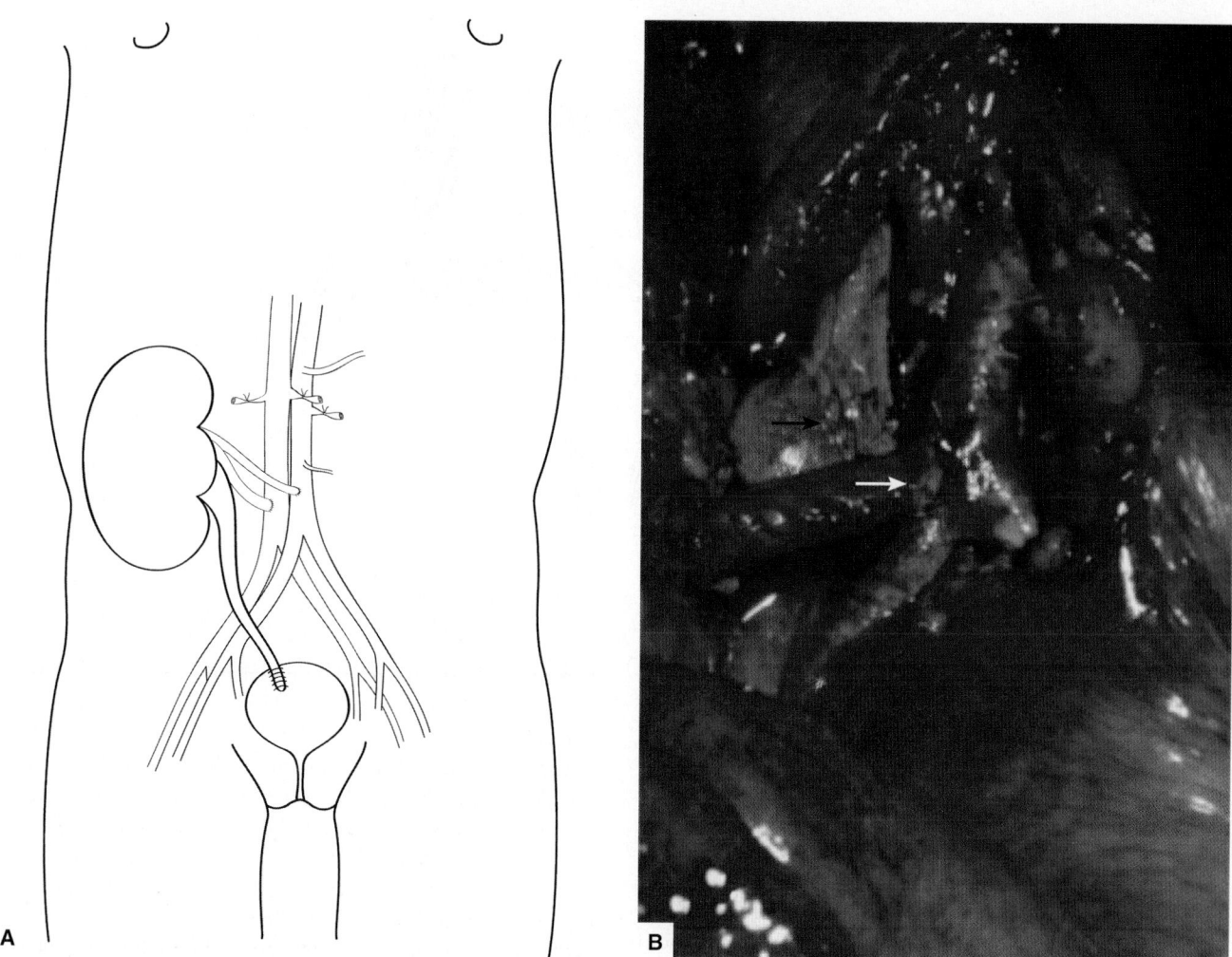

**FIGURE 98-7** **A.** End-to-side vascular anastomosis of the renal vessels to the distal aorta and vena cava in infants and small children in which the renal graft is placed in an intraabdominal position. We prefer to use a transperitoneal approach in these cases. (Reprinted with permission from Vakili K. Pediatric kidney transplantation. In: Klein A, Lewis C, Madsen JC, eds. *Organ Transplantation: A Clinical Guide*; 2011.) **B.** Intraoperative photo with end-to-side anastomoses of renal vein to inferior vena cava (black arrow) and renal artery to distal abdominal aorta (white arrow).

can certainly be performed first. Constant communication between the surgeon and the anesthesiologist is important to ensure satisfactory circulating volume and blood pressure prior to unclamping and re-perfusion of the allograft. Furosemide at 1 mg/kg and mannitol at 0.5 g/kg is administered prior to graft re-perfusion.

**Intra-Abdominal, Trans-Peritoneal Approach.** In patients weighing less than 20 kg, we prefer to place the graft in an intraabdominal position through a transperitoneal approach. The target vessels are usually the recipients' distal aorta and IVC. In this approach, either a midline or transverse abdominal incision can be used. An important consideration in deciding the type of incision is not only the access to the recipient vessels but exposure of the urinary reservoir or conduit. If indicated, either approach also allows for native nephrectomy prior to implantation of the graft. Generally, the kidney allograft is placed on the right side of the abdomen. The right colon and mesentery of the small intestine are mobilized to expose the distal IVC and abdominal aorta. Systemic heparinization (70 units/kg) is administered prior to clamping of

the recipient vessels. An end-to-side anastomosis is performed between the donor vessels and the recipient IVC and aorta using running 5-0 or 6-0 non-absorbable monofilament suture.

**Ureteral Implantation.** After satisfactory reperfusion of the kidney and appropriate hemostasis, the ureteral anastomosis is performed. The most commonly used technique for ureteral anastomosis to the bladder is the Lich extra-vesicle technique (Fig. 98-8). The bladder is distended with saline through the Foley catheter. The muscular layer of the bladder is carefully incised with electrocautery down to the level of the mucosa. The length of the muscular division which should be about 3 times the width of the spatulated ureter. The mucosa of the bladder is then incised with a knife and the fluid is suctioned out of the bladder. The ureter is anastomosed to the mucosa at the distal end of the tunnel with interrupted 5-0 absorbable monofilament sutures. The muscular layer is then closed over the ureter with interrupted 3-0 absorbable sutures. Ureteral stents are not routinely used. If the native bladder is small and non-compliant, uretero-ureterostomy/pyelostomy to the

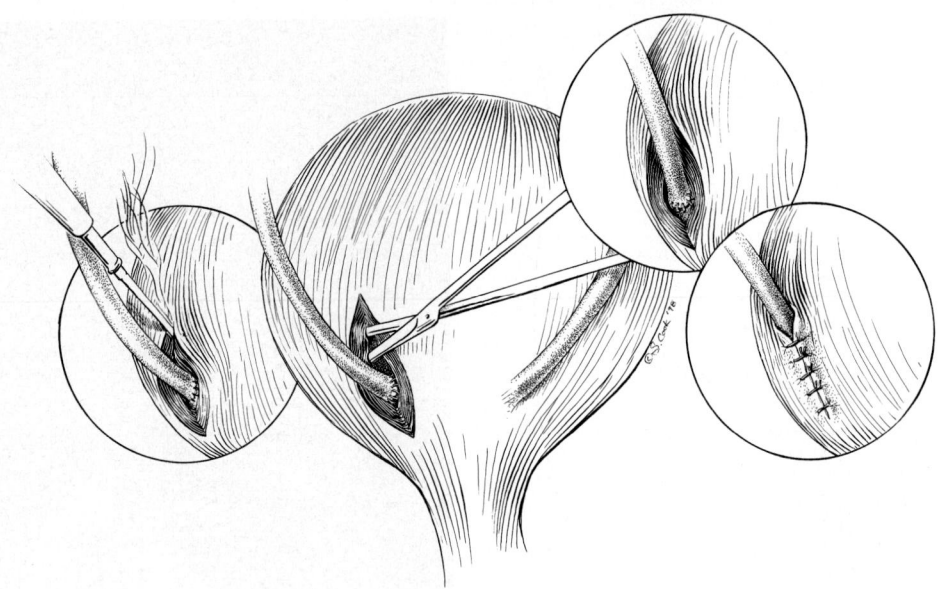

**FIGURE 98-8** Lich extravesical neoureterocystostomy.

ipsilateral native ureter/renal pelvis across a ureteral stent may be considered as long as there is no evidence of vesicoureteral reflux on the pretransplant work-up.

## Postoperative Management

It is important to maintain adequate circulating volume and perfusion pressure following renal transplantation. CVP can be used to guide fluid management with a target range of 5 to 12 mm Hg. Excessive volume overload in the operating room or in the early postoperative period, especially in small recipients, can result in pulmonary edema and the requirement for prolonged mechanical ventilatory support. Intravenous dopamine infusion can be used in the early postoperative period to maintain adequate perfusion pressures (mean arterial pressure >60-65 mm Hg) in the setting of adequate circulating fluid volume. In addition to replacement of insensible losses, urine output should be replaced for the first 1 to 3 days following transplantation to prevent hypovolemia. Output is generally replaced with ½ normal saline but adjustments can be made to the electrolyte balance based on urine and blood studies. Dextrose should be included in the insensible fluid replacement until the patient is able to tolerate enteral intake. Particular attention should be paid in patients requiring large fluid replacement due to early brisk renal allograft diuresis since they can develop substantial electrolyte abnormalities. One must be cautious about adding potassium to the urinary replacement solution to avoid the dangers of hyperkalemia. Hyperphosphatemia may be observed until normal graft function is achieved, requiring treatment with phosphate binders. However, once the graft begins to function well, the resulting diuresis may cause hypophosphatemia and hypomagnesemia which will usually require repletion of these electrolytes. Most centers perform a baseline imaging study (ultrasound or MAG3 scan) within the first 24 hours following transplantation. Further imaging is usually dictated by the clinical course.

An increase in blood creatinine concentration or a decrease in urine output in the postoperative period may be secondary to acute tubular necrosis, hypovolemia, vascular compromise, ureteral obstruction, or rejection. Based on the overall clinical scenario, appropriate diagnostic work-up should be initiated. Duplex ultrasound should be obtained to evaluate blood flow through the renal artery and vein. Ureteral obstruction with consequent hydronephrosis may also be evident on ultrasound. A nuclear medicine scan (MAG3) can also be used to assess perfusion, excretory function, or the presence of urine leak. If no mechanical cause is found for the decrease in urine output, other causes should be considered.

Post-operatively, the bladder is decompressed with an indwelling catheter for the first 4 to 6 days following operation. Patients with intestinal bladder augmentation may require longer catheterization or frequent intermittent catheterizations in order to remove the mucus from the bladder. A surgical closed suction drain is routinely placed at the time of operation. It is monitored for quality and quantity of output. If a urine leak is suspected, the creatinine concentration in the drain fluid should be assessed.

One should be aware of the relative size of the adult renal allograft to the infant recipient as depicted in Fig. 98-9.

Pretransplant peritoneal dialysis may enlarge the abdominal cavity and lessen the risk for acute compartment syndrome. However, more prolonged ventilatory and/or nutritional support may still be required.

**Immunosuppression (See also Chapter 97, "Immunology and Transplantation").** Transplant programs vary in their immunosuppression protocols. However, the majority of immunosuppression protocols involve both induction and maintenance regimens. The goal of induction therapy is to prevent T-cell activation and is initiated in the immediate perioperative or intraoperative period. Induction is usually achieved by either depleting circulating T-cells (Thymoglobulin®-rabbit derived antithymocyte globulin, Atgam®-horse-derived antilymphocyte globulin, Alemtuzumab (Campath®)-humanized anti-CD52 antibody) or blocking their activation signaling via the IL-2 receptor (basiliximab or daclizumab). IL-2 antibodies are currently the most commonly used agents for induction

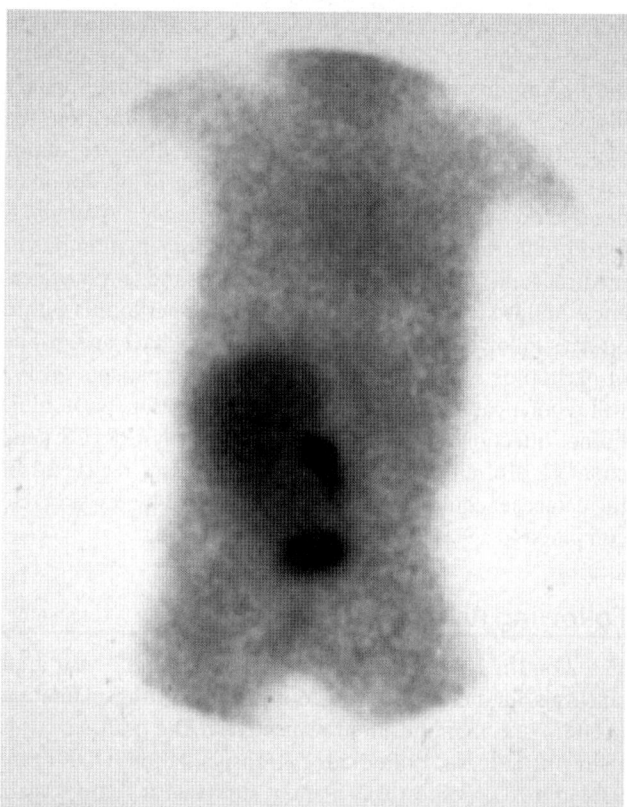

FIGURE 98-9 Postoperative renal scan of infant who received adult-sized allograft.

therapy for both living donor (51%) and deceased donor (50%) transplants.

Maintenance immunosuppression consists of a combination of agents to target several different pathways in the immune response. Traditionally, steroids have been a major part of immunosuppression following transplantation. However, with the introduction of more specific immunosuppressive agents there has been an effort to minimize or avoid steroids altogether. This trend is especially important in the pediatric population since steroids can have a profound negative impact on growth in addition to the other troublesome side effects including glucose intolerance, hypertension, aseptic bone necrosis, and impaired wound healing. The combination of prednisone, tacrolimus, and mycophenolate mofetil is still used for the majority (about 30%) of renal transplants. However, according to the NAPRTCS 2008 report, the use of prednisone has decreased from 95% in 1996 to 61% in 2007. Many pediatric centers have strategies to wean patients off of steroids within the first 1 to 2 years following transplantation. In our program, most patients are currently weaned off steroids within 7-14 days following transplantation.

## Postoperative Complications

**Delayed Graft Function.** Generally, renal allografts will achieve excellent function within the first 1 to 3 days after transplantation with normalization of serum creatinine concentration. Delay in satisfactory graft function is usually secondary to ATN; however, other causes must also be excluded. Delayed graft function (DGF) is generally defined as a recipient requiring dialysis within the first week following transplantation. Based on NAPRTCS data, DGF can be seen in 5% of living donor and about 16% of deceased donor transplants.

**Graft Thrombosis.** Vascular thrombosis of the renal vessels is a devastating event which is encountered in about 2% to 3% of pediatric renal transplant recipients. Vascular thrombosis usually occurs within the first several days following operation. The clinician should be alerted to the possibility of vascular compromise if there is a sudden decrease or cessation of urine production. The diagnosis can be established by obtaining an urgent duplex ultrasound of the kidney to evaluate patency of the vessels. In most cases, vascular thrombosis results in graft loss, requiring removal of the graft. Re-operation and thrombectomy within the first few hours following thrombosis provides the only chance for graft salvage.

**Hemorrhage.** Postoperative hemorrhage resulting in a large hematoma, especially in the retroperitoneal space, may result in compression of the renal parenchyma and renal vasculature, compromising graft function. If a compartment syndrome develops, it can place the graft at risk of ischemia, infarction, and eventual failure. Early recognition of clinically significant bleeding and prompt return to the operating room for control of bleeding and evacuation of hematoma is necessary in order to minimize graft compromise.

**Urologic Complications.** Urologic complications occur in approximately 5% to 10% of renal transplants. They include ureteral anastomotic leak, stricture, kinking, extrinsic compression, or clinically significant vesicoureteral reflux. Obstruction of the urinary flow results in decreased urine output with hydronephrosis. It may be secondary to edema at the ureterovesicle anastomosis, kinking of the ureter, or extrinsic compression from a lymphocele or hematoma. Ultrasound or MAG3 renal scan may aid in diagnosis. Depending on the cause of obstruction, insertion of a ureteral stent or percutaneous drainage of the lymphocele may be necessary to resolve the obstruction. If the above interventions do not resolve the obstruction, surgical revision of the anastomosis may be necessary. In general, pre-existing bladder or ureteral pathology will increase the risk for post-transplant urologic complications. For example, recipients with previous bladder augmentation procedures are at higher risk of developing urinary tract infections. If an intestinal segment has been used for augmentation, metabolic acidosis can develop secondary to absorption of urinary ammonia and ammonium chloride along with secretion of bicarbonate.

In the pediatric patients with ESRD and lower urinary tract dysfunction, preoperative planning and meticulous operative technique are required to minimize the risk of post-transplant urologic complications. Our patients are routinely evaluated by a pediatric urologist preoperatively who also assists in operative ureteral implantation, especially in patients with prior bladder reconstruction. We believe that this strategy is important in achieving optimal results in patients with complex urologic problems.

**Graft Rejection.** About 40% to 50% of all kidney grafts undergo an episode of rejection. The probability of rejection within the first post-transplant year has decreased over the past 25 years due to improved immunosuppression regimens. According to recent data (NAPRTCS), the probabilities of first rejection within 12 months after living donor and deceased donor transplants are 8.7 and 17.7%, respectively. Analysis of the United Network for Organ Sharing Database has revealed that about 21% of both DDKT and LDKT were treated for rejection within the first 6 months following transplantation. Risk factors for rejection following deceased donor transplantation include black race, two HLA-DR mismatches compared to no mismatches, and no induction therapy. In living donor recipients, age, HLA-DR mismatches, and post-operative ATN have been implicated as risk factors for rejection.

Graft rejection may be classified according to the mechanism of graft injury or the timing of the injury. The recipient immune system may damage the graft via cell-mediated (T cells), antibody mediated (humoral rejection), or a combination of both mechanisms. Acute rejection may manifest as a rise in serum creatinine level, decreased urine output, and in some cases, fever and graft tenderness. Once other causes of graft dysfunction are ruled out, definitive diagnosis of graft rejection can be made by graft biopsy with histological and immunohistochemical evaluation. Graft biopsy is usually performed percutaneously under ultrasound guidance.

## PATIENT OUTCOMES

### Undergoing Dialysis

Patients undergoing dialysis have worse overall survival in younger age groups. Based on NPRTCS, 3-year survival of patients on dialysis over 12 years of age is 89% compared to a 65% survival rate of patients less than 1 year of age. The most common cause of death on dialysis is cardiopulmonary disease. Within the first 6 months of dialysis initiation, the majority of patients will be either on the deceased donor list (24%) or in the process of undergoing living donor or deceased donor workup (32%). The remainder of patients is found to be unsuitable candidates for transplantation due to medical contraindications (75%) or patient and family preference. About 11% of patients on PD develop peritonitis within 30 days following initiation of PD and 50% have an episode of peritonitis within 2 years. About 20% of patients on PD will require catheter revision due to malfunction, peritonitis, tunnel infection, or leakage. Based on the NAPRTCS data, about 82% of all of the hemodialysis accesses registered in the database required a revision. AVF had a 34% revision rate compared to a 90% revision rate for AVG.

### Following Renal Transplantation

Based on the NAPRTCS 2008 report, the 1- and 5-year graft survivals for pediatric living donor kidney transplantation (LDKT) are 95% and 85%, respectively. The graft survivals following deceased donor kidney transplantation (DDKT) are 93% and 75%, respectively. Patient survivals at 1 and 5 years following transplantation are 98% and 95%, respectively. Infants younger than 24 months of age receiving a deceased donor organ have had lower survival rates in the past, but this disparity has improved significantly over the past 20 years such that the 5-year graft survival is fairly uniform across all pediatric kidney recipients.

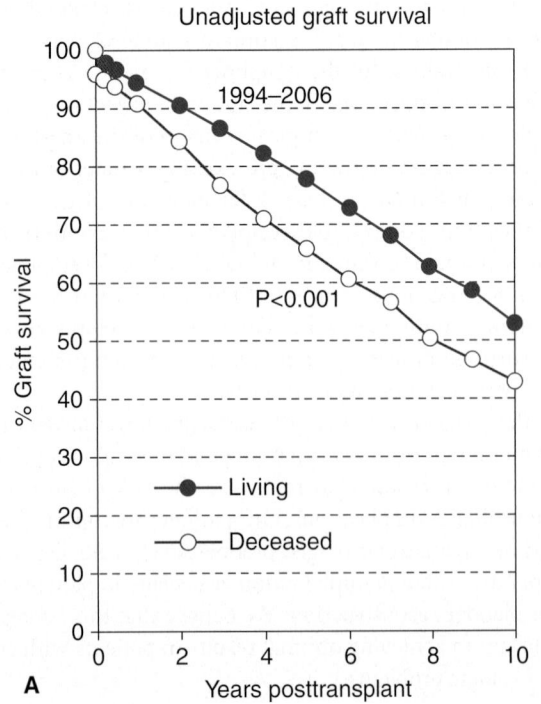

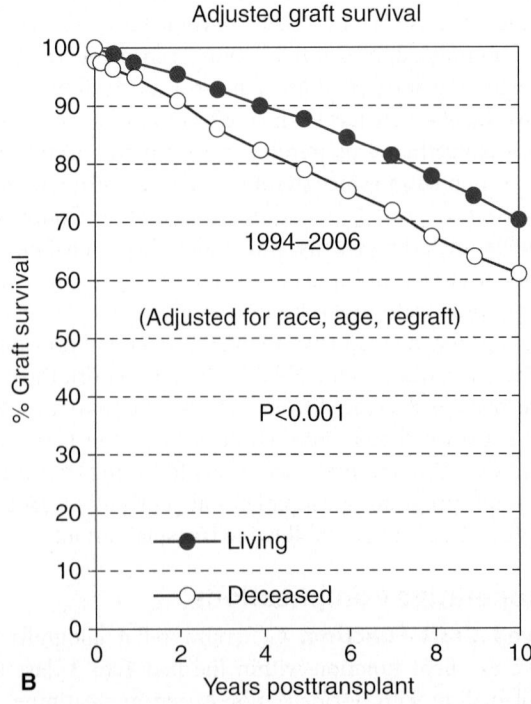

**FIGURE 98-10** (A) Unadjusted and (B) adjusted graft survival rates following LDKT and DDKT based on UNOS data. (From Hardy BE, Shah T, Cicciarelli J, et al. Kidney transplantation in children and adolescents: United Network for Organ Sharing Database. *Transpl Proc* 2009;1533–1535.)

Based on NAPRTCS data, the leading causes of death (percent of all causes) following transplantation are: cardiopulmonary (15.4%), bacterial infection (12.6%), malignancy (10.6%), viral infection (8.1%), and nonspecified infection (7.9%). The rate of malignancy is about 2.4%, with post-transplant lymphoproliferative disease comprising the majority (80%).

Chronic allograft nephropathy (CAN) is the most common cause of eventual graft failure in the pediatric transplant population (35% of all causes of graft failure). It is clinically manifested by a steady decline in renal function over several months to years. The term CAN has replaced what was previously referred to as chronic rejection. At this point, the pathophysiology of CAN is not fully understood and there are no effective treatments for its prevention or reversal.

Noncompliance increases as children enter adolescence with an incidence of 2% to 3% in the 10-14 year old age group which may result in graft failure. The frequency of noncompliance is slightly lower in LDKT compared to DDKT.

In some cases, the initial disease process leading to ESRD may recur in the renal allograft. The diseases most likely to recur and their recurrence rates include: focal segmental glomerulsclersosis (FSGS, 14-50%), atypical hemolytic uremic syndrome (20-80%), typical hemolytic uremic syndrome (0-1%), membranoproliferative glomerulosclerosis type 1 (30-77%), membranoproliferative glomerulosclerosis type 2 (66-100%), systemic lupus erythematosus (0-30%), IgA nephritis (35-60%), Henoch–Schönlein nephritis (31-100%), and primary hyperoxaluria type 1 (90-100%). Based on NAPRTCS 2008 data, recurrent disease is one of the top four causes of graft failure (6.8%). Disease recurrence may present subclinically or as a full-blown process which ultimately will lead to graft failure.

UNOS data analysis has demonstrated a 9% adjusted 5-year higher graft survival for LDKT compared to DDKT (Fig. 98-10). Based on the difference between long-term graft survivals, most clinicians recommend LDKT over DDKT whenever possible.

## SUMMARY

Most pediatric patients with ESRD will undergo multiple surgical procedures. Patients in need of dialysis require thoughtful surgical planning with regard to the choice of dialysis modality as well as its long-term maintenance. Kidney transplantation has become the optimal treatment for pediatric patients with ESRD since it provides improved long-term survival compared to dialysis as well as improved growth and development. Over the past several decades, advances in immunosuppression medications, surgical technique, and postoperative care have combined to improve both graft and patient survival. However, CAN, disease recurrence, and complications secondary to immunosuppression remain significant causes of morbidity and mortality in children following renal transplantation.

## SELECTED READINGS

Adams J, Mehls O, Wiesel M. Pediatric renal transplantation and the dysfunctional bladder. *Transpl Int* 2004;17:596–602.

Capizzi A, Zanon GF, Zacchello G, et al. Kidney transplantation in children with reconstructed bladder. *Transplantation* 2004;1113–1116.

Chand DH, Valentini RP, Kamil ES. Hemodialysis vascular access options in pediatrics: considerations for patients and practitioners. *Pediatr Nephrol* 2009;24:1121–1128.

Cochat P, Fargue S, Mestrallet G, et al. Disease recurrence in paediatric renal transplantation. *Pediatr Nephrol* 2009;24:2097–2108.

Fine RN, Martz K, and Stablein D. What have 20 years of data from the North American Pediatric Renal Transplant Cooperative Study taught us about growth following renal transplantation in infants, children, and adolescents with end-stage renal disease? *Pediatr Nephrol* 2010;25:739–746.

Hardy BE, Shah T, Cicciarelli J, et al. Kidney transplantation in children and adolescents: United Network for Organ Sharing Database. *Transpl Proc* 2009;41(5):1533–1535.

Harmon WE. Pediatric kidney transplantation. In: Avner ED, Harmon WE, Niaudet P, Yoshikawa N, eds. *Pediatric Nephrology*. 6th ed. Springer, Berlin Heidelberg, 2009.

Hijazi R, Abitbol CL, Chandar J, et al. Twenty-five years of infant dialysis: a single center experience. *J Pediatr* 2009;155:111–117.

Humar A, Matas AJ. Kidney transplantation. In: Humar A, Matas AJ, and Payne WD, eds. *Atlas of Organ Transplantation*. Springer, London, 2009.

North American Pediatric Renal Trials and Collaborative Studies (NAPRTCS) Annual Report (2008). Available at: *https://web.emmes.com/study/ped/annlrept/annlrept.html* (Accessed 1 March 2010).

Seikaly MG. Recurrence of primary disease in children after renal transplantation: An evidence-based update. *Pediatr Transpl* 2004;8:113–119.

Sheldon C, Shumyle A. Urological issues in pediatric renal transplantation. *Curr Opin Urol* 2008;18:413–418.

Strippoli GF, Tong A, Johnson D, Schena FP, Craig JC. Catheter type, placement and insertion techniques for preventing peritonitis in peritoneal dialysis patients. *Cochrane Database Syst Rev* 2004;18(4).

U S Renal Data System, USRDS 2009 Annual Data Report: Atlas of Chronic Kidney Disease and End-Stage Renal Disease in the United States, National Institutes of Health, National Institute of Diabetes and Digestive and Kidney Diseases, Bethesda, MD, 2009.

Washburn KK, Currier H, Salter KJ, Brandt ML. Surgical technique for peritoneal dialysis catheter placement in the pediatric patient: a North American survey. *Adv Peritoneal Dialysis* 2004;20:218–221.

# Liver Transplantation

# CHAPTER 99

*Greg M. Tiao*

## KEY POINTS

1. Though liver transplantation remains a technically challenging operative procedure and patients are complex in their perioperative management, the use of whole organ, reduced size, split liver, and even living donors has resulted in an overall improved patient survival approaching 90% for infants and children alike. These techniques have also reduced waiting list mortality.

2. The indications for liver transplantation have become somewhat more liberal and have improved outcomes for children with hepatoblastoma, a pediatric disease with a here-to-fore dismal prognosis.

3. Improved immunosuppression includes multiple drugs and in some centers even steroid-free immunosuppression. These protocols have limited the adverse impact of allograft rejection while minimizing the complications of immunosuppression including infection and PTLD. Chronic rejection awaits a better solution.

Over the past 30 years, orthotopic liver transplantation (OLT) in the pediatric population has evolved from a heroic last ditch intervention to become the current standard of care. The pioneering development of surgical procedures such as reduced-size, living donor (LD), and split liver transplantation along with the evolution of immunosuppressive management has improved 1-year survival rates to more than 90%. Because short-term outcomes have improved so dramatically, attention is now focused on the long-term, optimizing quality of life and cognitive development.

## INDICATIONS FOR TRANSPLANTATION

Table 99-1 reviews primary diagnoses leading to pediatric transplantation. These disease entities define the bimodal age distribution of pediatric transplant recipients. Infants and children in the first few years of life represent patients with biliary atresia unresponsive to portoenterostomy, unresectable

hepatoblastoma and, occasionally, rapidly progressive hepatic failure secondary to metabolic abnormalities such as neonatal tyrosinemia or neonatal hepatic vascular tumors. Older children and adolescents present with metabolic disturbances, fulminant liver failure, and cirrhosis from underlying chronic liver disease.

## Biliary Atresia

Children with extrahepatic biliary atresia constitute at least 50% of the pediatric liver transplant population. Successful biliary drainage via Kasai portoenterostomy is the most important factor governing preservation of liver function and long-term survival (See also Chapter 56—"Biliary Atresia and Choledochal Cyst"). Primary transplantation without portoenterostomy is not recommended in patients with biliary atresia unless the diagnosis is made at an age greater than 120 days and a liver biopsy shows advanced cirrhosis. Patients with progressive disease after a portoenterostomy are offered OLT. The sequential use of these 2 procedures optimizes overall survival and organ utilization. Patients diagnosed with biliary atresia who require transplantation form two cohorts: (1) infants with a failed portoenterostomy have recurrent bacterial cholangitis, ascites, rapidly progressive portal hypertension, malnutrition and hepatic synthetic failure require OLT within the first 2 years of life and (2) children with an initial successful portoenterostomy have an improved prognosis but develop cirrhosis with eventual manifestations of end-stage liver disease and require OLT in late childhood and adolescence. It is estimated that 15% to 20% of all biliary atresia patients who have a successful portoenterostomy may survive without eventual OLT.

## Alagille Syndrome

Alagille syndrome (angiohepatic dysplasia) is an autosomal dominant genetic disorder manifest as bile duct paucity leading to progressive cholestasis and pruritus, xanthomas, malnutrition, and growth failure. Occasionally, severe growth retardation, hypercholesterolemia, and pruritus can compromise the patient's overall well-being to the point that transplantation is valuable. Evaluation must include assessment for congenital cardiac disease and renal insufficiency, both of which are associated with this syndrome. Hepatocellular carcinoma also has been reported in these patients.

| TABLE 99-1 | Indications for Liver Transplantation at CCHMC from 2000 to 2010 | |
|---|---|---|
| Primary Diagnosis | Number of Patients | % of Total |
| **Neonatal cholestasis** | | |
| Biliary atresia | 84 | 31.3 |
| Alagille syndrome | 10 | 3.7 |
| Idiopathic | 1 | 0.4 |
| Primary sclerosing cholangitis | 9 | 3.4 |
| TPN-induced | 5 | 1.9 |
| **Metabolic Disease** | | |
| Alpha1 anti-trypsin deficiency | 16 | 6.0 |
| Tyrosinemia | 3 | 1.1 |
| Glycogen storage disease—IV | 3 | 1.1 |
| Hyperoxaluria | 1 | 0.4 |
| Wilson disease | 2 | 0.8 |
| Cystic fibrosis | 2 | 0.8 |
| Urea cycle disorders | 11 | 4.1 |
| **Acute Liver Failure** | | |
| Untyped | 30 | 11.2 |
| Drug-induced | 2 | 0.8 |
| Other | 2 | 0.8 |
| **Hepatitis** | | |
| Neonatal | 2 | 0.8 |
| Autoimmune | 11 | 4.1 |
| Hepatitis C | 1 | 0.4 |
| **Tumors** | | |
| Hepatoblastoma | 20 | 7.5 |
| Hepatocellular carcinoma | 3 | 1.1 |
| Vascular | 3 | 1.1 |
| Other | 4 | 1.5 |
| **Retransplantation** | | |
| Primary nonfunction | 3 | 1.1 |
| Hepatic artery thrombosis | 8 | 3.0 |
| Chronic rejection | 9 | 3.4 |
| Biliary tract complications | 2 | 0.8 |
| **Other** | 21 | 7.8 |
| **Total** | **268** | |

Experience using external biliary diversion or internal ileal bypass accompanied by ursodeoxycholic acid therapy has demonstrated a significant decrease in both pruritus and complications of hypercholesterolemia. Both of these procedures may ameliorate the ongoing liver destruction and cirrhosis, further decreasing the need for liver transplantation. The vast improvement in growth and nutrition and the resolution of pruritus, hypercholesterolemia, and xanthoma results in quality-of-life issues to be criteria for consideration for OLT.

## Metabolic Disease

The leading indication for hepatic transplantation in older children is hepatic-based metabolic disease. In these patients, OLT not only is lifesaving but also accomplishes phenotypic and functional cure. A review of these diseases is given in Table 99-2. Hepatic replacement to correct the metabolic defect should be considered before other organ systems are affected and before the development of complications that would preclude transplantation. Although results of transplantation are excellent in the metabolic disease subgroup, replacement of the entire liver to correct single enzyme deficiencies is an inefficient but presently necessary procedure. Current research efforts may show that orthotopic partial hepatic replacement, hepatocyte transplantation, or gene therapy may better serve this patient population. Patients with extrahepatic manifestations of their disease, such as cystic fibrosis, are occasionally helped by liver transplantation, although their prognosis is a function of their primary illness.

## Fulminant Hepatic Failure

Patients with fulminant acute hepatic failure (ALF) without recognized antecedent liver disease present diagnostic and prognostic difficulties. Rapid clinical deterioration frequently makes establishment of a definitive diagnosis

| TABLE 99-2 | Transplantation for Metabolic Disease |
|---|---|
| Wilson disease | |
| $\alpha_1$-Antitrypsin deficiency | |
| Crigler–Najjar syndrome (type I) | |
| Tyrosinemia | |
| Cystic fibrosis | |
| Glycogen storage disease-IV | |
| Branched-chain amino acid catabolism disorders | |
| Hemophilia A | |
| Protoporphyria | |
| Homozygous hypercholesterolemia | |
| Urea cycle enzyme deficiencies | |
| Primary hyperoxaluria | |
| Iron storage disease | |

Modified from Ryckman F. Pediatric Liver Transplantation. In Blasitreri WF, Ohi R, Todani T, Tsuchida Y, eds. Hepatobiliary, pancreatic and splenic disease in children: medical and surgical management. Elsevier, 1997:395–399.

impossible before urgent transplantation is needed. Causes of ALF include untyped acute viral hepatitis, drug toxicity, toxin exposure, and immune natural killer cell dysfunction. The prognosis for these patients is difficult to predict with potentially a suboptimal neurologic outcome.

Use of intracranial pressure (ICP) monitoring in patients with progressive encephalopathy has allowed early recognition and treatment of increased ICP. Monitoring should be instituted for patients with advancing grade III encephalopathy. Intracranial monitoring is continued intraoperatively and for 24 to 48 hours after OLT because significant increases in ICP have been identified throughout the entire clinical course. Failure to maintain a cerebral perfusion pressure (mean blood pressure—ICP) of greater than 50 mm Hg and an ICP less than 20 mm Hg has been associated with poor neurologic recovery. Efforts to identify and perform transplantation in children before encephalopathy develops are of utmost importance. When candidates are identified before irreversible neurologic abnormalities develop, the results of transplantation are dramatic. Hepatocyte transplantation can provide neurologic protection during organ acquisition or while awaiting spontaneous recovery.

## Malignancy

Transplantation in children for primary hepatic malignancy has increased markedly as multiple recent studies have demonstrated efficacy. Transplantation for hepatoblastoma is recommended for individuals with a neoplasm confined to the liver that after adjuvant chemotherapy remains unresectable by conventional means. In selected instances, individuals with isolated resectable metastatic lung disease or those in whom adjuvant chemotherapy has induced resolution of metastasis can be considered. Factors associated with a favorable prognosis include an absence of prior surgical resection attempts and unifocal rather than multifocal involvement. A favorable response to pretransplant chemotherapy also suggests a more favorable prognosis. In our experience, transplantation and postoperative chemotherapy has led to an overall survival of 88%. Recurrent disease has historically accounted for most of the postoperative mortality.

Transplantation for hepatocellular carcinoma is complicated by less successful chemotherapy options and frequent extrahepatic involvement. The reported 2-year survival rates of 20% to 30% are markedly different from the experience with hepatoblastoma. Most deaths are due to recurrent disease within the allograft or extrahepatic spread. When a hepatocellular carcinoma is discovered incidentally within a cirrhotic liver at the time of hepatectomy, the prognosis is unaffected by the tumor.

Patients with vascular tumors represent a group with diffuse pathology who can benefit from transplantation. Children with progressive, intractable high output heart failure caused by nonneoplastic vascular malformations/hemangioendotheliomas of the liver offer a unique opportunity for complete removal of the diseased liver and correction of congestive heart failure. In our experience, transplantation offers better long-term survival when compared with hepatic artery embolization, which can precipitate widespread hepatic necrosis. Pretransplant biopsy is essential to exclude angiosarcoma.

## CONTRAINDICATIONS

Contraindications to transplantation include: (1) primary unresectable extrahepatic malignancy, (2) progressive terminal nonhepatic disease, (3) uncontrolled systemic sepsis, and (4) irreversible neurologic injury. Relative contraindications to transplantation that must be individually evaluated include: (1) serology positive for human immunodeficiency virus (HIV), (2) advanced or partially treated systemic infection, and (3) severe psychosocial abnormalities.

## PREOPERATIVE PREPARATION

Efforts to correct abnormalities noted during candidate evaluation decrease both the operative risk and postoperative complications. Complications of portal hypertension and malnutrition are vigorously treated. Assessment of prior viral exposure and meticulous attention to the delivery of all normal childhood immunizations, particularly the live-virus vaccines, are imperative, if time allows, before OLT. Additionally, patients receive a one-time inoculation with pneumococcal vaccine, as well as appropriate administration of hepatitis B vaccine. Preoperative assessment of specific cardiopulmonary reserve and hepatic vascular anatomy is also necessary.

## OPERATIVE CONSIDERATIONS

### Donor Options

The largest single factor that limits the availability of OLT is an inadequate supply of donor organs. The number of patients awaiting liver transplantation continues to increase while available donor resources have not kept pace. The limited supply of available donor organs has driven the advancement of many innovative surgical procedures. The development of reduced-size liver transplantation allowed significant expansion of the donor pool for infants and small children. This not only improved the availability of donor organs but also allowed access to donors with improved stability and organ function. Evolution of these operative techniques allowed the development of both split-liver transplantation and LD transplantation (Fig. 99-1). In the hands of experienced transplant teams, these technical variant grafts have success rates similar to that of whole organ transplantation.

### Donor Selection

Assessment of donor organ suitability is undertaken by evaluating clinical information and biochemical tests of hepatocellular function. The clinical factors reviewed identify donors who are at the limits of age, have had prolonged intensive care hospitalization with potential sepsis, and have vasomotor instability requiring excessive vasoconstricting inotropic agents. Donor liver biopsy is helpful in questionable cases to identify preexisting liver disease or steatosis.

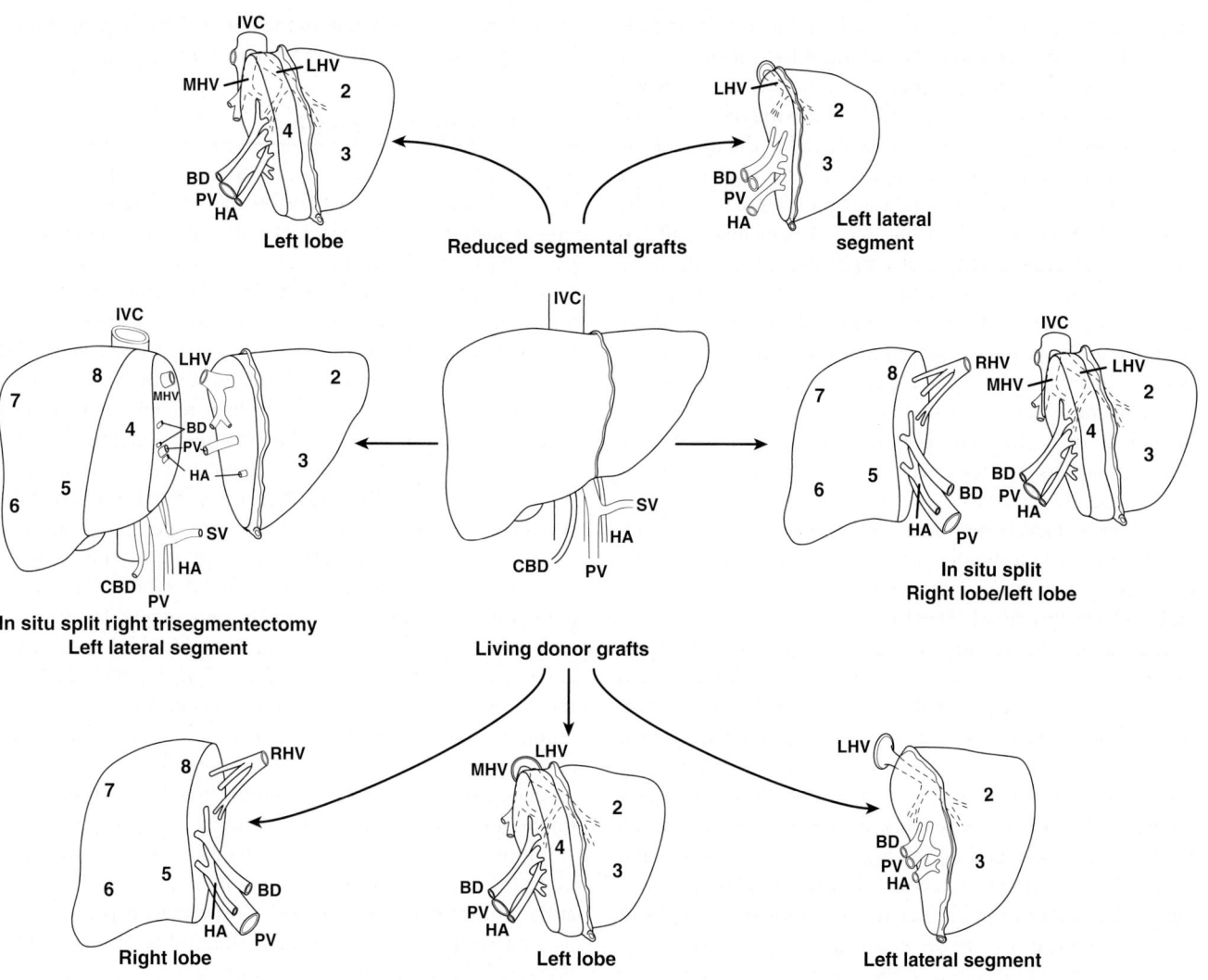

**FIGURE 99-1** Anatomic variants for liver transplantation.

Anatomic replacement of the native liver in the orthotopic position requires selection or surgical preparation of the donor liver to fill but not to exceed available space in the recipient. When using full-sized allografts, a donor weight range 15% to 20% above or below that of the recipient is usually appropriate. Surgical preparation of reduced-size liver allografts is based on the anatomy of the hepatic vasculature and bile ducts. Prolonged cold ischemic preservation allows the safe application of the extensive hypothermic bench surgical procedure necessary for reduction technology. The need for this preparation prolongs cold ischemia time which limits the acceptability of "marginal donors." The 3 reduced-size allografts used clinically, prepared ex vivo, are the right lobe, the left lobe, and the left lateral segment. The right lobe graft, using segments 5 to 8, can be accommodated when the weight difference is no greater than 2:1 between the donor and the recipient. The thickness of the right lobe makes this allograft of limited usefulness in small recipients. Similar right lobe anatomic grafts from LDs have become widely used in adults. The left lobe, using segments 1 to 4, is applicable with a donor-to-recipient (D/R) disparity from 4:1 to 5:1, and a left lateral segment (segments 2 and 3) can be used with up to a 10:1 D/R weight difference. For a left or right lobe graft,

the parenchymal resection follows the anatomic lobar plane through the gallbladder fossa to the vena cava. The middle hepatic vein is retained with the graft in all left lobe and many right lobe preparations. The bile duct, portal vein, and hepatic artery are divided and ligated at the right or left confluence. The vena cava is left incorporated with the allograft in both right and left lobe preparations. Vena caval reduction by posterior caval wall resection and closure is only occasionally necessary. When using left lateral segment allografts, the parenchymal dissection follows the right margin of the falciform ligament, with preservation of the left hilar structures. Direct implantation of the left hepatic vein into the combined orifice of the right and middle/left hepatic veins in the recipient vena cava is preferred; the donor vena cava is not retained with this segmental allograft.

Split-liver grafting involves the preparation of 2 allografts from a single donor. The ex situ split procedure divides the right lobe allograft (segments 5 to 8) from the left lateral segment allograft (segments 2 and 3) after the whole donor organ has been procured. Because this division is undertaken under vascular hypothermic conditions without hepatic perfusion, the vascular integrity of segment 4 is difficult to assess, and it is on occasion discarded. Conventional techniques for implanting the respective allografts are then used. The successful experience with in situ division of the LD organ left lateral segment is a basis for the in situ split procedure. In most cases, the left lateral segment is prepared identically to a living related donor. The viability of segment 4 can be examined at the time of the division, and it is usually incorporated with the right lobe graft to increase the cellular mass of the allograft. More recently, the proven effectiveness of the living related right lobe graft has resulted in in situ splits in which a right and left lobe grafts are prepared. Under these circumstances, the right lobe is implanted in a smaller adult recipient while the left lobe is utilized in an older child. Because these procedures add considerably to the donor procurement time, and increase the skills required of the donor operative team, it is more demanding and occasionally difficult to orchestrate successfully. Despite these challenges, this approach is the preferred method for split-liver donor preparation. The benefits of split-liver transplantation are best achieved when ideal donors are selected. The results from both in situ and ex situ techniques are similar, with both techniques now having patient survival for both allografts of 90% to 93% and graft survival rates of 86% to 89%.

The use of LDs has increased greatly in last years, with the safety and success of this procedure now well established (Fig. 99-2). In most pediatric cases, the left lateral segment donated from an adult is used as the graft. In situ dissection of the left lateral segment, preserving the donor vascular integrity until the parenchymal division is completed, is undertaken. At the time of harvest, the left hepatic vein is divided from the vena cava, and the left branch of the portal vein and proper hepatic artery are removed with the allograft. Vascular continuity of the hepatic arterial branches to segment IV is maintained if possible. Recently, increased experience has been gained in using the right lobe as an LD allograft for larger recipients such as adolescents and adults. This more extensive operation has proven to be a challenge to the donor and recipient alike, with complication and mortality rates significantly exceeding that of left lateral segmentectomy. Despite these risks, the number of right lobe LD recipients now greatly exceeds the number of children receiving LD grafts. Recent appreciation of the donor risk of this operation has moderated the early rapid rise in operative cases.

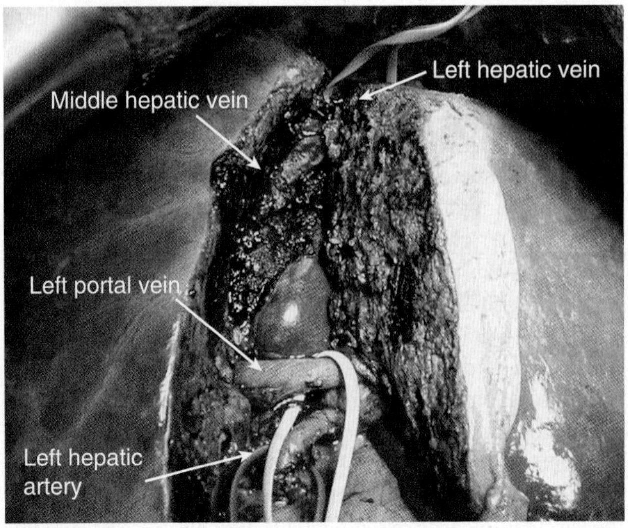

## The Recipient Procedure

The transplant procedure is carried out through a bilateral subcostal with midline extension incision. Meticulous ligation of portosystemic collaterals and vascularized adhesions is necessary to avoid slow but relentless hemorrhage. Dissection of the hepatic hilum, with provision for division of the hepatic artery and portal vein above their bifurcation, allows maximal recipient vessel length. The bile duct, when present, is divided high in the hilum to preserve the length and vasculature of the distal duct in case it is needed for later reconstruction. Preservation of the Roux-en-Y in biliary atresia patients who have undergone portoenterostomy simplifies biliary reconstruction. Complete mobilization of the liver, with dissection of the suprahepatic vena cava to the diaphragm and the infrahepatic vena cava to the renal veins, completes the hepatectomy. In children with serious vascular instability who cannot tolerate caval occlusion or in patients undergoing transplantation using a left lateral segment, "piggy-back" implantation is required. In this procedure, the recipient vena cava is left intact, and partial caval occlusion allows end-to-side implantation of a donor hepatic vein patch. Access to the infrarenal aorta to implant the celiac axis of the donor liver or iliac artery vascular conduits, provided by mobilizing the right colon and duodenum, is our preference for arterial reconstruction.

Use of venovenous bypass is reserved for recipients weighing more than 40 kg who demonstrate hemodynamic instability at the time of caval interruption. Venovenous bypass is rarely necessary in patients who weigh less than 40 kg. Removal of the diseased liver is completed after vascular isolation is achieved. Retroperitoneal hemostasis is achieved before implanting the donor liver. The donor liver is implanted by using conventional vascular techniques and monofilament suture for the vascular anastomosis. In small recipients, interrupted suture techniques, monofilament dissolving suture material, and a "growth factor" knot have all been used to allow for vessel growth. When left lateral segment reduced-size grafts are used, the left hepatic vein orifice is anastomosed directly to the anterolateral surface of the infradiaphragmatic IVC. The left lateral segment allograft is later fixed when necessary to the undersurface of the diaphragm to prevent torsion and venous obstruction of this anastomosis. Fixation is un-necessary with right/left lobe grafts or with a whole organ.

Before completing the vena caval anastomosis, the hyperkalemic preservation solution is flushed from the graft by using 500 to 1000 mL of hypothermic normokalemic intravenous (IV) solutions. When using full-sized grafts in older patients, we prefer to complete all venous anastomoses before reconstructing the hepatic artery. In reduced-size allografts and in small recipients in whom we prefer direct aortic vascular inflow reconstruction, the hepatic arterial anastomosis is completed before reconstructing the portal vein to improve visibility of the infrarenal aorta without placing traction on the portal vein anastomosis. We prefer to complete all anastomoses during vascular isolation before organ reperfusion, although some transplant teams reperfuse after venous reconstruction is complete.

Middle hepatic vein
Left hepatic vein
Left portal vein
Left hepatic artery

**FIGURE 99-2** Living-related left lateral segment graft.

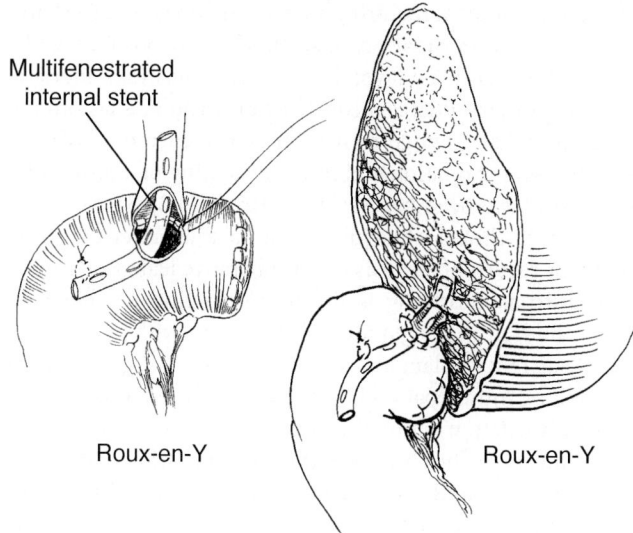

Multifenestrated
internal stent

Roux-en-Y                    Roux-en-Y

**FIGURE 99-3** Bile duct reconstruction.

Before re-establishing circulation to the allograft, anesthetic adjustments must be made to address the large volume of blood needed to refill the liver and the presence of hypothermic solutions released at reperfusion. Inotropic support with dopamine (5-10 mg/kg/min) is begun. Calcium and sodium bicarbonate are administered to combat the effects of hyperkalemia from any remaining preservation solution and systemic acidosis after aortic and vena caval occlusion. Sufficient blood volume expansion, administered as packed red blood cells to increase the central venous pressure (CVP) to 15 to 20 cm $H_2O$ and the hematocrit to 40%, minimizes the development of hypotension on unclamping and prevents dilutional anemia. Communication between the surgical and anesthesia teams facilitates a smooth sequential reestablishment of vena caval, portal venous, and then arterial recirculation to the allograft.

Biliary reconstruction in patients with biliary atresia or in those weighing less than 25 kg is achieved through an end-to-side choledochojejunostomy by using interrupted dissolving monofilament sutures. A multifenestrated polymeric silicone (Silastic) internal biliary stent is placed before completing the anastomosis (Fig. 99-3). In most cases, the prior Roux-en-Y can be used, with a 30- to 35-cm length being preferred. Primary bile duct reconstruction without stenting is used in older patients.

When closing the abdomen, increased intra-abdominal pressure should be avoided. In many cases, avoidance of fascial closure and the use of mobilized skin flaps and running monofilament skin closure are advisable. Musculofascial abdominal closure can be completed before patient discharge.

## IMMUNOSUPPRESSIVE MANAGEMENT

Most centers use an immunosuppressive protocol based on the administration of multiple complementary medications (See also Chapter 97, "Immunology and Transplantation"). All use

corticosteroids and cyclosporine or tacrolimus. Additional antimetabolites (azathioprine, mycophenolate) are used when more antirejection treatment is needed. The use of polyclonal or monoclonal induction therapy is less frequent because of a better understanding of immunosuppressive potency.

## POSTOPERATIVE COMPLICATIONS

### Primary Nonfunction

Primary nonfunction (PNF) of the hepatic allograft implies the absence of metabolic and synthetic activity after transplantation. Complete nonfunction requires immediate retransplantation before irreversible coagulopathy and cerebral edema occur. Lesser degrees of allograft dysfunction occur more frequently and can be associated with several donor, recipient, and operative factors. The status of the donor liver contributes significantly to the potential for PNF. Ischemic injury secondary to hypotension, hypoxia, or direct tissue injury is critical in donor assessment. Donor liver steatosis has been recognized as a factor contributing to severe dysfunction or nonfunction. Macrovesicular steatosis on donor liver biopsy is somewhat more common in adult than in pediatric donors and when severe, is recognized grossly by a yellow, greasy consistency of the donor liver. The risk of PNF increases as the degree of fatty infiltration increases. Microscopic findings are classified as mild if less than 30% of the hepatocytes have fatty infiltration, moderate if 30% to 60% are involved, and severe if more than 60% of the hepatocytes have fatty infiltration. Livers with severe fatty infiltration should be discarded, and donors with moderate involvement are used with caution, with the degree of steatosis and the condition of the recipient dictating allograft use. Microvesicular steatosis does not predict PNF.

### Vascular Thrombosis

Hepatic artery thrombosis (HAT) occurs in children 3 to 4 times more frequently than in adults, occurring most often within the first 30 post-operative days. Factors influencing the development of HAT are listed in Table 99-3. HAT has a variable clinical picture that may include (1) fulminant allograft failure, (2) biliary disruption or obstruction, or (3) systemic sepsis. Doppler ultrasound (US) imaging has been accurate in identifying arterial thrombosis, and it is used as the primary screening modality to assess blood flow after transplantation. Acute HAT with allograft failure often requires urgent retransplantation. Successful thrombectomy and allograft salvage is possible if reconstruction is undertaken before allograft necrosis. Biliary complications are particularly common after HAT. Ischemic biliary disruption with intraparenchymal biloma formation or anastomotic disruption is seen with cholestasis associated with systemic sepsis. Percutaneous drainage and biliary stenting may control bile leakage and infection. Late postoperative thrombosis can be asymptomatic or be seen with slowly progressive bile duct stenosis. Rarely, allograft necrosis occurs. Arterial collaterals from the Roux-en-Y limb can provide a source of revascularization of the thrombosed allograft through hilar

| TABLE 99-3 | Factors Influencing Hepatic Artery Thrombosis |
|---|---|
| Donor/Recipient age/Weight allograft type | |
| Whole organ > reduced size | |
| Living donor ≥ reduced size | |
| Anastomotic Anatomy | |
| Primary hepatic artery > direct aortic | |
| Allograft edema—Increased Vascular Resistance | |
| Ischemic injury secondary to prolonged preservation; prolonged implantation | |
| Rejection | |
| Fluid overload | |
| Recipient hypotension hypercoagulability | |
| Administration of coagulation factors, fresh-frozen plasma | |
| Procoagulant factor deficiencies | |

collaterals. These collateral channels develop during the first postoperative months, making late thrombosis a silent clinical event. Conversely, disruption of this collateral supply during operative reconstruction of the central bile ducts in patients with HAT can precipitate hepatic ischemia and parenchymal necrosis. When HAT is asymptomatic, careful follow-up is indicated.

Portal vein thrombosis is uncommon in whole organ allografts unless prior portosystemic shunting has altered the flow within the splanchnic vascular bed or unless severe portal vein stenosis in the recipient has impaired flow to the allograft. Preexisting portal vein thrombosis in the recipient can be overcome by thrombectomy, portal vein replacement, or extra-anatomic venous bypass. In biliary atresia recipients, preexisting portal vein hypoplasia is best corrected by anastomosis to the confluence of the splenic and superior mesenteric veins in the recipient. When inadequate portal vein length is present on the donor organ, iliac vein interposition grafts are used. Early thrombosis after transplantation requires immediate anastomotic revision and thrombectomy. Discrepancies in venous size imposed by reduced-size allografts can be modified to allow anastomotic construction. Deficiencies of anticoagulant proteins, such as protein C and S, and antithrombin III deficiency in the recipient also must be excluded as a contributing cause for vascular thrombosis. Failure to recognize portal thrombosis can lead to either allograft demise or, on a more chronic basis, significant portal hypertension with hemorrhagic sequelae or intractable ascites.

## Biliary Complications

Complications related to biliary reconstruction occur in approximately 10% of pediatric liver transplant recipients. Their spectrum and treatment are determined by the status of the hepatic artery and the type of allograft used. Although whole and reduced-size allografts have an equivalent risk of biliary complications, the spectrum of complications differs. Primary bile duct reconstruction is the preferred biliary reconstruction in adults, but it is less commonly used in children. It has the advantage of preserving the sphincter of Oddi, decreasing the incidence of enteric reflux and subsequent

cholangitis, and not requiring an intestinal anastomosis. Early experience with primary choledochocholedochostomy without a T-tube has been favorable. Late complications after any type of primary ductal reconstruction include anastomotic stricture, biliary sludge formation, and recurrent cholangitis. Endoscopic dilation and internal stenting of anastomotic strictures have been successful in early postoperative cases. Roux-en-Y choledochojejunostomy is the preferred treatment for recurrent stenosis or postoperative leak. Roux-en-Y choledochojejunostomy is the reconstruction of choice in small children and is required in all patients with biliary atresia. Recurrent cholangitis, a theoretical risk, suggests anastomotic or intrahepatic biliary stricture formation or small bowel obstruction within the Roux or distal to the Roux-en-Y anastomosis. In the absence of these complications, cholangitis is uncommon. Reconstruction of the bile ducts in patients with reduced-size allografts is more complex. Division of the bile duct in close proximity to the cut-surface margin of the allograft, with careful preservation of the biliary duct collateral circulation, decreases but does not eliminate ductal stricture formation secondary to ductal ischemia (Fig. 99-3). Operative revision of the biliary anastomosis and reimplantation of the bile ducts into the Roux-en-Y is necessary. Percutaneous transhepatic cholangiography is essential to define the intrahepatic ductal anatomy before operative revision, and temporary catheter decompression of the obstructed bile ducts allows treatment of cholangitis and elective reconstruction. Operative reconstruction is accompanied by transhepatic passage of exteriorized multifenestrated biliary ductal stents, which remain in place until reconstructive success is documented and late stenosis is unlikely. Dissection remote from the vasobiliary sheath in the donor has significantly decreased the incidence of this complication.

Biliary complications have been seen with an increased frequency after living donation in pediatric recipients. The left lateral segment 2 and 3 bile ducts are frequently separate at the plane of parenchymal division. The need for individual drainage of these small biliary ducts makes the development of late anastomotic stenosis more frequent. Individual segmental strictures may not lead to jaundice in the recipient but rather are identified by elevated g-glutamyl transferase enzymes or through US surveillance. Reoperation after ductal dilatation is necessary.

## Acute Cellular Rejection

Allograft rejection is characterized by the histologic triad of endothelialitis, portal triad lymphocyte infiltration with bile duct injury, and hepatic parenchymal cell damage. Allograft biopsy is essential to establish the diagnosis before treatment. The rapidity of the rejection process and its response to therapy dictate the intensity and duration of antirejection treatment. Acute rejection occurs in approximately two-thirds of patients after OLT. The primary treatment of rejection is a short course of high-dose steroids. Bolus doses administered over a period of several days with a rapid taper to baseline therapy is successful in 75% to 80% of cases. When refractory or recurrent rejection occurs, antilymphocyte therapy with the monoclonal antibody OKT-3 or Thymoglobulin is successful in 90% of cases.

## Chronic Rejection

Uniform diagnosis and management of chronic rejection is complicated by the lack of a consistent definition or clinical course. Chronic rejection occurs in 5% to 10% of transplanted patients. Its incidence appears to be decreasing in all transplant groups, perhaps related to better overall immunosuppressive strategies. Some suggestion has been made that the use of primary Tacrolimus-based immunosuppression is a key element in this apparent decrease. Risk factors for the development of rejection are many, and no factor predicts the outcome of treatment. The chronic rejection rate was significantly lower in recipients of LD grafts than in recipients of cadaveric grafts; African-American recipients had a significantly higher rate of chronic rejection than did white recipients; and the number of acute rejection episodes, transplantation for autoimmune disease, occurrence of post-transplantation lymphoproliferative disorder (PTLD), and cytomegalovirus (CMV) infection also were significant risk factors for chronic rejection. The primary clinical manifestation is a progressive increase in biliary ductal enzymes (alkaline phosphatase, g-glutamyl transferase) and progressive cholestasis. Retransplantation is occasionally necessary but rarely an emergency.

## Infectious Complications

Infections remain a common source of morbidity and mortality after transplantation. Multiple-organism infection is common, as are concurrent infections by different infectious agents. Bacterial infections occur in the immediate post-transplant period and are most often caused by gram-negative enteric organisms, enterococcus, or staphylococcus species. Intra-abdominal abscesses or infected collections of serum along the cut surface of the reduced-size allograft are best addressed with extraperitoneal or laparotomy drainage; percutaneous drainage has been less successful in our experience. Intrahepatic abscesses suggest hepatic artery stenosis or thrombosis, and treatment is directed by the vascular status of the allograft and associated bile duct abnormalities. Sepsis originating at sites of invasive monitoring lines can be minimized by replacing or removing all intraoperative lines soon after transplantation. Antibacterial prophylactic antibiotics are discontinued as soon as possible to prevent the development of resistant organisms.

Fungal sepsis represents a significant potential problem in the early post-transplant period. Aggressive protocols for pretransplant prophylaxis are based on the concept that fungal infections originate from organisms colonizing the GI tract of the recipient. Selective bowel decontamination was successful in eliminating pathogenic gram-negative bacteria from the GI tract in 87% of adult patients; in all cases, Candida was eliminated. These regimens are commonly used in the preoperative preparation for combined liver/small intestinal transplantation. Fungal infection most often occurs in patients requiring multiple operative procedures and in those who have had multiple antibiotic courses. Development of fungemia or urosepsis requires retinal and cardiac investigation and a search for renal fungal involvement; antifungal therapy should be promptly undertaken. Severe fungal infection has a mortality rate greater than 80%, making early treatment essential. All patients undergoing OLT should receive antifungal prophylaxis with fluconazole.

The majority of early and severe viral infections are caused by viruses of the Herpesviridae family, including Epstein–Barr virus (EBV), CMV, and herpes simplex virus (HSV). CMV transmission dynamics are well studied and serve as a prototype for herpes virus transmission. The likelihood that CMV infection will develop is influenced by the preoperative CMV status of the transplant donor and recipient. Seronegative recipients receiving seropositive donor organs are at greatest risk, with seropositive D/R combinations at the next greatest risk. Use of various immune-based prophylactic protocols including IV immunoglobulin G (IgG) or hyperimmune anti-CMV IgG, coupled with acyclovir or ganciclovir/valganciclovir, have all achieved success in decreasing the incidence of symptomatic CMV infection, although seroconversion in naive recipients of seropositive donor organs inevitably occurs.

EBV infection occurring in the perioperative period represents a significant risk to the pediatric transplant recipient. It has a varying presentation including a mononucleosis-like syndrome, hepatitis-simulating rejection, extranodal lymphoproliferative infiltration with bowel perforation, peritonsillar or lymph node enlargement, or encephalopathy. In small children, its primary portal of entry is often the tonsils, making asymptomatic tonsillar hypertrophy a common initial presentation. EBV infection can occur as a primary infection or after reactivation of a past primary infection. When serologic evidence of active infection exists, an acute reduction in immunosuppression is indicated. It has become clear that continuous surveillance is necessary, as the presentation is often nonspecific, and the prognosis is related to early diagnosis. Screening by determination of EBV blood viral load by quantitative polymerase chain reaction (PCR) appears to be the best present predictor of risk. However, viral loads have been identified in asymptomatic patients and patients recovering from PTLD, limiting the specificity of this test. The balance between viral load measured by quantitative PCR and specific cellular immune response, perhaps mediated by CD8 T cells specific to EBV, may explain this lack of specificity to viral load alone. Many pediatric transplant centers now use serially measured quantitative EBV-DNA PCR as an indication for primary immunosuppression modulation. We recommend monthly EBV-DNA PCR counts to monitor increased genomic expression. Increasing viral load levels warrant more frequent monitoring. In the EBV seronegative pretransplant patients, increasing EBV viral load warrants a 50% reduction in immunosuppression. We institute antiviral therapy with ganciclovir and CMV-IgG. Treatment should be continued until symptoms of lymphadenopathy have resolved and viral EBV-DNA PCR has returned to baseline. It should, however, be cautioned that PTLD can develop and progress without increases in EBV-PCR viral load. PTLD, a potentially fatal abnormal proliferation of B lymphocytes, can occur in any situation in which immunosuppression is undertaken. The importance of PTLD in pediatric liver transplantation is a result of the intensity of the immunosuppression required, its lifetime duration, and the absence of prior exposure to EBV infection in 60% to 80% of pediatric recipients. PTLD is the most common tumor in children after transplantation, representing 52% of all tumors compared with 15% in adults. About 80% occur within the first 2 years after transplantation. Multiple studies analyzing immunosuppressive therapy and the development of PTLD have shown a progressive increase in the incidence of PTLD with (1) an increase in total immunosuppressive load, (2) the EBV-naïve recipients, and (3) intensity of active viral load. No single immunosuppressive agent has been directly related to PTLD, although high-dose cyclosporine, tacrolimus, polyclonal antilymphocyte sera (MALG, ALG), and monoclonal antibodies (OKT-3) have all been implicated. Active EBV infection, whether primary or reactivation, involves the B-lymphocyte pool, causing B-cell proliferation. A simultaneous increase in cytotoxic T-cell activity is the normal primary host mechanism preventing EBV dissemination. Loss of this natural protection as a result of the administration of T-cell–inhibitory immunotherapy allows polyclonal B-cell proliferation to progress. Most tumors seen in children are large cell lymphomas, 86% being of B-cell origin. Extranodal involvement, uncommon in primary lymphomas, is seen in 70% of PTLD cases. Extranodal sites include central nervous system, 27%; liver, 23%; lung, 22%; kidney, 21%; intestine, 20%; and spleen, 13%. Allograft involvement is common and can mimic rejection. T-cell and B-cell immunohistochemical markers of the infiltrating lymphocyte population define the B-cell infiltrate and assist in establishing an early diagnosis.

Treatment of PTLD is stratified according to the immunologic cell typing and clinical presentation. Documented PTLD requires an immediate decrease in or discontinuation of immunosuppression and institution of anti-EBV therapy. We prefer to use IV ganciclovir for initial antiviral therapy owing to the high incidence of concurrent CMV infection. The development of newer antiviral alternatives such as valganciclovir may offer better long-term treatment options in the future. Patients with polyclonal B-cell proliferation frequently show regression with this treatment. If tumor cells express B-cell marker CD 20 at histology, the anti-CD 20 monoclonal antibody rituximab can be given in 4 weekly infusions of 375 mg/m². Although it is associated in many cases with significant reduction in tumor mass, patients have frequently experienced reversible neutropenia requiring granulocyte colony-stimulating factor (G-CSF) and hypogammaglobulinemia requiring supplementation. Acute liver rejection has frequently been seen during rituximab treatment. Patients with aggressive monoclonal malignancies have poor survival even with immunosuppressive reduction, acyclovir, and conventional chemotherapy or radiation therapy.

## OUTCOME AFTER TRANSPLANTATION

Although the potential complications after liver transplantation are frequent and severe, the overall results are rewarding. Most successful transplant programs have reached overall 1-year survival rates of 90%, with greatly decreased risk thereafter. Similar if not better results are associated with LD transplantation, especially for small recipients. Infants younger than 1 year or weighing less than 10 kg have historically had reported survival rate of 65% to 88% overall, an improvement over initial reported rates of 50% to 60% during the early era of OLT development. Survival rates in infants now equal those seen in older children. Improved survival in these small recipients is consistent throughout all levels of medical urgency and results from a decrease in life and graft-threatening complications, such as HAT and PNF, in the reduced-size donor organ (Fig. 99-4).

The increased donor availability for small recipients achieved through the use of surgically reduced, split, or LD organs also brought about a significant decrease in waiting-list mortality. Efforts to enhance donor availability, allowing transplantation in children before they reach a critical status, are essential before major improvements in postoperative survival rates can occur. The significant success now achieved after liver transplantation cannot overshadow the need for improved management of post-transplant consequences of immunosuppression and pre-OLT chronic disease. The most significant factors contributing to long-term failure of the allograft or patient death in our program and

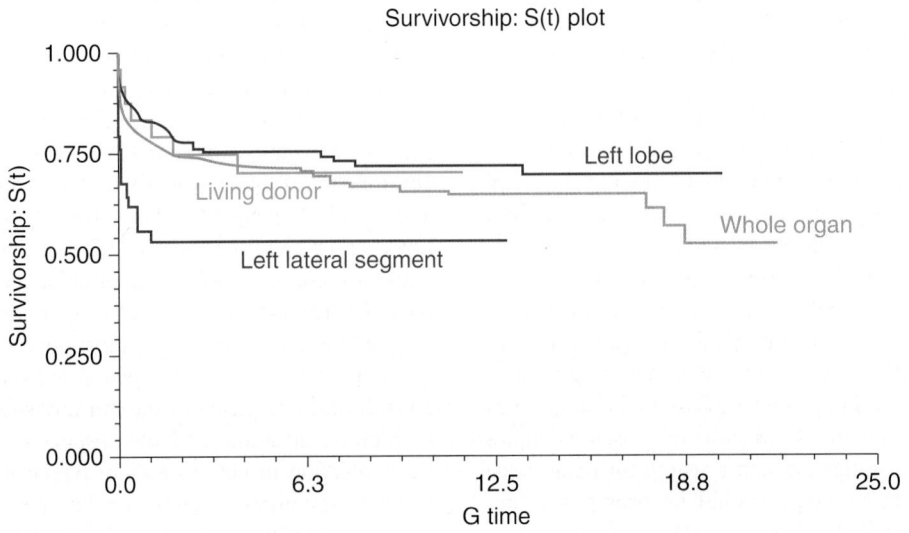

**FIGURE 99-4** Patient outcomes at CCHMC following transplantation using different graft types— overall survival since 1986.

others are consequences of immunosuppressive medications, such as late infection, and PTLD, and chronic rejection of the allograft. Our ability to address these challenges successfully will determine the life-long success of transplantation for our youngest recipients.

## SELECTED READINGS

Adams DH, Neuberger JM. Treatment of acute rejection. *Semin Liver Dis* 1992;12(1):80–88.

Al-Qabandi W, et al. Orthotopic liver transplantation for unresectable hepatoblastoma: a single center's experience. *J Pediatr Surg* 1999;34(8):1261–1264.

Andrews W, Siegel J, Renaro T. Prevention and treatment of selected fungal and viral infections in pediatric liver transplant recipients. *Clin Transpl* 1991;5:204–207.

Awan S, et al. Angiosarcoma of the liver in children. *J Pediatr Surg* 1996;31(12):1729–1732.

Axelrod DA, et al. Limitations of EBV-PCR monitoring to detect EBV associated post-transplant lymphoproliferative disorder. *Pediatr Transpl* 2003;7(3):223–227.

Azoulay D, Samuel D, Adam R, et al. Paul Brousse Liver Transplantation: the first 1,500 cases. *Clin Transpl* 2000;273–280.

Azoulay D, et al. Split-liver transplantation. The Paul Brousse policy. *Ann Surg* 1996;224(6):737–746; discussion 746–748.

Ben-Haim M, et al. Hepatic epithelioid hemangioendothelioma: resection or transplantation, which and when? *Liver Transpl Surg* 1999;5(6):526–531.

Broelsch CE, et al. Application of reduced-size liver transplants as split grafts, auxiliary orthotopic grafts, and living related segmental transplants. *Ann Surg* 1990;212(3):368–375; discussion 375–377.

Broelsch CE, et al. Liver transplantation in children from living related donors. Surgical techniques and results. *Ann Surg* 1991;214(4):428–437; discussion 437–439.

Broelsch CE, et al. Living donor liver transplantation in adults. *Eur J Gastroenterol Hepatol* 2003;15(1):3–6.

Broelsch CE, et al. Living related liver transplantation: medical and social aspects of a controversial therapy. *Gut* 2002;50(2):143–145.

Broughton S, et al. The effectiveness of tonsillectomy in diagnosing lymphoproliferative disease in pediatric patients after liver transplantation. *Arch Otolaryngol Head Neck Surg* 2000;126(12):1444–1447.

Bueno J, Ramil C, Green M. Current management strategies for the prevention and treatment of cytomegalovirus infection in pediatric transplant recipients. *Paediatr Drugs* 2002;4(5):279–290.

Busuttil RW, et al. Analysis of long-term outcomes of 3200 liver transplantations over two decades: a single-center experience. *Ann Surg* 2005;241(6):905–918.

Cardona J, et al. Liver transplantation in children with Alagille syndrome—a study of twelve cases. *Transplantation* 1995;60(4):339–342.

Colombo C, et al. Effects of liver transplantation on the nutritional status of patients with cystic fibrosis. *Transpl Int* 2005;18(2):246–255.

Cox K, et al. Liver transplantation in infants weighing less than 10 kilograms. *Transpl Proc* 1991;23(1 Pt 2):1579–1580.

Czauderna P, et al. Guidelines for surgical treatment of hepatoblastoma in the modern era—recommendations from the Childhood Liver Tumour Strategy Group of the International Society of Paediatric Oncology (SIOPEL). *Eur J Cancer* 2005;41(7):1031–1036.

D'Alessandro AM, et al. The predictive value of donor liver biopsies on the development of primary nonfunction after orthotopic liver transplantation. *Transpl Proc* 1991;23(1 Pt 2):1536–1537.

Deshpande RR, et al. Results of split liver transplantation in children. *Ann Surg* 2002;236(2):248–253.

Emond JC, et al. Reconstruction of the hepatic vein in reduced size hepatic transplantation. *Surg Gynecol Obstet* 1993;176(1):11–17.

Fan ST, Lo CM, Liu CL. Technical refinement in adult-to-adult living donor liver transplantation using right lobe graft. *Ann Surg* 2000;231(1):126–131.

Fishbein TM, et al. Use of livers with microvesicular fat safely expands the donor pool. *Transplantation* 1997;64(2):248–251.

Fox AS, et al. Seropositivity in liver transplant recipients as a predictor of cytomegalovirus disease. *J Infect Dis* 1988;157(2):383–385.

Fridell JA, et al. Causes of mortality beyond 1 year after primary pediatric liver transplant under tacrolimus. *Transplantation* 2002;74(12):1721–1724.

Fujimoto M, et al. Hepatic arterial complications in pediatric segmental liver transplantations from living donors: assessment with color Doppler ultrasonography. *Clin Transplant* 1997;11(5 Pt 1):380–386.

Genyk YS, et al. Liver transplantation in cystic fibrosis. *Curr Opin Pulm Med* 2001;7(6):441–447.

Gupta P, et al. Risk factors for chronic rejection after pediatric liver transplantation. *Transplantation* 2001;72(6):1098–1102.

Hanto DW, et al. Epstein–Barr virus, immunodeficiency, and B cell lymphoproliferation. *Transplantation* 1985;39(5):461–472.

Harper PL, et al. Protein C deficiency and portal thrombosis in liver transplantation in children. *Lancet* 1988;2(8617):924–927.

Heffron TG, et al. Hepatic artery thrombosis in pediatric liver transplantation. *Transplant Proc* 2003;35(4):1447–1448.

Hertl M, Cosimi AB. Liver transplantation for malignancy. *Oncologist* 2005;10(4):269–281.

Hoffenberg EJ, et al. Outcome of syndromic paucity of interlobular bile ducts (Alagille syndrome) with onset of cholestasis in infancy. *J Pediatr* 1995;127(2):220–224.

Holmes RD, Sokol RJ. *Epstein–Barr virus and post-transplant lymphoproliferative disease. Pediatr Transplant* 2002;6(6):456–464.

Holmes RD, et al. Response of elevated Epstein-Barr virus DNA levels to therapeutic changes in pediatric liver transplant patients: 56-month follow up and outcome. *Transplantation* 2002;74(3):367–372.

Horslen SP, et al. Isolated hepatocyte transplantation in an infant with a severe urea cycle disorder. *Pediatrics* 2003;111(6 Pt 1):1262–1267.

Imber CJ, et al. Hepatic steatosis and its relationship to transplantation. *Liver Transpl* 2002;8(5):415–423.

Iwatsuki S, et al. Role of liver transplantation in cancer therapy. *Ann Surg* 1985;202(4):401–407.

Jain A, et al. The absence of chronic rejection in pediatric primary liver transplant patients who are maintained on tacrolimus-based immunosuppression: a long-term analysis. *Transplantation* 2003;75(7):1020–1025.

Jan D, et al. Liver transplantation in children with inherited metabolic disorders. *Transplant Proc* 1995;27(2):1706–1707.

Kaneko J, et al. Prediction of hepatic artery thrombosis by protocol Doppler ultrasonography in pediatric living donor liver transplantation. *Abdom Imaging* 2004;29(5):603–605.

Kasai M, Mochizuki I, Ohkohchi N, Chiba T, Ohi R. Surgical limitation for biliary atresia: indication for liver transplantation. *J Pediatr Surg* 1989;24(9):851–854.

Kirsch JP, et al. Problematic vascular reconstruction in liver transplantation. Part II. Portovenous conduits. *Surgery* 1990;107(5):544–548.

Klein AS, et al. Organ donation and utilization in the United States, 1999–2008. *Am J Transplant* 2010;10(4 Pt 2):973–986.

Koneru B, et al. Liver transplantation for hepatoblastoma. The American experience. *Ann Surg* 1991;213(2):118–121.

Kusano T, et al. The use of stents for duct-to-duct anastomoses of biliary reconstruction in orthotopic liver transplantation. *Hepatogastroenterology* 2005;52(63):695–699.

Langnas AN, et al. Hepatic allograft rescue following arterial thrombosis. Role of urgent revascularization. *Transplantation* 1991;51(1):86–90.

Langnas AN, et al. The results of reduced-size liver transplantation, including split livers, in patients with end-stage liver disease. *Transplantation* 1992;53(2):387–391.

Lidofsky SD, et al. Intracranial pressure monitoring and liver transplantation for fulminant hepatic failure. *Hepatology* 1992;16(1):1–7.

Merion RM, et al. Hospitalization rates before and after adult-to-adult living donor or deceased donor liver transplantation. *Ann Surg* 2010;251(3):542–549.

Molmenti EP, et al. Treatment of unresectable hepatoblastoma with liver transplantation in the pediatric population. *Am J Transplant* 2002;2(6):535–538.

Mor E, et al. Acute cellular rejection following liver transplantation: clinical pathologic features and effect on outcome. *Semin Liver Dis* 1992;12(1):28–40.

Ng VL, et al. Long-term outcome after partial external biliary diversion for intractable pruritus in patients with intrahepatic cholestasis. *J Pediatr Gastroenterol Nutr* 2000;30(2):152–156.

Nio M, et al. Current status of 21 patients who have survived more than 20 years since undergoing surgery for biliary atresia. *J Pediatr Surg* 1996;31(3):381–384.

Otte JB, et al. Liver transplantation for hepatoblastoma: results from the International Society of Pediatric Oncology (SIOP) study SIOPEL-1 and review of the world experience. *Pediatr Blood Cancer* 2004;42(1):74–83.

Patel R, et al. Cytomegalovirus prophylaxis in solid organ transplant recipients. *Transplantation* 1996;61(9):1279–1289.

Peclet MH, et al. The spectrum of bile duct complications in pediatric liver transplantation. *J Pediatr Surg* 1994;29(2):214–219; discussion 219–220.

Penn I. Hepatic transplantation for primary and metastatic cancers of the liver. *Surgery* 1991;110(4):726–734; discussion 734–735.

Penn I. Post-transplant malignancy: the role of immunosuppression. *Drug Saf* 2000;23(2):101–113.

Perilongo G, Shafford E, Plaschkes J. SIOPEL trials using preoperative chemotherapy in hepatoblastoma. *Lancet Oncol* 2000;1:94–100.

Pimpalwar AP, et al. Strategy for hepatoblastoma management: Transplant versus nontransplant surgery. *J Pediatr Surg* 2002;37(2):240–245.

Reily D. Familial intrahepatic cholestasis syndromes. In Suchy FJ, ed. *Liver Disease in Children*. St. Louis: CV Mosby; 1994:443–459.

Reyes J. Adaptation of split liver grafts in pediatric patients. *Pediatr Transplant* 2001;5(3):148–152.

Reyes JD, et al. Liver transplantation and chemotherapy for hepatoblastoma and hepatocellular cancer in childhood and adolescence. *J Pediatr* 2000;136(6):795–804.

Ryckman F, et al. Improved survival in biliary atresia patients in the present era of liver transplantation. *J Pediatr Surg* 1993;28(3):382–385; discussion 386.

Ryckman, FC, Alonso MH, eds. Transplantation for hepatic malignancy in children. 1st ed. In: Busuttil RW, Klintmalm G, eds. *Transplanatation of the Liver*. Philadelphia: WB Sanders; 1996:216–226.

Ryckman FC, Schroeder T, Pedersen S. Use of monoclonal antibody immunosuppressive therapy in pediatric renal and liver transplantation. *Clin Transpl* 1991;5:186–190.

Schnater JM, et al. Surgical view of the treatment of patients with hepatoblastoma: results from the first prospective trial of the International Society of Pediatric Oncology Liver Tumor Study Group. *Cancer* 2002;94(4):1111–1120.

Serinet MO, et al. Anti-CD20 monoclonal antibody (Rituximab) treatment for Epstein–Barr virus-associated, B-cell lymphoproliferative disease in pediatric liver transplant recipients. *J Pediatr Gastroenterol Nutr* 2002;34(4):389–393.

Smets F, Sokal EM. Epstein–Barr virus-related lymphoproliferation in children after liver transplant: role of immunity, diagnosis, and management. *Pediatr Transplant* 2002;6(4):280–287.

Smets F, et al. Characteristics of Epstein–Barr virus primary infection in pediatric liver transplant recipients. *J Hepatol* 2000;32(1):100–104.

Smets F, et al. Ratio between Epstein-Barr viral load and anti-Epstein–Barr virus specific T-cell response as a predictive marker of post-transplant lymphoproliferative disease. *Transplantation* 2002;73(10):1603–1610.

Snover DC, et al. Orthotopic liver transplantation: a pathological study of 63 serial liver biopsies from 17 patients with special reference to the diagnostic features and natural history of rejection. *Hepatology* 1984;4(6):1212–1222.

Sokal M, et al. Liver transplantation in children less than 1 year of age. *J Pediatr* 1990;117(2 Pt 1):205–210.

Stieber AC, et al. The spectrum of portal vein thrombosis in liver transplantation. *Ann Surg* 1991;213(3):199–206.

Strom S, Fisher R. Hepatocyte transplantation: new possibilities for therapy. *Gastroenterology* 2003;124(2):568–571.

Strom SC, et al. Hepatocyte transplantation as a bridge to orthotopic liver transplantation in terminal liver failure. *Transplantation* 1997;63(4):559–569.

Strom SC, et al. Transplantation of human hepatocytes. *Transplant Proc* 1997;29(4):2103–2106.

SPLIT Research Group. Studies of Pediatric Liver Transplantation (SPLIT): year 2000 outcomes. *Transplantation* 2001;72(3):463–476.

Tiao GM, et al. The current management of hepatoblastoma: a combination of chemotherapy, conventional resection, and liver transplantation. *J Pediatr* 2005;146(2):204–211.

Tzakis AG, et al. Liver transplantation for Alagille's syndrome. *Arch Surg* 1993;128(3):337–339.

Van der Werf WJ, et al. Infant pediatric liver transplantation results equal those for older pediatric patients. *J Pediatr Surg* 1998;33(1):20–23.

Verran D, et al. Clinical experience gained from the use of 120 steatotic donor livers for orthotopic liver transplantation. *Liver Transpl* 2003;9(5):500–505.

Wiesner RH, et al. Selective bowel decontamination to decrease gram-negative aerobic bacterial and *Candida* colonization and prevent infection after orthotopic liver transplantation. *Transplantation* 1988;45(3):570–574.

Zamboni F, et al. Effect of macrovescicular steatosis and other donor and recipient characteristics on the outcome of liver transplantation. *Clin Transplant* 2001;15(1):53–57.

Zitelli BJ, et al. Evaluation of the pediatric patient for liver transplantation. *Pediatrics* 1986;78(4):559–565.

# CHAPTER 100

# Intestine Transplantation

*Jorge Reyes*

The intestine has been the last solid organ to be successfully transplanted, a journey spanning over 60 years which had seen the development of clinical kidney, liver, heart, and lung transplantation. During this time, life-saving support of patients losing function of their intestine came in the form of Total Parenteral Nutrition (TPN) similar to hemodialysis for kidney failure, as well as the development of several forms of corrective surgery for short gut; however, a comprehensive vision of outcomes, challenges, and future direction was lacking. Indeed, for the most part it was the individual patient's failing due to TPN-induced liver failure and the searching care at established liver transplant centers which promoted the continued research and clinical development of intestine transplantation. This process had been a series of trial and error case studies which paralleled immunosuppressive milestones in other organs and that was reported in historical summaries as "pre and post cyclosporine eras." Except for one pediatric recipient in Paris, these pioneer cases failed quickly due to acute rejection, sepsis, and multisystem organ failure. By the late 1980s the successful outcomes with cyclosporine and the transplantation of other organs, advances in organ preservation and procurement techniques, and improvements in perioperative care and prevention of infection provided the clinical platform for the introduction of a new immunosuppressive drug FK 506 (now known as Tacrolimus). These factors formed the essential components for the initiation in 1990 of an experimental trial of intestine transplantation in children under FK 506, the success of which fostered the development of multidisciplinary care teams managing a heretofore poorly defined malady now known as intestinal failure. In October 2000, intestine transplantation was recognized by the Center for Medicare and Medicaid Services (CMS) as an established treatment for patients with intestinal failure; since then there has been an increasing number of patients referred for intestinal transplantation. There are now nearly 700 patients alive with a functioning graft in the United States as of December 2007.

Interestingly, the development of the field of intestinal failure management has been one of the most important successes of intestine transplantation and is based on the work of multidisciplinary teams caring for acute and chronic loss of bowel function. Because of this, patients with intestinal failure have experienced a change in clinical outcomes. As such the indications for intestine transplantation continue to evolve. Also, national allocation of organ policies have required important modifications to address long wait times and a high wait list mortality (particularly for infants and adults with concomitant liver failure). Long-term functional/nutritional outcomes, information on quality of life after intestine transplantation, and cost information will further define the role of intestine transplantation. The present status of these areas will be the substance of this chapter.

## INTESTINAL FAILURE

Intestinal failure is the inability to maintain normal fluid and nutritional autonomy due to the loss of bowel length or function. Patients with intestinal failure require management with TPN through a catheter placed in a central venous location (6 principle sites: bilateral internal jugular, subclavian, and iliac veins) (See Chapter 9, Vascular Access Procedures). The evolution of intestinal failure varies with etiology and severity of disease and may be lifelong. The adaptive capacity of the remaining intestine (in cases of short gut) and the severity of functional disorders (motility or absorption) will dictate the rehabilitative capacity and need for intestinal transplantation. Intestinal transplantation may be lifesaving in a group of patients who cannot be rehabilitated or who have such severe forms of intestinal failure that they are committed to lifelong TPN with its inherent risks and complications. As with renal failure, intestinal failure manifests satellite complications that include catheter infections and sepsis, cholestatic liver disease or liver failure, foregut dysmotility, pancreatitis and glucose intolerance and insulin dependent diabetes insipidus, vascular thrombosis, and renal failure. The physiopathology of this "intestinal failure syndrome" is multifactorial, and though for the most part unclear, may be related to drug toxicity of TPN, abnormal neural/immunologic responses in short gut, and sepsis.

A multidisciplinary approach has been the key to improved outcomes with the development of innovative approaches in the management of intestinal failure. This includes a thorough clinical and nutritional history including surgical procedures, number and types of infections, previous central venous catheters, history of venous thrombosis, and a focused physical examination. Securing a road map to the residual bowel may include simple upper and lower gastrointestinal contrast studies, computerized tomography (CT) or magnetic resonance (MRI) scans, and assessment of patency of venous access sites and the abdominal vasculature through Doppler ultrasonography. Tissue assessments of the intestine (eg, Hirshsprung disease), and the liver are essential if there is evidence of portal hypertension with preserved function or if there is suspicion of another etiology in the development of liver failure. All of these tests may assist in the development of a clinical/surgical plan.

Management of the patient with intestinal failure focuses on the optimization of gut adaptation principally by trials of enteral feeding (feed the bowel), and addressing bacterial/fungal overgrowth and dysmotility. Corrective surgery focuses on addressing obstructions, functional dilations, and reestablishment of intestinal continuity. The use of serial transverse enteroplasty (STEP) has been an important procedure in the accomplishment of improved bowel function. With all patients, and particularly with extreme short gut or uncorrectable functional disorders, the overarching management focuses on the prevention of satellite complications and the consideration of intestinal transplantation when management is failing.

The most serious satellite complication of intestinal failure remains the TPN-induced liver disease. Infants are most susceptible to this complication, perhaps because they suffer life-threatening abdominal complications, sepsis, and associated failure in other organ systems around their loss of intestine; this scenario carries a 1-year mortality which exceeds 80%. The above-mentioned comprehensive strategies of intestinal failure management, in association with minimization of TPN (not always feasible) and advancement of enteral nutrition, may improve cholestasis. Other strategies include preventing overfeeding, structuring "off hours" by cycling

TPN, and providing taurine to neonates. Sludge and cholelithiasis in the intrahepatic biliary system and gallbladder may require cholecystectomy; however, its benefit has not been established. The removal of soy-based lipid solutions or their substitution with Omegaven (a fish-oil based, intravenous lipid solution rich in omega-3 fatty acids) has shown some evidence of retarding or potentially reversing the progression of liver disease.

Catheter-associated sepsis is the other satellite complication of TPN; such a complication often necessitates removal of the catheter, and this may result in venous thrombosis with loss of this site for future venous access. The "severity" of the loss of access sites has led to a threshold which would warrant consideration of intestinal transplantation; and generally it is perceived as a loss of 3 of the 6 standard sites.

## INDICATIONS FOR TRANSPLANT

Acute intestinal failure is never an indication for intestine transplantation since alternative supportive care with TPN usually allows the patient to stabilize and define their rehabilitative potential, and it will permit the management of satellite complications seen with the syndrome of intestinal failure. It is the presence of life-threatening complications which may exhaust the rehabilitative potential. In addition, the presence of extreme short gut or irreversible functional disease with the specter of lifelong need for TPN in some patients may also indicate the need for intestinal transplantation.

The disease processes which lead to intestinal failure have been classified as either surgical (due to resection leading to short gut) or functional (due to dysmotility or malabsorptive disorders). Table 100-1 lists the most common disease entities seen in pediatric or adult patients with intestinal failure.

| TABLE 100-1 | Indications for Intestinal Transplantation |
|---|---|
| **Children** | **Adults** |
| Volvulus | Superior Mesenteric Artery Thrombosis |
| Gastroschisis | Crohn Disease/IBD |
| Necrotizing Enterocolitis | Desmoid Tumor |
| Pseudo-Obstruction | Volvulus |
| Microvillus Inclusion Disease | Trauma |
| Intestinal Polyposis | Familial Polyposis |
| Hirschsprung's Disease | Gastrinoma |
| Trauma | Budd–Chiari Disease |
| Pseudo-obstruction | |
| Radiation Enteritis | |

A recent expert consensus panel recommended the following criteria for intestinal transplant evaluation: (1) extreme short gut; (2) severely diseased bowel and unacceptable morbidity; (3) continuing prognostic or diagnostic uncertainty; (4) microvillous inclusion disease or intestinal epithelial dysplasia; (5) persistent cholestasis (>6 g/dL); (6) thrombosis of 2 of 4 upper body central veins; (7) request by patient or family.

The type of graft to be used in a particular patient with intestinal failure is determined by the comprehensive evaluation of the function and anatomy of the remaining bowel. Whether to perform simultaneous hepatic replacement depends on the severity of portal hypertension and parenchymal liver dysfunction. Persistent cholestasis and jaundice, hypersplenism, and coagulopathy warrant consideration for a liver and intestinal transplant; some patients with motility disorders may warrant replacement of the foregut as in a multivisceral transplant (which includes the stomach, duodenum/pancreas, and liver). Patients with mild portal hypertension and preserved liver function may be considered for isolated intestinal transplantation.

## TRANSPLANT PROCEDURES

The multivisceral organ procurement forms the basis for all types of abdominal grafts and is conceptualized as the core cooling of all abdominal organs with the infusion of preservation solutions through the infra-renal aorta and into the celiac, superior mesenteric, and renal arteries. This surgical strategy has allowed the development of various types of organ grafts which address the unique and varied types of intestinal failure seen in this patient population.

### Isolated Intestine (Fig. 100-1)

This transplant includes the jejunum and ileum and is based on the superior mesenteric vein which is transected below the pancreas (respecting the inferior pancreatic veins in order to allow the use of the pancreas graft in another patient). It also is based on the superior mesenteric artery which is taken at the aorta or below the pancreas if there is an accessory right hepatic artery coming off the superior mesenteric artery going to the liver which must be preserved. The implantation hinges on vascular inflow and outflow, and usually involves placing donor vascular homografts of the iliac vein to the patients infra renal vena cava and the donor iliac artery to the patients infra renal aorta. These serve as interposition vascular conduits which are anastomosed to the graft's superior mesenteric vein and artery, respectively. In cases where recipient enterectomy of the intact dysfunctional intestine is performed at the time of transplant, direct anastomosis of the donor and recipient superior mesenteric artery and vein may also be feasible.

The intestinal reconstruction involves a proximal and distal connection with native residual intestine. If the patient has no functional distal colon, a permanent end-graft ileostomy is fashioned; if the recipient has remaining colon, this is connected leaving a short portion of the allograft distal to the

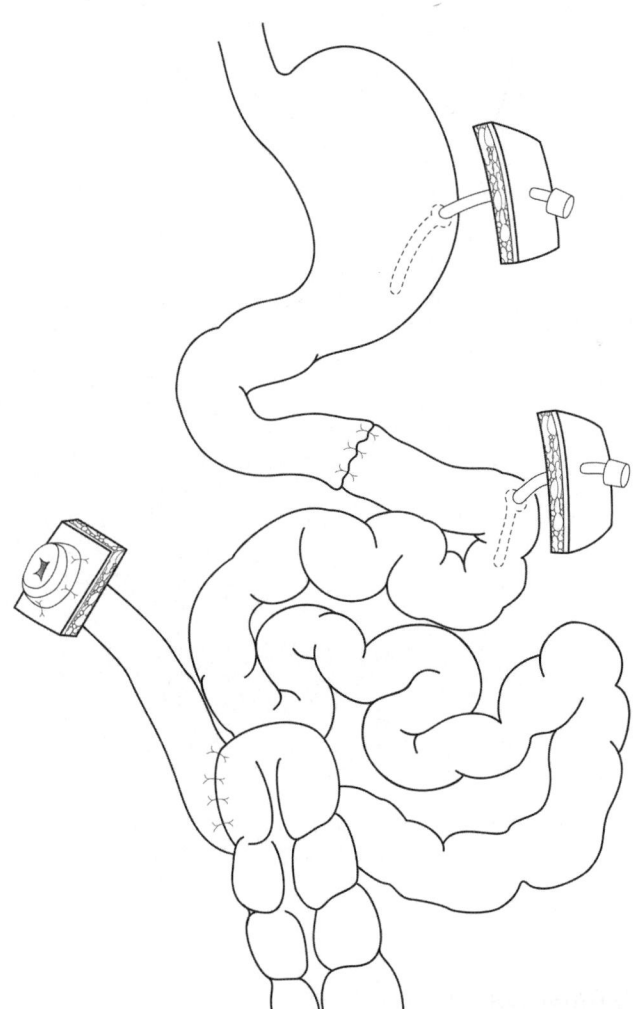

**FIGURE 100-1** Isolated intestinal transplant showing connections with native intestine, stoma, and feeding tubes.

enterocolic anastomosis which is brought out as a temporary end ileostomy. This allows access to the graft for endoscopic surveillance and mucosal biopsies. Feeding tubes are placed routinely in the stomach and graft jejunum; this allows for immediate use of the allograft (feed the bowel) and the introduction of enteral immunosuppressive agents.

### Liver and Intestine (Fig. 100-2)

The recipient's liver is removed preserving the native retrohepatic inferior vena cava and foregut (stomach, pancreas, and proximal duodenum); the venous drainage of the native foregut organs is re-directed to a permanent end-to-side porto-caval shunt. The composite donor graft includes the liver, small bowel, duodenum, and pancreas; this allows for maintenance of the graft hepatobiliary continuity. Arterial inflow to this type of composite graft is achieved using an interposition conduit of donor thoracic aorta to the patient's infra-renal aorta. The venous outflow is through the liver graft hepatic veins to the patient's inferior vena cava. Intestinal reconstruction and placement of feeding tubes is fashioned as described for the isolated intestine transplant.

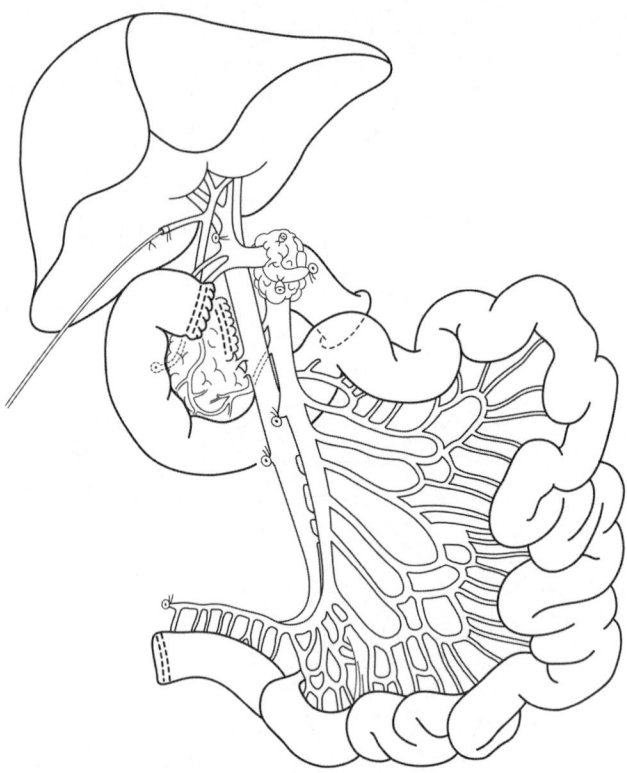

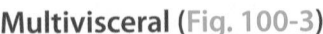

**FIGURE 100-2** Combined liver and intestinal transplant showing preservation of hepatic hilus with graft duodenum and pancreas.

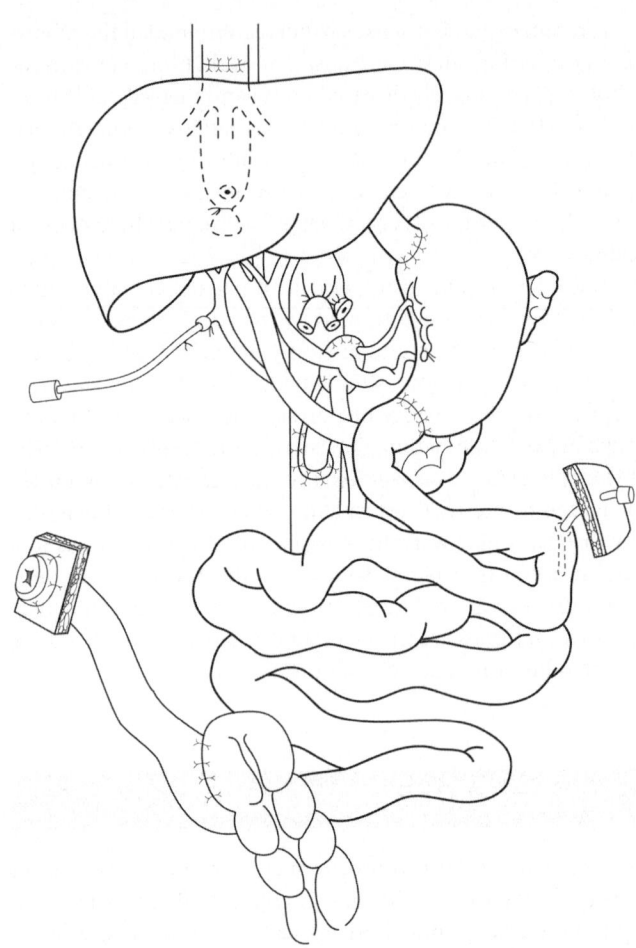

**FIGURE 100-3** Multivisceral transplant showing graft stomach and aortic conduit connected to native aorta.

## Multivisceral (Fig. 100-3)

The concept of a multivisceral transplant inherently involves removal of all of the patient's gastrointestinal tract, including the liver and stomach (leaving a cuff of fundus); the replacement graft of liver, stomach, duodenum, pancreas, and intestine are implanted in a similar fashion as in a liver–intestine transplant. The graft spleen is removed from the composite allograft on the back-bench, which will leave the patient asplenic. Intestinal reconstruction is performed proximally with a recipient gastric fundus to graft stomach anastomosis; the distal anastomosis is similar to previously described intestinal transplants. A Heineke–Mikulicz pyloroplasty is routinely performed on the graft as a backbench procedure. A "modified multi-visceral transplant" excludes the liver from the composite graft, since the recipient's normal liver is preserved.

## IMMUNOSUPPRESSION (SEE CHAPTER 97, IMMUNOLOGY AND TRANSPLANTATION)

Tacrolimus (Prograf, Astellas, Tokyo, Japan), a calcineurin inhibitor, is the cornerstone of long-term immunosuppressive therapy and is used in conjunction with various types of antibody induction (given only at the time of transplant) as well as "other" adjunctive medications which work in a different site of the antigen recognition/response chain.

Induction with depleting anti-lymphocyte antibody therapies include rabbit anti-thymocyte globulin (rATH, Thymoglobulin, Genzyme Corp., Cambridge, MA) and alemtuzumab (Campath-1H, Genzyme Corp., Cambridge, MA). The use of these agents by high-volume single centers has resulted in improved short- and long-term survival, with decreased rejection and infection rates. Induction with nondepleting interleukin-2 receptor antibody antagonists' daclizumab (Zenapax) and basiliximab (Simulect) has also been used successfully. Perioperative antibody induction is used in 60% of transplants and has allowed the development of steroid free therapy as well as minimization of Tacrolimus in the long term. This strategy may be responsible for the improved long-term outcomes, with less morbidity and mortality from infection and toxicity.

### Immunologic Monitoring

Endoscopic surveillance of the graft with biopsy remains the gold standard of intestine graft evaluation; this is performed weekly for the first 3 to 4 weeks, then at gradually decreasing frequencies depending on clinical need. The development of immunologic assays or markers of graft function remain investigational and not in clinical use; they include serologic, proteomic, and genomic markers which may identify patients at risk for rejection or excessive immunosuppression.

Preformed or de-novo anti-donor-specific antibodies may be of assistance in determining the risk of rejection. The use of fecal calprotectin or serum citrulline as markers of graft rejection has been helpful in center specific trials.

## POSTOPERATIVE CARE

### Infection Control

Intestinal transplant recipients will routinely receive prophylactic broad-spectrum antibiotics for 48 hours, and then specific antibiotic therapy is used based on a history of previous infections. The use of oral nonabsorbable antibiotics to achieve selective bowel decontamination, though routinely performed, has not been substantiated as therapeutically necessary; similarly, surveillance stool cultures are performed on a weekly basis post-transplant and provide information which may be helpful in cases of severe graft damage from ischemia/reperfusion or rejection.

### Antiviral Prophylaxis

Viral infections can cause significant disease and include CMV, EBV, herpes simplex virus (HSV), adenovirus, and influenza viruses. Since many pediatric patients do not have prior protective exposure to these viruses, a primary infection in an already immunosuppressed patient can be serious. Prophylaxis and pre-emptive therapy have decreased morbidity and mortality with EBV and CMV. Prophylaxis for CMV/EBV includes a 2-week course of intravenous ganciclovir with concomitant administration of cytomegalovirus-specific hyperimmune globulin (Cytogam).

### Nutritional Support

Enteral feeding is begun immediately postoperatively and advanced as tolerated (feed the bowel), concomitantly weaning the TPN and intravenous fluids as indicated. Because many patients are not able to eat normally before or immediately after the transplant (oral aversion), tube feeding may be necessary for prolonged periods.

### Assessment of Intestinal Allograft

Immediately upon reperfusion, the intestinal graft will appear pink, non-edematous, and occasional contractions will be seen. Varying severities of ischemia reperfusion damage may produce changes which include edema, venous congestion, and bleeding of the graft.

Routine endoscopic surveillance of the intestine graft allows for assessment of ischemia reperfusion and rejection (Fig. 100-4). Common changes to the normal appearance of an intestinal allograft include edema, cyanosis, congestion, ulceration, and rarely exfoliation of the mucosa.

The output through the stoma is assessed for volume, consistency, blood, or tissue. Normal/standard outputs of 1 to 2 L/day or 40 to 60 mL/kg/day for adult and pediatric recipients are thresholds which guide management. In order to control the volume of output, paregoric, loperamide, pectin, somatostatin, or oral antibiotics have been used alone or in combination. The presence of blood in the stool is a signal of significant pathology and warrants immediate endoscopy.

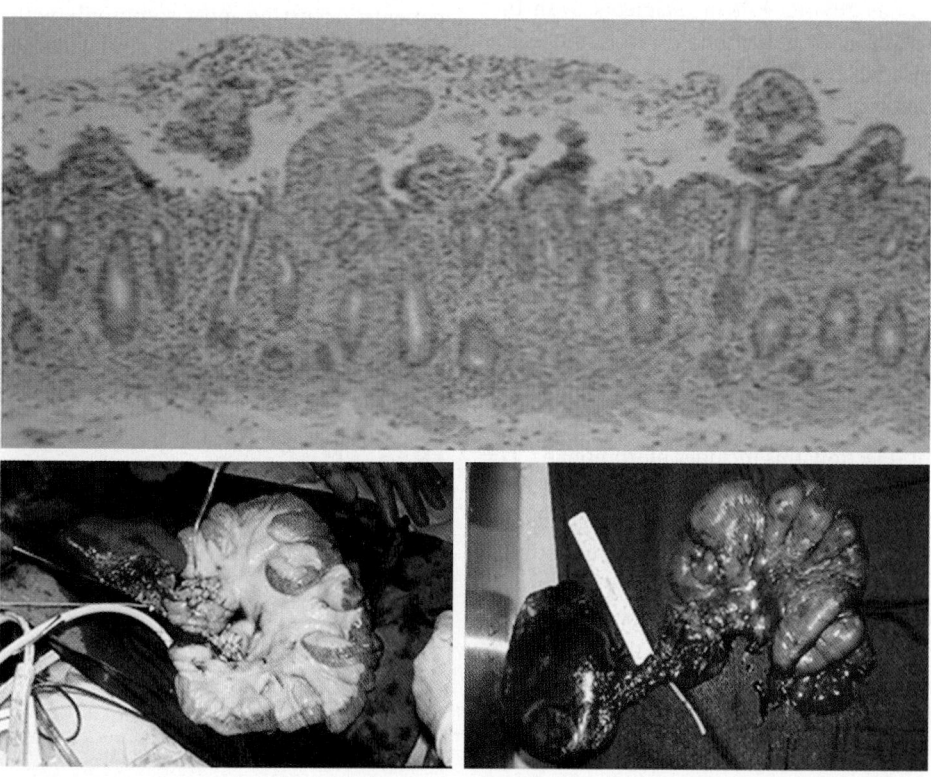

**FIGURE 100-4** Ischemia-reperfusion injury showing histologic picture with gross normal graft on the left, and severely damaged graft on right (at the time of graft removal).

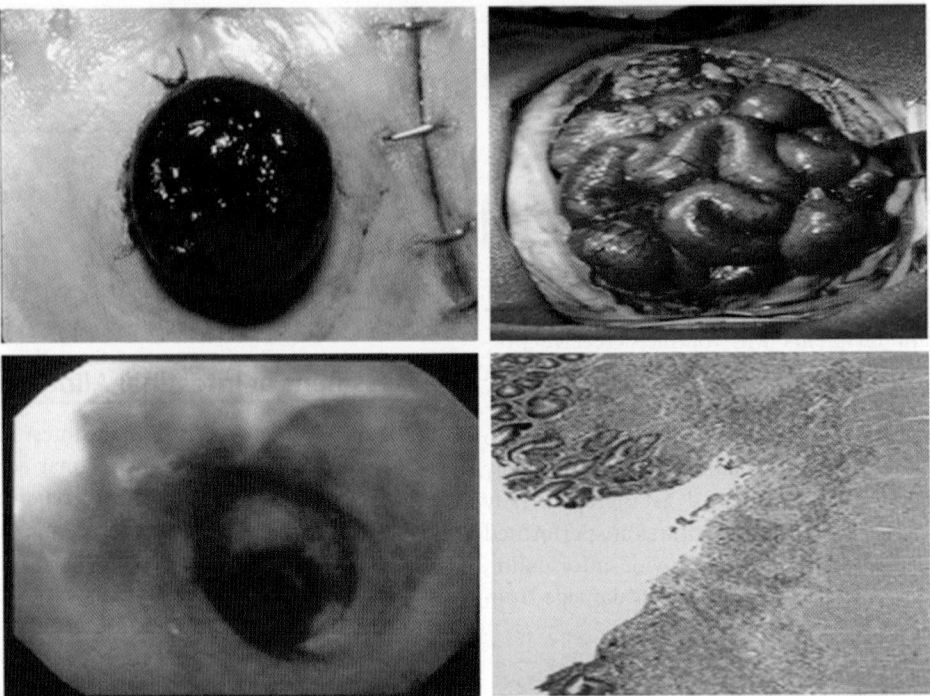

**FIGURE 100-5** Acute cellular rejection of intestinal graft showing (clockwise) severe stomal changes, inflamed bowel at graft enterectomy, endoscopy showing loss of mucosa, and histologic picture of severe rejection with loss of mucosal lining.

## REJECTION

Early rejection of the intestinal graft (Fig. 100-5) is associated with graft loss and death; until recently it remained a significant barrier to achieving long-term success. Historically reported in as many as 70% to 90% of recipients, with the recent application of antibody induction protocols, the rejection rate has decreased to 30% to 40%.

Clinical signs and symptoms of acute rejection are nonspecific and include diarrhea, fever, and abdominal pain. The stoma may become red and friable; endoscopy may demonstrate normal to very abnormal mucosa and evaluation of the proximal graft via an upper endoscopy may be necessary. The pathology of rejection may reveal the presence of edema in the lamina propria, villous blunting, varying degrees of mononuclear cell infiltrates, intestinal crypt apoptosis, and regeneration.

The treatment of acute intestinal allograft rejection includes high doses of steroids and then antilymphocyte antibodies for steroid-resistant rejection; this includes muromonab CD3 (OKT3, a murine, monoclonal anti-CD3 antibody) and antithymocyte globulin (rATG, rabbit-derived, Thymoglobulin). During and after the treatment of acute rejection, tacrolimus whole blood levels are maintained around 10 to 15 ng/mL, with maintenance steroid therapy being added (usually 1-2 mg/kg/day of oral prednisone). The addition of other agents such as mycophenolate mofetil (MMF, CellCept, Roche) or sirolimus (Rapamune) may be indicated for refractory or recurrent rejection or in the presence of toxicity to high levels of Tacrolimus.

Antibody-mediated rejection of the intestine is characterized by intestinal dysfunction, diffuse C4d staining on allograft biopsy, and usually identification of donor specific antibodies. Treatment consists of plasmapheresis in combination with intravenous immunoglobulin (IVIG) and steroids. Rituximab or bortezumib can be used in selected recipients.

Chronic rejection (Fig. 100-6) is observed in 10% to 15% of patients, occurring most commonly with isolated intestinal grafts. The presence of a liver graft with the intestine graft may provide protection from acute and chronic rejection when compared with isolated intestinal recipients. Risk factors for chronic rejection include type of allograft and retransplantation. The pathology of chronic rejection includes villous blunting, focal ulcerations, epithelial metaplasia, scant cellular infiltrates, and obliterative thickening of arterioles.

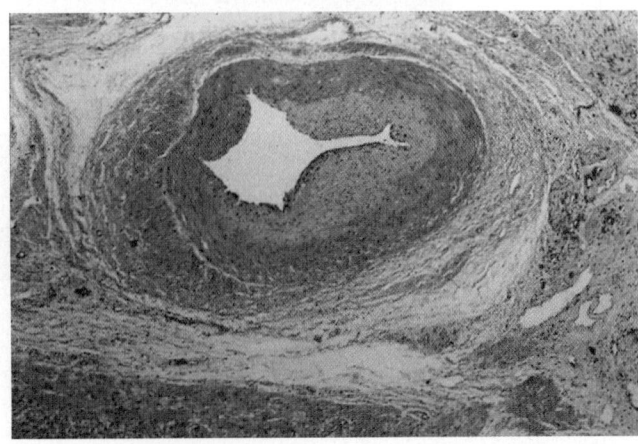

**FIGURE 100-6** Chronic rejection of the intestinal graft showing a histologic picture of vasculopathy.

## COMPLICATIONS

### Vascular Complications

Thrombotic events with these transplants are rare, however, the standard anticoagulation regimen as in isolated liver transplantation is generally used. Thrombosis will result in necrosis of the intestine which will require removal, or in cases of composite grafts which include the liver, urgent re-transplantation. Routine Doppler evaluations post transplant are followed throughout the perioperative period.

### Gastrointestinal Complications

Intestinal leaks seem to occur at a higher frequency with intestinal transplantation due to the effects of ischemia reperfusion syndromes with edema and residual ischemia, as well as because of technically very challenging procedures with long operative times. Diagnosis is comparable to that of any acute abdomen, operative repair is required, and sometimes innovative approaches with the construction of stomas as well as open abdomen management become applied options.

### Post-Transplant Lymphoproliferative Disorder

The development of EBV generated post-transplant proliferative disorder (PTLD) is an ominous sign of an uncontrolled balance between the control of rejection and an over immunosuppressed state (Fig. 100-7). Early experience with intestinal transplantation resulted in a PTLD risk over 40%; however, recent induction protocols which have facilitated less rejection and long-term minimization of Tacrolimus, as well as the introduction of EBV viral load monitoring with preemptive anti-viral therapy have resulted in an improved cumulative PTLD-free survival for intestinal transplant recipients undergoing induction immunosuppression to nearly 90%. Evaluation of PTLD is done by contrast-enhanced CT scanning of

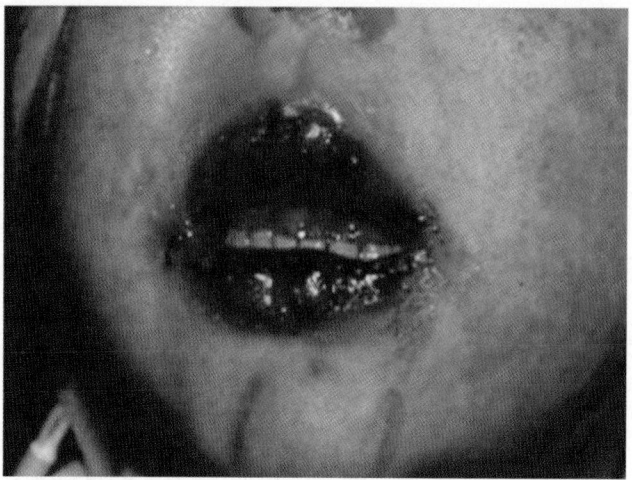

**FIGURE 100-7** Intestine recipient with obvious herpetic lesions around mouth, and with tongue lesions which on biopsy revealed PTLD.

the head, neck, chest, abdomen, and pelvis, with tissue diagnosis of lesions secured by whatever means is necessary to make the diagnosis. Specimens should be submitted for staining with the EBER-1 probe and CD20. Both stains may help guide diagnosis and management.

Treatment of PTLD includes cautious minimization of immunosuppression (unlike liver-transplant patients where immunosuppression can be stopped). Because many lesions stain positive for CD20, they can be treated with an anti-CD20 monoclonal antibody, usually rituximab. Refractory disease may benefit from low-dose cytotoxic chemotherapy and steroids.

### Graft-Versus-Host Disease

Graft-versus-host disease (GVHD) may occur when immunocompetent donor T-cells damage recipient tissues. GVHD can occur in as many as 5% of transplants (Fig. 100-8).

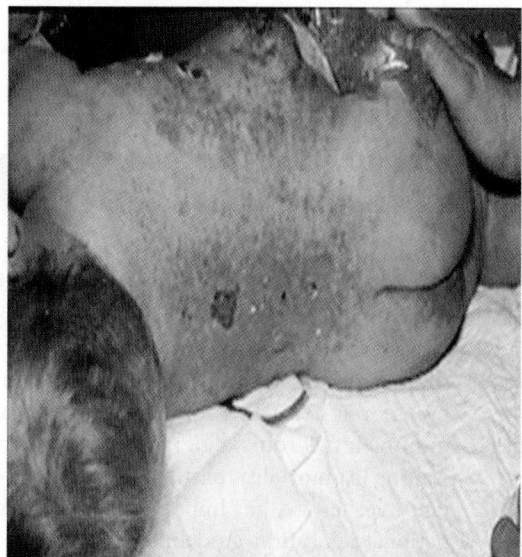 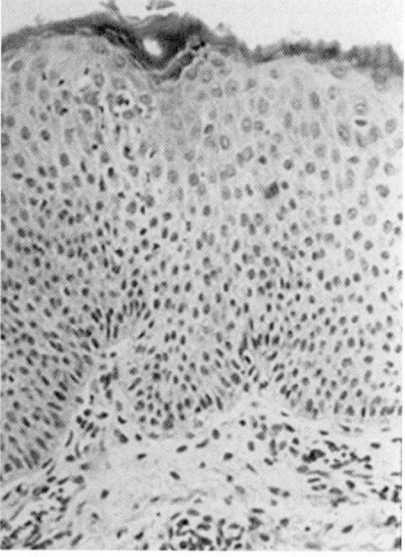

**FIGURE 100-8** Intestine recipient with GVHD lesions of skin, and histopathology showing inflammatory changes in dermis and skin appendages.

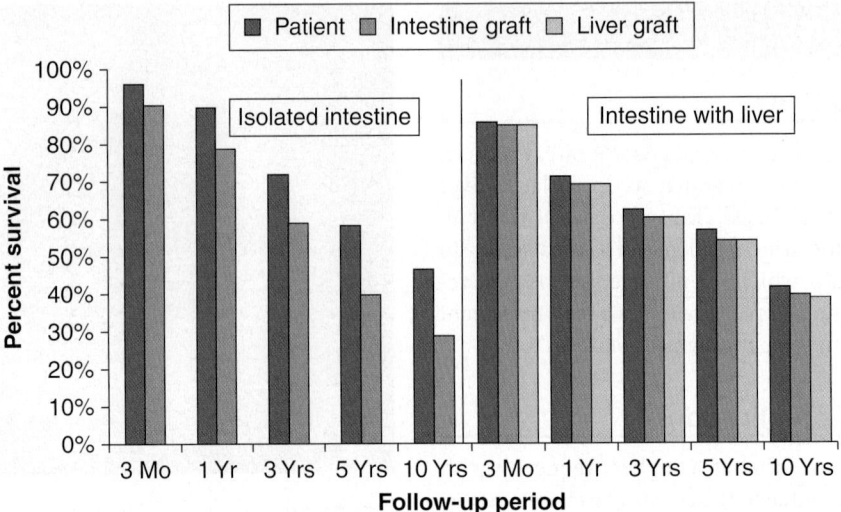

**FIGURE 100-9** Unadjusted patient and graft survival for isolated intestine and combined liver and intestine recipients. (Reprinted with permission from Mazariegos GV, Steffick DE, Horslen S, et al. Intestine transplantation in the United States, 1999–2008. *AJT* 2010;10:1020–1034.)

Presenting signs and symptoms include fever, a maculopapular rash on the upper torso, neck, or palms of hands and feet, blisters, or diffuse erythema. Oral lesions, diarrhea, intestinal ulcerations, liver dysfunction, lymphadenopathy, and bone marrow suppression with pancytopenia have been described.

The diagnosis of GVHD hinges on histological confirmation; chimeric studies to detect donor cells in peripheral blood or tissues have not been helpful in diagnosis of this pathology. Treatment is based on corticosteroids to control epithelial inflammation and it is effective in most cases. Unresponsive disease has been controlled by reduction of calcineurin-based immunosuppression, thereby allowing for recipient immunologic competency to balance out the donor immunocyte population causing the GVHD. Treatment with antilymphocytic agents (eg, Thymoglobulin and OKT3), as well using anti-interleukin therapy (eg, Zenapax and Simulect), and anti-TNF antibody therapy (eg, Remicade) has had disappointing results, likely due to advanced disease at the time of therapy.

## OUTCOMES

### Patient and Graft Survival

The introduction of antibody induction therapy, steroid free therapy, and early minimization of Tacrolimus has resulted in significant improvements in early patient and graft survival after intestinal transplantation. One-year patient and graft survivals (Fig. 100-9) reach 89.3% and 78.9% for intestine-only recipients and 71.5% and 69.0% for liver–intestine recipients, respectively. These outcomes are now comparable to those following pancreas, lung, and liver transplantation. Contributing factors also include improvements in intestinal failure management, better patient selection, and increased experience of transplant teams.

Long-term survival after isolated intestinal transplantation, however, has remained disappointing with 10-year patient

and graft survivals of 46% and 29% for isolated intestinal transplantation, and 42% and 39% for intestine with liver grafts, respectively. Though this cohort of long-term cases represent results from previous immunosuppressive strategies, they compare unfavorably to kidney, liver, and heart transplantation where 10-year patient and graft survivals exceed 50%.

### Long-Term Rehabilitation and Quality of Life

There is a paucity of information on long-term functional outcomes after intestinal transplantation; however, a small preliminary study in pediatric recipients with functioning intestinal allografts found that quality of life was perceived by recipients to be comparable to that of their peers, while parental proxy assessments compared less favorably in terms of physical functioning, general health, and family activities. This supports reports that demonstrate improvement with the transition from parenteral nutrition to post-transplant TPN independence.

## SUMMARY

Significant improvements in outcomes with intestinal transplantation have been achieved through advances in multi-disciplinary care of intestinal failure, organ preservation/procurement/and implantation, and innovative immunosuppressive strategies which presently include minimization of long-term Tacrolimus. The challenge of preventing or minimizing chronic allograft rejection remains elusive. The waiting list mortality, particularly for children with concomitant liver failure, has improved following recent revisions of national allocation guidelines. Long-term studies on intestinal function and nutritional outcomes promise to clarify further the role of intestinal transplantation in children with intestinal failure.

## SELECTED READINGS

Abu-Elmagd K, Costa G, Bond G, et al. Five hundred intestinal and multivisceral transplantations at a single center. *Ann Surg* 2009;250:567–581.

Abu-Elmagd K, Costa G, Bond GJ, et al.. Evolution of the immunosuppressive strategies for the intestinal and multivisceral recipients with special reference to allograft immunity and achievement of partial tolerance. *Transpl Int* 2009;22(1):96–109.

Abu-Elmagd K, Fung J, Bueno J, et al. Logistics and technique for procurement of intestinal, pancreatic, and hepatic grafts from the same donor. *Ann Surg* 2000;232:680–687.

Akpinar E, Vargas J, Kato T, et al. Fecal calprotectin level measurements in small bowel allograft monitoring: a pilot study. *Transplantation* 2008;85:1281–1286.

ASPEN Board of Directors and Clinical Guidelines Task Force. Guidelines for the use of parenteral and enteral nutrition in adult and pediatric patients. *JPEN* 2004;28(6):S39–S70.

Beath S, Pironi L, Gabe S, et al. Collaborative strategies to reduce mortality and morbidity in patients with chronic intestinal failure including those who are referred for small bowel transplantation. *Transplantation* 2008;85:1378–1384.

Berg CL, Steffick DE, Edwards EB, et al. Liver and intestine transplantation in the United States 1998–2007. *Am J Transplant* 2009;9:907–931.

Ching YA, Fitzgibbons S, Valim C, et al. Long-term nutritional and clinical outcomes after serial transverse enteroplasty at a single institution. *J Pediatr Surg* 2009;44:939–943.

Diamond IR, Sterescu A, Pencharz PB, et al. Changing the paradigm: omegaven for the treatment of liver failure in pediatric short bowel syndrome. *J Pediatr Gastroenterol Nutr* 2009;48:209–215.

Goulet O, Baglin-Gobet S, Talbotec C, et al. Outcome and long-term growth after extensive small bowel resection in the neonatal period: a survey of 87 children. *Eur J Pediatr Surg* 2005;15:95–101.

Grant D, Abu-Elmagd K, Reyes J, et al. 2003 Report of the intestine transplant registry: a new era has dawned. *Ann Surg* 2005;241:607–613.

Gura KM, Lee S, Valim C, et al. Safety and efficacy of a fish-oil-based fat emulsion in the treatment of parenteral nutrition-associated liver disease. *Pediatrics* 2008;121:e678–e686.

Kocoshis SA, Beath SV, Booth IW, et al. Intestinal failure and small bowel transplantation, including clinical nutrition: Working Group report of the second World Congress of Pediatric Gastroenterology, Hepatology, and Nutrition. *J Pediatr Gastroenterol Nutr* 2004;39:S655–S661.

Mazariegos GV, Abu-Elmagd K, Jaffe R, et al. Graft versus host disease in intestinal transplantation. *Am J Transplant* 2004;4:1459–1465.

Mazariegos GV, Steffick DE, Horslen S, et al. Intestine Transplantation in the United States 1999–2008. Am J Transplant (2010 Special Issue: The 2009 SRTR Report on the State of Transplantation) 2010;10: 1020–1034.

Nishida S, Levi DM, Moon JI, et al. Intestinal transplantation with alemtuzumab (Campath-1H) induction for adult patients. *Transplant Proc* 2004;38(6):1747–1749.

Reyes J, Mazariegos GV, Abu-Elmagd K,et al. Intestinal transplantation under tacrolimus monotherapy after perioperative lymphoid depletion with rabbit anti-thymocyte globulin (thymoglobulin). *Am J Transplant* 2005;5(6):1430–1436.

Sudan D, Horslen S, Botha J, et al. Quality of life after pediatric intestinal transplantation: the perception of pediatric recipients and their parents. *Am J Transplant* 2004;4:407-413.

Sudan D, Vargas L, Sun Y, et al. Calprotectin: a novel noninvasive marker for intestinal allograft monitoring. *Ann Surg* 2007;246:311–315.

Wiles A, Woodward JM. Recent advances in the management of intestinal failure-associated liver disease. *Curr Opin Clin Nutr Metab Care* 2009; 12:265–272.

Wu T, Abu-Elmagd K, Bond G, Demetris AJ. A clinicopathologic study of isolated intestinal allografts with preformed IgG lymphocytotoxic antibodies. *Hum Pathol* 2004;35:1332–1339.

Zeevi A, Britz JA, Bentlejewski CA, et al. Monitoring immune function during tacrolimus tapering in small bowel transplant recipients. *Transpl Immunol* 2005;15:17–24.

# Index

*Note:* Page numbers followed by *f* indicate figures; and page numbers followed by *t* indicate tables.

## A

AAP. *See* American Academy of
    Pediatrics
Abbreviated injury scale (AIS),
        1034, 1035
Abdominal abuse, 1047
Abdominal aortic aneurysms, 953
    diagnosis, 953
    repair, 953
    symptoms, 953
Abdominal compartment syndrome
        (ACS), 76
    large infantile hemangioma, 1232*f*
Abdominal cystic lesion, 664
    in newborn, 664
Abdominal cystic structure, 654*f*
Abdominal injuries, 1044–1048.
            *See also* Abdominal trauma
    abdominal abuse
        characterized by, 1047
    blows/kicks, abdomen
        predictable injuries, cause of, 1044
    blunt abdominal injuries, 1044
        duodenal hematoma, 1044, 1045*f*
        duodenal perforation, 1044, 1045*f*
        include gastric rupture,
            1044, 1045*f*
    common explanations, 1047, 1048
    common injury, abused
            children, 1048
    death, cause of, 1048
    inflicted abdominal injuries
        fatal child abuse, 1044
    intentional trauma
        common solid organ injured
            liver, 1047*f*, 1048, 1049*f*
        gender incidence, 1046
    intestinal shearing injuries,
            1044, 1045
        abdominal distension and
            bruising, 1045, 1046*f*

    chylous ascites, 1045, 1046*f*
    most common site of, 1045
    pancreatic contusion/transection,
            1045, 1046*f*, 1047*f*
    late presentation, 1046, 1047
    Ledbetter series, 1048
    less-common solid organ injuries
        laceration, 1048
        renal contusion, 1048
    mechanism of blunt injury
        liver, pancreas, and duodenum,
            1045, 1047*f*
    mechanism of injury
        spleen, 1045, 1047*f*
    midline injuries
        characteristics, 1045
    noninflicted injuries, 1046
        *vs.* inflicted injuries, 1046
    observed patters of injury, 1044
        duodenal and jejunal
            rupture, 1044
        duodenal and pancreatic
            hematomata, 1044
        major solid visceral injuries, 1044
        minor solid visceral
            injuries, 1044
    pancreatic pseudocysts, 1045
    severe internal injury
        susceptibility, 1044
    spleen injury, 1048, 1049*f*
    unintentional trauma, 1046
        lower abdominal injuries, 1046*f*,
            1048, 1048*f*
Abdominal mass, 620
    contrastenhanced CT scan, 620
    CT-guided drainage, 620
    nontoxic, 620
    pediatric patients, 620
    phlegmonous mass, 620
*Abdominal Surgery of Infancy and
        Childhood,* 10

Abdominal trauma, 1082
    colonic injuries, 1097
    diaphragm injury, 1083–1084,
            1083*f*–1084*f*
    distal pancreatic ductal injury,
            1091–1092, 1092*f*
    duodenum injury, 1094
        hematoma, 1094, 1094*f*
        laceration/perforation, 1094
        repair, 1095*f*
    jejunoileal injuries,
            1094–1095, 1096*f*
    lacerations, 1088, 1089*f*–1090*f*
        Pringle maneuver, 1089*f*
    laparotomy, 1083
    liver injury, 1087, 1088*f*
    mesenteric injury, 1095, 1096*f*–1097*f*
        hematoma, 1095
    operative management, 1082
        FAST examination, 1082
        history, 1082
        indications, 1082–1083
    pancreatic ductal injury
        combined duodenal, common
            bile duct, 1093–1094
        management, 1094*f*
        proximal, 1092–1094
        repair injury, 1093*f*
        Roux-en-Y
            pancreaticojejunostomy,
            1093*f*
    pancreatic injury, 1091, 1091*f*
    perihepatic venous injury,
            1088–1090
    rectal trauma, 1097
    splenic injuries, 1084–1087,
            1084*f*–1088*f*
    stomach injury, 1090, 1090*f*
    tract injuries, 1088, 1088*f*
Abdominal viscera, 451
    herniation, 464

INDEX

Abdominal wall defects, 11, 13, 471–482
  associated anomalies
    intestinal atresia, 471
  chromosomal defects, 471
  embryologic etiology, 471
  epidemiology, 471
  trocar placement in suprapubic
    position, 585f
  umbilicus, 471
  vitelline artery, 471
Abnormal fluid, 56
ABS. See American Board of
  Surgery (ABS)
Abscess
  cervical, 238f
  drainage, 197
  epidural/subdural, 1056
  gluteal, 695, 696
  intraabdominal, 204, 206, 621
  intrahepatic, 1313
  intraosseous, 203
  lung, 422, 432, 433
  painful deep dermal, 197
  pelvic, 1254
  perianal, 212
  perirectal, 662, 1021
  pilonidal, 198
  spinal, 1014
  splenic, 748
  subphrenic, 750
Abuse. See Child abuse
Accreditation Council on Graduate
  Medical Education
  (ACGME), 9
Acetaminophen, 100, 161
  nonopioid analgesics, 159t
Achalasia
  cardinal feature of children with, 360
  childhood achalasia, 360–361
  complications, 361
  diagnostic workup, 360
    esophagogram, 361f
    lateral chest radiograph, 361f
  impact on growth and
    development, 359
  laparoscopic Heller myotomy with
    Dor fundoplication, 361
    operative technique, 361–362
    preoperative preparation, 361–362
  operative technique, 362, 362f–364f
  postoperative management, 362
  thoracoscopic Heller myotomy,
    362–364, 364f, 365f
  outcome of treatments, 364
    Dor fundoplication in children
      with achalasia, 364
    myotomy, 364–365
  overview, 359–360
  pathophysiology, 359–360
  pneumatic dilation in children, 361

Acidosis, 80, 85, 106, 174
Acquired cystic masses, 1233f
Acquired immunodeficiency
  syndrome,. See also Human
  immunodeficiency virus
Acquired lesions, 217
Acquired respiratory distress
  syndrome (ARDS), 78
  changes in FRC and compliance
    seen with, 107f
ACS. See Abdominal compartment
  syndrome (ACS); American
  College of Surgeons (ACS)
Activated partial thromboplastin time
  (aPTT), 175
Acute bilirubin encephalopathy
  (ABE), 45
Acute chest syndrome, 174
Acute gastroenteritis, 614
Acute pancreatitis (AP), 733, 734
  children, etiology in, 734t
  recurrent, 735
Acute tumor cell lysis syndrome
  (ATLS), 1268
  hyperuricemic nephropathy, 1268
  renal shutdown, 1268
Adams–Oliver syndrome, 274
Adenocarcinoma, 831
Adenosine triphosphate (ATP), 52
Adjuvant antibiotic therapy,
  mycobacterial infections, 238
Adjuvant therapy
  benefits, 1174
  specific pediatric cancer,
    1174–1176
Adolescents. See also Pediatric and
  adolescent gynecology
Adolescent young adults (AYA), 1260
  adolescents aged, 1260
  nodular sclerosis, 1260
  socioeconomic status, risk
    factors, 1260
Adrenal glands, 1157–1164
  anatomy, 1157
    anatomic relationships, associated
      organs, 1157, 1158f
    axial view, 1157, 1158f
    left adrenal gland, anatomic
      relationship
      pancreas and spleen.,
      1157, 1159f
    left adrenal vein drains into
      left renal vein, 1157, 1158f
    located superior to kidneys
      bilaterally
      derive arterial supply, inferior
        phrenic artery, 1157, 1158f
    right adrenal vein drains into
      inferior vena cava, 1157, 1158f
  diagnosis essentials, 1157

  embryology, 1157
  adrenal medulla arise
    from, 1157
  arise from, 1157
  indications, 1160
    adrenal cortical lesions, 1160
      adrenal cortical carcinoma
        (ACC), 1160
      adrenal-dependent
        hypercortisolism, 1160
      benign adenoma, 1160
      complete resection,
        best cure, 1160
      cushing syndrome, 1160
      diagnosis, 1160
      ectopic adrenocorticotropic
        hormone (ACTH)
        secretion, 1160
      hyperaldosteronism/Conn
        syndrome, 1160
      hypersecretion, 1160
      signs, 1160
      symptoms, 1160
    adrenal masses, 1160, 1161t
      coagulopathy, 1160
      metastatic lesions, 1160
      myelolipoma, 1160
    adrenal medullary lesions, 1160
      imaging, diagnosis, 1160
      $^{131}$I metaiodobenzylguanidine
        (MIGB) scan, 1160
      neoplasms, 1160
      pheochromocytomas, 1160
      pre-resection, 1160
      survival rate, 1160
    hyperfunction, 1160
    malignant adrenal disease
      vs. benign adrenal disease, 1160
    medulla lesions, 1160
      secrete, 1160
    onset, mean age, 1160
    other adrenal masses, 1160
    primary malignancies, in
      children, 1160
  operative techniques,
    1161–1164
    adrenalectomy approaches, 1161
    bilateral adrenalectomy, 1164
      bilateral disease, utilized
        for, 1164
      laparoscopic anterior
        approach, 1164
      lateral approach, 1164
      posterior minimally invasive
        approach, 1164
      procedure, 1164
    laparoscopic left adrenalectomy,
      1162, 1163
      EndoCatch bag, 1163
      Harmonic scalpel, 1163

inferior-medial aspect, adrenal gland, 1163
initial trocar, technique preferred, 1163
port placement, patient in lateral decubitus position, 1163, 1163f
positioning, patient, 1162
procedure, 1162, 1163
laparoscopic right adrenalectomy, 1161, 1162
complications, 1162
EndoCatch bag, 1161
endoscopic retroperitoneal, 1162
general endotracheal anesthesia, performed under, 1161
Harmonic scalpel, 1161
inferior vena cava (IVC), 1161
instruments setup, 1161
port placement, patient in lateral decubitus position, 1161, 1161f
right colon mobilization, 1161
right lobe, liver, 1161
surgeon position, 1161
open left adrenalectomy, anterior approach, 1163
approaches include, 1163
hyperfunctioning neoplasms, 1163
left adrenal vein drains, left renal vein, 1158f, 1163
multiple incisions, 1163
positioning, patient, 1163
retroperitoneal fat, 1163
splenic flexure, 1163
utilized for, 1163
open left adrenalectomy, posterior approach, 1163, 1164
positioning, patient, 1164
utilized when, 1163, 1164
open right adrenalectomy, anterior approach, 1162
anterior trans-peritoneal approach, 1162
general endotracheal anesthesia, use of, 1162
inferior vena cava (IVC), 1162
malignancy suspicion, 1162
transabdominal approach, 1162
open right adrenalectomy, posterior approach, 1162
Hugh–Young paraspinous incision, 1162
incision, location, 1162, 1162f
utilized when, 1162
Valsalva, 1162

postoperative considerations, 1164
anterior approaches, pitfalls, 1164
hemorrhage, 1164
physiology, 1157–1160
adrenal cortex, 1157
hormone synthesis, cholesterol, 1157, 1159f
adrenal medulla
catecholamine, synthesis of, 1159, 1159f, 1160
aldosterone
regulation, 1157, 1158
zona fasciculate, adrenal cortex, 1158
glucocorticoids, produce, 1158
zona reticularis, adrenal cortex, 1159
androgens
dihydroepiandrosterone (DHEA) androstenedione, sex hormones, 1159
Adrenal hyperplasia, 247, 904
congenital, 791, 903t, 905f, 908t, 924
Adrenocortical insufficiency, 85
Adrenogenital syndrome, 904
*Advances in Endoscopy of Infants and Children*, 10
Air embolism, 123–124
Airway
anatomy, 293
distress
diagnostic guidelines, 295–298
pathophysiology, 294–295
laryngeal cysts, 295f
laryngeal papilloma, 295f
lesions of larynx and upper airway, 295f
patient assessment, 295–298
bronchoscopic evaluation, with increasing stridor, 296f
computed tomography, 298f
foreign bodies in airway, 297f–298f
endoscopy, 292
history, 292–293
narrowing, visualization, 320
Airway obstruction
congenital high airway obstruction syndrome (CHAOS), 34
indications for a tracheotomy, 303f
infant/pediatric trachea, 317
management, 319
persistent, 324
proximal, 945
severe or progressive, 299
tumors causing, 1201

Alagille syndrome, 1306
Alanine, 62
Alanine aminotransferase (ALT), 569
Albumin, 65, 91, 94–95
Alexander disease, 51
Algorithms, for various treatment/ management
in acute cardiopulmonary arrest, 90f
airway management of the burned child, 1119f
anticoagulant treatment in children with documented venous thromboembolism, 99f
approach for lung biopsy in children, 424f
assessment of hyponatremia, 58f
blunt cardiac trauma investigation, 1077f
for CCAM, 26f
criteria for peritoneal drainage and laparotomy in infants, 602f
cryptorchidism: diagnostic and treatment algorithm, 777f
decisional algorithm for primary hypospadias repair, 792f
decision-making algorithm
female newborns with an anorectal malformation, 677f
male newborns with an anorectal malformation, 676f
diagnosis and management of bronchiectasis, 431f
diagnosis and management of lung abscess, 433f
diagnosis and treatment
pediatric patient with acute severe bradycardia, 91f
pediatric patient with tachycardia, 92f
diagnostic algorithm to differentiate Crohn disease from ulcerative colitis, 634f
diagnostic and therapeutic approach for child with empyema, 427f
diagnostic and treatment algorithm for cervical lymphadenitis, 200f
diagnostic and treatment algorithm for various umbilical disorders, 487f
evaluation and early management of flame burn, 1123f
hot-water (scald) burn, 1125f
evaluation and treatment algorithm for primary repair of pectus excavatum, 257f
evaluation of patient with suspected hidradenitis, 198f
imaging of pediatric chest trauma with CT, 1068f

Algorithms, for various treatment/
    management (*continued*)
  management algorithm based on
      laparoscopic findings, 778*f*
  management of a congenital
      inguinal hernia, 494*f*
  management of a spontaneous
      pneumothorax, 440*f*
  management of chylothorax, 444*f*
  management of Crotalinae
      snakebites, 1132*f*
  management of fetal CDH, 26*f*
  management of fetal MMC, 33*f*
  management of fetal SCT, 29*f*
  management of fetal TTTS, 30*f*
  management of patients with
      prenatal ultrasound
      suspicious for MI, 560*f*
  management schemes for
      diaphragmatic hernia, 457*f*
  pediatric patient with acute severe
      bradycardia, 91*f*
  pediatric patient with
      tachycardia, 92*f*
  resuscitation algorithm for the
      pediatric patient in acute
      cardiopulmonary arrest, 90*f*
  in resuscitation of pediatric patient
      in acute cardiorespiratory
      arrest, 89*f*
  selection of an antireflux operation
      in infants and children, 383*f*
  stepwise procedures in resuscitation
      of pediatric patient in acute
      cardiorespiratory arrest, 89*f*
  surgical management of patients
      with dumbbell spine
      tumors, 1023*f*
  treatment algorithm for central
      line associated bloodstream
      infection (CLABSI), 147*f*
  treatment algorithm: infantile
      hepatic hemangioma, 1231*f*
  treatment of children with
      pneumonia, 428*f*
  treatment of child with a
      mediastinal mass, 1263*f*
  treatment of NEC depending on
      extent of disease, 603*f*
Alpha fetoprotein (AFP), 1229
  germ cell tumors, 1229
  level, 1229
  malignancy, 1229
  mesenchymal hamartoma, 1229
  treatment, 1229
  tyrosinemia, 1229
5-Alpha-reductase deficiency, 900
Alternate continent urine
      drainage, 869
  complications, 876–878

Mitrofanoff principle, 870–872
  inconspicuous umbilical stoma,
      easily catheterized, 872*f*
  neourethra brought to
      perineum, 872*f*
  procedure, 870*f*–871*f*
  typical Mitrofanoff neourethra
      with catheter, 871*f*
  physiologic considerations, 869–870
    flap valves, 870*f*
    nipple valves, 870*f*
Alveolar pressures, 78
Alveolar rhabdomyosarcoma (ARMS),
      1211–1212
  either PAX3 (chromosome 2), 1212
  PAX 7 (chromosome 1) transcription
      factor genes, 1212
  tumors, older children, 1212
AMA. *See* American Medical
      Association (AMA)
Amenorrhea, 925
American Academy of Pediatrics
      (AAP), 4, 7–8, 17
American Board of Surgery (ABS), 6–7
  certification by, 6–7
  description, 6
American College of Surgeons
      (ACS), 8–9
American Medical Association
      (AMA), 9
American Pediatric Surgical
      Association, 20
  obligations, 20
American Pediatric Surgical
      Association (APSA), 8
Aminoglycosides, 93
Amiodarone
  for child with ventricular tachycardia/
      ventricular fibrillation, 88
Amputation
  CAVLM patients, 996
  digital, 278
  extremity injuries management,
      1114–1116
  limb, 953
  in management of
      nonrhabdomyosarcoma soft
      tissue sarcomas, 1223*f*
  mangled extremity and, 1114–1116
  techniques, 1115
Amrinone, 86
Amylase, 44
Amyloid protein, 191
Anabolic hormone resistance, 131
Analgesia, 100
  titration, 100
Analgesia in office setting, 208
  administering digital nerve block
      anesthetic, 209*f*
  digital block, 209

local anesthesia, 208
  maximum dosages for tissue
      infiltration, 209*t*
  penile block, 209
  procedural sedation,
      209–210
  topical anesthesia, 208
Anal/rectal myectomy
  operative technique, 583
    transanal approach, 583
    transsacral approach, 583
  treatment options, 583
Anal/rectal myotomy. *See* Anal/rectal
      myectomy
Anaphylactic shock, 83
  diagnosis and treatment, 84*f*
Anaphylaxis, 85, 150, 152, 192,
      1134, 1135*t*
Anaplastic large cell lymphoma,
      1268–1269
  local, systemic disease, 1268
Anatomic scales, 1034–1037
  abbreviated injury scale (AIS),
      1034, 1035
    Association for the Advancement
        of Automotive Medicine
        (AAAM), owned by, 1034
    dictionary, 1035
    group injuries
      based on body regions,
        1034, 1035
  anatomic profile (AP),
      1035, 1036
    A Severity Characterization of
        Trauma (ASCOT), 1036
    uses, 1035, 1036
  ICD-9 codes and ICD-9 derived
      scores, 1036
    bayesian logistic injury severity
        score (BLISS), 1036
    ICD-9 injury severity score
        (ICISS), 1036
    injury scaling methods
        comparison, 1036*t*
    international classification of
        diseases, 1036
    patient's traumatic ICD-9
        codes, 1036
    survival risk ratios (SRR)
        calculation, 1036
    trauma mortality prediction
        model (TMPM-ICD9), 1036
  injury severity score (ISS), 1037
    blunt trauma, 1037
    calculation, 1037
    flaws, 1037
    new injury severity score
        (NISS), 1037
    odd sum-of-squared-scores
        method, 1037

organ injury scale (OIS), 1035
  developed by, 1035
  organ-specific scales grade
    injuries, 1035
  renal OIS, 1035, 1036f
  *vs.* abbreviated injury scale, 1035
Androgen insensitivity syndrome
  (AIS), 899
Anemia, 152, 173
  blood transfusion volume, 174
  chronic, 173
  erythropoietin, preoperative
    administration of, 174
  hematocrit levels, 173
  hemolytic, 174
  iron-deficiency, 177
  preoperative transfusion, 174
Anesthesia, 67, 476. *See also specific*
  *procedure* American Society
  of Anesthesiologists physical
  status classification, 133
  local, 208
  topical, 208
Anesthetic risks, 150
  latex sensitivity, 152
  malignant hyperthermia (MH), 151
Anesthetics, inhalational, 155
Aneurysm, 929
  rate, 939
Angiogenesis inhibitors, for putative
  therapy of diseases, 6
Angiography, 75
Angiohepatic dysplasia, 1306
Angiosarcoma, 1246
  prognosis, 1247
Animal assaults, 1129
  animal bites, 1135
    cat bites, 1136–1137
    dog bites, 1135–1136
    human bite, 1137
      *Eikenella corrodens*
        contaminant, 1137
  bite injuries, 1129
    degree of injury, 1129
    snakebites, 1130
      algorithm for management of
        Crotalinae snakebites, 1132f
      clotting factor abnormalities to
        guide FabAV redosing, 1132t
      coral and exotic snakes, 1133
      epidemiology, 1130
      evaluation, 1130–1131
      FabAV administration, 1131t
      management, 1131–1133
      outdated and unproven
        treatments, 1131t
    spider bites, 1133
      black widow *(Latrodectus),* 1134
      brown recluse *(Loxosceles),*
        1133–1134

epidemiology, 1133
evaluation, 1133–1134
treatment of acute
  anaphylaxis, 1135t
venomous spiders in the
  United States, 1133t
treatment, 1129
  administration of
    antivenin, 1130
  antibiotic therapy, 1130
  systemic treatment, 1129
type of bite, 1129
insect stings, 1134
  fire ants, 1135, 1135f
  scorpions, 1135
  stings of bees and wasps, 1134–1135
Annual pediatric trauma volume
  United States, 1029, 1030t
Anorectal malformation (ARM), 885
  associated defects, female, 674, 675
    gynecologic, 675
    other associated defects, 675
    sacral defects, 675
      hemisacrum, 675
      sacral ratio, normal
        individual, 675f
    spinal, 675
    urologic, 674, 675
  definitive reconstruction, 678–693
    females, 685–691
      rectoperineal fistula, 685
      rectovestibular fistula, 685, 686
      (*See* Rectovestibular fistula)
    laparotomy, 679
    males, 679–685
    PSARP (*See* Posterior sagittally
      using a posterior
      anorectoplasty (PSARP))
  diagnosis, 675–678
    female newborn
      anoplasty, 677
      cloaca, diagnosis, 678
      cutback procedure, 678
      decision-making algorithm,
        677, 677f
      morbidity, 678
      perineal fistula, presence, 677
      posterior sagittal
        anorectovaginourethroplasty
        (PSARVUP), 678
      single perineal orifice, 678
      therapeutic-decision,
        correct, 677
      treatment strategies, 677, 678
      ureterostomies, 678
      vestibular fistulas, 678
    male newborn, 675–677
      colostomy, 677
      decision-making algorithm,
        676, 676f

important questions to be
  answered, 675
meconium, 676
newborn anoplasty, 677
radiologic evaluation, 677
sphincter muscle, 676
type of defect
  determination, 675
ultrasound, 675
MRI image, with cloaca and
  hydrocolpos, 676f
historic review, 669, 670
types, 670
  female defects, 672–675
    complex malformations, 674
    imperforate anus without
      fistula, 673
    persistent cloaca, 673, 674
    rectoperineal fistula, 672
    rectovestibular fistula,
      672, 673
  male defects, 670–672
    imperforate anus without
      fistula, 671, 672
    rectal atresia/stenosis, 672
    rectobladderneck fistula, 671
    rectoperineal fistula, 670
    rectourethral fistula, 670, 671
Anorectal myectomy, 584f
Anterior diaphragmatic rim, clamp
  marks, 459f
Antibiotics
  cephalosporins, 95
  IgG or IgM antibodies, 191
  minimum inhibitory concentration
    (MIC), 95
  prophylactic, 95
  time-dependent killing, 95
  usage, children admitted to ICU, 95
  vancomycin, 95
Anticardiolipin antibodies, 177
Anti-CD3 monoclonal antibody, 1289
Anticoagulation therapy, 97, 177–178
  heparin, 177
  sodium warfarin, 178
  vitamin K dose, 178
  white clot syndrome, 178
Antimicrobials, 95
  appropriate use of, 95
  basic principles, use in critically ill
    child, 96t
  in critically ill child, basic
    principle, 96f
  overview of empiric therapy
    for select hospital-acquired
    infections in PICU, 97t
  pharmacodynamics, 95
    minimum inhibitory
      concentration (MIC), 95
  selection and duration, 95–96

Antiphospholipid antibodies, 177
Antiseizure medications, 175
Antisepsis, 138
Antithrombin III (ATIII), 177
$\alpha^1$-Antitrypsin, 61
Antral web, 512–513
  acquired, 513
  diagnosis, 513
  symptoms, 512
  treatment, 513
Anuria, 939
Anus
  imperforate, 14, 612f, 656, 1020
    malformations, 670
    without fistula, 661, 671, 673, 685
  mobilized colon, 587f
Anxiolysis, 208
Aortic and great vessel injuries,
    1077–1079
  aortic disruption, 1077
    mechanism, includes, 1077
  chest CT angiography, 1079
  chest x-ray, 1079
  clam-shell incision, 1078
  diagnostic testing, 1078
  main associated risk, 1078
  mortality rate, 1077
  operative intervention, 1078
  patient management, 1077
  radiographic marker, reliable
    funny looking mediastinum, 1077
  radiographic signs include, 1077
  surgeries necessities, 1078
  thoracic trauma, different
    approaches
    depending on location of injury,
      1078, 1079f
  thoracic vascular injury
    blunt trauma, 1077
    clinical signs, 1077
  trap-door incision, 1078
  traumatic brain injuries, 1078
Aortic and mitral hypoplasia, 941
Aortic arch
  developmental embryology of, 944f
Aortic coarctation, 937
  combined repair, 941
  definition, 938
  diagnosis, 939
  etiology, 938
  mortality with coarctation
    repair, 942
  paraplegia, 942
  patch aortoplasty, 940f, 941
  postcoarctation abdominal
    pain, 942
  presentation, 939
    MRI demonstration, juxtaductal
      aortic coarctation, 939f
    resected coarctation segment, 938f

resection with end to-end
    anastomosis, 939–940, 940f
resection with graft insertion, 941
risks and outcomes, 941
  pseudoaneurysm, 941–942
  recurrence, 941–942
subclavian flap repair,
    940–941, 940f
treatment, 939, 940f
Aortic cross-clamping
  with cardioplegia, 936f
Aortic narrowing, 938
Aortic stenosis, 72
Aortic thrombosis, 952
  complications, 952
  diagnosis, 952
  long-term morbidity, 952
  mortality, 952
  symptoms, 952
  treatment, 952
Aortopexy, 324–326
  surgical procedure, 325f
AP. See Acute pancreatitis (AP)
Apical bullae, wedge resection, 441f
Apnea
  diagnosis of, 47
  idiopathic, 47
  obstructive sleep, 152
  postanesthesia, 505
  prematurity, 47, 105t
APO regimen, 1269
  doxorubicin, 1269
  prednisone, 1269
  vincristine, 1269
Appendectomy, 621–628
  approach, 621
  gynecologic pathology, 621
  Inversion-ligation, 625f
  laparoscopic, 621
    children
      widespread popularity in, 621
  methods, 624–626
    endoloop or suture ligature,
      624–626
    stapled, 624
  open techniques, 621–624
    anterior superior iliac spine, 621
    cecal taeniae, 622
    cecum, 622
    cephalad gridiron, 622
    iliac fossa, extract from, 622
    Mayo scissors, 621
    peritoneal incision, 621
    rectus abdominus, 621
    sigmoid colon, 621
  pelvic surgery, 621
Appendicitis, 613–631
  acute, 614–616
    abdominal ultrasound (US),
      depicting, 616f

adhesions, 620
GI obstruction, 620
peritonitis, 620
  complication of, 620
  fecalith, 620
  walled-off abscess, 620
clinical diagnosing
  success rate of, 614
clinical presentation, 614
  paramount symptom, 614
  periumbilical location, 614
  symptomatology, 614
  urologic symptoms, 614
    dysuria, 614
    frequency, 614
    urgency, 614
  visceral afferents, 614
complicated, 619–620
diagnoses
  not require operation, 619
    acute rheumatic fever, 619
    constipation, 619
    diabetic ketoacidosis, 619
    hemophiliac, 619
    lead poisoning, 619
    porphyria, 619
    ureterolithiasis, 619
    urinary tract infection,
      pyelonephritis, 619
  require operation, 618
    choledochal cysts, 618
    Crohn disease,
      618–619, 629
    ectopic pregnancy, 618
    GI perforation, 618
    gonads, 618
    intussusception, 618
    pancreatitis, 619
    sickle cell disease, 619
    sickle cell disease/
      cholelithiasis, 619
    small bowel obstruction, 618
  require operation, pancreatitis
    anatomic abnormalities, 619
    childhood, 619
    serum amylase, 619
diagnostic imaging for, 617t
diarrhea associated with, 614
differential diagnosis, 617–619
  acute gastroenteritis, 617
  epiploic appendagitis, 617
  lymphocytosis, 617
  mesenteric adenitis, 617
    appendectomy, 617
  primary omental torsion, 617
  primary peritonitis, 617
  profuse watery diarrhea, 617
etiology of, 613–614
history, 613
  anatomic drawings, 613

imaging, 616–617
  abdominal radiographs, 616, 630
  appendicoliths, 616
  computerized tomography
      (CT), 616
  hemolytic uremic syndrome, 616
  Henoch–Schönlein purpura,
      616, 618
    hematuria, 618
  immunocompromised oncology
      patients, 616
  scoliosis, 616
incedence, 614
  abdominal condition, 614
  pediatric population ranges, 614
laboratory studies, 615–616
  C-reactive protein (CRP),
      level, 616
  pneumonia, 615, 619
  polymorphonuclear leukocytes
      (PMN), values, 616
  white blood count (WBC), 615
neonatal, 614
other considerations, 629–631
  acute typhlitis, 629
  carcinoid, 629
  incidental appendectomy, 629
  laparotomy, 629
pathophysiology, 613–614
  appendectomies, 613
  appendiceal colic, 613–614
  appendiceal luminal obstruction,
      concept, 613
  Enterobius vermicularis
      (pinworm), 613
  fecalomas, 613
  fecalomas, association of, 613
  fibrosis, 613
  lymphoid hyperplasia, 613
perforated, 619–620
  associated abscesses,
      percutaneous drainage, 620
  broad spectrum antibiotic
      coverage
    longer course of, 621
  conservatively, intravenous
      antibiotics, 620
  safely-accessible abscess
      amenable, 620
physical examination, 614–615
  abdominal muscle spasm, 615
  inflammation, 615
  involuntary guarding
      associated, 615
  psoas sign, 615
  Rovsing sign, 615
postoperative complications,
    628–629
  fecal fistula, 629
  intraabdominal abscess, 628

pylephlebitis, 629
  small bowel obstruction, 629
  wound infection, 628
preoperative considerations, 620–621
  antibiotics, 621
    ampicillin gentamicin
        metronidazole, 621
    ampicillin–sulbactam, 621
    Bacteroides fragilis, 621
    cefoxitin, 621
    Escherichia coli, 621
    piperacillin tazobactam, 621
    therapy, 621
  in-house observation, 620
    negative appendectomy
        rates, 620
  resuscitation, 620–621
    intraoperative catastrophe, 620
    isotonic fluid boluses, 620
prognosis, 631
  mortality, 631
  secondary multiorgan system
      failure, 631
Appendicostomy, 595, 610, 1011
  bowel lavage, 1011
  catheterizable cutaneous cecal
      stoma, 610
  Malone, 691
Appendix, 613–614
  anorexia, 614
  blood supply of, 615f
  central inflamed
    phlegmon with, 620
  clamp
    crushed with, 622f
  clamped distally, 623f
  classic pelvic computerized
      tomography (CT), 617f
  crushed base of, 623f
  gangrene develops, 614
  luminal obstruction of, 613–614
  mesentery
    endovascular stapler passed
        through, 627f
  nausea, 614
  pelvic, 615
  removed
    purse string appendectomy,
        622–624
    simple ligation, 622
  retrocecal position, 615
  sutures placed, endoloops
    base of, 628f
  visualized delivered, in wound, 622f
  wall of, 613
    edematous, 613
    mucosa, ischemia of, 613
  window created, mesentery
    avascular plane of, 627f
  A Z-stitch, 623f

APSA. See American Pediatric Surgical
    Association (APSA)
APSA Education Committee, 9
ARDS. See Acquired respiratory
    distress syndrome (ARDS)
ARM. See Anorectal malformation
    (ARM)
Arrhythmias, 77
  contributing to the hypoperfused
      state, treatment, 85
  treatment, 77
  types, 85
  ventricular, 78t, 151, 1076
Arterial access, 147–148
  alternative, 148
Arterial catheters
  complications, 75
  placement, 72
Arterial malformations, 992–993
Arterial puncture, 142
Arteriovenous fistulae (AVF),
    1295–1296, 1296f–1297f
Arteriovenous grafts (AVG),
    1295–1296, 1296f–1297f
Arteriovenous malformations,
    992–993
  arteriovenous connections, 992
  congenital vascular lesions, 992
  embolization techniques, 993
  face, neck, 993f
  head, 992
  neck, 992
  normal precapillary anastomosis,
      size, 992
  PTEN gene, 992
Artery
  cannulations in children, 73
    methods, 73
  femoral, 75
  radial, 74
    insertion of catheter, 73f, 74f
  umbilical, 73–75
    insertion of a catheter, 74f
Artificial bladder, 862, 865
Ascorbic acid, 66
A Severity Characterization of Trauma
    (ASCOT), 1039
Aspiration prophylaxis, 154
Aspirin, 175, 930
Assent, 17
  characteristics, 17
Asthma, 152, 155, 318, 438, 543, 728
ATP-regulated potassium channel, 1141
Atresias, 549. See also Biliary atresia;
    Colonic atresia; Duodenal
    atresia; Intestinal atresia;
    Jejunoileal atresia; Pyloric
    atresia; Vaginal atresia
  development, theories, 549
  types, 549

Atrial tachyarrhythmias, 85
Atropine, 86, 88
    administered via endotracheal
        tube, 88
    increase heart rate, conduction
        velocity, and contractility, 86
Attenuated FAP (AFAP), 1255
    endoscopic screening, 1255
    FAP, variant, 1255
    ileal pouch anal anastomosis, 1255
    reduced, colonic polyps, 1255
Autoimmune disorders, 745
    autoimmune hemolytic anemia, 745
        coombs test, 745
        result from, 745
        treatment, 747
            immunosuppression, 747
            plasmapheresis, 747
        warm agglutination, 745
    idiopathic thrombocytopenic
        purpura (ITP), 745
        diagnosis, 745
        IgG autoantibodies, 745
        result in, 745
        treatment, 747
            life-threatening
                hemorrhage, 747
            self-limiting, 747
            splenectomy, 747
Autologous intestinal reconstruction
        surgery, 647–649
    autologous reconstruction, 649
    Bianchi procedure, 647
        technical challenges, 647
    important conclusions, 649
    intestinal transplantation, 649
    longitudinal intestinal lengthening
        and tailoring (LILT)
        liver disease, 647
        patients analyses, 647
        procedure component
            anastomosis, bowel segments,
                647, 648f
            bowel, longitudinal division,
                647, 648f
            division, mesentery into 2
                separate leaflets, 647, 648f
            separation, 2 leaflets, 647, 648f
        published results, 647, 648t
    mortality, predictive factors, 648
    serial transverse enteroplasty
        (STEP), 647
        procedure, 647
        published results, 647
        redo-STEP operation,
            intraoperative
            photograph, 648f
    vs. LILT, 647
    weaning from PN, 647
Automatic blood pressure devices, 71

Avulsion fractures, 1100
Axillary nerve block, 167, 168f
Azathioprine, 402, 633, 734t, 1288,
        1291, 1311

B
Babinski response, 1063
Bacitracin
    antimicrobial creams, 1125t
    for facial burns, 214
Bacteria, 598
    aerobic and anaerobic, 237, 1136
    Clostridia, 598
    commensal, 195
    encapsulated, 194
    Enterobacteriaceae, 598
    gram-positive and gram-negative,
        146, 1313
    pathogenic, 43
    Staphylococcus, 598
Bacterial endocarditis, 930
Bacteriuria, 876
Bacteroides, 195, 201
BAL. See Broncho-alveolar lavage
        (BAL)
Bannayan–Riley–Ruvalcaba
        syndrome, 1257
    characterized, macrocephaly, penile
        pigmentation, 1257
    hamartomatous polyp
        disorder, 1257
    PTEN gene, mutation, 1257
Barbiturates, 155, 1064
Bariatric adolescent patients, 18
Bariatric surgery, 17, 523
    energy homeostasis, 526
    obesity, defined, 523–525
    obesity epidemic quantified,
        525–528
        medical comorbidities, 525
        morbidly obese adolescent, 526
        obese adult, 526
        psychosocial comorbidities, 525
        societal comorbidities, 525–526
    surgical decision protocol, 529f
    weight loss vs. weight gain, 526–527
        cholecystokinin (CCK), 527
        ghrelin, 527
        glucagon-like peptide-1
            (GLP-1), 527
        leptin, 527
        oxyntomodulin (OXM), 527
        peptide YY, 527
        special challenges, 528
        visceral fat, 527–528
    weight management team, 528
Baroreceptors, 48
Barotrauma, 416
Bartholin glands, 882
    cyst, 882

Bartonella henselae, 199
Bartonella henslae, 1137
Battery ingestion, 329–331, 515
B cells, 193, 1261, 1266, 1267, 1285,
        1286, 1314
B cell tumors, 1267
    malignant transformation, 1267
    plasma cells, 1267
Benign epithelial tumors, 1233–1234
    focal nodular hyperplasia,
        1233–1234
    hepatic (hepatocellular)
        adenoma, 1234
    nodular regenerative hyperplasia
        (NRH), 1234
Benign tumors, 1229–1235
    benign epithelial tumors, 1233
        focal nodular hyperplasia,
            1233–1234
            variable radiographic
                appearance, 1234f
        Hepatic (hepatocellular)
            adenoma, 1234
        nodular regenerative hyperplasia
            (NRH), 1234
    hepatic hemangioma, 1229–1232
    hepatic teratoma, 1235
    hepatobiliary cystadenoma, 1234
    infancy, 1229
    mesenchymal hamartoma, 1232
Benzodiazepines (BZDs), 100
    commonly used in PICU, 101t
    features of withdrawal, 103t
    GABA receptors, 163
    pain control, 154, 163
    prolonged administration of, 103
Bernard–Soulier syndrome, 175
Beta-cell dysfunction, 1141
Bezoars, 515
Bicarbonate, 56, 63, 88, 716, 735, 877,
        1303, 1311
Bifidobacterium bifidus, 195
Bifidobacterium breve, 195
Bifidobacterium infantis, 195
Bifidobacterium lactis, 195
Bifidobacterium longum, 195
Bilateral oophoropexies
    abdominal radiotherapy, 1263
Bilateral wilms tumor, 1184
    bilateral nephron-sparing
        surgery, 1184
    biopsy, 1184
    chemotherapy
        initiation, 1184
    cure
        high probability, 1184
    double-J ureteral stent, 1184
    genetic syndromes, 1184
        associated with, 1184
    metachronous tumor, 1184

neoadjuvant therapy, 1184
3-drug chemotherapy (regimen
DD-4A), 1184
operative intervention, 1184
renal failure, increased risk, 1184
Biliary atresia, 715
classification, based on biliary
obstruction, 710
Type I—distal obliteration, hilar
bile cysts, 710, 711f
Type III—complete obliteration,
extrahepatic ducts, 710, 711f
Type II—proximal obliteration,
distal patency, 710, 711f
definition, 710
diagnosis, 711, 712
$\alpha_1$-antitrypsin (AAT), 711
biochemical tests, 711
results, 711
cholangiography, 712, 713f
operative cholangiogram,
712, 713f
diagnostic algorithm, 711, 712f
endoscopic retrograde
cholangiography, 711
fluid-filled gallbladder, 711
hepatobiliary imaging, 711
infancy cholestasis
myriad causes, 711
jaundice, infants, 711
obstructive mechanical
causes, 711
Kasai portoenterostomy, 711, 713f
liver, 711
histological changes, 711, 712
magnetic resonance (MR)
cholangiography, 711
nucleotide uptake, 711
percutaneous liver biopsy, 711
polysplenia anomalies, presence
of, 711
serologic tests, 711
triangular cord sign, 711
ultrasound, 711
extrahepatic, 1306
hepatic portoenterostomy, 713, 714
ductal remnants, transected at
level of posterior portal vein,
713, 714f
fibrous biliary duct widens,
cone-shaped mass, 713, 713f
gallbladder, mobilization, 713
Kasai portoenterostomy,
713, 713f
operative procedure, 713
Roux-en-Y, intestinal
reconstructions, 714
Roux-en-Y limb of jejunum,
creation, 714, 714f
Roux limb, 714

laparoscopic techniques, 715
laparoscopic
cholecystocholangiography,
715
laparoscopic
portoenterostomy, 715
controversy, 715
prospective trial, European
Biliary Atresia Registry, 715
purported advantages, 715
liver transplantation, 714, 715
immunosuppression, 715
infancy, 715
Kasai operation, 715
adverse effects, 715
nasogastric decompression, 715
pathophysiology, 710, 711
atresias, gastrointestinal tract, 710
biliary remnant, 710
disease caused by, 710
extrahepatic biliary tree
embryological development, 710
hepatic ducts
development, 710
intrahepatic bile duct
development
process, 710
pathologic findings, 710
characteristics, 710
primitive bile duct cells, 710
portal hypertension, 716
cholangitis, 716
complications, 716
esophageal variceal
hemorrhage, 716
hepatic decompensation, 716
hepatic fibrosis, 716
hypersplenism, 716
portal pressure, increased, 716
portocholecystostomy, 714
proximal amputation, 714
temporary catheter
decompression, 714, 715f
prognosis, 716
hepatoportoenterostomy, 716
age, survival determinant, 716
cholangitis, 716
Kasai operation, 716
treatment, 712, 713
surgical, 712
Biliary rhabdomyosarcoma, 1246
Biliary tract, 1217
metastases, 1217
Biliopancreatic diversion procedure
(BPD), 529
Bilirubin, 44, 65
Bilirubin metabolic pathway, 46
Biotin, 66
Bishop-Koop distal chimney
enterostomy, 566f

Bites wounds
animal bites, 1135
cat bites, 1136–1137
Cat-scratch disease, 1136
*Pasturella* multilocida, 1136
dog bites, 1135–1136
human bite, 1137
bite injuries, 1129
degree of injury, 1129
snakebites, 1130
algorithm for management of
Crotalinae snakebites, 1132f
clotting factor abnormalities to
guide FabAV redosing, 1132t
coral and exotic snakes, 1133
epidemiology, 1130
evaluation, 1130–1131
FabAV administration, 1131t
management, 1131–1133
outdated and unproven
treatments, 1131t
spider bites, 1133
black widow
(Latrodectus), 1134
brown recluse (Loxosceles),
1133–1134
epidemiology, 1133
evaluation, 1133
treatment of acute
anaphylaxis, 1135t
venomous spiders in the
United States, 1133t
treatment, 1129
administration of antivenin,
1130
antibiotic therapy, 1130
systemic treatment, 1129
type of bite, 1129
Bladder capacity/compliance, 857
complications, 876–878
acute abdominal surgical
illness, 876
altered gastrointestinal
function, 878
hematuria–dysuria syndrome,
877–878
malignancy, 877, 878f
metabolic complications,
876–877
reconstructive failure, 876
urolithiasis, 876
inadequate, compensating
for, 857
autoaugmentation, 861
gastric segment procedures,
860–861
gastrocystoplasty, 861f
ileocecal segment procedures,
859–860
large-bowel procedure, 860

Bladder capacity/compliance
(*continued*)
  physiologic considerations,
      857–859
    inflated surgeon's glove, 858*f*
    urodynamics of cecal
        reservoir, 858*f*
  small-bowel procedures, 859
    bladder augmentation
        employing an intestinal
        segment, 859*f*
    Camey enterocystoplasty, 860*f*
    Kock pouch, 860*f*
  ureteral augmentation, 861
    operative stages, 863*f*
Bladder closure, 850
Bladder exstrophy, 828, 829*f*
  anatomy, 831–832
  bilateral iliac osteotomy, 829
  Coffey ureterosigmoidostomy, 828
  cystectomy, 828
  diagnosis, 832
  evolution, 828
  exstrophy patient as adult, 843
    bladder cancer, 844
    sexual function, 843–844
  gender ratio, 830
  incidence, 830
  inheritance, 830
  Leadbetter technique, 829
  management of complications, 842
    bladder prolapse or dehiscence, 842
    complications of epispadias
        repair, 842
    small capacity bladder/failed
        bladder-neck plasty, 842–843
  modification of Young continence
      procedure, 828
  pathophysiology, 830–831
  primary bladder closure, 832
    bladder closure, 833–835, 834*f*
      complete anatomic closure,
          834*f*, 835
      Mitchell epispadias repair, 836*f*
      types of osteotomies, 833*f*
    continence surgery
      bladder-neck
          reconstruction, 838
    epispadias repairs, 837
      Cantwell–Ransley epispadias
          repair, 837, 838*f*–839*f*
    herniorrhaphy, 835
    incontinent period, 837
    Mitchell Modified bladder-neck
        plasty, 840–841
    osteotomy, 832–833
    outcomes of reconstruction
        stages, 841
      results following bladder
          closure, 841

results following bladder-neck
    reconstruction, 842
results following the epispadias
    repair, 841–842
pelvic immobilization, 835–837
staged approach, 832
umbilicoplasty, 835
Young–Dees–Leadbetter–Jeff
    s–Gearhart procedure, 838,
    840, 840*f*–841*f*
treatment
  goals of, 832
urinary collecting devices, 829*f*
Blood gas monitoring
  transcutaneous, 72
Blood pressure, 71
  diastolic, 71, 75
  noninvasive, 80
  systolic, 71, 75
    lower limit of normal pressure in
        children, 84
Blood transfusion, 34, 39, 87, 178, 747,
    1252, 1286
Blount disease, 525
Blue rubber bleb nevus syndrome,
    983–984
  blue venous nodules, 984*f*
  disorder, 983
  morbidity, 984
  mortality, 984
Blunt cardiac injuries (BCI),
    1075, 1076
  commotio cordis
    injury pattern, 1076
  complications, 1076
  diagnosis, 1076
    electrocardiogram (EKG), 1076
  greatest risk factor
    force applied to thoracic
        cage, 1076
  hemodynamically stable
      patients, 1076*t*
  investigation algorithm, 1076, 1077*f*
  lung contusion
    associated problems, 1075
  most common mechanism
      of injury, 1075
  myocardial contusion, 1075, 1076
    myocardial infarction,
        mimic, 1076
  other consistent problems, 1076
  pathognomonic
      consequences, 1076*t*
  rib fracture
    associated problems, 1075
Blunt dissection, 148
BMI chart, 524*f*
Bochdalek hernias, 449
  diagnosis, 451
    antenatal, 45!

management, 449
  antenatal, 453
operative repair, 449
presentation, 451
surgical management, 449
  history of, 449
    delayed operation, 449
    infants and children,
        survival, 449
surgical repair, 459
Body temperature, 68, 71, 77, 131
Bombesin, 359
Bone graft, 437
Bonnevie–Ullrich syndrome, 274
Boston School of Pediatric
    Surgery, 5–6
Botulinum toxin, 197
Bovie cautery, 579, 583
Bowel injury, 823
Bowel lumen
  intraoperative interrogation of, 635*f*
Bowel-management program, 693
  colon, 693
    hypermotility, 693
  contrast enema study, 693
  enemas, 693
    use of, 693
  implementation, 693
  main problem, 693
  megasigmoid, 693
    degree of, 693
BPD. *See* Bronchopulmonary
    dysplasia (BPD)
BPS. *See* Bronchopulmonary
    sequestration (BPS)
Brachial plexus block, supraclavicular
    approach, 167
Bradyarrhythmias, 86
Bradycardia, 34, 43, 91, 102, 203, 762,
    931, 972, 1034
Branchial apparatus, 217
  anomalies, 217
Branchial cleft lesions, 218
Branchio-oto-renal [BOR]
    syndrome, 228
Breastfeeding, 633
Breast(s)
  adolescent girl with debilitating
      macromastia, 247*f*
  conditions
    apparrent at birth, 244–245
    in boys, 244*t*
    in children unrelated to age,
        250–252
    in first few weeks of life, 245–246
    in girls, 244*t*
    in prepubertal
      boys, 246
      girls, 246
    in pubertal girls, 247

developmental anomalies of
adolescent female, 247–248
disorders in children, 243
embryology, 243
extremely large fi broadenoma, 248*f*
infections of adolescent female,
249–250
male pubertal gynecomastia
Grade 1, 250*f*
Grade 2, 250*f*
mild Poland syndrome, 248*f*
neonatal mastitis, 246*f*
neoplastic diseases of adolescent
female, 248–249
normal development, 243–244
operative technique
for subcutaneous mastectomy
for male pubertal
gynecomastia, 251*f*
reduction mammoplasty for
macromastia, 247*f*
tanner stages of breast development
in pubertal girls, 245*f*
Bronchiectasis, 428
diagnosis, 430, 430*f*, 431*f*
essentials of diagnosis, 428–429
etiology, 429–430
management, 430–431, 431*f*
outcome, 431
pathophysiology, 429–430
Broncho-alveolar lavage (BAL), 422, 458
infants
fluid of, 458
Bronchogenic cysts, 403, 405, 416
computed tomography
thin-walled apparently cystic
lesion, 405*f*
mediastinal, 417*f*
minimally invasive technique,
418–419, 419*f*
muscle-sparing thoracotomy,
418–419, 419*f*
posteroanterior chest radiograph
for evaluation, 405*f*
resection technique, 406
thoracoscopic visualization, 418*f*
Bronchopulmonary dysplasia (BPD),
47, 64, 66, 115, 152, 416,
930, 937
Bronchopulmonary malformations, 407
Bronchopulmonary sequestration (BPS)
categories, 407
extralobar sequestration (ELS), 407
artery, clip process, 409*f*
chest radiograph of a female
infant, 408*f*
systemic artery, dissected out
using, 409*f*
intralobar sequestration (ILS),
407–409

intraoperative death, 409
lesions, 407
minimally invasive technique,
418–419, 419*f*
muscle-sparing thoracotomy,
418–419, 419*f*
newborn with intraabdominal, 409
resection of intralobar, 409
surgical approach, 409
Bronchoscopy, 344, 347, 416,
436, 950
with BAL, 423
flexible, 299, 300
laser, 302
lung, 436
rigid, 301, 320, 1074
Browne, Denis, 4–5
Brunner's glands, 42
Burkitt lymphoma
hematoxylin, eosin stained
slide, 1267*f*
Burn
care, 1118
early hospital care, 1123–1124
first-degree burns, 1119
injury causing serious, 330
management
algorithm for evaluation and early
management
flame burn, 1123*f*
hot-water (scald) burn, 1125*f*
antimicrobial creams, 1125*t*
nutrition and hypermetabolic
response, 1128
hyperglycemic control, 1128
oxandrolone, 1128
propranolol, 1128
pharmacologic agents, 1128
mortality rate, 1118
normal anatomy of skin, 1121*f*
resuscitation (*See* Resuscitation)
skin grafts, 1124–1126
obtain partial-thickness graft,
1126*f*
wound, 1121
deep dermal burn, 1122*f*
full thickness burn, 1123*f*
Button battery ingestion, 329

C
CACs. *See* Children's Advocacy
Centers (CACs)
Caloric delivery, excess, 132
Cancer. *See also* Carcinoma;
Neoplasms
FIGO staging classification for
ovarian cancer, 894*t*
Cancer cachexia, 131
Cantwell–Ransley epispadias repair,
837, 838*f*–839*f*

Capillary arteriovenous fistulae,
995–996
hypertrophic cardiomyopathy, 996
Capillary-arteriovenous malformation,
995–996
Parkes Weber syndrome, 995*f*
*RASA-1* gene, mutations, 996
skeletal hypertrophy, 995
soft tissue, association with, 995
Capillary malformations, 979–981
arteriovenous, 979
birth, 979
macular capillary stain, 979
management of, 980
hypertrophied lip, 980
laser therapy, 980
Nd:YAG laser, 980
pyogenic granulomas, 980
reduces complications, 980
surgical debulking, 980
neonatal, 979*f*
port-wine stains, 979
Wyburn–Mason syndrome, 979
Carbohydrate metabolism, 64–65
Carbohydrates, in breast milk, 45
Carbon dioxide, monitoring,
71–72, 72*f*
Carbon monoxide, 71
as leading cause of death
in fire, 1118
Carboxyhemoglobin, 71, 1118
Carcinoid tumor, 1258–1259
described
stomach rectum, GI tract, 1258
5-hydroxyindoleacetic acid
(5-HIAA), 1258
metastatic survey, 1258
octreotide scintigraphy, 1258
serosa, 1258
symptoms
cutaneous flushing, 1258
diarrhea, 1258
respiratory distress, 1258
Carcinoma. *See also* Cancer;
Neoplasms
Cardiac arrest, 38, 88, 151, 318,
1048, 1243
Cardiac catheterization, 939
Cardiac cycle, 72, 76, 1002
Cardiac insufficiency, 85
agents commonly administered in
setting, 86*t*
Cardiac malformations, 317
Cardiac output, 72
enhancement, associated with
improvement in SvO$_2$ and
the DO$_2$/VO$_2$ ratio, 87
measurement, 78–79
Fick equation, 79
optimization, 83

Cardiac output (*continued*)
  suprasternal Doppler ultrasound, 72
  thermodilution, 78
  thoracic electrical bioimpedance, 72
  transesophageal/transtracheal
      Doppler ultrasound, 72
Cardiac tamponade, 72, 85, 88
Cardiogenic shock, 83
Cardiopulmonary bypass, 929, 933
Cardiopulmonary collapse, 77
Cardiopulmonary resuscitation,
      acute, 83
Cardiovascular collapse, 439
Cardiovascular system, 48
  circulatory changes at birth, 49–50
  embryology of, 48
  fetal/neonatal, physiology of, 48–49
Care bundles, 104
  evidence-based intervention, 104
  used in critical care setting, 104
C-arm fluoroscopy, 436
Carotid arteriotomy, prepared for
      arterial cannulation, 121f
Carotid artery, 73
Cartilage, 228
Catecholamines, 67, 85, 131
Catheter, 439
  5 and 7-French catheter, 76
  hemothorax, 439
  position, 75
  pulmonary artery (PA) catheters, 76
    placement, 77f
  sizes for arterial cannulation, 73
Catheterization, 857
  bladder, 791
  cardiac, 255, 286, 939
  intermittent, 690, 852, 855,
      857, 869, 1299
  postoperative urethral, 825
  prolonged, 75
  umbilical artery, 952, 959
  umbilical vessel, 144
Catheter-related infection, 145
Catheter tip placement, 135
Cat scratch disease, 239
Caudal agenesis, 1020
  sacral agenesis, 1020
    Sagittal T1-weighted weighted
      MRI, child, 1020f
  syndrome, 1020
Caudal block, epidural nerve
      block, 165
Caudal cell mass, multipotent
      cells, 1008
Caudal neural tube, failure of, 50
Caustic ingestions, 328
Caustic injury, esophageal, 337
  corticosteroids/mitomycin-C
      in conjunction with
      bougienage, 340–341

dilation, 338–339
esophageal stenting, 340
management, 338
  caustic esophageal injury
    acute phase, 338
    management of chronic
      strictures, 338
    recovery phase, 338
  pathophysiology, 337–338
  replacement, 340–341
  segmental resection, 340
CBPFM. *See* Congenital
      bronchopulmonary foregut
      malformation (CBPFM)
CCAM. *See* Congenital cystic
      adenomatoid malformation
      (CCAM)
CD. *See* Crohn disease (CD)
CD4 cells, 192, 1286
CD8 cells, 192, 1286
CDH. *See* Congenital diaphragmatic
      hernia (CDH)
Cecum
  foramen, 1016f, 1147
  seromuscular suture, 623f
  taenia, 615f
  tubularized, 871
Celiotomy, 567
Central line associated bloodstream
      infection (CLABSI)
  treatment algorithm for, 147
Central venous access, 141
  complications of
    infection, 145–146
    venous thrombosis, 146
  external jugular vein, 141–142
  percutaneous access, 143
  saphenofemoral vein, 142, 142f
Central venous access, percutaneous.
      *See* Percutaneous central
      venous access
Central venous anatomy, 143
Central venous catheter
      placement, 141
Central venous complications, 1005
  endocarditis, 1005
  glomerulonephritis, diffuse, 1005
  thrombosis, 1005
  ventriculoatrial catheters, 1005
Central venous hemodialysis catheters,
      1294–1295
  catheter diameter sizes, 1295
  complications associated with, 1295
  dialysis catheters, 1295
  numerous advantages, 1295
  placement of a tunneled
      catheter, 1295
Central venous pressure, 75
Cephalic veins, 138
  antecubital fossa and serves, 139

Cerebral palsy (CP), 52, 937
Certification
  American Board of Surgery, 6–7
  description, 6–7
Cervical lymphadenitis, 238f
CF. *See* Cystic fibrosis (CF)
Chemical matrixectomy, 212
Chemical pleurodesis, 440–441
  caustic agents, 440
  doxycycline, 440
    lung transplant patients, 441
    thorax, 441
  symphysis, 440
  tetracycline, 440
Chemotherapy, 1167–1172, 1215,
      1221–1222, 1233, 1239–1240
  adjuvant *vs.* neoadjuvant
      chemotherapy, 1169
    adjuvant chemotherapy, use of
      post tumor resection, 1169
    disadvantages, neoadjuvant
      chemotherapy, 1169
    neoadjuvant administration, 1169
    nonmetastatic osteosarcoma,
      surgical resection
    survival benefit, 1169
  administration, dosing, and
      response, 1168, 1169
    chemotherapy courses, 1169
    complete response (CR), 1169
    dose-limiting toxicities, 1168
    hematologic toxicity, 1168
    maximum dose delivery
      small shortcomings, 1169
    nephrotoxicity/
      hepatotoxicity, 1168
    osteosarcoma, 1169
    partial response (PR), 1169
    supportive therapy measures, 1169
      granulocyte colony-stimulating
      factor (G-CSF), 1169
  biologic agents, 1172
    biologic response modifiers, 1172
      muramyl tripeptide
        phosphatidylethanolamine
        (MTP-PE), 1172
      patient's innate immune
        response, enhance, 1172
    cellular signalling pathways,
      inhibition, 1172
      Avastin, 1172
      Gefitinib, 1172
    intracellula signalling pathways,
      inhibition, 1172
  chemotherapeutic agents,
      1169–1172, 1171t
    action mechanism, within cell
      cycle
      different therapeutic agents
        classes, 1170f

alkylating agents, 1169
  cyclophosphamide, nitrogen-mustard derivative, 1169
  cytotoxic nature, 1169
  ifosfamide, 1169
antibiotics, 1169–1172
  anthracyclines, 1169
  antineoplastic activity, 1169
  bleomycin, 1169
  cardiomyopathy, 1169
  dactinomycin, 1169–1172
antimetabolites, 1169
  fluorouracil, 1169
  function as, 1169
  maximal cytotoxic effect, 1169
plant alkyloids, 1172
  etoposide, 1172
  neurotoxicity, 1172
  vinblastine, 1172
  vinca alkaloids, 1172
  vincristine, 1172
platinum agents, 1169
  carboplatin, 1169
  cisplatin, 1169
cisplatin, introduction, 1239
cyclophosphamide, 1216
cytotoxic, 1222–1223
  adriamycin, 1222
  dactinomycin, 1222
  ifosfamide, 1222
  vincristine, 1222
dose–response curve, 1169
first successful treatment, 1167
ototoxicity, 1239
standard therapeutic regimens, 1215
  actinomycin-D, 1215
  cyclophosphamide (VAC), 1215
  vincristine, 1215
surgical resection, 1239
therapeutic agents, development, 1167, 1168
tumor relapse, reduce, 1239
CHEOPS. See Children's Hospital of Eastern Ontario Pain Scale (CHEOPS)
Chest pain, 340
Chest radiographs, 77, 329f. See also Radiographs
  bilateral chylothorax, 443f
  parapneumonic effusion suggesting empyema, 426f
  visceral pleura., 439f
Chest wall
  defects, 347
  structural abnormality, 254
Child abuse
  diagnostic principles, 1050, 1051
    abdominal trauma, 1050
      symptoms and signs, 1050

abusive rectal injury, 1051
  patulous anus, 1051
  rectal vault, blood, 1051
based on, 1050
bruises, 1050
forensic concerns, 1050
historical background, 1050
inflicted extremity trauma, 1051
major blunt abdominal trauma, 1050, 1051
  peritonitis, 1050
medical report, 1050
pediatric surgeons
  identifying child abuse, role, 1050
  primary concern, 1050
physical findings
  immediate photographs, 1050
  meticulous documentation, 1050
physical signs, 1050
rib fractures, 1050
unexplained alteration, mental status, 1050
epidemiology, 1042, 1043
  child battering, 1043
  Gallup poll, 1042, 1043
  largest trauma registry based study, 1043
  maltreated children, 1042
expert testimony, 1053
  pretrial preparation, 1053
  voir dire, 1053
history, 1042
  battered child syndrome, 1042
  The Bible, 1042
  medico-legal study
    cruelty and brutal treatment inflicted on children, 1042
    infanticide, 1042
imaging studies, 1051, 1052
  Advanced Trauma Life Support® (ATLS®) guidelines, 1051
  angiography, 1052
  diagnostic approach, advocates, 1052
  diagnostic imaging, course of, 1052
  double contrast CT, 1052
  excretory urography (EUG), 1052
  gastrointestinal contrast examination, esophagogram, 1052
  hemodynamically unstable child, 1052
  hollow viscus injury, 1052
    diagnosis depends upon, 1052
  Image Gently® protocols, 1052
  invasive radiologic studies, 1051
  lateral chest radiographs, 1052
  liver–spleen scintigraphy, 1052

magnetic resonance imaging (MRI), 1052
noncontrast computed tomography (CT), 1051, 1052
  head, 1051
pancreatic injury, 1052
photographs, 1051
  documentation, 1051
postero-anterior radiographs, 1052
radiographic survey fractures, 1051
sonography, 1052
  Focused Assessment by Sonography in Trauma (FAST), 1052
  role of, 1052
ultrasonography, 1052
laboratory tests, 1051
  child abuse series, 1051
  coagulogram, 1051
  hematocrit, 1051
  urinalysis, 1051
pathophysiology, 1043–1050
  abdominal injury (See Abdominal injury)
  burn injury, 1044
    burn patterns, 1044
    inflicted burns, 1044
    scald burn, unusual location, 1044
  caregiver fabricated illness, 1049, 1050
    catheters, 1050
    cause of, 1049
    life-threatening manipulation, central line, 1050
    Munchausen syndrome, 1049
    reflux symptoms, 1049, 1050
  common pattern, abusive injuries, 1043
  head injury, 1044
    abusive head trauma, 1044
    benign enlargement of the subarachnoid space (BESS), 1044
    bilateral subdural hematomas, 1044
    blunt head trauma, 1044
    depressed skull fractures, 1044
    fragile bridging veins, 1044
    shattered eggshell pattern, 1044
    skull fractures, 1044
    violent shaking, 1044
  rectal injury and sexual abuse, 1049
    anorectal injury, 1049
    intravaginal injury, 1049
    noninflicted wounds, 1049
    observed injury patterns, 1049
    rectal abuse, 1049
    symmetric wounds, 1049

**Child abuse** (*continued*)
skeletal injury, 1043, 1044
callus formation, 1044
conditions mimicking child abuse, 1044
inflicted fractures, 1043
occult bony injuries, 1043
paraspinal fractures, lower ribs, 1043
proximal humerus acromion process, fractures, 1043
scapula acromion process, fractures, 1043
spiral extremity fractures, 1043
soft tissue injury, 1043
bite marks, 1043
bruises, 1043
cauliflower ear, 1043
lacerations, 1043
multicolored bruises, 1043
slap and grip marks, 1043
strangulation marks, 1043
whip marks, 1043
thoracic injury, 1048, 1049
abusive bear hug, 1049
chest injuries include, 1048
inflicted injuries, less-common, 1049
mechanism of injury, 1048
rib fractures, 1048
subcutaneous emphysema, unexplained, 1049
typical abusive injuries, 1043
treatment options, 1052, 1053
abusive intrathoracic injuries, most common, 1053
thoracotomy, 1053
abusive perineal injuries, 1053
Advanced Trauma Life Support® (ATLS®) guidelines, 1052
blunt traum injuries, 1053
child abuse pediatrician, 1052, 1053
Children's Advocacy Centers (CACs), 1053
cognitive dysfunction, 1053
duodenal hematoma
total parenteral nutrition (TPN), managed by, 1053
intestinal shearing injury, 1053
mesenteric biopsy, 1053
primary anastomosis, 1053
major traumatic brain injury, 1053
Brain Trauma Foundation (BTF) protocols, 1053
pancreatic pseudocysts
total parenteral nutrition (TPN), managed by, 1053
penetrating abdominal trauma, 1053
exploratory laparotomy, 1053

**Childhood Hodgkin lymphoma (HL), 1260**
children, 1260
exposure, Epstein-Barr virus (EBV), 1260
increasing, family size, 1260
lower, socioeconomic status, 1260
**Childhood obesity, 525**
**Children's Advocacy Centers (CACs), 1053**
**Children's Cancer Group (POG), 1198**
**Children's Hospital of Eastern Ontario Pain Scale (CHEOPS), 158**
*Chlamydia trachomatis*, 882
**Cholangiography, 703, 704f**
abdominal sonogram
hyperechoic gallstones, 703f
choledocholithiasis, evaluate for, 703
cholelithiasis, 703
fluoroscopy, 703
intraoperative, 703
Kumar clamp technique, 703, 704f
**Cholangitis, 715, 716**
broad-spectrum antibiotics, treatment, 715
development, 715
occurs in, 715
pyrexia, 715
development, 715
refractory, 715
ursodeoxycholic acid (UCDA), 715, 716
**Cholecystectomy, 174**
**Cholecystokinin (CCK), 527**
**Choledochal cyst, 716**
cystic lesions classification, 716, 717
Alonzo-Lej classification
Todani modification, 717, 717f
Type II deformities, 717
Type III lesions, 717
Type I malformations, 717
Type IVa deformity, 717
Type IVb lesions, 717
Type V anomalies, 717
diagnosis, 718
anatomic definition, ERCP, 718
biliary cystic disease
environmental basis for, 718
classic triad, 718
hyperamylasemia, 718
imaging techniques, 718
laboratory findings, 718
magnetic resonance pancreaticocholangiography (MRCP), 718
obstructive jaundice, newborn, 718
pancreatitis, 718

patients, two distinct populations, 718
adult form of disease, 718
infantile group, 718
surgical biliary obstructions, 718
ultrasonography, 718
operative technique, 719–722
cyst excision, 719, 720
CBD, identification, 719, 719f
common hepatic duct, transection, 720, 720f
completed reconstruction, 720, 721f
distal choledochal cyst, identification, 719, 719f
gallbladder, mobilization, 719, 719f
hepaticojejunostomy, construction, 720, 720f
operative procedure, 719, 720
operative therapy, 719, 719f
patient position, 719
posterior mucosectomy, 719
retrocolic Roux-en-Y jejunal limb, 720, 720f
second-generation cephalosporin, 719
internal approach, 720, 721
mucosectomy, 721, 722f
pericystic inflammation, 720, 721f
Roux-en-Y reconstruction, completed, 721, 722f
submucosal plane, lateral development, 721, 721f
laparoscopic approach, 721, 722
choledochal cysts excision, 721
complications, 722
hepaticojejunostomy, 721
Roux-en-Y hepaticojejunosotomy, 721
outcome, 722, 723
pathophysiology, 717, 718
choledochal cystic disease development of, 717
etiology, 717
neonatal lamb model, 717
ductal epithelium, immaturity of, 718
pancreaticobiliary ductal system, 717
anomalous drainage, 717
treatment, 718, 719
biliary carcinomas, 718
caroli disease, 718, 719
choledochocele (Type III), 718
management, 718
choledochocystduodenostomy, 718
definitive therapy, 718
duodenal-based cysts, 718A

fruste choledochal cyst, 719
hepaticoduodenostomy, 719
hepaticojejunostomy
    reconstructions, 718
medical therapy, 718
pancreatitis, 719
Roux-en-Y cyst jejunostomy, 718
surgical therapy
    arliest forms, 718
surgical treatment, 718
Choledocholithiasis, 702, 703
    decision analysis, 703
        algorithm, 703f
    laparoscopic, 703
        cholecystectomy, 703
        choledochal exploration, 703
    preoperative endoscopic retrograde
        cholangiopancreatography
        (ERCP), 702, 703
Christopherson, E. H., 6
Chronic anticoagulant therapy, 177
Chronic appendiceal pain, 630
    appendiceal colic, 630
    chronic appendicitis, 630
    recurrent appendicitis, 630
Chronic granulomatous disease, 1229
Chronic pancreatitis (CP), 733
    associated pain, 733
    complications, 733
    diagnosis, 735–737
        clinical presentation, 735, 736
            abdominal pain, 735
            intermittent attacks, epigastric
                pain, 735
            other symptoms, 736
            pancreatic insufficiency, 736
            steatorrhea, 736
        diagnostic challenge, 735
        endoscopic assessment, 736, 737
            endoscopic retrograde
                cholangiopancreatography
                (ERCP), limitations, 736
            endoscopic ultrasound
                (EUS), 736
            endoscopic ultrasound
                criteria, chronic pancreatitis
                diagnosis, 737t
            work-up, children with chronic
                pancreatitis, 737
        laboratory studies, 736
            amylase elevation, 736
            genetic testing, 736
            pancreatic function, indirect
                studies, 736
            predictive testing, use of, 736
        radiologic studies, 736
            advantages, computed
                tomography (CT), 736
            computed tomography
                (CT), 736

diffusion-weighted images, 736
        disadvantages, computed
            tomography (CT), 736
        limitations, ultrasound use, 736
        magnetic resonance imaging
            (MRI), 736
        ultrasound, pediatric diagnosis
            of pancreatitis, 736
    etiology, 734, 735
        autoimmune, 735
            auto antibodies, 735
            IgG4
                hypergammaglobulinemia,
                735
        congenital anatomic
            anomalies, 734
            anatomic pancreaticobiliary
                anomalies, 734, 735t
            congenital anatomic variants, 734
            annular pancreas, 734
        genetic susceptibility, 734 (See
            Genetic susceptibility)
        risk factors, 735
            choledocholithiasis, 735
            idiopathic fibrosing
                pancreatitis, 735
            metabolic diseases, 735
            pediatric-specific
                conditions, 735
        TIGAR-O classification system,
            734, 735t
    pathogenesis
        acute pancreatitis (AP), 733
        disease, 733
            advanced stage, 733
        mitogen-activated pathway
            (MAP) kinase system, 733
        pathogenesis
            acute pancreatitis (AP), 733
            basic fibroblast growth factor
                (bFGF), 733
            pancreatitis, results from, 733
            pathogenesis, 733
            platelet-derived growth factor
                (PDGF), 733
            recurrent pancreatitis, 733
            sentinel acute pancreatic event
                (SAPE), 733
            transforming growth factor
                (TGF) β, 733
        sentinel acute pancreatic event
            (SAPE)
            activates, 733
    treatment, 737–740
        combination procedures
            Beger procedure, 740
            Berne modification, 740
            duodenum-preserving
                pancreatic head
                resection, 740

DuVal procedure, 740
        Frey procedure, 740
        pancreaticobiliary
            anomalies, 740
        Roux limb, 740
        side-to-side
            pancreaticojejunostomy, 740
    ductal drainage procedures, 738
        longitudinal
            pancreaticojejunostomy
            (LPJ), 738
        puestow procedure, 738, 739f
        Roux limb, 738
    endoscopic therapy, 738
        benefits, children with CP, 738
        CP complications, 738
        post-ERCP pancreatitis, 738
    laparoscopy, 740
        cystogastrostomies, 740
        laparoscopic
            pseudocystgastrostomy, 740
    medical management, 737, 738
        antioxidants
            administration, 737
        CFTR mutations, 737
        cholecystokinin (CCK), 737
        enteric stimulation,
            pancrease, 737
        hereditary pancreatitis
            (HP), 738
        narcotics, parental, 737
        octreotide, use of, 738
        pancreatic enzyme
            replacements,
            formulations, 737
        postpyloric feeding tube, 737
        proton pump inhibitors, 737
        total parental nutrition
            (TPN), 737
    pancreatic resections, 738–740
        Berne modification, Beger
            procedure, 738
        clinical data, 739
        coring of head, pancrease,
            738, 739f
        Frey procedure, 740
        maximal resective procedure,
            CP, 739
        pancreaticoduodenectomy, 738
        side-to-side
            pancreaticojejunostomy,
            738, 739f
        total pancreatectomy, 739
    surgical therapy, 738
        body mass index (BMI), 738
        preoperative diagnostic
            imagining, 738
        preoperative planning, 738
Chronic ulcerative colitis, 639
    refractory pancolitis, 639

Chyle, 442
  cysterna chyli, 442
  diagnostic characteristics, 444*t*
  intestinal lacteal system, 442
  lymphatics, 442
  thoracic duct, 442
    anatomical illustration,
        pathway, 443*f*
  thoracic duct transports, 442
  venous system, 442
Chylothorax, 76, 442–445
  anatomy, 442–443
  diagnosis, 443
  etiology, 443
    congenital abnormalities, 443
    nontraumatic causes, 443
  lymphatic system transports
      lipids, 442
  management, 444
    medium-chain triglyceride
        (MCT)
      gut-barrier protection, 444
    treatment algorithm, 444*f*
  medical management, 444
    enterocytes, 444
  physiology, 442–443
  presentation, 443
  surgical management, 445
Chylous drainage, 444
Circumcision, technique, 784
  anesthesia, 784
    general anesthesia, 784
    neonatal circumcision, 784
    penile block, 784
    sensory blockade, penis, 784, 785*f*
  complications, 788, 789
    bleeding, postoperative, 788
    foreskin, 788
      excessive removal, 788
      insufficient removal, 788
    glans, damage, 789
    indirect cautery, 789
    postoperative infection, 789
      Fournier gangrene, 789
      generalized sepsis, 789
    rare morbidity, 788
    rare mortality, 788
  dorsal slit, 784–786
    hemostasis, 784
    Metzenbaum scissors, 784
    operative procedure, 785*f*, 786*f*
    ventral slit, 786
  Gomco clamp circumcision, 786
    cautery, 786
    Plastibell®, 786
      disposable device, 786
      technique representation, 787*f*
    protective bell, 786
    representation, 786*f*
    skin edges, suturing, 786

operative techniques, 784
    postoperative care, 787, 788
      antibiotic ointment, 787
    sleeve resection, 786, 787
      advantage, 786
      circumferential incision, 787
      foreskin, 787
        excision, 787
      free-hand sleeve circumcision
          representation, 787*f*
Circumferential fibrotic cicatrix, 613
    appendiceal lumen, 613
Cirrhosis, 79
Citrate toxicity, 176
"Clatworthy Committee," 9
Clavicle, 1072
  clavicular fracture, 1072
  medial fractures, 1072
  midclavicular fracture, 1072
  patient immobilization, 1072
  treatment, depend on
      age, 1072
    fracture location, 1072
CLE. *See* Congenital lobar
        emphysema (CLE)
Clindamycin, 92, 197
Clinical
  immunosuppression, 1286
  innovation, 20
  research, 20
Cloacal exstrophy, 846
  anatomy, 846
  characterization, 847*f*
  classification, 847*t*
  coding symbols, 847*t*
  diagnosis, 848–849
  embryologic basis, 848*f*
    correlation with surface pattern,
        of bladder and bowel, 849*t*
  management, 849–850
  operative procedure, 854, 855*f*–856*f*
  pathophysiology, 846
  patient outcome, 854–855
  spectrum of anomalies, 847–848, 849*t*
  treatment effectiveness, 854–855
  treatment options, definitive, 850
    gender reassignment, 853–854
    myelodysplasia, 854
    primary closure, 850–851
    staged closure, 851
    urinary reconstruction, 851–853
    vaginal reconstruction, 853
*Clostridium difficile*
  colitis, 206
*Clostridium perfringens,* 189
Cloves syndrome, 996
  congenital lipomatous overgrowth
      anomalies, constellation of, 996
  infant with, 996*f*
  truncal lipomatous masses, 996

Coagulase-negative *Staphylococcus,* 146
Coagulation disorders, 175–176
  acquired disorders, 176
  disseminated intravascular
      coagulation (DIC), 176
  factor IX deficiency, 176
  factor VIII deficiency, 176
  hemophilia A, 176
  inherited disorders, 176
Coagulation factors, 176
Coagulopathy, 176
Coarctation, of aorta, 938
Codeine, 161
  oral opioids in infants/children, 160*t*
Coe, Herbert E., 4
Cohen cross-trigonal technique, 823
Collagen type I, 185
Collectins, 191
Colloids, 94
Colon. *See also* Intestine(s)
Colon biopsy
  open seromuscular, 574*f*
Colonic atresia
  diagnosis, 557
  etiology, 556
  mortality, 557
  pathophysiology, 556
  treatment, 557
Colonic disease, 637–638
  colocolostomy, 637
  Hartmann pouch, 637
  ileorectostomy, 637
  mild-to-moderate rectal disease, 637
  proctocolectomy, 637
  segmental colonic resections, 637
Colonic duplications, 659–662
  associated conditions, 661
    gastrointestinal anomalies, 661
    spinal anomalies, 661
    urologic anomalies, 661
  barium enema, 661
  complications, 661
  CT scan, 661
  diagnosis, 661
    essentials, 659
  laparotomy, 661
  presenting signs, 660, 661
  symptoms, 660, 661
    rectal duplications, 660
    types, 660
      appendix duplication, 660
      colon cystic duplications,
          660, 661*f*
      tubular duplications, 660,
          661*f* (*See also* tubular
          duplications)
  treatment, 661, 662
    resection, 661
      adjacent colon, 661
  ultrasound, 661

Colonic injuries, 1097
Colon interposition, 350
  postoperative management,
    352–353, 352*f*
    gastroesophageal reflux, 353
    nil per os (NPO), 352
  preoperative management, 350
    cefoxitin, 350
  surgical technique, 351, 352
    isoperistaltic retrohilar
      descending colon
      interposition, 351*f*
Colorectal cancer, 1257
  Burkitt lymphoma, 1257
  common pediatric tumor,
    colon, 1257
  diagnosis, 1257
    abdominal X-ray, 1257
    computed Tomography
      (CT), 1257
    magnetic resonance Imaging
      (MRI), 1257
  pediatric population, 1257
  presentation, abdominal pains, 1257
  presentation, change,bowel
    habits, 1257
  treatment, 1257
    chemotherapeutic regimen, 1257
Colostomy, 678
  abnormal communication, 678
    between colon and genitourinary
      tract, 678
  anterior wall colostomy, 577*f*
  definition, 678
  distal colostomy, 678
  ideal, 678, 678*f*
  transverse colostomy, 678
Combined spina bifida, 1018*f*
Combined vascular malformations,
    993–996
  capillary-lymphatico-venous
    malformations, 993–994
    angiogenic growth factor gene
      *AGGF1,* 993
    capillaryarteriovenous lymphatic
      malformation (CAVLM),
      993, 994*f*
    capillary-arteriovenous
      malformation (CAVM), 993
    Klippel–trénaunay syndrome, 993
    Klippel Trénaunay Weber
      syndrome, 993
    MR venography (MRV), 994
    Parkes Weber syndrome, 993
  management, 994
    D-dimer levels, 994
    low fibrinogen levels, 994
    low-grade coagulopathies, 994
  procedural management,
    994–995

Common short-term toxicities
  alopecia, 1173
    associated chemotherapeutic
      agents, 1173
  anthracyclines use, associated with
    acute cardiac toxicity, 1173
    long-term cardiac toxicity, 1173
  cardiotoxicity
    anthracyclines, 1173
  cardiotoxicity, anthracyclines, 1173
  hemorrhagic cystitis
    alkylating agent, 1173
  highly-emetogenic agents, 1173
  myelosuppression, 1173
    associated with, 1173
    effects, 1173
  nausea, 1173
    bacterial infection, risk of, 1173
    fungal infection, risk of, 1173
  neutropenia, 1173
  oral mucositis, 1173
  recombinated G-CSF (filgrastim),
    use of, 1173
  supportive care, 1173
  toxicity, normal cells, 1173
  vomiting, 1173
Community-associated methicillin-
    resistant *Staphylococcus
    aureus* (CA-MRSA), 210
Compartment syndrome, 1103
  clinical symptoms, 1103–1104
  decompression of lower leg, 1104
  diagnosis, 1103–1104
  pathophysiology, 1103
  patient management, 1104
  treatment and outcomes, 1104
  wound aftercare, 1104
Compensatory sweating (CS), 434–436
Complement system, 191–192
  pathways for activation, 191*f*
Complete androgen insensitivity
    syndrome (CAIS), 901
Composite scores, 1038, 1039
  pediatric risk indicator (PRI), 1039
    calculated as, 1039
    pediatric-specific injury
      measurement tool, 1039
  a severity characterization of trauma
    (ASCOT), 1039
    age indexes, 1039*t*
    blunt and penetrating weights, 1039*t*
    pitfalls, 1039
    survival probability ($P_s$),
      calculation, 1039
  trauma and injury severity scores
    (TRISS), 1038, 1039
    derived from, 1038
    logit model, 1038
    pediatric patients, 1038
    survival probability ($P_s$), 1038

Computed tomography (CT), 197,
    593, 1212
  abdomen and pelvis, 1179
  acute suppurative
    lymphadenitis, 238
  bone erosion, evaluation, 1212
  ECMO monitoring, 122
  hemangiomas, 966
  large anterior mediastinal
    mass with pleural
    effusion, 1262*f*
  malignant thymoma, 401*f*
  noncontrast, head, 1051
Computing technology, 80
Conference Committee on Graduate
    Education in Surgery, 9
Conference on the Biology of
    Neuroblastoma, 10
Congenital, 1233*f*
Congenital abdominal aortic
    coarctation, 955
  diagnosis, 956
  Hallett anatomic classification, 955*t*
  management, 956
  surgical treatment, 956–957
    complications following
      surgical repair,
      957–958, 958*t*
    operative strategies, 957*f*
  symptoms, 955
Congenital adrenal hyperplasia,
    904, 924
Congenital anomalies, 16
Congenital bronchopulmonary
    foregut malformation
    (CBPFM), 408
Congenital craniospinal malformations,
    1006–1022, 1010
  central nervous system
    abnormalities, 1006
    myelocystocele, 1006
    spinal lipomas, 1006
  dysraphic malformations,
    1010, 1020
  gastrointestinal system,
    malformations, 1006
  neuroectoderm, juxtaposition, 1006
  occult malformations, 1010
  posterior mediastinum, neurenteric
    cysts, 1006
Congenital cystic adenomatoid
    malformation (CCAM),
    23–25, 408, 410
  algorithm for management of fetal
    SCT, 29*f*
  coronal section on MRI of fetus
    with large SCT, 29*f*
  fetal, algorithm for management, 28*f*
  fetal ultrasound, demonstrating
    echogenic microcystic, 28*f*

Congenital cystic adenomatoid
    malformation (CCAM)
    (*continued*)
  lobar resection, 37, 37*f*
    fetal thoracotomy and CCAM
        resection, 37
    outcomes, 38
    planned delivery, 37
    rationale, 37
    specific postoperative
        considerations, 37
Congenital cystic lung lesions, 23
  echogenic microcystic, 28*f*
Congenital diaphragmatic hernia
        (CDH), 23, 105, 447–449
  antenatal intervention, 453
  chromosomal anomaly, 453
  featal, algorithm for
        management, 26*f*
  fetal diagnosis, 454
    special considerations, 454
  fetal management, 453, 454*t*
  history, 449*t*–450*t*
  infants, 462
    ECMO technique, 462
      repair of CDH during, 463
    immediate resuscitation, 459
  Karyotypic investigation, 453
  posterolateral defects, 448
  prenatal diagnosis, 454
  surgery, 453
  technique, 462
  video-assisted thoracoscopic repair
        thoracoscopic procedures, 462
Congenital heart disease, 85
Congenital hemoglobinopathies, 173
Congenital lobar emphysema
        (CLE), 407, 413
  acquired form, 416
  characterization, 413
  chest radiograph in infant
        with, 414*f*
  differential diagnosis, 414
  intraoperative photograph
        of child, 414*f*
  lesions, 413
  lobectomy, 415*f*, 416
  minimally invasive technique,
        418–419, 419*f*
  muscle-sparing thoracotomy,
        418–419, 419*f*
  occurrence, 414
  resection, 416
  right upper lobectomy, 415*f*
  timing of surgery, 416
  treatment
    asymptomatic patient, 414
    symptomatic patient, 414
Congenital microgastria, 513
  asplenia, associated with, 513

Hunt–Lawrence reconstruction, 513*f*
  newborns with, 513
  surgical therapy, 513
Congenital pulmonary airway
        malformation (CPAM),
        407, 410
  associated malignancies, 412
  asymptomatic, 412
  chest CT scanning, 412
  differential diagnosis, 411
  hamartomatous lesions, 410
  infant with type I, II, or IV, 412
  MRI of fetus with, 411*f*
  transthoracic inspection of lobar, 413
  treatment, 412
  types, 410
Congenital spinal cord malformations,
        1020–1022
  cloacal exstrophy, 1020–1021
  currarino triad, 1020–1021
    unusual case of, 1021*f*
  imperforate anus, 1020–1021
  meningoceles, 1021
  OEIS (omphalocele, exstrophy,
        imperforate anus, and spinal
        defects), 1021
Congenital tracheal stenosis, 317
  anesthetic consideration, 321
  bronchoscopy, 320–321
  common types, 318*f*
  diagnostic principles, 319–320
  preoperative echocardiogram, 320
  radiological imaging, 320, 320*f*
  treatment options, 321
    dynamic obstruction, 324
      aortopexy, 324–326
      intraluminal airway stenting,
        326–327, 327*f*
      VR repair with or without
        concomitant CTS repair, 324
    fixed obstruction, 321
      repair associated with VR, 324
      tracheal resection, 321
      tracheal transplantation, 324
      tracheoplasty, 321–324
    vascular compression, 318–319
Congestive heart failure, 930
Conjoined twins
  classification by types, 753–757
    based on anatomy, shared area,
        754, 754*f*, 755*f*
    based on union orientation, 755
      dorsal to dorsal, 755
      ventral to ventral, 755
    cephalopagus (head) twins, 754
      characteristics, 755, 756
    craniopagus (helmet) twins, 754
      characteristics, 756
      frontotemporal/
        frontoparietal, 757

occipital/occipitoparietal, 757
      parietal, 757
    depends on, 753
    infants
      twin on the left, 754
      twin on the right, 754
    ischiopagus (hip) twins, 754
      characteristics, 755, 756
      development, 756
      dorsal structures, 756
      female tetrapus twins, 756
      genitourinary system, 756
      internal anatomy, 756
      internal rotation, *z* axis, 756
      male tetrapus twins, 756
      undeveloped appendage, 756
      *vs.* parapagus twins, 756
    naming convention, 754
    omphalopagus (umbilicus)
        twins, 754
      characteristics, 755, 756
    parapagus (side) twins, 754
      characteristics, 755, 756
      contiguous lateral anlagen,
        aplasia, 756
    pygopagus (rump) twins, 754
      anatomical features, 757
      characteristics, 756, 757
    rachipagus (spine) twins, 754
      characteristics, 756, 757
    thoracopagus (chest) twins, 754
      atrial conjunction, 756
      characteristics, 756
      shared heart, 756
      *vs.* omphalopagus twins,
        755, 756
    ventrally united twins, 753
  diagnostic principles, 759, 760
    anatomic problems, 760
    evaluation, 760*t*
    ex utero intrapartum (EXIT)
        procedure, 760
    fetal echocardiogram (ECHO), 760
    magnetic resonance imaging
        (MRI), 759
    postnatal evaluation, 760
      routine checkup, 760
    prenatal evaluation, shared
        organs, 760
    ultrasound evaluation, 759
      findings, 759
  embryology, 753
    cephalopagus twins, 753
      Janus type, 753
    characteristics, 753
    diamniotic omphalopagus, 753
    embryonic discs, 753
      orientation, 753
    parasitic/atypical twin
        development, 753

INDEX

pseudohermaphrodites, 753
spherical theory of
    development, 753
theories, twin development, 753
theory of fusion, 753
    postulates, 753
    twins joined at, 753
incidence, 752, 753
    circumscribed geographic
        area, 753
    dizygotic twins, 752
    frequency, world, 753
    monozygotic twins, 752
        frequency, 753
possible unions, 757t
postnatal management, 758, 759
    anesthetic management, 759
    differential growth rates, 759
    dress rehearsal, toy dolls, 759
    elective separation, 759
        delay, 759
    emergent surgery, 758
        echocardiography, 758
        plain skeletal films, 758
    feeding tubes, 759
    media attention, 759
    O'Neill, 758
    operation recording, 759
    operative procedures, 758, 759
    psychologic aspects, twins, 759
    pygopagus twins, 759f
    security, 759
    surgery timeline, 759
    surgical intervention, 758
surgery timing, 758, 759
treatment options, 760–764
    anesthesia, 761
        adrenal insufficiency, 761
        cross-circulation, 761
        general, 761
        management, 761
    cardiovascular system, 761
        actual anatomy,
            determining, 761
        blood source, identification, 761
        cardiac evaluation, 761
        CT angiography, 761
        defects, 761
        echocardiography, 761
        electrocardiography, 761
        ischiopagus tripus twins,
            angiogram, 761
        omphalopagus twins, 761
        Spencer, review, 761
        thoracopagus twins, 761
        three-dimensional magnetic
            resonance angiography, 761
        twin-reversed arterial
            perfusion (TRAP)
            sequence, 761

respiratory system, 761, 782
    cardiac anomalies,
        frequency, 782
    lobulation abnormalities,
        761, 782
    surgical team, 760
Constipation, 690–692
    abdomino-perineal pullthrough, 692
    causes of, 691
    define, 690
    diet to control, 691
    Hirschsprung disease, 692
    imperforate anus repair, 691, 692
    laxative requirements, 691
    nonmanageable severe
        constipation, 691
        poor prognosis, type of defect, 691
        treatment, 691
    rectal biopsy, 692
    results of
        distal colostomy, 690
        loop colostomy, 690
        transverse colostomies, 690
    sigmoid resection, 691, 692f
    transverse colostomies, 690
    types of defects, 691t
Continuous positive airway pressure
    (CPAP), 47
Contraceptives, 246, 701, 1233,
    1234, 1244
Contralateral pneumothorax, 459
Conventional anticoagulation therapy,
    for documented venous
    thrombolembolism in
    children, 98t
Copper accumulation, 66
Core temperature monitoring, 70
Cori cycle, 62, 131
Corticosteroids, 175, 180, 246, 955, 1287
Cortisol, 67
Cotting times, activated, 120
Coumadin®, 178
Cowden syndrome, 1256–1257
    breast cancer, risk, 1256
    gastrointestinal, diagnosis, 1256
    Management of, 1257
    mucocutaneous, diagnosis, 1256
    potential internal malignancy,
        treatment, 1257
    presentation
        hamartomatous gastrointestinal
            lesions, 1256
    PTEN gene
        chromosome 10q23, 1256
    thyroid cancer, risk, 1256
CP. See Cerebral palsy (CP); Chronic
        pancreatitis (CP)
CPAM. See Congenital pulmonary
        airway malformation
        (CPAM)

C-reactive protein (CRP), 61, 62, 64,
        91, 129, 191, 202
    serum prealbumin levels, 134
Creatine phosphokinase
        (CPK), 151
Crepitance, 330
Crohn disease (CD), 197, 632–635,
        637–638
    colonic disease, 633, 635
    diagnostic algorithm
        differentiate, 634f
    ileocolonic disease, 633
    mesenteric lymph
        resection of, 636
    nonpericryptal granulomas,
        demonstration of, 633
    serum biomarkers
        prevalence of, 635t
Cryptorchidism, 270
    absent testis, 777
        diagnostic algorithm, 777f
        treatment algorithm, 777f
    ascending testis, 777
    canalicular testis, 776
    classification, 776
    definition, 775
        ectopic testis, 775
        orchidopexy, 775
    diagnosis, 778
        imaging, 778
            computed tomography
                (CT), 778
            magnetic resonance imaging
                (MRI), 778
            ultrasonography, 778
        laparoscopy, 778
            management algorithm, 778f
        physical exam, 778
            diagnostic algorithm, 777t
            physiologic postnatal
                testosterone surge, 778
            testis position, 778
            treatment algorithm, 777t
            undescended testis, clinical
                examination, 778
    ectopic testis, 777
    embryology, 775
        calcitonin gene related
            peptide (CGRP),
            neurotransmitter, 775
        follicle stimulating hormone
            (FSH), 775
        human chorionic gonadotropin
            (hCG), 775
        Leydig cells, 775
        primitive gonad, begining, 775
        sex-determining region (SRY)
            human Y chromosome, 775
    emergent testis, 776
    incidence, 776

Cryptorchidism (*continued*)
  intra-abdominal testis, 776
    anatomical position, cryptorchid
      testes, 776*t*
  nomenclature, 776
  superficial inguinal pouch testis,
    776, 777
  testes descent, 775, 776
    abdominal wall malformation, 74
    androgen insensitivity
      syndrome, 776
    biphasic model, 775
      inguinoscrotal phase,
        second, 775
      transabdominal phase, first, 775
    congenital malformation
      syndromes, 776*t*
    cryptorchidism, 776
    hypothalmo-pituitary-testicular
      axis, 776
    normal testicular descent,
      factors, 775
    mechanical, 775
    neural, 775
    undescended testis, 775, 776
  treatment, 778–782
    anesthesia
      loco-regional anesthesia, 779
    complications, 782
    hormonal therapy, 778
    indications for, 778
    laparoscopic orchidopexy, 782
      difficult undescended
        testis, 782
      difficult undescended testis
        treatment, 782
      30° 3/5–mm transumbilical
        laparoscope, 782
      scrotum passage, 782
      testis mobilization, 782
    open inguinal orchidopexy,
      779–782
      blunt clamp "kelly" scrotal
        wound, 781*f*, 782
      blunt retractor, 781
      brought down, testis, 781*f*, 782
      conitnued dissection, 781
      external oblique
        aponeurosis, 779
      external oblique aponeurosis
        incision, 779*f*
      gubernaculum, 779
      high ligation, sac, 780*f*, 781
      ilioinguinal nerve, to avoid
        injury, 779
      inferior epigastric vessels
        ligation, 780*f*, 781
      meticulous blunt dissection,
        separate hernia sec from vas
        deferens and vessels, 779, 780*f*

      mobilization, spermatic cord,
        779, 780*f*
      mobilization, testis, 779, 780*f*
      scrotal skin, horizontal
        incision, 780*f*, 782
      skin crease incision, 779, 779*f*
      spermatic cord, 779
      sub-Dartos pouch, 781*f*, 782
      subdartos pouch creation,
        blunt dissection, 780*f*, 782
      transversalis fascia ligation,
        780*f*, 781
    orchidopexy, timing for, 778, 779
      spontaneous testicular
        descent, 779
    outcomes, 783
      fertility after orchidopexy, 783
      testicular cancer after
        orchidopexy, 783
      testicular size, 783
    pain management, 779
      postoperative pain, 779
    surgical technique, 779
      laparoscopic technique, 779
      orchidopexy, basic steps, 779
      prophylactic perioperative
        antibiotics,
        administration, 779
  vanishing testis, 777
Crystalloids, 94
C-shaped tracheal cartilages, 317
CTS. *See* Congenital tracheal stenosis
CT scan
  apical subpleural bullae, 439*f*
  exposure, 439
  radiation, 439
    evaluating, patients, 439
  standard diagnostic test, 439
Currarino-Silverman syndrome, 270
Cushing syndrome, 1291
Cutis marmorata telangiectatica
        congenita (CMTC), 981
  cutaneous atrophy, 981
  limb hemihypertrophy, 981
  newborn child, 981*f*
  phlebectasia, 981
  skin pigmentation, 981
  telangiectasia, 981
  violaceous skin marbling, 981
3′,5′-Cyclic phosphate (cAMP)-
        induced chloride
        channel, 559
Cystic adenomatoid malformation
        (CCAM), 451
  differential diagnosis, 451
Cystic fibrosis (CF), 438, 518, 558
  CFTR mutation testing, 561
  genotype–phenotype
        correlation, 559
Cystoscopy, 916, 916*f*

Cyst(s), 665–668
  adrenal, 667
  bartholin gland, 882
  bronchogenic, 403, 405, 416
    computed tomography
      thin-walled apparently cystic
        lesion, 405*f*
    mediastinal, 417*f*
    minimally invasive technique,
      418–419
      muscle-sparing thoracotomy,
        418–419, 419*f*
    posteroanterior chest radiograph
      for evaluation, 405*f*
    resection technique, 406
    thoracoscopic visualization, 418*f*
  cervical thymic, 223–224
  choledochal (*See* Choledochal cysts)
  dermoid and epidermoid, 229, 230*f*
    embryology, 229
    treatment, 230
      excision, 230
  dermoid cysts, 230
    midline nasal bridge, 230*f*
  embryology, 225
  enteric, 403, 406
  hepatic, 667
  hydrocolpos, 668
  introital, 883
  laryngeal, 295*f*
  lymphatic malformations, 666
  meconium, 668
  mediastinal, 393
  mesenteric, 665, 666, 666*f*
  neuroenteric, 406
  omental, 666
  pancreatic, 667
    pseudocysts, 1045
  pyriform sinuses and, 223
  skene glands, 882
  splenic, 667, 667*f*
  thymic, 394
  thyroglossal duct, 224, 226*f*
  urachal, 668
  ventriculoperitoneal shunt
        pseudocysts, 666, 667
Cytochrome P-450 isoenzyme (CYP)
        system, 93
  genetic polymorphisms, 93
Cytokine-induced counterregulatory
        hormones, 133
Cytomegalovirus [CMV], 194, 238,
        560, 1291, 1313, 1321

**D**
Dacron cuff, 144
Dacron, graft material, 941
Dandy–Walker syndrome, 50
Dantrolene
  malignant hyperthermia (MH), 151

D-dimer, 176
Decision
  making for infants and children
      with uncertain prognosis, 18–19
  moral problem, 18
Deep venous thrombosis (DVT), 96, 176
  in adolescence, 177
  pediatric, annual incidence, 96
  prophylaxis with subcutaneous
      heparin/sequential
      compression devices, 177
β-Defensins, 190, 191
Deflux®, 826
Dehydration, 174
Delirium, 100
  acute, 103
  categories, 103
  defined, 103
  hyperactive, 103
Denys–Drash syndrome, 903
Dermal sinus tracts, 1014–1017
  cerebral hemispheres, 1015
  coccygeal dimple, 1014
  cranial, 1016
  epithelial cells, desquamation, 1014
  foramen cecum, 1015
  frontonasal, 1015
  gadolinium-enhanced sagittal, 1016
  lumbar spine, MRI, 1015
  lumbosacral, 1016
  neural tube, dysjunction, 1014
  occipital, 1015
  ostium, 1014
  sacral region, 1015f
Dermal tissue repair, 188
Dermoid cysts, 230
Desflurane, anesthesia maintenance, 156
Desmoid tumors, 1225–1227, 1255
  colonic resection, 1255
  desmoplastic small round cell
      tumors (DSRCT), 1225
  familial adenomatous polyposis
      (FAP), 1225
  fibromatous tissue,
      proliferation, 1255
  general treatment protocol, 1227f
  mesenchymal neoplasm, 1225
  microscopic margin, 1225
  multivariate analysis, 1225
  non steroidal anti inflammatory
      drugs (NSAID), 1225
  operative resection, 1227
    critical neurovascular
        structures, 1227
    external beam radiation
        therapy, 1227
    intra-operative radiation
        therapy, 1227
    negative microscopic margin,
        achievement, 1227

Desmopressin, 175
Dexamethasone
  antinausea prophylaxis, 170
  postoperative nausea and vomiting
      (PONV), 157
Dexmedetomidine, 102
  usage, in children, 102
  vagotonic effect, 102
Dextran, 95
Diabetes mellitus, 181, 201
Dialysis, 94
Diaminotetra-ethyl-pentaacetic acid
      (DTPA), 820
Diaphragm
  embryologic anatomy, 451f
  gastric bubble, 451
  imbrication technique, 467f
  intraabdominal visceral protrusion
      thoracic space loss secondary, 466f
  localization, 467
Diaphragmatic eventration, 465–467
  diaphragm plication
    central portion of, 467f
  eventration repair
    operative techniques for, 467f
  fetal β-hemolytic streptococcal
      infection, 466
  hemidiaphragm
    elevation of, 466
  β-hemolytic streptococcal
      pulmonary infection, 466
  plain x-rays, 466
  surgical management, 466
    complications of plication, 467
    fibromuscular disruption, 467
    inferior pulmonary ligament, 466
    infradiaphragmatic structures, 466
    muscle-sparing thoracotomies, 466
    prolene sutures, 466
  transthoracic exposure, 466f
Diaphragmatic hernias, 11, 448–449
  chest radiographic diagnosis, 453f
  childhood, 453
  classification, 448
    acquired traumatic hernias, 448
    anterior subcostal hernias, 448
    central, paraesophageal
        hernias, 448
    posterolateral hernias, 448
  congenital, 449
    history of, 449t–450t
    predictors of outcome and
        survival for children
        with, 455t
  embryology, 448–449
    bilateral pleuroperitoneal
        membranes, 448
    diaphragm, 448
    embryologic sequence, 448
    mesenchyme, 448

    mesoderm, 448
    neuromuscular component, 448
    septum transversum, 448
  gastrointestinal tract, 452
  infancy, 453
  intrathoracic, 452
  neonatal period, 452
  outcome for congenital, 463–464
  phrenic nerve, 467
  polyhydramnios, 452
  postnatal management, 456
    newborn,treatment, 456
  preferred management schemes
      algorithm depicting, 457f
  preoperative stabilization, specific
      measures for, 458
  primary transabdominal repair
    surgical procedure, 459–461
  prognosis, 451
  prosthetic repair, 460f
  right-sided visualized, 459f
  through the foramen of Morgagni
    epigastric pain, 465
    peritoneal sac, 464
    sternocostal hiatus, 464
  traumatic, 465
    hernias posterior, 465
      intraabdominal injuries, 465
    operative repair, 465
      transthoracic repair, 465f
  visceral reduction, 459f
Diaphragmatic injuries, 1080
  blunt diaphragmatic rupture, 1080
  diagnosis, 1080
    chest x-ray, 1080
    laparoscopy, 1080
    thoracoscopy, 1080
  intra-abdominal injuries, 1080
  penetrating injury, 1080
  presenting signs, 1080
Diaphragm injuries, 1083–1084,
      1083f–1084f
Diarrhea, 133
Diazepam, 101
Diffuse large B-cell lymphoma
      (DLBCL), 1267
  NF kappabeta pathway, genes, 1267
  peripheral lymphoid organs
    mature B cells of, 1267
Digital dilatations, 571, 582
Digitalis, 85
Digital nerve block, 168
5α-Dihydrotestosterone (DHT), 904
Dilated intestinal loops
  decompression of, 605f
Dimercaptosuccinic acid (DMSA), 819
Diskectomy, technique, 437f
Dislocations, 1100
  lower extremity (See Extremity
      injuries)

Disorder of sexual differentiation (DSD), 899–902
diagnostic evaluation, 906–907
conditions, diagnostic and management strategy, 908t–909t
contrast genitogram, 910f
newborn evaluation of intersex infant, 907t
T2-weighted contrast MRI image, 910f
female, 904
46, XX child with congenital adrenal hyperplasia, 905f
male, 904–905
46, XY child with symmetric descended gonads, 906f
ovotesticular, 906
perioperative positioning, 907
treatment effectiveness/patient outcomes, 922
congenital adrenal hyperplasia, 924
neoplasia arising in dysgenetic gonads, 925, 925f
psychologic implications, 922, 924
vaginal atresia, 924–925
treatment options, 907
clitoral treatments, 907, 910
clitoral recession, 911f–912f
clitoral reduction, 914f–915f
glanuloplasty and reconstruction, 913f
operative view of clitoral shaft dissection, 913f
postoperative appearance, 913f–914f
wedge glanuloplasty, 914f
46, XX female adolescent, with CAH and clitoral hypertrophy, 913f
vaginoplasty, 916
absent vagina, 920, 922, 923f
cystoscopy, 916, 916f
high vaginal atresia repair, 917, 918f–920f
low vaginoplasty, 916, 916f, 917f
posterior approach, 917, 920, 921f–922f
preoperative preparation, 916
vaginoscopy, 916
2,3-Disphosphoglycerate, 178
Disseminated intravascular coagulation (DIC), 176
Distal anterior rectal wall anterior wall anastomosis, 580f
Distal colonic polyps, 1249
Distal mucous fistula, 604f, 607
Distal rectal mucosa, 587f
Distal rectum, dissection, 579

DLBCL. See Diffuse large B-cell lymphoma (DLBCL)
DNA polymerases, 66
Dobutamine, 86
for patients in cardiogenic shock, 86
Docosahexanoic acid (DHA), 65
Dopamine, 103, 1143
enhancement of renal and splanchnic blood flow, 86
myocardial contractility, 86
Doppler ultrasonography, 452, 729, 956, 1179, 1318
Dorsal lithotomy positioning on skis, 575f
suspension position, 572
for rectal biopsy, 572f
Double-stapled anal anastomosis intracorporeal view of, 640f
Down syndrome, 294, 443, 560
Drug biotransformation, 93
Drug clearance, 93
Drug disposition
alterations, 91
domains, 89
Drug–drug interactions, 89, 93, 101
Drug resistance, 95
Drug selection, 100
Drug therapy, oral absorption of, 91
Drug toxicity, 94
Drug withdrawal
features of, 103
features of opioid and benzodiazepine, 103
management strategies, 103
DSD. See Disorder of sexual differentiation (DSD)
Duane retraction syndrome, 274
Ductal recanalization, 929
Ductus arteriosus, 929
Duhamel, 584
pull-through, development of the retrorectal space for, 575f, 586
technique, 575
operative technique, 575–577
preoperative preparation, 575
Dumbbell tumors, 396, 1022–1024, 1022f
algorithm, surgical management of patients, 1023f
diagnosis, 1022
treatment, 1022–1024
Duodenal atresia, 549
complications, 554
diagnosis, 551
mortality, 554
pathophysiology, 549–551
treatment, 551–554
circumumbilical incision for repair, 552f
diamond-shaped anastomosis, 553f

periumbilical approach, 554
tapering duodenoplasty, 553f
Type I, 550f
Type II, 551f
Type III, 551f
Duodenal duplications, 655, 656
complications, 656
diagnosis, 656
endoscopic retrograde cholangiopancreatography (ERCP), 656
magnetic resonance cholangiopancreatography (MRCP), 656
diagnosis essentials, 655
located within "C-loop" of duodenum, 656f
presenting sign, 655, 656
symptoms, 655, 656
treatment, 656
cyst resection, 656
Roux-en-Y cystojejunostomy, 656
advantage, 656
Duodenal obstruction, 549
Duodenum injury, 1094
hematoma, 1094, 1094f
laceration/perforation, 1094, 1095f
DVT. See Deep venous thrombosis (DVT)
"Dynamic" tracheal obstruction, 318
Dyslipidemia, 527
Dysphagia, 330, 340, 944
lusoria, 947
Dysphoria, 163
Dysrhythmias, 70

E
EA. See Esophageal atresia (EA)
EA-tracheoesophageal fistula (TEF), 11
Echocardiography, 72, 77
ECMO. See Extracorporeal membrane oxygenation (ECMO)
Ectopia cordis, 277
case reported, 277
diagnosis of, 279
modern classification system, 279, 279t
prenatal diagnosis
midline thoracic defects, 281
simple sternal clefts, 279, 280f
thoracic/true ectopia, 281
thoracoabdominal ectopia cordis, 279, 280f, 281
documented historical cases of repair, 286–287, 290
embryology, 277
extrathoracic anomalies associated with, 278t
history, 277

management, 282–286
  repair techniques for larger
    thoracoabdominal
    defects, 288f
  second-stage thoracic ectopia
    cordis repair, 290f
  staged repair for extensive
    thoracoabdominal ectopia
    cordis, 289f
  steps in repairing a pentalogy of
    cantrell, 287f
partial, 277
pathophysiology, 278–279
preoperative evaluation, 281–282
thoracic and cardiac anomalies
  associated with, 278t
thoracoabdominal, 277
Ectopic ureter, 809, 810
operative technique, 809
  anastomosis, 809
    7-0 Maxon (Covidien)
     suture, 809
    7-0 Vicryl (Ethicon)
     suture, 809
  distal ureteroureterostomy, 809
  endoscopy, 809
  Gibson incision, modified, 809
  laparoscopic approach, 809
  open-ended ureteral catheter, 809
  Pfannenstiel incision, 809
  ureter
    lower-pole, 809
    upper-pole, 809
  uretero-ureterostomy, 809
  upper-pole nephroureterectomy,
    809, 810
    anterior approach, 810
    lower-pole ureter, 810
    renal capsule, incision, 810
    upper-pole moiety, 809
     excision, 810
    upper-pole ureter, 810
Ehlers–Danlos syndrome, 185, 953
5,8,11-Eicosatrienoic acid, 65
Electrocardiographic monitoring
  (ECG), 70
Electrocardiography
asystole, 85f
coarse ventricular fibrillation, 85f
fine ventricular fibrillation, 85f
sinus tachycardia, 85f
supraventricular tachycardia, 85f
ventricular tachycardia, 85f
Electrolyte imbalance, 85
Electrolyte physiology, 56
composition of gastrointestinal
  secretions, 56t
disorders of
  potassium, 57–58
  sodium, 57, 58f

hyperkalemia, 58
  treatment of, 58t
hyponatremia
  algorithm for assessment, 58f
  symptomatic, treatment of, 58t
normal, 55
  chloride, 56
  potassium, 56
  sodium, 56
Electrolytes. See also specific electrolyte
Elevated intraabdominal pressure
  (IAP), 76
Embolization, 76, 937
Embryonal rhabdomyosarcoma
  (ERMS), 1211–1212
botryoid subtypes, 1211
  hollow viscus, filling lumen
    of, 1211
histology, 1211
rich stroma, 1211
spindle-cell, 1211
  paratesticular lesions, 1211
tumors
  head, neck region, 1211–1212
Emergency Medical Services Act,
  1973, 1029
Empyema, 424
diagnosis, 426, 426f
  algorithm approach, 427f
essentials of diagnosis, 424
etiology, 426
management, 427, 428f
  operative, 427–428, 429f
pathophysiology, 426
Endocrine effects, 132
Endocrinologic shock, 83
diagnosis and treatment, 84f
Endorectal dissection, 579, 579f, 590
Endorectal pull-through, 577
operative technique, 578–580
preoperative assessment/
  preparation, 578
Endoscopic retrograde
  cholangiopancreatography
  (ERCP), 656, 657, 667, 702,
  703, 734, 737, 738
Endoscopic subureteric injection
  technique, 826f
Endoscopic third ventriculostomy (ETV)
arachnoid granulations, 1006
basilar tip, 1006
endoscope, aid of, 1006
fenestration, 1006
infundibular recess anteriorly, 1006
mammillary bodies posteriorly, 1006
small burr-hole, 1006
Endoscopic treatment of
  vesicoureteral reflux
right-grade IV VUR and left-grade
  V VUR, 826f

Endoscopy, 292, 328, 510
rigid, technique for insertion into
  esophagus, 335f
End ostomy
closed-loop anatomy, 610, 611f
mucous fistula, 611, 611f
proximal bowel end
  exteriorization, 610f
Endotracheal intubation, 88
Endotracheal tube, 436
placement, 72
Endovascular stents, 326
Endstage renal disease (ESRD), 1293
hemodialysis, 1294
  arteriovenous fistulae, 1295–1296
  arteriovenous grafts, 1295–1296
  central venous catheters,
    1294–1295
pathophysiology, 1293–1294
patient characteristics, 1293–1294
peritoneal dialysis (PD), 1296–1298
  proper location of the cuffs, 1298f
End-to-side ostomy
distal bowel
  exteriorization of, 610, 610f
Energy
homeostasis, 527
metabolism, 62–64
requirements in healthy humans, 61t
Enteral motility, 134
Enteral nutritional delivery, 134
Enteric nervous system (ENS), 43
Enterobacteriaceae, 195, 201
Enterostomy
hemorrhage, 612
prolapse of, 612
Enzyme capacity, 91
Enzyme defects, 744, 745
glucose-6-phosphate dehydrogenase
  (G-6-PD) deficiency, 744
pyruvate kinase deficiency, 744
treatment, 747
Epidural anesthesia
lateral position for, 165
Epigastric hernia, 485
anesthesia induction, 485
chronic cough, 485
linea alba, 485
obese children, 485
young adults, 485
Epigastrium
transverse colon, 593f
Epimorphin, 448
Epinephrine, 86, 88, 152, 208, 515
administered via endotracheal
  tube, 88
increase heart rate, conduction
  velocity, and contractility, 86
to provide potent α- and
  β-adrenergic effects, 86

Epithelial metaplasia, 348
Epstein–Barr virus (EBV), 1266
    african Burkitt lymphoma (BL)
            cells, 1266
    congenital immunodeficiencies, 1266
    lymphoproliferations, 1266
ERCP. *See* Endoscopic retrograde
            cholangiopancreatography
            (ERCP)
ERMS. *See* Embryonal
            rhabdomyosarcoma (ERMS)
*Escherichia coli*, 44, 194
Esophageal atresia (EA), 11, 342, 449
    anastomotic stricture and
            balloon dilatation, under
            fluoroscopic control, 347*f*
    associated malformations, 343
    bronchoscopy/esophagoscopy, 344
    chest radiograph, 343*f*
    classification, 343
    diagnosis, 343
    embryology, 342–343
    esophageal replacement, 346
    pathogenesis, 342
    postoperative chest radiograph
            after thoracoscopic EA repair, 347*f*
    postoperative treatment, 346
    success rate/complications, 346
    treatment, 344
            thoracoscopy, 345–346
            thoracotomy, 344–345
Esophageal duplications, 651–653
    associated conditions, 652
            vertebral lesions, 652
    complications, 652
            Holcomb series, 652
    diagnosis, 652
            chest x-ray, 652
            computed tomography (CT)
                scan, 652
            essentials, 651
    distribution, 652*t*
    esophagus, 652
            parts, 652
    midesophageal duplication cyst, 653*f*
    presenting signs, 652
    symptoms, 652
    treatment, 652, 653
            complications, 653
            marsupialization of cyst, 653
            resection, 652
            thoracoscopic resection, 652
Esophageal injuries, 1079, 1080
    diagnosis, 1080
    esophageal trauma, 1079
    esophagram/esophagoscopy, 1079
    hemodynamically stable patient
            pneumomediastinum
                chest CT, 1079
                initial chest x-ray, 1079

    intrathoracic, 1079
    repairing, 1080
    thoracic exploration, 1080
    treatment, 1079
            depend upon, 1079
Esophageal replacement
    advantages/disadvantages of various
            methods, 350*t*
    colon interposition, 350
            postoperative management,
                352–353, 352*f*
            gastroesophageal reflux, 353
            *nil per os* (NPO), 352
            preoperative management, 350
            cefoxitin, 350
            surgical technique, 351, 352
                isoperistaltic retrohilar
                    descending colon
                    interposition, 351*f*
    gastric transposition, 355
            postoperative management, 357
            and outcomes, 357
            preoperative management, 355
            surgical technique, 355–357
    gastric tube placement, 353
            postoperative management, 355
            success rate, 355
            preoperative management,
                353, 353*f*
            surgical technique, 353–355
    general considerations, 350
            anatomic considerations, 350
            VACTERL association, 350
    jejunal interposition, 357
            free jejunal grafts, 357, 357*f*
            postoperative management, 357
            success rate, 357
            preoperative management, 357
            surgical technique, 357
    overview, 349–350
Esophagoplasty, 341
Esophagus
    battery-induced local injury to, 330
    caustic injury, 337
    injury due to lithium-based
            batteries, 330
    nonopaque esophageal foreign body
            radiograph, 330*f*
    replacement (*See* Esophageal
            replacement)
    stenting, 340
    technique for insertion of rigid
            endoscope into, 335*f*
ESRD. *See* Endstage renal disease
            (ESRD)
Ethernet communications, 83
Ethical considerations, conjoined
            twins, 757, 758
    decision-making process
            important part, 758

    decision, to separate infants, 758
    ethically challenging situation, 758
    Great Ormand Street Ethical
            guidelines
            conjoined twin separation, 758
    Hippocratic Oath, 758
    neonatologist, 758
    obstetrical management, 758
            C-section/transvaginally
                born, 758
    prenatal diagnosis, 757
    prenatal evaluation, 758
Ethics, responsibilities of pediatric
            surgeon, 16
Etomidate
    disadvantage, 102
    dose, 102
    sympathetic nervous system, 155
Etoposide and bleomycin (PEB), 1198
ETV. *See* Endoscopic third
            ventriculostomy (ETV)
Excess weight loss (EWL), 526, 531
Extended field radiotherapy
            (EFRT), 1263
Extensive lesions, 666
Extracellular matrix (ECM)., 183
Extracorporeal membrane oxygenation
            (ECMO), 11, 116, 148, 449
    air embolism, 123–124
    anesthetic management, 459
    bridge to transplant, 125–126
    cannulation site bleeding, 124
    caring for patient, considerations, 118
    complications, 123
    growth restriction, 127
    indications, 117
    infectious complications, 124–125
    left CDH
            elective repair of, 459
    limb ischemia, 124
    mechanical dislodgement of
            cannulas, 124
    membrane dysfunction, 124
    methods, 118–122
    monitoring, 122–123
    neurologic sequelae, 126–127
    nutrition on, 123
    outcomes, 126
    physiology/circuit design, 117–118
    raceway tubing rupture, 124
    renal failure, 125
    respiratory complications after, 127
    risk of intracranial hemorrhage, 123
    second course, 126
    stabilization, 449
    use of E-CPR, 125
Extramucosal pyloroplasty, 534
Extremity injuries, 1098
    avulsion fractures, 1100
    bone remodeling, 1100

compartment syndrome, 1103
  clinical symptoms, 1103–1104
  decompression of lower leg, 1104
  diagnosis, 1103–1104
  pathophysiology, 1103
    Volkmann ischemic
      contracture of forearm, 1103*f*
  patient management, 1104
  treatment and outcomes, 1104
  wound aftercare, 1104
dislocations, 1100
fractures, 1104
  hand fractures and dislocations,
    1109, 1109*f*
  humeral shaft fractures, 1104–1105
  lateral condyle fractures,
    1106, 1106*f*
  medial epicondyle fractures,
    1106–1107, 1107*f*
  Monteggia fracture-dislocation,
    1106–1107, 1108*f*
  proximal humerus
    fractures, 1104
  radius and ulna fractures,
    1107–1109, 1108*f*
  supracondylar humerus fractures,
    1105–1106
  type III, 1105*f*
fractures and dislocations of lower
    extremity, 1109
fractures and dislocations of
    femur, 1110
  distal femur, 1110–1111, 1111*f*
  femoral neck fractures, 1110
  femoral shaft fractures,
    1110, 1110*f*
  intertrochanteric and
    subtrochanteric
    fractures, 1110
fractures and dislocations of hip,
    1109–1110
fractures of the tibia and
    fibula, 1112
  distal tibia and fibula physeal
    fractures, 1114
  foot injuries, 1114
  proximal tibia metaphysis
    fractures, 1113
  proximal tibia physeal
    fractures, 1113
  tibia intercondylar eminence
    fractures, 1112–1113, 1113*f*
  tibial shaft fractures,
    1113–1114
  vascular injuries in pediatric
    knee trauma, 1111–1112,
    1111*f*–1112*f*
intra-articular fractures, 1100
mangled extremity and
    amputation, 1114

amputation, 1115
  mangled extremity severity
    score variables, 1115*t*
  techniques, 1115
  Lawn Mower injuries, 1114–1115
  nonaccidental trauma, 1116
  prosthetics, 1115–1116
multiple injuries, 1098–1099
open fractures, 1100
  Gustilo classification of open
    fractures, 1100*t*
patient evaluation, 1098
physeal fractures, 1099–1100
  Salter–Harris classification of
    epiphyseal injuries, 1099*f*
stress fractures, 1100
vascular injuries, 1101
  diagnostic considerations, 1101
  diagnostic pitfalls, 1101
  overview, 1101
  patient management,
    1101–1102, 1102*f*
  pseudoaneurysm, 1102*f*
  penetrating extremity trauma, 1101

**F**
Facial vein
  intraosseous access, 140
Fallopian tubes, 897
  broad ligament cyst, 897
  hydrosalpinx/hematosalpinx/
    pyosalpinx, 897
  paratubal cysts, 897
  torsion, 897–898
Familial adenomatous polyposis,
    1252–1255
  adrenocortical, 1255
  APC (Adenomatous Polyposis Coli)
    gene, 1252
  desmoid tumors, 1252
  family member, 1252
  hepatoblastoma, 1255
  mucosectomy, 1255
  pancreatic, 1255
  patient
    colon specimen, 1254*f*
  retinal pigmentation (CHRPE),
    congenital hypertrophy, 1252
  thyroid malignancies, 1255
Familial polyposis syndromes,
    1252–1256
  bowel obstruction, 1254
  familial adenomatous polyposis,
    1252–1255
  diagnosis, 1254
    colonic polyps, 1254
    *de novo* mutations, patients, 1254
  presentation, 1252, 1254
    genetic testing, 1252
    symptoms, 1252

surveillance, 1255
treatment, 1254–1255
  cyclooxygenase inhibitor, 1254
  end-ileostomy, 1254
  pelvic sepsis, 1254
  rectal mucosa, 1254
FAMM syndrome (Familial atypical
    mole and melanoma), 1271
Fatal arrhythmia, 62
Fat malabsorption
  fat-soluble vitamin deficiency, 716
    cholestatic infants, 716
    fat malabsorption, 716
    intraluminal bile, 716
    medium-chain triglycerides, 716
Fatty acids, 65
Fecal elastase (FE) test, 568
Fecal incontinence, 692, 693
  accurate diagnosis, 692
  bowel control, 692
    valuable prognostic signs, 692
  bowel-management program, 693
    (See also Bowel-management
    program)
  prognosis type of defect, 692
    bad, 692
    good, 692
  soiling, 692
Federal Food and Drug
    Administration (FDA), 19
Feeding access, 517
  laparoscopic gastrostomy, 517
  open gastrostomy (Stamm
    gastrostomy), 517
  open jejunostomy, 517
  PEG, 517
  percutaneous radiologic
    gastrostomy, 517
    jejunostomy, 517
Feeding adjuncts, 646
  common clinical scenario, 646
    postreversal PN, 646
    reanastomosis, 646
    rectal tube feeding, 646
  refeeding, 646
    practical aspects, 646
  refeeding distal mucous fistulas, 646
  stoma placement, 646
    careful consideration, 646
    complications, 646
  stomas, 646
    initial abdominal operation,
    creation of, 646
  management, 646
Feeding intolerance, 134
Femoral artery, 73
  cannulated using Seldinger
    technique, 73
  cannulation, with antegrade distal
    perfusion catheter, 125*f*

Femoral hernias, 508–510
Femoral nerve block, 168, 169f
Femoral vein, 76, 142
Fentanyl, 101, 161
Fetal breathing, 46
Fetal cardiac output
   regulation of, 48
Fetal circulation, schematic
      diagram, 49
Fetal disease, 25
  diagnostic principles, 25
    congenital cystic lung lesions, 27
    congenital diaphragmatic hernia,
      25–27, 26f
    myelomeningocele, 30–31
    sacrococcygeal teratoma, 27
    twin-to-twin transfusion
      syndrome, 27, 30
  fetal imaging modalities, 25, 26f
Fetal hemoglobin, 48
Fetal surgery, 22
  developments, 22–23
  efficacy and future, 40–41
Fetal surgical anomalies, treatment
    options, 31
  ethical considerations, and
    preoperative management, 31
  invasive procedures, 31, 34
Fetal surgical disease, 23
  congenital cystic lung lesions, 24
  congenital diaphragmatic
    hernia, 23–24
  myelomeningocele, 25
  pathophysiology, 23
  sacrococcygeal teratoma, 24
  twin-to-twin transfusion syndrome,
    24–25
Fetal tracheal occlusion, 454
Fetal ultrasound
  left diaphragmatic hernia, 451f
  MRI depicting, 451f
Fetal wound healing, and scar
    formation, 188
Fetal wound repair, 188
α-Fetoprotein, 848
Fiber-optic bronchoscope, 293
Fiber-optic instruments, 292
Fibrin degradation products, 176
Fibrinogen, 61, 176
Fibrinolytic therapy, 75
Fibroadenomata, 248
  extremely large, 248f
Fibroblast growth factor (FGF), 183
Fibromuscular dysplasia (FMD), 953
Fingertip injuries, 212
  avulsions, 212
  nail bed injuries, 212–213
  subungual hematoma, 213
Fistulagram, 218
"Fixed" tracheal obstruction, 317

FKHR transcription factor gene
  translocations of, 1212
FLACC scale, 158
Flail chest, 1072
  intubation, requirement of, 1072
Flexible pediatric bronchoscopes, 293f
  sizes, 294t
  utility and limitations, 299–300
Fluid physiology, normal, 55
  conditions alter estimate of
    insensible fluid loss, 55t
  total body water (TBW), 55
Fluid replacement, 55
Fluid therapy, 55
Fluoroscopy, 77
Focal disease, 602–604
  anti-mesenteric borders, 603
  Bishop-Koop technique, 603, 605f
  coagulopathy, 604, 606
  distal mucous fistula, 603
  ileostomy, 603
  infants
    cohort of, 604
  mesenteric vessels, 603
  Mikulicz enterostomy., 605f
  primary anastomosis, 604
  Santulli procedure, 604, 605f
  seromuscular layer, 603
  spur-crushing clamp, 603
  terminal ileum, 603
Focal nodular hyperplasia, 1233–1234
  bile ducts, architecture, 1233
  diagnosed, 1233
  hemochromatosis, 1233
  Klinefelter syndrome, 1233
  lesions
    asymptomatic incidental, 1233
  portal vein, Abernathy
    syndrome, 1233
Fogarty catheter, 436f
Folate, 66
Foley catheters, 285, 578
Folkman, Judah, 6
Follicle-stimulating hormone, 246
Foreign bodies, 328
  balloon-tipped catheter, 336–337
  bougienage, 335
    bougie size as determined by
      patient's age, 336t
    criteria for application, 335t
    technique for pushing using a
      mercury-weighted
      bougie, 336t
  chest radiographs, 334f
  complications, 337
  disease pathophysiology, 328
  esophageal foreign bodies, clinical
    symptoms caused by, 332t
  esophagoscopy, 332–333
    flexible, 333

    mechanism causing airway
      compromise, 332t
  National Battery Ingestion Hotline
    treatment algorithm for button
      battery ingestion, 330
  operative procedure, 337
  radiograph of a nonopaque
    esophageal, 330
  rigid endoscopy, 334–335
    technique for insertion of
      rigid endoscope into
      esophagus, 335f
  success rates for removal of, 337
  treatment options for removal, 332
  types, in aerodigestive tracta, 329t
Foreign body. See also Airway
    obstruction
Fractures, 1104
  fractures and dislocations of
    femur, 1110
    distal femur, 1110–1111
    femoral neck fractures, 1110
    femoral shaft fractures, 1110
    intertrochanteric and
      subtrochanteric
      fractures, 1110
  fractures and dislocations of hip,
    1109–1110
  fractures of tibia and fibula, 1112
    distal tibia and fibula physeal
      fractures, 1114
    foot injuries, 1114
    proximal tibia metaphysis
      fractures, 1113
    proximal tibia physeal
      fractures, 1113
    tibia intercondylar eminence
      fractures, 1112–1113
    tibial shaft fractures, 1113–1114
  hand fractures and
    dislocations, 1109
  humeral shaft fractures, 1104–1105
  intra-articular fractures, 1100
  lateral condyle fractures, 1106
  medial epicondyle fractures,
    1106–1107
  Monteggia fracture-dislocation,
    1106–1107
  open fractures, 1100
  physeal fractures, 1099–1100
  proximal humerus fractures, 1104
  radius and ulna fractures,
    1107–1109
  stress fractures, 1100
  supracondylar humerus fractures,
    1105–1106
Frazier suction tip, 140
5-French catheter, 76
Frontonasal dermal sinus tract
  infant, 1016f

Functional endocrine neoplasms, 1147
Functional residual capacity (FRC), 46
Funnel-shape stenosis, 318

**G**
Gabapentinoids, pain control, 163
Galactorrhea, 245
Gallbladder disease, 699
  etiology, 699–701
    acalculous conditions, 701
      acute acalculous
        cholecystitis, 701
      biliary dyskinesia, 701
        CCK injection, 701
        cholecystectomy, 701
        Chronic cholecystitis, 701
        follow-up study, 701
        laparoscopic
          cholecystectomy, 701
        symptom, 701
    cholelithiasis condition, 699
    gallbladder polyps, 701
      laparoscopic
        cholecystectomy, 701
    gallstone formation, 699, 700
      bile, major chemical
        components, 699
      cholesterol crystal
        precipitation, 699
      lecithin—bile acid—cholesterol
        micelles, 699
      macroscopically detectable
        gallstones, formation, 699
      obesity, risk factor for, 699, 700
    hemolytic disease, 700
      conjugation, enzymatic
        process, 700
      gallbladder sludge, 700
      major hereditary hemolytic
        diseases, 700t
      red blood cells,
        composed of, 700
      result, 699
      reticuloendothelial system, 700
      sickle-cell disease (SCD), 700
      unconjugated
        hyperbilirubinemia, 700
    hereditary hemolytic
      diseases, 700
      acute chest syndrome, 700
      cholecystectomy, postoperative
        complications, 700
      elective splenectomy, 700
      hemolytic cholelithiasis, 700
      hereditary spherocytosis, 700
      laparoscopic approach, 700
      sickle-cell disease (SCD), 700
        (See also Sickle-cell disease
        (SCD))
      thalassemia, 700

hydrops, 701
  characterized by, 701
  conservative treatment, 701
  Kawasaki disease, 701
  nonhemolytic cholelithiasis,
    700, 701
  biliary ductules,
    obstruction, 701
  common cause of, 700
  cystic fibrosis, 700, 701
  enterohepatic circulation, 700
  gallstones, possible cause in
    older children, 701
  total parenteral nutrition
    (TPN), 700 (See also Total
    parenteral nutrition (TPN))
  nonhemolytic disease, 699
management, 702, 703
  cholangiography (See
    Cholangiography)
  choledocholithiasis (See
    Choledocholithiasis)
  cholelithasis, 702
  laparoscopic
    cholecystectomy, 702
    major advantages, 702
  nonoperative therapies, 702
  prophylactic
    cholecystectomy, 702
  semiurgent laparoscopic
    cholecystectomy, 702
  splenectomy, 702
radiographic evaluation, 701, 702
  hepatobiliary iminodiacetic acid
    scan (HIDA scan), 701, 702
  cholecystokinin-assisted
    cholescintigraphy, 702
  hepatobiliary
    cholescintigraphy, 701
  Lipomul-challenged
    cholescintigraphy, 702
  technetium-99m-labeled
    iminodiacetic acid
    (IDA), 702
  inflammatory changes, 701
  plain abdominal radiograph,
    radio-opaque gallstones,
    701, 702f
  real-time ultra sonograph (US), 701
Ganglionated bowel, 576f
Ganglion cells
  colon biopsy, open seromuscular, 574f
  frozen section, 591f
  loop colostomy, creation of, 574f
Ganglioneuromas, 396–397
Ganglionic colon, 582
Gans, Stephen L., 10
Gardner syndrome, 1255–1256
  epidermoid cysts, 1255
  extra-colonic osteomas, 1255

extraintestinal symptoms, 1255
  bone, 1255
  skin abnormalities, 1255
  fibromas, 1255
  lipomas, 1255
  malignant tumors, 1255
Gastric acid hypersecretion, 569
Gastric duplications, 514, 654–656
  associated conditions, 655
    pancreatitis, 655
  complications, 654
  diagnosis, 514
    abdominal CT image, 654
    abdominal ultrasound exam, 654
    essential, 654
    pancreatic pseudocysts, 654
  duodenal duplications
    (See Duodenal duplications)
  etiology, 514
  operative therapy, 514
  presenting signs, 654
  pyloric duplications, 655
    large pyloric duplication, 655f
    ultrasound, common diagnostic
      modality, 655
  symptoms, 514, 654
    gastrointestinal hemorrhage, 654
  treatment, 655
    cyst excision, 655, 655f
    technique of White, 655
Gastric foreign bodies, 515
  bezoars, 515
  button batteries, 515
Gastric inflammatory myofibroblastic
  tumor (IMT), 514
Gastric inhibitory peptide, 359
Gastric motility, 43
Gastric surgery, in children, 510
Gastric transposition, 355
  postoperative management, 357
  and outcomes, 357
  preoperative management, 355
  surgical technique, 355–357
Gastric tube placement, 353
  postoperative management, 355
    success rate, 355
  preoperative management,
    353, 353f
  surgical technique, 353–355
Gastric tumor, 510
Gastric volvulus, 510–511
  anatomic types, 511f
  associated abnormalities of
    diaphragm, 510
  coexisting abnormalities, 511
  diagnosis, 511
  laparoscopic approaches, 511
  recurrence prevention, 510
  symptoms, 511
Gastrin, 359

INDEX

Gastroesophageal reflux disease
        (GERD), 43, 45, 153, 347, 366
    complications of childhood, 366
    descriptions of childhood, 366
    diagnosis in children, 367
        clinical history, 367
        diagnostic studies, 367, 371t
            endoscopic evaluation of
                esophageal mucosa, 368
            esophageal mucosal biopsy, 368
            extended esophageal pH
                monitoring, 368
        physical examination, 367
        sequence for diagnostic workup
            in infants and children
            with irritability suspected to be
                caused by GERD, 373f
            with respiratory symptoms, 372f
            with suspected GERD and
                excessive emesis, 371f
    diagnosis of, 45
    impedance plethysmography,
        369–370
    incidence of corrected gastric
        emptying vs. reflux
        pattern, 367t
    normal functions of
        gastroesophageal
        junction, 366
    operative treatment, complications
        and side effects, 382–383
    patterns of reflux episodes, 368–369
        clinical findings in infants, 369t
        reflux episodes following apple
            juice feedings, 369f
    surgical intervention for
        childhood, 366
        antireflux operations, 374f
            common side effects and
                complications, 375t
            general algorithm, 383f
            selection of, 383–384
            Boerema gastropexy in children,
                380–382, 380f–381f
            incision for open laparotomy and
                port sites, 376f
            steps used to perform a Thal
                fundoplication in children,
                378f–379f
            steps used to perform Nissen
                fundoplication, 376f
    symptoms associated with, 366
    treatment, 370
        according to complications in
            children, 384, 390t
        advanced esophagitis, 386–388
        asymptomatic children with
            GERD, 390–391
        Barrett epithelium, 386–388
        medical therapy, 370, 374t

    operative therapy, 370–371
    peptic esophageal stricture,
        386–388
    recurrent emesis, 384–385
    respiratory symptoms/
        disease, 385–386
Gastrografin, 564
Gastrointestinal adenomatous polyps,
        1255–1256
    colon, 1255
    small bowel, 1255
    stomach, 1255
Gastrointestinal anastomosis (GIA)
        device, 577
Gastrointestinal blood flow, 50
Gastrointestinal endoscopy, 328
Gastrointestinal (GI) fluids, 549
Gastrointestinal markers (Nkx2.1 and
        Sox2), 342
Gastrointestinal polyposis syndromes
    hereditary, 1251t
    surveillance recommendations in
        patients, 1253t
Gastrointestinal (GI) secretions, 564
Gastrointestinal secretions,
        composition, 56t
Gastrointestinal stromal tumor
        (GIST), 1258
    cajal, cells, 1258
    platelet-derived growth factor
        receptor alpha
        overexpression, 1258
    surgical specimen, diagnosis, 1258
    symptoms
        abdominal mass, 1258
        gastrointestinal bleeding, 1258
        intestinal obstruction, 1258
    treatment
        adjuvant imatinib mesylate
        adult protocol of, 1258
Gastrointestinal system, embryology of
    digestion/absorption, 45
    enteric nervous system (ENS), 43
    gastroesophageal reflux disease, 45
    hollow organs, 42–43
    intestinal microflora, development
        of, 44
    intestinal motility, 43–44
    intestinal mucosa/immunologic
        development, 43
    liver/biliary tree, 44
    neonatal jaundice, 45–46
    pancreas, 44–45
Gastrointestinal tract, 598
Gastrojejunostomy, 534
Gastroschisis, 132, 471–472
    causative factors, 471
    management, 472
    outcomes, 481–482
        intestinal ischemia, 481

    intestinal transplant
        children, 481
    parenteral nutrition
        development of, 481
    perinatal management, 473
        amniotic fluid, effect, 473
        cesarean delivery, 473
        endotracheal intubation, 473
        neonates, 473, 481
            peripherally inserted central
                catheter (PICC), 474
            total parenteral nutrition
                (TPN), 474
        obstetric indication, 473
        pulmonary standpoint, 473
    postoperative management, 481
        abdominal compartment
            syndrome, 481
        enterocolitis clinical picture, 481
        pneumatosis intestinalis, 481
        postoperative antibiotics, 481
        prophylaxis, 481
    prenatal diagnosis, 472
        Intrauterine growth retardation
            (IUGR), 472
        MRI technology, 472
        serum α-fetoprotein, 472
        ultrasound, 472
    surgical management, 473–474
        loops of bowel, 476
        primary closure, 475–477
            intraabdominal pressure, 476
            proximal intestinal dilation, 477
        reduction, intestines, 475
        staged closure, 474
        silo placement with, 474–477
    umbilical cord, 472
    visceral protrusion
        variable degrees of, 474f
Gastrostomy
    indications, for placement of
        feeding access (See Feeding
        access)
    contraindication, 518
    jejunostomy, 520–521
    laparoscopic gastrostomy, 517, 520
        single-site, 520
    morbidity, 517
    open, 518–519
        complications, 518
    patient selection, 522
    percutaneous endoscopic
        gastrostomy, 519–520
    percutaneous radiologic
        gastrostomies and
        jejunostomies, 521–522
        complications, 521
    perioperative management, 518
    Stamm gastrostomy, 517
    treatment options, 518–522

Gastrostomy access, 517
Gastrostomy tube, 517
Gastrulation
    ectoderm, 1007
        neuroectoderm, 1007
    embryo, 1007
    endoderm, 1007
    mesoderm, 1007
    normal human, 1007f
    trilaminar structure, 1007
Gender assignment, 899
Gender-based basal energy
        expenditure data, 133
Gender dysphoria, 899
Gene expression, 1267
    activated B-cell (ABC), 1267
    germinal center B-cell like (GC), 1267
Generalized lymphatic anomaly, 990
    macrocystic lymphatic
        malformations, 990
    visceral involvement, 990
Genetic susceptibility, 734, 735
    chronic pancreatitis (CP), 734, 735
        cystic fibrosis (CF)
            transmembrane conductance
                gene (CFTR), 735
            mutations, 735
        hereditary pancreatitis (HP), 734
            autosomal dominant, 734
            complications, 734
            diagnosis, 734
            PRSS1 mutation, associated
                with, 734
            pancreatic trypsin, 734
            regulation, 734
            SPINK1 mutation, 734
                vs. PRSS1 mutations, 734
        tropical juvenile pancreatitis, 734
GERD. See Gastroesophageal reflux
        disease (GERD)
Germ cell tumors, 399
gestational age, 451
    cystic, 451
        fetal thorax, 451
Gestational age (GA), 45
Gestational amniotic fluid, 449
Giant cell arteritis, 953
Gianturco coils, 929
GIA stapler, 578f, 588f
GIST. See Gastrointestinal stromal
        tumor (GIST)
gland(s)
    montgomery, 244
    parotid
        metastatic neoplasms
            involving, 236
    submandibular, exposure of, 236f
Glanzmann thrombasthenia, 175
Glomerular filtration rate, 84
Glucagon, 67, 131

Glucagon-like peptide-1 (GLP-1), 527
Glucocorticoids, cause muscle
        proteolysis, 131
Gluconeogenesis, 62, 67, 131
Glucose, 62, 67
Glucose–alanine cycle, 62
Glutamine, 61, 62
Glycoprotein, 61
$\alpha_1$ Glycoprotein, 91
Glycopyrrolate, in intramuscular, 154
Glycosaminoglycans, 185f, 186
    tissue distributions, 186t
Gonadectomy, 851
Gorham disease, 989–990
    anti-osteoclastic medications, 990
    chylothoraces, 990
    chylous pericardial, 990
    clinical presentation, 990
    histopathologic examination, 990
    pleural effusions, 990
Graft -versus-host (GVH) disease, 178
Granuloma annulare, 214
Granulomatous inflammation, of
        aorta, 954
Grob, Max, 5
Gross, Robert E., 5
Group B streptococcus (GBS)
        capsule, 194
Growth hormone, 67
Gut associated lymphoid tissue
        (GALT), 614
    secretory immunoglobulin, 614
Gynecomastia, 249
    causes of, 249t
    neonatal, with galactorrhea, 245f

H
Haemophilus influenzae, 426, 1004
Haloperidol
    in hyperactive delirium, 103
Halothane–nitrous oxide, 67
Halothane–nitrous oxide anesthesia, 67
Hamartomatous polyps, 1256–1257
Haptoglobin, 61
Hartmann pouch, abdominal
        cavity, 603
HB. See Hepatoblastoma (HB)
HCC. See Hepatocellular carcinoma
        (HCC)
Head
    lesions in children, 217
    typical locations for dermoid
        cysts, 230f
Head injury
    cephalohematomas, 1056
        accumulate at, 1056
        birth trauma, result of, 1056
        calcified, 1056
        local surgical removal, 1056
        operative treatment, 1056

        subperiosteal hematomas, 1056
        treatment, 1056
    clinical evaluation, children
            sustaining head trauma,
            1061–1063
        asymmetric reflexes, 1063
        bulging fontanelle, infants,
            1061, 1062
        child's neurologic status, 1062
        deep-tendon reflexes, 1063
        direct trauma, orbit, 1062
        external signs, head injury, 1061
        focal neurologic deficits, 1062
            indicates, 1062
        Glasgow coma score (GCS),
            1062, 1062t
            postresuscitation, 1062
        initial assessment, 1061
        initial examination, 1061
        neurological assessment
            confounding factors, 1062
        nonincidental trauma, 1063
        overall prognosis, 1061
        pupillary response, 1062
        radiographic evaluation, 1063
        unilateral mydriasis, blown
            pupil, 1062
        unresponsive/comatose
            patient, 1062
        examination, 1062
    epidemiology, 1055
        all-terrain vehicle (ATV)
            accidents, 1055
        falls/drops
            caregivers' arms, 1055
            intracranial injuries, 1055
            cause of, 1055
            minor injuries, 1055
        motorbike accidents, 1055
        non-accidental trauma
            (NAT), 1055
        predominant mechanism,
            pediatric, 1055
        transportation-related
            incidents, 1055
    nonaccidental head injury,
            1064–1066
        abusive injury, 1065
            characteristic findings, 1065
        acute brain injury, 1066
            medical treatment, 1066
            surgical treatment, 1066
        classic triad, findings, 1064
        consciousness
            varying levels, 1065
        decompressive craniectomy, 1066
        inflicted injury, 1064
        inflicted neurotrauma, 1064
            syndrome, young
                children, 1064

1355

Head injury (*continued*)
   intracranial injury
      most common, 1065
   neurocritical care, 1066
      general principles, 1066
   parenchymal hypodensities
      MRI, 1065, 1065f
   perpetrators, 1064
   physical examination, initial, 1065
   presenting symptoms, 1065
   retinal hemorrhages, 1065
   seizures, 1066
   trivial blunt trauma, 1065
  primary brain injury (*See* Primary
      brain injury)
  secondary brain injury, 1060, 1061
   common examples, 1060
   intracranial processes, 1060, 1061
     black brain, 1060
     blood–brain barrier (BBB), 1060
     cerebral edema, 1060, 1061
     CT examination, cerebral
       edema, 1060, 1061f
     cytotoxic edema, 1060
     expanding intracranial mass
       lesion, compensation,
       1061, 1062f
     intracranial hypertension,
       1060, 1061
     intracranial pressure (ICP),
       1060, 1061
     Monro–Kellie doctrine, 1060
     uncontrolled cerebral
       edema, 1060
     uncontrolled intracranial
       hypertension, 1061
     vasogenic edema, 1060
   physiologic alterations, multitude
      of, 1060
   systemic processes, 1061
     definitive algorithms, 1061
     early hypotension, 1061
     factors, 1061
     hyperglycemia, 1061
     hypoxemia, 1061
     late hypotension, 1061
   *vs.* primary brain injury, 1060
  severe traumatic brain injury,
      treatment, 1063, 1064
   age-appropriate neurocritical
      care, 1063
   basic neurophysiologic principles,
      resuscitation, 1063
     adequate oxygenation, 1063
     apnea, 1063
     autopsy, evidence, 1063
     CBF, 1063
     cerebral ischemic injury, 1063
     cerebrospinal fluid (CSF)
       buffering, 1063

CNS injury, 1063
CNS-protective sedatives, 1063
fever, aggressive
   controlling, 1063
hypercarbia, 1063
hyperventilation, 1063
hypotension, 1063
hypotonic fluids, 1063
hypovolemia, 1063
normal pressure
   autoregulation, 1063, 1064f
rapid sequence intubation, 1063
seizures, 1063
intracranial pressure monitoring/
   treatment, 1063, 1064
barbiturates, administration
   of, 1064
elevated ICP, medical
   management, 1064
EVDs, therapeutic
   capability, 1063
intact pressure
   autoregulation, 1064
mannitol, 1064
pentobarbital, 1064
post-resuscitation GCS ≤8,
   children, 1063
severe traumatic barin injury
   (TBI), 1063
steroids use, 1064
ventriculostomy catheters, 1064
multidisciplinary team, trauma
   providers, 1063
skull fractures, 1056
depressed, 1056, 1057f
   absorbable craniofacial fixation
      plates, 1056
   associated
      complications, 1056
   bone flap, 1056
   compound fractures, 1056
   epidural bleeding, controlling
      of, 1056
   high-speed drill, 1056
   infectious risk, 1056
   operative elevation, 1056
   permanent titanium fixation
      plates, 1056
   silk sutures, 1056
   surgery procedure, 1056
   visible depression, patient's
      forehead, 1056
detected by, 1056
linear, nondepressed, 1056
   commonly occur in, 1056
   CT scan, 1056
   healing process, 1056
subgaleal hematomas, 1056
   collect in, 1056
   hemodynamic instability, 1056

percutaneous aspiration, 1056
   result of, 1056
traumatic brain injury (TBI), 1055
Heart block, 86
Heart rate, 70, 71
Hegar dilator, 582, 589
Heimlich valve, 440
Heineke–Mikulicz stricturoplasty
   fibrotic segment of bowel, 636f
*Helicobacter pylori,* 515
Hemangiomas, 963–967
  beard distribution, 970–971
   airway, 971
   airway involvement,
      endoscopy, 970f
   laryngotracheobronchoscopy, 971
   patients, cervicofacial, 970
   segmental facial hemangioma,
      infant, 970f
   subglottic hemangioma
      surgical resection of, 971
   tracheotomy, 971
   T2-weighted contrast (gadolinium)
      images, 970f, 971
  clinical course, 965
   complications, variety of, 965
   endothelial cell hyperplasia, 965
   ulceration, 965
  combined, 964–965
  congenital hemangiomas, 963
   noninvoluting congenital
      hemangiomas (NICHs), 964
   rapidly involuting congenital
      hemangiomas (RICHs), 964
  deep, 964–965
  diagnosis, 966–967
   computed tomography
      (CT), 966
   fast-flow pattern by ultrasound
      (US), 966
   magnetic resonance angiography
      (MRA), 966
   magnetic resonance imaging
      (MRI), 966
   proliferating infantile hemangioma
      lateral
      CT image of, 966f
  differential diagnosis, 967
   angiosarcoma, 967
   biopsy, 967
   infantile fibrosarcoma, 967
   neuroblastoma, 967
   rhabdomyosarcoma, 967
  hemangiomas of infancy, 963
   GLUT-1, marker for glucose
      transport, 964
  incidence, risk factors, and
      associations, 964
   chorionic villus sampling, 964
   familial transmission, 964

placenta previa, 964
pre-eclampsia, 964
lesions, 964
localized convex surface, 975f
localized infantile
　spectrum of, 964f
MRI of, 966f
pathogenesis, 965–966
　endothelial cells, clonal
　　proliferation of, 965
　infantile hemangiomas, 966
　mechanisms of, 965
　placental theory, 966
presentation, appearance, 964–965
　localized telangiectasia, 964
　lymphatic vascular
　　malformations, 964
　red macule, 964
problematic facial, 971
　amblyopia, 971
　bony malformation, 971
　corneal exposure, 971
　optic atrophy, 971
　strabismus, 971
segmental facial hemangioma,
　963–967
superficial, 964
Hematologic malignancies, 175
hepatic involvement, 1247
　hemophagocytic
　　lymphohistiocytosis, 1247
　　diagnostic, 1247
　megakaryoblastic leukemia, 1247
　　congenital acute
　　　megakaryoblastic leukemia
　　　(AMKL), 1247
Hematoma
duodenal, 1044, 1045f
duodenum injury, 1094, 1094f
mesenteric injury, 1095
subungual, 213
Hematopoietic stem cell transplantation
　(HSCT), 1173
bone marrow
　transplantation, 1173
human leukocyte antigen
　(HLA)-matched donor
　(allogenic), 1173
pediatric malignancies, 1173
Hematuria–dysuria syndrome,
　877–878
Hemicords, 1017
Hemodialysis, 175
Hemodynamic decompensation,
　81–82
identification patients at greatest
　risk for CV collapse, 83
LBNP model, 81–82, 81f
as primary outcome variable, 81
Hemodynamic monitoring, 80

Hemoglobin, 85, 173
abnormal, 174
and cardiac index to oxygen
　delivery, 87
estimation, 71
fetal, 71, 173
oxygen–hemoglobin dissociation
　curve, 173
Hemoglobinopathies, 174
Hemoglobin–oxygen dissociation
　curve, 72
Hemoglobin S, 174
Hemolysis, 174
Hemolytic uremic syndrome, 97, 619
microangiopathic (renal) hemolytic
　anemia, 619
　Colicky abdominal pain, 619
　flu-like syndrome, 619
　renal failure, 619
Hemoptysis, 77
Hemorrhage, 516
compensatory phase, 82
detection, 80
intracranial, 123
severe, 175
subclavian artery puncture
　leading, 76
Hemorrhagic shock, 80
risk for, 83
Hemostasis, 176, 177, 572, 931
inherited disorder, 175
Hemothorax, 140, 1074, 1075
chest tube, 1074
　placement, 1074
　urgent, 1074
pulmonary/pleural bleeding, 1075
　rib fractures, result of, 1075
thoracostomy tube size by
　weight, 1075t
trauma-related, 1074
Hendren, W. Hardy, 6
Heparin, 75, 177, 953
Hepatic (hepatocellular) adenoma, 1234
birth control hormonal therapy, 1234
cross-sectional imaging
　techniques, 1234
hepatocellular adenom, 1234
young women, 1234
Hepatic function, 93
Hepatic hemangiomas, 969–970,
　1229–1232
abdominal compartment syndrome,
　970, 1232
angiogenesis inhibitor interferon-
　alpha, 1232
arteriovenous shunting, 969
biopsies
　Glut-1 negative staining of, 970
clinical symptoms, 1229
deiodinase enzyme, 970

diagnosis of, 970, 1229
　screening antenatal US, 970
　treatment, child, 970
　visceral hemangiomas, risk, 970
diffuse, 969, 969f
echocardiogram, 970
focal, 969, 969f
hepatic parenchyma, 969
hypothyroidism, 970
intraperitoneal hemorrhage, 1232
medications, 1232
multifocal, 969, 969f
radiographic appearance, 1229
subtypes, 1229
　diffuse, 1229
　focal, 1229
　multifocal, 1229
symptomatic tumors, 1232
thyroid hormone, 970
Hepatic sarcomas, 1246
Hepatic teratoma, 1235
chronic infections
　mycobacterium avium
　　intracellulare, 1235
Hepatitis A, 180
Hepatitis B, 180
immune globulin, and
　vaccination, 1137
Hepatitis C, 180
Hepatobiliary cystadenoma, 1234–1235
found, middle aged women, 1234
mucin hypersecreting hepatobiliary
　cystadenoma, 1235
Hepatoblastoma (HB), 1228–1229,
　1232, 1234–1236, 1239,
　1241–1244
COG staging, risk stratification,
　AHEP 733, 1238t
cooperative trials, summary
　results, 1239t
current COG, protocol (AHEP-733)
　treatment scheme, 1240f
epidemiology, biology, genetics, 1235
examples PRETEXT
　hepatoblastoma risk
　　stratification, 1238f
outcome, 1243
pathologic classification
　histolic subtype, 1235t
pathology, 1235
risk group stratification, imaging,
　staging, PRETEXT,
　1235–1238
　metastatic lesions, 1236
staging risk stratification, 1237t
surgery, 1240–1243
　liver transplant, 1240–1241
　preoperative tumor rupture, 1242
　resection, resectability technical
　　aspects, 1240

Hepatoblastoma (HB) (*continued*)
  surgical complications, 1242
    bile leak, 1243
    bleeding major vessel injury, 1242–1243
    cardiac arrest, 1243
    liver failure, 1243
    major liver resection, 1242*t*
    trans arterial chemoembolization (TACE), 1242
    tumor biopsy, 1240
    tumor relapse liver, 1242
Hepatocellular carcinoma, 1243–1246, 1306
  chemotherapy, 1244–1245
  cooperative trials, 1245*t*
  epidemiology, 1243–1244
  pathology, 1244
    fibrolamellar hepatocellular carcinoma (FL-HCC), 1244
    transitional liver cell tumor (TLCT), 1244
  PRETEXT staging, 1244
  surgery, 1245
    liver transplantation, children, 1245
    new agents, treatment modalities
      percutaneous ablative therapies, 1246
      sorafenib, 1245–1246
      theraspheres, 1246
Hepatocellular carcinoma (HCC), 1229
  fibrolamellar carcinomas, 1229
  metabolic, cirrhotic liver disease, 1229
  transitional cell tumors, 1229
Hereditary spherocytosis, 174
Hermaphrodite, 899, 900
Hernias
  direct inguinal hernia, 508
  femoral hernias, 508–510
  incarcerated, 503–505, 503*f*–505*f*
  inguinal hernias
    indications, 494–495
    indirect, 489
      clinical presentation, 492–494
      congenital, 491
      diagnosis, 492–494
      embryology, 490–491
      incidence and associated conditions, 491–492
      overview, 489–490
      pathogenesis, 490
    laparoscopic technique (RAC), 495, 498–500, 499*f*
      advantages, 495–496
      disadvantages, 495–496
    open approaches, 495
      advantages, 495
      disadvantages, 495
    operative technique, 500–503, 501*f*–502*f*

pediatric, 489
  preparation and anesthesia, 496
  repair options, 495
    conventional or "open" procedure (MWLG), 495, 496–498
  timing of operation, 494–495
postoperative complications, 507–508
repair, 490
special considerations, 505
  adrenal rests, 506
  cystic fibrosis, 507
  intersex, 507
  peritoneal dialysis, 506
  premature infants, 505
  sliding hernias, 506
  transverse/crossed testicular ectopia, 507
  undescended testis, 505–506
  unusual intestinal segments in hernia sacs, 506
  ventriculoperitoneal (VP) shunts, 506
unusual groin hernias, 510
Herniorrhaphy, 835
Heterotaxia syndromes (HS), 540, 547–548
HHI. *See* Hyperinsulinemic hypoglycemia of infancy (HHI)
Hidradenitis suppurativa, 197
  algorithm for evaluation of a patient with suspected, 198*f*
Hirschsprung disease, 14, 21, 571–591
  chronic problems, 584
  constipation, 584
  Duhamel technique, 575–577
  laparoscopic-assisted pull-through, 584
    duhamel pull-through, 586–588
    endorectal pull-through, 584–585
    historical background, 584–585
    operative technique, 585
  leveling colostomy, 572–574
  loop colostomy, 609
  operative technique, 589
  procedures, 583
  pull-through techniques, 572*f*
  rectal biopsy, 571–572
  second pull-through, 584
  Soave procedure, transanal 1-stage, 589
  stooling issues, 584
  surgical outcomes, 588
  surgical outcomes/ongoing controversies, 589–591
  Swenson, 580–582
  treatment effectiveness, 588–589
  treatment options, 582

Hirsutism, 924
Histopathologic picture, interval appendectomy specimens, 613
Hodgkin disease, 1291
Hodgkin lymphoma, 239, 1260–1265
  adolescent young adults (AYA), 1260
  bimodal distribution, 1260
  chamberlain procedure, technique, 1264*f*
  childhood HL, 1260
  classical, 1260–1261
    CD30 positive Reed–Sternberg cells, 1260
      activated B, T-lymphoid cells, 1260
    subtypes, 1260–1261
      classical lymphocyte rich, 1260
      lymphocyte depleted, 1260
      mixed cellularity, 1260
      nodular sclerosing, 1260
  clinical presentation, 1261–1262
    lymphadenopathy, 1262
  diagnosis, 1262
    thoracoscopic biopsy, 1262
  eosin stained slide, patient, 1261*f*
  Epstein–Barr virus exposure, 1261
  high-power hematoxylin, 1261*f*
  histological subtype, 1260
  histology, 1260–1261
  Immunomarkers, diagnosing, 1260
  incidence, epidemiology, 1260
  lymphocyte predominant (LPHD)
    High-power hematoxylin, eosin stained slide, 1261*f*
  lymphocyte predominant hodgkin lymphoma, 1260
  older adult HL, 1260
  Reed–Sternberg cells
    germinal center B cells, 1260
  staging, 1262–1263
    Bone marrow (BM), 1262
    complete blood cell count, 1262
    C-reactive protein (CRP), 1262
    lactate dehydrogenase (LDH), 1262
    magnetic resonance imaging (MRI), 1263
  staging Ann Arbor classification
    cotswolds modification, 1262*t*
  surgery, 1263
    cytogenetics, 1263
    flow cytometry, 1263
    immunohistochemistry, 1263
    immunophenotyping, 1263
  treatment, 1263
    chemotherapy, radiation therapy, 1263–1264
    high-risk disease, therapy, 1264
      pediatric oncology group (POG), 1264

intermediate risk disease, therapy, 1264
low risk disease, therapy, 1264
  better event-free survival (EFS), 1264
  overall survival (OS), 1264
lymphocyte-predominant hodgkin disease, therapy, 1264
  clinical-pathological entity, 1264
  pediatric patients, 1264
risk classification, 1263
  high-risk disease, 1263
  intermediate, 1263
  low, 1263
toxicities, 1264
Hormonal stress, 67
Hormone and substrate responses, to illness and operation compared to starvation, 68t
Horner syndrome, 436
  T1 ganglion, 436
Host defenses, 190
  adaptive immunity, 192–193
  epithelial barriers, 190
  immune response, 190–191
  innate immunity, 191–192
HS. See Heterotaxia syndromes (HS)
Human immunodeficiency virus (HIV), 180
Human leukocyte antigen (HLA) class I, 179
Human neuroepithelium photomicrographs, 1009f
Human papilloma virus (HPV), 885
Hyaluronic acid, 186
Hydroceles, 490, 508
  examination, 508
  laparoscopy, 508
  management, 508
  postoperative reaccumulation, 508
  types, 508
Hydrocephalus, 76, 1001–1006
  cerebrospinal fluid (CSF), 1001
  CT scan, infant, 1002f
  diagnostic studies, 1002
    computed tomographic (CT), 1002
    cranial ultrasound, 1002
    magnetic resonance imaging (MRI), 1002
  etiology, 1001–1002
    aqueduct of Sylvius, 1001
    bloodstream, 1001
    cerebral subarachnoid spaces, 1001
    foramen of Monro, 1001
      colloid cysts, 1001
    fourth ventricle, 1001
    lateral ventricles, 1001
    syndrome, 1002
    tectum, 1001
    third ventricle, 1001

ventricular system, 1001
X-linked disorder, 1002
intracranial pressure (ICP), 1001
MRI scan, anatomic detail, 1002f
signs, symptoms, 1002
  anterior fontanelle, 1002
  child, age, 1002
  cranial vault, size, 1002
  lethargy, 1002
  sixth nerve palsy, 1002
treatment, 1002–1003
  central venous system, 1002
  distal catheter, 1002
  distal shunt catheters, 1002
  furosemide, 1002
  gallbladder, 1002
    distal catheter, placement of, 1003f
  neurosurgeons, 1002
  peritoneal cavity, 1002
  peritoneum, 1002
  pleural cavity, 1002
  preoperative ultrasound, 1002
  proximal catheter, 1002
  Seldinger technique, 1002
  ventricular shunt, 1002
Hydrocodone, 161
Hydrocodone, oral opioids in infants/children, 160t
Hydrogen–potassium ATPase pump, 99
Hydromorphone, 101, 161
Hydromorphone, oral opioids in infants/children, 160t
Hydrothorax, 76
tris-Hydroxymethylaminomethane (THAM), 86–87
Hymenal abnormalities, 883–885
  imperforate hymen, 884f
  microperforate, 884f
  prepubertal child, 883f
  septated hymen, 884f
  sign of estrogen stimulation, 883f
  unestrogenized, 883f
Hymenectomy, 880
Hyperbilirubinemia, treatment of, 46
Hypercalcemia, 86
Hypercarbia, 86, 106
Hypercholesterolemia, 1291
Hyperglycemia, 67, 129, 132, 133
Hyperhidrosis, 434
Hyperinsulinemic hypoglycemia of infancy (HHI), 1141
  causes in pancreatic beta-cell, schematic representation, 1142
  diagnosis, 1142–1143
  medical therapy for, 1143
    octreotide, 1143
    somatostatin analogue, 1143
  postoperative care, 1145

surgical intervention, 1143
  pancreatectomy, 1143
surgical technique, 1143, 1144f
  laparoscopic approach, 1145
  open procedure, 1143
  preoperative preparation, 1143
  subtotal (95%) pancreatectomy, 1144–1145
  success rate, 1145–1146
Hyperkalemia, 58, 86
  treatment of, 58t
Hyperkinetic (high-flow) portal hypertension, 727
  associated with, 727
  congenital arterial-venous fistula, 727f
Hypermagnesemia, 86
Hypernatremia, 87
Hyperosmolarity, 174
Hyperplasia, 394
Hyperpolarization, 101
Hypersalivation, 330
Hypersplenism, 179
Hypertension, 526, 939, 942
  hyperkinetic (high-flow) portal, 727
  portal, 177
  posthepatic portal, 726, 727
  prehepatic portal, 726
  rebound, 942
Hypertrophic pyloric stenosis (HPS), 534
Hypervolumia, 86
Hypocalcemia, 88, 176
hypocapnia, 458
Hypoglycemia, 52, 86, 156, 1142, 1146
Hyponatremia
  algorithm for assessment, 58f
  symptomatic, treatment of, 58t
Hypoperfusion, 84
  in children, 84
Hypoplasia, 412, 448, 943
  cardiac, 448
  pulmonary, 448
    lung-to-head ratio, 456
    ultrafast magnetic resonance imaging (MRI), 452
Hypospadias
  anatomic anomalies, 790
  associated disorders, 791
    cryptorchidism, 791
    disorder of sexual development (DSD), 791
    inguinal hernia, 791
  classification, 791
    according to position of urethra, 791
  cosmetic appearance, 798
    sexual outcome, 798
  epidemiology, 790
    diethylstilbestrol (DES), maternal estrogens, 790
    estrogen pollutants, 790

Hypospadias (*continued*)
frequency, 790
genetic virilization disorders, 790
larger gene pool, 790
human chorionic gonadotropin
(hCG)
insufficient production, 790
registry data, 790
risk factors, 790
in vitro fertilization, 790
genetic factors, 791
androgen
metabolism abnormalities, 791
receptor defects, 791
congenital adrenal hyperplasia
(CAH), 791
dihydrotestosterone (DHT), 791
enzymatic defects, 791
masculinization, urogenital sinus
androgen dependent, 791
proximal hypospadias
exam finding, 791*f*
treatment, 791–793
chordee correction, 792, 793
chordee, causes of, 792
Gittes artificial erection test, 792
graft, 793
Heineke–Mikulicz principle, 793
mild-to-moderate degrees,
chordee, 793
Nesbit technique, 793
neurovascular bundles, 793
12 o'clock position, 793
penile chordee, 792
small intestinal submucosa
(SIS), 793
tunica albuginea plication
(TAP), 793
general surgical principles, 791, 792
bipolar electrocautery, 792
broad-spectrum intravenous
antibiotic, single dose, 792
epinephrine, use, 792
hemostasis, 792
initial surgical repair
timing, 791
monopolar electrocautery, 792
operative procedure, 792
prophylactic antibiotics, 792
urethroplasty, 792
urinary diversion, 792
surgical algorithm, 792
decisional algorithm, primary
hypospadias repair, 792, 792*f*
tubularized incised plate
(T.I.P.) urethroplasty, 792
two-stage repairs, 792
Hypotension, 85
Hypothalamic–pituitary–gonadal
axis, 246

Hypothermia, 70, 71, 176, 942
pediatric patient at risk for, 71
Hypothyroidism, 246
Hypoventilation
administration of sodium
bicarbonate, 86
Hypovolemia, 81, 84, 88
Hypovolemic hypotension, 81
Hypoxemia, 85
Hypoxia, 85, 174
Hypoxia inducible factor-1$\alpha$
(HIF-1$\alpha$), 183

**I**

Ibuprofen, 100, 159*t*
Idiopathic thrombocytopenic purpura
(ITP), 175
IGF-1 inhibitory binding protein, 132
Ileocolonic disease
laparoscopic, 637
assisted, 637
singleincision laparoscopic
procedures, 637
Ileus, 158
Ilioinguinal/iliohypogastric nerve
block, 170*f*
Immune defenses, 1284
active humoral immunity, 1285
cellular immune defenses, 1285
B lymphocytes, 1285
T lymphocytes, 1285–1286
humoral components, 1284
passive humoral immunity,
1284–1285
Immune responses, 1283
Immune system, 190
human, 190
Immune system components, 1284*t*
Immunity
adaptive, 192–193
in infants and children, 193–194
innate, 191
Immunodeficiencies, 1286
common disorder, 1287*t*
congenital, 1286
laboratory evaluation, 194
primary, 194
secondary, 194
treatment for patients with, 195
Immunoglobulins, 195
immunoglobulin E, 1285
immunoglobulin G, 175,
1283–1285
immunoglobulin M, 1283, 1285
Immunosuppression
anti-CD3 monoclonal
antibody, 1289
Orthoclone OKT3, 1289
antithymocyte globulin, 1289
azathiaprine (Imuran), 1288

calcineurin inhibitors, 1288
cyclosporine (Sandimmune,
Neoral), 1288
sirolimus, 1289
tacrolimus (Prograf), 1288–1289
clinical, 1286
complications, 1290–1291, 1291*t*
corticosteroids (Solumedrol,
Medrol), 1287–1288
drugs classification, 1287*t*
effects of, 1291
IL-2 receptor antibodies, 1289
mycophenolate mofetil
(Cell-Cept), 1288
treatment
antirejection strategy, 1290
induction therapy, 1289
infection prophylaxis, 1291*t*
maintenance therapy, 1289–1290
protocols, 1290*t*
Imperforate anus, 14
without fistula
female, 673
characteristics, 673
male, 671, 672
presenting signs, 671
Inadequate bladder outlet resistance,
compensating for, 865
bladder-neck suspension and
fixation, 866
endoscopic bladder-neck
suspension, 868
fascial sling procedures, 868
open bladder-neck suspension,
866, 868
direct urethral compression by
foreign body, 868
artificial urinary sphincter,
868–869
American Medical Systems
model 802, 869*f*
periurethral injection, 868
urethral lengthening
procedures, 865
Kropp procedure, 866
detrusor flap valve, 867*f*
Pippi Salle procedure, 866
Young–Dees–leadbetter
procedure, 865–866
bladder incision, 865*f*–866*f*
posterior detrusor tube
suspended from, 866*f*
Inadequate ureteral length,
compensating for, 872
complications, 876–878
intestinal ureter, 874, 876
tapered intestinal ureter, 874*f*–875*f*
nephropexy, 872
Psoas hitch and Boari flap, 873–874
vesicopsoas hitch, 874*f*

renal autotransplantation, 874
transureteroureterostomy, 872–873, 873f
Incarcerated hernia, 503–505, 503f–505f
Incidental lesions, 1147
Indirect inguinal hernia, 489
    embryology, 490–491
    overview, 489–490
    pathogenesis, 490
Indomethacin, 106, 930
Indwelling T-tube ileostomy technique, 566f
Infant. *See also* Newborn
Infantile fibrosarcoma (IF), 1221–1222
    chromosome 12p13, 1222
    *ETV6 (TEL),* fusion, 1222
    helix loop helix, 1222
    TGF-beta receptor signals, inhibition, 1222
Infantile hemangioma
    periorbital involvement
        impact, visual acuity, 971f
    rapidly proliferating, 973f
Infantile hepatic
        hemangioendothelioma
        (IHEE), 1230
Infantile hepatic hemangioma
    diffuse, 1231f
    focal, 1231f
    multifocal, 1231f
    treatment algorithm, 1231f
Infections, 193–194
    atypical mycobacterial, 238f
    bone in children, 202 (*See also* Osteomyelitis)
    central venous access
        complications of, 145–146
    inflammatory responses
        definitions, 195
        inflammatory cytokines, 196
    involving deep tissues and body cavities, 201
        muscle compartment infections, 202
        necrotizing infections, 201–202
        osteomyelitis, 202–203
        peritonitis, 203
            associated, 203
            secondary, 203–204
    as leading cause of pediatric morbidity, 1283
    life-threatening neonatal bacterial, 194
    MRSA infection, 1133, 1134
    *Mycobacterium tuberculosis,* 238
    perioperative (surgical site) infections, 204
        definitions, 204
        incidence, 204

prevalence and cost, 204
prevention, 204
    antimicrobial prophylaxis, 204
    preoperative/intraoperative management, 204–206, 205t
    probiotics, 206
treatment of surgical site infections, 207
pleural cavity, 204
empyema, 204
prophylaxis, 1291t
risk factors for, 194
    colonization of newborn, 195
    immunodeficiencies, 194–195
    microbial virulence, 194
shunt infection, 1004
    gramnegative rods, 1004
    *Haemophilus influenzae,* 1004
    intravenous antibiotics, treated with, 1004
    *Propionibacterium acnes,* 1004
    *Staphylococcus aureus,* 1004
    *Staphylococcus epidermis,* 1004
skeletal muscle, 202
skin and soft tissue infections (SSTI), 210
skin and subcutaneous tissue, 196–197
    breast abscess, 199
    hidradenitis suppurativa, 197–198
    lymphatic infections, 199–201
    perianal infections, 199
    pilonidal abscess, 198–199
superficial, 210
    felon, 211
        management, 211f
    onchocryptosis/ingrown toenails (IGTN), 211–212
    paronychia, 210
    perianal abscess (PA), 212
    *Staphylococcal aureus,* 210
systemic inflammatory response syndrome (SIRS), 196
Inflammatory bowel disease, 632–637
    abdominal pain, 632
    clinical presentation, 632–633
        colonic disease, 632
        dizygotic twins, 632
        genetic predisposition, 632
        HLA haplotypes, 632
        inflammatory bowel diseases (IBD), 632
        monozygotic twins, 632
    diagnosis, 633
        anti-*Saccharomyces cervisiae* antibodies (ASCA), 633
        enterography, 633
        enteroscopy, 633
        standard barium small-bowel follow-through, 633

diagnostic algorithm, 634, 634f
functional outcome, 642
    etrograde ejaculation, 642
    fecundity rates, 642
    stool frequency, 642
indeterminate colitis, 642
    restorative proctocolectomy for patients, 642
    therapeutic challenge, 642
indications for operation, 639
    bloody bowel movements, 639
    colectomy, 639
    fulminant colitis, 639
    ileal-pouch anal anastomosis, 639
    long-term corticosteroid therapy, 639
    refractory disease, 639
laparoscopic technique, 640–641
    fulminant colitis, 640
    hand-sewn anastomosis
        Rectal mucosectomy with, 641f
    hand-sewn technique, 640
    ileostomy, 640
    mucosectomy, 640
    omentum, 640
    pelvic floor, 640
    Pfannenstiel incision, 640
    sphincteric complex, 640
medical therapy, 633–634
    corticosteroids
        osteoporotic effects of, 633
    enteral nutrition, 633
    osteoporotic effects of, 633–634
    studies of infliximab, 634
operation, choice of, 639
    laparoscopic-assisted, 639
    lithotomy position
        ileal-pouch anal anastomosis, 639f
operation, indications
    anti-saccharomyces cervisiae antibodies (ASCA) seropositivity, 634
    refractory illness, 634
operative principles, 635–637
    anastomosis, 636
    bowel mesentery, 635
    Finney stricturoplasty
        used for longer strictures, 636, 636f
    preserve bowel length, 635
    short bowel syndrome, 635
    side-to-side isoperistaltic stricturoplasty, 636
    widely patent anastomosis, 635
postoperative course
    chronic pouchitis, 642
    oral ciprofl oxacin, 641
    perioperative complications, 641

Inflammatory bowel disease (*continued*)
pouchitis
nonspecific mucosal
inflammation, 641
probiotics, 642
retained rectal segment
(cuffitis), 642
thrombocytosis, 641
pouch design, 641
J-pouch, 641
lateral pouches, 641
linear staplers, using, 641
S-pouch, 641
small-bowel mobilization, 641
hand-sewn anastomosis
mucosectomy with, 641
ileal pouch, reach of, 641
steroid therapy, shortened
mesentery from, 641
Inflammatory disorders, 954
Informed consent, 16–18
components, 17
cross-cultural study of parental
involvement, 18
guidelines for resolution of moral
problem, 18
patient- and family-centered
approach, 18
pediatric patients with chronic
illnesses, 17
specific issues about bariatric
surgery, 17–18
team members, role, 18
Infraclavicular incision, 144
Infraclavicular nerve block, 167
Inguinal hernias
direct, 508
indications, 494–495
indirect, 489
clinical presentation, 492–494,
492f–494f
congenital, 491
management, 494f
diagnosis, 492–494
differential, 492–494
embryology, 490–491
incidence and associated
conditions, 491–492,
491f–492f
overview, 489–490
pathogenesis, 490
manifestations of processus
vaginalis, 490f
laparoscopic technique (RAC), 495,
498–500
advantages, 495–496
disadvantages, 495–496
open approaches, 495
advantages, 495
disadvantages, 495

operative technique, 500–503
pediatric, 489
preparation and anesthesia, 496
repair options, 495
conventional or "open" procedure
(MWLG), 496–498, 496f–499f
special considerations, 505
adrenal rests, 506
cystic fibrosis, 507
intersex, 507
peritoneal dialysis, 506
premature infants, 505
sliding hernias, 506
transverse/crossed testicular
ectopia, 507
undescended testis, 505–506, 506f
unusual intestinal segments in
hernia sacs, 506
ventriculoperitoneal (VP)
shunts, 506
timing of operation, 494–495
Inhalational anesthetics, 155
Injuries
abdominal, 1044–1048, 1047
bite injuries, 1129
degree of injury, 1129
snakebites, 1130
algorithm for management of
Crotalinae snakebites, 1132f
clotting factor abnormalities to
guide FabAV redosing, 1132t
coral and exotic snakes, 1133
epidemiology, 1130
evaluation, 1130–1131
FabAV administration, 1131t
management, 1131–1133
outdated and unproven
treatments, 1131t
spider bites, 1133
black widow (*Latrodectus*), 1134
brown recluse (*Loxosceles*),
1133–1134
epidemiology, 1133
evaluation, 1133
treatment of acute
anaphylaxis, 1135t
venomous spiders in the
United States, 1133t
treatment, 1129
administration of
antivenin, 1130
antibiotic therapy, 1130
systemic treatment, 1129
type of bite, 1129
blunt abdominal, 1044
burn, 1044
fingertip, 212
head, 1044
multiple, 1098–1099
nail bed, 212

negative pressure wound therapy
(NPWT), 1126, 1128
rectal and sexual abuse, 1049
skeletal, 1043, 1044
soft tissue, 1043
telltale sign of full-thickness
injury, 1122
thoracic, 1048, 1049
vascular, 1101
diagnostic considerations, 1101
diagnostic pitfalls, 1101
overview, 1101
patient management, 1101–1102
penetrating extremity
trauma, 1101
wounds, 189, 1121
alternative wound coverage,
1126–1128
acticoat on arm, 1127f
biobrane, 1127
wound closure using
Integra, 1127f
dressing, 189
puncture, 213
VAC therapy, 207
Injury description, future directions,
1039, 1040
advanced imaging
pediatric trauma measures, 1040
anatomic injury
highly pixelated pictures, 1039
black-box regression methods, 1040
children
different patterns of injury, 1039
prediction models,
comparison, 1040
computerized medical records, 1040
*de facto* standards, 1040
mortality risk comparison
different injury scoring systems,
1039, 1040f
physiological injury
highly pixelated pictures, 1039
physiological measures, 1039
physiological reserve, 1040
severity of illness
calculation, 1040
weight jiggling, 1039
Injury prevention, 1040, 1041
classical approach, 1040
Haddon conceptual
framework, 1041t
Haddon postulates, 1040
matrix, 1040
motor vehicle-related mortality, 1041
prevention initiatives, 1041
education, 1041
enforcement, 1041
engineering, 1041
prevention measures, 1040

INDEX

Injury scales, 1033, 1034
  interval scales, 1033
  nominal scales, 1033
  ordinal scales, 1033
  ratio scales, 1033
  rely on, 1034
Injury scores, 1033, 1034
  composites of, 1033
  data acquisition, *post hoc* nature, 1034
  major injury scoring tools, timeline, 1034*f*
  nebulous concept, 1034
  outcome after injury, function of injury severity/ physiologic reserve, 1034
  physiological scaling effects, 1034
  regression method, 1034
  rely on, 1034
Injury severity scoring tools, 1034
  relationships between
    clinical data and common scores and scales, 1034, 1035*f*
    scoring systems, 1034, 1035*t*
Innominate artery compression syndrome, 949
  anatomy, 949
  bronchoscopy, 950
  contrast CT/MRI imaging modalities, 950
  embryology, 949
  evaluation, 949–950
  presentation, 949–950
  surgical intervention, 950
    aortopexy with complete/partial thymectomy, 950
    surgical intervention/management complications, 950
    pulse oxymetry/blood pressure monitoring, 950
    reimplantation of innominate artery, 950
Insulin
  dysregulation of beta-cell production and release of, 1141
  KATP regulating secretion, 1142
Insulin-like growth factor 1 (IGF-1), 67–68, 131, 181
Integrated platform, 83
Intelligent alarm algorithms, 83
Intelligent patient monitoring systems, 83
Intensive care unit (ICU), 70
  etCO$_2$ monitoring, 71
  new antimicrobials for, 96
  PA catheters in, 76
Intercostal muscle, 440
Intercostal nerve block, 166
Interleukin-1 (IL-1), 68
Interleukin-6 (IL-6), 68
Interscalene approach, 166

Intersex disorder, 899, 900. *See also* Disorder of sexual differentiation (DSD)
  defined, 899
  ethical considerations, 901–902
  gender assignment, 899, 900
  in literature, 900
  in military, 901
  newborn evaluation of infant, 907*t*
  in other societies, 900
  in pop culture and the media, 900
  in religion, 900
  in sports, 901
    Barr Body detection, 901
Intervertebral space, 436, 437
  electrocautery use, 437
  incise pleura, 437
  overlying fascia, 437
Intestinal atresia, 13, 477, 481, 549
Intestinal duplications, 651
  distribution, 652*t*
  embryogenic cause, 651
Intestinal failure, 1317
  management of patient, 1318
    serial transverse enteroplasty (STEP), 1318
    TPN, 1318
  physiopathology, 1318
  satellite complication, 1318
    catheter-associated sepsis, 1318
  total parenteral nutrition (TPN), 1317, 1318
Intestinal malrotation, 540, 542*f*
Intestinal rotation, 540, 542*f*
  associated abnormalities, 541
  children with heterotaxia syndromes, 540
  clinical presentation, 541–543
  definitions of abnormalities, 540–541
  embryology
    expression of *Nodal*, 540
    *Pitx2* and *Isl1*, asymmetric expression, 540
    *Tbx18*, asymmetric expression, 540
  fundamentals of operative correction, 545
  management
    asymptomatic rotation abnormalities, 547
    controversies, rotation abnormalities, 545
    heterotaxia syndromes, 547–548
    role of laparoscopy, 545–547
  normal, 542*f*
  occurence, 541
  operative correction
    fundamentals of, 545
    Ladd procedure, 545
    operative steps of ladd procedure, 546*f*

sensitivity and specificity of whirlpool sign, 545
  radiologic diagnosis, 543–545, 543*f*–544*f*
    findings, 547
Intestinal transplantation, 1318
  complications, 1323
    gastrointestinal complications, 1323
    graft -*versus*-host disease (GVHD), 1323–1324
    post-transplant lymphoproliferative disorder, 1323, 1323*f*
    vascular complications, 1323
  criteria for evaluation, 1319
  immunosuppression, therapy for, 1320
    basiliximab (Simulect), 1320
    daclizumab (Zenapax), 1320
    immunologic monitoring, 1320–1321
    tacrolimus, 1320
  indications, 1318*t*
  outcomes, 1324
    long-term rehabilitation and quality of life, 1324
    patient and graft survival, 1324, 1324*f*
  postoperative care, 1321
    antiviral prophylaxis, 1321
    assessment of intestinal allograft, 1321, 1321*f*
    infection control, 1321
    nutritional support, 1321
  rejection of the intestinal graft, 1322
    chronic rejection, 1322*f*
  transplant procedures, 1319
    combined liver and intestinal transplant, 1320*f*
    isolated intestine, 1319, 1319*f*
    multivisceral, 1320*f*
Intestine(s). *See also* Colon; Duodenum; Jejunum; Small intestine
Intraabdominal pressure (IAP), 76
Intrahepatic disease, 722
  cystic dilation, 722, 723*f*
Intralipid, 132
Intraoperative bowel irrigation technique, 565
Intraosseous access, 139
Intrathoracic herniation, 452
Intravascular volume expanders, 94*t*
Intravenous (IV) cannulation, 208
Introital masses, 881
  Bartholin gland cyst, 882
  other introital cysts, 883
  prolapsed ureterocele, 881
  Skene cyst, 882, 882*f*
  urethral prolapse, 881, 881*f*

Intussusception, 592–596
  children
    majority of cases, 592
  clinical presentation, 592
    abdominal colic, 592
      older children, 592
    full-blown clinical sepsis
      picture of, 592
  etiology, 592
    adjacent distal bowel, 592
    proximal bowel, 592
    viral-induced lymphoid
      hyperplasia, 592
  evaluation, 593
    hydrostatic reduction, 593
    pseudokidney, 593
    radiologic studies, 593
  ileocolic
    distal small bowel
      opacifying multiple loops of, 595f
    fluoroscopic image
      during air enema, 595f
    hemicolectomy, 595
    ileocecectomy, 595
    mesenteric vessels, 593f
    proximal transverse colon, 595f
    RLQ ultrasound demonstrates
      axial view of, 594f
    RUQ ultrasound demonstrates
      cross-sectional view of, 594f
    Supine x-ray of a child, 593f
  ischemia in, 593f
  manual reduction of, 595f
  nonoperative management, 593–594
    air column
      pressure of, 594
    decreased oral intake, 593
    fluoroscopically, 594
    intravascular volume, 594
    pediatric surgical consultation, 594
    pneumatic reduction, 594
    third space losses, 593
    vomiting, 593
  operative management, 594–595
    laparoscopic, 596
      atraumatic graspers, 596
      Length of stay (LOS), 596
      peritonitis, 596
      technique of, 596
      traditional open surgery, 596
    open surgery
      infraumbilical transverse right-
        sided incision, 594
      proximal ileal edge, 594
  pathologic, 592
    Meckel diverticulum, 592
  pathophysiology, 592
  postoperative, 596
    etiology, 596
    reexploration, 596

small bowel
  by polyp, 593f
  symptoms, 593
Invasive monitoring procedures, 72
  abdominal pressure, measurement
    of, 76
    pulmonary arterial catheters,
      76–78
  central venous catheters, 75–76
  mixed venous oximetry monitoring,
    79, 79f
  pulmonary artery pressure,
    measurement of, 78
  cardiac output, 78–79
  systemic arterial catheters, 72–75,
    73f–75f
Involved field radiation therapy
  (IFRT), 1263
Involved node radiation therapy
  (INRT), 1263
Iontophoresis, 208
Ischemia, 75
Isolated juvenile polyps, 1249–1250
  diagnosis, 1249
    colonoscopy, 1249
    juvenile polyposis syndrome
      (JPS), 1249
  Hill–Ferguson rectal retractor
    exposure, 1250f
  presentation, 1249
    chronic blood loss, 1249
    intermittent abdominal pain, 1249
  surveillance, 1250
  treatment, 1249–1250
    chronic blood loss, 1249
    dysplasia, 1250
    endoscopic polypectomy, 1249
    malignant transformation, 1250
    polypectomy, 1249
Isoproterenol, 86
  increase heart rate, conduction
    velocity, and contractility, 86
IV antibiotic therapy, 145
IVH, clinical signs, 53

J

Jarcho–Levin syndrome, 275
Jejunal interposition, 357
  free jejunal grafts, 357, 357f
  postoperative management, 357
    success rate, 357
  preoperative management, 357
  surgical technique, 357
Jejunoileal atresia, 554
  complications, 556
  laparoscopic/periumbilical
    incision, 556
  mortality, 556
  pathophysiology, 554
  resection of dilated bowel, 556f

survival rate, 556
Type I, 555f
Type II, 555f
Type III, 555f
Type IIIb, 555f
Type IV, 555f
Jejunoileal injuries, 1094–1095, 1096f
Jejunostomy, 520–521
  complications, 521
  contraindications, 521
  laparoscopic, 521
Joubert syndrome, 50
Journal of Pediatric Surgery, 10
Jugular vein, 75
  catheterization, 76
Jugular vein, external, 140f,
  141–142
Jugular vein, internal, 142–143
  intraosseous access, 140–141
Jugular venous pressure, 930
Juvenile polyposis syndrome,
  1249–1252
  BMPR1A gene
    chromosome 10q23, 1251
  colorectal polyp, 1249
  diagnosis, 1251
    lamina propria expansion, 1251
  familial syndromes, 1249
  gastric lesions, 1250
  gastric mucosa, 1252
  gastric polyps, 1252
  genetic basis, 1251
  hamartomas, 1249
  intestinal epithelium, 1249
  isolated juvenile polyps, 1249–1250
  large bowel, 1250
  presentation, 1250
    diffuse form, 1250
    infantile form, 1250
    Juvenile polyposis coli, 1250
  SMAD4 gene, 1251
    chromosome 18q21, 1251
  submucosa, 1249
  surgically excised colon specimen
    patient diagnosed, 1252
  surveillance, 1252
  treatment, 1252
    endoscopic polypectomies, 1252
    pouch-anal anastomosis, 1252
    psychosocial consequences, 1252
Juvenile polyps. See Juvenile polyposis
  syndromes
J-wire, 143

K

Kaposiform hemangioendothelioma
  (KHE), 977f
kaposiform hemangioendotheliomas
  (KHEs), 970
  interchangeably, 1230

Kaposiform lymphangiomatosis, 990
  lymphatic endothelial
        proliferation, 990
Kaposi sarcoma, 1291
Karyotypic abnormalities, 449
Karyotyping, 22, 31, 243, 247, 449,
        453, 473, 889, 904–907, 906,
        925, 1178
Kasabach–Merritt phenomenon, 970
  intravascular coagulopathy
        secondary, 970
  platelet trapping, 970
Kawasaki disease, 619, 953
  mucocutaneous lymph node
        syndrome, 619
Kelly clamp, 579
Ketamine, 102, 209
  bronchodilator effects, 102
  effect on CNS, 102
  effect on PVR, 102
  metabolism, 102
  properties, 102
Ketamine, pain control, 154, 163
Ketogenesis, 65
Ketorolac, 100, 159t, 163
Ketorolac, pain control, 163
$\Delta^4$-3-Ketosteroid-5$\alpha$-reductase
        (5$\alpha$-reductase), 904
Kidney transplantation, 1293
  children undergone, 1294t
King-Denborough syndrome, 151
Kingella kingae, 202
King syndrome, 270
Kirchner wire, 436
  intervertebral space, identified, 436
Klinefelter syndrome, 249, 899, 901
Klippel–Trenaunay syndrome, 885
Kommerell diverticulum, 943, 944
Koop, C. Everett, 6, 10
KTP laser, 302
Kyphoscoliosis, 270

L
Lacerations
  abdominal, 1049f
  arterial, 886, 1136
  bony prominences, 1043
  chylothorax and cardiac, 1049f
  diaphragm, 1084
  duodenal, 1094, 1095f
  fingertips, 212
  grade III splenic, 1033
  hepatic, 1088
  liver, 1089
  lower-pole splenic, 1086
  lung, 1075
  membranous trachea, 1074
  nail bed, 213, 1109
  pancreatic ductal, 1091
  pericardial, 1076

peripheral splenic, 1085
  renal contusion and, 1048
  scalp, 1046f, 1056f
  spleen, 1032, 1036t, 1136
  superficial, 212
β-Lactams, 93
Lactic acid, 80
Lactic acidosis, 86
Lactobacillus BB-L, 195
Lactobacillus GG, 195
Lactobezoars, 515
Lactococcus acidophilus, 195
Ladd operation, 13
Ladd, William E., 3–4
Laparoscopic adjustable gastric band
        (LAGB), 528
Laparoscopic appendectomy
  techniques, 624–628
    curvilinear infraumbilical, 624
    Hasson approach, 624
    nasogastric tube, 624
    three different approaches,
        depicted, 627
    transumbilical approach, 624
    umbilical port, 624
Laparoscopic-assisted Duhamel
        pull-through, 585
Laparoscopic cholecystectomy,
        703–707
  children's mercy hospital experience,
        708, 709
    choledocholithiasis, 708
    common duct stones (CBD), 709
    ductal injury, 708
    patients undergoing laparoscopic
        cholecystectomy, 708, 709t
    postoperative hemorrhage, 709
    reported complications, 708
    severe inflammation
        obliterating, 708
    symptomatic cholelithiasis, 709
  complications, 707, 708
    bile leakage, 707
    common complications, 707
    ductal injury, 707
      rate of, 707
    hepaticojejunostomy, 707
    infectious complications, 708
    significant, 707
    sphincter of Oddi, 708
  Ethicon disposable cannulas, 703
  four-port technique, 704–706
    bupivacaine, 706
    2-cannula technique, 704
    Credé maneuver, 704
    epigastric port, 704
    gallbladder
      detachment, 706
      extraction, 706
    herniation, prevention, 706

lateral retraction, infundibulum,
        704, 706, 706f
    operation procedure, 704
    orogastric tube, 704
    parallel orientation, 706
    pneumoperitoneum, 704
    port site location
      adolescent, 705f
      baby, 705f
      depends on, 704
      youth, 705f
    reverse Trendelenberg
        position, 704
    2 stab incision technique, 704
    triangle of Calot, 706
    two clips, placing of, 706, 706f
  2 right-sided incision, 703, 704f
  single-site umbilical, 706, 707
    advantage, 706
    cystic duct/artery ligation,
        707, 708f
    electrocautery, 707
    endoscopic clips, 707, 708f
    gallbladder
      extraction, 707
      mobilization, 707
    natural orifice transluminal
        endoscopic surgery
        (NOTES), 706
    complications, 706
    nice cosmetic result, 707, 708f
    SILS port, 706, 707, 707f
    single-site umbilical laparoscopic
        surgery (SSULS), 706
    TRIPORT, 706, 707, 707f
    umbilical fascia, 707
    used in children for, 706
    vs. 3/4-port/incision laparoscopic
        surgery, 706
  stab incision technique, 703
Laparoscopic Duhamel technique, 588
Laparoscopic leveling biopsies, 573
Laparoscopic pyloromyotomy, 534
Laparotomy, 601–602
  abdomen, exploratory
        laparotomy, 76
  enterostomy, 602
  fatal hemorrhage, 602
  infants, 602f
  subcapsular hematoma, 602
  transverse supraumbilical, 601–602
Laryngeal cleft, posterior, 307
  anatomic classification, 307, 308f
    subtypes, 307
  coexistent anomalies, 309
  concurrent tracheoesophageal
        fistula, 307
  diagnosis, 308–309
  embryology, 307
  history, 307

Laryngeal cleft, posterior (*continued*)
mortality rate, 307, 315
operative intervention, 309
presurgical considerations, 309
presentation, 308–309, 309f
surgical procedures, 310
endoscopic repair, 312–314
interposition grafts, 314
open repair, 310–312
type III posterior laryngeal
cleft repair, 310f–312f
revision surgery, 314
success rates for cleft repair, 315
type IV (long) clefts, 314–315
Laryngobronchoscopy, 299
airway foreign bodies, 300–301
layout for rigid
bronchoscopy, 301f
significant risks involved in
removing, 301
endoscopic evaluation, 299, 299f
indications, 299
KTP laser, 302
laser bronchoscopy, 302f
treatment with laser therapy,
301–302, 301f
YAG laser, 302
Laryngospasm, 156
Laser bronchoscopy, 302f
LATS. *See* Local anesthetic, toxicity
syndrome (LATS)
Left atrial pressure (LAP), 78
Left ventricular end-diastolic volume
(LVEDV), 78
Leptin, 526
Leptin resistance, 527
LES. *See* Lower esophageal
sphincter (LES)
Lesions, 393, 978–984
acquired, 217
benign lesions, 233
diagnosis and surgical treatment,
233–236
high-grade malignancies, 233
low-grade malignant
neoplasms, 233
metastatic neoplasms involving
parotid gland, 236
ranula, 236–237
salivary gland lesions, 233
in children, 233t
torticollis, 231–233
embryonic origin, 217
inflammatory, 237
acute cervical
lymphadenitis, 237
subacute/chronic lesions, 237
cat scratch disease, 239
cervical lymphadenitis,
chronic, 237–238

cervical lymphadenopathy,
causes, 239
mycobacterial lymphadenitis,
238–239
labial, 886
larynx and upper airway, 295f
malignant, 394
neoplastic, 239
pigmented lesions in childhood, 1270
differential diagnosis, 1270
salivary gland, 217
superficial lesions, 982
vulvar, 885
Leukemia, 175
Leukocyte-depleted RBCs, 178
Leveling colostomy, 572
operative technique, 573–574
postoperative care, 574
preoperative preparation, 573
treatment options, 572–573
Leydig cells, 905
L-hook electrocautery, 435
Liaison Committee on Graduate
Medical Education, 9
Lich–Gregoir technique, 822
Lidocaine, 88, 208
administered via endotracheal
tube, 88
Life-threatening thoracic
injuries, management,
1069, 1070
emergency thoracotomy, 1069
clamping of aorta, 1069, 1071f
emergency department, 1069
incision location
left resuscitative thoracotomy,
1069, 1069f
left anterolateral thoracotomy to
the right, extension
clam shell thoracotomy,
1069, 1071f
meta-analysis
patients undergoing ED
thoracotomy, 1069t
operative procedure, 1069
penetrating injury, 1069
pericardial tamponade,
evacuation, 1069, 1070f
emergent intubation
required in trauma bay, reasons
for, 1069
Glasgow coma scale (GCS), 1069
inline capnography, 1069
pericardial tamponade, 1069, 1070
echocardiography, 1069
expeditious subxiphoid
pericardotomy, 1069
pericardial fluid, detection, 1069
potential sternotomy
operating instruments, 1070

subxiphoid approach
pericardial fluid, 1070, 1072f
pericardial window, placement,
1070, 1072f
trauma setting, 1069
transesophageal approach, 1069
transthoracic approach, 1069
pulse oximetry, 1069
securing airway, 1069
endotracheal intubation, 1069
treatment priorities, order of, 1069
Li Fraumeni disorder, 1212
Ligamentum arteriosus, 943
Ligation, 929
Lingual duplications, 651
Linoleic acid, 65
Lipase, 44
Lipid, 61
metabolism, 65
overfeeding, 132
rescue therapy, 164
Lipogenesis, 132
Lipolysis, 132
Lipoma, 214
Liquid ventilation, 116
extensive animal studies, 116
extracorporeal membrane
oxygenation (ECMO), 116
caring for patient,
considerations, 118
complications, 123
indications, 117
methods, 118–122
monitoring, 122–123
nutrition on, 123
physiology/circuit design,
117–118
perfluorocarbon-assisted gas
exchange (PAGE), 116
perfluorocarbons, 116
total (tidal) liquid ventilation, 116
Lithium batteries, 330
Liver transplantation, 732
benefits, 732
contraindications to
transplantation, 1308
improved survival rates, 732
indications, 1306–1308, 1307t
alagille syndrome, 1306–1307
biliary atresia, 1306
fulminant hepatic failure,
1307–1308
malignancy, 1308
metabolic disease, 1307
transplantation for, 1307t
limitation, 732
long-term risks, 732
management, 1311
immunosuppressive
protocol, 1311

operative considerations, 1308
donor options, 1308
anatomic variants for liver
transplantation, 1308t
donor selection, 1308–1310
living-related left lateral
segment graft, 1310f
recipient procedure
bile duct reconstruction, 1311f
outcome after ransplantation,
1314–1315, 1314f
postoperative complications, 1311
acute cellular rejection, 1312
biliary complications, 1312
chronic rejection, 1313
infectious complications,
1313–1314
primary nonfunction
(PNF), 1311
vascular thrombosis, 1311–1312
preoperative preparation, 1308
primary transplantation, 732
progressive intrinsic hepatic
disease, 732
Liver tumors, 1228–1229
differential diagnosis, 1228–1229
acquired non-neoplastic
masses, 1228
alpha fetoprotein (AFP),
level, 1229
benign tumors, 1228
congenital, 1228
fatty infiltration of liver, 1230f
hemophagocytic
lymphohistiocytosis
(HLH), 1228
infantile hepatic
hemangioma, 1229
Langerhans cell histiocytosis
(LCH), 1228
malignant tumors, 1228
megakaryoblastic leukemia, 1228
Local anesthetic
maximum dosages for tissue
infiltration, 209t
maximum doses of, 164t
toxicity syndrome (LATS), 164
Location of cysts, diagnosis
fetus, 664
infants, 664
Long chain fatty acids, 442
Long-chain triglyceride (LCT)
formulations, 132
Long-term sequelae, pediatric cancer
therapy, 1173, 1174
childhood cancer survivor study
result, 1173
cranial irradiation, use of, 1173
central nervous system (CNS)
side effects, 1173

diminished fertility, 1174
females, 1174
infertility associated agents, 1174
males, 1174
cyclophosphamide
treatment, 1174
secondary neoplasm, 1174
severe/debilitating renal failure, 1173
incidence, 1173
severe growth retardation, 1173
Lorazepam, 101
half-life, 103
use of, 102
Lower body negative pressure (LBNP),
81–82, 81f
humans exposed to, 82
live LBNP experiment, 82f
Lower esophageal sphincter (LES), 359
Low-molecular-weight heparin
(LMWH), 97, 98, 178
LPS-binding protein, 191
Lumbar epidurals, 165
Lumbar plexus nerve block, 167
Lung
development, 104, 105t
response to injury, 107
functional residual capacity
(FRC), 107f
mediators, 107
Lung abscesses, 422, 431
diagnosis, 432
algorithm, 433f
essentials of diagnosis, 431–432
etiology, 432
management, 432, 433f
outcome, 432–433
pathophysiology, 432
Lung immaturity, 416
Lung infections, 422
Lung injuries, 1072, 1073
blunt injuries to the lung,
1072, 1073
pulmonary contusion, 1072, 1073
associated intrathoracic
injury, 1072
chest CT, 1072
chest x-ray, chest trauma
evaluation, 1072
external signs of injury, 1072
lung ventilation, 1073
management, 1072, 1073
Lung maturity, 46
Lung-to-head circumference ratio
(LHR), 452
Lupus anticoagulant, 177
Lymphangiectasias, 990–991
congenital pulmonary
lymphangiectasia, 991
diffuse dysplasia, 991
Down syndrome, 991

extracorporeal membrane
oxygenation (ECMO), 991
Noonan syndrome, 991
Ulrich Turner syndrome, 991
diffuse lymphangiectasia, 990–991
primary intestinal
lymphangiectasia, 991
lymphoma, 991
Waldmann disease, 991
Lymphangiomatoses, 988–990
diffuse lymphangiomatosis, 989f
lymphatic vessels, 989
Lymphatic infections, 199
algorithm for cervical
lymphadenitis, 200f
chronic lymphadenitis, biopsies, 201
diagnosis, 199
laboratory tests, 199
surgical treatment, 200
ultrasonography (US), 200
Lymphatic malformations, 984–992
common cystic lymphatic
malformations, 985–988
arteriovenous malformations
(AVMs), 985
children, 985
cystic hygroma, 985
diagnosis, 985–986
complications, 986
fiberoptic endoscopic
intubation, 985f
large cervicofacial lymphatic
malformation (LM),
microcystic
components, 986f
postnatal, 986
prenatal, 985–986
treatment, 986–988
diffuse lymphangiomatosis, 989f
homeobox gene Prox 1, 985
lymphatic development, 984–985
embryonic lymphatics, 984
endothelial sprouting, sacs, 985
slow-flow lesions, broad range
of, 984
Lymphedema, 991–992
autosomal dominant pattern, 991
congenital, 992f
genetic syndromes, 991
cerebrovascular
malformations, 991
distichiasis, 991
Turner syndrome, 991
yellow-nail syndrome, 991
interstitial protein-rich fluid, 991
Milroy disease, 991
Lymph node biopsy, 1263f
Lymphocytic and histiocytic (L&H)
cells, 1261
LymphomA, 236

Lymphoma, 397–399, 1258, 1260–1266
  adult small intestinal lymphomas
        diffuse large B-Cell
           lymphoma, 1258
  anaplastic large T-cell lymphoma
        (ALCL), 1266
  anterior mediastinotomy, 1262
  Burkitt-like lymphoma (BLL), 1266
  chemotherapy, treatment, 1258
  infection, *Helicobacter pylori,* 1266
  intestinal intussusception, 1258
  lymph node analysis, diagnosis, 1258
  lymphoblastic lymphoma (LL), 1266
  mucosa-associated lymphoid tissue
        (MALT), 1266
  non-Hodgkin Lymphoma, 1258
        Burkitt lymphoma, 1258
  supraclavicular
        lymphadenopathy, 1261
Lysozyme, 191

**M**
Macrocephaly-capillary malformation
        syndrome, 981
  Chiari malformations, 981
  congenital syndrome, 981
  hydrocephalus, 981
  macrocephaly, 981
  vascular lesions, 981
  Wilms tumor, 981
Macrocystic cervical lymphatic
        malformation
  CT image demonstrating extensive
        macrocystic lesions, 988f
  12 months postsurgery, 988f
  preoperative photo, 988f
Macrocystic lymphatic lesion
  fetus, Prenatal MRI, 985f
Macrocystic lymphatic malformation
  left anterior chest wall, axilla
        2-month-old infant, 987f
Macrophages, 182
Maffucci syndrome, 984
  bone union, 984
  chondrosarcomas, 984
  enchondromas, 984
Magnetic resonance angiography
        (MRA), 953
Magnetic resonance imaging (MRI),
        197, 939, 1212
  primary tumor, 1212
        Imaging of, 1212
  surrounding structures, 1212
Major histocompatibility complex
        (MHC), 1286
  class I alleles, 191
Major perianal disease, 696–698
  rectal prolapse, 696–698
        anatomical findings, adult
           prolapse, 696

complication of, 696
demographics, 696
dignostic procedures, 697
  contrast enemas, 697
  video defecography, 697
forms, 696
incidence, 696
major cause of, 696
presentation, 696, 697
  eversion, mucoepidermoid
        junction, 697, 697f
  mucosal mass, 696, 697
treatment, 697, 698
  Frykman–Goldberg
        operation, 698
  hypertonic saline, 697
  invasive abdominal
        procedures, 698
  perianal cerclage, technique, 697
  Ripstein operation, 698
  sclerotherapy, 697
  Thiersch wire technique, 697
Malformation, 342
Malignant hyperthermia (MH)
  anesthetic risks, 151
  clinical presentation, 151
  treatment for, 151
Malignant Hyperthermia Association
        of the United States
        (MHAUS), 151
Malignant liver tumors, 1229
  HCC, 1229
  undifferentiated sarcoma, 1229
Malignant peripheral nerve sheath
        tumor (MPNST), 1222
  Neoadjuvant radiotherapy, 1222
  neurofibrosarcoma, 1222
  neurovascular involvement, 1222
  schwannoma, 1222
  treatment, 1222
Malignant thymomas, 394
Malignant tumors, 1229, 1235–1246
  hepatoblastoma (HB), 1235–1238
  neonates, 1229
        biliary rhabdomyosarcoma, 1229
        rhabdoid tumor, 1229
        teratoma, 1229
Malinosculation, 407
Malnutrition, 131, 134, 181
Marfan syndrome, 270, 438, 953
Maryland-style dissector, 435
Mastitis
  lactation, 244t
  neonatal, 244t, 246, 246f, 249
McCune–Albright syndrome, 246
MCT-oil–containing formulas, 568
Measured energy expenditure (MEE)
        values, 129
Meatal stenosis, 800, 801
  diagnosis, 800

meatotomy, operative technique,
        800, 801, 802f
  Emla cream, advent of, 800
        effects, 801
  hemostasis, 800, 801
  puralube, ophthalmic Vaseline, 801
  Tegaderm dressing, 800
pathophysiology, 800
  result of, 800
  urethral meatus normal size,
        boys, 801t
presentation, 800
surgical outcome, 801
Mechanical ventilation, 111
  adverse effects, 115
        barotrauma, 115
        bronchopulmonary dysplasia, 115
        permissive hypercapnia, 115–116
  conventional, 111
        pressure-controlled/pressure-
           limited ventilation, 111–113
  high-frequency ventilation, 114–115
  volume-controlled, 113–114
Meckel diverticulum,
        complications, 618
Meconium, 481
Meconium ileus (MI), 13–14, 558
  abdominal distension in infant, 562f
  abnormal intestinal motility, 559
  algorithm for patients
        management, 560
  antenatal diagnosis/
        management, 559–560
  chronic obstruction and
        infection, 558
  cystic fibrosis (CF), postnatal
        diagnosis of, 567
        nutritional management, 567–568
        pulmonary management, 569
  cystic fibrosis (CF), prenatal testing
        for, 561–562
  distended loop of ileum, 562f
  microcolon of disuse, 563f
  nasogastric (NG) tube, 564
  non-CFTR genetic factors, 559
  pathophysiology of, 559
  postnatal management, 562
        clinical presentation, 562
        nonoperative management,
           563–564
        operative management, 564–567
        postoperative care, 567
        radiologic features, 562–563
  prenatal ultrasound suspicious, 560
  prognosis, 569
  rabbit pellets/*scybala,* 564
  radiologic findings, 563
  soap bubble appearance, 563f
  sonographic evaluation, 560–561
Mediastinal cysts, 393

Mediastinal masses, 393
  computed tomography scan
    pleural effusion, 1262f
  diagnostic techniques, guidelines for
      use, 394
    bronchoscopy, 395
    chest radiographs, 394
    computed tomography (CT)
        scans, 394
    esophagoscopy, 395
    magnetic resonance imaging, 394
    mediastinoscopy, 395
    positron emission tomography, 395
    ultrasound, 395
  incidence data, 394t
  simplified algorithmic approach
      treatment, child, 1263f
  treatment priorities for children
      with, 393
Mediastinal tumors
  evaluation of children with, 394
Mediastinum, 393
  compartments, 393
    visceral contents, as redefined for
        pediatric population, 394t
Medical error, 19
Medium-chain fatty acids, 442
Medium-chain triglycerides (MCTs), 130
α-Melanocyte stimulating hormone
    (MSH), 527
Melanocytic nevi, 1270
Melanoma, 1270
  Becker melanosis, 1272
  blue nevus, 1272
  characteristics, 1271t
  classic clinical signs, 1277
    ABCDE checklist, 1277
  congenital melanocytic nevus,
      1273–1274
  evaluation of suspected
      melanoma, 1279
  FAMM syndrome (Familial atypical
      mole and melanoma), 1271
  giant congenital melanocytic nevus,
      1274–1276, 1274f–1275f
  halo nevi, 1272
  malignant melanoma
    subtypes, 1276
    transplacental, 1276
  management
    of primary site, 1279
    of regional lymph nodes, 1279
  melanocytic nevus
    acquired, 1271, 1271t
    atypical, 1271, 1271t
  moderate, large, and giant nevi,
      1274f–1275f, 1277–1279,
      1278f
  neurocutaneous melanosis, 1276
  nevus of Ota, 1272

nevus sebaceous of Jadassohn,
    1273, 1273f
  tumors associated with, 1273t
nevus spilus, 1272–1273
pathophysiology, 1270, 1271
small nevi, 1277, 1277f
spitz nevus, 1271–1272, 1271f
systemic adjuvant therapy, 1279
treatment, 1277
Mendelian genetic disorder, 50
Meningoceles, 50
Meperidine, 101
Mesenchymal hamartoma, 1229, 1232
  cavernous lymphangiomatoid
      tumor, 1232
  marsupialization, 1232
  palpable mass, 1232
  pathogenesis of, 1232
  pseudocystic mesenchymal
      tumor, 1232
  school aged children, 1229
  theories, 1232
    abnormal embryologic
        development, 1232
    blood supply, abnormal
        development, 1232
    embryologic hepatic
        mesenchyme, abnormal
        proliferation, 1232
  toddlers, 1229
Mesenteric adenitis, 614
Mesenteric injury, 1095,
    1096f–1097f
  hematoma, 1095
Mesenteric vessels, 585, 586f
Mesoappendix
  divided, ligated, 622f
  endovascular stapler,divide, 628f
  Hook cautery, divide, 628f
Metabolic abnormalities, 70
Metabolic acidosis, 76, 88, 930
Metabolic imaging
  F-fluorodeoxyglucose positron
      emission tomography
      (FDG PET), 1213
Metabolic response mechanisms, 66
  hormones, 67–68
  inflammatory mediators, 68
  neural pathways, 66–67
Metabolic stress, acute, 132
Metabolism
  anaerobic, 80
  carbohydrate, 64–65
  energy, 62–64
  lipid, 65
  nutrient, 61
  protein, 61–62
  vitamin and trace mineral, 66
Metabolizable protein, 130
Metalloenzymes, 66

Metastatic disease, 1223
  computed tomography (CT), 1223
  lung metastasis, 1223
  sentinel lymph node biopsy, 1223
Metastatic liver tumors, 1247
  desmoplastic small round cell
      tumor, 1247
  gastric epithelial, 1247
  hepatic metastasectomy, 1247
  neuroblastoma, 1247
  osteogenic sarcoma, 1247
  Wilms tumor, 1247
Metastatic wilms tumor, 1185
  combined chemotherapy, 1185
  pulmonary metastases, 1185
  radiation therapy, 1185
  regimen DD-4A, 1185
  resecting pulmonary lesions, 1185
  response-based approach, 1185
  stage IV favorable histology
      tumors, 1185
Methadone, 162
Methemoglobinemia, 71
Methicillin-resistant Staphylococcus
    aureus (MRSA), 1133
Methylprednisolone, 1287
Metoclopramide, dopamine receptor
    antagonist, 170
MI. See Meconium ileus (MI)
Microcephaly, 51
Microspheres, 569
Midazolam, 101
  biotransformation, 102
  properties, 102
Midazolam, intravenous preparation
    of, 154
Midline skin markers, 1010
  spinal cord anomaly, 1010
Mikulicz double-barreled enterostomy,
    565, 566f
minimally invasive surgery (MIS), 459
Minor perianal disease, 694–696
  anal fissure
    demographics, 695
    diagnostic procedures, 695
    incidence, 694, 695
    outcome, 695
    presentation, 695
    treatment, 695
  fistula-in-ano/perianal abscesses,
      695, 696
    demographics, 696
    diagnostic procedures, 696
    incidence, 696
    outcome, 696
    presentation, 696
    treatment, 696
  hemorrhoidal disease, 694
    demographics, 694
    diagnostic evaluation, 694

Minor perianal disease (*continued*)
  incidence, 694
  outcome, 694
  presentation, 694
  treatment, 694
Mitomycin-C
  with bougienage, 340
5-mm access trocar, 435f
5-mm telescope, 435f
Mobile lesion, 664
Modified Heller esophagomyotomy
    (EM), 359
Montgomery glands, 244
Morphine, 92, 101, 161
Morphine, oral opioids in infants/
    children, 160t
Motilin, 359
Motor neurons, 51
Mucosal flap, 583, 583f
Mucosal–submucosal tube, 579
Mucosal tube, incision, 580
Mucosectomy
  laparoscopically mobilized
      rectosigmoid colon
      prolapses, 587f
Mucous membranes, 70
Mullerian inhibiting substance
    (MIS), 904
Müllerian-inhibiting substance
    (MIS), 15
multifocal disease, 604–606
  clip and drop-back approach, 606
  intestinal continuity
      restoration of, 606
  jejunostomy, 604
  necrotic intestine, 604
  short bowel syndrome, 604, 606, 607
    intestinal transplantation for, 606
Muscle fibers, 51
Muscle relaxants, use of, 156
Mutations
  in the *ABCC8* and *KCNJ1* genes,
      1141, 1142
  F508del mutation, 559
  gene within DSS locus, 904
  G544X mutations, 559
  KATP channel, 1142
  p53, germline mutation, 1212
Myasthenia gravis, 393, 401
  Osserman classification of, 402t
  pulmonary artery on postoperative
      chest radiograph, 405f
  treatment, 402–403, 403f–404f
Mycobacterial lymphadenitis, 238–239
*Mycobacterium avium-intracellulare*
    *scrofulaceum* (MAIS)
    complex, 238f
*Mycobacterium tuberculosis,* 199, 239
Mycophenolate mofetil, 1290
Myelination, 51

Myelodysplasia, 854
Myelomeningocele, 30–31, 1010–1013
  Chiari malformation, 1012
    cervicomedullary
        decompression, 1012
    foramen magnum, 1013
    Sagittal T1-weighted MRI
        showing, 1012f
    syringomyelia, cystic collection
        spinal fluid, 1012f, 1013
  child, photo, 1011f
  distal neurologic function, 1012
  fetal, algorithm for management, 33f
  gastroesophageal reflux, 1012
  hindbrain, 1012
  MRI, 33f
  myeloschisis, 1010
  primary neurulation, failure, 1010
  spinal fluid, accumulation, 1010
  swallowing dysfunction, 1012
  technique of fetal MMC repair, 39
    efficacy and future, 40–41
    fetal MMC repair, 39, 40f
    maternal morbidity, 40
    outcomes, 40
    rationale, 39
    specific postoperative
        considerations, 40
  therapeutic intervention, 1012
Myelomeningocele (MMC), 848
Myocardial contractility, 88
Myocardial ischemia, 70
Myositis, 202
Myotonia congenita, 151

**N**

Naproxen, 160
nasogastric tube, 481
Nasojejunal tubes, 134
National Button Battery treatment
    guidelines, 331t
National Highway Safety Act, 1966, 1029
National Institute of Diabetes and
    Digestive and Kidney
    Diseases (NIDDK), 532
National Institutes of Health (NIH), 524
National Study on the Costs and
    Outcomes of Trauma
    (NSCOT) project, 1030
National Surgical Quality
    Improvement Program,
    Pediatric (NSQIP-P), 9
Natural killer (NK) T-cell
    lymphomas, 1266
Neck
  anterior, anatomy, 226f
  lesions in children, 217
  scrofula, 239f
  typical locations for dermoid
      cysts, 230f

Necrotizing enterocolitis, 132, 930
  Modified Bell's Stages of, 598t
Necrotizing enterocolitis (NEC), 43, 195
necrotizing enterocolitis (NEC), 597
  Abdominal radiographs of
      infants, 599f
  clinical manifestations, 598–599
    extremely low birth weight
        (ELBW), infant, 598
    premature, low-birth-weight
        infants, 598
  cyanotic heart disease, 597
  diagnostic studies, 599–600
    differential diagnosis, 600
      focal intestinal perforation
          (FIP), 600
      radiographic findings, 600
    laboratory findings, 599
      hypercapnea, 599
      hypoxia, 599
      leukocytosis, 599
      thrombocytopenia, 599
    radiographic studies, 599
  gastrointestinal emergency, 597
    newborn, 597
  medical management, 600
    broad-spectrum antibiotics, 600
    coagulopathy, 600
    hypovolemia, 600
    metabolic acidosis, 600
    orogastric tube (OGT), 600
  mesenteric vessels, 603f
  pathogenesis, 597–598
    antigens, 598
    hypoxic, 598
    immature intestinal
        epithelial, 597
    inflammatory mediators, 598
      platelet activating factor, 598
      TNF-alpha, 598
    intestinal epithelium, 598
    lumenal bacteria, 598
    mucosal epithelial layer, 598
    transmucosal passage, 597
  postoperative management
    antibiotics, 607
      data conflicting, optimal
          duration of, 607
      positive blood cultures, 607
    feeding, 607
      total parenteral nutrition
          (TPN), 607
    ostomy management of intestinal
        continuity, 607
      distal ileostomies, 607
    resuscitation
      anemic, 607
      dopamine, 606
      hemodyamic status, 606
      thrombocytopenic, 607

prognosis, 607
  chronic complications
    strictures, 607
  colon, 607
  mortality, patients, 607
  surgical management, 600–606
    abdominal wall erythema, 600
    gangrenous bowel, 600
    intestinal necrosis, 600
    pneumoperitoneum, 600–601
  surgical techniques for
    treatment of, 603f
Necrotizing fascial infections, 201
  diagnostic studies, 201
  morbidity, 201
  surgical exploration, 201
  symptoms, 201
  treatment, 201
Necrotizing infections, 201
Negative pressure wound therapy
    (NPWT), 189
Neisseria gonorrhoeae, 882
Neonatal hyperbilirubinemia,
    treatment of, 46
Neonatal intensive care unit (ICU), 195
Neonatal intensive care unit (NICU),
    43, 140
Neonatal torticollis, 217
Neonate
  fat digestion, 45
Neoplasms, 400–401. See also Cancer;
    Carcinoma
  laboratory "markers" for ovarian
    neoplasms, 894t
Neorectal spur, 588f
Nephroblastomatosis, 1184, 1185
  bilateral Wilms tumor, 1185
  metachronous contralateral Wilms
    tumor, 1185
  nephrogenic rests, 1184
    perilobar, 1184
  term used in cases, 1185
  unilateral Wilms tumor, 1185
Nephropexy, 872
Nephrotic syndrome, 97
Nephrotoxicity, 95
Nervous system, 50
  central nervous system, development/
    disorders, 50–51
  cerebral blood flow, 52
  intracranial pressure, 52
  intraventricular hemorrhage (IVH),
    52–53
  metabolism/metabolic disorders, 52
  neuromuscular system, development/
    disorders, 51–52
  normal development, 1006–1010
    bilaminar structure, 1006
    caudal nervous system, 1008
    conus medullaris ascends, 1008

  conus medullaris, ascent,
    1008, 1011f
  epiblast, 1006
  hypoblast, 1006
  neural tube closure,
    abnormalities, 1007
  notochordal process, 1007
  primary neurulation, 1007
  secondary neurulation, 1008
    chick embryos, 1010f
Neural crest cell, 42
neural defects, 449
  anencephaly, 449
  encephalocele, 449
  hydrocephalus, 449
  myelomeningocele, 449
Neural tube defects, 343
Neural tube defects (NTD), 50
Neural tumors, 395
Neuraxial blocks, 164
  epidural blockade, 165–166
  paravertebral blockade, 166
  peripheral nerve blockade, 166
  subarachnoid blockade, 164–165
Neuraxium, 166
Neuroblastoma, 239
  chemotherapy, 1195, 1196
    autologous stem cell transplant
      (ASCT), 1196
      complications, 1196
    13-cis-retinoic acid (RA)
      mucocutaneous recovery, 1196
      multicourse regimen, 1196
    commonly used agents,
      1195, 1196
    high-dose, 1196
    high-risk neuroblastoma, 1196
    123iodine-metaiodobenzyl-
      guanidine (MIBG), 1196
    131iodine-metaiodobenzyl-
      guanidine (MIBG), 1196
    limitation, 1195
    maintenance therapy, 1196
    multiagent, 1195
    myeloablative consolidation
      therapy, 1196
    persistent disease, 1196
    primary tumor
      surgical resection, 1196
    therapy, total length of, 1196
    tumor resistance
      chemotherapeutic agents, 1196
      decreasing risk of
        developing, 1196
  classification, 1191
    disease progression, risk factors
      for, 1191
    favorable histology (FH), 1191
    histopathologic
      characteristics, 1191

  international neuroblastoma
    pathology classification
    (INPC), 1191, 1192f
  microscopic evaluation of
    neuroblastoma, depends
    upon, 1191
  mitosis-karyorrhexis index
    (MKI), 1191
  peripheral neuroblastic
    tumor, 1191
  Shimada classification, 1191
  tumor pathology, fundamental
    basis for, 1191
  clinical presentation, 1188, 1189
    advanced-stage disease, 1188
    clinical manifestations, 1188
    diagnosis, 1188
    frequently found in, 1188
    Horner syndrome, 1188
    intra-abdominal
      neuroblastomas, 1188
    presenting symptoms, 1188
  metastatic dissemination, 1188
  paraneoplastic conditions, 1189
    biologically active substance,
      secretion of, 1189
    corticosteroid therapy, 1189
    dancing eye syndrome, 1189
    endocrine tumor, 1189
    immune-mediated
      response, 1189
    occurrence, 1189
    opsoclonus-myoclonus
      syndrome (OMS), 1189
    surgical excision, 1189
    vasoactive intestinal peptide
      (VIP), 1189
  paraspinal neuroblastomas, 1188
  pelvic neuroblastomas, 1188
  periorbital ecchymosis
    raccoon eyes, 1188
  4S disease, 1189
    blueberry muffin, 1189
    characterized by, 1189
    clinical conditions, 1189
    diagnostic tissue biopsy, 1189
    liver metastases, 1189
    low-risk group category, 1189
    occurrence, 1189
    treatment, 1189
  sympathetic chain, may
    occur at, 1188
  symptoms
    initial, 1188
    severe, acute, 1188
  thoracic neuroblastomas, 1188
  epidemiology, 1187, 1188
  clinical incidence, 1187
    North America, 1187
    United States, 1187

Neuroblastoma (*continued*)
  diagnosis, 1187
    initial age, 1187
    median age, 1187
  disease expression, degree of, 1188
  event-free survival (EFS), 1188
  extra-cranial solid tumor, most
      common, 1187
  familial neuroblastoma, 1188
  high-risk group, 1188
    survival rate, 1188
  inheritance pattern, 1187
    study of, 1187, 1188
  low-risk group, 1188
    survival rate, 1188
  race predilection of, 1187
  exist as, 1187
  laboratory testing, 1190
    neuroblastomas, secretes, 1190
      biologically active
          products, 1190
      catecholamine, 1190
      homovanillic acid (HVA), 1190
      vanillylmandelic acid
          (VMA), 1190
    serum biomarkers
      lactate dehydrogenase
          (LDH), 1190
      neuron-specific enolase
          (NSE), 1190
      prognostic indicators, 1190
  operative considerations, 1194, 1195
    abdominal cavity
        exploration, 1195
    hemodynamic monitoring, 1194
    hemorrhage, 1195
      prevention, 1195
    laparoscopic adrenalectomy, 1195
    laparoscopic biopsy, 1195
    midline/transverse abdominal
        incisions, 1195
    nephrectomy, 1195
    thoracoabdominal approach,
        1195, 1195f
    tumor features, consideration, 1194
  radiographic studies, 1190, 1191
    computed tomography (CT), 1190
      characteristic image
          features, 1190
      intravenous contrast, use
          of, 1190
      large central neuroblastoma,
          scan, 1190f
    magnetic resonance imaging
        (MRI), 1190
      *vs.* computed tomography
          (CT), 1190
    plain radiograph, 1190
      abdomen, 1190
      chest, 1190

scintigraphy, 1190, 1191
  [123]iodine-metaiodobenzyl-
      guanidine (MIBG),
      radiolabeled, 1190, 1191
  lymph node metastase
      detection, 1191
  ultrasonograph, 1190
radiotherapy, 1196, 1197
  external-beam radiotherapy
      (EBRT), 1196
  focused, 1196
  20 Gy, 1196
  21 Gy, 1196
  for high-risk
      neuroblastomas, 1196
  for intermediate-risk
      neuroblastomas, 1196
  intraoperative radiation therapy
      (IORT), 1196, 1197
    benefits, 1196
staging, 1191–1193
  based on, 1191
  children's oncology group, 1192
    risk stratification, 1192
  event-free survival, based on
      risk-group categorization, 1193f
  image-defined risk factors
      (IDRFs), 1193
  international neuroblastoma risk
      group classification system
      (INRGCS), 1192, 1193, 1193f
  international neuroblastoma
      risk group staging system
      (INRGSS), 1193
    patients classification, 1193
  international neuroblastoma
      staging system (INSS),
      1191, 1192t
    fundamentally based on, 1192
  stage III tumors, 1191
    classification, 1191
  stage II tumors, 1191
    classification, 1191
  stage I tumors, 1191
  stage IV tumors, 1191, 1192
    classification, 1191, 1192
  tumor, node, and metastasis
      (TNM) system, 1191
surgery, 1194
  chemotherapy, 1194
  complete curative resection, 1194
  complete gross resection, 1194
  complete surgical excision
      primary tumor, 1194
  early surgical intervention, 1194
  incomplete resections, 1194
  *MYCN* amplification, 1194
  near-complete excision, 1194
  operation post-
      chemotherapy, 1194

    operation timing, 1194
      high-risk groups, 1194
      intermediate risk groups, 1194
      low-risk groups, 1194
    role, based on, 1194
    stage III tumors, 1194
      resection, 1194
    stage IV tumors, 1194
      resection, 1194
  tissue evaluation, 1189, 1190
    bone marrow biopsy, 1190
    histopathological assessment, 1189
      definitive diagnosis, 1189
      open/laparoscopic biopsy, 1189
    tissue sampling, 1189
    trephine biopsies, 1190
    US-guided core needle biopsy,
        1189, 1190
Neuroblastomas, 236, 394, 395–396
Neurocutaneous melanosis, 1276
  asymptomatic patients, 1276
  defined, 1276
  screening, 1276
  symptomatic, 1276
Neurocutaneous syndromes, 953
Neurofibroma, 250
Neurofibromatosis, 953
Neurofibromatosis I disorder, 1212
Neurofibrosarcoma, 1222, 1224
  surgical excision, 1224
  upper extremity, failed
      chemotherapy, 1225f
Neurogenic shock, 85
Neuromuscular system, development/
    disorders, 51–52
Neuropeptide Y, 359
Neurotransmitters, 103
Neutrophils, 182
Newborn. *See also* Infant
Newborn gastric perforation, 514
Newborn intestinal obstructions, 13
Niacin, 66
NIBP waveform data, 82
Nicotinamide adenine dinucleotide
    phosphate (NADPH), 44
Nitinol silicone, 340
Nitric oxide (NO), 87
nitrofen-treated animals, 448
Nitrous oxide, 67
Nodular regenerative hyperplasia
    (NRH), 1234
  Budd–Chiari syndrome, 1234
  celiac disease, 1234
  chronic granulomatous
      disease, 1234
  hepatopulmonary syndrome, 1234
  inflammatory bowel disease,
      treatment, 1234
  mimicking metastatic
      nodules, 1234

noncirrhotic liver
    multiacinar regenerative nodular
        lesion, 1234
    portal hypertension, children, 1234
Nodule(s)
    eyebrow soft tissue nodule, 229f
Nonairway anomalies, 314
Non-hodgkin lymphoma, 1265–1269
    anaplastic large cell lymphoma,
        1266, 1268
    Burkitt lymphoma, 1266
    chemotherapy, 1268
        acute tumor cell lysis syndrome
            (ATLS), 1268
        granulocyte colony-stimulating
            factor (G-CSF), 1268
    clinical classification, 1265t
    clinical presentation, surgery, 1266
        excisional biopsy, 1266
        fluorescence
            situ hybridization, 1266
        mediastinal disease, 1266
        pleural effusions, 1266
        polymerase chain reaction
            (PCR), 1266
        Superior vena cava syndrome, 1266
    cyclophosphamide, 1266
    epidemiology, classification, 1266
        natural killer (NK) T-cell
            lymphomas, 1266
    Epstein–Barr virus (EBV), 1266
    genetic differences, 1265
    human herpes virus 8 (HHV-8), 1266
    human lymphotropic virus type 1
        (HTLV-1), 1266
    immunophenotypic, 1265
    lymphoblastic lymphoma (LL), 1268
    morphologic, 1265
    pathogenesis, 1266
    precursor B, 1266
    radiation therapy, 1268
    staging, 1266
        St Jude Murphy system, 1266
    St. Jude Murphy staging system, 1266t
    T-lymphoblastic lymphoma, 1266
    toxicites, 1268
    treatment, outcome, 1268
        Berlin–Frankfurt–Münster
            (BFM), 1268
        COMP, 1268
        high-dose methotrexate
            (MTX). L-Asp
            difference, 1268
        LSA2-L, 1268
    world health organisation
        (WHO), 1265t
non-Hodgkin lymphoma, 1291
Non-Hodgkin lymphomas, 239
Noninvasive monitoring procedures, 70
    carbon dioxide monitoring, 71–72

cardiac output, 72
    echocardiography, 72
    pulse oximeters, 71
    transcutaneous blood gas
        monitoring, 72
nonneural tube defects, 449
    cardiovascular system, 449
        ventricular septal defects, 449
Nonopioid analgesics, 159t
nonpalpable testis
    surgical management, 782, 783
        diagnostic laparoscopy, 782
            findings, 782, 783
            follicular stimulating hormone
                (FSH), 782
                base level, 782
            hCG stimulation test, 782
            important question, 782
Nonrhabdomyosarcoma soft tissue
    sarcoma (NRSTS), 1221–1227
    chemo-insensitive, 1222
    flow chart
        management of, 1223f
    neoplasms
        heterogeneous group of, 1227
Nonrhadomyosarcomas, 1221–1227
    clinical characteristics, 1221–1227
Nonspecific (nonimmune) host
    defenses, 1283
    cellular components, 1283
    humoral components, 1283
Nonsteroidal antiinfl ammatory
    (NSAID), 106
Nonsteroidal antiinflammatory
    drugs, 515
Nonsteroidal antiinflammatory drugs
    (NSAIDs), 160, 884
Norepinephrine, 103
Normal appendiceal anatomy, 615f
Normal frontonasal development, 1016f
Normeperidine, 101
Notochordal development, 1008f
Nutrient metabolism, 61
Nutrition, 582
    and hypermetabolic response to
        burn patients, 1128
    strategies, 644, 646
        adolescence, 646
        breast milk, 645
        catheter-related infections
            (CRI), 644–645
        enteral feeds, initiation, 645
        feeds, 645
        fluid losses, 645
        gastrojejunal (GJ) tubes, 645
            vs. antireflux surgery, 645
        gastrostomy tubes (GT), 645
        initial feeds, 645
            oro/nasogastric (NG) routes, 645
            oro/nasojejenal (NJ) routes, 645

lipid-reduction protocol, 644
        meta-analysis, 645
        multidisciplinary approach, 644
        omega-3 fatty acids, 644
        oral feeds, initiation, 645
        PEG vs. laparoscopic
            placement, 645
        sepsis, 644
        skin breakdown, 645
        ultimate goal, 644
Nutritional strategies, 644, 646
    adolescence, 646
    breast milk, 645
    catheter-related infections (CRI), 644
        catheter salvage treatment, 645
        peripherally inserted central
            catheters (PICCs), 644
        prevention, 645
        treatment, 645
    enteral feeds, initiation, 645
    feeds, 645
    fluid losses, 645
    gastrojejunal (GJ) tubes, 645
        vs. antireflux surgery, 645
    gastrostomy tubes (GT), 645
        placement, 645
        techniques, 645
    initial feeds, 645
        oro/nasogastric (NG) routes, 645
        oro/nasojejenal (NJ) routes, 645
    lipid-reduction protocol, 644
    meta-analysis, 645
    multidisciplinary approach, 644
    omega-3 fatty acids, 644
    oral feeds, initiation, 645
    PEG
        vs. laparoscopic placement, 645
    sepsis, 644
    skin breakdown, 645
    ultimate goal, 644
Nutritional supplementation, 129–135
    energy metabolism/energy
        requirements, factors
        modifying, 131
    energy requirements, 130
    metabolic stress, acute
        anabolic hormone resistance,
            131–132
    metabolic stress response, acute, 131
    nonprotein caloric requirements,
        130–131
    overfeeding, 132–133
    overview of, 129–130
    postinjury setting, resuscitation,
        133–135
        delivery, 134
        enteral nutrition, 134–135
        parenteral nutrition, 135
        parenteral vs. enteral nutrition, 135
    protein requirements, 130

# O

Obesity, medical comorbidities, 525f
Obesity, psychosocial
        comorbidities, 525f
Obstructed megaureter, 810
    ureteral tailoring and
            reimplantation, operative
            technique, 810
        long submucosal tunnel, 810
        massively dilated megaureter, 810
        megaureters, antenatally
                detected, 810
        mid-line vertical cystotomy, 810
        Pfannenstiel incision, 810
        representation, 811f
Obstructive lesions, of stomach, 510
    antral web, 512–513
    congenital microgastria, 513
    gastric volvulus, 510–511
    pyloric atresia, 511–512
Odynophagia, 330
Oliguria, 939
omphalocele, 449, 471
    amniocentesis
        determine, chromosomes, 473
    antibiotic ointment, 481f
    Cantrell, exposed heart
            pentalogy of, 471f
    cardiac, 471
    cephalic end, prominent
            pulsation, 472f
    chromosomal defects, 472
    classic cloacal extrophy
            bladder plates of, 472f
    cloacal exstrophy, 471
    defect
            musculofascial margin of, 480f
    epithelialization, allowing, 481f
    giant
            definition of, 477
    hidden mortality, 472
    infants, 471
    intestinal loops, failure, 471
    lateral body wall closure, 471
    membrane-intact medium-
            sized, 476f
    midaxillary line, dissection, 480f
    neonatal reduction, 480f
    outcomes
        gastroesophageal reflux, 482
        pulmonary hypoplasia, 482
            chromosomal abnormalities, 482
    perinatal management, 473
        amnion lined sac, 473
        saline-soaked gauze, 473
        vaginal delivery, 473
    physiologic herniation, 471
    postoperative management, 481
        anomalies, impact, 481
        antibiotics, 481

Intestinal dysmotility, 481
    repair
        type of, 481
    povidone–iodine solution, 481f
    ruptured, 479–481
        bowel bag
            temporary coverage with, 479
    staged closure of, 480f
    surgical management, 477–481
        delayed repair, 478–479
            abdominal viscera, 478
            epithelialization, 478
            nonoperative techniques, 478
            ventral hernia, 479
            ventral hernia, closed, 480f
        Immediate Repair, 477–478
            absorbable material, 477
            bowel ischemia, 477
            hemodynamic status, 478
            intraabdominal pressure, 477
            umbilical vessels, 477
            umbilicoplasty, 477
            urachus, 477
        infant with, 477
        membrane
            removal of, 478f
        neonatal period, 478
        staged neonatal repair, 478
            amnion inversion technique, 478
            minimal skin flaps, creation
                of, 478
            prosthetic materials, 478
Ondansetron
    postoperative nausea and vomiting
            (PONV), 157
Ondansetron, 5HT serotonin receptor
            antagonist, 170
ontogeny, 448
Open fetal surgery, general
            principles, 34
    anesthesia, 34
    equipment, 34
    gravid uterus
        closure, 35, 36f
        opening, 35, 36f
    incision and exposure, 35
    personnel, 34
    positioning and draping, 34–35
    postoperative care, 35
    tocolysis, 35
open thoracotomy, 441
    latissimus dorsi muscle, 441
    serratus anterior muscle, 441
Operative repair after progressive
            and monitored
            (ECHO), 459
Opiate medications
    intravenous administration of, 162
Opiate therapy, adjuncts
    benzodiazepines, 163

    gabapentinoids, 163
    ketamine, 163
    ketorolac, 163
    tramadol, 163
Opioids, 101
    administered to CI patients, 101
    commonly used opioids in
            PICU, 101t
    features of withdrawal, 103t
    fentanyl, 101
    morphine, 101
    process of discontinuing, 103
    prolonged administration of, 103
    receptors, 101
    remifentanil, 101
    semisynthetic, 101
    tolerance, 101
Opioids, intravenous
    for infants and children, 162t
Opitz-Frias syndrome, 314
Oral duplications, 651
Oral intake, 134
Oral opioids in infants/children, 160t
Organ dysfunction, 174
Organoaxial volvulus, 510
orthopedic instruments, 436
    diskectomies, perform, 436
    rib interspaces, 436
Osteogenesis imperfecta (OI), 185
Osteomyelitis, 139, 202–203
    laboratory evaluation, 202–203
    radiographs, 203
    treatment, 203
Ostomies, 569
ostomy
    closure
        leakage, 612
        stricture formation, 612
    distal exteriorization, 611f
    parenteral nutrition
        infants with, 477
    prolapse, 612
Ovary, 892
    ovarian autoamputation, 893
    ovarian cyst, 892–893
    ovarian neoplasms, 893–897
    ovarian torsion, 893
Overfeeding, 132
Oversedation, 158
Oxycodone, 161
Oxycodone/acetaminophen, 161
Oxycodone, oral opioids in infants/
            children, 160t
Oxygen
    consumption monitoring, 79, 79f
    delivery at tissue level, 79
    hemoglobin saturation, 79
    kinetics, 87
    oxygen-carrying capacity of the
            blood, 87

Oxygen toxicity, 416, 937
Oxyhemoglobin, 71
Oxyntomodulin (OXM), 527

**P**

Pain
    management, 214
    postcoarctation abdominal, 942
    tramadol, for pain control, 163
Pain control, 157–159
    ambulatory analgesia, 170
    antiemetic agents, 170–171
    body wall blocks, 168
        ilioinguinal–iliohypogastric
            block, 168–169
    local anesthetics, 164
    local anesthetic toxicity syndrome
        (LATS), 164
        treatment of, 164
    lower extremity blocks, 167–168
    medication in children, 159
        acetaminophen, 160
        intravenous analgesics, 161–162
        nonopioid analgesics, 160
        nonsteroidal antiinflammatory
            drugs, 160–161
        opiate therapy, delivery systems
            of, 162–163
        oral opioids, 161
        pharmacology, 159–160
    neuraxial blocks, 164
        epidural blockade, 165–166
        paravertebral blockade, 166
        peripheral nerve blockade, 166
        subarachnoid blockade,
            164–165
    opiate therapy, adjuncts
        benzodiazepines, 163
        gabapentinoids, 163
        ketamine, 163
        ketorolac, 163
        tramadol, 163
    over/under-treatment, risks
        of, 158
    physiologic effects of, 157–158
    postoperative analgesia, monitoring
        developmentally delayed older
            children, 159
        drug research, in children, 159
        infants, 158
        pain scales and assessment, 158
        school-aged children, 158–159
        teenagers, 159
    regional analgesia techniques,
        163–164
    transverse abdominis plane block,
        169–170
    upper extremity blocks, 166–167
Pallister–Hall syndrome, 51
Palmaz stents, 326

Pancreatic ductal injury
    combined duodenal, common bile
        duct, 1093–1094
        management, 1094f
    proximal, 1092–1094
        repair injury, 1093f
        Roux-en-Y pancreaticojejunostomy,
            1093f
Pancreatic enzyme microtablets, 569
Pancreatic enzyme replacement
        therapy (PERT), 564
Pancreatic proteases, 45
Pancreatitis duplications, 656–658
    complications, 657
    diagnosis, 657
        CT scan, 657
        ECRP, 657
        ultrasound, 657
        upper GI study, 657
    diagnosis essentials, 656
    presenting signs, 657
    symptoms, 657
        duodenal duplication,
            communication to
            pancreatic duct, 657, 657f
    treatment, 657, 658
        operative intervention, 657
        Puestow procedure, 658
        simple cystectomy, 657
        Whipple procedure, 657
panintestinal disease, 606
    gastrostomy tube, 606
Pantothenate, 66
PAOP. *See* Pulmonary artery, occlusion
        pressure (PAOP)
Papavarin, 75
Paralyzing agents, 156
Parameningeal, 1216
    pterygopalatine, 1216
Paraplegia, 942
Paraspinal, 1217
    neurovascular bundles, 1217
Parathyroid glands, 1154–1157
    anatomy, 1154, 1155
        ectopic gland, 1154
            possible locations, 1154
        located in, 1154
        total 4 glands, 1154
            2 inferior parathyroid
                glands, 1154
            2 superior parathyroid
                glands, 1154
    diagnosis essentials, 1154
    embryology, 1154
    operative technique, 1156, 1157
        cervical exploration, 1156, 1157
            anatomic location
                variance, 1156
            benign parathyroid tissue,
                autotransplanting, 1157

half-life, parathyroid
        hormone, 1156
    hyperplastic parathyroid gland,
        vascular pedicle, 1156, 1156f
    inferior parathyroid glands,
        development, 1156
    intraoperative parathyroid
        hormone assay, 1156
    large parathyroid adenomas,
        identification, 1156
    minimal access approach, 1156
    minimal access
        parathyroidectomy, 1156
    multiple adenomas/
        hyperplastic glands, 1157
    superior parathyroid glands,
        development, 1156
    thyroid lobectomy, 1157
    thyroid, mobilization, 1156
positioning, 1156
    cervical exploration,
        appropriate neck extension,
        1151f, 1156
    intra-operative parathyroid
        hormone assay, 1156
    major caveat, 1156
postoperative considerations, 1157
    risk of recurrence, 1157
    serious potential
        complications, 1157
parathyroidectomy, indications for,
        1155, 1156
hypercalcemia
    associated end-organ
        damage, 1155t
    causes, 1155t
    symptoms, 1155t
primary hyperparathyroidism, 1155
    causes of, 1155
    diagnosis, 1155
    ectopic parathyroid hormone
        (PTH) secretion, 1155
    familial hypocalciuric
        hypercalcemia (FHH), 1155
    MEN syndrome, 1155
    parathyroid adenomas, 1155
    persistent/recurrent, 1155
    serum calcium level, 1155
    sestamibi nuclear subtraction
        scan, 1155
    ultrasonography, 1155
secondary hyperparathyroidism,
        1155, 1156
    end-stage renal disease
        (ESRD), 1155
    hypocalcemia, chronic
        state, 1155
    renal osteodystrophy, 1155
    supplementary nutrition,
        treatment, 1155

Parathyroid glands (*continued*)
  tertiary hyperparathyroidism,
      1155, 1156
    end-stage renal disease
        (ESRD), 1155, 1156
    kidney transplantation, 1156
  physiology, 1155
    parathyroid hormone (PTH), 1155
    primary function, 1155
parenchymal cellular proliferation, 449
Parenteral nutrition, 65
Parenteral nutrition (PN), 644
  after surgery, 645
  feed control, 64
  hepatic dysfunction, 644
  related complications, 646
Parenteral nutrition associated liver
      disease (PNALD), 132
Parotid gland
  metastatic neoplasms involving, 236
Parry–Romberg skin syndrome, 274
Partial androgen insensitivity (PAIS),
      905, 908t
Patent ductus arteriosus (PDA), 929
  clinical features, depend on, 930
  closure, complications of, 937
  closure from inside pulmonary
        artery, 935
    balloon catheter occlude
        PDA, 936f
    from inside pulmonary
        artery, 936f
    interrupted sutures, placed on
        pulmonary artery, 936f
    using interrupted pledgeted
        mattress sutures and a
        Dacron/Gore-Tex patch, 936f
  closure from midline sternotomy,
        933, 935, 935f
    encircle with ligatures of silk, 935f
    ligate just before institution of
        cardiopulmonary bypass, 935f
  diagnosis
    chest radiograph, 930
    echocardiogram with Doppler
        color flow imaging, 930
  division, 931
    straight vascular clamps
        application, 932f
  etiologic factors, 929
  ligation, 931
    aorta cross-clamped, 933f
    close to pulmonary artery, 932f
    lumen of PDA completely
        abolished, 932f
    obliterated using suture ligation
        technique, 934f
  morbidity, 929
  mortality, 929–930
  natural history, 929

percutaneous catheter closure,
      936–937
  using double umbrella device, 937f
  in premature infants, 930
  robotic ductal ligation, 937
  surgical closure, 930–931
    left thoracotomy through fourth
        intercostal space, 931f
    right angle clamp placement, 931f
    stay sutures placement, 931f
  thoracoscopic closure, 937
Patent processus vaginalis (PPV), 489
pathogenic Gram negative bacteria, 598
Patient-controlled analgesia (PCA), 101
PCA dosing recommendations, 162t
Peak inspiratory pressures (PIPs), 87
Pectoralis major, 274
Pectoral muscles, 277
Pectus carinatum, 270
  associated defects and syndromes, 270
  asymmetric chondrogladiolar
        deformity, 271f
  clinical presentation, 271
    deformities, classification and
        descriptions, 271
    symptoms, 271
  diagnostic evaluation, 272
  etiology, 270
  indications for intervention, 272
  management, 272
    nonoperative, 273
    operative, 272
  with Poland syndrome and Marfan
        syndrome, 270
Pectus excavatum, 20, 254
  cardiac impairment from, 255
  characterization, 255
  CMR protocol, 255
  complications, of repair, 267–268
  etiology, 254
  evaluation and treatment algorithm
        for primary repair, 257f
  intraoperative transesophageal
        echocardiography (TEE), 255
  noninvasive testing, 255
  plethysmography, 255
  preoperative assessment, 256
    Nuss procedure, 257
    surgical technique, 257–258,
        267f, 268f
      bar removal, 260
      bar stabilization and
          fixation, 259
      creation of the transthoracic
          tunnel, 258–259
      "open" pectus excavation
          repair, 262f–266f
      open surgical repair, 261–267
      pectus bar insertion, 259
      postoperative care, 259–260

  pulmonary function testing,
        255–256
  recurrent, 268
  surgical repair, 255, 256–257
  symptoms, 254
  pediatric, 436–437
  patients, 437
  surgeons, 436
Pediatric anesthesia
  anesthetic management, 156
    fluid management, 156–157
    intravenous induction, 155–156
    mask induction, 155
    monitoring, 156
  goals of, 150
  preoperative evaluation, 152
    family history, 153
    laboratory evaluation, 153
    NPO status, 153
    patient history, 152–153
    physical examination, 153
  preoperative preparation
    induction area, parental
        presence, 154
    premedication goals, 154
    sedation, premedications, 154
      intramuscular, 154
      nasal route, 154
      oral, 154
Pediatric cancers
  epidemiology, 1167
    cancer types distribution
      children less than age 15 years,
          1167, 1168t
    major tumor types, 1167
    occurence, 1167
    relative 5-year survival rates,
        trends
      cancer in children less than age
          15 years, 1167, 1168t
      pediatric cancers in children
          less than age 20 years,
          1167, 1168f
    graph shows survival
        statistics, 1261f
    survival statistics, 1167
Pediatric cancer therapy
  long-term sequelae, 1173, 1174
*Pediatric Endosurgery and Innovative
    Techniques,* 11
Pediatric gynecologic disorders, 881
  external anatomy, 880–881, 881f
  hymenal abnormalities, 883–885
    imperforate hymen, 884f
    microperforate, 884f
    prepubertal child, 883f
    septated hymen, 884f
    sign of estrogen
        stimulation, 883f
    unestrogenized, 883f

internal anatomy, 887–898
fallopian tubes, 897
broad ligament cyst, 897
hydrosalpinx/hematosalpinx/
pyosalpinx, 897
paratubal cysts, 897
torsion, 897–898
ovary, 892
ovarian autoamputation, 893
ovarian cyst, 892–893
ovarian neoplasms, 893–897
ovarian torsion, 893
uterus, 891
cervical anomalies, 891–892
rudimentary uterine horn, 891
vagina, 887
complete vaginal agenesis,
889–891
congenital absence of
vagina, 890*f*
distal vaginal agenesis, 888–889
Frank procedure for
neovagina, 889*t*
longitudinal vaginal septum,
887–888
malignancy, 891
transverse vaginal septum, 888
trauma, 887
vaginoscopy, 887*t*
introital masses, 881
Bartholin gland cyst, 882
other introital cysts, 883
prolapsed ureterocele, 881
Skene cyst, 882, 882*f*
urethral prolapse, 881, 881*f*
labial lesions, 886–887
agglutination of vulva, 886*f*
labial adhesions, 886
labial hypertrophy, 886–887
vulvar lesions, 885–886
genital condylomas,
885–886, 885*f*
lipomas, 885
trauma, 886
vascular anomalies, 885
Pediatric inguinal hernias, 489
Pediatric injury scoring, 1031–1033
decision support, 1031, 1032
Glasgow Coma Scale (GCS), 1032
injury measurements, 1031, 1032
injury scales, 1032
Organ Injury Scale (OIS), 1032
epidemiology, 1033
hospital quality improvement
(QI), 1032
observed/expected (O/E)
outcomes, 1032
injured-ness, degree of, 1031
survival, probabilistic estimate, 1031
utilization, 1033

Pediatric intensive care unit (PICU), 89
antimicrobial overview of empiric
therapy for select hospital-
acquired infections in, 97*t*
genetic variability on drug dosing
in, 93
multisystem organ, 89
Pediatric liver masses
differential diagnosis of, 1230*t*
Pediatric Oncology Group (POG), 1198
Pediatric patients, with complicated
peptic ulcer disease, 515
Pediatric surgery
certification, 6
history, 3
chronological table, 12*t*–13*t*
pioneers in, 3–5
pediatric surgical publication, 10
Pediatric trauma centers, 1030
access to care, 1030
pediatric-focused analysis, 1030
adult-only study
mortality comparison, 1030
annual injury-related mortality
pediatric population, 1990 to
2007, 1031*f*
limitations, 1030
National Study on the Costs and
Outcomes of Trauma
(NSCOT) project, 1030
statewide trauma system,
analysis, 1030
*vs.* non trauma center, 1030
Pediatric trauma epidemiology, 1030
injury body region, children
selected trauma centers, United
States, 1032*f*
injury mechanism, children
case-fatality rate, 1032*f*
selected trauma centers, United
States, 1031*f*
pediatric population, 60-minutes
access, 1033*f*
Pediatric wounds, 187
laparoscopy, 187
Pelizaeus–Merzbacher disease, 51
Pelvic inflammatory disease (PID), 618
cervical tenderness, 618
PELVIS syndrome, 885
Penetrating injuries, heart, 1076, 1077
clinical manifestations, 1076
depend upon, 1076
definitive treatment, 1076
sternotomy, 1076
thoracotomy, 1076
digital occlusion and laceration,
closing
nonabsorbable mattress sutures
over Teflon pledgets,
1077, 1078*f*

FAST examination, 1076
hemopericardium detection, 1076
gunshot wounds, 1076
*vs.* stab wounds, 1076
larger penetrating cardiac injuries
Foley catheter inserted into the
heart, 1077, 1078*f*
often related to, 1076
parasternal entrance wound, 1076
cardiac box, 1076, 1078*f*
stab wounds, 1076
Penetrating injuries, lung, 1075
ED thoracotomy, 1075
gunshot wounds, 1075
high-velocity injuries, 1075
pneumo/hemo-thorax
chest x-ray, assessment, 1075
quick surface echocardiogram
(FAST), evaluation
heart, 1075
mediastinum, 1075
hemothorax, 1075
hilum, 1075
rapid control, 1075
Satinsky/Debakey clamps, 1075
massive bleeding
lung/ pulmonary vessels, 1075
nonsimple chest injury, 1075
examples, 1075
operative intervention, 1075
result of, 1075
simple chest injury, 1075
examples, 1075
stab wounds, 1075
asymptomatic, 1075
chest x-ray, 1075
low-velocity injuries, 1075
tracheobronchial tree, 1075
diagnosis, 1075
Pentraxins, 191
Peptic ulcer disease, 515–516
bleeding patients, 515
children with primary ulcer
disease, 516
gastrotomy/duodenotomy, 516
operative interventions, 515
pediatric patients, 515
secondary ulcer disease, 515
treatments, 515
*Peptostreptococcus*, 201
Percutaneous balloon
angioplasty, 941
Percutaneous central venous
access, 142
femoral vein, 142
internal jugular vein, 142–143
subclavian vein, 143–144
umbilical vein, 144–145
Percutaneous endoscopic gastrostomy
(PEG), 517

Perfusion
  impaired, 83
  reduced, 71
Perianal disease, 638–639
  anal fissures, 638
  distal rectum
    endoscopy of, 638
  draining setons, 638f
  fistula-in-ano, 638
  hypertrophy, 638
  persistent fistulae, 638
  rectal mucosal flaps, 638
Peripheral intravenous catheter (PIV),
    137–138
Peripheral ischemia, 86
Peripherally inserted central catheter
    (PICC), 138
Peripheral vein cutdown, 138–139
Peritoneal complications, 1004–1005
  abdominal pain, 1004
  abdominal symptoms, 1004–1005
  CSF protein, 1005
  debris, 1005
  fever, 1004
  infections, 1004
  peritoneal serous membrane, 1005
  pseudocysts, 1005
  scrotum, 1005
  s. epidermidis, 1005
  ventriculoperitoneal shunt
    (VPS), 1004
Peritoneal dialysis (PD), 1296–1298
peritoneal drainage
  algorithm outlining criteria for, 602f
  concept of, 600–601
  extremely low birth weight (ELBW)
    infants, 601
  hemodynamically, 601
  history of, 600–601
  neurodevelopmental impairment
    (NDI), 601
  surgery
    indications for, 600t
  technique, 601–602
    half-inch penrose with, 602f
    penrose, 602
      anterior abdominal wall, 602f
peritoneum, 612
Persistent cloaca, 673, 674
  cloaca, 673, 673f
    definition, 673
    2 hemivaginas, 674, 674f
    hydrocolpos, 673, 674f
    long common channel, 673, 673f
    very high rectum, 673, 674f
  complications, 674
  defects, 674
  definitive reconstruction, 686–691
    cloaca repair, incision, 686, 687f
    cloaca types, 688t

colostomy closing, 690
complete separation, vagina, 688
contrast cloacagram, 686
Foley catheter, 686
functional results, 690, 691
  clinical results, 690
  constipation, type of defects,
    690, 691t
  defect types, 690t
  laxative therapy, 690
  soiling, types of defects,
    690, 690t
  totally continent patients,
    690, 691t
  urinary control, 691
  voluntary bowel movements,
    690, 690t
hemivagina, 688
laparotomy, 688
operation procedure, 686
preoperative cloacagram, 686
total urogenital mobilization,
    686, 688f
  advantage, 687
  mobilized urogenital
    complex, 688
  urethra, 686
  vagina, 686
urogenital sinus, 686, 687
vaginal switch, 688–690, 689f
Persistent Mullerian duct syndrome
    (PMDS), 905
Persistent pulmonary hypertension, 106
Persistent pulmonary hypertension of
    the newborn (PPHN), 106
  causes, 106
  development, 106
Peutz–jeghers syndrome, 1256
  autosomal dominant syndrome, 1256
  benign tumors, 1256
  gastrointestinal polyps, 1256
  hamartomatous polyp
    syndromes, 1256
  malignancy, increased risk, 1256
  malignancy, risk, 1256
  mucocutaneous pigmented
    lesions, 1256
  polyp-related symptoms, reduce, 1256
  potential benefit, metformin, 1256
Pharmacokinetic alterations, during
    various phases of critical
    illness, 93t
Pharmacotherapy, 972–976
  corticosteroids, 972–974
    intralesional corticosteroids,
      973–974
    systemic corticosteroids, 973
      sulfamethoxazole, 973
      synergistic effect, 973
    topical corticosteroids, 974

interferon, 974
propranolol
  beta fibroblast growth factor
    (bFGF), 972
  therapy, 972
  trigger apoptosis, 972
surgical management, 974
  hepatic hemangiomas, 974
    arteriovenous shunting, 974
    hepatic vascular
      embolization, 974
    laser therapy, 974
    surgical excision, 974
      fibrofatty residuum, 974
vincristine, 974
Phenothiazines, 175
Phentolamine, 86
Physical examination, 70, 196
Physiologic, 1037, 1038
  Glasgow coma scale (GCS),
    1037, 1037t
    level of consciousness (LOC)
      measure, 1037
    main advantages, 1037
    modified pediatric, 1037t
    pitfalls, 1037
  pediatric physiologic score, critical
    care, 1038
    nonspecific physiologic injury
      prediction models, 1038
    pediatric risk of mortality
      (PRISM), 1038
  pediatric trauma score (PTS), 1038
    age-specific PTS (AS-PTS), 1038
    logistic regression equation, 1038
  revised trauma score (RTS), 1038
    calculated as, 1038
    code values, 1038, 1038t
    logistic regression function, 1038
    shortcomings, 1038
    trauma score (TS), modification
      of, 1038
Phytobezoars, 515
Pigmented lesions, 1270
Pilonidal disease, 198
  complication, 199
  diagnosis, 198–199
    differential, 199
  etiology, 198
  incision and drainage, 199
Pituitary–ovarian axis, 247
Plain abdominal radiograph
  infant, 664, 665f
Plasma expanders, clinical use, 94–95
Plasminogen activator inhibitor 1
    (PAI-1), 527
Platelet
  ABO compatibility, 179
  aggregation, 175
  antiplatelet agents, 175

autoimmune destruction, 175
congenital causes of dysfunction, 175
dysfunction, 175
function, disorders of, 175
transfusion, 175
Platelet count, 174, 175
Platelet-derived growth factor
 [PDGF], 181
Pleural complications, 1005
 pleural catheter, insertion of, 1005
 pleural effusions, 1005
 pleural shunts, 1005
 pneumothorax, 1005
 Valsalva maneuver, 1005
pleural effusion
 cardiothoracic, mediastinal
  surgery, 443
 clinical presentation, 443
Pleur-Evac drainage system, 441
pleuroperitoneal shunt
 position, 445, 445f
Pneumothorax, 76, 140, 142, 1073
 adult trauma literature, 1073
 blunt traumarelated
  pneumothoraces
  associated hemothorax, 1073
  result from, 1073
 chest tube
  air leak, 1073
  removal, 1073
 imaging, 1073
 prospective studies
  chest tube removal, 1073
 size, expression of, 1073
 small pneumothoraces
  asymptomatic, 1073
 traumatic pneumothorax
  standard treatment, 1073
 tube thoracostomy, 1073
 volume loss calculation, 1073
pneumothorax, 436, 438–441
 diagnosis, 438–439
 etiology, 438
  apical subpleural bleb, 438
  lung disease, 438
  thorax increases, 438
 intercostal catheter, 439
 observation, needle aspiration, 439
 percutaneous technique, 438
 *Pneumocystis carinii*, 438
 presentation, 438–439
 primary spontaneous, 440
 secondary spontaneous, 440
 treatment, 439
POG. *See* Children's Cancer
 Group (POG)
Poland syndrome, 270
 associated defects and syndromes, 274
 clinical presentation, 274–275
 etiology, 274

management, 275
 breast reconstruction, 275
 replacement of aplastic ribs, 275
 surgical intervention, 275
 overview, 273–274
Politano–Leadbetter technique, 823
Polyarteritis nodosa, 953
Polymorphonuclear cells, 182
Polymorphonucleocytes (PMN), 1284
Polyostotic fibrous dysplasia, 246
Polypropylene suture, 931, 933
Polyps, 1250
 GI tract, 1256
 proximal rectum, colon, 1250
 sporadic lesions, 1251
Polysplenia, 314
Polytetrafl uorethylene (PTFE)
 nasogastric stent, 340
Polytetrafluoroethylene (PTFE), 284
Polytetrafluoroethylene (PTFE), graft
 material, 941
Portal hypertension, children
 diagnosis, 727
  clinical examination findings, 727
  doppler examination, 727
  hypercoagulability, 727
  imaging tests, 727
  liver biopsy, 727
  magnetic resonance
   venography, 727
  upper gastrointestinal
   endoscopy, 727
  valuable in, 727
 esophageal varices, endoscopic
  intervention, 728
  endoscopic band ligation
   (EBL), 728
  endoscopic sclerotherapy
   (EST), 728
  esophageal ulceration, 728
  recurrent hemorrhage, 728
  variceal sclerotherapy, 728
 etiology, 725, 726
  collateral circulatory
   pathways, 725
  collateral communications, less
   threatening, 725
  collateral vessels
   favorable, 725
   progressive development, 725
   superficial submucosal, 725
  esophageal varices, 725
  hyperdynamic circulatory state, 725
  pediatric diseases, 726t
  portal hypertension
   associated with, 725
   complications, 725
   definition, 725
  portal pressure, 725
  portal venogram, 725f

evaluation, 727
 hypercoagulability, 727
  evaluation, 727
 historical overview, 724, 725
  devascularization, 725
  distal splenorenal shunt, 725
  Eck, Nikolai
   surgical treatment, principle,
    724, 725
  end-to-side shunt, humans, 725
  esophagogastrectomy, 725
  H-graft, portal-systemic
   circulation bridge, 725
  liver transplantation, evolution, 725
  mesocaval shunt, 725
  portal hypertensive state,
   definiton, 724, 725
  splenectomy, 725
  splenic artery inflow
   reduction, 725
  thoraco-abdominal
   technique, 725
 hyperkinetic (high-flow) portal
  hypertension, 727
 improved survival, patients, 724
 intrahepatic causes of, 726
  chronic liver disease
   etiology, 726
  development basis
   cirrhosis, associated
    complications, 726
   portal hypertension, 726
  hepatic synthetic failure, 726
  related to, in children, 726
 liver transplantation (*See* Liver
  transplantation)
 mechanical tamponade, 728
  balloon catheter tubes, 728
  complications, 728
 nonshunt procedures, 731
 pharmacologic treatment, 728
  beta blocker, 728
   primary prophylaxis,
    treatment, 728
   therapy goal, 728
   variceal hemorrhage, β
    blockade, 728
  octreotide, 728
  vasopressin, 728
   action, 728
 portosystemic shunts (*See*
  Portosystemic shunts)
 posthepatic portal hypertension,
  726, 727
 prehepatic portal
  hypertension, 726
 transjugular intrahepatic
  portosystemic shunt (*See*
  Transjugular intrahepatic
  portosystemic shunt (TIPS))

Portal hypertension, children
  (*continued*)
  treatment, 727, 728
    gastrointestinal hemorrhage, 727
    hepatic synthetic dysfunction, 728
    intrinsic liver disease, 727
      therapeutic choices, 727
    portal hypertensive
      complications, 727
    postulated natural history, 727
    prognosis, 727
      related to, 727
    proton pump inhibitor, 728
Portal venous system, 76
Portosystemic shunts, 728–731
  children to be candidates for, 729
  classification, groups, 729
    direct reconstructions, 729
    nonselective shunts, 729
      advantage, 730
      Clatworthy shunt, mesocaval
        shunt, 730
      constructed to, 730
      disavantages, 731
      H-type mesocaval shunt,
        730, 731f
    selective shunts, 729
      constructed to, 729
      distal splenorenal shunt
        (DSRS), 729, 730f
  complex vascular reconstruction
    portal system, 730
  Doppler ultrasonography, 729
  hepatic vein outlet obstruction
    treatment, 731
  indications for, 729
  magnetic resonance angiography, 729
  mesentericoportal shunt (Rex
    shunt), 729, 729f
    conditons to fullfill, candidates, 729
    construction, 729
    intraoperative photo, 730f
    solution, adequate portal venous
      decompression, 729
  neuropsychiatric disturbances,
    incidences, 729
  nonsurgical shunt
    options, 729
  portal hypertension surgical
    options, 731t
  shunt patency, 730
  vascular reconstruction
    pediatric, 729
Positive end-expiratory pressures
  (PEEP), 75, 78, 87
Postanesthetic care/postoperative
  follow-up
  monitoring, 157
  nausea, 157
  postextubation croup, 157

stridor, 157
vomiting, 157
postcardiac surgery, 443
Posterior laryngeal clefT. *See* Laryngeal
  cleft, posterior
Posterior sagittally using a posterior
  anorectoplasty (PSARP)
  basis of approach, 679
  males, 679–685
    imperforate anus without
      fistula, 685
    rectal atresia, 685
    rectobladderneck fistula,
      laparoscopy/laparotomy,
      684, 685
      colostomy, 684
      distal rectum, 685
      rectal pull-through, 685, 685f
      total-body preparation, 684, 685f
    rectoperineal fistula, minimal
      PSARP for, 679
      areolar tissue, 679
      circumferential dissection, 679
      degree of rectal disscetion, 679
      dilatations, after surgery, 679
      dilations, protocol for, 679, 680t
      Foley catheter, 679
      lacrimal probe, 679
      operative complication, 679
      size dilators according to age,
        679, 679t
    rectourethral fistula, 679–683
      anoplasty, closure of, 682, 684f
      circumferential dissection,
        rectum, 682
      distal colostogram, 680
      exposure of the rectum,
        680, 681f
      foley catheter, 679
      gaining rectal length, tapering
        the rectum, 682, 683f
      incision, closure of, 682, 684f
      levator complex sutures,
        682, 684f
      muscle complex sutures,
        682, 684f
      parasagittal fibers, 679, 680
      placing the rectum, 682, 683f
      posterior sagittal incision,
        679, 680f
      rectobladderneck fistula,
        680, 681f
      rectobulbar fistula, 680, 681f
      rectoprostatic fistula,
        680, 681f
      rectum separation, from
        urinary tract, 682, 682f
  malformations anatomic
    characteristics,
    recognition, 679

Posterior urethral valves, 801–806
  diagnosis, 801–804
    broad-spectrum antibiotics, 804
    fetuses renal functions
      predictive parameters,
        803, 803t
      stratify, 803
    prenatal ultrasound, 803f
    pulmonary hypoplasia, 801
    suspected valve, newborn, 804
      Coude catheter, 804
    symptoms, 803, 804
    vesicoamniotic shunts, 803
    voiding cystourethrogram, 804
      posterior urethral valves,
        804, 804f
      vesicoureteral reflux, 804, 804f
  embryology, 801
    posterior urethral valve
      classification, 801
      type III valves, 801, 803f
      type II valves, 801, 803f
      type I valves, 801, 803f
    valve development theories, 801
  endoscopic valve ablation, operative
    technique, 804, 805
    appropriate prepping, genitalia, 804
    circumcision, medical
      indications, 804
    7.5-French infant
      cystourethroscope, 804
    8.5-French resectoscope, cold
      knife, 804, 805f
    options, 804
      cold knife, 804
      Holmium laser, 804
      hot knife, 804
    urethral meatus, calibration, 804
  presentation, 801–804
  surgical outcome, 805, 806
    azotemia, 805
    feeding tube, initial placement, 806
    postoperative problems, 805
    upper tract imaging
      bladder ultrasonography, 805
      renal ultrasonography, 805
    valve bladder syndrome, 806
    VCUG study, 805
    voiding cystourethrogram,
      805, 806f
posterolateral defect
  Bochdalek hernia
    foramen of, 451f
Posthepatic portal hypertension,
  726, 727
  caused by, 726
  hepatic vein obstruction, 726
    causes, 726, 727
Postoperative nausea and vomiting
  (PONV), 157

postreatment extent of disease (POST-TEXT)
  liver involvement
    after pre-operative chemotherapy, 1237f
Posttransplant lymphoproliferative disorders (PTLD), 1268
  EBV-induced monoclonal, 1268
  primary EBV infection, risk, 1268
  solid organ transplantation (SOT), 1268
  transmural necrosis, 1268
Potassium disorders, 57–58
Preauricular anomalies, 228
Preauricular sinuses, 228, 228f
  clinical aspects, 228
  embryology, 225–228
  incidence, 228
  operative technique used to excise, 228f
  preauricular skin tags, 229
  treatment, 228–229
Preauricular skin tags, 229f
Precocious puberty, 246
Prednisone, 1287
Prehepatic portal hypertension, 726
  embryological malformations, 726
  extrahepatic portal vein obstruction (EPVO), 726
    children with, 726
  inherited abnormalities, 726
Pre-made silastic silo
  wire-ring covered base, 474f
Preoperative portal venous embolization, 1242
  alcohol thrombosis, 1242
  cannulated percutaneously, 1242
  hypertrophy, 1242
  polyvinyl alcohol, 1242
Pre-treatment extent of disease (PRETEXT)
  cross-sectional imaging assessment, 1236
  liver, 4 main sections, 1236
  tumor involvement of 4 liver sections, 1236f
Pretreatment re-excision (PRE), 1215
  trunk lesions, 1215
Prilocaine cream (EMLA cream), 208
Primary brain injury, 1057–1060
  cerebral contusions, 1057
    blossom, 1057
    cause of, 1057
    intracerebral hematomas, 1057
    intracranial pressure (ICP) elevated, 1057
    intraparenchymal hematomas, 1057
    loacted in, 1057
    occur at, 1057
    penetrating trauma, setting, 1057

represents, 1057
risk management
  mild to moderate-sized contusions, 1057
diffuse axonal injury (DAI), 1059, 1060
  cerebral anoxic insult, 1060
  clinical management patient, 1060
  extensive shear injury, neurons, 1059
  external ventricular drain (EVD), 1060
  initial CT scan findings, 1060
  MRI, 1060
    T2 and FLAIR imaging, 1060, 1060f
  neurologic exams, 1059
  pathophysiologic mechanism, proposed, 1059
  result of, 1059
  traumatic subarachnoid hemorrhage, 1060
diffuse primary injury, 1057
epidural hematomas (EDH), 1057, 1058
  acute
    characteristics, 1057
    clot, mass effect, 1057
  asymptomatic children, 1057
  classic formation mechanism, 1057
  craniotomy, 1058
  CT scan, 1058f
  generous craniotomy, 1058
  injury mechanism, severity, 1057
  lucid interval, 1057
  meticulous hemostasis, 1058
  occurence, 1057
  postoperative CT scan, 1058
  question mark incision, over hematoma, 1058
focal primary injuries, 1057
refers to, 1057
subdural hematomas (SDH), 1058, 1059
  acute, 1058
  asymptomatic patients, 1059
  characteristic CT appearance, 1058
  CT scan, 1059f
  malignant cerebral edema, 1059
  meticulous hemostasis, 1059
  mortality rate, 1059
  neurocognitive deficits, 1059
  open craniotomy, 1059
  operative procedure, 1059
  optimal treatment strategies, 1059
  parenchymal ICP monitor, 1059
  pathophysiology, 1058
  postoperative management, 1059
  post-traumatic seizures, 1059

specific mechanism, injury, 1058
  subdural hemorrhage, 1058
    bridging veins, 1058
    tearing of cortical, 1058
    vs. epidural hematomas, 1058
Primary liver tumors
  age presentation, childhood, 1230t
Primary lung tumors, 412
Primary palmar hyperhidrosis (PHH), 434
Primary pediatric malignant tumors, 1228
  rhabdoid tumors, 1228
  sarcomas, 1228
primary pulmonary hypoplasia, 448
Prolactin, 67
Prolapsed ureteroceles, 881
Propionibacterium acnes, 1004
Propofol
  contraindication, 103
  formulation, 103
  metabolism, 103
Prostaglandin, 182, 938, 939
Protamine, 175
Proteases, 44, 190
  breast milk, 45
Protein
  administration, 62
  degradation, 61
  metabolism, 61–62
  requirements in healthy humans, 61t
Protein accretion, 130
Protein binding sensitivity, 91
Protein C, 177
Protein digestion, 45
Protein S, 177
Prothrombin time (PT), 176
Proximal ganglionated bowel
  residual muscular sleeve, 580f
proximal stoma, 604f, 607
Pseudoaneurysm, 941
pseudocysts, 666, 667
Pseudomonas aeruginosa, 44, 194
Pseudo precocious puberty, 246
Pseudorheumatoid nodule, 214
Pubic diastasis, 832
Pull-through procedures
  treatment options, 574–575
Pulmonary arterial catheter
  placement, 85
Pulmonary arterial catheters, 77
  placements, 77
  placements, complications, 77–78, 78f
  valvular damage, 78
Pulmonary artery, 78, 929, 943
  catheter placement, 77f
    complications of, 78t
  measurement of pressure, 78
  occlusion pressure (PAOP), 78
  rupture, 77

Pulmonary artery occlusion pressure (PAOP), 78
Pulmonary artery sling, 947
  anatomy, 947
  bronchoscopic examination, 948
  contrast CT angiogram/MRI, 949f
  diagnosis, 948
  embryology, 947
  infants with LPA sling, evaluation, 948
  left, relationship to trachea, 948f
  surgical management, 949
    and outcomes, 949
    reimplantation, 949, 950f
    restenosis/late hypoplasia, 949
    survival rate, 949
Pulmonary blood flow, 50
Pulmonary capillary wedge pressure assessment, 75
Pulmonary edema, 86
Pulmonary embolism (PE), 96
Pulmonary hypertension, 412
Pulmonary hypoplasia, 105
  fixed explanted specimen bilateral nature of, 463f
  outcome limiting, 463f
  autopsy, 463f
Pulmonary lymphangiectasia, 76
pulmonary parenchymal cell populations, 448
  type II pneumocytes, 448
Pulmonary parenchymal disease, 945
Pulseless electrical activity (PEA), 88
Pulse oximeters, 71
  assessment of hemoglobin saturation, 71f
Pulse oximetry, 157
Pyloric atresia, 511–512
  anatomic variants, 512f
  coexistence of epidermolysis bullosa, 511
  etiology, 511
  technical correction, 512
Pyloric atresia (PA), 510
Pyloric stenosis, 534
  diagnosis, 534
    critical pathway for, 536
  pathogenesis, 534
    theories, 534
  treatment effectiveness/patient outcome, 539
  treatment options, 535
    circumbilical approach, 535, 538
    circumbilical/transumbilical laparoscopic incision, 535
    laparoscopic approach, 538–539
    muscle-sparing (Rickham) incision, 535
    muscle-splitting (Robertson "gridiron"), 535

operative techniques for open pyloromyotomy, 537f–538f
  Ramstedt extramucosal longitudinal pyloromyotomy, 535
Pyogenic granuloma, 214
Pyomyositis, 202
Pyridoxine, 66
Pyruvate oxidation, 65

R
Radial arterY, 73
  cut-down technique, insertion of a catheter, 74f
  percutaneous insertion of catheter, 73f
Radial artery, 73, 148
  catheterization of, 148
Radiation therapy, 1172, 1173, 1216
  compliance, 1216
  Group II (microscopic residual), 1216
  Group III (gross residual) disease, 1216
  pediatric cancers, goal in, 1172
  principles, dosing, and administration, 1172, 1173
    absorbed dose, unit Gray (Gy), 1172
    apoptosis, 1172
    aspects, 1173
    dosing, design, 1172
    early-responding tissues, 1172
    fractionation, radiation dose, 1172
    impaired DNA repair mechanism, tumor cells, 1172
    mode of action, 1172
    total dose, radiation, 1172
    toxic dose, 1172
Radiographic features, 1230
  arteriovenous shunt, 1230
  central necrosis, thrombosis, 1230
  central varix, 1230
  diffuse hemangiomatous, 1230
Radiographs, 436, 439, 593. See also Chest radiographs
  chest, parapneumonic effusion suggesting empyema, 426f
  chest radiograph demonstrating, 329f
  chest radiograph in a baby with EA and vertebral anomalies, 343f–344f
  child with chondromanubrial pectus carinatum deformity, 272f
  child with Jeune syndrome, 276f
  collapse, lung, 439
  left lateral decubitus, 593
  monitor resolution, 439
  nonopaque esophageal foreign body, 330f

skull depicting a cranial bone defect beneath a scalp soft-tissue nodule, 230f
  supine frontal, 593
Radiologic reduction technique of, 594
Radiotherapy, 1225
  non-steroidal anti-infl ammatory drugs (NSAID), 1225
  suilindac combination, 1225
  systemic therapies, 1225
  tamoxifen, 1225
Randomized clinical trials (RCTs), 20, 23
  fetoscopic laser separation vs. amnioreduction of monochorionic (MC) twins, 23
  in multi-institutional settings, 20
RCT. See Randomized clinical trials (RCTs)
Rectal atresia/stenosis, 672, 672f
  diagnosis, 672
  presenting sigs, 672
Rectal biopsy
  dorsal lithotomy suspension position, 572f
  indications, 571
  operative technique, 571–572
  preoperative preparation, 571
  single layer anastomosis, 577f
  traction sutures, 573f
Rectal canal
  mucosal tube, 580f
Rectal cuff, 585, 587f
Rectal defect, 572
Rectal dissection, 586f
Rectal duplications, 662, 663
  diagnosis essentials, 662
  presenting signs, 662
  symptoms, 662
    diagnosis, 662
    lesions, 662
      representation factors, 662
    sagittal view, posterior rectal duplication cyst, 662f
  treatment, 662, 663
    marsupialization, 663
    midline posterior sagittal, retrorectal cystic duplication, 662, 662f
    transanal resection, 662, 663f
Rectal neobladder, 862
  augmented and valved rectum, 864f
Rectal prolapse, 831
Rectal trauma, 1097
Rectal wall, dissection, 581f
Rectobladderneck fistula, 671, 672f
  presenting signs, 671

Rectoperineal fistula
  female, 672, 672f
  male, 670, 671f
    presenting signs, 670
Rectourethral fistula, 670, 671
  bulbar, 670, 671f
  defects, 671
  prostatic, 670, 671, 671f
  treatment, 671
Rectovestibular fistula
  definitive reconstruction, 685, 686
    cloaca repair, incision, 686, 687f
    levator mechanism, 686
    rectum separation from vagina,
      686, 687f
    sutures placed, fistula site,
      686, 686f
  refractory hypoxia, 452
    pulmonary hypertension
      (PPHN), 452
Remifentanil, 101
removed, silo
  newborn, 475
Renal anomalies, 831
Renal blood flow, 84
Renal elimination of drug, 93
Renal embryology, 54
Renal failure, 93, 102, 930
Renal function, 54–55, 857
  glomerular filtration rate
    (GFR), 54–55
Renal insufficiency, 70, 930
Renal replacement therapy, 94
Renal replacement therapy (RRT), 1293
  choice, depend on factors, 1294
  hemodialysis, 1293, 1294
    central venous catheters,
      1294–1295
    complications associated
      with, 1295
Renal transplantation, 1298
  contraindications, 1298
  evaluation, 1298–1299
  indications, 1298
  native nephrectomy
    indications and approach, 1299
  patient outcomes, 1304
    following renal transplantation,
      1304–1305
    cause of eventual graft
      failure, 1305
    NAPRTCS data, mortality
      rate, 1305
    noncompliance, 1305
    UNOS data analysis, 1304f
  undergoing dialysis, 1304
  postoperative complications, 1303
    delayed graft function, 1303
    graft rejection, 1303–1304
    graft thrombosis, 1303

hemorrhage, 1303
urologic complications, 1303
postoperative management, 1302
  immunosuppression, 1302–1303
pretransplant urologic
  considerations, 1299
surgical technique, 1300
  end-to-side vascular anastomosis,
    1300f, 1301f
  extra-peritoneal iliac fossa
    approach, 1300–1301
  intra-abdominal, trans-peritoneal
    approach, 1301
  and intraoperative
    management, 1300
  ureteral implantation, 1301–1302
    Lich extra-vesicle
      technique, 1302f
Renin-angiotensin system, 939
Renin–angiotensin system, 50
Renovascular hypertension, 958
  diagnosis, 959–960
  optimal outcomes in children, 962
  percutaneous transluminal renal
    angioplasty (PTRA), 960, 960f
    complications, 960–961
  primary nephrectomy, 962
  surgical revascularization, 961
    complications, 961–962
    direct aortic reimplantation of left
      renal artery, 961f
    ostial renal artery lesions,
      resection of stenosis, 961f
  surveillance, 962
  symptoms, 958–959
  treatment, 960
Residency Review Committees
  (RRCs), 9
Resistin, 527
Respiratory distress, 317, 411
Respiratory distress syndrome
  (RDS), 47, 104
  diagnosis, 106
  long-term effects of severe
    cases, 106
  lungs, characterized by, 106
  mortality, 106
  pathology, 106
  reduction, 106
  risk of development, 106
  surfactant administration, 106
Respiratory failure, 104
  acute, 104
  interventions, improving survival
    rates, 104
  medical therapy, 107
    continuous positive airway
      pressure, 107–108
    nonpharmacologic respiratory
      care, 107

in neonatal and pediatric
  population, 104
pathophysiology, 104
persistent pulmonary
  hypertension, 106
pharmacologic therapy, 108
  bronchodilators, 109
  caffeine, 111
  corticosteroids, 109
  diuretics, 111
  nitric oxide, 109–110
  oxygen therapy, 108–109
  prostanoids, 111
  pulmonary vasodilators, 109
  sildenafil, 110
  surfactant, 111
of prematurity, 105–106
pulmonary development, 105t
pulmonary hypoplasia, 105
Respiratory insufficiency, 72
Respiratory muscle activity
  anesthesia, effects of, 152
Respiratory symptoms, 330
Respiratory syncytial virus (RSV), 412
Respiratory system
  apnea of prematurity, 47
  bronchopulmonary dysplasia
    (BPD), 47, 48
  changes at birth, 46–47
  embryology of, 46
  respiratory distress syndrome
    (RDS), 47
Resuscitation, 76, 85
  burned child, 1118
    absolute and relative
      indications for endotracheal
      intubation, 1119t
    algorithm for airway
      management, 1119f
    Parkland formula for burn
      injury, 1120t
    "rules of nine" to estimate burn
      size, 1120f
    sites used for escharotomy, 1120f
  cardiopulmonary, acute, 83
  IV fluid, 94
Reticular endothelial system
  (RES), 1284
retinoic acid pathway, 448
Retrorectal pull-through, 576f
  distal rectum, traction sutures, 576f
Reverse Bishop-Koop, 566f
Rhabdoid tumor, 1246
Rhabdomyosarcoma, 1211–1219
  asymptomatic mass, 1212
  classification of, 1212
  clinical group, 1213
    RMS patient, 1213t
  diagnosis of, 1212
  evaluation, 1212–1213

Rhabdomyosarcoma (*continued*)
  bone marrow aspirate, 1212
  bone scan, 1212
  complete blood counts
      (CBC), 1212
  distant lymph nodes, 1212
  electrolytes, 1212
  liver function tests (LFTs), 1212
  urinalysis (UA), 1212
  familial syndromes, 1212
  histologic subtypes, 1211
    alveolar (ARMS), 1211
    embryonal (ERMS), 1211
  Improvement in survival, 1212f
  malignant tumor, 1211
  Pathogenic roles, 1212
    MET proto-oncogene, 1212
  presentation, 1212
    extremities, 1212
    genitourinary tract, 1212
  pretreatment clinical
      staging, 1213
    TNM classification system, 1213
  prognosis, 1218–1219
  p53 tumor suppressor gene,
      inactivation, 1212
  RAS oncogene,
      hyperactivation, 1212
  risk stratification, 1214
    risk group, categorization of
        patients, 1214t
  RMS patient demographics, 1211
  RMS tumor biology, 1211–1212
    primitive neuroectodermal
        tumors (PNET), 1211
  skeletal muscle, 1212
  specific anatomic sites, 1216–1219
    biliary tract, 1217
    extremity, 1217–1218
    genitourinary
        bladder, prostate, 1218
        vulva, vagina, uterus, 1218
    metastatic disease, 1218
    parameningeal, 1216
    paraspinal, 1217
    paratesticular, 1218
    perineum, perianal, 1217
    retroperitoneum/pelvis, 1217
    superficial
        nonparameningeal, 1216
    trunk, abdominal wall, chest wall,
        1216–1217
  surgical approach, 1215
  surgical resection, 1214f
  treatment, 1214–1216
    assessment of response, 1216
    biopsy
        radiographic positive lymph
            nodes, 1214
    chemotherapy, 1215–1216

    lymph node sampling/
        dissection, 1215
      failure free survival (FFS), 1215
      ipsilateral supraclavicular
          (scalene) nodes, 1215
      overall survival (OS), 1215
      sentinel node mapping, 1215
    mass, resection, 1214–1215
    radiation therapy, 1216
    recurrence, second-look
        operations resection, 1215
      disease, resection, 1215
Rhabdomyosarcomas, 236
Rh-alloimmunization, 179
Rib fractures, 1070, 1071
  commonly fractured ribs, 1070
  first and second ribs, fracture, 1070
    high-impact mechanism
        of injury, 1070
  intentional injuries, 1070
  managing children
      important principle, 1071
  motor vehicle-related injuries, 1070
  ninth through 12th ribs, fracture
      concerns, 1070
  nonaccidental trauma
      prompting, 1070
Riboflavin, 66
right paramedian opening
  extended, vertical incisions, 475
Rigid endoscopy
  technique for insertion into
      esophagus, 335f
Rigid Storz bronchoscopes, 294t
  utility and limitations, 299–300
RNA polymerases, 66
Robotic surgery, 395
Robotic surgical systems, 937
*Rochalimaea henselae*, 239
role of prenatal therapy, 456
  fetoscopic tracheal occlusion
      (FETO), 456
Roux-en-Y gastric bypass
    (RYGB), 528
Roux limb, 529
Rubinstein–Taybi syndrome, 51
rudimentary rectus abdominis muscles
    approach, 483
RyR1 channels, 151

S
*Saccharomyces boulardii*, 195
SACRAL syndrome, 885
Sacrococcygeal teratoma, 27
  coronal section on MRI of fetus
      with, 29f
  debulking procedure, 38
    debulking of fetal SCT, 38
    outcomes, 39
    rationale, 38

    specific postoperative
        considerations, 38–39
  fetal, algorithm for management, 29f
Salivary gland lesions, 217
Saphenofemoral vein, 142, 142f
Sarcomas, 394
  extremity soft tissue sarcoma
      operative resection
        incisions, orientation, 1224f
Scapula, 1072
  aortic disruption, uncommon
      injury, 1072
  associated injuries, 1072
  common sites of fracture, 1072
Scarring, 188
  burn, 188
  hypertrophic scars, 188
  keloids, 188
Schwann cells, 51
Schwartz-Jampel syndrome, 151
Sciatic nerve block, 168
Scopolamine, anticholinergic
    medication, 170
Scrotal swelling, acute, 769, 771, 1050
  diagnostic principles, 771
    blue dot sign, appendages
        torsion, 771
    etiology, determination, 771
    incarcerated inguinal hernia, 771
    physical exam, 771
    radioisotope scrotal scanning, 771
        disadvantages, 771
    symptoms, 771
    testicular ischemia, 771
    torsion–detorsion episodes, 771
    ultrasonography, 771
  disease pathophysiology, 769–771
    bell-clapper anomaly, 770, 770f
    conditions responsible for, 769
    cremasteric muscles,
        contraction, 770
    epididymal inflammation,
        770, 771
    epididymitis, 770
    hydroceles, 771
    idiopathic scrotal edema, 771
    incarcerated hernias, 771
    infection
        bacterial, 770
        viral, 770
    peak incidence, 770
    systemic viral syndromes, 770
    testicular appendages, 770
    testicular/spermatic cord
        torsion, 769
    testicular torsion, 769
        extravaginal, 770, 770f
        intravaginal, 770, 770f
    testicular trauma, 771
        results, 771

patient outcome, 773, 774
    clinical studies, 774
        results, 774
    experimental studies
        results, 774
    nonexploration policy, 774
    spermatogenesis, abnormality, 774
    testicular atrophy, 773, 774
    testicular salvage rates, 773
treatment options, 771–773
    contralateral testis, fixation, 773
    detorsion direction, 772
    manual detorsion, 772
    nonsurgical treatment
        testicular appendages
            torsion, 771
    nontorsion causes, treatment, 771
    perinatal testicular torsion, 772
        treatment, 773f
    scrotal exploration, 772
    secondary testicular torsion, 772
    surgical procedure, 772f
    testicular teratoma, 773
Secretin, 359
Sedation, 100, 208
    assessment tools, 100
        COMFORT score, 100
        FLACC score, 100
        Oucher, 100
        State Behavioral Score (SBS), 100
    Bispectral Index (BIS), 100
    drawback to scoring systems, 100
Seldinger technique, 142
Sensor technologies, 80
Sentinel lymph node biopsy, 1224–1225
    extremity RMS, 1224
    flank lesions, 1224
    lymphatic mapping, 1224
    lymphazurin blue (LZB), 1224
        diphenhydramine, 1225
    lymph node, 1225
    melanoma, 1224
    nodal basin, location, 1224
    Operative technique of, 1226f
    radioactive counts, 1225
    sentinel lymph node excision, 1225
Sepsis, 75, 85, 174, 330, 644, 930
    management with antibiotic
        therapy, 76
    related to arterial catheters, 75
Septic shock, 76, 83
    diagnosis and treatment, 84f
septum transversum, 448
seromuscular nonabsorbable purse-
        string suture
    ligated appendiceal stump., 626f
Serotonin, 103
Sertoli cells, 904
Serum glucose concentrations, 132
Sevoflurane, anesthetics, 155

Sexual determination, 902
    normal process, 902
        molecular biology, 902–904
    pathophysiology, 904
        female DSD, 904
        gonadal ambiguities
            resulting from chromosomal
                abnormalities, 906
        male DSD, 904–905
Sexual differentiation, 899
    female differentiation, 904
    genes involved in, 902t–903t
    historical perspectives, 899–900
        Romans view, 900
    internal/external, 904
    male sex differentiation, 903
    perspectives on disorders, 899–902
SF-1 (steroidogenic factor one)
        gene, 903
Shone complex, 941
short bowel syndrome, 472, 481
Short bowel syndrome (SBS),
        643, 644
    careful placement of
        distal mucous fistulas, 644
        intestinal stomas, 644
    causes of, 643, 644f
    enteral nutrition, 644
    ischemia, 643
    necrotizing enterocolitis (NEC), 643
        clip-anddrop approach, 643
    potential complications
        avoidance, 644
Short gut syndrome, 132
short rectal stump
    EEA stapler inserted through, 640f
Sickle cell anemia, 173
Sickle cell disease, 174
    elective surgical procedures, 174
    SCD-related complications, 174
Sickle-cell disease (SCD), 700
    acute chest syndrome, 700
    laparoscopic approach, 700
    postoperative complication rate, 700
    preoperatively transfusion, 700
Sigma rectum, 862
sigmoid fistula
    Ileal CD, 638f
Silastic® intraluminal shunt, 941
silo
    amnion left intact, inverted, 480f
    membrane sheets, 479f
    neuromuscular blockade, 479f
    silastic, 478
    skin closure
        removal, fascial, 479f
Silvadene
    for extremities burn, 214
sinuses, 485
Sinus tachycardia, 85

Skin
    skin grafts
        obtain partial-thickness graft,
            1126f
    and soft tissue infections (SSTI), 210
small-bowel disease, 637
    duodenum
        fibrostenotic disease of, 637
    flexible sigmoidoscopy, 637
Small-bowel duplications, 658, 659
    complications, 659
    diagnosis, 659
        CT scan, 659
        Meckel scan, 659
        preoperative diagnosis, 659
        ultrasound, 659
            prenatal, 659
    diagnosis essentials, 658
    ectopic gastric mucosa
        frequency, 658f
    presenting signs, 658
    symptoms, 658
        cystic duplications, 658
            ileal duplication, 658f
        malignant degeneration, 658
        tubular duplications, 658, 658f
    treatment, 659
        end-to-end anastomosis, 659
        enucleation, 659, 659f
        long tubular duplications,
            659, 660f
            gastroduplication, 659, 660f
        operative resection, 659
        Wrenn method, 659
Small bowel malignancies, 1257–1258
    presentation, nonspecific
        symptoms, 1258
Small-for-gestational-age (SGA), 130
Small intestinal tumors, 1257–1259
    diagnosis, 1258
        double balloon enteroscopy, 1258
        inflammatory Bowel Disease, 1257
        small bowel malignancies,
            diagnosis, 1257
Soave–Boley anastomosis, 591f
Soave pull-through. See Endorectal
        pull-through
Sodium disorders, 57, 58f
Sodium nitroprusside, 86
Soft tissue infections, 210
Soft tissue sarcoma, 1221, 1223–1224
    adipose tissue, 1224
    core biopsy, 1223
    suction drains, 1224
    surgical resection, 1223, 1227
    vascular reconstruction, 1224
    verified, 1223
    vessel loop, 1224
Soft tissue tumors, 1223–1224
    operative resection, 1223

Sonic hedgehog [Shh] expression, 342
SOX gene family, 903
Specific cystic lesions, 665–668
  adrenal cysts, 667
    associated conditions, 667
    diagnosis, 667
    etroperitoneum, cystic lesion, 667
    symptoms, 667
    treatment, 667
    Waterhouse–Friedericksen
        syndrome, 667
  hepatic cysts, 667
    diagnosis, 667
      computed tomography (CT)
          scan, 667
      ultrasound guidance, 667
    future risk, 667
    presenting signs, 667
    symptoms, 667
    treatment, 667
      drainage, 667
      marsupialization, 667
  hydrocolpos, 668
    disgnosis, 668
    presenting signs, 668
    treatment, 668
  lymphatic malformations, 666
    complications, 666
    external impression, bulging flanks
        intra-abdominal mass, 666f
    large mesenteric lymphatic
        malformation, 666f
    symptoms, 666
    treatment, 666
      immunotherapy (OK-432), 666
  meconium cysts, 668
    diagnosis, 668
    presenting signs, 668
    symptoms, 668
    treatmenta, 668
  mesenteric cysts, 665, 666, 666f
    diagnosis, 665, 666
    presenting signs, 665
    symptoms, 665
    treatment, 666
  omental cysts, 666
    associated conditions, 666
    symptoms, 666
    treatment, 666
      laparoscopic resection, 666
      marsupialization, 666
  pancreatic cysts, 667
    associated conditions, 667
    diagnosis, 667
    symptoms, 667
    treatment, 667
  splenic cysts, 667, 667f
    diagnosis, 667
    presenting signs, 667
    symptoms, 667

  treatment, 667
    laproscopy, 667
    ligation, main splenic artery, 667
    percutaneous drainage, 667
  urachal cysts, 668
    diagnosis, 668
    presenting signs, 668
    symptoms, 668
    treatment, 668
  ventriculoperitoneal shunt
      pseudocysts, 666, 667
    associated conditions, 666
    diagnosis, 666
      imaging studies, 666
    symptoms, 666
    treatment, 666, 667
      methods, 666, 667
Specific pediatric cancer
  adjuvant therapy, 1174–1176
  hepatoblastoma, 1175
    chemotherapeutic regimens, 1175
    complete surgical excision
        primary tumor, 1175
    liver tumors, children, 1175
  neuroblastoma, 1174 (See
      Neuroblastoma)
    children's oncology group (COG)
        risk-assessment scheme, 1174t
    high-risk, 1174
    intermediate-risk, 1174
  pediatric malignancies, other, 1176
    adjuvant chemotherapy, 1176
      consists of, 1176
    Ewing sarcoma, 1176
      occult micrometastatic
          disease, 1176
      radiotherapy, 1176
    osteosarcoma, 1176
      treatment, 1176
  rhabdomyosarcoma, 1175
    common sites, 1175
    prognosis of, 1175
      factors associated with, 1175
    recurrent, 1175
    survival rate, 1175
      high-risk patients, 1175
      intermediate-risk patients, 1175
      lowest-risk patients, 1175
    treatment protocols, 1175
      childhood
          rhabdomyosarcoma, 1175
  Wilms tumor, 1174 (See Wilms
      tumor)
    current adjuvant treatment
        guidelines, 1174, 1175t
    nephroblastoma, 1174
    surgical procedures, 1174
sphincter mechanism, 483
Sphygmomanometry, 71
Spinal block, 164

Spinal cord. See also Craniospinal
    malformations
  dermoid tumors, 1014–1015
  dorsal aspect, 1014
  lipoma, 1013–1014
  scarified area of skin, 1015f
  sensorimotor deficits, 1014
    urologic changes, 1014
  symptoms, 1018
  symptoms, signs, 1013
  tethering, 1014
Spinal deformities, 347
Spinal developmental malformations
  embryogenetic Classification, 1011t
Spinal dysraphism, 850
Spinal lipomas (lipomyelomeningocele),
    1013–1014
  child with, 1014f
  closed congenital spinal cord
      malformations, 1013
  hyperintense lesions, 1014
  prophylactically, 1014
  T1-weighted images, 1014
Spleen
  abscess, 745
    causing organisms, 745
    morbidity, 745
    presenting
        signs, 745
        symptoms, 745
    treatment, 748
      high-dose antibiotics, 748
      image-guided drainage, 748
  anatomy, 741, 742
    ligamentous attachments, 741
    located in, 741
    odd number, mnemonic of
        Harris, 741
  benign tumors, 745
    treatment, 748
      partial/total splenectomy, 748
  cysts, 745
    acquired, 745
    congenital, 745
    parasitic cysts, caused by, 745
      Echinococcus, 745
    treatment, 748
      echinococcal disease, 748
      laparoscopic unroofing, 748
      multiple treatments, 748
      partial/total splenectomy, 748
      recurrent epidermoid cyst,
          748, 748f
  disorders, 742–744, 745, 746f, 747f
    accessory spleen, 742, 743, 745
      occurrence, 742
      rare locations of, 742
      result of, 742
      thrombocytopenia purpura
          (ITP), 743

agenesis and asplenia, 742
  absence of spleen, 742
  classifications, 742
  complications, 742
  Polhemus–Schafer–Ivemark
    syndrome, 742
  congenital and acquired
    disorders, 742t, 743t
  polysplenia, 743
    associated with, 743
    preduodenal portal vein, 743
  splenogonadal fusion, 743, 744
    clinical presentation, 743
    linked to, 743
    varieties, 743
  wandering spleen, 744, 745–747
    asymptomatic, 744
    complications, 744
    diagnosis, 744
    operative approach, 745
    risk for, 745
    vagabond spleen, 744
embryology, 741, 742
  incomplete fusion
    accessory spleen formation, 741
function, 741, 742
  blood cells (RBC), 741
  functional segments, 741, 742t
  Howell–Jolly bodies, 741
  immunoresponsive functions, 741
  phagocytic function, 741
  red pulp, 741
    function, 741
  source of IgM, 741
  ultrastructure
    key to its function, 741
  white pulp, 741
    function, 741
hemoglobinopathies, 744
  sickle cell disease, 744
    multiple sequential infarcts, 744
    occurs primarily in, 744
  thalassemia, 744
    caused by, 744
    major heterozygote, 744
    minor heterozygote, 744
    RBC destruction, 744
  treatment, 747
    major indications, sickle cell
      disease, 747
    preemptive vaccination, 747
    splenectomy, 747
    symptomatic treatment, 747
hereditary hemolytic disorders, 744
  autosomally inherited
    conditions, 744
  erythrocytes, increased
    destruction of, 744
  hereditary hemolytic anemias, 744
  result in, 744

surgery
  decision to perform, 744
hypersplenism and splenomegaly,
    treatment of, 748
  laparoscopic splenectomy, 748
  portal hypertension, 748
  splenomegaly
    compressive symptoms, 748
malignancies, 745
  Hodgkin lymphoma, 745
  primary splenic malignancies, 745
  splenic involvement
    systemic symptoms, 745
  treatment, 747
    chemotherapy, 747
    splenectomy, 747
membrane defects, 744
  hereditary hemolytic
    elliptocytosis, 744
    basic pathogenesis, 744
    Mendelian-dominant trait, 744
    splenectomy, 747
    treatment, 747
  hereditary hemolytic
    spherocytosis (HHS), 744
    definition, 744
    laparoscopic splenectomy, 747
    spherocyte's lifespan, 744
    spherocytic RBC, 744
    splenectomy, 747
    surgery timing, depends
      on, 747
    symptoms, 744
    treatment, 747
minimal access splenic surgery,
    750, 751
  laparoscopic splenic surgery, 750
    portal placement options, 751f
  single-site laparoscopic
    splenectomy, 751f
open total splenectomy, 749, 750
  celiotomy, 749
    elective splenectomy, 749, 749f
  incision
    splenorenal ligament,
      abdominal wall, 749, 749f
    preemptive epidural analgesia, 749
    splenic artery and vein, branches
      individual ligation, 750, 750f
    splenorenal, mobilization, 749
partial splenectomy, 750
  transverse incision, 750, 750f
  vertical mattress sutures
    hemostasis, 750, 750f
splenectomy, potential
    complications, 748, 749
  chronic thromboembolic
    pulmonary hypertension, 749
  adverse vascular events, 749
  morbidity, 748, 749

postsplenectomy infection, 749
  appropriate vaccination
    therapy, 749
  associated organisms, 749
  mortality rate, 749
  overwhelming
    postsplenectomy infection
      (OPSI), 749
  septic death rates, 749
splenic trauma, 750
  damage control trauma
    laparotomy
    principles, 750
  inspection, spleen, 750
  midline celiotomy, 750
  splenectomy/splenorrhaphy, 750
trauma, 745
  blunt force trauma, 745
  commonly injured intraperitoneal
    organ, 745
  focused abdominal ultrasound for
    trauma (FAST) exam, 745
  initial laboratory testing, 745
    hematuria, 745
  injury mechanism, 745
    includes, 745
  presentation, 745
  treatment, 748
    absolute indication,
      operation, 748
    coexisting injuries, 748
    CT imaging, 748
    hemodynamic stability, 748
    isolated splenic injury,
      guidelines, 748t
Splenectomy, 174, 175
Splenic injuries, 1084–1087,
    1084f–1088f
Split cord malformations, 1017–1019
  accessory neurenteric canal,
    formation, 1018
  axial metrizamide myelogram, type
    I, 1017f
  Axial T1-weighted MRI scan,
    type II, 1017f
  cutaneous stigmata, 1018
  dorsal enteric cyst, 1017
  double dural sac malformations, 1017
  endodermal–ectodermal
    adhesion, 1018
  posterior mediastinal cysts, 1017
  prophylactic repair, 1019
  radiographic evaluation, 1019
  single dural sac malformations, 1017
  split notochord syndrome, 1018
Spondylocostal dysplasia, 276
Spondylothoracic dysplasia, 275
Spontaneous pneumomediastinum, 1080
spontaneous pneumothorax
  treatment algorithm, 440f

INDEX

Squamous carcinoma, 831
Squiggle maneuver, 144
SRMD. *See* Stress-related mucosal damage (SRMD)
standard curets, 437
*Staphylococcus aureus, 202,* 426, 1004
*Staphylococcus epidermidis,* 145
*Staphylococcus epidermis,* 1004
Sterile probe, 145
Sternal clefts, 277
    embryology, 277
    pathophysiology, 278–279
    surgical treatment, 282
        repair in newborn age group, 284*f*
        sabiston technique for repair, 283*f*
Sternocleidomastoid muscle, 218
Sternocleidomastoid muscle (SCM), 76
Sternum, 254, 1071
    associated injuries, 1071
    chest x-ray, diagnosis, 1071
    common mechanism of injury, 1071
    electrocardiogram (EKG), 1071
    fractures, 1071
    operative stabilization, 1071
stoma
    single proximal, 606
Stomach, 510
    obstructive lesions, 510
    tumors of, 514
        inflammatory myofibroblastic tumor, 514
        teratomas, 514
Stomach injury, 1090, 1090*f*
stomas, 609–612
    antegrade colonic enemas (ACE procedure)
        children, 610
    bony prominences, 609
    children, 609
    closure, 612
        surgical procedure, 612
    complete obstruction of, 611
    complications of enterostomies, 611, 611*t*
        necrotizing enterocolitis, 611
        portal hypertension, 612
        venous stasis, 611
    function of, 612
    indications, 609, 610*t*
        basic intestinal disorder, 609
        primary anastomosis, 609
    necrosis from
        insuffi cient blood supply, 611
    techniques, 609–611
        cystic fibrosis, 610, 610*f*
        enterostomal therapist, 609
        loop enterostomy, 609
        loop ostomy, 609, 610*f*
            distal limb, 612
            sigmoid, 611*f*

meconium, 610
necrotizing enterocolitis, 609
    multiple ostomies, newborn, 611*f*
    solitary small bowel, 609
    transverse upper abdominal incision, 609
temporary soft rubber tube, 611*f*
umbilicus, 609
*Streptococcus pneumoniae, 202,* 426
*Streptococcus thermophilus,* 195
*Streptomyces hygroscopicus,* 1289
Stress-related mucosal damage
    acid reduction therapy, 100
    prophylaxis, 98–100
Stress-related mucosal damage (SRMD)
    comparative trials between H2RAs and PPIs, 98–99
    pediatric risk of mortality score, 98
    prevention, 98
    prophylaxis, 98–99
stretch-dependent cell cycle gene transcription, 449
Stridor, 330
Sturge weber syndrome (SWS), 979–980
    brain, leptomeningeal involvement of, 980
    environmental factors, 979
    facial port-wine stain, 979
    glaucoma, 980
    mutation, RASA1 gene, 979
    neurocutaneous disorder, 979
    neurologic problems, 979
    patient, cranial MRI documenting intracrania, 980*f*
    patient, left facial asymmetry, 980*f*
    seizures, 980
Subclavian artery, 929, 944
    aberrant, 947
Subclavian vein, 143–144
Subcutaneous mass
    RICH with pale, 964*f*
subcutaneous tissue, 440
Submandibular gland
    excision, 235*f*
    exposure, traversing platysma, 236*f*
Substance P, 359
Succinylcholine, 153
Sulfa antibiotics, 175
Sulfonylurea receptor gene, *SUR1,* 1141
Superficial nonparameningeal, 1216
    buccal, 1216
    head, 1216
    laryngeal, 1216
    neck, 1216
    oropharyngeal, 1216
    parotid areas, 1216
Superior mesenteric artery (SMA), 540
Superior mesenteric vein (SMV), 541

Supportive care
    common short-term toxicities, 1173
Suppurative lymphadenitis, acute, 238*f*
Supraclavicular block, 167
Supraumbilical disease, 483–488
Supraventricular tachycardia, 85
Surgical complication, 592
    cystic fibrosis, 592
    familial polyposis, 592
    Henoch–Schonlein purpura., 592
    nephrotic syndrome, 592
    Peutz–Jeghers syndrome, 592
Surgical error, 19
    role of pediatric surgeon, 19
Surgical intervention, 441
    ruptured bleb, 441
    video-assisted thoracoscopic techniques (VATS), 441
Surgical options, diagram of, 529*f*
Surgical research/investigation, 14–15
Surgical site infections (SSIs), 190
Sven-Ivar Seldinger technique, 142
SWS. *See* Sturge weber syndrome (SWS)
Sympathectomy, 434
    palmar temperature, 435
    sympathetic chain, 435
    technique, 435
    upper thoracic, 434
Syndrome
    Zollinger–Ellison syndrome, 515
Syndrome of inappropriate antidiuretic hormone (SIADH), 57
Syndromes, 471
    Beckwith–Wiedemann, 471
    pentalogy, 471
    prune belly, 471
Synovial sarcoma, 1222
    fusion gene, 1222
    malignant peripheral nerve sheath tumor (MPNST), 1222
Syphilis, 199
Syringomyelia, 1013
    laminectomy
        syrinx, largest portion of, 1013
Systemic inflammatory response syndrome (SIRS), 196

T
Tachyarrhythmias, 85
Tachycardia
    ventricular, 77
Tachypnea, 174
Tacrolimus, 1290
Takayasu arteritis, 953, 954
    diagnosis, 954
    outcomes of surgical revascularization, 955
    postoperative complications, 955
    symptoms, 954
    treatment, 954–955

Talc, 440
  acute respiratory failure, 440
T-cells, 194, 1285–1286
T cell tumors, 1267–1268
  anaplastic large T cell lymphoma
      (ALCL), 1267
    big cytoplasm, 1268
    CD30-positive, 1268
    hallmark cells, 1268
    horseshoe, 1268
    lymph nodes, involvement, 1267
    systemic (ALK + and ALK −), 1268
    T cell cancer, 1267
  lymphoblastic lymphoma (LL)
    acute lymphoblastic leukemia
        (ALL), 1267
    childhood NHL, 1267
    hepatosplenomegaly, 1267
    intrathoracic tumor, 1267
    lymphoblastic leukemia-type
        regimen, 1267
    precursor lymphoblast
        phenotype, 1267
    superior vena cava
        syndrome, 1267
    T-cell immunophenotype, 1267
TEF. See Tracheoesophageal fistula (TEF)
Temperature
  change in blood temperature, 79
  monitoring, 71
Temporalis fascia, 228
Teratogenic experiments, 448
Teratoma, 514
  abdominal and retroperitoneal, 1204
    AFP level, 1204
    histologic pattern, malignant
        tumors, 1204
    infantile choriocarcinoma, rare
        tumor, 1204
    postchemo resections, 1204
    presenting symptoms, 1204
    primary resection, 1204
      hazardous nature, 1204
  cervicofacial, 1205, 1206
    consists of, 1205
    ex-utero intrapartum treatment
        (EXIT), 1206
    presenting symptoms, 1206
  children's cancer group (CCG), 1198
  children's oncology group
    current study, 1198, 1200f
  developmental schema
    germ cell tumors, 1199f
  embryonal carcinoma, 1198
  etoposide and bleomycin
      (PEB), 1198
  event-free survival (EFS), 1199f
  gastric, 1206
    obstructive symptoms, 1206
    presenting symptoms, 1206

genital (vaginal), 1204, 1205
  CT scan findings, 1205, 1206f
  surgical procedure, 1205
  vaginal bleeding, 1205, 1206f
  vaginal mass, 1205, 1206f
malignant germ cell tumors
  survival, 1198
mature teratomas, 1198
mediastinal germ cell tumors,
    1200–1204
  Chamberlin procedure, biopsy
      anterior mediastinal tumor,
      1201, 1205f
  diagnostic procedure, 1201
    alternatives, 1201
  large tumors, 1201
    associated problems, 1201
    neoadjuvant chemotherapy
        treatment, 1201, 1205f
  located in, 1200
  median sternotomy/thoracotomy
      tumor resection, 1201
  survival rate, 1204
  symptoms, 1201
ovary, 1207–1209
  chemosensitive nature,
      tumors, 1208
  COG ovarian staging system,
      1208, 1208f
  cystic component, decompression
      retrieval bag, 1208, 1208f
  germ cell tumors, common site
      for, 1207
  gluing a bag to cyst, technique of
      decompression of cyst, 1208,
      1209, 1209f
  intergroup study
    results, 1208, 1209f
  laparoscopic approach, 1208
  neoadjuvant chemotherapy, 1208
  ovarian staging procedure,
      1208, 1208f
  preoperative assessment, 1208
  presenting symptom
    pain, most common, 1208
pediatric oncology group
    (POG), 1198
risk-based treatment schema, 1199f
sacrococcygeal tumors, 1199, 1200
  Altman's American Academy,
      classification based on,
      1199, 1200f
  buttocks contouring closure,
      Fishman et al, 1199, 1203f
  clinical presentation, 1199, 1200f
  controlling aorta, method of
      allow temporary vascular
      occlusion, high-flow tumors,
      1199, 1201f
  Currarino triad, 1200

event-free survival (EFS)
  malignant extragonadal
      tumors, 1200, 1205f
  extensive unresectable lesions,
      older infants, 1200, 1204f
  post chemotherapy resection,
      1200, 1204f
follow-up procedure, 1199
  importance, 1199
  long-term, 1199
germ cell tumors
  extragonadal tumor,
      neonates, 1199
initial biopsy, 1200
neurosurgical assistance,
    requirement of, 1200
surgical excision, primarily
    external lesions
  basic steps, 1199, 1202f
seminoma/dysgerminoma
  primitive germ cell tumor, 1198
testes tumors, 1206, 1207
  AFP
    preoperative, 1206
  COG testes staging system,
      1206, 1207f
  diagnosis, 1206
  intergroup study
    results, 1207f
    treatment schema, 1207f
  intersex disorders, 1206
  large tumor, 1206
  malignancy risk, 1206
    intraabdominal location, 1206
    undescended testes, 1206
  malignant yolk sac tumor, 1206
  prepubertal boys, 1206
    nongerm cell tumors, most
        common, 1206
  presenting signs, 1206
  retroperitoneal adenopathy,
      presence of, 1206, 1207
  surgical approach
    inguinal incision, 1206, 1207f
  yolk sac tumor, 1198
Terminal myelocystocele, 1019–1020
  caudal spinal cord
      malformation, 1019
  closed myelomeningoceles, 1020
  double compartment sac, 1019f
Testis
  absent testis, 777
  ascending testis, 777
  canalicular testis, 776
  ectopic testis, 777
  emergent testis, 776
  intra-abdominal testis, 776
  superficial inguinal pouch testis,
      776, 777
  vanishing testis, 777

Testosterone, 904
  metabolism, 904
  secretion, 904
Tetanus immunization, 214
Thalassemia, 173, 174
Theinopyridines, 175
Therapeutic decision support, 83
Therapeutic hardware devices, 83
*The Surgery of Childhood, Including Orthopaedic Surgery*, 10
*The Surgery of Infancy and Childhood*, 10
Thiamine, 66
Thickened filum terminale, 1019
  conus, 1019
  distal thecal sac, 1019
  fatty filum, 1019
Thiopental, 155
Thoracic aorta, 943
Thoracic deformity syndromes, 275
  treatment, 275–276
Thoracic epidurals, 165
Thoracic injuries
  diagnosis, 1067, 1068
    cardiac injury
      parasternal wounds, 1067
    chest CT, 1068
      controversies, 1068
      identifying underlying injuries, 1068
      imaging algorithm, pediatric chest trauma, 1068*f*
    focused assessment with sonography for trauma (FAST) examination, 1068
    helical CT angiography, 1068
    initial assessment
      chest x-ray, 1067
      physical examination, 1067
    intubated patient, 1067
    penetrating injuries, 1067
    thoracic aorta injury, 1068
    ultrasound, 1068
  epidemiology, 1067
    blunt trauma, 1067
    mortality rates, 1067
    most common injuries, 1067
    occurence, 1067
    penetrating chest injuries, 1067
Thoracic resistance, 72
Thoracoabdominal duplications, 653
  associated conditions, 653
  complications, 653
    abdominal connection to gastric antrum, 654*f*
  diagnosis essentials, 653
  presenting signs, 653
  symptoms, 653

treatment, 653
  laminectomy, 653
  resection, 653
Thoracoport trocars (Covidien, Norwalk, CT), 436
Thoracoscopic biopsy
  surgery, 1263
Thoracoscopic lung biopsy
  algorithm outlining an approach in children, 424*f*
  diagnostic algorithm, 423
    algorithm, 424*f*
  essentials of diagnosis, 422
  indications, 422–423, 423*t*
  operative procedure, 423, 425*f*
  outcome, 423, 430*t*
Thoracoscopic spine exposure, 436–437
  complications, 437
  patient positioning, 437*f*
  pitfalls, 437
  posterolateral thoracotomy, 436
  videoassisted thoracoscopic surgery (VATS), 436
    bronchial blocker, 436, 436*f*
    operative approach, 436–437
Thoracoscopic sympathectomy, 434
  anesthesia monitor, 435
  complications, 436
  operative approach, 435–436
    ganglions, 435
    hemithorax., 435
    patient positioning, 435
    Trendelenburg position, 435
  patient positioning, 435*f*
  pitfalls, 436
Thoracoscopy, trauma, 1080
  chest-wall bleeding, 1080
  single-lung ventilation, 1080
  video-assisted thoracoscopy, 1080
  *vs.* thoracostomy, 1080
Thoracotomy, 441, 459
Thrombectomy, 75
Thrombocytopenia, 98, 142, 174–175, 176
  refractory, 175
Thrombocytosis, 177
  defined, 177
  primary, 177
  secondary, 177
Thrombolytic therapy
  via catheter, 75
Thrombosis, 73, 75, 177, 937, 1005
  asymptomatic vascular, 177
  disorders of, 176–177
  Factor V Leiden, 177
  renal vein, 177
  risk for postphlebitic syndrome, 177
Thromboxane A2, 175, 182
Thymomas
  staging of, 401

Thymus, 950
  cysts, 400
Thyroglossal duct cysts, 230
Thyroid cartilage, 303
Thyroid gland, 1147–1154
  anatomy, 1147, 1148
    bilobed structure, 1147
    inferior thyroid artery, 1147
    recurrent laryngeal nerve (RLN), 1147, 1148
      inferior thyroid artery, relationship with, 1147, 1148
      left RLN, 1148
      non-RLN, 1148
      right RLN, 1148
      thyroid surgery, importance in, 1148
    superior laryngeal nerve, 1148
    superior thyroid artery, 1147
    venous drainage, 1148
  diagnosis essentials, 1147
  embryology, 1147
    ligament of Berry, 1147
    para-follicular C-cells, 1147
  operative technique, 1150–1154
    operative procedure, 1151–1154
      autotransplant, 1153
      devascularized gland, 1153
      downward traction, placing, 1151
      hemostasis, 1154
      inferior thyroid artery and vein, identifying, 1152, 1152*f*
      Kocher incision, 1151
      lateral dissection, identifyingsuperior thyroid artery and vein, 1151, 1152*f*
      left inferior parathyroid gland, 1153, 1153*f*
      ligament of Berry, 1153, 1153*f*
      malignancy suspicion, 1154
      minimally invasive techniques, 1154
      neuropraxia, 1153
      opening deep cervical fascia, exposing thyroid gland, 1151, 1152*f*
      parathyroid glands, preserving of, 1153
      parathyroid glands, preventing devascularizing, 1152
      postoperative hypoparathyroidism, 1153
      preoperative ultrasound, 1154
      recurrent laryngeal identification, dissection, 1152, 1152*f*
      RLN, 1152, 1153

self-retaining retractor, facilitating exposure, 1151, 1151*f*

silk suture, marking incision, 1151, 1151*f*

skin retractors, raising subplatysmal flaps, 1151, 1151*f*

superior lobe mobilization, 1152

thyroid lobectomy, 1151

thyroid vessels ligation, vascular supply preservation, 1153, 1153*f*

tracheo-esophageal (TE) groove, 1152

positioning, 1150, 1151

cervical exploration, appropriate neck extension, 1150, 1151*f*

postoperative considerations, 1154

cervical hematoma, 1154

hoarseness, 1154

hypocalcemia, 1154

hypoparathyroidism, 1154

patient's voice assessement, 1154

serum calcium, checking, 1154

other thyroid disorders, 1149, 1150

goiter, 1149

Hashimoto thyroiditis, 1149, 1150

subacute thyroiditis, 1150

thyroiditis, 1149

thyroiditis in children, characteristics, 1150*t*

toxic diffuse goiter, 1149

physiology, 1148

para-follicular C-cells, 1148

calcitonin, 1148

thyroid stimulating hormone (TSH), 1148

thyroxine (T4), 1148

production, 1148

regulation, negative feedback loop, 1148

triiodothyronine (T3), 1148

production, 1148

regulation, negative feedback loop, 1148

preoperative considerations, 1150

ultrasound-guided fine needle assessment (FNA), 1150

vocal cord, check, 1150

thyroidectomy, indications, 1148–1150

thyroid malignancies, 1149

anaplastic thyroid cancers, 1149

follicular adenocarcinoma, 1149

follicular thyroid carcinoma, 1149

MACIS score, based upon, 1149

medullary thyroid cancer (MTC), 1149

multiple endocrine neoplasia syndromes, characteristics, 1149, 1150*t*

papillary thyroid cancer, 1149

thyroid nodule, work-up of, 1148, 1149

cytologic evaluation, 1149

differential diagnosis, categorization, 1148, 1148*t*

multiple endocrine neoplasia (MEN), 1148

occurence, 1148

physical examination, 1148

primary thyroid malignancies, characteristics, 1149, 1149*t*

radiation exposure history, 1148

thyroid function tests, 1148

thyroid lobectomy, 1149

ultrasonography, 1148

ultrasound-guided fine needle aspiration (FNA), 1148

T lymphocytes, 188

TNM Pretreatment Staging Classification, 1213*t*

Total bicarbonate deficit, 86

Total parenteral nutrition (TPN), 13, 129, 135, 545, 700, 701

amino acids, deleterious effects, 700

associated

cholestasis, 700

gallstone formation, 700

liver disease, 700

cholecystikinin (CCK), 700

mediated bile flow, 700

use of, 700

cholelithiasis, 700

development, 700

factors responsible, 700

cholestatic effects, 701

dependent children, 700

long-term, 700

primary lithogenic effect, 700

Toxoplasmosis, 199

Trachea

diagnostic evaluation of child with suspected tracheal obstruction, 319*f*

Tracheal stenosis, 943. *See* Congenital tracheal stenosis

Tracheobronchial injuries, 1073, 1074

bronchial injuries, 1073

lung collapse, 1074

chest tube placement, 1073

air leak, 1073

early diagnosis, 1074

flexible/rigid bronchoscopy, 1074

intrathoracic, 1073

left thoracic approach

left bronchial injuries, 1074, 1074*f*

primary reconstruction, 1074

primary repair, 1074

right thoracic approach

tracheal and right bronchial injuries, 1074, 1074*f*

standard posterior lateral thoracotomy, 1074

tracheal injury, penetrating trauma, 1073

common site of injury, 1073

tracheobronchial disruption

common associated radiographic findings, 1074

common presenting signs, 1073

Tracheoesophageal fistula (TEF), 342

Tracheomalacia, 317–319, 347, 949, 950

diagnostic principles, 319–320

Insertion of intratracheal expandable metallic stent for, 327*f*

preoperative echocardiogram, 320

radiological imaging, 320, 320*f*

Tracheoplasty

for CTS, 321

surgical technique for slide, 324*f*

surgical technique of pericardial patch, 323*f*

Tracheotomy, 302

diagnostic principles, 302–303

disease pathophysiology, 302

endotracheal/tracheotomy tube size, formula for prediction, 304

evaluation, 302

indications, 303*f*

morbidity, 305

preparation for elective, 303, 303*f*–305*f*

retention sutures, use of, 304

surgical history, relevant, 302

treatment effectiveness, and patient outcomes, 305, 306

treatment options, 303

Tramadol, 163

Transanal mucosectomy, 586*f*

Transanal Soave pull-through, 589*f*

Trans arterial chemoembolization (TACE), 1242

chemotherapeutic cocktails, 1242

doxorubicin eluting beads, 1242

lipiodol, 1242

mitomycin, 1242

pirarubicin, 1242

tumor necrosis, 1242

Transducer, 75

Transferrin $\alpha^1$-acid, 61

Transforming growth factor β [TGF-β], 181

Transfusion medicine, 178–179
  massive transfusion, 179
    protocol for pediatric patients, 179*f*
  transfusion reactions, 179–180
    ABO incompatibility, 179
    febrile nonhemolytic
      reactions, 180
Transfusion-related GVH disease, 180
Transfusions in neonates, 178–179
Transfusion therapy, 174
Transjugular intrahepatic
      portosystemic shunt
      (TIPS), 731
  advantages, 731
  benefit, 731
  interventional radiologic
      techniques, 731
  introduction, 731
  long-term decompression, 731
  principal long-term
      complications, 731
  Roux-en-Y limb, 731
  technical difficulties, 731
Transplantation immunology, 1286
Transureteroureterostomy,
      872–873, 873*f*
Trauma, 80
  abdominal, 1050
  *Advanced Trauma Life Support*®
      *(ATLS*®*)* guidelines, 1052
  blunt, 886
  Focused Assessment by Sonography
      in Trauma (FAST), 1052
  identification of patients, 82
  inflicted extremity, 1051
  intentional, 1048
  major blunt abdominal, 1050, 1051
  minor, 212
    fingertip injuries, 212
      fingertip avulsions, 212
      nail bed injuries, 212–213
      subungual hematoma,
        213, 213*f*
    hair tourniquet, 213–214
      embedded circumferential
        hair, 213*f*
    indicators of malignant risk, 214
    minor scald and contact
      burns, 214
    puncture wounds, 213
    subcutaneous foreign bodies, 213
    superficial lacerations, 212
  mortality, 80, 94
  nonaccidental, 1116
  unintentional, 1046
Trauma centers
  categorization, based on resources
      available, 1030
    level 2, 1030
    level 1, highest category, 1030

Trauma mortality prediction model
      (TMPM-ICD9), 1036
Trauma systems, 1029, 1030
  federal legislation, developed
      through, 1029
  modern organized care, 1029
    injured child, 1029
  organized systems, 1029
  pediatric emergency care, 1029
    Institute of Medicine,
      1029, 1030
Trendelenburg position, 143
Trichobezoars, 515
Trisomy 13/18, 51
Tube, catheter thoracostomy, 440
  Atropine, 440
  child, 440
  intercostal space, 440
  neonates, 440
  Pleur-Evac drainage system, 440
  pulmonary edema,
      reexpansion, 440
Tuberous sclerosis, 953
Tubular duplications, 660, 661
  groups, 660, 661
    duplication in females with
      fistula(e), 660, 661
    duplication in males with
      fistula(e), 661
    duplication without fistula with
      imperforate anus, 661
    single perineal anus
      with communicating
      duplication, 661
    two perineal ani, 660
Tumor necrosis factor (TNF), 68
Tumors, 1212–1219, 1233*f*
  computed tomography (CT), 1212
  dysgerminomas, 896
  endodermal sinus tumor, 896
  epithelial cell tumor, 896
  gastric tumor, 510
  germ cell tumor, 895
  granulosa cell tumor, 896
  immature teratomas, 895
  location, 1216
  magnetic resonance imaging
      (MRI), 1212
  mature teratoma, 895
  mediastinal, 394
  negative tumors, 1212
  neoplastic ovarian tumors, WHO
      classification, 895*t*
  nevus sebaceous of Jadassohn,
      associated with, 1273*t*
  PAX/FKHR fusion positive, 1212
  Sertoli–Leydig tumor, 896
  sex cord stromal tumor, 896
  of stomach, 514
Tunneled central venous catheter, 144*f*

Turcot syndrome, 1256
  central nervous system, 1256
    ependymoma, 1256
    glioblastoma, 1256
    medulloblastoma, 1256
  intestinal polyps, 1256
  neoplasms, 1256
Turner syndrome, 899
Twin-to- twin transfusion syndrome
      (TTTS), 23
  fetal, algorithm for management, 30*f*
  fetoscopic laser coagulation, 39
    laser coagulation, 39
    outcomes, 39
    rationale, 39
    specific postoperative
      considerations, 39
  quintero staging of, 31*t*
  types of vascular communications, 30*f*
Two-stage orchidopexy
      (fowler-stephens), 782
  Fowler–Stephens procedure, 782
  retroperitoneal dissection
      laparoscopy, 782
Type III secretion system (TTSS), 194

U
Ulcerated hemangioma
  before, after PDL treatment, 972*f*
Ulcerations, 967, 995*f*
  focal, 1322
  gastric/duodenal, 727
  intestinal, 1324
  lip, 971
  painful, 1173
  peptic, 346
  treatment, 972
Ulcerative colitis (UC), 632–633
  ileitis, mucosal inflammation, 633
  serum biomarkers
    prevalence of, 635*t*
Ulcers, of stomach and duodenum,
      515–516
  gastrotomy/duodenotomy, 516
  operative interventions, 515
  secondary, 515
  treatment, 515
Ultrasonography, 449
Ultrasound-guided central venous
      access, 145
Ultrasound, large palpable
      abdominal mass
  infant, 664, 665*f*
Umbilical artery, 74, 148
  catheter, 75
  catheters, 73
Umbilical disease, 483–488
  anatomic considerations, 483
    apoptotic cell death, 483
    epidermis, transition, 483

epithelium, 483
 fascial mesoderm, 483
 umbilical ring, 483
  abdominal cavity, 483
   somatopleure, 483
   sphincter mechanism, 483
  urachus, 483
  vitelline duct, 483
 diagnostic, 487f
 epigastric hernia, 485
 treatment algorithm, 487f
 umbilical hernia, 483–485
 urachal remnant, 485
 vitelline duct abnormalities,
   485–488
Umbilical hernia, 483–485
 abdominal binders, 483
 Bowel incarceration, 483
 button hole, injury, 484
 dermis/cicatrix, 485f
 fascial defect, closure of, 483, 484f
 liquid adhesive, 485f
 omentum, 484
 seroma formation, 485
 smile incision, 484f
 steri-strips, 485f
 surgical repair of, 484f
 syndromes, 483
  Beckwith–Wiedemann
    syndrome, 483
  Down syndrome, 483
  exomphalos–macroglossia
    syndrome, 483
  hypothyroidism, 483
  mucopolysaccharidosis, 483
 umbilical cicatrix, 484
 umbilicus and associated structures
   embryology, 484f
 visible protrusion, 483
 young children, 483
Umbilical vein, 144–145
 cannulation of, 144
Umbilical vessel catheterization, 144f
Umbilicoplasty, 835
Umbilicus
 towel clips, toothed forceps
   everted with, 626f
Undifferentiated embryonal
   sarcomas, 1246
Unfractionated heparin (UFH),
   97, 98
Urachal Remnant, 485
 cystoscopy, 485
 fistula, 485, 486f
 granulomas, 485
  pink friable tissue, 485
 infraumbilical approach, 485
 omphalomesenteric duct, 485
 radiographic views
  fistulography with, 485

symptoms
  periumbilical granulation, 485
 tulography, 485
 ultrasonography, 485
 umbilical pathology
  urachal anomalies, 486f
 urachal sinus, 486f
 vitelline remnants, 485
Ureteric orifice, 823f
Ureterocele, 810–813
 ectopic, 812
 excision of, operative technique,
   810–813
  antibiotic prophylaxis, 812
  decompression, 812
  detrusor defect, 812
  endoscopic approach, 810
  factors considered, 810
  7.5-French infant cystoscope, 810
  8.5-French resectoscope beak, 810
  needle electrocautery, 812
  operative repair, 813f
  prenatal identification, 810
  pre-operative appearance, 812f
  reconstruction, 812
  VCUG study, 810
  4-0 Vicryl sutures, 812
 orthotopic, 812
Ureteropelvic junction obstruction,
   813–817
 diagnosis, 814, 815
  differential renal function
    calculation, 814
  DTPA Lasix renogram, 814
  giant multicystic dysplastic
    kidney, 814
  hydronephrosis
   prenatal detection, 814
  Lasix, 814
   administration, 814
  Mag III Lasix renogram, 814
  magnetic resonance urography,
    814, 815f
   functional analysis, 814
   functional parameters use, 814
  prenatal ultrasonography, 814
  radiographic studies, 814
   incidental findings, 814
  renal ultrasonography, 814
   different parameters, 814
  VCUG study, 814
 dismembered pyeloplasty, operative
   technique, 815–817
  Anderson–Hynes dismembered
    pyeloplasty, 815, 816f
   anterior subcostal incision,
     815–817
  conservative approach, 815
  surgical intervention timings, 815
   depends on, 815

pathophysiology, 813, 814
  intrinsic obstruction, cause of, 813
  Östling folds, 814
   retrograde pyelogram, 814f
  UPJ obstruction, 813
  result of, 813
 presentation, 814, 815
 surgical outcome, 817
  complications, 817
  focal stricture, 817
  Penrose drain, 817
  postoperative stricture, 817
  redo pyeloplasties, 817
  robotically assisted laparoscopic
    procedures, 817
Ureterosigmoidostomy, 861
Ureterovesical junction (UVJ), 819, 824
Ureterovesical junction obstruction,
   806–813
 diagnosis, 807–809
  dilated ureter ends, cystic dilatation
    radiograph, 808f
  filling defect, bladder, 808
  intravesical component,
    ureterocele
    radiograph, 808f
  Mag III Lasix renogram, 807
   renal scan, 808f
  magnetic resonance urography
    (MRU), 807
  obstructed ectopic upper-pole
    ureter, hydronephrosis, 807
   radiograph, 808f
  prenatal ultrasonography, 807
   hydroureteronephrosis, 807
  radiographically, 807
  ureterocele, 807
  voiding cystourethrography, 807
   right ureterocele, 809f
 pathophysiology, 806
  bladder development, 806
  ectopic ureters, 806
   bilateral single-system, 806
  embryological development, 806
  primary obstructed
    megaureter, 806
   caused by, 806
  ureterocele
   caused by, 806
   cecoureterocele, anatomical,
     806, 807f
   duplicated intravesical/ectopic,
     806, 807f
   single intravesical/ectopic,
     806, 807f
   sphincteric, anatomical,
     806, 807f
   sphincterosphincteric,
     anatomical, 806, 807f
   stenotic, anatomical, 806, 807f

Ureterovesical junction obstruction (*continued*)
presentation, 807–809
primary obstructed megaureter, 806
surgical outcome, 813
long-term-follow-up, 813
postoperative problems, 813
upper-pole nephrectomy, 813
ureteral tailoring and reimplantation
success rate, 813
surgical techniques, 809–813
ectopic ureter (*See* Ectopic ureter)
operative technique, 809
upper-pole nephroureterectomy, 809, 810
obstructed megaureter (*See* Obstructed megaureter)
ureteral tailoring and reimplantation, 810
ureterocele (*See* Ureterocele)
excision of ureterocele, 810–813
Urethral prolapse, 881
Urethral repositioning, 795–798
complications, 796, 797
balanitis xerotica obliterans (BXO), 797
early, 796
fistula, 796
intraurethral hair growth, 797
late, 796
meatal stenosis, 796
persistent chordee, 796, 797
urethral stenosis, 796
urethrocele, 797
glanuloplasty, 795
Heineke–Mikulicz principle
vertical incision transversely, closing, 795
meatal advancement and glanuloplasty (MAGPI), 795
meatal-based flap, 795
circumferential incision inner preputial skin, 795
vascularized pedicle flap, 795
onlay island flap, 795
anastomosis, 795
dartos tissue, 795
circumferential incision inner preputial skin, 795
glanuloplasty, 795
graft, 795
technique based on, 795
tubularized preputial island flap (TPIF), 795
outcomes, 797, 798
MAGPI, 797
Mathieu, 797
micturation, 797, 798
onlay island flap, 797

tubularized incised plate, 797
two-stage repair, 797
two-stage repair, 795
proximal hypospadias patients, 795
repair, first stage, 795
degloved penis, 795, 796*f*
harvesting free graft, dorsal hood, 766*f*, 795
quilting sutures, free graft is sewn, 766*f*, 795
repair, second stage, 795
tubularization, urethra, 795, 796*f*
Urethroplasty, 793, 794
hypospadias repair, 793
Duplay-type tubularization, 793
one-stage operation, 793
two-stage operation, 793
tubularized incised plate, 793, 794
circumferential subcoronal incision, penis, 793, 794*f*
glans wings created degloved penis, 793, 794*f*
glanuloplasty, 793, 794*f*
running subepithelial stitch, urethral stent, 793, 794*f*
skin closure, 793, 794*f*
tubularization, 793
vascularized pedicle flap mobilization
buttonholing, inner preputial skin, 793, 794*f*
Urinary continence, 857
via an intact anorectal continence mechanism, 861
artificial bladder, 862, 865
complications, 876–878
internal diversion, 861
rectal neobladder, 862
augmented and valved rectum, 864*f*
sigma rectum, 862
ureterosigmoidostomy, 861
Urinary incontinence, 693
Urinary reconstruction, 857
Urinary tract function, 857
Urinary tract reconstruction, 857
preoperative evaluation, 857
Urine pregnancy tests, 153
Urolithiasis, 876
Uterus, 891
cervical anomalies, 891–892
rudimentary uterine horn, 891

V
Vagal stimulation, 86
Vagina, 887
complete vaginal agenesis, 889–891
congenital absence of vagina, 890*f*
distal vaginal agenesis, 888–889
Frank procedure for neovagina, 889*t*

longitudinal vaginal septum, 887–888
malignancy, 891
transverse vaginal septum, 888
trauma, 887
vaginoscopy, 887*t*
Vaginal atresia, 924–925
Vaginal introitus, 881
Vaginoplasty, 916
absent vagina, 920, 922, 923*f*
cystoscopy, 916, 916*f*
high vaginal atresia repair, 917, 918*f*–920*f*
low vaginoplasty, 916, 916*f*, 917*f*
posterior approach, 917, 920, 921*f*–922*f*
preoperative preparation, 916
sigmoid, 920, 923*f*
vaginoscopy, 916
Vaginoscopy, 916
Vagus nerve, 359
Valsalva effect, 831
Vancomycin, 95, 96
antibiotic regimens for, 600
empiric therapy for select hospital-acquired infections, 97*t*
parenteral antimicrobial prophylaxis, 204
treatment for acute osteomyelitis, 302
Vascular access
arterial access, 147–148
arterial access, alternative, 148
central venous access, 141
external jugular vein, 141–142
saphenofemoral vein, 142, 142*f*
central venous access, complications of
infection, 145–146
venous thrombosis, 146
devices, 141
intraosseous access, 139
common facial vein, 140
internal jugular vein, 140–141
pediatric care, acute, 137
percutaneous central venous access, 142
femoral vein, 142
internal jugular vein, 142–143
subclavian vein, 143–144
umbilical vein, 144–145
peripheral intravenous catheter (PIV), 137–138
peripheral vein cutdown, 138–139
radial artery, 148
technical complications, 146–147
ultrasound guidance, 145
umbilical artery, 148
Vascular anomalies, 963–982
classification of, 964*t*
vascular malformations, 978–996
vascular tumors, 963–978

Vascular compression, 318–319
  syndromes, 943
Vascular endothelial growth factor
    (VEGF), 183
Vascular injuries, 1101
  diagnostic considerations, 1101
  diagnostic pitfalls, 1101
  overview, 1101
  patient management, 1101–1102
  penetrating extremity trauma, 1101
Vascular lesions, 399–400
Vascular malformations, 978–996
  arterial, 992–993
  capillary, 978–981
  combined, 993–996
  lymphatic, 984–992
  venous, 981–984
Vascular rings, 943
  anatomy, 943–944
    axial view, 945f
    computed tomography (CT)
        image, 945f–946f
    barium swallow method for
        detection, 945
    chest x-ray, 945
    embryology, 943–944
      aortic arch, 944f
    evaluation, 944, 945
    imaging modalities for anomalies,
        945–946
    physical examination, 945
    presentation, 944
    surgical management, 946–947
      and outcomes, 946
      surgical images of double
          aortic, 947f
    symptomatic, 945
Vascular smooth muscle relaxation
  biochemical pathways, 110f
Vascular thrombus formation, 76
Vascular tumors, 963–978
  kaposiform hemangioendothelioma,
      976–978
    infant, 977f
    Kasabach–Merritt phenomenon
        (KMP), 977
    treatment of, 978
      endovascular management, 978
      pharmacotherapy,
          vincristine, 978
      sirolimus, 978
      surgical management, 978
      VEGFR-3 receptor, 978
  management strategies, 971–978
  presentation, problematic patterns,
      967–969
  pyogenic granuloma, 976
    chemocautery, 976
    electrocautery, 976
Vasoactive intestinal peptide, 50, 359

Vasodilator, 86
VeinViewer, 138
Venipuncture cannulation, 208
Venoarterial extracorporeal life-
    support circuit, 117f
Venous lymphatic malformation
  MRI demonstrates, 996f
Venous malformations, 981–984
  coagulation disorders, 982
  coagulation profile, 982
    complete blood count (CBC), 982
    partial thromboplastin time
        (PTT), 982
    platelet count, 982
    prothrombin time (PT), 982
  diffuse ectatic veins, 981
  endothelial-specific receptor
      tyrosine kinase TIE2, 982
  genetic polymorphisms, 982
  glomuvenous malformation, 982–983
    foot, painful glomuvenous
        malformation of, 983f
    loss-of-function mutation,
        glomulin gene, 983
  Klippel–Trenaunay syndrome, 982
  manifestation, chronic pulmonary
      emboli, 982
  MRI demonstrating multiple
      enhancing, 983f
  phleboliths, 982
  prophylactic
      antithromboembolic, 982
  Sclerotherapy of, 983f
  symptomatic, 981
  thromboembolic events, 982
  treatment of, 982
    bleomycin, 987
    chemotherapeutic agent, 987
    debulking, 988
    doxycycline concentration, 987
    leakage, 988
    lymphatic cysts, 986–987
    MRI image of, 983f
    noticeable deformity,
        psychological impact of, 982
    sclerosant effect, 986
    sclerosing agent, 982
    sclerotherapy, 982, 986
    Streptococcus pyogenes, 987
    surgical excision, 987
Venous thromboembolism (VTE),
    hospital-acquired, 96
  anticoagulant treatment
      algorithm in children with
          documented, 99
  in children, 96
  compression stockings/intermittent
      compression device, 97
  conventional anticoagulant
      therapies, 98t

criteria for initiating prophylaxis, 97
critical care setting, risk of, 97
Venous thrombosis, 146
Ventilation
  measurements, 72
  mechanical, 112f
  modes of gas transport during high-
      frequency, 114f
Ventricular septal defects (VSD), 941
  patching, 941
Ventricular shunts, 1004
  complications of, 1004
  shunt infection, 1004
    gramnegative rods, 1004
    haemophilus influenzae, 1004
    intravenous antibiotics, treated
        with, 1004
    propionibacterium acnes, 1004
    staphylococcus aureus, 1004
    staphylococcus epidermis, 1004
  shunt malfunction, 1004
    choroid plexus, 1004
    distal catheter, occlusion of, 1004
    ependymal tissue, 1004
    flulike illness, 1004
    proximal catheter, occlusion
        of, 1004
    radionuclide, 1004
Ventricular tachycardia, 86
Ventriculogallbladder shunt
  infant, 1003f
Ventriculoperitoneal shunt
  intra-abdominal surgery, 1005–1006
    fundoplication, 1006
    gastrostomy tube, 1006
    laparoscopic intra-abdominal
        operations, 1006
    laparoscopic procedures
        surgery, 1006
Vertical banded gastroplasty, 530
Vesicoureteral reflux (VUR), 818–826
  clinical presentation, 820
  diagnosis of
    antenatally diagnosed reflux, 819
    prenatally diagnosed
        vesicoureteral reflux, natural
        history of, 819–820
  embryology, 818–819
  international classification of, 821f
  male infant showing grade V, 821f
  medical management, 821–822
  radiological investigations, 820
    DMSA scan, 821
    ultrasound, 820
    voiding cystography, 820–821
  renal scarring, mechanism of, 819
  surgical treatment
    cohen cross-trigonal
        technique, 822
    detrusorraphy, 823–824

Vesicoureteral reflux (VUR) (*continued*)
 extravesical approach, 823–824
 intravesical approach, 822–823
 laparoscopic ureteral
  reimplantation, 824
 open antireflux procedures, 822
 politano–leadbetter procedure,
  822–823
 vesicoureteral reflux, endoscopic
  treatment of, 824–826
 urinary tract infection (UTI), 818
Vessel loops encircle
 arteries, 1225f
 nerves, 1225f
 veins, 1225f
Vicryl sutures, 575, 582
Video-assisted thoracoscopic surgery
 (VATS), 395, 422
Video-assisted thoracoscopy, 441
 apical bulla, 441f
 blebectomy, 441
 Bullectomy, 441
 double-lumen endotracheal tube, 441
 mechanical pleurodesis, bovie
  scraper, 442f
Virginal hypertrophy, 247
Virulence
 GBS capsule, 194
 K1 capsule, 194
 microbial pathogen, 194
 PapG P-pili, 194
 Type III secretion system, 194
Vitamin and trace mineral
  metabolism, 66
Vitamin $B_{12}$, 66
Vitamin K, 176, 178
 deficiency, 176
Vitelline duct abnormalities
 curvilinear infraumbilical skin
  incision
   surgical excision through, 488
    fetal gut, 485
    Meckel diverticulum, 486
    umbilical sinus, 487f
    umbilico-intestinal fistula, 487f
    yolk sac, 485
 cyst infection, 488
 subumbilical cyst
  rupture of, 487f
Vomiting, 133, 330
von Willebrand disease, 175
von Willebrand factor (vWF), 175, 181
VUR. *See* Vesicoureteral reflux (VUR)

**W**
Warfarin therapy, 177
Waterhouse-Friedericksen
  syndrome, 667
Water-soluble vitamins, 66
Waveform analysis techniques, 81

Weight loss, 330
 surgical approaches, 528–532
  in adolescents, 531–532
  bariatric surgery, surgical
   decision protocol, 529
  collaborative efforts, 532
  malabsorptive/restrictive
   procedures, 531
  Roux-en-Y gastric bypass
   (RYGB), 528
  surgical options, diagram of, 529f
West Nile virus, 180
Wheezing, 330
Wilms tumor, 1177–1184
 adjuvant therapy, 1182–1184
  anaplastic Wilms tumor, 1184
   focal anaplasia, 1184
   Stage IV diffuse anaplasia, 1184
  favorable histology, patients, 1183
  histopathologic tumor
   classification, 1182
  metastases, 1183, 1184
  pulmonary disease, 1183
  risk factors
   clinical, 1182, 1183
   genetic, 1182, 1183
  risk stratification and treatment
   study assignment, 1183, 1183f
  standard risk therapy, 1183
   DD-4A, 1183
  surgery, definitive treatment for
   children, 1183
  survival statistics
   Wilms tumor treated on
    NWTS-4, 1182t
 diagnosis, 1179, 1180
  evaluation, 1179
   computed tomography
    (CT), 1179
   intravascular tumor extension,
    specific investigation of, 1179
   magnetic resonance imaging
    (MRI), 1179, 1179f
   metastatic spread, Wilms
    tumor, 1179
   real-time ultrasonography, 1179
   tumor histology,
    determination, 1179
  presentation, 1179
   associated signs, 1179
   associated symptoms, 1179
   asymptomatic abdominal
    mass, 1179
   physical examination, 1179
   Wilms tumor *vs.*
    neuroblastoma, 1179
  staging, 1179, 1180
   regional lymph node
    sampling, 1180
   system, 1179, 1180f

 epidemiology, 1177
  intra-abdominal cancer, 1177
  national Wilms tumor study
   group (NWTSG), 1177
  occurrence, 1177
 molecular biology, 1178
  Beckwith–Weidmann syndrome
   (BWS), 1178
  candidate genes, 1178
  congenital WAGR
   syndrome, 1178
   symptoms, 1178
  familial Wilms tumor, 1178
   linkage analysis, 1178
   occurs at, 1178
  loss of heterozygosity
   (LOH), 1178
  *p53* gene, 1178
   mutation, 1178
  sporadic Wilms tumor, 1178
  syndromes related to
   WT1/WT2 loci, 1178t
  tumor-suppressor gene, 1178
  Wilms tumor gene,
   location clue
    DNA cytogenetic
     analysis, 1178
  Wilms tumor therapy, 1178
  *WT1* gene, 1178
   Denys–Drash syndrome,
    1178
   expression, pattern, 1178
   mutation, 1178
   WT1 protein, 1178
 outcome, treatment, 1184
  adverse side effects, 1184
   therapy, 1184
  radiation therapy, 1184
   refinement, 1184
  survival statistics, NWTS-IV,
   1183f, 1184
 pathology, 1177
  anaplasia, 1177
  classic Wilms tumor, 1177
   appearance, 1177
  favorable histologic group, 1177
  mortality, 1177
  neoplastic cells, 1177
  unfavorable histologic
   group, 1177
   clear-cell sarcoma of the kidney
    (CCSK), 1177
   malignant rhabdoid tumor,
    kidney, 1177
 preoperative planning, 1178
  blood pressure, assessment, 1178
  clinical assessment, 1178
  genetic testing, appropriate, 1178
  neoadjuvant therapy, 1178
  radical nephrectomy, 1178

resection, 1178
   delayed, 1178
   stage I/II, 1178
   Wilms tumor-predisposition
      syndrome, 1178
surgery, 1178
   surgeon, role of, 1178
surgery timing, 1178, 1181
   controversies, main,
      1178, 1181
   preoperative chemotherapy, 1181
      proponents of, 1181
surgical approach, 1181, 1182
   bloody peritoneal fluid
      rupture sign, 1181
   complications, 1182
   dissection, 1181
      tumor/kideny, posterior
        surface of, 1181
   formal hepatectomy, 1182
   hilar vesse
      identification, 1181
   inferior tumor dissection, 1181
   intraoperative inspection, 1181
      liver, 1181
   invading surrounding
      structures, 1181
   lymph nodes, 1181
   nephrectomy
      central venous access device,
        1181, 1182
      laparoscopic, 1182
      radical, 1181
      unilateral partial, 1182
   preoperative chemotherapy, 1182
   primary tumor
      biopsy, 1181

renal vein
   palpation, 1181
spillage, 1181
   diffuse, 1181
   local, 1181
thoracic extension, 1181
tumor resections
   complications, 1181, 1182
typical transabdominal
   incision, 1181
tumor thrombus, 1182
   intravascular tumor
      extension, 1182
   IVC, 1182
      distal control, 1182
      proximal control, 1182
   primary resection, tumors, 1182
   tumor extension, 1182
Wilm tumor, 925
Wounds, 1121–1123
   alternative wound coverage,
      1126–1128
   acticoat on arm, 1127f
   wound closure using Integra,
      1127f–1128f
dressing, 189
healing, 181
   collagen formation, 184, 184f, 185t
   cytokines and growth factors
      implicated in tissue
      repair, 183t
   delayed healing, 189
   extracellular matrix, 184
      components, 184t
   fibroblasts infiltrate wound
      site, 184f
   hemostasis at wound site, 182f

phases, 181
   hemostasis, 181
   increased vascular
      permeability, 181–183
   inflammatory, 181, 182f
   proliferative phase, 183–184
   remodeling phase, 186
   timeline of events, 182f
schematic depiction
   delayed primary wound
      healing, 188f
   primary wound healing, 187f
   secondary wound healing, 187f
infections, 189
puncture, 213
repair
   types of
      delayed primary, 186
      primary, 186
      secondary, 186
VAC therapy, 207
WT1 (*Wilms tumor suppressor*)
   gene, 903
Wyatt, Oswald S., 4

**X**
X chromosome, 903, 906
45, XO gonadal dysgenesis, 925
XY karyotype, 905

**Y**
YAG laser, 302
Y chromosome, 903, 906, 925

**Z**
Zinc metalloenzymes, 66
Zollinger–Ellison syndrome, 515